CURRENT

Med Talk

A Dictionary of

Medical Terms, Slang & Jargon

CURRENT

Med Talk

A Dictionary of Medical Terms, Slang & Jargon

Joseph C Segen, M.D.

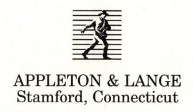

APPLETON & LANGE
Stamford, Connecticut

Copyright © 1995 by Appleton & Lange
A Simon & Schuster Company

95 96 97 98 99 00 / 10 9 8 7 6 5 4 3 2 1

Prentice Hall International (UK) Limited, *London*
Prentice Hall of Australia Pty. Limited, *Sydney*
Prentice Hall Canada, Inc., *Toronto*
Prentice Hall Hispanoamericana, S.A., *Mexico*
Prentice Hall of India Private Limited, *New Delhi*
Prentice Hall of Japan, Inc., *Tokyo*
Simon & Schuster Asia Pte. Ltd., *Singapore*
Editora Prentice Hall do Brasil Ltda., *Rio de Janeiro*
Prentice Hall, *Upper Saddle River, New Jersey*

ISBN 0-8385-1464-2

9 780838 514641   90000

Acquisitions Editor: Cheryl L. Mehalik
Cover Designer: Libby Schmitz

PRINTED IN THE UNITED STATES OF AMERICA

PREFACE

Much has changed in the world and in medicine since the standard medical dictionaries were compiled at the beginning of the 20th century. A well-educated physician was versed in the classics (ie Greek and Latin), specialization in medicine consisted of a one-to-three year apprenticeship in one of a handful of disciplines, often in some of the great medical centers of Germany or France, and subspecialization was virtually nonexistent. The diagnostic armamentarium consisted of a microscope, a stethoscope, and rudimentary x-ray devices; virology, genetics, and immunology were primitive, and other disciplines, eg molecular biology and computer science were decades in the future. Disease processes were poorly understood, bacterial infections were often fatal; other diseases did not exist or were not recognized, and little effective therapy was available. The average person's life span was less than 55 years.

The world, medicine, physicians, and their patients have changed considerably in the intervening years. Specialization and subspecialization are expected of today's physician and require six to nine years after medical school. English has become the lingua franca in medicine and in the world at large. Today's cornucopia of diagnostic modalities and therapeutic options would have left our predecessors breathless. Patients have become "clients" and have life spans of more than 75 years. Disease mechanisms are being dissected by molecular biologists, immunologists, and other scientists using a bewildering array of techniques. Medical information doubles every seven to ten years. Computers have been standard tools, and communication occurs by fax, e-mail, and the Internet. Physicians now share many decisions with patients, bureaucrats, ethicists, and lawyers. The changes in medicine have engendered a new vocabulary and a medical dictionary should have its finger on the pulse of those changes.

This work is not designed to replace traditional dictionaries, but rather to complement them. This is a compilation of terms, many of recent vintage that are integral to the language of modern medicine, a language replete with acronyms, jargon, neologisms, and the argot of new disciplines, diseases, their diagnoses, and therapies.

Joseph C Segen MD
Manhasset, New York
October, 1995

Introduction

THE PURPOSE OF A LANGUAGE IS TO TRANSMIT INFORMATION OR IDEAS The purpose of a dictionary is to catalog the structural units (words and phrases) used in a particular language. The formulation of a language's vocabulary is an imperfect exercise validated by colloquial usage and the passage of time—rarely by logical parameters. In a dynamic language such as medicine, new terminology is constantly being added; some terms undergo subtle changes in use or meaning or require redefinition; other terms are simply deleted from the working vocabulary without due notice. A key indicator of a contemporary medical dictionary's usefulness is whether it contains the terminology used in the working parlance, and whether it is relevant to a particular field of medicine, or to the world at large. The present work is an attempt to catalog the newer terms that have entered the medical lexicon in the recent past.

CHANGES IN MEDICINE HAVE DIRECTLY AND INDIRECTLY AFFECTED ITS VOCABULARY These changes are related to

1) TECHNOLOGY The use of increasingly sophisticated tools for studying pathophysiologic mechanisms of diseases have led to a greater understanding of biomedical phenomena and improvements in both diagnostic and therapeutic modalities. New data often invalidate older classification schema, which were based largely on observations by light microscopy,[1] a primitive tool by today's standards, and clinical observations.[2]

2) SPECIALIZATION Virtually every physician undergoes the further rigors of an additional four to seven years of training after finishing medical school. Each area of specialization and sub-specialization has its own vocabulary.

3) "PLAYERS" The practice of medicine is no longer that of a simple doctor–patient relationship. An increasing number of parties, each with an "agenda," is involved in patient management, including allied health professionals, various levels of government, the legal profession, reimbursement agencies, educators, ethicists, and others.

4) SHIFT IN THE "LINGUISTIC" ROOTS OF MEDICINE The major medical dictionaries currently used in English-speaking countries (and widely translated in other countries) were assembled at the beginning of the 20th century (Dorland's, 1900, Stedman's, 1911), when the 'classic' languages of Latin and Greek were core requirements in premedical education, and fluency in German and/or French were virtually required of those who spoke and wrote in medicine. Few physicians in the current generation have more than a passing familiarity with the 'classic' languages and English has become the lingua franca of medical communication.

CRITERIA FOR SELECTION Any dictionary that covers anything less than an entire field of endeavor must of necessity be selective. The terms included herein are largely

1) NEW A major thrust of the present work is to provide information and/or definitions on terms that have yet to appear elsewhere. Therefore while *Streptococcus pneumoniae* is not included, human herpes viruses 7 and 8 (the latter being known to some workers as Kaposi sarcoma-related herpesvirus—see New England Journal of Medicine 1995; 332:1181, 1186)

---

[1]The pituitary adenoma was traditionally divided into chromophobe (null cell), acidophil and basophil types. According to Rosai, '...*classification of pituitary adenomas into (these) varieties correlates so poorly with the specific cell types and the corresponding pattern of hormone secretion that there is little use in maintaining it*', based on work published in 1972 [2]It is difficult to infer the current equivalent of the syndromes described by the great European neurologists of the last century. Without the benefits of modern diagnostic modalities, the cases described by each may have included such diverse nosologies as vitamin B_{12} deficiency, neurosyphilis, various forms of meningitis, heavy metal poisoning, leukoencephalopathies and other conditions. Of these, perhaps the most confusing term is Schilder's disease, a designation first applied to diffuse sclerosis, and characterized by induration of the cerebral gray matter. The term lost its specificity as it was subsequently applied indiscriminately to gliosis, adrenoleukodystrophy, lymphoma, Krabbe's disease, metachromatic leukoencephalopathy and others.

are. Timeliness then is a common thread that requires the inclusion of recent references. Because of this selectivity, the reader must view this work as a supplement (albeit necessary) to his/her working medical library that would include the venerated medical lexicons, to wit, the Stedman's and/or Dorland's medical dictionaries.

2) "FASHIONABLE" The author believes that a pool of data of this nature should to some degree reflect the attention being paid to a particular "malade du jour." In the early 1990s, cystic fibrosis stepped to center stage, and the discovery of the cystic fibrosis transmembrane conductance regulator "stole the spotlight" in the biomedical sciences. In an earlier work by the author, that disporportionate attention was reflected in the length of the entry; a practice that continues with the present work. Therefore the reader should not be surprised to find greater coverage for "topical" areas, eg AIDS and HIV, euthanasia, or transesophageal echocardiography, than for sarcoidosis, nonsteroidal anti-inflammatory drugs, or conventional imaging modalities.

3) INTERESTING A number of entries included herein are droll (see Twinkie™ defense), fascinating (see Ballistics), disturbing (see Chemical warfare), or of general interest (see Nobel Prize). American slang has insinuated itself into modern "Medtalk," which is hardly surprising given that the United States is the planet's largest English-speaking country. While the purist in medical lexicography might disapprove of the inclusion of such entries, the author justifies this transgression as a vehicle to make the entire work more 'user-friendly' and palatable.

HISTORY AND COMMENTS The database from which the CMM is derived began life 11 years ago as a study aid to help the author pass the pathology boards examination. What was to have required six months first appeared after seven years in the form of the gratifyingly well-received Dictionary of Modern Medicine (Parthenon Publishing Group, Carnforth, UK, 1992). The present work continues in the tradition of that work with innumerable enhancements. Assembling a database of this size has been labor-intensive, with an estimated 15 000 person-hours having been thus far invested. There have been innumerable frustrations in the form of computer lock-ups, crashes, and premature death of equipment—one of the eight laptop computers thus far used for this project literally went up in smoke. Although many hurdles have been passed to reach the point of producing a viable dictionary, much more is already in the pipeline. It is the author's hope that this work will prove useful to the reader.

Acknowledgments

The author leads, as do most other physician-authors, a "double life," working in medicine during the day, and at night, at what has often seemed the impossible task of compiling a lexicon of the working language of medicine. The time has been "stolen" from family (Susan, Joseph, Monica, David, Pete, Pretty, and Wolfgang), and friends (too few mention) who have patiently waited for "the book" to be finished. Thanks to Jamie Kircher, my initial contact at Appleton & Lange, for her early support of this project. Thanks also to Mike Kelley, Cheryl Mehalik, Ginny Allen, and John Williams at Appleton & Lange for streamlining the production process.

FOREWORD

When I was younger and just discovering the pleasures of the written word, the best advice I ever received was to read with a trusty dictionary by my side. So I was delighted when one of my first gifts upon entering medical school was a dictionary, no doubt to keep me company through the long hours of reading I would have to endure. Too bad that dictionary could not have been this one. *Medtalk* is a compilation of terms that far surpasses its peers in relevance and scope.

Medicine of 1995 is a far cry from the medicine practiced by my grandfather, who would have been 100 this year. It is even vastly different from the medicine my father was trained in 30 years ago. Health care today is a world of HMOs, RFLPs, and MRIs—in short, a rapidly evolving lexicon which often has the effect of separating the supposedly enlightened from those in the dark.

So it is now more important than ever that physicians be conversant in the social issues which impact on their practices and on their patients. Consider that the volume you hold before you contains, among its more than 20,000 entries, a definition of "political correctness." Political correctness? In a medical dictionary?

This is a dictionary which finally puts to rest, in medical terms anyway, what defines "primary care." And, for good measure, defines a Picasso phone and a MAAC. More than simple definitions, this volume outlines many current treatments and suggests up-to-date references in the literature for further reading. Just as medicine is in a state of constant flux, so is the language we use to describe it. Lewis Thomas, in his book *The Youngest Science: Notes of a Medicine Watcher*, was perhaps the most prominent physician of this century to express his fascination for the evolution of our language. Dr. Thomas would have loved this dictionary, for it accomplishes a synthesis of so many of those links, roots, and riveting details which hold together our means of expression.

Enough of my words. The thousands contained herein are far more important.

Ivan Oransky, Senior Editor
"Pulse," the medical student section of the
Journal of the American Medical Association

tail coverage MEDICAL LIABILITY An umbrella of malpractice insurance protection that a physician is obliged to retain until the 'statute of limitations' (a period of two to three years) has been completed... ns that may be initiated after a physician has moved to another state or retired (the so-called tail period); equal to at least one year of malpractice premium... tiples thereof; see Malpractice, Statutes of limitations Cf 'Going bare', Nose coverage

Note: In the US, malpractice insurance costs from $2000 to $200,00 (Florida, California, and New York State are highest) and the relative... orthopedic surgery, and obstetrics are often the most expensive); the standard claims-made malpractice insurance policies are less expensive, but do not cover tail periods

Tangier disease Analphalipoproteinemia A rare AR [MIM 205400] condition caused by a deficiency in α-lipoprotein, first described on Tangier Island (Chesapeake Bay, Maryland) CLINICAL General... tonsils, other lymphoid tissues... splenomegaly, mild proximal peripheral neuropathy, intermittent diarrhea, corneal opacification LABORATORY Absent HDL, ↓ cholesterol 1.6-120 g/dl) ... phospholipids, ↓↓ apoA-1 an... enlarged yellow-orange tonsils, lymphoid tissues and rectal mucosa and storage of cholesteryl esters in foamy macrophages in BM, lymph nodes, thymus, spleen, skin, tonsils PROGNOSIS Usually benign, rarely coronary artery disease

tanning PUBLIC HEALTH A sedentary activity in which a person bastes him/herself in a beached whale-like fashion under a UVA... 15-30 minute dollops to achieve a natural look; evidence that tanning may prove ultimately fatal has been lacking; rare cases of benign (eg keratoa-... pre- (eg actinic keratosis) or malignant lesions (eg basal or squamous cell carcinomas, Bowen's disease) linked to 'recreational' tanning (due to UVA light) are reported (N Engl J Med 1995; 332:1450c)

T cell maturation The sequence of events through which the thymus become competent and is exported to peripheral l... divided into a conceptual stages
STAGE I The earliest T cells (10% of thymic lymphocytes)... marker and non-T stem-cell markers, including CD38 (T10) and transferrin (T9); the cells then acquire a thymocyte antigen, CD1a (T6) that reacts with Langerhans cells and CD4 (the 62 kD MHC class II-restricted antigen) and CD8 (the 76 kD MHC class I-restricted antigen)

Tarasoff* v *Regents of the University of California FORENSIC PSYCHIATRY A landmark legal case regarding patient-psychotherapist confidentiality that was initiated by the estate of Tatiana Tarasoff who was murdered by a P Podder, a psychiatric outpatient who had previously informed one of his therapists of his intent to kill Tarasoff; her estate claimed that the physician

Callout labels:
- ENTRY NAME
- AREA OF HEALTH CARE
- CROSS-REFERENCES
- FOOTNOTES AND COMMENTS
- SYNONYM(S)
- OFFICIAL DESIGNATIONS, eg EC. DSM-IV, MIM, NA, SI
- PATIENT INFORMATION
- SYMBOLS & ABBREVIATIONS
- ENTRY'S TEXT
- REFERENCES
- CLASSIFICATIONS, TYPES, OTHER SCHEMA

Ⓓⓔⓢⓘⓖⓝ ⓔⓛⓔⓜⓔⓝⓣⓢ

TYPEFACES

TEST	Eurostil ExtendedTwo for illustrations
TEST	ITC Century Bold for entry names
TEST-	ITC Century Light for entry text
TEST-	Univers Condensed for all tables
TEST-	Univers UltraCondensed for references
TEST-	Univers LightUltraCondensed for DSM-IV, EC, MIM, and NA catalog names
αβ	Symbol for various entries

STYLES

TEST	Small capitals, to indicate relevant area of medicine or science (eg Cardiology, Radiology) OR aspects of the disease process (eg Clinical, Treatment)
Test	Italics for word types (eg *noun, verb*), quotations ('*...while I pondered, weak...*'), pronunciations, and definitions of words or root forms, eg from Greek, Latin, or other languages
T^{est}	Superscripts, to indicate internal footnotes
Test	8 pts for body of tex
Test	7 pts for special notes
Test	6 pts for foonotes

NOMENCLATURE SYSTEMS

[DSM-IV] Diagnosis and Statistical Manual for Psychiatric diseases, 1994

[EC x.x.x.x] Enzyme Commission for Enzymes

[MIM xxxxxx] Mendelian Inheritance in Man (10th ed, 1992) for hereditary disease or gene sequence catalogued by VA McKusick et al

[NA6] Nomina Anatomica, 6th edition for anatomic terminology

[NH3] Nomina Histologica, 3rd edition for histological terminology

[NE3] Nomina Embryologica, 3rd edition for embryological terminology

[SI] System Internationale etc (International System) for laboratory data

ABBREVIATIONS

Abbreviations used in this work are indicated by textboxes (below) found on pages 248, 449, and 928.

2-D Two-dimensional **3-D** Three-dimensional **±** About, approximately, circa **‡** see there **aa** Amino acid **ACE** Angiotensin-converting enzyme **AD** Autosomal dominant **AFB** Acid-fast bacillus **AIDS** Acquired immunodeficiency syndrome **aka** also known as **ALL** Acute lymphocytic (lymphoblastic) leukemia **ALS** Amyotrophic lateral sclerosis **ALT** Alanine aminotransferase (formerly GPT) **AMA** American Medical Association **AML** Acute myelocytic (granulocytic, myeloid, myelogenous) leukemia **ANLL** Acute nonlymphocytic leukemia **apo** Apolipoprotein **aPTT** Activated partial thromboplastin time **AR** Autosomal recessive **ARDS** Acute respiratory distress syndrome or adult respiratory distress syndrome **AST** Aspartate aminotransferase (fomerly GPT) **AV** Atrioventricular **BCC** Basal cell carcinoma **BM** Bone marrow (or basement membrane) **BUN** Blood urea nitrogen **CAD** Coronary artery disease **cAMP** Cyclic adenosine monophosphate **CBC** Complete blood count **CDC** Centers for Disease Control and Prevention **cDNA** Complementary DNA **CEA** Carcinoembryonic antigen **CHF** Congestive heart failure **CIE** Counter-immunoelectrophoresis **CIN** Cervical intraepithelial neoplasia **CK** Creatinine phosphokinase **CML** Chronic myelocytic (granulocytic, myelogenous, myeloid) leukemia **CNS** Central nervous system **COD** Cause of death **COPD** Chronic obstructive pulmonary disease **CPR** Cardiopulmonary resuscitation **CSF** Cerebrospinal fluid **CT** Computed tomography **CVA**

CURRENT

Med Talk

A Dictionary of
Medical Terms, Slang & Jargon

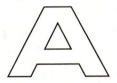

A Symbol for: 1) Absorbance 2) Adenosine 3) Admittance (electricity) 4) Alanine 5) Alveolar gas 6) Ampere 7) Area 8) Mass number 9) Radioactivity

a Symbol for: 1) Absorptivity 2) Acceleration 3) Activity (chemical activity) 4) Arterial blood gas 5) atto- 10^{18}

aa Amino acid

a/A ratio PHYSIOLOGY The ratio between the O_2 in the arterial blood and the alveoli, which serves as an estimate of the pulmonary gas exchange; in normal subjects, the ratio is relatively constant (> 0.75) for 21% to 100% O_2 in inspired air, and becomes increasingly variable in those with pulmonary disease

A_1AT see α_1-antitrypsin

A4 see Amyloid β peptide

A68 A neuronal antigen (recognized by a monoclonal antibody Alz-50) present in the developing fetus by 32 weeks of development, which disappears by age two; it is present in brain tissue and cerebrospinal fluid, is a major subunit of paired helical filaments of Alzheimer's dementia and is derived from low molecular weight tau protein (possibly Tau 69), but is more phosphorylated

A-64077 An experimental therapeutic agent under development which inhibits the 5-lipoxygenase pathway of arachidonic acid metabolism that attenuates the bronchoconstrictive response by asthmatics to cold air and allergen-induced nasal constriction, a response largely due to the eicosanoids produced by 5-lipoxygenase, including sulfidopeptide leukotrienes, 5-HETE, and leukotriene B4

A antigen A major blood group (ABO) antigen which defines the blood type A, assuming the codominant allele at the ABO locus is A or H; A antigens are highly immunogenic; when an A unit of packed red cells is transfused into a B or O recipient, the natural antibodies present in the recipient are capable of evoking a severe or fatal hemolytic transfusion reaction; Cf B antigen, Bombay phenotype, H antigen

AABB American Association of Blood Banks A professional, non-profit organization established in 1947 and dedicated to the education, delineation of standards, policy and other facets of the field of transfusion medicine and is responsible for collecting one-half of the blood supply in the US and transfusing 80%; the AABB is involved in accreditation of transfusion facilities, maintains a rare donor supply and serves as a reference laboratory

AαC see Heterocyclic amine

abandonment LEGAL MEDICINE Negligent termination of a physician-patient relationship either without the patient's consent or without giving adequate notification, so that the patient may continue his/her care with another physician, and under circumstances where continuing medical care is required; any denial of the patient's full benefit of the physician-patient relationship, eg not seeing a hospitalized patient as frequently as due care in treatment requires, also constitutes abandonment MEDICAL MALPRACTICE A physician's unilateral severance of a professional relation with a patient, without reasonable notice and at a time when the necessity for continuing medical attention remains; acts of abandonment include refusal, or more commonly, alleged refusal to treat after he has seen a person needing care, refusal to attend to a case in which the physician has already assumed responsibility, eg visit while the patient is in the hospital, failure to provide follow-up attention and failure to arrange for a competent substitute in times of absence; see Malpractice

abbreviated injury scale EMERGENCY MEDICINE A numerical scoring system for rating organ damage sustained during trauma, which is based on physical examination, operative reports, and autopsy results; a score of six is consistent with a fatal head injury (**N Engl J Med 1994; 331:1105oA**) see Injury Severity Score

abbreviated new drug application CLINICAL PHARMACOLOGY An application made in the US by a pharmaceutical company requesting authority to market a 'new' drug for which both its therapeutic indications and formulation have been previously approved by the FDA in another similar drug; if the previous drug is deemed safe and effective, the Office of Health and Human Services is required to approve or disapprove the new drug within 180 days; see Me too drug

A-B-C sequence EMERGENCY MEDICINE The first level of life support measures used in cardiopulmonary resuscitation according to the 'American school' of cardiology, is the simple mnemonic of 'airway, breathing and circulation'; advanced life support then continues as the D-E-F for 'drugs, electrocardiogram, fibrillation'; see C-A-B

A-B-C/D-E-F SEQUENCE	
AIRWAY	Ensure airway patency (clear bronchotracheal tree)
BREATHING	Ensure breathing by intermittent positive pressure ventilation
CIRCULATION	Compress chest at 60/minute
DRUGS/FLUIDS	Place intravenous line
EKG*	Monitor cardiac rhythms
FIBRILLATION	Defibrillate
*Electrocardiogram	

ABC method Avidin biotinylated horseradish-peroxidase complex, see there

ABC Aneurysmal bone cyst, see there

ABC superfamily ATP-binding cassette transporters A family of oligopeptide permease proteins, which includes the multi-drug resistance protein and a series of bacterial and eukaryotic transporters; these proteins are selective for a wide range of substrates including short oligopeptides, which transport them across membranes; the PSF (peptide supply factor) gene product has structural homology with the ABC transport proteins and the gene has been identified within the class II MHC (major histocompatibility complex) on chromosome 6, where it is thought to play a key role in antigen presentation

ABCD A simple mnemonic for the clinical features of early malignant melanomas, where A refers to asymmetry, B to border irregularity, C to variegation of color, and D to a diameter greater than 6 mm (N Engl J Med 1992; 326:1706c)

abciximab CLINICAL THERAPEUTICS A monoclonal antibody (ReoPro®, Eli Lilly & Co) with antiplatelet activity that was recently approved by the FDA as an adjunct for percutaneous transluminal coronary angioplasty or atherectomy to prevent acute coronary artery ischemia secondary to post-therapy vessel closure, a complication that occurs in up to 30% of those undergoing angioplasty (JAMA 1995 273:982, N Engl J Med 1995; 332:1553RV)

abdominal angina Chronic mesenteric ischemia, see there

abdominal aortic aneurysm A condition defined as a focal dilation of the aorta of ≥ 50% increase in diameter EPIDEMIOLOGY Incidence is rising $12/10^5$ (1951); $36/10^5$ (1980); ♂:♀ ratio 2:1; results in 15 000 deaths/year (US 1988, population ± 230 x 10^6); overall mortality rate from AAA rupture is circa 90% PATHOGENESIS Uncertain whether atherosclerosis is primary or secondary phenomenon DIAGNOSIS 100% accuracy with 1) Ultrasonography (disadvantage, difficult in obese subjects, or with excess bowel gas, periaortic disease, technique does not document proximal or distal ends of aneurysm for surgery 2) CT (disadvantage, ionizing radiation) 3) MRI (disadvantage, expensive) TREATMENT ≥ 5 cm in diameter AAAs should be repaired; therapy of smaller AAAs is controversial; contraindications to elective aortic reconstruction include MI within last 6 months, intractable angina pectoris or congestive heart failure, severe pulmonary insufficiency owith dyspnea at rest, severe renal insufficiency, life expectancy of ≤ 2 years PROGNOSIS Treatment mortality is ± 6%; 25--40% of untreated cases rupture in 5 years, with a 90% mortality if ≥ 5cm (N Engl J Med 1993; 328:1167RV)

abdominal apoplexy A virtually extinct term for intra– or retroperitoneal hemorrhage secondary to intestinal infarction or a ruptured aortic aneurysm, resulting in acute hemoperitoneum; in which small amounts of blood in the peritoneal cavity produce hyperosmolar irritation when RBCs lyse; when a visceral artery ruptures (splenic artery more commonly than the hepatic); the hyperosmolar irritation becomes clinically import, causing acute 'peritonitis', abdominal pain, diminished bowel sounds and an increased leukocyte count

abdominal bath RADIOTHERAPY A treatment field extending from the diaphragm to the pelvis, which is used to treat abdominal lymphomas or ovarian carcinoma; lead (Pb) blocks are used to shield the right hepatic lobe during the initial 15 Gy whole abdominal dose, given by antero-posterior opposed fields; horizontal decubitus (cross-table) lateral fields are then used to bring the para-aortic and mesenteric lymph node radiation dose to 30 Gy, followed by another 14 Gy through antero-posterior ports, thus totalling 4400

abdominal cocoon Idiopathic sclerosing peritonitis A colloquial term for a condition secondary to peritonitis, said to be common in those treated with a LeVeen shunt where reactive fibrosis encases the small intestine TREATMENT Surgical lysis of adhesions

abdominal-perineal resection SURGICAL ONCOLOGY The surgical excision of the lower rectum and anus with loss of the anal sphincter; APR has been largely replaced by RT for small lesions with the use of external beam treatment or with radioactive implants, eg ^{198}Iridium seeds, which achieve local control of 60-80% and 60-90% 5-year survival; for larger lesions a combination of RT and fluorouracil and mitomycin are used (N Engl J Med 1995; 332:371RV)

abdominal thrust maneuver EMERGENCY MEDICINE A maneuver of potential use in drowning victims that attempts to remove fluids from the upper respiratory tract; there are no controlled studies to prove its efficacy; arterial oxygen tension, intrapulmonary shunting of blood, and amount of residual water in the lungs do not differ significantly between animals subjected to ATM and those in which no active maneuver was used to remove fluids; ATM may moreover cause regurgitation, and aspiration of gastric contents; the American Heart Association recommends the use of ATM only in situations where obstruction of a foreign body in the upper airway is suspected, or in those patients who do not respond to mouth-to-mouth ventilation (N Engl J Med 1993; 328:253RA) see Drowning

abdominoplasty Tummy tuck ESTHETIC SURGERY A procedure in which a large ellipse of skin and fat is excised from the anterior wall of the lower abdomen, and the upper abdominal flap is stretched to the suprapubic incision and sewn in place; the umbilicus is exteriorized through an incision in the flap at the proper level; spinal anesthesia is used in some cases; hospitalization for a few days and/or blood transfusions may be required; the results are usually satisfactory

ABER Auditory brainstem evoked response A time-consuming (and costly) method for evaluating infants at high risk for hearing loss that in part depends on the infant's maturity; ABER yields a low false negative rate when screening for early deafness

Abelson leukemia virus A retrovirus carrying the v-*abl* oncogene that is capable of transforming immature B lymphocytes to pre-B lymphocytes (class switching), causing B cell leukemias in mice

aberrant claims HEALTH CARE REIMBURSEMENT A euphemism for medical claims submitted by physicians and other health care providers for reimbursement from private insurers that have the potential for being financially abusive or frankly fraudulent; the health insurance industry estimates that fraud and abuse costs up to $100 x 10^9/year (US), but it has been historically difficult to determine whether a particular physician's pattern of claims is aberrant, as the methods for checking claims were largely manual, ie cumbersome and haphazard; with the availability of increased computing power at lower prices and the growth of electronic claims, newer algorithms* for evaluating claims patterns can be applied, to reduce this financial burden (Am Med News 10 October 1994 p 3)

*Based on the structural constructs of artificial intelligence with fuzzy logic, and neural networks, and based on massively parallel computer processing

abetalipoproteinemia Bassen-Kornzweig syndrome A rare AR [MIM 200100] disease most common in Askanazi Jews CLINICAL Acanthocytosis, cerebellar ataxia, peripheral neuropathy, retinitis pigmentosa, steatorrhea, chronic diarrhea, anemia, failure to thrive LABORATORY Low cholesterol, absent apolipoprotein B TREATMENT Diet high in medium-chain triglycerides and high levels of water-miscible vitamin E (N Engl J Med 1992; 327:628CPC)

abl A proto-oncogene first identified in mice and located on human chromosome 9q34, which in CML, translocates to chromosome 22 adjacent to the 'breakpoint cluster region', bcr, forming the Philadelphia chromosome; this hybrid gene encodes a protein with tyrosine kinase activity; the normal (non-mutated) c-*abl* proto-oncogene is apparently critical in normal myelopoiesis as it inhibits myeloid colony formation; contrariwise it is mutated in 90% of those with CML, implying that c-*abl* is an active inhibitor of myeloid clonal expansion, and has been identified in acute myelogenous and lymphocytic leukemias; see Proto-oncogene

abl p210 see P210$^{bcr/abl}$

abnutzung pigment German, worn away The brownish, 'wear and tear' pigment ceroid, which is deposited with aging in cardiac muscle, liver, brain and other organs

ABO system TRANSFUSION MEDICINE The major alloantigen system in humans, based on three carbohydrate antigens expressed on red blood cells; individuals with A, B and AB phenotypes express glycosyltransferase activities that convert the 'H antigen' into A and/or B antigens, while O(H) individuals lack this enzyme; the genes controlling expression of either 'A-ness' or 'B-ness' differ in a few single-base substitutions which translates into A or B transferase specificity, while 'O-ness' results from a single base substitution in the O gene, which encodes an inactive transferase incapable of modifying the H antigen; virtually all humans form natural (ie without previous exposure) antibodies to the non-self ABO antigens, thus an O(H) individual can only be transfused O blood, as he forms antibodies to both the A and B antigens, but his blood can be transfused to anyone; see Lewis antigen, Transplantation, Universal donor

An AB individual is a 'universal recipient,' who can receive any blood, as he forms antibodies to neither the A nor B antigens

abortion Although the term abortion is generic and implies a premature termination of pregnancy for any reason, the lay public understands the word 'miscarriage' for involuntary fetal loss or fetal wastage, and abortion for the intentional elimination of gestational products STATISTICS Rate: 0.5% of women age 15 to 44 Netherlands; 1.4% in UK; 2.7% US; 5.8% Cuba; 18.1% former Soviet Union; where abortions are illegal, the rate of complications are much higher Glossary **COMPLETE ABORTION** An abortion is considered complete only if a curettage has been performed, given the possibility of necrotizing decidual tissue remaining in the uterus, which may act as a nidus for infection **CRIMINAL ABORTION** Deliberate termination of pregnancy under illegal circumstances; although prior to the Roe *vs.* Wade decision, see there, physicians regularly performed 'criminal' abortions, in the usual parlance, criminal abortion implies a clandestine termination of pregnancy under non-sterile and unsuitable conditions, predisposing the mother to sepsis and death by exsanguination through mutilation of the uterus and perineum **EARLY ABORTION** An abortion performed before the 12th week of gestation **ELECTIVE ABORTION** An interruption of pregnancy prior to fetal viability that is performed voluntarily at the request of the mother for reasons unrelated to concerns for maternal or fetal health or welfare **HABITUAL ABORTION** A third (or more) consecutive abortion, related to stress, nutritional status, an event occurring in up to 1:200 women **INCOMPLETE ABORTION** Partial expulsion of fetus and placenta with pain and bleeding, which is potentially fatal for the mother **INDUCED ABORTION** The voluntary termination of pregnancy, which can be either by dilatation and curettage when performed in the first trimester or a saline abortion when performed later **INEVITABLE ABORTION** The 'terminal' stage of threatened abortion where there is dilatation of the cervix and rupture of membranes **LATE ABORTION** An abortion performed after the 12th week of gestation **MISSED ABORTION** The retention of a fetus known to be dead for ≥ 4 weeks **SALINE ABORTION** Voluntary termination of pregnancy during the second trimester by replacing 200 ml of amniotic fluid with 200 ml of 20% saline solution, stimulating uterine contraction, followed by fetal delivery within 12-24 hours **SEPTIC ABORTION** Fetal loss due to a bacterial infection of the uterus, which is 50 times more common in intrauterine device-users; bacteria implicated include the native vaginal flora, including *Clostridium perfringens*, aerobic and anaerobic streptococci and gram-negative bacilli **SPONTANEOUS ABORTION** 'miscarriage' SAs occur at any time and for a wide variety of reasons; ± 20-50% of all conceptuses spontaneously abort, ½ are attributed to aneuploidy, often loss of a sex chromosome and trisomy, especially 16 **THREATENED ABORTION** Vaginal bleeding at any time within the first 20 weeks of pregnancy, accompanied by colicky pain, backache and a bright red to brownish discharge, occurring in up to 20% of early pregnancies of which ½ progress to inevitable abortion

Abortion Act Legislation passed in Britain in1967 that provides the legal framework for abortions performed in the UK, most of which are performed under clause C of the Act; abortions may be performed if '...*the pregnancy has not exceeded its 24th week and that the continuance of pregnancy would involve risk, greater than if the pregnancy were terminated, or injury to the physical or mental health of the pregnant woman.*' (N Engl J Med 1995: 332:983₀A)

abortion trauma syndrome '...*a medical syndrome that does not exist.*' ABS is a 'nonentity' presumed to have been created by 'pro-life' (anti-abortion) activists, and alleged to occur in women who have undergone abortion, who allegedly suffer deleterious physical and emotional consequences after abortion.

'Scientific studies indicate that legal abortion results in fewer deleterious sequelae for women compared with other possible outcomes of unwanted pregnancy. There is no evidence of an abortion trauma syndrome.' (JAMA 1992; 268:2078COM)

abortion pill RU-486, see there

above the knee amputation AKA An 'elective' procedure used for severe (gangrenous) peripheral vascular disease, an operation commonly required in older diabetics; the AKA is preferred to a below the knee amputation in treating peripheral vascular disease if the gangrene extends above the malleoli, as the AKA has a higher healing rate (85-100%), better rehabilitation with a prosthesis and fewer complications

A box D loop MOLECULAR BIOLOGY A highly conserved (ie DNA nucleotide sequence similarity among many eukaryotic species) region located between base pairs +10 and +20 'upstream' on the tRNA gene, having the dual role of encoding functional tRNA and promoting tRNA transcription, acting as a site of receptive protein binding

ABPA Allergic bronchopulmonary aspergillosis

'abracadabra therapy' A therapeutic modality that may effect a cure in certain conditions in mentally impressionable subjects; it is not known why warts in children may occasionally regress with the physician simply touching the wart and murmuring 'abracadabra', the classic incantation uttered by magicians (prestidigitators)

absence NEUROLOGY Petit mal epilepsy A form of epilepsy characterized by episodic arrest of sensation and voluntary activity CLINICAL Transient loss of contact with the environment, decline in school performance DIAGNOSIS A 3-minute hyperventilation test may elicit an 'absence' TREATMENT Trimethadione, ethosuximide; Cf Grand mal seizure

absence attack Absence, see there

absinthism Intoxication with an alcoholic beverage popular in fin-de-siècle France; the active toxin, thujone, is extracted from wormwood (*Artemisia pontica*, a plant used for de-worming, hence the trivial name); absinthe's neurological effects (mental deterioration, loss of time/space orientation and hallucinations) eventually led to its ban in 1915

absolute alcohol Ethanol that contains ≤ 1% water by weight; it is a critical working reagent in certain areas of the clinical laboratory, in particular histopathology, where it is required in certain steps of embedding tissues in paraffin

Because of its considerable potential for abuse as an inebrient, AA not uncommonly 'disappears' from storage areas and must be kept under lock and key-Author's note

absorbable suture see Catgut, Synthetic absorbable suture

absorbed dose RADIATION PHYSICS The energy imparted by ionizing radiation per unit mass of irradiated material, defined in the SI (International System) unit, the gray (Gy), which corresponds to the 100 rads, the rad being the old unit of absorbed dose

absorptiometry RADIOLOGY A technique that measures the degree to which radiation emitted by a radioisotope is completely dissipated in a tissue; absorptiometry is used to measure bone mass and is of two types: single photon and dual X-ray; see Bone mineral density

absorption IMMUNOLOGY A laboratory technique that consists of either 1) Removal of antibody from serum by adding an antigen or 2) Removal of an antigen by adding an antibody; absorption allows an antiserum to be purified by removing unwanted immunoglobulins or may be used to 'fish' for an antigen or antibody of interest

abstract RESEARCH A brief synopsis of research data, which may be presented at scientific meetings, and subsequently published in a peer-reviewed journal, although the abstracts themselves may not be subjected to the same rigorous review required of those writing 'lead' articles for the same journal SCIENTIFIC JOURNALISM The leading paragraph(s) that introduces a report of scientific information; the New England Journal of Medicine has adopted a structured format which has 1) Background 2) Methods 3) Results, and 4) Conclusions; the purpose of the abstract is to enable the reader to efficiently grasp the essence of the article

abstract 'creep' SCIENTIFIC JOURNALISM Growth in the length of abstracts, especially those longer than that stated in a journal's instructions for authors, some 'creep' occurs when authors attempt to provide as much information as possible, under the assumption that only the abstract will be read; a second, major cause of abstract 'creep' results from the advance of medical science, where the complexity of the physiology, molecular pathology, experimental design or procedure requires greater details for the reader to grasp the question being addressed

ABT-538 AIDS An inhibitor of HIV-1 protease (which carves functional proteins from a large precursor molecule) which when administered to HIV-infected individuals ↓ viral load by 2 orders of magnitude; and ↑ CD4 T cell levels 3-fold (**Bio/Technology 1995; 13:206**) see L735,524

abtröpfung German, dropping-off DERMATOPATHOLOGY A term used by histopathologists referring to the 'falling off' of epithelioid cells in a junctional nevus as they 'penetrate' the superficial dermis

abuse A behavior that may be formally defined as '...*the willful infliction of physical pain, injury, or mental anguish, or willful deprivation by a caretaker of services necessary for physical and/or mental well being.*' (**State of Connecticut. General Statutes. Chapter 319. Sect. 17A–430; in N Engl J Med 1995; 332:437RA**) see Battered wife syndrome, Child abuse, Domestic violence, Elderly abuse

ABVD ONCOLOGY A combination chemotherapy regimen consisting of doxorubicin-adriamycin, bleomycin, vincristine, and dacarbazine (**N Engl J Med 1993; 328:1045c**) 6-8 months of ABVD is as effective as 12 months of MOPP-ABVD; both are more effective than MOPP alone (**N Engl J Med 1992; 327:1478oa**) see CHOP, MOPP

abzymes Hybrid catalytic molecules designed to have a certain specificity; the hybrid is generated by combining an antibody with an enzyme; although these two molecules have different functions, both bind molecules in a specific manner and thus the 'marriage' of the two functions is logical; the 'ab-' portion corresponds to the highly specific binding sequence, analogous to an immunoglobulin's variable region and the '-zyme' portion incorporates catalytic machinery; the spin-off will be 'custom-made' catalysts for use in biology and medicine; there are two general types of 'abzymes' 1) Catalytic antibodies, which take advantage of an antibody's ability to selectively stabilize transitional state configurations or overcome entropic barriers by aligning reaction partners, accomplished by adding a catalyst that is either synthesized or a polypeptide with enzymatic activity, eg lipolytic abzymes and 2) Hybrid enzymes, which exploit a natural receptor with a designated specificity, accomplished by either redesigning an existing active site of enzyme action (Method: oligonucleotide-directed mutagenesis) or by adding or replacing an entire catalytic domain, thereby generating a hybrid enzyme, eg selective fusion of nucleic acid-specific binding domains to the non-specific phosphodiesterase enzyme, resulting in sequence-specific DNA (analogous to that of restriction enzymes) or RNA-cleaving molecules

aca LABORATORY MEDICINE The world's first automated discrete random-access analyzer, which when introduced by DuPont Chemical Diagnostics division in 1968 could perform 8 tests; the current generation of devices can handle up to 85 different assays (**CAP Today July 1993**)

academic boycott A concerted political effort by physicians and/or scientists that indicates their displeasure with a country's prevailing policy regarding fundamental human rights, eg the academic boycott of South Africa, which developed in the wake of the death of Steve Biko, or the boycott of the International conference on AIDS originally scheduled to meet in Boston, which was held in Amsterdam in 1992 due to the US government's policy about not allowing visas to HIV-positive individuals; such efforts may prove instrumental in causing a change in policy, although the academicians in the boycotted country may suffer the consequences of various forms of government pressure (**JAMA 1991; 266:501**) see Biko

academic medical center Academic hospital, academic institution A health care organization (numbering from 120 to 380 in the US, depending on the criteria of the definition) that is linked to a hospital or hospital complex that carries out the three missions of teaching, research, and (tertiary) patient care in close affiliation or as part of a degree-granting university; given the rapidly mounting momentum toward health care reform in the US, the AMC is unlikely to survive in its present form; possible transitions include 1) Parceling out of certain academic functions (eg research, teaching) to organizations better able to perform these functions 2) Splitting AMCs into two tiers, a large group of community-oriented AMCs that perform clinical investigations and focus on the production of primary care physicians and basic specialists and the provision of secondary and tertiary care, and a small group of 'super-tertiary' AMCs that concentrate on biomedical research, training of researchers and subspecialists and management of patients with extraordinarily complex conditions and 3) Full integration of AMCs into the reformed health care system (**N Engl J Med 1993; 329:1812sb**)

'academic pork' RESEARCH FUNDING A permutation of 'pork barrel' or earmarked funding for research (US), in which the equitable system of peer review for funding grant proposals is bypassed by pressures from legislators, constituencies or lobbyists (**Science 1992; 255:24n&v**)

academic detailing THERAPEUTICS The use of educational 'props' to improve drug prescribing practices (**JAMA 1990; 263:549; N Engl J Med 1992; 327:163oa**) Cf Detailing

academician An inhabitant of the medical ivory tower, usually referring to a health care provider who sees a minimal number of patients and spends more of his/her time advancing the science of medicine*; Cf Clinician

*Or his/her career by publishing findings that may be greater in volume than value

***Acanthamoeba* infection** An amebic infection that when disseminated, which is characterized by granulomatous lesions of the skin and brain, most commonly occurs in debilitated or immunocompromised subjects, often leading to death AT-RISK GROUPS AIDS, alcohol abuse, DM, immunosuppressive therapy (transplantation-related), malignancy (leukemia, lymphoma), malnutrition TREATMENT Uncertain; a case of *A rhysodes* was successfully treated with topical chlorhexidine and ketoconazole combined with systemic pentamidine (IV) and oral itraconazole (N Engl J Med 1994; 331:85CR)

AcAP *Ancylostoma caninum* anticoagulant peptide A small peptide produced by *A caninum* that has anticoagulant properties, which blocks the activity of coagulation factor Xa (Sci Am 1995; 272/6:70)

ACAT Acyl-coenzyme A:cholesterol *o*-transferase, sterol *o*-acyltransferase The enzyme [EC 2.3.1.26] responsible for forming cholesteryl esters from cholesterol, by transferring acyl groups with a single *cis* bond

acatalasemia Takahara's disease An AD [MIM 115500] condition of early onset first described in the Japanese, caused by a deficiency in tissue and erythrocyte catalase, the enzyme responsible for reducing peroxide to water and oxygen; as peroxide accumulates, malignant alveolar pyorrhea and oral gangrene ensue, requiring removal of all teeth

acclerated hypertension Malignant hypertension, see there

acceleration-deceleration injury A major cause of cerebral morbidity, related to abrupt movement and deformation of the brain within the cranial cavity ACCELERATION The head suddenly accelerates, eg a blow to the head, and the stationary brain is struck by the accelerated cranium at the site of the blow DECELERATION A rapidly moving skull is abruptly stopped, eg an auto accident, while the brain continues forward and impacts directly below the site where the skull stops; the immediate loss of consciousness is thought to be due to deformation of the brainstem and reticular activating system, with concomitant shearing, stretching, diffuse neuronal and axonal injury; tissue destruction is most marked in the inferior frontal gyri and anterior temporal lobes; the mechanism of acceleration-deceleration injury is the same as Contrecoup lesions, although the former term addresses the clinical aspects of the kinetics, while the latter addresses the pathological effects of abrupt movements on the brain

'access' The ability of a person or group to obtain health care, which is a function of 1) Geographic or logistic factors, eg rural communities have poor access to medical attention, due to a relative lack of providers, 2) Finances or ability to pay for services and 3) Other factors including ethnic, social and psychiatric aspects of the individual(s) seeking health care

accessory cell A macrophage that aids in immune recognition by binding circulating antigens, processing them and presenting them on the cell surface, in order for the immune recognition cascade to proceed, which in addition, secrete a broad palatte of cytokines and biological response modifiers‡; see Antigen-presenting cell

Note: Binding of an antigen to a self cell is a *sine qua non* for T cell response to an antigen, as the T cell receptor requires a self major histocompatability complex class II molecule with a bound foreign antigen before it can respond to an antigen

accessory spleen (*splen accessorius*) [NA6] Any of a number of small aggregates or masses of encapsulated splenic tissue that are located adjacent to the spleen or along the gastrosplenic ligament; they are common, are identified in up to 1/3 of all postmortem examinations, and may become clinically important in hematologic diseases (eg hereditary spherocytosis, TTP, and hypersplenism) for which splenectomy represents the definitive therapy, and for which accessory splenic tissue must be removed

accident PUBLIC HEALTH An unintentional and/or unexpected event or ocurrence that may result in injury or death; the most common cause of accidental death in developed countries is the automobile; after many years in the US,

the highway speed limit of 90 km/hr (55 mph) was increased to 110 km/hr (65 mph), resulting in a doubling of fatal accidents to 2.9/161 million vehicle-kilometers

accident-prone An adjective referring to a person's real or percieved tendency to suffer from accidents of various types

accident-proneness The state of being 'accident-prone'; see above

accidental hypothermia A condition defined as '...*an unintentional decline in the core* (body) *temperature below 35°C, a temperature at which thermoregulatory systems begin to fail, as compensatory responses intended to reduce heat loss through conduction, convection, evaporation, radiation, and respiration are limited* (N Engl J Med 1994; 331:1756RV)

accordion sign A periodic 'crumpling' of 2 distinct radiologic densities EMERGENCY RADIOLOGY Compression and medial displacement of a calcified splenic artery, which, when seen on the plain abdominal film of trauma victims, has been fancifully likened to an accordion and is suggestive of splenic rupture or hematoma formation GI RADIOLOGY A finding in upper gastrointestinal radiocontrast studies, described in advanced progressive systemic sclerosis*, where the jejunum is dilated and foreshortened with mural fibrosis and the valvulae conniventes are of normal thickness, thus imparting an accordion-like corrugated appearance to the contrast column PEDIATRIC RADIOLOGY Crumpling and shortening of long bones, especially the femurs, seen in type II osteogenesis imperfecta, a disease accompanied by low birth weight, beading of the ribs, early death due to respiratory insufficiency resulting from a defective thoracic cage, softened skull, fragile skin with defective type I collagen; heredity is variable, affecting 1:60 000 live births; ½ are stillborn

Note: Other radiologic findings in the GI tract in progressive systemic sclerosis include pneumatosis intestinalis, pseudo-obstruction, intussusception, sacculations and volvulus of the small intestine

accountability MEDICAL ETHICS The extent to which individual(s) are answerable to a higher authority; physicians are held accountable before the law, the Hippocratic oath and their patients; scientists are accountable before the law, their peers and grant-giving agencies; more recently, the physician's accountability to the patient has been broadened to include accountability to the public in general, insurance carriers, and government agencies at all levels (Lab Medicine 1994; 25:355; Ach Pathol Lab Med 1992; 116:602OA)

accountability 'fever' 'Dingellization', see there

accountable health partnership HEALTH CARE ENVIRONMENT A competing economic or for-profit unit (eg physicians considered in aggregate, or competing hospitals) that has been proposed as a key component of the Clinton Health plan; an AHP would contract with insurance-purchasing partnerships to provide standardized packages of medical benefits for fixed per capita rates; such partnerships would hasten the demise of the fee-for-service form of healthcare reimbursement, and place providers at financial risk for their performance (N Engl J Med 1993; 328:1208ED) see Managed competition

accreditation GRADUATE MEDICAL EDUCATION The process required of a hospital or health care center that allows it to act an accredited training program for interns, residents, and fellows HOSPITAL ADMINISTRATION The validating process that determines whether a body or facility (eg a hospital) meets a series of standards of quality in terms of physical plant, administration and professional staffing; most US hospitals are accredited by non-profit, professional 'policing' organizations, eg the Joint Commission on Accreditation of Health Care Organizations (see JCAHO) created to assure the public that a facility has met the accrediting organization's standards

accumulation theory see 'Garbage can' hypothesis

accuracy LABORATORY MEDICINE The extent to which a value obtained from a test reflects or agrees with the true value of the analyte being tested, measured statistically by standard deviations

Note: Precision The degree of reproducibility of test results, regardless of whether or not they are accurate, are measured statistically by the coefficient of variation

ACD-CPR Active compression-decompression cardiopulmonary resuscitation, see there

ACE Angiotensin-converting enzyme

ACE Angiotensin-converting enzyme (BIOCHEMISTRY) see there; Cf ACE inhibitors, also 1) Acute Care for Elderly (N Engl J Med 1995; 332:1338OA) 2) Alcohol, chloroform, ether (an obsolete aesthetic mixture) 3) American College of Epidemiology

ace of clubs appearance Cloverleaf appearance, see there

ACE inhibitors Angiotensin-converting enzyme inhibitors A group of drugs, eg captopril, enalapril that supplant β-blockers and diuretics in the treatment of essential hypertension, which act by blocking ACE; the total mortality and morbidity due to congestive heart failure is reduced by AIs* (JAMA 1995; 273:1450)

*Specifically, captopril, enalapril, lisionopril, quinapril, ramipril

ace of spades appearance GI RADIOLOGY 1) The normal appearance of the duodenal bulb in a radio-contrast study of an upper GI series; Cf Cloverleaf appearance 2) see Bird's beak appearance

acetaldehyde The major metabolic product of ethanol, which is generated by ethanol dehydrogenase and subsequently metabolized to acetate by aldehyde dehydrogenase; it is postulated that the hepatic injury induced by ethanol is the result of tissue responses to acetaldehyde, including acetaldehyde-induced fibrogenesis, acetaldehyde-induced lipid peroxidation enzyme inhibition and formation of antibodies against acetaldehyde adduct proteins, eg serum albumin, hemoglobin and cytokskeletal proteins, including tubulin

acemannin A complex sugar from the aloe vera plant, administered as a concentrate or injected, which is anecdotally reported to have antiretroviral activity (Am Med News 21 Nov 1994 p13) Cf AIDS fraud

acenocoumarol A fast-acting oral anticoagulant of the vitamin K-antagonist type; in patients with proximal vein thrombosis, acenocoumarol can be co-administered with full-dose heparin (N Engl J Med 1992; 327:1485OA)

Acer cluster A cluster of six cases of HIV seroconversion that allegedly shared only one feature in common–during an 18-month period they had all been treated by the same dentist, Dr DJ Acer; although each of the patients had one or more HIV risk factors, eg sexual activity or blood transfusion, the weight of epidemiological, laboratory (including analysis of HIV DNA sequences), and statistical evidence favors transmission from the dentist to the patients; the mechanism by which the transmission occurred is highly speculative, ranging from poor hygiene to homicide (New York Times 5 July 1994; C3) see Bergalis

acetowhite lesions GYNECOLOGY A whitish patch seen on the uterine cervix when it is 'painted' with 5% acetic acid (vinegar); most condylomatous lesions of the uterine cervix are white, the whiter the lesion, the greater the hyperkeratosis; given their premalignant potential, especially when positive for HPV types 16, 18 and 33, all acetowhite lesions warrant biopsy; see HPV

acetylcholine A neurotransmitter, which when bound to its cognate receptor, mediates synaptic transmission between nerve and muscle; the nicotinic acetylcholine receptor is located on the post-synaptic membrane and is a heterotetrameric polypeptide complex with the stochiometry of $\alpha_2\beta\gamma\delta$

acetylcholine receptor The nicotinic acetylcholine receptor is a 250 000 M_r glycoprotein arranged in a barrel-stave-like fashion around a central channel, which is composed of five subunits, two α subunits, a β subunit, a δ subunit, and a γ or ε subunit; each α subunit has an extracellular acetylcholine binding site located near amino acids 192 and 193; ARs undergo continuous turnover and renewal, which explains the complete recovery of ARs damaged by autoimmune antibodes as occurs in myasthenia gravis (N Engl J Med 1994; 330:1797RA, Sci Am 1993; 269/5:58) see Myasthenia gravis

Note: The most commonly used experimental source of AR is the electric organ of the marine ray, *Torpedo aplysia*

acetylcholine receptor antibodies AChR antibodies A group of antibodies that are reactive with epitopes other than the binding site for acetylcholine or α-bungarotoxin; AChR binding antibodies are present in up to 88% of patients with active myasthenia gravis, which wax and wane as a function of disease severity; AChR

acetylcysteine An agent that prevents hepatic necrosis in patients with fulminant hepatic failure induced by acetaminophen and other noxious stimuli; acetylcysteine acts by improving oxygen delivery and consumption through replenishment of glutathione stores

Acheulean tool kit PALEOANTHROPOLOOGY A group of stone hand axes circa ± 1.4 million years old, found near fossilized *Homo erectus* bones in Africa, which have been thought to be the tools necessary for *H erectus* to migrate from Africa (Scientific American 1994; 270/5:31)

Achilles' heel cleavage MOLECULAR BIOLOGY A method that allows a segment of DNA to be cut precisely at the desired location and nowhere else

BACKGROUND: Restriction endonucleases have been and continue to be the workhorses of molecular biology for gene cloning, hybridization analysis and gene sequencing; they cleave DNA at specific discrete sites, ie each time a specific 4-to-6 oligonucleotide sequence is 'seen' on the DNA molecule, a restriction endonuclease clips the DNA into pieces ranging from 2.5 (or smaller) to 35 kD, with 45 kD being near the limit of resolution of conventional electrophoretic gels

PROBLEM: Even the most selective of restriction endonucleases ('rare choppers') cut the DNA into too many small pieces, a major obstacle in handling large DNA segments required for the Human genome project (see there)

SOLUTION: Use a bacterial DNA-binding protein, the lac repressor, which recognizes a 20 base sequence, the lac operator (synthesized according to the needs of the investigator, containing the recogition sites for two commonly used restriction endonucleases; when the *lac* repressor is added to the yeast cell, the repressor finds the operator and binds it, covering up the two restriction sites (like Thetis' hand over Achilles' heel, see below note); then a methyltransferase is added, inactivating the restriction sites, except for the two 'hidden' below the lac repressor; removal of the *lac* repressor then leaves the genome with one recognition site for each of two enzymes; thus like Achilles' heel, a genome may be made to be vulnerable to cutting in only one site; Cf Triplex DNA; Achilles' heel has been used in other contexts: 1) The terminus of a DNA helix is related to Achilles' heel, given its lability when it is not 'capped' by a telomere (J Theor Biol 1973; 41:181) and 2) Psychological vulnerability to a degree sufficient to undermine a subject's character development; Achilles' mother, Thetis, dipped him into the River Styx which made him invulnerable to arrows except at the one place on the heel where she had held him

achoo syndrome Photic sneeze reflex An AD [MIM 100820] condition affecting ± 25% of the population causing sneezing upon passing from dark to bright light, also known as the helico-cilio-sternutatogenic reflex

acid aerosol ENVIRONMENT Colloidal suspensions of hydrogen ion-containing particles that form the so-called 'summer haze' generated by sulfur dioxide (SO_2) and nitrogen dioxide emissions from coal-burning electrical power plants; acid aerosols are transformed into ammonium bisulfate, sulfuric and nitric acids and coupled to low level ozone, where they are inculpated in pulmonary dysfunction in those who exercise during the warm weather

Note: Acid 'rain' derives from the same sources

'acid blob' activation domain MOLECULAR BIOLOGY A

structural motif that has been identified in various transcription factors that function by stimulating either RNA polymerase II or another general transcription factor

acid elution TRANSFUSION MEDICINE The use of a buffered solution of HCl to remove (elute) antigens from the surface of erythrocytes in order to identify those antigens which have potential for producing an hemolytic reaction or agglutination

acid-fast stain A generic term for any of a number of special histological stains (Ziehl-Neelsen, Kinyoun, and others), used to identify *Mycobacterium* species, which are acid-fast due to the mycolic acid content in the outer capsule; at an increased temperature, the basic fuchsin in phenol penetrates the capsular wax, hardens, and retains the dye during treatment with acid alcohol; acid-fast stains may adhere to free hydroxy and carboxi- group of mycolic acid, explaining the acid fastness of pine pollen, keratohyaline, lead inclusions, histoplasmosis and lipofuchsin, as well as *Nocardia* species and certain propionic bacteria; the Fite acid-fast uses a xylene-oil combination to partially 'restore' the acid-fastness lost in routine processing and is used to identify *M lepra*

acid phosphatase An enzyme [EC 3.1.3.2] with broad specificity that also catalyzes transphosphorylations

acid phosphatase stain A histochemical stain used in hematology to identify enzymes that hydrolyze organic phosphate esters at pH 5.0; acid phosphatase is present in normal lymphoblasts, neutrophils, mast cells, and pathologically in Gaucher's disease, histiocytosis X, hairy cell and ALL

acid rain ENVIRONMENT Precipitation laced with the detritus of developed nations' profligacy, produced predominantly by power plants that burn coal of variable purity, generating sulfur dioxide and nitrous oxide, which lower the pH of precipitation; the summary report from the National Acid Precipitation Assessment Program (NAPAP) on the effects of acid rain in the US (which cost $570 million, required 10 years, and accumulated 6000 pages of data), concluded that acid rain 1) Adversely affects aquatic life in 10% of lakes and streams in the eastern US 2) Contributes to the decline of certain trees at high elevations by reducing their tolerance to the cold weather and 3) Contributes to soil erosion and corrosion of buildings and materials

acid-reflux disorder A generic term for any of a number of conditions caused by the reflux of gastric secretions, on the esophageal mucosa (GI reflux disorder–GERD), as well as the laryngeal mucosa (reflux laryngitis) and lungs ('reflux pneumonitis') PATHOPHYSIOLOGY Transient relaxation of the lower esophageal sphincter, often after meals, and more common when there is fat in the duodenum, and accompanied by hiatal hernia DIAGNOSIS Post-prandial heartburn relieved by antacids, endoscopy (± biopsy), pH monitoring TREATMENT-MEDICAL Change lifestyle (eg raise head of bed, ↓ bedtime snacks, ↓ fatty foods, quit smoking, ↓ alcohol, use of antacids or alginic acid); histamine-receptor blockers, eg cimetidine, ranitidine, omeprazole TREATMENT-SURGICAL Nissen fundoplication (widely preferred), Hill gastropexy, Belsey fundoplication (**N Engl J Med 1994; 331:656cc**)

acid tide PHYSIOLOGY A long-term fall in the pH of the blood and urine which occurs in those on a prolonged fast; Cf Alkaline tide

acid vesicle system PHYSIOLOGY Subcellular structures in all nucleated mammalian cells formed as a result of receptor-mediated endocytosis, in which the ligand (molecule being internalized) is bound to receptors that cluster in specialized submembranous regions known as coated pits, ie 'coated' by the protein clathrin; once internalized, the vesicles are acidified; at pH 5-5.6, the ligand dissociates from its receptor; subcellular structures may also form as a result of lysosomal enzyme targeting, similar to receptor-mediated endocytosis, but is poorly understood; intracellular acid vesicles include coated vesicles (receptor-mediated macromolecule transport from the cell surface), endosomes (macromolecule sorting), lysosomes (degradation of internalized macromolecules), and the Golgi complex; defects in the acid vesicle system are implicated in familial hypercholesterolemia, myotonic dystrophy, I-cell disease, type III mucolipidosis and infections, including chlamydial, *Legionella* species, nocardiosis, toxoplasmosis and chloroquine-resistant malaria; see Clathrin, Coated pits, CURL

acidophilic body Any densely acidophilic, eosinophilic (ie pink), often 5-15 μm in diameter mass seen by light microscopy with H&E GYNECOLOGIC PATHOLOGY Dense pink, rounded, PAS-positive 2-8 μm in diameter masses, also known as hyaline globules, composed of basement membrane material seen intra- and extracellularly in ovarian endodermal sinus tumor HEPATOPATHOLOGY Individual condensed and necrotic hepatocytes with dense pink cytoplasm and a pyknotic nucleus, often multiple with periportal distribution, partially surrounded by a 'round cell' infiltrate, a finding characteristic of acute viral hepatitis RENAL PATHOLOGY Rounded intranuclear and intracytoplasmic inclusions with ragged edges composed of protein, lead and occasionally iron, seen in the renal tubular cells and hepatocytes of those with chronic lead exposure, often accompanied by aminoaciduria and glycosuria

acinic cell carcinoma A low-grade malignancy of the salivary glands, which has granular cytoplasm and which usually is adequately treated with wide local excision

acne mechanica SPORTS MEDICINE A '...*superficial occlusive folliculitis that results in a chronic acneiform eruption in athletes in areas of mechanical pressure, heat, and/or friction.*' (**JS Dover, in TB Fitzpatrick et al, Eds, Dermatology in General Medicine, 4th ed, McGraw-Hill, New York, 1993**) While football players are particularly prone (hence the synonym, football acne), other sportspersons are not immune to AM and it may be seen in hockey players and in those in aerobic and exercise classes who stuff more blubber than otherwise advisable in occlusive synthetic leotards

acorn deformity Spinning top deformity A descriptor for the radiocontrast findings in distal urethral stenosis, in which there is pre-stenotic widening of the urethra, fixation and narrowing of the bladder neck, forcing of large volumes of urine through a thin-walled urethra; the deformity is seen by voiding cystourethrography and is most commonly symptomatic in young males

acoustic coupler Modem, see there

acridine orange An immunologic fluorochrome (fluorescent dye) that non-specifically binds to RNA (red fluorescence), DNA (green fluorescence), proteins, polysaccharides and glycosaminoglycans; AO also acts as a non-specific tissue stain that 1) Detects increased mitotic activity (implying cancer in the proper setting) or 2) Is more sensitive (but less specific) than the Gram stain for detecting bacteria in wound swabs; because it is carcinogenic, intercalating itself within replicating DNA causing insertional or deletional mutations, acridine orange is not routinely used in most histological laboratories

acrocephalosyndactyly type III An AD [MIM 101400] condition with clinical features of Apert and Crouzon syndromes, characterized by a typical facies with a parrot-beaked nose, jaw hypoplasia, antimongoloid slant of the eyes, hypertelorism, deformed ears (long prominent crus), hydrophthalmos, acrocephalysyndactyly and cleft palate, as well as leukoderma, musculoskeletal contractions of elbows and knees, cardiac malformations, pseudohermaphroditism; other parrot noses have been described Rubenstein-Taybi disease and Pierre Robin disease; see Bird face

acroeponym An acronym that began life as an eponym, where the letters of the author's name can be used to form a relevant acronym, eg APGAR/Apgar score, MOHS/Mohs score; Cf Autoeponym

acromegaloidism A condition with the clinical features of acromegaly, see below, normal serum levels of growth hormone and insulin-like growth factor I (IGF-I), insulin resistance and defective IGF-I binding; some patients produce a poorly characterized erythroprogenitor growth factor

acromegaly An endocrinopathy of adults due to excess growth hormone secretion, of pituitary or extra-pituitary origin; acromegaly may also result from excess secretion of growth hormone-releasing hormone by hypothalamic tumors or be due to ectopic production by small cell carcinoma of the lungs, carcinoids, islet cell tumors, adrenal adenomas or other 'endocrine' tumors CLINICAL Coarsening of facial features, bony proliferation, soft tissue swelling, hyperhidrosis, macroglossia, headache, amenorrhea, impotence, glucose intolerance, hypertension, heart disease, carpal tunnel syndrome, sleep apnea

Note: Excess hormone production that precedes the closure of the epiphyseal growth plates results in gigantism in afflicted children and adolescents

act of smoking 'factor' PUBLIC HEALTH A generic term of recent vintage for those acts, eg fumbling for a cigarette or a 'light', flicking ashes from clothing, tossing the cigarette butt out the window, and so on; while AOSFs are rarely implicated factors in motor vehicle accidents, they have been shown in computerized driving simulators to significantly increase the likelihood of rear-end collisions (**JAMA 1995; 273:1334c**)

ACTH A 39-amino acid polypeptide hormone that regulates adrenal cortical function, stimulating the release of cortisol, mineralocorticoids, and adrenal androgens; pituitary ACTH* is in turn regulated by corticotropin-releasing hormone (CRH); ACTH is increased in pituitary-dependent Cushing syndrome

*Although ACTH is an abbreviation (abbreviations are in general frowned upon as standard terms in lexicography), its use appears to solve the dilemma of orthography (adrenocorticotrophic hormone—1994 Biomeda catalog and elsewhere, adrenocorticotropic hormone, and multiple other names that have enjoyed periods of popularity, to wit corticotropin, currently popular among some endocrinologists, as well as older terms including acortan, adrenocorticotrophin, adrenocorticotropic peptide, adrenocorticotropin, adrenotrophic hormone, adrenotrophin, adrenotropic hormone, adrenotropin, and corticotrophin

actin A major muscle protein, which with myosin, is responsible for muscle contraction and has an active mechanicochemical role in cell function; actin is an ATPase that binds to adenine nucleotides and is a filamentous protein divided into a 46-kD monomeric form, G-actin and a mature contractile form, F-actin, formed from G-actin polymers, capable of functioning in absence of myosin

β-actin MOLECULAR DIAGNOSTICS A molecule, the mRNA of which is constitutively produced by all cells; β-actin primers can be used to monitor the efficiency of RNA extraction from cells, the lack of genomic DNA contamination of an RNA preparation, and the success of cDNA synthesis

actin filaments Long and slender chains of G-actin that transmit tension in muscles, participate in cell protrusion, act as scaffolding for the binding of dozens of different molecules; these filaments are able to withstand molecular forces but are highly sensitive to gelsolin which cleaves them with almost surgical precision; gelsolin-actin cleavage is strictly regulated; micromolar concentrations of Ca^{2+} or a low pH activate gelsolin to sever; certain phosphoinositides inhibit severing and may release gelsolin and allow actin filament growth (**Nature 1993; 364:685; 675n&v**) by elec-

tron microscopy, AFs appear attached to the Z bands and at the other interdigitate with myosin filaments

acting out PSYCHIATRY A form of displacement in which the behavior is a response to a current situation; AO is a manifestation of masked adolescent depression, where desperation is denied or somatized, indicating a need for psychiatric intervention; acting-out behaviors include school truancy, substance abuse and somatization (headaches or abdominal pain)

'actinic' cancer A generic term for any cutaneous malignancy attributable to excess exposure to solar radiation, most commonly arising in the head and neck, followed by the legs and trunk; in one study, the incidence of squamous cell carcinoma of the skin in ♂ rose from 42 to $106/10^6$ between 1960 and 1986 and in ♀ from 10 to $30/10^6$; malignant melanoma in ♂ rose from 5 to $20/10^5$ between 1960 and 1986 and in ♀ from 5 to $17/10^6$; see Melanoma

actinic keratosis Solar keratosis A premalignant lesion of sun-exposed skin which is clinically characterized by scaly erythematous plaques, and histologically by changes which include hyperkeratosis, atrophy, and cellular atypia; in subjects with AK placed on a low-fat diet, the incidence of new lesions fell to ⅓ that of the control (non-dietary intervention) group (**N Engl J Med 1994; 330:1272oa**)

actinomycosis A chronic infection by *Actinomyces israelii*, a filamentous, slow-growing, facultative anaerobic gram-positive bacterium; it is characterized by indolent suppurative lesions of the cervicofacial region (40-60% of cases), lungs and thoracic region (15%), abdomen and other regions, often accompanied by draining sinus tracts and abscesses containing yellow aggregates ('sulfur granules') Note: Actinomycosis is often associated with intrauterine devices that have been in place for prolonged periods of time TREATMENT Penicillin IV (**N Engl J Med 1993; 329:264cpc**)

activated charcoal CLINICAL TOXICOLOGY Charcoal in a granular form that has been heated to 200°C with removal of volatile gases; AC is used for early management of oral intoxications and is effective against most toxic substances except mercury, iron, lithium and cyanide; if the drug has an enterohepatic cycle, as do barbiturates, glutethimide, morphine and other narcotics and tricyclic antidepressants, charcoal administration may be repeated for up to 24 hours; usual adult dose 50-100 g INDUSTRIAL HYGIENE AC can be used to purify gases, as a deodorant, decolorant, and filtering agent

activated macrophage IMMUNOLOGY A mononuclear phagocyte that has been 'turned on' (ie has enhanced activity) by lymphokines; activated macrophages are twice the size of resting macrophages, have increased lysozymes and surface expression of MHC class II antigens and are pivotal in defending against microorganisms that grow well in histiocytes and other cells, eg *Listeria* spp and *Salmonella* spp

activated protein C resistance APC resistance A condition caused by an inherited defect in the anticoagulant response to APC and clinically characterized by ↑ venous thrombosis; it is responsible for 20-50% of cases of deep vein thrombosis PATHOGENESIS Protein C, a key regulator of coagulation, circulates in the inactivated form and becomes activated by the binding of thrombin to thrombomodulin receptors on vascular endothelial cells; once activated, protein C lyses coagulation factors Va and VIIIa; APCR may be due to a selective defect in factor V coagulant function (**N Engl J Med 1994; 330:517oa**); the most common cause of APCR is a mutation of the factor V gene in residue 506 (Arg→Gln), which results in familial thrombosis (**N Engl J Med 1994; 331:1559oa**)

activated smooth muscle cell see Smooth muscle cell

activation BIOCHEMISTRY The conversion, often enzymatic, of a molecule to a functionally reactive form, eg activation of the complement or coagulation cascades IMMUNOLOGY see Lymphocyte activation

activator MOLECULAR BIOLOGY A protein that binds to genes at enhancer sites, helping to determine which genes will be transcribed, speeding the rate of transcription (Sci Am 1995; 272/2:56) see Transcription activator

active compression-decompression-cardiopulmary resuscitation A novel method for CPR in which the passive relaxation phase is converted into an active phase by a hand-held suction device (Ambu CardioPump); preliminary data indicates that ACD-CPR improves the rate of initial resuscitation, survival at 24 hours, and neurologic outcome after in-hospital cardiac arrest (N Engl J Med 1993; 329:1918OA) in a prospective randomized clinical trial with a crossover group design there was no reported difference (see Graph) in various parameters of survival and health states between ACD-CPR and standard CPR (JAMA 1995; 273:1261) see CPR; Cf Vest CPR

Note: The prototype for the ACD-CPR device was a toilet plunger; despite early reports of success, the device does not appear to be particularly effective in improving the outcomes of cardiac arrest (JAMA 1995; 273:1299)

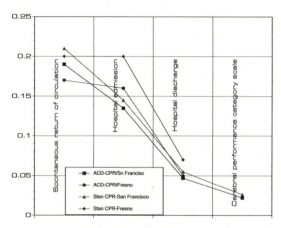

ACD-CPR vs Standard CPR

active immunotherapy The administration of substances that are capable of eliciting an immune response that protects a host organism from a potential pathogen; Cf Passive immunotherapy, Vaccine

active noise control The use of energy-consumptive systems to reduce 'white' noise by applying new algorithms and computer-controlled digital processors, generating sounds that are opposite that of the undesired noise(s), effectively canceling their effects (Science 1991; 252:508rv)

activin Any member of the transforming growth factor β superfamily, which are dimeric (βAβA, βAβB, βBβB) proteins that are widely expressed in murine development and highly conserved throughout vertebrate evolution; activins were first identified in *Xenopus* spp, and have diverse biological roles, including differentiation of erythroid precursors, promotion of the survival of nerve cells, stimulation of insulin and anterior pituitary hormone secretion, modulation of granulosa cell differentiation (activin binds to follistatin, an FSH release inhibitor), differentiation of certain erythroleukemia cell lines; activins were thought to act on the early mesoderm (notochord and segmented myotomes), either inducing the development of a rudimentary axial pattern with anteroposterior polarity at high concentrations and dorsoventral polarity at low concentration or revealing preexisting patterns, triggering tissue transition from a blastula to mesoderm,

ectoderm and endoderm; more recent data suggest that activin does not appear to play role in mesodermal development (Nature 1995; 374:354, 356, 360, 311) see Mesoderm-inducing factors

activity RADIATION PHYSICS The rate of disintegration (decay or transformation) of radioactive material, defined in the SI (International System) unit, the becquerel (Bq), which corresponds to 2.70×10^{-11} curies (Ci)

actomyosin A G actin-like contractile protein complex found in platelets, which consists of actin and myosin in a actin:myosin ratio of 100:1 (muscle has a ratio of 7:1), which appears with platelet activation

ACT-UP AIDS Coalition to Unleash Power A New York-based political activist organization with an AIDS-targeted agenda

actuarial (disease-free) survival STATISTICS

acuity EMERGENCY MEDICINE Acuteness, usually referring to the intensity of the emergency, see Triage OPTHALMOLOGY The sharpness of vision, which is expressed as a ratio, eg 20/100, where a subject can see at 20 meters what a person with perfect vision can see at 100 meters

acumentin A motility protein present in neutrophils and macrophages that regulates the length of actin filaments by binding to the slow-assembly end of the actin molecule

acupuncture A method of healing, which is used to treat pain and disease and to produce surgical anesthesia; acupunture has been practiced in China for more than 2000 years, in which fine needles are placed in one or more of 800 sites on the skin; acupuncture has been used for conditions as diverse as analgesia, arthritis, hypertension and gastric ulcers; when genuine acupuncture is compared to sham acupuncture in the control of moderate stable angina, there is no significant difference

acute *adjective* Of abrupt onset, or shortened duration, usually hours or days in duration, used in reference to a disease or set of symptoms

acute abdomen A relatively non-specific symptom complex, in which a patient is first seen in a 'toxic' state, complaining of incapacitating abdominal pain, variably accompanied by fever and leukocytosis; AA may also be defined as an acute intra-abdominal inflammatory process that

---

ACUTE ABDOMEN Etiology

INFECTION Amebiasis, hepatitis, falciparum malaria, pneumococcal pneumonia, rheumatic fever, salmonella gastroenteritis, staphylococcal toxemia, syphilis in 'tabetic crisis', trichinosis, TB, typhoid fever, viral enteritides, herpes zoster, infectious mononucleosis, Whipple's disease

INFLAMMATION Appendicitis, cholangitis, cholecystitis, Crohn's disease, diverticulitis, gastroenteritis, hepatitis, lupus erythematosus, mesenteric lymphadenitis, pancreatitis, peritonitis due to organ perforation, perinephric abscesses, pyelonephritis, ulcerative colitis, intestinal obstruction, rheumatoid arthritis, polyarteritis nodosa, Hennoch-Schoenlein disease

INTOXICATION Black widow spider bites, heavy metals, mushrooms

ISCHEMIA Renal infarction, mesenteric arterial thrombosis

MALIGNANCY Pain due to organ infarction, Hodgkin's disease ('classically' associated with alcohol ingestion), leukemia, lympho-proliferative disorders

METABOLIC DISEASE Adrenal insufficiency (Addisonian crisis), diabetic ketoacidosis, familial hyperlipoproteinemia, familial Mediterranean fever, hemochromatosis, hereditary angioneurotic edema, hyperparathyroidism, hyperthyroidism, acute intermittent porphyria, uremia, withdrawal from drug abuse

OBSTETRICS/GYNECOLOGY Twisted ovarian cyst, ectopic pregnancy, endometriosis, pelvic inflammatory disease

REFERRED PAIN Pneumonia, myocardial infarct, pleuritis, pericarditis, myocarditis, hematomata of the rectal muscle, renal colic, peptic ulcer, nerve root compression

TRAUMA Perforation, ruptured aortic aneurysm, ruptured spleen, ruptured bladder

may require surgical intervention; while appendicitis is the most common cause of an acute abdomen, nearly 100 other conditions may present in a similar fashion, in particular, ruptured ectopic pregnancy in a fallopian tube, ruptured acute diverticulitis and acute mesenteric lymphadenitis (table)

acute AIDS syndrome Acute HIV syndrome, see there

acute bacterial meningitis see Bacterial meningitis

acute chest syndrome A clinical complex occurring in patients with sickle cell anemia (SCA); it is characterized by fever, tachycardia, chest pain, leukocytosis, and pulmonary infiltrates; it is the single most common cause for hospitalization in SCA and is due to infection and/or vascular occlusion; in children, it is often due to bacterial pneumonia, most commonly *Streptococcus pneumoniae* (preventable by pneumococcal vaccine), *Mycoplasma pneumoniae*, and others; risk factors for early death in patients with SCA include acute chest syndrome, renal failure, seizures, baseline leukocyte count >15 x 10^9/L (15 000/m^3), low fetal hemoglobin (**N Engl J Med 1994; 330:1639OA**)

acute disseminated encephalitis An acute complication of viral infection (1:1000 cases of measles) or vaccination (1:10^6 measles vaccinations), involving the entire brain and spinal cord or focally affecting a nerve or cord root PATHOGENESIS Unclear, but may be an immune reaction to cerebral proteins (eg myelin basic protein), and is considered to be the human equivalent of experimental allergic encephalomyelitis CLINICAL Meningial signs and, if serious, coma and death TREATMENT None

acute effects of overexposure OCCUPATIONAL SAFETY A generic term for any adverse effects that are evident at the time of, or shortly after exposure to, a hazardous material

acute fatty liver of pregnancy see Fatty liver of pregnancy, acute

acute HIV syndrome A transient flu-like syndrome representing an early response to HIV-1, which occurs 1-6 weeks after exposure to HIV-1 in 50-70% of those with primary HIV infection; the syndrome presents as an acute infectious mononucleosis-like complex and is accompanied by viremia and an immune response to HIV within 1 week to 3 months (**N Engl J Med 1993; 328:327RV**) CLINICAL Sore throat, lymphadenopathy, anorexia, nausea, vomiting and a maculopapular rash; less commonly, diarrhea, lightning-like pain, major weight loss, abdominal cramping, palmoplantar desquamation LABORATORY Mild leukopenia, occasionally inversion of the CD4:CD8 ratio (see Flow cytometry), antibodies to HIV products (gp120, gp160, p24 and p41) first appear six months or more after infection; the acute syndrome affects $\frac{1}{3}$ of previously healthy subjects but is distinctly uncommon in homosexuals; see AIDS, HIV-1

acute intermittent porphyria An AD [MIM 176000] condition caused by a deficiency of porphobilinogen deaminase* CLINICAL Recurrent colicky abdominal pain, constipation, fever, leukocytosis, postural hypotension, peripheral neuritis, paraplegia, urinary retention, respiratory paralysis, behavioral changes and episodic organic psychosis

*The trivial name of hydroxymethylbilane synthase [EC 4.3.1.8] is preferred by the Nomenclature Committee of the International Union of Biochemistry and Molecular Biology

acute low back pain REHABILITATION MEDICINE A nonspecific symptom of abrupt onset or an exacerbation of chronic low back pain of less than 3 weeks in duration TREATMENT Continuance of normal activities within the limits allowed by the pain leads to more rapid recovery than either bedrest or back-mobilizing exercises (**N Eng J Med 1995; 332:351OA**)

acute lymphocytic leukemia Acute lymphoblastic leukemia* A malignant lymphoproliferative process that most commonly affects children and young adults affecting ± 1800/year (US) CLINICAL Abrupt onset with usually a < 3 month history of fatigue, fever, and hemorrhage from multiple sites, lymphadenopathy, hepatomegaly, and splenomegaly CLASSIFICATION According to the FAB classification, ALLs are L1 (little cells), L3 (big cells), and L2 (those that can't decide) MOLECULAR PATHOLOGY Most are B cells and express CD19; 60% have karyotypic abnormalities PROGNOSIS The prognosis for children with ALL (data, St Jude's Children's Hospital) has improved from ± 9% long-term disease-free survival (1962-66) to ± 71% (1984-88), and 90-95% achieving remission; the improved cure rate is attributed to prophylaxis for meningeal leukemia and intensification of systemic chemotherapy (**N Engl J Med 1993; 329:1289OA**)

*The term currently preferred for ALL is acute lymphoblastic leukemia; in the author's view, use of the term lymphoblastic is less intuitive than lymphocytic, eg acute lymphocytic leukemia, and makes the formulation of standards in terminology more difficult; for other malignancies, the terms acute megakaryocytic leukemia, acute monocytic leukemia, and acute myelocytic leukemia are widely accepted; moreover, for lymphomas, the adjective lymphocytic is also prefered, as in for example well-differentiated lymphocytic lymphoma

acute massive pulmonary embolus A condition defined as '...*obstruction or significant filling defect involving two or more lobar pulmonary arteries, or the equivalent amount of emboli in smaller or other arteries.*' (**Laboratory Medicine 1995; 26:330OA**)

acute mountain sickness see Mountain sickness, acute

acute myocardial infarction EPIDEMIOLOGY: ± 1.5 million myocardial infarctions occur/year (US), 75 000 of AMI occur after strenuous physical activity, of which $\frac{1}{3}$ die TRIGGER FACTORS Heavy exertion is reported in 4.4% of patients in the hour before the onset of MI and is inversely related to the patient's level of habitual physical activity; those who exercised ≥ 5 times/week have a relative risk (RR) of 2.4; 3-4 times/week RR = 8.6; 1-2 times/week RR = 19.4; <1 times/week RR = 107 (**N Engl J Med 1993; 329:1677OA**); in patients with thrombolytic therapy and first MIs, age was the best predictor of mortality: 1.9% mortality < age 40; 32% > 80; cardiac rupture 19% ≤ age 60; 86% ≥ 70 (**N Engl J Med 1993; 329:1442OA**) PREVENTION AMI is declining in the US AMI-reducing factors ↓ Smoking, ↓ serum cholesterol, ↓ hypertension; ↑ aerobic exercise; the influence of other factors (eg maintenance of normal body weight, maintenance of normoglycemic state in diabetics, estrogen-replacement therapy, mild-to-moderate alcohol consumptions, prophylactic low-dose aspirin) on the incidence of AMI is less clear (**N Engl J Med 1992; 326:1406RV**)

acute necrotizing ulcerative gingivitis Trench mouth A condition characterized by progressive necrosis of the intra-oral tissues, seen in those with poor oral hygiene and suboptimal nutrition CLINICAL Pain, edema, punched-out oral ulceration, pseudomembrane formation, halitosis; anaerobic flora, including *Fusobacterium* species and spirochetes possibly related to *Treponema pallidum* (**N Eng L Med 1991; 325:539**), which also cause Vincent's angina (which affects the soft palate and tonsils), cancorum oris and upper respiratory abscesses TREATMENT H_2O_2, antibiotics, eg tetracycline, if fever or lymphadenopathy is present, saline rinse and local anesthetics; non-response may indicate presence of another condition, eg erythema multiforme, lichen planus, pemphigus and pemphigoid; Cf Periodontal disease

Note: 'Trench mouth' is a coinage of World War I vintage which attributed ANUG to living in close quarters, ie trenches

acute neurologic illness A condition defined by the National Childhood Encephalopathy Study (Great Britain) as

1) Acute or subacute encephalitis, encephalomyelitis, encephalopathy (including postinfectious encephalitis but not pyogenic infections)

2) Unexplained loss of consciousness

3) Convulsions lasting > ½ hour, or followed by coma lasting 2 hours or more or by paralysis or other neurologic signs not previously present

4) Infantile spasms

5) Reye syndrome (JAMA 1994; 272:1087MN&P)

acute otitis media A middle ear inflammation that is most common in children, which presents with a rapid onset of pain, irritability, anorexia, or vomiting MICROBIOLOGY *Streptococcus pneumoniae, Haemophilus influenzae* TREATMENT Amoxicillin, erythromycin-sulfisoxazole, T-S (N Engl J Med 1995; 332:1560RV)

acute pancreatitis Inflammation of the pancreas of abrupt onset, often associated with gallstones and alcohol ingestion EPIDEMIOLOGY 109 000 hospitalizations and 2251 deaths (USA, 1987); 10-fold ↑ from 1960s to 1980s (reason unclear-possibly alcohol abuse, possibly widened diagnostic criteria); ± 250 admissions/10^6 population/year, higher in certain populations, eg 4-22% in AIDS patients ETIOLOGY Obstruction, toxins or drugs, trauma, metabolic abnormalities, infection, vascular abnormalities, idiopathic, and others PATHOPHYSIOLOGY Hypotheses abound, but still unkown CLINICAL Abdominal pain, nausea, vomiting, hypotension PATHOLOGY Edema, hemorrhage, necrosis DIAGNOSIS Clinical findings of typical abdominal pain, ↑ amylase, ↑ lipase, ultrasonography, contrast enhanced CT imaging PROGNOSIS Ranson's criteria, modified Glasgow criteria, APACHE II NATURAL HISTORY 25% have complications, up to 9% mortality, due to pancreatic infection, sepsis, pulmonary failure and others TREATMENT Supportive, bowel rest with parenteral nutrition (N Engl J Med 1994; 330:1198RV) see Chronic pancreatitis

acute phase reactants APR Proteins that migrate in the α_1 and α_2 regions of a serum electrophoresis gel, rising and falling with acute inflammation; APRs traditionally include α_1-antitrypsin, α_1 acid glycoprotein, amyloid A and P, antithrombin III, C-reactive protein, C1-esterase inhibitor, C3 complement, ceruloplasmin, fibrinogen, haptoglobin, orosomucoid, plasminogen, transferrin; screening tests for acute phase reaction include ESR, plasma viscosity, and zeta sedimentation ratio; reference ranges ↑ and the values themselves ↓ with age (Arch Pathol Lab Med 1993; 117:906OA)

Note: Some of the above do not meet the criteria defined by the French Society for Clinical Chemistry but are designated as APRs for convenience

acute phase response APR The constellation of non-specific host responses to cytokines*; the APR is associated with tissue injury, infection, inflammation and rarely malignancy, eg Hodgkin's disease and renal cell carcinoma, and causes functional changes in the liver (↑ synthesis of acute phase proteins), endocrine system (abnormal glucose tolerance, ↑ gluconeogenesis, thyroid dysfunction, altered lipid metabolism), immune system (left shift leukocytosis, hypergammaglobulinemia), metabolic system (↓ albumin synthesis, energy consumption, ↑ ceruloplasmin, ↓ iron and zinc levels) and CNS (lethargy); the most measured molecule in the response is the highly nonspecific C-reactive protein, which may rise 10- to 1000-fold within hours from a normal of 100 µg/L; intercellular communication is mediated by either direct cell-to-cell contact, or by soluble signaling molecules including hormones, eicosanoids, neurotransmitters, and to cytokines*, which appear to play the most central, albeit complex role in inducing the APR; acute phase reactants have other specific roles, eg as endogenous pyrogens (see there) and somnogens; other 'co-factor' molecules involved in the APR include corticosteroids, insulin, thrombin, histamine, and others (Perspect Biol & Med 1993; 36:611)

*Biological response modifiers, eg IL-1α, IL-6, TNF-α, TGF-β-1, and IFNs

acute phase response factor

acute promyelocytic leukemia A type leukemia that comprises 10% of acute myelocytic leukemia CLINICAL Presents with bleeding diathesis (fatal in 8-47%), often exacerbated by cytotoxic chemotherapy and related to thrombocytopenia and hypofibrinogenemia PATHOLOGY 5-20/cell Auer rods arranged in bundles (faggots) MOLECULAR PATHOLOGY Balanced reciprocal translocation between the long arms of chromosomes 15 and 17 t(15;17); the gene encoding the retinoic acid receptor-alpha (RAR-α) maps to chromosome 17q21 (the site of the breakpoint in APL); this finding, in addition to the clinical response of APL to therapeutic all-*trans*-retinoic acid has prompted studies on the potential role of the RAR-α gene in the t(15;17) reciprocal translocation TREATMENT Induction treatment with all-*trans*-retinoic acid, followed by conventional chemotherapy, commonly an anthracycline combined with cytarabine (N Engl J Med 1993; 329:177RV) see Retinoic acid syndrome

acute radiation injury syndrome Atomic bomb disease A complex described in highly exposed victims of the Hiroshima and Nagasaki bomb blasts (JAMA 1946; 131:504), as well as nuclear reactor accidents CLINICAL 5-25 centiGray (cGy); the symptoms are a function of level of exposure < 75 cGy Asymptomatic with chromosomal aberrations < 125 cGy Asymptomatic with a mild decrease in leukocytes and platelets < 200 cGy Anorectic with anorexia, nausea, vomiting, fatigue, leukopenia and thrombocytopenia and transient symptoms; leukopenia occurs in 50% of those exposed to < 350 cGy, who have a 50% mortality with severe marrow depression; at > 500 cGy, GI complications of hemorrhagic gastroenteritis occur within two weeks, causing death in most of those exposed Hyperacute radiation disease is extremely rare and the doses may be in excess of 5000 cGy, causing fulminant cardiovascular, gastrointestinal and CNS collapse with death in 24-48 hours

acute salicysm see Aspirin

acute skin failure The potentially fatal systemic consequences of widespread injury to the skin as may occur in extensive second- and third-degree burns—these now known as deep partial or full-thickness burns or in toxic epidermal necrolysis (see N Engl J Med 1994; 331:1272RV) see Toxic epidermal necrolysis

acute tubular necrosis The histopathological finding in acute renal failure and seen in shock, crush injuries, hemoglobinuria, toxic nephrosis, ischemic injury of transplanted kidneys (cold ischemia is tolerated for up to 48 hours, warm ischemia, only several hours) PATHOLOGY Morphological changes are scant, ranging from hydropic changes to ATN; ATN in transplanted kidneys is managed in an expectant fashion as renal function may resume spontaneously within 2-4 weeks

acute tumor lysis syndrome Tumor lysis syndrome, see there

acyclovir

acyclovir 9[2-Hydroxyethoxy-methyl]guanine A nucleoside analogue with antiviral activity that inhibits herpes simplex virus-2 (HSV-2, genital herpes); acyclovir is activated by HSV thymidine kinase by monophosphorylation and then triple phosphorylated by host enzymes, producing a potent inhibitor of HSV-2's DNA polymerase; HSV-2 resistance to acyclovir is increasingly reported, frustrating

HSV-2 ulcer therapy; foscarnet (trisodium phosphormate), a pyrophosphate analogue, also inhibits DNA polymerase and may circumvent resistance; acyclovir suppresses genital HSV infection, reducing the recurrence rate from 12/year to 1/year, but has no effect on viral latency; it is considered safe for pediatric chickenpox (varicella-herpes zoster), if instituted within the first 24 hours of rash, although it is unclear if it reduces the rare serious complications of chickenpox and it is more effective than vidarabine in reducing viral shedding by HSV-infected infants, but equally effective as a therapeutic agent; effective and safe drug for treating herpes simplex type 1 (HSV-1) and type 2 (HSV-2); viral resistance to acyclovir has been reported in both immunocompromised, eg HIV-infected patients, and immunocompetent hosts (**N Engl J Med 1993; 329:1777**BR); in patients with herpes zoster, increasing acyclovir therapy to 21 days and/or addition of prednisolone results in only a marginal benefit and does not reduce the frequency of postherpetic neuralgia (**N Engl J Med 1994; 330:896**OA) Cf Foscarnet, Gancyclovir

acylated plasminogen streptokinase complex APSAC, see there

AD Autosomal dominant (GENETICS) also 1) Adenovirus 2) Admitting diagnosis 3) Alcohol dehydrogenase 4) Alzheimer's disease 5) Androstendione

1) Abdominal diameter 2) Accident dispensary 3) Adult 4) Allergic disease 5) Anterior deltoid 6) Antidiarrhea 7) Antigenic determinant 8) Auris dextra (right ear) 9) Axiodistal

ADA 1) Adenosine deaminase, see there 2) Americans with Disabilities Act, see there

Adam Ecstasy, see there

Adam's apple Laryngeal prominence, *prominentia laryngea* [NA6], anterior prominence of the thyroid cartilage, immediately inferior to the superior thyroid notch and most prominent in males, which is used as a landmark in performing the now-rare emergency tracheostomy

*In the tradition of folk physiology, the body of the first man, Adam, was wiser than his soul; when Adam took a piece of the forbidden fruit from Eve it stuck in his throat, as his 'wise' throat was telling him not to swallow the apple

Adam complex PSYCHIATRY A guilt complex of a person who breaks a parental 'law' that the subject, often a child, did not previously know was forbidden; eg incestuous relations; this form of guilt is likened to Adam and Eve's 'fall from grace' in the garden of Eden

ADAM complex Amniotic band syndrome, see there

ADAMHA Alcohol, Drug Abuse and Mental Health Administration

ADAP see Alzheimer's disease-associated protein

adaptin(s) A family of proteins that is critical to clathrin-coated vesicle-mediated intracellular transport of proteins; Cf COP(s)

adaptive filtration NEUROPHYSIOLOGY A process thought to be mediated by neurons of the inferotemporal cortex, in which new or unexpected visual information is processed, for future storage in long-term memory (**Science 1991; 254:1275**)

adaptive gridlock Stabilizing selection EVOLUTIONARY BIOLOGY A steady state that characterizes a particular species, which results from multiple selective pressures for the organism to evolve in different directions, eg *'If a shellfish could reduce the weight of its shell...it might have a better chance of escaping from some fast-moving predators. But ...a light, thinner shell would also decrease its resistance to other predators that bore into their victims* (**Science 1995; 267:1421**RN) see Punctuated equilibrium

ADAS Alzheimer's disease assessment scale, see there

ADC AIDS dementia complex, see there

ADCC Antibody-dependent cell-mediated cytotoxicity A mechanism for eliminating bacteria, viruses, tumors and foreign cells, mediated by cells with Fc receptors, eg T cells, NK cells, large granular lymphocytes, macrophages and neutrophils; ADCC is a model of the relationship between antibodies, usually IgG and thymus-independent lymphocytes, where target cells with attached specific antibodies are lysed by 'killer' cells having Fc receptors for the attachment of IgG, triggering target cell lysis; see CD 16

ADD Attention deficit disorder, see Attention deficit-hyperactivity disorder

addict SUBSTANCE ABUSE A person who is vulnerable to the compulsive heavy consumption of substances with abuse potential; in order of risk of addiction, cocaine and amphetamines have greater abuse potential than opiates and nicotine, which in turn have greater addictive potential than alcohol and related drugs (benzodiazepine, barbiturates), which are greater than cannabis, hallucinogens and caffeine; see Controlled drug substance, –holic, Substance abuse

addiction A physiologic, physical, or psychological state of dependency on a substance, which is characterized by tolerance, and a withdrawal syndrome when intake of the substance is reduced or stopped; the most common addictions are to alcohol, caffeine, cocaine, heroin, marijuana, nicotine (the tobacco industry argues that nicotine's addictive properties are unproven), and amphetamines; criteria that define an addiction (per **WHO and American Psychiatric Association, in New York Times 2 August 1994:C3**)

1) Taking the drug more often or in larger amounts than intended

2) Unsuccessful attempts to quit, persistent desire to use the agent, craving for drug

3) Excessive time spent in procuring drug

4) Intoxication or withdrawal symptoms at inappropriate times

5) Sacrifice of other activities or things for the drug

6) Continued use of drug despite knowledge of its harm

7) Marked tolerance for the drug

8) Typical withdrawal symptoms

9) Use of drug to avoid or alleviate withdrawal symptoms

addiction specialist Substance abuse specialist A generic term for a health care professional, eg a psychiatrist* who is called upon to treat and/or reduce a person's dependence on various substances of abuse, eg alcohol, cocaine, opiates, tobacco

*Or surrogate, eg a general practitioner thrust in the role, when one of his/her patients suffers an addiction, or an allied health care professional, eg a nurse or psychologist functioning the context of an 'outreach' program

addisonian crisis Adrenal crisis, see there

add-on LABORATORY MEDICINE A generic term for any test that is ordered after a specimen (usually of blood) has been submitted to the laboratory; add-ons tend to create logistic problems, eg in the form of ↑ paperwork; because most laboratories retain the specimen for up to 5 days, unless the original specimen was a 'short draw', most add-ons can be performed (**Am J Clin Pathol 1995; 103:718**)

addressin A homing protein, peptide or other molecule that provides a form of message indicating a molecule's destination, eg ELAM-1

adduct *noun* A molecule that is the product of a reaction in which the major axes are parallel; adducts may include molecules attached to DNA or proteins after exposure to air pollution, cigarette smoke and other environmental contaminants, eg polyaromatic hydrocarbons

ADE 1) Acute disseminated encephalomyelitis 2) Adverse drug event, see there

adenoacanthoma A rare glandular (adeno-) carcinoma with (benign) squamous metaplasia that may occur in the ovary Note: It is of great interest to differentiate these tumors from the far more pernicious adenosquamous carcinomas, in which both the glandular and squamous cell components are malignant, the latter component is marked by cellular immaturity, squamous pearl formation, and accompanied by high-grade (ie poorly-differentiated) glandular elements

adenoma malignum Minimal deviation adenocarcinoma of the uterine cervix, see there

adenomatoid odontogenic tumor ORAL PATHOLOGY A tumor that is more common in the anterior female jaw; most common in the second decade of life in association with impacted teeth PATHOLOGY Tubular and ductal areas, calcification and hyaline material TREATMENT Simple excision; Cf Ameloblastoma

adenomatoid tumor A rare benign tumor of mesothelial origin that arises in the epidydimis that requires simple excision when symptomatic

adenomatous hyperplasia of uterus Endometrial hyperplasia, see there

adenomyosis Endometriosis of subendothelial tissues, including the myometrium, which is often accompanied by diffuse and symmetric enlargement of the uterus

adenosine CARDIOLOGY An endogenous nucleoside composed of adenine linked to D-ribose, resulting from hydrolysis of adenylic acid; it is of therapeutic use as an alternative to the calcium channel blocker verapamil, in treating both narrow- and wide-complex supraventricular tachycardia (N Engl J Med 1991; 325:1621RV)

adenosine deaminase The enzyme [EC 3.5.4.4] that catalyzes the hydrolysis of amino group of adenosine yielding inosine and ammonia; the ADA gene is located on chromosome 20q13-ter and encodes a 38-kD deaminating enzyme, without which there is accumulation of adenosine, deoxyadenosine, adenosine triphosphate (ATP), S-adenosyl homocysteine and deoxyATP; deoxyATP is a potent inhibitor of ribonucleoside-diphosphate reductase, an enzyme involved in purine synthesis; excess adenosine also inhibits intracellular DNA-methylation (called 'suicide inactivation' as this causes cell death) Note: ADA's structure is intimately linked to its function, with a pivotal role being played by the Glu and Asp residues, which fold ADA into an α/β-barrel motif with a zinc atom in the active site (Science 1991; 252:1278)

adenylyl cyclase Add is the prototypic second messenger generator, which is regulated by one or the other arm of the phospholipase C pathway, and are further regulated by cyclic changes in the cAMP and internal Ca^{2+} levels (Nature 1995; 374:421P)

ADA deficiency A uniformly fatal AD [MIM 102700] disease, comprising 40% of patients with severe combined immunodeficiency MECHANISM dATP inhibits ribonucleotide reductase in S phase of growth cycle, aborting DNA synthesis and incorporation of dATP into polyadenylated RNA; dATP accumulation inhibits RNA synthesis and single-strand separation of DNA; the lymphocytes are also relatively deficient in 5'-nucleotidase; increasing ADA levels inhibit the synthesis of S-adenosylmethionine which donates methyl groups to DNA; ADA is defective or absent in AIDS, anemia and lymphoproliferative disorders CLINICAL Cellular immune dysfunction, oral candidiasis, intractable diarrhea, failure to thrive, severe diaper rash, pseudoachondrodysplasia, death before age 2 LABORATORY ↓↓↓ Lymphocytes (< 0.5 x 10⁹/L, US: < 500 mm³), especially T cells; eosinophilia; ↑ adenosine and deoxyadenosine in serum and urine TREATMENT ADA deficiency rarely responds to bone marrow transplantation; given the prognosis of all such patients, workers at the NIH chose to treat one such patient by inserting the absent gene with a retroviral vector, a ploy that has proven successful, logistically, ethically and medicolegally paving the way for future gene therapy (JAMA 1991; 266:2193n&v) see Cartilage-hair syndrome

adenosis of prostate SURGICAL PATHOLOGY A lesion characterized by a well-circumscribed proliferation of benign glands, which is of clinical interest as certain histological features (eg infiltrative growth pattern, single cells, prominent nucleoli, and mitotic figures) mimic low-grade adenocarcinoma (Am J Surg Pathol 1994; 18:863OA)

The diagnosis of prostatic adenocarcinoma on 'skinny needle' biopsies of the prostate is particularly difficult because of these features–Author's note

adenotonsillar disease A generic term for any pathology of nasopharyngeal lymphoid tissues, eg chronic or recurrent infection and obstructive hyperplasia

adenovirus E1a protein E1a protein, see there

adenylate cyclase 3'-5'-cyclic AMP synthetase An enzyme [EC 4.6.1.1] that catalyzes ATP to form 3',5'-cyclic AMP and inorganic pyrophosphate; AC is intimately linked to the receptor-G protein machinery on the cytoplasmic face of the cell membrane, which generates the second messenger, cAMP (cyclic adenosine monophosphate) when stimulated by an extracellular message in the form of receptor binding of a hormone or other ligand, light or odors; G proteins dissociate into GTP-bound α subunits (activating adenyly cyclase, retinal phosphodiesterase, phospholipase C and ion channels) and a complex of β and γ subunits (selectively activating certain forms of adenyly cyclase) following interaction with the cell receptors (Science 1991:254:1500)

ADFR therapy Activate, depress, free and repeat A therapeutic modality (phosphorus, followed by calcitonin and calcium, administered in three-month cycles), used to attenuate post-menopausal bone loss in women for whom estrogen therapy is contraindicated or unacceptable

adhalin A 50-kD dystrophin-related glycoprotein that may be linked to autosomal recessive muscular dystrophy (see N Engl J Med 1994; 331:1162C)

ADHD Attention deficit/hyperactivity disorder, see there

adhesion filter TRANSFUSION MEDICINE Adsorption filter A 'third-generation' blood component filter that removes 99-99.9% of leukocytes (by adhesion) in units of packed red cells and platelets (Arch Pathol Lab Med 1994; 118:392OA) see Blood filters, Leukocyte reduction

adhesin Any of a number of bacterial components (pili in *Pseudomonas aeruginosa*, lipotechoic acid in group A streptococci) that bind to glycoprotein or glycolipid receptors on epithelial cells; the existance of adhesins explains the pulmonary morbidity due to *P aeruginosa* seen in intubated ICU patients, and renal tract infections caused by *Escherichia coli* are mediated by MS and MR adhesins, which may be inhibited by fruit juices; see Cranberry juice

adhesion SURGERY A collagen-rich fibrous band that forms after any intervention in a surgical field, classically occurring in the peritoneal cavity; adhesions may be related to a focal decrease in the plasminogen activator in the mesothelial lining or to local inflammation or infection; gentle manipulation of the organs and removal of blood minimizes adhesive band formation, which may be severe enough to cause intestinal obstruction; nothing effectively prevents adhesions

adhesion proteins MOLECULAR BIOLOGY A group of 'sticky' proteins found in the extracellular matrix that facilitate vascular egress of circulating leukocytes, eg ELAM-1 (endothelial leukocyte adhesion molecule-1), located on vascular endothelium stimulated by inflammatory lymphokines (eg IL-1 and tumor necrosis factor), attracting neutrophils to sites of inflammation; lymph node homing receptor found on the membranes of B and T cells, which transmigrate in the high endothelial venules and the 140-kD GMP-140 granule membrane protein; adhesion proteins have a 'mosaic' structure, composed of tandem arrays of sequences adopted from other proteins, incorporating functional domains into 'homing' molecules; dissection of these functions may determine the susceptibility of certain sites to metastases and 'engineering' of the receptors may direct neutrophils to, or away from, inflammatory targets

adhesion receptors A group of membrane-bound proteins responsible for interaction of cells and matrix molecules that regulate adherence and chemoattractant gradients responsible for directing cell migration; the adhesion receptors have been divided into three groups: 1) The immunoglobulin superfamily of adhesion receptors, including T cell receptor/CD3, CD4, CD8, MHC class I, MHC class II, CD2/LFA-2, CD58/LFA-3, ICAM-1/CD54, ICAM-2 and VCAM-1, 2) The integrin family, including LFA-1 and Mac-1 (CD11a and CD18), p150,95 (CD11c and CD18), VLA-5, VLA-4/LPAM-1, LPAM-2 and 3) The selectin family, including Mel-14/LAM-1, ELAM-1 and CD62/GMP-140

adhesive interaction CELL BIOLOGY A generic term for any interaction between molecules that '...*play critical roles in directing the migration, proliferation, and differentiation of cells; aberrations in such interactions can lead to pathological disorders.* (AI) *mediated by cell surface receptors that bind to ligands on adjeacent cells or in the extracellular matrix, also regulate intracellular signal transduction pathways that control... changes in cell physiology*.' (**Science 1995; 268:233**) see Integrin-mediated adhesive interactions

ad hoc committee A committee formed with the purpose of addressing a specific issue or issues that theoretically is disbanded once it fulfills its raison d'etre

adipocere Gravewax Hardened waxy adipose tissue seen in an unembalmed body lying a year or more in cold wet ground (or cold acidic water, which inhibits tissue hydrolysis); see Bog bodies

adipostat A set-point region that is thought to reside in the ventromedial, lateral, and paraventricular nuclei of the hypothalamus, and possibly elsewhere, which is thought to be intimately linked to the control of obesity; the adipostat's function appears to be to maintain the metabolic status quo, and adjust the rate of metabolism, thereby frustating the efforts of the obese wishing to lose weight; while at present purely speculative, the adipostat may modify behaviors traditionally perceived as voluntary, eg eating and physical activity, as well as metabolic activity to compensate for changes in diet (**N Engl J Med 1995; 332:673ED**) see Melanoma

adipsin A serine protease secreted by adipocytes into the circulation that is deficient in some animal models of obesity; adipsin has activities similar to and 61% sequence homology with complement factor D

adjectival eponym An eponym that has been so long in common usage that it has passed into public 'domain' and in so doing, is most commonly written in lower case (a convention apparently borrowed from German); thus fallopian tubes, gram-positive organisms, mendelian genetics and müllerian ducts are no longer capitalized; see Eponym; Cf Autoeponym

adjunct Something joined or added to another thing but which is not an essential part thereof, eg radiotherapy is an important adjunct to surgery and may represent appropriate adjuvant therapy

adjunct staff The body of physicians, dentists, osteopaths, or other independent medical practitioners who have achieved a certain level of professional distinction, who participate in educational or research programs in a hospital or health care institution, but in general do not provide or supervise the provision of direct patient management or medical care, and do not admit patients

adjunctive therapy A generic term for any therapeutic maneuver(s) that play an ancillary role in the treatment of a disease by reducing mortality and morbidity, but is not part of the immediate therapy required to stabilize the patient; in acute MI, AT includes aspirin, b-adrenergic blocking agents, angiotensin-converting agents, heparin, nitrates, calcium channel blockers, prophylactic antiarrhythmic agents, magnesium sulfate, morphine, warfarin, and hypolipidemic agents (eg simvastin) (**Mayo Clin Proc 1995; 70:453**) Cf Adjuvant therapy

adjuvant IMMUNOLOGY A non-specific immune enhancer, eg Freund's adjuvant, composed of particulate-containing oily substances that promote protein aggregation which, when mixed with an antigen, acts as a tissue depot, slowly releasing antigen and activating the immune system

adjuvant chemotherapy The use of chemotherapeutic agents in addition to a traditional modality, eg surgery for treating a malignancy; additon of AC to therapy for breast cancer is reported to improve the disease-specific survival, overall survival, and seven-year survival (**N Engl J Med 1994; 330:805OA, 1253OA**); it is uncertain if this improvement is due to lead-time bias (**N Engl J Med 1994; 331:402c**) AC for colorectal cancer (fluorouracil 500 mg/m²/day, radiotherapy circa 5040 cGy) may prevent more than 10 000 deaths annually (US) Note: Other combinations and modalties of AC for colorectal cancer have proven essentially useless (**N Engl J Med 1994; 330:1136OA**)

adjuvant disease An animal model for rheumatoid arthritis, consisting of an acute aseptic synovitis, induced in rats by injection of Freund's complete adjuvant, which consists of an oil-water emulsion containing killed *Mycobacterium tuberculosis* CLINICAL Granulomas, iritis, arthritis, and other symptoms similar to chronic connective tissue disease in humans (**CAP Today August 1993**) Cf Human adjuvant disease

adjuvant therapy ONCOLOGY Any treatment given after surgical resection of a tumor, in an effort to prevent recurrence at distal sites, or when residual malignancy is thought to remain after excision; AT is used in malignancy after one or more of the conventional therapeutic arms (surgery, chemotherapy and radiotherapy) has failed; ATs include immunotherapy (BCG, IL-2-stimulated lymphokine-activated killer cells, IFN-α) and regional hyperthermia with chemotherapy; see IL-2/LAK cells; AT is recommended for ♀ with axillary lymph node-positive breast cancer, eg hormonal manipulation and chemotherapy; but does not improve survival in lymph node-negative women; a gain of four months of life costs $5-7000 COLON CANCER Adjuvant therapy for stage III adenocarcinoma, using 5-FU and levamisole (side effects: Nausea, diarrhea, leukopenia), has a reported 32% improvement in 5-year survival, and may be appropriate also for stage II carcinoma LUNG CANCER Adjuvant therapy may actually decrease survival

administration The sum total of management and direction of health care organizations (personnel, budgets and logistics) and the implementation of health care policy; management requires a chain of command, proper organization, assignment of responsibility, positive worker interaction and feedback; administration is an ever-increasing component of physician activities and includes responsibilities in quality assurance and record keeping; in laboratory medicine, administration requires management of physical and human resources

administrator A bureaucrat or pencil-pusher

administrative costs The costs incurred by the 'business' component of health care facilities or universities, which includes staffing and personnel costs, nursing home and hospital administration, insurance overhead and overhead expenses; the per capita health care administration cost in the US of $400-500 contrasts to a per capita cost in

Canada of $100-150; it has been noted that if the US were as efficient as the Canadian health care bureaucracy, the $70 billion of annual savings would fund health care for the estimated 35 million Americans who are uninsured and underinsured; in fiscal 1990, administration costs in the US accounted for 24.8% of hospital expenditures, more than 2-fold greater than in Canada; in 1968 in the US, 1 378 000 in-patients were cared for by 435 100 managers and clerks; by 1990, 853 000* in-patients were cared for by 1 221 600 administrators and clerks (**N Engl J Med 1993; 329:400OA**) see Indirect costs

*The reduction in in-hospital patients is related to the 'DRG' (diagnosis-related group, see there) form of reimbursement, in which patients are often discharged 'quicker and sicker'

administrative intervention A generic term for any intervention on the part of an administrative body, which is intended to influence a habit, eg overordering of tests in patient management; AIs come in three flavors 1) Hassle factor, in which burdensome paperwork makes it difficult to order the tests 2) Redesign of requisition forms to encourage ordering the least amount of tests and 3) Providing ready access to computerized information on previously ordered tests, which prevents re-ordering a test that has always been performed (**CAP Today June 1995, p20**)

administrative responsibility A generic term for any task or duty that is related to the management of an institution; Cf Clinical responsibility

admissible evidence FORENSIC MEDICINE Any item, exhibit, object or materials which a local, district or federal court will accept as linking a person(s) with the commitment of an act; eg 1) A knife belonging to the accused, covered with the victim's blood 2) The killer's name uttered by a dying victim is accepted as admissible evidence in Michigan, California, Washington DC and the State of Washington

admission hyponatremia LABORATORY MEDICINE Serum sodium levels of < 130 mmol/L, a finding which, in older persons (> age 64) has been associated with two-fold increase in in-hospital mortality (**Ann Int Med 1994; 57:933**)

admit *noun* A highly colloquial term for a person who has been admitted to a hospital or ward *verb* To arrange for a person's ingression into a hospital

adolescent crisis PSYCHOLOGY An encompassing term for the relatively abrupt changes that the physical and emotional rigors of the adolescent period places on its 'victim'

adoption The care and nurturing of a child by a non-blood-related adult who assumes the roles, rights, and obligations of a natural parent; 2% of children < age 18 in the US are adopted (± 1 million); these children comprise 5% of children in psychotherapy, 6-9% of those in school with learning disabilities, 10-15% of those in residential treatment or psychiatric hospitals (**Science News 1994; 146:104**); infertility continues to be the major reason that a couple (or more recently, single adults) wishes to adopt and raise a child; 8000 babies enter the US annually because of the reduced availability of US-born babies, coming from less developed countries; 57% of internationally-adopted children in one study (**N Engl J Med 1991; 325:479**) were found to have at least one major medical condition, many of which could have been detected by a screening test; the most common medical problems in international adoptees are infections and parasitic infections, most commonly *Giardia lamblia, Trichuris trichiura, Blastocystis hominis* and others, tuberculosis and hepatitis B, followed by neurological, hematological, renal, metabolic and other diseases; ± 6000 children were adopted from orphanages in Romania, Russia, and other former Eastern Bloc countries by Americans and others from developed countries; the medical problems of these children included malnutrition and rickets, chronic diarrhea, hepatitis B, poor oral hygiene; the psychosocial and neurological problems suffered by

these children are regarded by the adopting parents as equally or more serious; many had suffered virtually complete sensory deprivation and/or physical abuse by caregivers (**NY Newsday 28 Nov 1994, A7**)

adoptive immunity The transfer of immunity from one organism to another by either injection of immune-competent cells, as in granulocyte transfusions or 'humors', as in passive immunity in neonates resulting from placental transfer of IgG across the placenta

adoptive immunotherapy An experimental therapeutic modality used to treat terminal malignancy consisting of the transfer of 'activated' anti-tumor cells, eg combining lymphokine-activated killer (LAK) cells or tumor-infiltrating lymphocytes (TIL) with IL-2 into patients with metastatic malignancy); about 10% of patients with terminal renal cell carcinoma and melanoma have achieved partial or complete remission with the LAK/IL-2 regimen Note: Passive transfer of immunologically-active cells; objective responses to LAK cells has been reported in advanced renal cell carcinoma, melanoma, colorectal carcinoma, and in Hodgkin's disease; the effects may be dose-dependent, non-MHC-restricted, and require the simultaneous administration of high-dose IL-2 MECHANISM Uncertain, possibly lymphocyte trafficking to the tumor site followed by local expansion and cytokine release under the baton of IL-2 (**Arch Pathol Lab Med 1994; 118:417RV**)

ADP Adenosine diphosphate

ADPKD Autosomal dominant polycystic kidney disease, see there

ADR Adverse drug reaction

adrenal-to-brain transplantation Brain-graft surgery, see there

adrenal crisis Addisonian crisis, acute adrenal insufficiency A state of acute adrenocortical insufficiency, induced by the stress of infections, trauma, surgery, dehydration with salt deprivation or evoked by replacing thyroid hormone in patients with hypothyroidism of hypothalamic or pituitary origin who have an underlying mild ACTH deficiency CLINICAL Hypotension, shock, fever, dehydration, anorexia, weakness, apathy LABORATORY ↓ Na$^+$, ↑ K$^+$, lymphocytosis, eosinophilia, hypoglycemia TREATMENT Pharmacologic doses of glucocorticoids

adrenal hyperplasia Congenital adrenal hyperplasia, see there

adrenal medullary transplantation Brain graft surgery, see there

adrenocorticotrophic hormone ACTH, see there

β_2-adrenoceptor agonists* β_2-agonists A family of anti-asthmatic agents (albuterol, formoterol, salmeterol, terbutaline) that induce bronchodilatation; β_2 agonists inhibit mast cell function, and histamine release after an allergen challenge in vivo; although the management of mild-to-moderate asthma is reported (**N Engl J Med 1992 327:1420OA**) to be superior with long-term agents, the prolonged use of β_2-adrenoceptor agonists may be ill-advised, given the potential for tolerance and deterioration in control of disease (**N Engl J Med 1992; 327:1198OA, 1204OA**)

*Note: Three terms are currently used for these compounds, the 'long' form, β_2-adrenergic receptor agonist, the mid-sized form, β_2-adrenoceptor agonist, and the increasingly popular 'short' form β_2-agonist

adrenoleukodystrophy An X-linked peroxisomal disease in which the impaired oxidation of saturated long-chain fatty acids is associated with Addison's disease and neurological impairment, and in the late-onset cases, adrenomyeloneuropathy (**N Engl J Med 1990; 322:13**)

Adriamycin ONCOLOGY Doxorubicin HCl An anthracycline antibiotic with antineoplastic activity, used to treat both leukemia and solid tumors; its therapeutic efficacy is hampered by cardiotoxicity that increases sharply as the cumulative dose administered rises above 500 mg/mm²; 23% of Adriamycin-treated (mean dose, 450 mg/mm²) patients in one study had late cardiac abnormalities, including cardiac failure, dysrhythmia and sudden death; post-mortem examination of the heart reveals myocardial fibrosis and 'Adria' cells

'Adria' cell A myocyte seen in patients with adriamycin cardiotoxicity characterized by central clumping of the nuclear chromatin by EM and mild cytoplasmic vacuolization

adsorption Removal of non-specific agglutinins by incubation in serum that does not contain the antigens to be measured

ADSOL® TRANSFUSION MEDICINE A proprietary red cell storage medium that permits greater plasma yields, eliminates certain restrictions on packed red cell hematocrits, and allows the addition of known volumes of diluting/preserving solution (ADSOL) to the RBCs, which allows ↑ component product flexibility; ADSOL-preserved RBC units have ↑ ATP, ↑ RBC recovery, and ↓ RBC lysis when compared with the formerly standard storage medium CPDA-1, at 35 days; ADSOL® preservation solution is FDA-approved for shelf-life storage of 42 days; Cf CPD

adsorption chromatography LABORATORY MEDICINE A technique in which molecules are separated according to their adsorptive properties, where a mobile (fluid) phase is passed over an immobile (solid) adsorptive stationary phase; Cf Affinity chromatography

adult immunization The administration of vaccines to prevent infection of adulthood; *'The contrast between the impact of vaccine-preventable diseases of adults compared with those of children is striking. Each year, fewer than 500 persons in the United States die of vaccine-preventable diseases of childhood. By comparison, 50 000 to 70 000 adults die of influenza, pneumococcal infections, and hepatitis B* (table); Cf Childhood immunization

ADULT IMMUNIZATION				
INFECTIONS	ANNUAL DEATHS	VACCINE EFFICACY	CURRENT VACCINE USE	PREVENTABLE DEATHS
Influenza	20 000	70	41	8260
Pneumococcal	40 000	60	20	19 200
Hepatitis B	5000	90	10	4050
Tet-diph[1]	<25	99	40	<15
MMR[2]	<30	95	variable	<30

[1]Tetanus-diphtheria [2]Measles-mumps-rubella From JAMA 1994; 272:1133

adult respiratory distress syndrome A clinical complex* affecting ± 150 000/year (US) characterized by acute pulmonary edema and respiratory failure, poor oxygenation, ↑ functional residual capacity, and ↓ compliance; ARDS may accompany a wide range of medical and surgical conditions that do not initially involve the lungs and are unrelated to cardiac failure, often associated with interstitial pneumonitides (usual, desquamative and lymphoid types) ETIOLOGY Gram-negative sepsis, pneumonia, shock, aspiration (of gastric content), trauma, drug overdose CLINICAL A 6-24 hour latency period is followed by hypoxia, ↓ aeration, dyspnea and 'stiff' lungs, ie ↓ pulmonary compliance RADIOLOGY Extensive, bilateral fluffy infiltrates PATHOLOGY Atelectatic, heavy (> 1000 g, normal < 400g) congested lungs filled with proteinaceous material, RBCs and occasionally, hyaline membranes and diffuse alveolar damage, which is characterized by widespread damage to the microvasculature and alveolar epithelium, related to fibrin deposition in the distal air spaces PATHOGENESIS Abundant fibrin and fibronectin in the exudative phase results in hyaline membrane formation and alveolar fibrosis, due to local urokinase deficiency or presence of urokinase inhibitors, eg plasminogen-activator inhibitor, PAI-1 ARDS is characterized by arterial hypoxia (due to intrapulmonary shunting), and acute pulmonary artery hypertension (due to vasoconstriction and occlusion of the pulmonary microvasculature), which contributes to pulmonary edema and may cause right ventricular dysfunction; vasodilators can be used to ↓ the increased pulmonary vascular resistance, thereby ↓ pulmonary artery resistance, and pulmonary capillary pressure, improving right ventricular function, promoting the resolution of pulmonary edema; a disadvantage of vasodilators is that they cause systemic vasodilation, leading to systemic hypotension, right ventricular ischemia, and resultant heart failure, as well as dilatation of pulmonary vasculature, increasing blood flow to areas of intrapulmonary shunt, leading to a ventilation/perfusion mismatch and further reduction of an already compromised partial pressure of arterial oxygen (PaO_2) TREATMENT Nitric oxide (NO, 18 ppm in one study) inhalation therapy results in a ↓ mean pulmonary artery pressure (37 to 30 mm Hg), ↓ intrapulmonary shunting (36% to 31%), ↑ ratio of partial pressure of arterial O_2 to the fraction of inspired O_2 (PaO_2/FiO_2), an index of arterial oxygenation efficiency (±152 to ±199) (**N Engl J Med 1993; 328:399**OA, **431**ED) PEEP, prayer Prognosis is a function of the underlying etiology MORTALITY ± 60%, the cause of death has shifted from hypoxia to multiorgan failure

*Synonyms include adult hyaline membrane disease, bronchopulmonary dysplasia, congestive atelectasis, DaNang lung, post-traumatic pulmonary insufficiency, pump lung, shock lung, stiff lung syndrome, transplant lung, traumatic wet lung, Vietnam lung, wet lung, and white lung syndrome

adult T-cell leukemia-lymphoma A rapidly-progressive lymphoproliferative malignancy of mature T lymphocytes, commonly associated with infection by the retrovirus, HTLV-I, first described in southeastern Japan, also seen in the Caribbean, Africa and in blacks in the southeastern USA, in whom the disease is aggressive with skin lesions, hypercalcemia, rapid enlargement of hilar, retroperitoneal and peripheral lymph nodes with mediastinal sparing, invasion of CNS, lungs, GI tract and opportunistic infections, eg *Pneumocystis carinii*; ATLL has been subdivided into five clinical forms: 1) Acute Median age 52, lymphadenopathy, hepatosplenomegaly, cutaneous lesions, up to a 20-year latency, often resistant to chemotherapy with poor prognosis following disease onset LABORATORY ↑ Ca⁺⁺, WBCs 10-500 × 10⁹ (US: 10-500 000/mm³), Sezary-like cells with CD3, CD4, CD2, and Tac+ surface antigens, causing a chronic, smoldering lymphoma 2) Chronic Clinically between acute and smoldering disease 3) Smoldering Characterized by erythematous skin nodules filled with lymphocytes that may undergo 'blast transformation' to the typical acute T cell leukemia (ATL) 4) Crisis When either 2) or 3) transform to ATL 5) Lymphoma Most common in US blacks with hypercalcemia, leukemia, hepatosplenomegaly, erythematous skin lesions and lytic bone lesions; see T-cell lymphoma

advance directive Self-determination MEDICAL ETHICS Instruction(s) providing competent persons the means by which they can influence their own treatment in the event of serious illness and/or loss of mental abilities; a person may clearly indicate in advance how treatment decisions are to be made regarding the use of artificial life support by either written directions (ie a living will) and/or by appointing a proxy to make the health care decisions; nursing homes are four times more likely than hospitals to override advance directives, as they may be simply ignored or prioritized by other considerations (**N Engl J Med 1991; 324:882, 889**) see DNR orders, Durable powers of attorney, Euthanasia, Living will

advanced glycosylation endproducts A group of glycoproteins are derived from the Amadori reaction induced by hyperglycemia and held responsible for the various manifestations of DM, including vasculopathy that causes leakage of proteins across vessels and progressive stenosis of small and large vessels; in diabetics, hyperglycemia causes proteins to combine with glycosylation endproducts in a reversible (early glycosylation endproducts) or irreversible (AGEs) fashion; hemoglobin (Hb) A is one of the AGEs formed in hyperglycemia and levels of HbA_{1c} correlate well with adequate glucose control in diabetics PATHOPHYSIOLOGY AGEs accumulate in vessels, forming covalent bonds with amino groups of vessel-based proteins (collagen IV, laminin and heparan sulfate proteoglycan), trapping transmigrating LDLs, enzymes, growth factors and other proteins, destroying the orderly self-assembled basement membrane 'system'; a macrophage receptor for the AGE-protein complex has been identified that induces secretion of TNF and IL-1, both of which release collagenases and proteases, stimulate proteoglycan degradation and induce proliferation resulting in 'sloppy' basement membrane synthesis; plaque formation may be initiated by lipoprotein deposition in a process of protein trapping and cross-linking; thus, the vessels are thicker than normal, but 'leaky'; AGEs are inculpated in diabetic cataracts, diabetes-induced atherosclerosis and diabetic nephropathy, the severity of which parallels the levels of AGE peptides in the circulation (**N Engl J Med 1991; 325:836**) knowledge of AGE levels is useful in long-term control of diabetics who require less hospitalization as they are recognized to be out of control earlier and are treated more aggressively TREATMENT Aminoguanidine may have currency in preventing the conversion of Amadori products to AGEs; more theoretical is the goal of stimulating the macrophage removal system

advanced life support EMERGENCY MEDICINE A generic term for any resuscitation effort that extends beyond basic CPR; ALS includes

1) ADVANCED VENTILATORY SUPPORT, eg tracheal intubation, pharyngotracheal lumen airway, esophageal obturator airway, and transtracheal catheter ventilation

2) IV ACCESS

3) CORRECTION OF ACIDOSIS

4) DIAGNOSTIC TESTS, eg EKG, arterial blood gases

5) CORRECTION OF ARRHYTHMIAS, either pharmacologic or electrical

6) ADVANCED PERFUSION SUPPORT Cf Basic life support

advanced-practice nurse A registered nurse with specialty training and education (usually a masters degree, ie 6+ years of formal college or university education) in primary care (eg nurse practitioner, midwife) or acute care of inpatients (eg clinical nurse specialist, intensive care specialist) who performs various examinations, eg flexible sigmoidoscopic examination; there are an estimated 100 000 nurse practitioners in US; in 21 states they may be reimbursed by private and commercial insurers; in 15 states, they have independent authority prescribed controlled drugs

Note: Advanced practice nursing has engendered considerable debate regarding its ability to lower total health care costs, relieve regional (eg inner city, rural) deficiency of primary health care providers, and to provide the same overall quality of health care with far less formal education (**N Engl J Med 1994; 330:204ED (con), 211ED (pro)**); as a specific example, if the American Cancer Society (and others) recommendations that asymptomatic adults ≥ age 50 should undergo screening by sigmoidoscopy to detect adenomas and early cancer are to be followed, there is a relative lack of specialists to perform this and other screening procedures usually performed by physicians--should more specialized physicians (when there already are too many) be trained, or should this role be filled by less costly but equally competent labor (**N Engl J Med 1994; 330:183SA**)

Advanced Technology Program A program sponsored by the National Institute of Standards and Technology that has as its specific agenda, the financial encouragement of projects that need development prior to bringing to the marketplace; the authorizing statute of the ATP requires that any patents arising from the work must belong to a profit-making company, ie not an institution of higher learning (**Sci Am 1994; 270/9:72**)

adverse drug event A generic term for any undesired or unintended response to a drug occurring at doses appropriate for a person's status, which can be divided based on the presence or absence of an immune mechanism; ADRs are common, occurring in 1-15% of all drug administrations, and may rarely be fatal; ADEs are therapeutic reactions that are noxious, unintended, and occur at doses used in man for prophylaxis, diagnosis, therapy or modification of physiologic functions; the definition of ADEs excludes therapeutic failures, poisoning or intentional overdoses (**WHO publication DEM/NC/84.153[E]**); ADEs occurred in 2% of hospitalized patients in one study (**JAMA 1991; 266:2847**) and were divided into type A (dose-dependent or predictable) or type B (idiosyncratic or allergic) reactions; clinical signs and symptoms of ADEs included pruritus, nausea, vomiting, rash, confusion, lethargy; ADEs are most commonly caused by analgesics (narcotics), antibiotics, cardiovascular agents, anticoagulants and psychotherapeutic agents

adverse drug reaction Adverse drug event, see there

Note: The term adverse drug reaction appears to be more popular in the spoken parlance

adverse event FORENSIC MEDICINE An injury caused by medical management (rather than by the underlying disease), which prolongs hospitalization, produces a disability at the time of discharge, or both; AEs occur in 0.2–7.9% of hospitalizations, 1–60% of which are due to negligence; 70% had a disability of less than six months, 2.6% were permanent and 14% resulted in death (**N Engl J Med 1991; 324:370, JAMA 1991; 265:3265**); AEs are caused by drug complications, wound infections and technical complications, and those due to negligence due to diagnostic mishaps, therapeutic mishaps and events occurring in the emergency room; one-half of AEs were related to an operation and are more common in older patients (**ibid, 324:377**) see Malpractice, Misadventure, Negligence

adverse experience Adverse drug event, see there

adverse selection HEALTH CARE ENVIRONMENT A stance adopted by health care insurers that fiercely compete to insure the healthiest of a particular population, leaving the sick, sicker, and sickest to whatever 'default' system or safety net is in place (**Am Med News 26 October 1992, p7**)

advertising The public notification of a product's availability and related activities for its promotion; in medicine, two forms of advertising have undergone ethical scrutinization, that of 1) Physician advertising, which, although traditionally considered beneath the dignity of the healing professions, which is being done with increasing frequency, see 'Yellow professionalism' and 2) Prescription drug advertising; in the US, the Food and Drug Administration is responsible for regulating the use of drugs and promotion of their use by the pharmaceutical industry and requires a 'fair balance' in advertising, such that all activities must present a balanced account of the clinically relevant information, ie the risks and benefits, that would influence the physician's prescribing decision; types of drug-related advertising 'COMING SOON' ADVERTISING A form of 'teaser' advertising that indicates the name of a drug without claims for potential indications, safety or effectiveness DIRECT-TO-CONSUMER ADVERTISING The use of mass media, eg television, magazines, to publicly promote drugs that by law require a physician's prescription; the intent of such advertising is to have patients and/or the lay public request their physician to prescribe drug 'X' INSTITUTIONAL ADVERTISING A form of 'teaser' advertising in which a drug company is linked to a field of research INTRODUCTORY ADVERTISING Promotional activities for a drug that has not yet been released PREAPPROVAL ADVERTISING see 'Teaser' advertising REMEDIAL ADVERTISING Advertising that attempts to rectify a situation in which a company has falsely misrepresented the drug's efficacy or approved uses REMINDER ADVERTISING Advertising that calls attention to a drug's existence in the market; any claims of efficacy in reminder activities requires that the promotional activities meet 'fair balance' and brief summary requirements 'TEASER' ADVERTISING Advertising for a product that has not yet come to market; under US regulations, a drug company must choose between either 'Institutional' or 'Coming soon' forms of 'teaser' advertising

Aedes albopictus A species of mosquito that is a vector of dengue, eastern equine encephalomyelitis, and yellow fever viruses that was introduced in Florida in 1985 (Science 1992; 257:526)

A end SUBCELLULAR PHYSIOLOGY One of two ends of microtubules that polymerize from α- and β- tubulin dimers; the rate of assembly at the A (net assembly) end is greater than the rate assembly at the D (net disassembly) end, thus microtubule formation and metabolism are analogous to a treadmill

aerobic exercise A generic term for cardiorespiratory-type exercise performed at a level of 60-70% of maximum heart-rate reserve for a period of 20-30 minutes, which improves circulation, controls weight, and glucose levels; it includes rapid walking, jogging, bicycling, swimming, and dancing; aerobic exercise can be initiated as early as 6-8 weeks pospartum and has no adverse effect on lactation (N Engl J Med 1994; 330:449oA); in AE, intense exercise results in re-synthesis of high energy compounds in the presence of oxygen, AE boasts the greatest health benefits as the energy expenditure is maximized while performing rhythmic contractions of large muscles over distance, eg jogging or against gravity, eg jazz-dancing, both of which are types of 'endurance' training, causing physiological cardiac hypertrophy and with time, a desirable physiologic bradycardia; some experts recommend at least three sessions of AE/week; see Exercise; Cf Anaerobic exercise

aerobic fitness A value obtained from exercise testing, expressed as either V_{O_2peak} (oxygen consumption at peak exercise), or W_{peak} (peak work capacity or tolerance, expressed as percentage of normal); AF has potential as a prognostic tool in cystic fibrosis, where 83% of patients with the highest levels of aerobic fitness ($V_{O_2peak} \geq 82\%$ of predicted) survived 8 years, compared to 28% survival at 8 years in those with the lowest aerobic fitness ($V_{O_2peak} \leq 58\%$ of predicted) (N Engl J Med 1992; 327:1785oA) see Physical fitness

aerobiology ALLERGY MEDICINE The formal study of living and nonliving atmospheric constituents of biological interest, eg airborne pollutants, microorganisms, and pollens

Intramural aerobiology is defined as the formal study of aerial hygiene and extramural aerobiology as the study of atmospheric constituents; aerobiology has been commandeered by allergy docs, for whom it is more elegant than a more plebian alternative, eg pollenology-Author's note

aerogel MATERIALS SCIENCE An ultralight subtsance composed of silica, alumina, zirconia and other substances that is transparent and has significant insulating and sound-attenuating properties, and which may have currency against ozone layer-depleting CFCs

aerosol A fine spray of liquid particles ranging from 10^{-6}-10^{-9} in diameter; commercial aerosols have various industrial, household and pharmaceutical applications

aerospace medicine 1) Aviation medicine, see there 2) Space medicine, see there

aerotolerant anaerobe An anaerobe that grows poorly in O_2 or CO_2 environments and is clearly 'happier' under anaerobic conditions, eg *Clostridium carnis, C histolyticum, C tertium*

AFB Acid-fast bacillus also 1) Aflatoxin B 2) American Foundation for the Blind 3) Aorto-femoral bypass

AFB₁ Aflatoxin B1, see there

Aflatoxin

afferent loop syndrome A variant of the postgastrectomy syndrome, caused by partial or complete obstruction of proximal portion (loop) of a Billroth II anastomosis between the stomach and jejunum CLINICAL Pain, bloating, abdominal tenderness, with bacterial overgrowth and malabsorption Note: In view of the vast change in the management of gastric ulcers, these and other postgastrectomy complexes are largely of historic interest

affiliation The association of a person, institution or organization with others, which in US hospital parlance, is the close tie of a health care institution to a medical school or university; in a typical symbiotic affiliation, the hospital gains prestige and a supply of resident physicians who provide patient care, while the medical school gains a clinical teaching facility

affinity IMMUNOLOGY The strength of the sum of the multiple binding sites between an antibody and an antigen, which increases the stability of the linkage, as measured by the association or affinity constant; the antibody recognizes the 3-D configuration of an epitope rather than a single specific binding site; low-affinity complexes may persist in the circulation, localize in the glomerular basement membrane and compromise renal function; see Avidity, Immune complexes

affinity chromatography LABORATORY MEDICINE A type of adsorption chromatography in which an antigen or antibody is purified based on a substance's highly specific and reversible adsorption by a complementary binding substance (ligand) and immobilized on an insoluble support (matrix) METHOD A fluid with an antigen of interest is poured through a column containing the corresponding antibody bound to a plastic bead (the solid phase); all nonbinding molecules flow through the column; in the second step, an elution buffer, eg acetate at pH 3.0 or diethylamine at pH 11.5, is poured through the column to remove the substance or ligand of interest; the advantage of affinity chromatography is that it allows the processing of large volumes of fluid, and is useful for purifying a substance of interest from a complex biological mixture, and for separating native from denatured forms of the same molecule

affinity maturation IMMUNOLOGY The ↑ in the average affinity of antibodies (to an antigen) produced after immunization, due to an increase of more specific and less heterogeneous IgG antibodies, following a more heterogeneous early response by IgM molecules

affirmative action A phrase popularized in the 1960s,

meaning the removal of artificial barriers to the employment of women and minorities; with time, the phrase has come to mean any effort to recruit and hire members of previously disadvantaged groups in an effort to erase past inequities; see Reverse discrimination; Cf Glass ceiling

affluent diet Western diet A diet characterized by ↑↑↑ fat, saturated fat, cholesterol, and ↑ calories; this regimen is held responsible for the marked ↑ in cardiovascular diseases typical of the US (N Engl J Med 1992; 327:52c) Cf Mediterranean diet

AFIP Armed Forces Institute of Pathology, see there

aflatoxin B1 A mold toxin derived from *Aspergillus flavus* and *A parasiticus* that may contaminate grains and is both mutagenic and a liver-specific co-carcinogen; dietary exposure to aflatoxin B1 in grains is inculpated in the high incidence of hepatocellular carcinomas HCC in Africa and China; AFB_1 appears to induce the p53 tumor suppressor gene mutation (AGG to AGT at codon 249), supporting the hypothesis that AFB_1 has an early causative role in the pathogenesis of HCC (Science 1994; 264: 1317RR) see p53

AFP α-fetoprotein, see there

Africa connection A catch phrase used before HIV-1 was implicated in AIDS, coined in an attempt to explain why the same disease that predominantly afflicted male homosexuals and drug abusers in the US[1] also afflicted heterosexual Africans[2]; Cf Monkey connection, Mosquito connection

[1]Now known as AIDS pattern I [2]Known as AIDS pattern II

Africanized bee 'Killer bee' A honey bee strain from Africa (*Apis mellifera* L) that has certain behaviors with adaptive value in the tropics, including swarming, absconding tendencies, defensive behavior and opportunistic use of resources; the Africanized bee has slowly migrated north and south from its tropical site of introduction in Brazil in the 1950s and has supplanted the European honey bee, although there is mixture of the races at the 'frontier' zones in both South America and the Northern Hemisphere

Note: The venom of the Africanized bee is no more allergenic or toxic that that of the European honeybee; the bee itself is simply more aggressive (N Engl J Med 1994; 331:523RV)

afterimage A visual sensation that is perceived when observing a homogenous neutral backgroup following visual stimulation; the afterimage is due to photochemical activity of the retina and may be negative, positive, or complementary

AG1343 AIDS An inhibitor of HIV-1 protease that is in phase I* trials and may ↓ viral load when administered to HIV-infected individuals (Bio/Technology 1995; 13:206) see L735,524

*Which determine drug safety and pharmacokinetics

age structure A characteristic of a population that reflects the historical trends in birth and death rates; until the 20th century, the human age structure had remained relatively constant and had a pyramidal appearance with a relatively large number of children at the base and due to a higher average mortality (30-50+/1000), a narrow apex of persons who had arrived to old age; with the improving health and decline in both infant mortality and birth rate; the age structure is undergoing a transition (see illustration) to an increasing columnar form, especially as developing nations achieve a balanced rate of reproduction (Sci Am 1993; 268/4:46)

age trend EPIDEMIOLOGY An age-specific change in the incidence of a particular condition, usually the age of onset of a particular disease, eg hypertension or cataracts (JAMA 1992; 268:3098cc) see Temporal trend

Agenda 21 GLOBAL VILLAGE A set of guidelines signed by the participants in the Rio de Janeiro summit that addressed issues of climatic changes and biodiversity; according to some workers, the enthusiasm to meet the possibly unrealistic goals delineated in A21 has waned, and some industrialized countries have already passed some of the goals to limit greenhouse gases, in particular CO_2 (Sci Am 1995; 272/6:36)

agent COMPUTERS A small mobile piece of computer software that can send itself across a computer network and perform a task on a remote machine (Sci Am 1995; 272/2:28) Cf Virtual critter

Note: A variation of the theme is that of the intelligent agent, where intelligence is not defined in human terms, but rather on a more primary level, ie that modicum of mental activity necessary for an insect to stay alive; it has been suggested that the term trainable ant is more appropriate

Agent Orange ENVIRONMENT A 50:50 mixture of 2,4-D n-butyl ester or 2,4-dichlorophenoxyacetic and 2,4,5-T n-butyl ester or trichlorophenoxyacetic acids in a diesel oil vehicle; AO was contaminated with 1 to 20 ppm of 2,3,7,8-tetrachlorodibenzo-p-dioxin (TCDD) that causes chloracne, cancer, affecting enzyme levels, porphyrin metabolism and immune dysfunction; because TCDD stores in adipose tissue, its long-term effects are currently unknown; the lawsuit brought by the exposed Vietnam veterans resulted in a $180 million settlement

AO was used as a general defoliant for forest, brush, broad-leafed crops, used in Southeast Asia by the American forces, as a tactic of warfare, for the purpose of destroying the jungle cover used by the Viet Cong guerilla forces during the Vietnam conflict as camouflage; experiments with defoliant chemicals as herbicides began during World War II and four agents of potential military use were weeded out of the 12 000 chemicals tested; the US defoliation effort in Vietnam began in late 1961 and by the time the aerial defoliation program (see Operation Ranch Hand) ended in 1968, 6603 square miles (17 300 km²) had been sprayed with defoliant, predominantly AO, mostly from fixed wing aircraft; see Times Beach

aggressive angiomyxoma A rare, locally aggressive, non-metastasizing tumor of the pelvis and/or perineum, usually of premenopausal ♀ PATHOLOGY Poorly circumscribed soft-tissue mass with a gelatinous consistency; by light microscopy, spindled cell in a myxoid background often with a prominent vascular component (Arch Pathol Lab Med 1993; 117:911oA)

aggregation toxicology An unusual, albeit well-established phenomenon in amphetamine research, where a dose of amphetamine that is not lethal in a solitary rat or mouse, is large enough to be fatal when an identical amount is administered to a group of rodents in a crowded cage (JAMA 1993; 269:1505MN&P)

aging see Geriatrics

'aging' pigment 1) Ceroid, see there 2) Lipofuscin, see there

agnogenic myeloid metaplasia HEMATOLOGY A chronic progressive panmyelosis characterized by variable fibrosis of the bone marrow, massive splenomegaly secondary to extramedullary hematopoiesis and a leukoerythroblastic anemia with dysmorphic red cells, circulating normoblasts, immature white cells and typical platelets CLINICAL Patients are often older than 50 and present with insidious weight loss, anemia, abdominal discomfort due to splenomegaly, often accompanied by hepatomegaly; 80% of cases are accompanied by non-specific chromosome abnormalities PROGNOSIS Average survival 5 years, often ending in acute leukemia; see Pseudonym syndrome

AgNOR Argyrophilic* nucleolar organizer region A loop of DNA in the nucleolus that encodes rRNA; AgNORs reflect proliferation and the number present correlates with the behavior of some tumors; in Kaposi sarcoma AgNOR staining of tissue ↑ as the tumors become more aggressive (Arch Pathol Lab Med 1995; 119:538) see Nucleolar organizing region

*aka Achromatic gap (argyrophilic, ie related to silver, chemical shorthand, Ag)

β_2-agonist* β_2-Adrenergic receptor agonist, see there

agonal biopsy A biopsy obtained at the time of terminal (or agonal) convulsions, which is procedure that may be necessary when the details about a dying patient's disease are needed by the managing physicians (as in the case of Ebola virus, or other potentially fatal viral infection), and the patient's religious beliefs (or next of kin) prohibit any form of postmortem examination (R Preston, The Hot Zone, Random House, New York, 1994)

A/G syndrome A disease complex characterized by amenorrhea and galactorrhea, seen in females with hyperprolactinemia caused by a microadenoma within the sella turcica

agrin A neuronal protein involved in forming clusters of acetylcholine receptors on muscle cells, which may play a role in development and in nerve regeneration; see ARIA

Agua de Tlacote Water from a spring in Querétero, Mexico, which is alleged to have curative properties, and which may be a carrier of *Entamoeba histolytica* (N Engl J Med 1995; 332:687c)

ague cake spleen A descriptor for any organ (liver, pancreas, spleen) that is blackened, brittle, dry and enlarged; the spleen may be 1000+g in *P falciparum* malaria

Ague, Middle English, malarial fever with shaking chills, (Chaucer, 1388)

'Aguecheek's disease' A fanciful synonym for the dementia seen in hepatic encephalopathy, coined after Sir Andrew Aguecheek, a timorous minor character in Shakespeare's *Twelfth Night*

AH$_{50}$ An assay that measures activity of the alternate pathway of complement-mediated hemolysis; the AH$_{50}$ serves as a screen for homozygous deficiencies of complement factors C3, factor I and factor H

AH interval CARDIOLOGY A period measured by electrophysiological studies of the heart equal to the time between the onset of the first rapid atrial deflection and the His bundle deflection; as the lower right atrium and the His bundle delineate the anatomic boundaries of the AV node, the AHI (usually 55-130 msec) is essentially equivalent to the AV nodal conduction time; the AHI is ↓ by atropine and isopreterenol, and ↑ by adenosine, digitalis, some Class I antiarrhythmic agents, eg moricizine (N Engl J Med 1992; 327:255OA), propranolol, rapid or premature atrial pacing, vagal maneuvers, and verapamil; Cf HV interval

Aha! phenomenon BASIC SCIENCE A flash of insight related to a problem, eg the integration of a complex set of data, that may result in a solution to the problem (New York Times 16 August 1994; C1)

Ahasuerus syndrome 'Wandering Jew syndrome', see there

AI Artificial intelligence, see there

AID 1) Agency for International Development 2) Artificial insemination by donor; see Artificial reproduction

AIDS Acquired immunodeficiency syndrome, see below also 1) Academy of International Dental Studies 2) Accident/Incident Data System

Also 1) Accretive Industrial Development Syndrome (a nonmedical term used in real estate) 2) All Individuals Deserve Support (a slogan used by an AIDS support group)

AIDS Acquired immunodeficiency syndrome A condition defined by criteria delineated by the CDC (see table) and intimately linked to the retrovirus, human immunodeficiency virus (HIV-1); although long-term survival after HIV infection is possible (see Nonprogressive HIV infection), when clinical AIDS develops, it is ultimately fatal, despite response for various lengths of time to a various therapeutic modalities **INCUBATION PERIOD** In homosexual and bisexual men, HIV infection precedes clinical AIDS by ± 11.0 years before clinical AIDS develops; 5 million are infected in Africa (WHO estimates, 1991); 10 million are positive worldwide **LABORATORY** Hyperkalemia 16-21% (N

Engl J Med 1993; 328:703OA) thrombocytopenia, possibly related to ↑ platelet-associated IgG, IgM, C3, and immune complexes on autologous platelets; there is also a ↓ platelet survival and production, possibly related to HIV infection of megakaryocytes, which may respond to zidovudine (N Engl J Med 1992; 327:1779OA) **NEUROLOGY** AIDS is associated with cryptococcal meningitis, dementia, lymphoma, neuropathy, progressive multifocal leukoencephalopathy, toxoplasmosis **RISK FACTORS** (1994) US) ♂ homosexual sex 47%; IV drugs 28%, heterosexual sex 9%, ♂ homosexual sex + IV drugs 5%, contaminated blood 1%, hemophilia 1%, undetermined 9% (Am Med News 10 October 1994 p 15) **STATISTICS** (1994, US) Number of cases 401 750; +3% (change 1992-1993); ♂ 347 770; ♀ 53 980; Mortality $^{401750}/_{243423}$ ie 61% (Am Med News 10 October 1994 p 15) deaths to date-243 423 (30 June 1994), 40 000 new cases/year (N Engl J Med 1994; 331:1451ED) AIDS is defined by the 'Revision of the CDC Surveillance case definition of AIDS'* **TRENDS** (1982-1993) In Los Angeles, PCP continues to be the most common cause of death; deaths from bacterial, CMV, *Mycobacterium avium* complex, and *Toxoplasma* infection ↓, while there was an ↑ in mortality due to fungal infections, TB, encephalopathy, and non-AIDS-related conditions (Arch Pathol Lab Med 1994; 118:884OA) THERAPY Some preliminary data suggest that cytokines (eg IL-1, IL-2, IL-4, IL-10, IL-12, and TNF-α) may be of use in treating AIDS (Science 1995; 268:205) see ARC, 'Dominant dozen', gp120, gp160, Hairy leukoplakia, HIV-1, HIV-2, *Isospora belli*, Patient zero, *Pneumocystis carinii*, VLIA (Virus-like infectious agent), Walter Reed classification

*In January 1992, the definition of AIDS was broadened to include any person seropositive for HIV-1 with CD4+ T lymphocyte ≤ 0.2 x 10^6/L

AIDS Beliefs Survey A survey of young subjects, in particular those who are sexually active (J Adolesc Health 1991; 12:434)

AIDS-belt A now-defunct term that referred to a group of tropical African nations reporting more than 1000 cases of AIDS, where the disease affected heterosexuals and related to sexual promiscuity; the 'belt' countries were: Burundi, Central African Republic, the Congo, Kenya, Malawi, Rwanda, Tanzania, Uganda and Zambia

AIDS-'case zero' see Patient zero

AIDS(-related) cholangitis A condition characterized by chronic abdominal pain, low-grade fever, cholestasis with bile duct ectasia and bile duct irregularities ETIOLOGY *Cryptosporidium* spp, CMV, and microsporidia *Enterocytozoon bieneusi* (**N Engl J Med 1993; 328:95oA**)

AIDS conspiracy HIV conspiracy, see there

AIDS-defining disease A disease which, when accompanied by evidence of HIV infection, fulfills the criteria necessary to diagnose AIDS; there has been a shift in ADDs since 1984, when 52% were due to *Pneumocystis carinii* pneumonia, 26% to KS, 10% to *Candida* spp esophagitis, and the remainder to *Cryptococcus* meningitis, HIV encephalopathy, HIV wasting syndrome, *Mycobacterium avium* complex bacteremia, lymphoma, *Toxoplasma* encephalitis, CMV retinitis; in 1992, HIV wasting syndrome caused 31% of ADDs, PCP 27%, HIV encephalopathy 23%, *Mycobacterium avium* complex bacteremia 8%, KS 8% and others, the remainder (**N Engl J Med 1994; 329:1962c**)

AIDS dementia complex An insidious (30% of asymptomatic HIV-positive subjects have electroencephalographic abnormalities ADC is characterized by progressive cognitive, motor and behavioral dysfunction, affecting up to two-thirds of AIDS patients, as HIV-1 remains latent in the macrophages of the CNS or microglia, serving as both a reservoir and a vehicle for dissemination, possibly related to HIV envelope glycoprotein gp120's structural similarity to neuroleukin; AIDS dementia may be complicated by infections, eg *Toxoplasma gondii* and CMV, and lymphomas CLINICAL Inability to concentrate, loss of memory, gait incoordination, dysgraphia, slowing of psychomotor functions and eventually, apathy PATHOLOGY Degeneration of subcortical white matter and deep gray matter, white matter vacuolization in the lateral and posterior columns of the spinal cord Note: gp120 blocks calcium channels, increasing intraneuronal calcium to toxic levels, suggesting possible response of the dementia to calcium channel manipulation with nimodipine

AIDS drugs see AIDS therapy

AIDS embryopathy An HIV-induced complex in children born to IVDA mothers, characterized by craniofacial defects including microcephaly, hypertelorism, box-like head, saddle nose, long palpebral fissures with blue sclera, a triangular philtrum and patulous lips

AIDS encephalopathy AIDS dementia complex, see there

AIDS enteropathy An AIDS-related condition, defined by the *absence* of a microorganism, which when seen in AIDS-related complex, may presage clinical AIDS CLINICAL Diarrhea, often worse at night, weight loss, occasionally fever and possibly malnutrition with impaired D-xylose absorption PATHOLOGY Partial villous atrophy with crypt hyperplasia in the small intestine, viral inclusions, ↓ plasma cells and ↑ intraepithelial lymphocytes in the large and small intestine

AIDS fraud A generic term for any form of health care fraud committed against patients with AIDS, conservatively estimated to have been perpetrated against 10% of those with AIDS; almost invariably for financial gain on the part of the perpetrator; this form of health care quackery is virtually identical to the various forms of unproven cancer treatment, differing only in the types of agents; AIDS therapies identified by the FDA as frankly fraudulent are CanCell‡, hydrogen peroxide‡, and ozone treatment‡; herb-based therapies have been anecdotally reported to

be effective in treating AIDS include acemannan‡, bitter melon‡ and its protein extract, MAP-30‡, curcumin‡, glycyrrhizin‡, megadoses of vitamins, and Chinese herbal formulae (**Am Med News 21 Nov 1994 p13**)

'AIDS-gate' An affair in which French authorities allegedly delayed the approval of the American ELISA test for detecting antibodies to HIV-1 for a period of months, awaiting the availability of an equivalent French test; the delay is believed by many to have resulted in exposure of countless hemophiliacs to HIV, an unknown number of whom became infected during this period (**Nature 1991; 353:197n**); a second aspect of the affair was that the major supplier of blood products in France is alleged to have decided to use its stock of existing unheated blood products even though authorities had been warned that 'probably all' of the pooled plasma from Parisian donors was infected with HIV Note: Similar scandals rocked the health care industries in other countries, eg in Japan, where an estimated 1800 hemophiliacs may have been infected by non-heat treated factor VIII during the critical period in the mid-1980s (**Nature Medicine 1995; 1:396**)

*The term AIDS-gate derives from the Watergate scandal that occurred during Nixon's presidency, which resulted in his resignation from the White House

AIDS Highway Kinshasa Highway, see there

AIDS litigation A generic term for any form of litigation initiated as a result of 1) An alleged wrongful infection with HIV, eg through negligence or criminal acts, or 2) Related to discrimination against an HIV-infected person who is guaranteed constitutional rights under the Americans with Disabilities Act and other relevant legislation

AIDS, long-term survival Up to 5% of those infected with HIV have survived 10+ years without developing clinical AIDS; although all have an increase in CD8 (cytotoxic) T lymphocytes, the reason is unclear; hypotheses regarding the reason for this resistance include a proposal that there are two distinct patterns of immune response to HIV, or the existance of 'benign' strains of HIV, or an increased host resistance to HIV (**Sci Am 1994; 270/5:20**)

AIDS-malaria connection A hypothetical linkage between the transmission of HIV and malaria, an association that had been assumed by some models; malaria is not more frequent or more severe in children with progressive HIV-1 infection nor does malarial infection appear to accelerate the rate of progression of AIDS

Note: The posit may have arisen from faulty interpretation of AIDS epidemiology in Africa, where the cost of screening blood for HIV antibodies is prohibitive, and unscreened blood (up to 20% of which is HIV infected) may be transfused to those with severe malaria-related anemia (N Engl J Med 1991; 325:105)

AIDS pathogensis It is unclear why there is prolonged period after HIV-1 infection and before the development of clinical disease; one explanation based on a mathematical model is that the HIV-1 viruses suffers multiple genetic mutations during replication; although the immune system recognizes (and destroys) most of the daughter viruses of each generation; however as 'escape mutants' accumulate, they eventually overcome the host's immune system by the vast diversity of antigenic epitopes that the 'escapees' represent (**Science 1991; 254:963, 941n&v**)

AIDS pattern I The pattern of AIDS epidemiology that is prevalent in developed nations, ie that is more common in male homosexuals and bisexuals, intravenous drug abusers, hemophiliacs and sexual partners or children born to HIV-positive women

AIDS pattern II The pattern of AIDS epidemiology that is prevalent in developing nations, ie Africa and Asia, ie that due to heterosexual promiscuity

AIDS precautions Those activities intended to minimize exposure to contaminated blood (and potentially bloody fluids, including extreme care, hand washing, use of face masks, double-gloving; see Universal precautions

AIDS quackery AIDS fraud, see there

Note: Since early 1988, labeling of specimens as potentially contaminated with HIV has been discouraged by the CDC, as it introduces a false sense of security that unlabeled specimens do not contain HIV-1

AIDS-RELATED COMPLEX (ARC)

CLINICAL FEATURES	LABORATORY
Temp. > 38 C	CD4 T-cells < 400/mL
Weight loss > 10%	CD4:CD8 T-cell ratio < 1.0
Lymphadenopathy	Anemia, leukopenia
> 3 months	Thrombocytopenia
Diarrhea > 3 months	Polyclonal gammopathy
Night sweats > 3 months	Anergy (to skin testing)
Fatigue	↓ Mitogenic response (PHA)

AIDS-related complex ARC A pre-AIDS condition with prodromal manifestations of AIDS where the criteria for defining a case as AIDS are not yet present; ARC is a 'Chinese menu disease', requiring two or more clinical features and two or more abnormal laboratory results; the patients may also have non-specific lymphadenopathy; see AIDS, Follicle lysis, HIV-1

AIDS statistics Incidence (US) 14/10⁵, higher in blacks and Hispanics Groups affected: Homosexuals, 56%; IVDAs, 23% Annual incidence (per 10⁵) Washington DC 81; New York 39; New Jersey 28; Florida 27; California 23; in the US, 100 777 people died of AIDS from 1981-1990, nearly ⅓ in 1990; AIDS is most common cause of death in young US adults, surpassing heart disease, cancer, suicide and homicide; ¾ of the deaths are of the 25-44 age group, 59% of the deaths have occurred in ♂ homosexuals, 21% in ♀ drug abusers; death rate (per 10⁵) 29 Blacks, 22 Hispanics, 9 Whites, 3 Asians and American Indians (**MMWR 1991; 40:41**) New cases per 10⁵ in US 1990: Washington 121, New York State 47, New Jersey 32, Florida 31, California 25 (**MMWR 1991; 40:55**) AIDS is the leading cause of ♂ death in the Ivory Coast (1447 deaths/10⁶) and is second in ♀ (340/10⁶) after pregnancy-related disease; 41% of ♂, and 32% of ♀ cadavers were infected

Note: Analysis of the AIDS epidemic has led some workers to postulate that AIDS would reach a plateau and may be on the decline in all risk categories except that of heterosexual transmission

AIDS therapy Various therapeutic modalities have been used to treat HIV-positive individuals; some may temporarily delay the progression of AIDS

EFFECTIVE (FDA-APPROVED) Zidovudine, ddC (dideoxycytidine), ddI (dideoxy-ionsine)

EXPERIMENTAL SUBSTANCES

∗ DAB/486IL-2, an IL-2 receptor-specific 'fusion' cytotoxin that selectively eliminates HIV-infected cells bearing high-affinity IL-2 receptors (**Science 1991; 252:1703**)

∗ PE40, a 40 kD *Pseudomonas* exotoxin linked to either IL-2 or the CD4 determinant with varying efficacy in vitro

∗ Ro24-7429, which targets the tat gene product

∗ U-81749 A synthetic peptide-like substance that blocks HIV-1's protease

INEFFECTIVE SUBSTANCES Compound Q (trichosanthin, GLQ 223), dextran sulfate, isoprinosine, lentinan (an extract of shiitake mushrooms), peptide T, TIBO derivatives, viroxan (an unsterilized mixture of uncertain nature); see HIV-1, *Pneumocystis carinii* pneumonia

AIDS vaccine As of 1995, there is no effective vaccine; any vaccine formulated must take into account 1) The rapid mutability of HIV 2) The mode of transmission, ie transmucosal and hematogenous 3) Its transmission as either an intra– or extracellular pathogen 4) The binding of the virus to the CD4 molecule on the surface of T lymphocytes and macrophages; at the beginning of HIV infec-

tion, the host produces type-specific neutralizing antibodies that appear to recognize a loop structure in the third hypervariable domain of the HIV envelope known as the V3-loop; the immune defense that develops later in HIV infection neutralizes a broader spectrum of HIV isolates and is mediated by antibodies that block the binding of the viral envelope to the CD4 binding region VACCINE Because the traditional or classic approaches to vaccination (immunization with either live attenuated viruses, or with inactivated viruses with adjuvant), other approaches have been proposed including use of recombinant or synthetic HIV proteins with adjuvant, use of live recombinant organisms (eg vaccinia, adenovirus, bacille Calmette-Guérin) as vectors for HIV proteins, and intramuscular inoculation with HIV genes VACCINE TRIALS Phase I trials are being carried out to determine safety (not efficacy); no candidate thusfar has elicited an effective immune response in the animal models (**N Engl J Med 1993; 329:1395SA; Science 1994; 264:1660N&C**) see HIV, V3 loop; see gp160 vaccine, HGP-30, Zagury

AIDS wasting syndrome HIV wasting syndrome, see there

AIL Angiocentric immunoproliferative lesions

AILA Angioimmunoblastic lymphadenopathy, see there

AIN Anal intraepithelial neoplasia, see Intraepithelial neoplasia

ainhum Black toe disease TROPICAL MEDICINE A possibly AD condition affecting young black males of Africa and Central America, in whom broad fibrous bands cause annular digitoplantar constriction, especially of the fifth toe, resulting in autoamputation; pseudoainhum is caused by neurologic disease and ectodermal dysplasia

air ambulance EMERGENCY MEDICINE A vehicle, often a helicopter, used to evacuate a person who requires immediate medical attention that cannot be provided in his/her current location; air ambulances, unlike their terrestrial counterparts, cannot be viewed as flying critical care units, as the most fundamental components of patient evaluation, eg assessment of breath, bowel and cardiac sounds are impossible because of the high noise levels (90-110 dB), which when accompanied by the vibrations and extreme space limitations, make the air transport of patients in critical condition 'scoop and run' operations (**JAMA 1991; 266:515C**); in one study, 62% of cases were medical-surgical, eg MI, 32% were trauma-related and 6% were neonates; the patients were transported circa 80 miles; the mortality was 16%

air bag PUBLIC HEALTH A device in a passenger vehicle in the US, which consists of a rubberized nylon bag that inflates 'instantaneously' in the event of a frontal impact in a motor vehicle accident; when first introduced ABs were placed only on the driver's side, although traditionally, the 'seat of death' is the front passenger side; more recently, passenger-side ABs are becoming 'standard' equipment, air bags are projected to reduce traffic fatalities by an estimated 6.5%, assuming that a shoulder belt is worn; a negative aspect of air bags relates to the mechanism used to inflate the bags, which hinges on spark ignition of sodium azide, nitrogen gas, ash and sodium hydroxide, potentially causing facial burns, chemical keratitis and photophobia related to intraocular deposition of powder (**N Engl J Med 1991; 324:1599C**), in addition to ocular contusions (**ibid, 325:1518C**) see Steering wheel injury

air meniscus sign A crescent-shaped radiolucency bordering a mass lesion, classically seen in pulmonary hydatid cysts, where air enters the cyst forming a radiolucency between the outer layer (host) and the inner layer (hydatid membrane of *Echinococcus granulosus*), the most common air meniscus sign in the US is caused by *Aspergillus fumigatus*

air monitor Xylene etc; Cf Film badge

air pollution PUBLIC HEALTH The presence of substances (listed below) in the air that are byproducts of human activities; in the South Coast Air Basin (Los Angeles) daily emissions of 1375 tons of hydrocarbons, 1208 tons of nitrogen oxides, 4987 tons of carbon monoxide, 134 tons of sulfur oxides, and 1075 tons of particulate matter (Sci Am 1993; 269/4:24); it is estimated that if the residents of Los Angeles (population 14 million, registered motor vehicles 10.6 million) were able to achieve the US federal standard for ozone and particulates, there would be an estimated $9.4 billion gain in health benefits, eliminating 1600 premature deaths in those with chronic respiratory diseases, 15 million workdays in those with respiratory disease, 18 million days of restricted activity, 65 million days of chest discomfort, 180 million days of sore throats, 190 million days of eye irritation; see London fog incident, Particulate air pollution

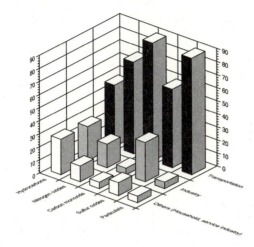

air pollution-contributers

airline food NUTRITION High-altitude fare is 'classically' inedible, but rarely dangerous; surprisingly, only 23 outbreaks of foodborne illness having been reported worldwide on commercial flights from 1947 to 1984; recognition of such outbreaks requires that the attack affects ≥ 20% of the passengers or crew, short incubation periods allowing in-flight recognition, or the occurrence of an epidemic illness, eg cholera or typhoid fever that is otherwise being investigated by public health officials; most cases have been attributed to food handling errors, in particular improper holding temperatures; a recent airline food-related outbreak of shigellosis was identified in a professional football team*, affecting 21 of 65 team players and staff (JAMA 1992; 268:3208oc)

*Giving new meaning to the phrase 'end runs'

Air Quality Standard PUBLIC HEALTH A benchmark of the quality of air based on the concentration of five ambient air pollutants

1) Carbon monoxide-9 ppm (eight-hour average)

2) Nitrogen dioxide-0.05 ppm (annual average)

3) Ozone-0.12 ppm (one-hour average)

4) Particulate matter (< 10 μm in diameter)-50 μg/m³ (annual arithmetic mean)

5) Sulfur dioxide-0.03 ppm (annual average)

The 1990, the US National AQS (N Engl J Med 1994; 331:1542oa)

air sickness A permutation of motion sickness, which occurs during ascent and/or descent in an airplane

airway responsiveness '...*the ease with which airways narrow in response to various allergic and nonsensi-*tizing *stimuli, including inhaled pharmacologic agents, such as histamine and methacholine, and physical stimuli, such as exercise...commonly assessed by measuring lung function before and after inhalation of increasing concentrations of an agent such as methacholine.*' (N Engl J Med 1992; 326:1540oa) see Asthma

AIS Abbreviated Injury Scale A classification of severity of injury formulated in 1985 by the American Association of Automotive Medicine; see Injury Severity Score

aka also known as, AKA, also above-the-knee amputatioin

AKA Above the knee amputation, see there

AKAP A-kinase-anchoring protein, see there

A kinase-anchoring protein AKAP A protein that binds (anchors) the regulatory subunit of cAMP-dependent protein kinase; anchoring is crucial in regulating synaptic function (Nature 1994; 368:853L)

Akureyri disease A clinical form of benign myalgic encephalomyelitis that occurred in 1948 in Akureyri, Iceland

Alar Daminozide ENVIRONMENT A pesticide extensively used by apple producers in the US with the added advantage of inducing a 'natural' red color and increasing shelf life; one of Alar's metabolic products, UDMH is carcinogenic with an estimated increased cancer risk of 1-4 per million exposed; when the data generated by the Natural Resources Defense Council was published, estimating the cancer risk in children at 24 cancer deaths/10⁵, a public outcry forced a temporary ban on its use, as 20-50% of apples tested were contaminated; in subsequent re-evaluation of Alar, the EPA concluded that the carcinogenic effect is about ½ of its previous estimate (Science 1991; 254:20n&v)

ALARA As low as reasonably achievable RADIATION SAFETY An acronym for a generic stance taken in reference to the exposure to radiation, ie the minimum possible and/or practical vis-à-vis the licensed use of the radioactive materials being used, and the economics of improvement in relation to the state of technology, the benefits to public health and safety and other socioeconomic considerations

albatross 'syndrome' Postgastrectomy-personality disorder A complex described in patients who continue to have abdominal pain, nausea, vomiting, drug dependency and poor food intake, despite successful surgery for upper GI ulcers

Note: This 'syndrome' was described nearly 30 years ago (Can Med Assoc J 1967; 96:1559) prior to the availability of H₂-blocking agents (cimetidine, ranitidine), and more recently the use of antibiotics (to treat ulcers that accompany infection by *Helicobacter pylori*) and is of largely historic interest; patients with the syndrome have been fancifully likened to the Albatross of *The Rime of the Ancient Mariner*, as they incessantly demand that the surgeon do something to alleviate their suffering

albinism A group of hereditary and congenital, often AR diseases that share a metabolic defect in the production of mature melanin, which translates clinically into hypopigmentation of the skin, hair, and eyes; albinism has been subdivided into three major groups: 1) Generalized or oculocutaneous albinism All six subtypes are AR; the most common, type IA is due to tyrosinase deficiency, which may be due to a missense mutation, oculocutaneous albinism also occurs in Chediak-Higashi, Hermansky-Pudlak and Cross syndromes 2) Partial albinism An autosomal-dominant condition with a focal white patch, similar to Waardenburg syndrome 3) Ocular albinism An X-linked recessive condition

albumin CLINICAL THERAPEUTICS A 66-kD protein produced by the liver, which acts as an osmotic regulator, stabilizer, binding and transport protein and, experimentally, as a growth media supplement; albumin levels in serum serve as a surrogate marker for various diseases of the liver; therapeutic albumin is prepared by current indications for use; see Colloids, Crystalloids; Cf Ovalbumin LABORATORY MEDICINE In the 'prehistoric' period of laboratory medicine, proteins were divided into two broad categories based on their solubility in various concentrations of ammonium sulfate (in water), to wit 1) Globulins, which precipitated in half-saturated ammonium sulfate, and 2) Albumin, which only precipitated in the face of complete saturation of ammonium sulfate; in this context, the term albumin is of historic interest only

ALC Alternate level of care, see there

Alcian blue stain A proprietary water-soluble phthalocyanin dye [CI 74240] used in histology, which can be modified at different pHs for identifying specific mucopolysaccharide families; at pH 2.5, the stain identifies sialomucins produced by gastric and small intestinal glands; at pH 1.0, the sulfomucins produced in the large intestinal glands are more prominent

alcohol CHEMISTRY Any of a broad category of organic chemicals with a –OH with a minimal tendency to ionize CLINICAL MEDICINE Ethanol **CARDIOVASCULAR EFFECTS** see Alcohol consumption **ELECTROLYTES/ACID-BASE** A wide range of transient renal tubular defects are present in chronic alcoholism, causing varying changes, including $\downarrow$ glucose due to $\downarrow$ in threshold, $\downarrow$ Ca^{2+}, $\downarrow$ Mg^{2+}, $\downarrow$ PO_4^-, $\downarrow$ K^+, $\uparrow$ fractional excretion of β_2-microglobulin, uric acid, and aminoaciduria, metabolic acidosis and respiratory alkalosis with a normal glomerular filtration rate (N Engl J Med 1993; 329:1927oA) **REPRODUCTIVE EFFECTS** In rats, a single exposure to inebriating levels of alcohol results in a 50% $\downarrow$ in pregnancy (Science News 1994; 146:6) **SOCIAL COST** Government revenues gained $14 x 10^9 vs $100-130 x 10^9 in life lost ($\pm$ 100 000/year due to accidents, liver disease, cancer, etc), illness, and intangibles (N Engl J Med 1994; 331:537rv); alcohol is responsible for 41% of deaths from unintentional falls, 47% of drowning in those < age 15, 69% of boating fatalities, 49% of interpersonal violence (eg homicide, attempted homicide), 39% of partner battering, 50% of reported rapes, and 39-58% of fire-related fatalities (JAMA 1992; 267:2289)

alcohol-related birth defect A generic term for any birth defect, eg pre- or postnatal growth retardation, facial dysmorphia (thin upper lip, poorly developed philtrum, short nose, and eye openings), CNS defects with mental retardation; ARBDs occur with $\uparrow$ frequency in mothers who abuse alcohol during gestation; when multiple ARBDs are present, the term fetal alcohol syndrome (see there) is appropriate (JAMA 1992; 268:3176nih)

Alcoholics Anonymous A self-help support group for alcoholics, which claims a high rate of long-term abstention

alcoholic cardiomyopathy A clinicopathologic state induced by chronic ethanolism, a major cause of dilated cardiomyopathy, characterized by severe left ventricular dysfunction and a 40-80% three-year mortality, presenting as sudden death or ventricular fibrillation; alcohol is directly cardiotoxic, decreasing inotropism or force of myocardial contraction due to decreased calcium and impaired excitability, resulting in mitochondrial damage with decreased oxidative enzyme activity and energy production and swelling of the endoplasmic reticulum; alcohol also interferes with myocardial lipid metabolism, protein synthesis and ATPase activity; acetaldehyde, alcohol's major metabolite, stimulates the release of norepinephrine; alcoholic cardiomyopathy may be associated with other overlapping conditions, related either to other substances of abuse, eg tobacco-related cardiac disease or to alcohol's effect on other organ systems, eg cerebrovascular accidents and hypertension

alcohol consumption It is being increasingly recognized that moderate alcohol consumption (1-2 drinks/day) is associated with $\downarrow$ cardiovascular mortality[1] (RR = 0.5) with an improvement of lipid profile, due to an $\uparrow$ in HDL_2 and HDL_3 (N Engl J Med 1993; 329:1829oa); there is a direct positive association between alcohol consumption and plasma levels of endogenous tissue-type plaminogen activator (tPA), which averages 10.9 ng/mL for those who consume alcohol daily, 9.7 ng/mL (weekly) 9.1 ng/mL (monthly) and 8.1 ng/mL, a finding that supports the hypothesis that changes in the fibrinolytic potential may be a mechanism whereby alcohol consumption decreases the risk of cardiovascular disease[2] (JAMA 1994; 272:929oc) moderate amount is associated with $\downarrow$ mortality in $\female$, in particular those at increased risk for coronary heart disease (N Eng J Med 1995; 332:1245oa)

[1]This being colloquially known as the French paradox, see there [2]Because of well-known deleterious effects of alcohol, the medical community has been understandably reluctant to condone the use of alcohol as a health-promoting activity; with the accumulating evidence that alcohol is beneficial in reducing cardiovascular disease, there is a pressing need to resolve this dilemma; assuming there is no history or potential for alcohol abuse or addiction, there are no underlying diseases (liver and/or pancreatic disease, porphyria, hypertriglyceridemia, and others) that would preclude alcohol consumption, and work-related functions are not being carried out at the time of consumption, ingestion of 30-50 g alcohol/day are thought to have a cardioprotective effect, and such a regimen may be initiated at a physician's discretion (see JAMA 1994; 272:967ed)

alcoholic cirrhosis Laennec, nutritional, or portal cirrhosis A clinicopathologic entity which (usually) evolves from the early lesion of alcoholic fatty liver, in which the liver is 'greasy' and weighs up to three kg, with intact lobules and veins, portal infiltration by neutrophils and prominent Mallory body formation to the end-stage alcoholic cirrhosis, characterized by collapse, bile duct proliferation, hemosiderin deposition, in which the liver is fibrotic and shrunken, weighing less than one kilogram; 'classic' cirrhosis is defined by the histopathologic triad of 1) Diffuse fibrosis with lobular collapse 2) Regenerative nodules of hepatocytes and bile duct proliferation and 3) Hepatocellular necrosis (and mild hemosiderin deposition); Cf Micromicronodular cirrhosis

alcoholic fatty liver A liver demonstrating acute and subacute, ie precirrhotic, changes induced by alcohol, a toxin that interferes with fatty acid oxidation, impairing the tricarboxylic acid cycle, resulting in incomplete β-oxidation products from fatty acids PATHOLOGY The liver weighs 2500 g or more (normal 1500 g); it is yellow and greasy EM Enlarged and distorted mitochondria, dilated smooth endoplasmic reticulum; see Fatty liver

alcohol flush syndrome A vasoactive phenomenon common among Orientals; restriction fragment length polymorphism (RFLP) analysis reveals a defective aldehyde dehydrogenase gene with inability of these subjects to metabolize acetaldehyde

alcoholic neuropathy Pseudotabes A nutritional neuropathy described in alcoholics, characterized by burning pain in the lower extremities, paresthesia, usually acral in distribution, $\downarrow$ tactile and position sensation, ataxia and weakness of the legs with atrophy and fasciculations, ulcerations of immobile parts TREATMENT Dietary

alcoholic paranoia Othello syndrome, see there

alcoholic rose gardener 'syndrome' Subacute and chronic mycosis due to the dimorphous fungus, a low-grade pathogen, *Sporotrichosis schenckii*, which is reportedly more common in alcoholics employed as gardeners; the association, if true, is probably related to the lesser caution exercised by alcoholics who have increased skin abrasions and less concern for early infections

alcoholic type I 'Maintenance-type' alcoholic An anxiety-prone or passive-dependent person who drinks to alleviate problems; the onset in either sex is after age 25; type I alcoholics have a high reward dependence and avoid harmful or novel situations; most have minimal (if at all) antisocial tendencies

alcoholic type II 'Binge' drinker The thrill-seeking alcoholic who enjoys the novelty of drinking; type II alcoholics may be antisocial, have a history of early violence, and be the biological sons of alcoholic fathers, becoming alcoholics by age 25

alcoholism A condition defined by the Joint Committee of the National Council on Alcoholism and Drug Dependence and the American Society of Addiction Medicine as a '...*primary, chronic, disease with genetic, psychosocial, and environmental factors influencing its development and manifestations. The disease is often progressive and fatal. It is characterized by ... distortions in thinking, most notably denial.*'; it is thought by some workers that denial is not integral to defining a person as alcoholic (JAMA 1993; 269:586l); alcoholism is characterized by the regular intake of 75 or more grams of alcohol per day CHRONIC EFFECTS In addition to the well-described co-morbidity associated with portal hypertension, hepatic failure, hyperestrogenemia, infections (especially pneumonia, which may be related to alcohol-induced suppression of various immune defenses) and psycho-social disruption, there is transient hyperparathyroidism that induces hypocalcemia, hypomagnesemia and osteoporosis (N Engl J Med 1991; 324:721); restriction fragment length polymorphism (RFLP) analysis of cerebral tissue in alcoholics suggested an association of some forms of alcoholism with the D_2 receptor gene, located on C-11q22-q23, although the association is controversial (ibid, 264:3156) see Blood alcohol levels, Standard drink

aldose reductase inhibitor CLINICAL THERAPEUTICS Any of a family of compounds (eg epalrestat, ponalrestat, sorbinil, tolrestat) that block aldose reductase, which catalyzes the reduction of glucose to sorbitol*; ↑ intracellular glucose leads to ↑ sorbitol, which competitively inhibits glomerular and neural synthesis of *myo*-inositol; the ↓ in *myo*-inositol synthesis depresses phosphoinositide metabolism, and ↓ in Na⁺K⁺-ATPase activity; ARIs have not proven effective in preventing the complications of IDDM (N Eng J Med 1995; 332:1210ʀᵥ)

*Accumulation of polyols through the aldose reductase pathway is believed to lead to microvascular and neurologic complications of DM

aleukemic leukemia A clinical variant of acute leukemia where the peripheral blood reveals pancytopenia and few discernible blast cells on peripheral blood smears; leukemic cells are seen only by a bone marrow biopsy

Aleutian mink disease A chronic fatal parvoviral infection of minks causing a polyclonal expansion of B lymphocytes, affecting minks that are homozygous for the Aleutian blue mink gene, and clinically characterized by anorexia, diarrhea, weight loss, and death

A-level An educational 'track' in Britain that focuses a student at circa age sixteen into one of several subjects in preparation for the material he plans on 'reading' while in the university

alexin Complement, see there

ALF Animal Liberation Front, see there

algae oil ENVIRONMENT An alternative fuel in an early stage of development; algae convert carbon dioxide and sunlight into carbohydrates and proteins, but in absence of nitrogen, produce oils; these oils can be converted to a diesel-like oil by esterification (Science 1994; 264:33m) see Biodiesel

alginate microsphere see Microsphere

alglucerase Ceredase® A monomeric 497 AA glycoprotein that is a modified form of β-glucerebrosidase, which catalyzes the hydrolysis of glucocerebroside in reticuloendothelial system lysosomes; alglucerase is the most effective therapy for type 1 Gaucher's disease[1]; alglucerase therapy results in ↓ hepatospenomegaly, hematologic defects, ↑ bone mineralization, and reversal of cachexia in Gaucher's disease COST Even when alglucase therapy is

optimized by ↑ frequency, and ↓ dose, the cost for a 70-kg person is $100 000/year, justifying its dubious honor as the 'world's most expensive drug'[2] (N Engl J Med 1992; 327:1632oa, 1676ed) see Gaucher's disease, 'Orphan drug'

[1]The costs of such expensive drugs are justified by their 'orphan drug' status
[2]Symptomatic anemia, hemorrhagic diathesis, bone disease, hepatosplenomegaly

algor mortis The cooling of a body at the time of death, a process that theoretically occurs at a rate of 1°C/hour, assuming the decedent is an adult of normal weight and the ambient temperature is circa 20°C; the rate of cooling is increased if the decedent is thin or malnourished, the environmental temperature is low and or windy; algor mortis is slower in the obese, or if the ambient temperature is high

algorithm Critical pathway A logical set of rules for solving problems of a specified type that assumes that all of the data is objective, that there are a finite number of solutions to the problem, and that there are logical steps that must be performed to arrive at each of those solutions; algorithms can be expressed in algebraic form, as lines of logic in a computer program, or in the graphic form as a branching tree, with each branch corresponding to a decision pathway; algorithms form the basis of traditional computing, defined by the parameters used in programming, eg the 'and' and 'or' gates that allow a sequence to proceed or to 'loop'; the use of algorithms in solving complex clinical problems is inherently attractive (see figure, below), but often fails as disease causes subjective signs and symptoms and thus 'logical' algorithms cannot substitute for clinical experience; see Back-propagation

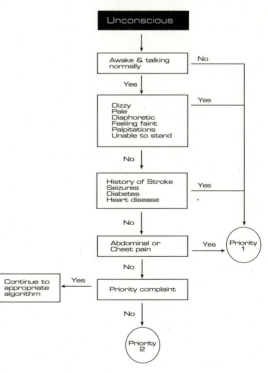

algorithm

ALI Annual limit on intake, see there

'Alice in Wonderland' changes A fanciful coinage for the cyclical, radiologically observed increases and decreases in the size of a prolactin-secreting pituitary adenoma, described in a patient receiving an ergot compound with dopaminic activity

Alice in Wonderland syndrome Bizarre perceptual distortions of the body image, space and size that may occur in 1) NEUROLOGY As a pre-epileptic aura or as a symptom preceding a migraine 2) PEDIATRICS Perceptual distortions as a presenting symptom of infectious mononucleosis that may be accompanied by convulsions, ataxia, nuchal rigidity, meningitis with mononuclear cells in the cerebrospinal fluid, encephalitis, transverse myelitis, Bell's palsy and Guillain-Barre syndrome 3) SUBSTANCE ABUSE Distortions of time, space and sensation associated with hallucinogens

Note: There is little reason to subdivide this 'syndrome' into types I and II as suggested by AE Rodin and JD Key, 1989

alien hand NEUROLOGY A type of dysfunction in which there is awkward assymmetical involuntary movement of the hand therefore interpreted by the internal sensors as 'alien'; the sign is nonspecific and occurs in infarction of the contralateral frontal cortex, or corpus callosum, or after corpus callosectomy (**N Engl J Med 1993; 329:1560cpc; J Neurol Neurosurg Psychiatry 1992; 55:806**)

ALK Actin receptor-like kinase A series of transmembrane serine-threonine kinases (six have been identified thus far) that are involved in signal transduction, forming heteromeric complexes upon binding their ligand (**Science 1994; 264:101r**)

alkaline phosphatase 'alk phos' A 69-kD homodimeric metalloenzyme [EC 3.1.3.1] A phosphatase with wide specificity that is widely distributed in nature, which has its optimal activity at an elevated ($\pm$ 10) pH; AP catalyzes the hydrolysis of phosphate esters, yielding alcohol and phosphate; serum AP is increased in hepatobiliary disease, eg obstructive jaundice, biliary cirrhosis, and intrahepatic cholestasis, as well as in bone disease, eg Paget's disease of bone (osteitis deformans), osteogenic sarcoma and others; AP is a commonly used indicator enzymes in enzyme immunoassays; see Immunoperoxidase; $\uparrow$ AP is a poor predictor of metastasis in breast carcinoma, and in one study was $\uparrow$ in only 27% of those with bone metastasis (**Am J Surg 1993; 165:221**)

alkaline tide PHYSIOLOGY A transient postcibal rise in the pH of the blood and urine, which is related to sequestration of hydrogen ions by the stomach during early digestion; Cf Acid tide

alkaptonuria Black urine disease, alcaptonuric ochronosis An AR [MIM 203500] defect in tyrosine metabolism, more common in males, that is due to homogentisic acid oxidase (HAO) deficiency; metabolic pathway of phenylalanine and tyrosine $\rightarrow$ ring opening of homogentisic acid $\rightarrow$ malylacetoacetic acid; without HAO, HA polymerizes into a blackened, oxidized, poorly soluble polymer, concentrating in the liver and kidney; BUD is first recognized by the mother who cannot clean the children's diaper as the urine oxidizes to pitch black upon exposure to air CLINICAL Arthritis due to homogentisic acid deposition in cartilage, tendons, as well as in the sclera, viscera and skin; when severe, pigment deposition can compromise cardiac, renal or pulmonary function, spilling into the urine as a melanin-like product; Cf Blue diaper syndrome

alkylating agent A generic term for any chemotherapeutic agent with unstable, highly reactive electrophilic rings that combine with tertiary nitrogens in purines and pyrimidines, as well as -NH$_2$, -COOH, -SH and PO$_3$H$_2$ groups forming stable covalent bonds; DNA, RNA and proteins each have one or more of these groups, but DNA damage at the N-7 position of the guanine ring is the most crippling to the proliferating, ie neoplastic cells; alkylating agents include busulfan, chlorambucil, cyclophosphamide, melphalan, nitrogen mustard and nitrosourea, administered intravenously or per os ADVERSE REACTIONS Stomatitis, nausea, vomiting, diarrhea, skin rash, anemia, alopecia; with cyclophosphamide, hemorrhagic cystitis and cardiac toxicity are not uncommon

alkyloidal cocaine Crack, see there

ALL Acute lymphocytic (lymphoblastic) leukemia, see there Also allergy

'all-American operation' A coinage from Dr Brunchwig's pelvic surgery service at Memorial Sloan-Kettering Cancer Institution (New York City), referring to radical surgery for a 'frozen pelvis,' consisting of total pelvic exenteration with radical en bloc resection of the rectum, uterus and urinary bladder; see Heroic surgery; Cf 'North American,' 'South American' operations

all-or-none law PHYSIOLOGY A rule that applies to the activation of individual muscle or nerve cells, where the response to stimuli (depolarization) only occurs above a certain threshold, usually -55 mV, and then a full-fledged action potential occurs which is maximal in intensity

all-or-none phenomenon CARDIAC PHYSIOLOGY The property of cardiac muscle in which stimulation of a single myocyte travels to the atrium and ventricle prior to contraction, resulting in a coherent and coordinated pump activity

allaylamine antifungal An antifungal antibiotic that inhibits squalene epoxidase which with oxidosqualene cyclase, cyclizes squalene to lanosterol, causing a depletion of ergosterol and squalene accumulation altering cell membrane and membrane functions, eg nutrient uptake (**Science 1994; 264:71p**)

all-payer system HEALTH CARE ENVIRONMENT A proposed health care system in which all insurers use the same fee schedule (**Am Med News 26 October 1992, p7**)

allele One of two or more variants of a gene present at a given locus (site) on a chromosome; alleles may differ in nucleotide sequence but not substantively in function or effect; in eukaryotic cells, alleles exist in pairs–one allele is contributed by each parent; the particular phenotypic expression is a function of whether the gene is dominant, in which case, only one allele is needed for phenotypic expression, or recessive, requiring that both alleles be the same for the phenotypic expression of a trait

allele-specific PCR MOLECULAR BIOLOGY A two-step nested PCR technique that allows detection of DNA with a point mutation in the presence of a 10^3-10^5 fold excess of normal DNA; AS-PCR '...based on the observation that Taq polymerase will extend primers with a 3' mismatch 10-3-10-6 fold less efficiently than perfectly matched primers. By choosing a primer that is complementary at its 3' end to a point mutation, selective amplification of (a) mutant allele can be achieved.' AS-PCR may be used to detect tumor-derived DNA in blood and plasma (**Am J Clin Pathol 1995; 103:404oa**)

allelic dropout A phenomenon may occur in the polymerase chain reaction, in which there is a failure to amplify one of the alleles and the specimen is interpreted as being negative for the presence of a segment of DNA of interest; AD occurs at specific temperatures (88–90°C) in the thermoregulator device

allelic exclusion GENETICS A phenomenon whereby one of the two genes for which an individual is a heterozygote is expressed, while the gene is excluded or not expressed, typically seen in the expression of immunoglobulin genes; this expression of one allele at a locus is characteristic of cells of the immunoglobulin 'superfamily', eg B and T cells, and is a mechanism that explains how a cell can express only one immunoglobulin or one specific T cell receptor

allele-specific expression assay MOLECULAR DIAGNOSTICS A strategy used to detect defective endogenous transcripts of DNA that has mutations in multiple sites (precluding for practical reasons the evaluation of each individual mutation by hybridization); the ASE assay requires isolation of RNA from a cell population, eg peripheral monocytes, conversion of the RNA transcript of interest (eg *APC*) to complementary DNA (cDNA) and amplification thereof by reverse transcriptase-PCR; the PCR products are then annealed with a common oligomer and allele-specific oligomer(s), which after ligation result in products corresponding to alleles of interest (**N Engl J Med 1993; 329:1982oa**) see Familial adenomatous polyposis

allergen immunotherapy see Desensitization therapy

allergic alveolitis see Farmer's lung, Hypersensitivity pneumonitis

allergic bronchopulmonary aspergillosis A condition characterized by episodic (asthmatiform) pulmonary obstruction, immune response to *Aspergillus fumigatus*, eg precipitating *A fumigatus* antibodies, and positive immediate skin reactivity to *A fumigatus* antigens CLINICAL Cough (± expectoration of brown plugs), fever, dyspnea, wheezing, malaise, chest pain, diaphoresis, hemoptysis RADIOLOGY Central bronchiectasis, atelectasis, transient or fixed pulmonary infiltrates, mucus plugging, hyperinflation LABORATORY Eosinophilia, ↑ serum IgE, *A fumigatus* in sputum TREATMENT Corticosteroids (**N Engl J Med 1993; 329:1484cpc**)

allergic contact dermatitis A condition resulting from an acquired cell-mediated immune reactivity secondary to contact with haptens, including nickel, chromates, ursodiols in poison ivy and poison oak, synthetic chemicals, drugs and cosmetics CLINICAL ACD is manifest as intense pruritus, erythema, intercellular edema, and papulovesicles, which with continued exposure is followed by vesiculation rupture and oozing dermatitis PATHOGENESIS Haptens (low molecular weight chemicals) bind to self protein carriers, are presented to the cutaneous macrophages (Langerhans' cell) which processes the complex and presents it to the T cells DIAGNOSIS Patch test (see there) TREATMENT Topical corticosteroids

allergic polyp Inflammatory polyp, see there

allergic rhinitis A condition that is the most common form of atopic (allergic) disease affecting 5–20% of the population; AR is initiated by exposure of the nasal mucosa to airborne foreign particles, evoking the production of IgE molecules; upon repeated exposure to the allergen, eg ragweed pollen and the release of histamine, leukotrienes C_4, D_4, E_4, B_4, PGD_2, kinins, and kininogen PATHOGENESIS Unclear; it is thought to be a hypersensitivity response to foreign allergens contained in pollen, animal danders, mites, insects, mold spores and foods; most patients have circulating IgE antibodies that bind to high-affinity receptors on mast cells and basophils and to low-affinity receptors on other cells, evoking the release of mediators of inflammation, including histamine, serotonin, leukotrienes, kinins and prostaglandin D_2 CLINICAL Paroxysms of sneezing, nasal congestion, and nasal and ocular pruritus (itching of nose and eyes), rhinorrhea, postnasal drip, partial or total obstruction of airflow, throat clearing, coughing, and allergic 'shiners' DIAGNOSIS Skin testing with appropriate inhalant allergens is of greater use than evaluation of the IgE levels TREATMENT Avoidance of provoking allergens, antihistamines, in particular H_1 receptor antagonists, sympathomimetic amines, anticholinergic agents, cromolyn, corticosteroids, decongestants, cromolyn sodium, glucocorticoids and immunotherapy (**N Engl J Med 1991; 325:860rv**) see H receptors, Immunotherapy, Sensitization

allergic 'salute' Frequent upward rubbing of the nose by the dorsal surface of a fisted hand, in an attempt to relieve itching, most often seen in children with allergies, which with time causes a central nasal groove

allergic 'shiners' Dark, discolored circles under the eyes, often accompanied by mouth breathing in children with allergic rhinitis which causes venous stasis due to imped-ed blood flow through the edematous nasal mucosa, while obstruction of the nasal passages obliges mouth breathing DIAGNOSIS Presence of eosinophils in the mucus

Note: 'Shiner' is an Americanism for a trauma-induced, often fisticuff-related, unilateral periorbital hemorrhage, also known as a 'black eye'

allergy unit AU An obsolete, arbitrarily assigned unit for allergen extracts, which has been replaced by bioequivalent allergy units BAU, see there (**JAMA 1992; 268:2491fda**) Note: AUs and BAUs *are not* interchangeable

allied health personnel All health care personnel who are 1) Not physicians, dentists, podiatrists and registered nurses and 2) Have received specialized training and require special licensure; these workers include dieticians, laboratory technologists, medical illustrators, technicians and transcriptionists, medial records technicians, occupational therapists, phlebotomists, physicians' assistants and practical nurses (**JAMA 1991; 266:964**); it is common practice in a formal health care setting, eg hospital, for AHPs to work under supervising physicians, and their duties are delineated by departmental director(s) after recommendations by the credentials and executive committees of the institution of employment

alligator boy A child covered with the indurated and laminated skin lesions of ichthyosis

allocation system A system for distributing a limited resource (eg kidneys for transplantation) in the most equitable fashion possible; allocation systems fall into three basic groups:

1) Physician-driven AS based on clinical parameters, see Pittsburgh criteria

2) Patient-driven AS, often driven by the 'squeaky wheel' principle, and private 'agendas'

3) Resource-driven AS, which attempts to maximize the organ's transplanted life

The UNOS (United Network for Organ Sharing) kidney-allocation point system incorporates elements of each; insertion of two new HLA-matching categories in the UNOS system would ↑ the number patients for whom donors could be found in local pools (**N Engl J Med 1994; 331:760sa**)

allogeneic That which is genetically dissimilar, but of the same species

allograft Allogeneic graft* A graft (organ, tissues or cells) donated from genetically distinct individual of the same species; renal allograft survival is a function of the degree of HLA matching and socioeconomic factors (**N Engl J Med 1992; 327:840oa**) see Renal transplantation; Cf Xenograft

*Other synonyms include homeograft, homeotransplant, homogenous graft, homograft, homologous graft, homoplastic graft, homotransplant

alloimmunization The development of an immune response to allogeneic antigens; an **alloimmunized** person is said to be **alloimmune**

allopatry EVOLUTIONARY BIOLOGY A mechanism of speciation that requires geographic separation from the rest of its kind (**Sci Am 1994; 270/8:25**) see Species; Cf Peripatry

allostery The cooperative interaction of two or more functional sites on a protein, or two or more proteins that results in ligand binding; allostery depends on dynamic interaction with a substrate or other molecule, eg heme-heme interactions

allosteric regulation The mechanism by which the individual polypeptides in a multimeric protein (protypically, hemoglobin) interact in order to transform into a functional state; in hemoglobin, the switch between the relaxed and tense states occurs whenever binding of a molecule at the heme site forms a tetramer with one or more ligand-binding subunit on each half of the hemoglobin (**Science 1992; 256:54**)

allotype A set of determinants or sequence of amino acids on immunoglobulin chains (and other proteins demonstrating heterogeneity) that is relatively specific for the individual and frequently more common in a racial group; Cf Idiotype, Isotype

ALP band 10 An isoform of alkaline phosphatase that is present at the isoelectric point of 4.73, obtained by isoelectric focusing; the 10 band (fraction) may derive from activated T lymphocytes (especially CD4 type); band 10 activity is present in serum from patients with aplastic anemia, childhood intestinal pseudo-obstruction, chronic liver disease, chronic pyelonephritis, chronic glomerulonephritis, DM, Hodgkin's disease, malignancy (breast, colon, lung, prostate, stomach), sarcoid, T-cell lymphoma, and ulcerative colitis; in absence of these conditions, its presence may be a useful surrogate marker for perinatal HIV-1 infection in children (Arch Pathol Lab Med 1994; 118:873oa) see Alkaline phosphatase, Isoelectric focusing

alpha (α) Symbol for: A band in serum electrophoresis

α₁-acid glycoprotein A 44-kD plasma protein of undetermined significance, which like haptoglobin, increases during acute inflammation, thus being an acute phase reactant; α-1-acid glycoprotein binds non-specifically to progesterone and vitamin B_{12}; see Acute phase reactants

α-amanitin A bicyclic 8-residue polypeptide derived from *Amanita phalloides* that inhibits transcription by RNA polymerase II and other RNA polymerases

3-alpha-androstanediol glucuronide 3-α-diol G   A metabolite of dihydrotestosterone, the levels of which in blood and urine reflect peripheral androgen action and which are decreased in androgen deficiency or testicular hypofunction

alpha₁-antichymotrypsin A 68-kD glycoprotein inhibitor of proteolytic enzymes, eg chymotrypsin and related serine proteases, which is produced by liver, macrophages and endothelial cells; the normal serum levels of 25-40 mg/dl are non-specifically increaed by inflammatory conditions, eg Crohn's disease, ulcerative colitis and burns, and it has been identified in the amyloid deposits of Alzheimer's dementia

alpha₂-antiplasmin A homogous protein of the serine protein inhibitor (serpin) family which controls the activity of plasmin through the rapid formation of stable plasmin complexes, and in addition, inactivates chymotrypsin

alpha₂-antiplasmin deficiency A rare AR [MIM 262850] condition characterized by fibrinolysis with early hemorrhages beginning at birth TREATMENT Antifibrinolysis, eg tranexamic acid

alpha₁-antitrypsin A 54-kD glycoprotein that inhibits proteolytic enzymes, including trypsin, chymotrypsin, elastase, plasmin, thrombin and others; the normal A1AT serum levels of 2-4 g/L rise non-specifically during inflammation and comprises one of the so-called acute phase reactants; the A1AT gene is inherited in a co-dominant fashion, located on chromosome 14 and encodes 25 different allelic forms classified according to electrophoretic mobility, of which the PiMM phenotype is normal; the most common A1AT deficiency phenotype is PiZZ, characterized by early-onset emphysema and cholestasis, cirrhosis, hepatic failure and a marked increase in hepatocellular carcinoma TREATMENT Prolastin in the face of COPD, IV or nebulized for direct delivery to the lungs; the gene for A1AT may be transferred via adenoviruses to the lung epithelium; following transfer, A1AT mRNA is expressed as functioning A1AT (Science 1991; 252:431)

alpha band see α rhythm

alphacarotene CLINICAL NUTRITION A carotenoid that is abundant in carrots, and has vitamin A and immunostimulatory activity, and is linked to a ↓ risk of lung cancer and cancer cell growth in vitro (New York Times 21 Feb 1995; C1) see Carotenoid

alpha chain disease Alpha heavy chain disease, see there

alpha decay RADIATION PHYSICS High energy, ie in the million electron volt range, radioactive decay products caused by the emission of α particles, which themselves are products of a disintegrating nucleus; see α particles

alpha effect ENDOCRINOLOGY The metabolic, hemodynamic and modulatory effects of epinephrine and norepinephrine are a function of the concentration of adrenergic receptors on the α and β cells of the pancreatic islets; α effects (epinephrine acting on β islet cells) include glycogenolysis, gluconeogenesis, inhibition of insulin-stimulated glucose uptake in skeletal muscle and arteriovenous vasoconstriction

alpha-fetoprotein A 70-kD protein, first synthesized by the embryonic yolk sac, later by the fetal GI tract and liver which has 40% homology with albumin; AFP's role in fetal development remains unclear; measurement of AFP levels in pregnant women serves to screen for open neural tube defects (incidence 1-2/1000 births); AFP levels in fetal serum are 150-fold greater than in amniotic fluid, which in turn are 200-fold greater than that of maternal serum; maternal serum levels are 3-400 µg/L in the third trimester; the levels in the fetal serum and amniotic fluid peak at 13 weeks, while the maternal levels peak at 30 weeks; increased AFP during pregnancy may be due to CNS defects (spina bifida and other open neural tube defects, hydrocephaly, cyclopia, microcephaly, sacrococcygeal teratoma), GI anomalies (esophageal and duodenal atresia with impaired fetal swallowing, omphalocele, due to transudation, gastroschisis, pseudo-obstruction and short bowel), hematology (fetomaternal hemorrhage, hydrops fetalis), immunodeficiency syndromes (severe combined immune deficiency and/or adenosine deaminase deficiency, combined T- and B-cell defects, ataxia telangiectasia), cardiovascular (Fallot's tetralogy) and other causes including cystic hygroma, Turner syndrome, fetal demise, twin gestation, congenital nephrotic syndrome; AFP is also increased in infants at high risk of subsequent fetal death up to four to five months after the screening, regardless of the presence of neural tube defects or multiple gestations ; AFP in adults is regarded as an 'oncofetal antigen' in adults and almost invariably increased in adults in hepatocellular carcinoma, and may also be elevated in endodermal sinus and Sertoli-Leydig cell tumors, pancreatic and gastric malignancies, teratomas, alcoholic and viral hepatitis, hypertyrosinosis; it has been reported that the sugar chains present in cirrhosis differ from that of liver cell carcinoma, a difference that can be exploited diagnostically (N Engl J Med 1993; 328:1802oa) see Liver cell carcinoma

alpha heavy chain disease Seligmann's disease The most common heavy chain disease or paraproteinemia, in which there is an excess production of an incomplete IgA1 molecule (partial heavy chain and no light chain), affecting Sephardic Jews, Arabs, and those living in the Mediterranean rim, South America and Asia CLINICAL Onset in childhood or adolescence as either a lymphoproliferative disorder confined to the respiratory tract or an enteric form (see IPSID) with severe diarrhea, malabsorption, steatorrhea, weight loss, hepatic dysfunction, hypocalcemia, lymphadenopathy, marked mononuclear infiltration which may eventuate into lymphoma (see Mediterranean lymphoma); α chain disease may remit spontaneously, respond to antibiotic therapy or if clearly monoclonal, may require combination chemotherapy, potentially causing death by ages 20-30 LABORATORY Increased alkaline phosphatase, hypocalcemia TREATMENT Antibiotics, or if advanced, chemotherapy

alpha helix A structural protein motif deduced by Pauling and Corey, where there are 3.6 amino acid residues per turn; the α helix of proteins has a right-handed 'screw' sense and is stabilized by intrachain hydrogen bonds between NH and CO groups, as well as the side chains of the amino acids, which themselves are partially helical; bundled together, α helices are found in keratin, myosin, fibrin and epidermin

α-interferon Interferon-α, see there

alpha particle A radioactive decay product, [4]He nucleus, composed of 2 protons and 2 neutrons with marked ionizing capacity (3-9 million electron-volts) but a short range (3-9 cm in air, 25-40 μm in water/soft tissue) derived from α decay, see there; α particles arising from radon, uranium and plutonium 'daughters' are implicated in inhalation-induced neoplasia of the respiratory tract; while α particles are highly tissue-destructive, they travel only short distances and are blocked by a thick piece of paper or skin

alpha rhythm ELECTROENCEPHALOGRAPHY A type of electrical activity in adults, recorded from the posterior regions, which may be abolished with visual stimulation and attenuated by thinking and is typically seen in relaxed adults with closed eyes; α rhythm occurs at 8-13 Hz, and has bihemispheric asynchrony, where the non-dominant hemisphere has a greater wave amplitude; focal central nervous system disease is accompanied by focally altered α rhythm, which becomes diffuse in coma; non-invasive diagnostic modalities of computed tomography and magnetic resonance imaging have relegated EEG to a diagnostic modality of lesser importance in localizing cerebral masses

alpha-satellite probe CYTOGENETICS A FISH probe containing DNA isolated from the centromeric region that is unique to each chromosome, which can be used to detect aneuploidy, eg trisomy 21, 18, 13, and others; see FISH probes

alpha testing The testing of a product with commercial potential by those who are knowledgeable about the product and closely associated with its design, but who are not part of the R&D staff; in the AT phase of product development, glitches (bugs, boo-boos, errors, faux-pas, etc) are identified that might cause software or hardware 'crashes' and corrected; under AT, the product is put through all its anticipated applications, and field product experts are brought in to provide a real-world dimension to the development process (**Am Lab Sept 1994 p24**) Cf Beta testing

α thalassemia Thalassemia, see there

Alpine Iceman ANTHOPOLOGY A mummified body of a prehistoric human (circa 5300 years old) from the Stone Age who was discovered frozen in ice at the Austrian-Italian border, and is providing information on the early settlers in Europe

Alport syndrome An AD **[MIM 104200]** condition characterized by hereditary nephritis, with hematuria, proteinuria, which evolves to nephrotic syndrome, hypertension and end-stage renal disease, variably accompanied by sensorineural deafness MOLECULAR PATHOLOGY Mutations in collagen α5(IV) gene TREATMENT Kidney transplantation may be successful if anti-glomerular basement membrane and anti-tubular antibody production can be avoided (**Arch Pathol Lab Med 1994; 118:728oa**)

ALS Amyotrophic lateral sclerosis, see there, also 1) Advanced Life Support 2) Alternate lifestyle, see there 3) Antilymphocyte serum

Also 1) Acetolactate synthase 2) Acute lateral sclerosis 3) Aldolase 4) Angiotensin-like substance 5) Anticipated lifespan

ALT 1) Alanine aminotransferase (glutamate pyruvate transaminase, GPT) 2) Acquisition lead time   2) Antilymphocyte therapy, see there 3) Autolymphocyte therapy

alternate complement pathway Properdin pathway IMMUNOLOGY A route of complement activation that occurs independently of complement-fixing antibodies; complement is a non-specific arm of the immune system, encharged with lysis of target organisms; the ACP is more complex than the classic pathway, requiring a 'priming' C3 convertase (C3,Bb) and an 'amplification' C3 convertase (C3b,Bb); in the presence of properdin, C3 convertase is stabilized, activating later complement components, leading to opsonization, leukocyte chemotaxis, increased vascular permeability and cytolysis; the ACP is activated by properdin, IgA, IgG, lipopolysaccharide and snake venom; both pathways are stimulated by trypsin-like enzymes

Note: C3b is continuously degraded when in contact with particulate activators; the surface provides protection from breakdown; C3b and factor B interact with serum protein factor D, cleaving factor B producing C3bBb, forming a positive feedback loop generating C3b; C3b + Bb + properdin form C5 convertase

alternate level of care A generic term for care, eg hospice, at-home nursing and so on, in which efforts are no longer made to cure or aggressively treat a disease process, but rather to prepare for death, as occurs in those who are terminally ill with cancer or AIDS

alternate site testing Point-of-care testing, see there

alternative birthing center An obstetrical unit or facility that provides a pleasant, 'friendly' atmosphere for women who are expected to have an uncomplicated vaginal delivery; these centers are staffed by obstetricians or midwives and located either within a hospital or are freestanding units; see Lamaze, Natural childbirth

alternative life-style Alternative lifestyle SOCIAL MEDICINE A generic, 'politically sensitive'[1] term for any form of living arrangements with a 'significant other'[2] in which sexual orientation differs from the usual male-female dyad, eg a male or female homosexual dyad

[1]Also known as politically correct [2]Close personal friend, lover, husband, wife, and so on

alternative medicine '...*a heterogeneous set of practices[1] that are offered as an alternative to conventional medicine for the preservation of health and the diagnosis and treatment of health-related problems; its practitioners are often called healers'* (**N Engl J Med 1992; 326:61**); these practices or alternative health care systems constitute a vast array of treatments and ideologies, which may be well-known, exotic or mysterious, or even dangerous, and are based on no common or consistent philosophy; the practitioners range from being sincere, well-educated and committed to their form of healing to charlatans (deprecatingly known in some circles as 'quacks') STATISTICS Estimated expenditures for AM $13.7 × 10[9] ($10.3 × 10[9] out-of-pocket); ⅓ of US citizens had used at least one form of alternative therapy in the previous year; ⅓ had made an average of 19 visits to alternative providers; the highest users of AM were upper-income whites, 25-49 years of age; 72% did not tell their physicians; most had sought relief for chronic, non-life-threatening conditions, eg allergies, arthralgias, back pain, insomnia, etc; by US congressional edict, the US National Institutes of Health established the Office of Alternative Medicine, see there; AM claims a 'whole body' approach to healing, and health maintenance, requiring integration of the body, mind and spirit, based on the holistic doctrine, which holds that the entire organism cannot be understood merely by studying lower levels of organization; holistic medicine 'disciplines' include acupuncture[2], aural analysis, biofeedback, chiropractic medicine[2], clairvoyant diagnosis, homeopathy, hypnosis, iridology, organicism, naturopathy, psychic healing, rolfing, tai chi and zone therapy

[1]Alternative terms for alternative therapies include complementary, fringe, holistic, natural, New Age, nontraditional, 'traditional', unconventional, and unorthodox medicine [2]Note: Acupuncture and chiropractic medicine are also

ALP
29

'holistic', but are generally regarded with less suspicion by mainstream medical practitioners as some data suggest they may be effective in certain types of diseases; alternative medicine is criticized as being more 'mystical' or magical than scientific in its approach to understanding disease; see Unproven methods of cancer therapy

alternative splicing MOLECULAR BIOLOGY The removal of varying lengths of DNA from precursor messenger RNA (mRNA), a mechanism for generating different proteins from the same DNA transcript and effecting gene control by serving as an on-off switch for variable expression of one gene in different organs (Science 1991; 251:33); in the basic splicing process, noncoding, intervening sequences of RNA are removed and exons are joined by two cleavage-ligand events requiring precise recognition of the 5' and the 3' splice junctions and assembly of a 'spliceosome' complex, involving interactions between the pre-mRNA and the small nuclear ribonucleoprotein particles (sNURPs) U1, U2, U5 and the U4/U6 particle; it is thought that the U1 sNRNP plays a critical role in selection of the 5' and 3' splice sites (Science 1991; 251:1045); AS is tissue-specific and related to the presence of stable double-stranded intron-exon (secondary structure) regions, the repression of which allows expression of the non-expressed exon, as in the alternative splicing of chicken tropomyosin, depending on whether the myogenic cells are in the myoblast (pre-differentiation) or myotubule (post-differentiation) stage (Science 1991; 252:1823, 1842); see Spliceosome

altitude sickness Mountain sickness, see there

Alu family MOLECULAR BIOLOGY A family of 150-300 base pair sequences of intermediate repeats (dispersed blocks of related non-identical DNA) of DNA that are often associated with introns, contain a recognition sequence for the restriction endonuclease Alu I, cap regions and a poly-A tail; about fifty of the highly homologous Alu regions have been identified; they are thought to play a role in initiating DNA synthesis, and may be transposed into human malignant cell lines; *Alu* has been identified with a novel mechanism of mutation, that of *Alu* retrotransposition into an intron, causing alternative splicing of the encoded precursor mRNA, clinically translating into a type 1 neurofibromatosis (Nature 1991; 353:864); see LINES, Tandem repeats

aluminum phosphide An inexpensive pesticide used to fumigate stored grains in India, which has proven to be a highly popular and effective agent for committing suicide in India, which when ingested, reacts with the hydrochloric acid in the stomach, releasing 1 gram of phosphine, ten times the lethal dose of this gas, causing the victim's death within two hours (Nature 1991; 353; 377n)

alveolar-capillary block syndrome A 'syndrome' of historical interest that was based on a concept that the distance that oxygen had to travel was increased in pulmonary interstitial disease and required extra diffusion time to reach equilibrium, thus explaining the hypoxia typical of these conditions, a value that is widely recognized as overestimated

alveolar soft part sarcoma A malignant tumor most commonly occurring in the soft deep tissues of the legs of young adults, especially ♀ PATHOLOGY Circumscribed firm, yellow-gray masses with areas of necrosis and hemorrhage; the fibrous tissue separates the tumor into nests composed of large cells with vesicular nuclei and prominent nucleoli HISTOGENESIS Uncertain PROGNOSIS Larger tumors are more aggressive TREATMENT Wide excision

Alzheimer's disease A degenerative brain disease characterized by progressive mental deterioration accompanied by disorientation, increasing defects in memory, confusion, leading to progressive dementia that may be accompanied by dysphasia, and apraxia; AD was defined in the DSM-III as '*a loss of intellectual abilities sufficient to interfere with social or occupational functioning,*' and in the DSM-IV '*...is currently a diagnosis of exclusion, and all other causes* (of) *cognitive defects ... must first be ruled out.*' AD affects 3% in those 65 to 74, 18% from 75 to 84 and 47% in those above age 85; AD is pathologically characterized by generalized frontal and parietotemporal cerebral atrophy (basal ganglia and reticular formation are less commonly affected) and a triad 1) SENILE (NEURITIC) PLAQUES, which consist of dilated, tortuous, presynaptic axon terminals, most common in the cortex 2) NEUROFIBRILLARY TANGLES, appearing as twisted fascicles of neurofilaments, commonly surrounding the nucleus in a neuron and 3) GRANULOVACUOLAR DEGENERATION, consisting of intracytoplasmic vacuoles within the neurons containing argyrophilic 'dots' of unknown origin; Hirano bodies, consisting of glassy eosinophilic inclusions composed of actin filaments located in the proximal dendrites are distinctly less common; a transgenic mouse has been bred that overexpresses a C-terminal fragment of the amyloid precursor protein demonstrates amyloid plaques, neurofibrillary tangles and neuronal loss; AD has been linked to a form of apolipoprotein E, those with one defective *APOE* ε4 gene (located on chromosome 19) are at an ↑ risk of suffering AD, and those with two copies have AD of early onset (Sci Am 1993; 269/5:29) MOLECULAR PATHOLOGY AD is not caused by a single genetically homogeneous gene (Nature 1991; 347:194); major molecules involved in Alzheimer's disease include 1) A 4.2-kD polypeptide (β-amyloid polypeptide, A4) isolated from senile plaques and neurofibrillary tangles of Alzheimer's brains, encoded by a gene on chromosome 21; APP had been linked to Down syndrome and associated with duplication of proto-oncogene *ets*-2, although this relation proved to be weak, given the genetic heterogeneity at 21q21; A68 protein is present in homogenates of Alzheimer brains, and implicated in the formation of neuritic plaques and neurofibrillary tangles (68 kD); one Alzheimer's type amyloid precursor may inhibit serine proteases, and is generated by alternative enzyme splicing, releasing an intact β fragment, possibly explaining the deposition of these fibrils in Alzheimer brains TREATMENT Tetrahydroaminoacridine (THA, an inhibitor of acetylcholinesterase), was claimed to improve the quality of life in Alzheimer's patients; see THA

Alzheimer's disease assessment scale A test that evaluates 1) The cognitive (memory, language, and praxis, 70 points) and 2) The noncognitive (mood and behavior, 45 points) components of Alzheimer's disease, up to a maximum score of 115 points (JAMA 1992; 268:2523oc)

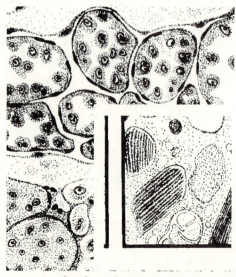

alveolar soft part sarcoma

Alzheimer's disease-associated proteins A group of three major protein subunits, eg A-68, identified by the ALZ-50 antibody, which are present in neuritic (senile) plaques and neurofibrillary tangles, the classic histological markers for Alzheimer's disease

ALZ-50 A monoclonal antibody that reacts against brain tissue from patients with Alzheimer's disease, that selectively binds to protein A-68 and is an early marker of Alzheimer's disease

ama Against medical advice The self-discharge of a patient from a health care facility, contrary to what the physician(s) perceive to be in the patient's best interests; a discharge 'ama' must be documented by the patient's signature, given the potential for lawsuit if the discharged patient dies before admission to another facility; in a follow-up of patients who sought care in a public hospital emergency department, and left 'ama' after waiting 6.4 hours without having been attended to, 46% needed immediate medical attention and 29% needed care within 48 hours (JAMA 1991; 266:1085)

Note: These statistics are thought to reflect the state of overcrowding in the 'safety net' hospitals which attend to the poor and uninsured in US inner cities

AMA American Medical Association, also 1) Aerospace Medical Association 2) Against medical advice 3) Alternative Medical Association 4) Antimitochondrial antibodies

Also, 1) Aminomalonic acid 2) Aminomethyl anthracene 3) Amyl acetate 4) Antimalarial agent

Amadori product A generic term for any molecule resulting from the steps in non-enzymatic 'glycosylation' of collagen, see Maillard reaction, Browning reaction, which begins when a glucose's aldehyde combines with a protein's amino group forming the unstable 'Schiff base' later undergoing an **Amadori rearrangement** forming a stable, but still reversible Amadori product, eg hemoglobin A1c, which with time, dehydrate and rearrange themselves into advanced glycosylation endproducts; free amino groups of proteins react with glucose aldehydes to form a Schiff base, resulting in an Amadori rearrangement; the resultant ketoamine structure is cyclized to form a hemiketal, forming the chemical basis of glycosylated hemoglobin (HbA$_{1c}$); see Advanced glycosylation endproducts

Amadori reaction A reaction that links the aldehyde group of a glucose and the amine group of a protein, eg Maillard reaction

amalgam Dental amalgam A silver-copper-tin alloy with varying amounts of mercury that has traditionally been used to fill teeth; although amalgam has been used by dentists for 150 years, it is unclear whether prolonged exposure to the relatively inert mercury in amalgam is entirely innocuous (JAMA 1991; 265:2934/FDA); some workers posit that the pulverization required to remove amalgam and substitute fillings with a non-toxic substance may actually increase a paient's exposure to mercury; see Cremation, Fluoridation, Mercury

amatoxin Any of a family of potentially lethal toxins present in certain mushrooms (most commonly *Amanita phalloides* was well as *Lepiota chlorophyllum* and others) which may cause accidental poisoning in amateur mushroom hunters PATHOGENESIS Amatoxins are thermostable cyclic octapeptides that bind to and inhibit RNA polymerase II, preventing the elongation of mRNA, thereby blocking protein production CLINICAL 12-hour latency, followed by nausea, vomiting, abdominal pain and diarrhea, which may be followed by an asymptomatic period prior to acute hepatic dysfunction TREATMENT Charcoal hemoperfusion (J Toxicol Clin Toxicol 1994; 32:715)

amaurosis fugax A transient loss of vision in one eye caused by hypoperfusion of the retinal circulation, of either embolic origin or due to vasospasm TREATMENT Calcium-channel blocker, eg nifedipine (N Engl J Med 1993; 329:396oa)

amber codon UAG One of three 'nonsense' codons (a triplet of DNA nucleotides, the others are ochre, UAA and opal, UGA) that terminates protein synthesis; amber suppressors are mutants that encode tRNAs, the anticodons of which respond to both UAG and to their usual codons

ambiguity MOLECULAR BIOLOGY The occurrence of errors in protein synthesis that is more common in vitro, where an incorrect amino acid is incorporated into a growing protein chain in response to a nucleotide triplet or codon for another amino acid; ambiguity represents a true error and thus contrasts to 'wobble', in which the degeneracy of the DNA code has only 20 different amino acids for 61 possible codons, where 'sloppy' translation is not uncommon event in the translation of messenger RNA from the DNA template; Cf Ambiquity, Wobble

ambiguous genitalia Male or female external genitalia that is indistinct or discordant with the genotype; the sex assigned to the infant is chromosomally incorrect, usually in the form of a male-to-female phenotype 'conversion', and the children adapt to their assigned sex

ambiguous sexuality Acquired sexual discordance in which the phenotype and genotype are correct, but as the 'psychotype' is incorrect, correction requires transsexual conversion; see Transsexuality

ambiquity A property of enzymes, where they exist either bound to a carrier protein or free in the circulation; Cf Ambiguity

ambivalence PSYCHIATRY The coexistence of two opposing emotions, usually referring to affective ambivalence, as in a 'love-hate' relationship with a person; according to some psychoanalysts, ambivalence first appears in the Freud's oral sadistic stage, and may be seen in bipolar I disorder (manic-depressive psychosis) or schizophrenia

'Ambu' bag EMERGENCY MEDICINE A self-refilling bag-valve-mask unit with a 1-1.5 liter capacity, used for artificial respiration which, although suboptimal for the non-intubated patient, is effective for ventilating and oxygenating intubated patients, allowing both spontaneous and artificial respiration

'ambulance chaser' American slang first used in 1897 for a lawyer or his/her agent who solicits accident victims as potential clients, by encouraging them to initiate a lawsuit against the party responsible for the accident, suing them for damages

ambulatory care center Walk-in clinic A free-standing facility that provides non-emergent medical, or less commonly, dental services; most visits to these centers occur outside of the regular work hours by patients who feel that their particular problem cannot wait until their private physician is available (Can Med Assoc J 1990; 143:740); because many such centers often have short waiting times, may not require appointments, and have a non-permanent or rotating medical staff, ambulatory care centers have been likened to 'fast food' restaurants, receiving facetious sobriquets, eg 'Doc-in-the-Box', 'McStitch'

ambulatory surgery center A free-standing center that performs various types of surgery; there are ± 1600 ASCs in the US, < 30% of revenues derive from Medicare, average charge/case is ± $1000 (Am Med News 2 Nov 1992, p 15)

ameloblastoma A locally aggressive tumor of the mandible that is most common in ♂ in the 4th decade, histologically characterized by stellate reticulum, epithelial metaplasia and polarization of tumor cell nuclei towards a lumen; patterns include acanthomatous, basal cell, follicular, granular, plexiform; Surgical excision is difficult and the tumor may recur

ameloblastoma An almost invariably benign (but locally infiltrative) arising from the odontogenic epithelium in a fibrous stroma, most commonly occurring in the mandible or maxilla TREATMENT NNN only do Radio and Rx

Americans with Disabilities Act Legislation passed by the US government in 1990 that was intended to remove the physical barriers and biases in places of public access and in the workplace, that had previously been responsible for preventing those with physical and mental disabilities (handicaps) from enjoying the full benefits of freedoms guaranteed by the US Constitution; compliance with the ADA has been somewhat problematic for employers given the vague wording of the language; the basic rule is that no entity[1] can discriminate against a covered[2] individual on the basis of disability; the ADA protects anyone with a physical or mental impairment that seriously limits one or more major life activities; to ensure compliance, the ADA has been given 'teeth' by the government in the form of injunctive relief from the EOEC and federal courts, attorney fees, and fines of up to $50 000/violation (see Advance/Laboratory May 1994) see Barriers, Disabilities

[1]Insurers, governments (municipal, or state), employers with 15+ employees, hospitals, or physicians [2]Areas of coverage include public services or public accomodations, employment, insurance, and services offered by private entities, including health care

American trypanosomiasis Chagas' disease, see there

Ames test TOXICOLOGY A bioassay that detects mutagenesis, used to detect and screen for toxic compounds with carcinogenic potential TECHNIQUE *Salmonella typhimurium*, TA100, which cannot synthesize histidine (and therefore requires histidine in the growth medium) is incubated in a histidine-poor medium with the compound of interest; if the chemical is mutagenic, then TA100 reverts to a form that can synthesize its own histidine (see New York Times 5 July 1994; C1)

AMF Autocrine motility factor, see there

AMI Acute myocardial infarction

amicus curiae FORENSIC MEDICINE A person or party with a strong interest or views on the subject matter of a legal action, but who is not a party to the action; the amicus curiae may petition the court for permission to file a brief that may suggest a rationale for a particular action on the part of either party; amicus curiae briefs are commonly filed in appeals of broad public interest, eg civil rights

amiloride An aerosolized sodium channel blocker that may slow the progression of pulmonary dysfunction in cystic fibrosis, a disease of excess sodium reabsorption, thickening of the mucus and decreased secretion clearance

amino acid The essential building block for polypeptides and proteins, which is abbreviated in a three-letter code, or for even more efficient communication by a single-letter designation, a convention of particular use among molecular biologists (table)

amino acid residue see Residue

aminoacyl transfer RNA synthetase MOLECULAR BIOLOGY Any of more than 20 enzymes present in living cells that bind the correct amino acid to its cognate transfer RNA in the presence of ATP, thereby ensuring the fidelity of translation of genetic information; the mechanism by which tRNA recognizes the appropriate amino acid was long a mystery and was incorrectly termed the 'second genetic code', where DNA is the first genetic code; aaRS ensures the proper conformation of tRNA (Science 1991; 252:1682)

2-aminopurine A specific protein kinase inhibitor that blocks the induction of the genes for β-interferon, c-*fos* and c-*myc* by virus or poly(I)-poly(C) at the level of transcription

amiodarone CARDIOLOGY A class III (blocks potassium channels, prolongs repolarization, ↓ automaticity, conduc-

amiodarone

tion, and prolongs refractoriness) antiarrhythmic drug which is indicated for refractory ventricular tachycardia and supraventricular tachycardia SIDE EFFECTS Pulmonary fibrosis, hypo– or hyperthyroidism, deposition in cornea and/or skin, hepatitis, ↑ digitoxin levels, neurotoxicity, GI toxicity

aminoglycoside CLINICAL THERAPEUTICS Any of a family of broad-spectrum antibiotics (amikacin, gentamicin, kanamycin, neomycin, streptomycin, and tobramycin) that are primarily used against (aerobic) gram-negative bacteria PHARMACODYNAMICS Poorly absorbed per os, poor penetration of CNS (BBB), rapid excretion if kidneys are normal TOXICIITY Given the relatively common dose-related toxicity to the kidneys, vestibular, auditory, and neuromuscular systems, which may be accompanied by minor skin rash, drug fever, hypomagnesemia, hypocalcemia, hypokalemia, it is common to monitor patients receiving aminoglycosides; see Therapeutic drug monitoring

aminoguanidine An agent that inhibits formation of advanced glycosylation end products (AGEs), and is reported to have a beneficial effect on the kidney, nerves, and retina of experimental animals; in the rat, aminoguanidine ↓ AGEs, BM thickening, mesangial proliferation, albumin excretion, and improves responses of peripheral nerves; aminoguanidine ↓ microaneurysm formation and intercapillary deposition of protein in the retina; results of human studies have not been reported (N Eng J Med 1995; 332:1210RV)

AML Acute myelocytic (granulocytic, myeloid, myelogenous) leukemia, see there

Also 1) Anterior mitral leaflet 2) Army Medical Library

Amnesty International An organization that works for the release of persons detained (anywhere) for their con-

AMINO ACID ABBREVIATIONS			
Alanine	Ala	A	
Arginine	Arg	R	‡
Asparganine	Asn	N	
Aspartic acid	Asp	D	
Arginine or Aspartic acid	Asx	B	
Cysteine	Cys	C	‡
Glutamine	Gln	Q	
Glutamic acid	Glu	E	
Glutamine or Glutamic acid	Glx	Z	
Glycine	Gly	G	
Histidine	His	H	‡
Isoleucine	Ile	I	Δ
Leucine	Leu	L	Δ
Lysine	Lys	K	Δ
Methionine	Met	M	Δ
Phenylalanine	Phe	F	Δ
Proline	Pro	P	
Serine	Ser	S	
Threonine	Thr	T	Δ
Tryptophan	Typ	W	Δ
Tyrosine	Tyr	Y	
Valine	Val	V	Δ

Δ Essential amino acids
‡ Amino acids essential during growth periods

sciously held beliefs, color, ethnic origin, sex, religion, or language, provided they have neither used nor advocated violence; AI opposes torture and the death penalty and was recipient of the 1977 Nobel Peace for Peace; 400 000 members; 7 networks include one for health professionals; see IPPNW, Red Cross, Médecins sans Frontières

AMPAC American Medical Political Action Committee The political arm of the American Medical Association (AMA) when certain public health issues (tobacco-export promotion, handgun control, 'gag rule') were examined, AMPAC campaign contributions favored the politicians who had opposed AMA's positions on these issures (**N Engl J Med 1994; 330:32sa**) see Political action committee

---

AMNIOCENTESIS-INDICATIONS FOR

Maternal age > 35

3+ spontaneous abortions

Previous history of

  Chromosomally abnormal child

  Metabolic disease

  Neural tube defect

Patient, father, or family history of chromosomal abnormality

Possible carrier of X-linked disease

---

amniocentesis OBSTETRICS A procedure in which fluid is obtained by an ultrasonographically-guided needle from the amniotic cavity (usually between weeks 15-17 of pregnancy) and analyzed for the presence of fetal abnormalities, which might be reasons sufficient for the mother to opt for an elective abortion; accuracy is reported to be 99.4%; complication rate < 0.5% above the background pregnancy loss of 2-3%; fetal loss minimal INDICATIONS See table DEFECTS IDENTIFIED BY AMNIOCENTESIS Cultured amniotic cells can be used for cytogenetic studies, DNA analysis, and enzyme assays; amniocentesis may not be necessary in women with ↑ alpha-fetoprotein and a normal fetus by ultrasonography (**N Engl J Med 1990; 323:557**); Cf Chorionic villus biopsy

amniotic band 'syndrome' OBSTETRICS A heterogeneous acquired complex that develops in utero; the ADAM complex, ie amniotic deformity, adhesions (Streeter bands) and mutilations, may be considered a 'sequence', and is associated with craniofacial defects, eg clefts, distortions, dislocations, limb deformities, amputations and secondary syndactyly; the syndrome consists of a complex collection of asymmetric congenital craniofacial, visceral, body wall and limb anomalies thought to be either related to idiopathic in utero formation of fibrous adhesion bands that encircle the fetus' fingers, limbs or head, causing autoamputation of the constricted part, or may be related to vascular interuption

amniotic fluid analysis LABORATORY MEDICINE A series of tests performed on the fetus' amniotic fluid obtained by amniocentesis, which 1) Detects isoimmunization of red cells by measuring bilirubin levels and and genetic defects by karyotyping of fetal cells and 2) Determines fetal maturity by measuring creatinine and lecithin/sphingomyelin ratio, and surfactant; see Amniocentesis

amniotic fluid embolism A clinical complex resulting from a traumatic delivery and 'injection' of amniotic fluid into the maternal circulation INCIDENCE 1:80 000 deliveries; maternal mortality approaches 80% ETIOLOGY Idiopathic, predisposed to by the high intrauterine pressure that allows amniotic fluid to pass into the maternal venous circulation, where the meconium is especially toxic to the mother, potentially causing disseminated intravascular coagulation

Note: The use of prostaglandin E_2 in obstetrics may facilitate amniotic fluid embolism

amphiregulin An 84 amino acid bifunctional cell growth-modulating glycoprotein that both inhibits the growth of certain tumors (eg epidermoid cancer) and stimulates the proliferation of fibroblasts; the carboxy-terminal half of amphiregulin has considerable structural homology with epidermal growth factor (EGF) and binds to its receptor

amok A culture-bound syndrome that occurs most commonly in males, which is characterized by a period of brooding precipitated by a perceived slight or insult, followed by an aggressive, violent, or if severe, homicidal rampage, with indiscriminate stabbing, shooting, or killing of anyone within reach of his weapon until he is overpowered or is himself killed; an episode may be accompanied by persecutory ideation, automatism, exhaustion, and post-event amnesia; the condition was first described in native populations of Malaysia (from DSM-IV), but has been described in other cultures; see Culture-bound syndrome

amorph GENETICS A 'silent' mutated allele with no effect on the phenotypic expression of a trait

amotivational syndrome SUBSTANCE ABUSE A condition induced by chronic marijuana abuse, affecting predisposed individuals who are often young, learning disabled and emotionally immature; in this psychologic background, marijuana, a drug that reinforces passivity and social withdrawal, causes a loss of interest in the environment, generalized apathy and passivity, loss of desire to work or perform adequately, loss of energy and generalized lassitude, moodiness, emotional lability, impairment of ability to concentrate and process new information, slovenly appearance and habits and a life-style that revolves in part around procurement of marijuana and other drugs; see 'Gateway' drugs

AMPA-kainate receptor α-amino-3-hydroxy-5-methyl-4-isoxazoleproprionate receptor A glutamate receptor that mediates the fast component of excitatory post-synaptic potentials; the AMPA-kainate receptors mediate a large fraction of excitatory transmission by neurotransmitters, and are regulated by cAMP-dependent protein kinase and phosphates (**Science 1991; 253:1133**)

amphipathic molecule A molecule that has hydrophobic and hydrophilic characters with positive, negative or no net charge at pH 7

amphotericin B A heptaene macrolide antibiotic that is administered IV as a systemic antifungal and is most effective against *Blastomycosis dermatitidis, Candida, Coccidioides immitis, Cryptococcus neoformans, Histoplasma capsulatum, Paracoccidioides braziliensis, Torulopsis glabrata* SIDE EFFECTS Fever, azotemia, nephrotoxicity, hypochromic normocytic anemia

amphotericin B

amplicon A segment of DNA to be amplified, eg as often occurs in PCR (polymerase chain reaction)

amplicon carryover The contamination of unwanted segments of nucleotides in a DNA amplification process, eg in

amplification MOLECULAR BIOLOGY An increase in the copy number of a gene sequence

amplification system PHYSIOLOGY A generic term for any group of proteins that function in coordinated sequences, forming positive feedback loops for expansion of the response to a signal of relatively low intensity; Amplification loops include 1) Coagulation, the best-described is factor Xa activating factor 'X' in the presence of factor VIII, Ca++ and phospholipid 2) Complement which augments the B-cell response, see Alternate and Classic pathways and 3) Cytokines, responsible for amplifying the T-cell response, interleukins, kinins, lipid mediators and mast cell products; see Gene amplification

amputation sign RADIOLOGY The descriptor for the sharp cut-off seen on air bronchograms, most commonly due to pulmonary thromboembolism, less commonly, carcinoma, tumor emboli, myxoma and intravascular sarcoma

Amsterdam dwarf see Dwarf

Amsterdam strategy POPULATION CONTROL The Amsterdam Forum world stabilization strategy A blueprint for limiting world population growth that was developed in 1989 and signed by 79 countries, which calls for developed nations to contribute 4% of their foreign aid budgets to international population programs (Science 1991; 252:1247n&v); see Contraceptives; Cf Mexico City policy, ZPG

amygdalin A β-cyanogenic glycoside that is structurally related to the semisynthetic laetrile, which is derived from the pits of certain fruits; see Laetrile

amyl nitrate 'Poppers' A substance of abuse that is similar in action to nitroglycerin, available in glass ampules; amyl nitrate decreases the blood to the brain, acting to enhance an orgasm

Note: In the early days of the AIDS epidemic, amyl nitrate was briefly inculpated in its pathogenesis

amylin A 37-residue polypeptide that has a 45% sequence homology with calcitonin; it is present in normal and diabetic pancreas and is a major component of islet amyloid in patients with non-insulin-dependent diabetes mellitus, in whom it is reported to be increased in the serum

amyloid β-fibrillosis A term coined in 1838 by Schleiden to describe starch-like constituents of normal plants; the term was later borrowed by von Rokitansky for a peculiar material in the liver and spleen that Virchow thought was polysaccharide; amyloid is a homogeneous, predominantly extracellular protein deposit with a fibrillary ultrastructure with a fibril diameter of 7-10 nm, which has an apple

green birefringence when stained with Congo red and viewed by polarization light; the various amyloids are unified by a common molecular theme, that of the β-pleated protein sheet, demonstrable by X-ray crystallography and responsible for amyloid's Congo red staining and its resistance to proteolytic digestion (Cardiovasc Pathol 1995; 4:79); a 28-residue polypeptide similar to β-amyloid enhances neuron survival in vitro, implying that amyloidosis may represent an aberration of the immune defense reaction; the nomenclature adopted for the fibril subunits is based on the finding that most forms of amyloidosis are associated with serum protein precursors, eg gelsolin (N Engl J Med 1991; 325:1780cr) Note: Focal accumulation of amyloid β protein in the brain, especially in the amygdala and the hippocampus of the temporal lobe is intimately linked to Alzhemier's dementia (Sci Am 11/91:68); Cf Alzhemier's disease

amyloid A protein An acute phase protein that may be ↑ at the time of admission and presage a poor outcome in patients with severe unstable angina, indicating an inflammatory component (N Engl J Med 1994; 331:417oa) see 'Kiss of death' test more things and X ref to KoD to here

NOMENCLATURE & CLASSIFICATION (AMYOID & AMYLOIDOSIS)
(WHO-IUIS Nomenclature sub-committee)

PROTEIN	PRECURSOR	CLINICAL SYNDROME/ASSOCIATION
AA	apoSAA	Inflammation (abscesses, arthritis, Hodgkin's disease, leprosy, IV drug use, TB); familial amyloid nephropathy with urticaria and deafness (Muckle-Wells syndrome); Familial Mediterranean fever
AL	κ or λ	Myeloma, macroglobulinemia, plasma cell dyscrasia, idiopathic, isolated pulmonary
ATTR	Transthyretin	Familial amyloid (FA) with neuropathy (several forms), eg FA cardiomyopathy, Danish type
ApoAI	apoAI	FA polyneuropathy, Iowa type
AGel	Gelsolin	Familial amyloidosis, Finnish type
ACys	Cystatin	Hereditary cerebral hemorrhage with amyloidosis, Icelandic type
Aβ	β precursor	Alzheimers's disease, Down syndrome, hereditary cerebral hemorrhage with amyloidosis, Dutch type
Aβ2M	β2-microglobulin	Chronic hemodialysis
AScr	Scrapie precursor	Creutzfeldt-Jakob disease, Gerstmann-Straussler-Scheinker sydnrome
ACal	(Pro)calcitonin	Medullary carcinoma of thyroid
AANF	Atrial natriuretic factor	Isolated atrial amyloid
AIAPP	Islet amyloid polpeptide	Islets of Langerhans, type II diabetes

(modified from Cardiovasc Pathol 1995; 4:79, and Bull World Health Organ 1993; 71:105)

amyloid β protein see beta-amyloid

amyloidosis Systemic amyloidosis is divided into 1) AL amyloidosis Primary amyloidosis An uncommon condition associated with plasma cell dyscrasias, where the accumulated amyloid fibers correspond to fragments of immunoglobulin light chains; the median survival in one study of 153 patients with primary AL amyloidosis as 20 months, less if they presented clinical signs of renal or cardiac amyloidosis and up to 40 months if neither system was involved; the other form of systemic amyloidosis is 2) AA (reactive or secondary) amyloidosis, which consist of a group of conditions seen in patients with chronic inflammatory conditions, in which the accumulated fibers derive from a circulating acute-phase lipoprotein, known as serum protein A; both types of amyloidosis contain amyloid P component, a non-fibrillary glycoprotein also found in the circulation; scintigraphy after injection of 123I-labelled serum amyloid P component can locate tissue deposition of amyloidosis and if the deposition is active, cytotoxic therapy may be instituted; focal amyloidosis commonly occurs in those organs most susceptible to aging, eg the heart and brain, and only is symptomatic if the amyloid deposition is significant

CLASSIFICATION (3rd Intl Symp. Amyloidosis, presented here for those more familiar with the older classification)

FAMILIAL
1) Amyloid polyneuropathy Fiber type: AFp (prealbumin)
2) Familial mediterranean fever Fiber type: AA
3) Familial amyloid syndrome Ostertag's disease

GENERALIZED
1) 'Primary' amyloidosis (the variable and of immunoglobulin light chains), affecting: Tongue, gastrointestinal tract, heart, kidneys, muscle, skin, nerves, ligaments and seminal vesicles: AL Fiber
2) Associated with plasma cell dyscrasia; most patients have an M component (amyloid deposits in the liver, spleen, kidneys and adrenal glands) and rarely, myeloma; survival is less than two years; AL fiber
3) Secondary to inflammation or infection Deposition of amyloid protein A (AA fibers) fibrils; in the pre-antibiotic era, secondary amyloidosis was most commonly associated with chronic infection, eg TB, chronic osteomyelitis and leprosy; in the current setting, sendary deposits are occur in chronic inflammation, eg Crohn's disease, ulcerative colitis and familial mediterranean fever, connective tissue disease, eg dermatomyositis, lupus erythematosus, rheumatoid arthritis and Sjogren syndrome, tissue destruction, eg bronchiectasis, malignancy, eg alpha heavy chain disease, Hodgkin's disease, leukemia, myeloma and Waldenstrim syndrome and heroin abuse, presenting with proteinuria and nephrotic syndrome

LOCALIZED
1) Lichen amyloidosis Fiber type: AD
2) Endocrine-related Fiber type: AEt Amyloid may occur with endocrine neoplasms, including pancreatic islet cell tumors, medullary thyroid carcinoma and parathyroid hyperplasia and adenomas seen in the MEN (Multiple endocrine neoplasia) syndrome
Senile types: Heart Fiber type: ASc
Brain Fiber: ASb
3) β-2 microglobulin derived amyloid cannot traverse the dialysis membrane, in patients on chronic dialysis, causing cystic bony lesions and carpal tunnel syndrome

amyotrophic lateral sclerosis Lou Gehrig's disease A motor neuron disease, characterized by upper limb weakness, atrophy and focal neurological signs EPIDEMIOLOGY Incidence, 0.5-1.5/10⁵, more common in ♂, usually > age 50; occurs randomly thoughout the world with local clustering on the Kii Peninsula of Japan and on Guam where it is associated with dementia and parkinsonism; 5% are autosomal dominant PATHOGENESIS Motor neuron death may be due to an aberrant accumulation of neurofilaments, and consequent disruption of axonal transport (Nature 1995; 375:61, 12); other possible mechanisms include mutant forms of superoxide dismutase, defect in high-affinity glutamate transport (N Engl J Med 1992; 326:1464oa); L-type voltage gated calcium channel autoantibodies are present in ALS and the levels correlate with disease severity, implying that ALS may be in part due to autoimmunity (N Engl J Med 1992; 327:1721oa) CLINICAL Loss of fine motor skills → by a triad of atrophic weakness of hands and forearms, leg spasticity, and generalized hyperreflexia MOLECULAR PATHOLOGY The gene defect is heterogeneous and located distal to the centromere on chromosome 21, specifically the superoxide dismutase (SOD) gene has been linked to ALS; a mouse ALS model has been created with mutations in the Cu,Zn SOD gene; *SOD1* mutations may not cause a loss of SOD activity, but rather a gain-of-function mutation which confers a neurotoxic property to the enzyme, possibly due to an interaction between the superoxide anion and nitric oxide to form the toxic free radical peroxynitrite (Science 1994; 264:1772r, 1663m, N Engl J Med 1994; 331:1091) TREATMENT Riluzole, an experimental drug that modulates glutamatergic transmission is reported in phase 1 trials to slow the progression of disease and possibly improve survival (N Engl J Med 1994; 330:585oa) Note: Only 5% of the cases are familial; see Motor neuron disease

Note: From 1924-1939, Lou Gehring, the Iron Horseman, started 2130 consecutive games with his baseball team, the New York Yankees, a record that is still unbeaten

amytal interview see Amytal test

amytal test Wada test A test that was introduced with the purpose of localizing speech function prior to the performance of temporal lobectomy in patients with medically refractory epilepsy; the test was subsequently used to to evaluate memory; this so-called 'Amytal interview', is carried out under the influence of Amytal, a sedative, which by causing full relaxation, with minimal sedation, attempts to elicit information from a subject who is voluntarily 'guarding' against its revelation; the interview is more specific if the Amytal is selectively injected into the posterior cerebral artery

ANA 1) Antinuclear antibodies 2) Antiviral nucleoside analogue, see there

ANA the 'gold standard' test for ANA is indirect immunofluorescence, which requires a certain amount of technical skill; in contrast, EIAs are easier to perform, are adequate for the usual clinical purposes, but suffer from markedly decreased sensitivity and lack of standardization among manufacturers (CAP Today April 1995 p1)

anabolic-androgenic steroids A group of 17-α-alkylated testosterone analogs, commonly abused by athletes (especially body builders) at various levels of professionalism, eg by international athletes 1-2%, college athletes 5%, 12th grade male athletes, 6% and professional football players 7-8% Lipid profile with abuse (more marked with oral stanazol than with IV testosterone) ↓↓↓ HDL-cholesterol (especially HDL₂) and ↑ hepatic triglyceride lipase (HDL catabolism) Therapeutic indications for anabolic steroids: Children and adolescents with delayed puberty, growth promotion, small penis and hypogonadism Other indications include the management of osteoporosis, aplastic anemia, endometriosis, angioedema and deficiency of testosterone ADVERSE EFFECTS ♂ Breast enlargement, testicular atrophy, sterility, sperm abnormalities, impotence and prostatic hypertrophy ADVERSE EFFECTS ♀ Clitoral hypertrophy, beard growth, baldness, deepened voice, decreased breast size ADVERSE EFFECTS, ♀/♂ Aggression and antisocial behavior, 'roid rage, see below; increased risk of cardiovascular disease, liver tumors, peliosis hepatis, jaundice, acne, accelerated bone maturation, resulting in short stature, liver tumors (hepatic adenomas and carcinoma) that may regress with steroid abstinence; high doses are thought to be physically addicting, as abrupt reduction in dose results in acute hyperadrenergic withdrawal symptoms (tachycardia, hypertension, nausea, vomiting, headaches, vertigo, diaphoresis and piloerection), paralleling other withdrawal syndromes, including those related to sedative, hypnotic and cocaine withdrawal; anabolic steroids act at the benzodiazepine/GABA receptor and may respond to benzodiazepine (JAMA 1990; 263:2049c); the use of stanozolol (manufactured for horses) LABORATORY Androgen analogues are detectable to levels 1 part per billion, four days after last use if the hormone is water-soluble, or 14 days after use in lipid-soluble compounds; one analog, nandrolone was detected up to 13 months after its alleged last use; anabolic steroids have been conferred 'schedule III' drug status in the US under the Controlled Substances Act, thus prescriptions may be scrutinized according to registration, reporting, record keeping and prescribing practices; anabolic steroid prescriptions may be refilled no more often than 5 times within six months (JAMA 1991; 265:1229); anabolic steroid abusers are at potential risk for HIV transmission, given the common practice of injecting these agents and 'fraternal' sharing of needles (N Engl J Med 1991; 325:357c) see 'Roid rage, 'Stacking'

anabolic-androgenic steroid

Note: The most flagrant abuse of anabolic steroids allegedly occurred in East Germany, where they were administered to Olympic athletes without regard to the potential effects; scientists became adept at creating formulations and delivery systems, eg intranasal spray, that eluded detection by Olympic drug-testing laboratories (Science 1991; 254:26n&v); use of an oral anabolic steroid resulted in forfeiture of a gold medal in the men's 100-meter sprint (world record of 9.79 sec) in the 1988 Seoul Summer Olympics; the athlete in question's testosterone levels were 15% normal, indicating significant short-term hormonal suppression

anaclitic depression PEDIATRICS A state of depression seen in children who have been separated from their mothers for prolonged periods of time, resulting in a disruption of the mother-child dyad; by six months, infants are strongly attached to the mother figure; when they are separated from the mother figure after 6 months by the mother's death or incarceration and a substitute mother figure is provided, the initial panic and searching reactions give way to anxiety, ending with apathy and withdrawal, accompanied by hypotonia and inactivity, a saddened facial expression, loss of appetite, weight loss, profound disturbances in motor, social and language development and, when the reaction is extreme, death

anaerobe A generic term for any organism (but in the usual context referring to bacteria) capable of living without air; anaerobic pathogens obtain their energy from fermentation; nonpathogenic anerobes in nature obtain their energy from anaerobic respiration in which nitrate or sulfate serve as electron acceptors; bacteria require from normal atmospheric pressure (21%) to less than 0.5% oxygen for optimal growth; the oropharynx, skin, colon and vagina harbor up to 10^{11} anaerobes/cm^3; these bacteria are common causes of infection, and may be associated with aerobic flora in infections and abscesses of the oral cavity, upper respiratory tract, colon, genital tract, skin and brain; factors controlling the virulence of anaerobic organisms are uncertain, as the most abundant anaerobes, *Veillonella*, *Eubacterium*, *Bifidobacterium*, and *Lactobacillus* virtually never cause clinical disease, while *Bacteroides fragilis* and *Fusobacterium* species are cultured from anaerobic infection far more often than expected given their low abundance PATHOGENESIS 'Noxins' produced by anaerobes include exotoxins, lipopolysaccharide endotoxin, superoxide dismutase, and the organism's capsule itself, which is capable of inducing abscesses, even in absence of viable organisms TREATMENT Penicillin for anaerobic infections above the diaphragm; clindamycin, metronidazole, chloramphenicol, or cephoxatin if the infection is below the diaphragm

Definitions **AEROTOLERANT ANAEROBE** grow poorly in O_2 or CO_2 environments and are clearly 'happier' under anaerobic conditions, eg *Clostridium carnis, C histolyticum, C tertium* **FACULTATIVE ANAEROBE** An anaerobe that grows in either completely anaerobic or microaerophilic environments, using oxygen as the terminal electron acceptor, yielding 38 ATP molecules when catabolizing a molecule of glucose, or in a 'pinch', utilizing glucose by the less energy-efficient fermentative metabolic pathway, yielding 2 ATP molecules, eg *Escherichia coli, Staphylococcus aureus* **MICROAEROPHILE** An anaerobe that requires oxygen as terminal electron acceptors but which grows in neither atmospheric nor in anaerobic environments, eg *Campylobacter jejuni* grows optimally in 5% O_2, 10% CO_2, and 85% N_2 **OBLIGATE AEROBE** Strict aerobe An aerobe that requires molecular oxygen as a terminal electron acceptor, resulting in the formation of water and does not obtain energy by fermentative pathways, eg *Micoccus* and *Pseudomonas* species **OBLIGATE ANAEROBE** Strict anaerobe Any of a group of anaerobic bacteria that may be either 1) Moderate, ie capable of growth in reduced oxygen (2-8%) environment, eg *Bacteroides fragilis, B melaninogenicus, Fusobacterium nucleatum, Clostridium perfringens* or b) Strict, ie incapable of growth in O_2 levels above 0.5%, eg *Clostridium haemolyticum, C novyi B, Selenomonas ruminantium, Treponema denticola*; see Oxygen toxicity

anaerobic exercise A generic term for exercise that strengthens muscles and increases joint mobility, reducing the risk of injury to the musuloskeletal apparatus; AE consists of slow rhythmic exercise, eg calesthenics (push-ups, sit-ups) and weight lifting, which result in a minimal increase in heart rate; Cf Aerobic exercise

anal cancer A generic term for any malignancy of the anal canal, which has been linked by some workers to anal intercourse PATHOLOGY Proximal anus = adenocarcinoma; transition zone = various pathologies, eg carcinoma, lymphoma, and malignant melanoma; Distal anus = squamous cell carcinoma PATHOGENESIS The diagnosis of anal cancer has been temporally (but not causally) associated with benign anal lesions (eg fissures, fistulas, hemorrhoids, perianal abscesses) which may be the first manifestation of a previously undetected anal cancer (**N Engl J Med 1994; 331:302oa**)

anal intraepithelial neoplasia A lesion that most commonly affects immunosuppressed male homosexuals who are commonly infected by human papillomavirus types 6/11, 31/33/35 and 16/18 , AIN is histologically characterized by irregular nuclear shape, hyperchromasia and chromatin; see CIN, Intraepithelial neoplasia

'anal-retentive' A colloquial term for a person with an 'anal personality', who, according to classic Freudian psychoanalysis, has traits that arose in the anal phase of psychosexual development, in which defecation constituted the primary source of pleasure, and retention of feces is held to represent defiance to the parent; the typical 'anal-retentive' is obstinant, rigid, meticulous, compulsive and overconscientious, which is a behavioral profile typical of many physicians and scientists

anal sphincter SURGICAL ANATOMY A hybrid structural unit composed of an internal sphincter (IS) and an external spincter (ES); the IS corresponds to the lowermost portion of the circular muscle of the rectum, the distal border of which is indicated by the interspincteric groove; the IS is surrounded by deep and superficial portions of the ES, and is innervated by the autonomic nervous system; the IS is not amenable to voluntary control; when under the normal state of maximal tone, the IS is closed, and relaxes in response to rectal distension; the ES is located below the pelvic floor and is formed from three muscular rings that act as a functional unit; the upper portions of the ES are continuous with the levator ani muscles, and it is innervated by branches from S2-S4; AS defects can be induced by forceps delivery (**N Engl J Med 1993; 329:1905oa**)

anal tag Swollen skin at the peripheral end of an anal fissure, often accompanied by pain on defecation and fresh bleeding

anal wink The cutaneo-anal contractile reflex, in which there is a visible puckering at the margin of the external anal sphincter, evoked by stroking the perianal skin with a pin; absence of an AW suggests a defect in either sensory or motor nerves or in the central pathways that mediate this reflex

analgesic drug 'ladder' CLINICAL PHARMACOLOGY An algorithm for managing cancer pain, ie the levels of intensity of therapy: **FIRST STEP** Non-opioids with/without adjuvants (neurolytic blockage, cordotomy, chemical hypophysectomy and others) **SECOND STEP** Weak opioids, with/without non-opioids and/or adjuvants **THIRD STEP** Strong opioids, with/without non-opioids and/or adjuvants

analgesic nephropathy Tubulointerstitial inflammation associated with papillary necrosis caused by ingestion of combinations of analgesics, including acetaminophen, aspirin and phenacetin which result in hematuria, renal colic and pyelonephritis; intravenous pyelogram reveals 'ring' shadows and multiple cavitations characteristic of papillary necrosis COMPLICATIONS Increased risk of future transitional cell carcinoma

analog COMPUTERS An adjective referring to data that is presented in the form of continuously variable (non-discrete) physical quantities, the mode in which most laboratory instruments produce information, where data is generated as non-discrete signals, as AC or DC current, voltage changes or pulse amplitudes; the analog data must be converted into a digital form before it can be manipulated by a computer, which, being a digital device, performs discrete mathematical operations; Cf Analogue

analog computer LABORATORY MEDICINE A computer in which the data is acquired in the form of continuous electrical variables across a continuum of temperature, pressure or flow; patient specimens evaluated by automated instruments in clinical chemistry and hematology yield analog data that must be converted into digital (discrete) information prior to its transfer to other sites in the hospital

analogue PHARMACOLOGY A drug or therapeutic substance which has structural or chemical homology to another substance, or which has effects mimicking that of another agent, but has a different chemical structure

analysand A victim of psychoanalysis, the human equivalent of analyte

analysis of variance see ANOVA STATISTICS An analytic method used for continuous variables, by determining whether the source of variability among data sets is due to true differences in the sets or due to random variations or 'statistical noise'; ANOVA compares the means of several random variables, assuming that each has a normal distribution with the same variance; these algorithms are quite complex and are usually computer-based

'ANA-negative' systemic lupus erythematosus A variant of systemic lupus erythematosus (SLE) characterized by the absence of antinuclear antibodies (which occurs in 5% of SLE patients), photosensitivity, features of Sjögren syndrome, a low incidence of lupus nephritis and lupus psychosis, presence of rheumatoid factor and antibodies to Ro/SSA antigen and La/SSB antigens and single-stranded DNA; see Antinuclear antibodies, Lupus erythematosus; Cf Antiphospholipid syndrome

anaphylactic reaction Anaphylaxis An antigen-induced, IgE-mediated release or formation of chemical mediators, the target of which are primarily blood vessels and smooth muscle; AR is an acute or excessive immune response in a previously sensitized host when re-exposed to an antigen; PATHOGENESIS The AR is a hypersensitivity (Gel and Coombs type I) reaction that occurs upon exposure to an antigen to which the body has previously formed an IgE antibody; within seconds of exposure to the antigen(s), which may be proteins, polysaccharides and haptens, IgE molecules cross-link on the surface of mast cells and basophils, stimulating the release of low molecular weight mediators of anaphylaxis; in the primary response, preformed molecules are released, including eosinophil chemotactic factor, heparin, histamine, serotonin and various enzymes; in the secondary response, acute phase reactants are produced and released; fatal and near-fatal ARs in children are most commonly evoked by peanuts > nuts > eggs, milk, fish and others (N Engl J Med 1992; 327:380oa) PATHOGENESIS Antigen is recognized by IgE on the surface of basophils and mast cells which degranulate, releasing histamine and other vasoactive substances CLINICAL Bronchospasm, dyspnea, edema, shock and possibly death TREATMENT Epinephrine STAT (N Engl J Med 1992; 327:380oa) see Acute phase reactants

anaphylactoid Anaphylaxis-like

anaphylactoid reaction An anaphylaxis-like reaction occurring without an allergen-IgE antibody event, caused by a nonimmune release, eg reaction to radiocontrast, chymopapain, aspirin of vasoactive and inflammatory mediators, including release of histamine

anaphylaxis see Anaphylactic reaction

anaplastic carcinoma An often aggressive malignancy of epithelial origin that lacks histological criteria required to confirm its embryologic lineage; these tumors lack architectural landmarks and are generally classified based on the cells types, often being divided into small cell, intermediate cell, giant cell, spindle cell and mixed cell types; anaplastic carcinomas occur in the lungs, thyroid and have been described in most sites in the form of case reports PROGNOSIS Often poor, as anaplasia implies that the tumor is 'primitive' and is commonly aggressive and responds poorly to excision and occasionally to chemo- and radiotherapy

anatomic snuffbox ANATOMY A triangular depression on the dorsal pollicar aspect of the hand when the thumb is fully extended; the AS on the radial aspect of the wrist that is produced by extending the thumb; the space bound posteriorly by the tendon of the extensor pollicis longus and anteriorly by the tendons of the extensor pollicis brevis and adductor pollicis longus; space is crossed superficially by the digital rami of the superficial branch of the radial nerve, and at the floor is crossed by the radial artery; the floor is formed by the trapezium and the scaphoid bone, a fracture of which can be identified by digital pressure in the anatomic snuffbox

Note: The sobriquet 'Tequila triangle' refers to the snuffbox's use when drinking tequila, a Mexican inebrient

ANCA Antineutrophil cytoplasmic antibody, see there

anchor disease CD11/CD18 leukocyte glycoprotein deficiency A rare disease of neonatal onset with delayed umbilical cord separation, leukocytosis and poor wound healing, accompanied by defects in neutrophil adherence, chemotaxis, secretion, phagocytosis and particle-stimulated respiratory burst, resulting in severe recurring bacterial infections of mucocutaneous regions that become systemic; anchor disease is due to defective 180 kD membrane glycoprotein, the α subunit of the heterodimeric protein Mo1, the C3bi receptor of neutrophils and monocytes

anchorage TISSUE CULTURE Adherence by cells, usually fibroblasts to a solid or semisolid support medium, which is required for optimal growth; the loss of anchorage dependence is a hallmark of cell (malignant) transformation that may be induced by oncogenic viruses; see Cadherin, CAM (cell adhesion molecule); Cf Cell senescence

anchovy paste appearance A fanciful descriptor for the olive-brown (less commonly, creamy white) grumous material seen in hepatic and cerebral amebiasis (*Entamoeba histolytica*), composed of autolyzed necrotic debris and hemorrhage, which is a lesion of middle-aged men

ancient DNA DNA derived from plants and animals that have been dead for a prolonged period of time, usually 100 or more years; analysis of ancient DNA by the polymerase chain reaction, which allows 'amplification' of minute amounts of DNA is of use in various fields, including archeology, anthropology, evolutionary biology, forensic pathology, paleontology and population genetics (Science 1991; 253:1354n)

ancient schwannoma Degenerated neurilemmoma A benign, potentially large tumor of peripheral nerve that is most common in the retroperitoneal space characterized by cyst formation, calcification, hyalinization and hemorrhage TREATMENT Simple excision; see Peripheral nerve sheath tumor(s)

ancillary service HEALTH CARE MANAGEMENT A generic term for any service (eg in-office laboratory, or mammography unit) provided by or available from a physician that is related to his/her practice of medicine; ASs may provide a source of increased revenues and facilitate the flow of information (Am Med News 24 April 1995 p11)

ANDA Abbreviated new drug application, see there

Andes' disease Mondor's disease; see Mountain sickness

androgen ablation A generic term for reduction of the androgens (testosterone and 5α-dihydrotestosterone) in the circulation by either orchiectomy or by an LHRH* agonist; AA is commonly used in metastatic prostate cancer and results in a response rate as high as 80%, althought the response is usually short-lived (12-18 months); AA can be augmented by flutamide, an androgen receptor antagonist that blocks the effect of androgens produced by the adrenal gland (N Engl J Med 1995; 332:1393oA) see Androgen-independent prostate cancer

*Luteinizing hormone-releasing hormone

androgen-independent prostate cancer A form of prostate cancer characterized by metastases, aggressive clinical behavior, and a poor response to androgen ablation; most AIPCs express high levels of androgen receptor gene transcripts, which may be linked to mutations of the androgen receptor itself (N Engl J Med 1995; 332:1393oA)

Andromeda strain A hypothetical virus* that would be spread by droplet (aerosol), highly virulent and result in a 'species-threatening event', ie capable of decimating the human population (R Preston, The Hot Zone, Random House, New York, 1994)

*Named after a science fiction novel by the same name; none are known to exist

'Andy Gump' A descriptor for a patient with a diminutive mandible, which may be congenital and seen in Pierre-Robin deformity and in otocephaly; in the latter, the mandibular hypoplasia and associated deformities are incompatible with extra-uterine life POST-SURGICAL Resection of the upper mandible as part of aggressive surgery in cancer of the floor of the mouth and POST-TRAUMATIC A fracture unique to elderly edentulous subjects, in which there is posterior mandibular displacement and airway obstruction, thus known as an 'Andy Gump fracture'

Note: Andy Gump was a syndicated comic strip character lacking a mandible

'anecdotal' Unsubstantiated, as in an anecdotal patient response to unproven cancer therapy, or anecdotal cause-and-effect relationship between a noxious environmental element and clinical disease; Cf Blinding

anemia of chronic disease A condition that accounts for ¼ of all anemia in hospitalized patients and is the predominant form of (hypoproliferative) anemia seen in patients with arthritis, chronic infections, and malignancy LABORATORY Mild-to-moderate anemia, often microcytic ± hypochromic PATHOGENESIS Possibly related to IFN-γ produced by activated macrophages and impaired iron utilization; ACD seen in malignancy may be due in part to chemo– or radiotherapy and exacerbated by tumor replacement of the bone marrow, by direct cytotoxic effect of chemotherapeutic agents or by indirect cytotoxic effect of platinum-based compounds TREATMENT Transfusion, erythropoietin (Arch Pathol Lab Med 1994; 118:417oa)

anemia panel A group of laboratory parameters that have been determined to be the most cost-efficient, sensitive, specific in evaluating a patient with anemia; the anemia panel includes the CBC (complete blood count) with indices, reticulocyte count; if the anemia is hypochromic and microcytic, the panel should include iron levels, iron-binding capacity, measurement of the levels and percent saturation of ferritin; if the anemia is macrocytic, then vitamin B_{12} and folate levels are measured; see Organ panel

anemia of prematurity Reduced erythrocyte mass most common in low- and very-low-birth-weight infants, characterized by low reticulocyte counts, and deficient erythropoietin production; this is often compounded by aggressive and frequent diagnostic phlebotomies; because of the need for adequate oxygenation, premature infants often recieve blood transfusions–average: 1.25 transfusions/infant, which can be reduced by administration of erythropoietin–0.87 transfusions/infant (N Engl J Med 1994; 330:1173oa)

anemic infarct White infarct A localized area of ischemic necrosis in a solid organ, due to abrupt arterial occlusion; while in the immediate post-insult period, blood may flow into the region yielding a false impression of a hemorrhagic infarct; by 1-2 days post-insult, the region is pale yellow-white and characteristic of occlusions in organs with one circulatory supply, eg kidney, spleen, heart; see 'White' graft; Cf Hemorrhagic (red) infarct

anemone cell villiform tumor A heterogeneous group of large cell malignancies with numerous circumferential or polar microvilli, an ultrastructural finding that usually implies epithelial origin; the lack of tonofilaments and intercellular junctions implies that some of these tumors may actually be large cell lymphomas

anencephalus An infant with anencephaly

anencephaly Congenital partial or complete absence of the cranial vault accompanied by absence of overlying tissues, including the brain, skull and scalp; anencephaly develops in the first month of gestation and affects 0.14-0.7/1000 live births; the primary abnormality is failure of cranial neurulation, the embryologic process separating the forebrain precursors from the amniotic fluid; since the neural tissue is exposed, the cerebral tissue is hemorrhagic, fibrotic and gliotic without functional cortex ETIOLOGY Usually idiopathic, possibly multifactorial or polygenic in origin; most anencephalics die within the first week and are of use as potential organ donors, although the ethical dilemmas intrinsic to the use of such human infants has made this a contentious issue; see Uniform Determination of Death Act

anergy IMMUNOLOGY Absence of immune response to an antigen to which the host was previously sensitive, a state in which viable T cells have a diminished or absent lymphokine secretion when the T cell receptor is engaged by an antigen; anergy can be induced in mature and differentiated CD4+ T cells by exposure to complexes of antigen and appropriate (self) major histocompatibility complex in absence of certain uncharacterized co-stimulatory signals on the antigen-presenting cells (Science 1991; 251:1228); anergy is usually tested by loss of delayed hypersensitivity, eg to PPD, *Candida* antigens, or to DCNB; in patients who have received blood transfusions, the resultant anergy is thought to be induced by the presentation of antigen by 'nonprofessional' antigen-presenting cells (Arch Pathol Lab Med 1994; 118:371oa) see Deletion

aneuploid Pertaining or referring to aneuploidy

aneuploidy GENETICS A congenital or acquired excess or deficient number of chromosomes in diploid cells that deviates from multiples of a diploid set of chromosomes, which in humans is 23 (normally present as a haploid complement multiplied by 2, ie 23 + 23); types of aneuploidy MONOSOMY Defined by the formula 2n-1, eg Turner syndrome HYPERDIPLOIDY Defined by the formula 2n+x, where x is greater than 1 HYPODIPLOIDY defined by the formula 2n-x, where x is greater than 1 TRISOMY Defined by the formula 2n+1, eg Klinefelter syndrome; the degree of aneuploidy in a dividing population of cells can be analyzed by flow cytometry and carries a negative prognostic significance in epithelial malignancies including breast carcinoma and endometrial carcinoma; Cf Polyploidy

aneurysmal bone cyst A tumor-like osteolytic lesion often located in the metaphysis of long bones of young patients, seen as a physalliferous (soap bubble-like) osteolytic cortical expansion; the term ABC is, like pyogenic granuloma and ganglion cyst, a misnomer that has withstood the sands of time and the dint of logic, as it is neither an aneurysm nor a cyst PATHOLOGY Blood-filled space partially lined by fibrous tissue, mixed with osteocytes, fibroblasts, histiocytes and giant cells TREATMENT Curettage of bone defects, optional filling with bone chips

'angel dust' PCP, see there

'Angel of Death' Josef Mengele (1911-1979), a German physician who performed pseudoscientific studies in the Auschwitz concentration camp and personally selected 400 000 prisoners to die in the gas chambers; Mengele eluded authorities and drowned in Brazil in 1979; Cf 'Death angel,' Dr Death

angel wing sign A pattern of symmetrical perihilar 'soft' radiodensities seen on a plain chest film in patients with simple silicosis, due to massive fibrosis where large masses are most prominent in the upper lobes; the term 'Angel wings' has also been used as descriptor for the findings of neonatal pneumomediastinum, see Spinnaker sail sign

Angelman syndrome Happy puppet syndrome A rare AR [MIM 234400] form of infantile epilepsy characterized by seizures, severe mental retardation, microcephaly, occasionally, unilateral cerebral atrophy, flattened occiput, large mandible, protruding jaw and tongue, a smiling vacuous open-mouthed facial expression, paroxysms of inappropriate laughter, gait ataxia and spastic puppet-like 'bouncing' movements of the extremities, likened to those of a marionette MOLECULAR PATHOLOGY Paternal disomy of chromosome 15 (15q11q13) accompanied by maternal deletion of chromosome 15, which contrasts with the Prader-Willi syndrome, in which there is maternal disomy of chromosome 15 (15q11q13) accompanied by paternal deletion of chromosome 15 (N Engl J Med 1992; 326:1599oa) see Prader-Willi syndrome

angina A generic term for an 'suffocatingly' intense pain, now almost always invariably refers to angina pectoris (the Latin adjective, *pectoris* has essentially disappeared) see Canadian Cardiovascular Society functional classification, Unstable angina

angina pectoris Angina, see there

angioedema Angioneurotic edema, see there

angiofollicular lymphoid hyperplasia Castleman's disease, see there

angiogenesis The growth of new blood vessels and capillary beds that sprout from existing vessels, which plays a fundamental role in embryonic development, tissue and wound repair, resolution of inflammation, and the onset of neoplasia; ischemia induces ↑ production of endogenous bFGF, which in turn leads to angiogenesis (Nature Medicine 1995; 1:453); integrin $\alpha v \beta_3$ is a necessary factor for angiogenesis induced by fibroblast growth factor, tumor necrosis factor-a, and human melanoma fragments (Science 1994; 264:569r); angiogenesis contributes to pathological conditions including cancer, diabetic retinopathy, and rheumatoid arthritis

angiogenic factors A group of substances present in the circulation, most of which are polypeptides, including angiogenin, fibroblast growth factor, transforming growth factors as well as some lipids; angiogenic factors may increase markedly following ischemic insults to the myocardium

angiogenin A 14-kD polypeptide with 35% homology to pancreatic ribonucleases, which induces angiogenesis in normal fetal development and wound healing as well as in cancer and in diabetes; its presence in the liver implies physiologic roles other than angiogenesis

angioid streaks Peripapillary, gray in non-whites to red-brown in whites, linear striations radiating from the optic fundus along stress lines or toward the equator in an abnormal Bruch's membrane; one-half of cases of angioid streaks occur in patients with pseudoxanthoma elasticum; angioid streaks also occur in fundi rendered brittle by calcium (tumor-related calcinosis), heavy metal, eg lead intoxication and occurs in acromegaly, a-β-lipoproteinemia, DM, hemochromatosis, hemolytic anemia, hypercalcinosis, hyperphosphatasia, ITP, myopia, neurofibromatosis, Paget's disease of bone, senile elastosis, sickle cell anemia, Sturge-Weber syndrome, tuberous sclerosis

angioimmunoblastic lymphadenopathy AILA A condition first described by Lukes (N Engl J Med 1975; 292:1) as a hyperimmune B-cell proliferation, characterized by a triad of histopathologic changes 1) Pleomorphic infiltrate of small and large immunoblasts and plasma cells with effacement of nodal architecture 2) Arborizing vascular proliferation with endothelial cell hyperplasia and 3) Interstitial deposits of amorphous eosinophilic PAS-positive, presumably cellular debris CLINICAL Polyclonal gammopathy, middle aged to elderly patients, hemolytic anemia, fever, night sweats, weight loss, generalized lymphadenopathy, hepatosplenomegaly, skin rashes MEDIAN SURVIVAL 15 months; some cases evolve to immunoblastic lymphoma or monoclonal gammopathy DIFFERENTIAL DIAGNOSIS AIDS, angiofollicular lymphoid hyperplasia, drug reaction, histiocytosis X, Hodgkin's disease, immunoblastic lymphoma, malignant histiocytosis, atypical or reactive lymphoid hyperplasia; CMV may play a role in the pathogenesis of AILA (Arch Pathol Lab Med 1992; 116:490oa)

angiomyolipoma A benign well-circumscribed and nonencapsulated tumor-like lesion (hamartoma) composed of a mixture of blood vessels, smooth muscle, and mature fat; angiomyolipomas are most commonly renal or paranephric lesions, but also occur in the fallopian tube, liver, nasal cavity, penis, skin, spermatic cord, and vagina IMMUNOHISTOCHEMISTRY Positive for antibodies to muscle-specific antigen and HMB-45 DNA CONTENT ANALYSIS Classic angiomyolipomas are diploid; multicentric angiomyolipomas are aneuploid (Arch Pathol Lab Med 1994; 118:735oa)

angioneurotic edema A chronic and potentially fatal condition characterized by episodes of subcutaneous and laryngeal edema, and abdominal pain; it is divided into an acquired form that is typically associated with paraproteinemia and/or malignant lymphoma and hereditary angioneurotic edema (HANE), which is subdivided into the more common type I HANE, in which the serum levels of an apparently normal complement 1 esterase inhibitor protein (C1 INH) are 5-30% of normal, and type II HANE, in which the serum levels of C1 INH are normal or elevated, but the protein itself is defective; in the hereditary form, the serum levels of the C1q subunit of complement are normal and decreased in the acquired form; see Episodic angioedema, HANE

angioplasty Percutaneous transluminal coronary angioplasty, see there

angiosarcoma An uncommon, usually aggressive mesenchymal malignancy, that may arise in the liver, as well as soft tissues and viscera PATHOLOGY Malignant endothelial cells forming variably sized anastomosing blood vessels with papillary infoldings; hepatic angiosarcoma is classically associated with exposure to thorium dioxide, an obsolete contrast medium, which is also associated with arsenic and vinyl chloride

angiostatin A recently identified protein factor that blocks the growth of primary and metastatic tumors by inhibiting angiogenesis; the worldwide license arrangement is with Entremed of Rockville, Md (from Cell Oct 21, 1994)

angiotensin I An N-terminal decapeptide produced when renin acts on angiotensinogen; A-I is the precursor of angiotensin II, but itself appears to have no known physiologic role

angiotensin II A-II Angiotensin An octapeptide produced when angiotensin converting enzyme (ACE, formally known as peptidyl-dipeptidase A [EC 3.4.15.1]) acts on angiotensin I by cleaving the C-terminal dipeptide; A–II is a potent vasoconstrictor (it is 4-8 **x** more potent that norepinephrine) and has a very short (1- 2 minutes) half-life in the circulation; it induces arteriolar constriction and increases systolic and diastolic blood pressure; A–II also acts directly on the adrenal cortex, increasing aldosterone secretion; it also facilitates norepinephrine release by direct action on the post-ganglionic sympathetic neurons, and acts on the brain, increasing blood pressure, water intake, and secretion of vasopressin and ACTH

angiotensin II receptor The cognate receptor for angiotensin II, which is unstable, present in low concentrations, has a transmembrane topology similar to G protein-coupled receptors, and is highly concentrated in the adrenal medulla, cortex and in the kidneys (Nature 1991; 351:230); the A-II receptor is divided into two forms, of which the AT1 receptor is held responsible for controlling blood pressure and volume (Nature 1991; 351:233)

angiotensin III A heptapeptide produced from A–II by aminopetidase which has 40% of the pressor activity of A–II, but 100% of its aldosterone-stimulating activity

angiotensin-converting enzyme A key enzyme* in the renin-angiotensin system, which converts the inactive decapeptide angiotensin I to the octapeptide, angiotensin II, which is a potent vasoconstrictor that also stimulates aldosterone secretion; ACE is also involved of the degradation of bradykinin; a deletion polymorphism of the *ACE* gene has been associated with left ventricular hypertrophy (**N Engl J Med 1994; 330:1634oa**), especially the *DD* genotype (**ibid 1994; 331:1097c**); in a large prospective study of US ♂ physicians, presence of the *D* allele of the *ACE* gene does not (contrary to results previously reported) ↑ the risk of ischemic heart disease or MI (**ibid 1995; 332:706oa**); ACE is encoded on chromosome 10 (**Nature 1991; 353:521**)

*The formal term for ACE recommended by the Nomenclature Committee of the IUBMB (International Union for BIochemistry and Molecular Biology) is peptidyl-dipeptidase A [**EC 3.4.15.1**]

angiotensinogen A glycoprotein found in the α_2 globulin fraction of plasma proteins; this 453-residue glycoprotein (13% carbohydrate) is synthesized in the liver, and is the source of angiotensin I, a decapeptide split from the N-terminal by renin, a proteolytic enzyme; angiotensinogen gene is located on 1q42-43; mutations thereof have been intimately linked to essential hypertension (**N Engl J Med 1994; 330:1629oa**) see Angiotensin, Renin-angiotensin system

angiotropic lymphoma Malignant angioendotheliomatosis A lesion first described as a neoplastic vascular proliferation that was shown to be either a B-cell, or less commonly, a T-cell lymphoma with a predilection for intravascular spaces CLINICAL Onset with multiple indurated and erythematous plaques or papules mimicking erythema nodosum, fever, neurological signs, minimal involvement of lymph nodes, BM, and spleen; see Lymphoma

angle du mort A common site of leakage in gastroenterostomy, specifically where the residual gastric pouch of a Hofmeister closure meets the anastomotic line with the small intestine

angular cheilitis Perleche A condition characterized by inflammation, exudation, maceration and fissuring at the angles of the lips, caused by multiple etiologies, most commonly candidiasis, but is also related to the decreased vertical dimension of the lower face in edentulous elderly with loss of alveolar bone, 'sagging' of cheeks due to myotonia (see Bloodhound face), sialorrhea, ariboflavinosis (with glossitis, keratitis and seborrhea-like dermatitis), malnutrition and streptococcal infection

angular momentum MRI A quantity given by the product of the momentum of a particle and its position vector; in absence of external forces, the AM remains constant, therefore a rotating body tends to maintain the same axis of rotation; when a torque is applied to a rotating body, the resulting change in angular momentum results in precession; atomic nuclei possess an intrinsic angular momentum referred to as spin, measured in multiples of Planck's constant; see Magnetic resonance imaging

anhidrosis The lack of sweat production in response to appropriate thermal or pharmacologic stimulation, which may become a medical emergency with hyperthermia, heat exhaustion, heatstroke, and death; anhidrosis may affect the entire body or be segmental in distribution and may be divided into structural defects, eg anhidrotic ectodermal dysplasia, sweat gland necrosis, or functional defects, often related to autonomic or thermoregulatory control which involve the central or peripheral nervous systems (**N Engl J Med 1994; 331:2259oa**)

animalcule Anton van Leuwenhoek's term for the first microorganisms he saw with his microscope

'Animal House fever' A limited outbreak of organic dust syndrome; the index report occurred in a college fraternity 'rush' party, which in the USA is an exercise in bacchanalian revelry; those who consumed more than ten drinks (see 'Standard drink') had more acute symptoms of pulmonary mycotoxicosis related to the fresh fungus-laden straw spread on the party floor which caused the air to be visibly thick with organic dust composed of fungal hyphae and spores CLINICAL Shaking chills or sweats, cough or shortness of breath and myalgia

Note: The term Animal House fever was coined after a motion picture about a college fraternity, entitled 'Animal House' (**JAMA 1987; 258:1219ed**) and is distinct from Silo-filler's disease, a chemical pneumonitis due to NO_2 exposure and Farmer's lung, an acute hypersensitivity pneumonitis, in which repeated exposure to organic dusts containing thermophilic fungi may progress to interstitial lung disease

Animal Liberation Front ALF An animal-rights activist group that allegedly includes violence (vandalism, arson, destruction of research data, and criminal assaults) in its repertoire of tactics for stopping the use of animals in any form in research (**JAMA 1992; 267:2577mn&p**) see Animal rights' activism, PETA

animal model An animal that has (usually) been highly inbred by selectively mating animals with a desired trait or group of characteristics that closely mimic a disease in humans, allowing the study of the disease mechanism and possibly its therapy, eg atherosclerosis in Watanabe rabbits or systemic lupus erythematosus in NZB/NZW

animals rights activism A movement that believes in and campaigns for humane treatment of animals; the organizations include ALF (Animal Liberation Front), a group listed as a terrorist organization by US Federal Bureau of Investigation and by Scotland Yard (**Nature 1991; 349:13c**), PAWS (Performing Animal Welfare Society) and PETA (People for Ethical Treatment of Animals); researchers have become victims of acts ranging from destruction of records and equipment to extreme violence; scientists have responded to this movement by reducing the number of animals used, refining procedures and replacement of animals, where possible, with alternate experimental models (**N Engl J Med 1991; 324:1640ed**) see PETA, Silver Springs monkeys, Toxicity testing

Note: 20 million animals are used in biomedical research in the US; the US Department of Agriculture, the responsible regulatory agency, considers dogs, cats and monkeys as animals, and mice, rats and birds as something else (**Nature 1991; 350:642n**)

Animal Welfare Act A legislative act by the US Congress in 1985 and re-written in early 1991 with the purpose that animals not be subjected to senseless pain and suffering; the Act required $800 million for the construction of newer facilities and an additional $200 million/year in operating expenses for improved sanitation and requiring humane treatment with 30 minutes of exercise and socialization and 60 minutes of *'positive physical contact with a human'*; compliance was re-estimated to cost $537 million (**Nature 1991; 349:641ed**)

anion gap LABORATORY MEDICINE A mathematical approximation of the difference between the unmeasured anions (PO_4^-, SO_4^-, proteins and organic acids) and the unmeasured cations (Ca^{2+}, Mg^{2+}); the unmeasured anions exceed the unmeasured cations; the AG is calculated as the difference between the sum of the most abundant measured serum anions (Cl^- and HCO_3^-) and serum cations (Na^+ and K^+), which is normally 8-16 mEq/L; ↑ AG is more common and occurs in renal failure due to defective renal tubular acidification with an ↑ in phosphate and sulfate; ↑ AGs also occur in diabetic ketoacidosis due to an accumulation of acetoacetate and β-hydroxybutyrate, in both disorders of amino acid metabolism and hyperglycemic nonketotic coma due to various organic acids and in lactic acidosis due to lactic acid; a decreased AG is less common and may occur in a GI loss of bicarbonate, in the nephrotic syndrome due to a loss of albumin which is anionic at a physiological pH, after lithium ingestion or in multiple myeloma due to an increase in cationic proteins; urinary AG is calculated as $Na^+ + K^+ - Cl^-$ and is a crude index of the levels of urinary ammonium and used to evaluate hyper-chloremic metabolic acidosis

anion paradox PHYSIOLOGY The finding that sodium chloride (NaCl) has a taste that is perceived as being 'saltier' than other sodium anions (eg sodium acetate or gluconate), despite the fact that the salty sensation is due to sodium and not chloride; the paradox is explained by a local effect of chloride ions which increase the sensitivity of the taste receptor cells to sodium (Science 1991; 254:724, 654n)

animism The belief that inanimate objects and forces of nature, eg sun, wind, storms, have inherent purposes and intent; see Gaia hypothesis

anisakiasis Infection of the upper GI tract (stomach, small intestine) mucosa by larvae of the family Anisakidae, which are common ascaroid parasites of marine fish; human infestation is a well-known complication of eating raw fish, eg sushi, see there

anismus GASTROENTEROLOGY A form of anorectal outlet obstruction of unknown etiology that affects older women and young boys, characterized by inappropriate contraction and typical electromyographic changes in the pelvic floor muscles and external anal sphincter CLINICAL Constipation, perineal pain, defecatory dysfunction PATHOGENESIS Anismus is thought to be a functional defects, as no organic cause has identified to date TREATMENT Biofeedback (Gut 1991; 32:1175)

Synonyms include abdominolevator incoordination, abdominopelvic asynchronism, abnormal anorectal expulsion dynamics, abnormal defecation dynamics (or pattern), outlet obstruction/constipation syndrome, paradoxic external sphincter contraction (or function), rectoanal dyssynergia, spastic pelvic floor syndrome, sphincteric disobedience syndrome

ankyrin A protein that binds spectrin to the erythrocyte anion exchanger, a defect of which may be cause a form of hereditary sphrocytosis; Cf Spherocytosis, Spectrin

ankyrin repeat MOLECULAR BIOLOGY A short repetitive sequence of amino acids that was first identified in ankyrin, that tethers different proteins, eg nuclear and cytoplasmic proteins, helping to regulate gene expression and embryonic development (Science 1991; 253:762, 789, 742ed)

ANLL Acute nonlymphocytic leukemia

Ann Arbor classification A system for staging Hodgkin's disease, thereby guiding therapy; clinical data is added based on A (absence) or B (presence) of associated symptoms, eg night sweats, fever or weight loss of > 10%; other symptoms of Hodgkin's disease include lethargy, fatigability, anorexia and pruritus

ANN ARBOR CLASSIFICATION
I   A single involved lymphoid region, organ or site
II Two or more involved lymphoid regions, or one extralymphoid site and a lymphoid region on the same side of the diaphragm
III Lymphoid regions involved on both sides of the diaphragm, variably accompanied by localized involvement of extralymphatic organs or spleen
IV Disseminated involvement of one or more extralymphatic organs or tissues, with or without associated lymphadenopathy

anneal Reanneal, see there

annealing The joining of complementary single-stranded chains of nucleic acid; Cf Denaturation

Anne Sexton MEDICAL ETHICS A confessional poetess with a multi-addiction disorder (alcohol and benzodiazepines) and a tempestuous life-style who rose to prominence as a feminist heroine and author, in part as a result of encouragement by her psychotherapist; her psychiatrist audio-taped the therapeutic sessions as a means by which the patient could assist in self-analysis, with the hope that she would develop a more stable self-concept and ability to function as a mother and wife (she subsequently committed suicide); because her therapist released the audio tapes to her biographer, as he felt this to be in accord with his patient's wishes, the 'Anne Sexton case' became a cause celebre regarding the issue of confidentiality in psychotherapy (N Engl J Med 1992; 326:1362c) see Confidentiality

Annex I nation GLOBAL VILLAGE An industrialized nation

Annex II nation GLOBAL VILLAGE A developing nation

annexin family A large group of calcium- and phospholipid-binding proteins and phospholipase A2- and blood coagulation inhibitors; because of the various approaches used to study these proteins, they have proven to be a nomenclatural 'nightmare', and it has been suggested that 'annexin' be used for proteins formerly designated as calphobindins, calpactins, chromobindins, endonexins, lipocortins, PAPs, synexin and VAC-α and VAC-β

anniversary phenomenon Sudden death related to psychological trauma that elicits an exaggerated autonomic nervous system response and fatal arrhythmia, inexplicably occurring on the anniversary of a past event; see Voodoo death; Cf Harvest Moon phenomenon

annual limit on intake ALI RADIATION SAFETY The derived limit for the amount of radioactive material taken into the body by inhalation or by ingestion of a given radionuclide by a worker in one year, which would result in a committed effective dose equivalent of 0.05 Sieverts (Sv or 50 rems) or a committed dose equivalent of 0.5 Sv (5 rems) to an individual organ or tissue

anomalad A dysmorphogenic complex characterized by a primary malformation and its derived structural defects (eg Pierre-Robin syndrome with cleft palate, glossoptosis and micrognathia); Cf Sequence

anodyne imagery ALTERNATIVE MEDICINE A '...technique that consists of conditioned relaxation, induction of a trance-like state, and guided processing of the patient's internal imagery...(which) allows patients to confront their fear and develop ways to mentally overcome their anxiety during interventional procedures, eliminating the need for intravenous sedation' (RT Image, 30 Jan, 1995) AI is believed by some radiologists to offer an alternative to sedation during radiologic procedures, which may depress cardiorespiratory function

anonymous sex Any form of sexual activity in which the partners' identities are unknown (often intentionally) to each other at the time of the activity's occurrance; anonymous sexual activity is more common among male homosexuals and may occur in various locations, eg in public restrooms (WCs), see Glory hole, or in quasi-public places, see Bathhouse

ANOVA Analysis of variance, see there

ANP Atrionatriuretic peptide, see there

anterior cleavage syndrome Mesodermal dysgenesis OPHTHALMOLOGY Anomalous development of the anterior segment of the eye with corneal opacification, abnormal anterior chamber angle, potentially glaucoma and abnormalities of the iris

anterior cord syndrome A spinal cord injury complex with loss of voluntary motor function, pain and temperature sense, and intact distal position, vibratory and light touch sense, dysfunctional anterior and lateral columns and intact posterior columns; the anterior cervical cord syndrome is a variation on this theme, caused by trauma to the relatively mobile cervical vertebrae, common in whiplash-type injury (spinal hyperextension)

anterior horn disease NEUROLOGY A group of conditions that predominantly affect the anterior horns of the spinal cord, including Werdnig-Hoffmann disease or infantile spinal muscle atrophy, the classic 'floppy infant' syndrome, characterized by hypotonia, symmetrical areflexic weakness with death by age two, amyotrophic lateral sclerosis, a distal disease of adults with fasciculations and wasting of 'bulbar' muscles and poliomyelitis, which is characterized by fever, asymmetric distal involvement, later becoming generalized, with muscle weakness of respiratory and bulbar muscles

anthracosis 1) A generic term for blackening of tissues, most commonly understood to mean the deposition of carbon dust in the lung and lymph nodes, which does not per se cause disease 2) Coal workers' pneumoconiosis

anthralin CLINICAL THERAPEUTICS A yellow crystal powder that is formulated in a paste and applied topically to psoriatic scales; although anthralin is the preferred topical treatment for psoriasis, it is easily oxidized to colored by-products that stain clothing purple or black, and may irritate pre-lesional skin given anthralin's formation of free radicals (N Engl J Med 1995; 332:581rv) see Psoriasis

anthropogenic Man-made, of human origin

anthropology The study of the origin of modern man; most of the major steps in human evolution occurred in Africa; the human ancestor appears to have split around 3 million years ago from am ancestor that had many anatomic and biochemical features in common with the African Great Apes Time table of the development of *Homo sapiens* 36 000 000 years BC *Dryopithecus* The hairy, tree-climbing herbivorous ancestor of all primates with a 200 cc cranial capacity (CC) 15 000 000 BC Orangutans and gorillas dropped out of the competition to become Earth's intelligent life and stopped evolving; *Ramapithecus*, the oldest hominid, with a 350 cc CC, was a vegetarian, walked on all fours with less dependence on the upper extremities, and spread from Africa to Southeast Asia 4 000 000 BC *Australopithecus africanus*, the earliest hominid from South Africa, had a 450-500 cc CC, measured 1.2 meters with bipedal locomotion, but had yet to make and use tools 2 500 000 BC *Australopithecus* split, one branch died, the other had by 1 500 000 BC begun to kill for meals Note: The 2-8 000 000 year period is important as man began to walk fully erect, had formed the primitive family unit of male breadwinner and female homemaker and women had developed continuous sexual availability, which was hormone-dependent,rather than seasonal, ie estrus cycling 2 000 000 BC *Homo habilis* had a 500-750 cc CC, was slightly under 1.5 meters tall, had an ape-like jaw, used tools, killed and ate raw meat 1 500 000 BC *H erectus* had a 900-1100 cc CC, was the first known human ancestor to walk fully erect, used and made tools, invented fire, wandered off to Southeast Asia into Indonesia as the Java man and into China as the Peking man 100 000 BC *H sapiens* had a 1400 cc CC, lived in caves; some of his paintings survive; at the time, the planet's population was 2 million; the swarthy, widely-regarded-as-pretty-stupid Neanderthal is thought to have lived from 250 000–30 000 BC, and may have co-existed with the tall, more gracile progenitor of modern man, the Cro-Magnon Note: Man's evolution is thought to have been that of australopithecine ape-men and/or *H habilis*, which evolved into *H erectus,* an arguably distinct species that later developed into *H sapiens*; see Homo erectus, Lucy, Mitochondrial 'Eve'

antiadhesive therapy A generic term referring to a therapy (as yet in the theoretical stage of development) that would interfere with the adhesion of WBCs to the vascular endothelium, preventing their egress from the circulation, thus having anti-inflammatory properties (Sci Am 1993; 268/1:82)

antiarrhythmic drug CARDIOLOGY A family of agents that counteract potentially life-threatening and refractory ventricular arrhythmias; the Vaughn Williams/Harrison classification divides antiarrhythmic agents into four groups (table)

antiarrhythmic therapy A generic term for any intervention designed to reduce cardiac arrhythmias and reduce mortality; β-adrenergic agents (eg propranolol, timolol, and metoprolol) effectively ↓ mortality; other antiarrhythmic agents have fallen short of expectations, clinical trials of these agents, eg CAST I (encainide, flecainide) and CAST II (moricizine) have shown an ↑ in mortality (N Engl J Med 1994; 331:785rv); Cf Proarrhythmic effect

antibiotic-associated colitis Pseudomembranous colitis, see there Note: Although the term pseudomembranous colitis continues to be widely preferred in the literature and among older physicians, it is less precise and is likely to be replaced by the above term

antibiotic bonding A technique that pretreats plastics to be used for indwelling devices, eg intravascular catheters, in order to prevent coating by bacterial glycocalyx, which counteracts opsonization, rendering systemic antibiotics ineffective METHOD Catheters are pretreated with a cationic surfactant material, tridodecylmethylammonium chloride, which enables subsequent bonding of anionic antibiotics, eg cephalosporins, penicillins (JAMA 1991; 265:2364)

antibiotic resistance The ability of a micro-organism (generally understood to be a bacterium) to conteract the desired (bacteriocidal or bacteriostatic) effect of an antibiotic; antibiotic resistance is affected by the microbe by 1) Membrane pumps, which may be specific for the antibiotic 2) Changing the cell wall proteins or by changing intracellular protein targets and 3) Production of enzymes that destroy or inactivate the antibiotic (Science 15 April 1994)

antibiotic-resistant bacteria A generic term for any bacterial species that has developed resistance to an antibiotic to which the species had previously been susceptible;

ANTIARRHYTHMIC DRUGS

CLASS I Sodium channel blockers, which are subdivided based on their effects on Purkinje fibers

CLASS IA AGENTS slow the rate of the action potential (V_{max}) and prolong its duration, slowing conduction and increasing refractoriness; class Ia agents, eg quinidine, disopyramide procainamide, moricizine, are indicated for supraventricular tachycardia, ventricular tachycardia, and symptomatic ventricular premature beats

CLASS IB AGENTS, eg lidocaine, phenytoin, tocainamide, mexiletine, shorten repolarization and are indicated for ventricular tachycardia, and symptomatic ventricular premature beats

CLASS IC AGENTS slow the rate of the action potential (V_{max}) and prolong its duration, slowing conduction and increasing refractoriness (similar to, but more intense than class Ia agents) class Ic agents, eg flecainide, propafenone, are indicated only for life-threatening ventricular tachycardia or refractory supraventricular tachycardia

CLASS II AGENTS (beta blockers) decrease automaticity and prolong both AV conduction and refractoriness; beta blockers, eg propranolol, acebutolol, esmolol, are indicated for supraventricular tachycardia and may be of use in preventing ventricular fibrillation

CLASS III AGENTS block K⁺ channels, prolong repolarization, ↓ automaticity, AV conduction, and prolong refractoriness; these agents, eg amidarone, bretylium, sotalol are indicated for refractory ventricular tachycardia and supraventricular tachycardia

CLASS IV AGENTS block slow Ca^{2+} channels, ergo ↓ automaticity and ↓ AV conduction; these agents, eg diltiazem, verapamil, are indicated for supraventricular tachycardia

CLASS V AGENTS, eg adenosine, digoxin, are indicated for supraventricular tachycardia

ARBs include *E coli* and *Klebsiella* spp, which are increasingly resistant to third-generation cephalosporins; 25% of *Staphylococcus aureus* isolates are resistant to ciprofloxacin; 18% of *Streptococcus pneumoniae* isolates are resistant to penicillin 8% of enterococci are resistant to vancomycin (CAP Today May 1995, p51)

antibiotic-resistant *Streptococcus pneumoniae* Any of a number of isolates of *S pneumoniae* that are resistant to one or more antibiotics, including penicillin (19%, Dallas 1993; 45%, South Africa 1989-1991); and cefotoxime (13%, Dallas 1993; 9%, South Africa 1989-1991); the isolation of these 'bugs' is increasing and requires judicious use of antibiotic therapy (N Engl J Med 1994; 331:377rv)

antibody Immunoglobulin, see there

antibody-dependent cell cytotoxicity ADCC, see there

antibody diversity V(D)J recombination, see there

antibody production The production of a specific antibody requires a series of responses in the immune system Antigen adheres the surface of B cells (or antigen-presenting cells) → Antigenic peptides are internalized by surface immunoglobulin → Peptides combine with class II MHC → epitope is externalized by MHC molcules → E cell receptor and CD4 of T cells recognize the MHC-epitope complex → Participation of ligands, eg LFA-1, ICAM-1, and TICCL → TICCL → Activation of T cell signals → Activation of B cells by TICCL → Secretion of IL-4 → Formation of IgE

antibody repertoire The total set of antigen-binding specificities that can be expressed in B cells, which is a function of the number of variable (V_H = 200-1500), diversity (D = 12), and J (J_H = 4 segment) of the Ig heavy chain, as well as those of the light chains; the preimmune (ie prior to exposure) antibody repertoire is designated as the primary repertoire and the immune subtypes as the secondary repertoire

antibody titer The level of a specific antibody that is present in the circulation, usually as a result of an acquired infection; titers usually rise abruptly at the time of infection and fall slowly; meaningful evaluation of a subject's exposure to an infection requires that the specimen be drawn at two different time intervals, as one 'draw' merely indicates exposure

anticardiolipin antibodies A family of antibodies that recognize an epitope on the cardiolipin molecule; ACA are prevalent in healthy subjects without clinical manifestations, represent natural antibodies, and are indicative of a normally functioning immune system; in one study, ACA levels measured on random and otherwise healthy blood donors revealed 6.5% had IgG ACA; 9.4% had IgM ACA; at followup, most ACAs had declined to undetectable levels (Thromb Haemost 1994; 72:209)

anticardiolipin antibody syndrome Antiphospholipid syndrome, see there

anticentromere antibody An antinuclear antibody that may be found in the circulation 22% of patients with systemic sclerosis, in particular those with limited scleroderma or CREST (calcinosis cutis, Raynaud phenomenon, esophageal dysfunction, sclerodactyly, telangiectasia) complex, either independently of, or in association with primary biliary cirrhosis; see Antinuclear antibody, CREST

anticipation MOLECULAR GENETICS The tendency of certain diseases to appear at an earlier age of onset and with increasing severity in each successive generation; one mechanism of anticipation occurs is unstable DNA fragments (restriction fragment length polymorphisms-RFLPs) that increase in length as they are passed from one generation to the next, through meiosis in both sexes, accompanied by an ↑ in disease severity (N Engl J Med 1993; 328:471oa) see CAG-repeat disease

anticipatory R&D Anticipatory research and development is the focusing of research agendas on areas of cutting edge technology, with the hope that they will provide new scientific insights, and/or commercially viable products

anticoding strand The strand of the native DNA double helix that is used as the template for the synthesis of complementary mRNA

anticontrol THEORETICAL MEDICINE A method for altering chaotic phenomena, eg heart rate, in which increased chaos is imposed on the system, which appears to cause an improvement in the system of interest; it is possible that seizure activity in patients with epilepsy can be reduced by anticontrol, ie increasing the randomness of signals (Sci Am 1994; 271/5:24) Cf Control

anticytoplasmic antibody Antineutrophil cytoplasmic antibody

'anti-dumping' laws Legislation that has been enacted in the USA to prevent the inappropriate transferral of patients who are medically unstable, eg in early labor or with impending rupture of aortic aneurysm, to other health care facilities; these laws were enacted in the wake of a case in Texas, where an indigent pregnant woman was transferred 240 km to another hospital, allegedly motivated by a financial decision (Am Med News 23 September 1991); see Dumping

anti-endotoxin monoclonal antibodies HA-1A therapy, see there

antiepileptic drug therapy A generic term for the use of any agent that is effective in treating seizure disorders; ADT is associated with changes in levels of sex hormones, causing an ↑ in serum concentrations of dehydroandrostendione, and sex hormone-binding globulin, with a resultant ↓ in androgen TREATMENT Valproate (N Engl J Med 1993; 329:1383oa)

antifolate chemotherapy The use of an antimetabolite, eg methotrexate to compete with folate, inhibiting dihydrofolate reductase, the enzyme responsible for reducing inactive dihydrofolate into the active tetrahydrofolate form; this block causes a buildup of toxic dihydrofolate, shutting down synthesis of purine nucleotides and thymidylate; antifolate therapy is used to treat malignancy; see Leukovorin rescue

anti-fungal azole see Azole

antigen-antibody complex The intimate association between an antigen and an antibody that recognizes (binds to) an epitope on the antigen; this interaction is due to conformation of the globular domains of the variable region of the heavy and light chains of the immunoglobulin molecule, which tightly interact by means of van der Waals forces and hydrogen bonds at multiple points on the antigen; see Immune complex

antigen capture assay An assay designed to detect low levels of antigen in sera or supernatants METHOD A solid surface is coated with purified high-titer antibodies to an antigen of interest; a fluid presumed to contain the antigen of interest is washed over the solid surface and the antigen, if present, is 'captured'; a second antibody with an attached 'marker', eg an enzyme, is then used to detect the presence of the captured antigen; this technique found temporary use for detecting HIV positivity, but is far less sensitive than the polymerase chain reaction

antigenic drift A relatively minor change that occurs every year or every several years in the genome of a virus, classically occurring in subtypes of influenza A, which are named based on the three different hemagglutinins (H1, H2, H3) and two different neuraminidases (N1, N2), and result from point mutations of the DNA encoding these proteins; see Influenza A; Cf Antigenic shift

antigenicity Immunogenicity, see there

antigenic shift A major change in a genome due to gene rearrangement(s) between two related organisms, eg that which occurs when two subtypes of influenza A simultaneously infect one cell; antigenic shift is rare but results in completely new antigens for which a population is immunologically 'naive', resulting in a potential for major epidemics; see Influenza A; Cf Antigenic drift

antigen-presenting cells A heterogeneous group of immune cells that present antigen (usually a peptide) to immune-responsive lymphocytes, eg CD4 helper T cells, an activity that is thought to be mediated by a peptide supply factor encoded by a transporter gene in the major histocompatability complex (**Nature 1991; 351:323, 271**); 'traditional' APCs include macrophages, Langerhans cells or dendritic reticulum cells that actively 'process' antigen; 'facultative' APCs include B cells, keratinocytes, endothelial cells and Kupffer cells, which are more passive antigen carriers; APCs are divided into: 1) APCs presenting exogenous antigen found in the extracellular fluid; these antigens are processed in the endosomal compartment of the APCs and displayed in association with MHC class II molecules, 2) APCs presenting endogenously synthesized antigen produced by all self cells processed in a distinct intracellular compartment and displayed in association with MHC class I molcules, and 3) APCs present exogenous antigen (usually octa- and nonapeptides) that is internalized, processed and presented in association with MHC class I molecules; antigens that are presented in a class II context are longer, eg 13-17 amino acid residues in length (**Nature 1991; 353:622, 605ed**)

antigen processing The sequence of steps pursued by the immune system resulting in the antigen being recognized as non-self or foreign, and thus requiring elimination; foreign proteins are encountered and internalized by macrophages, dendritic cells, B lymphocytes or other antigen-presenting cells (APC), where they undergo unfolding and proteolysis into short linear segments which constitute the antigenic determinants, fitting into the antigen-binding groove of class II major histocompatibility comple (MHC), an event that is thought to occur prior to extrusion from the cell in a subcellular lysosome-like compartment (**Nature 1991; 349:669, 655ed**); bound antigen fragments then attract the attention of passing T cells which are triggered to lyse the hapless APCs; class I MHC molecules process and present peptides generated from self antigens or viral proteins synthesized within the cells and either travel to the surface of the antigen-presenting cells 'encased' in a class I MHC molecule or are extruded from the cell and bind directly to preformed MHC molecules that are already expressed on the surface of these cells

antiglobulin test Coombs' test A test used to detect the presence of incomplete antibodies, eg anti-Rh_0 to red cell antigens; after washing away other serum proteins, the anti-Rh_0 IgG remains attached to the red cell surface; these erythrocytes may then be agglutinated by the addition of rabbit anti-human IgG raised in the direct antiglobulin test (DAT or direct Coombs' test); red cell antigens are either IgM (causing direct in vitro agglutination—due to the multiple binding sites on IgM) or IgG (which due to its small size and few binding sites is incapable of bridging the gap between two erythrocytes, due to the repulsive electrostatic forces); true positive DAT occurs in hemolytic anemia, non-specific uptake of protein on the red cell surfaces and transfusion reactions; false positive DAT occurs with insufficiently washed cells, absence of the antibody in the Coombs serum, high dissociation due to loss of antigen from the red cell membranes and low levels of IgG coating the red cells; the indirect antiglobulin test (IAT) is performed on commercial (reagent) group O cells to detect antibodies in the serum capable of causing a transfusion reaction; IAT is also used in crossmatching,

antibody screening and identification, red cell typing, determining antibody titers and D^u testing

anti-HIV hypothesis A hypothesis championed in particular by P Duesberg of the University of California, that the human immunodeficiency virus' role in the pathogenesis of AIDS is unproven; the anti-HIV hypothesis has received little support among mainstream scientists (**Nature 1994; 369:265ed**) although it has been supported by a recent Nobel laureate (discoverer of the polymerase chain reaction (PCR)

anti-idiotype antibody An antibody that binds to an epitope on a second antibody that is reacting to an antigen

anti-Jo-1 antibody RHEUMATOLOGY An autoantibody that is highly specific* for myositis; it is more common in polymyositis than in dermatomyositis, commonly associated with interstitial lung disease and is virtually absent in normal subjects or those with other rheumatic diseases
*With low sensitivity–it is positive in 20-30%

antikickback law HEALTH CARE FINANCING Legislation that was enacted in the US to prevent industries from having an unfair advantage in obtaining government contracts, where a company 'X' would offer a illegal 'kickback' fee to a person who was instrumental in ensuring that company 'X' would get a potentially lucrative contract for a service performed; in the US healthcare environment, antikickback law applies to physicians who demand illegal payments from hospital and other facilities for referring cases, as well as to hospitals that extract illegal fees from hospital-based physicians in the form of endowment, equipment and capital improvement fund contributions and non-reimbursement for part A services performed (**Am Med News 18 November 1991**)

antilymphocyte serum An antiserum 'raised' in one species against the lymphocytes of another species, which, upon injection, causes profound lymphopenia; Antilymphocyte serum formerly had currency in immunosuppression for ameliorating graft rejection

anti-metabolite Antimetabolic agent A generic term for any chemical compound that is structurally similar to a native cell metabolite, which either inhibits the enzymes of a particular metabolic pathway or is incorporated during synthesis to produce defective product; anti-metabolites are used for chemotherapy, treating viral infections, and as immunosuppressants, and include analogs of purine (eg azathioprine, see there), pyrimidine (of experimental interest), and folic acid (eg aminopterin, methotrexate, see there)

antimicrobial sensitivity test Antimicrobial susceptibility test, see there

antimicrobial susceptibility test CLINICAL MICROBIOLOGY A generic term for a laboratory procedure that is used to determine the susceptibility of a microorganism, usually a bacterium, to antibiotics; the most commonly used AST in the clinical laboratory is the so-called diffusion test in which the organism of interest is growth to confluence (ie a 'lawn') on a culture plate, usually Mueller-Hinton agar, and paper disks impregnated with standardized concentrations of various antibiotics are placed on the culture plate; the amount of growth inhibition (ie, the diameter of the inhibition) is measured; the laboratory then generates a list of antibiotics to which the 'bug' is susceptible in vitrol (and usually in vivo—Author's note)

antimitochondrial antibodies A family of antibodies that react mitochondrial antigens; the M2 antimitochondrial antibody is present in 90-95% of patients with primary biliary cirrhosis, some of whom also have scleroderma, and is directed against the ATPase lipoprotein present on the inner mitochondrial membrane; see Primary biliary cirrhosis

antimongoloid slant Antimongolic fissure A descriptor

for a downward slant of the eyelid in the horizontal plane that is opposite that of mongoloids; the finding is non-specific and may be seen in various congenital syndromes, including: Franceschetti or oculomandibulofacial syndrome, accompanied by a bird facies and in Treacher-Collins syndrome

antimongoloid syndrome An inherited disease caused by a partial deletion of chromosome 21 characterized by mental retardation, antimongoloid palpebral slant, craniofacial dysmorphia, pyloric stenosis, retarded skeletal growth, cryptorchidism and hypospadias

anti-müllerian hormone Meiosis activating sterol, see there, formerly Müllerian-inhibiting substance

antimyocardial antibodies An autoantibody commonly associated with Dressler syndrome, acute rheumatic fever and post coronary bypass surgery patients, which rarely occurs in the normal population

antineoplaston Either of two substances isolated from urinary peptides that are alleged to have antineoplastic activity and claimed to inhibit the growth of osteosarcoma and myeloblastic leukemia; the National Cancer Institute (USA) has concluded that these agents have no effect in treating malignancy

antineutrophil cytoplasmic antibody ANCA anticytoplasmic antibody One of a class of autoantibodies that are directed against certain components of granulocytes; ANCA are most common in certain forms of systemic vasculitis*, eg necrotizing vasculitis, active generalized Wegener's disease (84-100% are positive), and polyarteritis nodosa (**Arch Pathol Lab Med 1994; 118:517oa,**), as well as unexplained renal failure; there are two major patterns of ANCA: 1) Cytoplasmic ANCA, which is specific for a protein designated PR3‡; cANCA is most commonly positive in Wegener's granulomatosis 2) Perinuclear ANCA is specific for myeloperoxidase and is most commonly positive in idiopathic crescentic glomerulonephritis (**N Engl J Med 1993; 329:2019cpc**) anti-NCA antibodies are quantified by flow cytometry and indirect fluorescent microscopy, and may also be elevated in inflammatory conditions of the lung and kidney, including crescentic glomerulonephritis, and in HIV-1 infection

*ANCAs are thought to cause vascular damage by forming reactive oxygen species

antinuclear antibodies Any of a group of circulating antibodies that are directed against a variety of antigens in the nucleus, including histone, double- and single-stranded DNA and ribonucleoprotein, ANA are commonly present in the serum of patients with SLE and other connective tissue diseases, detected by immunofluorescence or immunoperoxidase; in the usual test for anti-nuclear

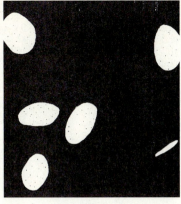

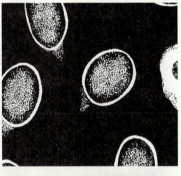

↑ **Homogeneous   Rim** ↓

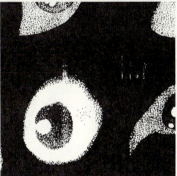

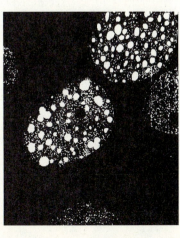

↑ **Nucleolar   Speckled** ↓

antibodies, the patient's serum is incubated with a standard tissue, eg Hep-2 cells, and the presence of ANA is detected by fluorescence microscopy (see figure); the homogeneous pattern is characteristic of ANA against ribonucleoprotein, seen in lupus erythematosus (SLE), rheumatoid arthritis, progressive systemic sclerosis (PSS) and others; the 'rim' or 'shaggy' pattern of staining is associated with antibodies to ribonucleoprotein and DNA and is most typical of SLE; the nucleolar pattern is typical of the anti-RNA ANA seen in PSS; the speckled pattern may be seen in all forms of connective tissue disease and thus is highly non-specific; see Speckled pattern

Note: Because there has been considerable variability in laboratory reporting of ANA levels, given the lack of standardized substrate cells and differences in technologist training and type of fluorescent microscopes being used, it has been suggested that ANA be reported in International Units (IU), recalibrating the standard curve each time the ANA is assayed

antinucleoside analogue Any of a family of compounds[1] that resemble natural nucleotide bases (which serve as building blocks in DNA; the pharmacologic efficacy of ANAs hinges on their selective interference with viral DNA replication, without major interference with cellular DNA replication[2] SIDE EFFECTS Short-term, minimal; long-term therapy has adverse effects on oxidative phosphorylation, which is widespread and has features of inherited mitochondrial diseases, resulting in myopathy, cardiomyopathy, neuropathy, lactic acidosis, and failure of the exocrine panceas, liver, and BM (**Nature Medicine 1995; 1:417**)

[1]Acyclovir, AZT (zidovudine), ddC, (zalcitabine), ddI (didanosine), 3TC (2'-deoxy-3'-thiacytidine
[2]Toxicity occurs when the cell's DNA polymerases are inhibited

antioxidant Any agent that is capable of reducing the highly histotoxic oxygen reduction products and reactive oxygen species, eg the hydroxyl radical, which derive from superoxide anion ($O_2\cdot^-$) and H_2O_2, the univalent and bivalent reduction products of oxygen generated during the normal intermediary metabolism of the respiratory chain; antixodants include glutathione, α-tocopherol (vitamin E), bilirubin; see Free radical, Superoxide dismutase

antioxidant therapy A generic term for the use of any agent (eg antioxidant vitamins, glutathione reductase, superoxide dismutase) to 'scavenge' oxygen free radicals (OFRs) or excited oxygen molecules, which are byproducts of normal metabolic reactions; excess OFRs have been linked to cancer secondary to OFR-induced DNA damage, and to cardiovascular disease secondary to OFR-induced oxidation of LDL-cholesterol to a more atherogenic form; in cardiology AT attempts to block the oxidative modification of low-density lipoprotein, which is thought to be an early step in fatty streak development, atherogenesis, and atherosclerosis-related pathologies, including coronary artery disease and cerebrovascular accidents; while antioxidant therapy has yet to be implemented, there is evidence in experimental animals that the antioxidant probucol may have an atheroreductive effect, and epidemiological evidence points a negative correlation between coronary disease and increased levels vitamin E and selenium, both of which have antioxidant activity

*Note: The jury is still out as to whether antioxidant therapy is effective in preventing cancer, and as of 1994, skepticism about such claims appears to be appropriate (**N Engl J Med 1994; 330:1080ed**)

antioxidant vitamin Any vitamin, eg beta carotene (provitamin A) or alpha-tocopherol (vitamin E) with antioxidant activity; data are equivocal as to whether AVs are effective in preventing cancer, with some recent data suggesting that it is not (**N Engl J Med 1994; 330:1029oa**) see Antioxidant therapy

antiparietal cell antibody An autoantibody that occurs in pernicious anemia (PA), severe atrophic gastritis and autoimmune thyroiditis, patients with PA may also have antithyroid antibodies; APCA is also found in 3% of the normal population and increases with age

antipersonnel An adjective referring or pertaining to any device or maneuver intended to disable, wound, maim, or kill persons, in particular military personnel

antiphospholipid antibodies see Anticardiolipin antibodies, Lupus anticoagulants

antiphospholipid antibody syndrome Circulating lupus anticoagulant syndrome, anticardiolipin antibody syndrome, lupus anticoagulant-antiphospholipid antibody syndrome A ' *thrombophilic disorder in which venous or arterial thrombosis, or both, may occur. The serologic markers are antiphospholipid antibodies (anticardiolipin antibodies, the lupus anticoagulant, or both)* **N Engl J Med 1995; 332:993oa**); the APAS is clinical condition characterized by the presence of circulating antiphospholipid antibodies (APA), in particular against cardiolipin (ACA, here used interchangeably), which overlap with lupus anticoagulants; APAs are identified in patients with SLE, and are associated with thromboembolic phenomena, which is classically accompanied by

1) HABITUAL ABORTION, with mid-pregnancy fetal wastage due to thrombosis of placental vessels, recurrent MI (coronary thrombosis), pulmonary hypertension, occasionally also renal infarction; less common manifestations include livido reticularis, valvular heart disease, labile hypertension, a positive Coombs' test, recurrent digital gangrene, often in a background of SLE; thrombosis may be related to the antibodies that inhibit PGI$_2$ (prostacyclin) production and interfere with the release of arachidonic acid from the cell membrane

2) NEUROLOGIC DYSFUNCTION (amaurosis fugax, cerebrovascular accidents, chorea, epilepsy, Guillain-Barré syndrome, migraines, multiple sclerosis-like disease, myelopathy, transient ischemic attacks); APA is thought to cause disease by acting on platelet membranes or vascular endothelia; high titers (> 7 standard deviations) of IgG ACA are reported to be 80% specific for this condition Note: In absence of previous spontaneous fetal loss, elevation of ACA was not a risk factor for fetal wastage (**N Engl J Med 1991; 325:1063**); ACAs cross-react with DNA, explaining the biological false positive serological test for syphilis commonly seen in SLE; increased APAs are found in the autopsy population with higher incidence of thromboembolism; APA occur in transient ischemic attacks and cardiac valve replacement (**Arch Pathol Lab Med 1994; 118:491oa**)

MANAGEMENT Long-term anticoagulation with warfarin, maintaining the INR (international normalized ratio, see there) ≥ 3 (**N Engl J Med 1995; 332:993oa**)

Note: ACAs and APAs are often associated with but are not identical to the lupus antibodies, ie an elevated ACA titer may not always coexist with a positive LA test (**Arch Pathol Lab Med 1993; 117:595oa**) Cf Lupus anticoagulant

antiplatelet therapy A generic term for any form of therapy intended to inhibit platelet adhesion and/or aggregation, platelet activities increase the complications of atherosclerosis

antiporter Na$^+$/H$^+$ antiporter, see there

antipromoter ONCOLOGY Any substance that blocks the action of a promoter molecule in carcinogenesis, potentially acting at any stage in the transformation sequence; these substances include dietary fiber, vitamins A, C and E, selenium, indoles, flavones and isothiocyanates; see Tumor promoter

anti-PRP antibody A serotype-specific antibody against the bacterial polyribosylribitol phosphate, which confers protection against invasive *Haemophilus influenzae* infection; anti-PRP antibody may be induced by vaccination with the *H influenzae* type b polysaccharide or the PRP-CRM vaccines, and is indicated for children and in the AIDS population (**N Engl J Med 1991; 325:1837**) see AIDS, Hib

anti-Purkinje cell antibody A circulating antibody that has been associated with subacute cerebellar degeneration and gynecologic, especially ovarian malignancy

anti-receptor antibody A generic term for an autoantibody directed against a substrate's receptor, which is capable of altering the cell's response to that substance; ARA are pathogenically linked to endocrine disorders, either increasing or decreasing hormonal activity, and are directed against the corticotropin, H$_2$, parathyroid, islet β cell, insulin, thyrotropin (TSH), gastrin and follicle-stimulating hormone; see Autoimmunity

Note: Other autoimmune antibodies occur in endocrine diseases, including anti-cytoplasmic antibodies that cause cell destruction and anti-trophic hormone antibodies that impact on a cell's growth or function

anti-reticulin antibodies An autoantibody that is highly specific (>98%), but relatively insensitive (25-30%) for the presence of celiac (coeliac) disease

anti-Scl-70 Anti-topoisomerase I antibody An autoantibody that occurs in 43% of patients with diffuse scleroderma and in 18% of those with limited scleroderma

antisense DNA A short sequence of that is complementary to messenger RNA (mRNA) and therefore capable of binding thereto BACKGROUND DNA is composed of two nucleotide helices; when a gene is transcribed, it encodes a chain of mRNA that is translated into a protein; the helix opens, revealing a 'sense' strand and an 'antisense' strand of DNA; the antisense strand of DNA acts as a template, yielding a sense mRNA; the other, *SENSE* strand of DNA encodes an *ANTISENSE* mRNA, which controls the production of certain enzymes; antisense mRNA can link to its mirror image sense mRNA, preventing translation; the possibilities for this technology, potentially representing a new therapeutic tool, direct antisense oligonucleotides against viral sequences and activated oncogenes; see Triple helix (**Sci Am 1990; 262/1:40**)

antisense oligonucleotides see Antisense DNA, Antisense RNA

antisense RNA A sequence of RNA nucleotides that is complementary to native or 'sense' mRNA transcribed from DNA; the combination of the sense and antisense RNA serve to block the translation of DNA into protein and thus serve to regulate DNA activity; antisense RNA may be produced from altered DNA for the packaging sequence of retroviral RNA, preventing it from binding with the packaging protein, thus yielding new (but empty) viral particles without the genetic information needed to infect other cells; such antisense strategies might be of use in protecting HIV-infected patients, possibly by introducing the antisense message into stem cells; Cf Antisense DNA

antisense therapy An as-yet hypothetical therapeutic modality for treating tumors and viral disease that would be based on antisense RNA, where complementary strands of nucleotides are used to turn off defective genes, and is of potential use in agriculture (Science 1991; 253:510ed); antisense therapy would consist of administering an antisense DNA or an RNA strand mirror-image of an oncogene's mRNA 'sense' strand; since the mRNA can only act in a single-stranded state, the oncogene cannot 'drive' tumor proliferation; interference with a regulatory gene could potentially evoke translational arrest, a goal being actively pursued in AIDS research, targeting HIV-1's rev (art/trs), using antisense phosphorothioate oligodeoxynucleotides

anti-sperm antibody Any of a group of antibodies produced against four distinct components of the sperm; low titers (< 1:8) of anti-sperm antibody are present in 90% of prepubertal boys and are of no significance; up to 50% of infertile females have anti-sperm antibody titers of 1:16 or greater, most commonly in the form of anti-sperm (immobilizing) tail IgG or IgA antibodies, while male homosexuals tend to develop anti-sperm head (agglutinating) IgM antibodies

'antistenotic' therapy CARDIOLOGY A generic term for any therapy or device designed to prevent or eliminate the complete blockage of a stenosed coronary artery at potential risk for an acute ischemic event; antistenotic approaches include dilation of sclerosed vessel by balloon catheterization, removal of atheromatous plaques by lasers or by mechanical atherectomy, or replacement of the stenosed vessels by metallic or bioabsorbable stents (JAMA 1991; 266:3397n&v)

antistreptolysin O assay A serologic test that monitors group A β-hemolytic streptococcal infection, ie 'strep throat' (90% positive) and acute streptococcal glomerulonephritis (± 25% positive); untreated patients have a 4-fold increase in IgM antibody titers (measured in Todd units, TU) within 3 weeks of onset; early penicillin suppresses and/or delays the ASO response, < 166 TU is the usual cutoff for 'normal'; > 250 TU in adults and > 333 TU in children is evidence of recent infection; ASO levels may also increase in acute rheumatic fever; the test is based on the principle of hemolysis inhibition; 1 unit of streptolysin O is added to serial dilutions of the patient's blood and incubated; the highest dilution that inhibits red cell lysis forms the basis for Todd units, the reciprocal of endpoint dilution; ASO titers are most useful for confirming the diagnosis of group A streptococcus-related acute rheumatic fever or acute glomerulonephritis; the standard method for measuring ASO levels has been the serological assay, which is complicated, labor-intensive and time-consuming; ASO may be more easily measured by rate nephelometry (Am J Clin Pathol 1995; 103:396oa)

Note: Cholesterol interference must be eliminated from the test sample

antistriational antibody An autoantibody found in 80-100% of patients with myasthenia gravis and thymoma, but in ≤ 18% of patients with myasthenia gravis without thymoma; 25% of rheumatoid arthritis patients treated with penicillamine also develop AStrA

antisubstitution laws Any form of legislation or regulations that prevent a pharmacist from substituting generic (almost invariably cheaper) alternative drugs for those prescribed by a physician when he/she specifies 'dispense as written'

Antitampering Act A US federal law (PL 98-127) that criminalizes tampering (changing the labeling or content)

of non-prescription ingestible consumer products; tampering with pharmaceuticals carries a fine of $25-100 000 and imprisonment of up to 20 years; see Cyanide

Note: The ATA legislation was enacted on the heels of an incident (the Tylenol® incident) in the early 1980s, in which a cyanide-bearing compound was placed by an unknown perpetrator in bottles containing a proprietary, over-the-counter acetaminophen, which resulted in 7 deaths in the Chicago area, a similar event subsequently occurred when a proprietary nasal decongestant was adulterated with cyanide, causing two deaths (MMWR 1991; 40:161); tampering with pharmaceuticals carries a fine of $25-100 000 and imprisonment of up to 20 years; see Cyanide

antithrombin III A 58 000 M_r α_2-glycoprotein with a single polypeptide chain that inactivates serine proteases (thrombin and other coagulation proteins including factor Xa, IXa, kallikrein and others) by an irreversible heparin-dependent reaction; decreased AT-III may be congenital, or acquired, occurring in disseminated intravascular coagulation and in hepatic disease

antithymocyte globulin ATG A therapeutic agent that has currency in treating aplastic anemia, especially in older patients and/or in those who lack a HLA-matched sibling donor; ATG is pooled monomeric horse IgG prepared from the plasma or serum of several healthy horses hyperimmunized with human thymic lymphocytes; commercial ATG contains 50 mg/ml of equine immunoglobulin and its therapeutic use is associated with 50% marrow recovery compared to no recovery without therapy SIDE EFFECTS Serum sickness occurs in most of those treated, rarely, anaphylaxis

antithyroid drugs A family of therapeutic agents, eg propyl-thiouracil and methimazole, containing thiourea's thiocarbamide radical, which inhibits thyroid hormone 'organification', ie the incorporation of oxidized iodide into tyrosine residues in the thyroid hormone precursor molecule, thyroglobulin; antithyroid agents are used to treat children, young adults and pregnant women with Graves' form of hyperthyroidism, but are not generally used for hyperfunctioning tumors or for Hashimoto's disease SIDE EFFECTS Occur in 1–5% and include rash, fever, urticaria, arthritis, transient leukopenia; agranulocytosis (0.5%), toxic hepatitis, and rarely aplastic anemia

antitrust laws Legislation and statutes that limit the ability of an organization or group of individuals to monopolize a service (or product), thereby controlling and restricting free trade; in the US, physicians may be prevented from certain vehicles of professional organization by antitrust laws, reducing the art of medicine to the equations of commerce; antitrust laws prohibit collective (or concerted) action that restrains trade unless an exception applies; antitrust analysis therefore addresses the issues of collective action, restraint of trade and exceptions; analysis is most complex in the issues of restraint of trade, in which the courts use 2 analytical methods, the 'per se' rule and the 'rule of reason'; the 'per se' rule is applied to types of conduct that clearly anticompetitive, eg agreements to allocate territory, economic group boycotts, and price-fixing; the rule of reason refers to any conduct that promotes competition or at least is competitively neutral is said to be reasonable (CAP Today 1994; 8:54)

antituberculosis drugs Isoniazid, rifampin, ethambutol, streptomycin, pyrazinamide, ethionamide, para-aminosalicylic acid, kanamycin, cycloserine, capreomycin, ciprofloxacin, amikacin; multidrug-resistant isolates of *Mycobacterium tuberculosis* are most commonly resistant to isoniazid and rifampin (Arch Pathol Lab Med 1993; 117:876oa)

anti-tumor necrosis factor-α monoclonal antibody TNF-α-MAb A murine IgG1 monoclonal antibody produced against TNF-α that has been used in clinical 'phase I' trials as a possible treatment of patients with sepsis syndrome (SS); a slight decrease in mortality has been reported with the use of TNF-α-MAb vis-a-vis placebos; the difference did not reach statistical significance (JAMA

1995; 273:942ₒₐ)

antler pattern Staghorn pattern, see there

ANUG Acute necrotizing ulcerative gingivitis, see there

⊞aortic arches EMBRYOLOGY *Arcus aorticus I-VI* [NE3] An array of six paired arteries that connect the dorsal and ventral aorta on each side; arise from the aortic sac in conjunction with the branchial arches formed in the fourth and fifth weeks of embryologic development, the vast bulk of which disappears shortly thereafter; the residuum of the 1st arch corresponds to the adult maxillary artery, the 2nd arch gives rise to the hyoid and stapedial arteries; the 3rd aortic arch forms the common carotid and the first segment of the internal carotid artery; the 4th arch persists on both sides of the embryo, forming part of the adult aortic arch on the left and the most proximal segment of the right subclavian artery on the right; the 5th arch is transient and disappears; the 6th arch gives rise to the proximal segment of the right pulmonary artery on the right and the ductus arteriosus on the left side; Cf Pharyngeal arches

aortic arch syndrome Takayasu's arteritis, see there

aortic dissection A condition occurring in an estimated 2000 people/year (US) it is characterized by the presence of a second (false) lumen within the aortic wall; dissection occurs when blood flows into a torn tunica intima of an aortic wall weakened by cysic medial necrosis, which follows degeneration of the elastic tissue and collage of the tunica media HIGH RISK GROUPS Older men, pregnant women, blacks, those with systemic hypertension, connective tissue diseases, vasculitis or congenital aortic coarctation; it may be induced by the trauma of the cardiac catheterization and exercise CLINICAL Hypotension asociated with loss of consciousness due to compromise of the brachiocephalic vessels, reactive hypertension, pulse-blood pressure dissociation and focal neurologic defects due to involvement of the spinal arteries RADIOLOGY Abnormal chest films with widening the mediastinal silhouette, an abnormal aortic contour, left-sided pleural effusion, a disparity of the luminal diameter between the ascending and descending aorta and separation of intimal calcification ≥ 0.5 cm from the outer edge of the soft tissue border of the aorta ('calcium sign'); other abnormalities may be seen by aortic angiography, as well as by echocardiography, CT, and MRI TREATMENT Sodium nitroprusside, β-blockers, ganglion blockers (eg trimethaphan camsylate), calcium blocker; blood flowing into a dissection may re-flow into the aortic lumen if there is a second intimal tear or may rupture into the pleural or pericardial cavities, with potential fatal consequences (Hosp Pract 28 Feb 1991) MORTALITY 21% of untreated AD die in the first 24 hours; 90% within 3 months

aortic nipple sign RADIOLOGY A normal variation of the cardiac shadow seen on a plain chest film at the aortic arch, causing the unwary to misdiagnose a tumor or lymphadenopathy; the 'nipple' corresponds to the left superior intercostal vein, enlarged when it serves as collateral circulation (Radiology 1970; 95:533)

AP-1 family MOLECULAR BIOLOGY A family of transcription factors that includes the proto-oncogene products c-Jun and c-Fos, which control the stimulation of cellular genes by growth factors and expression of oncogenes, eg *src* and *ras*; the AP-1 family binds to the DNA binding site TGACTCA, an 'enhancer' region incriminated in tumor induction by tumor promoters; AP-1 may be an intermediate in transmitting information from the cell surface via protein kinase C to the nucleus; homodimeric c-Jun can bind directly to the AP-1 recognition site, but the homodimeric c-Fos only participates in the binding as heterodimeric cFos/cJun, joined by a leucine zipper motif, explaining how heterologous proto-oncogenes function; recent studies suggest that signal transduction may increase c-Jun's and AP-1's transcriptional activity by interrupting the c-Jun:inhibitor interaction (Nature 1991; 352:165); see Leucine zipper

AP-2 A mammalian transcription factor, ie a retinoic acid inducible, sequence-specific DNA-binding protein, which when dimerized, binds to cAMP and the phorbol ester inducible sequence motif found in the cis-regulatory regions of various viral and cellular genes (Science 1991; 251:1067)

APACHE II Acute Physiology & Chronic Health Evaluation INTENSIVE CARE MEDICINE A 'second generation' system of objective criteria for predicting the outcome of critically ill patients in an ICU based on age, physiologic status and underlying health; it acts as a tool for scoring the severity of illness in patients admitted in an intensive care unit; the APACHE II scores total 71 points and are derived from age (maximum, 6 points), physiologic status based on 12 physiologic parameters (maximum, 60 points), chronic health problems (maximum, 5 points) and reasons for admission to the intensive care unit, yielding a weighted diagnostic component; according to one study, APACHE II offers little advantage over the simple 'eyeballing' of patients by ICU residents (physicians in training) and attendings in predicting patients' outcome; see Medisgroups, Prognostic scoring systems

APACHE III INTENSIVE CARE MEDICINE A 'third-generation' system* for estimating the probability of hospital mortality in adult ICU patients based on physiological assessments of most severely affected values during the first 24 hours in the ICU and subjecting the results to logistic regression modeling techniques; APACHE III contains more variables (27 vs 17) than SAPS II, stressing the inclusion of as much information as possible to characterize the patients; SAP II, APACHE III, and MPM II are well-researched systems for collecting ICU-related data, can be used to assess prognosis, and to stratify patients as to severity of disease for clinical trials (JAMA 1994; 272:1049cecc) see APACHE III, MPM II

*The others are MPM II and SAPS II

apartheid medicine The health care system practiced until recently in the Republic of South Africa, which was historically a 'soft' extension of the government's policies of racial discrimination; health care professionals who protested about the tortures or treated former detainees were regularly harassed or inexplicably committed suicide while in police custody; see Academic boycott, Biko, Torture; Cf 'Functional apartheid'

APARTHEID MEDICINE		
	BLACK	WHITE
Per capita health care expenditure	$51	$201
Hospitals	Overcrowded	Underutilized
Infant mortality	Black 5.6-fold > whites	
Life expectancy	13 years < white males	
Tuberculosis	Black 15-fold > whites	
Cause of death	Infections	Cancer
	Parasites	Cardiovascular

apathetic hyperthyroidism A masked hyperthyroidism, most commonly seen in depressed older patients, where the hypermetabolic state is manifest by weight loss and congestive heart failure, complicated by supraventricular tachyarrhythmias

APC Activated protein C, allophycocyanin, Antigen-presenting cells

APC gene A gene located on chromosome segment 5q21

that encodes a protein with tumor suppressor activity; it is mutated in familial adenomatous polyposis‡, and in most colorectal neoplasms, and thus may be of use as a screening tool for colon cancer (**N Engl J Med 1993; 329:1982oa, CAP Today March 1994, p1**) see Tumor suppressor genes; Cf hMSH-2

APC resistance Activated protein C resistance, see there

APECED Autoimmune polyendocrinopathy-candidiasis-ectodermal dystrophy An AR [MIM 240300] disorder characterized by 1) Various combinations of failure of parathyroid and thyroid glands, adrenal cortex, gonads, pancreatic β cells, gastric parietal cells and hepatitis, 2) Chronic mucocutaneous candidiasis and 3) Dystrophy of the dental enamel, nails, alopecia, vitiligo and keratopathy CLINICAL Hypoparathyroidism, adrenocortical failure, gonadal failure, candidiasis, malabsorption

apex beat Apical thrust, cardiac impulse CARDIOLOGY A pulsation of the heart that corresponds to the impact of the apex (left ventricular) as it rotates forward during systole; the AB is palpable or visible on the anterior chest wall in the 5th left intercostal space, and may be displaced by cardiac (eg an enlarged right ventricle or aortic aneurysm) or pulmonary (eg dilated pulmonary artery) disease

APGAR score OBSTETRICS A bedside test to evaluate a neonate's post-partum status and potential for survival in the neonatal period, based on an acronym of Virginia Apgar's name, where each of five parameters: Appearance or color, Pulse, Grimace-reflex, Activity or muscle tone and Respiratory effort, is give a value of 0 to 2, the higher the score, the better the infant will fare during the neonatal period (**Anesth Analg 1953; 32:260**)

apheresis Hemapheresis, see there

aphrodisiac Any agent, eg rhinocerous horn, that is alleged to increase libido or the duration of sexual activity, none of which has survived scientific scrutiny; agents that have a 'positive' effect on libido, eg testosterone, yohimbine and bupropion, have side effects that make any amorous gain a Pyrrhic victory; see Spanish fly, Yohimbine

apical cap sign RADIOLOGY 1) A subtle blush or shadow on a plain chest film in the left lung apex caused by blood leaking from a traumatically ruptured aorta into the pleura, indicating a need for emergency aortic aortography and surgery 2) Dunce cap sign A finding on a plain abdominal film in pheochromocytomas; the enlarged rounded tumor located in the adrenal medulla forms the 'head' and the triangular dunce-cap representing the normal residual cortex which may be pushed superiorly

apnea monitor PEDIATRICS An impedance-type device that monitors both the respiratory rate and heart rate and sounds an alarm alerting the care-givers of the possible need to perform CPR in the event of either apnea or a marked ↑ or ↓ in the heart rate; AMs are used for infants believed to be at high risk for prolonged apnea or prolonged bradycardia, which are assumed to be both life-threatening events, and high risk factors for developing SIDS; it is reported that the incorporation of event recording capacity into the device increases their cost-effectiveness (**Pediatrics 1995; 95:378**)
Note: It is not clear how many lives these devices actually save

apo- A prefix indicating the protein component of a conjugated molecule, eg apoferritin, apolipoprotein

apolipoproteins A family of molecules that comprise the protein moiety of lipoproteins; the ABC designation for apolipoproteins was first used in 1971 and subsequently popularized; coronary artery disease and myocardial infarction are associated with decreased HDL-cholesterol, in particular HDL₃-cholesterol, decreased ApoA-I and ApoA-II, and increased levels of cholesterol and ApoB-100 (**N Engl J Med 1991; 325:373**) see HDL-cholesterol

apoA The major protein (60% total) component of HDL; both ApoA subtypes are synthesized in the liver and intestine and catabolized in the liver and kidney

apoA-I A 28-kD single chain protein that activates LCAT (lecithin:cholesterol acyltransferase) and comprises 75% of the ApoA in HDL

apoA-II A 17-kD protein of unknown function composed of two identical disulfide bond-linked polypeptides that constitutes 20% of HDL

apo A-IV A 46-kD plasma apolipoprotein synthesized by the small intestine during fat absorption

apo A-IV A gene that encodes apo A-IV; allelic polymorphism in *apo A-IV* results in the substitution of histidine for glutamine at position 360 near the COOH terminus, generating the isoform apo IV-2, which attenuates the hypercholesterolemic response to dietary cholesterol (**N Engl J Med 1994; 331:706oa**) see Apolipoprotein A-IV

apoB A protein that is the major component (95%) of LDL and comprises 40% of chylomicrons and VLDL; apoB is divided into apoB-100 and apoB-48, which share the amino terminal sequences and 'kringle' domains

apoB-48 A 250-kD protein that is a major chylomicron component synthesized in the intestine, the transcription of which terminates shortly after an organ-specific RNA stop codon (UAA; a certain amount translates beyond UAA, producing a protein similar to hepatic Apo B-100); ApoB-48 has an obligatory role in the synthesis of chylomicrons and is essential for the intestinal absorption of dietary fats and fat-soluble vitamins

apoB-100 A 550-kD protein synthesized in the liver that is the major component in lipoproteins of endogenous origin (LDL, VLDL, IDL), provides the recognition signal targeting LDL to the LDL (apoB, E) receptor and is considered to be the l'enfant terrible of atherosclerosis; a mutation in ApoB-100 prevents LDL from binding to the LDL receptor, causing an elevation of cholesterol (**JAMA 1991;265:78**); ApoB-100's sequence is similar to plasminogen, thereby linking thrombosis with atherosclerosis

apoC A major component of VLDL and a minor component of HDL and LDL, divided into apoC-I and apoC-II

apoC-I A 6.5-kD protein that is a minor component of VLDL, HDL and LDL

apoC-II An 8.8-kD protein that is a minor constituent of VLDL and HDL, which activates lipoprotein lipase and is essential for the clearance of chylomicrons and VLDL

apoC-II deficiency An AR condition [MIM 207750] characterized by recurring pancreatitis; with time, DM LABORATORY Absent apoC-II, 50% ↓ apoA-I, ↓ A-II, and ↓ apoB, ↓↓↓ LDL, ↓↓↓ HDL; ↑ triglyceridemia, ↑ cholesterol; ↑↑↑ chylomicrons, ↑↑↑ VLDL, ↑ apoE TREATMENT Dietary

apoC-III A 8.7-kD protein inhibitor of lipoprotein lipase, a major constituent of chylomicrons and VLDL; apoC-III over-expression induced in transgenic mice, results in

---

APOLIPOPROTEINS

TYPE	CONC*	MW‡	COMPONENT OF:
A-I	40/110	28 kD	HDL, band 1.21, chylomicrons)
A-II	25/40	17 kD	HDL
B-100	1.7/90	250 kD	LDL, VLDL
B-48	Trace	120 kD	Chylomicrons
C-I	8.5/5.5	6 kD	Chylomicrons, VLDL, HDL, LDL
C-II	6/5.5	9 kD	Chylomicrons, VLDL, HDL, LDL
C-III	3/13	9 kD	HDL, VLDL, chylomicrons, LDL
E	1.2/4.5	37 kD	VLDL, chylomicrons, HDL, LDL

*Concentration, serum levels SI (μmol/L)/US (mg/dL)
‡Molecular weight in kilodaltons

hypertriglyceridemia

apoE A 34-kD cholesterol-binding glycoprotein that serves as a ligand for receptor-mediated* clearance of several classes of lipoproteins, including chylomicrons, VLDLs, and lipoprotein remnants; apoE has various functional subtypes; apoE3 is required to help the protein tau maintain neuronal microtubules intact; subjects with the inherited form, apoE4 are 3 times more likely to develop Alzheimer's disease as apoE4 binds poorly to tau (from **US News & World Report 22 November 1994:61**); apoE is encoded on chromosome 19, secreted by macrophages that mediates the uptake of lipoproteins (VLDL, HDL, LDL and cholesterol esters) into cells by virtue of different binding domains for each receptor

*Two receptors are thought to be involved in this clearance, the LDL-receptor and a putative remnant receptor, probably the LDL receptor-related protein

apolipoprotein E deficiency A rare cause of type III hyperlipoproteinemia, a condition characterized by ↑↑↑ serum cholesterol and ↑ triglycerides, accumulation of β-migrating remnants, and development of premature atherosclerosis; treatment of ApoE-deficient mice with transplants of normal bone marrow provides complete protection from diet-induced atherosclerosis (**Science 1995; 267:1034R**)

APOE ε 4 The type 4 allele of the apolipoprotein E gene locus located on chromosome 19, which appears to ↑↑↑ the risk of late-onset Alzheimer's disease, and has been associated with ↓ cerebral parietal metabolism (**JAMA 1995; 273:934OA**); possession of an *APOE* ε4 allele is a strong predictor of clinical progression of dementia (**ibid; 273:1274**)

Note: Specific mutations in apoE prevents the binding of chylomicrons and VLDL to the LDL-receptor (which has a leucine zipper motif), resulting in type III hyperlipoproteinemia

apopnea-hypopnea score The average number of episodes of apopnea and hypopnea per hour of sleep; a score of ≥ 5 is associated with sleep apnea syndrome (**N Engl J Med 1993; 328:1230OA**)

apoptosis Programmed cell death MOLECULAR BIOLOGY An intrinsic 'program' of cell death which is being increasingly recognized as a cellular process as complex and important as cell proliferation; it is characterized by chromatin condensation and DNA degradation and is a mechanism used by the immune system for antigen-induced clonal deletion of cortical thymocytes, ie immune tolerance; apoptosis is the most common form of eukaryotic cell death in embryogenesis, metamorphosis, tissue atrophy and tumor regression; it is induced by cytotoxic T cells, NK and killer cells, lymphotoxins, calcium glucocorticoids, withdrawal of interleukins, heat shock, viral infection, oxidants, free radicals, by some monoclonal antibodies (eg APO-1), chemotherapeutic agents (eg bleomycin, cisplatin, cytosine arabinoside, methotrexate, vincristine, and others), gamma radiation, UV light ; it is inhibited by physiologic factors (growth factors, extracellular matrix, CD40 ligand, neutral amino acids, zinc, and sex hormones), viral genes (eg adenovirus *E1B*, baculovirus *p35*, EBV *LMP-1* and others), and pharmacologic agents (eg inhibitors of calpain and cysteine protease, and tumor promoters including PMA and phenobarbital); multifocal single cell death may also occur in various pathologic states, eg water-selective channel that is responsible for the constitutively high water permeability in the proximal renal tubule and in the descending thin loop of Henle (**J Cell Biol 1993; 120:371**); there is considerable evidence that the mechanism of apoptosis is relatively conserved throughout animal evolution; in the nematode *Caenorhabditis elegans*, there are 4 steps, ie decision to die, execution of death, engulfment, and degradation (**Science 1995; 267:1445OA**); derangements of apoptosis have been pathogenically linked to AIDS, Alzheimer's disease and other neurodegenerative phenomena, autoimmune disease, cancer, ischemic injury, liver toxicity (eg by alcohol), myelodys-

plastic syndrome, viral infections, and others (**Science 1995; 267:1456RV**)

apoptotic cells Dense, eosinophilic, pyknotic cells surrounded by a thin clear space, often lying within epithelium; see Apoptosis

APP Amyloid β protein precursor A membrane-spanning glycoprotein expressed in many mammalian tissues, encoded by a gene located on chromosome 21 Note: A 40-amino acid fragment of APP, known as A4 is a major component of amyloid and accumulates in Alzheimer's diseased brains, as well as a recently devised mouse model ; of the possible alternately spliced APP transcripts, the most commonly expressed APP contains 56- and 19-residue exons; the 56-residue exon has 50% homology to the Kunitz serine proteinase inhibitors (KPI), and like KPI, inhibits trypsin; see Alzheimer's disease, β-amyloid

apparent agency MEDICAL MALPRACTICE A stance that may hold a hospital liable for alleged negligent acts on the part of independent contractors, eg ER physicians (**Am Med News 15 May 1995, p20**)

apparent volume of distribution (aVD) CLINICAL PHARMACOLOGY The ratio of the total amount of drug in the body to the concentration of the drug in the plasma, or the 'apparent' volume necessary to contain the entire amount of a drug, if the drug in the entire body were in the same concentration as in the plasma; the aVD doesn't correspond to any fluid volume per se and in the case of those drugs stored in adipose tissues, the aVD may be hundreds of times larger than the body's volume; a large aVD (eg amitriptyline, digoxin, imipramine, lidocaine, nortriptyline, procainamide, propranolol, thiopental) occurs when the majority of a drug is stored in tissue, while drugs with a small aVD (eg acetyl salicylic acid, aminoglycosides, valproic acid) are not stored in tissues; the aVD for any one drug is a constant, allowing correlation of the plasma to tissue levels; Cf Therapeutic drug monitoring

appetite center Feeding center, see there

apple core appearance Napkin ring lesion, see there

apple core erosions Circumferential narrowing of the femoral neck caused by erosion initiated by extrinsic pathological processes in the hip joint, seen in synovial osteochondromatosis, pigmented villonodular synovitis, rheumatoid arthritis, amyloidosis and multicentric reticulohistiocytosis

apple jelly nodule A finding classically associated with tuberculosis or 'lupus vulgaris', which may also be seen in sarcoidosis and other granulomatous processes; the finding consists of a small, soft, yellow-brown, 'glassy' cutaneous papule which, when compressed with a glass slide (a bedside test known as diascopy) oozes to one side (likened to apple jelly); the lesions heal with a central scar as the lesion extends outward and are thought to be sites at risk for future squamous cell carcinoma

'apple peel' syndrome Jejunal atresia A fanciful term for an AR [MIM 243600] condition characterized by jejunal atresia which becomes symptomatic at birth with vomiting of bile, which may be related to in utero obstruction of the superior mesenteric artery PATHOLOGY Twisting of the stenosed distal small intestine around the marginal artery has been likened to an apple peel TREATMENT Resection of stenosed intestine

applesauce sign PEDIATRIC RADIOLOGY A finding in infants with cystic fibrosis; the sticky meconium admixed with gas produces 'lumpy' or granular masses fancifully likened to applesauce visualized by plain abdominal films

applied kinesiology ALTERNATIVE MEDICINE The evaluation of muscles to identify weaknesses in specific muscle groups, which when stimulated or relaxed, can reduce the 'health imbalances' in the body's organs and glands AK is allegedly useful in determining a person's health status, to restore posture, improve gait, and range of motion, and normalize digestive, endocrine, immune, neural, and other systems (Alternative Medicine, Future Medicine Pub, Puyallup, Wash, 1994) Note: There is no data on the efficacy of AK in peer-reviewed journals; see Alternative medicine

applique red cell Marginal form A virtually pathognomonic morphology of the early ring form of *Plasmodium falciparum* trophozoites which appear 'plastered' on the RBC surface; Cf Banana form, Ring form

approach-avoidance (conflict) PSYCHOLOGY Any situation in which there is both an attraction towards something and repulsion therefrom, eg a compelling attraction towards a strongly disliked person, or a strong desire to view a horrifying automobile accident

appropriateness HEALTH CARE The use of a resource or service in the most suitable, or efficient manner possible; the definition of appropriateness of medical care (AMC) has not been standardized, given the differing vantage points of the persons or parties defining AMC; in defining appropriateness, a worker must 1) Define a medical intervention, eg carotid endarterectomy and its possible indications (up to 100 or more) must be listed, often by meta-analysis 2) Convene a panel of experts who rank the indications on a scale from most appropriate to least appropriate (most inappropriate) 3) Enlist a group of investigators and ancillary staff to abstract patient records looking for information relevant to previously defined indications 4) Match the abstracted patient record to the closest possible indication; studies of AMC suffer from a number of intrinsic problems, eg they do not factor in patient preferences (even though the indication for performing the procedure might have been inappropriate), they only study interventions that have already occurred (but not inappropriate failure to perform an intervention), they reflect the opinions of experts who may not practice in the 'real' world of clinical medicine, and finally, 'Methods used to study inappropriateness can lead to biased estimates of the rates of inappropriate treatment that may differ markedly from the true rates.' (N Engl J Med 1993; 329:1241sa) see Inappropriate; Cf Practice guidelines

'approved but not funded' A research proposal or grant application that is considered technically feasible by the major US grant-giving body, NIH, but which, given budgetary constraints, cannot be funded (less than 25% of grants in the US are funded, although 95% are considered technically feasible); approved but unfunded proposals are often excellent, innovative and performable (Science 1991; 250:1198n&v)

A protein A protein located on the U1 small nuclear ribonucleoprotein particle (snRNP) that harbors an 80-amino acid RNA-recognition motif (RRM) required for sequence-specific RNA binding

A/P ratio The ratio of actual to predicted mortality, a parameter that some authors feel is related in an inverse fashion to the quality of care provided by a health care facility, a posture that may be more a function of a populations' degree of sickness

aprotes PHYSIOLOGY Elementary ions that are either positively charged cations (Na^+, K^+, Ca^{++}, Mg^{++}) or negatively charged anions (Cl^-, SO_4^-), which neither donate nor accept protons; since they are neither acids, nor bases, they cannot act as buffers

aprotonin A bovine protease inhibitor with antifibrinolytic activity, is added to fibrinogen in 'fibrin glue', theoretically enhancing the persistence of the fibrin seal, although this effect is controversial; see Fibrin glue

APSAC Acylated plasminogen streptokinase complex A thrombolyic agent prepared from streptokinase and pasteurized human plasminogen, the active site of which is acylated to block activation by other plasma proteins, while its ability to bind fibrin is retained; although APSAC's half life in the circulation is increased (and has a longer $T_{1/2}$, than tissue plasminogen activator) APSAC is not fibrin-specific and may be associated with systemic proteolysis (Lab Med 1995; 26:323oa) see Thrombolytic therapy

APUD (Amine Precursor Uptake & Decarboxylation) system A morphological and functional subgroup (Nature 1966; 211:598) of the endocrine system, encompassing the C cells of the thyroid and ultimobranchial body, type I cells of the carotid body and paraganglia, norepinephrine and epinephrine-producing cells of the adrenal medulla, melanoblasts, pineal gland and posterior pituitary cells: APUD cells take up tryptophan, converting it to 5-HT (serotonin), which is later converted to MAO, 5HIAA; 'APUD' tissue is visualized with: Silver stains (Fontana-Masson, an argentaffin stain or Bodian, an argyrophilic stain), bichromate, diazo salts, formaldehyde-induced autofluorescence, immunoperoxidase, EM (dense-core neurosecretory granules)

APUDoma A tumor producing small peptide hormones from the APUD system; APUDomas include small (oat) cell carcinoma of the lung, carcinoid tumors of the lung, thymus, gastrointestinal tract and prostate, medullary carcinoma of the thyroid, pancreatic islet cell tumors, malignant melanomas and ganglioneuroma CLINICAL Heterogeneous, reflecting the functional nature of the tumor and/or metastases PATHOLOGY APUDomas are tumors with a 'neuroendocrine' appearance characterized by sheets of intermediate and relatively monotonous 'blue cells', and which by EM demonstrate dense core or neurosecretory granules; see MEN

aquaporins A family of structurally-related water channel proteins that regulate the movement of water across cell membranes; aquaporins-1, 2, and 3 are highly expressed in the kidneys, aquaporin-4 in the brain, and aquaporin-5 in salivary, lacrimal, and respiratory tissues (N Engl J Med 1995; 332:1575ed)

aquaporin-1 CHIP28 A water-selective channel that is responsible for the constitutively high water permeability in the proximal renal tubule and in the descending thin loop of Henle (N Engl J Med 1995; 332:1540oa)

aquaporin-2 A 29-kD water-selective channel protein that is located in the apical portion of the collecting ducts and encoded by a gene on chromosome 12; aquaporin-2 is essential for vasopressin-dependent concentration of urine and was found to be defective in a patient with nephrogenic diabetes insipidus (Science 1994; 264:92oa); A-2 is detectable in the urine and can be used as an indicator of vasopressin's effect on the kidney (N Engl J Med 1995; 332:1540oa) see Nephrogenic diabetes insipidus

aquaporin-3 A water channel protein that is thought to regulate the efflux of water at the basolateral membrane of the collecting duct cells of the kidney(N Engl J Med 1995; 332:1575ed)

aquifer ENVIRONMENT A generic term for a body of water located in the ground; see Plumes

AR Autosomal recessive, also 1) Acoustic reflex 2) Active resistance (rehabilitation medicine) 3) Adrenergic receptor 4) Allergic reaction 5) Allergic rhinitis 6) Aortic regurgitation 7) Apical rate 8) Autoradiographic

Also 1) Amphiregulin 2) Amrinone 3) Analytical reagent 4) Anaphylactoid reaction 5) Androgen receptor 6) Anterior resection 7) Aortic root 8) Applied research 9) Arabinoside 10) Arcuate (anatomy) 11) Argyll Robertson pupil 12) Arrested relaxation 13) Arsphenamine 14) Artificial respiration 15) Asthma rhinitis (allergic rhinitis) 16) At risk

Ara-C Cytarabine, see there

AraC family MICROBIOLOGY A family of virulence factor regulators present in various pathogenic bacteria that activate transcription (Science & Medicine 1995; 2/3:16) see LysR family, Virulence factor

ARAT Acyl coenzyme A:retinol acyltransferase An intestinal enzyme that esterifies retinol (vitamin A) absorbed in chylomicrons

Arato v Avedon FORENSIC MEDICINE A legal decision from the California Supreme Court on informed consent that revolves around the patient's right to a truthful prognosis; in July, 1980, M Arato, a 43-year old electrical contractor was operated on to remove a nonfunctioning kidney, at which time cancer was discovered in the tail of the pancreas and resected; because of the extremely poor prognosis, neither his surgeon, oncologist, nor other physicians told him of his expected survival of less than one year; after he died in July 1981, his family brought a lawsuit against the physicians of record; his wife believed that had Mr Arato known of the prognosis, he would have made final arrangements for his business affairs, which he did not, resulting in the failure of the business, and substantial tax losses after his death (N Engl J Med 1994; 330:223lim, 331:810c)

arbor vitae uterus A descriptor for a developmental anomaly of the uterus characterized by two longitudinal ridges in the endocervical mucosa, oriented antero-posteriorly with complex secondary branches

arbovirus see California encephalitis, Eastern equine encephalitis, St Louis encephalitis, Western equine encephalitis

ARC AIDS-related complex, also 1) American Red Cross, see there 2) Association pour Recherche du Cancer A private French charity founded and directed by J Crozemarie that is the largest single source of funds for cancer research in France and provides partial support for 2000 research groups, raising $60 million in 1990

Also 1) Addict rehabilitation counselor 2) Addiction Research Center 3) Aggregate of red (blood) cells 4) Alcohol rehabilitation center 5) American Refugee Committee 6) Anomalous retinal correspondence 7) Antigen-reactive cell 8) Arcuate nucleus (neuroanatomy) 9) Arthritis rehabilitation center 10) Arthritis and Rheumatism Council for Research (British) 11) Asbestosis Research Council (British) 12) Asthma Research Council (British)

architectural barrier Any structure or design feature that makes a building inaccessible to a person with a disability, eg lack of ramps, narrow elevator doors, signs not also written in braille; see Americans with Disabilities Act

arctic anemia Polar anemia A form of idiopathic anemia secondary to the exposure to cold which is usually microcytic then later normocytic

ardeparin sodium A formulation of low-molecular-weight heparin (LMWH), which like other LMWHs is reported to reduce the incidence of DVT in patients undergoing prosthetic replacement of the hip or knee (Am J Clin Pathol 1995; 103:642oA)

ARDS see Adult respiratory distress syndrome

ARESLD Alcohol-related end-stage liver disease

ARF Acute respiratory failure An acute $\downarrow$ in PaO_2 to < 50 mm Hg or an acute $\uparrow$ in $PaCO_2$ with a resultant fall in arterial pH to < 7.30, due to hypoventilation, shunting or a ventilation/perfusion mismatch

Arf proteins PHYSIOLOGY A family of small G proteins that is involved in vesicular trafficking, so named for their ability to support adenosine diphosphate-ribosylation of the trimeric G protein, G_s, which is catalyzed by cholera toxin; APs function by vesicle budding from Golgi cisternae and presumably from other membrane compartments, and mediate GTP-dependent stimulation of phospholipase D (Science 1995; 268:221)

Argentine hemorrhagic fever A viral illness caused by the Junin arenavirus, named in 1953 after its city of isolation EPIDEMIOLOGY Transmitted by contact with rodent urine; 23 epidemic outbreaks have been recorded, occurring in the maize-producing region of Argentina; the high (15-45%) mortality may be reduced to 1-4% by using con-valescent serum RODENT VECTORS *Akodon arenicola, Calomys laucha,* and *C musculinus* CLINICAL 1-2 week incubation, followed by mucocutaneous hemorrhage, fever, anorexia, nausea and vomiting, fluid losses (with oliguria, hypotension, shock), severe myalgia, leukopenia, thrombocytopenia, and transient hypocomplementemia TREATMENT Rehydration and specific Junin virus immune plasma that reduces the mortality

argentaffin reaction A histological staining reaction based on the reduction of ammonical silver to metallic silver, which while relatively nonspecific, is of use in identifying APUD cells, producers of polypeptides, classically, serotonin

argentophil reaction A histologic stain, which is similar to the argentaffin reactioin, but modified by pretreatment with a reducer (which makes it more sensitive (and less specific)

arginine butyrate HEMATOLOGY A butyric acid analogue that was identified as a possible therapy for the β-hemoglobinopathies (sickle cell anemia and β-thalassemia), as these substances cause a delay in the normal switch from the production of γ globin to β globin; in one clinical trial with AB, a slight $\uparrow$ of fetal hemoglobin was observed in only 2 of 10 of those treated (N Engl J Med 1995; 332:1606oA) see Hydroxybutyrate

arginine fork An arginine-rich structural motif present on RNA-binding proteins, eg Tat protein from human immunodeficiency virus that binds to a bulged region of RNA, an interaction required for RNA transcription; it is thought that the electrostatic charge provided by the arginine is more critical to RNA binding and activation than the actual protein sequence (Science 1991; 252:1167)

L-arginine-nitric oxide pathway A physiologic pathway in which the substrate L-arginine is catalyzed by nitric oxide synthase, releasing nitric oxide, which reverses some of the changes of atherosclerosis, and hypertension (N Engl J Med 1993; 329:2002cc)

ARIA Acetylcholine receptor-inducing activity A neuronal protein involved in forming clusters of acetylcholine receptors on muscle cells, which may play a role in development and in nerve regeneration; see Agrin

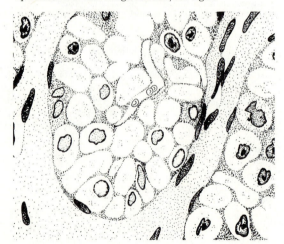

Arias-Stella reaction

Arias-Stella reaction GYNECOLOGIC PATHOLOGY A dysmorphic change in the endometrial glands that closely simulates a secretory adenocarcinoma, which is hormonally induced, and regarded as a typical endometrial reaction in ectopic pregnancy, which may be seen in trophoblastic disease, as well as in normal intrauterine pregnancies

Armed Forces Institute of Pathology A section of the

US military that opened in 1862 as the Army Medical Museum, and now comprises a collection of 2.2 million pathological specimens; the AFIP currently employs 125 pathologists and 575 ancillary staff, generates 350 publications per year, handles 350 consults/day, spends an estimated 60 000 hours/year training pathologists and has an operating budget of $35 million

armed macrophages Macrophages capable of antigen-specific cytotoxicity, 'armed' by cytophilic antibodies (IgG or IgM) or arming factors, ie cytokines from T-cells

aromatherapy ALTERNATIVE MEDICINE The use of 'essential' oils extracted from herbs, flowers, and other plants to treat various diseases MECHANISM FOR ALLEGEDLY BENEFICIAL EFFECT Aromatic molecules are thought to interact with appropriate receptors at the cribriform plate, stimulating the limbic system OILS USED Eucalyptus (*Eucalyptus radiata*), lavender (*Lavendula angustifolia*), peppermint (*Mentha piperita*), lemon oil, and others ROUTES OF ADMINISTRATION Vapor, topical (baths, lotions), or internal DISEASES ALLEGEDLY TREATED Bacterial and viral infections, herpes (simplex and zoster), dermatopathies, myopathies, arthritis (Alternative Medicine, Future Medicine Publishing, Inc, Puyallup, Washington, 1994) Note: There is no data on the efficacy of aromatherapy in peer-reviewed journals; see Alternative medicine

ARP-1 Apolipoprotein AI (apoAI) regulatory protein-1 A member of the steroid receptor superfamily that has various effects on lipid metabolism and cholesterol homeostasis; ARP-1 binds to DNA, down-regulating the apoAI gene and in addition binds to the thyroid hormone-responsive element and the regulatory regions of apoB, apoCIII and insulin gene (Science 1991; 251:561)

arrestin A vision-related protein, maximally activated by high levels of light, eg midday sun; arrestin binds to opsonin, blocking activation of transducin, shutting down rod-cell activity

arrhythmogenic right ventricular dysplasia Right ventricular dysplasia, see there

arrowhead body An organelle seen by ultrastructure, the presence of which serves to mark the transition of a *Babesia* trophozoite to gametocyte

arrowhead complex A structure seen by EM formed from heavy meromyosin, which has ATPase activity, and actin filaments; arrowhead complexes are a normal component of fibroblasts, myofibroblasts, chondrocytes, nerve and epithelial cells, and are seen in infantile digital fibromatosis

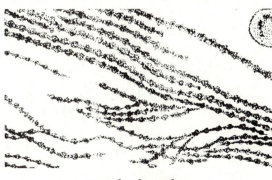

arrowhead complex

arrowhead sign RADIOLOGY Segmental dilatation of bile ducts, with sharp, conical tapering; first described in Chinese immigrants with relapsing pyogenic cholangitis

ARS Autonomously repeating sequence, see there

arsenic A toxic trace metal that is a key component of herbicides, insecticides, rodenticides, wood preservatives, and used in manufacturing glass and paints; usual fatal dose is 100-200 mg; there are ± 1900 arsenic intoxications/year (US), 85% of which are accidental by children under age 6, with the remainder being suicidal in adults CLINICAL Vague GI and neurological symptoms, and the classic clinical sign of 'garlic' breath, followed by dysphagia, severe abdominal pain and bloody diarrhea, then by renal and cardiac failure and circulatory collapse PATHOGENESIS Unlike other toxic heavy metals (eg lead and mercury), the inorganic forms of arsenic are more toxic than organic forms, with the trivalent arsenites being more soluble and toxic than the pentavalent arsenates; arsenic both uncouples mitochondrial oxidative phosphorylation, causing spontaneous decomposition of high-energy phosphate bonds, and arsenic reversibly binds to and inhibits enzymes with sulfhydryl groups TREATMENT Dimercaprol (BAL); see Heavy metals

arterial gas embolism Air embolism The entry of air into the arteries ETIOLOGY Traumatic chest injury, during various medical or surgical procedures, or secondary to distension and barotraumatic rupture of alveoli due to trapped gases in otherwise healthy scuba divers; in divers with arterial gas embolism, creatine kinase levels increase and correlate well with eventual neurologic outcome (N Engl J Med 1994; 330:190A) see Decompression sickness

arterial switch operation The surgical corrective procedure of choice for the relatively common (5-8% of all congenital cardiac malformations) transposition of the great vessels, a condition accounting for 25% of deaths due to cardiac malformations occurring in the first year of life; the 'switch' operation should be performed early to prevent development of pulmonary vascular disease

---

FORMS OF ARTERIOSCLEROSIS

ARTERIOLOSCLEROSIS, which may be
  a) Benign, associated with hyaline arteriolosclerosis
  b) Malignant, associated with myofibroblast hyperplasia, 'onion-skinning' of the endothelial basement membrane and deposit of fibrinoid material in the vascular wall

ATHEROSCLEROSIS Formed by cholesterol and cholesterol esters, covered by a fibrous plaque which, with time becomes calcified, ulcerated and causes thromboembolism of the coronary artery disease (cerebral 'strokes', myocardial infarcts, lower leg ischemia—especially in diabetics, ischemia of the large intestine)

MÖNCKEBERG'S SCLEROSIS Idiopathic and often asymptomatic annular calcified bands occurring in the muscular media of medium to small blood vessels of the extremities that have been fancifully likened to a goose's neck

---

arteriosclerosis A generic term for arterial 'hardening' (calcium deposition, thickening by fibrous tissue deposition with loss of elasticity) forms of arteriosclerosis including atherosclerosis (in which there is lipid deposition), Mönckeberg's sclerosis, and arteriolosclerosis; see Atherosclerosis

arteriovenous malformation A potentially fatal congenital intracranial anomaly with large arteries feeding in a mass of communicating vessels which empty into large draining veins filled with 'arterialized' blood; AVMs present as subarachnoid hemorrhage and mass effects potentially producing hydrocephalus; 7% of subarachnoid hemorrhages are due to cerebrovascular malformations, including capillary and venous angiomas and capillary telangiectasias

artesunate A qinghaosu derivative that rapidly clears *Plasmodium falciparum* but up to 50% relapse, unless mefloquine is added to the regimen (Lancet 1992; 339:821)

arthritis mutilans Mutilating arthritis A generic term for an end-stage destruction of the joints accompanied by osteolysis, which is typical of advanced psoriatic arthritis, as well as rheumatoid arthritis, and mixed connective tissue disease

arthritis panel LABORATORY MEDICINE A standard (CPT-4 code 80072) panel of laboratory tests used to evaluate possible causes of arthritis; for Medicare or Medicaid reimbursement, it must include fluorescent antibody screen, quantification of rheumatoid factor and uric acid, nonautomated erythrocyte sedimentation rate (see **CAP Today March 1993**)

artifact A substance or signal that interferes with or obscures the interpretation of a study, or a structure that is not representative of a specimen's in vivo state, or which does not reflect the original sample, but which is rather the result of the isolation procedure, its handling or other factors; artifacts occur in electronic readout devices, eg EEG, EKG and EMG, due to loose leads or electrical contacts HISTOLOGY Tissue processing artifacts, see 'Floaters' RADIOLOGY The artifact seen depends on the procedure, eg Barium enema, where zones of inconstant segmental contractions of the colon may be confused with organic constrictions or anatomic variations, due to mucosal or intramural tumors

artificial blood Artificial oxygen carrier A substance that is used to transport oxygen; while blood (ie erythrocytes) is the ideal vehicle for transporting oxygen, it 1) May transmit infection, eg HIV, hepatitis B, and others, 2) Is immunologically foreign to the recipient, potentially eliciting an immune reaction, and 3) Is unacceptable to certain religious groups, eg Christian Scientists, Jehovah's Witnesses*; in most situations, a blood loss of 20-25% is well tolerated and crystalloids, eg dextrose, are adequate to raise the blood volume to acceptable levels; the ideal artificial blood should 1) Be nontoxic, 2) Have an oxygen on- and off-loading or P_{50} similar to red cells, 3) Have a reasonable serum half-life, 4) Maintain adequate oncotic pressure; few substances have these properties and none have FDA approval; some candidates include: perfluorochemicals (**Fluosol, Green Cross, Osaka Japan**), synthetic chelaters of oxygen and polymerized, stroma-free pyridoxylated hemoglobin (**Poly SFH-P, Northfield, Northfield, Illinois**); the major impediment to the use of hemoglobin as an oxygen carrier is that removal of the whole molecule from the erythrocyte causes dissolution of the polypeptide tetramer, resulting in molecules that filter through the kidneys, causing renal failure

Note: Transfusion without permission in the US risks a felonious charge of assault and battery

artificial dermis Artificial skin, see there

artificial eye Ocular prosthesis An artificial device used as a cosmetic surrogate for an eye removed due to a tumor of the eye; AEs had been traditionally produced from glass (hence the often used, and now incorrect synonym, glass eye), in a limited number of sizes, shapes, and colors; they are now custom-made from a combination of plastics and resins, lacquer paints, thread, and wax (**NY Newsday 21 Feb 1995; B4**)

artificial heart see Jarvik-7, Penn State heart, Ventricular assist device

artifical insemination see Assisted reproduction

artificial intelligence A philosophical format of computer programming that attempts to simulate human 'intelligence'; the AI community has been divided into those who feel computers are capable of a form of thinking, ie that human thought is virtually equivalent to a complex computer program, and those who feel computers will always be incapable of thinking, but programs can be designed to contain dynamics with components of intelligence; traditional AI programming was based on vast stores of arcane information in the form of expert systems, which may require a supercomputer; newer AI systems are based on break-away groups such as Massachusetts Institute of Technology's 'Insect lab' that use integrated intelligence systems that act with perception and are imbued with a quasi-automatic ('knee-jerk') type of common sense; the new having an impact on machine vision and sensing, automated reasoning, planning, knowledge representation and the understanding of natural languages (**Sci Am Dec 1991, p125**) see Expert system, Neural networking

artificial insemination The instillation of sperm-bearing semen in the vagina, cervix, or endocervical canal with the purpose of fertilizing an egg, and carrying a pregnancy to term; ± 75 000 ♀/year (US) undergo the procedure; AI-related infections include *Chlamydia trachomatis*, CMV, genital herpes, gonorrhea, HBV, HIV—2 cases of AI-associated HIV infection have been identified (**JAMA 1995; 273:854, 890ED**), *Trichomonas vaginalis*; see Artificial reproduction

artificial life INFORMATICS A simulation process in which purposeful entities (aka cellular automata) compete, cooperate, interact, and evolve as an artificial ecosystem (**Forbes ASAP Oct 25, 1993**) see MOO

artificial liver A cartridge containing cloned human liver cells through which the blood flows for the purpose of removing waste products; the AL may provide an alternative therapy in the face of liver failure, serving as either a 'bridge' until a donor liver becomes available for transplantation, or to support a patient with acute hepatic failure until the liver regenerates (**New York Times 15 Nov 1994; C6, Science & Medicine 1995; 2/3:58**) see Liver dialysis

artifical pancreas Any device designed to control glucose levels and optimally deliver insulin to a patient whose pancreas' beta islet cells secrete inadequate amounts of insulin; closed-loop devices, or so-called artificial beta cells, are feedback-controlled instruments with glucose sensors that adjust the release of insulin in accordance with the glucose levels; the open loop systems sacrifice the self-adaption inherent in feedback-controlled systems for the advantage of portability; see Biohybrid artifical pancreas

artificial reproduction Assisted reproduction, see there

artificial 'skin' A synthetic material designed to have the fundamental physicochemical properties of skin, including optimal 'wetting' and 'draping', leading to adherence, control of bacterial invasion and fluid loss, while eliciting cellular and vascular invasion which would synthesize a dermal matrix while biodegrading the artificial graft; artificial dermis is composed of a porous mat of collagen-chondroitin 6-sulfate strands covered by a thin skin of silastic; burn sites covered with artificial dermis heal more rapidly and have better cosmetic results than the usual grafts; Cf Split-thickness graft, Spray-on-skin

artificial sweeteners A group of substances that have a taste similar to the usual dietary sugars, glucose and sucrose, but are metabolized incompletely or not at all, resulting in a minimal net gain of calories; given the known, albeit minimal, potential for the induction of bladder cancer in the saccharine and cyclamates, aspartame is recommended for use in pregnant women; see Aspartame, Cyclamates, Sugar substitutes, Sweet proteins

artificial tears A solution containing 0.5% carboxymethyl cellulose or 5% polyvinyl alcohol, used to treat xerophthalmia, which is classically associated with Sjögren syndrome, which may also be due to sarcoidosis, senile lacrimal gland atrophy, acute or chronic infectious dacryoadenitis, eg gonococcal and trachoma or tumors, including lymphomas, pseudolymphoma, primary or metastatic carcinoma

artistic temperament PSYCHOLOGY, PERFORMING ARTS MED-

ICINE A personality 'profile' that is well-described in creative writers, artists, and composers, which in the extreme case borders on a mental illness; *'Men have called me mad, but the question is not yet settled, whether madness is or is not the loftiest intelligence-whether much that is glorious-whether all that is profound-does not spring from disease of thought-from moods of mind exalted at the expense of the general intellect.'*–Edgar Allen Poe; many artists have been afflicted by major depression[1], bipolar disorder[2], cyclothymia; and die by their own hand[3]; episodes of hypomania or mania (which are characterized by an expansion of mood, increased self-esteem, insomnia, abundant energy, irritability, rapid movement of thought and fluid movement from one subject to another) may form the 'substrate' for the creative bursts[4] (**Sci Am 1995; 272/2:63**)

[1]Which is characterized by apathy, lethargy, hopelessness, insomnia, slowed movement and thought, and total anhedonia (lack of pleasure for otherwise enjoyable life events) [2]Manic-depressive disease, which with cyclothymia is thought to be 10-20 times more common among artists than in the general population [3]The suicide rate among artists is up to 18 times the rate of the general population [4]Robert Schumann, the composer, produced the majority of his musical works in 1840 and 1849, both of which were years during which he was described as hypomanic

ASAP As soon as possible A generic term for a level of immediate need that is less urgent than 'stat' (a term that is often abused by attending physicians, who may view everything that they require for managing their patients as being extremely urgent)

asbestos A generic commercial name for finished products containing a type of mineral fiber; the USA has used 30 billion (10^9) tons of asbestos since 1900 and asbestos is a component of an estimated 3000 manufactured products; maximum exposure levels by 1976 OSHA standards are 2 fibers/cc[3]/8 hour period CLINICAL Disease is graded according to the severity of peribronchial fibrosis, although fibers may not be found within the plaques PATHOLOGY Calcified fibrous plaques on serosal surfaces, benign or malignant mesotheliomas Note: Mesotheliomas, although characteristic of asbestos exposure, may also be induced in experimental models by nickel, viruses, and radiation; asbestos may induce gastrointestinal, hematopoietic, kidney and ovarian neoplasia, pleural calcification and non-malignant respiratory disease and peritoneal mesotheliomas; at highest relative risk for mesothelioma are workers exposed to fibers with the greatest length-to-diameter ratio, eg crocidolite which affects miners in South Africa and western Australia Note: These fibers were once used in a cigarette filter-making process and the exposed workers had an 8-fold increase in cancer and 14-fold increase in non-malignant respiratory disease; amosite fibers are known high-risk fibers, causing mesothelioma in miners, insulators and factory workers; tremolite fibers mined in Greece and inculpated in the 'Metsovo lung' are associated with a moderate risk for future mesothelioma and chrysotile fibers; 'Canadian' (white) asbestos, which have a low risk of malignancy; anthophyllite fibers and serpentine fibers have no known malignant potential; fibers are quantified based on bleach digestion of wet formaldehyde-fixed tissue, which reveals a broad range of asbestos fibers and related ferruginous bodies; control subjects have less than 10 bodies per gram of tissue; patients with asbestosis and mesothelioma have from 0 to 2000/gram

asbestos standards OCCUPATIONAL MEDICINE A set of rules and standards promulgated by the OSHA that limits exposure to asbestos fibers; under the new regulations, the PEL (permissible exposure limit) for all types of asbestos fibers is 0.1 fiber/cm[3]; building owners must disclose the presence of asbestos in the buildings, and put into place a worker protection scheme that attempts to link the most stringent controls with the hazardous working conditions; the rules are designed to protect the 4 million US workers how are employed in construction, general industry, and shipbuilding, and are estimated to cost $360 million

ascertainment The means by which a person or population with a particular trait is selected for inclusion in a genetic study, where certain factors, eg whether or not a proband has a smoking spouse, are considered as criteria for inclusion or exclusion

ASCII American Standard Code for Information Interchange COMPUTERS A 7-bit computer code used to encode a set of 128 characters, including the upper– and lowercase letters of the English and other alphabets, various special, numeric and control characters and symbols; ASCII files are used by most computer systems to transmit raw data

ascites A pathological accumulation of fluid in the peritoneum, most commonly a complication of a decompensatory phase of previously asymptomatic chronic liver disease; ascites develops in 50% of those with compensated hepatic cirrhosis; once it develops in a cirrhotic background, it has a 50% two-year survival ETIOLOGY-HEPATIC ORIGIN Cirrhosis, alcoholic hepatitis, massive metastases to liver, fulminant hepatic failure, vascular compromise (cardiac failure, Budd-Chiari syndrome, portal vein thrombosis, veno-occlusive disease, fatty liver of pregnancy) EXTRAHEPATIC ORIGIN Peritoneal carcinomatosis, peritoneal TB, biliary or pancreatic ascites, nephrotic syndrome, serosal inflammation CLINICAL Abdominal distension which, if extreme, causes dyspnea, portal hypertension, retention of water and sodium LABORATORY Hypoalbuminemia, ascitic fluid has a specific gravity of 1.010 and a protein content of $\leq$ 3% TREATMENT Paracentesis, reduced sodium diet and diuretics, liver transplant, peritoneal shunt, transjugular intrahepatic porotosystemic shunt (TIPS), extracorporeal ultrafiltration and reinfusion (**N Engl J Med 1994; 330:337**OA)

ascorbate-cyanide test HEMATOLOGY A sensitive measure of increased susceptibility paired with those from identical blood enriched with glucose or ATP prior to incubation, allowing the stratification of hemolytic anemias (glucose-6-phosphate dehydrogenase, pyruvate kinase, hereditary spherocytosis and others) into three abnormal patterns; because it is cumbersome, it is rarely used; Cf Autohemolysis test

ASCP American Society of Clinical Pathologists A voluntary agency in the US that certifies laboratory technologists–title: MT(ASCP); the quality of laboratory services based on scores in proficiency examinations is higher in laboratories that employ greater percentages of MT(ASCP) technologists (**Arch Pathol Lab Med 1992; 116:820**OA)

ASCUS Atypical squamous cells of undetermined significance, see there

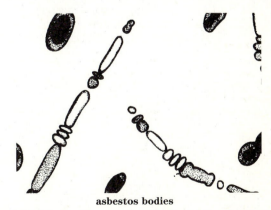

asbestos bodies

ash leaf lesion DERMATOLOGY An oblong hypopigmented cutaneous macule, simulating the leaf of the green ash (*Fraxinus lanceolata*), seen by a Wood lamp in children with tuberous sclerosis, where the presence of three or more such lesions is diagnostic; Cf Oak leaf configuration, neurofibromatosis

ASIA motor score American Spinal Injury Association motor score A clinical tool used to evaluate neuromuscular dysfunction in patients with spinal cord injury, in which the strength of 20 specific muscles in the body is assigned a value from 1 to 5 for a total of 100 in absence of motor dysfunction to 0 in complete quadriplegia (**N Engl J Med 1991; 324:1849**)

'Asian esophageal cancer belt' A region of Central Asia extending from the Caspian littoral region in Iran to the northern provinces of China with a very high (prevalence/100 000) 110 ♂, 184 ♀ (Mazandaran province of Iran) incidence of esophageal carcinoma; in contrast, the US prevalence of esophageal carcinoma ranges from 1.2 in white ♀ to 15.6 in black ♂

ASO 1) Allele-specific nucleotide hybridization 2) Antistreptolysin O, see there

aspartame Nutrasweet® An artificial sweetener that is a dipeptide ester of aspartic acid and phenylalanine, discovered in 1965, approved by the FDA in 1983, which appears to be safer than saccharin (with the notable exception of patients with phenylketonuria), although some 'soft' experimental data has indicated an association with brain tumors ADVERSE REACTIONS Symptoms rarely reported with ingestion of large amounts of aspartame include mild depression, headaches, insomnia, loss of motor control, nausea, seizures and others (**Quarterly report on Adverse Reactions Associated with Aspartame; US FDA, April 1 1988**) see Artificial sweeteners

aspartame

aspartate aminotransferase Formerly GOT, glutamate oxaloacetate transaminase AST A cytoplasmic and mitochondrial transaminase enzyme [**EC 2.6.1.1**] that catalyzes the reaction of aspartate and 2-oxoglutarate yielding glutamate and oxaloacetate; AST is increased in hepatic, myocardial, renal and cerebral infarction, hepatic and skeletal muscle disease

asphyxiant A generic term for any gas or vapor that compromises the availability of O_2 for breathing, either by displacing O_2, eg CO_2, or by replacing O_2, eg CO (carbon monoxide)

aspiration biopsy Fine-needle aspiration biopsy The removal of minute tissue fragments by a needle and syringe under suction to prepare a smear for cytological examination or to make a cell block

aspiration cytology Diagnostic cytologic material from internal organs, eg AC of breast, liver, lymph node, prostate, salivary gland, thyroid, and other relatively inaccessible sites, obtained by fine needle aspiration; Cf Exfoliative cytology

aspiration pneumonia A condition characterized by the inhalation of highly acidic gastric content, a clinical event

most often occurring in the comatose or obtunded, and has a mortality of up to 70%; after the insult, there is progressive respiratory depression, hypoxia, tachypnea and tachycardia; the tracheobronchial tree 'sweats' thin frothy fluid while the parenchyma is acutely inflamed, hemorrhagic and edematous with atelectasis and necrosis

aspirin A widely used analgesic that is also recommended for 'thinning' the blood in patients at risk for coronary artery disease; aspirin use is linked to childhood onset Reye syndrome, and thus is an inappropriate antipyretic in children with viral infection; aspirin use during pregnancy is no longer thought to increase the incidence of congenital cardiac malformations MECHANISM OF ACTION Aspirin induces a long-term functional defect in platelets, by permanently inactivating prostaglandin G/H synthase, which catalyzes the conversion of arachidonate to prostaglandin H_2; this effect is detected clinically as a prolonged bleeding time

aspirin

assassin bug Any of the cone-nosed arthropods of the hemipteran family Reduviidae, order Hymenoptera (true bugs), the trivial name refers to their insect predatory activity; those of the subfamily Triamtominae are vectors for *Trypanosoma cruzi* (Chaga's disease)

assault and battery FORENSIC MEDICINE ASSAULT The unlawful placing of an individual in apprehension of immediate bodily harm without his consent BATTERY The unlawful touching of another individual without his consent; one incident of assault and battery may elicit two lawsuits 1) A criminal action by the state against the assailant and 2) A civil action for monetary compensation by the plaintiff claiming injury; formal (ie written) documentation of informed consent prevents routine accusation of assault and battery

assault weapon An automatic or semiautomatic weapon that holds up to 30 or more rounds of ammunition; there is little justification for allowing these firearms to be in general circulation; the broad access that Americans have to weapons of virtually any firepower is rooted in the Second Amendment of the United States Constitution, the 'right to bear arms'; recently the US Congress banned the sale of AWs

Note: Opponents of this ban, most vocally, the National Rifle Association, held (among other arguments including that of restriction of constitutional rights) that these weapons have recreational value, a claim that citizens of civilized countries with far less access of firearms might find surprising

assay A generic term for the quantification of a substance of interest by a specific chemical, enzymatic, or immunological reaction, or by detecting its biological effect in a live tissue or organism

assembler COMPUTERS A special 'low-level' computer program that translates assembly language instructions into machine language for execution

assent A term* used to distinguish the agreement of a minor (≥ 7 years of age) to treatment or research from an adult's (informed) consent to treatment or research; the concept of assent is based on the assumption that while a child has sufficient capacity to understand a procedure and agree with parental decisions, he/she does not have sufficient autonomy to request and consent to a procedure on his/her own (**JAMA 1994; 272:875OA**); the elements of assent are similar to that of informed consent, see there

*Recommended by the National Commission for the Protection of Human Subjects; a child's objection to participation in research should be binding

assigned risk   A risk that insurance companies are required by law to take, eg insuring cigarette smokers; assigned risk insurance, eg malpractice insurance for physicians, is written by an insurance company only because it is compelled to do so by law

assignment   The transfer by an insurance beneficiary (ie, the patient) to the provider (ie, the physician) of the right to receive payment from a 'third party' (ie, the insurance company); in assignment, the patient is still liable for physician fees that are in excess of that provided (usually 80%) by the insurance company; see Participation

assisted reproduction   Non-coital and/or non-natural manipulation of the reproductive processes such that one (or rarely both) of the child's genetic parents is not the rearing parent(s); methods of AR include artificial insemination of the natural, the gestational or the rearing mother by the husband or a sperm donor, ovum donation into a gestational and rearing mother, in vitro fertilization, surrogate motherhood (surrogacy), cryopreserved embryo transplantation, gamete intrafallopian transfer, and induction of ovulation with exogenous gonadotropins, and permutations of the above; multiple-gestation pregnancy occurs in 15-30% of some forms of assisted reproduction, to wit, in vitro fertilization; use of exogenous gonadotropins, alone or in combination with intrauterine insemination, is reported to increase health care costs (**N Engl J Med 1994; 331:244OA**) in addition to the issues of anonymity of donors, donor screening (as a form of eugenics) and possible commercialization of surrogacy, the legal, ethical, social and psychological ramifications of AR are extraordinarily complex as a child may theoretically have up to five (six) parents—a genetic mother and father, a gestational mother (and her husband), and a rearing mother and father; see Baby M, in vitro fertilization, Surrogate motherhood

Note: While the adjective 'assisted' is more 'politically correct', artificial is preferred in the working parlance

association constant   LABORATORY MEDICINE A value that describes the equilibrium state of a reversible reaction, eg an enzyme-substrate or antigen-antibody reaction

assisted suicide   see Physician-assisted suicide

assumption of risk doctrine   MEDICAL MALPRACTICE *Volenti non fit injuria* A legal doctrine that states that those individuals who knowingly expose themselves to hazards with potential for bodily harm cannot hold others liable if harm occurs; under the rubric of the AOR doctrine, a person who consents to a medical procedure (or alternatively, who decides to forego a therapy that has been recommended by his physician or other health care provider) with knowledge that injury is a reasonably forseeable (albeit uncommon) result, waives the right to future complaint that injury (if it does occur) was caused by the physician's negligence, assuming medical treatment was performed with proper care, and res ipsa loquitor cannot be evoked; the AOR doctrine may be invoked when a hospital employee is injured in the normal performance of his duties, or when a blood recipient becomes infected with HIV, if the blood was properly tested (and the donor was in the 'window period'), the indications for transfusion were correct, and the recipient knew of the potential risk for infection; see 'Blood shield' statutes; Cf Contributory negligence

AST Aspartate aminotransferase, see there, fomerly GPT

Also 1) Absolute sensation threshold   2) Angiotensin sensitivity test   3) Antisyphilitic therapy   4) Audiometry sweep test   5) Ayres space test (psy-

chology)

asterisk sign   An early finding by computed tomography of ischemic necrosis of the femoral head (Legg-Perthes' disease), where a star-shaped structure is formed by thickened bony trabeculae

asteroid body   A term applied to any structure with a stellate appearance MICROBIOLOGY A descriptor applied to the centrally located chlamydospores of *Sporotrichum schenckii* that are surrounded by a stellate eosinophilic material thought to be represent antigen-antibody complexes SURGICAL PATHOLOGY Nonspecific delicate, acidophilic and stellate cytoplasmic striations of intermediate filaments seen in multi-nucleated giant cells of sarcoid granulomas, berylliosis, necrobiosis lipoidica and rarely in granular cell tumors

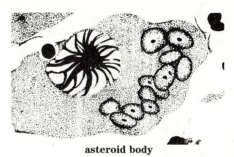

asteroid body

asteroid hyalinosis   OPHTHALMOLOGY A form of vitreous humor degeneration characterized by multiple whitish 'dots' floating in the vitreous humor corresponding to particulate calcium-lipid complexes

asthma   A chronic disease characterized by episodic dyspnea, wheezing, and cough, often related to bronchoconstriction PATHOGENESIS Exogenous allergens may cause exogenous asthmatiform attacks, reported by one group after the release of soybean dusts while filling a grain silo in Barcelona (**N Engl J Med 1993; 329:1760OA**) PATHOLOGY Bronchial and bronchiolar occlusion by plugs of thick, tenacious mucus, accompanied by Curschman spirals, Charcot-Leyden crystals, thickening of the bronchial epithelium, edema and inflammatory infiltrate with abundant eosinophils, increased size of submucosal glands, hypertrophy of bronchial wall muscle TREATMENT Bronchodilators (in particular β_2-adrenoreceptor agonists), antiinflammatory agents (especially glucocorticosteroids); others include anti-T-cell agents, phosphodiesterase inhibitor, potassium channel activators, thrombaxane antagonist

asthma triad   Bronchospasm, nasal polyps and increased sensitivity to aspirin (acetylsalicylic acid, but not sodium salicylate), to indomethacin, aminopyrine and yellow food additives, eg tartrazine yellow, FD&C yellow, #5; the triad is described in 10% of typical asthmatics and the accompanying reaction (severe bronchospasm, urticaria and hypotension) is attributed to defective prostaglandin metabolism, unmasked by these agents, some of which inhibit cyclo-oxygenase, perhaps diverting arachidonic acid metabolism towards production of spasmogenic leukotrienes; the triad may be inherited or due to environmental factors

astral fibers   MOLECULAR BIOLOGY Microtubules arising from the centrioles during mitosis, radiating from the mitotic poles toward the periphery of a dividing cell

astrovirus   A small, non-enveloped (28-30 nm in diameter) RNA virus with a cubic symmetry, that is less pathogenic than the Norwalk agent; it most often infects children, in whom it is more common than enteroviruses and one half as common as rotaviruses as a cause of gastroenteritis (**N Engl J Med 1991; 324:1757**) CLINICAL Diarrhea, headache, malaise, nauses and vomiting

asynchronous transfer mode INFORMATICS ATM A communication format that allows the isochronous transfer of multi-media type information over a network, smoothly handling videoconferencing, document transferral and sharing, and other groupware functions (Forbes ASAP Oct 25, 1993)

ATA 'box' Adenine-thymine-adenine MOLECULAR BIOLOGY A triplet of nucleotides identified as having promoter activity in transcribing the β-hemoglobin gene; single nucleotide substitutions in the ATA box result in decreased β-hemoglobin production and these mutations may appear in some patients with β-thalassemia

ataque de nervios A generic term used primarily among Latinos of the Caribbean for a culture-bound symptom complex characterized by uncontrollable shouting, crying, trembling, verbal, or physical aggression, fainting episodes, and suicidal gestures; an ataque de nervios most commonly follows a stressful life event, eg death of family member, divorce, or conflict with spouse or children; while it has features of a panic attack defined by the DSM-IV, an 'ataque' usually follows a precipitating event, occurs in absence of acute fear or apprehension, and is accompanied by amnesia for the 'ataque'; see Culture-bound syndromes

atavistic mutation EVOLUTIONARY BIOLOGY A mutation that results in the re-emergence of a trait that had been suppressed in evolution, eg extension of the coccyx into a tail in humans

atavism Any of a number of normally dormant traits, eg the presence in humans of multiple nipples, appearance of vestigial hind limbs in whales, or possibly hereditary hypertrichosis in humans (New York Times 31 May 1995; C10)

ataxia-telangiectasia Louis-Bar syndrome An AR [MIM 208900] condition that is associated with sinopulmonary infections, choreoathetosis, slurring of speech and muscular atrophy PATHOGENESIS Uncertain in genetic recombination is postulated LABORATORY ↓↓ IgG4 and IgA2, ± also ↓ IgE CLINICAL Progressive cerebellar ataxia, oculocutaneous telangiectasia, thymic aplasia or hypoplasia (cellular defect), increased susceptibility to radiation-induced chromosomal damage and carcinoma and rearrangements due to defective DNA repair; immune complexes deposit in glomeruli, choroid plexus, heart valves and synovium; increase in vasoactive amines (histamine, serotonin), IgE, platelets; presence of macrophages; antigen and antibody valences, class of antibody, antibody:antigen ratio, affinity of antibody:antigen, types of vasculature through which the ICs are passing, response of the reticuloendothelial system to the ICs; see phakomatosis

ATCC American Type Culture Collection The oldest repository of cell lines in the US (Rockville, Maryland), which contains 50 000 strains of biologicals in its regular collection, 2800 cell lines from 75 animal species; the ATCC is an invaluable resource for biomedical researchers who purchase the cells for use in toxicity assays, recombinant DNA experiments and production of human proteins Budget $12 million/year Annual shipments 35 000; the ATCC has been called the 'Swiss bank' of biology as it is a repository of biological material, including cell lines and DNA probes from researchers seeking patents and who are required to submit a sample and yet still want those secrets protected (ATCC will not release material unless explicitly instructed to do so by the researcher once a patent is issued, and then charges a small handling fee); ATCC is a center for standardization and exchange, it accepts US patent deposits and is recognized under the 1981 Budapest treaty as an international agency; the ATCC has 10 000 items in its protected inventory

Note: The proprietary rights over ownership of cell lines with commercial potential have become an issue since the case of the 'Mo' cell line, derived from a patient whose HTLV-2-infected cells (obtained from his spleen, removed as part of the treatment protocol for hairy cell leukemia) produce GM-CSF in large quantities

ATF Activating transcription factor A cellular protein that stimulates transcription of the adenovirus E4 transcription unit, acting early in infection at any of several 'enhancer' binding sites

ATG Antithymocyte globulin, see there

atherectomy The removal of atheromatous plaques from the lumen of a blood vessel, eg by coronary angioplasty (N Engl J Med 1993; 328:608oA)

atherosclerosis A condition caused by intramural deposition of LDL and calcium, secondary to exposure of smooth muscle to lipid, resulting in platelet-induced smooth muscle proliferation, see Atherosclerotic plaque; 'hard' risk factors: Hypertension (> 160/95 mm Hg), increased LDL-cholesterol (total cholesterol > 265 mg/dl), smoking (> one pack/day), DM; 'soft' risk factors include maleness, family history of previous atherosclerotic heart disease, ↑ apoB, ↑ apoC-III, ↑ total cholesterol, ↑ triglycerides, ↓ HDL-cholesterol, as well as ↑↑↑ homocysteinemia—high levels of homocysteine, a highly reactive amino acid, are toxic to vascular endothelium and may potentiate the auto-oxidation of LDL-cholesterol, promoting thrombosis (N Engl J Med 1991; 324:1149) PATHOLOGY, EARLY Fatty streaks, common in children; flat, lipid-rich lesions consisting of foamy macrophages and smooth muscle PATHOLOGY, LATE Fibrous plaque, calcification, increased intimal smooth-muscle cells, in a connective tissue matrix, containing intracellular and extracellular cholesterol Complications within atheromatous lesions: Aneurysms (dissecting and fusiform) of arterial wall subjacent to atheroma, bleeding into plaque, calcifications and thrombosis Note: The degree of atherosclerosis may be reduced by regular exercise, a vegetarian diet, fish substituted for meat and eggs, one alcoholic drink/day, and possibly various bio-feedback modalities, eg yoga TREATMENT: MEDICAL see Cholesterol-lowering drugs TREATMENT: INTERVENTION-AL (CONSERVATIVE) Balloon angioplasty, plaque scraping and plaque 'grinding' TREATMENT: INTERVENTIONAL (CONVENTIONAL) Bypass surgery

atherosclerotic plaque The core lesion of atherosclerosis, which begins as a fatty streak, an ill-defined yellow lesion that develops well-demarcated edges, then known as a fatty plaque; these evolve to become fibrous plaques, whitish lesions containing grumous lipid-rich core, which with time, becomes a complicated plaque (Arch Pathol Lab Med 1992; 116:1281oA) the AP is the initial lesion of atherosclerosis and is composed of lipid, leukocytes, smooth muscle cells and extracellular matrix in the intima of the large arteries; the plaque stage is preceded by the adherence of circulating monocytes and lymphocytes to the endothelium, with accumulation of foam cells (lipid-laden macrophages); the adhesion is thought to be mediated by a protein highly homologous to VCAM-1, a cell adhesion molecule (Science 1991; 251:788); smooth muscle cells isolated from plaques in culture, produce platelet-derived growth factor (PDGF)-like mitogens, which are thought to act as autocrine stimulators of atherosclerosis; chemically reactive lipids, eg malondialdehyde, are released from peroxidation, altering low-density lipoprotein, resulting in receptor-mediated deposition of a cholesteryl ester in the foamy macrophages of incipient atheromatous plaques; see Complicated plaque

athlete diseases see Sports medicine

athlete's foot Tinea pedis A malodorous dermatophytosis of the toe webs and soles of the feet of athletes, most common in adolescent males, resulting in maceration, erosion and pruritus due to *Trichophyton rubrum, T mentagrophytes* and *Epidermophyton floccosum* TREATMENT Drying, if recalcitrant, haloprogin and tolnaftate, if refractory, griseofulvin

athlete's heart Athletic heart A heart typical of highly trained athletes characterized by an increased left ventricular diastolic volume and increased thickness of the left ventricular wall, as seen by 2-D echocardiography; the upper limit of 'physiologic' ventricular hypertrophy is 16 mm for canoeists and rowers (and 13 mm for other athletes); ventricular walls greater than 16 mm indicate concomitant pathologic hypertrophy, eg hypertrophic cardiomyopathy (N Engl J Med 1991; 324:295); arrhythmias seen in athletes' hearts are usually benign and include sinus bradycardia, wandering pacemaker, cardiac blockages, nodal rhythm, atrial fibrillation, ST segment and T-wave changes, increased P wave amplitude and right ventricular hypertrophy

athlete drug testing LABORATORY MEDICINE Analysis of the use by athletes of substances that enhance or stimulate performace, or substances of abuse; drug classes and compounds tested include stimulants (eg amphetamine, caffeine, cocaine, pemoline, phentermine, strychnine), narcotics (eg buprenorphine, codeine, meperidine, methadone, morphine), anabolic steroids (eg boldenone, fluoxymesterone, methyltestosterone, oxandrolone, stanozolol), and others, including beta-blockers, and diuretics (CAP Today April 1992) see 'Roid rage

atomic absorption spectrophotometry LABORATORY MEDICINE A highly sensitive (to 1 ng/L) technique used to analyze various elements, especially metals, including aluminum, antimony, arsenic, beryllium, calcium, copper, iron, lead, lithium, nickel, selnium, thallium, tellurium, and zinc, which are present in trace amounts PRINCIPLE Atoms are excited above a ground state by flame vaporization, and the radiation emitted as the molecules return to a ground state is measured in unexcited non-ionized molecules

atomic force microscope A type of scanning probe microscope that is of use in visualizing DNA (Am Biotech Lab March1995, p65); AFM can be used to facilitate 3-D imaging and measurement of structures ranging from atomic to micron scale; AFM measures topography by moving (dragging) a probe across the sample to evaluate the contours of the surface similar to that of a phonograph needle, or in the case of soft biological materials which cannot tolerate the dragging, the scanning device taps its way across the surface; one commercially available AF microscope has a magnification range from 25 x to 10 000 000 x (!!!) and can be used in conjunction with brightfield, fluorescence and other optical techniques; AFM is user-friendly and allows imaging of the interaction of DNA, proteins, cell surface antigens, receptors and ligands, and other macromolecules at near-native conditions (Am Biotech Lab September 1994, p 67) see Scanning probe microscope

atopic dermatitis Atopic eczema A chronic dermatopathy affecting 1-3% of the pediatric population which is characterized by severe pruritus of early (usually in infancy) onset, and a familial tendency; it may be associated with IgE-mediated skin reactions, and allergic rhinitis and/or asthma CLINICAL In infancy, AD tends to be a weeping, papulovesicular, and intensely pruritic inflammation of the cheeks and inguinal region; in later childhood, it is more lichenified and is most prevalent in antecubital, popliteal, and collar regions TREATMENT AD is controllable, not curable; several strategies form the core of therapy, to wit:

1) Control of pruritus, eg antihistamines, and prevention of scratching

2) Identification of allergens (eg milk, eggs, wheat legumes, fish), and avoid

3) Use of anti-inflammatory agents, in particular corticosteroids

4) In older subjects, keratolytic agents can be used to treat the lichenification

atopy A state of increased sensitivity to common antigens, eg house dust, animal dander, pollen, with ↑ production of specific IgE; atopy is thought to have a hereditary component as there is increased susceptibility to hay fever, asth-ma, and eczematoid dermatitis; adjective **atopic**

atovaquone 566C80 A drug recently approved to treat PCP in AIDS patients, which is effective in patients who cannot tolerate trimethoprim-sulfamethoxazole that is also reported to be less toxic

atrial fibrillation A common type of arrhythmias, affecting ± 4% ≥ age 60, ± 11.6% ≥ age 75; ± 1 x 10⁶ (US) have atrial fibrillation, 80% also have cardiovascular disease PATHOGENESIS AF is characterized by a loss of coordinated electromechanical activity, resulting in blood stasis, and formation of atrial thrombi (AF is responsible for ± 50% of systemic thromboembolism of cardiac origin) which often 'seed' to the brain; in the Framingham study, non-rheumatic AF was associated with a 5-fold ↑ in strokes (rheumatic AF with a 17-fold ↑), and is responsible for ± 75 000 strokes/year (US) DIAGNOSIS Transesophageal echocardiography identifies those patients with atrial emboli who require short-term anticoagulation with heparin prior to cardioversion (N Engl J Med 1993; 328:750oa) TREATMENT Cardioversion

atrial 'kick' CARDIOLOGY An abrupt notch in the pressure curve in the ventricular outflow tract that is typical of idiopathic hypertrophic subaortic stenosis

atrial myxoma The most common primary cardiac neoplasm, age of onset 25-55 CLINICAL Symptoms may be obstructive (right-sided congestion, ± ascites), contstitutional (fever, fatigue, weight loss, arthralgias, myalgias, weight loss, Raynaud's phenomenon, skin rash, clubbing of digits), and related to embolism (dyspnea, pleuritic chest pain, and hemoptysis) DIAGNOSIS 2-D and transesophageal echocardiography PATHOLOGY Microcyst formation, blood vessels, nests of benign stellate and oval cells in a weakly basophilic background PROGNOSIS Excellent after complete excision (N Engl J Med 1994; 330:1143cpc; 328:640cpc)

atrial standstill A transient or permanent electrical atrial failure described in patients with familial amyloidosis and facioscapulohumeral dystrophy, possibly realted to perineural infiltration (N Engl J Med 1992; 327:1570oa) Cf Atrial systolic failure

atrial systolic failure Atrial failure A marked decline in late diastolic atrial transport, classically associated with primary amyloidosis, with most atrial filling occurring in early diastole; ASF has a characteristic transmitral Doppler spectral velocity profile and often presages a poor prognosis in patients with primary amyloidosis, possibly related to the generation of thromboembolism (N Engl J Med 1992; 327:1570oa) Cf Atrial standstill

atrionatriuretic peptides Peptide hormones derived from atriopeptigen, released from cardiac myocyte storage granules that alter 1) The electrical activity at cell membranes, suppressing ion flow at the sodium channel and increasing calcium channel permeability, a change attributed to conformational change in the channels and 2) The contractile activity of the heart; when vascular volume is increased, atriopeptin is released, increasing the glomerular filtration rate, renal blood flow, urine volume, and sodium excretion, while decreasing the plasma renin activity; when the vascular volume is decreased, a negative feedback loop suppresses atriopeptin release; ANP acts through cGMP as a second messenger, inhibiting sodium absorption across the inner-medullary collecting duct and cGMP-kinase inhibits the channel via a G protein pathway

atrioventricular block CARDIOLOGY A-V block Any delay in conduction or failure of the electrical impulse to reach the ventricular conducting system, which may arise in the atrium, at the A-V node, in the bundle of His, or in the bundle branches; A-V blocks are of 3 types:

1) FIRST DEGREE A-V BLOCK P-R intervals are > 0.20 seconds but all the P waves are conducted to the ventricle

2) SECOND DEGREE A-V BLOCK A) MOBITZ I P-R intervals increase in length until

a beat is 'dropped' B) MOBITZ II P-R intervals are constant but occasionally the P fails to conduct an impulse; Mobitz II blocks have potentially serious clinical implications

3) THIRD-DEGREE A-V BLOCK No atrial beats conduct to the ventricle

atrioventricular dissociation The independent depolarization of the atria and ventricles where the rate of the ventricular pacemaker is faster than that of the atrial pacemaker; in contrast to a pathologic A-V or third-degree block, normal conduction may occur once electrical conditions return to normal

atrioventricular nodal reentrant tachycardia AVNRT The most common form of paroxysmal supraventricular tachycardia PATHOGENESIS The cardiac reentrant circuit contains a 'fast' AV nodal pathway connecting the atrium to bundle of His, which corresponds to the normal pathway of AV conduction, and a 'slow' pathway, which has no known function; in ± 90% patients with AVNRT, the slow pathway provides the antegrade limb of the circuit, and the fast pathway the retrograde limb (thus being known as the 'slow-fast' or common form of AVNRT); this circuit is reversed in the 'fast-slow' form or uncommon form of AVNRT TREATMENT Antiarrhythmic drugs are rarely successful; catheter ablation of the fast pathway causes complete heart block in 10%, requiring placement of a pacemaker; selective catheter ablation of the atrial end of the slow pathway using radiofrequency current is reported to eliminate AVNRT with little risk of AV block (N Engl J Med 1992; 327:313OA)

'at-risk' pregnancy A pregnancy at risk for spontaneous abortion (an event occurring in 20-60% of all pregnancies); various factors weigh in 'at-risk' gestation including maternal factors, eg ↑ age, anticardiolipin antibodies, and thyroid autoantibodies

atrophic vaginitis A postmenopausal inflammatory condition characterized by pruritus ± burning sensation, prominent ↓ in vaginal secretions, dyspareunia, ± bacterial infection TREATMENT Topical (intravaginal) estrogen, which is contraindicated in those with previous breast or endometrial cancer

atrophoderma vermiculata Honeycomb atrophy A rare AR [MIM 209700] symmetric skin lesion characterized by cutaneous atrophy with sharply demarcated 'pits', variably accompanied by cardiac defects, mental retardation and neurofibromas

attending Attending physician

attending physician The physician who is on the medical staff of a hospital or health care facility and who is legally responsible for the care given to a patient while he/she is in the hospital; a patient's 'attending' is also regarded as a person's private physician if that physician cares for the person on an individual and/or outpatient basis; see Private physician

attention-deficit/hyperactivity disorder The most common neurobehavioral disorder[1] of childhood, which affects 2-6% of school children, characterized by impulsiveness, distractibility, variably accompanied by hyperactivity and/or aggressiveness, immaturity and emotional lability; although AD/HD is considered idiopathic[2], neurochemistry and genetics may play a role DIAGNOSIS PET imaging, the glucose metabolism of adults diagnosed in childhood as having AD/HD is lower, especially in the premotor cortex and the superior prefrontal cortex, cerebral regions involved in control of attention and motor activity Note: AD/HD has been associated (circa 3-fold more common) with generalized resistance to thyroid hormone (N Engl J Med 1993; 328:997OA), a disease caused by mutations in the thyroid receptor-β gene located on chromosome 3; phenylethylamine excretion may serve as a diagnostic marker TREATMENT Stimulants, primarily methylphenidate HCl (Ritalin) as well as dextroamphetamine and magnesium pemoline; see Breuning affair

[1]Designated as 314, by DSM-IV [2]Family stresses, eg divorce, parental death, depression and sickness must be evaluated prior to diagnosing a child as 'hyperactive'

attenuation A generic term for a reduction or diminution of activity, intensity, power, or virulence of a reaction, effect, or organism's ability to grow and/or multiply MICROBIOLOGY Decreased virulence of a microorganism, eg that of bacille Calmette-Guerin (BCG), a strain of *Mycobacterium bovis* that has been attenuated by multiple (238) subcultures on a bile-glycerine medium; the resulting bacterium is immunogenic, ie capable of eliciting antibody formation, but is non-virulent; live attenuated organisms are used to produce the poliomyelitis vaccine but may occasionally revert to a wild type RADIOLOGY Attenuation is the reduction of the intensity of a beam by either absorption or scattering

attestation HEALTH CARE REIMBURSEMENT A document signed by a physician stating that he or she performed the diagnostic or therapeutic procedures on a patient for which a bill is being submitted

atypical adenomatous hyperplasia (prostate) SURGICAL PATHOLOGY A well-defined lesion that occurs in the transition zone of the prostate, and is distinguished from well-differentiated carcinoma by a relative lack of nuclear or nucleolar enlargement, infrequent crystalloids, and a fragmented but partially intact basement membrane; AAH is more common in older patients with heavier and more voluminous prostates with more nodular hyperplasia, greater amounts of cancer, and (if malignant) with higher Gleason scores; a definitive association of AAH with carcinoma has not been made, but when identified in a specimen, warrants further tissue evaluation to rule out presence of malignancy (Am J Surg Pathol 1995; 19:506)

atypical carcinoid An intermediate form of neuroendocrine tumor between low-grade malignant (typical) carcinoid and high-grade malignant small cell carcinoma; in a series of 27 patients, 13/28 had regional LN metastases, distal metastases developed in 5/28; 10-year survival for an AC was 49% vs 84% for those with typical carcinoid; adjuvant therapy is recommended for those with stage III disease or metastases (Ann Thorac Surg 1995; 59:78)

atypical lymphocyte Downey cell An enlarged dysmorphic lymphocyte seen in various non-neoplastic conditions, classically in infectious mononucleosis (<20% of circulating leukocytes are atypical), as well as toxoplasmosis, CMV infection and viral hepatitis; these cells have abundant cytoplasm, a monocyte-like nucleus with basophilic condensations where they abut erythrocytes; ALs, have been divided into

TYPE I Monocyoid or prolymphocytic kidney-shaped or lobulated nuclei, with densely homogeneous hypergranular chromatin, more similar to mature lymphocytes than plasma cells; the cytoplasm is bubbly, pushed to one side and basophilic

TYPE II Cytoplasmic radiations from the nucleus ('ballerina skirt' cells); the cells have one or more nucleoli, the nuclear chromatin is less dense and the cytoplasm is less foamy than type I, containing occasional azurophilic granules, and has basophilic 'scallops' around adjacent red cells

TYPE III The nuclei are coarse, spanning the cell's breadth, have clumped red-to-purple chromatin with 1-4 nucleoli; the cytoplasm is abundant, basophilic and 'scallops' around adjacent erythrocytes (H Downey, Arch Int Med 1923; 32:82)

atypical measles A virulent form of measles affecting children vaccinated with an inactivated measles vaccine (available between 1963 and 1967), which followed exposure to natural measles CLINICAL High fever, pneumonia, pleural effusion, obtundation and an atypical maculopapular, petechial and vesicular rash with very high measles antibody titers; AM is due to the inability to form antibodies to the F protein, see there

atypical mycobacterium Any *Mycobacterium* spp exclusive of *M lepra*, *M tuberculosum*, or *M bovis* (the latter two of which cause 'typical' tuberculosis); AM are so designated because they grow more rapidly, produce no niacin, fail to reduce nitrates, produce heat-stable catalase and are highly resistant (usually, see Multidrug-resistant tuberculosis) to isoniazid; of particular interest is *M avium-intracellulare*, which is associated with AIDS and *M marinum*, seen in the Chesapeake Bay region, affecting fishermen and aquarium keepers, and *M ulcerans*, endemic to the banks of the upper Nile

atypical squamous cell of undetermined significance CYTOPATHOLOGY A cell seen in a pap smear (of the uterine cervix) that fulfills some of the criteria (eg nuclear enlargement and irregularity, cytoplasmic clearing, and thickened cell membranes) used to define cells typical of either a condyloma or a neoplasm; 12% of pap smears with ASCUS have HPV DNA (**CAP Today May 1992 p51**)

AU Allergy unit, see there

augmentation mammoplasty COSMETIC SURGERY A generic term for any of a number of surgical procedures intended to increase the size of the breasts; until recently, the standard procedure consisted of creation of a pocket above or below the pectoralis major muscle and the insertion of a silicone bag implant filled with a silicone gel, air, or saline, with the intent of modifying or enhancing the breast's contours COMPLICATIONS Capsule contraction (20% of cases), hematoma, infection, implant exposure, deflation or rupture of the implant, breast asymmetry, external scars; the complaints (and associated lawsuits) linked to rupture, and/or collagen disease-type responses, caused one implant manufacturer, Dow Corning, to file for bankruptcy (**New York Times 16 May 1995; A1**) Cf Reduction mammoplasty

'Aunt Millie' approach Pattern recognition CLINICAL DECISION-MAKING An unsound (albeit usually correct) sequence of clinical logic (**N Engl J Med 1987; 316:738cpc**), from the quip:

'HOW DO I KNOW IT IS AUNT MILLIE? BECAUSE IT LOOKS LIKE AUNT MILLIE

Pattern recognition is the traditional model for teaching pathology and radiology, both of which are visual 'arts'; although it allows molding of future generations in an accepted paradigm, exceptions to any 'rules' are generally relegated to wastepaper basket categories, as exceptions cannot be explained or understood in an arbitrarily defined context; Cf Heuristic method, Stochastic process

aura ALTERNATIVE MEDICINE see Chakra NEUROLOGY A subjective (illusionary or hallucinatory) or objective (motor) event marking the onset of an epileptic attack or a migraine

Australia antigen Hepatitis B viral antigen, first isolated from an Australian aborigine, which is located in the hepatocyte cytoplasm and in scattered mesenchymal cells; early stages of hepatitis B are characterized by sublobular involvement of all cells, later stages by scattered antigen-positive hepatocytes; the presence of HBV antigen within a population's livers correlates epidemiologically with an increased incidence of hepatocellular carcinoma in that population; Cf Dane particles

Australian X syndrome Murray Valley encephalitis, see there

Austrian syndrome A subgroup of patients (usually alcoholics) with pneumococcal pneumonia, meningitis and endocarditis with rupture of the aortic valve who present with bacteremia and despite adequate antibiotic therapy have a high (80%) mortality

author 'inflation' The growth in number of people receiving authorship credit on published reports in biomedical sciences Note: Scientific advances require multiple expertises, and credit may be shared by clinicians, molecular

biologists, laboratorians and statisticians, thus single-author papers in science are increasingly anachronistic (**N Engl J Med 1990; 323:488c**) see Mega-author paper

authority figure PSYCHIATRY A person who is or is perceived to be in a position of power or authority, eg parent, spouse; in the transference phase of psychoanalysis, the analyst plays the role of AF

authorship The state of being an author; the credits for a publication in the sciences are problematic; the advantages of being an author on published reports in the literature are considerable, and include peer respect, conferral of 'expert' status and career advancement, which is often a function of how many publications a person has generated, see CV-weighing; sharing authorship credits has the potential disadvantage of being the co-author on a report later deemed fraudulent; Dr A Relman, emeritus editor of the New England Journal of Medicine, delineated four criteria (table), at least two of which must be met to legitimately share authorship credits (**Science 1988; 242:658**)

AUTHORSHIP ('RELMAN'S CRITERIA')
1. Conception of idea and design of experiment
2. Actual execution of experiment; hands-on experience
3. Analysis and interpretation of data
4. Writing the manuscript

---

authorship misconduct A generic term for the listing of a person as an author of a journal article or contribution in which the 'author' did not personally participate; perhaps the most '...*egregious form of authorship misconduct is the practice of a prominent professor's accepting money to allow his or her name to be attached to articles written by ghost authors. Frequently...sponsored by a pharmaceutical company to write a review article favorable to that company's product. The editors of the JAMA have called this practice "deceptive and disgraceful"'* (**JAMA 1995; 273:115c**)

autoantibody IMMUNOLOGY Any antibody that is produced by an organism against one of its own (self) antigens, which include anti-glomerular basement membrane antibodies, anti-parietal cell antibodies, and others

autoantigen IMMUNOLOGY Any of an organism's own (self) antigens, eg glomerular basement membrane, mitochondria, muscle, parietal cells, thyroglobulin and others, which may evoke the production of antibodies

autoclaving PUBLIC HEALTH A method for treating medical waste to render it noninfectious to humans, by heating it to 140°C (284°F), after which the waste can be disposed of in landfills (**Laboratory Medicine 1995; 26:323ᴀ**); while autoclaving is as effective as incineration in eliminating the health risk of medical waste, the latter is viewed by some as being more energy efficient; see Medical waste

autocrine loop A type of interaction between growth factors and cytokines and target cells, in which a cell produces the same growth factors and cytokines for which it has receptors, allowing the cell to stimulate itself, as occurs with smooth muscle cells and their production and response to interleukin-1 (IL-1)

autocrine motility factor MOLECULAR BIOLOGY A cytokine that stimulates random and directed tumor cell motility and generation of inositol triphosphate; both of these activities are inhibited by pertussis toxin, implying that AMF acts by a guanine nucleotide-binding protein (G protein) pathway; a 78-kD glycoprotein acts as an AMF receptor on melanomas and may have a role in melanocyte locomotion (**Cancer Res 1990; 50:409**); see also Scatter factor

autoeponym A term reserved for a condition affecting the author who described it and/or who died from the disease named in his honor; Cf Acroeponym **CARRION'S DISEASE**

DA Carrion, a medical student who inoculated himself with a skin lesion from verruga peruana (*Bartonella bacilliformis*) to prove that the agent was both infectious and the agent of Oroya fever that killed 7000 of those who built the railroad from Lima to La Oroya; he died within 23 days **HUNTINGTON'S DISEASE** George Huntington, his father and his father's father all studied their own disease that was traced back to an index case in 1649 in Bures, England **LEWIS SYNDROME** Autosomal dominant synostosis of the first metacarpophalangeal joint of the thumb or stiff thumb 'syndrome' **JONES FRACTURE** A diaphyseal fracture of the fifth metatarsal, which Jones incurred '...*whilst dancing*...' and who considered it a stress fracture **PRAUSNITZ-KÜSTNER (PASSIVE TRANSFER) TEST** A clinical assay that measures allergic response to foreign proteins that was identified by Küstner who was allergic to fish, injected his serum into Prausnitz's skin, which, when followed by a 'challenge' fish extract injection into Prausnitz's skin, causing a typical wheal and flare reaction **RICKETTSIA SPECIES** Named for Howard Ricketts, who in 1906 identified the organism responsible for Rocky Mountain spotted fever (*Rickettsia rickettsii*); Ricketts died in 1910 in Mexico City while investigating typhus (*Rickettsia prowazekii*) **THOMSEN'S DISEASE** A benign autosomal dominant myopathy, described by Julius Thomsen (who had it), which is first seen in childhood, characterized by tonic rigidity and spasticity, which is overcome by repeated voluntary contraction of the muscles to reduce the clinical and muscular 'stiffness' of these patients (the 'warm-up' effect) **TROUSSEAU SIGN** Superficial petechial hemorrhage and thrombophlebitis, occurring secondary to visceral malignancy, described by Trousseau prior to his own death from gastrointestinal malignancy

autohemolysis test HEMATOLOGY A measure of the amount of spontaneous hemolysis that occurs after incubation of defibrinated blood at 37°C at 48 hours; the results obtained are compared with those from identical blood enriched with glucose or ATP prior to incubation, allowing the stratification of hemolytic anemias (glucose-6-phosphate dehydrogenase, pyruvate kinase, and others) hereditary spherocytosis) into three abnormal patterns; because it is cumbersome, it is rarely used; Cf Ascorbate-cyanide test

autoignition temperature OCCUPATIONAL SAFETY The minimum temperature needed for self-sustained combustion in absence of a spark or flame at which the vapors from a volatile liquid will ignite spontaneously; the AT is a datum of interest to OSHA, which requires listing of ATs in its Materials Safety Data Sheets‡

autoimmune disease A condition that is pathogenically linked to the production of antibodies against self antigens, affecting ± 5% of adults (⅔ are ♀) in North America and Europe; criteria used to define a disease as being autoantibody mediated:

1) An antibody is present
2) The antibody interacts with a target (self) antigen
3) Passive transfer of serum reproduces features of the disease
4) Immunization with the antigen reproduces the disease
5) Reduction of the antibody ameliorates the disease

ADs include Goodpasture's disease, Hashimoto's disease, multiple sclerosis, myasthenia gravis, rheumatoid arthritis, SLE (**N Engl J Med 1994; 330:1797RA**), pernicious anemia

autoimmunity The reaction of an organism's immune system to self antigens as if they were non-self or foreign; like alloimmunity, autoimmunity is characterized by the activation of T cells, clonal expansion and antibody production; why autoimmunity occurs is unclear; postulated mechanisms include immune dysregulation, normal inflammatory response to a virus or other foreign antigen expressed in a self tissue, and molecular mimicry, in which there is cross reactivity of foreign haptens with structurally similar self antigens; autoimmunity increases with age and is intimately linked to connective tissue disease and endocrinopathies; in one autoimmune model, experimental allergic encephalitis of mice, there is a trimolecular complex formed from myelin basic protein (BP), MHC, and T-cell receptor; the autoimmune proliferative response may be blocked by an antibody raised against the BP-MHC complex, implying that autoimmunity may ultimately respond to specific 'magic bullet' therapy (**Nature 1991; 351:147**) see Anti-nuclear antibodies, Anti-receptor antibodies, Clonal anergy, Superantigen

autologous blood transfusion see Autologous transfusion

autologous bone marrow transplantation A therapeutic modality for leukemic patients who are in relapse, and thus likely to die of their disease in which a suitable (HLA-matched) donor cannot be found; the bone marrow is removed during the second remission, treated in vitro to remove the leukemic cells, and is then cryopreserved; the patient then receives supralethal chemoradiotherapy and the marrow is reinfused; ABMT in acute lymphocytic leukemia yields a 20-30% survival rate

autologous chondrocyte tranplantation ORTHOPEDIC SURGERY A procedure for treating defects of articular cartilage BACKGROUND Defects of articular cartilage are not uncommon sequelae of articular trauma; if these defects are of sufficient size and depth, they may lead to pain and joint dysfunction followed by osteoarthritis, eventually requiring replacement of the joint by an artifical prosthesis; total knee replacement (see there) is commonly performed on those > 60 years of age, but is increasingly problematic in younger patients, as prosthetic devices have a limited lifespan ACT is more physiological approach to treating defects of articular cartilage–a biopsy of healthy cartilage is obtained and enzymatically digested to release chondrocytes; these are cultivated in growth media for 10-21 days, resulting in a 10-fold increase; the condrocytes are then injected in the site of interest under a periosteal flap (**N Engl J Med 1994; 331:889OA**)

autologous transfusion Collection and re-infusion of the patient's own blood and/or blood products, which despite a slight inconvenience of surgical delay and vasovagal reactions, is the preferred transfusion option for appropriately-selected patients; the blood volume available for AT can be increased using recombinant erythropoietin and iron supplements; although in principle, AT can be used for any elective surgical procedure, blood is most often needed for orthopedic (total hip replacement) and cardiovascular surgery; AT represents 2.5% of all transfusions; as many of 23.5% of units collected for autologous transfusion are unwarranted; current thinking is that AT is not superior to allogeneic blood in terms of reduced hospital stay or cancer recurrence, although if infections are the ONLY consideration they may be warranted (**Arch Pathol Lab Med 1994; 118:333ED**); AT in elective surgical procedures reduces the use of homologous transfusion in cardiac surgery from a peak of 82% to as low as 27% (**JAMA 1991; 265:86**); AT may also be considered in selected pediatric, geriatric or occasionally obstetric surgery; although most surgery does not require transfusions, some procedures are especially 'bloody', and place an enormous strain on a blood bank's resources, eg an average of 13 units of packed red cells are used in a liver transplantation, ⅓ of which may be provided by blood salvaged from the operative field; in view of the improved safety of the blood supply available for allogeneic donation, the ↑ protection provided by preoperative donation of autologous blood is minimal; the cost effectiveness values range from $235 000 to 23 million per quality-adjusted year of life saved (**N Engl J Med 1995; 332:719**) see Intraoperative 'autologous' blood transfusion; types of autologous donation:

1) PREOPERATIVE PHLEBOTOMY Drawing of blood prior to an elective or anticipated surgical procedure; up to 5 units can be made available in the 20 days preceding surgery, using a 'piggie-back' method

2) IMMEDIATE PREOPERATIVE PHLEBOTOMY or acute normovolemic hemodilution

3) INTRAOPERATIVE SALVAGE

4) POSTOPERATIVE SALVAGE

AT ↓ the risk of most types of transfusion reactions, except clerical errors, contamination and low transfusion temperatures, and is increasingly popular as it substantially ↓ the number of homologous (ie, non-autologous) units transfused; up to 60% of all blood products required in elective surgical procedures can be fulfilled by the patient's own blood; 50% of those who donate autologous units for specific medical indications (rare blood types or presence of multiple blood cell alloantibodies) utilize the blood; 21% of those who donate autologous units without specific medical indications utilize that blood

autologous unit A unit of red blood cells or other blood product to be transfused into a donor at the time of elective or anticipated surgery, see Autologous transfusion

autolymphocyte therapy A form of immunotherapy for treating metastatic renal carcinoma, in which a patient's leukocytes are removed, stimulated by monoclonal antibodies, causing the leukocytes to produce and secrete cytokines; the cytokine supernatant is then removed and readministered with an aliquot of the patient's own leukocytes; despite an early report of success with this modality, conservative oncologists are awaiting further, more definitive reports of success

automated cytology LABORATORY MEDICINE A series of evolving technologies that are intended to automate the labor-intensive process of screening cervical cytology smears; it is uncertain which, if any, of the diverse commercial approaches currently available will be most effective in ultimately replacing the human eye for differentiating normal from abnormal cells (Anal Quan Cytol Histol 1994; 16:52abstr)

autonomic failure A generic term for any of a number of conditions characterized by sympathetic, and usually parasympathetic failure, with orthostatic hypotension and ↓ sympathetic activity; AF contrasts with the severe vasomotor lability typical of baroreflex failure, see there (N Engl J Med 1993; 329:1449OA) FORMS AF can be divided into primary, secondary, and drug-induced forms with considerable overlap and may be caused by or associated with aging, alcohol imbibition, carcinomatous autonomic neuropathy, CNS disease, dopamine β-hydroxylase deficiency, familial dysautonomia (Riley-Day syndrome), idiopathic orthostatic hypotension, Parkinson's disease, Shy-Drager syndrome CLINICAL Syncope, orthostatic hypotension

autonomic triad Dilated pupils, moist palms and tachycardia, a characteristic finding in schizophrenics that may be accompanied by ↑ systolic pressure of 10-20 mm Hg

Note: Schizophrenics are reported to be hypersensitive to all stimuli: noise, odor, touch and light

autonomous proliferation The autonomous activation of DNA synthesis, an event in leukemogenesis that is linked to an aggressive clinical course, with ↓ response to chemotherapy, ↓ between relapse, and ↓ survival; in one study 3 year survival was 36% in those with low proliferation, and 3% in those with high levels of proliferaiton (N Engl J Med 1993; 328:614OA)

autonomously replicating sequence MOLECULAR BIOLOGY A sequence of DNA that serves as an initiation site on a gene for replication; Cf Transcription unit

autopoietic Gaia ENVIRONMENT A theory advanced by L Margulis that organisms evolve in symbiotic systems, eg humans filled with *Escherichia coli* evolved through mutually driven ('symbiotic') mutations rather than by random mutation of either organism, in a 'vacuum'; autopoietic (self-maintaining) systems can range from the size of bacteria to that of the entire planet and are composed of living organisms and environments that are codependent and interactive; Gaia analyses requires integration of data and concepts from fields that have not traditionally overlapped or interacted (Science 1991; 252:378); see Gaia; Cf Neo-darwinism

autopsy PATHOLOGY postmortem, necropsy A postmortem examination of a body Types of autopsies **BIOPSY ONLY** A minimalist post-mortem examination, in which, although the prosector has permission to enter body sites and fully examine the organs, he may only keep fragments ('biopsies') for histologic examination **CHEST ONLY** An autopsy in which the family members have only given permission to examine the lungs and heart, in anticipation of identifying an occluding thrombus in the coronary arteries or finding massive pulmonary thromboembolism **COMPLETE** A complete autopsy in which the chest, abdominal and cranial cavities are examined **HEAD ONLY** A postmortem examination in which the pathology of interest is presumed to reside entirely in the cranial cavity **NO HEAD** An autopsy examining the chest and abdominal cavity without violating the cranial cavity; despite the concern, the autopsy rate continues to fall (JAMA 1995; 273:96MN&P) in one study of nearly 2500 autopsies, 40% had major unexpected findings (ie undetected while the patient was alive) at autopsy that contributed to death (CAP Today March 1995 p41) Cf Psychological autopsy

autopsy rate The frequency (in percent) with which nonforensic deaths are subjected to postmortem examination; in the US, the AR has fallen within the last 30 years from 60-80% to an average of 13%* nationwide to ≤ 5% in private nonteaching institutions (Arch Pathol Lab Med 1994; 118:871ED, 1992; 116:1147OA); in other regions of the world the rate continues to be ± 80%; perceived reasons for the decline in autopsy rate include

1) The often incorrect belief that all of a patient's relevant and treatable diagnoses were known before death

2) Fear of litigation or of misdiagnosis by the attending physician, who may have missed a treatable disease

3) Hospital certification, eg by the JCAHO, no longer requires specific autopsy rates for accreditation

4) Pathologists have lost interest in performing autopsies (due in part to lack of financial incentive, as autopsies are non-reimbursable procedures) and the paperwork associated therewith is burdensome (Arch Pathol Lab Med 1992; 1161128OA)

*With some notable exceptions, eg University of Nebraska ≥ 45%

autoradiography A technique that detects the presence of radioisotopes, usually immobilized on a nylon or nitrocellulose membrane when exposed to a radiation-sensitive medium, eg unexposed radiologic film; autoradiography is used in molecular biology to detect radioactive probes which have bound to segments of DNA or RNA of interest; autoradiography allows visualization of Southern and Northern blot hybridizations

autosomal dominant polycystic kidney disease ADPKD A common (1:400-1:1000) autosomal dominant [MIM 173910] condition, which is responsible for 6-9% of end-stage renal disease in the USA and Europe, caused by the defective gene, PKD1, on the short arm of chromosome 16, close to the α-hemoglobin complex; a second defective gene with identical clinical features is responsible for 4% of cases, but is thought to cause a milder disease PATHOGENESIS The cyst walls are composed of renal tubular epithelium, although most are not connected to glomeruli; the accumulation of fluid in cysts is an active process of transepithelial secretion (rate = ± 21 µl/cm² of surface area) which is mediated by cyclic AMP that may be amenable to pharmacologic intervention (**N Engl J Med 1993; 329:310oₐ**) MOLECULAR PATHOLOGY 85% of AFPKD have a mutation in the *PKD1* gene localized to human chromosome 16p13.3; autosomal recessive form (ARPKD) 1:10 000 (up to 1: 370 in stillborns); a candidate gene has been identified for ARPKD; a complementary DNA derived from this gene predicts a peptide containing a motif first identified in some genes involved in the cell cycle (**Science 1994; 264; 1329ᴿᴿ**) CLINICAL Acute or subacute onset of azotemia and hypertension, related to increased activity of the renin-angiotensin-aldosterone system, possibly related to the ischemic pressure induced by the expanding cysts; ADPKD first appears in adults with upper quadrant tenderness; extrarenal disease is due to defective extracellular matrix, with hepatic cysts, diverticulosis, berry and abdominal aneurysms, annuloaortic ectasia, valvular regurgitation, anemia, very high erythrocyte sedimentation rate and leukocytosis DIAGNOSIS Ultrasonography; see Polycystic kidneys

autotransfusion Autologous transfusion, see there

AV Atrioventricular, also 1) Anteversion 2) Aortic valve 3) Arteriovenous 4) Audiovisual

Also 1) Adriamycin and vincristine 2) Anterior ventral neuron (neurophysiology) 3) Avoirdupois (obsolete) 4) Auriculoventricular

A-V block Atrioventricular block, see there

A-V dissociation Atrioventricular dissociation, see there

AVEC microscopy Allen video-enhanced contrast or Dynamic microscopy A television camera that distinguishes weak contrasts by amplifying differences in brightness; AVEC microscopy studies the direction of transportation of materials along microtubules, which are packaged in vesicles and 'walked' along the microtubule by projections in the axons; see Kinesin

aviation medicine In-flight emergencies Federal Aviation Agency regulations require that an 'enhanced' medical kit (stethoscope, sphygmomanometer, airway tube, syringes, epinephrine, nitroglycerin, 50 ml 50% dextrose, diphenhydramine injectable) be carried on any airplane with more than 30 seats TYPES OF IN-FLIGHT EMERGENCIES Syncope 29%, cardiac/chest pain 16%, asthma/shortness of breath 10%, allergic reactions 5% In-flight deaths, DISEASE TRANSMISSION The resurgence of TB has made the aerosol transmission through aircraft ventilation systems a real health hazard of currently unknown epidemiologic significance (**MMWR 1995; 44:137**) STATISTICS 0.31 deaths/million passengers-regardless of flight length; 125 deaths/billion passenger kilometers; 25 deaths per million departures; the average victim was male, age 53.8; physicians were available in 43% of cases CAUSE OF DEATH Cardiac 56%, terminal cancer 8%, respiratory 6%, miscellaneous and no cause, remainder; Cf Airline food

aviator's astralagus ORTHOPEDICS A generic term referring to various permutations of fracture and fracture-dislocations of the talus; the term was coined in 1919 when the fracture was related to aviation accidents in pilots whose aircraft had been descending too rapidly and which had a rudder bar which caused the above fracture at the time of the airplane's impact

avidin A 68 kD tetrameric glycoprotein found in egg white that has an high affinity for biotin, an association used in immunology for the avidin-biotinylated immunoperoxidase method, see ABC; when eggs are eaten in excess, the avidin-biotin avidity may cause biotin deficiency

avidin biotinylated horseradish-peroxidase complex method A commercial method for detecting antigen or antibody in tissues; avidin, a 68 000 egg white glycoprotein with a very high natural affinity (and multiple binding sites) for biotin, a vitamin readily bound covalently to an antibody; the ABC system allows amplification of antigen 'signal' obtained by the multiple binding sites available on

the avidin; the avidin:biotin linkage can be used for gene mapping, double label studies, DNA in situ hybridization, hybridoma screening, Southern blotting, radioimmunoassay, solid phase ELISA, immune electron microscopy, studies of neuronal transport and as a means of controlling enzymatic reactions METHOD The tissue containing the antigen of interest is frozen, air-dried and acetone fixed, incubated with a primary antibody, washed, then incubated with a secondary antibody bearing attached biotin, washed, re-incubated with fluorescently or enzyme-tagged avidin, and finally counterstained

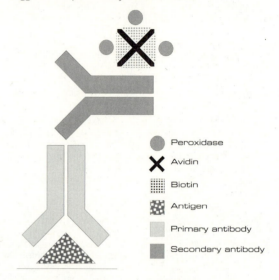

Peroxidase

Avidin

Biotin

Antigen

Primary antibody

Secondary antibody

avidin-biotin method

avidity IMMUNOLOGY The degree of stability of an antibody with its antigen, a function of the number of shared binding sites; Cf Affinity

AVM see Arteriovenous malformation

a wave A positive a wave is a component of a normal jugular phlebogram produced by retrograde transmission of the pressure pulse, corresponding to atrial systole; the a wave begins before the first heart sound peaking at the moment the first sound begins; abnormalites of the a wave indicate cardiopulmonary disease; it may disappear in atrial fibrillation, be 'swallowed' in the v-y descent of a prolonged P-Q interval, it may be very large (giant) when the atrium is contracting against resistance (eg tricuspid valve stenosis or atresia, pulmonary hypertension or pulmonary edema) or bear a presystolic 'notch' (pulmonary edema); Cf Cannon wave

axial centrifugation LABORATORY MEDICINE A method for separating serum and plasma from cells in the clinical laboratory, where the separation is achieved by spinning a specially designed tube lengthwise, ie on its own axis; AC is regarded as a major advance in technology, as centrifugation is much more rapid, requiring as little as 1 minute, and thus has the potential for significantly reducing turnaround times for specimens of critical interest, and is less 'robotics-hostile' (**CAP Today October 1994 p1**)

axillary tail Axillary fat pad The fibroadipose tissue in the axilla that contains the lymph nodes (numbering from 12 to 25) and lymphoid drainage from the breast and arm; in carcinoma of the breast, the number of positive lymph nodes in the axillary tail constitutes the single most important prognostic indicator of survival, where a breast carcinoma with no positive lymph nodes is associated with a greater than 80% five-year survival, while a patient with 20 or more positive lymph nodes is associated with a less than 20% five-year survival

axon hillock NEUROPHYSIOLOGY A conical protuberance that surrounds the axon at its point of departure from the neuron's body, as which point the Nissl substance is minimal and there is specialized plasmalemma

ayur-veda Sanskrit, Life knowledge The oldest existing medical system, practiced primarily in the subcontinent of India; ayur-veda holds that disease is caused by an imbalance of homeostatic and immune mechanisms related to three physiological principles known as 'doshas'

VATA DOSHA represents fluid and motion, corresponding to the Western concepts of circulation and neuromuscular activity

PITTA DOSHA directs all metabolic activities, energy exchange and digestion

KAPHA DOSHA represents structure, cohesion and fluid balance and when deranged, predisposes toward respiratory disease, DM, atherosclerosis and tumors

Ayur-veda's therapeutic modalities include transcendental meditation, a 'healthy' life style, herbal compounds and behavior modification (JAMA 1991; 265:2633)

azacytidine A nucleoside analogue that may useful in treating β-thalassemia as it stimulates fetal globin production; azacytidine's mechanism of action is unknown, but may hinge on its ability to inhibit methylation of newly synthesized DNA in cognate regulator regions, ie hypomethylation of fetal globin gene promoters that participate in the switch in expression from fetal to adult globin; it may also enhance fetal globin synthesis by impacting on the kinetics of of erythroid-precursor maturation (N Engl J Med 1993; 329:844OA)

azathioprine Imuran A purine analog that is the most potent and popular immunosuppressive agent used in clinical transplantation; azathioprine is 6-mercaptopurine with a side chain to protect the labile sulfhydryl group, which is split off in the liver; full metabolic activity follows addition of ribose 5-phosphate from phosphoribosyl pyrophosphate that is metabolized to the cytotoxic derivative 6-mercaptopurine; azathioprine acts primarily on T cells and is of use in myasthenia gravis

azo dye A group of dyes produced from amino compounds by diazotization and coupling the reactants; the reactions are a function of the number of –N=N– groups in the molecule; the dyes are used for plastics, rubber and in the cat-tle industry; the carcinogenicity of these substances is related to the ortho-hydroxylated metabolites complexed with sulfates and glucuronic acid

azole One of a family of synthetic broad-spectrum antifungal antibiotics (including ketoconazole, fluconazole, itraconazole) that inhibit the C-14 demethylation step, a cytochrome P450-dependent reaction of ergosterol biosynthesis, preventing the conversion of lanosterol to ergosterol; ergosterol depletion has a net fungistatic effect (Science 1994; 264:71P); unlike amphotericin B, azoles can be administered orally, wherein lies their advantage CLINICAL INDICATIONS Various azoles have established efficacy in treating blastomyocosis, candidiasis, coccidioidomycosis, cryptococcosis, histoplasmosis, paracoccidoidomycosis, and in sporotrichosis ADVERSE EFFECTS Nausea, vomiting, anorexia, rash, pruritus, nonspecific ↑ liver enzymes, anemia, leukopenia, thrombocytopenia, headache, and others DRUG INTERACTIONS Plasma levels of azoles are ↓ by antacids, H_2-receptor antagonists, sucralfate, isoniazid, phenytoin, rifampin (N Engl J Med 1994; 330:263OA)

Azorean neurologic syndrome Machado-Joseph spinopontine atrophy syndrome

AZT 3'-azido-3'-deoxythimidine see Zidovudine

azurophilic granules Primary granules, primary lysosomes Membrane-bound organelles in neutrophils that act as reservoirs for digestive and hydrolytic enzymes prior to their delivery to a phagosome, appearing as large, coarse, non-specific blue-purple granules within progranulocytes, myelocytes and neutrophils containing myeloperoxidase (causing oxygen-dependent bacteriolysis), lysozyme (which destroys the bacterial wall), neutral proteases (cathepsins C and G and elastase which destroy inflamed tissue), acid hydrolases (glycosidases, phospholipases, acid proteases, β-glucuronidase, α-mannosidase, N-acetyl-glucosaminidase, which degrade material ingested), α-naphthyl acetate, α-butyrate esterase, naphthol ASD chloracetate esterase, cationic proteins, defensins, bactericidal or permeability-increasing protein (BFI), C5a inactivating factor and sulfated mucosubstances

Note: The other major granulocytic granules are secondary or specific granules, which contain alkaline phosphatase, aminopeptidases, lysozyme and basic proteins, and tertiary granules

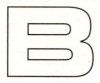

B Symbol for: 1) Asparagine, aspartic acid 2) Bacillus 3) Bel 4) Blood 5) Boron 6) 5-Bromouridine 7) Magnetic induction, expressed in teslas

b Symbol for: 1) Base 2) Inconvertible enzyme

B19 A parvovirus that infects humans causing fifth disease (erythema infectiosum, which affects ± 40% of teachers and day-care workers, hydrops fetalis (due to intrauterine infection), and pure red cell aplasia and chronic anemia in immunocompromised patients; this seemingly disparate group of diseases is explained by the finding that the cell receptor for B19 is the blood group P antigen (globoside) that is found on the surface of erythrocytes, megakaryocytes, endothelial cells, placenta, fetal liver and heart cells; those subjects lacking the P antigen (p phenotype) are naturally resistant to B19 infection (**N Engl J Med 1994; 330:1192OA**); see Fifth disease

B complex IMMUNOLOGY A designation for the major histocompatibility complex (MHC) in chickens with loci encoding class I and II MHC antigens as well as red blood cell antigens

B complex NUTRITION An obsolete and incorrect term for the water-soluble vitamin B1 and B2 isoforms

33B3.1 A monoclonal antibody raised against the interleukin-2 receptor, which is reported to be effective in preventing graft-versus-host disease in renal transplantation as rabbit antithymocyte globulin with fewer side effects and infections

B-72.3 A proprietary (Oncoscint) FDA-approved radiolabeled murine antibody that labels TAG-72 (tumor-associated glycoprotein-72), an antigen present on 97% of ovarian and 83% of colonic carcinomas; B-72.3 scans are used to detect primary and recurrent cancer of the ovaries and colon, and is reportedly useful in differentiating metastatic from primary liver cancer (**Arch Pathol Lab Med 1994; 118:930OA**)

babbling Quasi-random vocalizations in infants that precede language acquisition; babbling is intimately linked to the abstract structure of language and not (contrary to prevailing opinion) a concrete specific linguistic structure, as language acquisition in the profoundly deaf is not hindered by the lack of auditory and verbal signals, indeed deaf infants born to deaf parents produce a manual version of vocalizations ('man-bling'), in which similar ('phonology', morphology, syntax and semantics) linguistic structures are acquired in the manual form (**Science 1991; 251:1493**)

babesiosis A systemic infection caused by *Babesia* spp, in particular *B microti* transmitted by *Ixodes dammini*; in Nantucket, an endemic region, circa 40% of *I dammini*

have *B microti* sporozoites in their saliva CLINICAL 1-4 week incubation, fever, shaking chills, malaise myalgias, fatigue, hemoglobinuria LABORATORY *B microti* in peripheral red cells; indirect fluorescent test titers ≥ 1:1024 TREATMENT Clindamycin, quinine (**N Engl J Med 1993; 329:194CPC**)

baby boomer Boomer An increasingly popular term (that began as slang) for a member of the post-World War II (WWII) baby boom generation, which corresponds to those (now in their 30s-50s) persons who were conceived from the time that WWII ended in 1945 until 1964; the population 'swell' caused by BBs has evoked major changes in virtually every facet of American society; the impact of BB demographics on medicine has been broad and promises to be greatest as BBs age and reach retirement*

*When the impact of an older population (with relatively few to care for them and a potentially bankrupt safety net of social services) is fully realized—Author's note

baby bottle syndrome Severe caries of deciduous dentition, due to prolonged use of milk or juice bottles as a sleeping aid for infants

Baby Doe An infant born in April, 1982 in Indiana who was diagnosed as having Down syndrome and a tracheoesophageal fistula that required surgery for the infant's prolonged survival; given the infant's anticipated poor quality of life; the parents decided to withhold treatment with the approval of the local court and the child died within six days; the ensuing ethical debate resulted in an interpretation of section 504 of the Rehabilitation Act of 1973 that contends it is unlawful to withhold nutritional support or necessary medical treatment from handicapped infants

Baby (Jane) Doe A female infant born in October, 1983 on Long Island, New York, with multiple birth defects, including spina bifida, microcephaly and hydrocephalus; the parents decided to withhold treatment; a complaint by an unidentified person designated as a 'private citizen', forced the US federal government to become involved via the Health and Human Services, which questioned whether a parent has the right to initiate or terminate the life-support for infants and children with overwhelming disease or conditions for a party that is underage and is unprotected; the two Baby Doe cases resulted in 1) The **BABY DOE LAW** Public Law 98-457 A legislative act in 1984, requiring states to establish mechanisms in their child-protection services responsive to reported medical neglect of disabled children and 2) The **BABY DOE REGULATIONS** Federal regulations promulgated in 1985 for implementing the 'Baby Doe Law', requiring that disabled infants with life-threatening conditions receive the '...appropriate nutrition, hydration and medication, which in the treating physician's....reasonable medical judgement will be most likely to be effective in ameliorating or correcting all such conditions' TREATMENT (but not nutritional support or necessary medication) may be withheld if the infant is 1) In an irreversible coma or 2) If the treatment is unlikely to prevent death in the near future

Baby Fae heart Hypoplastic left heart syndrome (HLHS) Pediatric cardiology A condition characterized by hypo- or agenesis of the left ventricle, aortic and mitral valves; the ascending and transverse aorta is narrowed with a diaphragm-like aortic coarctation at the preductal aortic isthmus; postnatal life hinges on adequate blood supply, ie is ductus dependent, unrestricted atrial shunting and a balance between the pulmonary and systemic vascular resistances; HLHS surgery is difficult as there are extensive malformations and thus carries a high mortality

Note: Baby Fae was a 2-week-old premature infant with HLHS who survived for 20 days in October 1984 when she received a walnut-sized heart from a 7½-month-old baboon, in an operation performed by L Baily in Loma Linda, California

baby 'farming' A popular term occasionally used in the UK and New Zealand for the illegal practice of accepting 'unwanted' babies, often from unwed mothers, and passing them (with various attached 'processing' fees) to would-be adopting parents

baby fat A popular term for two poorly studied clinical forms of fat deposition in ♀

1) The fat that marks a girl's preadolescent (hence baby 'fat') contour of the body and face

2) The extra poundage or 'lipobulk' that a ♀ may accumulate during pregnancy (hence 'baby' fat), ne'er again to lose

Baby K BIOMEDICAL ETHICS An anencephalic infant in persistent vegetative state born in 1992 in the state of Virginia; anencephaly was diagnosed prenatally, and the mother chose to continue the pregnancy against advice from her obstetrician and a neonatologist; the courts have upheld the mother's decision to continue life-support (N Engl J Med 1994; 330:1542ED) Cf Baby Theresa

Baby L A 36-week, 1970-g baby girl, born in the mid-1980s to a young mother of 3 healthy live children, who developed oligohydramnios and hydronephrosis during the last trimester; decelerations in the fetal heart rate and thick meconium below the umbilical cord were noted at delivery; APGAR scores were low and resuscitation efforts allowed weaning of an infant responsive only to pain; consultation among members of the nursing and medical staff and nearly two years of intensive care led to the unanimous opinion that the child's condition was hopeless and the medical team declined further efforts to salvage a child who was deaf, blind, quadriplegic, in a permanent vegetative state and required 16 hours/day of intensive nursing care, contrary to the wishes of the mother (although physicians usually abide by the wishes of patients, family members or guardians in resuscitation efforts); the Baby L case is a 'charged' issue in which both parents and a health care system must resolve the ethical dilemma of whether to allow one child to die and spend those resources elsewhere; Baby L was transferred to another facility and has the mental status of a 3-month-old

Baby Lance The 'Minnesota Baby Doe' A 7-month-old baby boy who was the first major legal test of the 'Baby Doe regulations,' see there; Baby Lance was beaten to unconsciousness and an irreversible coma by a care-giver; the higher Minnesota court ruled that heroic measures were not required, given his hopeless condition

Baby M A female infant born in mid-1980s in New Jersey by a surrogate mother contract; at the time of birth, the gestational and natural mother decided to renege on the contract and the ensuing court battle became a cause celebre on the issue of surrogate parenthood; on one side was the natural father, a biochemist and his wife, a pediatrician with multiple sclerosis; on the other side was a woman who was the gestational and natural (genetic) mother, who received $10 000 in expenses for providing use of her uterus in a surrogate contract; at the close of the case, the court ruled for the natural father who was allowed to retain the child; see Assisted reproduction, Surrogate motherhood

Note: The Baby M case was not true surrogacy, as the gestational mother was also the genetic mother

'babysitter' A person, often an intelligent family member, who stays by the bedside of a patient respirating by mechanical ventilation, ensuring that no malfunctions or other problems arise

Baby Theresa BIOMEDICAL ETHICS An anencephalic infant born in 1992 whose parents wanted her declared dead at birth (she lived 10 days) in order to donate her organs; the two courts to which the parents appealed rejected their request as 1) Florida law defines brain death as the cessation of brain activity, including the brain stem, which the baby had, and 2) It would become a license to prematurely kill an infant for the express purpose of harvesting the organs (Am Med News 21 September 1992 p5) Cf Baby K

BAC Blood alcohol concentration (or content)

Also 1) Bachelor of Acupuncture 2) Bacterial antigen complex 3) Bacteriology (rarely used) 4) Bile acid concentration 5) Biological activated carbon 6) Biospecific affinity chromatography 7) Biotechnology Advisory Committee 8) bis(aminomethyl)cyclohexane 9) Breath alcohol concentration 10) Bronchial allergen challenge 11) Bronchoalveolar cells 12) Buccoaxiocervical (dentistry)

Bach remedy Flower remedy, see there

bacillary angiomatosis Epithelioid angiomatosis A distinct vascular proliferative disorder of the skin and lymph nodes seen in HIV-positive subjects, which may be associated with disseminated visceral disease, eg bacillary peliosis hepatis ETIOLOGY *R quintana* is the most common cause of BA; *Rochalimaea henselae* is less common, but may also cause bacteremia in immunocompromised and immunocompetent hosts, as well as bacillary peliosis hepatis, and splenitis (N Engl J Med 1992; 327:1625RV) CLINICAL Erythematous papules and nodules, fever and bacteremia PATHOLOGY Lobular capillary proliferation composed of protuberant atypical endothelial cells containing clusters of curved Warthin-Starry positive curved bacilli which may also be gram-negative TREATMENT Erythromycin, other antibiotics; tissue analysis with an oligonucleotide primer complementary to the 16S ribosomal RNA genes of eubacteria and DNA sequence by the polymerase chain reaction amplification, reveals that bacillary angiomatosis is due to a previously uncharacterized rickettsia-like organism, most (98.3% sequence homology) related to *Rochalimaea quintana*; see Peliosis hepatitis

bacillary bodies Iron-containing cytoplasmic inclusions in bone marrow precursors of the erythroid series that are increased in hemolytic anemia or after splenectomy

Bacillus cereus A non-anthrax *Bacillus* that is a rare cause of epidemic gastroenteritis due to ingestion of food contaminated with one of two enterotoxins that cause nausea and vomiting, or abdominal pain and diarrhea (Sci & Med Nov/Dec 1994 p9)

back bleeding CARDIOVASCULAR SURGERY An unreliable* test to determine the completeness of thrombectomy of an occluded artery; for an operation to be considered successful, a test of arterial integrity, eg intraoperative angiography, is required

*Unreliable in that it gives a false sense of security since back bleeding may occur through the nearest arterial branch while a major arterial 'distad' remains occluded

back calculation EPIDEMIOLOGY An approach used to quantify the magnitude of the AIDS epidemic and forecast future trends, BC requires only AIDS incidence data and an estimate of the incubation period distribution; although BC suffers from such features as the limited knowledge of the incubation period, the effects of therapy on the incubation period, errors in the AIDS incidence data, it is more attractive than alternative approaches including simple extrapolation of the AIDS incidence curve, surveys of HIV prevalence and a mathematical model, which requires an enormous amount of often uncertain data (Science 1991; 253:37) see 'Look-back' programs

back extensor strength BES A parameter used to evaluate elderly patients with lower back pain and osteoporosis that may be measured by using a back isometric dynamometer (Mayo Clin Proc 1991; 66:39)

background A baseline of minimal 'chaos' in any study, eg radioactivity in sample that may be due to cosmic radiation, instrument noise and radioactive contamination

background radiation Electromagnetic radiation (often referring to ionizing radiation) originating from 'natural' sources, including 'natural' radon, cosmic radiation, and fallout in the environment from anthropogenic sources

back-propagation COMPUTERS A learning algorithm used in a three layer (inner, middle correctional and outer) neural network (a computer simulation of neurological connections), which allows the system to 'learn' from errors by altering the strength of neural connections, ie allowing the system to teach itself; some workers consider the brain to be the biological correlate of back-propagation; see Neural network

backscatter CYTOMETRY One of two parameters measured in flow cytometry, which is detected at a 90° angle to the laser's light beam and corresponds to the fluorescence of individual cells or intracellular components stained with rhodamine- or isothiocyanate-labelled monoclonal antibodies Note: The other parameter used in flow cytometry is forward scatter, measured at 180° angle to the light, ie directly in front of the laser, and is a function of the cell's size; see FALS, Flow cytometry PHYSICS Any electromagnetic radiation (usually referring to photons, but also ultrasonic waves, etc) that reflects more than 90° from the source, or back in the general direction of the source

back-to-back pattern A 'soft' histologic criterion seen in well-differentiated adenocarcinomas that separates malignant lesions from premalignant hyperplasia or atypical lesions; when glands are arranged in a back-to-back fashion, the intervening stroma (and by extension, the basement membrane) disappears, a finding characteristic of gastrointestinal, endometrial and ovarian adenocarcinomas

back typing Reverse typing TRANSFUSION MEDICINE A 'cross-match' in which a person's serum, which may contain antibodies, is tested against a panel of commercially available erythrocytes (the antigens of which are well characterized) to determine whether a person has antibodies to any red cell antigens; Cf Front typing, Major cross-match, Minor cross-match

backward failure Cardiac failure attributed to elevated filling pressure of the ventricles, due to obstruction, as occurs with mitral or tricuspid stenosis, which causes increased venous pressure with congestion, ie backward failure; the term is a physiologic concept of dubious importance and thus has decreasing clinical currency; Cf Forward failure

backwash ileitis The contiguous mucosal involvement of the terminal ileum, extending proximally, seen in 10-15% of cases of ulcerative colitis as a 'spillover' phenomenon; unlike Crohn's disease which may involve the entire gastrointestinal tract, ulcerative colitis is usually confined to the colon and rectum and occasionally, a 'backwashed' segment of ileum

baclofen A γ-aminobutyric acid (GABA) antagonist that may be administered per os or intrathecally to reduce recalcitrant spinal spasticity in patients with multiple sclerosis or spinal-cord injury

m-BACOD ONCOLOGY A 'second-generation' combination chemotherapy regimen (methotrexate, bleomycin, doxorubicin, cyclophosphamide, vincristine, and dexamethosone); despite extensive clinical research, CHOP is considered better than m-BACOD for non-Hodgkin's lymphoma as it is less expensive, less complicated to administer, and has fewer fatal toxic side effects (**N Engl J Med 1993; 328:1002oa, 1992; 327:1342oa**)

BACOP ONCOLOGY A 'third-generation' combination chemotherapy regimen (bleomycin, doxorubicin, cyclophosphamide, vincristine, and prednisone), used for non-Hodgkin's lymphoma; esc-BACOP (escalated doses of doxorubicin) regimens have increased toxicity but do not improve rate of response or survival when compared to standard doxorubicin doses (s-BACOP) (**N Engl J Med 1993; 329:1770oa**), see CHOP

bacterial count PUBLIC HEALTH A generic term for any of a number of tests used to evaluate the level of contamination of drinking and recreational waters; the drinking water is assumed to be safe if no coliform organisms (bacteria normally present in the human GI tract) are found ($\leq$ 5% of the samples collected); for recreational marine or fresh waters, the EPA has suggested a geometric mean of 35 enterococcus or *Escherichia coli*/100 ml for the water to be considered safe

Note: This is lower than the former standard of 200 organisms/100 ml which was widely used until 1986

bacteriophage A virus that infects bacteria; of interest in the study of human disease are the temperate phages of *Escherichia coli*, in particular the lambda bacteriophage, a double-stranded 48 500 base pair DNA virus that is commonly used as a vector for molecular cloning; upon entry into the bacterial host, it replicates either by 1) Lysis The phage's circular DNA replicates many times, independently of the bacterium, causing the cell to burst or by 2) Lysogeny The phage DNA integrates itself within the bacterial chromosome per se and is carried to future generations of the bacterium

bacterial endotoxin Endotoxin The liposaccharide on the outer coat of gram-negative bacteria, including those causing cholera, some forms of meningitis, pneumonia, plague, whooping cough and others* STRUCTURE Endotoxin has an outer polysaccharide with an O-specific chain linked to an outer core, which in turn is linked to an inner core containing unusual molecules, to wit heptose, ethanolamine and Kdo; the polysaccharide is linked to an anchoring lipid, lipid A, which is responsible for endotoxin's clinical effects PATHOGENESIS Endotoxin acts primarily on macrophages resulting in the production of cytokines (TNF, IL-1, IL-6, and IL-8), oxygen free radicals (O_2^-, H_2O_2, NO), and lipids (PGE$_2$, TXA$_2$, PAF) CLINICAL Leukopenia, thrombocytopenia, fever, chills, and shock (**Sci Am 1992; 267/2:54**) Adjective: **endotoxic**

*Endotoxins are integral to the family Enterobacteriaceae, eg *Escherichia* spp, *Salmonella* spp, *Shigella* spp, etc

bacterial overgrowth LABORATORY MEDICINE A term referring to the multiplication of contaminating bacteria in a specimen (eg blood, urine) when either there is inadequate fixative, or it is not processed in an appropriate or timely fashion; overgrowth is rarely confused with a true infection of the urinary tract or sepsis, as it is not accompanied other criteria suggestive of an in vivo infection, in particular PMNs

'bad' cholesterol LDL-cholesterol Cholesterol that is carried in the circulation by low-density lipoprotein, the elevation of which is directly related to the risk of coronary artery disease and cholesterol-related morbidity (**New York Times 8 February 1994; C1**) see LDL-cholesterol; Cf Good cholesterol

BAD operon MOLECULAR BIOLOGY A group of 3 genes (B, A and D) that encode three enzymes, an isomerase, a kinase and an epimerase, respectively, requiring in addition the presence of the positively acting protein AraC for transcription of the ara operon into BAD mRNA

BADS syndrome Ermine phenotype An AR [MIM 227010] condition characterized by Black locks, Albinism and Deafness, Sensorineural type, which has certain features of oculocutaneous albinism but which is not true albinism; the melanocytes in BADS are reduced or absent

'bad trip' SUBSTANCE ABUSE A hallucinogenic drug-induced experience in which the desired pattern of time-space disorientation causes a varying amount of anxiety on the person taking the 'trip'; see Flashbacks, 'High'

Baecke questionnaire A survey of habitual physical (ie sports) activity, ranging from 1 (low level of activity) to 5 (high level) which is of use in epidemiological studies (**Am J Clin Nutr 1982; 36:936, from Engl J Med 1993; 329:1069oa**)

BAER Brainstem auditory evoked response A clinical method for evaluating hearing by using scalp electrodes; the early responses reflect electrical activity at the cochlea, cranial nerve VIII and brainstem; late responses are due to cortical activity

bagassosis A hypersensitivity pneumonitis seen in cane sugar workers, who are sensitive to *Thermoactinomyces sacchari*, a fungus that grows well in sugar cane pressings; the term derives from the cellulose-rich olive husks, bagasse, remaining after olives are pressed to extract oil, and is generic for various 'pressings'; see Farmer's lung

bag cell neuron A neuron of the gastropod mollusk, *Aplysia californica*'s nervous system that serves as a model for studying the neuroendocrine system

bag of worms appearance Any lesion or density that has a polyvermiform pattern or one in which the activity is fancifully likened to a quivering mass of live elongated organisms CEREBRAL ANGIOGRAPHY The appearance of arteriovenous malformations in which there is little interposed cerebral tissue; this finding may also be mimicked by intracranial tumors, although the irregular and bizarre vessels may be separated by a mass GASTROENTEROLOGY An uncommon descriptor for the gross appearance of the stomach in Menetrier's disease in which the stomach is soft, smooth and enlarged and the mucosa has large, swollen, inelastic worm-like rugal folds, separated by deep valleys NEUROLOGY Asynchronous, involuntary quivering and squirming of multiple skeletal muscle fascicles of the tongue, which disappear during sleep and may be suppressed with rest, sedation or volition, characteristically seen as a manifestation of Sydenham's chorea SURGICAL PATHOLOGY The quasi-pathognomonic gross appearance of a plexiform neurofibroma seen in von Recklinghausen's disease, where a major nerve trunk is transformed into a redundant convoluted serpentine mass of tumorous nerves UROLOGY The tactile sensation of a varicocele lying within the scrotal sac

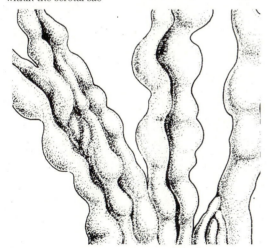

bag of worms appearance

'bags' Bags under the eyes Loose suborbital skin caused by inflammation and edema, associated with vasodilation (the prominence of the blood vessels impart the dark color); bags occur with lack of sleep, smoking, and other aerosolized irritants; 'bags' occur in allergic 'shiners', various dermatitides and in aging

Baghdad button An indurated lesion of cutaneous leishmaniasis caused by *Leishmania tropica*

Bairnesdale ulcer A necrotizing skin ulcer caused by *Mycobacterium ulcerans*, first described in Australia; see Buruli ulcer

Bak *Bak* A recently identified member of the *bcl*-2 family which is expressed in a wide range of cells, and when overexpressed in NGF (nerve growth factor)-deprived sympathetic neurons accelerates apoptosis, and counteracts the apoptosis-protecting effects of Bcl-2 (Nature 1995; 374:731, 733, 736)

Bak^a An antigen present on the platelets of most normal subjects; immune-mediated neonatal thrombocytopenia may be due to an IgG anti-Bak^a antibody, produced in women who are Bak^a negative and passively transferred to the fetus

Baker scale COSMETIC SURGERY A grading system (from grades 1 to 4) used by plastic surgeons to quantify the degree of capsular contraction surrounding a breast implant in patients with augmentation mammaplasty; breasts with grade 1 contractions are soft and compressible; higher grades are correspondingly less pliable (JAMA 1992; 268:1913oc)

Bakke v Regents of the University of California A lawsuit initiated by a white student in California in response to an affirmative action in 1973 by the University of California Medical School at Davis that admitted a number of black students who had lower grades and test scores than white students; the case went before the state Supreme Court which ruled for the student's accusations of 'reverse discrimination'; Bakke was admitted to medical school in 1978 and is today an anesthesiologist in Minnesota (NY Times Magazine 11 June 1995, p36; Med Educ 1978; 53:776) see Affirmative action, Project 3000 by 2000, Reverse discrimination, Underrepresented minorities

BAL 1) Blood alcohol level; useful values > 100 mg/dl, legal intoxication, most states in the US; > 200 mg/dl narcosis, > 300 mg/dl, stupor and coma 2) Broncho-alveolar lavage A 'wash' of the upper respiratory tract to obtain cells representative of any inflammatory or neoplastic process in the lungs; BAL material is used for 1) Cytopathologic analysis 2) Analysis of the CD4:CD8 ratio and (rarely) 3) To obtain cells for gene rearrangement, ie Southern blot hybridization, to diagnosis lymphoma; like acetylcholinesterase levels and gallium scans, flow cytometry of the BAL is useless in diagnosing hilar sarcoidosis, although increased CD4 T cells and decreased neutrophils in a BAL may be suggestive of sarcoidosis in certain patients; flow cytometry has a relatively low diagnostic value in hypersensitivity (increased CD8 T cells and normal to increased neutrophils) and idiopathic pulmonary fibrosis (increased neutrophils)

balance billing HEALTH CARE REIMBURSEMENT A bill submitted for payment from a billing agent(s) to a patient whose insurance only pays for part of the service(s) rendered by the physician or hospital, dunning him for the unpaid portion

balanced (reciprocal) translocation Must put in

BALB/c mouse IMMUNOLOGY A strain of inbred white mice that develops a myeloproliferative response to intraperitoneal injection of mineral oil and complete Freund's adjuvant

bald sac sign A myelographic finding caused by lateral migration of nerve roots to the periphery of and adherence to the dural sac occurs in a background of arachnoiditis with clumping of nerve roots

bald spot MOLECULAR BIOLOGY An area on a hybridization blot (Southern, Northern, Western) that does not hybridize and which represents a technical artifact due to inadequate bathing of hybridization fluid in the bag containing the radiolabelled or biotinylated probe

bald tongue Complete atrophy of lingual papillae, seen in pernicious or iron-deficiency anemias, pellagra (specifically known as the bald tongue of Sandwith), syphilis

CLINICAL Pain, burning, and a beefy red color

Balkan nephropathy An tubulointerstitial nephropathy endemic to the littoral regions of the Danube river, affecting the Balkan countries of Bulgaria, Romania and Yugoslavia ETIOLOGY Although uncertain, the environmental effects of Eastern Bloc progress make the recently implicated aromatic hydrocarbon leachate out of the low-grade coal, lignite, into local water supplies more likely than the previously suggested possibility of fungal nephrotoxins (which had been related to high regional rainfall or genetic factors) CLINICAL Most patients die within 10 years of onset PATHOLOGY Prominent cortical involvement with interstitial fibrosis, amyloid deposits, chronic inflammation, marked loss of renal tubules and atrophy

balkanization The subdivision of a department in a hospital or academic institution, eg internal medicine into specialized fields, eg cardiology, dermatology, nephrology, neurology, and so on, each having its own separate administration and staff, with the disadvantage that one might lose sight of the individual patients and the stated goals of medicine as the 20th century closes, ie an increased emphasis of primary care (N Engl J Med 1994; 330:1453ED, 1456ED)

ballerina skirt cell Downy type II cell HEMATOPATHOLOGY A fanciful term for the morphology of one of the three types of atypical lymphocytes seen in infectious mononucleosis, in which there are cytoplasmic radiations extending from the nuclear membrane

ball-and-chain model NEUROPHYSIOLOGY A model first proposed in 1977 for the physical conformation of the potassium ion channel; this ion channel is constructed of a 19-20 residue peptide (ball) domain tethered by a 17 residue (chain) to the cytoplasmic face of the cell and 'pops out' of a transmembrane pore upon electrical activation, allowing the channel to gate for potassium in either a resting, an open or an inactivated state (Science 1991; 252:1092; 250:533); the model was corroborated using a combination of site-specific mutagenesis and patch-clamping; see Voltage-gated channels

ball-and-socket Ball in socket An adjectival descriptor for a morphology in which there is a sharply circumscribed round mass surrounded by a clear or lucent space followed by a density similar to the first central 'ball' BONE RADIOLOGY A sequel of epiphyseal fractures with a primary fusion of the central portion of the epiphysis, appearing as a ball within a relatively radiolucent 'socket', seen in infantile scurvy, battered child syndrome, and acromelic dwarfism PARASITOLOGY A 'ball-and-socket' appearance is typical of the trophozoites and occasionally the cysts of *Endolimax nana* and *Iodamoeba buetschlii* where there is a large, deeply staining karyosome lying in an empty space; the nuclear membrane is not visualized as the chromatin is not peripheral RHEUMATOLOGY A descriptor for the compressive erosions in the interphalangeal joint of rheumatic diseases, where a central sclerotic zone is surrounded by an osteoporotic 'ring'

ball-in-claw pattern DERMATOPATHOLOGY A descriptor for the histopathological appearance of the dermal-epidermal junction in lichen nitidus, characterized by epidermal flattening, hydropic degeneration or absence of basal cell layer, varying degrees of epidermal detachment, abundant lympho-histiocytic infiltration in the upper dermis, occasional multinucleated giant cells; the lateral margins (rete ridges) form a pincer around the infiltrate; see Collarette CLINICAL Flat-topped, flesh-colored papules located on the penis, arms and abdomen

Note: The ball and claw or ball in talon is an ending to the cabriole leg where a bird of prey's or lion's claw grasps a ball, a style thought to have developed between 1690-1730 in the English school of furniture design, inspired by the dragon's claw grasping a pearl, a motif originating in China

ball valve obstruction A partial endobronchial obstruction allowing facile entry but not free egress of air, result-

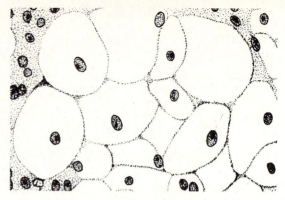

balloon cells

ing in the build-up of pressure in the terminal airways and potential rupture of alveoli; air percolates into soft tissues causing interstitial emphysema; if extreme, ball-valve air leaks may cause a tension pneumothorax with increased positive pressure in the hemithorax, shifting the mediastinum and compromising the circulation

ballistics FORENSIC MEDICINE The science of the motion of projectiles in flight, and as regards disease, the motion of said projectiles as the flight is slowed or stopped by a body or tissues; the energy imparted to tissue is calculated as E = mv² (m = mass; v = velocity) (JAMA 1988; 259:2730)

Relevant terms **CALIBER** The diameter of a bullet measured in hundredths of an inch (in the US and English-speaking countries); commonly used bullets are .22, .25, .30, .32, .38, and .45; in other ('metric') countries, calibers are measured in millimeters, eg .38 caliber corresponds to 9 mm **CAVITY** The permanent cavity along a bullet's trajectory is caused by the bullet per se, the temporary cavity is related to tissue stretching up to 11 times the diameter of the bullet (in contrast to the 30- to 40-fold increased diameter stated in older literature); the kinetic energy transferred during the short life of the temporary cavity is about 4 atmospheres (previously stated to be 100 atmospheres) **CHOKE** The narrowing of the cylinder bore of a shotgun at the muzzle, which is intended to minimize the spread of shot as it leaves the barrel; it is usually expressed as the percentage of shot that falls within a 30 inch (76 cm) circle at 40 yards (36.5 m); ± 70% for a full choke, ± 60% for a medium choke weapon **GAUGE** The inside diameter of a shotgun's bore; gauge is an obsolete unit based on the number of round lead balls, each having the same diameter of the bore, which will in toto weigh 1 pound (454 g); thus each lead ball in the most commonly used shotgun, the 12 gauge, weighs ¹⁄₁₂ of a pound (37.3 g or 1⅓ ounces) **VELOCITY** The difference in tissue destruction between high or low velocity projectiles is likely caused by the fragmentation of the bullet itself (as in the M-16 semiautomatic weapon) **YAW** The angle between line of flight and the bullet's long axis; bullets enter tissue and tumble once they are inside, rotating 180°, exiting with the base forward, explaining the large size of some exit wounds

ballistic movement NEUROPHYSIOLOGY An extremely rapid movement of the limbs which, once initiated, cannot be modified, eg striking a nail with a hammer, throwing a ball, and to be effective, require a great deal of practice and skill; BMs are of interest to anthropologists as they are integral to the manufacture and use of tools and hunting weapons, reflecting a level of sophistication in early humans and hominids (Sci Am 1994; 271:4:101)

ballistic stretching Bouncing stretching SPORTS MEDICINE Rapid, jerking movements in which the body part is moved with a momentum that would stretch the muscles to a maximum; during the bouncing motion, the muscle responds by contracting to protect itself from overstretching (JC DeLee, D Drez, Jr, Eds, Orthopedic Sports Medicine WB Saunders, Philadelphia, 1994)

balloon angioplasty A generic term for a minimally invasive procedure in which use of a catheter with an inflatable balloon is 'snaked' to a previously identified (by angiography) zone of arterial stenosis or occlusion; once in place, the balloon is inflated, expanding the lumen of the occluded vessel, BA is used for coronary and carotid arteries, and may be used for other vessels; see Percutaneous transluminal coronary angioplasty

balloon cell A non-specific term for any cell with abundant clear cytoplasm, which may be benign or malignant, of any embryologic origin and store any histologically clear material in the cytoplasm; ballooned cells include carcinoid cells, ependymal cells (myxopapillary ependymoma), hepatocytes, see ballooning degeneration, histiocytes storing glycosaminoglycans and mucopolysaccharides, neurons (Farber's disease, lipogranulomatosis, mannosidosis) and pigmented cells either benign (balloon cell nevus) or malignant (balloon cell melanoma); Cf Signet ring cell

balloon form A morphologic variant of *Trichophyton rubrum* and *T mentagrophyte* microaleuriospores, which are responsible for superficial dermatoses, tinea pedis and tinea corporis

ballooning BONE RADIOLOGY Biconcave compression of the end-plate of the vertebral body caused by pressure in the intervertebral discs, most commonly in the lumbar spine, a feature characteristic of osteoporosis; Cf Fish vertebrae

ballooning degeneration HEPATIC PATHOLOGY A histologic change seen in hepatocytes infected with HAV and HBV; the cells have abundant pale granular cytoplasm; the 'ground-glass' granularity of the cells is due to the accumulation of viral particles NEUROPATHOLOGY A descriptive term for the changes seen in vincristine therapy-induced peripheral neuropathy, enhanced by VP-16 PATHOLOGY Vacuolization, vesicle formation, unraveling of the myelin lamellae and electron-opaque material within and adjacent to the axon

balloon tamponade EMERGENCY MEDICINE A hemostatic procedure for upper gastrointestinal bleeding using a Sengstaken-Blakemore tube and a larger round tube, inflated in the stomach, which anchors the device in the desired location; balloon tamponade is indicated for bleeding esophageal varices or persistent hemorrhage of the esophagus for any reason

balloon valvoplasty A method used to treat stenotic cardiac valves, including 1) Pulmonic valve, where balloon valvoplasty is considered the optimal therapeutic modality 2) Mitral valve The results may be suboptimal if the valve ring is extensively calcified, but good if the valve is pliable or 3) Aortic valve Valvoplasty is considered the optimal therapy only for frail, elderly patients who are otherwise poor surgical candidates; recurrence of symptoms, restenosis and death occur in 50%; see Inoue balloon

Ballot Measure 16 see Death With Dignity Act

BALT Bronchiole-associated lymphoid tissue see MALT

Baltic myoclonus An autosomal recessive form of light-sensitive myoclonic epilepsy which at autopsy reveals loss of Purkinje cells TREATMENT Valproic acid

Baltimore affair A full-scale investigation by the US Congress, headed by representative Dingell that was initiated when a Nobel Laureate (discoverer of reverse transcriptase) at Massachusetts Institute of Technology was one of a number of co-authors, on a report (*ALTERED REPERTOIRE OF ENDOGENOUS IMMUNOGLOBULIN GENE EXPRESSION IN TRANSGENIC MICE CONTAINING A REARRANGED MU HEAVY CHAIN GENE* Cell 1986; 45:247), in which irregularities of data were alleged; see 'Dingellization', qui tam lawsuit, 'Whistle blowing'

Dr Baltimore was exonerated and requested that the paper be retracted and apologized for his role, albeit quite peripheral to the events; it is unclear whether scientifically unsophisticated juries and politicians should be allowed to evaluate complex data Time table of the events: Nature 1991; 351:95n&v; Bottom lines: Science 1991; 253:24 n&v

bamboo hair Trichorrhexis invaginata Dry, fragile, poorly growing hair with a 'ball-in-cup' invagination of the distal into the proximal hair shaft, related to a transient defect in keratinization, which improves by puberty, a finding central to the Netherton syndrome

bamboo vertebrae Universal syndesmophytosis that may be associated with osteoporosis and bony ankylosis, a finding typical of ankylosing spondylitis

banana form Crescent form A fanciful term for the morphology of the macrogametocyte, which corresponds to the female sexual intraerythrocytic form of *Plasmodium falciparum* which also has compact chromatin

banana sign An ultrasonographic finding when a major neural tube defect accompanies the Arnold-Chiari malformation with herniation of the cerebellar tonsils and midbrain structures into the foramen magnum, causing ventriculomegaly due to compression of the outflow from the third and fourth ventricles; the 'banana' corresponds to the compressed cerebral hemisphere

band HEMATOLOGY A region on an SDS-PAGE gel electrophoresis of the 'ghost' (membrane devoid of hemoglobin) of RBCs, when subjected to a hypoosmolar (low-ionic strength) solution; electrophoresis divides the membrane into bands 1 and 2 (spectrins), bands 2.1 and 2.2 (ankyrin), band 3 (a 90-kD glycoprotein dimer forming part of the erythrocyte ion channel, which is involved in anion transport, band 4.5 (a glucose transporter) and band 5 (actin) MOLECULAR BIOLOGY Any 'spot' on an electrophoretic gel, corresponding to the distance of migration of a molecule of interest (DNA, RNA or protein) which is the combined function of molecular weight and ionic charge (pI); bands are detected by a radioactive or biotinylated complementary probe of DNA (Southern blot), RNA (Northern blot), or protein (Western blot)

band Band cell, band form An immature neutrophil with a nucleus lacking the segmentation typical of mature polymorphonuclear leukocytes, having one continuous nuclear membrane 'band'; more than 5% of the neutrophils in the peripheral blood implies increased neutrophil production; see Left shift

Band-Aid™ MILITARY MEDICINE A medical corpsman (JE Lighter, Historical Dictionary of American Slang, Random House, New York, 1994)

Band-Aid™ is a trademark name for the first adhesive tape and gauze device devised in 1920 by Earle Dickson of the Johnson & Johnson company of New Brunsick, New Jersey; an estimated 1 x 10¹¹ Band-aid™ have been sold (C Panati, Extraordinary Origins of Everyday Things, Harper&Row, New York, 1987)

Band-Aid™ solution A highly colloquial generic term for any partial or 'cosmetic' solution to a problem, often referring to a treatment that falls far short of that demanded by the disease being treated

band form A mature trophozoite intraerythrocytic form of *Plasmodium malariae*; see Applique form, Ring form; Cf Band form

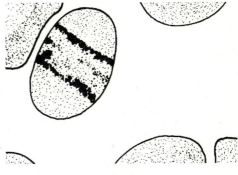

band form

la 'bandera' see Torture

banding CARDIAC PATHOLOGY Zonal changes of cardiac muscle due to myocardial ischemia, characterized by opaque transverse bands within myocytes adjacent to an intercalated disc, accompanied by shortening and scalloping of the sarcomere, fragmentation of Z bands, distortion of myofibrils and displacement of mitochondria away from intercalated disc; see Contraction band necrosis; Cf Wavy changes CYTOGENETICS A group of techniques for evaluating chromosomal 'landmarks', which allows identification of gross chromosomal defects that are regularly associated with either congenital conditions, eg trisomies, monosomies, aneuploidies, or with acquired disease, or translocations in lymphoproliferative disorders

---

CHROMOSOMAL BANDING

C Centromere banding The chromosomes are pretreated with strong bases, eg NaOH or strong acids, eg HCl, followed by Giemsa staining, which selectively highlights the centromeres

G Giemsa banding The chromosomes are pretreated with either concentrated salt, eg NaCl at high temperature or with proteolytic enzymes and then Giemsa stained

Q Quinacrine banding The chromosomes are stained with fluorescent dyes, then Giemsa stained

R Reverse banding The chromosomes are pretreated with alkaline solutions and analyzed at high temperature with controlled pH; the image seen is opposite that of G and Q banding

---

band keratopathy OPHTHALMOLOGY A broad deposit of opaque calcium phosphate in vertical lines parallel to, within and often lateral to the limbus on Bowman's membrane, which is seen by slit lamp examination; bands in absence of phosphate elevation may presage the onset of renal failure; although band keratopathy is classically associated with hyperparathyroidism, it may occur in hypercalcemia of any etiology, eg in subcorneal calcium deposition in chronically inflamed eyes (chronic iridocyclitis of juvenile rheumatoid arthritis or Still's disease), increased vitamin D absorption, uveitis, pilocarpine therapy, glaucoma and laser-induced injury; non-calcific band keratopathy occurs with elastotic degeneration

band ligation A therapeutic modality used to treat potentially fatal esophageal varices associated with portal hypertension, which may be more effective than the widely accepted sclerotherapy used to obliterate varices (JAMA 1991; 266:187n&v)

bandpass width LABORATORY INSTRUMENTATION The range of wavelengths between two points used by a spectrophotometer or colorimeter, at which point the transmittance is ½ the peak value, where the remaining wavelengths were blocked by a bandpass filter

band 3 protein An anion-exchange protein that in the kidney is restricted to a subpopulation of collecting duct-intercalated cells; the expression of band 3 protein in renal oncocytomas is interpreted as evidence that these tumors are histogenically unrelated to renal cell carcinomas, which are derived from the metanephric blastema (Arch Pathol Lab Med 1994; 118:702oa)

band regularity CYTOGENETICS A term that connotes constancy of DNA-protein interactions; chromosomal bands are presumed due to folding of the chromosomes, where each band represents approximately 5% of any one chromosome

bandshifting MOLECULAR BIOLOGY A difference in the rate in DNA band migration in gel electrophoresis that occurs despite equal size of the fragment or band of DNA; the amount of bandshifting migration is relatively small, in the range 1-4%, which may become significant in forensic DNA analysis; the faster migration is corrected for by running a 'monomorphic' probe that attaches to a fragment of DNA similar in all persons; bandshifting is a function of the actual size (in number of nucleotides) of the band, the concentration of the gel (ie concentration of the agarose) and the actual running time (speed of the run); one way to eliminate this problem is to run a sequencing gel, in which the actual 'signature' of the entire hypervariable (unique to the individual in question) has been previously amplified by a PCR technique; see DNA fingerprinting

band test Lupus band test IMMUNOPATHOLOGY Immune deposition of IgG, accompanied by varying amounts of IgM, IgA, C3 at the dermal-epidermal junction in discoid (DLE) and systemic lupus erythematosus (SLE); the band test is negative in the uninvolved areas of DLE; 90-95% of lupus erythematosus patients have bands in clinical lesions, 80% have bands in sun-exposed skin and 50% of non-sun-exposed skin; the presence of dermal bands is poorly reflective of renal disease, although DLE and SLE patients with a negative band test or IgM deposits alone may have a better prognosis or less intense renal involvement, hypocomplementemia and anti-DNA antibodies; 'bands' also appear in acne rosacea, anaphylactoid purpura, atopic and contact dermatitides, autoimmune thyroiditis, early bullous pemphigoid, cold agglutinin syndrome, dermatomyositis, facial telangiectasia, hypocomplementemic vasculitis, lepromatous leprosy, polymorphous light eruption, primary biliary cirrhosis, procainamide and hydralazine-induced lupus erythematosus, pyoderma gangrenosum, rheumatoid arthritis and scleroderma; a band is also seen in NZB/NZW mice, the animal model for lupus erythematosus; Cf Antinuclear antibodies

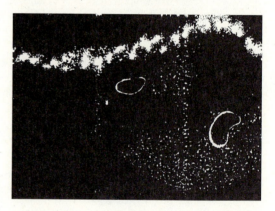

band test

bandwidth COMPUTERS A measure of transport (speed and throughput) of data between connected computers; at the low end are current modems with the industry-standard V.32bis, which transfers uncompressed data at 14.4 kilobytes/sec (Kbps); Switched 56 at 56 Kbps; ISDN (Integrated Services Digital Network) at 64 Kbps to 1.54 Mbps (megabytes/sec); the Asynchronous Transfer Mode will transfer data at 45 Mbps to 1.2 Gbps (gigabytes/sec) and be available by the mid-1990s

BANF Bilateral acoustic neurofibromatosis, Neurofibromatosis, type II, see there

bangungut Sudden unexplained nocturnal death, see there

B antigen A major blood group (ABO) antigen which defines the blood type B, assuming the codominant allele at the ABO locus is B or H; B antigens are highly immunogenic; when a B unit of packed red cells is transfused into an A or O recipient, the natural antibodies present in the recipient are capable of evoking a severe or fatal hemolytic transfusion reaction; Cf A antigen, Bombay phenotype, H antigen

B-antigen-acquired TRANSFUSION MEDICINE A modified antigen found on the membranes of A1 red blood cells that agglutinates as though it were a group B erythrocyte, due to enzymatic modification of the normal A1 into a B-like antigen, caused by bacteria, including *Escherichia coli*, *Clostridium tertium* and *Bacteroides fragilis*, associated with GI pathology, eg carcinoma or severe infection

BAO Basal Acid Output, see there

bar code Machine-readable identifier LABORATORY MEDICINE A printed pattern of vertical bars of varying widths corresponding to the numbers 0-9 which represent numeric or alphanumeric codes in a machine-readable format; bar codes may be 'scanned' by a device detecting variations in light patterns, allowing the symbols to be recognized directly by a computer's central processing unit; bar coding allows automated entry of test and patient information; originally used in supermarkets, bar coding is becoming standard in the medical environment as a means of reducing error rates to a minimum (Am Clin Lab August 1994) by providing the patient with a unique identifier, eg for laboratory specimens, x-rays and medical records, preventing incorrect transferral of data and to facilitate documentation

barbed ends MEMBRANE PHYSIOLOGY The portion of the nonmuscle actin filament which points towards the membrane or sites of attachment

barber pole pattern A fanciful descriptor of the angiographic appearance of the 'supercoiled' superior mesenteric artery and vein as seen in a midgut malrotation with volvulus

barbell tumor Dumbbell tumor, see there

barbiturate coma BIOMEDICAL ETHICS The use of barbiturates, eg pentobarbital to produce a loss of consciousness, which has a secondary ('double') effect of inducing hypoxia and ultimately respiratory failure; barbiturate comas have been used in executions to prepare prisoners for lethal injection, by Dutch physicians in performing euthanasia, and in assisted suicides in the US; the use of the barbiturate coma to hasten the death of patients who are terminally ill is an ethically charged issue, and viewed as either fulfilling the basic tenets of the physician's moral duty to care for the patient, or as a first step on the 'slippery slope' of physician-assisted 'murder' (N Engl J Med 1992; 327:1678SB)

bare see Go bare

bare-bones health plan HEALTH CARE ENVIRONMENT A colloquial term for low-cost, no-frill, stripped-down health insurance policy that is designed for small businesses, which often has large deductibles, co-payments, low policy limits, and minimal hospitalization benefits (Am Med News 26 October 1992, p7)

barefoot doctor A term originating in and being phased out of the Republic of China, referring to countryside health aides who were neither barefoot nor doctors (JAMA 1988; 259:3561)

bare lymphocyte syndrome An AR [MIM 209920] immune deficiency disorder described in several North African kindreds due to non-expression of HLA-A, -B or -C (Class I) major histocompatibility complex, caused by a defect in surface expression of β_2-microglobulin; in some cases, the HLA-Dr determinant is also not expressed CLINICAL Variable, from asymptomatic to mucocutaneous candidiasis, respiratory tract infections, opportunistic infections, chronic diarrhea and malabsorption, poor response to antigens, aplastic anemia and leukopenia with normal or increased B cells with decreased T cells MOLECULAR BIOLOGY The condition is thought to be due to a defect in gene activation and/or a defect in accessibility of the promoter protein (Science 1991; 252:709)

BARI Bypass Angioplasty Revascularization Intervention (Circulation 1991; 84:Suppl V:V-1–V-27)

barium burger test A method for evaluating increased gastric retention of food as occurs in the gastric outlet obstruction (GOO), where the 'burger' is 'flavored' with barium contrast; GOO is diagnosed if barium is retained for more than 6 hours in an intact stomach or for more than 3 hours in a resected stomach (Am J Gastroenterol 1972; 58:411)

barium enema A barium-rich fluid used to visualize the colonic lumen, of greatest utility in delineating colonic neoplasia

barium peritonitis A rare complication of a barium enema, in which there is a high (50%) mortality, due to intraperitoneal perforation with leakage or spillage of radiocontrast material, variably accompanied by feces, release of histamine and vasoactive substances into the peritoneum with activation of coagulation pathways causing fibrinous peritonitis

barium 'sandwich' A mixture of solid food and barium contrast used to evaluate esophageal deglutition by fluoroscopy, obtaining information beyond the capabilities of the plain 'barium swallow'

β-ARK β-adrenergic receptor kinase A membrane (protein) enzyme that phosphorylates agonist (ie hormone)-bound receptor, turning off the signaling pathway initiated by the hormone-G protein ligand coupling (Science 1995; 268:247); β-ARK down-regulates (desensitizes) cellular sensitivity to sensory, neurotransmitter and hormonal stimulation, mediating stimulatory effects of catecholamines on the adenylyl cyclase system and by extension regulating intracellular cAMP levels; the β-ARK gene sequence is similar to protein kinase C and cAMP-dependent protein kinase

barn RADIATION PHYSICS A unit of area ($10^{-24}cm^2$) for the effective cross-section of atomic nuclei, so named as it is the droll opposite of a large area, 'big as the side of a barn'

BARN Bilateral acute retinal necrosis A herpes virus-induced anterior and posterior uveitis, papillitis with retinal detachment occurring 1-3 months after onset, of which only 50% are bilateral

Barney Clark see Clark, Barney

baroreflex A vasomotor reflex that originates in the baroreceptors and sends information about distention of the vessel walls of great vessels of the head and neck, transmitting the information to the commissural, dorsolateral, and medial portions of the solitary tract nucleus of the brain stem; baroreceptor information passes to the brainstem from the carotid sinus via the glossopharyngeal nerve, from the aortic arch and great vessels of the thorax via the vagal nerves (N Engl J Med 1993; 329:1449OA)

baroreflex failure A constellation of clinical findings characterized by marked lability of blood pressure with systolic and diastolic hypertension and tachycardia (± headache, diaphoresis, emotional lability, and refractoriness of heart rate in response to exogenous vasoactive substances) alternating with hypotension and bradycardia PATHOGENESIS Damage to the glossopharyngeal or vagal nerves by surgery, regional irradiation, or degenerative changes of the corresponding solitary tract nuclei in the brainstem MANAGEMENT Clonidine suppresses pressor and tachycardic surges, diazepam, stress reduction (N Engl J Med 1993; 329:1449OA, 1494ED) Cf Autonomic failure

Barr body Sex chromatin A condensed clump of chromatin located adjacent to the nuclear membrane which is best seen in somatic cells in interphase; in humans, BBs correspond to an inactivated X chromosome, and the number of BBs/cell is one less than the number of X chromosomes

barrel An adjectival descriptor occasionally used in medicine referring a morphology or pattern likened to a barrel

Rounded bulging vessel constructed of wooden staves, bound with metal hoops with flattened ends, designed to hold liquid or grains, whose length is slightly greater than its diameter

barrel cervix GYNECOLOGY A descriptor for the rounded thickening seen in the rare lymphoma of the uterine cervix

barrel chest RESPIRATORY MEDICINE A broad chest with hyperinflated, poorly aerated lungs, typical of emphysema; a similar short, but broadened chest of a different etiology occurs in Morquio syndrome or mucopolysaccharidosis, type IV

barrel staves pattern An ultrastructural finding in clear cell sarcoma (malignant melanoma of soft parts) that simulates flattened and curved barrel staves, corresponding to the internal structures of premelanosomes

Barrett's esophagus A condition* estimated to occur in up to 2 million in the US; that develops in patients with GERD and defined as the replacement of the normal stratified squamous epithelium with metaplastic potentially premalignant intestinal columnar epithelium lining a segment of the distal esophagus, occasionally accompanied by peptic ulceration; it is postulated that BE is a defensive reaction of GERD, as gastric mucosa is more resistant to the refluxate ENDOSCOPY The changes of BE include a proximal migration of the squamocolumnar Z-line, and patchy areas that correspond to single layered columnar cells that are in intimate contact with underlying blood vessels and pink; although most patients are adults, it may affect children, leading to speculation that the condition has a congenital component; Barrett's esophagus places a patient at an estimated 35-40-fold increased risk of suffering adenocarcinoma of the esophagus, which is almost invariably accompanied by dysplasia, and has a prognosis similar to that of epidermoid carcinoma of the region (14.5% five-year survival) PATHOLOGY Barrett's epithelium is of three broad types: atrophic gastric fundus with parietal and chief cells, cardiac (junctional type), consisting of mucus glands and specialized columnar glands, possibly representing a form of intestinal metaplasia; in one report, 9/13 patients with aneuploidy or ↑ G2 or tetraploidy by flow cytometry progressed to high-grade dysplasia or adenocarcinoma; no cases without these findings advanced to higher-grade lesions (Gastroenterology 1992; 102:1212; see Sci & Med Nov/Dec 1994 p16RV)

*The terms, eg Barrett's epithelium, Barrett syndrome, and Barrett's ulcer, that refer either to the lesion per se or the disease have been essentially deleted from the medical lexicon

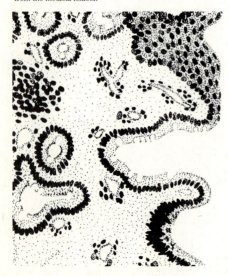

Barrrett's esophagus

barrier An impediment to access to a service or activity, defined in the context of the Americans with Disabilities Act (ADA, see there), which may be architectural (eg requiring widened doors, wheelchair ramps, and others) or barriers to communication (eg linguistic barrier, defects of vision, which according to the ADA may require reasonable accomodations in the form of obtaining an interpreter or braille forms (paperwork); see Americans with Disabilities Act, Disability

barrier-free Pertaining or referring to structural or architectural design that does not represent an impediment for use by individuals with special physical needs (NY Newsday, 25 Nov, 1994, D1)

barrier method Contraceptives (condom or diaphragm) that attempt to prevent the boy-meets-girl-make-baby sequence; the theoretical effectiveness of barrier methods is 2.5 pregnancies/100 woman-years, the actual effectiveness is closer to 15/100; see Pearl index

barrier precautions INFECTION CONTROL Any method or device used to reduce the contact with potentially infectious body fluids, including facial masks, doubled gloves and fluid-resistant gowns

Bartonella henselae *Rochalimaea henselae* A slender fastidious coccobacillary bacterium first identified in both HIV-infected and in immunocomptent patients with persistent or relapsing fever; both *B henslae* and *B quintana* have been linked to bacillary angiomatosis (N Engl J Med 1995; 332:463ED)

Bartonella quintana *Rochalimaea quintana* A slender fastidious coccobacillary bacterium that is the agent of trench fever, transmitted by the body louse; *B quintana* infection also causes bacillary splenitis, bacteremia, endocarditis, cat-scratch disease, and cutaneous bacillary angiomatosis, in chronic alcoholics, and in the homeless DIAGNOSIS Blood culture, direct immunofluorescence, DNA-hybridization, PCR-amplified RFLPs, serology TREATMENT Nafcillin, ceftriaxone, and others in an empirical fashion (N Engl J Med 1995; 332:419, 424)

basal acid output BAO Production of gastric H+ under baseline conditions, normal: 0-10 mmol/hr; BAO serves to measure the completeness of vagotomy; patients with Zollinger-Ellison syndrome have a ratio of basal to maximal acid output (BAO/MAO) of greater than 60%; BAO is also increased in pernicious anemia, gastric carcinoma, myxedema and rheumatoid arthritis; Cf MAO, PAO

basal cell carcinoma A relatively indolent epithelial malignancy of the skin that is most common in the sun-exposed regions of the head, neck and upper body in older individuals PATHOLOGY The cells are often arranged in nests with a peripheral pallisading, often in a background of solar elastosis; subtypes include adenoid, solid, and cystic variants TREATMENT Local excision; if areas where tissue border may compromise function or appearance, eg angle of eyes, eyelids, nose, Mohs surgery may be indicated

basal cell nevus syndrome Nevoid basal cell carcinoma syndrome, basal cell carcinoma syndrome, Gorlin-Goltz syndrome A rare AD [MIM 109400] disease characterized by the childhood onset of multiple nevoid basal cell carcinomas associated with abnormalities of the skin ('pits' in the hands and feet in the form of 2-3 mm in diameter cells occasionally filled with carcinoma, milia, sebaceous cysts, lipomas, fibromas), lymphomesenteric cysts, CNS disease (mental retardation, electroencephalographic abnormalities, calcification of the dura, medulloblastoma and schizophrenia), endocrine system (ovarian cysts or fibroma, male hypogonadism, female escutcheon, scanty facial hair), eyes (canthal dystopia, hypertelorism, coloboma of nerve, congenital blindness), typical facies (hypertelorism, lateral displacement of medial canthi, frontoparietal bossing, mandibular prognathism, accentuated supraorbital ridges, jaw cysts and a broad nasal root), skeleton (spina bifida occulta, fused, absent or cervical ribs, kyphosis, scoliosis, cervical and thoracic vertebral fusion, bridging of sella turcica, frontal and temporoparietal bone 'bossing', spina bifida occulta, shortened 4th-5th metacarpals, epithelial-lined cysts of the jaws (N Engl J Med 1960; 262:908, ibid, 314:700cpc)

basal energy expenditure The amount of oxygen consumed while resting and fasting, extrapolated to 24 hours, roughly equivalent to 25 kcal/kg; see Basal metabolic rate

basal factor MOLECULAR BIOLOGY A protein that responds to signals from activators and positions RNA polymerase at the beginning of a protein-coding region of a gene, sending the RNA polymerase on its mission; BFs include the *TATA* binding protein and factors A, B, E, F, and H (Sci Am 1995; 272/2:56) see Transcription activator

basal metabolic rate BMR A value which may be calculated with formula for calculating a person's proteo-caloric requirements; the most commonly used is that of Harris and Benedict:

BMR, ♂: 66 + (13.7 x WEIGHT) + (5 x HEIGHT) – (6.8 x AGE)
BMR, ♀: 655 + (9.6 x WEIGHT) + (1.8 x HEIGHT) – (4.7 x AGE)

basaloid carcinoma Cloacogenic carcinoma A histologic variant of epidermal carcinoma arising at the anorectal transition zone, which comprises 20% of all carcinomas of this region; although this tumor histologically mimics basal cell carcinoma (from whence its name), it often displays mucin production and squamous differentiation and behaves clinically like a 'garden variety' anal carcinoma, the distinction appears to be unwarranted Note: Anal carcinoma may be associated with lesions of sexual partners, eg squamous cell carcinoma of the uterine cervix, condyloma acuminatum and with the practice of receptive anal intercourse in the male homosexuals, thus indirectly inculpating human papillomaviruses

baseball finger Mallet finger A flexion deformity at a 30° angle of the distal phalanx, produced by a blow to the tip of the finger, in US most often associated with catching a baseball thrown at high speed, with forced flexion of the distal phalanx and separation (by rupture or avulsion fracture) of the common extensor tendon from its insertion in the base of the distal phalanx; accompanied by inability to extend the fingertip

baseball stitch A type of surgical repair used to close the uterus in the classic Cesarean section incision, an incision more cephalad than the now-preferred lower uterine segment incision, as it is associated with greater immediate and remote morbidity; the baseball stitch closure is continuous, not locked, with 2-0 chromic and each needle 'bite' begins on the raw surface of the wound, exiting through the serosa a few millimeters from the cut edge, infolding the cut edge, bringing the serosal surface over to cover the uterus

baseline A generic term for any basal, null, or unstimulated state, often represented as a horizontal line, hence the name

basement membrane An organized multi-molecular layer composed of collagens, predominantly type IV, glycoproteins, eg laminin and fibronectin, and proteoglycans, eg dermatan sulfate, which is subjacent to epithelium and endothelium; basement membranes are dynamic structures involved in cell growth, adhesion and differentiation; dissolution of the basement membrane is a final step in the development of metastasizing carcinoma

base pair A pair of hydrogen-bonded bases that link to each other; in the DNA double helix, purines (adenine and guanine) or pyrimidines (cytosine and thymine) link to each other

base pairing The complementary binding of the bases in a nucleic acid, between two strands of DNA or a strand of DNA and RNA; see Hybridization

BASIC Beginners' All-purpose Symbolic Instruction Code A high-level symbolic computer programming language that is commonly used to write programs for mini- and microcomputers

basic life support EMERGENCY MEDICINE The emergency procedures necessary to ensure a person's immediate survival, including cardiopulmonary resuscitation, control of bleeding, treatment of shock and poisoning, stabilization of injuries and/or wounds, and basic first aid; Cf Advanced life support

Note: BLS is a generic term that overlaps considerably with and is virtually synonymous with CPR (cardiopulmonary resuscitation)

basket cell NEUROHISTOLOGY A cell of the cerebellar cortex, the axons of which give off splays of fine branches that enclose the Purkinje cells in a basket-like fashion HEMATOLOGY A fragmented and degenerated leukocyte in a peripheral blood smear with a bare nucleus partially surrounded by a coarse network of splayed, red-purple nucleoplasm which may be seen in normal subjects and which is increased in atypical lymphocytosis, chronic lymphocytic and acute leukemias, thus being similar in origin to 'smudge' cells

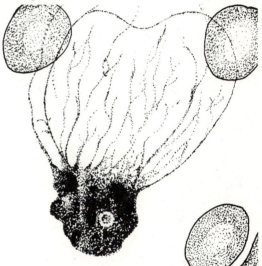

basket cell

basophil A granular leukocyte bearing distinctly basophilic secondary granules containing heparin, histamine, platelet-activating factor and other mediators of the immediate hypersensitivity, released when IgE cross-links to the high affinity Fc receptors on the cell's surface

basophilic stippling Punctate stippling HEMATOLOGY A finding in Wright-Giemsa-stained erythrocytes that appears as 'blue' dots, spots and blots within erythrocytes consisting of 1) RNA granules (coarse stippling) due to RNA instability in young red cells, seen in lead poisoning (lead inhibits ALA dehydrogenase and ferrochetolase, impairing heme incorporation and inhibiting nucleotidase), defective hemoglobin C or hemoglobin E synthesis, sideroblastic or megaloblastic anemia, thalassemia major and minor, preleukemic states, pyrimidine 5'nucleotidase deficiency 2) Aggregates of precipitated ribosomes (fine stippling), resulting in diffuse polychromasia secondary to increased erythrocyte production in thalassemia, malabsorption and pernicious anemia

Bassen-Kornzweig syndrome Betalipoproteinemia, see there

BAT Blunt abdominal trauma

bathing suit distribution A pattern of truncal skin involvement in rheumatic heart disease (erythema marginatum) characterized by flattened, slowly enlarging maculopapules that undergo central healing; the pattern is also seen in X-linked lipidosis, Fabry's disease (angiokeratoma corporis diffusa, accompanied by punctate to macular, non-blanching telangiectasia), glycosphingolipidosis, fucosidosis and sialidosis

bathing trunk nevus Garment nevus, see there

battered baby Battered child, see there

battered buttock 'syndrome' A rare complex described in females which consists of fracturing of fat or traumatic lipomas, in which tissue is sheared between the dermal anchorage of the skin and the deep fascia

battered child Abused child PEDIATRICS A young child often under the age of three who has been repeatedly neglected by his/her caretakers; BCs have signs of multiple episodes of trauma, eg subdural hematomas, fractures, and bruises in various stages of healing, often in combination with failure to thrive and chronic malnutrition (**N Engl J Med 1995; 332:1425RV**)

battered child syndrome Child abuse, see there

battered prize fighter face A descriptor of the facies seen in the X-linked or autosomal dominant otopalatodigital syndrome of Taybi, which is characterized by frontal bossing, a broad nasal bridge, flattened facies, accompanied by a cleft palate and micrognathia, deafness, mental and growth retardation, deformities of the hands and feet and pectus excavatum

battery MEDICAL MALPRACTICE The unauthorized touching of another; a patient's visit to a physician for a consultation or '...*treatment implies consent to reasonable physical contact necessary for the examination...more than such customary contact, as in surgery, invasive diagnostic procedures, and drug treatment* (requires specific consent). *In the absence of such consent, treatment by the physician would be battery...*' as would operating at a site different from that specified in the consent form (**LW Way, Ed Surgical Diagnosis & Treatment, 10th ed, Appletone & Lange, Norwalk, 1994**) see Malpractice

battle-axe appearance see Halberd bone

Battle's sign Bruising over the mastoid bone, a finding typical of basilar fracture of the skull (see **N Engl J Med 1992; 327:1507RA**)

battledore placenta A morphological placenta variant where the umbilical cord is placed at the margin, which is not thought to have clinical significance

Battledore: Old English, a flat, wooden paddle used in the game of battledore, an ancestor of badminton

batwing distribution Butterfly distribution RADIOLOGY A descriptor for shaggy, bilateral perihilar lung opacifications, seen on an antero-posterior chest film, due to intraalveolar fluid exudation, first described in uremia, but more typical of pulmonary edema and may occur in pulmonary alveolar proteinosis

BAU Bioequivalent allergy unit, see there

baud A unit of velocity of electronic transferral of data, where one baud is equal to 1 bit/second; standardized transmissions are 300, 1200, 2400 and 9600 baud; see Computers, Modem

bay region EXPERIMENTAL ONCOLOGY The site on benzo(a)pyrene (Figure), an indirect carcinogen that is metabolically activated by the P-450 system at the 7, 8 double bond, leading to a 7, 8 oxide, which is rapidly converted to a 7, 8 dihydrodiol and later epoxidated near the bay region at the 9, 10 double bond; the resulting product, a diol-epoxide is a poor substrate for epoxide hydratase and is released from the mitochondria into the cell as a highly reactive electrophil, becoming an 'ultimate' carcinogen, as it reacts with negative charges in DNA; P-450 reactions at the K region (see there) yield a non-reactive non-carcinogenic inert molecule

bay region

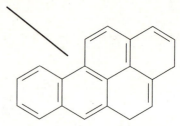

Bayesian analysis An analysis that '...*permits the calculation of the probability that one treatment is superior based on the observed data and prior beliefs...subjectivity of beliefs is not a liability, but rather explicitly allows different opinions to be formally expressed and evaluated.*' (**JAMA 1995; 273:871**) RISK FACTORS Nonblanchable erythema, lymphopenia, immobility, dry skin, low body weight, and activity limited to bed or chair (**JAMA 1995; 273:865**)

Bayesian belief network 'An inference technique that provides a framework for reasoning while working under the uncertainty principle, based on the theory of probability...in a BBN, each fact or assertion is in the knowledge base is represented by a node. A linkmatrix of conditioned probabilities represents the dependence of of assertions and outcomes between nodes. The knowledge-engineering process for these networks consists of identifying relevant variables...represented by the nodes, and determining the links as the causal relationship between them.' (**Anal Quan Cytol Histol 1994; 16:29abstr**)

Bayesian logic A type of reasoning in which the likelihood of an event occurring can be described in quantitative (ie probabilistic) terms; Bayes' rules incorporate prevalence (eg of a disease), a range of possible relations (eg differential diagnoses), and can be modified as new information becomes available; Bayes' rules may be used in computer-based diagnostic systems (**N Engl J Med 1994; 330:1824ED**)

Bayh-Dole Act A legislative act passed in 1980 (US Congress) that allowed industry and universities to retain control of the intellectual property (eg patents) from government-supported grants and research (**Sci Am 1994; 270/9:72**)

bayonet hairs A developmental defect of the hairshaft with excess keratinization of the upper third, thought to be common in ichthyosis and seborrhea and occasionally seen in normal scalps

bayonet hand A deformity described in hereditary multiple exostosis (diaphyseal aclasis) characterized by ulnar deviation of the carpus and subluxation of the radius

bayonet incision An elongated S-shaped incision used to treat lacerations and for providing access in reconstructive surgery to the wrist bones; the bayonet incision is not indicated in the rheumatoid wrist where the distal skin flap may slough, requiring an abdominal pedicle flap

BBB syndrome Hypertelorism-hypospadias syndrome, see there; aka G syndrome

BCC Basal cell carcinoma, also 1) Balanced calorimeter chamber 2) Behavior Classification Checklist (psychology) 3) Birth control clinic

B cell B lymphocyte‡

B-cell lymphoproliferative syndrome An uncommon, life-threatening complication of bone marrow or organ transplantation caused by profound immunosuppression, which may be induced by Epstein-Barr virus; BLS occurs in 0.23 to 0.45% of the recipients of HLA-identical bone marrow, especially in those patients who suffered severe graft-versus-host disease and were treated with anti-CD3 antibodies CLINICAL Ranges from self-limited, spontaneously-resolving infectious mononucleosis to oliclonal or monoclonal proliferations and aggressive lymphomas PROGNOSIS 80-90% mortality in bone marrow recipients; 60% survival in those receiving other organs; one 'magic bullet' modality uses anti-B cell antibodies (monoclonal antibodies to CD21 and CD24 antigens) to suppress the B-cell lymphoproliferative syndrome and is well-tolerated, although its efficacy remains unproven (**N Engl J Med 1991; 324:1451**)

BCG bacille Calmette-Guerin A strain of *Mycobacterium bovis* that has been grown for multiple generations on potato, bile glycerine agar to a point where it has retained its immunogenicity but lost its virulence; BCG is an effective vaccine for TB and has been used to non-specifically stimulate the immune response in patients with certain malignancies, eg melanoma; because of its long-term persistence in the body, it has potential use as a vector for genes encoding HIV proteins including Gag, Pol, Env, reverse transcriptase, gp20, gp40 and tetanus toxin (**Nature 1991; 351:479, 442**); extrachromosomal and integrative expression vectors carrying the regulatory sequences for major BCG heat-shock proteins (hsp60 and hsp70) allow the expression of foreign antigens present in BCG (**Nature 1991; 351:456**), and may be used as a live recombinant vaccine vehicle to induce immune response to the pathogen's protein

BCGF B cell growth factor

B chain therapy CLINICAL THERAPEUTICS A potential therapeutic modality in the early stages of development, which may be of use in treating autoimmune disease; in BCT, the B chain* of cholera toxin is linked to an antigen evoking autoimmune antibody production, which in animals is reported to evoke immune tolerance to the antigen (**Science News 1995; 147:247**)

*Which anchors cholera toxin to the intestinal cells and evokes a strong immune response; in contrast, the A toxin is responsible for the disease state evoked by *Vibrio cholera*

B chromosome GENETICS Supernumerary ('extra') segments of DNA that are present in many species, which appear to be driven to self-duplication, as they are transmitted at higher rates than otherwise expected from classic Mendelian genetics

bcl The B cell leukemia/lymphoma gene family has traditionally been written in a lowercase italic (*bcl*), and in many regions continues to be so written, with its protein product being written in simple lowercase (bcl); many authors now prefer using uppercase italic (*BCL*) for the gene and uppercase (BCL) for the gene product; as this conversion is fragmented and incomplete, the author will use the lowercase italic

bcl-1 A gene located on chromosome segment 11q13 that is involved in the t(11;14) translocation, in which chromosome 11 sequences join in the J region cluster of the IgH gene locus on chromosome 14q32; mtc (major translocation cluster) is the predominant breakpoint region; this translocation is characteristic of mantle zone-derived B-cell lymphomas

bcl-1 The protein encoded by *bcl-1*, most commonly known as CyclinD1, see there

bcl-2 MOLECULAR BIOLOGY The B-cell leukemia/lymphoma proto-oncogene which is associated with follicular lymphoma; it is located on chromosome segment 18q21, the site of t(14;18) translocations; increased expression of bcl-2 is an early event in certain lymphomas, and when

present in diffuse or nodular large cell lymphomas, indicates a poor prognosis (those with a *bcl-2* rearrangement survive less than 3 years; those with a duplication of chromosome 2 survive less than 1 year *bcl-2* protects the cell from programmed cell death, and is a member of the same gene family as the *ced-9* gene of the nematode *Caenorhabditis elegans*; a single (Gly→Glu) mutation in the *ced-9* gene prevents cell death, an event that may also occur in the human *bcl-2*, the protein product of which, bcl-2 is overexpressed in follicular lymphomas; a point mutation* in the BH1 domain of *bcl-2* abrogates its death repressor function by blocking the production of Bcl-2/Bax heterodimers (**Nature 1994; 369:318, 321,272OA**); the translocation of *bcl-2* to chromosome 14* juxtaposes it with the immunoglobulin heavy chain gene, and brings it under the control of the heavy chain gene's promoter; this results in $\uparrow$ production of Bcl-2 protein, protecting the affected cells from programmed cell death; $\uparrow$ *bcl-2* expression in certain lung malignancies is associated with $\uparrow$ survival, in particular those > age 60 and those with squamous cell carcinoma (**N Engl J Med 1993; 329:690OA**) *bcl-2* mutations $\uparrow$ with age, < $0.3/10^6$ at age 20, $3.93/10^6$ at age 65 (**G Coropassi et al, Proc Nat Acad of Sci (US) 13 Sept, 1994**)

*The 14;18 translocation t(14;18) is present in 31-74% of follicular and 20% of diffuse B-cell lymphomas ; it had been reported to be positive in reactive lymphoid hyperplasia, but only with enhanced PCR techniques (**Arch Pathol Lab Med 1994; 118:791OA**)

bcl-2 A 25-kD protein encoded by the *bcl-2* miniprotooncogene and located on the inner mitochondrial membrane, which blocks programmed cell death, an event that occurs by apoptosis

bcl-6 A proto-oncogene located on chromosome segment 3q27 with structural similarities to transcription factors that participate in the control of cell proliferation and differentiation and organogenesis; *bcl-6* rearrangements occur in ± 30% of diffuse lymphomas with large cell components, and may serve as a marker of a favorable prognosis in terms of an independent prognostic marker for improved survival and freedom from disease (**N Engl J Med 1994; 331:74OA**)

BCNU Carmustine A member of the nitrosurea family of chemotherapeutic agents (related compounds include lomustine-CCNU and semustine) that partially overlap the range of activity and toxicity of alkylating chemotherapeutic agents, which is of particular use in Hodgkin's disease, and may be used in NHL, malignant melanoma, multiple myeloma, brain neoplasms, GI carcinomas; BCNU crosses the blood-brain barrier and is thus useful in treating both meningeal leukemia and brain tumors SIDE EFFECTS Nausea, vomiting, $\downarrow\downarrow\downarrow$ platelets, $\downarrow\downarrow\downarrow$ WBCs, secondary leukemia, pulmonary fibrosis, renal failure

bcr Breakpoint cluster region A 5.8-kilobase DNA segment on chromosome 22 that is related to malignant transformation of pluripotent hematopoietic stem cells in chronic myelogenous leukemia (CML); in CML there is a reciprocal translocation between chromosome 9, band q34 (a site containing the human homolog of the Abelson viral oncogene, c-*abl*) and chromosome 22 band q11 (the location of the breakpoint cluster region); this translocation results in formation of the 'Philadelphia' chromosome (named after the city of its discovery), which transcribes a hybrid mRNA encoding a protein with tyrosine kinase activity

BCS theory A theory* that explains the concept of superconductivity, where *two electrons* (a Cooper pair) *of opposite spin and momentum are bound together so that they have zero net spin and momentum. The attractive force behind this pairing is a subtle interaction between the negative charge of electrons and the positive charge of ion cores in the superconducting material. These ion cores are simply atoms that have lost one or more of their outermost electrons, which*

become free to conduct electricity. The ion cores are pulled in toward an electron as it moves through the lattice of a solid, creating a region of enhanced positive charge' (Sci Am 1994; 270/8:46) see SQUID, Superconductivity
*J Bardeen, LN Cooper, JR Schreiffer (1957)

BCYE agar MICROBIOLOGY L-Cysteine-buffered charcoal-yeast extract agar (BCYEα-L Cys) An agar used to grow *Legionella pneumophila*

BDNF Brain-derived neurotrophic factor A member of the nerve growth factor family that selectively elicits growth in the retinal ganglion, evokes increased secretion of dopamine in the substantia nigra and GABA in the forebrain; in the MPTP-induced model of Parkinson's disease, 75% of dopamine neurons are lost, an effect prevented by addition of BDNF, implying that loss of this trophic factor may have a role in Parkinson's disease (Nature 1991; 350:230, 195); see MPTP, Neurotropin-3, Nerve growth factor

B-DNA A sequence-dependent local variation in the structure of the DNA helix, seen in states of high hydration, which influences groove width, helical twist, mechanical rigidity, bending and resistance to bending; each segment of DNA has its own molecular surface 'signature', critical for specific recognition by proteins that repress and enhance DNA transcription; see DNA forms

beaded hair disease Monilethrix, see there

beaded ureter Corkscrew ureter, see there

beading CARDIOVASCULAR PATHOLOGY Luminal irregularity of arteries supplying regions affected by electrical injury; beaded vessels are at risk for subsequent thromboses RADIOLOGY Diffusely distributed dilated divisions and diverticular outpouchings of the common bile duct punctuated by short annular fibrotic strictures seen by direct cholangiography in primary sclerosing cholangitis ORTHOPEDICS Multiple post-fracture tumefactions of the ribs, characteristic of osteogenesis imperfecta, type II; see Accordion, Rosary

'beads on a string' see Solenoid structure

beak sign UROLOGIC RADIOLOGY A gently curved outward bulging of renal cortex adjacent to a well-circumscribed renal mass in the late or nephrogram phase of selective renal angiography, indicating the presence of a slowly expanding, usually benign avascular renal cyst with smooth inner walls, typically seen in arterionephrosclerosis, but also in renal cell carcinoma

beaking PEDIATRIC RADIOLOGY A finding in lateral films of the spine in mucopolysaccharidoses and mucolipidoses where there is a bird-beak-like tapering of the anteroinferior or anterosuperior margin of the lumbar vertebrae; a 'beak' is also described in the medial aspect of the proximal tibia at the epiphyseal plate in Blount's disease or coxa vara, the functional correction of which may require osteotomy

BEAM Brain electrical activity mapping‡

bean bag cells Histiocytes filled with phagocytosed leukocytes, erythrocytes, and cellular debris, seen in histiocytic phagocytic panniculitis

'bean counter' A colloquial expression for an administrator or functionary in any institution's finance department, who 'counts beans', an ancient form of exchange

bearskin rug appearance A descriptor for the gross pathology of the small intestinal mucosa in Whipple's disease, in which the villi are distended with macrophages; the serosa is dull, the intestinal wall is thickened, and the mesentery indurated

'bear tracks' OPHTHALMOLOGY A descriptor for blotchy congenital pigmentation seen in the ocular fundus, without known clinical significance

beaten brass/silver RADIOLOGY A fanciful descriptor for the variably-sized rounded zones of bony attenuation of the cranial bones caused by pressure from the cerebral cortical gyri, resulting from premature closure of the cranial sutures and by extension, increased intracranial pressure

beat knee Coal miner's knee Prepatellar bursitis caused by prolonged kneeling often associated with trauma and/or infection, either acute, associated with serous effusions or chronic with hemorrhage, loose bodies and calcifications

Beaver body MICROBIOLOGY A stool contaminant confused by the inexperienced with helminth eggs, corresponding to an alga, *Psorospermium haeckelii*, found in crayfish tissues and in the stool following a typical Creole meal, described by PC Beaver in 1984

Beck Depression Inventory A 21-item questionnaire designed to assess the severity of depression, which evaluates self-dissatisfaction, indecisiveness, work difficulty, and fatigability (N Engl J Med 1992; 327:1041oa)

Beckwith-Wiedemann syndrome A rare AD [MIM 130650] condition characterized by overgrowth with visceromegaly (which may be asymmetrical resulting in hemihypertrophy), macroglossia, omphalocele, hyperinsulinemic hypoglycemia and embryonal tumors including Wilms' tumor, hepatoblastoma and rhabdomyosarcoma MOLECULAR PATHOLOGY Genomic imprinting has been identified in the *WT2* gene, in which there is constitutional duplication of the paternal chromosome segment 11p15.5 (trisomy at 11p15), or loss of maternal genes in this region (uniparental isodisomy) (N Engl J Med 1994; 331:586oa); see Imprinting

becquerel The SI (International System) unit for measuring radioactivity, equal to one disintegration/sec; 1 Bq = 3.70×10^{10} Ci

bed HOSPITAL ADMINISTRATION A unit of 24-hour patient occupancy in a hospital or other inpatient health care facility, which is a measure of the hospital's size; licensure and certificates-of-need are based on the number of beds, allocated according to intended use or duration of stay and designated as an obstetric bed, oncology bed, outpatient bed, ie less than 24-hour use, resident bed, ie long-term stay for persons requiring custodial and personal, but not medical or nursing care and temporary bed, ie that which is allowed when a hospital temporarily exceeds its legally allowed capacity; see Certified bed, 'Swing' bed

bedbug Chinch A blood-sucking arthropod that is either cosmopolitan (*Cimex lectularius*) or relatively confined to the tropics (*C hemipterus*); the bedbug elicits pruritus and in sensitive individuals, urticaria, vesiculo-bullous lesions, arthalgia and asthmatic symptoms

bedside manner The degree of compassion, courtesy, sympathy displayed by a physician towards a patient in a clinical setting
*A major criticism of modern medicine has been the waning of 'bedside skills', which are rooted in a number of factors, to wit, quantum leaps in technology (requiring close scrutinization of laboratory and other diagnostic data), patients' willingness to initiate lawsuits or change physicians (erecting a barrier against a long-term patient-physician relationship), and changes in the financial environment (in which intangible and time-consuming services are not reimbursed); while the ability to 'schmooze', hold hands, and establish rapport with patients is being lost, it is being replaced by more therapeutically efficacious medicine

bedside testing LABORATORY MEDICINE Evaluation of analytes in the immediate vicinity of a patient, often in a relatively critical state; devices used are often less accurate than the machines used in a hospital's laboratory, but have the advantage of short 'turn-around' time, eg two minutes, facilitating therapy, using minimal volumes, eg 250-500 µl; bedside testing may be used for pH, PO_2, PCO_2, sodium, potassium, hematocrit, glucose, calcium and chloride (JAMA 1991; 266:382); the most commonly performed BTs are blood glucose (44% of all BTs), blood gas (15%), electrolytes (13%), coagulation studies (12%), pregnancy (8%), and others (**Advance/Laboratory Feb 1995**) Cf Stat testing

bedsore Pressure ulcer, see there, more widely known as decubital ulcer

BEE Basal energy expenditure, see there

beef growth hormone An anabolic steroid used by the cattle industry to increase the muscle mass, the safety of which has been seriously questioned, to the point that some countries have banned importation of such meat; Cf Bovine somatotropin

beef tapeworm *Taenia saginata*

beehive on the bladder RADIOLOGY A fanciful term for a biconvex triangular deformity, the apex of which corresponds to the bladder end of a colovesicular fistula; the colon becomes fixed to the peritoneal surface of the bladder, resulting in restricted bladder contraction, stasis and focal cystitis with necrosis of the fibromuscular tissue between the bladder and the colon, causing a fistula (**Ann R Col Surg Eng 1982; 63:195**)

beep *verb* To contact by portable pager, eg *Dr. Kildare was beeped while on rounds*

Note: The synonym, page is more formal and is the more commonly used written form

beeper A portable paging device that allows a person to contact ('beep' or page) its wearer by calling a specific telephone number; depending on the device's sophistication and capacity, a person[1] contacting the person wearing the beeper[2] may send a message[3] of various length at a range of up to 100 kilometers (62 miles) from the 'home base'

[1]The beeper's beeper [2]The beepee [3]eg, *'Patient died of complications, flee country'*

beer drinker cardiomyopathy A disease complex of historical interest that occurred when cobalt was added to the malt as a 'frothing' agent, affecting those consuming 2 or more liters of cobalt-treated beer/day CLINICAL Cardiomegaly, congestive heart failure, tachycardia, hypotension, hepatomegaly, dyspnea PROGNOSIS 50% fatality

behavior modification PSYCHOLOGY The use of operant conditioning models, ie positive and negative reinforcement as espoused by BF Skinner to modify behavior

behavioral genetics A rapidly evolving field that attempts to understand the genetic basis of behavior; the progress of BG to a state of scientific 'legitimacy' has been hampered by various reports linking specific chromosomal defects to certain diseases, including the alleged association of an extra Y chromosome with ↑ aggression in ♂ (in 1993, the US National Academy of Science dismissed the linkage as unproven), schizophrenia to a gene on chromosome 5, psychosis to chromosome 11, manic-depressive disorder (bipolar disorder) to chromosomes 11, and the X chromosome, dyslexia to chromosome 15 *'All were announced with great fanfare, all were greeted unskeptically in the popular press; all are now in disrepute.'* More recently, a link was reported between alcohol and the dopamine receptor gene (DRD2); subsequent linkage of DRD2 to attention-deficit hyperactivity disorder, autism, drug abuse, pathological gambling, post-traumatic stress disorder, and Tourette syndrome; the DRD2-pleasure center linkage has not been replicated by other groups; the research data of behavioral genetics is criticized as being prey to the misuse of statistical methods, failure to properly define the trait being studied, bias in selection of cases and controls, and inadequate sample size (**Science 1994; 264:1686-1739**)

behavioral teratology A postulated form of teratogenesis in which drugs or toxins induce permanent behavioral 'damage'; it is difficult to verify behavioral changes given the subtlety of teratogenic effects and the subjectivity of interpretation; functional neurotransmitters appear early in fetal development and may be vulnerable to teratogenic agents during periods of fetal or postnatal immaturity

behaviorism A school of psychology that holds that only overt or 'external' behaviors can be reasonably analyzed, and internal constructs, developmental stages, and psychoanalysis is in essence poppycock; modern behaviorism is exemplified by BF Skinner's school of operant conditioning

beige mice A mutant murine model for Chediak-Higashi disease characterized by pigmentary abnormalities, defective natural killer cell activity and an increased incidence of malignancy

BEIR studies Biological effects of exposure to low levels of ionizing radiation A series of studies from the National Research Council (UK) that periodically analyze the cancer data from Japanese atomic bomb blast survivors and from those with long-term exposure to low levels of radiation; BEIR IV studied the long-term effects of short-range α radiation, primarily from radon gas in the home and in uranium mines; BEIR V was released in 1989 and indicated that those with low-level exposure were 3-4 times more likely to get cancer

bejel A non-venereal infection by a strain of *Treponema pallidum* that is virtually indistinguishable from venereal *T pallidum* (syphilis); bejel affects children in Saharan Africa and the Middle East CLINICAL, EARLY Lymphadenitis, condyloma-like oropharyngeal and anogenital lesions CLINICAL, LATE Lesions mimic those of tertiary syphilis, including gumma, bony deformities and nodular skin ulcers TREATMENT Penicillin, erythromycin and tetracycline

bel ACOUSTIC SCIENCES A unit expressing the logarithm of the ratio of power of a sound (P_1) to that of a reference sound (P_2)*, ie $log_{10}P_1/P_2$; in practice, the unit decibel is used

*The reference sound is usually 10^{-16} watts/cm^2, which approximates the threshold of sound of the human ear at 1000 Hz

bell clapper testicle Congenital lengthening of the tunica vaginalis or mesorchium; the testicle lies horizontally in the scrotum, predisposed to torsion and infarction; the testicle has been likened to the clapper of a bell

The Bell Curve SOCIOLOGY A controversial book by C Murphy and R Herrnstein that presents data supporting the argument that there are fundamental differences in IQ among various racial groups with the Orientals being at the top and blacks at the bottom, as much as 60% is genetically predetermined; the book further argues against a status quo in the welfare system in the US, and represents a bellwether for a fundamental shift towards conservative politics* (**NY Newsday, 5 Jan 1995;B4**); see Affirmative action, Bakke decision

*This in turn is reflected in the types of biomedical research that may not be funded, eg human embryo-related projects, and whether abortions will become once again illegal, as they were before the *Roe* v *Wade* decision, this being the case as the 'Right-to-Life' movement is both conservative and has an anti-abortion philosophy

Belle Glade The largest city in western Palm Beach County, a rural agricultural area in Florida that has one of the highest HIV seroprevalence rates(52/1011 pregnant ♀, rate in non-Hispanic and non-Haitian blacks, 48/575) in the US; initially the high HIV seroprevalence was attributed to transmission of blood by local mosquitoes (the mosquito connection), but has been shown to be due to heterosexual contact; a greater percentage of HIV-infected ♀ who also used crack-cocaine had a higher incidence of syphilis (**N Engl J Med 1992; 327:1704OA**)

la belle indifference Conversion disorders, see there

'belly' tap Abdominal tap CRITICAL CARE MEDICINE A rapid method for differentiating the 'surgical' abdomen, ie that requiring surgery, from a 'non-surgical' abdomen, avoiding an unnecessary laparotomy; the tap consists in either a bilateral flank or four-quadrant cytologic sampling along the peritoneal gutter with a 20- or 18-gauge spinal needle; the yield is about 80%, demonstrating unclotted blood or if delayed, florid acute inflammation, both requiring immediate intervention; 'belly' taps are indicated in: Blunt abdominal trauma alone or in combination with injuries to the head, thorax or the extremities or with concomitant substance abuse, acute pancreatitis, post-operative peritonitis or peritonitis in children with a second disease process

belt Any broad geographical region with an increased incidence of a particular disease; see AIDS belt, Asian esophageal cancer belt, Lymphoma belt

bench A long worktable; a colloquial term for the site where hands-on experimental research, ie 'benchwork', is performed

Bendectin An antinausea drug that had been prescribed to 33 million pregnant women over a period of 27 years; it was withdrawn from the market in 1983 by its manufacturer, because of the mounting lawsuits alleging that it was a teratogen; of the 38 cases thus far brought to trial, the manufacturer won judgements in 36 (30 more are pending); one case in particular is of broad interest as the experts called by plaintiff J Daubert (who was born with limb-reduction defects) introduced epidemiological evidence that contradicted the published studies, none of which found Bendectin to be a human teratogen; the trial court dismissed the case, concluding that the plaintiff's scientific evidence was inadmissible as it was essentially invalid (N Engl J Med 1994; 330:1018LIM) see *Daubert* v. *Merrell Dow Pharmaceuticals*, Frye rule

the 'bends' Acute decompression sickness, the chokes A clinical complex caused by rapid whole body decompression, with intravascular 'boiling' of nitrogen and resultant morbidity or mortality in scuba divers and high-altitude pilots or workers in high-pressure environments, eg caissons (in chronic decompression sickness) CLINICAL Headache, nausea, vomiting, vertigo, tinnitus, dyspnea, tachypnea, convulsions and shock, joint and abdominal pain; nitrogen gas in the brain causes 'boxcar' air bubbles in leptomeningeal vessels separating the blood 'column', potentially causing death; Cf Caisson disease

'benefits not provided' clause A generic term for any clause in a health insurance policy that indicates a lack of provision of certain, eg preventive (childhood vaccinations, mammography, Pap smears) or surveillance (office visits, well-baby care) services (N Engl J Med 1992; 327:275)

benign familial leukopenia A relatively common condition in blacks, West Indians, and Yemenite Jews, characterized by a low-normal leukocyte count; leukocytes rise to 'normal' range after immune 'challenges' by bacteria, (8630/µL, which is below the leukocytosis seen in normal controls, 13 600/µL), pregnancy, exertion, and stress; leukocytosis does not occur in response to viral infections (Acta Haematol 1992; 87:126)

benign lymphadenopathy Any non-malignant regional or generalized enlargement of lymph nodes, which may be divided into histological patterns (table)

benign lymphoepithelial lesion Mikulicz disease A lesion of the salivary and lacrimal glands, clinically related to Sjögren's syndrome and thought to be autoimmune in nature PATHOLOGY Clusters of epithelial cells (epimyoepithelial cells) and abundant lymphocytic infiltration with occasional germinal centers; BLEL may demonstrate transition to carcinoma, implying that the lesion arises in the epithelium (Am J Clin Path 1989; 92:808); Cf 'Eskimoma'

benign 'metastasis' Presence of non-malignant non-lymphoid tissue in lymph nodes, eg thyroid follicles in regional lymph nodes of the neck, potentially confused with carcinoma (Cancer 1969; 24:309); when thyroid follicles are seen, microscopic size, lack of stromal proliferation or psammoma bodies, presence of round-to-oval follicles that are not papillary or crowded, bland, uncrowded nuclei with fine chromatin and small nucleoli militate against malignancy; see Lymph node inclusions

benign neglect A philosophical stance that a clinician may adopt in the face of certain lesions and clinical conditions that are well known for their tendency to be either stable over time, eg verruca vulgaris or to actually regress, eg capillary hemangioma; because these lesions do not undergo malignant degeneration and at most represent cosmetic problems, an appropriate 'therapy' is that of benign neglect; Cf Watchful waiting

benign paroxysmal positional vertigo A very common vestibular end organ disorder resulting in positional vertigo PATHOGENESIS ? Caused by free-floating particles in the endolymph of the posterior semilunar canal; cupulolithiasis DIAGNOSIS Hallpike maneuver TREATMENT Particle repositioning maneuver; occlusion of affected canal using a bone chop:fibrinogen glue plug

benign Triton tumor Neuromuscular choristoma; see there, aka neuromuscular hamartoma; Cf Triton tumor

bentiromide test GASTROENTEROLOGY A 'tubeless' pancreatic function test in which bentiromide (N-benzoyl-L-tyrosyl-p-aminobenzoic acid) is cleaved by chymotrypsin, yielding p-aminobenzoic acid which is measured in the urine FALSE POSITIVITY Hepatic disease, renal failure, intestinal malabsorption (N Engl J Med 1995; 332:1482RA) see Pancreolauryl test, Tubeless test

benzene TOXICOLOGY A volatile hydrocarbon by-product of the destructive distillation of coal, present in coal tar; it is

---

BENIGN LYMPHADENOPATHY PATTERNS

NODULAR AIDS, giant lymph node hyperplasia (Castleman's disease), reactive hyperplasia, rheumatoid arthritis and in secondary syphilis

PARACORTICAL Dermatopathic lymphadenitis, nodular paracortical hyperplasia, immunoblastic response to viruses and drugs

SINUSOIDAL Sinusoidal hyperplasias, histiocytic medullary reticulosis, histiocytosis X, sinus histiocytosis with massive lymphadenopathy (Rosai-Dorfman disease), sinusoidal lipogranulomas and as a reactive pattern in certain malignancies, eg Kaposi sarcoma, metastatic carcinoma, melanoma

DIFFUSE OR OBLITERATIVE Post-vaccinial or other viral lymphadenitis, eg herpes zoster, phenytoin hypersensitivity, dermatopathic lymphadenopathy, atypical reactions to metastatic carcinoma and melanoma, lupus erythematosus, angioimmunoblastic lymphadenopathy, infectious mononucleosis

GRANULOMATOUS Lymph nodes draining joint and breast (silicon) prostheses, intravenous drug abuse, *Yersinia*, lymphogranuloma venereum, tularemia, tuberculosis and atypical mycobacteria, cat scratch disease, sarcoidosis, sarcoid-like changes seen in lymph nodes draining tumors, fungal, brucellosis, toxoplasmosis, syphilis, leshmaniasis

MIXED Metastatic carcinoma, allergic eosinophilic granulomatosis; cat scratch disease, granulomas, infectious mononucleosis, lymphogranuloma venereum, sarcoidosis, toxoplasmosis and

DEPLETED AIDS-related complex; see Lymph node necrosis

the simplest aromatic compound; serves as an organic solvent, and is both toxic, in particular to mucocutaneous surfaces, and carcinogenic, as chronic exposure to benzene has been linked to BM depression, aplastic anemia, and acute leukemias, usually of myeloid lineage, ¼ of which were accompanied by preceding pancytopenia and/or peripheral neuropathies

benzene ring ORGANIC CHEMISTRY An aromatic hydrocarbon composed of six carbon atoms linked with alternating single and double bonds (2 atoms in the σ orbital and 1 atom in the π orbital)

benzodiazepine receptors BZ-1, BZ-2 Two different receptors for benzodiazepine have been tentatively identified in the brain; BZ-1 receptors may affect neural pathways involved in normal sleep patterns, while BZ-2 receptors are involved in memory and motor functions

benzoylecgonine The major metabolite of cocaine, which is the molecule most often measured in the toxicology laboratory; see Cocaine

bereavement The loss of a 'significant other' or other loved one, or as is more commonly used, the act of bereaving or mourning the loss of said person; bereavement is generally accompanied by a transient (usually less than several months) period of depression; bereavement may become the focus of clinical attention and can be diagnosed as a pathological state

Bergalis, Kimberly A young woman who became infected with HIV-1, reportedly by her dentist (JAMA 1990; 264:2018), the first case of this route of transmission known to AIDS epidemiologists; the 'Bergalis case' has heightened the debate on whether 1) HIV-infected health care workers should provide 'hands-on' health care, potentially endangering the lives of patients and 2) Whether physicians and other health care workers should be regularly tested for HIV-1, and whether the results of those tests should be available to the public; see Acer cluster

Bergherr v Sommer LABORATORY MEDICINE A seminal legal case that in part addressed the increasingly common practice of sending diagnostic specimens, eg blood, Pap smears, to a site at a considerable distance from the patient's location and legal jurisdiction; in *Bergherr*, the husband of a woman who died of cancer of the uterine cervix initiated a lawsuit against a referral laboratory that had read 10 of her Pap smears, diagnosing them as atypical; according to Minnesota state law, the rules of jurisdiction did not prevent the plaintiff from initiating a legal action for negligence (CAP Today April1995 p3)

Berlin Conference GLOBAL VILLAGE An international congress held in Berlin in April 1995 on issues of how to minimize increases in greenhouse gases; a major issue addressed was the inequities in the amount and types of gases produced between developed and underdeveloped countries (Nature 1995; 374:483)

Berlin Mandate An agreement reached at the Berlin Conference to negotiate a new set of targets for reducing greenhouse gas emissions that would try to set specific targets within specified time frames, eg 2000, 2005, 2010 (Science 1995; 268:197)

Bernard-Soulier syndrome Giant platelet syndrome An AR [MIM 231200] condition with mucocutaneous and visceral hemorrhage due to deficiency of glycoprotein Ib, the receptor for von Willebrand factor (vWF), as well as GP 1s (glycocalicin), both of which are involved in the interaction between vWF and the platelet membrane, which is critical for normal platelet adhesion in the early phases of primary hemostasis CLINICAL Moderate to severe bleeding of the purpuric type, eg bruising, epistaxis, menorrhagia LABORATORY Prolonged bleeding time (due to poor platelet adhesion to subendothelium), no platelet aggregation with ristocetin; platelet abnormalities in BSS include ↑ size,

basophilia of membrane, aggregation (or absence) of cytoplasmic granules, pseudopod formation and cytoplasmic vacuolization

berry aneurysm A 0.2-0.5 cm saccular dilatation of arteries at the base of the brain, at or adjacent to the circle of Willis (95% of berry aneurysms) or at the vertebrobasilar arteries (5%), due to a developmental or congenital weakness in the medial muscle layer of the cerebral arteries; 30% of aneurysms are multiple, located at bifurcations, often anterior and appear in 1-2% of all autopsies; most berry aneurysms rupture when they exceed 1 cm in diameter and are more likely to rupture under stress, due to acutely increased systemic blood pressure, eg coitus, athletic competition, but not related to trauma; berry aneurysms may be associated with aortic coarctation, polycystic renal disease, collagen disorders, eg Ehlers-Danlos and Marfan syndromes, arteriovenous malformation and fibromuscular dysplasia

berry picking operation SURGICAL ONCOLOGY A colloquial term for the practice of removing multiple metastatic malignancies from an organ or body cavity; for colorectal carcinoma metastatic to the liver, most authors believe resection of up to four metastases (preferably less than 5 cm in diameter) is reasonable; Cf Cherry picking

BES Back extensor strength, see there

BESS Brain edema severity score, see Hepatic encephalopathy

BEST A T1-weighted inversion recovery sequence, a variant of the echo-planar technique of MRI, developed by P Mansfield of Nottingham, used for ultra-high-speed imaging of the brain; Cf MBEST, MRI

bestiality Zooerastia A form of paraphilia (sexual deviancy) in which animals are the primary or only vehicle for sexual excitement

BESWL Biliary extracorporeal shock-wave lithotripsy

beta-3 A subunit of vitronectin receptor integrin that is reported to absent on day 19-20 in most (86% accuracy) endometrial biopsies of infertile ♀ with endometriosis, implying that a simple test can be used to detect this condition (Science News 1994; 146:118)

β–amyloid A4 A 4 kD polypeptide encoded on chromosome 21 that is derived from altered processing of amyloid precursor protein*, an integral membrane glycoprotein secreted as a carboxyl-terminal truncated molecule; β-amyloid may also accumulate in Down syndrome, infectious encephalopathy and cerebral amyloid angiopathy EM Haphazardly arranged fibrils 8-10 nm in diameter by 30-100 nm length; crystallographic analysis demonstrates β-pleating; ABP may be found in skin, intestine and adrenal gland (JAMA 1991; 265:309n&v); it is unclear whether β-amyloid causes Alzheimer's disease or is a 'passenger' protein produced by damaged neurons, although patients with early onset Alzheimer's disease have a highly specific point mutation in the APP gene (Nature 1991; 353:844), a transgenic mouse with the amyloid precursor has been generated (Science 1991; 253:323, 266n&v) see Amyloid

*APP is deposited in small vessels of the leptomeninges and cerebral cortex in Alzheimer's disease, is a major component of neurofibrillary tangles and senile plaques, and may be of vascular origin

beta carotene CLINICAL NUTRITION A carotenoid that is abundant in broccoli, cantaloupe, and carrots, and has vitamin A and immunostimulatory activity, and is linked to a ↓ risk of bladder, colon, lung, and skin cancer and cancer cell growth in vitro (New York Times 21 Feb 1995; C1) see Carotenoid

betacryptoxanthin CLINICAL NUTRITION A carotenoid that is abundant in mangos, orange, papaya, and tangerines, and has vitamin A activity (New York Times 21 Feb 1995; C1) see Carotenoid

β-decay Low-level radioactive decay in which β particles (usually an electron with an antineutrino, less commonly a positron with an antineutrino) are emitted; Cf α decay, Electron capture

β effect Hormonal action of epinephrine and norepinephrine resulting in metabolic, hemodynamic and modulatory changes, a function of the concentration of adrenergic receptors on the α and β cells of the pancreatic islets; β effects (epinephrine acting on α islet cells) include: lipolysis, ketogenesis, stimulation of glucagon secretion, β_2 arterial vasodilatation and β_1 increases in myocardial rate, contractility and conductivity

β emitter A radioisotope that decays with the emission of an electron (β particle), designated as 'soft' if the electron emitted is of low energy and has a short distance of penetration, or 'hard' if the electron is high-energy with a great penetrating distance

β-enolase An enzyme, two forms of which are present in skeletal and cardiac muscle, that catalyzes glycolysis of 2-phosphoglycerate to phosphoenolpyruvate; in acute myocardial infarction, the rapid peak of β-enolase at 12 hours is potentially more specific and of more use than that of creatine kinase; Cf Cardiac enzymes

beta-gamma bridge IMMUNOLOGY A 'spanning' of the usually well-defined peaks in the β and γ regions in serum protein electrophoresis, seen in chronic hepatopathies, classically in alcoholic liver disease; the β-γ bridge also occurs in chronic infections and connective tissue disease and is due to polyclonal production of proteins that migrate in the region, which may 'bury' small monoclonal expansions or the clone may produce polymeric forms of the protein resulting in differences in electrophoretic mobility, causing a 'pseudo-polyclonal' expansion Normal β migrating proteins: Transferrin and β-lipoprotein Normal γ migrating proteins: IgG, IgA, IgM

β-glucuronidase A lysosomal hydrolase that is increased in the cerebrospinal fluid of 75% of patients with metastatic intracranial carcinoma and in 25% of patients with intracranial myelogenous leukemia

β-lipotropin β-LPH A 91-residue peptide derived from the carboxy-terminal portion of pro-opiomelanocortin (POMC), the precursor molecule for corticotropin-related peptides, eg ACTH, MSH and others which arrive through the mechanism of alternative slicing; see POMC

β_2 microglobulin Thymotaxin An 11.8-kD polypeptide produced by the thymic epithelium and expressed on the surface of antigen-presenting cells, providing one of two immunoglobulin-like domains, in part participating in the selection of MHC I peptides, and which, by ensuring the proper folding of class I molecules, is a key non-antibody member of the immunoglobulin superfamily; β_2M is noncovalently linked to MHC class I proteins, and is a component of the class I trimer (peptide antigen/class I/β_2-microglobulin) and that presents antigens to cytotoxic T cells; while the highly polymorphic class I MHC proteins determine the immune response, β_2M is chemotactic and stimulates T-cell maturation; as a free molecule, β_2M markedly increases the generation of antigenic complexes capable of T-cell stimulation (Nature 1991; 349:74); β_2M is coexpressed with CD1 thymocyte glycoproteins and intestinal IgG receptor; disruption of the gene in a mouse embryonal stem cell line through homologous recombination with a nonfunctional β_2M gene results in an unexpectedly healthy mouse that lacks CD4$^-$8$^+$ T cells with defective T-cell-mediated cytotoxicity and thus β_2M is not critical to survival

β-pleated sheet A protein structural motif elucidated by Pauling and Corey, so called as they had previously delineated the α-helix; the polypeptide chains in β sheets are almost completely extended, with an axial distance of 35 nm, versus an axial distance of 15 nm in the α helix); the β-pleated sheet is stabilized by hydrogen bonds between NH and CO groups of different polypeptide strands; adjacent molecules may run in the same direction (parallel) or in the opposite (antiparallel) direction, eg silk fibroin; the β-pleated sheet is a tertiary structure elucidated by X-ray crystallography and seen by EM, which can be produced experimentally by treating Bence-Jones proteins with enzymes and is a structure typical of amyloidosis PATHOLOGY The β-pleated structure may be appreciated by the Congo red stain using polarizing light to reveal the characteristic apple-green birefringence EM Extracellular 700-1000 nm in diameter, fine complex non-branching fibrils

Betaseron A biopharmaceutical that is reported to be useful in the treatment of multiple sclerosis (Bio/Technology 1995; 13:319)

beta testing The testing of a vendor's product (a device, equipment, hardware or software) by applications-knowledgeable users, who are familiar with the product's use but not with its design; BT provides both a different perspec-

---

BETHESDA SYSTEM (1991)

ADEQUACY OF SPECIMEN
Satisfactory for evaluation

Satisfactory for evaluation, but limited by ... (specify reason)

Unsatisfactory for evaluation...(specify reason)

GENERAL CATEGORIZATION (OPTIONAL)
Within normal limits

Benign cellular changes: see descriptive diagnoses

Epithelial cell abnormality: see descriptive diagnoses

DESCRIPTIVE DIAGNOSES

BENIGN CELLULAR CHANGES
INFECTION
Trichomonas vaginalis

Fungal organisms morphologically consistent with *Candida* spp

Predominance of coccobacilli consistent with shift in vaginal flora

Bacteria morphologically consistent with *Actinomyces* spp

Cellular changes associated with herpes simplex virus

Other

REACTIVE CHANGES ASSOCIATED WITH:

Inflammation (includes typical repair)

Atrophy with inflammation (atrophic vaginitis)

Radiation

IUD (intrauterine contraceptive device)

Other

EPITHELIAL CELL ABNORMALITIES
SQUAMOUS CELL

Atypical squamous cells of undetermined significance: Qualify

Low grade squamous intraepithelial lesion (LGSIL) encompassing HPV and mild dysplasia/CIN 1

High grade squamous intraepithelial lesion (HGSIL) encompassing moderate and severe dysplasia, CIN 2 and CIN 3/CIS

Squamous cell carcinoma

GLANDULAR CELL

Endometrial cells, cytologically benign in postmenopausal ᵀᴹ

Atypical glandular cells of undetermined significance: Qualify

Endocervical adenocarcinoma

Endometrial adenocarcinoma

Adenocarcinoma, NOS

Predominance of coccobacilli consistent with shift in vaginal flora

OTHER MALIGNANT NEOPLASMS Specify which neoplasms

HORMONAL EVALUATION
Hormonal pattern compatible with age and history

Hormonal pattern incompatible with age and history: Specify

Hormonal evaluation not possible due to: Specify

†Acta Cytologica 1993; 37:115A

tive and a 'reality check' on the product's performance under working conditions, as it will be put through various unanticipated uses and applications that the vendor had not anticipated; BT offers the advantage to an end-user of being at the 'cutting edge' of a technology, and allows the user to add specific features in the marketed version of the product (**Am Lab Sept 1994 p24**); beta testing is usually performed on-site under the same working conditions for which it was designed, in order to identify potential problems associated with its use, colloquially known as 'working out the bugs'; Cf Alpha testing

betatron RADIATION ONCOLOGY A doughnut-shaped device with a circular pathway that accelerates electrons by a pulsating magnetic field to provide electrons with up to 20 MeV of energy

betel nut chewing A habit popular among Javanese, Malayan and Indian men; the 'chew' is composed of ground betel nut, slaked lime, ground spices including ginger and pepper wrapped in a betel leaf; Indians add tobacco to their chew and have a high incidence of oral cancer (comprising 36% of all cancers in this group), whereas the Javanese and Malayans who don't add tobacco have a very low incidence of cancer, exonerating betel nuts as carcinogens; see Khaini cancer

Bethesda System A system (see table) for reporting cervical and vaginal cytologic diagnoses that was developed to replace the aging, oversimplistic and inadequate Papanicolaou system; the BS provides a uniform format for reporting results for cervical cytologic specimens, classifying the noninvasive lesions* and offers a standardized lexicon for cervical/vaginal cytopathology reports, emphasizing communication of clinically relevant information (**Acta Cytologica 1993; 37:115**)

*As atypical squamous cells of undetermined significance, low-grade squamous intraepithelial lesions, or high-grade squamous intraepithelial lesions

Bethesda unit BU HEMATOLOGY A unit measuring factor VIII (F8) inhibitory activity in plasma; 1.0 BU reduces F8 in 1.0 ml of plasma from 1.0 to 0.5 units; BUs are measured when F8-dependent hemophiliacs become refractory to F8 therapy, caused by a circulating inhibitor or an F8 antibody

betulinic acid AIDS A triterpene extracted from plane tree bark that is reported to block HIV-1 infection at a post-binding step, specifically after HIV's gp120 binds to the host cell CD4 molecule, possibly due to conformational changes in the gp120-gp41 complex (**Proc Nat Acad Sci (US) 1994; 91:3564OA**)

beziehungswahn PSYCHIATRY A paranoid state with a prominence of delusions of (self-) reference

bezoar Any concretion or conglomerate mass of foreign material in the stomach, facilitated by partial or complete gastrectomy, as acid hydrolysis of gastric content is diminished; bezoars remain undigested in stomach, causing discomfort or frank pain, halitosis, gastric wall erosion or ulceration, and potentially peritonitis, hemorrhage, obstruction, nausea, vomiting, a palpable mass, more easily palpable in tricho- than in phytobezoars; vegetable (phyto-) bezoar may result from ingesting the persimmon *Disopyros virginiana*, which contains phlobantanin, a substance that coagulates on contact with dilute acid, the dissolution of which requires per os enzyme treatment, a low-fiber diet and decreased intake of high-fiber fruits (persimmons, pears, citrus) in bezoars due to gastrectomies; trichobezoars are seen in trichophagic neurotics; anecdotal association with gastric carcinoma is probably a statistical artifact

Note: Aggregates of *Candida* species within the renal collecting ducts have also been termed bezoars Note: Bezoar is a translation of the Arabic 'Badzehr' for antidote or anti-poison; bezoars from the Middle East were from the stomachs of goats and gazelles, those from South America, the vicuna, each thought to have medicinal value in the treatment of aging, snakebites, evil spirits and the plague

BFP Biological false positive, see there

BFU Burst-forming unit, see there

BH₄ Tetrahydrobiopterin cofactor Synthesized from GTP, BH_4 is a cofactor for tyrosine and tryptophan hydroxylase, both of which are required for dopamine and serotonin synthesis; deficiency of BH_4 may result from three different enzyme defects; without BH_4, phenylalanine cannot convert to tyrosine and thus accumulates, accounting for 2% of cases of phenylketonuria

BHA Butylated hydroxyanisole, see there

bHLH Basic helix-loop-helix, a structural motif, see Helix-loop-helix

Bhopal ENVIRONMENT An environmental disaster occurring in India in late 1984, caused by methyl isothiocyanate (MIC) used in the production of carbaril pesticides; water leaked into a tank containing MIC, resulting in a heat-producing reaction that vaporized 30-40 tons of gas covering an area of 80 km² (30 square miles), exposing up to 600 000; the official body count was 2500; the unofficial count *begins* at 7000 CLINICAL Acute toxicity consisting of respiratory distress, attributed to cyanide toxicity, including dyspnea, cough, throat irritation, chest pain and hemoptysis; with time the lesions evolved to interstitial pulmonary fibrosis; ocular effects include burning, edema, erythema, tearing, pain, photophobia and corneal ulceration; negative impact of MIC is reported in gestation, in the immune, neuromuscular and other systems; nearly 10 years after it occurred, those exposed continue to suffer from respiratory (40-93% of those exposed), ophthalmic (eg blindness), intestinal, reproductive (43% miscarriage, birth defects), neurologic (eg paralysis) disease (**Sci Am 1995; 272/6:16**), and malignancy; toxicologic data is minimal as MIC is regarded as too dangerous (according to some workers, even more than phosgene, the poison gas used as a chemical weapon during World War I) see Disaster; Cf Chemical warfare

Note: In 1978, the US National Institute for Occupational Safety and Health (NIOSH) indicated MIC had poor warning properties, eg smell, and thus had been considered a dangerous chemical

BHT Butylated hydroxytoluene A food preservative used to prevent fats and oils from becoming rancid, which is also added to packaged foods; BHT is alleged to be teratogenic in mice, resulting in a significant ↓ in cholinesterase activity, ↑ aggressiveness, cause sleep disturbances, and weight disturbances (**Alternative Medicine, Future Medicine Pub, Puyallup, Wash, 1994**) see Alternative medicine

$$[CH_3]_3C \qquad \overset{OH}{\bigcirc} \qquad C[CH_3]_3$$
$$CH_3$$

BHT

bicarbonate loading SPORTS MEDICINE The administration of sodium bicarbonate (baking soda) prior to competing in a particular sporting event with the purpose of neutralizing the lactic acid produced during anaerobic metabolism; BL is of little use in extremely short events, eg sprints, but is reportedly useful in anaerobic activities of intermediate duration, usually of 5 minutes or more in duration, eg 800+

meters (JC DeLee, D Drez, Jr, Eds, Orthopedic Sports Medicine WB Saunders, Philadelphia, 1994) Cf Carbohydrate loading, Phosphate loading

biclonality A generic term for the rare occurrence of an uncontrolled expansion of two (or more) clones of neoplastic cells, as would be biclonal expansion of two B-cell lines or B- and T-cell lines; this contrasts to the more common, uncontrolled clonal expansion of a single, often hematopoietic progenitor cell line; Cf Composite lymphoma

BIDS syndrome Hair-brain syndrome An AR [MIM 234050] condition characterized by Brittle hair (and fingernails), Intellectual impairment, mild Decreased fertility and Short stature, which affects the Amish kindred of Pennsylvania

bighead Infection by *Clostridium novyi* and *C sordelli* in rams, which results in acute inflammatory edema

bigjaw Actinomycosis in cattle

bigleg Sporadic lympangitis VETERINARY MEDICINE A non-contagious disease of horses characterized by fever, lymphangitis, and swelling of one or both hindlegs TREATMENT Penicillin, sedative, hot fomentation, massage

'big science' A term that refers to large, long-term, multi-center and often multinational research efforts that are goal-oriented, initiated by consensus committees, rather than an individual investigator and costly, ie multiples of billions ($, US), eg Human genome project, the 'War on Cancer', the Space station and Superconducting super collider; Cf 'Little science'

'big spleen disease of Africa' Tropical splenomegaly, see there

Biko, Steve A black human rights activist from the Republic of South Africa (RSA) who was tortured to death while in prison and under medical supervision, six days after being detained by police for questioning; see Academic boycott, Apartheid medicine

Note: Although torture and murder by police in RSA was common before and after Biko's death in 1977, the case brought to fore issues of apartheid medicine and physician involvement in activities clearly against the tenets of the Hippocratic Oath; one of the physicians involved in the Biko case lost his license to practice medicine

bile cytology The formal study of material obtained directly from the biliary tract by percutaneous biliary drainage, used to determine the etiology of biliary obstruction; cytologic criteria favoring the diagnosis of adenocarcinoma include loss of polarity and/or the usual honeycomb arrangement of cells, enlarged and/or flattened nuclei, cell-in-cell arangement, or a bloody background (Acta Cytologica 1994; 38:51OA)

bile lake HEPATIC PATHOLOGY An extravasated pool of bile lying outside of partially necrotic liver cell plates, caused by peripheral (extrahepatic) biliary obstruction and rupture of the bile canaliculi

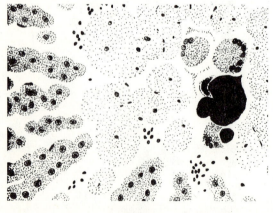

bile lake

bile reflux syndrome A post-gastrectomy complex characterized by retrosternal pain, anorexia, nausea, bilious vomiting TREATMENT Roux-en-Y anastomosis

bilis A generic term used by Latinos of Central America for symptoms induced or presumed to be induced by anger or rage, which include nervous tension, screaming, trembling, gastric dysfunction, or if extreme, loss of consciousness (from DSM-IV); see Culture-bound syndrome

bill stuffer MEDICAL MARKETING A generic term for any form of literature that is sent to a client along with a bill for services; a BS often provides information that might be of use in increasing the sender's revenues by encouraging the use of the sender's services (Am Med News 25 May 1992 p16)

billable test LABORATORY MEDICINE A unit of productivity in the clinical and hospital (where it is known as 'ordered' test) laboratory that has replaced the Workload unit*; the billable test unit is easily understood, requires no special methods for its determination, it is understood and accepted by non-laboratory management, is easily tracked through the financial system of most institutions, and is not subject to manipulation by laboratory management or by section personnel (CAP Today June 1993); Cf Workload unit

*A virtually extinct unit of productivity formerly sanctioned by the College of American Pathologists

billiard ball effect FORENSIC PATHOLOGY That which occurs after a second shotgun blast to the same body site, where the original shotgun pellets are struck from the rear by the incoming pellets, splaying deeper into the body at multiple angles, likened to the opening shot or 'breaking' in a game of billiards

Bill of Patient Rights A statement of the ethical principles used by a health care facility that obligates all members of the professional, operational and voluntary staff working in that facility to respect a patient's dignity and rights

binaural fusion NEUROPHYSIOLOGY The process by which the brain compares auditory information received in each ear and translates the differences into a unified perception of a single sound coming from a specific region of space; the cues used by the brain are the differences in signal timing and intensity, which travel by different routes to the point of central integration in the midbrain auditory area; if the signals arriving at each ear are identical, eg as occurs when the source is directly ahead, localization becomes difficult (Sci Am 1993; 268/4:66)

binder Granulator CLINICAL PHARMACOLOGY An inert agent used to impart cohesive qualities to a powdered drug or other material, ensuring that a drug tablet will remain intact after compression; binders include starch, gelatin, gums, methylcellulose and sugars including sucrose, dextrose, molasses and lactose; see Inactive ingredient

binding domains MOLECULAR BIOLOGY Structural motifs present on DNA-binding regulatory proteins that govern gene expression, either enhancing or repressing mRNA synthesis; 'binding proteins' recognize sequence specific sites 'binding domains' on the DNA and often share sequence homology with each other, eg Leucine zipper motif and protein products of the myc, fos and jun proto-oncogenes; see DNA-binding proteins, Transcription factors

binding protein Carrier protein CHEMISTRY A generic term for a circulating protein that reversibly binds a variety of small molecules, including amino acids, sugars, inorganic ions, vitamins and others NEUROPHYSIOLOGY An as-yet-unresolved dilemma of what mechanism(s) transform the firing of the neurons scattered throughout the visual cortex into a unified perception; the binding problem is considered by some to be a holy grail in the neurosciences (Sci Am 1994; 270/7:92)

binge PSYCHIATRY A component of bulimia nervosa, which

consists of an episode of hyperpolyphagia, in which up to 15 000 calories may be consumed in one hour; binges are commonly followed by self-induced emesis or 'purging' COMPLICATIONS Gastric rupture (Mallory-Weiss syndrome), vascular compression, pancreatitis, aspiration pneumonia, ipecac-induced myocarditis, cardiac failure, refeeding edema, hypokalemia, hypochloremia, and metabolic alkalosis; see Bulimia nervosa SUBSTANCE ABUSE A session of cocaine snorting that is repeated as often as every 10 minutes over a period from 12 hours to an entire week; with time, cocaine-induced euphoria deteriorates to neuropharmacological dependence; compulsive abuse ensues in up to 20% and actual addiction occurs in 5% which may reach a point of excluding all else but obtention of more drug

binge drinking An early phase of chronic alcoholism, characterized by episodic 'flirtation' with the bottle by binges of drinking to the point of stupor, followed by periods of abstinence; bouts of heavy alcohol consumption are accompanied by alcoholic ketoacidosis (accelerated lipolysis and β-hydroxybutyric acid production due to impaired insulin secretion), decreased food consumption and recurrent vomiting; see 'Eyeopener'

binge eating see Binge, bulimia nervosa

binge-purge syndrome see Bulimia nervosa

binging SUBSTANCE ABUSE A phenomenon described in IV cocaine abuse, where the subject may inject the cocaine up to 5 times/hour for up to 48 hours without sleeping or eating, since in cocaine, the 'high' (burst of euphoria) is shorter and the craving for more cocaine is very intense; cocaine 'bingers' are often too paranoid to share their needles and thus less likely to spread HIV; with 'Ice', a substance of abuse of recent vintage, binging occurs cyclically, with 4-5 days of binging, followed by a 2-3 day period of rest; see Ice

Note: Animal models for cocaine abuse become 'bingers'; given unlimited access, rats 'binge' to death within 2 weeks, dying of cardiorespiratory failure;

bioaccumulation An accumulation of chemicals or nutrients against an inorganic background, which is the result of a high partition coefficient and resistance to degradation on the part of the bioaccumulating organism

bioaeration PUBLIC HEALTH The bubbling of air through sewage sludge as a means of purification Note: In practice, the prefix bio- may be dropped

bioartificial liver Artificial liver, see there

bioartificial organ TRANSPLANTATION MEDICINE An evolving artificial organ design in which the cells needed to replace the function of a failing organ (eg liver) are placed in a synthetic receptacle, eg a hollow-fiber dialysis cartridge, allowing contact of the donor cells with host fluids, while eliminating contact of the donor cell antigens with the host immune system, thereby minimizing rejection phenomena; the bioartificial liver and pancreas are currently in various stages of development (N Engl J Med 1994; 331:268ED)

bioassay Any quantification procedure that measures either 1) The functional or effective amount of a substance (eg antibiotic, drug, hormone, vitamin, and so on) or 2) Toxicity of a substance (eg a pollutant) or organism (eg a pathogen) of interest in an in vivo system, ie within a cell or test animal

bioavailability The in vivo presence of a substance in a form that allows it to be metabolized, serve as a substrate, bind a specific molecule or participate in biochemical reactions; bioavailability depends on the pI or ionic form, presence of side chains or the conformation of the epitope; bioavailability is affected by the route of administration, rate of metabolism, lipid solubility and binding proteins

biochemical biopsy LABORATORY MEDICINE A diagnostic maneuver of uncertain clinical utility, in which diagnostic chemical analyses are performed on small tissue samples (or alternatively on fluid content from cysts) to quantify analytes (eg hormones, metabolites) that would be consistent with either a benign or malignant lesion; in thyroid cysts, cytological evaluation is more efficient diagnostically than the biochemical biopsy (Arch Pathol Lab Med 1993; 117:625OA, 593ED)

biochemical convergence A series of 'simplification' events seen in cells evolving toward malignancy; the cells lose such features of differentiation and organ specificity as microvilli, desmosomes, intermediate filaments and suffer down-regulation of 'differentiated' enzymes

biocompatibility The extent to which a foreign, usually implanted, material elicits a immune and/or nonimmune response in a recipient (Science & Medicine 1995; 2/3:73)

biocomputing A somewhat nebulous term referring to computing activities and research on biochemical or biological phenomena, eg neural networking, biosensors and molecular design (BIOCOMPUTERS, Kaminuma, Matsumoto, Chapman & Hall 1991); Cf Computers, Medical informatics

biocontrol ENVIRONMENT The use of natural products or engineered microorganisms to protect food crops against insects, circumventing the use of chemical pesticides; biopesticides include *Bacillus thuringiensis* (Bt), an organism that has been endowed with a wide range of activity thanks to recombinant engineering of a gene that encodes a chimeric Bt protein toxic to a wide range of insects, or by splicing the Bt toxin gene into other organisms; other biocontrol products include baculovirus-derived toxins and pheromones (Science 1991; 252:211n&v)

biocybernetics *The science of communication and control in animals* (Dorland's Medical Dictionary, 28th edition, WB Saunders, Philadelphia, 1994) or *The science of biologic feedback control mechanisms and communication in living organisms* (International Dictionary of Medicine, J Wiley & Sons, New York, 1986)

biodegradability ENVIRONMENT The capacity of a molecule or substance to be degraded by an enzyme system of a living organism, without leaving toxic residue in the environment; see Bioremediation

biodegradable Pertaining or referring to biodegradability

biodegradation The breakdown of any organic material in a simpler form, usually understood to be a process effected by bacteria

biodetritus Dead organic matter

biodiesel ENVIRONMENT An alternative fuel used for the internal combustion engine which is produced from soybean and rape seed oils PROS Less sulfur fumes, particulate matter, and carcinogens than petroleum-based fuels CONS Unlikely to replace petroleum products given the potential demand (Science 1994; 264:33RN) see Algae oil

biodiversity ENVIRONMENT The existence of multiple flora and fauna in an ecosystem; it is widely accepted that the loss of biodiversity, ie a reduction in the number of species, subspecies and strains is dangerous and could have disastrous consequences for humans, as well as the planet's ecosystem; an example would be growing a crop food, eg corn or rice, from only one highly productive, rapid-growing, spoil-resistant strain; while seemingly having all the desirable features, should the strain then become susceptible to a particular pathogen, all those dependent on the crop could face famine; marine biodiversity is thought by some biologists to be in a state of ecological crisis due to a combination of coastal development (eg destruction of estuaries), motorized marine vessels, ocean dumping, oil spills, overfishing with trawling of the ocean flood, and subsequent disruption of bottom communities and coral reefs, overwhaling with loss of the nutrients they may provide to the ocean floor, pollutant runoffs, and toxic tides due to eutrophication (Sci Am 1994; 270/8:16); in prairie ecosystems stressed by drought, recovery to a normal state of productivity was more rapid in experimental plots of vegetation with the greatest biodiversity, a finding that supports the need to maintain biodiversity (New York Times 1 Februrary 1994; C4)

bioenergetic medicine Energy medicine, see there

bioengineered tissue TRANSPLANTATION SURGERY A neologism for any tissue created by hybrid technologies of molecular biology (eg biochemistry and tissue culture) and materials science that is intended to replace a failed or failing tissue; an early BT being developed is a bioengineered heart valve in which cells grown in culture are placed on a biodegradable polymer (polyglycolic acid) scaffold; once the cells grow, the scaffold dissolves, leaving normal valve tissue; after 10 weeks the new valve is implanted, at present in the sheep, the 'guinea pig' for these experiments, possibly in the forseeable future, in humans (Sci Am 1995; 272/6:46)

bioequivalent allergy unit A unit based on quantitative skin testing using standardized extracts of various allergens; BAUs replace but are not equivalent to allergy units, in which the value of the units was arbitrarily assigned (JAMA 1992; 268:2491FDA)

bioethics An evolving field of allied health care that examines ethical issues ranging from the doctor-patient relationship to the medical decision-making process in general; bioethicists debate such diverse topics as futility of medical care for certain patient groups, rationing of health care, patients' rights issues, physician-assisted suicide, or may be directly involved in specific cases that require an unbiased patient advocate (Medical Economics 25 April 1994 p 33)

biofeedback A form of operant conditioning in which the patient learns to control certain deranged physiologic functions; components of these dysfunction have been 'translated' into perceivable stimuli, such that the patient is made aware of the nature of the dysfunction by watching or listening to an instrument that records or measures the deranged process; as an example, control of fecal incontinence may be increased by watching the recorder of a balloon manometer, control of constipation in the elderly by watching an anal-plug electrode, reduction of pulse rate by listening to amplified pulse sounds; biofeedback may be successful in controlling hypertension, Raynaud's phenomenon, seizures and pain

biogeneric A generic term for a (proposed) generic biopharmaceutical that has emerged from patent protection; BGs are of particular interest in developing nations, given the prohibitive prices of proprietary products; BGs would require more efficient manufacturing processes (eg the methylotrophic yeast, *Hansenula polymorpha*) for producing recombinant proteins; the first BGs planned are IFN-α and hepatitis B vaccine (Bio/Technology 1995; 13:535)

biohazardous waste Waste products including body fluids and tissues that may carry dangerous human pathogens; these waste products often originate from health care facilities and/or research laboratories, and place a relatively small or confined group of people at risk for infection during the time necessary for the infectious agent to desiccate or otherwise become inactive; these materials are indicated by an internationally recognized biohazard symbol (figure); see Biosafety, Regulated waste, Sharps

Note: Biohazardous waste became a 'media epidemic' in the mid-1980s when vials of blood with HIV-1 washed up on beaches in metropolitan New York

biohybrid artificial pancreas A therapeutic device currently being developed as an optimal insulin delivery system, which is constructed of a selectively permeable tubular membrane containing xenogeneic pancreatic islets that lock out molecules larger than 50 kD, which is coiled in a protective housing and connected to the vascular system; the low kD of the membrane prevents access of the immune system to the foreign islets; six of ten pancreatectomized dogs maintained good control of the fasting glucose with long-term implantation of the biohybrid (Science 1991; 252:718) see Organoid; Cf Insulin pump, Islet cell transplantation

biohybrid organ CLINICAL THERAPEUTICS Any hybrid device that marries a biological unit, eg a cell, with a synthetic delivery vehicle with the intent of circumventing (through a process known as immunoisolation) the immune system which attacks and destroys transplanted (non-self) tissues; three major types of BOs have been attempted, to wit, the perfusion shunt, the diffusion chamber, and that which is most promising, the microsphere (Science & Medicine July/August 1995, p16)

'biolistics' CELL BIOLOGY A technique that 'shoots' DNA of interest at a high speed directly into organelles, using a 1-µm tungsten projectile coated with a nucleic acid of interest, shot from a specialized 'gun'; biolistics developed as a solution to the problem of directly transforming, ie introducing foreign DNA into chloroplasts and mitochondria, which is difficult as these organelles are invested with a double membrane envelope that prevents nucleic acid entry

biologicals Therapeutic agents (eg antitoxins, sera, and vaccines) that derive directly from the pools of various living organisms (usually mammals or other humans); biologicals are thus not amenable to chemical or physical standardization steps required of pharmaceuticals, are potentially impure chemically and their safety cannot be assumed; biologicals are regulated by the FDA and include vaccines, anti-toxins and blood plasma products prepared from donor pools

Note: 'Therapeutic agents' prepared by recombinant DNA technology, eg lymphokines and other biological response modifiers are also biologicals and regulated by the FDA, but are considered safe as they derive from non-pathogenic recombinant viruses and their doses can be standardized

biological clock Circadian rhythm

biological dentistry ALTERNATIVE MEDICINE A field that '...*treats the teeth, jaw, and related structures with specific regard to how treatment will affect the entire body.*' BD addresses a diverse array of dental problems including problems with specific teeth related to acupuncture meridians and the autonomic nervous system, toxicity and/or toxicity from dental restoration materials, electrogalvanism and ion migration, and temporomandibular joint dysfunction (Alternative Medicine, Future Medicine Pub, Puyallup, Wash, 1994) Note: There is no data on the efficacy of BD in peer-reviewed journals; see Alternative medicine

biological determinism A theory that seeks to explain the concept of free will as a rationalization, artifact or epiphenomenon that is biochemically or genetically predetermined; if BD is supported by data, the impact on society and the legal system will be enormous, as a person's faults and faux pas will be attributed factors beyond his/her control, and not a manifestation of dysfunction and maladjustment (JAMA 1993; 269:1485MIN&P)

biological false positive A laboratory result that is positive in a subject known to be a true negative for the substance being measured; the classic BFP is a positive result with the VDRL serological test for syphilis, seen in 10-20% of patients with lupus erythematosus; BFPs are common cause of the 'Ulysses' syndrome, see there

biological gradient A broadly applicable posit that holds that the higher the concentration of a noxious agent, eg *Helicobacter pylori*, the more severe the resultng pathology, eg acute and chronic inflammation (see Am J Clin Pathol 1992; 98:549)

biological response modifiers A broad family of molecules that modulate the immune response; BRMs include interferons, interleukins, (hematopoietic) colony-stimulating factors and tumor necrosis factor, B-cell growth factor and differentiating factors, eosinophil chemotactic factor, lymphotoxin, macrophage chemotactic factor, macrophage-activating factor, macrophage-inhibiting factor, osteoclast-activating factor, and others, many of which are generated after a T cell recognizes an antigen present on the surface of a self antigen-presenting cell), which, once activated, produces a 'catalog' of lymphokines (cytokines); many BRMs are commercially available, produced by recombinant DNA technology; the first FDA-approved agent was α-interferon, used to treat hairy cell leukemia, and although BRMs have already been called the 'fourth therapy' in the anti-cancer armamentarium (the first being surgery, radiotherapy and chemotherapy), BRM therapy is in its infancy and most of the agents are not fully characterized or available for clinical use, although many are in early stages of the drug development process; the therapeutic effects of BRMs include

1) Regulation and/or increased immune response
2) Cytotoxic or cytostatic activity against tumor cells
3) Inhibition of metastasis, or cell maturation and
4) Stimulation of BM stem cells, required for recuperation from cytotoxic insult secondary to chemotherapy

The adverse reactions vary according to the agent, dose schedule and route of administration SIDE EFFECTS Flu-like with fever, chills, malaise, arthralgia, myalgia, anorexia, headache, symptoms that often decrease with time, despite a continued high dose (a phenomenon known as tachyphylaxis); the optimal route of administration for each BRM is at present empirical

COLONY-STIMULATING FACTOR Any of five myelopoietic cytokines that bind to specific cell receptors and orchestrate growth and differentiation of hematopoietic cells; granulocyte-macrophage colony-stimulating factor (GM-CSF) is produced by activated T cells and NK cells; erythropoietin, granulocyte-CSF and macrophage-CSF are produced by monocytes and other cells; CSFs have a role in recuperation of hematopoiesis after bone marrow transplantation or toxic chemotherapy, mitigating the effects of chemotherapy, allowing higher than usual doses of chemotherapeutic agents to be given and/or stimulating the phagocytic activities of macrophages and granulocytes SIDE EFFECTS are similar to, but less intense than those of other BRMs, eg flu-like and GI symptoms, dyspnea and hemorrhage INTERFERON IFNs were the first BRMs to be identified (in 1957) and are divided into IFN-α (20 subtypes) and IFN-β (2 subtypes), both produced by macrophages and bind to a type I membrane receptor and IFN-γ, produced by T and NK lymphocytes, which binds to a different receptor; IFNs are 1) Antiviral, causing those cells playing host to certain viruses (eg rhinovirus, papillomavirus and retrovirus) to produce proteins capable of interfering with intracellular viral replication 2) Antiproliferative, acting by unknown mechanisms, possibly decreasing the translation of certain proteins, slowing the cell cycle and 3) Immunomodulation, stimulating or increasing certain immune effects (T cell activation, maturation of pre-NK cells and increased phagocytosis and cytotoxicity by macrophages SIDE EFFECTS Flu-like symptoms, GI (nausea, vomiting, anorexia, diarrhea, dysgeusia, xerostomia), neurologic (confusion, somnolence, poor concentration, seizures, transient aphasia, hallucinations, paranoia, psychoses), cardiopulmonary (tachycardia, dyspnea, orthostatic hypotension, cyanosis), hepatorenal (↑ transaminases, ↑ BUN, proteinuria) and hematological (neutropenia, thrombocytopenia); IFN-α has FDA approval for treating hairy cell leukemia, AIDS-related Kaposi sarcoma and condylomas, and is active in hematopoietic malignancies, as well as malignant melanomas, renal and transitional cell carcinomas INTERLEUKIN The best studied in clinical applications is IL-2, which is not directly cytotoxic, acting

rather as an immune modulator and immune regulator; IL-2 is produced by activated T cells in response to macrophage-processed antigen and IL-1 in the medium, and 1) Facilitates T-cell proliferation by binding to 'high-affinity' receptors on activated T cells, enhancing T cell cytotoxicity, 2) Facilitates the secretion of and enhances the functions of other cytokines (interleukins, suppressor factors and colony-stimulating factors), increased B-cell production via T helper cells, facilitates proliferation and activation of NK cells; IL-2 and LAK (lymphokine-activated killer) cell combination may induce partial or (rarely) complete remissions in metastatic renal cell carcinoma, malignant melanoma and colonic adenocarcinoma SIDE EFFECTS Flu-like, GI, and neurologic symptoms (as above), cardiovascular (capillary leak syndrome, peripheral edema, ascites, arrhythmias, orthostatic hypotension), bronchopulmonary (nasal congestion, cough, dyspnea, tachypnea, pulmonary edema), hepatorenal (↑ transaminases, ↑ BUN, proteinuria, oliguria) and hematological (anemia, thrombocytopenia) MONOCLONAL ANTIBODY An immunoglobulin produced by fusing an immortal mouse cell line (eg myeloma) with a mouse plasma cell that produces antibody against an antigen of interest, forming a mouse 'hybridoma' that is an immortal antibody-producing factory; theoretically, monoclonal antibodies (MoAbs) could target a specific antigen on a tumor cell's surface, initiating an immune-mediated tumor-lysis or toxins linked to the constant end of a MoAbs heavy chain, being directly toxic to tumor cells; viable anti-tumoral products for use in human malignancy have been hindered because the human recipients of MoAbs react immunologically against various epitopes on the mouse immunoglobulin, producing human anti-mouse antibodies, see HAMA; one solution is to 'humanize' the antibodies, using only the portion of the mouse immunoglobulin absolutely required for immune recognition TUMOR NECROSIS FACTOR TNF is produced by macrophages and other cells and is directly toxic to tumor cells or may cause vascular endothelial damage, causing necrosis in the vessels supplying tumors; TNF may increase production of immune cells (NK and B cells, neutrophils), increasing NK cytolytic activity SIDE EFFECTS Similar to other BRMs; see Colony-stimulating factors, Interferons, Interleukins, T cells and Tumor necrosis factor

Biological Stain Commission A nonprofit organization that provides specifications for standardization of biological stains, and evaluates the performance of commercially marketed stains

biological thyroid hormone Thyroid hormone preparations that derive from slaughterhouse animals, which contain both thyroxine (T_4) and triiodothyronine (T_3), in proportions that differ according to the animal species, iodine content in the diet of the animal, season of the year, and other factors; BTH is available as either crude desiccated thyroid or thyroglobulin; endocrinologists do not use these preparations as their potency and bioavailability is uncertain, making them difficult to measure and titrate

Note: BTH continues to have currency for self-proclaimed nutritionists and holistic health practitioners who reason that the more 'natural' the product, the safer it is (JAMA 1989; 261:2694ed)

biological variability LABORATORY MEDICINE The variability in a laboratory parameter due to physiologic differences among subjects, known as interindividual BV, and in the same subject over time, known as intraindividual BV

biological warfare The use of infectious agents as a weapon of mass destruction; agents of potential use as biological weapons include, in addition to anthrax, botulinum toxin and the agents for Argentine hemorrhagic fever, Q fever, Rift Valley fever and tularemia; deployment of such weapons is prohibited by the Biological and Toxin Weapons Convention (1972), supplementing the Geneva Protocol of 1925

The first known deployment of biological weapons was in 1347 by the Tartars who catapulted their dead (from bubonic fever) into the beseiged city of Caffa, spreading the disease to the Genovese defenders; a similar result was obtained by the British who gave smallpox-infected blankets to the American Indians; during World War II, the British experimented with (but never deployed) biological weapons, detonating bombs filled with *Bacillus anthrax*-laced cattle cakes on the uninhabited Gruinard Island in 1942, an island declared habitable in 1988; a 1979 accident in a biological weapons plant in Ekaterinburg (formerly Sverdlovsk) resulted in the deaths of 68 people, when an estimated one gram of concentrated anthrax spores escaped from compound 19 (a germ warfare research center) of the Microbiology and Virology Institute (NY Newsday, 24 Nov. 1994, A17); biological warfare research was alleged to have been responsible for an anthrax outbreak due to an explosion in a weapons plant in Sverdlovsk; the 'Yellow rain' incident is equally unclear, alleged to have been due to deployment of biological weapons, alternately explained as having been induced by bee pollen

bioluminescence Chemiluminescence, see there

biomagnetism The formal study of magnetic fields associated with life functions is a new 'discipline' of biomedicine, the boundaries of which are not yet delineated; it potentially offers a new tool for localizing electrical activity seen in normal and abnormal cortical and cardiac functions; the EEG and EKG 'average' the impulse throughout large regions of measured organ's electrical activity, magneto-cardiogram and magnetoencephalogram sample the magnetic field produced by the ion flow inside the cell itself; biomagnetism is an intradisciplinary 'hybrid' with roots in quantum mechanics, superconductivity, and bioelectricity

biomass ENVIRONMENT The sum total of living (biota) and dead organisms and organic detritus (biodetritus, ie dead organic matter) in an ecosystem or on the planet

biomaterial Any synthetic material or device that is intended to replace an aging or malfunctioning (or cosmetically unacceptable) native organ, in the form of an implant or prosthesis; a critical factor to be weighed in the use of biomaterials is biocompatability, ie the ability to be implanted without evoking an immune response against the implant see Breast implants, Hybrid artificial pancreas, Shiley valve, Teflon, Total hip replacement

biome An ecosystem which is named based on the principal form of vegetation, eg grassland, deciduous forest, marsh

biomechanics A generic term for the application of the principles of mechanic engineering to living structures, in particular to the musculoskeletal system and locomotion; biomechanics has provided the forum for solving many of the problems inherent in designing prosthetic devices with moving parts, eg artificial hips and knees, which must successfully address issues of fluid pressure, mechanical stress, and friction

BioMOO see MOO

bion A generic term for any living (flora or fauna) organism present in an ecosystem

biopesticides Biocontrol, see there

biophysical profile OBSTETRICS Measurement of five fetal activities that usually identify a fetus at risk for potentially poor outcome, except for the non-stress test, the other parameters may be measured simultaneously by dynamic ultrasound imaging: Fetal breathing movement, a non-stress test, fetal muscle tone, fetal movement and amniotic fluid volume

bioprospecting The collecting of biological units, eg bacteria, fungi from various sources in an attempt to identify those with commercial or therapeutic potential (Sci Am 1994; 270/6:105) see Biodiversity, Ethnobotany

bioprosthesis An implanted device of natural (ie nonsynthetic) origin designed to replace a defective body part, eg a porcine heart valve; bioprosthetic valves are less thrombogenic than mechanical valves, they are more prone to structural degeneration, limiting their durability (N Engl J Med 1993; 328:1289oa, 329:517oa) see Heart-valve prosthesis

bioprosthetic Pertaining or referring to a bioprosthesis

bioreactor MOLECULAR BIOLOGY A device that is in essence a large reaction chamber, which is used for the large-scale (commercial) production of cells, which are of interest either by themselves or because they synthesize a product of interest; bioreactors provide a means of automatically regulating the flow of oxygen, (culture) medium, and other nutrients, maintaining the temperature, and pH; they minimize the potential for contamination and are capable of producing a higher density of cells than can be produced in traditional cultures; because of the limited midprocedure cell access, bioreactors are of limited use in producing cells destined for cell therapy, for which culture bag systems have been more popular (Bio/Technology 1995; 13:449)

bioremediation ENVIRONMENT The addition of microorganisms and/or nutrients to supplement a process of biodegradation, as may occur in an oil spill Note: The release of organic chemicals to water and soil may have long-term consequences to the integrity of an ecosystem; assessment of the extent of biotic remediation of soil contaminated by polyaromatic hydrocarbons, eg mineralization of naphthalene and phenanthrene by bacteria requires that abiotic attenuating processes (chemical dilution, migration, volatilization and sorption) be considered in the model (Science 1991; 252:830) see Iron hypothesis

bioremediation by consortium The use of multiple bacteria to perform bioremediation of soils contaminated by various man-made toxins; the use of multiple agents allows the digestion of various toxic metabolites produced in the initial round of detoxification

biosafety Any activity related to safeguarding a population from the untoward effects of biologic materials or infectious agents, and minimizing their environmental impact; because of the legal ramifications of exposure to these agents, biosafety has generated a new administrative bureaucracy in hospitals, academic and research facilities, the function of which includes risk assessment and waste management; see Biohazardous waste

biosafety levels INFECTIOUS DISEASES Classification for the degree of caution that must be exercised when working with infectious agents; see Maximum containment facility

BIOSAFETY LEVEL 1 Organisms are relatively innocuous and are not known to cause infection in healthy human adults, eg *Bacillus subtilis* and *Naegleria gruberi*

BIOSAFETY LEVEL 2 Organisms are 'moderate risk' agents that may cause human disease of varying severity, potentially affecting healthy adults; often good microbiologic technique, such as minimizing exposure to aerosols is a sufficient precaution for these agents, eg Creutzfelt-Jakob agent, hepatitis B, *Salmonella* spp and *Toxoplasma* spp

BIOSAFETY LEVEL 3 Organisms are indigenous or exotic and may infect personnel by aerosols, autoinoculation or ingestion, resulting in disease with potentially serious or lethal consequences, eg human immunodeficiency virus, *Mycobacterium tuberculosa*, St Louis encephalitis virus and *Coxiella burnetii*

BIOSAFETY LEVEL 4 Organisms are dangerous and exotic, require a maximum containment facility, and pose a high individual risk of exposure and risk to laboratory personnel, eg Lassa fever virus (US Dept Health and Human Services Publication [NIH] 88-8395, May 1988)

biota A generic term for all living (flora or fauna) organisms that are present in an ecosystem

biotechnology GENETIC ENGINEERING The methodological components of molecular and cell biology that consists of the application and modification of biological systems and reactions, eg fermentation, monoclonal antibody production and agritechnology, providing the tools and framework for dissecting cellular and subcellular function and dysfunction, immunologic mechanisms, membrane physiology, cell signalling, oncogenesis, virology and others; the tools of biotechnology include recombinant DNA and monoclonal antibody techniques

Biotechnology Index A group of biotechnology companies that American Stock Exchange (AMEX) regards as representative of the biotech industry as a whole in terms of growth and investment potential; the AMEX BI currently includes Amgen Inc, Biogen Inc, Calgene Inc, Centocor Inc, Cephalon Inc, Chiron Corp, Cor Therapeutics, Gensia Inc, Genzyme Corp, The Immune Response Corp, Protein Designs Lab Inc, Scios Nova Inc, Synergen Inc, and Vertex Pharmaceuticals Inc

biotelemetry A generic term for locating and tracking of an animal by an electronic device with the recording of data at a peripheral site

biotin deficiency syndrome A nutritional deficiency syndrome which may be induced by excess consumption of raw egg whites which contain avidin that chelates biotin, resulting in enteritis and dermatitis; biotin is a coenzyme in carboxylation reactions; sources include egg yolks, milk, tomatoes and yeast

biotrodes Food-based electrodes Many plants contain enzymes that can be integrated directly into an electrode, thereby measuring molecules of interest, eg bananas contain polyphenol oxidase and can measure dopamine; corn kernels contain pyruvate decarboxylase and can be used to measure pyruvate, sugar beets contain tyrosine and jack beans contain urease

biparental inheritance Inheritance of one maternal and one paternal allele of a gene (normal Mendelian inheritance) (from Glossary, N Engl J Med 1992; 326:1599OA)

bipedality ANTHROPOLOGY The ability to walk on two feet, a characteristic that is regarded as the definitive characteristic of the earliest homonids

biphenotypic leukemia A clonal expansion of two or more leukocyte populations which may occur in 21-35% of adult leukemias having both lymphoid and myeloid markers; a finding associated with fewer complete remissions (29% for biphenotypic and 71% for pure lymphocytic leukemias) and decreased survival (8 months vs 26 months); ALL that co-express myeloid antigens has a poor prognosis (N Eng J Med 1991; 324:800)

biphosphonate Any of a number of compounds, eg etidronate, pamidronate that are carbon-substituted analogues of pyrophosphate, an endogenous physiologic inhibitor of bone mineralization, which are as potent inhibitors of bone resorption that bind tightly to the hydroxyapatite crystals; biphosphonates are being examined for possible therapeutic potential in osteoporosis (N Engl J Med 1992; 327:620RV)

biplane (intraoperative) transesophageal echocardiography BTEE A permutation of TEE in which there are two (longitudinal and transverse) imaging planes allowing real-time detection of residual cardiac lesions during the perioperative management of patients with congenital heart disease (Mayo Clin Proc 1995; 70:317:OA) see Transesophageal echocardiography

bipolar cells DERMATOPATHOLOGY Elongated, wavy, slender melanocytes filled with fine melanin granules, having long branching dendritic processes, grouped in irregular bundles, often located in the superficial dermis, characteristic of the common type of blue nevus HEMATOPATHOLOGY Primitive or 'early' cells found in the bone marrow that have yet to terminally differentiate and are thus capable of giving rise to erythroid and megakaryocytic daughter cells, depending upon the type of locally produced cytokines NEUROHISTOLOGY A generic term for a neuron with two processes that leave the body in two opposite directions, eg in the vestibular and cochlear ganglia, and in the retina (**bipolar retinal cell**) NEUROPATHOLOGY Elongated, well-differentiated cells, thought to be a feature dictated by the pre-existing fibers; bipolar cells are seen in the pilocytic astrocytoma (bipolar spongioblastoma), a relatively common pediatric tumor found in the third ventricle and cerebellum; in adults, the tumor most commonly affects the temporal lobe

bipolar disorder Manic-depressive disease A psychiatric disorder affecting 1% of the US population, first appearing by age 30; ½ of patients have two or three episodes during their lives, each from 4-13 months in duration; an AD form was linked to chromosome 11 (the linkage has not survived subsequent scientific scrutiny) CLINICAL Bipolar disorders are divided by the authors of the DSM-IV (American Psychiatric Association, Washington, DC, 1994) into

BIPOLAR I DISORDER (296.0x, DSM-IV) is characterized by a occurrence of one or more manic episodes or mixed episodes, and one or more major depressive episodes, and an absence of episodes better accounted for by schizoaffective, delusional, or psychotic disorders

BIPOLAR II DISORDER (296.89, DSM-IV) Recurrent major depressive episodes with hypomanic episodes Bipolar II is characterized by one or more major depressive episodes, one or more hypomanic episodes, and an absence of manic or mixed episodes or other episodes better accounted for by schizoaffective, delusional, or psychotic disorders

TREATMENT Lithium salts prevent or attenuate manic and depressive episodes, maintained at 0.8-1.0 mmol/L; if a manic episode is unresponsive to therapy, electroconvulsive therapy may be effective

Famous manic-depressives include Paul Gauguin, Ernest Hemingway, Herman Hesse, Gustav Mahler, Edgar Allen Poe, Franz Schubert, Mark Twain, Vincent van Gogh, Tennessee Williams, Virginia Woolf (Sci Am 1995; 272/2:63)

bipolar traits Personality traits that represent extreme opposites of expression, eg dominance-submission, extroversion-introversion, passive-aggression

bird arm A virtually extinct colloquial term of uncertain clinical utility for an arm that is greatly reduced in diameter secondary to muscular atrophy

bird's beak sign A radiologic descriptor for GI tract findings by barium studies COLON 'Ace of spades' appearance A sharply delineated, voluptuously-curved, cut-off of the enema column in a volvulus of the sigmoid colon; if the barium passes proximally, 2 kissing 'bird beaks' are seen, known as an Omega loop ESOPHAGUS The over-distended esophagus of achalasia tapers into a pointed beak corresponding to the non-relaxing lower esophageal sphincter, seen by an upper gastrointestinal radiocontrast study (barium 'swallow'), also known as a 'sigmoid' esophagus ILEOCECAL VALVE The contour of the normal ileocecal valve seen by radiocontrast studies of the lower gastrointestinal tract

bird breeder's lung A hypersensitivity reaction to aspirated avian feather and proteins, occurring in those raising budgerigars, chickens, ducks, parakeets, pigeons and turkeys

bird facies A facial dysmorphia characteristic of the Pierre-Robin anomalad, consisting of high-arched, cleft palate, micrognathia and glossoptosis resulting in a bird-like face (the mandibular growth may normalize with time); similar facies may appear alone or associated with Franceschetti (oculomandibulofacial), Hallermann-Streiff, Seckel ('bird-head'), and Strickler (cerebrocostomandibular) syndromes

bird-headed dwarfism Seckel syndrome An AR [MIM 210600] condition characterized by growth and mental retardation, a beak-like nose, micrognathism, microcephaly, prominent maxilla and eyes, hypertelorism, strabismus, antimongoloid slant of the palpebral fissures, premature balding, short trunk, variable musculoskeletal changes, eg kyphoscoliosis, joint dislocations, clubbing of fingers and genitourinary anomalies, eg cryptorchidism; see Parrot beak syndrome

bird leg A colloquial term for a leg that is greatly reduced in diameter secondary to muscular atrophy

bird's nest filter see Inferior vena caval filter

birdshot calcification Buckshot calcification, see there

Bird sign A region of dullness to percussion overlying hydatid cysts of the lungs

BI-RG-587 AIDS PHARMACOPOEIA A dipyridodiazepinone that is a potent inhibitor of human reverse transcriptase, capable of in vitro inhibition of HIV-1 replication; BI-RG-587 may be of use as an adjunct to nucleoside analogs, eg zidovudine, ddC, ddI or when HIV-1 becomes refractory to them; see AIDS

birefringence Polarization, see there

BIRRU Benign idiopathic recurrent rectal ulceration; see Solitary rectal ulcer syndrome

birth canal Parturient canal A somewhat colloquial term for the passage through which the fetus travels during the travails of parturition, to wit, the uterus, the vagina, and the vulva

birth cushion OBSTETRICS A prepartum pillow provided to parturients allowing them to assume a partially squatting, au naturelle position for delivery; 'squat' deliveries appear to require fewer forceps deliveries and shorter second stages of labor

birth defect Congenital malformation, see there

birthing chair OBSTETRICS A device that places a woman in labor in a position that is more erect than that of the usual Western delivery position (head and shoulders up 30°); the BC pretends to simulate the 'squatting' delivery position which had been reported by some authors to ↑ the pelvic outlet by 20-30%; when compared with the standard delivery, BC offered no 'mechanical' advantages, no changes in the subjective component of the childbirth experience as reported by the mothers, and a slight ↑ in hemorrhage in the second phase of the delivery

birthing room Alternate birthing center, see there

bisalbuminemia A polymorphism of serum albumin, characterized by a double albumin peak corresponding to both normal and abnormal albumins, as measured in the serum protein electrophoresis; transient bisalbuminemia may occur with DM, nephrotic syndrome, hyperamylasemia, or penicillin therapy

biscuit DENTISTRY Fired porcelain prior to glazing

BISH Borderline isolated systolic hypertension, see there

bisexual *adjective* Having both male and female sexual characteristics or orientation, usually referring to a person who engages in both homo– and heterosexual activity

bisferiens pulse A double-beat pulse palpated over the carotid or brachial arteries, characteristic of idiopathic hypertrophic subaortic stenosis (obstructive cardiomyopathy) and aortic regurgitation; the ascending limb (percussion wave) initially arises rapidly and forcefully, producing a systolic pulse peak, followed by a dip or trough and a second slower and broader positive (tidal) wave; in some patients, the pulse is intermittent, and may be evoked by mechanical (Valsalva) or pharmacologic (nitroglycerin or catecholamines) maneuvers; Cf Spike-and-dome Note: The other double beat pulses are dicrotic and anacrotic pulses

bismuth encephalopathy A subacute neurologic condition linked to ingestion of bismuth subgallate CLINICAL Fluctuating confusion, somnolence, loss of concentration, tremor, occasionally hallucinations and delusions; with continued ingestion, the symptoms worsen and are accompanied by diffuse myoclonic jerks, seizures, ataxia and inability to walk or stand TREATMENT Discontinuation

bismuth subsalicylate A virtually insoluble basic salt containing 58% bismuth by weight which is of use in treating intestinal disorders MECHANISM OF ACTION Unknown, possibly antimicrobial (prevention of attachment of microorganisms, inactivation of enterotoxins, inhibition of rotavirus replication), antisecretory, and antiinflammatory; in children with watery diarrhea, BS therapy (100-150 mg/kg/d) results in a ↓ stool output, ↓ intake of oral rehydration solution, and ↓ hospitalization (N Engl J Med 1993; 328:1653oA)

bit COMPUTERS The basic linguistic unit of the binary system, corresponding to an 'on-off' signal in a computer's memory or logic circuit

bite cell HEMATOLOGY Keratocyte When hemoglobin dena-tures (as in α-thalassemia or G6PD deficiency), it precipitates into clumps (Heinz bodies) that stick to the red cell membrane; the spleen 'pits out' a fragment of membrane with precipitated hemoglobin as the cells pass through the splenic sinusoids and the cells appear as if a central piece had been removed and are then called blister cells; when the blister(s) rupture, the RBCs are called keratocytes or horn cells

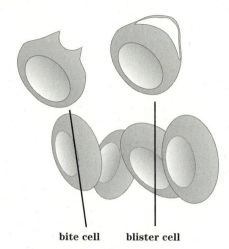

bite cell   **blister cell**

bitter ALTERNATIVE MEDICINE *noun* A medicinal preparation, usually of herbal origin that is characterized by a bitter taste, which is alleged by some alternative health care practitioners to trigger a sensory CNS response, resulting in cascade of responses, including stimulation of the appetite, ↑ flow of gastric and bile juices, hepatic detoxification, and stimulating intrinsic repair (?) of the GI tract

Bitterfeld ENVIRONMENT An industrial city in former East Germany considered by some to be 'Europe's dirtiest city' due to a combination of 1) Lack of treatment of industrial waste water containing aluminum, zinc, copper, mercury, chlorine, phenols, and insecticides 2) Air pollution caused by use of low-quality brown coal as an energy source and by untreated pollutants from 80 factories manufacturing film, dyes, pesticides, polyvinyl chlorides and other chemicals and 3) Soil erosion due to strip mining; a pre-unification study commissioned by Communist authorities found that Bitterfeld's children were immunocompromised, suffered retardation of bone growth and respiratory disease; the clean-up of Bitterfeld is projected to cost DM 20×10^9

bitter melon A plant from Asia administered as an extract in tea, capsules or in retention enemas; it is claimed to 'purify' blood, prevent infections, and anecdotally reported to have antiretroviral activity (Am Med News 21 Nov 1994 p13) Cf AIDS fraud

BKA Below the knee amputation An 'elective' procedure often required for peripheral vascular disease; while preferred by the patient (since their sense of loss is lessened), the BKA often requires re-amputation, an important factor related to mortality; furthermore, the prosthetic device fits less satisfactorily to the BKA than the AKA, see there

B-K mole syndrome see Dysplastic nevus syndrome

BK virus A small human polyomavirus which, like the JC virus, is capable of transforming infected cells in culture; primary BK virus infection is usually subclinical, occurs most commonly in early childhood, persists in the renal epithelium and may be reactivated in the face of immune compromise, potentially causing severe tubulo-interstitial nephritis and cystitis in recipients of bone marrow transplants, or in the immunocompromised patients, eg those with hyper-IgM immunodeficiency syndrome; Cf JC virus

black adenoma An extremely rare, often nonfunctional tumor of adrenal cortex (associated with Cushing syndrome) arising between the reticular and fasciculate zones; the color is due to lysosomal accumulation of lipofuscin PATHOLOGY Polygonal cells with microvilli and desmosomes DDx Hematoma, hemangioma, melanoma, myelolipoma

blackbird Black bomber, see there

black & blue Bruised, contused

black bomber SUBSTANCE ABUSE American slang for black-and-white capsule containing biphetamine, a recreational drug of abuse popular in the 1970s

black cardiac disease of Ayerza A condition characterized by asthma, bronchitis, cyanosis (hence the name), causing secondary polycythemia, dyspnea, emphysema, fibrosis, pulmonary arterial sclerosis, right cardiac ventricular dilatation and hypertrophy, clubbing of fingers, congestive hepatosplenomegaly, and reactive BM

BLACK'S CLASSIFICATION

I	Cavities that begin as structural defects (pits & fissures)
II	Proximal surfaces of bicuspids & molars
III	Proximal surfaces of cuspids and incisors, not involving the incisal angle
IV	As in III, requiring work on the incisal angle
V	Cavities on gingiva of labial, buccal or lingual surfaces of teeth
VI	Cavities on the incisal edges and cusp tips

Note: Class VI is not a true Black group

Black's classification A system used for stratifying severity of cavities (table)

black cataract A colloquial term of uncertain clinical utility for an advanced cataract with brown-black color

black death Black plague, see there

'black diaper' disease Black urine disease, see there

black disease Black fever, see there

black dot UROLOGY An early transillumination finding in the scrotum in torsion of the testicular appendix, which is a normal persistent embryologic remnant; the black dot may be visualized before major edema appears

black dot ringworm A non-inflammatory endothrix form of tinea capitis involving the hair shaft, with minimal folliculitis; the 'black dot' designation refers to the patchy baldness where the hair breaks at the surface of the scalp resulting in black ('polka') dots; the spores in the hair shaft measure 5-8 µm and do not fluoresce with Wood's light; fungi implicated: *Trichophyton tonsurans, T violaceum,* and African dermatophytic fungus, *T yaoundei;* Cf Ectothrix

'black eye' 1) see Raccoon eyes 2) A blackened conjuntival nodule in patients using norepinephrine eye drops caused by an adrenochrome pigmented metabolite; other causes of black eyes include choroidal melanoma and melanocytoma of the optic disc and other drugs, eg Atabrine, minocycline

Blackfan-Diamond see Diamond-Blackfan syndrome

black fever Hindi, Kala azar Invasion of the reticuloendothelial system by *Leishmania donovanii,* with accumulation of histiocytes in the spleen, lymph nodes, BM, lungs, GI tract, kidneys and testes; when the disease is fulminant, it is accompanied by hepatosplenomegaly, lymphadenopathy, pancytopenia, fever, weight loss, hemorrhage and hyperpigmented skin

black fly Buffalo gnat *Simulidium* spp flies which measure 1-5 mm, suck blood and cause hemorrhagic oozing papules accompanied by edema and lymphadenopathy, in tropical Africa, Central and South America; black flies are vectors for *Onchocerca volvulus,* see River blindness

black gallstone A type of gallstone composed of polymers of bilirubin mixed with mucin glycoprotein matrix which is most common in a background of cirrhosis and chronic hemolysis, as occurs in sickle cell anemia or thalassemia (**N Engl J Med 1993; 328:412oA**) BGs comprise from 10-90% of all gallstones, depending on the population being studied, and have more calcium, carbonate and unmeasured residue, but less cholesterol and fat; see Gallstone; Cf Brown gallstone

black hairy tongue A variant of hairy tongue, characterized by hyperkeratosis of the filiform papilla and secondary hemosiderin deposition; the lesion is anterior to the circumvallate papillae, related to prolonged antibiotic therapy, resulting in overgrowth of chromogenic bacteria on the papillae, or due to oral bismuth therapy; see Black tongue, Hairy tongue; Cf Hairy leukoplakia

black heel Talon noir, see there

black light A lamp that emits electromagnetic radiation invisible to the human eye, commonly understood to be ultraviolet radiation, Cf Wood's lamp

black lipid membrane A lipid bilayer that is constructed from either natural or artificial lipids, with holes small enough to force the membrane to remain flat (which would otherwise spontaneously form rounded liposomes), as flattened membranes are necessary to study lipid membrane and partition characteristics

black-listing HEALTH CARE ENVIRONMENT A colloquial term for the refusal of insurers to cover high-risk individuals (eg those with heart disease, family histories of malignancy, and so on) or high-risk occupations, the latter being a practice also known as industry screening (**Am Med News 26 October 1992, p7**)

'black liver disease' A blackened liver characteristic of the rare AR [MIM 237500] asymptomatic Dubin-Johnson disease, which is caused by defective conjugated bilirubin excretion; bilirubin levels are usually ≤ 120 µmol/L (US ≤ 7 mg/dl), 60% conjugated (direct); estrogens should be avoided as they may intensify the jaundice

black lung disease INTRODUCTION Anthracosis is present in the lungs of all urban dwellers and these minimal deposits of carbon dust have no clinical significance; in coal miners, early and significant peribronchiolar deposition of aggregates of pigmented macrophages ('coal dust macules'), are diagnostic for 'coal workers' pneumoconiosis (CWP), and with time, convert to firm blackened 'miliary' nodules with scarring, emphysema, especially in smokers, fibrosis and thickening of the pulmonary arteries, causing obliterative vasculitis, the end stage of which is termed progressive massive fibrosis; the conversion of pneumoconiosis to massive fibrosis may be related to the burden of dust, presence of concomitant silica, underlying tuberculosis, obliterative vascular disease and immune mechanisms; in the US, certain medical benefits are available (**Public Law 92-303**) to those with black lung disease

'black measles' A descriptive term for the darkened hemorrhagic cutaneous spots seen in Rocky Mountain spotted fever, which has been likened to the rash of hemorrhagic measles (rubeola)

black molly SUBSTANCE ABUSE American slang for black capsule containing amphetamine, a recreational drug of abuse

blackout A sign of early chronic alcoholism (or substance abuse) characterized as an episode of amnesia totalis lasting from hours to days after a period of intense drinking or alcoholic binge; blackouts may be due to alterations in central serotoninergic neurotransmission, as these patients also have decreased plasma levels of tryptophan TREATMENT Zimelidine (a serotonin-reuptake inhibitor) may improve the memory in moderate intoxication

black pain disease Black urine disease, see there

black palm Tâche noire A condition that is most common in young adults, seen on the thenar eminence of climbers, gymnasts, golfers, tennis players, weight lifters, and others; the lesion is the result of lateral shearing stress of epidermis against the rete pegs of the papillary dermis, resulting in rupture of capillaries, intraepidermal and intracorneal hemorrhage which translate into multiple symmetrical black spots (JS Dover, in TB Fitzpatrick et al, Eds, Dermatology in General Medicine, McGraw-Hill, New York, 1993) see Sports dermatology, Talon noir

black patch delirium A transient clinical complex most common in the elderly who have had both eyes patched following surgery of the eyes CLINICAL Restlessness, anxiety, disorientation in time and space, persecutory delusions, hallucinations, suicidal ideation TREATMENT Time

black piedra A superficial phaeohyphomycosis of the tropical Americas and Indonesia, affecting the stratum corneum with little or no deep tissue response CLINICAL Fragile hair with hardened and gritty nodules of *Piedraia hortae*, often affecting scalp hairs; Tinea nigra is another form of superficial phaeomycosis, due to *Exophiala wernickii* and *Stenella araguata*; Cf White piedra

black plague Bubonic plague, black death The black (bubonic) plague is an infection that in the full-blown fulminant form with explosive *Yersinia pestis* growth may be fatal in 24 hours, destroying normal tissue architecture; after 3 days of incubation, patients suffer high fever, black blotchy rashes (disseminated intravascular coagulation plus petechial hemorrhage) and become delirious; the bursting of a bubo (a massively enlarged, painful lymph node) is excruciatingly painful enough to 'raise the dead' EPIDEMIOLOGY *Y pestis* is transmitted by the oriental rat flea (*Xenopsylla cheopis*), which bites the rat, ingesting *Y pestis* that rapidly reproduces in the flea's gut forming a 'plug' of obstructing bacteria in the flea's GI tract, whereupon the flea becomes ravenously hungry, goes into a feeding frenzy, repeatedly biting the host and regurgitating *Y pestis*, as the usual hosts (the rats) start dropping like flies, the flea becomes less discriminating and attacks any warm-blooded animal; once in the human population, aerosol becomes the most common mode of transmission, the bacteria's fraction I glycoprotein is antiphagocytic, the endotoxin is responsible for DIC and shock, and thus is well-armed against the host's counterattack

Note: The black plague arrived with the Tartars in Sicily in late 1347, reaching Paris by the following winter, and within 3-4 years of its debut, 25 million had died, 20-35% of Europe's population at the time

black rage PSYCHOLOGY/SOCIOLOGY A psychological state triggered in a non-white by living in a predominantly white, racist society.

black rage defense FORENSIC PSYCHIATRY An argument recently introduced as a highly controversial legal tack for disadvantaged blacks accused of crimes occurring in a race-related substrate; lawyers for the alleged perpetrator of the 'Long Island Rail Road Massacre'[1], may use the argument that black rage[2] caused their client to mentally 'snap' and become temporarily insane, as an explanation for his crime (Vanity Fair January 1995, p30-49)

[1]In which there were 6 deaths and 19 wounded, on the 5:33 train to Hicksville, Long Island, December 7, 1993; Weapon: Ruger 9-mm. semi-automatic pistol, using Black Talons bullets that are very devastating, as they spread on impact
[2]Experts have expressed concern that if this argument is successful, other permutations of the 'rage' theme will appear in the US legal system, eg American Indian rage, Jewish rage, white rage and so on

black rain ENVIRONMENT Precipitation colored by soot, incompletely combusted petroleum products and other industrial pollutants; the health effects of drinking intensely 'black' rain water, eg from the burning of Kuwait oils, is uncertain

black rose STD American slang of Vietnam conflict vintage for a putative STD that was alleged to affect those who frequented Vietnamese prostitutes

black spot Tache noir, seen at the tick or mite bite sites of spotted fevers

black stool A clinical finding often caused by malignancy-related 'occult' hemorrhage; tar-colored or 'tarry' stools appear with as little as 50-75 cc of blood, usually above the ligament of Treitz (as oxidation of the heme by the combined action of enzymes and bacteria requires a number of hours), but may also be due to drugs, eg salicylates, steroids, rauwolfia, phenylbutazone, indomethacin, all known to cause gastrointestinal blood loss in normal subjects and even more in those with underlying digestive tract anomalies; black stool may also be iatrogenic (charcoal, iron and bismuth)

Note: The closer the initial point of bleeding is to the rectum, the more likely there will be fresh blood (hematochezia) versus melena (partially metabolized blood); melena evokes a clinical work-up for the source of bleeding to include upper gastrointestinal tract radiocontrast studies (upper 'GI'), barium enema, endoscopy and biopsies

black sunburst pattern OPHTHALMOLOGY A darkened stellate 'lesion' seen in the optic fundus of patients with sickle cell-hemoglobin C (SC) retinopathy due to the high rate of glycolysis in the end arteriolar system

black thyroid gland syndrome Intense black pigmentation of the thyroid gland which is benign and associated with minocycline therapy (Arch Otolaryngol Head Neck Surg 1990; 116:735)

black tobacco A pungent, relatively crude air-cured tobacco, which contrasts to the flue-cured blond or Virginian tobacco; BT was once thought to be less carcinogenic as the incidence of lung cancer in countries consuming BT was once lower, a finding that was probably a statistical artifact due to slowly increasing exposure; BT may be even more malevolent than blond tobacco, as the incidence of bladder cancer in BT smokers is 2.5-fold greater than in blond tobacco smokers and the urine of BT smokers contains twice the mutagenic activity (see Ames assay) as blond tobacco; when skin surfaces are painted with the two tars, the latency prior to cancer formation in the black tobacco was shorter; in the lungs there is no difference in the incidence of cancer between blond and black tobacco

black toe disease Ainhum, see there; Cf Blue toe disease

black urine A clinical finding due to pathologic excess of various pigments, including homogentisic acid, see Black urine disease, methemoglobin, hemoglobin; nonpathologic causes of black urine include cascara, iron-sorbitol-citric acid complexes, levodopa, radiocontrast media, methocarbamol, naphthol, phenols, pyrogallol, salicylates, diatrizoates

black urine disease Akaptonuria, see there

black vomit The 'vomito negro' typical of the 'intoxication' period of group B arbovirus yellow fever may be intense, recurrent and fatal; the darkened color is from altered blood, accompanied by hiccupping, tarry stools, anuria, wild delirium, coma and death

blackwater fever A rare, often fatal complication of *Plasmodium falciparum* malaria CLINICAL Fever, severe hemolysis with hemoglobinuria, marked jaundice, thrombosis as the parasitized RBCs agglutinate, adhering to the vascular endothelium causing occlusive thrombi and local ischemia, a sequence facilitated by concomitant DIC or related to a drug-dependent, eg quinine, hypersensitivity reaction; renal thrombosis may beget renal failure, with parasitized RBCs plugging glomerular capillaries and red cell and epithelial cell casts in urine

the 'Black Widow' FORENSIC PSYCHIATRY A sobriquet for a woman in the US Midwest who had been married 11 times to 9 men, and who was recently convicted of killing husband number 9 (New York Times 19 March 1995; 31)

black widow spider *Lactrodectus mactans* A venomous spider indigenous to North America, measuring 13 mm in length with a leg spread of 40 mm that bites with anterior fangs and is potentially fatal in the very young or old; the bites are more common in summer in those using an outdoor privy (WC), explaining why most bites are on the buttocks and genitalia CLINICAL Immediate sharp cramping and/or burning pain, dizziness, weakness, spreading to the entire body, activation of the autonomic nervous system (nausea, vomiting, sweating, salivation, tremors, muscle cramping, muscle spasms, twitching, paresthesias) if severe, accompanied by rapid shallow breathing, tachycardia and systolic hypertension, acute nephritis and hemoglobinuria in small children

Blacky pictures PSYCHIATRY A series of 12 pictures in the family life of a dog named Blacky, developed in 1946 for analyzing psychosexual development of children; while the validity has been questioned, they continue to have some analytic currency

bladder training A biofeedback technique used to treat urinary incontinence, which affects ⅓ of ♀ ≥ age 60 based on a combination of behavior modification, a schedule of voluntary micturition, and patient education that emphasizes neurological control of lower urinary tract function; BT reduces the episodes of incontinence by 57% and the volume loss by 54% in women with urinary incontinence who had been urodynamically classified as having either urethral sphincteric incompetence and those with detrusor instability (JAMA 1991; 265:609)

blade of grass sign An elongated radiolucency extending over a long bone, ending in a sharply demarcated curvilinear 'margin', seen in the destructive phase of Paget's disease of the bone

bland diet A mechanically soft diet that is commonly prescribed in peptic ulcer disease as it has no spices or gastric irritants, despite its dubious efficacy; see Diet, Histamine (H2) receptor, Spicy foods

blank LABORATORY MEDICINE A negative control specimen required for immunoassays and quality assurance in many laboratory tests; a blank is processed in tandem with the test serum or tissue, differing therefrom in that a primary antibody is not added in the first step; blanks assure a true negative result, allowing comparison of a possibly positive result with a known negative

BLARS β-lactam antibiotic-resistant staphylococci A term that correctly refers to the mechanism of antibiotic resistance, ie β–lactamase production by *Staphylococcus* spp), rather than to the antibiotic (methicillin) in which this resistance was first recognized; nevertheless, 'methicillin-aminoglycoside-resistant *Staphylococcus aureus*' (see there), has more currency in the literature Note: Bacteria resistant to methicillin are often also resistant to nafcillin and oxacillin and respond poorly to cephalosporins

blast cell Blast* A generic term for the earliest identifiable precursor of any cell line (erythroblast, lymphoblast, megakaryoblast and myeloblast); blasts are relatively large (15-20 μm), with fine chromatin, actively synthesize DNA, have a prominent nucleolus and abundant RNA

*The colloquial or spoken term; blast cell is the formal written form

blast crisis ONCOLOGY A term* widely understood to mean the conversion of a chronic myelocytic (myeloid) leukemia to an acute decompensated phase of increased aggressiveness; BC may refer to any abrupt transition of a chronic, relatively indolent but malignant lymphoproliferative disorder into an accelerated phase, with a marked ↑ in blast cells, where > 30% of the circulating cells are blasts CLINICAL Progressive leukocytosis, thrombocytosis or thrombocytopenia, anemia, lymphadenopathy, hepatosplenomegaly, splenic and bone pain, fever and thromboses TREATMENT Response to the accelerated blast phase of leukemia is usually short-lived; myeloid blastic transformations are commonly treated with hydroxyurea; 25% of lymphoblastic transformations respond to prednisone with vincristine; Cf Blast transformation, Relapse

*'In the typical patient, the hematologic picture converts rapidly to a predominance of myeloblasts, promyelocytes, myelomonocytes and/or erythroblasts in the blood and marrow;...the term (blast crisis) is not ideal because 'blasts' may not predominate in some patients....(the term) Accelerated phase of CML might better encompass the range of changes observed' (JW Athens in GR Lee, et al, Eds, Wintrobes Clinical Hematology, 9th ed, Lea and Febiger, Philadelphia, 1993)

blast injury An injury due to explosions or rapid decompression, the severity of which is a direct function of the intensity of the blast wave; death is caused by exsanguination from ruptured pulmonary vessels with hemorrhage, hemoptysis, air embolism, hypoxia and respiratory failure; other lesions include cardiac contusion, causing arrhythmia, rupture of hollow organs, cerebral injuries (parenchymal hemorrhage and air embolism), and rupture of tympanic membranes TREATMENT Supportive; if air embolism is present, hyperbaric oxygen is indicated; other facets of blast injuries include impinging flying objects and whether the subject was submerged or freestanding at the time of the explosion; Cf Nuclear war

blast transformation HEMATOLOGY The activation of lymphocytes by nonspecific mitogens[1]; BT requires the binding of the mitogen to the appropriate receptor, followed by cross-linking of the receptors, changes in the flux of monovalent cations (Na^+ and K^+), and activation of membrane-associated methyltransferases; this is accompanied by a simultaneous increase in phospholipid[2] synthesis and turnover, and an influx of calcium ions[3]; within hours of mitogen binding, protein synthesis increases, peaking at 48-72 hours of transformation; PHA-transformed lymphocytes are large (10-20 μm) with dark blue nuclei, mitotically active and have increased RNA content; Cf Blast crisis

[1]In this context, a mitogen is defined as any substance that is capable of inducing cell division by mitosis; the most commonly used 'experimental' mitogens are phytohemagglutinin (PHA) which activates T cells, and pokeweed mitogen (PWM), which triggers Ig secretion by B cells in the presence of T cells [2]especially phosphatidylinositol [3]the exact role of which is unclear, but which may be related to the phosphorylation of critical enzymes or proteins

blastomycosis A suppurative granulomatous infection caused by *Blastomycosis dermatitides* EPIDEMIOLOGY ± $4/10^5$ symptomatic, many more asymptomatic (US) CLINICAL-SYSTEMIC Usually acquired by inhalation; usually begins as a respiratory infection accompanied by cough, peluritic chest pain, ARDS, chills, malaise, anorexia, and weight loss, which may spread to bone and internal genitalia TREATMENT Amphotericin B (N Engl J Med 1993; 329:1225OA)

bleed MOLECULAR BIOLOGY see Gel penetration SURGERY Traditionally used as a verb, 'bleed' has acquired nominative status in the highly colloquial synonym for an 'episode of hemorrhage'

bleeder An extension of the noun bleed as used in surgery, which refers to either 1) A patient who is hemorrhaging from acute trauma, or one whose BM has been virtually destroyed by the miraculous vicissitudes of chemotherapy or 2) A blood vessel in an operative or endoscopic field that is overtly hemorrhaging; Cf 'Clotter'

bleeding time test LABORATORY MEDICINE A tool of waning popularity for evaluating the effectors of primary hemostasis, ie platelets and vascular endothelium, by means of an incision into the skin (eg Duke and Ivy BTTs); data from the literature suggest that the BTT is widely misused and only 1-5% of those ordered are actually warranted; the BTT is neither an accurate device for surgical bleeding, nor is it specific as an in vivo indicator of platelet function (Arch Pathol Lab Med 1994; 118:965DA)

bleep see Beep

BLEL Benign lymphoepithelial lesion, see there

blepharoplast Basal body Any of the fine, dark, occasionally argentophilic dots seen in the cytoplasm of normal ependymal epithelial cells; they are positive with PTAH, iron hematoxylin and glial stains, and correspond to the basal bodies of the cilia; when ependymal cells are displaced from the ventricles, blepharoplasts aggregate around the nucleus

blighted ovum An ovum with arrested development, which may appear as a fluid-filled sac with amorphous embryonic rests; blighted ova are typical of grossly abnormal or anembryonic pregnancy and may occur in a background of inevitable spontaneous abortion PATHOLOGY Edema of villi with hydropic swelling and an absence of blood vessels, causing confusion with gestational trophoblast disease; see 'Grapes on a plate', Mole

blinding CLINICAL PHARMACOLOGY The process of making patients unaware of whether a drug (or therapeutic modality) being administered is a placebo/sham treatment, ie the control group or the drug or treatment being investigated; studies are blinded with the intent of removing patient subjectivity **DOUBLE BLINDING** is when the clinical investigator(s) are also unaware of the drug's identity, removing interpretive subjectivity **TRIPLE BLINDING** is when the patients, the clinical investigators and those encharged with interpreting the data are unaware of the 'therapeutic arm' in their data set; see Double blinded studies, 'Nocebo', Placebo, Triple blinded studies; Cf Control

blind loop syndrome Stagnant or afferent loop syndrome A complication of Billroth II subtotal gastroenterostomy (end-to-side enteroenteric anastomosis) that may be seen years after the surgery; the afferent loop consists of duodenum and a variable portion of jejunum, a loop that is a temporary reservoir for 1-1.5 liters of biliary and pancreatic secretions; after a fatty meal, the contents of a partially obstructed afferent loop increase and 'explosively' enter the stomach and can be regurgitated as greenish bilious fluid Note: In the rare complete obstruction, the vomitus is free of bile; blind loopness may be accompanied by gastric atrophy, hypochlorhydria and the clinical manifestations of bacterial overgrowth, commonly anaerobes, eg *Bacteroides* species and anaerobic lactobacilli, as well as enterobacteriaceae, enterococci, clostridia and diphtheroides, accompanied by vitamin B_{12} malabsorption, the result of bacterial competition for B_{12}; other symptoms include intermittent diarrhea due to disaccharidase deficiency, abdominal 'colic', hemorrhage vitamin deficiencies and neurologic symptoms; with prolonged partial obstruction, the stool becomes steatorrheic (bulky, gray and greasy) accompanied by weight loss; complete blind loop obstruction may be a medical emergency with rapid deterioration, shock and perforation peritonitis TREATMENT Antibiotics, eg T-S, loop shortening, afferent-to-efferent or Roux-en-Y anastomoses or gastrojejunostomy

blind spot 'syndrome' of Swan A periodic compensatory diplopia or squint that is not a syndrome per se, has no clinical significance, and responds to simple optical correction

blindness see Legal blindness

blister beetle An arthropod from which the substance popularly known as Spanish fly (SF) originates; (SF) has been held by some members of the lay public to have

aphrodisiac qualities, and is prepared from the hemolymph or coelomic fluid from the blister beetle, *Lytta vesicatoria*, member of the family Meloidae; when applied to mucocutaneous surfaces, it causes erythema, urticaria, and vesiculation; per os, it causes GI irritation, nausea, vomiting, diarrhea, cramping and collapse; as little as 60 mg of this highly nephrotoxic agent may be fatal; the active component is cantharidin, a rubifacient; ammonia may partially ameliorate the pruritus induced by the blister fluid and corticosteroids may relieve the pain

blister cells Bite cells, see there

blobs NEUROPHYSIOLOGY Clusters of cells measuring 0.2 mm in diameter that are located in layers II and III of the visual cortex that have a high content of mitochondrial cytochrome oxidase and are involved in color perception

BLOBs COMPUTERS Binary Large OBjects A tool facilitated by object-oriented relational databases that allow an information system to compress and compact highly dense objects, eg images and voice files, and store them for subsequent retrieval and display (CAP Today September 1993)

block ANESTHESIOLOGY Regional anesthesia to ameliorate locoregional pain; in obstetrics, blocks are used to eliminate parturitional pain, without compromising uterine contractility; blocks used in obstetrics:

CAUDAL BLOCK Extradural anesthesia, which may be administered as a single injection or as a continuous drip; they are technically demanding and require more anesthetic **EPIDURAL BLOCK** The most popular locoregional obstetric anesthesia, which is administered as a single injection or intrathecal 'drip', inserted in the L2-L3 or L3-L4 interspaces; little local anesthetic is used and the bearing-down reflex is not abolished **PARACERVICAL BLOCK** Locoregional obstetric anesthesia that is used in the first stage of labor and consists of injecting a local (< 2 hour in duration of action) anesthetic in the lateral paracervical region; $1/2$ of infants experience post-anesthetic bradycardia; paracervical blocks are ill-advised if the placental circulation is already compromised **PUDENDAL BLOCK** Locoregional obstetric anesthesia that is used in the second stage to relieve episiotomy-related pain, by transvaginally injectiong local anesthetics into the pudendal nerve **SPINAL BLOCK** Subarachnoid block Locoregional anesthesia that is rapid with effective with very low doses; spinal block is not commonly used in obstetrics as it abolishes the bearing-down reflex and the mother cannot cooperate in expulsion of the infant

'blocked pipe' appearance A descriptor for the eosinophilic casts within distal renal tubules and collecting ducts, characteristic of 'myeloma kidney', a finding thought to be more common in lambda light chain myeloma; see Myeloma kidney; Cf Tubular 'thyroidization'

blocking IMMUNOLOGY Reduction or elimination of non-specific binding of an antibody to an epitope, accomplished by washing with the serum of a mammal other than one used in the assay system; blocking is the first step in enzyme-linked immunosorbent assay, see ELISA

blocking antibody Any immunoglobulin that competes with another for an antigenic binding site; BAs may appear in malignancies, preventing a tumor's destruction by cytotoxic T cells CLINICAL IMMUNOLOGY A protective venom- or allergen-specific IgG present in high titers in those exposed to anaphylaxis-producing substances; the IgG successfully competes with IgE, blocking the allergenic epitope, preventing mast cell degranulation TRANSFUSION MEDICINE An often incomplete antibody, usually an IgG that when diluted, adheres to erythrocyte antigens, blocking agglutination; since agglutination is used to detect red cell antigens, BAs may cause incorrect blood group typing, appearing in Rh, -K and -k blood groups; their presence may be corrected for by pre-treating test erythrocytes with enzymes or suspending them in colloid solutions when performing the agglutination reaction

bloodborne pathogen A generic term for pathogenic microorganism(s) present in the human blood that include but are not limited to viruses (eg HIV, HBV, HCV, and others), parasites (eg malaria, *Leishmania*, *Babesia*) PROPHYLAXIS After HBV exposure, HBV hyperimmune globulin is reported to be of use in preventing clinical disease (N Engl J Med 1995; 332:445RV)

blood–brain barrier PHYSIOLOGY A structural and functional barrier that exists between the capillaries and the brain; water, O_2 and CO_2 readily cross the BBB, glucose is slower, Na^+, K^+, Mg^{++}, Cl^-, HCO_3^- and HPO_4^- require 3-30-fold more time to equilibrate with the cerebrospinal fluid than with other interstitial fluids; urea penetrates very slowly; catecholamines and bile salts essentially do not cross the BBB (kernicterus is due to accumulation of bile salts in the brains of neonates whose BBB is yet immature); integrity of the BBB is impaired in hepatic encephalopathy

blood component filter Blood filter, see there

blood 'doping' SPORTS MEDICINE Induced erythrocythemia, where an athlete places a unit of autologous blood in storage to be transfused immediately prior to an endurance event, eg long-distance running, resulting in increased athletic performance due to better oxygen delivery to the tissues

Note: Long distance runners have physiological anemia, which allows an elevated velocity of circulation, dissipation of heat generated while running and rapidly delivery of O_2 to tissues; blood doping results in polycythemia, sluggish red cell circulation and predisposition towards thrombosis, and has been inculpated in at least one race-related fatality

blood component therapy Component therapy The therapeutic use of specific portions (components) of blood, eg factor VIII concentrates, packed red cells, or platelets rather than whole blood (see Arch Pathol Lab Med 1994; 118:411OA)

blood filters TRANSFUSION MEDICINE A device attached to a unit of blood or components designed to retain blood clots and debris, which are divided into 1) First-generation filters that have a screen (pore size 170-260 μm) that traps the most clinically significant particles, ie gross debris and sludge; because it is used with all components, it is also known as a 'standard' blood filter, and is used for platelet concentrates and cryoprecipitates 2) Second-generation (aka microaggregate) filters have a micropore screen (pore size 20-40 μm) to remove 75-90% of leukocytes; these filters are used for RBC transfusions as they trap degenerated platelets, leukocytes and fibrin; routine use of micropore filters to reduce the incidence of transfusion-related adult respiratory distress syndrome is controversial and slows the rate of flow, making them unpopular in urgent care 3) Third-generation filters function by adhesion to remove 99-99.9% of leukocytes, and may be used for transfusing RBCs and platelets (Arch Pathol Lab Med 1994; 118:392OA) see Leukocyte reduction

blood gas analyzer LABORATORY MEDICINE A device used to measure the partial pressure of gases (P_aO_2 and P_aCO_2) and pH in the blood, which can be used to determine respiratory or metabolic acidosis and alkalosis

Bloodgood syndrome see Blue domed cyst

bloodhound face A descriptor for the facies characteristic of cutis laxis, in which the infant has an 'aged' face and sagging jowls, accompanied by a hooked nose, everted nostrils, a short columella, a long upper lip and everted lower eyelid; the entire cutis is loose, resembling a poorly-fitted suit

blood irradiation The subjecting of blood components to ionizing (gamma) radiation for the purpose of inactivating WBCs capable of causing transfusion-associated GVHD CLINICAL INDICATION BI is indicated for BM transplant recipients, congenital immunodeficiency states, intrauterine transfusions and post-natal exchange transfusions, prematurity, high-dose chemotherapy, ALL, Hodgkin's disease and directed donations; BI is relatively indicated for ANLL, CLL, CML, aplastic anemia, cytoxan therapy, massive transfusion (Laboratory Medicine 1995; 26:315OA)

blood mole The retained blood-covered product of a missed abortion that forms a firm, nodular fleshy mass

blood oxygen saturation Oxygen saturation, see there

'Blood Shield' statutes TRANSFUSION MEDICINE Those laws that protect the health care team from liability for transfusing blood products that subsequently prove to be from an individual infected with hepatitis B, HIV-1 or other pathogen, when the indications for transfusion were appropriate for the patient's condition and the unit was tested to be negative for infections by widely used tests in accordance with the blood bank's own standard operating procedures and 'industry standards'; THESE LAWS REGARD BLOOD AS A SERVICE, in the widely accepted landmark case of *Perlmutter* vs *Beth David Hospital*, RATHER THAN A PRODUCT, as in the earlier *Cunningham* vs *MacNeal Memorial Hospital* decision, which would therefore be subject to product liability, based on warranty theory

blood shortage TRANSFUSION MEDICINE A relative deficiency in the supply of blood and blood products available for transfusion in a particular region; in the US, the number of people donating blood has dropped precipitously, due to a relative increase in demand and shrinkage of the donor pool; many cities have made emergency appeals for donations (New York Times 1 February 1994 A1)

blood storage lesions TRANSFUSION MEDICINE Those reversible changes that occur in a unit of packed red cells while stored at 4°C until time of transfusion: ↑ K^+, inorganic phosphate; ↓ pH, Na^+, 2,3 DPG

blood and thunder appearance OPHTHALMOLOGY A fanciful term for the fundoscopic appearance that follows retinal central vein occlusion; the veins are dilated and tortuous, the nerve head is hyperemic, accompanied by superficial retinal hemorrhages and soft exudates with only slightly impaired visual acuity

blood warmer A device that warms blood stored at 4°C to body temperature and indicated for

1) Rapid infusion of cold blood at rates in excess of 50 ml/kg/hour in adults and at rates in excess of 15 ml/kg/hour in children

2) Exchange transfusion in children

3) Massive transfusion directly into a central venous line and

4) Transfusion into patients with cold agglutinins

bloodworm A popular term for 1) Blood flukes, eg *Schistosoma* spp and 2) A nematode, *Elaeophora schneideri*, which causes elaeophoriasis (filarial dermatitis) in sheep

bloody show OBSTETRICS Cervical discharges of prelabor and early labor, consisting of pink nonhemorrhagic discharge preceding the onset of labor by hours to days, but is not itself an indication for admission to the labor and delivery unit

'blooming' see Virilization

blot Blotting MOLECULAR BIOLOGY A nitrocellulose or nylon membrane bearing a molecule of interest, eg DNA, RNA or protein, transferred to the membrane from an electrophoretic gel by either osmosis or vacuum; following transfer of the molecule of interest, the membrane is bathed in a solution that contains a 'mirror-image' molecule to the one that is already on the membrane, producing a 'hybridization blot' SOUTHERN BLOT A technique for identifying the presence (or absence) of a segment of DNA in a sample; the procedure begins by partial enzymatic digestion of nucleic acids, cutting the DNA at specific sites by a restriction endonuclease, each of which recognizes and cuts at a five or six nucleotide sequence; for example, *Hind*III, from *Haemophilus influenzae* cuts DNA at all sites bearing the nucleotide sequence A/AGCTT (at the mirror image sites on the two DNA chains between the two adenines A/A), resulting in a mixture of DNA fragments of varying lengths measuring up to 30 kD that is then electrophoresed in an agarose gel and transferred to a membrane; because the DNA on the membrane is single-stranded, it has a high affinity for its complementary strand; the final step in the blot is to radioactively 'tag' the complementary DNA (a Southern blot after Dr E Southern) or RNA (Northern blot), protein (Western blot), and RNA-protein hybridization (Northwestern blots) ;

Note: The various blots were named by molecular biologists who thought it droll to base the names of further, non-DNA hybridization blots on directions of the compass, and thus these techiques were not described by Drs Northern or Western; see Southern blot, Western blot

blotter's blister MOLECULAR BIOLOGY Photo-reactivation of orofacial herpes simplex virus following exposure to an artificial source of UV light, specifically a transilluminator used by molecular biologists when examining DNA fragments in an ethidium bromide-stained agarose gel (N Engl J Med 1992 327:1462DA)

Note: The term blotter's blister, while easily remembered is not entirely accurate, as the blotting step (in blot hybridization) follows gel electrophoresis and exposure to UV light

blowback phenomenon FORENSIC PATHOLOGY A finding in close-contact ('execution-type') gunshot wounds where the muzzle of the weapon is in direct contact with the victim's skin; the gases accompanying the explosion expand inside the victim and push some of the subcutaneous tissue back outside of the wound; the blowback pressure plus the heat of the muzzle itself burns the muzzle's 'signature' onto the victim's flesh if no clothing is worn at the point of contact, aiding in identification of the weapon

blow-out fracture A fracture of the floor and medial walls of the orbit caused by a blunt object, eg baseball, fist, rock) with herniation of the orbital contents (fat, inferior oblique and inferior rectus into the maxillary sinus), accompanied by diplopia, enophthalmos and limitation of the upward gaze; see LeFort fractures

blow-out fracture (hip) Dashboard fracture, see there

blow-out metastases An osteolytic bone metastasis, seen as an expansile, marginated, trabeculated lesion, characteristic of metastatic thyroid and renal carcinomas and also seen in liposarcoma, melanoma, pheochromocytomas, lung and breast carcinoma

blue atrophy Focal attenuation of the skin with scarring and degeneration of the subdermal collagen, which imparts a bluish color, a finding seen in those who inject narcotics, eg heroin

blue baby A generic term for any infant or child with a neonatal onset of cyanosis of any etiology, which is most common in transposition of the great vessels and in the tetralogy of Fallot

blue belly Cullen's sign Periumbilical bluish discoloration due to intraperitoneal hemorrhage, seen in acute pancreatitis

blueberry muffin appearance PEDIATRICS Multiple blue-brown cutaneous nodules, corresponding to aggregates of leukocytes, seen in infants with CMV infections, as well as in other 'TORCH' (toxoplasmosis, rubella, and herpes) infections, in the rare congenital leukemia and in neonates with multiple blue-brown nodular metastases of neuroblastoma to the skin; 'blueberry infants' under age six months have a good prognosis even without therapy; a useful clinical sign is to press lightly on the skin, causing them to blanch, surrounded by an erythematous halo, probably due to the release of catecholamines

Note: Given the neuroblastoma's tendency to regress in very young children, tumor extension to lymph nodes, liver and skin is not a harbinger of death or disaster, unlike bone metastases which carries a poor prognosis

blueberry muffin baby Dermal erythropoiesis A generalized rash characterized by multiple raised 2-7 mm in diameter dark blue-magenta nodules corresponding to foci of erythropoiesis which regress within 3-4 weeks after birth due to the presence of generalized hemorrhagic-purpuric eruptions

bluebird Bluejay, blue bullet, blue heaven SUBSTANCE

ABUSE A blue capsule, in particular one containing sodium amytal

'blue bloater' A patient with COPD who has the symptoms of chronic bronchitis, a normal to ↓ lung capacity, increased residual volume with air-trapping, decreased expiratory flow, and characteristic arterial blood gas parameters (↓ PO$_2$, ↑ PCO$_2$, despite normal diffusing capacity), cyanosis and right-sided congestive heart failure, due to sleep apnea and inexorably progressive chronic pulmonary hypertension; with time, it may be impossible to distinguish this from other forms of COPD; see 'Pink puffer'

blue blobs Blue globules, see there

blue bodies GYNECOLOGIC CYTOLOGY, see Blue globules PULMONARY CYTOLOGY Laminated, extracellular, birefringent and ovoid 15-20 μm structures composed of calcium carbonate adjacent to or surrounded by macrophages; by H&E staining, they are blue-gray, by PAS staining, red-purple; blue bodies were described in diffuse interstitial pneumonia but may occur in any accumulation of alveolar macrophages

blue bone An early lesion of otosclerosis characterized by repeated cycles of lacunar resorption and replacement of the otic capsular bone in a background of immature vascularized spongy neo-osteogenesis with basophilic (bluish) cementum, which with time, evolve to bony mosaics

'blue book' see TTAPS

'blue cell' tumor SURGICAL PATHOLOGY Any neoplastic, usually malignant tumor, the cells of which share several histologic features in common; they are arranged in nests, sheets and masses and composed of relatively monotonous, round to oval, 8-15 μm in diameter cells with poorly defined cytoplasmic borders and strongly basophilic (blue by H&E staining) nuclei; the embryologic origin of the cells may not be recognizable by conventional LM, but is required information for guiding therapy and thus requires ancillary information that may be provided by histological pattern, immunohistochemistry, ImPx for presence of intermediate filaments and EM

BCTs OF CHILDREN Neuroblastoma, Ewing sarcoma, NHL, embryonal rhabdomyosarcoma

BCTs OF ADULTS APUDoma, mesenchymal chondrosarcoma, hemangiopericytoma, large cell lymphomas, Merkel cell tumor, small cell osteosarcoma, small/oat cell carcinoma, alveolar rhabdomyosarcoma

blue cheer SUBSTANCE ABUSE American slang for a blue pill containing LSD and methedrine, named after the laundry detergent with the same name

Blue Cross A Chicago-based national (US) not-for-profit health care insurer involved in hospital reimbursement; Cf Blue Shield

Blue Cross and Blue Shield Association The largest health insurance association in the US, which is a non-profit fiscal intermediary for the government (under contract with the Health Care and Financing Administration) for payment of Medicare costs; the BCBSA administers and approves BCBS health care plans, provides services related to the bureaucracy of providing health care, and represents the BCBS plans in issues of national interest; Blue Cross is the bureaucracy involved in hospital reimbursement, while Blue Shield is the reimbursement intermediary for physicians; see 'Major medical', Wrap-around policy

blue diaper syndrome Tryptophan malabsorption syndrome, see there

blue disease A nonspecific term for 1) Cyanotic heart disease 2) Rocky Mountain spotted fever

blue domed cyst A variant of fibrocystic breast disease which affects perimenopausal women, and is characterized by cysts filled with light brown (post-hemorrhagic) fluid with benign stromal and epithelial hyperplasia; tenderness is exacerbated prior to menstruation; see Fibrocystic disease of the breast

Note: The blue color of the cysts is due to the Tyndall effect, see there

'blue dot' tumor Acinic cell carcinoma of salivary glands, so designated because of the abundance of clear cells with basophilic cytoplasmic granularity, due to glycogen and hormones; it comprises 1-3% of all salivary gland tumors, is more common in young males, and is often located in the parotid gland TREATMENT Complete surgical excision is paramount PROGNOSIS Relatively good: 12% recur, 8% metastasize

blue ear A consequence of external ear trauma, where the green-brown hemosiderin coupled with the Tyndall effect imparts a bluish tinge to the ear

blue eye OPHTHALMOLOGY An ocular infection seen in Australian aborigines due to conjunctival granulomata from infection by the equine gastric nematode Habronema; Cf Red eye

blue globules GYNECOLOGIC CYTOLOGY Round to oval masses of blue-staining mucus, measuring about the size of an epithelial cell seen in late menopausal vaginal smears, which may simulate a hyperchromatic (ergo malignant) nucleus; an alternate view is that the globules represent degenerated parabasal cells; either way, they are benign

bluejay Bluebird, see there

blue nevus A sharply circumscribed black-blue in color intradermal nevus presenting at birth or which develops with time; it is most common on the acral parts and buttocks of females, appearing as elevated sebaceous yellow, smooth plaques on the scalp, face, < 1 cm in diameter that may be seen in the oral cavity, uterine cervix and prostate PATHOLOGY Aggregates of deeply pigmented, spindled bipolar dendritic melanocytes in the deep dermis and skin appendages and islands of large closely packed cells with oval nuclei and abundant cytoplasm filled with finely granular melanin; a variant, the cellular blue nevus, is more common on the buttocks, often pigment-poor, may undergo malignant transformation and, if the cell clusters penetrate lymph nodes, may be confused with melanoma

'blue people' A colloquial expression for the clinical appearance of subjects who have been exposed to high levels of sodium nitrite, which oxidizes hemoglobin to methemoglobin, resulting in a dusky blue-gray appearance of the skin surface; those persons with congenital methemoglobinemia are at particular risk for hemoglobin oxidation by nitrites; other risk groups include dynamite workers, amyl nitrite 'poppers', cardiac patients treated with nitroglycerin, newborns (erythrocyte cytochrome b5 reductase is low)

Note: Up to 40% of hemoglobin can be methemoglobin with minimal symptoms of mild fatigue and dyspnea (Eleven blue men, Little Brown, Boston, 1953)

blue ribbon A colloquial adjective for highly-qualified, derived from the blue ribbons that may be awarded to the first-place winners in in a competition

blue ribbon committee A committee of experts who may be selected to serve a particular function; such a BRC was convened by Bernadine Healy, former director of the National Institutes of Health for a trial of HIV vaccines (in Sci Am 1993; 269/5:107)

blue-ringed octopus *Hapalochlaena maculosa* and *H lunulata*; both produce tetrodotoxin, an inhibitor of action potentials by sodium channel blockage, with the potential for respiratory shut-down; Cf Puffer fish

blue rubber bleb nevus syndrome An AD condition [MIM 112200] characterized by multiple compressible cavernous hemangiomas of the skin, mucosal membranes, gastrointestinal tract and liver that are blue-purple and rubbery, measuring up to several centimeters in diameter with a

bleeding tendency, rarely, painful and disfiguring, producing hypochromic anemia; the hemangiomas may also be located in the spleen, adrenal gland, central nervous system, penis, liver and lung DIAGNOSIS Angiography

the 'blues' Transient mental depression, often related to exogenous events

the Blues see Blue Cross, Blue Shield

blue sclera Sclera of variable thickness that retain the normal fetal transparency so that the blue uvea is visible; blue sclera occur alone or with brittle bones and deafness, many of which are AD; variants of blue sclera/brittle bone diseases include

1) Eddowes-Lobstein syndrome (ELS), aka osteogenesis imperfecta tarda, characterized by brittle bones, multiple fractures, dislocation and hypermotility of joints, onset in late childhood or adolescence, with blue sclera, keratoconus, cataracts, dysodontogenesis

2) van der Hoeve syndrome (vdHS), which is similar to ELS with osteosclerosis and deafness

3) Vrolik syndrome, which is similar to vdHS, but which lacks blue sclera

4) Blegvad-Haxthausen syndrome, which is similar to vdHS and has cutaneous atrophy and zonular cataract

Blue sclera may also be seen in AIDS embryopathy, Bloch-Sulzberger syndrome, Crouzon syndrome, Cornelia de Lange syndrome, Ehlers-Danlos syndrome, Foelling syndrome, Laron dwarfism–Loja type, Lowe syndrome, Marfan's disease, pseudohypoparathyroidism, Turner syndrome, and Werner syndrome

the Blue Sheet A specialized weekly publication that provides business and US governmental information on health policy and biomedical research (produced by FDC Reports, Inc Chevy Chase, Md)

Blue Shield A Chicago-based national (US) not-for-profit health care insurer which is the reimbursement intermediary for physicians; Cf Blue Cross

blue skin Bluish discoloration of the skin is abnormal and the result of various toxins, including cyanide, gold (therapeutic), or silver-based drugs, amiodarone or photosensitivity to tetracycline, sulfonamides, phenothiazines or exposure to blue dyes

blue sky Heroin

'blue spell' An episode of hypoxia, cyanosis, dyspnea, restlessness and syncope with acutely decreased arterial PO_2 and decrease of an already compromised pulmonary blood flow, characteristic of Fallot's tetralogy, but which also appears in other cyanotic congenital heart disease; see Shunts (right-to-left)

blue stone Cupric sulfate

blue stroma PATHOLOGY A colloquial term for the low-power morphology of any inflamed tissue by LM, first described in endometrial stroma

blue suit Chemturion space suit, see there

blue tags TRANSFUSION MEDICINE Given the significance of transfusing an incorrect blood unit in the ABO blood group system, California state law requires color coding of ABO units, where O units are blue (group A is yellow, group B is pink and group AB is white)

blue toe syndrome Atherothrombotic microembolism of the lower extremities due to recurrent cholesterol embolic 'showers' with painful cyanotic discoloration of the toes and embolism to other sites that completely resolve between attacks (hence the mnemonic, pain, purple, and painful pulses); despite the gangrene-like appearance, blue toes may respond to conservative therapy without amputation DIAGNOSIS Arteriography MEDICAL TREATMENT Dypyridamole plus aspirin SURGICAL TREATMENT Thromboendarterectomy of aorta; see Black toe disease

blue tongue sign A strikingly blue tongue due to selective D_2 dopamine antagonism, as seen in metoclopramide therapy, causing a dystonic reaction, accompanied by trismus, torticollis, facial spasms, opisthotonus and oculogyric crises, a reaction occurring in 1:500 young women treated with metoclopramide; blue tongue has been anecdotally associated with haloperidol

blue top tubes CLINICAL CHEMISTRY 4.5-ml tubes containing sodium citrate as an anticoagulant, used to collect specimens for coagulation factor assays, fibrinogen, glucose-6-phosphate dehydrogenase, partial thromboplastin time, prothrombin time, thrombin time

blue valve syndrome A descriptor for the bluish, vaguely translucent and hypermobile[1] cardiac[2] valves that have been removed from patients with Marfan disease(s), which demonstrate mucoid degeneration

[1]Floppy [2]Most prominently the mitral valve

'blue velvet' SUBSTANCE ABUSE The 'street' name for an IV drug of abuse, consisting of paregoric and triphenamine-HCl mixed with talc DESIRED EFFECTS Euphoria, excitement UNTOWARD EFFECTS Depression, tachycardia, systolic murmur, rales, hepatomegaly with centrilobular hepatic necrosis, sudden death

blunt end ligation MOLECULAR BIOLOGY The joining of two double-stranded tailless DNA molcules at their ends

blunt trauma A generic term for any injury sustained as a result of blunt force, which may be related to motor vehicular collisions, or mishaps, falls or jumps, blows or crush injuries from animals, blunt objects or unarmed assailants (JAMA 1993; 269:1525c) Cf Penetrating trauma

B lymphocyte B cell One of the two major classes of lymphocytes of the immune system (so-named given its similarity to the analogous cell originating from the avian bursa of Fabricius, the human equivalent of which have proven impossible to identify, although some workers believe it to be in the fetal liver); B cells comprise 30% of the circulating lymphocytes and are concentrated in the follicular zones of lymphoid tissue, while the T cells are located in the deep cortex; B cells are responsible for antibody production, immune defense against viruses and bacteria, surveillance (cytolysis of potentially malignant 'self' cells), mediation of antibody-dependent cell cytotoxicity, allergic reactions, formation of antigen-antibody complexes and production of cytokines; surface and cytoplasmic antigens indicate the degree of B-cell maturation and function; cytoplasmic IgM is present in pre-B cells and surface immunoglobulin and complement receptors are seen in mature cells B-cell markers include CD9, CD10, CD19, CD20, CD24, the Fc receptor, B1, BA-1, B4 and Ia

BM Bone marrow, also 1) Bachelor of Medicine 2) Basal metabolism 3) Basement membrane 4) Black male 5) Body mass 6) Bowel movement 7) Buccomesial

Also 1) Basal medium (microbiology) 2) Basilar membrane 3) Buccal mass 4) Bureau of Medicine (agency of the FDA)

bmi-1 DEVELOPMENTAL BIOLOGY An oncogene that was first linked to B– and T–cell lymphomas, which encodes a protein, Bmi-1; Bmi-1 is thought to belong to the so-called Polycomb complex that regulates segmental identity by repressing homeobox (*Hox*) genes during development (Nature 1995; 374:724)

BMI Body mass index, see there

B-mode see Ultrasound

BMR Basal metabolic rate, see there

BO Body odor, see there

board-certified An adjective for a US or Canadian physician (or other health care professional) who has both 1) Completed the minimum years (ranging from four to eight years) of post-medical school residency training, ie a physician who is 'board-eligible' and 2) Passed an examination, commonly called the 'Boards' that tests his/her theoretical knowledge in the area of specialization; board-certification is often required for appointment to a hospi-

tal's medical staff; Cf Board-eligible

Note: Approximately 250 000 physicians in the US are certified by one of 23 specialty boards and 12 000 are certified by more than one specialty board

board-eligible An adjective for a US or Canadian physician (or other health care professional) who has completed the minimum years (4-8 years) of post-medical school residency training and is eligible to sit for an examination (the 'boards') that tests his/her theoretical knowledge in the area of specialization; Cf Board-certification

board of health A governmental body responsible for coordinating public health activities in a specified city, county, or state

'boarded' Board-certified, see there

board-like rigidity Spastic rigidity of the abdominal wall muscles induced by acute peritonitis, classically elicited by a perforated peptic ulcer although any fulminant peritonitis may elicit the same reaction; see Hippocratic facies

board of medical examiners A body that is recognized by a state's government, which may if necessary, exercise its authority to place a physician on probation, to suspend or to revoke his license to practice medicine; the infractions which would cause a state board to initiate punitive actions against a physician include drug abuse, irregular subscription practices regarding 'controlled drugs', ie those drugs with addictive potential and various other major deviations from the tenets of the Hippocratic Oath

bobbittize A highly colloquial term for the performance of an unscheduled penectomy outside of a hospital or other health care environment, using suboptimal equipment (eg 12-inch kitchen knife), and in absence of known medical indications; of 100 bobbittizations documented in Thailand (performed by the wives for the husbands' adultery); in the 1970s few penises were successfully reattached; recovery of function requires microsurgical techniques that allow the sewing of vessels and nerves of 1 mm or less (New York Times 13 July 1993; C3) see Penile reattachment

'bobble-headed doll syndrome' A neurologic symptom complex described in children with a cyst in the third ventricle, or hydrocephalus, characterized by bobbing of the head in three-second cycles and rhythmic flexion and extension of the extremities that may be controlled voluntarily, and which ceases during sleep, accompanied by mental retardation, generalized fine tremor, hydrocephalus, obesity and visual impairment

body bag A popular term for the zippered black bag (known to cognoscenti and morticians as a body pouch) that is used to transport a dead body from point A (hospital, nursing home, crime scene) to point B (funeral home, crematorium, coroner's office) prior to burial Note: For in-house transportation of a cadaver, a white plastic sheath, known as a shroud, may be used

body image The concept of one's body or self in space

body language PSYCHOLOGY An informal often culture-independent form of communication in which emotions, feelings, motives, and thoughts are expressed by changes in facial expression, gesture, posture, and other nonverbal signs

body mass index BMI A clinical parameter used to determine obesity, defined by the formula Weight (kg)/height (m)^2; a BMI of less than 25 is considered obese

body odor An odor that is

1) Apparent only to the owner of the nose, thus being defined as a disorder of perception only, which may occur in an aura prior to a seizure, in schizophrenia and in the olfactory reference syndrome (see there), or

2) Apparent to others, emanate from various orifices and derive from urine, feces, saliva, skin, breasts, sex organs, and sweat glands; the major contributor to and 'classic' cause of BO is the combined activity of eccrine and apo-

crine sweat glands, especially of the axillae and anogenital regions, with lesser contributions from the sebaceous glands; the quasi-rancid smell of well-aged BO is due in large part to volatile fatty acids, steroids, and amines of apocrine gland origin, which may be intensified by aerobic (eg micrococci and diphtheroids) and anaerobic bacteria and fungi which secrete isovaleric, butyric, carbonic, and other volatile acids and indoles; sweat gland secretions ↑ after puberty and begin to ↓ at menopause (JAMA 1995; 273:1171)

'body packing' SUBSTANCE ABUSE A method for smuggling narcotics in which a 'courier' swallows condoms or other impermeable containers filled with pure cocaine or heroin in order to escape detection by customs agents and specially trained dogs; the body packer 'syndrome' consists of a constellation of medical complaints including intestinal obstruction and rupture of the bags, the latter being almost invariably fatal DIAGNOSIS, ULTRASONOGRAPHY Sickle-shaped echo with a dorsal echo deficit; most 'packs' are in the stomach at the time of examination (Dtsch Med Wochenschr 1990; 114:1865) DIAGNOSIS, SCOUT FILMS, see 'Double condom' sign, Drug mules

Note: Body packing began in the mid-1980s with cocaine (pretax street value $18 000/kg), originating from South America; more recently, the couriers are from Africa, carrying heroin (street value $200 000/kg) originating from Afghanistan, Pakistan, and the 'Golden Triangle' (Thailand, Laos and Burma), these 'sherpas' swallow between 55 and 100 doubly wrapped 'balloons', totalling 700-1.5 kg, making as many as 3 'runs' per month, for $5-10 000 per shipment (Personal communications,NYPD Organized Crime Unit; SS, DEA, New York Field Office, JFK Intl Airport)

body rocking NEUROLOGY Monotonous rhythmic movements, which can be seen in a wide range of conditions, including autism, mental retardation, psychiatric disorders, and institutionalization; the phenomenon is thought to provide a means of relieving tension and blocking external stress by maintaining a pleasurable whole-body 'mantra'; body rocking-type flexion and extension of the trunk may be seen in tardive dyskinesia, a complication of antipsychotic therapy, which is more common in the elderly and in women, which may persist indefinitely

body sculpting A highly colloquial term for cosmetic surgery intended to change the contours of a person's body to achieve what he or (more commonly) she perceives to be a perfect physique; the analogy to sculpting with clay is not inappropriate as BS can subtract tissue by liposuction, and add mass by variably-sized synthetic implants

body snatching The illegal (and ghoulish) removal of a body from its grave with the express purpose of providing material to medical students for the study of human anatomy; Cf Burking

BS had its heyday in the UK in the 18th and 19th Centuries; it allegedly continues unabated in Transylvania

body substance isolation A system of precautionary measures taken to reduce the nosocomial transmission of pathogens in a health care environment; BSI requires that gloves be worn at every contact with mucous membranes, secretions and moist body substances which includes oral secretions, stool and others (that BSI ignores air-borne pathogens is acknowledged by its advocates); the term universal precautions is a set of principles developed by the CDC to protect hospital personnel, *not to prevent the transmission of nosocomial infections* (N Engl J Med 1992; 327:120ED) Cf Universal precautions

body weight fluctuation Weight cycling, see there

bodywork ALTERNATIVE MEDICINE A generic term for the use of touch[1] to either improve bodily structure and function[2], or as a therapeutic modality, to reduce pain, and heal damaged musculoskeletal units (Alternative Medicine, Future Medicine Publishing, Inc, Puyallup, Washington, 1994) see Alexander technique, Alternative medicine, Feldenkrais method, Rolfing®

[1]eg massage, deep tissue manipulation, movement awareness, energy balancing and others [2]eg stimulate circulation and promote relaxation

bog body ANTHROPOLOGY A human body that has been 'pickled' by the acidic water in bogs and marshes, nearly 700 of which have been catalogued from Scandinavia and Britain, and who died 10-1000 years prior to their discovery; most were victims of violent death; the best studied of bog bodies is the Lindow man, 'Pete Marsh'

boiled lobster appearance Erythema neonatorum A brilliant red vasomotor flush of no clinical significance that may transiently (up to 24 hours) cover the entire infant mimicking inflammation; Cf Harlequin changes

boilerplate COMPUTERS A standard passage of text or other material that is used repeatedly; boilerplate dictations are a standard tool used in voice recognition systems that may be used by radiologists and pathologists

The term was first used in journalism (in 1893) for any ready-to-print copy provided by a news agency

Bolam principle A 1957 ruling from British case law, which states that the law imposes a duty of care, but the standard of that care is a matter of medical judgement (Lancet 1992; 340:1399c)

Bolivian hemorrhagic fever A viral infection that is clinically similar to Argentine HF affecting the cardiovascular, hematopoietic, and renal, as well as the central nervous system; BHF is endemic to the grain-producing province of Beni in Amazonian Bolivia, caused by the Machupo virus (an arenavirus) excreted in the urine of the rodent vector, *Calomys callosus* CLINICAL High pediatric mortality, with early fever, anorexia, nausea, vomiting, myalgia, neurologic signs (50% have intention tremor, 25% develop convulsive encephalopathy), and a 10-20% mortality; Cf Haverhill fever

bolus A generic term for either a large mass of food, or a large often spherical preparation or dose, of a drug administered to achieve an immediate effect; in treating malignancy, prolonged IV infusions may be more effective than intermittent bolus injections (N Engl J Med 1994; 331:502OA)

Bolus may be used colloquially to indicate a hyperinfusion of information, eg a crash-type review course prior to a boards examination (CAP Today March 1993)

bomb Crash COMPUTERS *verb* An abnomal termination of a program being executed, which requires that the computer be re-booted

bombard RADIATION PHYSICS To expose to a beam of ionizing radiation or highly charged particles

Bombay phenotype TRANSFUSION MEDICINE A very rare phenotype of erythrocyte first described in Bombay (Lancet 1952; 1:903); the O_h phenotype is a variant of the ABO antigens on red cells; for A or B antigens to be expressed on RBCs, the cells must have a precursor substance (H antigen) encoded by the H gene; O_h type red cells do not agglutinate with antisera containing anti-A, anti-B, or anti-H type antibodies as they lack the H gene, and therefore H substance; O_h subjects do have anti-A, anti-B, and anti-H antibodies in their serum, which may cause problems when cross-matching donors and recipients Note: The condition was identified in Bombay (Lancet 1952; 1:903)

bombesin A 14-residue neuropeptide that is analogous to gastrin-releasing peptide, which is produced in the GI tract, from the gastric antrum, stimulating GI smooth muscle contraction, release of gastric acid and most GI hormones except secretin, with which bombesin has a yin-yang effect; bombesin also acts on vasculature, gallbladder, pancreas lung, and urinary tract; see Secretin; when administered into the cerebral cisterna, bombesin evokes hypothermia, analgesia, hyperglucagonemia and hyperglycemia; bombesin also stimulates proliferation of bronchial epithelial cells, pancreas, small cell carcinoma; anti-bombesin antibodies have theoretical potential for treating small cell carcinoma of the lung, since these tumors both secrete bombesin and have bombesin-like receptors

bond The 'glue' that maintains the molecules in their three-dimensional configuration **COVALENT BOND** Electron pair bond Electrons are shared between two atoms, classified as polar or nonpolar when the sharing is uneven; covalent are the strongest bond in biological systems; the bond strength of a single covalent bond is 50-110 kcal/mol, a double bond, 120-170 kcal/mol and a triple, 195 kcal/mol; the molecular structure is stabilized by weaker bonds **ELECTROSTATIC BOND** Ionic bond The attractive force that exists between an anion and cation **HYDROGEN BOND** A weak association between an electronegative atom (the acceptor atom) and a hydrogen atom covalently bound to a donor atom; the greater the length between atoms, the weaker the bond strength (4-5 kcal/mol) **HYDROPHOBIC INTERACTION** The attractive force between nonpolar or polar molecules in an aqueous solution **NONCOVALENT BOND** Any bond between molecules that don't share pairs of electrons, eg electrostatic bond, hydrogen bond, hydrophobic interaction **VAN DER WAALS BOND** A weak attraction when two atoms approach each other, the result of fluctuating dipoles, occurring in both polar and nonpolar atoms (1 kcal/mol)

bonding NEONATOLOGY The emotional ties formed between the infant and mother that occur in the early post-partum period, considered analogous to imprinting in animals; Cf Anaclitic depression

bone-in-bone pattern PEDIATRIC RADIOLOGY A descriptor for a morphology seen under different circumstances

1) Normal A 'double bone' appearance in the infant vertebral body, seen at 1-2 months of age, with peripheral decrease of bone density and retention of a sharp cortical outline, thought to represent postnatal bone remodelling

2) Pathological A symmetrical increase in bone density accompanied by a lack of 'tubulation'; when limited to the end-plates of the vertebrae, the radiological appearance results in a sandwich vertebra (see there) or if more extensive, a miniature 'Vertebra within a vertebra', classically associated with osteopetrosis, but also seen in osteomyelitis, sickle cell infarction with periosteal elevation, osteolysis, endosteal absorption and neo-osteogenesis along the inner cortex of the medullary space, Gaucher's disease, cleidocranial dysostosis, late post-irradiation changes in young children, or Thorotrast-related

bone densitometry The measurement of bone mass or density; all of the current methods (single-photon absorptiometry, dual-energy photon absorptiometry, dual-energy X-ray absorptiometry) are based on a tissue's absorption of photons derived from either a radionuclide or an X-ray tube, the latter of which have an increased accuracy and shorter scan time; bone densitometry objectively determines the risk of suffering fractures, by quantifying osteoporosis, which with dementia, constitute the two most common morbid conditions of the elderly; other methods to evaluate osteopenia include 'eye-balling' of a plain film of a bone requires a bone loss of at least 30% before osteoporosis can be diagnosed with certainty and the 'feel' of the bone when it is drilled by the surgeon at the time of joint replacement is even cruder; other indications for performing bone densitometry analyses include indirect evaluation of estrogen deficiency, osteopenia, long-term glucocorticoid therapy and primary asymptomatic hyperparathyroidism (N Engl J Med 1991; 324:1105ʀᴠ) see Osteoporosis

bone glue ORTHOPEDICS A formulation of calcium and phosphate* that hardens into dahllite within 5 minutes after mixing and serves as 'instant bone', which is injected at the site of fractures; BP is in clinical trials and is reported to be a marked improvement over the locoregional use of bone chips and hydroxyapatite to heal fractures, as it serves as internal fixation to maintain proper bone alignment while healing occurs; early results suggest that operations using BP are performed more quickly, require less hardware (screws and plates), and allow the patients to resume normal activities more quickly (Science 1995; 267:1796, 1772) see Dahllite

*Based on the mineralization process of coral, which is a physicochemical process, in contrast to bone formulation in vertebrates, which is slower and directed by proteins

bone graft A 'raw material' often of cadaveric origin, used in orthopedic surgery to fill defects and/or 'sculpt' plains; common indications for bone grafting include spinal fusion, revision of failed articular prostheses, and filling of traumatic or malignancy-related bone defects, or periodontal defects (CAP Today May 1992) see Tissue bank

bone hunger see Hungry bone(s) disease

bone/joint panel A group of laboratory tests that have been determined to be the most cost-effective, sensitive, specific (and 'efficient') in evaluating a patient with bone and joint complaints; the B/J panel includes measurement of uric acid, calcium, phosphorous, alkaline phosphatase, total protein and albumin; see Organ panel

bone marrow transplantation The IV infusion of hematopoietic progenitor cells to re-establish marrow function in a person with damaged or defective bone marrow (N Engl J Med 1994; 330:827ʀᴠ); BMT is used to treat aplastic anemia (5-year survival, 80%), acute nonlymphocytic leukemia (ANLL, 50%) and acute lymphocytic leukemia (ALL, 25%); the 750 ml of marrow required for BMT is 'harvested' from the iliac crests, a painful procedure; in ALL, BMT of an HLA-matched or preferably, an identical donor, is an option generally reserved for those in second or subsequent remissions, or used to induce first remissions in 'high-risk' ALL; see Autologous BMT; in ANLL, BMT may induce first remissions in 50-60% of younger (< 20 years old) patients; see Chemotherapy, Relapse, Remission; BMT survival in leukemia 32-48%, depending upon chronicity and cell type; BMT survival in non-neoplastic conditions 63-75+%; minor HLA mismatching does not ensure failureCOMPLICATIONS Acute or chronic graft-versus-host disease (35-60%), interstitial pneumonia, idiopathic or viral (CMV, herpes simplex, varicella-zoster), rarely, post-BMT leukemic relapse or acute myeloid leukemia from donor into an HLA-identical sib for chronic myelocytic leukemia CAUSE OF DEATH Opportunistic infections 17% of BMTs suffer CMV-associated interstitial pneumonia (85% mortality); prophylactic gancyclovir reduces the incidence of this complication (N Engl J Med 1991; 324:1005); these infections are due to immune defects; other causes of interstitial pneumonia include *Pneumocystis carinii* or radiation CLINICAL GVHD with skin rash, hepatic defects, diarrhea, infections and autoimmune phenomena Cost $75-150 000 (1990 dollars) INDICATIONS BMT is appropriate and often successful therapy for leukemia and aplastic anemia, but less so in treating lymphoma, thalassemia major, osteopetrosis, inborn errors of metabolism, congenital immune deficiencies, eg Wiscott-Aldrich disease and severe combined immune deficiency Note: 75% of post-BMT leukemic relapses occur in the first two years; in ANLL, 50-60% of those transplanted in the first remission survive, 25% survive in the second remission; adjuvant therapy includes cyclophosphamide and busulfan access to BMT is not compromised by single-payer financing, global budgeting, and universal coverage (N Engl J Med 1994; 331:1067sᴀ)

bone mineral density A measurement of bone mass, expressed as the amount of mineral (in grams) divided by the area scanned (in square centimeters); calcium supplementation increases peak bone mineral density if given prior to puberty (N Engl J Med 1992; 327:820ᴀ)

bone paste PODIATRY A colloquial term for the fragmented bone and fibro-osseous tissue removed in various forms of surgery to the foot

bone pearls Small rounded osseous masses seen in electrical injury, due to actual melting of the bone by intense heat, eg lightening; adjacent bone may have rarefaction, periostitis and fractures

bone pointing 'syndrome' Hexing phenomenon A reaction described in primitive aboriginal societies where a witch doctor points a bone at someone during a ritual and that person becomes ill and dies shortly thereafter; an analogous situation in modern society is a patient being told that he/she has little time to live from a terminal disease upon which he/she lapses into a state of apathy and dies; see Anniversary phenomenon, Voodoo death; Cf Harvest Moon phenomenon

bone & stone disease see Stone, bone and groan disease

bone spicule appearance OPHTHALMOLOGY Fundoscopic appearance of retinitis pigmentosa seen as jagged, jet-black pigmented patches at the equator, often accompanied by bilateral nyctalopia

Bonner v Moran An early landmark case regarding the ethics of human experimentation, in which Bonner, a 15-year-old boy, was recruited in an attempt to graft some of his skin to a burned relative, keeping it attached as part of a living tube of flesh (Nature 1995; 374:827BR)

Böök syndrome PHC syndrome An extremely rare AD [MIM 112300] condition characterized by premolar aplasia, hyperhidrosis, and premature canities (gray hair), described in a single Swedish family in 1950

boomer Baby boomer, see there

BOOP Bronchiolitis obliterans organizing pneumonia A disease formerly considered a form of interstitial pneumonia ETIOLOGY Obscure, but may be associated with toxic fumes, infection, connective tissue disease PATHOGENESIS The role of the eosinophil in idiopathic BOOP is uncertain (Mayo Clin Proc 1995; 70:137OA) CLINICAL Cough, dyspnea, 'flu' symptoms, 50% recovery, 12% BOOPs eventually die of the disease, many develop usual interstitial pneumonia; obstructive symptoms are limited to smokers, most of whom have restriction disease and impaired diffusing capacity, remission may follow use of corticosteroids RADIOLOGY Patchy ground-glass appearance on a plain antero-posterior chest film PATHOLOGY Patchy, polypoid masses of intraalveolar granulation tissue in small airway lumina and alveolar ducts with preservation of the alveolar architecture and uniform intrabronchiolar fibrosis (N Engl J Med 1991; 324:1195cpc)

Boophilus microplus FOOD INDUSTRIES A widely distributed hematophagous tick that debilitates cattle in the tropics and subtropics through blood loss and transmission of several arboviruses and bacterial disease, eg anaplasma and babesiosis; in Australia, where *B microplus* causes estimated annual losses of greater than $100 million, an injectable vaccine has been developed using as an antigen, a tick protein that coats the gut lining; if effective, the vaccine would be of economic importance, where *B microplus*-related annual losses exceed $1 billion (Science 1994; 264; 1398); Cf Dipping

booster Booster dose Re-exposure to an antigen usually as a deliberate, often iatrogenic attempt to induce a secondary immune response months to years after a primary response to an antigen, 'boosting' the response

booster phenomenon An increase in the size of the tuberculin reaction (> 6 mm, or from less than to greater than 10 mm) after a second PPD skin test for tuberculosis; persons with a booster phenomenon are thought to have enhanced immunologic 'recall', due to either 1) Previous infection with *M tuberculosis* or 2) Infection with a non-TB mycobacterium; this phenomenon is most common in the elderly previously infected with *M tuberculosis*, who usually do not convert to active disease

booster 'shot' A second immunization dose, administered after an appropriate time interval, allowing the body to mount an immune response; when a person is exposed, eg to 'dirty' wounds, or plans potential exposure, eg travel to regions endemic for certain infectious agents, the booster shot provides a rapid anamnestic response that outpaces the development of disease, eg tetanus

boot COMPUTERS Initiation of an automatic routine in a computer that clears the random access memory (RAM), loads the operating system (eg DOS), and prepares the computer for use; a PC-type computer is booted at the time of it being turned on, or when restarted; the term boot originates from bootstrap, since the computer is pulling itself up by its bootstraps in a figurative sense (B Pfaffenberger, Computer User's Dictionary, Que Corporation, Indianapolis, 1993)

BOR Branchio-oto-renal syndrome, see there

borderline An adjectival expediency widely use in medicine for any condition that cannot be neatly placed in one of usually two categories, each of which has a distinct clinical significance, therapy and prognosis

borderline hypertension That range of systolic and diastolic blood pressures in which there is no unequivocal benefit obtained by therapy

borderline isolated systolic hypertension A distinct subtype of hypertension, defined as a systolic blood pressure between 140 and 159 mm Hg and a diastolic blood pressure below 90 mm Hg(US); BISH is the most common type of untreated hypertension in adults ≥ age 60; after 20 years of followup, 80% had progressed to definite hypertension (versus 45% of normotensives) and are at increased risk for developing cardiovascular disease (N Engl J Med 1993; 329:1912OA)

borderline leprosy Dimorphous leprosy The spectrum of leprosy is broad: in tuberculous leprosy, there are adequate host defenses resulting in reactive granulomatous disease with scattered large, sharply demarcated, hairless anesthetic plaques; lepromatous leprosy carries a relatively poor prognosis, in which there are multiple skin nodules filled with innumerable bacilli; between these two extremes are the borderline lesions, borderline tuberculous leprosy and borderline lepromatous leprosy

borderline malignancy Borderline tumor, see there

borderline personality PSYCHIATRY A personality disturbance that may be defined in terms of constitution, ie one that lies between a neurotic, who is capable of coping with his environment and a psychotic, who has lost contact with reality, or a person who is neither clear-cut schizophrenic nor non-schizophrenic; the borderline personality may be also be defined in adaptability, ie one who is not clearly beyond the reach of classical analytic techniques, but who responds poorly thereto, ie neither analyzable nor nonanalyzable

borderline personality disorder PSYCHIATRY A disorder of adult onset that is characterized by instability in interpersonal relationships, self-image, and affect, accompanied by impulsivity that occurs in various contexts; BPD is a 'Chinese menu' disease in the sense that it is defined by five or more criteria from a menu (see table, page 102)

borderline tumor SURGICAL PATHOLOGY A term of considerable use in evaluating neoplasms with many (but not all) of the histological criteria of malignancy, as the future behavior of these tumors cannot be reliably predicted; the borderline concept has currency in epithelial tumors of the ovary and stromal tumors of the uterus (see below); the Virchowian paradigm of morphological changes predicting the true nature of disease is problematic as some borderline lesions may evolve toward frank malignancy, while other morphologically identical lesions are stable or regress; the borderline dilemma is relatively common in

Borderline Personality Disorder

1) Frantic efforts to prevent real or imagined abandonment

2) A pattern of intense and unstable interpersonal relationships that swing between extremes of idealization and devaluation

3) Unstable self-image

4) Impulsivity in 2+ areas with self-destructive potential, eg binge eating, driving, gambling, sexual relations, substance abuse

5) Recurring suicidal or self-mutilating gestures or behaviors

6) Marked lability of moods and affect

7) Chronic feeling of 'emptiness'

8) Inappropriate anger and inability to control anger

9) Transient stress-related paranoid ideation or dissociative symptoms

Modified from Diagnostic and Statistical Manual of Mental Disorders, 4th ed, Washington, DC, American Psychiatric Association, 1994

the 'borderline tumor' or 'cystadenocarcinoma of low malignant potential' of the ovary, which has a behavior between an innocuous cystadenoma and a frankly malignant cystadenocarcinoma; these tumors may have serous, mucinous or endometrioid differentiation, and are characterized by complex oligocellular piling-up ('tufting') of the superficial cells Serous 'borderline' tumors comprise 15% of serous tumors (benign or malignant) of the ovary, ½ of which are unilateral; 20% are extraovarian; 5-year survival is 100%; 10-year survival is 75% versus 50% and 13% for malignant serous cystadenocarcinomas Mucinous 'borderline' tumors comprise 6-13% of all mucinous tumors of the ovary; 90% are unilateral; 10-year survival is 68% versus 34% for mucinous cystadenocarcinomas; endometrioid 'borderline' tumors are rare; other tumors of 'borderline' malignant potential affect 1) Epithelium, eg adenomatous hyperplasia of the endometrium with atypia, adenomatous colonic polyps with atypia 2) Mesenchymal cells, eg 'smooth muscle tumors of uncertain malignant potential' (STUMP), tumors that affect the uterus and the stomach; other mesenchymal tumors with 'borderline' behavior include epithelioid hemangioendothelioma and low-grade chondrosarcomas 3) Hematopoietic cells, eg pseudolymphomas, monoclonal gammopathies of uncertain significance, refractory anemia/myelofibrosis, lymphomatoid papulosis and cells of uncertain lineage, eg giant cell tumors of bone

Borg scale A system for scoring the perception of dyspnea, consisting of a linear scale ranking the degree of difficulty in breathing, ranging from 0 (none) to maximal (10) (N Engl J Med 1994; 330:1329oa)

Borna disease A viral encephalopathy of domestic horses and sheep that occurs in Central Europe, which is characterized by neurological disease in the form of behavioral disorders (aggression, eating disorders, hyperactivity, disrupted social and sexual activity)

Bornholm disease A coxsackievirus infection now preferably known as epidemic pleurodynia (see there) that was first described on the Danish island of Bornholm

boron therapy Boron neutron capture therapy RADIATION ONCOLOGY A form of radiotherapy in which a patient with a malignancy ingests a boron compound and then is exposed to a stream of neutrons from a nuclear reactor; the compound concentrates in the tumor, and itself becomes radioactive, delivering the highest radiation directly into the tumor; the 'first generation' of BT was in clinical trials from 1951 to 1960, but abandoned when it was held responsible for a number of deaths; the current BT uses a different boron compound that concentrates better in tumors and is the early clinical trial stage as a treatment for brain tumors (Science 1995; 267:956N&c)

Borrelia burgdorferi A spirochete that is the agent of Lyme disease; PCR (polymerase chain reaction) can be used on synovial fluid specimens to detect persistence of *B burgdorferi* (N Engl J Med 1994; 330:229oa)

borrowed servant An employee (eg a nurse) who is paid by one person or organization (eg a hospital) and who is temporarily employed by another person (eg a surgeon); in the usual medico-legal context, the temporary employer is responsible for the actions of the 'borrowed servant'; see Captain of the ship doctrine, Respondeat superior

borrowed servant doctrine MEDICAL MALPRACTICE A principle under which the party usually liable for a person's actions, eg the hospital being responsible for a nurse, is absolved of that responsibility when that person is asked to do something, eg by a surgeon, which is outside of the bounds of hospital policy; see 'Captain of the Ship' doctrine, Malpractice

Note: A hospital is only liable if the plaintiff can prove that the hospital was negligent in removing a physician or employee known to be incompetent

bossing Frontal bossing Rounded prominence of the frontal and parietal bones in an infant's cranial vault, due to various etiologies, including 1) Untreated vitamin D-induced rickets, causing a thickened outer table (alternately, Boxhead, Caput quadratum) with permanent enlargment of the head 2) Congenital anemia, eg thalassemia with massive hematopoiesis in an expanded marrow space, also known as 'hot cross bun skull' and 3) Others, including conditions associated with 'gargoyle' facies, acromesomelic dysplasia of Maroteaux, anhydrotic ectodermal dysplasia, craniometaphyseal dysplasia of Pyle, frontodigital syndrome, Kenney's tubular stenosis syndrome, nevoid-basal carcinoma syndrome, Taybi syndrome, thanatophoric dwarfism and, recently, AIDS embryopathy; see Hot-cross bun skull

Boston exanthem An exanthematous roseoliform salmon-colored maculo-papular face and chest rash caused by echovirus 16, preceded by a high 1-2 day fever which subsides with the onset of the rash; both last a week, more common in children in the late summer; epidemic or sporadic

the Boston Strangler see Serial killers

botanical medicine Herbal medicine, see there

botox Botulinum toxin, see there

bottleneck GENETICS A marked qualitative reduction in gene pool diversity due to low number of genetically distinct individuals in the population, ie a population bred from two individuals has far fewer variables on the allelic loci (a bottleneck) than a second population bred from hundreds of individuals; the variability of allelic loci in bottlenecks increases, a finding that is discordant with theoretical models; despite the presumed advantage to species survival of increased variability of genetic loci at such bottlenecks, inbred populations are less fit, having increased juvenile mortality; see Consanguinity, Inbreeding; Cf Biodiversity

bottom line A generic and highly colloquial term borrowed from accountancy for the final result of a complex process or ultimate conclusion (JAMA 1992; 268:3143)

botulinum toxin Any of several toxins produced by *Clostridium botulinum*, of which the 150-kD type A toxin has been purified and used to treat various neuromuscular junction diseases MECHANISM OF ACTION BT binds to presynaptic cholinergic nerve terminals; it is then internalized and inhibits exocytosis of acetylcholine, which is followed by sprouting of new terminals that re-innervate the muscle fibers; BT injection is effective for treating certain conditions characterized by skeletal muscle spasms, to wit, strabismus and various dystonias, eg blepharospasm, spasmodic torticollis, hemifacial spasm, tremors, task-specific dystonia and spasmodic dysphonia (a speech disorder with loss of voice, pitch breaks and hoarseness); injection of BT into the lower esophageal sphincter by endoscopy is reported to be a safe, effective, simple method for treating achalasia, the effects of which may last up to several months (**N Engl J Med 1995; 332:774OA**)

botulism A paralyzing disease caused by a potent toxin produced by *Clostridium botulinum* under anaerobic conditions, which is either foodborne or is acquired via wounds CLINICAL Progressive dizziness, blurred vision, slurred speech, dysphagia, nausea, decreased gag reflex TREATMENT Botulism antitoxin (**MMWR 1995; 44:200**)

boufée delirante A French term for a culture-bound symptom complex described in West Africa and Haiti characterized by an abrupt onset of agitated and aggressive behavior, confusion, and psychomotor excitement, which may be accompanied by auditory or visual hallucinations or paranoid ideation, which has features of a psychotic episode (from DSM-IV); see Culture-bound syndrome

bougienage A technique introduced 60 years ago for treatment of corrosive burns of the esophagus; following stabilization, an intraluminal silicon splint is left in place for 2-3 weeks, followed by daily bougienage, tapered to once every two days and finally once/week for many months; early bougienage increases complications

bound water Water of hydration, see there

boundary violation A reversal of roles in the relationship between a professional and his/her client, where the client becomes the caretaker; boundary violation dilemmas (BVDs) occur when a professional places his/her needs first in the relationship, twisting the ethics of providing care (**JAMA 1992; 268:3142**); BVDs are of critical concern in the doctor-patient relationship, and 'crossing the line' may result in sexual misconduct, see there

bouttonneuse fever Fièvre Bouttonneuse, see there

boutonniere deformity RHEUMATOLOGY Flexion of the proximal interphalangeal PIP joint and hyperextension of the DIP, caused by the detachment of the extensor tendon from the middle phalanx, volar displacement and resultant action as a flexor, associated with lupus erythematosus, Jaccoud's (post-rheumatic fever) arthritis, rheumatoid arthritis and camptodactyly; likened to a carnation secured in a lapel

bovarism PSYCHIATRY A condition with sexual overtones, that appears to most commonly affect older single women, in which the fantasized world overlaps and becomes confused in the patient's mind with the real world; the term derives from the principal character in Gustav Flaubert's Madame Bovary

bovine growth hormone Bovine somatotropin, see there

bovine somatotropin A 190-amino acid protein produced by the bovine pituitary gland that evokes somatic growth (partially mediated by insulin-like growth factor) and increased milk production, for which BST use in cows is approved by the FDA; recombinant or genetically engineered BST is regarded as completely safe and is distinct from 'beef growth hormone', an anabolic steroid used in the cattle industry, the safety of which is being seriously questioned (some countries are moving to ban importation of such meat); the bioengineered product was approved by the US FDA for use in boosting milk production in cows; there are some reports that some cows so treated may suffer reproductive losses, chronic mastitis and other chronic toxic effects (**JAMA 1991; 265:1391c, 1423**)

bovine spongiform encephalopathy A disease of cattle, popularly known as 'mad cow' disease for the presentation of the cows with high-stepping or staggering gait, anxiety, increased sensitivity and kicking while being milked, less commonly exhibiting frenzy and aggression; BSE was first described in the UK in cows fed with sheep offal and is a 'prion' disease and therefore similar to kuru and Creutzfeldt-Jakob disease in that there are prominent vacuolar (spongiform) lesions in the brain and disease-specific fibrils derived from the normal glycoprotein PrP and is related to transmissible mink encephalopathy, which similarly results from infected feed; the BSE brouhaha resulted in a British beef ban by the rest of the European community; see Prions

bowlegs Genu varum External deviation of the knee(s), a certain degree of which is normally present in infants and which corrects itself by 12-18 months, coinciding with bipedal ambulation; when the degree of bowing falls outside of a standardized curve, rickets must be considered as vitamin D-induced osteomalacia allows bending of the femoral shaft that bears the mechanical brunt of ambulatory kinetics; when combined with anterior curvature of the tibia and fibula, the children may have a 'saddle-sore' stance; anterior or antero-lateral bowing of the tibia may occur in neurofibromatosis as a prelude to fractures, which are commonly complicated by pseudoarthrosis

bowler hat sign GI RADIOLOGY Spreading of barium contrast material around an adenomatous or villotubular colonic polyp, at the base of which there is a recess between the stalk and the polyp 'body', forming the 'crown' of the bowler hat; the sign cannot differentiate between benign (leiomyomas, lipomas, 'garden variety' polyps) and malignant (leiomyosarcomas, lymphomas, metastatic melanomas), but merely signals their presence

bowel 'prep' A preoperative enema, often used in conjunction with prophylactic oral and parental antibiotics to purge the large intestine of food and feces prior to intestinal surgery; the most popular agent for preparing the large intestine for surgery is polyethylene glycol for mechanical cleansing; the remaining surgeons use conventional enemas, dietary restriction and cathartics

bowler's thumb SPORTS MEDICINE A nerve compression syndrome due to pressure of the ulnar and radial digital nerves of the thumb on the edge of the bowling ball's thumb hole CLINICAL Numbness, paresthesias, hypesthesia of skin distal to the nerve; BT may lead to perineural fibrosis and the formation of a painful nodule TREATMENT Rest, thumb guard, change grip, rounding off edge of hole in bowling ball; surgery is not indicated

bowel toxemia see Colon therapy

box MOLECULAR BIOLOGY A repeated oligonucleotide 'motif' that appears in multiple sites along the DNA and which functions as a signal for gene transcription or gene regulation; see Homeobox

boxcar An adjectival descriptor used for any periodically interrupted series of elongated objects with parallel lateral sides CARDIOVASCULAR PATHOLOGY Boxcar nuclei are typical of hypoxic myocytes, following ischemic insult of any kind FORENSIC MEDICINE Columns of intravascular blood interrupted by air in the small blood vessels and capillaries of the brains in scuba divers who died of air embolism due to rapid ascent and intravascular expansion of gases; see Caissons' disease MICROBIOLOGY 'Boxcar'-like organisms are arranged in long parallel chains of bacteria in an end-to-end arrangement, characteristic of *Clostridium perfringens* and *Bacillus anthracis* MYCOLOGY Arrangement of arthrospores of *Geotrichum* and *Trichosporon* species and *Coccidioides immitis* (alternating bands of pigmentation frequently cause rudimentary bodies arthroderma, described in *Fusarium solani* hyphae stained by safranin; *Geotrichum* species have a morphology of hockey sticks OPHTHALMOLOGY Boxcar pattern is seen in vascular stasis with segmentation of the venous column (of blood) in the retinal vein, a sequela of central retinal artery occlusion

boxer fracture A fracture of the fifth metacarpal neck following a direct blow impacting on the fifth metacarpal head with the fist clenched, causing dorsal angulation of the fracture line and volar displacement of the head

Boxgrove PALEOANTHROPOLOGY An archeological excavation site located in West Sussex, England that dates with reasonable certainty using the 'vole clock' (see there) the first human habitation of Europe (by *Homo* cf *heidelbergensis*) at 500 000 years ago, later than that suggested by data from Italy (730 000 years ago) and up to 2 million years ago (Czechoslovakia, France, Spain) (Nature 1994; 369:311; 275N&V)

box-head Bossing, see there

box jellyfish *Chironex fleckeri* and *Chiropsolmus quadrigatus* are lethal coelenterates, which have been held responsible for 74 documented deaths (countless unconfirmed), due to a high-molecular-weight dermatonecrotic venom, the nature of which is as yet unknown

boxing SPORTS MEDICINE A contact sport that causes major neuropsychological defects in its long-term practitioners when tested by the Wechsler and Bender Gestalt test, causing variable organic mental disease with impaired recent memory, dysarthria, nystagmus, computed tomographic evidence of cortical atrophy and a cavum septum pellucidum **ACUTE BOXING INJURIES** Cerebral edema, ischemia and (temporal or uncal) herniation; see 'Punchdrunk' syndrome

Note: The 'knock-out' punch causes generalized flaccidness, apnea, bradycardia, dilated pupils, unresponsiveness to light, rarely accompanied by a seizure; recovery occurs within 30-60 seconds; MRI is better able than CT in evaluating boxing injuries as it excels in detecting hematomas, white lesions, ie atrophy, contusion, and early hydrocephaly

---

BOXING: MECHANISMS OF NEUROLOGICAL SEQUELAE

ROTATIONAL (ANGULAR) ACCELERATION Subdural hematomas, intracerebral hemorrhage and diffuse axonal injury (rupture of individual axons)

LINEAR ACCELERATION Focal ischemia and retinal detachment

CAROTID INJURY Potential dissection of arteries, thrombosis or initiation of hypotensive or bradycardic reflexes

IMPACT DECELERATION Hitting the mats or ropes results in 'contrecoup' injuries and subdural hemorrhage

---

B protein A 25-kDal protein contained within snRNPs (small ribonuceloprotein particles); the variability of this and other (A and C) proteins may explain the differential splicing and polyadenylation as variations in pre-mRNA processing machinery

brachytherapy A modality of radiation therapy in which implanted beads or seeds containing iridium-192, radium-226 and other radioisotopes are used to treat certain carcinomas with high amounts of local radiation, eg as in invasive carcinoma of the uterine cervix

brady-tachy syndrome see Sick sinus syndrome

brain bank Any of a limited number of repositories (in the US and in the UK) of formalin-fixed or frozen brains and/or other brain tissue, which can be used for research on Alzheimer's disease, bipolar disorder, dystonia, HIV infection, Huntington's disease, multiple sclerosis, Parkinson's disease, schizophrenia, seizure disorder(s), SIDS, Tourette syndrome, and others (Science 1995; 267:1764; MT Today 1995; 5/6:5) see Transesophageal echocardiography

brain-bone-fat syndrome An AD condition with progressive neurologic disease leading to death, accompanied by developmental cysts on acral parts and bones PATHOLOGY Narrowed cerebral blood vessels, gliosis, calcified basal ganglia, demyelinization and senile plaque formation

brain dead *adjective* Pertaining or referring to the complete loss of brain activity above the medulla

brain death see Multiorgan donation

brain-derived growth factor see BDGF

'brain drain' A colloquialism for the migration of highly trained and/or skilled workers, especially physicians and scientists from underdeveloped countries to countries offering better working conditions and/or life styles Note: While the USA has been a favored mecca for drained brains, there is increasing emigration to Europe and Japan, as the US budget deficit reduces the funding of innovative research

brain fag An idiom for a symptom complex described in former British colonies of West Africa that affects secondary school and university students whose brains are 'fatigued' from the stresses and challenges of formal and regimented study; is relatively nonspecific and characterized by loss of concentration, memory, and 'focus', accompanied by tightness in the chest, and blurring of vision (from DSM-IV); see Culture-bound syndrome

Brain fag is not confined to any culture and has been experienced in some form by virtually anyone who has undergone the rigors of education-Author's note

brain-graft surgery A neurosurgical procedure for treating Parkinson's disease, in which chromaffin adrenal cells are transplanted into the caudate nucleus; the early Swedish cases were discouraging, but in the animal model, the MPTP-treated monkey, promising results were reported by grafting fetal substantia nigra into the caudate; the success reported by the Mexican team in 1987 has not been reproduced elsewhere and the neurosurgical community has taken a 'wait-and-see' policy; of one small series, one patient had significant improvement, ½ of the remainder required less levodopa and dopaminic agonists TECHNIQUE Implantation of fetal mesencephalic cells unilaterally into the putamen of one patient, resulting in focal dopamine production, replacing that missing in parkinsonism, verified by PET scanning; clinical improvement was most marked contralateral to the implantation side, evidence of a positive benefit from the surgery

brain-heart infusion agar MICROBIOLOGY An agar used for the primary recovery of fungi from clinical specimens, eg *Actinomyces* spp, *Cryptococcus neoformans*

brain oscillation NEUROPHYSIOLOGY A wave of neuronal excitation ('firing') that is sustained either by (according to Hebb and others) reverberation of electrical activity in neuronal loops or (proposed more recently) based on activity-dependent increase in membrane excitability; BOs may correspond to a timing mechanism for controlling the serial processing of short-term memories (Science 1995; 267:1512OA)

brainstem The central axis of the 'lower' functional components of the CNS which includes the medulla oblongata, pons, midbrain, and for some, also the diencephalon

brainwashing A generic term for any psychologic technique used to change, and ultimately control the mind of another person, who is usually held against his/her free will

Brainerd diarrhea An epidemic of diarrhea in Minnesota that immortalized a town and immobilized its populace, beginning in 1984; BD is presumed to have been due to an infectious agent, although none was identified; 2-3 weeks after ingestion of raw milk from one of the local dairies in this community of 14 000, 8% of those exposed had diarrhea which slowly improved with time

'brake' drugs SPORTS MEDICINE Steroid hormones used by female athletes to delay body growth and minimize body fat, thereby preventing the center of gravity from shifting, giving them a competitive 'edge', allowing a 15- to 18-year-old to compete as a prepubertal gymnast; medroxyprogesterone (estrogen) and cyproterone (antiestrogen) delay puberty by suppressing ovulation and menstruation SIDE EFFECTS Premature closure of the epiphyseal plate, resulting in short stature as adults

bran A product derived from grain that contains a water-soluble fiber with a high content of β-glycan, a substance which, by an unknown mechanism, reduces LDL-cholesterol by 5-15% (JAMA 1991; 265:1833) Note: Rice bran may be more effective in reducing cholesterol than oat bran as it may be defatted, further reducing cholesterol by 25%; see Dietary fiber

branched chain amino acids Valine, leucine, isoleucine The amino acids that accumulate in maple syrup urine disease, which is due to a deficit in oxidative decarboxylation of the keto-acid derivatives of these amino acids

branched chain ketonuria see Maple syrup urine disease

brancher deficiency Glycogen storage disease IV, see there

branchial cleft cyst A cyst that arise from one of the branchial clefts, usually the second, which most commonly presents as an asymptomatic fluctuant mass posteroinferior to the angle of the jaw

branching enzyme A generic term for an enzyme that catalyzes the addition of branches and side chains to a polymer; the term usually refers to amylo-1,4 →1,6 transglucosidase [EC 2.4.1.18], which packs sugar molecules onto starch, the enzyme that is defective in type IV glycogen storage disease, Cf Debranching enyme

branching snowflake test A crude but useful bedside test using a glass microscopic slide for differentiating amniotic fluid (positive) from maternal urine (negative), based on the radiating 'fern-like' pattern of amniotic fluid

branchio-oto-renal syndrome An AD [MIM 113650] condition characterized by mixed hearing loss accompanied by a Mondini-type cochlear malformation, bilateral renal dysplasia with abnormalities of the collecting ducts, and bilateral branchial clefts and/or cysts; the defect has been tentatively linked to breakpoint mutations on chromosome segment 8q

brassy cough A descriptor for the non-productive 'metallic' cough heard in children with acute bacterial or viral laryngotracheitis, often accompanied by inspiratory stridor and respiratory distress; Cf Whooping cough

BRAT diet Bananas, rice, apples, toast A bland diet prescribed for viral gastroenteritis that, with water, replenishes liquids and electrolytes lost in pediatric diarrhea; other foods appropriate for diarrhea include plain chicken, crackers and potatoes

Brat, noun A spoiled, tedious, ill-mannered child

Bravo The code-name for an atmospheric nuclear test in which a 15-megaton thermonuclear device was detonated on March 1, 1954 on the Bikini Atoll of the northern Marshall Islands; in Bravo, most of the 253 inhabitants of the Rongelap and Utrik Atolls suffered from acute radiation sickness and many later developed neoplasia of the thyroid in the form of nodules or carcinoma, due to exposure to β radiation from radioiodines; Cf Smoky

brawny edema Cutaneous changes characteristic of chronic venous insufficiency with thickening, induration, liposclerosis and non-pitting edema; the brawny color is due to hemosiderin from lysed erythrocytes; with chronic ischemia, the skin undergoes atrophy, necrosis and stasis ulceration, surrounded by a rim of dry, scaling and pruritic skin

BRCA1 MOLECULAR PATHOLOGY A very large gene with exons spread over 100 000 base pair of genomic DNA; the BRCA1 mRNA is 7.8 kb in length; the BRCA1 protein sequence contains a zinc-finger motif that is often found in transcription factors, but otherwise appears to be unrelated to previously described proteins (N Engl J Med 1994;

331:1523sa); candidate gene for hereditary breast cancer, which represents 5% of all breast cancers; ♀ who carry the gene have an 85% chance of developing breast cancer before age 65 (New York Times 16 July 1994; C1); the patent for commercial products derived from BRCA1 is jointly held by the U of Utah, NIH, and Myriad Genetics, Inc (JAMA 1995; 273:833MN&P)

breach FORENSIC MEDICINE An infraction or violation of the law, which is either intentional (an act of comission) or unintentional (an act of omission, often the same as negligence); see Malpractice, Negligence, Standard of care

breach of contract Abandonment, see there

'bread and butter' disease A catch-phrase for routine maladies treated by each specialty that comprise a large part of the physician's work-load and present little intellectual challenge; 'bread and butter' surgical pathology includes routine specimens, eg hernia sacs, gall bladders, appendices, cataracts and tonsils

bread and butter lesion CARDIAC PATHOLOGY Diffuse fibrinous and serofibrinous 'stringy' adhesions or plaque-like thickening on the chronically inflamed pericardium of rheumatic heart disease; similar lesions occur in connective tissue disease, eg SLE, viral pericarditis, post-acute MI, neoplasia, uremia, trauma, radiation and fusobacterium infection; the end-result may be restrictive pericardial fibrosis, which compromises the inflow of blood to the ventricle

bread crumb appearance MICROBIOLOGY A descriptor for the gross morphology of cultures of *Blastomyces dermatitidis* grown at 37°C, *Streptomyces madurae*, *Fusobacterium nucleatum* and *M tuberculosis*, which have been fancifully likened to broken pieces of French or Italian bread OPHTHALMOLOGY see Granular dystrophy

breakage syndromes GENETICS A group of autosomal recessive disorders characterized by congenital chromosomal breaks and rearrangements that increase the risk for malignancy, including Bloom and Fanconi syndromes, ataxia-telangiectasia and xeroderma pigmentosum; Cf Fragile X

Note: Acquired diseases may also have chromosomal breakages, structural rearrangement and aneuploidy caused by viral infections, eg chickenpox, hepatitis, measles and malignancy, often lymphoproliferative, with translocations that juxtapose oncogenes with functional genes, encoding hybrid proteins that 'drive' expansions and leaving the cells locked in a 'turned-on' position, eg AML t(8;21) and CML t(9;22)

breakeven analysis LABORATORY MEDICINE A method used to evaluate the cost-effectiveness of purchasing a new piece of equipment or 'buying into' a new technology; BA demonstrates the relationship between fixed costs (F) and variable costs (V), number of tests (Q) and profit; determination of the breakeven point (Q_{BE}) provides the number of tests needed to achieve profitability, ie to 'break even' (Advance/Laboratory July/August 1994) Cf Replacement analysis

$$Q_{BE} = F/(P - V)$$

'breaking' EMERGENCY MEDICINE A maneuver used in drowning and near-drowning victims to clear the pharynx of water and vomitus; the victim is turned prone (on his/her stomach), the hands of the person rendering cardiopulmonary resuscitation are locked together under the abdomen, and the fluid-filled body is lifted to expel the water and gas; Cf Flake maneuver, Heimlich maneuver

breakthrough INFECTIOUS DISEASE A positive blood culture for an infectious agent after adequate therapy, eg 72 hours for *Candida krusei* after fluconazole therapy (N Engl J Med 1992; 327:644c)

breakthrough bleeding GYNECOLOGY A nebulous term applied to various types of gynecologic bleeding, usually referring to mid-cycle bleeding in oral contraceptive users, thought to be the result of insufficient estrogenic stimulation; the term is not applicable to abnormal bleeding in oral contraceptive users

'breakthrough organism' Progenote, see there

breast augmentation see Breast implants

breast conservation therapy ONCOLOGY A generic term for any therapy of breast cancer in which the minimum possible amount of tissue is removed at the time of excising the tumor Stage I and II breast cancer treated with breast conserving therapy (lumpectomy, axillary node dissection, and irradiation) and modified radical mastectomy offer similar results at 10 years of followup (N Engl J Med 1995; 332:907OA) see Breast reconstruction

breast feeding Reduces risk of subsequent cancer of the breast; lactation and breast feeding (≥ 6 months) before age 20 is associated with a relative risk of 0.54 (N Engl J Med 1994; 330:81OA)

breast implant An inert sac filled with silicone, some of which are covered by polyurethane foam, used to augment cosmetically the female contour; with time, the implants covered by polyurethane (composed of long chains of isocyanate monomers joined together in ester linkages), are hydrolyzed in vivo, yielding various breakdown products (eg toluene 2,4-diisocyanate, and toluene 2,6-diisocyanate diamines) from the polyurethane sponge covering the implants which were thought to have carcinogenic potential in humans, as these products are known to cause sarcomas in rats; the relationship of BIs with breast cancer is uncertain, and probably close to 'unity' (N Engl J Med 1995; 332:1535OA); an expert panel of the Canadian Medical Association concluded that 'surgical removal of polyurethane-foam-covered breast implants solely for reasons of potential risk of cancer is not indicated' (N Engl J Med 1992; 326:1649OA, 1695ED, 1696ED) STATISTICS 1-2 million US women had breast implants since the early 1960s, when the silicone gel-filled elastomer envelope-type breast prosthesis was introduced until the moratorium placed in January 1992 by the US FDA on breast implants pending further evaluation of safety (see DA Kessler, N Engl J Med 1992; 326:1713OA); implantation was performed for either cosmetic reasons (ie augmentation) or for post-mastectomy recostruction; breast implants may not be associated with an ↑ incidence of connective-tissue diseases (see there) or other diseases including autoimmune disorders, eg Hashimoto's thyroiditis or primary biliary cirrhosis, sarcoidosis, or cancer (N Engl J Med 1994; 330:1697OA) PATHOLOGY Fibrous scarring, with dense collagen, fibroblasts, macrophages, giant cells, lymphocytes and plasma cells (Arch Pathol Lab Med 1994; 118:686OA); asymptomatic rupture is estimated (by manufacturers) to occur in 0.2-1.1%; preliminary findings presented at the FDA's advisory panel (February, 1992) suggested that 4-6% had ruptured; rupture may be detected by ultrasound mammography (N Engl J Med 1993; 328:733C), as well as by X-ray mammography; see Biomaterials, Silicone

breast (cancer) markers Any of a number of antigens variably present in breast tissue that may be of use in either differentiating between benign or malignant lesions of the breast, or in identifying the breast as the site of origin in tumor metastases; breast markers include estrogen receptor, zinc-α_2-glycoprotein, GCDFP-15 (gross cystic disease fluid protein 15), casein, α-lactalbumin, lactoferrin, B73.2, TAG-12, MAM-6, MCA b-12, MMTV-related antigens (Arch Pathol Lab Med 1992; 116:1181OA)

breast milk NEONATOLOGY Human milk is similar to cow milk in the water content (88%, specific gravity, 1.030), fat content (3.5%), energy value (0.67 kcal/ml), and type of sugar (lactose); mom's milk has less protein (1.0-1.5% vs. 3.3% cow's milk, the latter due to a 6-fold increase in casein), more carbohydrate (6.5-7.0% vs 4.5%), less min-

erals and different vitamins (more vitamins C and D, less thiamine and riboflavin and equivalent amounts of vitamins A and B and niacin); maternal milk is usually sterile, provides IgA and is more easily digestible, as reflected in rapid transit time; breast-fed infants have a better response to vaccines than formula-fed infants; BM also contains bradykinin, epidermal growth factor, gonadotropin-releasing hormone, insulin-like growth factor, melatonin, mammotropic growth factor, nerve growth factor, oxytocin; it is considered unethical to feed children anything but human milk in Sweden, where there are banks of human milk for those cannot breast-feed (New York Times May 24, 1994; C1) Cf Necrotizing enterocolitis, White beverages

breast pump A tubular mechanical device that provides gentle suction, allowing extraction of milk, used when the breasts are engorged or when direct infant feeding is not possible for various physical (eg prematurity) or logistic (eg mommy has to work) reasons

breast reconstruction SURGICAL ONCOLOGY A generic term for any surgical revision of the anterior chest wall following mastectomy for breast cancer, which may be performed at the time of the initial therapy or as a second procedure; BR should be offered to any ♀ who is not a candidate for or does not wish breast-conserving surgery with radiation therapy; immediate BR avoids a second procedure, minimizes the psychological trauma, and helps coordinate the therapeutic team; BR is a function of available donor skin, the ♀ expectations, and the size and shape of the contralateral breast

breast self-examination The periodic palpation by a ♀ of her own breast, which is intended to detect new growths; although there is little evidence of the effectiveness of BSE (VT DeVita, Jr, S Hellman, SA Rosenberg, Cancer, The Principles and Practice of Oncology, JB Lippincott, Philadelphia, 1993), it is the only means by which neoplasms can be detected between examinations by health care personnel; data suggest that BSE results in an ↑ the incidence of cancer, and possibly and overall ↓ in mortality

'breathing' BIOCHEMISTRY A local unfolding of a polypeptide to allow the exchange of one isotopic molecule for another MOLECULAR BIOLOGY A local unwinding of the DNA double helix to allow formation of transcription bubbles; alternately, the 'chaotic' transient rupture and reforming of interchain hydrogen bonds that facilitates the interaction with the regulatory DNA-binding proteins; Cf Premelting

breath test Any of a number of clinical tests used to evaluate malabsorption, in which a food containing a substance emitting low levels of radioactivity is ingested and, if malabsorbed, is exhaled through the lungs; BTs include the ^{2}H-lactose test‡, for detecting lactase deficiency, and the ^{14}C-xylose test‡ for general malabsorption

breech position OBSTETRICS Buttocks presentation at the time of delivery, a position that carries a 3-6-fold increased mortality due to complications, including umbilical cord prolapse, tentorial tearing, and cerebral hemorrhage of the after-coming head; in the US breeches are usually delivered by cesarean section; TYPES OF BREECH: FRANK BREECH Thighs are flexed over the abdomen and the legs extended COMPLETE BREECH legs are flexed on the thighs and the fetus sits like Buddha INCOMPLETE BREECH: SINGLE OR DOUBLE FOOTLING One or both feet are the presenting parts

bremsstrahlung German, braking radiation A broad spectrum (rather than an energy peak) of electromagnetic radiation that is generated by the rapid deceleration of a photon or electron when it hits the electron cloud of the atomic nucleus; most X-rays generate a significant amount of bremsstrahlung, which deeply penetrates organic tissues, as these are formed of molecules with low atomic weights

brick Inclusion body VIROLOGY US military slang for a crystalloid structure corresponding to packed viral particles present within host cells

brick dust appearance LABORATORY MEDICINE Granular red-brown crystalline material corresponding to amorphous urates seen in a normal acid urine, composed of calcium urate, magnesium urate, sodium and potassium urates which crystallize when the urine is acidified

brick-red sputum A thickened mixture of blood, bacteria, necrotic lung tissue and mucus, characteristic of *Klebsiella pneumonia*

bridge TRANSPLANTATION SURGERY A generic term for any organ or surrogate device used to stabilize a patient prior to definitive transplantation; organ bridges may be synthetic, eg the now abandoned Jarvik-7, an artifical heart of historic interest or nonhuman, eg pig liver (**N Engl J Med 1994; 331:234OA**) or an organ surrogate (eg hemodialysis prior to kidney transplantation)

bridging CARDIOLOGY A designation for systolic narrowing of the left anterior descending coronary artery seen by angiography as an isolated finding during cardiac catheterization or in patients with coronary artery disease, left ventricular hypertrophy or hypertrophic cardiomyopathy; Cf Rat-tail, Sawfish patterns TRAUMATOLOGY The 'spanning' of breaks in the skin by blood vessels, seen after a blunt object strikes tightened skin, rupturing the epidermis and dermis whilst the blood vessels (being more mobile) remain intact, 'bridging' the gap

bridging fibrosis HEPATOPATHOLOGY The loose spanning of hepatic lobules by broad bands of fibrous tissue and collagen, seen by light microscopy in the healing phase of cirrhosis

bridging necrosis HEPATOPATHOLOGY A finding seen by low-power light microscopy, consisting in spanning of hepatic vessels by confluent necrosis, linking portal tracts to centrilobular veins and to each other; the 'bridge' is necrotic, with broad bands of apoptotic hepatocytes and fibrotic condensation of 'stroma'; presence of bridging necrosis is considered to be the only reliable criterion for establishing the diagnosis of chronic active hepatitis, a disease which may evolve to cirrhosis or be a precursor of hepatocellular carcinoma

Brief Pain Inventory A brief, relatively simple, self-administered questionnaire for evaluating pain, which addresses the relevant aspects of pain (history, intensity, timing, location, and quality) and the pain's ability to interfere with the patient's activities; in the BPI, the patient locates the pain by shading in on a diagram, and rates the pain on a scale of 0 (no pain) to 10 (worst imaginable pain), including details as to their ability to function when in pain; the BPI has been translated into several languages and appears to be valid in diverse cultural and linguistic settings (see **N Engl J Med 1994; 330:592OA**) see Pain

bright plaque An optical fundoscopic finding consisting of a light-reflecting fragment of atherosclerotic plaque lodged in a retinal arteriole that may be associated with amaurosis fugax

brilliant cresyl blue A high pH histological dye with affinity for nucleic acids used to delineate platelets, immature red cells and Heinz bodies

brilliant green agar MICROBIOLOGY An agar used for the isolation of *Salmonella* spp other than *S typhi*

brim Thickening of the iliopectineal line in the pelvic bone, a radiologic finding suggestive of Paget's disease of the bone that may also be seen in osteoporosis and osteoblastic metastases

bris *pron* Briss The traditional religious rite (commonly

written as Brith Milah) of circumcision as practiced by Jews; it is performed by on the eighth day of life, not by a physician, but rather by a mohel (*pron* moyel) see Circumcision

Note: The word bris (aka brith) translates from Hebrew as covenant (**L Rosten, The Joys of Yiddish , 1968**)

British anti-Lewisite Dimercaprol 2,3-dimercaptopropanol A sulfhydryl compound that was developed in World War II as an antidote to the vesicant arsenical war gas, which may be used as a therapeutic chelator for arsenic and mercury

British fetal hemoglobin A congenital hemoglobinopathy due to a regulatory defect in postnatal γ chain synthesis; 20% of the hemoglobin in homozygotes and 3.5-10% in heterozygotes is hemoglobin F, which is of clinical importance as it may mimic massive feto-maternal hemorrhage and thereby possible overdosage of Rh immune globulin

brittle bones Bones with increased osseous fragility, a phenomenon seen in osteogenesis imperfecta, caused by various genetic defects, eg point mutation in collagen, type I

brittle cornea syndrome An uncommon disease reported among Tunisian Jews, which is characterized by red hair, blue sclera and brittle corneas with spontaneous perforation

brittle diabetes IDDM in which the blood glucose fluctuates widely, swinging rapidly from the hypoglycemia to hyperglycemia despite frequent 'titration' of the insulin dose

brittle hair syndrome Trichothiodystrophy A condition characterized by brittle, sulfur-poor hair, mental and physical retardation, onychodystrophy and ichthyotic skin, which is caused by an inherited defect in the 'excision repair' pathway; see Excision repair syndromes, Xeroderma pigmentosum; Cf Kinky hair syndrome

'brittle & shallow' A descriptor for the sleep of the elderly who are easily aroused (brittle) and do not fall into a deep sleep (shallow); see REM, Sleep disorders

BRM see Biological response modifiers

broadcast storm COMPUTERS A generic term for a network-wide failure that is usually hardware-related, less often software-related

Broadcast storms on Ethernet may be caused by 'rogue' devices known as screamers that talk at high rates, not allowing the other devices to get a 'word in edgewise' (see **CAP Today November 1993**)

Broad Street pump A pump used to draw drinking water from the Thames in the London cholera epidemic in 1855; Dr John Snow painstaking tracked down the cases of cholera and found that evidence pointed to the BS pump , which drew its water downstream from sewage; JS frustrated by the BS bureaucrats, himself removed BS handle, and virtually eliminated the cholera; to 'remove the Broad Street pump handle' is therefore to identify a cause and take action for the common good (**N Engl J Med 1993; 329:1807ED**)

broken ring sign A finding by magnetic resonance imaging (that consists in disruption of the lateral wall of the superior vena caval 'ring', seen in anomalous pulmonary venous connection to the superior vena cava

broken straw sign SURGICAL PATHOLOGY Bent, elongated, eosinophilic cells with occasional cross-striations seen by light microscopy in embryonal rhabdomyosarcoma

brominated vegetable oil A food additive that is used as an emulsifier in some foods, and as a clouding agent in some soft drinks, which is alleged to be extremely dangerous by alternative health care advocates; see Alternative medicine

Brompton mixture An oral analgesic 'cocktail' of morphine, cocaine, chloroform water, alcohol and flavored syrup first formulated at the Brompton Chest Hospital;

'Brompton mixture' is currently is a generic term for an alcoholic solution containing an opioid (heroin or morphine) and either cocaine and/or a phenothiazine and is used to treat the pain of terminal cancer

'bronch' A highly colloquial verb for performing bronchoscopy, as in 'to bronch' (pronounced bronk) a patient

bronchial hyperresponsiveness A exaggerated bronchial constriction* of unknown pathogenesis that occurs in response to various nonspecific provocative stimuli, a finding that is so characteristic of asthma that it is virtually part of the case definition of asthma; BH is demonstrable by inhalation of various pharmacologic bronchoconstrictors, but also occurs with various 'physical' challenges in the form of exercise, dry or cold air, hypertonic or hypotonic aerosol
*Synonyms include bronchial hyperactivity, bronchial hyperexcitability, bronchial hypersensitivity

bronchiole-associated lymphoid tissue BALT The lymphoid tissues of the hilar region and that surrounding the bronchioles, which is associated with production of IgA specific for inhaled antgens; see Gut-, Mucosa-, and Skin-associated lymphoid tissue

bronchopulmonary dysplasia A chronic lung disease affecting circa 7000 premature infants/year (US) treated for respiratory distress syndrome with supplemental oxygen and mechanical ventilation; the diagnosis is clinical and is made at one month of age in premature infants who have undergone mechanical ventilation for $\geq$ one week, who have symptoms of persistent respiratory distress, who are dependent on supplemental oxygen and who have rounded radiolucencies on a plain film of the chest LABORATORY $\uparrow\uparrow$ Leukotrienes C_4, D_4, and E_4 in lavage fluid PATHOLOGY 40% of the infants die and microscopy of the lungs reveals necrotizing bronchiolitis, alveolar fibrosis, emphysema and arterial changes of pulmonary hypertension PROGNOSIS Those who survive infancy have pulmonary dysfunction in later life, in the form of airway obstruction, airway hyperreactivity and hyperinflation

bronchopulmonary sequestration An uncommon congenital condition related to developmental abnormalities of the embryonic foregut, in which nonfunctioning pulmonary tissue is detached from the normal lung, and does not communicate with the bronchopulmonary tree; sequestered lung tissue is supplied by an anomalous systemic artery, usually arising from the aorta or one of its tributaries and contains normal elements in a disorderly array with variable amounts of cartilage, alveolar parenchyma and bronchial glands, the secretion from which leads to the formation of fluid-filled cysts; communication with functional pulmonary tissue accounts for the not uncommon development of bacterial infections; although there is considerable overlap, BSs are subdivided into

1) Intralobar bronchopulmonary sequestration 85% of cases, bilateral, usually supplied by a branch of the thoracic aorta and

2) Extralobar bronchopulmonary sequestration More common in ♂, associated with other congenital abnormalities, may communicate with the foregut; 90% are left sided (N Engl J Med 1993; 329:1873CPC) Cf Pseudosequestration

bronze baby syndrome A complication of phototherapy (used for infants with clinical jaundice and indirect hyperbilirubinemia), which is characterized by dark gray-brown skin discoloration that may persist for many months, significant elevation of direct bilirubin, mixed hyperbilirubinemia and evidence of obstructive liver disease; other complications of phototherapy include rashes, overheating, overcooling, and dehydration

bronze diabetes A clinically (but not pathologically) distinct form of diabetes mellitus that occurs in association with hemochromatosis, in which there are yellow-red hemosiderin deposits in the skin

Brookhaven Protein Data Base '*The PDB archives the experimental findings describing protein structures to atomic resolution, the 3D structures of more than 3000 proteins, nucleic acids, and other biological macromolecules. Each one of these data entries is an annotated ASCII text file...average size of a typical entry is over 4000 lines or 300 kb, and the entire database...is doubling in size every two years.*' (Nature 1995; 374:572PRV)

Brotherton v Cleveland FORENSIC MEDICINE A case (923 F2d 477 (6th Cir 1991)) tried in Ohio that challenged certain aspects of the Uniform Anatomical Gift Act, a legislative act that has been instrumental in increasing organ procurement; S Brotherton died in an automobile accident, was pronounced DOA at the local hospital, and his body was transported to the coroner's (medical examiner's) office where an autopsy was performed, and the decedent's corneas removed*; Brotherton's wife had (at the hospital) denied authorization for an anatomical gift and subsequently filed suit in federal court against the related parties, as she had 'property interests' in her husband's corneas; the ***Brotherton*** decision is regarded as a setback in efforts to expand the number of organs available for transplantation (CAP Today March 1992); see Cadaveric organ, Organ procurement, Uniform Anatomical Gift Act
*Under Ohio state law, a coroner performing an autopsy may remove the corneas from a decedent if the coroner 'has no knowledge of an objection to the removal'

brown adipose tissue Brown fat, see there

brown atrophy ANATOMIC PATHOLOGY A brownish pigmentation due to the accumulation of lipofuscin in certain organs (eg heart, liver, and others), which may occur in the organs of older subjects; the organs are smaller and flabby; by light microscopy there is extensive accumulation of lipofuscin ('aging' pigment)

brown bowel syndrome Melanosis coli, see there

Brown-Brenn stain A variant of the gram stain used to identify bacteria in histological section

brown fat Brown adipose tissue A special form of mesenchymal tissue that generates heat by nonshivering thermogenesis, so designated as it is rich in mitochondria, which imparts a brown hue; BF is rich in sympathetic nerve endings and vessels and its metabolic activity and development is regulated by norepinephrine, and it is normally located in the axillary, subscapular, and interscapular regions, along the large thoracoabdominal vessels, and around the heart, kidneys and adrenal glands; BF is $\uparrow$ Chagas' disease, CHF, Duchenne's muscular dystrophy, malignancy, pheochromocytoma, SIDS, and in malnutrition (Arch Pathol Lab Med 1992; 116:1152OA); although human adults essentially lack this 'superfat', thermogenesis from BF is crucial to infant survival as well as hibernating animals; in brown fat mitochondria, an inner-membrane protein acts as a natural uncoupler of oxidative phosphorylation, causing transmembrane transportation of H^+, short-circuiting the membrane's usual proton gradient, directly converting the energy released by NADH into heat; the glucose utilization index in brown fat is a function of the amount of available food (Biochemistry 1991; 273:233)

brown gallstone A type of gallstone that is most common in Asians and composed of calcium salts of unconjugated bilirubin with varying amounts of protein and cholesterol; BGs commonly arise in the bile ducts, often associated with infection MECHANISM Bacteria in the biliary system release β-glucuronidases, which hydrolyze glucuronic acid from conjugated bilirubin; the resulting unconjugated bilirubin precipitates as its calcium salt and may be associated with decreased IgA in the bile (see N Engl J Med 1993; 328:412OA) see Gallstone; Cf Black gallstone

brown heroin SUBSTANCE ABUSE A contaminated form of heroin imported from Mexico in 1974 that was linked to folliculitis and subcutaneous nodules, noninfectious musculoskeletal hypersensitivity, fever, paraspinal myalgias, arthralgias, periarticular tenderness; the color was due to 'additives', including procaine and opium-processing contaminants (noscapine, papaverine) imparting a brown tinge and a viscid consistency to the heroin SIDE EFFECTS Hypergammaglobulinemia, biological false positive serological reaction for syphilis

brown induration Chronic passive pulmonary congestion A gross finding in any chronic condition with long-standing transalveolar leakage of blood, often accompanied by increased pulmonary venous pressure ETIOLOGY CHF, Goodpasture's disease, hemosiderosis, mechanical obstruction of pulmonary vein, mitral valve stenosis PATHOGENESIS Chronic hemorrhage and edema within thickened alveolar walls results in fibrotic induration accompanied by brawny discoloration of the soggy lungs

brown oculocutaneous albinism An autosomal defect in pigment production seen in Africa and New Guinea characterized by hyperkeratosis, photophobia, pachydermia and a relatively low amount of pigment

brown lung disease see Byssinosis

brown journal A colloquialism of uncertain utility for the American Journal of Kidney Disease

Brown-Pearce tumor A transplantable anaplastic carcinoma originating in a syphilitic scar in the rabbit scrotum; the tumor metastasizes to spermatic cord and the peritoneum

Brown-Sequard syndrome A clinical complex characterized by hemiparaplegia caused by hemilateral compression or destruction of the spinal cord associated with ipsilateral (homolateral) motor paralysis, loss of vibratory, joint and tendon sensation and diminished tactile discrimination with contralateral anesthesia and loss of temperature sensation; the syndrome occurs with traumatic spinal cord injuries, tumors, as a complication of spinal irradiation or herpes zoster

brown spider *Loxosceles reclusa* and *L laeta* are secretive spiders that seek secluded sites and bite when bothered LOCAL SYMPTOMS Cyanosis, necrosis, pustule or bullae, rimmed by ischemia and erythema expanding to 20 cm over weeks and months SYSTEMIC SYMPTOMS Fever, chills, nausea, vomiting, dizziness, myalgia, arthralgia and potentially fatal intravascular hemolysis with hemoglobulinuria and acute renal failure

'brown stains' SURGICAL PATHOLOGY A colloquial term for immunoperoxidase (special) stains, which are used to detect antigens, eg leukocyte common antigen, cytokeratin(s), S-100, in tissues by linking monoclonal antibodies raised against the antigen(s) of interest to an enzyme in the last of several antigen-antibody linking steps; if the antigen X is present, the enzyme digests a colorless substrate into a a brown pigmented product

brown stool The normal fecal color is due to the content of mesobilifuscin dipyrrole, a byproduct of heme synthesis which does not react as either bilirubin or blood

Brown-Symmers disease Acute fulminant, often postviral encephalitis in children, accompanied by fever, vomiting, irritability, eventuating in bulbar and cerebral disturbances with respiratory difficulties, strabismus, nystagmus, hemiplegia; the condition may be fatal within days

Brown syndrome Neural crest syndrome NEUROLOGY Congenital analgesia with neurogenic anhidrosis, loss of deep and superficial pain sensation, dental dysplasia, meningeal thickening with cystic degeneration, hyperreflexia, mild mental retardation LABORATORY Abnormal homovanillic acid and vanilmandellic acid assays OPHTHALMOLOGY Restriction or loss of ability to elevate the eye in adduction, often associated with down-turning of the affected eye, a compensatory tilt of the head associated with congenital fibrosis and shortening of the anterior sheath of the superior oblique tendon sheath of the trochlear muscle ETIOLOGY Idiopathic or associated with inflammation, possibly related to forceps delivery TREATMENT Surgical

brown teeth of Capdepont An AD [MIM125490] dysodontogenesis characterized by small, yellow-brown teeth TREATMENT Remove teeth, replace with prostheses

brown tonic Hoxsey method, see there

brown tumor Osteitis fibrosa cystica A hyperparathyroidism-induced tumor-like mass of bony tissue characterized by fibrosis, cyst formation, marked osteoclastic resorption, multinucleated giant cells and hemosiderin (which imparts the brown color) deposits and rounded, cyst-like radiological defects; brown tumors also occur in secondary hyperparathyroidism and may be the first sign of renal osteodystrophy in patients with end-stage renal disease who are maintained alive by renal dialysis and have sufficient time to develop the osseous reaction

Brown-Vialetto-van Laere sydrome see Bulbar palsy

browning reaction Any of a group of complex enzymatic (eg oxidization) and non-enzymatic (eg caramelization, degradation of ascorbic acid and Maillard reaction) reactions that affect foods when processed or stored

Brueghel syndrome A fanciful term[1] for prolonged forceful spasms of the facial, tongue, and neck muscles which may be seen as a rare complication of treatment with phenothiazines and butyrophenones[2]; the syndrome is characterized by grotesque involuntary facial movements seen in later adult life, most common in women, characterized by forceful opening of the jaw, retraction of the lips, spasm of the platysma and protrusion of the tongue (alternately, the jaw may be clamped shut and the lips may purse)

[1]The name derives from Brueghel's painting, *De Gaper* [2]Both neuroleptics, which are more commonly linked to orofacial dyskinesia (choreoathetotic chewing, lip smacking, and licking movements)

bruit CARDIOLOGY An arterial 'thrill' caused by atherosclerosis; when auscultated over the carotid arteries, bruits predict future cerebrovascular accidents; it is unclear whether surgical correction actually helps, as the ischemic event often occurs at a distance from the identified 'danger zone'

brujeria Rootwork, see there

brush border PHYSIOLOGY A specialized portion of the free or apical aspect of certain epithelial cells, consisting of closely packed microvilli that facilitate absorption; brush border cells line the luminal surface of the intestine and proximal convoluted tubules of the kidneys; the BB contains absorptive microvilli and glycocalyx, which is rich in hydrolytic enzymes; BB antibodies were first described in rodents with Heymann nephritis and occur in ulcerative colitis (50% of patients) and *Yersinia* enterocolitis (20%)

brutal beginning INFECTIOUS DISEASE A descriptor for the abrupt onset of disease (often within 1-2 hours) seen in half of the cases of leptospirosis CLINICAL Fever, headache, myalgia, nausea, vomiting, pain, hepatomegaly

'B' symptoms ONCOLOGY Systemic disease associated with leukemia and lymphoma, including significant fever (in Hodgkin's disease, the classic, but uncommon Pel-Ebstein fever), night sweats and unintentional weight loss of > 10%; 'A' symptoms represent the absence of clinical manifestations of malignancy

BSE 1) Breast self-examination, see there 2) Bovine spongiform encephalopathy, see there

BSL Biosafety level, see there

B-type virus A virus enzootic to macaques and Old World monkeys that is closely related to herpes simplex and displays a similar clinical pattern characterized by intermittent shedding and reactivation during periods of stress and immunosuppression, occasionally proving fatal to human handlers of monkeys; B-type viruses are oncogenic and have an eccentric core of nuclear material, similar to MMTV (mouse mammary tumor virus; see C-type virus

'bubble and hole disease' Subacute spongiform encephalopathy Creutzfeldt-Jakob disease A colloquial descriptor for the spongiform changes seen by light microscopy in the cerebral cortex and basal ganglia, resulting in neuronal loss and fibrillary gliosis EM The 'holes' correspond to intracytoplasmic membrane-bound vacuoles within neuronal and glial processes

'bubble boy' David X, a child with severe combined immunodeficiency who had been kept alive in a gnotobiotic environment at the U of Texas since birth; at the age of 12 he received a BM transplant from a histoincompatible sibling to reconstitute his immune system; to prevent GVHD, the donor marrow was treated with monoclonal antibodies and complement to reduce alloreactive T cells; the child died of an EBV-induced polyclonal gammopathy that evolved into a monoclonal proliferation, ie a lymphoma

'bubble boy' disease Severe combined immunodeficiency, specifically caused by adenosine deaminase deficiency

bubble gum cytoplasm A fanciful descriptor for massive cytoplasmic vacuole(s) that may be seen in endocervical cells obtained from a routine Papanicolaou-stained smear in a subject with an intrauterine device

bubble hypothesis Prebiotic origin of organic molecule hypothesis A theoretical component in the evolution of life on earth, which posits a role of bubbles as means of facilitating the incubation of the primordial ooze into viable organic molecules; in the scenario proposed by L Lerman, a geophysicist at Lawrence Berkeley Laboratory in California, 1) Air and sea water come together 2) Organic materials, clay particles and metallic ions are attracted to the surface of the bubbles 3) Energy to drive the reactions is provided by solar radiation, lightning and thunder, and the mechanical action of the wind, waves, and water currents 4) The enriched surface foam dissolves, sending the molecules through new cycles in the water, atmosphere, or at the depths of the ocean, each of which may result in different changes in the evolving molecules (New York Times 6 July 1993; C1) Cf Origin of life experiment

bubble signs Three radiologic signs related to accumulated gas in the upper GI tract in neonates secondary to atresias at different levels **SINGLE BUBBLE SIGN** A gas pocket in the upper left quadrant, seen in complete stenosis at or proximal to the pyloris, or in complete gastric atresia **DOUBLE BUBBLE SIGN** Two upper abdominal gas pockets in neonates with duodenal atresia, annular pancreas (which wraps around the duodenum causing luminal stenosis) or the ultrarare midgut volvulus; the smaller bubble on the right corresponds to the duodenum and the larger to the left, the stomach Note: In atresia, there is no passage of gas to the intestine; thus intestinal gas militates against atresia **TRIPLE BUBBLE SIGN** A trio of upper abdominal gas pockets considered pathognomonic for jejunal atresia, where the upper right bubble corresponds to gas in the stomach, the left bubble corresponds to gas in the duodenal bulb and the lower right bubble corresponds to gas in the pre-atretic jejunum

bubble stability test Foam stability test, see there

bubble stretcher A portable biocontainment pod used to transport a patient infected with a potentially lethal (ie level 4) virus

'bubbly' lung PEDIATRIC RADIOLOGY A vaguely vacuolated pattern seen on a plain chest film in infants with hyaline membrane disease or in Wilson-Mikity syndrome

bubbly vacuolization SURGICAL PATHOLOGY A Swiss cheese-like appearance of the cytoplasm of lipoblasts, malignant melanoma, Burkitt's lymphoma and malignant fibrous histiocytosis

bubo Soft, matted, plum-colored lymph nodes measuring 4-5 cm in diameter, seen in lymphogranuloma venereum

bubonic plague see Black plague

'bucket handle' fracture FORENSIC RADIOLOGY Fragmentation of the distal end of one or both femurs appearing at the bone margins as a crescent-shaped osseous density paralleling the metaphysis, seen radiologically when the growth plate is oblique to the radiographic beam; incomplete 'bucket handles' are characteristic of child abuse-related injuries, which may also be associated with subperiosteal neoosteogenesis (trauma of recent origin), distal transverse dense lines (previous growth disturbance), and cortical thickening (evidence of remote trauma); see Battered infant syndrome, Child abuse

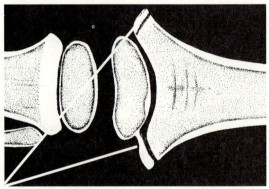

bucket handle fracture

bucket handles Folds of the skin of undetermined significance that may occur in low (anal agenesis, stenosis or incomplete rupture of the anal membrane) or high (complete failure of invagination of the proctodeum) obstructions of the terminal large intestine

'bucking' RESPIRATORY THERAPY Violent resistance by a patient to intubated ventilation that may cause asynchronous breathing, ergo V/Q mismatching and risk of barotrauma, cardiac arrhythmia and increased intracranial pressure; the newer ventilatory support devices rarely evoke this reaction, but patients may still require sedation, or narcotics

buckminsterfullerene see Fullerene(s)

buckshot pattern A pattern of multiple minute lesions, radiodensities or cell clusters, likened to the innumerable pellets from a shotgun blast HEMATOLOGY Scattered subcutaneous aggregates of lymphocytes seen in nodular lymphoid hyperplasia

buckshot calcifications RADIOLOGY Widely spread and minute ('miliary') calcifications that correspond to partially calcified (healing) granulomas in pulmonary, splenic and lymphoid histoplasmosis; in the lungs the granulomas may erode into the bronchi and be expectorated as broncholiths: Cf Miliary calcification

buckyballs Fullerene(s), see there

Budd Light MILITARY MEDICINE An anti-fratricidal device designed by Budd* Croley of the US Army Matériel Command to reduce 'friendly fire' (firing of weapons against one's own side) in military conflicts which consists of a 9-volt battery topped with a blinker that produces timed flashes of infrared light visible by night-vision goggles (**New York Times 18 May 1993; C1**) see Friendly fire

*The term Budd Light is a facetious play-on-words of a popular low-calorie ('light') beer, Bud Light® produced by Anheuser-Busch, St Louis, Missouri

'buddy' taping TRAUMATOLOGY Immobilization of fingers or toes adjacent to one that is fractured or otherwise injured; buddy taping is used for injuries of the proximal interphalangeal joint with incomplete collateral ligament tearing, where the affected finger is taped to an adjacent 'buddy' and immobilized for two weeks, or more if there is also distal dislocation

budesonide A synthetic glucocorticosteroid structurally related to 16α-hydroxyprednisolone which has high topical antiinflammatory activity and low systemic activity; nebulized budesonide is of use in mild-to-moderate croup (**N Engl J Med 1994; 331:285OA**) and long-term control of mild asthma (**ibid 331:700OA**); it may also be used to treat inflammatory colitides, eg ulcerative colitis, and Crohn's disease (**ibid 331:836OA, 42OA, 73ED**)

buffalo hump Gibbus A mass of adipose tissue present at the lower cervical and upper thoracic vertebrae, characteristically seen in long-standing Cushing's disease/syndrome; a gibbus may also accumulate in the thoracolumbar regions of black South Africans with achondroplasia (possibly related to their practice of carrying infants on their backs), mucopolysaccharidoses and chronic osteomyelitis induced by coccidioidomycosis and *Mycobacterium tuberculosis*

buffer CHEMISTRY A chemical system that minimizes the effects, in particular the pH, of changes in the concentration of a substance COMPUTERS A storage zone that 'resides' temporarily in the RAM (random access memory) and contains either input or output data, remaining there while waiting for an output (less commonly an input) device, eg a printer, to allow it access to perform a function Note: Buffer sizes can be increased with 'spooling' software or by increasing the printer's random access capacity

buffer theory CLINICAL NUTRITION A theory on the regulation of food intake and weight autoregulation that holds that only changes in the original equilibrium or rapid fluctuations in the food intake or body weight are opposed; the set point is easily disturbed, with rapid weight loss when food is not available, or rapid gain when ingestion is acutely increased

'buffy' coat LABORATORY MEDICINE The flavescent band of cells and cellular debris that forms between the upper layer of plasma and the lower layer of red cells when whole blood is spun at 5000 RPM, corresponding to leukocytes; the 'buffy-crit' is usually 1-2% and is often increased in leukemia and leukocytoses

'bug' COMPUTERS Any defect in a system, often a software problem MICROBIOLOGY A highly colloquial term that is used interchangeably with bacteria

'bugeyes' ENDOCRINOLOGY A colloquialism for marked bilateral exophthalmos with proptosis, caused by the infiltrative ophthalmopathy, which is seen in more than ½ of Graves' thyrotoxicosis, but which is less common in non-Graves' hyperthyroidism; other ocular signs in Graves' disease include upper lid spasm and lid retraction, external ophthalmoplegia, easy tearing with a gritty sensation of the eyes, supra- and infra-orbital swelling, congestion, edema and weakness of the extrinsic ocular muscles; when severe chemosis and inflammation are present, it is designated as malignant exophthalmos PATHOGENESIS Hypersecretion of a LATS-like (long-acting thyroid stimulator-like) substance

buggery A colloquial term of waning popularity for anal intercourse (sodomy), see there

bulimia An eating disorder consisting of binge eating,

accompanied by frequent fasting, laxative use, or induced vomiting; bulimia is either primary (bulimia nervosa, see there) or a component of other diseases, eg schizophrenia, oral contraceptives, Kluever-Bucy and Kleine-Levin syndromes; see Binge; Cf Scarlet O'Hara 'syndrome'

bulimia nervosa *bulimia*, Greek, to eat like an ox A compulsive eating disorder (table), characterized by binge eating and inappropriate compensation to prevent weight gain; BN usually affects women at a slightly later (age 17-25) onset than anorexia nervosa, but similar in its preoccupation with food; bulimics may consume enormous quantities of food, a 'binge', followed by self-induced emesis, a 'purge'; bulimics may have concomitant impulsive behavior (alcohol and drug abuse), poor peer and parental relations; sexual promiscuity and stealing may be required to financially support the eating 'addiction'

BULIMIA NERVOSA (DSM 307.51)-CRITERIA

A Recurrent episodes of binge eating characterized by
1) The consumption in a defined timespan of a quantity of food that is clearly in excess of what a normal person could (or would) consume in that same time or
2) A subjective lack of control over eating during the episode

B Recurrent inappropriatecompensatory action pursued to prevent weight gain, eg self-induced vomiting, misuse of laxatives, fasting, or excess exercise

C Criteria A and B both occur, on average twice/week for three months

D Self-image is excessively influenced by body shape and weight

E The disturbance does not occur exclusively during episodes of anorexia nervosa

DSM-IV™, American Psychiatric Association, Washington, DC, 1994

---

bulky SPORTS MEDICINE *adjective* A colloquial adjective pertaining or referring an increased muscle mass linked to weight lifting

bulky disease ONCOLOGY A term for a malignancy with a considerable tumor burden ('bulk'); bulky disease generally has a poorer prognosis independent of the histological grade, and a major priority in oncology is to debulk a tumor in order to optimize chemo- or radiotherapy; see Debulking operation

bulldog scalp see Cutis verticis gyrata

bulldog syndrome An X-linked dysmorphia complex described by Simpson, characterized by a large, square protruding jaw, a broad nasal bridge, an upturned nose tip, macroglossia and broad short limbs, resulting in a physiognomy fancifully likened to that of a bulldog

'bulldozing' invasion SURGICAL PATHOLOGY A colloquialism for a broad elephant-foot-like front of tissue invasion characteristic of 1) Squamous cell carcinomas of low aggressiveness, eg verrucous carcinoma of the oral cavity and external female genitalia, a relatively 'bland' malignancy that evokes little inflammatory response, which may be underdiagnosed as verrucous or pseudoepitheliomatous hyperplasia and 2) Hepatocellular carcinoma as it invades into the diaphragm and lungs, usually seen in a terminal stage of disease; Cf 'Stabbing' invasion

bull neck INFECTIOUS DISEASE Prominent and acute cervical lymphadenopathy associated with soft tissue edema that has a brawny color, demonstrates 'pitting', is warm and tender and affects children over age 6; the change may be so extensive as to cover the sternocleidomastoid muscle's border; the 'bull neck' is seen in children with epiglottitis who present with agitation, a muffled cry, labored respiration, cyanosis, drooling and dysphagia, due to *Hemophilus influenzae* type B, *Corynebacteria diphtheriae* and rarely, *Streptococcus pneumoniae* and *Staphylococcus aureus*

bullet 399 see 'Magic bullet' theory

bullet nose deformity Canoe paddle deformity, see there

'bulletproof' mentality A highly colloquial term for a mindset regarded by some as typical of men, who as a species tend not to seek medical advice until absolutely necessary; the BM of men is linked to underuse of preventive health care and screening for diseases and a ↓ in life-span (NY Times 14 June 1995; C14)

Bullis fever Camp Bullis fever An epidemic illness related to a bite from the Lone Star tick, *Amblyomma americanum* that occurred in a military 'boot' camp in 1942 CLINICAL Fever, headache, nausea, rash, neutropenia, thrombocytopenia and persistent lymphadenitis; although historically attributed to *R rickettsia*, it may have been caused by *Ehrlichia canis*

Bull's-eyes' appearance Targetoid appearance A common descriptor for a rounded lesion or mass that is circumferentially rimmed by two or more distinct densities or colors; the inner circle is often dark (or radiopaque), rimmed by a lighter (or radiolucent) ring that in turn is surrounded by a third, dark or radiopaque circle; the opposite (light-dark-light) has been called a Doughnut pattern

bull's-eyes granules HEMATOLOGY Dense core (α) granules of platelets

bull's-eyes lesion DERMATOLOGY The morphology of erythema multiforme, a lesion mediated by circulating immune complexes, elicited by infections, drugs, collagen vascular disease; the skin may also have erythematous plaques and vesiculo-bullous lesions; bull's-eyes lesions are also a classic lesion of Lyme's disease that is seen 1-3 weeks before the onset of the arthritic symptoms; mucosal involvement has been designated as Stevens-Johnson syndrome ENDOSCOPY A finding within the gastrointestinal lumen, in which edematous folds surround a central depression (mass lesion with a central ulcer), non-specific finding seen in solitary amebomas, actinomycosis, amyloidosis, appendiceal disease, TB; single endoscopic 'bull's-eyes' include submucosal carcinoid, primary carcinoma, KS, leiomyoma, leiomyosarcoma, lipoma and lymphoma; multiple 'bull's-eyes' occur in neoplasia: metastases from primary breast, lung and renal carcinoma, lymphoma and mastocytosis OPHTHALMOLOGY A fundoscopic finding described in chloroquine-induced retinopathy, where a depigmented lesion surrounds the macula, surrounded by another ring of relative hyperpigmentation, with possible permanent loss of visual acuity GI RADIOLOGY The bull's-eyes lesions are similar to those seen by endoscopy, are caused by centrally ulcerated lesions, suggestive of malignancy, where the central zone is hypodense, ie necrotic, implying a rapidly growing lesion that has outgrown its vascular supply; multifocal bull's-eyes are suggestive of malignant melanoma; unifocal bull's-eyes occur in carcinoma metastatic to the GI tract, benign or malignant smooth muscle tumors of the intestinal wall, KS and other sarcomas, eosinophilic granuloma and ectopic pancreatic tissue SURGICAL PATHOLOGY An uncommon histological finding in breast carcinoma, where vacuoles have a central spot that variably stains with Giemsa, H&E, or PAS, possibly a processing artifact

bumper fracture FORENSIC MEDICINE Compression fracture of the lateral tibial plateau with separation of the plateau's margin or depression of the central articular surface, due to abduction of the leg caused by an automobile bumper striking the lateral aspect of an extended leg and fixed foot, where the valgus stress forces the two bones into a close contact; bumper fractures are often bilateral and involve both the tibia and fibula; while the height of the bumper fracture on the victim's leg may determine the intensity of the driver's braking effort at the time of impact but the amount of bony and soft tissue destruction is a poor determinant of vehicular speed at impact

BUN Blood urea nitrogen In the US, urea concentrations in the blood are expressed as BUN (normal adults, 8-26mg/dl); SI expresses nitrogen as urea (normal adults, 2.9-8.2 mmol/L); BUN/creatine ratio normally is 20:1; ↑ BUN or azotemia may be

1) Prerenal, due to ↓ renal blood flow (with ↓ glomerular filtration rate) and/or excess urea production, seen in dehydration, shock, ↓ blood volume, and CHF

2) Renal, with ↓ decreased glomerular filtration caused by acute or chronic renal failure; see Uremia

3) Postrenal, due to urinary tract obstruction or perforation with extravasation of urine; ↓ BUN occurs in pregnancy (due to ↑ GFR), malnutrition, high fluid intake, severe liver disease (decreased protein production)

bundle of His SURGICAL ANATOMY *Fasciculus atrioventricularis* [NA6], atrioventricular bundle A bundle of specialized cardiac muscle fibers that carries the electric impulses required for the coordinated contraction of the heart; the AV bundle begins at the AV node located at the inferior interatrial septum, and passes in the subendocardium through the right fibrous trigone to the interventricular septum after which it divides into right and left limbs that pass along either side of the septum branching to the walls of the ventricles; see Atrioventricular nodal reentrant tachycardia

bundling CLINICAL PHARMACOLOGY An attempt by one pharmaceutical company to link the availability of a drug to a mandatory (and for-profit) monitoring system, in order to reduce the liability from a well-known and potentially fatal side effect of the drug; the only drug that has been thus far 'bundled' is clozapine, an agent that has proven more effective than other neuroleptic agents in treating schizophrenia, as it offers better control of psychotic symptoms and is used when patients don't respond to the usual therapeutic neuroleptic agents (1-2% of clozapine-treated patients develop potentially fatal agranulocytosis)

The drug's manufacturer had made the drug available at a cost of $9000/year in one-week supplies, to be released only after blood had been drawn from the patient, in order to closely monitor the white cell count; an obvious concern with 'bundling' is that the practice would spread to other drugs, increasing the price of therapeutics Note: In response to protests from the American Medical Association, the manufacturer unbundled itself from the monitoring system and reduced the price, which is three-fold more expensive in the US than Europe (JAMA 1991; 265:837n&v)

HEALTH CARE FINANCING The combining of multiple surgical procedures under one fee schedule, such that the sum of the fees is less than each individual fee alone, eg excision of a lipoma, hernia sac repair and scar removal would be combined under one fee schedule and the surgeon paid less than for each individual procedure; Cf Unbundling INFORMATION SCIENCE The practice of combining a number of 'electronic journals', usually produced by one publisher for one reduced price; see Electronic journal

bungarotoxin NEUROPHYSIOLOGY An anticholinergic neurotoxin derived from venom of the snakes of the genus *Bungarus*, which binds in a non-covalent fashion to nicotinic-type acetylcholine receptors, preventing depolarization at the postsynaptic membrane of the neuromuscular junction

buprenorphine An opiate analog that substitutes for methadone in heroin addicts SIDE EFFECTS Sedation, constipation

Burgundy red urine A deep red urine produced in porphyria caused by uroporphyrin in the urine, a consistent finding in those with congenital erythropoietic porphyria, intermittently so in those with hepatic porphyria

Burkholderia cepacia Formerly *Pseudomonas cepacia* A bacterium that causes one of the most common infections in patients with cystic fibrosis MODE OF TRANSMISSION Direct physical contact from contaminated environmental sources, possibly also by aerosol (**Thorax 1994; 49:1157; N Engl J Med 1995; 322:819c**) EPIDEMIOLOGY The strains of *B cepacia* seen after lung transplantation are of endogenous origin, ie persistence of a strain present prior to transplantation (**N Engl J Med 1994; 331:981oa**)

burking FORENSIC MEDICINE Homicidal suffocation, accomplished by sitting on the victims' chest with a hand placed over the mouth and nose; see Body-snatching

In pre-Victorian Scotland, bodies for the study of anatomy were supplied by grave-robbing at a price of 10 guineas; W Hare who ran a boarding house in Edinburgh's Tanner Row and W Burke formed a partnership circumventing the unpleasantries of grave-robbing, for which they stood trial for 'burking' 15 victims; Burke was hanged

Burkitt's lymphoma A high-grade extranodal lymphoma of children and young adults EPIDEMIOLOGY African BL is most common in regions with endemic malaria; Epstein-Barr virus infection is intimately linked to the African BL, but not to nonendemic BL PATHOLOGY The African form is more common in the mandible and maxilla; the non-African form arises in abdominal sites (eg distal ileum or cecum, mesentery, ovary, kidney, breast); BL is composed of a monotonous sea of cells of intermediate (10-25 μm) size punctuated by benign macrophages, known as the 'starry sky' pattern MOLECULAR PATHOLOGY Translocation of c-*myc* from chromosome 8 to the immunoglobulin heavy chain region on chromosome 14, and less commonly translocations to light chain loci on chromosomes 2 [t(2;8)] or 22 [t(8;22)]; in the African (endemic) form, the breakpoint on chromosome 14 involves the heavy chain joining region, implying that the B cell is earlier in ontogeny than the nonendemic form in which the breakpoint on chromosome 14 involves the heavy chain switch region, implying that the B cell in which the translocation occurs is more developed (**N Engl J Med 1994; 331:107cpc**)

burn cancer A malignancy, usually squamous cell carcinoma that arises in a background of burns (especially in radiant energy-induced burns)

Note: A healing wound, when examined by LM may mimic the malignant fibrosarcoma, as it is characterized by markedly atypical fibroblasts, nuclear hyperchromatism and bizarre mitotic figures

burn rate The speed at which a non-income-producing company consumes the monies invested in it by venture capitalists (**Bio/Technology 1995; 13:313**)

'burned-out' germinal centers Morphologically distinct germinal centers that are typical of angioimmunoblastic lymphadenopathy; BOGCs are composed of loose aggregates of pale histiocytes and scattered immunoblasts or epithelioid cells mixed with amorphous eosinophilic and PAS-positive intercellular material, thereby resembling granulomas; see Germinal centers

'burned out' mucosa A gross anatomic finding in severe, long-standing cases of ulcerative colitis, with virtually complete mucosal denudation and scattered residual pseudopolyps

'burned-out' phase 'Spent' phase HEMATOLOGY A desirable end-stage of polycythemia vera, where hyperproduction of erythrocytes settles down and much of the bone marrow is replaced by reactive fibroblasts which produce the collagen typical of myelofibrosis

burning feet syndrome Gopalan syndrome A nutritional sensory polyneuropathy; well described in prisoners of war and thought to be due to deficiency of B vitamins; it is characterized by intense burning pain of the feet with hyperesthesiae, increased skin temperature and vasomotor changes, occasionally accompanied by scotoma and amblyopia; the lightning foot is of uncertain etiology, but

may be due to a combination of vitamin B and protein deficiency and/or a toxin present in polished rice, a condition reported in late Colonial India

burnout DENTISTRY '...*the elimination, by heat, of an invested pattern from a set investment in order to prepare the mold to receive casting metal.*' (**Stedman's Medical Dictionary, 25th ed, Williams & Wilkins, Baltimore, 1990**) MATERIALS SCIENCE A 'stress' pattern seen in solid materials when subjected to red heat

'burnout' A feeling of hopeless frustration often accompanied by depression, experienced by workers in certain fields; in the health care field, without an active, self-renewing support group, nurses and social workers assigned to AIDS units, oncology and geriatrics, in which there is an endless parade of dementia, deterioration and death, tend towards callousness and desire to change fields

burnout syndrome Compassion fatigue A form of chronic stress in which the subject gives of himself or herself 'until it hurts', described as a sensation of depletion without time for psychological 'replenishment'; these subjects (usually health care givers) suffer chronic fatigue, have muscle tension, may engage in substance abuse, usually alcohol also Old Soldier syndrome

burning feet syndrome Causalgia with excessive perspiration, slight weakness and changes in the reflexes

burning tongue 'syndrome' Transient glossodynia related to eating Hot foods, see there

burr cell Echinocyte *echino*, Greek, sea urchin HEMATOPATHOLOGY Erythrocytes with regular spines or bumps on the surface, seen after venomous snake (crotalids/pit viper) bites, uremia, pyrokinase deficiency (mechanism: decrease of cellular ATP), erythrocytes low in potassium (as may occur after transfusion of very old blood which may be close to its 42-day maximum shelf limit), gastric ulcers and carcinoma; similar cells (with longer spines) may be seen in acanthocytosis typical of a-β-lipoproteinemia; more attenuated spines are designated as 'created' erythrocytes with an undulating cellular membrane associated with exposure to hypertonic saline

Burt affair Sir Cyril Burt, a British mathematician cum psychologist credited with accumulating data on a group of identical twins raised separately; although Burt had been considered the greatest British psychologist, after his death in 1971, it became apparent that some of the studies probably had not been performed at all, and many of the research associates named in publications were probably fictitious; Cf Breuning case

Buruli ulcer A deeply penetrating ulcer caused by *Mycobacterium ulcerans* seen in Central Africa, New Guinea, Malaysia and Australia TREATMENT None is consistently effective

burst BIOCHEMISTRY An abrupt onset of a reaction VIROLOGY The rupture of cell filled with viral progeny

burst-forming activity IL-3, Interleukin-3

burst-forming unit HEMATOLOGY A small, partially differentiated lymphocyte-like progenitor cell that arises from a pluripotent stem cell, the CFU-GEMM (colony-forming unit for granulocytes, erythrocytes, megakaryocytes and monocytes) in the bone marrow, giving rise to either erythrocytes (BFU-E) or megakaryocytes (BFU-Meg)

burst-forming unit BFU, erythron A self-renewing cell giving rise to a cluster of erythroid clones, known as the burst unit, which in turn gives rise to the colony-forming units (CFU); 'bipolar' BFUs have either erythroid or megakaryocytic differentiation

burst MRI Frequency shifted burst imaging IMAGING A non-isotopic permutation of MRI that allows imaging of the entire brain in 2 seconds, which detects areas of low blood flow that may correspond to neuritic plaques and neurofibrillary tangles and thus is of potential use as a diagnostic tool for Alzheimer's disease (Sci Am 1995; 272/2:12) see MRI

burst therapy A relatively high dose (administered over a short period) of a drug which has untoward side effects when therapy with the agent is prolonged; burst therapy is used for corticosteroids, in which a typical 'burst' dose consists of 50-150 mg/day of prednisone for several days, followed by a rapid drop to 10-20 mg/day, followed by discontinuation if the patient can be 'weaned'

Büschke-Loewenstein tumor Giant condyloma acuminatum A verrucous carcinoma (squamous cell carcinoma of low histologic aggressiveness) of the ♀ anogenital region, demonstrating HPV types 6 and 11 TREATMENT Early lesions require radical local excision, while recurrent or metastasizing lesions require abdominoperineal resection

Buschke-Ollendorff syndrome Osteopoikilosis, see there

buserelin A gonadotropin-releasing hormone analogue that down-regulates the pituitary-gonadal axis, used to treat metastatic prostatic carcinoma; see Disease flare

bush tea see Jamaican vomiting sickness

butter yellow A fat-soluble yellow dye formerly used in food, that proved to be a hepatic carcinogen in rodents

'butterfly drug' CI-911 A drug whose distinct molecular structure has earned it this interesting appellation

butterfly effect THEORETICAL MEDICINE A situation in which a minute dynamic movement (eg the beating of butterfly's wings) in a particular direction might be randomly amplified, such that a butterfly could in theory cause a typhoon on the other side of the world (Sci Am 1994; 271/5:24)

butterfly fragment ORTHOPEDICS A wedge-shaped fragment of bone which is split off the main fragments, seen in a comminuted (more than two fragments) fracture, usually of long bone

butterfly needle A short needle with flexible plastic handles that fold for insertion and lay flat for stabilization with tape; alternately known as scalp vein needles as they are the most practical and commonly used intravenous needles for infants

butterfly pattern RADIOLOGY The fine diffuse infiltrates seen by a plain chest film that radiates bilaterally from the hilum to the lung periphery, characteristic of pulmonary alveolar proteinosis

Note: The 'Bat wing' pattern is more radiodense, sharply defined, prominent in the hilum and associated with pulmonary edema Bat wing and Butterfly wings; some authors have considered the two terms synonyms

butterfly rash An often photosensitive facial rash typical of lupus erythematosus, consisting of an erythematous blush or scaly reddish patches on the malar region, extending over the nasal bridge (the facial 'seborrheic' region), potentially becoming bullous and/or secondarily infected; 'butterfly' region rashes have been described in AIDS, ataxia-telangiectasia, Bloom syndrome, Cockayne syndrome, dermatomyositis, erysipelas (St Anthony's fire, accompanied by waxy guttate indurations of the nose and cheeks that are red, hot, tender and painful with raised borders, a streptococcal skin infection of warm climates, often due to β-streptococcus group A (rarely also group C), pemphigus foliaceus, pemphigus erythematosus (an autoimmune vesiculobullous disorder with immune deposition of IgG and C3), riboflavin deficiency, tuberous sclerosis with smooth, red-yellow papules (adenoma sebaceum), appearing by age four at the nasolabial fold

butterfly scheme A graphic representation of control loops found in regulation of serum calcium under physiological and pathological conditions and the potential for adaption in each situation

'butterfly' tumor The trivial name for the aggressive bilateral, often bifrontal and symmetrical growth pattern of grade III and IV astrocytomas (glioblastoma multiforme), in which there is leaf-like tumor growth on both sides of the corpus callosum with extension along the white tracts, mixed with hemorrhage and necrosis CLINICAL More common in men with a vague familial tendency, accompanied by hemorrhage causing a stroke-like clinical picture and potentially, sudden death PATHOLOGY Butterfly gliomas are poorly demarcated macro- and microscopically

butterfly vertebra A congenital anomaly of a vertebra with persistence of the fetal notocord remnant due to incomplete embryologic notocord regression, or chorda dorsalis; sagittal clefts appear, causing a characteristic 'pinching' of the superior and inferior aspects of the body and compensatory overgrowth of the vertebral bodies above and below the affected bone

buttock cell HEMATOPATHOLOGY A small lymphocyte with deep central nuclear cleavage, seen in lymphosarcoma cell leukemia, mixed cell malignant lymphoma or nodular or diffuse poorly differentiated lymphocytic lymphoma; Cf Cerebriform nuclei

button TRANSFUSION MEDICINE An aggregate of erythrocytes adherent to the bottom of a test tube after centrifugation, if with gentle shaking of the test tube, the cells remain adherent, agglutination is assumed to have occurred, implying presence of both an antigen (on the erythrocyte) and a specific antibody (immunoglobulin in the serum)

button hole stenosis Fishmouth stenosis, see there

'buttonholing' A clinical finding in cutaneous neurofibromatosis in which compressed tumors seem to 'pop' through an opening in the deep dermis, likened to a button; other skin tumors (eg lipomas and fibroepithelial polyps) generally do not 'button-hole'

button sequestrum A preserved island of bone (sequestrum) lying within a 'punched-out' osteolytic lesion of the skull, well-described in eosinophilic granuloma of the diploë (skull), also seen in infections (M tuberculosis, staphylococcal infection), metastatic carcinoma, multiple myeloma, radiation necrosis, meningioma, benign osseous tumors and secondary to a ventriculoatrial shunt

buttressing effect FORENSIC PATHOLOGY The reduction in the size of a projectile's exit wound caused by compression or 'shoring' of the skin by clothing, seating materials or by any externally placed deformable object (JAMA 1993; 269:1544sc)

butylated hydroxyanisole BHA A preservative used in food processing industry to prevent fats and oils from becoming rancid, which is also added to packaged foods; a BHA-rich diet in pregnant mice is alleged to significantly reduce cholinesterase activity in offspring, and impact on the animals' level of aggressiveness, sleep patterns, and weight (Alternative Medicine, Future Medicine Publishing, Inc, Puyallup, Washington, 1994) see Alternative medicine

butylated hydroxytoluene BHT, see there

butyrate A fatty acid that stimulates the promoter of the fetal hemoglobin gene, leading to an increase in γ-globin gene expression; butyrate increases fetal hemoglobin production to levels sufficient to ameliorate the symptoms of β-hemoglobinopathies (β-thalassemia) (N Engl J Med 1993; 328:81oA)

B-virus B-type virus, see there

'bypass' HEALTH CARE ADMINISTRATION The re-routing of patient to be admitted to facility A (eg emergency ward, pediatric intensive care unit) to an equivalent facility B, when facility A is filled to capacity (Am Med News 16 Nov 1992 p1)

bypass obstruction A partial occlusion of the mainstem bronchus resulting in hyperdistension of an entire lobe,

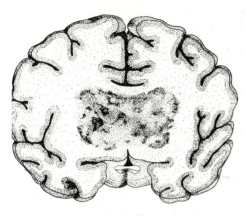

butterfly tumor

with potential for interstitial emphysema and rupture, in a fashion identical to that of the ball-valve phenomenon

bypass surgery Coronary artery bypass graft, see there

byssinosis Brown lung An occupational lung disease, secondary to inhalation of airborne cotton, hemp, linen; the early stages of disease are attributed to endotoxin, characterized by coughing, wheezing, airway obstruction; the

later stages by chronic bronchitis, emphysema and interstitial lung disease, and long-term disability; see Farmer's lungs

byte COMPUTERS Eight binary bits, a unit for measuring computer memory and storage capacity; in perspective, two kilobytes is roughly equivalent to one type-written page; the current generation of personal (desktop) microcomputers built around Intel's Pentium microprocessor (chip) or Motorola's 68040/PowerPC chips are configured with 2-256 Megabytes of random access memory and 240 megabytes to 1+ gigabytes of hard drive storage capacity; see Computers, RAM

BZ-1, BZ-2 receptors see Benzodiazepine receptors

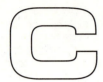

C Symbol for: 1) Calorie 2) Carbon 3) Celsius 4) Centigrade 5) Closure 6) Complement 7) Cysteine 8) Cytidine 8) Cytosine

c Symbol for: 1) calorie (1/1000 of a Calorie) 2) centi- 3) Complementary (molecular biology) 4) cum (Latin, with) 5) Molar concentration 6) Speed of light

C_{max} CLINICAL PHARMACOLOGY Maximum concentration of a therapeutic agent

C-peptide A biologically inactive moiety of proinsulin* produced endogenously, and stored in secretory granules in a 1:1 ratio with insulin; unlike factitious hypoglycemia, which is induced by insulin of exogenous origin, an ↑ in C-peptide (≥ 0.2nmol/L, as well as ↑ insulin, ≥ 42 pmol/L) is characteristic of insulinoma (J Clin Endocrinol Metab 1993; 76:655) C-peptide measurement is of use in detecting fictitious insulin injection and in diagnosing insulin-secreting tumors in diabetics, where > 7 ng/ml of C-peptide after induced hypoglycemia supports a diagnosis of insulinoma

*A polypeptide that connects proinsulin with insulin

C-peptide suppression test ENDOCRINOLOGY A test that may be used to identify the causes of hypoglycemia, which '...is based on the observation that that beta cell secretion (as measured by levels of C peptide) is suppressed during hypoglycemia to a lesser degree in persons with insulinomas than in normal persons.' The test requires that the serum glucose be ≥ 60 mg/dL and that the data be adjusted for body-mass index and age (N Engl J Med 1995; 332:1144RA)

CA 15-3 A group of mucin-like 300–450-kD glycoproteins that are increased in ± ⅓ of all patients with breast cancer (from 5% of those with stage I to 95% with stage IV) have serum levels > 25 U/mL, which correlates with tumor bulk; CA 15-3 is detected by immunoradiometric assay (IRMA) and is most useful to monitor post-operative tumor recurrence

Because 2% of normal healthy subjects and 9% of those with benign breast disease have serum levels > 30 U/mL, CA 15-3 is not used as a screening test

CA 19-9 A tumor-associated carbohydrate antigen that is an epitope located on the sialylated Lewis A blood group antigen (subjects who are genotypically Lewis a-b- comprise 5% of the population and cannot synthesize the antigen); serum levels > 37 U/mL are found in 72-100% of patients with pancreatic carcinoma (97% of those with levels above 1000 U/mL), in ⅔ of those with hepatocellular carcinoma, over ½ of those with gastric carcinoma and ⅕ of those with colorectal carcinoma; although the monoclonal antibody to CA 19-9 cannot be used to screen for pancreatic cancer, it can be used to detect post-surgical recurrence and to differentiate between benign and malig-

nant disease of the pancreas

Because 0.6% of healthy blood donors and 18% of those with benign pancreatic disease have serum levels > 37 U/mL, CA 19-9 is not used as a screening test

CA-125 A cell surface glycoprotein first identified in mucinous ovarian carcinomas that is also expressed on adenocarcinomas of the uterine cervix, endometrium, gastrointestinal tract and breast, measured in the serum, where rising levels indicate a poor prognosis, but low levels are of little clinical utility; CA-125 is normally expressed on the cell membrane of normal ovarian tissue and ≥ 80% of nonmucinous (usually serous type) epithelial ovarian cancers; CA-125 may also be ↑ in non-gynecologic cancers, liver disease, acute pancreatitis, renal failure, occasionally in normal ♀ (N Engl J Med 1993; 329:1531OA), and lymphoma (Arch Pathol Lab Med 1995; 119:371OA)

CA 549 A cancer marker that is ↑ in breast cancer stage I-5%; II-14%; III-32%; IV-74%; CA 549 is nonspecific and ↑ in nonbreast malignancies eg liver-45%, ovary-39%, as well as benign diseases of the liver-24%, lung-19%, prostate-14% (D Chan et al, Am J Clin Pathol April, 1994OA)

CAA Cerebral amyloid angiopathy, see there

CAAT box MOLECULAR HEMATOLOGY A semi-conserved 'box' of DNA with the 'consensus' sequence GG(T/C)CAATCT, located approximately 80 nucleotides upstream (ie, in the 5' direction) from the start site for transcription of α and β globin genes, forming part of the promoter site for RNA polymerase II

C-A-B sequence The order of emergency life support, where C Chest compression is followed by A Airway maintenance and B Breathing; CAB is preferred by the Dutch school of cardiology, while the 'American' school prefers the A-B-C sequence, see there

cabergoline A selective, potent, long-acting dopamine antagonist that suppresses prolactin secretion and restores gonadal function in ♀ with hyperprolactinemic amenorrhea; cabergoline is more effective and better tolerated than bromocriptine, which must be injected 2-3 times/day vs 1-2 weekly for cabergoline (N Engl J Med 1994; 331:904OA)

CABG pronounced cabbage Coronary arterial bypass graft, see there

cabin fever 1) Relapsing fever, see there 2) Also, a highly colloquial term referring to a heightened sense of restlessness that follows a period of prolonged time confined to a particular place, often, one's own home

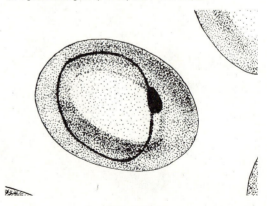

Cabot ring

Cabot ring HEMATOLOGY An attenuated annular, loop-shaped or figure-of-eight structure seen in Romanovsky (eg Wright stain) stained erythrocytes that is thought to correspond to residual microtubules from a mitotic spindle; CBs may be seen in the RBCs of pernicious anemia, lead poisoning, and other defects of erythropoiesis, are accompanied by reticulocytosis, polychromatophilia, basophilic stippling, and appear in accelerated erythropoiesis

CAC cart Crashcart, see there

CACA box MOLECULAR BIOLOGY The DNA oligonucleotide, CCACACCC contains CACA, a conserved sequence or 'box' located 93 residues upstream from the the β globin gene; base pair substitutions in the ACA box 31 residues upstream, the CAT box 76 residues upstream, or the duplicated CACA box cause inaccurate and inefficient transcription by RNA polymerase, which is linked to the pathogenesis of thalassemia

cachectin Tumor necrosis factor-α, see there

CAD 1) Cold agglutinin disease, see there 2) Computer-aided design (or drafting) 3) Coronary artery disease 4) Cyclophosphamide, adriamycin, dacarbazine

Also 1) Collision-activated dissociation (spectrometry) 2) Computer-aided design (or drafting) 3) Computer-assisted diagnosis 4) Council on Anxiety Disorders 5) Cytarabine, daunorubicin

cadaver A dead body

cadaveric organ Any organ transplanted after the death of its owner; transplanted organs of cadaveric origin are less optimal than allografts from living often related donors, having 5-15% less graft survival and overall survival, as cadaveric organs are usually less HLA-matched, and the time between procurement ('harvesting') and transplantation may cause subtle ischemia-related changes; organs are retrieved from only 15-20% of 15-20 000 eligible cadaveric donors; because of the continued shortage of organs resulting in potentially preventable deaths, the AMA's Council on Ethical and Judicial Affairs has suggested two proposals, mandated choice‡, and presumed consent‡, for increasing the supply of cadaveric organs (**JAMA 1994; 272:809CR**)

cadherins MOLECULAR BIOLOGY A family of 118-135 kD single-pass transmembrane glycoproteins that are specific Ca⁺⁺-dependent cell-cell adhesion molecules crucial for tissue differentiation, structure and cell sorting; cadherins are divided into neural cadherin (N-CAM), which binds to neurons, epithelial cadherin (E-cadherin) or uvomodulin, liver cadherin (L-CAM), and placental cadherin (P-cadherin) which have 50-60% sequence homology with each other; they are thought to mediate their many activities by means of a cell-adhesion zipper motif, a structure that mirrors the linear structure of cadherin's intercellular filaments (**Nature 1995; 374:327, 306N&V**) N-cadherin is involved in neural tube formation, functions in morphogenesis and CNS homeostasis; they form a complex with the cytoskeleton, colocate with the tyrosine kinases of the *src* family, and thus cadherin-mediated cell-cell junctions may play a role in intercellular signalling; cadherin down-regulation is associated with tumor cell invasion (**Science 1991; 251:1451**) see also CAM (Cell Adhesion Molecule)

Caenorhabditis elegans A small nematode that has proven to be a major 'workhorse' model in experimental biology, providing key information in embryology, as the exact lineage of each of the worm's adult cells is known, and neurology, where the connections of each of the *C elegans'* 302 neurons has been determined; it has provided the basis for key discoveries in programmed cell death, heterochronic genes, sex determination and neuronal guidance; the goal of the nearly 100 research groups that are studying *C elegans* is to map its 100 million DNA (the human genome has 3×10^9) base pairs by the year 2000, an effort known as the 'worm project'

cafe-au-lait spot A generic term for large smooth ('coast of California'), sharply-demarcated cutaneous macules which are light brown in whites, dark-brown in blacks, due to increased epidermal melanocytes and melanin; while up to 10% of the population has these spots, six or more spots

larger than 1.5 cm is virtually diagnostic of von Recklinghausen's disease; cafe-au-laits spots also occur in Albright's disease (see Coast of Maine appearance), Russell-Silver syndrome, congenital syphilis, and Jaffee-Campanacci disease

café coronary Vallecular dysphagia Complete and abrupt upper airway obstruction by a bolus of food, often meat, resulting in occlusion of both the esophagus and larynx, so named as the sudden onset of symptoms simulates an acute myocardial infarction; the victims are speechless, breathless, and without help (eg Heimlich maneuver), lifeless; cafe coronaries occur in the inebriated, bedentured, mentally retarded, demented, or in those who simply like to eat CLINICAL Violent coughing, cyanosis, collapse and death; Cf Steakhouse syndrome, Sushi syncope

Note: Although a cafe coronary was the alleged cause of death at age 33 of the corpulent siren of the 60s, (Mama) Cass Elliot, according to Dr K Simpson, forensic pathologist and G Thurston, Coroner of London, she in fact died of atherosclerotic heart disease

cafeteria diet Snack diet, 'Trash' diet An experimental system for studying obesity that allows rats free or cafeteria-style access to cookies, candy, cake ('junk-food'); if the diet is begun in prepubertal animals, they remain lean despite excess intake; if the diet is begun as adults, they become obese, due to insufficient thermogenesis; this serves as a non-genetic animal model for obesity of the pure over-feeding type, in which adipsin levels (a serine protease analog synthesized by adipocyte), are normal; genetically obese rats have low adipsin levels

caffeine A methylxanthine compound that has become the most widely used psychoactive substance in the world; sources of caffeine include coffee, tea, maté, soft drinks, cocoa, kaola nuts, guarana products; low doses of caffeine (20-200 mg) produce mildly positive subjective effects, feelings of well-being, alertness, energy; higher doses may result in negative effects, eg nervousness, anxiety (**JAMA 1994; 272:1043OC**) its use during pregnancy has NOT been linked to an increased risk of spontaneous abortion, intrauterine growth retadation, or microcephaly (**ibid, 1993; 269:593OC**)

caffeine dependence syndrome SUBSTANCE ABUSE A clinical complex that can be defined based on fulfilling 3 of 4 generic criteria for substance dependence from the *Diagnosis and Statistical Manual of Mental Disorders*, 4th edition (DSM-IV); 16 of 99 subjects in an early report (**JAMA 1994; 272:1043OC**) were diagnosed as being caffeine dependent; Cf Caffeine withdrawal syndrome

1) Tolerance (DSM-IV substance dependence criterion 1, occurring in 75% of cohort)

2) Symptoms of withdrawal in absence of the use of caffeine (criterion 2, in 94%)

3) Persistent desire or unsuccessful attempt to reduce or control use of caffeine products (criterion 4, in 81%)

4) Continued use despite knowledge of a persistent or recurrent problem that is likely to have been caused or exacerbated by substance abuse (criterion 7, in 94%)

Criteria 3, 5, and 6 were excluded from the definition of caffeine dependence as they are not applicable (**JAMA 1994; 272:1043OC**)

caffeine withdrawal syndrome A complex of findings associated with cessation of caffeine consumption of doses as low as 100 mg/day (equivalent to one cup of coffee/day); CWS is a defining criterion for the caffeine dependence syndrome, see there CLINICAL Headache, lethargy, muscle pain or stiffness, decreased performance, dysphoric mood changes including depression, occasionally nausea and vomiting (**N Engl J Med 1992; 327:1109OA, 1160ED**)

CAG repeat CAG trinucleotide expansion A trinucleotide that is repeated a certain number of times in a gene; in Huntington's disease, CAG repeats on the affected allele on chromosome 4p16.3 range from 40 to 55 or more, versus 10 to 29 in the unaffected controls; excess CAG repeats have also been identified in hereditary dentatorubral-pallidoluysian atrophy, and spinocerebellar ataxia type 1 (**N**

Engl J Med 19934; 330:1401oA) TREATMENT None

CAG-repeat disease Any of a group[1] of triple-repeat[2] diseases that are caused by a gene that accumulates changes with each successive generation, with an expansion of the CAG triplet of nucleotides; once the CAG repeats pass a certain threshold (eg more than 40 repeats), a genetic Götterdämmerung unfolds and the disease of interest[1] has an earlier age of onset with each passing generation, which serves to explain the phenomenon of anticipation (Science News 1995; 147:360) see Anticipation

[1]Which includes dentatorubral and pallidoluysian atrophy, Huntington's disease, Kennedy's disease, and spinocerebellar ataxia type 1 [2]Fragile X disease is characterized by repeats of CCG

caged ATP EXPERIMENTAL BIOLOGY An ATP molecule bound to $CH_7(CO)NO$, which in this form, can neither serve as a substrate for myosin ATPase, nor bind to myosin head-pieces

CAGUGX A loop of nucleotides corresponding to the iron-responsive element in the messenger RNA for ferritin; CAGUGX is located in the 5' direction (upstream) and is not translated into protein but is sensitive either to iron or to an iron-induced protein-linked substance that binds to the CAGUGX stem-and-loop structure, increasing ferritin synthesis

Cain complex PSYCHIATRY A destructive sibling rivalry, in which one of the sibs resents the other for perceived favoritism from a parental figure; so named after the biblical Cain, son of Adam and Eve, who killed his brother Abel

'caine family CLINICAL PHARMACOLOGY A colloquial term for a group of essentially interchangeable local anesthetics which includes carbocaine, lidocaine, xylocaine, and others

caisson disease Chronic decompression sickness A clinical complex caused by long-term whole body decompression, with repeated 'boiling' of nitrogen and resultant morbidity of workers in high-pressure environments, eg caissons PATHOGENESIS The cause of the 'classic' findings of ischemic necrosis of bone is uncertain, but may be linked to platelet activation, intravascular coagulation, and hypoxic damage to marrow fat, resulting in a narrowing of small vessels in the marrow spaces CLINICAL Dysbaric (ischemic) osteonecrosis with medullary infarcts of the femoral, humoral, and tibial heads and rarely, malignancy (malignant fibrous histiocytoma) arising in the site of bone infarction ; Cf the Bends

Note: Caissons are air compression chambers used for underwater construction; Roebling, engineer of the Brooklyn Bridge (an engineering 'triumph' of the 19th century) was among the first to suffer from the late deforming arthritic effects of caisson disease

Cak Cdk-activating kinase, see there

cake kidney Clump kidney Congenital fusion of both renal anlage at the midline into a solid, irregularly lobed mass located caudad to the usual site or as far south as the pelvic floor; the blood is supplied by the lower aorta or common iliac arteries; the ureters are anterior and short, but may enter the bladder normally CLINICAL Lower abdominal pain, caused by stretching of the vascular pedicle, obstruction, infection, calculus formation and nephritis; Cf Horseshoe kidney

'cake' omentum The exceedingly rare diffuse omental involvement by malignancy, usually of epithelial origin, including carcinomas of the colon, stomach, pancreas and ovary

Calabar swelling A transient, one week in duration allergic response to microfilarial infestation by *Loa Loa* as well as *Dipetalonema perstans*, described in West and Central Africa; Vector *Cryosops silacea* and *C dimidiata*, biting flies of the rain forest

calanolide A A compound derived from a Malaysian tree (*Calophyllum lanigerum*) which may have potential as a

therapy for AIDS, reported to be active against AZT-resistant HIV-1 (Sci Am 1993; 268/1:142)

calbindins One of two (calbindin-D_{28k}, and calbindin-D_{9k}, or possibly more) vitamin D-induced calcium-binding proteins located in the intestine that play a major role in the intracellular transportation of calcium (Arch Pathol Lab Med 1994; 118:633oA)

calciferol A molecule with vitamin D activity, derived from steroids by breaking the B ring's 9-10 bond, eg cholecalciferol and ergocalciferol

calcifying aponeurotic fibroma Juvenile aponeurotic fibroma, Keasbey's tumor A benign tumor of fibrous tissue of the hand or wrist in children or adolescents PATHOLOGY Fibrous tissue, calcification, and cartilage TREATMENT Although ½ recur locally, local surgical incision is curative

calcifying epithelial odontogenic tumor Pindborg's tumor A slow-growing lesion of the oral cavity, mandible and maxilla, that affects any age group, population and sex; although the CEOT is locally invasive, radical therapy is not required PATHOLOGY Polyhedral epithelial cells with minimal stroma; the cells may demonstrate nuclear pleomorphism; intracellular degeneration results in amyloid-like eosinophilic material that may with time become calcified

calcineurin Ca^{2+}/calmodulin-dependent phosphatase 2B A phosphatase protein that binds both Ca^{++} and calmodulin, inhibiting the latter's activity; calcineurin alters proteins by removing phosphate groups, shortening the duration of NMDA channel opening (Nature 1994; 369:235L) resulting in the synaptic desensitization of NMDA receptors (Science 1995; 267:1510oA); it is present in highest concentrations in the CNS and is inhibited by tacrolimus (FK 506), an immunosuppressive drug

calcipotriene DERMATOLOGY A topically applied analogue of vitamin D (with minimum effects on vitamin D metabolism) that is approved for treating mild-to-moderate psoriasis, which is similar in efficacy to topical corticosteroids of medium strength (N Engl J Med 1995; 332:581RV) see Psoriasis

calcisome A subcellular organelle involved in pumping Ca^{++} in permeabilized neutrophils

calcitonin A 32-residue polypeptide (plasma levels 100 pg/mL) produced by the parafollicular or 'C' (ultimobranchial) cells, cleaved from the larger molecule, katacalcin, circulating as polymers joined by disulfide bonds; calcitonin is rapidly secreted in response to small increases of plasma Ca^{++}, pentagastrin, glucagon, β-adrenergics and alcohol and is the physiological antagonist of PTH; although excess or deficient PTH and vitamin D cause clinical disease, fluctuation of calcitonin levels is asymptomatic; see C cells

calcium channel blocker CARDIOLOGY BACKGROUND: The extra- to intracellular calcium ratio is usually 10 000:1, a ratio crucial to normal neuromuscular function; during hypoxia, calcium accumulates in the cytoplasm and mitochondria, causing post-insult vasospasm (possibly also lipid peroxidation and free radical damage); thus in the early re-perfusion stages after a hypoxic event, calcium is capable of wreaking havoc and while it is philosophically sound to administer calcium channel blocking agents (eg verapamil), it is unclear whether this strategy is as effective in practice as it is in theory for preventing post-ischemic vasospasm of the coronary and cerebral arteries

calcium hypothesis A hypothesis that explains neuronal release of neurotransmitters, positing that membrane depolarization is required only to open the calcium channels and increase internal calcium concentration near the membrane transmitter release sites

calcium paradox A phenomenon in chronically ischemic (and hypocalcemic) smooth and cardiac muscles which, when re-exposed to normal calcium levels, become over-loaded with calcium, enter a sustained contracted state and die, thought the result of 1) Calcium loading by hypoxic mitochondria and 2) Exacerbation of ischemia by hypercalcemia-induced vasospasm, triggering thromboxane and prostaglandin release; a similar but less understood event is known as the oxygen paradox

calcium shock EXPERIMENTAL BIOLOGY A 'trick' used at the research bench to facilitate passage of substances into cells and bacteria; excess calcium in a cell culture medium causes cells to enlarge and membranes to become 'leaky', allowing transmembranous passage of relatively large molecules, eg plasmids

calcium soap A descriptive term for the often numerous chalky, white-to-pale yellow, rounded lenticular precipitates caused by lipase-induced fat necrosis, which cover the peritoneum and pancreas; these millet seed-sized masses are classically associated with acute pancreatitis, seen on gross examination of the peritoneal surface of the abdominal cavity

*Free fatty acids complex with calcium, producing opaque chalky-white deposits ('soap')

calcofluor white LABORATORY MEDICINE A fluorochrome stain that binds with chitin in the thick electron-lucent endospore layer of microsporidial cell walls; CW is used to identify the presence of yeast, filamentous fungi, and *Pneumocystis carinii* and *Acanthamoeba* spp in clinical specimens; it is not widely used in view of its nonspecificity (Am J Clin Pathol 1995; 103:656oA)

caldesmon An 83-kD protein that binds both actin and calmodulin-inhibiting actomyosin ATPase, preventing the binding of myosin; myosin dissociates from microfilaments during mitosis, an action thought to be mediated by transient caldesmon phosphorylation, possibly explaining the profound changes in the cell shape during mitosis (Nature 1990; 344:675)

caliber FORENSIC PATHOLOGY The diameter of a bullet measured in hundredths of an inch (in the US and English-speaking countries); commonly used bullets are .22, .25, .30, .32, .38, and .45; in other ('metric') countries, calibers are measured in millimeters, eg .38 caliber corresponds to 9 mm; see Ballistics

calibration LABORATORY MEDICINE The matching of a measurement against a standard; CLIA-67 regulations require routine calibration using three points and a minimum or zero for linear procedures and five points for nonlinear procedures

calibrator LABORATORY MEDICINE A solution of a known amount (concentration) that is weighed or determined by repetitive testing using a reference or definitive method that spans the reportable range (Arch Pathol Lab Med 1992; 116:739oA)

calicheamicin/esperamicin ONCOLOGY A family of antitumor antibiotics derived from *Micromonospora calichensis* and *Actinomadura verrucosospora*, respectively that have 4000-fold greater antitumoral activity than adriamycin, and which share a molecular motif of a double-triple-double carbon bond, known as an enediyene; this motif rearranges to form two chemically active radical sites which extract critical hydrogen atoms from DNA's sugar-phosphate backbone, resulting in double strand breakage; this new class of anti-tumoral agents is in phase I trials (Nature 1991; 349:566n&v)

California disease A trivial name for coccidioidomycosis

California encephalitis A viral infection by any of four California Bunyaviridae; most CE is by the LaCrosse virotype, occurring in the summer in north central US; in endemic regions, CE causes 20% of acute childhood meningitides with a very low mortality rate; the infectious cycle is maintained in the mosquito vector, *Aedes trise-*

riatus CLINICAL Non-specific viral prodrome, followed by a 3-8 day meningismus with spontaneous resolution, excellent prognosis with possible psychological residua

California relative value studies (scale) HEALTH CARE REIMBURSEMENT A numerical coding system for all diagnostic and therapeutic procedures performed by or directly under the supervision of a physician; the system is used by physicians to determine a procedure's level of difficulty, which in part determines the fee; Cf RBRVS (Resource-based relative value scale)

call The responsibility (usually 'after hours') that a physician has for evaluating already hospitalized patients or admitting new patients to a particular service or to the hospital per se (PL Fine, The Wards, Little, Brown and Co, Boston, 1994)

Call syndrome An acquired vasospastic disorder condition that is most common in ♀ with migraine, and tends to occur during puerperium; it is characterized by reversible segmental vasoconstriction of multiple cerebral arteries CLINICAL Headache, seizures, transient or persistent multifocal brain signs, accompanied by brain edema and ↑ intracranial pressure DIAGNOSIS Alternating zones of vasoconstriction and vasodilation (N Engl J Med 1995; 332:452cPc)

cALLA Common acute lymphocytic leukemia antigen CD10 antigen A marker for non E-rosette-forming pre-B lymphoblasts that comprise the most common cell type (65%) of childhood acute lymphocytic leukemia (ALL), which when accompanied by the Ia antigen indicates a relatively good prognosis; cALLA is also positive in B cell lymphomas, Burkitt's lymphoma and 40% of T cell lymphoblastic lymphomas; ALL affects both adults and children, with a pronounced peak between ages two and six; ALL blasts are often cALLA, TdT and Ia positive; white cell count is often < 100 x 10^9/L (US: < 100 000/mm^3) PROGNOSIS With treatment, 90% achieve complete remission and have a prolonged survival

calmodulin A ubiquitous 148-residue protein subunit of erythrocyte and other plasma membrane calcium channel ATPases, which reversibly binds calcium in response to various stimuli, eg contraction and relaxation of smooth muscle; when complexed to Ca^{++}, calmodulin binds cAMP phosphodiesterase, hydrolyzing it, acting on protein kinases, releasing hormones, catalyzing biochemical reactions, triggering microtubule catabolism; calmodulin is also involved in DNA repair, activating synthase-phosphorylase kinase, catalyzing activation of phosphorylase b, mediating the degradation of glycogen to glucose

caloric restriction The deliberate reduction in the intake of calories to levels that are as up to 30% below a 'usual' diet; calorically restricted experimental animals live longer, remain healthier, and maintain better phyiologic and behavioral functions than their well-fed counterparts; animals subjected to CR from birth are smaller, mature later, have lower blood levels of insulin and glucose, have ↑ daytime activity; hypotheses to explain the anti-aging properties of CR include altered glucose utilization, ↓ oxygen radical damage, ↓ glycation of macromolecules, changes in patterns of gene expression and in levels of stress hormones (Nature Medicine 1995; 1:414)

caloric test NEUROLOGY A test of vestibular function in which the ear canal is irrigated with cold and hot water, which often identifies an impairment or loss of thermally induced nystagmus on the involved side*; the presence, direction, and type of nystagmus seen in CT can be used to reliably determine whether the vestibular end-organs react, and comparison of the responses indicates which is paretic

*The patient's head is tilted forward 30° from horizontal, which brings the horizontal semicircular canal into a vertical plane, this being the horizontal canal's position of greatest sensitivity for thermal stimulation; each canal is irrigated separately for 30 sec, first at 7ºC below, and then 7ºC above body temperature, separating each maneuver by 5 minutes; in normal subjects there is a tonic

deviation of the eyes to the side being irrigated, followed by nystagmus to the opposite direction (RD Adams, M Victor, Principles of Neurology, 5th ed. McGraw-Hill, New York, 1993)

calpain A proteolytic enzyme present in red cells and platelets that is activated by high intracellular concentrations of calcium, which in the platelets cleaves calmodulin-binding proteins during platelet activation, serving to terminate Ca^{++}-dependent signal transduction

calpain II A calcium-activated protease [EC 3.4.22.17] involved in mitosis that changes its intracellular location during various phases of mitosis: it is plasma membrane-bound during interphase, migrating with the dividing chromosomes, perinuclear in anaphase and mid-cell in telophase

calretinin A neuron-specific calcium-binding protein present in the retina, and in subsets of neurons in the brain, spinal cord, and sensory ganglia; calretinin has a 55% sequence homology with calbindin; both are resistant to excitotoxicity

calsequestrin A soluble, acidic Ca^{++}-binding glycoprotein in sarcoplasmic reticulum vesicles with 43 calcium ions, serving as a reservoir for intracellular calcium when the cytoplasm is overloaded

CAM Cell adhesion molecule Any of a family of calcium-independent intercellular adhesion proteins that are cell selective; the three forms of (neuronal) N-CAMs are produced by alternative splicing, modified by different polysaccharide groups, and are presumed to direct cellular traffic during embryonal development, appearing during neuroepithelial morphogenesis, disappearing during migration and reappearing during ganglionogenesis; see Selectin

CAM 5.2 IMMUNOLOGY A monoclonal antibody raised against keratins 8 and 18, which are present on secretory epithelium, but not on stratified squamous epithelium; anti-cytokeratin reacts with all adenocarcinomas tested and mesotheliomas

cambium layer ANATOMIC PATHOLOGY A dense zone of primitive undifferentiated mesenchymal cells immediately below a mucosal lining, seen in 1) Botryoid rhabdomyosarcoma, where the cambium cells are malignant and the tissue below the cambium layer is loose and myxoid and in 2) Mesenchymal cystic hamartoma where the cells are benign, the layer averages 1-2 mm in thickness and is separated from the respiratory epithelium by a collagen layer of < 0.2 mm

Cambrian explosion PALEONTOLOGY A burst of evolutionary activity during which the diverse life forms that now exist on the planet evolved; the 'explosion' occurred circa 525 million years ago, and spanned a period of 1-12 million years (New York Times & September 1993; C8)

camel back curve Double quotidian febrile 'spikes', ranging from 38-40° C; infections with a characteristic twice daily peak in fever, include gonococcal endocarditis, measles, visceral leishmaniasis and Rift Valley fever; Cf 'Saddleback' curve

camel nose Tapir nose, see there

CAMP Continuous air monitoring program A system of monitoring air pollution in the US

cAMP cyclic adenosine monophosphate, see there

cAMP-dependent protein kinase PKA An enzyme that has two regulatory and two catalytic domains, and multiple isoforms; type II PKA associates with microtubules, and is thought to be involved in peptide binding in cells (Science 1995; 268:247)

CAMP test MICROBIOLOGY A culture plate test for the presumptive identification of group B streptococci, which exhibit clearing when grown adjacent to β-lysin-producing staphylococci TECHNIQUE *Streptococcus agalactiae*, a group B streptococcus that produces the CAMP factor, is streaked on a sheep blood agar plate perpendicular to a streak of β-lysin-producing *Staphylococcus* forming a cleared 'arrowhead' of hemolysis pointing towards the *Staphylococcus*; see Reverse CAMP test

Note: CAMP is an acronym of Christie, Adkinson, and Munch-Peterson, the 3 Australian public health workers who recognized the reaction on agar plates while investigating an outbreak of scarlet fever

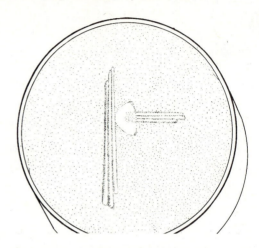

CAMP test

Campath-1 antigen CDw52 An antigen present on most lymphocytes and monocytes but not on other cells; Campath-1H is a 'humanized' antibody raised against this antigen

camphor PHARMACOLOGY Any of a family of alcoholic or ketonic bicyclic terpenes obtained from *Cinnamomum camphora* in the form of whitish crystals; camphor is used topically as an analgesic, antipruritic, rubifacient, and as a counterirritant for inflamed joints; internally it is a carminative, mild decongestant, and expectorant TOXICITY Nausea, vomiting, delirium, coma, respiratory arrest

20(S)-camptothecin A chemotherapeutic plant alkaloid isolated from *Camptotheca acuminata* that targets DNA topoisomerase I (a 100-kD protein, that relaxes supercoiled DNA, acting in semiconservative replication of double-stranded DNA), which is responsible for the breakage-reunion reaction of coiled DNA; since there are increased levels of topoisomerase I in colonic carcinoma, camptothecin has potential in otherwise recalcitrant metastatic colonic carcinoma

campus The physical environment of a large medical center with multiple buildings; those areas or sections that are located in the on-site complex of buildings are 'on campus'; off-site affiliates of the medical center are said to be 'off campus'

Campylobacter A genus of gently-curved gram-negative rods that are common zoonotic commensal organisms found in the gastrointestinal tracts of a wide variety of wild and domesticated animals, and cause three types of human disease—enteric, eg diarrhea, typically by *C jejuni*, extraintestinal, most often by *C fetus*, and gastric, due to *C pylori*, re-classified as *Helicobacter pylori*; most human infections have been attributed to consumption of contaminated water or food, and it has been suggested that some cases of human *C jejuni* infection may be due to magpie and jackdaw (bird) attacks on milk bottles; see *Helicobacter pylori*

Canadian Cardiovascular Society functional classification CARDIOLOGY A system (see table) used to stratify the severity of angina pectoris (see JAMA 1992; 268:2537oc)

Canadian plan HEALTH CARE ENVIRONMENT Canada's

national health insurance system that covers the cost of both the hospital and out-patient care, and some prescription drugs; 38% of the system is financed by national taxation, and 62% by provincial taxation; private physicians in fee-for-service practices submit bills on a monthly basis to the Provincial Health Ministries and trustee- or community-owned hospitals negotiate annual budgets with the provincial governments, which in turn set limits on the fees that the physician providers may charge for their services (**Congressional Quarterly, 1993, in Clin Lab Sci 1994; 7:141**); Canadian acute care hospitals have more admissions, outpatient costs, and inpatient days/capita than the US, but spend less, which may be due to the lower administrative costs and greater use of centralized equipment and personnel (**N Engl J Med 1993; 328:772OA**); the pros and cons of the Canadian plan are hotly debated by all players in the health care scene (**N Engl J Med 1993; 328:1778ED, ibid 329:804ED, ibid 329:806C**); it is reported that Canadian patients with myocardial infarcts had more cardiac symptoms, and a worse functional status at the one year mark than those in the US; Canadians underwent fewer invasive cardiac procedures and had fewer specialist visits related to their MIs, suggesting that the aggressive treatment plan in the US may improve the post-MI quality of life (**N Engl J Med 1994; 331:1130SA**) see Primary care

Note: If US hospitals followed the same spending patterns as the Canadians, the savings would have been an estimated $30 x 10^9 (1985 dollars)

canalplasty OTORHINOLARYNGOLOGY A procedure used to repair abnormalities of the external auditory canal by removing abnormal bone growth, eg anterior overhang or exostosis, removal and replacement of intractably infected mucocutaneous tissue in the canal and enlargement or straightening of a stenotic or tortuous external auditory canal

CanCell A 'therapy' consisting of water 'energized' by a plant, which was promoted as a cure for AIDS, arthritis, cancer, DM, and SLE, administered per cutaneously or per rectum, and determined by the FDA to be fraudulent (**Am Med News 21 Nov 1994 p13**) see AIDS fraud, Quackery; Cf Unproven forms of ccancer therapy

cancer A generic term for malignancy of any embryologic origin, which was defined by WH Clark, Jr (**Human Pathol 1990; 21:1197**) as a '*...population of abnormal cells showing temporally unrestricted growth preference (continually increasing number of cells in the population) over normal cells. Such abnormal cells invade surrounding tissues, traverse at least one basement membrane zone, grow in the mesenchyme at the primary site, and may metastasize to distant sites. It is the totality of properties that determines whether a given lesion should be designated as a cancer*

Note: The lay public and many health professionals use the term 'cancer' interchangeably with 'carcinoma', a malignancy of epithelial and occasionally neuroepithelial origin

CANADIAN CARDIOVASCULAR SOCIETY FUNCTIONAL CLASSIFICATION

CLASS I Usual physical activity, eg walking or climbing stairs, does not cause angina; angina is evoked by strenuous and/or rapid work or recreation

CLASS II Slight limitation of ordinary activities, eg after walking two blocks, climbing one flight of steps, under normal circumstances, after meals, in the cold, wind, in the morning, or when under emotional stress

CLASS III Marked limitation of ordinary activities, eg walking 1-2 blocks or climbing stairs under normal circumstances

CLASS IV Inability to carry out any physical activity without discomfort–anginal syndrome may be present at rest

Circulation 1976; 54:522

cancer clusters EPIDEMIOLOGY A cancer that occurs in a group of people living or working in a geographically defined region who appear to share one or more environmental factors, eg DES, and a characteristic lesion, eg vaginal adenocarcinoma in common; see Clusters

cancer family A genetically-linked family in which malignancy occurs with greater than expected frequency; when the cancer occurs in older subjects, the investigation may suggest exposure to an environmental agent that all family members have in common with a minimal genetic contribution; when members of a family develop neoplasms (especially if the tumors are malignant) when they are young, a significant genetic component is presumed to act with minimal environmental contribution, and are known as 'cancer families'; family members of patients with early-onset malignancy, especially of the colon and breast, may have a 20- to 30-fold ↑ risk of malignancy, the cancer often being of one or at most a few 'restricted' histological types, eg an association of colonic and endometrial adenocarcinoma, or ovarian and breast carcinomas; analysis of heredity and the potential contributions by environmental (dietary, viral, electromagnetic radiation and other) exposures is complex; see Dysplastic nevus syndrome, Li-Fraumeni syndrome

Cancer and Leukemia Group B CALGB, see there

cancer phobia An excessive fear of suffering the ravages of malignancy, a 'condition' that more commonly affects those who have directly cared for a loved one who suffered marked pain or disfigurement for a protracted period before death; cancer phobia is considered an appropriate indication for a simple mastectomy in patients with a diagnosis of carcinoma-in-situ, which may be treated more conservatively by close observation and periodic mammograms and breast examination

cancer-prone personality A person who is alleged to be at an ↑ risk of suffering malignancy due to ill-defined and nebulous internal conflicts; it is unclear whether this state actually exists as evaluation of 'proneness' is based on non-objective personal data (**Prof Ed Pub, Am Cancer Soc**) Cf Psychoneuroimmunology

cancer screen Any measurable clinical or laboratory parameter that can be used to detect early malignancy; although these tests are relatively non-specific, they are highly sensitive, and detect the vast majority of subjects who are 'abnormal' for the parameter being measured; the most common cancer screens are those that detect occult blood in the stool as a screen for colon cancer and mammography for identifying microcalcifications and geographic densities for detecting breast carcinoma; logistically viable cancer screens must be viewed in the context of a cost-benefit ratio, and are not available for many of the more common malignancies, eg lung cancer, which theoretically could be detected by annual chest films, although this has not been recommended; Japan has responded to its 'epidemic' levels of gastric carcinoma by recommending periodic gastroscopy for its population

cancer screening The testing of a large group of people for malignancies that are common to the group; screening tests must be inexpensive and, in order to detect all people who are abnormal for the analyte, highly sensitive

cancer screening guideline A generic term for any rule of thumb, often promulgated by an authoritative organization (eg American Cancer Society) for the early detection of a malignancy that is relatively common in a particular population, the diagnosis of which in initial stages of development results in a complete cure or improved long-term survival

BREAST CANCER Self-breast examination on a monthly basis, a baseline mammogram at age 40 and mammography every 1-2 years thereafter, depending on risk factors;

see Breast self-examination

COLON CANCER Recommendation by the National Cancer Institute, American Cancer Society and Americal College of Physicians for colorectal carcinoma is annual fecal occult blood test after age 40 and flexible sigmoidoscopy every three to five years after age 50 (N Engl J Med 1991; 325: 37)

PROSTATE CANCER Annual digital rectal examination after age 40, and measurement of prostate-specific antigen or acid phosphatase in the serum

UTERINE CERVIX CANCER Annual pap smear (Papanicolaou test) and pelvic examination after initiation of sexual activity; after three normal years, the test may be reduced in frequency at the discretion of the patient's physician

cancer surgery Surgical treatment of a malignancy, a relatively routine procedure in most body sites; not all malignancies are amenable to surgical therapy, as 1) Some tumors respond better to non-surgical treatment, eg lymphoma, which often responds to multiagent chemotherapy, choriocarcinoma, which responds to a single agent, methotrexate or seminoma, which responds to radiotherapy 2) The lesion may have extended to or beyond vital structures, eg intracranial glioma or pericardial involvement 3) The site is a surgical 'danger zone'; eg, esophagus and tail of the pancreas, associated with poor surgical salvage; see Operable cancer, Resectable cancer

cancer-to-cancer metastasis A rare event in which there is metastatic penetration of one malignancy into another (Cancer 1968; 22:635); 'donor' cancers include bronchogenic 33%, breast 10%, gastrointestinal 10%, prostate 10%, thyroid 10%; 'recipient' cancers include hypernephroma 60%, lymphoproliferative 12%, and others

cancerization Carcinogenesis, see there

'cancerization' SURGICAL PATHOLOGY A relatively specific term that traditionally refers to extension of a ductal carcinoma-in-situ into lobules ('lobular cancerization'), although this may represent a morphological variant of ductal carcinoma in situ; the term has been used by some surgical pathologists for a visible transition zone between an epithelial lesion with marked atypia and well-differentiated carcinoma, as in 'cancerization' of a villous adenoma of the colon

candela The SI (International System) unit of luminous intensity in a given direction from a source emitting monochromatic radiation of a frequency of 540×10^{12} hertz, where the energy in that direction is 1.464×10^{-3}/steradian

candida enolase A 48-kD antigen present in the serum of many patients with invasive candidal infection, an event usually associated with terminal cancer; detection of candida enolase complements blood cultures, but does not replace them (N Engl J Med 1991; 324:1026)

Candida krusei A *Candida* species that has emerged as a major systemic pathogen in patients with BM transplantation who have received prophylactic fluconazole therapy, administered to prevent infection by *Candida albicans* and *C tropicalis* (N Engl J Med 1991; 325:1274) see Bone marrow transplantation

candidate gene method MOLECULAR BIOLOGY A technique used to identify a gene possibly involved in a disease process by picking a cloned gene known to have a physiologic role in the diseased tissue; one then searches for mutations in the gene (often point mutations) in patients who have the disease in question; this method is considered more scientific than the 'serendipitous' technique of finding a mutated gene by 'reverse genetics' (N Engl J Med 1994; 330:930OA)

candidate hormone An incompletely studied substance with hormone-like activity, eg enteroglucagon, urogastrone

candidemia The systemic dissemination of *Candida* spp TREATMENT In patients without neutropenia and/or major immunodeficiency, amphotericin B and fluconazole are equally effective (N Engl J Med 1994; 331:1325OA)

candidiasis hypersensitivity syndrome Yeast connection A complex, the very existence of which is controversial, said to occur in women, due to an overgrowth of *Candida albicans* on mucosae, especially the vagina and gastrointestinal tract ETIOLOGY CHS has been linked to various agents, ranging from broad-spectrum antibiotics to oral contraceptives, and pregnancy CLINICAL Chronic GI symptoms, eg bloating, heartburn, constipation and diarrhea, as well as depression, loss of concentration, poor memory, fatigue, irritability, nasal congestion TREATMENT Nystatin had been recommended by certain health professionals; in a randomized study of oral and/or vaginal nystatin versus placebo, there was no difference in response of symptoms (N Engl J Med 1990; 323:1717)

candle flame appearance CARDIOLOGY A finding by Doppler color flow imaging consisting of a central blue color, corresponding to a zone of high velocity, surrounded by a yellow-orange blush, corresponding to a turbulent zone of lower blood flow; the 'candle flame' sign is typical of mitral stenosis, other morphological permutations in mitral stenosis have been described as having scimitar, mushroom and bifid jet shapes

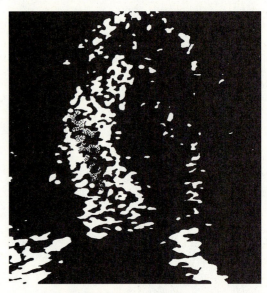

candle flame appearance

candlestick appearance BONE RADIOLOGY A sharply marginated 'cut-off' of the terminal phalanges with a central depression, seen in burns, diabetes mellitus, gout, leprosy, malabsorption, occlusive vascular disease, porphyria, psoriasis (Cf Pencilling), Raynaud's disease, rheumatoid arthritis, scleroderma

candle wax bone Melorheostosis, see there

candle wax drippings A descriptor for a morphology likened to the pearlescent gutterings of melted candle wax NEUROPATHOLOGY Smooth pinpoint-to-thumbnail-sized rounded elevations on the lateral ventricular walls or cerebral cortex in patients with tuberous sclerosis HISTOPATHOLOGY Architectural distortion, gliosis and bizarre, often enlarged neurons OPHTHALMOLOGY Fundoscopic changes in which the vascular sheath is surrounded by preretinal inflammatory exudates, appearing as bulbous perivascular dilatations, a finding suggestive of sarcoidosis

C&S Culture and sensitivity MICROBIOLOGY A set of tests performed on a clinical specimen, where isolation of a potentially pathogenic bacterium is followed by antibiotic susceptibility testing; see MIC

candy cane sign PEDIATRIC CARDIOLOGY Infrahepatic interruption of the inferior vena cava with continuation in the azygous or hemizygous vein, an angiographic finding associated with congenital heart disease

canker sore Aphthous ulcer A painful, recurrent ulcer of the oral cavity or vermilion border, preceded by tenderness and pruritus, beginning as an erythematous indurated papule that rapidly erodes, leaving an ulcerated base, covered with grayish exudate; although associated with Behçet syndrome and inflammatory bowel, the condition is idiopathic and may be of allergic, autoimmune, drug-related, endocrine, hypersensitive, infectious (viral), stress-related or traumatic origin, with secondary bacterial infections that respond to topical tetracycline; the ulcer itself responds poorly to treatment, eg oral rinses with benadryl, xylocaine and corticosteroids

cannabinoid see Marijuana

cannabinoid receptor THC receptor, see there

cannibalism The eating of the flesh of another, which can be

1) A symbolic act in which surrogate flesh, eg bread wafers, is consumed (Western-style cannibalism[1])

2) A ritualistic act in which actual flesh is consumed, divided in

a) Endo-cannibalism, the consumption of a blood relative[2], who was respected and loved in life, see Morbid affection

b) Exo-cannibalism, in which the flesh of those outside of one's tribe were eaten, the most popular donors being '...*fallen warriors, medicine men, and virgins, to gain, respectively, bravery, wisdom, and purity.*' (C Panati, Extraordinary Endings of Practically Everything and Everybody, Harper&Row, New York, 1989)

3) An imperitive and desperate act of survival

[1]Although not known as cannibalism, the 'eating' of the body of Christ, as practiced by Christians, derives from certain practices by the ancient Greeks, in which blood or body parts from priests were consumed; the sacrament of the Eucharist, is believed by some to originate in *eucharistia*, Greek, gratitutde
[2]Pun potential duly noted and nobly ignored

cannon 'a' wave An abnormal jugular venous pressure curve with an accentuated a wave, of sufficient intensity to cause the earlobes to 'flap', due to reduced right ventricular compliance, tricuspid stenosis or an arrhythmia in which the atrium contracts against a closed or stenosed tricuspid valve; a less 'explosive' but still prominent 'a' wave may by associated with pulmonary hypertension; CAWs may be regular, as are atrioventricular junctional rhythms, where a CAW occurs every second beat in a 2:1 block, or irregular, which are more common and may occur in complete heart blocks without atrial fibrillation, ventricular tachycardia and atrioventricular dissociation

cannonball metastases One or several large, well-circumscribed metastatic nodules within the lungs, classically seen in renal cell carcinoma, also seen in choriocarcinoma

cannonball pattern Death star, see there

canoe paddle rib A rib deformity described in Hurler and Hunter types of mucopolysaccharidoses, with a spatula-like narrowing at the vertebral origin and widening of the middle of the ribs, ending in a 'bullet-nose' broadening at the anterior end; canoe paddles also occur in craniocarpotarsal dysplasia or Freeman-Sheldon syndrome, or may refer to the distal femur in Pyle's disease

canonical correlation analysis STATISTICS A maneuver that defines covariation for two groups of variables

canthaxanthin B,B-carotene-4,4'-dione A highly lipid-soluble synthetic carotenoid, which in humans cannot be converted to vitamin A; it is used as a 'natural' food coloring (to dye jellies, salad dressings, tomato juice) and added to animal feed to 'enhance' the colors of chicken skin, egg yolks, and rainbow trout flesh; it is not approved for prescription nor as an over-the-counter drug, but has been marketed as an oral tablet for skin tanning under various names, is available in combination with β-carotene and has been implicated in aplastic anemia CLINICAL NUTRITION It is linked to a ↓ risk of skin cancer and cancer cell growth in vitro, and associated with an improved immune response (New York Times 21 Feb 1995; C1) see Carotenoid

canyon hypothesis VIROLOGY A possible site for virus-receptor binding that is present in rhinoviruses and picornaviruses, in which the target is bound while prohibiting anti-viral antibody interaction as the narrowness of the 'canyon' renders the pathogen inaccessible to the immune system (Science 1991; 251:1456)

c'ao gio Coining A Vietnamese folk therapy consisting of rubbing coins over warm, oiled skin to draw out fever, appearing as darkened erythematous zones, which when seen in feverish children in the emergency room, erroneously raise the question of child abuse

cap DENTISTRY A popular ('layman's') term for a crown HEALTH CARE ENVIRONMENT A limit on reimbursement for a health care service or therapy imposed by an insurance company or governmental agency; see Capitation MOLECULAR BIOLOGY A complex methylated structure at the 5' end of mRNA and hnRNA, consisting of a terminal 7-methylguanylate nucleotide in a 5'-5' linkage to the initial mRNA molecule, possibly having a role in mRNA synthesis after translation HEALTH CARE ENVIRONMENT A limit on reimbursement for a health care service or therapy imposed by an insurance company or governmental agency; see Capitation

CAP 1) Catabolite activator protein MOLECULAR BIOLOGY A cAMP-binding molecule responsible for positive feedback control of the lac (gene cluster in *Escherichia coli* required for lactose metabolism) and ara (gene cluster in *E coli* required for arabinose metabolism) operons, that attracts RNA polymerase, facilitating the initiation of transcription; CAP is required for the transcription of many genes; see BAD operon   2) College of American Pathologists, see CAP Survey   3) Community-acquired pneumonia

CAP survey College of American Pathologists survey An organized program from the CAP survey that provides information on proficiency and productivity among clinical laboratories, comparing techniques and instruments, the work load performed per technician, the total number of tests performed and the cost per test; CAP's interlaboratory comparison program is the largest in the world and serves to satisfy the regulatory requirements of most accrediting agencies

CAPD Continuous ambulatory peritoneal dialysis; see Peritoneal dialysis

capillary electrophoresis High-performance capillary electrophoresis A highly-sensitive (in the picomolar range, which is 10 000-fold more sensitive than conventional electrophoresis) and efficient technique that allows separation of proteins, nucleic acids and carbohydrates; CE is used for analytical chemistry, biomedical research, clinical diagnosis, environmental science, food science, forensic science, toxicology, and others (Am Clin Lab May 1994) for separating peptides using a polar bonded phase CE column (Am Biotech Lab Feb 1995, p80)

capillary electrophoresis-laser-induced fluorescence LABORATORY MEDICINE A technique that combines the highly efficient separation capacity of CE, the affinity and specificity of antibody and antigen binding with the high sensitivity of LIF; CE-LIF may be used for simultaneous immunoassays of multiple analytes in biologic fluids, eg to screen urine for the presence of drugs of abuse; in one report, CE-LIF was used to simultaneously detect morphine, a heroin and codeine metabolite, phencyclidine, THC, a marijuana metabolite, and benzoylecgonine, a cocaine metabolite (Am Clin Lab Feb 1995, p27)

capillary fragility test A crude test for vitamin C (ascorbic acid) deficiency that is based on the number of petechiae that appear on the forearm after application of a blood pressure cuff (sphygmomanometer) inflated to the person's mean arterial pressure

capillary gel electrophoresis A technology that can be used to identify single base deletion products or failure sequences from full-length product in the analysis of synthetic oligonucleotides (Am Lab July 1994, 30)

capillary ion analysis ENVIRONMENT A highly sensitive separation method that is of particular use for analysis of organic acid anions in groundwater; the samples require little preparation, low sample volume with minimal reagent consumption (Am Lab May 1993)

capillary leakage syndrome A toxic side effect consisting of progressive dyspnea and pericarditis that may occur in therapy with GM-CSF (granulocyte-macrophage colony-stimulating factor), which has been used to treat metastatic solid tumors; a similar response may occur in IL-2 therapy, where large amounts of fluid (10-20 liters) are held hostage in peripheral tissues, accompanied by high fever, confusion and disorientation

capital budget HOSPITAL ADMINISTRATION Any financial allocation for the purchase of fixed and durable goods; in hospitals, capital includes beds, buildings, equipment and other items that are not operating expenses

capital punishment Punishment by death for a crime; CP is legal in 36 states of the US and is used for certain crimes, usually homicides, which are almost invariably tried by the jury in a public, and often well-publicized trial; STATISTICS The US is the only major industrial nation to retain execution as a form of punishment, and uses it in record numbers (it is also the only nation that allows its citizens free access to firearms—Author's comment) the state of Virginia has the record (2049) for most executions; New York State follows at 1361 (New York Times 19 March 1995; 37); physicians are extremely polarized about participating in CP; some are dead against it, while others feel it is both an ethical and civic duty; the American Medical Association has denounced certain types of physician participation (PP) in CP; PP in CP may be divided into stages, only the first of which is broadly accepted:

STAGE I–provision of medical care for prisoners on 'death row'

STAGE II–preparing for the execution itself, designing protocols for lethal injection, estimating the length of rope necessary for a prisoner to die instantly without losing his head (ie decapitation)

STAGE III–participation in the execution per se; there have been a number of well-documented mishaps in which executions were inefficiently performed

STAGE IV–pronouncing the prisoner dead

STAGE V–certifying the death

STAGE VI–harvesting organs after death (a procedure that has not been successful)

*'The participation of physicians in capital punishment is a longstanding phenomenon. During the French Revolution, the physician Joseph Ignace Guillotin developed a device now known as the guillotine as a more humane and efficient method of execution. In recent years, lethal injection has become an increasingly popular method of execution. It is less expensive than the alternatives; it is more acceptable to those who must witness the execution; it may increase the willingness of judges and juries to apply the death penalty; and it is generally seen…as more humane and less painful than other methods.' (N Engl J Med 1993; 329:1346ss)

capitate HEALTH CARE ENVIRONMENT A term referring to the payment or acceptance of payment for persons enrolled in a health plan on a per capita basis such that each person pays a predetermined monthly fee for the medical service, regardless of whether it is used on not, and if it is used, the payment remains fixed regardless of how much a particular person uses the service

capitated payment see Capitation

capitation Capping HEALTH CARE FINANCING A form of payment for health care services in the US in which physician(s) are paid a fixed fee per person (ie per capita) served, regardless of how often the services might be used, in exchange for which the physician takes complete responsibility for the patients' physician services; 'Capitated' care is typical of health maintenance organizations and of some preferred provider organizations

***Capnocytophaga canimorsus* sp nov** DF-2 A gram-negative bacterium found in the oral cavity of healthy dogs introduced into humans by bites; *C canimorsus* causes necrosis of soft tissues and skin with disseminated purpuric lesions, and fulminant sepsis in patients with cirrhosis or those who have undergone splenectomy (N Engl J Med 1994; 331:1362cPc)

***Capnocytophaga cynodegmi* sp nov** DF-2-linked organism A gram-negative bacterium that is similar to, but less virulent than *C canimorsus*, see there

capnography The measurement and graphic display of CO_2 levels found in the airway, which can be performed by infrared spectroscopy; capnography facilitates patient management by providing 1) Continuous and noninvasive monitoring of ventilation in critically ill patients and 2) Early detection of clinically significant changes in respiratory status by displaying changes in the a) amount of CO_2 and b) abnormal CO_2 waveforms; capnography can be used to detect a wide range of clinical conditions, eg extubation of respiratory support, hypotension or massive blood loss, emphysema, COPD, pulmonary embolism, and others

capnometry 1) The measurement and numerical display of CO_2 levels found in the airway 2) The science of measuring atmospheric concentrations of smoke, eg in smoke plumes or in flue gas

capping IMMUNOLOGY An energy-consuming contractile filament (actin and myosin)-mediated process occurring on the lymphocyte surface that 'strips' the cells of immunoglobulin receptors, functions as the initial signal for activation of the lymphocyte; after antigens are bound by surface, often divalent immunoglobulins, there is initial focal coalescence, followed by migration of the cross-linked antigen-immunoglobulin complexes toward one pole, forming a 'cap' that is internalized by the B cell; an analogous phenomenon also occurs in T cells and in prolymphocytic leukemic cells; cross-linking is the mitogenic signal that triggers cell differentiation MOLECULAR BIOLOGY Addition of a methylation cap to eukaryotic mRNA; Cf Methylation MUSCLE PHYSIOLOGY The binding of protein, eg gelsolin to the barbed end of F-actin to prevent further polymerization

capsaicin A chemical derived from hot peppers that may be used to treat painful dysesthesias of herpes and diabetes; topical capsaicin triggers release of the neuropeptide, substance P from the type C nociceptive fibers, opens the calcium and sodium channels causing the initial pain associated with 'hot' foods; substance P is not replenished (due to a combination of early sodium channel inactivation and later calcium buildup that inactivates voltage-gated channels and/or mediates degradation of neurofilaments, preventing axonal transport of substance P), thus pain sensation is reduced after the initial pain; capsaicin's effectiveness as a topical agent for painful peripheral neuropathy is unclear and requires up to a month of use before the reduction of pain occurs; topical capsaicin is reported to be effective in ↓ the pain-related symptoms of painful diabetic neuropathy (Diabetes Care 1992; 15:159) see Blister beetle, Spicy foods

capsular drop RENAL PATHOLOGY An exudative glomerular lesion seen light light microscopy in end-stage diabetic glomerulosclerosis, which consists of PAS-positive focal thickenings of Bowman's capsule that 'hang' into the urinary spaces

capsid VIROLOGY The protein envelope of a virus that is composed of protein subunits known as capsomers

'captain of the ship' The legal principle that is an adaptation of the 'borrowed servant rules' as applied to an operating room in a hospital; the COTS doctrine arose from *McConnel* v. *Williams* (Pennsylvania, 1949; Thomas v Hutcjhinson, 442. Pa. 118, 275 A.2d. 23,27) that holds the person in charge (eg a surgeon) to be ultimately responsible for all those under his supervision or command, regardless of whether the 'captain' is directly responsible for an alleged error or act of alleged negligence, and despite the assistants being employees of a hospital; see 'Borrowed servant', Respondeat superior

captopril An angiotensin-converting enzyme inhibitor used for hypertension, in IDDM, and in patients with post-MI left ventricular dysfunction, long-term administration of captopril is associated with ↑ survival, and ↓ cardiovascular mortality and morbidity, possibly by attenuating ventricular dilatation and remodeling (N Engl J Med 1992; 327:669OA) WARNING Angioedema of upper airways may prove fatal ADVERSE EFFECTS Neutropenia, agranulocytosis, proteinuria, rash with/without pruritus, hypotension, dysgeusia

caput medusae Medusa head, see there

caput succedaneum NEONATOLOGY A yarmulka-like edematous bulge that forms on that portion of the infant scalp immediately overlying the cervical os in a vertex presentation; CS is most prominent in prolonged labor and an incompletely dilated cervix and disappears within a few days after birth

cap Z protein PHYSIOLOGY A heterodimeric protein located in the Z line of skeletal muscle, composed of 2 subunits (32 kD and 36 kD) that selectively binds to the '+' ends of actin filaments, stabilizing them and preventing depolymerization

CAR syndrome Cancer-associated retinopathy A paraneoplastic complex due to autoantibodies reactive against retinal components, in particular, a 23-kD protein, the CAR antigen, with loss of visual acuity due to retinal nerve demyelinization, described in pulmonary small cell carcinoma

carapace pattern NEUROLOGY A broad pattern of sensory loss affecting the very short nerves of the upper body (trunk and thorax)

carbamazepine Divalproex sodium NEUROLOGY An antiepileptic drug which is a standard drug for treating partial or secondarily generalized tonic-clonic seizures; in contrast to valproate which is as effective (as carbamazepine in treating generalized tonic-clonic seizures), carbamazepine therapy is associated with better seizure control and seizure-rating score, ↓ number of seizures, and time to first seizure SIDE EFFECTS Rash, hair loss, tremor (N Engl J Med 1992; 327:765OA) Cf Valproate

carbohydrate loading Pasta loading SPORTS MEDICINE The ingestion of a meal high in carbohydrates and low in fats and proteins (after previous depletion of the hepatic stores of glycogen) with the intent of maximizing the amount of the glycogen stored in muscle; as fuel, carbohydrate is more versatile than fat or proteins as it can be used anaerobically, its consumption is more efficient, and provides a more efficient aerobic substrate than fat stores (JC DeLee, D Drez, Jr, Eds, Orthopedic Sports Medicine WB Saunders, Philadelphia, 1994) Cf Bicarbonate loading, Phosphate loading

carbon-14 dating PALEOANTHROPOLOGY A method for determining the age of life forms that have died in the relatively recent past, having a limit of less than 40 000 years (Science 1990; 247:798N&c) see Potassium-argon dating

carcinogen A chemical or other substance that has been shown to cause cancer in humans, or in experimental animals (ie a potential human carcinogen); a chemical is regarded as carcinogenic if it has been found to be a carcinogen or potential carcinogen by 1) The (US) National Toxicology Program or 2) The International Agency for Research on Cancer (IARC); the IARC classifies human carcinogens as

DNA-REACTIVE Aflatoxins, benzidine, betel quid with tobacco, chlorambucil, coal tars, cyclophosphamide, hexavalent chromium compounds, melphalan, MOPP, nickel compounds, thiotepa, vinyl chloride

EPIGENETIC Azathioprine, cyclosporine, diethylstilbestrol (DES), estrogens, oral contraceptives

UNCLASSIFIED Alcohol, arsenicals, benzene, mineral and shale oils

carcinogenesis ONCOLOGY A series of genotypic and phenotypic changes that occur in cells that are ultimately identified as being malignant, by virtue of having metastatic potential; the carcinogenic (cancerization) process is difficult to dissect as the genomic events, eg gene amplification, chromosome translocations, deletions, and point mutations, don't always translate into recognizable phenotypic changes; one model holds that cancer results from inducers and promoters in the form of chemicals, toxins, radiation and unknown environmental influences that impact on a genome that develops increasing susceptibility to environmental 'hits', responding with ↓ production of tumor suppressor proteins and ↑ production of proteins that 'drive' cell proliferation, often derived from proto-oncogenes; this multistep or multi-'hit' process requires genetic alterations in the form of anti-proto-oncogenes (dominant alterations) and inactivated tumor suppressor genes (recessive alterations), requiring up to ten distinct genomic mutations before malignant changes occur; in the well-characterized cancerization cascade for familial adenomatous polyposis, the first step involves a mutation of the MCC (mutated in colorectal cancer) gene on chromosome 5q21 (Science 1991; 251:1366), resulting in increased cell growth, followed by the loss of methylated sites, a mutation of the c-*ras* gene, loss of the DCC gene on chromosome 18 and the p53 gene on chromosome 17, during which time the cell morphology is transforming from an increasingly aggressive adenoma, carcinoma in situ, to eventually become malignant; see Cancerization, Inducer, One-hit/two-hit model, Proto-oncogenes, Tumor promoter, Tumor suppressor

carcinoid syndrome A symptom complex caused by carcinoids arising from the enterochromaffin system, most concentrated in midgut that release vasoactive substances, including bradykinin, histamine, prostaglandin, substance P and serotonin; serotonin and its metabolite, 5-HIAA, cause most of a carcinoid's symptoms, which usually arise in metastases, often from a primary ileal carcinoid metastatic to the liver CLINICAL Episodic cutaneous flushing beginning on the face, spreading to the trunk, later becoming telangiectatic; these symptoms are precipitated by alcohol, food, stress or liver palpation; other findings include diarrhea or obstructive symptoms, bronchospasms, pleural, peritoneal, retroperitoneal and endocardial fibrosis, the last involving the right valves and right ventricular wall, potentially evoking cardiac failure LABORATORY 5-HIAA in urine as high as 1000 mg/24 hours (normal, 2-8 mg/24hours)

carcinoma A malignancy of epithelial and occasionally neuroepithelial origin, a term that is often incorrectly equated to the more encompassing term 'cancer', which is used by the lay public for malignancy; carcinomas are subdivided according to the type of tissue in which they arise, eg glands (ergo adenocarcinoma), squamous epithelium (squamous cell carcinoma), and bladder epithelium (transitional cell carcinoma); Cf Cancer

carcinoma-associated antigens Antigenic alterations that result from the direct or indirect effects of certain malignancies on native antigens, transforming the epitopes to a form that is no longer recognized as self, eg 1) T antigen The precursor molecule of the blood group MN, enzymatically unmasked by sialidase-producing bacteria which do not occur in vivo and 2) Tn antigen The result of somatic mutation at the pluripotent hematopoietic stem cell level due to the blockage of the transfer of galactose to N-acetyl-D-galactosamine; Cf CA 15-3, CA19-9, CA 125, Tumor associated antigens

Note: Most subjects have naturally occurring antibodies directed against T and Tn antigens that may be exposed in carcinomas as well as T-cell lymphomas

carcinoma en cuirasse A markedly indurated ('scirrhous') carcinoma, involving a broad expanse of skin and subcutaneous breast tissue that is covered by papules and nodules evolving into morphea-like plaques PATHOLOGY Exuberant desmoplasia and few tumor cells; the cuirasse pattern is usually associated with carcinoma of the breast, but may also occur with carcinoma of the stomach, prostate, lung, uterus, and pancreas; see Scirrhous carcinoma

Cuirasse, French, Breast plate used in suits of armor during the Middle Ages

carcinoma ex-mixed tumor ORAL PATHOLOGY An epithelial malignancy arising in a pre-existing untreated mixed tumor of the salivary gland; metastases arise from the malignant component; ⅔ arise in the parotid gland; average age at diagnosis, 60; average age at diagnosis of 'benign' mixed tumor, 40 TREATMENT Surgical, often radical neck dissection; local recurrence occurs in ½; 5-year survival is 60%

carcinoma in situ SURGICAL PATHOLOGY A carcinoma in which all of the cytological and pathological criteria used to define malignancy have been met, but which has not yet invaded; CIS may regress or may be stable for a long period of time; although the cervix was one of the first locations where CIS was recognized, most other epithelia in the human economy have CIS lesions; in sexual epithelia, the term 'intraepithelial neoplasia' (IN), the least severe of which, grade I, corresponds to the popular term, mild dysplasia, which is followed by grade II IN (moderate dysplasia) and grade III IN (severe dysplasia), which is generally equated to carcinoma in situ; CIS is widely regarded as the lesion that immediately precedes microinvasive carcinoma; see Cervical intraepithelial neoplasia (aka CIN), Intraepithelial neoplasia, Microinvasive carcinoma; Cf Borderline tumors

carcinomatosis A preterminal condition characterized by the presence of disseminated, fulminant extension of multiple metastatic carcinomas

carcinosarcoma A malignancy of dual, ie epithelial and mesenchymal embryologic origin; although the term is firmly entrenched in the medical literature, the vast majority of these highly aggressive tumors are carcinomas and the cells display marked sarcoma-like spindling, thus the terms spindle cell carcinoma or sarcomatoid carcinoma are often more appropriate; the epithelial nature of the cells can often be confirmed by immunoperoxidase staining of cells or by electron microscopy; see Spindle cell carcinoma; Cf Pseudosarcoma

cardiac amyloidosis The infiltration of cardiac tissues with various types of amyloid proteins, often resulting in progressive heart failure; at autopsy, the infiltration of the atrium is universal resulting in atrial septal thickening recognized antemortem by echocardiography

cardiac 'cirrhosis' A hepatopathy characterized by hepatocellular atrophy, centrilobular necrosis and extensive fibrosis (the end-stage is virtually identical to posthepatitis cirrhosis), caused by repeated and/or prolonged congestive heart failure with increased venous pressure and reduced hepatic blood flow; see Nutmeg liver

cardiac concussion see Steering wheel injury

cardiac 'cripple' A person who has had an innocent cardiac murmur or normal physiologic variant of an EKG pattern that is misinterpreted as indicating cardiac disease or failure, whose physical activity is subsequently restricted and/or who receives various cardiac medications; see Innocent murmurs

'cardiac' enzymes A group of three enzymes used to monitor suspected myocardial ischemia, including creatine phosphokinase (CPK), for which the isoenzyme CK-MB has the greatest clinical import, although β-enolase may be equally useful; the rise in CPK is followed by aspartate aminotransferase (AST, formerly GOT-glutamate-oxaloacetate transaminase) and lactate dehydrogenase (LDH); following myocardial infarction, these three enzymes rise and fall in the same order over a period of a week; see β enolase, CK-MB, Flipped pattern, Troponin(s)

cardiac index The cardiac output of blood (in liters)/minute/m² surface area

cardiac injury panel A cost-effective, abbreviated battery of parameters for evaluating patients who may have suffered an acute myocardial infarct, measuring lactate dehydrogenase, creatine kinase and creatine kinase isoenzymes; see Organ panel

cardiac risk evaluation panel A group of tests determined to be cost-effective in stratifying a subject according to his risk for suffering atherosclerosis-related morbidity that measure serum levels of cholesterol, triglycerides, HDL-cholesterol and glucose; see Organ panel

cardiac sarcoidosis A relatively common finding in sarcoidosis occurring in 25% of patients, 5% of which is deemed of clinical importance; onset age 25-55; the changes include first-degree heart block, or bundle branch block, complete heart block, ventricular ectopy, myocardial disease with heart failure, and sudden death (N Engl J Med 1993; 328:792cPc)

cardiac series RADIOLOGY A group of four plain chest films (postero-anterior, lateral, right and left anterior oblique views) obtained after a 'barium swallow', used to evaluate the relative contribution of the chambers and vascular structures to the cardiac boundaries per se

cardiac tamponade An elevation of the mean right atrial pressure and near-equalization with the intrapericardail pressure; CT is a serious manifestation of pericardial effusion with a wide range of clinical and hemodynamic findings HEMODYNAMIC FINDINGS None to ↑↑↑ intrapericardial and intracardiac pressures, ↑ systemic vascular resistance, and ↓↓↓ cardiac output; CT may be associated with hypertension, which falls after pericardiocentesis (N Engl J Med 1992; 327:463oA)

cardiogenic shock The inability of the heart to deliver sufficient blood to the tissues to meet resting metabolic demands due to impaired pump function; when hemodynamic monitoring is available, cardiogenic shock is defined by a systolic blood pressure < 30 mm Hg, increased arteriovenous oxygen difference (> 5.5 ml/dL), and a depressed cardiac index (< 2.2 L/min/m² body surface) in the presence of an increased pulmonary capillary wedge pressure (>15 mm Hg) (N Engl J Med 1994; 330:1724Rv)

cardiolipin Diphosphatidyl glycerol A phospholipid present in mitochondrial and bacterial membranes that comprises the major antigen component of the Wasserman reaction for syphilis; see Anticardiolipin antibodies

cardiomyoplasty see Dynamic cardiomyoplasty

cardiopulmonary bypass CARDIOTHORACIC SURGERY A procedure in which the flow of blood through the heart is circumvented via a heart-lung machine, which is used in modern open heart surgery; aortic cannulation is used for arterial inflow and a single right atrial cannula is used for venous return to the pump; after the ascending aorta is clamped, cold potassium cardioplegia solution is infused into the oartic root, which both arrests and protects the heart during the heart surgery PLATELET DYSFUNCTION Exposure of blood to the extracorporeal circuit causes a transient ↑ in bleeding time and the release of α-granules which contain platelet factor 4 and β-thromboglobulin (**Arch Pathol Lab Med 1994; 118:411**OA)

cardiopulmonary resuscitation The restoration of cardiopulmonary function, usually following a cardiac arrest; components of CPR include chest compression and artificial ventilation and defibrillation Note: The success of CPR depends on where it occurs (in or out of hospital), underlying condition, and age of CPR victim; if an elderly person is informed of a relatively poor prognosis, they are less likely to chose CPR (**N Engl J Med 1994; 330o:545**SA, ibid 1992; 327:1075RV) METHODS Manual CPR, active compressioin-decompression-cardiopulmary resuscitation (ACD-CPR), vest CPR; see ABC method, CAB method

cardiovascular fitness A parameter used to determine a subject's cardiovascular 'reserve', which is commonly assessed using some form of exercise testing; improved cardiovascular fitness is associated with a reduced risk of myocardial infarction (**N Engl J Med 1994; 330:1550**OA) see Thallium (exercise) stress test

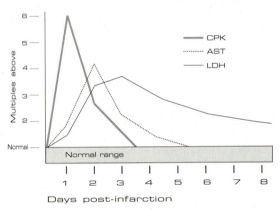

cardiac enzymes

cardioversion The conversion of a cardiac arrhythmia, usually a tachyarrhythmia to normal; the myocardial damage is directly proportional to the amount of applied energy, and the minimum (usually 25-50 joules) should be used; the synchronixed shock is delivered during the QRS complex; electrical cardioversion are most effective in terminating tachycardias due to defective reentry, eg atrial flutter and fibrillation, AV nodal entry, WPW syndrome, ventricular tachycardia, flutter, and fibrillation; the electric shock depolarizes all excitable myocardium, prolongs refractoriness, interrupts rentry circuits, and establishes electrical homogeneity; it is attempted in patients with atrial fibrillation in order to improve cardiac function, relieve symptoms, and ↓ the risk of thrombus formation; transesophageal echocardiography identifies patients with atrial emboli requiring short-term anticoagulation with heparin prior to cardioversion (**N Engl J Med 1993; 328:750**OA)

cardiovocal syndrome Hoarseness due to compression of the left laryngeal nerve between the aorta and dilated pulmonary artery, often first seen in infancy CLINICAL Symptoms are those of the underlying cardiac conditions including lesions of the aortic arch and congenital cardiac defects, mitral valve stenosis, coronary artery disease and hypertension

care map Critical pathway, see there

care path Critical pathway, see there

caries A destructive disease affecting the enamel and dentine linked to infection by *Streptococcus mutans* and microaerophilic organisms that thrive when protected by a layer of hardened dental plaque; caries is most common in the young who have refined carbohydrate-rich diets, especially when they 'snack' excessively (as this increases the oral pH); caries affects specific older population groups, including those with diabetes mellitus, cancer or other forms of immunocompromise; see Fluoridation, Periodontal disease, Plaque

carjacking A recent phenomenon in which a criminal steals an automobile and its driver, a crime similar to hijacking (hence the name). Its impact on public health and safety is not known, although it has been responsible for a number of deaths and injuries

carmustine BCNU, see there

carnal knowledge Coitus

L-carnitine β-hydroxy-γ-N trimethylammonium butyrate An amino acid required for the transport of long-chain fatty acids across the mitochondrial membrane for catabolism to CO_2 or ketone bodies, acting as an acyl (fatty acid) carrier; carnitine is endogenous (synthesized in the liver and kidney) or exogenous (red meat and dairy products) in origin

carnitine deficiency A deficiency state that may be caused by absence of carnitine palmityl transferase, or may occur in cobalamin deficiency, electron transfer flavoprotein deficiency, renal Fanconi syndrome, isovaleric acidemia, medium chain acylCoA dehydrogenase deficiency, methylmalonic and propionic acidemias and valproate therapy for seizure disorders may develop a toxicity syndrome with associated carnitine deficiency CLINICAL Myoglobinuria, renal failure, hypoglycemia, hypotonia, hepatomegaly, hepatic coma, congestive heart failure, neurologic changes (progressive myasthenia, lethargy, encephalopathy, coma, death), cardiomegaly, cardiac arrest, impaired growth, and development

carnosinase The enzyme [EC 3.4.13.4*] that hydrolyzes carnosine to histidine and β-alanine, without which there is toxic accumulation of carnosine

*Formally known as X-His dipeptidase, per the Nomenclature Committee of the International Union of Biochemistry and Molecular Biology

carnosinase deficiency Carnosinemia An AR [MIM 212200] condition characterized by severe psychomotor retardation, accompanied by myotonic and grand mal seizures TREATMENT Low-protein diet

carnosine A dipeptide of β-alanine and histidine that is concentrated in skeletal muscle of unknown function that may act as a buffer, stabilizing the pH of anaerobically contracting muscles

carob The sweet pulp of a Mediterranean evergreen leguminous tree, *Ceratonia siliquia*, which is a chocolate surrogate that is consumed by those who are either truly allergic to chocolate or who adhere to the tenet that chocolate is inherently evil; carob is high in palm kernel oil, ie a 'tropical oil' and therefore atherogenic; it is also high in sodium, and thus linked to hypertension; Cf Chocolate

carotid endarterectomy A surgical technique for relieving carotid artery stenosis by removal of atheromatous plaques from the carotid artery with the purpose of reducing the morbidity and mortality of cerebral ischemia; the technique was introduced in 1954 and has waxed and waned in popularity (107 000 performed in 1985, 68 000 in 1990); the NASCET* concluded that surgery plus medical therapy was superior to medical therapy alone in patients with ≥ 70% stenosis when compared to the diameter of the artery beyond the stenotic site (**N Engl J Med 1993; 328:221**oa**, 276**ED); in the US, 500 000 new strokes occur annually, with a total of 1.8 million long-term survivors, 60% of whom require assistance; 40% of first stroke victims remain permanently dependent; carotid endarterectomy is a procedure of scientific and cognitive uncertainty as to its ultimate benefit

*North American Symptomatic Carotid Endarterectomy Trial

carotid sleeper FORENSIC MEDICINE A form of restraint used to subdue overactive, unruly, violent or inebriated subjects with the intent of preventing them causing physical harm to themselves and others; the carotid sleeper consists of compression of the carotid baroreceptor resulting in asystole or marked slowing of the ventricular rate, a fall in the blood pressure and syncope; under controlled conditions, non-combative subjects lose consciousness within 6-10 seconds; see Neck hold; Cf Choke hold

Note: The carotid baroreceptor is located at the bifurcation of the internal carotid, the nerve endings of which join Hering's sinus nerve and the glossopharyngeal nerve, terminating in the cardio-inhibitory and vasomotor center in the medulla

β-carotene A natural retinoid, the increased intake of which induces benign xanthochromia and decreases photosensitivity in patients with protoporphyria; beta carotene is not as effective as isotretinoin (after high-dose tretinoin induction) in preventing the progression of oral leukoplakia (**N Engl J Med 1993; 328:150**oa) see Carotenoid

carotenoid CLINICAL NUTRITION Any of a family of nutrients that are precursors of vitamin A and have antioxidant activity; although beta carotene[1] is the best known, 600 carotenoids have been identified; 40 are common in fruits and vegetables[2]; high carotenoid[3] consumption is associated with a reduced incidence of bladder, colon, lung[4] and skin cancers and growth of cancer cells in general (**New York Times 21 Feb 1995; C1**)

[1]It had been long assumed that beta carotene was the major carotenoid responsible for the reduced incidence of strokes, cardiovascular disease, and cancers linked to the increased consumption of vegetables [2]Tomato juice is highest in carotenoids, followed by kale, collard greens, spinach sweet potato, chard, watermelon, carrots, and pumpkin [3]which include alpha carotene, beta carotene, betacryptoxanthin, lutein, and lycopene [4]The cause-and-effect relationship is not so clear; in one recently reported and well-designed study from Finland, men who were heavy smokers and received beta carotene as a vitamin supplement had an INCREASE in both the incidence of lung cancer (18% ↑) and an overall mortality (8% ↑)

carpal tunnel SURGICAL ANATOMY *Canalis carpi* [NA6], carpal canal A fibro-osseous tunnel on the volar surface of the wrist where the carpal bones form a concavity bridged by the flexor retinaculum; the carpal tunnel is formed anteriorly by the flexor retinaculum and posteriorly by the carpal bones and ligaments, which is the conduit for flexor tendons of the hand and median nerve from the forearm to the hand

carpal tunnel syndrome A syndrome of painful paresthesiae of the median nerve, affecting the hands and fingers, in particular the index, long, and ring fingers; it is most common in pregnant or post-menopausal ♀; if prolonged, it may result in partial atrophy of the lateral half of the thenar eminence with weakness of abduction and opposition of the thumb; it is either as a chronic idiopathic flexor tenosynovitis or as part of systemic conditions, eg acromegaly, amyloidosis, DM, granulomatous disease, hypothyroidism, mucopolysaccharidosis I-S, myxedema, obesity, pregnancy, or local processes (ganglia, bone dislocations, lipoma, exuberant callus formation in wrist fractures, eg Colles or Smith fractures, gout, pseudogout and rheumatoid arthritis causing flexor tenosynovitis EXAMINATION Phalen‡ and Tinel‡ signs CLINICAL Most symptomatic at night, hypesthesia of median nerve region, thenar muscle atrophy, slowing of nerve conduction and EMG studies; the median nerve is a 'mixed' nerve and sensory loss precedes motor dysfunction, affecting sensation in the palmar aspect of the radial 3½ fingers DDx Proximal sites of nerve entrapment, eg Pancoast tumor, pronator

teres syndrome TREATMENT, EARLY Wrist splint, injection of corticosteroids, eg β-methasone TREATMENT, LATE Longitudinal section of the epineurium and flexor retinaculum in the face of thenar atrophy DIAGNOSIS Electromyography is the 'gold standard' test, which detects ↓ conduction velocity

carpet tack appearance DERMATOLOGY A descriptor for the multiple small keratin plugs (corresponding to the follicular openings) attached to the underside of scales removed from skin affected by discoid lupus erythematosus, or pemphigus foliaceus

Carr-Purcell sequence MRI A sequence of 90° radiofrequency pulses followed by repeated 180° radiofrequency pulses, producing a train of spin echoes that is used to measure T2; see Magnetic resonance imaging

Carr-Purcell-Meiboon-Gill sequence MRI A modification of the Carr-Purcell radiofrequency pulse sequence with 90° phase shift in the rotating frames of reference between the 90° pulse and subsequent 180° pulses, reducing the accumulating effects of imperfections in the 180° pulses; suppression of effects of pulse error accumulation can also be achieved by alternating the phases of the 180° pulses by 180°; see Magnetic resonance imaging

carrot cells A colloquial term for the elongated angulated cells seen in granulosa cell tumors of the ovary, which is a 'soft' criterion differentiating these tumors from the far less common ovarian lymphoma

carry-over artefact SURGICAL PATHOLOGY An artefact consisting of tissue fragments from an unrelated specimen or area of the same specimen, which is carried into a section of tissue being examined by the pathologist; carryovers are introduced at the time of the gross examination and are largely due to suboptimal technique by the 'grosser'; once introduced, they may lead to misinterpretation of histological findings

cartilage-hair hypoplasia syndrome Metaphyseal chondrodysplasia, McKusick type An AR [MIM 250250] form of short-limbed dwarfism, common in the Amish, an ethnic group of German descent located in Pennsylvania CLINICAL Bone dysplasia, bradycarpia, redundant skin, sparse hair, defective pigment, malabsorption, and death by age 20 IMMUNE DEFECTS Neutropenia with defective T-cell-mediated immunity, potentially fatal vaccinia, progressive vaccine-related poliomyelitis, defective antibody production and severe combined immunodeficiency, related to defective adenosine deaminase activity TREATMENT Antibiotics, IFN, bone marrow transplantation; see Adenosine deaminase deficiency

cartoon Any schematic, usually in color, representation of a biological process or molecule, presented either in a journal or in a lecture; Cf 'Nettergram'

Note: Cartoon is traditionally defined in the US as either a panel in a comic strip, or a satirical drawing with a caption commenting on public or political matters or an animated 'short' film with such characters as Elmer Fudd, Popeye and Tom and Jerry

cartwheel *adjective* Pertaining or referring to a pattern that has a vague roundness, from which short curved radiations appear to emanate **CARTWHEEL NUCLEUS** Peripheral chromatin clumping, characteristic of plasma cell nuclei **CARTWHEEL PATTERN** 'Whorled' cellular arrangement described in neurogenic tumors, less commonly in astroblastomas*; see Pinwheel pattern, Storiform pattern **CARTWHEEL PIGMENTATION** Ocular fundus A non-specific 'whorling' of pigment in the fundus, seen in tyrosinase positive albinism, yellow-mutant albinism, Chediak-Higashi syndrome and Hermansky-Pudlak syndromes

Note: A cartwheel pattern is virtually identical to 'pinwheel' and 'storiform' patterns; separation of tumors based on these highly subjective criteria is unsatisfying exercise

carving out HEALTH CARE ENVIRONMENT A colloquial term for questionable and/or frankly illegal practice of allowing

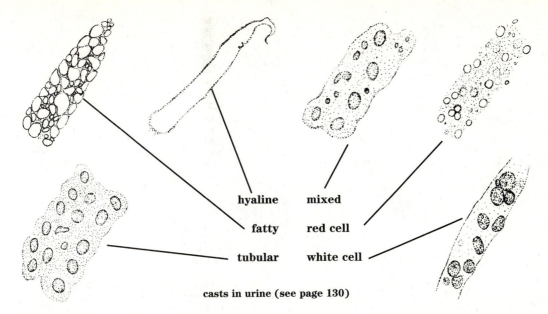

hyaline   mixed

fatty   red cell

tubular   white cell

casts in urine (see page 130)

healthy individuals in small-employer groups to buy lower cost health insurance policies, while workers who are sicker must purchase more expensive high-risk pool coverage (Am Med News 26 October 1992, p7)

cascade A generic term for any of a number of molecular systems that is capable of self-propagation or amplification; once a cascade is initiated, it may continue to be amplified through positive feedback loops and pathways until it is downregulated by local mechanisms often in the form of proteolytic enzymes; cascades in humans include the coagulation, complement, kinase and electron transport (mediated within the mitochondria via cytochrome oxidases) cascades

cascade effect HEALTH CARE A constellation of adverse effects that may be triggered by diagnostic testing; while the result of a false-positive test may ultimately prove to be benign, false positivity evokes a cascade of progressively more invasive, and expensive diagnostic tests evoking what has been called the Ulysses syndrome, see there (N Engl J Med 1992; 327:424oA)

cascade testing LABORATORY MEDICINE The sequential use of a group of tests to establish the diagnosis of a disease or process, eg fetal lung maturity; the use of a testing cascade is required when the 'gold standard' methodology is technically demanding and/or costly and the diagnosis can under most circumstances be established by simpler or more cost-effective strategies (Mayo Clin Proc 1995; 70:183RV)

case-control study EPIDEMIOLOGY A study that begins with a disease and searches for past differences in exposure (or other characteristics) between groups of affected and non-affected individuals; this retrospective study method is useful when few clues exist as to causation or when the evidence implicating a particular agent is strong but the actual number of patients is too small to allow a prospective study; see Epidemiology

case-fatality ratio EPIDEMIOLOGY A value calculated as 100 cases of a disease 'X', divided by the number of persons with the disease who died in a given period of time; the resulting ratio is equal to the rate of a disease's occurrence; see Cause-fatality ratio

case manager HEALTH CARE ADMINISTRATION An individual, usually a nonphysician, who is employed by a managed care organization to coordinate medical care and benefits in cases (eg head injuries, malignancy) that have the potential for incurring high cost (N Engl J Med 1995; 332:581RV)

Note: Because CMs are employed by a managed care organization, their loyalties may lie with minimizing costs at the expense of the patient's long-term welfare; some physicians have expressed concern that CMs have acquired too much power, and may impede quality health care

case mix The characteristics of a health care facility's patient population for a given period of time, classified by disease, diagnostic or therapeutic procedures performed, method of payment, duration of hospitalization, intensity and type of services provided; in the US, a hospital's case mix is based on the diagnosis-related groups, see DRGs

case-mix adjustment HEALTH CARE FINANCING The placement of patients in groups according to the anticipated use of health care resources based on the diagnoses recorded during one year of care; the failure to adjust for case-mixes in a physician's practice profile may result in an overestimate of variation and misidentification of patient outliers (JAMA 1994; 272:871oA)

case-mix group HEALTH CARE FINANCING A classifier used in the Canadian health care system to stratify reimbursement for a particular set of helalth care services (eg diagnosis, therapy) based on the costs of its actual costs; CMGs are similar to the American DRG (diagnosis-related group)

case-mix index HEALTH CARE REIMBURSEMENT An average of the relative weights assigned to its patients' diagnosis-related groups and is a measure of the complexity of illness in a hospital's discharged patients; hospital populations with more complex illnesses have higher case mixes and thus receive higher Medicare reimbursement; see 'Creep', DRGs and 'Optimization'

caseous debris Caseation Cheesy, dry yellow-white grumous material, resulting from combined coagulation and liquefactive necrosis, classically associated with TB, but also seen in histoplasmosis

Note: The keratinaceous debris within epidermal inclusion cysts has a similar consistency

cassette A segment of eukaryotic DNA that can be substituted for by another sequence by transposition; the cassette model serves to explain the expression of various mating types of primitive organisms

cassette mutagenesis MOLECULAR BIOLOGY A technique where point mutations are induced in oligonucleotide segments of DNA or tRNA that are then analyzed for loss or gain of functional properties (generally with repressor or enhancer proteins) to determine 'allowable' substitutions in the nucleotide structure

Note: Three-dimensional analysis of molecular surfaces helps understand biological interactions; the protein sequence bears the information needed to determine its three-dimensional structure

CAST Cardiac arrhythmia suppression trial A long-term multicenter study that examined the question of whether suppression of asymptomatic or mildly symptomatic post-MI ventricular ectopia and arrhythmia reduces the incidence of sudden death; some class I-C antiarrhythmic agents, eg encainide and flecainide, actually increase post-MI mortality (N Engl J Med 1992 327:1818c)

CAST-II A second study (see CAST-I) that evaluated the suppression of asymptomatic or mildly symptomatic ventricular premature depolarizations in survivors of myocardial infarction using moricizine; CAST-II was halted when 14-day treatment with moricizine, as delineated by the study protocol was associated with a five-fold increase in mortality (N Engl J Med 1992; 327:227oA)

cast A translucent proteinaceous mold of the renal tubules seen in the urine, which is markedly increased in renal disease, the nature of which is a crude indicator of the type of renal disease; the matrix of all casts is composed of albumin, small (< 50 kD) globulins and glycoprotein secreted by Henle's ascending loop and the distal tubule together forming Tamm-Horsfall protein, uromodulin; casts are classified according to type of

1) MATRIX, eg hyaline or waxy

2) INCLUSIONS, eg crystals, fat, granules, hemosiderin and melanin

3) PIGMENTS, eg bilirubin, drugs, hemoglobin, myoglobin and

4) CELLS, eg bacteria, red cells, leukocytes, tubular epithelial cells; in general, red cell casts are associated with glomerular injury, white cell casts with parenchymal injury and broad casts with dilated collecting ducts, as occurs in chronic pyelonephritis

cast syndrome Superior mesenteric artery syndrome, see there

Castleman's disease A heterogeneous group of multicentric lymphoproliferative disorders of unknown etiology EPIDEMIOLOGY A disease of young adults LABORATORY ↑ IL-6 in circulation and in tissue CLINICAL Lymphadenopathy, hepatosplenomegaly, anemia, hypoalbuminemia, hypergammaglobulinemia PATHOLOGY Hyaline-vascular type, and plasma cell type, localized or multicentric TREATMENT Anti-IL-6 antibodies may alleviate symptoms (N Engl J Med 1994; 330:602oA); surgical resection is definitive therapy

Note: Clinically aggressive forms of lymphoid hyperplasia may have features of Castleman's disease, and may be 'driven' by EBV and accompanied by clonal rearrangements of DNA (Diagn Mol Pathol 1993; 2:57)

castor oil An oil that is cold-pressed from the kernel of the seeds of *Ricinus communis**, which contains glycerides of ricinoleic and isoricinoleic acids, eg dihydroxystearin, isoricinolein, palmitin, and triricinolein; it has been used externally as an emollient and internally as a laxative

*The *R communis* seed contains the highly toxic principles, ricin and ricinine

CAT 1) Children's apperception test; see Psychologic testing 2) Chloramphenicol acetyl transferase, a 'reporter' gene 3) Cholesterol acyl transferase 4) Computerized axial tomography

cat *Felis catus* A mammal of medical interest that is

1) A model for some human diseases, eg dermatosparasix, a defect in the conversion of type I procollagen to collagen, or mannosidosis, a condition affecting the short-hair cat and Niemann-Pick disease, type I, which affects Siamese cats

2) A vector for a) Bacteria, eg *Pasteurella multocida*, *Yersinia pestis*, *Campylobacter jejuni*, *Francisella tularensis* b) Fungi, eg *Microsporum canis*, *Sporothrix schenckii* c) Parasites, eg *Ancylostoma braziliense*, *A caninum*, *Brugia pahangi**, *Clonorchis sinensis*, *Cryptosporidium* spp, *Dipylidium caninum*, *Dracunculiasis medinensis**, *Echinococcus vogeli*, *E multilocularis*, *Gnathostoma spinigerum*, *Isospora belli*, *Leptospira* spp, *Opistorchis felineus*, *Sarcoptes scabiei*,

Toxoplasma gondii, Trypanosoma cruzi*, Wuchereria bancrofti ; see Cat scratch disease

*Parasites that have part of their life cycle in humans

cat-bite fever An infection by *Pasteurella multocida*, an oral saprobe of felines, forming an abscess at the inoculation site, potentially causing focal arthralgia (other complications are rare); Cf Cat scratch disease

CAT box see CACA box

cat-cry syndrome Cri du chat syndrome, see there

cat eye syndrome Anal atresia-coloboma of iris syndrome An AD [MIM 115470] condition characterized by vertical iris coloboma (hence, 'cat eye'), microphthalmia, pale optic discs, ocular hypertelorism, downward slanting of palpebral fissures, preauricular fistula, anal atresia, umbilical hernia, mental retardation and variable cardiac and renal defects MOLECULAR PATHOLOGY A small extra acrocentric chromosome is typical, possibly from chromosome 14; most have 1+ extra copies of chromosome fragment 22q11

cat's-eye reflex Leukocoria A white reflection seen through the pupil in 1) Retinoblastoma (due to the tumoral deformity of the fundus) 2) End-stage retrolental fibroplasia (caused by a flattened to nodular scarred white retrolental membrane that is nonreactive to light; salvage of vision in either is rare with a persistent anterior persistent hyperplastic primary vitreous humor, due to noninvolution of the fetal hyaloid artery and accompanying fibrovascular tissue; leukocoria also occurs in visceral larva migrans due to *Toxocara* species

cat's paw sign A fanciful term for the radiocontrast findings of intramural hemorrhage of the small intestine, in which there is short length of splaying in the radiocontrast column; see Stacked coin sign; Cf Coiled spring

CAT-signal bioassay VIROLOGY An assay in which an indicator cell contains long terminal repeats (LTR) of a retrovirus, eg HIV-1, linked to chloramphenicol acetyltransferase (CAT); when HIV-1 is added, CAT increases in the medium

cat scratch disease A self-limited regional lymphadenitis of children and adolescents, caused by close contact with or being scratched by household pets; 95% are due to cats, 5% to dogs EPIDEMIOLOGY ± 22 000/year (US) 2 000 hospitalizations; most cases occur in those under age 20, more common in ♂, often in fall and winter; CSD is associated with owning a kitten; fleas may be the vector of transmission CLINICAL Erythematous papules at the inoculation sites, eg hands and forearms, anorexia, malaise, fever, parotid swelling, maculopapular rashes, regional or generalized lymphadenopathy, splenomegaly, encephalopathy; the agent was identified at the Armed Forces Institute of Pathology (Science 1983; 221:1403) as a small, pleomorphic gram-negative bacillus and later cultured in a biphasic (broth then agar) brain-heart infusion medium at 30-32°C PATHOLOGY Lymphoid hyperplasia, granuloma and abscess formation DIAGNOSIS History, indirect fluorescent antibody test for antibodies to *Rochalimaea henselae* is 88% sensitivity; 94% specificity (N Engl J Med 1993; 329:8oA) skin-test TREATMENT Gentamycin, ciprofloxacin (JAMA 1991; 265:1563); Cf Bacillary angiomatosis, Cat bite fever

catalytic antibody A biologically selective enzyme in which catalytic activity is introduced into the highly selective binding site of a monoclonal antibody, allowing enzymatic catalysis of pre-determined specificity; the specificity is achieved by site-directed mutagenesis (ie substitution of an amino acid into a combining site thereby introducing a catalytic residue); other strategies for producing specific catalysts include genetic modification of active enzyme sites and chemical modification of biological or synthetic receptors bearing catalytic groups; see Abzymes

catalytic motif One of a family of oligopeptides, eg Asp-

His-Ser and Asp-His-Zn that correspond to specific catalytic sites in an enzyme, which can be studied by site-directed mutagenesis to probe the chemical function of the amino acid residues or by transplanting the catalytic motifs into antibody combining sites (Nature 1990; 348:589c)

catalytic RNA An RNA molecule that can act as its own enzyme, ie a 'ribozyme', cutting out introns, splicing and assembling itself without the aid of protein enzymes

Note: The discovery of this unexpected mechanism of RNA action netted its discoverers (T Cech, University of Colorado and S Altman, Yale University) the 1989 Nobel prize in Chemistry (Science 1989; 246:325)

catastrophic benefits HEALTH CARE INDUSTRY The second tier of health insurance or a health care plan, where the basic (usually non-hospitalization) medical services form a first tier of coverage; once the benefits have been exhausted from the first tier, coverage is provided under the catastrophic portion of the policy or plan, where 'deductible' fees must be paid and co-payment requirements met; see Wrap-around policy

catastrophic health insurance A health insurance plan proposed by US Congressman Pepper that would include all the coverage provided in the Pepper Commission plan (see there) as well as providing long-term care and medical coverage for all US citizens who are currently uninsured; while the plan is noble, the cost would be very high

catastrophic illness Any morbid condition that results in health care costs exceeding a person's income and/or compromising his financial independence, reducing him to subsistence or near-poverty levels; such illnesses are usually life-threatening and may leave significant residual disability, eg AIDS, major burns, trauma with residual paralysis or coma and preterminal malignancy

catastrophe theory A purely mathematical formulatiion that was claimed by its developer René Thom to explain a broad range of phenomena displaying abrupt discontinuities, from the metamorphosis of caterpillars into butterflies and the collapse of civilization; by the 1970s CT had run its course, and essentially discredited (Sci Am 1995; 272/6:104)

catchment area HEALTH CARE INDUSTRY A region served by a health care facility or health care plan that is delineated by population distribution, geographic boundaries, or transportation patterns

Note: A facility's catchment demographics is modified by whether it provides secondary (in which case the traditional boundary definitions are valid) or tertiary care where referral patterns often define the catchment area

category X drug CLINICAL PHARMACOLOGY A therapeutic agent that has a confirmed teratogenic effect that is contraindicated for use during pregnancy, eg vitamin A congeners used for severe recalcitrant acne, which causes a characteristic clinical complex in neonates; see Retinoic acid embryopathy

catenins A family of proteins that are thought to have a major role in regulating cell-cell adhesion because of their interaction with E-cadherin and the actin cytoskeleton (N Engl J Med 1994; 330:1580RA)

caterpillar cell A descriptor for a cell with an elongated vesicular nucleus, central wavy chromatin and finger-like projections to the nuclear membrane, a morphological variant of the Anitschkow cardiac histiocyte, 'owl eye' cell, aggregates of which are known as Aschoff nodules

caterpillar dermatitis An allergic reaction evoked by contact with the urticariogenic hairs of the larvae and spines of larvae of brown-tail, flannel, Io, tussock, and other moths

caterpillar hump artery A fanciful descriptor for a variant of the right hepatic artery that may be mistaken surgically for the cystic artery

catgut SURGERY An absorbable suture material obtained from the submucosa of bovine intestine, which both evokes considerable inflammation and tends to potentiate infections; it loses its strength quickly and unpredictably in sutured intestine and in infected wounds due to hydrolysis; catgut is not widely used in modern surgery; Cf Silk

cathartic colon A colon affected by long-term abuse of cathartics and laxatives CLINICAL Intractable diarrhea with hypokalemia, protein-losing enteropathy, cachexia, hypogammaglobulinemia, finger-clubbing and potentially increased constipation, resulting in a vicious cycle of increased use of purgatives by the patient RADIOLOGY Barium studies may be normal or have complete loss of haustral markings, or mimic ulcerative colitis PATHOLOGY Flattening of the mucosa without epithelial destruction, loss of haustra, a mucosa likened to shark skin (as well as snake, lizard and toad skin) and melanosis coli if the agent is of the anthracene group, eg cascara, senna; chronic inflammation and fatty infiltration of the submucosa, hypertrophy of the muscularis mucosa, occasionally, degeneration of Auerbach's plexus and lipofuscin deposits

cathepsin(s) A group of lysosomal proteinases or endopeptidases that function optimally at an acidic pH, stored within the azurophilic granules of neutrophils; cathepsin B functions at an acidic pH and degrades matrix glycoproteins; cathepsin D functions at acidic pH and is a heterodimeric 34-kD and 14-kD estrogen-induced lysosomal protease produced in breast tissue; a 52-kD cathepsin D precursor molecule is increased in hormone-dependent breast carcinoma, the serum levels of which are predictive of early recurrence and death in node-negative cases; high levels have an increased risk of 2.6 for recurrence and a relative risk of 3.9 for death; Cf Metastasis

catheter ablation therapy CARDIOLOGY A nonsurgical technique in which an electrode catheter is introduced into the veins of the arms or legs and advanced into the heart; if an abnormal electric pathway of depolarization is identified in the conduction system, as is commonly the case with supraventricular tachycardia or WPW syndrome, the defective pathway is 'zapped' with a high intensity (> 25 joules) radiofrequency wave to permanently neutralize it.

cathode ray tube see Video display terminal

caudal block OBSTETRIC ANESTHESIOLOGY Extradural anesthesia that is administered as a single injection or as a continuous drip; CBs are technically demanding and require more anesthetic than other forms of locoregional anesthesia

cauliflower ear An external ear deformity caused by inadequate treatment, ie through-and-through stitches, of an otohematoma, commonly due to contact sport-related trauma in adolescents or falls in the elderly and children, which occurs as the natural evolution of hematomas in this site is towards granulation tissue and exuberant fibrosis; primary cauliflower ear occurs in polychondritis

cauliflower lesion A generic term for any broad-based pedunculated polypoid mass that grows freely into a lumen or hollow viscus, including sclerosing stromal tumor of the uterus, colonic adenocarcinoma, papillary transitional cell carcinoma of the urinary bladder, villous adenoma of the colon

causation MEDICAL MALPRACTICE The establishment of a cause-and-effect relation between the allegedly negligent act and the purported injuries; see Malpractice

cause-facility rate EPIDEMIOLOGY The number of deaths due to a disease per unit of time (usually one year) divided by either 1000 or 10 000 people with the disease; see Case-fatality rate

cause of death FORENSIC MEDICINE The reason or event that precipitates a person's death, which is divided for medicolegal purposes into **PROXIMATE CAUSE OF DEATH** The most important, immediate, direct or actual cause, or last event or act that occurred prior to the chain of events leading to death **IMMEDIATE CAUSE OF DEATH** The concluding or final event that actually produces death; see Death

cavalry fracture A crushing plantar-flexion fracture of the tarso-metatarsal joint that occurs when a violent force is applied to the heel along the axis of the foot when the toe is fixed; such fractures were common in the battlefield when a cavalryman was thrown from and then had his foot pinned under his fallen horse; tarso-metatarsal fractures are now more commonly associated with automobiles, stepladders, or in misguided steps

cave disease A trivial name for pulmonary histoplasmosis that affects explorers of bat-infested caves, as bat dung is an ideal growth medium for *Histoplasma capsulatum*

CAVEAT Coronary Angioplasty versus Excisional Artherectomy Trial (see N Engl J Med 1993; 329:273ED, 1891c)

caveola MEMBRANE PHYSIOLOGY A 50-100 nm flask-shaped invagination in the plasma membrane which functions as a membrane-bound organelle (plural = caveolae) that opens into the cytosol; caveolae contain a wide range of proteins, eg CD36, caveolin, glycosylphosphatidylinositol, protein kinase C, and over 25 others, some of which have been implicated in human diseases, including atheromatosis, DM, and Duchenne muscular dystrophy (Science News 1994; 146:4); caveolae are most prominent on the surface of endothelial cells, smooth muscle cells, and fibroblasts, but are presumed to present on all cells; caveolae are formed from three different proteins: 1) Folate receptor, 2) Caveolin, and 3) An IP3 (inositol 1,4,5-triphosphate) receptor-like molecule (Science & Medicine 1995; 2/3:80) see Endocytosis

caveolin MEMBRANE PHYSIOLOGY A 22-kD protein component of caveolae that is a substrate for tyrosine phosphorylation, eg by v-*src*, and is thought to play a role in cell signal transduction (Science & Medicine 1995; 2/3:80) see Caveola, Endocytosis

cavernous sinus syndrome NEUROLOGY Parasellar syndrome, orbital apex syndrome A condition caused by mass lesions of the cavernous sinus and/or parasellar region resulting in pressure on cranial nerves III, IV, part of V, and VI CLINICAL Oculomotor nerve paralysis (ophthalmoplegia, ptosis, mydriasis, and anesthesia of the eyeball, characerized by the loss of the corneal reflex), ophthalmic branch of the trigeminal nerve, often accompanied by blindness and cortical analgesia DIAGNOSIS CT, MRI scans PATHOLOGY Aneurysms, cysts, infection, inflammation, thrombosis, trauma, and tumors, vascular (see N Engl J Med 1993; 328:266cpc) see Tolosa-Hunt syndrome

cavity BALLISTICS The permanent cavity along a bullet's trajectory is caused by the bullet per se, the temporary cavity is related to tissue stretching up to 11 times the diameter of the bullet (in contrast to the 30- to 40-fold increased diameter stated in older literature); the kinetic energy transferred during the short life of the temporary cavity is more destructive to parenchymal tissues, eg spleen, liver than deformable tissue, eg muscle, lung and fat; the explosion-related pressure generated in the temporary cavity is about 4 atmospheres (previously stated to be 100 atmospheres); see Ballistics

'cayenne pepper' lesion A descriptor for the hyperpigmented and petechial lesions of the lower legs, arms and trunk, due to idiopathic capillaritis, seen in Schamberg's disease (pigmented purpuric dermatitis) or secondary to drug reactions

CBAVD Congenital bilateral absence of vas deferens, see there

CBC Complete blood count LABORATORY MEDICINE The automated analysis of certain parameters of the cells in the circulation, often performed by a Coulter counter; the CBC includes a count of the red cells, white cells and platelets, hemoglobin, hematocrit, mean corpuscular hematocrit, hemoglobin and volume in the red cells, and a differential count of white cells, dividing them into lymphocytes, monocytes, granulocytes, basophils and eosinophils

Also 1) Carbenicillin 2) Cerebro-buccal commissure 3) Children's behavior checklist (or characteristics)

CCAAT Box MOLECULAR BIOLOGY One of the cis-regulatory elements that mediates transcription; the CCAAT and GGGCG ('promoter-proximal') sequences are located 60-120 nucleotides upstream from the transcription start site and necessary for optimal promoter activity; a family of proteins bind to the CCAAT and the SP1 protein binds to the GGGCG

CCAM Congenital cystic adenomatoid malformation, see there

CCAT Canadian Coronary Artherectomy Trial (see N Engl J Med 1993; 329:273ED)

C cells Neuroectodermal calcitonin-secreting cells that are derived from the APUD system, located laterally in the thyroid, and in the appropriate setting, give rise to medullary carcinoma of the thyroid; in submammalian beasts, C-cells are in a separate organ, the ultimobranchial body; see Calcitonin

CCHF see Crimean-Congo hemorrhagic fever

CCK Cholecystokinin

CCNU Cyclonexyl-chloroethyl-nitrosourea A highly toxic chemotherapeutic agent that is used in adjunctive therapy of high-grade astrocytomas and may be used in NHL, malignant melanoma, multiple myeloma, brain neoplasms, GI carcinomas SIDE EFFECTS Nausea, vomiting, ↓↓↓ platelets, ↓↓↓ WBCs, secondary leukemia, pulmonary fibrosis, renal failure; see BCNU, Nitrogen mustards

CD Cluster(s) of differentiation A nomenclature system for surface antigens of human leukocytes, which have been characterized by monoclonal antibodies, allowing leukocytes and other hematopoietic cells to be categorized the expression on the cell surface of one or more to be classified according to lineage, where most cells express more than one surface antigen; the 'w' (workshop) designation that follows some CDs indicates an incompletely characterized antigen

CD1 A family of major histocompatibility complex class I-like molecules expressed on the surface of immature thymocytes, Langerhans cells, and certain B cells; CD1 is a ligand for T-cell subpopulation, is present in the intestinal epithelium adjacent to the gut-associated lymphoid tissue (GALT) and may be involved in epithelial immunity

CD1a A 49-kD thymocyte antigen associated with the 12-kD β_2 microglobulin; CD1a is present on 60-90% of thymocytes and the Langerhans cell of the skin, and may be expressed on some T-cell leukemias and lymphomas

CD2 T11 A 50-kD molecule involved in cell adhesion, which is the receptor that binds to the leukocyte function associated antigen-3 (LFA-3) or CD58; CD2 is a 'pan-T' cell marker, ie is found on most T cells and corresponds to the E-rosette receptor; CD2 is present on ± 80% of normal lymphocytes, and reacts with virtually all peripheral lymphocytes and with a subset of NK cells

CD3 T3 A 'pan-T' cell antigen, ie an antigen present on virtually all T cells (60-85% of peripheral T cells, 20-85% of thymocytes), consisting of multiple 16- to 28-kD in length polypeptide chains, designated gamma, sigma, epsilon, and eta, which are closely associated with each other and the T-cell receptor (CD4); most antibodies against the CD3 antigen are directed against the 20-kD epsilon chain; see

Pan-T cell markers; CD3 is also present on Purkinje cells in the cerebellum; it is a constant component of the T-cell receptor, and is noncovalently linked to polymorphic structure designated Ti

CD4 A 59–62-kD surface glycoprotein antigen present on T helper/inducer cells (60% of peripheral T cells), 80-95% of thymocytes, and monocytes; CD4 participates in adhesion of T cells to target cells and is involved in thymic maturation and transmission of intracellular signals during T cell activation by the class II major histocompatibility complex; CD4 has inducer or helper activity for T cell, B cell and macrophage interactions and evokes T-cell proliferation in response to soluble antigens or autologous non-T cells, providing appropriate signals for B-cell proliferation and differentiation into immunoglobulin-secreting cells; CD4 is also a high-affinity receptor for HIV-1's gp120, binding at amino acid residues 42 to 55 of the NH_2 terminal domain, which has an immunoglobulin-like fold similar to the complementarity-determining region of the kappa light chain; CD4 also binds immunoglobulins independently of the Fc receptor , and is an accessory to the T-cell receptor and a receptor for p56Ick, a cellular tyrosine kinase receptor with immunoglobulin-like domains

CD4/CD8 ratio The ratio of circulating T lymphocytes with 'helper cell' determinants (CD4 antigen) on the cell surface to T lymphocytes with 'suppressor cell' determinants (CD8 antigen); the maturational step or partition between CD4 and CD8 cell lines is regarded as irreversible, although a small percentage of circulating CD3 cells coexpress both CD4 and CD8 molecules); the explanation for this coexpression is that in most CD8 T cells the CD4 genes are methylated and therefore 'terminally' repressed, while in the CD4 and CD8 coexpressing cells, the CD4 genes are not methylated and CD4 expression is inducible by IL-4 (**Nature 1991; 349:533**)

CD4 cell CD4+ lymphocyte A circulating T lymphocyte with a 'helper' phenotype; in AIDS patients, the levels of CD4+ cells is a crude indicator of immune status and susceptibility to certain AIDS-related conditions, and these patients may suffer Kaposi sarcoma as the CD4+ cells fall below 0.3 X 10^9/L (US: 300/mm³), non-Hodgkin's lymphoma below 0.15 X 10^9/L (US: 150/mm³), *Pneumocystis carinii* below 0.1 X 10^9/L (US: 100/mm³) and MAIS (*Mycobacterium avium-intercellulare*) below 0.05 X 10^9/L (US: 50/mm³)(**N Engl J Med 1991; 324:1332**); the absolute number of CD4+ T cells in the peripheral circulation is a critical decision point for beginning certain prophylactic therapies in patients with AIDS: Antiretroviral prophylaxis is < 500/mm³, *Pneumocystis carinii* pneumonia < 200/mm³, *Mycobacterium avium* complex, and cytomegalovirus < 100/mm³; the gold standard method for enumerating CD4+ lymphocytes is flow cytometry DISADVANTAGES (of measuring CD4 cell levels) Low specimen throughput (± 40/day), high cost prevents its use in developing nations; alternate methods for quantifying CD4+ cells are in development or implementation, including those that lyse the cells and measure the total CD4+ (including that on monocytes) by an enzyme immunoassay (**CAP Today October 1993**)

CD4 immunoadhesin A molecule formed by fusing CD4 (the receptor for HIV) with an immunoglobulin that both binds gp120 and blocks HIV; this synthetic molecule has therapeutic potential as it mediates ADCC towards HIV-infected but not uninfected cells and is easily transported across the primate placenta

CD4+ T-lymphocytopenia Idiopathic CD4+ T-lymphocytopenia, see there

CD4 T cells Helper T cells, see there

CD4(178)-PE40 A recombinant protein that consists of the HIV envelope glycoprotein-binding region of CD4

linked to the translocation and ADP-ribosylation domains of *Pseudomonas aeruginosa* exotoxin A; this hybrid toxin ('magic bullet') selectively binds to and destroys HIV-1-infected human T cells (in vitro) after productive infection of T cells has occurred, an event signaled by the presence of viral gp120 at the cell surface, and thus has potential currency as an HIV-virostatic agent

CD5 T1 antigen A 67-kD glycoprotein with receptor activity that is present on most T cells and on a subpopulation of B cells, as well as in chronic lymphocytic leukemia, which binds to the B-cell surface protein CD72/Lyb-2 (**Nature 1991; 351:662**)

CD6 T12 antigen A 100-kD antigen present on most T cells and a subset of B cells, which is similar in distribution to CD3

CD7 A 40-kD antigen present on 85-95% of peripheral T cells and most NK cells, which may correspond to the Fc receptor for IgM; the antigen is expressed throughout T-cell differentiation

CD8 T8 antigen A 33-kD heterodimeric protein that is a marker for T cells with suppressor and cytotoxic activity; it binds to class I MHC antigens on antigen-presenting cells and is physically associated with a p56 tyrosine kinase that phosphorylates adjacent proteins; see Cytotoxic T cells

CD8 cells T lymphocytes with CD8 antigen on the cell surface, which are suppressive, lack inducer functions and are responsible for suppressing mitogen-induced and antigen-specific antibody production, requiring CD4 cooperation for this activity

CD9 A 24-kD protein present on pre-B cells, monocytes, granulocytes and platelets, which has protein kinase activity

CD10 A 100-kD membrane-associated neutral endopeptidase* [EC 3.4.24.11] the CD10 antigen is a zinc metalloproteinase expressed on early B and T cells, and germinal center cells and is present on many other normal (eg renal epithelium, fibroblasts, and granulocytes) and neoplastic (eg acute lymphoblastic leukemia, lymphoma, melanoma, and glioma) cells; CD10 mediates the enkephalin-mediated inflammatory response

*The formal term preferred by the IUBMB (International Union of Biochemistry and Molecular Biology) is neprilysin, a term unlikely to win many converts in the face of the firmly entrenched alternative terms CALLA (common lymphoblastic leukemia antigen) and neutral endopeptidase, other less used synonyms include endopeptidase 24.11, enkephalinase, and kidney brush border neutral peptidase

CD11 A group of three different α chains CD11a (180 kD), CD11b (170 kD) and CD11c (150 kD) leukocyte adhesive antigens (LFA/Mac-1) that are associated with an invariant 95 kD β-glycoprotein (CD18); the CD11/CD18 family (Leu-CAM integrin family) of leukocyte adhesive glycoproteins is present on neutrophils and monocytes, eg Mo1 (CR3:iC3b), LeuM5 (p150,95) and LFA-1; CD11 requires the associated CD18 β chain, without which neutrophils fail to migrate to sites of infections, and cannot adhere in vitro to endothelial cell monolayers; see CD18, Leukocyte adhesion deficiency

CD11a LFA-1α The 180-kD α subunit of LFA-1 (leukocyte function-associated antigen-1), which is a member of the subfamily of integrin receptors that bind to an intracellular cell adhesion molecule (I-CAM); CD11a is expressed on virtually all peripheral WBCs, and is essential for immune responses requiring cell-cell contact, eg lymphocyte adhesion, NK- and T-cell-mediated cytolysis, and T cell proliferation; its expression is up-regulated by IFN-gamma

CD11b Leu-15 C3bi complement receptor CR₃ The 165-kD α subunit of CD11b/CD18 heterodimeric antigen; CD11b is expressed on 30% of peripheral lymphocytes, including most NK cells, and a subset of T cells, and is present on mature neutrophils, eosinophils, and monocytes

CD11c Leu-M5 C4 complement receptor CR_4 The 150-kD α subunit of CD11c/CD18 heterodimeric antigen; CD11c is expressed on monocytes, macrophages (eg 'starry sky' macrophages of germinal centers, sinus histiocytes, Kupffer cells, alveolar macrophages, elongated intratubular renal cells) and in low density on granulocytes and NK cells, as well as hairy cell leukemia, and some acute myelocytic leukemia

CD13 Aminopeptidase N A 150–170-kD integral membrane glycoprotein [EC 3.4.11.2] involved in metabolism of regulatory peptides that is present on mast cells, monocytes, macrophages, granulocytes, enteric and renal tubular epithelial cells, synaptic membranes of CNS origin and connective tissue; CD13 is expressed pathologic conditions, eg AML and SLE

*The term recommended by the Nomenclature Committee of the IUBMB (International Union of Biochemistry and Molecular Biology) is membrane alanyl aminopeptidase

CD14 My23 A 53–55-kD glycoprotein expressed by monocytes and on 70-95% of peripheral monocytes, pleural, peritoneal and synovial macrophages; it is weakly expressed on granulocytes; CD14 is a cell surface receptor, which when it binds its ligand, lipopolysaccharide-binding protein-soluble lipopolysaccharide (LBP-LPS), releases tumor necrosis factor (Science 1991; 252:1321)

CD15 LeuM1 Hapten X A myelomonocyte carbohydrate antigen* present in the secondary granules of ≥ 95% of mature eosinophils and neutrophils, Reed-Sternberg cells, and in AML and CML; see CD30

*The structure recognized by monoclonal antibodies to CD 15 is 3-fucosyl-N-acetyllactosamine

CD16 Low-affinity Fc receptor, IgG Fc receptor III A 50–65-kD receptor antigen that is expressed in various forms on virtually all NK cells, granulocytes, on activated macrophages, is present on ± 15% of peripheral lymphocytes and participates in antibody-dependent cell cytotoxicity; in some cells CD16 may serve merely as a binding site for IgG complexes, while in others (eg NK cells) interaction of a ligand with CD16 may unchain a cascade resulting in the transcription of lymphokines and trigger cell-mediated cytotoxicity

CD18 A 95-kD glycoprotein β chain that is non-covalently linked to specific α chains of the CD11 family of molecules; a genetic defect in the CD18 gene results in Leukocyte adhesion deficiency syndrome, see there

CD19 A 95-kD (71-kD after deglycosylation) transmembrane polypeptide with two immunoglobulin domains, which is expressed on B cells from earliest pre-B cells to plasma cells; CD19 expression is lost with terminal differentiation of B lymphocytes in the form of plasma cells

CD20 A 35-kD–37 transmembrane ion channel, the gene for which is located on chromosome 11q12-13; CD20 is expressed on B cells late in ontogeny at the same time as the expression of surface IgM; it is present on both resting and activated B cells, but is lost prior to differentiation into plasma cells; CD20 is present in the mantle zone and in the germinal center, and may be expressed on follicular dendritic cells

CD21 Complement receptor 2 CR_2 A 140-kD protein encoded by chromosome 1q32 that is a receptor for C3d component of complement and EBV, which is expressed in early B cells and dendritic reticulum cells

CD22 A 130–135-kD protein with five extracellular immunoglobulin-like domains that has significant sequence homology with neural cell adhesion molecule (N-CAM); CD22 is expressed in the cytoplasm of early B cells and on the cell surface of mature B cells with surface immunoglobulins, but is lost on fully mature plasma cells and may be expressed in most B-cell lymphoproliferative

disorders; CD22 is not expressed on benign or malignant T cells, monocytes, or macrophages

CD23 Low-affinity IgE receptor A 45–50-kD receptor for B-cell growth factor, which is expressed in increased amounts on B cells that have been activated with IL-4, as well as EBV-transformed cells, tonsillar B cells, and in CLL

CD24 A 42-kD glycoprotein present on B cells and granulocytes, an expression that is lost following activation; CD24 is expressed on the surface of many B cell leukemias and lymphomas

CD25 Tac antigen A 55-kD glycoprotein that is the α chain of the interleukin-2 receptor, which complexes to the β chain, both of which are encoded on chromosome 10, and is expressed on activated B and T cells and activated macrophages

CD26 Dipeptidyl aminopetidase IV A T cell activation molecule that is the binding site for HIV's Tat protein, which may be the manner in which HIV suppresses antigen-induced T-cell proliferation (P Nat Acad Sci (US) 1994; 91:6594)

CD28 A disulfide-liked homodimeric 44-kD glycoprotein CAM (cell adhesion molecule) present on 60-80% of peripheral T (CD3+) cells, 50% of CD8+ T cells, and 5% of immature CD3+ thymocytes; T cell signaling by CD28 requires binding by phosphatidyl-inositol-3-OH kinase (Nature 1994; 369:327oA); CD28 is expressed as a homodimer on the surface of most T cells, and is the initial point in a signal transduction cascade, which when stimulated, increases IL-2 enhancer activity with secretion of IL-2 as well as TNF-α, GM-CSF, IFN-γ, and lymphotoxin (Science 1991; 251:313)

CD30 Ki-1 antigen A 105-kD glycoprotein present on activated T cells, B cells, embryonal carcinoma cells, Reed-Sternberg cells, and anaplastic large cell lymphoma, nodular small cleaved-cell lymphoma, peripheral T-cell lymphomas, and in Lennert's lymphoma (Arch Pathol Lab Med 1992; 116:1197oA)

CD30 lymphoma Ki-1 lymphoma, see there

CD31 PECAM-1 A 130-140 kD glycoprotein member of the Ig superfamily that is expressed on the surface of platelets, certain subsets of WBCs, and at the endothelial intercellular junction; CD31 is involved in myelomonocytic differentiation and present on granulocytes, monocytes, platelets, and endothelial cells; CD31 has 6 extracellular Ig-like homology units typical of other cell-cell adhesion molecules and has properties that suggest its involvement in angiogenesis, thrombosis, and wound healing (Am J Clin Pathol 1995; 103:443oA)

CD33 A 67-kD transmembrane glycoprotein that is strongly expressed on monocytes and weakly on granulocytes; it is expressed on CFU-Mix, CFU-GM, CFU-Meg, on some BFU-E, and early myeloid cells; CD33 is also expressed in ≥ 85% in AML and occasionally in ALL

CD34 A 105–120-kD transmembrane glycoprotein expressed on immature hematopoietic cells and endothelial cells

CD35 CR1, Complement C3b receptor A 160–220-kD group of antigens expressed on RBCs, B cells, monocytes, granulocytes, some NK cells, and dendritic cells

CD36 gpIIIb, gpIV A 90-kD membrane glycoprotein that acts as the receptor for thrombospondin and collagen, as well as for *Plasmodium falciparum*; CD36 is expressed on monocytes, platelets, endothelial cells, and weakly on B cells; CD36 serves as a docking site for oxidized LDLs which are concentrated in caveolae (Science News 1994; 146:4)

CD37 A 40–45-kD glycoprotein expressed on mature B cells

CD38 A 45-kD integral membrane glycoprotein (with a 35-kD protein core) that is expressed during early T- and B-cell differentiation, with ↓ expression on resting cells, and

↑ expression with cell activation; CD38 is expressed on pre-B cells, plasma cells, T-cell subsets, thymocytes, NK cells, monocytes, myeloblasts, and very early erythroblasts; CD38 is also expressed in lymphoproliferative disorders, eg ALL, AML, Burkitt's lymphoma, and multiple myeloma

CD39 An 80-kD antigen present on the surface of B cells, T cells and macrophages, but not on pre-B cells or plasma cells

CD40 A 45–50-kD transmembrane glycoprotein that is expressed on B cells, epithelial cells and some carcinoma cell lines; cross-linking of CD40 to a monoclonal anti-CD40 antibody in the presence of IL-4 results in the production of a long-lived human B cell line; the CD40 ligand is expressed on the surface of activated T cells and forms a complex with the CD40 receptor on B cells, an interaction that can induce B-cell proliferation and, in the presence of the appropriate cytokines, can promote switching of immunoglobulin isotypes; infants with hyper-IgM immunodeficiency syndrome (see there) have heterogeneous point mutations or deletions throughout the coding region of the CD40 ligand (**N Engl J Med 1994; 330:962**0A)

CD40L CD40 ligand, aka T-BAM, gp39, TRAP A surface protein that is most abundant on CD4+ (helper) T lymphocytes in lymphoid follicles; CD40L delivers a contact-dependent signal that stimulates B-cell survival, growth, differentiation, and class switching; signaling via CD40 re-routes B cells from programmed cell death (apoptosis) induced by Fas protein (CD95) or by cross-linking of the IgM complex; defective CD40L results in X-linked hyper-IgM syndrome, which is characterized by an absence of IgG, IgA, and IgE, elevated IgM, and no lymphoid follicles (**Science 1995; 267:1494**0A); CD40L also has antiviral activity (**Nature Medicine 1995; 1:437, 409**)

CD41 Platelet glycoprotein IIb/IIIa A glycoprotein that is a Ca++-dependent complex between the 110 kD gpIIIa (CD61) and the heterodimeric 135-kD gpIIb; CD41 is the receptor for fibrinogen, von Willebrand factor, collagen and fibronectin; it is present on the surface of megakaryocytes and platelets, and absent in Glanzmann's thrombasthenia

CD42 A surface antigen on platelets and megakaryocytes that is divided into CD42a (glycoprotein IX), a 23-kD antigen and CD42b or glycoprotein Ib, a 170-kD heterodimeric antigen, either of which may be reduced or absent in Bernard-Soulier disease

CD42a Glycoprotein IX CD42a antigen forms a noncovalent complex with CD42b (glycoprotein Ia); the CD42a/CD42b (or gpIX/gpIa) complex functions as the von Willebrand factor receptor, and is involved in vWF-dependent adhesion of platelets to exposed vascular subendothelium; the complex also serves as the attachment site for the platelet plasma membrane to the submembrane cytoskeleton; CD42a is present on platelets and megakaryocytes and is absent in Bernard-Soulier syndrome

CD44 H-CAM (homing cell adhesion molecule) A 37-kD cell surface glycoprotein that is present in multiple isoforms, which when glycosylated is converted to an 80–95-kD form; in combination with LFA-3 and CD45, CD acts as a physiologic trigger for the release of TNF-α and IL-1 from monocytes; CD44 is present on 90% of lymphocytes, monocytes, and granulocytes, with lesser expression on thymocytes, fibroblasts and RBCs; it mediates various cell functions, eg T-cell adhesion to RBCs, leukocyte-endothelial cell binding, 'homing' of lymphocytes to specific lymphoid microenvironments which bind to cell adhesion glycoproteins; CD44 is surface receptor for hyaluronic acid; CD44 is up-regulated early in T-cell activation by the CD3/T cell receptor complex

CD45 Leukocyte common antigen T-200 A family* of 180–220-kD transmembrane glycoprotein receptors expressed on most hematopoietic cells; CD45s are structurally similar to tyrosine phosphatase, have phosphotyrosine phosphatase activity, and are present on all WBCs and leukocyte precursors; T lymphocytes express various forms of the CD45 antigen, resulting from the use of different CD45 exons during transcription, eg the CD45R+ T-cell subset is involved in graft-versus-host reactions and interleukin-2 activity, which may interconvert into the CD45RO+ T-cell subset that responds to recall antigens; CD45 may also regulate signal transduction by modulating the phosphorylation state of B-cell antigen receptors (**Science 1991; 252:1839**)

*Which includes CD45RA, CD45RB, and CD45RO

CD45RA A 220-kD isoform of leukocyte common antigen corresponding to a protein tyrosine phosphatase present on 50% of CD4+, and 75% of CD8+ T lymphocytes, virtually all B and NK cells; CD45RA is expressed on naive T cells; antigen density decreases with activation

CD45RA A high molecular weight form of CD45; the recovery of the CD4+ T lymphocyte population in patients with HIV infection, BM transplantation, and chemotherapy correlates quantitatively with the appearance of CD45RA+ CD4+ T cells, which are regenerated from the BM via a thymus-dependent pathway (**N Engl J Med 1995; 332:143**0A)

CD45RO A low-molecular-weight (180-kD) isoform of CD45 (leukocyte common antigen) derived from a thymus-independent pathway (**N Engl J Med 1995; 332:143**0A), which is a protein tyrosine phosphatase present on 40% of resting peripheral T cells, including both CD4+ and CD8+ subsets, most thymocytes, and activated T lymphocytes; it is also expressed on monocytes, macrophages, and granulocytes; its level of expression is low early in the T-cell maturation cycle (unlike CD45RA which is well-expressed in naive cells), and high when activated T cells are rechallenged

CDw52 CAMPATH-1 antigen, see there

CD54 ICAM-1 A 90-kD antigen that is the ligand for CD11a/CD18 (aka LFA-1) affecting LFA-1-dependent leukocyte-endothelium adherence and cell-cell contact-related immune activities; after mitogenic stimulation CD54 expression increases on B and T cell, macrophages, and lymphocytes, and is inducible on fibroblasts, epithelial, and endothelial cells

CD56 A 140-kD isoform of N-CAM (neural cell adhesion molecule) that is extensively glycosylated resulting in a mature antigen of up to 220 kD; CD56 is present on 10-25% of peripheral lymphocytes and on all NK cells; CD3+CD56+ T lymphocytes comprise a unique subset of cytotoxic T cells that mediate MHC-restricted cytotoxicity

CD57 A 110 kD carbohydrate antigen linked to myelin-associated glycoprotein; it is present on 15-20% of peripheral mononuclear cells, subsets of NK and T lymphocytes, and cells of the central and peripheral nervous system

CD59 A 65 kD membrane-anchored[1] complement-neutralizing protein[2] that is expressed on most leukocytes and erythrocytes(see **N Engl J Med 1994; 330:249**0A) CD58 may be absent in some forms of paroxysmal nocturnal hemoglobinuria

[1]Glycosyl-phosphatidylinositol-anchored [2]Synonyms include H19, HRF20 (20-kD homologous restriction factor), MACIF (membrane attack complex inhibitory factor), MEM-43, MIRL (membrane inhibitor of reactive lysis)

CD61 Glycoprotein IIIa A 110-kD antigen that is the β-subunit (integrin β_3 chain) for both the gpIIb/IIIa complex and the vitronectin receptor, which are integrins involved in cell; in combination with CD41, CD61 acts as a receptor for fibrinogen, von Willebrand factor, vitronectin, and fibronectin on activated platelets; in combination with CD51 (the vitronectin α chain), CD61 forms the vitronectin receptor-mediating activation-dependent cell adhesion to fibrinogen, thrombospondin, vitronectin, and vWF; CD61 is expressed on all normal and activated platelets, megakaryocytes, endothelial cells, some myeloid, and erythroid cells, and T cell leukemia cell lines; see CD41

CD62 GMP-140, PADGEM, P-selectin A 140-kD single-chain polypeptide of the selectin family of cell adhesion molecules, which mediates the attachment of activated platelets to neutrophils and monocytes during hemostasis; CD62 is associated with the α-granules of platelets and megakaryocytes, and expressed on the surface of activated platelets and endothelial cells when these cells are stimulated by thrombogenic agents, allowing these cells to bind neutrophils and monocytes at the site of tissue injury (**Nature 1991; 349:196n&v**) CD62 is associated with the Weibel-Palade bodies of endothelial cells

CD68 Macrophage-associated antigen A highly nonspecific 110-kD glycoprotein that is associated with lysosomes; CD68 was first found on histiocytes, but is also found in a wide range of neoplasias, eg lymphomas, sarcomas, carcinomas, melanomas and other tumors (**Am J Clin Pathol 1995; 103:425QA**)

CD69 A disulfide-bonded 60-kD homodimeric polypeptide which is expressed on activated B, NK, and T cells, peaking at 18 hours post activation, preceding the appearance of HLA-DR, IL-2 receptor, and CD71 (transferrin receptor); CD69 is also expressed on platelets

CD71 Transferrin receptor A 190 kD receptor that is essential for the transport of iron into proliferating cells, eg activated lymphoblasts; CD71 expression occurs in early erythroid cells, but is lost with maturation

CD72/Lyt-2 A cell surface protein that is only expressed on B cells which serves as a ligand for CD5 receptor; see CD5

CD73 Ecto-5'-nucleotidase An antigen that is a marker of T- and B-cell maturation

CD90 Fas protein, see there

CDC Centers for Disease Control and Prevention, see there, also 1) Calculated date of confinement (obstetrics) 2) Cancer detection center 3) Capillary diffusion capacity 4) Caudodorsal cells (neuroanatomy) 5) Cell division cycle 6) Chenodeoxycholate (chenodeoxycholic acid) 7) Child development center 8) Child development consultant 9) Communicable disease center (uncommonly used) 10) Crohn's disease of the colon

CDC group DF-1 *Capnocytophaga gingivalis, C ochracea,* and *C sputigena*

CDC group DF-2 *Capnocytophaga canimorsus* and *C. cynodagmi*

CDC proteins Cell division cycle proteins Proteins of the cell cycle, some of which have been linked to chromosomal DNA replication, see MCM

CDC6 MOLECULAR BIOLOGY A protein produced late in G$_1$ in budding yeasts that is essential for DNA replication and prevents mitosis until DNA replicationis complete (**Nature 1994; 372:497n&v**) see Cyclins

CDC18 MOLECULAR BIOLOGY A protein produced late in G$_1$ in fission yeasts that is essential for DNA replication and prevents mitosis until DNA replicationis complete (**Nature 1994; 372:497n&v**) see Cyclins

CDC25 protein A protein required to dephosphorylate a specific tyrosine residue in p34cdc2, a key protein in the biochemical engine that controls the eukaryotic cell cycle, which activates p34cdc2/cyclin B kinase, triggering the onset of mitosis (**Nature 1991; 351:194c**)

CDC46 MCM5, see MCM

CDE diet A choline-deficient, ethionine-supplemented diet used to produce experimental pancreatitis in rodents; in this diet, the normally discrete lysosome and zymogen granules fuse (a process called crinophagy) into bodies which extrude across the basolateral wall of the acinar cell, delivering digestive and lysosomal enzymes to the interstitial and peripancreatic adipose tissue; cathepsin B is also recruited, activating trypsinogen and trypsin, which in turn activate other protease precursors

CDI Cartilage-derived inhibitor A peptide isolated from stromal tissue that inhibits angiogenesis (proliferation and migration of capillary endothelial cells), explaining why cartilage is resistant to ingrowth of capillaries (Science 1990; 247:1408)

Cdk-activating kinase A 62-kD subunit of human transcription factor IIH (TFIIH), which is a positive regulator of Cdc2 and Cdk2, and thought to play a role in the regulation of transcription and in cell cycle control (**Nature 1995; 374:280L, 283L**)

CDK Cyclin-dependent kinase, see there

cDNA MOLECULAR PATHOLOGY DNA that is complementary to an mRNA actively translating various proteins; cDNA fragments are inserted into a viral gene coding for the β-galactosidase enzyme; by extension, bacteria containing the virus with an altered β-galactosidase will contain the protein fragment encoded by the cDNA, which is identified on a cell culture plate by radioactively 'tagging' a monoclonal antibody to the desired protein and performing autoradiography

Steps in production of cDNA

1) Beginning with an mRNA template, an enzyme (eg tobacco acid pyrophosphatase) is used for decapping the RNA prior to RNA template construction, followed by preparation of well-defined sequence RNA template using an RNA ligase

2) Synthesis of full-length first-strand cDNA (see 3, below) using reverse transcriptase, followed by DNA polymerase to construct the second cDNA strand

3) Removal of RNA from first-strand cDNA using a ribonuclease

cDNA library MOLECULAR BIOLOGY A living repository of genetic material raised in a bacteriophage-infected *Escherichia coli* (or, less commonly, other bacteria) that contains only inserted segments of DNA, ie introns, which is created by making complementary DNA (cDNA) from a full set (hence, the term library) of mRNAs in a cell, using reverse transcriptase (RNA-dependent DNA polymerase) that converts single-stranded cDNA to double-stranded DNA, then carrying out the steps required to establish a gene library; see Human Genome Project, STS mapping

CD-ROM Compact disk-read only memory

CDS Controlled Drug Substance, see there

CEA Carcinoembryonic antigen A glycoprotein present in the circulation in nanogram amounts first described as relatively specific for detecting occult primary adenocarcinomas; CEA is ↑ in up to 30% of colorectal, lung, liver, pancreas, breast, head and neck, bladder, cervix, prostatic and medullary thyroid carcinomas, and may be ↑ in lymphoproliferative disorders, malignant melanoma and in heavy smokers; although elevation is not a reliable cancer screen, it is useful for monitoring recurrent colon cancer; a 35% ↑ of CEA above a patient's post-resective surgery baseline may indicate need for a 'second look' operation to rule out metastases; CEA is ↑ in 60-90% of metastatic lung cancer; CEA is normally found in the fetal gut; in smokers or in inflammatory bowel disease; any gain in overall survival by CEA monitoring is small; possibly ≤ 1% can be salvaged after resection of liver metastasis (**CAP Today April 1994**); in HIV-infected patients with PCP, ↑ CEA (8.8 vs 2.7 ng/mL in normals) is associated with a poor short-term prognosis and a mortality of ± 80% with a CEA > 20 ng/mL (**Scand J Infect Dis 1992; 24:309**); if elevated prior to colonic surgery, it is a poor prognostic sign and may identify patients at ↑

risk of cancer recurrence (Am Surg 1994; 60:528)

c7E3 Abciximab, see there

C/EBP A DNA-binding protein, first thought to bind to the **CC**AAT boxes, later shown to act as a viral **E**nhancer **B**inding **P**rotein; C/EBP is present at high levels in hepatocytes, adipocytes, intestinal mucosal cells and in neurons, binding to DNA as a dimer, joined by a leucine 'zipper' motif; see DNA-binding, Helix-turn-helix, Zinc finger

ced-9 A gene of the nematode *Caenorhabditis elegans*, which is a member of the same gene family as the human *bcl-2* proto-oncogene; both protect cells from programmed cell death; see *bcl-2*

celery stick sign PEDIATRIC RADIOLOGY A descriptor for a disorganized diaphysis and metaphysis with osteitis of long bones, seen in the distal femur and proximal tibia, where longitudinal radiolucent striations alternate with sclerotic bands; 'celery stick' changes are typical of children with rubella embryopathy, infected during the first trimester, but also occur with other transplacental infections, including cytomegalovirus, herpes simplex, syphilis, toxoplasmosis (see TORCH), malignancy, eg leukemia, neuroblastoma, systemic disease, scurvy, hypervitaminosis D, osteogenesis imperfecta, osteoporosis

ceiling principle MOLECULAR BIOLOGY A guideline proposed by the US National Academy of Science for calculating the odds of a spurious match in forensic DNA fingerprinting that arises due to racial (white European, African-American, etc) subgroups; population studies would be used to determine how often a particular allele appears in the different subgroups; the allele would then be assigned the highest frequency observed in a subgroup or a value of 10%, whichever is highest, a DNA match using five different alleles would thus have $\leq 1/10^5$ chances of occurring by chance (Sci Am 1994; 271/4:33)

celiac disease Production of copious fatty stools, abdominal distention and wasting Jejunal biopsy reveals flattening of villi PATHOGENESIS Most common in those of Western European extraction, and is strongly associated with expression of HLA-B8, DR3, and DQ(α1*0501,β1*0201) Celiac disease predisposes to malignancies including intestinal lymphoma, and carcinoma of the oral cavity, esophagus and small intestine (N Engl J Med 1994; 331:383cPc)

celiac sprue Gluten-sensitive enteropathy A malabsorptive syndrome resulting from hypersensitivity of intestinal mucosa to α-gliadin, a gluten extract composed of glutamine and proline-rich proteins, present in wheat, barley, rye and, to a lesser degree, oats PATHOGENESIS Uncertain, although some data implicates viral infection, eg the α-gliadin peptide of gluten has considerable homology with the E1B protein of human adenovirus 12; antibodies to E1B cross-react with α-gliadin and celiac disease is more common in those previously exposed to adenovirus 12 CLINICAL Diarrhea, weight loss, anemia, hemorrhage, osteopenia, muscular atrophy, peripheral neuropathy, central nervous system and spinal cord demyelination (sensory loss, ataxia), amenorrhea, infertility, edema, petechiae, dermatitis herpetiformis, especially if the patient has an HLA B27 haplotype PATHOLOGY Mucosal flattening, lengthening of the crypt with crypt hyperplasia, loss of villi and nuclear polarity, causing local and systemic changes Note: Crypt hyperplasia and villous atrophy may transiently occur in GI hypersensitivity reactions to milk, fish, rice and chicken and should be ruled out TREATMENT Eliminate gliadin from diet; poor response is due either to non-compliance or incorrect diagnosis; without treatment, 10-15% develop lymphoma (immunoblastic lymphoma, less commonly, T cell lymphoma), a risk that increases with disease duration; the otherwise rare small intestinal adenocarcinoma is up to 80-fold more common in sprue patients; Cf Tropical sprue

CE-LIF Capillary electrophoresis-laser-induced fluorescence, see there

cell adhesion molecules CAM(s), see there

cell block CYTOLOGY A paraffin-embedded specimen derived from dried mucus, sputum or debris found in clear fluids of pleural, pericardial, endobronchial and other sites that cannot be processed in the usual fashion for cytological analysis; cell blocks are suspended in formaldehyde, centrifuged at 2500 rpm and processed as per routine for histological specimens

cell-in-cell pattern Partial molding of one cell into another, sometimes such that one cell seems to engulf another; the pattern is a typical cytopathological feature of small (oat) cell carcinoma of the lung; usually the nuclei of pulmonary small cell carcinomas are hyperchromatic and fragile and some have a morphology likened to pulled taffy candy; confusion arises if the dense nuclei are surrounded by eosinophilic cytoplasm, thus mimicking the squamous pearls of epidermoid carcinoma of the lungs; this distinction is of practical importance as small cell carcinomas may respond

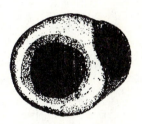

cell-in-cell

to radiotherapy, while squamous cell carcinomas are unsalvageable if surgically unresectable; the cell-in-cell pattern may also be seen in reactive mesothelial cells obtained from washings of serosal, eg pleural and peritoneal surfaces

cell junction PHYSIOLOGY An intercellular zone of adherence between and contributed by two cells, functionally divided into **ADHERING JUNCTION** A mechanical junction that holds cells in place, eg spot desmosome, belt desmosome, hemidesmosome **COMMUNICATING JUNCTION** A junction that mediates the passage of small molecules between cells, eg gap junction, synaptic 'junction' **IMPERMEABLE JUNCTION** A tight impermeable junction that seals two cells allowing no leakage, eg septate junction, tight junction

cell junction molecule A protein, similar in function to cell adhesion molcules and surface adhesion molecules (SAMs) but which is a component of complex intercellular junctions, including belt, gap, spot and tight junctions

cell-mediated immunity The arm of the immune system that acts through the 'direct' cell action, commonly equated to T-cell immunity (humoral or B-cell immunity is 'indirect', mediated by antibodies) Postulated route of CMI An antigen arrives on the 'scene' and is processed by a specialized macrophage, the antigen-presenting cell (APC), which presents the antigen to a T cell within the self MHC (major histocompatibility complex) class II protein complex present on the APC surface; antigen is then presented to T cells, activating various T cells having helper, suppressor and cytotoxic functions; the 'activated' T cells then produce cytokines that 1) Autoamplify T cell reactivity 2) Activate macrophages or 3) Facilitate immunoglobulin production, thus facilitating the action of killer cells; CMI is pivotal in host defense against tuberculosis, fungi, tumor cells and plays a key role in allograft rejection; see ADCC, APC

cell therapy ALTERNATIVE MEDICINE *'the injection of cellular material* from organs, fetuses, or embryos of animals to stimulate healing, counteract the effects of aging, and treat a variety of degenerative diseases such as arthritis, Parkinson's disease*, atherosclero-*

sis, and cancer. ...methods include the use of live cells, freeze-dried cells...cells from specific organs, and whole embryo preparations.' (**Alternative Medicine, Future Medicine Publishing, Inc, Puyallup, Washington, 1994**) Note: There is no data on the efficacy of CT in peer-reviewed journals; it is not approved for use in the United States, but is regionally popular in other countries; see Alternative medicine

*There is a vast difference between the therapeutic use of cells in a legitimate (ie 'mainstream') medical context and the pseudoscience that is intimately linked to 'cell therapy'; in conventional medical practice, the indications for such therapy are controlled by ethical 'standards of practice' if it is part of the accepted medical armamentarium (eg for BM transplantation from a person from whom an HLA profile has been defined), or strictly delineated if it is part of an experimental protocol (eg the use of LAK–lymphokine activated killer cells, or fetal mesenchymal cells for the treatment of Parkinson's disease); moreover, the cells used in conventional medical practice are 'biologicals', the quality of which is regulated by the US Food and Drug Administration; the use of cells as therapy by both conventional and nonconventional practitioners of medicine lends to considerable confusion—Author's note

cellular oncogene Proto-oncogene, see there

cellular telephone CARDIOLOGY Preliminary data suggests that CTs using digital technology inhibit the function of cardiac pacemakers, with the greatest interference occurring when the CT's antenna was next to the pacemaker's pulse generator (**Am Med News 15 May 1995, p22**)

'cellulite' A term used by the lay public for cosmetically undesirable subcutaneous layer(s) of adipose tissue that causes peau d'orange-like dimpling of the skin surface; cellulite is not an accepted medical term, either clinically or pathologically, as histologic examination reveals nothing more than 'garden variety' adipocytes, although billions of dollars are spent annually in the US alone to rid the body of this physical manifestations of dietary excess

cement *cementum* [NH3] An attenuated layer of calcified fibrous tissue that covers and is firmly attached to the dentin of the tooth root, and is either cellular or acellular

censorship Endopsychic censor PSYCHIATRY A generic term for the internalized 'braking' system's ability to critically evaluate any outgoing actions or verbalizations; the ego and superego have censorship activity that alters the original drive and/or action

censorship phenomenon PUBLIC HEALTH A term referring to the anecdotal evidence that advertising revenue-dependent media sources, eg magazines sold to the general public, restrict their discussion of a health issue, in particular that of smoking, out of fear of the loss of revenues related to the potentially unhealthy product being advertised (see **N Engl J Med 1992; 326:305SA**)

centiGray see Gray

census 1) The number of inpatients (ie occupied beds) in a service, unit, ward, or in the entire hospital or health care facility, exclusive of newborns 2) A list of the patients in a service, unit, ward, or in the entire hospital; see Bed

centenarian GERIATRICS A person who has lived 100 or more years; the number of centenarians in developed countries has increased exponentially, eg in the 1950 US census, there were 4475, in 1990 there were 54 000 (**JAMA 1995; 273:1319MN&P**) see Gerontology

Centers for Disease Control (and Prevention) CDC The pre-eminent epidemiologic agency of the world, located in Atlanta, Georgia, established in 1946 from the Office of Malaria Control in War Areas (at the time, CDC meant Communicable Disease Center); the Epidemic Intelligence Services was established in 1951; the CDC's successes have included the description of Lassa fever (1969), proof of sexual transmissibility of HBV (1971), documentation of an epidemic of Reye syndrome (1973), identification of Legionnaire's disease (1976), playing a pivotal role in the eradication of smallpox (1977), and the first reports of AIDS (1981); CDC future directions include: Adolescent health, chronic disease and epidemiology of violence

Note: In recognition of its responsibility for adressing illnesses and disability before they occur, the CDC's new name is Centers for Disease Control *and Prevention*, in a law signed by the US President on October 27, 1992 (**MMWR 1992; 41:830**)

centiMorgan GENETICS A unit of physical map distance on a human chromosome, equivalent to a 1% crossover frequency

central cord syndrome A post-traumatic condition affecting the spinal cord, in which a lesion spreads from the central gray matter peripherally to the myelin; voluntary myelinated motor fibers to the arms are more central and those to the legs more peripheral; in CCS, lower motor neuron changes occur in the arms and are accompanied by leg spasticity; sensory defects are a function of the degree of anterolateral and posterior column destruction, often accompanied by altered pain and temperature sensation in hands; cases of acute onset may be accompanied by urinary retention and incontinence

central core myopathy Shy-Magee disease An AD myopathy causing hypotonia in infancy and non-progressive proximal weakness, with sparing of the cranial muscles PATHOLOGY Central muscle fiber zone lacking oxidative or glycolytic enzyme activity EM Decreased numbers of mitochondria with disorganized myofibrils

central dogma MOLECULAR BIOLOGY The pedagogical tenet held in the infancy (circa 1960s) of molecular biology that translation of a protein invariably follows a chain of molecular command, where DNA acts as the template for both its own replication and for the transcription to RNA (and with subsequent maturation, to messenger RNA), which then serves as a template for translation into a protein; although this represents the usual flow of molecular information, it is now well-established that RNA may also act as its own RNA polymerase and may serve as a template (via reverse transcriptase and formation of a complementary DNA strand) for its own replication; see RNA polymerase

Note: The identification of prions, infectious particles composed only of protein, complicates this once simple scheme; see Prion

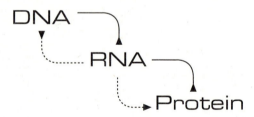

central dogma

central (reparative) giant cell granuloma ORAL PATHOLOGY A predominantly osteodestructive lesion of uncertain pathogenesis that is most common in the young female mandible, and more osteodestructive than the peripheral giant cell granuloma RADIOLOGY Radiolucent destructivelesion with faint trabeculation and loculation PATHOLOGY Loose fibrillar connective tissue, fibroblast proliferation, hemosiderin pigmentation and variably-sized giant cells DDx Giant cell tumor of bone, parathyroid hormone-induced 'brown' tumor (hyperparathyroidism) TREATMENT Curettage Note: It is unclear whether this condition is neoplastic or reactive

central nervous system leukemia Involvement of the CNS by leukemia, which is defined per 'modified' Rome Workshop criteria (**N Engl J Med 1993; 329:314oA**) as

GROUP 1 No blast cells detectable by cytocentrifuge

GROUP 2 < 5 leukocytes/mL, blasts detectable by cytocentrifuge

GROUP 3 > 5 leukocytes/mL, blasts, cranial nerve palsies

central pontine myelinolysis NEUROPATHOLOGY A condition that is characterized by softening of the base of the brain at the pons, related to aggressive correction of hyponatremia, first identified in alcoholics; CPM has also been described in AIDS, infection, lymphoproliferative disorders (eg AML), malnutrition, and local venous obstruction PREVENTION Slow correction of electrolytic imbalance

central retinal artery occlusion OPHTHALMOLOGY A fundoscopic finding often due to embolization, appearing as arteriolar narrowing and stasis with segmentation of the venous blood column, resulting in a 'boxcar' appearance; regional infarction of the superficial retina and accompanying edema results in a cherry red appearance; with time, the edema resolves and the fundoscopic findings mimic the usual type of retinal atrophy

central serous retinopathy Serous retinal detachment A condition characterized by fluid accumulation in the subretinal area with loss of adherence of the retinal epithelial basement membrane to Bruch's membrane; CSR is thought to be more common in subjects with psychological dysfunction, and may be related to adrenergic stress ETIOLOGY Detachment may occur in corticosteroid therapy, Crohn's disease, fungal infection, leprosy, leukemia, periarteritis nodosa, SLE, toxoplasmosis, TTP, ulcerative colitis (see N Engl J Med 1992; 326:1762cpc)

central supply The department in a hospital or health care facility that stores, distributes and assures the availability of sterile materials, equipment, instruments, reusable and disposable items

central venous catheterization A generic term for the placement of a 'central' IV line* specifically used for critically ill patients; CVC is indicated for three specific reasons

1) Administer solutions that cannot be given through peripheral veins, eg total parenteral nutrition, and certain chemotherapeutic agents

2) Obtain venous access in patients with poorly accessible veins

3) Insert monitoring devices, eg Swan-Ganz catheter for determination of central venous blood pressure (N Engl J Med 1994; 331:1769ED) see Subclavian venous catheterization

*As the vast majority of central venous catheters are placed in the subclavian vein, the terms central venous catheter and subclavian vein catheter, and related terms have been used interchangeably

centrocytic lymphoma Mantle-zone lymphoma, see there

centrosome MTOC (microtubule organizing body), see there

centronuclear myopathy Myotubular myopathy, see there

CEOT Calcifying epithelial odontogenic tumor, see there of Pindborg A slow-growing lesion of the oral cavity, mandible and maxilla, that affects any age group, population and sex; although the CEOT is locally invasive, radical therapy is not required PATHOLOGY Polyhedral epithelial cells with minimal stroma; the cells may demonstrate nuclear pleomorphism; intracellular degeneration results in amyloid-like eosinophilic material that may with time become calcified

cephalad march CRITICAL CARE MEDICINE The slow progression of weakness and loss of sensory perception seen in an acute epidural hematoma

cephalic index A ratio calculated as the maximum width of the head x 100 divided by its length, which is of some use when classifying odd skulls, eg turricephaly, dolichocephaly, brachycephaly, and so on

cephalosporin see Third-generation cephalosporin

c-erbB-2 HER-2/neu An oncogene of the *erb*B oncogene family, which is related to epidermal growth factor; c-*erb*B-2 is amplified 2–20-fold in ⅓ of breast cancer and is associated with decreased survival and shortened time to relapse[1]; a significant dose-respone effect of adjuvant chemotherapy (cyclophosphamide, doxorubicin [adriamycin] and fluorouracil) has been reported in patients with node-positive early breast carcinoma in whom c-*erb*B-2 is overexpressed (N Engl J Med 1994; 330:1260OA) c-*erb*B-2 expression is associated with an unfavorable prognosis in gastric carcinoma (308-day survival vs 763-day survival without expression, Arch Pathol Lab Med 1994; 118:235OA) Note: Although the nomenclature has not been completely standardized[2], c-*erb*B-2 is widely preferred

[1]Note: The prognosis of breast cancer is best predicted based on tumor size, number of lymph nodes involved and estrogen and progesterone receptor status [2]Note: Many names exist for the same gene or gene product and the choice about whether to write a gene, oncogene, or proto-oncogene in upper- and lowercase, italic or nonitalic forms, is often arbitrary—Author's note

cerebral amyloid angiopathy A sporadic disease that is present in an estimated 5-10% of primary nontraumatic cerebral hemorrhage, in which extensive vascular deposition of amyloid β protein is inculpated in recurrent and extensive intracerebral hemorrhages, resulting in neurotrophic and neurotoxic effects that are reversed by tachykinin-type neuropeptides CLINICAL Dementia is characteristic of CAA DIAGNOSIS Cerebral edema by CT, leukoencephaly and petechial hemorrhages by MRI (Mayo Clin Proc 1995; 70:477); CAA is idiopathic or may be associated with human hereditary cerebral hemorrhage with amyloidosis, Dutch type, see HCHWA-D

cerebral cysticercosis A CNS infestation by intermediate-stage larva (metacestode) of *Taenia solium* (pork tapeworm) EPIDEMIOLOGY Cysticercosis is acquired by ingesting taenia eggs shed in the feces of human carriers of pork tapeworms, and may occur in people who have not ingested or have contact with pork; this contrasts with taeniasis, an intestinal tapeworm infection acquired by eating undercooked pork contaminated with cysticerci CLINICAL Aphasia, seizures, late-onset epilepsy, hydrocephalus DIAGNOSIS Identification of cysts by CT, MRI; serum antibody measurement by ELISA TREATMENT Praziquantel, albendazole (N Engl J Med 1992; 327:692OA, 696OA; 727ED)

cerebral gigantism Sotos syndrome, see there

cerebral granulomatous angiitis An inflammatory reaction of multiple etiologies defined histologically by giant cell or epithelioid cell granulomatous inflammation of the cerebral blood vessels; CGA is heterogeneous with regard to caliber, location, and type of vessels involved, degree of necrosis, and presence of systemic vasculitis

cerebral malaria A severe complication of *Plasmodium falciparum* infection, more common in young children; it has a 15-50% mortality and leaves 10% of its survivors with gross neurologic sequela; CM is diagnosed when asexual forms of *P falciparum* are identified in the peripheral blood accompanied by diffuse acute symmetric encephalopathy PATHOLOGY Parasitized RBCs are sequestered in CNS microcirculation, accompanied by perivenular ring hemorrhages TREATMENT Iron chelation therapy is reported to clear parasitemia and enhance recovery from deep coma in cerebral malaria; these somewhat surprising data await confirmation by other workers (N Engl J Med 1992; 327:1473OA)

cerebral palsy A symptom complex affecting 0.4% of all term births; 75% of quadriplegic cerebral palsy has a known etiology—53% are congenital, 14% due to intrapartum asphyxia and 8% are due to other identified causes; 40% of non-quadriplegic cerebral palsy have known causes—35% are congenital, 5% are due to other causes

cerebral performance category scale EMERGENCY MEDICINE A scale that grades response to cardiopulmonary resuscitation, based on a scoring system from 1 to 5 (JAMA 1995; 273:1261) Cf Glasgow coma scale

CPC SCORE 1 A return to normal cerebral function and normal living

CPC SCORE 2 Cerebral disbility but sufficient function for independent activities of daily living

CPC SCORE 3 Severe disability, limited cognition, inability to carry out independent existance

CPC SCORE 4 Coma

CPC SCORE 5 Brain death

cerebriform nuclei Twisted, convoluted nuclei with a cerebral gyri-like appearance, classically seen in the atypical T cells of mycosis fungoides, Sezary syndrome and lymphomatoid papulosis; although cerebriform cells are usually T lymphocytes, they may also be B lymphocytes

cerebroma A virtually extinct generic term for any mass of brain tissue, which is now designated as 'cerebral mass'

cerebrospinal fluid leak CSF leak ETIOLOGY Trauma, cranial base surgery DIAGNOSIS Suspicious drainage, imaging studies (MRI, CT, CT cisternography, radioisotope scans), β-transferrin assay, endoscopic fluorescein technique TREATMENT Soft tissue and mucosal flaps, biomaterial grafting

cerebrovascular accident Stroke, see there

Ceredase An orphan drug (Genzyme Corp, Boston) product that is available under a treatment IND protocol for Gaucher's disease, which acts to replace the missing glucocerebrosidase

ceride A wax ester formed from a long-chain fatty acid and a long-chain aliphatic alcohol

ceroid Alcohol-insoluble, oxidized polyunsaturated lipid pigment(s) that results from the peroxidation of unsaturated lipids, which are similar or identical to lipofuscin; ceroid accumulates in macrophages of the heart, liver, GI tract, and brain in the elderly and is thus termed 'wear and tear' pigment and has been inculpated in age-related organ dysfunction, see 'Garbage can' hypothesis, in hypovitaminosis E, in cathartic colon and in hereditary conditions, eg Batten's disease, and sea-blue histiocytosis

ceroid 'granuloma' A finding in chronic cholecystitis, in which there are focal aggregates of neutral fat and lipofuscin-laden macrophages, contrasting with cholesterosis, which also occurs in chronic cholecystitis and is a diffuse process with cholesterol-laden macrophages accumulating immediately subjacent to the mucosa, imparting a macroscopic appearance, fancifully termed 'strawberry' gall bladder

certifiable *adjective* Capable of being certified, as in either an infectious disease* or a mental disorder, the latter being by far the most common use in American 'English'

*Reportable is more widely used in the US—Author's note

certificate of death Death certificate, see there

Certificate of Need A document often required by state law in the US and issued by a governmental body to an individual or organization proposing to a) Construct or modify a health care facility b) Make major capital equipment purchases or c) Offer a new health care service; CONs can be used by government to prevent duplication of services or excess regional development of facilities or services; if a major purchase, eg a magnetic resonance imager (MRI), is made by a health care facility without an approved CON, the sponsoring institute's 'part A' costs may not be reimbursed

certified bed A 'legal' bed in a health care facility that has been approved for use by patients on a permanent basis, which the governing body (usually the state board of health) has deemed to have sufficient staffing to support its unqualified use; see Bed; Cf 'Swing' bed

certifying death The act of confirming that an individual is dead after another person (or physician) has pronounced or determined that the individual is dead (see N Engl J Med 1993; 329:1346SB) Cf Pronouncing death

cerumen Wet cerumen, see there

cervical 'collar' An erythematous rash affecting the second and third cervical nerve roots in reactivated varicella-zoster

cervical disk syndrome NEUROSURGERY A condition caused by cervical cord or root displacement or compression (often at multiple levels), which is characterized by radicular (suboccipital, cervical, interscapular, and thoracic) pain that radiates into the upper extremities and is aggravated by movement, accompanied by pain, paresthesias, and dysesthesias in cervical dermatomes; CDS may be accompanied by muscle fasciculations, spasms, and atrophy, lower extremity spasticity with extensor plantar sign, and spastic bladder DIAGNOSIS Narrowed disk spaces, osteophytes or spinal stenosis by radiology, myelography, CT, MRI TREATMENT-MEDICAL Immobilization, mild traction in a neutral position, transcutaneous injection of enzymes (eg collagenase) to dissolve cartilage TREATMENT-SURGICAL Decompression with laminotomy, foraminotomy, total diskectomy through bilateral laminotomy followed by interbody fusion

cervical intraepithelial neoplasia A malignancy arising in uterine cervical epithelium and confined thereto; CIN represents a continuum of histologic changes ranging from well-differentiated CIN 1, (formerly, mild dysplasia) to severe dysplasia/carcinoma in situ, CIN 3; the lesion arises at the squamocolumnar cell junction at the transformation zone of the endocervical canal, with a variable tendency to develop invasive epidermoid carcinoma, a tendency that is enhanced by concomitant human papillomaviral infection, of which HPV 6 and 11 are associated with the 'garden variety', ie benign condylomas; HPV types 16, 18 occur in CIN 3, while types 31, 33, 35, 52, 56 may appear in CIN; 78% of ♀ who are positive for HPV, especially HPV 16 and 18 develop CIN 2-3 (N Engl J Med 1992; 327:1272OA) PROGRESSION see table facing page TREATMENT Cone biopsy, laser vaporization or excision, loop electrosurgical excision, cryotherapy (N Engl J Med 1993; 328:856RV) see Carcinoma in situ, Intraepithelial neoplasia

cervical neck syndrome Cervical disk syndrome‡

cervical rib A uni- or bilateral congenital anomaly of the first thoracic rib, affecting up to 1% of the population, 15% of whom have an associated thoracic outlet syndrome (see there); cervical ribs range from type I, a short bar extending from the transverse process to type IV, which is a complete extra rib articulating with the sternum

cervical ripening The stromal response of the uterine cervix that occurs in phase 1 of parturition, which precedes the onset of labor, in which the cervix becomes softer and more dilatable; during CR the collagen fibers break down and undergo rearrangement and there is an alteration of the proportion of the glycosaminoglycans, with ↓ dermatan sulfate and a marked ↑ in hyaluronic acid, the latter of which helps the tissues retain water; PE$_2$ gel can be used to ripen the cervix prior to the induction of potentially difficult inductions (Can Med Assoc J 1991; 145:1249)

cervical zygapophysial joint ORTHOPEDIC ANATOMY One of a pair of synovial joints between the neural arches of the cervical vertebrae which is a common site of chronic post-traumatic neck pain, classically caused by whiplash injury

cervix mark NEONATOLOGY A fluid-filled vesicle of no clinical significance, that lies atop the caput succedaneum, the edematous 'mass' at the presenting aspect of the head in a vaginally delivered infant

cesarean section C-section OBSTETRICS Surgical extraction of a product of conception, which has become the single most commonly performed invasive procedure in many nations STATISTICS Brazil has the world's highest rate of C-sections at 32/100 hospital deliveries; Japan and Czechoslovakia have the lowest at 7/100; US, non-Hispanic Caucasians, 20.6/1000, Hispanics, 13.9/1000; frequency, post-C-section vaginal delivery, 5% in USA, 43% in Norway; private patients are more likely to have C-sections than clinic patients

C-section is the oldest of all surgical operations; royal law (lex regia) by Numa Pompilius (715-672 BC) decreed that children be excised from any woman dying late in pregnancy, later known as lex caesarea under the rule of the Caesars; some scholars maintain that the name derives from the Latin caedere, to cut, an abdominal birth would thus be partus caesareus

CETP Cholesteryl-ester transfer protein, see there

CF Complement fixation, see there

CFCs Chlorofluorocarbons ENVIRONMENT A family of stable non-toxic, non-flammable, non-corrosive chemicals used as coolants, foaming and cleaning agents, and aerosol propellants; in 1988, 10^6 metric tons of CFCs were consumed on the planet, 730 000 metric tons of CFC-11 and CFC-12, resulting in a net addition of 100% to the atmospheric gases, since this last group requires many decades to naturally disappear; CFC-related goods and services generate $28 x 10^9/year and employ 700 000 workers in the US, where refrigerants comprise 30% of CFC use; foam-blow-

PROGRESSION OF CERVICAL INTRAEPITHELIAL NEOPLASIA			
	CIN I	CIN II	CIN III
Regression (←)	60%(50%)	40%(43%)	33%
Persistence	30%(41%)	40%(48%)	55%
Progression (→) to CIN III	10%(9%)	20%(9%)	N/A
→ to squamous carcinoma	± 1%	5%	≥ 12%

¹Int J Gynecol Pathol 1993; 12:186 (Modern Pathol 1990; 3:679)

ing agents for polystyrene and polyurethane 28% (rigid foam is used for insulation; non-rigid for cushions) and industrial solvents and cleaning agents 19% (in 1978, aerosol CFCs were banned in the US); CFCs are largely responsible for depleting the ozone layer and are minor contributors to the greenhouse effect; CFC-12 (CF_2Cl_2) is the most widely used coolant which is targeted for replacement by the less ozone-depleting HCFC-134a; international treaties plan to reduce CFC use to one-half the current levels by 1999; industry retooling to less ozone-depleting CFCs will cost $10 x 10^9; the Montreal Protocol assumes that certain substitutes, eg HCFC-22, for 'hard' CFCs (CFC-11, -12, -113, -114, -115) are less damaging, although the terms 'ozone-depleting potential' and 'halocarbon global warming potential' are not equivalent; potential CFC substitutes for refrigerant, CFC-12: HCFC-134a (CF_3CFH_2), HCFC-22 (CHF_2Cl); potential CFC replacements, blowing agent, CFC-11 ($CFCl_3$): HCFC-141b (CH_3CFCl_2), HCFC-123 (CF_3CFCl_2), HCFC-22 (CHF_2Cl); potential CFC replacements for cleaning agents, CFC-113 ($CF_2ClCFCl_2$); see Greenhouse effect, Montreal protocol, Ozone layer

Note: Bromocarbons (halons) CF_3Br and CF_2ClBr fire extinguishers have an atmospheric half-life of 10- and 2-fold greater than that of a proposed substitute, CHF_2Br, which has a seven year half-life (Science 1991; 252:693)

CFS see Chronic fatigue syndrome

CFTR Cystic fibrosis transmembrane conductance regulator A cyclic-AMP-regulated chloride channel, encoded by the *CFTR* gene; there are a wide array of mutations seen in the *CFTR* gene, eg that which occurs in intron 19, in which there is cystic fibrosis-like lung disease but normal sweat chloride levels (N Engl J Med 1994; 331:974OA) see Cystic fibrosis

CFU Colony-forming unit

CFU-GEMM A colony-stimulating factor for all cell lines

(granulocytes, erythroid, megakaryocytes, macrophages); complete absence of CFU-GEMM is implicated in the pancytopenia of Fanconi's disease and myelodysplasia and its production can be suppressed by chemicals, drugs, radiation, malnutrition, viral and bacterial infections

CFU-S Colony-forming units, spleen A heterogeneous population of cells that are thought to contain the ultimate stem cell, as the putative cells have the key capabilities of proliferation, pluripotentiality and self-renewal

CGD Chronic granulomatous disease, see there

CGRP Calcitonin gene-related peptide A 37-residue polypeptide produced by alternate splicing of pre-mRNA from the calcitonin gene; CGRP is a potent vasodilator that functions by activation of K^+/ATP channel, acting as a positive feedback signal for acetylcholine synthesis, increasing the number of acetylcholine receptors in cultured cells; it is secreted by the thyroid C cells and by the sensory nerve endings at the same site of secondary and tertiary calcification in bone, increasing the cAMP levels in osteoblasts; CGRP is structurally related to N-proCT, see there

Cg/Sg family Chromogranin/secretogranin family, see there

CHAD Cold hemagglutinin disease(s) see Cold agglutinins

Chagas' disease American trypanosomiasis A parasitic disease caused by the protozoan, *Trypanosoma cruzi*, and is a major cause of morbidity and mortality in Latin American countries EPIDEMIOLOGY Circa 17 x 10^6 have chronic CD in Latin America; *T cruzi* is transferred in the feces of hematophagous triatomine insects (reduviid bugs) which may contaminate the bite itself, the conjunctiva or a mucosal surface; less common routes of transmission include blood transfusion (20 000 transfusion-related cases/year, Brazil), maternofetal (vertical), accidental (laboratory workers) CLINICAL-ACUTE CD Mild with 5% mortality; fever, malaise, edema of face and lower extremities, lymphadenopathy, hepatosplenomegaly; rarely muscle or CNS invasion CHRONIC CD 10-30 years latency; severe cardiomyopathy with biventricular enlargement, thinning of ventricular walls, mural thrombi, interstitial fibrosis, conduction defects, eg right bundle branch block, or complete AV block; GI disease with megaesophagus and/or megacolon due to either local denervation or possibly to an autoimmune mechanism LABORATORY Acute CD Parasites in peripheral blood smear; chronic CD Serological to identify IgG by ELISA, complement fixation, or by indirect immunofluorescence TREATMENT: Therapeutic armamentarium (benzidazole, nifurtimox) is inadequate; parasitologic cures are achieved in 50% but at a highly toxic price to the patient (N Engl J Med 1993; 329:488CPC, 329:639RA)

chain growth and synthesis MOLECULAR BIOLOGY DNA synthesis in vivo occurs in the 5'→3' direction; in vitro (chemical) synthesis of DNA occurs in the 5'→3' direction; peptide synthesis in vivo occurs from amino terminus towards the carboxy terminus; in vitro (chemical) peptide synthesis starts at the carboxyl terminus, working toward the amino terminal

chain-like thickening NEPHROPATHOLOGY A histologic feature of stage III membranous glomerulonephritis, best seen with a PAS stain, a finding that follows the 'spike stage' and corresponds to a variable corrugated pattern of thickened glomerular basement membrane with a few recognizable projections

chain of custody Chain of evidence FORENSIC MEDICINE The path that objects (eg bullets, knives) or clinical specimens (eg semen specimen in alleged rape) must take for these materials to be legally accepted as evidence in a court of law; emergency room physicians and pathologists often find themselves part of the chain and have a responsibility to document all pertinent details regarding the specimen and to turn these materials into the appropriate authorities

chain of lakes appearance A descriptive term for a finding by ERCP seen in chronic pancreatitis where the main pancreatic duct measures 1.0 cm in average diameter and is 'punctuated' by scattered focal obstructions; other ERCP features of chronic pancreatitis include strictures, cysts and ductal calculi

chain of survival CARDIOLOGY A sequence of steps that the American Heart Association emphasizes to successfully treat cardiac arrest, which depends on community-wide emergency cardiac care and includes early access to emergency services, early initiation of CPR, early defibrillation, and early advanced life support (N Engl J Med 1993; 329:604ₒₐ)

chair see Endowed professorship

'chair' A non-sexist sobriquet for the chairman, -woman or -person, ie the presiding officer in an organization; in academics, the 'chair' is often a full professor who is responsible for the academic, clinical, administrative and research activities of the department; Cf Endowed chair, Professor

chairman The head of an academic department; see 'Chair', Cf Chief

chairman of staff Chief of staff, see there

chair rung appearance A descriptive term for a morphologic patern seen by light microscopy, which consists of periodic constrictions in asbestos fibers that are focally surrounded by protein-mineral complexes

chakra ALTERNATIVE MEDICINE An energy center allegedly present in the body that is believed by some advocates of alternative forms of health care to create a luminous energy field known as an aura, which is alleged to be a manifestation of the total body energy; disease or malfunction of the body is believed by 'esoteric healers' to be the result of a block or restriction in the flow of the body's energy (The New Age Catalog, Island Publishing Co, Dolphin, Doubleday, New York 1988) see Alternative Medicine, 'New Age'; Cf Aura

chalasia chair A device formerly used to treat GI reflux in young children; in infants less than 6 months of age, the device may exacerbate reflux

'chalk bone' disease Osteopetrosis (Albers-Schönberg disease), see there

chalk streaks Verkalkung Short whitish striations seen on gross examination of intraductal carcinomas of the breast, tumors that are often 'gritty' to cutting, the result of desmoplasia with microcalcifications; chalk streaks are rarely seen in other epithelial malignancies

challenge IMMUNLOGY The administration of an antigen or allergen to a person who has been previously exposed to the antigen, specifically to evoke an immune response

challenge stock IMMUNOLOGY A precisely calibrated dose of an antigen that is administered after previous exposure to an infectious agent, eg HIV-1 that is used to test a vaccine's efficacy

chalone A target organ or tissue-specific (but not species-specific) inhibitor of cell proliferation or other activity, which, unlike true hormones, are not produced by a specific organ

champagne bottle legs NEUROLOGY Marked distal peroneal muscle atrophy with tapering of the distal extremities and hypertrophy of the proximal muscles, imparting an inverted champagne bottle or 'stork leg' appearance; this appearance is typical of advanced Charcot-Marie-Tooth type of chronic familial peripheral neuropathy; pes cavus may be the only early finding, which is followed by foot drop (leading to a high 'steppage' gait); walking is difficult given the combination of sensory ataxia and muscu-

lar weakness; EMG reveals ↓ conduction velocity and ↑ distal latency; see Onion bulb, Piano playing

champagne glass appearance RADIOLOGY A fanciful descriptor for the inner pelvic contour with narrowed sacrosciatic notches typical of achondroplasia, where the pelvic width exceeds the depth due to an increased iliac base; in contrast, the 'brandy snifter' contour is normal and 'wine glass' contour occurs in Morquio syndrome

chance node The initial branch in a clinical decision-making algorithm at which a particular diagnostic or therapeutic intervention is performed; based on the results (eg response, nonresponse), further procedures or interventions are planned at each subsequent decision node; see Decision node, Decision tree, Outcome node

'chandelier' sign GYNECOLOGY A highly colloquial term for the extreme hypersensitivity to pain in women with pelvic inflammatory disease; an internal examination in afflicted women evokes pain of such intensity that the patient seemingly leaps out of the examination stirrups 'for the chandelier'

channeling PARAPSYCHOLOGY The alleged communication with a dead person, either directly or through a physically 'embodied' person from a source that is alleged to exist on a level or dimension of reality other than the physical reality as accepted or recognized by mainstream science; channeling has been anecdotally reported by 'entities' known as Lazaris (channeled via J Pursel), Ramtha (via JZ Knight), and Seth (via Jane Roberts) (The New Age Catalog, Island Publishing Co, Dolphin, Doubleday, New York 1988) see Alternative Medicine, 'New Age', Parapsychology

chaos Non-linearity THEORETICAL BIOLOGY Unpredictability arising from dynamic instability such that initially neighboring trajectories develop differently; chaos is complex, non-linear, yet completely deterministic order that is present in all living systems, which is extremely sensitive to initial conditions and perturbations, such that minute changes impact on a ground state, potentially leading to large differences in an end state; all healthy physiological systems have innate variability or chaos, the loss or reduction of which leads to a less complicated and more ordered state, signaling an impaired system; although the mathematics of non-linear dynamics is arcane, it is present in biological systems by design, appearing in normal fluctuations of the heart rate, blood flow and blood pressure; the chaos phenomenon has been studied in and appears to influence such diverse fields as cardiology, epidemiology, immunology, neurology, psychiatry and other fields (JAMA 1991; 266:12ᵣᵥ)

CHAP Cyclophosphamide, hexamethylmelamine, doxorubicin, cisplatin, a chemotherapeutic regimen that has had some currency in treating ovarian cancer

chaperones A class of proteins that facilitate the correct assembly or disassembly of oligomeric protein complexes, participating in the transmembrane targeting of certain proteins; chaperones include nucleoplasmins, chaperonins (see there), heat shock proteins 70 and 90 classes, signal recognition particle, trigger factor and BiP, an immunoglobulin heavy chain-binding protein

chaperonins A group of 60-kD cytosolic proteins, eg heat shock protein 60, hsp60, that use the energy from ATP hydrolysis to maintain proteins in the necessary folded configuration for proper function, thus having 'foldase' activity; other postulated roles for chaperonins include protein transport, oligomer assembly, DNA replication, mRNA turnover and protection of the cell from various stresses; some chaperones have auto-foldase activities; Cf Chaperones, Heat shock, hsp70

character Personality, see there

character education SOCIAL MEDICINE A formal initiative

that '...*represents an effort to teach moral behavior to primary- and secondary-school students in a time percieved to be morally rudderless and to be without such teaching in the local communities or in the home.*' (New York Times Magazine 30 April 1995, p36)

Charcot's joint Neuropathic arthropathy, see there

Charcot-Leyden crystals A crystalline structure composed of lisophospholipase of unknown function produced by eosinophils, and classically seen in the sputum cytology of patients with asthma

Charcot-Marie-Tooth disease A clinically heterogenous condition that is the most common (1:2500) inherited peripheral neuropathy CLINICAL Slowly progressive atrophy of distal muscles, especially those innervated by the peroneal nerve, leading to muscular atrophy of hands, feet, and legs with pes cavus deformity, claw-hand and stork-leg appearance PATHOLOGY Hypertrophic neuropathy with 'onion-bulb' formation lowly HEREDITY CMT disease is genetically heterogeneous with AD [MIM 118200, 118210], AR [MIM 214400], and X-linked [MIM 302800] forms being described MOLECULAR PATHOLOGY The most common form, CMT 1A is AD and is characterized by a 1.5 Mb (megabase) duplication in 17p11.2p12 (which leads to a gene-dosage effect) with a spontaneous point mutation in the *PMP22* gene, which is similar to the *trembler* mutation of mice (N Engl J Med 1993; 329:96OA)

CHARGE complex A disease complex of probable neural crest origin, diagnosed when infants have four of the seven components of the CHARGE acronym Coloboma, Heart defects (conotruncal or septal), Atresia of the nasal choanae, Retarded growth and development, Genital hypoplasia, and Ear anomalies and/or deafness; other findings in the CHARGE complex include facial palsy, renal anomalies and cleft lip/palate

charlatan see Quack

Charley Horse A colloquial term for leg pain caused by a contusion injury to the thigh involving the quadriceps muscle; without immediate compression, the ensuing hematoma and pain can be substantial; the term is being increasingly applied to painful injuries to other muscle groups

The origin of this American colloquialism for muscle stiffness is unknown, but it is anecdotally related to a horse named Charley who walked with a limp, drawing a roller to flatten the playing field in the Chicago White Sox baseball park in Chicago during the 1890s

Charlie Chaplin gait A gait that occurs in bilateral external torsion of the tibia, caused by faulty sitting or sleeping habits, as in prolonged maintenance of the 'spread-eagle' or frogleg position TREATMENT Early, change sleeping habits, brace, and if too late, osteotomy

The deformity results in a form of ambulation that has been fancifully likened to the waddling gait affected by Charlie Chaplin's silent film character, *The Little Tramp*

chart *noun* A formal document that includes relevant data and records from a person's medical history *verb* To place orders, progress notes or information in a person's medical record (chart)

chart war A highly colloquial term for a patient management-related skirmish between two physicians or services that occurs in writing on the pages of a patient's chart with parries and thrusts in the form of progress notes, with each party questioning the other's justification for performing a particular procedure; in a CW, one 'combat-ant' may impugn another's intelligence at least, and competence at most, literature is quoted freely, and the language used may be arcane and obtuse; there is no justification for CWs regardless of how elegant the thrusts and parries are, as the chart is a document that can be quoted in a court of law

chase A term that can be either a noun or verb, which refers to the halting of a chemical or dynamic reaction, in which a so-called 'pulse' incorporation of a labelled or radioactive compound is 'chased' by a non-labelled compound; this sequence of events allows evaluation of the kinetics of a reaction; Cf Pulse-chase experiment

'chatterbox' syndrome Cocktail party syndrome, see there

chauffeur fracture An oblique fracture of the distal radius extending radially from the articular margin with separation of both the styloid process and a triangular portion of attached bone; these fractures were seen forty or more years ago when all automobile engines were started mechanically by a crank and the engine 'backfired', and therefore is an injury most likely to occur in antique car enthusiasts

Note: The last automobile to have a hand crank (for emergency starting) was Citroen's venerable 2CV, which was produced until July 1990

Chauvenet's criterion method STATISTICS A method that allows the rejection of statistical outliers in a data set; Chauvenet's criterion states that an observation ('outlier') should be rejected if the probability of obtaning the value is less than $\frac{1}{2}n$, where n equals the number of values in a data set; the method is reapplied until no more outlying data can be excluded (Arch Pathol Lab Med 1993; 117:704OA)

CHD 1) Congenital heart disease 1) Coronary heart disease

Also 1) Centre for Human Development (British) 2) Chediak-Higashi disease 3) Childhood disease 4) Chronic hemodialysis 5) Cyclohexadiene

checkerboard Punnett square CLINICAL GENETICS A grid chart used to determine the possible genotypes at a particular locus and the relative frequency with which they occur in progeny, when the parents' alleles are known; the haploid gametes of one parent are indicated in rows of the matrix, and of the other parent in the columns; the matrix squares contain the progeny's genotype

'checkerboard' nucleus Tortoise shell nucleus, see there

checkerboard pattern HISTOLOGY The normal interspersing of dark (type I) and light (type II) skeletal muscle fibers which develops by the 30th fetal week, a pattern that is directly controlled by the CNS and which is lost in many myopathic diseases, as may occur in proliferative myositis, mitochondrial myopathies and neurogenic atrophy

checkerboard titration A laboratory method used to study the effect of varying any one parameter on the sensitivity and specificity of, eg a staining system while the other parameters of the system are held constant; the equilibrium is called the plateau titer

check valve obstruction Ball valve obstruction, see there

cheese disease see Tyramine-induced hypertension

chelation therapy ALTERNATIVE MEDICINE A '...*method for drawing toxins and metabolic wastes from the bloodstream.*' CT consists of administration of chelating agent, eg EDTA (ethylenediaminetetracetic acid) usually IV, or penicillamine administered orally; its only FDA-approved indication is for the treatment of lead and other heavy metal poisoning; it is claimed by practitioners of alternative medicine that CT may be used to remove calcium from atherosclerotic plaques, and by extension is a viable alternative to bypass surgery and angioplasty; it has been also claimed that CT can be used to treat arthritis, and connective tissue diseases, and can be used to improve vision, hearing, sense of smell, and memory (Alternative Medicine, Future Medicine Publishing, Inc, Puyallup, Washington, 1994) Note: There is no data on the efficacy of CT (other than for FDA-approved indications) in peer-reviewed journals; see Alternative medicine

chem6 LABORATORY MEDICINE A battery of basic tests that measures six components in the serum, which are commonly ordered as part of a routine 'stat' profile, and include Na^+, K^+, Cl^-, CO_2, glucose, urea nitrogen

chemabrasion Chemical peel, see there

chemical colitis An acute inflammatory colitis that develops hours after self-administration of a 'cleansing' enema containing soap or other inappropriate agents, eg hydrogen peroxide, vinegar and potassium permanganate, resulting in hypertonic, detergent or directly toxic effects CLINICAL Effects range from vague pain to cramping, anaphylaxis, serosanguinous diarrhea, hypovolemia and acute hemoconcentration; when the mucosal damage is severe, bacteria may penetrate the mucosa, causing sepsis, hypokalemia, pseudomembrane formation, hemorrhagic necrosis, intestinal gangrene, and acute renal failure; see Soap colitis

chemical carcinogenesis The induction of malignancy by a **chemical carcinogen** (or putative carcinogen), which can be occupation-related (eg aromatic amines, arsenic, benzene, cadmium, chrome ores, soots, tars, vinyl chloride), environmental (eg aflatoxin, asbestos, tobacco), or iatrogenic (eg alkylating agents, anabolic steroids, phenacetin) PATHOGENESIS Initiation of the carcinogenic 'cascade' occurs when an electrophilically reactive chemical (initiator), or more often, one or more of its metabolites interacts with DNA, and repair of the damaged DNA is unsuccessful; this is followed by a sequence of events known as tumor promotion

chemical diabetes mellitus A subclinical or preclinical form of DM characterized by DM-like response curves to glucose tolerance tests or other provocative tests; it is controversial whether therapy is beneficial for these patients

chemical disinfection PUBLIC HEALTH A method for treating medical waste to render it noninfectious to humans, by treating it with chlorine dioxide, after which the waste can be disposed of in landfills (Laboratory Medicine 1995; 26:323OA) see Medical waste

'chemical McCarthyism' A colloquial phrase coined in reference to the US government-sponsored drug abuse testing of employee urine, which in the USA, smacks of infringement of constitutional rights, and to be reliable, would require trained micturition observers, represents an invasion of privacy

The McCarthyism refers to US Senator Joe McCarthy who during the early 1950s led zealous and often unfounded campaigns of defamation against various suspected communists

chemical 'mumps' 'Iodine mumps', see there

chemical peel DERMATOLOGY A technique in which phenol or (which is more popular) trichloroacetic acid (TCA) is 'painted' on elderly sun-exposed skin with extensive actinic keratoses (a pre-malignant condition); CPs can be of superficial, medium-depth, or deep*; TCA treatment results in chemical exfoliation of the epidermis and upper dermis, and ↓ future incidence of basal and squamous cell carcinoma in the treated region and removes fine wrinkles; chemical peels are used to rejuvenate sun-damaged and aging skin, and has both cosmetic and therapeutic applications in managing rhytides, actinic lesions, and pigmentary changes; Cf Mohs' surgery

*Which is indicated for skin wrinkling, moderate actinic keratosis, and for various (benign) pigmentary abnormalities

chemical pollutant ENVIRONMENT A chemical substance that enters the environment through industrial, agricultural or other human activities, which poses an immediate or potential hazard to plant, animal or human life; the major chemical pollutants are heavy metals, eg mercury and lead, aromatic hydrocarbons, eg benzene and other petrochemicals, organic solvents, eg toluene and xylene, organo-halogens, eg polychlorinated biphenyls (PCBs), polybrominated biphenyls (PBBs), dioxins, and others, eg

nitrogen and sulfur dioxides; Cf Hazardous chemical

chemical shift (delta) MRI The change in the Larmor frequency of a given nucleus when bound to different sites in a molecule, due to magnetic shielding effects of the electron orbitals; chemical shifts are responsible for the differences among various molecules and different sites within the molecules in high-resolution magnetic resonance spectra; the amount of shift is proportional to strength of the magnetic field strength and is usually specified in parts per million of the resonance frequency relative to a standard; see Magnetic resonance imaging

chemical shift to the left see Neuroblastoma

chemical spill PUBLIC HEALTH A generic term for the inadvertent release in a liquid form of a chemical that is regarded as hazardous to human health, which in the workplace are identified with hazardous materials labels, see there

chemical 'splenectomy' Therapeutic immune paralysis A method that inhibits splenic endocytosis of opsonized, ie immunoglobulin or complement-coated cells or microorganisms by blocking Fc receptors; the targets are thus bound, but not endocytosed; chemical splenectomy is a state inducible by high-dose corticosteroids or IV immunoglobulin; the effect lasts as long as the therapy and is an alternative to surgery in immune-related hypersplenism, eg autoimmune hemolytic anemia, autoimmune neutropenia, and Felty syndrome

chemical transfection GENE THERAPY A method of gene insertion in which foreign genes are inserted into a cell of interest by a chemical means, eg by use of calcium phosphate, liposomes, and molecular conjugates (Bio/Technology 1995; 13:222) Cf Physical transfection, Viral transduction

chemical warfare The use of chemicals as weapons of war, usually deployed as gases; the tremendous morbidity caused by these weapons of mass destruction, used in World War I against ± 1.3 million soldiers led to their ban under the 'Geneva Protocol' of 1925[1] AGENTS Phosgene, nerve agents (sarin, soman, tabun), which are chemical mixtures, including diisopropylfluorophosphate that react with the serine hydroxyl group of acetylcholinesterase, inhibiting neural transmission, hydrogen cyanide, blistering agents (mustard gas) and thionyl chloride, which are gases that are intended be fired from long range artillery CLINICAL Mustard gas, the prototypic chemical weapon, causes marked irritation of the skin, eyes, upper respiratory and GI tracts; the skin lesions heal in 'geographic' waves, leaving residual hyperpigmentation or induration; at the time of Glasnost, the US stockpile had a global overkill for chemical weapons of 4000 (in contrast, the overkill for nuclear weapons was estimated at 10-20); ½ of the US chemical weapon stockpile was in the form of nerve agents; although the Soviets reported they had 45 000 tons of chemical weapons, the actual amount was estimated to be as high as 270-360 000 tons; see Biological warfare, Weapons of mass destruction; Cf Zyklon B

[1]Despite the ban, in World War II poison gas was reportedly used by the Italians against the Ethiopians, and by the Japanese against the Manchurians; the Germans developed the chemicals tabun and sarin during the war for this purpose, and had packaged these potent cholinesterase inhibitors into bombs, but never deployed them [2]Because of the relatively transient nature of the injuries, the remoteness or difficulty of access to a site of an attack, language barriers between the victims and the interviewers and the deterioration of the chemicals themselves with time, allegations of the use of chemical weapons may be difficult to corroborate; chemical weapons were allegedly deployed in 1) The 'Yellow rain' incident in the 1970s, in which the Laotian and Kampuchean governments attacked Hmong villages with trichothecane and 2) In August 1988 by Iraqi troops under Saddam Hussein against the Kurds in northern Iraq

chemiluminescence LABORATORY MEDICINE A reaction in which chemical energy is converted into light by an oxidation reaction, where a precursor molecule reacts in the presence of peroxide and an alkali to form a high-energy peroxide intermediate (luminol, lophine, lucigenin); when specially designed peroxides, eg AMPPD, AMPGD are used, very low molar amounts, 10^{-18} of a substance of interest, eg DNA and RNA probes, oligonucleotides and immune molecules may be detected

chemoembolization see Hepatic artery embolization

chemonucleolysis NEUROSURGERY The injection of an enzyme, eg chymopapain as an alternative to laminectomy in certain cases of intervertebral disc rupture, 10-40% meet the criteria; the stated advantages of chemonucleolysis include earlier ambulation and ability to perform the procedure on an outpatient basis

chemoprevention The use of a substance or chemical in the diet or drugs to prevent or reduce the incidence of a disease, usually referring to cancer; among the agents with chemopreventive effects (as supported by 'soft' data) are vitamins A, C, and E, bran and other dietary fibers, and cruciferous vegetables; Cf Chemoprophylaxis

Statistical support for the efficacy of chemoprevention continues to be weak; use of vitamin A or β carotene does not prevent secondary non-melanoma skin cancer; high doses of the vitamin A analog, isoretinoin reportedly prevent second primary malignancies in the head and neck region

chemoprophylaxis The use of a chemical, usually a therapeutic drug, to prevent the occurrence of a disease, usually infectious, eg malaria or tuberculosis; Cf Chemoprevention

Note: While the terms chemoprevention and chemoprophylaxis are by definition synonymous, they differ in usage; chemoprevention is generally used for the use of a 'natural' substance to reduce the risk of a constellation of diseases, ie malignancy, while chemoprophylaxis refers to a specific agent's efficacy in treating a particular disease

chemoreceptor trigger zone Area postrema NEUROANATOMY The emetic center is located in the floor of the fourth ventricle, receiving vagal afferents or stimulated directly by apomorphine, cardiac glycosides, ergot compounds, chemotherapeutic agents, staphylococcal enterotoxin, salicylate and nicotine, and other circulating chemicals; in contrast to the adjacent but distinct vomiting center, the CTZ does not respond to electrical stimulation

chemosensitivity The sensitivity of chemoreceptors to hypoxia and hypercapnea; reduced chemosensitivity to hypoxia has been linked to fatal asthma attacks (N Engl J Med 1994; 330:1329OA)

chemosurgery Mohs' micrographic technique A technique used in plastic surgery for excising superficial, locally invasive, tumor microfingerlets of primary skin cancers, which yields a cure rate of more than 98% for these tumors; the technique is of use in treating skin tumors that are broad, but not deep, eg basal and squamous cell carcinomas, but not malignant melanomas, optimally designed for lesions > 1-2 cm, recurrent skin tumors, cancer recurrence-prone sites (nose, eyes, ears) and aggressive histologic subtypes, eg morphea-like or metatypical basal cell carcinoma TECHNIQUE The surface of the lesion plus 3-5 mm margin of normal tissue is coagulated with dichloroacetic acid, overlaid with a 20% zinc chloride paste and covered with an occlusive dressing; the $ZnCl_2$ fixes the tissue similar to formaldehyde; after from 1 to 48 hours, a 'saucer' of tissue is removed and submitted for frozen section analysis to determine sites, if any, of deep tumor extension; although the procedure is tedious in short-term, Mohs' surgery reduces future recurrences while preserving uninvolved tissue; Cf Chemical peel

chemotaxis IMMUNOLOGY A stimulus that is exerted along a chemical's concentration gradient; chemotaxins are usually small molecules and in vivo act to attract macrophages and other cells along a concentration gradient

chemotherapy 1) A virtually extinct synonym for antituberculous therapy 2) The use of various agents, most of which are toxic to cells undergoing division, to induce tumor cell lysis; successful chemotherapy is a function of tumor responsiveness, which most predictably occurs in lymphoproliferative malignancies, eg leukemias and lymphomas as well as in small cell carcinoma, an undifferentiated carcinoma; because these agents are most effective against rapidly proliferating cells, 'collateral damage' to the dividing cells in skin and hair, BM, and GI tract are predictable, causing reversible hair loss, myelosuppression, nausea and vomiting is the norm; the most feared late effect of chemotherapeutics, especially in successfully treated pediatric leukemias, is the induction of a second malignancy, which is usually refractory to therapy; see Combined modality therapy, Damocles' syndrome; popular therapeutic formulations include

BACOD Bleomycin, Adriamycin (doxorubicin), cyclophosphamide, vincristine (Oncovorin), dexamethasone

BACOP Bleomycin, Adriamycin (doxorubicin), cyclophosphamide, vincristine (Oncovorin), prednisone

CHOP Cyclophosphamide, hydroxydaunomycin (doxorubicin), Oncovorin (vincristine), prednisone

COP Cyclophosphamide, Oncovorin (vincristine), prednisone

COP-BLAM Cyclophosphamide, Oncovorin (vincristine), prednisone, bleomycin, Adriamycin (doxorubicin), Matulane (procarbazine)

COPP Chloramphenicol, Oncovorin (vincristine), procarbazine, prednisone

m-BACOD Methotrexate/citrovorin rescue, bleomycin, Adriamycin (doxorubicin), cyclophosphamide, Oncovorin (vincristine), decadron

MOPP Mechlorethamine, Oncovorin (vincristine), procarbazine, prednisone

PROMACE Prednisone, methotrexate/citrovorin rescue, Adriamycin (doxorubicin), cyclophosphamide, etoposide

chemotherapy-induced emesis Chemotherapy-induced nausea and vomiting, which is mediated by dopamine D_2 receptors and serotonin receptors in the chemoreceptor trigger zone of the area postrema and in the GI tract; CIE is a side effect of certain chemotherapeutic agents, which while often the most anxiety-provoking of the toxic effects of chemotherapy, is self-limited and rarely life-threatening HIGHLY EMETOGENIC DRUGS Cisplatin, carmustine, dacarbazine, dactinomycin mechlorethamine HCl (nitrogen mustard), streptozocin MODERATELY EMETOGENIC DRUGS Azacitidine, arparginase, carboplatin, cyclophosphamide, doxorubicin, mitomycin TREATMENT Dopamine D_2 high-dose metoclopramide, and serotonin (5-HT_3) receptor antagonists, eg ondansetron (N Engl J Med 1993; 329:1790RV) see Ondansetron

chemotherapy-induced leukemia see Secondary malignancy

Chemturion space suit Blue suit A pressurized, bright blue heavy-duty biological suit used in Biosafety Level 4 containment areas (R Preston, The Hot Zone, Random House, New York, 1994) Cf Racal space suit

chemzymes A group of small, soluble organic molecules that catalyze chemical reactions in a fashion similar to that of natural enzymes catalyzing biochemical reactions; chemzymes copiously produce innumerable copies of the same three-dimensional and chiral form of a desired molecule; chirality is a feature essential to biological systems, since the incorrect isomeric, ie dextro- or levo- form is not recognized by the body and cannot be metabolized; chirality has plagued drug companies, as separation of a biologically useful chiral form from the afunctional chiral form may be tedious or impossible and often the drug is packaged as a 1:1 mixture of right- and left-handed forms; Corey (Nobelist, 1990) et al of Harvard modified a boron-containing organic compound, resulting in the first chemzyme, dubbed the 'CBS' (Corey, Bakshi, Shibata) enzyme that favors production of one chiral form over the other in a 20:1 ratio; 20 chemzymes have been described; see Chirality

Chernobyl The site of a nuclear reactor accident occurring in April 1986 at a power plant near Kiev in the Ukraine, caused by a steam explosion, exposing 200 people to significant total-body doses of radiation; a team performed BM transplants in 13 people exposed to doses of

5.6-13.4 Gy; two survived with recovery of endogenous hematopoiesis; the others died of burns, interstitial pneumonitis, graft-versus-host disease and combined acute renal and respiratory failure; a 30-fold ↑ in incidence of thyroid cancer in children has been reported in the geographic regions surrounding the Chernobyl meltdown, which is thought to be due to the release of ^{131}I (**Nature 1995; 375:465**) see Acute radiation injury, Goiana, Pilgrim plant, Sellafield, Three Mile Island

Note: Although two critical populations (the emergency clean-up crews and the 10^6 residents evacuated from the 30 km zone around the reactor) were not studied epidemiologically, a five-year post-blast study revealed little excess cancer in those exposed to the radiation; the Hiroshima studies revealed 700 excess cancers in a 110 000 exposed survivors over a period of 45 years (**Nature 1991; 351:335n**)

cherry angioma Senile angioma, De Morgan spot A ruby red, 1-3 mm in diameter papule surrounded by a pale halo, common on the trunk and extremities of older adults, located in the superficial corium, consisting of dilated, thinned capillaries, causing superficial bumps **cherry blossom appearance** A descriptive term for the punctate cavitary radiocontrast-filled defects that percolate directly through the salivary gland ducts, a sialologic appearance described in Sjögren's disease; the contrast material may persist for up to a month

cherry hemangioma Cherry angioma, see there

cherry-picking Cream skimming HEALTH CARE ENVIRONMENT 1) A colloquial term for the practice by insurers of selling policies to those who don't need the policies, then dropping those insured when they do need the policies (**Am Med News 26 October 1992, p7**) 2) A highly colloquial term for the acceptance of patients based solely on their ability to pay (ie with insurance or hard cash) while turning away those who are indigent or unable to pay; Cf Berry picking

cherry red color Mucocutaneous discoloration classically associated with carbon monoxide poisoning; 'cherry red' also refers to oropharyngeal discoloration in acute epiglottitis

cherry red spot myoclonus syndrome Sialidosis, type I, neuraminidase deficiency An AR [MIM 256550] condition characterized by a deficiency of α-N-Acetylneuraminidase, most common in the Japanese of preadolescent onset CLINICAL Coarse facies, dysostosis multiplex, hearing loss, mental deterioration, cherry red-colored macules in the optic fundus, lenticular opacification, gradual visual failure, myoclonus and tonic-clonic seizures, peripheral neuropathy with burning feet

cherry spot Bright red macules in the optic fundus of patients with Tay-Sachs syndrome (GM2-gangliosidosis type 1), Niemann-Pick diseases, Sandhoff's disease (GM2-gangliosidosis type 2), generalized gangliosidosis (GM1-gangliosidosis type 1), cherry red spot myoclonus syndrome or sialidosis, type 1, sialidosis type 2, Goldberg syndrome, mucolipidosis type 1, metachromatic leukodystrophy and retinal vasculopathy PATHOGENESIS 1) Storage disease-type cherry red spots Ganglion cell lysosomes are engorged with lipid, the retina is pale and the central vascularized fovea is prominently red 2) Vascular-type cherry red spots are caused by central retinal arterial occlusion or microaneurysms, the retina is edematous and the ganglion cells are swollen from hydropic degeneration, causing retinal opacification; the central fovea being free from ganglion cells, appears bright red against the background

cherubism An AD [MIM 118400] condition, 100% penetration in males, with a cherub-like physiognomy, first recognized by age 5 with puffed-out cheeks, agenesis of permanent teeth, dental dysgenesis, exophthalmos and progressive bilateral soap-bubble expansile lesions at the angle of the mandible, submandibular lymphadenopathy PATHOLOGY Giant cell reparative granuloma onset

Cheshire cat 'syndrome' A name that dignifies one of two clinical dilemmas, where either the patient 1) Has the 'classic' signs and symptoms of a well-defined and often treatable disease that cannot be confirmed by histologic or laboratory criteria or 2) Has the disease with few of the characteristic findings

In either case, the clinician is left with an 'animal' fancifully likened to that seen by Alice in Wonderland, who saw the Cheshire cat's grin without the cat, making it difficult to convince others of the cat's existence

chevron pattern Christmas tree pattern, see there

'chew' Chewing tobacco; see Smokeless tobacco

chewing gum diarrhea An osmotic diarrhea caused by excessive intraluminal sorbitol in 'sugarless' chewing gum Note: The hexitol-type sugar alcohols, sorbitol and mannitol, are major constituents of sugar-free dietary foods, which are not used by bacteria as substrates and thus by remaining in the intestinal lumen may cause osmotic diarrhea; the amount consumed may be large, eg 50-100 sticks of gum/day, translating into 85-170 g sorbitol/day

CHF Congestive heart failure

Also 1) Chick heart fibroblast 2) Coalition for Health Funding 3) Cyclophosphamide, hexamethylmelamine, fluorouracil

chewing tobacco Smokeless tobacco, see there

CHH syndrome Cartilage-hair hypoplasia syndrome, see there

Chicago disease Infection with *Blastomyces dermatitidis*, blastomycosis

chicken breast deformity Pigeon breast deformity, see there

chicken fat clot A descriptor for a slowly formed post-mortem blood clot, composed mainly of leukocytes that settled to dependent parts of the vasculature PATHOLOGY Yellow, rubbery, and non-adherent to vascular walls Polymorphous cell population with abundant neutrophils, few red cells and fibrin; chicken fat clots may occur in fulminant bacterial endocarditis; Cf Currant jelly clots

chicken footprint eggs A descriptor for the eggs of *Taenia* species (*T solium* and *T saginatum*) that have a thick, bile-stained, radially striated shell enclosing a six-hooked embryo (oncosphere); these eggs are indistinguishable from each other, from the eggs of *Echinococcus granulosus* and from those of other animal taeniid tapeworms; absolute identification requires that the embryo's six hooks be seen; Cf Prince Charles looking to the left

chicken footprint nucleus A large nucleus with radiating striations, seen in the convoluted T-cell lymphoma of Lukes and Collins, a tumor of adolescents and young adults that is thought to be of thymic origin as 50-75% are mediastinal and often display markers typical of primitive intrathymic T-cells; these tumors are mitotically active and have a 'starry sky' pattern

'chicken liver era' A facetious term for the 'new age' in the study of gastric physiology, which began in 1976; ^{99m}Tc is bound to sulfur colloid, injected into a chicken where it concentrates in the Kupffer cells; the chickens are then killed, the liver resected, diced up and served in the stew as part of a radionuclide meal; gastric emptying is then studied by scintiscans of the supine patient

chickenpox Varicella, human herpesvirus type 3 An acute HHV-3 infection, most common before age 10; in the US, 50 children die/year of chickenpox; 9000 are hospitalized CLINICAL 2-week incubation, followed by a scarlatiform prodromal rash, low-grade fever, anorexia, malaise, crops of reddish papules that become intensely pruritic vesicles, increasing in number for 3-4 days, the itching and excoriation of which causes extensive scarring COMPLICATIONS Secondary bacterial infection, viral pneumonia (1:400 require pneumonia-related hospitalization), thrombocytopenia, purpura fulminans, encephalitis (5-15% mortality,

15% with permanent neurological sequelae), myocarditis, glomerulonephritis, hepatitis, myositis; after resolution of clinical disease, HHV-3 becomes latent, integrating its DNA into the dorsal root ganglion cells VACCINE A vaccine that is 70-90% effective has been approved by the FDA (**NY Newsday 18 March 1995; C2**)

Note: Chronic HHV-3 infection is the recrudescence form of herpes zoster or shingles

chicken soup A fowl broth that has long had currency as a home remedy for upper respiratory tract infections, despite its uncertain efficacy; in older literature, CS is reported to mobilize nasal mucus and inhibit the growth of pneumococci in vitro (**JAMA 1994; 272:1104c**)

Notes: 1) In some regions, fish soup is regarded as the universal elixir 2) A scientifically stringent systematic study of the efficacy and the molecular components of chicken soup might prove enlightening '

'chicken soup' A highly colloquial term for any drug, maneuver, or device that has virtually no recognized (or at most, minimal) efficacy, which may be used in absence of a efficacious product (**JAMA 1992; 268:1987MN&P**) see Band-Aid® therapy; Cf Placebo

chicken wing appendage A descriptor for a form of phocomelia with foreshortened arms and forearms, flexion contraction at the elbows, a proximal thumb and short, tapered fingers; the finding is typical of the Cornelia de Lange syndrome, which may be accompanied by a low hairline, hirsutism, bushy eyebrows, an antimongoloid slant of the eyes, and various cardiac defects, eg ventricular septal defect

chicken wire pattern A descriptor applied to a delicate plexiform or reticulated pattern imposed on that of another density LIVER PATHOLOGY A pattern of fibrosis associated with alcoholic hepatitis; Cf Bridging fibrosis SOFT TISSUE PATHOLOGY The arrangement of the capillaries in myxoid liposarcoma RADIOLOGY A descriptor for the pattern* of calcification in chondroblastoma, a pediatric tumor

*Also seen in chondroblastoma is the 'fluffy cotton wool' pattern

chiclero's ulcer A clinical form of cutaneous leishmaniasis caused by *Leishmania mexicana* which occurs in the ear of chicle workers in Central America

chief 1) Chief of service, see there 2) Chief of staff, see there

chief cell hyperplasia A pathologic state of primary or secondary increase in the production of parathyroid hormone; the primary form is a constant feature of MEA types I and IIa (but not type IIb) PATHOLOGY All glands are enlarged; the cells are arranged in nodular aggregates; the secondary form is caused by peripheral disease, eg renal dysfunction, chronic malabsorption; the glands display from minimal to florid hyperplasia, weighing up to 5 g, where small uniform cells with finely granular and transparent cytoplasm completely replace the fat typical of a normal parathyroid gland

chief complaint The principle reason for that a person seeks medical attention; CCs include acute abdomen, colicky pain, crushing chest pain, hip or other fracture, and so on; see Complaint

chief of service The head of a department or section of a clinically oriented service in a health care facility Note: The term has various uses, although perhaps the most common use equates a 'chief' to the department head of a non-academic institution, or when used in the context of academic medicine, the director of a service, who is subordinate to the chairman

chief of staff The physician or other health care professional who is in charge of the medical staff in a hospital or health care organization

chief 'syndrome' A condition that most often occurs after the admission of a 'very important person' (V.I.P.) to a major medical center or university hospital; since the chief of a service may be more involved in the department's administration than in 'hands-on' practice of his specialty, he may be unfamiliar with the location of where essential equipment is located and be out of practice with routine procedures; because a V.I.P. is deemed worthy of nothing less than the best, the chief of service is pressed into service and the V.I.P. may receive less than optimal care; see V.I.P. 'syndrome'

chilblains Pernio A cutaneous inflammation due to cold, damp climates, ie in the UK; presumed due to prolonged arteriolar vasoconstriction CLINICAL, EARLY Pallor and coolness of acral parts, often due to 'underdressing' CLINICAL, LATE The skin displays patches of painful pruritic erythema, variably accompanied by blistering, swelling and encrusted ulceration; light microscopy reveals acute, occasionally necrotizing angiitis in a background of chronic inflammation TREATMENT Proper clothing, cessation of smoking and corticosteroids

The term Chyll blayne is of Welsh origin, where the treatment for prolonged exposure to cold was warm wine

child abuse Battered child syndrome, trauma 'X' PUBLIC HEALTH A tragedy that claims 2-5000 lives/year in the US, often first recognized radiologically by certain characteristic findings, consisting of metaphyseal fragmentation, due to repeated subperiosteal contusions with hemorrhage, which heals with a thickened cortex, incomplete 'bucket handles' (avulsed metaphyseal fragments torn from the periphery of the cartilage-shaft junction), old fractures, sub-periosteal hematomas due to 'wringing' of extremities with epiphyseal dislocations, metaphyseal cupping, shortening of the shaft and a ball-and-socket configuration); pelvic fractures (which rarely occur by falling, as the child's caretakers may claim, and are always of a suspicious nature); fractures of posterior ribs (often at the articulation between the transverse process and the rib tubercle), spine and sternum, a post-mortem radiological survey may be indicated in order to convict the caretaker/parent of manslaughter; see Child maltreatment; see also Battered child, Emotional abuse, Neglect, Physical abuse, Sexual abuse, Shaken-baby syndrome

child labor PUBLIC HEALTH A generic term for the employment of a child (usually defined as under the age of 15) in a workplace setting that employs adults functioning in equal or similar functions; although there are major gaps in labor information in and outside of the US, the International Labor Organization in Geneva estimates that 200 million children work in developing nations, and may be increasing (**Sci Am 1993; 269/4:14**) see Sweatshops; Cf Terms of Engagement

child maltreatment '*...intentional harm or threat of harm to a child by someone acting in the role of a caretaker, for even a short time. maltreatment is commonly divided into four categories: physical abuse, sexual abuse, emotional abuse, and neglect.*', the last of which, neglect, is most common STATISTICS 2-3% of the US population < age 18 (ie 1.4 million children) suffer some form of maltreatment each year; ± 160 000 suffer serious or life threatening injuries; ± 2000 die of CM, of whom 80% are ≤ age 5 and 40% are ≤ age 1; '*When they become adults, abused children have two or three times as many problems with substance abuse and depression as members of the general population, and many* (circa 30%) *abuse their own children...these outcomes may be related in part to changes mediated by abuse, in the neuroendocrine systems influencing arousal, the pain threshold, learning, and growth* (**N Engl J Med 1995; 332:1425RV**)

child sexual abuse see Sexual abuse

CHILD syndrome An X-linked [MIM 308050] congenital lethal complex* that is fatal in ♂; ♂:♀ ratio 19:1 CLINICAL Unilateral ichthyosis, limb malformation, accompanied by ipsilateral hypoplasia of paired organs, eg lung, thyroid,

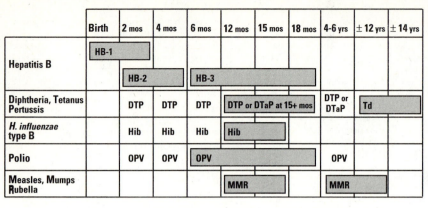

	Birth	2 mos	4 mos	6 mos	12 mos	15 mos	18 mos	4-6 yrs	± 12 yrs	± 14 yrs
Hepatitis B		HB-1								
			HB-2		HB-3					
Diphtheria, Tetanus Pertussis			DTP	DTP	DTP	DTP or DTaP at 15+ mos			DTP or DTaP	Td
H. influenzae type B			Hib	Hib	Hib	Hib				
Polio			OPV	OPV	OPV				OPV	
Measles, Mumps Rubella						MMR			MMR	

childhood immunization schedule

psoas muscle, CNS, and cranial nerves

CHILD-Congenital Hemidysplasia-Ichthyosiform erythroderma-Limb Deformity

childhood immunization Recommended childhood immunization schedule, US, current as of Jan 1995; bars indicate acceptable ages for vaccinations; Cf Adult immunization

childhood trauma The mental result of a sudden external blow or series of blows, rendering the child temporarily helpless and breaking past ordinary coping and defensive operations (Am Med News 27 May, 1991) see Child abuse

chikungunya An acute alpha-virus infection of the Sahara, tropics and subtropics, afflicting children in the rainy months, with fever, arthralgia and rash, which may be likely a 'spillover' from the cycle maintained in wild primates; VECTORS _Aedes aegypti, A africanus, A furcifer_

chili pepper A condiment used in certain cuisines, in particular Mexican, that is particular high in capsaicin; in a case-control study with 220 gastric cancers and 752 population-based controls, ↑ consumption of 'hot' (ie spicy) chili pepper was associated with ↑ risk of gastric cancer, with an odds-ratio of up to 17:1 in those with the highest consumption (Am J Epidemiol 1994; 139:263)

chimera 288 Sted

chimera Any individual or molecule that derives from two or more species CLINICAL GENETICS An organism with two or more cell lines, genotypes, or karyotypes descended from at least two zygotes (a very rare phenomenon seen only in twins), resulting from chorionic vascular anastomoses, transplantation, or double fertilization, and subsequent participation of both fertilized meiotic products in one developing embryo; all hermaphrodites should be karyotyped to evaluate possible chimerism, a finding confirmed by the presence of two distinct blood groups, due to an exchange of primordial blood cells between non-identical twins early in fetal development, prior to development of an immune system capable of rejection; Cf Freemartin, Mosaic

Note: The chimera of Greek mythology was a female monster that breathed fire, had the head of a lion, the tail of a serpent, and the body of a goat (Iliad 6.181-82, Theogony 319ff)

chimney sweeps' cancer MEDICAL HISTORY The oldest occupation-related malignancy, corresponding to a squamous cell carcinoma of the scrotum induced by carcinogens deposited in the region

China paralytic syndrome An acute flaccid paralysis of unknown etiology affecting children in northern China during the summer, which has been recently described in epidemic proportions in Latin American children; the condition shares certain features of polio and, like polio, attacks the motor neurons of the spinal cord (Science 1991;

253:26n&v)

'China white' 3-Methylfentanyl A synthetic ('designer') drug of abuse derived from the anesthetic, fentanyl, which has opiate properties and is 1000-fold more potent than morphine; it has been held responsible for more than 100 overdose deaths in California since 1979, and recently caused an 'epidemic' of overdosage in Pennsylvania (JAMA 1991; 265:1011) Cf Designer drug, Ecstasy, 'Ice', Rave party

Note: China white is a generic 'street' term for white powdered agents, either natural, eg heroin or synthetic, eg above that have opiate effects ANALYSIS Solid-phase radioimmunoassay

Chinese character appearance Any visual pattern that to the occidental eye simulates Chinese ideographs or kanji, where a relatively monotonous background is punctuated by short, curved well-circumscribed and complexly-arranged densities BONE PATHOLOGY Haphazardly arranged trabeculae in woven and immature bone, a LM finding characteristic of fibrous dysplasia MICROBIOLOGY Loosely cohesive clustering of _Corynebacterium_ colonies seen by LM, aka a 'picket fence' arrangement PEDIATRIC DERMATOLOGY A pattern of blisters seen in incontinentia pigmenti (Bloch-Sulzberger and Goltz-Gorlin syndromes), appearing at birth in bizarre linear arrays, almost exclusive to females, associated with congenital ocular anomalies, cerebral malformations and severe neurological defects; the skin lesions heal by crusting, leaving a 'splashed' appearance in their wake

Chinese hamster ovary cell A cell line isolated in 1958 used in research that grows well in culture and spontaneously transforms to a malignant morphology, due to cytoskeletal disorganization; CHO cells can be induced to revert to a normal morphology, and CHO's resistance to DNAse I can be reverted to normal with the addition of cAMP

Chinese hamster ovary cell assay A tissue culture assay to detect a bacterium's production of enterotoxin, where exposure to a toxin-bearing fluid results in cell damage causing the cells to form round clusters (syncytia)

Chinese herbal formula A generic term for any of a number of concoctions (eg Enhance, Composition A) from plants of Asian origin that may be anecdotally reported to have antiretroviral activity (Am Med News 21 Nov 1994 p13) Cf AIDS fraud

Chinese lantern sign PEDIATRICS A finding in hydranencephaly and poroencephaly seen by transillumination of the infant skull, consisting in a lack of opacification as there are no cerebral hemispheres, although the brain stem and basal ganglia are well-formed; intellectual or voluntary motor development is impossible and most infants die by age 1

'Chinese menu' disease A highly colloquial term for any condition, the diagnosis of which is based on the presence of major and minor criteria in the patient; these diseases include AIDS-related complex, Behçet disease, Carney syndrome, chronic fatigue syndrome, polymyositis, rheumatic fever (Jones' criteria), rheumatoid arthritis, SLE, and tuberous sclerosis (Gomez classification)

Note: The coinage refers to a type of menu that was formerly popular in Chinese restaurants where the meals were selected based on one choice of dish from column A and one from column B

Chinese restaurant syndrome An abrupt allergic reaction, the susceptibility to which is an autosomal recessive trait, caused by sensitivity to monosodium glutamate (MSG, a seasoning used in Chinese restaurants and soy sauce) CLINICAL Severe headaches, numbness, palpitations, vertigo (especially with chronic MSG exposure), thirst, abdominal and chest pains, sweating, and flushing Onset: ½ hour postcibum, lasting up to 12 hours

CHIP28 Aquaporin-1, see there

chip COMPUTERS An integrated circuit that contains a million or more microscopic components etched on a silicon wafer; the term is a generic synonym for microprocessor and is the key component of computers

chipmunk face A descriptor for the expanded globular maxilla with marrow hyperexpansion into facial bones, combined with prominent epicanthal folds, a physiognomy characteristic of severe β thalassemia; chipmunk facies may also refer to soft tissue swelling, eg diffuse parotid gland swelling, accompanied by xerostomia and reddened eyes, described in Sjögren syndrome

chipper A colloquial term for a person who smokes fewer than five cigarettes/day; chippers are thought to be resistant to nicotine dependence or addiction, as they are often offspring of non-smoking parents (N Engl J Med 1994; 331:1530c)

chirality Handedness The left– or right–sidedness of virtually all members of the physical universe, from elementary particles, eg electrons and molecules to highly complex organisms ORGANIC CHEMISTRY The 3-D conformation of a molecule[1], referring to whether the molecule has a left-handed[2], levo– or L– orientation, as do most molecules in functioning biological systems or a right-handed, dextro– or D– orientation; single entantiomer synthesis has long been a goal for industrial chemists as chiral chemicals tend to acts in completely different manners depending on whether they are left– or right–handed, eg one entantiomer of limonene smells of oranges, the other of lemon, one entantiomer of ibuprofen has a three-fold greater analgesic effect than its mirror-image; a tragic reminder of the effects of chemical chirality is thalidomide; one form is effective in treating morning sickness in pregnancy, and the other interferes with fetal development; it has been reported that the form of entantiomer being produced can be controlled by the simple application of a magnetic field, the confirmation of which is awaited by industry (Science 1994; 264:908N&v) see Chemzymes, Thalidomide

[1]The existence of chirality was first discovered by Pasteur in 1848 in tartaric acid salts [2]Handedness is the term increasingly preferred when referring to this phenomenon in living organisms; chirality continues to be preferred in chemistry

chiropodist Podiatrist, see there

chiropractic ALTERNATIVE MEDICINE A system of health care founded in 1895 based on the concept that the nervous system is the single most important determinant of a person's state of health; abnormal nerve function may result in musculoskeletal derangements and aggravate pathological processes in other body regions or organ systems; chiropractic treatment consists of adjustment and manipulation of the vertebral column and extremities, which some chiropractors supplement with physiotherapy, nutritional support and radiography (for diagnostic purposes only), but do not perform surgery or prescribe drugs; there are 30 000 licensed chiropractors in the US; chiropractors have a four-year post-secondary school education in one of 16 schools of chiropractic; see Alternative medicine; Cf Osteopathic medicine

Mainstream medical practitioners are not as a general principle, opposed to patients seeking chiropractic manipulation when indicated, or under the Hippocratic principle of *primum non nocerum*; the difficulty lies when chiropractic physicians claim to treat such diverse clinical conditions as bladder infections, anginal chest pain, sexual dysfunction, dysmenorrhea, disorders of speech, and mental disorders ranging from mild depression to schizophrenia—Author's note

chisel fracture An incomplete fracture of the head of the radius where the fracture line extends distally from the center of the articular surface

chi-square test STATISTICS: A statistical maneuver used to evaluate categorical variables, eg differences in patient characteristics

chi-squared distribution STATISTICS A theoretical frequency distribution representing the sum of the squares of number n (the degrees of freedom), where the normally distributed variables have a mean of zero and a standard deviation of one, thus assuming a Gaussian distribution

chitterlings An ethnic food popular especially among the blacks in the American South which, if improperly prepared, may result in infections by *Yersinia enterocolitica* O:3

Chitterlings consist of the external seromuscular layer of the large intestine of the pig, prepared by boiling several times in spices and finally baked to a crisp consistency and served

chiufa An acute gangrenous colitis of unknown etiology, which is accompanied by high fever and in ♀, vulvovaginitis, which is described in southern Africa and South America at high altitudes

Chlamydia pneumoniae An organism that has been linked to coronary artery disease and acute MI, based on the finding of increased *C pneumoniae*-specific IgA, IgG, immune complexes, antigens, elementary bodies, and DNA by PCR in those with CAD and acute MI (Sci & Med Nov/Dec 1994 p9)

Chlamydia trachomatis A species restricted to humans; it is the most common sexually-transmitted organism in the US; it is present in 1-3% of all ♀ and 15-40% of ♀ seen in STD clinics CLINICAL Inclusion conjunctivitis, lymphogranuloma venereum, mucopurulent cervicitis, urethritis, bartholinitis, endometritis, and salpingitis (*C trachomatis* has been implicated in 40-60% of salpingitis and PID); infection may also be asymptomatic DIAGNOSIS Direct fluorescent antibody staining, solid phase immunoassay, ELISA, cell culture, nucleic acid probe, PCR (Arch Pathol Lab Med 1994; 118:483oa; JAMA 1994; 272:868) TREATMENT Doxycycline, azithromycin (Sci & Med Nov/Dec 1994 p9)

chloasma Melasma, see there

chloramphenicol acyltransferase gene MOLECULAR BIOLOGY A widely used reporter gene in expression studies that assess the activity of promoters and other upstream transcription-regulating sequences; conventional CAT assays provide an indirect measurement of the upstream sequences, as it is the enzyme (CAT) that is measured and not the mRNA, an issue that can be resolved by use of a ribonuclease protection assay (Am Biotech Lab September 1994, p 108)

chloride channel An ion channel in the plasma membrane of most cells with roles in regulating cell volume, transepithelial transport and stabilization of membrane potential in muscle; there is a wide diversity of chloride channels; their importance is most evident when the channels are defective, as in cystic fibrosis (where the gene defect translates into a block in cAMP activation of the chloride channel), or in certain forms of myotonia

chloroquine-resistant malaria Backgound *Plasmodium falciparum*, the parasite responsible for the malignant tertian form of malaria is increasingly resistant to the previously effective chloroquine, a pharmacologic 'staple' used as malaria prophylaxis in visitors to highly endemic regions of western Africa; the exact incidence of chloroquine-resistant *P falciparum* malaria is unknown, but may exceed 25% which may be prevented by 250 mg/week of mefloquine (JAMA 1991; 265:361)

chlorination PUBLIC HEALTH The addition of various chlorinated compounds to water as a disinfectant; although liquid chlorine (Cl_2) is the most commonly used compound given its ease of transportation, it is being increasingly replaced by sodium hypochlorite (NaOCl) solution, as Cl_2 is also highly toxic; chlorination has been linked to an ↑ in cancer of the bladder, lower GI tract; ozonation had been proposed as an alternative, but appears to be no less carcinogenic than chlorination (**Science 1995; 267:1771**) Cf Ozonation

2-chlorodeoxyadenosine ONCOLOGY A chlorinated purine analogue of vidarabine used to treat CLL, that is reported to be less effective than fludarabine (**N Engl J Med 1994; 330:319OA, 1828C**) see Fludarabine

chloroma *chloro*, Greek, green A variant of granulocytic leukemia, remarkable for the greenish color (due to neutrophil myelo- or verdoperoxidase) seen in freshly sectioned tissue; notably, a 'green tumor' may precede marrow and peripheral blood involvement by years; chloromas were first described in 1811 as a retro-orbital, paranasal and lacrimal tumor composed of masses of immature (primitive) granulocytes; since the color is not always present, the term granulocytic sarcoma is preferred, see there

chlorosis Virgins' disease, green sickness A term first used in 1681 for iron-deficiency anemia, named for the yellow-green skin pallor of its young female victims; other findings included koilonychia and increased jugular venous pressure; in adult women, iron deficiency is associated with hypochlorhydria and premature graying **CHO cell** see Chinese hamster ovary cell

chocolate A comestible prepared from ground and roasted beans of the cacao plant, native to South America, *Theobroma cacao* and composed of cocoa butter, a substance high in stearic acid, converted in vivo to oleic acid, possibly lowering cholesterol levels; ⅓ of cocoa butter is palmitic acid, which elevates cholesterol; chocolate craving is thought to be more intense in females and may be associated with increased progesterone levels; theobromine may be the chemical in chocolate responsible for the intense cravings in those people who are facetiously known as 'chocoholics'; Cf Carob

Note: Chocolate was the ceremonial brew of Aztecs, Mayas and Toltecs and returned with Columbus to the Royal Court of Spain, where it remained a state secret until it was stolen by the Italians in 1606; chocolate was first consumed in the solid form in 1847

chocolate agar Chocolatized agar Blood agar that has been heated to open the pyrrole ring, forming hemin, a required growth medium for bacteria not possessing hemolysins, usually grown in a microaerophilic (3-10% CO_2) environment, providing an ideal growth medium for *Haemophilus influenzae*, *Neisseria* spp, and fastidious anaerobes

chocolate cyst Endometrioma GYNECOLOGY A periadnexal or ovarian cyst filled with thick, inspissated, old and unclotted blood, seen in endometriosis that grossly is likened to chocolate

Note: Carcinoma occurs in approximately 0.5% of ovarian endometriosis and is usually of the endometrioid or clear cell types, more often seen in ♀ younger than those with 'garden variety' ovarian carcinomas

choke FORENSIC PATHOLOGY The narrowing of the cylinder bore of a shotgun at the muzzle, which is intended to minimize the spread of shot as it leaves the barrel; it is usually expressed as the percentage of shot that falls within a 30-inch (76 cm) circle at 40 yards (36.5 m); ± 70% for a full choke, ± 60% for a medium choke weapon; < 20% for a sawed-off shotgun; see Ballistics

Note: Shotguns are responsible for the 'messiest' firearms-related homicides and suicides, with the tissue devastation increasing as the distance from the muzzle to the target decreases

the 'chokes' Sudden onset of respiratory distress occurring in caisson's disease which is associated with pulmonary edema, hemorrhage, atelectasis, and emphysema, thought due to an increase in platelet adhesion to gas bubbles that release vasoconstrictors and platelet factor 3, causing coagulopathy

choke hold Bar arm control FORENSIC MEDICINE A form of restraint used to subdue overactive, unruly, violent, or inebriated subjects with the intent of preventing them causing physical harm to themselves and others; the choke hold consists of occlusion of the upper airway by compressing the thyroid cartilage and displacing the tongue posteriorly, a hold that is considered more dangerous than the carotid sleeper; see Neck hold; Cf Carotid sleeper

choked disc OPHTHALMOLOGY Papilledema with swelling of the nerve head, caused by increased intracranial pressure with edema-induced blurring of the disc margins and obliteration of the optic cup, elevation of the nerve head, capillary congestion, hyperemia, venous engorgement, loss of venous pulse, peripapillary exudates, retinal wrinkling, and punctate nerve fiber layer hemorrhage; if the pressure is reduced, the fundus returns to normal without loss of vision; increased intracranial pressure is due to meningoencephalitis, hemorrhage, metabolic disease, toxins, trauma and tumors; see also Pseudotumor cerebri

cholangiocarcinoma A rare malignancy arising in the bile ducts that presents with jaundice (71%), abdominal pain (49%), and weight loss (44%); cholangiocarcinoma, unlike hepatocellular carcinoma, is not associated with alcohol abuse PROGNOSIS 53% 1-year, 9% 3-year, and 4% 5-year survival (**Mayo Clin Proc 1995; 70:425**)

LAPAROSCOPIC VS OPEN CHOLECYSTECTOMY

	LAPAROSCOPIC	OPEN
Bile duct injuries	13/1518	1/1200
Hospital stay/recovery time	1 day/<1 week	5 days/4-6 weeks
Source of costs	↑ Surgeon fee/OR time	↑ Inpatient costs

¹Am Med News May 4 1992

cholecystectomy A surgical procedure used to remove the gallbladder, the storage receptacle for gallstones INDICATIONS Gallstones, cholecystitis, gallbladder cancer Note: Although the increasingly popular laparoscopic cholecystectomy has a lower death rate than open cholecystectomy, the total mortality related to cholecystectomies has not ↓ as the number of procedures performed has ↑ (**N Engl J Med 1994; 330:404SA**)

cholecystokinin Pancreozymin* A 33-residue peptide, the activity of which resides in the 8 N-terminal amino acids (CCK-8), CCK is released from the small intestinal mucosa by certain amino acids, eg tryptophan and phenylalanine and medium- to long-chain fatty acids; CCK stimulates gall bladder contraction, pancreatic acinar cell secretion, relaxes the sphincter of Oddi and induces satiety in food-deprived rats; see Hormone families

*This name is increasingly preferred among the cognoscenti; cholecystokinin is used here for the hoi polloi (among whom the author is included) who are not yet 'up to speed'

cholera cot Hybrid hospital equipment, consisting of a cama-commode combo, required in *Vibrio cholera* infection, as the victims are flat on their backs with no place to go

Note: In the late 20th century, cholera epidemics have become vanishingly rare, with the notable exception of the recent South American epidemic (**MMWR 1991; 40:108**)

cholera toxin A heat-sensitive enterotoxin produced by *Vibrio cholera* composed of five 11.6-kD cell-binding B subunits forming a ring around a finger-like 27-kD (**Nature 1991; 351:371, 351**) catalase that transfers ADP-ribose to a G protein, locking adenyl cyclase in the 'on' position; cholera toxin's functional properties are shared by pertussis toxin, diphtheria toxin and exotoxin A

cholesterol BIOCHEMISTRY Cholesterol levels are closely linked to atherosclerosis and thus incriminated in cardio- and cerebrovascular disease; total cholesterol > 6.21

mmol/L (US: > 240 mg/dl) is associated with a high risk, 5.17-6.18 mmol/L (US: 200-239 mg/dl) is associated with a 'borderline' risk and < 5.17 mmol/L (US: 200 mg/dl) is associated with a low risk for atherosclerotic heart disease; other high risks include: LDL-cholesterol > 160 mg/dl, HDL-cholesterol < 35 mg/dl; Low risks LDL-cholesterol < 130 mg/dl, HDL-cholesterol > 55 mg/dl Note: All subjects in high and borderline groups should have LDL-cholesterol levels measured and other atherosclerosis risk factors determined; LDL-cholesterol > 130 mg/dl, requires dietary control; LDL-cholesterol that remains > 160 mg/dl after 3-6 months of diet, requires drug therapy, especially in those with HDL-cholesterol < 35 mg/dl (Am J Cardiol 1990; 65:7F) Note: Cholesterol levels undergo a slow decline in evolving colonic carcinoma, thus serving as a 'soft' criterion for cancer Note: transgenic mice that over-express LDL-receptors have reduced cholesterol levels; see Hypercholesterolemia Note: Elderly ♂ with a low serum cholesterol (< 4.14 mmol/L or 160 mg/dL) are reported to have a RR of 6.7 for depression in contrast to those with normal cholesterol levels (Lancet 1993; 341:75)

cholesterol-lowering drugs The most cost-efficient agents for ↓ LDL-cholesterol are nicotinic acid (niacin) and lovastatin; the most efficient for ↑ HDL-cholesterol are nicotinic acid and gemfibrozil Types of drugs available

1) BILE ACID SEQUESTRANTS Colestyramine, cholestipol are used to treat hypercholesterolemia, enhancing hepatic catabolism of cholesterol to bile acids

2) NICOTINIC ACID Niacin NA suppresses hepatic synthesis of lipoprotein Note: Both NA and bile acid sequestrants are poorly tolerated and may cause hepatitis (Mayo Clin Proc 1991; 66:23)

3) FIBRIC ACIDS Clofibrate, gemfibrozil, fenofibrate; fibric acid's mechanism of action is unknown; these agents cause a modest (10-20%) reduction in serum cholesterol

4) PROBUCOL reduces cholesterol by enhancing the clearance of LDLs, but also reduces serum HDL, an undesired effect; long-term probucol therapy delays the onset of atherosclerosis in Watanabe rabbits, an animal model of atherosclerosis

5) INHIBITORS OF 3-HYDROXY-3-METHYLGLUTARYL-COENZYME A (HMG-CoA) **REDUCTASE**, a rate-limiting step in cholesterol synthesis; this family of compounds was isolated in 1976 from *Penicillium citrinum* (Compactin or mevastatin, lovastatin) and first approved by the FDA (1987); lovastatin with gemfibrozil may cause severe myopathy and life-threatening rhabdomyolysis with renal failure and is a combination discouraged by the FDA

cholesterol pneumonia Lipoid pneumonia, see there

cholesterol-raising fatty acids Exogenous dietary lipids that increase total and/or LDL-cholesterol, eg palmitic acid, myristic acid, trans-monounsaturated fatty acids and probably also lauric acid; see Tropical oils

cholesteryl-ester transfer protein A 74-kD hydrophobic plasma glycoprotein that facilitates the transfer of cholesteryl esters from their site of synthesis in HDL to lipoproteins containing apolipoprotein B; CETP deficiency has only been described in Japanese cohorts, possibly due to a 'founder effect' as the mutation is the same in all the identified persons with the defect which is associated with increased longevity, possibly related to the antiatherogenic effect of CETP deficiency

cholestyramine resin A bile acid-sequestering drug used as a first-line LDL-cholesterol-reducing drug, which acts by increasing hepatic catabolism of cholesterol

Note: Some 'soft' data suggest that long-term therapy is associated with a two-fold increase in malignancies of the GI tract

chondroid lipoma A recently-described benign neoplasm that is most common in the subcutis, superficial muscular

fascia, or skeletal muscle of the extremities; the tumors are yellowish, usually encapsulated, and average 4 cm in greatest dimension LM Nests, strands, and sheets of eosinophilic and vacuolated cells (hibernoma-like), in a background of mature adipose tissue admixed with a fibrinous to hyalinized myxoid stroma IMMUNOHISTOCHEMISTRY S-100, vimentin, CD68/KP1 DDx Myxoid liposarcoma, myxoid chondrosarcoma (Am J Surg Pathol 1993; 17:1103)

chondroid syringoma Mixed tumor of the skin An almost invariably benign 0.5-3.0 cm in diameter skin tumor usually of the head and neck that recapitulates the histologic features of mixed tumor of the salivary gland PATHOLOGY Ductal and secretory lumina, eccrine differentiation with fibrocollagenous stroma and chondroid elements with chondrocytes (Acta Cytologica 1993; 37:535oA)

cholinergic crisis see Myasthenic crisis

CHOP ONCOLOGY A 'first-generation' regimen of combination chemotherapy consisting of cyclophosphamide, doxorubicin, vincristine, and prednisone; despite extensive clinical research, CHOP is considered better than second- and third-generation chemotherapy regimens (to wit, m-BACOD, MACOP-B and ProMACE-CytaBOM) for treating non-Hodgkin's lymphoma; overall survival with all is the same; fatal toxic reactions occur in 1% of CHOP patients, and in 3-6% of those treated with other protocols (N Engl J Med 1993; 328:1002oA); the outcome of patients with aggressive NHL who respond poorly to first-line CHOP is not improved by early high-dose myeloablative chemotherapy with autologous BM transplantation (N Engl J Med 1995; 332:1045oA) see Chemotherapy, Remission

chordoma A malignant tumor derived from the fetal notochord that appears most commonly in 5th-6th decade, arising in the sacrococcygeal region and sphenooccipital regions, the latter is more common in younger patients PATHOLOGY Chordomas are soft, gelatinous and hemorrhagic, having a microscopic appearance fancifully likened to soap bubbles (physaliferous cells) with cleared glycogen-filled cytoplasmic vacuoles TREATMENT Surgery, radiotherapy PROGNOSIS Recurrence is common, often years after adequate therapy

chorea gravidarum Choreiform movement that may appear in the first trimester of pregnancy, occasionally reappearing with subsequent pregnancy TREATMENT None (given the teratogenic potential of anticonvulsants); if severe, terminate pregnancy

chorionic villus biopsy A method for early (first trimester) prenatal diagnosis of fetal chromosomal anomalies and other disease; tissue is obtained at 9-11 weeks (vs 16th week for amniotic fluid analysis) from the developing placenta by ultrasound-guided transcervical catheter aspiration biopsy; the tissue obtained is from the chorion frondosum, the layer which develops chorionic villi; the diagnostic yield of CVB is 97.8%; the yield of amniocentesis performed at 16 gestational weeks is 99.4%, CVB has a 30% greater (7.2 % loss vs 5.7%) wastage of normal fetuses; the unanticipated fetal loss attributed to CVB is 6-8/1000; there are two approaches for CVB, the transcervical and the transabdominal, which is reported to be better as it is easier to learn, carries a lower risk of infection, uses a needle that can be aimed with more accuracy (versus a plastic catheter used in the transcervical approach), and has a lower rate of spontaneous fetal loss (2.5% vs 2.3% in transcervical approach (N Engl J Med 1992; 327:594oA); CVS may be associated with a slight to 11-fold ↑ in defects of the extremities and/or digits (Science News 1994; 146:21)

choristoma Non-specialized tissue that develops in utero corresponding to microscopically normal cells and tissues located in abnormal sites, eg ectopic breast tissue

choroideremia Tapetochoidal dystrophy A form of X-linked [MIM 303100] hereditary retinal degeneration (other hereditary retinal degenerations include Refsum's disease, gyrate atrophy, and a-β-lipoproteinemia), characterized by centripetal loss of visual fields due to a gene mutation localized to chromosome Xq21

Christchurch chromosome A defective chromosome 1 with loss of the short arm in the cultured cells of a New Zealand family, associated with lymphoproliferative disorders, eg CLL

Christian Science A religious doctrine established in 1879 by MB Eddy in which therapy in the form of so-called 'healings', consisting of *'heartfelt yet disciplined prayer'* by members of the Christian Scientist Church are administered to the sick in lieu of drugs or most standard measures normally used to alleviate pain; while anecdotal 'healing' testimonials available from the Christian Science Church imply that their form of therapy is better than conventional medical therapy for the care of children, which has not been supported by some peer-reviewed reports (JAMA 1989; 262:1657); Christian Scientists do not smoke or drink; Christian Science has major impacts on American medicine:

1) Christian Scientist parents may override the physician's control in the care of underage minor children with potentially fatal consequences

2) Christian Scientists may be difficult to treat (especially as unconscious victims of trauma), as they may refuse therapy deemed appropriate by conventional medical thinking, eg blood transfusion; if such therapy is administered, the medical team may be held liable for committing acts of assault and battery

3) Religious exemption statutes allow healers to perform their services ('healing') without liability and at standards of practice that are variance for those expected of physicians and

4) 'Healing' therapy can be billed to an insurance company, Medicare or Medicaid (JAMA 1990; 264:1379)

Christian's triad A 'classic' but rarely observed trio of symptoms in histiocytosis X, consisting of lytic bony lesions, diabetes insipidus and exophthalmos

Christian syndrome An X-R [MIM 309620] condition characterized by skeletal dysplasia (short stature, fusion of cervical vertebrae, scoliosis), mental retardation and abducens palsy, and glucose intolerance; the responsible mutation is located in Xq28-qter

Christian-Weber disease Relapsing non-suppurative panniculitis Focal painful aggregates of subcutaneous fat necrosis with erythematous, ulcerating and eventually atrophic skin, seen in corpulent middle-aged women CLINICAL The condition may be acute or chronic, fulminating or transient, systemic or confined to the skin and variably associated with polyserositis and fever ETIOLOGY Unknown, possibly related to trauma, cold, drugs, chemicals, and may occur in patients with SLE, rheumatoid arthritis, DM, sarcoidosis, after corticosteroid withdrawal, in acute and chronic pancreatitis, and in pancreatic carcinoma LABORATORY ↑ Lipase, ↑ amylase

Christmas 'blues' A colloquial term for depression that is most common in those who are alone (without family, friends, or otherwise 'disenfranchised') during Christmas, a holiday that is traditionally shared with family members

Christmas disease Hemophilia B, Factor IX deficiency

Christmas tree bladder Pine cone bladder A broad, flat and smooth-walled atonic bladder with a flaccid base and a jagged superior funneling into the posterior urethra, described as characteristic of spastic neurogenic bladder, a finding by cystography that may be mimicked by outlet obstruction with superimposed urinary tract infection; diagnosis of neurogenic bladder based on radiologic findings may therefore prove difficult PATHOLOGY The bladder is markedly trabeculated, with a peaked dome and attenuated epithelium

Christmas tree deformity PEDIATRIC SURGERY A severe form of jejunoileal atresia in which only a single branch of the superior mesenteric artery fully develops, supplying in a retrograde fashion, a markedly shortened ileum arranged in pattern fancifully likened to a reversed 'Christmas tree'

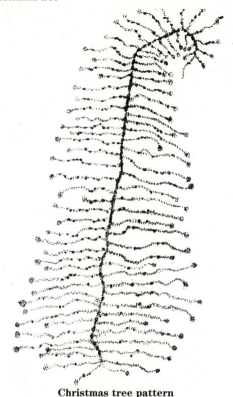

Christmas tree pattern

Christmas tree pattern Chevron pattern DERMATOLOGY A clinical finding in pityriasis rosea; the lesions are oval, 1 cm pink-brown papules covered by fine keratinaceous scales, corresponding to parakeratosis, which are aligned parallel to the skin cleavage lines of the trunk; the lesions last 2-12 weeks before fading MOLECULAR BIOLOGY A descriptor for appearance seen when a complex of multiple transcribing pre-mRNA molecules arise from a single chain of DNA; see Feather pattern

Christ-Siemens-Touraine syndrome Hypohidrotic ectodermal dysplasia An X-linked [MIM 305100] ectodermal dysplasia with anhidrosis, heat intolerance, hypoplasia of sebaceous and sweat glands, resulting in dry smooth and glossy skin, gonadal hypoplasia, ageusia, anosmia, upper respiratory tract infections, absent nipples, partial anodontia or peg-teeth, hypotrichosis, saddle nose, dysphagia, physical and mental retardation, feminine appearance and cleft palate, almost invariably affecting males MOLECULAR PATHOLOGY The defect is thought to be located on the X chromosome, 10 cM distal to DXS1 on proximal Xq

chromatin puff Chromosome puff, see there

chromatography A laboratory technique in which mixtures of complex molecules are separated along a gradient of pressure or solubility between a mobile (either liquid or gas) and stationary (solid or liquid) phase; the molecules are separated by absorption, gel filtration, ion exchange or partitioning or a combination of these priciples; see Gas-liquid chromatography, High-performance liquid chromatography, Ion exchange chromatography, Partition chromatography, Thin-layer chromatography

chromatoid body Any of a number of darkly staining, elongated, relatively well-circumscribed masses, 1-4 in number that are located in amoebic cysts in *Entamoeba* *histolytica, E hartmanni, Entamoeba coli* and *Endolimax nana*

chromogen Any compound that can be used to detect the presence of a substance of interest by changing its color; chromogens are critical components of immunoenzyme reactions

chromogranins A family of 20–100-kD acidic glycoproteins present in the soluble fraction of neurosecretory granules, serving as 'pan-endocrine' markers for neuroendocrine tumors, eg small cell carcinoma; Chromogranins A, B and C have been characterized; the latter two are also known as secretogranin I and II

chromogranin/secretogranin family Cg/Sg family A group of acidic proteins (chromogranins A and B, secretogranins I and II) that are present in secretory granule-laden endocrine cells and tumors, eg of pancreatic islets and tumors, eg gastrinomas; the Cg/Sg profile changes during the maturation sequence neuroblastoma → ganglioneuroblastoma → ganglioneuroma (Diagn Mol Pathol 1992; 1:155)

chromophobe carcinoma NEPHROLOGY A recently described neoplasm that is thought to arise in the normal intercalated cells of the collecting ducts; CC represents ± 4% of all renal epithelial neoplasms and affects the middle aged population PATHOLOGY CDCs average 8 cm and are pathologic stage T2 or T3 at presentation; CC has a solid tumor growth pattern with central or slightly eccentric cytoplasm and either reticular or eosinophilic cytoplasm SPECIAL STUDIES Antimitochondrial antibodies, hypodiploidy, aneuploidy by flow cytometry, allelic imbalance, abundant cytoplasmic vesicles on EM (Am J Clin Pathol 1995; 103:624OA) see Renal epithelial neoplasms

chromosomal RNA Oligonucleotide segments of RNA that serve to 'prime' the growth fork of DNA in the lagging strand after DNA duplication; Cf Okazaki fragment

chromosome A morphologic gene-bearing unit of the genome that is most readily recognized during mitosis; chromosomes are present in the eukaryotic nucleus that consists of one or more (23 in humans), usually paired, very long (100 to 300 million base pairs each in humans) DNA molecules that are associated with RNA and histone proteins; the complete complement of chromosomes contain the complete genetic information present in a living organism; chromosomes are classified into groups sharing structural similarity in terms of length from the centromere, divided into group A (chromosomes 1-3), group B (chromosomes 4 and 5), group C (chromosomes 6 to 12 and the X chromosome), group D (chromosomes 13 to 15), group E (chromosomes 16 to 18); group F (chromosomes 19 and 20); group G (chromosomes 21, 22 and the Y chromosome); see Banding, Flow cytometry, Human genome project, Ploidy analysis

chromosome analysis Karyotyping GENETICS A laboratory procedure in which cells of fetal origin are obtained either in the first trimester by chorionic villus biopsy or later in pregnancy by amniocentesis and grown in a tissue culture medium to detect major chromosomal defects (table); the technique is indicated for mixed congenital anomalies with mental or growth retardation, infertility, in cryptorchidic testes, ambiguous genitalia, repeated neonatal death, advanced maternal age and in analysis of neoplasia; see Banding; Cf DNA hybridization, Polymerase chain reaction

chromosome breakage syndromes A group of inherited diseases in which the chromosomes have an increased fragility, eg ataxia-telangiectasia, Bloom, Fanconi, Louis-Bar syndromes, and xeroderma pigmentosum, resulting in a marked increase in susceptibility to certain malignancies

chromosome 'jumping' MOLECULAR BIOLOGY Cloning and mapping of large segments of DNA; see Jumping library

chromosome mapping A generic term for the process of determining the position of a specific gene on a chromosome and its relationship with other genes on the chromosome being mapped; methods of CM include familial studies with statistical analysis to determine lod scores, somatic cell hybridization, and deletion mapping

chromosome painting CYTOGENETICS A technique in which specially developed fluorescent dyes are used to stain chromosomes for rapid identification of chromosomal abnormalities

chromosome painting probe CYTOGENETICS A FISH probe containing a complete set of DNA fragments from one chromosome, which can be used when the banding pattern suggests a rearrangement, but does not provide enough information to determine from whence it came; see FISH probes

chromosome puff A localized separation of polytene chromosomes, eg chromosomes of *Drosophila melanogaster*, which represents a site of active RNA synthesis, ie transcription, which when very large, is known as a Balbiani ring

chromosome 'walking' MOLECULAR BIOLOGY A time-consuming method that sequences (ie, determines the sequence of) segments of DNA located on either side of a region of a fully characterized (ie, 'sequenced') segment of DNA, 'walking' out in overlapping short fragments of DNA, each 15-20 000 bases in length, from a point of known sequence, enabling one to sequence (ie, determine the sequence of) DNA that is far removed from the marker gene; see Cystic fibrosis gene, Chromosome jumping

chronic active hepatitis Chronic viral hepatitis

chronic disease EPIDEMIOLOGY A generic term for XXXX ; three common risk factors identified across racial/ethnic groups and education levels are cigarette smoking, sedentary lifestyle, and obesity (MMWR 1994; 43:894; JAMA 1995; 273:102)

chronic effects of overexposure OCCUPATIONAL SAFETY A generic term for any adverse effects that develop slowly over a long period of time or after repeated prolonged exposure to a hazardous material without regard to severity of said effects

chronic eosinophilic pneumonia A clinical condition with a group of characteristics (see table) PATHOLOGY ↑↑↑ Eosinophils in interstitium and airspaces with ↑ histiocytes in airspaces (Mayo Clin Proc 1995; 70:137OA); some features overlap clinically and histologically with BOOP

CHROMOSOMES: KARYOTYPING TERMS	
:	Break without union
::	Break and join
cen	Centromere
chi	Chimerism
del	Deletion
der	Unbalanced karyosome
dic	Dicentric
dmin	Double minute
dup	Duplication
i	Isochromosome
inv	Inversion
mos	Mosaicism
p	Short arm (petit)
q	Long arm (the letter in the alphabet after p)
r	Ring
ter	Termination
+	A gained chromosome or segment thereof
–	A lost chromosome or segment thereof
→	Site of origin of transfer of a segment of chromosome to another

Comparison of CEP and BOOP[1]

Factor	CEP	BOOP
Age	Young, often < 30	Older, often > 50
Clinical course	Subacute/chronic	Acute/subacute/chronic
Radiology	Nonspecific peripheral infiltrates in 25%	Groundglass airspace 50% are peripheral
PFTs[2]	Mild restriction, ± obstruction	Mild restriction
Pathology	Airspace eosinophils, histiocytes, PMNs	Interstitial fibrosis, cells, few eosinophils
Clinical response	Improvement in days	Improvement in weeks
Outcome	Usually good (>95%)	Variable (75% reponse)

[1]Chronic interstitial pneumonia, bronchiolitis obliterans and organizing pneumonia [2]Pulmonary function tests; Modified from Mayo Clin Proc 1995; 70:137 oa

chronic fatigue syndrome Yuppie disease, Chronic Epstein-Barr syndrome, Postviral syndrome A condition first described in the mid-1980s in California, which shares clinical features with epidemic neuromyasthenia, Iceland or Royal Free Hospital disease; CFS often follows viral infections, eg herpes, hepatitis, CMV, or may be induced by an unrecognized virus; the polymerase chain reaction reveals enteroviral RNA sequences in muscle, possibly also in the brain in 53% of CFS, in contrast to 15% of controls (Br Med J 1991; 302:692) Note: Although CFS had been associated with EBV infection, more than half of those with the CFS improve without a change in EBV titers TREATMENT None; the 'cures' reported are thought to be due to placebo effect or spontaneous remission

Chronic Fatigue Syndrome (CDC case definition)
Major criteria (required)

1) Recent onset of debilitating or recurring fatigue of > 6 months duration and

2) Exclusion of clinically similar conditions

Minor criteria (eight of ten required)

1) Low-grade fever (< 38.6° C) or chills

2) Sore throat (or pharyngitis)

3) Painful anterior and/or posterior cervical and axillary lymphadenopathy

4) Unexplained muscular weakness

5) Myalgia

6) Generalized fatigue of > 24 hours for previously tolerated exercise

7) Severe generalized headache

8) Migratory arthralgia

9) Neuropsychological complaints, eg photophobia, irritability, inability to concentrate, depression and

10) Sleep disturbance

chronic granulomatous disease(s) A heterogeneous group of inherited (²⁄₃ are X-linked and ⅓ AR) phagocytic defects characterized by recurrent and potentially fatal pyogenic infections of early onset; the neutrophils ingest pathogens, but fail to produce superoxide and related microbicidal oxygen intermediates (the respiratory 'burst') due to defective NADPH oxidase, resulting in recurrent bacterial, eg *Staphylococcus aureus* and *Enterobacteriaceae,* and fungal, eg *Aspergillus* species infections with sinusitis, pneumonia and abscess formation; ♂:♀ ratio 4:1 PHYSIOLOGY A phagocyte's microbicidal properties hinge on its ability to produce toxic compounds, eg superoxide, with the reduction of molecular oxygen by a specific membrane-bound NADPH oxidase, aka respiratory-burst oxidase; at rest the enzyme system is disassembled into a membrane-bound part, cytochrome b_{558}, a heterodimer composed of a 91-kD glycoprotein and an 11-kD protein; cytosolic components include 47-kD and 67-kD proteins, and possibly others MOLECULAR PATHOLOGY CGD may be due to mutations of genes that encode any of the 4 major proteins, usually point mutations, which in X-linked CGD lie in the gp91-phox gene and in AR CGD in the p47-phox gene DIAGNOSIS Nitroblue tetrazolium test (see there) is negative due to defective NADPH oxidase*; other tests include assays that directly measure superoxide production, or fluorescent substrate oxidation TREATMENT IFN-γ may be used to reduce the incidence of serious infection (N Engl J Med 1991; 324:509), the mechanism of which may be related to a 'boost' in other components of the immune system

A multicomponent complex of a membrane-bound heterodimeric cytochrome b, composed of glycosylated heavy 91-kD (gp91-phox) and light 22-kD (gp22-phox) components of the enzyme and two or more cytosolic proteins (p47-phox and p67-phox)

chronic idiopathic diarrhea A self-limited condition defined as the presence of persistently loose stools for ≥ 4 weeks without identifiable cause, occurring in absence of systemic illness; the diarrhea is secretory in nature and does not respond to antibiotics, but resolves within several months (N Engl J Med 1992; 327:1849oa); the absence of inflammation seen on colonic biopsy, fecal leukocytes and intractable disease is alleged to distinguish CID from Brainerd diarrhea (see there), although this is uncertain (N Engl J Med 1993; 328:1713c)

chronic mesenteric ischemia Abdominal angina A condition characterized by intermittent severe ischemia resulting in colicky abdominal pain, beginning 15-30 minutes post-prandially 1-2 hours in duration, which appears when two or all three (superior and inferior mesenteric and celiac) major abdominal arteries have severe atherosclerosis; since the intestine's oxygen demand increases with meals, the patients avoid the pain by not eating and thus lose weight; malabsorption may occur since absorption is oxygen-dependent TREATMENT Bypass, endarterectomy, vascular reimplantation, percutaneous transluminal angioplasty

chronic mucocutaneous candidiasis see APECED

chronic obstructive pulmonary (or lung) disease COPD, see there

chronic persistent hepatitis Chronic viral hepatitis

chronobiology Need May 1994 issue of Laboratory Medicine for glossary The formal study of circadian rhythms on an organism's function and dysfunction; certain hormones have their peak secretions at specific times of the day, eg thyrotropin when falling asleep, growth hormone 1-2 hours after onset of sleep, ACTH immediately prior to waking (circa hours), and prolactin prior to waking (Lab Med 1994; 25:372)

chronodesm A time-specific range of an acceptable hormone level that takes into account the difference in the levels of certain hormones at different times of the day (Lab Med 1994; 25:372)

chronotherapy ONCOLOGY A form of administering cancer chemotherapy in which the doses are synchronized with the body's circadian rhythm; chronotherapy has been reported to allow an increase in doses, reduction in tumor burden, and in chemotherapy-related side effects (New York Times May 17, 1994; C5)

chubby puffer syndrome A sleep apnea complex affecting obese, prepubescent males resembling those with Pickwick syndrome, caused by primary alveolar hypoventilation; although temporarily ameliorated by tonsillectomy, the condition is more central, possibly arising in the reticular activating system TREATMENT Weight loss or tricyclic antidepressants; Cf Pink puffer

chunking NEUROPHYSIOLOGY A process in short-term memory in which seemingly disparate elements are combined so as to minimize the required 'space', eg individual letters A, I, L, S, T, U, W would be in a single chunk, LAWSUIT

church spire pattern DERMATOPATHOLOGY Irregular epidermal acanthosis and hyperkeratosis simulating church spires; classically seen in seborrheic keratosis, but also occurs in: Acanthosis nigricans, actinic keratosis, papillary intradermal nevi, 'stucco' keratosis, verruca vulgaris and erythrokeratoderma variabilis

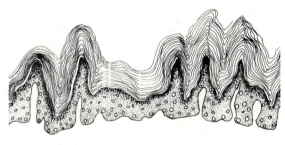

church spire pattern

Churg-Strauss syndrome Allergic granulomatosus and angiitis A triphasic condition characterized by an initial phase of allergy, asthma, or atopic disease, peripheral eosinophilia and vasculitis (fibrinoid necrosis, or perivascular inflammatory infiltrate), involving the heart, lungs, skin, GI tract, CNS (N Engl J Med 1993; 329:1639cpc), and neurologic involvement is common, often as peripheral neuropathy (Mayo Clin Proc 1995: 70:337:341oA)

churning INSURANCE A colloquial term first used in 1953 on Wall Street*, which has been modified by some members of the health and life insurance industry to encompass the act of convincing of a consumer to buy more life insurance with the promise that it would be paid for with built-up values on old policies

*Defined as the repeated buying and selling of stocks to increase the broker's commissions, presumably derived from the act of churning milk, which eventually is converted into a more desirable product, butter

chutta A heat-induced squamous cell carcinoma of the palate linked to the practice in some countries of Southeast Asia of smoking cigarettes with the lighted end inside the mouth

chylomicronemia syndrome A clinical complex characterized by marked chylomicronemia with plasma triglyceride levels in excess of 225 mmol/L (US: 2000 mg/dL) CLINICAL Abdominal and chest pain, pancreatitis, memory defects, carpal tunnel-like paresthesiae, hepatosplenomegaly, chronic eruptive xanthomata, and insulin-resistant diabetes, possibly related to marked hypertriglyceridemia; symptoms are exacerbated by alcohol, β-adrenergic blockers, diuretics, estrogens and glucocorticoids

CIC Circulating immune complexes, see Immune complexes

CID Cytomegalic inclusion disease, see CMV

cidofovir A nucleotide analog that is reported in early clinical trials to have a potent long-acting effect against a

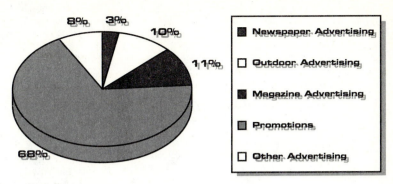

cigarette marketing expenditures

broad spectrum of herpesviruses, which may be of use in treating CMV retinitis, but limited by its nephrotoxicity (JAMA 1995; 273:1458)

CIE Counterimmunoelectrophoresis, see there, aka crossed immunoelectropheresis

cigar bodies A descriptor for short, finger-like structures MICROBIOLOGY A descriptor for the morphology of the yeast form of *Sporothrix schenckii*, seen microscopically with a lactophenol cotton blue stain; see Alcoholic gardener syndrome VETERINARY PATHOLOGY A descriptor for the ultrastructural morphology of insulin granules in the β cells of the canine pancreas

cigarette marketing PUBLIC HEALTH A practice in which a manufacturer promotes or otherwise makes the public aware of a product, here a product with known deleterious effects (Sci Am 1995; 272/5:44)

Note: In the evolving ethics of business, the laws that protect a person or organization's right to free trade through product promotion confront the moral dilemmas inherent in promoting products known to be harmful to the health

cigarette paper scales A descriptor for the flattened, flaked keratotic scales found on the trunk of patients with pityriasis rosea, which are round to oval, salmon-colored and peripherally attached patches that follow the lines of cleavage, fancifully likened to a Christmas tree; see Chevron pattern

cigarette-paper skin A descriptor for the markedly attenuated skin with a shiny, velvety surface seen in Ehlers-Danlos syndrome, type I (less commonly also in type II), caused by defective synthesis, processing or stability of types I and III collagen CLINICAL Premature rupture of membranes, tearing out of sutures, and poor wound healing EM Irregular and enlarged collagen fibers

cigarettes see Fetal tobacco syndrome, Passive smoking, Smoking

ciguatera poisoning The ciguatera, a coral reef fish, in his battle to remain a coral reef inhabitant, secretes ichthyosarcotoxin (ciguatoxin, a lipid-soluble, heat-stable substance isolated from bottom-dwelling fish in temperate and tropical zones), which is produced by the reef dinoflagellate, *Gambierdiscus toxicus,* and concentrated, unchanged up the food chain by herbivores and carnivores; ciguatera poisoning is the most common marine intoxication in the US; 400 species are implicated, including barracuda, grouper, red snapper, amberjack, surgeonfish, sea bass and (unlike scombroid poisoning) may cause morbidity regardless of the form of preparation CLINICAL Onset 6-12 hours after ingestion with nausea, vomiting, cramping, diarrhea, paresthesias, reversal of temperature sense, arthralgias, myalgias, cranial nerve palsies, pruritus with alcohol ingestion, chills, hypotension, bradycardia, respiratory paralysis or death, average duration 8 days DIAGNOSIS RIA, ELISA TREATMENT IV mannitol completely and rapidly reverses symptoms; Cf Scombroid poisoning

cilia Whiplike, motile structures that extend from the plasma membranes, comprising a major structural 'motif' in eukaryotes consisting of a 9 + 2 pattern (see illustration) of nine peripherally-placed doublets and a centrally-placed doublet of microtubular filaments; in contrast, centrioles and basal bodies have a 9 + 3 motif; the ciliary motif is found at all phylogenic levels, from bacterial flagella to the human cilia of the upper respiratory tract, choroid plexus, axial thread of the chromosome, spermatozoa and fallopian tubes; cilia movement occurs in either a metachronous or isochronous fashion; human diseases affecting cilia include 1) Choroid plexus carcinoma and papillomas, which have a 9 + 0 configuration 2) Immotile cilia syndrome, in which the dynein arms are absent CLINICAL Recurrent sinopulmonary infections, decreased female fertility and sperm motility 3) Kartagener syndrome, which is similar to the immotile cilia syndrome, but has in addition, situs inversus, sinusitis, and bronchiectasis and 4) Young syndrome

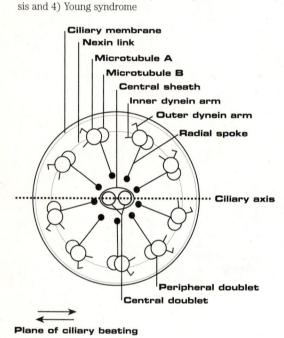

Ciliary membrane
Nexin link
Microtubule A
Microtubule B
Central sheath
Inner dynein arm
Outer dynein arm
Radial spoke
Ciliary axis
Peripheral doublet
Central doublet
Plane of ciliary beating

cilia

ciliary neurotrophic factor A small polypeptide of neuronal origin that promotes in vivo survival of motoneurons (Science 1991; 251:1616)

CIN Cervical intraepithelial neoplasia, see there

Also 1) Cerebriform intradermal nevus (rarely used term, possibly *ad hoc* in nature—Author's note) 2) Chronic interstitial nephritis

cinchonism A mild toxic state that develops when the plasma levels of the antimalarial agent quinine exceed 10-12 mg/L CLINICAL Flushed and sweaty skin, tinnitus, blurred vision, dizziness, nausea, vomiting and diarrhea; truly toxic levels are associated with skin rashes, somnolence, blindness and profound hypotension

'Cinderella' A colloquialism of minimal utility for a relatively neglected area of medicine, a 'forgotten' disease or organism

Cinderella is the rag-beclad heroine in the children's story from Perault's Mother Goose tales

'Cinderella dermatosis' A fanciful synonym for erythema dyschronicum perstans (ashy dermatosis), a term originating from its analogy to Cinderella, who was covered in ashes while she carried out menial tasks

Cinderella delusion A colloquial term for the delusional belief on the part of some medical students that once they graduate from medical school, they will, on the first day (or shortly thereafter, depending on the intensity of the delusion) of their graduate medical education (internship or residency) '...*suddenly be able to develop succinct differential diagnoses, make accurate diagnostic and treatment plans and sign medication orders ...without a senior physician's countersignature controlling for error*' (JAMA 1992; 268:3143) see July phenomenon

Cip1 see *WAF1*

CIP1 p21, see there

Cipollone v. Liggett Group PUBLIC HEALTH A 'landmark' product-liability lawsuit against cigarette manufacturers filed by Mrs Rose Cipollone in 1983* that resulted in a trial by jury and an award of $400 000 to her estate (Cipollone vs Ligett group, 693 F Supp (D.N.J. 1988)); Cipollone is considered important because of the relevant decisions by the US Supreme Court as it set rules for future product-liability lawsuits of a similar nature, and illustrates the difficulties faced by injured smokers seeking retribution from manufacturers of tobacco products known to be harmful; the key question addressed by the US Supreme Court is: 'Does the pre-emption language in the 1965 US Federal Cigarette Labeling and Advertising Act and the Public Health Cigarette Smoking Act of 1969 bar smokers and and their families from suing cigarette manufacturers on the basis of state tort laws.' (N Engl J Med 1992; 327:1604ᴜᴍ)

*and continued on her behalf by her husband after her death, in 1984 from metastatic lung cancer, and after his death, by her estate

CIR Calcium inward rectifier, see I_{KACh}

circadian pacemaker Zeitgeber A small group of neurons in the hypothalamus, the activity of which increases and decreases in ± 24 hour cycles; 'photoperiodic' information from the eyes synchronizes the pacemaker with the light-dark cycle; the pacemaker influences the pineal gland, which produces melatonin at night (Lab Med 1994; 25:372)

circadian rhythm The diurnal cadence; without cyclical cues provided by light, man's daily rhythm is 25.4 hours; the internal clock may reside in the pineal gland, derived embryologically from the ependyma at the roof of the third ventricle, an aggregate of parenchymal cells surrounded by a neuroglial network, weighing 100-180 mg, with direct retinal innervation (retinohypothalamic tract), which is thought to act by secreting melatonin; in rats, the 'biogenic oscillator' resides in the ventral hypothalamus, in hamsters, in the suprachiasmatic nucleus; the CR affects drug metabolism, production of substances measured to detect and monitor disease, myocardial ischemia and oxygen demand (JAMA 1991; 265:386), psychosomatic disease and sleep disorders, which may be thrown out of synchronization by shiftwork, and may be reset or completely suppressed by a light stimulus at a critical time and at a critical strength (Nature 1991; 350:59, 18); daily peaks are described for hormonal secretion, eg adrenal gland, drug metabolism, eg antacids, halothane, physiologic activities, eg blood pressure, cell division, hematopoiesis, natural killer cell activity; see Insomnia, Jet lag, Melatonin, Shift work

circle of Willis ANATOMY: *Circulus arteriosus cerebri* [NA6] A conduit of anastomosed arteries that encircle the optic chiasm and hypophysial region at the base of the brain composed of parts of each internal carotid, anterior, middle, and posterior cerebral arteries, and the anterior and posterior communicating arteries; it plays a pivotal role in cerebral infarction; a small (<1 mm in diameter) or absent ipsilateral posterior communicating artery is a risk factor for ischemia or infarction in subjects with internal carotid artery occlusion (N Engl J Med 1994; 330:1565ᴏᴀ) see Berry aneurysm

circular A-21 A document generated by the US Office of

Management and Budget that prescribes general guidelines for (indirect) costs, eg 'overhead' that may be charged to the recipients of federally funded grants and contracts by educational institutions (Science 1991; 252:636n&v); see Indirect costs

circular DNA A 65-200 kilobase fragment of DNA formed by a process of 'looping out and deletion', containing a constant region of the μ heavy chain (Cμ) and the 3' part of the μ 'switch' region joined to the 5' part of the switch segment for the class to which the cell has switched; circular DNA is a normal product of rearrangement among gene segments encoding the variable regions of immunoglobulin light and heavy chains, as well as the T-cell receptor

circulating lupus anticoagulant syndrome The association of recurrent thromboses (including cerebral), repeated spontaneous abortions and renal disease frequently in ANA-negative lupus patients has been termed the circulating lupus anticoagulant syndrome with repeated fetal wastage and an IgM gammopathy

circulating nurse A nurse who participates in a surgical procedure, coordinating, planning and implementing all the nurse-related activities during an operation, who has not scrubbed with the surgical team itself; see Scrub nurse

circumcision Surgical removal of the foreskin, either by an obstetrician, or as a part of a religious rite (eg, a bris, performed by a rabbi in the Jewish religion at birth and Moslems in preadolescence); the American Academy of Pediatrics recommends (Pediatrics 1989; 84:388) circumcision as it reduces the incidence of balanitis, balanoposthitis, phimosis, colonization by fimbriated pyelonephritogenic *Escherichia coli*, and other bacteria, urinary tract infection (urinary tract infections are 10-20 times more common in uncircumcised boys); the lifetime risk for penile cancer in uncircumcised males is 600-fold greater than that of circumcised males; the risk for cancer of the uterine cervix is closely linked to HPV infections (HPV-16 in 50% and HPV-18 in 10%) in uncircumcised male partners; the incidence of STDs, eg genital herpes, syphilis, gonorrhea, chancroid, and HIV-1 is lower in the circumspect and circumcised (N Engl J Med 1990; 322:1308, 1312)

'circumcision', female Female circumcision, see there

circumoral pallor A rim of pale perioral skin seen in scarlet fever

circumoval bodies Granulomas in schistosomal infections that surround the eggs (or ova, hence the name); circumoval bodies are found histologically in the bladder, caused by *S haematobium* or in the liver due to *S mansoni* PATHOLOGY Schistosomal egg partially or completely rimmed by a foreign-body giant cell reaction with concentric fibrosis and a lymphocyte and plasma cell response; with time, the liver develops marked fibrosis, whereupon it is termed 'pipestem fibrosis'

circumstantial homosexuality The practice of homosexual acts when there are no opportunities for heterosexual activity, most commonly occurring in adolescents in detention centers, youth prisons and residential treatment centers, which may be accompanied by sadism and sexual exploitation; Cf Latent homosexuality

Note: Homosexual experimentation is not thought to predict future homosexual behavior

circumstatiality PSYCHIATRY A feature of certain mental disorders, where the loss of a normal 'filtering mechanism' results in a nonselectivity of thoughts and speech, such that an excessive amount of detail ('circumstances', hence the name) is provided regardless of how tangential or irrelevant the information being provided actually is; circumstantiality is typical of schizophrenia, and may occur in obsessional disorders

circus movement Reentry or reciprocal movement

CARDIOLOGY Circus movement forms the basis for some (if not all) supraventricular tachycardia and requires that there be

1) An available circuit of conducting tissue

2) A difference in refractoriness in the two limbs of the circuit and

3) A rate of conduction through the tissue that is slow enough in the less refractory limb so that the more refractory limb has had time to recover when the circus impulse approaches a second time; supraventricular flutter and fibrillation are likely due to an ectopic pacemaker

cirrhotic glomerulonephritis A form of renal disease related to liver failure, characterized by subendothelial and mesangial thickening of glomerular basement membrane, with fusion of the epithelial foot processes seen in patients with micro- or macronodular cirrhosis; Cf Hepatorenal syndrome

CIS Carcinoma-in-situ, see there

cis MOLECULAR BIOLOGY A mutation that is active only when it is on the same chromosome, but not when it is on the opposite chain is said to be cis-active; if the mutation is active at another chromosome site or on another chain, it is trans-active

***cis*-acting locus** A region of the DNA molecule affecting genes located on the same, ie not opposite or trans molecule; Cf trans-activation

cis-platinum Diaminedichloride A chemotherapeutic agent that forms covalent bonds and crosslinks with DNA, which is used to treat head and neck, ovarian, testicular, and bladder cancers SIDE EFFECTS 1) Nephrotoxicity, requiring adequate hydration to maintain renal flow and high chloride concentration 2) Nausea is a constant feature of cisplatinum therapy, which responds to Ondansetron, a selective antagonist of serotonin S_3 receptors and 3) Neurotoxicity, with peripheral neuropathy with features similar to vitamin E toxicity

CISS hybridization MOLECULAR GENETICS A technique for high-resolution physical mapping of chromosomes based on the suppression of fluorescent hybridization signals from ubiquitous repeated sequences, eg Alu and Kpn elements by addition of competitor DNAs to a probe mix; CISS hybridization is of use as a supplementary tool in generating a 1-3 centiMorgan map of the human genome; it permits direct visualization of the presence or absence of a genomic DNA sequence in the face of a specific deletion or duplication, or determination of its position relative to a translocation breakpoint

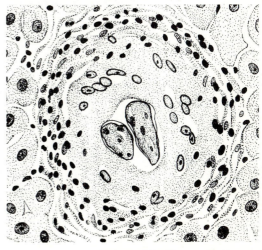

circumoval body

cistron Structural gene MOLECULAR BIOLOGY A unit of genetic information or an independent transactive complementation unit of DNA that was thought to encode one polypeptide; the term is no longer used as it lends to confusion, as it is defined by techniques that have fallen into disuse

citation classic An article or abstract in a scientific journal that has been cited in the subsequent biomedical literature more than four hundred times, an objective criterion specified by the Institute for Scientific Information (J Lab Clin Med 1990; 116:755); Citation classics are often examined by the Nobel committee as a benchmark of original work; see Landmark article; Cf Uncitedness index

citation impact A major parameter for measuring the importance of a scientific report is the frequency with which it is cited in subsequent scientific literature; CI is a datum generated by the ISI (Institute of Scientific Information, Philadelphia) from their science indicators database, which generally ignores laboratory techniques; the highest citation impact is produced by the workers at Harvard, where each paper was cited an average of 24.63 times discounting methodology papers; the CI is used by the Nobel institute for evaluating future candidates for Nobel prizes

Note: Of the 894 most cited papers in biology identified by the ISI, the 220 researchers sponsored by the Howard Hughes Medical Institute accounted for 82, while the 3000 scientists of the National Institute of Health (USA) accounted for 84; the disadvantage of the CI is that some papers may win a high citation score because they are erroneous or use poorly designed studies, attracting critical citations, as occurred with cold fusion (Science 1991; 252:639n&v)

cited scientist Most cited scientist A scientist whose research is considered by his peers to be of sufficient merit to cite in bibliographies of their own research reports; for the decade from 1981-90, the 35 papers from J Messing (molecular biology, Rutgers U) were cited 18 229 times; the 93 papers of MJ Berridge (biochemistry, U of Cambridge) were cited 16 004 times and the 81 papers of T Maniatis (molecular biology, Harvard U) were cited 11 167 times (Science 1991; 254:28n)

Note: A technique that represents major advances in methodology (eg Southern blot hybridization) may result in frequent citation, but unless it is coupled with a major theoretical advance (eg monoclonal antibody production, Nobel prize 1984; polymerase chain reaction, Nobel prize 1993), may not be considered of Nobel prize-winning potential

Citrus Red 2 [CI 12156] A dye used to color orange skins a bright orange color, which induces chromosomal damage and is carcinogenic in animals when administered in extremely high doses; the impact that the low levels to which humans eating dyed oranges are exposed is uncertain, and probably minimal, although alternative health care advocates and organically grown food aficionados often make broad sweeping statements to the contrary (Alternative Medicine, Future Medicine Publishing, Inc, Puyallup, Washington, 1994) see Alternative medicine

Citrus Red 2

Civatte bodies Cytoid bodies, see there

civil commitment Involuntary hospitalization, see there

CJD Creutzfeldt-Jakob disease, see Prions, Spongiform encephalopathy

CJM Cell junction molecule, see there

CK Creatinine phosphokinase, also 1) Choline kinase 2) Cyanogen chloride (US Army) 3) Cytokeratin 4) Cytokine

CK-MB Creatine phosphokinase [EC 2.7.3.2], MB isoenzyme LABORATORY MEDICINE An isoform of CK that is typically increased in myocardial infarction, which may also be increased in muscular dystrophy, polymyositis, myoglobinuria, occasionally in malignancy, eg lung cancer, all possibilities that must be considered in the face of an elevated CK-MB without myocardial infarction; Cf Troponin

CK-MB subform A form of CK-MB; $CK-MB_2$ is present in myocardial tissue, and when released into the blood is acted upon by lysine carboxypeptidase which cleaves the positively charged terminal lysine from the M subunit, resulting in the more negatively charged $CK-MB_1$; measurement of the CK-MB subunits ($CK-MB_2 \geq 1.0$ U/L and a ratio of $CK-MB_2$ to $CK-MB_1 \geq 1.5$) is more sensitive (95.7% vs 48%), and more specific than the conventional CK-MB assay in identifying patients with acute MI, and can be obtained within 6 hours of hospitalization, reducing admission to the coronary care unit, thereby reducing costs (N Engl J Med 1994; 331:561oA) Cf Troponin I, Troponin T

Note: It is as yet unknown whether assays of serum levels of troponin I and troponin T (see there) are superior to the immunoinhibition test for CK-MB subunits

CLA A conjugated dienoic derivative of linoleic acid (an 18-carbon essential polyunsaturated fatty acid), in which the two pairs of double bonds are separated by a single carbon instead of a pair of carbons (like normal linoleic acid); the double bond position shift may be induced by heating, free-radical oxidation and enzymatic reaction; CLA is present in cheese and cooked meat and may be anti-carcinogenic, incorporating itself directly into the protected cells, quenching oxygen free radicals and singlet oxygen; Cf PUFAs

clade MOLECULAR EPIDEMIOLOGY A genetic diversity grouping in which member genomes share a certain level of pattern of nucleic acid 'homology' (sequence similarity); 'cladograms' can be constructed to identify geographic distribution of the members (Science & Medicine 1995; 2/3:38) see Phylogenic tree

clang association NEUROLOGY A shift in the conversation or flow of ideas based on the sound of the words being used, eg feed and read, where a converstation might shift from that about pets to spare time activities

claims made policy MALPRACTICE A malpractice insurance policy in which coverage is provided for any claim that occurs while the policy is in force, regardless of when the alleged malpractice, negligence, or injury actually occurred; Cf Tail coverage

clamp-derived insulin-sensitivity index An index of the effect of changes in the insulin concentration on glucose clearance (glucose uptake rate divided by plasma glucose concentration) per unit of body surface area, which is obtained by means of the glucose-clamp technique; the CDIS index is calculated as

$$CDISI = \frac{\Delta GDR}{\Delta I} \times G$$

where GDR (glucose-disposal rate) is expressed in mg/m²/min, I (insulin) is expressed in mU/mL, and G (glucose) is expressed in mg/dL (N Engl J Med 1994; 331:1188oA) Cf Insulin-sensitivity index

'clap' STD A colloquial sobriquet for gonorrhea

The term clap is of murky parentage, derived from either 1) Provençal, clap, a heap of stones, from which rabbits made their homes, evolving in Old French to rabbit's burrow, arriving in Middle English as clap(er) a brothel or 2) Middle French, clapoir, a bubo Note: Since buboes are not seen in gonorrhea, the latter origin is unlikely according to JE Lighter (**Historical Dictionary of American Slang, Random House, New York, 1994**), its use in the New World dates to 1587

Clark, Barney A dentist who was the first patient to receive a completely artificial heart, the Jarvik 7, in an operation performed by cardiovascular surgeon, Wm de Vries at the University Hospital in Salt Lake City; Clark later died of renal failure and on postmortem examination had pseudomembranous colitis; see Artificial heart, Jarvik 7

CLAS 1) Cholesterol-Lowering Atherosclerosis Study A randomized, placebo-controlled trial using colestipol and niacin in men with previous coronary artery bypass surgery; in treated subjects, elevated triglyceride-rich lipoproteins have a major role in atherogenesis; CLAS/CLAS-II at the four-year mark continue to demonstrate the benefits of this regimen on blood lipids, lipoprotein-cholesterol and apoprotein and nonprogression of atherosclerotic lesions and/or regression 2) Circulating lupus anticoagulant syndrome; see Anticardiolipin antibody syndrome, Lupus anticoagulant

clasp knife phenomenon NEUROLOGY A manifestation of corticospinal spasticity in which there is increased tone in either flexion or extension with sudden relaxation as the muscle continues to be stretched, imparting a sensation fancifully likened to that of an opening clasp knife; this effect is often accompanied by weakness of the affected extremity, increased tendon reflexes and a Babinski sign; Cf Cogwheel phenomenon, Gegenhalten

class action (lawsuit) A legal action undertaken by one or more plaintiffs on the behalf of themselves, and all other persons with an identical interest in an alleged wrong; in the US, a number of medically-related class action suits have appeared, resulting in prolonged legal battles with settlements by the product manufacturer(s) allegedly at fault costing hundreds of millions of dollars to settle the claims; see Agent Orange, Dalkon shield, Shiley valve

Class I recall The recall of an FDA-regulated medical device or product the use of or exposure to which a reasonable probability exists for adverse health effects or death (**MDDI reports, The Gray Sheet 1995; Jan 2; 12**); Class I devices are low-risk products, that are minimally regulated by the FDA; the manufacturers of class I products are required to adhere to general guidelines and good manfacturing practices, and are prohibited from misbranding and adulteration; these devices include elastic bandages and tongue depressors; Class II devices are products that are considered to have a medium risk to patients, and are required to adhere to performance standards to assure safety and effectiveness; manufacturers of Class II devices must notify the FDA prior to marketing a product through the so-called 510(K) process; Class II devices include hearing aids and syringes; Class III medical devices are considered to pose high risks to patients and are subject to premarket approval by the FDA and verification of safety and efficacy of the device through review of clinical and other relevant data prior to marketing; special controls are required to ensure the safety and effectiveness of these products; Class III devices include life-support or life-sustaining devices such as pacemakers and heart valves (**Special Communication, College of American Pathologists, April 3, 1995**)

class switching PHYSIOLOGY A step in the normal maturation of hemoglobin during fetal development requires switching from embryonal zeta chain, which is structurally similar to the α chain, and occurs on chromosome 16 to mature α chain production; β chain production is a two-stage maturation process with early loss of the ε chain, the presence during fetal and early post-natal life of a γ chain, the decrease of which coincides with increased expression of the β chain

classic pathway IMMUNOLOGY The usual route of activation of the complement cascade (the non-specific arm of the immune system, which is responsible for lysis of target organisms and cells); the classic pathway is initiated by C1q binding to either IgM or to two adjacent IgG molecules; the resulting conformational change of C1q autoactivates C1r2, in turn activating C1s2, cleaving C4 (C4b) followed by C2 (C2a); C4b,2a, the C3 convertase of the classic complement pathway, initiates opsonization, leukocyte chemotaxis, increased vascular permeability, and finally cytolysis; the classic complement pathway is activated by IgG, IgM, DNA, staphylococcal protein A and C-reactive protein; both the classic and alternate pathways are stimulated by trypsin-like enzymes; see Common pathway; Cf Alternate pathwat

clathrin MEMBRANE PHYSIOLOGY A heterodimeric membrane transport protein, composed of one heavy (80-kD) and several light (20–40-kD) chains that polymerize three-legged protein complexes, termed triskelions, which aggregate into 'patches' at the internal face of the cell membrane forming a cage-like polyhedral lattice around the coated pits and vesicles and mediate selective transport events; clathrin is pivotal in transport vesicle biogenesis, facilitating receptor transport by concentrating and sorting the receptors into specific intracellular compartments, eg Golgi apparatus and endosomes, while retaining Golgi membrane protein within the cell; clathrin thus acts as a shuttle molecule, endlessly cycling between the membrane and lysosome; see Endocytosis; Cf Golgi-derived coated vesicle

claw finger deformity A deformity that results from combined paralysis of the median and ulnar nerves, characterized by hyperextension of the metacarpophalangeal joint and hyperflexion of the proximal interphalangeal joints TREATMENT Tenodesis, capsulodesis, or arthrodesis

claw foot A foot deformity due to atrophic paralysis of the intrinsic foot muscles, allowing the long extensors of the toes to dorsiflex the proximal phalanges and the long flexors to shorten the foot, heighten the arch and flex the distal phalanges, pulling the foot into talipes equinus; claw foot occurs in chronic polyneuropathies and is characteristic of Charcot-Marie-Tooth disease; Cf Lobster claw deformity

clawhand Main en griffe The hand deformity may follow the claw foot deformity of Charcot-Marie-Tooth disease, where the atrophy is usually confined to the distal arm and may occur in Dejerine-Sottas' hypertrophic polyneuropathy, leprosy, and Refsum's disease; a similar 'stiff hand' occurs in mucopolysaccharidosis, type I-S; Cf Lobster claw deformity

claw toes A deformity characterized by metatarsophalangeal joint hyperextension and interphalangeal joint flexion, usually associated with neuropathic conditions, eg Friedrich's ataxia, poliomyelitis and spinal cord injury, which may occur in a familial setting PATHOGENESIS Although paralysis of the intrinsic muscles of the foot is a commonly evoked explanation, the muscles are functionally and histologically normal CLINICAL Incapacitating and painful callosities at the 'new' pressure points, especially of the great toe TREATMENT Conservative, tendon resection, joint resection

clean *adjective* Free of dirt or pollution; clean is used colloquially for an organ or tissue lacking pathological findings, eg 'clean' coronary arteries and aorta are typically seen at autopsy in persons dying with terminal cancer or alcoholism

Clean Air Act A legislative act passed in California that mandates drastic reductions in the pollutants produced by various industrial, commercial and private sources; while the emissions in the Los Angeles basin are 75% less than that of the mid-1950s, the pollutants in Los Angeles' air exceeded US federal health standards on 143 days in 1992; by the year 2010, hydrocarbons are to be reduced by 90%, nitric oxides by 70%, and carbon monoxide by 45% The current levels of air pollution cost an estimated $10 billion/year in the form of increased health care costs, reduced crop yields, and lowered industrial productivity; this contrasts with the Environmental Protection Agency's estimates of the cost for implementing the Clean Air Act of $4-6 x 10⁹/year (Sci Am 1994; 270/5:113)

clean-catch urine LABORATORY MEDICINE A specimen of 'midstream' urine for bacterial culture that is obtained from women after cleansing the perineum and meatus with CCCC; although this technique continues to be a standard practice for collecting urine for bacterial culture, studies do not support its efficacy (N Engl J Med 1993; 328:289c)

clean-contaminated wound A wound that involves transection of nonsterile mucocutaneous surface

clean wound A superficial wound produced by uncontaminated sharp objects, either electively, eg surgical procedure or by accident, being cut by sharp glass or metal, eg broken glass; clean wounds theoretically do not require antibiotic coverage or tetanus prophylaxis, although it is commonly administered, often as an act of 'defensive' medicine; Cf Clean-contaminated wound, Dirty wound

clear cell Light cell HISTOLOGY A finely vacuolated, cholesterol-filled cell with central dark nuclei arranged in clusters and located in the midzone or zona fasciculata of the adrenal cortex; these cells are the major reserve for glucocorticoid and sex hormone production when the adrenal gland is stressed; see Compact (dark) cells

clear cell acanthoma Pale cell acanthoma DERMATOLOGY A benign sharply demarcated, solitary lesion of the legs that mimics seborrheic keratosis and pyogenic granuloma PATHOLOGY Enlarged clear, glycogen-filled basal cells, mild spongiosis, elongated intertwining rete ridges, parakeratosis with few granular cells and weak DOPA positivity

clear cell adenocarcinoma A malignancy of the vagina and uterine cervix, two-thirds of which cases have occurred in young women who were exposed in utero to estrogen analogues, especially diethylstilbestrol (DES) as well as hexestrol or dienestrol; relative risk for those exposed, 0.014; 5-year survival, 80+% with local recurrence PATHOLOGY Tubes and cysts lined by clear cells, admixed with solid areas and papillary formations

clear cell carcinoma 1) ENDOMETRIUM A tumor of elderly women, of presumed müllerian origin PATHOLOGY Solid, papillary, tubular and cystic arrangement of glycogen-filled 'hobnail' cells, once described as 'mesonephric carcinomas', histologically similar to DES-induced clear cell adenocarcinoma of the vagina, but not aoociated with DES PROGNOSIS Poor; 5-year survival of 0% if the lesion is greater than stage I 2) LIVER A tumor comprising 5% of hepatocellular carcinomas, cytologically mimicking metastatic renal cell and adrenal cortical carcinomas PATHOLOGY 'Alveolar' pattern of clear cells PROGNOSIS Similar to usual hepatocellular carcinoma 3) OVARY A tumor of presumed müllerian origin that may be associated with endometriosis, comprising up to 10% of primary ovarian carcinomas, affecting women circa age 55 PATHOLOGY Yellow with cystic degeneration LM Tubules lined by 'hobnail' cells PROGNOSIS Five-year survival, 40%

clear cell chondrosarcoma A radiolucent low-grade sarcoma of the epiphysis of long bones, especially of the proximal femur, affecting all ages ♂:♀ ratio, 2.5:1, metastases occur to other bones and lungs TREATMENT en bloc resection and wide margin Prognosis 15-20% mortality

clear cell myeloma A monoclonal plasma cell expansion, clinically similar to the 'garden variety' of myeloma, which has vacuolated cytoplasm and clonally increased IgA and kappa chains and lytic bone lesions

clear cell sarcoma Malignant melanoma of soft parts A sarcoma of young, often female adults, of the lower extremities and acral regions, intimately bound to tendons as circumscribed but unencapsulated melanin-bearing tumors of neuroectodermal origin PROGNOSIS 45-60% mortality, late recurrence; see Barrel-staves appearance

clear cell tumor A generic term for a neoplasm composed of clear cells that may be of any embryologic (endo-, ecto-, meso- or neuroectodermal) origin; the cytoplasmic clearing may be real (lipid, mucopolysaccharide and mucosubstance) or artifactual due to post-fixation shrinkage of cytoplasmic content away from an intact and rigid cell membrane; clear cell tumors include balloon cell melanoma, carcinoma, eg signet ring cells, seen in carcinomas of the stomach as well as in renal cell, adrenal, ovary, parathyroid and thyroid, clear cell tumors of tendons and aponeuroses, germ cell tumors (seminomas, dysgerminoma), histiocytosis X, lymphoma (B- and T-cell clear cell lymphomas), myeloma, clear cell type, myxoid lesions (benign and malignant), paraganglioma, xanthoma; see Clear cell carcinoma

clear-glass appearance RADIOLOGY A descriptor for the 'empty' holes, spaces and clefts seen in osteoporosis, compared to the ground-glass graininess characteristic of osteomalacia

clearance The theoretical volume from which the drug is totally removed in a unit time; see Therapeutic drug monitoring

cleaved cell A malignant lymphocyte that has one or more deep clefts, linear infoldings of the nucleus, condensed chromatin and indistinct nucleoli, typically seen in the follicular small cleaved cell lymphoma, an intermediate grade lymphoma, which despite widespread disease at the time of diagnosis follows a relatively prolonged and non-aggressive course; large cleaved cells are typical of immunoblastic (Rappaport's diffuse histiocytic) lymphoma, in which the cells are slightly larger than the small cleaved cells and somewhat more mitotically active, having a slightly more aggressive clinical course, falling between an intermediate and a high-grade lymphoma by the Working Formulation, see there

clenched fist syndrome A cutaneous abscess most often infected by *Eikenella corrodens* due to a traumatic laceration, typically over the 3rd and 4th metacarpophalangeal joints, the result of striking someone in the teeth; with improper management, local osteomyelitis may develop TREATMENT Debridement, broad-spectrum antibiotics to 'cover' for the often-present anaerobic bacteria

CLIA '88 Clinical Laboratory Improvement Amendments of 1988 Legislation passed by the US Congress that promulgates quality assurance practices, and requires clinical laboratories to measure performance at each step of the total testing process from the beginning to the end-point of a response to a test result (Arch Pathol Lab Med 1994; 118:601); part of CLIA '88 raison d"être was to bring the previously poorly regulated physician office laboratories (POLs) under strict federal regulation with the purpose of improving the reliability of POL testing; the regulations took effect 1 July 1991 (Arch Pathol Lab Med 1992; 116:681sA); there are 300-600 000 labs that require CLIA scrutinization; the Health Care Financing Administration is responsible for ensuring compliance with the CLIA regulations; see HCFA, POLs, Waived tests

client/server computing COMPUTERS An architectural philosophy that can be constructed in various ways using different types of computers; in the simplest form, a C/S system is composed of a PC-based server and various PC clients; when large, C/S systems provide massively distributed cooperative processing, as evidenced by the C/S system in the Brigham and Women's Hospital in Boston, which has 4000 PC clients, 130 servers, and supports 70 applications including those for the clinical laboratory, accounts receivable, and general accounting; the advantages of C/S systems are that they are scalable* and performance bottlenecks can improved by migrating to faster (eg RISC-based) microprocessors, splitting the work among servers, more efficient use of cache, and altering the load processing between client and server; the ultimate goal of a C/S system is become completely independent of the hardware, operating system, and database environment (CAP Today Nov 1994 p1)

*ie the system architecture and applications programs can support a 50-bed hospital or a 1000-bed hospital, allowing for incremental growth

climacteric The perimenopausal period of functional ovarian involution, characterized by vasomotor lability, eg hot flashes, dysmenorrhea, redistribution of fat, dyspareunia, hormonal changes, eg increased FSH and LH, decreased PGE_2, estrogen and progesterone; postmenopausal ovaries continue to secrete androgens, which are peripherally converted into postmenopausal estrogens, incipient osteoporosis and decreased skin elasticity

climatological disaster PUBLIC HEALTH A generic term for a natural disaster caused by climatological disturbances, which may be linked to global phenomena (eg El Niño, La Niña) that impact on local weather; CDs include floods and storms, which may be land-based (tornadoes) or water-based (cyclones, hurricanes, typhoons) (JM Last, RB Wallace, Eds, Public Health and Preventive Medicine, 13th ed, Appletone & Lange, Norwalk, 1992) see Earthquake; Cf Geological disaster

'climbing up on oneself' Gower sign NEUROLOGY A clinical sign referring to the manner in which children with well-developed Duchenne's muscular dystrophy (DMD) rise from a sitting to a standing position, by grasping and pulling in order on body parts from the knees to hips until they are in an erect position

Note In DMD, ambulation is often lost by age 12; 75% die by age 20 secondary to respiratory paralysis

clinic A location where patients are seen on an out-patient basis, either as a first-time visit or as a follow-up to some form of previous therapy

Note: The term clinic also encompasses a clinical lecture in which a patient is present, or instruction of students at the bedside, both uses of which have largely fallen into disuse (in the US)

clinical alert Clinical update Prepublication release of information from federally-funded research that may have an immediate effect on patient care; the format and criteria for clinical alerts was pending consensus as of early 1991, but have included alerts on the use of immunoglobulins to reduce the incidence and severity of bacterial infections in children with AIDS and the benefits of performing carotid endarterectomy on symptomatic patients with 70-99% occlusion of one or both carotid arteries (Am Med News 11 March 1991) see Ingelfinger rule; Cf Embargo arrangement

clinical algorithm see Algorithm, Critical pathway

clinical decision analysis A quantitative approach to complex decisions first used by the military and industry and increasingly popular in medicine; despite early objections that the models created would distort reality, or need to include every possible condition, action, and outcome, clinical decision analysis (the adjective clinical is often dropped) has reached a stage of maturity that it allows creation of useful decision-making models; vague descriptor, eg sometimes, almost never, can be replaced by quantifiers; dimensionless numerical quantifiers of outcome have been replaced by life expectancy, and the subjectivity inherent in evaluating patient preferences has been replaced by factoring in quality of life 'yardsticks', eg quality-adjusted life years (N Engl J Med 1994; 330:562ED)

clinical ecologist A non-traditional practitioner of medicine who claims to have special expertise in the diagnosis and treatment of 'environmental illness', a condition that is not thought to exist by many mainstream medical practitioners; see Environmental hypersensitivity syndrome

clinical equipoise Equipoise BIOMEDICAL ETHICS A state of genuine uncertainty of the ultimate benefits or disadvantages of both therapeutic arms in a clinical trial; because the clinical investigator may become biased as a study progresses, due to the perceived benefit of one of the therapeutic regimens being evaluated, he may enroll fewer and fewer patients in the perceived less beneficial arm, due to ethical considerations, and may ultimately defeat the very purpose of the study for lack of patients in the control arm; a moral exit to this dilemma, known as 'clinical equipoise' is possible, since genuine uncertainty exists in the 'expert' medical community at large; the investigator may thus continue to enroll control patients 'blindly', despite his bias

clinical faculty An unpaid member of a medical school staff who regularly practices his specialty in a private setting privately, and devotes less than 50% of his time to the institution; the responsibilities of 'voluntary track' faculty include participation in teaching efforts, administrative functions and/or research efforts; clinical faculty members receive the titles of clinical instructor, clinical assistant professor, clinical associate professor, and professor, in increasing rank of accomplishments

clinical feedback The act of providing a physician with information re: his/her own use of tests in order to influence them, and hopefully reduce unnecessary testing (CAP Today June 1995, p20)

Clinical Global Impression of Change A 7-point subjective scale that rates a patient's change in psychological status from the time of initial screening (JAMA 1992; 268:2523oc)

clinical laboratory test A generic term for any test that is regarded as having value in assessing health or disease states; CLTs may be divided into those that 1) Define risk and/or disease, eg detection of hyperglycemia, or hypercholesterolemia 2) Classify a subject into a disease or nondisease state in which the population is bimodal with overlapping parameters, eg above normal without disease, high normal with disease 3) Monitor a disease, eg glucose, cholesterol (CAP Today, 1994; 8:34)

clinical pathology The field of pathology dedicated to the measurement and/or identification of substances, cells, or microorganisms in body fluids, and encompasses clinical microbiology (bacteriology, mycology, parasitology, and virology), clinical immunology, clinical chemistry, hematology, and immunohematology (blood banking); definition of clinical pathology adopted by the Board of the College of American Pathology (CAP Today July 1993)

'...the branch of pathology that involves

1) Analysis and medical interpretation of the results of laboratory testing of blood, body fluids, and certain other specimens from an individual patient and correlation of those results with the patient's medical history, physical examination, and anatomic pathology findings to arrive at a diagnosis of the clinical condition of the patient. In order to be certified in clinical pathology by the American Board of Pathology, a physician must successfully complete 4 years of medical school,

2) 3-5 years of medical training specializing in the selection, performance, and medical interpretation of laboratory tests and analysis, and

3) An intensive examination. The definition also identifies 10 medical services that a clinical pathologist performs, including analyzing and reporting on the clinical significance of laboratory test results on patient specimens, consulting with physicians on the medical interpretation of test results, and determining the appropriateness of blood and blood products for transfusion. '

clinical practice guidelines see Algorithm, Critical pathway

clinical responsibility A generic term for any task or duty involving the professional capabilities of a practitioner that requires the exercise of clinical judgement with respect to patient care; Cf Administrative responsibility

clinical rotation MEDICAL EDUCATION A time period[1] in which a medical student in the clinical part[2] of his/her education passes through various 'working' services[3] in 1 to 4 month blocks of time; a CR provides the student with a panoramic view of medicine, allowing him/her to put career choices in perspective and helps him/her to begin to translate the knowledge gained in the basic sciences[4] into the practice of medicine

[1]Usually one or more years [2]The last two years of a four-year program of education in the US [3]eg OB/Gyn, surgery, pediatrics [4]The first two years of a four-year program of education in the US

clinician A generic term for a health care professional involved in active patient management; Cf Academician

clinicopathological conference A formal discussion of a patient's clinical, radiological, laboratory data, usually in front a large group of junior and senior colleagues; the CPC is often presented as an 'unknown' problem case, and in the first portion of the presentation does not include (for the sake of didactics) the confirmed pathological diagnosis; the presentation of the patient's baseline data is then followed by discussion of the case as an unknown by an expert, to view the steps he would have taken in arriving at a diagnosis; the final stage of a CPC is a discussion by the pathologist who usually is the ultimate arbiter regarding the diagnosis; Cf Professorial rounds

Clinton plan A proposal to reform the US health care system delineated by Presidents Bill and Hillary Clinton and crystallized in the American Health Security Act of 1993 *'The Clinton Plan, as presented in an initial draft was an ingeneous amalgam of regulation and market competition* ('managed competition') ...(which)...*called for the formation of a National Health Board that would ...bring health care costs into line with general inflation by 1999. The states would be required to set up purchasing cooperatives* ('regional alliances') *that would enroll all residents within a given area and purchase insurance on their behalf from at least three competing groups of providers* ('health plans').' (**N Engl J Med** 1993; 329:1569ED) see Health care reform

Note: Some analysts feared that the Clinton plan (in particular the 'pay-or-play' component) could result in the closing of businesses, loss of jobs, a marked ↑ in expenses for the private sector and the taxpayer, and a complex new government bureaucracy; as of early 1995, the Clinton plan had been emasculated by a complex interplay of 'agendas' and if it succeeds at all, will be an effete shadow of its promising beginning (Author's note)

CLIP Corticotropin-like intermediate lobe peptide One of the peptides released from Pro-opiomelanocortin (POMC); CLIP's precursor is the 39 residue ACTH that splits into two peptides, α-MSH (residues 1-13) and CLIP (residues 18-39); see POMC

clipase Intracellular proteolytic enzyme(s) that remove the pre- and pro- portions of hormones, eg for para-thyroid hormone (PTH), a 25-residue polypeptide is 'clipased' from the 115-residue pre-pro-parent, yielding a 90-residue pre-PTH; a 6-residue segment is then removed by tryptic 'clipase' from the pre-PTH yielding the mature 84-residue PTH

Clipper chip COMPUTERS An encryption device that is being proposed for installation in Internet that has engendered controversy vis-à-vis the potential misuse by the US government which would have the ability to tap into private or priviledged communications on Internet; in the earliest forms of electronic communication, a secret key or coding method was agreed upon by the parties involved in the exchange; because of the vulnerability inherent in communicating the coding methods, three workers at MIT delineated how a public key coding system might work; once such a device becomes readily available, the government would lose its ability to listen to any conversation or monitor any communication which is what the Clipper effectively counteracts (**Atlantic Monthly** June 1994:46)

clipping NEUROSURGERY A routine and definitive therapy for intracranial aneurysms, which consists of the direct obliteration of the aneurysmal neck by a clip of the proper strength, shape, and size that prevents the flow of blood into the dome of the aneurysm, while preserving the parent artery; clipping is problematic in sclerosed arteries as the clip may further compromise a vessel with a suboptimal baseline of blood flow (**Mayo Clin Proc** 1995; 70:153RV) Cf Interventional neuroradiology, Trapping

clitoridectomy A type of female circumcision that has been divided into type I, in which part or the entire female clitoris is removed, a procedure that has been likened to amputation of the penis and type II in which in addition to clitoridectomy, part of the labia minora is removed, with the wound being closed by various threads, grasses or other suture materials, or by use of a poultice; the procedure is deeply rooted in the culture of certain African countries and symbolizes the society's control over the woman's sexual pleasure (**N Engl J Med** 1994; 331:712SA) see Female circumcision, Cf Infibulation

CLL Chronic lymphocytic leukemia

cloacogenic carcinoma Basaloid carcinoma, see there

cloasma Melasma A rash caused by the hormonal effects of pregnancy or birth control pills, which is exacerbated by the sunlight CLINICAL Irregular flat symmetrical light brown areas on the malar region, cheeks and forehead; this 'pregnancy mask' tends to fade with delivery or discontinuation of birth control pills

clock theory CELL BIOLOGY A hypothetical explanation for the events involved in somatic cell duplication, which holds that the production of mitotic progeny are the work of an oscillating biological metronome that alternately swings between mitosis and interphase, a concept championed by marine biologists; research data supports a merging of the clock theory with the domino theory; Cf Domino theory

clomiphene OBSTETRICS An ovulation-induction agent that causes marked ↑ in the frequency of multiple gestations; use of clomiphene is associated with twins in 7-13%, triplets in 0.5%, quadruplets in 0.3%, and quintuplets in 0.1%; clomiphene ↑ the risk (RR = 2.3) of a borderline or invasive ovarian tumor (**N Engl J Med** 1994; 331:771OA)

clonal analysis Any of a number of techniques used to determine whether a tissue is polyclonal–and therefore reactive, or monoclonal, ie arising from a single cell, thereby fulfilling a major criteria for defining a process as malignant; clonal analysis of lymphoid proliferations hinges on identifying rearrangement of antigen receptor genes; in females, cell line clonality can be determined in most females by molecular analysis of the patterns of X chromosome inactivation; clonal analysis has been performed with X-linked polymorphic loci, of which *HUMARA* the human androgen receptor gene has proven most useful given the high rate (> 90%) of heterozygosity seen at this locus, which is accompanied by consistent patterns of methylation (**N Engl J Med** 1994; 331:154OA) see Clonality

clonal anergy IMMUNOLOGY Inactivation of immune cells encountering an antigen in absence of a second antigenic signal; since a second signal is normally required for response to an infectious agent (or other antigen); clonal anergy can be reversed by incubating the anergic cells in IL-2

clonal deletion Negative selection IMMUNOLOGY A maturation process occurring in the context of the major histocompatibility complex (MHC) in which the T cells that recognize self antigens are eliminated in the thymus; clonal deletion is a normal component of the natural self-tolerance; self antigens expressed in the thymus result in physical elimination of autoreactive thymocytes prior to complete maturation; most peripheral circulating CD4+ T cells (which survived intrathymic clonal deletion) are unresponsive to any stimulus, indicating that suppression of autoimmunity also involves clonal anergy; clonal deletion is an important mechanism for eliminating autoreactive T cells, effected by the minor lymphocyte stimulation (Mls) family of antigens, which by interacting with the Vβ portion of the T cell receptor, mimic bacterial superantigens; clonal deletion and functional inactivation of self-reactive cells explains intrathymic as well as peripheral tolerance in T cells, the latter explains clonal anergy (**Nature 1991; 349:245**) see Superantigen

clonal expansion The proliferation of cells (arising from a single cell) that are virtually identical in structure and function to the progenitor cell; clonal expansions can be 1) Physiological or defensive if the expanding clone is capable of responding to down-regulatory mechanisms, ie can be turned off or 2) Non-physiologic as they don't respond to down-regulating mechanisms; although often malignant, clonal expansions may be clinically benign (eg, lymphomatoid papulosis, composed of large atypical histologically malignant T lymphocytes with clonal rearrangement of T-γ or T-β receptor genes); B-cell clonality is detected by gene rearrangements with Southern blot hybridization or by the polymerase chain reaction

clonal selection IMMUNOLOGY A theoretical model that holds that the antigenic stimulation of preexisting clones of lymphocytes accounts for the main characteristics of the humoral immune response; antigen X interacts with several clones, initiating antigen-dependent differentiation leading to clones of memory cells and plasma cells; clonal selection occurs in two phases 1) The antigen-independent phase in which innumerable B cells 'mindlessly' proliferate and 2) The antigen-dependent phase where a circulating B cell encounters a recognized antigen, becomes activated, divides and secretes antibody

clonality A distinguishing feature of a proliferating tissue is its cell or cells of origin; daughter cells arising from multiple cells (ie polyclonal) of origin are reactive in nature; daughter cells arising from a single cell (ie monoclonal) of origin are neoplastic in nature; differentiating a reactive from a neoplastic process is important both in order to treat a disease, and to understand its physiopathology; clonality can be assessed in cell lineages in most females by molecular analysis of the patterns of X chromosome inactivation (**N Engl J Med 1994; 331:154OA**)

clone An organism or cell arising from a single parent that is an exact genotypic (and phenotypic) duplicate thereof; clones occur in nature in the production of multiple daughter cells in a monoclonal gammopathy, or can be created in the laboratory as an 'engineered' process using the methods of recombinant DNA technology

clonidine suppression test A test in which the inability of clonidine, an α_2-agonist to suppress catecholamine secretion is suggestive of a pheochromocytoma; a normal response to clonidine is ↓ plasma norepinephrine to ≤ 500 pg/mL; the CST is of use if a pheochromocytoma is suspected, plasma catecholamines are ± ↑, urinary excretion of catecholamines is ± normal, and norepinephrine levels are < 2000 pg/mL; CST's accuracy is 92%; CST is not needed when the norepinephrine levels are > 2000 pg/mL (**Arch Int Med 1992; 152:1193**)

cloning MOLECULAR BIOLOGY Synthesis of multiple copies of a segment of DNA Principle: A sequence of DNA of interest is inserted by recombinant techniques into a 'vector', a circular fragment of DNA capable of independent or autoreplication within a bacterium, eg bacteriophages, cosmids and plasmids, which are introduced into *Escherichia coli*, grown within the bacteria in culture media and after the appropriate growth, vectors removed and the segments of DNA of interest are isolated; cloning of genes for a human disease is usually based on chromosomal assignment by 'reverse genetics', where the first step is the labor-intensive identification of DNA probes close (ie within several hundred kilobases) to the gene of interest, followed by the construction of a restriction map surrounding the probe's sequence which is followed by a search for mRNA transcripts derived from the region, often by finding a probe sequence in the 'mapped' region that has been conserved during evolution; genes that are defective in human disease and identified by this method include the genes responsible for chronic granulomatous disease, cystic fibrosis, retinoblastoma and Wilms' tumor; see cDNA library

Note: DNA amplification by the polymerase chain reaction is an updated and more sensitive method for producing multiple copies of segments of DNA of interest

cloning vector A plasmid into which foreign DNA (up to 40+ kb, depending on the type) of interest may be inserted for cloning

clonotypic vaccine A product in the early stages of development that attempts to use the variable region (idiotype) of an antibody to produce cytotoxic anti-idiotypic T cells capable of destroying malignant cells; alternatively a clonotypic vaccine could (theoretically) be designed to treat therapeutically refractory autoimmune phenomena (**N Engl J Med 1992; 327:1209OA, 1236ED**)

closed loop system CRITICAL CARE MEDICINE A 'state of the art' electronic system used in intensive care units that monitors multiple patient parameters, eg pulse and respiratory rate, and regulates and controls everything by computer, including the rate of infusion of IV drugs and fluids

closet A term derived from Middle French (*clos* enclosure, a small room for privacy), which is widely used in reference to homosexual orientation, as indicated by the phrases 'to be in the closet'[1], 'to come out of the closet'[2], or the highly colloquial and derogatory 'closet queen'[3] (see **N Engl J Med 1994; 331:923SA**)

[1]To not have openly declared to colleagues, friends, or family a person's homosexual attitude, [2]To openly declare one's homosexual orientation, also known as 'coming out'[3]A homosexual who has not 'come out' Note: Use of closet in this context as a verb (eg to 'closet') or an adverb (eg subject X is 'closeting' his homosexuality) are unwieldy and somewhat counterintuitive, but have no currently viable alternatives

***Clostridium difficile* colitis** A generic term for colonic infections caused by *C difficile**, which includes the 'classic' pseudomembranous, and 20% of antibiotic-associated diarrhea without colitis PATHOGENESIS Disruption of normal colonic flora by broad-spectrum antibiotics, especially clindamycin, colonization by *C difficile*, and release of toxins A and B, which cause mucosal damage and inflammation DIAGNOSIS Stool-cytotoxin assay is sensitive (≥94%) and specific (≥99%) but expensive; enzyme assays are more cost-effective but less sensitive; latex agglutination assays are essentially useless TREATMENT Metronidazole(98% response rate), vancomycin (96%), bacitracin (83%), cholestyramine (68%) (**N Engl J Med 1994; 330:257RV**) see Pseudomembranous colitis

*Although most of the *C difficile*-induced colitides are 'pseudomembranous', and most pseudomembranous colitides are intimately linked to *C difficile* infection, they are not synonymous and in this work are regarded as separate but broadly overlapping conditions

***Clostridium difficile* toxin A** A 308-kD enterotoxin produced by *C difficile* that causes fluid secretion, mucosal damage, and intestinal inflammation in rodents; toxin A is a chemoattractant for human neutrophils, induces the release of cytokines from monocytes, and is lethal when injected parenterally; toxin A has a specific G protein-linked receptor, and once it enters the cells alters the cytoskeleton, leading to cell rounding; it is measured by cytotoxicity assay and enzyme immunoassay

***Clostridium difficile* toxin B** A 250–270-kD molecule that is 1000-fold more cytotoxic than toxin A

'clotter' A colloquial term for a hematologist specialized in disorders of coagulation

cloud baby A popular term for an infant with an infection that spreads by aerosol, who releases 'clouds' of the evil humor (ie virus, bacterium) into the air, thus acting as a vector for miniepidemics

cloudy swelling A descriptor for the histopathologic changes seen in the dilated, flabby beri-beri myopathic hearts, where myocytes are pale and swollen due to hypoxia-induced hydropic degeneration of mitochondria resulting in uncoupling of oxidative phosphorylation, ↓ ATPase activity, Na$^+$-K$^+$ pump failure and intracellular accumulation of K$^+$

clove cigarettes A cigarette made of a mixture of tobacco leaves and cloves, spice prepared from the dried flowers of the tropical tree, *Eugenia aromatica*, produced in Indonesia, where they are the preferred smoking product, 30-40% of which is shredded clove buds, and the remainder, tobacco

Importation of clove cigarettes to the US began in 1970, peaked in the mid-1980s and is on the decline; eugenol is the main (85%) constituent of clove oil; while not carcinogenic or mutagenic in test animals, clove cigarettes cause respiratory depression, atelectasis, alveolar edema, bronchopneumonia and may exacerbate asthma (**JAMA 1988; 260:3641**)

cloverleaf A morphological descriptor for a multilobed pattern that appears to emanate in a two-dimensional plane from a single point, likened to the low leguminous herb of the genus, *Trifolium*

Note: When a multilobed pattern is three dimensional, the commonly used adjective is 'popcorn'

cloverleaf anemia German, Kleeblattanämie, 'neurocirculatory edema' of liver A pattern of patchy paleness admixed with hyperemia due to irregular transhepatic blood flow; the edematous Disse's spaces are pale, compromising the hyperemic capillary circulation, classically associated with cranial injuries

cloverleaf cell A hyperconvoluted lymphocyte seen in diffuse large cell lymphoma, similar to the 'popcorn cells' of Hodgkin's disease

cloverleaf duodenal bulb 'Ace of clubs' sign RADIOLOGY A finding in upper GI barium studies, where the duodenal bulb is extensively scarred by multiple previous ulcers with central pinching of the duodenal bulb; Cf Ace of spades sign

cloverleaf skull Kleeblattschädel PEDIATRIC RADIOLOGY Severe deformation of the cranial vault in which a frontal film demonstrates a tri-lobed appearance caused by premature closure of the sutures accompanied by hydrocephaly, seen in thanatophoric dwarfism and accompanied by a prominent forehead, depressed nasal bridge, shortened limbs, bowing of the femora, epiphyseal cupping, flattening of the vertebral bodies, an achondroplasia-like pelvis, and mental retardation

cloverleaf structure Cloverleaf diagram MOLECULAR BIOLOGY The normal planar representation of transfer RNA which folds back upon itself to allow the maximum stability through formation of multiple hydrogen intrachain bonds at the 'arms' of the cloverleaf; the segments of RNA that are not hydrogen bonded are termed 'loops'

clozapine A dibenzodiazepine antipsychotic agent that is the most efficacious agent for treating refractory schizophrenia; unlike other neuroleptics, clozapine does not cause dystonia, parkinsonism, tardive dyskinesia, or elevate prolactin levels; clozapine has been associated with agranulocytosis (73 of 11 555 patients treated), which may be fatal (2/73); agranulocytosis may be monitored by

aggressive surveillance (**N Engl J Med 1993; 329:162oA**); the drug became the center of controversy regarding its manufacturer's practice of Bundling, see there

Club of Rome ENVIRONMENT An informal group of academics, civil servants, and business leaders that met in the early 1970s, and proposed the 'limits to growth' hypothesis based on computerized simulations of human activities on the planet; the hypothesis held that the limits to population growth would be breached within a century and that at that point, there would be an uncontrollable decline in the population and industrial capacity (**New York Times 5 May 1992; C1**)

clubbing The terminal expansion of a relatively short cylindrical object, simulating the tip of a drumstick or a caveman's club

clubbing of the fingers Expansion of the fingertips, often accompanied by underlying hypertrophic osteitis, associated with chronic 'central' (pulmonary origin) hypoxia due to infection, congenital heart disease, cystic fibrosis, bronchogenic carcinoma, bronchiectasis, pneumoconiosis, interstitial pulmonary fibrosis; clubbing may rarely occur in nonpulmonary disease including Crohn's disease, ulcerative colitis, cirrhosis, thyroid acropathy, Graves' disease

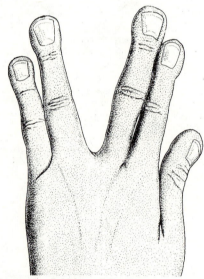

clubbing of the fingers

clubbing of the hand PEDIATRIC ORTHOPEDICS Absent radius or less commonly, the ulna, resulting from soft tissues acting as tension bands, pulling the wrist entirely off the end of the ulna; the defect may be associated with congenital heart disease and blood dyscrasia, eg Fanconi's anemia; Cf TAR syndrome

clubbing of kidneys Focal, finger-like expansion of renal calices, accompanied by cortical scarring, seen by tomography during intravenous pyelography, a finding characteristic of chronic pyelonephritis; see 'Thyroidization'

clubfoot Talipes varus A congenital deformity of the foot, formed from a combination of equinus (plantar flexion of the forefoot), calcaneus (dorsiflexion of the forefoot, the cacaneus forms the plantar prominence), varus (the heel and forefoot are inverted, the plantar surfaces medially) and valgus (eversion of the forefoot and lateral facing of the plantar surface) ETIOLOGY Unknown, possibly related to muscular dysplasia, anomalous insertion of tendons, arthrogriposis, congenital constriction bands, in utero compression, central nervous system disease (spina bifida, poliomyelitis, Friedrich's ataxia), in the 'whistling face' syndrome of Sheldon-Freeman and in the Moebius syndrome

'Club Med' dermatitis A photodermatitis consisting in linear, mirror-image, hyperpigmented, tender patches with scalloped edges, located on the inner thighs; this entity arose in a subject who played a 'drinking game' in which participants rolled limes up and down their thighs: furocoumarin (present in citrus fruits, celery, parsley) elicits erythema and vesiculation if the exposed skin is subsequently exposed to light

Note: This phototoxic reaction was first described in 1916 in women wearing oil of bergamot (N Engl J Med 1986; 314:319c)

clue cell GYNECOLOGICAL CYTOLOGY A superficial squamous epithelial cell with peripheral clumps of gram-negative *Gardnerella* (formerly *Haemophilus*) *vaginalis*, which imparts a stippled, granular appearance on a 'wet mount' of a cervical smear TREATMENT Metronidazole

cluster EPIDEMIOLOGY A disease process occurring in a group of people living or working within one stratum (physical, social or economic) of society, who appear to share one or more environmental factors in common, as in a cancer 'cluster'; while cluster studies occasionally bear the fruit of a legitimate cause-and-effect relation (DES and vaginal adenocarcinoma, PVC production and use in the packing industry and angiosarcoma, thalidomide and phocomelia), the ratio of reports to actual associations is very low (100:1) in terms of proving a relation between a putative cause and the effect and the CDC has relegated the study of clusters to state departments of health

cluster headache A short-lived (30 minutes to two hours) intense unilateral cephalalgia that has a 'clock-setting' predictability, often occurring with spring to fall seasonality, of 3-8 weeks duration, later disappearing for months to years; the headaches cause a knife-like intranasal or retrobulbar pain; unlike migraines (in which the patients prefer to lie still in a darkened room), cluster victims restlessly pace, bang their heads against the wall and have suicidal ideation; cluster headaches are thought to be of vascular origin TREATMENT Prevention (ergotamine tartrate, methysergide) is more effective than the use of analgesics once an acute attack has begun

Note: 'The relationship of the cluster headache to migraine remains conjectural. No doubt certain headaches have some of the characteristics of both migraine and cluster headaches, hence the migrainous neuralgia and cluster migraine (Kudrow)...however (there are) differences that seem important...flushing of the face on the side of a cluster headache and pallor in migraine; increased intraocular pressure in cluster headache, normal in migraine, increased skin temperature over the forehead, temple, and cheek in cluster headache, decreased in migraine; and notable distinctions in sex distribution, age of onset, rhythmicity, and other clinical features...' (RD Adams, M Victor, Principles of Neurology, 5th edition, McGraw-Hill, New York, 1993)

cluster of grapes appearance PATHOLOGY The gross morphology of a hydatidiform mole, a trophoblastic disease in which the chorionic villi undergo massive swelling ranging from 1-30 mm in diameter (total weight, 200 g) with hydropic degeneration; a complete mole usually occurs without identifiable embryonal tissue; choriogonadotropin levels are markedly increased

cluster of grapes sign Septation sign PEDIATRIC RADIOLOGY A finding in infants with congenital polycystic kidney disease, in whom an excretory urogram reveals an afunctional non-visualized kidney, the walls of which contain viable vessels visualized in the vascular or opacification phase of urography RADIOLOGY A finding consisting of multiple round-to-oval radiological shadows seen by a plain chest film in mucoid impaction of the bronchi in bronchiectasis

cluttering SPEECH PATHOLOGY A condition characterized by an excessive rate of speech and irregular rhythm, often with collapsing of sounds and words, ranging in severity from garbled but generally intelligible to virtually unintelligible; cluttering may co-exist with stuttering, see there TREATMENT Bethanechol may be beneficial (N Engl J Med 1993;

329:753oA)

CME Continuing medical education Professional education that physicians participate in on a part-time basis following completion of formal post-medical school specialty training, eg residencies and fellowships; CME may be required for maintaining state licensure, eg New York State requires 150 hours of accredited CME every two years and takes the form of lectures, seminars, refresher courses, workshops, audio- and video-tapes and may be sponsored by medical schools, professional organizations and hospitals Note: It was increasingly common for the pharmaceutical industry to sponsor CME and symposia; according to the ethical guidelines adopted by the American Medical Association (JAMA 1991; 265:501); these companies can no longer directly or indirectly provide for travel, lodging, honoraria, or personal expenses incurred during continuing medical education; 'The hardest conviction to get into the mind of a beginner is that the education in which he is engaged is not a college course, not a medical course but a life course, for which the work of a few years under teachers is but a prepration.' Sir Wm Osler (Arch Pathol Lab Med 1992; 116:602oA)

CMF regimen ONCOLOGY An adjuvant combination chemotherapy protocol using cyclophosphamide, methotrexate, and fluorouracil, which is administered after modified radical mastectomy in patients with lymph node-positive breast cancer; in a 20-year follow-up study of premenopausal ♀ treated with the CMF regimen, relapse-free survival was 37% for CMF (vs 26% for controls; overall survival was 47% for CMF (vs 22% for non-treated controls); with 10+ lymph nodes, 17% of CMF ♀ survived, vs 0% in the untreated controls (N Engl J Med 1995; 332:901oA)

CMG Case-mix group, see there

CML Chronic myelocytic (granulocytic, myelogenous, myeloid) leukemia, also 1) Clinical Medical Librarian 2) Clinical microbiology laboratory

Also 1) Cell-mediated lymphocytolysis 2) Collimated monochromatic light

CMO I, II Corticosterone mixed (function) oxidases CMO II deficiency is an autosomal recessive enzymopathy accompanied by a marked decrease in aldosterone and its metabolites, increased plasma renin activity and 18-hydroxicorticosterone with hyponatremia, hyperkalemia, early onset metabolic acidosis, growth retardation and occasionally spontaneous amelioration with maturation

CMU10 A monoclonal antibody of murine origin that is reported to mark an antigen in the mucin of pathological lesions, benign (eg hyperplastic polyps, ulcerative colitis), premalignant (adenomatous polyps), and malignant (colonic adenocarcinoma) of the colon; CMU10 did not identify normal colonic epithelium (Arch Pathol Lab Med 1995; 119:454A)

c-myc A cellular oncogene that translocates in Burkitt's lymphoma from its normal site on chromosome 8 to chromosome 14 within the immunoglobulin heavy chain gene, at different sites, either in the switch region or within the variable region; this translocation leads to oncogene activation at a transcriptionally active site and lymphoma-genesis; see *myc*

CNRS Centre National de la Recherche Scientifique A French government-based research organization created in 1939, whose stated purpose is to conduct and encourage basic research in the whole of science; life science is one of its seven subdivisions; over 40% of the 26 000 employees are researchers 1990 BUDGET FF10 330 million DIRECTOR F Kourilsky (Nature 1990; 346:127n&v); see SERC; Cf INSERM

CNS Central nervous system, also Clinical Nurse Specialist, see Advanced practice nurse

Also 1) Child neurology service   2) Congress of Neurological Surgeons   3)

CNTF Ciliary neurotrophic factor, see there

coagulation factors A brief reminder for the forgetful, see table

COAGULATION FACTORS	
I	Fibrinogen
II	Prothrombin
III	Thromboplastin
IV	Calcium (obsolete term)
V	Proaccelerin (obsolete term)
VI	Accelerin (obsolete for Factor Va)
VII	Proconvertin (obsolete term)
VIII	A composite of three separate proteins
VIII:C	Low weight component with coagulant activity, deficient in classic hemophilia
VIII:Ag	Antigenic portion of molecule
VIIIR:RCo	Supports ristocetin-initiated platelet aggregation
VIII:vWF	von Willebrand factor, platelet adhesion
IX	Christmas factor, plasma thromboplastin
X	Stewart-Prowel factor
XI	Plasma thromboplastin antecedent
XII	Hageman factor
XIII	Laki-Lorand factor; fibrinoligane

coagulation necrosis A type of necrosis that results from the denaturation of cellular proteins in response to severe injury, eg hypoxia, infection, ischemia, toxins and trauma PATHOLOGY Nuclear pyknosis, karyorrhexis, karyolysis, hypereosinophilia of cytoplasm, and preservation of cell outlines (Arch Pathol Lab Med 1993; 117:1208oa) Cf Colliquative necrosis

coagulation panel A group of assays designed to efficiently identify a probable cause of hemorrhage in a patient who is bleeding, including prothrombin time, activated partial thromboplastic time, platelet count and bleeding time; see Organ panel

coactivator MOLECULAR BIOLOGY Any of a poorly understood family of 'adaptive' molecules that integrate signals from activators and possibly also repressors, relaying the results to the basal factors (Sci Am 1995; 272/2:56) see Transcription activator

coal miner's elbow Student's elbow Olecranon bursitis caused by prolonged pressure, friction or trauma to the elbow; Cf Beat knee

coal tar CLINICAL THERAPEUTICS A blackish semisolid byproduct of the destructive distillation of bituminous coal, which contains benzene, naphthalene, phenols and other organic compounds; CT has a time-honored role in the treatment of psoriasis, and when used alone may induce the clearance of psoriatic plaques, but is limited by its unpleasant odor, and its reported ability to induce skin cancer; CT is usually used in combination with UVB light (N Engl J Med 1995; 332:581rv) see Psoriasis

coal workers' pneumoconiosis An occupational lung disease affecting those with prolonged exposure to carbon dust, which accumulates in the macrophages of peribronchiolar tissues CLINICAL Early pneumoconiosis is often a 'pathologist's disease', ie the diagnosis can only be established by histological examination; with time, dyspnea, pulmonary hypertension and respiratory failure develop PATHOLOGY The early lesion is the 'coal macule', a pigmented parenchymal nodule that undergoes massive fibrosis, producing stellate contracted lesions TREATMENT None; see Anthracosis

coamplification The simultaneous (and unwanted) amplification of multiple DNA target sequences using PCR; see Amplicon carryover

Coast of California pattern DERMATOLOGY Smooth, gently curved borders of the macular cafe-au-lait skin lesions seen in patients with neurofibromatosis, likened to the smoothly contoured Pacific coastline of the US state of California

Coast of Maine pattern DERMATOLOGY Jagged contours of the macular (Cafe-au-lait color) skin lesions in McCune-Albright disease (polyostotic fibrous dysplasia, precocious puberty and multiple endocrine dysfunctions), usually 3-4 in number, often unilateral, located on the buttocks or neck, likened to the convoluted and craggy contoured Atlantic coastline of the US state of Maine

coatamer A cytosolic complex containing the same coat proteins (COPs) as those of the Golgi transport vesicles, one of which, β-COP, resides exclusively within complex (Nature 1991; 349:248); Cf GERL

coated pit A specialized depression in the cytoplasmic face of the cell membrane that is lined by the scaffolding protein, clathrin, which is pivotal in down-regulating hormonal activity, as the coated pits internalize and degrade receptors for vasoactive intestinal polypeptide, insulin and other hormones, playing a role in hormone receptor-mediated endocytosis; see Clathrin

cobblestone A widely used descriptor for multiple, equally-sized rounded densities that project from a single linear surface, when the image is two-dimensional or that rise above a flattened plane when viewed in three dimensions, a pattern likened to pre-infernal combustion engine roadways, paved by multiple similarly-sized 'cobbled' stones GI DISEASE Characteristic radiologic and gross appearance (figure) of the intestinal mucosa in Crohn's disease due to submucosal involvement; to the endoscopist, cobblestoning refers to the uniform nodules (due to the submucosal edema), while the pathologist refers to severe ulcerative disease with crisscrossing of the ulcers through inflamed but intact mucosa; intestinal 'cobblestoning' may also occur in ulcerative colitis (where ulcers alternate with regenerating mucosa), ischemic colitis, lymphoid hyperplasia of common variable immunodeficiency, amyloidosis, mucoviscidosis, pneumatosis cystoides intestinalis, multiple lymphangiomas and polyposis coli; in the intestine, the mucosal rugosities may correspond to polyps or be filled with air, lymphoid tissue and amyloid GYNECOLOGY A roughened appearance rarely seen by colposcopy of the uterine cervix infected with *Neisseria gonorrhoeae* OPHTHALMOLOGY Multiple sharply demarcated non-elevated, lesions with prominent choroidal vessels, located between the ora serrata and the equator, seen in peripheral chorioretinal atrophy, a common aging phenomenon, seen in one-fourth of all autopsies, ⅓ of which are bilateral ORAL DISEASE Multiple, closely-set intraoral papilloma-like fibromas that impart a pebbly tactile sensation in Cowden's premalignant multiple hamartoma syndrome SOFT TISSUE PATHOLOGY Multiple 'hobnail' projections of malignant endothelial cells into the vascular lumina seen in angiosarcoma, a pattern mimicked by Kaposi sarcoma and spindle cell hemangioendothelioma

COBRA Consolidated Omnibus Budget Reconciliation Act of 1985 HEALTH CARE ENVIRONMENT A legislative act that entitles ex-employees of companies with 20+ workers to continued coverage for 18 months after leaving the place of employment (Am Med News 26 October 1992, p7)

COBRA legislation EMTALA, see there

cobrahead sign The pattern seen by an excretory urogram of the ureterovesicular junction, in a urinary bladder ureterocele; a thin outer membrane corresponding to the ureteral walls, seen as a dark halo, encloses a cystically dilated distal intravesicular ureter that protrudes into the bladder, where opacified urine collects in both the dilated segment and the bladder; simple ureteroceles of adults are associated with stenosis of the ureteral orifice and prolapse of the distal ureter into the bladder, possibly due to the persistence of Chiralla's membrane and blockage of the ureteral orifice

cobweb pattern Lacy neurofibrillary material present in the center of the rosettes of neuroblastomas, ganglioneuroblastomas and benign ganglioneuromas which ultrastructurally corresponds to 6-10 nm cytoplasmic filaments, cell processes with microtubules, rare dense core granules, synaptic vesicles and cell junction material

Coby H A seven year-old boy with ALL who died while awaiting a potentially life-saving BM transplant, a procedure that was not at the time funded by public monies in the state of Oregon; see Health care rationing, Oregon plan, 'Rule of rescue'

Note: The Coby 'case' sparked a growing debate on two fronts, financial and ethical; regarding finances, the question is being increasingly asked whether a human life has become 'too expensive'; in the case of a bone marrow transplantation, will society accept a cost of $200 000 to save one life, when the same money would pay for the Pap smear screening of thousands of women, potentially saving a dozen lives; the pecuniary issue is intimately linked to ethical dilemma of which life is worth saving, and what rules will be applied to decide the value of the lives being saved

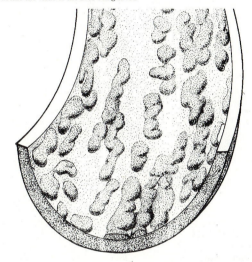

cobblestone appearance

cocaethylene A cocaine metabolite produced by an alternate metabolic pathway in the presence of alcohol, which is associated with a marked increase in coronary artery spasm and commonly present in post-mortem body fluids from those who have died while simultaneously abusing cocaine and alcohol; cocaethylene can be measured in meconium to detect combined fetal exposure to cocaine and alcohol (**J Toxicol Clin Toxicol 1994; 32:697**)

cocaine

cocaine SUBSTANCE ABUSE A powder[1] (benzoylmethyl-ecgonine $C_{17}H_{21}NO_4$) derived from *Erythoxylon coca* that evokes intense physical and psychological addiction STATISTICS Three million US citizens use cocaine regularly

(600 000 use heroin), 10-15% of the entire US population has tried cocaine (40% of those between age 25-30) and 10-15% of experimenters eventually become addicted; cocaine is implicated in 5/1000 deaths in ages 25-30; up to 25% of motor vehicle accident fatalities in drivers aged 15-45 in New York City had cocaine in their system PHARMACOLOGY Cocaine's presumed site of action is the nucleus accumbens and the 'high', like that of amphetamine, is attributed to cerebral 'flooding' with dopamine, where it blocks the re-uptake of dopamine by the cell producing it; the increased dopamine in the synaptic cleft is also held responsible for cocaine's addictive properties; cocaine receptors are located on dopamine transporters CLINICAL Cardiovascular symptoms are most prominent, with dysrhythmia, eg ventricular tachycardia and fibrillation, myocarditis, myocardial infarction, sudden death, convulsions, hyperpyrexia, cerebral vasculitis, loss of sense of smell and (due to collapse of nasal mucosa and matrix) a nose to smell with, decreased oxygen diffusing capacity, spontaneous pneumomediastinum, eating disorders, eg bulimia and anorexia; with chronic abuse, there is increased sensitivity ('reverse tolerance') to the non-euphorigenic effects of cocaine, including hyperactivity and anesthesia CLINICAL FEATURES OF COCAINE ABUSE Chronic rhinitis, rhinorrhea, ulceration of nose, perforation of the nasal septum and madarosis (singeing of eyebrows and eyelashes due to hot vapors associated with smoking crack) CARDIOVASCULAR The deleterious effects of cocaine on the myocardial oxygen supply are exacerbated by concomitant cigarette smoking, increasing the heart's metabolic demand for oxygen, while simultaneously the diameter of diseased coronary artery segments (**N Engl J Med 1994; 330:454OA**) CHRONIC ABUSE Seizures are common in habitual abusers, who have diffuse cortical atrophy, seen by CT and diffuse slowing of waves, seen by EEG DRUG TESTING Urine and serum may be screened for benzoylecgonine, cocaine's major metabolite, by enzyme-labelled competitive immunoassay (see EMIT), and confirmed for legal purposes by the 'gold standard' method, gas chromatography-mass spectrometry, see GC-MS; cocaine's plasma $T_{1/2}$ is 90 minutes; cocaine-induced euphoria lasts 45 minutes PATHOLOGY-BRAIN Subarachnoid hemorrhage, cortical atrophy GI TRACT Intestinal ischemia due to a adrenergic vasoconstriction HEART Mononuclear cell inflammation of myocardium with myocytic necrosis LUNGS Congestion, spontaneous pneumothorax ORAL CAVITY Cocaine's pH of 4.5 causes dental erosion, and has been implicated in ↑ caries in cocaine abusers, although this may be related to a change in eating habits PREGNANCY Abruptio placentae, premature onset of labor, vaginal bleeding after intravenous injection, placental vasoconstriction, spontaneous abortion, congenital malformation, ↑ perinatal mortality, neurologic and behavior defects, tachycardia, and hypertension PSYCHIATRIC DISORDERS Dysphoria, paranoid psychosis, severe depression SEXUAL DYSFUNCTION Cocaine's myth as an aphrodisiac derives from its ability to delay ejaculation and orgasm, causing temporary mood elevation, and heightened sensory awareness may be undeserved[2]; chronic cocaine abuse evokes impotence, subfertility, eg low sperm counts, low motility and increased abnormal sperm forms TREATMENT & REHABILITATION Cocaine-induced acute rhabdomyolysis may respond to dantrolene, a drug used in malignant hyperthermia; experimental drugs for treating cocaine addiction include buprenorphine (a mixed opiate agonist-antagonist), desipramine and flupenthixol (both antidepressant), carbamazepine (antiseizure), buspirone (anxiolytic) bromocriptine (dopamine antagonist) and mazindol (dopamine blocker) CAUSE OF DEATH Arrhythmia due to ventricular fibrillation and cardiovascular collapse, respiratory arrest with pulmonary edema, cerebrovascular insults associated with hypertension; see Binge, Crack,

[1]Street names Bolivian marching powder, coke, flake, snow, toot [2]One subject inserted cocaine intraurethrally to heighten his sexual experience and developed priapism, paraphimosis, DIC, gangrene, massive necrosis of the extremities, resulting in the loss of nine fingers, the penis and both legs below the knees (JAMA 1988; 259:3126/8) Notes: Cocaine was found in the tombs of Western Hemisphere Indians circa 600 AD; Sigmund Freud was a major advocate of cocaine's beneficial effects, and later became addicted thereto; ½ of the US supply is from Peru's Huallaga Valley; several 'epidemics' of cocaine and stimulant abuse have occurred in the US, in the 1890s, the 1920s ('drug madness'), early 1950s and late 1960s (amphetamines), and now in the 1980s; patients with pseudocholinesterase deficiency are at increased risk of sudden death as this enzyme is part of cocaine's metabolic route

'cocaine nose' A constellation of findings in chronic intranasal abusers of cocaine CLINICAL Frequent rubbing of nose RHINOSCOPY There is a range of findings from unremarkable mucosa to visible perforation PATHOLOGY Granulomas, inflammation, massive mucosal edema, erosion and necrosis of the nasal mucosa Surgical complications Localized septal collapse, poor mucosal healing, inadequate correction of septal deflection TREATMENT Rhinoplasty may be performed on highly selected patients, although the results are often poor; submucosal resection and septoplasty should be avoided

cocaine withdrawal syndrome Abstinence from cocaine results in a triphasic response consisting of 1) 'Crash' Paranoia, hypersomnia followed by hyperphagia 2) Withdrawal with prolonged anhedonia and cocaine craving and 3) Extinction (Science 1991; 251:1580rv)

cocarcinogen Tumor promoter, see there

coccal lesions OPTIC FUNDOSCOPY A descriptor for the black hemorrhagic dots that float in the vitreous humor, caused by small hypertension-induced leakage of blood

coccidioidomycosis An infection by air-borne arthroconidia of the soil fungus *Coccidioides immitis* which is endemic to the southwestern US and Western Hemisphere CLINICAL 60% of those infected are asymptomatic or have disease that is indistinguishable from upper respiratory tract infection; in the rest, there is a 1-3 week asymptomatic period followed by a lower respiratory tract infection with fever, sweating, anorexia, weakness, arthralgias, cough, chest pain, erythema nodosum, erythema multiforme DIAGNOSIS The mycelial form is easily cultured on artificial media, is highly infectious, but cannot be definitively identified; serological testing for IgM antibodies is transiently detected in 75% TREATMENT IV amphotericin B; oral fluconazole, itraconazole, ketoconazole (N Engl J Med 1995; 332:1077rv)

coccoon A descriptor for the fibrotic encasement of the entire small intestine seen in sclerosing peritonitis, a spontaneous idiopathic process in young women, following peritoneovenous shunting, practolol therapy, peritoneal dialysis and chemotherapy, in which unknown toxins may stimulate fibroblastic proliferation and reactive fibrosis

cochlear implant An electronic prosthetic device designed to replace the cochlea's acoustic functions by translating sound waves into electrochemical signals, stimulating surviving neuronal elements in the inner ear of a patient with profound (auditory threshold > 90 dB, normal ± 25 dB) hearing impairment (nerve deafness), providing some degree of auditory sensation; unlike hearing aids, which amplify sound and deliver it to the external ear, CIs transduce sound into electrical signals, delivering them to cells of the spiral ganglion, or to the axons of the cochlear nerve; CIs have been FDA-approved for adults since 1984, and for children since 1990, with 4800 having been implanted in adults, and 2000 in children; CIs cost $14-18 000 and implantation and rehabilitation costs $6-10 000; CIs may have a single channel[1] or multiple channels with multiple electrodes[2]; CIs may be implanted deeply or shallowly in the cochlea, or applied to the surface of the inner ear; CI electrodes may be stimulated in a mono- or bipolar fashion, and multiple electrodes may be stimulated either simultaneously or sequentially, either by analogue or by digital signals; speech is processed by either filter-bank encoding, or by speech-feature encoding; transmission between the hardware and the CI occurs either transcutaneously through induction or percutaneously via a plug protruding through the skin (N Engl J Med 1993; 328:233OA, 281ED)

[1]A pathway through which the information is transmitted from the implant to the auditory nerve, with a monopolar electrode stimulating all areas simultaneously [2]With bipolar electrodes stimulating discrete areas of the cochlea, a design that is clearly superior, given its increased discriminatory capacity; ⅔ of patients with multichannel CIs are able to understand open-set speech (speech without referential cues)

Cochran-Mantel-Haenzel test STATISTICS An analytic method used for categorical variables

Cockayne syndrome An AR [MIM 216400] condition characterized by dwarfism, microcephaly, 'salt and pepper' choroidoretinitis, optic atrophy, cerebral calcifications, mental retardation, intention tremor, tottering gait, deafness, small trunk, long extremities, attenuated subcutaneous fat, sexual infantilism, hepatosplenomegaly, atherosclerosis and early death; Cf Hutchinson-Gilford syndrome

cockroach A largely nocturnal insect (order Blattaria) that ranges from 5 mm (*Attaphila*) to 10 cm (*Megaloblatta*) in length, of which 3500 have been catalogued; in the US, the most familiar roaches include *Periplaneta americana*, *Blattella germanica*, and *Blattella orientalis* and are of medical interest as they are potential vectors for bacteria, especially *Salmonella* spp; other organisms cultured from cockroaches include *Shigella*, *Proteus*, *Mycobacterium* spp, *Escherichia coli*, *Klebsiella pneumoniae*, and *Pseudomonas aeruginosa*, but their relative contribution as vectors for infections is unknown and difficult to study, but they have been implicated in hepatitis; 97.5% of low-income housing has them, with an average of 33 600/dwelling; their presence in an environment is associated with poor sanitation

cockscomb cervix Collar, Hood, Pseudopolyp formation A transverse ridging of uterine cervix and upper vagina, described in one-fourth of females exposed in utero to diethylstilbestrol (DES), a finding of no known pathological significance PATHOLOGY Core of fibrous tissue, lined by metaplastic squamous epithelium, or occasionally tubal or endometrial epithelium; see Clear cell adenocarcinoma, DES

cocktail MIXOLOGY Any multicomponent concoction[1] of often partially-related substances that may be touted as having complementary activities towards the same goal, named in the tradition of the alcoholic beverage[2], eg analgesic cocktails (Brompton's mixture), fluor cocktail (liquid scintillation counting), immunosuppressive cocktail (a Gemisch of agents used to suppress GVHD) or a keratin 'cocktail', a mixture of antibodies to a two or more of the 19 different well-defined subclasses of keratins with molecular weights between 40 and 68 kD

[1]Amalgamation, Chinese menu, combination, conglomeration, gallimaufry, hodge-podge, mish-mash, mélange, medley, minglement, olla-podidar, omnium-gatherum, pasticcio, potpourri, salmagundi [2]Le cocktail

cocktail party effect NEUROPHYSIOLOGY The interference with a single signal (eg a conversation) by multiple background signals (eg multiple conversations), fancifully named because of its occurrence in cocktail parties; the deciphering of a meaningful signal from background ('white') noise is an acquired skill that may be dissected mathematically, possibly using neural networks (Nature 1994; 369:517N&V)

cocktail party 'syndrome' Chatter-box 'syndrome' A descriptor for the behavior of children with arrested hydrocephalus, who are highly sociable, hyperloquacious, pseudointelligent (speaking in a seemingly erudite fashion on subjects about which they have no true understanding), scanning dysrhythmic speech; cocktail party chatter is also a symptom of Williams 'elfin face' syndrome with mild mental retardation, congenital cardiac defects (valvular stenoses and septal defects) and, due to hypercalcemia, nephrosclerosis and bony sclerosis; see Elfin face syndrome

cocktail purpura An unusual form of thrombocytopenic purpura, induced by the quinine in tonic water, due to ingestion of 'gin & tonic(s)'

cocktail sausage appearance Diffuse periosteal swelling of a toe, a rare radiological finding seen in rheumatoid arthritis

'cocktail' therapy Any mixture of drugs to produce a therapeutic effect may be considered a 'cocktail', eg antibiotics, chemotherapeutic agents, or immunosuppressive agents administered in combination

The term has had most currency in immunology as a mixture of immunosuppressive agents for controlling rejection; one early immune cocktail had azathioprine and steroids, and was used to counter early renal transplant rejection, having various side effects, including osteoporosis, anemia, diabetes, cataracts, hearing loss, gout and reduced growth in younger transplant victims; when cyclosporine was added to the cocktail in 1983, the one-year survival for transplanted kidneys rose to 90%, for transplanted hearts to 80% and for transplanted livers to 70%; despite this improvement, 20% require a second transplant due to graft failure, rejection or drug-related complications; tacrolimus (formerly FK-506), a new immunosuppressive promises further improvement in graft survival

COD Cause of death

Also 1) Chemical oxygen demand 2) Coefficient of oxygen delivery 3) Consortium of Doctors 4) Cyclooctadiene

code *noun* A widely used (albeit highly colloquial) term for a cardiopulmonary arrest which is invariably accompanied by a frenzied fracas and frenetic fray *verb* To suffer a cardiac arrest in a hospital environment

'code blue' Code EMERGENCY MEDICINE A message announced over a hospital's public address system indicating that a cardiac arrest requiring medical attention is in progress; in a similar context, to be 'coded' is to undergo cardiopulmonary resuscitation

code of ethics see Hippocratic Oath

Code of Hammurabi A code of laws promulgated by Hammurabi, the great Amorite king of Babylon in Mesopotamia; specifically the physicians in this culture which flourished circa 2000 BC were known as asu, skilled in herbal medicine, mineral cures, snakebites, fractures and visible sores; the asu were under strict government regulation; the scale of fees was fixed by law, based on the patients ability to pay and the seriousness of the disease; payment was made only upon recovery of the patient and the physican was severely punished for failure, eg loss of a nobleman's sight would translate into loss of the physician's hand, and so on

code status The formally indicated (often through signed documents) status of a patient in a hospital with respect to his/her desire for resuscitative (ie CPR) efforts, should the need arise; unless the patient specifically requests that he/she *NOT* be resuscitated, ie DNR (do not resuscitate) status, CPR will be performed

codec Coder/decoder COMPUTERS/TELEMEDICINE A device that compresses data from 10- to 100-fold, which can be used to transmit information in the evolving field of telemedicine; the codec is far more efficient than a modem in transferring information and allows the use of existing copper wire telephone lines; however, the speed requirements for transmitting high-resolution images for teleradiology and telepathology are too high to make the codec anything but than a 'band-aid solution' (**Am Med News 1995; 17 April 1995 p19**) see Asynchronous transfer mode switching, T-1, Telemedicine

codependency SUBSTANCE ABUSE The concomitant presence of two or more states of drug dependency, eg alcohol and substance (marijuana, heroin, barbiturates)

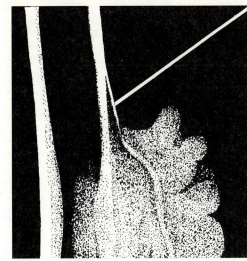

Codman's triangle RADIOLOGY A wedge-shaped elevation of periosteal bone seen on a plain film of the long bones, a 'classic' finding of Ewing sarcoma, which may also be seen in osteosarcoma, metastases to bone, hematomas, syphilis, and TB

codominance CLINICAL GENETICS A clinical state in which each allele of a gene expresses an effect in a heterozygous individual; eg α-1 antitrypsin deficiency, which has 25 different allelic forms, or red cell blood groups MN(Ss), where there are 3 possible expressions: M, MN, and N, or the ABO blood group, where there are three possible states, eg A, B, or AB (in addition to the 'null' genotype, O)

codon A triplet of RNA nucleotides derived from DNA that symbolizes each amino acid; because there are four possible nucleotides in each of the three positions, there are 4 x 4 x 4 = 64 possible combinations of RNA triplets, which translate into one start codon, three stop codons and 20 amino acids, resulting in redundancy or 'degeneracy' of the genetic code and many amino acids have more than one codon and some have up to six codons; this redundancy allows for considerable error to occur in translation while still encoding functional proteins

coefficient of variation LABORATORY MEDICINE The standard deviation expressed as a percentage of the mean; the CV is of use when evaluating and comparing methodologies and instruments; the lower the CV, the greater the precision; a general rule is that nonenzymatic chemistries should have CVs of < 5%, and CVs from enzyme assays should be < 10%

$$CV = {}^{SD}\!/_{x} \times 100$$

SD = standard deviation and x = the mean STATISTICS A calculation that compares two different analytic methods, which assumes a Gaussian distribution of data, quantitating the 'between-run' precision of an analytic procedure when a stable control product is analyzed with each run of patient sample, defined by formula as 100 x standard deviation divided by the mean CV

coercion The use of some form of force to force a person into a form of therapy, most commonly psychiatric, eg child psychiatry and treatment of substance abuse (**N Engl J Med 1994; 331:1533BR**)

Note: The use of therapeutic coercion raises ethical issues on multiple levels; a critical question is whether a positive result justifies the means used, even if it means that personal freedom and civil rights have been compromised or ignored, transiently or otherwise

coffee A beverage made from dried, roasted beans[1] of the coffee tree (*Coffea arabica*), a moderate stimulant causing mild physical dependence; annual US consumption: 1 million metric tons (33 million gallons/day) coffee is of medical interest for its postulated negative impact on the cardiovascular system and for an ↑ risk of malignancy[2] reported in heavy coffee drinkers Note: When each 'association' is rigorously examined with properly designed studies of large populations, the relative risks (RR) fall below levels of statistical significance CARDIOVASCULAR SYSTEM ≥ 5 cups/day was associated with a 2.5-fold ↑ in coronary artery disease, arrhythmia, ↑ LDL-cholesterol and apolipoprotein-B; a later study of the relation of coffee to acute MI and strokes revealed an RR of 1.04 (not significant), in 4+ cups/day and a RR of 1.63 (marginally significant), for decaffeinated coffee, a beverage reported to ↑ LDL-cholesterol

[1] Regular coffee is made from arabica beans, decaffeinated coffee from robusta beans [2]Coffee's role as a carcinogen is heuristically logical as coffee derivatives can be used in thymidine-poor culture media to increase breaks or gaps in certain 'fragile sites' of the chromosomes, in particular, 3p14.2, 6q25.3, 16q23.2, an effect attributed to caffeine's inhibition of DNA repair in replicating cells, 20 of the sites cited in one study are associated with human malignancy and caffeine may be used to enhance the expression of chromosomal damage in the 'Fragile X' (Xq27) syndrome; in one small cohort, there was a marked increase in pancreatic cancer in heavy coffee drinkers, a conclusion repeatedly refuted by subsequent studies; the risk for colorectal carcinoma may be decreased (RR, 0.6-0.8) in heavy (> 5 cups/day) coffee consumption; the increase in pancreatic carcinoma (RR: 1.03) is not statistically significant

coffee bean appearance A descriptor for an oval cell often invested with a linear groove GYNECOLOGIC PATHOLOGY A descriptive term for coelomic epithelial cells often seen in Brenner tumor of the ovary; similar cells are described in granulosa cell tumors which, when multi-nucleated, may appear as 'florettes', considered a degenerative phenomenon MICROBIOLOGY A descriptor for *Pneumocystis carinii* trophozoites, which have also been likened to a 'folded envelope'

coffee enema An enema that uses coffee to stimulate bile and hepatic glutathione-SH production, both of which are claimed to assist in detoxifying the body in cancer patients; coffee enemas are a major component of Gerson therapy, an unconventional form of cancer treatment based on a program of 'detoxification' (JAMA 1992; 268:3224sc) see Gerson therapy, Unproven forms of cancer therapy

coffee grounds appearance A descriptor for the color and consistency of gastric hemorrhage that is associated with both benign or malignant ulcers; 'coffee grounds vomitus' is characteristic of yellow fever

coffin RADIATION SAFETY A heavily-leaded container used to transport relatively large amounts of radioactive material, eg from the manufacturer; see Pig

coffin lid crystals A descriptor for the three- to six-sided colorless prism-shaped crystals that may be seen in 1) Synovial fluid, associated with acromegaly, hyperparathyroidism, hemochromatosis, hypomagnesemia, hypophosphatasia, myxedema, ochronosis and Wilson's disease; the crystals may complicate other arthritic conditions, eg gout, osteoarthritis, rheumatoid arthritis, chondrocalcinosis 2) Urine Ammonium magnesium phosphate (triple phosphate) crystals in neutral or alkaline urine, associated with urinary tract infections; see Struvite concrements

cognitive death Persistent vegetative state, see there

cogwheel phenomenon NEUROLOGY Circular jerking rigidity in flexion and extension in a background of a tremor that continues throughout the entire range of movement, a finding characteristic of parkinsonism; this jerky movement is due to an underlying tremor rhythm; it is less commonly 'smoothly' rigid, fancifully termed lead pipe rigidity; Cf Clasp knife phenomenon, Gegenhalten

coherence therapy ADFR therapy, see there

cohoba A hallucinogen used in Central America that is obtained from the bark of *Anadenanthera* tree, *Acacia niopo*, *Piptadenia peregrina*, and other plants, which is ingested as a snuff or as an enema

cohort A group of persons with a defined disorder

cohort effect ADOLESCENT PSYCHIATRY Those influences that a peer(s) exercises on an individual, including drug abuse, sexual mores and suicide

cohort study EPIDEMIOLOGY A longitudinal study of a specific group or cohort sharing a selected, often morbid condition, with the purpose of identifying features unique to the cohort that may be related to the morbid condition; see Cluster, Epidemiology

cohort trend EPIDEMIOLOGY A change in the incidence of a particular condition among individuals who are defined by a shared and continued temporal experience, eg year of birth, marriage (JAMA 1992; 268:3098oc) see Temporal trend

cohorting EPIDEMIOLOGY Separating of patients, eg infants in a neonatal unit, into small groups, such that the patients are treated by a limited number of health care workers; in infants, cohorting and frequent hand-washing results in a reduced incidence of respiratory syncytial virus infection (Arch Dis Child 1991; 66:227)

coiled coil MOLECULAR BIOLOGY A structural motif in proteins formed by two or three α helices in parallel and in register that cross at a 20° angle, are strongly amphipathic with hydrophobic and hydrophilic residues that repeat every seventh residue; coiled-coil domains are thought to be critical for a number of as-yet unknown biological activities and may be found in flagellins, β chains of G proteins, heat shock proteins, keratins, myosins, tropomyosins and in α and β tubulins, and may coexist with other structural motifs, including leucine zippers and zinc finger domains (Science 1991; 252:1162)

coiled spring appearance RADIOLOGY A descriptive term for a finding seen by radiocontrast studies of the upper GI tract, caused by posttraumatic intramural hematoma of the third segment of the duodenum, where the folds over the mass are stretched; a similar finding may be seen in intussusception; see Stacked coin appearance

coin lesion RADIOLOGY A rounded, circumscribed nodule measuring less than 4 cm that may be surrounded by well-aerated pulmonary parenchyma, appearing as an incidental finding in an otherwise unremarkable plain chest film; in the US, coin lesions are often malignant and details of importance include age, smoking history, geography and previous malignancy ETIOLOGY Infection (abscesses, aspergilloma, bacteria, coccidioidomycosis, echinococcal cysts, *Dirofilaria immitis*, histoplasmosis, TB), benign masses (bronchial adenoma, chondroma, diaphragmatic hernia, benign mesothelioma, neurogenic tumor, sarcoidosis, sclerosing hemangioma, Wegener's granulomatosis, rheumatoid nodules); malignant masses (primary lung carcinomas, which comprise 35% or more, metastases approximately 10%, sarcoma, myeloma, Hodgkin's disease and choriocarcinoma)

coining ETHNOMEDICINE The practice of rubbing the edge of a coin across the skin or body part which is performed as part of a traditional Southeast Asian therapy, used to treat migraine headaches and other conditions; body regions subjected to 'coining' demonstrate linear microecchymoses that may confused with various forms of abuse (N Engl J Med 1995; 332:1552icm)

COLA Commission of Office Laboratory Assessment A coalition group formed by the American Medical Association, College of American Pathologists and the American Association of Family Practitioners for the purpose of accrediting physician office laboratories, see POLs; also, Cost of living adjustment An increase in salary given to those who move to a more expensive region of the country

COLD Chronic obstructive lung disease, see COPD

cold abscess Focal, well-circumscribed acute inflammation without the usual signs of a 'hot' abscess, eg dolor, calor, rubor and functio laesa; cold abscesses may occur in normal individuals infected by an attenuated organism or as a result of inadequate antibiotic therapy, classically a paravertebral tuberculotic cold abscess; cold abscesses are also characteristic of the hyperimmunoglobulin E syndrome; see Job syndrome

cold agglutinin disease Cold agglutinin syndrome An immune disorder characterized by IgM autoantibodies that optimally agglutinate red cells at very low temperatures, eg 4°C; low titers (< 1:32) of cold agglutinins are detectable in many normal subjects; polyclonal cold agglutinins increase after certain infections, eg mycoplasma, CMV, EBV, trypanosomiasis and malaria, peaking within 2-3 weeks and are of no significance if non-hemolytic; cold agglutinins should be ruled out in all patients with acquired hemolytic anemia and a positive direct Coomb's test and certain antibodies have been implicated, eg anti-I, -i, -Pr, -Gd, Sdᵃ; cold agglutinin syndrome occurs in 1) Elderly patients with a monoclonal kappa proliferation or concomitant lymphoma, often large cell (Rappaport's 'histiocytic') type or 2) Younger patients with a polyclonal proliferation induced by *Mycoplasma pneumoniae* infection (anti-I antibodies) or infectious mononucleosis (anti-i antibodies); the cells are coated with C3d (C3d is also increased in up to 40% of patients with *Mycoplasma* infections, 20% of adenovirus infections); cooling of acral parts results in intravascular agglutination and complement fixation; elevation of the complement-bearing red cells to body temperature evokes mild, self-limited hemolysis; Cf 'Room temps'

cold chain A colloquial term for the continuous maintenance of low temperature that is required for biologicals (eg vaccines) from the time they are manufactured to the time they are shipped, warehoused and stored prior to being administered; the CC may break down when vaccines are being transported to remote parts of the world where refrigeration can sometimes be sporadic or even nonexistent

cold hemoglobinuria Paroxysmal cold hemoglobinuria, see there

cold hypersensitivity An excess autonomic nervous system reaction to low ambient temperature, characterized by bradycardia and a local wheal-and-flare reaction; when familial in nature, the reaction is dignified as 'cold urticaria'

cold laser Excimer laser, see there

cold nodule RADIOISOTOPIC IMAGING THYROID A focus of reduced radioisotope uptake on a ¹²³I or ⁹⁹ᵐTc scintillation scan of the thyroid, seen in either cystic (seen in follicular adenomas that have outgrown their vascular supply resulting in cystic degeneration) or solid, often nonfunctional lesions; when the mass is solid by ultrasound, a biopsy is warranted as most carcinomas are cold nodules Note: Benign lesions, eg non-functional follicular adenomas are usually 'cold' as well; hepatic lesions that may be 'hot' or 'cold' include abscesses and tumor nodules; each warrants a biopsy, best visualized by ¹⁹⁸Au and ⁹⁹ᵐTc; Cf Hot nodules, Warm nodules

cold scan RADIOLOGY A rounded non-imaging region in a solid organ, eg the liver, when viewed by immunoscintigraphy; in one such protocol, anti-CEA monoclonal antibody was labeled with ⁹⁹ᵐTc and whole body and SPECT scans performed; the significance of a 'cold' vs a 'hot' scan is uncertain (Croatian Med J 1994; 35:233)

cold sore A popular term for a lesion of the perioral tissues that is caused by herpes simplex and characterized by the formation of vesicles that rupture. leaving weeping ulcers

Cold Spring Harbor laboratory One of the premier institutes of molecular biology in the world, located on Long Island, New York; it was home to 3 Nobel laureates: JD Watson, A Hershey, B McClintock; 120 scientists from 18 countries work in the CSHL; on-going research projects include tumor viruses, eukaryotic genetics, cell biology, ultrastructure, protein chemistry, X-ray crystallography, yeast genetics, neuroscience, HIV gene regulation; CSHL is involved in education from grade-school to the post-graduate level (35 annual conferences) and publications (two journals, 140 titles in print) BUDGET $26 million

'cold turkey' SUBSTANCE ABUSE American slang* for the acute opiate withdrawal syndrome, usually referring to heroin withdrawal CLINICAL Rhinorrhea, lacrimation, perspiration, yawning, followed by restlessness, anxiety and irritability, dilated pupils, anorexia, nausea, vomiting, abdominal cramps, tremors, convulsions and shock if severe; the reaction may be precipitated by naloxone, a pure opiate antagonist

*The first documented use of the term cold turkey (thus defined) was in 1925; JE Lighter (Historical Dictionary of American Slang, Random House, New York, 1994) recorded two further definitions for the term cold turkey, to wit 1) The most basic level, bedrock, first documented in 1927 and 2) An easy target, a helpless victim, first documented in 1928; both uses of the term have been essentially abandoned

'cold turkey' method SUBSTANCE ABUSE A cessation technique used for narcotic or nicotine addiction, where the symptoms of withdrawal are treated as little as possible, with the hope that once the addict has passed through the 'cathartic' trauma of withdrawal, he would be unwilling to re-initiate drug abuse

cold-(induced) urticaria-angioedema Autonomic nervous system reactivity to low temperatures CLINICAL forms, Acquired After cold exposure, the patient suffers a pruritic urticarial eruption, potentially evolving into angioedema, accompanied by headaches and wheezing; if the whole body is cooled (swimming in winter), hypotension, collapse and death may ensue Hereditary, immediate-type erythematous maculopapules accompanied by a burning sensation, pyrexia, arthralgias, and leukocytosis Hereditary, delayed-type erythematous swelling 9-18 hours after a cold 'challenge' **colera** Bilis, see there

Coley's toxin IMMUNOLOGY A 'cocktail' of bacterial products, including hemolytic streptococcal proteins, eg streptokinase and streptodornase, formulated by Wm Coley, New York in 1893, that was occasionally successful in treating cancer or evoking tumor regression; the first case was an inoperable head and neck sarcoma that regressed with each attack of erysipelas; the toxin caused high fevers related to endogenous tumor necrosis factor production

colic PEDIATRICS A symptom complex affecting young infants, in which paroxysmal abdominal pain of presumed intestinal origin is accompanied by severe crying, lasting until the infant is completely exhausted; in absence of organic causes (strangulated hernia, intussusception, pyelonephritis and others), no therapy gives consistent relief and parents are often obliged to wait until the infant outgrows it, often by six months of age

colipase A trypsin-activated proenzyme secreted by the exocrine pancreas that acts on fat droplets, binding at the bile salt-triglyceride-water interface, providing a recognition site for lipase

collaborative care HEALTH CARE ENVIRONMENT A (Bill) Clinton euphemism for managed care, see there (Am Med News 26 October 1992, p7)

collagen PHYSIOLOGY Any of a family of abundant proteins that are integral to the extracellular matrix, which form fibril of considerable tensile strength; the core shape of collagen is rod-like, composed of a triple helix of core proteins described by the generic formula –Gly-Pro-Xaa–, each chain of which is ± 1000 amino acids in length, cross-

COLLAGEN MUTATIONS

MUTATION	DISEASE
COL1A1, COL1A2	Osteogenesis imperfecta
COL2A1	(some) Chondrodystrophies
COL3A1	Ehlers-Danlos syndrome (a severe form)
COL4A1/COL4A2	Alport syndrome (autosomal dominant)
COL4A3/COL4A4	Alport syndrome (autosomal recessive)
COL4A5/COL4A6	Alport syndrome ((X-linked)
COL7A1	Epidermolysis bullosa
COL10A1	Metaphyseal chondrodystrophy of Schmid
COL11A1	Uncertain, possibly Stickler syndrome

Science & Medicine 1995; 2/3:58

linked to each other by covalent bonds; collagens are bound at each end by globular domains that either promote folding or or serve as sites for interaction with other proteins; the structures have been resolved for 12 (figure) of the 19 known collagens; mutations of collagen genes have been linked to an increasing number of hereditable diseases (table) (Science & Medicine 1995; 2/3:58) see Extracellular matrix, Fibrillin

Collagens

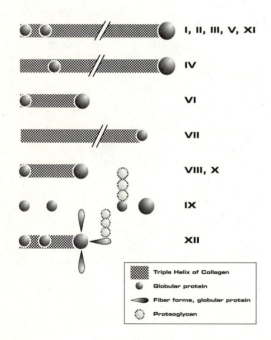

I, II, III, V, XI

IV

VI

VII

VIII, X

IX

XII

Triple Helix of Collagen
Globular protein
Fiber forms, globular protein
Proteoglycan

collagen structures

collagen disease & arthritis panel LABORATORY MEDICINE A group of tests that are designed to establish the diagnosis of rheumatic disease in the most cost-effective manner possible, which entails measurement of the erythrocyte sedimentation rate, rheumatic factor (by latex agglutination), uric acid levels, antinuclear antibody and C-reactive protein; see Organ panel

collagenase type IV (72 kD) Matrix metalloproteinase-2

collagenous colitis A rare condition first described in 1976 characterized by watery diarrhea and the case-defining but patchy histologic finding of ↑ collagen in the upper lamina propria of the intestinal mucosa, which obscures the lower border of the epithelial basement membrane, accompanied by mononuclear inflammation of the lamina propria; fecal WBCs occur in 55% TREATMENT Uncertain, clinical response has been reported with 5-aminosalicylic acid, cholestyramine, corticosteroids, sulfasalazine (Mayo Clin Proc 1995; 70:430)

collagenous micronodule SURGICAL PATHOLOGY A microscopic aggregate of paucicellular eosinophilic fibrillar stroma that impinges on glandular lumina in prostatic adenocarcinoma (PA); although CMs are regarded as specific for PA, they are an infrequent finding and are not known to have prognostic significance (Arch Pathol Lab Med 1995; 119:444OA)

collagenous spherulosis SURGICAL PATHOLOGY Rounded aggregates of hyalin-like material produced by myoepithelial cells in benign breast lesions and salivary gland tumors, which are composed of acidic mucins, collagens I, III, IV, elastin, and laminin (Arch Pathol Lab Med 1992; 116:649OA)

collagenous stalk motif Collagen is characterized by the repeating triple helix of amino acid residues, Gly-X-Y, a motif also found in secretory proteins, eg complement C1q, pulmonary surfactant apoprotein, asymmetric acetylcholinesterase and serum mannose-binding protein and non-secretory proteins, eg macrophage scavenger receptor

collagen vascular diseases A group of 'rheumatic' diseases characterized by arthropathies, immune complex deposition, renal involvement, and partial or complete temporary response to corticosteroids, including dermatomyositis, mixed connective tissue disease, polyarteritis nodosa, rheumatoid arthritis and systemic lupus erythematosus

collar sign RADIOLOGY A radiolucent band of edema surrounding a benign peptic ulcer, seen by radiocontrast studies of the upper GI tract

collar button abscess An advanced abscess of the finger that forms on the palmar and dorsal surfaces, commonly located at the metacarpophalangeal joint; the infection tends to spread beneath the palmar fascia or into the dorsal compartment opposite the web space, later filling the web space, extending along the synovial tendon sheath into the midpalmar or thenar spaces TREATMENT Palmar and dorsal incision and drainage

collar button lesions Numerous small deep ulcers with narrow necks, paralleling a barium-filled large intestinal lumen affected by ulcerative colitis; the 'button' surface corresponds to the eroded ulcer base and the 'button neck' corresponds to the sides of the islands of preserved mucosa; a similar phenomenon occurs in colonic amebiasis ulcers; see Flask lesion

collarette A rim of thickened epidermis in pyogenic granuloma, morphologically similar to the pincer-like surrounding epidermis of lichen nitidus, Cf Ball in claw lesion

collar-stud abscess An abscess of the ocular orbit present beneath the skin and constricted in a 'collar stud'-like fashion by the orbital septum TREATMENT Enlarge the septum with an artery forceps to provide effective drainage

collateral damage A colloquial term* for any undesired but unavoidable co-morbidity associated with a therapeutic modality, eg chemotherapy-induced collateral damage to the BM and GI tract as an expected but unwanted side effect of destroying tumor cells

*Borrowed from the military and popularized during the Gulf War in reference to unintentional, but inevitable loss of life and destruction of civilian property and non-military facilities when these are adjacent to military targets (N Engl J Med 1991; 324:1746c)

collecting duct carcinoma Bellini duct carcinoma NEPHROLOGY A rare tumor that arises in the collecting duct epithelium of middle-aged persons with a ♂:♀ ratio of 4:1, which represents ± 1% of all renal epithelial neoplasms PATHOLOGY CDCs average 5 cm and are firm and gray-white; the architecture is papillary, the cells have either granular or eosinophilic cytoplasm arranged in a 'hobnail' fashion around luminal spaces and a fibrovascular stroma SPECIAL STUDIES HMW keratins, CD15, vimentin PROGNOSIS Uncertain, some cases have been highly aggressive (Am J Clin Pathol 1995; 103:624oA) see Renal epithelial neoplasms

collection HEALTH CARE FINANCING The obtention of fees for services rendered; the collection period is the average number of days required to collect professional fees (Am Med News 2 November 1992, p 16)

collective dose RADIATION SAFETY The sum of individual doses received after exposure to a specified source of radiation in a specified time period by a specified population type

collimation RADIATION ONCOLOGY The formal process in which the beam or field of radiation is reduced by means of a lead diaphragm, tube. or cone

colliquative necrosis A type of necrosis in which the tissue is rapidly 'liquified; due to a relative paucity of proteins, due either to the tissue involved, eg the brain, or due to previous insult, eg due to hydrolytic enzyme activity related to acute inflammation (Arch Pathol Lab Med 1993; 117:1208oA) Cf Coagulation necrosis

collision COMPUTERS A garbled communication between two devices in a local area network (LAN) that results when both attempt to transmit data simultaneously; after a collision, each device waits for a random period of time and retry; the more devices on the LAN, the greater the likelihood that collisions will occur (CAP Today November 1993) see Ethernet OBSTETRICS A mechanical obstruction to the birth of twins such that the lay of one fetus impedes the engagement of the other; the most extreme of collisions is known as interlocking, see there RADIATION PHYSICS The interaction between two molecules, eg a proton and an electron; see Compton effect

collision tumor The extremely rare merging of two originally separate (primary) tumors from two organs, most often seen clinically at the esophago-gastric junction, where a squamous cell carcinoma of esophageal origin merges with an adenocarcinoma of gastric origin; diagnosis of a 'collision' tumor requires that the colliding tumors be histologically distinct; Cf Composite tumor, Mixed tumor

collodion baby An infant covered with thickened, taut, parchment paper-like skin that is cyclically shed as a manifestation of lamellar type ichthyosis; the tightened skin results in a flattened nose, ectropion, fixation of the lips into an O-shape, 'cracking' of the skin with respiratory effort; hair may be absent or may penetrate the membrane PROGNOSIS Uncertain TREATMENT High humidity

Note: Collodion was a solution of gun-cotton, a highly explosive compound prepared by steeping cotton in nitric and sulfuric acids in ether that was supplanted by dynamite; collodion formed a colorless gummy liquid that dried in air, used in photography for covering plates and in surgery for covering wounds

colloid bodies (skin) Cytoid bodies, see there, Civatte bodies

colloid carcinoma Mucinous carcinoma SURGICAL PATHOLOGY A gelatinous subtype of secretory adenocarcinoma, histologically appearing as clusters of tumor cells floating in pools of pale mucin; colloid carcinomas occur in 1) Breast Although focal colloid features may occur in 'garden variety' breast carcinomas of ductal and lobular types, tumors with predominantly colloid features comprise only 2% of all cases; colloid carcinomas of the breast occurs in slightly older women, has a lower incidence of lymph node metastases, an excellent short-term prognosis (most deaths 12 years or more after diagnosis) and may have neuroendocrine features Note: Juan Rosai feels the benign behavior is related to its status as an in situ ductal carcinoma 2) Colon The colloid type adenocarcinoma of the colon is viewed as a subtype of mucinous carcinoma in

which the mucin is extracellular (while in the signet ring carcinoma, the mucin is intracellular) comprises about 5-15% of colonic carcinoma and is thought to have a slightly worse prognosis that the 'garden variety' of adenocarcinoma of the colon; see Mucin lakes

colloid droplets Homogeneous masses of eosinophilic debris seen in the renal tubules in bismuth and mercury poisoning

colloid solution TRANSFUSION MEDICINE A suspension of particles that are so small (1 nm to 1 μm in diameter) that they do not settle out of solution in absence of external force, eg centrifugation; colloid solutions are used to provide prolonged volume expansion and include 5% albumin, 25% albumin, plasma protein fraction (which contains 83% albumin and 17% globulins, less commonly used as rapid infusion may induce hypotension), dextran 40 (Rheomacrodex), dextran 70 (Macrodex), and hydroxyethyl starch (HESPAN), a polymer synthesized from amylopectin Note: The albumin-containing solutions are heated for 10 hours at 60°C, which inactivates any viral contaminants; Cf Crystalloid solutions

colloidal gold curve see Gold curve

colon cut-off sign RADIOLOGY Gaseous distension of the right and transverse colon with decreased or absent air beyond the splenic flexure, characteristic of acute pancreatitis; the inflamed transverse mesocolon (which is attached to the anterior pancreas) 'cuts off' the barium flow, causing mesenteric arterial thrombosis and ischemic colitis (Radiology 1962; 79:763)

colonic irrigation 1) ALTERNATIVE MEDICINE A controversial procedure in which a series of enemas are administered over a short period by a gravity-dependent device; the technique is practiced by chiropractors, 'colon therapists', 'nutrition therapists', naturopaths and 'homeopaths' with the nebulous purpose of 'detoxification'; the use of a wide variety of detoxifying enemas is an integral component of 'metabolic therapy'; see 'Holistic' medicine, Unproven treatments for cancer 2) SURGERY An intraoperative procedure for antegrade cleansing of the large intestine in an emergency colon resection, which can be used in elective left-sided colonic surgery in patients who are clinically stable, circumventing the need for a temporary colostomy; see Bowel prep(aration)

colon therapy ALTERNATIVE MEDICINE A generic term for the use of various permutations of enema, which are alleged to '...balance body chemistry, eliminate waste, and restore proper tissue and organ function.' (Alternative Medicine, Future Medicine Pub, Puyallup, Wash, 1994); in contrast to enemas, which irrigate the sigmoid colon, CT bathes the entire colon to the cecum, using 2-6 liters of herbs and oxygen in a filtered water solution; CT is reported to reduce the body's burden of impacted feces, microorganisms, and dead cellular debris, which cause the condition known to alternative health practitioners as 'bowel toxemia'; in addition to impacting on bloating and constipation, CT is claimed to be effective in relieving backache, fatigue, halitosis, headaches, loss of concentration, dermatopathies, sinusitis, pulmonary congestion, and other conditions; see Alternative medicine

Note: There is little (if any) peer-reviewed data to support many of the claims for the efficacy of CT

colonoscopic polypectomy A generic term for the removal of any polyp (hyperplastic, adenomatous, villous adenoma), or polypoid (eg lymphoid hyperplasia) by endoscopy; timely removal of adenomatous polyps virtually eliminates the incidence of colorectal cancer, reducing its incidence by 76 to 90% (N Engl J Med 1993; 329:1977oA); in general, polyps measuring less than 1.0 cm in greatest dimension are of little clinical significance

colony bank Gene library, see there

colony-forming unit HEMATOLOGY A cluster of cells consisting of a hematopoietic stem cell and its progeny; the most likely candidate cell with potential for giving rise to all hematopoietic lineages has been regarded as the CFU-S (spleen) that forms undifferentiated heterogeneous colonies containing pluripotent stem cells; all terminally differentiated or end-stage hematopoietic cells in the circulation theoretically arise from one CFU, although the role of CFU-S as the most primitive hematopoietic stem cell has been challenged; other contenders for the title of the most primitive cell complex include CFU-blast, CFU-D (CFU, Diffusing chamber), CFU-GEMM (CFU, granulo-cyte-erythroid-macrophage-megakaryocyte), and CFU-LM (CFU, lymphoid-myeloid)

colony-stimulating factor A generic term for any of a number of glycoproteins that control the production, differentiation and function of granulocytes and mono-macrophage systems; see Biological response modifiers

COLONY-STIMULATING FACTORS

GRANULOCYTE-CSF Encoded on chromosome 17, produced by endothelial cells, fibroblasts and macrophages that stimulates granulocyte formation and act synergistically with IL-3 to form megakaryocytes, granulocyte-macrophages, and colonies with a high proliferative potential; G-CSF may successfully 'drive' myeloid leukemia into terminal differentiation, forcing it to become a less aggressive disease

GRANULOCYTE-MACROPHAGE-CSF Encoded on chromosome 5, produced by endothelial cells, fibroblasts and T cells that stimulates formation of granulocyte and macrophage colonies, acting synergistically with other factors to stimulate megakaryocyte blast cell and BFU-E colonies

COLONY-STIMULATING FACTOR-1 Encoded on chromosome 5, produced by endothelial cells, fibroblasts and macrophages that stimulates formation of macrophage colonies and acts synergistically with other factors

MULTI-CSF Interleukin-3 Encoded on chromosome 5, produced by T cells that stimulates formation of granulocyte, macrophage, eosinophil and mast cell colonies and acts synergistically with other factors to stimulate BFU-E colonies and hematopoietic precursor colonies

ERYTHROPOIETIN Encoded on chromosome 7, produced by renal interstitial cells that stimulates formation of erythroid colonies, acting synergistically with IL-3 to form BFU-E colonies; see Erythropoietin

Colorado tick fever An acute tick-borne (vector *Dermacentor andersoni*) RNA reoviral infection occurring in the early spring in the Rocky Mountains CLINICAL Chills, biphasic ('saddleback') fever, myalgias of the back and legs, headache, retro-orbital pain, photophobia, malaise and nausea Prognosis Excellent with little residua

color blindness Most color blindness is X-linked; it is tested by using the Ishihara pseudoisochromic charts; more than 90% occur in males; color blindness is subdivided into: 1) Incomplete achromatopsia, defective vision of blue color which worsens with age 2) Deuteranopia or daltonism, defective vision of blue and green 3) Partial protanopia, defective red vision (uncertain heredity pattern) and 4) Partial tritanopia

colorectal cancer EPIDEMIOLOGY 152 000 new cases, 57 000 deaths (estimates, 1993, US) SURVEILLANCE (annual) Fecal occult blood testing is reported to decrease mortality by 33% (N Engl J Med 1993; 328:1365oA) see Colorectal adenoma MOLECULAR PATHOLOGY Colorectal cancers develop as distinct genetic alterations accumulate, in the form of alterations of the K-*ras* oncogene on chromosome 12, and the tumor-suppressor genes on chromosomes 5, 17p (which encodes p53) and 18q (*DCC* gene); the status of chromosome 18q has strong prognostic value in stage II colorectal cancer; 5-year survival in those with no loss of 18q is 93% (similar to those in stage I) in contrast to 54% of those with 18q loss (N Engl J Med 1994; 331:213oA)

'Columbus theory' The theory that syphilis originated in the New World and was brought back to Europe by Columbus' crew from venereal contacts with natives of Hispaniola, causing the 'great pox' epidemics among the sexually promiscuous in the 16th and 17th centuries

column chromatography A technique for separating a variety of different sized molecules, in which the mobile phase is poured through a glass or plastic column containing a stationary phase, which is a solid, commonly Sephadex beads of different porosities, which will retain molecules with certain characteristics; the molecule of interest is then washed out or eluted using a solvent

coma depassé A long-standing coma in which there is no sign of higher cerebral activity or cortical function, ie 'brain-dead' NEUROPATHOLOGY The classic 'respirator brain' reveals global softening of noble tissue, microscopically corresponding to autolysis and/or necrosis

coma panel LABORATORY MEDICINE A group of tests that has been shown to be the most cost-effective means (under the diagnosis-related group [DRG] system for health care reimbursement in the US) of determining tha etiology of a coma; the panel includes assays for alcohol, ammonium, calcium, creatinine, glucose, lactic acid, osmolality, phenobarbital and a general toxicology screen of the blood and urine; see Organ panel

coma vigil NEUROLOGY Extreme dementia with degeneration of the cerebral white matter that may accompany apparently uncomplicated head injuries PATHOLOGY Petechial hemorrhages, especially in the corpus callosum, ventricular dilatation, chalky white discoloration in the spinal cord and extensive wallerian degeneration

combat fatigue Battle fatigue A condition affecting soldiers following long tours of combat duty, characterized by a loss of self-esteem, anxiety, tremulousness, depression, extreme emotional lability, dyspepsia and dyspnea; see 'Burn-out syndrome', Old soldier's heart, Post-trauma stress disorder

combination therapy REPRODUCTIVE PHARMACOLOGY The most common form of steroid contraception, where the tablets contain both an estrogen (ethinyl estradiol, 30-35 µg) and a progesterone analog (norethindrone, norgestrel or levonorgestrel, 0.5-1.5 mg) taken for three weeks with a one week 'rest' period to allow 'break-through' bleeding

combinatorial chemistry A chemistry-based technology platform that generates vast arrays of screenable compounds for rapid drug discovery; '...the strategy is to assemble every possible combination of a given set of chemical building blocks while simulataneously recording which ones have been used and in what order, then assay the resulting molecules all at once–and refer to the record to determine the identity of any that look promising.' (Science 1994; 264; 1399RN); drugs developed by 'classic' synthetic chemistry require an average of 12 years at a cost of $359 million; combinatorial compounds of potential interest may be identified within a month; most combinatorial compounds thus far created include peptides and oligonucleotides; in the pharmaceutical industry, combinatorial 'libraries' of millions of compounds may be produced by smaller biotechnology companies (eg Affymax, Selectide), which may purchased in their entirety by larger companies seeking leads for newer therapeutic agents (Bio/Technology 1995; 13:310, 351)

combined modality therapy The use of more than one

broad class of therapeutic modalities, eg radiotherapy and chemotherapy to treat a disease, usually malignant; the use of combined therapies is a function of the stage of a disease; lower stage malignancies respond to a single modality, eg early carcinomas respond to surgery and localized lymphoproliferative disease responds to chemo-surgery, while more advanced or extensive disease requires multimodality therapy; combination chemothera-py may be of use in treating AIDS as the commonly-used agents, eg zidovudine and ddI attack different sites in HIV viruses (Science 1991; 253:1557)

combustible liquid OCCUPATIONAL SAFETY A liquid with a flash point ≥ 37.8ºC (100ºF) but below 93.3ºC (200ºF); in the US the use of CLs in the workplace is monitored by OSHA

comet cell Comma cell, decoy cell An atypical transition-al epithelial cell with elongated cytoplasmic wisps or tails seen in bacterially infected urine; the nucleus is normal in size, without nuclear atypia and filled with dense degener-ated chromatin, mimicking a cell with transitional cell car-cinoma in situ

COMET surgical technique Combined microscopic and endoscopic technique An alternative to the technically demanding endoscopic sinus surgery for surgical manage-ment of chronic sinus diseases, which allows less experi-enced operators to manage these disorders with a low rate of complications

comet tail sign RADIOLOGY A curvilinear soft tissue densi-ty extending from the lateral pleura to the hilum, caused by contracted fibrous scarring, seen in the folded lung syndrome, see there

comfort care Palliative and supportive treatment for patients who are suffering from a terminal illness (eg AIDS, cancer) or who have refused curative or life-sus-taining treatment; CC is aimed at relieving the symptoms, enhancing the quality of the patient's remaining life, and easing the dying process; when CC becomes inadequate, some workers feel that physician-assisted suicide should be an available next step, which it currently is not (N Engl J Med 1994; 331:119ED) see Euthanasia, Initiative 119, Kevorkian, Physician-assisted suicide

coming out Part of the phrase, 'coming out of the closet', see Closet

'coming soon' advertising A form of 'teaser' advertising that indicates the name of a drug without claims for poten-tial indications, safety or effectiveness; see Advertising

commensal organism MICROBIOLOGY An organism that lives on or in another without benefit or harm to the host; commensal sites include the skin, oral cavity, external genitalia, and intertriginous zones

comma cell CYTOLOGY see Comet cell SURGICAL PATHOLOGY A morphological variant cell of unknown significance seen in neurofibromas

commando operation A term first used by Hayes Martin, a pioneer in head and neck surgery, for the en bloc removal of an advanced primary malignancy of the oral cavity, usually squamous cell carcinoma (lymphoma is amenable to radio- or chemotherapy); the 'commando' is one of the most aggressive of all surgical procedures, and entails partial removal of the mandible, floor of the mouth and/or tongue accompanied by a radical neck dissection; see Heroic surgery, Radical neck dissection

The operation was named after the British Commandos, a special strike force that crossed the English Channel carrying out raids against the German U-boats; the analogy is apropos given the high risk of not safely returning home by either the commando or the patient

'commitment' HEMATOLOGY An irreversible maturation step by plasma cells which have terminally differentiated, ie have undergone heavy chain rearrangement and thus are 'clonal' and capable of producing only one specific

immunoglobulin; cell specificity or idiotype is conferred by the heavy and light variable regions

committed donor program TRANSFUSION MEDICINE Dedicated donor program A permutation of directed donation in which a donor recruited by a recipient under-goes repeated phlebotomy to provide red cell support for the recipient; unlike directed donations, 'minimal expo-sure' programs reduce the risk of allogeneic immunization (Arch Pathol Lab Med 1994; 118:380OA); the risk to the donor is uncer-tain, as multiple closely spaced donations cause ↓ NK cell activity (Transfusion 1993; 33:368) see Directed donation

committed dose equivalent H_{T50} RADIATION PHYSICS The dose equivalent to reference tissue (T) that will be received from an intake of radioactive materials by a per-son during the 50 years after the intake

committed effective dose equivalent H_{E50} RADIATION PHYSICS The sum of the products of the weighting factors applicable to each irradiated tissue or organ and the com-mitted dose equivalent to the tissue or organ $H_{E50} = \Sigma(W_T H_{T50})$

committed step A point of no return in a synthetic reac-tion or in cellular differentiation, after which a cascade of reactions occurs or a cell undergoes terminal and irre-versible 'specialization'

commodity test LABORATORY MEDICINE Any test in a clini-cal laboratory that can be performed in terms of economy of scale, ie the higher the volume of tests of a particular type being performed, the lower the cost per unit; in gen-eral, commodity tests do not require a rapid turnaround, and thus the price per unit test can be reduced to a mini-mum (CAP Today October 1994)

common acute lymphocytic leukemia antigen see CALLA, CD10

common cold Acute nasopharyngitis Rhinitis and coryza that is usually spread by aerosol, caused by any of a num-ber of viruses: Rhinovirus has 111 serotypes and is incul-pated in 15-40% of common colds, coronavirus in 10-20%; other viral causes of the common cold include influenza A, B, C, parainfluenza, respiratory syncytial virus, aden-ovirus, rarely coxsackie and enterovirus; group A β-hemolytic streptococci cause 2-10%; in 30-50% no etiolog-ic agent is identified Incidence, common cold 41/100 annual cases (US) the CC is responsible for 23 million days of lost work, and 161 days of restricted activity (1985), and loss of $12 billion (Bio/Technology 1992; 10:502) CLINICAL Influenza-like syndrome

Note: When the symptoms are protracted, antibiotics may be indicated to 'cover' for bacterial infections including Group A streptococcus, *Haemophilus influenzae*, *Corynebacterium diphtheriae*, *Mycoplasma pneumoniae*, *S pneumoniae*, *Staphylococcus aureus*, and *Neisseria meningitidis*

common pathway PHYSIOLOGY The final route in a molec-ular 'cascade' in which there is a complex interplay among enzymes, substrates, activators and inactivators, and a rel-atively small signal is 'amplified' by a positive feedback loop to produce an effect; the common pathway of coagu-lation is initiated by either the extrinsic or intrinsic path-way, either of which activates factor X (Xa), which in turn activates factor II, converting it into thrombin in the pres-ence of factor V, Ca++, and membrane phospholipid, acti-vates prothrombinase producing thrombin from prothrom-bin; prothrombin then converts fibrinogen into fibrin, forming a blood clot that becomes irreversible when factor XIII is activated; the common pathway of complement is initiated by either the alternate or the classic pathways, either of which activates C3 convertase, which is the first in the common pathway of complement activation; see Amplification, Cf Cascades

common variable immunodeficiency A heterogeneous, often AR group of primary immune dysfunctions affecting 20-90/10^6 live births, characterized by a decrease in most immunoglobulin isotypes (B-cell precursors are present but don't differentiate into plasma cells) and T-cell defects without major defects in cell-mediated immunity; the disease is usually limited to intrinsic B-cell defects, but in most patients, there are also abnormalities of T-cell activation and ↓ secretion of IFN-γ, IL-2, IL-4, IL-5, and B-cell differentiation factor CLINICAL Average age at diagnosis is 12 years, by which time the patients have suffered recurrent bacterial infections, chronic otitis, sinusitis, bronchiectasis, pneumonitis, diarrhea, malabsorption, sprue-like enteritis, achlorhydria, pernicious anemia, cholestasis and giardiasis, which affects up to 50% of patients PATHOGENESIS CVID is caused by various blocks in B-cell maturation, possibly induced by EBV infection, which may turn off B cells, ↓ Ig production or nonglycosylation of secreted antibodies or T-cell suppression of Ig production LABORATORY ↓↓↓ Igs, ↓ serum IgG, IgA, and usually IgM, impaired antibody response to antigens, ↓ 5'-nucleotidase in lymphocytes these patients have a 50-fold ↑ risk for gastric cancer, 70% of whom have ↓ gastrin secretion in response to bombesin (a clinical marker for CVID patients at risk for gastric carcinoma) TREATMENT IV gammaglobulins, polyethylene glycol-conjugated IL-2* injected subcutaneously once/week is reported to ↑ serum IgG up to 4 times above baseline and may allow the weaning of patients from immune globulin infusions (N Engl J Med 1994; 331:918OA)

*Covalently bound PEG increases the half-life of IL-2 by a factor of 10

communicating hydrocephalus Enlargement of cerebral ventricles due to an imbalance between production and absorption of cerebrospinal fluid, where the ventricular pathway is open and the fluid moves freely into the spinal subarachnoid space, but is blocked by obliteration of the subarachnoid cisterns around the brainstem or subarachnoid spaces over the cerebral convexities ETIOLOGY Arnold-Chiari malformation, infections, eg bacterial meningitis, toxoplasmosis, CMV, or other viral meningitides, subarachnoid hemorrhage, increased production of cerebrospinal fluid, eg choroid plexus papilloma, Hurler syndrome due to fibrosis in the subarachnoid space, hypervitaminosis A

community care network HEALTH CARE ENVIRONMENT A system for reforming the US health care system that was proposed by American Hospital Association; in a CCN, local hospital-organized groups of physicians and clinics would compete for contracts with group insurers and would provide care to those enrolled in the plan; the fees would be capitated and the rates determined by an independent regulatory board (Am Med News 26 October 1992, p7) see Capitation

community cell borders CYTOLOGY Cell borders shared in common by clusters of malignant epithelial cells, a 'soft' criterion for cytological diagnosis of malignancy; Cf Party wall appearance

community hospital Voluntary hospital A nonfederal short-term general or other specialty* hospital, the services of which are available to the public; in the US there are 5342 community hospitals (3175 private not-for-profit, 1429 public, and 738 for-profit), which have 924 000 beds, circa 173 beds/hospital, 31 x 10⁶ admissions/year, 22.4 x 10⁶ operations/year, 7.2 days length of stay (N Engl J Med 1993; 329:372SR)

*Obstetrics and gynecology; eye, ear, nose, and throat; rehabilitation and orthopedic

community medicine An informal division of general medicine defined as the care of patients in the context of their daily lives (Am Med News 2 November 1992, p 30)

community rating (of insurance premiums) HEALTH CARE FINANCING A method for determining the cost of health insurance premiums, in which the amount that an individual should pay for insurance coverage is based on the experience of the community; the premium is based on the average medical cost for all people who are covered (insured) in a particular geographic region, without regard to any one person's medical condition, claims experience, and risk of injury or illness; this method tends to reduce health care costs as it includes a large pool of individuals in the premium equation (CAP Today March 1993; Congressional Quarterly, 1993, in Clin Lab Sci 1994; 7:141) Cf Experience rating

comorbidity The simultaneous presence of two or more morbid conditions or diseases in the same patient, which may complicate a patient's stay in the hospital; in the US health care environment, comorbidity is a term of considerable importance when determining the length of reasonable hospitalization under the diagnosis-related group system of classification, see DRGs

compact (dark) cells HISTOLOGY Clusters of non-vacuolated, darkly acidophilic, lipochrome-laden cells, located in the inner zone (zona reticularis) of the adrenal cortex; compact cells are thought to be the major source of glucocorticoid and sex hormone production under normal circumstances; Cf Clear (light) cells

comparative negligence A type of negligence in which both the plaintiff and the responible professional or health care provider can be viewed as partly responsible for the adverse outcome, eg a patient who does not return for the recommended follow-up visit after cancer screening, and who cannot be reached by telephone; in such cases, the law would view the plaintiff as partly responsible for the outcome

*Whose 'contribution' to an adverse outcome resulting in the lawsuit is known as contributory negligence

compartment syndrome A condition that is caused by ischemia, trauma or infection of the forearm's deep flexor compartment, resulting in ↑ tissue pressure due to venous occlusion, followed by arterial occlusion of the anterior interosseous artery (which has little collateral reserve space); when untreated, chronic ischemia converts the forearm musculature into fibrous tissue, causing Volkmann's ischemic contraction with a severe flexion deformity of the wrist and fingers; early therapy (fasciotomy) is crucial as end-stage disease requires major reconstructive surgery for salvage of function

compartmentation Compartmentalization CELL BIOLOGY The division of a cell into 'compartments', eg organelles, eg mitochondria, Golgi apparatus, membrane compartments MUSCLE The division of muscle groups according to which ones act together in reflexes PSYCHIATRY A subconcious fragmentation of components of the personality or thought process **compassion fatigue** Burn-out syndrome, see there

compassionate investigational new drug (IND) protocol A protocol that allows physicians to obtain experimental drugs (or drugs in development) from a manufacturer in order to treat patients for whom conventional therapies have failed or for whom no other drug exists; although these protocols cannot generate data regarding drug efficacy, they can generate data regarding dosage and potential side effects; see IND

compensation CELL BIOLOGY An adjustment in physiologic responses of a cell, tissue, or organism to an impairment or defect to counterbalance the resulting changes

compensation package The combination of salary, contributions to retirement funds, payment for continuing medical education activities, bonuses, state licensing fees, malpractice and other components with monetary value, eg automobile leasing, that comprise the financial arrangement being offered to a physician or other professional for providing his/her services to a hospital or health maintenance organization

compensatory damages MEDICAL MALPRACTICE A monetary sum determined by a court of law and awarded to a party injured by negligence that pretends to restore the victim to the state he would have been in had the 'wrong' not occurred, ie lost wages, pain and suffering, permanent disabilities, mental anguish and loss of consortium (conjugal fellowship, exchange of body fluids); see Damages, Malpractice; Cf Punitive damages

competence MEDICAL MALPRACTICE The ability of a trained physician or other health care professional (who may also be certified by a corresponding specialty board) to perform procedure(s) and practice his specialty in a skilled fashion; see Board certification, Malpractice; Cf Impaired health care provider **competency** CARDIOLOGY The functional adequacy of a valve IMMUNOLOGY The ability of the immune system to mount a response to an antigen; Cf Anergy MEDICAL MALPRACTICE Competence, see there PSYCHOLOGY A constellation of abilities possessed by a person that are needed for adequate decision-making; competency is a measure of a person's autonomy and ability to give permission for either diagnostic tests or for dangerous, but potentially life-saving procedures; the difficulty in legally defining competency is the subjectivity that enters in trying to determine whether a person is too rigid or is flexible enough to evaluate the advantages and disadvantages of his options; Cf Autonomy

competitive binding assay LABORATORY MEDICINE A generic term for a method that quantifies the amount of an unknown substance X in a solution based on the variable binding of labeled and unlabeled substance X to a carrier molecule with a limited (and known) number of binding sites; in the first step, the unknown substance (and unlabeled) X is incubated with the binding molecule; in the second step, the remaining sites are bound with the labeled substance X, and the amount of bound sites is determined

complain *verb* To indicate verbally or otherwise indicate a symptom

Note: This does not carry the same negative connotation that complaining carries in a nonmedical context (PL Fine, The Wards, Little, Brown and Co, Boston, 1994)

complaint *noun* A generic term for a symptom of which a person is aware or which causes discomfort; see Chief complaint

complement activation The initiation of one of the non-specific arms of the immune system that follows assembly of a molecular complex on the cell surface, ultimately leading to lysis of the target cells; complement activation may result in tissue injury including immune-complex-mediated vasculitis, glomerulonephritis, hemolytic anemia, type II collagen-induced arthritis, myasthenia gravis, and non-immune-mediated forms of tissue damage, burns, and ischemia

complement cascade IMMUNOLOGY A complex, multimolecular biological system with more than 20 different proteins that self-assemble on cell surfaces functioning in concert with the specific immune defenses to mediate host defense reactions and anti-microbial defense; the coup d'grace to the hapless target cell is the polymerization of C9 on its surface forming a transmembrane 'doughnut' that facilitates the egress of ions, resulting in cell death; Cf Alternate pathway, Classic pathway, Common pathway

complement fixation test LABORATORY MEDICINE An assay of broad clinical application, which depends on the ability of serum complement to interact with antigen-antibody (Ag-Ab) complexes; in the first stage of the CFT, complement is incubated with a solution that may contain the Ag and Ab of interest; if an an Ag-Ab complexes are formed, they interact with complement, the complement is consumed ('fixed'); in the second stage, sensitized sheep red

(EA) cells are added to the milieu and incubated at 37°C for one hour; if the serum contained the antibody of interest, the complement was previously consumed ('fixed') and not available to lyse the EA cells; therefore the absence of lysis indicates a positive test; CFT can be used to detect Ag-Ab complexes, soluble and particulate Ags, Abs, bacteria, fungi, and gamma globulins

complementarity BIOCHEMISTRY The matching and mutual compliance of two surfaces or molecules to each other, eg the adaption of an enzyme's active site to its substrate, ie the 'induced fit' model or the adherence of two complementary strands of nucleic acids to each other, as in hybridization; see Hybridization, Induced fit model MOLECULAR BIOLOGY The specific matching capability between a nucleic acid and an opposite-stranded partner, eg that demonstrated between DNA and/or RNA

complementary medicine An alternative term for alternative medicine, see there

complementary physician A generic term for a physician who practices alternative medicine

complete abortion An abortion is considered complete only if a curettage has been performed, given the possibility of necrotizing decidual tissue remaining in the uterus, which may act as a nidus for infection

complete carcinogen A carcinogenic substance or agent, eg UV-B light, that acts as both an initiator and promoter

complex disease A generic term for any condition that arises from a multifaceted interaction of environmental and inherited factors, which includes hypertension, ischemic heart disease, and obesity (N Engl J Med 1995; 332:679CHBR)

complexity A term that has proven difficult to define; it has been defined as the disorder of a system, the amount of thermodynamic resources required to assemble the system 'from scratch', the time (or computer memory) needed for a computer to describe a system, the diversity displayed at different levels of a hierarchically structured system, the degree of detail a complex system displays at ever smaller scales (Sci Am 1995; 272/6:104)

compliance The capacity or ability to yield to a pressure or force without disruption or dysfunction; compliance is a measure of tissue distensibility, eg of an air- or fluid-filled organ CLINICAL MEDICINE Patient compliance, see there PHYSIOLOGY Flexibility, or ability to yield to pressure, a term applicable to internal organs

complicated plaque An advanced lesion of atherosclerosis, defined as one or more of the following: rupture or fracture of the fibrous cap of the fibrous plaque, hemorrhage into the plaque, mural thrombosis, and prominent fibrosis (Arch Pathol Lab Med 1992; 116:1281OA) see Atherosclerotic plaque

component therapy Blood component therapy, see there

composite tumor A tumor, eg a lymphoma that involves the sequential emergence of different chromosomal rearrangements (heuristically implying a worsened prognosis with each transition, as predicted in the multistage carcinogenesis model); a composite lymphoma present with one histological form, eg follicular lymphoma and a chromosomal rearrangement, eg t(14;18), which juxtaposes the *bcl-2* oncogene on chromosome 18 with the immunoglobulin heavy chain genes on chromosome; this may then be followed by a second translocation, eg t(8;14) which results in the activation of the c-myc oncogene, which may be accompanied by an aggressive lymphoblastic lymphoma; Cf Biclonal lymphoma, Collision tumor, Compound tumor, Mixed tumor

compound Q A purified form of the plant protein tricosanthin, derived from Chinese cucumber root and imported from China as an unproven therapy for AIDS;

compound Q has also had currency as an 'underground' agent for inducing second trimester abortions and treating choriocarcinoma

compound tumor A neoplasm in which two or more histologically (and embryologically) distinct components, eg follicular and medullary (parafollicular) carcinomas of the thyroid merge, such that future clinical behavior cannot be determined; Cf Biclonal lymphoma, Collision tumor, Composite tumor, Mixed tumor

compressed gas OCCUPATIONAL SAFETY A gas or mixture of gases having in a container 1) An absolute pressure of ≥ 40 pounds/inch² (2.86 kg/cm²) at 21.1°C (70°F) 2) An absolute pressure of ≥ 104 pounds/inch² (7.43 kg/cm²) at 54.4°C (130°F) or 3) A flammable liquid with a vapor pressure ≥ 40 pounds/inch² (2.86 kg/cm²) absolute pressure at 37.8°C (100°F), as determined by the Reid method (American National Standard Method of Test for Vapor Pressure for Petroleum Products); in the US the use of CGs in the workplace is monitored by OSHA

compression ultrasonography A permutation of 'garden variety' ultrasonography which is used to diagnose deep vein thrombosis; the PPV (positive predictive value) of an abnormal impedance plethysmography for the presence of deep vein thrombosis is 83%; the PPV for an abnormal compression ultrasonography is 94% (**N Engl J Med 1993; 329:1365**ₒₐ)

Compton effect RADIATION PHYSICS The interaction between a photon and an electron (a Compton electron) in the outer shell, which is either unbound or weakly bound; the photon is deflected and loses some of its energy to the electron; in the process, the electron changes direction, which is known as Compton scattering

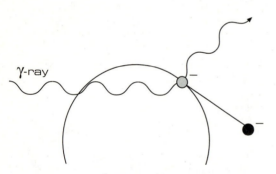

γ-ray

Compton effect

compulsion PSYCHIATRY A behavior defined as

1) Repetitive behaviors, eg handwashing, double-checking), mental acts (praying, repeating words silently) that person feels compelled to perform in response to an obsession, or in accord with rules that must be applied strictly

2) Behaviors or mental acts aimed at preventing or reducing distress or preventing some dreaded event or situation, which are not realistically connected with what they are intended to neutralize or prevent, or behaviors that are clearly excessive (**modified from DSM-IV, 1994**) Cf Obsession, Obsessive-compulsive disorder, Obsessive-compulsive personality disorder

compulsive buying PSYCHIATRY A behavior disorder that is characterized as 1) Uncontrollable 2) Markedly distressing, time-consuming, and/or resulting in familial, social, vocational, and/or financial difficulties 3) Not occurring in the context of hypomanic or manic symptoms; 19 of 20 compulsive shoppers in one study had a lifetime diagnosis of major mood disorder, 16 had anxiety disorders, 8 had impulse control disorders, and 7 had eating disorders; thymoleptic agents may ameliorate acute exacerbations of 'shoppingosis' (**J Clin Psychiatry 1994; 55:242**)

computer An electronic device that follows programmed instructions written in a logical language and processes the information in binary code; computers were formerly classified into three types, to wit 1) Mainframe computers, capable of simultaneously manipulating large blocks of data, 2) Minicomputer which is capable of performing several logical 'conversations' virtually simultaneously, and 3) Microcomputer, traditionally the slowest, with the storage and memory capabilities Note: The advances in technology and design have erased may of the differences between the microcomputer and the minicomputer, as well as between the minicomputer and a mainframe, leaving the divisions nebulous and of decreasing utility; see AI (artificial intelligence), Buffer, Clone, Database, DOS, Dumb terminal, Electronic publishing, Icon-driven, IBM clone, INIT, Menu, Modem, Mouse, PC, RAM, ROM, RISC chip, SIMM, Smart terminal, Video display terminal, Windows, WYSIWYG

Glossary **AND** A word used in programming that restricts the available logical choices, as both of two conditions must be met for a sequence of logic to be allowed **BAUD** A unit of data transmission equalling 1 bit/sec, named after the French inventor, JME Baudot **BIT** Binary digit A unit of binary system measurement, in which all information is based on the logic of a switch being 'on' or 'off' **BOOT** To load the software into the computer's random access memory **BYTE** 8 bits, equivalent to one typed character **CAD** Computer-assisted design **CHIP** see Microprocessor **COMPILER** A computer program that translates high-level (people) language into bits (machine language) **CPU** Central processing unit; the 'thinking' part of a computer, in microcomputers, the CPU is incorrectly equated to the 'box', which also contains the logic board, the hard and floppy drives **CURSOR** The flashing point on a computer monitor, located at the point of data entry **INTEGRATED CIRCUIT** An electronic circuit mounted on a silicon crystal (chip), which forms the basic unit of a microprocessor **I/O DEVICE** In/Out device Hardware that allows both data input and output, eg modems, disk drives; input only devices include the mouse, keyboard or scanning devices; output only devices include printers and dummy terminals **MACRO** see Programmable key **MAGNETIC CORE MEMORY** The earliest form of computerized data storage, in which each bit of information was represented by a change in the direction (clock- or counterclockwise) of a magnetic field, memory that has long been replaced by semiconductors which are several orders of magnitude smaller **MONITOR** The video display unit for a computer's activity **MS/DOS** Microsoft's disk operating system, the standard disk operating system used in IBM microcomputer models PC, PC/XT and AT and the IBM 'clones' **NUMBER 'CRUNCHING'** A colloquial term for intense and complex mathematical computations, eg three-dimensional rotation of complex molecules and images **OPERATING SYSTEM** The internal system that oversees movement of information between the CPU and the input-output devices **OR** A word used in programming that expands the available logical choices, such that either of two conditions may be met for a sequence of data flow or processing to be allowed **PARALLEL INTERFACE** A port that sends or receives 8 bits at a time **PERIPHERALS** Accessory hardware components including printer, modem, flat-bed scanner, mouse **PORT** The computer gate to the outside world **PROGRAMMABLE KEY** One of the keys, usually an 'F' key, on a microcomputer's standard keyboard, that has been defined or modified to suit the needs of the user, aka 'Macro' **PROMPT** The caret on its side (>) that indicates the drive being accessed **SERIAL INTERFACE** A port that sends out information one bit at a time, as do modems **SPREADSHEET** A software program which provides a flexible format of rows and columns of numerical values for various calculations **VIRTUAL MEMORY** Open-ended random access memory that is 'borrowed' from space on the hard drive

computer-assisted diagnosis A generic term for any use of computer hard- and software to arrive at a diagnosis; while no system is expected to replace the diagnostic acumen of an experienced and well-trained physician, CAD has been used to address specific clinical questions, eg acute abdominal pain, resulting in a 20% improvement of diagnostic accuracy, and a 50% reduction in the rates of perforation and negative laparotomies (**N Engl J Med 1994; 331:1238**c)

computer-based diagnostic system Any of a number of comercially available software programs, eg Dxplain, Iliad, Meditel, QMR that attempt to simulate the clinical decision-making process and provide a diagnosis (**N Engl J Med 1994; 330:1792**ₒₐ)

computer languages BASIC Beginners' all-purpose symbolic instruction code A high-level symbolic computer programming language well-suited for writing programs for mini- and microcomputers; BASIC is a compiled or interpreted language which is both user-friendly and relatively high level **COBOL** Common business-oriented language A slower language, standard in the industry **FOR-TRAN** Formula Translation language A fast, high-level computer language, used for science and math, but less user-friendly than BASIC **MUMPS** Massachusetts General Hospital utility multiprogramming system High-level language program designed to handle large, complex databases

computer virus A short, self-replicating computer program that 'infects' other programs by insinuating its logic into existing programs, known as a 'Trojan horse' virus, then forcing the host program to bear the 'offspring'; a computer virus modifies host programs to include a version of itself, carrying its 'genetic code' in the form of machine language and telling the 'host' system to insert the 'virus' into its main memory—the hard memory; computer viruses can consume memory, execute unwanted operations or delete material ranging from a small file in a microcomputer to wreaking havoc in a mainframe; such viruses may 'infect' corporate, military and hospital networks, destroying vital information; some viruses have been implanted as 'time bombs' destroying information when a sequence of specific commands is given on or after a certain date

computer worm A computer program which is self-contained, that 'lives' off weaknesses in the computer host's logic; the worm may do nothing more than reproduce, ie consume memory and slow the processing of data, but is incapable of 'reinfection'

computerized immunoquantification The use of a computerized image analysis system to quantify an immune reaction, eg that of estrogen and progesterone immunocytochemical assays (ER-ICA, PR-ICA); in contrast to the subjective nature of traditional ER– and PR-ICA analysis, CIQ provides objective and consistent results, with a more rapid turnaround time and is well-suited for use on FNA aspirates of breast carcinoma (Anal Quan Cytol Histol 1993; 15:274)

CON Certificate of need, see there

conantokins *antokin*, Tagalog, sleepy A family of pepides isolated from cone snails that induce local anesthesia and which may be specific for the NMDA receptor; see Conotoxins, 'King-Kong' peptide

concanavalin A IMMUNOLOGY A lectin from the jack bean (*Concanavalin ensiformis*) which is used to stimulate the proliferation of certain subsets of T lymphocytes; Cf PHA and PWM

concentration camp syndrome A psychological complex representing the residual effects of persecution, mental and physical stress, most specifically referring to the survivors of the Nazi concentration camps, although the complex may also be seen in the survivors under the dictatorships of the Khmer Rouge, Pinochet, Idi Amin and others CLINICAL Chronic tension, vigilance, irritability, depression, fear, disordered sleep, nightmares, headaches, fatigue, excess sweating and potentially, complete withdrawal from human contact; see Post-traumatic stress disorder, Survivor syndrome, Torture

concentric contraction SPORTS MEDICINE Muscular contraction that occurs while the muscle is shortening; Cf Eccentric contraction

concept-based routing A format of 'intelligent' computer logic that allows identification of the type of incoming information, eg a patient record that 'belongs' to various areas of the health care system, and sends the relevant parts of the patient record in the appropriate format to the right areas or departments (CAP Today November 1993)

concerted evolution MOLECULAR BIOLOGY The production and maintenance of homogeneity or loss of heterogeneity within repeated multi-gene families that occurs in the genes of individuals and populations, resulting from 'biased' gene conversion, switching genes to a dominant form, rather than having a 'permanent hybrid' genome (Science 1991; 251:308)

concertina nucleus A fanciful descriptor for the large, oval nucleus (figure) with multiple sharp, transverse lines punctuating the cleared nucleoplasm, which is highly characteristic of nuclei in smooth muscle tumors, ie leiomyomas of the GI tract and uterus; CNs may also be seen in diverticulosis coli

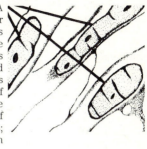

concordance CLINICAL GENETICS The presence of a particular trait in two closely related individuals, eg HLA profile in monozygous twins

concurso ACADEMICS The system of awarding tenured academic positions in Italy which is based on success in a national competition (concurso) which is organized every few years by the ministry of research and universities in Rome; the concursi are a two-stage process in which the applicant's academic achievements are considered by a subject committee; those candidates who are successful in 'round one' are then subjected to an oral examination after which they are assigned to a university by the ministry; the concurso system has been criticized as being open to abuse, as there are no fixed criteria for either stage and members of the assessment committees may use personal influence to support a particular candidate; this translates into too many people with poor publication records being given posts, while making it difficult for expatriate researchers to re-enter the Italian University system and infuse it with new blood (Nature 1994; 369:512N); in the face of the mounting scandal, 8 academics were suspended (Nature 1995; 374:756N)

condition *verb* To subject a person or organism to a set of circumstances that increases functionality

condom A diaphanous device for decreasing STDs; in a longitudinal (20 months) study of couples in which one partner was HIV-positive, use of condoms prevented transmission to the other partner (episodes of intercourse ± 15 000, 124 couples); in 121 couples, condom use was sporadic, and HIV seroconversion occurred at a rate of 4.8/100 person-years (N Engl J Med 1994; 331:341OA, 391ED)

Note: The name condom was first used in English in 1705 by the Duke of Argyll who used a 'Quondam for debauching ladies', although earlier history is murky, as it is unclear whether a Dr Condom existed, nor, despite the Gallic 'amour d'amour' and the ville de Condom in southern France, is there evidence linking the appliance, also known as a 'French letter' with a French origin

condyloma acuminatum An epithelial proliferation induced by HPV of low malignant potential, eg types 6, 11; condylomata may be precursors to malignancy, especially types 16, 18, 31, are at a high risk for future squamous cell carcinoma, but are uncommon in the usual vulvar condylomata TREATMENT IFN-α-2a (JAMA 1991; 265:2684)

cone biopsy GYNECOLOGY A conical biopsy of the uterine cervix that encompasses the ectocervix and endocervical tissue, which is performed as definitive therapy for cervical intraepithelial neoplasia (from CIN1 to CIN3) PROCEDURE A CB is performed under local or general anesthesia, with a scalpel ('cold knife') or with a CO_2 laser COMPLICATIONS Bleeding, infections, cervical stenosis or incompetence; Cf LEEP

coned cecum A concentric fibrotic tapering of the cecum with a grossly patent ileocecal valve, a radiocontrast finding in chronic amebiasis

confection CLINICAL PHARMACOLOGY A generic term for any

pharmacologic preparation that incorporates sugar, honey, or other sweeteners as a means of easing the ingestion of a bitter medicine

confetti lesions DERMATOPATHOLOGY A descriptor for the innumerable, small, scattered hypopigmented macules seen in 96% of patients with tuberous sclerosis, best seen in a darkened room by Wood's UV light

confidence interval STATISTICS A range of values (calculated from observations) of a random sample within which will lie (with a prespecified degree of probability) the true value of a parameter being studied in a given population

confidence limits STATISTICS The endpoints of the confidence interval, a range over which it can be stated with a given probability or 'degree of confidence', that a parameter of interest, eg a mean or standard deviation will be present

confidence profile method STATISTICS A technique used in meta-analysis that allows a worker to examine sources of error or bias, eg lack of subject participation, dropouts, and differences in distributiion of demographic variables (JAMA 1992; 268:2109BR)

confidentiality MEDICAL MALPRACTICE An implied agreement between the physician and patient that all information related by a patient is to be held in the strictest of confidence unless it is illegal and/or dangerous to society; see Anne Sexton, Doctor-patient relationship, Hippocratic oath, Malpractice

The issues of confidentiality extend to the person after death, and include relevant data (eg HIV status) obtained at the time of autopsy; according to the American Medical Association's Council on Ethical and Judicial Affairs, confidentiality should only be violated in cases where there is an ethical obligation to potentially endangered third parties, eg sexual or needle-sharing partners, or those encharged with procuring organs for transplantation (Arch Pathol Lab Med 1992; 116:1120RV)

configurable *adjective* COMPUTERS Pertaining or relating to a computer system that is relatively easy to set-up and implement, administer, and trouble-shoot (Am Lab March 1995, p46)

confined space OCCUPATIONAL MEDICINE A vertically or horizontally limited space in which an employee carries out a specified task, eg boilers, furnaces, manholes, pipelines, pits, vesels, sewers, silos, storage tanks, and utility vaults; because of the high risks associated with working in confined spaces (hundreds of workers die/year, US), OSHA has proposed regulations (29 CFR 1910.146) governing how an employee can work in confined spaces

Note: ½ of those dying are would-be rescuers who attempt to rescue the stricken worker

confirmation LABORATORY MEDICINE Verification of the results obtained from a screening method; a **confirmation method** is more sensitive and usually more expensive, labor-intensive and complex than a screening method; confirmation methods are 'gold standards' for detection, and may have medicolegal import, as they can in a court of law be used to determine liability in accidents, homicide, to terminate employment; in toxicology, confirmation methods include gas chromatography, and high-performance thin-layer chromatography; in infectious disease, Western blot hybridization is widely regarded as **confirmatory** for HIV infection; Cf Screening

conflict 1) '*An emotional tension resulting from incompatible inner needs or drives.*' (Webster's New Collegiate Dictionary) 2) Collision, clash 3) War, battle

conflict of interest ETHICS The actual (or potential for) compromise of decision-making capacities because a party has a vested interest in etc; physicians have a conflict of interest when their interests or commitments compromise their independent judgement or loyalty to patients; there are 6 conflicts of interest areas in the current medical environment–all offer physicians self-serving incentives to generate services and channel referrals: 1) 'Kickbacks' for referrals 2) Physician investment and self-referral 3) Dispensing drugs, selling medical products and performing ancillary medical services 4) Hospital purchase of physicians' practices 5) Hospital payments to recruit and bond physicians 6) Gifts from medical suppliers or drug companies (N Engl J Med 1993; 329:892OA) see Kickbacks, Safe harbor rules RESEARCH That which occurs when a person is presumed to be unduly compromised in his objectivity as he has a vested interest or bias in the analysis of data that might affect him financially Note: When a researcher has commercial ties with a business that would benefit from his research, the potential for bias is significant; Harvard University's guidelines (Science 1990; 248:154) are the most stringent, delineating both the conflict of interest and conflict of commitment, where no more than 20% of a working week should be dedicated to an outside interest; see Harvard's guidelines, Krimsky index

confocal microscope A variant of light microscopy in which the light is focused in one plane allowing the organelles to be viewed in vivo below the cell membrane, producing high-resolution 2- and 3-dimensional images with light, allowing imaging of cells in vivo; in confocal microscopy, light is focused by an objective lens into an hourglass-shaped beam so a bright waist of light strikes the object at a selected depth of a specimen; then the light reflected from the waist of light is focused to a point and allowed to pass and allowed to pass in its entirety through a pinhole opening in a mask positioned in front of a detector; the opaque regions surrounding the pinhole block most of the light rays reflected by illuminated parts of the specimen above and below the plane of interest (which would obscure the resulting image); the light is moved rapidly through various points in the specimen until the entire plane is imaged (Sci Am 1994; 270/8:40) see Microscopy

conformation MOLECULAR BIOLOGY The 3-D configuration of a molecule in space, which is a function of the molecule(s), whether they are arranged in a chain, the types of bonds, the energy of the system, and the presence of other molecules in the system; see Protein folding

confounding variable Confounder A factor that distorts the true relationship of the variables being examined in a study with the end-point changes in those same variables, by virtue of being related in a nonlinear fashion to those variables, extraneous to the study question and unequally distributed between the study groups

confronting cisternae An ultrastructural finding consisting of lamellar layering of Golgi-related structures, which had been described as specific for HIV-infection, but which is also found in herpes-infected cells, sarcomas, hepatomas, giant cell tumor of bone and multiple sclerosis; Cf Tubular reticular structures

congener Any member of a family of related molecules

congenic mice Inbred strains of mice that are genetically identical except at one locus or well-defined group of loci; a line of congeneic mice is produced by eliminating those mice with background genes of less interest while at the same time backcrossing the progeny bearing the characteristics and by extension, the gene(s) of interest

congenic strain MOLECULAR BIOLOGY A strain of organisms, eg mice that differs from another in the region of a single genetic locus, which is produced by 10 or more backcrosses or intercrosses to the control strain; congenic strains can be used to evaluate a mutation or allelic variant of against an inbred strain background of interest (Science 1994; 264:1725) Cf Inbred strain

congenital (lipoid) adrenal hyperplasia An group of AR conditions characterized by a partial or complete defect of enzymes (most commonly steroid 21-hydroxylase) involved in the synthesis of cortisol by the adrenal cortex; the lack of cortisol results in an ↑ in ACTH (due to a loss of feedback inhibition), which in turn leads to hypertrophy and hyperplasia of the adrenal cortex and ↑ production of mineralocorticosteroids and androgenic steroids, which explains the clinical findings of virilization, salt loss, and hypertension MOLECULAR PATHOLOGY Dissecting the pathogenesis of CAH had proven difficult, as the absence of P450scc activity was functional (not structural); it now believed that the defect lies in StAR, an acutely regulated mitochondrial protein that activates steroidogenesis in heterologous systems, which is intimately linked to the mobilization of cholesterol from lipid stores to the vicinity of the side chain cleavage enzyme P450scc in the inner mitochondrial membrane (Science 1995; 267:1828, 1780) see StAR

congenital agranulocytosis Congenital neutropenia, see there

congenital bilateral absence of vas deferens CBAVD A condition that is responsible for 1-2% of ♂ infertility and 6% of obstructive azoospermia; CBAVD is present in ± 95% of ♂ with cystic fibrosis MOLECULAR PATHOLOGY In most patients there is a mutation of the *CFTR* (cystic fibrosis transmembrane conductance regulator) gene, with a copy of the *5T* allele in one copy of the *CFTR* gene and a cystic fibrosis-type mutation in the other copy of the *CFTR* gene (N Engl J Med 1995; 332:1475oa)

congenital cystic adenomatoid malformation PEDIATRIC PATHOLOGY A rare developmental defect of the lungs characterized by abnormal cystic spaces; CCAM has been divided into three types; most are type 1, which has a good prognosis and large (3-10 cm) cysts lined by ciliated columnar epithelium (Arch Pathol Lab Med 1994; 118:1034oa)

congenital diabetes Fetal diabetic 'syndrome', see there

congenital dyserythropoietic anemia A group of inherited conditions characterized by multinuclearity of erythroblasts, nuclear budding, karyorrhexis, mitotic abnormalities, premature extrusion of nucleus, internuclear bridging, nuclear-cytoplasmic maturational dyssynchrony, cytoplasmic vacuolization, basophilic stippling and siderotic granules CLINICAL Lifelong familial mild-to-moderate anemia and ineffective erythropoiesis

CDA, type I Megaloblastosis, Cabot type AR condition characterized by macrocytic anemia, binuclearity, internuclear bridging, Cabot rings and anti-I antibodies

CDA, type II HEMPAS, Degas type AR condition that comprises 65% of CDA characterized by normocytic anemia, bi- and multi-nuclearity of erythroblasts, pluripolar mitoses with karyorrhexis, anti-I antiantibodies; see HEMPAS

CDA, type III Swedish or Bjoekman type AD condition characterized by erythroid gigantoblasts, less than 12 nuclei and macrocytic anemia

'CDA, type IV' Inherited dyserythropoiesis that does not fall into neat categories

congenital gout *gutta*, Latin, droplet A usually acquired condition that the ancients considered to occur 'droplet by droplet'; congenital gout is linked to 2 X-linked enzymes

1) Hypoxanthine-guanine phosphoribosyl transferase (HGPRT), which is defective in Lesch-Nyhan disease and

2) 5-phosphoribosyl-1-pyrophosphate (PRPP); gout is intimately linked to ↑ serum uric acid, often ≥ 410 μmol/L (US: 7.0 mg/ml), a level found in a significant minority of ♂ (90% of gout occurs in ♂); the indigestible monosodium urates in the synovium stimulate the release of lysosomal enzymes from neutrophils, the crystals of which remain undigested, causing a vicious cycle, in which crystals are ingested but not digested, although lytic enzyme is released, the end-result of which is joint destruction; family history can be evoked in ± ½ of cases; ½ of cases present with the classic 'podagra' (first metatarsophalangeal joint) and up to 90% will suffer podagra at some time during their disease ACUTE TREATMENT Colchicine, NSAIDs, corticosteroids INTERVAL TREATMENT Dietary CHRONIC TREAT-

MENT Allopurinol, sulfinpyrazone, salicylates

congenital generalized hypertrichosis Wolfman syndrome A rare X-R [MIM 307150] condition characterized by hair everywhere that spares only the palmoplantar area; it is postulated that the condition represents an atavistic mutation, ie one that has been suppressed during the course of evolution (New York Times 31 May 1995; C10)

congenital iodine deficiency disorder Endemic cretinism, see there

congenital malformation Birth defect A generic term* encompassing a heterogenous group of structural abnormalities usually identified at birth including clubfoot, genital, limb, or cardiac defect, cleft lip and/or palate, spina bifida and others; in one report 2.5% of first-born children have CMs; mothers of first-borns with CMs are 2.4-fold more likely to have a second infant with a CM, and a 7.6-fold increased risk of having the same defect; in women who lived in the same municipality during both pregnancies, the relative risk of having a second infant with the same defect was 11.6 compared to 5.1 in those who had moved to another muncipality between pregnancies (N Engl J Med 1994; 331:1oa)

*The informal term is birth defect, formal written form is congenital malformation; other synonyms include congenital abnormality, defect, or deformity

congenital malignancy Neoplasia that appears at or shortly after birth; as spontaneous remission is not uncommon in these tumors, some of these 'malignancies' may represent hyperplastic reactive albeit monotonous proliferations; examples: Leukemia (often an aggressive disease), sarcoma (although histologically malignant, clinically benign), melanoma (potentially transplacental), and neuroblastoma

congenital melanoma A rare lesion that develops in utero, arising in melanocytic nevi, in large or giant congenital nevi. or less commonly is acquired transplacentally; CMs may grow rapidly, ulcerate, and bleed; nodal metastases and visceral involvement should be ruled out; absence of metastases at the time of initial examination correlates poorly with survival; the behavior of CMs is unpredictable (N Engl J Med 1995; 332:656rv) see Melanoma

congenital neutropenia Congenital agranulocytosis, Kostmann's disease A rare AR [MIM 202700] disease characterized by ↓ neutrophils in the circulation and arrested maturation of myeloid precursors CLINICAL Recurring bacterial infections and mucocutaneous ulcers MOLECULAR GENETICS A nonsense mutation in the G-CSF receptor gene results in production of a truncated G-CSF receptor that confers a growth signal but not a differentiation signal to the transfected cells PROGNOSIS Poor; most die in first decade of life THERAPY G-CSF may prove useful (N Engl J Med 1994; 330:839rv) see Hematopoietic growth factor receptor

congenital nevus An uncommon (1:1-20 000 neonates) lesion that is often larger than acquied melanocytic nevi; extremely large CNs, known as garment nevi, occur in 1:500 000 newborns; ⅓ of prepubertal melanomas arise in large CNs; rarely other neuroectodermal neoplasms arise in CNs, eg neuroblastomas (N Engl J Med 1995; 332:656rv) see Garment nevus, Melanoma

congenital rubella syndrome A malformation complex in a fetus infected in vitro by a mother with active rubella ('German measles'); the malformations are consonant with the embryologic stage at the time of infection, with developmental arrest affecting all 3 embryonal layers, inhibiting mitosis, causing delayed and defective organogenesis of involved tissues; maternal infection in the first eight weeks of pregnancy causes embryopathy in 50-70% of fetuses; the susceptible period extends to about the 20th week; infection in late pregnancy is associated with little fetal morbidity CLINICAL Cardiac malformations, eg patent ductus arteriosus, pulmonary valve stenosis, ventricular septal defect, hepatosplenomegaly, interstitial pneumonia, low birth weight, congenital cataracts, deafness, microcephaly, petechia, purpura, and CNS symptoms including mental retardation, lethargy, irritability, dystonia, bulging fontanelles and ataxia LABORATORY Viral isolation, detection of specific IgM antibodies in the fetus by hemagglutination inhibition VACCINATION Attenuated live virus vaccine is administered to all children between the ages of 15 months and puberty; effective antibodies develop after immunization in 95% of patients; in 1986, 11 cases of congenital rubella were reported in the US; see Extended rubella syndrome

congenital toxoplasmosis A transplacental infection with the protozoan *Toxoplasma gondii* affecting ± ⅓ of fetuses of ♀ with acute acquired toxoplasmosis, most severely if the infection occurs in 1st trimester; often normal at birth, blindness and mental retardation may ensue INCIDENCE 1-10/10 000 CLINICAL Hydrocephalus, microcephaly, cerebral calcifications, cerebral atrophy, chorioretinitis, uveitis and vitritis, convulsions, hyperbilirubinemia, hepatomegaly DIAGNOSIS PCR of amniotic fluid to detect 35-fold repeat *B1* gene of *T gondii* Sensitivity 97.4% (vs 89.5% with conventional parasitologic methods); PCR may be done in a day (**N Engl J Med 1994; 331:695oa**) LABORATORY Serological screening (see TORCH) with toxoplasma-specific IgM immunoassay TREATMENT Pyrimeth-amine, sulfadiazine, leukovorin (**N Engl J Med 1994; 330:1858oa**)

congestive heart failure '...*a complex clinical syndrome characterized by abnormalities of left ventricular function and neurohormonal regulation, which are accompanied by effort intolerance, fluid retention, and reduced longevity.*' (**M Packer, via E Braunwald, Heart Disease, 4th ed, WB Saunders, Philadelphia, 1992**) TREATMENT Inotropic agents that increase intracellular sodium, eg vesnarinone (**N Engl J Med 1993; 329:149oa**); vesnarinone appears to have a narrow therapeutic range FUTURE DIRECTIONS Enhanced myocardial function has been demonstrated in transgenic mice that overexpress the β_2-adrenergic receptor, resulting in an increase in myocardial adenylyl cyclase activity and increased ventricular function, suggesting that a gene therapy approach may be of use in treating CHF (**Science 1994; 264:582r**)

conglutinin IMMUNOLOGY A collagen-rich polymeric plasma protein produced by Bovidae, which has been found to be a specific ligand for 1C3b, and therefore agglutinates complement-bound cells and particles, only in the presence of calcium ions

Congo-Crimean hemorrhagic fever A tick-borne infection by Bunyaviridiae, seen in Eastern Europe, Central Asia, Middle East, Africa CLINICAL After a 3-6 day incubation, abrupt headache, myalgia, fever, chills, nausea, watery stools, anorexia; conjunctivitis, leukemia, severe thrombocytopenia PROGNOSIS 10-50% mortality

conicotine A metabolite of nicotine that may remain at detectable levels in the circulation for up to a week after a last cigarette; measurement of urinary conicotine is used by insurance companies to determine whether subjects applying for health and/or life insurance are indeed non-smokers and entitled to lower premium costs, as non-smokers are in general healthier; see Nicotine, Smoking

Conidiobolus coronatus A rarely pathogenic fungus that most commonly causes nasal (eg chronic rhinofacial zygomycosis) and soft tissue infections in the tropics and subtropics, which may on occasion infect immunocompromised hosts (**Am J Clin Pathol 1992; 98:559oa**) PATHOLOGY Focal necrosis, granulomata, prominent eosinophilic sleeves (Splendore-Hoeppli phenomenon), and fibrosis

conization GYNECOLOGY The surgical excision of a conical portion of the uterine cervix to treat CIN (cervical intraep-

ithelial neoplasia), circumscribed foci of carcinoma in situ, microinvasive squamous cell carcinoma, occasionally, condylomas*; the excised cone includes any grossly identifiable lesions of the ectocervix, and extends into the endocervix, which usually encompasses the majority of squamous cell neoplasias of the cervix

*Because condylomas are known to undergo spontaneous regression, it is not common practice to excise them

conjugal malignancy Neoplasia affecting marriage partners is low; the risk of suffering rare malignancy, eg glioma in non-related persons living together is extremely low $1/10^8$; in the face of such events and the absence of consanguity, environmental factors, eg carcinogens and/or viruses weigh heavily in the etiologic 'equation'

connectin Titin, see there

connective tissue disease Autoimmune disease, collagen (vascular) disease* A generic term for a group of diseases that have in common widespread immunologic and inflammatory alterations of connective tissue CLINICAL Arthritis, connective tissue defects, endocarditis, myositis, nephritis, pericarditis, pleuritis, synovitis, vasculitis LABORATORY Antinuclear antibodies, direct antiglobulin (Coombs') test positive hemolytic anemia, leukopenia, thrombocytopenia, ↑ or ↓ Igs, rheumatoid factors, biological false positive test for syphilis TYPES Ankylosing spondylitis, dermatomyositis, inflammatory bowel disease-related arthritis, polychondritis, polymyalgia rheumatica, polymyositis, psoriatic arthritis, rheumatoid arthritis, Sjögren syndrome, SLE, systemic sclerosis, and vasculitis (**N Engl J Med 1994; 330:1697oa**)

*A universally accepted name for this family of conditions does not exist; autoimmune disease is preferred by some authors, but not all the members of the group have identifiable autoimmune phenomena; connective tissue disease, while somewhat more ecumenical, is not applicable to all; and finally, the term collagen disease is problematic, in that acquired 'collagen diseases' are synonymous with other members of this group, while inherited diseases of collagen (eg Marfan disease, Ehlers-Danlos disease) are designated (**Dorland's Medical Dictionary, 28th edition, WB Saunders, Philadelphia, 1994**) 'collagen disorders', which might be viewed by some medical lexicographers as an absurdity

connexins A family of at least 12 proteins, each of which is the product of a distinct gene, and which form the intercellular membrane channels of gap junctions; all have 4-membrane spanning domains and cytoplasmic NH2 and COOH termini; accumulating data indicates the connexin family is important in physiologic and developmental process (**Science 1995; 267:1831**)

connexin 37 A protein that is abundant in the lungs and belongs to a family of transmembrane proteins that form intercellular hydrophilic channels, the gap junctions; other connexins may act as tumor-suppressor genes and down-regulated in breast carcinomas (**Nature 1994; 369:67l**)

connexin43 A gene that encodes connexin43, a major protein of the cardiac gap junctions that forms membrane-spanning hexameric hemichannels (connexons), which in conjunction with apposed cell membranes forms a hydrophobic channel through which ions, metabolites and other molecules involved in signal transduction can move from one cell to another; mutation in the gap junction gene, *connexin43* leads to defective regulation in cell-cell communication and is associated with visceroatrial heterotaxia (**N Engl J Med 1995; 332:1323oa, Science 1995; 267:1796, 1772**)

connexon see Gap junction

conotoxin Any of a family of 10-30 residue in length toxic peptides that act as high affinity ligands for various receptors and ion channels, produced by cone snails (*Conus*, of which there are 500 known species, each producing a unique assortment of toxins); conotoxins have a wide variety of effects, including inhibition of acetylcholine receptors, local anesthesia and blockage of ion channels that regulate the flow of potassium, sodium and calcium ions; the diverse spectrum of venomous peptides may result from a 'fold-lock-cut' synthetic pathway, one toxin binds a type of glutamate receptor (NMDA receptor, see there); the snails appear to have evolved a battery of toxins as a necessity to simultaneously act on multiple subclasses of ion channels in order to quickly stop their prey

consanguinity A state of close genetic relationship, affecting the progeny of a mating and marriage between close blood relatives, eg first cousins, an event accounting for 20-50% of marriages from Asia and Africa, which is associated with increased gross fertility due to younger maternal age at first live birth, and increased morbidity and mortality in the offspring; adverse effects of inbreeding are uncommon (**Science 1991; 252:789**); see Bottleneck, Inbreeding

CONSENSUS II Cooperative New Scandinavian Enalapril Survival Study II (see**N Engl J Med 1992; 327:678oa**) see Enalapril, SOLVD

consent A voluntary yielding of a person's free will to that of another; in medicine, the term refers to either a formal document or verbal agreement* by the patient that gives permission to perform a therapeutic or diagnostic procedure; any operation or intervention performed without consent constitutes assault and battery, see 'ghost surgery'; even if an operation is successful, punitive damages may be awarded, as lack of consent constitutes an intentional invasion of another's rights; thus all elective diagnostic or therapeutic procedures require an 'informed consent' document

*Given the medicolegal ramifications of a verbal agreement that may be later contested in a court of law, verbal consent is facing 'extinction'

conservative *adjective* Pertaining or referring to that which is not aggressive (eg conservative therapy), experimental or innovative, excessively high (eg estimation of data), or radical (eg conservative surgery)

conservative therapy The management of a clinical nosology with the least aggressive of therapeutic options, often equated with 'medical' as opposed to 'surgical' treatment, eg drug, diet, and lifestyle management of severe but asymptomatic coronary atherosclerosis, in contrast to aggressive management of the same condition with coronary artery bypass surgery; see Benign neglect, Palliative therapy; Cf 'Heroic' therapy, Radical surgery

consistent with CLINICAL DECISION MAKING A widely used term among practitioners of the 'visual arts' of medicine (ie pathology and radiology) in which diagnoses are based on the subjective interpretation of various types of images

Note; The statement 'consistent with' is used when the pathologist or radiologist is relatively (but not absolutely) certain of the diagnosis for a particular lesion, but at the same time wishes to 'cover himself' for the potential legal ramifications should the lesion prove to be something else

consolidation chemotherapy ONCOLOGY A phase of therapy for leukemia or other lymphoproliferative malignancies that follows the initial 'intensification' phase of chemotherapy, in which a patient is given (as an example), several cycles of 3 days of daunorubicin followed by 7 days of cytarabine (ara-C), separated by a resting period of 2-3 weeks; objective response is then 'consolidated' by one or two more identical cycles of chemotherapy, which in turn is followed by the maintenance phase Note: In AML, both autologous and allogeneic BM transplantation result in better disease-free survival than intensive consolidation chemotherapy with cytarabine and daunorubicin (**N Engl J Med 1995; 332:217oa**)

constant region IMMUNOLOGY The highly conserved portion of an immunoglobulin molecule that can be separated from the whole molecule by partial digestion with either papain or pepsin, forming a crystallizable fragment (Fc), for which certain cells, eg macrophages have a specific Fc receptor; see Fc, Variable region

constellation PSYCHIATRY A group of related thoughts that surround a core idea, or a 'universe' of factors that result in a particular action or effect

Note: Although this term was preferred by Jung, it is essentially equivalent to the more widely preferred term 'complex' (eg Oedipus complex)

constitutional 1) Involving the entire organism, ie systemic 2) Biologically fixed or immutable, which in genetics refers to an inherited genotype that is present in all tissues

constitutional disease 1) A virtually extinct term for any disease of the 'constitution', usually understood to be inherited 2) A disease '...that involves a system of organs or one characterized by widespread symptoms.' (**Dorland's Medical Dictionary, 28th edition, WB Saunders, Philadelphia, 1994**)

constrictive pericarditis A condition characterized by a chronic fibrous thickening of the wall of the pericardial sac which is so contracted to the point that normal diastolic filling of the heart does not occur ETIOLOGY Infections, connective-tissue disorders, malignancy, trauma, metabolic disorders, eg uremia, radiation therapy, sarcoidosis, asbestosis, previous myocardial infarction (**N Engl J Med 1994; 330:127cpc**)

consult *noun* 1) A formal consultation from another health care professional on the diagnosis, therapy, or prognosis of a disease, see Consultation 2) A physician's office *verb* To engage in a formal tête-á-tête with another health care professional

consultant A respected individual or practitioner who is well qualified to render an opinion in the field in which his opinion is sought; the consultant's status is determined by his/her training, experience, and competence; the consultant has an advisory role only, and his/her recommendations may or may not be accepted by the physician of record, and has no formal relation with patient; see Second opinion; Cf Expert witness

consultation Consult A formal (or less commonly, informal) second opinion obtained from a consultant, which is sought by an attending physician regarding a diagnosis or therapeutic plan being considered in the context of patient management

consultation staff The body of physicians, dentists, osteopaths, or independent medical practitioners who have attained a certain level of professional distinction (ie status of consultant), who maintain private or other practices outside of the hospital or health care institution for which they are consultants

consumer choice Market-based approach HEALTH CARE ENVIRONMENT A component of proposed health care reform in the US that is modeled after the Federal Employee Health Benefits Program proposed by the conservative Heritage Foundation; CC gives the consumer opportunity and incentive to 'shop around' for insurance; everyone gets a tax credit for purchasing insurance, which is mandatory; there is no tax credit for companies that provide insurance (**Am Med News 26 October 1992, p7**)

contact sport SPORTS MEDICINE Any sport in which body contact is either an integral component of the sporting activity per se (eg boxing, football, martial arts, rugby, wrestling) or commonly occurs while engaged in the sporting activity (eg basketball, hockey, lacrosse); a major concern of contact sports in the current environment is the possibility of trauma-induced abrasions and cuts might result in hemorrhage and blood contact among players, who might have blood-transmissible infections

contact inhibition The inhibitory effect of normal cells on each others' growth, such that lateral contact prevents further cellular expansion, a feature of normal cells grown in tissue culture medium

contact inhibiting factor A factor that induces reversion of certain growth characteristics of cancer cells to a more 'normal' appearance in tissue culture media; CIF induces contact inhibition (once normal cells have spread out in a monolayer, further growth is inhibited), anchorage dependence (normal cells will not grow in a suspension), and dependence on serum-based 'growth factors'; CIF may induce tumor regression in hamsters with melanomas

contact lenses 18.2 million people in the USA (FDA estimate) wear contact lenses, 50% wear soft contacts, 25% hard contacts and 25% use extended-wear soft lenses that cause a 4-fold increase in ulcerative keratitis; disposble soft type ↑ the risk of ulcerative keratitis (Arch Ophthalmol 1992; 110:1555)

contact ring FORENSIC PATHOLOGY A funnel-shaped depression of the skin with marginal abrasion and bruising of the epidermis caused by a zero range or 'execution' type gunshot wound that leaves a 'fingerprint' of the firearm's muzzle; see Execution

contagion INFECTIOUS DISEASE A term of waning popularity for 1) *The transmission of an infectious disease from one person to another...*' (International Dictionary of Medicine, J Wiley & Sons, New York, 1986) and 2) An infectious disease

containment PUBLIC HEALTH The confining or prevention of further dissemination of a potentially hazardous, eg biologic, radioactive or toxic, agent(s)

PRIMARY CONTAINMENT Protection of personnel and immediate environment from the agent, use of proper safety equipment and for some biologic agents, the use of vaccines

SECONDARY CONTAINMENT Protection of the environment external to the 'contained' area which is provided by a combination of facility design and operational practices see Biosafety levels, Regulated waste

contaminated data RESEARCH ETHICS A set of data some of which is flawed, either inadvertedly ('sloppy science') or intentionally (fraudulent)

contaminated sharp Any contaminated (by blood, pathogenic organisms, and so on) object that can penetrate the skin including, but not limited to, needles, scalpels, broken glass, broken capillary tubes, and exposed ends of dental wires (Federal Register Dec 6, 1991, p 64175)

contamination CLINICAL RESEARCH A bias that is introduced in a double-blinded study when one or more components of an intervention in the study arm is unitentionally introduced in the 'negative' or control arm; as an example, geriatricians' advice may be unconsciously integrated into the knowledge base of nonintervention arm physicians in a blinded study of the effects of geriatric interventions (N Engl J Med 1995; 332:1377ED) PUBLIC HEALTH The presence of any foreign or undesired material in a system, eg toxic contamination of the ground water in an ecosystem or viral contamination of a tissue culture plate

contiguity theory A theory that attempts to answer why the spread of malignancy in the lymph nodes of Hodgkin's disease occurs in a distinctly nonrandom fashion; it is postulated that the lymphoma spreads from an initial focus to adjacent lymph nodes, transmigrating to more distal organs, leaving no trace in the initial sites of spread; this theory is tenuous as 1) The often-involved spleen has no lymphatic vessels and 2) All peripheral nodes may be involved without intervening mediastinal involvement

continence Self-control with regard to defecation, sexual activity, and urinatioin

continent Pertaining or referring to continence

continental scale metro-agro-plex ATMOSPHERIC SCIENCES A neologism referring to one of three regions (eastern North America, Europe, eastern China and Japan) that are characterized by their large size and the intimate intermingling of agricultural and urban industrial activities; these regions comprise 23% of the earth's land, consume 60% of the world food production and food exports; the CSMAPs consume 75% of the fossil fuels and fertilizer, which accounts for more than one-half of the atmospheric nitrogen oxide (NO_x) emissions with a consequent increase in ground-level ozone (O_3) pollution which reduces crop yields (Science 1994; 264:33RN)

contingency fee LEGAL MEDICINE A fee arranged between a client and attorney, whereby the attorney represents a client with compensation based on a percentage of the money being recovered in a lawsuit, eg 25% if the case is settled (out-of-court), 30% is the case goes to trial; the contingency fee system allows a person with limited finances to seek just retribution for legitimate claims (N Engl J Med 1994; 330:11236C), but is alleged to foster greed and avarice for large settlements on the part of attorneys

contingency table STATISTICS A classification of data points which are divided according to two qualitative attributes, each of which may be divided into two or more subgroups; one attribute may be represented by rows, the other by columns

continuing medical education CME, see there

continuous ambulatory peritoneal dialysis Peritoneal dialysis, see there

continuous positive airway pressure A type of artificial ventilation in which the lung pressure is maintained above atmospheric pressure through the entire respiratory cycle; CPAP has proven effective in both salt water drowning, and in fresh water drowning, where the improvement of the V/Q ratio is most reliable when combined with mechanical ventilation (N Engl J Med 1993; 328:523RA, Mayo Clin Proc 1994; 69:244)

continous quality improvement An organization-wide process in which all individuals (leaders, workers, and clients) and activities (resources, processes, and outcomes) strive to achieve a common goal; CQI is regarded as the next level for improving products and processes after quality assurance (see there) and total quality management (see there) (CAP Today November 1993)

continuous-read blood culture system MICROBIOLOGY A recently developed device in the clinical microbiology laboratory that monitors the growth of microorganism, allowing the early detection of potential pathogens (eg *Bacteroides fragilis, Candida albicans, Clostridium perfringens, Pseudomonas aeruginosa, Haemophilus influenzae, Torulopsis glabrata*) and initiation of therapy, while reducing the hands-on time required of manual or semiautomatic batch processing (CAP Today May, 1994)

continuous-read device LABORATORY MEDICINE An instrument that makes multiple (eg every 10-15 minutes) measurements of a particular parameter, eg production of CO_2 in blood cultured for bacteria or fungi, which is detected either by a photodetector, or by a pressure detector; these instruments improve turnaround time for certain laboratory results, and offer greater hand-off capability (CAP Today May 1993)

contraceptive Any method for preventing a fertilized, term product of conception, including barrier methods (condoms, diaphragm), hormone combinations, spermicides, implantable hormonal contraceptives, RU-486 and others; population growth is having an increasing impact on the health of society and its control is being addressed on international fora, see Amsterdam strategy, although not all governments believe this is a problem, see Mexico City policy; contraceptives under development include spermicides with antiviral properties, a reliable ovulation predictor, reliable and reversible male sterilization, male contraception, an antifertility vaccine once-a-month pill, designed to induce menses at a designated time, without disturbing subsequent menstrual periods; see 'Litogen', Pearl index, Wrongful birth

Note: The US litigation system is considered by some to be the primary impediment to development of anything beyond well-intentioned rhetoric, given the claims of unforeseen embryopathy

contractile smooth muscle cell see Smooth muscle cell

contraction alkalosis A reduced extracellular fluid compartment with increased extracellular bicarbonate and increased bicarbonate resorption in the renal tubules, a finding characteristic of chronic furosemide therapy TREATMENT Discontinue therapy and substitute acetazolamide (carbonic anhydrase inhibitor) until metabolic derangement is corrected

contraction band necrosis A nonspecific finding in irreversibly ischemic myocytes, which is often the only, albeit unreliable histologic change seen in hyperacute myocardial infarction, where central coagulated cells are arrested in the relaxed state and reperfusion around the infarct results in cell death 'frozen' in a hypercontracted state, spanning the cell's width (figure) PATHOLOGY Hypercontracted, structureless masses of contractile protein and transverse eosinophilic bands span the myocyte in ischemic zones, early mononuclear inflammation is followed by acute inflammation EM Thickened and 'compacted' Z bands PATHOGENESIS ↑ Ca++ in cells due to increased sarcolemmal permeability with irreversible anoxia and shock, probably catecholamine-mediated

Note: Contraction bands also occur in cardiac muscle in selenium deficiency in Keshan disease and in skeletal muscle in Duchenne and Becker types of muscular dystrophy

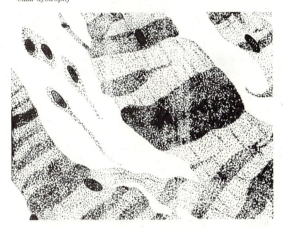

contraction band necrosis

contragestion Any contraceptive method that specifically prevents the gestation of a fertilized egg, eg the 'morning after' pill or RU-486, either by making viable implantation uninhabitable or by promoting the fertilized product's expulsion; the term was introduced by E-E Baulieu, the 'father' of RU-486, specifically in reference to postfertilization interruption of the gestational process (**Science 1989; 245:1351RV**) see Contraceptive, RU-486

contraindication A generic term for any reason or circumstance that would preclude the use of a particular form of therapy; contraindications may be relative–eg abdominal surgery in acute pancreatitis, formerly regarded as a 'kiss of death' or absolute–eg the use of thrombolytic therapy in active internal bleeding, recent head trauma or intracranial neoplasia, suspected pregnancy, and others

contrast bath SPORTS MEDICINE A bath designed to produce alternating vasodilation and vasoconstriction or to reduce subacute or gravity-dependent edema; in a typical CB, the water temperature is cycled between 40-43°C (5 minutes) and 10-15° (1-2 minutes), ending on a cold cycle (**JC DeLee, D Drez, Jr, Eds, Orthopedic Sports Medicine WB Saunders, Philadelphia, 1994**)

contrast-induced nephropathy Acute renal failure that occurs in 2-16% of those who have had radiocontrast studies of the kidney; diabetics do not appear to be at higher risk than other subjects, although those with diabetic nephropathy, pre-existing renal insufficiency and congestive heart failure are at higher risk for nephropathy and

studies suggest that the incidence of this condition would be reduced by use of non-ionic, low-osmolality contrast agents

contrast medium RADIOLOGY A substance with a density differing from that of the organ or structure being imaged, which allows delineation of abnormalities of contour; contrast media that are more radiopaque (usually containing barium or iodine) than the organ or structure being analyzed may be designated as positive contrast media, while those that are less radiopaque, eg air, are known as negative contrast media

contrecoup TRAUMATOLOGY A cerebral 'bruise' diametrically opposite the site of the impinging blow to the cranium; the head is in motion and the brain lags behind by a split-second; a blow to the back of the head results in lesions of the frontal lobes and horns of the temporal lobes; a blow to the top of the skull results in contrecoup lesions to the hippocampus and the corpus callosum; in 'Coup' lesions, the head is stationary and receives a blow; the brain lesion is directly below the site of the injury

Note: Contrecoup injury also occurs in blunt pulmonary trauma, and is characterized by subpleural capillary disruption, hemorrhage, edema, infiltration by leukocytes, protein, and fluid obstruction of the small airways

Contreras method A proprietary form of unproven cancer therapy based on the use of laetrile and administered in a private 'clinica' in Tijuana, Mexico; see Laetrile, Tijuana, Unproven forms of cancer therapy

contributory negligence Contributory neglect MEDICAL MALPRACTICE Conduct on the part of the plaintiff, which occurred after he/she came under the physician's care, that falls below that which a reasonable person would exercise for his own protection, thereby contributing to the alleged act of negligence; see Malpractice

control CLINICAL RESEARCH A group of subjects with features similar to an experimental or treatment group, in whom no intervention is undertaken; a control population is required in order to assure validity of the results; see Double blinding, Zelen design LABORATORY MEDICINE A specimen having known or standardized values for an analyte that is processed in tandem with an unknown specimen; the 'control' specimen is either known to have the substance being analyzed, ie 'positive' control or known to lack a substance of interest, ie 'negative' control THEORETICAL MEDICINE A method for altering chaotic phenomena, eg heart rate, in which exact periodicity is imposed on the system, which appears to cause a dynamic deterioration of chaotic systems (**Sci Am 1994; 271/5:24**) Cf Anticontrol

control measurement points see Energy medicine

controllable life-style specialty 'Regulated' specialty A field of medical specialization that can be scheduled in terms of work hours, CLSs include anesthesiology*, dermatology, emergency medicine, physical medicine, support specialties (pathology, radiation oncology, radiology), and surgical specialties* (**JAMA 1992; 268:2060sc**) Cf Noncontrollable life-style specialty

*With the obvious exception being unscheduled emergency procedures

controlled drug substance A generic term for a drug or therapeutic agent with potential for abuse or substance with potential for addiction, held under strict governmental control, delineated by the Comprehensive Drug Abuse Prevention and Control Act and passed by the US Congress in 1970, requiring that such substances be prescribed only by a licensed physician, with stringent control of registration, reporting, record keeping, prescribing these substances; misuse or questionable practices of prescribing controlled substances may lead to investigation, penalties and potential punitive action(s)

Note: The Drug Enforcement Administration, a branch of the Department of Justice, was created to enforce the Controlled Substances Act, gather intelligence and conduct research in the area of dangerous drugs and drug abuse;

the Act classified these potentially addicting drugs into five groups or 'schedules' (table) that differ on the stringency of control, conditions of record keeping and prescribing forms (paperwork) required for their use

CONTROLLED DRUG SUBSTANCES

SCHEDULE I DRUGS High abuse potential, no accepted medical use in the US, eg Acetorphine, bufotenine, dextromoramide, etorphine, hashish, heroin, LSD (N,N-diethyl-D-lysergamide or lysergic acid diethylamide), marijuana, mescaline, PCP (Phencyclidine), peyote, phenampromide

SCHEDULE II DRUGS High abuse potential, potentially leading to severe psychologic or physical dependence, a currently acceptable medical use, eg narcotics (cocaine, codeine, hydromorphone, meperidine, methadone, morphine and oxymorphone) and non-narcotics (amphetamine, amobarbital, methaqualone, nalorphine, paregoric, pentobarbital, percodan phencyclidine and secobarbital)

SCHEDULE III DRUGS High abuse potential, moderate to low physical dependence and high psychologic dependence potentials, with acceptable medical uses, eg amphetamines, barbiturates, codeine formulations, doriden, paregoric, Noludar

SCHEDULE IV DRUGS Minimal abuse potential, limited physical or psychological dependence, potential eg chloral hydrate, Dalmane, Equanil, Librium, Miltown, paraldehyde, phenobarbital

SCHEDULE V DRUGS Very low abuse or dependence potential, eg Lomotil, some formulations of Robitussin, diazepam

conundrum A problem with no satisfactory solution

convergent therapy CLINICAL THERAPEUTICS The use of two or more drugs (eg ABT-538 and MK-639, which are both are HIV-1 protease inhibitors) that target the same protein, in particular of a highly mutable virus; the thinking with CT is that the mutations induced by drug 1 may sensitize the virus to the second drug (Nature 1995; 374:494N&v)

conversion disorder Hysteria A group of psychiatric reactions in which the patient 'converts' mental problems into a physical manifestation, including the sensation of something being stuck in the throat, 'globus hystericus', recurrent abdominal pain without physical findings, hysterical blindness, gait disturbances, paralysis, sensory loss, seizures and urinary retention, often reporting disturbing symptoms with indifference, 'la belle indifference'; see Factitious diseases

convertase Prohormone convertase, see there

'cookbook' medicine A colloquial term for the practice of medicine in strict accordance with practice guidelines, which are not regarded as an appropriate substitute for clinical judgement (JAMA 1995; 273:1534ED)

cookie bite cell Bite cell, see there

cookie cutter An adjectival descriptor for a sharply circumscribed or punched-out lesion with minimal complexity of the scalloped, vertical margins

cookie cutter border DERMATOLOGY A descriptor for the gross morphology of the scalloped ulcerated margins of squamous cell carcinoma

cookie cutter estimate An approximation of the number of deaths that would occur in a nuclear exchange, based on knowledge of the population of a particular location and the assumption anyone within a certain distance from 'ground zero' would be killed

cookie cutter etching FORENSIC PATHOLOGY A descriptor for the sharply demarcated but ragged or scalloped edges of a wound in a close range (4-5 feet) shotgun wound, where the charge enters the body in a conglomerate mass

cookie cutter technique EXPERIMENTAL BIOLOGY A propri-

etary process for selecting subpopulations of cells growing on film-lined culture dishes by cutting around the cell(s) of interest using an ACAS interactive laser cytometer that 'welds' the plastic film to a dish allowing one to strip away the unwanted cells and film, permitting isolated cells to proliferate (Meridian Instruments, Okemos MI)

cooking RESEARCH ETHICS A 'soft' method of altering scientific data, which consists of the selection of data to achieve agreement (C Babbage, Reflections on the decline of Science, London, 1830); as an example, 7 runs of a particular experiment are performed; 3 or 4 are inconclusive, while the remainder are vaguely suggestive of a trend; the equivocal results are 'cooked' out; while not blatantly fraudulent, such tampering with data is unethical; see Fraud in science, Trimming

Coombs' test Antiglobulin test, see there

Cooper pair A pair of electrons that are the central actors in superconductivity, see there

cooperative learning EDUCATION THEORY A student-centered instructional strategy in which heterogeneous groups of students work to achieve a common academic goal, eg completing a case study or a evaluating a QC problem; CL is thought to enhance the learning process, as the students learn and retain more, improve problem solving skills, gain peer support, enjoy the subject material, and develop a rapport with the instructor; the major features of CL are positive interdependence, individual accountability, fomenting of group efforts, and improving of social skills (Clin Lab Sci 1994; 7:166F) see Problem-based learning

Cooperative Research and Development Agreement CRADA, see there

coordinated care HEALTH CARE ENVIRONMENT A (George) Bush euphemism for managed care, see there (Am Med News 26 October 1992, p7)

cootie A colloquial term for a body louse (*Pediculus humanus*), thought to have derived from the Malay term, kutu for louse

Note: 'Cooties' is most commonly used by the layperson for any disagreeable substance, eg sputum or organism, eg 'germs' in the environment, and is thus of little utility

COP 1) Coat proteins A family of proteins that are present in Golgi-derived coated vesicles, including α-COP (160 kD), β-COP (110 kD), γ-COP (98 kD), δ-COP (61 kD), at least one of which, β-COP has sequence similarity to β-adaptin proteins of clathrin-coated vesicles (Nature 1991; 349:215); see Coatamer; Cf Adaptin 2) Colloid oncotic pressure, see there

COP-1 Copolymer I A mixture of 14-23 kD myelin-like polymers synthesized from L-alanine, L-glutamic acid, L-lysine, and L-tyrosine, which suppresses experimental allergic encephalomyelitis, the animal model of multiple sclerosis (MS), and reported to be useful in treating MS; COP-1 may act as a decoy protein, attracting WBCs that would otherwise attack the myelin sheath; it is possible that a combination of COP-1 and IFN-β might be more effective in treating MS than either agent alone (New York Times 11 October; C5 1994) see Myelin basic protein

COP-BLAM III A 'third-generation' chemotherapeutic regimen (cyclophosphamide, Oncovin [vincristine], prednisone with bleomycin, Adriamycin [doxorubicin] and methotrexate) used for advanced lymphoma; although 5% of patients die from COP-BLAM's toxicity, 60-70% have a prolonged disease-free survival, methotrexate decreases tumor spread to the central nervous system Note: The use of multiple non-cross-resistant drugs circumvents the tumor's anti-chemotherapeutic 'defense' mechanisms, which include amplification of the MDR (multi-drug resistance) gene

copayment HEALTH CARE FINANCING A generic term for a shared payment by both the recipient and the insurance provider for a rendered health care service, eg mammography; a typical copayment is 20% of the service's cost; copayments are thought to limit the frivolous abuse of services when such are available without charge (N Engl J Med 1995; 332:1138oa)

MANAGEMENT OF COPD

MINIMIZING AIRFLOW RESTRICTION
    Reduced production of secretions
    Increased elimination of secretion
    Bronchodilatation
    Sympathomimetic agents, eg inhaled b_2-adrenorecep-
    tor agonists
    Anticholinergic agents, eg ipratropium, nebulized
    atropine
    Theophyllin
    Corticosteroids

CORRECTING SECONDARY PHYSIOLOGIC ALTERATIONS
    Hypoxemia
    Pulmonary hypertension and cor pulmonale
    Hypercapnia

OPTIMIZING FUNCTIONAL CAPACITY
    Exercise conditioning
    Upper extremity training
    Respiratory muscle training
    Respiratory muscle rest
    Dyspnea
    Nutrition
    Physical and occupational therapy
    Psychosocial rehabilitation

OTHER ISSUES OF MANAGEMENT
    α_1-antitrypsin augmentation
    Bullectomy
    Lung transplantation

from N Engl J Med 1993; 328:1017

COPD Chronic obstructive pulmonary disease An umbrella term for pulmonary diseases with partially overlapping signs and symptoms, including asthma, bronchiectasis, chronic bronchitis and emphysema; COPD, usually associated with a long history of cigarette smoking, is the fifth most common cause of death (65 000 annual deaths), the third most common (after heart diseases and schizophrenia) cause of chronic disability of older individuals, and the most common cause of pulmonary hypertension and cor pulmonale in the US; the major COPD lesions, chronic bronchitis and emphysema, commonly coexist; the former is responsible for the alveolar hypoxia, ↓ PO_2, ↑ CO_2, and ↓ pH that lead to pulmonary hypertension, which is seen in 65% of males at autopsy and 15% of females, and is due to the unopposed effect of elastases in the lungs; patients with COPD have been divided into type A, ie those with emphysema, fancifully known as Pink puffers and type B, ie chronic bronchitis, known as Blue bloaters; respiratory function and dyspnea in severe COPD may improve with theophylline therapy, which improves respiratory-muscle function PREVENTION ↑ Dietary n-3 polyunsaturated fatty acids may be protective against COPD, possibly by interfering with the production of inflammatory mediators, including leukotrienes, platelet-activating factor, IL-1 and TNF (N Engl J Med 1994; 331:2280a) TREATMENT Based on meta-analysis of the literature, there appears to be a small but statistically significant improvement in the clinical course when antibiotics are used for exacerbations of COPD (JAMA 1995; 273:957oa)

Copper-7 An intrauterine device (IUD) that was withdrawn from the US market in 1986 by its manufacturer, when the 'trickle-down' phenomenon of lawsuits (see Dalkon shield) threatened to make the product an economic liability; see Litogen

coping DENTISTRY A metal covering attached to a tooth root or base which serves as an accomodation or platform for a crown or bridge abutment PSYCHIATRY A constellation of conscious and unconscious mechanims that a person uses to adjust for external demands without changing the direction or intensity of his/her goals

copper penny appearance Sclerotic body, see there

copper line A rarely-observed blue-black line on the gingiva caused by copper poisoning linked to the inhalation of copper salts in the form of dust

copper sulfate test A rapid test for determining the specific gravity of blood that serves as an indirect measurement of hematocrit and used in transfusion medicine to determine blood donor acceptability; specific gravity of 1.053, which corresponds to a hematocrit of 125 g/L (US: 12.5g/dl), a level adequate for blood donation in females, specific gravity of 1.055, which corresponds to a hematocrit of 135 g/L (US: 13.5g/dl), adequate for male donation

copper wire appearance A descriptor for the fundoscopic appearance in grade III arteriolosclerotic retinopathy, in which the arterial wall is opacified to a degreee that the blood column is only seen perpendicularly, ie through the vessel wall, yielding a burnished copper wire appearance due to light reflection; Cf Silver wire appearance

coprolalia The use of 'colorful' language and phraseology punctuated with the 'F' and the 'S' words; Cf Telephone scatologia

Note: While scatologia and coprolalia are synonyms according to the International Dictionary of Medicine (J Wiley & Sons, New York, 1986), in practice, the former is more commonly used in the context of inappropriate use of obscene language as occurs in Gilles de la Tourette or in stroke victims, while scatologia is preferred for the use of obscene language in an erotic context, as in 'telephone scatologia', as preferred by the American Psychiatric Association in DSM IV

coprophilia A condition classified in the DSM-IV as 302.9 paraphilia (sexual deviancy), not otherwise specified, which is defined as 1) A period of at least 6 months in which there are recurrent, intensely sexually arousing fantasies, sexual urges, or behaviors involving the use of feces* in various ways, and 2) The fantasies, sexual urges, or behaviors cause clinically significant distress or impairment in social, occupational, or other important areas of functioning
*Hideous, after N Grismanelli

copy-editing JOURNALISM The correction of various errors on a final copy or 'proof'; in general, the exercise of copy-editing is the responsibility of a work's publisher and is intended to address grammatical, semantic, syntactical and typographic errors; errors of content are usually considered to be the responsibility of the work's author(s) MOLECULAR BIOLOGY Proof-reading, see there

coral reef lesion A macroscopic descriptor for tortuous, ectatic submucosal veins that may rupture in colonic angiodysplasia, a disease so difficult for the surgeon to document in vivo and the pathologist to verify ex vivo that it has been called the 'Emperor's new clothes' syndrome

cor bovinum CARDIOLOGY A heart affected by tertiary syphilis, in which aortitis and consequent aortic valve insufficiency results in circumferential stretching of the valvular leaflets and rolling of the free margin, causing massive cardiomegaly, with weights of 600-1000 g being recorded (normal 275 g female, 325 g male); see Tree barking

cord blood Umbilical cord blood A therapeutic medium used to reconstitute the hematopoietic (stem) cells of patients whose bone marrow has been depleted ('wiped out') by disease, eg anemia, leukemia, lymphoma, or chemotherapy, or radiotherapy; 40 transfusions had been performed as of May 1994

cord-blood stem cells HEMATOLOGY A therapeutic 'medium' containing substantial numbers of hematopoeitic stem cells, which is of use in transplantation and BM reconstitution; CBSCs are collected at birth from the umbilical cord, mixed with an equimolar concentration of DMSO (dimethylsulfoxide) and frozen in liquid nitrogen; they are ideally transfused into HLA-identical siblings and have been successful in reconstituting the BM of patients with Fanconi's anemia, aplastic anemia, leukemia, X-linked lymphoproliferative disorder, and severe thalassemia (N Eng J Med 1995; 332:367oA)

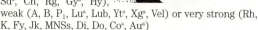

cord cells TRANSFUSION MEDICINE Red blood cells obtained from the neonatal circulation via the umbilical cord; the potency of the antigens expressed on the fetal erythrocytes can be very weak (I, Le^a, Le^b, Sd^a, Ch, Rg, Gy^a, Hy), weak (A, B, P$_1$, Lu^a, Lub, Yt^a, Xg^a, Vel) or very strong (Rh, K, Fy, Jk, MNSs, Di, Do, Co^a, Au^a)

cordite An explosive compound containing nitroglycerine, which may produce headaches, nausea, and vomiting in those working with it; the transient tolerance to cordite is lost over the weekends, resulting in the so-called Monday death, see there

cordocentesis Percutaneous umbilical blood sampling, see there

corduroy cloth appearance RADIOLOGY A fanciful descriptor for the vertically oriented, finely reticulated loss of bony density seen in vertebrae affected by hemangiomas, best seen on a lateral film

core decompression ORTHOPEDIC SURGERY A procedure for treating nontraumatic osteonecrosis in which the bone marrow is decompressed by removing a core of medullary bone, which is then reinserted to support the weakened cortical bone; while the core decompression is reported to be successful in stage I and II osteonecrosis, not all studies have supported this contention (N Engl J Med 1992; 326:1473RV)

core-lipopolysaccharide immune globulin A preparation of IV immunoglobulin containing high titers of antibodies against the core lipopolysaccharide of gram-negative bacilli, in particular lipid A, which is primarily responsible for the biological effect seen in gram-negative sepsis; in practice, CLIG may not be effective in preventing gram-negative infections or their systemic complications (N Engl J Med 1992; 327:234oA)

core promoter MOLECULAR BIOLOGY A discrete sequence of DNA nucleotides that control the ability of RNA polymerase to initiate transcription in all eukaryotes (from the lowly yeast, *Saccharomyces cerevisiae* to complex multicelled organisms), acting as the site where RNA polymerase begins its activity, serving as an 'ignition switch' (Sci Am 1995; 272/2:56) see Transcription activator

core window That timespan in which a hepatitis B-infected patient has detectable hepatitis core antigen (HBc) in the serum but has yet to produce detectable levels of hepatitis B surface antibody; thus 'core window' period in hepatitis B differs from the 'window' period; see Hepatitis serology, Window period

corkscrew esophagus The radiocontrast image of an esophagus with periodically spaced, high-amplitude spastic peristaltic contractions of the lower esophagus (figure, left), attributed to increased responsiveness to neurotransmitters or hormones, clinically characterized by the 'corkscrew esophagus triad', which consists of retro-sternal pain, increased intraluminal pressure and uncoordinated muscle contractions, as well as dysphagia and weight loss, but it may also be asymptomatic; in the lower esophagus, the contractions may increase the intraluminal pressure, producing transient pseudodiverticuli, thus the aliases of 'rosary bead', nutcracker, and 'supersqueezer' esophagus

corkscrew hairs Kinking of the individual hairs, a 'classic' clinical finding in vitamin C deficiency that may be associated with perifollicular hemorrhages; Cf Kinky hair, Wooly hair

corkscrew mesentery GI RADIOLOGY A descriptor for the appearance by mesenteric arteriography of a volvulus in which the main vessel is twisted upon itself

corkscrew metaplasia A term for the microsocopic findings in bile reflux-induced gastritis; although erythema, friability and bleeding may be seen at endoscopy, the correlation of clinical disease with histology is poor

corkscrew ureter A 'curlicue' appearance of the distal ureters due to extrinsic compression as may occur in the uncommon ureteral varices

corkscrew vessels Tight tortuosity of blood vessels seen in the liver of patients with advanced micronodular, often alcoholic cirrhosis, a logical result of collapse of the hepatic parenchyma without loss of vascular length, resulting in 'crimping' of vessels; this appearance has become a radiologic curiosity as hepatic arteriography is rarely used to analyze hepatic masses, this role being now filled by CT and MRI and is only rarely indicated, eg in the rare vascular tumors

cork worker's syndrome A form of hypersensitivity pneumoconiosis due to exposure to moldy cork dust; see Farmer's lung

corneal graft A 'raw material' of cadaveric origin, used to treat herpetic scars, keratoconus, and corneal edema (CAP Today May 1992) see Tissue bank

corneal ring An annular superficial ulcer of the corneal limbus, which is a coalescence of several marginal ulcers in a background of marginal keratitis ETIOLOGY Infections (bacillary dysentery, brucellosis, dengue, gonorrhea, hookworms, influenza, TB), connective tissue disease (gold intoxication, SLE, periarteritis nodosa, rheumatoid arthritis, scleroderma, Sjögren syndrome) and others, eg ischemia, lethal midline granuloma, leukemia, porphyria, ulcerative colitis, Wegener's granulomatosis PATHOLOGY PMNs, eosinophils, plasma cells

cornflake appearance CYTOLOGY An artefact 94-53296 MICROBIOLOGY A descriptor for the yellow-tan, bread crumb-like colonies of the scotochrome (Runyon group II) *Mycobacterium szulgai* when grown on a Lowenstein-Jensen agar slant, fancifully likened to a breakfast cereal

coronary arterial bypass graft A procedure in which vascular grafts, usually saphenous, less commonly cephalic veins are anastomosed end-to-side to the internal mammary arteries, bypassing atherosclerotically stenosed coronary arteries; some work suggests that the internal mammary artery is a better donor conduit, given its relative resistance to collapse; internal mammary procedures are associated with longer survival, better long-term patency and lower rate of reoperation; it is unclear whether medical therapy (diet, exercise and cholesterol-lowering drugs) is more beneficial than surgery, although the so-called 'triple bypass' is indicated in unstable angina

STATISTICS In the US, each year 800 000 survive an acute MI (another 200 000 do not) 175 000 undergo CABG, ⅔ of whom may benefit from the procedure; CABG is indicated in patients with chronic stable angina who are medical 'failures', patients with 2-vessel disease and left anterior descending coronary arterial stenosis; CABG is also indicated in patients with 2- or 3-vessel disease and ischemia detected by an exercise stress test; in one study, the annual mortality in surgically-treated patients with single, double and triple vessel disease was 0.8%, 0.8% and 1.2% and for medically treated patients, 1.1%, 0.6% and 1.2%, respectively; medical therapy is preferred in those without evidence of myocardial ischemia and in those with 1- or 2-vessel disease without significant left anterior descending coronary arterial stenosis COMPLICATIONS Progression of atherosclerosis, recurrent angina (see Angina), arrhythmia, sudden death, which occurs in ± 2% of surgically and ± 6% of medically treated patients followed for 5 years; Cf Percutaneous transluminal angioplasty; Thallium imaging, Treadmill exercise test

Note: Moderate alcohol consumption reduces the serum cholesterol, raises HDL-cholesterol and may reduce the risk of coronary atherosclerosis

coronary artery steal Like other steal syndromes, the CAS is characterized by the shunting of all relatively well oxygenated blood from a critical area of low perfusion to an area of higher perfusion; it is unique in that it may be iatrogenic and occur in pharmacologic stress imaging (see there) using dipyridamole to induce vasoconstriction, causing a fall in the blood flow to the subendocardium distal to the site of the stenosed coronary artery

coronary perfusion pressure A pressure gradient that exists between aortic and right atrial pressures during the relaxation phase in cardiopulmonary resuscitation; CPP correlates well with myocardial blood flow and serves to predict outcome during cardiac arrest; a minimum pressure of 15 mm Hg is required for spontaneous return of circulation; in evolving myocardial infarcts, multiple 1-mg doses (high-dose regimen) of epinephrine (adrenalin) improve survival when arrested patients do not respond to low-dose regimens (JAMA 1991; 265:1139)

coronary revascularization Any of a number of procedures intended to increase coronary arterial blood flow, including coronary artery bypass surgery, angioplasty

coronary stent Intracoronary stent A tubular device left in a lumen to maintain its patency; clinical and angiographic outcomes are better with intracoronary artery stent implantation than with standard balloon angioplasty, at a cost of ↑↑↑ vascular complications and ↑ hospital stay (N Engl J Med 1994; 331:489OA), a lower rate of restenosis and need for revascularization (N Engl J Med 1994; 331:496OA)

coronary vasodilator reserve The ratio of maximal to basal coronary blood flow, which can be used as a functional index of the severity of coronary artery stenosis; the CVR also correlates with the geometry of the stenosis by quantitative arteriography (see N Engl J Med 1994; 330:1782OA, ibid; 331:222OA)

coronary vasodilator response see Coronary vasodilator reserve

coroner FORENSIC MEDICINE An elected or appointed public official whose chief responsibility is to investigate and provide official interpretation regarding the manner and possible cause(s) of deaths occurring 1) Suddenly, 2) Violently, 3) Without explanation or natural cause, 4) for which the stated causes conflict with the findings at the scene of death or at postmortem examination and 5) Due or potentially due to foul play

Note: The office of the coroner in the US is a political appointment, a custom that dates to English common law, where the representative of the crown (coroner) determined whether the king would share in the deceased's worldly goods; in the USA, because of the political aspects of the office, the pathologist is often a victim of the machinations of an elected government and may be forced to choose between ethics and his own continued employment; pol-

itics were allegedly responsible for the dismissal of forensic pathologists of international renown in Los Angeles, New York City and Michigan

corpora amylacea Ovoid, lamellated and sharply-circumscribed masses of pale to darkly eosinophilic structures, likened to starch granules, have been described in the brain, prostatic duct lumina and lungs which have no known clinical significance

corpora arenaceus Brain dust NEUROPATHOLOGY Intra- and extracellular, PAS (periodic acid Schiff)-positive basophilic masses seen by LM in the cerebral white matter, thought to be an aging phenomenon, correspond to axonal degradation endproducts, composed of glycoproteins and mucopolysaccharides, which have been described in Huntington's and Parkinson's diseases, and herpes simplex-induced encephalopathy

corporal punishment The use of physical punishment as a means of discipline, generally by striking the perpetrator/victim with a ruler, paddle, hand, etc; corporal punishment is more often administered to boys, racial minorities, students in rural districts, or the southern US, and to children with emotional or learning disorders; it had been a standard practice in many school systems but is being deleted; corporal punishment was banned in Poland in 1783, and the rest of Europe by 1982; in the US it was banned in New Jersey in 1867; over 20 states still allow it (Am Med News 9 March 1992)

corps ronds DERMATOPATHOLOGY Degenerated double-contoured dyskeratotic squamous cells with large, round basophilic masses surrounded by a clear halo, located in the spinous layer of the epidermis, classically described in Darier's disease, also found in: benign familial pemphigus, keratosis follicularis, and warty dyskeratoma; Cf Colloid bodies

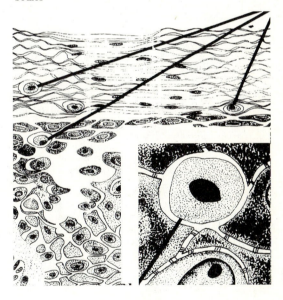

corps ronds

corpus delecti FORENSIC MEDICINE The substantial and fundamental fact(s) and material evidence necessary to prove the commission of a crime; since the vast majority of cases of medical malpractice do not imply deliberate acts or criminal intent, these cases are tried in civil and not in criminal court; see Chain of evidence

cor pulmonale A heart affected secondarily to pulmonary disease, resulting in right ventricular hypertrophy (ventricular wall thicker than 5 mm or autopsy weight of the right ventricle of greater than 65 g); primary lung diseases evoking cor pulmonale include pulmonary vascular disease, parenchymal defects, an abnormal ventilatory drive, defects in the thoracic cage or defective pumping mechanism; in chronic cor pulmonale, there is a combination of cardiac hypertrophy and dilatation, while in acute cor pulmonale, there has only been time sufficient for cardiac dilatation; in the older population, chronic cor pulmonale is the third most common cardiac disorder after atherosclerotic and hypertensive heart disease; because of its relation to cigarette smoking, cor pulmonale is more common in ♂, a datum that is likely to change MEDICAL TREATMENT Supplementary oxygen, corticosteroids, anticoagulants, vasodilators and other therapy to address underlying lung disease SURGICAL TREATMENT Selected patients are candidates for lung and heart-lung transplantation

correctional facility Prison, jail, gaol, pokey, slammer An institution for incarcerating persons arrested for, or convicted of various crimes; as of 1992, 0.5% of the US population was incarcerated at any given time (the highest rate in the world), due in part to the 'zero tolerance' policy towards drug abuse; US prisons are operating at 18 to 51% over capacity (JAMA 1992; 268:3176MN&P); the severe overcrowding, inadequate ventilation, and altered host susceptibility are an ideal milieu for incubating pulmonary infections, in particular TB (N Engl J Med 1994; 331:643OA)

corrosive material OCCUPATIONAL SAFETY A chemical liquid or solid that causes visible destructioin or irreversible alteration of mucocutaneous surfaces at the site of contact, or one that causes slow destruction of steel

corrupted file COMPUTERS A generic term for any file, usually stored on magnetic media (eg floppy disks, hard drive), which contains scrambled or unretrievable data, which may be due to bad sectors (surface flaws on the disk, software errors, or failures of the disk drive controller (B Pfaffenberger, Compuer User's Dictionary, Que, Indianapolis, 1993)

cortical oscillations NEUROLOGY Cortical rhythms that range from 4-7 Hz theta waves during sleep to 14-60 Hz waves while aroused are generated and synchronized by layer 5 pyramidal neurons from the neocortex (Science 1991; 251:432); see Chaos

corticotropin-releasing factor CRF, see there

Corvac™ tube LABORATORY MEDICINE A proprietary* blood collection tube available in sizes from 1 to 15 ml that contains a silicone-based material; after collection, the specimen is spun at 2500-3000 rpm for 10 minutes; the cells and sludge in the blood are 'driven' through the silicone and the serum is easily removed for analysis of a wide range of chemical components DISADVANTAGES Specimens that have been inadequately separated have an ↑ in K+ and LDH, and ↓ in glucose; exposure of Corvacs to direct sunlight (as may occur in the courier services provided by commercial laboratories) may cause a separation of the silicone into the specimen, which has been reported to interfere with RIA and clinical chemistry instrumentation
*The equivalent tube produced by Becton-Dickinson is known as an SST tube

COS cell COS-1 cell An altered African green monkey kidney cell line that has been transformed by the SV40 virus and used in transfection experiments for efficient vector expression

co-sign *verb* To authorize or approve in writing, requisitions for diagnostic or therapeutic procedures that have ordered by a subordinate or one who is not in a position of authority at a particular institution

co-sleeping PEDIATRICS, SOCIAL MEDICINE The habit by a young child of sleeping in the parents' bed for all or part of the night, a custom that occurs in 20% of Hispanic households in the US versus 6% of white households and is more common in single parent families and in those living in multiple households; regular co-sleeping is associated with increased sleep disorders

Cosgrove v Sullivan A federal class action lawsuit that hinged on overpayment by Medicare for services rendered by physicians during the mid-1980s; some Medicare beneficiaries were found to be eligible for refunds (CAP Today Jan 1993 p42)

cosmetic surgery ESTHETIC SURGERY That branch of plastic and reconstructive surgery that is dedicated exclusively to sculpting an Adonis or Venus from a lump of mortal clay; CS techniques include chemical peels, dermabrasion, facial sculpturing, fat injections, liposuction, and plastic surgery

cosmid MOLECULAR BIOLOGY A large recombinant plasmid which has an inserted lambda phage cos site that allows the plasmid to be packaged in vitro in a phage coat and efficiently introduced into bacteria; cosmids are designed to carry 35-45 kilobase 'inserts' of DNA and are used to clone large DNA fragments and construct genomic libraries; see Plasmid, Cf YAC cloning

cosmid cloning vector A genetically engineered plasmid into which up to 42 kb of foreign DNA, eg large genes of interest may be inserted for cloning

cost containment HEALTH CARE ENVIRONMENT *'An assemblage of strategies–including cost-sharing approaches, benefit designs, provider contracts, volume of services to be provided, discounts or set charges, and benefit and payment incentives and disincentives–used to control the cost of health care services.'* (Dictionary of Health Care Management, Facts on File, New York, 1988); costs are regarded as being contained when the price of the health care services does not increase faster than the price of other consumer services; CC devices used in the 1990s include managed care, managed competition, regulation by insurance companies, reimbursement of services based on diagnosis-related groups, global budgets, and expenditure caps (JAMA 1993; 269:631c)

cost-effectiveness analysis HEALTH CARE ENVIRONMENT Economic analysis related to the effectiveness of therapies or interventions and their associated costs; CEA requires the development of a model of alternative therapies using published data on the probabilities of various outcomes, identifying the expenses associated with each type of intervention or therapy (eg drug, use of device, or procedure) and comparing the results (often in the form of money spent/year of life saved, and wages lost or gained) with those of benchmark (or 'standard') therapies; CEA has acquired increasing importance and in some countries may be required before a drug or therapy is approved for use (N Engl J Med 1994; 331:669ED; 1993; 329:1517OA)

cost-sharing HEALTH CARE FINANCING A generic term for any maneuver or format by which a person's principal reimbursement agent or vehicle, eg Medicare or primary insurance carrier, shares a portion of the financial burden of incurred health care costs; CS includes supplementary insurance (eg 'medigap'), balance billing, copayments, and deductibles (N Engl J Med 1995; 332:1138OA)

cost shifting HEALTH CARE ENVIRONMENT A practice by which a health care provider (ie physician) may offset his/her losses from treating one group of patients by charging other patients more; eg if a certain health insurance company pays only a specific amount for a particular procedure, the physician (or other healthcare worker) may bill another patient a higher fee for the same procedure (Congressional Quarterly, 1993, in Clin Lab Sci 1994; 7:141, JAMA 1995; 273:1223); CS is the primary method of paying for indigent care in the US (Am Med News 26 October 1992, p7)

cot curve COT curve analysis MOLECULAR BIOLOGY That relation defined by the equation $Ct = 1/(1 + K C_0 t)$, which quantifies the rate of reassociation of DNA as a function of an organism's genomic complexity and when plotted, yields a sigmoid-shaped curve; 10-15% of mammalian genomic DNA reassociates immediately and is regarded as simple sequence DNA as it is composed largely of different sets of repeated oligonucleotides arranged in long tandem repeats; Cf Zoo blot

cot-sides 'syndrome' Hospital bed 'syndrome', see there

cotinine A urinary metabolite of nicotine which can be used to monitor exposure to environmental tobacco smoke (ETS); in one report, urinary cotinine levels in children not known to have been exposed to ETS was 5.6 ng/mL, with home exposure to one smoker, 13 ng/mL, and with two or more smokers (N Engl J Med 1993; 328:1665ₒₐ)

cotton An adjectival descriptor for a pattern characterized by wispy radiopacities or whitish patches

cotton ball patches BONE RADIOLOGY Irregular, rounded, 'fluffy' patches of sclerotic bone seen by a plain skull film in the thickened diploe of advanced Paget's disease, associated with exuberant chaotic bone formation in a background of osteosclerosis; cotton wool patches may also occur in metastases, hereditary hypophosphatasia and chondroblastomas PULMONARY RADIOLOGY A descriptor for multiple rounded fluffy nodules seen on a plain chest film in patients with pulmonary histoplasmosis

cotton candy lung A descriptor for the gross findings of endstage panlobular or panacinar emphysema, in which residual fibrosed septae have been likened to cotton candy, a wispy, sugar-based snack traditionally consumed in county fairs, carnivals and circuses

cotton wool patches OPHTHALMOLOGY A descriptive term for the fluffy exudates and axoplasmic debris seen in the retinal nerve fiber layer, that accumulate after microinfarcts in the retinal nerve fiber layer, typical of grade III hypertensive retinopathy, but also occurs in collagen vascular disease, DM (nonproliferative retinopathy), immune suppression, infections (*Babesia microti*, CMV, *Pneumocystis carinii*), ischemia, pheochromocytoma, and BM transplant recipients PATHOLOGY, see Cytoid bodies; Cf Cotton ball patches

---

'COTSWOLDS' STAGING CLASSIFICATION

STAGE I Involvement of a single lymph node or lymphoid tissue, eg spleen, thymus, Waldyer's ring

STAGE II Involvement of a two or more lymph nodes or lymphoid tissues on the same side of the diaphragm, the number of sites involved are indicated by a subscript, eg II₃

STAGE III Involvement of a two or more lymph nodes or lymphoid tissues on both sides of the diaphragm

III₁ With or without splenic hilar, celiac, or periportal lymph nodes

III₂ With para-aortic, iliac, or mesenteric lymph nodes

STAGE IV Involvement of extranodal sites with 'bulky' disease

> ⅓ widening of mediastinum

> 10 cm greatest dimension of mediastinum

Semin Oncol 1990; 17:696

Cotswolds Staging System HEMATOLOGY The most recent staging system for Hodgkin's disease, which adds the definition of bulky disease and presence of multiple sites of disease (table), based on data provided by staging laparotomy and CT imaging; Cf Ann Arbor classification, Rye Staging System

The Rye System was supplanted by the Ann Arbor System, delineated in 1971, which recognized that identification of extranodal involvement was a parameter of prognostic value, which at the time was based on staging laparotomy

'couch potato' A facetious American colloquialism for sedentary individuals, usually males, whose predominant non-work activity consists in lying on a couch, watching television; anecdotal evidence suggests that these subjects may represent an evolving clinical entity; typical of the

couch potato 'syndrome' is a diet of high-carbohydrate, salt-laden foods, eg pretzels, potato chips (potato 'crisps'), popcorn and other forms of 'junk' food, decreased physical activity and a psychological state of suggestibility and decreased environmental interaction; see Television intoxication 'syndrome'

Note: It is uncertain whether a passive lifestyle predisposes a person to increased atherosclerotic heart disease, hypertension and other nosologies, as it has yet to be formerly studied, although preliminary data suggests that children who spend prolonged periods of time watching television have higher cholesterol levels, and a tendency towards obesity, related to a combination of snacking on high-calorie foods and inactivity

'cough CPR' EMERGENCY MEDICINE Subjects who develop sudden ventricular fibrillation can maintain consciousness for over 90 seconds with an arterial pulse by vigorous coughing in rapid sequence with a physiological staccato rhythm; cough cardiopulmonary resuscitation (CPR) has two components: 1) Vigorous inhalation, causing negative intrathoracic pressure ('thoracic diastole' or Mueller's maneuver) and 2) Explosive coughing, causing positive intrathoracic pressure ('thoracic systole' or Valsalva maneuver)

Coulter™ A proprietary cell counter that functions on the principle of the electrical impedance of particles; the Coulter counter (Hialeah, Florida) has become an 'industry standard' instrument used in clinical hematology laboratories to determine a wide range of parameters of the cells in the circulation, allowing automated loading of specimens and electronic classification of broad categories of conditions, including the relative increase or decrease of erythrocytes, leukocytes and platelets in the circulation

counterimmunoelectrophoresis LABORATORY MEDICINE A rapid immunoassay capable of detecting nanogram quantities of an antigen by the formation of a precipitin line in a gel between an antibody and antigen of different electrophoretic mobilities, CIE is of use in the early diagnosis of bacterial meningitis, for identifying *Streptococcus pneumococcal* serotypes, *Haemophilus influenza* type b and *Neisseria meningitidis* groups A, C, D, W135, X, Y and Z

counterstain HISTOLOGY A stain of a different color (eg red) after a primary stain (eg blue) that is used in a differentiate among various cellular elements

countersuggestion PSYCHIATRY A technique used in 'negativistic' patients, where the therapist deliberately suggests the opposite of what is intended

countersuit MEDICAL MALPRACTICE A lawsuit initiated by the defendant, who alleges that the original malpractice suit (see Frivolous lawsuit, below) was without reasonable or probable cause, was actuated by malice (improper motive), or the lawsuit ended in the physician's favor or the physician suffered damages (to reputation or otherwise); see Malpractice

countertransferrance PSYCHIATRY An emotional reaction evoked in the psychotherapist by the patient; alternatively, the effects of the therapist's internal conflicts and needs that impact on his/her ability to treat a patient

coup see Contrecoup

coup de sabre appearance A curved, sharply demarcated, depressed and hyperpigmented linear groove, often seen on the frontoparietal scalp, accompanied by linear alopecia and dermal atrophy, which is seen in localized scleroderma, an appearance fancifully likened to that of a saber blow

couplet CARDIOLOGY A pair of successive premature ventricular contractions (PVC); sporadic PVC may occur in young subjects, increase with age and are of no clinical significance unless there is underlying cardiac disease, in which PVC are a risk factor for sudden cardiac death; PVC may result from medication (digitalis, quinidine and tricyclic antidepressants) and are ample indication for discontinuing the drugs

Note: The term 'ventricular premature depolarization' is more semantically and physiologically correct than 'premature ventricular contraction'

courtesy Professional courtesy, see there

couvade Sympathy pregnancy, see there

covariate *'a variable that is related to a secondary variable.'* (Dorland's illustrated Medical Dictionary, 28th ed, WB Saunders, Philadelphia, 1994); possibly less confusingly, a covariate may be defined as a potentially confounding factor or datum that is regarded as being of minimal importance in a particular study, but which must be considered in both the study's design and in the collection of data, to allow the elimination of statistical 'noise'; depending on the study, covariates may include sociodemographic factors, eg adequacy of health care, education level, and marital status

cover *verb* To administer antibiotics as a prophylaxis for a person at increased risk of suffering bacterial infections after surgery or open trauma

coverage 1) The extent of insurance or benefits afforded by an insurance policy, eg typical 'coverage' for medical malpractice insurance ranges from $1-3 million per incident and $3-5 million for complete liability coverage; these values depend on the state (of the US) where the physician is practicing medicine; for individual health insurance, coverage is the amount and type of benefits that would be paid by the policy 2) The provision of medical services by one physician for another, who is usually board certified in the same specialty as the physician for whom he is 'covering'; in the US, a physician is compelled to ensure that 'coverage' is provided should he take a vacation, otherwise he may be legally liable for 'abandonment', should one of his patients need his services in his absence

cow RADIATION MEDICINE A colloquial term for a device used to generate radioactive isotopes with a short half-life, which are separated by elution or separation ('milking') a short-lived daughter from a parent with a longer half-life (eg ^{99m}Tc from ^{99}Mo; ^{113m}In from ^{113}Sn)

'cow method' TRANSFUSION MEDICINE A highly colloquial term of occasional currency referring to the sub-subdivision of a unit of blood, such that one unit can be processed either into a 'quad' pack of 125 ml each, which have a normal shelf-life or transferred into two to four smaller aliquots with a 24-hour shelf-life or apportioned at the time of use into pediatric transfer packs that outdate in 24 hours, providing twelve ml aliquots of blood and four 'mini-units' of fresh frozen plasma; see Quad pack

Cowden's disease see Multiple hamartoma syndrome

Cox (proportional-hazards) regression analysis see Proportional-hazards regression analysis

Coxsackie A family of picornaviruses from the genus *Enterovirus*, named for a city in New York State where they were first identified; there are 23 virotypes* of Coxsackie A virus types based on pathogenicity in newborn mice and 6 types of Coxsackie B CLINICAL Syndromes Herpangina (Coxsackie A), hand, foot and mouth disease (group A16), summer grippe, aseptic meningitis (both A and B), epidemic pleurodynia, acute nonspecific pericarditis and myocarditis (group B)

*Virotype A23 was reclassified as echovirus 9

CP-96,345 A potent highly-selective nonapeptide antagonist of substance P's NK1 receptor, a receptor that in the guinea pig is concentrated in the locus ceruleus (Science 1991; 251:435, 437); see NK receptors, Substance P

CPAP Continuous positive airway pressure, see there

CPC 1) Chronic passive congestion, see Nutmeg liver 2) Clinicopathologic conference

CPD Citrate phosphate dextrose TRANSFUSION MEDICINE A storage medium that allows preservation of packed red cells for up to 21 days at 4°C **CPDA-1** Citrate phosphate dextrose-adenine, which supplies ATP, extending the shelf life of blood to 35 days, yielding a higher ATP level **CPDA + ADDITIVE SOLUTIONS** In addition to the substances provided in the CPDA preservation fluid, additive solutions containing saline, dextrose, adenine and other additives allow a maximum shelf life of packed red cells of 42 days, see ADSOL®

Note: CPDA-1 is no longer used at the New York Blood Center, which as of early 1995 switched to collection of whole blood in ADSOL® bags

CPE Cytopathologic effect, see there

CPFs N-carbomethoxycarbonyl-prolyl-phenylalanyl benzylester(s) A family of molecules derived from the dipeptide prolyphenylalanine that bind to gp120, the envelope protein of HIV-1, which is involved in the pivotal first step in HIV-1 infection, binding directly to the host cell's CD4 receptor; the CPF(DD) isomer is highly specific for gp120 and in an in vitro model system, prevents the spread of infection by binding to gp120, preventing HIV's binding to the CD4 receptor, while still preserving CD4's ability to function in the class II major histocompatibility complex

CpG A dinucleotide of cytosine base followed by a guanine base

CpG effect A 'senseless'* B cell-mediated immune response to DNA that is stimulated by an unmethylated dinucleotide of cytosine and guanine; that the immune system can be stimulated directly by DNA has critical implications in infectious diseases, pharmacology, and rheumatology (Nature Medicine 1995; 1:407)

*Here 'sense' refers to the mRNA transcription; 'antisense' to the hybridization to the sense or coding strand of DNA

CpG island MOLECULAR ONCOLOGY One of multiple cytosine-guanine dinucleotides on double stranded DNA that are the site of frequent mutations (a mutational 'hot spot') in the p53 gene (Science 1991; 253:49); see p53; these sites are susceptible to methylation, which represses the expression of a structural gene; CpG islands may exist in clusters, fancifully termed 'CpG archipelago' as in the transcripts of Wilms' tumor, which are variably expressed and explain the pathogenic heterogeneity characteristic of Wilms' tumorigenesis

cpm Counts per minute NUCLEAR MEDICINE A unit of measurement indicating the energy released by a gamma ray emitting isotope, eg ^{125}I, detected by a scintillation counter; see RIA; Cf ELISA

CPM Central pontine myelinolysis, see there

CPPT Calcium pyrophosphate dihydrate see 'Coffin lids'

CPR Cardiopulmonary resuscitation Those activities performed on a person in order to revive him from apparent death, ie one whose heart and/or lungs are apparently not functioning; as a facet of DNR orders, CPR in the elderly may be considered a futile exercise, as septuagenarians subjected to CPR rarely survive to hospital discharge, despite 'successful' CPR; see A-B-C sequence, C-A-B sequence, Cough CPR

Also 1) Cardiopulmonary reserve 2) (cerebral) Cortical perfusion rate 3) Cerebro-pedal regulator (neurobiology) 4) Cold pressor response test 5) Cold protective response 6) Cortisol production rate

C-protein HISTOLOGY A minor muscle protein of unknown function MOLECULAR BIOLOGY A protein that associates with hnRNA (heterogeneous nuclear RNA) that may be involved in spliceosome assembly; Cf C-peptide, C-reactive protein, Protein C

CPT Current procedural terminology HEALTH CARE REIMBURSEMENT A systemic listing and coding of procedures and services performed by physicians in the USA, each of which is identified by a five-digit number: 00100-01999 and 99100-99140 are anesthesiology services; 10000-69999 are surgical procedures; 70000-79999 are radiology (nuclear medicine and diagnostic ultrasound) services; 80000-89999 are pathology and laboratory medicine services; 90000-99999 are medical services; CPT terminology was developed to serve as free-standing descriptions of medical procedures, eg 25105 corresponds to an arthrotomy of the wrist joint for synovectomy (CAP Today December 1992)

CPU Central processing unit COMPUTERS The hardware that comprises the 'thinking' part of a computer; although the CPU is one microprocessing chip on the logic or 'mother' board, for microcomputers, the simple-minded often equate the CPU to the entirety of the electronic circuitry in the box containing the hard and floppy drives; thus defined, the CPU contains various components including

1) ROM BIOS, which stores all the information programmmed into the computer on 'read-only memory' chips and circuits; the ROM bios sets the CPU's limits in terms of RAM memory, eg 4 megabytes and hard drive capacity, eg 200 megabytes

2) TIMER CHIP, which places the commands or activities of the microprocessor in a sequence so that they can be carried out in order

3) MATH-COPROCESSOR and

4) CACHE MEMORY A memory-containing circuit built into the mother board that accelerates accession of information more quickly than is possible with the floppy or hard drive, acting in a sense as a fast-access hard drive; see Computer

CR Complement receptor

CR1 A 30-kD receptor on the surface of B cells that binds to complement C3b with high affinity, and with lesser affinity to complement C4b, ligands which, once bound, modulate B-cell activity

CR2 A 140-kD receptor on the surface of B cells that binds to complement C3d and modulates B-cell activity

CR3 A heterodimeric receptor for complement C3bi, which is a composite of CD11a (α chain) and CD18 (β chain)

CR3 deficiency syndrome Leukocyte adhesion deficiency syndrome, see there

Crabtree effect An anomalous response observed in malignant cells in tissue culture; when a glucose-containing substrate is added to a cell-culture medium, normal cells respond by an increase in both glycolysis and respiration, while malignant cells respond with increased glycolysis and inhibition of respiration

crack SUBSTANCE ABUSE A 'free-base' form of cocaine, prepared by sodium bicarbonate extraction of cocaine-HCl, resulting in inexpensive yellowish crystals, which when smoked in a pipe produce a brief, very intense 'high'; crack is considered the most addicting substance of abuse in existence and may cause addiction within one week; crack appeared on the drug scene in the USA, circa 1985 and already out-competes other drugs of abuse in producing human tragedy in the form of loss of family structure and 'crack' babies; see Binging, Cocaine, Crack 'smile', Free base cocaine

*Study population, socially and economically 'disenfranchised', inner-city young adults aged 18-29; for crack ethnography, see Science 1989; 246:1377

crack baby An infant born to a crack‡-addicted mothers are at high risk for prematurity, low birth weight, birth defects, respiratory, and neurological defects; up to 30% of babies admitted to neonatal ICUs in some US inner city hospitals have crack-abusing mothers and these infants are feared to fare far worse than 'cocaine babies' and have a characteristic trembling likened to a delicately shaking cup of tea; they are four times more likely to be premature, more commonly suffer SIDS, and given the high mortality and morbidity of the mothers, are often in foster care*; see Crack, Neonatal withdrawal syndrome

*In 1980, 19% of children in certain zones of the urban US had foster parents; by 1990, this figure had risen to 50%, largely attributed to crack

'cracked dermis' DERMATOPATHOLOGY A soft histologic criterion seen in Kaposi sarcoma where the dermal collagen is haphazardly dissected, forming bizarre clefted spaces

cracked ice pattern BONE RADIOLOGY Poorly defined, patchy, mottled appearance due to tumoral replacement of medullary bone, characteristic of Ewing sarcoma; the preferred descriptor is 'moth-eaten'

cracked pot sign of MacEwen A finding of late hydrocephalus, where increased intracranial pressure leads to palpable separation of the cranial sutures; percussion of the skull evokes a 'jagged' sound, unlike the clear sound when a normal noggin is knocked, a noise likened to a 'cracked vessel' CLINICAL The skin is thin and shiny, the veins prominent and the cry high-pitched; see Hydrocephalus, Setting sun sign

cracker sign RHEUMATOLOGY Extreme difficulty in eating dry foods, eg salted crackers, a clinical finding typical of xerostomia, a component of Sjögren syndrome

cracking artifact HEMATOPATHOLOGY A cleared space seen by low-power light microscopy, which surrounds germinal centers or nodules in lymph nodes; it is a 'soft' criterion supporting the diagnosis of nodular lymphoma and is related to the differences in density between the compact nodule of the homogeneous tumor cells in lymphoma and the surrounding uninvolved tissues; the difference in density between the nodules and surrounding tissue in benign reactive hyperplasia, which may mimic nodular lymphoma is less marked and thus 'cracking' is less common in benign lymphadenopathies

crack 'smile' 'Life mark' Traumatic lacerations inflicted by a razor or knife extending from the tragus to the oral commisure, often involving the facial nerve and less commonly the parotid duct, that are inflicted on drug pushers or other addicts who have been responsible for a 'bad deal' TREATMENT End-to-end anastomosis of facial nerve, cannulation with stent if the parotid gland is affected (JAMA 1991; 265:1528c)

CRADA Cooperative Research And Development Agreement A component of the US Federal Technology and Transfer Act of 1986, that allows business to invest in ongoing government-funded research, eg National Institute of Health activities, providing extra capital with the hope that the businesses will be able to transfer any technology 'spun off' into commercially viable products, patents or inventions; see 'Krimsky index'

cradle cap NEONATOLOGY Diffuse or focal, greasy encrustation of the scalp in infants that occurs at about six months of age that may be the presenting or only manifestation of seborrheic dermatitis; the lesions may contiguously involve other 'seborrheic' regions, ie ears, nasal alae, eyebrows and eyelids

cranial base surgery A generic term for what is possibly the most complex areas of surgery, given the anatomic complexity of the deep intra- and extracranial structures and the wide range of diseases that affect the boundary regions, eg acoustic neuroma (which occurs between the ear and the brain), pituitary tumor (between the roof of the nasal cavity and the base of the brain) and meningiomas; CBS requires a multidisiciplinary approach involving neurosurgeons, ENTs (otorhinolaryngologists), ophthalmologists, head & neck surgeons, oral surgeons, neurologists, interventional radiologists, radiotherapists, and various support staff

cranial osteopathy see Craniosacral therapy

cranial vault OBSTETRICS Those bones that form the movable part of the fetal skull (two frontal, two parietal and occipital bones), and mold themselves to the female birth canal, allowing passage of the cephalic-presenting infant

craniosacral therapy ALTERNATIVE MEDICINE A form of alternative therapy in which the bones of the skull are manipulated, a maneuver that is allegedly effective in treating a wide range of conditions including autism, cerebral palsy, dyslexia, ear infection, edema, epilepsy, headache, hypertension, hypotension, mood disorders, recurrent infections, spinal cord injury, stroke, temporomandibular joint syndrome, tinnitus, and others; CT's claimed benefits are linked to the alleged ability to affect the circulation of the cerebrospinal fluid; CT has three approaches, the sutural (aka cranial osteopathy), in which the sutures between the cranial bones are manipulated, the meningeal, and the reflex (Alternative Medicine, Future Medicine Publishing, Inc, Puyallup, Washington, 1994) see Alternative medicine

craniotabes NEONATOLOGY Softening of the cranial bones to such a degree as to allow them to be indented by digital pressure, most often at the vertex of the parietal bone near the sagittal suture; craniotabes occurs in neonates, especially in premature infants and in those exposed to abnormal intrauterine pressures and is usually of no clinical significance, although persistence beyond the first few months of life warrants investigation; occipital bone softening is of more concern, as the irregular calcifications typical of craniotabes may also be seen in osteogenesis imperfecta, cleidocranial dysostosis, lacunar skull, congenital hypothyroidism, Down syndrome and rickets

CRAO Central retinal artery occlusion, see there

crank A 'street' name for methamphetamine

crash COMPUTERS The abrupt malfunction of a computer, due either to a 1) Software crash, in which a software malfunctions for any of a number of reasons, eg opening a 'system' file and changing the program's instructions; these crashes are often resolved by simple exercises, including rememorizing the system software or by using a 'utility' program, eg Norton utilities to circumvent the problem or 2) Hardware crash, which is usually far more serious and can be due to wear or 'trauma' to the machinery, eg dropping; the lost data may be recuperated in harddisk crashes, if the magnetic storage disk is intact and can be opened in a 'safe' (clean and dust-free) environment, and the data downloaded to another storage device CRITICAL CARE MEDICINE An abrupt decompensation of a patient's clinical status

crash and bleed out VIROLOGY US military slang for shock-related death, accompanied by hemorrhage from multiple orifices, which has been described in some cases of human Ebola virus infection, in which there is intense proliferation of viral particles to such degree that much of the host tissue is converted into viral particles (R Preston, The Hot Zone, Random House, New York, 1994)

'crash' diet A semi-starvation type of fad diet which has a wide variety of formulations that is followed for a short period of time by a person wishing to rapidly lose weight; such radical approaches to rarely result in the desired permanent loss of weight

crashcart CAC cart EMERGENCY MEDICINE A cart that is readily accessible to health care workers and strategically placed in sites in a hospital where patients most commonly 'crash', ie undergo acute cardiovascular decompensation, including the recovery and emergency rooms and intensive care units; a crashcart contains both equipment, eg syringes, gloves, tongue depressors, tubes and airways, as well as medications, eg aminophylline, calcium chloride, digoxin, ferosemide, heparin, naloxone, phenytoin, propranolol, and verapamil, required for resuscitation of a person who has 'arrested'

craving A strong desire to consume a particular substance; craving is a major factor in relapse and/or continued use after withdrawal from a substance of abuse and is both imprecisely defined and difficult to measure (JAMA 1992; 267:2293ADAMHA) Cf Addiction, '–holic'

crazing DENTISTRY The development of minute cracks on plastic prosthetics and restorations, eg filling materials, teeth, or base

'crazy pavement' appearance A descriptor for mottled zones of pigmented and depigmented skin, reminiscent of cobblestone pavement, seen in the children suffering from the kwashiorkor-marasmus disease 'complex'

C-reactive protein LABORATORY MEDICINE A 120-kD polypeptide produced in the liver so named for its ability to bind the C polysaccharide of the *Streptococcus pneumoniae* cell wall; CRP is an 'acute phase reactant', whose functions include complement activation, binding of T cells, inhibition of clot retraction, suppression of platelet and lymphocyte function and enhancement of phagocytosis by neutrophils QUANTIFICATION Latex agglutination, rate nephelometry; CRP serves as a biological marker for inflammation and necrosis, it is useful as a monitor of early deterioration or development of complications of therapy, eg empyema after pneumonectomy (Ann Int Med 1994; 57:933); an ↑ in CRP at the time of admission may presage a poor outcome in patients with severe unstable angina, indicating an inflammatory component (N Engl J Med 1994; 331:417OA)

'cream cheese' appearance GYNECOLOGY Thickened, whitish, caseous or tree bark-like exudate that adheres in plaques to the vaginal mucosa, a colposcopic appearance seen in vaginal candidiasis

CREB protein Cyclic AMP response element binding protein A 43-kD protein which, after phosphorylation, activates nuclear transcription, binding as a dimer to consensus cAMP response elements (CRIe 5'TGACGTCA3') by a 'leucine zipper' motif; see Leucine zipper motif

Note: Transcription of some genes is activated by second messengers, eg cAMP that act through specific protein kinases and requires both the cAMP response element and the 'A' kinase

creatine kinase An enzyme [EC 2.7.3.2] that catalyzes the reaction ADP + phosphocreatine = ATP + creatine, in which there is an exchange of high-energy phosphate and maintenance of ATP; see CK-MB, CK-MB subunit

creationism EVOLUTIONARY BIOLOGY The philosophy based on the Judeo-Christian concept that all forms of life, in particular, the human, were created out of 'nothingness', ie de novo, a theory that is diametrically opposite that of Darwinism or evolution, in which all organisms evolved from a previous ancestor; despite the lack of valid scientific evidence supporting creationist theories, creationist 'science' has accrued widespread sympathy in some states of the Southeastern US; Cf Darwinism, Gaia hypothesis

credentials The sum total of all the documentation of a practitioner's formal undergraduate (college or university and medical school) and graduate (internship, residency, fellowships) education, relevant board certifications, and state licenses

credentials committee A formal committee of a hospital or health care institution's medical staff that has a legal onus to the parent institution to verify a practitioner's credentials when he/she applies for appointment to the medical staff

'creep' DRG creep, see there

creep MATERIALS SCIENCE Cold flow A time-dependent strain or deformation of a material in response to a continuous force or constant stress; creep is of particular interest to those physicians who place prosthetic devices in weight-bearing regions, as in the case of polyethylene components of artificial joints PHYSIOLOGY A slow, continued lengthening of a muscle following a first phase of muscle lengthening

creeping fat GASTROENTEROLOGY The delicate circumferential extension of the mesenteric fat around the small and large intestinal serosa, characteristic of Crohn's disease, but also described in renal transplant patients

CREM cAMP-responsive element modulator CELL BIOLOGY A gene that is highly expressed in a rhythmic fashion in neuroendocrine cells, which encodes a potent repressor of cAMP-induced gene transcription; CREM is also hormonally regulated during spermatogenesis (Nature 1993; 365:314)

crenation artefact HEMATOLOGY Distortion of erythrocytes, appearing as echinocytes in peripheral blood smears due to hyperosmolar fixative, or water contamination of the Wright-Giemsa stain

creosote A mixture of phenols, especially guaiacol and creosol, which is obtained by the fractional distillation of wood tar; it is used as a disinfectant, a deodorant; internally, creosote has had some currency as an expectorant

crepitation 'Crunching' of tissue caused by the presence of gas, due to a 1) Spontaneous rupture of small pulmonary blebs (most common in young men, causing mediastinal or apical emphysema, of little clinical significance) and 2) Gas-producing microaerobic or anaerobic bacteria (requiring a low red-ox potential, eg *Clostridia perfringens, C sporogenes, C tertium, Bacteroides* spp, peptostreptococci and peptococci), potential inoculums in open trauma, causing cellulitis, myonecrosis, foul odor and abundant gas production with minimal systemic disease

crescendo angina Unstable angina, see there

crescent A commonly used adjectival descriptor (alternately termed 'Quarter moon') for a sharply circumscribed, smoothly curved radiolucent or light-colored mass in a dark background, which converges at both ends

crescent BONE RADIOLOGY A curvilinear subcortical radiolucency corresponding to a fracture line and bony collapse, seen in early ischemic necrosis of the epiphysis of the femoral head, a finding that may also be seen in the humoral head, and may be accentuated by traction RENAL PATHOLOGY Epithelial crescents are curved, semilunar lesions seen by low-power light microscopy, which correspond to extracapillary proliferation of Bowman's (glomerular) capsule epithelium, acquiring a fibroblast-like spindled morphology, possibly stimulated by release of fibrinogen from basement membrane; crescents may be accompanied by collagen and fibrin deposition, mononuclear cell proliferation; crescents may be seen in primary and secondary glomerular disease RENAL RADIOLOGY A scalloped curvilinear radiolucency seen in the kidneys secondary to chronic lower urinary tract obstruction, eg concrement-induced obstruction, seen in the early phases of urography; the crescent is due to accumulation of radiocontrast material within flattened collecting tubules and thus indicates residual renal function in contrast to the rim sign, in which there is no renal function, best seen by angiography

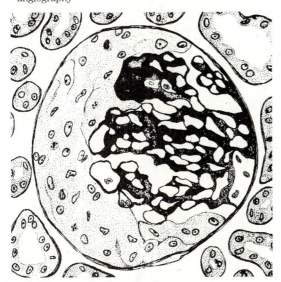

glomerular crescent

crescentic glomerulonephritis A glomerulopathy that may be associated with diabetes mellitus, characterized by heavy proteinuria, microaneurysms and hypertension; without therapy, 80-90% eventually require regular dialysis; CGN may be idiopathic or primary, a condition which, in absence of an infection, multisystem disease or other primary glomerulopathy reveals extensive (greater than 50% of glomeruli are involved) crescents, divided into Type I Anti-glomerular basement membrane antibody without pulmonary hemorrhage Type II Immune complex crescentic glomerulonephritis and Type III Idiopathic; CGN may also be superimposed on other primary glomerulopathies, including membranoproliferative (mesangiocapillary) glomerulonephritis, membranous, IgA nephropathy and focal and segmental glomerulosclerosis; CGN may be secondary to infection, eg Post-streptococcal GN, infective endocarditis, sepsis, hepatitis, multisystem disease, cryoglobulinemia, Goodpasture's disease, relapsing polychondritis, Henoch-Schönlein purpura, SLE, disseminated vasculitis, polyarteritis nodosa, Wegener's disease, lung cancer, lymphoma, and other malignancy

CREST complex An acronym for the pentad of clinical signs seen with mixed connective tissue disease, including Calcinosis, Raynaud's phenomenon, Esophageal dysmotility with eventual stricture, Sclerodactyly, Telangiectasia; CREST has a slightly better prognosis than other connective tissue disorders, but is susceptible to late complications, eg biliary cirrhosis and pulmonary hypertension LABORATORY Anticentromere antibodies are characteristic of CREST, but may also be seen in progressive systemic sclerosis, older women or in those with HLA-DR1

cretin Congenital hypothyroidism A condition caused by defective thyroxine or thyroglobulin synthesis, associated with a goiter, iodine deficiency or thyroid gland defects (aplasia, hypoplasia or dysgenesis) CLINICAL Cold intolerance, serosal effusions, myxedema, low metabolic rate, increased cholesterol and profound mental retardation (hypothyroid idiocy); when detected in neonatal screening and treated early, these children have normal school performance at age 10 (J Pediatr 1990; 116:27)

Note: Cretin is from French for Christian, as these children are so profoundly retarded that they were considered to be incapable of sinning and therefore the purest of God's creatures, ergo the most perfect Christians

Creutzfeldt-Jakob disease A disease caused by an aberrant protein, the prion CLINICAL Pyramidal tract disease with Babinski sign; cerebellar dysfunction is manifest by ataxia, and intention tremor, myoclonus; involvement of the basal ganglia is manifest by rigidity, bradykinesia, tremor, dystonic postures, and choreoathetosis (N Engl J Med 1993; 328:1259CPC) DISINFECTION The agent is highly contagious and

IS inactivated by autoclaving for 1 hour at 132°C and 20 psi, 5% hypochlorite, and 0.03% permanganate solutions

IS NOT inactivated by boiling water, 10% formalin, 70% alcohol, or ultraviolet light (CAP Today March 1993)

crewcut appearance Hair on end appearance, see there

CRF Corticotropin-releasing factor, see CRH

CRH Corticotropin-releasing hormone A potent neuropeptide that stimulates synthesis and secretion of proopiomelanocortin-derived peptides, which is released in the median eminence of hypothalamus into the portal circulation of the pituitary gland, regulating (via cAMP and Ca⁺⁺ as intracellular messengers) ACTH secretion; CRH injection evokes hormonal, metabolic, circulatory and behavioral biological stress response; CRH is markedly increased in pregnancy and its activity is turned off by a 37-kD binding protein (Nature 1991; 349:423)

CRH stimulation test ENDOCRINOLOGY A stimulation test used to evaluate pituitary response to corticotropin-releasing hormone; in general, pituitary (adrenohypophysis) tumors causing Cushing's disease response to CRH, while ectopic ACTH-secreting tumors do not RESULTS Plasma ACTH ↑ 2-4-fold in most patients with CD (see N Engl J Med 1994; 331:629oA)

crib death Sudden infant death syndrome, see SIDS

cribriform *adjective* Relating or pertaining to a sieve-like histologic pattern, in which sheets of epithelial cells are punctuated by gland-like spaces; the cribriform pattern is highly suggestive of adenoid cystic carcinoma

cri-du-chat syndrome Lejeune syndrome An embryopathic complex that is more common in females due to the loss of the short arm of chromosome 5, occasionally due to a ring chromosome CLINICAL High-pitched feline mewing which often diminishes with age, low birth weight, mental and physical retardation, hypertelorism, hypotonia, microcephaly, micrognathia, epicanthal folds, a moon-like facies, low-set ears, congenital cardiac defects, short metacarpals and metatarsals, pes planus, and partial syndactyly PROGNOSIS Lifespan relatively normal

crime against humanity GLOBAL VILLAGE A generic term of uncertain origin for crime(s) committed against other persons that reflects depravity (serial killing with body mutilation) or fanaticism (eg ethnic 'cleansing', genocide, terrorism)

crime gene BEHAVIORAL GENETICS A putative gene or family of genes based on the controversial concept that criminal acts have genetic underpinnings; epidemiological data or chromosomal candidates have been proposed for a hereditary component in criminal acts, eg the Jukes family‡ in the 1870s, and the 'XYY hypothesis' that surfaced in the 1970s, and subsequently resubmerged due to lack of valid data; there is no known cancer gene (New York Times 15 Sept 1992; C1)

criminal abortion Deliberate termination of pregnancy under illegal circumstances; prior to the *Roe* v. *Wade* decision‡, physicians regularly performed 'criminal' abortions, in the usual parlance, criminal abortion implies a clandestine termination of pregnancy under non-sterile and unsuitable conditions, which predisposes the mother to sepsis and death by exsanguination through mutilation of the uterus and perineum

criminal homicide Murder, see there

criminal insanity Insanity, see there

criminal intent FORENSIC MEDICINE Intent to do harm, either by demonstration of the mindset to perform a criminal act, or by the commission of such an act

criminal negligence see Negligence

'criminal' nerve of Grassi A branch of the right posterior vagus which passes to the left behind the esophagus, terminating in the cardia

Note: The sobriquet 'criminal' derives from the significant potential for ulcer recurrence if the nerve is not severed during surgery

criminal victimization SOCIAL MEDICINE A social condition most common in women who are single mothers and suffer physical and mental abuse from boyfriends; in general, the victims have ↓ sense of well-being and ↑ greater levels of stress; victims incur 2.5-fold greater inpatient costs than non-victims (Arch Int Med 1991; 151:342)

criminology 1) The study of criminal behavior, more commonly known as forensic psychiatry 2) The study of the nature, causes, and means of handling criminal acts

crisis CLINICAL MEDICINE 1) An abrupt change in the course of a disease, either for better or for worse, eg an acute exacerbation of adrenal insufficiency, Addisonian crisis 2) An abrupt intensification of a symptom or other manifestation of a disease, paroxysm INFECTIOUS DISEASE Abrupt improvement ('breaking' of a fever) of untreated lobar pneumonia, most often due to *Streptococcus pneu-*

moniae, occurring at the end of the first week, at the time when the production of antibodies rises and successful phagocytosis of the bacteria occurs, a clinical finding common in the pre-antibiotic era TISSUE CULTURE The self-imposed limit on the growth of cultured, non-neoplastic fibroblasts and other cell lines; after 50-100 generations, these cells undergo a series of agonal changes in the genome, including the shortening of telomers, lose their ability to divide and die

crisis intervention PSYCHIATRY The counseling of a person who is suffering from a stressful life crisis (AIDS, cancer, death, divorce) by providing mental and moral support

crisscross heart Superoinferior heart, upstairs-downstairs heart A rare cardiac malformation in which the AV spatial relation places each ventricle in a position contralateral to its corresponding atrium, characterized by a horizontal interventricular septum, with complex cardiac plumbing; one-third have AV discordance CLINICAL Cyanosis and heart failure TREATMENT Palliative rather than corrective surgery

crit Hematocrit

crithidia assay LABORATORY MEDICINE A direct immunofluoresence test for quantifying anti-DNA antibodies in the serum of patients with SLE using *Crithidia luciliae*, a hemoflagellate, the kinetoplast of which is a modified mitochondrion containing abundant double-stranded DNA

critical care YD critical care of patients is optimal in the controlled environment of intensive care unit; in the hospital environment, critical care is often provided in the OR suite, recovery room, and in the emergency department

critical mass RESEARCH A generic term for the minimum threshold number of individuals working in related fields in a particular location, below which creative thinking and interaction is believed to be suboptimal; as an example, in the laboratories of a number of well-funded world-class, part of the 'fun' intrinsic to 'doing' science may be related to being in a milieu of similarly-minded persons, which like a nuclear reaction (from whence the name), requires a critical mass of fissionable material

critical pathway Care path A standardized sequence of diagnostic and therapeutic protocols, and interventions that are conducted on a patient with a certain set of symptoms from the time of admission by a hospital's ancillary staff to the end of the patient's stay; CPs attempt to achieve the most efficient and effective outcome in patient management; an example of a CP for the management of a needle stick injury is presented on the facing page; CP 'algorithms' are being developed with the pretext of improving operations, total quality management, and ultimately to reducing the costs of health care by promoting a specific outcome within a predetermined timeframe (CAP Today February 1994)

Note: The most popular of the many synonyms for critical pathway is algorithm or clinical algorithm, which continues to be widely used; other synonyms include care pathway, clinical algorithm, clinical pathway, clinical practice guidelines, care map, and patient standards; it is uncertain which will ultimately prevail

CRNA Certified registered nurse anesthetist

crocodile tear 'syndrome' A clinical analog of gustatory hyperhidrosis, in which the peripheral autonomic pathways for lacrimation and salivation are misdirected or short-circuited, usually following facial nerve injury, where food or chewing induce unilateral or inappropriately abundant tearing, due to faulty regeneration of nerve fibers which originally supplied the salivary glands are routed to the lacrimal gland via the petrossal nerve

Crohn's disease activity index An index based on the patient's symptoms, requirement for antidiarrheal drugs, presence of abdominal masses??, hematocrit, and body weight with scores from 0 to 700; a score of 151-400 is associated with disease that is mild to moderately active; higher scores indicate more intense disease activity (see **N Engl J Med 1994; 331:836oA**)

Cro-Magnon PALEOANTHROPOLOGY Tall slender hominids that first appeared in the fossil record ± 30 000 years ago

cromolyn sodium Used for asthma and allergic rhinitis An anti-inflammatory that acts to to reduce airway hyperresponsiveness, and early and late asthmatic responses

crossbite ODONTOLOGY A form of malocclusion in which there is a reversal of the normal relation of the mandibular with the maxillary teeth, with lateral displacement of opposing teeth; in normal dentition, the mandibular teeth lie inside the maxillary teeth and the outside mandibular cusps (incisal edges) meet the central portion of the opposing maxillary teeth

cross-bridge HISTOLOGY A finding by light microscopy characterized by several parallel fiber-like structures that extend from the cell membrane of one epithelial cell* to its nearest neighbor; cross-bridges are an artefact of shrinkage during fixation and correspond to desmosomes as seen by electron microscopy

*Most prominently seen in the squamous epithelial cells of the skin

'cross country' pattern SURGICAL PATHOLOGY A descriptor for the manner in which the polymorphic infiltrates of pulmonary lymphomatoid granulomatosis destroys the lung, 'spilling over' into the interstitium

Note: Originally described as benign, lymphomatoid granulomatosis is viewed as premalignant or frankly malignant, as the average patient survives 14 months and often involves extrapulmonary sites, eg skin, central nervous system and kidney, extending in a lymphoma-like fashion, often causing a septic death

cross-cover *noun* A physician who 'covers' for another physician and provides patient care when the other physician is not available *verb* To provide health care for another physician's patient (**PL Fine, The Wards, Little, Brown and Co, Boston, 1994**)

cross eyes Convergent strabismus A process affecting 3%

of all children; once recognized, strabismus should be treated immediately to allow maximum development of visual acuity, binocular function and cosmetic results

Note: In general, children do not outgrow strabismus

cross-feeding MICROBIOLOGY The growth of two or more organisms in the region, as each is dependent on the waste or synthetic products of the other organism; see CAMP test

cross infection A converging pattern of infection in which person A is infected with microorganism A; person B with microorganism B; upon person-to-person contact, microorganism B infects person A, microorganism A infects person B; both patients must be treated with the appropriate antimicrobial agent for both infections, otherwise a 'ping-pong' infectious sequence may develop

cross-linkage theory A biologic model for aging that assumes that post-translation cross-linking of normally translated intra- and extracellular proteins is responsible for aging, eg glycosylation end-products causing cataracts and collagen degeneration causing atherosclerosis; while not central to the pathogenesis of aging, the cross-linkage theory provides a valid framework for aging process; see Garbage can theory

crossed syndrome(s) NEUROLOGY Cranial nerve lesions that are opposite to the side of a hemiplegia, which may occur in transient occlusion of the basilar artery

(serologic) crossmatch TRANSFUSION MEDICINE An agglutination test that determines donor-recipient blood compatibility; cross matches are of two types: 1) Major crossmatch Patient serum (which may contain antibodies) is cross-reacted against the donor's red cells and 2) Minor crossmatch Patient erythrocytes are incubated with donor serum, this is of lesser clinical significance and reveals donor antibodies against low incidence antigens (eg C^w, -Wr^a, -Li^a); Cf Electronic crossmatch

cross-match/transfusion ratio TRANSFUSION MEDICINE The C/T ratio is the ratio of units of packed red blood cells that are cross-matched (in the blood bank for potential infusion during surgical procedures) to the number of units actually transfused; under optimal conditions, this ratio is 2.5 or less for general surgery and somewhat higher for obstetrics and gynecology; a high C/T ratio may indicate excess caution by the surgeon or overordering, while low ratios indicate effective prediction of actual usage

crossover CLINICAL STUDY DESIGN The switching of a subject or patient in a clinical trial from one arm (eg therapeutic or placebo) of the study to another; crossing-over of patients may be either part of the original study protocol (crossover study) or a decision motivated by ethics as the patient might be deteriorating in the less

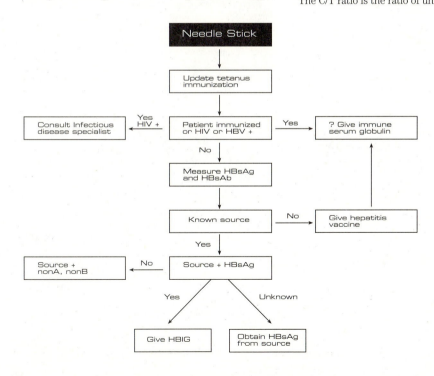

critical pathway (clinical algorithm)

effective therapeutic arm

crossover tendinitis SPORTS MEDICINE Inflammation of the adductor pollicis longus and extensor pollicis brevis tendons in rowers, a form of overuse injury

'crossover' unit TRANSFUSION MEDICINE A unit of autologous blood product(s) that is made available for general use after the donor's surgery and potential need for the blood has passed; the FDA has recommended against using cross-over units, reasoning that 1) Donor criteria are less stringently applied when accepting a donor for transfusion of his own blood and 2) The unit has a greater potential for being infected

cross-reaction IMMUNOLOGY A partial reaction or 'recognition' of an epitope by an antibody that was generated in response to another antigen

cross-sectional study EPIDEMIOLOGY A survey that determines the difference in the prevalence of disease among various segments of the population at a particular time, which may be used to infer a causitive relation; Cf Epidemiology

crosstalk Self-inhibition CARDIOLOGY The inappropriate detection of the atrial stimulus by the ventricular channel in a cardiac pacemakers; crosstalk depends on amplitude of the atrial stimulus and the ventricular channel's sensitivity; maneuvers used to eliminate crosstalk include reduction of the atrial output and/or ventricular sensitivity, and requires a ventricular blanking (refractory) period of 10-60 msec that coincides with the atrial stimulus; in absence of spontaneous rhythm, crosstalk may cause asystole, which with appropriate pacemaker programming and ventricular safety pacing mechanisms is rarely problematic

cross-talk ENDOCRINOLOGY An alternative action effected by a ligand when it binds to a receptor other than its own, blocking the activity stimulated or evoked by the binding of the receptor's cognate ligand; an example of cross-talk is testosterone binding to the estrogen receptor, resulting in an antiestrogenic effect

croup Acute laryngotracheobronchitis PEDIATRICS A generic term for a heterogeneous group of relatively acute, often infectious conditions; croup is a common cause of acute upper-airway obstruction of childhood, with an incidence of 3/100 children < 6 years, up to 1.3% of whom require hospitalization; it is characterized by a brassy, seal-like barking or 'croupy' cough accompanied by inspiratory stridor and hoarseness, resulting from intense edema, laryngeal mucus, subglottic stenosis, accompanied by dyspnea, tachypnea, cyanosis, sternal and intercostal retractions; a common form is viral laryngotracheitis with progressive subglottic edema, affecting children age 3 months to 3 years, commonly due to respiratory syncytial virus and parainfluenza virus; bacterial laryngotracheitis is most common in ages 3 to 7 and is due to *Haemophilus influenzae* and *Corynebacterium diphtheriae* CLINICAL Progressive dyspnea, dysphagia, low-grade fever, chills and an upper respiratory tract infection in the recent past RADIOLOGY see Gothic arch TREATMENT Dexamethasone-IM, prednisolone-oral, budesonide-nebulized, the last of which is also effective for mild-to-moderate croup (**N Engl J Med 1994; 331:285oA**), mist tents, antibiotics

Note: 'Croupy' coughs may occur with upper airway obstruction due to aspiration of a foreign body, retropharyngeal abscess, intraluminal masses (angioedema, hemangioma), extrinsic compression, eg hematoma secondary to neck trauma, spasms initiated by endotracheal intubation, hypocalcemic tetany and asthma

crowding SOCIAL MEDICINE Excess population density; rhesus monkey colonies respond to crowding by increasing 'coping' behaviors (**Science News 1994; 146:20**) which militates against a widely-held theory that there is a direct relation between crowding and aggressiveness, a posit supported by data from rodent studies; under long-term crowding conditions, the behavior of individual mice in colonies of mice begins to 'autodestruct' two-to-four generations after passing twice the optimal population density; maternal instincts fail, juvenile behavior extends into adulthood, younger animals become aggressive and males huddle together in small 'gangs'

Note: Correlating rodent data to the human social fabric is fraught with error, despite the disturbing implications

crowing PEDIATRICS Cantus galli, laryngismus stridulus Noisy respiratory 'cawing', stridor and severe respiratory distress, heard in infants with 1) Congenital laryngeal stridor Crowing may be the first sign of congenital epiglottic and supraglottic deformity or flabbiness (laryngomalacia and tracheomalacia) with collapse and partial inspiratory airway obstruction, a condition more common in males; during the paroxysms, the children are hoarse, aphonic, dyspneic, have inspiratory muscle retractions and if prolonged, fail to thrive 2) Double aortic arch and 3) Others, including branchial cleft cysts, chondromalacia, congenital goiter, croup, intraluminal webs, laryngeal masses, lymphangioma, macroglossia, mandibular hypoplasia, mucus retention cysts, Pierre-Robin syndrome, and thyroglossal duct remnants

crow's feet appearance A fanciful descriptor for short linear striations radiating from one point or a short line NEURORADIOLOGY Angiographic morphology of cerebellopontine angle hemorrhages RADIOLOGY Vague linear opacifications radiating from the pleura into the pulmonary parenchyma, seen on a plain chest film in pleural asbestosis Note: Crow's feet on a chest film are usually benign, but may also appear in malignant mesotheliomas and other tumors SURGICAL ANATOMY A fanciful term for the terminal branches of the left (anterior) vagus nerve, which are preserved in highly selective vagotomy for surgical therapy of peptic ulcer disease

CRT Cathode ray tube; see Video display terminals

cruciferous vegetables CLINICAL NUTRITION A group of indole-rich vegetables, eg broccoli, brussels sprouts, cabbage, cauliflower and mustard that have anti-tumor promoting activity in laboratory animals; crucifer consumption is decreased in patients with colonic cancer; see Tumor promoter

cruciform DNA Foldback DNA An unstable, non-double helix form of DNA, consisting of a pair of hairpin oligonucleotide palindromes, generated either as an intermediate in homologous genetic recombination, resulting in a transient 'Holliday' junction or as a supercoiled palindromic sequence; the binding protein that recognizes cruciform DNA is an evolutionarily conserved nuclear protein, the non-histone high mobility group protein 1, HMG-1; cruciform DNA is useful for in vitro studies of DNA kinetics and structural analysis, but is thought to be a 'forbidden' structure under natural conditions

cruise *verb* A colloquialism defined as the seeking, watching, or flirting with potential sexual partners, used primarily by homosexual ♂ (as in 'to cruise the bars'), but also by prostitutes searching for clients (**JE Lighter, Historical Dictionary of American Slang, Random House, New York, 1994**)

crumbled bone disease Osteogenesis imperfecta, type IIA An often lethal AD (**MIM 120150.0027**) condition (50% are stillborn), with low birthweight, beading of ribs with multiple fractures and an accordion-like collapse of shortened, bent and deformed long bones with potentially fatal neonatal respiratory insufficiency in those who survive birth

crumpled tissue paper appearance A descriptor for the faintly striated eosinophilic cytoplasm in the foamy 20-80 μm Gaucher histiocytes, best seen by a PAS (periodic acid Schiff) stain; the striations are due to bilayered stacks of glucosyl ceramide within lysosomes EM Twisted tubules arranged in rod-shaped, 125 nm in diameter membrane-bound fascicles; cytoplasmic striation may be seen in the pseudo-Gaucher cells of thalassemia, lymphomas, and type II dyserythropoietic anemia

crush preparation Squash prep* A rapid cytologic smear that is prepared by crushing (ie squashing) small tissue fragments between two glass slides, which are then either fixed in 95% ethanol and stained with H&E, or air-dried and stain with Diff-Quik®; the squash prep is of particular use in evaluating the 3-D morphology of various brain tumors, including meningiomas, neurilemomas, and astrocytomas (**Acta Cytologica 1993; 37:884**0A, 9130A)

*The formal (written) form is crush preparation; the informal (spoken) form is squash prep

crush syndrome Traumatic rhabdomyolysis A condition[1] that results from prolonged and continuous pressure on the limbs, which reflects the disintegration of muscle and influx of myolytic products into the circulation LABORATORY ↑ K+, purines, phosphates, lactic acid, myoglobin, thromboplastin, creatine kinase, creatine and BUN, hemoglobinuria and myoglobinuria PATHOPHYSIOLOGY CS was first thought to be due to blockage of the distal convoluted renal tubules by myoglobin, but later shown to result from post-anoxic acute tubular necrosis with local renal vasoconstriction due to stimulation of the autonomic nervous system, a pathogenic 'cascade' that also occurs in drug-induced (eg heroin) coma; also implicated in the syndrome is the so-called reperfusion injury (**N Engl J Med 1991; 324:1417**) ; IM pressure in patients with compressed limb injuries may increase to 240 mm Hg, resulting in rhabdomyolysis independent of ischemia and anterior compartment syndrome

[1]First described during the Battle of Britain (**Br J Med 1941; 1:427**), when it was induced by massive trauma caused by air-raid and rocket (V-1 and V-2) bombings; the victims went into shock only after they had been released from entrapment by crushing objects, despite initial response to wound care and intravenous therapy [2]Note: Rhabdomyolysis, myoglobinuria, and renal failure with hypocalcemia is due to a shift of extracellular Ca++ into injured muscle and impaired Na+-K+-ATPase activity

'crushed cranberry' appearance MICROBIOLOGY A fanciful descriptor for the gross appearance of cultures of *Actinomadura pelletieri*, where the colonies are blood red and glistening

Cruzan, Nancy Beth A 32-year-old woman who was in a prolonged unconscious (vegetative) state since an automobile accident in 1983, despite her parents' efforts to disconnect her life support; according to the Supreme Court of Missouri, *'The state's interest is not in quality of life, but rather in life itself, an interest that is unqualified'*; in the US, 10 000 patients are in a persistent vegetative state, each at an annual cost of $130 000

Note: This 'right-to-life' case ended in December 1990 with the removal of life support and Ms Cruzan's death; see Persistent vegetative state

cruzin A highly specific neuraminidase inhibitor isolated from *Trypanosoma cruzi* which is identical both functionally and molecularly to HDL; when *T cruzi* epimastigotes are grown in a lipoprotein-depleted medium, addition of HDL and cruzin restores multiplication; cruzin binds to *T cruzi*, inhibiting neuraminidase produced in the infective trypomastigote

cry for help PSYCHOLOGY A colloquial expression for any verbalization (eg telephone call to crisis intervention hotlines) or action (eg standing on outer ledge of tall building, notes left in conspicuous places) that indicates a person's state of extreme mental distress or anguish and the potential for suicide

'cryo' Cryoprecipitate, see there

cryoglobulinemia A clinical condition caused by proteins, especially polymeric IgG3 that precipitate in vivo on cooling of acral parts, often associated with immune complex-related disease, which has been divided into three clinical forms (see table) CLINICAL Arthralgias, vascular purpuras,

cold intolerance, hypertension, congestive heart failure LABORATORY Decreased C4 and other complement proteins

The response of HCV-associated cryoglobulinemia to IFN-α-2a is a function of the titers of HCV (**N Engl J Med 1994; 330:51**0A)

cryocrit A crude, rapid method for quantifying cryoglobulin; a hematocrit tube of serum is cold-incubated, spun, and the percentage of precipitate determined

cryoprecipitate 'Cryo' TRANSFUSION MEDICINE A product derived from a unit of whole blood, which has a volume of 15 ml and provides a minimum of 80 units of factor VIII:C procoagulant (for hemophilia A), factor VIII:vWF (for von Willebrand's disease), factor XIII, fibronectin and fibrinogen (for DIC, dysfibrinogenemia)

cryopreservation The freezing of tissue Certain human tissues, eg packed red cells and pre- and post-fertilization products can be reversibly frozen by using glycerol, which 1) Lowers the freezing point of fluids by increasing the number of molecules in solution and 2) Transforms water into a glass-like solid instead of ice crystals which would rupture the cells; in animals, hyperglycemia allows subfreezing survival; see Frozen cells, in vitro fertilization

Note: In California, whole body cryopreservation has been offered commercially, although no body has been successfully thawed

cryopreservatives TRANSFUSION MEDICINE Agents that allow long-term storage of packed red cells for up to a projected 40 years, with 85% viability of erythrocytes 24 hours after transfusion; the agent of choice is 40% glycerol, which is stored at -80°C, requires post-thaw washing to reduce the glycerol to 1% and which tolerate wide fluctuations of temperature during transportation; other cryopreservatives include 20% glycerol which is stored at -150°C and is therefore difficult to transport, 14% hydroxyethyl starch, and 15% DMSO-dimethylsulfoxide; see Frozen blood, HES

cryostat SURGICAL PATHOLOGY A device that houses a microtome, maintaining it at -20°C to -30°C, for the purpose of providing the surgeon relevant information, eg an intraoperative diagnosis of malignancy for a breast lesion, or whether the margins are involved in a basal cell carcinoma of the skin, on how to best continue a procedure, while the patient is under anesthesia; see Frozen section

cryosurgery A surgical technique that uses liquid nitrogen to freeze and destroy malignant tissues, eg carcinoma of the uterine cervix; cryosurgery is an increasingly popular modality for treating cancer of the prostate PROS In contrast to radical prostatectomy, cryosurgery is less painful,

---

CRYOGLOBULINEMIA

TYPE I Monoclonal cryoglobulinemia Underlying disease is often malignant; IgG (Malignant myeloma), IgM macroglobulinemia or lymphoma/chronic lymphocytic leukemia, rarely others (eg IgA nephropathy), benign monoclonal gammopathy

TYPE II Poly-monoclonal cryoglobulinemia A complex of immunoglobulins including mixed IgM-IgG, G-G, A-G or other combinations that may be associated with lymphoreticular disease or connective tissue disease (rheumatoid arthritis, Sjögren syndrome, mixed essential cryoglobulinemia)

TYPE III Mixed polyclonal-polyclonal cryoglobulinemia Mixtures of IgG and IgM, occasionally IgA, associated infections; rheumatoid arthritis, SLE, Sjögren syndrome, EBV and CMV viruses, subacute bacterial infections, poststreptococcal, crescentic and membranoproliferative glomerulonephritides, DM, chronic active hepatitis, biliary cirrhosis

CRU
199

requires less cutting, and has a shorter recuperation period CONS Incomplete removal of cancer is thought to be relatively common, and the incidence of impotence is ± 60% (Science News 1994; 146:13) see Radical prostatectomy

crypt abscess GI PATHOLOGY Aggregates of neutrophils, eosinophils, fibrin and sloughed epithelial cells within a partially ruptured colonic glandular lumen; this histologic finding (figure) is highly characteristic of ulcerative colitis, but may be seen in Crohn's disease, inflammatory bowel disease, radiation colitis, and infection by *Helicobacter* spp

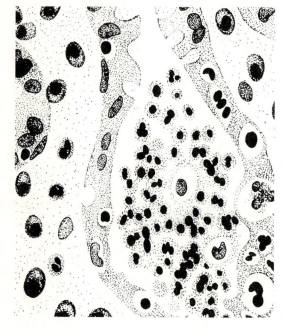

crypt abscess

crypto-nuclear power GLOBAL VILLAGE A coinage of recent vintage for any nation[1] that has the capacity to build, or already has nuclear weapons[2] that it will not admit to possessing in a public forum[3] as this might compromise its perceived options (Nature 1995; 374:579) see Nuclear Nonproliferation Treaty, Third nuclear age

[1]eg according to some specialists in the field, Israel [2]and often the capacity to deliver the nuclear device over a distance [3]eg the Nuclear Nonproliferation Treaty

Cryptosporidium A genus of protozoan parasites that may cause watery diarrhea, variably accompanied by abdominal cramping, nausea, vomiting, and fever; in the immunocompetent the diarrhea is self-limited, while in the immunocompromised (eg cancer or immunosuppressive therapy), HIV infection, radiation therapy or renal dialysis) it may be severe and intractable; '*Crypto*' may be associated with outbreaks when it passes through the filtration system in a municipal water supply (N Engl J Med 1994; 331:161oA)

crystal healing ALTERNATIVE MEDICINE The use of certain types of crystals, in particular quartz, as a therapeutic modality, which is alleged to be of use in treating a wide range of mental, physical or emotional problems; CH enjoys virtually no support in mainstream medical practice

crystallin(s) A large family of homologous water-soluble proteins that form the major structural component of the ocular lens, divided into α, β and γ crystallins, ranging from the 28-kD monomeric γ crystallin to the larger oligomeric and polymeric crystallins; crystallins are diverse and taxon-specific; while some crystallins are specialized for the lens, others have been found to be identical to enzymes found in other tissues, which are structurally related to heat shock proteins (Science 1991; 252:1078ed)

crystallized memory Long-term memory, see there

crystalloid solution A balanced isotonic solution, eg Ringer's lactate or saline fluid solution which may be used for volume expansion; because of the low osmotic pressure of these solutions, within minutes of administration, 80% of the crystalloid migrates to the interstitial space, while 20% remains in the vessels; there is thus a controversy in transfusion medicine whether blood volume should be expanded with colloid solutions (which are composed of high-molecular-weight substances, and therefore retained within the vessels and not associated with peripheral edema) or crystalloid solutions (which are less expensive, easily excreted and do not induce allergic reactions; Cf Colloid solutions

CSF Cerebrospinal fluid, also colony-stimulating factor

Also 1) Canadian Schizophrenia Foundation 2) Contrast sensitivity foundation (retina) 3) Cytostatic factor (cytology, obsolete)

CSF leak Cerebrospinal fluid leak, see there

CSIF Cytokine synthesis inhibitory factor; see IL-10, interleukin-10

CT Computed tomography, also 1) Carpal tunnel 2) Chemotherapy 3) Chest tube 4) Connective tissue 5) Continue treatment 6) Crossmatch:transfusion 7) Cytotechnologist

Also 1) Carbon tetrachloride 2) Cardiac type 3) Cardiothoracic ratio 4) Carotid tracing 5) Cellular telephone, see there 6) Cellular therapy 7) Cerebral thrombosis 8) Cerebral tumor 9) Chemical test 10) Child trends 11) Chlorothiazide 12) Cholera toxin 13) *Chorda tympani* [NA6] 14) Chymotrypsin 15) Ciguatoxin 16) Circadian time (circadian rhythm) 17) Circulation time 18) Clotrimazole 19) Clotting time 20) Coated tablet 21) Collecting tubule 22) Colloidal thorium (obsolete) 23) Compressed tablet 24) Confirmatory test 25) Constitutive transcript 26) Contraceptive technique (gynecology) 27) Contrast 28) Conventional therapy 29) Coombs' test 30) Corneal transplant 31) Coronary thrombosis 32) Corrected transposition (Cardiology) 33) Corrective therapist 34) Cortical plate thickness (anatomy) 35) Corticosterone 36) Cover test (ophthalmology) 37) *crista terminalis* [NA6] 38) Cystine-tellurite (medium, microbiology)

CTCL Cutaneous T cell lymphoma, see there

CTD 1) Connective tissue disease 2) Cumulative trauma disorder, see there

Also 1) Carboxy-terminal domain 2) Carpal tunnel decompression 3) Congenital thymic displasia

CTL Cytotoxic T lymphocyte, see there

C/T ratio Cross-match/transfusion ratio, see there

C-type virus A single-stranded RNA retrovirus with a central nucleoid, which has oncogenic potential, ie capable of acting as a proto-oncogene, first appearing in the infected cells as immature 'A' particles; see B-type virus, Retrovirus

CTZ Chemoreceptor trigger zone, see there

cul-de-sac French, blind pouch An anatomic 'blind alley', seen in

1) Pouch of Douglas, the most dependent (ie lowest) extension of the free peritoneal cavity, located between the anterior rectal serosa and posterior uterine serosa, gravity makes this a favored site for accumulation of acute inflammatory debris and tumor aggregates

2) Conjunctiva The reflexion of the cornea and conjunctiva

3) Dura The end of the spinal canal and

4) Colonic cecum, Latin for cul-de-sac

Culex A globally-distributed genus of mosquitoes (family Culicidae) with over 2000 species, including the common mosquito of temperate climates, mosquitoes that are vectors for Togavirus, Bunyavirus, eastern equine encephalitis, St Louis encephalitis, microfilariases, ie *Wuchereria bancrofti*, *Dirofilaria immitis*, and avian, but not human, malaria; the genus *Aedes* has intermediate hosts for *Wuchereria bancrofti*, and vectors for togaviral infections, including dengue and yellow fever; *Anopheles* is the only genus of mosquitoes that is a vector for human malaria

culling HEMATOLOGY The removal of abnormal, aged or damaged cells from the circulation by the spleen due to its unique circulation, which allows selective 'harvesting' of antibody-coated red cells and platelets as well as removal of deformed or defective erythrocytes; Cf Pitting

cult PSYCHIATRY An organization that may be religious (often with bizarre or unorthodox beliefs), psychotherapeutic, political, or commercial; they engender conflict between the group and society, and make extensive use of unethical manipulative techniques of persuasion and control to advance the leader's goals (JAMA 1994; 272:979BR)

cultural competence SOCIAL MEDICINE The ability to understand, appreciate, and interact with individuals from cultures and/or belief systems other than one's own (Am Med News 9 November 1992, p 27)

cultural genocide A term attributed to the National Association of Black Social Workers (US) referring to the adoption of black children by white parents (and applicable to virtually any other seemingly disparate adoptee-parent/guardian dyad); 500 black-by-white adoptions occur annually in the US (Science News 1994; 146:104) Cf Ethnic cleansing

cultural psychosis A generic term for any acting-out behavior that is unique to certain, often primitive societies, often accompanied by a strong component of superstition; one classification divides these reactions into 'taxa' which appear to have some validity; see Amok, Latah, Piblokto, Zombies

cultural reformulation The redefinition of an object or activity in a completely different cultural context, as might occur when a drug of abuse is used in a different social setting by a different group of individuals (JAMA 1993; 269:1505MN&P) see Ecstasy

culture-bound syndrome PSYCHIATRY A generic term for any of a number of '...recurrent, locality-specific patterns of aberrant behavior and troubling experience...', many of which cannot be linked to a particular DSM-IV diagnostic entity; they '...are generally limited to specific societies or culture areas and are localized, folk, diagnostic categories that frame coherent meanings for certain repetitive, patterned, and troubling sets of experiences and observations...' (DSM-IV, American Psychiatric Association, Washington, DC, 1994) see Amok, Ataque de nervios, Bilis, Boufée delirante, Brain fag, Dhat, Ghost sickness, Hwa-Byung, Koro, Latah, Locura, Malocchio (mal-de ojo), Nervios, Pibloktoq, Qi-gong psychotic reaction, Rootwork, Sangue dormido, Shenjing shuairuo, Shenkui, Shin-byung, Spell, Susto, Taijin kyofusho, Zar

culture-negative endocarditis CARDIOLOGY Endocarditis in which attempts to identify a causative microorganism are unsuccessful, for one of three reasons

1) The bacteria that typically cause infective endocarditis are not detected, usually because of antibiotic therapy; other causes for negative cultures when the 'usual' organisms are present include the presence of mural thrombi, right-sided endocarditis, and uremia

2) Slow-growing[1] and/or fastidious[2] bacteria with special growth requirements and

3) Nonbacterial pathogens, including fungi (eg *Candida* spp, *Aspergillus* spp), rickettsial disease, eg *Coxiella burnetii*, *Chlamydia psittaci* (N Engl J Med 1995; 332:1015CPC)

[1]Slow-growing gram-negative bacilli, eg *Actinobacillus actinomycetemcomitans, Cardiobacterium hominis, Eikenella corrodens, Haemophilus aphrophilus* [2]Anaerobes, corynebacteria, nutritionally-deficient streptococci, and others, eg acid-fast organisms, brucella, neisseria

culture shock A generic term for the suboptimal response to a constellation of altered external factors when a person is 'transplanted' to a completely different culture, in which there are major differences in language, social cues, mores, environment

cumulative meta-analysis A type of meta-analysis‡ in which the results of clinical trials are cumulated as they are published; this technique would in theory would identify any significant difference between an existing (standard) treatment and an experimental one as the information from such trials accumulate; CMAs might be useful in deciding whether continued study of a problem is needed (N Engl J Med 1992; 327:273)

cumulative trauma disorders Any of a group of often repetitive conditions that have psychological and/or physical ramifications, eg avoidance personality disorder, carpal tunnel syndrome, and others which should be critically examined in the working environment, to assure that a business is complying with the mandates of the Americans with Disabilities Act; CTDs are the most common reason for workers' compensation claims in the US (Advance/Laboratory May 1994)

cupid's bow shape A morphology with two convex curves joined at the midpoint, likened to the mythical Cupid's bow ORAL DISEASE A descriptor for a double lip anomaly, characterized by redundancy of tissue on the inner mucosal aspect of usually the upper lip, that is either congenital or acquired through trauma or in a background of nontoxic thyroid enlargement (Ascher syndrome), the bow is seen when the lips are 'pursed' RADIOLOGY The normal smooth parasagittal biconcavity of the caudal face of the 3rd, 4th, and 5th lumbar vertebrae, with the bow pointing anteriorly

cupping PEDIATRIC RADIOLOGY A widened, metaphyseal concavity caused by muscular and ligamentous pulling on softened bone, which may occur at the sternal ends of the ribs, the proximal tibia and humerus, and the distal radius and ulna; cupping was first described as radiological evidence of repeated trauma to the growth plates of long bones and thus is suggestive of child abuse, but also occurs in achondrogenesis, cretinism, congenital syphilis, diastrophic and thanatophoric dwarfism, hypervitaminosis A, homocystinuria, hypophosphatasia, infarction, infection, leukemia, metaphyseal dysostosis, phenylketonuria, scurvy, sickle cell anemia, thermal injury, trauma, vitamin D rickets

CUPS Carcinoma of unknown primary site, see Occult primary malignancy

curare A generic term for a quaternary neuromuscular-blocking alkaloid first used as an arrow poison by the Indians on the Amazon and Orinoco rivers, obtained from plants of the *Strychnos* species; curare and related compounds are used as adjuvants in surgical anesthesia for relaxation of skeletal muscle and to prevent trauma in electroconvulsive therapy

curbside (consultation) Sidewalk consultation An informal and unofficial consultation obtained in one of two different contexts, either by

1) A lay-person who may 'corner' any physician seeking an opinion about a medical condition, diagnostic modality, or therapeutic option; this form of consultation is particularly dangerous for the physician offering the opinion, as a) the physician being cornered may not have expertise in the area, eg a plastic surgeon being questioned about minutiae related to the complications of chemotherapy b) the person may be asking for information about another person, eg Aunt Gertrude with gallstones, in which case the information being provided to the consultant is confusing (to both the consultant and the messenger) and/or becomes complete gibberish by the time that Aunt Gertrude receives the second-hand consultation, and c) The consultant is potentially liable for a lawsuit for misinformation that a damaged party may allege that he/she

provided in an informal context

2) A physician asking a colleague in another specialty for the best method for managing a particular clinical problem (N Engl J Med 1995; 332:474c)

curbstone sign UROLOGY Sharp intravesicular pain occurring as a patient with urinary calculi descends a staircase or steps down from a curbstone/kerbstone, caused by calculi bouncing on the trigone

curcumin A chemical extract from the food spice turmeric that has been anecdotally reported to have antiretroviral activity by inhibiting critical sequences in viral replication (Am Med News 21 Nov 1994 p13) Cf AIDS fraud

cure ONCOLOGY Restoration to one's usual state of health; although this is the ideal goal of all fields of health care, oncologists are often reluctant to use the term in reference to malignancy, especially lymphoproliferative disorders, given the known tendency of these tumors to recur ten or more years after therapy; it is thus common practice by oncologists to substitute the more guarded terms, 'no evidence of disease' or 'remission' for what non-cognoscenti call 'cure'; Cf Remission

curie An obsolete unit of radioactivity equal to 3.7×10^{10} disintegrations/sec of a radioactive nuclide, which has been replaced by the International System (SI) derived unit for radioactivity, the becquerel, which equals 2.70×10^{-11} curies

curing A process in which a semisolid thermosetting plastic is transformed into a solid form by the application of heat

CURL Compartment of uncoupling of receptor and ligand MEMBRANE PHYSIOLOGY A fusion vesicle in the cell characterized by a low (circa 5) pH that facilitates the separation of LDL and other ligands from their respective receptors, allowing the recycling of the receptor to the cell surface

CURL technology Cybernetic unmanned remote laboratory LABORATORY MEDICINE An evolving technology on the 'cutting edge' of clinical laboratory medicine in which remote laboratory testing stations, either automated (equipped with robotics) or nonautomated (in which a technician, acting as a surrogate robot, introduces specimens into an analyzer) are interfaced with the central laboratory computer for both results review and QC; in the automated or robotic station, the user selects appropriate patient and test information from a touchscreen, a door opens, the specimen is inserted, and the user is then free to move on to other tasks (CAP Today, 1994; 8:1)

curlicue ureter A ureter that has herniated either into the inguinal region (male) or sciatic region (female); the horizontal loops imply loop herniations with development of a hydrocele (JAMA 1952; 149:441)

curly toe A congenital deformity in which one or more toes are deviated plantarward, medially and rotated laterally at the distal interphalangeal joint; the twisting of the terminal pulp may cause the toe to curl under the adjacent toe; curly toes are often bilateral and symmetrical with familial tendencies TREATMENT Surgery

currant jelly An adjectival descriptor for a tissue or material with a rubbery, elastic consistency, usually replete with erythrocytes, which impart a deep violet or magenta hue, fancifully likened to jelly

currant jelly clot A red-black, gelatinous and non-adherent coagulum composed of red cells with scattered leukocytes, a type of postmortem intravascular blood clot, that develops more rapidly than the slowly sedimenting chicken fat clot

currant jelly sputum An endobronchial secretion composed of blood admixed with sputum, mucus and scattered debris, 'classically' described in untreated *Klebsiella pneumoniae* pneumonia

currant jelly stools Dark red, gelatinous stools composed of blood and mucus, passed by 60% of children with intussusception; similar stools are passed in those with juvenile 'retention' polyps RADIOLOGY Contrast studies reveal a coiled spring appearance

current procedural coding CPT coding, see there

curriculum EDUCATION A formal organized didactic program for teaching a particular subject

curvilinear profiles Farber bodies A virtually pathognomonic finding of Farber's disease, a glycosphingolipidosis that consists of comma-shaped rods within vacuoles, seen by EM (N Engl J Med 1991; 324:395) PATHOLOGY Wispy, PAS-positive structures; similar (if not identical) material occurs in the cytoplasmic inclusions in peripheral lymphocytes or skin fibroblasts in juvenile lipofuscinosis (Batten-Mayou-Spielmeyer-Vogt disease, amaurotic familial idiocy, Batten's disease, Kufs disease, Jansky-Bielschowsky syndrome, and Spielmeyer-Vogt disease), Cf Fingerprint profiles CLINICAL Intellectual deterioration, progressive loss of motor function, ataxia and retinal pigmentary degeneration; death commonly occurs in the teens to twenties

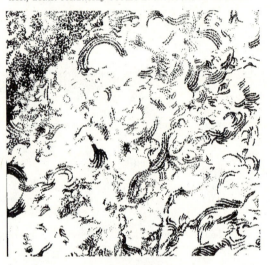

curvilinear profiles

Cushing's disease A form of Cushing syndrome (CS, see there) due to a pituitary adenoma, or rarely, hyperfunction of the anterior pituitary (adenohypophysis) which is most common in ♀ (♀:♂ = 3-8:1), usually in the childbearing years; CD accounts for ± 70% of endogenous (spontaneous) CS; unique to CD is the relative excess of neuropsychiatric dysfunction, including depression, bipolar disease, and psychosis; CD is also characterized by menstrual abnormalities related to ↑ androgen production in ovaries driven by ↑ ACTH of central origin TREATMENT Transsphenoidal microadenoidectomy (N Engl J Med 1995; 332:791RA)

Cushing syndrome A condition characterized by an excess of corticosteroids, due either to an hypersecretion of cortisol by a hyperfunctioning or neoplastic adrenal cortex, or due to exogenous corticosteroids* CLINICAL Amenorrhea, hirsutism, hypertension, impotence, muscular wasting, neuropsychiatric dysfunction, osteoporosis, truncal obesity LABORATORY Persistent hypersecretion of cortisol, loss of the usual circadian rhythm of ACTH and cortisol, and loss of suppressibility of cortisol production by administration of dexamethasone, a synthetic corticosteroid used for this purpose Note: CS is rare in children, clinically manifest as ↑ weight and growth retardation, diagnosed by corticotropin-releasing hormone stimulation and imaging studies, and usually responsive to therapy (N

Engl J Med 1994; 331:629OA) A condition caused by the long-term exposure to glucocorticoids (N Engl J Med 1995; 332:791RA) see Ectopic hormone syndrome; Cf pseudo-Cushing syndrome

*When the excess corticosteroid production is of central (adrenohypophysis) origin it is known as Cushing's disease, see there

Cushing's ulcer An acute gastric ulcer linked to severe CNS disease in the form of head trauma or tumor

cushingoid appearance An alteration in patients with Cushing syndrome consisting of 'moon' faces, truncal obesity, abdominal striae, thin skin and hyperpigmentation of skin folds

custodial care Non-medical care provided to a person who is able to function in a relatively independent fashion, but who needs environmental protection or who needs to have medical attention readily accessible; individuals requiring custodial care include the elderly, the moderately handicapped and those with later stages of malignancy or AIDS; see Hospice; Cf Home health care industry

cusum statistics CUmulative SUMmation statistics are used to (qc) quality control laboratory values, calculated by adding the observed values to the assumed values based on an idealized Gaussian distribution, serving to compare two different analytic methods; see Westgard's multirule

cut-corner configuration PEDIATRIC RADIOLOGY A rounding of the 90° angle at the distal metacarpals of Hurler syndrome

cutdown EMERGENCY MEDICINE A small surgically created incision made over a major blood vessel, usually a vein (hence, venous cutdown) that facilitates rapid and direct venous access for situations where percutaneous placement of a venous cannula is not possible, there is no 'good vein', emergent situations or global venous sclerosis (as in intravenous drug abuse); any peripheral vein can be used, the most commonly used include the cephalic vein at the shoulder, the basilic vein above the elbow, the saphenous vein at the ankle or when extremely urgent, the external jugular vein

cut effect SURGICAL PATHOLOGY The loss of a signal or reduction of signal intensity (eg by immunohistochemistry or FISH analysis) which occurs when tissue is sectioned by a microtome*, leading to an underestimation of the amount of a substance of interest (see Diagn Mol Pathol 1993; 2:94)

*Cells range from 5-25 μm; in general, examination of a tissue by light microscopy requires sectioning, usually at a thickness of 4-6 μm, meaning that larger cells will have a lesser signal

'cut-off' ANESTHESIOLOGY The point at which elongation of the carbon chain of the 1-alkanol family of anesthetics results in a precipitous drop in the anesthetic potential of these agents, eg at greater than 12 carbons in length, there is little anesthetic activity, beyond 14 carbons, none; this phenomenon was studied by Fourier transform IR spectroscopy and shown to be due to a change in the hydrogen bond-breaking activity LABORATORY MEDICINE The term cut-off most commonly refers to either 1) A time after which a specimen cannot be processed due to logistics or the necessity for 'batching' specimens to reduce the labor in performing certain assays and 2) A critical value for an analyte which is two or more standard deviations above or below a mean or 'cut-off' and therefore is abnormal

cut-off sign Colonic cut-off sign RADIOLOGY An abrupt 'amputation' of the colonic gas column occurring at the splenic flexure, characteristic of acute pancreatitis but also seen in ischemic colitis or thrombosis of the mesenteric vasculature

cut & patch repair Patch and cut repair, see there

cutaneous horn A focal hyperproduction of keratin seen in various keratoses (solar, seborrheic or inverted follicular keratoses), in marsupialized tricholemmal or epidermoid cysts and verruca vulgaris; cutaneous horns are very rarely seen in squamous cell or sebaceous gland carcinoma

Cutie-pie A type of handheld Geiger-Mueller radioactivity detector that measures α and β radiation energetic enough to pass through the mica window; the drawbacks of these radiation detectors are that they 1) Do not distinguish between types of particles or energy levels 2) Lose their sensitivity above 10 000 cpm and 3) Detect a minuscule fraction of γ radiation

cutis anserina Goose-flesh, see there

cutis marmorata Skin with a lacy reticulated red-to-bluish vascular pattern extending over most of the body, a vasomotor reaction to low ambient temperature, occurring either transiently in neonates or as a persistent change, seen in Cornelia de Lange, Down or trisomy 18 syndromes; in Cutis marmorata telangiectatica congenita (van Lohuizen's disease), the skin findings are similar but more intense and restricted to one limb; the lesion becomes more pronounced with changes in the ambient temperature or with physical activity and may spontaneously involute during adolescence

cutis verticis gyrata Bulldog or washboard scalp An alteration of the scalp, more common in males that often develops in adolescence as redundant 1-2 cm folds of scalp skin which cannot be flattened by traction; when primary (idiopathic), cutis gyrata is associated with mental retardation, ocular defects, seizures, spasticity and cranial dysmorphia; cutis verticis gyrata may be secondary to chronic inflammatory diseases, tumors (eg cylindromas, see Turban tumor), giant congenital pigmented nevus, melanocytic nevi, acromegaly and pachydermoperiostosis

'cutting edge' A highly colloquial adjective, equivalent to 'state of the art', as in 'cutting edge research'

cuvette LABORATORY TECHNOLOGY A clear receptacle that has stringently specified parameters in terms of dimensions (ie thickness) and optical properties that is used in the laboratory to measure substances at various wavelengths; quartz cuvettes are traditionally used in spectrophotometers

CV see Coefficient of variation

CVA Cerebrovascular accident, also costovertebral angle

Also 1) Cardiovascular accident (rarely used in view of potential for confusion) 2) Cyclophosphamide, vincristine, adriamycin

C value paradox EVOLUTIONARY BIOLOGY The heuristically incongruous finding that the mass of DNA or 'C value' does not reflect the evolutionary complexity of the organism, thus some small primitive organisms have a high C value, while other relatively 'sophisticated' organisms have a low C value; the paradox is partially resolved by the presence in the latter of abundant redundant or functionless DNA, the latter which is known as 'junk DNA'

CVID Common variable immune deficiency, see there

C-virus C-type virus, see there

c-v wave CARDIOLOGY An abnormally prominent pulsation of the jugular vein in tricuspid valve insufficiency, variably accompanied by systolic pulsations of the liver and a blowing systolic murmur in the 4th and 5th left parasternal spaces, which is more intense with inspiration

c wave The wave in the normal jugular phlebogram corresponding to early ventricular systole caused by bulging of the tricuspid valve into the right atrium

'CV-weighing' ACADEMIA The evaluation of a candidate for an academic appointment, based on the thickness ('weight') of his curriculum vitae (CV); 'CV-weighing' equates quality with quantity and may pressure a researcher to either 1) 'Unbundle' the research, ie separate various aspects of the experimental question(s) and report them individually, in order to 'fatten' his CVs or 2) Compromise the scientific ethic, which ranges in degree from the seemingly innocuous 'fixing' of data, to the extremely rare overt fabrication of data; to resolve this dilemma, some academic centers are evolving towards using the Institute of Scientific Information's 'Citation impact', or evaluating a researcher's innovativeness to determine whether an appointment and promotion is merited; see Authorship, Citation impact, Uncitedness index; Cf 'Hot' paper

Note: A creative report in a 'cutting edge' journal eg, Cell, Nature or Science outweighs many reports in highly specialized (often a euphemism for 'second-string') journals

CWP see Coal workers' pneumoconiosis

14C-xylose test A test for general malabsorption METHOD 1.0 g (5-10 µCi) of 'hot' xylose is administered per os; increased breath radioactivity at 30 min indicates overgrowth in the small intestine by gram-negative anaerobes

'CYA' see Defensive medicine

cyanobacterium-like bodies *Cyclospora* spp

cyberdoc A colloquial term for any computer-based interactive program that fills some of the roles traditionally filled by a physician, eg explaining to patients the risks, potential benefits, and possible negative and positive outcomes of various diagnostic or therapeutic interventions; cyberdoc software is of interest to both malpractice insurance carriers, that recognize that more informed patients tend to sue less, and by health insurance companies, as patients when faced with a menagerie of options, tend to chose the least intensive (ie least expensive) intervention (LP GRIFFIN IN SCIENCE NEWS 20 MAY 1995, p315)

cybernetics A formal comparitive study between the circuitry in the brain and electronic devices, eg computers

cyberpunk An on-line informaniac

cybersickness Simulator sickness, cyber side effects A constellation of clinical findings that affect 14-40% of those subjected to 'total immersion' virtual reality (VR), in which external audio, visual, and possibly (when using a 'virtual glove') also tactile sensation are replaced by computer-generated information; the term encompasses the autonomic symptoms (eg cold sweats, nausea, vomiting) and motion sickness which occur while 'plugged in' to the VR devices, as well as the post-session residua in the form of altered perceptions and flashbacks (Technology Rev July 1995, p14)

Note: Because of the concern for the potential ramifications of cybersickness, one video game manufacturer, Sega, decided not to sell its VR system

cyberspace INFORMATICS A virtual environment in which on-line information can be accessed and manipulated (Forbes ASAP Oct 25, 1993) see MOO

cyclamates A family (calcium cyclamate and its metabolites, cyclohexylamine, cyclamic acid, sodium cyclamate) of artificial sweeteners banned by the US Food and Drug Administration in 1970, when a study revealed increased bladder carcinoma in rats given extremely high doses; subsequent studies have failed to reveal direct, intrinsic genotoxicity of cyclamate, although when added to saccharin (another artificial sweetener), there is an additive tumorigenic effect, causing increased growth potential of focal areas of bladder epithelium; see Artificial sweeteners

cyclic AMP Cyclic adenosine monophosphate An intracellular mediator (second messenger) of hormonal action, produced from ATP by adenylate cyclase; cAMP acts on 1) Hormone receptors 2) The guanine nucleotide regulatory system 3) The catalytic unit of the cyclase itself and 4) Ion channels, modulating their activity by phosphorylation or by direct interaction with the channels on the cytoplasmic face (Nature 1991; 351:145); binding of a hormone to its cognate receptor induces a conformational change in the regulatory G (guanosine) protein, binding GTP, forming cAMP from ATP by adenylate cyclase, either increasing (ACTH,

β-adrenergic agonists, calcitonin, corticotropin-releasing factor, dopamine, FSH, glucagon, LH, PGE1, parathyroid hormone, serotonin-5HT, TSH and vasopressin V1) or decreasing (acetylcholine, α_2-adrenergic agonists, angiotensin II, insulin, opiates, oxytocin, somatostatin) intracellular substances; cAMP action is terminated by degradation to 5'AMP through phosphodiesterase, which in turn may be inhibited by various drugs, eg theophylline, and is regulated by Ca++; cAMP modulates protein kinase activity, regulates synaptic transmission, hormonal secretion, urinary osmolality, phosphate excretion, osteolysis, glycogenolysis and synthesis, lipolysis, activation of cAMP-dependent smooth muscle protein kinase phosphorylates target proteins throughout the cell; see Second messengers

3'-5'-cyclic AMP synthetase Adenylate cyclase, see there

cyclic edema A transient condition affecting women who work on their feet, possibly of psychogenic origin, as it occurs in the emotionally labile; cyclic edema is a diagnosis of exclusion, to be considered after ruling out angioneurotic edema, IgE-dependent or complement-mediated urticaria and other immune-related nosologies

cyclic neutropenia A disorder characterized by periodic episodes of severe neutropenia occurring in 3-4 week cycles, accompanied by maturational arrest of myeloid precursors in the bone marrow CLINICAL Fever, oral ulceration, cervical lymphadenopathy and multiple acute local infections that, while severe, are rarely fatal TREATMENT If symptomatic, antibiotics, eg aminoglycosides and penicillin Note: Cyclic neutropenia occurs in the collie dog

cyclin(s) A family of cell cycle control proteins synthesized during each cell cycle, controlled by a serine-threonine protein kinase p34^{cdc2}; cdc2 encodes the catalytic subunit of maturation-promoting factor, inducing the transition of G2 to M phases of the cell cycle; cyclin A is a 33-kD protein identical to an adenovirus-associated protein (E1A p60); cyclin B is a 58-kD protein that is regulated post-transcriptionally and post-translationally in the cell cycle (Nature 1990; 346:760); cyclins regulate the cell cycle and fluctuate according to the phase of the cycle; cyclin catabolism marks a cell's exit from mitosis, an event that occurs when cyclin is recognized by the ubiquitin-conjugating system (Nature 1991; 349:132)

cyclic AMP

cyclin D1 *PRAD1*, bcl-1 A proto-oncogene that plays a critical role in regulating the eukaryotic cell cycle; CD is activated by chromosome inversion, which places it under the influence of the regulatory region of the parathyroid hormone gene; it is implicated in the pathogenesis of some benign parathyroid tumors (N Engl J Med 1994; 330:757oA) and is overexpressed in various tumors, including parathyroid adenoma, carcinoma of the breast, in squamous cell carcinoma of the head and neck, and in mantle zone lymphoma, but rarely in other low-grade lymphomas MOLECULAR PATHOLOGY Cyclin D1 overexpression is the result of bcl-1 rearrangement, t(11;14)(q13;q32), which is not expressed in normal or reactive lymphoid tissues (Am J Clin Pathol 1995; 103:756) Cf RB

cyclin-dependent kinase CDK MOLECULAR BIOLOGY Any of a large family of enzymes that are key cell cycle regulators, which are themselves tightly regulated by extra- and intracellular signals in the form of four highly conserved biochemical mechanisms that forms a web of intricate and 'elegant' regulatory pathways; '*CDK-activation requires cyclin binding and phosphorylation of a conserved threonine by the CDK-activating kinase...The active CDK-cyclin complex can be inhibited by phosphorylation of a conserved threonine-tyrosine pair or binding to CDK inhibitory subunits* (Nature 1995; 374:131)

cyclooxygenase pathway A major pathway of arachidonic acid metabolism, giving rise to prostaglandins (PG); the first product is the unstable PGG_2, which absorbs oxygen and kicks out a free radical forming PGH, which is then metabolized in the individual cells forming PGE_2, $PGF_{2\alpha}$, PGD_2, PGI_2 (prostacyclin) and thromboxane A_2; other arachidonic acid metabolic pathways include lipooxygenase (forming HETE and leukotrienes) and the epoxygenase pathways (cytochrome P450 microsomal enzyme pathway); the pathway is involved in the early, non-specific response to trauma and injury (vasoconstriction and platelet aggregation)

cyclopia Cryptophthalmos, see Fraser syndrome

cyclophilin An abundant and ubiquitous 18 kD cytoplasmic protein with peptidyl-prolyl isomerase activity, catalyzing the interconversion of *cis*- and *trans*-rotamers; cyclophilin's high-affinity binding to the cyclosporin A explains cyclosporin's immunosuppressant activity; Cf Immunophilins

***Cyclospora* spp** A recently-described protozoon 8-10 μm in diameter acid-fast pathogen that causes diarrhea in both immunocompromised and immunocompetent hosts; the organism's lifecycle is incompletely characterized but undergoes both sporulation and encystation (N Engl J Med 1993; 328:1308OA, NY Times 3 Jan 1995; B13)

cyclosporin A A cyclic endecapeptide of fungal origin that induces potent T cell suppression (possibly in the G_0 or G_1 phase of mitosis) by binding to calmodulin, blocking gene activation and mRNA transcription, inhibiting cytotoxic T cell production of IL-2 and other T lymphocyte-activating cytokines; cyclosporin has ushered in a new era of transplantation, without which the success rate in liver, heart-lung (see Domino-donor), kidney and bone marrow (given the high incidence of graft-versus-host disease) transplantation would be much lower; cyclosporin is of potential use in other immune-related disorders, eg Crohn's disease, although diseases with autoimmune underpinnings, eg IDDM, do not respond; cyclosporin mouthwash is effective therapy for oral lichen planus, markedly reducing erythema, erosion, reticulation (whitish lesions) and pain; cyclosporin may be of use in aplastic anemia, in combination with antilymphocyte globulin and methylprednisone (N Engl J Med 1991; 324:1297) or for treating psoriasis (ibid 324:277); cyclosporin A exerts its immunosuppressive effect by preventing the transcriptional induction of the expression of IL-2; CsA also ininhibits the growth of autocrine tumor cells by destabilizing IL-3 mRNA (Nature 1994; 369:239L) TOXICITY Kidney (atrophy, sclerosing glomerulonephritis, tubulointerstitial fibrosis and reduced glomerular filtration rate), hypertension, anemia, anaphylaxis, nausea, tremor, paresthesias, ↑ EBV infection, lymphomas, pseudolym-

phomas, fluid retention, thromboses, encephalopathy, seizures, coma, hirsutism, and liver toxicity LABORATORY ↑ Creatinine, ↑ uric acid, ↑ bilirubin, ↑ cholesterol QUANTIFICATION HPLC, RIA, fluorescence polarization assay USES May be of use in ulcerative colitis in non-responders to corticosteroids (N Engl J Med 1994; 330:1841OA), but not in patients with Crohn's disease (N Engl J Med 1994; 330:1846OA) Nephrotoxicity: Focal interstitial fibrosis, tubular atrophy, renal arteriolar changes, including smooth muscle necrosis, intimal hyalinosis and nodular protein deposition in the walls of afferent glomerular arteries; most renal transplant recipient tolerate long-term cyclosporine therapy without progressive toxic nephropathy (N Engl J Med 1994; 331:358OA) cyclosporine-induced nephropathy is associated with ↑ production of thromboxane A_2, and leukotrienes C_4 and D_4; addition of 6 g of dietary fish oil to cyclosporine therapy in renal transplant victims reduces the episodes of rejection, but appears to have no effect on survival (N Engl J Med 1993; 329:769OA)

cyclosporin

cylindroma DERMATOPATHOLOGY A skin adnexal tumor[1] that consists of well-circumscribed epithelial 'islands[2] composed of 1) undifferentiated, palisaded and peripherally-oriented cells with small dark nuclei and 2) central lighter staining cells with larger nuclei differentiating towards glands that may focally demonstrate secretion; cylindromas are usually solitary, smooth, variably shaped nodules on the face, trunk and extremities, corresponding to skin appendage proliferations; when extensive and on the scalp, known as Turban tumors, see there; apocrine, rarely merocrine differentiation; some cylindromas are autosomal dominant, they may be associated with trichoepitheliomas and may undergo malignant degeneration

[1]the term was formerly used for adenoid cystic carcinoma of the salivary glands (named for its typical 'Swiss cheese' pattern of growth) [2]aka the jigsaw puzzle tumor, a colloquialism that refers to its histological pattern

***Cynomolgus* monkeys** A primate that is imported for use in many areas of research from AIDS vaccine development to behavioral sciences; the shipments to the US were strictly reduced in late 1989, when the CDC in Atlanta isolated filovirus (a virus related to the potentially devastating Ebola virus) in some of the monkey shipments, which to date has proven to be of no human consequence; see AIDS vaccine

CYP1A1 The major polycyclic aromatic hydrocarbon (PAH) inducible-cytochrome P4501A1 gene, which is thought to have a role in pulmonary carcinogenesis and toxicology, the product of which, CYP1A1-dependent monooxygenase, transforms certain xenobiotics, eg PAH procarcinogens in tobacco smoke to potent carcinogenic metabolites; active cigarette smoking causes the gene to remain in a 'turned-on' state and its expression is increased in certain lung cancers (J Natl Cancer Inst 1990; 82:1333)

CYP21 The gene that encodes a microsomal cytochrome

P-450 responsible for steroid 21-hydroxylation (adrenal 21-hydroxylase P-450c21); mutation of the CYP21 gene in the form of deletions or transfers of the deleterious sequences from the adjacent pseudogene CYP21P resulting in gene conversion, is usually responsible for 21-hydroxylase deficiency (N Engl J Med 1991; 324:145)

CYP2D6 A liver cytochrome P-450 enzyme that is largely responsible for the elimination various drugs*; polymorphism of the gene encoding CYP2D6 (and therefore its absence) occurs in 7% of the white population and explains the increased side effects seen in some people being treated with fluoxetine (Prozac), which is a potent inhibitor of CYP2D6 (N Engl J Med 1994; 331:1354RV)

*eg antiarrhythmic agents, β-adrenergic antagonists, neuroleptics, some selective serotonin reuptake inhibitors, and tricyclic antidepressants

cyproheptadine Periactin SPORTS MEDICINE A substance that has transient currency with some atheletes as it was believed to stimulate the appetite (JC DeLee, D Drez, Jr, Eds, Orthopedic Sports Medicine WB Saunders, Philadelphia, 1994)

cystic fibrosis An AR [MIM 219700] disease that is most common in those of Celtic stock (1:2000 births, US; carriers 1:25 white, 1:250 blacks) in which excessive chloride and sodium in secretions causes thickening of mucus and decreased clearance of secretions, in part related to defective cAMP-dependent phosphorylation of a chloride selective channel of both epithelial cells and lymphocytes PHYSIOLOGY Both the cAMP-dependent protein kinase and protein kinase C fail to activate otherwise normal chloride channels CLINICAL Progressive lung disease, pneumonia (*Pseudomonas aeruginosa* or *P cepacia*), exocrine pancreatic insufficiency, impaired growth, increased sweat electrolytes, especially chloride, as well as meconium ileus, nasal polyposis and hepatobiliary disease SCREENING The ΔF508 deletion is present in 68% of all cases of CF (76% of US whites but less common in other races, eg 30% in Ashkenazic Jews); more than 20 different gene mutations cause CF; the sensitivity of a CF test in the average white couple in the US is a mere 56% (76% x 76%), every successfully avoided case of CF would cost ± $2.2 million, assuming that all parents informed of a CF gestational product would opt for an abortion; screening is not thought to be cost-effective DIAGNOSIS Sweat chloride test, see there TREATMENT Pancrease, a porcine-derived enzyme concentrated within microspherules, coated by an acid-resistant polymer (McNeil), designed to reduce the degree of malabsorption; aerosolized α1-antitrypsin to counteract the excess production of neutrophil elastase and aerosolized DNAse, which digests the partially degraded neutrophils that accumulate in the alveoli; see Passive smoking; a potential therapeutic modality would involve the activation of chloride channels by a multifunctional calcium/calmodulin protein kinase (Nature 1991; 349:793) Diagnosis early in childhood because of meconium ileus, failure to thrive, chronic sinus and bronchopulmonary infections; other features include sterility, deafness and intraocular damage, and different mutations produce different symptoms (New York Times 16 Nov 1993; C1) SCREENING Given that more than 350 mutations have been identified, and even when a person inherits one mutated gene from each parent, he/she may not develop CF, effective screening for CF remains an elusive goal TREATMENT Recombinant DNAse (the high viscosity of the pulmonary secretions is due in part to the high concentration of DNA–10.2% of dry weight) reduces the exacerbations of respiratory disease, resulting in a slight improvement in pulmonary function (N Engl J Med 1994; 331:637OA) PROGNOSIS Prognosis has improved from a median survival of 10.6 (1966) to 28 years (1989); prognosticators in CF (arranged from least to greatest statistical significance in terms of P value) are ♀ sex (P value = 0.300), ↑ age (P = 0.200), poor nutritional status (body mass index (P = 0.016), impaired pulmonary function

(FEV₁, P < 0.001), respiratory tract colonization with *Pseudomonas cepacia* (P < 0.001), and degree of aerobic fitness (P < 0.001); in a cohort of 109 CF patients age 7-35, the 8-year survival was 83% in those with highest levels of aerobic fitness vs 51% and 28% of those with middle and lowest levels of aerobic fitness (N Engl J Med 1992; 327:1785OA) those with the R117H/ΔF₅₀₈ genotype are at ↑ risk for pancreatic insufficiency (N Engl J Med 1993; 329:1308OA)

cystic fibrosis transmembrane conductance regulator MOLECULAR BIOLOGY A 1480-residue protein involved in chloride transport in the lungs, pancreas, and sweat glands that is encoded within the J3.11 and met oncogene markers, which has a deleted phenylalanine at position 508; CFTCR was identified by chromosome 'walking' and 'jumping' by LC Tsui (Children's Hospital, Toronto) and F Collins (then at U of Michigan), locating the defective 250 kilobase gene on the long arm of chromosome 7, CFTCR has five functional domains, two transmembrane domains, two nucleotide binding domains and a regulatory domain; the 508 deletion induces changes in the nucleotide binding domain (Science 1991; 251:555)

cystinosis An AR [MIM 219750, 219800, 219900] condition characterized by impaired transport of cystine across across lysosomal membranes; the accumulation of cystine in lysosomes results in crystal formation in various tissues, in particular the kidneys; early renal tubular involvement results in Fanconi syndrome with failure to thrive, dehydration and acidosis in infancy; cystal-related loss of glomerular function leads to uremia and death by age 10 CLINICAL Growth retardation, photophobia, hypothyroidism, and in later survivors visual impairment, corneal ulcerations, pancreatic insufficiency, distal myopathy, dysphagia, and CNS involvement TREATMENT Cysteamine (β-mercaptoethylamine) or the more palatable phosphocysteamine effectively remove the cystine crystals (N Engl J Med 1993; 328:1157OA)

cystosarcoma phyllodes see Phyllodes tumor

cytapheresis TRANSFUSION MEDICINE The collection of cells for therapeutic transfusion; although by definition, cytapheresis could refer to any collected cells, it is understood in the more restricted sense of a procedure for 'harvesting' either platelets, or less commonly, granulocytes; in each, the donor is often a friend or family member of a patient requiring the cells on a regular basis; the frequency of donation is limited by loss of erythrocytes (ideally, less than 25 ml/week), plasma loss (less than 1000 ml/week) and in granulocytapheresis, the accumulation of hydroxyethyl starch, see there; the most common indication for platelet apheresis is transient thrombocytopenia caused by chemotherapy for malignancy when the patient's platelet count fall below 10 x 10⁹/L; the indications for granulocytapheresis are less clearly defined

cytarabine Ara-C, cytosine arabinoside An antimetabolite analog of deoxycytidine, used synergistically with antifolates, alkylating agents and cis-platinum for treating leukemia, causes nausea, vomiting, myelosuppression, and in high doses, cerebral dysfunction and ataxia

cytochrome-c oxidase A heme enzyme [EC 1.9.3.1] with copper group that catalyzes the oxidation of cytochrome c; cytochrome oxidase is highly sensitive to cyanide

cytochrome P450 3A4 A compound that is responsible for the biotransformation of human sex hormones as well as various drugs, to wit, astemizole, cyclosporine, some benzodiazepines, dihydropyridine calcium channel blockers, nifedipine, terfenadine, and some macrolide antibiotics, eg erythromycin (JAMA 1993; 269:1513OC)

cytoid bodies Cell-like bodies DERMATOPATHOLOGY Civatte, colloid or hyaline bodies Densely eosinophilic, dyskeratotic cells that are often surrounded by a cleared space due to retraction of viable squamous epithelium away from the dead cells, a finding characteristic of lichen

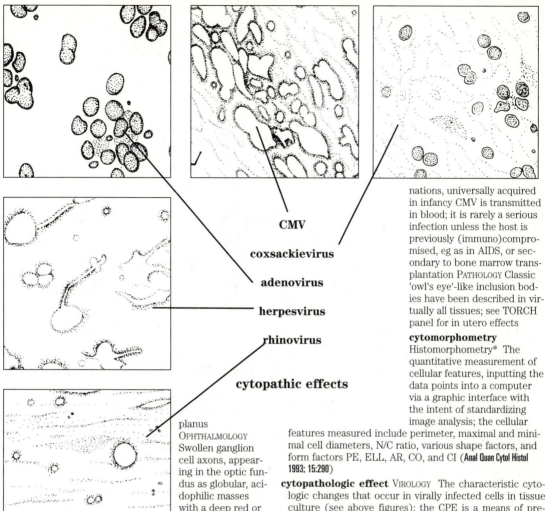

CMV

coxsackievirus

adenovirus

herpesvirus

rhinovirus

cytopathic effects

nations, universally acquired in infancy CMV is transmitted in blood; it is rarely a serious infection unless the host is previously (immuno)compromised, eg as in AIDS, or secondary to bone marrow transplantation PATHOLOGY Classic 'owl's eye'-like inclusion bodies have been described in virtually all tissues; see TORCH panel for in utero effects

cytomorphometry Histomorphometry* The quantitative measurement of cellular features, inputting the data points into a computer via a graphic interface with the intent of standardizing image analysis; the cellular features measured include perimeter, maximal and minimal cell diameters, N/C ratio, various shape factors, and form factors PE, ELL, AR, CO, and CI (Anal Quan Cytol Histol 1993; 15:290)

cytopathologic effect VIROLOGY The characteristic cytologic changes that occur in virally infected cells in tissue culture (see above figures); the CPE is a means of presumptive identification of a virus obtained from a clinical specimen, eg Adenovirus produces grape-like clusters in HEK cells; rhinovirus produces irregular, rounded 'dewdrop' changes in culture cells; rubella is diagnosed by exclusion, as it interferes with the CPE of other viruses

cytoredutive surgery Debulking surgery, see there

cytotoxic T lymphocyte (CTL) A T cell with a CD8 receptor on the surface that recognizes (via the T-cell receptor), interacts with and lyses malignant or virally infected native cells bearing self, ie 'haplotype restricted', class I major histocompatibility complex (MHC) molecules; once recognition occurs, CTLs react to the MHC class I 'restricted', antigen-bearing cell, by secreting a) lymphokines, recruiting other lymphocytes to the region and b) proteinases and proteins (perforins) that form nonspecific ion channels in the target cell membrane, cause a rapid loss of osmotic pressure and bursting of the target; CTLs downregulate the immune response and one CTL may attack many targets; see Helper cells, Perforin, Suppressor cells

cytotrophoblast The inner cell of the trophoblast; cytotrophoblasts are of variable size with clear cytoplasm, large hyperchromatic nuclei with irregular nuclear contours and finely granular chromatin; cytotrophoblasts are difficult to distinguish from endometrial and decidual cells (Acta Cytologica 1993; 37:451OA) Note: Cytotrophoblasts in a cervicovaginal smear are rare in a normal pregnancy and are commonly associated with threatened abortion

planus OPHTHALMOLOGY Swollen ganglion cell axons, appearing in the optic fundus as globular, acidophilic masses with a deep red or blue 10-20 µm in diameter nucleoid, seen in microinfarcts of the inner retinal layer, the histological translation of cotton-wool patches, seen in grade III hypertensive retinopathy

cytokines Polypeptide signaling proteins of the immune system, aka biological response modifiers which 1) Coordinate the interaction between the humoral and cellular immune 'systems' and 2) Augment the immune response; by convention, they are released by activated cells; cytokines are produced by many cells in response to multiple stimuli, and have many targets and multiple functions (Perspect Biol & Med 1993; 36:611); cytokines are divided into 1) Monokines, produced by macrophages eg α and β interferons, interleukin-1, tumor necrosis factor, and several colony-stimulating factors and 2) Lymphokines, produced predominantly by activated T cells and natural killer cells eg γ-interferon, interleukins (IL-2 to IL-6), granulocytemacrophage colony-stimulating factor and lymphotoxin; see also Biological response modifiers, Colony stimulating factor(s), Fibroblast growth factor, Interferons, Interleukins, Platelet-derived growth factor, Transforming growth factor β, Tumor necrosis factor molecules

cytokine synthesis inhibitory factor see IL-10

cytomegalovirus A member of the herpes (DNA) virus group, which is global in distribution and in developing

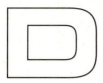

D Symbol for: 1) Aspartic acid 2) Dalton 3) Deuterium 4) Diopter 4) Dose 5) Duration 6) Dorsal

d Symbol for: 1) Day 2) deci- (in SI units) 3) Deoxyribose 4) dextro- 5) Dextrorotary

D_1, D_2, D_3 receptors see Dopamine receptors

DAB Diaminobenzene

Also 1) Deutsches Artzneibuch 2) Devereux Adolescent Behavior (rating scale, psychology) 4) Diaminobenzidine 5) Diaminobutanoic acid 6) Diaza-butadiene 7) Dimethylaminoazobenzene 8) Dysrhythmic aggressive behavior

D17S74 A highly polymorphic gene located on the long arm of chromosome 17 (17q21) that is closely linked to an early-onset form of familial breast cancer which is accompanied by proliferative breast disease (Science 1990; 250:1684)

dacarbazine An agent that is indicated for treating metastatic malignant melanoma; when the antiestrogenic agent tamoxifen was added to the protocol, the response rate was 38% in ♀ (vs 19% ♂) and length of survival was 69 weeks for ♀ (vs 31 weeks for ♂) (N Engl J Med 1992; 327:516OA)

Dachau hypothermia experiments see Unethical medical research

DAD Diffuse alveolar damage* The histological findings in adult respiratory distress syndrome, see there RADIOLOGY Acute onset of diffuse pulmonary infiltrates PATHOLOGY The acute exudative phase with edema and hyaline membrane formation is followed by a subacute proliferative phase at one week, ending with fibrosis by the second or third week ETIOLOGY AIDS, air embolism, cardiopulmonary bypass, connective tissue disease (SLE, rheumatoid arthritis, scleroderma), drugs (therapeutic or of abuse), eosinophilic granuloma, heat injury, hemosiderosis, high altitude, iatrogenic (PEEP), infections, molar pregnancy, noxious inhalants and gases, acute pancreatitis, shock, uremia; see Adult respiratory distress syndrome

*Also 1) Depression after delivery (obstetrics, more commonly known as postpartum blues) 2) Dispense as directed (pharmacology) 3) Donor-acceptor-donor (physiology)

DAF Decay accelerating factor A complement-regulating glycoprotein that is covalently anchored to the cell membrane by a glycophospholipid at the protein's COOH terminus; DAF binds activated C3b and C4b, inhibiting the assembly of C3 convertase (C3bBb) at cell surfaces, thereby preventing amplification of the classic pathway of the complement cascade on the host cell membrane; it is defective in paroxysmal nocturnal hemoglobinuria, see there

DAG Diacylglycerol, see there

dagger sign Ossification of the posterior longitudinal liga-

ment with spinal cord compression due to a dense, vertical ossified 1-5 mm wide strip or plaque at the posterior margin of the vertebral body and intervertebral disks; although usually located in the cervical spine, the ossification may appear at T4 to T7 DIAGNOSIS CT, Tomography, or myelography Note: OPLL may be a disorder, distinct from spondylosis deformans and ankylosing spondylitis, or merely a permutation of the DISH complex, see there

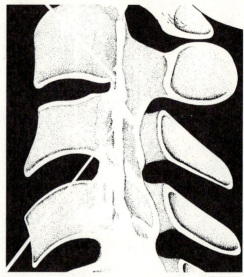

dagger sign

dahllite Carbonated hydroxyapatite (with some substituted acidic phosphate) which is reported to be of use as an 'instant bone' that is administered in a paste form, hardening within 12 hours to provide 55 megapascals of compressive strength (Science 1995; 267:1796, 1772) see Bone paste

daily census see Census

daisy An adjectival descriptor for a pattern in which a central mass is surrounded in a rosette-like fashion with oval structures that abut the central mass at one end

daisy form HEMATOLOGY A colloquial term for the segmented rosette-like intraerythrocytic form of mature schizonts of *Plasmodium malariae*

daisy pattern HEMATOLOGY A rosette-like intraerythrocytic pattern of HISTOPATHOLOGY Radiating stellate fibrillary forms, corresponding to tyrosine crystals seen in pleomorphic adenoma when stained with Mayer's hemalum and tartrazine MYCOLOGY A descriptor for the microscopic morphology of *Sporothrix schenckii* cultured at 20°C, the hyphae of which simulate the petals of a daisy, a pattern that may also be seen in *Candida* species

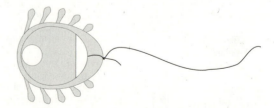

Dalkon Shield

Dalkon shield An intrauterine device produced by AH Robins, Inc, that was withdrawn from the market in 1974 after it was implicated in seven maternal deaths, 110 cases of septic abortion, increased pelvic inflammatory disease and salpingitis; it was found that minute breaks in the shield allowed ascending bacteria continuous access from the vagina into the endometrial cavity; as a direct result of the mounting costs of settling the lawsuits; see Pelvic inflammatory disease; Cf Copper-7, intrauterine devices

Note: In 1989, the manufacturer filed for bankruptcy, setting aside a trust fund of $2.5 billion (US) to settle the claims of those alleged to have been damaged by the Dalkon shield (Wall Street Journal 70:A3, Nov 7, 1989)

Dallas criteria Those criteria established by a group of internationally renowned cardiac pathologists in Dallas in 1984 and 1987 that set standards for the diagnosis of myocarditis (as obtained in an endomyocardial biopsy), subdividing them into: No myocarditis, borderline myocarditis or lymphocytic myocarditis

DALM Dysplasia-associated lesion or mass An acronym indicating an increased incidence of adenocarcinoma in a colon with ulcerative colitis when the pathologist finds dysplasia and the endoscopist finds a tumor mass; DALM alone may be a sufficient criterion for performing a proctocolectomy

dam Rubber dam, see there

damages MEDICAL MALPRACTICE A generic term for a monetary sum that reflects financial losses and/or compromise in the quality of life incurred by an injured party as a result of an allegedly negligent act; see Compensatory damages, Malpractice, Punitive damages

Damocles' syndrome Stress and anxiety experienced by the patients and families of those 'successfully' treated for childhood leukemia, as 1) the cure rate averages 50% and 2) 2-10% of treated patients with leukemia suffer future (often lymphoproliferative) malignancy; this state of long-term uncertainty is likened to that of Damocles

Note According to Cicero, Damocles was a courtier under Dionysius I, tyrant of Syracuse who lavished praise on his king in order to ensure his own survival; Dionysius invited Damocles as guest of honor at a magnificent banquet, at which Damocles was seated directly beneath a naked sword suspended by a single horsehair; a sword of Damocles therefore implies imminent danger

damping The reduction or elimination of oscillations in a resonating system by dissipation of stored energy, eg muffling of normal lung sounds by the presence of pleural fluid; in ultrasonography, damping refers to the mechanical or electrical loading of the piezoelectric transducer to minimize the echo duration

DAN see Diabetic autonomic neuropathy

danazol A non-virilizing androgen that increases the resistance of erythrocytes to osmotic lysis; danazol is the most effective agent available for treating endometriosis, and may be of use in treating autoimmune hemolytic anemia and autoimmune thrombocytopenia (Acta Haematol 1990; 44:286), although it may itself mediate immune thrombocytopenia

dancing eyes NEUROLOGY Prominent nystagmus with rapid changes in all directions (rotary, vertical, horizontal, and diagonal); DE was first described in glycogen storage disease, type VIII, but may occur in normal subjects; there is no demonstrable enzymopathy, although inactived hepatic phosphorylase is implicated CLINICAL CNS accumulation of α-granular glycogen in axons and in synaptic spaces causes truncal ataxia, nystagmus, 'dancing eyes', neurologic deterioration, spasticity, swallowing difficulties and possibly aspiration pneumonia PROGNOSIS Hypotonia, decerebration and death

dancing eyes-dancing feet syndrome Opsoclonus-myoclonus 1) Infantile myoclonic encephalopathy A rare idiopathic (or due to occult retinoblastoma) encephalopathy of early childhood onset, which may follow respiratory infections, and follow a benign but protracted course CLINICAL Irregular, rapid jerking spasms of the trunk and limbs (myoclonus) and eye (opsoclonus) with gait ataxia, intention tremor and nystagmus TREATMENT ACTH and cortisone may induce remissions 2) Paraneoplastic opsoclonus-myoclonus syndrome, see there

dander A mixture of microorganisms, desquamated epithelium, hair and sebum from domestic animals (dogs and cats) that evokes allergic reactions in atopic individuals

dandruff Exfoliative dermatitis of the scalp

Dane particle A particle seen by EM in the acute infective stage of hepatitis B, which measures 42 nm and has an inner icosahedral 27 nm in diameter core, composed of DNA polymerase (Lancet 1970; 1:695) see Hepatitis B

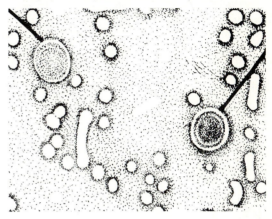

Dane particle

'danger' space SURGICAL ANATOMY A region that is posterior to the retropharyngeal space, and descends in the posterior mediastinum to the diaphragm

danger space infection A potentially life-threatening infection of the 'danger' space by extension from the retropharynx, causing dysphagia, dyspnea, high fever, nuchal rigidity and esophageal regurgitation TREATMENT Immediate open drainage

dangle NURSING A colloquial term for the first movement a patient is allowed either after a surgical procedure under general anesthesia, or before and after surgery 'under local', where the recuperee allows his/her feet to dangle over the side of the bed (MLO April 1995)

Daniel Webster forehead A fanciful descriptive term for the high, squarish forehead typical of the Smith-Lemli-Opitz syndrome, see there

3,4-DAP 3,4-Diaminopyridine NEUROLOGY A substance which in experimental animals blocks the fast K^+ channels and improves conduction in regions of nerve demyelination; 3,4-DAP therapy is not effective therapy for stable chronic demyelinating polyneuropathy (Mayo Clin Proc 1995; 70:532)

dapsone Diaminodiphenyl sulfone A sulfa drug classically used for leprosy, which has therapeutic currency for treating dermatitis herpetiformis, and some dermatopathies, eg erythema elevatum diutinum, therapeutically refractory acne, and subcorneal pustular dermatosis, as well as for malaria prophylaxis; Cf Thalidomide

dark adaptation PHYSIOLOGY The decline in visual threshold as the eye grows accustomed to reduced lighting conditions (± 20 minutes), which corresponds to the adjustment of the retina from primarily cone vision ('color vision', range of luminance from 10^2-10^7 lux) to rod vision ('black & white vision', 10^{-2}-10^{-6} lux) after passing through a transition zone (10^2-10^{-2} lux); Cf Light adaptation

dark (basal) epithelial cells Dedifferentiated cells seen in preneoplastic epithelia (skin, respiratory tract) as electron-dense cells with large nuclei, prominent nucleoli, scant cytoplasm and abundant free ribosomes

dark cells Compact cells, see there

darkfield microscopy A variant of light microscopy, in which a condensor is used to illuminate an object at an oblique angle, which appears bright against a dark background (all light reaching the eye is reflected); darkfield microscopy is the preferred method for identifying spirochetes; Cf Serological tests for syphilis

dark reactivation MOLECULAR BIOLOGY The enzymatic repair of DNA damaged by ultraviolet light, which causes thymine dimerization; repair occurs via excision, recombination or SOS repair mechanisms

darmbrand Pigbel, see there

Darsee affair A major scandal that affected the departments of internal medicine and cardiology at two major US universities, which among other 'casualties' in the medical literature, was held responsible for invalidating a multicenter study on cardiovascular disease; the physician allegedly responsible began fabrication and manipulation of data as a university undergraduate, and later generated multiple published reports and abstracts at Emory University and at Harvard University, generating 116 publications between 1978 and 1982; many of the publications shared authorship with researchers of renown, who were compelled to retract the papers once they were aware of the allegations of fraud (N Engl J Med 1983; 308:1415; JAMA 1983; 2867) see Authorship, Fraud in science, Honorary authorship, Slutsky affair

darting motility The characteristic 'falling leaf' pattern of movement of flagellated parasites, eg *Trichomonas vaginalis;* Cf Tumbling motility

Darwinian cloning A neologism for a process defined as '...the process of selecting random collections of combinatorially synthesized molecules,' which has been called molecular evolution, a term that had been previously defined as the change in the molecular (as opposed to bone) structure of organims as they evolve (Bio/Technology 1994; 12:433c)

Darwin's theory The basic premises of Darwin's theory of evolution by natural selection are that organisms vary, the variation is inherited, and the variation is subject to selection

Darwinism The currently accepted paradigm of evolution, which holds that the cumulative changes in successive generations of organisms, ie the evolution of species, results from mutation and selection of organisms that are best adapted phenotypically to survive in their environment, ie 'survival of the fittest'; see Autopoietic Gaia, Neodarwinism; Cf Creationism, Lysenkoism

dashboard fracture A shear fracture with hip dislocation that occurs when a seated (usually front seat) passenger is thrown forward, striking his knee against the dashboard transmitting axial force to a flexed and adducted femur, with dislocation of the hip through a rent in the posterior capsule or where posterior rim of the acetabulum is sheared off by the femoral head

dashboard perineum A descriptor for the appearance of an elongated perineum, resulting from an overzealous perineal repair at the time of delivery or during posterior colpoplasty; the dashboard defect may be surgically corrected by transverse repair of a longitudinal incision made through the mucosa and underlying perineal body

DASI Duke Activity Status Index, see there

DAT Direct antiglobulin test, see Coomb's test, direct

data Factual information in the form of measurements or statistics

FRAGILE DATA Unexpected or unusual results obtained from a study, which because of either the small size of the cohort studied and therefore low statistical power or the unexpected results, may reach conclusions that do not withstand the rigors of scientific scrutiny HARD DATA Tangible data of any nature, eg blood levels of an analyte, persons in a defined region with a certain type malignancy INCONCLUSIVE DATA Results from the study of a phenomenon that fall far below that required for statistical significance, eg p > 0.05; alternately, data from multiple studies that consistently reach opposite conclusions of low statistical power SOFT DATA Those results from a study or series of studies that demonstrate a consistent trend, eg the risk of suffering a morbid condition, but which falls short of statistical significance

Data Bank National Practitioner Data Bank, see there

database COMPUTERS A pool of computer-stored information that allows information to be accessed or retrieved by any of the parameters or 'fields' used for the data's entry, eg patient name, medical record number, date of admission, date of surgery, and so on

Note: For MS/DOS-based microcomputers, dBASE III, IV, and VI have been 'gold standard' software programs

data compression COMPUTERS Any technique (either hardware or software) that exploits redundancies to recode data, resulting in the same kind of information in a minimum space; DC is a way to reduce (in a compression ratio of up to 15:1 or more) the amount of information that must be transmitted over a communications network, and to reduce the amount of memory required to store an image; under most DC schemes, repeated strings of data are replaced by a single symbol called a token; there are two types of DC: 1) Loss-less compression, which uses an algorithm that allows the information to be retrieved in its original form, a requirement for medical, scientific and legal purposes; the disadvantage is that more memory is required 2) Lossy compression, which uses an algorithm that simplifies the data during compression; decompressed data from lossy compression is not an exact replica but an approximation, and is useful for imaging and full-motion video

date rape A permutation of rape*, an event that may affect 20% or more adolescent girls, peaking at age 16-19; DR is the end-point of sexual play in which the female is an active participant, but which advances to forced and unintended coitus (N Engl J Med 1995; 332:234RV) see Rape, Spousal rape; Cf Statutory rape

*Defined as '*a nonconsensual act of sexual intercourse carried out by force or other means of duress.*' (International Dictionary of Medicine, J Wiley & Sons, New York, 1986)

DATTA A (Diagnostic And Therapeutic Technology Assessment) program sponsored by the American Medical Association that polls opinions on issues of clinical interest that are rendered by consultants selected from a panel of 1700 experts, nominated by their respective medical specialty societies

Note: DATTA data is usually at the end of each issue of the Journal of the American Medical Association

Daubert v. Merrell Dow Pharmaceuticals A lawsuit initiated by plaintiff J Daubert, who was born with limb-reduction defects, and who claimed that the culprit was Bendectin, produced by Merrill Dow Pharmaceutical; the plaintiff introduced an 'overwhelming body of epidemiological evidence' that contradicted the 30 published studies involving 130 000 subjects, none of which found Bendectin to be a human teratogen; the trial court granted Merrell Dow summary judgement (ie dismissed the case), concluding that the plaintiff's scientific evidence was inadmissible as it was not sufficiently established to have general acceptance; based on this case, the US Supreme Court ruled that federal judges should admit all relevant scientific testimony and evidence that is 'reliable' (Daubert v Merrell Dow Pharmaceuticals, Inc, 113 S Ct 2786 (1993), N Engl J Med 1994; 330:1018LM) the 'Daubert case' has had a wide impact in the US legal system regarding the validity of scientific data in the courtroom; see Frye rule, Litogen; Cf Expert witness

dauernarkose Continuous sleep therapy

daughter NUCLEAR MEDICINE A radionuclide formed from the radioactive decay of a parent molecule; see Radon

Davis v. Davis A legal dispute over the custody of frozen embryos that had been conceived by in vitro fertilization, which arose when the parents got a divorce; the court designated the embryos as 'children in vitro', providing them with legal protection (N Engl J Med 1990; 323:1200) see Surrogacy

dawn phenomenon DIABETOLOGY Early morning hyperglycemia, that is not preceded by hypoglycemia, which is related to increased insulin requirements in insulin-dependent DM, possibly the result of nocturnal pulses of growth hormone; the phenomenon also occurs in 'insulin-pump' users receiving continuous subcutaneous insulin infusion who are supposed to be euglycemic and thus is an effect attributed to residual endogenous insulin or insulin-like molecules; Cf Subcutaneous insulin resistance syndrome

Note: In contrast, the Somogyi phenomenon is a 'counter-regulatory' hyperglycemia, where insulin therapy causes hypoglycemia, stimulating the release of counter-regulating hormones to increase the glucose levels; the two phenomena are responsible for 'brittle diabetes'

day care PEDIATRICS, SOCIAL MEDICINE A facility in which infants and pre-school children are supervised and their needs attended to while the parent(s) works; because of the childrens' proximity to each other, miniepidemics of GI and respiratory tract infections are common in these centers (JAMA 1991; 265:2212) see 'Quality time

dazzling OPHTHALMOLOGY The constellation of ocular responses to light intensity that is in excess of the eye's adaptability, which is best addressed by tinted glasses

D&E Dilation and extraction GYNECOLOGY A method used to terminate pregnancy in the second trimester, which is an alternative to the more popular prostaglandin-induced abortion (PIA); D&E consists of surgical dilation of the cervix, followed y instrumental fragmentation and evacuation of the fetus in parts; D&E is more rapid and less painful than PIA, and can be performed on an outpatient basis; despite its advantages, D&E yields pathologic specimens that are suboptimal for evaluation and may be contaminated by microbes, precluding growth of fetal cells in culture; the complication rate for D&E is 2.9%; death rate $5/10^5$ (Am J Clin Pathol 1995; 103:415oA) Cf Prostaglandin-induced abortion

dbl protooncogene A gene first isolated in a human diffuse lymphoma that is also expressed in several types of neoplasms; it encodes a 66-kD cytoplasmic phosphoprotein with transforming properties, the exact function of which is unknown (Diagn Mol Pathol 1993; 2:160)

DCB1 A unique bacterium capable of detoxifying highly chlorinated aromatic compounds, including toxic polychlorinated biphenyls PCBs; in the detoxification scheme formulated by J Tiedje at Michigan State University; DCB1 removes chlorine from chlorobenzoate, producing benzoate, then a benzoate-oxidizing bacterium transforms benzoate to acetate; finally a methanogen finishes the process by converting the end-products into methane; see PCBs

DCC DCC gene A gene deleted in colorectal cancer (hence the name) and located on chromosome 18 that was the first identified tumor suppressor gene; DCC encodes a protein with structural features of certain types of cell-adhesion molecules and thus the DCC protein may be involved in cell-cell and cell-extracellular matrix interactions; loss of chromosome segment 18q may result in impaired intercellular contacts, contributing to tumor growth and invasion (see N Engl J Med 1994; 331:213oA)

dDAVP 1-deamino, 8-D-arginine vasopressin A long-acting antidiuretic analog of vasopressin, administered as a nasal spray, which is the current drug of choice in treating diabetes insipidus

ddC dideoxycytidine A reverse transcriptase inhibitor that is being used in an AIDS therapeutic trial, which is similar in most aspects to ddI, below

ddI 2',3'-dideoxyinosine A purine analog that inhibits HIV-1 in vivo and is converted by a complex metabolic pathway to a triphosphorylated moiety, ddA-TP, which inhibits HIV reverse transcriptase and suppresses HIV replication by blocking the synthesis of viral DNA; ddI is associated with an ↑ in CD4 (T-helper) cells, and ↓↓↓ p24 antigen (an indicator of HIV activity) in the blood; ddI is better tolerated than zidovudine and causes less myelosuppression than AZT SIDE EFFECTS Painful peripheral neuropathy, pancreatitis LABORATORY Hyperuricemia, asymptomatic ↑ of serum aminotransferases PHASE I RESULTS Weight gain of 2+ kg and/or clinical improvement and promising antiretroviral activity in children with AIDS (N Engl J Med 1991; 324:137); see AIDS, Zidovudine

DDDR pacing Dual-chamber, rate-modulated pacing An optimized rhythm for an implantable cardiac pacemaker, which requires periodic reprogramming as a function of a patient's activities

D-dimer HEMATOLOGY A term that refers to the site of covalent cross-linkage between the D domains of adjacent fibrin monomeric subunits in a polymer of fibrin; disruption of the D-dimer cross-links by factor XIIIa results in stabilization of the fibrin clot

D-dimer screening test LABORATORY MEDICINE A generic term for any of a number of tests used to detect fibrin breakdown products using latex beads coated with monoclonal antibodies to the D-dimer; the D-dimer test has become increasingly popular as it is performed with plasma, and does not have the disadvantages of the FDP test, which may be false positive with heparinized specimens and requires a special tube for collection (CAP Today August 1993 p57)

DDS syndrome A hypersensitivity reaction seen in 1:5000 leprosy patients treated with dapsone (DDS, 4,4'-diaminodiphenylsulfone, which blocks the p-aminobenzoic acid condensation reaction required for folate synthesis) CLINICAL Hemolysis, hypoalbuminemia, agranulocytosis and a potentially fatal combination of hepatitis and exfoliative dermatitis TREATMENT Discontinue dapsone, high-dose steroids, eg > 100 mg/day of prednisone

DDT Dichloro-diphenyl-trichloroethane ENVIRONMENT A highly hepatotoxic and potentially neurotoxic insecticide that accumulates in fat; DDT is non-biodegradable and concentrates up the food chain; because of its genotoxicity to wildlife and unknown effects on humans, its use as a pesticide was banned in the USA in 1971, but continues to be used elsewhere for control of arthropods, including body lice and vectors of typhus fever and malaria

DDT

de lunatico inquierendo FORENSIC PSYCHIATRY '*The name of a writ directed to the sheriff, directing him to inquire by good and lawful men whether the party being charged is a lunatic or not.*' (Black's Law Dictionary, West Pub Co, St Paul, Mn, 1990)

'de minimis' doctrine A philosophical stance of ancient common law, '*de minimis non curat lex*', ie the law does not concern itself with trifles; the 'de minimis' rule seeks to avoid overburdening the legal system with lawsuits of little merit, eg a lawsuit against a pathologist who opens the cranial cavity (without specific permission) in a medically indicated autopsy; see Malpractice-Frivolous lawsuit

'DEAD box' proteins A family of proteins that share the tetrapeptide, Asp-Glu-Ala-Asp, abbreviated DEAD (in the single letter code of amino acids) and DEAH (H for Histidine) and have roles in splicing, translation, development and cell growth; the prototypic DEAD-box protein is eIF4A, which uses the energy generated from ATP hydrolysis to unwind mRNA secondary upstream, facilitating the attachment of 40S ribosome (**Nature 1991; 349:487ed**) see Spliceosome; Cf RGD superfamily

dead fetus 'syndrome' Macerated 'fetus syndrome' The clinical complex due to intrauterine death with retention of the fetus for greater than 48 hours (missed labor), which occurs after the 20th gestational week; the philosophy in the US is to await spontaneous onset of labor for up to two weeks, then induce labor (barring fetal or maternal dystocia), using either prostaglandin E_2 in a vaginal or cervical gel, or oxytocin; intraamniotic saline injection is no longer recommended COMPLICATION Disseminated intravascular coagulation

dead space CLINICAL THERAPEUTICS That portion of a syringe's tip and needle that contains medication that cannot be administered; dead space is of considerable importance in insulin therapy and in those medications where the syringe has < 0.5 cc capacity PULMONARY PHYSIOLOGY All non-air exchanging spaces of the upper respiratory tract, ± 2.0 ml of 'dead space' per kilogram of body weight, ie a 70 kg person has 140-150 ml of 'dead space' in the oronasopharynx, bronchi and bronchioles Note: Anatomic dead space (respiratory system volume exclusive of alveoli) and physiologic dead space ('wasted ventilation' or volume of gas not equilibrating with blood) are the same in healthy subjects, clinically measured by single breath nitrogen curve; the relation of ventilation (V) to blood flow (Q), V/Q ratio may be substantially altered in disease states; see Lung, physiological volumes, V/Q ratio

'dead wood' ACADEMIA A person, eg a professor, or other tenured academe whose function has been served but who cannot be elimated from their position or deleted from a payroll (eg because of tenure) to free the position for a more qualified often younger person

deaf and dumb An obsolete and politically incorrect term attributed to Aristotle for a person who is both deaf and unable to speak (ergo to the ancients, 'dumb')

deaf-mute A person with deaf-mutism

deaf-mutism The inability to speak due to deafness

dean ACADEMIA The top banana in the hierarchy of a college, university, or medical school, to whom all professorial faculty and academics are ultimately responsible

dean's tax ACADEMIC MEDICINE A portion of the revenues (from 5-20%) obtained from a faculty* practice plan that is allocated to the affiliated medical school for educational purposes (**N Eng J Med 1995; 332:407oa**)

*An organized group of physicians that treats patients who are referred to an academic medical center, which is often a unit of the medical school

'Dear Doctor' letter A remedial communication required by the Food and Drug Administration (USA), when a pharmaceutical company has advertised a drug with incomplete or misleading information about a product's effectiveness or safety; see Advertising; Dear Doctor letters are also used to warn physicians about important drug prescribing information or unanticipated drug interactions; the efficacy of 'Dear Doctor' warnings regarding the alteration of physician prescribing habits is unknown (**JAMA 1993; 269:1513oc**)

death The Uniform Determination of Death Act passed by the US Congress, 1981 states that an individual is dead if there is

1) Irreversible cessation of circulatory and respiratory functions or

2) Irreversible cessation of all functions of brain, including the brain stem, a concept endorsed by the American Medical Association and the American Bar Association; see Cause of death, Harvard criteria

'Death Angel' A nurse in Nevada accused of killing patients on her service and running a 'book-making' operation, allegedly placing odds (and bets) on a patient's potential for survival; the patient around whom the accusations hovered was an elderly man dying of the complications of alcoholic cirrhosis; none of the allegations were verified, the nurse was exonerated and the sobriquet was considered an example of news media malpractice; Cf Angel of death

death certificate A document in which the certifying physician formally states, to the best of his/her knowledge, the immediate, intermediate, and underlying cause of death; the DC is generally filled out by the decedent's attending physician if the death is deemed natural, and by the local medical examiner or coroner in the case of an unnatural death; the DC is used by health statisticians and policymakers as a marker of morbidity and to determine the prevalence of disease in a population; it has legal ramifications and may be the catalyst for a lawsuit initiated by the decedent's family, which may allege 'wrongful death' if a morbid process that resulted in death was not identified while the patient was alive (**Arch Pathol Lab Med 1995; 119:1230a**) Cf Unnatural death

'Death with Dignity' A campaign slogan for the State of Washington's failed Initiative 119, see there

Death With Dignity Act An initiative passed by voters in late 1994 in the State of Oregon as Ballot Measure 16, which permitted physician-assisted suicide (**MT Today 1995; 5/6:8:0a**)

'death list' A highly colloquial term for a list produced by the US HCFA (Health Care Financing Administration) that names the 'statistical outliers' in Medicare's database of 6000 hospitals, ie those that exceeded the range of predicted mortality; many of the nearly 200 hospitals on the list have been on the list more than once and have included large urban hospitals, eg Harlem Hospital (New York City) and Martin Luther King, Jr-Drew Medical Center (Los Angeles)

death rattle A sound characteristic of end-stage lung disease, eg terminal lung cancer or pulmonary edema that occurs when the clearance of large airway secretions becomes nearly impossible; as air moves to and fro in the bronchi, the sound acquires a gurgling or rattling quality, often presaging death

Death Star pattern CYTOLOGY A fanciful descriptor for the morphology of the rounded aggregates of malignant cells obtained from fine needle aspiration biopsies from breast carcinoma, which often connote a poor prognosis; 'death stars' may occur in various forms of ductal carcinomas of the breast, deriving name (and significance) from a secret weapon used in the science fiction film, Star Wars

Although this has also been referred to a cannonball pattern (**Acta Cytologica 1993; 37:483oa**), it is best to reserve the adjectical cannonball for its widely accepted use, ie that of one or more 5-10 cm in diameter masses of malignant cells metastatic to the lungs, most commonly from renal cell carcinoma

debrancher disease Glycogen storage disease type III

debrancher enzyme An enzyme with both amylo-1,6-glucosidase [EC 3.2.1.33] and oligo-1,4-1,4-glucantransferase [EC 2.4.1.25] activity

debridement Surgical cleansing of wounds, which consists of wide excision of potentially contaminated wounds, making fresh margins, removing necrotic tissue and foreign debris

Note: Although debridement has been credited with a decreased incidence of clostridial myositis in dirty wounds (5% in World War I vs 0.08% in the Korean conflict), this decrease is more likely the result of antibiotic therapy

debrisoquin CLINICAL PHARMACOLOGY A drug used to evaluate a major pathway for the metabolism of wide variety of drugs, including tricyclic antidepressants; 7% of the population is deficient in the debrisoquin enzyme and thus have high or even toxic levels of certain drugs

debug A term first used in the computer industry, referring to the removal of 'bugs' or minor defects in a product, eg a program or a process that prevent its optimal performance or function

debulking operation Cytoreductive surgery SURGICAL ONCOLOGY Excisional reduction of large malignant tumor masses; debulking serves three purposes, it 1) Reduces tumor 'load' (bulk) 2) Oxygenates tissues (malignant cells often survive well in low oxygen environments and oxygen may be toxic to them) and 3) Allows malignant cells the 'space' necessary to freely proliferate, at which time they become susceptible to chemotherapeutic agents that act optimally at various steps in the cell growth cycle, eg only 10% of the cells in larger tumor masses are actively proliferating and quiescent cells are not susceptible to chemotherapy; in gynecologic oncology, debulking is performed in extensive metastatic ovarian carcinoma, a tumor in which implants may virtually cover the peritoneum; debulking attempts to excise all tumor implants > 1.0 cm in diameter, followed by radiation and chemotherapy, after which, if the tumor has 'melted' sufficiently, a second, hopefully definitive operation may be performed; this combined modality approach yields a 50% five-year survival; DS significantly increases the length of progression-free and overall survival; after adjusting for various prognostic factors, the risk of death is reduced by ⅓ (**N Engl J Med 1995; 332:629**0A); the patient is then 'followed' with serial measurements of CA-125, a serum marker for recurrent malignancy Note: Debulking procedures may be of use in aggressive high-grade lymphomas; see Second-look operation

decavitamin A multivitamin preparation containing the ten most 'common' vitamins, vitamins A, B_1, B_2, B_6, B_{12}, C, D, E, folic acid, niacinamide and calcium pantothenate; see Multivitamins

decay-accelerating factor DAF, see there

decay disaster Decay catastrophe NUCLEAR MEDICINE The radioactive disintegration of an atom, eg ^{125}I, in a sample that results in radiolabeled molecular fragments of free iodide with decreased immunoreactivity in the remaining iodine when measured by radioimmunoassay; see RIA

deceleration Dip OBSTETRICS The periodic and transient slowing of the fetal heart rate in response to uterine contractions, ie stress

UNIFORM DECELERATION The fetal heart rate response to uterine contractions is symmetrical and has a uniform temporal relation thereto; uniform decelerations are DIVIDED INTO 1) EARLY DECELERATION TYPE I DIP Due to vagal stimulation elicited in the first stage of labor by fetal head compression and 2) LATE DECELERATION TYPE II DIP Due to uteroplacental insufficiency, potentially associated with a less favorable outcome and may signal early vasomotor lability VARIABLE DECELERATION The fetal heart rate response is asynchronous with respect to uterine contractions; the curves on the fetal heart monitor are more angulated and saw-toothed and may be related to compromise in placental blood flow, eg umbilical cord compression, and like late decelerations may signify parturition-related difficulties; see Fetal heart monitor

deceleration injury EMERGENCY MEDICINE A motor vehicle accident-related injury, where the freely-mobile heart in the pericardial cavity is thrown forward and either tears the fixed ligamentum arteriosum or if the deceleration is extreme, ruptures the aorta, causing massive fatal hemopericardium

decentralization ADMINISTRATION A process in which specific duties are assigned to each worker or area of a particular type of operation, defining areas of responsibility but not giving unlimited autonomy

decerebrate rigidity NEUROLOGY A rare clinical condition characterized by hyperextension of extremities, pronation of the arms and hyperflexion of the hands; decerebrate rigidity is evoked in experimental animals by transection of the brain at the superior border of the pons; decerebrate posturing in humans implies tentorial herniation, often associated with paralysis of the contralateral third cranial nerve; Cf Decorticate posturing

decibel 10 $\log_{10}$ (P/P$_o$) A measurement of relative potency of a sound, defined as a power ratio equal to 0.1 bel; see Noise-induced hearing loss

Note: The loudest human sounds according to the Guiness' book of world records: Loudest snore 87.5 dB; loudest whistle 122.5 dB; loudest shout 123.2 dB; other loud sounds: Race cars 125 dB; rock & roll concerts 130 dB, toy guns, up to 170 dB; whales 188 dB; prolonged levels above 150 cause hearing loss or deafness

decidua GYNECOLOGY Endometrial tissue that has been transformed by pregnancy; 'decidualization' begins at the inception of conception and is complete by the end of the first month **DECIDUA BASALIS** The layer immediately external to the embryo, forming a compact layer adherent to the chorion frondosum, constituting the maternal vascular 'socket' in which the placenta is plugged **DECIDUA CAPSULARIS** The layer that covers the endometrium around the remainder or non-basalis portion of the embryonic sac, covering the chorion laeve, eventually expanding to fuse with the **DECIDUA PARIETALIS** That portion of the decidua seen at the fallopian tube junction with the endometrium, or 'corners' of the endometrium

decidual cast The entirety of the decidual components with some hypersecretory endometrium that is characterized by Arias-Stella changes

decidualized cell A modified endometrial stromal cell seen in pregnancy, which is round to polygonal with abundant eosinophilic or basophilic cytoplasm and vesicular nuclei with one or more nucleoli, and may be confused with atypical squamous or neoplastic cells; the presence of decidual cells in the cervicovaginal smear of a pregnant woman is not as clearly associated with abortion as the finding of trophoblasts (**Acta Cytologica 1993; 37:451**0A)

'deciduous tree in winter' sign RENAL PATHOLOGY A fanciful descriptor for the discrete granules and clumped deposits of IgA, seen by immunofluorescence microscopy in the glomerular mesangium in Berger's disease (IgA nephropathy), in which there may be subsequent deposition of IgG and IgM; the vasculocentric deposits also appear in the dermis, supporting an immune complex origin of this condition

decision analysis Clinical decision analysis An analysis in which '...*a problem is stated, assumptions concerning probabilities and utilities are made, and a conclusion is reached based on the results. If the reader* (of the analysis) *agrees with the structure, assumptions, probabilities of the analysis, then he or she must agree with its conclusion.*' (**JAMA 1995; 273:1173**)

decision level(s) LABORATORY MEDICINE An alternative to reference values, representing values for laboratory test results, which when exceeded, require a response by the clinician, eg a total serum calcium level above 2.55 mmol/L (US: 10.2 mg/dl) or below 1.75 mmol/L (US: 7.0 mg/dl); Statland, the principal champion of decision levels, delineated a list of 100 commonly ordered analytes; see Panic values

Note: 'Panic values' are conceptually similar but more extreme in degree of the deviation of the value from the norm, and require that the laboratory report the results immediately to the clinician, given the pernicious portent of the results; examples of decision levels include the point for beginning certain prophylactic therapies in patients with AIDS: Antiretroviral prophylaxis < 500/mm³, *Pneumocystis carinii* pneumonia < 200/mm³, *Mycobacterium avium* complex, and CMV < 100/mm³

decision node A point in a clinical decision-making algorithm at which the effect of a particular diagnostic or therapeutic intervention is evaluated, and further procedures or interventions planned; see Chance node, Decision tree,

decision tree A schematic representation of the major steps taken in a clinical decision algorithm, which begins with the statement of a clinical problem that can be followed along branches based on presence of certain objective features eventually arriving at a conclusion (**JAMA 1995; 273:1173**)

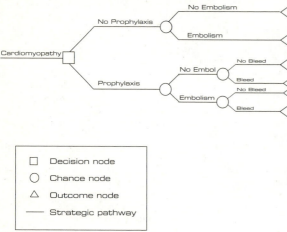

	Decision node
○	Chance node
△	Outcome node
—	Strategic pathway

decision tree

decoction ALTERNATIVE MEDICINE A medicinal preparation of herbal origin in which a ground substrate (eg cinnamon bark, ginger root, nuts, or seeds) is hard or ligneous, making its extraction difficult, and thus requires boiling to extract the volatile oil or substance of interest

decompression sickness A clinical complex caused by rapid whole body decompression, with intravascular 'boiling' of nitrogen and resultant morbidity or mortality in scuba divers and high-altitude pilots or workers in high-pressure environments CLINICAL, ACUTE the 'Bends' Headache, nausea, vomiting, vertigo, tinnitus, dyspnea, tachypnea, convulsions and shock, pain in the joints and limbs (the bends), chest (the chokes) and abdomen; nitrogen gas in the brain causes 'boxcar' air bubbles in leptomeningeal vessels separating the blood 'column', potentially causing death CLINICAL, CHRONIC Caisson disease Dysbaric (ischemic) osteonecrosis with medullary infarcts of the femoral and humoral heads and rarely, malignancy (malignant fibrous histiocytoma) arising in the site of bone infarction

Note: Caissons are air compression (ie pressurized) chambers used for underwater construction; Roebling, engineer of the Brooklyn Bridge (an engineering 'triumph' of the 19th century) was among the first to suffer from the late deforming arthritic effects of Caissons' disease; synonyms include aerobullosis, aeroemphysema, the bends, caissons' disease, caissons' sickness, the chokes, compressed air sickness, decompression disease, tunnel disease

decontamination The use of physical or chemical means to remove, inactivate, or destroy bloodborne (or other) pathogens on a surface or item to the point where they are no longer capable of transmitting infectious particles, and the surface or item is rendered safe for handling, use, or disposal (**Federal Register Dec 6, 1991, p 64175**)

Note: The term decontamination was formerly used for non-infectious agents, eg 'the freeing of a person or an object of some contaminating substance such as war gas, radioactive material, etc.'(**Dorland's Medical Dictionary, 25th ed, WB Saunders, Philadelphia, 1974**)

'decorate' IMMUNOLOGY A verb referring to the positive staining by the immunoperoxidase method; when a cell or tissue has an antigen of interest, eg cytokeratin, it is said to be 'decorated' when stained with (usually) monoclonal antibodies to cytokeratin; the substrate for most ImPx methods yields a red-brown color and thus these techniques are drolly known as 'brown stain'* methods; see Avidin-biotinylated complex, Immunoperoxidase

*or Red stain methods, depending on the color of the digested substrate

decorin A small chondroitin-dermatan sulfate proteoglycan consisting of a single glycosaminoglycan chain and a core protein containing 10 repeats of a leucine-rich 24 amino acid sequence (repeats that also occur in other proteoglycans including biglycan and fibromodulin); decorin binds TGF-β and is involved in down-regulating TGF-β's autocrine functions (Nature 1990; 346:281)

decorticate posture A clinical sign elicited in deep coma, indicating severe diffuse cortical dysfunction, as may occur in a deep coma, where primitive reflex posturing prevails after loss of higher cortical control, characterized by fisted hands, arms flexed on the chest, extended legs, often in response to painful stimuli, a sign of midbrain dysfunction; Cf Decerebrate posture

decoy cells Comet cells URINARY CYTOLOGY Small, exfoliated epithelial cells with scant cytoplasm, large dense, degenerated nuclei and coarse chromatin; decoy cells mimic those of bladder carcinoma but lack nuclear detail and structure (Acta Cytologica 1971; 15:303)

decubitus ulcer see Pressure ulcer

dedifferentiation The loss of cellular characteristics of a terminal differentiation, a feature often associated with increased aggression of a neoplastic process

deductible HEALTH CARE INDUSTRY The amount of out-of-pocket expenses an insured individual must pay before the benefits of a insurance policy or a health care plan begin; after the deductible has been paid, the insurer assumes any further costs; the amount of the deductible is defined by the insurance policy, where the higher the deductible, the lower the cost of the insurance

deeming authority Deemed status A surrogate authority or judicial power granted to a body that is viewed as being equivalent to a formal authority; deeming authority may be granted to certain organizations, eg the College of American Pathologists' (CAP) Commission of Laboratory Accreditation (CLA) when the organization has activities that overlap a governmental function; eg inspection of laboratories in terms of proficiency and quality (CAP Today August 1994)

deep dose equivalent H_d RADIATION PHYSICS The dose equivalent at a tissue depth of 1 cm (1000 mg/cm²) as applied to external whole-body radiation

deep hypothermia CARDIOVASCULAR SURGERY The reduction of a patient's core body temperature, with the purpose of slowing the metabolism to a minimum; DH is coupled to either total circulatory arrest (TCA) or low-flow bypass (LFB); in children undergoing major heart surgery, those with TCA were at a higher risk of delayed motor and cognitive development than thos who had LFB (N Engl J Med 1995; 332:549oa)

deep shave biopsy (skin) see Saucerization biopsy

deep vein thrombosis A postoperative condition in which there is clotting of blood within veins, most often of the lower extremity, which may give rise to emboli; DVT occurs in ½ of total hip replacements without prophylactic anticoagulation, 2-3% of which evolve to fatal pulmonary thromboembolism; acute DVT occurs in 1:1000 of the general population; 92% are idiopathic, approximately 8% are due to isolated deficiencies of protein C, protein S, antithrombin III and plasminogen PATHOGENESIS Idiopathic DVT is associated with subsequent diagnosis of malignancy; overt cancer develops in up 17% of those with recurrent idiopathic DVT (N Engl J Med 1992; 327:1128oa) RISK FACTORS

↑ Age, immobilization, previous DVT, anestheisa, surgery, pregnancy, malignancy, hypercoagulable states (↓ antithrombin III, ↓ protein C, ↓ protein S, activated protein C resistance (which is relatively common) (**N Engl J Med 1994; 331:1559oa**), antiphospholipid syndrome, polycythemia vera, erythrocytosis), tissue trauma (with activation of coagulation cascade) DIAGNOSIS Phlebography, impedence plethysmography, compression ultrasonography (real time B mode), Doppler flow velocity, magnetic resonance venography, radionuclide venography, thermography TREATMENT Anticoagulation, eg heparin or warfarin or thrombolytic therapy, eg alteplase or streptokinase, vena caval filters, surgical thrombectomy (**N Engl J Med 1994; 331:1630ra**)

deepers HISTOTECHNOLOGY A colloquial term for additional tissue that is cut from a paraffin block, usually requested by the pathologist when light microscopic examination of the original stained tissue fails to demonstrate the anticipated pathology or architectural landmarks

'deepest pockets' MEDICAL MALPRACTICE A colloquial adjective referring to the party that will ultimately be responsible for paying an injured plaintiff when multiple parties, eg the physician(s), health care facility, manufacturer of an allegedly defective device or dangerous or teratogenic drug, are named in a successful lawsuit for malpractice, ie the party with the 'deepest pockets'

deer tick *Ixodes scapularis*, see there

deet *N,N*-diethyl-*m*-toluamide An insect repellent that reduces exposure to ticks, carriers of Lyme disease and Rocky Mountain spotted fever Note: Deet may cause seizures and should be used with caution in children

defamation MEDICAL MALPRACTICE An intentional tort which consists of '...*injury to reputation by means of slanderous (oral) or libelous (written) statements to another person that diminish the respect in which the plaintiff is held by others and lessen his or her standing in the community. The extent of the injury caused by verbal defamation must be proved by the plaintiff except in the case of slander involving the accusation of criminal conduct, loathsome disease (eg syphilis, leprosy), acts incompatible with one's business, trade, or profession, or unchastity of a woman.*' (**Surgical Diagnosis & Treatment, 10th ed, Appleton & Lange, Norwalk, 1994**) see Malpractice

defecography GASTROENTEROLOGY A technique for evaluating rectoanal function in which a small amount of barium is injected into the rectum and lateral radiographs are made as the patient relaxes or strains while seated on a special commode; see Videodefecography

defensive innovation HEALTH CARE INDUSTRY A stance taken by manufacturers or providers of health care services or products in which the research monies shift from the goal of advancing medical science to that of anticipating lawsuits; such defensive innovation may cause medical advances or innovations to die in early stages of development for fear that the risk of liability and of irrational lawsuits exceed a reasonable return on investments (**CAP Today 4/1994**)

Note: This form of reverse innovation has been held to be responsible for the decline of birth control modalities in the US

defensive medicine A style of patient management defined as those '...*objective measures taken to document clinical judgement in case there is a lawsuit* (costing ± $7 billion/year US)...*can be expected not only to continue, but also probably to increase.*' (**N Engl J Med 1993; 329:1733sb**) DM is practiced by an estimated 84% of US physicians, eg ordering of extra tests to protect themselves from potential malpractice-related lawsuits (**Am Med News 25 May 1992 p3**) in the US, anything less than a perfect outcome is unacceptable to the consumer, for whom the threshold for litigation appears to decrease as medical technology increases, despite the known risks for certain procedures; defensive practice is designed to minimize lawsuits and includes such 'devices' as

1) INFORMED CONSENT A document that indicates that a patient should understand the intended outcome and potential risks of a procedure Note: The disadvantage of providing a list of potential complications (each of which may be extremely rare) may overwhelm the patient, causing him to forego a needed procedure, resulting in 'Misinformed consent'

2) DOCUMENTATION The formal paperwork by a physician which may be used to justify his reasoning when managing a patient, which may be considered to be 'unreasonably excessive' and

3) MEDICAL WORKUP Over-ordering of diagnostic tests to rule out 'zebras' (unusual diseases that are not seriously considered as diagnoses, but have been known to occur in rare circumstances), as a form of the highly prevalent CYA (Cover your ass)*

although defensive medicine is virtually a standard of practice in the US, its financial impact is difficult to quantify, and is estimated by some to increase the cost of the health care system by 20-40%

*This highly colloquial and vulgar abbreviation is commonly used at all levels of medical practice and training, and has appeared in at least one major medical journal; 'CYA', ie diagnostic 'overkill', has acquired a mystical overtone, in that the physician may be advised to 'CYA' to ward off the evil humors of litigation

deferiprone 1,2-Dimethyl-3-hydroxypyridin-4-one An iron-chelating agent that is administered orally (unlike deferoxamine B mesylate, which is administered IM) to reduce the iron load in patients with severe thalassemia; deferiprone's narrow therapeutic range due to its association with agranulocytosis may limit its use to thalassemic patients who are unable or unwilling to use deferoxamine (**N Engl J Med 1995; 332:918oa**)

deferment Delaying of an obligatory activity; see Medical student debt; Cf Forbearance

deferoxamine Deferoxamine mesylate A naturally occurring trihydroxamic acid that is produced by *Streptomyces pilosus* that ↑ urinary iron excretion; it is the only iron-chelating agent FDA-approved for clinical use; early use of deferoxamine in thalassemia major reduces the transfusion-related iron overload and helps protect against DM, cardiac disease, and early death (**N Engl J Med 1994; 331:567oa**) TOXICITY Auditory and visual symptoms of neurotoxicity are rare, as is the pulmonary syndrome associated with ≥ 10 g/day of therapy

defibrillator CARDIOLOGY A device used to synchronize electrical signaling through the heart that is so erratic as to prevent efficient pumping by the ventricles; according to some experts, the lack of ready access to defibrillators is a major cause for mortality in sudden cardiac arrest; in New York City, where the average response time for an ambulance is 12 minutes following an emergency call, there is a 2% survival of sudden cardiac arrest; in Seattle, the response time is 7 minutes; there is a 20% survival of sudden cardiac arrest (**NY Times 27 Dec 1994, C3**)

deficiency LABORATORY MEDICINE A generic term for any inadequacy in procedure, record-keeping, policy or implementation thereof that has been identified by a regulatory agency

deficiency disease Any clinical condition that results from the inadequate availability of an essential nutrient, including protein, minerals or vitamins

definitive *adjective* DEVELOPMENTAL BIOLOGY Having, pertaining, or referring to a structure or organ that has final and/or adult features although growth has not been completed growth THERAPEUTICS Referring or pertaining to a treatment intended to be curative, complete, or final

definitive radiation RADIATION ONCOLOGY The administration of radiation as the sole or primary therapeutic modality, usually for malignancy, with curative intent; the doses used for DR average 40-50 Gy (4-5000 rads); higher doses may be administered with if 3-D computer-controlled radiotherapy devices are used; DR is commonly used to treat Hodgkin's disease, non-Hodgkin's lymphoma, seminoma, retinoblastoma, choroidal melanoma, cancers of the anus, brain, (uterine) cervix, head & neck, prostate, in unresectable cancer of the lung and pancreas, and unresectable sarcoma (N Engl J Med 1995; 332:371RV)

defloration Rupture of the hymen, which often occurs at the time of the first sexual intercourse, or during digital vaginal examination, masturbation, or through the use of tampons

degeneracy GENETICS see Hereditary degeneration MOLECULAR BIOLOGY The presence of two or more 'synonym' codons for a single amino acid, ie redundancy PSYCHIATRY An obsolete term for 'moral bankrupcy', now included under the rubric of psychotic disorders, formerly deviant behavior, degenerate behavior

degenerate code MOLECULAR BIOLOGY Any coding system in which each piece of information is encoded by two or more different symbols; although there are 64 RNA nucleotide triplets or codons, there are only 20 amino acids and three stop codons; there is therefore, redundancy or 'degeneracy', indeed, three amino acids, leucine, serine, arginine may be translated from six different RNA codons; the survival advantage to this redundancy is that it allows a wide margin of error to occur, where 'sloppy' translation of an incorrect base pair will nevertheless encode a normal protein; thus point mutations may exist without yielding a defective protein, although a point mutation in a situation of 'alternative splicing' may yield 'stop' codons; see Wobble

degenerin(s) An as-yet poorly characterized class of proteins that have been associated with late-onset neuronal deterioration, acting either as membrane receptors or transmembrane channels (Nature 1991; 349:588)

degloving injury EMERGENCY MEDICINE An avulsion-type injury in which the skin and subcutaneous tissue of the hand is torn off in a glove-like fashion, leaving the muculofacial plane intact TREATMENT Clean, debride, sew any clean flaps, light compressive dressing, antimicrobial, eg cefazolin, hospitalize

degmacytes see Bite cells

degrees of freedom STATISTICS The total number of ways in which a set of data, observations, and means can vary independently, given by the number of independent measurements minus the number of restrictions

DEHP bis(2-ethylhexyl)phthalate A plasticizing agent that is responsible for the toxic effects of polyvinyl chloride (PVC), see there

dehumanization A generic term for the removal of human qualities from people or from situations involving people; dehumanization is a expediency that allows policy makers to justify untenable situations, as the person(s) of interest are 'less than human'; dehumanized situations include the virtual incarceration of those with mental disorders in warehouse-like institutions, and ethnic cleansing and genocide

'dehydration fever' Increased temperature in a neonate due to inadequate fluid intake, most severe in high ambient temperatures or when the infant is overclothed

déjà French, already, previously PSYCHIATRY A group of paramnesias in which there is a perception of being familiar or having had previous experiences which have not occurred (deja) or complete absence of memory (jamais) for events known to have been experienced by the subject, each of which has been associated with neurotic depersonalization and temporal lobe epilepsy

DÉJÀ ENTENDU Intense feeling of having previously heard something, that he/she had never in fact previously (STH/SHNIFP) heard DÉJÀ EPROUVÉ Intense feeling of having previously experienced STH/SHNIFP experienced DÉJÀ FAIT Intense feeling of having previously done STH/SHNIFP done DÉJÀ PENSÉE Intense feeling of having previously thought STH/SHNIFP thought DÉJÀ RACONTÉE Intense feeling of having previously related, ie having told someone STH/SHNIFP related DÉJÀ VÉCU Intense feeling of having previously experi-

enced STH/SHNIFP experienced DÉJÀ VOULU Intense feeling of having previously wished STH/SHNIFP wished DÉJÀ VU Intense feeling of having previously seen STH/SHNIFP seen; see Jamais

Delaney clause A legislative addition to the US Food, Drug and Cosmetics Act, proposed by JJ Delaney (NY-Democrat) in 1958 prohibiting use of food additives that are known to be carcinogenic in experimental animals or in humans; in 1986, the US Congress recognized that state-of-the-art techniques could detect nano- and picogram amounts of potential carcinogens, posing little risk for malignancy (1:10 000 000), and reasoned that 'risk assessment' is the best way to determine the likelihood for malignancy; see Alar, Ames test, Risk assessment

delayed response gene Any of a number of genes that are regulated by changes in intracellular Ca^{2+}; DRGs are induced slowly and usually require the synthesis of new proteins for their transcription, possibly those encoded by immediate early genes (IEGs); the proteins encoded by DRGs more directly influence cell physiology than those encoded by IEGs (Science 1995; 268:244) Cf Immediate early gene

deletion IMMUNOLOGY One of two mechanisms of T cell tolerance, which occurs during intrathymic maturation of T cells, resulting in programmed cell death; see Anergy MOLECULAR BIOLOGY The loss of genetic material ranging from a single base for RNA or base pair for DNA to a large portion of a chromosome

deletion polymorphism A deletion polymorphism has been found in the ACE gene that links it to left venticular hypertrophy (N Engl J Med 1994; 330:164OA)

deletion syndrome CLINICAL GENETICS A generic term for any of number of hereditary disease complexes due to the loss of major chromosome segments; all are rare, often have microcephaly and an IQ < 50

4P- DELETION SYNDROME Wolf-Hirshhorn syndrome Low birth weight, hypertelorism, cleft palate, micrognathia, hypospadia, cryptorchism 5P- DELETION SYNDROME see Cri du chat syndrome 9Q- DELETION SYNDROME Antimongolic palpebral slanting, epicanthal folds, low-set ears, micrognathia, short and webbed neck, mammary hypertelorism, arachnodactyly 11Q- DELETION SYNDROME Growth retardation, aniridia, Wilm's tumor, gonadoblastoma, ambiguous genitalia in males 13Q- DELETION SYNDROME Rare, low birth weight, failure to thrive, holoprosencephaly, large deformed ears, microphthalmia, retinoblastoma, hypertelorism, broad protuberant nose without bridge, hypoplasia of the hands, syndactyly, atrial and ventricular septal defects; ambiguous genitalia, cryptorchism, hypo- and epispadias, hypoplastic kidneys and anal atresia 18Q- DELETION SYNDROME Rare, seizures, hypotonia, midfacial hypoplasia, deep-set eyes, visual abnormalities, (glaucoma, strabismus, nystagmus, optic atrophy), external auditory canal atresia, fish-shaped mouth, cleft lip or palate, patellar dimples, supernumerary ribs, arachnodactyly, talipes equinovarus, cardiac malformations, cryptorchism, hypoplastic external genitalia, survival to adolescence 18P- DELETION SYNDROME Rare, low birth weight, Turner syndrome-like features, holopros-encephaly, low-set floppy ears, hypertelorism, epicanthal folds, strabismus, ptosis, hypotonia, stubby hands, partial webbing of toes, normal lifespan 21Q DELETION SYNDROME Rare, growth retardation, skeletal malformation, large low-set ears, prominent nasal bridge, micrognathia, downward slanting palpebral fissures, high-arched cleft palate or lip, hypotonia, pyloric stenosis, hypospadias and cryptorchism 22Q- DELETION SYNDROME Rare, hypotonia, high arched palate, large low-set ears, epicanthal folds, syndactyly of the toes

Delilah syndrome PSYCHIATRY A clinical complex seen in the daughters of domineering aggressive men, characterized by marked sexual promiscuity, related to fear and dislike of the father and an unconscious switching of roles with the father figure, such that they seduce and overcome men, allegorically as the biblical Delilah seduced and overcame the powerful Samson; see Diana complex, Wild woman phenotype; Cf Don Juan syndrome

delirium An acute defect in cognate functions, due to toxins, substance abuse, acute psychosis and metabolic disease states, a state which can either progress or regress; Cf Dementia

dell HEMATOLOGY The central cleared area of a normal erythrocyte

dellen OPHTHALMOLOGY Foci of stromal degeneration with reversible corneal attenuation, caused by a break in the tear film layer due to a local elevation of the cornea, eg pterygium, filtering blebs, suture granuloma or limbal tumor

delphi method A multi-stage survey technique intended to produce a consensus from a target group of experts regarding therapy for a particular nosology or other point of clinical interest METHOD Published data and unpublished information are obtained, integrated then submitted anonymously to the experts and feedback is obtained; the data is then reevaluated and re-submitted to the experts, conclusions are reached, the data is then re-re-evaluated, re-re-submitted to the experts and so on until either their stamina is exhausted or a consensus is reached

delta agent Hepatitis D virus, HDV A virus causing a form of hepatitis that was first described in southern Italy (**Gut 1977; 18:997**); the delta agent is a 1.7 kilobase, circular single-stranded non-enveloped incomplete RNA virus similar to virioids and the satellite RNA of plants; HDV has a small and highly conserved domain with replicational features and a larger, less conserved domain, bearing antigenic determinants; although HDV has little sequence homology with HBV, it is a subviral satellite of HBV, and is dependent on HBV for packaging its genome into viral particles; thus HDV requires that the patient be previously infected by HBV, as HDV is ensconced in HBV surface antigen or HBsAg; patients with delta viremia are positive for HBsAg, anti-HBc and usually HBe; HDV is found in IV drug abusers (73% in Los Angeles are positive for HDV), hemophiliacs and AIDS patients; HDV is often associated with fulminant hepatitis and is endemic in many parts of the world; see Hepatitis

delta bilirubin Biliprotein A bilirubin fraction tightly bound to albumin with a serum $T_{1/2}$ of 17 days, detected only in patients with conjugated hyperbilirubinemia in whom it is a substantial fraction of the direct-reacting bilirubin; the existence of this fraction explains the slow resolution of hyperbilirubinemia after hepatitis or after surgical correction of biliary obstruction

delta cell tumor Somatostatinoma, see there

delta check LABORATORY MEDICINE A technique for quality control of clinical specimens in which patient results are compared to his previous values; the delta check is easier in theory than in practice, as it is cumbersome, requires a great amount of computer time and increases the rate of false positivity for analytes

Delta Dental Plan of California v. Banasky The first court decision to grant physicians and dentists who contract with managed health care plans a 'common-law right to fair procedure', ie that practitioners can challenge an HMO's internal review process in court; the appellate court's ruling provides doctors with new grounds to challenge the deselection decisions (**Am Med News 21 Nov 1994 p1**)

ΔF508 Cystic fibrosis, see there

delta heavy chain disease A single case has been reported in an elderly man with osteolytic lesions, marrow infiltration by abnormal plasma cells, who died in renal failure

delta osmolality LABORATORY MEDICINE That value representing the difference between the calculated and the measured (by freezing point depression) osmolality; a DO of > 40 mosmol/kg often presages a poor clinical course, indicating accumulation of osmotically active metabolites or toxins including: ethanol, ethylene glycol, isopropanol, ketoacids, lactic acid, azotemia, methanol; see Osmolarity

delta sign NEURORADIOLOGY A descriptive term for a filling defect in cerebral venous sinus thrombosis, seen by CT, accompanied by hemorrhage, hyperdensity along the straight sinus and linear hyperdensity corresponding to the thrombosed veins

delta wave CARDIOLOGY An EKG finding in the Wolff-Parkinson-White (WPW or pre-excitation) syndrome, characterized as a slow upstroke of the QRS wave in a background of short P-R intervals

Note: WPW syndrome pre-disposes patients to re-entrant tachycardia and occurs in normal hearts, Ebstein's anomaly, corrected transposition (ventricular 'inversion') and in cardiomyopathy

delusion of grandeur PSYCHIATRY A popular term for what is designated by the American Psychiatric Association as 'delusional disorder, grandiose subtype' [DSM-IV 297.1], which is characterized by '*delusions of inflated worth, power, knowledge, identity, or special relationship to a diety or famous person.*' (**Diagnostic and Statistical Manual of Mental Disorders, 4th ed, Washington, DC, American Psychiatric Association, 1994**)

demand model HEALTH CARE POLICY A simplistic model for determining the existance of 'units' (eg pathologists) in a system that is based on supply dynamics as well as environmental factors (**CAP Today 1995; 9:5**) Cf HMO (extrapolation) model, Needs model, Supply model

dematiaceous fungi A group of environmental saprobic fungi (about 20 species) that produce a melanin-like pigment and may cause clinical conditions, eg chromoblastomycosis, and phaeohypomycosis; phaeohypomycosis results in diseases ranging from the benign tinea nigra, caused by *Exophiala werneckii* and *Stenella araguata*, to the pernicious fungal sepsis, caused by *Cladosporium, Curvularia, Exophiala, Mycocentrospora* species

dementia The end stage of mental deterioration, characterized by a loss of cognitive capacity*, leading to impaired social and/or occupational activity; dementia's prevalence in the general population is a function of age, and affects ± 10.5% of those 80-85; 12.6-47.2% ≥ 85 (**N Engl J Med 1993; 328:203ED**) ETIOLOGY 47% Vascular-type (potentially amenable to therapy), 44% Alzheimer's type; other causes of dementia include alcohol, schizophrenia, subdural hematoma, normal pressure hydrocephalus, vitamin B_{12} deficiency (**ibid; 328:153OA**) and repeated trauma ('punch-drunk' syndrome, torture victims) Note: Dementia is a component of senility that should be, but rarely is, separated from 'Alzheimer's disease', a term that has long lost its original specificity, which was described (**Zbl Nervenkh 1906; 25:1134; 1907; 30:177**) as an idiopathic, early, or presenile form or pre-senile dementia

*Note: It is common practice to refer to the loss of cognitive function as dementia if the cause is organic, and as mental illness if the loss is due to psychologic decompensation

demic diffusion ANTHROPOLOGY A theory of the spread of ancient culture, which modifies the more general diffusion theory by postulating that the farmers advanced at a rate of one kilometer per year, assimilating the hunter-gatherers' gene pool (**Nature 1991; 351:143, 97**); see Diffusion; Cf Migration

demographics The objective characteristics of a population, including age, racial origin, religion, income and education, often referring to the patient population served by a health care facility, eg Patient demographics; Cf Epidemiology

denaturation CHEMISTRY The alteration of a substance in such a way as to render it unsuitable for consumption, eg alcohol MOLECULAR BIOLOGY A process in which non-covalent, eg hydrogen bonds and disulfide bonds are broken, either reversibly or irreversibly, resulting in a change in the native conformation of a protein or a nucleic acid, leaving the primary structure; denaturation is a critical step in many processes involving nucleic acids and consists of separating double-stranded nucleic acids into a single-stranded ones

dendrite NEUROLOGY *dendritum* [NH3] A branching protoplasmic process of a neuron; the dendrite is now known to play an active role in transporting signals to and from neurons, and are actively involved in formation of action potentials, and in 'back-propagation', which is a feedback signal from the dendrites to the synapse (**Science 1995; 268:200rn**)

dendritic keratitis Linear and arborescent ulcerations on the anterior corneal surface seen in the relatively mild keratitis caused by herpes simplex or herpes zoster; Cf Geographic ulcer

dendritic reticular cells Cells of the mononuclear phagocytic system (MPS) located in the skin (Langerhans cells), lymph nodes (interdigitating cells of the paracortex), marginal sinus of afferent lymphatics (veiled cells), and spleen that present antigen to T cells; these cells are characterized by nonspecific esterase, endogenous peroxidase, Birbeck granules, a tennis racquet-like structure seen by electron microscopy, a 15-kD antigen recognized by the M1-8 monoclonal antibody, and depending on their maturation, may have CD1 surface antigen, Fc receptors and complement receptors CR1 and CR3; the Langerhans cells express class MHC I as well as abundant MHC class II HLA-DR determinants, and are thought to migrate in a 'veiled' fashion via the afferent vessels into the paracortical regions of the draining lymph nodes and into the thymus where the cell processes interdigitate with T cells, coercing them into maturation

dendritic reticulum cell sarcoma A nonlymphoid neoplasm, thought to arise from reticulum cells native to the lymph nodes Histopathology Interfollicular storiform proliferation of oval or spindled tumor cells with bland nuclei Prognosis Unknown, given this tumor's rarity, although it may recur and metastasize to the liver

dendritic ulcer A herpetiform corneal ulcer seen in tyrosinemia (Richner-Hanhart syndrome) Clinical Self-mutilation, mental retardation, punctate palmoplantar hyperkeratosis, multiple lipomas Treatment Early dietary restriction of tyrosine and phenylalanine prevents mental retardation

dendrogram Molecular epidemiology A diagram used to represent the phylogenic or evolutionary relatedness of molecular species of organisms which is based on allelic variations of a specific gene or sequence of DNA

dengue Tropical medicine A flavivirus infection* caused by the flavivirus, a group B arbovirus, transmitted by the mosquito, *Stegomyia Aedes aegypti*; there are four serotypes (DEN-1 to DEN-4), all of which have been identified in the Western hemisphere (**MMWR 1995; 44:21**) Clinical forms Benign dengue fever, seen in the African and American tropics and malignant dengue hemorrhage shock syndrome, causing severe bone pain or 'break bone fever', accompanied by a biphasic or 'saddleback' fever curve, arthralgia, nausea, vomiting, prostration, headache, myalgia, lymphadenopathy, a morbilliform maculopapular truncal rash that spares the palmoplantar regions Laboratory Lymphocytopenia, thrombocytopenia

*The name is Spanish, via Swahili, kadingapepo *ka*, a kind of; *dinga*, sudden cramp-like seizure; *pepo*, evil spirit, plague

dengue hemorrhagic fever A dengue virus induced condition defined by WHO criteria: 1) Fever 2) Hemorrhagic manifestations 3) Thrombocytopenia ($\leq$ 100 000/mm³) 4) Objective criteria of increased capillary permeability, eg hemoconcentration (hematocrit $\geq$.20% above normal), pleural effusions (by chest radiography), or hypoproteinemia (**MMWR 1995; 44:21**)

dengue shock syndrome A dengue virus-induced condition, which in addition to the criteria of dengue hemorrhagic fever (*vide supra*) is defined by the presence of hypotension or narrow pulse pressure ($\leq$20 mmHg) (**MMWR 1995; 44:21**) Clinical Prolonged high fever, petechiae, hepatomegaly, severe hypotension and a narrow pulse pressure Laboratory ↑↑↑ hematocrit, ↓ platelets; DSS is a medical emergency requiring rapid fluid expansion,

heparin, sodium bicarbonate, sedation, and oxygen Mortality Up to 44%

denial Psychiatry A primitive (ego defense) mechanism used by a person to consciously or unconsciously negate the existence of a disease or other stress-producing reality in his environment

dens in dente Oral pathology A maldeveloped tooth with invaginated outer enamel epithelium of the odontogenic germ layer; in its mildest form occurs in 5% of the population; the tooth is grossly and radiologically malformed appearing as a tooth within a tooth

dense core granule Neurosecretory granules, see there

dense deposit disease Type II membranoproliferative glomerulonephritis A glomerulopathy in which electron-dense material (usually complement C3) is deposited in the glomerular capillary basement membrane, with decreased serum C3 due to alternate complement pathway activation in the face of normal C4; there is patchy mesangial proliferation in Bowman's capsule, and accumulation of basement membrane material in the peritubular capillaries and arterioles Prognosis Poor; see 'Tramtrack' appearance

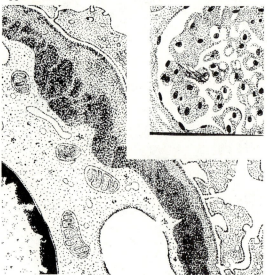

dense deposit disease

dense granule A spherical storage vesicle in platelets that houses ADP, ATP, calcium, pyrophosphate and serotonin Note: ADP is considered the key player in platelet activity and held responsible for propagating the primary platelet response and enlargement of the hemostatic plug; Cf α granules, Storage pool disease

density gradient centrifugation Immunology see Ficoll Molecular biology Centrifugation of large molecules, eg RNA and DNA, in a solution with a density gradient molecule, eg cesium chloride, a commonly used medium for ultracentrifugation

dental amalgam A filling material that contains up to 50% mercury, as well as silver and other metals, which has been used in dental restoration since the early 1800s; more recently, the wisdom of using a toxic heavy metal in the mouth has been questioned; some data suggest that a single amalgam can release 3-17 μg of mercury/day; in some Northern European countries, eg Germany, Sweden, the use of DAs has been either prohibited or severely restricted, with health insurers paying for the cost of replacement of the amalgams with a less toxic alternative, eg composite amalgam

Note: According to alternative health care providers, DAs can be responsible for chronic fatigue syndrome, chronic inflammation (eg rhematoid arthritis, phlebitis, fibromyalgia), numbness, lowering of pain threshold, defects in the immune system (Alternative Medicine, Future Medicine Publishing, Inc, Puyallup, Washington, 1994)

dental dam DENTISTRY Rubber dam A thin sheet of rubber latex punctuated with small holes that are stretched around the crown of the teeth, which is used to isolate the teeth from the mucosal secretions during dental procedures and prevent the aspiration of various materials used in or resulting from oral surgery; dental dams may also be used to protect the buccal cavity during oral sex (Am Med News 18 May 1992 p24)

dental implant Osseointegrated implant A dental prosthesis that is implanted in the maxilla or mandible allowing subsequent placement of artificial teeth; the procedure is performed in a three-step process: 1) A titanium anchor is 'screwed' into a threaded hole made in the bone of the oral cavity by a low-speed drill and covered with soft tissue and allowed to 'fuse', ie osseointegrate 2) After a 3–6-month healing process, some of the gum overlying the anchor is removed and an abutment post is placed 3) A tooth, bridge, or entire jaw is fitted by a restorative dentist

dentatorubral and pallidoluysian atrophy A CAG repeat-disease (see there) characterized by selective destruction of cerebellar neurons (Science News 1995; 147:360)

Denver developmental screening test A psychological screening test for assessing a child's neurodevelopmental maturation

Denver shunt A peritoneo-venous shunt that relieves ascites and improves renal function

2'-deoxycoformycin ONCOLOGY A purine analogue used in chemotherapy, eg hairy cell leukemia (Ann Int Med 1993; 119:278oA)

deoxyribonucleic acid see DNA

department head The director of a service (ie a specialty field, eg surgery) who is usually appointed by the chief of the medical staff; his/her function is to foster, facilitate, and participate in institutional activities, coordinate departmental activities, maintain the quality of medical care rendered by the department; arbitrate intradepartmental disputes, and interact with administration, nursing, and other departments in the institution, and serve as a liaison with the community

dependence SUBSTANCE ABUSE A psychological or physiological compulsion for a person to use a substance (usually a narcotic) on a chronic and repeated basis; the dependence on the drug may become overwhelming, compelling the abuser to sacrifice his quality of life in exchange for the drug

dependent *adjective* ANATOMY The lower-most aspect of a body part or cavity; decubital ulcers occur on the dependent parts, eg sacrum and abscesses and tumor masses tend to collect in the most dependent regions of a cavity, eg in the cul-de-sac in acute peritonitis PSYCHIATRY see Dependent personality disorder *noun* Any person, eg wife, children, and occasionally, grandparents and other significant others, who relies on someone else for the majority of their financial support; see Extended family, Most significant other, Nuclear family

dependent personality disorder PSYCHIATRY A condition of onset in early adulthood which is characterized by a '...pervasive and excessive need to be taken care of (by others) that leads to submissive and clinging behavior and fears of separation.' (**DSM-IV**) subjects with DPD have difficulty in making everyday decisions (eg fish or cut bait); DPDers tend to be passive, allowing others to make decisions for them and assume responsibility for their life activities

depersonalization PSYCHIATRY Any of a group of personality disorders in which the patient thinks that either he or those in his environment have been changed into other

people or life-forms, depersonalization is calssically associated with schizophrenia, but may also occur in hysteria, depression, drug-induced states, temporal lobe epilepsy, and in fatigue

> **DEPERSONALIZATION DISORDER (DSM-IV 300.6)**
> A Persistent or recurrent sensation of detachment from one's own body, as if one were in a dream
> B During the depersonalization experience, the subject's reality testing remains intact
> C The depersonalization results in significant distress or impairment of social, occupational, other function
> D The experience does not occur exclusively during the course of another mental disorder
> DSM-IV™, American Psychiatric Association, Washington, DC, 1994

depersonalization disorder PSYCHIATRY A compelling delusional state characterized by persistent of recurrent episodes of depersonalization (see table) formally described DDs include

1) PHANTOM DOUBLE SYNDROME OF CAPGAS, a delusion that impostors have replaced friends and relatives; it is more common in women who deny knowing their spouse

2) CLERAMBAULT-KANDINSKY SYNDROME, a delusion in which a person thinks that his mind is controlled by outside influences

3) PRESENILE DERMATOZOON PSYCHOSIS OF EKBOM, a delusion that parasites are crawling over the body

depolarizing bipolar cells Retinal neurons that are hyperpolarized by glutamate and L-2-amino-4-phosphonobutyrate, decreasing membrane conductance by increasing the rate of cGMP hydrolysis by a G protein-mediated process

Depo-Provera Medroxyprogesterone acetate A synthetic progestin that is an FDA-approved injectable contraceptive, which is administered every three months; it has also been used to treat female precocious puberty, dysfunctional uterine bleeding, dysmenorrhea, endometriiosis, threatened abortion, and to suppress postpartum lactation SIDE EFFECTS Weight gain, menstrual abnormalities, fatigue, vertigo, nervousness, headaches, and abdominal pain

deposition ENVIRONMENT The fallout or precipitation of airborne pollutants in an ecosystem FORENSIC MEDICINE An oral or written testimony that is obtained under oath from a witness or expert outside of a court of law; the deposition can be subsequently used in a court of law METABOLIC DISEASES The accumulation of crystallizable or nonmetabolizable material in certain organs

depraved FORENSIC PSYCHIATRY An inherent deficiency of moral sense and rectitude, equivalent to the statutory term, 'depravity of heart', defined as the highest grade of malice, or with indifference to the lives of others, a requirement (in the US) for a person's conviction of second-degree murder; see Mad dog

depraved heart murder FORENSIC PSYCHIATRY The killing of a person by extreme atrocity, with malicious intent inferred by the nature of the act; a depraved heart murder may also be defined as one in which there was extremely negligent and unjustifiable conduct carrying a high degree of risk of bodily harm or death to others, which may be unaccompanied by any intent to kill, but nevertheless result in death; see Manslaughter, Murder, Serial murder

deprenyl Selegiline phenylisopropylmethylpropynylamine A selective irreversible inhibitor of type B monoamine oxidase that reportedly delays the onset of disability in patients with early untreated Parkinson's disease MECHANISM Unknown, it may ↑ dopamine levels by inhibiting monoamine oxidase, thereby preventing Parkinson's disease, as dopaminergic regions of the substantia nigra are destroyed in PD (**N Engl J Med 1993; 328:1760A**) see MPTP

depression A condition* characterized by attenuation of mood accompanied by psychogenic pain, diminution of self-esteem, retardation of thought processes, psychomotor sluggishness, disturbances of sleep and appetite, and not uncommonly, suicidal ideation; depression can be divided into **ENDOGENOUS DEPRESSION**, which is characterized by pervasive sadness, hopelessness, loss of interest in activities, and physical symptoms, eg weight loss, and sleep problems and **REACTIVE DEPRESSION**, which is viewed as an exhuberant response to stressful life events; in both forms, a stressful life event has occurred in the relatively recent past; in endogenous depression, there may be an increased 'threshold' that requires little external input to initiate recurrence (**Science News 1994; 146:52**); see Depressive disorders

*The term depression is too nonspecific, despite the adjectival modifiers, eg endogenous and reactive, indicated above, and has been replaced by the generic term depressive disorder when it refers to a condition in which depression is a major component

depressive disorder PSYCHIATRY A generic term for any of a number of conditions characterized by one or more depressive episodes (major depressive disorder[1]), depressed mood (dysthymic disorder[2] and adjustment disorder with depressed mood[3]) and those that do not fit the criteria of others conditions, known as depressive disorder not otherwise specified[4]

[1]296.2x, 296.3x in DSM-IV [2]300.4 in DSM-IV [3]309.x in DSM-IV [4]311 in DSM-IV

dereism PSYCHIATRY A generic term for thought processes and mental activities that ignore reality, logic, or actual experience; deiristic thought is characteristic of schizophrenia

derived air concentration RADIATION PHYSICS The concentration of a radionuclide in the air, which if inhaled by the reference man for a working year of 2000 hours under light (ie not heavy) working conditions (inhalation rate 1.2 m³/hour) results in the intake of 1.0 ALI (annual limit on intake)

derived protein A protein derived from a larger molecule by digestion, alteration of the pH, or by heating

derived standardized score see Z score

dermabrasion A technique in which a dermatome or abrading device* is used to remove the epidermis and superficial layers of the dermis allowing regeneration of the epithelium to occur from underlying adnexal structures (eg pilosebaceous unit); dermabrasion was developed to treat postacne scarring, as well as scars caused surgery, trauma, or varicella; dermabrasion may be used to treat actinic keratosis, nevi, rhinophyma, seborrheic hyperplasia, seborrheic keratosis, solar elastosis, and tattoos; it is contraindicated as a therapy for radiodermatitis, as radiation damages adnexal structures and blood supply

*Dermabrasion was first used in 1550 BC (!) by Papyrus Ebers of Egypt who used papyrus and pumice to remove blemishes

dermatoglyphics A term that refers to both 1) The formal study of the combined patterns of skin ridges on the fingers and toes, palms and soles and 2) The patterns per se; because of the uniqueness of the patterns in an individual person and that certain motifs may be shared by those in a particular racial group, dermatoglyphics are of interest to criminologists, anthropologists, and to geneticists; dermatoglyphic patterns have been studied in conditions as diverse as autism, celiac disease, congenital cataracts and dislocation of the hip, Prader-Willi syndrome, SLE, and von Recklinghausen disease, to name a few, and used to differentiate among various races, although its main, albeit uncommon use, is in the study of trisomies, 13, 18 and 21; see Simian crease, Triradius

dermatographism Dermographism, see there

dermatomyositis A distinct form of collagen vascular dis-

ease characterized by rash, edema (eyelids, back of hands) and IM complement-mediated microangiopathic muscle fiber destruction, leading to loss of capillaries, muscle ischemia, muscle fiber necrosis, and perifascicular atrophy RISK OF CANCER Increased TREATMENT Various agents, including azathioprine, cyclophosphamide, cyclosporine, methotrexate, and prednisone are unsuccessful; high-dose IV immune globulin has been reported to ↑ muscle strength and ↓ neuromuscular symptoms in refractory dermatomyositis, requiring long-term therapy (**N Engl J Med 1993; 329:1993OA**)

Dermatophagoides farinae House dust mite, see there

dermographism Dermatographism A wheal-and-flare reaction evoked by stroking the skin

DES Diethylstilbestrol A synthetic estrogen that is more potent than natural estrogens; between the 1940s and 1970s, DES was prescribed to 2-3 million ♀ as it was thought to prevent certain complications of pregnancy; ≥ 1 million US ♂ were exposed prenatally to DES, DES's use during pregnancy was banned in 1972 as in utero exposure before the 18th gestational week results in a 3-fold ↑ in congental abnormalities (but no impairment of fertility or sexual function-**N Engl J Med 1995; 332:1411OA**) with vaginal wall adenosis in 35-70% of exposed ♀ infants, see Cockscomb cervix and vagina; 0.14% of cases progress to vaginal adenocarcinoma, and are thought to have a better prognosis than non-DES clear cell adenocarcinoma (which may be a function of increased surveillance, rather than a difference in tumor biology); DES acts as a carcinogen by forming transient covalent bonds to the DNA of rapidly dividing cells, having a five-fold greater affinity for female DNA than male DNA; other DES changes include obliteration of vaginal fornices, microglandular hyperplasia of the cervix (cervical ectropion, and transverse ridging (cock's-comb appearance) and a 2.5-fold increase in primary infertility TREATMENT Surgery for the carcinoma is aggressive, including vaginectomy, hysterectomy and lymphadenectomy; a postulated relation between prenatal DES exposure and neoplasia of müllerian remnants of males remains undetermined

desalting LABORATORY MEDICINE The removal of inorganic salt ions from a sample by dialysis, ion-exchange chromatography and electrophoresis, without which the assay may be significantly affected

descending perineum syndrome A clinical condition that partially overlaps the symptoms of anismus, which is characterized by prolonged inhibition of the pelvic floor muscles and, like anismus, occurs in a background of constipation; it is possible that DPS is a end stage of anismus, resulting from denervation, although longitudinal studies have not been performed

desensitization ALLERGY MEDICINE A therapeutic modality that attempts to reduce IgE-mediated hypersensitivity to various substances by administering ever-increasing amounts of an antigen, eg urushiol in poison ivy, sumac and pollen, with the purpose of evoking the formation of blocking antibodies

desert rheumatism San Joaquin fever A clinical condition caused by *Coccidioides immitis*, a pathogenic fungus endemic to the arid Southwestern US CLINICAL Subclinical disease during childhood exposure with malaise, fever, chills, headache, backache, chest pain, dry cough, fine macular erythema and rarely, meningitis

DESI Drug Efficacy Study Implementation The 1962 Kefauver-Harris amendment to the Food and Drug Act that required drug manufacturers to prove both safety and efficacy of a marketed drug; with the aid of the National Academy of Science and the National Research Council, thousands of drugs were reviewed for thousands of indications, 40% of which had equivocal effects and were considered to be 'less-than-effective'; in 1982, the HCFA stopped reimbursement for less-than-effective agents that had been recommended for various acute and chronic conditions, eg peripheral or cerebral vasodilators, combinations of asthma therapies with sedatives, gastrointestinal antispasmodics with sedative, steroid with antibiotic creams, diuretics with potassium, phenylbutazone with antacids, cerebral 'stimulants' and others

designated driver PUBLIC HEALTH A person at a social function[1] who either volunteers or is 'volunteered' to act as the chauffeur to ensure that all revellers arrive home safely; the designated driver campaign[2] is credited with changing public awareness about drinking and driving, and may be partly responsible for the 25% ↓ in drunk driving-related accidents in the US since 1989 (**Am Med News 19 Sept 1994**) Cf Squash it

[1]In which the consumption of 'industrial' quantities of alcohol is anticipated
[2]The term designated driver has been incorporated into the popular culture, largely through the efforts of workers at the Harvard School of Public Health in persuading Hollywood producers to incorporate the concept into television and film story lines

designer antibody A generic term for an immunoglobulin that has been genetically engineered for a specific purpose, forming chimeric antibodies by combining for example, the gene segments encoding a mouse immunoglobulin's variable region with a human constant region, reducing the hybrid molecule's antigenicity, since the 'mousier' the molecule, the more likely its various epitopes will elicit an immune response in humans; see Humanized antibody

'designer' drug A substance of abuse produced in a clandestine laboratories, eg an analogue of fentanyl (a short-acting narcotic analgesic used in surgery that is 1000-fold more potent than morphine), that are often methylated, thereby escaping detection by standard drug screens; because many DDs have not categorized and specifically outlawed, they are in a sense, not illegal; DDs of high analgesic potential include sufentanil and alfentanil, which are up to 2000-fold more potent than morphine; DDs include analogs of meperidine (MPPP, PEPAP, PCP) and amphetamine (phenyl-ethamine); DDs are most popular in California, where they comprise up to 20% of that state's substances of abuse; see Adam, 'Ice'

'designer' lymphocytes A lymphocyte containing inserted genes that enhance the cells' tumorlytic activity, endowing it with desirable characteristics, eg tumor-infiltrating lymphocytes, resulting in 'adoptive immunotherapy'

'desktop' hypoglycemia An erroneous diagnosis of hypoglycemia due to errors in collection or handling of a blood specimen Note: If a prolonged delay between time of collection and analysis of glucose levels is anticipated, the specimen should be collected in sodium fluoride, which in the US are often 'grey top' blood collection tubes, as NaF paralyses the red cells' glycolytic system, preventing falsely low levels of glucose

desmin A 55 kD muscle-type intermediate filament present in mesenchymal cells, including vascular endothelial cells, smooth and skeletal muscle cells and possibly also myofibroblasts; desmin is of greatest use in identification of muscle tumors

Note: Malignant tumor cells often 'forget' their embryological lineage and display more than one intermediate filament; see also Intermediate filaments

desmoid Aggressive fibromatosis A nonencapsulated mass on the anterior abdominal wall of postpartum females, often related to trauma,which according to some anecdotal reports, may regress with local progesterone injection

desmolase An obsolete term for the enzyme (cytochrome P-450$_{scc}$

17,20-desmolase P-450$_{c17}$ hydroxylase/17,20-lyase

20,22-desmolase (Cytochrome) P-450$_{scc}$ side-chain cleaving enzyme, see there

desmoplakin Either of two membrane-bound proteins, desmoplakin I (250 kD) and desmoplakin II (215 kD) that are present in the desmosomes of all epithelia, and serve as markers for the presence of cell junctions, and which have homology with the bullous pemphigoid antigen

desmoplasia Desmoplastic response SURGICAL PATHOLOGY A dense stromal reaction in which malignant epithelial cells are compressed into single cell layers ('Indians in a file'), a pattern that is highly characteristic of infiltrating ductal carcinoma of the breast, which may be due to stromalysin-3, a secreted matrix metalloprotein; see Stromalysin-3

desquamative interstitial pneumonitis A nonspecific interstitial pulmonary reaction; DIP is often idiopathic but may be associated with inhalation of inorganic particulates (**N Engl J Med 1993; 328:869cPc**) DIP is most common in adults and characterized by the filling of alveoli with large mononuclear macrophages, minimal interstitial changes and no necrosis, hyaline membrane formation and fibrin deposition RADIOLOGY Bilateral ground-glass opacifications TREATMENT Corticosteroids

detailing HEALTH CARE INDUSTRY An educational activity of sales representatives ('detailers'), eg from pharmaceutical companies or manufacturers of medical devices, in which legitimate attempts are made to provide details or scientific information on the product's potential uses, benefits, side effects and adverse effects; detailing information is often packaged with a subtle bias towards the product's good results; in one university teaching hospital-based study, 11% of the statements made by pharmaceutical representatives contradicted the information readily available to them; these errors are rarely recognized by physicians (**JAMA 1995; 273:1296**)

detached ciliary tufts CYTOLOGY Small apical fragments of ciliated cytoplasm without nuclei, which have been identified in cytologic specimens from various sites, including upper respiratory tract, peritoneal washings, seminal fluid, endometrium, and from ovarian and paraovarian cysts; DCTs generally originate from normal tissue or benign lesions, and their presence in an ovarian cyst rules out the diagnosis of follicular cyst (**Acta Cytologica 1993; 37:489oA**)

detection bias CLINICAL RESEARCH Any confounding factor that ↑ or ↓ the likelihood that a disease will be detected in a particular population (**JAMA 1992; 268:1900oc**)

detector INSTRUMENTATION Any component of a quantification device that recognizes an incoming chemical or physical signal; these signals include changes in gas pressure, particle number, pH, substrate or product concentration (eg organic compounds eluted from a column in gas-liquid chromatography), or wave transmission (eg radiation in Geiger counter)

detergent CHEMISTRY A generic term for an amphipathic molecule, eg a long-chain hydrocarbon that has at one end a charged polar group that makes the whole molecule water-soluble; detergents allow non-polar molecules, eg fats and lipids to be suspended in water and function as cleaning agents MOLECULAR BIOLOGY A surface-active emulsifying agent used to lyse cells and solubilize membranes

determinism A philosophical stance that assumes that all natural phenomena including human behavior are the results of preceding causes; if the preceding events are known, a person's subsequent actions can be predicted

deterministic effect Nonstochastic effect, see there

detoxication therapy ALTERNATIVE MEDICINE A generic term for any maneuver that is intended to rid the body of the myiad of environmental toxins and pollutants (eg food preservatives and additives); detoxification is a 'metabolic therapy' that includes such unproven maneuvers as enemas with coffee, soapsuds, herbs, and hydrogen peroxide, fasting, specific diets (eg water fast, alkaline detoxification), colon therapy, vitamin C (ascorbic acid), chelation therapy (with wheat grass or ethylene diamine tetraacetic acid-EDTA, hyperthermia (heat stress detoxification), and others (**Alternative Medicine, Future Medicine Pub, Puyallup, Wash, 1994**) see Alternative medicine INTERNAL MEDICINE A generic term for the removal of a toxic excess of any agent, including overdosage of a therapeutic agent, drug of abuse or toxic agent, eg pesticides and heavy metals from the body by induction of vomiting, administration of activated charcoal, hemodialysis, peritoneal dialysis or use of metabolic interference, eg treating methanol intoxication with ethanol overloading; the term often refers to medically supervised withdrawal from a substance of abuse and treatment of the symptoms of the withdrawal syndrome; see 'Cold turkey' method

Note: There is little (if any) data in peer-reviewed literature to support the claims that DT may be useful in treating acne, allergies, arthritis, back pain, food allergies, headaches, hemorrhoids, insomnia, joint pain, moodiness, psoriasis, recurrent respiratory problems, sinus congestion, ulcers, and other conditions

Detroit case BIOMEDICAL ETHICS A secretly planned but never implemented project to perform experimental amygdalotomies with destruction or removal of temporal-lobe brain tissue on mentally ill patients who had been imprisoned for various violent crimes (**N Engl J Med 1987; 316:114c**); see Tuskagee study, Willowbrook State School

Detroit fibrinogen Fibrinogen Detroit, see there

deuteranopia OPHTHALMOLOGY A form of red-green color blindness that is due to a lack of middle wavelength (MW, 530 nm) photopigment MOLECULAR PATHOLOGY The genes for both MW and LW (long wavelength, 560 nm) photopigments are composed of six coding regions (exons) and changes that result in color blindness are attributed to illegitimate pairing between highly homologous genes followed by crossing-over (**Science 1995; 267:984A, 1013R**)

development gap The time period between the development of products and processes with commercial potential in academia and the utilization thereof by industry in the form of licensing agreements, or spin-off companies (**Nature 1993; 364:659N**)

developmental biology The field of biology that attempts to understand the regulation of gene activity in time and space, and determine the mechanisms by which an organism's three-dimensional structure and diverse and complex functions derive from the fertilized egg; this requires knowledge of how the embryo's body plan is established and evolves, and how morphogenetic processes (eg cell-cell interactions and cell migrations) give rise to the mature organism (from **Nature 1994; 369:11N**)

developmental delay A generic term for a lag in reaching developmental milestones by the expected age; developmental delays may be due to 1) Biological factors, eg chromosomal defects or in utero infection or 2) Environmental factors, eg maternal mental malady or marital malaise, but are generally viewed in a 'transactional' context, ie an interplay between biological and environmental factors; DD can be identified by developmental screening tests and identification of developmental red flags (**N Engl J Med 1994; 330:478cc**)

developmental milestone PEDIATRICS Any of a series of activities, eg, raising the head, rolling over, walking or other significant points in a child's physical and/or mental development that may be used to assess maturation and detect developmental delay

developmental noise EVOLUTIONARY BIOLOGY Random events in development of an individual organism that results in uncontrolled phenotypic variation, eg color of eyes in Drosophila or the morphology of facial features

developmental 'red flag' PEDIATRICS Any of a number of objective findings that indicate a delay in achieving developmental milestones; DRFs in the assessment of infants, toddlers, and preschoolers fall into five major areas:

1) Gross motor skills, eg does not roll over (5 months), can't hop (4 years)

2) Fine motor skills, eg doesn't hold rattle (4-5 months), can't copy a circle (4 years)

3) Language skills, eg not babbling (5-6 months), doesn't understand prepositions (4 years)

4) Cognitive skills, eg does not search for dropped object (6-7 months), doesn't know colors or any letters (5 years)

5) Psychosocial development, eg does not smile socially (5 months), in constant motion, resists discipline, does not play with other children (3-5 years) (**N Engl J Med 1994; 330:478cc**)

developmental screening test Any of a number of tests or questionnaires for evaluating a child's achievement of developmental milestones; the Denver Developmental Screening Test II is the most popular of these tests because of its brevity and ease of administration, and has been widely translated (**N Engl J Med 1994; 330:478cc**)

devil's grip see Epidemic pleurodynia

devil's nips Petechial and ecchymotic patches seen on easily traumatized sites of the body, seen in purpura simplex, a heterogeneous disease of older women, possibly representing milder forms of vascular, platelet or platelet factor disorders, a reaction enhanced by aspirin

devitalization DENTISTRY The destruction of the pulp in the root of a tooth

dewdrop (on a rose petal) appearance CARDIOLOGY A descriptive term for the minute rounded nodules of amyloid seen by gross examination of the heart, and occasionally seen in cardiac amyloidosis PEDIATRICS A fanciful but accurate description of the appearance of fresh vesicles of chickenpox

dewlap jowls Wattles Bilateral median, hanging folds of loose tissue on the ventral aspect of the neck seen in cutis laxa, which may be accompanied by a bloodhound-like face

dexamethasone suppression test A clinical test that measures the ability of dexamethasone (a potent synthetic glucocorticoid) to suppress ACTH and cortisol secretion; the DST is performed in two stages: the low-dose DST (1.0 mg of dexamethasone per os is followed by plasma cortisol measurement, where > 5.0 μg/dl) confirms increased corticosteroid production; the high-dose DST locates the site of hyperproduction in the 'steroid axis' and is suggestive of Cushing's syndrome (false positives range from 5% in the ambulatory subjects to 25% in the chronically ill, anorectics, alcoholics, uremics and others); in the high-dose DST, having established the presence of a Cushing's syndrome, 8 mg of dexamethasone is given per os; suppression of cortisol to < 50% of baseline values is consistent with either an adrenal tumor that is not under pituitary control or an ectopic ACTH-producing tumor; the DST was reported to have moderate sensitivity (40-50%) and high specificity (90-95%) for the diagnosis of depression, a claim later proven incorrect; see Metapyrone test

dexfenfluramine PHARMACOLOGY A derivative of amphetamine that has been evaluated by the FDA as an appetite suppressant; despite its potential as an antiobesity drug, some data suggest that it might be neurotoxic, casuing a pruning of axons and axon terminals, resulting in depleted serotonin levels in the brain (**JAMA 1994; 272:1087MN&P**)

dextran A high MW, branched-chain polysaccharide polymer of D-glucose that is permeable to water and forms a viscid gelatinous material, that is synthesized commercially or naturally by glycosyl transferases on the surface of certain bacteria AIDS Dextran sulfate was reported to inhibit HIV-1 and HIV-2 binding to CD4+ cells; therapeutic trials proved disappointing DENTISTRY Dextrans formed from sucrose by *Streptococcus mutans* are intimately linked to dental plaque and caries, as they form a 'shell' trapping lactic acid adjacent to teeth MICROBIOLOGY Dextran is abundantly present in yeasts and bacteria, serving as a source of energy and a component of the bacterial capsule MOLECULAR BIOLOGY Dextrans form the solid phase, eg Sephadex, for molecular sieve chromatography, which separates molecules according to size, based on the number of cross-links formed in the dextran TRANSFUSION MEDICINE Various weights of dextrans are produced by *Leuconostoc mesenteroides* in preparing commercial colloid substances, dextran 40 (40 kD) and dextran 70 (70 kD); these substance have the desired properties of being sticky, viscid and gelatinous, exerting oncotic pressure to retain fluids within vessels and are widely used as replacement fluids and volume expanders; see Colloid solutions, Crystalloids

dextrin A partial lysate of intermediate lengths of polysaccharide (starch) by hydrochloric acid or amylase, which is composed of glucose, maltose and short dextrin polymers

dextrocardia A heart misplaced into the right chest, with the apex in the left; the cardiac function is normal if there is concomitant situs inversus of the abdominal organs (mirror-image dextrocardia); if the dextrocardia is due to immotile cilia, sinusitis and bronchiectasis (Kartagener syndrome) may also be present; the EKG demonstrates mirror-image electrical activity with P, QRS and T waves in leads I, aVR and aVL that are the reverse of normal and the right activity resembles that normally seen in the left side of the chest; if the abdominal organs are not reversed, dextrocardia may be associated with ventricular inversion, single-chamber ventricle, pulmonary valve stenosis and anomalies of the venous return

dextrose Obsolete for D-glucose

DF-2 Dysgonic fermenter-2 INFECTIOUS DISEASE A fastidious gram-negative bacillus native to the canine oral cavity that causes infections of dog-bite wounds, resulting in cellulitis, septicemia (potentially serious with Waterhouse-Friderichsen-type adrenal cortical collapse), endocarditis, gangrene, malar purpura (a finding that is quasi-pathognomonic of generalized Schwartzman reaction); the patients are weakened or have had splenectomies, some of whom (3/17 of the initial cohort) die with disseminated intravascular coagulation Note: DF-2 has been formally named *Capnocytophaga canimorsus* sp nov, see there

DF-2-like organism *Capnocytophaga cynodegmi* sp nov

dhat PSYCHIATRY A diagnostic term of uncertain validity described in the subcontinent of India, for a subjective sensation of anxiety, weakness, exhaustion, and hypochondriasis that may accompany the discharge of semen or whitish discoloration of urine (from DSM IV); see Culture-bound syndrome

DHFR Dihydrofolate reductase, see there

DHT Dihydrotestosterone, see there

'diabesity' A colloquial term for the relatively common clinical association of NIDDM (adult-onset diabetes mellitus) and obesity, a subgroup of which has been dignified by the term 'Syndrome X', see there

diabetes-dermatitis syndrome Dermatopathy accompanying α-cell tumors (glucagonomas) of pancreatic islet cells CLINICAL Necrotizing migratory erythema; glucagon inhibits intestinal motility, causing ileus, constipation or diarrhea and may have associated glossitis, angular cheilitis, venous thrombosis, black-outs

Note: The syndrome may rarely be caused by insulinoma

diabetes mellitus EPIDEMIOLOGY: Affects 5-10% of population in most countries; both the insulin-dependent (IDDM) and non-insulin-dependent (NIDDM) forms are heterogeneous PATHOGENESIS Mechanisms include autoimmune destruction of β cells in the pancreas in IDDM, mutations in the insulin gene, the insulin receptor gene, a adenosine deaminase gene-linked gene, and the glucokinase gene in NIDDM; a gene mutation (A→G, ie a guanine for adenine substitution, which encodes leucine transferase RNA*) has been identified in mitochondrial DNA which occurs in a subset of patients with both IDDM, and NIDDM (**N Engl J Med 1994; 330:962OA**) PROGNOSIS DM is not a risk factor for pancreatic cancer (**N Engl J Med 1994; 331:81OA**)

*This mutation is within the mitochondrial DNA-binding site for a protein that promotes the termination of transcription between the 16S RNA and tRNA$^{Leu(UUR)}$ genes, interfering with synthesis of tRNA$^{Leu(UUR)}$ and binding of the transcription termination factor

diabetes panel A battery of cost-efficient laboratory tests that are used to evaluate patients with a 'working diagnosis' of DM, determine the level of long-term glucose control and co-morbid conditions; the panel includes carbon dioxide, cholesterol, chloride, creatinine, fasting glucose, hemoglobin A_{1c}, potassium, sodium, triglycerides; see Organ panel

diabetic autonomic neuropathy A neuronal dysfunction seen in long-standing IDDM, thought to be the result of various insults including ischemia, impaired neuronal protein synthesis, abnormal axoplasmic transport, polyol or myo-inositol metabolism and microangiopathy

diabetic embryopathy A complex of major congenital anomalies affecting 8-12% of children born to diabetic mothers; these changes occur early (between the 5th and 8th week of gestation) in embryologic development, eg sacral agenesis, holoprosencephaly, atrioventricular septal defects, tetralogy of Fallot and other cardiac, genitourinary and gastrointestinal defects and can be reduced to the normal 'background' levels (1-2%) by prenatal counselling and aggressive maintenance of normoglycemic levels during gestation (**JAMA 1991; 265:731**) see Honeybee syndrome

diabetic foot A generic term for the constellation of pathological conditions that impact on the lower extremity and may lead to amputation of and/or death due to complications; in most cases, the initial lesion leading to amputation is a nonhealing skin ulcer induced by regional pressure, which is pathogenically linked to sensory neuropathy, ischemia, and infection (**N Engl J Med 1994; 331:854CC**)

diabetic ketoacidosis A hyperglycemia-induced clinical crisis that is most common in IDDM CLINICAL Vomiting, nausea, thirst, diaphoresis, hyperpnea, drowsiness, fever, prostration, coma, and possibly death LABORATORY ↑↑↑ Glucose, often > 33.6 mmol/L (US: > 600 mg/dl), ↑ ketone bodies, relative ↑ in protein, albumin, Ca^{++}, bilirubin, alkaline phosphatase, aspartate aminotransferase, creatine kinase, and anion gap, acidosis, dehydration, ↓ K^+, Na^+, and phosphate TREATMENT Insulin, fluid and electrolyte replacement, treatment of initiating factors, eg leukocytosis or hypothermia, avoidance of complications, eg hypokalemia, late hypoglycemia, rebound CNS acidosis and CNS deterioration

diabetic microangiopathy Microvascular disease A generic term for any clinical or pathological changes resulting from diabetic microangiopathy PATHOGENESIS Early in the evolution of DM, there is an ↑ in capillary blood flow and pressure, followed by impaired blood flow and loss of autoregulation in the microvascular beds of the skin and subcutaneous tissues, eye, and kidney MEASUREMENT Capillary hypertension can be measured directly by microcannulation of nailfold capillaries with a glass micropipette PROGNOSIS Progression of microvascular disease can be slowed by metabolic control (**N Engl J Med 1992; 327:760OA**), in particular with the use of long-term intensified insulin therapy (**N Engl J Med 1993; 329:304OA**)

diabetic nephropathy A generic term for any renal alteration attributed to DM, including Armanni-Ebstein lesion, arterionephrosclerosis, arteriolonephrosclerosis, chronic interstitial nephritis, diabetic glomerulosclerosis, fatty changes in renal tubules, glomerulonephritis, Kimmelstiel-Wilson disease (focal and segmental glomerulosclerosis), nephrotic syndrome, papillary necrosis, pyelonephritis and tubulointerstitial nephritis; DN is the most common cause of end-stage renal disease in the West, and accounts for ⅓ of all nw cases of ESRD; it occurs in 30% of those with IDDM and 4-20% of those with NIDDM; incidence of DN has ↓, possibly due to better control of the disease (N Engl J Med 1994; 330:15oa) DIAGNOSIS Microalbuminuria PREVENTION Intensive management, ACE inhibitors TREATMENT Antihypertensive therapy, eg ACE inhibitor therapy (eg captopril) protects the kidneys against further deterioration in IDDM, and results in a 50% ↓ risk in the end points of death, dialysis and transplantation (N Engl J Med 1993; 329:1456oa); if renal failure is in an early stage, the patients are good transplant candidates, while terminal renal failure requires dialysis; protein restriction (N Eng J Med 1995; 332:1210rv)

diabetic neuropathy NEUROLOGY A neuropathy that affects up to 50% of those with DM have either slowing of nerve conduction and/or symptoms of neuropathy, eg distal, bilateral, usually symmetrical often sensory polyneuropathy with hyperesthesiae of the hands and feet, focal and multifocal neuropathy, and trophic changes of the extremities, including loss of hair, thinness of skin, disorders of sweating and sensation of cold; clinical syndromes falling under the rubric of DN include diabetic ophthalmoplegia, thoracoabdominal radiculopathy, acute mononeuropathy, mononeuropathy multiplex–a painful, asymmetrical, multiple neuropathy TREATMENT No drug has proven effective; aldose reductase inhibitors are 'promising' and are in early clinical trials

diabetic retinopathy A condition characterized by the progressive changes of the retina with microaneuryms, hemorrhage, and neovascularization; DR is the most important cause of visual impairment in the US in those under age 60; at 20 years, 40% of those with IDDM and 20% of those with NIDDM have proliferative type DR (N Eng J Med 1995; 332:1210rv); the first lesions of DR are microaneurysms (< 100 µm in diameter with the escape of RBCs resulting in dot-and-blot hemorrhages; with ↑ severity, the abnormal vessels become occluded leading to retinal ischemia with infarction in the nerve layer, appearing as soft ('cotton wool') exudates corresponding to preproliferative retinopathy; in response to ischemia, there is neovascularization of the disk and elsewhere (N Engl J Med 1993; 328:1676rv); DR is divided into GRADE I Generalized arterial narrowing due to vasoconstriction and hyaline deposition in blood vessels GRADE II As above with arterial thickening and arteriovenous 'nicking' known as copper or silver wiring due to vascular thickening GRADE III As above with hemorrhage, exudation or cotton wool changes; diabetic retinopathy is related to poor diabetic control, as measured by glycosylated hemoglobin

1,2-diacylglycerol An intracellular 'second messenger' that is released from the cytoplasmic face of a cell membrane after a ligand, eg a hormone interacts with a cognate receptor on the cell's external surface and activates a G protein; DAG acts on protein kinase C, increasing the secretion or production of hormones, enzymes, neurotransmitters, vasoactive compounds and other molecules; see PIP2, Second messenger

diagnosis of exclusion A disease or clinical nosology that is extremely rare, and often unresponsive to therapy, the diagnosis of which should only be considered and seriously entertained when all other possible (potentially treatable) conditions have been completely ruled out, eg 'growing pains' or idiopathic midline granuloma

diagnosis-related groups see DRGs

diagnostic accuracy The closeness of the results of a diagnostic test to the actual clinical state, which is reflected in high sensitivity, high specificity, high positive and negative predictive values (Acta Cytologica 1993; 37:870oa)

diagnostic 'overkill' The use of excess or overlapping tests that merely confirm a diagnosis, eg the ordering of a magnetic imaging study of the brain when a previous computed tomography has already identified an intracranial mass (JAMA 1991; 265:2229) Cf Defensive medicine

DO may be more common in academic medicine, where tests can be ordered 'out of curiosity' and with relative disregard for cost-efficiency

dialysis The separation of molecules in solution based on differences in size; in clinical practice dialysis is used to separate macromolecules from low molecular weight molecules by use of a semipermeable membrane; see Hemodialysis, Peritoneal dialysis

dialysis ascites Exudative peritonitis related to chronic dialysis PATHOGENESIS Unknown, but related to infections, stress or protein catabolism in a background of fluid overload and poor nutrition TREATMENT Some success has been reported with a LeVeen shunt

dialysis dementia Dialysis encephalopathy Aluminum toxicity affecting those with terminal renal failure requiring long-term dialysis; aluminum is present in the dialysate solutions and in the oral $AL(OH)_3$ required to control terminal renal failure and accumulates in the brain and serum in these patients CLINICAL Speech disturbances, myoclonus, apraxia, seizures, mental deterioration, bone pain, osteolysis (fractures, pseudo- fractures), microcytic anemia, porphyria cutanea tarda and delta wave patterns by EEG similar to those of metabolic encephalopathy TREATMENT Chelation (desferroxamine); recognition of the association has led to decline of the disease

dialysis membrane The critical component of hemodialysis devices that allows the removal of metabolic waste products; DMs can be cellulose, composed of either cotton fibers (cuprophane) or synthetic composed of polymethyl methacrylate (PM); the PM membrane is associated with improved recovery from acute renal failure, as it is less prone to complement and leukocyte activation, and thus is more biocompatible (N Engl J Med 1994; 331:1338oa)

Diamond-Blackfan syndrome Congenital hypoplastic anemia An AR [MIM 205900], occasionally consanguinous condition associated with pure red cell aplasia of early infancy onset with anemia, pallor and failure to thrive, accompanied in 30% of cases by minor physical abnormalities, including short stature, thumb deformities and ocular changes PATHOGENESIS Possibly related to a stem-cell defect, given the ↓↓↓ of colony-forming units (CFU-E) and burst-forming units (BFU-E); corticosteroids may stimulate the proliferation of the structurally and functionally abnormal erythroblasts, resulting in 'immature' RBCs (fetal hemoglobin, presence of the 'i' surface antigen and a fetal enzyme 'profile') TREATMENT Transfusion, corticosteroids, BM transplantation, growth factor therapy

diamond skin A rhomboid urticarial skin reaction described in swine infected by *Erysipelothrix rhusiopathiae*, a zoopathic infection of those occupationally exposed by cuts and superficial abrasions (butchers, fishmongers); other human disease induced by *E rhusiopathiae* includes septicemia and endocarditis (with high mortality)

Diana complex PSYCHIATRY A reversal of roles by a woman, such that she affects the mien, appearance, and dress of a man; see Delilah syndrome, Wild woman phenotype

The name derives from Diana, the virgin Greek goddess of the hunt, sister of Apollo who was known as a huntress and for her vigor or 'male' qualities

Dianetics® A component of the Scientology® philosophy

defined as the manner in which the soul affects the body, and is the means of handling life's energy to enable a greater efficiency in the organism and in the spiritual life of an individual person; see Scientology®

diaper dermatitis A dermatopathy of early infancy due to prolonged contact with soiled diapers, soaps or topical lotions, resulting in secondary maceration of a skin that is scaly and erythematous with papulovesicular or bullous lesions, which may be extensive, often sparing the crural folds; secondary bacterial and yeast (especially *Candida* spp) infections may complicate recalcitrant cases; chronic diaper dermatitis may undergo papular induration

diaphragmatic flutter Rapid, rhythmic diaphragmatic contractions that have a cogwheel pattern of respiration, likened to hiccups, lasting for a period of seconds to weeks and if intense, interfere with gas exchange TREATMENT Empirical, as with hiccups

diaphragmatic hernia A relatively common (1:2000 live births) congenital malformation, due to a defective closure of the pleuroperitoneal membrane (through the foramen of Bochdalek), resulting in a common cavity, with the abdominal organs (usually left-sided) prolapsing into the chest cavity, compromising respiration; morphological permutations may be discovered later in life, eg parasternal hernias or membranous defects; less common sites of herniation include those occurring through the esophageal hiatus or through Morgagni's foramen TREATMENT With peri- and postoperative ventilatory support and bicarbonates, the formerly reported 90% mortality has been reduced to 40%

diarrhea A daily stool weight of > 200 g; acute diarrhea is < than, and chronic diarrhea is > than 4 weeks in duration (N Engl J Med 1995; 332:725RV)

diarrhea of undetermined origin A rare phenomenon, which is a diagnosis of exclusion; the majority of DUOs are due to laxative abuse, inflammatory bowel disease, irritable bowel syndrome, anal sphincter dysfunction, bacterial overgrowth; the cause of DUO may require inpatient evaluation (N Engl J Med 1995; 332:725RV)

diathermy SPORTS MEDICINE The use of high-frequency electromagnetic waves to induce an ↑ in temperature of deep tissues due to resistance to the passage of energy; diathermy is used either as an adjunct to physical therapy or in the context of surgery, where high-frequency currents are used to coagulate or cauterize tissues; diathermy's beneficial effects are similar to any other form of regional heat, and include vasodilation, ↑ filtration and diffusion, ↑ capillary permeability, ↑ blood flow, and ↑ rate of metabolism; the main clinical forms are microwave diathermy and shortwave diathermy (JC DeLee, D Drez, Jr, Eds, Orthopedic Sports Medicine WB Saunders, Philadelphia, 1994) see Microwave diathermy, Shortwave diathermy

*Or other physical agents (electric current or ultrasound) to induce a focal ↑ in temperature

diazo reaction A method described in 1883 by Ehrlich that continues to be widely used for measuring bilirubin, which consists in mixing bilirubin with diazotized sulfanilic acid (the diazo reagent) to produce reddish-purple azodipyrroles; the diazotization reaction of unconjugated bilirubin can be accelerated using alcohol (the van der Bergh reaction), which measures the so-called indirect bilirubin

diazo salt Diazonium salt A salt with a diazonium group that is prepared from an arylamine by diazotization

diazo stain A histochemical stain that uses stables salts of a diazonium salt of a dye, eg fast red B or fast red GG to detect enterochromaffin granules as seen in carcinoid tumors within formalin-fixed paraffin-embedded tissues

dibucaine number ANESTHESIOLOGY An assay used to determine a person's susceptibility to cholinesterase BACKGROUND Succinylcholine (SC) is a potent muscle relaxant, used in anesthesiology for tracheal intubation that has a rapid onset of action (30-45 seconds post-IV injection) with a short (5-10 minutes) duration of action, given its rapid metabolism by plasma cholinesterase; prolonged apnea following IV SC may occur in inherited (frequency 1:2500) or acquired deficiency of cholinesterase caused by liver dysfunction, pregnancy, neostigmine, IMAOs and organophosphate pesticides; given the importance of identifying these subjects, several assays were devised, of which the dibucaine test has proven the most useful; dibucaine inhibits PC, which in turn inhibits the normal cholinesterase by 80%, but atypical cholinesterase by only 20%; the percent of cholinesterase inhibition is calculated by a formula, yielding the Dibucaine number

DIC Disseminated intravascular coagulation, see there, also diisopropylaminoethylchloride

Also 1) Days in culture (tissue culture) 2) Dissolved inorganic carbon

Dice coefficient of similarity STATISTICS A method for comparing small populations with multiple parameters, eg quantitative pairwise comparison of RFLP patterns (see N Engl J Med 1994; 331:981SA)

$$D = {2n_{xy}}/{n_1 + n_2}$$

n_{xy} is the number of identical fragments, n_1 is the number of DNA fragments from strain X, n_2 is the number of DNA fragments from strain Y; D value ≥ 0.90 represents closely related strains; unrelated strains have values ≤ 0.60

dichloroacetate An agent that ameliorates lactic acidosis by increasing myocardial glucose oxidation and contractility and by inhibiting glycolysis, thereby reducing lactate production; dichloroacetate also stimulates oxidation of lactate to acetyl coenzyme A and CO_2 in peripheral tissues; dichloroacetate treatment of patients with severe lactic acidosis results in statistically significant (but clinically unimportant) changes in the pH and the arterial blood lactate and does not alter the hemodyanimcs or survival (N Engl J Med 1992; 327:1564OA)

dicing TRAUMATOLGY Multiple 0.5-1.0 cm, cube-like lacerations of the skin seen in motor vehicle accident victims who strike shattered tempered glass car windows

dicumerol A polycyclic aromatic compound derived from sweet clover that is an anticoagulant analog of vitamin K which uncouples oxidative phosphorylation; see Warfarin

didanosine 2',3'-dideoxyinosine A nucleoside analogue that inhibits HIV reverse transcriptase; didanosine was approved in 1991 for treating HIV-positive individuals who were either zidovudine-intolerant, or whose strain of HIV was zidovudine-resistant; didanosine may be more effective than zidovudine and may be an anti-retroviral nucleoside of first choice (N Engl J Med 1992; 327:581OA)

dideoxynucleoside A family of compounds including zidovudine, didanosine, and zalcitabine used to treat HIV-positive patients; see ddC, ddI

DIDMOAD syndrome Wolfram syndrome An AR condition characterized by the acronym's symptoms diabetes insipidus, diabetes mellitus, optic atrophy and neural deafness (DIDMOAD), which may be accompanied by ischemic muscle contractures, autonomic dysfunction, neurogenic bladder and hypertension

diener *dienen*, German, to serve PATHOLOGY An attendent who maintains and cleans the hospital morgue and who may assist in performing autopsies

diet To eat and drink either sparingly or according to a prescribed regimen; diets are either for supplementation, ie weight gain or restriction, ie weight loss; in restrictive diets, the intent is to limit one or more dietary components, eg gluten or oxalate, or to globally reduce caloric intake; high-fat diet has been associated with an increased incidence of cancers of the breast, colon, ovary, prostate, and more recently, with actinic keratosis* (N Engl J Med 1994; 330:1272oA); the mechanism is unclear; excess calories are thought to be restricted to tumor initiation, and excess fat to tumor promotion and growth; low-fat, high-fiber causes an increase in the fibrinolytic activity of plasma, and a biphasic decrease in factor VIIc (Arteriosclerosis and Thrombosis 1993; 13:505)

Diet types **BLAND DIET** A mechanically soft diet that is commonly prescribed in peptic ulcer disease as it has no spices or gastric irritants, despite its dubious efficacy; see Histamine (H2) receptor, Spicy foods **BRAT DIET** see there **'CRASH' DIET** A semi-starvation type of fad diet which has a wide variety of formulations; in general crash diets may be followed for a short period of time by a person wishing to rapidly lose weight; such radical approaches rarely result in the desired permanent loss of weight **ELIMINATION DIET** A regimen used in individuals, especially children with atopy, suspected of being allergic to certain foods, where one food or major food group is eliminated at a time to determine whether there is reduction of the symptoms attributed to allergy; Cf Desensitization diet **FAD DIET** Any of a number of diets that either eliminate one or more of the essential food groups or recommend consumption of one type of food in enormous excess, often reducing the consumption of other foods; fad diets rarely follow modern dietetic principles of weight loss, which hinge on the combination of 1) Eating less or 2) Consuming more energy through exercise, and are thus rarely endorsed by the medical profession **LIQUID DIET** A variant of the very low calorie diet that fulfils the daily fluid requirements and places little functional demand on the gastrointestinal tract; liquid diets have little fiber and do not provide adequate protein or calories, circa 1000 kcal/day **MACROBIOTIC DIET** see Macrobiotics **NOVELTY DIET** Fad diet, see there **ORNISH REGIMEN** Beans, bean curd, grains, maximum of two ounces of alcohol, fruits, vegetables, weekly sessions of 'meditation' and stress management PROHIBITED Meat, poultry, fish, egg yolks, caffeine and all dairy products (except one cup of fat-free); no fat or oil added to foods) RESULT Weight loss; 39% decrease in total cholesterol, 59% drop in LDL-cholesterol **PRITIKIN DIET** see Pritikin diet **RESTRICTION DIET** A diet intended to reduce the incidence of various conditions, eg 1) Atherosclerosis Reduction of body weight, decreased consumption of saturated fat, cholesterol and increased consumption of bran 2) Hypertension Salt restriction Note: Only one-half of patients have a pressor response to salt restriction 3) Cancer Fat is epidemiologically linked to cancer of the breast, colon, prostate and possibly also ovaries; polyunsaturated fats are a substrate for peroxidative reactions and thus should be reduced; increased fiber and cruciferous vegetables in the diet are linked to decreased colonic carcinoma, an effect thought to be due to decreased contact of the colonic mucosa with carcinogens; alcohol consumption is associated with hepatoma, oropharyngeal and esophageal cancer with very low cholesterol, 4) Renal failure A low protein regimen that slows the progression of renal failure **STARVATION DIET** see Very low calorie diet **VERY LOW CALORIE DIET** A potentially dangerous diet that provides 300-700 kcal/day, which must be supplemented with high quality protein given the risk of death through intractable cardiac arrhythmias and which should be limited to 3-6 months; side effects of this form of crash diet include orthostatic hypotension, due to loss of sodium and decreased norepinephrine secretion, fatigue, hypothermia and cold intolerance, xeroderma, hair loss, dysmenorrhea; see Elemental diet, TPN

*As well as basal cell and squamous cell carcinomas, but with less statistical significance

---

DIETARY GUIDELINES-AMERICAN HEART ASSOCIATION

1　Fat comprises < 30% of total calories

2　Saturated fat comprises < 10% of total calories

3　Polyunsaturated fat consumption < 300 mg/day

4　Carbohydrates (especially complex type) should constitute ½ of calories in diet

5　Protein constitutes the remainder, ie 100% - (#1% + #3%) = #5

6　Sodium should be < 3 g/day

7　Alcohol consumption should be ≤ 60 g (2 oz)/day[1]

8　Calories should be sufficient to maintain the body weight[2]

9　A wide variety of food should be consumed[3]

[1]This recommendation is likely to be changed in the near future-author's note, see the French paradox [2]see Caloric restriction [3]see Food pyramid

---

'diet pills' Therapeutic agents that either suppress appetite or increase the basal metabolic rate, including amphetamines, available only by prescription and over-the counter dietary aids, including phenylpropanolamine, ephedrine and caffeine, which in high doses may cause marked agitation, hypertension, seizures and potentially death due to cerebral hemorrhage; see Artificial sweeteners, Diet

dietary fiber Indigestible plant-derived residues composed predominantly of cellulose, hemicellulose, and cell wall polymers; DF eg bran, provides stool 'bulk', ↑ the transit time for nutrients in (surgically) shortened GI tracts and ↓ the transit time in long or constipated GI tracts; ↑ dietary intake of fiber is associated with ↓ colonic malignancy and with tumor regression in the premalignant familial adenomatous polyposis and diverticulosis; fiber improves the plasma lipid ratios, evoking a 10-17% ↓ in cholesterol (including reduced HDL-cholesterol) as well as a reduced dietary intake of energy, fat and cholesterol-rich foodsthe DF common to all plants, lignin, is found in most plants, and pectin is present in fruits; ↓ DF intake has been linked to colorectal cancer, diverticulitis, ↑ cholesterol, gallbladder disease, constipation, and appendicitis; see Bran, Water-soluble fiber

dietary guidelines CARDIOLOGY A series of dietary recommendations from the Nutrition Committee of the American Heart Association that promote cardiovascular health

'diff' White blood cell differential (count) HEMATOLOGY A colloquial term for the differential count of circulating leukocytes, which is usually generated by 'Coulter counter'-type multichannel instrument; the results are provided qualitatively, where 42-75% of circulating white cells are granulocytes, 20-50% are lymphocytes and 2-10% are monocytes, as well as quantitatively, where the absolute count of granulocytes is 1.4-6.5 x 10⁹/L, that of lymphocytes is 1.2-3.4 x 10⁹/L; monocytes 0.1-0.6 x 10⁹/L

differential *noun* A datum or consideration in a differential diagnosis for a particular process or condition, eg acute cholecystitis is in the differential for acute abdomen

differential brushing CYTOLOGY A technique for localizing radiographically occult lung cancer by obtaining the specimens individually from each branch of the tracheobronchial tree (Acta Cytologica 1993; 37:879oA)

differential diagnosis 1) A list of conditions that may cause a particular clinical sign or symptom (PL Fine, The Wards, Little, Brown and Co, Boston, 1994) 2) The arrival at a diagnosis by means of comparing the similarities and differences in various clinical signs

differential growth medium MICROBIOLOGY A bacterial growth medium that has a variety of integrated organic compounds and salts that favor the growth of certain organisms

differential pivot CLINICAL DECISION MAKING A key step in arriving at a patient's diagnosis, which consists in finding a 'pivot' or the key finding that is at the center of the patient's disease; once a pivot is found, a list of viable or reasonable differential diagnoses is created from which most likely causes are considered and either validated or discarded; Cf Artificial intelligence, Expert systems

differential splicing see Alternative splicing

differentiation antigens see Oncofetal antigens

differentiation therapy ONCOLOGY A therapeutic strategy used to treat malignancies in which there is block in the normal cell differentiation by driving the malignant cells into a mature nonproliferating state of remission (see N Engl J Med 1992; 327:385oA); in acute promyelocytic leukemia, tretinoin reverses the 15;17(q22;q12-21) translocation; the breakpoint on chromosome 17 occurs in the region that encodes the retinoic acid receptor-α, a receptor involved in the growth and differentiation of myeloid cells

'difficult' patient LEGAL MEDICINE A patient who is troublesome, paranoid, or refuses to follow instructions; termination of a relationship with such patients requires that they be given reasonable advance notice, often an open-ended length of time, a list of competent board-certified physicians who treat the same condition; all communications with difficult patients must be documented in a legally acceptable form; see ama; Cf 'Good' patient

Diff-Quik® DIAGNOSTIC PATHOLOGY A proprietary stain that uses three dyes-triarylmethane, xanthene, and thiazine, yielding results on cytological and pathological specimens that are similar to that of Wright-Giemsa stain; the Diff-Quik stain can be performed in ± 15 seconds, making it a method of choice for procedures requiring a rapid turn-around time, eg evaluation of cytological preparations of tissue aspirates during a surgical procedure (**Acta Cytologica 1994; 38:37OA**)

diffuse axonal injury A type of brain damage caused by head trauma that is a major cause of neurologic disability in survivors PATHOLOGY Retraction balls, or axonal swellings; quantification of DAI is facilitated by staining for the presence of ubiquitin (**Arch Pathol Lab Med 1994; 118:168OA**) see Retraction balls

diffuse laminar endocervical glandular hyperplasia DLEGH An incidental pseudoneoplastic lesion of the uterine cervix that occurs during child-bearing years (mean age = 37), is often associated with hormonal therapy, and characterized histologically by a diffuse proliferation of moderately-sized, evenly spaced endocervical glands; the importance of DLEGH is its potential for confusion with adenoma malignum (minimum deviation carcinoma) of the uterine cervix, from which it differs by its lack of cytologic atypia, stromal invasion and desmoplastic stomal response (**Am J Surg Pathol 1991; 267:1123**)

diffuse panbronchiolitis A condition largely studied in Japan, characterized by chronic relapsing bronchiolitis with bacterial infection, slowly progressing peripheral airways destruction by granulation tissue and ending in respiratory failure (**Arch Pathol Lab Med 1994; 118:975OA**)

diffusion ANTHROPOLOGY A general theory of the spread of ancient culture that holds that social, economic and political change occurred by learning, ie by slow diffusion of cultural parameters; see Demic diffusion; Cf Migration

diffusion chamber CLINICAL THERAPEUTICS A biohybrid device in which cells of interest (pancreatic islet cells) are placed in tubular chamber and implanted via trocar or incision in the peritoneum or subcutis; the DC is like the perfusion chamber before it, and the currently preferred microsphere, a type of encapsulated cell therapy, which in some cases. achieves adequate glucose control (**Science & Medicine July/August 1995, p16**) see Biohybrid organ

digest *noun* A mixture of molecules obtained by chemical or enzymatic hydrolysis of larger molecules, eg DNA digest obtained from restriction endonuclease hydrolysis of a DNA macromolecule

digital computer A computer that performs mathematical and logical operations on discrete blocks of data in the form of bits; Cf Analog computer

digital imaging spectroscopy A technique combining optical spectroscopy and digital image processing so that a spectrum can be obtained from each pixel or cluster of pixels located in two dimensions; commercial digital imaging spectrophotometers have been developed that incorporate charge coupled device detectors (CCD) and diffuse light sources in transmission and reflectance modes; DIS can be used to study microbial colonies directly on Petri dishes, dispensing with the weeks-long labor-intensive tasks of picking colonies of interest, resuspending the colonies in a medium, cellular disruption, centrifugation and finally analyzing the samples one at a time by conventional spectrophotometry; potential applications include clinical microbiology where microbes could be plated on a complex indicator medium (**Nature 1994; 369:79L**)

digital mammography The production of mammographic images without film, which results in greater resolution and clarity than that obtained by conventional fil-screen mammography; faster earlier and more accurate detection of early breast abnormalities (**NY Newsday 9 Jan 1995; C1**)

digital rectal examination The insertion of a gloved index finger into the rectum by a physician or other examiner, in order to palpate the prostate (and detect ↑ firmness), and the mucosa of the rectosigmoid colon; given its efficacy as a screening tool for identifying both lower rectosigmoid lesions and prostatic lesions (benign hypertrophy or, less commonly, adenocarcinoma) contrary to previously held beliefs, it is not necessary to have subjects return for a separate drawing of PSA specimens, as DRE does not significantly ↑ serum PSA levels during the immediate (ie 5-20 minutes) post-examination period (**JAMA 1992; 267:2227**)

A regionally popular clinical aphorism is '*...the only reasons not to perform a DRE is that patient has no rectum or the examiner has no fingers.*'

digital subtraction angiography RADIOLOGY A computerized enhancement of images obtained with conventional angiography, used primarily to study the carotid, aortic arch and vertebral circulation, as well as that of the lower extremity; DSA uses less contrast, reduces radiation exposure, enhancing the contrast image at a sacrifice of the spatial resolution

dihydrofolate reductase An oxidoreductase enzyme [EC 1.5.1.3] essential for DNA synthesis that catalyzes reactions involving one-carbon transfers from a donor molecule X to an acceptor molecule Y; the effect of methotrexate, the prototypic folic acid antagonist used to treat malignancies, is linked to paralysis of DHFR; deficiency of DHFR results in megaloblastic anemia

dihydrotestosterone A potent C19 androgen produced from testosterone by 5α-reductase, which is the predominant androgen in skin, prostate, seminal vesicles, and epididymis (testosterone is the main androgen in the brain, pituitary, kidney, muscle, bone, and testes); DHT is reported to be a surrogate marker for sexual activity, and ↑ DHT may be linked to an ↑ in prostate cancer (**C Mantzoros in May 20 Brit Med J in Science 1995; 268:1381**)

'dilapidated brick wall' appearance DERMATOPATHOLOGY A fanciful descriptor for marked acantholysis, with scattered preserved intracellular bridges, seen in the overlying epithelium in benign familial chronic pemphigus or Hailey-Hailey disease, that may occasionally be seen in other acantholytic processes including pemphigus vulgaris

dilated cardiomyopathy The most common cardiomyopathy (in the US); it is usually idiopathic and is characterized by ↑ ventricular size ETIOLOGY Infectious (eg coxsackievirus, CMV, HIV, diphtheria, trichinosis), inflammatory (eg collagen vascular disease, sarcoidosis), metabolic (eg hypothyroidism, thyrotoxicosis, DM, Cushing's disease, thiamine or selenium deficiency), or toxic (eg cocaine, antiretroviral agents, lead, cobalt, ethanol, phenothiazines) insults PROGNOSIS Often progressive with heart failure, accompanied by mitral and tricuspid valve insufficiency COMPLICATIONS Atrial and ventricular tachyarrhythmias and fibrillation, and conduction abnormalities (**N Engl J Med 1993; 329:1639CPC**) TREATMENT Supportive therapy (rest weight control, cessation of smoking, ↓ physical activity during periods of exacerbation); active therapies that are effective in most patients are ACE inhibitors, anticoagulation, digoxin, diuretics, implantable defibillators nitrates, potassium and magnesium repletion INVESTIGATIONAL MODALITIES Amiodarone, amlodipine, betablockers, dual-chamber pacing, felodipine, pimobendan, vesnarinone (**ibid 1994; 331:1564**)

diltiazem HCl A calcium channel-blocker indicated for the control of atrial flutter or fibrillation, paroxysmal supraventricular tachycardia, and hypertension; diltiazem may prevent the usual reduction in coronary artery diameter after heart transplantation (N Engl J Med 1993; 328:164OA; IBID,) WARNING: Diltiazem may prolong AV nodal conduction and refractoriness, possibly causing second- or third-degree AV block in sinus rhythm, congestive heart failure, hypotension, acute hepatic injury, and premature ventricular beats ADVERSE EFFECTS Atrial flutter, tachyarrhythmias, pruritus, sweating, constipation, nausea, vomiting

diluent CLINICAL PHARMACOLOGY An inert substance added to a drug formulation, increasing its bulk in order to make the tablet a practical size for use; diluents include dicalcium phosphate, calcium sulfate, lactose, cellulose, kaolin, dry starch and powdered sugar; see Inactive ingredient

dilution end point IMMUNOLOGY A value, measured in titers, that corresponds to the minimum amount (titer) of an antibody in a system of interest, determined by serial dilution of a serum or other fluid with the antibody, while holding the antigen constant

dilutional anemia A 'pseudoanemia' due to a relative $\uparrow$ of plasma, usually occurring in a health care setting, which results in a relative (but not absolute) $\downarrow$ in hemoglobin concentration, RBC count, or hematocrit

D-dimer HEMATOLOGY A fibrin split product that can be used in a sensitive assay of plasmin activity, which is often but not invariably elevated in systemic consumptive coagulopathy, ie DIC

dimethyl sulfate protection MOLECULAR BIOLOGY A method used to identify protein-binding regions of DNA regions, which do not allow methylation of adenine and guanine nucleotides in the presence of a bound protein; subsequent digestion of a treated DNA molecule by a restriction endonuclease will not be allowed in sites that have been 'protected' by dimethyl sulfate; see Footprinting

dimorphism MYCOLOGY A property of fungi capable of producing two different forms depending on whether the organism is being cultured (25°C) or is at body temperature (37°C)

1)) Yeasts at 37°C, mycelia at 25°C *Blastomyces dermatiditis, Histoplasma capsulatum, Paracoccidioides brasiliensis, Sporotrichum schenckii*

2) Spherules at 37°C, mycelia at 25°C *Coccidioides immitis*

3) Yeasts and hyphae at both 37°C and 25°C, *Candida* species

dimorphic anemia A dual population of RBCs in the peripheral blood smear, in which there are both microcytic hypochromic and normocytic macrocytic red cells, a finding in combined iron deficiency and B_{12}/folic acid deficiency, as well as idiopathic acquired sideroblastic anemia with B_{12}/folic acid deficiency

dimple sign Pinching of a subcutaneous lesion results in a central dell or dimple, seen in well-circumscribed, often benign superficial dermal tumors, including dermatofibromas, inclusion cysts, lipomas and neurofibromas; Cf 'Tent' sign

'Dingellization' ACCOUNTABILITY FEVER A colloquial term for zealous investigation of purported cases of scientific misconduct and/or fraud, coined in reference to a US legislator who has chaired 'fraud in science' committees that have investigated alleged research-related improprieties of several key scientists who had received federal grant monies (N Engl J Med 1993; 329:725SB) see Baltimore affair, Gallo probe, 'Whistle blowing'

dinitrophenol TOXICOLOGY Any of a family of substituted compounds used in weed control (and, at one time as a slimming agent) may cause fatal poisoning, as it uncouples oxidative phosphorylation in mitochondria, which results in body temperature, rapid breathing, tachycardia, nausea, flushed skin, fever, cyanosis, collapse, and coma; the clinical course of poisoning is rapid, with death or recovery occurring in 24 hours TREATMENT Ice baths, O_2, correction of fluid and electrolyte imbalances

dinner fork appearance ORTHOPEDICS A descriptor for the clinical deformity seen in fractures of the distal radius with dorsal angulation (Colles fracture), a fracture common in osteoporotic post-menopausal women who fall on outstretched hands, where the distal fractured ends of the radius and ulna (and hand) are deviated in a palmar direction

Dioctophyma renale Giant kidney worm A 35 cm ($\male$) to > 100 cm ($\female$) nematode most common in mammals, in particular in minks and dogs, which concentrate in and eventually destroy of the kidneys; human acquisition of *D renale* may result from eating raw fish, frogs, or from drinking water containing infected annelids from reservoir hosts (mink, dog, jackal, coyote, wolf)

Diogenes' cup NEUROLOGY A fanciful term for the palm of the hand in certain myopathies, which is deepened by muscular contraction

Diogenes syndrome Senile neglect GERIATRICS A dementia-related lassitude in which a subject allows his home and personal environment to deteriorate, and may begin to collect objects of little value, eg milk cartons, string

Diogenes (412-323 BC) was a Greek philosopher who taught that a virtuous life was a simple one, proving his point by living in a bathtub; he condemned the excesses of his contemporaries and wandered about Athens with a candle, looking for an honest man

dioxin

dioxins ENVIRONMENT A family of highly toxic chlorinated hydrocarbons in which two benzene rings are linked by two oxygen atoms, which includes dibenzodioxins and dibenzofurans (Nature 1995; 375:353); the prototypic dioxin is 2,3,7,8-tetrachlorodibenzo-*p*-dioxin (TCDD), a chemical byproduct of the herbicide, 2,4,5-trichloro-phenoxy-acetic acid, Agent Orange; other dioxins include polychlorinated dibenzo-p-dioxins (PCDD) and polychlorinated dibenzofuran (PCDF); dioxin came to public attention in the late 1970s in Times Beach, Missouri, where dioxin-contaminated waste oil had been sprayed on the ground since 1971 to control dust, and associated with the deaths of horses and a general deterioration of the local human population's health; the clean-up of Times Beach has cost mega-millions and its residents were forced permanently to evacuate; dioxin and Agent Orange have been implicated in soft tissue sarcomas and lymphomas; the liver (acute toxicity and hepatoma) and immune system (thymic atrophy and defective cell-mediated immunity) are the most severely involved in animal studies; in humans, intense chronic exposure causes weight loss, myalgias, insomnia, dyspnea, cold intolerance, irritability, peripheral neuropathy, hepatomegaly, hemorrhagic cystitis, chloracne, actinic elastosis, loss of libido and impotence LABORATORY $\uparrow$ Prothrombin time and lipid levels; dioxin was released in an industrial accident in Seveso, Italy, 1976 at a factory producing 2,4,5-trichlorophenol; the total TCDD released was less than 1.3 kg; there were no fatalities; some suffered chloracne; the levels of TCDD may rise to 4 **x** baseline levels (8 pg/g of plasma lipid) in those who eat contaminated fish, eg in the Baltics (N Engl J Med 1991; 324:8); dioxin exposure of > than one year with a latency of greater than 20 years is associated with a 46% increase of all cancers and 42% increase in cancers of the respiratory tract (N Engl J Med 1991; 324:212); dioxin's toxic and carcinogenic effects may be due to membrane receptor binding (**Science 1991; 251:524n&v**); see Agent Orange; Cf Bitterfeld

dip see Deceleration

DIP Desquamative interstitial pneumonia, see there

dip/peak pattern see Harvest Moon festival

diplomate A physician who is board-certified (see there) in a particular specialty, and thus holds a diploma from a specialty board

dipping SUBJECT Blood and Radostits

dipstick Reagent strip LABORATORY MEDICINE A blotting paper impregnated with enzymes or chemicals sensitive to various parameters of clinical interest, which when dipped in urine, undergoes a color change allowing a substance to be semiquantitatively measured, including bilirubin, glucose and reducing substances, hemoglobin, nitrates, ketones, pH, protein, hemoglobin, specific gravity and urobilinogen; reagent strip methodology was born in part out of the relatively low diagnostic yield of routine urinalysis

Note: Some interfering substances may alter the strip's reactivity for a particular analyte (strip manufacturers provide lists of substances most likely to cause interference); if the clinical suspicion is strong for the presence of a disease, a proper quantitative analysis of the specimen should be performed; in urinary dipsticks for protein, clinically significant proteinuria may occur in a high percentage of those with negative to trace dipstick results; 12% of those with 1+ to 2+ dipstick results had normal 24-hour urine as did 4% of those with 3+ to 4+ results; ≥ 1+ has a positive predictive value of 92% for identifying proteinuria ≥ 300 mg/24 hours; ≥ 3+ has a positive predictive value of 36% for identifying proteinuria ≥ 5 g/24 hours (**Am J Obstet Gynecol 1994; 170:137**); dipsticks for hematuria have a 86% sensitivity and 85% specificity (**Br J Urol 1993; 72:594**)

diphtheria toxin A 62-kD protein that is responsible for *Corynebacterium diphtheriae*'s cardio– and neurotoxic effects, as well as for mucosal damage; DT is activated by proteolysis into a 39-kD binding fragment B which is required for entry of A into the cell, and an enzymatically active 21-kD fragment A, which blocks protein synthesis by transferring ADP-ribose from NAD to elongation factor-2, leading to EF-2's inactivation

dipole moment see Magnetic resonance imaging

dipyridamole-thallium scintigraphy A diagnostic procedure that permits the assessment of myocardial perfusion in patients who are unable to undergo exercise testing; see Dipyridamole-thallium SPECT

dipyridamole-thallium SPECT A diagnostic procedure (dipyridamole-thallium single photon-emission computed tomography) that is a refinement of dipyridamole-thallium scintigraphy; DT SPECT allows assessment of myocardial perfusion without requiring exercise testing; the data supporting the use of this diagnostic modality is tenuous and suggest that its use for predicting adverse cardiac outcome prior to abdominal aortic surgery may not be justified (**N Engl J Med 1994; 330:663OA**); cardiac risks were more accurately determined based on previous clinical evidence of coronary artery disease and advanced age

direct access The immediate access to health care services provided by both nonphysicians (eg nurse practitioners, physician assistants) and physicians, ranging from a routine phlebotomy to midwifery and endoscopy (**Clin Lab Sci 1994; 7:72F**); direct access is a key component for reducing the healthcare costs in the Clinton Plan (see there), which contains the phrase

'No state may, through licensure or otherwise, restrict the practice of any class of health professionals beyond what is justified by the skills and training of such professionals.'

direct billing HEALTH CARE FINANCES The submission of bills for services rendered (eg laboratory work) directly to the party (ie patient, or responsible third party) for whom the service was performed rather than to the physician who ordered the test; physician billing promotes the practice of marking up (ie increasing) the bill for services the physician submits to the patient, resulting in increased costs of health care (**Clin Lab Sci 1994; 7:72F**)

direct consumer advertising see Direct-to-consumer advertising

direct costs HEALTH CARE ADMINISTRATION Those costs that are incurred as a direct result of patient management, including salaries, reagents and supplies, equipment costs, heating, lighting and water; Cf Indirect costs, Sunk costs

direct diagnosis MOLECULAR BIOLOGY The diagnosis of a disease based on well-established and relatively constant mutations that are directly detectable in the DNA molecule, eg sickle cell anemia and α_1-antitrypsin, both of which have point mutations that are identical in all patients; direct diagnosis can be used when there are large gene deletions, insertions or nonsense mutations

direct fluorescent antibody method IMMUNOLOGY A technique in which a molecule of interest is detected directly by an antibody labelled or tagged with a fluorochrome, eg FITC (fluorescein-isothiocyanate); the direct test is most often used for detecting the presence of immune depositions in a histologic section, eg IgG or C3 complement deposits in an epithelial basement membrane or in glomeruli; Cf Indirect immunofluorescence

direct-to-consumer advertising The use of mass media, eg television, magazines, newspapaers, to publicly promote drugs that by law require a physician's prescription; the intent of such advertising is have patients and/or the lay public request their physician to prescribe drug 'X'; see Advertising

directed donation TRANSFUSION MEDICINE The donation of blood products intended for use by one specified recipient; pre-AIDS directed donations were carried out in the context of 1) Donor-specific transfusions prior to renal transplantation 2) Platelet pheresis transfusions and 3) Transfusions of rare blood types; directed donation has increased in the recent past due to public concern about the safety of the blood supply and the general feeling that a friend or family member is less likely be infected by the HIV virus than an anonymous donor (although the available data does not support this conclusion) placing the selection of the allogeneic donor in the hands of the transfusion recipient has certain disadvantages, eg use of a husband or his close relatives increases the risk of delayed hemolytic reaction and may cause maternal sensitization to a paternal antigen that could lead to hemolytic disease of the newborn (**Arch Pathol Lab Med 1994; 118:380OA**) Cf Autologous donation, Intraoperative autologous donation

DIRECTIONAL CORONARY ATHERECTOMY VS BCA		
	DCA	BCA**
↓ Stenosis < 50%‡	89%	80%
Immediate ↑ vessel diameter‡/†	1.05/1.45 cm	0.86/1.16 cm
Early complications‡/†	11%/5%	5%/6%
In-hospital costs‡	$11 904	$10 637
Restenosis at 6 months‡/†	50%/46%	57%/43%
Death or myocardial infarction‡	8.6%	4.6%
Success rate†	94%	88%

*Directional coronary arthrectomy **Balloon coronary angiography
†N Engl J Med 1993; 329:221OA ‡N Engl J Med 1993; 329:228OA

directional coronary atherectomy A technique of coronary revascularization in which an atherosclerotic plaque is excised and retrieved from a target lesion; DAC was approved in 1990 by the FDA for coronary revascularization; by 1992, 33 000 procedures had been performed

PROS: DAC results in a larger luminal diameter and a slight reduction in angiographically evident restenosis (especially of the proximal left anterior descending coronary artery); when compared to balloon coronary angioplasty (BCA)

CONS: DAC had a higher rate of early complications, increased cost and no apparent benefit after 6 months of follow-up (**N Engl J Med 1993; 329:221OA**) see Coronary revascularization

directly observed therapy A clinical maneuver that specifically addresses the lack of patient compliance to medical regimens; in patients with *Mycobacterium tuberculosis* infection, DOT (versus unsupervised therapy) reduces primary drug resistance from 13% to 6.7%, acquired drug resistance from 14% to 2% and relapse rate from 21% to 5.5% (N Engl J Med 1994; 330:1179oA, 1993; 328:576sB)

director of laboratories A physician who is a licensed doctor of medicine or osteopathy (MD or DO), and who is acceptable to an accrediting agency, eg the JCAHO (Joint Commission of Accredited Hospitals Organization); a person with a PhD may act as director of one section of the clinical laboratories but may not render opinions regarding patient management

'dirty background' A finding in Papanicolaou-stained smears of uterine cervix which consists of cell debris and necrosis often associated with inflammation, due to *Gardnerella* or *Trichomonas* species, pregnancy, post-partum, post-menopause, in oral contraceptive users and cervical carcinoma; a 'dirty background', then has no specific clinical significance

'dirty' bomb A weapon of mass destruction in which highly radioactive (but subnuclear weapons-grade) material is added to a conventional bomb that would contaminate a wide area with radioactivity (US News & World Report 17 April, p39)

'dirty' chest of Simon RADIOLOGY Patchy radiopacities on a plain chest film due to mucus gland hyperplasia, seen in bronchiectasis, which is often associated with bronchitis

DIS 1) Digital imaging spectrophotometer 2) Digital Imaging Spectroscopy, see there

disability Handicap A limitation in a person's mental or physical ability to function in terms of work, learning or other socially required activities, to the extent that the person might be regarded as having a need for certain benefits, compensation, exemptions, special training because of said limitations; disabilities include impairment of hearing, mobility, speech, and vision; infection with TB, AIDS, or other contagion, malignancy, past history of alcohol or drug abuse, or mental illness; see Americans with Disabilities Act

disappearing bone disease A progressive disease of unknown pathogenesis that most often affects subjects $\geq$ age 30 following trauma, characterized by extensive bone resorption variably associated with hemangiomas or lymphangiomas, pain, progressive weakness and elevated alkaline phosphatase

disaster PUBLIC HEALTH Any usually unanticipated event that requires urgent response, bringing people and/or property out of harms way in order to minimize loss of life or destruction of property; disasters are described by certain parameters

NATURE, ie either a) Natural, eg geophysical (earthquakes, volcanoes) and weather-related (floods, hurricanes) or b) Man-made origin (transportation-related, structural collapse, war, hazardous materials, explosions, fires)

LOCATION single site, eg explosion or multiple sites, eg hurricanes

PREDICTABILITY, eg hurricane 'season' vs toxic spill

ONSET, ie gradual vs acute

DURATION, ie brief vs extended

FREQUENCY, eg hurricanes vs mass intoxication (N Engl J Med 1991; 324:815rv)

see Natural disaster RADIATION PHYSICS Decay disaster, see there

disaster committee A hospital committee that is responsible for developing, coordinating, and implementing emergency disaster plans that would enable the hospital to meet the community's emergency medical needs within the confines of the hospital's resources

Only when the hospital is faced with a true emergency does it become clear whether it was a disaster or disastrous committee–Author's note

disaster 'syndrome' PSYCHOLOGY A response in survivors of major natural or man-made disasters that has been subdivided into four chronologic stages: MINUTES TO HOURS Stunned apathy, disorientation DAYS Inefficiency while attempting to help other victims in worse condition than self, onset of guilt at having survived WEEKS Euphoria and enthusiasm at rebuilding and renewing activities, sense of communality with co-victims MONTHS Resolution; Cf Concentration camp syndrome

DISC Diffuse inflammatory salmon-patch choroidopathy Birdshot retinopathy An idiopathic condition characterized by a 'quiet eye' in children and adolescents due to posterior segment inflammation, symmetrical retinal vascular leakage, macular edema and multiple depigmented spotting with narrowing of retinal arterioles

discharge CLINICAL MEDICINE *noun* Any secretion or material eliminated from a wound or orifice *verb* 1) To release a secretion or material from a wound or orifice 2) To release of a patient from a hospital or health ENVIRONMENT *noun* Any material released in effluents, generally of human origin *verb* A generic term for the release of materials (eg radioactive, biohazardous waste, and sundry anthropogenic detritus) in effluents to the air, water, or sanitary facilities HEALTH CARE ADMINSTRATION *verb* The formal act of terminating a person's care in a hospital or other health care facility

discharge summary A document prepared by the attending physician of a hospitalized patient that summarizes the admitting diagnosis, therapy received while hospitalized, prognosis and plan of action upon the patient's discharge

disclosure RESEARCH ETHICS A formal statement about a person's or institution's financial relationship with a company or other commercial enterprise by means of employment, consultancy, or through ownership of stock, or other significant equity; disclosure of such relationships of authors and/or institutions with commercial organizations (ie a potential for financial gain) is required for manuscripts submitted to peer-reviewed journals, and in a sense is a public statement about the potential bias(es) that may be introduced into the study of a process, product, or therapy (N Eng J Med 1995; 332:262sB)

discovery FORENSIC MEDICINE A legal term that is variously defined as 1) The ascertainment of that which was not previously known 2) The disclosure or coming to light of what was previously hidden 3) The acquisition of knowledge of given facts or acts (Black's Law Dictionary, 6th ed, West Publishing, St Paul, Mn, 1990); the discovery process may impact on physicians in a court of law, as discovery is a pre-trial device used by one party to prepare itself in the prosecution or defense of a case; certain types of information, eg privileged communication in a doctor-patient relationship are not discoverable

'discovery rule' LEGAL MEDICINE A rule that expands the Statute of Limitations (which usually limits a plaintiff's right to initiate a lawsuit to 2-3 years after an alleged tort occurred), such that the time period during which a lawsuit may be initiated begins from the moment the victim of the tort or plaintiff becomes aware of the act of malpractice; see Emancipated minor

discriminant analysis STATISTICS A device used in statistics that allows an individual observation to be assigned to one or more categories with a minimum probability of error; DA takes advantage of a discriminant function that was previously derived from a large number of observations of individuals of known categories

disease flare-up A generic term for a transient $\uparrow$ in the severity of the clinical manifestations of a disease

disease-free survival ONCOLOGY The amount of time that a person with a disease[1] lives without known recurrence[2]; DFS is major clinical parameter used to evaluate the efficacy of a particular therapy, which is usually measured in 'units' of one or five years

[1]Usually understood to be malignant [2]As measured by the usual means used to detect or monitor that disease

disease of regulation Any clinical nosology, the symptoms of which are attributed to the loss of homeostatic mechanisms responsible for maintaining in balance a hormone, eg parathyroid hormone or the autonomic nervous system, eg blood pressure

disease of the week 'syndrome' A hypochondriacal symptom complex described in medical students, who, as they learn about a disease, discover that they, too, have all of the symptoms of the disorder being described

disenfranchised An adjective referring to any person, or cultural group that has no political, social, or economic power

disenfranchized population SOCIAL MEDICINE Any group of people who are without a home or a political voice and who live at the whims of their host; disenfranchized populations include the homeless or refugees of war and natural disasters and suffer from a wide variety of illness, low-grade malnutrition and inability to educate themselves and integrate themselves into the host population; see Refugee

DISH Diffuse idiopathic skeletal hyperostosis of Forester RHEUMATOLOGY A disease complex affecting the middle-aged and elderly, characterized by florid neo-osteogenesis (bone spurs and potentially spinal fusion) at ligamentous insertions in numerous sites; severe complications may arise if the cervical spine is involved, potentially causing dysphagia; the process may more prominent on the right side; DISH may be associated with impaired glucose tolerance, DM, and obesity

dishface deformity A concave face that occurs in an unrepaired midface fracture, characterized by a protruding forehead, prominent jaw, depressed nose and malar prominences (with loss of direct contact with the anterior teeth) seen in the LeFort III fracture, which extends bilaterally through the frontozygomatic suture lines, the base of the nose and the ethmoid region; the lateral rims of the orbits are separated and the infraorbital rim may be fractured; in this most severe type of LeFort fracture, cerebrospinal rhinorrhea may occur, indicating 'violation' of the cranial vault

dishwater pus A fanciful descriptor for the seropurulent discharge typical of synergistic necrotizing cellulitis due to an anaerobic bacterial infection, which is most commonly associated with cardiorenal dysfunction, diabetes mellitus, obesity and perirectal infections CLINICAL After a 3-14 day incubation, there is abrupt development of a malodorous lesion with sloughing of skin, gas production in the wound, muscle involvement and marked systemic toxicity TREATMENT Opening and aeration of the wound kills bacteria through oxygen toxicity

disinfection Elimination of the ability of a surface or material to act as a vector for an infectious agent; objects may be disinfected by a variety of methods including chemicals (alcohol, chlorine, hexachlorophenes, iodines, phenols or quaternary ammonium compounds), high dry heat or 'wet' autoclaved heat; 'high-level' disinfectants are used for instruments that will penetrate the body cavities, eg surgical instruments and include ethylene oxide, glutaraldehyde (2%), formaldehyde (8%), alcohol (70-90%), stabilized hydrogen peroxide (6%), phenolic compounds (3%), iodophors (500 ppm), bleach (1000 ppm) and pasteurization at 75°C; see Biosafety level, HIV-active decontaminating agents

Note: The Creutzfeldt-Jakob disease agent, a prion is extremely resistant to disinfection in the form of boiling, chemicals (alcohol, β-propiolactone, formalin) and irradiation and requires Biosafety Level 2 practices

disintegrin Any of a family of peptides (eg albolabrin, bitistatin, echistatin, eristostatin) that that have been isolated from viper venoms and are potent inhibitors of ligand binding to the glycoprotein IIb/IIIa (integrin $\alpha_{IIb}\beta_3$) receptor, and inhibit platelet aggregation (in Clin Lab Sci 1994; 7:147) ; because of their antigenicity, disintegrins are used primarily as a basis for the design of low-molecular weight antagonists (N Engl J Med 1995; 332:1553RV)

disk kidney Cake kidney, see there

diskectomy 1) Laminectomy, see there 2) Microsurgical laminectomy, see there

dismember *verb* To remove the members or limbs from a body; see Jeffrey Dahmer

dismemberment The removal of members or limbs from a body, which has been used as an expediency by some mentally unbalanced serial killers to store body parts for future use; see Mad dog

disomic gamete A gamete containing an extra copy of a specific allele, gene, or chromosome; Cf Nullisomic gamete

disomy The inheritance of both haploid chromosomes from one parent, either the father, paternal disomy or mother, maternal disomy

disposable *adjective* Pertaining or relating to that which can be discarded or disposed of *noun* Any item used in health care-related patient contact that is discarded following use, which includes masks, gloves, gowns, needles, paper products, syringes, wipes; care must be exercised in proper disposable disposal, as contaminated or presumably contaminated disposables must be treated as biohazardous waste and 'red bagged' (ie placed in properly labeled biohazardous bags or containers)

disruption OBSTETRICS The in utero destruction of a previously formed normal fetal body part, caused either by 1) 'Amputation', the result of pressure-induced strangulation by an amniotic band or 2) Interruption of regional blood supply, causing ischemia, necrosis and sloughing of the dead part; see Dysmorphology

disseminated intravascular coagulation An acquired bleeding diathesis that translates into a pernicious clinical event in which the balance between coagulation and fibrinolysis tips toward coagulation; 30-65% of DIC is caused by infection; DIC is divided into a 'fast' DIC, which presents as an acute, fulminant, uncompensated consumptive coagulopathy with clinical manifestations of bleeding due to abruptio placentae, septic abortion, amniotic fluid embolism, toxemia, malignancy, massive tissue injury, as occurs in burns, surgery, trauma, infections, gram-negative sepsis, meningococcemia, Rocky Mountain spotted fever, incompatible blood transfusion and purpura fulminans; 'fast' DIC requires replacement of deficient or consumed factors; 'slow' DIC occurs in diseases that are chronic, indolent and compensated, for which there is little overt manifestation of bleeding; the clinical picture is rather painted by thrombosis, microcirculatory ischemia and end-organ infarction, due for example, to acute promyelocytic leukemia, dead fetus syndrome, transfusion of coagulation factor concentrates, neoplasia (adenocarcinoma of the pancreas, prostate, lung, stomach), aortic aneurysm, cocaine, MAOI, giant hemangioma (Kasabach-Merritt syndrome), liver disease, vasculitis, chronic and/or low-grade infections, eg histoplasmosis, aspergillosis, malaria and compensated obstetric conditions, (eg, hemolysis, eclampsia, infection, hypoxia, acidosis, respiratory distress); 'slow' DIC may respond to heparinization PATHOGENESIS 1) Endothelial cell damage by endotoxins, hypoxia and acidosis or immune complexes; endothelial damage results in a thrombogenic surface that activates platelets and the intrinsic coagulation pathway 2) Release of tissue factor (factor III, thromboplastin) by neoplasia, trauma or complications of pregnancy (leading to extrinsic pathway activation) LABORATORY ↑ PT, aPTT, FDPs, and fibrinopeptide A; ↓ fibrinogen, prothrombin, platelets, factor V, factor VIII, antithrombin III, plasminogen, and lesser decreases in factors VII, IX, X, and XI PATHOLOGY Kidneys demonstrates diffuse cortical necrosis, necrotic columns of Bertini with acute ischemic infarct

dissociative identity disorder Multiple personality disorder* The '*presence of two or more distinct identities or personality states...that recurrently take control of behavior.*' DID is accompanied by an inability to recall important personal information that is well beyond ordinary forgetfulness; there are estimated 20 000 patients with DID in the US (Nature Medicine 1995; 1:490)

*Although this is the term preferred in the Diagnosis and Statistical Manual for Mental Disorders, the term multiple personality disorder is far more widely used

distributable *adjective* COMPUTERS Pertaining or relating to a computer system in which the workload can be spread over an entire network with increased efficiency (Am Lab March 1995, p46)

disuse atrophy A generic term encompassing the degenerative changes that tissues undergo when not carrying out their normal functions or are doing so at suboptimal levels; DA of the musculoskeletal unit is characterized by atrophy of muscles, contractions of the tendons, and osteoporosis; diversion of the intestinal flow in the GI tract results in a DA-type phenomenon known as diversion colitis

DIT 3,5-diiodotyrosine The iodinated molecular precursor for either T_3 or T_4

dithiocarb Dithiocarbamate A drug with potent antioxidant capacity and chelating activities that improves the depressed immune responses of newborn and aging mice, mice immunosuppressed through chemotherapy of radiotherapy or those with a murine retrovirus-induced immunodeficiency; dithiocarb has a similar effect in AIDS and appears to improve survival (JAMA 1991; 265:1538)

divalent metal ions Divalent cations Metal ions that have major roles in metabolic functions, including Ca^{++}, Mg^{++}, Cu^{++}, Mn^{++}, Co^{++}, and Zn^{++}, the physiologic levels of which in the human economy range from gram to trace quantities

dive bomber sound An adjectival descriptor for the sound heard by electromyography corresponding to the myotonic response (delayed relaxation of the muscle following a maintained contraction or twitch), elicited by movement of the needle electrode within the muscle as well as percussion; in the myotonias (dystrophia myotonica, paramyotonia and myotonia congenita), prolonged trains of potentials occur in great profusion in response to movement of the electrode, producing a sound likened to that of the Junkers Ju-87 (Stuka) bomber when diving

diversity see Gene diversity

diversion colitis A condition characterized by inflammation in bypassed segments of the colorectum after surgical diversion of the fecal stream; DC may be asymptomatic or appear as a bloody discharge, colicky anorectal pain, tenesmus, purulent or hemorrhagic discharge, and occurs in the majority of diverted colons from one month to years after the procedure ENDOSCOPY Friable, erythematous and granular mucosa that mimicks both Crohn's disease, and ulcerative colitis PATHOLOGY Diffuse follicular lymphoid hyperplasia, expansion of the lamina propria by plasma cells, lymphocytes and PMNs, cryptitis, reactive epithelium and mucin depletion, variably accompanied by crypt abscesses, aphthous ulcers, architectural distortion and Paneth cell metaplasia (Human Pathol 1993; 24:211) PATHOGENESIS Possibly due to local nutritional deficiency of the mucosa TREATMENT Local application of short-chain fatty acids

divide-and-dump HEALTH CARE ENVIRONMENT A colloquial term for a philosophical stance that may be adopted by insurance companies in which they identify low-risk and high-risk individuals and find a means to 'dump' the latter (Am Med News 26 October 1992, p7)

dizygotic twins Fraternal twins Twins resulting from two separate fertilized eggs liberated simultaneously from the ovaries that develop in separate or partially fused chorionic sa; Cf Monozygotic twins

Both terms are in active use, fraternal is more colloquial, dizygotic more formal

DKA Diabetic ketoacidosis, see there

DM Diabetes mellitus

Also 1) Daunomycin 2) Deciduous (primary) molar (dentistry) 3) Deletion mutation (genetics) 4) Dental Mechanic (British Royal Navy) 5) Dermatomyositis 6) Dextromorphan 7) Diabetic mother 8) Diastolic murmur 9) Dioxane-methanol (a scintillation fluid) 10) Diphenylaminechloroarsine 11) Diseased mucosa (rarely used) 12) Doctor of medicine (MD is the abbreviation used in the US) 13) Double minute (cytogenetics) 14) Vomiting gas (abbreviation used in the US Chemical Corps)

DMSO Dimethylsulfoxide A substance that occurs naturally in minute amounts in certain foods, and which has been used as an industrial solvent for making paper since the 1940s DMSO is of potential use for treating familial amyloidotic polyneuropathy, acetaminophen hepatotoxicity; human trials suggest it may have analgesic and anti-inflammatory properties; DMSO reduces the ice crystals formed in frozen section tissues from the operating suite, and may be an effective cryopreservative medium Note: DMSO has been used (without proven efficacy) to treat arthritis, mental illness, emphysema and cancer

DNA Deoxyribonucleic acid DNA's conformation is a function of 1) The types of bonds and the stacking of the nucleotides, which is deduced by diffraction analysis and 2) The medium, in particular, the state of hydration, which can facilitate or hinder certain three-dimensional configurations **A-DNA** Right-handed, double-stranded, stable at intermediate relative hydration of the medium, 11 bases per turn of the double helix, contains major and minor grooves; the phosphate groups face each other across the major groove; A-DNA is less common than B-DNA **B-DNA** The most common form of DNA in living cells (aka Watson-Crick DNA); it is right-handed, double-stranded, stable at high relative hydration of the medium, contains 10.6 bases per turn of the double helix, a pitch of 34, and has major and minor grooves; the twist improves the stacking of the bases along each backbone chain **cDNA** Complemenatry DNA, see cDNA **C-DNA** Right-handed, double-stranded, stable at low relative hydration of the medium, 9.3 bases per turn of the double helix **H-DNA** A convoluted configuration of DNA that contains adjacent triple-stranded and single-stranded regions with sharply-angled hinging and kinking; H-DNA requires intense supercoiling to maintain this structure, which is a function of the acidity of the pH of the medium; it is unknown whether the H-DNA configuration exists in vivo **J-DNA** A unique and convoluted configuration of DNA that exists in mildly alkaline solutions; it is unknown whether the J-DNA configuration exists in vivo **k-DNA** Extranuclear DNA contained within kinetoplasts, which exists in the form of maxicircles and minicircles; analysis of k-DNA by buoyant density, DNA hybridization or polymerase chain reaction is of use in speciating organisms with kinetoplasts, eg *Leishmania* species (N Engl J Med 1991; 324:476cpc) **mtDNA** see Mitochondrial DNA **rDNA** Any segment of DNA that encodes ribosomal RNA **Watson-Crick DNA** B-DNA, see there **Z-DNA** DNA that is expressed in vivo as a regulator of function; it is left-handed, has a zig-zag (hence Z-DNA) configuration, a ptich of the helix of 44.6, and contains multiple CGCGCG nucleotides; a configuration in which the phosphate groups face each other across a deep minor groove; see Left-handed DNA

DNA amplification MOLECULAR DIAGNOSTICS A generic term for any method used to increase the copy number of a sequence of DNA; see Cycling probe technology, Gap

LCR (gap ligase chain reaction), NASBA (nucleic acid sequence-based amplification), PCR (polymerase chain reaction), SDA (strand-displacement amplification), TMA (transcription-mediated amplification); see Gene amplification

DNA analysis Any of a vast array of techniques are used to analyze genes and DNA; see Chromosome walking, Fingerprinting, Footprinting, in situ Hybridization, Jeffries' probe, Jumping libraries, PCR, RFLP (restriction fragment length polymorphism) analysis and Southern blot hybridization

DNA bending MOLECULAR BIOLOGY A loco-regional transformation of the secondary structure of DNA that is mediated by activator proteins that have no obvious activation domains; DB changes the physical conformation of DNA and is a prerequisite for transcription; a transcription factor, MerR, can mediate both repression as well as activation of bending through stereospecific modulation of the DNA structure; activator-induced unbending coupled to operator untwisting, remodels the promoter and it a better template for the waiting RNA polymerase (**Nature 1995; 374:371**); DNA bending factors include the testes-determining factor, HIV and other viruses (**New York Times 4 August 1992; C1**)

DNA binding protein Any of a group of proteins that form dimers and bind at specific sites on DNA, often located near highly positively charged regions of amino acids interacting with negatively charged DNA, either activating or quenching gene expression, acting during cell growth and differentiation or during normal cell function; three structural motifs capable of binding DNA are well recognized a) Helix-turn-helix motif, seen in MyoD protein b) Leucine zipper motif, see in the protein products of the *fos, jun* and *myc* oncogenes and c) Zinc finger motif, seen in growth signal-regulating proteins; see Helix-turn-helix motif, Leucine zipper motif, Zinc finger motif

DNA chip A glass chip that carries an array of short DNA segments representing all the possible sequences of a given length of DNA, which is used to rapidly sequence DNA in a process known as DNA sequencing by hybridization (**Science 1994; 264; 1265**)

DNA cleavage MOLECULAR BIOLOGY The breaking of a DNA bond, an event that is essential for replication, transcription, recombination, and repair of DNA, which is carried out by

1) Topoisomerases, which catalyze DNA relaxation by cleavage, strand passage, and reunion

2) Recombinases, which catalyze DNA rearrangements by concerted cleavage and exchange of DNA ends

3) Endonucleases, which catalyze the cleavage of single- and double-stranded DNA (**Science 1995; 267:1817**)

DNA clock MOLECULAR PHYLOGENY The use of DNA hybridization studies to infer relatedness of organisms and their points of evolutionary divergence from each other Method DNA is melted and hybrids are allowed to form, comparing the degree of hybridization from homoduplexes (duplexes of DNA strands from the same species) and heteroduplexes (duplexes of DNA strands from different species) see 'Homology', Mitochondrial 'Eve'

DNA conformation The three-dimensional configuration of DNA with respect to coiling and supercoiling, which is classified as Form I Native DNA in its supercoiled form Form II DNA subjected to partial DNAse digestion, which introduces a single nick and thus has a relaxed conformation Form III DNA that has been incubated with DNAse and because both of DNA's helices have been broken, ie, double 'nicked', has a linear form; see Cruciform DNA; Cf DNA structural types, DNA supercoiling

DNA dosimeter ENVIRONMENT A device containing human DNA used to measure exposure to ultraviolet B radiation; the mutation rate is an indirect monitor for the carcinogenic effects caused by depletion of the ozone layer; DNA dosimeters cost ± $ 1.0 to produce, absorb UV light in a 360° arc, are 2-fold more sensitive than spectroradiometers, and measure the number of cyclobutane rings formed between adjacent nucleotides (**New York Times 25 May 1993; C4**)

DNA fingerprinting MOLECULAR BIOLOGY DF may be defined in terms similar to that of RNA fingerprinting, ie oligonucleotide sequence pattern-matching; DNA fingerprinting currently refers to a technique based on short, tandem-repeated (or hypervariable) genomic sequences (minisatellites) that are highly specific; the likelihood that two individuals have the same DNA fingerprint is ± 1:30 billion, and thus is more specific than RFLP (restriction fragment length polymorphism) analysis; the insert-free wild-type M13 bacteriophage detects these hypervariable minisatellites, which have an accordion-like length since the number of 'repeats' varies with each person; the DNA sequence that detects these differences is located to two clusters of 15 base pair repeats translating to (Glu, Gly, Gly, Gly, Ser)n in the bacteriophage's protein III gene; the probe's ('**Jeffries' probe, Nature 1985; 314/316:67**) specificity makes it useful in paternity testing, in human genome mapping and forensic medicine, where it is being increasingly used in criminal law (**JAMA 1988; 259:2193, Science 1989; 244:1033, ibid 246:1558**); see Bandshift, Fingerprinting; Cf Protein fingerprinting, RNA fingerprinting

DNA folding Folded DNA The native DNA configuration that results from the interplay between the DNA itself (the 'internal message') and its regulatory proteins (the 'external message'); this dynamic conformation is pivotal in understanding the effects of DNA; establishment of 'ground rules' for DNA-protein interactions requires knowledge of DNA's 'surface morphology', obtained by complex mathematical and biophysical modeling; see DNA-binding proteins

DNA footprinting A technique in which a DNA molecule is 'incubated' with a binding protein, which binds to a specific site along the double helix, and then subjected to restriction endonuclease digestion, which reduces the entire DNA to mono- and oligonucleotide fragments except for the portion of the DNA molecule that was 'protected' from digestion by the binding protein; removal of the protein by simple chemical means, eg by gel electrophoresis, allows study of DNA and binding protein interaction

DNA forms see DNA

DNA gyrase A type II prokaryotic topoisomerase that catalyzes the negative supercoiling of DNA ahead or downstream from the advancing replicating fork (structure, Nature 1991; 351:624); see DNA supercoil

DNA hybridization A technique for determining the presence of a target DNA in a sample of tissue or cells Method A sample of cells is lysed, the protein is removed by digestion with proteinase K and the DNA extracted using phenol, chloroform and isoamyl alcohol; the DNA is then denatured with a salt, sodium hydroxide, separating one of DNA's chains; the single-stranded or denatured DNA may be immobilized on a blotting paper as in Southern blot hybridization or present in a tissue as in in situ hybridization; the final step adds a ^{32}P-labeled probe or a biotinylated probe that is visualized by either autoradiography, as in the ^{32}P-labelled probe or by adding avidin-biotin acid phosphatase, which evokes a color change in the substrate upon digestion; uses of DNA hybridization Rapid diagnosis of infection, eg in tissue, using in situ hybridization

1) Virus, eg CMV, EBV, HPV, herpes simplex virus, adenovirus, HIV-1

2) Bacteria, eg enterotoxin-producing *Escherichia coli* and gonococcus and

3) Detection of neoplasia

a) Specific DNA mutations (point mutations, deletions, translocations), clonal expansions of rearranged immunoglobulins (B-cell lymphomas) or T-cell receptors (T-cell lymphomas) and other specific mutations associated with various neoplasms

b) Detection of integrated viral DNA and

c) Detection of oncogenes Diagnosis of genetic diseases

see HLA analysis, Paternity testing, RFLP analysis

DNA index DI An expression of the relative DNA content (ploidy) of a cell population, which is calculated by dividing the DNA content of the $G_{0/1}$ peak of a specified population by the peak channel number of the $G_{0/1}$ peak of a known, standard diploid population, usually a fresh or frozen lymphocyte population; the DI of a haploid population is 0.5, of a diploid population 1.0, and of a tetraploid population 2.0; aneuploidy refers to any non-multiple of 0.5; Cf Ploidy, Proliferative index, RNA index

DNA instability syndromes see DNA repair syndromes

DNA library see Library

DNA ligase An enzyme that links strands of DNA during repair and replication, catalyzing the formation of phosphodiester bond between the 3'-OH and the $5'-PO_4$ of DNA's phosphate backbone

DNA methylation Methylation, see there

DNA ploidy analysis The determination of the number of single copies of a complete haploid (n) set of chromosomes present in a particular cell population; for most organisms, a diploid set (2n) is normal, and is a 'soft' criterion that supports a cell population's relative normalcy, and is some malignancies is regarded as positive prognostic feature in cancer of the bladder, colon, kidney, and ovary, but not small cell carcinoma of the lung (Science 1994; 264; 1265) DNA ploidy analysis is most efficiently performed using a flow cytometer; see DNA index, Flow cytometry, Ploidy analysis, Proliferation index

DNA polymerases A group of enzymes involved in DNA replication, forming two distinct complexes acting in sequence 1) DNA-polymerase α-primase complex, which first initiates DNA synthesis at the replication origin, acting as the polymerase for the lagging strand, opposite the Okazaki fragments, followed by 2) DNA polymerase sigma complex, which initiates replication on the leading strand template; see Replication

Note: Some prokaryotic DNA polymerase complexes can replace the DNA polymerase sigma complex; prokaryotic DNA polymerases I, II and III (pol I, pol II, pol III) correspond to the eukaryotic DNA polymerases α, β and γ, designated as pol α, pol β and pol γ

DNA polymorphism A condition where more than one normal but different nucleotide sequences exist at a particular site in DNA; these inherited differences in DNA sequences are normal variations of an individual's DNA, also known as restriction length polymorphisms and can be exploited to document the pattern of inheritance of genes associated with certain diseases; the term polymorphism requires that the less frequent of two loci be found in more than 1% of the population; see RFLP (restriction fragment length polymorphism) analysis

DNA probe A small single-stranded fragment of cloned, biotin-labelled or radiolabelled DNA that is complementary to a DNA molecule of interest; this complementary can be detected 1) Semiquantitatively by the Dot-blot technique 2) When located in a tissue of interest by in situ hybridization and 3) Immobilized on a nitrocellulose or nylon membrane, see Southern blot hybridization

DNA repair syndrome DNA instability syndrome A heterogeneous group of diseases with damaged genomes, chromosomal 'instability', hypersensitivity to irradiation and mutagenic chemicals and an increased risk of suffering malignancy, including ataxia-telangiectasia, Bloom syndrome, dyskeratosis congenita, Fanconi's anemia, progeria and xeroderma pigmentosum

DNA restriction site polymorphism see DNA polymorphism, RFLP (restriction fragment length polymorphism)

analysis

DNAse protection assay Any method for studying DNA, in which the parent double-stranded DNA is 'protected' from DNAse digestion by virtue of being bound by a protein TECHNIQUE A segment of DNA is subjected to digestion by a restriction endonuclease (a DNAse), which will reduce the entire DNA chain to mono- and dinucleotides, except for the segment of DNA protected by a bound protein; the protein is then removed from the DNA and the sequence is determined by either the Maxam-Gilbert or Sanger technique; see Achilles heel cleavage, Dimethyl sulfate protection assay, Footprinting

DNA sequencing by hybridization A novel approach to DNA sequencing in which the pattern by which a particular unknown sequence of DNA binds to a DNA chip (see there) is observed with high-resolution fluorescent light microscopy (Science 1994; 264; 1265)

DNA structures see DNA forms

DNA supercoil A circular double helix of DNA that has been twisted into a supercoil by a DNA gyrase, rendering it more compact, resulting in rapid sedimentation by ultracentrifugation and rapid migration by gel electrophoresis; reversal of the supercoil is accomplished by topoisomerase, which 'nicks', opens and closes the strands; see Topoisomerase

DNA topoisomerase see Topoisomerase

DNA topology The surface properties of a DNA molecule, which are a function of linking number (the number of times one strand of the double helix crosses over the other), twist (the periodicity of winding of one strand around another), and writhe (the supercoiling of the overall helical structure in space)

DNA vaccine IMMUNOLOGY An at-present not yet available vaccine consisting of the gene encoding a protein responsible for the immune reaction against the pathogen of interest, which may be directly injected into the muscle (Bio/Technology 1995; 13:420)

DNAR Do not attempt resuscitation, see DNR

DNCB Dinitrochlorobenzene A compound used to measure a person's ability to mount a de novo cell-mediated reaction; the skin of a subject not previously exposed to DNCB is 'painted' with DNCB, a substance that acts as a hapten; in normal subjects, re-exposure to DNCB 2 weeks later elicits a type IV hypersensitivity reaction

DNR Do not resuscitate MEDICAL ETHICS An order written in a patient's chart that explicitly and unequivocally states that cardiopulmonary resuscitation should not be initiated if a patient is found in cardiac arrest; DNR orders may be written at the request of the patient, or if incompetent, at the request of the patient's family; although in theory, DNR or 'No code' orders may be written by the physician if he feels that CPR will not be successful in restoring meaningful life to the patient, see Baby L, most physicians are disinclined to 'play God'; DNR orders do not preclude treating airway obstruction, congestive heart failure, arrhythmias and metabolic derangements, although it is a fine line between this type of 'supportive care' and resuscitation DNR generally is understood to mean not intubating not using a defibrillator or minimal efforts at resuscitation; 22% of patients participate in DNR decisions and the family, 86% of the time; it has been argued that objective evaluation of medical futility in quantitative or qualitative terms must be integrated into the ethics of DNR orders (JAMA 1995; 273:1240A) see Medical futility; Cf Advanced directives, Euthanasia, Living will

DOA 1) Date of admission 2) Dead on arrival

Also 1) Defeat Opiate Addiction (an organization) 2) Dioctyladipate

DOB Date of birth

DOC Date of confinement or delivery

'doc-in-a-box' A deprecative sobriquet for a physician who provides primary health care, usually at an hourly rate and in the setting of a free-standing ambulatory care clinic

docking protein see Signal recognition particle

'Doctor Death' Dr. Jack Kevorkian, a retired pathologist and self-proclaimed 'obitiatrist' (a physician who assists patients wishing to commit suicide), who invented a 'self-execution machine' allowing a patient to switch an intravenous saline line to thiopental and from there to potassium chloride, thereby causing a painless and fatal arrhythmia; the first client to use the device was a middle-aged woman suffering from Alzheimer's dementia, who preferred death to the slow inexhorable deterioration of mental function; see Euthanasia; Cf Angel of death; Doctor death II, Dr 'X'

Dr Kevorkian was barred by court injunction from allowing others to use the device; in October, 1991, the same physician provided the expertise and equipment for two assisted suicides

Doctor Death (II) In addition to Kevorkian, Dr John Kitzhaber, MD of Portland Oregon, has also been called Dr Death in view of his role as chief architect of the so-called Oregon Plan*, a bipartisan coalition effort to develop a framework for fundamental resource allocation; the Oregon Plan attempts to address the financial limits on health care spending in the state of Oregon by providing the most health care value for the most people (**Am Med News 16 Nov 1992 p7**)

*It was the Oregon Plan's guidelines that denied coverage of a bone marrow transplantation to a 7-year-old boy Coby Howard, resulting in his death, hence Dr Kitzhaber's unofficial anointment as Dr Death

Doctor Feelgood American slang for an unscrupulous physician who prescribes controlled mood-altering drugs, eg amphetamines in absence of clinically valid indications for their use

'Doctor-nurse game' The complex 'pas de deux' between physician and nurse(s); in the US, nurses have begun to demand complete equality and the autonomy to make decisions about patient management, the wisdom of which is questionable (**N Engl J Med 1990; 323:201c**) as the education differs substantially (3-5 years for a nurse, 11-14 years for a physician) and the medico-legal responsibility is ultimately born by the physician

doctor of osteopathy D.O., see Osteopathy

doctor-patient interaction The doctor-patient 'game' comprises the social aspects of a confidential relationship shared by the physician and his patient; several models of this relation have been described and each 'player' in the dyad has an appropriate role:

1) ENGINEERING MODEL The physician distances himself from the moral dilemmas of the relation per se, merely providing all the facts, allowing the patient to make his own decisions

2) PRIESTLY (PATERNALISTIC) MODEL The physician guides the patient through both various disease processes and the moral dilemmas of his life

3) CONTRACTUAL MODEL The physician and the patient each share in the moral responsibilities of the medical decisions; see 'High touch'

'Doctor X' A surgeon suspected of causing the untimely demise of 30-40 patients from 1963 to 1968 at a now-defunct hospital in New Jersey, who was indicted on five counts of murder, allegedly administering curare as part of his modus operandi; after losing his medical license in the US, he returned to Mar de la Plata, Argentina, where he died in 1984

document *noun* INFORMATICS A bundle of information that is a common 'currency' for groupware communication including text and relevant formatting details, graphics, audio, and video *verb* To fomally record information, usually in a permanent legally acceptable fashion; see Documentation

documentation A generic term for any formal record, in particular of patient-physician contact of with dates (and

often times) that 'document'* various aspects of patient management; in certain types of patient care, eg cosmetic surgery, photographs are used as documentation of such interactions

*Providing 'An instrument on which is recorded, by means of letters, figures, or marks, the original, official, or legal form of something, which may be evidentially used.' (Black's Law Dictionary, St Paul, Minn, West Publishing Co, 1990)

DOD Dead of disease

DOE Dyspnea on exertion

dog The canine is the vector for many microorganisms capable of causing human disease, including arthropods and mites (*Cheyletiella yasguri, Sarcoptes scabei,* var hominis, var canis), bacteria (*Brucella abortus, B suis, B melitensis, B canis, Campylobacter jejuni,* CDC-designated bacteria, including DF-2, IIj, EF-4, M-5, *Francisella tularensis, Leptospira canicola, Pasteurella multocida, Yersinia pestis*), parasites (*Ancylostoma brasiliense, A caninum, Babesia microti, Dirofilaria immitis, Dipetallonema perstans, Dipylidium canum, Echinococcus granulosa, E multilocularis, Giardia lamblia, Gnathostoma spinigera, Multiceps multocida, M senilis, Spirometra (Diphyllobotrium) mansonoides, Toxocara canis, Toxoplasma gondii*), rickettsia, eg *Ehrlichia canis,* virus (rabies)

dog-ear appearance PLASTIC SURGERY A one-sided mound of redundant tissue, which is seen after the repair of certain skin lesions and defects; 'dog ears' may be inevitable in complex wounds, occurring when the long axis of an elliptical incision is too short (the general rule being a 4:1 length-to-width ratio) and may appear at both ends of the surgical incision; excision requires either lengthening of the wound, creating an oblique limb at the incision or loosening with a Y-shaped incision, repairing by shortening (excising) the long side and lengthening the short side RADIOLOGY A fanciful descriptor for the symmetrical settling of free blood or fluid on either side of the bladder at the posterior pelvic floor, visualized in the supine victim of massive trauma to organs, fractures and rupture of organs

doigt-en-lorgnette Telescoped fingers, see there

doll face PEDIATRICS A face with chubby cheeks and prominent chin, described as typical of glycogen storage disease type Ia or von Gierke's disease, further characterized by hepatomegaly, enlarged kidneys, growth retardation LABORATORY Hypoglycemia, lactic acidosis, ↑ uric acid and hyperlipidemia PROGNOSIS Good; Cf Cherubism

doll's head maneuver NEUROLOGY A clinical sign for evaluating brainstem function in a comatose patient; in the normal subject, as the head is turned rapidly to one side, the eyes conjugately deviate in the direction opposite to the head's movement; loss of this reflex implies dysfunction of the brainstem or of the oculomotor nerves; infero-lateral deviation of the eyes in combination with pupillary dilatation and implies dysfunction of the third cranial nerve, possibly due to tentorial herniation

dolomite A generic term for a specific form of calcium-magnesium carbonate that may used as a calcium supplement to ensure healthy bones, which is mined in the Dolomite mountains of Northern Italy (and elsewhere); some of the mineral deposits may be contaminated with heavy metals (lead, cadmium and others), for which there is a maximum ceiling of 5 parts per million allowed by the US Food and Drug Administration

Note: Dolomite has been claimed by some advocates of 'holistic' health, to be the most natural (and therefore 'healthiest') calcium supplement available; ironically one of the most vocal of the advocates of dolomite's use died of a malignant bone tumor

domain A generic term for any structurally (eg α-helix, β-pleated sheet) or functionally (eg antigen-antibody or receptor-ligand binding site) significant region on a macromolecule MOLECULAR BIOLOGY A discrete block of 40-

400 amino acid in length region of a protein or polypeptide chain that folds spontaneously into a characteristic relatively globular shape under a defined set of conditions, which presents a spatially distinct 'signature', often allowing it to interact in a specific fashion with other proteins or receptors; the term 'domain' is also used for 1) The functional disulfide bond-linked polypeptide loops on the constant and variable regions of both the light and heavy chains of the immunoglobulin molecule 2) A chromosome region in which the supercoiling is independent of the rest of the molecule and 3) A long segment of DNA bearing a functional gene that is highly-susceptible to DNAse degradation; Cf Motif

domain knowledge MEDICAL EDUCATION A format for acquiring medical knowledge based on memorizing the characteristics of a particular disease process (**N Engl J Med** 1995; 332:1507ED)

dominant dozen A transiently popular and colloquial term for the 12 most common conditions clinically associated with AIDS, which includes *Pneumocystis carinii* pneumonia, Kaposi sarcoma, *Toxoplasma* encephalitis, candidiasis of the upper GI tract, and others

domino donation Transplantation of heart and lungs of cadaveric origin into patient A, who has suffered from long standing lung disease, eg cystic fibrosis, but who has a heart suitable for donation, while transplanting patient A's heart into patient B; it is estimated that optimal domino-donation in the USA would free an extra 50-75 hearts for transplantation

domestic violence PUBLIC HEALTH Physical abuse by a person's 'significant other' (boy– or girlfriend, lover, spouse) occurring in the home environment; domestic violence is the cause of 100 000/year of hospitalization in the US; 18% of American ♀ have been victims of physical abuse; 12% of Americans believe that some ♀ may deserve to be hit by their husbands or boyfriends; 29% believe that some ♂ may deserve to be hit by their wives or girlfriends (**US News & World Report** 10 January 1994:8)

domino theory A hypothetical explanation of cell duplication that holds that the daughter of a somatic division is produced by a series of linear metabolic pathways where the initiation of a new pathway hinges on completion of a previous pathway, a concept championed by yeast biologists, in contrast to the 'clock theory' that postulates the existence of a series of 'switches'; accumulated data supports a merging of the two theories; Cf Clock theory

domoic acid An excitatory kainic acid analogue that is a neurotoxic glutamate agonist that ↑ neuronal activity; it is produced by marine plants (*Nitzschia pungens*), concentrates in mussels, and causes seafood-related envenomation

An outbreak in Prince Edward Island in 1987 was clinically characterized by vomiting, abdominal cramps, diarrhea, incapacitating headache, seizures, hemiparesis, ophthalmoplegia and loss of short-term memory, which may prove useful in developing a model for Alzheimer's disease

Don Juan syndrome Male hypersexuality, satyrism PSYCHIATRY A form of male sexual deviancy in which the subject masks his feelings of insecurity regarding his own masculinity and/or latent homosexuality by myriad sexual liaisons with the opposite sex; to the Freudians, this represents an Oedipus complex in which the sexual promiscuity represents a search for maternal love; male hypersexuality is considered a sociopathy, as there is no emotion attached to the relations and up to 50% of subjects are impotent; Cf Delilah syndrome

Donath-Seifert tumor Epithelial-myoepithelial carcinoma, see there

donor One who donates tissue(s), an organ, blood or blood products; in the usual parlance, a donor is an altruistic individual who contributes blood products, often on a reg-

ular basis; formerly, a 'two-tier' system of quality of blood products existed in North America, where the 'better' blood was from voluntary donation in non-urban environments, while the less-desirable blood, ie more commonly infected with hepatitis virus and other pathogens, came from paid donation (often from a 'disenfranchised' population, eg drug addicts or the homeless, who exchange blood for money) in urban regions DONOR REQUIREMENTS The donor must have a body temperature of < 37.5°C, pulse 50-100, blood pressure of 100 to 180 mm Hg systolic, and 50 to 100 mm Hg diastolic, hematocrit of > 41% for men and 38% for women, no skin lesions, 48 hours passed since last plasmapheresis or platelet donation, more than 12 months passed since receiving hepatitis B immunoglobulin DONOR REJECTION see Donor exclusion criteria DONOR BLOOD TESTS Alanine aminotransferase, HBV surface antigen, HBV core antigen, HCV antibody, HIV-1, HTLV-I, serological test for syphilis

donor deferral The nonacceptance of a potential donor based on lifestyle criteria or previous exposures; see Donor exclusion criteria

donor dominance DERMATOLOGY The property of a hair-bearing autograft to maintain the characteristics of the donor site, including continued hair growth when transplanted to a different recipient site; see Hair transplantation

donor exclusion criteria A potential donor is excluded if he has received therapy for malaria within the past 3 years (or travelled to a malaria endemic area within last 6 months), has ever had hepatitis B surface antigenemia, or lives with a hepatitis B carrier, has a 'high-risk' life style, has donated blood within the last 8 weeks, has a temperature > 37.5°C, or has, within the last six months: Delivered a term-infant, received Rho-GAM or blood products, had surgery or a tattoo, is being treated with antihistamines, steroids, tetracycline, barbiturates; there are four-week deferrals for tetanus, typhoid, and oral polio vaccines (**Arch Pathol Lab Med** 1994; 118:333ED) see Blood shortage

donor fatigue A generic term for the unwillingness of people to contribute to charitable causes on an ongoing basis (**Science** 1995; 267:11), a phenomenon that may affect those whose research monies are provided by charitable foundations that are funded by private contributors

Do not resuscitate DNR, see there

'don't ask, don't tell' MEDICAL ETHICS A colloquial term for a philosophical stance that might be applicable to various aspects of medicine, eg the practice of various resuscitative techniques (intubation, catheterization) on the recently dead; DADT skirts the ethical issues of violation of the human body without prior permission (which in the deceased, might prove difficult to obtain), and justifies such violation as it would seem to be better than practicing resuscitative techniques on live patients (**N Engl J Med** 1995; 332:1424C)

DOOR Deafness, onycho-osteodystrophy, mental retardation A rare AR [MIM 220500] or AD [MIM 124480] condition in which sensorineural deafness is accompanied by aplasia or hypoplasia of finger- and toenails, digital anomalies and epilepsy LABORATORY ↑ Plasma and urinary 2-oxoglutarate

dopamine receptors Dopamine's diverse physiological activities are mediated by G protein receptors; D_1 and D_2 receptors are considered together, as they are both located in the brain and endocrine tissues and have a variable response to neuroleptics agents that are used to treat schizophrenia; D_1 receptors have a viable response to neuroleptics, and when stimulated, increase the levels of adenylyl cyclase, while D_2 receptors respond to low (nanomolar) doses of these agents by decreasing adenylyl cyclase activity; the reported association between the D_2 receptor gene and alcoholism (**JAMA** 1991; 265:2667c) has not withstood rigorous scrutiny; D_1 receptor mRNA is most abundant in the caudate, nucleus accumbens and olfactory tubercle and D_1 receptors may mediate behavioral changes, modulate D_2 receptor activity and regulate neuron growth and differentiation; the D_1 receptor is encoded by a long intronless gene on chromosome 5; both D_1 and D_2 receptors are potential therapeutic targets for psychomotor disorders, eg Parkinsonism, schizophrenia and drug and alcohol abuse D_3 receptor is a recently characterized receptor that is both autoreceptor and post-synaptic receptor, located in the limbic system and associated with cognitive, emotional and endocrine functions; the D_3 receptor appears to mediate some of the effects of antipsychotic and anti-Parkinson's disease drugs that had been previously attributed to D_2 receptors

dope INDUSTRY *verb* A generic term for the use of an additive to improve a chemical compound's performance; see Doping SUBSTANCE ABUSE *noun* A generic and colloquial term for any recreational drug, almost invariably referring to a narcotic

doping COMPUTERS The deliberate introduction of impurity into a material eg a semiconductor to improve its performance

doppelgänger PSYCHIATRY A delusion that a double of a person or place exists elsewhere, which is related to other defects in recognition and suggests organic disease in the nondominant parietal lobe

Doppler color flow imaging CARDIOLOGY A noninvasive two-dimensional Doppler technique which provides a real-time image of the blood flow 'jet', allowing the severity of valvular stenosis to be determined, see Candle Flame, Mushroom, and Scimitar signs

Doppler effect A physical principle based on the decrease in oscillation frequency of an object emitting sound or energy waves as it passes a point of measurement; this principle is applied in the Doppler flowmeter used to evaluate blood velocities, which are distinctly abnormal in atherosclerotic arteries

Doppler sonographic imaging Any of a group of imaging modalities that takes advantage of the Doppler shift, a change in pitch resulting from the relative motion between an ultrasound source and an observer, which is directly related to the velocity of the moving object (red cells) and the cosine of the angle (Doppler angle) between the direction of blood flow and the ultrasound beam (the ideal Doppler angle is the rarely achievable 0°; it usually ranges from 45° to 60°)

Doppler velocimetry CARDIOLOGY A technique used to analyze blood flow wave forms, allowing accurate noninvasive measurement of volume and velocity of blood flow; DV is of use in assessing preterm fetuses with growth retardation, reducing the need for repeated fetal-blood monitoring, which is invasive and carries a risk of hemorrhage, bradycardia (6.6%), premature rupture of membranes (0.4%) and death (0.8%) (N Engl J Med 1993; 328:6892A)

DORA Directory of Rare Analyses A book published by the American Chemical Society that catalogs uncommonly ordered clinical tests and details on the laboratories performing them; the major criteria for inclusion in the DORA is that the test of interest is not performed by more than two laboratories; DORA tests include forensic ABO grouping, acetylcholinesterase, chymopapain, quantitative hepatitis C, lead in paint, latex-specific IgE platelet typing, meconium drug screening selenium, silicon *Giardia lamblia* antibodies, and 1900 others (DORA '94-96, AACC Press Washington DC)

DOS COMPUTERS Disk operating system Programmed information that is loaded into the computer's random access memory at start-up, which tells the machine what it can and cannot do

dosage compensation DEVELOPMENTAL BIOLOGY The equalization of the X-linked expression between animals with one and two X chromosomes; dosage compensation is nearly universal among animals with heteromorphic chromosomes; mammalian dosage compensation results in the inactivation of all but one X chromosome in diploid individuals, with the other X chromosome being inactive and visible cytologically as Barr bodies (Science 1994; 264:924oA)

dosage effect TRANSFUSION MEDICINE The presence of different quantities of an antigen on the red cell surface depending on whether the allele encoding the antigen is homo- or heterozygous, resulting in variability in the agglutination reaction in certain red cell antigens, including Kidd, MNS (but not s), Kell, Jk[a], Xg[a], Rh-C, Rh-c, Rh-E, Rh-e

dose A generic term for a quantity of a substance, medication, or radiation, that is administered or absorbed during a specific time period

dose equivalent H_T RADIATION PHYSICS The product of the absorbed dose in tissue, quality factor, and other modifying factors at the location of interest, which is measured in Sieverts (Sv or 100 rems)

dose-response curve A graphic representation of the effects that a series of dosage levels of an agent, eg ionizing radiation or a chemotherapeutic agent, has on a given parameter, eg cell viability, mutational frequency, DNA damage, tumor growth or metastasis or other behavior

dosimetry The formal science that measures and calculates the doses and format of radiation to be administered to a patient with a disease requiring radiotherapy, in particular malignancies; see Definitive radiation

dot blot MOLCULAR BIOLOGY Add in the clinical environment, can be used to quantify the copy numbers of multidrug resistance gene (Am Biotech Lab Jan 1995, p36)

dot (and blot) hemorrhages OPHTHALMOLOGY Relatively small hemorrhages seen in the inner nuclear layer that extend to the outer plexiform layer, typical of the retinal fundi of patients with diabetic retinopathy, which when seen in three dimensions, are anointed as 'serpiginous' hemorrhages

dot blotting MOLECULAR BIOLOGY A rapid ('quick and dirty'), hybridization technique for semiquantifying a specific RNA and DNA fragment in a specimen without performing the more time-consuming Northern and Southern blots METHOD The DNA is serially diluted and 'spotted' on a nitrocellulose or nylon membrane, denatured (ie one of the DNA strands is separated) with NaOH, then bathed in a solution containing a heat-denatured, presumably complementary DNA fragment (a 'probe') that is 'tagged' with a radiolabel, eg ^{32}P or ^{35}S, or a non-radioactive label, 2-acetyl-aminofluorene, which attaches to the guanine nucleotides; complementarity between the two single strands results in 'hybridization' that is detected by virtue of the probe's radiolabel through autoradiography or if biotinylated, by enzymatic digestion of a substrate, resulting in a color change detectable by spectrophotometry; see 'Quick and dirty'

dot-DAT Dot blot-direct antiglobulin test A variant of the Coombs test in which IgG is immobilized on a nitrocellulose membrane or solid phase; the patient's red cells are co-incubated on the membrane; subjective interpretation is essentially eliminated as the test need not be placed on a scale (1+ to 4+) as for the usual DAT, thereby reducing false positivity and negativity to a minimum

dot dystrophy OPHTHALMOLOGY A pattern of microcystic dystrophy occurring in healthy individuals, characterized macroscopically by groups of tiny, round or comma-shaped, gray-white opacities in the pupillary zones, uni- or bilaterally, corresponding to minute cystoid spaces

dot-ELISA Dot-enzyme linked immunosorbent assay A semiquantitative assay tused to detect the presence of a particular antigen by 'dotting' it on support medium and probing it with an antibody raised against the antigen, followed by the use of a detection system, eg 3,3'-diaminobenzidine (Arch Pathol Lab Med 1994; 118:1007oA)

dot hybridization Dot blotting see there

dot plot diagram Depiction of test results as a special type of scattergram in which the horizontal axis represents discrete categories rather than a continuous scale and the vertical axis is assigned values falling in a range; dot plots can depict many clinical states over a wide spectrum of health and disease, allowing projection of disease-positive and disease-negatives states, forming a basis from which multiple studies of diagnostic performance may be compared

double aorta A congenital cardiovascular defect of the aorta in which both of the dorsal embryonic aortae persist and encircle the trachea and esophagus; after birth, and consequent to the aorta's growth in a region with limited space, the ring produces a relative constriction, resulting in stridor and dysphagia; Cf Double-barrelled aorta

double-barrelled aorta An aorta with a second vascular lumen formed in the media of the aortic wall connecting the proximal and distal intimal tears in an aorta with a dissecting aneurysm; Cf Double aorta

double billing A form of health care fraud in which both a third-party payer and the patient or a second third-party payer are charged for the same service

double bind Any situation wherein both option A and its alternative option B have considerable disadvantages (Am Med News 19 Sept 1994) PSYCHIATRY An interpersonal dilemma in which an individual is presented with mutually contradictory messages by another person, usually one who is respected by or who has authority over the person receiving the 'mixed message'

double blinded study A clinical study in which both the patients and researchers are unaware of whether a patient is in the treatment or experimental drug arm or in the placebo arm of the study; see Blinding, Triple blinding; Cf Anecdotal

double 'boarded' An adjective referring to a physician who is board-certified by two separate specialty boards

double bolus approach CARDIOLOGY A regimen currently (mid-1995) under investigation, in which t-PA (tissue plasminogen activator, alteplase) is administered shortly after vascular occlusion in patients in the early stages of myocardial ischemia; DBA is believed by some authors to improve coronary artery revascularization and may minimize the size of myocardial infarcts (N Engl J Med 1995; 332:1443ED)

double bubble sign RADIOLOGY A radiographic sign in which there are two distinct gas pockets in an upper GI radiocontrast study in atresia of the second segment of the duodenum, 20-30% of whom have Down syndrome; the larger left bubble corresponds to gastric gas; the smaller right corresponds to gas in the duodenal bulb; the double bubble may also occur in an annular pancreas with or without duodenal atresia, duodenal stenosis, peritoneal bands and volvulus Note: The duodenal bubble is correspondingly smaller if there is passage of air; see Bubble

double condom sign SUBSTANCE ABUSE A finding seen by barium enema in body packers, who swallow doubly and triply wrapped condoms filled with heroin and cocaine in order to escape detection by the US customs when deplaning from Nigeria, Colombia and elsewhere; the condoms at the time of packaging, trap annular air pockets, revealing the 'double condom'; see 'Body packing'

double contrast studies RADIOLOGY A technique used to enhance visualization of the intestinal mucosa; after a cleansing enema of tap water, administered with atropine to prevent potential volume overload-induced vaso-vagal syncope, the patient ingests a suspension of a milkshake-like radiocontrast solution, eg 1 g of Barosperse, Intropaque or others per 2 ml water; the contrast is allowed to flow to the splenic flexure in the prone patient and followed by insufflation of air and rotation of the patient to his back, maintaining the left side elevated; further manipulation of the patient occurs under fluoroscopic control and spot films are taken to monitor the study; single contrast studies identify 77% of colonic lesions > 1.0 cm and 18% of those < 1.0 cm, compared to 98% in > 1.0 cm lesions by double contrast and 78% in lesions < 1.0 cm; it is less commonly used for colitis, given the high correlation with endoscopy and facile access of the endoscope

double diffusion IMMUNOPATHOLOGY A semiquantitative method for detecting an antibody (or antigen) in a system; a known antigen is placed in a well cut in a block of agar; a test serum which may have the antibody is placed in a second well; the two molecules migrate in a centrifugal fashion; if an antibody and its antigen are present in the system, eg Ouchterlony technique a precipitation line occurs that is detectable by Coomassie Blue staining

double dipping see Antikickback law

double discordance PEDIATRIC CARDIOLOGY Corrected transposition of the pulmonary arteries and aorta The major cardiac arteries are in a mirror-image of their normal location, ie the aorta arises from the anterior left heart and the pulmonary artery from the right posterior heart, the blood from the morphologic right atrium reaches the pulmonary trunk by traversing a mitral valve and morphologic left ventricle; blood from the morphologic left atrium traverses the tricuspid valve and morphologic right ventricle reaching the aorta; the coronary arteries are similarly reversed, ie the right is anterior, the left, posterior; many of those with this complex have other cardiac malformations including conduction and ventricular septal defects, requiring surgical repair and carrying an operative mortality of 25% and a 60% ten-year survival

double duct sign GI RADIOLOGY Irregular, nodular, 'rat-tailed' obstruction or interruption of both the common bile duct and pancreatic duct, seen by endoscopic retrograde cholangiopancreatography (ERCP), a finding suggestive of pancreatic adenocarcinoma, especially if the remaining pancreatic duct is normal

double effect ETHICS The use of a dose of sedatives and anagesics in critically or terminally ill patients that is large enough to both relieve pain and suffering (the 'good' effect) and hasten their demise (the 'bad' effect); four criteria are required to ethically justify the use of a treatment with a double effect: 1) The act per se must be morally good 2) Only the good effects (ie relief of suffering or pain) of the act are intended 3) The good effect (relief of suffering) must not be brought about by the bad effect (death) 4) There must be a compelling reason for permitting the bad effect (JAMA 1992; 268:1858L)

double gloving The use of two gloves when performing medical interventions in which there is contact with bio-hazardous materials; the use of two gloves is a practice that minimizes the hazards inherent in contact with body fluids, as latex gloves are prone to perforation*; the inner glove of a two-glove set is perforated in 3% (Am J Roentgenol 1992; 159:131)

*1% of unused gloves have defects; the perforation rate is circa 7% in gloves worn < 2 hours and 23% when worn > 2 hours

double helix A structural motif described by Watson and Crick and classically associated with DNA* which consists of paired nucleobases attached to a deoxyribose phosphate backbone; the importance of nucleobases in the double helix is obvious, but that of the deoxyribose phosphate backbone is not; peptide nucleic acids may also form a DNA-like double helix (Nature 1994; 368:561oa), raising interesting questions in terms of the evolution of the primordial soup

*So much so that the two terms DNA and double helix are often used interchangeably

double immunodiffusion IMMUNOLOGY A technique used to identify the presence of an antigen (Ag) in a solution by placing it and its cognate antibody (Ab) in separate wells cut in an immunologically inert gel and allowing the Ag and Ab to diffuse toward each other; the region of Ag-Ab contact is indicated by a line of precipitation; partial identity is indicated by a spur

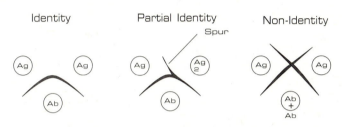

Double immunodiffusion

double knockout technique A generic term for the disruption (eg by homologous recombination) of two normal, but presumably related cellular genes in an animal model, most commonly in mice to evaluate the phenotypic effect of the absence of the genes of interest (Nature 1995; 374:159, 118N&v) see Knockout mice

double-labeled water method CLINICAL NUTRITION A technique used to measure the total energy expenditure which is accurate to within ± 5%; DLW method is based on the calculation of CO_2 production from the differential disappearance rates of two stable radioisotopes (^{16}O and ^2H) from the body and is of use in identifying whether diet resistant obesity is due to a discrepancy between the actual caloric intake and exercise a defect or alteration in thermogenesis (N Engl J Med 1992; 327:1893 oa,1947ED) see Eye-mouth gap

double labeling study IMMUNOLOGY A technique in which a cell or tissue is labeled with two or more different antibodies each of which is linked to an different immunofluorochrome, allowing the simultaneous detection of two antigens of interest (Arch Pathol Lab Med 1992; 116:622oa)

double minutes MOLECULAR BIOLOGY Redundant doublet and tetrad fragments (minutes) of chromosomes that may be seen when normal cells are exposed to methotrexate or which appear in malignant cells as localized reduplications of DNA, see HSR (homogenously staining regions) or as independent paired chromosomal fragments seen in a quinacrine-stained chromosome preparation

double pneumonia An obsolete term for bilateral lobar pneumonia, a vanishingly rare condition; double pneumonia also refers to combined viral-bacterial pneumonias which may follow each other, eg an initial *Staphylococcus aureus* infection, causing a one hundred-fold enhancement of infectivity and increased multiplication rate of influenza viruses through production of a hemagglutinin-cleaving enzyme

double parenthesis structure INFECTIOUS DISEASE A popular descriptive term for the LM morphology of a structure found in the cysts of *Pneumocystis carinii* which have a redundant curved lamination; DPSs in a bronchoalveolar lavage and other similar specimens are reported to be 100% specific for *P carinii*; the exact nature of DPS is

uncertain, although it is thought by some authors to correspond to redundant membrano-tubular extensions (Arch Pathol Lab Med 1995; 119:142oa)

double reading A generic term for the interpretation of any form of visual image, eg from pathology (cytology, surgical pathology) or radiology (CT, MRI, mammography) by either a second 'pair of eyes' (ie pathologist or radiologist) or by the same physician at a different diagnostic session; in Sweden, DR results in a 10-15% ↑ in cancer detection (N Engl J Med 1994; 331:1521sa)

double ring appearance OPHTHALMOLOGY A small pale double-contoured spot corresponding to the retinal nerve head surrounded by a pigmented or pale ring, seen in optic nerve hypoplasia, attributed to a primary defect in retinal ganglion cell or axonal differentiation, resulting in visual field defects varying in severity from blindness to virtually normal vision; asymmetrical hypoplasia presents as deviation (strabismus) towards the good eye, not often recognized early enough to reverse the commonly associated visual loss

double set-up examination OBSTETRICS A two-team approach for a high-risk, eg placenta previa, vaginal delivery, where the first team is prepared for a normal, ie uneventful, vaginal delivery, while the second team, including an anesthesiologist and gynecologist, is on alert should the delivery 'go sour', ready to perform an immediate cesarean section; see Cesarean section

double wall sign EMERGENCY MEDICINE A radiological finding on a plain supine abdominal film caused by rupture of a hollow gastrointestinal viscus, eg stomach, duodenum or colon, where free air (pneumoperitoneum) outlines the falciform ligament and enhances visualization of loops of small intestine; see inverted 'V' sign

double whammy 'syndrome' The ability to propulse the eyeball out of its socket, performed by simultaneously contracting the superior and inferior oblique external ocular muscles and orbicularis while relaxing the rectus muscles, with some assistance by external digital pressure; this 'condition' is not associated with pathology and may be performed as a parlor trick

double zone of hemolysis MICROBIOLOGY A finding on a blood culture plate consisting of an inner zone of complete β-hemolysis and an outer zone of partial hemolysis, a finding characteristic of *Clostridium perfringens*; see Hemolysis

doubling time A parameter used to determine tumor aggressiveness, serving to prognosticate, objectively measure therapeutic success, quantify growth kinetics and growth rate of a malignancy; tumor doubling time tends to be characteristic for a particular tumor: 1.5-5 days for Burkitt's lymphoma, 4 days for ALL, 25 days for early breast cancer, 125 days for advanced breast cancer (the growth rate is slower due to the central necrosis); 135 days for pulmonary adenocarcinoma; often by the time a tumor reaches a clinically detectable size of about one cm, it comprises a mass containing 10^9 cells and has undergone 30 doublings; 10 further doublings result in a one-kg tumor mass, which, given the hypermetabolism of most malignancies, may be sufficient to make most patients very sick or cause death; the tumor doubling rate does not truly reflect tumor growth since an increasing proportion of daughter cells enter the G_o or resting phase of the growth cycle; in large malignancies, only 10% of the tumor's cells may be proliferating at any one time; successful chemotherapy hinges on the proportion of cells actively proliferating and therefore susceptible to these agents; Cf Gompertzian growth curve

doughnut *adjective* A commonly used descriptor referring or pertaining to a targetoid lesion or radiodensity in which the central and peripheral fields are relatively more radiodense or darker that the middle field *noun* GENERAL SURGERY A sleeve of tissue that is excised after a major GI tract resection, often of the distal colon, when a carcinoma extends close to the margin of the original segment Note: Doughnut excisions are most commonly used for infiltrating adenocarcinomas of the lower rectum, where salvage of sphincter function is a function of the length of the tissue available for anastomosis

Note: Today's doughnuts originated from sweet breads in 16th century Holland and acquired the hole in the early 1800s, an innovation claimed by both the Pennsylvania Dutch and a sea captain, Hanson Gregory

doughnut granuloma 'Fibrin ring' A lipid granuloma composed of epithelioid histiocytes, neutrophils, mononuclear or 'round' inflammatory cells, giant cells and a central cleared lipid vacuole; while a characteristic finding in Q fever (*Coxiella burnetii*), it occurs in less than ½ of cases and is located in the bone marrow and liver

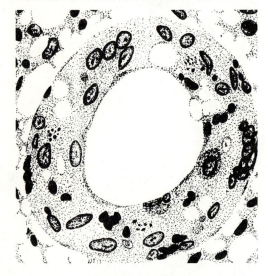

doughnut granuloma

doughnut kidney A rare congenital renal malformation, formed by the fusion of the renal anlagen prior to its rotation and caudal migration; the kidneys are located on the sacral prominence or in the pelvic floor; the ureteropelvic junctions emerge anteriorly and the blood vessels enter posteriorly; Cf Disk and Horseshoe kidneys

doughnut sign CARDIOVASCULAR IMAGING A descriptor for the radionuclide image of a large anterior wall myocardial infarction in which there is decreased uptake of 99mTechnetium stannous pyrophospate in the central infarcted zone, surrounded by a zone of intermediate uptake; the doughnut sign is seen in larger infarcts and is associated with a poor prognosis GI ENDOSCOPY see Bull's-eye sign PULMONARY RADIOLOGY A well-circumscribed mass (coin lesion) with a central, rounded hypodense area corresponding to central tumor necrosis, usually associated with bronchogenic carcinoma, less commonly also seen in abscesses but these are often accompanied by a fluid level

doughnut structure IMMUNOLOGY A multimeric assembly of C9 complement protein monomers that are inserted into cells, forming a transmembranous pore through which a cell targeted by the complement cascade disintegrates, an event that follows the common pathway of the complement activation and the previous reversible assembly of a leaky patch MEMBRANE PHYSIOLOGY A homopolymeric protein contained within the outer wall of gram-negative bacteria and the outer membrane of mitochon-

dria that is freely permeable to small, < 10-kD molecules

dough sign HEMATOLOGY A morphological descriptor suggestive of monocytes, where the 'dough' represents the nuclei of blasts and promonocytes which have been squashed in the middle

doula OBSTETRICS According to the original Greek usage, a doula is an experienced woman who guides and assists a new mother in her infant-care tasks; in an early study in the US, the term doula was defined as a woman who provides emotional support to primiparous women during labor and delivery; adding a doula to the obstetric team is believed by some to reduce the need for a cesarean section, epidural anesthesia, use of oxytocin and duration of labor (**JAMA 1991; 265:2197**)

dowager's hump Dorsal kyphosis caused by multiple wedge fractures of the vertebral bodies as seen in type II (age-related) osteoporosis

Dowager, Old French for a widow with a title or property from her husband

downgrading reaction A subacute deterioration in the clinical and immune status in patients with leprosy accompanied by increased load of organisms, due either to poor drug compliance or to the emergence of a drug-resistant strain of *Mycobacterium leprae*; Cf Upgrading reaction

downregulate GENETICS To decrease the activity of a gene's transcriptional machinery usually by a protein that acts on a ??? region

downregulation PHYSIOLOGY The reduction of a cell's response to a hormone or other ligand by internalization of its cognate receptor and degradation within a coated pit; see Clathrin, Coated pit

downstream MOLECULAR BIOLOGY A descriptor for a location on a molecule of interest, eg protein or DNA that is 'before' or in front of a reference point DNA transcription Downstream refers to nucleotides located on the transcribed DNA strand from the 3' to 5' direction; the term downstream differs according to the system involved

DNA TRANSLATION: Direction on the messenger RNA strand from the 5' to 3' direction

ELECTRON TRANSPORT SYSTEM: Direction from the highest to the lowest level of energy

POLYPEPTIDE CHAIN: Direction of the linkage of the amino acids from the N- terminal to the C- terminal

REPLICATION: Direction of the replicating fork

downtime INSTRUMENTATION The amount of time an information system or other device is nonoperational, due to failure, malfunction, servicing, or shut-down; during the 1970s hospital and laboratory information system vendors guaranteed downtimes of < 5% (438 hours annually); in the current environment, unexpected downtimes of less than 0.25% (22 hours annually) are the norm (**CAP Today November 1993**) see Mean time between failure

'downward' negotiations The practice by grant-giving bodies of reducing the number of grants after they have been approved with the purpose of saving money; see 'Approved, but not funded'

doxorubicin Adriamycin An anthracycline antibiotic used to treat lymphoproliferative malignancies, including leukemia and solid tumors; it is associated with dose-dependent cardiotoxicity (those receiving more than 228 mg/m² have an increased incidence of ventricular failure, **N Engl J Med 1991; 324:808**), due to either free radicals or uncoiling of DNA secondary to DNA-binding by drug; see Chemotherapy

2,3 DPG Diphosphoglycerate An inorganic phosphate produced in red cells by the Rapoport-Luebering shunt; 2,3 DPG binds to the β chain of reduced hemoglobin, lowering hemoglobin's affinity for oxygen and by extension, facilitating oxygen release to the tissues, causing a 'right shift' of the oxygen dissociation curve; DPG further shifts the curve to the right by lowering the erythrocyte's pH; when transfused, red cells regain 50% of the 2,3 DPG within 3-8 hours and 100% within 24 hours; see Storage lesion

dpm Disintegrations per minute

DPT 1) see DTP vaccination 2) An analgesic-sedative 'cocktail' of Demerol, Phenergan and Thorazine

Dr Doctor, for most entries, see under Doctor

Dr Acer see Acer cluster

Dr Doe A surgeon who contracted HIV when he suffered a needle stick from an HIV-infected patient; he was fired (dismissed) from the hospital where he was working when he refused to give up his surgical practice (**Am Med News 24 April 1995 p10**)

D receptors see Dopamine receptors

dragged disc phenomenon A finding seen in advanced retrolental fibrodysplasia (retinopathy of prematurity), in which the scar in the optic fundus 'drags' the disc and retinal vessels, displacing the macula; when severe, a 'V'-shaped or funnel-shaped detachment of the retina may occur; see also Cat's-eye reflex

draw-a-person test PSYCHOLOGY A clinical test in which a person's character traits are inferred from the manner in which he/she drawsa human figure

dread disease rider A clause in a health insurance policy that pays additional benefits for certain diseases known to incur high financial costs, eg extensive burns or cancer and/or cause significant and permanent residual morbidity, ie loss of eyes or limbs; Cf Catastrophic illness, Trolley car policy

dread risk A risk (eg of HIV infection from transfused blood) over which a person has no control and which may have catastrophic consequences (**N Engl J Med 1995; 332:740ED**) Cf Unknown risk

dream A series of images and thought processes that occur during sleep, which in the framework of psychoanalysis, dreams are believed to have latent and manifest content Eyelid movement and REM sleep coincides; dreaming is more common in REM sleep; while it is uncertain how dreams occur, the most widely accepted paradigm of dreaming is the Hobson model*; as a person goes to sleep, the adrenergic system shuts down, and the cholinergic system gears up, uncoupling the neural networks integral to cognition and behavior; and becoming sensitive to random thoughts resulting in juxtaposed images that may be contradictory; the cholinergic system fires in bursts known as pontine-geniculate-occipital waves, see there (**New York Times 16 July 1994; C1**)

*Dr Alan Hobson, Harvard University

dream team A generic term for any group of people involved in same field of endeavor, eg sports, scientific research, belles artes, who are widely regarded as being the top in their respective areas of expertise, and who, when their talents are pooled in an activity would be expected to achieve synergistic results that can only be dreamed about (**Science 1995; 268:191**)

DREZ Dorsal root end zone One of the central nervous system pathways that may be surgically sectioned to relieve chronic pain (other sites include the anterolateral cord and the trigeminal tract); DREZ lesions are produced by thermal coagulation or laser and relieve 65-70% of the intractable pain associated with brachial and lumbar plexus avulsion and spinal cord trauma

DRGs Diagnosis-related groups A system of classifying patients according to diagnosis, length of hospital stay and therapy received that was developed in the US in the 1970s by a group at Yale University as a mechanism of utilization review; the DRGs are derived from all of the possible diagnoses in the International Classification of Disease (ICD-9-CM) system, classifying them into 23 major diagnostic categories based on organ systems, then further breaking them down into 470 distinct groups; DRGs are used as a form of cost containment intended to limit the wastage of medical services and were adopted in 1983 by Medicare as a mechanism of paying hospitals, changing from a cost-based, retrospective-reimbursement system to a prospective payment system, giving hospitals a financial incentive for reducing health care costs; numerical coding and accuracy have become crucial for both the hospital and reimbursement agencies; the coding error rate is about 20% and approximately 60% of these errors favor the hospital; Cf CPT coding

DRG creep 'Creep' HEALTH CARE REIMBURSEMENT A method of coding of diagnosis-related groups (DRGs) under Medicare's prospective payment plan in a fashion that does not conform to the 'optimization' rules governing coding DRGs, usually erring in favor of the hospital, ie paying the hospital more than it is entitled to; causes of 'creep' include mis-specification, miscoding and resequencing (**N Engl J Med 1988; 318:352**) see Case-mix index, DRGs, Optimization

drift see Antigenic drift

drift parameter EPIDEMIOLOGY A coefficient that reflects the long-term forces (eg period and cohort trends) acting on the rates of major depression over time (**JAMA 1992; 268:3098oc**)

drinking water see Maximum contaminant levels, Tapwater

'drip' A colloquial term for the purulent penile discharge beginning 2-5 days after *Neisseria gonorrhoeae* infection, caused by neisserial endotoxins, and seen in other neisserial infections, including *N meningitidis, N catarrhalis,* as well as *N flava, Mima polymorpha, M polymorpha* var *oxidans* and *Chlamydia trachomatis*; chronic thin mucopurulent discharges are colloquially known as 'gleet'

drive-by shooting A phenomenon of recent vintage in the US in which one or more persons (commonly members of street gangs) open fire à la Al Capone from moving vehicles, often in retaliation for an alleged wrong-doing by a rival gang, catching various innocent victims in the crossfire DATA OF INTEREST In one study, 677 adolescents and children were shot at, 429 had gunshot wounds (mostly in arms and legs), 36 (5.3%) died of the wounds; 71% were members of gangs, handguns were used in 73%, and 31% of these were semiautomatic (commonly 9mm); shotguns were used in 13%; use of assault weapons was rare; in 15 incidents, multiple weapons were used; all homicide victims were African-American or Hispanic; 97% were male; the most popular month was August (data from Los Angeles, 1991)

Note: In 1991, in Los Angeles, there were a total of 1548 drive-by shootings in which 2222 people were shot at, including the 677 adolescents and children studied by HR Hutson et al (**N Engl J Med 1994; 330:324oA, 1833c**)

driving while intoxicated PUBLIC HEALTH Motor vehicle accidents are the leading cause of non-disease-related death in the US (± 35 000, 1992); ½ are attributed to alcohol; the risk of a fatal accident is linked to ↑ blood alcohol levels (BAL); a person with a BAL of 22 mmol/L (100 mg/dL) is 7-fold more likely to be involved in a fatal motor vehicle accident; and a person with a BAL of 33 mmol/L (150 mg/dL) is 25-fold more likely to be so involved; those arrested once for DWI have an ↑ risk (4.3-fold if 21-35; 11.7-fold if > 35 years old) of being subsequently involved in a fatal alcohol-related accident (**N Engl J Med 1994; 331:513sA**); it is estimated that for every arrest, 1000 episodes of drunk driving are not discovered (**New York Times May 22, 1994; A1**)

Note: Over ½ of the reckless drivers who are not intoxicated with alcohol were found to be intoxicated with other drugs, eg marijuana and cocaine (**N Engl J Med**

1994; 331:537⊞)

drooping lily sign RADIOLOGY A descriptor for a pattern seen in intravenous pyelography, caused by obstruction with eventual development of hydronephrosis of the superior pelvis in renal duplication (not visualized), causing inferior and lateral displacement of the renal pelvis; the normal renal pelvis has an oblique line paralleling the psoas muscle—here the renal pelvis runs inferior and medially)

drop attack NEUROLOGY An episodic and precipitous loss of motor function, where the victim is either standing or walking and suddenly the legs give way and the subject plummets, fully conscious to the floor; the idiopathic form is most common in middle-aged to elderly women, attributed to age-related defects in reflexes; drop attacks may also occur in vertibrobasilar ischemia, acute labyrinthine vertigo, cataplexy, 'plateau waves'; drop attacks with loss of consciousness occur in syncope and seizures

droplet nuclei EPIDEMIOLOGY 1-3 μg in diameter particles of liquid that contain single or small clumps of bacteria; droplet nuclei are considered the infective unit for airborne respiratory infections

drowning A mechanism of death that claims 7000 lives annually in the US, comprising 15% of the non-motor vehicle-related accidental deaths; death occurs by asphyxia due to submersion, especially in water with aspiration of fluid in 90% of cases accompanied by hypoxemia **FRESH WATER DROWNING**, hypo-osmolar water affects the surface tension of alveolar surfactant, resulting in an imbalance in the V/Q ratio with a collapse of some alveoli, resulting in both true or absolute and relative intrapulmonary shunting; the V/Q abnormality is further compromised by pulmonary edema; the shifts of fluids and electrolytes in fresh water drowning result in hemodilution, hemolysis, circulatory overload, and hyponatremia **SALT WATER DROWNING**, sea water aspiration results in fluid-filled but perfused alveoli, accompanied by a V/Q abnormality due to pulmonary edema; the shifts of fluids and electrolytes in salt water drowning result in hemoconcentration, CHF, and hypernatremia; in both forms, hypercapnia is corrected quickly, while hypoxemia and metabolic acidosis tend to persist MANAGEMENT The 'standard' ABC of CPR are recommended, accompanied by intubation, placement of a venous line, if necessary, and use of continuous positive airway pressure (CPAP), treatment of hyperthermia; the abdominal thrust maneuver (see there) is no longer recommended for routine use PROGNOSIS The main priority in near-drowning is the prevention of brain injury; parameters that adversely influence 'intact' survival include delays in initiating CPR, severe metabolic acidosis (pH < 7.1), asystole on arrival to the hospital, fixed and dilated pupils, and a low (< 5) Glasgow score (**N Engl J Med 1993; 328:6254**RA) PATHOPHYSIOLOGY 'DRY' DROWNING Asphyxiation secondary to prolonged glottic spasm that persists beyond apnea; the lungs demonstrate little water IMMERSION SYNDROME Cardiac arrest due to an intense vasovagal discharge, the 'diving' reflex 'Secondary' drowning Death occurs 15 minutes to 72 hours after rescue, caused by intense pulmonary edema and adult respiratory distress syndrome 'WET' DROWNING Laryngospasm followed by relaxation and aspiration of copious amounts of fluid (the most common form); the site of drowning death may be determined by analysis of the lung fluids, eg in brackish water, microscopy reveals diatoms; the mechanism of death is a function of the type of water MECHANISM OF DEATH (MOD)–FRESH WATER DROWNING Ventricular fibrillation with a rapid increase in potassium (> 8 mg/dl) secondary to osmotic hemolysis of red cells in the lungs, with death occurring 2-4 minutes after submersion MOD-ICE-COLD WATER 'DROWNING' DEATH Vaso-vagal cardiac arrest, and thus does not per se represent drowning MOD-SALT-

WATER DROWNING Myocardial ischemia, and occurs 6-7 minutes after submersion MOD-SWIMMING POOL DROWNING Massive pulmonary edema related to chlorinated water

DRPLA Dentatorubral and pallidoluysian atrophy, see there

drug abuse see Substance abuse

drug of abuse A generic nonspecific term for virtually any agent that can be used (usually self-administered) outside of context for which it was originally intended; although this definition is usually synonymous with illegal 'recreational' drugs (eg marijuana, cocaine, heroin), it may also encompass controlled prescription drugs that are abused for various reasons, as well as alcohol and nicotine

drug-baby case Legal medicine *An expectant mother is protected by a constitutional right to privacy and bodily integrity which the state may not violate without showing a compelling state interest* (**NY Newsday; A29, 22 March 1995**)

drug challenge The administration of a drug suspected of causing an adverse drug reaction in order to determine its culpability in the adverse effect; drug challenges are used in detecting aspirin sensitivity, and for identifying adverse reactions to contrast media, and local anesthetics

drug of choice CLINICAL THERAPEUTICS A generic term for any drug or medication that is regarded as being the best agent or first agent to use when treating a particular disease; in general, DOCs have the lowest toxicity and the widest therapeutic range of the drugs, Cf Second-line drug

drug-drug interaction A generic term for any interaction between two therapeutic agents

drug holiday A time period in which a prescribed drug is proscribed; DHs are regarded as being a means by which the total dose of antipsychotic drugs can be reduced, thereby decreasing the incidence of tardive dyskinesia; it is unknown whether DHs actually achieve this goal

'drug lag' CLINICAL THERAPEUTICS A term analogous to the 'missile gap' of the Cold War, coined by the pharmaceutical industry indicating its disapproval of the prolonged delays that occur before a new pharmaceutical agent is allowed in the US drug marketplace; see NDA (New drug application)

drug monograph A document promulgated by the US Food and Drug Administration specifying the ingredients and composition a prescription drug may contain, the conditions for which it may be prescribed, directions for its use, warnings concerning potential side effects and other relevant information; once a drug monograph is released, any company that meets the drug's monograph requirements may produce and market the drug under its own name without seeking special approval from the FDA, as long as there are no current applicable patents on the drug's formula

drug mule SUBSTANCE ABUSE A generic term for any living or nonliving vehicle used to smuggle illicit drugs, usually from the country of origin to a country where they will be purchased for a substantial profit; DMs include batteries, busts, concrete fence posts, dead parrots*, dog kennels, fishes, horses, ice cream cones, mannekins, snakes, surfboards, vegetables, and a menagerie of other devices (**NY Times Magazine 11 June 1995, p44**) see Body packer syndrome
*Monty Python afficionados take note

drug recognition PUBLIC HEALTH A rigorous, standardized 'discovery' program for recognizing and analyzing suspected drug abuse that may endanger public health or safety; DR is being implemented law enforcement officers to overcome the limits of devices (eg the breathalyzer) and physical examinations (eg walking a straight line) that identifiy drivers under the influence of alcohol, but not of substances of abuse, eg cocaine, marijuana, cocaine, or others; parameters used in the DR process include pupil reactivity, blood pressure, examination of conjunctiva; the DR program divides substances into 7 categories: CNS depressants eg alcohol; CNS stimulants eg cocaine, amphetamines hallucinogens eg LSD; narcotic analgeics eg heroin, Demerol, codeine; phencyclidine (PCP) and its relatives; *Cannabis*, eg marijuana, hashish; inhalants, eg glue (New York Times 5 Dec 1993; 49)

drug-resistant tuberculosis Multidrug-resistant tuberculosis, see there

drug screening CLINICAL TOXICOLOGY A generic term for any rapid method for identifying the presence of one or more drugs of abuse, usually in the urine, by one of several widely stat methods, including EMIT (enzyme-mediated immunologic technique), FPIA (fluorescence polarization immunoassay), and TLC (thin-layer chromatography); DS is used in emergency departments, or in the context of preemployment testing and is used to identify commonly abused substances, eg cocaine, opiates, tranquilizers, sedatives (barbiturates), and hallucinogens (PCP, LSD, tetrahydrocannabinol)

drug tapering The gradual discontinuation or reduction of the dose of a drug required by the patient over a prolonged period of time, but which either have toxicity sufficient to make 'permanent' therapy undesirable or have a deleterious cumulative effect; for certain drugs, eg corticosteroids, antiepileptic medications, abrupt disocontinuation may be a shock to the system, or cause a recurrence in the disease being treated, eg recurrence of seizure activity; it was thought that antiepileptic drugs required up to nine months before the drug continuation; it has been reported that drug tapering over six weeks is equally effective (N Engl J Med 1994; 330:1407OA)

drumstick appendages CYTOGENETICS A mass of X chromatin that is attached to one of the lobes of a polymorphonuclear leukocyte; in accord with the Lyon hypothesis, cells demonstrate one 'drumstick' (or Barr body) less than the karyotype number, a characteristic of sexual dimorphism, ie normal; thus an XY male has none, an XX female or XXY Klinefelter syndrome each have one, an XXX 'superfemale' has two and so on

drumstick fingers see Clubbing

drumstick spores see Tennis racquet spores

drunkenness The state of acute alcohol-induced inebriation, which is a factor in ½ of the 35 000 motor vehicle accidents that occur per year in the US; it plays a critical role in domestic violence, drownings, falls, fires, homelessness, homicides, and suicides (N Engl J Med 1994; 331:537ED)

drusen OPHTHALMOLOGY Yellow-white, occasionally confluent nodules composed of aggregated abnormal glycoproteins and glycolipids produced by and adjacent to the basal cells of the retinal pigment epithelium; drusen are the earliest stage of senile degeneration of the macula and is a finding suggestive of retinitis pigmentosa; by low-power light microscopy, drusen appear as nodules filled with homogeneous wispy debris, corresponding to basement membrane material

dry chemistry LABORATORY MEDICINE YD Dry chemical technology (eg Ektachem, Eastman Kodak Co) is generally more costly per test, but claims certain advantages including automation and biosafety, ↑ productivity of laboratory workers, better turnaround time, and as it does not require a water source or drainage, is amenable to point-of-care testing of the same quality and virtually the same menu of tests* as that provided by the central laboratory (Am Clin Lab June 1994)

*Acid phosphatase, albumin, alcohol, alkaline phosphatase, ALT, ammonia, amylase, AST, BUN, calcium, CO_2, chloride, cholesterol, cholinesterase, CK, CKMB, conjugated bilirubin, creatinine, GGT, glucose, HDL-cholesterol, iron, lactate, LDH, lipase, magnesium, phosphorus, potassium, salicylate, sodium, theophylline, total bilirubin, total iron-binding capacity, total protein, TGs,

unconjugated bilirubin, uric acid

dry drowning A phenomenon described in 90% of successfully resuscitated drowning victims, in whom aspirated water is minimal, presumably the result of reflex laryngospasm with airway obstruction and asphyxia; a rapid return of spontaneous ventilation is typical if CPR is begun early and the period of anoxia brief; see Drowning; Cf Wet drowning

dry gangrene A condition caused by chronic occlusion that slowly progresses to severe tissue atrophy and mummification, often associated with peripheral vascular disease, eg diabetes mellitus, atherosclerosis; see Gangrene

dry pleurisy Plastic pleuritis A complication of acute bacterial pneumonia, tuberculosis or rheumatic fever CLINICAL Pain and guarding on inspiration, with patients lying on the affected side to 'splint' HISTOPATHOLOGY Multiple serofibrinous adhesions on the visceral pleura, which may, if intense, cause a fibrothorax

dry socket Alveolar osteitis ODONTOLOGY A complication seen in 1-2% of all tooth extractions, most commonly in molar tooth extraction wounds consisting of focal osteomyelitis in which the clot in the socket disintegrates prematurely and becomes a nidus for oral bacteria, characterized by severe pain and foul odor without purulence; once established, the condition responds poorly to therapy and must be aggressively prevented and treated with tetracycline, either locally or systemically at the time of extraction

'dry tap' HEMATOLOGY A needle biopsy of bone marrow, usually obtained from the iliac crests, in which either only blood without clot or no material at all is obtained (a true 'dry tap'); dry taps are due to reticulum fibrosis, marrow necrosis or an extremely packed marrow, occurring in 5-10% of all marrow biopsies; at least 60% of dry taps are malignant; most are lymphoproliferative disorders, including hairy cell leukemia, acute myelocytic leukemia, myelofibrosis, lymphoma and myeloma, the remainder are metastatic carcinomas, with benign disease accounting for the remainder, eg iron deficiency, marrow hypoplasia, hemosiderosis, granulomas and pernicious anemia of dry taps

***Dryopithecus* spp** PALEOANTHROPOLOGY The first discovered of the large fossil apes, which is among the best-known of the apes from the Miocene (± 10-12 million years ago) period, which is thought to be more closely related to great apes and humans than to gibbons (Nature 1993; 365:543, 494)

DSAP Disseminated superficial actinic porokeratosis A benign condition of sun-exposed skin, in particular of the extremities that affects light-skinned individuals living in sunny climates, which is characterized by horny papules arising in an erythematous base; it is thought to occur in a substrate of immunocompromise

DSM Diagnostic and Statistic Manual of Mental Disorders A document produced by the American Psychiatric Association in Washington, DC that standardizes the criteria required for establishing the diagnosis of psychiatric nosologies; the DSM terminology conforms to that of the ICD-10 (10th edition of the International Classification of Diseases, published in 1992); DSM-I was released in 1952, DSM-II in 1968, DSM-III in 1980, which was subsequently revised in 1987 as the DSM-III-R; the most recent edition, DSM-IV was released in 1994*

*DSM-IV terminology has been (where possible) incorporated in the present work–Author's note

DSM-IV The most recent of edition of the DSM, released in 1994 CRITICISM Strict adherence to DSM-IV guidelines for defining diseases means that many healthy people could be redefined in some fashion as having one or more mental disorders, such reductions ad absurdum include poor spelling or illegible penmanship*, which would be listed as Disorders of Written Expression (code 315.2); a tomboy could be diagnosed as having a gender-related personality disorder, or a student imbibing an excess of alcohol in a socially-appropriate situation in college or university as being an alcoholic (Sci Am 1994; 270/9:17)

*Facetiously regarded in some parts as being a sine qua non physcian 'skill'

DSM-IV MULTIAXIAL CLASSIFICATION

AXIS I Clinical disorders or other specific conditions, eg depression, neurosis that may be the focus of attention

AXIS II Specific personality disorder (PD), eg paranoid PD, narcissistic PD, obsessive-compulsive PD, OR mental retardation (eg reading or language disorder)

AXIS III General medical conditionsedical or physical conditions that may contribute to disease

AXIS IV Psychosocial stressors, eg marital status

AXIS V Highest level of adaptive function within the past year, eg functiioning in the workplace must rework table

*Diagnostic and Statistical Manual of Mental Disorders, American Psychiatric Association, Washington, DC, 1994

DSS gene DSS = Dosage-sensitive sex reversal A gene located on the X chromosome, which when two copies are present is capable of feminizing an otherwise chromosomally ♂ fetus; if the DSS gene is completely absent, some ♂ have abdominal testis; ♀ are may be unaffected as they usually have at least one normal X chromosome (New York Times 30 August 1994; C1)

d4T AIDS Stavudine A recently approved drug that inhibits reverse transcriptase (RT), which may be used in patients who are refractory to therapy with other RT inhibitors, eg AZT, ddI, ddC (New York Times 28 June 1994)

DTAA di-tryptophan aminal acetaldehyde; see Eosinophilic myalgia syndrome

DTPA 99mTc diethylenetriamine pentaacetic acid A radionuclide used to evaluate renal perfusion for bilateral comparison of blood flow

DTP COMPUTERS Desktop publishing INFECTIOUS DISEASE Diphtheria, tetanus, poliovirus (vaccine) NEUROLOGY Distal tingling on percussion

DTP vaccine An immunizing vaccine against diphtheria, tetanus and pertussis, containing a mixture of formaldehyde-inactivated diphtheria and tetanus toxoids and a sterile suspension of killed *Bordetella pertussis*; the recommended schedule for administration is at 2, 4, 6 and 15 months, a booster at 4-6 years and a repeat of the tetanus and diphtheria toxoids at ages 14-16; CONTRAINDICATIONS Acute febrile or during suspected evolving neurological illness or when a previous DTP resulted in an allergic reaction; although lifelong protection is not conferred by natural disease or immunization, most cases are prevented by the DTP vaccine Note: The pertussis component of the DTP vaccine may cause neurologic complications, which are uncommon (Pediatrics 1988; 81:345); a genetically engineered mutant for use in a vaccine is under development (Science 1989; 246:497)

Dᵘ TRANSFUSION MEDICINE A recently retired (AABB Standards, 15th ed, 1993) designation for a type of Rh antigenicity defined as 'agglutination by some, but not all, anti-Rh antigens;' Dᵘ was subdivided into low-grade Dᵘ, ie those cells that agglutinate only in the indirect antiglobulin (Coombs') test, and high-grade Dᵘ, defined by the older slide versus saline test; Dᵘ is now known as 'weak D'

dual degree A generic adjective referring to the earning two advanced degrees, eg MD (medical doctor), MBA (masters' of business administration); MD, MPH (masters' of public health); MD, PhD (doctor of philosophy)

dual diagnosis disease PSYCHIATRY A popular term for the combined findings of both a psychiatric disorder and a substance-abuse disorder (N Engl J Med 1994; 331:750BR)

dual relationship PROFESSIONAL ETHICS Any situation in which a physician-patient relationship may be 'contaminated' by the existance of a second relationship, eg business or financial relationships, romantic involvement, or blood or marital relatedness; the ancient tradition of a physician not treating his own family stems from the concern that in maintaining both relationships, the physician's decision-making capacity may be jeopardized and his/her objectivity compromised (JAMA 1995; 273:1445) see Professional boundaries

dual relationship ETHICS Any situation in which a physician-patient relationship may be 'contaminated' by the existance of a second relationship, eg business or financial relationships, romantic involvement, or blood or marital relatedness; the ancient tradition of a physician not treating his own family stems from the concern that in maintaining both relationships, the physician's decision-making capacity may be jeopardized and his/her objectivity compromised (JAMA1995; 273:1445) see Professional boundaries

dualism HEMATOLOGY The posit that all cells in the general circulation derive from either a lymphoid or myeloid precursor or stem cell

DUB Dysfunctional uterine bleeding, see there

Duchenne muscular dystrophy An X-linked recessive disease [MIM 310200] caused by a deficiency of the muscle protein dystrophin[1], which affects 1:3500 males[2], resulting in progressive muscular atrophy and wasting with death by age 20 often related to respiratory (due to compromised diaphragm activity) or cardiac failure; the calf and deltoid muscles display the typical finding of pseudohypertrophy; when *mdx* mice (the model for DMD, which also has a defective dystrophin gene) express a recombinant gene (full length complementary DNA) encoding dystrophin, muscle destruction is prevented, muscle fiber morphology and function normalizes, leading to normal power and force of the diaphragm (Nature 1993; 364:725; 673N&V) see Climbing up on oneself, Dystrophin, Pseudohypertrophy

[1]Lesser degrees of loss or alteration of the dystrophin gene results in the clinically more benign Becker's muscle dystrophy, which has a longer survival
[2]Manifest by males, carried by females

Duesberg, P A well-respected molecular biologist from the University of California who has taken the unusual position that the cause-and-effect relation between AIDS and infection by human immunodeficiency virus (HIV), remains unproven (Nature 1991; 350:10c)

Dugas, Gaetan see Patient 'Zero'

Duke Activity Status Index CARDIOLOGY A measure of functional capacity based on a 12-item questionnaire that correlates well with peak oxygen uptake during exercise testing; the DASI varies from 0 to 58.2, with higher scores indicating greater functional capacity (JAMA 1995; 273: 1187)

Dukes classification A system for prognosticating colorectal carcinoma (table) that has been modified with time: Dukes' original classification of intestinal wall invasion (J Pathol 1932; 35:323) recognized only three categories: 1) Limited to the bowel wall, 2) Through the bowel wall, and 3) Regional lymph node involvement by tumor; the most widely used permutation of the 'Dukes' is that of Astler and Coller, in which the carcinoma is divided into depth of invasion of the mucosa, muscularis propria and serosa (Ann Surg 1954; 139:846), with addition of a D distal metastasis group, (Ann Surgery 1967; 166:4290) and tallying of involved lymph nodes (N Engl J Med 1984; 310:737)

Note: The TNM classification of colonic adenocarcinoma is increasingly preferred by surgical pathologists; see TNM classification

dumbbell Barbell An adjectival descriptor applied to a tubular structure with terminal bulbous enlargement and central constriction

dumbbell bones A descriptor for the shortened and terminally enlarged long bones seen in the hyperplastic metaphysis in metatropic dwarfism; the descriptor has also been applied to the end-stage of subperiosteal hemorrhages with calcification of the periosteum as may occur in resolving scurvy

dumbbell gallbladder see Hourglass gall bladder

dumbbell tumors A nonspecific term for any of a variety of tumors, most of which are benign, all of which have a central constriction 1) Carcinoid 'Iceberg' tumor A submucosal tumor located in the large bronchi, 15% of which metastasize 2) Ganglioneuroma A tumor located in a vertebral body that may cause bony resorption or erosion of the pedicles 3) Leiomyoma A tumor of the gastrointestinal tract with both intra- and extraluminal components 4) Neurofibroma A tumor located on either side of the intervertebral foramina impinging on the spinal cord, usually thoracic with central constriction or 'pinching' of the tumor by the thick fibers of the intervertebral discs 5) Paraspinal neuroblastoma A tumor with intraspinal extension that has a central constriction by the spinal ligaments 6) Pleomorphic adenoma A tumor that extends through the gap between the ascending ramus of the jaw and the styloid process and stylomandibular ligament, entering the parapharyngeal space interfering with phonation, obstructing the nasal choanae and eustachian tube in the deep tissue, seen in 10% of pleomorphic adenomas

dum-dum FORENSIC PATHOLOGY An irregularly weighted bullet that tumbles upon entry into the body, causing massive tissue destruction as it adds a rotational component to a bullet's trajectory; see Ballistics, Caliber

dummy terminal Dumb terminal A peripheral unit connected to a mini- or mainframe computer that consists of a keyboard, a monitor and cables to allow accession of a database without the option to input data, alter the database or interact with the computer's central processing unit; see Computers; Hospital information system

dumping Patient dumping The practice, often by private, for-profit hospitals, of transferring indigent, uninsured patients to other, usually public hospitals for economic reasons; patient-transfer guidelines and laws are generally limited to cases of 'unstable' emergencies and women in active labor; Cf 'Anti-dumping' laws

'dumping' FORENSIC MEDICINE A term used in two contexts regarding a subject's untimely demise and disposal of a body 1) Homicide Dumping is an expedient for removing the bodies of execution victim(s), often in the context of organized crime or drug wars; in New York City, favored 'dumping grounds' include the long-term parking lot of JFK International Airport and the marshes off the West Shore expressway in Staten Island, where the victims are

Class	Depth of invasion	5-year*
A	Limited to mucosa	100.0%
B1	Muscularis propria, negative nodes	66.4%
B2	Penetrates muscularis propria, negative nodes	53.9%
C1	Limited to wall, positive nodes	42.8%
C2	Through wall, positive nodes	22.4%
(D)	Non-Dukes designation for distal metastases	3.0%

*5-year survival

often found in the trunk (boot) of an abandoned automobile 2) Accidental death When a drug abuser overdoses and dies, his friend(s), fearing the legal consequences of acknowledging drug abuse per se, or the potential accusa-

tions of homicide, may remove (dump) the body after having first attempted resuscitation, resulting in changes to the body which themselves may mimic 'injuries' of a homicidal nature

dumping syndrome(s) GASTROENTEROLOGY A disease complex confusing to both those who read about it and to those who write about it, seen in about 20% of those subjected to gastric surgery, including resection, gastroenterostomy with total gastric vagotomy and gastric bypass; most inculpated in 'dumping' are pyloric ablation and bypass CLINICAL Diaphoresis, palpitations, colicky abdominal pain and diarrhea, due to rapid movement (dumping) of gastric contents into the small intestine **early dumping syndrome*** A condition affecting 5-10% of those with sub-total gastrectomies, caused by the release of vasoactive substances, eg serotonin, bradykinin, glucagon CLINICAL Onset 20-30 minutes after meals with early satiety, upper gastric discomfort and vasomotor phenomena (flushing, diaphoresis, palpitations, tachycardia and hypotension), resolving in one hour, weakness, nausea, diarrhea, cramping and borborygmi, flatulence, aerophagia, vomiting, anemia; when prolonged malabsorption, steatorrhea, weight loss and osteomalacia may ensue LABORATORY Increased glucose (worse with high carbohydrate meals), increased hematocrit and decreased blood volume, related to dehydration, decreased serum K+ **late dumping syndrome** A less common condition that is more polymorphous clinically; most symptoms are due to reactive postcibal hypoglycemia, as the rapid entry of glucose releases GIP (gastroactive intestinal polypeptide), inhibiting the hyperglycemic response to glucagon; spontaneous remission may occur 3-12 months after surgery TREATMENT, MEDICAL Decrease carbohydrate intake, smaller meals, pectin (a dietary fiber), acarbose, anticholinergics, L-dopa and opiates TREATMENT, SURGICAL 2-5% are medical failures, requiring surgical conversion to a Roux-en-Y Note: Other post-gastrectomy syndromes include the small capacity, afferent and efferent loop syndromes, bile gastritis, anemia, postvagotomy diarrhea and metabolic bone disease

*Synonyms include afferent loop syndrome, bilious vomiting syndrome, early post-prandial postgastrectomy syndrome and small stomach syndrome

dunce mutation A mutation in the experimental model, *Drosophila melanogaster*, which under normal circumstances, can be trained to avoid noxious stimuli; fleas bearing the dunce mutation cannot, due to a defective cAMP phosphodiesterase gene; the mechanism is unclear

duodenal 'sweep' GASTROENTEROLOGY A term used by both radiologists and endoscopists that refers to the first and second segments of the duodenum as it sweeps superiorly and posteriorly past the gastric antrum

duplication (9p) syndrome A rare condition of which about 60 cases have been reported, normal birth weight, circa 50 IQ, microcephaly, flappy ears, 'beady' eyes, bulbous nose, 'worried' look, unilateral grin, clinodactyly, long carpal bones with short metacarpal bones

duplicative drug 'Me too' drug, see there

durable power of attorney An 'advance directive' document that allows patients to appoint a substitute decision maker to implement their preferences for continued life support in the event of incapacitation; see Advanced directive, Living will

dust mite House dust mite, see there

DVT Deep vein thrombosis, see there

dwarfism Nanosomia A generic term for excessively short stature; the term 'dwarf' is less preferred than dysplasia, dysostosis, eponyms and others; 35% of nanosomia is familial, 25% is idiopathic, 10% is due to pituitary failure, 10% to hypothyroidism, 10% to congenital gonadal aplasia and the remainder due to various causes; proper classification of the more than 55 congenital conditions associated with nanosomia, allows determination of the likelihood of conceiving a second similarly afflicted child

LETHAL DWARFISM A generic term for any form of nanosomy accompanied by premature death, including achondrogenesis, eg Fraccaro-Parenti and Houston-Harris syndromes, homozygous achondroplasia, chondrodysplasia calcificans congenita punctata, campomelic syndrome, hypophosphatasia, osteogenesis imperfecta, thanatophoric dwarfism

NONLETHAL DWARFISM A generic term for any form of nanosomy that is compatible with a normal lifespan, including achondroplasia, diastrophic dwarfism, fibrous dysplasia, spondyloepiphyseal dysplasia congenita, metatrophic dwarfism, chondroectodermal dysplasia (Ellis-van Crevald syndrome), asphyxiating thoracic dysplasia, Laron dwarfism, metaphyseal chondrodysplasia (cartilage-hair hypoplasia), mesomelic dwarfism (Langer and Reinhard-Pfeiffer type); see Bird-headed dwarfism (Seckel syndrome), Bird face, Cherubism, Elfin face syndrome, Leprechaunism, Progeria, 'Walt Disney' dwarf

dwarf megakaryocyte 1) Micromegakaryocyte, see there 2) A misnomer for a fragment of cytoplasm from a megakaryocyte

dwarf tapeworm *Hymenolepsis nana* The only human tapeworm that has no intermediate host; it is most common in warm, dry climates; infection is by direct subject-to-subject transmission, often among children, families and in institutions; the eggs hatch in the stomach and small intestine, penetrate the villi and metamorphose into cercocysts; recalcitrant infections are maintained by autoinfection CLINICAL Irritability, headache, convulsions, vertigo, anorexia, abdominal pain, weight loss, nasopharyngeal and anal pruritus and intermittent diarrhea TREATMENT Praziquantel, niclosamide

DWI Driving while intoxicated, see there

dyad symmetry Palindrome, see there

dying A poorly understood phenomenon that becomes a terminal event in the elderly even in absence of identifiable disease; in the traditional 'Western' construct, death and the dying process require a pathology caused by injury or disease, which once identified, should or at least can (theoretically) be treated; it has been argued that dying is a process a sui generis which should b accepted rather than fought by the medical community; when a person is undergoing the natural process of dying, the role of the physician and nurse is that of medical stewardship to prevent overtreatment (JAMA 1995; 273:1032)

dying-back gliopathy NEUROLOGY A common pathway result of primary destruction of myelin seen in multiple sclerosis that begins at the distal extension of the oligodendrogliocyte, the myelin sheaths

dying-back neuropathy A pattern of neuropathy seen in 'toxic' damage to large diameter peripheral sensorimotor nerves, affecting the long axons, eg lower extremities, before the short, eg cranial nerves; the condition, also known as distal axonopathy is a generic reaction to beriberi, pontocerebellar atrophy, spastic paraplegia and thallium intoxication

dynamic cardiomyoplasty CARDIOVASCULAR SURGERY A technique for treating moderately severe (New York Heart Association class III) heart failure in which a skeletal muscle, usually the latissimus dorsi is transplanted from its usual insertions from the proximal humerus to the chest wall, and from the fascia to the pericardium (Sci & Med Nov/Dec 1994 p68)

dynamic graciloplasty SURGERY A procedure for treating intractable fecal incontinence in which the gracilis muscle is transposed into the anus, with implantation of stimulat-

ing electrodes and a pulse generator; in one study 38 of 52 patients with severe fecal incontinence treated with DG remained continent two or more years after therapy (N Engl J Med 1995; 332:1600oA)

dynamin MOLECULAR BIOLOGY A 100-kD microtubule-bundling GTPase that is capable of self-assembly in helical arrays and rings, which facilitates endocytosis of surface membrane in wide range of cells; dynamin wraps itself around the neck of membrane vesicles and helps pinch them off from the plasma membrane (Nature 1995; 374:186, 190, 116N&V) see Endocytosis

dynein CELL BIOLOGY A ubiquitous mechanicochemical 500 kD ATPase that forms the arms of the axoneme in cilia and flagella, which requires a divalent cation, eg Ca^{++} or Mg^{++} for its action; dynein is responsible for movement of cilia, located on the subfiber A of the ciliary microtubules; according to the 'dynein-walking' model, the dynein arms on the A subfiber of one doublet push the B subfiber on the adjacent doublet toward the tip of the axoneme; the force produced by the sliding of adjacent doublets is the result of repeated formation and breaking of the cross-bridges between the dynein arm of one doublet and the subfiber of the adjacent doublet; dynein powers various forms of intracellular organelle transport, eg minus-end (retrograde) movement* of vesicles along microtubules and various membrane-trafficking events molecular motor protein (Science 1995; 267:1834) see Cilia

*Plus-end (anterograde) movement of vesicles is directed by kinesin

dynorphin One of three opioid neuropeptides (endorphins) in the gastrointestinal tract (the others are met-enkephalin and leu-enkephalin), which are antisecretory, inhibiting plexus neurons, causing constipation and eating disorders in rats and possibly also in humans

dyserythropoiesis A generic term for any abnormality of erythrocyte production characterized by morphologic abnormalities of the nuclei and cytoplasm in the bone marrow, which may be acquired (eg pernicious anemia, sideroblastic anemia, secondary to myeloproliferative disorders or erythroleukemia) or congenital (eg thalassemia, or congenital dyserythropoietic anemia, see there)

dysfibrinogenemia A generic term for qualitative, usually AD fibrinogen defects [MIM 134820], first described in 1958 that now includes 140 different families; disease severity ranges from innocuous to hemorrhagic diathesis; most are asymptomatic and detected by presurgical screens, given the abnormalities in coagulation parameters; these subjects suffer frequent spontaneous abortion, bleeding, poor wound healing, arterial and venous thromboses LABORATORY Fibrin levels and clotting times are normal; increased prothrombin time, thrombin time, reptilase time

Note: Each type is designated by its city of origin, followed by a Roman numeral; five cities have four types each, Baltimore-IV, London-IV, Oslo-IV, New York-IV, Paris-IV

dysfunctional uterine bleeding Excess menstrual hemorrhage of hormonal origin, related to 'breakthrough bleeding' or estrogen withdrawal, often occurring in anovulatory cycles; no organic genital or extra-genital cause can be found in 75% of cases, although adolescent DUB is attributed to immaturity of the hypothalamic-pituitary-ovarian axis; peri- and post-menopausal DUB often occurs in endometria that are deaf to the ovary's curtain call; DUB in the elderly requires curettage to rule out malignancy

dysgammaglobulinemia A generic and imprecise term of waning popularity for a defect in the production of one or more classes of gamma-globulins; the classification scheme of dysgammaglobulinemias, eg dysgammaglobulinemia type I (now known as hyper-IgM syndrome) has fallen into disfavor

dysgenic gonadoma Gonadoblastoma

dyslexia Impaired reading ability, which is either developmental, related to receptive aphasia or word blindness, or acquired, due to a lesion of the dominant parietal cortex; new data suggest that the difficulty may be due to miscomprehension of information, in particular fast sounds, eg the 'stop' consonants, including ba, pa, ga, ka, da, and ta NEUROPATHOLOGY Dyslexic brains have a predominance of smaller neurons in the medial geniculate nucleus, a relay point in the auditory circuit essential for processing sounds; dyslexic brains also have malformations of Brodmann's area 45 (New York Times 16 August 1994; C1)

dysmorphology The systemic study of structural defects of prenatal onset, a complex field in which single or multiple primary malformations are idiopathic or related to chromosome defects (recurrence rate of 2-5%), drugs, chemicals, toxins or radiation; the most common single primary defects are congenital hip dislocation, talipes equinovarus, cleft lip and/or palate, septal defects, pyloric stenosis and neural tube defects

Relevant definitions **deformation** An alteration in the shape or structure of a part that differentiates normally, but cannot develop fully due to in utero constraints, eg compression, or oligohydramnios **disruption** Destruction of a previously normal part, either through interruption of a vascular supply or by entanglement and/or tearing of the structure (often a digit) by floating amniotic bands **malformation** An isolated defect which, if surgical correction is possible, has an excellent prognosis **Sequence** An array of multiple congenital anomalies resulting from an early single primary defect of morphogenesis that unleashes a 'cascade' of secondary and tertiary defects see Multiple malformation syndrome, Sequence

dysmyelopoietic syndromes A group of hematologic malignancies and premalignancies: Idiopathic sideroblastic anemia, refractory anemia with excess 'blasts (RAEB), subacute and oligoblastic leukemia, chronic myelomonocytic leukemia, preleukemias, for which there is considerable overlap; most predictive of the lesion's future behavior is the presence of excess blasts in the bone marrow and circulation, neutropenia and thrombocytopenia

dysplasia A term that signifies defective growth, used by pediatricians for the altered growth of tissues or an extremity and by pathologists for a histologic lesion that has premalignant potential PEDIATRICS The more common dysplastic syndromes include anhidrotic ectodermal dysplasia (Christ-Siemans syndrome), atridigital dysplasia (Holt-Oram syndrome), chondro-ectodermal dysplasia (Ellis-van Creveld syndrome), hidrotic ectodermal dysplsia (Clouston syndrome), metaphyseal dysplasia (Pyle's disease), oculoauriculovertebral dysplasia (Goldenhar syndrome), oculodentaldigital dysplasia (ODD syndrome), olfactogenital syndrome (Kallmann syndrome) and progressive diaphyseal dysplasia (Camurati-Engelmann syndrome) SURGICAL PATHOLOGY A histological lesion with premalignant portent, affecting epithelial linings, in particular squamous epithelium of the uterine cervix, oral cavity, upper respiratory tract, penis, anus and elsewhere; epithelial dysplasia may be induced by HPV, especially types 16, 18, 31 and 33 and is similar (if not identical) to intraepithelial neoplasia, a term that has become integrated in the pathologist parlance

dysplastic nevus A skin lesion often regarded as premalignant, which is characterized by irregular, > than 5 mm in diameter macules numbering from a few to hundreds with a central papule, variegated dark color and lenticular changes PATHOLOGY A 'moth-eaten' Malpighian layer with features of dysplastic nevus superimposed on a junctional or compound nevus and 1) Basilar melanocytic hyperplasia with elongation of rete ridges 2) Cytologic atypia with enlarged hyperchromatic melanocytic nuclei 3) Spindled or epithelioid, horizontally arranged melanocytes, aggregated in variably-sized nests, fusing with adjacent rete ridges ('bridging') 4) Lamellar or concentric dermal fibroplasia and 5) Patchy or diffuse superficial dermal lymphocytosis CLINICAL classification (of congenital nevi): Small

(< 1.5 cm diameter), medium (1.5 to 20 cm), both of which lack hair, but have homogeneous pigmentation and a smooth surface and large (> 20 cm in diameter), eg garment nevi, which have grossly irregular surface, hypertrichous and variegated pigmentation, 10% of which evolve toward malignancy; congenital nevi are either located in the lower dermis or reticular dermis, associated with appendages, nerves and vessels or appear as single or single-file cells between collagen fibrils; DNs tend to affect the horse-collar region of the torso and buttocks, are larger than congenital nevi, have fuzzy indistinct borders, are multicolored with shades of tan, brown, pink, and black, and require annual surveillance (N Engl J Med 1995; 332:656RV)

Note: At least one authority on pigmented lesions has rejected the term 'dysplastic' nevus, as pathologists often disagree on the term dysplasia, the clinical presentation of common, dysplastic nevi and frank melanomas overlap considerably, only 10-20% of melanomas arise from preexisting neval clusters and it is thought that any melanocyte is capable of giving rise to a melanoma

DYSPLASTIC NEVI, CLASSIFICATION	
Type A	Sporadic dysplastic nevus without melanoma
Type B	Familial dysplastic nevi without melanoma
Type C	Sporadic dysplastic nevi with melanoma
Type D1	Familial dysplastic nevi with 1 melanoma in family
Type D2	Familial dysplastic nevi with ≥ 2 melanomas in family (relative risk, 150 if the family member has dysplastic nevi or 500 if they have had a previous melanoma but no risk if he/she has no dysplastic nevi

N Engl J Med 1986; 315:1615

dysraphism A term of waning popularity for defects in the fusion of the primitive neural tube (rachischisis), for which the term neural tube defect is increasingly popular

dyssomnology The study of sleep disorders, see Sleep disorders

dysthymic disorder Minor depression PSYCHIATRY A condition characterized by '...*a chronically depressed mood that occurs for most of the day more days than not for at least 2 years*...(persons so afflicted) *describe their mood as sad or 'down in the dumps*' (300.4 DSM-IV) it is generally accepted that childhood depression of any form (minor depression or dysthymic disorder, or major depression) increases the likehood of same occurring adulthood (New York Times 11 January 1994; C1)

dystrophic calcification The combination of fat necrosis and caseating necrosis, resulting in the focal deposition of hydroxyapatite crystals in previously damaged tissues, eg heart valves, scars, foci of tuberculosis and atherosclerotic blood vessels (arising in mitochondria), calcification in hyperparathyroidism which develops in the basement membrane of the renal tubules; DC may occur in absence of hypercalcemia and abnormalities of calcium metabolism

dystrophin A 427 kD protein, present in low amounts (0.002% of the total muscular protein) as an intracellular component of the transverse tubular system in normal muscle; complete absence results in Duchenne muscular dystrophy, partial absence in Becker muscular dystrophy; dystrophin is most abundant in the neurons of the cerebral and cerebellar cortices, concentrated at post-synaptic membrane specialization; it is postulated that in Duchenne's muscular dystrophy, the role in neurons differs from that of muscle and the cognitive impairment may be due to an alteration of dystrophin at the synaptic level; dystrophin may stabilize cultured myotubes and isolated mature muscle fibers it is detected by immunoblotting and immunofluorescence and shares homology with cytoskeletal proteins α-actinin and spectrin, is localized at the plasmalemma, and is required to anchor certain integral membrane proteins, eg dystrophin-associated glycoproteins (DAGs) which may control calcium flux at the plasma membrane (**Nature** 1993; 364:725; 673N&V) see Duchenne muscular dystrophy, Nebulin

common abbreviations: 2-D Two-dimensional **3-D** Three-dimensional **±** About, approximately, circa **‡** see there **aa** Amino acid **ACE** Angiotensin-converting enzyme **AD** Autosomal dominant **AFB** Acid-fast bacillus **AIDS** Acquired immunodeficiency syndrome **aka** also known as **ALL** Acute lymphocytic (lymphoblastic) leukemia **ALS** Amyotrophic lateral sclerosis **ALT** Alanine aminotransferase (formerly GPT) **AMA** American Medical Association **AML** Acute myelocytic (granulocytic, myeloid, myelogenous) leukemia **ANLL** Acute nonlymphocytic leukemia **apo** Apolipoprotein **aPTT** Activated partial thromboplastin time **AR** Autosomal recessive **ARDS** Acute respiratory distress syndrome or adult respiratory distress syndrome **AST** Aspartate aminotransferase (fomerly GPT) **AV** Atrioventricular **BCC** Basal cell carcinoma **BM** Bone marrow (or basement membrane) **BUN** Blood urea nitrogen **CAD** Coronary artery disease **cAMP** Cyclic adenosine monophosphate **CBC** Complete blood count **CDC** Centers for Disease Control and Prevention **cDNA** Complementary DNA **CEA** Carcinoembryonic antigen **CHF** Congestive heart failure **CIE** Counter-immunoelectrophoresis **CIN** Cervical intraepithelial neoplasia **CK** Creatinine phosphokinase **CML** Chronic myelocytic (granulocytic, myelogenous, myeloid) leukemia **CNS** Central nervous system **COD** Cause of death **COPD** Chronic obstructive pulmonary disease **CPR** Cardiopulmonary resuscitation **CSF** Cerebrospinal fluid **CT** Computed tomography **CVA** Cerebrovascular accident **DAD** Diffuse alveolar damage **DDx** Differential diagnosis **DIC** Disseminated intravascular coagulation **DM** Diabetes mellitus **DNA** Deoxyribonucleic acid **DOA** Dead on arrival **DSM-IV** Diagnostic and Statistical Manual, fourth edition **DWI** Driving while intoxicated *E coli* *Escherichia coli* **EEG** Electroencephalogram, electroencephalographic **eg** *exempli gratia*, for example **EGF** Epidermal growth factor **EKG** Electrocardiography **ELISA** Enzyme-linked immunosorbent assay **EM** Electron microscopy, ultrastructure **EMG** Electromyography **EMT** Emergency medical technician **ENT** Ears, nose, and throat, otorhinolaryngology **EPA** Environmental Protection Agency **ER** Emergency room, emergency ward **ERCP** Endoscopic retrograde cholangiography **ESR** Erythrocyte sedimentation rate **ESRD** End-stage renal disease **FDA** United States Food and Drug Administration **FDP** Fibrinogen degradation product(s) **FISH** Fluorescence in situ hybridization **FNA** Fine-needle aspiration (biopsy or cytology) **FSH** Follicle-stimulating hormone **FUO** Fever of unknown origin **GABA** gamma-aminobutyric acid **GC-MS** Gas chromatography-mass spectroscopy **GFR** Glomerular filtration rate **GGT** Gamma-glutamyl transferase **GI** Gastrointestinal **GM-CSF** Granulocyte-macrophage colony-stimulating factor **GMS** Gomori-methenamine-silver **GN** Glomerulonephritis **GNP** Gross National Product **GVHD** Graft-versus-host disease **HAV** Hepatitis A virus **HBV** Hepatitis B virus **hCG** Human chorionic gonadotropin **HCV** Hepatitis C virus **HDL** High-density lipoprotein **H&E** Hematoxylin & eosin **HHV** Human herpesvirus (HHV-1, HHV-etc) **HIV** Human immunodeficiency virus **HLA** Human leukocyte antigen (the major histocompatibility complex of humans) **HMO** Health maintenance organization **HPLC** High-performance liquid chromatography **HPV** Human papillomavirus **HSV** Herpes simplex virus **HTLV-I** Human T cell leukemia/lymphoma virus **ICU** Intensive care unit **IDDM** Insulin-dependent diabetes mellitus **ie** *id est*, that is (to say) **IFN** Interferon **Ig** Immunoglobulin **IL** Interleukin **IM** Intramuscular **ImPx** Immunoperoxidase **IQ** Intelligence quotient **IR** Infrared **ISH** in situ hybridization **ITP** Idiopathic thrombocytopenic purpura **IUD** Intrauterine (contraceptive) device **IV** Intravenous **IVDU** Intravenous drug use/user **JCAHO** Joint Commission of Accredited Hospitals Organization **K⁺** Potassium **kD** Kilodalton **KS** Kaposi sarcoma **LDH** Lactate dehydrogenase **LDL** Low-density lipoprotein **LGV** Lymphogranuloma venereum **LH** Luteinizing hormone **LM** Light microscopy **LN** Lymph node **MAOI** Monoamine oxidase inhibitor **MEN** Multiple endocrine neoplasia **MHC** Major histocompatibility complex **MI** Myocardial infarction **mo/ma** Monocyte/macrophage (tissue histiocyte) **MPS** Mucopolysaccaride(s), mucopolysaccharidosis **MRI** Magnetic resonance imaging **mRNA** Messenger RNA (ribonucleic acid) **MS** Multiple sclerosis **MVA** Motor vehicle accident **MW** Molecular weight **Na⁺** Sodium **N/C ratio** Nuclear/cytoplasmic ratio **N-CAM** Neuronal-cell adhesion molecule **NGF** Nerve growth factor **NHL** Non-Hodgkin's lymphoma **NIH** National Institutes of Health **NHL** Non-Hodgkin's lymphoma **NIDDM** Non-insulin-dependent diabetes mellitus **NK cell** Natural killer cell **NO** Nitric oxide **NSAID** Nonsteroidal anti-inflammatory drug **OR** Operating room, operating suite **OSHA** Occupational Safety and Health Administration **PAF** Platelet activating factor **PAS** Periodic acid-Schiff **PCBs** Polychlorinated biphenyls **PCP** *Pneumocystis carinii* pneumonia **PCR** Polymerase chain reaction **PDA** Patent ductus arteriosus **PG** Prostaglandin **PID** Pelvic inflammatory disease **PMN(s)** Polymorphonuclear neutrophil(s) or leukocyte(s), segmented neutrophil(s) **ppm** Parts per million *pron* Pronounced **PT** Prothrombin time **PTE** Pulmonary thromboembolism **PTH** Parathyroid hormone **aPTT** (activated) Partial thromboplastin time **QA** Quality assurance **QC** Quality control **RA** Rheumatoid arthritis **RBCs** Red blood cells, erythrocytes **RDS** Respiratory distress syndrome **REM sleep** Rapid eye movement sleep **RFLP** Restriction fragment length polymorphism **RIA** Radioimmunoassay **RR** Relative risk **rRNA** Ribosomal RNA (ribonucleic acid) **RSV** Respiratory syncytial virus **RT** Radiation therapy, reverse transcriptase **SD** Standard deviation **sec** Second (time) **SI** International System (of units), see there **SIDS** Sudden infant death syndrome **SLE** Systemic lupus erythematosus **STD** Sexually-transmitted disease **TAH-BSO** Total abdominal hysterectomy with bilateral salpingo-oophorectomy **TB** Tuberculosis **TDM** Therapeutic drug monitoring **TGF-β** Transforming growth factor-β **TIA** Transient ischemic attack **TIBC** Total iron-binding capacity **TLC** Thin-layer chromatography **TNF** Tumor necrosis factor **tRNA** Transfer RNA (ribonucleic acid) **T-S** Trimethoprim-sulfamethoxazole **TSH** Thyroid-stimulating hormone **TTP** Thrombotic thrombocytopenic purpura **TX** Thromboxane **U** 1) Unit 2) University **UK** United Kingdom **URI** Upper respiratory tract infection **US** United States **UTI** Urinary tract infection **UV** Ultraviolet **VDRL** Venereal disease research laboratory (test) for syphilis **VIP** Vasoactive intestinal polypeptide **VLDL** Very low density lipoportein **V/Q** Ventilation/perfusion **vs** versus, in contrast to, in comparison with, in contrast to **VSD** Ventricular septal defect **VZV** Varicella-zoster virus **WBCs** White blood cells, leukocytes **WHO** World Health Organization **X-R** X-linked recessive **↓** Decrease, decreased, decreases, decreasing **↑** Increase, increased, increases, increasing **♀** Female, women **♂** Male, men

E Symbol for: 1) Electromotive force 2) Energy 3) Enzyme 4) Glutamic acid 5) Redox potential

e Symbol for: 1) Electrical potential 2) Electron 3) Natural logarithm (2.7187818285)

ε (epsilon) Symbol for: 1) Hemoglobin ε, an 'early' hemoglobin chain that disappears by the 3rd month of fetal development 2) Immunoglobulin E heavy chain 3) Molar absorptivity

E7 A protein derived from bovine papillomavirus that is of experimental interest as it enhances the cellular immune response (Sci Am 1993; 268/4:115)

E5531 A stabilized endotoxin antagonist based on the proposed structure of the nontoxic *Rhodobacter capsulatum* A, which protects mice from lipopolysaccharide-induced lethality, and in conjunction with an antibiotic, protected them from lethal infection with *Eschericia coli*; E5531 is being eyed as a possible therapy for gram-negative bacterial sepsis (Science 1995; 268:80)

e-mail Electronic mail COMPUTERS The use of a local or wide-area computer network to send and recieve messages; unlike a telephone call (Cf Voice mail), the recipient(s) need not be present to recieve the message, as the message will be displayed when the recipient(s) next log on to the system; e-mail's advantages include

1) More efficient communication, by eliminating social niceties-do you really want to know how well Throckmorton's son is doing at Harvard Medical School

2) Eliminates distance-a team can work together even if most some members are in a different country, and allows flexibility-an e-mail based team can continue to function, despite changes in address or assignments

3) Can be used to tap into unknown expertise with such devices as a network-wide help message, eg 'does anybody know...' (B Pfaffenberger, Compuer User's Dictionary, Que, Indianapolis, 1993)

E rosettes Nonimmune rosettes IMMUNOLOGY The spontaneous clustering of sheep erythrocytes around T-cells; Erythrocyte rosettes are formed by lymphocytes with abundant CD3 receptors, which are 'pan-T' cell markers

E sign Figure 3 sign, see there

E5 therapy E5 murine antiendotoxin monoclonal antibody therapy INFECTIOUS DISEASE An experimental therapy consisting of anti-endotoxin monoclonal antibodies, reportedly of use in treating patients with gram-negative sepsis (JAMA 1992; 267:2325L) Cf HA-1A therapy

E26 virus An avian acute leukemia virus that induces a mixed erythromyelocytic leukemia in chickens and carries two oncogenes, v-*myb* and v-*ets* that are structurally related to the human oncogene, *erg*

E1a protein A 289-residue promotion and transcription activating protein required for the efficient expression of early viral, eg adenovirus genes; E1a's activating region is structurally distinct from other transcription activators and may interact directly with the cell's transcription 'machinery' E1a is a transcription activator that can act in a 'promiscuous' fashion, ie stimulate the transcription of adenovirus as well as other viral and cellular genes, and interact with several classes of cellular DNA-binding domains (eg homologous basic/leucine zipper of c-Jun, the zinc-finger DNA-binding of Sp1, and the basic/helix-loop-helix DNA-binding domain of USF) and thereby be recruited to different promoters (Nature 1994; 368:520A)

EA rosettes Eythrocyte-antibody rosettes IMMUNOLOGY Clusters of sheep erythrocytes around monocytes and macrophages sensitized with sheep erythrocyte hemolysin, which occurs when the Fc portion of the hemolysin molecule attaches to the Fc receptor on the surface of the M cell

EAC rosettes Erythrocyte-antibody-complement rosettes IMMUNOLOGY Cell clusters formed by B cells, monocytes and macrophages when sheep erythrocytes have been sensitized with a heterophile antibody in the presence of complement

EAE see Experimental allergic encephalomyelitis

EAEC Enteroadherent *Escherichia coli*, see there

earlobe crease A deep furrow on the earlobe, the number of which was reported to correlate with the incidence of coronary artery disease; both increase with age and are probably unrelated

early abortion An abortion performed before the 12th week of gestation

early dumping syndrome see Dumping syndrome‡

early gene VIROLOGY A gene produced by a host cell shortly after integration of a virus into the host's genome, which encodes enzymes of interest to the virus; see Late genes

earmarking 'Pork-barrel' funding, see there

ears Bladder ears UROLOGY Transient, bilateral extraperitoneal herniation of the bladder, occurring in a reported 10% of infants, often less than 6 months of age; bladder ears are of clinical interest, as these children may also have inguinal hernias

Eastern equine encephalitis A rare, sporadic and aggressive enzootic infection by a single-stranded RNA Toga family virus that primarily affects birds VECTOR The ornithophilic mosquito, *Culiseta melanura* is largely confined to the US Northeast, especially Massachusetts; infection of horses and humans is an accidental 'dead-end' occurring when the virus is transmitted to other mosquitos, eg *Aedes vexans*, *Aedes sollicitans* and *Coquillitidia perturbans*; ± 5 human cases/year occur in the US, carrying a 30-70% mortality and severe neurological sequelae CLINICAL Presents with meningismus, lethargy, stupor, high fever, and spinal pleocytosis; Cf St Louis equine encephalitis, Western equine encephalitis

Earth Day ENVIRONMENT An annual 'memorial day' celebrated each year in mid-April, in which those interested parities assess the progress that has been made in reducing man's (negative) impact on the environment in terms of air and water pollution, protecting and preserving species, and general stewardship of the land and oceans (NY Times March 18 1995, C1)

earthquake prediction The divining of when and where the next 'big one' will occur, an exercise that most seismologists believe is virtually impossible, although attempts are made to analyze foreshocks, bulges and creeps, electric resistivity, magnetic fields, and ultra-low frequency electromagentic waves (Science 1994; 264:1656N&C) see Geological disaster; Cf Climatological disaster

EBNA Epstein-Barr nuclear antigen

Ebola disease A hemorrhagic fever syndrome caused by an RNA virus that is similar to that of Marburg disease CLINICAL Onset with GI symptoms, arthralgias, intractable diarrhea, and high mortality; infection is thought to be by direct contact rather than aerosol TREATMENT Interferon, convalescent serum

Ebola virus An extremely virulent ('hot', ie biosafety level 4) virus of the filovirus family that was first isolated in 1976 in devastating epidemics that occurred in Zaire and Sudan; EV has three serotypes *Ebola Zaire*, *E Sudan*, and *E Reston*; *E Reston* was identified near Washington DC in a group of primates imported from Africa in 1989 (R Preston, The Hot Zone, Random House, New York, 1994) INFECTIOUS DISEASE Add a small (< 100 cases) outbreak occurred in Zaire in mid-1995, which carried a 90% mortality; at this writing (18 May 1995), it is unkown if it has been contained (NY Times 16 May 1995, C3)

ebullism Air embolism at high altitude, the last of which was isolated where the total ambient pressure is 47 mm Hg or less (> 20 000 meters); in addition to acute hypoxia, the body fluids boil/evaporate causing widespread air bubble formation in vessels and tissue; in experimental mammals at high altitudes, vaporization occurs at the entrance of the great veins into the heart, blocking venous return, which is rapidly fatal due to abrupt cardiac failure

eburnation A marbled appearance of weight-bearing joints with complete cartilaginous erosion, leaving polished, sclerotic bone as the new articular surface; cross-section of the articulation reveals a narrowed joint space, osteosclerosis and cystic changes overlying the affected bone, which is surrounded by bony and cartilaginous overgrowths (osteophytes/exostoses)

EBV Epstein-Barr virus, see there

EBV-associated lymphoproliferative disorder CLINICAL IMMUNOLOGY A lymphoproliferative process associated with Epstein-Barr virus infection, which may complicate chronic immunosuppressive therapy for organ transplantation; when first recognized, up to 40% of those surviving heart transplantation developed malignant lymphoma; with lesser amounts of immunosuppression, 1-13% of those with solid organ transplants develop malignant lymphoma (30–60-fold greater than general population); these lesions range from an infectious mononucleosis-like syndrome in younger patients to a monoclonal B cell proliferation (usually lymphoma); absence of immunoglobulin gene rearrangement (see Southern blot) and lack of EBV detection implies that the process being observed is reactive and not neoplastic in nature; EBV-associated lymphoma is a complication of BM transplantation that responds poorly to standard forms of therapy, but responds to infusions of unirradiated T cells from the BM donor (N Engl J Med 1994; 330:1185OA, 1231ED); some cases of polyclonal EALPD evolve into monoclonal lymphoproliferative disorders (Arch Pathol Lab Med 1995; 119:409OA)

EC Enzyme Commission, see there

eccentric *noun* PSYCHOLOGY A person who is not regarded as average or 'normal' by his peers, friends, or family; while some workers find little evidence to connect eccentricity to mental illness*, data supporting such a posit is scanty, and hampered by the lack of universally accepted case definition and populations for study (Nature 1995; 374:419BR)

*30-45% have at least mild forms of delusional thinking, including paranormal, religious, and persecutory delusions; the incidence of hypomania and substance abuse in eccentrics is unknown

eccentric contraction SPORTS MEDICINE Muscular contraction that occurs while the muscle is lengthening; Cf Concentric contraction

eccentric training SPORTS MEDICINE The lengthening of the muscle tendon unit while it is active, resulting in a negative movement required under conditions of rapid deceleration; eccentric forces are required to reverse the body's trajectory after a particular athletic move, eg jumping and throwing (JC DeLee, D Drez, Jr, Eds, Orthopedic Sports Medicine WB Saunders, Philadelphia, 1994)

ECFMG Educational Commission for Foreign Medical Graduates An organization formed by the American Hospital Association, American Medical Association, American Board of Medical Specialties, Association of American Medical Colleges and others for the purpose of establishing standards and evaluating the qualifications of graduates of foreign medical schools

echocardiography A noninvasive group of two-dimensional imaging techniques using Doppler ultrasonography; these methods provide information on pressure differences and blood flow in the heart and great vessels; the principle common to these methods is that blood flowing to (and through) the heart produces sound, some of which is reflected back by each acoustic interface the blood encounters, ie the Doppler effect, which is received by a transducer; the time elapsed between the sound's transmission to the time that the echo is received is converted to a display; when a number of depth samples are taken in sequence, an imaging plane is created, allowing construction of a two-dimensional echocardiogram, a procedure of considerable use in evaluating pericardial and myocardial disease, ischemic and congenital heart diseases and infectious endocarditis

echo planar imaging MRI A technique of planar imaging in which a complete planar image is obtained from one selective excitation pulse; see Magnetic resonance imaging

echovirus A virus[1] with 30 types[2], of the picornavirus (small single-strand RNA) family, genus Enterovirus; echoviridæ produces a characteristic cytopathic effect in cell culture CLINICAL Upper respiratory tract infections, exanthema, diarrhea, viremia, and less commonly, viral meningitis and poliomyelitis

[1] The name derived originally as the acronym ECHO (enteric cytopathogenic human orphan), subsequently written in lower case [2] Of the original 34 serotypes described, 1 and 8 are identical, 10 was reclassified as rreovirus 1, 28 as rhinovirus 1A, and 34 is a variant of coxsackie 24

'eclipse' The period between the time a cell is infected by a virus and the production of intracellular viral progeny

'eclipsed' antigen IMMUNOLOGY Any non-self antigen, eg that of a parasite, which so closely mimics the host antigen that it doesn't elicit an immune response

ECM Extracellular matrix, see there

ECMO see Extracorporal membrane oxygenation

ECOG Eastern Cooperative Oncology Group

eco-labeling Green labeling ENVIRONMENT A seal that is affixed to a product based on its environmental 'correctness'; criteria for eco-labeling include whether the item is produced from recycled materials, how much energy is consumed during its production or use, what by-products its creation entails, or whether the product contains pollutants; there are now 30 eco-labeling programs in the world, which started in 1978 with the Blue Angel seal from Germany (Sci Am 1994; 270/5:115)

E coli O157:H7 see *Escherichia coli* O157:H7

economic credentialing HEALTH CARE ENVIRONMENT The use of factors other than quality of care, eg ability to generate revenue, to decide whether to credential a physician, ie to allow him/her to become affiliated with a hospital (Am Med News 21 September 1992 p3)

economics '... *the study of how men* (sic) *and society end up choosing, with or without the use of money, to employ scarce productive resources that could have alternative uses, to produce various commodities and* *distribute them for consumption now or in the future among various peoples and groups in society. It analyses the costs and benefits of improving patterns of resource allocations.'* (Science & Medicine 1995; 2/3:4)

economy of scale LABORATORY MEDICINE A principle of business, which in essence states: As the number of 'widgets' produced in one site increases, the effect of operating costs (utilities–heating and lighting, leasing of building, ancillary staff, and basic core of workers to run widget-making machinery) on each widget decreases

***Eco*RI, *Eco*RII** MOLECULAR BIOLOGY Restriction endonucleases from *Escherichia coli* that are used to cut double stranded DNA at specific sites on the DNA double strand, G*AATTC (G*CCTGG for EcoR II); EcoR I is a major 'workhorse' used in DNA analysis to cut DNA down to size

ecstasy 3,4-Methylenedioxymethamphetamine A 'schedule I' controlled substance analogue ('designer drug'[1]) of amphetamine, potentially causing fatal overdose, which is selectively neurotoxic to serotonergic nerve fibers and manufactured in clandestine laboratories; it had been promoted as a safe, nontoxic (albeit illegal) vehicle for relaxation, and was a popular 'recreational' drug of abuse during the 1980s, most often used by individuals (or in small groups) who reported that it imparted a sensation of euphoria, warmth, and closeness to loved ones (hence its synonym, 'love drug'); when used in 'old' cultural context[2], ecstasy was rarely fatal, and then only related to cardiac arrhythmias, or due to exacerbation of various underlying diseases; it has recently undergone a 'cultural reformulation' and has become a popular pharmacologic 'lubricant' for large all-night dance parties known as 'raves', where the combination of heat and poor ventilation, sweating, low fluid intake and frenetic pace of the dancing may induce a severe, potentially fatal MDMA-related toxic reaction with high temperatures (43.3°C, 110°F), tachycardia, convulsions, hypotension, rhabdomyolysis, acute renal failure, and despite aggressive therapy[3] may die in a state of hyperthermia and DIC TOXICITY At high levels, MDMA causes serotonin neurotoxicity, agitation, hallucinations, sweating, dilated pupils, tachycardia, fever, spasticity, hypotension, bronchospasm and acidosis; contribution to the fatal response to a low ('recreational') dose of MDMA of the phenomenon of aggregation toxicology (see there) is uncertain (JAMA 1993; 269:1505MN&P) see Designer drugs, 'Ice', Rave parties; Cf Eve

[1] aka Adam, MDM, MDMA, XTC [2] The drug was developed but never marketed in 1914 as a dietary suppressant and languished until the 1970s, when a small group of psychiatrists used it as an adjunct to insight-oriented psychotherapy, during which time the drug enjoyed a 6-month legalized hiatus so that the psychiatric community could use it experimentally; by 1983 it had become a recreational drug on college campuses (cost: $10-40 per 100 mg 'hit'), producing a pleasant nonhallucinogenic 'high' in low doses, with sensory components of amphetamine, mescaline and amphetamine, but is hallucinogenic above 150 mg [3] eg control of convulsions, eg with dantrolene, ↓ body temperature, rapid rehydration

ECT Electroconvulsive therapy, see there

ectoderm EMBRYOLOGY The most external layer of the embryo that gives rise to epidermis, the teeth, tongue, palate, salivary glands, anogenital region, hypophysis, nervous system and sensory organs, eg eyes, ears and nose

ectopic hormone A hormone is considered ectopic if there is 1) Biochemical or clinical evidence of abnormal endocrine function, eg increased hormone levels or an endocrine 'syndrome' 2) Disappearance of the endocrine abnormality with tumor resection or persistence of the syndrome despite resection of the gland normally responsible for that hormone's production and 3) Presence of hormone in greater than normal amounts and/or presence of an arteriovenous gradient of the hormone and/or hormone synthesis by the tumor in tissue culture Note: Ectopic hormone production is most common in malignancy and may cause a paraneoplastic syndrome

MECHANISM Unknown, possibly due to amplification of genes that are not expressed under the usual circumstances, de-repression of previously inactive genes or dedifferentiation or abortive attempts towards differentiation

ectopic hormonal syndrome Any of a variety of conditions caused by the long-term exposure to various hormones produced in abnormal sites; the ectopic corticotropin and ectopic CRH syndromes are clinically indistinguishable and are characterized by a rapid onset of hypertension, edema, hypokalemia, and glucose intolerance; both are often caused by carcinoid and other neuroendocrine tumors; the acute ectopic corticotropin syndrome is classically caused by small cell lung carcinoma (N Engl J Med 1995; 332:791SA)

ectopic pregnancy The implantation of an embryo in sites not designed to accommodate the massive vascular supply required by a growing fetus, an event that cost the US health care system an estimated $462 million in 1985; EP is most common in fallopian tubes scarred by gonococcal salpingitis, and has a recurrence rate of 10-30%; relative risk (RR) for suffering an ectopic pregnancy include current intrauterine device use (RR, 13.7), prior tubal surgery (RR, 4.5), history of pelvic inflammatory disease (RR, 3.3), history of infertility (RR, 2.6), douching, and infection with *Chlamydia trachomatis*, or douching with an infected douche solution (JAMA 1991; 265:2670c); hCG levels are often lower in ectopic than in intrauterine pregnancy, a fact complicating early management of ectopic pregnancy PATHOLOGY Endometrial curettings demonstrate the 'classic' Arias-Stella phenomenon, a histologic mimic of endometrial carcinoma; EP accounts for 10% of maternal deaths in the first trimester of pregnancy, represent 0.3% of all pregnancies increased from 4.5/1000(1970) to 16.8/1000 (1987) CLINICAL Lower abdominal pain, nausea, vomiting, amenorrhea MORBIDITY-SHORT-TERM Hypovolemia, transfusions, emergency surgery MORBIDITY-LONG-TERM Repeated EP, chronic pelvic pain, infertility WARNING EP may occur in the face of termination of pregnancy (by endometrial currettage), as the shaggy and spongy decidual tissue obtained during termination of pregnancy, may be misinterpreted as being definitive products of conception (chorionic villi) with fatal concequences; follow all questionable cases with serial hCG determination (Arch Pathol Lab Med 1993; 117:698OA)

ectothrix A form of tinea capitis involving the hair shaft, which may be inflamed; the spores surrounding the hair shaft are small (2-3 µm) and fluoresce bright green with Wood's light, as with *Microsporum canis, M audouinii, M distortum, M ferrugineum*, or are large (5-10 µm) and do not fluoresce, as with *Trichophyton verrucosum, T mentagrophytes, T megninii, T gallinae, M gypseum, M fulvum*, and *M nanum*; Cf Endothrix

EDC/EDL Expected date of confinement or labor An estimate of the 'usual' duration of pregnancy; gestational or menstrual age is estimated from the first day of the last menstrual period (ie 2 weeks before ovulation and fertilization); in general, ± 280 days (40 weeks) elapse between the first day of the last menstrual period and delivery of the infant, ie 9⅓ or 10 lunar months; obstetricians calculate gestational age; embryologists are more correct as they calculate the ovulation or fertilization age (280 days minus roughly two weeks)

edge artifact IMMUNOPATHOLOGY The nonspecific peripheral staining of paraffin-embedded tissue by immunoperoxidase methods, caused by tissue drying

editing Proofreading MOLECULAR BIOLOGY A generic term for any activity that allows correction of errors that occur during replication, transcription, translation or other processing of genetic information, eg that displayed by the α and delta DNA polymerase complexes in eukaryotic cells, in which mismatched double-stranded DNA, ie incorrectly hydrogen-bonded bases are removed by the 3'→5' exonuclease activity of DNA polymerases

Edman digestion MOLECULAR BIOLOGY A technique used to determine the sequence of a protein's amino acids; a peptide of interest is treated with phenylisothiocyanate (Edman reagent), which attaches at the N-terminal residue, making the first peptide bond in the protein labile to digestion by a mild acid; the first amino acid is removed and determined by chemical means; repetition up to 20-30 amino acids can be accomplished automatically by the sequenators; see Sequencing

EDRF Endothelium-dependent relaxing factor A substance produced by endothelium, now known to be nitric oxide (Nature 1990, 346:69) that causes hyperpolarization and relaxation of arterial smooth muscle; see Myocardial infarction; see Nitric oxide

EDTA Ethylenediaminetetraacetic acid, edetic acid A chelating agent that binds divalent, eg arsenic, calcium, lead and magnesium and trivalent cations and is used to treat lead and other heavy metal intoxication; EDTA is added to specimen tubes to transport specimens in laboratory medicine for analysis in 1) Chemistry, eg carcinoembryonic antigen, lead, renin 2) Hematology where it is the preferred anticoagulant for blood cell counts, coagulation studies, hemoglobin electrophoresis and sedimentation rate and 3) Transfusion medicine where it prevents hemolysis by inhibiting complement binding

EEC syndrome An often AD [MIM 129900] dysplastic syndrome characterized by ectrodactyly, ectodermal dysplasia and cleft lip and/or palate, variably accompanied by attenuated, dry, poorly pigmented skin, sparse hair, eyebrows, defective skin adnexae, eg nail hypoplasia, poor dentition, syndactyly and/or 'clawing' of hands and feet, urinary tract and ocular (blepharophimosis, atretic lacrimal punctata, strabismus) anomalies, granulomatous perleche and candidiasis; see Tabby mutation

EEE Eastern equine encephalitis, see there

EEL Emergency exposure levels

EEO Equal employment opportunity, see there

EF-1, EF-2 Elongation factors, see there

EF13 *Vibrio hollisae*, CDC Enteric Group 42 An organism that inhabits the US gulf coast and Chesapeake Bay, which has been isolated from some patients with diarrhea and gastroenteritis who had ingested raw seafood

E2F MOLECULAR BIOLOGY A transcription factor that interacts with Rb (the retinoblastoma gene product) that is involved in the expression of genes necessary for entry into the growth cycle (Nature 1995; 374:114N&V)

E-ferol syndrome Vitamin E overdose, see there

effect modification EPIDEMIOLOGY An interaction among multiple possible cause-and-effect relationships, where the estimate of the effect of one factor on a (disease) process depends on another factor in the study base (see N Engl J Med 1993; 329:377OA)

effective dose equivalent H_E RADIATION PHYSICS The sum of the products of the dose equivalent to a tissue (H_T) and the weighting factors (W_T) applicable to each irradiated tissue $H_E = \Sigma W_T H_T$

effector inhibition model EXPERIMENTAL IMMUNOLOGY A model that explains the ability of NK cells to differentiate between self and nonself cells based on absence of a critical self peptide within surrounding class I MHC molecules (Science 1995; 267:976P)

efficiency LABORATORY MEDICINE The relative ability of a test to detect a person with a disease, while maintaining the rate of false positive results to a minimum; the efficiency of a test is defined as the number of true positives

and true negatives multiplied by one hundred, divided by the sum of true positives, true negatives, false positives and false negatives

effort syndrome Neurasthenia, see there

effort thrombosis A blood clot that forms within a vessel of a muscle group (eg axillary vein) that was subjected to strenuous exercise; ET may also occur in thoracic outlet syndrome

EF hand PHYSIOLOGY A secondary protein structural motif (α-helix-loop-α-helix) that is typical of sites that bind ions, eg Ca^{++}, which is derived from aspartic and glutamic acid side chains and carbonyl groups and contains six-to-eight oxygen molecules; EF hands are present in calmodulin and diacylglycerol kinase; see Recoverin

EGCG (–)-Epigallocatechin gallate, see Green tea

EGF see Epidermal growth factor

egg-shaped heart 'Pumpkin' heart PEDIATRIC CARDIOLOGY A globoid cardiac shadow seen on a plain chest film of young children with transposition of the great vessels where there is a large ventricular silhouette and a small 'waist' due to the abnormal location of the aorta directly in front of the pulmonary artery, associated (by physiological necessity) with a ventricular septal defect; these defects evolve toward congestive heart failure

Note: A similar radiologic finding is seen in the hypoplastic left heart syndrome, especially in the face of congestive heart failure

eggshell skull principle FORENSIC MEDICINE A colloquial term for a legal principle referring to a minor injury that causes grave harm and/or death because of a preexisting medical condition, eg a person with a markedly thinned (eggshell) cranial vault may die from minor trauma to the skull, for which a defendent would be liable (N Engl J Med 1995; 332:1450C)

eggshell calcification Fine peripheral rimming of calcium in the enlarged hilar and peribronchial lymph nodes, characteristic of silicosis

egg white injury 'syndrome' see Biotin deficiency syndrome

ego identity The sense of connection (belonging) between an individual and a particular social (religious, or political) group, the values of which a person shares; the ego identity is formed by early adulthood and is rooted in early developmental experiences; a person's sexual orientation is a facet of ego identity (N Engl J Med 1994; 331:923SA)

EHEC Enterohemorrhagic *Escherichia coli*(s), see there

Ehrlichia chaffeensis A bacterium of the family Rickettsiaceae that may infect humans, causing systemic disease, fever, headache VECTORS *Amblyomma americanum* (Lone Star tick), *Dermacentor variabilis* (American dog tick) DDx Rocky Mountain spotted fever, gastroenteritis, influenza, upper respiratory tract infection LABORATORY Leukopenia, thrombocytopenia TREATMENT Tetracycline (Science News 1994; 146:44)

ehrlichiosis A rare tick-borne infection of humans caused by *Ehrlichia canis*, that usually affects dogs CLINICAL Fever, chills, rigors, malaise, nausea, myalgia, anorexia, acute respiratory failure with infiltrates, acute renal failure with ↑ creatinine and encephalopathy LABORATORY Leukopenia or lymphocytosis of T cells expressing the γδ heterodimer T-cell receptor and the not the usual αβ heterodimer (Am J Clin Pathol 1995; 103:761), thrombocytopenia, ↑ transaminases TREATMENT Chloramphenicol, tetracycline

EHS tumor Engelbreth-Holm-Swarm tumor A tumor of experimental rodents that prolifically produces basement membrane material, serving as a source for laminin, fibronectin and proteoglycans

EIA 1) Enzyme immunoassay, see ELISA, EMIT 2) Exercise induced anaphylaxis, see there

eicosanoid A 20-carbon cyclic fatty acid derived from arachidonic acid, synthesized from membrane phospholipids; eicosanoids and other arachidonic acid metabolites, eg HETE, HPETE, leukotrienes, prostaglandins, and thromboxanes are site-specific, increased during shock and after injury, and have diverse functions, including bronchoconstriction, bronchodilation, vasodilation, and vasoconstriction

EIEC Enteroinvasive *Escherichia coli*, see there

eIF-4F A specific initiation factor mediating the activity of the 5' cap structure (m7GpppX), located on eukaryotic mRNA, required for efficient translation; one of eIF-4F's subunits, eIF-4E, is present in limiting amounts and is regulated by phosphorylation; decreased eIF-4E phosphorylation results in decreased DNA translation; overexpression of eIF-4E in some tumor cell lines may evoke tumor transformation

Einstein sign EMERGENCY MEDICINE A ruptured aortic aneurysm mimicking biliary colic; Albert Einstein was admitted to a New Jersey hospital in 1955 with a diagnosis of acute cholecystitis, despite a 10-year history of aortic aneurysm and pulsations typical of impending rupture; he died three days later (**N Engl J Med 1984; 310:1538c**)

Eisenmenger syndrome Pulmonary hypertension at systemic level due to a high pulmonary vascular resistance (> 800 dynes sec/cm) with reversed or bidirectional shunt at the aortopulmonary, ventricular or atrial level CLINICAL Cyanosis, dyspnea on exertion, hemoptysis, atypical chest pain or angina pectoris, syncope, congestive heart failure, arrhythmia, cerebrovascular accident due to paradoxical embolism and gout

ejaculation center PHYSIOLOGY A region of the lumbosacral spinal cord that coordinates the sympathetic and parasympathetic activity of ejaculation; Cf Erection center

ejection click A cardiac sound heard in early systole, related to cardiac dilation or hypertension in the great vessels (aorta and pulmonary artery); ejection clicks may be so close to the first heart sound that they simulate a splitting thereof; aortic clicks are constant and best appreciated at the left lower sternal border, occurring in aortic dilation (aortic stenosis, Fallot's tetralogy, truncus arteriosus); pulmonary ejection clicks occur with pulmonary stenosis, are best heard at the left midsternal and disappear with inspiration; a midsystolic ejection click heard at the apex, preceding a late systolic murmur is suggestive of mitral valve prolapse

ejection fraction CARDIOLOGY The volume of blood in the ventricles that is effectively propulsed forward during systole; the ejection fraction is measured dynamically by injecting a bolus of 99mTc and is heard as a high-pitched click

ELAM-1 Endothelial leukocyte adhesion molecule An endothelial glycoprotein that mediates neutrophil adhesion; ELAM-1's primary structure has a lectin-like domain, an epidermal growth factor-like domain, 6 tandem-repeated motifs and amino acid homology shared by complement-regulating proteins; its production is induced by IL-1, TNF, and substance P and is immune-regulatory, recruiting neutrophils to sites of inflammation, mediating cell adhesion by a carbohydrate ligand, sialyl-Lewis X, and serves as an adhesion molecule ('addressin') for skin-homing T cells, acting in addition to VLA-4 and LFA-1 integrins (**Nature 1991; 349:796, 799**)

elastin A fibrous protein that is similar to collagen in that ⅓ of the amino acids are glycine with abundant proline, valine and arginine, and it is formed by cross-linking small globular subunits to lysine residues; elastin's elasticity is ideally for its prominent role in arterial walls, vocal cords, alveolar septa, and ligaments, having an amorphous wavy appearance by LM; defects in the cross-linking in elastin's unique β spiral as well as increases or decreases in elastin are implicated in atherosclerosis, emphysema, Ehlers-Danlos, type V, Menke's kinky hair syndrome, pseudoxanthoma elasticum and X-linked cutis laxa

elderly abuse A generic term for a clinically entity which is an act of commission, defined in an arbitrary and somewhat nebulous fashion; given the current absence of a consensus definition, it is best to delineate features that would constitute EA in the eyes of a reasonable person

---

ELDERLY ABUSE-

PHYSICAL VIOLENCE with intent to cause bodily harm: Hitting, slapping, or striking with objects, resulting in bruises, abrasions, fractures, burns

EMOTIONAL/PSYCHOLOGICAL ABUSE with intent to cause mental or emotional pain or injury: Verbal aggression, statements that humiliate or infantilize, insults, threats of abandonment or institutionalization

MATERIAL EXPLOITATION -an 'optional' form of EA: Includes misappropriation of money or property, theft of social security checks, changing the older person's will, and so on
N Engl J Med 1995; 332:437RA

Some experts prefer to use alternative terms, eg inadequate care of the elderly or mistreatment of the elderly, which include acts of commission and omission, do not assign blame and at the same time are 'politically correct'

elderly neglect The failure for a caregiver to meet the needs of a dependent elderly person, which may be intentional, eg withholding of food, medications, failure to clean or bathe, or unintentional, resulting from genuine ignorance of or physical inability to address a particular need (**N Engl J Med 1995; 332:437RA**)

'elderly' primigravida A woman who delivers her first child after age 35; these women are often professionals who delay childbearing to pursue a career; there is no increased risk to the pregnancy per se, although the medical risks due to increased age may cause increased pregnancy-induced complications

elective *adjective* Pertaining or referring to that which is undertaken by choice and without urgency, as in elective surgery

elective abortion An interruption of pregnancy prior to fetal viability that is performed voluntarily at the request of the mother for reasons unrelated to concerns for maternal or fetal health or welfare; most abortions fall into this group; there is one EA for every three live births in the US

elective surgery Any operative procedure that can be performed with advanced planning, eg cholecystectomy, hernia repair, colonic resection, coronary artery bypass, in contrast to emergency surgery that is required by trauma or impending organ rupture, eg appendicitis or rupture of an aortic aneurysm

Electra complex PSYCHIATRY The female equivalent of the Oedipus complex, in which the daughter perceives the mother as a rival, while the father is the psychosexual source of nourishment; Cf Delilah syndrome, Diana complex, Oedipus complex

Electra of Greek mythology, with the help the help of her brother Orestes, killed both her mother Clytemnestra and her mother's lover in retaliation for their murder of Electra's father

electrical alternans CARDIOLOGY Marked swings in the amplitude of the QRS complex that occur every 2 to 3 beats, caused by 'circus movement' in the myocardium, due to various causes, including tamponade, pericardial effusion, pneumopericardium, cardiac muscle dysfunction and paroxysmal supraventricular tachycardia; EA may presage sudden cardiac death, and may precede ventricular fibrillation in patients undergoing coronary angioplasty or those with Prinzmetal's angina, congenital prolonged QT syndrome, acute myocardial infarction, catecholamine excess, and electrolyte derangements; EA affecting the ST segment and T wave is a common event in patients at risk for ventricular arrhythmias (VAs) and may represent a noninvasive marker of susceptibility to VAs (N Engl J Med 1994; 330:235oA)

electrically enhanced drug delivery see Iontophoresis

electroacupuncture biofeedback ALTERNATIVE MEDICINE A technique that '...*makes use of the acupuncture meridian system to screen for infections in the body...a screening tool for alternative health care practitioners...involves placing an electrode...then applying a small electric current and recording the response. Any deviation from the normal reading indicates that there is an infection or disturbance...*' (Alternative Medicine, Future Medicine Publishing, Inc, Puyallup, Washington, 1994) Note: There is no data on the diagnostic utility of EB in peer-reviewed journals; see Alternative medicine, Energy medicine

electrocerebral inactivity see Brain death

electrocochleography A test for measuring sound-evoked cochlear potentials, which is part of the battery of auditory evoked potential tests used to diagnose inner ear disease and for intraoperative monitoring; ECOG comes in three flavors: 1) Transtympanic, performed with a needle electrode placed through the tympanic membrane onto the promontory of the middle ear is useful for intraoperative auditory monitoring 2) Tympanic, performed with a needle electrode on the tympanic membrane, which has the advantage of being noninvasive 3) Extratympanic, performed with a needle in the ear canal, which has significant drawbacks, including patient discomfort and poor response quality; ECOG is useful for diagnosing endolymphatic hydrops in Meniere's disease, sudden hearing loss, and detecting perilymphatic leaks; despite its utility, some ENTs are circumspect in its use, as it is invasive, time-consuming, requires a local anesthetic, and the placement of the recording electrode with an operating microscope

electroconvulsive therapy Electroshock PSYCHIATRY A form of therapy for major depression which consists in the iatrogenic induction of generalized tonic-clonic seizures, which if of adequate duration has an antidepressant effect CLINICAL INDICATIONS Lack of response or intolerance to antidepressant medication, a compelling need for rapid clinical response (inanition/starvation, psychosis, suicidality), or history of previous response to ECT METHOD Succinylcholine is used during anesthesia to attenuate seizure activity, utilizing a sine wave shock pattern or a brief pulse; unilateral therapy is associated with less severe post-therapeutic cognitive impairment (eg retrograde amnesia about personal information); ↑ electrical dosage (eg 2.5 × greater than seizure threshold) ↑ the efficacy of right unilateral ECT, but not to the level of bilateral therapy (N Engl J Med 1993; 328:839oA); 5-10 sessions are often needed to treat depression (85-95% of cases of severe depression are effectively ameliorated), bipolar disease, manic type, schizo-affective disorders or catatonic schizophrenia; chronic disease requires longer therapy; ECT mechanism of action is unclear; some evidence points to an answer from neurochemistry, neuroendocrinology and neurophysiology; contraindications are few, although patients with intracranial masses, tumors, hematomas and evolving strokes respond poorly, due to the transient breakdown in the blood brain barrier and ↑ intracranial pressure; the use of ECT in young patients (eg with Tourette syndrome or post-traumatic stress disorder) is a questionable practice (Nature Medicine 1995; 1:199ED), for which further data is needed; the relation of long-term ECT to cerebral atrophy remains unresolved; an uncommon and feared complication is ECT psychosis, which is characterized by loss of memory, attenuation of affect and hallucinations

*The technique was formulated in the 1930s by the Hungarian psychiatrist Meduna, who observed that some schizophrenic patients improved after insulin-induced comas

electrofocusing Isoelectric focusing, see there

electrogalvanism ALTERNATIVE MEDICINE A term referring to the electricity generated by a person's own dental amalgams, where saliva acts as a conductant and the dissimilar metals in the mouth form electric circuits to neutralize the ionic charge; electrogalvanism is allegedly responsible for the slow leaching of metals from amalgams, the most important of which is mercury, which according to alternative health care providers is responsible for a plethora of ill-defined 'evil humors', including lack of concentration and poor memory, insomnia, psychological defects, tinnitus, vertigo, seizures, hearing loss, and eye problems (Alternative Medicine, Future Medicine Publishing, Inc, Puyallup, Washington, 1994) see Biological dentistry

electroimmunodiffusion Rocket electrophoresis, see there

electrolysis DERMATOLOGY A procedure for removing ill-placed and/or undesired hair, in particular on the face, which consists of insertion of an electrode and zapping the skin with electricity; removal is complete and permanent if the follicular papilla is destroyed; Cf Wax epilation

electrolyte/fluid balance panel A group of assays used to detect and diagnose, in the most cost-efficient way possible, the most common imbalances of electrolytes and fluid, including measurement of sodium, potassium, chloride, pH, PCO_2, CO_2 content, osmolality in the plasma and urine and BUN; see Organ panel

electromagnetic field PUBLIC HEALTH An invisible field of electromagnetic radiation of the spectrum of energetic particles that move as quanta (radiowaves, infrared, visible light, UV light, and gamma radiation); EMFs are generated by moving electrical charges that propagate outward from any object carrying electrical current and result from an electric field that pushes or pulls charged particles or ions in the direction of the field; electric fields are stopped by most objects from skin to concrete having a strength of 1 mV/m^2 (similar to the strength of cells' intrinsic electrical activity; the second component of EMF is a magnetic field that acts on moving particles, pushing them perpendicular to their direction of motion, passing through most matter without losing strength; the actual power generated by a magnetic field is a few milligauss (1% of the strength of the earth's magnetic field); tumor cells exposed in vitro to extremely low electromagnetic fields (ELF) of 60 Hz electromagnetic radiation from electrical distribution systems (powerlines, video display terminals, household appliances) have increased mitotic activity; some reports have suggested that ELF radiation may be associated with a 1.5–2.5-fold increase in leukemia, lymphoma and intracranial malignancy, especially in children living close to either 765-kV power lines or 15-kV distribution lines; nonetheless, the relation of ELF with malignancy continues to be controversial; with breast cancer (as with others), the significance of data that is not statistically significant is unclear, moreover poor design hampers valid conclusions (Science 1994; 264:1658N&C)

Note: ELF increases ornithine decarboxylase activity or cell membrane resistance to spontaneous lysis

electromagnetic spectrum The spectrum of energy in the physical universe which is measured in Hertz* and which has an inverse relationship with the length of the wave of energy (Science & Medicine July/August 1995, p68) see EMF radiation

*An informal subjective classification of pre-World War II vintage exists, where ELF corresponds to extremely low-frequency waves, LF to low-frequency

waves, VHF to very high high-frequency waves, and EHF to extra high-frequency waves

electromechanical dissociation CARDIOLOGY Mechanical failure with adequate, albeit occasionally bizarre electrical activity; while the pathogenesis is unknown, pump failure may be due to depletion of high-energy phosphates, acidosis and cytoplasmic accumulation of calcium; two-thirds of sudden cardiac deaths are attributed to electromechanical dissociation

electromotility AUDITORY PHYSIOLOGY The cyclical elongation and contraction of outer hair cells of the organ of Corti, a process that is assumed to be responsible for high sensitivity and frequency selectivity of amplification in the mammalian cochlea; at low frequencies, electromotility is due to mechanical stimulation, and at high frequencies it is driven by extracellular potential gradients across the hair cell (Science 1995; 267:2006R)

electron capture NUCLEAR MEDICINE A type of radioactive decay; the radioisotope captures an inner shell electron, converting a proton to a neutron (decreasing the atomic number, without changing the atomic mass); a neutrino is emitted as well as (depending on the isotope's energy) either γ radiation or an Auger electron

electron microscopy A technique based on theories formulated by the French physicist, L de Broglie (Nobel prize, 1929), where electrons have shorter wavelengths than light and therefore a higher resolution; the first electron microscope was constructed in 1937 in Canada at 7000 magnifications; the three major types of electron microscopes are scanning electron microscopy‡, scanning tunnel microscopy‡, and transmission electron microscopy‡; see Microscopy

electron-spin resonance PALEOANTHROPOLOGY A method from solid-state physics that measures time by testing for minute radiation-induced damage to crystals, which increases with age; in ESR the sample is placed in a magnetic field and bombarded by finely tuned microwaves, exciting the electrons in the crystal lattice; a sensor detects a response, the intensity of which correlates with the age of the sample; unlike thermoluminescence, the sample can be tested repeatedly; ESR has been instrumental in providing the oldest dates for anatomically modern human beings in the Near East and Africa, as it is accurate in the periods that cannot be measured by standard* dating methods; Cf Thermoluminescence

*Carbon-14 dating methods reach only 40 000 years in the past, and potassium-argon dating begins counting at 300 000 years

electromagnetic spectrum

		Wavelength		DC power
AC Power		1000 km	ELF	1 Hz
Voice Sound Ultrasound AM radio		1 km	LF	1 kHz
FM radio Cellular phones		1 m	VHF	1 MHz
Satellite link Microwave ovens		1 mm	EHF	1 GHz
		1 µm		1 THz
		1 nm		1 PHz
		1 pm		1 EHz
gamma rays				

InfraRed / TV Range / Visible Light / UV / X-rays

electron spin resonance spectrometry A technique for measuring the mobility of cell membrane lipids in which synthetic phospholipids containing a nitrogen group are introduced into an otherwise normal phospholipid membrane; the technique measures the energy absorbed by the unpaired electron of the nitroxide group; these studies have demonstrated that natural membranes have a low viscosity and are fluid-like; see Photobleaching

electron tunneling BIOCHEMISTRY A quantum mechanical effect that allows electrons to overcome energy barriers, eg as occurs in photosynthesis

electronic billing Electronic claims processing, see there

electronic claims processing The submission of a bills for services rendered by a physician to third-party payers by modem, which are usually paid within 15 days of filing claims; it is estimated that by the year 2000, Medicare's electronic billing system will process 1 billion claims/year, saving the government ± $200 million/year in administrative costs (CAP Today March 1994 p57)

electronic crossmatch TRANSFUSION MEDICINE A process whereby a computer operating with FDA-approved blood banking software evaluates several parameters in the donor and recipient ABO and Rh blood types and permits the release of the donor unit if there is concordance between donor and recipient data (Laboratory Medicine 1995; 26:315QA)

electronic data interchange The electronic exchange of data and payments, a process that impacts on all aspects of the health care environment, serving to both cut costs and improve cash flow; EDI users include insurance carriers, medical products supplies, pharmaceutical companies, hospitals and physicians; in the US, the major driving force behind EDI is the Health Care Financing Administration, a branch of the US federal Human and Health Services, which has a powerful incentive to reduce paperwork in claims and fund transfers as it issues 500×10^6 checks and process 4×10^9 claims/year (InfoWeek/8 Feb 1993)

electronic data publishing A type of formal scientific communication in which data, eg DNA sequences by GenBank, are gathered, processed, and distributed electronically, serving to complement and support printed publications; in contrast to electronic journal publishing, scientific conclusions that are supported by the data are published in the 'hard copy' or paper journal, while the data itself is published via a network-accessible database (Science 1991; 252:1273)

electronic journal An 'on line' journal that allows immediate access to a researcher's findings; the first users of EJs include libraries in response to the consolidation or 'bundling' of major and minor journals

electronic mail e-mail, see there

electronystagmography A battery of neurologic and neuro-otologic examinations that record eye movements electro-oculographically; these test are of use in separating vestibular and oculomotor deficits of the CNS from deficits of the peripheral vestibular system

electroporation BIOCHEMISTRY A technique used to gain access to cells by creating transient pores with short controlled electric pulses, either exponential decay pulses, or 'square wave' pulses; electroporation allows incorporation of drugs, proteins, nucleic acids, or other molecules into the cell after it reseals, or can be used to integrate molecules in cell structures or insert them into the cell membrane; electroporation has traditionally been used for the transfection and/or transformation of prokaryotic and eukaryotic cells in vitro, but may have clinical applications, eg insertion of recombinant CD4 into RBC membranes, which blocks the transcription of HIV from patient isolates (Am Biotech Lab Jan 1995, p18)

electrothermal deactivation PUBLIC HEALTH A method for treating medical waste to render it noninfectious to humans, by treating it with low-frequency radiowaves, after which the waste can be disposed of in landfills (Laboratory Medicine 1995; 26:323QA) see Medical waste

elemental diet A basic diet composed of oligopeptides and amino acids, disaccharides or partially hydrolyzed starch and minimal fat; these diets provide proton neutralization sufficient to maintain gastric pH above pH 3.5; in patients with severe burn injury, only 3% of patients maintained on an elemental diet had major upper gastrointestinal hemorrhage compared to 30% fed with a regular diet; commercial elemental diets include Precision, Travasorb and Vivonex

elementary body A 300-nm extracellular infective form of *Chlamydia* spp; it is uniform, acidophilic, coccoid and once within the cell, perinuclear; EBs attach to specific membrane receptors on the host cell and are endocytosed; after six hours in a phagosome, the EB reorganizes into larger (800-1000 nm) particles known as reticulate bodies

elephant ear appearance PEDIATRIC RADIOLOGY A descriptor for flaring of the iliac wings, flattening of the acetabular roofs and ischial tapering; the iliac index, which is ½ the sum of the iliac and acetabular angles, is characteristically reduced in Down syndrome

elephant feet invasion Bulldozing, see there

the Elephant man Joseph Merrick   A 19th century Londoner who suffered from a severe deforming disease that had been diagnosed by medical historians as von Recklinghausen's disease, and subsequently re-diagnosed as Proteus syndrome, see there (Br Med J 1986; 293:683)

'elephant policy' see Trolley car policy

elephant skin Subcutaneous edema with redundancy of the skin and dermal thickening with elephantiasis, seen in *Onchocerca volvulus*

elephantiasis Pachydermoid cutaneous induration elicited by chronic lymphatic blockage, a clinical event that may occur in 1) The legs, causing edema, chronic inflammation and eventually pachydermia, due to lymphatic plugging by microfilaria, eg *Wuchereria bancrofti, Brugia malayi, Onchocerca volvulus*; the scrotal lymphedema may extend cranially to the renal lymphatics and rupture into the renal pelvis, causing chyluria 2) The penis and scrotum due to lymphogranuloma venereum 3) The arm, often secondary to axillary lymph node dissection in a modified radical mastectomy

elevator testicle see Migrating testicle

ELF see Electromagnetic radiation

elfin face syndrome Williams syndrome, see there

elimination diet A dietary regimen in which foods are eliminated in turn, in order to detect the cause(s) of a food allergy, commonly implicated causes of which include milk, egg, and others; an ED is used in individuals, especially children with atopy, suspected of being allergic to certain foods, and is used to determine whether there is reduction of the symptoms attributed to allergy; elimination are time-consuming, onerous, and costly, and may not necessarily identify a specific detary allergen; if the symptoms continue while the subject is the diet, the symptoms are unlikely to be due to the eliminated foods; Cf Desensitization diet

ELISA Enzyme-linked immunosorbent assay A heterogeneous immunoenzymatic assay that approaches the sensitivity of RIA and has the advantage of lower cost, simpler equipment, faster 'turn-around time', and none of the problems and inconvenience inherent in handling radioactive substances; ELISA may be used to measure virtually any antigen and antibody, although radioimmunoassay continues to be preferred in research, given its ease of performance PRINCIPLE An antigen of interest is incubated in a medium containing an antibody (usually monoclonal) raised against the antigen and bound to a 'solid' phase, ie either attached to a bead or to the wall of plastic plate with multiple wells; a second incubation is carried out with a detector antibody raised against the monoclonal antibody, often with an attached indicator enzyme, eg peroxidase or alkaline phosphatase, see Avidin-biotin method, EMIT

Note: The detector antibody is linked to an enzyme, eg peroxidase; a final step is addition of a substrate that is digested by the detector's enzyme, producing a color measured by spectrophotometry; ELISA is used in the clinical laboratory to detect viral antigens including cytomegalovirus, various hepatitis A and B viral antigens and antibodies, eg to HIV gp120, as well as *Neisseria gonorrhoeae*, choriogonadotropic hormone, thyroid-stimulating hormone and others

'Elisha method' Mouth-to-mouth artificial respiration

ELK Ears (nose and throat), lungs, kidneys An acronym for the organs involved in Wegener's granulomatosis (WG); limited WG spares the kidneys and lacks signs of systemic vasculitis; generalized WG involves the kidneys and/or has signs of systemic vasculitis; disease exacerbation is best monitored by measuring titers of antineutrophil cytoplasmic antibodies by indirect immunofluorescence

ellipse sign An oblong 'mass' seen in an upper GI radiocontrast study corresponding to simple (non-malignant) pooling of contrast material in an ulcer base

elliptocytosis Hereditary elliptocytosis, see there

ELM test PEDIATRICS An abbreviated outcomes-based test that measures an infant's expressive, receptive, and visual language abilities; in the ET, the parents are questioned about certain components of the infant's speech, and the infant is asked to carry out certain simple tasks; serial ELM testing can be used to monitor response to various interventions intended to improve communication

El Niño PUBLIC HEALTH A large interannual climate variation* of the Pacific Ocean-atmosphere system which corresponds to a warming of the east equatorial water of the Pacific Ocean occurring in 3-6 year cycles; the El Niño-Southern Oscillation cycling model is consistent with a low-order chaos mechanism (Science 1994; 264:70, 72R) a recent theory posits that EN may be initiated by volcanic activity ('hot vents') on the ocean floor, resulting in warming of the overlying waters (New York Times 25 April 1995, pC1) see Climatological disaster; Cf La Niña

Note: The term El Niño (Christ child) originates from Peruvian fishermen who recognized that the coastal changes associated with El Niño occurred around Christmas

elongation MOLECULAR BIOLOGY Any synthetic reaction which proceeds by adding one component per synthetic cycle, as in elongation of a protein chain; see Translation

elongation factors MOLECULAR BIOLOGY Eukaryotic proteins, eg eEF-1, eEF-2 that are similar to the TuTs complex of prokaryotes, which facilitate the binding of the amino-acyl-tRNA to ribosomes and subsequent transfer to the peptidyl-tRNA complex Note: For the growth of a peptide chain, two sites on the ribosome are required, the A site, which accommodates the incoming amino-acyl-tRNA, holding the tRNA until the next codon has arrived and the P site, containing the Peptidyl-tRNA complex, the tRNA linked to the amino acids added to a nascent peptide chain

EM Electron microscopy, also 1) Electromagnetic 2) Electromechanical 3) Emergency medicine

Also 1) Ejection murmur 4) Electrophoretic mobility 5) Embden-Meyerhof pathway (of glycolysis) 7) Emmetropia (ophthalmology) 8) Endosteal marrow 9) Environmental monitoring 10) Erythrocyte mass 11) Exact match

emancipated minor A person under the age of 'majority' or adulthood who is regarded in the eyes of the law as being old enough (usually by virtue of marriage or financial independence) to make adult decisions; an EM may make decisions about termination of pregnancy, countermand his/her parents religious beliefs, in particular those that may be viewed as possibly life-threatening, eg the refusal of blood transfusion or certain forms of therapy

'emasculated' hormone CLINICAL PHARMACOLOGY A drug designed to simulate a target hormone molecule involved in a receptor-hormonal ligand interaction, which may be partial agonists or antagonists of the target hormone; these substances include propranolol, a β-adrenergic receptor antagonist, an 'emasculated' adrenaline and cimetidine, a histamine H2-receptor antagonist, which might be regarded as an 'emasculated' histamine

EMB agar MICROBIOLOGY A bacterial growth medium containing eosin, methylene blue, peptones, and lactose, used as a differential growth medium to differentiate lactose and non-lactose fermenting enterobacteriaceae

embargo arrangement MEDICAL JOURNALISM An unwritten agreement between the news media (newspapers, television, radio) and scientific and medical journals, in which 'newsworthy' stories about major therapeutic advances or diseases are not publicly disseminated until physicians or scientists receive the journal(s) and have had sufficient time to evaluate the results of the trial; once a member of the media breaks the silence, as occurred in the 'Reuters News Agency/aspirin' case (**N Engl J Med 1988; 318:918ed**), the rest of the media 'breaks herd', and 'stampedes' with the story; articles from the New England Journal of Medicine are not reported by the electronic news media until Wednesday afternoon, and by the paper news media Thursday morning; when the Ingelfinger rule has been waived (because the information is deemed important, ie of potential benefit for patient management), the authors may choose to either report or not report the information in accordance with the NEJM's policies (**N Engl J Med 1994; 330:1608ED**) see Ingelfinger rule

embedded objectives A secondary benefit of a stated or overt objective, eg development of new technologies while attempting to solve a particularly difficult scientific problem, eg the Human Genome Project (**N Engl J Med 1993; 329:585BR**)

EMBO European Molecular Biology Organization

embolism The presence of extraneous material within vessels **AIR EMBOLISM** The presence of gas is of greatest importance when it is in the coronary and cerebral arteries; although difficult to quantify, 100 cc is considered sufficient to cause death; to document its presence at autopsy, the organ must be opened underwater (to detect bubbling) **AMNIOTIC FLUID EMBOLISM** An embolus containing lanugo, squames, mucus and debris which occurs when the opened maternal circulation communicates with amniotic fluids **FAT EMBOLISM** An embolic event that follows long bone fractures, and less commonly hepatic trauma; embolic fat 'metastasizes' to the lungs, causing dyspnea, shock to the brain causing coma, to the kidneys causing lipiduria **NITROGEN EMBOLISM** An embolic event that shares certain features in common with air embolism, which is directly responsible for the 'bends' or Caisson's disease, occurring in divers who surface too rapidly, where the nitrogen 'boils' in the vessels, causing joint and abdominal pain, or if it affects the brain, may prove fatal **PARADOXICAL EMBOLUS** An embolus that migrates in the direction opposite, ie 'paradoxical', to the blood flow, a potential complication of right-to-left shunt in congenital heart disease where septic or other vegetations from the right side of heart (or from peripheral veins) pass through a patent foramen ovale to the systemic circulation

embryoid body A histological component of a germ cell tumor containing an embryonal disk, an amniotic sac and an amniotic cavity; rare germ cell tumors with abundant embryoid bodies are known as 'polyembryoma'; occasionally, the semantically incorrect 'embryonal' body or the distinct 'glomerular' body is used interchangeably with embryoid body, which may be partially mimicked by cellular aggregates seen in the neuroectodermal tumor of infancy, Wilms' tumor or the Schiller-Duval bodies of the yolk sac tumor; see Glomeruloid body

embryoma An outmoded, imprecise term implying a structure that recapitulates an undifferentiated primitive, often mesenchymal tumor; although embryoma is still used by some pathologists, the preferred term is blastoma, as in pulmonary blastoma, neuroblastoma or nephroblastoma

Note: Embryoma is still an accepted term when referring to the ultra-rare parotid embryoma

embryonic testicular regression syndrome Vanishing testes syndrome A heterogeneous group of male pseudo-hermaphrodites resulting from the cessation of testicular function during the mid-portion of male sex differentiation (weeks 8-14) resulting in the absence of gonads in an XY person

Note: It is likely that with time, the adjective embryonic will be deleted in the working parlance, resulting in the simpler term, testicular regression syndrome, as already used in the Mendelian Inheritance in Man catalogs

embryoscope A narrow-bore device used to perform embryoscopy, which is a modification of an arterioscope

embryoscopy An imaging technique in which a ultrasound-guided small-bore needle with an endoscope is inserted through the abdominal wall into the uterus (without violating the amniotic cavity) to view a living embryo; unlike fetoscopy, which can only be performed in the second and third trimesters of pregnancy and carries a not insignificant risk of fetal wastage, embryoscopy can be performed as early as 6 weeks after fertilization, and appears to be safer, and is more informative than ultrasonography; embryoscopy is in early stages of development, but is likely to replace fetoscopy as both a diagnostic tool (eg to identify gross physical defects), and therapeutic tool for performing fetal surgery and delivering gene therapy (**New York Times 6 July 1993; C1**) Cf Fetoscopy

EMD Electromechanical dissociation, see there

emergency doctrine A guiding principle that grants permission to health care providers to perform a procedure under circumstances where it is impossible or impractical to obtain consent; this allows the surgeon to repair other potentially life-threatening situations at the same time he is performing a procedure for which there is appropriately documented consent; the emergency doctrine is a component of fully informed consent; see Informed consent; see Good Samaritan laws; Cf 'Rule of rescue'

emergency medical service An organized system, created by the US government in 1973 (Public Law 93-154) that provides emergency care, intimately linked to the universal emergency telephone number, 911; the care is provided from vehicles, ie ambulance or helicopter, by certified and licensed personnel, eg emergency medical technicians, in restricted geographic regions; services provided by the EMS system include: Emergency medical communications, transportation, disaster plans and consumer training programs; see Air ambulance

Emergency Medical Treatment and Active Labor Act HEALTH CARE ADMINISTRATION A law passed as part of the Consolidated Omnibus Budget Reconciliation Act of 1986 that was enacted to protect against patient dumping*; the EMTALA has created a legislative morass due to its vague wording and lack of interpretive guidelines, opening it to broad judicial interpretation; it has been broadly applied to include patients who were either never admitted to a hospital, or could not be, as the ward to which they were to be admitted was filled to its legal capacity, and thus was 'bypassed' (Am Med News 16 Nov 1992 p1) see COBRA legislation

*The transfer or 'bypass' of indigent or uninsured patients from private, ie for-profit, hospitals to public hospitals for financial reasons

emergency psychiatric commitment The temporary admission of a person with an acute psychotic reaction to a mental institution for a period of observation, not to exceed seven working days; beyond this time, the patient must be formally committed or released; the patient must be dangerous, intoxicated or inebriated to justify commital; see Malpractice

emergency response Fight-or-flight response, see there

emerging pathogen PUBLIC HEALTH Any of a number of pathogens (eg *Cryptosporidium*, *Escherichia coli* O157:H7, *Hantavirus*, multidrug resistant pneumococci, vancomycin-resistant enterococci) that are regarded as increasing in incidence (Arch Pathol Lab Med 1995; 119:397ED)

emerging virus PUBLIC HEALTH Any of a number of viruses that is regarded as increasing in incidence

emeritus staff The body of physicians, dentists, osteopaths, or other independent medical practitioners who have retired from active medical practice; emeritus staff fulfill roles in teaching and consultation but usually do not admit patients

EMG Electromyography

EMIT Enzyme-multiplied (or mediated) immunoassay technique A proprietary immunoassay (Syva Corp, Palo Alto) that consists of a homogeneous (one phase) enzyme-labeled competitive immunoassay, used for therapeutic drug monitoring, eg antiepileptic, antiasthmatic, antineoplastic and cardioactive agents, detection of 'abuse' drugs, eg cannabinoids and cocaine metabolites and hormones, eg thyroxine

emollient CLINICAL THERAPEUTICS A generic term for a hydrating agent that is applied topically with the purpose of softening the skin, in particular laminated keratin or hyperkeratotic scales, eg of psoriasis; aqueous emollients (eg yellow paraffin or aqueous cream) are widely preferred to greasier (eg petrolatum, aquaphor cream) for cosmetic and comfort reasons (N Engl J Med 1995; 332:581RV)

emotion NEUROPHYSIOLOGY One of most human of attributes, defined as a strong feeling of any kind, which includes anger, excitement, fear, grief, joy, hatred, love; emotion is not the product of a single emotional center, but rather the integration of interconnecting pathways; in happiness, the right prefrontal and temporal-parietal cortex are most active; in sadness, the anterior limbic system and the left prefrontal cortex are most active (NY Times March 28 1995, C1)

emotional abuse PEDIATRICS '*...coercive, demeaning, or overly distant behavior by a parent or other caretaker that interferes with a child's normal social or psychological development.*' (N Engl J Med 1995; 332:1425RV) see Child abuse, Elderly abuse, Psychological abuse

emotional distress MEDICAL MALPRACTICE Intentional infliction of emotional distress The 'outrage' tort A legal action initiated against a defendant who allegedly said or did something so completely absurd (medically) or insulting to the plaintiff that he suffered emotional damage; see Damages, Malpractice; Cf Punitive damages

emotional memory NEUROPHYSIOLOGY A recently-identified type of memory that is imprinted at the time of emotionally-charged events, in particular by information received during 'fight or flight' phenomena (FoF) in contrast to the usual form of memory that requires repetition to become permanent, emotional events are thought to 'burn' a permanent mental image into the core memory; the same hormones, adrenaline (epinephrine) and norepinephrine that cause the FoF response are responsible for burning the image and response sequence into the core

memory, the intensity of which is proportional to the intensity of the emotion; control of EM is thought to be under the baton of the amygdala, and may be blocked by propranolol (New York Times 25 Ocotober 1994; C1)

emperipolesis Active intrusion of viable hematopoietic cells in the cytoplasm of histiocytes, a histological finding typical of sinus histiocytosis with massive lymphadenopathy, that may also be seen in histoplasmosis, rhinoscleroma and salmonellosis

'Emperor's New Clothes' syndrome A facetious sobriquet for angiodysplasia of the right colon, which consists of a convoluted mesh of dilated, tortuous submucosal veins seen by the radiologist with selective mesenteric angiography, but which is invisible to both the surgeon and the pathologist, as the dilated vessels collapse upon resection (N Engl J Med 1974; 291:569, 573cpc); post-resection injection of silicon rubber into the arteries is required to visualize angiodysplasia, a disease of the elderly, which may be congenital or neoplastic or secondary to fecal impaction

Note: Gastric angiodysplasia causes a 'Watermelon appearance', see there

employer mandate HEALTH CARE ENVIRONMENT A regulation that requires employers to provide insurance coverage or face stiff penalties (Am Med News 26 October 1992, p7) EMs include health insurance obtained through an individual person's employer (either current or former), union, or family member, and are the mechanism by which 60% of US citizens (with insurance) obtain healthcare coverage (from Congressional Quarterly, 1993, in Clin Lab Sci 1994; 7:141)

'empty calorie' CLINICAL NUTRITION A unit of food-derived energy, usually in the form of carbohydrates, which is essentially devoid of nutritive value, ie lacking protein, vitamins, dietary fibers; empty calories are typical of 'junk' or snack foods, including potato chips (potato crisps), pastries, cakes and soft drinks; see Cafeteria diet, Couch potato, Junk food

empty nest syndrome PSYCHOLOGY A popular term of uncertain origin for the constellation of symptoms described in middle-aged women whose children have left home (the 'nest') for various reasons (college and university, pursuit of career, marriage); symptoms of this understudied phenomenon include depression, loss of self-esteem, and loneliness, which are due to the mother having lost her principle raison d'etre, ie raising children, who are no longer dependent on her for their basic needs

empty sella syndrome NEURORADIOLOGY The finding of a moderately enlarged sella turcica that may not translate into clinical findings, caused by a partial or complete absence of the sellar diaphragma, most commonly seen in obese, middle-aged ♀; the compression of the hypophysis against the floor and posterior wall by the extended suprasellar cisterns in not invariably accompanied by pituitary hypofunction, although thyroid-stimulating hormone, gonadotropin and prolactin levels may be diminished and/or accompanied by diabetes insipidus; primary empty sella syndrome is due to chronically elevated intracranial pressure or secondary to regional surgery or irradiation CLINICAL The patients may complain of vague headaches, systemic hypertension, pseudotumor cerebri and if secondary, CSF rhinorrhea, but it is most often asymptomatic

empty scrotum syndrome Functional prepubertal castrate syndrome Bilateral absence of functional testicular tissue in a genotypically and phenotypically normal male; the absence of müellerian-derived tissue implies that functional testicular tissue was present in the fetus, which was followed by prepubertal atrophy CLINICAL Eunuchoid habitus, delayed puberty, but in marked contrast to true eunuchs, subjects with this syndrome are short in stature TREATMENT Androgen to induce secondary sex characteristics and a penile prosthesis

EMS see Emergency medical service

EMT EMERGENCY MEDICINE An abbreviation* for any of a number of grades of Emergency Medical Technician which are based on the number of hours of formal training

*Also 1) Electromagnetic team 2) Electromagnetic technology 3) Electron microscope tomography 4) Emergency medical tag 5) Emergency medical treatment 6) Evaluation monitoring team

EMT-A Basic EMT A level that requires at least 81 (up to 140) hours of training which is standardized by the Department of Transportation; EMT-As constitute the backbone of the EMT workforce in the US and known the basic principles of patient care, how to identify clinical signs that are central to patient assessment and care and how to treat specific emergencies; see EMT; Cf First responder

EMT-D A basic Emergency Medical Technician (EMT-A) who is trained in automatic or manual defibrillation, but is not authorized to perform any other advanced life support skill; see EMT

EMT-I Intermediate EMT A level that requires at least 110 (up to 1000) hours of training; in addition to the skills and knowledge base of basic levels of emergency care, EMT-Is also have advanced life support skills including the insertion of IV catheters, administration of certain emergency medications, noninvasive airway management, and use of automatic or manual defibrillators; see EMT

EMT-P Paramedic or advanced EMT A level that requires at least 1000 hours of training and all advanced life support skills ranging from the assessment of all organ systems, insertion of IV catheters, administration of emergency fluids and medications, noninvasive airway management, and use of automatic or manual defibrillators, to management of the emotionally disturbed and obstetric emergencies; see EMT

EMTALA Emergency Medical Treatment & Active Labor Act, see there

ENA see Extractable nuclear antigens

enabling technology A component of a developing market (for anything from a new technology, eg multimedia, cellular telephone communication) which includes protocols, (eg NetWare, PostScript), operating systems (eg MS-DOS), services (eg CellularOne), and others that corresponds to the 'glue' that allows something of significance to be performed with the infrastructure that has been put into place ((Sci Am 1994; 270/9:72, Forbes ASAP 27 Feb 1995, p42) see Infrastructure

enalapril maleate CARDIOLOGY An angiotensin-converting enzyme inhibitor used as an antihypertensive agent, and reportedly useful in ameliorating the remodeling phenomenon[1]; in SOLVD[2], enalapril therapy in patients with asymptomatic left ventricular dysfunction ↓ the incidence of heart failure, and the rate of cardiovascular hospitalization (N Engl J Med 1992; 327:685OA); in CONSENSUS II[3], enalapril therapy was not found to improve survival and was associated with an ↑ deaths due to heart failure in patients with myocardial infarction, despite a slight but significant beneficial effect on the progression of congestive heart failure (N Engl J Med 1992; 327:678OA)

[1]The progressive left ventricular dilation that follows a myocardial infarction, a finding that has prognostic import [2]Studies of Left Ventricular Dysfunction [3]Cooperative New Scandinavian Enalapril Survival Study II

en bloc French, entirety Surgical en bloc resection is performed in certain malignancies with the hope of removing the entire primary lesion, the contiguous draining lymph nodes and everything lying between, as in a modified radical mastectomy; in autopsies, the brief form, 'en bloc' refers to complete evisceration of the thoracic and abdominal cavities

encainide MJ 9067 An analog of lysergic acid with antiarrhythmic activity, which with flecainide, was entered in the CAST (Cardiac Arrhythmia Suppression Trial) study evaluating the effect of such agents in patients with asymptomatic or mildly symptomatic arrhythmia; the treated group mortality had a 3.5-fold greater incidence of death with arrhythmia than with the placebo-treated group; encainide is not thought to be an appropriate prophylactic agent for arrhythmia (N Engl J Med 1991; 324:781); Cf CAST, Flecainide

encapsulated bacteria A generic term for bacteria that are enclosed in an extracellular polymeric substance that is usually composed of polysaccharides; in general, capsules inhibit phagocytosis and adherence, and encapsulated strains of bacteria (eg *Streptococcus pneumoniae*, or *Haemophilus influenzae*) are more virulent that their nonencapsulated brethren; the response of the immune system to infection by EBs is poor in HIV-infected children; the risk of serious bacterial infections in children with advanced HIV disease is ↓ by either IV immune globulin (N Engl J Med 1994; 331:1181OA) or prophylactic T-S

encapsulated cell therapy CLINICAL THERAPEUTICS A generic term for the enclosing of cells capable of producing some desired substance (eg pancreatic islet cells that produce insulin) in a semipermeable nonimmunogenic sheath, with the purpose of restoring a lost function; ECT is still experimental, but is approaching clinical application; it is being driven by the need for a viable means of circumventing (through a process known as immunoisolation) the immune system which attacks and destroys transplanted (nonself) tissues in the absence of long-term immunosuppressive therapy; three major types of biohydrid 'organs' have been attempted, to wit, the perfusion shunt, the diffusion chamber, and that which is most promising, the microsphere (Science & Medicine July/August 1995, p16) Note: While the most obvious and immediate need for ECT is for treating DM, the use of implantable 'bioreactors' that produce hormones, biological response modifiers, and growth factors is likely to follow the first successes with biohybrid organs

encode MOLECULAR BIOLOGY The process of reading a message from a segment of DNA nucleotides, transcribing that message into code for a messenger RNA from a structural gene, with the ultimate step being a mature protein

en coup de sabre Coup de sabre appearance, see there

end-labeling MOLECULAR BIOLOGY The addition of a label (usually radioactive) to either the 3' or the 5' end of a DNA probe

end-piece EXPERIMENTAL BIOLOGY An obsolete term for a fraction of guinea pig serum now known to correspond to C2 (complement) HISTOLOGY *pars terminalis* [NH3] The terminal part of the tail of a spermatozoon, which consists of the axoneme and the flagellar membrane

end-stage renal disease The decompensated stage of chronic renal failure, which is defined as renal insufficiency of a degree requiring dialysis or kidney transplantation for survival (MMWR1992; 41:834) EPIDEMIOLOGY DM (30% of cases are directly related to DM) and hypertension are the most common causes of ESRD; 1 in 400 of the 2 million (US) new hypertensive patients/year eventually develop ESRD (Sci & Med Nov/Dec 1994, p8) and ESRD may be seen in kidneys subjected to chronic dialysis; 27% of ESRD in the USA occurs in blacks (who have an increased incidence of DM, glomerulopathies and hypertension); in the US, blacks have a reduced rate of transplantation of kidneys (and other organs) and a reduced rate of survival when transplanted (N Engl J Med 1991; 324:302) COSTS ESRD program for 200 000 patients (0.08% of US population), cost $6 x 10^9 (0.8% of total health care expenditures) (N Engl J Med 1993; 329:1395SA) PATHOLOGY Intravascular smooth muscle proliferation, evoked by ischemia, venous thrombosis, proliferation of arterial granular cells and Bowman's epithelium COD Infection is a frequent complication of ESRD and may be due to impaired macrophage Fcg-receptor function (N Engl J Med 1990; 322:717)

endemic cretinism A condition that affects up to 10% of isolated populations, which is caused by severe endemic iodine deficiency and characterized by deaf-mutism, mental retardation, rigid-spastic motor disorder, and occasionally hypothyroidism; iodine therapy prevents EC when administered before the last trimester of pregnancy (N Engl J Med 1994; 331:1739OA)

endocardial fibroelastosis A rare idiopathic condition of early childhood onset with focal or global cartilage-like fibroelastic endocardial thickening, most prominently affecting the left ventricle; the heart may be dilated, hypertrophic or both PATHOGENESIS Uncertain; postulated mechanisms include hypoxia, hemodynamic pressure overload (⅓ of cases have congenital cardiac malformations), lymphatic obstruction, fetal endomyocarditis of viral origin, metabolic or enzymatic defects or autoimmune phenomena PATHOLOGY ↑ in collagen and elastic fibers parallel to the surface PROGNOSIS EF may cause sudden cardiac arrest in children or slow congestive heart failure in adolescent or adult survivors; Cf Endomyocardial fibrosis

endocervical brush A device used to obtain cytological specimens from the endocervical canal, which has virtually replaced wooden spatulas, and cotton swabs; EBs increase the yield of endocervical cells at the price of an ↑ in 'reactive' artefacts, in particular herpes-like changes in the form of multinucleation, and margination of nuclear chromatin; the findings of ground-glass chromatin, and intranuclear inclusions in difficult cases favor the diagnosis of herpes (Acta Cytologica 1994; 38:51OA)

endocytosis MOLECULAR BIOLOGY The uptake of materials from outside of a cell, which involves three steps: Clustering of membrane proteins by clathrin and associated proteins, invagination of the membrane into a clathrin-coated pit, and pinching off of the neck, resulting in a coated vesicle (Nature 1995; 374:186, 190, 116N&V)

endod Soapberry plant PARASITOLOGY A plant, the dried berries of which are used in Ethiopia as a laundry detergent, which contains a group of oleanic acid glucosides known as lemmatoxin, which make endod toxic to schistosome-bearing snails (JAMA 1991; 265:2650)

endoderm The innermost of the embryo's primary germ layers, which gives rise to the lining of the mouth, pharynx, gastrointestinal and respiratory tracts, liver, gall bladder and pancreas

endodermal sinus tumor Yolk sac tumor An ovarian tumor of female children and adolescents, characterized by elevated α-fetoprotein levels, a large tumor mass (average 15 cm in diameter) composed of a meshwork of cuboidal cells arranged in pseudopapillary structures that recapitulate the embryonal yolk sac PROGNOSIS Untreated, 3-year survival 13%; with multidrug regimen, 50%; see Germ cell tumor

endogenous depression PSYCHIATRY Melancholia A clinical form* of depression that occurs either de novo, or in absence of external events that would justify the degree of depression; ED is characterized by pervasive sadness, hopelessness, loss of interest in daily activities, and physical symptoms including weight loss, insomnia, and reduced libido; in ED, there may be an increased 'threshold' to stressful life events that requires little external input to initiate recurrence (Science News 1994; 146:52) see Depression; Cf Reactive depression

Note: The terms used in this condition may be confusing; a possible equivalent term used by the American Psychiatric Association is 'Dysthmic disorder' (300.4 in DSM-IV, 1994) or an alternative, minor depressive disorder

endogenous pyrogens Any of a number of compounds, usually cytokines, eg IL-6, IL-1α, TNFα, INFγ, and macrophage inflammatory protein-1 that induce a febrile reaction, typically in a background of an acute phase response (Perspect Biol & Med 1993; 36:611) Cf Intracellular signaling

endometrioid cancer An adenocarcinoma that histologically mimics that of primary endometrial carcinoma, which occurs in 1) The ovary, where it comprises 10-25% of epithelial malignancies and in 10-20% of cases is accompanied by endometriosis, a condition which may precede the tumor; the prognosis is two-fold better than that of serous or mucinous cystadenocarcinomas of the ovaries 2) The prostate A histologic variant of the usual type of prostatic adenocarcinoma that has a similar clinical behavior and prognosis

endometrial hyperplasia Adenomatous hyperplasia of endometrium GYNECOLOGY A potentially premalignant endometrial lesion of older women, that is divided (per the International Society of Gynecological Pathologists) into

1) HYPERPLASIA WITHOUT ATYPIA Glands are crowded without cytologic atypia; these have a < 2% chance of progressing to carcinoma and are further divided

A) SIMPLE HYPERPLASIA Glands are not back-to-back

B) COMPLEX HYPERPLASIA Glands are back-to-back

2) HYPERPLASIA WITH ATYPIA Glands are crowded with cytologic atypia; ± 23% progress to carcinoma

endometriosis A condition affecting up to 50% of ♀, defined as the presence of functioning endometrial glands and stroma outside of the uterine cavity which is often accompanied by dysmenorrhea and pain; ectopic sites in

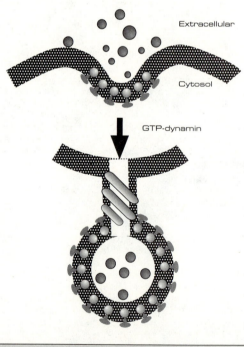

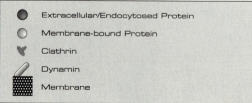

endocytosis

descending order of frequency include ovaries, broad ligaments, rectovaginal septum, umbilical scars, intestine, lungs, and elsewhere; endometriosis is often associated with cyclical pain and regional swelling linked to vicarious ectopic bleeding that parallels the menstrual period in the uterine cavity EVALUATION Diagnostic laparoscopy TREATMENT Medical therapy is ineffective; surgical therapy may be of use when pelvic anatomy is distorted; TAH-BSO is the definitive treatment (Mayo Clin Proc 1995; 70:453)

endomyocardial biopsy A biopsy of the endocardium and subjacent myocardium, a procedure used to detect inflammation, anthracycline cardiotoxicity or the rare presence of cardiac tumors; see Dallas criteria

endomyocardial fibrosis A restrictive cardiomyopathy that affects relatively young patients and causes the death of 15-25% of those in equatorial Africa, which is less common elsewhere; EMF is characterized by dense fibrotic thickening of the inflow tracts of both the right and left ventricles, causing tricuspid and mitral valve regurgitation, while sparing the outflow tracts, resulting in a defect in diastolic filling with intact systolic function, which often progresses to decreased cardiac output and congestive heart failure PATHOGENESIS Uncertain, although fruits rich in serotonin (plantain) are implicated as EMF resembles the lesions of carcinoid syndrome; althernately, carnitine deficiency TREATMENT Surgical excision of the fibrosed area and valve replacement may be effective; Cf Fibroelastosis

endonuclease A generic term for any of a group of hydrolytic enzymes that attack specific internal DNA and RNA oligonucleotide sequences; bacterial restriction endonucleases are major tools in molecular biology and used for hybridization and probe analysis; see EcoR I, HindIII

endorphin A generic term for endogenous opioid peptides that include endorphin, leu-enkephalin, met-enkephalin and dynorphin, each of which binds to a cognate receptor; endorphin is divided into α-, β- and γ-endorphins, which have the same N-terminal amino acid sequences but are cleaved at different C-terminal sites from the precursor protein β-lipotropin; see Enkephalin and POMC

Note: Endorphin research has focused on delineating the pathogenesis of addiction disorders and the perception of pain

β-endorphin β-endorphin is derived from proopiomelanocortin POMC via β-lipotropin, and is linked to hypophyseal secretion and pain perception; β-endorphin is present in the CNS, pituitary gland, and peripheral tissues, and is linked to various physiologic and pathological conditions, including responses to pain and stress, endotoxic shock, opiate addiction, premenstrual syndrome, childbirth, exercise, mental disorders and hypertension; β-endorphin can be measured in body fluids using RIA; specimens not processed immediately should be frozen (Arch Pathol Lab Med 1992; 116:827OA)

endoscopic biliary drainage A procedure in which a distended gallbladder is decompressed (either by endoscopic papillotomy, or by placement of a prosthesis) without extraction of gallstones; EBD is used as emergency therapy for severe acute cholangitis; following resolution of the acute attack, definitive therapy is performed in the form of cholecystectomy or completion of endoscopic papillotomy (N Engl J Med 1992; 326:1582OA)

endoscopic hemostasis The treatment of bleeding vessels measuring up to 2 mm in dimeter, eg of the stomach by either 1) Injection of a hemostatic solution (eg absolute ethanol, a 1:10 000 diluted solution of epinephrine, or polidocanol, a sclerosing agent) or by 2) An endoscopically guided device that generates heat by either a) Electrical energy (with bipolar electrocoagulation) generating a maximal temperature of 100° C or by b) Thermal energy (with a heater probe) that generates up 250° C of heat;

although the comparitive data is preliminary, all three methods appear to be equally effective (N Engl J Med 1994; 331:717SA)

endoscopic ligation The treatment of esophageal varices (EVs) by endoscopically ligating the veins with small O-shaped elastic rings; endoscopic ligation (EL) is superior to endoscopic sclerotherapy (ES) in terms of ↓ recurrent hemorrhage (36% vs 48% for ES), ↓ mortality (28% vs 45%), complication rate (2% vs 22%), and required fewer treatment sessions for definitive therapy (4 vs 5) (N Engl J Med 1992; 326:1527OA) see Endoscopic sclerotherapy

endoscopic papillotomy The use of a duodenal endoscope to dilate and treat defects of the ampulla of Vater, eg impaction of stones, and ascaris; the timely removal of ductal stones is believed to prevent progression of edematous pancreatitis to hemorrhagic necrotizing pancreatitis, thereby reducing mortality; the endoscpic approach has certain advantages over surgical therapy, as it allows documentation by ERCP, and the removal of the stone(s) at the time of endoscopy circumvents the subsequent need for general anesthesia and a surgical procedure (N Engl J Med 1993; 328:228OA, 279ED)

endoscopic sclerotherapy The treatment of esophageal varices (EVs) by endoscopically injecting a sclerosant (sodium tetradecyl sulfate) into the veins; ES is an accepted treatment for acute and for definitive management of bleeding EVs and is superior to medical management in terms of control of active bleeding, prevention of recurrences, and improved overall survival; ES also appears to be equal or superior to non-medical management of EVs, eg insertion of a portacaval shunt, or selective splenorenal shunt in term of survival and preservation of hepatic function DISADVANTAGE Complications occur in up to 40% of patients treated with ES is the form of pulmonary and renal effects, as well as ulcers, structures, and perforations of the esophagus; death occurs in 1-2% (see N Engl J Med 1992; 326:1527OA) see Endoscopic ligation

endoscopic sphincterotomy Endoscopic papillotomy, see there

endoscopic ultrasonography A technique in which an echoendoscope is used to identify masses that are below the limits of resolution of conventional imaging modalities; in one report of patients who had negative results on CT and abdominal ultrasonography, EU identified 32 of 39[1] pancreatic endocrine tumors[2] measuring 0.5-2.5 cm in 37 patients (N Engl J Med 1992; 326:1721OA); if all else fails to identify a tumor evident biochemically, intraoperative ultrasonography becomes the ultimate arbitrar (N Engl J Med 1992; 326:1770ED)
[1]82% sensitivity vs 6/22 identified by angiography [2]31 insulinomas, 7 gastrinomas, 1 glucagonoma

endosymbiont hypothesis CELL BIOLOGY A theory that holds that mitochondria have lost the autonomy of their prokaryotic ancestors, as they are required to import most of their proteins from the cytosol since the mitochondrial genome encodes only a small percentage of the poplypeptides and proteins residing in the mitochondrion

endothelial cell Endotheliocytus [NH3] A flattened cell lining vascular luminae; ECs have either a 'normal' permeability (Endotheliocytus nonfenestratus), or are fenestrated (Endotheliocytus fenestratus) to facilitate passage of various substances; fenestrated ECs are present in renal glomeruli, intestinal villi, and endocrine glands; endothelial cells respond to a wide range of stimuli, especially of platelet origin, express receptors for inflammatory mediators (cytokines) and adhesive proteins, and by the release of substances that prevent platelet aggregation and affect fibrinolysis (N Engl J Med 1993; 328:628RV)

endothelin Any of a family of 21-amino acid peptides encoded on chromosome 6 that are synthesized as a 203 residue preprohormone and propeptide, cleaved to form 'big' endothelin, and then further cleaved to form active peptides; endothelin-1 is formed in vascular endothelium, endothelin-3 in neural tissue; endothelin-2 is somewhat mysterious as its site of production is unknown and it cannot be measured in the plasma; the intense renal vasoconstriction of hepatorenal syndrome (potentially irreversible form of acute renal failure caused by chronic liver disease) may be partly due to ↑↑↑ endothelin-1 (36 ng/L vs 4 ng/L in normal subjects) and endothelin-3 (43 ng/L vs 18 ng/L) (**N Engl J Med 1992; 327:1774oA**); ↑ endothelin-1 may contribute to the vascular abnormalities seen in pulmonary hypertension (**N Engl J Med 1993; 328:1732oA**); endothelins were first isolated from aortic endothelial cells; endothelins are the most potent known vasoconstrictor, causing prolonged pressor response, stimulating aldosterone release, impairing renal hemodynamics and excretory functions and inhibiting renin release; endothelin is increased in cardiogenic shock, myocardial infarction, pulmonary hypertension, major abdominal surgery, liver transplantation, uremia, and hypertension and may play a role in the pathogenesis of congestive heart failure, vasospasm, vasculitis, sepsis, cyclosporine nephrotoxicity, and toxemia of pregnancy; endothelin excretion is increased in patients treated with cisplatin, due to renal tubular damage

Note: The structure of endothelins has been determined by X-ray crystallography (**Nat Struc Biol 1994; 1:311**)

endothelin receptor Two distinct G protein-linked endothelin receptors have been identified, one of which is highly specific for ET-1, the other binds all three; the ER cDNA has been cloned and expressed various drug companies are targeting the therapeutic potential of an endothelin antagonist, the first of which is phospharamidon, a neutral protease inhibitor

endothelium-derived growth factor Nitric oxide, see there

endothrix Black dot ringworm, see there

endotoxin Bacterial endotoxin, 'lipid A' A heat-stable lipopolysaccharide derived from gram-negative bacterial cell walls, which induces the release of pyrogens from neutrophils, potentially causing hemorrhagic shock and altering resistance to infection

endovascular stent-graft Stent graft A prosthetic intravascular graft that is placed transluminally as an alternative to invasive surgical replacement of an artery with an aneurysmal dilatation; in aneurysms of the thoracic aorta, surgical interposition of a synthetic graft carries a 50% mortality if performed as an emergency procedure, and a 'mere' 12% mortality when performed electively; ESGs are less invasive, less expensive, and carry a lower risk than standard operative repair (**N Engl J Med 1994; 331:1729oA**), and have been used to treat aneurysms of the abdominal aorta, thoracic aorta, subclavian artery, arteriovenous fistula, and femoral occlusive disease

endowed professorship Chair An academic appointment that is supported fully or partially by the income of an endowment, which is usually awarded to an individual who is already a fully-tenured professor; see Professor; Cf 'Chair'

endoxin Endogenous digoxin A low weight molecule, ie < 500 kD that is antigenically related to and cross-reactive with digoxin; it is a physiologic inhibitor of ATPase, causing contraction of vascular smooth muscle and is increased in states of chronic volume expansion, renal failure, essential hypertension, and acromegaly

endurance SPORTS MEDICINE *'The ability to perform repetitive submaximal contractions.'* (**JC DeLee, D Drez, Jr, Eds, Orthopedic Sports Medicine WB Saunders, Philadelphia, 1994**); Cf Eccentric contraction

enema see Barium enema, Colonic irrigation

energy balance A state in which the caloric intake equals the energy comsumed, such that the body weight is stable

energy medicine ALTERNATIVE MEDICINE A generic term for *'...therapies that use an energy field—electrical, magnetic, sonic, acoustic, microwave, infrared—to screen for or treat health conditions by detecting imbalances in the body's energy fields and then correcting them.'* In EM, patient evaluation is based on 'electroacupuncture biofeedback', in which a device measures electrical resistance at acupuncture points that correspond to specific organs and tissue, known as 'control measurement points'; therapy is effected by instruments with such colorful names as the cymatic device, Diapulse™, electro-acuscope, infratonic QCM, MORA, sound probe, TENS unit, Teslar Watch (**Alternative Medicine, Future Medicine Publishing, Inc, Puyallup, Washington, 1994**); there is little data in peer-reviewed literature to support the claims that ET can detect diseases as diverse as aflavatoxin B_1 intoxication, chronic fatigue syndrome, failure to thrive (infants), Hashimoto's disease, lung cancer, schistosomiasis and others; the author is unaware of scientifically valid data that supports claims of ET's efficacy in treating allergies, angina (pectoris), circulatory defects, dermatopathies, headaches, infections (bacterial or viral), migraines, myopathies, myalgias, rheumatoid arthritis, sore throats, tendinitis; see Alternative medicine

Engel's phenomenon PUBLIC HEALTH *'As income falls, foods characteristic of higher earnings disappear until the poorest have to support life on foods providing the most calories* (low protein) *for the least money'* (**JAMA 1985; 254:3178c**), a phenomenon that occurs wherever there is poverty

engineering controls OCCUPATIONAL SAFETY A term defined by OSHA in reference to blood-borne pathogens as controls (eg sharps disposal containers, self-sheathing needles, and others) that are intended to isolate or remove the blood-borne hazard from the workplace (**Federal Register Dec 6, 1991, p 64175**)

engrailed A homeobox gene that was first discovered in *Drosophila melanogaster*, and thought to be 600 million years old, having been found in most organisms, from worms to humans; 'engrailed' controls formation of the nervous system in all animals and segmentation in the lower animals (arthropods) but not in higher animals (annelids, vertebrates)

Note: A homeobox is a gene triggering a cascade of structural and developmental changes in embryos

engrailed protein(s) A group of homeodomain proteins that are conserved in mice and other vertebrates and which play a role in establishing muscle identity during embryogenesis and in enabling neuromuscular target recognition (**Science 1991; 251:1239**)

enhancer MOLECULAR BIOLOGY A sequence of DNA, which, regardless of orientation (either in the 3' or the 5' direction) or position (ie, up to thousands of base pairs distant from), is capable of increasing the amount of RNA produced (transcribed) in a cell

enkephalin(s) A family of endogenous pentameric opioids that are produced in the CNS and GI tract, first isolated in 1975, which share amino acid homology with each other, having in common the first 4 amino acids (H-Tyr-Gly-Gly-Phe-); see Endorphin, POMC

enkephalinase CD10, see there

enolase A 90 kD neuroendocrine enzyme* [**EC 4.2.1.11**] that catalyzes the formation of high-energy phosphoenolpyruvic acid during glycolysis, which is composed of dimeric combinations of α, β and γ chains, yielding five isoenzymes; see Neuron-specific enolase

*Phosphopyruvate hydratase is the term recommended by the Nomenclature Committee of the International Union of Biochemistry and Molecular Biology

enoxaparin A formulation of low-molecular-weight heparin, see there

en plaque A generic adjective pertaining or referring to a flattened lesion that is often whitish and fibrous in consistency, which is located on an organ's surface, as in 'en plaque' meningioma, 'en plaque' mesothelioma and so on; since the term is a descriptor of gross morphology that may not correlate with histological findings, when used alone it is non-specific and of little diagnostic utility

enriched food A comestible or food product to which various nutrients, eg vitamins and minerals, have been added to compensate for those essential nutrients removed by the rigors of refinement; see Fortified food, Refined food

enrichment design A design for clinical trials in which patients are chosen for their potential to respond to a particular intervention or a therapeutic drug; enriched population designs may be warranted when clinical, biochemical, and pathological heterogeneity of a disease (eg Alzheimer's disease) suggests that not all patients would respond to any single treatment, and those who do respond, might do so in a limited dose range (see **N Engl J Med 1992; 327:1253oa**)

ENT Ears, nose and throat A commonly used colloquial abbreviation for the specialty, otorhinolaryngology, also environmental test

enteritis necroticans Pigbel, see there, aka darmbrand

enteroadherent *Escherichia coli* EAEC Any of a number of *E coli* serotypes implicated in a certain rare form of chronic diarrhea in infants with failure to thrive; EAEC serotypes implicated in traveler's diarrhea include O55, O111, O119, O125-128, O142

Enterobacteriaceae MICROBIOLOGY A family of oxidase-negative often nonmotile gram-negative bacilli (rods) with relatively simple growth requirements, which includes both normal flora of the GI tract and potential pathogens, eg *Citrobacter, Edwardsiella, Escherichia, Enterobacter, Erwinia, Hafnia, Klebsiella, Proteus, Salmonella, Serratia, Shigella*, and *Yersinia* spp

Enterococcus faecium A nosocomial pathogen of increasing importance in the US as it is resistant to available antibiotics, including penicillin, teicoplanin, vancomycin, and more recently, aminoglycosides and glycopeptides; identification of *E faecium* in a clinical specimen requires that the patient be placed in isolation with barrier precautions (**JAMA 1992; 268:2563ED**)

enteroclysis A small bowel radiocontrast study, administered as an enema that specifically studies the post-duodenal small intestine, requires greater interpretive skills and increased radiation exposure without improving the diagnostic yield

Enterocytozoon bieneusi PARASITOLOGY The most frequently reported microsporidial infection of of humans; in AIDS, *E bieneusi* infects the mucosa of small intestine, hepatobiliary tract, and the gallbladder; it has been implicated in previously unexplained (ie pathogen-'negative') cases of AIDS-related cholangitis (see there) PATHOLOGY May-Grünwald-Giemsa staining identifies free forms (**N Engl J Med 1993; 328:95oa**) in one case report, the prolonged production of intra- and extracellular spores was not associated with systemic dissemination (**Arch Pathol Lab Med 1995; 119:424oa**)

enteroglucagon A generic term for any proglucagon-derived peptide originating from the gut, eg glucagon-like insulinotropic peptide (GLIP), and glucagon-like peptide (GLP-1) that increase after the oral intake of glucose and fat, and have regulatory pathways that differ from that of pancreatic glucagon (**N Engl J Med 1992; 326:1352sB**)

enterohemorrhagic *Escherichia coli* EHEC Any of a group of *E coli* serotypes (implicated are O29, O39, O145) that produce shiga-like toxins resulting in bloody inflammatory diarrhea, evoking a hemolytic uremic syndrome; see Escherichia coli O157:H7

enteroinsular axis The structural and functional network between the GI tract and pancreatic islets consisting of the interaction of nutrients, enteric hormones

enteroinvasive *Escherichia coli* EIEC Any of a group of relatively uncommon *E coli* serotypes, including O28ac, O29, O42, O112a and others that produce a *Shiga*-like toxin CLINICAL Inflammatory dysentery

enteropathic *Escherichia coli* EPEC An agent causing epidemic diarrhea Note: The serotype system is based on the Kaufman-White O, H and K antigen system; of the 140 O serotypes of *E coli*, O55, O111, O119 are most often associated with EPEC, a more often sporadic than epidemic condition TREATMENT Symptomatic

enterotoxic *Escherichia coli* ETEC A group of *E coli* serotypes (implicated are O6, O8, O15, O20, O25 and others) which, like *Vibrio cholerae* and *Yersinia* species, cause secretory or 'traveller's' diarrhea, due to an 80-kD heat-labile toxin that 'locks' the adenylate cyclase into the 'on' position; other ETECs produce diarrhea by a heat-stable toxin which locks guanylate cyclase in the 'on' position, produced by serotypes O20, O27, O63 and others

enterotoxins A toxin that has a direct effect on the intestinal mucosa, eliciting net fluid secretion; the 'classic' toxin is choleratoxin, which evokes intestinal fluid secretion by activating adenylate cyclase; other true enterotoxins are produced by noncholera vibrios, *Escherichia coli* (LT, STa, and STb toxins), *Salmonella, Klebsiella, Clostridium perfringens, Shigella dysenteriae*, and *Bacillus cereus*; see Endotoxin, Exotoxin

enterprise liability MEDICAL MALPRACTICE An innovative system in which the burden of malpractice liability is shifted from the physician to the organization in which the physician works; theoretically, under this system, the risk-prevention measures would be stronger and the defense against the malpractice claims better managed DISADVANTAGES Physicians affiliated with an organization are unduly controlled in their clinical activities and are required to provide some of the funds for insurance; physicians not affiliated with an organization are not encompassed by the system (**N Engl J Med 1993; 329:1733sB**)

enthesopathy Inflammation at the enthesis (zone of a ligament's insertion into the bone), seen in certain rheumatic diseases, typically, HLA-B27-linked ankylosing spondylitis TREATMENT NSAIDs

enthusiasm hypothesis A term that seeks to explain the tendency of physicians in a geographic region to become enamored with a particular type of therapy or diagnostic modality because of the effect of influential (ie enthusiastic) personalities (**N Engl J Med 1994; 331:1017ED**)

entomophagy NUTRITION The dietary consumption of insects, which although unpopular with the Western palate is a major source of nutrition in the rest of the world; insects provide up to 60% of the protein in the diet of rural Africa, and are rich in vitamins and lysine, an amino acid deficient in the diet of those subsisting primarily on grain; insect delicacies include chocholate cricket torte, honeypot ants, mealworm ganoush, roasted crickets, and wax worm fritters with plum sauce; cockroaches have not been popularized as menu items (**Sci Am 1992; 267/2:20**)

entrance wound FORENSIC PATHOLOGY The first lesion that a bullet or other projectile causes when entering the body; analysis of the EW can provide useful information on the range of the weapon (close-range EWs may be surrounded by powder burns) used to fire the bullet, the angle of the discharge, what the victim was wearing, and the caliber of the weapon used; Cf Exit wound

entrapment neuropathy OCCUPATIONAL MEDICINE A neuropathy usually of a single peripheral sensorimotor nerve caused by its compression in a bony or fibrous canal, eg carpal tunnel syndrome‡, thoracic outlet syndrome‡, ulnar neuropathy; EN are characterized by numbness, painful tingling, or weakness (N Engl J Med 1993; 329:2013RV; N Engl J Med 1994; 330:1389c)

entrapment syndromes A group of neuromuscular disorders caused by anatomic restriction or compression of peripheral nerve(s) CLINICAL Pain, especially at night, paresthesia, muscle weakness which if not relieved, evolves into atrophy of the innervated muscle group; the most common of the entrapment syndromes is that affecting the carpal tunnel; others include the obturator canal and tarsal tunnel syndromes

envelope appearance see Sealed envelope appearance

env A retroviral gene that encodes envelope glycoprotein, ENV; see HIV-1, HTLV(s), Retrovirus

EnviroChem A proprietary green liquid that is an effective virucide used as a disinfectant in air-lock chemical showers (R Preston, The Hot Zone, Random House, New York, 1994)

environmental hypersensitivity 'syndrome' A poly-symptomatic condition* believed by so-called 'clinical ecologists' to result from immune dysregulation induced by common foods, allergens and chemicals, resulting in various physical and mental disorders; the medical community has remained largely skeptical of the existence of this 'disease', given the plethora of symptoms attributed to environmental illness, the lack of reproducible laboratory abnormalities and the use of unproven therapies to treat the condition; the incidence of psychiatric disorders, eg depression, anxiety and somatization is 2.5-fold greater in those with environmental illness (JAMA 1990; 264:3166) see Clinical ecologist, Candidiasis hypersensitivity syndrome

*Synonyms include environmental illness, immune dysregulation syndrome, total allergy syndrome

environmental medicine ALTERNATIVE MEDICINE A field that '...*explores the role of dietary and environmental allergens in health and illness...Virtually any chronic physical or mental illness may be improved by the care of a physician competent in this field.*' EM is claimed by its practitioners to address a diverse array of conditions including allergies, cardiovascular disease (angina, arrhythmia, thrombophlebitis, vasculitis), pediatric disease (bedwetting, chronic otitis, learning disabilities, gastritis), endocrine disease (autoimmune thyroiditis, hypoglycemia), ENT (allergies, sinus headaches, vertigo), GI disease (bloating, constipation, gastritis, inflammatory bowel disease, irritable bowel syndrome), gynecologic disease (dyspareunia, premenstrual syndrome), skin disease (angioedema, eczema), and neuromuscular disease (epilepsy, headaches, migraines, myalgias), psychiatric disease (anxiety, attention deficit-hyperactivity disorder, bipolar disorder, schizophrenia, sexual dysfunction), rheumatoid arthritis, SLE, and others (Alternative Medicine, Future Medicine Publishing, Inc, Puyallup, Washington, 1994); the intent of EM is to identify a toxin(s) in the environment by means of elimination diets, skin testing, provocation/neutralization testing, electroacupuncture biofeedback, and RAST (radioallergosorbent test), and to eliminate the allegedly noxious agents in the environment; a person's susceptibility to an adverse environment is alleged by 'environmental physicians' to be ↑ by hereditary, poor nutrition, infection, chemicals (eg pesticides, petrochemicals) and physical and psychological stress; see Alternative medicine, Environmental hypersensitivity syndrome

Note: Although there is little data to support the efficacy of EM in peer-reviewed journals, the concept that low levels of noxious components in the environment may cause disease has been attractive to some workers

environmental physician see Environmental medicine

Environmental Protection Agency A US federal agency created to facilitate coordinated and effective government action on the part of the environment; the EPA's current priorities include health risk assessment, air pollution, both 'criteria' type, eg smog and particulate and 'toxic' type, eg benzene, drinking water contamination, indoor air pollution, occupational exposure to chemicals, pesticide exposure, radon, ecological risks, global climate change, habitat alteration, ozone depletion, species extinction, and loss of biodiversity (Science 1990; 249:616n&v); see Superfund, Toxic dump; Cf Bitterfeld, OSHA

environmental terrorism Deliberate and wanton destruction of natural resources and the environment to serve a political or military end; the term was coined during the '100-hour war', in which Iraqi forces 1) Caused the largest oil spill on record, jeopardizing water-desalination facilities and 2) Used high-explosives to ignite ± 600 oil wells in Kuwait, which released major amounts of sulfur dioxide and partially combusted hydrocarbons (Nature 1991; 350:11c), and required nearly nine months to extinguish; see Greenhouse effect; Cf Nuclear terrorism

environmental tobacco smoke The smoke from burning tobacco products to which one is unintentionally exposed, in particular in public places (ie restaurants, hospitals, government buildings, aircraft); ETS is directly linked to an ↑ in acute exacerbations of asthma in children, measured by urinary cotinine levels (N Engl J Med 1993; 328:1665OA) see Second-hand smoke

Enzyme Commission A body of the International Union of Biochemistry and Molecular Biology (IUBMB) that periodically* convenes and makes recommendations on classification and nomenclature of enzymes and definitions of units; natural enzymes are designated 'EC' followed by four digits, separated by periods that serves to classify an enzyme according to main division (see table), subclass, sub-subclass and serial number within the sub-subclass eg EC 3.1.21-31.X, an enzyme that corresponds to a family of hydrolases

*The most recent list of recommendations were published in 1992 by Academic Press

> **ENZYMES MAJOR CLASSES**
> EC 1 OXIDOREDUCTASE catalyzes oxidation/reduction reactions
> EC 2 TRANSFERASE catalyzes the transfer of one molecular species to another
> EC 3 HYDROLASE catalyzes hydrolytic cleavage
> EC 4 LYASE catalyzes the removal or addition of a group to a double bond, or other cleavages involving electron rearrangement
> EC 5 ISOMERASE catalyzes intramolecular rearrangement
> EC 6 LIGASE catalyzes a reaction joining two molecules

enzyme enhancement TRANSFUSION MEDICINE The change in the agglutinin of erythrocyte antigens when red cells are exposed to enzymes, which is increased with C^w, i, Jk^a, Kidd, Rh-Hr, P system; decreased with Ch^a

enzyme induction The stimulation of the increased production of an enzyme by a drug or other compound, a process in which the inducing substance combines with the repressor, preventing its continued blockage of the gene by its operator

enzyme-linked immunosorbent assay ELISA, see there

enzyme-multiplied immunoassay technique EMIT™, see there

enzyme replacement therapy A generic term for any therapeutic modality in which a congenitally defective or absent enzyme is administered, either 1) Directly, by coupling the enzyme to a carrier molecule or by organ transplantation or 2) Indirectly, by introducing the gene into the recipient; see Adenosine deaminase deficiency

enzyme therapy ALTERNATIVE MEDICINE A form of alternative health care in which enzymes of plant or pancreatic origin are administered '...*in complementary ways to improve digestion and absorption of essential nutrients*.' (Alternative Medicine, Future Medicine Publishing, Inc, Puyallup, Washington, 1994); in ET, enzymes are co-administered with food in order to predigest it and preserve internal enzymes '*for the important work of maintaining metabolic harmony*', and are allegedly effective in breaking down circulating immune complexes as they pass through the kidneys; ET is alleged by its advocates to be effective in treating a wide range of conditions including cancer, chronic degenerative diseases, infection of the lungs and teeth, inflammation, multiple sclerosis, scarring, and others; the author is unaware of any reports in peer-reviewed literature that confirm ETs claim health benefits; see Alternative medicine, Environmental hypersensitivity syndrome; Cf Starch blockers CLINICAL MEDICINE A generic term for a therapeutic modality in which an enzyme that is present in adequate amounts under normal conditions, is supplemented with a related or identical enzyme to perform a specific task, eg rapid lysis of blood clots in evolving myocardial infarction by streptokinase, tissue plasminogen activator or urokinase

EOE Equal opportunity employer, see there

eosinophil cationic protein Eosinophil protein X A protein with a ribonuclease-like that is a potent neurotoxin, measurement of ECP in the circulation may be useful in estimating eosinophil activity

eosinophil-derived protein A 22 000 M_r (19 000 M_r as an intracellular storage product) protein with a ribonuclease-like structure that is 10-fold more potent than major basic protein's parasiticidal effect; ECP is thought to form canals in leukocytes allowing entry of biological response modifiers

eosinophil peroxidase A heterodimeric 71-77 000 M_r protein formed of a heavier glycosylated chain and a lighter nonglycosylated chain; in the presence of H_2O_2 (formed by the eosinophil), EP may represent the most potent mechanism by which the eosinophil can kill parasites and some leukocytes

eosinophilic peroxidase deficiency LABORATORY MEDICINE A finding of undetermined significance that occurs in 1:14 000 routine CBCs performed/year; EP deficiency has a nonsignificant association with allergic conditions (Am J Clin Pathol 1992; 98:615OA)

eosinophilic fasciitis A disorder with scleroderma-like changes in the trunk and extremities LABORATORY Eosinophilia, hypergammaglobulinemia PATHOLOGY Inflammation of the skin, subcutaneous tissue, fascia, and muscle, reflecting the during of clinical disease TREATMENT Corticosteroids

eosinophilic gastroenteritis A rare idiopathic condition, ½ of which occur in a background of allergy and atopy, which may be associated with autoimmune connective tissue diseases CLINICAL Abdominal pain, fever, rebound tenderness, mesenteric inflammation PATHOLOGY Mucosal, submucosal, mural and serosal forms are recognized (N Engl J Med 1993; 329:343CPC)

*Note: The search for a specific allergen is usually fruitless

eosinophilic granuloma A term for a relatively benign clinical form of histiocytosis X characterized by circumscribed cystic osseous lesions occurring in children and adolescents composed of eosinophile and histiocytes; the histiocytoses X are no longer considered to be reactive but rather clonal neoplasms (N Engl J Med 1994; 331:154OA); it would appear that a unifying term that connotes both the interrelation of these entities while recognizing their specificity, eg Langerhans' cell histiocytosis, eosinophilic type would represent a viable alternative; see Langerhans' cell histiocytosis

eosinophilic major ('basic') basement membrane pro-

tein An abundant 14-kD arginine residue-rich protein that is a major cationic (from whence, 'basic') constituent of eosinophils, which, while devoid of enzymatic activity, displays non-specific toxicity to helminths, tumor and 'tagged' host cells

eosinophilic-myalgia syndrome An 'epidemic' intoxication that occurred in North America in the late 1980s, attributed to a chemically altered form of L-tryptophan* EPIDEMIOLOGY 1500 cases of EMS were described in 1990 in subjects who had allegedly ingested this particular form of L-trytophan CLINICAL Myalgia, myopathy, arthralgia, alopecia, angioedema, dermatoglyphism, morbilliform rash, sclerodermoid lesions, oral ulcers, restrictive lung disease, dyspnea, fever, lymphadenopathy and edema of extremities LABORATORY Eosinophilia > 1 x 10⁹/L (US: > 1000/mm³), ↑ creatinine phosphokinase PATHOLOGY Sclerosing dermatopathy, arteriolitis; the responsible agent was an altered amino acid, DTAA (di-tryptophan aminal acetaldehyde) a contaminant introduced during tryptophan's manufacturing process (Nature 1991;349:5n) see 'peak E', and EMS was linked to a new strain of *Bacillus amyloliquefaciens* used to produce high-dose tryptophan, while reducing the amount of powdered charcoal used in purification; Cf Eosinophilic fasciitis; high-dose L-tryptophan was recalled by the FDA in April 1990 (see JAMA 1992; 268:1828FDA)

*This essential amino acid is ingested in adequate amounts in the diet, but is believed by some to be of use in treating insomnia, neurasthenia, premenstrual syndrome, and other conditions, and thus may be self-administered by 'health advocates'; tryptophan's subsequent metabolism to serotonin, gave rise to some claims that it could ameliorate obsessive-compulsive disorders and depression

EPA Environmental Protection Agency, see there, also 1) 1) Eicosapentaenoic acid, see n-3 fatty acids (biochemistry, aka omega-3 fatty acids) 2) Environment Pollutions Agency (British) 3) Epidermolysis bullosa acquisita

Also 1) Eastern Psychological Association 2) Electron probe analyzer 3) Erect posterior-anterior (radiology) 4) Erythroid potentiating activity 5) Ether-isopentane-ethanol 6) Europaeisches Patentamt (now known as the European Patent Office, see there) 7) Extrinsic plasminogen activator

epalrestat see Aldose reductase inhibitor

EPEC Enteropathic *Escherichia coli*, see there

ependymal rosettes NEUROPATHOLOGY Structures that recapitulate features of the normal ependymal cavity, which have a small central rounded-to-elongated lumina, optional cilia and blepharoplasts (distinct basally oriented granular corpuscles in the cytoplasm)

ependymoma A relatively indolent ependymal cell tumor arising in the walls of the ventricles (lateral, 3rd, 4th) and central canal of the spinal cord PATHOLOGY The tumor cells form rosettes, pseudorosettes, and spaces; grooves in cell nuclei is reported to be relatively specific for this tumor (Arch Pathol Lab Med 1994; 118:919OA) see Myxopapillary ependymoma

ephelis Freckle The most common pigmented lesion of young light-skinned Caucasians, often of Celtic stock, consisting in light brown 1–10-mm macules that fade in winter and become accentuated in summer PATHOLOGY The melanocytes are normal in number but contain hyperplastic and elongated melanosomes

epibolin Vitronectin, see there

epidemic pleurodynia An acute viral infection, most commonly caused by coxsackievirus (usually B1-6, but also A4, A6, A10 and enteroviruses 1, 6, 9, 19); a summer, early fall disease first described on the Danish island of Bornholm CLINICAL Paroxysms of crushing, 'vise-like' pain, in the chest of adults or upper abdomen of children, shortness of breath; ± ½ of patients have multiple recurrences COMPLICATIONS Septic meningitis 5%, orchitis

*Synonyms include Bamle disease, Bornholm disease, Bornholm syndrome, Daae's disease, Daae-Finsen disease, Dabney's disease, devil's clutch, devil's grip, devil's grippe, Drangedal disease, epidemic benign dry pleurisy, endemic myalgia, epidemic diaphragmatic pleurisy, epi-

demic myalgia, epidemic pleurisy, epidemic transient diaphragmatic spasm, myalgia endemica, myositis acuta epidemica, Silvest's disease, Sylvest syndrome

epidemic vomiting Intestinal flu, winter vomiting disease A generic term for any gastroenteritis* that is presumed to be of viral in etiology and epidemic in nature, which is most common in children, occurs in the winter months, and resolves in 1-3 days CLINICAL There are 2 typical patterns: 1) Nonfebrile and confined to the GI tract and 2) Febrile and systemic ETIOLOGY 1) Norwalk and Norwalk-like agents (eg Hawaii, Snow Mountain, Montgomery agents) 2) Caliciviruses 3) Astroviruses 4) 'Also-rans', including Cockle, Paramatta, Wollan, et al TREATMENT None

Note: The most popular synonym is intestinal flu; other synonyms include acute epidemic nonbacterial gastroenteritis, acute infectious nonbacterial gastroenteritis, acute nausea and vomiting, Bradley's disease, epidemic collapse, epidemic nausea, epidemic nonbacterial gastroenteritis, epidemic vomiting and nausea, epidemic vomiting syndrome, nausea epidemica

epidemiologic necropsy EPIDEMIOLOGY A method for studying the incidence of a morbid condition in a population that is designed to minimize the bias introduced by selection for autopsy (necropsy); criteria for eliminating the selection bias include 1) Exclusion of patients who did not die in the hospital 2) Standardization of the population being autopsied and the population being compared and 3) Reduction of the clinical selection bias (JAMA 1991; 265:2085)

epidemiology The science of public health; epidemiology studies the frequency, distribution, and causes of infectious and noninfectious diseases in a population rather than in the individual; epidemiology examines the impact of social and physical factors in the environment on morbid conditions; 'types' of epidemiology **ANALYTIC EPIDEMIOLOGY** Causative epidemiology The study of diseases distributed in a seemingly non-random fashion, attempting to identify factors in the disease-bearing population A that differ from the non-diseased population B; analytic epidemiology is divided into cross-sectional, prospective and retrospective forms **CASE-CONTROL EPIDEMIOLOGY** see Retrospective epidemiology **CLINICAL EPIDEMIOLOGY** A decision-making process applied by an individual practicing physician, where decisions are based on the likelihood of a patient having disease process X or Y, given a patient's age, previous state of health, family history, the season, the previous appearance of similar diseases in the community and other parameters **CROSS-SECTIONAL** Study of 'slices' of the population and disease prevalence in each over time **DESCRIPTIVE EPIDEMIOLOGY** An epidemiological study that tabulates the incidence of various types of disease process, providing details on mortality, morbidity, demographics and other relevant information **EXPERIMENTAL EPIDEMIOLOGY** Clinical trials in which a preventive or therapeutic measure is compared to the usual negative control population in order to determine or compare response rates **PROSPECTIVE EPIDEMIOLOGY** A study over time of a cohort of individuals having a feature of clinical or other interest, eg hypertension, exposure to an environmental toxin and so on; this population is compared in a parallel population of individuals presumed not to be exposed to the same factor **RETROSPECTIVE EPIDEMIOLOGY** Case-control study An epidemiological study that begins with a disease process in a population and searches for differences in exposures or features of that population which might have put it at risk for the disease in question

Epidemiology Intelligence Service A branch of the Centers for Disease Control and Prevention (CDC) that was founded in 1951 to 1) Train field epidemiologists 2) Assist the CDC in preventing and controlling communicable diseases and 3) Provide public health services to state and local health departments, thereby improving national (USA) disease surveillance; see CDC

epidermal growth factor A 53-residue (tri)sulfated polypeptide[1] of the tyrosine kinase family of growth stimulators (related to the *erb* oncogene) that acts on the membrane receptor; EGF serum levels are 0.016 nmol/L (US: 100 pg/ml); EGF stimulates mitogenic response, increasing transportation, phosphatidyl inositol turnover, bulk endocytosis, ruffling of the plasma membrane, glycolysis, activity of ornithine decarboxylase, synthesis of DNA, RNA, proteins, macromolecules, and accelerates wound healing [2]

[1]S Cohen shared the 1986 Nobel prize for his work on EGF with R Montalcini-Levi who worked on neuronal growth factor [2]EGF is abundant in rodent saliva; the phrase 'licking of one's wounds thus becomes a logical activity after trauma

epidermal growth factor-like domain Calcium 'two finger' domain A calcium-binding polypeptide motif present within EGF-like domains of various proteins including coagulation factors IX and X, which contain a consensus region, Asp/Asn, Asp/Asn, Asp*/Asn*, Tyr/Phe (the asterisk denotes β-hydroxylated residues), that is critical to ligand binding (Nature 1991; 351:164)

epidermal growth factor receptor A 400-amino acid protein having significant amino acid homology with the low-density lipoprotein receptor and coagulation factors, which is present in carcinomas, cornea, fibroblasts, glia, neurons, T cells, vascular endothelium, liver and placenta; measurement of EGFR may be useful in prognosticating malignancy, as breast cancer is more aggressive in EGFR-positive than EGFR-negative patients

epidermoid pearl Squamous pearl, see there

epidermolysis bullosa A heterogeneous group of rare inherited diseases characterized by an abnormal fragility of the skin; in patients with EB, minor trauma to the skin translates into blisters prone to secondary infection and scarring EM EB can be subdivided into simplex, junctional, and dystrophic types; see Recessive dystrophic epidermolysis bullosa

epidural block OBSTETRIC ANESTHESIOLOGY The most popular locoregional obstetric anesthesia, which is administered as a single injection or intrathecal 'drip', inserted in the L2-L3 or L3-L4 interspaces; little local anesthetic is used and the bearing-down reflex is not abolished

epifluorescence microscopy LABORATORY MEDICINE A technique that uses a single objective lens and a dichroic beam splitter to filter out wave lengths of light that cause an image to appear out-of-focus; the advantages of epi-fluorescence: high sensitivity, improved contrast and image quality

epigenetic An adjective referring to phenotypic alterations (eg due to imprinting or environmental effects) of a gene that are not attributed to a mutation

epigenetic defects Alterations that are present at certain sites or epigenetic 'switch regions' along DNA that control gene expression in higher organisms; a gene's expression is related to the pattern of cytosine nucleotide methylation and may be altered when the DNA is damaged, resulting in defective gene expression, related to oncogenesis and aging; demethylation defects may be repaired by recombination during meiosis or transmitted to the offspring Note: Methyl groups act as recognition sites for regulatory proteins; see CpG Island, Methylation

epiligrin A glycoprotein thought to be associated with the anchoring filaments of the basement membrane of the skin

epimutation A neologism referring to hereditable changes based on DNA modification, which is distinguished from classic DNA mutations, ie base substitution, insertion, deletion, or rearrangement (Science 1987; 238:163)

epimyoepithelial carcinoma Epithelial-myoepithelial

carcinoma, see there

epinephrine A sympathomimetic catecholamine hormone synthesized in the adrenal medulla and released into the general circulation in response to hypoglycemia, stress, and splanchnic nerve stimulation; epinephrine acts on both α– and β-receptors resulting in vasoconstriction or vasodilation, ↓ peripheral blood flow, ↑ heart rate, ↑ force of contractility, ↑ glycogenolysis, ↑ lipolysis; the pharmaceutical preparation is used as bronchodilator for acute asthma, and to raise blood pressure; epinephrine has been used in cardiac arrest (acute MI) to improve myocardial and cerebral blood flow; high-dose epinephrine (0.2 mg/kg vs standard 0.02 mg/kg) in cardiac arrest may actually worsen measurable outcomes, including rate of return of spontaneous circulation, survival to hospital admission or discharge, and neurological outcome (**N Engl J Med 1992; 327:1045OA, 1051OA**)

episode of care HEALTH CARE FINANCING A proposed unit of health care services bundled as a package, which is larger in value than a DRG (diagnosis-related group) payment, but smaller than an annual capitation payment

epithelial collarette A rim of crusted epidermis partially or completely surrounding the raised, red, pedunculated nodule in pyoderma gangrenosum; Cf Ball in claw appearance

epithelial displacement SURGICAL PATHOLOGY A histologic artefact that occurs when tissues, in particular breast, has been 'violated' by various needling procedures* immediately prior to or following surgical excision; ED is of interest as it may be misdiagnosed as stromal invasion; the actual incidence of the artefact is unknown (**Am J Surg Pathol 1994; 18:896OA**)

*eg fine needle aspiration, core-needle biopsy, needle localization (for mammography), suture placement, or infiltration with local anesthetic

epithelial membrane antigen A glycoprotein present in human milk fat globule membranes that is a marker for normal and neoplastic epithelia and perineurial cells; EMA can also be expressed by meningioma, mesothelioma, various mesenchymal tumors, and some lymphomas

epithelial-myoepithelial carcinoma Intercalated duct carcinoma A rare neoplasm accounting for 1-2% of all salivary gland tumors; peak incidence is in the 7th-8th decades; ♀:♂ ratio 2:1; 85% occur in parotid gland PATHOLOGY EMC is characterized by two morphologically distinct cell types, dark PAS-positive inner duct-forming epithelial cells, surrounded by clear outer S-100 and actin-positive myoepithelial cells PROGNOSIS EMC behaves as a low-grade tumor; flow cytometric data and immunostaining for tumor markers is of little prognostic utility (**Am J Clin Pathol 1995; 103:432OA**)

epithelioid Epithelial-like An adjective applied to cells, in particular histiocytes, whose morphology mimics large epithelial cells; epithelioid histiocytes are negative by immunoperoxidase stains for cytokeratin, a marker for epithelial differentiation and positive for the Mac-387 antigen, a histicyte marker

epithelioid angiomatosis see Bacillary angiomatosis

epithelioid granuloma A granuloma in which multiple histiocytes fuse into giant cells in a background of mononucleated histiocytes and chronic inflammatory cells; the granuloma may be accompanied by caseating necrosis, as in tuberculosis, or may be 'naked' as in sarcoidosis; granulomas occur in 1) Non-malignant conditions including angioimmunoblastic lymphadenopathy, cat scratch disease, Langerhans' cell histiocytosis (histiocytosis X), sarcoidosis, sinus histiocytosis, atypical SLE, toxoplasmosis, TB and 2) Malignant conditions including Hodgkin's disease and Lennert's lymphoma (diffuse lymphoma with high content of epithelioid histiocytes)

epithelioid hemangioendothelioma SURGICAL PATHOLOGY

A tumor of medium-to-large veins, composed of plump-to-spindled endothelial cells that bulge into vascular spaces in a tombstone-like fashion; EH is thought to have 'borderline' aggression-⅓ develop local recurrences, but few metastasize; it is unclear whether the epithelioid hemangioendothelioma is truly neoplastic or an exuberant tissue reaction, nor is it clear if it is the same as Kimura's disease IMMUNOHISTOCHEMISTRY EH is often positive for factor VIII-related antigen, vimentin, and may stain focally with *Ulex europaeus* PROGNOSIS Despite often ominous clinical, radiological, and pathological features, EHs of the anterior mediastinum (and of other sites) pursue a rather indolent course and may be adequate controlled with surgery (**Am J Surg Pathol 1994; 18:871OA**)

epithelioid sarcoma A low-grade, soft tissue sarcoma of the upper extremity, ♂:♀ ratio, 2:1, of the young (age 10-35), which may be linked to previous trauma PATHOLOGY Central geographic necrosis, positive staining for cytokeratin, epithelial membrane antigen, vimentin PROGNOSIS Recurrence is common; 45% metastasize, eg to lung, regional lymph nodes, scalp TREATMENT Wide local excision or amputation DDx-BENIGN Fibromatosis, fibrous histiocytoma, nodular fasciitis, infectious granuloma, necrobiosis lipoidica, rheumatoid nodule DDx-MALIGNANT Synovial sarcoma, fibrosarcoma, malignant melanoma

epitope IMMUNOLOGY Any site on a molecule (an antigenic determinant) that is capable of eliciting antibody formation; the minimum size of a molecule capable of evoking antibody formation is approximately 1 kD; if the molecule is smaller, as in haptens, it may evoke an immune response by virtue of its association with a carrier protein; large non-polymeric molecules may have many epitopes; when the van der Waals surfaces of proteins are constructed by X-ray crystallography, epitopic sites appear to require prominently exposed regions ('hills' and 'ridges') with surface rigidity; the more flexible sites being less antigenic; see Idiotype, Immunogenicity

EPO 1) Erythropoietin, see there 2) European Patent Office, see there

epoietin beta Recombinant human erythropoietin, see erythropoietin

eponym Any syndrome, lesion, surgical procedure or clinical sign that bears the name of the author who first described the entity, or less commonly, the name of the index patient(s) in whom the lesion was first described; despite a movement toward eliminating the possessive 's for eponyms, in the present work, the 'McKusick rule' (**JAMA 1984 252:1041**) is used, in which the **'s** is eliminated if it occurs in

1) A hyphenated eponym, eg Blackfan-Diamond syndrome, Lesch-Nyhan syndrome

2) Precedes a sibilant, eg Hodgkin cell or Cushing syndrome, which would then acquire the **'s**, should the eponym then modify a non-sibilant noun, as Hodgkin's disease and Cushing's disease or

3) Itself ends in a sibilant, eg Wilms' tumor; this rule allows retention of commonly used nomenclature without sacrifice of euphony as would occur in His and Her's diseases

Cf Acroeponym, 'Autoeponym', Eponymic adjective (adjectival eponym)

Note: Other spoken languages resolve the possessive dilemma more gracefully, with 'da', 'de' and 'di' in the Romance languages, 'no' in Japanese, and 'sche' in German (**JAMA 1986; 255:1879c, 256:1295c**)

epoxygenase pathway An arachidonic acid metabolic route with omega and omega-1 oxidation by cytochrome P450 microsomal enzymes with formation of EETs (epoxy-eicosatetraenoic acids), vasotonic effectors and inhibitors of platelet aggregation in experimental models, although it is unclear whether EETs are produced in humans

epsilon ε, see E

Epsom salts Magnesium sulfate

Epstein-Barr immunodeficiency syndrome An X-linked [MIM 308240] or less commonly AR [MIM 226990] condition accompanied by congenital cardiovascular and CNS defects associated with fatal infectious mononucleosis IMMUNOLOGY Poor response to EBV infection with BM aplasia, agranulocytosis, agammaglobulinemia, poor B-cell response to antigens and mitogens, ↓ NK cell activity, T-cell subset abnormalities CAUSE OF DEATH Hepatitis, immune suppression, B-cell lymphomas

Epstein-Barr nuclear antigen A molecule that is the earliest indicator of Epstein-Barr virus infection, appearing in B lymphocytes before the detection of virus-directed protein is detectable within the infected cells' nuclei

Epstein-Barr virus Human herpesvirus-4 A double-stranded DNA virus; the immature viral particles measure 75-80 nm and are found in the cytoplasm and nucleus; the mature fully infectious particles measure 150-200 nm and are cytoplasmic; associated with aplastic anemia, Burkitt's lymphoma (usually African type), chronic fatigue syndrome, (the connection between EBV and the chronic fatigue syndrome is uncertain), hairy cell leukemia, histiocytic sarcoma in renal transplantation and immune compromise; EBV may facilitate development of various lymphoproliferative disorders including Hodgkin's disease and NHL, infectious mononucleosis, Izumi fever, undifferentiated nasopharyngeal carcinoma, which occurs in mainland China, and thymic carcinoma; in model systems, expression of EBV's latent membrane protein elicits cell changes similar to those seen histologically in nasopharyngeal carcinoma, representing a block in terminal differentiation; post-transplantation lymphoproliferative disorder (PTLD), a complication of 1-10% of organ transplant recipients; post-transplantation patients at risk for PTLD can be identified by detecting expression of the EBER-1 gene (N Engl J Med 1992; 327:1710OA)

epulis Giant cell reparative granuloma, see there

equal employment opportunity A job or position that is not subject to adverse exclusion based on a candidate's race, sex, religion, or national origin; see equal opportunity employer

equal opportunity employer An employer who does not discriminate against or subject a candidate for a position of employment to adverse exclusion based on the candidate's race, sex, religion or national origin; theoretically, in the US, all publicly offered positions, especially in academics, are based on the principle of equality of opportunity; see EEO

equilibrium constant K A value (constant) that reflects the concentrations of the reactants and products of a chemical reaction when it has reached a steady state (equilibrium), which varies with the temperature and is related to the free energy in the reaction; the 'K' value of a reaction equals the mathematical product of the concentrations of the chemical reactants, each raised to a power (usually 2) equal to the coefficient of the product in the equation, divided by the product of the concentrations of the reactants, each raised to its coefficient

equilibrium radionuclide angiocardiography ERNA CARDIOLOGY A technique in which an objective signal, eg the EKG is used to 'gate' or physiologically control the otherwise static imaging of the cardiac blood pool; ERNA uses EKG '...events to define the temporal relationship between the acquisition of nuclear data (using ^{99m}Tc to achieve equilibrium blood pool labeling) and the volumetric components of the cardiac cycle. Sampling is performed repetitively over several hundred heartbeats with physiological segregation of nuclear data according to occurrence with within the cardiac cycle

(BL Zaret etal, in E Braunwald, Heart Disease, 4th ed, WB Saunders, Philadelphia, 1992) ERNA is of use in evaluating the right and left ventricles (hence the synonym equilibrium radionuclide ventriculography) in terms of volumes, as well as systolic and diastolic function, and regional or global myocardial performance (eg myocardial infarction); Cf First-pass radionuclide ventriculography

equipoise BIOMEDICAL ETHICS A state of genuine uncertainty of the ultimate benefits or disadvantages of both therapeutic arms in a clinical trial; because the clinical investigator may become biased as a study progresses, due to the perceived benefit of one of the therapeutic regimens being evaluated, he may enroll fewer and fewer patients in the perceived less beneficial arm, due to ethical considerations, and may ultimately defeat the very purpose of the study for lack of patients in the control arm; a moral exit to this dilemma, known as 'clinical equipoise' is possible, since genuine uncertainty exists in the 'expert' medical community at large; the investigator may thus continue to enroll control patients 'blindly', despite his bias

ER Emergency room, emergency ward, also 1) Ejection rate 2) Electrical resistance 3) Endoplasmic reticulum 4) Erythrocyte rosette 5) Estrogen receptor 6) Evoked response 7) Exchange ratio 8) Extended release (pharmacology) 9) External rotation

Also 1) Early release 2) Ego resiliency (psychology) 3) Embryo replacement 4) Emergency rescue 5) Environmental resistance 6) Equivalent Roentgen (obsolete) 7) Erythrocyte (rarely used, RBC is more common) 8) Estradiol receptor 9) Eye research

E/R Exercised/repositioned (sports medicine)

ERAP160 A 160-kD estrogen receptor-associated protein that may mediate estradiol-dependent transcriptional activity by the estrogen receptor; see Estrogen receptor, Tamoxifen

***erb*A, *erb*B** Oncogenes with tyrosine kinase activity that have structural homology to the avian erythroblastosis retrovirus and encode proteins located at the cell membrane; erbB is an NH_2-terminal truncated form of epidermal growth factor receptor expressed in various malignancies, eg breast and salivary gland carcinomas; gene amplification (increased copy numbers) of the c-erbB-2 (HER-2/neu) gene may indicate poor prognosis in breast carcinoma due to a lower disease-free interval and lower survival rates

ERBB2 NEU protein, HER-2, MAC 117 The gene product of the c-erbB-2 (*neu*) proto-oncogene, a membrane-bound receptor, which has extensive homology with epidermal growth factor; amplification of the c-erbB-2 gene (*neu* gene) expression occurs in breast cancer, but not in ductal carcinoma in situ; tumors with neu amplification are larger but increased expression of neu has little bearing on the prognosis **ERCP** Endoscopic retrograde cholangiopancreatography A clinical procedure in which an endoscope is inserted through the ampulla of Vater with the injection of radiocontrast material to delineate the bile and pancreatic ducts; ERCP is used to detect bile stones, seen as a frank blockage of the duct(s) or findings suggestive of pancreatic adenocarcinoma; see Rat tail tapering

erectile dysfunction UROLOGY A generic term for the inability to achieve and/or maintain penile tumescence, which may be due to medical, psychological, or surgical disease; ED may respond to penile injection therapy, penile implant surgery, and microvascular bypass surgery

erection center PHYSIOLOGY A region at S2-4 spinal cord that coordinates the efferent parasympathetic activity mediated by the nervi erigentes, which cause vasodilation of the penile arterioles and subsequent compression of the veins; erection is terminated by sympathetic vasocontriction; Cf Erection center

erg A human oncogene located on chromosome 21, first identified in a colonic tumor cell line that is closely related to the v-*myb* and v-*ets* oncogenes of the chicken E26 virus

ergogenic drug Performance-enhancing drug, see there

ergonomic standards OCCUPATIONAL MEDICINE A series of guidelines being developed (NY Newsday 21 March 1995; A35) by the OSHA (US) that will address activities in the workplace that carry a high risk for injury, including

Repetitive motion over prolonged periods of time of up to 4 hours

Maintaining a fixed or awkward position for a prolonged period of time

Use of vibrating or impact tools for a prolonged period of time

Lifting of heavy loads frequently during a shift

ergonomics The formal study of work situations, which attempts to evaluate, and if necessary, reconfigure a workplace by taking into account the anatomic and psychological variables of those working in the environment

ergotype A T cell in the process of activation; the development of autoimmunity in animal models, eg experimental autoimmune encephalitis (EAE) can be circumvented by injecting anti-ergotype T lymphocytes to prevent full-scale T-cell activation; see EAE

ERISA Employee Retirement Income Security Act of 1974 HEALTH CARE ENVIRONMENT A legislative act that exempts from state regulations those companies that provide self insurance, or those that fund their own insurance plans (Am Med News 26 October 1992, p7)

ERK Extracellular signal-regulated kinase, also known as MAP kinase, see there

Note: Although the acronym ERK is both more exact and 'efficient', the term MAP kinase is firmly entrenched in the literature

Erlenmeyer flask deformity A morphological descriptor for a deformity, lesion, or mass that is broad-based and tapers to a relatively narrow neck, likened to the flask used in organic chemistry BONE RADIOLOGY The Erlenmeyer flask change corresponds to undertubulation of the distal femur and a loss of the usual constriction, due to ischemic necrosis; this non-specific finding may be seen in healing fractures, rickets, scurvy, cystic fibrosis, extra- and intrahepatic biliary atresia, enchondromatosis, chronic lead poisoning, Gaucher's disease, adult hypophosphatasia, osteopetrosis, diffuse osteosclerosis, Pyle's disease (craniometaphyseal dysplasia or dysostosis), dysosteosclerosis, thalassemia major, von Gierke's disease GASTROENTEROLOGY The Erlenmeyer flask appearance refers to the colonic pathology seen in patients with fulminant *Entamoeba histolytica*-induced amebiasis; gross examination reveals mucosal ulcerations with a narrow neck and a flask-like broad base; the extensive submucosal lesion may be covered by a relatively intact-in-appearance mucosa; the organisms invade the crypts, spread laterally in a background of necrosis and are best seen by a diastase-resistant periodic acid Schiff stain

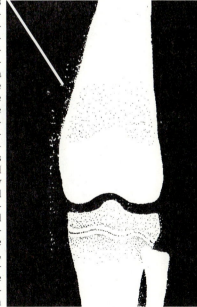

Erlenmeyer flask deformity

ERNA Equilibrium radionuclide angiocardiography, see there

erotomania 1) Hypersexuality, a pathologic obsession with sexual thoughts or activities 2) A virtually extinct term for delusion that one is the object of another's sexual desires

error An unintentional deviation from standard operating procedures or practice guidelines LABORATORY MEDICINE An erroneous result from a patient sample, the frequency of which reflects the laboratory's quality control procedures and adherence to well-designed procedure manuals **ALLOWABLE (ANALYTICAL) ERROR** A systemic error that is 'acceptable', both statistically and analytically, eg 95% limit of error **PRESYSTEMIC ERROR** An error that occurs prior to the specimens' analysis, eg specimen mislabeling, operator-related inconsistencies in performing tests, different volume 'draws' into a blood collection tube, varying the concentration of anticoagulant, altering coagulation studies **RANDOM ERROR** An error that cannot be corrected, which is intrinsic to a properly designed analytical system, eg anything beyond two standard deviations of a statistical mean **SYSTEMIC ERROR** A defective statistical analysis or equipment-related problem that consistently yields erroneous results, which is detectable and correctable by quality assurance and quality control procedures MEDICAL MALPRACTICE see Misadventure STATISTICS see Type I error, Type II error

error catastrophe GERIATRICS A theoretical explanation of the process of aging, which holds that the decline of bodily function typical of later life is due to ↑ 'sloppiness' in protein synthesis, resulting in the accumulation of defective and non-functioning products that eventually prove to be incapable of maintaining normal cell function; see 'Garbage can' hypothesis

error-prone repair see SOS repair

Erysichthon syndrome A condition characterized by overeating, insatiable hunger and indiscriminate dietary indulgence, despite repeated warnings of the dangers by cardiologists and other health care providers, eg a patient who has suffered myocardial infarction; see Morbid obesity; Cf Bulimia nervosa

Erysichthon of Greek mythology angered the Gods, who instilled in him an insatiable hunger that ultimately caused him to eat himself

erysipeloid An infection by the microaerophilic gram-positive *Erysipelothrix rhusiopathiae*, which is almost exclusive to those who occupationally handle animal products, manifested as sharply demarcated red maculopapular lesions of the hands, which may spontaneously heal COMPLICATIONS Arthritis, Endocarditis

erythema toxicum (neonatorum) 'Fleabite' dermatitis A benign condition characterized by generalized macular, papulovesicular, and occasionally pustular, slightly erythematous waxing and waning rash seen on the trunk and extremities of neonates, disappearing by the end of the first week of life, possibly induced by histamine condition; ET affects 4-77% of all neonates in the first week after delivery and may be accompanied by intraoral erythema (red gum disease) and tissue eosinophilia TREATMENT Unnecessary, as spontaneous resolution is the rule

The condition was first described in ancient Mesopotamia between the Tigris and the Euphrates rivers

erythrocyte sedimentation rate 'sed' rate, ESR A simple laboratory test that measures the rate at which red cells in well-mixed venous blood settle to the bottom of a special test tube, which serves as a non-specific indicator of inflammation; the ESR is ↑ in collagen vascular disease, neoplasia, pregnancy, anemia, and hyperproteinemia, and ↓ in polycythemia, microcytosis and in sickle cell anemia

erythroid differentiation factor see Activin

erythromelia A clinical condition more commonly affecting older women, characterized by episodic, vasodilation-induced erythema of the acral parts, accompanied by burning pain; erythromelia may be idiopathic or secondary to hypertension, obstructive vascular disease or polycythemia TREATMENT Most cases respond to aspirin, methysergide, or epinephrine

erythropoietin A 46-kD glycoprotein growth factor produced predominantly by cells adjacent to the proximal renal tubules in response to signals from an oxygen-sensitive substances in the kidneys, eg heme; erythropoietin (EP) binds to receptors in erythroid precursors that mature into red cells; it is increased by hypoxia or by ectopic production from tumors, eg cerebellar hemangioblastoma, hepatoma, pheochromocytoma, uterine leiomyoma and renal cell carcinoma; it may not be increased in anemic premature infants and is ↓ in secondary anemia, chronic inflammation, polycythemia vera, and certain cancers and may be useful in myeloma-related anemia; the EP gene is regulated by a carbon monoxide-inhibitable heme protein that acts as the oxygen sensor; EP production is modulated by adenosine that is increased in renal transplants and is inculpated in the erythrocytosis seen in 10-15% of renal transplants; theophylline, a non-specific adenosine antagonist, attenuates both the production of EP and the erythrocytosis; recombinant EP improves the anemia and quality of life parameters, ie energy, functional abilities, sexual activity, and happiness in patients on hemodialysis, and ameliorates zidovudine-induced anemia in AIDS patients if the endogenous EP is less than 500 U; EP therapy is indicated for anemia of renal failure and prematurity, and may be beneficial for ↑ the number of units of autologous red cells that may be donated prior to surgery, for ↑ the number of units that may be phlebotomized in patients with hemochromatosis, and in ↑ the units that may be drawn from a person with a rare blood type; recombinant human EP (epoietin beta) reduces the transfusion needs of infants with anemia of prematurity (**N Engl J Med 1994: 330:1173₀ₐ**); the erythropoietic response to EP may be blunted by iron deficiency, folic acid deficiency, infection, inflammatory disease, myelofibrosis, aluminum-induced microcytosis, and severe hyperparathyroidism (**N Engl J Med 1993; 328:171₀ₐ**); erythropoietin levels differ in the polycythemias; in polycythemia vera 2.1 U/L (vs 6.7 U/L), in relative polycythemia 7.0 U/L, and secondary polycythemia 121.7 U/L (**Br J Haematol 1992; 81:603**)

escalation situation PSYCHOLOGY A set of circumstances in which the individuals or organizations involved in a project tend to persist in 'failing courses of action'; escalation situations are due to variables of the project itself, as well as psychological, social and organizational variables

escape beat CARDIOLOGY An automatic beat occurring after an interval longer than the dominant cycle length, ie a normal ventricular contraction occurring when the usual cardiac pacemaker, the sinoatrial node, defaults

Note: The AV node, which has an intrinsic rhythm of 35-60 beats/min, allows a slower pacemaker to take over, thus acting as a safety mechanism; since escape beats are a defense mechanism, they should not be pharmacologically suppressed

escape mutant INFECTIOUS DISEASE A generic term for any microorganism, eg virus (eg HIV-1 variants), bacteria, that escapes the modality, eg therapy or vaccine intended to eradicate it or prevent its attachment to a host, by undergoing mutation, thereby 'sidestepping' the host's natural or acquired defense (**NY Newsday 21 Feb 1995; C1**) see AIDS pathogenesis

'escapees' A highly colloquial term for older relatives of those at risk for Huntington's disease (see there) who did not develop the disease

***Escherichia coli* 0157:H7** A shiga-like verotoxin-producing serotype of *E coli* inculpated in outbreaks of hemorrhagic diarrhea, linked to eating undercooked meat in 'fast-food' restaurants; the 0157:H7 agent is a relatively common stool isolate; of pathogens in one series in Minnesota, O157:H7 was the fourth most common isolate after, in order, *Campylobacter* species, *Salmonella* spp, *Aeromonas* spp and it was more common than *Yersinia* spp CLINICAL Colicky pain, bloody diarrhea RADIOLOGY Submucosal edema and 'thumbprinting'

escutcheon The patch of pubic hair; the normal female escutcheon is a triangle pointing downward, sharply cut off at the level of the pubic symphysis; the male escutcheon is diamond-shaped with both downward and upward angles; a male pattern in a female may indicate pathological excess of androgen or be a familial trait without significance

Note: An escutcheon is a heraldic shield on which a coat of arms is depicted and in a broader sense, the shield itself

eskimoma Lymphoepithelioma-like carcinoma, malignant lymphoepithelial lesion A colloquial term for a poorly differentiated squamous cell carcinoma with non-malignant lymphoid stroma, formerly affecting the salivary glands and esophagus of Eskimo women, related to the manner in which these women prepare mukluks, ie by chewing sealskins covered by ashes (a source of lye and potential co-carcinogen)

esophageal ring A partially encircling intraluminal mass in the esophagus, also known as Schatzki's ring, is actually a web; to be semantically correct, a ring is composed of mucosa, submucosa and muscle (which the esophageal ring lacks); the literature is sparse on the clinical and pathological differences between the esophageal rings and webs, and the distinction may be of little practical use; see Webs

esophageal web A two-to-three mm in thickness stricture composed of mucosa and submucosa only (the term 'ring' is used when muscle is present, thus Schatzki's 'ring' is a misnomer), located anywhere along the length of the esophageal lumen; upper esophageal webs occur in the upper 2-4 cm of the esophagus, are lined by squamous epithelium, often associated with the Plummer-Vinson (-Paterson-Brown-Kelly) syndrome and after years may evolve into postcricoid carcinoma; webs in the body of the esophagus may be multiple, possibly representing embryonal remnants and may be associated with esophageal reflux; the lower esophageal web (or ring) of Schatzki is a thin membrane marking the squamocolumnar junction that is seen in about 10% of normal subjects; symptomatic subjects may suffer intermittent dysphagia and impaction of a bolus of bread or meat TREATMENT Intraluminal balloon dilation

esoteric testing LABORATORY MEDICINE The analysis of 'rare' substances or molecules that are not within the realm of the routine clinical laboratory; see DORA

esperamicin Calicheamicin, see there

espundia Mucocutaneous leishmaniasis caused by *L braziliensis*, a natural infection of large rodents that may be transmitted to humans by the sandfly, causing severe ulcerating lesions of the nasal cavities, see Tapir nose, with scarring and secondary bacterial infections, accompanied by fever, anemia and weight loss; in advanced cases, the prognosis is poor

ESR 1) Electron spin resonance spectroscopy, see there 2) Erythrocyte sedimentation rate, see there

Also Extrahepatic shunt ratio

ESRD see End-stage renal disease

essential amino acids A group of eight amino acids, isoleucine, leucine, lysine, methionine, phenylalanine, threonine, tryptophan and valine that are essential for normal growth and development of humans; the absence of an essential amino acid results in a negative nitrogen balance; in premature infants, histidine, arginine and cystine are also required; see Amino acids

essential dietary component CLINICAL NUTRITION A requirement in the diet, without which a deficiency state or syndrome will develop, including water (1-2 liters/day), calories (2000 to 3500 kcal/d) carbohydrates, fat, protein, vitamins, minerals and fiber; see Essential amino acids, Essential Fatty acids, Fiber, Trace minerals, Vitamins

essential fatty acids Fatty acids that humans cannot synthesize, which contain double bonds more distal than the COOH end of the 9th carbon atom; EFAs include 1) Linoleic acid (18:2 *cis*-delta 9, delta 12), which has two unsaturated carbon bonds, the first of which is attached at the methyl end to the 6th carbon (hence, n-6 or omega-6) and 2) Linolenic acid (18:3 *cis*-delta 9, delta 12, delta 15)

essential hematuria A condition that causes symptomatic episodic gross hematuria, most commonly affecting male children between age 2 and 11, often in a background of chronic glomerulopathy, 'nil' disease or Berger syndrome PROGNOSIS Spontaneous resolution

essential hypernatremia A disease complex characterized by increased secretion of anti-diuretic hormone (ADH) in response to volume contraction, but lack of response of ADH to hyperosmalarity, which may be seen in sodium retention and in burn patients with central pontine myelinolysis

essential hypertension Primary hypertension A condition comprising 90% of all cases of hypertension; it is associated with impaired endothelium-mediated vasodilation, which may play an important role in the functional abnormalities of resistance vessels; based on twin studies, 20-40% have a genetic basis; one study found a sgnificant link between the angiotensinogen gene located on q142-43 and EH (N Engl J Med 1994; 330:1629OA) EH requires long-term drug therapy, in contrast to secondary hypertension, eg that due to unilateral renal artery stenosis (Goldblatt kidney), pheochromocytoma and primary aldosteronism, which may respond to surgery

essential nutrient see Essential dietary component

essential oil ALTERNATIVE MEDICINE An oily preparation of herbal origin that is distilled or extracted from various plants, eg citrus fruits or eucalyptus

essential thrombocythemia A primary myeloproliferative disorder of upper middle-aged adults (50-75), or less commonly of young ♀s, in which the platelet count is consistently > 600 × 10^9 /L; ET has many clinical features of polycythemia vera, affects the same age group, and is accompanied by splenomegaly, similar BM findings and intensity of leukocytosis; the Polycythemia Vera Study Group has delineated criteria to establish the diagnosis of essential thrombocythemia (table) TREATMENT Long-term therapy with hydroxyurea, a myelosuppressive drug, prevents recurrent thrombotic phenomena (N Engl J Med 1995; 332:1132OA)

Synonyms include DiGuglelmo II syndrome, Epstein-Goedel syndrome, idiopathic thombocythemia, primary hemorrhagic thrombocythemia, primary thrombocythemia, thrombocythemia

essential thrombocytopenia A condition of young adults with thrombotic complications occurring in less than ½ of cases, associated with vasocclusion-induced headaches and erythromelalgia TREATMENT Conservative, anegrelide if symptomatic (Mayo Clin Proc 1991; 66:149)

esthesioneuroblastoma Olfactory neuroblastoma A tumor arising in the nasal cavity, retrobulbar region or the

middle cranial fossa that affects all ages from 3 to 79 PATHOLOGY The tumor is red-gray, hemorrhagic and composed of uniform small cells arranged in Homer-Wright rosettes DDx Lymphoma, plasmacytoma, embryonal rhabdomyosarcoma PROGNOSIS Five-year survival 50-60%; late recurrence is common

esthetic rehabilitation A branch of cosmetology that is dedicated to covering wounds, burns, and scars, with silicone-based prostheses and makeup, which are seen in victims of trauma, violence, crashes, and fires (NY Daily News 7 May 1995, p20)

estrogen dermatitis A recently described entity, characterized by severe premenstrual exacerbations of papulovesicular eruptions, urticaria, eczema, or generalized pruritus ETIOLOGY Sensitivity to endogenous (ie self) or exogenous estrogens DIAGNOSIS Intradermal tests for sensitivity to estrogens TREATMENT Antiestrogen therapy with tamoxifen, or elimation of estrogen (J Am Acad Dermatol 1995; 32:25)

estrogen receptor A member of a superfamily of nuclear receptors for small hydrophilic ligands including steroid hormones, thyroid hormone, vitamin D, and retinoids; these receptors are transcription factors regulated allosterically by ligand binding; extracellular estradiol diffuses across the cell membrane, binding to the ER, leading to its dimerization and binding of ER to the estrogen responsive element, ER's specific DNA target; a 160-kDal estrogen receptor-associated protein (ERAP160) appears to mediate estradiol-dependent transcriptional activation by the ER; the ability of antiestrogenic agents, eg tamoxifen to block estrogen receptor-ERAP 160 complex formation may explain their therapeutic effects in breast carcinoma (Science 1994; 264; 1455R); in humans, mutation of the ER gene is not lethal, and a case report of a male was associated with tall stature (due to delayed skeletal maturation) and osteoporosis (N Engl J Med 1994; 331:1056OA) see Tamoxifen

estrogen receptor assay The estrogen receptor is a protein found in high concentrations in the cytoplasm of breast, uterus, hypothalamus and anterior hypophysis cells; the ER levels are measured by oncologists to determine a breast cancer patient's potential for response to hormonal manipulation (60% of breast cancers are 'estrogen positive'); one-half of ER-positive patients respond favorably to anti-estrogen (tamoxifen citrate) therapy, in contrast to less than one-third of ER-negative patients respond to tamoxifen; see 'Flare' phenomenon Note: Breast carcinoma induced by the *ras* oncogene is not hor-

---

ESSENTIAL THROMBOCYTHEMIA-DIAGNOSTIC CRITERIA

1) Platelets > 1 x 10^9 /L (US: < 1000/mm³)

2) Hemoglobin < 2.05 mmol/L (US < 13.0 g/dl)

3) Iron in the marrow or if absent, little increase in hemoglobin after one month of oral iron therapy

4) Absent marrow fibrosis by biopsy and

5) Absent Philadelphia chromosome

Polycythemia Vera Study Group

---

monally-dependent, implying a multistep progression from benign to dysplastic to malignant LABORATORY ER levels > 10 fmol/mg of protein are positive; the estrogen receptor levels may be quantified by biochemical means and semiquantified by immunocytochemical, immunohistochemical methods, gel electrophoresis and protamine sulfate precipitation

estrogen replacement therapy Estrogen administered to postmenopausal women, often in the form of a vaginal cream, which ameliorates the effects of lost ovarian function, reducing the progression of osteoporosis, asserting a cardiovascular protective effect (decreased LDL-cholesterol and increased HDL-cholesterol), reducing hot flashes, urogenital symptoms, including vaginal dryness, burning, itching, dyspareunia, bleeding, and skin changes as well as depression; the increased risk of endometrial cancer is partially offset by adding progestational agents to the regimen Note: By meta-analysis, ERT is associated with a 3.4-fold increased risk in women with a family history of breast cancer ± 3 million ♀ (US) receive ERT MECHANISM OF ACTION Uncertain; ERT may modify the risk of coronary heart disease by altering plasma concentrations of lipoproteins, hemostatic factors, glucose, insulin, and blood pressure LABORATORY Hormone replacement results in ↑ HDL_2– and HDL_3-cholesterol, ↑ apoA-I, and↓ LDL-cholesterol, apoB, lipoprotein(a), fibrinogen, antithrombin III, fasting glucose and insulin; users of estrogen alone had higher factor VII, protein C, and triglyceride levels than either nonusers or those using estrogen and progesterin, inferring that further benefit is accrued by adding progestin to the replacement regimen, thus making the term estrogen-replacement therapy less preferred than hormone-replacement therapy (N Engl J Med 1993; 329:1069oa); in ♀ < 75 years with ERT ≥ 7 years had bone mineral density 11.2% > than ♀ who had not taken estrogen; ♀ > 75 years with ERT ≥ 7 years had bone mineral density only 3.2% > than ♀ who had not taken estrogen (N Engl J Med 1993; 329:1141oa); intravaginal estriol prevents recurrent UTI, probably by modifying the vaginal flora, ↑ lactobacilli and ↓ Enterobacteriaceae (N Engl J Med 1993; 329:753oa) NEUROLOGY ERT is associated with improved neurologic function, ↑ performance on cognitive tests, and ↓ incidence of Alzheimer's disease, possibly due to the estrogen's ability to ↑ neuronal sensitivity to nerve growth factor (NGF) by ↑ production of NGF receptors, or due to estrogen's ability to ↑ production of choline acetyltransferase (New York Times 8 March 1994; C3)

état glacé A neuropathological finding characterized by cerebellar pallor with conglutination of the granular cell layer neurons, occurring without a gliotic reaction, possibly representing postmortem autolysis

état lacunaire Lacunar state, see there

état marbré Status marmoratus A neuropathological condition associated with the athetoid form of cerebral palsy or Little's disease PATHOLOGY Hypermyelination of the striatum and basal ganglia, figure; the myelin is arranged in coarse perivascular bundles, fancifully likened to veined marble, which by LM corresponds to moderate fibrillary gliosis

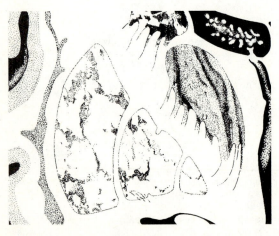

état marbré

ETEC Enterotoxic *Escherichia coli*, see there

ETF syndrome(s) A rare and polymorphous group of clinical conditions characterized by a defect in electron transfer flavoprotein or related enzymes, resulting in sarcosinemia, variably accompanied by mental and growth retardation and acute metabolic dysfunction, including vomiting, hepatic enlargement and hypertension

ethanolaminosis METABOLIC DISEASES A condition characterized by decreased ethanolamine kinase activity and increased phosphatidyl ethanolamine in the liver and urine, with cardiomegaly, hypotonia, cerebral dysfunction, and a gamut of clinical findings similar to type II glycogen storage disease, with death occurring by age two

Ethernet COMPUTERS A high speed LAN (local area network) hardware standard (developed by Xerox) for communicating among personal computers that is capable of linking up to 1024 nodes in a bus network; Ethernet is capable of transferring raw data at 10 megabits/sec and 'real' data at 2-3 megabits/sec; because it uses a single-channel (baseband) communication technique, it is prone to collision, ie the simultaneous transmission of data (CAP Today November 1993) see Broadcast storm, Collision, Screamer

ethical value A core 'unit' that determine ethical behavior; unlike the objective and measurable units used for example in the clinical laboratory, EVs are not amenable to standardization; MS Josephson, an expert in ethics, lists six EVs that he calls the 'pillars of character' upon which all people, regardless of cultural, ethnic, or socioeconomic background agree: Trustworthiness, respect, responsibility, justic and fairness, caring, civic virtue and citizenship (CAP Today March 1994 p68)

ethics committee A multidisciplinary committee in a health care facility that is composed of a broad spectrum of personnel, eg physicians, nurses, social workers, priests and others, which addresses the moral and ethical issues within the hospital, eg forming policies regarding the institution's obligations for care of the indigent, developing 'do not resuscitate' protocols and resolving on-going moral conflicts; see DNR, Institutional review board

ethidium bromide A planar molecule that is a 'workhorse' reagent in molecular biology; EB intercalates itself between base pairs on a 'closed' circular double-stranded DNA molecule, generating positive superhelical coils; since natural closed DNA is negatively supercoiled, the amount of ethidium bromide required to achieve zero supercoiling is a measure of the density of the DNA's original negative supercoils; since EB fluoresces in ultraviolet light, it has the added advantage that is facilitates 'tracking' of bands of DNA during gel electrophoresis; see Intercalation

ethnic cleansing HUMAN RIGHTS A permutation of genocide in which one population systematically kills another based on differences in ethnic origin; see Eugenics, Genocide

ethnobotany The field that formally studies the relationship between plants and a population, in particular the medicinal use of plants by an ethnic group; the ethnobotanical approach to drug discover is more efficient than random searches for plant-derived agents of therapeutic interest (Sci Am 1994; 270/6:82); drugs discovered by the ethnobotanical approach include aspirin (*Filipendula ulmaria*), codeine (*Papaver somniferum*), ipecac (*Psychotria ipecacuanha*), pilocarpine(*Pilocarpus jaborandi*), reserpin (*Rauvolfia serpentina*), theophylline (*Camelia sinensis*), and vinblastine (*Cantharanthus roseus*)

ethnomedicine Folk medicine Any of a number of 'traditional', often aboriginal, medical systems that combine the use of native plants and herbs administered by a medicine man, witch doctor, curandero or shaman who recieves his education through a long apprenticeship and who may administer the therapy by a ritual, verbally evoking the help of a deity; ethnomedicine is practiced with decreasing frequencies in cultures ravaged by 'civilization', despite the finding that a number of medications have been shown to have therapeutic value in the context of Western medicine; see Hot-cold syndrome, Shaman; Cf Alternative medicine, 'Folk' medicines

ethylene glycol A chemical used as an antifreeze, as ink and paint solvents, and in the manufacture of polyesters; antifreeze is an inebriating and highly toxic (50-100 ml may be fatal) ethanol surrogate occasionally used by alcoholics MECHANISM OF TOXICITY Ethylene glycol is converted by alcohol dehydrogenase to glycolic acid (causing metabolic acidosis and the glycolate is further metabolized to oxalate (causing renal toxicity); 4-methylpyrazole inhibits alcohol dehydrogenase, forming a basis for therapy; clinical intoxication with ethylene glycol develops in three stages 1) CNS symptoms, occurring within the first 24 hours 2) Cardiovascular symptoms, up to 72 hours in duration 3) Respiratory arrest and renal failure with anuria LABORATORY Anion-gap metabolic acidosis, increased measured serum osmolality and osmolar gap, hypocalcemia; urinalysis reveals double-refractile envelope-shaped calcium oxalate dihydrate or needle-shaped calcium oxalate monohydrate crystals in the urine or proximal convoluted tubules, protein, erythrocytes and epithelial casts DIAGNOSIS GLC, fluorometric, colorimetric methodologies TREATMENT Gastric lavage, emesis, charcoal and catharsis, calcium gluconate for symptomatic hypocalcemia

ethylene oxide OCCUPATIONAL MEDICINE A gas used to sterilize medical supplies and other materials; approximately 270 000 workers in the US are exposed to ethylene oxide, with high levels of exposure occurring in 96 000 hospital workers and 21 000 workers in commercial sterilization of medical supplies, pharmaceuticals and for spices (NIOSH data); exposed workers are at ↑ risk for hematopoietic malignancy (N Engl J Med 1991; 324:1402), as well as renal and gastric malignancy

etidronate disodium An organic biphosphonate that inhibits osteoclast-mediated bone resorption; when administered cyclically, it increases spinal bone density and decreases the incidence of new vertebral fractures in the elderly; as a therapeutic agent, it slows accelerated bone turnover and is of use in Paget's disease of bone (osteitis deformans), heterotopic ossification, hypercalcemia of malignancy, and osteoporosis; see Coherence therapy, Osteoporosis

EtOH Ethanol

etoposide VP-16-213 A semisynthetic chemotherapeutic agent that derives from podophyllotoxin, extracted from the root of the American mandrake *Podophyllum pelatatum*, which blocks cells in the late S-G2 phase of mitosis, possibly by its effect on topoisomerase (DNA degradation), inhibiting nucleoside transport and mitochondrial electron transport; it is active against monocytic leukemia, lymphoma, small cell carcinoma, testicular cancer and KS and may be co-administered with cyclophosphamide and doxorubicin (Cancer 1991; 67:215)

etretinate CLINICAL THERAPEUTICS A derivative of retinoic acid that stimulates epithelial differentiation and inhibits the malignant transformation of skin and mucosa; etretinate is a second line agent used to treat psoriasis, used in combination with PUVA, to ↓ the dose of methoxsalen (N Engl J Med 1995; 332:581RV) see Psoriasis

eucalyptus oil Steam-distilled oil from *Eucalyptus globulus*, used as an expectorant and antiseptic; an overdose of as little as 3.5 ml may be fatal CLINICAL Epigastric pain, nausea, vomiting, vertigo, ataxia, myasthenia, pallor,

cyanosis, stridor, delirium, convulsions, stupor, transient coma or death

euchromatin Nuclear chromatin that is completely uncoiled, which is seen in interphase as a ground-glass clearing of the nucleoplasm

eugenics A movement that was popular in pre-WWII (to borrow from the Nazi propaganda, Author's note)

eugenetics see Eugenics

eugenics Eugenetics MEDICAL ETHICS A movement that was popular from 1905 until the early 1930s in the US, UK, and Northern Europe, which lost favor with the advent of the Nazi pseudoscientific eugenics program, which included elimination of 'lives not worth living' (Nature 1995; 374:303) and its justification for anti-Semitic genocide (Science 1994; 264:1686-1739); the concept that heredity may play a major role in behavior is reborn in the rapidly evolving field of behavioral genetics, see there

eumelanin The pigment that is native to skin and hair, which is composed of cross-linked tyrosine polymers

eunuchoidism A condition characterized by androgen insufficiency of pre-pubertal onset with infantile genitalia and secondary sexual characteristics, aspermia, lack of male hair pattern, high-pitched voice, infertility, lack of libido, poor muscular development, 'female' fat pattern, increased long bone growth with an arm span 4 cm > height, small testes (< 2 cm, normal ± 4 cm); see 'Fertile' eunuch syndrome, Hypogonadotropic eunuchoidism

Euroblood TRANSFUSION MEDICINE A generic term for a unit of packed RBCs, which in certain regions of the US comprise a significant minority (up to 30% in metropolitan New York) of the units transfused; Euroblood is in a sense, a 'waste' product, as the blood is collected for the serum, in order to purify various plasma proteins, including coagulation factors and fibrinogen

European Patent Office The official agency involved in delineating the parameters of the European Patent Convention (EPC), an agreement that has been signed by the EC (European Commission) member states, Austria, Sweden, and Switzerland; under the provisions of the EPC, before a patent is granted, the EPO must consider requirements of novelty, inventive step, disclosure of the invention (sufficiency), industrial application, and (most difficult to delineate) morality; this provision excludes inventions likely 'to induce riot or public disorder, or to lead to criminal or other generally offensive behaviour' (Nature 1994; 369:589s&L)

eusocial behavior Eusociality A constellation of behavioral characteristics including reproductive altruism (ie restricted reproduction, often one or a severely limited number of reproducing female(s)), multiple generations living together, and a strong division of labor; eusocial behavior occurs in a wide range of animals from insects, eg ants, honeybees, termites, and ants to vertebrates, the most studied of which is the naked mole rat (Sci Am 1992; 267/2:72); other eusocial vertebrates include the African wild dog, the dwarf mongoose, and the Florida scrub jay; components of eusocial behavior are present in tribes and aboriginal populations living in extremes of climate

euthanasia The induction of death or painlessly putting to death those who are suffering from incurable diseases; euthanasia has also been defined as the deliberate administration of medication (eg narcotics or barbiturates) to an ill patient at his/her own request with the primary intent to end his/her own life; after publishing a story by a gynecology resident who 'killed' a young terminally ill woman with ovarian cancer (It's Over, Debbie-anonymous JAMA 1988; 259:272) and the ensuing debate about euthanasia, G Lundberg, editor of the *Journal of the American Medical Association* offered a classification of the types of euthanasia (table) in the Netherlands, an estimated 2% of the population dies by euthanasia, which is defined as the active killing of a patient by a physician at the patient's own request; to be legally acceptable by Dutch law, three conditions must be met: 1) The act must be voluntary and initiated by the patient 2) The life situation must be hopeless, where both the physician and patient recognize that recovery is impossible and 3) The decision must be corroborated by a colleague who agrees with the appropriateness of the request (JAMA 1989; 262:3316); only 10% of the Dutch public is frankly opposed to the concept of euthanasia (JAMA 1995; 273:1411); 54% of physicians believe that euthanasia should be legal in some situations, 48% believe that it is never ethically justified, only 33% would be willing to perform euthanasia; hematologists and oncologists are more likely to oppose physician-assisted suicide and euthanasia; psychiatrists are more likely to support these practices (N Engl J Med 1994; 331:89SA) see Initiative 119, Kevorkian, Physician-assisted suicide

Note: The pros and cons of the euthanasia debate will reverberate until society agrees to either completely reject the concept of euthanasia, or to accept the inevitable need to perform euthanstia in a legitimate context (N Engl J Med 1992; 326:197OA, 327:201C)

EUTHANASIA

VOLUNTARY EUTHANASIA

PASSIVE EUTHANASIA The physician chooses not to treat a condition, eg pneumonia in a terminal cancer or Alzheimer's diease, or treat the condition in a non-aggressive fashion; see Slow code

SEMIPASSIVE EUTHANASIA Nutritive support is withheld in a comatose patient; see Cruzan, Nancy

SEMIACTIVE EUTHANASIA A life support 'line' from a comatose patient is disconnected, see Quinlan

'ACCIDENTAL' EUTHANASIA Double effect A narcotic intended to relieve pain depresses respiration enough to cause either immediate death or secondarily induces a fatal pneumonia; see It's over, Debbie

SUICIDAL EUTHANASIA Intentional overdose by alcohol or barbiturates by the terminally ill patient, facilitated by the physician who makes the lethal dose available; see Dr Death

ACTIVE EUTHANASIA Administration of a fatal overdose of morphine or potassium by the physician

PASSIVE EUTHANASIA The forgoing of life-sustaining therapy, which corresponds to any of the first five above delineated forms of euthanasia; see Advance directive, DNR orders

INVOLUNTARY EUTHANASIA

CRYPTEUTHANASIA Without patient consent

ENCOURAGED EUTHANASIA Chronically ill are pressured into choosing death to spare their families the emotional and financial strain

SURROGATE EUTHANASIA The patient is incompetent to make such a decision

DISCRIMINATORY EUTHANASIA Vulnerable groups, eg the elderly, poor, disabled and racial minorities, are assisted more than others

euthyroid sick syndrome LABORATORY MEDICINE A complex of deranged laboratory parameters found in patients who are critically ill with nonthyroid diseases that alter the serum levels of thyroid hormones and which in absence of the underlying nonthyroid illness would be correctly interpreted as indicative of disease of the thyroid 'axis' LABORATORY Peripheral decrease or inhibition of 5'-deiodinase, the deiodination enzyme, resulting in decreased peripheral 5'-monodeiodination of thyroxine (T_4), reversed, free and total T_3; TSH, TRH and (usually) the free thyroxine levels are normal; in absence of suggestive thyroid symptomatology, thyroid function tests in sick patients may prove fruitless and not require treatment for hypothyroidism, but rather for their underlying condition, eg anorexia nervosa, chronic obstructive pulmonary disease, fever of unknown origin, infection, malignancy, myocardial infarction and trauma

eutrophication ENVIRONMENT The release of excess nitrogenous material in the form of nitrates and ammonia into the ocean, the air (Nature 1995; 374:117), major rivers, and into lakes, eg Lake Okeechobee, Florida, which are the result of 'run-offs' of fertilizers from farming and treated sewage products, causing massive overgrowth of vegetation and algae that consume the oxygen dissolved in the water, asphyxiating the lowest organisms in the food chain, major alteration of the local estuarial ecosystems and loss of higher organisms; see Nitrates, Red tide

Eve 3,4 Methylenedioxyethamphetamine; see Ecstasy

'event' 1) Error, see there 2) Misadventure, see there

evernomicin A member of a family of antibiotics in the early stages of development that may be effective against multi-drug resistant gram-positive bacteria; it is nephrotoxic in experimental animals

evoked response NEUROPHYSIOLOGY Evoked potential* Any stimulus-evoked electrical potential recorded by EEG, which varies according to intensity, modality, location and level of consciousness; the response is detectable over the appropriate cortical receptive areas by EEG after stimulation of sense organs or peripheral nerves, eg brainstem auditory, transcortical motor, pattern shift visual, and somatosensory ERs; averaging methods introduced by Dawson improve the resolution of waveforms allowing them to be recognized above the background electrical activity (white noise)

*Although the noun potential is more correct, response is widely preferred

evolution Any time-related change in the genetic composition of a population, described in terms of allelic frequencies that change in response to

1) Mutations There are an estimated 10^4 mutations per gene per generation

2) Selection Survival to reproductive age of the 'fittest', ie those best adapted to their environment

3) Genetic drift Gene frequencies of progeny differ from their parents and

4) Migration Shift of populations causes allelic 'drift'

evolutionary clock Molecular clock, see there

evolutionary medicine A new discipline that pretends to bridge the gaps between medical anthropology, paleoanthropology, and modern medicine, using as its tools the study of genetic relationships between hunter-gatherers and various Stone Age surrogates, eg the !Kung San of Botswana (JAMA 1993; 269:1477MN&P)

Ewing family of tumors A subgroup of small round cell tumors (usually of children) which includes osseous Ewing sarcoma, atypical Ewing sarcoma, and peripheral primitive neuroendocrine tumors (PNET, pronounced 'peanut'); EFTs are phenotypically similar, and most have the chromosomal translocation t(11;22)(q24;q12), and express high levels of the $MIC2p^{30-32}$ antigen; in most cases, an in-frame hybrid transcript* has been identified, making it likely that the presence of specific fusion transcripts is a defining criteria for the Ewing family of tumors (N Engl J Med 1994; 331:294OA)

*The N-terminal part of the *EWS* gene on chromosome 22 is linked to either the DNA-binding domain (Ets domain) of the *FLI1* transcription factor gene or to ERG, a member of the Ets gene family, closely related to *FLI1* forming a *EWS-FLI1* or *EWS-ERG* fusion transcript

Ewing sarcoma A primitive neuroectodermal tumor of bone that is closely related (if not biologically identical) to peripheral neuroepithelioma; although they differ by light microscopy, both share the cytogenetic translocation abnormality, t(11;22)(q24;q12); in both, neural markers (eg neuron-specific enolase, S100 protein, neurofilaments triple protein, and HNK-1/Leu-7) can be detected, and ultrastructurally, both have constant pools of glycogen, cytoplasmic processes with neurofilaments and dense core granules (Arch Pathol Lab Med 1994; 118:608OA, 606ED) CLINICAL Locoregional bone pain, or pathological fractures see Peripheral neuroepithelioma

exchange proteins Phospholipid-transfer proteins, see there

exchange plasmapheresis Plasmapheresis, see there

exchange transfusion NEONATOLOGY A therapeutic procedure for reducing 'immunotoxins' in the neonate; exchange transfusion is appropriate in 1) Hemolytic disease of the newborn, caused by maternal IgG antibodies against fetal antigens 2) Neonatal hyperbilirubinemia, due to red cell and bilirubin metabolic defects 3) Lesser indications, including hematomas, prematurity, perinatal infection, RDS, hyaline membrane disease, DIC, marked (often iatrogenic) hypermagnesemia, adenosine deaminase deficiency with SCID, congenital ITP, hypovolemia or anemia, cardiovascular surgery and necrotizing enterocolitis COMPLICATIONS Thrombocytopenia, iron-deficiency

excimer laser Cold laser CARDIOLOGY A laser used in coronary artery angioplasty that delivers pulsating ultraviolet light to excise atherosclerotic plaques within stenosed arteries; in contrast, balloon coronary angioplasty has a 30-40% restenosis rate, while 'hot-tip' lasers (constant pulse infrared radiation) have been abandoned as there is a 20-30% incidence of vessel perforation, the 'bed' left after hot laser therapy is roughened and charred, and forms a nidus for future atherosclerotic lesions, creating a false intramural channel rather than a true lumen; in one report, 90% of patients treated with excimer lasers had reduction of the stenosis from 81% to 37%; 20% had complications in the form of restenosis that required a conventional semi-invasive procedure, eg balloon angioplasty; Cf Percutaneous transluminal coronary angioplasty

excision repair Cut-and-patch repair MOLECULAR BIOLOGY A mechanism by which damaged DNA is repaired, which involves the removal of damaged nucleotide(s), either through nuclease-catalyzed single-nucleotide base excision (short patch) or segmental excision (long patch) of the damaged region, followed by DNA synthesis with a DNA polymerase, which uses the intact DNA strand as a template, followed by joining to the intact strand with a DNA ligase; mutagens affect each pathway differently, eg methotrexate inhibits the short patch repair system

excision repair syndrome(s) A group of conditions characterized by a defect in the excision repair pathway, eg xeroderma pigmentosum, Cockayne syndrome, and trichothiodystrophy (Nature 1991; 350:190N&V) see Brittle-hair syndrome, Xeroderma pigmentosum

excitability protein A generic term for any membrane protein, including membrane receptors, ion channels and ion pumps that is activated by electrical activity and often the site of action of therapeutic agents; EPs have been exploited therapeutically, as non-specific 'ligands' and include β-adrenergic receptor blockers, eg propranolol, an anti-hypertensive, dihydropyridine, calcium channel blockers, nifedipine for angina pectoris, GABA receptor potentiator, eg benzodiazepine for status epilepticus, dopamine receptor blockers, phenothiazine, Na^+, K^+-ATPase blockers and digoxin for congestive heart failure; since all drugs have undesirable side effects and the expression of these proteins varies according to the tissue, it is theoretically possible to identify mRNAs specific for a target tissue, producing more specific drugs with fewer side effects

excitotoxicity A postulated final pathway for neuronal injury from diseases caused by a wide range of phys-

iopathologic mechanisms; neuronal injury (excitotoxicity) is caused in part by overstimulation of receptors for excitatory amino acids which occurs in diverse neurologic diseases that may be acute (eg hypoglycemia, seizures, stroke, or trauma) or chronic (eg AIDS-dementia complex, amyotrophic lateral sclerosis, Huntington's disease and possibly also Alzheimer's disease; exicitotoxicity is largely mediated by an excessive influx of calcium into neurons triggered by the activation of glutamate receptors (N Engl J Med 1994; 330:613OA)

exclamation mark hairs Short (3 mm in length) irregularly thickened and terminally dilated hairs with tapered proximal ends, seen in alopecia areata

exclusion colitis Diversion colitis, see there

exclusion criteria AIDS see Donor exclusion criteria Any objective parameter that would invalidate the inclusion of a set of data or population in establishing reference values and/or normal distribution curves; possible exclusion criteria in humans include substance abuse (alcohol, illicit drugs, tobacco, vitamin abuse), abnormal blood pressure, obesity, transient conditions (nonfasting state, recent hospitalization, illness, surgery, transfusion, or use of prescription or nonprescription drugs), ♀ factors (lactation, use of oral contraceptives, pregnancy), environmental, genetic, or occupational factors (Arch Pathol Lab Med 1992; 116:710OA) see Partitioning factor, Reference values

exclusion map GENETICS A schematic representation of each of a haploid complement of chromosomes, which is formed by pooling negative data from linkages analyses for a particular disease, which allows 'unsuccessful' studies to provide useful information where a particular will not be found

execute COMPUTERS *verb* Do FORENSIC MEDICINE *verb* Kill

'execution' wound FORENSIC MEDICINE A gunshot wound intended to kill the victim, carrying the legal implication of premeditation, ie first-degree manslaughter; in close-range executions, handguns are used, the entrance wound is often in the parieto-occipital region and the gun's muzzle is in direct contact with the victim's head; when the victim is mobile, other weapons are preferred by the 'executioner', eg a 'sawed-off' shotgun; see Murder one

Note: The crime-scene at an 'execution' differs from that of gun-related crimes of passion and suicides in that there is a deliberate attempt at 'efficiency'; in the crimes of passion, multiple erratic shots may have been fired throughout the scene or into the victim and the scene itself may show more signs of struggle and violence that crescendo into homicide; in suicides, the crime-scene is often quite neat (except for pieces of the tissue adjacent to the exit wound), the angle of the entrance wound implies complete knowledge of the act and only one fatal shot can possibly be fired

executive monkey An experimental model of uncertain validity; the 'executive' role is (for non-human primates) a stress-producing situation in which the 'executive' is forced to decide whether a nearby monkey would receive an electric shock; these primates developed stress ulcers occasionally resulting in fatal perforation (Psychosom Med 1958; 20:379)

Note: Although the concept that non-human primates (which are phylogenically and physically proximous to man) should react like humans when placed in related situations, subsequent studies only weakly corroborated the original 'executive monkey' studies

executive profile A broad battery of laboratory parameters that may be measured annually on specimens from quasi-important people, ie 'executives', in order to detect any potentially morbid condition that may require early intervention; one commercially available executive profile measures the A/G ratio, albumin, alkaline phosphatase, direct and indirect bilirubin, BUN, BUN/creatinine ratio, calcium, chloride, cholesterol (HDL-, LDL- and total), triglycerides, creatinine, glucose, iron, lactate dehydrogenase, 'liver' enzymes (alanine aminotransferase, aspartate aminotransferase, γ-glutamyl transferase), phophorous, potassium, total protein and immunoglobulins, sodium, uric acid, STS-RPR, thyroxine (T_4), urinalysis, CBC with differential count of leukocytes and platelet count; see Organ panel

exercise Substantial literature supports the benefits of exercise; although it is heuristically logical that exercise would reduce the incidence of ischemia, poor adherence to exercise regimens, the number of subjects required to achieve statistical significance and other factors make it difficult to confirm these benefits CARBOHYDRATE METABOLISM Exercise ↑ removal of glucose from the circulation by replenishing depleted glycogen in the muscles and ↑ the sensitivity of insulin receptors, allowing more efficient glucose metabolism CARDIOVASCULAR Exercise ↑ coronary artery collateralization, oxygenation of the heart, the diameter of the proximal coronaries and ↓ myocardium oxygen demand by ↓ the heart rate and systolic blood pressure; the incidence of acute MI is inversely related to the patient's level of habitual physical activity; exercise ≥ 5X/week have a relative risk (RR) of 2.4; 3-4X/week RR = 8.6; 1-2X/week RR = 19.4; <1X/week RR = 107 (**N Engl J Med 1993; 329:1677OA**) LABORATORY ↑↑↑ Creatine kinase (6000 U/L, normal 200 U/L) 4-5 days after intense exercise, with smaller ↑ in LDH, AST, and ALT (**J Lab Clin Med 1992; 119:183**) COAGULATION ↑ Fibrinolytic activity with ↑ platelet factor 4, β-thromboglobulin and ↑ sensitivity of platelets to prostaglandin I_2 (inhibitory to ADP-induced platelet aggregation) HYPERTENSION Exercise is reported to be more effective than drug therapy in ↓ blood pressure LIPID PROFILES ↑ HDL and ↓ cholesterol are seen only when exercise occurs 75% or above the maximal heart rate METABOLIC EXPENDITURE see table OSTEOPOROSIS Exercise ↓ bone mineral loss PSYCHOLOGY Exercise is widely thought to promote a sense of well-being, help people to cope better and be mentally healthier; see Vigorous exercise

Note: It is difficult to separate the benefits of exercise from the lifestyles of 'healthy' people, in that those who exercise regularly tend to have a more balanced diet and, if they abuse drugs and tobacco and drink alcohol at all, do so in extreme moderation

exercise-associated amenorrhea A finding described in female long-distance runners; in prospective studies, although menstrual irregularities occur in the form of anovulatory cycles, irregular cycles and decreased endogenous production of progesterone with shortened luteal phases, true amenorrhea does not occur; the menstrual dysfunction may be accompanied by osteopenia, osteoporosis and hypoestrogenic amenorrhea; see Running

exercise-induced anaphylaxis A distinct form of allergy manifest by a sensation of cutaneous warmth, pruritis and secondary erythema, urticaria, hypotension and upper airway obstruction DIFFERENTIAL DIAGNOSIS Cholinergic urticaria and anaphylaxis; see MK-571

exercise-induced asthma A condition* in which intense physical exertion results in acute airway narrowing in subjects with airway hyperreactivity PATHOGENESIS EIA is closely linked to thermal provocation that occurs when large volumes of air are 'conditioned' (heated and humidified), a scenario that is most common in winter; the limit of airflow is most intense with running, less so with jogging, and least with walking; the obstruction is greatest with cold dry air, and least with warm humid air CLINICAL Cough, wheezing, dyspnea, cough, chest tightness, hyperinflation, airflow limitation, and hypoxia TREATMENT Cromolyn and $β_2$-agonist (**N Engl J Med 1994; 330:1329OA**)

*Although exercise-induced bronchospasm is the most correct term for this condition, exercise-induced asthma is firmly entrenched in the literature; other synonyms include exercise asthma, exercise-induced bronchial lability, and thermally induced asthma

exercise pyramid A proposed schematic diagram that recommends the types and amount of exercise that should be performed for optimal health; at the bottom are non-structured physical activities, eg walking the dog and

EXERCISE-KCAL CONSUMED/HOUR	
Distance running (15 km/hour)	1000
Contact sports (wrestling, karate)	900
Bicycling (25 km/hour)	800
Swimming, freestyle	800
Basketball, volleyball	700
Jogging (9 km/hour)	600
Tennis	500
Coitus	450
Walking	400

climbing stairs; higher on the pyramid are active recreational activities, eg basketball, swimming, tennis, and others; at the peak of the EP is vigorous exercise, which should be performed at least three times/wk for at least 30 min each session (**N Y Times 29 March 1995, C1**) see Exercise, Vigorous exercise

exercise test CARDIOLOGY A generic term for any clinical method used to evaluate a person's cardiovascular responsiveness (ie tolerance) to exercise; see Treadmill exercise test

exertional rhabdomyolysis Azoturia, Monday morning sickness VETERINARY MEDICINE An acute condition characterized by sweating and paralysis of the hindquarter muscles accompanied by myoglobinuria, which follows a period of rest, usually the weekend

exfoliatin An exotoxin produced by *Staphylococcus aureus* strains that carry a group II phage

exfoliative cytology Diagnostic cytologic material from 'accessible' organs, ie uterine cervix, urinary bladder, breast and nipple discharges, GI tract, respiratory tract, which is obtained noninvasively from hollow or tubular organs; Cf Aspiration cytology

exit wound FORENSIC PATHOLOGY The lesion that a bullet or other projectile causes when leaving the body; EWs are often larger that the entrance wound, which is the result of tumbling and deformation of the bullet; Cf Entrance wound

exodus ball GYNECOLOGICAL CYTOLOGY A rounded cluster of endometrial cells seen in a vaginal smear from 6-10 days after menstruation, which has no pathological significance

exodus ball

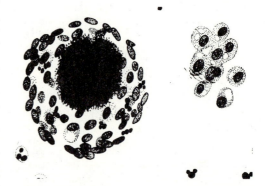

ex officio From office, ie by virtue of one's office or position; ex officio refers to privileges or services that are implied without being officially delineated

exon MOLECULAR BIOLOGY A coding sequence of DNA that is transcribed into mature mRNA and later translated into proteins; exons form functional and folding regions, domains and subdomains; introns (unused or 'junk' DNA) are spliced out DNA segments and mark the turns or edges of secondary structures; the DNA contained in the

46 chromosomes is sufficient in theory to produce ± 3 million proteins; that there are only 30-100 000 proteins begs the question of whether all of the remaining is 'junk' and how is it accounted for in the genome; the tens of thousands of proteins are derived from a finite number, possibly from 1000 to 7000 exon motifs, which have existed for about two billion years

exon amplification An alternate means for determining a gene's location that takes advantage of a natural feature of transcribed sequences of DNA, to wit, RNA splicing* (Sci & Med Nov/Dec 1994 p48)

*In RNA splicing, the 'raw' transcript of DNA is 'edited' to delete the intervening segments (introns) of DNA that do not encode peptides

exon trapping Exon amplification, see there

exonuclease An enzyme that catalyzes the hydrolysis of the nucleotides, beginning at either the 3' end or the 5' end of the DNA molecule; 3' to 5' exonuclease activity is present in DNA polymerases I, II and III, removes mismatched nucleotides from the 3'-end of a growing strand of DNA, thus having a proof-reading or editing role; 5' to 3' exonuclease activity is present in DNA polymerase I and III and removes RNA priming molecules

exotoxin MICROBIOLOGY A bacteria toxin, prototypically, *Vibrio cholera* that increases cAMP production by intestinal mucosal cells and flow of water and ions into intestinal lumen, ie diarrhea; there are two broad categories of exotoxins, to wit, 1) Enzymatic toxins that chemically modify host proteins, eg cholera and diphtheria toxins, or are proteolytic, as is the tetanus toxin and 2) Pore-forming toxins, most commonly produced by gram-negative bacteria that insert themselves into host cells, forming a channel that allows free flow of ions and cytolysis (Science & Medicine 1995; 2/3:16) see MECHANISM Cholera exotoxin transfers the ADP-ribose moiety from NAD to the α subunit of the Guanine-nucleotide membrane-bound (G) protein, reducing GTPase activity, leaving adenylate cyclase in the 'on' position; *Escherichia coli* enterotoxin, inculpated in traveler's diarrhea may act similarly; see Endotoxin, Traveler's diarrhea, Virulence factor

expanded rubella syndrome A complex of symptoms that may affect infants with the congenital rubella syndrome in addition to the 'classic' findings of congenital heart disease, corneal clouding, microcephaly, mental retardation and deafness; the 'expanded' symptoms include hepatosplenomegaly, thrombocytopenic purpura, intrauterine growth retardation, interstitial pneumonia, myocarditis and metaphyseal bone lesions; see Congenital rubella syndrome, TORCH

experience hypothesis A posit that the outcome in term of survival and complications of certain procedure (eg transplantations of heart, kidney, and liver) is a function of frequency with which the procedure is performed and the experience of the team performing the surgery, and the physicians caring for the patient after the procedure (N Engl J Med 1993; 328:514c)

experience rating HEALTH CARE ENVIRONMENT A system used by commercial insurers for determining risks and health insurance premiums based on the costs of a group's medical claims; groups with the sickest workers and largest claims may eventually be dropped by the insurers (Am Med News 26 October 1992, p7) Cf Community rating

experimental allergic encephalomyelitis An acute neurological disease of mice that is an ideal model system for studying autoimmune phenomena of the central nervous system, which are mediated by CD4+ T lymphocytes reactive against myelin basic protein, in which the immune reaction causes myelinolysis, wasting and paralysis; see Autoimmunity

'experiments of nature' see 'Inborn errors of metabolism'; Cf Natural experiment

expert laboratory A rarely-used term for a laboratory that is regarded as having a particular expertise Note: Because of overlapping definitions, the more understood terms, reference laboratory or specialized laboratory, appear to be preferable (Author's note)

expert shell MEDICAL INFORMATICS A set of software with a core design that lacks information and domain, which once it is fed the appropriate data, becomes an expert system in a particular field

expert system An artificial intelligence system that is designed to help in a particular decision-making process; the key component of such a system is a knowledge base, which combines a database of facts, beliefs and an algorithm based on heuristic logic, eg expert systems of internal medicine, CADUCEUS, INTERNIST; see Artificial intelligence, Neural networking

expert witness see Physician expert witness

exploding HEALTH CARE FINANCING The practice of expanding into individual units, a group of diagnostic or procedural test codes (based on the 4th edition of the Current Procedural Terminology promulgated by the American Medical Association) that might have been previously included as a 'panel', in order to maximize the reimbursement (see CAP Today March 1993)

explosive OCCUPATIONAL SAFETY A chemical that causes a sudden, virtually instantaneous release of pressure, gas, and heat when subjected to sudden shcok, pressure, or high temperature

explosive syndrome PSYCHIATRY Episodic outbursts of verbal abuse and physical violence in response to minor provocation, which occurs in organic brain disease, after cerebral trauma, related to psychiatric disease, metabolic dysfunctions, including hypoglycemia, Wilson's disease, uremia, hyperammonemia, ↑ androgens ('roid rage), premenstrual syndrome, Cushing's disease; the patients are usually pleasant between outbursts and apologetic for the explosions TREATMENT Some patients respond to propranolol

ex post facto A really neat way of saying 'retroactive'*

*Or for those who have an even more poverty-stricken vocabulary, 'after the fact'

exposure RADIATION PHYSICS The amount of ionizing radiation at a specific point in space, which is defined as the ratio between the total charge of ions divided by the mass that would completely stop that radiation; the SI (International System) unit is coulomb per kg (C/kg); in human terms, exposure refers to the amount of ionizing radiation to which an individual is subjected

expression cloning A technique of molecular biology in which pools of clones from a cell line's complementary DNA (cDNA) library are transfected into another cell that is capable of expressing a protein of interest, eg the noradrenaline transporter (Nature 1991; 350:351)

expression vector MOLECULAR BIOLOGY A cloning vector that contains all the elements, eg promoter, enhancer, splicing signals, and poly(A) tail for transcription and translation; EVs direct programmed protein synthesis, allowing an experimenter to utilize a bacterium's genes to increase mRNA synthesis and produce large quantities of a protein of interest, eg hormones (eg insulin and hGH), and enzymes (eg tissue plasminogen activator) by the biotechnology industry; the form of expression is dependent in part on the host cells, which can range widely to include bacterial, yeast, or animal cells

extern A student in his third or fourth year of medical school (in North America), who attends ward rounds of a university or teaching hospital, and learns clinical medicine by example and quasi-active participation in patient management; a common complaint of externs is their common role as a go-fer' (*pronounced* gopher, as in 'go *for this...', go for that...'*), performance of menial 'scut' duties, and other subtle forms of psychological abuse; see Pimping; Cf Intern

external cranioplasty Head shaping, see there

extended family SOCIAL MEDICINE A family unit that is related by blood or by marriage that extends over 3 or more generations, which may include 'collateral' relatives, spouses, and progeny; an EF may also be defined as one composed of a core nuclear family unit of mother, father, children, and any other blood relative who lives either in the same household or closely proximous thereto, including in-laws, cousins and grandparents; the EF provides an interactive system of moral, and often economic support; dissolution of the extended family 'unit', like the disintegration of the nuclear family, through the forces of divorces and economics, has been held responsible for loss of moral cohesion and increase in certain forms of mental illness in advanced societies; see 'Significant other'; Cf Nuclear family, Single-parent family

extended haplotypes HLA associations with allelic loci that exist in linkage disequilibrium*; EHs may be the result of crossover suppression by environmental factors in conjunction with certain HLA types, producing autoimmune phenomena, eg B-27 associated with *Klebsiella*, DR2 associated with lepra, and increased cellular immune response

*eg B8/DR3/SC01/GL02 is associated with membranoproliferative glomerulonephritis and A25/B18/DR2 is associated with complement C2 deficiency

extension of life A generic term for any maneuver intended to reduce the morbidity of various conditions in the elderly, thereby increasing the lifespan

external version OBSTETRICS An active intervention consisting of gentle external rotation of the fetus from the undesirable breech position to the more easily deliverable cephalic position; the potential procedure must be weighed against the danger of premature separation of the placenta, rupture of membranes or of the uterus and potential litigation; such a risk often proves too great; in the US, most breech presentations are delivered by cesarean section; see Cesarean section; Cf Internal version

extinction BIOLOGY The disappearance of a species GENETICS The loss of an allele from a gene pool OPTICS Absorbance PSYCHOLOGY A facet of operant (classical) conditioning in which there is weakening and eventual disappearance of a conditioned response through nonreinforcement

extinguishing medium OCCUPATIONAL SAFETY Any of a number of 'standard' materials, including alcohol foam, CO_2, dry chemical, foam, and water fog, used to extinguish a 'standard' fire (ie one that does not requires special equipment); the EM is of interest to OSHA, which requires that the EM for a particular material be indicated in its Materials Safety Data Sheets‡

extracellular matrix A complex, self-assembling network of proteins and glycoproteins which interact with cell surfaces, consisting of two major components: interstitial stroma and basement membranes; components of the extracellular matrix include collagens, types IV and VII, heparan sulfate proteoglycan and glycoproteins, the most abundant of which is laminin

extracellular signal-regulated kinase MAP (mitogen-activated protein) kinase, see there

extracorporeal membrane oxygenation A form of artificial oxygenation of blood, in which a cannula in the jugular vein is connected to a small reservoir, into which the blood drains by gravity; the blood is then pumped from the reservoir through a membrane oxygenator and heat exchanger and returned to the patient via the right carotid artery cannula; ECMO is considered a vital part of the surgical repair of congenital diaphragmatic hernia in infants

ECMO is considered standard therapy for many full-term infants with inadequate pulmnary function, which has had limited success in older children and adults (see **N Engl J Med 1993; 329:354**SB)

extracorporeal photochemotherapy Photochemotherapy, see there

extracorporeal shock-wave lithotripsy see Lithotripsy

extractable nuclear antigens A group of antibodies that react against the Sm antigen, a nonhistone nucleoprotein devoid of nucleic acid (after Smith, a propositus with the antigen) and ribonucleoprotein (RNP), an antibody now known as anti-U1 small nuclear RNP; anti-Sm antibodies are relatively specific for lupus erythematosus, RNP are common in mixed connective tissue disease, demonstrating a 'speckled' pattern of immunofluorescence

extralobar pulmonary sequestration Bronchopulmonary sequestration, see there

extraordinary treatment A permutation of 'heroic treatment', defined as *'Treatment or care that does not offer a reasonable hope or benefit to the patient, or which cannot be accomplished without excessive pain, expense, or other great burden; (extraordinary treatment is) an ethical determination about rendering care depending upons the patient's condition and prognosis.'* (**JC Rhea, JS Ott, JM Shafritz, Dictionary of Health Care Management, Facts on File, New York, 1988**)

extrapolation model HMO model HEALTH CARE ENVIRONMENT A model for determining the needs for health care providers (eg anesthesiologists, internists) that is based on changes in patient demographics, utilization rates, and the outsourcing of services (**CAP Today 1995; 9:5**) Cf Demand model, Needs model, Supply model

extreme amplification VIROLOGY An intense proliferation of viral particles, to such degree that much of the host tissue may be converted into viral particles (**R Preston, The Hot Zone, Random House, New York, 1994**)

extreme thrombocytosis A laboratory abnormality defined as a platelet count of $> 10^6/mm^3$; in one review of 280 cases, the age ranged from 12 days to 92 years (mean age 31), and were reactive, related to myeloproliferative disorders, or idiopathic (see table) the peak platelet count (1.2 vs 1.8 x $10^6/mm^3$) and bleeding and/or vasocclusive symptoms (4% vs 56%) were lower in the reactive than in the myeloproliferative cases (**Am J Med 1994; 96:247**)

extremely low birth weight see Limits of viability

extremozyme An enzyme that functions at extreme con-

EXTREME THROMBOCYTOSIS (PLATELETS $> 10^6$/MM^3)
REACTIVE (82.5%)
Infection (31%)
Postsplenectomy hyposplenism (19%)
Malignancy (14%)
Trauma
MYELOPROLIFERATIVE DISORDERS (13.6%)
Chronic granulocytic leukemia (42%)
Primary thrombocythemia (29%)
UNKNOWN (3.9%)

ditions, eg high or low temperatures, pHs, salinity, or other harsh conditions that are suboptimal for 'idealized' enzymes; Taq polymerase, the key enzyme in the polymerase chain reaction is the first commercially viable extremozyme (**Am Biotechn Lab, August 1994**)

extrication EMERGENCY MEDICINE The process of removing a person from a condition of entrapment, usually from a motor vehicle, often requiring the use of special tools, eg heavy metal or bolt cutters or powered spreading devices;

extrication requires considerable skill as partial removal may release pressure on critical vascular supplies and the 'prisoner' being extricated may exsanguinate before he/she is accessible to emergency therapy

extrinsic factor inhibitor Tissue factor pathway inhibitor, see there

extrinsic pathway The arm of coagulation activation that, like the intrinsic pathway, converges on the common pathway, ie factor X activation; the extrinsic pathway is activated by exposure of blood to tissue factor, circulating factor VII, Ca^{++} and phospholipid; Cf Common and Intrinsic pathway

ex vivo cell therapy MOLECULAR MEDICINE A generic term for the transplantation of living cells (previously grown outside of the body or other living system) to treat a particular disease; EVCT is currently understood to mean BM or stem cell transplantation; with advances in technology, other cells may in the future be transplanted eg bone, cartilage, nervous system cells, pancreas, and skin; most EXCT is not yet available as a clinical option, but is in the advanced planning stages; one of the main obstacles to successful growth of cells is the absence or inadequacy of a suitable microenvironent, interaction with which has proved necessary for the replication of the cells of interest (Bio/Technology 1995; 13:449) see Bioreactor

ex vivo gene therapy MOLECULAR MEDICINE A generic term for the transfer of genes into cells (transduction) as a means of treating inherited diseases of the genome, eg adenosine deaminase deficiency; EVGT has recently aroused considerable controversy as a broad-reaching

patent covering its key components has been awarded (some say unfairly) to a group of three workers at the NIH (Science 1995; 265:1899N&c)

eyeless A gene found in fruit flies that is similar to the *Small eye* gene of mice and the *Aniridia* gene of humans, all of which, when mutated, result in defects of the iris, lens, cornea, and retina; *eyeless* is thought by some workers to be a 'master control gene'*, which singlehandedly triggers the formation of an organ or structure; the protein encoded by *eyeless* has features of a transcription factor, which turns genes on or off(Science 1995; 267:1788, 1766)

*A 'holy grail' gene long sought in developmental biology

eye-mouth gap The discrepancy between the actual caloric intake and exercise and that reported by a subject, usually with an eating disorder; this misreporting is not thought to represent conscious deception on the part of the subject, but may result in the diagnosis of 'diet-resistant obesity', a dilemma that can be resolved with the double-labeled water method, see there (N Engl J Med 1992; 327:1947ED)

'eye-opener' SUBSTANCE ABUSE A highly colloquial term for the first drink in the day of an alcoholic, which he/she requires to steady him/herself or to 'treat' his/her hangover (JAMA 1992; 268:3183NIH)

eye rolling Rhythmic eye movements which accompany rotation of the head, seen in the Pelizaeus-Merzbacher form of leukodystrophy

'eye structure' Replication bubble, see there

eye teeth A highly colloquial term for the maxillary canine teeth

F Symbol for: 1) Degrees Fahrenheit 2) Factor 3) Farad, the SI (International System) derived unit of capacitance 4) Faraday constant 5) Fertility factor (bacteriology) 6) Fluorine 7) Force 8) Fragment (of antibody) 9) Inbreeding coefficient 10) Phenylalanine 11) Variance ratio

f Symbol for: 1) Breathing frequency (pulmonary function testing) 2) femto-, the SI (International System) abbreviation for 10^{-15} 3) Frequency 4) Friction coefficient

F508 see Cystic fibrosis

F-actin A filamentous double helical polymer of G-actin units which, with the tropomyosin-troponin regulatory complex, forms the thin filaments of skeletal muscle; Cf G-actin

F_1 hybrid GENETICS The progeny that result from mating two different inbred strains of the same species; the F_1 hybrid is capable of accepting allografts from either of the inbred parents, but cannot accept an allograft from a non-self F_0 generation, since the entire complement of the MHC is distinct and thus capable of evoking an immune reaction in the graft recipient

F_2-isoprostane Any of a number of arachidonic acid-derived compounds (regioisomers I and II shown in figure) that undergo free radical-catalyzed peroxidation, which are produced independently of cyclooxygenase and are two- to six-fold ↑ in the circulation of cigarette smokers; these data support the hypothesis that smoking causes oxidative damage to important biological molecules (N Eng J Med 1995; 332:1198oA) implying that anti-oxidative maneuvers may be of use

F_2-isoprostane

1/f noise Pink noise A form of temporal fluctuation that has a power density that is inversely proportional to the frequency (power ~ $1/f$), which varies with a predictability intermediate between that of white noise (no correlation in time, power ~ $1/f^0$) and Brownian motion (no correlation with increments, power ~ $1/f^2$); $1/f$ is present in a wide variety of physical systems and may be a typical marker of complexity (Science 1995; 267:1837)

F protein A protein produced by the measles virus, which is responsible for viral penetration, cell fusion (syncytium formation), and hemolysis, resulting in cell-to-cell spread of the virus

Fab fragment IMMUNOLOGY The papain-digested fragment of a molecule of immunoglobulin that is cleaved at the hinge region and bears the variable domains of the light and heavy chains (V_L and V_H) and the constant domain of the light chain and the first constant domain of the heavy chain (C_L and C_H1), a cleavage that occurs at residue 224 in IgG1 and near this site in the other immunoglobulins and yields two Fab fragments and an Fc fragment

F(ab')$_2$ fragment Fab" fragment A pepsin-digested fragment of the immunoglobulin molecule, which in IgG1 is cleaved between residues 234 and 233, yielding a Fab" fragment containing the heavy and light chain variable domains (V_H and V_L) and the light chain constant domains, as well as the first domain of the heavy chain's constant region (C_L and C_H1), as well as an Fc' fragment

FAB classification French-American-British classification of acute leukemia (table) which are divided into cells with lymphoid (ALL) or myeloid (AML) differentiation; of childhood ALL, 70% are predominantly L1, 27% are L2 and 3% (or less) are L3 or Burkitt cell type (N Engl J Med 1991; 324:800); in adults with ALL, 30% are L1, 65% are L2 and 5% are L3

Fab therapy CLINICAL THERAPEUTICS The use of antibody fragments (Fab fractions) against certain antigens, eg digoxin, may be used to treat poisonings with that agent; in a report of pediatric patients with digoxin intoxication 27/29 responded to treatment with digoxin-specific antibody fragments (N Engl J Med 1992; 326:1739oA); monoclonal Fabs may ultimately prove useful in treating viral pneumonia, eg due to RSV (New York Times 18 May 1993; C3), colchicine-specific Fab fragments to treat severe colchicine OD (N Engl J Med 1995; 332:642oA) see Psoriasis

Fabian Bridges An indigent male homosexual who, despite his diagnosis of AIDS, continued to have anonymous sex, nomadically migrating to various cities in the US, presumably infecting multiple others; health officials were unable to quarantine him, arrest him on any vice charges or institutionalize him on the grounds of incompetency; eventually, the gay community charitably provided him with shelter and supervision until he died (JAMA 1987; 257:344) see High disseminator, Patient zero; Cf Typhoid Mary

face-bow DENTISTRY A caliper-like device attached to the teeth or occlusal rim that is used to document the positional relationship between the maxillary arch and the temporomandibular joint and to orient dental casts to the opening (hinge) axis of the jaw, transferring it to an articulator

facelift Rhitidectomy* COSMETIC SURGERY A surgical procedure in which the wrinkles and sagging soft tissues of the face and neck are 'tightened', imparting a more youthful appearance OPERATION The procedure may last 2-4 hours and requires extensive incisions in front of and behind the ear, and in the temporal scalp; the skin is dissected free and the excess removed, often in conjunction with the removal of regional fat, which may be by liposuction COMPLICATIONS Asymmetry, hematoma, injury to nerves (facial, great auricular), scars, sloughing of skin; the signs of aging may recur in as little as one year

*While the term rhitidectomy is preferred by esthetic surgeons, its use is confined to specialists in the field

facet syndrome ORTHOPEDICS A low back syndrome in which the pain is attributed to osteoarthritis of the inter-articular vertebrae CLINICAL Low back pain that increases on extension that irradiates to the posterior thigh and ends at the knee; x-ray and CT imaging reveals narrowing of the disk space and osteophyte formation TREATMENT NSAIDs, intra-articular injections with anesthetics, low back fusion of cases with degeneration

facial sculpturing COSMETIC SURGERY A technique of recent vintage which is used to erase superficial wrinkles* in which the proprietary material Gore-tex is layered below the skin surface (NY Newsday 20 March 1995; B15)

*ie a new wrinkle in wrinkle removal

FAB CLASSIFICATION, ACUTE LEUKEMIAS

ACUTE LYMPHOCYTIC LEUKEMIA (**ALL**)

L1	Small monotonous lymphocytes
L2	Mixed L1- and L3-type lymphocytes
L3	Large homogeneous blast cells

ACUTE MYELOID LEUKEMIA (**AML**)

M1	Myeloblasts without maturation
M2	Myeloblasts with maturation (best AML prognosis)
M3	Hypergranular promyelocytic leukemia (Faggot cells)
M3V	Variant, microgranular promyelocytic leukemia
M4	Myelomonocytic leukocytes
M5	Monocytic, subtype
	a) Poorly differentiated monocytic leukemia
	b) Well-differentiated monocytic leukemia
M6	Erythroleukemia or DiGuglielmo syndrome
M7	Megakaryocytic leukemia Pleomorphic undifferentiated cells with cytoplasmic blebs; myelofibrosis or ↑ marrow reticulin; positive for platelet peroxidase antifactor VIII

---

facilitated communication A form of behavioral therapy that has been reported to be successful in treating some cases of autism; in FC, a helper holds or braces the hands or arms of person with autism, who uses one finger to type words on a keyboard, a task that initially is impossible in autistics; with time the facilitator reduces his control over the autistic person's movement, the expectation being that the autistic will eventually initiate movement and activities spontaneously; despite some enthusiasm for the method, many experts are unconvinced that FC is truly effective, and its reported success may be more related to 'wishful thinking' than with any form of therapeutic breakthrough (New York Times 13 July 1993; C1)

facilitator cell HEMATOLOGY A cell in the bone marrow that improves the 'taking' of grafts between species (New York Times 19 July 1994; C3)

facioscapulohumeral dystrophy Landouzy-Dejerine muscular dystrophy An AD [MIM 158900] limb-girdle dystrophy of childhood onset and variable presentation CLINICAL The dystrophic changes begin in the face with hypomimia and pouting lips, then extend to the shoulder girdle; other disorders with a major 'limb-girdle' component include Emery-Dreifuss dystrophy, endocrine myopathies, congenital myopathies (central core, myotubular and nemaline types), mitochondrial myopathies, polymyositis, progressive muscular atrophy, scapuloperoneal syndrome and 'slow-channel' myasthenia

FACS 1) Fellow, American College of Surgeons 2) Fluorescence-activated cell sorter A device attached to a flow cytometer that allows separation of a relatively pure population of cells by 'tagging' them with a monoclonal antibody raised against a component in the cell of interest;

the monoclonal antibody and therefore the desired cell is stained with a fluorescent dye; the cells are then sent through the flow cytometer, a device that allows only one cell to pass at a time; the stained cells fluoresce and the machine's computer then sends every cell with fluorescence greater than a 'gated' cut-off level of scattered light down chute A, the remaining cells are diverted to chute B which may have defined a second parameter of interest or may be waste; see Flow cytometry

factitious 'diseases' PSYCHIATRY Self-produced lesions or biochemical changes produced by neurotics in order to gratify various self-motivated needs, including sympathy and narcotics; these conditions share the same raison d'etre, differing only in the site of injury and the agent used to produce the lesions; see Munchhausen syndrome, Self-mutilation **FACTITIOUS DERMATOPATHY** A skin condition produced by sharp objects, thermal or chemical agents, the gross and histologic appearance of which reflects the damaging agent **FACTITIOUS DIARRHEA** The spurious increase in fecal production due to either excess use of laxatives, or dilution of the 'product' (N Engl J Med 1994; 330:1418OA); the condition is most common in ♀, and is related to excessive and inappropriate use of laxatives, occurring in 1) Anorectics, who are often ♀ age 18-40 with an altered self image, for whom weight control is a central focus and laxatives are an alternative to vomiting or 2) Older ♀, who are perimenopausal and emphatically deny the abuse; here the motives for laxative abuse are complex and may be related to secondary gain of attention or may be a component of hysteria; side effects of prolonged laxative abuse include chronic diarrhea, colicky abdominal pain, nausea, vomiting, weight loss, weakness, hypokalemia, skin pigmentation, arthralgia, cyclic edema, nephrolithiasis (ammonium urates); see Cathartic colon **FACTITIOUS FEVER** An FUO described in either young ♀ health professionals, which occurs after a legitimate disease or in older neurotic ♀ who are prone to self-mutilation **FACTITIOUS HYPOGLYCEMIA** Surreptitious ingestion of hypoglycemic agents, eg sulfonylureas or insulin; often by ♀ ages 30-40, employed in the health professions who have highly variable levels of glucose DIAGNOSIS Measurement of oral hypoglycemics, insulin antibodies, and C-peptide; the C-fragment of the insulin molecule is present in the serum of normal subjects at a ratio of 5-15:1; it is ↓↓↓ in those who inject insulin **FACTITIOUS KIDNEY DISEASE** Spuriously altered parameters of renal function or kidney-related clinical history (N Engl J Med 1992; 327:388OA) **FACTITIOUS PANNICULITIS** A condition characterized by diffuse indurated subcutaneous nodules, due to auto-injection of mineral and cotton seed oil, liquid silicones (see Sexual reassignment), drugs, eg meperidine, morphine, pentazocine, tetanus toxoid, milk and feces CLINICAL Acute inflammation evolving into end-stage fibrosis, avascular necrosis and when infected, ulceration **FACTITIOUS PURPURA** Devil's pinches Patchy self-inflicted lesions that may be produced by pinching flesh; see Conversion disorders

factor A molecule or substance that is known to exist in a system, but which are poorly characterized when the system is first described; with time, the molecules are characterized and/or sequenced, such that the 'factor' designation falls into disfavor and retains historic interest Noncoagulation factors

factor B Complement C3 proactivator, a protein of the alternate complement pathway

factor D Protein activator of factor B of the alternate pathway of complement activation

factor F Fertility-bearing plasmid; see Factor IF

factor H A complement glycoprotein that inactivates C3b (alternate pathway)

factor I A protein that degrades C3b (alternate pathway)

factor R 1) Antibiotic resistance-bearing plasmid 2) Release factor (any proteins that release a polypeptide chain from the ribosome)

factor S A component produced with serotonin by sleep-deprived experimental models, which induces non-REM or slow-wave sleep, composed of muramyl peptide, a normal component of bacterial walls, possibly serving to explain why bacterially 'naive' newborns don't have slow-wave sleep; Cf S factor

factor T Elongation factor, a protein that participates in the elongation of prokaryote polypeptides

factor V HEMATOLOGY A coagulation factor, which when activated, is a cofactor with activated factor X (factor Xa) in the formation of thrombokinase; see Factor V deficiency MICROBIOLOGY Nicotinamide adenine dinucleotide (NAD) or NADP A requirement for growth of certain bacteria (eg most *Haemophilus* species); NAD is supplied by the co-cultured *Staphylococcus aureus*

factor V HEMATOLOGY The coagulation factor that in the activated form is a cofactor of factor Xa in the formation of prothrombinase (Nature 1994; 369:64oa, 14n&v)

factor V deficiency Parahemophilia A condition characterized by mild bleeding or petechial hemorrhage or menorrhagia that is either congenital, due to the AR [MIM 227400] defect in the gene for factor V or acquired due to the development of IgA or IgG antibodies to factor V LABORATORY Increased partial thromboplastin time and prothrombin time TREATMENT Fresh plasma

factor VIII A coagulation protein encoded by a 186-kb, 26 exon gene located on the X chromosome; factor VIII is a 2351 amino acid protein with a globular core comprising 70% of factor VIII's mass, and has heavy and light chains; it is synthesized as a single chain, but undergoes several cleavage activation steps by thrombin, factor Xa, and others to form the mature heterotrimer (44 kD, 54 kD, and 72 kD) factor VIIIa which has been separated from von Willebrand (N Engl J Med 1994; 330:38rv); recombinant factor VIII (rF VIII) therapy is an effective treatment of hemophilia A (factor VIII deficiency); transient or low levels of factor VIII inhibitors do not appear to interfere with response to treatment (N Engl J Med 1993; 328:453oa)

factor VIII inhibitor An abnormal endogenous component, usually an antibody to factor VIIIc that inhibits coagulation; anti-factor VIIIc antibodies occur in 5-21% of patients with hemophilia A, and are most common in the most severely affected; transient or low levels of FVIs develop in ± 20% of pediatric patients with factor VIII deficiency and do not appear to interfere with response to factor VIII therapy (N Engl J Med 1993; 328:453oa) factor VIII antibodies may arise spontaneously in a menagerie of inflammatory diseases, to wit, rheumatoid arthritis, SLE, and ulcerative colitis, or with ↑ age, in the post-partum period, and in a background of a drug reaction

factor X Hemin MICROBIOLOGY A group of heat-stable tetrapyrrole compounds provided by several iron-containing molecules, eg heme and hematin, which are required for synthesis of catalase, peroxidase and the cytochrome electron transport system; bacteria dependent upon factor X include *Hemophilus influenzae*, *H haemolyticus*, *H aegyptius*, *H ducreyi* cannot synthesize protoporphyrin from delta-aminolevulinic acid, a reaction that aids in speciating *Haemophilus*

Note: *H influenzae*, *H hemolyticus* and *H aegyptius* require both factors V and X; 'the term 'factor X' was once used for vitamin B_{12} and biotin

factor X OPHTHALMOLOGY A hypothetical (the existence of which was posited in 1948) substance that is elaborated in the retina and stimulates neovascularization in DM; factor X appears to be a growth factor, most probably vascular endothelial growth factor (VEGF), possibly with contributions from basic fibroblast growth factor (bFGF), insulin-like growth factor-1 (IGF-1) (N Engl J Med 1994; 331:1519ed)

facultative anaerobe An anaerobe (usually understood to be bacterial) that grows in either completely anaerobic or microaerophilic environments, using oxygen as the terminal electron acceptor, yielding 38 ATP molecules when catabolizing a molecule of glucose, or in a 'pinch', utilizing glucose by the less energy-efficient fermentative metabolic pathway, yielding 2 ATP molecules, eg *Escherichia coli*, *Staphylococcus aureus*

faculty practice plan ACADEMIC MEDICINE An organized group of physicians and other health care professionals that treats patients referred to an academic medical center; FPPs are often units of a medical school (with the notable exceptions of Harvard and Tufts), and may set their own priorities, business plans, and bill the patients separately, resulting in an autonomy of such degree that FPPs may be infelicitously known as fiefdoms (N Eng J Med 1995; 332:407oa)

'fad' diet Any of a number of diets that either eliminate one or more of the essential food groups or recommend consumption of one type of food in enormous excess, often reducing the consumption of other foods; fad diets rarely follow modern dietetic principles of weight loss, which hinge on the combination of 1) Eating less or 2) Consuming more energy through exercise, and are thus rarely endorsed by the medical profession; see Diet

Fagan test of infant intelligence PEDIATRIC NEUROLOGY A test designed to assess visual recognition memory, based on the time that an infant can spend looking at a novel stimulus (Pediatrics 1986; 78:1021)

faggot cells   **faggots**

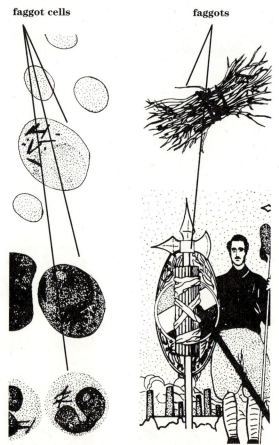

faggot cells HEMATOPATHOLOGY A fanciful term for the leukemic cells of French-American-British class M3 (acute promyelocytic leukemia), characterized by bundles of Auer rods, hence the name

The trans-Atlantic translation has transformed the adjectival 'faggot' into the bulkier, but less confusing, 'bundle of kindling wood' cell; a faggot or fagot is a bundle of sticks, twigs or small branches, to be used as kindling wood, or a bundle of iron or steel rods

failed disk syndrome see Laminectomy

failure to thrive PEDIATRICS The inability of a child to gain weight or one who loses weight without discernible cause, which may be due to: 1) Environmental deprivation, the more common cause of failure to thrive, in which children have poor appetites, are apathetic and withdrawn; this constellation of findings is typical of abused children, offspring of schizophrenics or in children with physical deformities or secondary problems causing the parents to subconsciously reject them or 2) Organic diseases, which include ill-defined cerebral lesions, chromosome defects, chronic infection or inflammation, cystic fibrosis, eclampsia, endocrinopathy, heart disease, idiopathic hypercalcemia, malabsorption, malignancy, renal insufficiency or tubular defects and the TORCH complex; see Child abuse; Cf Infanticide

faith healing An alternative form of health care lying outside of the mainstream of medical practice, in which therapy consists of trusting in a 'higher' or other power(s) without active medical or surgical intervention; Cf Christian science, Psychic surgery

FAK Focal adhesion kinase A tyrosine kinase that localizes to sites of focal adhesion by means of a COOH-terminal FAT (focal adhesion targeting) domain; FAK is activated by β-integrin cross-linking and associates with other tyrosine kinases (Csk, Src), SH2-SH3 signaling molecules (Grb2, Pl-3K), paxillin, and β_1 integrin peptide (Science 1995; 268:233)

'falanga' see Torture

fall PUBLIC HEALTH A precipitous drop from a height or coming down from a higher position, which may be accompanied by injuries; falling is a major problem among the elderly, given 1) The ability to recuperate from fall-related injuries is less than that of younger subjects, and 2) The frequency and the costs ($\pm$ $10 x 10^9) of the morbidity associated therewith; EPIDEMIOLOGY 30% of those > 65 years old fall/year, and sustain injuries therefrom; it is the 6th leading cause of death in this age group; 10-15% result in injuries including fractures of the hip (1%) and other sites (5%), and soft tissue injuries (5%) RISK FACTORS Postural hypotension, use of sedatives, use of 4+ prescription medicines, and impairment of arm or leg movement, strength, balance, or gait; intervention in the form of exercise programs, behavior modification, and adjustment of medications may reduce the risk of falling in the elderly (N Engl J Med 1994; 331:821oA); fall survivors suffer from functional decline in the activities of daily living and have a high risk of subsequent institutionalization; the risk of falls can be ↓ with exercise and endurance, flexibility, dynamic balance, and resistance training (JAMA 1995; 273:1341oc)

fallen arch A popular term for a flattening of the longitudinal and transverse tendinous arches of the foot

'falling leaf' motility Darting motility, see there

falling-out PSYCHIATRY A culture-bound episode described in the southern US, and regionally in the Caribbean characterized by sudden and often unexpected collapse, which may be preceded by feelings of dizziness; it is thought to be a type of conversion reaction; see Culture-bound syndrome

fallout Radiation that settles out of the atmosphere following a nuclear explosion, see Nuclear war; more colloquially, 'fallout' refers to the broad consequences of an error or action

FALS Forward angle light scatter, see there

false aneurysm A blood-filled pseudo-vascular space that parallels the native vessel lumen and which may carry blood if there is a site of exit and re-entry; the 'vessel' wall is formed by reactive connective tissue; false aneurysms are secondary to trauma, transmural rupture of the vessel wall or dehiscence of vessels

false imprisonment MEDICAL MALPRACTICE An intentional tort which consists of a violation of the personal interest in the freedom from restraint of movement; the physician (often a psychiatrist) who places a patient in physical restraints or uses pharmacologic restraints to the point of immobility without a viable medical reason may be accused of FI; see Pharmacologic restraint, Physical restraint

false memory PSYCHOLOGY A set of suggestions and cues that cause a person to believe an event occurred which in fact did not; the mechanism by which this occurs is known as source amnesia (New York Times May3, 1994; C1) see Repressed memory, Source amnesia

Falstaff snore A loud snore heard in the sleeping obese, named after the portly Falstaff, a minor character in Henry IV, part I, Act II, who was a '...fat-kidneyed rascal...fast asleep and snorting like a horse'; the snore may occur in the sleep apnea syndrome (Br Med J 1987; 294:371c)

FAM 5-Fluorouracil, adriamycin (doxorubicin), mitomycin C ONCOLOGY A chemotherapeutic regimen used with varying degrees of failure to treat advanced gastric carcinoma

familial adenomatous polyposis An AD [MIM 175100] condition affecting $\pm$ 50 000 (US) characterized by the progressive development of hundreds of adenomatous colorectal polyps, some of which progress irrevocably to cancer MOLECULAR PATHOLOGY The APC gene located on chromosome segment 5q21 is mutated in FAP and may also be mutated in sporadic colorectal tumorigenesis DIAGNOSIS Use of both allele-specific expression assay (see there), and in vitro synthesized protein assay (see there) successfully identifies 87% of cases (N Engl J Med 1993; 329:1982oA) TREATMENT Sulindac, an NSAID is reported to ↓ the number and size of colorectal adenomas in FAP, an effect that is incomplete and thus unlikely to replace colectomy as a primary therapy (N Engl J Med 1993; 328:1313oA)

familial combined hyperlipidemia A common (1:300) AD [MIM 144250] disorder in which there is ↑ triglyceride and/or cholesterol-the common denominator is ↑ hepatic synthesis of apoB, ↑ LDL and/or VLDL, and a mild ↓ in HDL-cholesterol and apoA1 CLINICAL Early coronary atherosclerosis with a first MI occurring as early as age 40; the patients are often overweight and hypertensive; smoking is forbidden as it exacerbates the arteriosclerosis

familial dysautonomia Riley-Day syndrome An AR [MIM 223900] condition most common among Jews, affecting neurons of the peripheral sensorimotor autonomic and CNS CLINICAL Failure to thrive, episodic vomiting, upper respiratory tract infection, autonomic dysfunction (skin blotching, lacrimation, defective temperature control, diaphoresis, hypertension and postural hypotension) and early demise

familial dysbetalipoproteinemia Broad beta lipoproteinemia A rare (1:10 000) AD [MIM 107741] condition with a defective apoE (the apoE$_{2/2}$ phenotype), poor 'remnant' catabolism, and overproduction of triglyceride-rich lipoproteins, eg VLDL CLINICAL Palmoplantar tuberoeruptive xanthomas, atherosclerosis < age 50, peripheral vascular and coronary artery disease; other conditions may be associated with FD, eg hyperthyroidism LABORATORY ↑ Triglyceride, ↑ cholesterol, presence of floating beta lipoproteins TREATMENT Diet, exercise, drugs, eg bile acid-binding resins, and nicotinic acid, and in post-menopausal women, low-dose estrogens

familial dyslipemic hypertension Williams-Hunt-Hopkins syndrome A complex that affects two or more siblings in a family, which may comprise up to 12% of hypertensives, and 25% of hypertensives diagnosed before age 60 LABORATORY HDL-cholesterol is < 10th percentile, LDL-cholesterol and triglyceride levels are > 90th percentile

familial erythrocytosis A heterogeneous group of rare congenital conditions characterized by an increase in red cell mass and low serum erythropoietin MOLECULAR GENETICS In one AD kindred of FE, a nonsense mutation in the erythropoietin receptor gene (which maps to chromosome segment 19p) results in production of a truncated erythropoietin receptor lacking 70 C-terminal amino acids containing a negative regulatory domain (**N Engl J Med 1994; 330:839RV**) see Hematopoietic growth factor receptor

familial focal facial dermal dysplasia An AD [MIM 136500] condition characterized by lesions devoid of hair with fingerprint-like puckering of the skin, especially at the temples, due to alternating bands of dermal and epidermal atrophy, one family described was cancer-prone and had gastric and familial polyposis (**Birth Defects 1971; 7:96**)

familial hypercholesterolemia A common (1:500) congenital AD [MIM 144400] defect in the LDL receptor gene, resulting in dysfunctional or absent receptor CLINICAL Early coronary atherosclerosis in ♂ and first MI by age 40 (♀ may remain asymptomatic throughout life), tendinous xanthomas, corneal arcus and xanthelasma LABORATORY Elevated LDL-cholesterol, circa 300-500 mg/dl (20% of cholesterol in this range is due to familial hypercholesterolemia) TREATMENT Smoking cessation, diet, exercise, drugs (bile-acid binding resins, eg cholestipol, cholestyramine and nicotinic acid, a low cholesterol and low saturated fat diet, liver transplant may provide LDL receptors; acquired hypercholesterolemia may be transient, due to dietary excess or related to acute intermittent porphyria and anorexia nervosa; congenital hypercholesterolemia is relatively common, often AR and polygenic, different alleles being affected in each cohort; in a French-Canadian cohort, a 10-kilobase deletion in the LDL receptor gene causes the loss of the promoter and the first exon, abolishing production of the LDL-receptor mRNA (**JAMA 1991; 265:780A**); see Cholesterol-lowering drugs

familial hypertriglyceridemia A common (1:200) AD [MIM 145750] disorder, due to ↑ in hepatic triglyceride, cholesterol and cholic acid synthesis, with ↑ VLDL and transportation of triglycerides by HDL CLINICAL ↑ Trglycerides in obesity, alcohol consumption, drug therapy (β-adrenergics, diuretics, estrogens and steroid therapy) TREATMENT Diet, exercise, drugs, eg clofibrate, gemfibrozil

familial hypertrophic cardiomyopathy A relatively uncommon (± 3/10 000) AD [MIM 160760] disease that is one of the most common forms of obstructive cardiomyopathy MOLECULAR PATHOLOGY 30% of FHC (and some cases of sporadic hypertrophic cardiomyopathy) are caused by missense mutations in the β-cardiac myosin heavy chain on chromosome 14; 15% of FHCs are due to mutations in troponin T, on chromosome 1; 3% are due to mutations in α-tropomyosin on chromosome 15 (**N Engl J Med 1995; 332:1058OA**); other point mutations occur on exons 13, 14, 16, and 23 in the β-myosin heavy chain, α/β-myosin heavy-chain hybrid gene CLINICAL Angina, arrhythmia, dyspnea, syncope, and possibly, sudden death in adolescents or young adults DIAGNOSIS EKG reveals asymmetric hypertrophy of the septum (usually of the left side), systolic anterior movement of the mitral valve, and midsystolic closure of the aortic valve

familial hypoparathyroidism A heterogeneous group of relatively uncommon conditions that can be X-linked [MIM 307700] or AD [MIM 146200]* and accompanied by other congenital abnormalities, including absence of thymus; some kindreds have distinct profiles, eg AD pattern of inheritance, sensorineural deafness, and renal dysplasia (**N Engl J Med 1992; 327:1069OA**)

*The 'autosomal recessive' cases [MIM 241400] reported in the literature may have been misinterpretations of autosomal dominant kindreds

familial hyperphosphatasemia A rare AR [MIM 239000] form of early-onset osteopetrosis* with multiple fractures, enlarged head, broadened diaphyses, bowed legs, ↓ height, ↑ alkaline phosphatase, histologically divided into Bakwin-Eiger syndrome and juvenile Paget's disease, a distinction of uncertain clinical utility; hyperphosphatasemia may also be seen with an ↑ in the intestinal isoenzyme of alkaline phosphatase, which causes no clinical disease unless the altered enzyme levels evoke an aggressive work-up for bone or liver disease, malignancy, pregnancy, resulting in a 'Ulysses syndrome', see there

Synonyms include Bakwin-Eiger syndrome, benign familial hyperphosphatasemia, chronic congenital idiopathic hyperphosphatasemia, chronic idiopathic hyperphosphatasemia, familial osteoectasia (with macrocranium), hyperostosis corticalis deformans juvenilis, juvenile osteitis deformans (Paget's disease), juvenile Paget's disease, osteochalasia desmalis familiaris

familial juvenile nephronophthisis An AR [MIM 256100] form of chronic interstitial nephritis condition which may accompanied by retinal dysplasia, hepatic fibrosis, and skeletal abnormalities CLINICAL Urinary concentration defect with polyuria and polydipsia, possibly due to a primary tubular defect, and often sodium wasting, persistent hypokalemia, and metabolic acidosis, possibly accompanied by growth retardation (**N Engl J Med 1994; 330:1072CPC**)

familial malignancy The development of a malignancy in two or more blood-related members of a cohort, eg hepatocellular carcinoma (**Cancer 1968; 22:142**)

familial Mediterranean fever Familial paroxysmal polyserositis An AR [MIM 249100] disease affecting eastern Mediterranean rim Jews, both Armenian and Sephardic (the latter comprise ½ of cases), as well as Arabs, Greeks, Turks, and other 'rim' inhabitants, causing episodic serosal (especially peritoneal) inflammation, more common in ♂ MOLECULAR PATHOLOGY The gene causing FMF in non-Ashkenazi Jews is located on chromosome segment 16p, specifically on the subtelomeric region of the short arm, in the centromeric direction of the marker D16S84 (**N Engl J Med 1992; 326:1509OA**) PATHOGENESIS Unclear, possibly due to a deficiency of an inflammatory inhibitor (of neutrophil chemotaxis by complement C5a) with abnormalities of suppressor T cells or defective arachidonic acid metabolism CLINICAL Onset by adolescence as recurring peritonitis, arthritis, pleuritis, diffuse abdominal pain due to serositis, episodic fever, sometimes complicated by amyloidosis, muscle 'guarding', leukocytosis and malabsorption that resolve within 24 hours; long-term prognosis is good in absence of renal amyloidosis which causes terminal nephropathy, an event preventable by colchicine therapy

familial multiple hamartoma syndrome Multiple hamartoma syndrome, see there

family cancer syndromes see Familial malignancy, Fetal overgrowth syndrome of Beckwith Wiedeman

family 'ganging' A form of health care provision that may be practiced by some physicians in less financially advantaged regions in the US, eg inner cities, in which a patient is encouraged to bring his entire family along for a check-up or other evaluation at the time of his return visit, regardless of whether it is indicated; 'ganging' is most commonly practiced when providing services to Medicaid patients, for whom the level of reimbursement to the physician is very low; see Medicaid

family history A summary of diseases that have occurred in close blood relatives; the FH is a datum of increasing importance as a broadening spectrum of evil humors, eg cardiovascular disease, DM, malignancy, and others are known to be linked to heritable DNA mutations (**N Engl J**

Med 1994; 331:1669oa) Cf Social history

family therapy Family psychotherapy A generic term for the treatment of a dysfunctional family as a unit in which the individual dynamics and relationships within the family are dissected and evaluated as to their ability to impact on the unit, eventually forming the basis for therapy

farcy An accidental infection of humans, linked to contact with domestic animals, especially horses, infected by *Pseudomonas mallei*, a strict aerobic gram-negative bacillus, a condition known as glanders CLINICAL Epithelioid granulomas in the skin and lymphatics ('farcy buds') with induration of the connective tissue of the head and neck; see Glanders

farmer's lung Farm worker's lung An IgG1-mediated form of extrinsic allergic alveolitis or hypersensitivity pneumonitis that occurs in non-atopic individuals, who after repeated exposure to organic dust and fungi, eg *Aspergillus* species, become allergic to thermophilic actinomycotic organisms; 90% of patients have antibodies to moldy hay, an ideal growth medium for the fungi implicated (*Microspora vulgaris*, *Thermoactinomyces vulgaris* and *Micropolyspora faeni*) PATHOGENESIS Unknown, possibly due to an immune complex deposition in the lungs causing a type III hypersensitivity reaction CLINICAL Attacks of several days duration between May and October (the growing season in the Northern Hemisphere), causing rales, cyanosis, fever, dry cough, rhonchi and dyspnea, beginning 4-8 hours after exposure to stored corn, barley and tobacco; with time, weight loss PULMONARY FUNCTION TESTS Reduced volumes and impaired gas exchange RADIOLOGY Normal or diffuse interstitial reticular pattern, occasionally with fine nodular shadows PATHOLOGY Chronic inflammation, peribronchiolar granulomatous response and foreign-body-type giant cell reaction, eventually fibrosis TREATMENT Corticosteroids COMPLICATIONS Pulmonary hypertension, right ventricular hypertrophy and failure; Cf 'Animal House fever, Silo filler's lung

Faroe Islands A small archipelago between Norway and Iceland (capital Torshavn, population 46 000, major industry, fishing), with an isolated population that is of medical interest as 1) The first cases of multiple sclerosis coincided with the landing of British troops in 1943, lending support to a slow viral etiology (Ann Neurol 1979; 5:6) and 2) The population had been devastated in 1846 when measles killed ¼ of the population of 8000

Farr's law of epidemics William Farr, an English statistician, who analyzed the mortality of a waning smallpox epidemic (1838-39) and demonstrated mathematically that the fall in mortality of an epidemic occurs at a uniformly accelerated rate; when applied to the current AIDS epidemic, some data suggested that the rate of increase in new cases may be slowing (at least in some developed nations) and a 'crest' in the incidence of AIDS would arrive by 1993–it did not

FARS Fatal accident reporting system

Fas MOLECULAR BIOLOGY A type-I membrane receptor that binds FasL (Fas ligand) a member of the TNF family; Fas-FasL interaction induces apoptosis, and is involved in down-regulation of immune reactions and T cell-mediated cytotoxicity; Fas-FasL system defects result in lymphoproliferative disorders and autoimmune responses; Fas hyperactivity results in tissue destruction (Science 1995; 267:1449oa); the Fas/APO-1 signal transduction receptor for apoptosis is activated by ICE (IL-1β-converting enzyme), an interaction that is critical for Fas/APO-1-mediated cell death (Nature 1995; 375:78, 81L)

fasciculin II A glycoprotein expressed on axonal subsets in the grasshopper that mediates selective fasciculation (a form of neuronal recognition), belongs to the immunoglobulin superfamily, is homologous in structure and function to N-CAM (neuronal cell adhesion molecule), myelin-associated glycoprotein and other cell adhesion molecules

fasciclin III A transmembrane glycoprotein with three extracellular immunoglobulin domains tht functions as a homophilic cell adhesion molecule in vitro; F-III is thought to act as a synaptic target recognition molecule for motor neuron RP3 (Nature 1995; 374:135)

FASEB Federation of American Societies for Experimental Medicine

fast CT imaging A technique using the same computed tomographic principle delineated by EMI in 1972; fast CT scanners are of greatest use in cardiac imaging, as the scan requires less than a fraction of a second, allowing the scanning of multiple slices, which can be repeated at frequent intervals for a specified period; fast CT provides information about cardiac anatomy, pulmonary and coronary arteries, myocardial perfusion and microcirculation; see Spiral CT

fast food Prepared food from a restaurant that specializes in providing a full 'meal', often consisting of a form of hamburger or permutation of chicken, French fries and a soft drink or a milk shake, in less than two minutes; an estimated ⅕ of the US population of 240 million purchases at least one 'fast-food' meal daily; a diet consisting solely of fast food overloads the body with protein, fat and calories and is low in vitamins, mineral and fibers (Consumer Reports 1988; 54:355); Cf 'Junk food'

'fast' hemoglobins A hemoglobin (Hb) with an electrophoretic mobility greater or faster than HbA on a pH 8.6 gel, including HbBart, HbI, HbH, HbA_{1a}, HbA_{1b} and HbA_{1c}, based on their order of elution from a column containing cation-exchange resin; see Glycosylated hemoglobin

'fast track' paper SCIENTIFIC JOURNALISM A publication in the sciences that is of such 'newsworthiness' that the journal, eg Cell, Nature, Science may choose to either bypass or accelerate the usual review and typesetting processes so that it will appear as little as two weeks after the manuscript's submission; the advantage to the journal is that it maintains a reputation for quality reporting, as the papers may have Nobel prize-winning potential; the disadvantage is that some 'hot' papers, eg 'cold fusion' (J Elect Chem, 1989), may ultimately prove to be inaccurate, causing the journal to lose credibility (Science 1991; 251:260n&v); Cf Citation impact, 'Hot paper'

fast twitch fibers White fibers, see there

fast-twitch muscle White fibers, see there

fastidious organism MICROBIOLOGY A term that is theoretically applicable to any living organism, as each has specific growth requirements, and therefore is 'fastidious'; in the clinical laboratory, although it is a fact that parasites and viruses have highly specific (and therefore, fastidious) growth requirements, 'fastidious' has come to be applied to bacteria that grow poorly or not at all on the usual growth media, under the usual conditions; such organisms may 1) Grow optimally at room temperature (25°C) or at 4°C 2) Grow very slowly, ie over the space of several weeks, whereas culture plates are generally discarded as 'no-growths' after one week of incubation 3) Require a microaerophilic or strictly anaerobic atmosphere 4) Require special growth media or 5) Require a combination of the above

fasting specimen LABORATORY MEDICINE A blood specimen that is drawn from a patient who has not eaten for 12 hours; fasting is an absolute requirement for a limited number of tests, eg glucose tolerance test; prolonged fasting causes a marked (240%) ↑↑↑ in bilirubin, ↑↑ plasma triglycerides, glycerol, and free fatty acids, without affecting cholesterol levels, and a marked (± 50%) ↓ in glucose

fat A generic term for any of a class of neutral organic compounds formed by a molecule of glycerol linked to three fatty acids (a glycerol ester); fats are water-insoluble, ether soluble, solid at ≤ 20°C, combustible, energy-rich (9.3 kcal/g); see Fatty acids, Fish oil, Olive oil, Tropical oil *adjective* **fatty**

fat consumption The amount of fats in any form consumed in the diet, the amount and type of which correlates directly with the incidence of coronary artery disease (CAD); fats comprise 34% of the US diet (down from 42% in the mid 1960s); saturated fats comprise 12% (16% in mid-1960s); cholesterol levels average 205 mg/dL (213 mg/dL in 1978); the reduction of fats in the diet are credited with the 40% ↓ in CAD-related mortality (US) since 1968 (New York Times 8 March 1994; C6)

fat distribution There are two patterns of distribution of corporal adipose tissue, as measured by the ratio of the corporal diameter at the hips and waist, waist:hip ratio, normal: 0.7-0.8; these patterns differ significantly in co-morbidity of obesity

GYNECOID PATTERN Female pattern, fat is deposited in the lower body (abdomen, buttocks, hips, thighs) by mesenchymal differentiation or hyperplasia

ANDROID PATTERN Male pattern, fat is deposited in the upper body, especially around the abdomen; (gut fat) adipocytes are more sensitive to insulin and catecholamines and fat accumulates by hypertrophy, possibly a function of membrane receptor density; the android pattern has greater lipolytic and lipogenic potential, and thus carries a greater risk for hypertension, cardiovascular disease, DM, and hyperinsulinemia; see Obesity; Cf Morbid obesity

FAT domain Focal adhesion targeting domain

fat embolism Emboli composed of fat are common, relatively innocuous and may occur in alcoholism, bone marrow biopsy, cardiopulmonary bypass, compression injury, diabetes, lymphangiography, pancreatitis, sickle cell anemia and steroid therapy; contrarily, the fat embolism 'syndrome' is neither a common nor a trivial condition; clinically significant fat emboli may be endogenous or exogenous and most are due to major fractures and trauma to parenchymal organs (most deaths in the immediate posttrauma period have significant fat embolism), burns, blast injury, severe infections, especially α-toxin-producing *Clostridium* species PATHOGENESIS Coalesced fat globules of up to 20 μm in diameter may circulate in the 'embolic' phase, possibly causing sudden death on entering the pulmonary microcirculation (the lung is the only site of embolism in most patients); the subsequent or 'ameboid' phase is characterized by emboli in the cardiac, cerebral, renal and other arteries, causing hypoperfusion due to mechanical obstruction by fat globules, platelets, erythrocytes and early non-specific immune mediators, eg serotonin and kinins; in the final or enzymatic phase, lipase enters the circulation, catabolizing the neutral fats into highly toxic free fatty acids, evoking inflammation, hemorrhage and chemical pneumonitis due to lipolysis and disruption of the surfactant CLINICAL Hypoxia (50% of femoral shaft fractures have reduced arterial PO$_2$ within the first few days), acute onset of dyspnea, tachypnea, cyanosis, tachycardia with sudden onset of right-sided cardiac failure, showers of petechiae, thrombocytopenia, cerebral embolism (with changes in personality, confusion, drowsiness, weakness, agitation, spasticity, defects of the visual field and rarely, extreme pyrexia) DIAGNOSIS It had been reported that fat droplets in a bronchoalveolar lavage was indicative of fat embolism, a finding that in one small (34) group of patients proved to have a low speci-

ficity of 26.5% (Am Surg 1994; 60:537) TREATMENT No therapy is consistently effective

fat/fiber hypothesis The posit that some aspects of a diet high in meat, fat, protein, and energy, and low in fiber are pivotal in the pathogenesis of colorectal carcinoma (JAMA 1992; 268:1573sc)

'fat-mobilizing hormone' A fanciful term for a non-existent 'factor', the production of which was claimed to be induced by the Atkin's diet; see Diets; Cf Starch blocker

fat necrosis Liquefactive necrosis that is initiated by trauma and effected by lipolytic enzymes; FN is relatively common in 1) The breast, where it is often well-circumscribed and by light microscopy demonstrates large epithelioid and bizarre cells, causing both clinical and (occasionally) histologic confusion with carcinoma and 2) Pancreas, where blockage of the ducts by concrements facilitates the breakdown of normal barriers, causing focal leakage of lipases and subsequent calcium 'soap' formation; see Soap

fat sickle cells A descriptor for plump variant drepanocytes, which are typical of hemoglobin SC that may be associated with target cells and 'Washington monument' crystals

'fat spurt' PEDIATRICS A temporary relative increase in subcutaneous adipose tissue occurring in preadolescence

fate map EMBRYOLOGY A schematic diagram that indicates the prospective fate of a particular region of a blastula or gastula

father 'factor' PSYCHOLOGY A colloquial term* for the ill-defined constellation of components that a father figure contributes to a person's personality development and psychologic maturation; in single-parent households headed by a mother, the FF may be provided by stepfathers, older brothers, uncles, grandfathers, male teachers; some soft data suggest that fatherless children are less likely to achieve their full potential and take on responsibility, and are more likely to succumb to peer pressures (NY Newsday 3 Jan 1995; B13) see Two-parent advantage

*From the book by the same title *Father Factor*, by H Biller, Pocket Books, 1994

fatigue fracture A stress fracture affecting the feet of formerly fit foot soldiers, caused by repeated, relatively 'trivial' trauma to normal bone, resulting in local bone resorption; among civilians, stress fractures are either occupational or afflict the so-called 'week-end warrior', who strenuously exercises an often untrained or sedentary skeleto-muscular system

fatigue syndrome see Chronic fatigue syndrome; Cf Compassion fatigue syndrome

fatty acids, diet The relative importance of saturation of the bonds in fatty acids remains unclear, although saturated animal-derived and 'tropical' oils are thought to have the greatest atherogenic potential, while the literature suggests that those high in monounsaturated fats, in particular olive oil have the least atherogenic potential

Note: The table from the US Department of Agriculture is provided to place these studies in context

fatty change The accumulation of droplets of neutral fat in various parenchymal organs, classically, the liver and most common in alcoholics; FCs may also be seen in other parenchyma organs, eg heart and kidney; with abstention, the fatty changes regress

fatty degeneration Accumulation of fat globules due to deterioration of lipid storage and metabolic pathways of intracellular origin; Cf Fatty infiltration

'fatty food attack' A colloquial term for severe transient colicky abdominal pain that occurs in response to ingestion of fried or fat-laden foods, which is considered a common clinical sign of cholelithiasis

fatty infiltration Intracellular accumulation of fat that is of extracellular origin; Cf Fatty degeneration

fatty liver A lipid-laden liver due to the accumulation of triglycerides of both intra- and extrahepatic origin; fatty change is the single most common biopsy finding in alcoholics and may be divided according to the size of the fat droplets LARGE FAT DROPLET FATTY LIVER The nucleus is displaced to the side and the cytoplasm is replete with large fat vacuoles, appearing in chronic alcoholics (see Alcoholic fatty liver), choline deficiency, obesity, steatosis, protein-calorie malnutrition (kwashiorkor, jejuno-ileal bypass), DM, and steroid therapy SMALL FAT DROPLET FATTY LIVER The nucleus is central and surrounded by mutiple bubbly vacuoles filled with globules of fat that may be seen in alcoholics as well, and occurs in acute fatty liver of pregnancy, eclampsia/pre-eclampsia, Reye syndrome, Jamaican vomiting sickness, IV tetracycline therapy, toxic shock syndrome and valproic acid therapy

fatty liver of pregnancy Acute fatty liver of pregnancy A rare (1:10-15 000) idiopathic complication of pregnancy, most often affecting primiparas with male infants or twin gestation, occasionally associated with pre-eclampsia CLINICAL Onset after 35th week, possibly progressing to fulminant hepatic failure with jaundice, encephalopathy, DIC, and death PROGNOSIS When this condition was first recognized in the 1970s, the reported mortality was 85%; more recently, fetal mortality is reported to be 23%, maternal, 18%, possibly representing recognition of earlier or milder cases PATHOGENESIS Estrogens are implicated and may act by altering the membrane fluidity PATHOLOGY Fine droplet fat deposition in hepatocytes, cholestasis TREATMENT Terminate pregnancy; the condition may respond to S-adenosyl-L-methionine

fatty metamorphosis of viscera White liver disease An AR [MIM 228100], rapidly fatal condition characterized by massive hepatic (and corporal) steatosis, progressive hypotonicity, lethargy, coagulopathy and jaundice LABORATORY ↑ triglycerides, chylomicrons, HDL-cholesterol, hypoglycemia, hypocalcemia

fatty streak A defect confined to the vascular lumen that is the earliest lesion of atherosclerosis, which has no respect for age, race, sex or social status, and occurs as early as one year of age PATHOLOGY Intimal lipid and foam cell (fat-laden histiocytes filled with cholesteryl esters) accumulation at the ostia of branches of the aorta and aortic valve rings; in advanced lesions, smooth muscle appears in the streak, later giving rise to fibrous plaques; fatty streaks are most prominent and extensive in those exposed to a westernized diet

DIETARY FATS (% SATURATION)

	A	B	C
Safflower Oil	9%	13%	72%
Sunflower Oil	11%	20%	69%
Corn Oil	13%	25%	62%
Olive Oil	14%	77%	9%
Soybean Oil	15%	24%	61%
Peanut Oil	18%	48%	34%
Cottonseed Oil	27%	19%	54%
Lard	41%	47%	12%
Palm Oil	51%	39%	10%
Beef Tallow	52%	44%	4%
Butterfat	66%	30%	4%
Palm-kernel Oil	86%	12%	2%
Coconut Oil	92%	6%	2%

A % Saturated fatty acids   B % Monounsaturated fatty acids
C % Polyunsaturated fatty acids

Faust complex The obsessive desire for knowledge to the exclusion of virtually all else; Cf Physician invincibility syndrome

The legend of Faustus was first related in a play by Marlowe in 1592 and has been retold in various forms by Goethe, Thomas Mann, and others; the essential feature is that of a scholar who sinfully trades his soul for knowledge and power; academic physicians often subconsciously feel they will be granted the power, knowledge (and health) and, like the later versions of the Faustus theme, their sins will ultimately be forgiven (JAMA 1966; 196:156)

favism A condition characterized by episodic hemolysis affecting subjects with glucose-6-phosphate dehydrogenase deficiency, type Gd/Med that occurs after ingesting fava beans (Italian broad beans), which are high in oxidating pyrimidine derivatives, divicine and isouramil, which are capable of destroying erythrocyte glutathione, an antioxidant

favus A disfiguring scalp dermatophytosis caused by *Trichophyton violaceum* and *Microsporum gypseum* resulting in destruction of hair follicles and alopecia

FBN1 A gene located on chromosome 15 that encodes fibrillin, an extracellular matrix glycoprotein; *FBN1* is both mutated in and responsible for Marfan syndrome, which has a wide range of clinical expression that varies according to the family, and each appears to have a unique mutation, which can be identified from a panel of intragenic microsatellite polymorphisms or genetic markers that allow determination of kindred- or family-specific haplotypes–combinations of polymorphic variants that are inherited as a unit and define single copies of *FBN1* (N Engl J Med 1994; 331:148OA) see Fibrillin, Marfan syndrome

FBI sign Fat-blood interface ORTHOPEDICS A semi-lunar soft tissue effusion, seen radiologically with a 'horizontal' beam in post-traumatic lipohemarthrosis; the FBI sign is most commonly seen in the knee and in the shoulder (because of increased marrow fat and blood in the joint space)

F body A fluorescent structure corresponding to the distal Y chromosome, seen in male interphase cells and spermatozoa when stained with quinacrine mustard dihydrochloride

FBS Fasting blood sugar levels Normal values in an adult: 3.9-5.8 mmol/L (US: 70-105 mg/dl); diabetes mellitus > 7.8 mmol/L (US: > 140 mg/dl)

F cell An erythrocyte in adults that contains (persistent) hemoglobin F, which is of no pathological significance, Cf Fetal erythrocyte

F⁺ cell A 'male' bacterium that donates an F plasmid to the F⁻ or 'female' bacterium and has the pilus to enact the exchange

Fc Fragment, crystallizable The portion of an Ig heavy chain's constant region remaining after papain digestion; prolonged papain digestion of Fc results in the smaller Fc' fragment; incubation with pepsin results in low molecular weight peptides and the pFc' fragment, which has a region for the Fc receptor on macrophages and monocytes

Fc receptor A cation permease receptor that is activated by binding of the immunoglobulin Fc fragment; binding of the Fc fragment is followed by an influx of Na+ or K+ which activates macrophage functions including phagocytosis, cell movement and generation of H_2O_2

FcγRIII IgG Fc receptor type III CD16, see there

FDA United States Food and Drug Administration

Also 1) Federal Drug Administration 2) Ferrocenedicarboxylinic acid 3) Fluorescein diacetate 4) Fronto-dextra anterior (obstetrics)

FDA Food and Drug Administration An agency of the US government established by the Federal Food, Drug and Cosmetic Act in 1938, that is encharged with determining the safety (and efficacy) of drugs and therapeutic devices before marketing and assuring that certain labeling specifications and advertising standards be met while marketing the product; see Investigational new drug

Note: The Durham-Humphrey Amendment of 1952 increased governmental control of drugs by restricting the number of allowable refills for prescriptions; the Kefauver-Harris Amendment of 1962, following in the wake of the thalidomide disaster, added that a product must be proven both effective and safe, requiring a series of clinical testing phase prior to marketing (Nature 1994;

369:27BR)

FDA classification of devices A system of stratifying devices used for various health care needs based on the potential for causing morbidity **CLASS I** Devices used by and easily accessible to the public that are regarded as having minimal potential for incorrect use when used in the context of health care **CLASS II** Must undergo an approval process that includes special controls, eg performance standards and general controls required of all devices **CLASS III** In addition to the above, the device or product must meet a rigorous premarketing approval standard, which may delay the release of the product by months or years (CAP Today July 1993)

FDA therapeutic drug rating Therapeutic rating, see there

FD&C yellow No. 5 Tartrazine A ubiquitous colorant used in foods and drugs that cross-reacts with aspirin, exacerbates asthma and may cause a life-threatening anaphylactic reaction

Note: In the US, the approved colorants are designated by numbers under the Food, Drug and Cosmetic Act, abbreviated as FD&C

FD&C Yellow No. 5

FD&C Yellow No. 6 CI 15985 Sunset Yellow FCF A food dye that has been used in candies and carbonated beverages, that in animals has been linked to adrenal and renal tumors, chromosomal damage, and in humans to allergic reactions

Fd fragment That portion of an IgG molecule that remains after papain digestion, consisting of two separate fragments of heavy chain joined to an intact light chain

Fd' fragment That portion of an IgG molecule that remains after pepsin digestion, consisting of two separate fragments of heavy chain joined to an intact light chain

FDP Fibrin degradation products, see there

Also 1) Financially disadvantaged person 2) Fixed dose procedure (toxicology) 3) *Flexor digitorum profundus* [NAG] 4) Food distribution program 5) Fronto-dextra posterior (obsolete, obstetrics) 6) Fructose diphosphate (biochemistry)

fear conditioning A conditioned response induced by linking an intense noxious stimulus to another unrelated stimulus, eg auditory stimulus; fear conditioning can be evoked at all phylogenetic levels at which it has been studied, from fruit flies to vertebrates, including mammals, primates and humans; fear conditioning has been used as a starting point in the study of emotion-related memory (Sci Am 1994; 270/6:50)

feather pattern Christmas tree pattern MOLECULAR BIOLOGY A descriptor for the ultrastructural pattern seen by the technique of rotary shadowing after gene activation by DNA polymerase, when multiple pre-rRNAs simultaneously initiate transcription on a single DNA molecule, where each of the feather's 'branches' corresponds to lengths of nascent rRNA, the chains of which are progressively shorter towards the initiation site

feathery degeneration HEPATIC PATHOLOGY A descriptor for the hepatocytic changes due to chronic cholestasis secondary to extrahepatic biliary destruction; the 'feathers' may represent phospholipids and bile acid crystals, which may be accompanied by an intracellular triad consisting of hydropic swelling, aggregation and reticulation of bile pigment and feathery cytoplasm, possibly related to the toxic effect of bile salts

feather-stitched pattern A descriptive term for the closely packed arrangement of connective tissue and stromal cells arranged in 'stitched' lines, characteristic of ovarian fibromas, often accompanied by hyaline bands (as seen in the related ovarian thecoma) and edema, seen by low-power light microscopy; Cf Herringbone

febrile lumbago Dull, ill-defined lower dorsal and lumbar pain occurring in spinal osteomyelitis, accompanied by low-grade fever and hematogenous 'seeding' of bacteria

febrile seizure A convulsion triggered by fever–the most common type of seizure (prevalence, 3-4%); febrile seizures occur in 2-4% of children, and recur in 33% of cases, and in 50% of cases if the first event occurs before one year of age, and may be associated with subsequent development of a febrile seizures, making the prevention of recurrences desirable; although phenobarbital had been the agent of choice, it may be no better than a placebo and has side effects including behavioral changes and decline in IQ; diazepam is now recommended (N Engl J Med 1993; 329:79OA) it '...*has been well established that that simple febrile seizures cause no neurologic morbidity in children. Such seizures have no effect on intelligence later in life...*' (N Engl J Med 1994; 331:1308C)

febrile torticollis A neck spasm accompanied by dull, ill-defined pain, low-grade fever and bacteremia seen in osteomyelitis of the cervical spine

FEBS Federation of European Biochemical Societies

fecal occult blood testing see Occult blood testing

Federal Register An official daily publication produced by the US federal government that serves to notify the public of any changes of federal regulations, rulings, legal notices, proclamations and documents generated by the executive branch of the government; the range of material published in the Federal Register includes activities regarding safety of products, occupational health, standards of foods and drugs; proposed changes in policies or rules published in the Register are accompanied by an invitation to citizens or others to participate in the decision-making process by submitting data or arguments regarding the proposal

Federal Rules of Evidence Rules that govern the admissibility of evidence at trials in the US Federal District Courts and before US magistrates; these rules provide that unless there is a specific exception, all relevant information is admissible (N Engl J Med 1994; 330:1018LIM); the Federal Rules of Evidence supersede the *Frye* rule, see there

feedback loop ENDOCRINOLOGY The loop 'classification' was established at a time when the pituitary gland and target organs were thought to control the secretion of releasing and stimulating hormones from the hypothalamus and hypophysis, respectively, a posit that has proven largely correct

LONG FEEDBACK LOOP Target organs produce hormones that act on the hypothalamus and the pituitary, modifying pituitary secretion, eg thyroid hormone inhibits the synthesis and secretion of thyrotropin-releasing hormone (TRH) from the hypothalamus and thyroid-stimulating hormone (TSH) from the pituitary

SHORT FEEDBACK LOOP There is negative inhibition of pituitary hormones at the hypothalamus, eg increased growth hormone results in decreased somatostatin secretion

ULTRASHORT FEEDBACK LOOP A term occasionally used referring to hypothalamic hormones that regulate their own secretion

PHYSIOLOGY Any control system, in particular those involving hormonal and receptor-ligand interactions, in which the output signal or effect, eg increase of the production of a hormone by an end-organ, is received by the early components of the system, causing an alteration in the subsequent output, either decreasing (negative feedback) or increasing (positive feedback) the production of an early-stage component of the system

fee-splitting MEDICAL REIMBURSEMENT A practice that is considered frankly unethical, in which physician A refers a patient to physician B and shares a portion of the professional fee of services received by physician B; Cf Finder's fee*

*Fee-splitting contrasts sharply with concept of a 'finder's fee' that compensates a referring physician for locating a certain type of patient for participation in clinical research protocols

feeding center Appetite center PHYSIOLOGY A region of the lateral hypothalamus at the junction of the medial forebrain bundle with the pallidohypothalamic fibers; stimulation of the FC (eg by low glucose) evokes eating behavior in conscious animals, and its destruction evokes fatal anorexia; Cf Satiety center

fehldiagnose German, Unclear diagnosis The inability to establish a diagnosis in a patient who is ill, despite an extensive work-up, and who is ultimately discharged without a primary diagnosis; in one study (Dtsch Med Wschr 1989; 114:1431), 1.5% of all hospitalized patients were discharged without a diagnosis, ie had a fehldiagnose, having presented with fever of unknown origin, syncope, chronic pain, nonspecific inflammation or hematological changes

FEIBA Factor VIII inhibitor (see there) or factor VIII bypassing activity; see Prothrombin complex concentrate

felbamate Felbatol, 2-phenyl-1,3-propandiol dicarbamate A second-line antiepileptic agent related to the tranquilizer meprobamate, which interacts with sodium and calcium ion channels, it ↓ seizures in Lennox-Gastaut syndrome, a severe form of epilepsy of childhood onset that is poorly controlled with other agents; it is reported to ↓ the frequency of tonic seizures by 34%, and total incidence of seizures by 19%; it may act by ↑ seizure threshold and by preventing the spread of the seizures SIDE EFFECTS Anorexia, nausea, vomiting, insomnia, headache, in 1/2000, aplastic anemia (Medico Interamericano 1995; 14:125), interaction with other antiepileptic agents (N Engl J Med 1993; 328:29ₒₐ; Science & Medicine Sept/Oct 1994) WARNING: The FDA and its manufacturer have issued a recommendation to immediately withdraw patients from felbamate because of reports of aplastic anemia (JAMA 1994; 272:995FDA)

'felinization' Transverse ridging of the esophagus occasionally seen by a barium 'swallow' in patients with longstanding reflux esophagitis, simulating the morphology of a normal feline esophagus; see Water brash appearance; Cf Leopard spotting

fellow A physician who is in fellowship, see there

fellowship A term that when defined in the usual context of US medical academics, a fellowship is a post-residency training period of one to two years in a subspecialty, eg interventional radiology, immunopathology and microsurgery of the hand, that allows a candidate to develop a particular expertise that may have a related subspecialty board; the time period of a fellowship is often used to prepare for the specialty boards examinations

felon Whitlow A purulent infection within the tight fascial plane adjacent to the terminal intraphalangeal joint of the fingers or toes, secondary to an open wound; as the inflammatory mass expands within the confined space, the vascular supply is compromised and a scenario is created that predisposes the site to osteomyelitis (most often, streptococcal or staphylococcal), pulp necrosis and sloughing of tissue; the pain is very intense and seemingly disproportionate with the scant amount of swelling and erythema clinically evident TREATMENT Drainage by an incision directly over the site of maximum swelling; the term has also been applied to a localized painful herpetic skin infection 'seeded' in an open abrasion by contact exposure

female circumcision HUMAN RIGHTS The disfigurement and/or removal of parts of the external female genitalia which is performed in many Central and West African countries and is required for tribal identity; circumcision has deeply rooted cultural significance; male circumcision is a symbol of religious and ethnic identity, female circumcision is linked to women's sexuality and reproductive role in society, and is usually performed from age 4-10, but may be performed as early as infancy and as late as after the delivery of the first child; FC is performed on 5-99% of ♀ in 26 African countries, with ± 100 million ♀ world-wide having undergone the mutilating procedure; FC may be classified into two broad categories, clitoridectomies (type I and II procedures) and infundibulations (type III and IV procedures) COMPLICATIONS-SHORT TERM The procedure is rarely if ever performed by trained physicians, but rather by unskilled and uneducated village healers, shamans, or by local women who are 'specialized' in the procedure, who may use old razors or broken glass; severe pain, hemorrhage, and potentially fatal shock may result; infection is common and may be accompanied by abscesses, gangrene, septicemia, and tetanus COMPLICATIONS-LONG TERM Disfigurement in the form of dermoid cysts, stitch ('suture') neuromas, splitting of scars; at the time of childbirth, if de-infibulation is not performed prior to childbirth, exit of the fetal head may be obstructed and the perineum torn; if the uterine contractions are relatively weak, and delay in delivery of the fetal head may result in fetal demise, necrosis of the vesicovaginal septum, fistula formation and/or urinary incontinence TREATMENT De-infibulation, psychotherapy ETHICAL ISSUES FC is regarded in developed nations as genital mutilation and, when performed in the very young, a form of child abuse (N Engl J Med 1994; 331:712SA) see Clitoridectomy, Infibulation; Cf 'Love surgery'

female condom Vaginal pouch An externally placed contraceptive device, which offers some protection against both pregnancy and sexually transmitted diseases, resulting in an annual rate of pregnancy of 21-26% (vs ± 15% with a latex condom); the pouch is a polyurethane sheath measuring 16.5 cm (6 ½) that is held in place by two plastic rings, one held at the cervix and one outside the body (New York Times 11 May 1993; C5)

*The first of which (Reality™) is marketed in the US by Wisconsin Pharmacal and in several European countries as Femidon™ (Chartrex Intl, Ltd, UK)

female genital mutilation see Female circumcision

female 'prostate' RADIOLOGY A filling defect occasionally seen in women where the levator ani muscle is more prominent than usual; associated with urethritis, and best visualized in the prone position, while the real prostate is less pronounced in prone position UROLOGY Paraurethral glands seen rarely in female humans, but are well-studied in rodents, homologous to the male prostate; the female prostate may contain psammoma bodies, and if enlarged, require transurethral resection

female pseudohermaphroditism A type of intersex, in which the ovaries and müllerian derivatives are normally developed, and the anatomical ambisexuality is limited to the external genitalia; masculinization is the result of prenatal exposure to androgens, which may be of fetal origin, eg congenital adrenal hyperplasia with virilization or due to placental P450 deficiency, or of maternal origin, eg ingestion of androgens, presence of virilizing tumors in the mother

feminine ethics The moralistic constructs focused on approaches to moral reasoning that are more common or unique to women (N Engl J Med 1993; 328:360BR) Cf Feminist ethics

feminism 1) Feminist movement, see there 2) Feminization, see there

feminist ethics The moralistic constructs focused on the general structures that oppress women in society (**N Engl J Med 1993; 328:360BR**) Cf Feminine ethics

feminization The development of ♀ secondary sex characteristics in a genotypic ♂, with regression of body hair and change to a female body contour

fenestration Laminotomy, see there

fenoldopan An investigational antihypertensive agent that is a dopamine (D₁) receptor antagonist with renal vasodilatory activity, administered by intravenous drip and has been reported to be as effective as nitroprusside with renoprotective effect

fentanyl A synthetic narcotic analogue that is 100 x more potent than morphine; it has recently been made available in lozenge form for children (**Sci Am 1994; 270/5:113**)

FEP Free erythrocytic porphyrin

ferning A term for two light microscopic patterns related to normal gynecologic physiology, in 1) Cytology Ferning is a palm leaf-like pattern seen in dried endocervical mucus, consisting of a branched heterogeneous network of crystallized glycoprotein, sodium and potassium chloride salts that forms a parallel canalicular system facilitating sperm penetration; the ferning reaction is induced by estrogen and seen from days 7-18, peaking on day 14 of the menstrual cycle, and 2) Endometrium Ferning corresponds to complex branching of endometrial glands, which is histological evidence that ovulation has occurred; other parameters corroborating ovulation include subnucleolar vacuolization with palisading of the gland cells, stromal 'decidualization', glandular necrosis, vascular thrombosis, inflammation and aggregates of stromal cells; see Spinnbarkeit

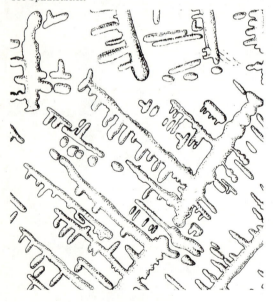

ferning

ferritin An 18.5-kD protein that is the major iron storage protein; when all available sites are filled, ferritin is 23% iron by weight; the only test needed to diagnose iron-deficiency anemia; serum levels ≤ 40 µg/L are consistent with iron deficiency in the general population, and ≤ 70 µg/L make iron deficiency likely in those with inflammatory or liver disease (**J Gen Intern Med 1992; 7:145**); a serum ferritin of ≤ 2500 ng/mL may be used as a parameter to monitor doses of defoxamine (iron chelation therapy) in patients with transfusion-related iron overload (**N Engl J Med 1994; 331:574OA**)

ferruginous body A generic term for asbestos fibers clad in iron, protein and mucopolysaccharides; the definition has been expanded to include any iron-covered elongated fiber that can't be digested by macrophages, including fiberglass, aluminum silicates and diatomaceous earth (**Arch Pathol Lab Med 1985; 109:849**); Cf Asbestos body

'fertile' eunuch syndrome A variant of Kallmann syndrome with selective LH deficiency and intact FSH production (ie normal 'equipment' with aspermatogenesis, thus, despite the name, these patients are infertile but may be rendered fertile with hormonal support) TREATMENT hCG, the luteinizing hormone-like activity of which stimulates spermatogenesis

the 'fertility' doctor A 55-year-old fertility specialist from Virginia who is alleged to have donated his own sperm for the artificial insemination of 70 women, in addition to fathering 8 children; he was convicted of 52 counts of fraud and perjury, fined $116 805, and sentenced to five years in prison (**Am Med News 25 May 1992 p2**)

FESS Functional endonasal sinus surgery, see there

festooning DERMATOPATHOLOGY A descriptor for the ribbon-like strands of epithelial cells that extend vertically from the basal cell layer to the epidermal canopy, periodically tethering the fluid-filled bullae to the dermis; festooning is a histologic finding characteristic of dermatitis herpetiformis, likened to festoons or party streamers

fetal alcohol syndrome A disease complex due to in utero exposure to alcohol EPIDEMIOLOGY 6% of babies born to alcoholic primiparas have FAS; up to 70% of infants of subsequent pregnancies also have FAS (**JAMA 1992; 268:3183NIH**) it is the most common cause of mental retardation in pregnancy (surpassing Down syndrome and spina bifida), affecting at least one-third of the infants born to women who are defined as alcoholics, ie those who consume greater than 50 grams of alcohol/day; FAS affects 1-2 per 1000 live births (US) and may to be related to the toxic effects of acetaldehyde, produced by both the mother and fetus; the alcohol may interfere with the placenta's ability to transfer amino acids and zinc, essential for normal growth, explaining the associated intrauterine growth retardation CLINICAL Prematurity, perinatal asphyxia, intrauterine growth retardation that may persist into adulthood, mild to profound developmental delays, mental dysfunction, microcephaly, cranial defects, atrial septal defect and facial dysmorphia (short palpebral fissure, epicanthal folds, short up-turned nose, thin upper lip, long smooth filtrum, micrognathia, maxillary hypoplasia), muscular hypotonia, bone anomalies (vertebral malformation and spina bifida) with joint contraction; when FAS children are re-examined as adolescents and adults, their IQ averages 68, with academic functioning at the second to fourth grade levels, poor mathematical abilities, maladaptive behavior, including poor judgement, distractibility and difficulty in perceiving social cues; the subjects tend to be short and microcephalic (**JAMA 1991; 265:1961**)

Note: The 50% decrease in alcohol consumption during pregnancy reported from 1985-88 is attributed to educational efforts (**JAMA 1991; 265:876**)

fetal brain grafting Fetal mesencephalic tissue transplantation, see there

fetal bovine serum MOLECULAR BIOLOGY A minor product of the cattle industry that has considerable value in the biotechnology industry; 500 000 liters are traded/year with a value > $100 million; the sales of biopharmaceuticals (eg erythropoietin, growth hormone, interferon) that use FBS as a raw material is > $2 billion/year; many cell lines grow much better in FBS than in either artificial media or in other sera obtained from older animals; the raw material for FBS consists of blood drawn from freshly killed pregnant cows, usually in an abattoir, which is then passed along a long chain of processes and middlemen, eg collectors, blenders, filters, importers, exporters, and distributors; a bottle of FBS costs from $50 to $300; the 'magic factor(s)' present in FBS that makes it an ideal culture medium is unknown, but it is superior to both artificial and calf serum (Bio/Technology 1995; 13:327)

fetal diabetic 'syndrome' A complex seen in the children born to diabetic mothers, who have a 3- to 5-fold increased incidence of various congenital and acquired anomalies, including visceromegaly, ↑ body fat, respiratory distress, and hyaline membrane disease, cardiomegaly, ventricular septal hypertrophy, skeletal anomalies, hypoplastic left colon syndrome (aganglionosis-like presentation), hypocalcemia and immaturity

fetal distress syndrome Intrauterine fetal hypoxia caused by prematurity or antepartum maternal infection, DM, eclampsia, hemolytic disease of the newborn, hemorrhage and others CLINICAL Tachycardia (>160/min) or bradycardia (<100/min, which carries a worse prognosis) and ↓ pH

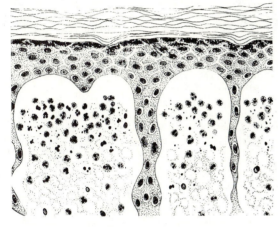

festooning

'fetal' erythrocyte Prolonged presence of hemoglobin F in neonatal erythrocytes, which is thought to have no pathological significance; Cf F cell

Note: At birth, RBCs contain 53-95% HbF that usually completely disappears by 45-70th day of life

fetal heart rate OBSTETRICS In the non-stressed fetus, the FHR is a reflection of cardioaccelerator and cardiodecelerator reflexes; proper analysis of the FHR requires evaluation of a baseline FHR occurring between uterine contractions or periodic changes in the FHR and non-periodic, short-term fluctuations in the FHR; see Deceleration

fetal hemoglobin An 'immature' hemoglobin (Hb) composed of two α and two γ chains that usually disappears in the neonatal period FETAL-TO-ADULT HB 'SWITCH' The β globin locus contains 5 different genes expressed in embryonic, fetal and adult erythrocytes as a function of the LAR (locus activation region), located 6-20 kilobases upstream of the genes, which turns the genes on, one at a time in predetermined sequence; hydroxurea may evoke an increase in Hb F levels and a decrease in sickle cell hemolysis; normally, the finding of red cells with fetal hemoglobin in the maternal circulation implies fetal-maternal hemorrhage, measured by the Kleihauer-Betke test (a test that determines the number of RBCs with fetal Hb, a value of importance if the infant is Rh-postive and the mother is Rh-negative and requires Rh immune globulin to prevent sensitization against the fetal red cell antigens); see hereditary persistence of fetal hemoglobin

Note: β Hb is not expressed in fetal erythrocytes, explaining why these cells, circulating in the fetus' 'hypoxic' environment, are not susceptible to sickling

fetal hydantoin syndrome A congenital complex caused by in utero exposure to anticonvulsants, affecting the infants of pregnant women being treated with these agents CLINICAL Growth retardation, microcephaly, midfacial hypo- or dysplasia, hypertelorism, short nose, broad depressed nasal bridge, cleft lip and palate, onychodigital dysplasia, cardiac malformations, mental retardation and rarely neuroblastoma Note: in utero exposure to carbamazepine affects the same organs and to a similar degree as hydantoin, causing craniofacial defects 11%, developmental delay 20% and fingernail hypoplasia 26%, which is not unexpected, given that both agents are metabolized by the arene oxide pathway, yielding an intermediate epoxide that may be a direct teratogen; see Fetal trimethadione syndrome

Note: Another anticonvulsant, valproic acid, when administered in the first trimester, is associated with spina bifida

fetal lung maturity OBSTETRICS A physiological parameter that determines the likelihood a neonate will develop respiratory distress syndrome (RDS); infants delivered at 40 ± 2 weeks have 0% incidence of RDS; at 36 weeks 0-2%, at 34 weeks 8-34% (depending on birthweight); biochemical test currently used to evaluate fetal lung maturity are lecithin to sphingomyelin (L/S) ratio by TLC, phosphatidylglycerol (PG) determination by TLC, PG determination by lipid agglutination, optical absorption at 650 nm, surface tension measurement, foam stability index, microviscosity, lamellar body number density (CAP Today 1993; 7:1)

Note: Given the medico-legal ramifications of FLM; a hospital's obstetric service must be aware of which tests the laboratory is capable of performing

fetal mesenscephalic tissue transplant The implantation of fetal dopaminergic neural tissue, eg from the ventral mesencephalon (adrenal gland or other tissues) into the caudate nucleus, or putamen to restore neurologic function in patients with Parkinson's disease; most of the patients undergoing the procedure demostrate significant improvement (amelioration of rigidity, bradykinesia, postural imbalance, gait disturbance and facial expression), in the form of improved disease control with lower doses of antiparkinsonian medication (N Engl J Med 1992; 327:1541-60A, 1589-92ED) long-term survival of transplanted tissue with restoration of dopaminergic innervation was documented in the brain of a patient with PD who died of unrelated causes (N Engl J Med 1995; 332:1118OA)Note: Post-surgical immunosuppression with cyclosporine and prednisone is common practice; see Parkinson's disease

*Parkinson's disease is characterized by the loss of mesencephalic dopaminergic neurons that innervate the caudate and putamen, in the pars compacta of the substantia nigra

fetal overgrowth syndrome Beckwith-Wiedemann syndrome, see there

fetal paralysis The intramuscular injection of short-acting agents, eg atracurium besylate, and vecuronium bromide into the thigh of a fetus during intrauterine transfusion in order to prevent fetal movement which may result in visceral injury (Arch Pathol Lab Med 1994; 118:421RV) see Hemolytic disease of the newborn, Intrauterine transfusion

fetal posture The position assumed by the fetus in the uterus, which may be adopted ex utero by those with severe mental retardation, or by a normal person when in a state of extreme mental stress

fetal rubella syndrome see Congenital rubella syndrome

fetal tissue transplantation BIOMEDICAL ETHICS FT is attractive as a transplantation 'donor' material; it grows readily, is capable of multilineage differentiation, and has reduced antigenicity; FTT into adults has been used in experimental protocols for treating immunodeficiency states, metabolic diseases, Parkinson's disease, DM (fetal pancreatic cells), infertility (eggs from fetal ovaries), and cardiac failure (cardiac muscle cells) (New York Times 5 April 1994; C3) see Fetal-brain grafting

Note: The use of human fetal tissues in research is ethically charged and has been hotly debated in Parliament, the US Congress, Germany and the governing bodies of other nations

fetal tobacco syndrome A malformation complex affecting infants born to ♀ smoking ≥ 1 pack of cigarettes/day during pregnancy; FTS neonates are 200 g lighter, infant mortality is 40% greater (and is indirectly responsible for 4000 excess infant deaths, in the form of ↑ spontaneous abortion, fetal wastage, perinatal mortality, SIDS) and the children have impaired cognitive and emotional development; by age 10, children born to actively smoking (as well as ⅔ of infants born to passively 'smoking') mothers are 1.0 cm shorter, with ↓ adult height, and are 3-6 months behind peers in measurable parameters of intelligence; tobacco is synergistic with other environmental toxins impacting on the fetus, eg benzene exposure to infants in utero or in early infancy is implicated in excess leukemia in later life, if one parent also smokes, there is a 2-fold increase, if both parents smoke, there is a 5-fold ↑ in leukemias; see Passive smoking, Smoking

Note: Tobacco smoke contains 4720 different compounds and is the most highly concentrated aerosol known to man and is the most powerful determinant of poor fetal growth in the developed world

fetal trimethadione syndrome A fetal dysmorphia complex described in 1970, affecting two-thirds of pregnancies in which the anti-convulsant, trimethadione was administered CLINICAL Brachycephaly, midfacial hypoplasia, upslanting eyebrows, saddle nose, prominent forehead, cleft lip and palate, cardiac (eg tetralogy of Fallot, septal defects), genital (eg hypospadias), simian crease, growth and mental retardation and other malformations; Cf Fetal hydantoin syndrome

fetal varicella syndrome An embryopathy affecting an estimated 2% of fetuses of mothers infected with herpes varicella-zoster in the first 20 weeks of pregnancy (**N Engl J Med 1994; 330:901ₒₐ**) CLINICAL Scarring along dermatomes, muscular and osseous hypoplasia, eye defects (cataracts, microphthalmia, chorioretinitis), and neurologic abnormalities (mental retardation, microcephaly, sphincter dysfunction)

fetal warfarin syndrome A fetal dysmorphia complex caused by in utero exposure to dicumarol (Warfarin) CLINICAL Developmental defects causing optic atrophy and affecting the CNS with fatal fetal bleeding, hypoplasia of the nose and extremities and diffuse epiphyseal 'stippling', which has features similar to Conradi-Hunermann chondrodysplasia punctata

Note: Heparin is not teratogenic but may cause stillbirth

fetal wastage Any loss of a gestational product, either voluntary or involuntary that occurs between the 20th week of pregnancy and the 28th day of life, a value known for epidemiological purposes, as 'total pregnancy wastage'

FETI Fluorescence excitation transfer immunofluorescence IMMUNOLOGY A laboratory method for measuring the serum levels of various substances, eg morphine, albumin, thyroxin-binding globulin and IgG, in which two fluorescent labels are used, one that fluoresces at a maximum at 525 nm and the other that fluoresces at a minimum at 525 nm; when the antigen is absent in the serum, fluorescence is quenched, as the two cancel each others' effect; when present, the antigen causes a proportionate increase in fluorescence

fetish A device (eg women's underpants, bra, shoes, or other wearing apparel) that is the object of sexual arousal, which may in extreme cases replace the need for a sexual partner for sexual arousal or orgasm

fetishism A paraphilia (sexual deviation) that involves the use of nonliving objects (fetishes) for sexual arousal; as defined by the DSM-IV, fetishism occurs over a period of six months or more, is distressful to the subject, and is not limited those articles of female clothing used in the context of cross-dressing, known as transvestic fetishism

fetomaternal hemorrhage Fetomaternal transfusion The passage of blood from the placenta (via the umbilical cord) into the mother at the time of delivery; FH is of considerable importance in Rh-negative ♀ who deliver Rh-positive babies, against which the mother may form antibodies, possibly resulting in 'rejection' of subsequent babies, greater (in the extreme of cases) hydrops fetalis

fetor hepaticus A sweet, musty odor on the breath of those with hepatic encephalopathy, due to mercaptans, the degradation products of sulfur-containing molecules

fetoscopy An imaging technique in which an ultrasound-guided 3 mm in diameter needle with an endoscope is inserted through the abdominal wall into the uterus to view a living fetus, a procedure that can be performed in the second and third trimesters of pregnancy and carries a not insignificant risk of fetal wastage, related to rupture of fetal membranes (**New York Times 6 July 1993; C1**) Cf Embryoscopy

Feulgen method HISTOLOGY YD used for staining DNA--mas cosas

FEV Forced expiratory volume The maximal amount of air that can be exhaled in a period of time, usually one (FEV_1) or less commonly, three (FEV_3) seconds; FEV_1 is usually reduced (and thus is a major parameter measured) in obstructive airways disease, a generic term that encompasses both asthma and COPD

fever A corporal temperature of ≥ 37.2°C (99.0°F) when taken in the early morning, or ≥ 37.8°C (100.0°F) when taken in the evening; the febrile reaction per se is a complex and coordinated adaptive response that is part of the reaction to immune challenge; this response is stereotyped and largely independent of etiologic agent; as with other integrated responses, eg regulation of energy metabolism, blood pressure and volume, and reproduction, fever depends on humoral cues and is orchestrated by the hypothalamus which coordinates autonomic, behavioral, endocrine and metabolic responses (**N Engl J Med 1994; 330:1880ʀᵥ**) when corporal temperature is raised by endogenous pyrogen, T-cell production increases 20-fold; endogenous pyrogen also shifts iron (needed by bacteria) away from plasma; hyperthermia (up to 40°C) has been associated with regression of malignancy, see Coley's toxin

*Also known as the sacred disease, Hippocrates considered fever the body's way of burning off toxins, which has proven conceptually correct; Sydenham, the 'English Hippocrates' called fever 'a mighty engine which Nature brings into the world for the conquest of her enemies'; modern appreciation of hyperpyrexia comes from the desert lizard (*Dipsosaurus dorsalis*), an ectotherm that controls its temperature by moving to hotter places in the cage; animals that are infected but unable to move to warmer areas of a cage, have a higher mortality, lending credence to fever's role in immune defense

fever blister One of possible multiple minute perioral vesicles caused by herpes simplex virus

fever of unknown origin A febrile state with temperature of ≥ 37°C for at least 2, preferably 3 weeks in duration, for which a cause cannot be identified despite thorough physical examination and aggressive and relevant laboratory work-up; the etiology ultimately proves infectious in 30-40%, collagen vascular in 15-20% for both children and adults; in adults, 20-30% of the remainder are due to malignancy, which comprises 10% of the remainder in children; other rare causes include sarcoidosis and colitis; hereditary FUOs are rare and appear in Fabry's disease, familial Mediterranian fever, type 1 hyperlipidemia and cyclic neutropenia

fever therapy A therapeutic modality that continues to intrigue cancer biologists, as hyperthermia is associated with enhanced immune function, related to the release of a wide variety of pyrogenic (and nonpyrogenic) cytokines; controlled hyperthermia may be used to enhance tumor cell lysis, and is most successful when combined with chemotherapy and radiotherapy; Cf BCG therapy

F₀F₁ ATPase ATPase synthase membrane protein complex MOLECULAR BIOLOGY A group of 15 proteins that form the enzyme system required to generate ATP from ADP + Pi; the complex is present at all levels of phylogenetic sophistication, from plant and animal; in higher eukaryotes, it is seen as knobby protuberances on the inner membrane of the mitochondrium

FFP Fresh frozen plasma, see there

FFP rule SCIENTIFIC INTEGRITY Fabrication, falsification, and plagiarism, see Misconduct

FGF Fibroblast growth factor, see there

FHR Fetal heart rate, see there

FIAU Fialuridine, see there

fialuridine FIAU An experimental agent intended to eliminate the carrier state of hepatitis B, which was associated with liver toxicity and death in early clinical trials (JAMA 1995; 273:1165MN&P)

fiber see Dietary fiber

fiber cells GYNECOLOGIC CYTOLOGY An elongated malignant epithelial cell with hyperchromatic nuclei and irregularly clumped chromatin that may be seen in Papanicolaou-stained smears of carcinoma-in-situ of the uterine cervix (figure); Cf Tissue culture appearance PULMONARY CYTOLOGY Elongated, twisted keratin-filled malignant cells seen in well-differentiated bronchogenic carcinoma cells, derived from the peripheral 'husks' of squamous pearls

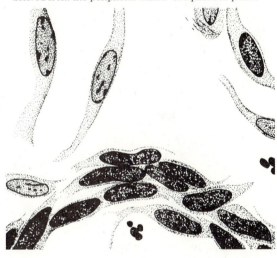

fiber cells

fibrillin A 350-kD glycoprotein of the extracellular matrix that is the main component of microfibrils, arranged in a head-to-tail fashion and contribute to the globular domains of matrix proteins; fibrillin microfibers are associated with elastin, connective tissue around blood vessels, in developing bone matrix, and are present as bundles in elastin-poor tissues, eg cornea and tendon which is encoded by the *FBN1* gene located on chromosome segment 15q21.1; *FBN1* is both mutated in (40 different mutations of *FBN1* are known to cause Marfan syndrome (Science & Medicine 1995; 2/3:58) and responsible for Marfan syndrome, which is characterized by a wide range of clinical expression that varies according to the family affected; each family appears to have a unique mutation, precluding the routine use of mutation screening for presymptomatic diagnosis of Marfan syndrome (N Engl J Med 1994; 331:148OA) see Collagen, Extracellular matrix, *FBN1*, Marfan syndrome

fibrin caps Exudative glomerular lesions seen in later stages of diabetic glomerulosclerosis composed of aggregates of plasma protein suspended between endothelial or epithelial basement membrane

fibrin degradation products FDPs, fibrin 'splits' Polypeptide fragments that are generated by unchecked primary fibrinolysis in 1) Intravascular lesions, associated with DIC, deep vein thrombosis and pulmonary embolism (ie, pathological fibrinolysis) or in 2) Extravascular conditions, eg hematomas, neoplasia, sepsis, allograft rejection, glomerular and severe liver diseases and obstetric complications, eg abruptio placentae, eclampsia, retained dead fetus

fibrin glue A commercial product used to seal operative wounds, by partially re-enacting the final stage of the coagulation cascade in which fibrinogen is converted to fibrin in the presence of thrombin, factor XIII, fibronectin and calcium ions; lyophilized and concentrated fibrinogen is reconstituted with aprotonin, a proteinase that theoretically enhances the persistence of fibrin, warmed to 37°C; thrombin and calcium chloride are mixed separately and then both are applied with a double-barreled syringe; fibrin sealants are of greatest use in cardiothoracic and general vascular surgery in controlling focal slow bleeding, diffuse oozing, puncture wounds, lymphatic leaks and diffuse parenchymal organ hemorrhage **fibrinogen** A 340-kD plasma glycoprotein that consists of three (α, β, and γ) subunits that is the molecular precursor of fibrin in coagulation; the conversion of fibrinogen into fibrin is orchestrated under the baton of thrombin; ↑ fibrinogen levels and ↑ blood viscosity in a stroke survivor is a risk factor for subsequent cardiovascular events, including strokes, myocardial infarction, and other atherothrombosis-related phenomena (Ann Intern Med 1992; 117:371OA); fibrinogen levels (2.00-4.00 g/L; US: 200-400 mg/dL) are strongly associated with severity of coronary artery disease (CAD), with 315 mg/dL indicating no CAD, 328 mg/dL indicating 'evident' CAD, and 333 mg/dL indicating totally occlusive CAD (Am J Heart 1993; 125:1601OA)

fibrinogen Detroit A congenital defect in fibrinogen, first described in a city well-known for acquired bleeding disorders; fibrinopeptide A is structurally normal and released normally by thrombin; an amino acid substitution close to the point of bond splitting prevents a conformational change necessary to expose the terminal domain, resulting in a ↑ thrombin time; PTT and coagulation time are usually normal; see Dysfibrinogenemia

fibrinoid necrosis 'Smudgy' eosinophilic fibrin-like deposits corresponding to degeneration of collagen or ground substance that may be seen in arterial walls in malignant accelerated hypertension and periarteritis nodosa, but which may also be seen in the Arthus reaction, acute rheumatic fever, subacute bacterial endocarditis, adjacent to peptic ulcers, rheumatoid arthritis, immune complex disease, hepatitis B, malignancy, complement C2 deficiency, Henoch-Schönlein purpura, SLE, and other collagen vascular disease

fibrinolysin An obsolete term for plasmin

fibroadenoma Fibroadenoma is reported to be a long-term risk factor for breast cancer (relative risk-RR = 2.17); the risk is greatest in women with complex fibroadenomas (RR 3.1), concomitant family history (RR 3.72) and benign proliferative changes adjacent to the fibroadenoma (RR 3.88) (N Engl J Med 1994; 331:10OA)

fibroblast growth factor family A family of growth factors with nine members (at most recent count) FGF-1 is linked to YD, and is mutated in Pfeiffer syndrome (New York Times 1 Nov 1994; C1); FGF-2 has been identified as a growth signal for chick limb development (Science 1994; 264:104R) and is mutated in Crouzon and in Jackson-Weiss syndromes (ibid 1 Nov 1994; C1) FGF-3 is mutated in achondroplastic dwarfism (ibid 1 Nov 1994; C1); FGFs undergo changes in regional expression that varies in accord with a higher organism's embryological development (Nature 1995; 374:217N&v)

fibrocystic disease SURGICAL PATHOLOGY A relatively common disease of the female breast, first appearing ± age forty, presenting as a diffusely indurated breast; there appears to be

NO RISK FOR FUTURE MALIGNANCY: FCD with adenosis (sclerosing or florid), apocrine metaplasia, cysts (macro- or microscopic), ductal ectasia, fibroadenoma, fibrosis, hyperplasia

MINIMAL RISK FOR FUTURE MALIGNANCY with glandular 'crowding', ie 2-4 epithelial cells in depth, mastitis, especially periductal, squamous metaplasia

1.5-2-FOLD ↑ RISK OF FUTURE MALIGNANCY with hyperplasia (moderate or florid, solid or papillary) or in a papilloma with a fibrovascular core

2-5-FOLD ↑ RISK OF FUTURE MALIGNANCY with atypical hyperplasia (borderline lesion), either ductal or lobular

8-10-FOLD ↑ RISK OF FUTURE INVASIVE CANCER Carcinoma-in-situ

fibrodysplasia ossificans progressiva Generalized myositis ossificans An idiopathic or AD [MIM 135100] condition of irregular penetration and pre-pubertal onset, in which interstitial tissues undergo extensive fibrosis and ossification; the lesions first appear in late childhood as firm tumor masses that later extend to globally to involve muscle, tendons, ligaments, fascia, aponeuroses and skin CLINICAL Microdactyly, focal, transient and occasionally painful ossifying tumors in the neck, back and extremities, with bony replacement of fasciae, ligaments and fibrotendinous tissue, associated with baldness, deafness, mental retardation, fever; tragically, the patients may find employment in circus 'freak' shows; in general, glossal, diaphragmatic, laryngeal and perineal musculature is spared and patients die of respiratory infections as the intercostal muscles become petrified DDx Osseous metaplasia, myositis ossificans, extraskeletal osteosarcoma; Cf Parana hard skin syndrome, Stiff man syndrome

fibroelastosis see Endocardial fibroelastosis

fibrolamellar carcinoma Polygonal cell hepatocellular carcinoma A rare low-grade hepatocellular carcinoma variant that is most common in acirrhotic young (age 5-35) females, possibly associated with use of oral contraceptives; 50% are resectable and 50% of the resectable cases are curable PROGNOSIS Excellent; the average survival is 32 months—the usual hepatocellular carcinoma is fatal within 6 months PATHOLOGY Nests of deeply eosinophilic neoplastic hepatocytes with cytoplasmic hyalin droplets or pale bodies, surrounded by broad lamellar bands of fibrosis

fibromatoses A family of benign fibrous tissue proliferations that have similar microscopic features and aggressiveness intermediate between benign fibrous lesions and low-grade fibrosarcoma, differing from the former in their marked tendency to recur, and from the latter as they do not metastasize; these lesions are either 1) Superficial (fascial), affecting the palm (Dupuytren's contracture), penis (Peyronie's disease), and knuckles or 2) Deep (aponeurotic), associated with desmoid tumors

fibronectin(s) A class of large dimeric glycoproteins that are abundant in the extracellular matrix and basement membrane and mediate the adhesion of cells (through a tetrapeptide, Arg-Gly-Asp-Ser) to fibrin, sulfated proteoglycans and collagens type I, II, III, V and VI; at least 20 different fibronectin chains have been identified, all of which are generated by alternative splicing of the RNA transcript from the fibronectin gene; fibronectin plays a major role in contact inhibition, in cell-substrate adhesion, migration of cells during embryogenesis, inflammation and in wound healing; malignantly transformed cells do not express fibronectin

fibrous dysplasia A non-neoplastic process affecting the bone that is divisible into 1) Monostotic fibrous dysplasia, a condition more common in the femur, tibia and ribs of children and older adolescents and 2) Polyostotic fibrous dysplasia, which is less common and associated with

endocrinopathy, precocious puberty and cutaneous hyperpigmentation (cafe-au-lait spots), the triad that defines Albright syndrome RADIOLOGY Long bones demonstrate a fusiform expansion with multiple loculations PATHOLOGY The tissue is gray-yellow and gritty to cutting and by light microscopy, demonstrates curved attenuated bony spicules, fancifully likened to fishhooks or Chinese characters (see there) in a fibroblastic background MOLECULAR PATHOGENESIS High levels of c-fos proto-oncogene are expressed in FD, which may be due to ↑ adenylate cyclase activity; the ↑ of c-fos may be due to an activating mutation of the gene encoding the stimulatory guanine-nucleotide-binding protein $(G_s\alpha)$ linked to adenylate cyclase (N Engl J Med 1995; 332:1546oA) TREATMENT Bone curettage

Note: Cafe-au-lait spots and fibrous dysplasia without precocious puberty corresponds to Jaffe syndrome

fibrous plaque The advanced lesion of atherosclerosis, composed of proliferated smooth muscle fibers, macrophages (foam cells or lipid-laden histiocytes) and lymphocytes; the plaque surface is covered by pancake cells overlying a dense connective tissue matrix that may 'prolapse' into the vascular lumen, compromising and deforming blood flow; calcium deposition in the plaque, cracking and ulceration results in a 'complicated' plaque; Cf Fatty streak

FICA Fluoroimmunocytoadherence IMMUNOLOGY A technique in which column chromatography is used to isolate antigen-binding cells

ficin TRANSFUSION MEDICINE A thiol proteinase used to remove sialic acid, thereby reducing the zeta potential and by extension, increasing the immunologic 'signal' of antigens on erythrocytes, by extension facilitating the detection of weak or non-agglutinating antibodies; ficin treatment enhances Ii, Kidd, Lewis and Rh agglutination and destroys Duffy, MNSs, Lutheran, Chido, Rogers, Tn, and others

ficoll IMMUNOLOGY A synthetic 400-kD, water-soluble sucrose and epichlorohydrin polymer used to prepare Ficoll-Hypaque, a proprietary density gradient medium used to separate and purify leukocytes by centrifugation, after the 'buffy coat' has been removed by pipetting from blood diluted in saline or Hanks medium; Ficoll-Hypaque separation provides optimal preparation of leukocytes and platelets for flow cytometric analysis

FICSIT Fraility and Injuries: Cooperative Studies of Intervention Techniques (*pronounced* 'fix-it') GERONTOLOGY A series of independent, randomized placebo-controlled clinical trials that assessed the efficacy of various interventions in reducing falls and frailty in elderly patients; a meta-analysis of the FICSIT trials revealed a ↓ risk of falls with ↑ exercise and training in the form of endurance, flexibility, and balance, dynamic balance (Tai Chi) and resistance (JAMA 1995; 273:1341oc); in another study, the subjects received either lower-extremity resistance training, multinutrient supplements (MNS), both, or placebo activity and MNS; one of FICSIT's major conclusions is that high-resistance exercise training (but not MNS) counteracts muscle weakness and physical fraility in the very elderly (age 85+) (N Engl J Med 1994; 330:1769oA) see Gerontology

fiddleback spider see Brown spider

fidelity MOLECULAR BIOLOGY The accuracy with which a segment of DNA is copied (replicated), translated or transcribed

fiefdom ACADEMIC MEDICINE A colloquial term for balkanized organization and autonomy that often characterize faculty practice plans in academic medical centers (N Eng J Med 1995; 332:407oA) see Faculty practice plan

field carcinogenesis ONCOLOGY The constellation of locoregional changes resulting from carcinogenic toxin(s) that induce frankly malignant changes in one site and concomitantly cause premalignant dysplasia or carcinoma-in-situ in the remaining organ, tissue or 'field'; thus despite adequate resection, the remaining field may be 'cancerized', despite a normal appearance, thus making it more susceptible to future malignancy; the effect occurs in tissue of any embryologic origin, and is easily recognized in epithelia of the colon, breast ducts, bladder, bronchial and laryngeal epithelium (eg entire aerodigestive tract in tobacco exposure and leukoplakia); in one venerated study (Cancer 1967; 20:699), 38 000 sections were obtained from 250 patients with bronchial carcinoma; using strict histologic criteria, 3.5% had a second primary carcinoma; in contrast, field cancerization is difficult to prove in non-epithelial tissues and its existence is implied by such terms as 'pseudolymphoma' and 'smooth muscle tumor of uncertain malignant potential'; Cf 'Cancerization'

field effect The action of an agent on an entire organ system EMBRYOLOGY The field effect refers to a combination of specific multisystem defects, eg in a renal/supermammary nipple defect

field inversion electrophoresis MOLECULAR BIOLOGY A gel electrophoresis technique that allows separation of large DNA molecules, which migrate at similar rates, despite large differences in length, due to 'reptation'; in FIE, the electric field is periodically inverted, such that the DNA makes large movements forward and small movements backward

fiery agent of the Israelites Filariasis

fièvre boutonneuse A benign rickettsial spotted fever caused by *Rickettsia coronii*, affecting visitors to the Mediterranean rim countries (natives develop permanent immunity) VECTOR Dog tick, *Rhipicephalus sanguineus* CLINICAL Initial lesion is a tache noire or primary eschar, followed by a diffuse maculopapular, later petechial rash with little systemic illness; agglutinin reactions to OX19 and OX2 are positive in the second week TREATMENT Doxycycline, tetracycline, chloramphenicol

fifth disease Erythema infectiosum A childhood exanthema caused by the moderately contagious B19 parvovirus; the condition was so named as it was the fifth childhood disease typically accompanied by a rash; the other nosologies classically associated with rashes in childhood are rubella, measles, scarlet fever and a mild, atypical variant of scarlet fever (Filatov-Dukes disease); see B19; Cf Fourth disease, Sixth disease

the 'fifth pathway' GRADUATE MEDICAL EDUCATION A route by which foreign, ie graduates of non-North American medical schools, may become eligible to begin internship or residency, ie specialty training in the USA, consisting of a year of supervised clinical training; the fifth pathway was created in response to one country's withholding of the medical school diplomas from the graduates until they had provided a year of rural service

fifth plague of Egypt An epidemic of ancient Egypt described in the Bible's Old Testament (Exodus 9:3); although the agent of the fifth plague is unknown, medical historians have postulated various nosologies including plague (*Yersinia pestis*), foot and mouth disease (picornavirus), rinderpest, anthrax and Rift Valley fever

fight bite A jagged laceration on the dorsum of the hand, often over the knuckles, seen when belligerent A's fist strikes belligerent B's teeth, causing abrasions, deep lacerations, puncture wounds and a sizeable inoculum of mixed oral flora, including staphylococci, 50% of which produce penicillinase, also β-hemolytic streptococci, *Eikenella corrodens*; without treatment, a fight bite may become complicated, resulting in the clenched fist 'syndrome'

fight-or-flight response General adaption 'syndrome' A generalized 'physiologic' reaction displayed by most mammals in the face of imminent danger or anticipated pain; this emergency response evokes a full-scale activation of the central nervous system and the release of 'stressors' by the adrenal medulla, eg epinephrine and norepinephrine and cortex, eg corticosteroids, mineralocorticoids, as well as renin and insulin CLINICAL Tachycardia, diaphoresis, tremor, pallor, increased inotropism, vasoconstriction, mydriasis, bronchodilation and hyperglycemia

FIGLU Formiminoglutamic acid A breakdown product of histidine that is ↑ in the urine in folic acid deficiency (which diminishes purine biosynthesis and is partially offset by the ability of accumulated 5-amino-4-imidazole carboxamide ribotide to slow purine degradation); ↑ urinary FIGLU after oral histidine ingestion favors a diagnosis of folic acid deficiency as the cause of a case of megaloblastic anemia, although ⅔ of patients with vitamin B$_{12}$ deficiency also have increased FIGLU excretion

FIGO International Federation of Gynecologists and Obstetricians A major contribution of this international body of experts has been to stage gynecologic malignancy, in particular, carcinomas of the ovary (table)

FIGO STAGING, OVARIAN CARCINOMA

I	Malignancy of one (Ia) or both (Ib) ovaries, without ascites: 5-year survival: 60%
II	Malignancy of one (IIa) or both (IIb) ovaries, with pelvic extension and ascites: 5-year survival: 40%
III	Malignancy involves one or both ovaries, intraperitoneal metastases outside pelvis and/or positive retroperitoneal lymph nodes: 5-year survival: 5%
IV	Involvement of one/both ovaries with metastases and histologically confirmed extension to pleural cavity or liver: 5-year survival, 3%

figure 3 sign PEDIATRICS A combination of pre- and post-stenotic aortic dilation seen on a plain chest film of patients with postductal coarctation of the aorta; when this same finding is viewed by a barium 'swallow' study, it is known as the 'letter E' sign due to two vertical indentations in a barium-filled esophagus; the higher indentation corresponds to the left subclavian artery and the aortic knob, the lower indentation corresponds to post-stenotic aortic dilatation; Cf Reverse 3 sign

figure 8 appearance MOLECULAR BIOLOGY A descriptor for the 'cartoon' model of two circles of DNA partially linked by a recombination event in progress

figure 8 sign see Snowman sign

filaggrin A structural protein that specifically binds to intermediate filaments

filaments see Intermediate filaments

filamin CELL PHYSIOLOGY A flexible homodimeric protein produced by smooth muscle cells and fibroblasts, composed of two 270-kD chains; filamin is involved in sol-gel transitions in vertebrate cells and links actin fibers, enabling them to form a three-dimensional network, and which in solution, forms a semisolid gel

filaria A generic term for nematodal worms of the superfamily Filarioidea that cause human disease, including *Wuchereria bancrofti, Brugia malayi, Loa loa*, microfilaria of *Mansonella* (formerly, *Dipetalonema*) *perstans, Mansonella ozzardi*, and *Onchocirca volvulus*; filarial vectors include the mosquito (*Aedes, Culex, Mansonia*), black fly (*Simulium*), midge (*Culicoides*), and tabanid fly (*Chryosops*)

filarial fever Acute, recurring, episodes of high-grade fever, often with shaking chills, edema, lymphadenitis with retrograde progression, caused by filarial permeation of lymphatic channels, by *Wuchereria bancrofti, Brugia malayi,* and *Loa loa*; filarial fever occurs 5-10 times/year and each 'attack' lasts about a week; microfilariasis per se is asymptomatic

file drawer problem STATISTICS A type of publication bias that attempts to estimate the number of negative studies of a phenomenon required to eliminate the observed statistical significance (JAMA 1992; 268:2515L)

file server COMPUTERS A dedicated computer in a LAN (local area network) that provides access to files for all the workstations or PCs in network; with a properly designed and functioning network oprating system, the files can be accessed from the client's workstation, as if from an adjacent hard disk (B Pfaffenberger, Compuer User's Dictionary, Que, Indianapolis, 1993)

filgrastim Recombinant granulocyte colony-stimulating factor, see Granulocyte colony-stimulating factor, G-CSF

film badge NUCLEAR MEDICINE A device that holds a photographic film capable of absorbing radiation, which is used to quantify a person's exposure to occupation-related X-rays and gamma-radiation; the maximum radiation exposure allowed by the NIOSH is 5000 mRad/year or 1500 mRad for any one quarter

filter hybridization MOLECULAR BIOLOGY A hybridization procedure in which single-stranded DNA or RNA immobilized on a nitrocellulose or nylon membrane is bathed (incubated) in a solution containing labeled probe that may be complementary to the immobilized single-stranded nucleic acid

fimbrin An actin-binding protein that cross-links adjacent filaments, forming parallel actin filaments

Final Exit A book (Final Exit: The Practicalities of Self-Deliverance and Assisted Suicide for the Dying, D Humphrey, Hemlock Society, Eugene, Oregon, 1991) written as a 'suicide manual' on how to end one's own life, which delineated several maneuvers on how to successfully commit suicide, eg using a plastic bag to induce asphyxia or self-poisoning by certain drugs, and the 'preferred' format for a suicide note; New York City's Medical Examiner's office examined the impact of *Final Exit* on suicides and found that while the overall suicide rate did not increase, plastic bag-related asphyxia increased by $\geq$ 300% (N Engl J Med 1993; 329:1508ON) see Euthanasia, Physician-assisted suicide, Werther effect

final solution A catch phrase of Nazi Germany--much more detail is needed who were the targets and what was the German word

financial conflict of interest A state which, unlike other conflicts of interest, is a condition and not a behavior; when clinicians or researcher might benefit financially from the outcome of their work, a financial conflict of interest is said to exist, regardless of whether the data, analysis or conclusions are in fact distorted; it is common policy for premier biomedical journals (the New England Journal of Medicine began the practice in 1984) to require authors to disclose any associations they had with businesses that could be affected by their work–including direct employment and consultancy, stock ownership and patent-licensing arrangements (N Engl J Med 1993; 329:570ED, 573SB)

financial triage HEALTH CARE FINANCING A highly colloquial term referring to the evaluation of a patient's ability to pay for hospitalization or anticipated medical services, in a fashion similar to that of a triage to determine the urgency of injuries (Am Med News 16 Nov 1992 p1) see Triage

finasteride Proscar® An inhitor of 5α-reductase, the enzyme responsible for converting testosterone to dihydrotestosterone (DHT); finasterid has been approved to ameliorate the symptoms of benign prostatic hypertrophy (↓ obstructive symptoms, ↓ prostatic volume, ↑ urinary flow); it binds with 5α-reductase type 2, inhibiting the preduction of DHT; its potential uses include male-pattern baldness, hirsutism, and acne SIDE EFFECTS ↓ Libido, impotence, ejaculatory defects (N Engl J Med 1994; 330:120OA); finasteride therapy ↓ PSA by 50%, therefore serum PSA levels of > 5 ng/mL are suspicious (but not diagnostic) for the presence of prostatic carcinoma (Urology 1994; 43:53) see Androgen ablation therapy

finder's fee Compensatory remuneration for the service of locating or finding a client, a common business practice; when used in a medical context, is a fee offered to a physician or other health care professional for his help in locating subjects for participation in clinical trials of diagnostic or therapeutic modalities, as an attempt to reduce the chronic problem of finding an adequate number of appropriate subjects for such trials; Cf Fee splitting

fine droplet fatty liver see Fatty liver

fine needle aspiration A method used in diagnostic cytology and pathology using a thin or even skinny (from 18- to 23-gauge) needle; FNA material sits squarely on the fence between the domain of the classic histopathologist (who is most comfortable when the tissues obtained are large enough to have architectural 'landmarks') and the cytopathologist (who lives by cells alone); thus the terms FNA biopsy and FNA cytology overlap considerably, evidenced by a recent title, *'Fine Needle Aspiration Biopsy Cytology of Sclerosing Hemangioma of the Lung'* (Acta Cytologica 1993; 37:933OA)

fine needle aspiration biopsy A specimen obtained by FNA; lesions identified children include thyroglossal duct cyst, sialadenitis, lymphangioma, granulomatous lymphadenitis, lymphomas, neuroblastoma, Wilms' tumor, sarcomas, eosinophilic granuloma, and others (CAP Today November 1993); in adults, virtually any lump or bump (especially of internal organs that cannot be readily biopsied by an open procedure, eg liver, periaortic lesions, etc) can be 'FNABed' to obtain diagnostic material (Acta Cytologica 1993; 37:943OA)

fine needle aspiration cytology A diagnostic cytology specimen using a 'skinny' (eg 22– or 23-gauge) needle; virtually any lesion can be aspirated and sufficient material obtained to establish a diagnosis (Acta Cytologica 1993; 37:879OA)

finger motif Zinc-finger motif, see there

finger fracturing A crude post-mortem technique for evaluating organ consistency, where increases or decreases in firmness are determined by simple 'pinching' of a 1-2 cm in thickness slice of tissue is suggestive of certain pathological nosologies; under normal circumstances, the liver fractures readily; in cirrhosis, the liver is markedly indurated due to intense fibrosis; contrarily, normal lung is resistant to fracturing and in acute necrotizing pneumonia, can be easily pinched, shredded, or torn

finger-in-glove appearance SURGICAL PATHOLOGY Focal glandular outpouchings seen within glands in mild endometrial hyperplasia, which may be secondary to chronic anovulation and/or associated with Stein-Leventhal syndrome and infertility RADIOLOGY 'Gloved finger' shadow of Simon A descriptor for a mucoid plug within a bronchiectatic segment of a fibrotically thickened bronchus or bronchiole, as seen on a plain film of the chest

finger nucleases Those enzymes secreted by the skin of the digits that are capable of digesting ribonucleic acid, especially RNA, thus requiring special precaution by molecular biologists who work with RNA

fingerprint CHEMISTRY The 'signature(s)' that a chemical compound and its metabolites have when analyzed by a highly sensitive technique, eg HPLC or GC-MS, which may be stored on a computer's hard disk and electronically matched ('fingerprinted') with an unknown specimen for the purpose of identification; see DNA fingerprint, Protein fingerprint DERMATOGLYPHICS Increased ulnar loops and decreased whorls and arches are seen in Alzheimer's disease, a pattern similar to that seen in Down syndrome; see Dermatoglyphics

fingerprint appearance RENAL PATHOLOGY A descriptor for the layered epithelial crescents, thrombi and hematoxylin material, accompanied by granular deposition of IgG, C3 and fibrin in diffuse glomerulonephritis EM Reticular aggregates in capillary endothelium, which in lupus erythematosus may represent a reaction of the endoplasmic reticulum to injury

fingerprint pattern OPHTHALMOLOGY A horizontally oriented, whorled filagreed layering with apposition and separation of linear densities of vacuolated ground substance, which occurs in corneal dystrophy; the pleomorphic gray opacities are slightly basophilic, amorphous intraepithelial material under the corneal basement membrane, composed of a protein-polysaccharide matrix, and is seen in microcystic or map-dot dystrophy EM Amorphous fibrillo-granular material

fingerprint profile A type of 'mixed' or irregular cytoplasmic inclusions composed of ceroid/lipofuscin, appearing as short curved lamellations, seen by electron microscopy in juvenile lipofuscinosis (Batten-Spielmeyer-Vogt disease) CLINICAL Intellectual deterioration, progressive loss of motor function, ataxia and retinal pigmentary degeneration; death commonly by early adulthood TREATMENT None; see Curvilinear profiles; Fingerprint profiles may also be seen in peripheral lymphocytes or skin fibroblasts in amaurotic familial idiocy, fucosidosis, Hermansky-Pudlak disease, Jansky-Bielschowsky syndrome and Kufs' disease

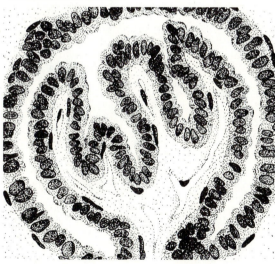

finger-in-glove appearance

Finnish congenital nephrotic syndrome An AR [MIM 256300] form of proliferative mesangial glomerulosclerosis that is frequent in Finns, often fatal, and associated with eclampsia and low birth weight PATHOGENESIS Absence of heparin sulfate anionic sites in the glomerular basement membrane with alteration of type IV collagen PATHOLOGY Microcystic changes in tubules at the corticomedullary junction and arteriolar hypertrophy TREATMENT None; Cf French congenital nephrotic syndrome

fire ant A non-winged hymenopteran arthropod of increasing importance in clinical medicine; the imported black fire ant, *Solenopsis saevissima richteri* and the imported red fire ant, *S invicta* are originally native to South America and have spread extensively in the south-eastern USA as they have no natural enemies; they are omnivorous, attacking livestock, crops and electrical insulation; the fire ant sting injects a venom causing a sterile pustule within 24 hours is typical (N Engl J Med 1994; 331:523RV) with intense burning and pruritus, due to the presence of necrotoxin or solenamine; the reactions range from a wheal-and-flare response, a sterile pustule to anaphylaxis-related death (32 have been reported); fire ant venom is 95% alkaloid with a small aqueous fraction containing soluble proteins Note: In contrast, the venom of wasps, bees and hornets is an aqueous solution containing proteins

firearm STATISTICS 330 000 deaths 1980-1989 (US); of 35 000 gun-related deaths in the US in 1989, 52% were suicides, 42% homicides; from 1960 to 1980, there was a 100% ↑ in homicide rate, and 150% ↑ in homicide by firearm; from 1933 to 1982, rate of suicides by firearms has ↑ 139% (Am Med News 16 Nov 1992 p3)

fireplace see PM_{10}, Wood smoke

fire wind Wind that is produced by air heated to 10^6°C by a nuclear explosion, which burns anything combustible, rising and sucking air into its vortex; the wind is most intense in metropolitan areas and less intense in rain see Nuclear war

first arch syndrome A sequence type of developmental embryopathy with anomalous development of the first branchial arch due to inadequacy of the stapedial artery, a function of maternal nutrition during early pregnancy CLINICAL Facial bone hypoplasia, including macrostomia, hemignathia and mandibular deformity

Note: These changes may be accompanied by hypertelorism, cleft lip and palate, deformities of the middle and inner ear or may accompany well-described clinical syndromes, eg Franceschetti-Klein, Goldenhar, Pierre-Robin and Treacher-Collin syndromes; see Sequence

first order kinetics The dynamics of a reaction system in which the rate of an enzyme reaction is determined by substrate concentration; this is difficult to define in closed systems since the rate changes as more substrate is consumed; see Michaelis-Menten equation; Cf Zero order kinetics

first pass elimination Presystemic elimination The rate at which circulating drugs are metabolized as they traverse the liver; first pass elimination kinetics assume the amount of parent drug arriving to the liver is proportional to its concentration in the circulation, and further assumes there is optimal blood flow, uncompromised hepatic function, free access of the drug to the liver's metabolic 'machinery', appropriate transportation by carrier molecules

first-pass radionuclide ventriculography CARDIOLOGY A technique in which there is a brief sampling of radionuclide data as the labeled bolus passes through the heart; it is assumed that the mixing of the label (usually ^{99m}Tc) with the blood is virtually complete and the changes in the count rates are directly proportional to volumetric changes; because all of the data is acquired in 8-10 cardiac cycles, the presence of rhythmic abnormalities would invalidate the data used to evaluate the right and left ventricles in terms of volumes, as well as systolic and diastolic function, and regional or global myocardial performance (eg myocardial infarction; Cf Equilibrium radionuclide ventriculography

First Responder EMERGENCY MEDICINE A person who has received > 40 hours of classroom instruction and clinical training in basic first aid and CPR; FRs include law enforcement officers, fire fighters, volunteer EMS (emergency medical service); FRs have basic emergency care equipment, oxygen and mask combinations, tools for extrication, and defibrillators; Cf EMT

first use syndrome An anaphylactoid reaction described in patients undergoing hemodialysis, which occurs with the first use of a dialyzer, attributed to various dialyzer substances or to residual ethylene oxide, which is used for sterilization (MMWR 1991; 40:147)

Fisch-Renwick syndrome A variant of Klein-Waardenburg syndrome characterized by congenital deafness, hypertelorism, high palatal arch, ocular heterochromia and a white forelock

Fish A 'high quality' source of protein and essential oil

HAZARDS OF FISH[1] 1) Fish oil Despite its cardioprotective effects, high levels of fish oil may cause nosebleeds due to impaired platelet function (J Pediatr 1990; 116:139) 2) Envenonation, see Ciguatera poisoning, Scombroid poisoning 3) Heavy metal poisoning, eg mercury, which concentrates up the food chain, especially in certain fish, eg tuna 4) Parasitosis, see Sushi

BENEFITS OF FISH[2] The beneficial effects of fish consumption are attributed to fish oil's omega-3 or n-3 fatty acids, including eicosapentanoic and docosahexanoic acids Note: Deep water trout has three-fold more n-3 oil than other fish; effects of fish oil on disease; fish oil's benefits may be a function of the length of the fatty acid acyl chain (C20 and C22) rather than polyunsaturation ATHEROSCLEROSIS n-3 oil inhibits production of platelet-derived growth factor (PDGF) in endothelial cell cultures; PDGF causes smooth muscle proliferation, a factor in atherogenesis, possibly related to free radical production CARDIOVASCULAR EFFECTS The incidence of myocardial infarcts in Danes and Americans is 10-fold greater than that of Greenland Eskimos, despite similar levels of dietary fat; Danes consumed twice the saturated fat and more n-6 polyunsaturated fat than Eskimos, who consumed 5-10 g/d of longchain n-3 polyunsaturated eicosapentanoic acid (C20:5n-3) and docosahexaenoic acid (C22:6n-3), essential fatty acids are concentrated up the food chain from phytoplankton to fish to marine mammals Note: ↑ consumption of fish from 1-2 to 5-6 servings/week does not substantially ↓ the risk of coronary heart disease in ♂ previously free of cardiovascular disease (N Engl J Med 1995; 332:977OA) DIABETES MELLITUS n-3 lipids prevent the insulin resistance induced in rats by non-'aquatic' fat (n-6 fat derived from vegetables and meats rather than fish), replacement of 6% of the vegetable oil with n-3 fish oil circumvents the insulin-resistance otherwise seen in the rats HYPERTENSION Marine oils are high in n-3 polyunsaturated fatty acids (PFA); salad oils are high in n-6 fatty acids; vegetable PFAs are reported to decrease platelet aggregation, vaso-occlusive events and blood pressure, evoking low-level decreases in both diastolic and systolic pressures, as well as decreasing the levels of thromboxane A_2 metabolites LONGEVITY When n-3 fish oil replaces corn oil or lard in the laboratory rodent diet, they live longer, have less atherosclerosis, arterionephrosclerosis and produce fewer autoantibodies

[1]Damned if you do [2]Damned if you don't

FISH Fluorescent in situ hybridization A technique for determining cell ploidy and for detecting the presence or absence of chromosome segments by evaluating interphase (non-dividing) nuclei; in FISH, fluoresceinated chromosome probes are used to perform cytological analysis and cytogenetic studies, and to detect intratumoral heterogeneity; FISH is a hybrid of three technologies, to wit cytogenetics, fluorescence microscopy, and DNA hybridization; in FISH DNA probes with fluorescent labels are applied to cell preparations on a slide; if the complementary DNA sequence is present, it binds to DNA and be detected under the microscope; FISH labels probes nonradioactively either directly with fluorochromes, or indirectly with biotin and fluorochrome-labeled avidin, with digoxeginin and fluorochrome-labeled anti-digoxeginin, or others; the use of multiple band-pass filters allows simultaneous viewing of numerous probes for different chromosomal sequences labeled with different fluorochromes;

FISH is of particular use in cytogenetic studies, where probes for particular chromosomes (eg chromosomes 13, 18, 21) or chromsomal regions (eg ABL and BCR genes in the Philadelphia translocation) can be used for the prenatal diagnosis of common aneuploidies or to detect early stages of lymphoproliferative disorders; FISH is still considered an investigational diagnostic tool by the FDA (CAP Today 4/1994) FISH is as sensitive as other analytical techniques, eg conventional cytology and flow cytometry, used to diagnose transitional cell carcinoma of the urinary bladder (Anal Quan Cytol Histol 1994; 16:1) the advantage of FISH is that it is simpler, less labor-intensive, and time-consuming (48 hours vs 2-3 weeks) than classic cytogenetics (karyotyping); FISH's major disadvantage is that only one question can be asked at a time, ie rather than asking 'global issues', eg what is the genetic composition of a population of cells, one determines whether there an extra chromosome 21

fish-eye disease A rare AD [MIM 136120] condition with intense corneal opacification and vague non-specific atherosclerosis-related cardiac disease LABORATORY ↓ HDL-cholesterol, ↑ triglycerides (2.8-4.0 mmol/L US: 250-350 mg/dl), ↑ cholesterol (8.7-13.8 mmol/L US: 340-540 mg/dl) PATHOGENESIS Defective esterification of free cholesterol into HD; Cf LCAT deficiency

Note: Similar corneal opacities occur in Tangier's disease and in combined apoA-I and apoC-III deficiency

fish facies A physiognomy characterized by antimongolic palpebral fissures, colobomata, fishmouth, total deafness and malformation of ears, fancifully likened to that of aquatic poikilothermic vertebrates; FF may be seen in mandibulo-facial dysostosis, Treacher-Collins syndrome and Franceschetti syndrome

fish flesh A descriptor denoting both the tactile sensation and gross appearance of mesenchymal tumors, seen in sarcomas, but also lymphomas and florid reactive lymphoid hyperplasia

fishhook sign RADIOLOGY An upwardly curved or J-shaped distal ureter, seen by cystography, characteristic of prostatic hypertrophy

fish-mouth deformity A facial deformity characterized by cleft lip or palate and accompanied by patellar dimples, supernumerary ribs, arachnodactyly, talipes equinovarus, cardiac malformations, hypoplastic external genitalia, hypotonia and seizures, findings typical of the Prader-Willi syndrome, as well as in the 18q- syndrome

fishmouth incision A wide horizontal incision made on the tip of the finger to provide drainage for a subungual abscess

fishmouthing CRITICAL CARE MEDICINE A clinical sign characterized by lower jaw depression with inspiration, an ominous sign of increasing medullary damage with apneic potential in the face of autonomic respiratory failure

fishmouth stenosis Buttonhole deformity CARDIOLOGY A flattened and stenosed mitral valve caused by fibrous bridging across valvular commissures, commonly associated with rheumatic heart disease

fish oil A product that enhances the immunosuppressive effects of cyclosporine in rats with heart transplants, and in these animals inhibits delayed hypersensitivity; fish oil also results in ↓ production of IL-1, IL-2, IL-6, TNF, and eicosanoids; cyclosporine-induced nephropathy is linked to ↑ production of thromboxane A_2, and leukotrienes C_4 and D_4; addition of 6 g of dietary fish oil to cyclosporine therapy in renal transplant victims reduces the rejection episodes, but appears to have no effect on survival (N Engl J Med 1993; 329:769OA) use of fish oil reportedly slows the progress of renal failure in IgA nephropathy (N Engl J Med 1994; 331:1105OA) see Fish

FISH probe Any of three different types (see alpha-satellite probe, chromosome painting probe, unique sequence probe) of fluoresceinated chromosome probes used in FISH (fluorescence in situ hybridization)

fish smell Fishy odor, see there

fish soup see Chicken soup

fishtail lesions OPHTHALMOLOGY Scattered pisciform yellow spots, seen in the optic fundus of young subjects with the autosomally inherited fundus flavimaculatus CLINICAL Bilateral, slowly progressive posterior pole degeneration, which overlaps with Stargardt's macular atrophy, and with time, causes a loss of visual acuity

fish tank granuloma An opportunistic infection by an 'atypical' mycobacteria, *M marinum,* after inoculation in contaminated fresh or salt water, that may occur in occupational exposure, and in *M avium-intercellulare-scrofulaceum* CLINICAL A solitary nodule develops at sites of abrasion (fingers and hands), later becoming indurated and ulcerated, resembling 'garden variety' cutaneous tuberculosis; occasionally developing satellite lesions, thus being clinically identical to the swimming pool granuloma

fish tapeworm *Diphyllobothrium latum* A tapeworm that parasitizes freshwater fish of temperate zones in the Northern hemisphere (*D pacificum* has been described in marine fish off Peru); the definitive hosts are humans, domestic pets and other mammals *D latum* is the largest known vertebrate tapeworm, measuring 10 meters in length with 4000 proglottids, the most distal of which disintegrate, releasing eggs into the feces that mature and hatch into ciliated coracium; the coracium are ingested by the first intermediate host, an aquatic arthropod, the copepod, which is then ingested by a second intermediate host, a freshwater fish, eg salmon, trout and whitefish; the eggs develop into procercoid larvae in the fish muscle and viscera and are eaten by man as raw fish and the cycle continues CLINICAL In general, infection is limited to one worm, causing CNS and GI symptoms, abdominal discomfort, weakness, loss of weight, malnutrition and megaloblastic anemia TREATMENT Niclosamide

fish vertebrae RADIOLOGY A descriptor for biconcave, fish-like vertebrae, resulting from infarction and central bone collapse secondary to thrombosis of the vertebral arteries, a finding typical of sickle cell anemia, which often occurs before the second decade; the peripheral perforating metaphyseal arteries are relatively spared, explaining the lesser involvement of the anterior and posterior faces of the vertebrum; fish vertebrae may also be seen in hereditary spherocytosis, homocystinuria, Gaucher's disease, osteoporosis and osteopenia, renal osteodystrophy or hyperparathyroidism, osteomalacia, and thalassemia major

Fisher, B see Poisson, R

Fisher's exact test STATISTICS A maneuver used in a four-fold contingency table for determining statistical independence, by providing the exact probability that the observed frequencies are statistically independent; Fisher's exact test is used when the number of samples or data points are small, and the chi-square method is not applicable

Fisher syndrome Ophthalmoplegia-ataxia-areflexia syndrome A variant of Guillain-Barré syndrome seen in middle-aged males after a viral infection of the upper respiratory tract CLINICAL Headache, fever, dyspnea, facial paralysis, and cerebellar ataxia; most resolve spontaneously within 3 months or progress to coma (**N Engl J Med 1956; 255:57**)

Fisher-Volavsek syndrome An AD condition characterized by syringomyelia, sparse facial and scalp hair, and thickened terminal digits

fishy odor A piscine odor described in wide variety of clinical conditions, eg vaginosis, caused by a newly described *Mobiluncus* genus, *Gardnerella vaginalis,* excretion of

trimethylaminuriae (due to large oral doses of L-carnitine, 'rotting' fish), di-*N*-butylamine, diethylamine, stools infected by *Vibrio cholera,* which have a 'rice-water' appearance, a rancid fish odor is described in tyrosinemia, which may occur in hereditary tyrosinosis (tyrosinemia type I) or in severe hepatic failure; see Odors

fisting A paraphilia (sexual deviancy) in which the closed hand (fist) is thrust into the rectum or further into the lower GI tract as a form of sexual gratification; the frequency with which this practice (largely confined to homosexual males) is associated with lesions in the form of mucosal tearing on the part of the fistee, or coliform dermatitis on the part of the fister is unknown, but is probably underreported

FITC Fluorescein-isothiocyanate A stable 'label' that binds both basic and acidic protein side chains at pH 8.0; FITC's absorption minimum is at 490-495 nm, and it emits its characteristic green color at 517 nm; FITC is a 'workhorse reagent' in immunology and is used to 'tag' proteins of interest and follow their movement in the cell or site(s) of deposition; it may be used clinically to evaluate complement and immunoglobulin deposits in 1) The skin in patients with vesiculobullous lesions and 2) The kidneys to detect immune complex deposition, both by direct immune fluorescence; see Flow cytometry, Immunofluorescence

fitness gadget A generic term for any device that is intended to convert a person's flab into firm muscle; FGs include rowing machines, treadmills, and proprietary devices, eg Dyna-bands, Nordic Track, Stairmaster, and Thigh Master; they are often purchased on impulse with the hope that one will obtain the advertised sleek physique sans travail (**N Y Times 29 March 1995, C1**)

fitness pyramid Exercise pyramid, see there

FIV Feline immunodeficiency virus A lentivirus that is similar to HIV-1 in many molecular and biochemical properties, which causes an immunodefiency state in cats that is similar to the five stages that occur in human AIDS (ie acute primary infection with generalized lyphadenopathy, an asymptomatic carrier state, persistent generalized lymphadenopathy, AIDS-related complex, and AIDS), making it an attractive model system for AIDS (**Nature Medicine 1995; 1:410**)

five day fever Trench fever, see there

five-factor model PSYCHIATRY A model that asserts that every personality has five dimensions that are heritable and relatively stable; these are neuroticism (worry or anxiety factor), extroversion (which contrasts with one's intrinsic introversion), openness (a function of one's flexibility and creativity), agreeableness (vis-á-vis other persons) and conscientiousness (versus one's own lack of discipline (from **N Engl J Med 1994; 330:1244BR**)

5p- syndrome Cri-du-Chat syndrome, see there

five Fs Food, fingers, fomites, flies, feces; a mnemonic for the most common mode of transmission of *Salmonella typhi*

fixed cost LABORATORY MEDICINE Any cost incurred regardless of whether a test is performed, including salaries of laboratory technicians, cost of an analyzer (with depreciation), service contracts, overhead including administration, and hospital charges (**Advance/Laboratory July/August 1994**) Cf Variable cost

fixed drug reaction A skin eruption of unknown pathogenesis that is more common in blacks, characteristically recurring at the same site each time a particular drug or a related congener is administered; the fixed reaction may also occur with chemically unrelated drugs or disappear with repeated administration of the same drug CLINICAL The FDR is a sharply circumscribed edematous red-brown or purplish plaque that may be surmounted by a bulla, most often located on the extremities, the hand and glans penis which with time becomes lichenified, scaly, and occasionally accompanied by hypermelanosis; common drugs and chemicals evoking the reaction include phenazone, barbiturates, sulfonamides, quinine, tetracycline, oxyphenbutazone, chlordiazepoxide, food dyes, toothpaste and mothballs PATHOLOGY Erythema multiforme-like changes, including hydropic degeneration of basal cell layer, pigmentary incontinence, and scattered dyskeratotic keratinocytes

fixed effects model STATISTICS A restrictive statistical regression formulation known as the covariance model, which is equivalent to including a dummy variable with each sample of a population (see N Engl J Med 1992; 326:305sa)

'fixover' SURGICAL PATHOLOGY A colloquial term for a specimen that is not processed on the day of surgery as it requires fixation in formalin prior to cutting, eg fatty tissue, in particular breast, or large specimens from the GI tract, which if sectioned prematurely are associated with 'rolling' of the mucosa away from the muscularis propria, making staging, ie evaluation of the depth of tumor invasion difficult; in contrast, some tissues, eg uterine leiomyomas become 'hardened' by prolonged fixation and brittle to cutting by a microtome

FK506 Tacrolimus, see there

FKBP FK 506 binding protein A rotamase enzyme and receptor for FK 506 and rapamycin (Science 1991; 252:836); FKBP's amino acid sequence is similar or identical to that of protein kinase C (Nature 1991; 351:195c)

flabby heart An atonic, dilated and fat-laden heart characteristic of *Corynebacterium diphtheriae*-induced myocarditis; the flabbiness of the heart is attributed to a diphtheria exotoxin that interferes with a translocating enzyme responsible for elongation of polypeptide chains; the same exotoxin inhibits carnitine metabolism, thereby interfering with the oxidation of long-chain fatty acids, with the consequent accumulation of triglycerides in the cardiac muscle

'flag' LABORATORY MEDICINE A determined value on a diagnostic test at or above which a certain action is taken; eg fasting glucose > 7.8 mmol/L (US: > 140 mg/dl), is a flag for notifying the attending physician; see Decision level, Panic value, Red flag

flagella The organelle responsible for bacterial locomotion; the average bacterial flagella measures 10-30 µg in diameter, and is best seen with a modified Leifson stain; flagella are classified according to location on the bacterium: peritrichous, polar and mixed; like eukaryotic cilia, prokaryotic flagella have the characteristic 9 + 2 arrangement of fibrils; Cf Cilia

flagellin A fibrous bacterial protein, which is the major component of flagella and which has structural homology with keratin, myosin and fibrinogen

flag sign CLINICAL NUTRITION The finding of sharply demarcated alternating bands of pigmented and depigmented hair, evidence of intermittent malnutrition, seen in kwashiorkor and marasmus type of malnutrition, or rarely, associated with chemotherapy, eg methotrexate

flail chest TRAUMATOLOGY The result of multiple anterior rib fractures; for 'flailing' to occur, there must be a two-point fracture involving at least two adjacent ribs; these fractures are usually symptomatic if four or more ribs are involved in one hemithorax; this causes instability of a large area of the anterior chest wall, paradoxic movement during inspiration, ie the free-floating 'flailed' part moves inward as the chest expands, in response to the negative intrathoracic pressure; the extent and location of the fractures determines the adequacy of ventilation, ranging from asymptomatic to severe dyspneic; hypoxemia is common, but not hypercapnia or alveolar hypoventilation; when conscious, the patient may 'splint' the involved region, causing the examiner to pass over the lesion; the inability to maintain adequate ventilation in concert with the paradoxic (and ineffective) respiratory effort and atelectasis, hypoxia and hypercapnia develop; posterior flail segments are less of a concern as the muscles and scapula provide 'scaffolding', and patients lie on their backs, supported by the mattress; flail chest is most often secondary to motor vehicle accidents or aggressive cardiopulmonary resuscitation

Flake maneuver EMERGENCY MEDICINE A variation of the Heimlich maneuver, in which the victim lies with his head down, eg on stairs and pumps his own diaphragm; the Heimlich maneuver has the considerable disadvantage of 1) Requiring two people to perform and 2) May worsen the situation by causing the food to pop up, then sink even further down the trachea as the patient gasps for air; Cf Cough CPR, Heimlich maneuver

'flaky paint' dermatitis A dermatopathy characterized by irregular, dry, hyperkeratotic, hyperpigmented psoriasiform lesions located on the face, extremities and perineum that may become excoriated and infected, seen in Kwashiorkor

flame cell Thesaurocyte A plasma cell with intensely eosinophilic (flaming) cytoplasm containing glycoprotein globules; although these cells were initially considered specific for IgA myelomas, flame cells also occur in Waldenström's macroglobulinemia and the leptomeningitis of African trypanosomiasis adjacent to clusters of neutrophils; Cf Mulberry cells, which are cytologically similar, although the material is membrane-bound

flame figure DERMATOPATHOLOGY Aggregates of smudged necrobiotic material from decomposed eosinophilic granules and nuclear debris and collagen, seen in eosinophilic cellulitis or Wells syndrome (Acta Derm Venereol (Stockh) 1986; 66:213) CLINICAL Episodic waves of pruritic cutaneous tumefactions (and eosinophilia) spreading over the body for 2-3 days, resolving within 1-2 months

flame photometry A laboratory technique used to identify elements, eg Na^+, K^+, Li, Ba^{2+}, Ca^{2+}, in the 5-100 ppm range in a solution, where a fluid of interest is atomized and sprayed into a flame produced from a mixture of gases including oxygen, hydrogen, natural gas and acetylene; the emission spectrum is analyzed as the electrons excited by the flame fall to a lower energy level

flame-shaped lesion Splinter lesion A hemorrhage in the nerve fiber layer of the optic fundus, seen in grade III hypertensive retinopathy, which resolves 4-6 weeks after acute hypertensive crisis, and may occur in anemia, leukemia, arteriolosclerotic retinopathy and DM

Note: Dot and blot hemorrhages, cotton-wool spots and waxy exudates are fundoscopic findings also seen in grade III hypertension

flammable aerosol A chemical substance or mixture that is dispensed as a mist, spray, or foam by a propellant under pressure and which under certain test conditions yields a flame projection of ≥ 4.6 cm (18 inches), at full valve opening, or a flash-back at any valve; see Flammable material

flammable gas A gas which, at atmospheric temperature and pressure, forms a flammable mixture with air when present at 13% or less; see Flammable material

flammable limits in air OCCUPATIONAL SAFETY The range (lower and upper limits) of concentrations of a flammable vapor or gas that will burn or explode or burn if an ignition source is present; the lower concentration is of particular interest, as it helps determine the volume of ventilation required in an enclosed space to prevent fires and explosions; a material's FLIA is of interest to OSHA, which requires listing of FLIAs in its Materials Safety Data

Sheets‡

flammable liquid A liquid with a flashpoint below 37.8ºC (100ºF); see Flammable material

flammable material OCCUPATIONAL SAFETY A chemical that can be ignited, including flammable aerosols, flammable gases, flammable liquids, and flammable solids; in the US the use of FMs in the workplace is monitored by OSHA

flammable solid A non-explosive solid that can be ignited by friction, absorption of mixture, spontaneous chemical change, or from heat absorbed from manufacturing procedures or other processing, or which can be easily ignited, and when ignited will continue to burn or to be consumed after removal of the source of ignition; see Flammable material

flanking DNA Any fragment of DNA that is immediately adjacent, either upstream or downstream of a DNA segment of interest

flap PLASTIC SURGERY A pedicle of tissue, used to cover a defect, usually of the skin; flaps are cut in such a way as to leave a well-vascularized base of the 'peninsula', and sewn at the site of the defect, allowing time for the free end to become vascularized before separating the tissue from the 'donor' site

flapping tremor Asterixis, Icarus sign HEPATOLOGY An abnormal, involuntary jerking tremor of wide amplitude elicited upon dorsiflexion of the pronated wrist and spreading of extended fingers; in full-blown flapping, there is abrupt flexion of the fingers at the metacarpophalangeal joint and flexion of the wrist, occurring asynchronously with each other every few seconds, due to exaggerated reflexes; bilateral flapping is quasi-pathognomonic for metabolic, often alcohol-related, hepatic encephalopathy seen in end-stage (post-fibrotic) cirrhosis due to ↑ blood ammonia NEONATOLOGY Coarse bilateral tremors, accompanied by limb rigidity, hyperreflexia, resistance to flexion and extension, described in infants born to heroin-addicted mothers who undergo 'withdrawal' at birth

flare OPHTHALMOLOGY A 'spume' of translucent proteins in the aqueous humor, appearing as a whitish shadow as a beam of light traverses the anterior chamber, the intensity of the flare is a function of the amount of protein in the anterior chamber, being faintly visible in the normal eye and prominent in anterior uveitis, accompanied by conjunctival hyperemia, inflammation and posterior corneal keratinization, congestion of the iris, neovascularization and band formation; see Band keratopathy RHEUMATOLOGY An acute exacerbation of the symptoms and disease activity of SLE LABORATORY ↑ (anti-)double-stranded DNA antibodies, plasma C3a, serum complex of complement 5b-9 and plasma Bb and ↓ serum levels complement C3 and C4 UROLOGY A worsening of clinical disease seen in the early stages of hormonal manipulation for metastatic prostate carcinoma; therapeutic gonadotropin-releasing hormone analog, eg buserelin, down-regulates the pituitary-gonadal axis and within one week of therapy, plasma levels of gonadotropin and later testosterone and dihydrotestosterone fall to castration levels; 'flare' affects 10% of patients in the first week of therapy, and is attributed to a surge in plasma gonadotropin and androgen levels, manifested by ↑ prostatic acid phosphatase levels, worsening of clinical symptoms and possibly, death; an anti-androgenic agent nilutamide (RU 23908) may prevent this complication

flare phenomenon NUCLEAR MEDICINE Pseudo-enlargement of tumor masses, in which a temporary increase in the radioisotope uptake by radionuclide scanning in advanced prostatic carcinoma may accompany the early stages of successful treatment; the flare phenomenon invalidates bone scans as follow-up vehicles in tumors with osteoblastic metastases

flash point OCCUPATIONAL SAFETY The temperature at which the vapors from a volatile liquid will ignite spontaneously; the FP is determined by either the open cup, or preferably the closed cup method, which differ from each other by a few degrees; the FP is a datum of interest to OSHA, which requires listing of FPs in its Materials Safety Data Sheets‡

flashback Hallucinogen persisting perception disorder SUBSTANCE ABUSE An involuntary recurrence of some aspect of an hallucinatory experience or perceptual distortion, often with negative overtones and accompanied by fear and anxiety; flashbacks are a classic adverse effect of psychedelic drugs, eg LSD and PCP that occur days to weeks after the last dose; flashbacks are most common in heavy users and disappear with time; the term also refers to non-drug-related repetition of frightening experiences or images, as may affect ex-soldiers, as is well-described in veterans of the Vietnam conflict

---

-FLASHBACK-HALLUCINOGEN PERSISTING PERCEPTION DISORDER (292.89*)

A The re-experiencing, after discontinuation of use of a hallucinogen, of 1+ perceptual symptoms experienced while intoxicated with the hallucinogen, eg geometric hallucinations, flashes of colors, macropsia, micropsia, and others

B Symptoms in A cause clinically significant distress or impairment of social, occupational, or other form of important function

C Symptoms are not due to a general medical condition, or otherwise accounted for another mental disorder

*DSM-IV™ American Psychiatric Association, Washington, DC 1994

---

flask-shaped heart A heart with an enlarged, water-bottle shaped cardiac silhouette, with loss of the usual 'signature' of the chambers when seen on a plain chest film, a finding characteristic of marked pericardial effusion

flask-shaped lesions Erlenmeyer flask deformity, see there

flat chest syndrome Straight back-flat chest syndrome, see there

flat face A non-specific group of facial dysmorphias of variable intensity characterized by attenuation of the malar prominences and a broadening of the facies, which may be due to achondroplasia, Apert, arteriohepatic dysplasia, camptomelic dysplasia, chondrodysplasia punctata (Conradi-Hunermann type, Down syndrome, Escobar syndrome, Kniest dysplasia, Larsen syndrome, lethal multiple pterygium syndrome, Marshall syndrome, partial 10q syndrome, rhizomelic chondrodysplasia, Stickler syndrome, trisomy 20p syndrome, XXXXX syndrome, XXXXY syndrome, Zellweger syndrome

flat foot Pes planus A common orthopedic complaint affecting many age groups; true flat feet are uncommon; often the parent will perceive flattening of the foot when a child first ambulates; laxity of the ligaments may result in collapse of the foot with valgus on the hindfoot and eversion or pronation of the forefoot; a valgus deformity of > 10% requires therapy; often a shoe will suffice as therapy; acquired flat feet may be

1) Ligamentous, due to tendino-ligamentous trauma

2) Muscular, due to poor control or incoordination, as in poliomyelitis or cerebral palsy

3) Osseous, due to trauma or degeneration and

4) Postural, due to internal tibial torsion as occurs in obesity, muscle fatigue, faulty footwear and footwork and

arthritis; flat feet are divided into four grades of disability, ranging from mere strain or tenderness to osseous rigidity: the peroneal spastic flatfoot variant is commonly due to abnormal coalescence between two or more tarsal bones, often at the calcaneocuboid, calcaneonavicular and talocalcaneal bars

'flat line' A colloquial term for complete lack of cerebral activity as measured by electroencephalography, a finding that is equated with 'brain death'; by extension, a 'flat liner' is a patient with a flat line; see Harvard criteria, Persistent vegetative state

flatulence Physicians rarely regard excess flatus rationally; one 'xylophonist' with numerous, noisy and noisome events (N Engl J Med 1976; 295:261) meticulously recorded a production of 35 detonations/day (control population, 13 events/day); despite use of antibiotics, simethicone, charcoal and *Lactobacillus acidophilus*, the fanfare of the flatteur's fecal flora continued unabated; gas chromatography revealed: CO_2 44%, H_2 38%, N_2 17%, O_2 1.3% and CH_4 0.3%, a production that partially responded to lactose elimination; borborygmi are associated with legumes (chick-peas, lentils, navy, string and soy beans, which contain indigestible polysaccharides with raffinose, stachyose and verbascose side chains, rendered digestible by soaking in water), nonabsorbable carbohydrates, eg fruits, vegetables, lactose, wheat, cryptococcal infection, and iron and vitamin E deficiencies; in most subjects, methane production is low, but increases dramatically in colon carcinoma, reflecting a change in the colonic flora (flatulographic screening assays have a lower yield than occult blood testing) Note: H_2 and CH_4 are explosive gases, and detonation may occur (Am J Surg 1952; 84:514) during electrocauterization or colonoscopic polypectomies, disasters are prevented by using bowel 'preps' containing nonfermentable agents; see 'Downwind of matters gaseous' (Western J Med 1986; 145:502) TREATMENT A fabis abstinetis; gastric gas may respond to simethicone, intestinal gas to activated charcoal

flat waist sign The loss of concavity of the left cardiac border, seen on a plain antero-posterior chest film corresponding to a slight rotation of the heart anteriorly, to the right and obliquely, that accompanies the left lower lobe collapse of the lung

Flaviviridae A large group of small (40 nm in diameter) viruses with a single-stranded 10–11-kilobase positive-sense RNA genome housed in a central nucleocapsid surrounded by a lipid envelope; the entire flaviviral life cycle occurs in the cytoplasm, without an intermediate DNA form; human flaviviruses include the dengue, Omsk hemorrhagic, St Louis encephalitis, West Nile, and yellow fever viruses (JAMA 1990; 263:3065)

Flavr Savr Antisense tomato A genetically engineered tomato produced by Calgene that is of broad interest as it is the first genetically engineered whole food to receive premarket scrutiny by the FDA , which ordinarily evaluates food additives; the Flavr Savr contains a two-part antisense gene construct; the gene of interest is blocked by one of the antisense constructs that encodes polygalacturonase (PG), which when active dissolves pectin, a polypeptide that imparts firmness to tomatoes, because the antisense constructs block PG production, the tomato can stay on the vine until ripe and flavorful but remains hard (for shipping); FDA's concerns about the safety of the kanamycin-resistance gene (*kan-r*) portion of the construct have been addressed; which is merely a marker to identify the presence of the gene (Bio/Technology 1994; 12:433c)

flea A wingless blood-sucking member of the order Siphonaptera, measuring 1-4 mm, vectors of the bubonic plague and rickettsial disease; fleas of medical interest include the human flea (*Pulex irritans*), oriental rat flea (*Xenopsylla cheopis*), and water flea (Cocepod)

flea-bite appearance A descriptor for multiple punctate hemorrhages of various sites, eg GI tract, a descriptor for the endoscopic findings of multiple lesions of KS within the lumen

'flea-bite' dermatitis Erythema toxicum, see there

'flea-bite' encephalitis A circumscribed influenza-induced hemorrhagic leukoencephalitis, with macroscopic cortical petechiae likened to flea bites

flea-bitten kidney A descriptor for the petechial hemorrhages and microinfarctions seen on the renal cortical surface, which are characteristic of malignant hypertension, arising secondary to thrombosis in the arcuate and interlobular arteries; the flea-bitten appearance has also been described in SLE, polyarteritis nodosa, leukemia and lymphoma

flecainide CARDIOLOGY An antiarrhythmia agent that has fallen into disfavor after the CAST trials demonstrated a 3.5-fold greater incidence of death due to arrhythmia in the treated subjects than those 'treated' with placebo (N Engl J Med 1991; 324:781); Cf CAST, Encainide

fleck dystrophy OPHTHALMOLOGY A hereditary (with various AR and AD patterns of transmission) condition characterized by bilateral variably sized, white-gray, wreath-like and non-progressive transcorneal opacities that do not interfere with vision Note: Family members may have other corneal abnormalities, atopy and pseudoxanthoma elasticum PATHOLOGY Swollen vacuolated keratinocytes filled with complex lipids and acid mucopolysaccharides

fleckmilz German, spotted spleen A spleen with a mosaic or 'shower' of scattered 1-5 mm in diameter yellow-white lesions, caused by septic infarcts, secondary to acute infections, which induce acute vasculitis and splenic vessel thrombosis and uremia PATHOLOGY Infarcted areas are bound by palisaded histiocytes and the vessels are 'cuffed' with lymphocytes

Fleck phenomenon Focal aggregation of cytologically similar leukocytes that may be seen in fever, pregnancy, inflammation, epilepsy, anaphylactic shock, cerebral edema, and cerebrovascular accidents; the finding has no known significance but is important as it may simulate a lymphoproliferative process

flesh-eating bacteria A variant of *Streptococcus* group A, which cause Toxic shock-like syndrome, see there, aka Jim Henson's disease

fleur-de-lis A stylized iris, used in heraldry to denote French royalty, and in medicine in reference to a trefoil pattern ORTHOPEDICS A stenotic pattern due to impingement of lumbar spinal canal by laminar fibrosis accompanied by anterior and posterior bony overgrowth PULMONARY PATHOLOGY A pattern of involvement of the pulmonary parenchyma seen in *Pseudomonas* pneumonia, which affects the terminal airways with a striking alternation between whitish necrotic and dark red hemorrhagic zones

FLEX exam Federal licensing exam An examination required of physicians who are licensed to practice medicine in the USA, consisting of a three day, written multiple-choice examination, which assesses a physician's knowlege in 'basic' and 'clinical' sciences

flexibility SPORTS MEDICINE The range of motion of a joint(s) as influenced by muscles, tendons, ligaments, bones, and periarticular structures; flexibility is influenced by age, sex (♀ are generally more flexible), and previous level and type of activity

Flexner report A study of US medical schools conducted by A Flexner in the early 1900s and commissioned by the Carnegie Foundation, which was largely responsible for the reform of medical education, in which an orientation towards research and education led to appointment of full-time faculty dedicated to the furtherance of medical science (JAMA 1991; 265:1555, see N Engl J Med 1993; 328:362BR)

Flexner-Wintersteiner rosette NEUROPATHOLOGY A structure that is virtually pathognomonic for well-differentiated retinoblastomas, consisting of 'bland' primitive round tumor nuclei arranged around a fibrillary background of axonal material

flexometry SPORTS AND REHABILITATION MEDICINE The measurement of joint flexibility in which a flexometer is strapped to the appropriate body segment, and the range of movement with respect to the perpendicular is determined (JC DeLee, D Drez, Jr, Eds, Orthopedic Sports Medicine WB Saunders, Philadelphia, 1994) Cf Goniometry

FLI1 A gene located on chromosome segment 11q24 that is the human counterpart of the murine *fli-1* gene (Friend leukemia virus integration site-1), which belongs to the *ETS* family of proto-oncogenes (Diagn Mol Pathol 1993; 2:141)

flight of ideas PSYCHIATRY A virtually continuous flow of accelerated speech in which a person abruptly changes from one to another topic, usually based on understandable associations; in extreme FOI, the speech is disorganized or incoherent (DSM-IV)

flip angle MRI The amount of rotation of the macroscopic magnetization vector produced by an RF pulse with respect to the direction of the static magnetic field; see Magnetic resonance imaging

flip-flap PLASTIC SURGERY A popular single-stage procedure for the repair of hypospadias; an incision is made in the glans and penile shaft; another incision releases the prepuce and a flip-flap of skin and soft tissue is molded to the distal urethra

flip-flop COMPUTERS A simple electronic logic circuit; a simple flip-flop is known as a toggle, where the input flips the toggle to 0 or 1; flip-flop devices may be connected to each other to yield complex circuitry MEMBRANE BIOLOGY The rotation of a transmembrane molecule through the lipid bilayer (membrane) at a 180° angle, such that the exterior portion of the molecule faces the cytoplasm or vice versa HEMATOLOGY A process in which active binding sites for PF-3 (platelet factor 3) are translocated from the internal to the external surface of the platelet membrane, an event that is abrupt and is activated by traces of collagen and thrombin

flippase MOLECULAR BIOLOGY A protein integral to certain biological membranes, eg endoplasmic reticulum that catalyzes the movement of small phospholipids through the lipid bilayer

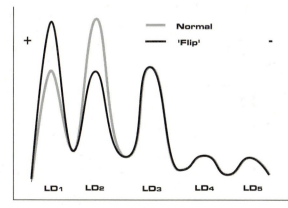

LDH 'flip'

'flipped' LDH CARDIOLOGY An inversion of the ratio of lactate dehydrogenase (LD) isoenzymes LD_1 and LD_2; LD is an enzyme composed of H and/or M subunits; LD_1 is a tetramer of four H (heart) subunits, is the predominant cardiac LD isoenzyme and migrates more rapidly at pH of 8.6 than LD_5, a tetramer of M subunits that is present in high concentrations in liver and skeletal muscle (tissues with predominantly anaerobic metabolism) Note: LD_2, LD_3 and LD_4 are present in differing amounts in other non-muscle tissues; normally the LD_1 peak is less than that of the LD_2, a ratio that is inverted (flipped) in 80% of myocardial infarcts within the first 48 hours; less common causes of LD flipping are: Renal infarcts, hemolysis, hypothyroidism and gastric carcinoma

flirting PSYCHOLOGY A behavior manifest in humans, in particular females, that is a nonverbal template used by Homo sapiens to attract and approach a prospective mate; according to some anthropologists and ethologists, flirting shares much in common with the courtship rituals of lower animals, in particular primates; the 'opening move' in flirting consists of the nonverbal message, 'notice me', which includes such behaviors as parading through a crowded room, walking with the hip swaying, and coy looks away from the 'target' male, once eye contact has occurred (New York Times 14 Feb1995; C1)

'FLK' Funny-looking kid PEDIATRICS A highly colloquial descriptor for non-specific facial dysmorphias that may be accompanied by growth and/or mental retardation; the term arose in the US in the 1950s and has been used in reference to children with facial features that are not typical of any particular condition

Note: The term is strictly confined to clinical parlance as there are no citations in the English language literature referring to 'funny-looking kids', presumably because of its derogatory nature

'float' *noun* A skilled and responsible person, eg house staff officer, resident physician or supervisory nurse, who 'floats' about an institution addressing various concerns, assuring continuity of care, allowing for breaks and relief of personnel

'floater' FORENSIC PATHOLOGY A popular term for a body that rises as a result of bacterial putrefaction and gas production, which is often accompanied by a malodorous nauseating stench; putrefaction is more rapid in fresh, stagnant water, slower in salt water and may not occur in very cold water Note: As a general rule, if there is no air trapped in the clothing, dead bodies sink HISTOLOGY Extraneous tissue fragments inadvertently introduced onto a histological glass slide of material from person B, which is derived from paraffin-embedded material floating on a water bath from patient A; floaters constitute a serious problem in surgical pathology, and may be classified according to the tissue processing step in which they are introduced into the diagnostic material or histologic slide: 1) Cutting board 'metastasis' Knife blade metastasis A cluster of malignant (or 'foreign') cells or tissue introduced at the time of initial gross (macroscopic) examination into a specimen being processed for histologic evaluation; these artefacts are usually 'carry-overs' from a malignant (or other) lesion being examined on the cutting board or on the gross examiner's knife immediately preceding the specimen with the 'metastasis' SOLUTION clean grossing instuments carefully between specimens 2) Embedding floater A cluster of malignant (or foreign) cells or tissue that is introduced into a specimen being processed for histologic evaluation at the time of embedding the tissue in paraffin SOLUTION None, see below 3) Water bath floater A cluster of malignant (or foreign) cells or tissue erroneously introduced into a specimen as the tissue ribbon is cut with a microtome from the paraffin block, floated on the water bath and picked up on the glass slide SOLUTION Cut deeper levels of tissues, the artifact is usually only on one level; in a certain percentage of cases, immunostains to the ABH blood group antigens can be used to identify tissues that do not belong to the patient (Arch Pathol Lab Med 1994; 118:293oa)

*While the term 'metastasis' is easily understood in this context, it indicates origin from a malignant lesion, and thus is not entirely correct, as not all cell and tissue floaters are malignant; placental villi may occasionally 'metastasize' into decidualized endometrial tissues from ♀ with ectopic pregnancies-Author's note

'floaters' Muscae volitantes Proteinaceous aggregates within the vitreous humor of the eye, corresponding to degenerative changes

floating β-lipoprotein An abnormal VLDL containing excess triglycerides, which is seen in the ultracentrifuge serum fraction (density < 1.006 g/ml), which contains the pre-β VLDL-migrating band; floating β-lipoprotein bands are associated with familial dyslipoproteinemia (hyperlipo- proteinemia, type III), have a β mobility by serum protein electrophoresis, are smaller and heavier than VLDL and have a cholesterol:triglyceride ratio of > 0.3 (a criterion for diagnosing type III hyperlipoproteinemia) CLINICAL Flat xanthomas on palmar creases, nodular xanthomas of elbows, knees, tendons and trunk, coronary artery disease, and peripheral vasculopathy, due to a mutation in the apolipoprotein E gene, causing defective binding of apo-E to its hepatic membrane receptor, retarding the uptake and clearance of chylomicrons and VLDL TREATMENT Diet, weight loss

floating gall bladder An abnormally positioned gall bladder with increased peritoneal covering, a finding of no known pathological significance

floating teeth Marked osteolysis surrounding mandibular teeth, imparting a radiographic appearance of teeth levitating atop cystic loculations; floating teeth are classically described in circumscribed Langerhans' cell histiocytosis (histiocytoses X, ie Hand-Schüller-Christian disease and eosinophilic granuloma), but may appear in Burkitt's lymphoma and neuroblastomas

float nurse 'Float', see there

flocculation IMMUNOLOGY An immune reaction between antigen and certain antisera (antibody in solution) in which precipitation occurs over a narrow range of antigen-antibody ratios; the term was originally used to describe the 'H' precipitation test; the term flocculation has also been applied to aggregation of lipids, eg cardiolipin and others in the serological tests for syphilis, although the term 'agglutination' is preferred

flocculent densities 'Fluffy' dense patches within mitochondria, seen by EM in infarction and mercuric chloride intoxication, considered a sign of early cell death

floor A generic term for any non-emergent or non-urgent care ward for patient management

floor plate EMBRYOLOGY *Lamina ventralis* [NE3] A specialized group of midline neuroepithelial cells that regulates cell differentiation and axonal growth in the vertebrate nervous system, which is induced by local signals from the notocord

floppy baby syndrome A rare condition thought to be the most common manifestation of botulism in the US (± 100 cases/year), resulting from intestinal colonization and production of neurotoxin by *Clostridium botulinum*, a bacterium that may be found in commercial honey, which may account for one-third of cases CLINICAL Lethargy, weakness, feeble cry, failure to thrive, loss of head control and later flaccid paralysis TREATMENT Supportive; antibiotics, antitoxin, and guanidine have little effect PROGNOSIS 2% mortality

floppy head syndrome A non-specific condition characterized by isolated weakness of the neck musculature, affecting the oropharynx and/or shoulder girdle and upper trunk, which may be idiopathic or seen in myasthenia gravis, motor neuron disease, and polymyositis

floppy infant PEDIATRICS A generic term for any neonate with poor muscular tone and/or response to stimulation of extremities caused by a heterogeneous group of neuromuscular and musculoskeletal disorders (table)

FLOPPY INFANT CAUSES

BONE DISEASE Osteogenesis imperfecta, rickets

CNS Atonic diplegia, cerebellar ataxia, cerebral lipidosis, kernicterus, chromosomal defects, Lowe's oculocerebrorenal syndrome, Prader-Willi syndrome, Zellweger's cerebrohepatorenal syndrome, cerebral lipidosis

MUSCLE DISEASE Central core disease, glycogen storage disease type IIa (Pompe's disease), mitochondrial myopathies, muscular dystrophy, myotonic dystrophy, nemaline myopathy

NEUROMUSCULAR JUNCTION DISEASE Botulism, myasthenia gravis

PERIPHERAL NERVE DISEASE Familial dysautonomia, Guillain-Barre syndrome, Oppenheimer's amyotonia congenita, anterior horn cell diseases, polyneuritis, congenital sensory neuropathy

SPINAL CORD DISEASE Poliomyelitis, spinal cord trauma and tumors, transverse myelopathy, Werdnig-Hoffmann disease

NON-NEUROMUSCULAR DISEASE Endocrinopathies, metabolic disease, vitamin deficiencies

floppy valve syndrome Mitral valve prolapse syndrome, see there

florette giant cells Multinucleated giant cells, with marginally placed, often overlapping nuclei and an eosinophilic center, characteristic of pleomorphic lipoma, a benign tumor of the upper back, most common in older men

the Florida dentist see Acer cluster

flotation method PARASITOLOGY A simple method for isolating parasite eggs, devised in 1906; when shaken with water, feces sink, hookworm and other parasite eggs float

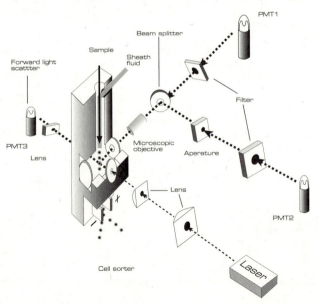

flow cytometry LABORATORY MEDICINE A procedure based on laser-induced excitation and fluorescence of cells that have been labeled with monoclonal antibodies raised against cell surface and intracellular antigens, and tagged with fluorochrome markers; the cells can be sorted by size, intensity, and type of fluorescence, and the DNA ploidy analyzed; see Backscatter, FACS, FALS; the clinical uses of the flow cytometer include

DIAGNOSIS OF CLONAL EXPANSION Marked increase of cells displaying only one set of surface or cytoplasmic markers confirms the presence of a monoclonal lymphoproliferation; Cf Gene amplification

MONITORING OF IMMUNE STATUS The helper:suppressor ratio, a measure of the ratio of the helper subset of T lymphocytes (CD4) to suppressor T lymphocytes (CD8), is a commonly used parameter in AIDS patients for titrating the dose of zidovudine; see Helper: suppresspor ratio

ANALYSIS OF DNA PLOIDY In general, more anaplastic tumors are more aggressive and display greater aneuploidy; see Ploidy analysis

DETERMINATION OF GROWTH CHARACTERISTICS OF A CELL POPU-LATION, a benchmark for aggression is the percentage of cells in the S1 growth phase (Anal Quan Cytol Histol 1993; 15:195)

flower remedy Bach remedy ALTERNATIVE MEDICINE A form of alternative health care in which flower are used to '...*directly address a person's emotional state to ...facilitate both psychological and physiological wellbeing...balancing negative feelings and stress, flower remedies can ...remove the emtional barriers to health and recovery.*' (Alternative Medicine, Future Medicine, Puyallup, WA, 1994) FRs consist of an infusion prepared from freshly picked sun-exposed flowers placed in spring water and brandy, which forms a so-called 'Mother Essence'; see Alternative medicine

The most widely used of the FRs is Dr Bach's Emergency Stress Formula, which is alleged to have a tranquilizing effect in acute situations, including anxiety, asthma, bereavement, hysteria, migraines, physical trauma, and when applied topically to be of use in bruises, burns, cuts, and insect bites; there is little peer-reviewed data to support the health benefits claimed by FR enthusiasts

flowerette appearance see Pilot's wheel appearance

flower-petal pattern A fanciful descriptor for the pattern of fluorescein leakage out of the vessels in cystoid macula, seen shortly after injection in a retinal angiogram in endogenous uveitis

fluconazole Diflucan® INFECTIOUS DISEASE An antifungal agent that has advantages over amphotericin B, the previous therapeutic mainstay, as it is far less toxic, has both oral and parenteral formulations, and is more effective in treating mucosal candidiasis; in patients without neutropenia and/or major immunodeficiency, amphotericin B and fluconazole are equally effective (N Engl J Med 1994; 331:1325OA); it is regarded by some workers as the antifungal agent of choice for cryptococcal meningitis and local or systemic candidiasis in AIDS patients; it has a long serum half-life and good penetration of CSF (N Engl J Med 1991; 324:580) WARNING Fluconazole is linked to nondose-related hepatotoxicity ADVERSE EFFECTS Occur in 16%, eg nausea, headache, skin rash; see *Candida krusei*

fludarabine ONCOLOGY A fluorinated purine analogue of vidarabine with a phosphate molecule attached to the arabinose moiety that is used to treat chronic lymphocytic leukemia; it requires phosphorylation for activation, is a substrate for DNA polymerase and when incorporated into growing DNA chains, inhibits further chain elongation; F also decreases the pool of intracellular nucleotides by inhibiting ribonucleotide reductase; in vitro, F induces morphologic and biochemical changes in the lymphocytes of CLL, causing them to re-enter the cell cycle and undergo programmed cell death (apoptosis) (N Engl J Med 1994; 330:319OA, 1828C)

fluffy infiltrate Patchy perihilar parenchymal infiltrates on a plain chest film, which corresponds to alveolar lesions of well-advanced pulmonary sarcoidosis

fluid memory Short-term memory, see there

fluid mosaic model The Singer-Nicholson 'fluid mosaic' is

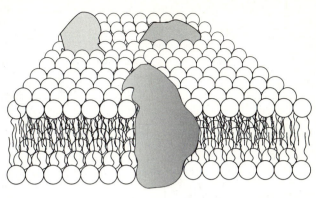

fluid mosaic model

the accepted model for cell membranes, which consists of a bilayer of phospholipids and glycolipids, with the hydrophilic portions of the molecules oriented either toward the exterior or interior of the cell, while the hydophobic lipid tails face the interior of the membrane; both amphipathic lipids and globular proteins are 'scattered' throughout the membrane, and its fluidity allows the relatively unrestricted lateral movement of the proteins, glycoproteins, receptors and other molecules embedded therein

fluid resuscitation The infusion of isotonic IV fluids to a hypotensive patient with trauma; for decades it had been standard practice in emergency medicine to administer fluids prior to stabilization and surgical control of bleeding; aggressive fluid resuscitation may disrupt thrombi, ↑ bleeding, and ↓ survival; in one report, delayed FR resulted in an ↑ survival (70% vs 62% in those receiving immediate FR), ↓ complication rate in terms of ARDS, acute renal failure, coagulopathy, wound infection, and pneumonia (23% vs 30%), and ↓ hospital stay (N Engl J Med 1994; 331:1105OC)

fluke A widely distributed family of Trematodes that infect man as either the definitive or accidental host, which includes genuses *Heterophyes, Metagonimus, Fasciola, Opisthorchis, Paragonimus, Schistosoma, Clonorchis*

fluorescein angiography OPHTHALMOLOGY A procedure for diagnosing chorioretinal disease, eg choroidal neovascularization, and light toxicity

fluorescence polarization A technique for studying molecular interactions; when fluorescent molecules are excited with polarized light, they emit polarized light in the same plane assuming the molecule being studied remains stationary during the period of excitation (4 nsec for fluorescein); if the molecule being studied rotates during the excited state, light will be emitted in a plane that differs from that of the plane of excitation; large fluorescently labeled molecules move little during the state of excitation, and what light is emitted continues to be highly polarized with respect to the plane of excitation; smaller molecules tend to rotate and the emitted light is depolarized relative to the plane of excitation; FP thus can be used to follow a biochemical reaction in which there is a change in the size of the reacting molecules, as with DNA-protein interactions, immunoassays, receptor-ligand interactions, and catalytic or degradation reactions ADVANTAGES Measurements can be made in real time without manipulation and can be performed in a single reaction phase (Am Biotech Lab September 1994 p 113)

fluorescence polarization immunoassay LABORATORY MEDICINE A highly sensitive homogeneous drug assay in which a drug of interest is linked to a fluorescent probe molecule; when a solution containing immune reactants is excited with polarized light, the fluorescent molecule will act as a fluorophore (ie it will emit polarized light) if it is 'stationary', ie not tumbling in solution, and locked in a complex with the drug and antidrug antibody

fluorescence recovery after photobleaching Fluorescence microphotolysis A method used to study the lateral movement of membrane-bound proteins and lipids in which a small area of a cell membrane is 'bleached' by light and the amount of time necessary for fluorescent marker-tagged proteins to reappear in the bleached site is a measurement of the cell membrane's fluidity

fluorescence spectrophotometry A powerful analytical tool with a sensitivity 2 orders of magnitude greater than traditional absorbance methods; in FS two wavelengths are used, one for excitation and one for emission, thus providing two spectra for a sample; a refinement of the technique is that of 3-D plotting in which 'fingerprints' of the analyte are produced; FS has been used to analyze materials as diverse as tamoxifen or the type of dye and cloth used in 1st Century BC; in the latter application, FS has the further advantage of being non-destructive (Am Biotech Lab Feb 1995, p22)

fluorescent microscopy A variant of light microscopy, in which a tissue or cell of interest is stained with a fluorochrome and illuminated by ultraviolet or short-wave visible light, eg by use of a laser; the light is projected onto the specimen by halogen-quartz, mercury or xenon lamps and re-emitted at another wavelength; FM thus contrasts with conventional microscopy as the tissue emits (fluorescent) light upon returning from an excited to a ground state; although many objects naturally fluoresce; the technique is used to detect the presence of antigens or antibodies PRINCIPLE A naturally fluorescing molecule, isothiocyanate (FITC) has a high affinity for the Fc fragment of immunoglobulins, which can be used to 'tag' a monoclonal antibody 'raised' against an antigen, 'X' of interest; if the antigen is present, the FITC tag allows detection in the tissue (the same principle is used in flow cytometry); FM is of use in 1) Detecting circulating autoantibodies 2) Differentiating vesiculo-bullous skin lesions 3) Delineating immune deposits in glomerulonephritides and 4) Karyotype analysis (quinacrine staining or 'Q-banding'); see Microscopy

fluoridation The addition of small amounts of fluoride to drinking water to reduce the incidence of cavities; although most data suggest that fluoridation reduces the incidence of caries, it remains unclear whether fluoride actually has this effect and soft data suggest possible carcinogenesis (Science 1990; 247:276); more than one-half of the US water supply has more than 0.7 ppm of fluoride, a level that is considered adequate to reduce the incidence of caries (JAMA 1991; 265:2934/FDA)

fluoride intoxication Fluoride poisoning, see there

fluoride poisoning TOXICOLOGY Excess fluoride may be fatal, given its affinity for calcium, notably causing one of the lowest serum calcium levels ever recorded, 0.85 mmol/L (US: 3.4 mg/dl) (Pediatrics 1976; 58:90) fluoride is present in some rodenticides, insecticides, fertilizers, industrial and anesthetic gases and may cause acute intoxication by inhalation (coughing, choking chills and fever), ingestion (nausea, vomiting, salivation, paresthesias, diarrhea and abdominal pain) or contact (hydrogen fluoride is similar to hydrogen chloride, causing severe, intense burns of the skin) fluoride-associated death may be either accidental or suicidal; acute intoxication can be due to excess in water supply (N Engl J Med 1994; 330:95oa) chronic fluoride poisoning results in weight loss, brittle bones, anemia, weakness, general ill health, and stiffness of joints; low level fluoride intoxication causes fluorosis

fluoroquinolone A member of a family of broad-spectrum antibiotics, eg ciprofloxacin HCl; see Quinolones

fluorosis Chronic fluoride poisoning A chronic low-level intoxication that occurs where the drinking water has fluoride in excess of 2 ppm CLINICAL Mottled enamel and chalky white discolored teeth that have a normal resistance to caries; fluorosis is common, given its availability in mouth rinses, toothpastes, the injudicious use of fluoride treatments

fluorocarbons see CFCs

fluorouracil 5-FU ONCOLOGY A pyrimidine antagonistic antimetabolite, derived from uracil that blocks demethylation of dUMP to dTMP, interfering with DNA synthesis, depriving DNA of functional thymidine; 5-FU is used in a wide range of malignancy, including carcinoma of the bladder and in terminal epithelial malignancies SIDE EFFECTS Bone marrow toxicity and mucosal inflammation

fluoxetine Prozac® A selective inhibitor of serotonin (5-hydroxy-tryptamine, that may also cause regional inhibition of dopamine synthesis) uptake approved by the FDA for treating clinical depression; during the early 1990s, Prozac gained popularity for treating non-FDA-approved conditions* and was viewed by some enthusiasts as a psychological panacea SIDE EFFECTS 5-30% experience side effects, including anxiety, nervousness, tremor, insomnia, diarrhea, nausea, anorexia, undesired weight loss, and sexual dysfunction Note: Fluoxetine inhibits CYP2D6, a liver cytochrome P-450 enzyme that is largely responsible for eliminating various drugs, is absent in 7% of the white population, explaining the increased side effects in some people being treated with Prozac; it is contradicted in those who also are receiving MAOI therapy (N Engl J Med 1994; 331:1354RV) as combination of these two agents may be fatal

*eg anxiety, binge eating, bulimia, obsessive-compulsive disorder, anorexia nervosa, obesity, panic disorder, diabetic neuropathy-associated pain, premenstrual syndrome, and alcohol abuse

flush method PEDIATRICS A method for obtaining the blood pressure in a restless infant; an appropriately-sized cuff is placed on the infant's upper arm or thigh and inflated until the skin blanches; the pressure is slowly released until a flush is seen; the pressure at the flush stage is slightly below that found by the direct auscultation method

flutter CARDIOLOGY A family of cardiac tachyarrhythmias **ATRIAL FLUTTER** occurs at 200-350 beats/min (with a 2:1 block, so that the ventricle fires at circa 150 beats/min); atrial flutter results from a circus pathway, occurs in atrial dilatation, primary myocardial disease or rheumatic heart disease and responds poorly to antiarrhythmic agents **VENTRICULAR FLUTTER** is characterized by a continuous and regular depolarization rate of greater than 200 beats/min and demonstrates high-amplitude zigzag pattern on the EKG, without clear definition of the QRS and T waves, a pattern that may revert spontaneously to a normal sinus rhythm or progress to ventricular fibrillation

FLV 23/A An AIDS drug derived from cyclohexane-based hexylene oxides, that was claimed in clinical trials to assist in a patient's recovery from AIDS (Nature 1990; 347:606n); FLV 23-A was used to treat children infected with HIV-1 in Romania; the trials were halted when the manufacturer failed to provide data regarding the drug's chemical formula, mechanism of action and efficacy

fly-catcher tongue NEUROLOGY A fanciful descriptor for the intermittent in-and-out darting of the tongue characteristic of tardive dyskinesia, a complication of chronic antipsychotic drug therapy; see Tardive dyskinesia

FMF Familial Mediterranean fever

FMG Foreign medical graduate, see there

Note: The 'politically correct' term is International Medical graduate

FMR-1 The gene responsible for the fragile X syndrome, see there

fMRI Functional magnetic resonance imaging

FNA Fine needle aspiration, see there

FNAB Fine needle aspiration biopsy, see there

FNAC Fine needle aspiration cytology, see there

FN-IMG Foreign national international medical graduate, see International medical graduate

foamy appearance A descriptor for the granular appearance of lymph nodes affected by lymphoma (a pattern described as more characteristic of T cell lymphomas), as seen by lymphography

foamy histiocyte Foam cell A generic term for a histiocyte filled with a wide variety of materials, in particular lipid, but also iron, and ceroid; in adults, lipid-laden foam cells in the vascular intima accompanied by injury of the microvasculature occur in 8% of patients with terminal atherosclerotic heart disease; morphologically identical cells are commonly seen in congenital lipid storage diseases, including cholesteryl ester storage disease, Farber's, Gaucher's, Niemann-Pick and Wolmann's diseases, Langerhans' cell histiocytosis (histiocytosis X), sea-blue histiocytosis, malignant histiocytosis, infectious mononucleosis, type I hyperlipoproteinemia, hyperlipemia, mineral lipidosis, DM, metachromatic leukodystrophy, thalassemia, sickle cell anemia, hypoplastic anemia, ITP, rheumatoid arthritis, corticosteroid therapy, ALL, AML, CML, and infections with *Mycobacterium leprae* or *Cryptococcus neoformans*

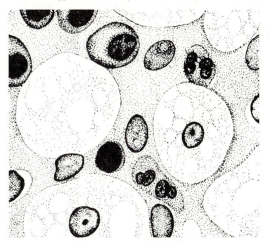

foam cells

foam stability index (test) Foam stability test, shake test OBSTETRICS A semiquantitative bedside test for determining fetal lung maturity, based on the stability of bubbles when amniotic fluid is shaken in test tubes with increasing concentrations of ethanol (which reduces the foaming or bubbling action of phosphatidyl choline, using 42% to 58% alcohol) in a series of amniotic fluid-filled test tubes; each is shaken vigorously; the higher the concentration of alcohol in which the bubbles are maintained, the more mature the lungs; see Surfactant

FOBT Fecal occult blood testing; see Occult bleeding

fodrin Non-erythrocyte spectrin A fibrous 475 kD actin-binding protein consisting of two similarly-sized subunits that is closely linked to CD45 (leukocyte common antigen) during leukocyte activation; fodrin mediates the association of actin filaments with the cell membrane and is structurally and functionally similar to spectrin, which cross-links adjacent actin bundles in the 'terminal web'

subjacent to the intestinal brush border; fodrin has been identified in leukocytes, sensory nerve cells, and keratinocytes

fogging RADIOLOGY Haziness or clouding of diagnostic X-ray films due to aging of unexposed film, or leakage of radiation or light prior to developing the films

foldase see Chaperonin

foldback DNA Any single-stranded DNA that folds upon itself and forms a hydrogen-bonded segment which is either a simple inverted repeat, ie a palindrome, aka hairpin DNA, or an interrrupted series of inverted repeats resulting in a structure known as stem-and-loop DNA, together forming cruciform DNA

'fold-lock-cut' PHYSIOLOGY A synthetic pathway for the production of the high-affinity conotoxins, a diverse family of venom peptides produced by the cone snail (*Conus geographicus* and others), which act on voltage-sensitive calcium channels, sodium channels, NMDA receptors, acetylcholine receptors and vasopressin receptors

folded lung syndrome Shrinking pleuritis with rounded atelectasis A condition that may be associated with asbestosis and pleural plaques RADIOLOGY see Comet tail sign PATHOLOGY Chronic fibrosing pleuritis, varying degrees of inflammation; asbestos fibers are conspicuously absent from the pleural plaque and effusions but may be seen in the subpleural lymphatic plexus

Foley catheter A pliable rubber catheter that is placed through the urethra and anchored in the bladder neck by an inflatable balloon, which can be left in place for prolonged periods

folie à deux PSYCHIATRY Shared psychotic disorder An exotic condition (297.3 in DSM-IV) in which two closely related people share a delusional system, eg a mother who believes her son to be a prophet of God, a belief shared by the son; '...*the essential feature...is a delusion that develops in an individual who is involved in a close relationship with another person* (the 'inducer', or primary case) *who already has a psychotic disorder with prominent delusions*' (Diagnostic and Statistical Manual of Mental Disorders, American Psychiatric Association, Washington, DC, 1994)

folie du doute PSYCHIATRY A manifestation of obsessive-compulsive disorder in which the person is constantly checking to determine whether he/she has performed a particular (compulsive) act

folk medicine Any system of health care practiced among the aborigines, see Ethnomedicine; Cf Alternative medicine

'folk' medicines Self-prescribed 'natural' drugs and products that are consumed in the US, and to a lesser degree in developed countries, by a segment of the population that has a categoric distrust of physicians and medical science and when sick, seek alternative therapeutic modalities, treating themselves with 'folk' or natural medicines, potentially causing significant co-morbidity, eg heavy metal poisoning with lead, mercury, arsenic and cadmium (JAMA 1990; 264:2212c); see Alternative medicine, Dolomite, Herbal medicine; Cf Unproven forms of cancer therapy

follicular lymphoma A heterogeneous group of lymphomas arising in follicular center cells, which comprises 50% of all non-Hodgkin's lymphomas in adults (US), more common in the elderly and distinctly uncommon in those under age 20 and in blacks; FLs are usually confined to lymph nodes, follicular lymphomas are histologically divided into those with predominantly small cleaved cells (large cells comprise < than 20% of cells), those with more than 50% large cells, and those with mixed, small cleaved and large cells MOLECULAR PATHOLOGY ± 85% are characterized by the t(14;18)(q32;q21) chromosomal translocation; the breakpoints involve the Ig heavy chain

(IgH) at 14q32[1] and the *bcl*-2 gene at q21[2] Note: The 8:14 translocation's accompanied by del 13q32 are more aggressive and may enter a leukemic phase DIAGNOSIS In one study, 115 cases were identified by LM, [104/115] by cytogenetic analysis and/or immunoglobulin gene rearrangements ,[91/102] by cytogenetics, [78/104] by Southern analysis, and [68/104] by PCR; the use of PCR in this clinical setting (using single primer sets for mbr and mcr) results in a high false negative rate (**Am J Clin Pathol 1995; 103:472oA**)

[1] Within the cluster of the joining segment J_H exons [2] Most commonly (60% of cases) in a major breakpoint region (mbr) located in the 3' untranslated segment of exon 3; in 20% of cases, in a minor cluster region (mcr) located > 20 kb in the 3' direction of the mbr

follicle lysis A finding by light microscopy consisting of invagination of small, mantle zone lymphocytes into and disruption of the germinal centers, which may be associated with hemorrhage; follicle lysis is a 'soft' histopathological criterion thus far unique to AIDS-related complex lymph nodes; see AIDS, Benign lymphadenopathy

follicular phase see Proliferative phase

follistatin A 30-35 kD glycosylated activin-binding protein (and activin antagonist in vitro) that is thought to function by presenting activins to their receptors; it is structurally distinct from inhibin but has similar activity, as both inhibit FSH release; follistatin is the binding site on the ovary for Activinfollistatin-deficient mice are growth-retarded, have ↓ mass of diaphragmatic and intercostal muscles, tight shiny skin, bone defects in the hard palate and ribs, apnea and death within a few hours of birth; follistatin appears to modulate the activity of other members of the transforming growth factor-β family, as the defects in these animals are more extensive than those seen in activin-deficient mice (**Nature 1995; 374:360**)

follow *verb* To maintain clinical surveillance on a patient

follow-up *noun* The constellation of future activities (eg return visits, imaging modalities) by a patient after hospitalization or therapy intended to ensure success return to a desired state health *verb* To participate in a follow-up

Fontan operation Fontan's procedure PEDIATRIC CARDIO-VASCULAR SURGERY A technique for functional correction of tricuspid valve atresia, eg to treat the hypoplastic left heart syndrome; the FO consists of anastomosis of the right atrium to the pulmonary artery, either directly, or via a conduit inserted to the outflow area of the right ventricle with closure of interatrial communication (eg atrial septal defect or foramen ovale); enteric protein loss is not a common comorbid process of FO (**Mayo Clin Proc 1994; 69:112oA**) see Hypoplastic left ventricle syndrome

food see Chinese restaurant, Ciguatera poisoning, Diet, Dietary fiber, Fats, Fish, Scombroid poisoning, Spicy food, Succotash, Sushi

food allergy A condition that is widely percieved to be a major health problem, the incidence of which (0.3-7.5%) has been obscured by controversial data and differing disease definitions; food-induced reactions of immediate-hypersensitivity type are well-recognized and include anaphylaxis, angioedema, and urticaria; food-induced reactions of delayed hypersensitivity type or those mediated by antigen-antibody complex formation is rarely documented, and includes a few specific reactions, eg gluten-sensitive enteropathy CLINICAL Edema and pruritus of oropharyngeal mucosae, followed by various responses in the GI tract as the offending and ultimately offensive content works through the system, including vomiting, colicky pain, abdominal distension, flatulence, diarrhea, and less commonly occult blood loss, malabsorption, protein-losing enteropathy, functional GI obstruction, and eosinophilic gastroenteritis DIAGNOSIS Diet (elimination or challenge, rotation, sublingual), in vivo (intradermal, multi-test, sublingual), and in vitro (IgE, IgG, IgG₄, RAST, cytotoxic, histamine release)

foodborne pathogen Any pathogenic organism for which the 'vector' is a comestible; although most pathogens are bacteria, eg *Listeria monocytogenes* (from dairy products) and *Vibrio* spp (from shellfish), parasites can waylay the owner of an adventuresome palate, classically sushiphiles

food irradiation PUBLIC HEALTH A generic term for the use of ionizing radiation (eg by ^{60}Co, or ^{137}Cs) to retard spoilage (1000 Gy prevents sprouting in potatoes, onions and garlic) and destroy pathogenic organisms (> 1000 Gy kills bacteria in cereals, poultry, frog's legs, and other foods) in foods without causing 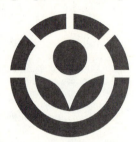 deleterious organoleptic or nutritional changes; as the process induces only a minimal ↑ in temperature, the qualities typical of raw unprocessed food are preserved; a major criticism of irradiated foods is that the effects of the chemical compounds produced during irradiation may themselves be toxic; low level irradiation is designated radurization, so named as it has the same effect as pasteurization, ie to improve shelf life and inactivate bacteria that cause food spoilage; higher dose irradiation of food intended to inactivate specific pathogens and parasites is termed radicidation; very high dose irradiation for producing commercial sterility is not commonly used, although it is approved and regarded in the same category as a food additive by the US FDA, which requires that foods so preserved carry a so-called radura label (figure) although irradiation is considered safe, irrational fears and mass hysteria prevent its broader use

food preservatives A group of chemical preservatives that the FDA classifies under a GRAS (generally regarded as safe) definition of food additive, first conceptualized in the 1958 Amendment to the FFD&C Act; GRAS preservatives include the antioxidants butylated hydroxyanisole (BHA) and butylated hydroxytoluene (BHT), propylparaben, sodium nitrate, sodium nitrite, benzoic acid, stannous chloride and others; see GRAS

food (diet) pyramid PREVENTIVE MEDICINE A diagrammatic representation (figure) promulgated by the US Department of Agriculture as an outline on the amounts of particular foods that should be consumed on a daily basis in a healthy diet (**USDA, Human Nutrition Information Service, Home and Garden Bulletin, number 252, August 1992**); dairy products include milk, yogurt, and cheese; proteins include meat, poultry, fish, eggs, dry beans, and nuts; Cf Exercise pyramid, Mediterranean pyramid

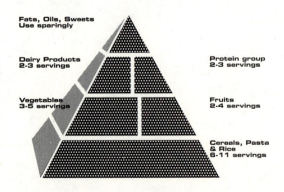

food pyramid

foot-and-mouth disease An infection of cloven-hoofed barnyard beasts, including cattle, goats, pigs and sheep by a picornavirus, genus Aphthovirus, or by a rhabdovirus, vesicular stomatitis virus, which has an RNA clothed in a naked icosahedral nucleocapsid CLINICAL After a 24-hour incubation, human infections are self-limited with fever, oropharyngeal and palmo-plantar vesicle formation; Cf Foot-in-mouth disease, Hand, foot, and mouth disease

football acne Acne mechanica, see there

football calf A term of historic interest referring to the boggy sensation imparted by a massive necrosis of the gastrocnemius muscles caused by arterial embolism

football sign PEDIATRICS A radiologic finding in massive pneumoperitoneum described in children with perforated hollow organs, due to free air accumulation in the supine upper abdomen, which gives rise to an ovoid increase in the radiolucent abdominal cavity

foot-drop NEUROLOGY A manifestation of peripheral neuropathy seen in diabetic mononeuropathy, Charcot-Marie-Tooth syndrome and severe vitamin B_{12} deficiency, which causes subacute combined degeneration of the spinal cord with symmetrical loss of myelin sheaths and (to a lesser degree), axons; the pathological changes are most prominent in the posterior and lateral columns and results in paresthesiae of the feet, loss of vibratory and position sensation, spasticity, and exaggeration of the tendon reflexes in the legs; see Wrist drop

'foot-in-mouth' disease American slang for the tendency to blunder when verbally ad-libbing; Cf Foot-and-mouth disease

The term for this non-medical condition was coined by W Safire in 1968, as a play-on words between hoof-and-mouth disease and to put one's foot in one's mouth

footprinting MOLECULAR BIOLOGY A method for detecting sites of interaction between regulatory or promoter proteins and DNA (DNA footprinting), DNA and RNA (RNA footprinting)

DNA FOOTPRINTING A DNA molecule is 'incubated' with a binding protein, which binds to a specific site along the double helix, and then subjected to restriction endonuclease digestion, which reduces the entire DNA to mono- and oligonucleotide fragments except for the portion of the DNA molecule that was 'protected' from digestion by the binding protein; removal of the protein by simple chemical means, eg by gel electrophoresis, allows the study of DNA and binding protein interaction RNA FOOTPRINTING A purified fragment of double-stranded DNA is labeled with an isotope at the 5' end of one strand and allowed to interact with RNA polymerase or histones; this same strand (with the attached RNA proteinase) is then subjected to scission by either DNAse I or by the synthetic reagent MPE (methidium propyl-EDTA) causing DNA to be cleaved at every base pair, except at those sites where 'protecting' proteins, ie promoter or regulatory proteins or histones prevent base pair cutting; the sites where DNA remains intact are the sites that are bound by the regulatory proteins and thus these experiments are known as 'DNA protection experiments'

footprints INFECTIOUS DISEASE A descriptor for the appearance of *Mycobacterium lepra*-laden macrophages seen in the absence of caseation necrosis, which may also occur in patients with AIDS and anergic Hodgkin's disease, infected by *M avium-intercellulare*

foot process fusion RENAL PATHOLOGY The foot process or podocyte is a cytoplasmic extension from the epithelial cell of the glomerulus that attaches to the basement membrane and it is diffusely effaced or fused in minimal change glomerulopathy or 'nil disease'; foot process fusion is seen by electron microscopy, is reversible and may be the only morphological change seen in this condition

FOP Fibrodysplasia ossificans progressiva, see there

forbearance Delaying of payment of a financial obligation with accrual of interest; see Medical student debt

forbidden clone theory A hypothesis that explains autoimmunity as a re-appearance (through mutation) of clones of lymphocytes that had been functionally deleted in the thymus during ontogeny; forbidden clones of lymphocytes are those that react against self antigens, which under normal circumstances are 'forbidden', ie against which an organism should not react

forced feeding A generic term for either 1) The administration of nutrients against the will of the recipient, or 2) The self-administration of excess quantities of food in the context of the binge-purge complex

Forced feeding per definition 1) represents an ethical dilemma in that, what is assumed by society to be in the patient's best interest (feeding) runs contrary to his/her personal freedom (fasting)-Author's note

forced vital capacity FVC The volume of air exhaled with maximum effort and speed after a full inspiration; FVC is usually reduced (and thus is a major parameter measured) in obstructive airways disease, a term that includes both asthma and COPD

foreign body A generic term for any object introduced into the human economy as the inevitable accompaniment of an invasive procedure (ie iatrogenic), by accident, or by intent; FBs may be microscopic or macroscopic in size

IATROGENIC, eg sutures, sponges, instruments left during surgery, metals and plastics that replace or enhance failing or non-functioning body parts, eg artificial joints, limbs and pacemakers

ACCIDENTAL (UNINTENTIONAL), eg from abrasions and open wounds in various accidents, or in gun shot wounds, which may elicit foreign body-type granuloma formation, or

INTENTIONAL, eg introduced in the context of sexual deviancy, for inflicting pleasure or pain, commonly, in the anorectum or vagina, including an array of 'jeux d'amour', eg vibrators, bottles, light bulbs, eggs and others; see Sexual deviancy

foreign medical graduate International medical graduate, see there A physician who graduated from a medical school outside of the US, Canada or Puerto Rico; FMGs may suffer discrimination resulting from poor linguistic skills or because of the perception of inferior education and skills; FMGs are either alien FMGs (non-North Americans) or USFMGs (North Americans who studied medicine outside the US, Canada, and Puerto Rico); see USFMG

forequarter amputation A major surgical procedure in which the upper extremity and a variable portion of the supporting shoulder girdle is amputated, to treat either advanced malignancy, eg malignant melanoma or for primary malignancy of the soft or bony tissues, eg chondrosarcoma or osteosarcoma; an alternative to forequarter amputation of an upper extremity with a sarcoma is the Tikhoff-Lindberg procedure, in which the distal clavicle, proximal humerus and the majority of the scapula is resected (Surg Gyn Obstet 1989; 169:1, Yonsei Med J 1990; 31:110); forequarter amputations of the leg and pelvis are generally considered more 'heroic' than those of the upper extremity and are not commonly performed, although they were once considered the treatment of choice for certain bone tumors, eg Ewing sarcoma; see Heroic surgery, Mutilating surgery

forensic anthropology The scientific study of human remains, usually with the express purpose of identifying the remains of the deceased and if the cause of death if unknown; the techniques of FA have been applied to tasks of identifying victims of mass disasters or 'los desaparecidos' in Argentina, Guatemala, and other totalitarian states that dispose of dissention

formaldehyde $H_2C=O$ Methanal A highly toxic, flammable gas that is highly irritating to the respiratory and conjunctival mucosa at concentrations above 2 ppm; formaldehyde is soluble in water and forms methylene bridges between denatured proteins; see Formalin

formaldehyde standards LABORATORY SAFETY Standards for formaldehyde exposure promulgated by OSHA: **permissible exposure level** (PEL) 0.75 ppm; short-term exposure level 2.0 ppm **action level** 0.5 ppm; respirators must be supplied and pulmonary function testing performed in those who work in areas exceeding PEL (the average exposure over 8 hours)

formalin A 37% solution of formaldehyde gas in water that reacts with the amine groups of proteins and DNA, serving as a disinfectant and when buffered, to denature ('fix') tissues for histological examination

formamide The amide of formic acid that reacts with adenine in DNA, disrupting the adenine-thymine base pairs and denaturation of DNA

forme fruste The aborted, attenuated or atypical expression of a clinical entity or pathological condition

forseeable emergency OCCUPATIONAL SAFETY A term which, in OSHA parlance refers to any potential occurrence of equipment failure, rupture of containers, failure of control of equipment, or other potentially anticipated contingency that could result in an uncontolled release of a hazardous chemical in the workplace

forskolin A nonspecific stimulator of adenylate cyclase, which is used experimentally to study modulation of 1) voltage-gated potassium ion channels, and 2) acetylcholine receptor that acts directly instead of via a second messenger

Fort Bragg fever Anicteric leptospirosis A condition first described in an outbreak of pretibial rashes in military recruits in Fort Bragg, Texas during World War II, caused by *Leptospiralis autumnalis*; in peacetime, leptospirosis is more common in children with an abrupt onset of a 'toxic' state, fever, shaking chills, headache, nausea, vomiting and severe myalgias (especially of the legs), lethargy, dehydration, photophobia, orbital pain, generalized lymphadenopathy and hepatosplenomegaly

Note: Because the various serotypes of *Leptospira* species do not produce clinically distinct syndromes (eg canicola fever, Fort Bragg fever, Weil's disease and others), it has been suggested that these diseases be referred to simply as leptospirosis

fortification The addition of a required dietary component to a food

fortification phenomenon 'Maginot line' phenomenon, see there

fortified food Any food, eg cereals that has been supplemented with essential nutrients, eg iron and vitamins, either in quantities that are greater than those present normally, or which are not present in the fortified food (this latter is considered the more correct usage of 'fortification'); Cf Enriched food, Refined food

fortified milk PUBLIC HEALTH Milk with added vitamin D; usually 400 IU of vitamin D_3/quart (0.94 L); there is little consistency in the amount of vitamin D that is actually added; in the US and Canada, only 20% of milk purchased contains 80-120% of stated vitamin D; the remainder are either low (or even absent), increasing the risk of rickets or too high (up to 3– 9-fold greater than stated vitamin D content) thus carrying a risk of toxicity (N Engl J Med 1993; 329:1507c)

FORTRAN COMPUTERS A high-level language used to program mainframe computers, ideally suited for complicated mathematical computations; see BASIC, Computers

forward angle light scatter LABORATORY MEDICINE The amount of light scattered by a particle in flow cytometry, which is a function of its size; in FALS, the detector is at 180° or directly in front (forward scatter) of the laser beam; see Backscatter, Flow cytometry

forward failure CARDIOLOGY A concept of uncertain value that refers to decreased cardiac output and inadequate perfusion of organs implying either 1) Symptoms of congestive heart failure, ie low cardiac output with easy fatigability, weakness and even shock or 2) A pathogenic mechanism of cardiac failure, in which ↓ cardiac output produces tissue edema and ↑ capillary permeability, secondary to tissue hypoxia, a mechanism that has proven conceptually incorrect; FF is best understood as ↓ cardiac output due to ↓ renal blood flow and altered glomerular filtration with retention of salt and water, causing a secondary ↑ in blood volume; Cf Backward failure

forward genetics MOLECULAR BIOLOGY A technique in which a phenotype is examined and attempts are make to identify a gene of interest causing the phenotypic changes (from Science 1994; 264:1724)

fos The *fos* oncogenes include the cellular *fos* oncogene, c-*fos*, which is the normal cellular counterpart or proto-oncogene of the viral oncogene, v-*fos*; c-*fos* encodes a 380-amino acid nuclear phosphoprotein that modulates the expression of other genes, requiring phosphorylation for efficient activity; c-*fos* is rapidly and transiently expressed in response to various stimuli, including epidermal, neural and platelet-derived growth factors (PDGF, EGF, and NGF), as well as by neurotransmitters, neuronal stimulation and the cancer promoter-phorbol ester; *fos* encodes a nuclear phosphoprotein with DNA-binding properties and is thought to function as a 'third messenger' molecule in signal transduction systems, coupling short-term intracellular signals elicited by a variety of extracellular stimuli, serving as a 'master switch', turning on other genes; see Serum response element

Note: The *fos* oncogene is named after the FBJ and FBR osteogenic sarcomas

foscarnet AIDS An experimental drug used in AIDS patients with CMV-induced infections, eg colitis, hepatitis, pneumonia, and retinitis who don't respond to or cannot tolerate gancyclovir, the usual drug of choice for CMV infections; Cf ddC, ddI, Zidovudine

fossil fuel ENVIRONMENT A fuel derived from decomposing fossilized organic material of fossilized plant or animal origin, including oil, coal and natural gas, the burning of which is widely regarded as the single greatest contributor to the Greenhouse effect, and a major contributer to Acid rain

foster care SOCIAL MEDICINE The care, nurture, and raising of a child by a person(s) other than the child's own natural, usually for a temporary period of time (often less than a year, although semipermanent arrangements are not uncommon); FC may be mandated officially by a state or local governmental agency to help alleviate a family crisis; the FC givers have no legal parental rights or permanent 'dibs' on the children

found experiment EPIDEMIOLOGY A natural experiment that was created by natural or social events beyond the researchers' control; FE have three characteristics in common (see table): 1) The independent variable has a marked change in brief period of time 2) The dependent variable displays a large and abrupt change in level and 3) Investigation seeks to link the independent and dependent variables (JAMA 1995; 273:1221)

Found Experiments

Event	Independent variable	Dependent variable
London smog-1952	Air pollution	↑ Mortality
Athens earthquake-1981	Psychological stress	↑ Fatal heart attacks
Imitation of suicide	Publicity of a suicide	↑ Suicides
Iraqi missile attacks-1991	Life-threatening stress	↑ Mortality

JAMA 1995; 273:1221

founder cell A cell that has undergone minimal differentiation, passing the primitive 'stem' cell stage, while retaining the ability to colonize an entire tissue, eg primitive hepatocytes or chondrocytes that could give rise to the liver or cartilage

founder effect CLINICAL GENETICS The result of a small subgroup of a species establishing itself as a separate and isolated entity in an ecosystem or location; the founder colony carries with it only a fraction of the gene pool of the parent population, which may result in an increased frequency of certain diseases, in particular autosomal recessive conditions; the founder effect is described in CETP deficiency in the Japanese, Tay-Sachs disease in the Jews, yellow mutant albinism in the Amish

Founier's gangrene A fulminant subcutaneous bacterial infection of the genital and anorectal regions characterized by necrosis (cellulitis, fasciitis, myositis) rapid progression, severe systemic toxicity, and lack of suppuration; virtually all patients are male, average age 50 MICROBIOLOGY In 70%, the flora is mixed (aerobic and anaerobic); the common bugs in FG are *E coli*, *Bacteroides melaninogenicus*, *Bacillus fragilis*, gram-positive cocci, and others ETIOLOGY Periurethritis with urinary extravastion, postsurgery, postinstrumentation, septic injection in the dorsal vein of the penis UNDERLYING DISEASES DM, IVDA, carcinoma CLINICAL Systemic toxicity, urinary retention, abdominal discomfort, regional necrosis, fever, leukocytosis TREATMENT Debridement, broad-spectrum antibiotics; controversial therapies include high-dose prednisone and hyperbaric oxygen

four cell diagnostic matrix LABORATORY MEDICINE A simple decision-making model (figure) for the evaluating the relative merits of a diagnostic test, which allows comparison of the ability of various methodologies to diagnose the presence of a disease, defining such terms as false negativity and positivity, sensitivity and specificity (**Ann Int Med 1981; 94:553**) see ROC curve

FOUR CELL DIAGNOSTIC MATRIX

	DISEASE PRESENT	DISEASE NOT PRESENT
Test positive	True positive (TP)	False positive (FP)
Test negative	False positive (FP)	True negative (TN)

Sensitivity	TP / TP + FN (Total patients with disease)
Specificity	TN / TN + FP (Total patients without disease)
False negative	FN / TN + FP (Total patients without disease)
False positive	FP / TP + FN (Total patients with disease)

four Fs Fat, female, flatulent and forty—a mnemonic with clinical currency as factors often associated with cholelithiasis and acute cholecystitis

four food groups NUTRITION A grouping of comestibles by the US Department of Agriculture that delineates in a simplefied form, its recommendations for eating priorities, graphically presented as a pyramid, at the base of which are carbohydrates with 6-11 portions recommended daily (group one), on top of which are fruits and vegetables with 5-9 portions, followed by dairy products, fish and meat 4-6; at the pyramid's peak are the 'discouraged' foods to be eaten sparingly, including fats, oils and sweets (**Science 1991; 252:917n**)

4p- syndrome see Deletion syndromes

Fourier transform A mathematical function that describes the amplitude (height of a sinusoid) and the phase (starting point) of a sinusoidal pattern of any fluctuating phenomenon in the physical universe (light, tidal and solar waves, molecular vibration); the transform states that any distribution (Fourier analyzed temperature) can be described mathematically in an equation and its higher frequency harmonics; the Fourier transform has had broad applications in biology and medicine; analysis of the X-ray crystallography data was pivotal in identifying the double helical nature of DNA, and has assisted in analysis of other molecules including viruses; the modified back-projection algorithm, universally used in CT-imaging is based on the Fourier transform; Cf Fractals, Wavelet theory MRI A mathematical procedure that separates the frequency component of a signal from its amplitude as a function of time or vice versa; the Fourier transform is used to generate the spectrum from the free induction decay in pulse MRI and is essential to most imaging techniques; see Magnetic resonance imaging

*Jean-Baptiste-Joseph Fourier was a French mathematician of post-revolutionary vintage who formulated the transform in 1807 Note: The merging of mathematics with biology may occur when DNA folding patterns are analyzed in the contexts of chaos, fractal analysis, Fourier transforms and knot and wavelet theories

fourth disease Parascarlatina, Filatov-Duke disease

'fourth therapy' A colloquial term for the next generation of therapies to treat malignancies BACKGROUND Cancer is traditionally treated with one or more of the three tumor-ablative modalities, ie surgery, radiotherapy and chemotherapy; the use of biological response modifiers (interferons, interleukins, monoclonal antibodies, colony-stimulating factors and tumor necrosis factor), is known as the 'fourth therapy', which attempts to take advantage of certain aspects of the immune system, including immunomodulatory, antiproliferative and tumorilytic activities; see Biological response modifiers

fourth ventricle 'syndrome' Symptoms that arise from expansile lesions (neoplastic or inflammatory) or infarction in the floor of the fourth ventricle, involving cranial nerves V-VII

Fourth World SOCIAL MEDICINE A colloquial term referring to the phenomenon of 'Third World' poverty within the borders of a developed, ie 'First World' country, as occurs among the homeless in the USA; see Homeless

Fowler's solution A potassium arsenite solution, formerly used to treat leukemia and various dermatological conditions; after a latency period of up to 43 years, malignancy may appear in those treated with or occupationally exposed to arsenicals, in the form of hepatic angiosarcoma, small cell, squamous cell and bronchoalveolar carcinomas of the lungs, esophageal and genitourinary carcinoma

Fox Chase Cancer Center An institute established in 1904 near Philadephia dedicated to the diagnosis and treatment of cancer and research into its mechanisms; it is the fourth largest (100 inpatient cancer beds) such center in the US

FCCC has been the site of new concepts and discoveries, eg the Philadelphia chromosome (1959), one-hit, two-hit mutagenesis model (1971), promotion insertion mutagenesis in carcinogenesis (1981), LINE-1 sequence mutation (1988), and is the site of more than 100 on-going diagnostic and therapeutic clinical trials, including immunotherapy, radiotherapy, and surgical oncology

FPIA Fluorescence polarization immunoassay, see there

F protein VIROLOGY A glycosylated surface protein that is critical in the infectivity and pathogenesis of respiratory syncytial virus; it is a 70-kD fusion protein consisting of 2 (50-kD-F_1 and 20-kD-F_2) disulfide-linked fragments; F protein is thought to initiate viral penetration by fusing viral and cellular membrane, and by fusing the membranes of infected to noninfected cells, resulting in the characteristic syncytial clusters of cells; see Atypical measles; Cf G protein

fractal THEORETICAL MEDICINE An invention of IBM mathematician Benoit Mandelbrot, which are 1) Self-symmetrical, ie an enlargement of a small part is similar to the whole and 2) Have fractional dimension; man has traditionally related nature to artificial and invalid geometric shapes (circles, squares, triangles); with fractals, a true representation of the natural universe can be reduced to a mathematical model; in the human economy, the ever-increasing number of branches in the blood vessels as they become capillaries, as well as the branching of the bronchi are each considered to be recapitulations of fractal geometry; see Chaos

fractal dimension The 'fuzziness' or complexity of a system, which is measured by the degree of detail it displays at ever smaller scales (Sci Am 1995; 272/6:104)

fractional kill hypothesis BACKGROUND Dosing of cancer chemotherapeutic agents is based on experimental studies where the tumor's size, kinetics and percentage of cells killed can be determined within reasonable limits; the hypothesis assumes a homogeneity of the tumor cell population and a constant percent decrease in tumor bulk with each course of therapy; in treating cancer, tumor populations are actually heterogeneous; although chemotherapy does kill a certain large percentage of actively dividing cells; cells not in a susceptible period of the growth cycle are not killed, while other cells are resistant, expressing the MDR (multi-drug resistance) gene; one way to reduce the tumor load is to debulk by surgery or radiation therapy, then 'consolidate' the treatment with chemotherapy or subject the patient to a 'second look' procedure

fracture threshold A theoretical cancellous bone density below which osteoporosis-related fractures occur Note: ♀ lose 50% of cancellous and 30% of their cortical bone during their lifetime ♂ lose 30% of cancellous and 20% of their cortical bone during their lifetime; cancellous bone is concentrated in the spinal column and at the ends of the long bones, the sites of most fractures; the skeleton is a reservoir of labile calcium and base (as alkaline calcium salts)

fragile data Unusual results obtained from a well-designed study, which because of either the small size of the cohort studied and therefore low statistical power, or the unexpected results, may result in conclusions that do not withstand the rigors of scientific scrutiny; because FD may result in unusual conclusions, a study's authors may present the data with caveats on the 'fragility' of the findings; see Data

fragile site MOLECULAR BIOLOGY Any of a number of specific chromosomal loci (of the 320 bands per haploid set) of a routine human metaphase chromosome preparation that may be expressed as gaps or breaks, which are co-dominantly inherited, eg those found on chromosomes 3p14.2, 6q25.3, and 16q23.2; cells grown in folic acid- and thymidine-deficient culture media have an increased expression of 13 of 16 common heritable (constitutive) fragile sites and increased spontaneous chromosomal breakage; extended haploid sets with 850 bands, when incubated in caffeine, an inhibitor of DNA repair in replicating cells, reveal that 20 of the 51 fragile sites in the human genome correlate with known chromosomal defects in leukemias, lymphomas and solid tumors

fragile X syndrome A condition related to mutation in a highly unstable 550-base pair locus on chromosome Xq27.3, which is susceptible to insertions, methylations, amplifications and varies in length across generations; insertions of less than 400 base pairs are not associated with phenotypic expression of a gene that requires the abnormal cytosine methylation of a single CpG island (Science 1991; 252:1097, 1070) Note: Fragile X is the most common (1:1500) cause of inherited mental deficiency in males (30% of female carriers are also mentally deficient); CLINICAL Moderate mental retardation, neuropsychiatric disorders (hypotonic or hyperactive state, autism), large forehead, macroorchidism, enlarged chin, jaw and ears MOLECULAR PATHOLOGY The defective gene *FMR-1* is located in chromosome segment Xq27.3; the defect appears in 10-50% of chromosomes tested and is diagnosed by growth in a folic acid-poor growth medium, which enhances chromosomal breakage; it is characterized by trinucleotide (CGG) repeats and abnormal methylation of the CpG cap island (Arch Pathol Lab Med 1993; 117:1121oA); the gene's methylation may explain both the pattern of inheritance

and the lack of expression, as methylation of a gene functionally stops its activity (Science 1991; 251:1236) Cf CAG repeat disease

frailty A non-medical term for the state of frailness or weakness; as the mean age of the population in developed countries rises, there is an increasing need for a formal (ie legally viable) definition of the term frailty; it is often understood in a medical context to encompass age-related fragility, in particular osteoporosis; see FICSIT

frameshift mutation MOLECULAR BIOLOGY The loss or gain of one or more nucleotide base pairs in a gene, which results in the 'misreading' of all codons downstream from the mutation, and the encoding of different amino acids or stop codons in the elongating polypeptide chain; see Point mutation

framework regions The regions of an immunoglobulin where the amino acid residues are relatively constant and β-pleated, forming the folding portion of the immunoglobulin molecule; FRs in the light chain are located at amino acid residues 1-28, 38-50, 56-89 and 97-107; FRs in the heavy chain are located at amino acid residues 1-31, 35-49, 66-101 and 110-117; Cf 'Hot spots'

Frankenfood A highly colloquial generic term of uncertain utility for any food product produced by recombinant DNA technology, eg the genetically engineered tomato, see Flavr Savr (Bio/Technology 1995; 13:540)
*Waggishly named in the tradition of Mary Shelley's Frankenstein

Frankenstein The central character of Mary Shelley's novel by the same name; 'Frankenstein' is used as an adjective in various biomedical contexts, eg
FRANKENSTEIN COMPLEX The fear that machines via artificial intelligence may replace physicians
FRANKENSTEIN FACTOR Any unforeseen consequence of genetic engineering
FRANKENSTEIN 'SYNDROME' The potential result of experimentation on humans; used as a noun, a Frankenstein is any enterprise that circumvents or expands beyond the mechanisms designed to control them, eg the health-care reimbursement system (Am Rev Respir Dis 1975; 111:689)

Frankfort (horizontal) line Reid's base line RECONSTRUCTIVE SURGERY An imaginary line that projects from the median line of the occipital bone and upper rim of the external auditory canal (the auricular point) to the lower rim of the orbit (the infraorbital point); the FHL divides the head into upper and lower halves from gnathion to trichion, and is used for craniometric studies (as it approximates the base of the skull) and may be used as a point of reference in otoplasty

FRAP see Fluorescence recovery after photobleaching

Fraser syndrome Cryptophthalmos with syndactyly cyclopia, cyclopism A severe AR [MIM 219000] form of holoprosencephaly characterized by fusion of the ocular globe and doubling of the normal ocular structures and arhinia GENETICS Chromosome defects described in cyclopia include 3p duplication, 2p deletion, balanced 3/7 translocation, anomalies of chromosome 7 and the most common defect, trisomy 18

fraternal twins Dizygotic twins Twins resulting from two separate fertilized eggs liberated simultaneously from the ovaries that develop in separate or partially fused chorionic sacs; 70-80% of twins are dizygotic Note: Both terms are in active use, fraternal is more colloquial, dizygotic more formal; Cf Identical twins

fratricidal fire Friendly fire, see there

fraud in science The intentional misrepresentation or manipulation of data; scientific fraud ranges from 'innocent correction' of data by the investigator (see Cooking, Trimming), to complete fabrication of data; in the US, misinterpretation of complex data in difficult niches of research has been scrutinized by non-scientists and 'whistle-blowers', see Qui tam lawsuit, engendering a label of fraud, despite commonly held opinions that such inquiries are best left to peer review; retraction of fraudulent data reduces subsequent citation by 35%

'freak out' SUBSTANCE ABUSE A highly colloquial verb, first used in North America in the 1960s, during which time the chief proponents of social changes were known as hippies or 'freaks', who used psychedelic drugs for 'mind expansion', which in excess, would cause hyperexcitation or 'freaking out' (**N Engl J Med 1991; 324:926**) see 'Bad trip', Flashback

freckles Ephilides Brown macules, often exacerbated on sun-exposed zones of the skin surface, disappearing during the winter; most commonly affecting the fair-skinned, especially of Celtic stock; freckles are not associated with atypical melanocytic hyperplasia, nor with malignancy PATHOLOGY ↑ Melanin and fewer but enlarged melanocytes

free base (cocaine) SUBSTANCE ABUSE An aqueous form of cocaine that allows it to be injected intravenously or smoked, producing a more intense 'high' (and more intense addiction) that is prepared through the chemical conversion of cocaine-HCl by alkalinizing and extracting through heated ether and organic solvents

Note: The danger of explosion at the ether extraction phase forced clandestine chemists to create a newer formulation of cocaine, crack, see there

free flap microsurgery A type of reconstructive surgery in which a flap of autologous 'donor' tissue is removed from a patient's back, abdomen, buttock, or thigh; it is then shaped, attached to the desired site and circulation restored by connecting the flap's vascular supply with that of the recipient site; **free flap breast reconstruction** is an option* for women who undergo mastectomy, or who require revision after breast implants have been removed for various reasons, including severe pain, deformity, rupture, and systemic complaints, informally known as Human adjuvant disease (**JAMA 1992; 268:2627MN&P**)

*Albeit time-consuming (4 hours for one, and 7 hours for both breasts) and expensive ($35-50 000)

Freeman surgery see Psychosurgery

freemartin Bovine intersex, stable chimera A heifer born as a co-twin to a ♂ calf (ie, dizygotic bovine twins that are of the opposite sex), the ♀ of which often has reproductive abnormalities (hypoplastic uterus, ovaries, and vagina); during gestation, the ovaries of the ♀ fetus lose their germ cells and may develop testicular structures; freemartins occur only if the twins share a common in utero circulation; they are immune tolerant to each other's red cell antigens; freemartins may rarely occur in sheep and in goats, but do not occur in higher mammals (**Nature 1995; 374:684BR**); the system of shared in utero circulation was reduced in size by Billingham, Brent, and Medawar (Nobel prize, 1959) to a mouse model

free induction decay MRI A transient MR signal produced by transverse magnetization of the spins, eg by a 90° pulse, which decays toward zero with a characteristic time constant T2 (or T2*); in practice, the first part of the FID is not observable due to residual effects of the powerful exciting radiofrequency pulse on the electronics of the receiver; FID is observed while periodically switching the y-gradient field in the presence of a static x-gradient field; the Fourier transform of the resulting spin-echo train can be used to produce an image of the excited plane; see Magnetic resonance imaging

free radical One of a highly reactive family of molecules containing an unpaired electron in the outer orbital, eg the excited variants of oxygen; free radicals cause random damage to structural proteins, enzymes, macromolecules and DNA and play major roles in inflammation, hyperoxidation, post-ischemic tissue damage, infarcts, and possibly also in carcinogenesis and tissue damage induced by organ transplantation; superoxide dismutase is the major 'scavenger' enzyme, catalyzing reduction of reactive oxygen

species to O_2 and H_2O; the havoc wreaked by radicals includes polyunsaturated fatty acid peroxidation of organelles and plasma membranes, oxidation and inactivation of sulfhydryl group-bearing enzymes, polysaccharide depolymerization and DNA damage; the action of free radicals on DNA in the form of hydroxylation of bases, crosslinking, nicking may block transcription and by extension, synthetic activities

Note: Free radical production by endothelial cells during coronary artery ischemia and inculpated in myocytolysis may be reduced in experimental systems by pre-treatment with superoxide dismutase

free radical inactivator Any molecule that reduces free radical-induced damage, including ceruloplasmin, cysteine, glutathione, superoxide dismutase, transferrin, vitamin E and D-penicillamine

free radical scavenger Any compound that reacts with free radicals in a biological system and provides protection against the indirect effects, ie free radicals, of ionizing radiation; see Antioxidant

free radical theory GERIATRICS A biological theory that assumes that the changes seen in aging cells and organisms result from the accumulation of molecules damaged by free radicals; the host cell's defenses against free radical damage include glutathione peroxidase, α-tocopherol (vitamin E) and superoxide dismutase; intracellular superoxide levels correlate well with lifespan; Cf Crosslinkage, Error catastrophe, 'Garbage can' hypothesis, Pacemaker theory

free-standing HEALTH CARE INDUSTRY An adjective referring to any physically and often financially discrete entity, eg a surgical center, that is separated from, but which may be affiliated with a hospital; free-standing facilities may provide ambulatory surgery, emergency or primary care; see Walk-in clinic

free thyroxine index FT_4I, T7 assay, T12 assay LABORATORY MEDICINE A clinical parameter measured by radioimmunoassay, used to evaluate thyroid function, calculated by T_4 x %T_3RU (resin uptake); the FTI is not susceptible to fluctuations of T_3/T_4 binding globulin and is more reliable than thyroxine when the binding proteins are altered; the FTI is ↑ in hyperthyroidism and factitious hyperthyroidism and ↓ in hypothyroidism; it is falsely ↑ in heparin therapy and falsely ↓ in phenytoin and valproic acid therapy and in the euthyroid sick syndrome

freeze-clamp technique A method used in experimental biology to analyze metabolic processes in quasiphysiological conditions, by immersing the tissue of interest in liquid nitrogen, abruptly stopping any in vivo reaction, allowing the study of concentrations of the metabolites in various intracellular compartments; Cf Patch-clamp method

freeze-fracture 'imaging' CELL BIOLOGY A technique that allows ultrastructural examination of membrane-bound proteins and subcellular particles as they appear within cells Method A cell or tissue of interest is frozen in nitrogen and 'fractured' with a blow from a sharp knife removing membranes interfering with visualization of organelle topography; the surface is then overlaid with carbon to form a continuous layer and then 'shadowed' with platinum, imparting a 3-D image of the organelles

freezing Freezing spells NEUROLOGY Eisodic immobility (the 'off' compenent of the on-off phenomenon) typical of later stages of Parkinson's disease (see **N Engl J Med 1992; 327:1541QA**) also defined as hesitation on gait initiation, ie start-hesitation, upon stopping, ie terminal hesitation or when walking in crowded places

French-American-British classification see FAB classification

French congenital nephrotic syndrome An often fatal autosomal recessive proliferative mesangial glomerulosclerosis of onset in early infancy HISTOPATHOLOGY

Atrophy of the tubules with interstitial fibrosis and increased mesangial matrix; Cf Finnish congenital nephrotic syndrome

the French paradox A term dignifying the epidemiologic shift in mortality in France, where there are lower rates of coronary heart disease, attributed to an increase of alcohol consumption; it has been postulated that the protective effect afforded by red wine is due to polyphenols in the grape skins; in one report, mixing of red wine with LDL resulted in a 70% reduction in LDL oxidation, which contributes to atherosclerosis; in contrast, white wine (in which the grapes skins are removed during processing) increased LDL oxidation (**M Aviram et al, Am J Clin Nutrition March, 1995**); the FP's benefits are in part offset by higher rates of alcohol addiction and alcohol-induced diseases (**JAMA 1994; 272:967ED**) see Alcohol

French sizes EMERGENCY MEDICINE The system for sizes of tubes used in endotracheal intubation, the use of which varies according to the age of the patient; at one month, size 4; at age 2, size 5.0; at age 6, size 6; at age 12, size 7.0

frequency shifted burst imaging Burst MRI, see there

fresh frozen plasma CLINICAL THERAPEUTICS A blood component separated from whole blood at 5°C by centrifugation at 4100 rpm (5000G, a so-called 'hard' spin) and frozen to –18°C within 6 hours of collection; FFP provides 80-120 mg of fibrinogen and at least 80 units each of factors VIII and XIII; FFP is indicated for prothrombin time > 16 seconds, acute hepatic decompensation, massive hemorrhage, massive transfusions where more than 10 units of packed red cells causes coagulation factor depletion; FFP is administered pre-operatively in patients with known coagulopathies, eg hemophilia B, in therapeutic apheresis, disseminated intravascular coagulation, idiopathic thrombocytopenic purpura and hemolytic disease of the newborn

fresh water drowning A type of drowning in which hypo-osmolar water compromises the surface tension of alveolar surfactant, causing an imbalance in the ventilation-perfusion (V/Q) ratio with a collapse of some alveoli, and both true (absolute) and relative intrapulmonary shunting; the shifts of fluids and electrolytes in fresh water drowning result in hemodilution, hemolysis, circulatory overload (and pulmonary edema that further compromises the V/Q abnormality), and hyponatremia; see Drowning

friction rub CARDIOLOGY A scratchy triphasic (occasionally, biphasic or monophasic) sound extending over the entire precordium, best heard along the left midsternum with the patient leaning forward, which changes in quality with inspiration and positional changes; the rub is considered pathognomonic for pericarditis and must be differentiated from to-and-fro or machinery-like murmurs and 'crunching' sounds heard in emphysema; the 3 phases of the triphasic rub are due to pericardial-epicardial contact during ventricular systole, diastole and atrial systole

fried egg appearance A descriptor for a pattern likened to eggs fried with an intact yolk* NEUROPATHOLOGY The appearance by light microscopy of oligodendrogliocytes, in which a large central nucleus is surrounded by cleared cytoplasm, a finding thought to be an artefact due to slow fixation of tissue; a similar finding may rarely occur in astrocytomas MICROBIOLOGY A descriptor for the colony morphology characteristic of *Mycoplasma hominis* and *M pneumonia* on Shepherd's differential growth medium, where the growth occurs in two planes, both deep to and on the surface of the agar; *M hominis* is further characterized by its ability to utilize arginine

*Note: Fried eggs may be either 'scrambled' or 'sunny side-up' (with the yolk intact), although the adjective usually refers to the latter

Friedenwald calculation An equation used in the clinical laboratory for estimating levels of LDL-cholesterol (the 'bad' cholesterol), where measured HDL-cholesterol and 'guestimated' VLDL-cholesterol (⅕ triglyceride) are subtracted from measured total cholesterol; the calculation loses validity in the face of high triglycerides (**CAP Today Nov 1994 p34**)

$$LDL\text{-}C = Total\text{-}C - HDL\text{-}C - {}^{TG}\!/_{5}$$

friendly fire Fratricidal fire MILITARY MEDICINE A generic term for any unintentional discharge or misdirection of firepower or other weapons of war, eg gunfire, dropping of bombs, and shelling by long-range weapons in an armed conflict against combatants of the same side; friendly fire is estimated to have caused 17% of casualties in the Gulf War, and 24% of casualties in the US beachhead defense of Bougainville Island in the Pacific theater of World War II; anti-fratricidal technology is in its infancy, and includes such specific devices as infrared light-reflecting thermal tape, GPS (Global Positioning System) receivers, and Budd lights, see there (**New York Times 18 May 1993; C1**), and technical advances as 'surgical' bombing

fringe medicine Alternative medicine, see there

frivolous lawsuit MEDICAL MALPRACTICE A groundless lawsuit in which injury did not occur or which was so negligible that it caused no damage, real or perceived, to the plaintiff; such lawsuits have little prospect for success and are brought with the purpose of annoying or embarrassing a defendant; see de minimus rule; see Malpractice

frogbelly PEDIATRICS A fanciful term for the pendulous abdominal fat of children with congenital hypothyroidism (cretins)

frogface The end-stage facial dysmorphia seen in long-standing angiofibromas (large, pedunculated gray-pink spongy fibrous 'tumors' with superficial ulceration) of the intranasal cavities which may ultimately protrude into the orbits, causing bilateral exophthalmos, associated with nasal congestion and a flat, croaking voice

frog leg position A descriptor for a position that may occur 1) As an incorrect sleeping position in infants with an 'out-toeing' deformity of the leg, which may evolve into a Charlie Chaplin-like gait, prevented by sewing together the legs of the pajamas 2) In infants with fulminant scurvy, where tenderness and irritability cause the children to assume the least painful position, resulting in a pseudoparalysis with the hips and knees semiflexed and the feet rotated externally, often accompanied by edematous swelling of the femoral shafts and occasionally, palpable subperiosteal hemorrhage, and 3) In children with congestive heart failure

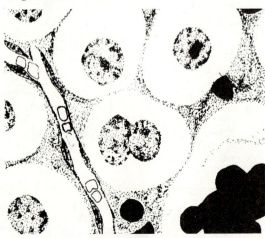

fried egg appearance

frog neck appearance A descriptor for a deep-set neck and hairline, regarded as characteristic of Klippel-Feil disease

front typing TRANSFUSION MEDICINE Use of known antibodies (from commercially available 'panels') to detect ABO antigens on the red blood cells; a discrepancy between front and back typing can be due to acquired group B or group B antigenic subtypes, cold or saline agglutinins, decreased immunoglobulins, polyagglutination of anti-B and anti-A$_1$ antibodies, rouleaux formation, the presence of Wharton's jelly, mosaicism or two different cell populations, as seen after transfusion

frontal bossing Bossing, see there

frost Uremic frost, see there

frostbite Tissue damage or destruction induced by temperatures below 0°C, which is divided into superficial (frostnip) and deep forms; in deep frostbite, subcutaneous tissue, muscle and bone are involved CLINICAL Numbness, prickling, itching, if severe paresthesia, stiffness, bulla formation, necrosis, gangrene TREATMENT-IMMEDIATE Rewarm in water 40-42°C (104-107.6°F) *never warmer* TREATMENT-POST EMERGENT Debride blister, topical aloe vera gel, tetanus prophylaxis, analgesia, NSAIDs, penicillin, hydrotherapy, physical therapy

'frosting' Finely granular salt deposits on the skin overlying sweat glands in children with cystic fibrosis

frostnip Superficial frostbite

frottage A form of sexual gratification in which the frotteur derives erotic pleasure from rubbing against the sexual object or person, usually with the clothes in place; frottage may be performed by mutually consenting individuals in the context of safe sexual practices; see Paraphilia, Safe sex

frotteur A person who performs frottage, see there

'frozen' Frozen section, see there

frozen blood TRANSFUSION MEDICINE A blood product that was a 'spin-off' of the Cold War, in anticipation of the need for transfusions in a world without donors, assuming that the only survivors of a total 'exchange' would be those living in nuclear submarines; in order to extend the shelf life of packed red cells, most of the plasma is replaced with glycerol; frozen red cells are licensed by the FDA for routine transfusion for up to 10 years after collection, when stored at -80°C in certain agents, eg 40% glycerol plus 15% DMSO-dimethylsulfoxide, allowing survival of viable red cells (80% recovery) for up to 40 years; upon rethawing, hemoglobin (due to rethawing lysis) is 100 mg/dl; inadequate removal of cryopreservatives may induce hemolysis; frozen erythrocytes may be used in 1) Rare blood types, eg Bombay phenotype 2) Paroxysmal nocturnal hemoglobinuria 3) IgA deficiency, with production of anti-IgA antibodies 4) Those with graft-versus-host transfusion reactions

frozen pelvis ONCOLOGICAL SURGERY A term for massive involvement of the pelvic floor by malignancy, usually carcinoma, often of the female genital tract, in which there is contiguous extension of the tumor from the bladder, female genital tract and sigmoid colon; adequate surgical resection of a frozen pelvis is virtually impossible, although surgery, chemotherapy, and radiotherapy are palliative at best CLINICAL The symptoms are related to compression and stenosis of pelvic floor organs, formation of fistulous tracts (which may unchain one of the common terminal events, sepsis), difficulty in defecation and dyspareunia; see All-American operation

frozen section SURGICAL PATHOLOGY A rapid diagnostic procedure performed on tissue obtained intra-operatively, where the tissue is frozen in a synthetic material, eg OCT (Miles Laboratories), sectioned with a cryostat, stained with hematoxylin and eosin and viewed with a light microscope, allowing a rapid diagnosis of a pathologic tissue; the technique provides the surgeon with information necesary to guide therapy and to determine the extent of further surgery at the time of surgical procedure; the information obtained from a 'frozen' includes 1) Differentiating between benign and malignant 2) Determining the type of malignancy, eg lymphoma versus carcinoma 3) Evaluating tissue margins for involvement by malignancy, eg basal cell carcinomas 4) Determining the adequacy of tissue for further studies after the patient is closed and 5) Determining the type of tissue, eg differentiating lymphoid tissue from parathyroid gland; 'quick sections' shorten the turn-around time for a diagnosis from 1-3 days to 15 minutes, with the disadvantage that the tissue is suboptimal, as it contains freezing artefact and is thus more difficult to interpret than paraffin-embedded tissue; in nonpalpable mammographically identified lesions of the breast, FS diagnosis has a sensitivity of 92% and specificity of > 99%; 3.3% of diagnoses were deferred to permanent section (Am J Clin Pathol 1995; 103:199)

frozen shoulder A generic term for a shoulder afflicted with incapacitating pain secondary to bursitis and marked inflammation, which may be due to primary or secondary osteoarthritis, rheumatoid arthritis, cuff tear arthropathy and the clinically similar 'Milwaukee shoulder', avascular necrosis and calcific tendonitis and tearing of the rotator cuff muscles

FRP Fusion regulatory protein, see there

fructose-3-phosphate A monosaccharide phosphate not present in normal lenses but found in the lens of diabetic rats, F-3-P glycosylates proteins and inactivates enzymes; its metabolic product, 3-deoxyglucosone is implicated in the visual defects of diabetes mellitus (Science 1990; 247:451)

fructose intolerance syndrome The AR [MIM 229600] deficiency of fructose-1-phosphate aldolase; the subject is asymptomatic until exposed to fructose (or sucrose) CLINICAL Hepatomegaly, jaundice, edema; with time, patients may develop cirrhosis TREATMENT Dietary, avoidance of fructose-containing foods

fruit-laden tree appearance Cherry blossom appearance, see there

fruit and vegetable PREVENTIVE MEDICINE A unit or bundle of food that has been widely regarded as healthful, given the high content of potassium and antioxidants; data has begun to accumulate suggesting that F&Vs are indeed 'good for you'*; in the population-based longitudinal Framingham study, there was a 22% ↓ in incidence of ischemic and hemorrhagic stroke for every 3-serving/day ↑ in F&V intake (JAMA 1995; 273:1113OA) see Food pyramid

*Mother may have been right

***Frye* rule** General acceptance rule A legal rule that was enunciated by a Federal Court of Appeals (United States v Frye, 293 F 1013 (DC Cir 1923)) in a criminal case in which the defendent sought to present evidence that a crude (and not scientifically valid or generally accepted) test showed that he was telling the truth; '...*abandonment of the general acceptance requirement could result in a free-for-all in which befuddled juries would be confounded by absurd and irrational pseudoscientific assertions*' (N Engl J Med 1994; 330:1018LIM); the *Frye* rule has been superseded by the Federal Rules of Evidence (see there); see Expert witness, Rule 702, Malpractice

FSH 1) Ffacioscapulohumeral 2) Follicle-stimulating hormone A 30 kD plasma (4-25 U/L, urine) glycoprotein that binds membrane receptors, activating adenyl cyclase and increasing intracellular AMP; FSH stimulates ovulation and spermatogenesis and is increased in primary gonadal failure, testicular or ovarian agenesis, Klinefelter syndrome, FSH-secreting tumors and decreased in anorexia nervosa, hypogonadotropic hypogonadism, panhypopituitarism, malignancy of the ovaries, testes and adrenal glands

FSI see Foam stability index

FSV Fujinami sarcoma virus A transforming virus that acts on rat fibroblasts, forming a fusion product from viral GAG and cell-derived FPS, encoding a chimeric protein with tyrosine kinase activity and oncogenic transforming capacity

FTA-ABS Fluorescent treponemal antibody-absorption A highly sensitive (circa 100%) and sensitive (96 to 97%) serological test for the diagnosis of congenital, secondary, tertiary and neurosyphilis; see VDRL

FTE Full-time equivalent, see there

F Test A statistical test that allows comparison of the standard deviations of two different sets of data or populations, defined as $F = s^2$ new data/s^2 old data; the smaller the standard deviation, the more precise or reliable the test or data being studied

FTI Free thyroxine index, see there

FTIR spectroscopy (open-path) Fourier transform infrared spectroscopy A method for identifying volatile organic compounds (VOCs) in the ambient air, which can be used for on-site air pollution analysis, and oxygenate and aromatic content of gasoline; FTIR spectroscopy can detect VOCs, eg dichloromethane, tetrachloroethylene, trichloroethane, in the 50-400 ppb (parts per billion) range (Am Lab Oct 1994)

FTT see Failure to thrive

ftz Fushi tarazu, Japanese, Insufficient segments A 2-kilobase gene of *Drosophila melanogaster* that controls the number of body segments during embryogenesis and cell fate during neurogenesis; *ftz* is transiently expressed in neuronal precursors, and when mutated, allows production of one half the normal body segments, resulting in death before birth, in the neurons, absence of *ftz* caused the cells to change identity

fugu Puffer fish A raw fish delicacy eaten in Japan that contains tetrodotoxin, a highly selective sodium channel blocker that is concentrated in the ovaries, liver, skin, and intestines; it is fatal when improperly prepared, causing about 100 deaths annually in Japan

fugue state NEUROLOGY A state in which the patient denies any memory of his activities for a period of time ranging from hours to weeks; to external appearances these activities were either completely normal or the patient disappeared and traveled extensively; most are of a functional nature although rare cases of short-lived fugues occur with temporal lobe epilepsy; Cf Jamais vu

'full house' syndrome A highly colloquial term for Familial focal facial dermal dysplasia, see there

Note: The name is inspired by poker, a card game in which a 'full house' is three cards of one value and two of another

full-time equivalent HEALTH CARE MANAGEMENT The amount of time worked by the combined full and part-time staff, divided by the time worked (in the USA, 40 hours) by a full-time employee; in hospitals, FTEs are calculated for services which provide 24 hour/day service, including the nursing staff and laboratory

fullerenes Hollow cage-like all-carbon molecules that are generated when carbon burns, including C60, C76, C84, C90, C94 and C70; fullerene variants include **BUCKYBALL** C60 or Soccer ball structure **HAIRYBALL** A C60 structure festooned with a dozen or more ethylene diamine molecules whose nitrogen groups have spare electrons **DOPEYBALL** C60 with boron inside, so named as it is a fullerene that has been 'doped' with another molecule; it is unclear what applications in biology and medicine this new class of compounds will have (Science 1991; 252:547, 548)

fulleride A C_{60} molecule that has various other ions incorporated into its structure

fulminant hepatic failure GASTROENTEROLOGY An acute and/or severe decompensation of hepatic function, which has been briefly defined as '...*the onset of hepatic encephalopathy within 2 months after the diagnosis of liver disease.*', which may be linked to brain edema (Mayo Clin Proc 1995; 70:1119 0A)

fumagillin A natural antibiotic from *Aspergillus fumigatus* that inhibits endothelial cell proliferation and tumor-induced angiogenesis; fumagillin also inhibits tumor growth but because it causes severe weight loss, fumagillin analogues ('angioinhibins') are designed to inhibit tumor growth without the side effects; see Neovascularization

fumonisin A toxin produced by the corn molds *Fusarium moniliforme* and *F proliferatur*, that causes fatal encephalopathy in horses and pneumonia-like disease in pigs, which may be linked to carcinoma of the esophagus in humans (Science News 1995; 147:254)

'function-way-result' test INTELLECTUAL PROPERTY A test of the 'doctrine of equivalents' in arbitrating disputes of patent infringement; '*A claim is infringed under the doctrine of equivalents if the accused product performs substantially the same FUNCTION in substantially the same WAY to achieve the same RESULT.*' (Bio/Technology 1995; 13:318)

functional assessment '...*the evaluation of the patient's ability to carry out the basic activities of daily living...*', which include eating, ambulation, and personal hygiene; FA can be broadened to encompass aspects of psychosocial functioning, eg cognition, behavior, and social interactions, as well as instrumental activities of daily living, eg cooking, shopping, using transportation, managing medications, and performing ordinary housework; as the population of industrialized countries ages, FA becomes important as a measure of the outcome of various interventions (as mortality data are too crude a yardstick of quality of care and quality of life); FA is also of use in planning patient care, in allotting resources and controlling costs, and as a predictive tool to be used in planning preventive programs (N Engl J Med 1995; 332:598ED)

functional (endonasal) endoscopic sinus surgery ENT A surgical procedure introduced in the US in the 1980s that is an effective therapy for diseases of the nasal cavity and paranasal sinuses, eg chronic and/or recurrent sinusitis in children and adults who have been therapeutic 'failures' with conventional medical therapy; FESS is also of use in treating suppurative sinusitis, and for asthmatics with aggressive disease; with FESS, the diseased tissue is removed and the mucociliary clearance restored, and thus is not ablative or exenterative, but rather functional in nature

functional exercise REHABILITATION MEDICINE The '...*restoration of strength and agility through dynamic exercise.*' (JC DeLee, D Drez, Jr, Eds, Orthopedic Sports Medicine WB Saunders, Philadelphia, 1994) in FE and functional rehabilitation, several muscle groups are exercised simultaneously, the set of exercises is usually sport specific, and there is virtually no need for special equipment, eg paddleball, skip rope, basketball, and badminton are effective for knee rehabilitation; other functional exercises include cycling, rowing, and swimming

functional illiteracy SOCIAL MEDICINE The inability to read and write with enough proficiency to effectively function in an office or business; in contrast, complete illiteracy is a major cause of 'disenfranchisement', where patients cannot use the health benefits available to them

funerary goods ANTHOPOLOGY Any item that is buried with a person, often in the context of cultural or tribal beliefs regarding the deceased journeys in the 'after-life'; funerary goods include religious icons, vessels, games, and other diverse items

fungible *adjective* Pertaining or referring to any product that is readily exchanged for another, eg plasma, generic drugs, sterile gloves, without compromise of function or inconvenience

fungoides Bacteria that mimic true fungi, both morphologically and clinically, eg *Actinomadura, Actinomyces, Nocardia* and *Streptomyces* species

fungus ball Aspergilloma, mycetoma A tumor-like mass of fungi, classically the saprobic form of *Aspergillus* species that colonizes a preexisting pulmonary cavity RADIOLOGY A solid rounded mass within a cavity, rimmed by an 'air density' crescent; surgical excision of large lesions carries a 5-10% intraoperative mortality rate and a 25-35% complication rate, but without surgery, potentially fatal hemoptysis occurs in 50-83%; radiologically similar lesions occur in abcesses, ankylosing spondylitis, congenital lung cysts, cystic bronchiectasis, emphysematous bullae, cavitary histoplasmosis, neoplasia, radiation fibrosis, sarcoidosis and AIDS (**N Engl J Med 1991; 324:654**)

funnel chest Pectus excavatum A congenital, often isolated, skeletal anomaly associated with upper airway obstruction or segmental bronchomalacia; surgical correction is not clearly beneficial and some cases may resolve spontaneously

funny looking kid see FLK

FUO Fever of unknown origin, see there

furanose A 5-carbon ring sugar that results from the reaction of the 5-hydroxyl group with the aldehyde in aldose, a Hayworth projection of which is shown in figure

furry tongue see Black hairy tongue, Hairy tongue

fused protein see Hybrid protein

fushi tarazu see ftz

fusion beat CARDIOLOGY The superimposition of an ectopic beat on an impulse arising in the sinoatrial node; an FB is usually narrower than a paced impulse and has various morphologies that reflect the relative contributions of the impulse to the venticular depolarization; Cf Pseudofusion beat

fusion peptide A strongly hydrophobic, highly conserved amino acid sequence contained in influenza viruses; at pH 7.0 the sequence is virtuously tucked away in a crevice of the hemagglutinin spike, at pH 5.0 (presumably intracellularly), the fusion peptide swings outward and pierces the cell membrane

fusion protein An 'unnatural' protein that is encoded when a segment of DNA is translocated to another site on a chromosome, resulting in a hybrid gene that may be transcribed into mRNA and subsequently translated into protein; disease-specific fusion proteins have been identified in acute myelocytic leukemia, acute promyelocytic leukemia (PML/RAR-α), chronic myelocytic leukemia, Ewing sarcoma (*EWS/FLI-1*), and others (**N Engl J Med 1993; 329:177RV**); as these products are presumably linked to the development of specific malignancies, the term fusion carcinogenesis may be appropriate

fusion regulatory protein Any of a family of proteins that regulate the viral-mediated cell fusion that are expressed on a wide range of tissue including epithelium, skeletal muscle sarcolemma, some stem cells, germ cells, and others; some data suggest FRPs may play a role in fertilization, multinucleated giant cell formation, and protein secretion (**Arch Pathol Lab Med 1995; 119:461oA**)

fusion transcript The transcript of an unnatural 'gene' that occurs when a segment of a gene, eg *FLI-1* gene on chromosome 11q24, is translocated to the site of a second gene, eg *EWS* gene on chromosome 22q12, forming a new hybrid transcript, eg *EWS/FLI-1* (**Diagn Mol Pathol 1993; 2:147**); see Fusion protein

futility Medical futility, futile resuscitation BIOMEDICAL ETHICS A subjective term that encompasses a range of probabilities that a patient will benefit from efforts designed to improve his life and will survive to discharge from a health care facility; see DNR orders; Cf Euthanasia

The definition for futility has proven to be a stumbling block on whether a person should be subjected to cardiopulmonary resuscitation if the likelihood for a 'meaningful existence' is minimal (**JAMA 1991; 265:1868**)

fuzz factor LABORATORY MEDICINE An appoximation of the line width in a data set used to establish linearity; the data are linear if the difference between two consecutive deltas (slopes between adjacent points on a line) is less than 1/50 of the range

(Solution 1 – Solution 5)/50 = Fuzz

The fuzz factor can be likened to the width of a pencil line, which if broad in a low-resolution linearity graph would correspond to a large fuzz factor (**Arch Pathol Lab Med 1992; 116:740oA**)

fuzzy space An intracellular, submembranous region in excitable tissue, eg heart muscle that acts as a calcium ion 'purgatory'; on one side, there is sodium-calcium exchanger located on the cell membrane and on the other side is sarcoplasmic reticulum that responds to the influx of calcium by contracting

fuzzy logic ARTIFICIAL INTELLIGENCE A tool for calculating the probability that activities or objects are related by assigning a weight to each factor and measuring them to reach uncertain conclusions linked to the probabilities of various conclusions being correct; fuzzy logic is being applied to a wide variety of fields, eg in the health insurance industry to identify fraud and abuse, and may have a return of $25 for each $1 invested in developing the modeling system (**Am Med News 10 October 1994**)

FVC Forced vital capacity, see there

FVIIc Factor VII coagulant activity

F waves CARDIOLOGY The waves of atrial flutter on the EKG, which appear as a 'sawtooth' pattern in leads II, III and aVF; less commonly, F waves are undulating, firing at a rate of 280-320/min; this rate is often associated with a 2:1 block and alternating F waves merge with the QRS or T wave NEUROLOGY F wave F response An undulation of the electromyogram that corresponds to time between the application of the stimulus to the axon of the α motor neuron as it propagates andromically to the anterior horn of the spinal cord, and then returns orthodromically along the same axon

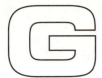

318

G Symbol for: 1) Gauss 2) giga-, the SI (International System) abbreviation for 10^9 3) Glycine 4) Gravitational constant 5) Guanine 6) Guanosine

g Symbol for: 1) Gram 2) Gravity/centrifugal force

G_1 Gap 1 A quiescent period in the cell cycle between the phases of mitosis and DNA synthesis; G_1 arrest of cells is a reversible process maintained by p53, a tumor-suppressor gene (**N Engl J Med 1994; 331:49RV**)

G7 The seven wealthiest and industrially advanced nations: Canada, France, Germany, Italy, Japan, United Kingdom, United States

G-actin A 42-kD globular form of monomeric actin that polymerizes spontaneously under physiological conditions; Cf F-actin

G deletion syndrome CLINICAL GENETICS A disease complex resulting from various anomalies of the G chromosome, eg partial deletion and ring formation CLINICAL Ptosis, epicanthal folds, flattened nasal bridge, growth and mental retardation

G6PD Glucose-6-phosphate dehydrogenase

G protein VIROLOGY 1) A protein that may be responsible for the neurotoxicity of the rabies virus (amino acid substitution of arginine at position 333 for valine or isoleucine eliminates rabies' neuropathogenicity); it is the only antigen produced by the rabies virus that evokes virus-neutralizing antibodies (T helper) cells (**Science & Medicine 1995; 2/3:48**) Cf G protein 2) An 84–90-kD surface glycoprotein involved in the pathogenesis of respiratory syncytial virus, which mediates attachment of the virus to the host cell; Cf F protein

G protein(s) Guanosine phosphate GDP, GTP-binding proteins A family of more than 20 different membrane-bound proteins that regulate ten or more different ion channels and as many enzymes; G proteins function as heterotrimers (α, β and γ subunits), transducing biological signals, including light, hormones and neural neural signals (table); according to the accepted model, a transmembrane receptor undergoes a conformational change, interacts with a G protein, which, depending on the ligand, either activates (as do ACTH, glucagon or epinephrine, left side of below figure) or inhibits (eg, prostaglandine E_1 or adenosine) adenylate cyclase, which is mediated by GTP and GDP; the α G protein subunit is thought to be the most central component of the complex and is linked to critical intracellular effectors including receptors via adenyl cyclase, effector enzymes, phosphoinositide cycle proteins, calcium and sodium ion channel proteins and transportation of proteins and sugars; subtypes of G-pro-

teins include G_s, stimulatory for adenylate cyclase; G_i, inhibitory for adenylate cyclase; G_o, otherwise, function unknown and G_t, a transducin or photoreceptor; G-protein diseases are processes that block G-protein activity at the membrane, eg pertussis and cholera, preventing signal transduction

G proteins '...have seven transmembrane domains with marked similarity, an extracellular N terminus with consensus sequences for N-linked glycosylation, sequence divergence in the connecting hydrophilic loops, a cytoplasmic carboxyl tail and/or a large intracellular loop rich in serine and threonine residues, which are sites for phosphorylation and conserved sites for post-translational modifications, including fatty acylation and disulfide bond formation; the diverse ligands appear to interact within a pocket created by some of the α-helical membrane-spanning regions, while other regions on the inner surface of the receptor interact with and activate specific G proteins, determining the nature of the biological response...' (**Nature 1991; 351:353**);

G protein receptors A family of membrane receptors including D_1, D_2, D_3 (dopamine) receptors, β, α_1 and α_2-adrenergic and muscarinic and serotonergic receptors that evoke intracellular responses by degrading GTP to GDP; see G proteins

G statistic A statistical device used to test for linearity, which is an F test of the ratio of the lack-of-fit and pure error variances (**Arch Pathol Lab Med 1992; 116:739OA**)

G syndrome An AR [MIM 145410] (formerly thought to be X-linked recessive) condition* of neonatal onset, characterized by pulmonary aspiration at birth due to a laryngotracheoesophageal cleft, stridor, ocular hypertelorism, a broad nasal bridge, cleft lip and palate, cardiac defects, imperforate anus and hypospadias, and mental retardation

*Synonyms include BBB syndrome, BBBG syndrome, hypertelorism-hypospadias syndrome, Opitz syndrome, telecanthus-hypospadias syndrome

GABA γ-aminobutyric acid An amino acid that is the major inhibitory neurotransmitter in the vertebrate gray matter; GABA-ergic neurons are classified according to the direction of the cell processes and the signal transmitted and received

TYPE I GABA-ERGIC NEURONS send and receive signals

TYPE II GABA-ERGIC NEURONS send messages to other neurons within adjacent gray matter

TYPE III ('PROJECTION') GABA-ERGIC NEURONS have axons that project from the gray matter to the white matter; benzodiazepines potentiate GABA's action by lowering the concentrations of GABA necessary to increase chloride permeability, but therapeutic stimulation or inhibition of GABA release is difficult to achieve, given the ubiquity of GABA's actions; see Stiff man syndrome; GABA is increased in the GI tract in hepatic failure and may have a role in hepatic encephalopathy

GABA receptors Membrane receptors which are composed of one or more α/β subunits, each capable of forming receptor-type ion channels; once the ligands bind to the receptor, chloride channels are activated

gabapentin 1-aminomethyl-cyclohexane acetic acid An antiepileptic agent that is a structural analogue of GABA, which binds to an as yet poorly characterized receptor in the brain; it was approved by the FDA in 1994 for treating

G PROTEIN-COUPLED LIGANDS
ARACHIDONIC ACID DERIVATIVES Thromboxane A2
BIOGENIC AMINES Acetylcholine, adenosine, dopamine, epinephrine, histamine, 5-hydroxytryptamine, norepinephrine
BRAIN/GUT PEPTIDE HORMONES Angiotensin, arginine, vasopressin, bombesin/gastrin releasing hormone, thyrotropin-releasing hormone, vasoactive intestinal polypeptide
HORMONES Choriogonadotropin (lutropin), follicle-stimulating hormone, parathyroid hormone, thyrotropin
SENSORY STIMULI Light (retinal), odorants
TACHYKININS Substance K, substance P, neuromedin K
MISCELLANEOUS: cAMP, cannabinoids, complement 5a, endothelins, platelet-activating factor, thrombin (see G protein receptors)

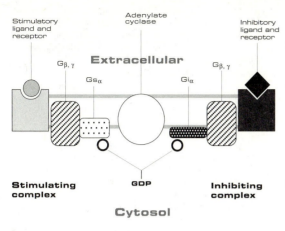

Stimulatory ligand and receptor

Adenylate cyclase

Inhibitory ligand and receptor

Extracellular

$G_{\beta, \gamma}$

Gs_α

Gi_α

$G_{\beta, \gamma}$

Stimulating complex

GDP

Inhibiting complex

Cytosol

G protein receptors

refractory complex partial and secondarily generalized seizures, and it is effective in treating convulsions with and without secondary generalization SIDE EFFECTS Vertigo, somnolence, headaches (**Medico Interamericano 1995; 14:125**); it has little interaction with other agents (**Science & Medicine Sept/Oct 1994**)

gadolinium A rare element (atomic weight, 157.25) used as a contrast medium for MRI of the CNS to enhance visualization of neoplasms, parenchymal and congenital lesions, infections and post-operative 'failed back' syndromes

gag A retroviral gene that encodes a structural protein within the virus core, which in HIV-1 corresponds to the heterogeneous p24 protein; see HIV-1, Retrovirus

'gag rule' A US Supreme Court decision in *Rust* v. *Sullivan* that prohibits physicians employed by the Title X projects, the federal family planning grant program initiated during the Reagan Administration, from fully counseling women who are unintentionally pregnant, thereby preventing them from offering nondirective advice on prenatal, infant, foster care, adoption and pregnancy termination; R Scaletter of the AMA felt that the 'gag rule' regulations would '*denigrate the integrity of the doctor-patient relationship and force health care professionals to violate established standards of medical care and professional ethics.*' (**N Engl J Med 1993; 330:32**SA) see Title X projects

Gaia hypothesis ENVIRONMENT Background: According to Darwin, evolution of the species, ie life, is driven by a static environment or nonlife; Gaia is the theoretical opposite of Darwinism, postulating that living organisms control and modify the relative compositions of the sea, air and environment, thus viewing all life (flora and fauna) on the planet as an interacting homeostatic macrocosm or organism driving mutual coordinated evolution of both the geophysical sphere and the diverse multitude of living organisms; Gaia is viewed by its chief architect, J Lovelock as not being endowed with the foresight to regulate the planet's temperature and composition, but rather to optimize it; Gaia-ists are often scientifically 'innocent', while non-Gaia-ists are often mainstream biologists; '....*We should be careful, however, not to pretend* (that) *Gaia is a testable hypothesis, much less a basis for managing the biosphere. The risk is this: a metaphor like Gaia, flexible enough to wrap around any data set, is also versatile enough to be invoked, ad hoc, to lend a spurious air of scientific legitimacy to almost any reckless conjecture.*' JW Kirchner, Cal Tech (**Nature 1990; 345:470**c) see Autopoietic Gaia, Creationism; Cf Darwinism, Neo-Darwinism

*Gaia, the Greek Goddess of the Earth, is an 'organism' from J Lovelock's book on a magical kingdom, Gaia, A New Look at Life on Earth, Oxford University Press, 1979

gain-of-function mutation Any mutation in a gene that results in a new activity, eg activation of an oncogene (see **Nature 1994; 369:318**0A); Cf Loss-of-function mutation

galactosialidosis Neuraminidase deficiency with beta-galactosidase deficiency AR [MIM 256540] condition due to a defective gene on chromosome 10, resulting in neuroaminidase and β-galactosidase deficiencies CLINICAL Neonatal onset with mental and physical retardation, seizures, visual defects, deafness, gargoyle facies, corneal clouding, a cherry red spot of the macula; see Cherry red spots

galanin A 29-residue neuropeptide/neurotransmitter produced in the GI tract that induces both contraction and inhibition of the circular and longitudinal smooth muscle and is thus involved in peristalsis; it is widely distributed in the central and peripheral nervous system; its highest concentration is in the median eminence of the hypothalamus, a key 'node' in neuroendocrine regulation through releasing and inhibiting factors

gale filarienne INFECTIOUS DISEASE Nodules located on the flanks tht correspond to subcutaneous lymphatic vessels plugged with *Ochocerca volvulus* microfilaria
Gale is French for scabies

gallium-67 lung scanning see Gallium scanning

gallium scan NUCLEAR MEDICINE Radioscintillation imaging method that uses ^{67}Gallium citrate ($T_{1/2}$, 25 days); once injected, the gallium binds primarily to transferrin and any tissue that concentrates lactoferrin also concentrates gallium; the gallium scan was formerly used to localize abscesses and osteomyelitis and is used for staging of lymphomas, lung carcinoma, hepatoma, melanoma, metastases (to bone, brain, lung), head and neck, gastrointestinal and genitourinary neoplasia

Gallo probe Robert C Gallo and Luc Montagnier were chiefs of the AIDS research teams at the National Institute of Health in Bethesda and the Pasteur Institute in Paris respectively (Gallo moved in 1995 to another institution); in 1984; Gallo et al, announced the discovery of the retrovirus held responsible for AIDS, which his group called HTLV-III (human T-cell lymphotropic virus, now known as human immunodeficiency virus-1 or HIV-1); it was alleged that HTLV-III had been isolated from a cell line designated H9 (or HUT78) that was inadvertently infected with LAV (lymphadenopathy-associated virus, now known as HIV-1) from Montagnier's laboratory, an event with commercial and academic ramifications in the primacy of HTLV-III's discovery; the 'Gallo probe' concluded that the event was the result of unintentional contamination of the tissue culture medium (**Science 1990; 248:1494, Nature 1990; 347:603**n) see HUT78

gallop(s) Cardiac auscultatory phenomena in which the tripling or quadrupling of heart sounds have been likened to the canter of a horse; although gallops may be the first sign of cardiac disease, they are often unrecognized, misinterpreted or ignored; gallops occur in diastole*; diastolic sounds are separated by the phase in which they occur; the ventricular (S3 or protodiastolic) gallop follows the normal first and second heart sounds, occurs in early diastole, coinciding with rapid ventricular filling, causing high-pitched vibrations of the ventricular wall as the blood is abruptly stopped; the S3 gallop connotes serious heart disease or decompensation and is associated with coronary, hypertensive, rheumatic, and congenital cardiac disease, but may be normal when found in young adults; once diagnosed, the average ventricular 'galloper' survives 4-5 years; the atrial (S4) gallop occurs during presystole or atrial systole and is characteristic of left ventricular hypertrophy or ischemia; if ventricular failure accompanies ventricular hypertrophy, an S3 gallop may also be heard; the S4 gallop may occur in absence of cardiac decompensation or in primary myocardial disease, coronary artery disease, hypertension and severe valvular stenosis, accompanied by an increased P-Q interval; if the P-R interval is prolonged or the heart rate sufficiently rapid S3 and S4 merge resulting in a 'summation' gallop

*The term 'systolic' gallop is considered incorrect and the appropriate descriptive terminology, eg ejection sound or systolic click is preferred Note: Traditionally both the three- and four-beat sounds are called gallops, after the footfall of horses; however, while a four-beat heart sound is properly known as a gallop, a three-beat heart sound is equivalent to the equine canter, which in French translates as 'le galop' (JAMA 1989; 262:352c)

galloping consumption Diffuse tuberculous bronchopneumonia

gallstones A major cause of morbidity and mortality; the diagnosis and treatment of gallstones cost ± $5 billion (US, 1990) EPIDEMIOLOGY 10% of adults have gallstones; this increases with age; ♀:♂ = 2:1; highest incidence in Scandinavia, Chile, Native Americans; ↑ risk with child-bearing history, estrogen-replacement therapy, oral contraceptives, obesity, rapid weight loss TYPES Gallstones are composed of cholesterol, bilirubin, calcium salts and other minor contributors; cholesterol gallstones constitute 75% of total in Western nations, and up to 80% of the volume is cholesterol; non-cholesterol gallstones are designated as either black or brown gallstones CLINICAL Biliary pain (colic), recurrent upper-quadrant pain; fatty food intolerance, while suggestive, is nonspecific; gallstones are often associated with acute cholecystitis which causes severe abdominal pain, nausea, vomiting, fever, and leukocytosis DIAGNOSIS Ultrasonography, cholescintigraphy (radionuclide scanning for uptake of iodinated radiocontrast), oral cholecystography TREATMENT 'The decades-long supremacy of open surgical cholecystectomy as therapy for gallstones was challenged by gallstone-dissolution techniques and shock-wave lithotripsy and has been overthrown by laparoscopic cholecystectomy.' (N Engl J Med 1993; 328:412oa)

gallstone pancreatitis Inflammation of the pancreas caused by common bile duct obstruction, which may be accompanied by acute inflammation of the gallbladder (Arch Pathol Lab Med 1995; 119:355oa)

GALT Gut-associated lymphoid tissue The GI immune system present in the mucosa and submucosa of the GI tract, but especially prominent in the oropharynx (tonsils), subjacent to the mucosa (Peyer's patches) and appendix; GALT's components include

1) M cells overlying Peyer's patches, the 'gatekeepers' for molecular traffic

2) Intraepithelial lymphocytes including CD8 T cells and IgA-producing B cells, which mediate T-cell cytotoxicity and immune recognition, and

3) Lamina propria lymphocytes including CD4 T cells, null cells and IgA-producing B cells

gamblegram A diagram that represents the cationic and anionic composition of the body, dividing each into rectangles

gamekeeper's thumb An avulsion fracture at the ulnar aspect of the base of the proximal phalanx, characterized by valgus instability, treated by a cast in adduction; if point instability is marked, open repair of the ligament is indicated; while now more common in 'week-end warriors', ie football or skiing injuries

Note: The original gamekeeper's thumb resulted from repetitive low-grade force, described in gamekeepers who used their thumbs to dislocate the necks of rabbits

gamma (γ) Symbol for: 1) Heavy chain of immunoglobulin G (IgG) 2) Hemoglobin monomeric chain 3) Photon 4) The third carbon in an aliphatic organic molecule

gamma camera NUCLEAR MEDICINE A device that evaluates the distribution of a radionuclide in the body following administration by injection or other means; in the GC a large sodium iodide crystal detects scintillations produced by the radionuclide which are amplified by photomultipliers behind the crystal; the photomultipliers send the information to a cathode ray tube which sends the amplified flash to the appropriate area of the CRT, which is recorded by a film based on time-lapsed photography

gamma-glutamyl transferase LABORATORY MEDICINE An enzyme [EC 2.3.2.2] that catalyzes the transfer of a γ-glutamyl group from glutathione or γ-glutamyl peptide to another peptide or amino acid; GGT is located on the cell membrane and microsomal fractions and is involved in amino acid transport across cell membranes; GGT is in highest in the kidney, but it is also present in the liver and pancreas; in hepatobiliary diseases, a 10-fold + ↑ in GGT is seen in primary liver cancer, hepatic metastases, and primary biliary cirrhosis; a 4-fold + ↑ in GGT is seen in chronic active hepatitis, intrahepatic cholestasis, alcoholic hepatitis, extraheaptic biliary obstruction, and in inactive cirrhosis; in nonhepatic disease, serum GGT is ↑↑ to ↑↑↑ (defined as 5-fold > upper reference limits, URL) in alcohol abuse, exocrine pancreatic disease, and malignancy; GGT is 2-5 fold > URL with analgesic (eg acetaminophen), anticonvulsants (eg phenytoin), antidepressants (eg tricyclics), barbiturates, hyperlipidemia, myocardial injury (CAP Today Nov 1994 p91) GGT concentrations are highest in liver, and it is the best single screening assay for detecting latent or chronic liver disease, including malignancy; elevated GGT often indicates continued imbibition in chronic alcoholics as it increases in response to microsomal enzyme induction; serum GGT levels ≥ 80th percentile in ♂ (80 U/L) correlated with alcohol intake of 51 g/day and comorbidity of liver disease, GI bleeding, and trauma; GGT levels ≥ 80th percentile in ♀ (37 U/L) correlated with alcohol intake of 12 g/day and comorbidity of hypertension and trauma (Clin Chem 1993; 39:2266)

gamma heavy chain disease Franklin's disease A disorder of older males, ranging from fulminant, ie death in weeks to prolonged, lasting 20 years, although usually death occurs in the first year, often due to infection CLINICAL Presents as a lymphoproliferation with fever, fatigue, anemia, angioimmunoblastic lymphadenopathy, hepatosplenomegaly, uvular and palatal edema, eosinophilic infiltrates, leukopenia, associated with autoimmune disease, TB and lymphoma LABORATORY ↑ IgG₁; most cases excrete < than 1 g/day of paraprotein, rarely up to 20g/day TREATMENT Cyclophosphamide, vincristine, prednisone

gamma 'hemolysis' MICROBIOLOGY Streptococci hemolyze blood by one of two hemolysins 1) The antigenic O₂-labile streptolysin O, which produces α or partial hemolysis and 2) The nonantigenic O₂-stable streptolysin S, which produces β or complete hemolysis; non-hemolytic streptococci were once designated as gamma-hemolytic, a misnomer of little practical utility

gamma-hydroxy-butyrate An agent that has been proposed as a possible therapy for narcolepsy; in Europe, GHB has been used as an anesthetic adjunct and experimentally to treat post-hypoxic cerebral edema and ethanol withdrawal; GHB has been marketed illicitly to body builders since mid-1990 as a sleeping aid, for weight control, as a replacement for L-tryptophan and for allegedly producing a 'high', acting on the endogenous opioid system TOXIC EFFECTS Potentially severe respiratory depression, seizure-like activity, nausea, vomiting, amnesia, vertigo, hypnagogic effect and coma; the FDA has issued a warning against potential complications when GHB is used outside of an experimental protocol (JAMA 1991; 265:1802)

gamma-interferon see Interferon-γ

gamma knife NEUROSURGERY, RADIATION ONCOLOGY A stereotactic radiotherapy device that contains 201 sources of ⁶⁰Co that destroys intracranial targets by 3-D focused beams of γ radiation with stereotactic precision; the GK and linear accelerators can be adapted to provide stereotactic irradiation to highly localized regions of the brain and have been used to treat arteriovenous malformations, and may be of use in treating primary and secondary tumors* (N Engl J Med 1995; 332:371ʀᵥ); thousands of patients have been treated worldwide with minimal intraoperative mortality for such diverse conditions as arteriovenous malformations, meningiomas, acoustic neuromas, pituitary adenomas, craniopharyngiomas and malignancy; the reported delayed morbidity is 3% versus 15% for helium beam therapy; the obliteration rate of arteriovenous malformations by the standard helium beam is 30%, while the γ knife has an 80-90% rate of obliteration with negligible recurrent hemorrhage

*The data comparing sterotactic techniques with surgery are scant at present

gammopathy An abnormal ↑ in immunoglobulin production; monoclonal gammopathies are usually malignant and include multiple myelomas, Waldenström's disease, CLL, heavy-chain disease, but may also be benign, appearing in amyloidosis and monoclonal gammopathy of undetermined significance; polyclonal gammopathies are usually benign and appear in inflammatory conditions, including angioimmunoblastic lymphadenopathy, cirrhosis, leishmaniasis, rheumatoid arthritis, SLE, TB Note: Polyclonal gammopathies may occur as epiphenomena in lymphomas, Hodgkin's disease, metastatic adenocarcinoma; see Monoclonal gammopathy of undetermined significance

gancyclovir (9-[2-hydroxy-1-(hydroxymethyl) ethoxymethyl] guanine An anti-viral agent used to treat CMV infections in immunocompromised patients with CMV-induced retinitis, gastroenteritis and hepatitis; gancyclovir eliminates CMV from the blood, urine and respiratory secretions CMV progression despite adequate therapy indicates drug resistance by CMV Side effects Changes in mental status, neutropenia, thrombocytopenia Note: AIDS patients and BM recipients may respond poorly to gancyclovir; Cf Acyclovir

gancyclovir

ganglion A mass of organized neural tissue

ganglion cyst A common soft tissue 'tumor' of the hand that is 1) Not a ganglion, ie it is not neural in origin and 2) Not a cyst, but rather represents mucoid degeneration of tendinous tissues; ganglion cysts are often located on the wrist in middle-aged women and may cause the carpal tunnel syndrome

ganglioneuroma A benign, embryologically differentiated tumor of the sympathetic nervous system which is associated with well-differentiated neurofibromatous elements

gangrene Tissue death most common in the distal lower extremities or internal organs, usually the large intestine; the type of gangrene is a function of the environment or host

Types of gangrene **Dry gangrene** A condition caused by chronic occlusion that slowly progresses to severe tissue atrophy and mummification, often associated with peripheral vascular disease, eg diabetes mellitus, atherosclerosis **Gas gangrene** A condition most common in open or poorly cleaned wounds infected by gas-producing gram-positive anaerobes, including *Clostridium perfringens, C histolytica, C septicum, C novyi* and *C fallax* that release histolytic enzymes, eg collagenase, fibrinolysin, hyaluronidase and lecithinase **Wet gangrene** A condition caused by relatively acute vascular occlusion, eg burns, freezing, crush injuries and thromboembolism, resulting in liquefactive necrosis, causing bleb and bullae formation with violaceous discoloration

GANT Gastrointestinal autonomic nerve tumor, see there

GAP GTPase-activating protein A 110-kD cytoplasmic protein that has a role in human cancer, acting as a growth signal, enhancing the GTPase activity of the N-ras p21 protein by interacting with the ras effector binding domain (Science 1988; 240:518); GAP has a 25% homology with the catalytic region of the neurofibromatosis gene

gap 1 see G₁

GAP-43 Growth-associated protein A neuron-specific protein associated with the membrane of the nerve growth cone, having a role in cytoskeleton and intermediate filament regulation

gap filling Molecular biology An activity that occurs on the discontinuous strand of DNA during replication, which entails joining of the gaps between the Okazaki fragments; see Okazaki fragments

gap junction A cluster of transmembrane channels or connexons, separated by a 2–4-nm space that allow communication between cells and the free passage of small (< 1.2 kD) molecules, including ions, water, amino acids and nucleoside phosphates; each connexon is composed of a six subunits, each containing 12 molecules of 28–32-kD connexin, arranged in a hexamer that opens as cellular calium ions fall; Cf Tight junction

gap LCR Gap ligase chain reaction Molecular diagnostics An probe amplification-type technique for detecting DNA; GLCR uses 4 probes and requires a denatured DNA template; the probes bind in pairs to complementary sequences on the 2 strands of the DNA template, such that the 2 probes on one strand are adjacent to each other and exactly across from the 2 probes on the opposite strand; the pair of probes on one strand is covalently joined by a thermostable ligase; repeated cycles of denaturation and ligation produce numerous copies of the ligated pair of probes, thus differing from other methods of DNA amplification in which the target sequence is amplified

Note: Because the probe pairs may join nonspecifically, without binding to the template, false-positive results may occur, which is eliminated by leaving a gap (hence the name) of 1-3 nucleotides between probes, which are then filled in by a heat-stable DNA polymerase (CAP Today May1995 p1)

GAPO syndrome An AR [MIM 230740] condition characterized by growth retardation, alopecia, pseudoanodontia (the teeth are present but unerupted) and optic atrophy, often in a background of parental consanguity; the few cases described have also had hydrocephalus, high palate, low-set ears

garbage Computers A colloquial term for 'nonsense' produced by a printer, eg incorrect ASCII characters versus text, often due to loose cables to the printer or due to use of an incorrect printer driver

'garbage can' hypothesis Accumulation theory A theory regarding the pathogenesis of senescence, which holds that as a cell line ages, it converts to a multigenerational wastebasket, where the older cells accumulate metabolic products capable of damaging the cell's macromolecules, eg proteins and nucleic acids, and are less efficient in repairing damage; the most critical intracellular 'garbage' accumulated are the oxygen free radicals; mechanisms designed to remove the free radicals include antioxidants and superoxide dismutase; another contributor to senescent 'garbage' is glucose, which attaches to proteins by non-enzymatic glycosylation, forming advanced glycosylation end products and decreased collagen elasticity; Cf Pacemaker theory

Note: Enzyme systems have been shown to be less efficient in aging cell lines, lending credence to this theory

garbage collector COMPUTERS A colloquial term for a program that condenses the scattered 'dead' storage space either on a hard drive or on floppy disks that is usually due to deleted files; the sum aggregate of the dead space is large enough to store extra files, despite 'insufficient memory' messages

garden hose appearance The appearance of tubular lumens with extensive transmural fibrosis and stenosis, seen in 1) The small intestine, usually affecting the terminal ileum in advanced Crohn's disease and 2) Esophagus in well-developed progressive systemic sclerosis

'garden variety' A highly colloquial adjective referring or pertaining to lesions or diseases that are both common and/or have relatively routine clinical, radiologic, or pathological findings, and which constitute the bulk of disease seen in medical practice, thus there is 'garden variety' appendicitis, 'garden variety' myocardial infarction, 'garden variety' colonic adenocarcinoma and so on

Gardner effect see Sellafield studies

Gardner syndrome An AD [MIM 175100.0006] condition characterized by condition of neonates characterized by colonic polyposis, which often undergo malignant degeneration, epidermoid cysts of the face, scalp, trunk, or extremities, multiple osteomas of the facial and occasionally of the long bones, and other mesenchymal tumors, eg lipomas, fibromas, and odontomas

gargoyle cell A nonspecific term for a cell engorged with mucopolysaccharide-laden (dermatan and heparan sulfate) lysosomes, seen in patients with Hurler syndrome (mucopolysaccharidosis type I-H), due to α-L-iduronidase deficiency

gargoyle face The characteristic facies seen in gargoylism, an obsolete term for mucopolysaccharidoses (MPS); the classic gargoyle face is seen in MPS type I-H (Hurler syndrome) and MPS type IV (Morquio syndrome) and characterized by thickening and coarsening of facial features due to subcutaneous deposit of MPSs, most commonly seen after the first year of age; the head is large and dolichocephalic, with frontal bossing and prominent sagittal and metopic sutures, with mid-face hypoplasia, depressed nasal bridge, flared nares and increased prominence of the lower ⅓ of the face, thickened facies, widely spaced teeth and attenuated dental enamel and gingival hyperplasia; similar facies may be seen in the cherry red spot myoclonus syndrome, Coffin-Siris syndrome, GM1 gangliosidosis, Goldberg syndrome, hyperimmunoglobulin E syndrome, hypothyroidism, Kniest syndrome, mannosidosis, type II, mucolipidosis (I-cell disease), MPS types I-S (Scheie syndrome), II (Hunter syndrome) and III (Sanfilippo syndrome), multiple neuroma syndrome, multiple sulfatase deficiency, Robinow syndrome, Rolland-Desbuquios syndrome, sialic acid storage disease with sialuria, sialidosis, type II, Sotos' syndrome, and Williams syndrome

Note: Gargoyles are grotesque spouts in the form of mythical animals, fantastic beasts or grotesque humans that project from the gutters of Gothic buildings; the term arrived to Middle English in 1412, via Spanish, gargola, throat

garlic *Allium sativum* A pungent herb used in cooking that has been used traditionally in medicine as a rubefacient and an antihelmintic; it has attracted more recent research interest given its positive systemic effects on metabolism, the immune and other systems; in experimental systems allicin, the active ingredient of garlic oil extract

1) Inhibits tumor growth and activity of tumor promoters and has chemopreventive activity against methylcholanthrene-induced carcinogenesis

2) Enhances defenses against systemic toxins, acting in antihepatotoxin, stabilizing liver microsomal membranes from lipid peroxidation and ameliorates cyclophosphamide toxicity in mice

3) Has non-specific anti-infectious activity, inhibiting growth of *Entamoeba histolytica*, lipid synthesis by *Candida albicans* and attachment of *Candida* species to buccal mucosa and

4) Inhibits platelet aggregation, inhibiting platelet release reaction; garlic owes its aroma to the high content of selenium, which is eliminated through the lungs and skin as volatile dimethyl selenide Note: Garlic's protective effect against upper respiratory tract infection may be an epiphenomenon as those with 'hypergarlicosis' may be given a wider berth by peers and are thus less exposed to infected aerosols; Cf Spicy foods

garlic clove fibroma A fanciful term for a benign, pedunculated tumor arising in the fingernail bed HISTOPATHOLOGY Either a fibroepithelial polyp or irritation fibroma

garment nevus Giant congenital melanocytic nevus* A congenital pigmented skin nevus covering any large area, thus also designated as 'stocking', 'cap' or 'coat sleeve' nevi; these nevi may be 20 cm or larger in greatest dimension with satellite lesions, deeply pigmented with moderate growth of hair, require multiple operations for excision and about 12% undergo malignant degeneration HISTOLOGIC PATTERNS Compound or intradermal nevus, neural nevus and blue nevus; involvement of the head and neck region may be associated with epilepsy, mental retardation and leptomeningeal malignant melanoma; the draining lymph nodes are often pigmented, corresponding to benign nevus cell aggregates within lymphoid tissue

*A wide range of terms have been used for this condition; Fitzpatrick et al prefer 'congenital nevomelanocytic nevus', of which the bathing suit nevus is but a large variant Note: A bathing trunk pattern also occurs in the neurocutaneous melanosis complex, or in lower 'girdle' mongolian spots, which may be extensive if the patient also has a bilateral nevus of Ota

gas-bloat syndrome GASTROENTEROLOGY The inability to vomit after gastric fundoplication for reflux esophagitis, a complication of the Nissen repair of a hiatal hernia, a procedure that corrects 96% of cases of esophageal reflux; the bloating is thought to be due to vagal injury and is characterized by post-operative dysphagia and an accumulation of gas

gas gangrene A necrotizing condition most often developing in open or poorly cleaned wounds contaminated by gas-producing gram-positive anaerobes, in particular *Clostridium perfringens* (formerly *C welchii*), *C histolytica, C septicum, C novyi, C welchii*, and *C fallax* that release histolytic enzymes, eg collagenase, fibrinolysin, hyaluronidase and lecithinase TREATMENT Most cases require surgical debridement

gas hydrate ENVIRONMENT A frozen form of methane that is held at high pressure 1500 feet below the ocean floor; the vast deposits of this potential fuel beg the question of whether it can be mined to provide a relatively clean fuel, and whether its use will significantly accelerate the greenhouse effect (New York Times 21 Feb 1995; C5)

gas-liquid chromatography INSTRUMENTATION A type of column partition chromatography in which the stationary phase is an inert vehicle covered by a nonvolatile gas and the mobile phase is volatile; GLC is a highly sensitive and specific analytic technique for quantifying volatile substances (and substances that can be transformed into volatiles) that is used in toxicology and in research, eg in microbiology to identify short-chain fatty acids, nonvolatile organic acids and alcohols produced by bacterial metabolism

gas-producing 'syndromes' Excess gas in the GI tract is due to aerophagia or increased production by intestinal bacteria which may be facilitated by a deficiency of pancreatic enzymes; gastric gas is accompanied by bloating, pain, eruction and flatulence; intestinal gas is often accompanied by abdominal distension, flatulence and hypomotility or hypermotility; see Flatulence

gas washout technique PHYSIOLOGY A method that uses inert gases (N_2, He, Ne, Xe) to measure the functional, freely-communicating airway and lung volumes; Fowler's 'single nitrogen wash-out test' measures the uniformity of ventilation throughout the lungs; the patient first expires to maximum residual volume, then fills the lungs maximally with 100% O_2; during the next breath, the concentration of nitrogen at the mouth is continuously recorded and plotted against the volume of expired gas

Fowler's initial measurements in 1949 concentrated on changing N_2 concentrations, addition of xenon to the mixture increases the test's utility as it provides information on functional size of the small airways or the closing volume, which in normal healthy young adults is about 10% of the vital capacity, a volume that increases with age and in smokers

GASA Growth adjusted sonographic age OBSTETRICS A sonographic estimation of fetal age based on two determinations of biparietal diameter, one at 26 weeks and one at 30-33 weeks; Cf Biophysical profile

gasoline pump appearance A descriptor for the apically-oriented eosinophilic secretory 'snouts' seen by LM in apocrine metaplasia of the breast, the presence of which suggests benign behavior in breast lesions, although 'snouting' may occur in the rare cases of apocrine carcinoma

Note: The term derives from the bulbous tops of gasoline (petrol) pumps of pre-1950s vintage

gasping syndrome NEONATOLOGY A condition due to toxic systemic accumulation of benzyl alcohol (used to clean neonatal skin), which because of the immaturity of their metabolic systems and relative fragility of their skin, is most severe in preterm infants CLINICAL Gradual neurological deterioration, severe metabolic acidosis, sudden onset of gasping respiration, hematological abnormalities including pancytopenia, hyperbilirubinemia and hyperammonemia, skin sloughing, hepatic failure, renal failure, hypotension, cardiovascular collapse and a 'negative' autopsy

gastric bubble of Garren A doughnut-shaped inflatable polyurethane cylinder designed to decrease the available stomach volume, a therapeutic modality for morbid obesity, reducing the gnawing hunger pangs by inflating a balloon in their stomachs; when the gastric bubble is placed for prolonged periods, it may induce hyperplasia of the G or gastrin-producing cells or rarely, pressure ulcers; see Diet, Ileal bypass operation, Morbid obesity

gastric 'cannonball' RADIOLOGY A descriptor for any smoothly contoured, large and non-ulcerated filling defect in the stomach, seen in radiocontrast studies; these filling defects are most often due to metastasizing hepatoma, but also seen with hematomas, multiple submucosal leiomyomas, lymphomas, neurofibromas, metastatic intraperitoneal malignancy and other lesions that deform the gastric mucosa; Cf 'Golfball' metastases

gastric inhibitory polypeptide see GIP

gastric outlet obstruction A manifestation of gastric dysmotility; the rate of gastric emptying is controlled by duodenal receptors for fat or acid GOO is diagnosed when there is 1) More than 50% retention of a barium 'meal' more than 4 hours after ingestion 2) An overnight fasting gastric residue volume of more than 200 ml or 3) Fractional emptying of a ^{99m}Tc-labelled liquid of less than 10%/min; GOO is due to ulcers, benign or malignant tumors, inflammation (cholecystitis, acute pancreatitis or Crohn's disease), caustic strictures, pyloric stenosis CLINICAL Vomiting (often daily), intermittent epigastric pain NEONATOLOGY GOO may occur in neonates associated with antral hyperplasia; it is attributed to therapy with prostaglandin E_1, used to maintain patency of the ductus arteriosus in the face of congenital heart disease (**N Engl J Med 1992; 327:505OA**)

gastrin G34 (34-amino acid residues, 'big' gastrin) is the circulating form in both patients with Zollinger-Ellison syndrome and in normal subjects; G17 (17 residues, 'little' gastrin) is the tissue-based form produced in gastrinomas, the normal gastric antrum, duodenum and jejunum; G13 or G14 (14 residues, 'minigastrin', formed from the carboxyl-terminal); a non-functional 13-residue amino-terminal fragment is also produced; gastrin is released by local (partially digested proteins and calcium salts) and neural

(bombesin) stimulation and inhibited by secretin, somatostatin and VIP; gastrin is the most potent stimulant of gastric acid secretion, and increases the mitotic activity of gastric mucosal cells, and blood flow through gastric mucosa SITE OF SECRETION G cells of gastric antrum, proximal duodenum, delta islet cells, small and large intestine STIMULANTS Eating, vagus nerve stimulation, hypoglycemia; liver metastasis was reported in 37% of patients with serum gastrin levels ≥ 150 pg/ml vs 12% of those with gastrin levels ≤ 150 pg/ml (**Dis Colon Rectum 1993; 36:497**); excess gastrin causes the release of calcitonin and insulin, spasm of the lower esophageal sphincter, hyperacidity with formation of multiple peptic ulcers, hypertrophy of the gastric mucosa, steatorrhea and secretion of water and electrolytes and enzymes; normal levels 100 pg/ml, occur while in the Zollinger-Ellison syndrome, levels of up to 60 000 pg/ml occur; gastrin is increased in antral or G-cell hyperplasia, atrophy of mucosa achlorhydria, gastric carcinoma, gastric outlet syndrome, pernicious anemia, pheochromocytoma, 'retained antrum' syndrome, short bowel syndrome and uremia

gastrinoma An often multicentric tumor of the pancreatic islet delta cells that arises spontaneously or may be associated with MEN-1 (multiple endocrine neoplasm, type 1); rarely the tumors may be very small, eg 2-6 mm and located in the duodenum and/or are associated with the Zollinger-Ellison syndrome; it is usually accompanied by gastrin hyperproduction PATHOLOGY Neuroendocrine tumor features, ie carcinoid- or islet cell tumor like

gastrinoma triangle The anatomic region defined by the junction of the cystic and common bile ducts superiorly, the junction of the second and third segments of the duodenum infero-laterally and the neck and body of the pancreas medially, a region that is the most common site of gastrinomas

gastrointestinal autonomic nerve tumor SURGICAL PATHOLOGY A rare vimentin-positive stromal (spindle-cell) tumor of the GI tract (and retroperitoneum), of middle-aged adults (± 58); size ≥ 10 cm and mitotic activity ≥ 5/10 high-power fields; GANTs are associated with aggressive behavior (**Hum Pathol 1993; 24:766**)

gastrointestinal stromal tumor SURGICAL PATHOLOGY GIST A term of recent vintage for nonmucosal tumors of the GI tract which are most common in the stomach; the behavior of GISTs ranges from benign (leiomyoma) to malignant (leiomyosarcoma), which is best determined histologically by the presence of ↑ mitotic activity and bizarre cells, findings that are typical of aggressive lesions

GATA-1 A zinc-finger transcription factor that binds to the GATA consensus elements in regulatory regions of the α- and β-globin gene clusters and other erythrocyte-specific genes and which is critical in differentiation of erythrocytes (**Nature 1991; 349:257**)

gate COMPUTERS An electronic circuit that performs an operation when the criteria for a logical relation, eg AND, or OR are fulfilled; see Computers

gate control theory NEUROPHYSIOLOGY The theory that holds that the amount and quality of nociception is determined by multiple physiologic and psychologic variables, modulated at the dorsal horns and at other levels of the ascending afferent pathway (**Science 1965; 150:971**); this theory attempts to explain why neural impulses generated by painful stimuli and transported by small A-delta and C fibers can be blocked at the synapse in the dorsal horn by simultaneous firing of large diameter, low-threshold myelinated A fibers, inhibiting nociception; it is also evoked to explain the effects of acupuncture and transcutaneous electrical nerve stimulation on recalcitrant pain; the gate control theory contrasts to the more widely accepted 'specificity' theory in which individual branches of peripheral nerves are thought to be devoted to carrying only one type of sensation, eg pain, touch or temperature

gated blood pool scanning A radionuclide technique used in cardiology to calculate various hemodynamic parameters including cardiac output, right and left ventricular ejection fractions; one parameter, stroke volume ratio, allowing quantification of valvular regurgitation at rest and during exercise; finally the technique detects abnormalities of regional wall movement

gatekeeper Any person, organization or legislation that selectively limits access to a service; in health care, primary-care physicians (eg family practitioner, general practitioner, internist, pediatrician (see **Am Med News 3 October 1994**), peer-review organizations and utilization review committees function as direct or indirect gatekeepers

gatekeeping *'Gatekeeping has come to imply the medically limited and bureaucratic function of opening or closing the gate to high-cost medical services. This simplistic view … is controversial, both because of its menial connotation and because of the implication that the physician is the agent of the third-party payers, not the patient.* (gatekeeping may also be defined as) *… matching patients' needs and preferences with the judicious use of medical services.'* (**N Engl J Med 1992; 327:424SB**)

gateway Interface engine, hub COMPUTERS A device that interconnects two or more dissimilar computer systems eg LANs (local area networks) to a WAN (wide area network), minicomputer, or mainframe computer; a gateway consists of a system of software programs designed to facilitate data exchange at both the communication protocol layer, and at the message format layer, and has its own processor and memory, and may perform both protocol and bandwidth conversions; interface engines are becoming an increasing necessity in health care and hospitals, given the proliferation of heterogeneous computer systems of different ages and architectures, each of which was designed to serve a particular function, application, and department; to be most effective a gateway design should incorporate concept-based routing, see there

gateway drug Any drug or addictive subtance, eg nicotine and alcohol that may be abused, and allegedly linked to subsequent abuse of illicit 'soft' drugs, eg marijuana and/or 'hard' drugs, eg cocaine and heroin; see Glue sniffing, 'White-out'

gating INSTRUMENTATION A process of electronic selection, in which the observer selects a level of an electronic signal above which a certain action is allowed, as in flow cytometry, where only those lymphocytes that fall within a 'gated' region are counted as such on the histogram, while those outside of this region are not PHYSIOLOGY The opening and closing of an ion channel in a cell membrane, which is caused by conformational change in one or more transmembrane proteins and regulated by transmembrane voltage and neurotransmitters; see Ball and chain model, Voltage-dependent calcium channel

Gaucher's disease A rare AR **[MIM 230800]** hereditary metabolic disease due to the absence of β-glucocerebrosidase CLINICAL Hematologic abnormalities with hypersplenism, hepatomegaly, bone lesions, skin pigmentation, pingueculae, growth failure, hypoglycemia, lactic acidosis, oral and anal lesions, inflammatory bowel disease, neutropenia, impaired neutrophil chemotaxis and metabolism TREATMENT Alglucerase is the most effective therapy for GD-I, resulting in a ↓ in hepatospenomegaly, hematologic defects, ↑ bone mineralization, and a reversal of cachexia DISADVANTAGE The annual cost for a 70-kg person is $100 000 (**N Engl J Med 1992; 327:1632OA**); liver transplantation ameliorates the pancellular enzyme deficiencies by the mechanism of microchimerism (**N Engl J Med 1993; 328:745OA**) BM trans-

plantation may also be effective

gauge FORENSIC PATHOLOGY The inside diameter of a shotgun's bore; gauge is an obsolete unit based on the number of round lead balls, each having the same diameter of the bore, which in toto weigh 1 pound (454 g); thus each lead ball in the most commonly used shotgun, the 12 gauge weighs 1/12 of a pound (37.3 g or 1⅓ ounces); see Ballistics

gausssian probability distribution Normal distribution STATISTICS A bell-shaped probability distribution of data points (figure) that is symmetic about a mean with the 'tails' indicating the '+' and '–' standard deviations extending to infinity; it is common practice to assume that random samplings of a phenomenon will result in a normal or gaussian distribution of data, and the tests commonly used in statistics, eg *t*-test or analysis of variation reflect this assumption; Cf Bell curve

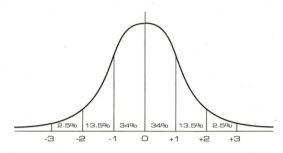

Standard deviations

gaussian distribution

gavage Nasogastric feeding of patients, eg premature infants with weak sucking reflexes or nasogastric hyperalimentation

gay Homosexual; in common parlance, when used as a noun, gay more commonly refers to male homosexuals and homosexuality; when used as an adjective, gay is generic for both male and female homosexual orientation, as in gay rights activism (**N Engl J Med 1994; 331:923SA**) see Homosexuality

gay bar A establishment that serves alcoholic beverages that is frequented by homosexuals of either sex; Cf Bath house

gay bashing To condemn or speak disparagingly of homosexuals; in the traditional parlance, GB is a generic term that encompasses 'passive' forms of homophobic behavior, but does not in general include acts of physical violence or destruction of property, but is rather confined to verbal abuse

gay bowel syndrome An array of infectious and non-infectious GI symptoms first described in homosexual males prior to the early reports of AIDS (**Am J Gastroenterol 1977; 67:478**) CLINICAL Proctalgia 80%, change in bowel habits 50%, condyloma acuminata 52%, cramping diarrhea, bloating, flatulence, nausea and vomiting, adenomatous polyps, fissures, fistulas, hemorrhoids, perirectal abscess, shigellosis, proctitis, rectal ulcers, giardiasis and STDs, including herpes simplex, syphilis, gonococcus and *Chlamydia trachomatis*; other 'gay bowel' organisms, include 'gay CLOs', ie *Campylobacter*-like organisms, eg *C fennelliae* and *C cinaedi*, HPV (associated with anal carcinoma and dysplasia), CMV, HAV, HBV, parasites, eg *Entamoeba histolytica, Entamoeba coli, Endolimax nana, Enterobius vermicularis, Strongyloides stercoraliz, Iodamoeba beutschlii* and bacteria (*N meningitis, Haemophilus ducreyi* and *Salmonella* species); other findings in GBD include rectal dyspareunia, pruritis ani, anal incontinence, trauma, eg secondary to 'fisting' that, like insertion of variably-sized and shaped foreign objects, may cause colorectal perforation and abscess formation TREATMENT Acute proctitis may require penicillin, probenicid and doxycycline, changing to specific agents if an organism is identified

Note: Anal cancer is more common in the male gay population and has been related to receptive anal intercourse; the relative risk for squamous cell anal cancer is 1.8; genital warts are often positive for HPV and may precede squamous cell carcinoma, but not transitional cell carcinoma

'gay' gene A putative gene reported to be located in chromosome segment Xq28 that has been linked by some workers to homosexuality (**N Engl J Med 1995; 332:1311BR**)

Gc Gc protein, vitamin D binding protein A 58-kD α_2-globulin of the albumin gene family (located on chromosome 4) that is structurally similar to albumin, and alphafetoprotein; Gc is present in plasma (6.25-9.8 µmol/L, 350-550 mg/L) and may be attached to cell membranes; it is the main protein involved in the transportation of vitamin D, although only ± 5% of Gc is so occupied; Gc also binds (in a stochiometric 1:1 ratio) and sequesters G-actin, as well as fatty acids (**N Engl J Med 1992; 326:1335RV**)

GC 1) Gas-liquid chromatography, see there 2) *Neisseria gonorrhoeae*, see Penicillinase-resistant *Neisseria gonorrhoeae*

GC box see GGGCGG box

G cells Flask-shaped gastrin-secreting cells thought to be of neural crest origin, which have features of APUD system; G cells are located in the gastric mucosa, especially in the pyloric antrum

G:C ratio MOLECULAR BIOLOGY The ratio of DNA nucleotide base pairs guanine and cytosine to adenine and thymidine BACKGROUND Guanine and cytosine in the double helix share three hydrogen bonds and denature at higher temperatures than adenine and thymine, which share two hydrogen bonds, therefore the higher the G:C base pair content of the double helix, the higher the temperature required for thermal denaturation of DNA; this occurs at 70°C when the double helix is composed entirely of adenine and thymine base pairs and at 110°C when the entire DNA molecule is composed of cytosine and guanine base pairs; the G:C ratio has been used to compare relatedness between various organisms, eg in microbiology for classifying bacteria

GCDFP-15 A marker of apocrine differentiation that is positive in pleomorphic lobular carcinoma of the breast (**Hum Pathol 1992; 23:655**)

G-CSF Granulocyte colony-stimulating factor A biological response modifier, the recombinant DNA-produced form of which, filgrastim (Neupogen®, Amgen Inc) was licensed in 1991 ACTIVITY G-CSF stimulates granulocyte production in bone marrow suppressed by chemotherapy and/or radiation, serving to reduce infections in patients with malignancy; in addition, it can induce terminal maturation of myeloid leukemia cell lines and suppress self-renewal, and is thus useful in some patients with leukemic relapses after allogeneic bone marrow transplantation; in one study, G-CSF induced a complete hematologic and cytologic remission in 3/7 patients (**N Engl J Med 1993; 329:757OA**) G-CSF is encoded on chromosome 17, produced by endothelial cells, fibroblasts and macrophages, and stimulates granulocyte production in the BM, acting synergistically with IL-3 to stimulate proliferation of other marrow cells; see Biological response modifiers, Colony-stimulating factors; Cf GM-CSF

GDNF Glial cell-derived neurotrophic factor, see there

geezer American slang for an offensive or dull-witted old person, especially a man (**JE Lighter, Historical Dictionary of American Slang, Random House, New York, 1994**); in the hospital environment, geezer is a highly derogatory term for an elderly, cantankerous, often poorly-educated male patient

gefilte fish A traditional Jewish dish eaten on Friday

nights, made from various fishes that are chopped, ground, mixed with eggs, salt, onions and peppers, often garnished with chrayn (horseradish), and then cooked; gefilte fish may be a vector for the fish tapeworm, *Diphyllobothrium latum*, which may be ingested while the chef is preparing the garnee prior to cooking and is well-described in Jewish mothers; see Fish, Sushi

The parasite is destroyed by cooking for 10 minutes at 56°C, or blast-freezing to -35°C for 15 hours or -23°C for 7 days; freezing for 24 hours, salting, smoking and pickling does not kill parasites

gegenhalten German, to hold against NEUROLOGY Paratonia Resistance to passive movement that increases with the velocity of movement and continues through the full arc of motion, thought to be due to diffuse forebrain dysfunction as occurs in anterior cerebral artery occlusion ('arteriosclerotic parkinsonism' or pseudoparkinsonism); gegenhalten may be accompanied by grasp reflex; Cf Clasp-knife phenomenon, Cogwheel rigidity

gel Agar gel A semisolid 'workhorse' medium made from the seaweed agar that is used as a support in various areas of the clinical and research laboratory; gels are primarily a liquid but also have some solid properties, as well as critical ionic and hydraulic properties, eg the ability to retard the flow of solvents, in a manner similar to a sponge retaining water; the elasticity and water-retention capacity of gel (concentrated in the cortex of 'crawling' cells) derives from the water-soluble polymers in the cell cytoplasm, which also serve as scaffolding, eg actin and actin-binding proteins needed to support contractile forces (**Sci Am 1994; 270/9:54**); see Cell crawling, Modulus of rigidity, Sol, Sol-gel transformation; gels are used in CLINICAL CHEMISTRY for serum protein electrophoresis for separating proteins into albumin and α, β and γ bands, see SPEP HEMATOLOGY for separating hemoglobins IMMUNOLOGY for antigen-antibody reactions MICROBIOLOGY where various nutrients are added to the agar to enhance or select for the growth of certain bacteria and fungi MOLECULAR BIOLOGY for separating DNA, RNA and proteins by electrophoresis

gel filtration chromatography Molecular sieve chromatography A column chromatographic technique in which gel particles of a certain size and porosity comprise the stationary phase, allowing the fractionation of a solution of molecules according to size, shape and rate of diffusion into the gel, where larger molecules pass through the column and are eluted before smaller molecules

gel penetration 'Bleed' The passing of microdroplets of silicone through the semipermable gel envelope of a breast implant; the amount is small, generally a few grams (which contrasts with 25-50 g that a person with insulin-dependent diabetes mellitus [IDDM] might inject over time)

gel shift analysis A method in which an altered ('shifted') band found on an electrophoretic gel, eg by single-strand conformation polymorphism analysis (a technique for screening possible mutations in DNA) is isolated and subjected to PCR (polymerase chain reaction) to amplify the DNA and determine its sequence of nucleic acids (see **Diagn Mol Pathol 1993; 2:23**)

gelastic epilepsy A form of complex partial seizure due to epileptic discharges in the temporal lobe characterized by inappropriate laughter as a manifestation of automatism

gelatinase-A Matrix metalloproteinase 2, MMP2

gelatinous infiltration Gray infiltration, see there

gelatinous transformation (bone marrow) SURGICAL PATHOLOGY An uncommon condition (aka serous atrophy) characterized by patchy or diffuse extracellular deposition of gelatinous material in the BM, and accompanied by marrow hypoplasia and fat atrophy; GT occurs in chronic wasting disease, including AIDS, anorexia nervosa, malabsorption, malignancy, and starvation

gelling Stiffness following rest, characteristic of rheumatic diseases, eg in juvenile rheumatoid arthritis (Still's disease) variably accompanied by polyarthritis and guarding of the joints against activity

gelsolin A multidomain protein produced by macrophages that has six similar domains of M_r 14 000, all of which may participate in various types of actin binding (for structure, see **Nature 1993; 364:685; 675N&v**) gelsolin-actin interactions include severing of actin filaments, binding of actin monomers, and promoting actin polymerization by accelerating the slow nucleation step; gelsolin participates in actin's assembly and dissembly and increasing the motility of some cells, eg fibroblasts in a concentration-dependent fashion (**Science 1991; 251:1233**); it is activated by calcium ions and inhibited by membrane polyphosphoinositides; precise regulation of actin assembly may result from an interplay between gelsolin and the related, structurally homologous gCap39 protein

Note: Gelsolin is so named as it was first identified as the factor liquefying (solating) gels formed by macrophage extracts

gemfibrozil A drug that inhibits VLDL synthesis, used to ↓ serum cholesterol, triglycerides and lipoproteins; in healthy volunteers, gemfibrozil causes a 30-40% ↓ in VLDL and IDL and 10% ↑ in HDL; in type V hyperlipoproteinemia, gemfibrozil is an agent of first choice for ↓ cholesterol and triglyceride; see Cholesterol-lowering drugs, Lovastatin

gemeprost OBSTETRICS A prostaglandin analogue administered vaginally that has been used in conjunction with mifepristone (RU 486) as an abortifacient; it is safe but expensive and requires specific conditions for storage and transportation (**N Engl J Med 1995; 332:983OA**) see Abortion, Mifepristone, Misoprostol, Sulprostone

GenBank A repository for nucleic acid sequence data created in 1982 from the Los Alamos (US) DNA sequence library, which currently accumulates 20 million nucleotide of DNA sequences per year in its database, providing a format for electronic publishing so that a sequence of nucleotides is published within 2 weeks of submission of the information rather than the one year required in usual (paper) publishing (**Science 1991; 252:1273**)

gender bias A generic term for any alteration in the amount of screening activities, diagnostic work-up, or aggressiveness of therapy based on a person's sex; some workers believe a gender bias is a cause for underdiagnosis and undertreatment of ♀ with high cholesterol and cardiovascular disease; in the US this issues is being addressed 14-year project involving 158 000 ♀ that will extend into the next century under the title of Women's Health Initiative, at a cost of $625 million (**CAP Today April 1993**)

gender identity Core gender identity *'The inner conviction that one is male, female, ambivalent, or neutral.'* (**Intl Dict Med, J Wiley & Sons, New York, 1986**) GI is a major personality trait that is thought to develop within the first two years of life, and become 'fixed' before the third year

gender identity disorder Transsexualism A clinical condition in which a person has a persistent desire to be of the opposite phenotypic sex[1] (cross-gender identification) and discomfort about his/her assigned sex; this desire may take the form of simple 'cross-dressing' or may be of such intensity to compel the person to seek sexual reassignment[2]; see Sexual reassignment

[1]Unrelated to perceived advantages of belonging to the opposite sex [2]Sought in circa 1:30 000 ♂, 1:100 000 ♀Note: ♂→♀ transition with protracted estrogen administration (x 14 years) induced a prolactin-producing pituitary adenoma (**Arch Pathol Lab Med 1994; 118:562OA**)

gene The classic mendelian definition of a gene as a unit of heredity carrying a single trait and recognized by its ability to mutate and undergo recombination is primitive; as currently defined, a gene is a segment of DNA nucleotides, comprised of 70 to 30 000 base pairs including introns,

that encodes a sequence of messenger RNA, capable of giving rise to a functional (enzyme, hormone, receptor) polypeptide; genes may be structural, forming cell components or functional, having a regulatory role

gene amplification The increase in copy numbers of a gene, an event associated with cellular oncogenes in malignancy, where the copy number is a crude benchmark of tumor aggression; chromosomal abnormalities typical of amplified genes include double minutes, C-bandless (fragments of DNA without centromers) chromosomes and homogenously-staining chromosomal regions; the precise mechanism of amplification is unknown, but may be due to multiple repeated unequal sister chromatid exchanges; an example of gene amplification au natural is that of the multi-drug resistance gene in tumors treated with methotrexate

Note: PCR (polymerase chain reaction) is a form of 'gene amplification', but given the potential for confusion, 'gene amplification' is best used for a phenomenon occurring in vivo in aberrant, often malignant cells that appear to be mounting a defense against a hostile environment; 'DNA amplification' is best reserved for an in vitro process in which the double helix of DNA is manipulated as per the desires of the researcher; see PCR

GENE DIVERSITY HOW IMMUNOGLOBULIN RESPONDS TO MANY ANTIGENS
Multiple germ-line V genes
VJ and VDJ recombinations (**Nature 1983; 302:575**)
Recombinational inaccuracies
Somatic point mutation
Heavy and light chain combinations
Signal sequence replacement
Science 1988; 242:261, Proc Nat Acad Sci 1976; 73:3628

---

gene diversity The breadth of immune response that an antigen is capable of evoking, based on a simple principle of mixing and matching of exons from gene segments designated as variable, diversity, joining and constant regions (table); elucidation of this mechanism of gene diversity (**Proc Natl Acad Sci 1976; 73:3628**) garnered its author, S Tonegawa, the 1987 Nobel Prize

gene expression The multistep (transcription of a segment of DNA to mRNA and translation into a protein) process by which a functioning protein product is produced

gene gun A device used to inject DNA-covered fragments of gold directly into host cells, resulting in an immune response that is reported to be protective against the antigen or organism of interest (**Proc Nat Acad Sci (US) 15 December 1993**)

gene jumping Gene shuffling MOLECULAR BIOLOGY A generic term for any form of movement that can occur or be induced in DNA, including DNA recombination, site-specific recombination, transposition, and translocation (**N Engl J Med 1995; 332:941OA**)

gene knockout technique An experimental technique used in yeast genetics in which a normal gene is replaced by a defective gene at the exact same chromosomal site (hence, the normal gene is 'knocked out' by the defective gene); in contrast, insertion of DNA in mammalian cells occurs in random sites

gene library A molecular 'database' created when the mRNA extracted from a given tissue is reverse transcribed into cDNA (complementary DNA) segments that in toto comprise the sequences of genes that are expressed in the tissue of interest; see Library

gene machine A colloquial term for a semi-automatic or automatic device that is capable of synthesizing high-quality chains of nucleic acids of up to 100 bases in length; Cf Sequenator

gene mapping Mapping, see there

gene 'pharming' A form of biotechnology in which genes that produce desired proteins (eg those used to treat cystic fibrosis, or cancer, or other therapeutic agents, eg antithrombin III) are transferred into the embryos of diary animals, eg sheep and goats; the technology may ultimately prove to be a more cost-effective method for producing large quantities of these proteins than the traditional tissue culture based methods (Science 1994; 264;902N&v)

gene pool The sum total of the type of genes and permutations of 'junk' DNA present in a sexually-reproducing population; see Consanguinity, Founder effect

gene product A polypeptide or protein encoded by a gene

gene promotion Induction or activation of genes, which is facilitated by breaks in the ordered arrays of nucleosomes, these sites being sensitive to DNase I

gene rearrangement The shuffling of genetic material, where introns (intervening sequences) are removed and exons are spliced together to form mRNA; GR is a process typical of antigen receptor genes in which gene segments are juxtaposed or rearranged; after which intervening DNA is looped out and excised, and the segments are juxtaposed, an activity carried out by a enzyme system known as recombinase; GR indicates a lymphocyte's commitment to production of one specific cell type, either immunoglobulin production by B-cells or a β-chain receptor in T-cells; lymphoproferative malignancies, then, may be viewed as irreversible clonal expansions that are detectable by changes in a cell's genotype; in lymphocytes, if the cell population is heterogeneous, as it is under normal circumstances, there will be no predominance of any one cell type and by extension, no 'signal' as detected by Southern blot hybridization; however if one clone of cells is expanding, ie malignant, a 1-5% ↑ in those cells is detectable by Southern blotting; for lymphoproliferative disorders, 1) T-cell malignancies, somatic rearrangement and clonal expansion of the T-cell receptor β-chain is diagnostic for T-cell lymphoma/leukemia and 2) B-cell malignancies, somatic rearrangement and clonal expansion of immunoglobulin genes (V, D, J and C regions) is virtually diagnostic for a B-cell lymphoproliferative disease

gene recombination Recombinant DNA, see there

gene shuffling 1) Gene jumping 2) Gene shuffling

gene splicing see Recombinant DNA technology, Splicing

gene targeting A generic term for a group of techniques of molecular biology in which a gene of interest is manipulated either by mutational inactivation, eg the 'knock-out mouse' or by replacement, if it is determined to be the cause of a particular disease process

gene therapy A generic term for any form of therapy that specifically targets hereditable diseases, either by affecting somatic cells or germline cells; GT encompasses a family of therapeutic modalities and products derived from recombinant DNA technology, which include tissue plasminogen activator and Alglucerase (for Gaucher's disease) the diseases targeted for gene therapy include inborn diseases of metabolism, where a defective gene cannot encode a crucial protein, usually an enzyme; the first disease placed in a formal protocol for gene therapy was adenosine deaminase (ADA) deficiency; strategies for gene therapy include 1) Introduction of a recombinant retrovirus bearing the missing gene, the promoter and the gene regulator sequence in the package or 2) Implant the colonies of cells producing the missing factor(s), eg $α_1$-antitrypsin deficiency with the missing enzyme introduced into 'carrier' fibroblasts

The debate about the ethics of manipulation of the human genome first evolved around whether such therapy amounted to 'playing God'; ultimately the groups representing patients with lethal genetic diseases replaced the romantic view with the idea that GT was no more than another therapeutic modality to be used to battle an otherwise lethal condition, and the issues were reduced to those in any form of possible therapy, ie safety, efficacy, and informed consent (Nature Medicine 1995; 1:181ED)

gene vaccine DNA vaccine, see there

general acceptance rule *Frye* rule, see there

general adaption 'syndrome' Fight-or-flight response, see there

general health panel LABORATORY MEDICINE A standard [CPT-4 code 80050] panel of laboratory tests used to evaluate a person's baseline health status, for Medicare or Medicaid reimbursement, it must include 12 or more automated chemistries, CBC with a differential white cell count, and thyroid-stimulating hormone [CAP Today March 1993] Cf General health screen

general health screen A battery of serum assays that are considered to be the most cost-effective in determining a person's basic state of health, including albumin, alkaline phosphatase, AST (GOT), BUN/creatinine, calcium, total bilirubin, cholesterol, glucose, K+, LDH, total protein, Na+, triglycerides, uric acid; see Executive profile, Organ panel; Cf General health screen

general practitioner A physician who practices 'general medicine', often an older physician who did not specialize in any field of medicine following graduation from medical school; in the current environment (US), to practice general medicine, a physician undergoes a three-year period of training in internal medicine, and thus is most commonly known as an internist **generalist** A physician who sees the patient as a whole 'unit', ie not as an 'organ system' (specialist); generalists include family practitioners, general internists, and general pediatricians

generalized anxiety disorder A syndrome characterized by unrealistic or excessive anxiety and worry about life circumstances CLINICAL Findings can be divided into those related to motor tension, autonomic hyperactivity, and vigilance and scanning (N Engl J Med 1993; 328:1398RV)

generalized cortical hyperostosis van Buchem's disease, hyperostosis corticalis generalisata, sclerosteosis An AR [MIM 239100] osteoporosis complex of early onset with bony overgrowth of 1) BM, resulting in chronic cytopenias and 2) cranial foramina, causing stenosis and paresthesia of the facial nerve, loss of vision and deafness LABORATORY ↑ Alkaline phosphatase

generally regarded as safe list CLINICAL PHARMACOLOGY An extensive list compiled by the FDA of compounds that are often used in foods, cosmetics and drugs and widely regarded as having little or no adverse effects on humans, first legally defined under the 1958 Amendment of the Federal Food, Drug and Cosmetics Act; GRAS compounds include food preservatives, coatings and films that may be used on fruits and vegetables, special dietary and nutritive additives, anticaking agents, eg sodium ferrocyanide, flavoring agents, gum bases and other multipurpose agents; see Food preservatives

generic Nonproprietary

GENESIS A computer program (Loomis & Gilpin, U California, San Diego) that has rules for DNA sequence duplications, deletions, exons and mutations

genetic anticipation A non-mendelian segregation ratio that results in an ↑ severity of disease in successive generations, with an earlier age of onset; the phenomenon occurs in the fragile X syndrome, where there is 9% mental retardation in first generation of the pedigree, 40% in the third, and 50% in the fourth generation (Arch Pathol Lab Med 1993; 117:1121OA) see CAG repeat disease

genetic code The 'words' and 'language' that governs the way in which genetic information (DNA) is 'written' in the genome and 'translated' into the proteins that perform the genes' activities; four nucleotides (adenine, cytosine, guanine, and thymine) are arranged in triplets (codons) which are translated into one of 20 amino acids, or one of three stop codons; there are two initiating codons (CAC and CAG) which also translate as amino acids (valine and methionine)

which genetic mapping can be performed

genetic counselor An allied health professional with an undergraduate (4 years of college or university) degree, usually in biology or psychology, who has in addition a master's degree in genetic counseling; GCs are trained to present data in simple language, in a nonjudgemental fashion, to allow clients to make informed decisions; there are an estimated 1200 GCs in the US (1993); as increasing number of genes associated with human disease (in particular those of adult onset) are identified, the need for trained GCs is expected to increase

genetic counseling The activity carried out by various health professionals regarding a person's susceptibility for either developing or passing on to his/her progeny a particular disease with hereditary underpinnings; GC is often performed by those with suboptimal training (eg nurses, primary care physicians), who have little understanding of the ethical, legal, and social aspects of genetic testing and molecular diagnostics; see Genetic counselor

genetic discrimination A generic term for any form of discrimination by insurance companies, employers, health maintenance organization (HMOs) and adoption agencies based on a person's genetic complement (gene pool) that is based not on the identification of diseases that have already developed, but rather on genetic defects that are likely to result in diseases, eg Alzheimer's disease, fragile X syndrome, Huntington's disease, neurofibromatosis, and others (Technology Rev July 1995, p16); although in theory, such discrimination might be illegal by the Americans with Disabilities Act of 1990, the Equal Employment Opportunity Commission, which enforces this act, has offered the opinion that healthy carriers of a genetic disease do not, in fact have a disability (Sci Am 1994; 270/6:88)

genetic disease A generic term for any (inherited) condition caused by a defective gene, most of which are known as an 'inborn error of metabolism'

genetic engineering Recombinant DNA technology The manipulation of the genome of a living organism, resulting in the modification of both 'domesticated' and wild-type bacteria by insertion of genes or by genetic selection; genetic engineering has broad potential applicability in

1) Agriculture, as natural enemies to crop parasites or by increasing nitrogen-fixing

2) Industry, for production of fuels, eg ethanol, chemicals, eg amino acids and for mineral processing, eg bioleaching

3) Environment, for the production of biodegradable plastics and treatment of municipal and industrial wastewater and

4) Medicine

genetic heterogeneity The presence of a variety of genetic defects which cause the same clinical disease, often due to mutations at different loci on the same gene, a finding common to many human diseases including Alzheimer's disease, cystic fibrosis, lipoprotein lipase and polycystic kidney disease

genetic marker A visible mutable site on a chromosome which when mutated, leads to gross changes to the host organism and on the chromosome itself

genetic mosaicism A condition in which there is a mixture of genetic distinct cell populations

genetic mother A woman who for various physical reasons, eg anatomic defects or antibody production, cannot herself carry a fertilized egg to full-term; under the usual scenario, the genetic mother's egg is fertilized in vitro and implanted into a surrogate (gestational mother‡) who carries the product to completion (N Engl J Med 1992; 327:286c)

genetic polymorphism RFLP, see there

genetic recombination The process by which blocks of homologous chromosomes exchange material by crossing over, an event that occurs during meiosis in sexually reproducing organisms and forms the mechanism by

genetic testing The analysis of a person's DNA or chromosomes to detect inheritance of a disease caused by a gene mutation; GT was formerly limited to the detection of rare inherited diseases of children, often by relatively crude and laborious techniques, eg karyotyping, in which photographs are taken of chromosomes in metaphase, and the resulting images of the chromosome pairs matched by cutting the pictures with scissors and gluing them on a chromosome spread preparation; GT is a major 'growth industry' as genetic mutations have been linked to an increasing number of diseases, eg amyotrophic lateral sclerosis (Lou Gehrig's disease), breast cancer, cystic fibrosis, familial colon cancer, Huntington's disease, subtypes of muscular dystrophy, retinoblastoma and others; GT has become more elegant, and in contrast to karyotyping in which major chromosome segments (or entire chromosomes) were absent or redundant before a disease could be linked to a particular gene defect; the tests now available are far more eloquent, and are capable of linking a disease to a gene by identifying a change as simple as a point (single base pair) mutation

Geneva Convention A protocol established in 1864 regarding the conduct of the military towards medical personnel and the obligations of medical personnel during acts of war; the first Geneva Conference of 1864 simply recognized the neutrality of medical personnel, acknowledged the need for common protection in time of battle, and agreed upon rules for the protection and exchange of wounded personnel; in the 1949 GC, 60 nations agreed upon conventions that bound all nations to the laws of humanity and to the dictates of public conscience; under the revision, medical personnel and treatment facilities are designated as immune from attack and captured medical personnel are to be promptly repatriated; see Helsinki Declaration, Nuremburg Code of Ethics, Unethical medical research

---

OBLIGATIONS & RESPONSILIBIES OF MEDICAL PERSONNEL (PER THE GENEVA CONVENTION)

As 'noncombatants', medical personnel are forbidden to engage in or be parties to acts of war

The wounded and sick, both soldier and civilian, both friend and foe, shall be respected, treated humanely and cared for by the belligerants

The wounded and sick may not be left without medical assistance, and only urgent medical reasons authorize any priority in the order of their treatment

Medical aid must be dispensed solely on medical grounds, without distinctions founded on sex, race, nationality, religion, opinion or any other similar criteria

No physical or moral coercion shall be exercised against protected personnel (civilians), in particular to obtain information from them or from third parties

---

Genie A girl who had been imprisoned by her parents from age 2 until age 13 when she was discovered by authorities in Southern California in 1970; her height was in the 10th percentile, she walked in a permanently stooped position, had little speech and had permanent calluses on the buttocks as she had been strapped to a potty seat for long periods; the case has raised various ethical and scientific issues and she was seen in a light similar to that of the 'wild child' of France; she has remained in a foster home for adults (N Engl J Med 1994; 331:1030BR OF *Genie*, R Rymer, HarperCollins) see Psychosocial dwarfism, '*The Wild Child*'

genital mutilation The destruction or removal of a portion or the entirety of the external genitalia, which may occur in the context of a crime of passion (see 'Bobbittize') or as part of a religious rite (see Female circumcision)

genital prolapse The prolapse of internal organs into a weakened pelvic floor, including uterine prolapse, cystourethrocele, enterocele, rectocele CLINICAL Pelvic pressure, urinary incontinence, rectal discomfort and discomfort related to irritation or ulceration of exteriorized mucosae MANAGEMENT Pessary with topical estrogens and exercise aimed at strengthening the pelvic floor; hysterectomy (N Engl J Med 1993; 328:856RV)

genocide Syematic killing of a population that is sanctioned by the leaders in a country constitutes a policy, and may have the implied support from the medical community wherein it is occurring; Cf Massacre

Genome Project Human genome project, see there

genomic imprinting A form of developmental gene regulation in which only one of the parent's alleles is expressed; how GI actually occurs in unknown, but may be *cis*-acting in nature, and act 90 kilobases upstream of the imprinted gene (Nature 1995; 375:34, 16, N Engl J Med 1992; 326:1599OA); Prader-Willi and Angelman syndromes are the clearest examples of genomic imprinting to be thusfar described in humans; see Imprinting

genote MOLECULAR EVOLUTION A term for an organism with modern translation machinery, based on the 'evolutionary clock', where organisms are phylogenically classified according to the evolving complexity of ribosomal RNA; Cf Progenote, Universal ancestor

genotypic method A generic term for any DNA-based method

gentleman scientist A term arising in post-Renaissance Europe, referring to a financially-independent gentleman who had the luxury of studying scientific phenomena as a hobby; see 'New scientist', Cf 'Lab rat'

Note: During most of the 20th century, science has been more egalitarian and any person who could do 'good science' would be able to support himself and his 'significant others' on his salary; in the 1980s and 1990s, budget deficits in developed nations have burgeoned, and monies to support new grants have receded (in the US and in part in Europe), with the result that many excellent grants are awarded the hollow accolade of *'approved but not funded'* (approximately 20% of grant proposals are ultimately funded), or suffer the lesser indignation of 'downward negotiation' and 'dunning fees' from their own institution in the form of bills for overhead costs Note: Given the current economic environment for scientists, independent wealth may become necessary in order to 'do science' and the gentleman scientist may once again become a fixture in academia

genu genuflectum Infrapatellar bursitis in clergy, which can be so intense (as with Saint Tekla Haymanot, 12th century) as to cause gangrene of the foot

According to legend, St Tekla was compensated for his lost legs by being given a pair of wings, ie alae neoplasticae post-gangrenosa eremeticum (N Engl J Med 1983; 309:561c)

geochronology A field under the rubric of geology, that dates a site, often in a paleoanthropologic context

geode Giant subchondral pseudocysts often of weight-bearing joints, with articular destruction, characteristic of rheumatoid arthritis, but also seen in osteoarthritis and hemophilia

geographic exclusion TRANSFUSION MEDICINE A ban on the collection or use of blood donated by subjects native to certain countries, eg Africa with the exception of Algeria, Egypt, Libya, Mauritania, Morocco, Sudan, Somalia, Tunisia and Western Sahara (Arab nations with a low incidence of AIDS)

Since the beginning of the AIDS epidemic, there has been a well-publicized, higher-than-expected incidence of HIV seropositivity in Haitians, leading the US FDA to ban blood donation from this population group, a ban that was lifted in 1990

geographic pattern A descriptor for lesions in which large areas of one color, histological pattern or radiological density with variably scalloped borders are superimposed on another color, pattern or density, likened to national boundaries and coastlines DERMATOLOGY A pattern of skin involvement in psoriasis FORENSIC PATHOLOGY A descriptor

for the variegated pattern of skin ulceration seen in drug addicts who inject heroin subcutaneously (skin popping), which may be surrounded by 'ameboid' rim of hyperkeratotic and inflamed skin PATHOLOGY Sharply defined 'fjord-like' histologic separation of one tissue morphology from another, seen at low-power (40 x) in 1) Lymph nodes affected by LGV, less commonly cat-scratch disease 2) Lungs of Wegener's granulomatosus where irregular necrotic patches are interspersed with scattered islands of preserved pulmonary parenchyma, also described in rare fulminant pulmonary infections 3) Soft tissue in epithelioid sarcoma (ES), in which geographic lesions may result from fusion of several necrotizing nodules, often accompanied by hemorrhage and cystic degeneration; the geographic islands have central necrosis and are rimmed by chronic inflammation; ES is a slow-growing tumor of young adults, often of the upper extremities; the prognosis is poor if necrotic RADIOLOGY Broad areas of patchy destruction, seen in such diverse conditions as Gaucher's disease, histiocytosis X, osteolytic tumors, eg metastatic bronchogenic carcinoma and osteosarcoma

geographic tongue Benign migratory glossitis ORAL DISEASE CLINICAL Idiopathic tender or irritated lesions, possibly related to emotional stress, more common in children and adolescents or asymptomatic inflammation with denudation of the filiform papillae (smooth bright red patches) in an irregular circinate pattern, surrounded by yellow, gray or white membranous frontiers which slowly extend, resolving spontaneously only to later recur PATHOLOGY Focal absence of granular and horny layers, mimicking psoriasis (hyperkeratosis and Kogoj's microabscesses) TREATMENT Empirical, eg vitamins, psychotherapy, not often successful DDx Lingual syphilis with dense white patches Note: In the pre-antibiotic era, 21% of oral cancer occurred in a background of syphilis

geographic ulcer OPHTHALMOLOGY A sharply demarcated corneal ulcer with scalloped margins caused by Herpes simplex, which arises in dendritic herpetic keratitis, approximately ½ of which respond to idoxuridine therapy

geological disaster PUBLIC HEALTH A generic term for a natural disaster linked to geological disturbances, often the result of shifts in tectonic plates and seismic activity; GDs include earthquakes, tsunami (seismic sea waves), and volcanic eruptions and avalanches (JM Last, RB Wallace, Eds, Public Health and Preventive Medicine, 13th ed, Appleton & Lange, Norwalk, 1992) see Earthquake; Cf Climatological disaster

geomedicine Global medicine *The branch of medicine concerned with the influence of environmental, climactic, and topographic conditions on health and the prevalence of disease in different parts of the world* (Intl Dict Med, J Wiley & Sons, New York, 1986)

It is likely that the alternative term Global medicine will eventually replace the term geomedicine-Author's note

geophagy Clay-eating A formerly common custom practiced in many cultures, still extant in some regions of the Southern US Note: Although clay may be beneficial during pregnancy, providing trace minerals, mainstream medical thinking considers geophagy a form of pica (ingestion of indigestibles as comestibles, itself is commonly associated with iron-deficiency anemia)

***Geotrichum* spp** A candida-like arthroconidia-producing imperfect fungus of the Cryptococcaceae family, which has a 'hockey stick'-like morphology, as it buds from the corners; *Geotrichum* grows well in corn meal agar and when isolated, is clinically significant as it often affects immunocompromised patients with lymphoreticular neoplasia; the arthroconidia have a 'box car'-like appearance

'gerbiling' see Sexual deviancy

GERD Gastroesophageal reflux disease, reflux disease Chronic reflux affects up to 20 million US citizens, 10% of whom are estimated to have Barrett's esophagus CLINICAL Burning upper abdominal pain, dyspepsia, regurgitation, and aspiration with coughing ENDOSCOPY 90% of those with GERD have endoscopic evidence of inflammation at the EG junction, aka squamocolumnar Z-line (see Sci & Med Nov/Dec 1994 p16RV)

geriatric abuse The physical or psychological mistreatment of elderly subjects, which like child abuse, most often occurs at the hands of family members and is difficult to diagnose, as it rarely suspected; between 0.5 and 2.5 million events are estimated to occur annually

geriatric intervention A generic term for any maneuver intended to improve the evaluation process, patient care, design of environment (ie physical plant), discharge, rehabilitation, and implementation of changes in health care provided for older patients (N Engl J Med 1995; 332:1338OA) GIs include specialized acute care units, emphasis on independence in self-care, detailed discharge planning, and avoidance of iatrogenic illness; early studies suggest on the efficacy of GIs suggest that there is two-fold improvement in functionality (ibid 1995; 332:1377ED)

geriatrics The medicine specialty involved in the care and management of the elderly; the life expectancy in the USA in 1900 was 45 years; the life expectancy in the USA in 1983 was 71 years in males and 78 years in females; Cf Gerontology, Todeserwartung

Geritol fix see Iron hypothesis

GERL Golgi-endoplasmic reticulum lysosome Transtubular network A hydrolase-rich region of the endoplasmic reticulum, which is the last compartment of the Golgi apparatus, representing the sorting site for proteins, where they are separated into membrane proteins, secretory proteins and lysosomal enzymes

germ cell gene therapy Germline therapy A type of gene therapy which has raised considerable ethical clamor as, unlike now widely accepted somatic cell gene therapy (which in its day also engendered ethical debates about the dangers of genomic manipulation) in which the therapy affects the genome of a single person, GT carries for some, Hitlerian overtones of eugenics, as the intent is to prevent the passing of the parents' diseases to their children (Nature Medicine 1995; 1:181ED) see Gene therapy

germ cell tumors A group of tumors arising from malignant degeneration of the germ cell epithelium, with an annual incidence rate of 3/10⁵; GCT mortality has doubled since the 1940s; 10% occur in cryptorchid testes and cryptorchid testes have a 33-fold increased incidence of these tumors; GCTs are common in males, comprising 90-95% of all testicular tumors and are the most common malignancy of men ages 25-35, but relatively less common in blacks; GCTs are classified by the Dixon and Moore ('American') scheme as either 1) Seminoma, the most common GCTs, which have a good prognosis (90-95% five-year survival) or 2) Non-seminomatous GCTs, which have a less favorable prognosis, and include embryonal carcinoma, mature and immature teratoma, teratocarcinoma and choriocarcinoma, the last of which has a 0% five-year survival; yolk sac tumor and mixtures thereof; GCTs are less common in females, comprising 20% of ovarian tumors, the majority of which are benign cystic teratomas; other female GCTs include immature (ie, malignant) teratoma, dysgerminoma (the female counterpart of the seminoma), the highly malignant endodermal sinus (yolk sac) tumor and others, including choriocarcinoma, embryonal carcinoma and polyembryoma; see Sex cord-stromal tumors

germ-line configuration A 'primitive' arrangement of genes that have not yet undergone the rearrangement required for cell maturation; the term is usually applied to genes of the immunoglobulin superfamily that are in a pristine state; these genes include those encoding the immunoglobulin heavy and light chains in B cells and the genes encoding the T-cell receptor in T lymphocytes; see Gene rearrangement

germline mutation An inherited mutation that is transmitted through the germline, eg that of a tumor suppressor gene, eg p53 (N Engl J Med 1992; 326:1309OA) which may thus increase a person's susceptibility for malignancy

germline therapy Germ cell gene therapy, see there

germ tube test MICROBIOLOGY The germ tube is a short projection on a germinating spore of either *Candida albicans* or *C stellatoidea* that appears after three hours of incubation at 37°C on an appropriate culture medium; the GTT is a rapid bench test that allows a rapid presumptive diagnosis of *C albicans* as *C stelloidea* is a rare clinical isolate

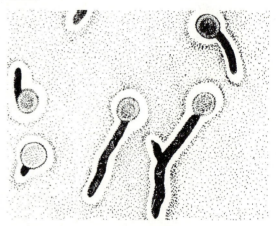

germ tube test

germ warfare Biological warfare, see there

German measles Rubella, see there

German-style system HEALTH CARE ENVIRONMENT The health care system extant in Germany in which ± 1200 Krankenkaße (sickness funds) are organized by employers, labor unions, and health care professionals; Krankenkaße are funded by equal payroll taxes on employers and employees; those workers who are self-employed and/or wealthy have the option to purchase private insurance, although few actually do; the monies in the funds are passed to regional physician networks that reimburse physicians in private practice and hospitals (which in turn pay staff physicians) and police utilization (Am Med News 25 October 1992, p7)

German syndrome see Fetal trimethadione syndrome

germinal centers Follicular centers The site in lymph nodes and lymphoid aggregates where normal B lymphocyte transformation occurs; the germinal center is composed of a mixed cell population composed of cleaved and noncleaved or transformed lymphocytes; when the lymphoid follicles are hyperplastic, the germinal centers are replete with tingible body macrophages; several terms are used by pathologists: '**BURNED-OUT**' **GERMINAL CENTERS** are morphologically distinct GCs typical of angioimmunoblastic lymphadenopathy, which are composed of loose aggregates of pale histiocytes, thereby resembling granulomas and scattered immunoblasts or epithelioid cells mixed with amorphous eosinophilic and PAS-positive intercellular material **PROGRESSIVELY TRANSFORMED GERMINAL CENTERS** are morphologically distinct, enlarged and reactive GCs that are often centrally located within the lymph node, with loss of the usually distinct frontiers between different cell types, accompanied by a 'starry sky' pattern, scattered epithelioid histiocytes, increased dendritic reticulum cells, mantle zone lymphocytes and increased T cells; PTGC is of particular interest as it may be associated with nodular lymphocyte-predominant Hodgkin's disease, but is not itself considered neoplastic **REGRESSIVELY TRANSFORMED GERMINAL CENTERS** are small, virtually devoid of lymphocytes and have an onion-skin layering of dentritic reticulum cells, fibroblasts, vascular endothelial cells and eosinophilic, hyalinized, PAS-positive intercellular material

germinoma Any neoplasm with the morphologic features of a germ cell tumor, eg seminoma; the term is reserved for midline tumors of germinal origin, including those of the CNS and pineal gland, mediastinum, retroperitoneum and thymus; see Germ cell tumor; Cf Teratoma

geroderma osteodysplastica A rare AR [MIM 231070] condition characterized by stunting of growth, marked senile changes of the skin with wrinkling, corneal opacification, osteoporosis with multiple bone fractures and deformities; the facial dysmorphia of these patients have a *'droopy, jowled, prematurely aged appearance'*, hence the highly colloquial alternative term, Walt Disney dwarfism*; see Progeria

*Named for the verisimilitude of these subjects' physiognomies to the protagonists of the classic Walt Disney animation, Snow White and the Seven Dwarfs, produced in 1939

gerontology The systematic study of the aging phenomenon as it affects cells and organisms; gerontologists have found that rodents are less 'instructive' than other 'unusual' animals, including lizards, bats, turtles and fish; senescence is thought to be the result of 1) Accumulation of degradation products, coupled with a cell's increasing inability to metabolize the products, see Garbage can hypothesis and/or 2) Activation of longevity-determining or aging genes which may be intimately linked to certain oncogenes, eg c-*fos*, which evokes uncontrolled cell proliferation; current data indicates that the agony of the human condition may be prolonged by 1) Eating less A 30% reduction in caloric intake decreases the incidence of cancer, autoimmunity, cross-linking of collagen, post-absorptive cholesterol levels, loss of striatal dopamine receptors and loss of lens γ crystallins; increased lipolysis in response to glucagon and epinephrine and the age-related changes in lipid levels and insulin are seen in rodents on low-calorie diets 2) Reduction of protein intake, especially tryptophan-rich products 3) Exercise When begun early in life and performed regularly, exercise retards or reverses age-related changes in lipid deposits, insulin levels, bone mineral loss, cardiovascular deterioration 4) Ingestion of antioxidants 'Soft' data implies that increased antioxidant ingestion, eg vitamin E, vitamin C, glutathione may increase longevity

gerovital A factor claimed (by Dr A Aslan, Institute of Geriatrics, Bucharest) to be present in procaine-HCl, and given the fanciful synonym of vitamin H₃; gerovital is alleged to have anti-aging and antineoplastic properties by some alternative health advocates and some self-proclaimed cancer specialists

Gerson therapy A system of unorthodox medical treatments of cancer that attempt to 'detoxify' the body with coffee enemas and 'sodium-poor, potassium-rich, poison-free' diets; scientific evidence supporting the claims made by proponents of the Gerson methods is virtually nonexistant, and has been summarized by S Green (**JAMA 1992; 268:3224sc**)

Claim 1: Anaerobic energy production causes cancer

Claim 2: Vital organs have been poisoned by toxic substances in processed foods and are detoxified by bile

Claim 3: Coffee enemas (see there) stimulates bile production

Claim 4: Cafestol and kahweol (compounds present in coffee enemas) enhance detoxification by stimulating liver GST

Claim 5: Enzymes from raw fruit, vegetables, and calves' liver restore normal function to poisoned organs

Claim 6: Once detoxified, the organs mount a tumoricidal allergic inflammatory reaction

geschlechtsverkehr Sexual traffic, Sexual activity

gestalt therapy German, Configuration A form of psychotherapy that focuses on the whole person, thus representing a 'holistic approach' to a patient's psyche, taking into account his perceptions and the effects of his environment and related stresses on his behavior; see 'Holistic' medicine

gestational diabetes (mellitus) A usually transient condition characterized by glucose intolerance coinciding with the onset of pregnancy, which is associated with 1) Increased perinatal complications for the mother, as well as the infant, see Fetal diabetes 'syndrome' and 2) Tendency to develop glucose intolerance in absence of pregnancy 5-10 years after gestational diabetes; based on ROC curve analysis, a fasting blood glucose of ≥ 4.88 mmol/L (≥ 88 mg/dL) has an 80% sensitivity in detecting GDM; fasting blood glucose requires less time, effort, and expense than the one-hour glucose screening test and may be more specific (**J Reprod Med 1992; 37:907**); the incidence of GD by criteria from the National Diabetes Data Group was 3.2%, and by modified criteria 5.% (see table); the 'expanded definition' increased the number of pregnant women with risk factors for DM, infant macrosomia, and cord hyperinsulinemia, with little loss of specificity (**JAMA 1993; 269:609oc**) see Glucose tolerance curve

Note: Early diagnosis of pregnancy in insulin-dependent diabetes mellitus allows optimal metabolic control, reducing the risk for spontaneous abortion, a common event in diabetic gestation (**N Engl J Med 1988; 319:1617**)

gestational mother SURROGACY A woman who carries a fertilized embryo to completion of pregnancy; in the 'pre-surrogacy era', the gestational and genetic mother were one and the same, an assumption which is no longer valid with the advent of in vitro fertilization and the surrogate uterus, which can be made available or even quasi-commercialized, so that a genetic mother whose gestational 'plumbing' (for various physical reasons, eg anatomic defects) prevents the carriage of a fertilized egg to full-term; under the usual scenario, the genetic mother's egg is fertilized in vitro and implanted into a surrogate (gestational mother) who carries the product to completion (**N Engl J Med 1992; 327:286c**) see Surrogacy; Cf Genetic mother

gestational thrombocytopenia Immune thrombocytopenic purpura (ITP) that first appears in pregnancy, which carries the risk of neonatal thrombocytopenia and intracranial hemorrhage; conservative management is appropriate when ITP (a not uncommon event in women of child-bearing years) first appears in pregnancy and no circulating antiplatelet antibodies are detected

GFAP Glial fibrillary acidic protein An intermediate filament characteristic of glial cells, which can be detected by immunohistochemical methods (eg immunopeoxidase); GFAP may be rarely co-expressed with S-100 protein in peripheral nerve tumors; see Intermediate filament

GGGCG box MOLECULAR BIOLOGY A highly conserved sequence of DNA, which like the CCAAT and TATA 'boxes', is located between 60 and 120 nucleotides upstream from the start site for gene transcription;these boxes are known as promoter-proximal sequences, which when mutated, result in lower rates of transcription, implying that they are DNA-binding sites

GGM see Glucose/galactose malabsorption

GGT γ-glutamyl transferase see Glutamyl transferase

GHB see GABA, γ-hydroxy-butyrate

ghost HEMATOLOGY The pale white membrane of a hemoglobin-depleted red cell, which is virtually identical to all other mammalian cell membranes (52% protein, 40% lipid, 8% carbohydrate), and is thus useful in studying cell membranes; erythrocyte membranes differ in that most of the membrane is attached to the proteins glycophorin and band 3, identified by gel electrophoresis; see Band

ghost cell A shadowy, light pink (by the H&E stain) cell wraith with a well-demarcated cytoplasmic border that may appear in the presence of coagulation, ie anoxic necrosis, accompanied by abolition of cell detail CYTOLOGY An anuclear yellow-orange squame seen in well-differentiated squamous cell carcinoma DERMATOPATHOLOGY see Shadow cells HEMATOLOGY Ghost, see there ORAL PATHOLOGY A pale, eosinophilic and swollen keratinocyte that lacks a nucleus but retains the cellular and nuclear contour, a finding characteristic of the calcifying odontogenic cyst PARASITOLOGY Hemoglobin-depleted RBC 'husks' that are infected with the schizonts of *Plasmodium ovale*; Cf Ghost

ghost sickness PSYCHIATRY A disease complex observed in Native Americans (American Indians), characterized by a preoccupation with death and the dead; symptoms include anorexia, asthenia, bad dreams, confusion, loss of consciousness, fainting, fear, feeling of futility, a sense of suffocation, and other (DSM-IV™); see Culture-bound syndrome

ghost surgery LEGAL MEDICINE A surgical procedure that Dr 'A' has the patient's permission to perform, which is performed by Dr 'B'; without the proper provisos for formally allowing substitution (as in university hospital residency training programs, where much of the surgery is performed by the residents) in the patient consent form, the patient may initiate a lawsuit for assault and battery, as he was operated on by someone other than the physician to whom he gave permission

ghost teeth Regional odontodysplasia An uncommon dental anomaly affecting predominantly the maxillary teeth, both deciduous and permanent, especially the central and lateral incisors and cuspids; the teeth while normally mineralized, are delayed or fail to erupt; the resulting deformity causes cosmetic defects necessitating tooth extraction

ghost villi OBSTETRICS Rounded pale eosinophilic masses seen by light microscopy that are surrounded by inflammatory cells and correspond to chorionic villi in a placental infarct; ghost villi may also be seen with retained products of conception (missed abortion)

GHRH Growth hormone regulatory hormone

GI Gastrointestinal, also

Also 1) Giant interneurons (neurophysiology) 2) Gingival index (dentistry) 3) Globin insulin 4) Glomerular index 5) Graded index (optics) 6) Growth inhibiting 7) Guidance inventory (psychology) 8) Guided imagery (psychology)

giant axonal neuropathy An AR disease of early onset characterized by symmetric distal polyneuropathy, mental retardation and tightly coiled kinky hair and segmental axonal dilatations packed with neurofilaments; a histologically identical neuropathy may be seen in N-hexane intoxication; Cf Kinky hair disease

giant cell Giant cells may occur in benign or malignant lesions and come in many forms; although they are highly nonspecific, their presence in the proper setting supports the diagnosis of certain diagnoses Epithelioid giant cells of Langerhans and Touton are associated with infections and other 'benign' processes, eg sarcoidosis, have abundant cytoplasm and a rim or clutch of enlarged histiocyte-like nuclei; giant cells in tumors are less inhibited by the rules of cytologic etiquette and are anointed with adjectival modifiers, eg bizarre, monster, osteoclastoma-like and Reed-Sternberg; in tumors, the nucleus and/or cytoplasm may be markedly enlarged and the cell mitotically active; a general rule is that the larger and 'uglier' the cell, the worse the clinical outcome

giant cell arteritis Temporal arteritis A self-limited disease of middle-aged women that evolves to systemic arteritis in 10-15% of cases, with blindness as a potential late complication PATHOLOGY Nodular transmural swelling of arteries, infiltration by neutrophils, eosinophils, mononuclear cells and giant cell granulomas

Note: Although the term giant cell arteritis is more correct from a pathologic (and often a clinical) standpoint, temporal arteritis is widely preferred

giant cell carcinoma A highly malignant epithelial tumor with fulminant clinical course, bizarre histologic appearance and poor prognosis that is most common in 1) Lung An aggressive, poorly differentiated carcinoma that arises peripherally, grows rapidly and is often too large for adequate therapy by the time of clinical presentation PATHOLOGY Bizarre pleomorphic multinucleated giant cells, large mononuclear cells in a background of neutrophils and 2) Thyroid An anaplastic carcinoma arising in a pre-existing well differentiated thyroid carcinoma CLINICAL Aggressive infiltration and compromise of vital neck structures with 100% mortality, most dying within six months PATHOLOGY Storiform infiltration, neutrophilic inflammation, vascularization and osteoclast-like giant cells; most tumors produce cytokeratin; the giant cell tumor of the pancreas does not behave as an anaplastic tumor, but rather like a 'garden variety' ductal carcinoma

giant cell fibroblastoma A benign mesenchymal tumor exclusive to children under the age of 10, often located in the superficial soft tissues of the back and thigh

giant cell glioblastoma A firm, well-circumscribed variant of grade III-IV astrocytoma or glioblastoma multiforme PATHOLOGY Highly cellular with abundant bizarre, multinucleated giant cells, hemorrhage and necrosis

giant cell granuloma see Central giant cell granuloma, Peripheral giant cell granuloma

giant hemangioma of Kasabach-Merritt A condition characterized by thrombocytopenia and 'giant' (± 5 cm in diameter) hemangiomas associated with disseminated intravascular coagulation TREATMENT Mild cases may respond to steroids, or spontaneously regress in five years

giant cell hepatitis Giant cell transformation of the liver NEONATOLOGY A nonspecific reaction of the newborn liver to increased conjugated hyperbilirubinemia of any etiology, that is most common in infants with intra- or extrahepatic biliary atresia, erythroblastosis fetalis, TORCH (toxoplasmosis, rubella, CMV, herpes simplex) and other in utero and neonatal infections, eg coxsackie, hepatitis, *Escherichia coli*, syphilis, metabolic defects, eg α1-antitrypsin deficiency, cystic fibrosis, hereditary fructose intolerance, galactosemia, parenteral nutrition and tyrosinosis, choledocal cysts, idiopathic, congenital hepatic fibrosis, Byler's disease, Lucy-Driscoll disease, Niemann-Pick disease, trisomy 18, and Zellweger's disease PATHOGENESIS Theories abound, but no simple explanation exists PATHOLOGY The liver is enlarged with dense bodies, lobular disarray, multinucleated hepatocytes, mononuclear cell infiltration and marked biliary stasis; the presence of bile-duct proliferation indicates exhepatic biliary atresia, a lesion that may be amenable to surgery Cf Syncytial giant cell hepatitis

giant cell myocarditis A severe idiopathic form of inflammatory heart disease of unknown etiology that may represent a virally-induced immune reaction, which is associated with underlying diseases including encephalitis, hepatitis, infection, intoxication, nutritional defects, thymoma, thyroiditis and Wegener's granulomatosis CLINICAL Rapid deterioration and high mortality PATHOGENESIS A recent report identified high titers of anti-heart antibodies reactive against cardiac myosin in a patient with GCM, suggesting that GCM may have an autoimmune component (Cardiovasc Pathol 1995 4:127) PATHOLOGY Focal granulomatous necrosis, multi-nucleated giant cells, epithelioid histiocytes, eosinophils, lymphocytes

giant cell (interstitial) pneumonia An idiopathic, interstitial pneumonia with lymphoid infiltrates, bizarre, actively phagocytic giant cells, associated with respiratory syncytial virus, influenza and other viral infections, easily confused with measles, or associated with bacterial or mycoplasmal infections, drugs (nitrofurantoin, chemotherapy, methysergide) and collagen vascular disease

giant cell pneumonia of Hecht A fulminant respiratory disease with tachycardia, dyspnea, which is most commonly due to fulminant measles infection that compromises the cellular and humoral immune response PROGNOSIS Poor with high mortality, especially in those with underlying leukemia, cystic fibrosis, immunodeficiency and persistent measles viremia; Cf Atypical pneumonia

giant cell reaction A nonspecific term for a reparative tissue reaction with multinucleated epithelioid histiocytes that may be due to exogenous material, eg sutures, or due to endogenous material, eg the sebaceous contents of a ruptured epidermal inclusion cyst, chalazion, or fat

giant cell reparative granuloma see Central giant cell granuloma, Peripheral giant cell granuloma

giant cell thyroiditis De Quervain's subacute (granulomatous) thyroiditis

giant cell tumor of bone A lesion comprising 5% of all osseous tumors, which is most common in the weight-bearing epiphysis of females over age 20, affecting the distal femur, proximal tibia and distal radius PATHOLOGY GCTs are red-brown with pale necrotic areas, with stromal mesenchymal cells and tumor giant cells that have nuclei identical to those of the mesenchymal cells and a high acid phosphatase content; 60% recur with curettage and 10% metastasize, an event that is far more common in deep (to the fascial planes) tumors DDx A GCT-like histopathologic lesion that may be seen in the brown tumor of hyperparathyroidism, chondroblastoma, giant cell reparative granuloma, benign and malignant fibrous histiocytoma, non-ossifying and chondromyxoid fibroma, unicameral bone cyst, aneurysmal bone cyst, fibrous dysplasia, osteoblastoma, osteosarcoma, osteoid osteoma and eosinophilic granuloma

giant cell tumor of tendon sheath A potentially recurring lesion of the acral flexor tendon sheath that is a variant of fibrous histiocytoma, which reaches a maximum of 3 mm in size and may erode into the bone PATHOLOGY Osteoclast-like giant cells with hyalinization, pseudo-glandular formation, lipid and hemosiderin accumulation (simulating malignancy)

giant condyloma acuminatum Büschke-Loewenstein tumor, see there

giant congenital melanocytic nevus* Garment nevus, see there

'giant' hairs Fusion of sensory hairs in the cochlea and vestibule, described in aminoglycoside-induced ototoxicity (guinea pigs), presumed to occur in humans but not searched for in post-mortem examinations

giant (pigmented) hairy nevus A large congenital melanocytic nevus measuring more than 5 cm in greatest dimension that has a 'garment-like' distribution (bathing trunk, cap, coat sleeve, stocking), often with scattered satellite lesions and is considered premalignant, as up to 12% develop melanoma; leptomeningeal involvement may be accompanied by epilepsy and mental retardation; the three histological patterns are compound and intradermal nevus, neural nevus and blue nevus

giant hypertrophic gastritis A condition characterized by rugal folds of the stomach and late development of parietal cell autoantibodies and gastric atrophy; giant hypertrophic gastritis is associated with Menetrier's disease (gastric mucosal hypertrophy, decreased acid secretion, protein loss in the stomach, edema, weight loss, abdominal pain, nausea), and hypertrophic hypersecretory gastropathy, morphologically similar to Menetrier's disease but with increased acid secretion, more common in men, age 30-50 TREATMENT Varying success is achieved with anticholinergics, cimetidine, vagotomy and pyloroplasty

giant metamyelocyte An atypical myeloid cell with clumped chromatin in a large, often bizarre, immature nucleus and relatively mature cytoplasm, typically seen in megaloblastic anemia, as the nucleus cannot properly mature without the single-carbon transport provided by the deficient vitamin B_{12} and folic acid

giant mitochondria Massively enlarged mitochondria that appear as pale rounded eosinophilic masses by LM, which mimic both red cells and Mallory's hyaline; the finding of giant mitochondria in hepatocytes is non-specific but characteristic of all phases of alcoholic liver disease ranging from fatty liver to cirrhosis

giant platelets A platetet that is larger than usual; up to 10% of normal platelets are 'giant', ie 'squashed' and oversized; when more than 20% of the platelets are giant, certain other conditions must be considered in addition to BSS, eg ITP, lympho- and myeloproliferative disorders, reticulocytosis, DIC, SLE, gray platelet syndrome, May-Hegglin anomaly, Montreal platelet syndrome, thrombopathic thrmobocytopenia

giant platelet syndrome Bernard-Soulier syndrome, see there

giant reparative granuloma see Central giant cell granuloma, Peripheral giant cell granuloma

giant T wave inversion CARDIOLOGY An EKG finding characterized as an inversion of the normal T wave, seen in the mid- to left precordial leads and suggestive of apical hypertrophic cardiomyopathy

Giardia lamblia The most common protozoan parasite affecting the human small intestine LABORATORY ↓ Intestinal load of trophozoites is associated with an ↑ in *G lamblia*-specific secretory IgA PATHOLOGY Pathologic changes induced by *G lamblia* infection of the small intestine range from near-normal to villus atrophy and/or crypt elongation with a variable inflammatory response (**Arch Pathol Lab Med 1994; 118:891oA**)

gibbus An anterior angular deformity of the lower back due to hypoplasia or 'wedging' of one or more lower thoracic or upper lumbar vertebrae, resulting in beaked projections on the infero-anterior aspects and hypoplasia of the upper portions of vertebral bodies, seen in mucopolysaccharidosis, type I-H Hurler syndrome, TB (Pott's disease) or trauma; the gibbus or 'buffalo hump' seen in Cushing's disease and syndrome is due to accumulation of soft tissue secondary to prolonged endogenous or exogenous corticosteroid and is located in the cervicothoracic region

GIFT Gamete intrafallopian transfer, see there

gigantism Sotos syndrome, see there

GIGO Garbage in, garbage out COMPUTERS An acronym referring to incorrect entry of data in a database, which cannot be coherently retrieved; GIGO has been colloquially borrowed by various fields, in particular, laboratory medicine for improperly obtained materials, eg stool cultures, urine and cytologic specimens for which a diagnosis cannot be rendered

The term GIGO is equally applicable to other fields of medicine and been used by cytotechnologists in reference to poor quality specimens that preclude diagnosis

ginkgolides ALTERNATIVE MEDICINE A large group of medicinal preparations from a tree in northern China *Gingko biloba* that has had currency among practioners of herbal medicine; gingkolides are alleged to be of use in treating a wide range of conditions, including cardiovascular disease, emotional lability, ocular defects, panic disorder, vertigo

ginkgolide B A chemical extracted from the ginkgo tree (*Gingko biloba*) of potential use for treating asthma and circulatory deficiency in the elderly

ginseng Any one of 22 different deciduous plants, usually of the Panax family eg Siberian giseng (*Eleintherococcus senticosus*), commonly Panax ginseng that are native to Southeast Asia, used in Chinese folk medicine as a tonic and restorative, consumed for its purported antifatigue, immunologic and hormonal effects, claimed to cure respiratory infections, GI disease, impotence, fatigue and stress; the active chemicals include panaxin, panax acid, panaquilen, panacen, sapogenin and ginsenin; the physiologic effects include ↑ testosterone, corticosteroid levels in experimental animals, and ↑ gluconeogenesis, CNS activity, blood pressure, pulse, GI motility and hematopoiesis and ↓ cholesterol levels; controversy has arisen as a result of ginseng's purported androgenic potential; in one study using castrated Sprague-Dawley rats, no androgenic activity was identified, as measured by lack of change in the weights of the seminal vesicles or the ventral prostate (JAMA 1992; 267:2329L); Cf Garlic

ginseng abuse 'syndrome' A clinical complex secondary to daily ingestion of 3 or more g/day of ginseng CLINICAL Diarrhea, nervousness, insomnia, eruptive dermatosis, increased cognitive and motor activity

GIP 1) see Giant cell (interstitial) pneumonia 2) Gastric inhibitory polypeptide A 43-residue insulinotropic polypeptide hormone of the incretin family produced by the pancreas, that is secreted in response to oral (but not parenteral) administration of nutrients, eg glucose and lipids; see Incretin

GIPP Gonadotropin-independent (ie nonpulsatile) precocious puberty A possibly familial condition due to a lack of suppression in response to LHRHa with non-cyclic steroidogenesis, CLINICAL Ranges from complete testicular immaturity to maturity; see Precocious puberty

GISSI-2 Gruppo Italiano per lo Studio della Streptochinasi nell' Infarcto Miocardico II (N Engl J Med 1992; 327:1oA) Gruppo Italiano per lo Studio della Sopravivenza nell' Infarcto Miocardico II (N Engl J Med 1993; 329:1442oA)

GIST Gastrointestinal stromal tumor, see there

gitterzellen German, lattice cells Cells seen in early CNS necrosis, where the normal microglia is converted from small round cells with fine branching processes to rounded plump macrophages filled with variably sized fat globules and disintegrating myelin

glacial acetic acid LABORATORY MEDICINE 99% absolute acetic acid A 'workhorse' reagent that is a component of various fixatives, to wit, Bouin's, Carnoy's, Zenker's, and formalin-alcohol-acid solution; because acetic acid causes cell constitutents to swell it is never used alone, but combined with reagents that cause shrinking, eg mercuric chloride, picric acid, ethyl alcohol; it does not fix lipids or carbohydrates

glairy material Greasy, clear yellow, fat-laden semi-fluid material, characteristically seen in mature cystic teratomas, which is often admixed with hair

glamour image PUBLIC HEALTH A generic term for an artificial media-driven portrayal of the 'good life' in which all participants are 'beautiful people', ie young, svelte, healthy, and vivacious, ie glamorous; the image is fueled in large part by the advertising industry, which in turn is subservient to corporate agendas; various subliminal messages* are incorporated into the 'image', and the consumer may unwittingly associate the use and consumption of these products with success and health (JAMA 1992; 267:2289MN&P)

*eg the use of certain products, eg cigarettes, soft drinks, alcohol, and others, not rarely with a backdrop of flashy red Italian cars

glanders An infection by *Pseudomonas mallei*, a gram-negative strict aerobic bacillus, which affects large domestic animals, most common in horses and is an entity distinctly uncommon in the US; human disease occurs in the form of acute septicemia (which is often fatal), chronic mucocutaneous disease (see Farcy), or pulmonary infection CLINICAL Ranges from cellulitis to necrosis and granuloma formation with draining mucosal ulcers, pleuritis, necrotizing lobar or bronchopneumonia, nasal septal necrosis, fever, chills, malaise, headaches, pustular rash, lymphadenopathy, splenomegaly; chronic disease is associated with hepatosplenomegaly, pulmonary abscess formation and granuloma formation TREATMENT Sulfadiazine, tetracycline, chloramphenicol, aminoglycosides

Glasgow coma scale CRITICAL CARE MEDICINE A method for evaluating the severity of central nervous system involvement in head injury that measures three parameters for a maximum score of 15 for normal cerebral function and zero for brain death; the parameters are

BEST MOTOR RESPONSE, ie the subject obeys commands 6, if none 0

BEST VERBAL RESPONSE, ie oriented 5, if no response 0 and

EYE OPENING, if spontaneous 4, if none 0; the system is of lesser use in children (N Engl J Med 1992; 327:1507RA) Cf Pittsburgh score

'glass ceiling' phenomenon ACADEMIA The constellation of barriers to career advancement that confront women who strive for leadership positions; glass ceilings are experienced by women in academic medicine, due in part because they are expected to juggle two major roles, to wit that of mother and of leader of a department (Am Med News 19 Sept 1994, JAMA 1995 273:1022) see Sticky floor phenomenon

glass eye Artificial eye, see there

'glass pusher' A highly colloquial and derogatory synonym for a 'service' surgical pathologist, whose primary function is to 'push glass', ie interpret the histology of biopsies and tissues removed during surgery, which have been embedded in paraffin, mounted on a glass slide and stained

glassy appearance An adjectival descriptor for a smooth or vitrioid grayish radiolucency or pale eosinophilic hyalinized cytoplasm or stromal tissue

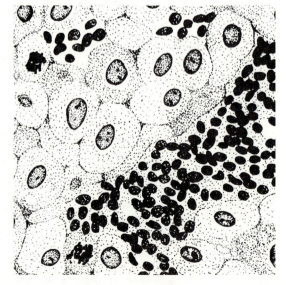

glassy cell carcinoma

glassy cell carcinoma A female genital tract malignancy

of 1) The uterine cervix, which comprises 1.2% of primary cervical cancers and is an aggressive, poorly differentiated adenosquamous carcinoma, originating from the subcylindric reserve cell; 5-year survival: 25% PATHOLOGY Large, mitotically active polygonal cells with abundant, finely granular amphophilic 'glassy' cytoplasm, distinct cell borders, large nuclei with one or more prominent nucleoli, or 2) The endometrium is also very rare and histologically similar to that of the cervix with an equally poor prognosis

GLC Gas-liquid chromatography, see there

PROSTATIC ADENOCARCINOMA
(Histologic Grades)

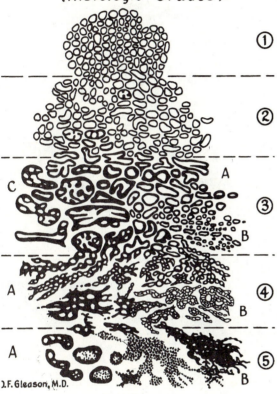

J.F. Gleason, M.D.

Gleason grades

Gleason grading system ONCOLOGY 'The histologic grade of prostate cancer is the strongest independent clinical variable predictive of outcome' (GE Hanks et al, in VT DeVita, Jr, et al, The Principles and Practice of Oncology, JB Lippincott, Philadelphia, 1993); the most widely used system* for stratifying the histologic features of prostate cancer is that delineated by Gleason, which divides the lesions into 5 groups of decreasing glandular differentiation

*Others include those described by Broders, Mostofi, and Brawn

Gleason score ONCOLOGY A value derived from the Gleason grading system that is the sum of the two most predominant histologic patterns seen in prostate cancer, eg a score of 7 (Gleason grade 4 + 3), which is relatively predictive of the clinical outcome

glial cell-derived neurotrophic factor A growth factor that reduces toxicity to dopaminergic neurons, enhances survival in neuronal trauma, and arrests apoptosis in developing cells (Nature in NY Times 31 January, 1995, C3)

gliding motility A pattern of movement typical of *Capnocytophaga* species, in which the yellowish colonies display finger-like projections that appear to glide on the primary isolation media; these gram-negative fusiform bacilli are indigenous to the oral cavity, are implicated in periodontal and oral infections and lack flagella, and thus are intrinsically motile; Cf Swarming

glioblastoma Astrocytoma, grade III-IV A highly aggressive tumor comprising 30% of the 5000 primary brain malignancies diagnosed annually (US); those at possible occupational risk include anatomists, pathologists, dentists, and ophthalmologists (N Engl J Med 1991; 324:1441) TREATMENT Glioblastoma is not affected by surgery, chemotherapy and radiotherapy, but may respond to genetically engineered viruses (Science 1991; 252:854)

GLIP Glucagon-like insulinotropic peptide, see there

glitter cells Neutrophils that are swollen in hypotonic (dilute) urine and contain granules in Brownian motion that 'glitter' when seen by low-power LM, a finding described as typical of pyelonephritis

global budget HEALTH CARE ENVIRONMENT A proposal for capping (setting the limits of) state or national health care expenditures, which is designed to force providers, patients, and reimbursement agents to chose among who is covered for what services (Am Med News 25 October 1992, p7)

global warming ENVIRONMENT The ↑ of average temperature on the planet, estimated to be ↑ 1.5-4.0° C by the year 2100 if drastic measures are not taken to ↓ the escalating emission of CO_2, and other 'greenhouse gases'; computer models of the effects of global warming project ↑↑↑ of hunger in developing nations and ↓ food production; the most significant impact of global warming for humans will be on agriculture, which may be either beneficial in the form of ↑ CO_2-related fertilization, longer growing seasons, and ↑ precipitation, or deleterious in the form of droughts, heat stress, and ↑ flooding of coastal regions and salinization due to fertilization (Sci Am 270/3:36; New York Times 18 January 1994; C4) INFECTIOUS DISEASE GW is likely to increase the range of infectious disease vectors, including mosquitoes (vectors for malaria, filariasis, denque fever, and yellow fever), flies (onchocerciasis, African trypanosomiasis) and snails (schistosomiasis) (Science 1995; 267:957N&C)

globalization The dissolution of national borders in all aspects of human endeavor; in science, this translates into international collaboration efforts, eg Human Frontier Science Project with funds being provided by funding agencies and/or private companies from different countries; the term represents a recognition that1) Changes in one part of the world have a broader impact, both regionally, eg the burning oil wells of Kuwait, or over the entire planet, eg CFC use by developed nations and ozone layer depletion and 2) Resolution of issues of international concern, eg environment, population, research, loss of human rights, requires participation of all members of the 'global village'; see G7

globi Masses of acid-fast staining *Mycobacterium leprae* present in histiocytes ('lepra cells') in advanced lepromatous leprosy lymphadenitis; globi are usually located in the subcapsular region of lymph nodes; when stained by H&E, the histiocytes are foamy with gray cytoplasm; similar globi-like masses occur in *M avium-intercellulare* infections in patients with AIDS

globoid cell leukodystrophy Krabbe's disease An AR [MIM 245200] defect in sphingolipid metabolism due to galatocerebroside β-galactosidase deficiency, causing in utero demyelination, and death in early infancy CLINICAL Spastic paralysis, seizures and pyrexia, vomiting, cortical blindness, deafness, dysphagia, pseudobulbar palsy, quadriplegia, mental deterioration NEUROPATHOLOGY The lesions are confined to the CNS (figure page 336) with a loss of myelin, fibrous gliosis and abundant, perivascular clusters of 20-25 µm rounded or globoid macrophages and multinucleated cells with faintly granular cytoplasm filled with galactosyl ceramide EM Hollow crystalline tubes or twisted tubular arrays similar to inclusions found in Gaucher's disease; autosomal recessive; Cf Leukodystrophy

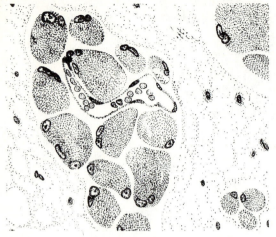

globoid cell leukodystrophy

globoside Ceramide-(glucose)m-(galactose)-N-(N-acetyl-hexosamine) A family of ceramide-based molecules, designated as GL-1, GL-2, and so on, according to the number of sugar residues added to the ceramide; globosides represent the predominant glycolipid in the red cell membrane and other plasma membranes

globoside dysfunction syndrome A group of enzymopathies characterized by defective addition of sugar residues to ceramide, eg Fabry's disease and Lactosyl ceramidosis

globular protein In the early days of clinical chemistry, proteins were separated into either albumin or 'globulins' (immunoglobulins, enzymes and other proteins) the latter calculated as 'total protein', determined by the Biuret method, minus albumin, separated by using a salt solution; the term is obsolete as electrophoresis is used to separate proteins into more clinically relevant groups

globulin LABORATORY MEDICINE In the 'prehistoric' period of laboratory medicine, proteins were divided into two broad categories based on their solubility in various concentrations of ammonium sulfate (in water), to wit 1) Globulins, which precipitated in half-saturated ammonium sulfate, and 2) Albumin, which only precipitated in the face of complete saturation of ammonium sulfate; in this context, the term albumin is of historic interest only

globus hystericus A subjective sensation of compression or a lump (bolus) in the throat, considered a symptom of psychoneurosis; see Factitial syndromes

Note: A bolus sensation is characteristic of carcinomas or strictures in the oropharynx or pharyngeal pouch, or may occur in pharyngeal paralysis, hypochromic anemia or cervical spinal disease, eg osteoarthritis

glomerular polyanion A negatively charged glycoprotein lining the glomerular foot processes of the epithelial cells of Bowman's capsule, responsible for the selective permeability of the glomeruli; loss of negative charges in the foot process region is responsible for increased filtration, ie loss of albumin and proteinuria, as occurs in minimum change nephrotic syndrome

glomeruloid bodies Glomerular bodies A loosely used term that refers to an organized cluster of often primitive cells that simulate primitive glomeruli; the classic glomeruloid body is a key histological feature of Wilms' tumor, a tumor accompanied by nests of primitive cells and a fibroblast-like stroma), and consists of a Bowman-like space, epithelial cell tufts and PAS-positive basement membrane material without a capillary lumen and lining

endothelial cells; the Schiller-Duval bodies, characteristic of endodermal sinus tumor and yolk sac tumors and clear cell carcinoma are sometimes also called glomeruloid bodies and contain a central capillary surrounded by loose connective tissue, rimmed by a layer of epithelial cells with scattered intracytoplasmic hyaline globules; Cf Embryoid bodies

glomerulonephritis see Capsular 'drops', Casts, Crescents, Deciduous tree in winter appearance, Dense deposits, Fingerprints, Fusion of foot processes, Humps, 'Shunt' nephritis, Spike, Tramtrack pattern

glomus tumor A neoplasm that is most common in age 20-40 that arises in the neuromyoarterial glomus, an arteriovenous shunt CLINICAL When located in the 'usual' subungual site, the abundant innervation makes the tumor exquisitely painful; when located elsewhere, eg middle ear, stomach, the glomus tumor is painless

glory hole 'A hole for the penis used for anonymous sexual encounters, especially made in a partition between toilet stalls in a public lavatory.' (JE Lighter, Historical Dictionary of American Slang, Random House, New York, 1994); see Anonymous sex, Bath-house

Note: The first known use of the term 'glory hole' (as above defined) was in 1949; less common uses of glory hole are 1) a gay bar (1966), 2) the vagina (1930), 3) shipboard quarters for stewards and stokers (1889), and 4) patch of clear sky in a bank of clouds (1987)

glossy skin Neuritic atrophoderma A term referring to the smooth skin that is characteristic of denervation atrophy

'glove' FORENSIC PATHOLOGY A colloquial term for a broad sheet of epidermis, especially of the hands and feet, which may include the fingernails that slough from bodies immersed in water for long periods of time, a phenomenon that occurs more rapidly in warm water; Cf 'Floater'

glove box MICROBIOLOGY A sealed glass or plastic chamber that has two or more pairs of rubber gloves for the manipulation of cells, microorganisms or mammals without physically violating the environment within the box; the box is designed to either maintain an atmosphere that a 'fastidious' organism requires for optimal growth, eg a strict anaerobe, or to protect an immune defenseless organism from all pathogens, see 'Bubble boy; alternatively, a glove box is used to protect the manipulators from toxic chemical or from dangerous pathogens

glove & stocking anesthesia NEUROLOGY A characteristic pattern of decreased sensation occurring in leprosy

gloved finger shadow of Simon RADIOLOGY A descriptor for retained plugs of mucopurulent secretion within ectatic bronchi in patients with chronic obstructive pulmonary disease (COPD), best seen by an air bronchogram; the thickened bronchial walls may be accompanied by atelectasis and pneumonitis

glucagon A 29-residue polypeptide hormone produced by the pancreatic islet α cells that activates hepatic phosphorylase, decreases gastric motility, secretion and muscle mass, increases ketogenesis and hepatic incorporation of amino acids and urinary excretion of K^+ and Na^+

glucagon-like insulinotropic peptide GLP-1 (7-36) amide A naturally-occurring fragment of glucagon-like peptide-1 (GLP-1) which in turn is a fragment of proglucagon; GLIP is antidiabetogenic and ↓ meal-related release of insulin, glucagon, and somatostatin; it ↓ postprandial insulin requirements and is of therapeutic potential in NIDDM (N Engl J Med 1992; 326:1316oA)

glucagonoma A pancreatic α cell tumor with two distinct clinical and histological patterns, presenting either as a benign tumor, not associated with the glucagonoma syndrome, which has a bland gyriform histologic pattern or a potentially malignant tumor associated with the glucagonoma syndrome

glucagonoma syndrome A symptom complex associated

with glucagonoma, a tumor of post-menopausal women who often have diabetes mellitus, blistering dermatitis (necrolytic migratory erythema, epidermal necrosis, subcorneal pustules, suppurative folliculitis, confluent parakeratosis, epidermal hyperplasia, and prominent papillary dermal hyperplasia), weight loss, normochromic anemia, ileus, constipation or diarrhea, glossitis, angular cheilitis, venous thrombosis, hypoproteinemia, neuropsychiatric disease PATHOLOGY Glucagonomas are small, solitary tumors with atypical neuroendocrine granules Note: ½ are malignant; many produce more than one hormone

glucocorticoid regulatory element see GRE

glucose-clamp technique ENDOCRINOLOGY A method used to determine the clamp-derived insulin-sensitivity index, see there (N Engl J Med 1994; 331:1188OA)

glucose clearance A value corresponding to the rate of glucose uptake divided by plasma glucose concentration

glucose-dependent insulinotropic polypeptide An incretin*, that is released from crypt cells of the proximal small intestine into the circulation after oral intake of glucose and long-chain fatty acids; GIP stimulates insulin secretion when the plasma glucose is > 5.6-6.1 mmol/L (100-110 mg/dL); pancreatic beta cells have a high-affinity receptor for GIP, the binding of which decreases the threshold of glucose-stimulated insulin secretion in vitro (N Engl J Med 1992; 326:1352SB) Cf Glucagon-like insulinotropic peptide (GLIP)

*Insulinotropic substance of GI tract origin released into the circulation by oral glucose

glucose/galactose malabsorption An AD [MIM 182380] condition of neonatal onset characterized by malabsorption of glucose and galactose, resulting in severe, potentially fatal diarrhea and dehydration if these sugars are not eliminated from the diet PATHOGENESIS Normal glucose absorption is mediated by the Na^+/glucose cotransporter, which is encoded by the SGLT1 gene on the distal q arm of chromosome 22; in GGM, there is a single missense mutation in the SGLT1 gene, resulting in a complete loss of Na^+/glucose transport (Nature 1991; 350:354)

glucose oxidase An enzyme [EC 1.1.3.4] that catalyzes the oxidation of glucose to glucuronolactone, which hydrolyzes spontaneously to gluconic acid, with simultaneous reduction of oxygen to hydrogen peroxide; GO is isolated from the mold *Penicillium notatum* and is used to measure glucose in serum

glucose paradox A physiologic phenomenon in which glucose appears to be incorporated into glycogen both directly, by passing through glucose-6-phosphate and uridine diphosphate glucose, and indirectly, by being metabolized first to the three-carbon precursors (glycerol, lactate, and alanine), then resynthesized to through the gluconeogenic pathway to glucose-6-phosphate and then glycogen (see N Engl J Med 1992; 327:707RV)

glucose-6-phosphate dehydrogenase deficiency Moth ball syndrome An X-R [MIM 305900] disease caused by the congenital deficiency of glucose-6-phosphate dehydrogenase, resulting in hemolytic crises when exposed to naphthalene (moth balls), sulfonamides, primaquine, nalidixic acid and others; it affects American blacks 11%, Kurdish Jews 50%, others of Mediterranean rim bloodlines and in Orientals CLINICAL Acute exposure by ingestion causes nausea, vomiting, diarrhea, hematuria, anemia, jaundice, oliguria and potentially renal shut-down

glucose tolerance Glucose uptake rate divided by plasma glucose concentration

glucose tolerance test A standardized test that measures the body's response to an oral (challenge) dose of glucose, used to diagnose diabetes mellitus; in the most commonly used GTT, 100 g of glucose is ingested per os in a fasting individual, which stimulates insulin secretion; the peak

glucose levels in normal subjects are reached within one hour; in diabetics, the peak is reached after 2-3 hours and the peak glucose level is much higher; in the below figure, Siperstein's (Adv Int Med 1975; 20:297) 'liberal' criteria are used, which recognize that the GTT differs with age

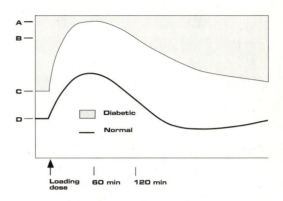

glucose tolerance test

glucosuria see Glycosuria

glue ear Secretory otitis media Chronic otitis media with effusion, a common cause of conduction-type deafness in school-age children CLINICAL Variable pain, accompanied by upper respiratory infection and tonsillitis TREATMENT Adenoidectomy plus bilateral myringotomy with grommet insertion for young children

glue-sniffing SUBSTANCE ABUSE A potentially fatal form of substance abuse practiced by young male adolescents, in which model airplane glue is placed in a paper or plastic bag and deeply sniffed in order to obtain the maximum desired effect, which consists of a combination of euphoria and CNS depression caused by toluene, an organic solvent; exposure to toluene vapors causes irritation of mucosae, lacrimation, arrythmias, nausea, vomiting, mental confusion, hallucinations, chemical pneumonitis, respiratory arrest and sudden death; direct contact may cause erythema, defatting dermatitis, skin paresthesiae, conjunctivitis and keratitis; see Gateway drugs; Cf 'White-out'

NIOSH recommendations for toluene exposure is 200 ppm at an 8-hour time-weighted average; abusers may be exposed to 1000 ppm for prolonged periods; toluene is also present in adhesives, explosives and dyes

GLUT A family of cell membrane-bound glucose transporting proteins, of which five isoforms have been identified; on the basis of hydropathy plots, all forms have 12 membrane-spanning domains, six exoplasmic loops and five endoplasmic loops; GLUT-1, GLUT-3, GLUT-4 and GLUT-5 all have low Km, which allows their facile transportation throughout the corporal economy and into various tissues; GLUT-2 regulates glucose homeostasis (Science 1991; 251:1200)

GLUT-2 Glucose transporter A protein with a high Km (Michaelis constant) that transports glucose into the β cells of the pancreatic islets, providing an essential signal for the normal insulin secretory response; GLUT-2 is ele-

100 G ORAL GLUCOSE TOLERANCE TEST (GTT)–mmol/L (mg/dl)		
HOUR	NDDG†	MODIFIED CRITERIA‡
0	5.9 (105)	5.3 (95)
1	10.6 (190)	10.1 (180)
2	9.2 (165)	8.7 (155)
3	8.1 (145)	7.8 (140)

†National Diabetes Data Group (Diabetes 1979; 28:1039)
‡Am J Obstet Gynecol 1982; 144:768

vated in those cells, eg pancreatic β cells, liver, basolateral aspect of the epithelial cells of the small intestine and renal tubules that participate in the regulation of blood glucose homeostasis; GLUT-2 is reduced in both insulin-dependent (autoimmune) and non-insulin-dependent DMs due to a down-regulation that is defective in NIDDM (Science 1991; 251:1200)

GLUT-4 Insulin-stimulated glucose transporter

glutamate cascade NEUROLOGY A sequence of events thought to be a major cause of ischemia-induced neuronal death in cerebrovascular insults (strokes) that can be topographically divided into a core region immediately adjacent to an occluded vessel, which is almost invariably doomed to infarction unless the thrombus is removed immediately (which is usually impossible) and a penumbral region, which receives some blood from non-occluded collateral vessels, the region in which the glutamate cascade is thought to occur in a three-step process

1) INDUCTION The cascade begins when the terminals of ischemic neurons oversecrete the excitatory neurotransmitter glutamate into the intercellular spaces, in response to which NMDA receptors open and allow the free passage of sodium and calcium ions, AMPA/kainate receptors allow passage of sodium ions and metabotropic receptors trigger the generation of intracellular messengers diacylglycerol (DAG) and inositol 1,4,5-triphosphate (IP3)

2) AMPLIFICATION The excess intracellular sodium activates a sodium-for-calcium transporter, which activates voltage-gated calcium channels; the excess IP3 releases calcium from intracellular stores, which may combine with DAG, activating enzymes and triggering the release of more glutamate

3) EXPRESSION Excess calcium activates enzymes that degrade DNA, proteins and phospholipids, the last of which is catabolized to arachidonic acid generating highly-destructive oxygen free radicals and eicosanoid molecules, which combine with activated platelet-activating factor, recruiting previously uninvolved vessels and widening the extent of the ischemia (Sci Am 1991; 265:1/56rv)

glutamic acid decarboxylase A protein on the surface of pancreatic beta cells that is thought to play a major role in the pathogenesis of IDDM, a condition attributed to an aberrant autoimmune response; GAD appears to be the first molecular target against which the host develops antibodies, an event that coincides with the development of insulinitis

glutamic acid decarboxylase autoantibody An autoantibody against a 64-kD antigen associated with IDDM and with the 'stiff man' syndrome

glutamyl transferase γ-Glutamyl transferase, see Gamma glutamyl transferase

glutathione γ-Glutamyl-cysteinyl-glycine A ubiquitous tripeptide involved in CNS metabolism, serving as a coenzyme for some enzymes of oxidation-reduction systems, transmembrane amino acid transport, maintenance of erythrocyte integrity and prevention of H_2O_2 accumulation in red cells

gluten A wheat endosperm protein composed of gliadin and glutelin, which is inculpated in the pathogenesis of celiac disease

glycated hemoglobin Glycosylated hemoglobin, see there

glycerol 1,2,3 propanetriol, trihydroxypropane A sweet oily liquid that is obtained from the hydrolysis of neutral fats, which is used as an industrial solvent, plasticizer, suppository, and emollient; it is hygroscopic, ie soluble in both alcohol and water; it is a component of neutral fats, phosphatides and cardiolipin, and is used in transfusion medicine for long-term storage of frozen red cells; like DMSO, glycerol is an intracellular cryopreservative; HES (hydroxyethyl starch) is extracellular

glycine An inhibitory neurotransmitter that acts primarily at the level of the spinal cord, the receptors for which are distributed in a heterogeneous pattern

glycocalicin A 135-kD hydrophilic glycoprotein split from the α-chain of platelet glycoprotein Ib that is markedly reduced (5-20% normal levels) in aplastic anemia or amegakaryocytosis; patients with peripheral-destruction type thrombocytopenia (and normal marrow precursors) have less than 50% normal levels

glycocalyx HISTOLOGY The 'fuzzy coat' formed by oligosaccharide side chains and the negatively-charged sialic acid; it is attached to membrane-bound proteins and lipids and located on the surface of secretory epithelial cells, eg of the gastrointestinal tract ULTRASTRUCTURE Granular extracellular 'fuzz'

glycogen granules Glycogen-filled 'organelles' that appear as granular dots by electron microscopy that may be seen in benign tumors, eg hepatic adenomas, parathyroid adenomas and 'sugar' tumor and malignant tumors, eg sarcomas, classically Ewing sarcoma as well as extraskeletal chondrosarcoma, clear cell sarcoma, leiomyosarcoma and rhabdomyosarcoma, clear cell carcinoma of the urogenital tract, endometrial carcinoma and choriocarcinoma

glycogen loading Carbohydrate loading, see there

glycogen rosettes Garland-like clusters of granular 'specks' seen by electron microscopy in the cytoplasm of malignant cells, classically seen in Ewing sarcoma

glycogen storage disease(s) Glycogenosis A group of 12 inherited defects in the ability to store glucose and/or retrieve glucose from intracellular storage depots, all of which have an AR pattern of heredity, resulting in the accumulation of glycogen in the liver, muscle, heart, kidney and other tissues enzyme defects, resulting in an array of symptoms, including hepatosplenomegaly, cardiomegaly, mental retardation, eg Dancing eyes syndrome (GSD VIII) or doll face syndrome (GSD Ia)

GLYCOGEN STORAGE DISEASE

TYPE	DEFICIENT ENZYME
0	Hepatic glycogen synthetase
I	Glucose-6-phosphatase
II	Lysosomal acid maltase alpha-1,4 glucosidase
III	Amylo-1,6 glucosidase ('debrancher' disease)
IV	Amylo-1,4-1,6-trans-glucosidase ('brancher' disease)
V	Myophosphorylase
VI	Hepatic phosphorylase
VII	Phosphofructokinase
VIII	Inactive hepatic phosphorylase is implicated
IX	Hepatic phosphorylase kinase
X	Cyclic 3'5'-AMP-dependent kinase
XI	No deficiency identified

glycogen synthase kinase-3 DEVELOPMENTAL BIOLOGY A mammalian kinase activity phosphorylating enzyme (with two genetically distinct isoforms) that mediates insulin regulation of glycogen synthesis, which is down-regulated by hormonal stimulation; GSK-3 is required for ventral differentiation in early development, while dorsal differentiation may required suppresion of GSK-3 activity by a *wnt*-related signal (Nature 1995; 374:617A)

*The Wnt family of secreted glycoproteins have features of dorsalizing signals

glycogenosis see Glycogen storage disease(s)

glycogen tumor A colloquial term for the glycogen-rich rhabdomyoma; see Spider cells

glycophorin A 131-amino acid sialoglycoprotein (60% carbohydrate, 40% protein) that spans and comprises a major component of the erythrocyte membrane and cytoskeleton

glycoprotein Ia/IIa Integrin $\alpha_2\beta_1$

glycoprotein Ic/IIa Integrin $\alpha_5\beta_1$

glycoprotein IIb/IIIa Integrin $\alpha_{IIb}\beta_2$

glycosaminoglycan GAG, mucopolysaccharide Any of a number of disaccharide polymers, one of which is either a

D-acetylglucosamine or a D-galactosamine, linked by ester or amide bonds; GAGs are the carbohydrate component of proteoglycans and include hyaluronic acid and chondroitin sulfate, dermatan sulfate, heparan sulfate, heparin sulfate and keratan sulfate; see Basement membrane

glycoside CLINICAL PHARMACOLOGY A molecule formed from the condensation of either a furanose or a pyranose with another molecule as an acetal, nitrogen glycoside or phosphate ester glycoside; cardiac glycosides include digitoxin, digoxin and ouabain

glycosuria Glucosuria The spillage of excess glucose into the urine, an event common in uncontrolled DM and in 'renal' glycosuria; it may be divided into Type A T_m mutation or V_{max} type, result of a lowering of the renal threshold for glucose Type B K_m or degree of splay mutation; as with the T_m mutation type, K_m may be inherited as an autosomal recessive

glycosylated hemoglobin hemoglobin A1c   see Advanced glycosylation endproducts, Fast hemoglobins

glycosyl-phosphatidylinositol Any of a number of glycosylated phosphatidylinositol (GPI) glycophospholipids, which are responsible for 1) Anchoring particulate cell-surface proteins to the membrane, eg alkaline phosphatase, 5'-nucleotidase, acetyl-cholinesterase, Thy-1, carcinoembryonic antigen, TAP, N-CAM, Decay accelerating factor and 2) Signal transduction for insulin, nerve growth factor and IL-2 (**Science 1991; 251:78**), where they act as 'second messengers'

glycyrrhizin A whitish crystalline extract from the root of the licorice plant that is composed of calcium and potassium salts of glycyrrhizic acid; it is used as a demulcent, expectorant, and flavoring agent for drugs, and is claimed to have antibacterial and antiretroviral activity (**Am Med News 21 Nov 1994 p13**) Cf AIDS fraud

glypiation MOLECULAR BIOLOGY A convoluted coinage referring to the anchoring of glycosyl-phosphatidylinositol residues to a protein or substrate, which serves as a signal for sorting glycoproteins

Gm An allotype of an IgG heavy chain, resulting from an inherited variation in the amino acid sequence Note: Allotypes exist for IgA heavy chain and kappa light chains, but not for IgM, IgD and IgE heavy chain or the lambda light chain

GM-CSF Granulocyte macrophage-colony stimulating factor A hematopoietic growth factor, which in the native form is produced by monocytes, lymphocytes, fibroblasts and endothelial cells; recombinant GM-CSF (sargramostim) may be of use in increasing leukocytes in AIDS patients, or stimulating hematopoiesis after high dose chemotherapy in autologous bone marrow transplantation; it may also be useful as an immune 'tonic' in cancer and AIDS patients, anemia, increasing the survival of bone marrow grafts and reducing infections in congenital neutropenia (**N Engl J Med 1992; 327:28RV**) see Biological response modifiers, Sargramostim; Cf G-CSF

GME Graduate medical education, see there

GM-1 ganglioside A complex acidic glycolipid that may be of use in reducing the morbidity and hastening the functional recovery in patients with spinal cord injury (**N Engl J Med 1991; 324:1829**)

GM-1 gangliosidosis A lysosomal disorder caused by β-galactosidase deficiency with accumulation of GM1 ganglioside, a monosialoganglioside of the gray and white matter, divided into Type I (infantile form), characterized by severe mental retardation and neurological, somatic and osseous defects, accumulation of β-galactoside and death by age two, and Type II (juvenile and adult form) is milder than type I, with death occurring by age ten

GM-2 gangliosidoses Type I Tay-Sachs disease, infantile

amaurotic idiocy An AR (carrier frequency, Ashkenazi Jews, 1:25) condition due to hexosaminidase A deficiency, resulting in a 100-fold increase in GM-2 ganglioside in the brain CLINICAL Onset in early infancy with generalized hypotonia, apathy and poor head control, 'cherry-red spots' in the optic macula Note: Genetic screening has virtually eliminated the disease **Type II** Sandhoff's disease An AR condition caused by a complete deficiency of hexosaminidase isoenzymes A and B, with the central nervous system changes of Tay-Sachs disease as well as visceral involvement; 100–200-fold increase in GM-2 gangliosides and a 50–100-fold in GA2, the asialo- derivative of GM-2 in the brain, liver, spleen and kidney; type II is not more common in eastern European Jews **Type III** Juvenile GM-2 gangliosidosis An AR condition of later onset (between ages 2 and 6), with ataxia and psychomotor retardation and death by age 5-15; it is not associated with organomegaly and, like type I, is more common in Ashkenazi Jews

GMP Granule membrane protein, G monophosphate

GMP-140 CD62, see there, formerly known as P-selectin, PADGEM

GMS Gomori-methenamine-silver

Also 1) Gas measurement system 2) General medical services (British) 3) Giant motor synapse (neurophysiology) 4) Glyceryl monostearate (organic chemistry)

GMS stain Gomori-Grocott methenamine silver stain A chromic acid, sodium bisulfite stain used in histology and cytopathology for identifying fungi and for *Pneumocystis carinii*; the glass slide with the tissue or cytologic smear is placed in a hot bath (58ºC) for the penetration of tissue, staining fungi a distinct black with sharp margins and a cleared center; see Sealed envelope appearance

This appearance that may be mimicked by RBCs, which also absorb silver and stain black, but are rounder and have a dark center

GN Glomerulonephritis, also 1) Gram-negative 2) Guanine nucleotide

Also 1) Ganglion nodosum 2) Graduate nurse

gnotobiotic Germ-free; gnotobiotic organisms are either experimental models, eg mice with naive immune systems or 'experiments of nature', in which the natural immune defense mechanisms are grossly defective, eg severe combined immune deficiency; prolonged survival of the host requires complete avoidance of exposure to pathogens; see 'Bubble boy'

GnRH Gonadotropin-releasing hormone, see there

GnRH analogue A generic term for any polypeptide analogue of gonadotropin-releasing hormone (GnRH) some of which are 15–200-fold more potent than GnRH in stimulating the release of gonadotropins; these analogs include leuprolide and histrelin, which can be administered in a pulsatile fashion, with the purpose of restoring lost GnRH, normalizing pituitary-gonadal function, as in congenital GnRH deficiencies, eg hypogonadotropic hypogonadism with anosmia (Kallmann syndrome) or without anosmia or in acquired GnRH deficiency secondary to irradiation of the central nervous system, pituitary tumors or panhypopituitarism; GnRH may be administered continuously in order to induce biochemical 'castration', by 1) Suppressing a pituitary-gonadal axis that at normal levels of activity is exacerbating an underlying medical condition, eg endometriosis or prostatic carcinoma or 2) Suppressing a pituitary-gonadal axis acting in pathological excess, eg polycystic ovarian disease or hyperthecosis (**N Engl J Med 1991; 324:93RV**) see Gonadotropin-releasing hormone

GNR Gram-negative rods MICROBIOLOGY An abbreviation for bacilli that do not absorb the gram stain, ie, pink in color; the most common GNRs of clinical importance are of the coliform family *Enterobacteriaceae*, eg *Escherichia, Proteus, Pseudomonas, Salmonella,*

Shigella, growth of GNRs usually implies fecal contamination, as in peritonitis induced by appendicitis, a ruptured diverticulum, or gunshot wound

go down COMPUTERS A verb for an interruption in the flow of information in a computer, eg to or from the central processing unit, usually referring to larger (ie mini–[1] or mainframe* computers); when the information flow is restored, it is said to be 'back up'[2]

[1]The distinction between microcomputers and either minicomputers or more recently mainframe computers has been essentially abolished as 'microcomputers' become increasing powerful [2]It is worthy to note the difference between the noun back-up, which in information science commonly refers to a copy of a set of data, often stored in a magnetic medium, eg a floppy disk and the verb back up, as indicated above, as their written form differs only in the presence in the former of a dash (–) between work segments

go live COMPUTERS A generic term for the initiation of the flow of data in a computer system, usually referring specifically to the first time the system has been up and running; the second and subsequent times that a system goes live (after 'going down', see there) is often expressed as 'back up'

'go sour' Go South CLINICAL MEDICINE Popular generic American slang for an abrupt and/or unanticipated deterioration of a patient's clinical status; it is used in a broad range of situations, eg an uncomplicated myocardial infarction that 'goes sour' with the development of intractable arrhythmia, or a routine hip replacement on an elderly patient that undergoes an abrupt and unanticipated intraoperative deterioration

goalie finger SPORTS MEDICINE An injury that results when the goalkeeper in soccer is wearing a ring and suffers partial or complete avulsion of the finger when the ring is caught by one of the hooks used to anchor the goal's net (J Hand Surg [Br] 1994; 19B:459)

Goals 2000 see Project 3000 by 2000

goblet appearance RADIOLOGY A radiolucent filling defect seen in tumors of the ureters, where the superior meniscus 'front' of the contrast outlines a goblet-shaped lower or upper margin of the tumor, best visualized by retrograde pyelography, an appearance fancifully likened to that of a wine goblet

goblet cells Caliceal mucin-laden cells, located in the lateral wall of the intestinal crypts and elsewhere in the GI tract

Goiania A city near Brazilia (Brazil) that was the scene of a civilian radiation accident second only in severity to that of Chernobyl; in 1987, some unemployed men entered a partially demolished radiotherapy unit and extracted the core cannister containing 1400 curies of ^{137}Cs, which was sold to a junk dealer, who distributed the glowing cesium as 'carnival glitter'; 10 people died, 54 were hospitalized, 244 received 'major league' exposure and a large region of the city required decontamination; the treatment administered was Prussian blue (to chelate the radioactive cesium and induce excretion) BM transplantation, and stimulation of BM recovery by GM-CSF; see Chernobyl

go 'bare' *Bare*, Old High German, without clothing LEGAL MEDICINE To practice medicine without malpractice insurance; the cost of malpractice insurance in the US is a function of 1) Specialty, ranging from a low of $1-2000/year in rehabilitation medicine, to > $100 000/year in neurosurgery, orthopedic surgery, plastic surgery and obstetrics and 2) Location Long Island (New York), Florida and California are most expensive; because of these costs, some physicians transfer all their financial assets to third parties, incorporate themselves and practice their specialty without insurance, ie 'go bare'; see Malpractice, Cf Surplus line companies

Note: This practice may prevent 'frivolous' lawsuits initiated through avarice, but also prevents truly damaged parties from recuperating compensation

the 'God committee' Seattle committee, see there

gold compound RHEUMATOLOGY A family of second-line anti-rheumatic agents administered intramuscularly (aurothioglucose, gold sodium thiomalate) or per os (auranofin) (N Engl J Med 1994; 330:1368DT) to treat rheumatoid arthritis and other arthritic conditions, acting to protect membrane proteins and lipids from oxidative degradation and quench singlet oxygen generated as free radicals SIDE EFFECTS GI tract, eg diarrhea, abdominal pain, nausea, and vomiting, partially relieved by cromolyn sodium, renal, eg nephrotic syndrome and proteinuria, skin rashes, blood dyscrasias, hepatitis PATHOLOGY IgG and C3 deposits in a 'moth-eaten' glomerular basement membrane and feathery crystals in the renal tubules

gold curve Gold-sol curve, see there

the Gold Sheet A specialized monthly publication that provides business and US federal regulatory information on quality control in the pharmaceutical and health care industry produced by FDC Reports, Inc, Chevy Chase, Md

gold-sol curve Lange's colloidal gold test An empiric, obsolete and nonspecific method for measuring protein in cerebrospinal fluid, where progressive dilutions of fluid are added to 10 test tubes containing colloidal gold solutions; precipitation within the tubes indicates the presence of gammaglobulin, causing a bright red colloidal gold color 0, to change to red-blue 1+, purple 2+, deep blue 3+, pale blue 4+ or colorless 5+; the highest concentration of protein in the fluid is on the left; a 'mid-peak' curve is normal 0001210000, a 'first zone' curve, eg 44332000000 is classically associated with neurosyphilis, but is now more common in multiple sclerosis (50% are positive), and may be seen in subacute sclerosing panencephalitis, central nervous system hemorrhage, meningitis and polyneuritis

gold standard The best or most successful diagnostic or therapeutic modality for a clinical condition, against which any new tests or therapeutic results and protocols are compared; a GS is loosely equivalent to a 'standard of practice' and may be delineated in textbooks, having withstood the test of time; deviation from such standards without reason may be considered malpractice, thus potentially forcing a physician to adhere 'to the book', even though he might believe that a newer therapy is appropriate, eg the X-ray venography for diagnosing deep vein thrombosis is considered to be a GS, although the diagnosis may be established using radionuclide venography, liquid crystal thermography, ultrasonography, and impedance plethysmography; laparoscopic cholecystectomy has been anointed with the GS seal of approval (Arch Surg 1992; 127:917)

Goldberg-Maxwell-Morris syndrome Testicular feminization, see there

Goldberg syndrome Galactosialidosis, see there; also known as neuraminidase deficiency with beta-galactosidase deficiency

Goldblatt kidney A classic model for studying renovascular hypertension; renal artery from kidney 'A' is partially obstructed by an atheromatous plaque (or less commonly, a factor external to the vessel, eg a tumor); the juxtaglomerular apparatus of kidney 'A' perceives decreased circulating blood volume and secretes renin, increasing the blood pressure (systemic hypertension) and, over time, inducing morphologic changes of malignant hypertension, ie arterionephrosclerosis in kidney 'B' due to increased activity of the RAA system; in contrast, kidney 'A' is 'protected' by first pass inactivation of renin and aldosterone; the 'Goldblatt kidney' effect allows separation between benign and malignant hypertension, as in the malignant form, the affected side has 1.5-fold more renin than the unaffected side

'goldbricking' Benign self-mutilation A condition in which a benign skin disorder, eg an occupational dermatosis, is exacerbated by self-induced excoriation prior to workman's compensation review in order to ensure that pension benefits will continue, rather than return to work

Note: This is a permutation of the noun goldbricker, defined as a malingerer or shirker, was first used in reference to loafers in World War I (JE Lighter, *Historical Dictionary of American Slang*, Random House, New York, 1994)

Goldenhar syndrome Oculoauriculovertebral dysplasia An AR [MIM 257700] condition characterized by multiple developmental defects CLINICAL Malar hypoplasia and dysplasia, macrostomia, micrognathia, cleft palate, vertebral body anomalies, eg spina bifida, scoliosis, epibulbar dermoids, external ear defects, antimongoloid slant, and less commonly, mental retardation, clubfoot and congenital heart defects

golden hour CRITICAL CARE MEDICINE A rarely used term for a timespan after a trauma victim's arrival to a health care facility, during which the physician has an opportunity to have a positive impact on the patient's outcome, ie order appropriate diagnostic tests and initiate patient management, either surgical or continued observation; Cf Golden period

Golden-Kantor syndrome Steatorrhea with the radiologic 'moulage' sign, small intestinal segmentation, colonic dilation, redundancy, osteoporosis and dwarfism

golden period CRITICAL CARE MEDICINE A term referring to a period of time during which an injury or other potentially urgent condition may go untreated without harmful effects; the 'golden period' differs according to the organ system or body site, eg revascularizaton of an extremity may be delayed up to six hours without compromising a limb's potential for functional recuperation; thrombolytic therapy with urokinase or streptokinase may be delayed up to 24 hours

golden pneumonia see Lipoid pneumonia

'golden shower' see Sexual deviancy

golden tongue A bright yellow lingual lesion, occasionally seen in an immunocompromised patient with ALL treated with chemotherapy, who became infected with the otherwise saprobic fungus, *Ramichloridium schulzeri*

Note: A general rule in mycology is that the brighter the colony of fungus, the less likely is the organism to be pathogenic

Golden Triangle SUBSTANCE ABUSE A region of Southeast Asia that produces high-grade heroin; see Body-packing syndrome

'goldrush effect' A term coined in a report about a mathematical proof of Johannes Keplers' sphere-packing problem, expounded in 1611; the proof is so complex that it is anticipated that other mathematicians would become involved in proving side theorems and other related geometric complexities; the term is applicable to any area of science in which a large conceptual leap forward is followed by those rushing to find 'gold', where none had been previously known to exist (*Science* 1991; 251:1028)

Goldscheider syndrome An AR dystrophic variant of Fox's disease with hemorrhagic, scarring, pigmented or depigmented bullous lesions due to loose anchoring of the epidermis to the upper dermis; the lesions are acral and accompanied by onychodystrophy, leukoplakia, clawhand, bony deformities and dwarfism

Goldstein's disease A cerebellar disease with defects of equilibrium, perception of time, space and weight (ergo, unsteady gait), adiadochokinesia, megalographia, hyperreflexia of joints and intention tremor

Note: The disease was described in 1915 and it is difficult to determine whether this entity was not a form of another disease, eg neurosyphilis or meningoencephalitis

G_{olf} A G protein involved in olfaction, a neural activity that is similar to vision in that it requires that external signals be converted to electrical signals recognizable by the brain; one model of olfaction proposes that the olfactory signal is transduced as follows: An odorant is received at the membrane receptor of the sensory dendrite, after which GTP is degraded to GDP by the inner membrane-bound G_{olf} protein, which activates adenylate cyclase, generating a cAMP from ATP, activating a Na^+/K^+ cation-conducting channel, generating a neural signal (*Nature* 1991; 350:16n&v)

golf ball bodies A fanciful descriptor for RBCs of severe α thalassemia that are filled with Heinz bodies, large rounded inclusions composed of precipitated hemoglobin H (four β chains) that has undergone oxidative denaturation; Heinz bodies are more prominent after splenectomy, best seen in peripheral blood smears stained with brilliant cresyl blue, and comprise more than ½ of the RBCs in these patients

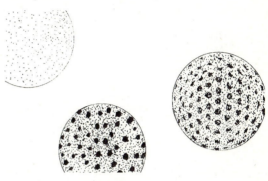

golf ball bodies

golf ball metastases A pattern of pulmonary metastases, seen on a plain chest film, where the nodules are between the size of the 'cannonball' metastases of renal cell carcinoma and the 'miliary' or millet-seed sized metastases of thyroid, lung and breast carcinomas, typically seen in sarcomas, clear cell carcinomas and seminomas and melanomas

golf elbow Medial epicondylitis SPORTS MEDICINE A sports injury characterized by pain and tenderness of the medial humeral epicondyle at the origin of the flexor tendons, caused by excessive golfing TREATMENT Rest, corticosteroid injection if severe; Cf Tennis elbow

Golgi-derived coated vesicle A vesicle involved in non-specific intracellular transport of biosynthetic molecules, mediated by non-selective 'bulk flow' carrier molecules, designated as COPs (coat proteins), one of which, β-COP, has sequence similarity to adaptin proteins of clathrin-coated vesicles (*Nature* 1991; 349:215) see COPs; Cf Clathrin

Gompertzian growth ONCOLOGY A growth curve expressed as an exponentially decreasing function, ie as the size increases (to a theoretical limit), the relative speed of the increase falls exponentially; the curve is named after an 18th century mathematician, and describes the growth of cell masses, eg a fetus or the growth dynamics of most malignancies; Cf Farr's law of epidemics

gonadal dysgenesis see Intersex syndromes

gonadotropin-releasing hormone GnRH A decapeptide synthesized in the hypothalamus and secreted in the anterior hypophysis via the hypophyseoportal circuit, where it stimulates release of the gonadotropins, FSH and LH; GnRH is secreted in 1) A pulsatile fashion (when the pituitary gland is under constant stimulation by GnRH or its analogs, the anterior pituitary becomes desensitized, with subsequent gonadal suppression) and 2) With peaks of secretion during the neonatal period followed by a quiescent phase, later reaching adult levels in puberty MECHANISM OF ACTION GnRH binds to a cell receptor that mobilizes calcium ions, with the subsequent release of gonadotropins; because of GnRH's short half-life (2-4 minutes) and its vital physiological role, GnRH analogs have been developed (**N Engl J Med 1991; 324:93rv**) see GnRH analogs

gonadal dysgenesis Underdeveloped or imperfectly formed gonads; the prototypic gonadal dysgenesis is Turner syndrome 45, X0, seen in 1/2-7000 ♀ births CLINICAL Short stature, webbed neck, cubitus valgus, micrognathia with high arched palate, epicanthal folds, lymphedema of the hands and feet, aortic coarctation, renal malformation, osteoporosis, diabetes, widely spaced nipples, sexual infantilism PATHOLOGY Ovaries are small and thin ('streak' ovaries); a variant, mixed gonadal dysgenesis is characterized by a mosaic phenotype 45,X/46,XY, and a streak ovary on one side and a testis or germ cell tumor on the other side, accompanied by intense virilization

goniometry SPORTS MEDICINE The measurement of joint flexibility in which a large protractor is used to measure the extreme points in a joint's range of motion (**JC DeLee, D Drez, Jr, Eds. Orthopedic Sports Medicine WB Saunders, Philadelphia, 1994**) Cf Flexometry

'good' cholesterol HDL-cholesterol Cholesterol that is carried in the circulation by high-density lipoprotein, the elevation of which is inversely related to the risk of coronary artery disease and cholesterol-related morbidity (**New York Times 8 February 1994; C1**) see HDL-cholesterol; Cf 'Bad' cholesterol

'good' patient A patient who provides reliable information to the physician, who follows the prescribed regimen, drug therapy or recommended change in lifestyle, if appropriate for the patient's condition, and who can be counted on to return for 'check-up' visits at appropriate intervals; Cf Difficult patient

Good Samaritan laws FORENSIC MEDICINE Legislation tailored to the needs of individual jurisdictions that applies to health care professionals and citizens providing emergency medical care in 'good faith'; these laws are designed to protect 'Good Samaritans' from civil liability while attempting resuscitation

Note: If the statutory requirements of 'acting in good faith' at the 'scene of an accident or emergency' are met, a plaintiff's lawsuit against a physician or other 'good samaritan' (for allegedly causing damage to the plaintiff) is often dismissed as 'frivolous'

goodness of fit STATISTICS The degree to which statistical data supports a specified theoretical model; a 'good fit' assumes that the probability model is valid

goose-flesh Cutis anserina Diffuse 1-3 mm bosselations or papules, fancifully likened to a goose's skin after the feathers have been plucked FORENSIC PATHOLOGY 'Goose-flesh' is an early postmortem finding caused by rigor mortis of the erector pili, especially common in drowning victims INFECTIOUS DISEASE Diffuse, finely papular rash of scarlet fever overlying an erythematous base SUBSTANCE ABUSE Horripilation, one of the early symptoms of heroin withdrawal or 'cold turkey', a reflection of marked sympathetic discharge, occurring about 8 hours after the last dose, accompanied by yawning, lacrimation, mydriasis, insomnia, hyperactivity of the gastrointestinal tract, diarrhea, tachycardia and systolic hypertension

gooseneck deformity The convoluted twisting of a short tubular structure, likened to a goose's neck has been used in two cardiovascular contexts, 1) 'Gooseneck' describes the distorted left ventricular outflow tract seen by selective left ventriculography in patients with partial AV canal defects (ostium primum and common AV valve), where the failure of the endocardial cushions to fuse produces an abnormally low AV valve with an abnormally high anterior position of the aortic valve and 2) The gooseneck lamp deformity is a nodularity palpated externally in Mönckeburg's arteriosclerosis, caused by dystrophic calcified rings within the media of the medium to small blood vessels, likened to the flexible 'gooseneck' lamps PATHOLOGY No inflammation, no involvement of the adventitia and intima

Gordon Research conferences A series of meetings held annually in New England (US) in which research scientists with common interests in chemistry and related sciences meet and interact for discussion and free exchange of ideas, stimulating advanced thinking at universities, research foundations and industrial laboratories; see Rs (the three Rs of research)

The conferences were first organized and chaired by Dr Neil Gordon of Johns Hopkins University; they began with one meeting in 1931 and have grown to 130 annual meetings; the camaraderie of these conferences is such that critics at one session may become collaborators by the next and are felt by some to represent the spirit of science practiced in its purest and most selfless form; current director A Cruickshank, U Rhode Is (Emeritus)

Gore-tex™ A proprietary form of expanded polytetrafluoroethylene that is a versatile synthetic material, which is biologically similar to fascia and used for abdominal and thoracic wall, pediatric and diaphragmatic reconstructions, rectal, vaginal and urethral suspension and hernia repair

gork American slang acronym[1] referring to a terminally comatose patient[2]; the term[3] has also been used in reference to patients with a difficult diagnosis; gork has a derogatory flavor and has been used by medical students and interns on the wards of some US teaching hospitals; Cf Gomer

[1]God only really knows [2]ie brain-dead or in irreversible coma [3]Which can be used as both a verb and a noun

goserelin A gonadotropin-releasing hormone analog that may be used to suppress testosterone activity in advanced prostate carcinoma; see Androgen ablation therapy

Note: The prognosis of prostatic adenocarcinoma is poor in the presence of bone pain, elevated testosterone and alkaline phosphatase levels (**JAMA 1991; 265:618**)

gossypol An aromatic triterpene derived from cotton (*Gossypum hirsutum*) seed oil that is 90% effective in reducing sperm counts to the level of infertility, thus having potential as a male contraceptive DISADVANTAGE Nephrotoxicity, hypokalemia, ¼ suffer irreversible sterility

GOT Glutamic oxaloacetic transaminase see AST (aspartate amino transferase)

gothic arch appearance Steeple sign ENT Narrowing of the glottis and subglottis due to edema and acute and chronic inflammatory cells in the soft tissue, seen in a lateral neck film of young children with croup infections, eg due to parainfluenza, other viruses and bacteria, an appearance fancifully likened to that of a gothic arch

goundou TROPICAL MEDICINE Osteoblastic periosteitis of the paranasal maxillae that is a sequela of yaws (infection by *Treponema pallidum* subsp *pertinue*) that occurs in rural and/or primitive tropical regions of Central and South America, Africa, Southeast Asia, and Oceania CLINICAL Purulent nasal discharge, headache, nasal swelling, orbital invasion and visual field defects

'gowns' ACADEMIA The academic faculty of a medical school; many US teaching hospitals are university-based and the teaching faculty may spend more time writing papers and in research than seeing patients; according to Sir William Osler '...to practice medicine without patients is to not sail at all'; Cf 'Towns'

Note: 'Gowns' are the ceremonial robes of education and learned professions

GP2 A homologue of the protein responsible for renal cast formation that, like lithostathine, is secreted by pancreatic acinar cells, and is abundant in pancreatic juice, ductal plugs, and stones (**N Engl J Med 1995; 332:1482ra**)

gp90mel see Selectins

gp120 A 120-kD glycoprotein on the surface of HIV-1 that binds to cells (T cells, macrophages) with the CD4 receptor; blockage of gp120 antigens by soluble synthetic CD4 peptides (sCD4) results in reduced infection of CD4 cells in a 'dose-dependent' fashion, implying that sCD4 may have a role in blocking HIV-1 infection; gp120 is divided into a 'loop region', which although readily accessible to the immune system, is the product of the highly mutable env gene, frustrating the host's attempts to produce effective antibodies; in vitro antibodies to this region block HIV's fusion to CD4-bearing cells and infection and a 'pit region'

gp130 MOLECULAR BIOLOGY A common component of receptor-ligand complexes through which the pleiotropic cytokines IL-6, IL-11, ciliary neurotropic factor, leukemia inhibitory factor, and oncostatin M transduce their signals (Science 1995; 265:1990R)

gp160 vaccine A vaccine prepared from a cloned fragment of HIV-1's envelope protein, which increases the cellular and humoral immunity to HIV products in patients with early HIV infection, slowing the rate of reduction of CD4 T cells, a major predictor of AIDS progression (N Engl JMed 1991; 324:1677) see AIDS vaccine

G protein see under G

graafian follicle GYNECOLOGY A fluid-filled cystic 'unit' containing the ovum, partially covered by a cap of granulosa cells (cumulus oophorus, discus proligerus) that measures 5-10 mm, is lined by an inner layer of granulosa cells and outer layer of theca cells (theca interna) and surrounded by an avascular capsule (theca externa), a structure that is partially recapitulated in the endodermal sinus tumor

grade-flation A neologism (derived from inflation) for the upward shift in the grades that has been observed in certain US academic institutions in the past few decades; in academic year 1968-1969; 35% of students at Stanford University received an A (highest mark), 4% a D and 1% an F (failure); in 1992-1993, 51% recieved an A, 0.7% a D (F was banned in the mid-1970's) (Science 1994; 264; 1255rs)

graduate medical education GME A generic term for any type of formal usually hospital-sponsored or hospital-based training and education that follows graduation from medical school, including internship, residency, or fellowship; there is a general consensus that in the US, GME has been too successful, resulting in an excess of specialists, a paucity of generalists, and too many doctors altogether; to meet the demands of the anticipated health care reform in the US projections call for an estimated increase to 50% (up from the current 30%) in generalists, a decrease in training of specialists, except general surgeons, psychiatrists, and specialists in preventive medicine, who are viewed as being in short supply (N Engl J Med 1993; 329:1810sb) Cf Continuing medical education (CME), Fifth pathway

gradient magnetic field MRI A magnetic field that changes in strength in a given direction; such fields are used in MR imaging with excitation that 'selects' a region for imaging and encodes the location of MR signals received from the object being imaged; the GMR is measured in teslas/meter; see Magnetic resonance imaging

gradualism EVOLUTIONARY BIOLOGY A formal term for Charles Darwin's concept of 'survival of the fittest', a widely accepted posit that has traditionally held that species change gradually over a period of millions of years of natural slection, until one subspecies is so different from its ancestor that it constitutes a new species; this contrasts sharply with the concept of punctuated equilibrium, which is now thought to be the predominant mechanism of speciation, where a species is stable for a period of 2-6 million years, then 'abruptly' in a period of 100-200 000 years splits to form a new species (Science 1995; 267:1421RN) see Adaptive gridlock

graft-versus-host disease A condition that is a major cause of morbidity and mortality in allograft transplants, in articular BM transplantation; GVHD is less problematic in transplantation of kidneys, heart, liver and skin; viable donor T lymphocytes react immunologically against the host, rejecting the hand that feeds them CLINICAL Fever, morbiliform skin rash (central erythematous maculopapular eruption that may spread to the extremities with bulla formation), anorexia, nausea and vomiting, severe watery or bloody diarrhea, lymphadenopathy, infections, hepatosplenomegaly, ↑ liver function tests, jaundice, and hemolytic anemia PATHOGENESIS For GVHD to exist, the graft must contain immunocompetent cells, the recipient must express antigens that are not present in the transplant donor, and the recipient must be incapable of mounting an effective response to destroy the transplanted immunocompetent cells (Billingham, 1966) PROPHYLAXIS Cyclosporin and methotrexate TREATMENT ½ of the 40% of patients who develop post-BM transplantation GVHD respond to high-dose corticosteroids (N Engl J Med 1991; 324:667); agents in development include tacrolimus (formerly FK506), rapamycin and anti-T-cell ricin (ricin conjugated to a monoclonal antibody against CD5, a pan-T-cell marker seen on the cell surface of 95% of all T-cells); see Bone marrow transplantation, Tacrolimus (formerly FK506), Rapamycin Note: An HLA mismatch is more compatible with graft survival than a blood group ABO mismatch; GVHD occurs in 1) Immature immune systems, eg runt disease of mice or 2) Immunodeficiency states, either a) Congenital, eg thymic alymphoplasia, severe combined immunodeficiency disease, Wiskott-Aldrich and T-cell defects and b) Acquired, due to cytotoxic drug therapy, BM transplantation, lymphoproliferative disease, eg acute lymphocytic or myelocytic leukemias, NHL, Hodgkin's disease as well as in neuroblastoma and glioblastoma Gradation of skin changes in GVHD 1) Vacuolization of the basal cell layer 2) Dyskeratosis 3) Subepidermal cleft formation and 4) Complete epidermal separation, which serves as a method for predicting GVH in bone marrow transplant victims PREVENTION Irradiation of the donated blood may prevent the functionally active leukocytes from rejecting recipient cells and tissues **ACUTE GVHD** is associated with rashes, elevated 'liver function' tests, diarrhea, dermatitis, hepatitis, 35-60% respond to immunosuppression; addition of MTX to cyclosporine and prednisone reduces the incidence of acute GVHD from 23% to 9%, but no significant change in disease-free survival (N Engl J Med 1993; 329:1225oA) **CHRONIC GVHD** Occurs in 20-40% of those who survive transplantation > 180 days; see Transfusion-associated graft-versus-host disease

Note: GVHD may also occur when maternal lymphocytes are transferred into a fetus with a congenital deficiency in the immune systems, ie intrauterine transfusion

graft-versus-leukemia effect The antitumor effect mediated by immunocompetent donor (from an allogeneic BM transplantation) cells; the GVL reaction (which is a form of GVHD) is associated with a lower rate of relapse, and patients in leukemia relapse may enter remission when GVHD follows the withdrawal of immunosuppression; thus formal induction of GVHD has potential as a therapeutic modality in patients with CML in relapse after bone marrow transplantation; GVHD is induced with interferon alpha-2a and infusions of mononuclear cells from the donor, in in one report, complete remission (defined by molecular genetic criteria, ie no cells with bcr/abl mRNA transcripts) was induced in 6 of 11 GVL treated patients (N Engl J Med 1994; 330:100oA), offering an alternative to a second bone marrow transplanatation in patients with CML

grain itch An ectoparasitosis-induced irritation of the skin of farmers caused by infestation of straw and grains by the mite *Pyemotes ventricosus*

gramicidin(s) A family of linear antibiotics produced by

Bacillus brevis that carry an N-terminal formyl group and a C-terminal ethanolamine group; gramcidins are active against gram-positive bacteria, acting by increasing ion permeability of the cells

gramicidin A An antibiotic composed of a dimer of hydrophobic amino acids with alternating L- and D-forms, used in membrane research as it is the simplest protein capable of forming transmembrane ion channels, which is selective for monovalent cations (NH_4^+, H^+, and others) (Science 1990; 250:1256)

gramicidin S An antibiotic that is a cyclic polypeptide, more properly named tyrocidin as it uncouples oxidative phosphorylation of tyrosine

Gram stain A stain formulated by a great Dane, HCJ Gram, used to identify bacteria; gram-positive bacteria (purple) have cell wall peptidoglycan and an inner cell membrane and are digested by lysosomal enzymes of macrophage origin; gram-negative bacteria are red, have a membrane similar to the above and in addition, an outer lipid bilayer with lipopolysaccharide which is destroyed by cationic proteins and complement (the 'fluid-phase'); once an organism is identified by its 'gram-ness' and morphology, laboratory algorithms may be followed to identify and speciate the organism

grand mal seizure A form of epilepsy with an onset between infancy and early adulthood, with attacks triggered by fever or unidentified environmental cues, eg psychological and emotional stress CLINICAL Prolonged tonic-clonic seizures with the risk of intra-ictal cerebral hypoxia; sequelae include intellectual impairment, behavioral changes or more rarely ataxia and spasticity EEG Tonic-clonic seizures demonstrate low-voltage fast (10 Hz or faster) activity during the tonic phase evolving to slower, larger, sharp waves associated throughout both hemispheres; during the clonic phase, the bursts of sharp waves are associated with rhythmic muscular contractions while the slow waves coincide with the pauses; between seizures, the EEG is usually abnormal demonstrating polyspike, spike or rarely, sharp and slow-wave discharges; Cf Petit mal epilepsy

grand rounds ACADEMICS The formal presentation of a specific aspect of clinical medicine, with discussion of pathogenesis, symptomatology and therapy; see Rounds; Cf Clinicopathologic conference

Note: Although the term was first used for the formal presentation of a patient's clinical, radiological and laboratory data in an academic setting, for review by colleagues, this latter is regionally known 'professorial rounds', while in grand rounds, the patient is a peripheral player to the topic being discussed

GRANDDAD syndrome An [MIM 138920] condition characterized by Growth Retardation, Aged facial appearance*, Normal Development, Decreased subcutaneous fat, and Autosomal Dominant inheritance

*With triangular facies, prominent forehead, thin or absent scalp hair, deep-set eyes, mid-facial hypoplasia, prominent nasal septum, hypoplasia of nasal alae, prominent ears and thin lips

'grandfather' clause A colloquial term for any policy or rule that exempts a group of individuals, organizations or drugs from meeting new standards or regulations; eg when a new subspecialty board in internal medicine is created, the physicians practicing in that area are 'grandfathered' into the subspecialty and not required to meet residency requirements

grandfather paradox QUANTUM PHYSICS A theoretical impossibility advanced by some physicists to argue that time travel is impossible; briefly stated, if a person from time period A were to travel backward in time and meet his/her grandfather in an earlier time B that preceded the time traveler's birth, and prevent his/her grandfather from meeting his future wife (and the traveler's grandmother), the traveler's birth would be prevented (Sci Am 1994; 270/3:68)

granisetron HCl A 5-HT_3 antiemetic and antinauseant used in patients treated with various chemotherapy agents including cisplatin, and cyclophosphamide ADVERSE EFFECTS Headache, asthenia, somnolence diarrhea, constipation

granular cell tumor Granular cell myoblastoma A small (< 3 cm) painless subepithelial tumor of the tongue, skin, breast and other epithelia and muscle, affecting older blacks with a ♂:♀ ratio of 2:1 PATHOLOGY Small round nests of large, polyhedral cells with pale pink granular cytoplasm, thought to be of Schwann cell origin, which are separated by bundles of mature collage, often covered by pseudoepitheliomatous hyperplasia of superficial epidermis EM Autophagocytic lysosomal vacuoles filled with cellular debris; the cells are positive by periodic acid Schiff/diastase resistant (PAS/dr) and neuron-specific enolase (NSE) stains DDx Any mass composed of enlarged cells with granular cytoplasm, eg oncocytoma, metastatic Hürthle cell tumor, rhabdomyosarcoma, hybernoma, xanthogranuloma; less than 2% become malignant (Virch Arch Path Anat 1926; 260:215)

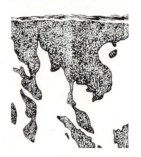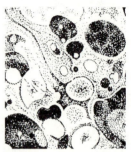
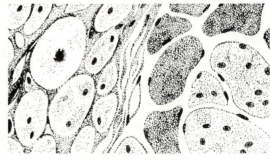

granular cell tumor

granulomatous angiitis of the central nervous system Isolated or primary angiitis of the central nervous system A condition that is most common in middle-aged persons which is diagnosed when angiitis (giant cell, lymphocytic, or necrotizing) is present in the leptomeningeal or less frequently in parenchymal vessels; when the diagnosis of GACNS is established by histologic criteria the ♂:♀ is 2:1; when angiography is used, the ♂:♀ is 1:2 (Arch Pathol Lab Med 1995; 119:334oA)

granular dystrophy An AD variant of early-onset corneal stroma dystrophy with central 'bread-crumb'-like opacities, episodic irritation, and photophobia

granulation tissue A post-inflammatory reaction characterized by edema, chronic (lymphocytes, macrophages, scattered plasma cells, neutrophils) inflammation and numerous proliferating endothelial cells and blood vessels

granules HEMATOLOGY Intracytoplasmic inclusions seen in myeloid cells, by LM that may be divided into

1) Primary azurophilic or immature granules in promyelocytes contain membrane-bound lysosomes filled with acid phosphatase, α-mannosidase, aryl-sulfatase, β-glucuronidase, cathepsin, elastase, esterase, lactoferrin, myeloperoxidase, 5'-nucleosidase, N-acetyl-β-glucosaminidase, sulfated mucosubstance, lysozymes and other basic proteins

2) Secondary (specific) granules contain lactoferrin and alkaline (but lack acid phosphatase and peroxidase and

3) Tertiary granules contain amino peptidase, lysozyme, collagenase and basic protein

granulocyte A mature cell of the myeloid series that comprises 25-40% of the circulating leukocytes or white cells; neutrophils, both the immature 'band' form and the mature polymorphonuclear neutrophil, have a multilobed mature nucleus, and comprise the majority of circulating granulocytes; eosinophils and basophils each comprise 1-3% of the circulating leukocytes

granulocytic sarcoma A variant of granulocytic leukemia, classically associated with AML (2.5-8.0% of which have granulocytic sarcoma); some data suggest the GS may be 2-fold more common in CML and associated with polycythemia vera and myelofibrosis with myeloid metaplasia CLINICAL, CHILDHOOD FORM Acute, often presenting as an orbital tumor mass with ocular proptosis with intracranial, soft tissue, GI tract, gonadal, mammary, cutaneous, nodal, paranasal sinusoidal masses; axial bones, eg skull and paranasal may be involved with subperi- and periosteal tumefactions and local bone destruction CLINICAL, ADULT FORM Chronic, often painful due to cranial and spinal cord compression, followed by motor dysfunction; ♂:♀, 2:1; a leukemic phase may develop 1-49 months after the onset of chloroma symptomatology LABORATORY Sheets of myeloblasts that are positive for naphthyl ASD and chloroacetate esterase enzymes DDx High-grade lymphoma LABORATORY CD13, CD33 expression, a lack of B- and T-cell markers (N Engl J Med 1993; 329:417CPC)

Some clinical forms of GS were known as chloroma (*chlor*, Greek, green, *oma* tumor), as they had a remarkable greenish hue (due to neutrophil myelo- or verdoperoxidase) seen in freshly sectioned tissue; notably, a 'green tumor' may precede marrow and peripheral blood involvement by years; chloromas were first described in 1811 as a retro-orbital, paranasal and lacrimal tumor composed of masses of immature (primitive) granulocytes; as the color is not always present, the term granulocytic sarcoma is preferred, see there

granuloma A nodular aggregate of epithelioid histiocytes (macrophages) with abundant endoplasmic reticulum, giant multinucleated epithelioid cells and scattered CD4 T cells in the center, which function in antigen recognition, surrounded by a rim of collagen, rare CD8 T lymphocytes and proliferating fibroblasts; granulomas are common in chronic infection, especially if the organism remains viable, has metabolic machinery allowing circumvention of the macrophage's phagocytic defense and is capable of residing in histiocytes; granulomas (with Langhans' giant cells) are characteristic of TB but occur in 1) Other infections, eg brucellosis, cat-scratch disease, glanders, fungal infections, leishmaniasis, lepra, listeriosis, mesenteric lymphadenitis, schistosomiasis, tularemia and 2) Noninfectious conditions, eg berylliosis, Crohn's disease, rheumatoid arthritis, sarcoidosis, silicosis, sprue; Cf Giant cells

granuloma gravidarum Pregnancy 'tumor', see there

granulosa cell tumor GYNECOLOGY A sex cord tumor of older women comprising 1-2% of ovarian neoplasms, which is 'driven' by unopposed estrogen stimulation; the endometria of patients with GCTs often has cystic hyperplasia and 5-25% of cases have a concomitant well-differentiated endometrial carcinoma PATHOLOGY GCTs measure up to 4-5 cm, 5% are bilateral and have cystic and solid areas, with a gross appearance fancifully likened to watered silk; 10% rupture, causing hemoperitoneum; 10% of GCTs are malignant, and these are histologically characterized by more prominent nucleoli; GCTs are divided into 1) Adult GCTs, which are more common with an onset after age 30, characterized by Call-Exner bodies and pale cells with grooved nuclei and 2) Juvenile GCTs occur in younger patients, and are characterized by irregular follicles, large, dark cells with ungrooved nuclei and common luteinization

granulovacuolar degeneration PATHOLOGY Lucent 3-5 μm in diameter vacuoles with a dense central granule, which comprise one of three cardinal neuropathological features seen in 10-50% of pyramidal neurons of the hippocampus in Alzheimer's disease, and are possibly of lysosomal origin; granulovacuolar degeneration may also occur in Down syndrome, Pick's disease, amyotrophic lateral sclerosis, Guam-type Parkinson's dementia complex, in the red and pontine nuclei in progressive supranuclear palsy and in cerebral nodules of tuberous sclerosis

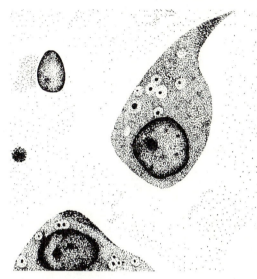

granulovacuolar degeneration

grape-like appearance A morphologic descriptor for massively enlarged, hydropically degenerated chorionic villi seen in hydatidiform mole (molar pregnancy); a similar morphology may be seen in benign cystic mesothelioma and in embryonal rhabdomyosarcoma

grape cell HEMATOLOGY A large (30-80 μm) variant 'reticulum cell' with a small nucleus, condensed chromatin and regular, rounded spaces filled with immunoglobulins separated by wisps of bluish cytoplasm, occasionally seen in the BM of multiple myeloma and other clinical states with ↑ Ig production, occasionally seen in bone marrow

graphic users' interface GUI, see there

GRAS Generally recognized as safe, see there

GRATEFUL MED MEDICAL INFORMATICS A low-priced and 'user-friendly' software package that facilitates literature searches and accession of the data at the National Library of Medicine's database, MEDLARS; MEDLARS' most popular database is MEDLINE

Graves' ophthalmopathy A potentially disfiguring, sight-threatening condition that occurs in 25-50% of patients with Graves' disease CLINICAL Gritty sensation in the eyes, diploplia, blurred vision, ↑ lacrimation, exophthalmos, extraocular muscle dysfunction, periorbital edema, lid edema and retraction, conjunctival chemosis and injection, exposure-type keratitis PATHOGENESIS GO may result from a cascade of events, initiated by T cells that recognize a thyroid follicle cell antigen that is also found in periorbital and pretibial fibroblasts; the T cells release IL-1α, IFN-γ, TGF-α, TGF-β, insulin-like growth factor I, leading to ↑ glycosaminoglycan (especially hyaluronic acid) production in fibroblasts or fibroblast proliferation, accompanied by edema, inflammation, and fibrosis; in the periorbital region, this accumulation results in compression of the extraocular muscles, atrophy and fibrosis (N Engl J Med 1993; 329:1468RV)

gravewax Adipocere Waxy induration of adipose tissue that occurs when an unembalmed body resides one or more months in cold wet ground, see Bog bodies

gray Gy The International system (SI) unit for radiation based on actual absorption as measured by a thermoluminescent dosimeter placed within a patient or a phantom; 1 Gy is equal to 1 joule/kg of the absorber (100 rads); because of the potential for confusion in the conversion of units, it is customary in some circles to use the unit centiGray (cGy), which is quantitatively interchangeable with the rad

Note: The formerly used unit for radiation exposure, the rad, is an 'indirect measurement' based on dosage measured in the air or on the skin surface and equated to a dose of radiation resulting in absorption of 100 ergs of energy/gram in the medium of interest, usually tissue

gray 'hepatization' A phase in lobar pneumonia, typically occurring at the first week of infection, at which time the lobe is covered with fibrin, the cut surface is gray, dry and granular, the alveoli are filled with fibrinous exudate composed of degenerating polymorphonuclear leukocytes and the inflammation is interconnected through the pores of Kohn

gray infant syndrome Gray syndrome, see there

gray infiltration PULMONARY MEDICINE The transformation of pulmonary parenchyma into a grayish semisolid mucoid ooze, a change occasionally seen in acute necrotizing tuberculous pneumonia

the 'Gray Journal' A colloquialism of little utility used in the US for certain journals that may be requested in a medical library by color; the classic 'gray journal' is the gray-green Annals of Internal Medicine; Cf Green journal

Note: There are many other widely circulated 'gray' journals, including the American Journal of Obstetrics and Gynecology, the American Journal of Surgical Pathology, the Journal of Pediatrics, and Radiology

gray lethal mouse The murine model for osteopetrosis, which has normal appositional bone growth without physiological resorption of bone; osteoclasts are present but nonfunctional

gray matter *substantia grisea* [NH3] Th component cells and circuitry that comprise the 'central processing unit' of the CNS and spinal cord, which is composed of neuronal cell bodies, initial axon segments, dendritic processes and arborizations, glial (neuroglial cells), and capillaries and vascular support; in the brain, the gray matter is peripheral, in the spinal cord, gray matter is central

gray-out A descriptor for faintness due to vasodepressor illness/vasovagal syncope that may be seen in cardiac disease, eg in idiopathic hypertrophic subaortic stenosis; 'gray-out' also refers to visual 'misting' seen in acceleration or deceleration injuries in high speed vehicles; Cf Graying out

gray patch ringworm Fungal folliculitis in children, caused by *Microsporum canis* and *M audouinii*, which progresses from an erythematous papule at the hair follicles, extends peripherally and forms annular lesions

gray platelet syndrome An AD [MIM 139090] condition in which the platelets lack alpha and dense granules and by extension, certain platelet proteins, eg von Willebrand factor, fibrinogen, fibrin, fibronectin, platelet factor 4 (PF4), β-thromboglobulin, platelet-derived growth factor, thrombospondin and contact-promoting proteins CLINICAL Lifelong bleeding diatheses with epistaxis, bruisability, petechiae LABORATORY Thrombocytopenia, enlarged platelets with a grayish hue on Wright-Giemsa stained peripheral blood smears, ↑ bleeding time TREATMENT DDAVP (desmopressin acetate)

gray scale see Ultrasonography

the Gray Sheet A specialized weekly publication that provides business and US federal regulatory information on medical devices, diagnostics and instrumentation; it is produced by FDC Reports, Chevy Chase, Md

gray syndrome A condition that may occur when chloramphenicol levels exceed 70 µg/ml; premature infants are most susceptible, given their limited capacity to glucuronidate and excrete chloramphenicol (the functional deficiency in glucuronyl transferase activity corrects itself within the first 3-4 weeks of life); high levels of chloramphenicol inhibit mitochondrial electron transport, disrupting energy metabolism CLINICAL Ashen gray skin (hence the name), vomiting, tachypnea, dyspnea, abdominal distension, cyanosis, diarrhea (pseudomembranous colitis), flaccidity, hypothermia, and potentially death due to circulatory collapse; in children under one month of age, doses should be ≤ 25 mg/kg LABORATORY Chloramphenicol may be quantified by colorimetry, GLC, HPLC, microbiological and radioenzymatic methods

gray top tube LABORATORY MEDICINE A blood collection tube containing powdered sodium fluoride and/or potassium oxalate, which inhibits glycolysis; 'gray tops' are used for glucose tolerance testing, as erythrocytic glycolysis would cause falsely-low glucose levels, as well as for measuring lactate (transported on ice) and lactate tolerance

gray zone Gray area EPIDEMIOLOGY A room or area located between the 'normal' nonbiosafety level world and a Biosafety Level 4 'hot zone' in which trained personnel are working with highly virulent infectious oragnisms, eg Ebola virus (R Preston, The Hot Zone, Random House, New York, 1994)

Note: Gray zone/area is commonly used in the lay parlance for anything that is not readily apparent, ie not 'black' or 'white'

'graying-out' Slow visual impairment accompanying papilledema caused by slow-growing intracranial masses, eg brain tumors and abscesses; Cf 'Gray-out'

GRE Glucocorticoid regulatory element(s) A group of steroid hormone-responsive DNA sequences that bind to the glucocorticoid receptor, enhancing DNA transcription from linked promoters in both mammals and yeasts, implying high conservation of biological mechanisms among species

great imitator A nonspecific term for any condition that is difficult to diagnose due to the polymorphous nature of its presentation; the classic 'great imitator' is syphilis, which has a broad palette of clinical manifestations, affecting in particular the skin and CNS; of more recent vintage are a host of lesser 'great imitators', including HIV infection, hypothyroidism, neuroborreliosis (tertiary Lyme disease), and pheochromocytoma*; Cf Internists' tumor

*Given the non-specificity of signs and symptoms, including hypertension, migraines, tachyarrhythmias, endocrine and CNS dysfunction that mimic both benign and malignant conditions

great pox Syphilis The first clinical descriptions of 'the mother of venereal disease' appeared when Charles VIII's mercenaries invaded Naples in the late 1400s; while the origin of the disease is uncertain, historical evidence vaguely implicates Haiti as the place where Columbus' sailors first contracted syphilis, anointed the 'great pox' to contrast to smallpox

Greek cancer cure An unproven cancer therapy involving blood tests of an undisclosed type that allegedly serve to diagnose the presence, stage and progression of malignancy; the treatment consists of injecting an unknown substance, possibly pure nicotinic acid that is purported to cure the cancer; the principal proponent of this therapy is a physician whose license to practice medicine had been twice suspended in Greece, who treated foreign tourists in various hotels in Athens; according to the evidence available to the American Cancer Society, this modality has no known effect in treating malignancy; see Unproven methods of cancer management

Greek helmet facies see Wolf-Hirschhorn syndrome

'green' *adjective* Environmentally 'correct'

green bottle fly A fly that is an opportunistic pathogen, causing a form of myasis, ie maggot infestation, pupating in open sores or purulent discharges

Green Book Directory of Graduate Medical Education Programs A book published annually by the American Medical Association that catalogs the accredited internships and residency training programs sponsored by university and teaching hospitals in the USA and Canada; 'Green book' is also a schedule of adult immunizations published by the American College of Physicians, Cf Red book

'green' card A white and salmon-colored document that identifies an alien as a permanent resident of the US, and in the case of physicians in specialty training, allows them the option of staying in the US after finishing their training, thereby contributing to the Brain drain, see there

'green foot' Verdant discoloration of the soles and toenails of those wearing sweat-dampened rubber-soled basketball shoes that are actively colonized by a pigmented strain of *Pseudomonas aeruginosa;* see Green nail syndrome

green hair SPORTS DERMATOLOGY A 'condition' affecting light- (blond, gray, white) haired individuals who frequent swimming pools due to assimilation of copper into the hair matrix; the copper may occur naturally in the water supply, leach from the pool's pipes, or derive from copper-based algicides; GH is of merely cosmetic concern, responds well to bleaching with H_2O_2 and can be prevented by maintaining the pool's pH at the alkaline side of 7.4 (JS Dover, in TB Fitzpatrick et al, Eds, Dermatology in General Medicine, McGraw-Hill, New York, 1993) see Sports dermatology

the 'Green Journal' A colloquial term of little utility, referring to commonly requested journals in medical libraries; the classic 'Green journal' is the American Journal of Medicine (British racing green); other green journals, include Obstetrics and Gynecology (Kelly green), Pediatrics (sherbet green), and American Journal of Psychiatry (forest green)

green monkey disease Marburg virus disease, see there

green nail syndrome Verdant discoloration of the fingernails, most often associated with *Pseudomonas paronychia,* seen in persons who regularly submerge their hands; the greenish discoloration is merely the result of diffusion of pyocyanin produced by *Pseudomonas* spp infection in the adjacent paronychia; Cf Green foot

'green paper' Parliamentary policy A 'discussion' document that is published when the British government has plans for or is considering reform in any field, eg Health policy or consolidation of funds allocated to basic sciences; after publication of a 'green paper', the issue becomes a matter for comment or open debate, which is then followed by a 'White paper', see there

the Green Sheet A specialized weekly report that provides business and US federal regulatory information in the pharmaceutical industry produced by FDC Reports, Chevy Chase, Md

green sickness Iron-deficiency anemia, formerly chlorosis

green soap Medicinal soap, soft soap A soap prepared from certain saponified vegetable (excluding coconut and palm kernel) oils and mixed with potassium hydroxide and glycerin

greenstick fracture An incomplete angulated fracture that causes bone bowing with rupture of the periosteum on the convex side of the bone, ie the opposite cortex is intact, without the fracture line traversing the bone, which is more common in vitamin D-deficiency rickets

Note: The small tender 'green' branches of trees when bent, buckle but don't break, leaving the internal wood intact

green stool syndrome Transient neonatal passage of thickened, bile-stained stools, thought to be caused by an unknown bacterium that alters urobilin metabolism, responding within 24 hours to penicillin

green tea A beverage alleged to be more carcinoprotective than black tea (which is produced from green tea by a fermentation process); both have (–)-epigallocatechin gallate, an antioxidant responsible for the alleged protective effect (Cancer Reseach 1 July 1994, in Science News 1994; 146:61)

green technology ENVIRONMENT The modification of energy consumption, manufacturing processes and products being produced and waste disposal to minimize or eliminate its impact on the environment; among the 'green tech' targets are substitutes for CFCs, bioremediation of soil and water contaminated by pollutants and biodegradable plastics; the most concerted effort in this vital arena is being spearheaded by the Japanese (Nature 1991; 350:266n)

green top tube LABORATORY MEDICINE A blood collection (test) tube with a green stopper containing sodium or lithium heparin that is used to obtain blood for ammonia (collected on ice), carboxyhemoglobin and oxygen saturation, cholinesterase, hemoglobin, methemoglobin, pH, as well as histocompatibility testing, including HLA-A, B, HLA-D (mixed lymphocyte culture), NBT (nitrotetrazolium blue) assay, phagocytosis, T- and B-cell studies surface markers

green tumor Granulocytic sarcoma, see there (formerly chloroma)

green urine disease Massive increase of verdohemoglobin in the urine which fluoresces with ultraviolet light, a sign of fulminant *Pseudomonas aeruginosa* infection; the finding of green urine in such patients may be accompanied by poor response to aminoglycosides

Greenberg v. H&H Music HEALTH INSURANCE A lawsuit initiated by F Greenberg, MD, on behalf of J McGann, a former employee of H&H Music, Inc whose allowable medical expenditures were capped at $5000 after his employer learned he had AIDS, and was likely to incur enormous health-related expenses; the legal arguments in the case revolve around interpretation of the anti-discrimination provisions of the Employee Retirement Income Security Act (ERISA) that governs how self-insurance plans may operate; the argument is that a self-insured employer has the right to modify or cut benefits to maintain a plan's 'structural integrity', and only acted illegally if the benefits were capped to retaliate an employee, or to deprive him/her of a pre-existing right (Am Med News 2 Nov 1992, p 1)

Greenfield filter see Inferior vena caval filter

Greenfield syndrome Metachromatic leukodystrophy, late infantile type (see there)

greenhouse effect ENVIRONMENT The ability of environmental gases to trap solar radiation, an effect likened to a greenhouse, and attributed to an imbalance of the $O_2:CO_2$ ratio; production of O_2 is $\downarrow$ by deforestation (rain forest destruction occurs at the rate of 100 000 km²/year), while production of CO_2 and other 'greenhouse' gases has $\uparrow$; CO_2 concentration has $\uparrow$ from 315 ppm in 1958 to 352 ppm in 1988; the global temperature has $\uparrow$ 0.6°C within the past 100 years-1990 was the hottest year on record (Science 1991; 251:274); a global rise of another 2-5°C would partially melt the polar caps, causing a one meter rise in the sea level, endangering coastlines, creating from 50 to 500 million 'environmental' refugees, leaving arable land inundated and much of the low-lying remainder susceptible to the elevated (salt) water table that would further deteriorate both the potable water supplies and croplands (in a worst-case scenario, there may be a rise of 5-10°C by the year 2100, with an inland migration of the oceans in a densely crowded, polluted and contaminated environment; sea level has $\uparrow$ 2.4 mm/year since 1920; while $\uparrow$ CO_2 may stimulate photosynthesis, the positive effect on plant growth is offset by the acid rain pollutants (SO_2 and NO_2), vegetation toxins (H_2S, NH_3, dimethyl sulfide), industrial NO_2, natural and industrial hydrocarbons and ↑ atmospheric ozone, explaining the dying forests of Europe; in addition to the direct effects of greenhouse gases, minor contributing gases eg NO_2 and CFCs (chlorofluorocarbons) are major actors in depletion of the ozone layer in the stratosphere that blankets the earth at 20-50 km, filtering out the 'hard' ultraviolet-B; the ozone holes at the polar caps may increase the UV-B to levels toxic to the phytoplankton that initiates the marine food chain; see CFCs, Iron hypothesis, Montreal protocol

greenhouse gases Those gases that are held responsible for causing the planet's warming, including CO_2, CH_4, NO_2, SO_4 and others; per capita emission of CO_2 Italy 2.01 tons per person, France 2.04 tons, Japan 2.45 tons, UK 2.97 tons, West Germany 3.45 tons and USA 6.14 tons; anthropogenic gas production in 1987 was estimated to be: 7.9×10^9 metric tons of CO_2 (due to changes in land use/deforestation, fossil fuel combustion and cement manufacture, resulting in a net addition of 47% to the atmospheric gases), 270×10^6 metric tons of CH_4 (from livestock, wet rice cultivation, solid waste and coal mining, caused a net addition of 18% to the atmospheric gases)

greenhouse index A method proposed by the IPCC (Intergovernmental Panel on Climate Change) for measuring a nation's contribution to the Greenhouse effect by comparing the infrared heating effectiveness of a greenhouse gas with CO_2 and multiplying the relative productions by the population Note: This index has potential for allowing an equitable reduction in global anthropogenic gases by fining the nations with high values

Greenwood-Yule method EPIDEMIOLOGY A method that attempts to resolve whether a disease process is related to the order of birth within a sibship

grenz radiation RADIATION ONCOLOGY Low-dose superficial radiation (10-kV range) that has been used to treat psoriasis, in which the positive effect is transient and the carcinogenic effect permanent; Cf Bremstrahlung

grenz zone *Grenz*, German, border, frontier DERMATOPATHOLOGY A well-demarcated zone of separation in the upper dermis (figure), delineated by the collagen of the flattened basal epidermis from the upper dermis, the latter of which often has a dense, usually lymphocytic infiltrate; a grenz zone is seen in granuloma faciale, lepromatous leprosy and lymphocytoma cutis and may separate a pilar tumor or leiomyoma from the atrophic overlying skin

Gresham's law A 'rule' for expensive health care, that holds that considerations of cost will drive out considerations of quality in administering a medical program (N Engl J Med 1994; 329:1395sa)

GRID Gay-related immune deficiency A transiently used acronym for the AIDS (acquired immunodeficiency syndrome), the first cases of which occurred in homosexual (gay) men; see AIDS

grind and find dilemma LABORATORY MEDICINE A diagnostic challenge encountered when performing procedures that require partial digestion or homogenization of cells or tissues in order to identify the presence of an increased amount of a substance or molecule of interest, eg estrogen receptors in breast cancer, or viral genome in a lymphoma; the dilemma revolves around the fact that while the presence of the substance of interest can be established, if it can't be proven from which cell(s) it exactly came, as the cellular 'context' is lost by grinding (homogenization); the G&F dilemma can be solved by in situ hybridization and in situ PCR (Arch Pathol Lab Med 1993; 117:1115oa)

griseofulvin An oral antifungal agent isolated from *Penicillium griseofulvum dierckx* and *P janczewski* with an affinity for skin, used for dermatophytic infections (*Epidermophyton* spp, *Microsporum* spp and

Trichophyton spp) MECHANISM Griseofulvin disrupts the mitotic spindle by interacting with polymerized microtubules SIDE EFFECTS Headache, nausea, diarrhea, vomiting, photosensitivity, fever, rashes, dysfunction of hepatic, nervous, hematopoietic systems; it is teratogenic and carcinogenic in rodents

GRK2 G-protein-coupled receptor kinase (Science 1995; 268:247) Note: The more commonly used term is βARK (β-adrenergic receptor kinase)

grommets see Tympanostomy tubes

groomed whisker appearance Sun ray pattern Hairlike periosteal projections perpendicular to bony trabeculae seen by radiology most commonly associated with Ewing sarcoma, but also seen in osteosarcoma, neuroblastoma, and renal cell carcinoma metastatic to bone

groove see Major groove, Minor groove

groove sign RHEUMATOLOGY Branched zone linear loss of dermal fibrosis overlying the veins in eosinophilic fasciitis; when the affected extremity is raised, the reticulated pattern of the intersecting veins seen has been likened to dry, merging river beds STD A finding characterized as linear fibrotic depressions parallel to the inguinal ligament, bordered above and below by enlarged and matted lymph nodes and covered by adherent, erythematous skin, seen in 10-20% of cases of LGV (*Chlamydia trachomatis*, serotypes L1, L2, L3)

grooved tongue Scrotal tongue, see there

gross negligence MEDICAL MALPRACTICE The reckless provision of health care that is clearly below the standards of accepted medical practice, either without regard for the potential consequences or with wilful and wanton disregard for the rights and/or well-being of those for whom the duty is being performed; see Malpractice

gross description SURGICAL PATHOLOGY A formal 'script' generated by a pathologist that describes surgically excised tissues, providing details on size, shape, morphology, color and consistency; 'grossing' serves to document the nature of surgery-removed tissues, from which representative sections are made and processed through aqueous and non-aqueous solutions, embedded in paraffin, sectioned with a microtome, placed on a glass slide, stained, (usually with H&E), and interpreted by LM; the pathologist may elect, in certain tissues, eg uncomplicated hernia sac or a fractured femoral head in an older person, not to submit tissue, which may be designated as 'gross only'; see Glass pusher

grossing see Gross description

ground glass A adjectival descriptor commonly used in medicine for a homogenous translucency, which is equivalent to the German, Milchglassartig BACTERIOLOGY A shadowy ground glass-like appearance on culture plates that is midway between the greenish hue of α hemolysis and the ochre-brown of β-hemolysis, incorrectly termed γ-hemolysis HEMATOLOGY Ground-glass histiocytes have 'washed-out' cytoplasm and are typical of reticulocytic granuloma HEPATOLOGY Ground glass cytoplasm is classically associated with hepatitis B virus and results from swelling of the smooth endoplasmic reticulum, see figure HISTOPATHOLOGY Uniform, finely granular eosinophilic (orcein and aldehyde fuchsin positive) cytoplasm with a peripheral clear halo; a similar morphology may be seen in dilated lysosomes in Gaucher's disease or in the lung with viral inclusions, which by electron microscopy, reveal spherules of HBsAg or Dane particles; similar PAS inclusions may be seen in alcoholics treated with alcohol aversion-inducing disulfiram (Antabuse), an acetaldehyde dehydrogenase inhibitor; see Pseudo-ground glass inclusion NEUROPATHOLOGY Ground glass cytoplasm is characteristic of gemistocytic cells in astrocytomas PANCREAS A ground glass appearance is typical of the abolished architectural details seen by low-power light microscopy in enzymatic fat necrosis or in postmortem autolysis OPHTHALMOLOGY Ground glass opacification of the cornea occurs in children in mucopolysaccharidosis (MPS) type I-H (Hurler) with global MPS deposition in the ocular structures, photophobia, retinal degeneration, attenuation of vessels, optic atrophy, loss of vision and hydrocephalus RADIOLOGY, ABDOMEN A ground glass appearance with haziness and erasure of organ silhouettes, which is typical of massive ascites, and related to an increased water density and peritonitis RADIOLOGY, BONE The ground glass appearance corresponds to a relatively uniform loss of osseous density which may be accompanied by intravascular calcification and subcutaneous ossification, seen in bones affected by fibrous dysplasia, scurvy (located at the epiphyses), osteomalacia, agnogenic myeloid metaplasia, osteoporosis RADIOLOGY, CHEST The ground glass appearance corresponds to an alveolar, acinar or amorphous pattern seen in bronchiolitis obliterans and obstructive pneumonia RADIOLOGY, PEDIATRIC Ground glass is a descriptor for poorly circumscribed radiopacifications of the right lower quadrant, mixed with fine trapped bubbles within the meconium 'plug', seen on a plain film in meconium ileus; Cf Applesauce VIROLOGY Ground glass-like appearance is seen in the nuclei of epithelia infected with herpes simplex

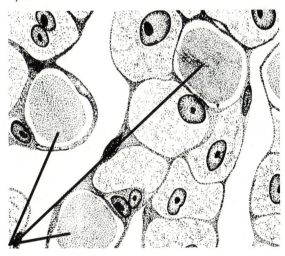

ground glass hepatocytes

ground itch A hypersensitivity reaction to hookworms, occurring in previously sensitized individuals CLINICAL Inflammation, erythema, blistering and intense pruritus at the larval penetration site (feet) AGENTS *Necator americanus, Ancylostoma duodenale*

group atrophy A light microscopic pattern seen in denervation, where the normal 'checkerboard' pattern of type I mixed with type II skeletal muscle fibers is lost and there is a histochemical 'regrouping', so that there are large bundles of each type, a change typical of reinnervation

group B streptococci *Streptococcus agalactiae* A streptococcus classified into 7 capsular serotypes (Ia, Ib, II, III, IV, V, and VI), which is the leading cause of sepsis and meningitis in neonates, affecting 1.8/1000 infants aged ≤ 90 days; it causes morbidity in ≥ 50 000 pregnant women/year (US), and has emerged as a major pathogen of nonpregnant adults, occurring in 2.4-4.4/10⁵ more commonly in blacks; in one study of nonpregnant adults, GBS caused localized skin, soft tissue and bone infections in 36%, bacteremia of unknown source in 30%, UTIs in 14%, pneumonia in 9%, and peritonitis in 7% with a total mortality rate of 21% (N Engl J Med 1993; 328:1807oa)

group C drug An investigational drug that has reproducible efficacy in one or more specific tumor types; these drugs alter or are likely to alter the pattern of treatment of a disease and can be safely administered by properly trained physicians without specific supportive care

group I intron MOLECULAR BIOLOGY A generic term for any of a family of unique introns that are capable of folding into very specific shapes capable of cutting and splicing RNA (being thus also known as group I ribozymes); in nature both the catalytic site and the substrate are formed from a single strand of RNA (Bio/Technology 1995; 13:323)

group practice A generic term for the practice of medicine as a team with physicians and administrators being 'players' who share various overhead costs and expertise; in 1965, there were 4289 GPs comprising 10.6% of all physicians; by 1991, there were 16 576 GPs comprising 32.6% of physicians with an average of 13 members (US); GP 'alliances' are often formed to gain 'clout' in the health care delivery system and to be able to successfully negotiate contracts with HMOs and insurers for providing health care services (Am Med News 1995; 17 April 1995 p1) Cf Solo practice

group psychotherapy Group therapy, see there

group therapy Group psychotherapy A generic term for the regular[1] treatment of a group of 2 to 20 people[2] who may share a similar problem; the techniques used in GT are as varied as the methods used in psychoanalysis, and are therapist-specific

[1]Usually weekly [2]Often with the same therapist in order to develop the maximum level of comfort with the 'clients'

growing fork MOLECULAR BIOLOGY Replication on double-stranded DNA is bidirectional, starting at one origin giving rise to two de novo synthesized DNA chains (replicons); the rate of replication is a function of the organism's complexity, the growing forks of *Escherichia coli* duplicates at a rate of 1000 base pairs/second (bp/s), while human cells duplicate at 100 bp/s; the human genome of 3×10^9 base pairs requires 8 hours to complete duplication and involves 10 to 100 thousand replicons; of the growing forks, the 'leading' strand is reproduced as an unbroken strand of new DNA growing continuously in the 5'→3' direction, while the 'lagging' strand forms short discontinuous segments also in the 5'→3' direction, which are primed by short segments of RNA; these short DNA-RNA primer sequences are known as Okazaki fragments, see there

growing pains Benign leg pains occurring in young children; experts disagree on whether this condition actually exists; if it does exist, it is a diagnosis of exclusion, requiring that trauma, infection, avascular necrosis of bone, tumors, collagen vascular disease, Lyme disease, psychosomatic nosologies, congenital and developmental abnormalities be ruled out CLINICAL Growing pain complaints are bilateral, intermittent, most often occurring after going to bed, thought to be due to edema of muscles encased within 'tight' fascia, often following a day of strenuous exercise, although a temporal or activity-relatable pattern may not be detected; the pain may be accompanied by restlessness and disappears with the cessation of growth TREATMENT Local heat, massage and if severe, quinine sulfate

growth see Mitosis

growth cone NEUROPHYSIOLOGY A bulbous expansion at the tip of an immature growing or regenerating axon which is directed and guided by neuronal growth factor and netrin, and confined by N-cadherin; growth cones from severed nerves find their amputated end by means of N-CAM, and mature to become an axon terminal; see Netrin

growth factors A broad family of cytokines that facilitate cell growth and proliferation, including epidermal growth factor (S Cohen, 1986 Nobel Prize), erythropoietin, fibroblast growth factor, insulin-like GF I, IGF II, nerve growth factor (R Montalcini-Levi, 1986 Nobel prize), platelet-derived growth factor, relaxin, somatomedin A and B, transforming growth factors (TGF-α and TGF-β)

growth hormone Somatotropin A 21.5-kD protein hormone that is under the hypothalamic control via growth hormone-releasing hormone (GHRH), acting via insulin growth factor-1 (IGF-I or somatomedin-C), increasing protein and glycogen synthesis, lipolysis, opposing the effect of insulin on muscle and 'priming' macrophages for superoxide production Note: Short children may respond to growth hormone therapy and are identified with stimulation (arginine-insulin) tests rather than baseline measurements; the use of human-derived growth hormone to treat these children was stopped when Creutzfeldt-Jakob disease developed in some recipients; recombinant growth hormone (rGH) is being used to treat reduced height; early data has linked the use of rGH to a 2-fold ↑ in childhood leukemia and slippage of the femoral head epiphysis Normal 5-10 µg/L (US: < 5 ng/ml, ♂; < 10 ng/ml ♀); growth hormone levels ↓ with age, reflected in the ↓ levels of IGF-I (< 350 U/L, normal for age: 500-1500 U/L), a ↓ that may result in ↓ bone density and lean body mass and ↑ adipose tissue mass typical of older subjects CIRCADIAN RHYTHM A daily growth hormone peak occurs in the first 2 hours of sleep, ↑ with stress, exercise, hypoglycemia, amino acid (arginine) and protein infusions, and may be 4- to 12-fold normal in acromegaly

growth hormone insensitivity syndrome Laron dwarfism Severe growth retardation and physical manifestations typical of one who is deficient in growth hormone, with low serum insulin-like growth factor-I (IGF-I), which responds to IGF-I infusion with increase in calcium excretion and decrease of serum and urea nitrogen, suggesting therapeutic potential for this agent (N Engl J Med 1991; 324:1483cr)

growth spurt PEDIATRICS A brief period of rapid growth that occurs in middle adolescence in which ♀ have an average increment of 8 cm/year at a mean age of 12 years, and ♂ have an average increment of 10 cm/year at a mean age of 14 years; the GS is further characterized by an orderliness in location, with the acral parts of the skeleton (ie the hands and feet) growing before the more proximal regions, explaining in part the clumsiness typical of this period of life

grübelsucht PSYCHIATRY A colloquial translation for hairsplitting, a feature of obsessive-compulsive neuroses Note: The literal translation of the root verb, grüben, refers to brooding, and thus imparts a melancholic Gefühl to this variant of neurosis

GSD Glycogen storage disease, see there

GSH Glutathione, see there

GTPase superfamily A family of conserved 'molecular switch' enzymes that bind and hydrolyze GTP, acting as 'on-off' switches for various intracellular activities; the switch is turned on when GTP is bound and off when GTP is hydrolyzed to GDP; GTPases sort and amplify transmembrane signals, direct the synthesis and translocation of proteins, guide vesicular traffic through the cytoplasm, control cell proliferation and differentiation and have a pivotal role in pathogenesis of malignancy and infectious diseases since they are targets of mutations and microbial toxins; GTPases are divided into three groups

1) 21K family, which includes the products of *ras* oncogenes and protooncogenes

2) GTPases involved in ribosomal protein synthesis and

3) The α subunits of the signal-transducing G proteins (Nature 1991; 349:117rv)

The high conservation of structural motifs across diverse species suggests that the family originates from a single primordial protein

GTT 1) Gastrostomy tube 2) Germ tube test 3) Glucose tolerance test, see there

GU-AG rule MOLECULAR BIOLOGY The finding that an intron begins at the guanine and uracil nucleotides at the 5'-end of the 'donor' junction and closes when the spliceosome reads an adenine and uracil at the 3'-end of the recipient junction

Guam An island in the Marianas (Oceania), the native inhabitants (the Chamorros) of which have had their brains poked and prodded by Japanese and American neuropathologists, who wonder why this population is so susceptible to the amyotrophic lateral sclerosis-Parkinson's-Alzheimer's dementia complex (ALS-P-A); a proposed explanation for the disease's decline since insidious 'Americanization' began 35 years ago is that the use of the plant *Cycas circinalis*, containing BMAA, an unusual amino acid (related to BOAA, a grass pea neurotoxin causing lathyrism in animals), a native medicine and food, is being used with decreasing frequency; Cycas-fed macaques develop corticomedullary dysfunction, the parkinsonian shuffle, behavioral and neuropathological manifestations that mimic ALS-P-A complex

guaiac-positive stool see Occult blood testing

guaranty (sic) fund HEALTH CARE ENVIRONMENT A pool that covers the benefits of insolvent insurers, which is designed to protect providers and consumers (Am Med News 25 October 1992, p7)

guarding Involuntary muscle spasm elicited by fulminant acute peritonitis, leaving the anterior abdominal muscles in a state of tonic contraction, imparting a board-like consistency to the rectus abdominis muscles, to be distinguished from voluntary guarding, seen in 'ticklish' patients

GUI Graphical users' interface A symbol-based visual interface with a computer, allowing a computer-'illiterate' person to use a computer as a tool for his/her particular needs without the need to understand how it actually works BACKGROUND Prior to the mid-1980s, knowledge of a minimum vocabulary of often arcane operating system commands was required to be able to use a PC (personal computer); this non-intuitive interface met with considerable resistance among the 'technically challenged' and made the introduction of PCs in the home and work environment difficult; with the advent of the GUI, first by Apple Computer (Cupertino, CA) with the Macintosh, and subsequently by Microsoft (Redmond, WA) with its software-based equivalent, Windows, end-users could easily learn and use software; GUIs share in common a number of features: They are mouse-driven; they have pull-down menus, and icons which are easily recognizable symbols of hardware, software, tools, and files created in a particular program; once an icon is selected on the screen, a file can be copied, deleted, transferred or opened, by a variety of intuitive clicks and drags; see User-friendly

guided imagery ALTERNATIVE MEDICINE A form of health care in which the power of the mind is used '...to evoke a positive physical response...reduce stress and slow heart rate, stimulate the immune system, and reduce pain.' (Alternative Medicine, Future Medicine Pub, Puyallup, WA, 1994); GI attempts to place 'mind over matter' for the relief of allergies, cancer, chronic pain, dysmenorrhea, headaches, hypertension, premenstrual syndrome, stress-related GI symptoms, functional urinary complaints; see Anodyne imagery, Alternative medicine

Note: There is little peer-reviewed data to support the health benefits claimed by guided imagery therapists

guillotine amputation A sharply defined loss of a portion or entire segments of extremities, ranging from digits to major amputations, seen in the congenital aglossia-adactylia syndrome

guinea pig A rodent occasionally used in research Note: The idiom in English '*to be a guinea pig*', which implies that one is being used as an experimental animal, is largely incorrect; the guinea pig, *Cavia cobaya*, is cuddly and resembles the human hormonally, immunologically and in reproductive physiology, but is a poor experimental model, comprising but 2% of the rodents in the research rat race; they are stupid, ie rather incapable of learning, have less complex immune systems than mice, have a long gestation period, produce small litters, are picky eaters, are susceptible to infections and are more costly to maintain than smaller rodents (**Handbook of Inbred and Genetically defined Strains of Laboratory Animals, Altman and Katz, 1979**), and thus, most research is performed on rats and mice, the choice differing based on the needs of the researcher; eg mice are of interest as their immune system (major histocompatibility complex is on chromosome 17 in mice and very similar to the human system located on chromosome 6; although guinea pigs, eg *C porcellus*, are traditionally classified as a New World hystricomorph rodent, phylogenetic analysis of the amino acid sequence data implies that the guinea pig diverged before the separation of the primates and artiodactyls from the myomorph rodents (**Nature 1991; 351:649**) see Rat

Gulf War syndrome Since returning from the Gulf, thousands of veterans have complained of symptoms including fever, headache, loss of short-term memory, deteriorating vision, shortage of breath, coughing, diarrhea, skin changes, bleeding gums, loss of hair and teeth, numbness, tingling, aching joints and fatigue; in absence of any diagnosis, the condition has been dubbed 'Gulf War syndrome' (**Nature 1993; 364:659N**); the US National Institutes of Health has rejected the idea that these symptoms constitute a single medical syndrome (**Nature 1994; 369:8N**)

gull wing pattern Seagull appearance A descriptor for a gull wing-like pattern with a broad, flattened and gently curved V-shape IMMUNOLOGY The presence of two distinct and connected, relatively flat precipitin arcs in the serum protein electrophoresis, typically seen in lambda light chain myeloma or IgD or IgE myelomas MICROBIOLOGY The classic high-power LM morphology of the gently undulated gram-negative *Helicobacter* and *Campylobacter* species RADIOLOGY A double curved shadow seen on a plain lateral film of the entire pelvis in either fracture-dislocation of the posterior acetabular rim or dislocation of the femoral head; the 2 wings are contributed by the intact and fractured acetabulum

gumboil Parulis A dental abscess, converted into a cyst with chronic drainage through a fistulous tract, seen by a plain film of the jaw

gumma Lentil-to-cherry-sized masses characteristic of tertiary syphilis, which represent a hypersensitivity response to treponemal products (the organism itself is rarely found) PATHOLOGY Central caseating necrosis surrounded by epithelioid histiocytes and multinucleated giant cells and vessels 'cuffed' with inflammatory cells; gumma also occur in the skin, liver, bones, testes, mucosal membranes and stomach

'gun barrel' vision Tunnel vision, see there

gun control FORENSIC MEDICINE The United States is unique in the easy access its citizens have to firearms, an anachronistic right guaranteed by the US Constitution, the consequence of which is that 1) Suicide rate by handguns is 5.7-fold greater in the US than Canada (adjusting for other methods, the US suicide rate ages 15-24 is 1.38-fold greater (**N Engl J Med 1990; 322:369**) HOMICIDE RATE (per 100 000 population) Philippines 38.7, Lesotho 36.40, Jamaica 18, US 8.6, France 4.05, Italy 1.52, Germany 1.5, UK 1.33, Ireland 0.54

Gunn rat Animal model for the study of jaundice due to this rodent's inherited deficiency of glucuronyl transferase (**J Heredity 1938; 29:137**)

gunstock deformity ORTHOPEDICS A reversal of the arm's carrying angle, resulting from 1) Inadequate correction of the medial angulation of the distal fragment of a supracondylar fracture of the humerus or 2) Stimulation of the lateral condylar epiphysis from the fracture itself (even when the fracture has not been displaced)

gustducin An intermediary protein messenger present in the taste buds that is activated in response to all sweet and some bitter taste stimuli that arrive to cell surface receptor (**New York Times 4 August 1992; C1**)

GUSTO Global Utilization of Streptokinase and Tissue plasminogen activator for Occluded coronary arteries trial An international initiative (41 021 patients, 1081 hospitals, 15 countries) that examined the effect of aggressive thrombolytic therapy (streptokinase and tissue plasminogen activator-t-PA) on survival in patients with acute MI; GUSTO concluded that t-PA (cost $2300) in combination with IV heparin provides a survival advantage (1%) over previous standard thrombolytic regimens, eg streptokinase (cost $320) (**N Engl J Med 1993; 329:673oA**); a seemingly logical conclusion of the GUSTO trial is that the more rapid and complete the restoration of blood flow through the infarct-related artery, the more improved the ventricular performance and the lower the mortality in MI survivors (**N Engl J Med 1993; 329:1615oA**) There is a slight survival advantage of t-PA vs streptokinase; if t-PA is administered early after an acute MI there is in an absolute ↓ of 1% in 30-day mortality (**N Engl J Med 1995; 332:1418oA**)

gut-associated lymphoid tissue GALT, see there

gut feeling Intuition, visceral sensation

GVH disease Graft-versus-host disease, see there

GVHD Graft-versus-host disease, see there

gynandroblastoma 'Yin-yang' tumor A rare ovarian sex-cord tumor with masculinizing (hirsutism, clitoral hypertrophy and deepening of the voice) and/or feminizing (vaginal bleeding due to endometrial hyperplasia) hormonal effects; it is believed by some authors to be an over-diagnosed term that should be reserved for when well-differentiated testicular and ovarian tissue is present in the neoplasm, requiring that at least 10% of the minor component be present PATHOLOGY Functionally active and mature masculinizing elements, granulosa-(Call-Exner body formation) thecal cells and Sertoli-Leydig (Reinecke crystalloids) cells CLINICAL The tumor presents in the second to the sixth decade as a unilateral cystic and solid pink-to-yellow 0.6-18.0 cm pelvic mass TREATMENT Excision

---

GYNECOMASTIA Etiology

ENDOCRINOPATHY Orchitis, hypogonadism (androgen deficiency), androgen resistance syndromes, tumors or hyperplasia of the adrenal gland, testes, eg Leydig cell tumors (hCG production), lung cancer, Klinefelter syndrome (increased risk of breast carcinoma) and thyroid hyperplasia

DRUGS Alpha-methyldopa, amphetamine, androgens, benzodiazepines, cimetidine, chemotherapeutic agents, digitalis, INH, marijuana, penicillamine, phenothiazine, reserpine, spironolactone, tricyclic antidepressants

OTHER CONDITIONS Starvation diet (mechanism: testicular and hepatic hypofunction) or on resuming normal feeding, hemodialysis, hepatopathies (cirrhosis, hepatomas, hemochromatosis, due to decreased hepatic metabolism of estrogens), mycosis fungoides, myotonic dystrophy with spastic paraplegia, leprosy

---

gynecomastia Benign enlargement of the male breast that most commonly affects boys and adolescents, often regresses at puberty; it is usually due to a proliferation of the glandular component; there are 3 age-related peaks in incidence: 1) Perinatal, occurring in 60-90% of ♂ at birth, related to the transplacental passage of estrogens 2) Pubertal, occurring in 4-69% (depending on the stringency of definition) of ♂ age 10-14 3) Involutional, in ♂ age 50-80% PATHOGENESIS 1) ↑ Estrogen 2) ↓ Androgen 3) Androgen receptor defects 4) Hypersensitive breast tissue TREATMENT Clomiphene, tamoxifen, testolactone have been reported to be effective in uncontrolled trials, and if ineffective, surgical excision (**N Engl J Med 1993; 328:490**ᴿᵛ)

gyrase Topoisomerase II An enzyme first isolated from *Escherichia coli*, cutting double-stranded DNA, passing a portion of double helix through the uncut double helix, resealing it on the other side, a maneuver that transforms a 'positive' supercoil into a 'negative' supercoil; in mammalian cells, the density of supercoiling is a function of histone binding; see Supercoiling

gyrate atrophy Ornithine aminotransferase deficiency An AR [MIM 258870] condition characterized by hyperornithinemia with gyrate atrophy[1] of the choroid and retina causing a slowly progressive loss of vision, myopia and nyctalopia, ↓ glutamate levels and minimal hepatic and renal tubular dysfunction; about 10% have proximal muscle weakness with variable histologic abnormalities of the type 2 skeletal muscle fibers LABORATORY 10-20-fold ↑ of ornithine and mild ↑ of lysine, glutamic acid and glutamine, due to deficiency of ornithine-δ-aminotransferase[2] [EC 2.6.1.13], the gene for which (OAT) maps to 10q26 TREATMENT Dietary and metabolic manipulation is unsuccessful

[1]Hence the transiently used synonym, HOGA syndrome [2]Also known as ornithine-oxo-acid transminase, the term recommended (1992) by the Nomenclature Committee of the IUBMB (International Union of Biochemistry and Molecular Biology)

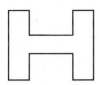

H Symbol for: 1) Hauch (microbiology) 2) Heavy chain 3) Henry, the term for derived SI (International System) unit for electrical inductance 4) Histidine 5) Hounsfield unit 6) Hydrogen 7) Hyperopia 8) Magnetic field strength

h Symbol for: 1) hecto- (10^2) 2) Hour

H1, H2A, H2B, H3, H4 Histones, see there

H antigen IMMUNOLOGY Histocompatibility antigen, see there MICROBIOLOGY A protein present in bacterial flagella TRANSFUSION MEDICINE The trisaccharide stem molecule chain of the ABO blood group, which islocated on red cell membrane surfaces; the enzyme, α-L-fucosyl-transferase is encoded by the H gene and produces the oligosaccharide structure

H blocker see Histamine receptor blocking agents

H bodies Heinz bodies (clumps of denatured hemoglobin); see Golf ball bodies

H-bomb sign RADIOLOGY A finding in a radiocontrast study of a stomach with atrophic gastritis, where the fundus appears as a 'bald' dome with thinned rugae and an attenuated gastric wall; the speckled background is due to poor mixing of gastric secretions with the barium; when erect and distended with air, the 'mushroom' appearance has been fancifully likened to the appearance of a hydrogen bomb explosion

H-2 complex The term for the major histocompatibility complex (MHC) in the mouse, which is located on chromosome 17 and analogous to the human HLA system on chromosome 6; the H-2 complex is 2-4000 kilobase pairs in length and contains the thousands of genes involved in immune recognition, each 600 base pairs in length; the H-2 subregions of K, D and L correspond to HLA's subregions A, B and C3, and the I-A and I-E regions correspond to the HLA-D region in humans

Note: The MHC was discovered in the 1930s in inbred mice by Gorer who was studying the effects of graft rejection on erythrocytes; the gene for histocompatibility that rejected the red cell antigen was designated as number 2 (ergo H-2)

H gene TRANSFUSION MEDICINE A gene that encodes the enzyme, α-L-fucosyl-transferase, which produces an oligosaccharide, the H antigen; homozygous deficiency of H gene results in a Bombay (or hh) phenotype individual who, lacking the above transferase, cannot attach the fucose to the galactose on the precursor H substance; when the H gene is present, ABO precursor molecule is encoded; when the A gene is also present, the 'A-transferase' is encoded, which adds N-acetyl-D-galactosamine to the H antigen, resulting in group A red cells; when the B gene is present, 'B-transferase' adds D-galactose to the H antigen, resulting in group B red cells; the amount of H substance on red cells differs according to the blood type, where group $O > A_2B > B > A_1 > A_1B >$ Bombay; see Bombay phenotype, H-antigen, Secretor, *Ulex europa*

H$_1$ receptor Histamine receptor, see there

H$_1$ receptor antagonist Histamine receptor antagonist, see there

H reflex NEUROLOGY An electrically induced spinal reflex thought to be monosynaptic that is used to diagnose S-1 radiculopathy and for studying nerve conduction, as in Guillain-Barré syndrome

H-shaped esophagus H type fistula, see there

H- or U-shaped vertebra PEDIATRIC RADIOLOGY A vertebrum with a flattened central body with mineralization of its posterior aspects , which may be seen in sickle cell anemia and in thanatophoric dwarfism

H-type fistula PEDIATRICS A congenital variant of esophageal atresia and tracheoesophageal fistula (EATF) that corresponds to Gross-Vogt's type E fistula, where the esophagus communicates with the stomach in the usual fashion and has a small fistulous tract to the trachea, causing recurrent aspiration pneumonia TREATMENT Surgical closure, nutritional support

Note: The most common EATF is type C, in which the upper esophagus ends in a blind pouch and the lower esophagus communicates with trachea

H wave H reflex NEUROPHYSIOLOGY A spikelike form seen on electromyography which represents a monosynaptic reflex response to the excitation of spindle 1a afferent axons by a single impulse stimulation of a muscle nerve; the H wave measures the sensitivity of the monosynaptic reflex pathway of the spindle 1a axons

HA-1A INFECTIOUS DISEASE A human monoclonal IgM antibody that binds to the lipid A domain of endotoxin and prevents death in laboratory animals with gram-negative bacteremia and endotoxemia; its efficacy in humans with septicemia (400 000 cases/year, US, 30% caused by gram-negative bacteria, mortality 20-60%) is less spectacular, but its use may be associated with a slightly improved clinical course (**N Engl J Med 1992; 327:889c**) Cf E5 therapy

habenula NEUROANATOMY A dorsomedial thalamic prominence that receives afferents from the amygdala via the medullothalamic striae and from the hippocampus via the fornix, forming a central point where olfactory, visceral and somatic afferent pathways are integrated, mediating GI secretion and deglutition, and possibly also thermoregulation

Haber-Weiss reaction A devastating intracellular event that occurs when superoxide dismutase and catalase in tissue are insufficient to degrade superoxides and peroxides and other toxic free radicals in the tissues: $H_2O_2 + O_2^- = OH^\bullet + OH^- + O_2$; see Free radical, 'Garbage can' hypothesis, Superoxide dismutase

habitual abortion A third (or more) consecutive abortion, related to stress, nutritional status, an event occurring in up to 1:200 women, many of whom may eventually have successful gestations; see Abortion

habituation An adaptive response characterized by a decreased reactivity to a repeated stimulus, eg a substance of abuse or repeated electrical stimuli of a nerve

habitually wandering patient see Wandering patient

habitus The general corporal type of the adult body; an asthenic habitus is seen in tall thin subjects whose organs are said to hang low in the body; the hyperthenic subject is plethoric and his organs are higher in the body and the hyposthenic habitus lies between the two

HACEK group An acronym for a group of bacteria that commonly cause infective endocarditis, to wit *Haemophilus, Actinobacillus, Cardiobacterium, Eikenella,* and *Kingella* species

Hachinski ischemic score NEUROLOGY A clinical scoring system for quantifying features common in multi-infarct dementia (MID); 2 points are given to each of the following: Abrupt onset, fluctuating clinical course, focal neurologic signs, focal neurologic symptoms, history of stroke; 1 point is given to: Stepwise deterioration, nocturnal confusiondepression, relative preservation of personality, somatic symptoms, emotional lability, hypertension, evidence of atherosclerosis; a score ≥ 7 supports the diagnosis of MID and ≤ 4 favors the diagnosis of primary degenerative dementia (N Engl J Med 1993; 328:153oA)

HADD Hydroxyapatite deposition disease, see there

Haff disease German, Bay, Harbor A disease of historic interest that occurred epidemic waves (1924, 1925, 1940) in Königsberg Bay in Lithuania CLINICAL Myalgia, dyspnea, dysuria and myoglobulinuria; death due to renal failure occurred in about 1% of the cases; HD was attributed to either ingestion of fish tainted with cellulose-derived toxic resins and/or arsine from paper-processing plants that discharged their waste into the Haff waters or ingestion of an unidentified toxin in certain eels and fish

Hafnia A motile, gram-negative, facultative anaerobic fecal saprobe of the Klebsiella tribe; formerly an Enterobacter, *Hafnia* is separated therefrom by DNA homology studies and has but one species, *H alvei* that is rarely pathogenic and responds to Enterobacter-type antibiotics

hair Types of hair ANAGEN HAIR Actively growing hair LANUGO HAIR Fine hair of the fetus, usually shed at birth TELOGEN HAIR Non-growing hair that is easily removed TERMINAL HAIR Coarse, deeply pigmented, stiff and thick, seen in the scalp and eyebrow, chest, facial and pubic hair; androgens typically induce transition of vellous to terminal hair, although there is marked variation in the response of different body regions to androgens VELLOUS HAIR Fine, soft and downy hair of children and women; see Hair replacement, Hirsutism, Minoxidil

Note: Except for the knuckles, elbows, knees, lips and palmoplantar regions, the body is covered with hair

HAIR-AN Hyperandrogenic insulin-resistant acanthosis nigricans A subtype of hyperthecosis affecting 5% of hirsute females, often associated with polycystic ovaries, characterized by 1) Hyperandrogenesis (increased testosterone, increased androstenedione; early, premenarcheal hyperandrogenism) 2) Insulin-resistance, where the patients are either normal or have clinical diabetes and 3) Acanthosis- nigricans, possibly an epiphenomenon TREATMENT Bilateral oophorectomy, contraceptives, corrects the hyperandrogenism, but often not the excess insulin

hair analysis The use of scalp hair as primary analytical specimen, the only legitimate diagnostic use of which is to detect chronic heavy metal intoxication, eg arsenic, lead and mercury TOXICOLOGY The use of samples of hair to detect chronic drug abuse* METHODS RIA, EIA, GC/MS AGENTS DETECTED Amphetamines, cocaine, heroin LEVELS OF DETECTION 10 pg/mg to 10 ng of hair CONFOUNDING FACTORS Differences in drug levels determined by the testing are based on race (Orientals absorb most, Causcasians less), hair color (dark-colored hair is worse) and environmental contamination (eg passive absorption of cocaine (which may occur in children of drug abusing parents (CAP Today June 1995, p14) Note: HA has been periodically reported (usually by providers of alternative forms of health care) to be of use in evaluating a person's health and nutritional status, but has been largely relegated to the domain of quackery

*The use of hair as a source for drug testing, has certain advantages, as it is nonintrusive, clean and difficult to cheat on, providing a long-term 'record' of drug ingestion

hair-brain syndrome BIDS syndrome, see there

hairbrush appearance A fanciful descriptor for the elongated periosteal bony spicules projecting from the femoral metaphyses in achondrogenesis, which may be seen radiologically and which focally have a hair-on-end appearance

hair-on-end appearance Crewcut appearance A radiologic pattern seen as calcified spicules perpendicular to the bone surface, corresponding to a periosteal reaction to disturbed bone repair with neoosteogenesis of the outer cranial table, marked calvarial thickening, external displacement and thinning of the inner table; it is classically seen in children and young adults with thalassemia; the 'crewcut' appearance may occur in periostitis of long bones in congenital syphilis (syphilitic periosteitis of the tibia, gives rise to Saber shins, see there); HOEA is also seen in congenital hemolytic anemias (pyruvate kinase deficiency, and hereditary elliptocytosis and spherocytosis), as well as in sickle cell anemia, metastatic neuroblastoma, iron-deficiency anemia, cyanotic (right-to-left shunt) congenital heart disease, osteomyelitis, early onset polycythemia vera, thyroid acropachy, hemangiomas; bone spiculation in malignant tumors of bone has three broad patterns 1) Hair-on-end Parallel spiculations, eg Ewing sarcoma 2) Sunburst Radiation from a central point, eg osteosarcoma and 3) Velvet-like low, slanting spicules, eg chondrosarcoma

hair replacement (surgery) A generic term for any form of surgical therapy intended to 'correct' baldness. including hair transplantation‡ (with use of standard grafts, minigrafts, and micrografts), scalp flaps‡, scalp-lifting procedures‡, scalp reduction‡, tissue expanders

hair transplantation Therapy used to correct baldness; HT is only successful using hair-bearing autografts from the patient (or from an identical twin); the earliest HTs (Orentreich, 1959) consisted of punch grafts, which were of a relatively large diameter and did not provide a natural appearance; see Baldness, Hair replacement

'...hair transplantation involves a redistribution of existing hair; the extent and density of the area that can be covered with transplants are limited by the amount of remaining permanent fringe hair. Attempts to circumvent a paucity of donor hair by using synthetic fiber or human hair implants have uniformly resulted in severe complications including fiber/hair rejection, infection, pruritus, and cicatricial alopecia.' (GJ Hruza, JL Fewkes, in TB Fitzpatrick et al, Eds, Dermatology in General Medicine, 4th ed, McGraw-Hill, New York, 1993)

hairpin loop MOLECULAR BIOLOGY DNA hairpin A short segment of inverted repeat DNA that forms under low-stringency denaturing conditions (low-stringency conditions allow 'sloppy' binding between complementary DNA strands), when the complementary segments are adjacent to each other on the DNA; if the regions of complementarity are distant to each other, they form heteroduplexes RNA hairpin A short segment of RNA transcribed from a DNA palindrome, which folds upon itself, forming a double strand; RNA hairpins are found within the nucleus and are an integral component of the 'cloverleaf' configuration of tRNA

hairpin vessels Minute blood vessels that are doubled upon themselves, seen at the metaphyseal-diaphyseal junction of normal bone

hairy cell leukemia Leukemic reticuloendotheliosis A low-grade B-cell leukemia that comprises 2% of adult leukemia, commonly affecting ♂ (♂:♀ ratio, 4:1) age 50-55 and leading to progressive pancytopenia CLINICAL Insidious onset with weight loss, bruising, abdominal fullness due to splenomegaly, pancytopenia with normocytic, normochromic anemia, rarely aplastic anemia due to infiltration of bone marrow, spleen, lymph nodes; 10% have platelet counts of < 20 x 10^9/L (US: < 20 000/mm^3), 20% have thrombocytosis; 1-80% of nucleated blood smear cells are hairy CAUSE OF DEATH Infections, gram-negative bacteria, atypical mycobacteria and fungal LABORATORY ↑ acid phosphatase, especially isoenzyme 5 (which is also ↑ in bone metastases and in children with Gaucher's disease), 'dry tap' from a BM biopsy and the cells (see figure) are positive for tartrate-resistant acid phosphatase (TRAP), an enzyme that may be weakly expressed in infectious mononucleosis, macroglobulinemia, prolymphocytic leukemia and Sézary syndrome; hairy cells measure 10-20 μm and are in late stages of B-cell ontogeny, have undergone Ig gene rearrangement and are positive for mature pan-B cell markers (CD19, CD20, CD22) and may co-express monocytic and T-cell markers B cells expressing eg CD11c, CD25, and B-Ly7 Note: The hairy cell gene may be X-linked and located close to the glucose-6-phosphatase D gene EM Villous processes and intracytoplasmic lamellar ribosomal complexes, zipper-junctions TREATMENT Purine analogues 2'-deoxycoformycin (pentostatin) and 2-chlorodeoxyadenosine (cladribine) (N Engl J Med 1994; 330:691DT), a purine nucleoside used in low-grade lymphoproliferative processes, eg CLL and NHL is more effective than IFN-α

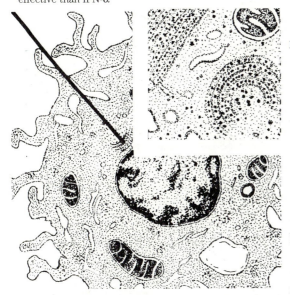

hairy cell

hairy leukoplakia ORAL PATHOLOGY An EBV-associated infection seen in HIV-infected subjects, characterized by a condyloma-like tongue mass (75% of patients have papilloma virus, 95% have EBV in epithelial cell nuclei) preceding the onset of clinical AIDS PATHOLOGY Koilocytosis with ballooned prickle cells, perinuclear halos, pyknotic, hyperchromatic and occasionally atypical nuclei, basal cell disorganization and increased mitotic activity; the hyper- and parakeratotic 'hairy' projections appear as a corrugated surface

hairy penis Pearly penile papules, see there

hairy polyp Teratoid tumor A benign congenital malformation of young, often female children arising from ecto- and mesodermal totipotent cells, located in the nasopharynx, oropharynx and tonsils DDx Intranasal glioma, rhabdomyosarcoma, meningoencephalocele, Rathke's pouch cyst, pharyngeal hypophysis and craniopharyngioma

hairy tongue A benign elongation of the tongue's filiform papillae and failure of the superficial layer to desquamate,

serving as a nidus for microorganisms, potentially resulting in halitosis; although idiopathic, hairy tongues may be associated with heavy smoking, alcohol abuse, radiotherapy to the head and neck, dehydration, systemic illness and antibiotic therapy, resulting in decreased flow of saliva, occasionally allowing unrestrained fungal growth

Note: When the papillae are stained deep brown or other colors by extrinsic substances, including tobacco and chromagens, the condition may be termed 'black hairy tongue'

Haiti see Geographic exclusion

halberd bone Battle ax bone PEDIATRIC RADIOLOGY Marked flaring of the iliac crests, typical of metatropic dwarfism, a rare metaphyseal dysplasia with bulbous joints and multiple, markedly deformed and shortened bones

Halcion PSYCHOLOGY A sleeping pill with serious side effects, eg paranoia and severe anxiety; it has been alleged that its manufacturer knew of these effects and chose to drop out evidence about these side effects in studies submitted to the FDA, the agency encharged with approving new agents

Haldane's rule DEVELOPMENTAL BIOLOGY The principle that if only one sex is sterile or inviable among species hybrids, it is the heterogametic sex (Nature 1994; 369:189N&V)

half & half nails An idiopathic onychopathy occasionally seen in chronic renal insufficiency (uremia), characterized by a transverse distal red-brown band occupying most of the nail with a dull, white proximal band

half-life ($T_{1/2}$) The amount of time required for a substance to be reduced to one-half of its previous level by degradation and/or decay (radioactive half-life), by catabolism (biological half-life) or by elimination in a system, eg half-life in serum HEMATOLOGY $T_{1/2}$ is the time that cells stay in the circulation, eg erythrocytes 120 days, which increases after splenectomy, platelets (4-6 days), eosinophils (3-7 hours), and neutrophils (7 hours) IMMUNOLOGY $T_{1/2}$ is the time an immunoglobulin stays in the circulation: 20-25 days for IgG, 6 days for IgA, 5 days for IgM, 2-8 days for IgD and 1-5 days for IgE PHYSICS $T_{1/2}$ is the time required for a radioisotope to decay to one-half of the original amount having the same radioactivity; a radioisotope's effective $T_{1/2}$ is either the time required to decay (physical $T_{1/2}$) or the time required for elimination from the biological system

half moon sign BONE RADIOLOGY A semilunar shadow that may disappear in posterior dislocation of the humerus with the glenoid capsule, as under normal circumstances, the medial humeral head overlaps the glenoid fossa

half-side trial CLINICAL THERAPEUTICS A trial of a topical agent for a systemic dermatopathy, eg ichthyoisis, where the agent with a putative therapeutic effect is placed on one half of the body and the other half acts as a control to monitor response or lack thereof

halfway house A semi-sheltered environment for subjects who are in rehabilitation for mental illness or addiction disorders including drug and alcohol abuse, who do not require in-patient hospitalization; HHs are often staffed by their own 'graduates' or professionals who provide guidance and if necessary, treatment; Cf Homelessness, Shelter

halfway technology A coinage by Lewis Thomas for a therapeutic approach to diseases that are incompletely understood, or for which appropriate therapy is beyond technological reach; halfway therapeutic modalities ameliorate or modify illness without curing, as incomplete understanding of the pathogenesis precludes prevention

halitosis Bad breath An offensive odor emanating from the mouth, which is caused by either oral pathology (eg poor dental hygiene with bacterial growth in plaques, acute or chronic gingivitis, or fungal overgrowth) GI pathology (eg food entrapment in Zenker's diverticulum

(JAMA 1995; 273:1171) see Body odor, Odors

halo appearance A descriptive adjective for a doughnut-shaped light density within and surrounded by a rounded darker dense zones DERMATOLOGY see Target lesions BONE PATHOLOGY The 'halo' is a rimming of osteocytic lacunae, seen by light microscopy in X-linked hypophosphatemia, caused by delayed maturation BREAST PATHOLOGY The halo is an annular rim of stromal edema seen in gynecomastia, due to acid mucopolysaccharides, eg hyaluronic acid, which surrounds ducts with epithelial hyperplasia; a similar effect is seen in fibroadenomas of the female breast CARDIAC RADIOLOGY A halo of radiolucency seen on a plain antero-posterior chest film in pneumopericardium GI RADIOLOGY The 'halo' may be seen either in duodenal ulcers, where the radiocontrast settles in a fixed location, typically occurring in an acute ulcer within a mound of radiolucent edema surrounding the crater; alternately, 'halo' refers to a saccular collection of radiocontrast surrounded by radiolucency, seen in the rare intraluminal duodenal diverticulum, which causes a windsock deformity GYNECOLOGIC RADIOLOGY The 'halo' or wall sign is a smooth-contoured delineation of one tissue density from another, seen in a mature cystic teratoma or dermoid on a plain abdominal film, that is enhanced by the firm fibrous capsule investing these usually benign tumors HEPATIC RADIOLOGY An avascular radiolucency surrounded by radiodensity, which corresponds to increased vascularity, seen by hepatic angiography in hemangiomas Note: CT and MRI have reduced the utility of hepatic angiography to very specific applications; a 'paradoxical' halo may appear as an extrahepatic density, simulating an intrahepatic mass OBSTETRIC RADIOLOGY Spaulding's halo sign is a semispherical shadow seen on a plain film of the maternal abdomen, corresponding to the skull of a dead infant that is covered by edematous skin and soft tissue overlying the skull RENAL RADIOLOGY The hypernephroma halo is a radiolucent rim surrounding perinephric fat caused by a diffuse renal mass, first described in renal cell carcinoma (hypernephroma) that may be seen in abscesses, hematomas, disseminated malignancy and, if left-sided, pancreatitis

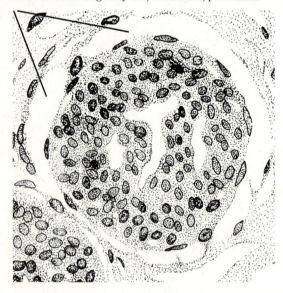

halo appearance

halo device An orthopedic device used to manage cervical spine injuries to minimize neurological damage, requiring long-term immobilization; in the halo device, pins are inserted on the outer skull for skeletal traction, using a 2-3-kg weight for upper cervical injuries and 10-15 kg for lower cervical injuries

halo effect The beneficial effect of a physician or other health care provider on a patient during a medical encounter, regardless of the therapy or procedure provided; see Hawthorne effect, Placebo effect, Physician invincibility syndrome

Note: A halo is a shimmering ring of light floating above the heads of angels of Judeo-Christian dogma, endowed with mystical healing powers, as in the 'healing hands' of the physician

halo nevus Leukoderma acquisitum centrifugum A pigmented melanocytic nevus surrounded by a peripheral zone of depigmentation (melanocytes absent with a lymphohistiocytic infiltrate), measuring ± 5 mm in diameter surrounding a common nevus, most often affecting adolescents on the back; when inflamed, it is called an inflammatory halo nevus; a halo phenomenon may also occur in congenital, blue, and Spitz nevi, neurofibromas, primary and metastatic melanomas

haloperidol A dopamine-blocking neuroleptic agent of the butyrophenone class that is the archetypal antipsychotic drug for schizophrenia; it is used to reduce hallucinations, delusions, thought disturbances and improves the symptoms of withdrawal and apathy, as maintenance therapy to control symptoms, and as long-term prophylaxis for preventing relapses Note: Haloperidol is useful for managing schizophrenia in the short term, but is less successful for long term therapy; negative symptoms do not respond to haloperidol; 10-20% of schizophrenics do not respond at all to haloperidol (see N Engl J Med 1994; 330:681ʀᵥ); haloperidol may also be used to treat Giles de la Tourette syndrome SIDE EFFECTS Sedation, weight gain, extrapyramidal signs (which may be be immediate, eg parkinsonism, akathisia and acute dystonia), or late with long-term therapy, eg tardive dyskinesia, 'rabbit' syndrome (see there), and orthostatic hypotension), cardiovascular and GI effects, and the potentially fatal neuroleptic malignant syndrome; see Clozapine, Neuroleptic malignant syndrome, Schizophrenia

halophyte Salicornia bigelovii, subspp Torr, see there

halothane hepatitis A carbon tetrachloride-related halocarbon, used as a maintenance-type anesthetic (thiopental is often used for induction); halothane is preferred for the ease of awakening patients, its relatively low toxicity, and low blood:gas partition coefficient; although classically, halothane causes hepatotoxicity (post-operative jaundice and hepatic necrosis), the incidence of this reaction is low (1/35 000 halothane administrations); hepatotoxicity occurs in 7-14% of hypoxic animals pretreated with phenobarbital

HALV Human AIDS/lymphotrophic virus, HIV-1 (human immunodeficiency virus-1), see there

Prior to settling on the acronym of HIV for human immunodeficiency virus, Montagnier favored LAV and Gallo preferred HTLV-III, in the spirit of collaboration, F Wong-Staal suggested (Nature 1985; 314:574c) a non-partisan acronym, as a '...perfect solution for the two groups to meet HALV (sic)-way'

halzoun TROPICAL MEDICINE An acute upper respiratory tract infestation by the sheep liver fluke, Fasciola hepatica that occurs in Lebanon and Syria, through ingestion of raw goat and sheep liver; improperly cooked liver may contain viable third stage larvae, which colonize the oropharyngeal mucosa causing deafness by blocking the eustachian tube, episodic sneezing and coughing, hemoptysis, dysphagia, dysphonia, and dyspnea, the last potentially fatal by closure of the nasopharynx

HAM HTLV-I-associated myelopathy see Tropical spastic paraparesis

HAM-1 and **HAM-2** Histocompatibility antigen modifier Two genes in mice that encode permeases that transport antigen (oligopeptides) from the cytoplasm into a membrane-bound compartment in which the antigen interacts with major histocompatibility complex (MHC) class I and

II molecules; the human equivalent of HAM-1 and -2 are designated ATP-binding cassette transporters, see ABC superfamily

HAM syndrome Hypoparathyroidism, Addison's disease and mucocutaneous candidiasis see MEDAC syndrome

HAMA Human anti-mouse antibody A family of antibodies that may be used in research protocols in which patients with advanced malignancy are treated with monoclonal antibodies directed against an epitope on the tumor cells; host production of HAMAs limits the amount of monoclonal antibodies that can be administered, causing adverse immune reactions including anaphylaxis, subacute allergic and delayed hypersensitivity reactions, flulike syndrome, GI symptoms, rash and urticaria, hypotension, dyspnea and renal failure; see Biological response modifiers, 'Humanized' antibody

Haman Tashen-induced opium intoxication Haman Tashen are cookies filled with poppy seeds traditionally consumed during the Jewish holiday of Purim; when consumed in excess, trace amounts of opium alkaloids may accumulate, resulting in clinical intoxication with vomiting, abdominal pain, pallor, hallucinations, sweating and pinpoint pupils, a possibly false positive tests for the presence of opioids; see Jewish traditions

hamartoma A tumor-like, non-neoplastic disordered proliferation of mature tissues that are native to a site of origin, eg exostoses, nevi and soft tissue hamartomas; although most hamartomas are benign, some histological subtypes, eg the neuromuscular hamartoma may proliferate aggressively

hamartosis Any of a number of congenital disease complexes with hamartomas often associated with benign or malignant neoplasms, including dyskeratosis congenita, incontinenti pigmenti, linear nevus sebaceous syndrome, von Recklinghausen's neurofibromatosis, tuberous sclerosis, xeroderma pigmentosa and the Gardner, Goltz, Klippel-Trenaunay-Weber, Mafucci, neurocutaneous (McCune-Albright), melanosis, multiple lentigines (LEOPARD), multiple neuroma, Sturge-Weber, and von Hippel-Lindau syndromes

Note: The 'formal' term is hamartomatosis; the brief form, hamartosis has insinuated into the literature

hamburger thyrotoxicosis An 'epidemic' form of exogenous thyrotoxicosis that occurred in the US in 1984-85 caused by the inclusion of bovine thyroid in ground beef peparations, which disappeared when the practice was discontinued

hammerhead motif MOLECULAR BIOLOGY A molecular configuration seen in ribozymes that has a unique secondary (possibly also tertiary) structure crucial for cleavage; this motif may have therapeutic potential for reducing HIV-1 tat gene's transcript

hammer toe Hallux valgus A lateral deviation of the great toe, common in middle-aged to elderly females in whom life-long use of high-heeled shoes may have played a causative role; with time, the deformity elicits callosities on the plantar surfaces of the second and third metatarsal heads TREATMENT Keller arthroplasty (which consists of removal of the exostosis and proximal phalangectomy)

hamstring muscles The muscles of the posterior thigh, consisting of biceps, semitendinosus and the semimembranosus muscles

H&D Curve Hurter and Driffield curve RADIOLOGY An exposure response graph, supplied with X-ray film for plotting absorbance (optical density) vs. log of relative exposure, used for quality control of the film

hand-arm vibration syndrome White finger syndrome A Raynaud phenomenon-like complex due to cold-induced vasospasm resulting from a prolonged use of vibrating hand-held tools, which may be seen in assembly line workers, grinders, mechanics, jack-hammer operators and others; plethysmographic studies demonstrate changes in digital blood flow

hand-foot syndrome Sickle cell dactylitis A 'crisis' in sickle cell anemia caused by sludging of RBCs in vessels and characterized by symmetric infarction of the small bones of the hand and foot, periosteal neoosteogenesis, pain and swelling that may occur as early as 18 months of age, often resolving spontaneously within 1-4 weeks

hand-foot-flat face syndrome An AD [MIM 139750] condition characterized by a flattened physiognomy, flexion and extension deformities of the hands and feet, mental and growth retardation

hand-foot-genital syndrome An AD [MIM 140000] condition characterized by minor digital anomalies of the hands and feet and uterine duplication extending into the cervix and vagina, causing increased stillbirth and perinatal death in the gestational products of afflicted mothers; the genital abnormalities in the affected males include hypospadias with chordee

hand, foot and mouth syndrome A clinical complex appearing in infants due to Coxsackievirus A16, A5, A9, A10, B2, B7 and enterovirus, resulting in vesicular stomatitis and exanthema, which occurs in summer-fall cycles CLINICAL After a 4-6 day incubation, most infected toddlers suffer a low-grade fever, 0.5 cm intraoral vesicular ulcers (sore throat and refusal to eat), vesicular lesions of the hands, buttocks and feet, resolving in a week Note: Hand, foot and mouth disease due to enterovirus 71 is more commonly associated with meningoencephalitis and paralysis

hand-foot-uterus syndrome Hand-foot-genital syndrome, see there

H&H Hemoglobin and hematocrit; see 10/30 rule, Transfusion trigger

hand mirror cell A lymphocyte with the nucleus at the 'mirror end' and an elongated cytoplasmic appendage or uropod mimicking a mirror's handle; HMCs may correspond to immature T lymphocytes, large granular lymphocytes, including NK cells and atypical lymphocytes, and are present in benign (eg infectious mononucleosis) or malignant hematopoietic conditions; HMCs are most common in ALL, FAB L1 or L2 subtypes, but may be seen in lymphosarcoma, multiple myeloma, Hodgkin's disease, CLL, and AML, FAB M5a subtype; the HMCs seen in AML may reflect locomotive disturbances while those of ALL may be related to immune defects; the hand-mirror morphology per se has no prognostic value

hand mirror cell leukemia A morphologic descriptor that has been used for two biologically distinct tumors a) A variant of acute monoblastic leukemia (FAB M5a), which is thought to have a better prognosis (than the 'garden variety' leukemia), a diagnosis that requires that 40% or more of the blasts have the hand-mirror morphology, average age of onset, 12, female:male, 2:1 b) An acute lymphoblastic leukemia seen as a blast crisis in chronic myelogenous leukemia

hand-washing A simple technique that remains the single most effective method for reducing nosocomial infections; despite its utility there and apparent simplicity, there is poor compliance with hand-washing procedures, especially in the intensive care units (ICUs); in one study, hand disinfection with chlorhexidine was more effective than isopropyl alchol in reducing the incidence of nosocomial infections (N Engl J Med 1992; 327:88oa), although an increase in compliance with hand-washing protocols might be equally effective; although hand-washing between draws by a phlebotomist is required by OSHA, it is rarely performed with the recommended frequency

handedness Chirality* The left– or right–sidedness or asymmetry of virtually everything in the universe from the 'lowly' molecule to highly complex organisms and has existed in primitive and now extinct life forms, eg trilobites circa 550 million years old (**New York Times 15 June 1993; C1**)

*Chirality is the more time-honored term and continues to be preferred in chemistry, handedness is increasingly popular outside of chemical circles

handicap SOCIAL MEDICINE Any of a broad range of physical and mental disabilities which substantially limit a person's major life abilities (**1974 Amendment, 29 USC S706(7)(B)**) Note: AIDS patients are legally considered to be handicapped and thus are protected from discrimination in the workplace, in housing and education; see Americans with Disabilities Act, Disability

'handicapped' health care provider A health care worker or physician who is impaired by physical limitations, usually of sufficient duration that he/she has learned to compensate for the defects; Cf 'Impaired' health care provider, 'Incapacitated' health care provider

Hand-Schüller-Christian disease A term for a clinical form of histiocytosis X (see below note) which is characterized by a childhood onset of osteolytic lesions of the skull and the sella turcica, loss of teeth, chronic draining ears; the histiocytoses X are no longer considered to be reactive but rather clonal neoplasms (**N Engl J Med 1994; 331:154OA**)

Note: A unifying term indicating both the interrelation of these entities while recognizing their specificity, eg Langerhans' cell histiocytosis, Hand-Schüller-Christian type is of lexicographic interest; see Langerhans' cell histiocytosis

HANE Hereditary angioneurotic edema, see there

HANES Health and nutrition examination survey A series of dietary surveys first carried out in 1971 by the NIH (US); HANES I determined that Americans consumed suboptimal levels of iron, calcium and vitamins A and C; HANES III is in progress and under the auspices of the National Center for Health Statistics and will determine the weights of the average American

'hang a shingle' A colloquial American phrase for the opening of a private office by a professional, eg physician, lawyer

The phrase derives from the name plate used, which is symbolically a roofing shingle, as the person is traditionally so impoverished when opening his own practice that he can't afford anything more luxurious

hanging drop technique MICROBIOLOGY A method for evaluating bacterial motility, where a flagellated bacterium is placed in a drop of clear physiologic or nutrient solution on a cover glass ('upside-down', therefore, 'hanging') and examined by LM

hangman's fracture A bilateral avulsion fracture through the neural arch (lamina or pedicles) of the axis (C2, without injuring the odontoid process), causing acute central cervical spinal cord damage with axial dislocation in the C3 vertebral body; major injury to the upper cervical vertebrae is a relative contraindication for surgical correction, unless the vertebral column is unstable or requires neural decompression; formerly, such fractures were seen when hangings used a submental knot; the classic hangman's fracture is now only seen in high speed trauma, eg automobile accidents; Cf Capital punishment

Note: Hanging as a form of capital punishment was introduced in England in the 5th century; early hanging caused death by strangulation; later technical refinements included a long drop of the body (ensured by the optimal length of rope) and a submental knot to effect the desired avulsion or 'Hangman's' fracture, the latter of which minimizes the unesthetic (yet strangely crowd-pleasing) writhing of a slowly strangling criminal

hangover headache Intense cephalgia and malaise upon awakening often prematurely after a night of binge drinking or with prolonged use of benzodiazepines, often accompanied by mental dulling, hyperacusia, mild incoordination, tremor and nausea, due to the toxic effects of alcohol and its metabolites, dehydration and decreasing blood levels of alcohol; see Eyeopener

Hank Gathers affair SPORTS MEDICINE Hank Gathers was a 23 year-old black senior who was a forward on the Loyola Marymount University basketball team; because he was the 1988-1989 US national leader in scoring and rebounds, he was likely to be a first draft choice in the 1990 National Basketball Association (NBA), and be offered a lucrative multimillion-dollar, multiyear contract for playing professional basketball; in part because of his court prowess, Loyola Marymount appeared to have a good chance at winning the National Collegiate Athletic Association (NCAA); during the NCAA's sixth game of the season in December 1989, Gathers had a syncopal episode, after which he was removed from the game and suffered an extensive cardiovascular workup that identified exercise-related ventricular tachyarrhythmias, for which propranolol was prescribed; an external defibrillator was made available at all his subsequent team games and practices; in March 1990, he collapsed, ventricular fibrillation was recorded; efforts at defibrillation were unsuccessful, and he was pronounced dead; in this background, BJ Maron comments (**N Engl J Med 1993; 329:55SB**)

In the highly visible Gathers case, who was accountable?…A large measure of responsibility may rest with society itself, which often attaches too much importance to sports…what does it say of our priorities and sense of moral responsibility when student athletes with heart disease are allowed to train and compete? Much of the Gathers affair is really about big-time college sport, its materialism and its excesses…In such a charged atmosphere, with public recognition and enormous sums of money at stake, elite athletes come to be viewed as high-priced commodities, not as patients…other catastrophes are likely to occur and strike to the core of our sensibilities. ..reminding us of our misplaced priorities

hantavirus Korean hemorrhagic fever, see there

hantavirus pulmonary syndrome A recently described often fatal respiratory infection caused by a newly recognized hantavirus; the first cluster of cases[1] occurred in the Four Corners region of Southwestern US[2]; EPIDEMIOLOGY: Mean age 32, 61% ♀, 72% Native American CASE DEFINITION Unexplained bilateral interstitial infiltrates on the chest film and arterial O_2 saturation < 90% CLINICAL, PRODROME Fever and myalgia (100%), cough or dyspnea (76%), GI symptoms, headache, tachycardia, tachypnea, hypotension LABORATORY Leukocytosis ($\pm$ 26 x 10^9/L), often with myeloid precursors, ↑ hematocrit, thrombocytopenia ($\pm$ 64 X 10^9/L), ↑ PT and aPTT, ↑ LDH, ↓ serum protein, and proteinuria; massive acute pulmonary edema is common at the time of death (**N Engl J Med 1994; 330:949OA**) PREVENTION A vaccine is under development, in which the hanta genes are inserted into a vaccinia virus vector (**New York Times 23 May1995; C6**)

[1]Until HPS was definitively linked to hantavirus, public hysteria increased, with some attributing HPS to the US Biological warfare program (**Sci Am 1993; 269/5:16**)
[2]The condition has also been described in New England and Europe (**N Engl J Med 1994; 331:545c; MMWR 1994; 43:548, 555**)

Hanukkah factor Granzyme A A trypsin-like serine protease encoded by the CTLA3 gene on chromosome 5 and produced by cytotoxic T lymphocytes and NK cells; HF is thought to be the enzyme responsible for the remarkable lytic capacity of these cells; Cf Christmas factor

The name derives from the similarities of the cDNA (complementary DNA) nucleotide sequence to that of coagulation factor IX (Christmas factor)

HAPC Hospital-acquired penetration contact, see there

HAPE High-altitude pulmonary edema, see there

haplotype A cluster of alleles that are located at the same locus on a chromosome and which are usually inherited together; assuming simple mendelian genetics, ie, without unexpected translocations, one in four siblings will share both haplotypes; see MHC

'–happy' A highly colloquial, commonly used adjective referring to a zealous inclination to perform a particular task or activity, eg 'scope-happy' referring to a gastroenterologist who uses an endoscope seemingly before exercising his clinical judgement, or 'trigger-happy' for an aggressive surgeon

happy letter A communication sent by a physician, hospital, laboratory, or other health care provider to a patient to inform him/her that the results of a test (eg 'Pap' test, thus being known as 'happy Pap' letter) or battery of tests indicate no abnormalities requiring therapy; Cf Recall letter

happy Pap letter see Happy letter

happy puppet syndrome Angelman syndrome, see there

hapten X CD15, see there

haptotaxis A type of chemotaxis in which the cells respond to a concentration gradient of an insoluble ligand (eg developing cells responding to various tissue concentrations of fibronectin)

hard clot An insoluble, usually intravascular thrombus in which the fibrin monomers have been terminally cross-linked by coagulation factor XIII in the presence of calcium ions

hard copy A term derived from 'computerspeak' that has been modified in various fields and come to be equated to any paper printout of a file in magnetic storage, eg hard or floppy disks or printout from devices as diverse as electrocardiographs, laboratory instruments or medical records retrieved from microfiche storage; see Smart card

hard data Tangible data of any nature, eg blood levels of an analyte, persons in a defined region with a certain type malignancy; see Data; Cf Soft dara

hard disk COMPUTERS A permanent or non-removable data storage device, which for microcomputers ranges from 80 to 600 megabytes or more; hard disk memory can be either 1) Magnetic, which has a faster access time and a practical ceiling of up to one gigabytes of memory and 2) Optical, which is currently slower than magnetic devices but may practically store 1 or more gigabytes of information and is less expensive

'hard' drug Any intensely addictive substance of abuse that may compel its user to commit crimes in order to obtain the drug, due to its high cost, eg heroin, or through loss of societal inhibitions, eg cocaine

Note: 'Soft drug' is an uncommonly used term for less addictive agents that may be legal, and thus viewed as less addicting and/or more socially acceptable, eg tobacco, alcohol and marijuana

'hard' liquor A colloquial term for beverages with a high, often greater than 30% alcohol by volume (60 proof), eg gin, rum, vodka, whiskey; hard liquors are preferred by alcoholics as a steady state of low-level inebriation is easier to maintain; see Standard drink

'hard' spin Heavy spin, see there

'Hard Times Report' A 38-page memo drafted by a group of 8 extramural program leaders at the National Cancer Institute (NCI), which recommended a comprehensive analysis that would define the problems confronting the NCI; the HTR was stimulated by budgetary constraints and identified a number of programs sponsored by the NCI that might be regarded as redundant, and proposed means by which overlapping research activities, eg on animal models, basic biology and carcinogenesis, and oncogenes, as well as coordination of clinical trials, gene transfection vctors, and tissue banking, and redundant administrative infrastructure could be reduced (Science 1995; 267:1412)

'hard' tubercle Naked granuloma, see there

hardening CLINICAL NUTRITION Hydrogenation of unsaturated fatty acids in triglycerides into saturated fatty acids; see Browning reaction, Tropical oils

hardware COMPUTERS The electronic and mechanical, non-software components of a computer, which include the central processing unit, monitor, disk drives, keyboard, and 'peripherals', eg printer, modem, scanning devices ORTHOPEDICS Any of a number of devices (eg nuts, bolts, pins, plates, screws, and wire) that are placed in a site of orthopedic surgical procedure performed to stabilize a fracture or to anchor a prosthetic joint; see Bone glue

hard water Water with a high content of calcium and magnesium salts (eg carbonates and sulfates), which may interfere with certain tests in the laboratory; Cf Soft water

hard water 'syndrome' A clinical complex seen when 'hard' water (which contains high levels of iron, calcium and magnesium) is used during hemodialysis, resulting in post-dialysis nausea, vomiting, asthenia, hypertension

hardwired COMPUTERS *adjective* Pertaining or referring to any processing function that is built into a computer system's electronic circuitry (hardware) rather than in the program (software) instructions

hardwiring NEUROPHYSIOLOGY Permanent neural connections between the sensory input and motor output that are present in the brain of infants after a critical period of perinatal rewiring; the hardwiring concept is part of neuroscience dogma, which holds that reorganization in an adult organism is minimal, although recent data from the Silver Spring monkeys indicates that reorganization occurs in the cerebral cortex, extending 10 to 14 mm into the somatosensory region formerly dedicated to the region of limbs that had been denervated (Science 1991; 252:1789n&v)

hard X-rays RADIATION ONCOLOGY Short wavelength, high-frequency and highly penetrating X-rays that may be used in radiotherapy or which may be generated by nuclear 'incidents'

harlequin chromosome technique GENETICS An experimental method used to demonstrate 'sister chromatid exchange' in chromosomes, where one of the 'sisters' is chemically altered and made to fluoresce more brightly than its twisted sister (figure); here there is no gain or loss of genes, only axial rotation of alleles

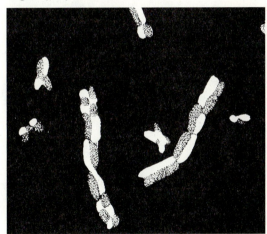

harlequin chromosomes

harlequin (skin) reaction PEDIATRICS A benign erythema that longitudinally 'sections' the prone infant into a pale upper and a vividly flushed lower half (most prominent from the forehead to the pubis), related to autonomic vascular lability; this color change is rare, occurring most commonly in premature or low birth weight neonates and, like erythema neonatorum, is a transient vasomotor phenomenon with no clinical significance

harlequin fetus Ichthyosis congenita A rare AR [MIM 242500] disease of infants in which the baby is encased in a thickened keratinaceous 'coccoon' with deep fissures, accompanied by ectropion; once thought a variant of lamellar ichthyosis, this is a severe dyskeratosis, the defect of which lies in lipid metabolism; there is massive hyperkeratosis; the stratum corneum is up to 30-fold thicker than the stratum malpighii; the stratum granulosa is reduced to a one-cell layer or absent

harlequin nail A fingernail in a subject who has abruptly stopped smoking; the proximal zone of new growth is pink while the outgrowing nail formed during nicotine exposure (the 'nicotine sign') is a dirty yellow-brown

harm reduction PUBLIC HEALTH A principle that recognizes that it is impossible to completely eliminate a high-risk activity, eg drug abuse, and thus combines efforts to prevent drug abuse with efforts to minimize the harm that a drug abuser will do to him/herself, the latter being known as secondary prevention (JAMA 1995; 273:1143OA)

harp player's thumb PERFORMING ARTS MEDICINE A nerve compression syndrome due to irritation of the ulnar and radial digital nerves of the thumb by the strings of the instrument CLINICAL Numbness, paresthesias, painful hypo– and hypersensitivity, which may lead to perineural fibrosis and the formation of a painful nodule TREATMENT Rest, change strumming and plucking patterns; surgery is not indicated

Harrison Narcotics Act of 1914 The first legislation in the USA that regulated importation, manufacture, sale and use of opium, cocaine and all related derivatives, and restricted their use to 'legitimate medical purposes', interpreted to preclude their use by physicians for treating those already addicted or dependent on these subtances; the act stood with many amendments, later encompassing marijuana, LSD and other hallucinogens until its replacement by the Controlled Drug Substances Act of 1970, see there

Hartmannella A genus of free-living protozoa found in fresh water and soil, once thought to be a causative agent in Primary aseptic meningoencephalitis, see there

Note: 'Because of the confusion that existed in the earlier literature with regard to the nomenclature of *Acanthamoeba* and *Hartmannella*, some workers in the field referred to these amebas as belonging to the *Hartmannella-Acanthamoeba* group. Since no true *Hartmannella* species has as yet been found to be pathogenic to humans, all references to *Hartmannella* in human tissues should be corrected to read as *Acanthamoeba*...' (A Balows, et al, Eds, Manual of Clinical Microbiology, 4th ed, American Society for Microbiology, Washington, DC 1991)

HARVARD CRITERIA FOR BRAIN DEATH-
Unreceptivity and unresponsiveness
No movement or breathing
No reflexes
Flat electroencephalogram (confirmatory)
IN ADDITION, THE FOLLOWING MUST BE PRESENT
Body temperature ≥ to 32º C
Absence of CNS depressants

Harvard criteria A series of four parameters delineated by the the Harvard medical school ad hoc committee for irreversible coma, see Table

Harvard guidelines A series of guidelines issued by Harvard University in 1988 intended to prevent scientific fraud, rather than act in response to it; in addition to guidelines on supervision of research trainees, care in gathering, record-keeping and analysis of data and establishment of criteria for authorship credits, see Relman's criteria, there is an objective limit on the number of publications reviewed for faculty appointment or promotion; five publications are reviewed for assistant professor, seven for associate professor and ten for full professor

Harvard law BASIC RESEARCH A colloquial rule on the predictability of experimental materials, '...*under optimal laboratory conditions of constant temperature, light, humidity and substrate availability, an organism will do as it damned well pleases...*'

Note: This colloquial term is well-known in some circles in the natural sciences;

the author has been unable to confirm its source

harvest TRANSPLANTATION Procurement of an organ from a cadaveric or live donor; because the word harvest connotes gathering of a mature crop, alternate terms, eg donation, 'procurement' or 'recovery' appear to be less degrading to the donor

Harvest Moon phenomenon A decrease in mortality in certain subjects prior to the occurrence of a symbolically meaningful event or occasion; epidemiologists usually examine the impact of external factors in establishing cause-and-effect relations to disease; cultural factors are rarely examined and usually viewed as having a negative impact on disease; one study (JAMA 1990; 263:1947) revealed a positive impact of culturally significant events on mortality to two populations, older Chinese women (event: Harvest Moon festival) and older Jewish men (event: Passover); each group proved itself capable of staving off death, especially of cardiovascular disease and cancer with mortality dipping 35% before the event and increasing by 34.6% thereafter

Hashimoto's disease Hashimoto's thyroiditis, see there

Hashimoto's thyroiditis Autoimmune thyroiditis A form of thyroiditis most common in ♀ age 30-50, often presenting as a diffuse firm thyroid enlargement and/or with a familial history of goiter, hypothyroidism, Graves' disease or circulating antithyroid antibodies; other diseases with autoimmune components are often associated with HT, eg chronic active hepatitis, DM, pernicious anemia, primary biliary cirrhosis, rheumatoid arthritis, Sjögren syndrome PATHOGENESIS Autoimmune, linked to the presence of antibodies against thyroid peroxidase (microsomal antibodies), thyroglobulin and colloid CLINICAL Goiter, and often little else, which, when extreme, may cause esophageal or tracheal compression LABORATORY Antimicrosomal antibodies (Arch Int Med 1993; 153:862OA); while euthyroid state is maintained, ↑ RAIU, ↑ TSH, normal T_3, normal T_4; with loss of response to TSH, ↓ RAIU, ↓ T_4, ↑ T_3 which reflects a maximally stimulated state PATHOLOGY Lymphocytic infiltration, oxyphilic changes of thyroid follicular epithelium, lymphoid follicles with prominent germinal centers, often accompanied by atrophy of the thyroid epithelium TREATMENT Hormonal replacement PROGNOSIS Excellent COMPLICATIONS Rarely, lymphoma

hashitoxicosis Hashimoto's thyroiditis (chronic autoimmune thyroiditis) presenting as hyperthyroidism

hassle factor HEALTH CARE REIMBURSEMENT A generic term for any time-consuming and/or paperwork-ridden maneuver that is required by physicians, pharmacologists (and other health care professionals) before a third party reimbursement agent/agency (eg Medicaid, Medicaid, insurance company) approves payment for a medical therapy, service or drug (N Engl J Med 1995; 332:1641SB)

HAT medium Hypoxanthine, aminopterin and thymidine A culture medium optimal for hybridoma (monoclonal antibody) production; aminopterin blocks de novo synthesis of GMP by the myeloma cells, while hypoxanthine and thymidine are nutrients required by both myeloma cells and the monoclonal antibody-producing cells; the cells producing the monoclonal antibodies have hypoxanthine guanine phosphoribosyl transferase, bypassing the aminopterin-induced blockage of GMP production that would otherwise kill the non-fused myeloma cell line; see Hybridoma

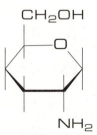

hatband sign A unilateral sweat stain on a hat, seen in Horner syndrome, associated with pulmonary carcinoma

hatchet face The characteristic physiognomy of advanced myotonic dystrophy; the face is drawn and lugubrious, with hollowing of the muscles around the temples and jaws; the eyes are 'hooded', the lower lip droops, and global weakness of facial muscles causes sagging of the lower face, accompanied by marked wasting of the neck muscles, especially the flexors imparting a 'swan-necked' appearance; a similar facies may rarely occur in amyotrophic lateral sclerosis, and Curschmann-Batten-Steiner syndrome

HAV Hepatitis A virus, see Hepatitis

Haverhill fever An epidemic disease first described in Massachusetts in 1925 (Bost Med Surg J 1926, 194:285) caused by *Haverhillia multiformis*, now known as *Streptobacillus moniliformis* (a non-motile, gram-negative rod of varible length, growing in liquid culture medium as 'puff-ball'-like colonies, transmitted in crowded urban slums by ingesting milk contaminated by rat excreta; *S moniliformis* is present in the nasopharynx of up to 50% of laboratory and healthy wild rodents CLINICAL 2-10 day incubation, then abrupt onset of an acute prostrating disease with shaking chills, spiking fever, upper respiratory symptoms, pharyngitis, vomiting, headache, myalgias, generalized, predominantly palmoplantar blotchy, maculopapular, morbilliform petechial rashes, nonspecific migratory polyarthritis MORTALITY 10% LATE COMPLICATIONS Endocarditis, pericarditis, pneumonia, abscesses, anemia, biological false positive tests for syphilis, urticaria TREATMENT Penicillin, tetracycline; see Rat-bite fever, Sodoku

hawkinsinuria An AD [MIM 140350] form of tyrosinuria, named after the index family, presenting in infancy with severe metabolic acidosis, ketosis, failure to thrive, transient tyrosinemia, excess excretion of *p*-hydroxyphenylpyruvic and *p*-hydroxyphenylacetic acids as well as unusual tyrosine metabolites, one of which is hawkinsin; the disease responds to dietary restriction of phenylalanine and tyrosine and resolves spontaneously with age without mental retardation or hepatopathy

Hawthorne effect A beneficial effect that health care providers have on the workers in virtually any environment when an interest is shown in the workers' well-being; the 'Hawthorne studies' were conducted in the 1930s at the Hawthorne plant of the Western Electric company and attempted to delineate the effects of improving the social environment and laborer-management relations in the workplace

Note: This phenomenon differs from both 1) The 'Halo' effect, in which the contact with health care personnel is personal and occurs in a legitimate medical context and 2) The placebo effect, in which the subject may believe a therapeutic effect is present, where none exists, ie *cogito ergo sum*; Cf 'Nocebo'

Haworth projection Biochemistry A convention used in chemistry to partially represent the three-dimensional configuration of cyclic sugars, in particular furanoses (cyclical five-carbon sugars, eg ribose and fructose) and pyranoses (cyclical six-carbon sugars, eg glucose and galactose); Haworth projections are shown as planar molecule with the oxygen bridge in the rear and the three carbon bonds in the front (see figure, facing page)

hay fever A popular term for allergic rhinitis

hazard risk rating OCCUPATIONAL HEALTH A scale defined by OSHA that quantifies the allowable exposure in ppm (parts per million) to chemicals in the workplace, designated per-

HAZARD RISK RATING	
PEL* > 500 PPM	1
PEL 200-500 PPM	2
PEL 100-200 PPM	3
PEL 10-100 PPM	4
PEL < 10 PPM	5
CARCINOGENIC	6
*Permissible exposure limit	

missible exposure limits (PELs); an HHR rating of 1 has the highest PEL > 500 ppm, a HHR of 6 correponds to any substance that is frankly carcinogenic (CAP Today Jul 1992)

hazardous chemical OCCUPATIONAL HEALTH Any chemical substance (as defined by OSHA) that is a physical hazard‡ (eg compressed gas, combustible, explosive, a strong oxidizer, or a pyrophoric material) or a health hazard‡ (eg carcinogenic, toxic, corrosive, irritant, sensitizing); HCs may be single agents or mixtures of multiple agents; OSHA requires recording of mixtures used in the workplace, if the mixture contains ≥ 1.0% of a noncarcinogenic HC, or ≥ 0.1% of a carcinogenic HC

hazardous material labeling OCCUPATIONAL HEALTH A labeling system that is required by OSHA for material that are recognized as dangerous to human health

HAZARDOUS MATERIALS WARNING LABEL				
	HEALTH HAZARD	FIRE HAZARD	REACTIVITY	SPECIFIC HAZARD
4	Deadly	FP < 73ºF	May detonate	OXY-Oxidizer
3	Very dangerous	FP < 100ºF	Shock and heat	ACID-Acid
2	Hazardous	FP > 100ºF	Violent chem. change	ALK-Alkali
1	Slightly hazardous	FP > 200ºF	Unstable if heated	Use no water
0	Normal material	Won't burn	Stable	® Radiation hazard
FP Flash point				

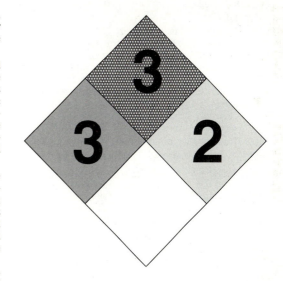

hazardous material label

▦	BLUE-Health hazard
▨	RED-Fire hazard
▢	YELLOW-Reactivity
☐	WHITE-Specific hazard

hazardous waste ENVIRONMENT, OCCUPATIONAL HEALTH Any unwanted product that poses a hazard or potential hazard to human health, which may be generated by a manufacturing process, eg radioactive gas cylinders, chemicals, pesticides, acids and liquid or by a health care facility, including regulated biohazardous waste; this contrasts with municipal solid waste, eg paper, plastics and metals; the health care industry is a major producer of HW, which includes infectious and chemical waste products, including formaldehyde, xylene, mercury-based fixatives, and radionuclides (**CAP Today June 1992 p46**) see Regulated waste, Toxic dump

haz-mat warning label Hazardous material labels, see there

H-1B visa A temporary visa issued by the US immigration service that allows alien (non-US citizen) physicians to function in an educational, research, and more recently in a clinical capacity; the H-1B visa is for foreign national international medical graduates who have both an offer of employment[1] and are eligible for state licensure[2]; the H-1B is granted initially for 3 years but may be extended for another 3, and has no 'return home' requirements (**JAMA 1995; 273:1521OA**) Cf Green card, J-1 visa

[1]From a hospital or other institution [2]Which means that they already have obtained some form of graduate medical education (GME), as GME is required for state licenses to practice medicine

HBA71 A 30–32-kD cell surface glycoprotein (p30/32[MIC2]) encoded by the pseudoautosomal *MIC2* gene on chromosomes X and Y which is present in most cases (41/43) of Ewing sarcoma, and is more useful in the diagnosis of these tumors than vimentin (29/43) or neuron-specific enolase (21/43) (**Am J Surg Path 1992; 16:746**) see Ewing family of tumors

HBGF Heparin-binding growth factor(s) A family of seven structurally-related polypeptide cytokines that are activated after binding heparin

HBGF-8 Heparin-binding growth factor-8, see Pleitrophin

HBIg Hepatitis B immunoglobulin A 3-5 ml preparation of antibodies to hepatitis B virus (HBV), derived from donor pools and administered at the time of and one month after presumed exposure to HBV; HBIG is heat-treated and negative for HIV-1 (and HIV-2); HBIG is available in low- (anti-HBs > 1:128 – $5/dose) or high titer (anti-HBs > 1:100 000 – $150/dose) forms; there is little evidence that the high-titer immune globulin is more effective

HBLV Human B-lymphotropic virus, see Herpesvirus-6

HBV Hepatitis B virus, also honey bee venom

HBx A hepatitis B regulatory gene that encodes the HBx protein that acts as a transcriptional transactivator of viral genes, altering the host gene expression and inducing the development of hepatocellular carcinoma in transgenic mouse induced hepatomas (**Nature 1991; 351:317**) see Hepatitis

HCA 1) Heterocyclic amine, see there 2) Hypothalamic chronic anovulation, see there

HCAM Homing cell adhesion molecule

HCFA Health Care Financing Administration A bureaucracy created by the US government 1977 from Medicare, Medicaid and the Office of Long-Term Care, which administers these programs at the federal level; the HCFA is also charged with ensuring compliance with the CLIA '88 standards for laboratory testing; in the face of noncompliance, the HCFA may impose intermediate (fines of up to $10 000/day) or principal (revocation of laboratory's license) sanctions or initiate civil action (**CAP Today April 1992**) see JCAHO, Medicaid, Medicare

HCFC Hydrochlorofluorocarbons, see CFCs, Ozone layer

hCG Human choriogonadotropic hormone A 36–40-kD dimeric glycoprotein hormone synthesized and secreted by the placenta composed of a 92-amino acid α subunit that is similar to pituitary hormones (TSH, FSH and LH) and a unique 145-amino acid β-subunit linked to lactose and hexosamine that is produced by the syncytiotrophoblast, β subunit that is used as an early diagnostic test for pregnancy as it indicates the presence of fetal liver and kidney and certain tumors; hCG's 3-D structure has been resolved (**Nature 1994; 369:455A, 438N&V**) and has a quasi-dyad

symmetry axis; the intermolecular interactions are of the β-sheet type, and a segment of the carboxy-terminal tail of the β-subunit embraces a long loop of the α-subunit in a 'seatbelt' like fashion; with complete evacuation of gestational products, hCG levels fall to ½ in ± 2 days, to ¼ in ± 13 days, persistent elevation of hCG = persistent trophoblastic disease (**Am J Obstet Gynecol 1993; 168:787**); hCG is released in a pulsatile fashion in normal pregnancy, peaks at the tenth gestational week with serum levels of 50-140 000 IU/L, thereafter falling to 10-50 000 IU/L Note: hCG levels during pregnancy are below 100 000; hCG may be low to undetectable in ectopic pregnancy or markedly elevated in multiple gestation, polyhydramnios, eclampsia, erythroblastosis fetalis or trophoblastic disease, eg hydatidiform moles, choriocarcinoma and placental site trophoblastic tumor; hCG levels may be extremely elevated in tumors producing either the β subunit or both α and β subunits, measured by ELISA or RIA; ectopic elevation of hCG may occur with carcinomas of the stomach, liver, pancreas, breast, kidney, lungs and adrenal cortex, as well as seminoma, leukemia, lymphoma and melanoma

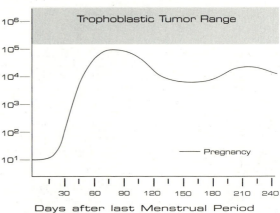

hCG in pregnancy/trophoblastic disease

hCG-like activity A term for any functional cross-reactivity of the α subunit of TSH, LH, and FSH with the α subunit of hCG, such that elevation of these hormones mimics an elevation of hCG when measured by RIA Note: The 18-kD α subunit of hCG has an 80% amino acid homology with these cross-reactors, which explains why the β subunit is used for analysis

HCHWA-D Hereditary cerebral hemorrhage with amyloidosis, Dutch type An AD [MIM 105150] form of cerebral amyloid angiopathy in which the patients develop recurrent intracerebral hemorrhages leading to death by the sixth decade of life; HCHWA-D has been described in four families from two coastal villages in the Netherlands; cloning and sequencing of the exons reveals a mutation causing an amino acid substitution in the amyloid protein; see Cerebral amyloid angiopathy

HCT Hematocrit

HCV Hepatitis C virus, see there, also Human coronavirus

HDC-ABMT High-dose chemotherapy with autologous bone marrow transplantation An experimental therapeutic modality used in patients with terminal malignancy, of currently unknown efficacy

HDL High-density lipoprotein A plasma lipoprotein with density of 1.063-1.210 kg/L (US: 1.063-1.210 g/dl); HDL is 33% protein (predominantly apoA-I and A-II), 29% phospholipid, 30% cholesterol and 8% triglycerides and transports cholesterol from the intestine to the liver; the larger the HDL molecule, the more efficient the lipid transport and by extension, lipolysis; HDL levels are the single most important predictor of coronary heart disease (CHD), given that 1) Several risk factors for CHD, eg smoking, obesity and lack of exercise may lower HDL 2) HDL has an inverse relation with VLDL and LDL, lipoproteins known to be atherogenic and 3) HDL may interfere with atherogenesis by promoting reverse cholesterol transport or prevent aggregation of LDL particles in the arterial wall; small HDL molecules (HDL$_3$) are metabolically 'early' forms and more prominent in alcoholics; increases in the larger HDL$_2$ molecule are associated with a ↓ risk of coronary heart disease; in sedentary older adults, HDL$_2$ is inversely related to truncal (waist-to-hip) fat, insulin levels and glucose intolerance; apoE may prove a better measure of atherosclerotic risk than HDL$_2$, as it correlates well with exercise; see Apolipoprotein

Note: Anabolic steroids eg stanozolol, testosterone reduce HDL$_3$, HDL-cholesterol and apoA-I, an effect partially ameliorated by oral rather than parenteral administration

HDL-cholesterol That cholesterol that is bound to high-density lipoprotein ↑ HDL-C and HDL-C:total cholesterol ratios are associated with ↑ longevity and ↓ morbidity and mortality from myocardial infarction; ↑↑↑ HDL-C levels (≥2.58 mmol/L, ie ≥100 mg/dl) may occur in genetic conditions, eg hyper-α-lipoproteinemia, hyper-β-lipoproteineinemia, deficiency of cholesteryl-ester transfer protein, deficiency of hepatic triglyceride lipase, and in structural changes in apoC-II and apoA-IV; ↑↑↑ HDL-C most commonly affects ♀ with hypertension or obesity, and may be related to environmental causes, eg alcohol consumption, or therapy with H$_2$-blockers or estrogens (**Arch Pathol Lab Med 1992; 116:831OA**) MEASUREMENT Until 1994, HDL-C measurement in the clinical laboratory required centrifugation (which blocks the flow of specimens), a situation that changed with commercial availability of a new method of precipitation using a standard dextran sulfate/MgCl$_2$ precipitation reaction enhanced with magnetic particles (**CAP Today Nov 1994 p36**)

HDL/LDL ratio The ratio of cholesterol carried by high-density lipoprotein to that carried by low-density lipoprotein, which allows a rapid risk stratification for atherosclerosis-related cardiac disease; the HDL/LDL ratio is decreased by saturated fatty acid

HDN Hemolytic disease of the newborn

HE 1) Hearing Examiner 2) Hemoglobin electrophoresis 3) Hereditary elliptocytosis 4) Human enteric

Also 1) Hall effect 2) Hematoxylin & eosin 3) Hepatic encephalopathy 4) Hepatic extract (rarely used formulation of hepatic 'juice') 5) High efficiency 6) Human engineering 7) Human enolase 8) Human exposure dose 9) Hydroxyecdysone (endocrinology) 10) Hygienic effect

H&E Hematoxylin & eosin, also 1) Hemorrhage and exudate 2) Heredity and environment

headbanger's tumor A lesion that may develop in children who bang their heads as part of a 'routine' for falling asleep, which consists of a mass of organizing fibrous tissue covered by hyperpigmented skin, identical in pathogenesis to the lump described on the foreheads of devout Moslems; headbanging occurs transiently in 3.5% of infants of normal intelligence and is 3.5-fold more common in boys, in 5% of whom it may be of longer duration, especially in the mentally retarded or psychiatrically disturbed

head of department The physician or scientist who is the person in charge of a department of a hospital or medical school Note: The director of a medical school department that provides clinical care is also known as chief of service

head drop sign NEUROLOGY A finding evoked by raising an infant's trunk at the shoulders; a head that drops backward suggests nuchal limpness typical of both paralytic and non-paralytic poliomyelitis

'head-hunter' A highly colloquial, but virtually standard term for a person (or employment agency) who recruits physicians, upper echelon executives or other professionals, matching potential employees with employers

head and neck cancer A generic term that can be broadly applied to any malignancy of the head and neck, including brain, ocular, salivary gland, skin, thyroid gland, as well as nonepithelial neoplasms including lymphomas and sarcomas; in practice, the term H&NC refers to squamous cell carcinoma of H&N mucosae (oral cavity, oropharynx, hypopharynx and larynx) STATISTICS ± 43 000 new cases (21 100 oral, 12 500 laryngeal, 9200 pharyngeal) per year (US, 1992) with 11 600 deaths, most often seen in ♂ > age 50; worldwide ± 500 000 new cases/year ETIOLOGY Tobacco (cigarette, cigar, and pipe, and smokeless tobacco) products, alcohol, woodworking, textile fiber exposure, nickel refining; dietary factors (eg carotenoids, ↑ fruit and vegetable consumption) may exert a protective effect; a specific type, nasopharyngeal carcinoma, has been associated with EBV infection MOLECULAR GENETICS 3p, 18p, and other nonrandom chromosomal deletions and rearrangements, amplification and overexpression of epidermal growth factor receptor, amplification of bcl-1, int-2, and other oncogenes, and p53 mutations–which may have prognostic significance CLINICAL Signs and symptoms are site-specific, eg in the oral cavity leukoplakia, erythroplakia, and in other sites, nasal obstruction, epistaxis, otalgia, serous otitis media, unilateral sore throat, cranial neuropathy TREATMENT Patients with stage I or II are treated with either surgery or radiotherapy with curative intent, which is achieved in 80% of stage I and 60% of stage II disease; chemotherapy is not a 'first-line' therapy and is added to surgery and radiotherpy to ameliorate symptoms, improve the quality of life, and prolong survival PROGNOSIS Patients with localized stage III and IV disease who continue to smoke while undergoing radiation therapy have a lower rate of complete response (45% vs 74%) and poorer 2-year survival (39% vs 66%) than nonsmokers and in pretreatment quitters (**N Engl J Med 1993; 328:159OA**) metastatic or recurrent disease is usually incurable (**N Engl J Med 1993; 328:184OA**)

head shaping External cranioplasty The intentional employment of external forces or devices to conform the head (of children) to a desired shape, producing permanent modifications of the craniofacial bony architecture; head molding was formerly widely practiced in various cultures as a sign of aristocracy and continues to be practiced in certain aboriginal tribes and cultures of North and South America; although head shaping may cause proptosis, epilepsy, mental retardation and even death when performed with excess diligence by the medically inept, the procedure is generally regarded as safe (**JAMA 1991; 265:1179**)

HEADSS An interviewing technique that addresses areas (Home, Education, Activities, Drugs, Sex, Suicide) of major psychological stress for adolescents, in a format that encourages development of rapport with the adolescent 'client', beginning with the least stressful (Home) and progressing to areas of increasing psychological stress (**JAMA 1992; 268:2628MN&P**)

head space analysis LABORATORY MEDICINE Gas chromatographic analysis of the air (head space) from a stoppered specimen tube warmed to 40-60°C, which detects the presence of volatile organic substances

healer One who heals; the term is used in several distinct contexts 1) Conventional (Western) medicine; healer is a romantic synonym for physician 2) Ethnomedicine; a healer (curandero) is one who uses various plants, concoctions (potingues), rites and rituals to treat various diseases or to rid the sufferer of various culture-bound syndromes (see there) 3) Alternative medicine; in general, a person (faith healer) who alleges to manipulate a person's internal forces to effect therapy

health A condition defined by the WHO as '*...a state of complete physical, mental, and social well-being and not merely the absence of disease or infirmity.*' INTENSIVE CARE MEDICINE A 'third-generation' system* for estimating the probability of hospital mortality in adult ICU patients based on physiological assessments of most severely affected values during the first 24 hours in the ICU and subjecting the results to logistic regression modeling techniques; APACHE III contains more variables (27 vs 17) than SAPS II, stressing the inclusion of as much information as possible to characterize the patients; SAP II, APACHE III, and MPM II are well-researched systems for collecting ICU-related data, can be used to assess prognosis, and to stratify patients as to severity of disease for clinical trials (**JAMA 1994; 272:1049cecc**) see APACHE III, MPM II

health advocacy Health promotion, see there

health care access SOCIAL MEDICINE The ability of an individual to receive health care services, which is a function of availability of personnel and supplies; in the US these are in chronic short supply in rural regions due to logistics and in the inner cities, due to financing and the ability to pay for those services; health care access ranges from universal access in socialized medicine to the 'free market' system prevalent in the US; each of these 'extremes' has considerable disadvantages, with the free market model becoming increasingly problematic as the cost of health care continues to spiral upward, such that it constitutes between 11 and 13% of the US gross national product, while more than 20% of the population has no access to health care, thus creating a two-tiered system of inequity, between the 'haves' and the 'have-nots' (**May 15, 1991, JAMA; summary: pp 2564-5**)

health care rationing The limitation of access to or the equitable distribution of medical services, through various 'gatekeeper' controls Note: The limitless expansion of technology, the aging population and the upward spiralling costs of health care (the health care industry expenditure was estimated at $5.5 x 10^{11}$ in 1990, representing 11.3% of the US gross national product) in the developed nations has brought to the fore the ethical issue of '*who is allowed to get how much of what*', and deciding, for example, between financing 5 liver transplantations or prenatal care for 1000 pregnancies, becomes a morally unsolvable conundrum, as the 5 will die without treatment, while the benefits of prenatal care are difficult to translate into concrete and immediate benefits; Cf Coby Howard, Oregon plan, Rule of Rescue, 'Squeaky wheel'

health care reform A plan ('Clinton Plan'*), ill-defined in the mode of implementation, that was proposed at the level of the federal government by US President(s) Bill and Hillary Clinton in 1993, intended to revamp the US health care (HC) system and address the inequities in the provision of HC in the US; although HC commands nearly 14% of the US gross national product, 39 million people have no HC insurance (**Clin Lab Sci 1994; 7:72f**); despite the political 'hoopla', the Clinton Plan never materialized; its failure was attributed to a combination of a lack of political leadership, manipulation of Congress and the electorate by special interest groups, and (by some cynics) corruption and incompetence on the part of politicians; the debate on HCR continues and may ultimately develop in some form at the state level or in the private insurance marketplace (**N Engl J Med 1995; 332:465ed**)

Which proved a '...tale ...full of sound and fury...signifying nothing...*'

health food A non-medical term defined by the lay public as a food that has little or no preservatives, which has not undergone major processing, enrichment or refinement and which may be grown without pesticides; health foods have been mystically endowed by certain segments of the

population with the ability to prevent the development of most diseases, including atherosclerosis, aging phenomena, rheumatic disease and cancer, as well as to treat malignancy and prolong life; see Food preservatives, Organic food; Cf Diet, Junk food

health fraud A generic term used in the context of either

1) Any form of financial finagling committed against third-party payer of health care; 43% of health fraud is in the form of services not rendered, 33% for fraudulent diagnoses or

2) Deceit for profit, including false representation of efficacy and concealment of adverse effects of medications or 'natural curatives; see Pseudovitamins, Unproven methods of cancer therapy

health hazard OCCUPATIONAL SAFETY Any agent or activity posing a potential hazard to health; in OSHA parlance, an HH is any chemical for which there is scientifically valid data that acute or chronic health effects may occur in exposed employees; HHs include carcinogens, toxic or highly toxic agents, reproductive toxins, mucocutaneous irritants and/or corrosives, and hepato–, nephro–, and neurotoxins; Cf Physical hazard

health insurance purchasing cooperative HEALTH CARE FINANCING A term developed in the context of managed competition (the 'Clinton Plan') for a not-for-profit entity that would negotiate contracts with accountable health partnerships to provide health care services; the cooperative would offer a menu of health coverage options for enrollment and for collecting premiums

health maintenance organization see HMO

health promotion Any activity that seeks to improve a person's or population's health by providing information about and increasing awareness of 'at risk' behaviors associated with certain diseases, with the intent of reducing those behaviors; in the USA, health promotion has met with success in reducing the incidence of cardiovascular and tobacco-related diseases

healthy food A generic term for those foods that are 'good for you', which encompasses those that are high in fiber, natural vitamins, fructose, and other (at present) unidentified 'factors'; see Fiber, Fruit and vegetables; Cf Health food

Note: While the terms healthy food and health food may refer to the same comestibles, the latter trm acquires a mystical overtone as they may be alleged by health food advocates (health food nuts, to their cynical detractors) prevent or cure diseases, despite current lack of even the most vaguely suggestive data to support such contentions

'Healthy People 2000' PUBLIC HEALTH A series of health goals (table) promulgated by the US Public Health Services that provides insight into the state of American health; the priorities include health promotion, ie targeting risk behaviors and health protection, which includes environmental or regulatory measures that confer broad-based protection, as well as preventative services and surveillance systems, addressing numerous specific issues (**JAMA 1995; 273:1123, NY Times 12 April 1995, C13**) see Mortality, YPLL

healthy worker effect The finding that death from disease is markedly reduced in certain occupations; the mortality in young men enlisted in the US Army is one-fourth that of civilian men of similar age, a fact attributed to self-selection, pre-enlistment screening (eliminating the less physically or psychologically fit), exercise, health care, and health promotion; see Hawthorne effect

health 'yuppie' An often egocentric 'yuppie' (young, upwardly-mobile professional) who is a physician, dentist, or other highly paid health care worker (**NY State J Med 1991; 91:43**); it has been alleged that the HY's goals tend to pivot around material gains rather than the altruistic principles that traditionally guide physicians and others in the health care field

'heaped-up' appearance GASTROENTEROLOGY The endoscopic morphology seen in malignant gastric ulcers where the margins of the lesion are irregular, with overhanging borders, and a 'dirty', necrotic base; Cf Punched-out appearance; see Meniscus sign of Carmen

'heartburn' Burning retrosternal, often postprandial discomfort due to reflux of gastric contents into the esophagus, associated with dysfunction of the lower esophageal sphincter; heartburn may be idiopathic or associated with Barrett's esophagus, duodenal ulcers, reflux, scleroderma and Zollinger-Ellison syndrome

heartcutting INSTRUMENTATION A method for improving the resolution of gas chromatography by switching a portion of the analyzed specimen into a second separation column with a different polarity, measuring a second parameter; thus is also known as multidimensional gas chromatography

heart failure cells Intra-alveolar hemosiderin-laden macrophages seen in the lungs of patients with compromised cardiac function that results in low-grade pulmonary hemorrhage, as in congestive heart failure; the cell content is confirmed by an appropriate iron stain, eg Prussian blue

'heart laws' OCCUPATIONAL MEDICINE Legislature that attempts to distinguish cardiovascular injury and consequences due to work-related physical exertion and/or psychologic stress from those due to the natural progression of underlying cardiac disease; HLs do not provide for workman's compensation if the disability is related to coronary artery disease or hypertension, ie naturally-progressing disease, except for certain 'favored' occupational groups, eg uniformed police and firefighters, whose death or disability may be presumed to have been suffered in the line of duty

heart-lung machine Extracorporeal circulation A device that consists of a pump and blood oxygenator, which is used during open heart (eg cardiothoracic and cardiovascular) surgery; in the HLM, the blood is pushed by a roller pump and gently separated into tubing, where the blood is then bubble-oxygenated, reheated, filtered, and pumped back into the body

---

HEALTHY PEOPLE PLAN

ALCOHOL ABUSE ↓ Alcohol-related motor vehicle accidents to < 8.5/10^5; reduce alcohol abuse to 13% in those < age 17

CHRONIC DISEASE 15% ↓ in chronic disease-related disability

DRUG ABUSE ↓ Drug-related deaths to 3/10^5, ↓ marijuana abuse to < 8% in those aged 18-25 and ↓ cocaine abuse in 18-25 to 3%

CONFINE HIV INFECTION to < 800/10^5 and new cases to < 98 000/year

IMMUNIZATIONS Eliminate measles; ↓ pneumonia and influenza-related death to 7.3/10^5; ↑ number of children immunized to 80%

OBSTETRIC CARE ↓ Infant mortality to 7/1000; ↓ low birth weight to less than 5%; extend first-trimester care to 90% of all pregnancies; ↓ teen pregnancies to < 50/1000 teen-aged girls

SEXUALLY TRANSMITTED DISEASE ↓ Gonorrhea to 225/10^5 and

---

heart-lung transplantation A procedure that is being successfully performed at specialized centers; post-transplant patients have adequate ventilation, despite a loss of innervation and increased tidal volume; heart-lung transplantation may be effective for 1) Primary respiratory disease with chronic disturbance in gas exchange and alveo-

lar mechanics and a secondary increase in pulmonary vascular resistance (those with primary vascular resistance fare poorly with heart-lung transplants) and 2) Pulmonary vascular disease with primary high-resistance circulatory disorder, for whom the procedure is beneficial as tracheobronchial and alveolar abnormalities are not present; Cf Domino donor transplantation, Lung transplantation, UNOS

heart rate The rate at which the heart pumps blood; the normal range is now defined as ranging between 50 and 90 beats/min (Science & Medicine 1995; 2/3:10)

heart sound see Third heart sound

heart-shaped face A descriptor for a physiognomy described in Turner syndrome (45,XO), characterized by prominent ears, broad malar bones and a small chin

heart transplantation An estimated 2000 patients per month (US) need hearts—the procedure is performed ± 100/month; when a heart fails to 'take' in one recipient, or that recipient dies, the heart or other organ can then be transplanted into another recipient (N Engl J Med 1993; 328:319oA) CAUSE OF DEATH Infection 17%, acute rejection 16%, chronic rejection 14%, embolism 14%, pancreatitis 11%, peptic ulcer 9%, and others 18%* (Arch Pathol Lab Med 1992; 1161137oA) Italian experience with 1068 transplants: Actuarial survival 74% at 6.5 years; mortality ↑ with ↑ age, is greater in ♂, more common in those who had not been transplanted for dilated cardiomyopathy (Virchow Arch A Pathol Anat Histopathol 1993; 422:453)

*Data 22 years of experience (171 transplants, 158 patients, 81 autopsies) at Groote Schuur, Cape Town—1967-1989

heart tumors Cardiac neoplasms are rare; most primary lesions are benign (myxoma > rhabdomyoma > osteoclastoma) although malignant tumors occur (angiosarcoma, rhabdomyosarcoma); secondary neoplasms are usually malignant and hone in on the pericardium, arising in the lung, or extend from a hilar-based lymphoma or melanoma

heart valve prosthesis A structure or device used to replace a damaged (stenosed or 'insufficient') cardiac valve, ± 50 000 of which are transplanted/year (US); there is no significant difference in the probability of death with either a mechanical (eg Bjork-Shiley tilting disk valve, the Starr-Edwards caged ball and St Jude's pivoting bileaflet valve) or bioprosthetic valve; mechanical valves are durable but thrombogenic and thus require long-term anticoagulant therapy; bioprosthetic valves are less thrombogenic, but have a limited lifespin related to tissue deterioration (N Engl J Med 1993; 328:1289oA); in addition to the porcine bioprosthesis, there is a commercially available cryopreserved human aortic valve see Shiley valve

heat intolerance SPORTS MEDICINE A generic term for any condition caused by thermal challenges of exercise, resulting in a range of responses from cramps and exhaustion to heat syncope, stroke, and even death; HT represents a failure of the physiologic mechanisms that offset increased body temperature including hypohydration and decreased sweat production (100 mL reduces the rise in core temperature by 1°C), increased body temperature and inability to increase the heat loss (which is limited by the body surface area (JC DeLee, D Drez, Jr, Eds, Orthopedic Sports Medicine WB Saunders, Philadelphia, 1994)

heat lamp Infrared lamp, see there

heat shock MOLECULAR BIOLOGY The inhibitory effect that high ambient temperatures have on transcription and translation; severe heat shock blocks gene splicing, blocking translation of intervening sequences (introns) of mRNA precursors; since the mRNA in the cytoplasm doesn't have the usual cuts at the 5' and 3' splice junctions and translation of the mRNA proceeds into the exons (which are usually spliced out), resulting in the production of abnormal proteins, therefore repression of normal transcription during heat shock is beneficial to the host cell or organism, as defective proteins are not produced

heat shock proteins A small group of highly-conserved proteins, containing a 'heat shock consensus' region, the production of which increases when a cell is subjected to various metabolic stresses, especially heat; hsp activities include assembly of proteins into protein complexes, correct protein folding, uptake of protein into organelles and protein sorting (**Nature 1991; 349:627**); the largest group of hsps has a molecular mass of about 70 kD; when cells are treated with antibodies to hsp70, they accumulate heat shock proteins and die by thermal stress; when the HSP104 gene of *Saccharomyces cerevisiae* is eliminated by deletion mutation, thermotolerance is lost, implying that the gene is required for thermotolerance; hsp70s stimulate translocation and folding of precursor proteins into the mitochondrial matrix and endoplasmic reticulum, and are thus thought to facilitate transport competence to precursors; hsp60 proteins have 'foldase' activities, see Chaperonins; hsp90 proteins are thought to act in the signal transduction pathway for steroid, eg glucocorticoid and estrogen receptors, facilitating response of the aporeceptor to the hormonal signal; hsp70 proteins that help cells recover after exposure to high temperatures are Ss1p and Ss2p, which increase the rates of translocation of proteins into microsomes and possibly salvage precursor proteins that prematurely fold into translocation-incompetent conformations during translation, allowing passage, possibly by binding and unfolding hydrophobic receptor sites of certain proteins produced outside of the cells where needed; two groups of hsps respond to different stressants, 1) Group I Ethanol which induces translational errors and amino acid analogs, eg puromycin causing production of abnormal proteins and 2) Group II Heat shock (protein unfolding), heavy metals and inorganic toxins (copper-chelaters, arsenite, iodoacetamide, *p*-chloromercuribenzoate, which causes conformational changes in the proteins by binding to sulfhydryl groups, recovery from anoxia, H_2O_2, superoxide ions and other free radicals (oxygen toxicity, free radical fragmentation of proteins), ammonium chloride (inhibition of proteolysis), others (inhibition of oxidative phosphorylation, changes in redox state, protein modification)

heat shock response A constellation of responses that occur when an organism is exposed to high temperatures, including repression of synthesis of some proteins, increased synthesis of other proteins and transcription and translation of genes to form 'new' proteins that are not produced at lower temperatures

heat-stable toxin MICROBIOLOGY Any of a number of short cysteine-rich polypeptides produced by various gram-negative bacteria, eg *E coli* that cause diarrhea by activating host guanylate cyclase* (**Science & Medicine 1995; 2/3:16**) see Virulence factor

*Of note and of interest to evolutionary biologists is the structural similarity of bacterial HSTs to guanylin, the endogenous activator of host guanylate cyclase

heat stress detoxification Hyperthermia* ALTERNATIVE MEDICINE The artificial induction of fever, often in a person whose fever responsiveness is viewed by holistic health care providers as being inadequate; HSD is by design a 'low-tech' exercise, and the ↑ temperature is induced by saunas, steam baths, local hot compresses, and friction, and is claimed to be of use either alone or as an adjunctive therapy in bladder and lung infections, cancer, HIV infection, and viral infections; while various forms of 'high-tech' hyperthermia (eg induced by diathermy, extracorporeal heating, IR, ultrasound) are being examined for possible effects, there is little evidence in peer-reviewed journals to establish the 'low tech' form of hyperthermia as an effective therapeutic modality; see Alternative medicine

heat stress disease CRITICAL CARE MEDICINE A group of conditions due to overexposure to or overexertion in excess environmental temperatures, of increasing severity, from 1) Heat cramps, which are non-emergent and treated by salt replacement 2) Heat exhaustion, which is more serious, treated with fluid and salt replacement and 3) Heat stroke, a condition most commonly affecting extremes of ages, especially the elderly, accompanied by convulsions, delusions, coma and treated with cooling the body and replacement of fluids and salts

Note: The body's reaction to heat is a function of controllable (use of anticholinergics, phenothiazines, alcohol, heavy exercise, clothing, obesity, direct exposure and acclimatization) and uncontrollable factors (high ambient temperatures or humidity, lack of air circulation, underlying fever, old age or infancy, ectodermal dysplasia

heavy chain disease Any of a family of monoclonal gammopathies or paraproteinemias that are characterized by excess production of an immunoglobulin Fc fragment that may be detected in the serum and/or urine, and accompanied by lymphoproliferative disease

ALPHA HEAVY CHAIN DISEASE Seligmann's disease The most common heavy chain disease or paraproteinemia, in which there is an excess production of an incomplete IgA1 molecule (partial heavy chain and no light chain), affecting Sephardic Jews, Arabs and Mediterranean rim inhabitants CLINICAL Onset in childhood or adolescence as either a lymphoproliferative disorder confined to the respiratory tract or an enteric form (see IPSID) with severe diarrhea, malabsorption, steatorrhea, weight loss, hepatic dysfunction, hypocalcemia, lymphadenopathy, marked mononuclear infiltration which may eventuate into lymphoma (see Mediterranean lymphoma); α chain disease may remit spontaneously, respond to antibiotic therapy or if clearly monoclonal, may require combination chemotherapy, potentially causing death by ages 20-30 LABORATORY ↑ Alkaline phosphatase, ↓ Ca^{++} TREATMENT Antibiotics, or if advanced, chemotherapy DELTA HEAVY CHAIN DISEASE A single case has been reported in an elderly man with osteolytic lesions, marrow infiltration by abnormal plasma cells, who died in renal failure GAMMA HEAVY CHAIN DISEASE A disorder of older males, ranging from fulminant, ie death in weeks to prolonged, lasting 20 years, most die in the first year, often due to infection CLINICAL Presents as lymphoproliferation with fever, fatigue, anemia, angioimmunoblastic lymphadenopathy, hepatosplenomegaly, uvular and palatal edema, eosinophilic infiltrates, leukopenia, associated with autoimmune disease, tuberculosis and lymphoma LABORATORY Increased IgG1; most cases excrete less than 1 g/day of paraprotein, rarely up to 20 g/day TREATMENT Cyclophosphamide, vincristine, prednisone MU CHAIN DISEASE A rare paraproteinemia that affects the middle-aged to elderly, most of whom have or slowly progress to CLL CLINICAL Lymphadenopathy, hepatosplenomegaly and BM infiltration by vacuolated plasma cells, often accompanied by ↑ kappa chain production TREATMENT As with CLL

'heavy guns' A highly colloquial term, most commonly used in the context of highly aggressive therapy, as in chemotherapy of an advanced malignancy that the oncologist 'hits with heavy guns', using multiple agents and several therapeutic modalities; see Induction

heavy-ion treatment A type of radiotherapy (RT) in which a large[1] (expensive[2], power-hungry[3]) ion accelerator[4] is used to deliver focused beams of positively charged nuclei stripped of their electrons to tumors; in conventional RT (X-rays or gamma radiation), there is lateral dispersion ('leakage') of ionizing radiation into adjacent non-tumorous tissues as the energy from the beam is lost slowly, heavy ion beams lose all their energy at once with little damaging leakage into surrounding healthy tissue; HIT is of greatest use in treating malignancies that occur in organs for which radiation 'leakage' can cause severe damage, eg the eye or spinal cord; the only dedicated HIT accelerator is the Himac (heavy-ion medical accelerator in Chiba) in Japan (**New York Times 21 Dec 1993; C3**)

[1]Circa two football fields [2]Circa $300 million; cost to maintain $50 million for 1000 patients/year [3]25 megawatts, enough to provide electricity to 8000 homes [4]Heavy ions, eg from carbon or neon are accelerated to 11% of the speed of light with the two accelerators, then brought to circa 85% of the speed of light with two synchrotrons, and beamed at the patient's tumor

heavy metal A generic term for a metal that is 5 times heavier than water, and often toxic, a feature that is linked to ability of the HM's tight cationic binding to proteins in the circulation; HMs include antimony, arsenic, bismuth, cadmium, copper, lead, mercury; cells respond by HMs by ↑ transcription of a variety of genes, including the eukaryotic heat shock system, metallothioneins, prokaryotic mercury resistance gene and iron uptake systems CLINICAL General, fine tremor, speech slurring, stomatitis, drooling, cataracts and neurasthenia TREATMENT Chelation with EDTA; see Mad Hatter, Minamata Bay disease, Queen of Poisons, Pink disease

heavy spin TRANSFUSION MEDICINE Hard spin A term referring to the intensity of centrifugation (5000 g) used in a blood bank for separating various blood components from a donated unit of erythrocytes; a heavy spin of 5-7 minutes is required for separation of red cells, platelets, plasma, cryoprecipitate and leukocyte-poor red cells

heavy water ^2H_2O Water formed from a stable radioisotope of hydrogen (deuterium); HW differs from normal water in that it freezes at 3.8°C, and boils at 101.4°C; it cannot support life, and is used as a moderator in nuclear reactors

Hebbian model A model proposed by DO Hebb (1904-1985), Canadian physiologic psychologist, that sought to explain memory on the basis of long-term potentiation of single synapses; this particular model was found to be inadequate in the face of the extracellular diffusion effect displayed by nitric oxide on neural pathways that are not directly connected (Sci Am 1994; 270/5:16); Cf Volume learning

'hectic-septic' fever An erratic fever pattern that, while uncommon and non-specific, may be seen in abscesses, as well as malaria, kala-azar and endocarditis

hedgehog genes EMBRYOLOGY A recently-identified family of genes that are critical in the structural and development of organisms from the stage of fertilized egg to that of an early embryo; hedgehog gene products act in a gradient fashion controlling the organization of the body shape and structures including limbs and digits, brain and spinal cord; the hedgehog* genes encode **hedgehog proteins** (also known as morphogens) a class of signaling molecules that may prove to be the most important molecules in vertebrate embryology; in humans, hedgehog genes are thought to switch on ± day 15 postfertilization, helping to shape the CNS, and are finished ± day 28 (New York Times 11 January 1994; C1) see Morphogen

*The term derives from the ability of these genes, when mutated to impart a bristly hedgehog-like appearance to the fruit fly (*Drosophila melanogaster*), the first model system in which these genes were recognized; nomenclature of the hedgehog genes may prove problematic; some authors favor an alpha- or numeric system; others prefer naming each new gene after the trivial name for a particular hedgehog, eg Indian hedgehog, moonrat hedgehog, and desert hedgehog, a system that might prove a boon to the playful and bane to those less so, given the recent identification of the most fascinating of the genes thus far identified, waggishly called Sonic Hedgehog after the character in a popular video game produced by Sega by R Riddle, a postdoctoral fellow in CJ Tabin's laboratory at Harvard Medical School (New York Times 11 January 1994; C1, 13)

heel-pad sign A characteristic clinical finding in acromegaly, where soft tissue under the heel is thickened to greater than 30 mm (normal < 23 mm)

Hegsted's score A formula for determining a diet's relative lipid composition, where a high value indicates increased saturated fatty acids and cholesterol and low polyunsaturated fatty acids

Heinz bodies Inclusion bodies seen in erythrocytes and occasionally in reticulocytes that correspond to denatured proteins, especially hemoglobin; the inclusions are the result of a chemical insult due to defects in the hexose monophosphate shunteg glucose-6-phosphate dehydrogenase deficiency, thalassemias, 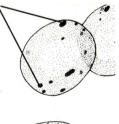 in unstable hemoglobin syndromes, and in irreversibly sickled cells; they are usually marginal in distribution, and can only be visualized with supravital dyes, eg brilliant cresyl blue or crystal violet; Heinz body-laden red cells may

be phagocytosed in the splenic sinuses

Heimlich maneuver A technique for removing a bolus of food stuck in the oropharynx potentially causing acute asphyxia; the Hiemlich-*er* stands behind the victim and clasps his hands around the Heimlich-*ee*, slightly above the umbilicus and abruptly pulls backwards, forcing residual air in the lungs out the trachea (JAMA 1975; 234:398) COMPLICATION Fatal aortic regurgitation; see Cafe coronary, Flake maneuver

Note: While the maneuver is often successful, the victim may have developed an air hunger so intense that the benefit of the expulsive rush of air dislodging the bolus is immediately offset by a gasp by the victim, that jams the food further down the traheobronchial tree, exacerbating the situation; to minimize this occurrence, the upper mouth should be lowered as much as possible

Hektoen enteric agar MICROBIOLOGY An agar used for isolation and differentiation of gram-negative enteric pathogens

HeLa cells TISSUE CULTURE An aneuploid epithelial cell line isolated by GO Gey (John Hopkins) from Henrietta Lack, a young Baltimore woman who died in 1951 of an anaplastic carcinoma of the uterine cervix; the Hela cell line has been in continuous culture in numerous laboratories around the world and is a 'gold standard' cell line widely used in experimental oncology, which has contributed much to the understanding of cancer

the Helga Wanglie case BIOMEDICAL ETHICS A legal case in Minnesota that tested the concept of 'futility' in which the husband of an 86-year woman in persistent vegetative state insisted that her life was to be maintained at all costs even though her physicians believed that the continued use of mechanical ventilation and intensive care was futile; when attempts to transfer Ms Wanglie to another health care facility failed, her physicians sought to have a court appoint an independent conservator with responsibility for making medical decisions on her behalf; the judge denied the petition and reaffirmed the authority of her husband as legal guardian–she died 3 days later (N Engl J Med 1992; 326:1509oA)

helical scanning Spiral computed tomography, see there

helical structure BIOCHEMISTRY The α helix is a major structural motif present in many proteins, eg myoglobin that is most stable in a right-handed conformation, which usually has 3.6 amino acid residues per 360° turn; the peptide bonds are parallel and side chains perpendicular to the helical axis of the α helix; each amino acid forms a hydrogen bond to the fourth amino acid above and to the fourth amino acid below at a distance of 0.29 nm; Cf β-pleated sheets

helicase An enzyme that binds DNA downstream of the replicating fork, catalyzing the unwinding of the DNA duplex; Cf Gyrase, Topoisomerase

Helicobacter A genus of bacteria originally designated as *Campylobacter*, and split therefrom when phylogenetic studies provided convincing data that certain organisms (eg *C pylori*, and *C mustelae*) are not true camplyobacteria, but rather more closely related to *Wolinella succinogenes*

Most changes of nomenclature in microbiology pass unnoticed by 'mainstream' medicine; in view of the 'trauma' in the literature that followed the name change from *Campylobacter* to *Helicobacter* at a time of high visibility, further change in nomenclature (eg to *Wolinella*) seems unlikely-Author's note

Helicobacter cinaedi *Campylobacter cinaedi* A gram-negative, spiral or curved bacillus that was first identified in gay bowel disease (see there, characterized by enteritis and proctocolitis); *H cinaedi* may also cause recurrent cellulitis, fever, and bacteremia, most commonly in immunocompromised hosts (Ann Int Med 1994; 121:90)

Helicobacter pylori A gently-curved gram-negative microaerophilic bacillus*; *H pylori* is held responsible for most cases of gastritis and is present in 10% of healthy young persons and up to 60% of those 60 years or older

Note: 90% of patients with intestinal-type gastric carcinoma have been infected by *H pylori*, which may be a co-factor for gastric cancer, acting either by stimulating the production of cellular mutagens or by inducing a high rate of proliferation following damage to the cells; *H pylori* may be spread by intrafamilial contacts and is increasingly implicated in duodenal ulcers which may respond to antibiotics; circa 50% of world's population is infected with *H pylori*; it has been linked to the development of gastric ulcer, duodenal ulcer, hypertrophic gastropathy, gastric adenocarcinoma, and more recently to gastric non-Hodgkin's lymphoma (**N Engl J Med 1994; 330:1267oA**); B-cell proliferation can be induced in response to *H pylori* antigens in the presence of *H pylori*–specific T cell (**Lancet 1993; 342:571**) *H pylori* has been isolated from domestic cats (**Infect Immun 1994; 62:2367**) TREATMENT Antibiotics, eg amoxicillin, metronidazole, tetracycline (**N Engl J Med 1993; 328:308oA**) (for non-NSAID-induced gastric ulcers) Bismuth subcitrate (**N Engl J Med 1995; 332:139oA**) see Duodenal ulcer, Gastric lymphoma*

*Note: Although the term hyperthermia is more popular among alternative health care practitioners than heat stress detoxification, hyperthermia is also widely used in conventional medicine and thus lends to considerable 'cross-cultural' confusion; the organism was first classified as a *Campylobacter*, but later separated therefrom (**Int J Syst Bacteriol 1989; 39:397**), due to major differences in ultrastructure, fatty acid content, respiratory quinines, growth properties, RNA sequence and enzymes, eg urease production

heliotrope rash The classic rash seen on the face of patients with dermatomyositis, so named for its purplish hue, likened to that of the fragrant herb, *Heliotropium peruvianum*

heliox CLINICAL THERAPEUTICS A mixture of helium and oxygen used to treat obstructive lung disease; *'Helium is one seventh the density of nitrogen. The drop in pressure across a site of convective acceleration is directly related to the density of the medium. Since convective acceleration occurs at loci of flow limitation, expiratory resistance may be reduced, and maximal expiratory flows have been shown to increase with heliox during induced bronchoconstriction.'*; heliox may be used as an adjuvant therapy for patients with rspiratory failure due to reversible lower airway obstruction (**N Engl J Med 1995; 332:192c**)

Helix MOLECULAR DIAGNOSTICS A computerized (US) national directory of DNA diagnostics laboratories that is funded by the National Library of Medicine and the National Center for Biotechnology Information; Helix is housed in the Children's Hospital and Medical Center in Seattle and (as of 1994) provides information on 160 laboratories that test for 190 diseases; access to Helix is limited to health care professionals—lay persons are referred to regional genetic counseling centers: Telephone (206) 538-2689; Fax (206) 528-2687 (**Directory of Rare Analyses 1994-1996, AACC Press, Washinton, DC, 1994**)

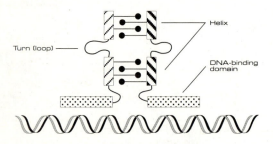

helix-turn-helix motif Helix-loop-helix motif MOLECULAR BIOLOGY A group of 20-residue peptides characterized by two α helices separated by a non-helical segment, of nearly invariant geometry but with considerable amino acid sequence variation, which have conserved amino acid residues at the points of contact with the repressor-operator complexes; like other DNA-binding motifs, eg the Leucine zipper and Zinc finger, the helix-turn-helix configuration regulates gene expression by binding in the major and minor grooves of the DNA; the motif occurs in the MyoD protein and myogenin

HELLP syndrome OBSTETRICS A clinical entity associated with eclampsia or severe pre-eclampsia, characterized by the acronym of Hemolysis, Elevated Liver function tests, Low Platelets, which may transiently worsen following delivery; other HELLP symptoms include blood pressure greater than 160 systolic and/or 110 diastolic, urinary volume less than 400 mL/24 hours, nonspecific cerebral abnormalities, pulmonary edema and/or cyanosis LABORATORY Proteinuria ≥ 5 g/24 hours, schistocytes (RBCs that have been sheared and fragmented by intravascular fibrin deposition), increased liver function tests (ALA, AST, ALT, bilirubin), increased prothrombin time; partial thromboplastin time and fibrinogen levels are normal

helmet PUBLIC HEALTH A device of hardened plastic worn on the head to reduce the severity of injuries MOTORCYCLE In one report, 63.3% of those involved in motocycle crashes were unhelmeted; helmet use in motorcycling ↓ accident-related skull fractures (0.2% vs 0.9%), brain injury (1.7% vs 4.8%) and brain injury-related hospital costs ($334 000 vs $2.4 million); use of helmets would have prevented 14 deaths, 60 brain injuries, 13 skull fractures, 8 concussions, as of 1994, 25 states in the US had not enacted laws requiring the use of helmets by motocyclists (**MMWR 1994; 43: 423, 431**)

helmet bodies Large compact, dense homogeneous, perinuclear inclusions in epithelial cells, surrounded by a mononuclear cell infiltrate (lymphocytes, plasma cells and macrophages), seen in mucocutaneous infections by *Chlamydia* species that may be identified by conjunctival scrapings stained with Romanovsky stain

helmet cells Schizocytes, see there

helmet field A radiotherapeutic field that covers parallel opposing lateral whole brain fields, reaching as low as C2 to include the meninges, of use in treating CNS lymphoma, either prophylactically (2400 cGy) or if the CNS is known to be involved (4000 cGy)

helmet skull A fanciful descriptor for the cranial deformity seen in craniometaphyseal dysplasia, which is characterized by brachycephaly, prominent forehead, ocular hypertelorism, and microstomia, as well as bilateral hip dislocations and muscle wasting

helmet vertebrum A descriptor for a vertebrum seen in spondylosclerosis, which has a hemispherical 'dome' above the body proper, end-plate erosions, neo-osteogenesis and narrowing of the disk space caudad to the affected vertebrum

Helms Amendment US Congressional legislation passed in1973 that prohibits US aid for pharmacologic agents that can induce menstruation after fertilization, ie abortifacients (**Sci Am 1993; 268/4:22**) see Contraceptives

helper T cell Helper T lymphocyte, CD4+ T cell A subset of T lymphocytes bearing the antigenic determinant CD4, which are presented with a foreign antigen in the context of both a self MHC class II antigen and IL-1; once immune recognition or response occurs, helper cells produce various cytokines, eg interferon-γ, IL-2 and osteoclast-activating factor, which are critical in hematopoietic differentiation, collagen synthesis and antibody formation; helper T cells lay a central role in normal and pathologic immune responses by secreting various cytokines, including IL-2, IFN-γ, and TNF are involved in cell-mediated immunity; IL-4 stimulates the production of IgE antibodies; IL-5 promotes the differentiation and activation of eosinophils CD4+ (helper) T cells are functionally divided into type 1, which produce IL-2 and IFN-γ, and are found in infectious granulomatous processes and type 2, which produce IL-4 and IL-5, and are found in atopic disorders, lepromatous leprosy, visceral leishmaniasis and as a clonal expansion in hypereosinophilic syndrome (**N Engl J Med 1994; 330∘:535**OA) see CD4, Flow cytometry, Suppressor cells, T cells

helper:suppressor ratio IMMUNOLOGY The ratio of CD4 helper T-lymphocytes to CD8 suppressor T-lymphocytes, normally 1.5-2.0; in AIDS; this ratio is the single best monitor for clinical deterioration, where less than 0.5 is commonly seen and values of 0.1 or less presage fulminant clinical deterioration; the helper:suppressor ratio is also decreased in other conditions, including viral infections (CMV, herpes, EBV, measles), GVHD, recuperation from BM transplantation, exercise, severe sunburn, burns, myelodysplasia, ALL in remission, sleep deprivation; the ratio is ↑ in atopic dermatitis, psoriasis, Sézary syndrome, chronic autoimmune hepatitis, primary biliary cirrhosis, rheumatoid arthritis, SLE (with or without renal involvement), and IDDM

Helsinki Declaration A document based on the Nuremburg Code of Ethics that offers recommendations for conducting experiments using human subjects; the HD was adopted in 1962, revised by the 18th World Medical Assembly (WMA) in Helsinki in 1964, and subsequently re-revised in the 29th WMA in Tokyo in 1975; see Geneva Convention, Nuremburg Code of Ethics, Unethical research

hemagglutination LABORATORY MEDICINE A serological test used to screen for the presence of various antigens PRINCIPLE A latex bead is coated with an antigen 'X' and coincubated with an antibody having a weak affinity for antigen 'X', but having a stronger affinity for the antigen X of interest; if X antigen is also present in the test serum, the linking antibody will preferably bind to X rather than 'X', thereby causing a non-agglutinating reaction, ie a positive reaction; a negative result appears as 'clumping' of the latex particles; hemagglutination is of use in 1) Transfusion medicine for detecting antigens on the red cell's surface and 2) Microbiology to identify hepatitis B virus, leptospirosis, rubella and others

hemagglutination inhibition reaction LABORATORY MEDICINE A generic term for an immune reaction in which an agglutination reaction is prevented or inhibited; therefore in HIR, a positive result results when an antigen-antibody reaction does not occur, because an antigen or antibody is present in the reaction systems that prevents red cell agglutination; HAI is used to diagnose

Viruses

1) Exanthematous viruses (rubella, rubeola, variola-vaccinia)

2) Herpesvirus (herpes simplex-1 and -2, H zoster, CMV, EBV)

3) Respiratory viridiae (Adenovirus, coronavirus, influenza, mumps, parainfluenza) and

4) Togaviridiae (Eastern, St Louis, Venezuelan and Western equine encephalitides)

Bacteria. eg *Neisseria gonorrhea, Streptococcus pneumoniae, Vibrio cholera, Rickettsiae*

Parasites

hemagglutinin A generic term for a protein that agglutinates erythrocytes VIROLOGY A glycoprotein located on the surface of a virus that has an intrinsic affinity for red cells, or other cells, eg respiratory epithelium at the receptors HEMATOLOGY An antibody that agglutinates RBCs, acting either at body temperature as 'warm hemagglutinins' or at subcorporal temperatures as 'cold hemagglutinins'

hemangioblastoma An uncommon vascular tumor of the cerebellum, representing 2% of all CNS neoplasms, appearing in the 3rd-4th decades, either alone or in association with von-Hippel-Lindau syndrome, pheochromocy-

toma, syringomyelia, and erythrocythemia PATHOLOGY Grossly, the tumor is well-circumscribed, yellow-brown and hemorrhagic PATHOLOGY Anastomosing network of capillaries and abundant plump stromal cells that are thought to represent the neoplastic component of the lesion TREATMENT Surgical PROGNOSIS Good

hemangiopericytoma A tumor of perivascular cells or pericytes appearing in the legs and retroperitoneum of adults; recurrence is common, one-half develop metastases PATHOLOGY Jagged endothelial channels with 'staghorn'-like blood vessels, best seen when the tissue is stained for reticulin or by PAS, which are variably surrounded by increased basement membrane DDx Synovial sarcoma, mesenchymal chondrosarcoma, fibrous histiocytoma, thymoma

hemapheresis Apheresis The removal of whole blood from a donor or patient, followed by its separation into components, retention of certain components and return of the recombined remaining elements to the patient; hemapheresis is a therapeutic modality for removing 1) Leukocytes in hyperleukemic leukostasis with > 100 x 10^9/L blasts 2) Platelets in thrombocytosis with > 1000 x 10^9/L platelets, if symptomatic 3) Defective red cells and replacement by normal red cells as in sickle cell anemia with sickle cell crisis 4) Immunoglobulins causing a hyperviscosity syndrome in macroglobulinemia or multiple myeloma 5) Autoantibody production in myasthenia gravis, Goodpasture syndrome, SLE, factor VIII antibodies and 6) Lipoproteins in patients with homozygous familial hypercholesterolemia; other conditions may respond to hemapheresis, including allograft rejection, Guillain-Barre syndrome, hemolytic disease of the newborn, autoimmune hemolytic anemia, ITP, post-transfusional purpura, glomerulonephritis (crescentic or rapidly progressive), Goodpasture's disease, HUS-TTP complex, intoxication from various agents and thyroid crisis; the devices used in apheresis include those with intermittent flow and continuous flow; see Cytapheresis, Hemodialysis, Leukapheresis, Plasmapheresis

hematin A chemical complex of porphyrin and hydroxide ion bound to Fe^{3+} that is isolated from hemoglobin in a dimeric form; hematin forms brown granular crystals that may be seen by LM in formalin-fixed tissue or tissue that is too acidic, or seen in fixed parasites that have ingested blood in vivo, thus also being known as malarial or schistosomal pigment; Cf Hematoidin

hematochezia Passage of bright red or maroon stool, usually due to blood; upper GI tract hemorrhage resulting in hematochezia implies a blood loss of ≥ 1000 ml, often accompanied by hypovolemia, hypotension, and tachycardia; lower GI or rectal hemorrhage may be guaiac-positive with as little as 25 ml, ie the blood is brighter red when it is more caudal

hematoidin A golden-yellow pigment chemically identical to bilirubin formed in tissues from hemoglobin under conditions of reduced oxygen

hematopoietic growth factor receptor HGFR Cytokine receptor A generic term for any member of a superfamily of receptors responsible for cell response to cytokines; HGFRs* typically have 4 conserved cysteine residues and a WSXWS (tryptophan-serine-X-tryptophan-serine) structural motif that is critical for proper folding of the extracellular region and for hormone binding; 3 types of HGFrs are recognized:

SUBFAMILY 1 are homodimers and are receptors for erythropoietin, G-CSF, IL-4, IL-7, growth hormone and prolactin

SUBFAMILY 2 are heterodimers (with the α unit providing the binding site and the β subunit carrying the signal-transduction activity) and are receptors for GM-CSF, IL-3,

IL-5, IL-6, leukemia inhibitory factor, oncostatin, and ciliary neutrophilic factor

SUBFAMILY 3 are heterotrimers with receptors for IL-2 (N Engl J Med 1994; 330:839RV)

*Except c-fms and c-kit which are HGFRs but are tyrosine kinase receptors

hematopoietin IL-3, interleukin-3, see there

hematoxylin HISTOLOGY A natural dye derived from logwood (*Hematoxylin campechianum*), that was the first major stain used to examine tissues by light microscopy, which continues to be the major 'workhorse' stain in histopathology, staining nuclei and calcium-bearing material a blue-purple color; hematoxylin is usually used in conjunction with eosin, the so-called counterstain, which stains other tissues and cell components in varying shades of pink

hematoxylin bodies RHEUMATOLOGY A virtually pathognomonic* finding of SLE that consist of homogeneous globular masses of nuclear remnants with nucleoproteins, DNA, and anti-DNA antibodies which are blue-purple when stained with hematoxylin; HBs may be seen in the atrial endocardium, kidneys, lungs, spleen, lymph nodes, serous membranes and synovium, are less common in fulminant cases of SLE and are thought to represent the tissue equivalent of the LE cell, see there

*LE cells have also been described in chronic active hepatitis, rheumatoid arthritis and in Sjögren syndrome

hemiballism NEUROLOGY A form of secondary chorea characterized by violent flinging movements of the limbs of one body half, often due to hemorrhage or infarction, or rarely tumors of the contralateral subthalamic nucleus; hemiballism develops after recovery from a stroke-induced hemiparesis and hemisensory defect; hemiballism (like other abnormal involuntary movements) disappears during sleep; in the usual scenario, hemiballism fades to hemichorea and finally extinction as the weeks pass; a mild form of hemiballism is hemichorea TREATMENT Persistent hemiballism may respond to reserpin or antipsychotic drugs

hemi '3' syndrome A form of hemihypertrophy occurring in females, possibly related to neural tube defects characterized by unilateral musculoskeletal hypertrophy, hyperesthesia, areflexia and progressive scoliosis

hemihypertrophy Hemimacrosomia A unilateral ↑ in some or all paired organs or tissues of the body; hemihypertrophy may be idiopathic, possibly related to neural, vascular, lymphatic, endocrine or chromosomal abnormalities and may occur in the Curtius, Klippel-Trenaunay, and Silver-Russel syndromes and in hepatoblastoma

hemilaminectomy ORTHOPEDIC SURGERY The unilateral excision of the vertebral lamina with removal of variable parts of the adjacent facet, a procedure used to treat a herniation of an intervertebral disk; see Laminectomy

hemin A hemoglobin-derived chemical complex composed of porphyrin, chloride, and iron

hemipelvectomy A form of 'heroic' surgery in which an entire lower extremity including the hemipelvis with disarticulation of the sacroiliac joint and symphysis pubis, and removal of all major muscles to the lower extremity except the iliopsoas; hemipelvectomy be required for large malignant soft tissue tumors of the buttock and anterior or lateral proximal thigh

hemivertebra A congenital vertebral body deformity arising from a simple, ie nondysplastic, nonmetabolic embryonal defect, in which the anterior half of a vertebral body is absent and adjacent vertebrae expand attempting to fill the vacated space, accompanied by preservation of the interspaces; Cf Butterfly vertebra

hemlock Any of a family of poisonous herbs of the carrot family; in particular, *Conium maculatum*, contains the alkaloid conine that first produces CNS hyperactivity, followed by medullary depression and respiratory failure TREATMENT Activated charcoal

Note: Socrates died from hemlock in 399 BC when he was tried and convicted for corrupting Athenian youth, two of whom, Alcibiades and Critias, betrayed Athens

the Hemlock Society EUTHANASIA MOVEMENT A nonprofit research and education organization based in Eugene, Oregon, the purpose of which is to increase public awareness of the options for terminally ill persons, as well as provide reference materials for interested parties, eg students, bioethicists, lawyers, and others (MT Today 1995; 5/6:80A) see Euthanasia

hemochromatosis An AR [MIM 235200] excess of GI iron absorption with progressive iron loading in parenchymal organs, the gene for which is linked to the HLA locus on the short arm of chromosome 6 EPIDEMIOLOGY 1-5:1000 (US) SCREENING Transferrin ≥ 50% ≥ 60% ; ferritin*; liver biopsy (N Engl J Med 1993; 328:1616OA; ibid 331; 460CPC) CLINICAL Cardiomegaly, 300-fold ↑, cirrhosis is 13-fold ↑ (once cirrhosis occurs, there is a 200-fold ↑ in hepatocellular carcinoma), gray-bronze skin pigmentation and DM with a 7-fold increase, 'bronze diabetes', arthropathy and hypogo-

---

CLINICAL FORMS OF HEMOGLOBINOPATHY

SICKLING PHENOTYPE, eg HbS, HbSC, HbS-Thalassemia

THALASSEMIC PHENOTYPE, eg Constant Spring, HbE, Lepore, Kenya, Vicksburg, Indianapolis

LOW OXYGEN AFFINITY PHENOTYPE, eg Bristol, Bucuresti/Louisville, Caribbean, Etobicoke, Hammersmith, Moscva, Okaloosa, Peterborough, Seattle, Torino

HIGH OXYGEN AFFINITY PHENOTYPE, eg Altdorf, Istanbul, Baylor, Belfast, Boras, Buenos Aires, Cranston, Duarte, Djelfa, Freiburg, Geneva, Hopkins II, Koln, Lyon, Niteroi, Nottingham, Pasadena, Sabine, Santa Ana, St Louis, Shepherds Bush, Tak, Tours, Toyoake, Tübingen, Zürich

---

nadism (impotence, testicular atrophy) LABORATORY Transferrin saturation > than 62% warrants a 'workup' SCREENING 1/3000 persons have undetected hemochromatosis, which if detected saves $845/year of life saved per patient, justifying the cost of serum iron screening (Gastroenterology 1994; 107:453)

*Normal levels ♂ 15-200 µg/L (US 15-200 ng/mL) ♀ 12-150 µg/L (US 12-150 ng/mL) Note: Other metals may accumulate in hemochromatosis, eg copper, lead, molybdenum (Am J Med 1991; 90:445rv, Am J Med Sci 1991; 301:47)

hemochromatosis triad Hepatomegaly, DM, and skin pigmentation seen in hemochromatosis, caused by the deposition of iron pigment that may also deposit in pancreas, heart, pituitary, glands (adrenal, parathyroid, thyroid), and joints

hemodilution CARDIOVASCULAR SURGERY A technique used during cardiopulmonary bypass to reduce the incidence of intraoperative thrombosis, by diluting the blood with crystalloid solutions, reducing the hematocrit index to 0.25-0.30 or less; by the time CPB is begun the activities of most coagulation system proenzymes has been reduced to 50% normal; factor VIII levels remain at normal levels throughout CPB as endogenous factor VIII is released in response to surgical stress (Arch Pathol Lab Med 1994; 118:411OA)

hemodynamic instability A condition requiring pharmacologic or mechanical support to maintain a normal blood pressure or adequate cardiac output

hemodialysis A therapeutic procedure for removing small-molecular-weight toxins by allowing the blood to flow past a semipermeable membrane where the toxins diffuse away from the blood down a concentration gradient, either via an external AV shunt, or a surgically placed AV fistula; hemodialysis is used in renal failure to reduce BUN, creatinine, hyperkalemia and correct metabolic acidosis; prolonged dialysis results in a poor quality of life with anemia, ↑ infections, myalgia, peripheral neuropathy, cerebral edema, myocardial infarcts, aluminum toxicity (see Dialysis dementia); thus renal transplantation is always the preferred long-term therapy COMPLICATIONS Pyogenic reactions due to gram-negative endotoxemia, with chills, fever, hypotension, nausea and myalgia, depressed natural killer cell activity, ↓ serum calcitriol; Cf Hemapheresis

Note: Reduction of dialysis time to < than 3.5 hours is associated with ↑ mortality (RR 1.17-2.18, JAMA 1991; 265:875)

hemoflagellate A flagellated parasite of the Kinetoplastidea family, characterized by kinetoplasts composed of mitochondrial DNA; hemoflagellates of human importance include *Leishmania*, *Trypanosoma*, *Leptomonas* and *Crithidia* spp

hemoglobin A tetrameric 64-kD protein that transports O_2 and CO_2 and which comprises 99% of the protein weight of erythrocytes; it is composed of two α chains, each 141 amino acids in length, encoded from the zeta chain gene on chromosome 16 and two β chains, each 144 amino acids in length, encoded from the contiguous eta, Gγ, Aγ and delta chain genes on chromosome 11

β hemoglobinopathy Sickle cell anemia or β-thalassemia (N Engl J Med 1995; 332:1606OA)

hemoglobinopathy A defect in production of either α or β hemoglobin, which may be quantitative or qualitative, congenital or (rarely) acquired; while the more common hemoglobin defects, eg HbS, HbC and the thalassemias, cause a characteristic clinical picture, '*rare hemoglobin variants are variously ignored, misunderstood, misdiagnosed, feared, shunned or rejected...*' and are not accompanied by clinical disease MOLECULAR PATHOLOGY Hemoglobinopathies are caused by various deletions, additions, and point mutations of the hemoglobin genes, or due to changes in the heme molecule per se

hemoglobin (Hb) nomenclature The first Hb described was HbA (normal Hb); HbB was proposed for sickle cell hemoglobin (but never assigned, as HbS was considered more euphonic); abnormal Hbs subsequently recognized in the 1950s were designated HbC, HbD, HbE, HbF (fetal Hb), HbG, HbH, HbI and HbJ, based on migrations on zone (paper) electrophoresis, a practice that stopped when more specific methods became available ; Hb variants subsequently received geographic names or names of cities, a practice that continues, with the disadvantage that some cities have up to four different Hbs and identical Hbs may be discovered in two different cities; most hemoglobinopathies are due to a single base substitution, eg a point mutation; as of early 1990, there were 119 α, 225 β, 32 γ and 14 δ chain variants that are divided into

FUSION HEMOGLOBIN eg Hb Constant Spring and Lepore

ELONGATED HEMOGLOBIN Chains are longer than normal-translation continues beyond the termination codon or

TRUNCATED HEMOGLOBIN Chains are shorter than normal-translation stops prior to the termination codon, all three of which may be due to point mutations, frame shifts and insertions

hemoglobin A$_{1c}$ see Advanced glycosylated endproducts, Glycosylated hemoglobin

hemolysis The destruction or lysis of erythrocytes (table) which may be immune-mediated or non-immune-mediated, due to defects intrinsic or extrinsic to the erythrocyte Clinical types of hemolysis: Immune hemolysis may be 1) Intravascular and is often more severe, IgM-mediated and requires complement activation, eg ABO blood groups LABORATORY ↑ free hemoglobin or 2) Extravascular, which is less severe, IgG-mediated and does not activate com-

plement, eg Rh, Kell, Duffy Note: Clinically significant hemolysis is usually detected by hemagglutination, less commonly by hemolysis, which detects anti-P, -P$_1$, -PP$_1$P^k, -Jk^a, -Le^a, occasionally also anti-Le^b and -Vel LABORATORY ↓ haptoglobin, ↓ half-life of circulating RBCs, ↑ indirect bilirubin as the hepatic capacity to conjugate bilirubin (forming direct bilirubin) may be overwhelmed if the hemolysis is massive, ↑ lactate dehydrogenase, hemoglobin in blood and urine, hemosiderinuria, methemoglobin and metalbumin, ↑ urobilinogen in urine and feces LABORATORY MEDICINE Even slight hemolysis is associated with substantial ↑ in acid phosphatase, K$^+$, LDH, and prostatic acid phosphatase (Clin Chem 1992; 38:575) MICROBIOLOGY Hemolysis is characteristic of certain strains of streptococci and is divided into α- and β-hemolysis; γ 'hemolysis' is a complete misnomer, see Gamma-hemolysis

hemolytic disease of the newborn Erythroblastosis A hemolytic condition due to an incompatibility of fetal antigens with the maternal immune system, caused by the production of maternal IgG antibodies in response to the fetal erythrocytes that innocently enter the maternal circulation; if the IgG response and the sharing of circulations (as in low-grade feto-maternal hemorrhage) is intense, erythroblastosis fetalis occurs; the most intense HDN occurs in incompatibilities of the RhD blood group antigen, which is responsible for 70% of all HDN; within the Rh group, anti-D causes 93% of anti-Rh reactions and anti-DC, -E, -Ce cause the remainder; Rh-induced HDN is reported in 11/10 000 births, but this figure is thought to be an underestimate of the actual incidence (JAMA 1991; 265:3270); routine screening for only anti-RhD and -D^u, causes a proportionate increase in anti-C, -c, E and -e related Rh disease, see RhIG; two other red cell antibodies potentially requiring exchange transfusions are anti-Fy^a and Kell Frequencies of HDN: ABO (mild, transient) > Rh-D > Rh-c > Rh-E > K (Kell); rarely incriminated in HDN are anti-PP$_1$, -Be^a, -K, -k, -Kp^a, -M, -S, -s, -U, -FAR, Mt^a, Js^a, Js^b, Jk^a, -Jk^b, -Fy^b, -Fy$_3$, Mv, -Lu^a, Di^a, -Di^{bm}, Yt^a, -Do^a, -Wr^a, -Jr^a, Cs^a; HDN has not been described due to anti-Le^a, -Le^b and anti-P$_1$ antibodies, as these are IgM and do not pass to the placenta; the serum half-life of IgG is 20-25 days and

---

HEMOLYSIS

INTRACORPUSCULAR HEMOLYSIS

Membrane defects, eg hereditary elliptocytosis, spherocytosis, stomatocytosis and paroxysmal nocturnal hemoglobinuria

Metabolic defects, eg G6PD, pyruvate kinase deficiency

Abnormal hemoglobins see Hemoglobin

EXTRACORPUSCULAR HEMOLYSIS

Immune reactions, primary, eg autoimmune hemolytic anemia

Immune reactions, secondary, due to

1) Infections, eg Bartonella, Clostridia, malaria, sepsis

2) Neoplasia, eg lymphoma, leukemias

3) Drug reactions due to the 'Innocent bystander' phenomenon (drug-antibody complex activates complement, causing intravascular hemolysis, eg quinidine), hapten-mediated (a protein-bound drug attaches to the red cell membrane, eliciting an immune response when the 'signature' of the hapten-protein complex is recognized as foreign, evoking an immune response, eg penicillin acting as a hapten

4) Induction of autoimmunity by red cells antigen alterations, eg Rh antigen

Physical, eg thermal, high concentrations of glycerol as in inadequate washing of frozen blood, bladder irrigation, cardiac valves

significant amounts of maternal immunoglobulin remain in the infant's circulation for up to 3 months after birth CLINICAL see Hydrops fetalis PATHOLOGY Placenta Large, edematous with immature red cells, lipid-laden pink Hofbauer cells in the stroma of the villi; basal ganglia kernicterus LABORATORY 'Panic' values of bilirubin are 16-20 mg/dl of indirect bilirubin; the immaturity of the blood-brain barrier allows penetration of bilirubin and deposition on the basal ganglia; in utero antibody titers above 1/32 may presage a difficult recovery period; prenatal Rh type can be determined prenatally by polymerase chain reaction in amniotic cells, a procedure of considerable use in the case of RhD-negative mothers who may be carrying RhD-positive fetuses against whose red cell antigens, the mother's immune system may form antibodies, leading in extreme cases to hydrops fetalis (**N Engl J Med 1993; 329:607oa**) Cf Hemorrhagic disease of the newborn

hemolytic-uremic syndrome A clinical complex often accompanied by a prodrome of bloody diarrhea, most commonly occurring in the summer and microangiopathic hemolytic anemia, thrombocytopenia and platelet abnormalities and not uncommon in infants < age two LABORATORY Impaired aggregation, depletion of platelet serotonin, ADP and β-thromboglobulin PATHOLOGY Renal arteries occluded by fibrin thrombi in the interlobular arteries, afferent arterioles and capillaries, widespread cortical necrosis, that may also involve the liver, brain, heart, islet cells and muscle PATHOGENESIS Uncertain, *Escherichia coli* O157:H7, which produces a 'verotoxin' has been implicated and in one enteric nursing home outbreak, 50% died

Note: HUS has been re-interpreted as a polar form of a clinical spectrum, at the other end of which is thrombotic thrombocytopenic purpura, see TTP-HUS

hemophagocytic syndrome HEMATOLOGY A clinically-defined condition characterized by the systemic proliferation of hemophagocytic histiocytes, often accompanied by fever, hepatosplenomegaly, and pancytopenia, most commonly in a background of angiocentric lymphoproliferative disorders, and occasionally lymphomas (**Arch Pathol Lab Med 1992; 116:1209oa**)

***Hemophilus influenzae* vaccine** see Hib

hemorrhagic disease of the newborn A neonatal condition caused by vitamin K deficiency, the combined result of a lack of unbound maternal vitamin K, immaturity of the fetal liver and lack of vitamin K-producing bacteria in the infant colon CLINICAL Abrupt early postpartum onset with spontaneous nasogastric or intracranial hemorrhage, affecting up to 1/1000 neonates and carrying a 5-30% mortality, if untreated; the condition is thought to be more common in breast-fed infants and is more severe and of earlier onset in infants of mothers receiving anticonvulsives (antagonistic to warfarin) during pregnancy LABORATORY Increased prothrombin time due to extrinsic factor depletion, inceased clotting time, decreased liver-dependent coagulation factors; Cf Hemolytic disease of the newborn

hemorrhagic fever with renal syndrome see Korean hemorrhagic fever

hemosiderosis An iron overload syndrome that is arbitrarily differentiated from hemochromatosis by the reversible nature of this accumulation in the reticuloendothelial system

hemostatic plug After tissue trauma and rupture of vessels, the platelets fill the gap, forming a plug; formation of a 'hemostatic plug' is an orderly process divided into stages

1) ADHESION Following tissue injury, collagen and basement membrane are exposed and serve as signals for platelets to 'huddle' about the open vessel

2) RELEASE Platelets come in contact with collagen and

are stimulated to release thrombin, epinephrine and ADP, releasing their granular contact

3) AGGREGATION ADP is released, promoting platelet aggregation that becomes irreversible as local ADP concentrations rise above $2 \times 10^{-6}M$

4) FUSION Fibrin, thrombin, ADP and Thromboxane A_2 cause coalescence of the plug

5) CLOT RETRACTION Fibrin threads contract, squeezing out the liquid caught in the meshwork

hemozoin An insoluble pigment formed from heme (Fe(II) protoporphyrin) by intraerythrocytic malarial parasites, which consists of Fe(III) protohematoporphyrin subunits that are formed by a chemical polymerization process in the parasites' digestive vacuole (**Nature 1995; 374:269L**)

HEMPAS Hereditary erythrocytic multinuclearity with

ETIOLOGY, HEMOLYTIC-UREMIC SYNDROME
1) Prototypic or 'classic' form
2) Post-infectious, eg *Shigella dysenteriae*-1, *Streptococcus pneumoniae*, *Salmonella typhi*, occasionally viruses
3) Hereditary forms: Autosomal dominant, or autosomal recessive associated with hypertension
4) Immune-mediated forms
5) Associated with other diseases, eg hypertension, connective tissue disease, immunosuppression or radiotherapy to kidneys
6) Related to pregnancy and oral contraceptives

---

positive acidified serum lysis Congenital dyserythropoietic anemia, type II An AR **[MIM 224100]** condition characterized by an IgM autoantibody directed against the red cell membrane i antigen ('anti-HEMPAS'), an antigen that is present in 1/3 of normal sera CLINICAL Mild or subclinical congenital dyserythropoietic anemia LABORATORY Normocytic aniso-poikilocytosis and multi-nucleated erythroblasts; ↑ agglutinability of serum with anti-i antibodies Note: A positive acidified serum lysis test may be seen in paroxysmal nocturnal hemoglobinuria TREATMENT None; splenectomy partially beneficial; see CDA

Henderson County epidemic An epidemic of chronic diarrhea that left an entire county on the edge of its seat that occurred in the 1980s, which was attributed to untreated water (**N Engl J Med 1995; 332:725rv**)

Henoch-Schönlein purpura An acquired form of small vessel vasculitis that is most common in younger age groups CLINICAL Raised red macules on the legs and buttocks, glomerulonephritis, abdominal pain that may be accompanied by infarction, diarrhea, fever, arthritis LABORATORY IgA deposits in the basement membrane of skin and glomerulus PROGNOSIS Generally self limited (**N Engl J Med 1994; 330:8347cpc**)

HEPA respirator High-efficiency particulate air filter respirator A device (cost/unit $7.51–disposable, $9.08–with replaceable filter) that filters particulate matter more effectively than simple isolation masks (SIM, cost/unit, $0.06) or dust-mist respirators (DMR, cost/unit, $0.92); because of the ↑ in multidrug-resistant TB, the CDC had proposed the use of HEPA respirators as part of isolation precautions against TB; a cost-effectiveness analysis at the U of Virginia concluded that adding by HEPA respirators to other methods used to prevent nosocomial transmission of TB, it would take 41 years to prevent a single case of occupationally acquired TB at a cost of $1.3-18.5 million (**N Engl J Med 1994; 331:169oa**)

Hepadnaviridiae A recently formed family of small DNA viruses with a circular genome that includes hepatitis B and hepatitis D (delta agent); Cf HHV

heparin A 4-30 kD, heavily-sulfated glycosaminoglycan anticoagulant that inhibits activated factors IXa, Xa, XIa, XIIa and thrombin, decreasing local anti-thrombin-III, promoting its inactivation by neutrophil elastase; the interaction of heparin with endothelial cells results in the displacement of platelet factor 4, which in turn inactivates heparin; heparin therapy is indicated for venous thromboembolism, coronary artery disease, and following acute MI (12 500 U bid) and pulmonary thromboembolism (10-15 000 U sid); heparinization is monitored by measuring aPTT, titrating heparin levels so that the aPTT is 1.5-2.0-fold normal SIDE EFFECTS Hemorrhage, thrombocytopenia, osteoporosis, skin necrosis, alopecia, hypersensitivity, hypoaldosteronism (**N Engl J Med 1991; 324:1565rv**); heparin prevents exercise-induced asthma without affecting histamine-induced bronchoconstriction, an effect attributed to modulation of mediator release rather than to a direct effect on bronchial smooth muscle (**N Engl J Med 1993; 329:900A**)

heparin-binding fibroblast growth factor(s) A family of seven related gene products with a broad range of biological activities including stimulation and inhibition of proliferative and secretory functions in hepatocytes (**Science 1991; 251:665**) see Pleiotrophin

heparin cofactor II A 66-kD protein produced in the liver which, like antithrombin III (heparin cofactor I), neutralizes thrombin and chymotrypsin, but not factor Xa or other coagulation factors; its activity is accelerated by dermatan sulfate and heparin; HC-II deficiency is associated with thromboembolic disease; HC-II is reduced in cirrhosis and DIC

heparin-induced thrombocytopenia An acquired thrombocytopenia affecting 1% of heparin-treated patients, which is induced by heparin-dependent antibodies against endothelial-bound heparin; HIT-like phenomena may occur in heroin addicts, in whom an IgG antibody induces thromboxane synthesis and platelet aggregation; the signs and symptoms of HIT appear 6-10 days after exposure to heparin and may be an immune response possibly with a precipitous drop in platelet count and/or thrombosis PATHOGENESIS The platelet-activating antibodies of HIT are either IgG or IgM and are specific for the heparin-PF4 (platelet factor 4) complex (**N Engl J Med 1995; 332:1374oA**); HIT is associated with thrombotic events and heparin-dependent IgG antibodies; HIT is less common in those treated with low-molecular-weight heparin ab initio (**N Engl J Med 1995; 332:1330oA**) DIAGNOSIS Aggregation studies using platelets from people known to be sensitive to the offending antibody; quantification of serotonin release from platelets radiolabeled with serotonin in an assay using patient serum (**Am Surg 1994; 60:26**)
*Also known as heparin-associated thrombocytopenia, heparin-induced thrombocytopenia and/or thrombosis

hepar lobatum A deformed lobated liver described in the currently rare end-stage tertiary syphilis PATHOLOGY Broad bands of fibrotic scar tissue coalesce and bridge poorly-healed small and large gummata, alternating with nodules and masses of well-normal preserved parenchyma, mimicking macronodular cirrhosis Note: Arsenic, the preantibiotic therapy for syphilis caused massive hepatic necrosis and obstructive cholangitis

hepatic ALTERNATIVE MEDICINE *noun* A medicinal preparation, usually of herbal origin that to 'tone' and strengthen the liver and ↑ the flow of bile and aid in hepatic detoxification CONVENTIONAL MEDICINE *adjective* Pertaining or referring to the liver

hepatic arterial infusion ONCOLOGY A transiently popular therapeutic modality used to treat liver metastases of various malignancies; the procedure requires major abdominal surgery to insert an expensive intra-arterial pump filled with the costly chemotherapeutic agent, floxuridine, allowing high concentrations of drug to be delivered directly to the metastatic tumors; while the frequency of tumor shrinkage is higher with HAI than with conventional systemic administration, the victory is pyrrhic in that the injury to the liver and bile ducts may be irreversible and accompanied by GI hemorrhage; HIA achieves neither substantive palliation nor improved survival in colorectal cancer and is essentially useless (**N Engl J Med 1994; 330:1136oA**)

hepatic encephalopathy NEUROLOGY A complication of hepatic failure that is linked to ↑ ammonia levels in the circulation, which may occur in a background of decompensated cirrhosis or portocaval anastomosis; the major morphologic change of HE is cerebral edema, which is associated with ↑ morbidity; the Mayo group has devised a CT-based system (the Brain Edema Severity Score) for classifying HE (**Mayo Clin Proc 1995; 70:119oA**); it is uncertain whether treatment of cerebral edema results in ↑ survival in patients with HE

hepatic fibrosis A common response to chronic liver injury caused by various agents, including alcohol, hereditary metal (copper, iron) overload, and infections (hepatitides and helminthiditides), and largely orchestrated by the hepatic lipocyte*; HF is characterized by an ↑ in extracellular matrix, forming a **hepatic scar** which consists of collagens I and III, and matrix glycoconjugates (proteoglycans, fibronectin and hyaluronic acid) (**N Engl J Med 1993; 328:1828oA**)
*aka Fat-forming cell, Ito cell, perisinusoidal cell, stellate cell; see Hepatic lipocyte

hepatic funtion panel LABORATORY MEDICINE A standard (**CPT-4 code 80058**) battery of laboratory tests used to evaluate the baseline status of the liver; for Medicare or Medicaid reimbursement, it must include a serum albumin, total or direct bilirubin, alkaline phosphatase, amino alanine transferase, and amino aspartate transferase (**CAP Today March 1993**)

hepatic panel Liver panel, see there

hepatic rickets Vitamin D-deficient rickets due to reduced bile salt secretion, resulting from inadequate absorption of fat-soluble vitamins, seen in extrahepatic biliary atresia, neonatal hepatitis and injury induced by parenteral nutrition, see Total parenteral nutrition LABORATORY ↓ Ca++, ↓ vitamin 25(OH)D, ↑ alkaline phosphatase

hepatic scar Hepatic fibrosis, see there

hepatitis A generic term for hepatic inflammation, classically caused by hepatitis A (HAV) and hepatitis B (HBV) viruses; HAV is usually acquired through the oral-fecal route, has a shorter incubation period and is rarely associated with long-term morbidity; HBV is usually acquired through parenteral contact, has a longer incubation period and is linked pathogenically to hepatocellular carcinoma ETIOLOGY Other viral hepatitides include hepatitis non-A, non-B (many of which are due to hepatitis C), hepatitis D (delta agent), hepatitis E, CMV, coxsackievirus, EBV, herpesvirus, infectious mononucleosis, measles, mumps, rubella, rubeola, bacteria, parasites and fungi Non-infectious hepatitides may be induced by hyperthermia, radiation, alcohol, toxins CLINICAL Anorexia, nausea, vomiting, malaise, jaundice, myalgia, arthralgia, photophobia, bleeding diathesis LABORATORY ↑ Transaminases (ALA, AST, GGT), bilirubin and immunoglobulins (specific if hepatitis is infectious) and decreased vitamin K- dependent coagulation factors, ergo prolonged prothrombin time

hepatitis A An acute rarely fatal disease of global distribution caused by a pironavirus; hepatitis A is a common cause of morbidity in both developing and developed (US cost ± $200 million) CLINICAL Fever, nonspecific GI malaise, hepatosplenomegaly, jaundice, pruritus LABORATORY ↑ Liver enzymes, dark urine AT-RISK GROUPS

Given the usual (oral-fecal) route of transmission, certain groups are at high risk, to wit, travelers, military personnel, institutionalized persons, day care center inmates, other children and adolescents, Native Americans, raw shellfish eaters, those engaging in 'high-risk' sexual practices VACCINE Formalin-inactivated hepatitis A vaccine is well tolerated; a single dose is effective against clinically apparent hepatitis A (N Engl J Med 1992; 327:453OA)

hepatitis B For 'conventional' details see standard texts MOLECULAR BIOLOGY Hepatitis B is a small DNA virus with four open reading frames: S gene encodes HbsAg, P gene encodes a DNA polymerase, an X gene and the core gene that encodes HBcAg and the pre-core region which encodes HBeAg; patients with fulminant hepatitis B have a point mutation that results in a stop codon in the pre-core region, implicating a mutant virus in non-self-limited hepatitis B (N Engl J Med 1991; 324:1699, 1705) SEROLOGY see Hepatitis immunopathology panel

hepatitis B vaccine Of the hepatitis B vaccines that became available during the 1980s, the human plasma-derived hepatitis B vaccine (Heptavax-B) proved unpopular, attributed in part to 'AIDS-phobia' and is no longer used; the yeast (*Saccharomyces cervesiae*)-derived recombinant DNA vaccine, (Recombivax™) has reported protective levels of close to 100% and those who do not respond initially may respond with intradermal vaccination by the same agent

hepatitis B virus protein X HBx, see there

hepatitis C The agent(s) responsible for most transfusion-induced hepatitides, which may play a role in the pathogenesis of hepatocellular carcinoma; EPIDEMIOLOGY In addition to blood-borne transmission, HCV can be transmitted vertically (from mother to infant), the risk of which is correlated with the titer of HCV RNA (N Engl J Med 1994; 330:744OA); cDNA from HCV was used to develop RIA for HCV antibodies, which detects ½ of cases; patients receiving HBC-positive blood products have a 20-fold ↑ of non-A, non-B hepatitis (NANBH); during the early or window period of primary HCV infection, the only evidence of disease may be HCV RNA in the serum; disappearance of HCV RNA from the serum correlates with the resolution of NANBH LABORATORY After screening for HCV (first with surrogate markers, then when available in 1990, screening for anti-HCV antibodies, the risk for seroconversion ↓ from 0.45%/unit transfused (UT) to 0.03%/UT (ibid 1992; 327:369OA) COMPLICATIONS Cryoglobulinemia, membranoproliferative glomerulonephritis, possibly related to intraglomerular deposition of immune complexes containing HCV, anti-HCV IgG, and IgM rheumatoid factors (ibid 1993; 328:465OA) MANAGEMENT IFN-α suppresses the TGF-β1-induced fibrosis typical of hepatitis C that could eventuate in cirrhosis in HCV-infected patients the response of HCV-associated cryoglobulinemia to IFN-α-2a is a function of the titers of HCV (ibid 1994; 330:51OA) EPIDEMIOLOGY ± 3.5 million people have chronic hepatitis C, of whom 8-10 000 die/year and 1000 have liver transplants (ibid 1995; 332:1509ED) TREATMENT 3 million units of IFN-α2b 3x/week x 18 months results in more significant histologic reversal and serum ALA response of NANBH (±90% of which are due to hepatitis C) than that seen with lower doses and/or shorter durations of therapy (ibid; 332:1457OA) PROGNOSIS 20% of people with post-transfusion hepatitis progresses to chronic hepatitis[1], cirrhosis[2], or hepatocellular carcinoma[3] (ibid; 332:1463OA)

[1]Time from transfusion to hepatitis, 10.0 years [2]Time to cirrhosis, 21.2 years [3]Time to hepatocellular carcinoma, 29.0 years (Hepatology 1990; 12:671) Note: Although they are not synonymous, many cases of nonA, nonB hepatitis are due to hepatitis C and there is considerable overlap between the two conditions; see nonA, nonB hepatitis

hepatitis D Delta hepatitis PATHOGENESIS HDV can reproduce in absence of HBV, but hepatic pathology may require HBV synergy (Am J Clin Pathol 1992; 98:554OA; 551ED); severe liver disease; cirrhosis develops in 60-70% of HDV-infected patients; it is rapidly progressive in 15% TREATMENT IFN-α-2a (9 million U, 3 x/week x 48 weeks) results in normalization of liver enzymes, disappearance of HDV RNA from serum, and histologic improvement; relapse occurs shortly after cessation of IFN therapy (N Engl J Med 1994; 330:88OA)

hepatitis D virus HDV A unique RNA virus that requires a helper function provided by hepatitis B virus (HBV); HDV is no longer considered a defective virus, as it can reproduce in absence of HBV coinfection, although production of hepatic disease may require HBV synergy (Am J Clin Pathol 1992; 98:554OA; 551ED)

hepatitis E virus HEV Enteric non-A, non-B hepatitis A virus with a highly conserved single-stranded RNA transmitted by the oral-fecal route and implicated in major epidemics where sanitation is poor, the drinking water contaminated and the population malnourished

hepatitis, giant cell neonatal see Giant cell hepatitis

hepatitis, non-A, non-B NonA, nonB hepatitis, see there

hepatitis panel LABORATORY MEDICINE A standard (CPT-4 code 80059) battery of laboratory tests that are the most efficient, ie cost-effective, in evaluating the clinical and immune status of a person with possible hepatitis; for Medicare or Medicaid reimbursement, the HP must include HBsAg, HBsAb, HBc-IgM, HBc-IgG, HAV-IgM, HAV-IgG and HCV Ab (see CAP Today March 1993); the acute HP includes hepatitis B surface antigen (HBsAg), anti-hepatitis B surface antigen (anti-HBs), antibody to hepatitis B core antigen (anti-HBc), anti-HBe, anti-hepatitis A (IgM) and anti-hepatitis C; the chronic hepatitis (carrier) panel includes the above but not anti-hepatitis A assay; Cf Organ panels

hepatitis serology Hepatitis B serological markers LABORATORY MEDICINE A generic term referring to hepatitis B antigens and antibodies to these antigens CORE ANTIGEN The HBc particle that contains double-stranded DNA and DNA polymerase, and is associated with the HBe antigen; HBc is not directly detected by currently-used assays; its presence indicates persistently replicating hepatitis B virus CORE ANTIBODY A long-term serologic marker for hepatitis B, that rises early and detectable as an IgM antibody, which remains elevated up to 20 years after infection, especially in those with active liver disease; partially protective anti-HBc antibody levels can be induced by recombinant vaccination, but are short-lived; IgM anti-HBc is the single best serological marker for acute hepatitis B infection e ANTIGEN An antigen that rises and falls parallel to HBsAg, and derives from the proteolytic cleavage of the nucleocapsid; its presence implies a carrier state e ANTIBODY anti-HBe An antibody that rises as HBe falls, appearing in convalescent patients, persisting for up to several years after resolution of hepatitis SURFACE ANTIGEN (HBs) is the first marker to appear after hepatitis B infection, preceding clinical disease by weeks, peaking with the onset of symptoms and disappearing six months post-infection ANTIBODY TO SURFACE ANTIGEN (anti-HBs, antibody to surface antigen) begins to rise as the HBsAg falls and may persist for life

hepatization A generic term for the transformation of a tissue that is normally fluffy to one with a liver-like consistency, classically described as an acquired firmness of the lungs, commonly seen in lobar pneumonia, especially that caused by *Streptococcus pneumoniae* types 1, 3, 7 and 2, as well as other streptococci, *Klebsiella* species, staphylococci, and gram-negative rods; hepatization occurs in the elderly and infants; in healthy adults lobar pneumonia is largely of historic interest that has been classically divided into

STAGE 1 Congestion

STAGE 2 Red hepatization, which occurs in early lobar pneumonia and is characterized by hemorrhage, fibrin accumulation and neutrophils within alveoli and fibrinopurulent pleural exudate

STAGE 3 Gray hepatization occurs before the first week, representing early resolution with leukocytes, indurated fibrinopurulent exudate and rare erythrocytes; the pleural surface is gray, dull and granular

STAGE 4 Resolution occurs after the first week

hepatoblastoma A malignant hepatic tumor almost exclusively found in infants that may be associated with hemihypertrophy, Wilms' tumor and glycogen storage disease DIAGNOSIS Hepatic angiography, computed tomography, elevated α-fetoprotein and ectopic hormone production PATHOLOGY The tumors are single, solid, well-circumscribed, with immature hepatocytic, fetal, embryonal, macrotrabecular or mixed patterns PROGNOSIS Better than hepatocellular carcinoma TREATMENT Surgery and adjunctive chemotherapy

hepatocellular carcinoma Hepatoma, liver cell carcinoma PATHOLOGY HCC displays cytoplasmic reactivity α1-antitrypsin, alpha-fetoprotein, and factor XIIIa; cholangiocarcinoma shows membranous and cytoplasmic reactivity for Le^x, and cytoplasmic reactivity for Leu-M1 and B72.3; tumors metastatic to the liver show and cytoplasmic reactivity for Le^x, and cytoplasmic and membranous reactivity for Leu-M1 and B72.3 (**Arch Pathol Lab Med 1994; 118:927OA**) RISK FACTORS 3-year cumulative risk for HCC is 12.5% in those with cirrhosis and 3.8% in those with chronic liver disease; HCC is 7-fold ↑ in those with HBsAg background, and 3-fold ↑ in those with hepatitis C antibody (figure may be low given the relative lack of sensitivity of the 'first-generation' assays) (**N Engl J Med 1993; 328:1797OA**) MOLECULAR PATHOLOGY Homozygous carriers of two functional *CYP2D6* genes are at ↑ risk of primary HCC (**N Engl J Med 1995; 332:1294ED**); postoperative recurrence by 5 years after resection reaches 80%, and is a function of adequacy of surgical margins, and detected by α-fetoprotein levels (**Arch Surg 1994; 129:738**) Cf V statistic

hepatocyte growth factor A plasminogen-like protein that is thought to act as a humoral mediator of hepatic regeneration; the HGF receptor is the protein product of the c-*met* proto-oncogene (**Science 1991; 251:802**)

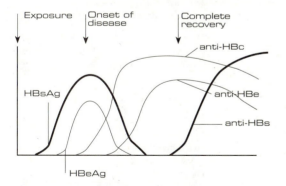

hepatitis serology

hepatocyte transplantation The grafting of hepatocytes in the liver to perform defective metabolic, immune, endocrine, and homeostatic activities; although in theory HT could be used to treat both acute and chronic liver failure, it appears to be bested suited for correcting genetic defects, eg alpha1-antitrypsin deficiency, biliary atresia, Dubin-Johnson syndrome, glycogen storage disease, hemochromatosis, Wilson's disease; HT has not (as of early 1995) been implemented in humans (**Sci & Med Nov/Dec 1994 p58**)

hepatoma Hepatocellular carcinoma, see there

hepatopulmonary syndrome A condition in which hypoxemia due to intrapulmonary shunting and/or a V/Q mismatch develops in a patient with liver cirrhosis; usually there is no apparent parenchymal lung disease, but patients may have orthodeoxia, an unusual finding of ↑ hypoxemia with a change from the supine to the erect position; the pathogenesis of HPS is uncertain but may be due to an ↑ production of endogenous nitric oxide; in one case, the pulmonary shunting of HPS responded to IV methylene blue (**N Engl J Med 1994; 331:1098c**)

hepatorenal syndrome A not uncommon complication of acute and chronic hepatic liver failure characterized by renal dysfunction without renal pathology, due to decreased renal perfusion, hypovolemia, and hyperaldosteronism, secondary to liver disease including acute liver failure due to cirrhosis, acute fatty liver, hepatic failure, obstructive jaundice, sepsis and infectious hepatitides Note: Kidneys from these patients may be used for transplantation; membranous nephropathy occurs in hepatitis B; ⅓ relentlessly deteriorate (**N Engl J Med 1991; 324:1457**) Cf Cirrhotic glomerulonephritis Note: The intense renal vasococonstriction (Vc) mediates a potentially irreversible form of acute renal failure; the Vc in HRS may be due in part to the marked elevation of endothelin-1 (36 ng/L vs 4 ng/L in normal subjects) and endothelin-3 (43 ng/L vs 18 ng/L) which are markedly elevated in HRS (**ibid 1992; 327:1774OA**); Vc may also in part be related to activation of the sympathetic and renin-angiotensin systems, endotoxin, and eicosanoid production

HEPES N-2-Hydroxyethylpiperazine-N'-ethanesulfonic acid An agent used to prepare biological buffers between pH 6.8 and 8.2

heptaspan A term recently proposed as a viable substitute for the unwieldy 'seven transmembrane spanning receptor' or the potentially confusing 'serpentine' receptor*; the author (**LL Brunton, University of California. San Diego**) proposes that all transmembrane spanning proteins be designated by the root form, –span, modified by a numerical prefix, as in monospan (adjective monospanning), a structural motif typical of many growth factor receptors, eg EGF receptor, heptaspan (adjective heptaspanning), a motif typical of G protein-linked receptors, eg β-adrenergic receptor, and dodecaspan (adjective dodecaspanning), eg adenylyl cyclase (**Nature 1994; 369:270c**)

*Dr Brunton observes, 'While this usage (ie serpentine receptor) conjures up the overall shape of such proteins, it does not distinguish among membrane proteins that may be equally serpentine, but that have other than seven transmembrane spans, it risks confusion with the mineral of the same name ($Mg_3Si_2O_5(OH)_4$), and it might even appear to suggest some devious receptor activity á la Satan and Eve of Biblical fame.'

HER-2/neu c-*erb*B-2 An oncogene of the *erb*B oncogene family, which is related to epidermal growth factor; HER-2 is amplified 2-20 fold in ⅓ of breast cancer and is associated with decreased survival and shortened time to relapse[1]; although the nomenclature has not been completely standardized[2], the term ERBB2 is increasing preferred

[1]Note: The prognosis of breast cancer is best predicted based on tumor size, number of lymph nodes involved and estrogen and progesterone receptor status [2]Note: Many names exist for the same gene or gene product and the choice about whether to write a gene, oncogene, or proto-oncogene in upper- and lowercase, italic or nonitalic forms, is often arbitrary-Author's note

herald bleed An episode of hemorrhage, often accompanied by abdominal pain, which may precede by hours to weeks a catastrophic hemorrhage; herald bleeds are characteristic of arterial-enteric fistulas with false aneurysms, often at the site of the proximal anastomosis of a prosthetic graft of the abdominal aorta

herald patch DERMATOLOGY A lesion typical of early pityriasis rosea consisting of a solitary oval, 1-10 cm annular macule with raised border and fine, adherent scales; the HP precedes by 7-10 days the other lesions, which are multiple, smaller, a dull red color and distributed along the lines of cleavage of the trunk in a Christmas tree or chevron fashion DDx Contact dermatitis, impetigo, secondary syphilis, psoriasis, and tinea corporis

herald state of leukemia A term referring to the nonspecific manifestations of dyshematopoiesis that precede the onset of AML, including anemia, which may be accompanied by weakness and pallor, malaise, exertional dyspnea and fever unrelated to infections

herald wave phenomenon EPIDEMIOLOGY The finding that the strains of influenza virus present in a population at the end of one season's epidemic are the same strains responsible for the next season's influenza syndromes

herbal medicine A somewhat nebulous term that can refer to alternative medicine‡, ethnomedicine‡, naturopathy‡, some unproven forms of herbal based-therapies, and unproven forms of cancer therapy, as well as the use of herbs as therapeutic agents

herb ALTERNATIVE MEDICINE A generic term for a plant or part thereof that may be used to produce a medicine[1], which encompasses roots, bark, stems, leaves, flowers, fruit, seeds, or other parts which can be used for its medicinal[2] value; according to the WHO, ¾ of the plant-derived pharmaceuticals are used in the same fashion as they were traditionally in the native cultures from which they were first identified (Alternative Medicine, Future Med Pub, Puyallup, WA, 1994) see Alternative medicine

[1]Flavor (eg spices) or fragrances [2]Flavoring or fragrance

herbal tea An infusion made from various plants, usually that do not contain caffeine; HTs are purported to have beneficial effect(s) on one or more organ systems in treating or ameliorating various conditions; some plants have toxic as well as tonic effects, affecting the cardiovascular system, GI tract, and CNS CHAMOMILE Anaphylactic shock, contact dermatitis COMFREY Veno-occlusive disease, hepatic failure, possible hepatic carcinogen FOXGLOVE (*Digitalis purpurea*) Malignant arrhythmia, cardiac arrest JIMSONWEED Atropinic and hallucinogenic effects, central nervous system intoxication, ataxia, blurred vision MANDRAKE Scopolaminic effect with anticholinergic blockade MATE Veno-occlusive disease with possibe hepatic failure POKE ROOT High saponin content causes gastroenteritis, bloody diarrhea POKEWEED Respiratory depression, mitogenic effects SASSAFRAS Hepatic carcinogen SNAKEROOT Reserpinic effect, causing CNS intoxication (Arch Environ Health 1987; 42:133) see Holistic medicine, Natural food, Organic food

hereditary angioneurotic edema HANE An immune complex-induced condition caused by a deficiency of C1q esterase inhibitor (C1q-INH) characterized by episodic consumption of activated C1, C4 and C2, triggered by physical stimuli (trauma, cold, vibration), histamine release, menstruation; fewer attacks occur in the last two trimesters of pregnancy CLINICAL Transient non-pitting, non-pruritic, non-urticarial swelling that peaks at 12-18 hours, affecting extremities, lips, face, fingers, toes, knees, elbows, buttocks, GI mucosa and oropharynx, causing potentially fatal epiglottic edema (33% mortality), often accompanied by abdominal pain with nausea and vomiting; angioneurotic edema has been divided into four types, two of which are congenital; HANE Type I Common (85%) with C1q-INH decreased to 30% of normal levels; HANE Type II Variant form The gene product is present but dysfunctional; type II may be 1) Acquired, associated with lymphoproliferative disorders, eg IgA myeloma, Waldenström's macroglobulinemia, CLL, and other B-cell proliferations or 2) Autoimmune associated with IgG1 autoantibodies, due to uncontrolled activation of C1s TREATMENT Androgens; see C1-INH

Note: Sir Wm Osler described the first case in a young woman over 100 years ago (Am J Med Sci 1888; 95:362)

hereditary cancer syndrome Any of a group of often AD conditions characterized by tumors that are often site-specific, of early onset and multiple and/or bilateral; these conditions include nevoid basal cell carcinoma syndrome, dysplastic nevus (B-K mole) syndrome, Cowden syndrome, familial polyposis, Gardner syndrome, Gorlin syndrome, Li-Fraumeni syndrome, MEN I, MEN II; see Hereditary neoplasms, Hereditary preneoplasia

hereditary degeneration BEHAVIORAL GENETICS An obsolete (circa 1857) posit that held that criminality, alcoholism, insanity, and feeblemindedness were all manifestations of a single 'traité des dégénérescences' (degenerative trait) that could originate in one generation (in a Lamarckian fashion, ie non-mendelian) through drink, poor working conditions, or lapses in morality (New York Times 15 Sept 1992; C1) see Crime genes

hereditary elliptocytosis An AD [MIM 130500] condition, affecting up to 1:2500 of the general population, in which 15% of the erythrocytes are ovoid; hemolysis is relatively uncommon, although it may be severe in 5% MOLECULAR PATHOLOGY The primary defect may lie in the protein scaffolding of membrane proteins, in particular spectrin (both α- and β-chains), which is quantitatively normal, but when isolated from cells, is present in the dimeric form, rather than tetramers, and higher order oligomers; defects have also been identified in proteins 4.1 and 3

hereditary hemorrhagic telangiectasia Rendu-Osler-Weber disease An AD [MIM 187300] condition characterized by telangiectases of mucocutaneous surfaces (tongue, nose, lips, hands, feet), resulting in episodic epistaxis in childhood, chronic GI hemorrhage, palmo-plantar, hepatic telangiectasias, and pulmonary arteriovenous malformations; telangiectasias may also be seen on the spleen, brain and spinal cord; rupture of the thin-walled vessels may result in hemorrhage of varying severity MOLECULAR GENETICS Candidate genes located on 9q33-34 include the gene for alpha-2 polypeptide chain of collagen V (*COLVA1*) and a member of the zinc-finger DNA regulatory-protein family (*ZNF79*) (Nat Genet 1994; 6:197, 205) TREATMENT Aminocaproic acid, an inhibitor of fibrinolysis (N Engl J Med 1994; 330:1789OA)

hereditary motor and sensory neuropathy A group of conditions dignified by eponym and subdivided into **TYPE I** CHARCOT-MARIE-TOOTH DISEASE, hypertrophic form An AD (type 1a [MIM 118220]; type 1b, [MIM 118200] or X-linked [MIM 302800]) condition that is the most common form of HMSN, characterized by a slowly progressive disease of childhood onset with predominantly motor symptoms, pes cavus, calf atrophy, very slow motor impulse conduction with segmental demyelination and remyelination with 'onion-bulb' formation **TYPE II** Roussy-Levy syndrome, or CHARCOT-MARIE-TOOTH DISEASE, neuronal form An AD [MIM 180800] condition characterized by slowly progressive disease of adolescent onset with predominantly motor symptoms, clubfoot deformity, calf atrophy, mild reduction in impulse transmission and 'onion-bulb' formation **TYPE III** DEJERINE-SOTTAS DISEASE A rare relentlessly progressive AD [MIM 145900] condition of infant onset with short stature, scoliosis, pes cavus, calf atrophy, very slow conduction of motor impulses with segmental demyelination and remyelination 'onion-bulb' formation; see Hereditary sensory neuropathy

hereditary neoplasia A generic term for any neoproliferation that appears to have a genetic component, which includes chemodectomas, medullary carcinoma of the thyroid, neurofibroma, pheochromocytoma, polyposis coli, retinoblastoma, trichoepithelioma; other tumors may occur more frequently in certain families, including leukemia and melanoma; see Hereditary cancer syndromes

hereditary neutrophilia A rare benign AD [MIM 162830] condition characterized by lifelong neutrophilia, hepatosplenomegaly, pseudo-Gaucher cells, thickened calvaria, ↑

leukocyte alkaline phosphatase (LAP score), ↑ vitamin B$_{12}$ (Am J Med 1974; 56:729)

hereditary nonpolyposis colon cancer Warthin-Lynch syndrome, Lynch I syndrome An AD [MIM 114500] form of cancer that may account for 5-10% of all colorectal carcinomas; it is thought to be a relatively distinct condition, which is most common in the proximal colon, and occurs more commonly at an early age and in multiple generations of a particular cohort MOLECULAR PATHOLOGY 2 genes are linked to HNPCC, the most important of which is hMSH-2, located on chromosome 2 (CAP Today March 1994, p1) see hMSH-2; Cf Familial adenomatous polyposis

hereditary palmoplantar keratoderma Tylosis A group of AD [MIM 148400] (the classic type was described by Unna and Thost) or AR [MIM 248300] (the classic type is known as Mal de Meleda) conditions characterized by palmo-plantar hyperkeratosis, the dominant form of which may be associated with oral leukoplakia and carcinoma of the lower ⅓ of the esophagus

hereditary persistence of fetal hemoglobin Hbα$_2$γ$_2$ An AD [MIM 142200] condition caused by a defect in the hemoglobin 'switch' mechanism, where the usual transition from γ to β chain production does not occur; in HPFH, the number of cells with Hb F in the maternal circulation is greater than the baby's total blood volume, and therefore the condition's presence may be suspected by mere calculations of maternal and fetal volumes; HPFH may be 1) Type I where there is uniform distribution of Hb F in all red cells, as in the Greek, Kenyan and Black American forms and 2) Type II where there is heterogeneous distribution of Hb F in all red cells, as in the British and Swiss forms; see Class switching, Fetal hemoglobin

hereditary preneoplasia A generic term for neoplasms that arise in the context of an underlying syndrome, including phacomatoses, eg Cowden's disease, multiple exostoses, Peutz-Jegher syndrome, von Hippel-Lindau syndrome, neurofibromatosis, tuberous sclerosis, genodermatoses, eg albinism, dyskeratosis congenita, epidermodysplasia verruciformis, polydysplastic epidermolysis bullosa, Werner syndrome, xeroderma pigmentosa, chromosome instability syndromes and immune deficiencies, eg ataxia-telangiectasia, common variable immunodeficiency, Wiskott-Aldrich syndrome, X-linked a-γ-globulinemia and X-linked lymphoproliferative syndrome; see Cancer families; Cf One-hit, two-hit model

hereditary pyropoikilocytosis HEMATOLOGY A rare AR [MIM 266140] congenital hemolytic condition that is most common in blacks, which is caused by impaired self-assembly of the spectrin tetramer in the red cell membrane; there are more dimers and defective forms and fewer multimers, resulting in increased membrane instability and susceptibility to thermolysis, occurring at circa 45°C, which in normal red cells occurs at 49°C; HP may represent a variant of hereditary elliptocytosis LABORATORY Anisocytes, elliptocytes, poikilocytes, schistocytes, microspherocytes and polychromasia, findings that resemble the peripheral blood smears in burn patients

hereditary sensory neuropathies A group of diseases with chronic pain, skin ulcers due to hypoesthesia, dyskinesis, autonomic dysregulation, loss of pain, touch-pressure and temperature sense, affecting the small nerves with degeneration of large myelinated nerves **TYPE I** AD [MIM 162400], characterized by perforating foot ulcers **TYPE II** AR [MIM 201300], characterized by early onset of mutilating ulcers, sensory loss and loss of tendon reflexes HSM **TYPE III** Riley-Day disease syndrome, familial dysautonomia AR [MIM 223900], affecting Jewish children, causing autonomic dysfunction, xerophthalmia, loss of temperature control, skin blotching, diaphoresis, hypertension, postural hypotension, pain insensitivity, poor feeding, vomiting, lung infec-

tions and early death, possibly related to defective nerve growth factor **TYPE IV** Familial dysautonomia, type II AR [MIM 256800], which overlaps features of type III; see Hereditary motor and sensory neuropathies

hereditary transmission EPIDEMIOLOGY The maintenance of an infection, usually viral, within the insect vector population through transovarial transmission; Cf Horizontal transmission, Vertical transmission

heritability The likelihood of suffering from a hereditary disease when the defective gene is in the patient's gene pool

hermaphroditic flukes Sexually self-contained worms that in humans may migrate and flourish in the

HEPATOBILIARY TRACT, eg *Clonorchis sinensis, Dicrocoelium dentriticum, Fasciola hepatica, Metorchis conjunctus, Opisthorchis* species

INTESTINE, eg *Echinostoma ilocanum, Fasciolopsis buski, Gastrodiscoides hominis, Heterophyes heterophyes, Metagonimus yokogawai*

LUNG, eg *Paragonimus westermani, P skrjabani* and

SYSTEMIC, eg *Alaria americana*

hermaphroditism A clinicopathological nosology characterized by the presence of both testicular tissue (ie seminiferous tubules) and ovarian tissue (ie follicular structures) in the same organ, yielding an 'ovotestis', in which the tissues are arranged end-to-end and may be accompanied by a left-sided ovary and a right-sided testis; 60% of patients are 46 XX, 12% 46 XY, the remainder are mosaics CLINICAL Most true hermaphrodites have asymmetrical external genitalia, eg labioscrotal folds; phenotypic males may have gynecomastia, phenotypic females may be amenorrheic or have successful gestation; 2.6% develop germ cell tumors; Cf Pseudohermaphroditism

herniated (intervertebral) disk Herniation of an intervertebral disk is most common in the lumbar region; the term herniation in this context has been loosely used to describe a broad spectrum of disk abnormalities; the following terms are used for MRI examinations of intervertebral disks

BULGE–circumferential symmetric extension of the disk beyond the interspace

PROTRUSION–focal or asymmetric extension of the disk beyond the interspace

EXTRUSION–more extreme extension of the disk beyond the interspace Note: Bulges and protrusions on MRI examination are common findings in normal subjects, and appear to be coincidental findings (N Engl J Med 1994; 331:69OA)

herniated disk 'syndrome' An acquired condition most commonly affecting active middle-aged adults, classically occurring after a minor trauma or tortion stress of the vertebral column, punctuated by the sensation of a 'snap', which corresponds to a prolapse of the nucleus pulposus into the nerve roots or spinal cord, causing progressive and distal radiation of pain; the backache subsides as the sciatica 'syndrome' develops with its sensorimotor consequences

'heroic' therapy Aggressive treatment of an often malignant disease that is regarded by a patient's care-givers as incurable with standard treatment at usual and prudent doses of toxic drugs; in **heroic surgery**, wider than normal resection margins are obtained, as a malignancy has spread beyond a resectable size, eg radical mastectomy; these therapies are performed in order to alleviate pain or improve the quality of life of the terminally ill; see All-American operation, Commando operation, Forequarter amputation

heroin Diacetyl morphine A semisynthetic narcotic drug that was formulated and commercially marketed in 1898, one year before aspirin was introduced; the adverse effects of heroin abuse include sepsis, shock and systemic pathology CARDIOVASCULAR *Staphylococcus aureus* endocarditis, especially right sided and tricuspid valve LIVER

Viral hepatitis (HAV, HBV, HCV/non-A,non-B hepatitis, HDV, HEV) Lungs Pulmonary edema, due to direct heroin toxicity to capillaries or myocardium, hypoxic endothelial damage, CHF, central vasomotor effect ($\uparrow$ protein in edema fluid) Skin Track marks and circular scars with necrotic ulcers Pathology Hypoxic endothelial damage and asteroid body formation (heart), non-specific anoxic changes (brain), focal membranoproliferative glomerulonephritis and glomerulosclerosis, periglomerular fibrosis, basement membrane thickening, nephrotic syndrome, IgM and C3 deposition within vessels (kidney), chronic nonspecific portal 'triaditis', chronic active hepatitis with septal fibrosis, piecemeal necrosis, lobular inflammation, chronic persistent hepatitis and non-specific hepatitis (liver), hypoxia, edema and talc granulomas (lung), musculoskeletal system (acute rhabdomyolysis, septic arthritis, chronic osteomyelitis) and regional lymphadenopathy with chronic non-specific hyperplasia due to injected contaminants; see Brown heroin, Opium

heroin

HERP index Human exposure/rodent potency index Risk assessment A formula that extrapolates the data obtained from toxicologic studies of potential carcinogens in food or other ingested substances in the rodent and attempts to determine the daily amount that must be ingested by humans to induce a similar carcinogenic effect; see Risk assessment; Cf Ames test

herpesvirus A family of DNA viruses with a central icosahedral (containing 162 capsomeres) core of double-stranded DNA, a trilaminar 100 nm in diameter lipoprotein envelope, a 30-43 nm in diameter nucleus and prolonged dormancy, lasting up to years; seven (and possibly eight) human herpes viruses (HHV) have been identified

(human) herpesvirus-1 HHV-1 Herpes simplex-1 A herpesvirus that typically affects the body above the waist, and is responsible for most cases of oral herpes and fever blisters, and is often accompanied by stomatitis, conjunctivitis, necrotizing meningoencephalitis, encephalitis Portal of entry Fibroblast growth factor receptor

(human) herpesvirus-2 HHV-2 Herpes simplex-2 A herpesvirus that most commonly is sexually transmitted (only 5% of venereal herpes is caused by HHV-1, and is uncommon under age 15) and predominantly affects the body below the waist, causing venereal, vulvovaginal and penile herpetic ulcers; HHV-2 is more often prevalent in multiply married, female, black city dwellers with lesser educations; HHV-1 and HHV-2 have a 50% homology and may bind to different membrane receptors, generally transmitted by contact; one form, Kaposi's varicelliform eczema herpeticum is potentially fatal and seen in atopic individuals Herpes in pregnancy Early gestational infection may cause spontaneous abortion, while the products of late gestational infection suffer microcephaly, mental retardation, retinal dysplasia and hepatosplenomegaly; recurrence rate in subsequent pregnancies approaches 70%; HS-2 causes most neonatal herpes, infecting via the birth canal; the infants are healthy at birth and become symptomatic 1-4 weeks post-partum Early neonatal herpes causes vesiculo-bullous lesions (absent in 20%), lethargy, irritability, hypotonia and loss of gag and sucking reflexes; late neonatal herpes may cause generalized seizures, jaundice, hypotension, DIC, acidosis, apnea, thrombocytopenia, and shock Diagnosis ELISA linked to an amplification culture system, complement fixation, RIA, culture in fetal fibroblasts, fluorescent antibody against membrane antigen; RFLP (restriction fragment length polymorphism) analysis allows epidemiologic tracking of sources of infection Cytopathology Stage 1 Granular chromatin Stage 2 Multinucleated giant cells with 'ground glass' chromatin, where the 'grains' correspond to viral particles, 50-200 000 viruses per infected cell Stage 3 Inclusion bodies surrounded by a halo, Cf HBLV Molecular biology The double-stranded DNA viral genome is 108 kD, with many guanine and cytosine nucleotides, having therefore a high GC:AT ratio; the herpes genome encodes 60-70 gene products divided into α, β and γ genes, based on the timing of their expression after infecting the host cell: the γ genes are 'late expressors', require previous production of the 'early' α and β proteins and encode structural proteins; HS-1 and HS-2 remain latent for years once the viral DNA is integrated into the host DNA, and are usually confined to the sensory nerves; the latency may be due to the presence of a mirror image of the viral protein ICPO (infected-cell protein zero) that 'commandeers' host cell replicative machinery, producing virions Treatment Antiviral agents, eg cytosine arabinoside (5-iodo-2'-deoxyuridine), adenine arabinoside (Acyclovir) and trifluorothymidine (Trifluidin) shorten the duration of an attack

herpesvirus-3 HHV-3 Herpes varicella-zoster has two clinical forms: Acute HHV-3 infection (chickenpox) and chronic HHV-3 infection (shingles)

herpesvirus-4 HHV-4 Epstein-Barr virus, see there

herpesvirus-5 HHV-5 Cytomegalovirus, see there

herpesvirus-6 HHV-6 Human B cell lymphotropic virus measures 200 nm and transforms infected B-cells into enlarged refractile mono- or binucleated cells, generating abundant extracellular virus from infected cells, seen as cytoplasmic and nuclear inclusion bodies; many HHV-6 isolates have been from AIDS patients and HHV-6 is synergistic with HIV-1 as both have affinity for CD4 T cells and activate HIV-1's long terminal repeat sequence; HHV-6 may be a co-factor in the pathogenesis of AIDS, as it both upregulates expression of the CD4 receptor in neoplastic T-cell lines and induces de novo expression of the CD4 receptor in CD8 cells, rendering them susceptible to HIV (Nature 1991; 349:533); although usually benign, HHV-6 may cause malignant fulminant hepatitis (N Engl J Med 1991; 324:1290c) and roseola (exanthema subitum) with acute infectious mononucleosis-like symptoms; HHV-6 is a major cause of febrile seizures, emergency department visits (10% of visits in first 2 years of life and 20% of visits age 6-12 months), and hospitalization; perinatal transmission may result in asymptomatic, persistent, or transient neonatal infection (ibid 1994; 331:432oa); it may be fatal in patients undergoing BM transplantation (ibid 1994; 330:1329oa); HHV-6 infects 90% of the US early in life, causing a fever and rash, it is a major cause of acute febrile illness in young children, and may be associated with varied clinical manifestations, and viremia; the persistence of HHV-6 in the DNA of mononuclear cells and saliva implies that infection is lifelong; increased concentration of HHV-6 DNA occurs in idiopathic pneumonitis in immunocompromised patients, eg bone marrow recipients with graft-versus-host disease, which may be due to reactivation (N Engl J Med 1992; 329:156oa)

herpes virus 7 An as-yet poorly characterized γ-type herpes virus with a $\pm$ 145 Kbp x 10^6 genome that has been associated with roseola infantum (exanthem subitum) and like HHV-6 (HHV-6A and HHV-6B), replicates within CD4+ T cells (GL Mandell, JE Bennett, R Dolin, Eds, Principles and Practice of Infectious Diseases, 4th ed, Churchill-Livingstone, New York, 1995)

herpes virus 8 see Kaposi sarcoma-related herpesvirus

herpes gestationis Duhring-Brocq disease A rare pruritic, polymorphic, subepidermal bullous dermatitis of preganancy, which occurs in 1:10 000 deliveries, and is associated with ↑ infant mortality; it tends to recur with subsequent pregnancies and may be activated by oral contraceptives PATHOGENESIS Uncertain, although probably immune-mediated PATHOLOGY Edema, hyperemia, ↑ eosinophils in dermis IMMUNOFLUORESCENCE Linear C3 (C1q, C4 and properdin) and IgG occur in 50% of cases TREATMENT Corticosteroids

herpes gladiatorum Trumatic herpes Herpes simplex-1-induced lesions of the eyes and skin of the head, neck, trunk, or extremities, accompanied by lymphadenopathy, sore throat, fever, chills and headache, described in modern 'gladiators', eg wrestlers and rugby players (see N Engl J Med 1992; 327:821c) Cf Tinea gladiatorum

herpes zoster Human herpesvirus-3 A condition caused by the (re)activation of the varicella-zoster virus which is latent in the sensory ganglia after primary infection CLINICAL Radicular neuralgic pain, varicella-like vesicular eruptions that follow the dermatomes; the lesions are more frequent and severe in the immunocompromised THERAPY ↑ Acyclovir therapy to 21 days and/or addition of prednisolone offers only a marginal benefit and does not reduce the frequency of postherpetic neuralgia (N Engl J Med 1994; 330:896OA)

herpetic giant cell A cell with multiple nuclei, due to cell fusion induced by infection with Herpes simplex that may be seen in a Tzanck preparation (smear of fluid obtained from a skin vesicle)

herpetic whitlow An acute herpes simplex-induced paronychia that may occur in occupationally-exposed health care workers, eg nurses on neurosurgical units, appearing as periungual blisters with a honeycombed appearance, later becoming purulent and accompanied by regional lymphadenopathy; see Whitlow

herringbone pattern A descriptor for the arrangement of malignant fibroblasts when viewed by low-power light microscopy, where the elongated nuclei are positioned at sharp angles to each other in linear arrays, a pattern characteristic of fibrosarcoma, which has also been seen in malignant schwannomas and in benign nodular fasciitis; a herringbone pattern is composed of rows of parallel lines with adjacent rows slanting in reverse direction

Her's disease Glycogen storage disease, type VI; Cf His disease

HES Hydroxyethyl starch TRANSFUSION MEDICINE A synthetic starch that is added to the input line during leukapheresis to promote red cell rouleaux formation, which facilitates their separation from leukocytes SIDE EFFECTS Minimal and limited to occasional urticarial and anaphylactoid reactions due to slow elimination, patients requiring granulocyte transfusions should be monitored with erythrocyte sedimentation rates; HES has been used as a cryopreservative for frozen packed red cells, but glycerol is preferred; see Colloid solutions; Cf DMSO (dimethylsulfoxide)

hetastarch Hydroxyethyl starch An artificial colloid that has been extensively used in Europe as an inexpensive and effective plasma expander and resuscitation medium; it has not been widely used in the US as it evokes anaphylactoid and anaphylactic reactions and because its long-term effects are unknown as it is retained in the reticuloendothelial system

HETE 8, 15-dihydroxyeicosatetraenoic acid PHYSIOLOGY A leukotriene precursor formed in the 15-lipoxygenase pathway of arachidonic acid metabolism within eosinophils that is similar in potency to leukotriene B_4 for neutrophil chemotaxis

heterochromatin GENETICS A cytologically visible form of condensed chromatin that remains tightly coiled during interphase, which is capable of repressing genes in eukaryotic cells; heterochromatin can be

FACULTATIVE, arising from inactivation or 'lyonization' of one of the X chromosomes, the Barr body that corresponds to a 'clump' of heterochromatin and

CONSTITUTIVE, where the heterochromatin is integral to each chromosome, located adjacent to the centromeres, telomeres, in the long arm of the Y chromosome and contains highly repeated DNA sequences

heterocyclic amine One of a family of potentially carcinogenic compounds present in grilled meat, which include PhIP and AαC, compounds that volatalize and may represent a risk factor for malignancy in 'short-order' cooks (Science News 1994; 146:103)

heterodisomy Inheritance of two different copies of an allele, gene, or chromosome from one parent

heterogeneous nuclear RNA A 5–15-kilobase segment of RNA that is confined to the nucleus and is the presumed precursor of messenger RNA; hnRNA and mRNA are similar in structure and both may be transcribed by RNA polymerase II; hnRNA is associated with proteins (hnRNP) and like snRNPs (small nuclear ribonucleic proteins) may have a role in splicing, an activity that results in mRNA maturation

heterophile antibody An antibody, usually an IgM 'agglutinin' that is produced in one species (of animals) and capable of reacting against the antigens (usually red cells) of another, phylogenically unrelated species; HAs are classically observed in humans with infectious mononucleosis (IM) where the antibodies react against sheep erythrocytes; high titers of HAs also occur in serum sickness; the two conditions are differentiated by adsorbing the serum with beef red cells (bearing the so-called Forsemann antigen) and retesting; the sera of infectious mononucleosis no longer react

Heterophyes A genus of minute (1-3 mm) intestinal trematodes (flukes) that may parasitize humans ingesting poorly or uncooked fish, eg sushi, occurring in Southeast Asia, Egypt and India; the worms adhere to the small intestinal mucosa by a ventral sucker CLINICAL Diarrhea and abdominal pain TREATMENT Praziquantel

heterosexism PSYCHIATRY The belief that heterosexual activities and institutions are superior to those with a genderless or homosexual orientation (N Engl J Med 1994; 331:923SA) see Homophobia

heterosexual *adjective* Pertaining or referring to heterosexuality *noun* An individual who is heterosexually oriented or sexually prefers those of the opposite sex

heterosexuality A state of sexuality directed to those of the opposite sex individual who is heterosexually oriented or sexually prefers those of the opposite sex

heterosis Hybrid vigor The greater fertility and strength of progeny obtained when highly inbred strains are crossed; the vigor is partially attributed to the elimination of homozygous traits that are deleterious to survival of each parent cell; Cf Bottlenecks, Consanguinity, Inbreeding

heuristic method A form of problem solving based not on scientific proof but rather on plausible, possible, or creative conclusions to questions that cannot be answered in the context of, or the 'logic' of which lies outside of, a currently accepted scientific paradigm; the heuristic process is of use as it may stimulate further research; Cf Aunt Millie approach, Stochastic method

HEXA gene A gene that encodes the α unit of hexosaminidase A, the enzyme deficient in Tay-Sachs disease; three different mutations account for 98% of Tay-Sachs disease (GM-2 gangliosidosis, type 1), two of which cause infantile Tay-Sachs, the third causing adult Tay-Sachs (79% have exon 11 insertion, 18% have intron 12 splice-junction mutation and 3% have the less severe disease characterized by an exon 7 mutation); DNA-based analysis of the HEXA gene is more specific and has a higher predictive value than the currently used enzyme test for hexosaminidase A

HEXB gene A gene that encodes the β chain of hexosaminidase A and both β chains of hexosaminidase B

hexachlorophene An antibacterial agent used as a preoperative scrubbing solution and as a detergent; its use is contraindicated in premature infants, as it is associated with neurotoxicity; Cf Gasping syndrome

Heymann glomerulonephritis A membranous glomerulonephritis animal model that is induced by immunizing rodents with proximal tubule brush border homogenates containing subepithelial antigen or the 330-kD Heymann factor in Freund's adjuvant; granular subepithelial (lamina rara interna) immune complex deposition may be detected on the glomerular basement membrane by immunofluorescence

HFC Hydrofluorocarbon ENVIRONMENT Any of a family of ozone-friendly compounds intended to replace the ozone-unfriendly CFCs (chlorofluorocarbons); the complete phasing-out of the use and production of CFCs will require development of alternative refrigerants and refrigeration systems; HFC substitution is likely to play a minor role (estimate, 15%) in the CFC replacement process, as will HCFCs (estimate, 11%) (New York Times 11 Jan 1994; C5) Cf CFC

HFG syndrome Hand-foot-genital syndrome, see there

Hfr cell High frequency of recombination MOLECULAR BIOLOGY A conjugating organism, eg *Escherichia coli* with its DNA-exchanging equipment in 'overdrive' because the episomal fertility factor is integrated into the bacteria's chromosome

HFU syndrome Hand-foot-uterus syndrome, see Hand-foot-genital syndrome

HGSIL High-grade squamous intraepithelial lesion, see there

HGBF see Heparin-binding fibroblast growth factor family

HGP-30 An experimental AIDS vaccine (based on a synthetic HIV core protein, p17); HGP-30 has been added to the growing list of failed AIDS vaccines

HGPRT see Hypoxanthine guanine phosphoribosyl transferase

HHH syndrome An AR [MIM 238970] condition of early childhood to late adulthood onset characterized by hyperornithinemia, postprandial hyperammonemia and homocitrullinemia, caused by a defect in ornithine transport from the cytoplasm into the mitochondria (where the urea cycle occurs) CLINICAL Chronic vomiting, repeated neurological 'attacks' after high-protein meals, resulting in seizures, failure to thrive, lethargy, ataxia, choreoathetosis, acute episodic hyperammonemia, or coma, moderate to severe growth and mental retardation PATHOGENESIS Unknown, although ornithine decarboxylase or mitochondrial transport of ornithine is possibly involved EM Bizarre, elongated mitochondria with crystalloid inclusions TREATMENT Protein restriction, dietary supplements with ornithine or arginine

HHHH syndrome Hereditary hemihypotrophy hemiparesis hemiathetosis syndrome An X-linked [MIM 306960] condition characterized by congenital hemiparesis, hemihy-

poplasia and athetoid posturing of same-sided hand

HHHO syndrome Hypomentia, hypogonadotrophic hypogonadism, muscular hypotonicity and obesity A clinical complex seen in Prader-Willi syndrome which is often accompanied by short stature, adult-onset diabetes mellitus, acromicria (small hands and feet), micrognathia, strabismus, fish-like or Cupid's bow mouth, clinodactyly, absence of auricular cartilage and hypoventilation with pulmonary hypertension

HHT Hereditary hemorrhagic telangiectasia, see there

HHV Human herpes virus, see Herpes virus

hiatal hernia Herniation of the esophagogastric junction affects up to 1% of the population, 5% of whom are symptomatic and is divided into

SLIDING HIATAL HERNIA 90% of cases, characterized by axial displacement of the esophagogastric (EG) junction in the cranial direction, where it slides in and out of the chest depending on changes in the intrathoracic and intraabdominal pressures; the sliding hernia is ensheathed in its own peritoneal sac TREATMENT Symptomatic cases are repaired by surgically returning the distal esophagus back to the peritoneal cavity with a valvoplasty

PARA-ESOPHAGEAL HIATAL HERNIA Less common and often accompanied by a sliding component; pure hiatal hernias are rare and associated with chronic hemorrhage and gastric volvulus, both indications for surgical repair

Hib *Hemophilus influenzae*, type b A bacterium responsible for 20 000 infection-related hospitalizations/year (US) most common < age 5, up to 5% mortality; prevalence in infants, 275/10⁶; the polysaccharide vaccine (HibVac) licensed in 1985 had a low efficacy attributed to its limited immunogenicity; anti-Hib vaccine composed of Hib's capsular polysaccharide covalently linked to a carrier protein (polyribosylribitol-diphtheria toxoid or PRP-D) provided 94% protection to a cohort of Finnish infants and 35% protection to Eskimo infants; the lower immunogenicity of the PRP-D has been surpassed by PRP-tetanus toxoid which provides up to 75% protection; the PRP-diphtheria toxoid vaccine is reported to be 88% effective (JAMA 1991; 265:987)

hibernation PHYSIOLOGY A state of winter dormancy that classically occurs in bears, as well as some rodents (eg chipmunks, ground squirrels), birds (eg nighthawks, swifts), and bats; most hibernating animals 'overfeed' in autumn, which serves to increase the amount of brown fat; some may store food nearby, as the periods of prolonged sleep (known as bouts) are punctuated by periods of wakefulness during which the stored food is consumed*; hibernation is characterized by hypothermia and occurs as part of the life cycle of both some warm-blooded animals, as well as many poikilotherms (eg frogs, turtles, snakes)

*Homo sapiens did not apparently invent the 'midnight snack'

hibernating myocardium Regional dysfunction of myocardial tissue due to prolonged local hypoperfusion, which is completely reversible upon restoration of adequate blood flow; hibernation occurs in patients with coronary artery disease and impairment of left ventricular function at rest ; Cf 'Stunned' myocardium, Thallium imaging

hibernoma A benign, well-circumscribed and asymptomatic tumor measuring 5-10 cm, consisting of a proliferation of brown fat cells, which occurs in neck and shoulder of young adults PATHOLOGY Lobules of rounded granular and/or vacuolated acidophilic cells PROGNOSIS No recurrence TREATMENT Excision

hiccup Hiccough, singultation An abrupt inspiratory muscle contraction, followed within 35 msec by closure of the glottis; the hiccup center is located in the spinal cord between C3 and C5; the afferent impulse is carried by the vagus and phrenic nerves and the thoracic sympathetic chain; the efferent impulse is carried by the phrenic nerve with branches to the glottis and accessory respiratory muscles; many conditions elicit hiccups, including gastric distension, GI hemorrhage or inflammation, abrupt temperature change, alcohol, inferior wall MI, irritation of tympanic membrane, diaphragmatic irritants, excess smoking, excitement or stress, toxins, metabolic defects, eg azotemia, hyponatremia, uremia, pharmacologics, eg general anesthesia, barbiturates, diazepam, α-methyldopa, tumors, pneumonia, herpes zoster, central and peripheral nervous system disease (encephalitis, brainstem infarcts, phrenic nerve compression); intractable hiccupping may result in inability to eat or sleep, may cause arrhythmia or reflux esophagitis, or may be compatible with a normal life*; no hiccup therapy gives consistent results, but chlorpromazine (a dopaminergic blocker) and diphenhydramine may be as effective as (and more dignified than) standing on one's head; other dopaminergic blockers include haloperidol, metoclopramide and apomorphine; rare cases may respond to amantidine, amitriptyline, carbamazepine, nifedipine, baclofen, ketamine, and phenytoin, and lidocaine, which has fewer side effects (N Engl J Med 1993; 329:890c)

*The most recalcitrant known case of hypersingultation occurred in an American pig farmer, which began in 1922, and continued to 1987

Hickman catheter NUTRITION An indwelling silicone elastomer device used to allow long-term IV access for the administration of total parenteral alimentation, hyperalimentation, blood products, drugs, or high-dose chemotherapy; the distal IV portion is inserted into the superior vena cava or right atrium via either the external jugular or cephalic veins; the extravascular portion exits outside the body via a tunnel between the nipple and sternum and is surrounded by a Dacron cuff intended to facilitate fibroblast ingrowth (thereby anchoring the catheter) and prevent microorganisms tracking from outside the body; infections occur at a rate of 0.14/100 catheter days (GL Mandell, JE Bennett, R Dolin, Eds, Principles and Practice of Infectious Diseases, 4th ed, Churchill-Livingstone, New York, 1995) Cf Port-A-Cath

'hide-bound' skin A descriptor for the smooth shiny indurated skin associated with adherent fibrosis and sclerosis that 'glues' the subcutaneous tissue to underlying structures, classically described in scleroderma

HIE Hyperimmunoglobulin E syndrome, see there

hierotherapy Prayer therapy; see Christian Science

HIG Human immune globulin, see there

'high' SUBSTANCE ABUSE A generic term for any state of pleasant and/or manic euphoria that is often a desired end-point for users of narcotics, hallucinogens or other potentially addicting substances of abuse; while a subject is high, he may experience megalomania and commit acts that may be in wanton disregard for the safety of himself and others; a 'high' may be evoked by alcohol, amphetamines, cocaine, heroin, LSD, marijuana and others; see Bad trip, 'Stoned'

high altitude acclimatization Höhendiurese, see there, Mountain sickness

high-altitude pulmonary edema A clinical complex caused by rapid ascent of unacclimatized individuals to altitudes above 2000-2500 meters that is accompanied by headache, insomnia, dyspnea and tachycardia; see Höhendiurese, Mountain sickness

high amplitude swelling PATHOLOGY An intracellular finding seen by electron microscopy indicative of irreversible hypoxia-induced cell death, which causes a shut-down of the calcium pump and consists of vacuolization of mitochondrial cristae, accompanied by aggregates of amorphous densities, disruption of the outer limiting membrane and nuclear pyknosis

'high-ceiling' diuretics see Loop diuretics

high disseminator EPIDEMIOLOGY A subject who is the carrier of a highly virulent and easily transmissible infectious agent, eg *Salmonella typhi*, transmitted by a cook infelicitously known as Typhoid Mary who was responsible for more than ten epidemics of typhoid fever; in the current AIDS epidemic, high dissemination is thought to be more common among heterosexuals and related to the virulence of the strain of HIV; see Typhoid Mary; Cf Fabian Bridges

high-dose epinephrine EMERGENCY MEDICINE A 'megadose' of epinephrine (15 mg vs 1 mg for standard therapy) used as an initial treatment of prehospital cardiac arrest (PCA); HDE significantly improves the rate of return of spontaneous circulation and hospital admission in patients in PCA, but the increase in (live) discharge rate is not statistically significant (JAMA 1992; 268:2667oA)

'high dry' field A colloquial term used by pathologists for 400X (of less commonly, to 600X) magnification, the combined result of a 10X ocular and 40X objective; 'high dry' fields are generally used to study nuclear details and to count mitotic figures; the maximum obtainable resolution by light microscopy without resorting to immersion oil is 1200X, using a 15X ocular and a 60X 'dry' objective; Note: 25-40x magnification is referred to as 'scanning power'; 100X is known as 'low power' and 1000X is termed 'oil power'

high-efficiency particular air filter respirator HEPA respirator, see there

high endothelial venules Postcapillary venules that are located in the paracortical region of lymph nodes and in the GALT (gut-associated lymphoid tissue, eg Peyer's patches); HEVs contain specialized columnar cells with receptors for antigen-sensitized lymphocytes, providing the main signal for the egress of lymphocytes from the circulation; lymph nodes have a 'homing' receptor for circulating lymphocytes involving ubiquitin; synovial HEV receptors are distinct from lymphoid HEV receptors, implying 'specialization' within the lymphoid tissue

high-energy bond BIOCHEMISTRY A covalent bond that serves as a ubiquitous intracellular 'storage battery', as hydrolysis of these bonds provides the energy necessary to activate various enzymatic reactions; high-energy bonds are most efficiently formed during aerobic glycolysis and are often attached to phosphate groups, eg ATP, ADP, NADP and NADPH and designated by a 'squiggle' ($\sim$) shape

high-energy phosphate Any phosphate (PO_4)-containing compound which has one or more energy-rich (21 to 54,400 J/mol) phosphate bonds, eg ATP, ADP, cyclic AMP, ITP, GTP, NADP, phospho-creatinine and acetyl phosphate; high energy phosphate bonds form during energy-releasing reactions, eg glycolysis, and serve as intracellular stores of energy required for synthetic reactions

high frequency antigen Public antigen TRANSFUSION MEDICINE An antigen present on the surface of erythrocytes in such a high percentage of the population that antibodies to these antigens are rare, thereby presenting difficulties in identification; high frequency antigens include AT[a], Co[a], Dib, Ge, Gy[a], Hy, K and Kell group antigens including Js[b], Kp[b], Kelly, Lan, Sc₁ (Sc₂ or Bu[a] is a low frequency, probably allelic), SD[a], Vel, Yk[a], Yt[a] and Yus

high-grade lymphoma A group of aggressive lymphomas that respond poorly to chemotherapy and comprise 20% of all lymphomas classified by the Working Formulation (Cancer 1982; 49:2112); high-grade lymphomas include diffuse large cell immunoblastic lymphoma, lymphoblastic lymphoma and the diffuse small, non-cleaved cell lymphoma, which includes the Burkitt's lymphoma and non-Burkitt's lymphomas Note: High-grade lymphomas have a mean survival of < one year without therapy, but may respond well to therapy; see Lymphoma, Working Formulation

high-grade squamous intraepithelial lesion GYNECO-LOGIC CYTOLOGY A lesion defined by an array of cytopathologic findings (cells occur singly or in syncytia-like sheets, increased nuclear:cytoplasmic ratio, nuclear hyperchromasia) that translate into moderate-to-severe dysplasia (CIN 2 to 3/carcinoma in situ) of the uterine cervix (a diagnosis made on histologic examination of biopsied tissue); in contrast to low-grade squamous intraepithelial lesion, the diagnosis of HSIL requires that the clinician take further action, usually to excise a portion of the cervix by cone biopsy, or by LEEP (RJ Kurman, D Solonmon, The Bethesda System, Springer-Verlag, New York, 1994) Cf Low-grade squamous intraepithelial lesion

high-impact sport SPORTS MEDICINE A generic term for any physical activity or sport in which there is intense and/or frequent wear and trauma of weight-bearing joints, in particular the foot, knee, and hip; HISs include baseball, basketball, football, handball, hockey, karate, racquetball, running, soccer, and waterskiing; participation is HIS activities is discouraged after hip and knee arthroplasty (Mayo Clin Proc 1995; 70:342OA) Cf Low-impact sport, Moderate impact sport, No-impact sport

high-level (radioactive) waste RADIATION SAFETY A specific form of (man-made) radioactive waste that includes the spent fuel from nuclear power plants, radioactive liquids and solids, and other highly radioactive materials; the global accumulation of 'hot' waste has become a 'hot' political issue, as there is no place to place the HLW[1], estimated at > 1100 metric tons[2] in long-term storage[3]; proposed solutions to the global HLW problem include burial in long-term storage, eg in the Yucca Mountains[4] or other geologic site, turning it into a glassy compound and burial, burning plutonium in highly efficient nuclear reactor, converting ^{239}Pu into other elements using particle accelerators, dumping it into the ocean-sealed in permanent titanium casings, and firing it off into space[5]-directly into the sun (NY Times March 14 1995, C1) see Plutonium, Radioactive waste; Cf Low-level waste

[1]Most of which is produced by nuclear reactors in the form of plutonium 239 [2]And expected to climb to 2000 tons in the next decade [3]Plutonium has a half-life of 24 360 [4]Nevada, US, which is composed of volcanic ash [5]The final frontier

high-mortality outlier A hospital that has been identified by the US Health Care Financing Administration (HCFA) as having a mortality rate far in excess of what is considered 'normal' for the remaining nearly 5500 health care facilities in the US; because these 'outliers' may be due to characteristics of the patient population, eg elderly (older than 85), 'high-risk' diagnoses or skewing of data by those who require nursing care upon discharge (JAMA 1991; 265:1843); it is thought that mortality rates are of little utility as a determinant of patient quality of care; see Hospital mortality rate

high-output cardiac failure Congestive heart failure due to a marked increase in circulating blood volume without functional myocardial abnormalities, where the demand outstrips the capacity, resulting in a hyperkinetic state; the cardiac pump activity is a function of preload (ventricular end-diastolic fiber tension), myocardial contractility, afterload and the heart cardiac rate; HOF may be a physiologic response to such 'insults' as anemia, cor pulmonale, exercise, fever, high humidity, systemic hypertension, obesity, pregnancy, emotional stress and temperature extremes, or non-physiological in Albright's disease (polyostotic fibrous dysplasia), carcinoid syndrome (serotonin-producing usually hepatic metastases), arteriovenous fistulas (trauma, Paget's disease of bone, hemangiomatosis, glomerulonephritis, hemodialysis, hepatic disease (alcohol-related thiamine deficiency decreases peripheral arterial resistance), hyperkinetic heart syndrome, polycythemia vera, and thyrotoxicosis (T_3 increases heart rate, cardiac sensitivity to epinephrine and causes peripheral vasodilation)

high-output gastrointestinal fistula An abnormal communication between the GI tract and another segment of intestine or other intraabdominal organ[1], or skin[2], caused by trauma, GI pathology or surgery, which produces > than 200 ml of fluid; HOGFs most often arise in the stomach, proximal small intestine and pancreas; the pancreas may produce up to 1500 ml of electrolyte-rich fluid/day; see Low-output gastrointestinal fistula

[1]Internal fistula [2]External fistula

high-performance liquid chromatography HPLC, see there

high power field A unit of measurement, usually understood to be a 'high dry' field (400X magnification); used by pathologists to assess a tissue's growth, which by extension is an indicator of tumor aggression; the number of mitotic figures per HPF serves to prognosticate certain tumors, in particular

HODGKIN'S DISEASE The number of classic Reed-Sternberg cells (RS) per single HPF allows subclassification of Hodgkin's lymphoma into lymphocyte predominance less than or equal to 5 RS/HPF (often far fewer), mixed cellularity 5-15 RS/HPF and lymphocyte-depleted, which is greater than or equal to 15 RS/HPF and

SMOOTH MUSCLE TUMORS of 1) Stomach These tumors are considered malignant if there are greater than five mitotic figures/10 HPF, although 40% of gastric leiomyosarcomas have less and 2) Uterus These tumors are regarded as frankly malignant if there are more than 10 mitotic figures/10 HPF; the diagnosis of 'smooth muscle tumor of uncertain malignant potential' (STUMP) or low-grade leiomyosarcoma (which has a low mortality, but often recurs) is rendered in smooth muscle tumors with less than 10 mitotic figures/10 HPF (in absence of cellular atypia), or 5 to 9 mitotic figures/HPF in the presence of atypia

'high power institution' ACADEMIA A colloquial term used in academic circles in the US for highly regarded (and therefore highly competitive) hospitals (eg Massachusetts General Hospital, the Mayo Clinic, National Institutes of Health), research institutions (eg Massachusetts Institute of Technology, the Whitehead Institute) and universities (eg U of Chicago, Harvard U, Stanford U, U of Utah, and others) that perform 'cutting edge' ('world class') science, and are highly selective in who they train

high-pressure liquid chromatography HPLC, see there

high-resolution computed tomography A CT study at slice (collimation scan interval) widths of 4mm or less, which is narrower than the usual 1-3 cm interval 'slices' obtained in conventional CT imaging; HRCT is the optimal technique for evaluating interstitial lung disease and emphysema and is preferred to conventional CT in detecting subpleural nodules, small linear densities, 'honeycombing' and bronchiectasis (Diag Imaging 1991; 13:102), and is of use in any body region where great detail is desired; Cf Spiral computed tomography

high risk INFECTIOUS DISEASE An adjective referring or pertaining to occupational groups at increased risk for exposure to blood-borne pathogens, eg blood bank technicians, dental professionals, dialysis unit staff, EMTs, ER staff, IV therapy teams, laboratory and medical technologists, morticians, OR staff, pathologists, phlebotomists, surgeons, and others

high-risk behavior INFECTIOUS DISEASE A generic term for a lifestyle activity, eg non-protected sexual activity, anal intercourse, IV drug abuse, that places a person at increased risk of being infected by certain pathogens, usually referring to AIDS; see Safe sex practices

high-risk infant NEONATOLOGY An infant at ↑ risk of suffering co-morbid conditions and potentially fatal complications due to fetal, maternal or placental anomalies FETAL HIGH-RISK FACTORS APGAR score of < than 4 at one minute, birth weights of < than 2500g or > than 4500g, gestational age < than 37 or > than 42 weeks, fetal malformation, fetal-maternal blood group incompatibility and twinning **MATERNAL HIGH RISK FACTORS** Previous in utero or neonatal death, infection, true DM (gestational diabetes is less risky to the infant), premature rupture of membranes, maternal age < than 16 and > than 40, alcohol, drug or tobacco use, gestation beginning within six months of previous delivery, poor prenatal care, severe emotional stress, accidents or general anesthesia, use of teratogenic medication **PLACENTAL AND INTRAUTERINE HIGH-RISK FACTORS** Placenta previa, short umbilical cord, single umbilical artery, abruptio placentae, oligohydramnios

high-risk group A group of people with a higher than expected risk for developing a particular disease, which may be defined on a measurable parameter, eg an inherited genetic defect, physical attribute, lifestyle, habit, socioeconomic and/or educational characteristic, as well as the environment to which they are exposed

high-risk pool HEALTH CARE ENVIRONMENT Any of a group of individuals who have been denied health insurance by insurers because of medical history that may include cancer, cardiovascular disease, emphysema, and others, placing them at high risk for future claims and medical costs (Am Med News 25 October 1992, p7)

high-risk sex Safe sex practices, see there

high-stringency hybridization MOLECULAR BIOLOGY Hybridization between two molecules capable of forming nucleotide base pair dimers, eg DNA with DNA or DNA with RNA under conditions that require virtually exact alignment of bases; the stringency of a hybridization can be controlled by titrating the temperature and salts; Cf Low-stringency hybridization

high-titer, low-avidity antibodies TRANSFUSION MEDICINE A group of antibodies that cause red cell agglutination at high dilutions in the antiglobulin test (Coomb's) phase, but which evoke weak aggregation and are rarely associated with clinically significant hemolysis; HTLA antibodies include anti-Ch, –Cs, –JMH, –Kn[a], –McC[a], –Rg, –Yk, and occasionally, anti–Hy, Lutheran group and leukocyte antibodies, eg anti-Bg[a]

high touch SOCIAL MEDICINE An adjective pertaining or referring to patient contact on a individual basis, in which there is physical and or direct emotional interaction, distinct from modern medicine's trend toward technological and innovative aspects of healing; 'high-touch' fields of health care include nursing, psychiatry, and family practice; see Doctor-patient interaction

higher multiple OBSTETRICS A term for multiple or higher order gestations greater than triplets, lumping together quadruplets and quintuplets; although traditionally, the frequency of triplets was considered the square of the 1:85 $(1:85^2)$ frequency of twins, ie, circa 1:7000 and that of quadruplets, the cube $(1:85^3)$ ie, circa 1:600 000, the use of fertility drugs, in vitro fertilization and other modalities has made higher multiples more common; differences in multiple gestations includes in-hospital stay for mothers: 1.4 days for mothers of singletons, 9.5 days for twins, 29.5 days for triplets and 54.5 days for quadruplets; in higher multiples, the incidence of lower birth weight is increasingly higher, and by extension the incidence of cerebral palsy; the more 'products', the greater the health care costs and the greater the puerperal complications for the mother including hemorrhage, anemia, infections and high blood pressure

highly toxic OCCUPATIONAL MEDICINE An adjective referring to a chemical that 1) Has a median lethal dose (LD_{50}) of ≤ 50 mg/kg when administered orally to 200-300 g albino rats 2) Has an LD_{50} of ≤ 200 mg/kg when administered by continuous contact for 24 hours on the shaved skin of 2.0-3.0 kg albino rabbits 3) Has an LD_{50} of ≤ 200 ppm of volume of gas or vapor, or ≤ 2 mg/L of mist or dust, when adminstered by continuous inhalation to 200-300 g albino rats

Hill-Burton Act A program that arose from US Public Law 79-725 (the Hospital Survey and Construction Act of 1946), which provided financial assistance for modernizing health care facilities in areas that had undergone a rapid post-World War II population growth; the Hill-Burton Act was superceded by US Public Law 93-641 of 1974, which attempted to reverse the migration of health providers and services to large population centers by supporting rural facilities or areas deficient in health services, eg inner-city

hilus cell An interstitial (Leydig) cell located in the ovarian hilum, associated with the rete ovarii, containing Reincke crystalloids (eosinophilic rods measuring 1-4 μm in length x 0.5 μm in diameter), without which the cells are indistinguishable from lutein cells or adrenocortical cells; hilar cells are present as unencapsulated aggregates in the embryonal ovary that disappear in childhood and reappear in puberty, increasing in number with pregnancy and aging and are abundant in postmenopausal women; hilar cells produce androstenedione, estrogen and progesterone; when 'driven' by hCG, hilar cells undergo mitosis and hypertrophy, and are an integral histologic feature of gonadoblastoma and androblastoma

hilus cell tumor SURGICAL PATHOLOGY A subtype of ovarian Leydig cell tumor (the other is the non-hilar Leydig cell tumor) CLINICAL Benign, autumn colored (red, yellow and brown) tumor, causing hirsutism or virilization in most cases, average age, 58 years TREATMENT Excision PROGNOSIS Excellent

Note: The other form of Leydig cell tumor is the ultrarare, non-hilar cell tumor, which behaves clinically like the hilus cell tumor

***Hind*II, *Hind*III** MOLECULAR BIOLOGY Two commonly used bacterial restriction endonucleases derived from *Hemophilus influenzae* that selectively hydrolyze or cut double-stranded DNA at the appropriate mirror-image or 'palindromic' sites; Cf *Eco*RI, RII, pBR 322

hinge region
IMMUNOLOGY A region of an immunoglobulin heavy chain that is often located between the first and second constant domains (CH1 and CH2) of the immunoglobulin chain and highly flexible due to the high content of proline residues (figure); C refers to the constant portions of the immunoglobulin, and V to the variable segments, which provide antibodies with their high degree of specificity

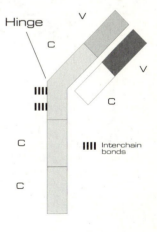

hip fracture A fracture usually of the head of the femur, which affects 1 in 6 white ♀ (US) during her lifetime EPIDEMIOLOGY see Total hip replacement RISK FACTORS ↑ risk for HF in tall and/or thin ♀ with ↓ bone density, previous fractures or stroke, white, use of aids in walking, ↑ consumption of alcohol or coffee, poor health, sedentary lifestyle, therapy with long-acting benzodiazepines or anticonvulsants (N Engl J Med 1995; 332:767oA); postmenopausal estrogen is protective for ♀ < 75 years of age (N Engl J Med 1994; 330:1555oA)

hip-pointer contusion SPORTS MEDICINE A bruise of the

iliac crest which occurs in contact sports due to a blow delivered by the knee, elbow, football helmet or other blunt object causing a subperiosteal hematoma and either avulsion of abdominal muscle or a fracture of the iliac crest

Hippocratic facies A physiognomy characteristic of advanced, untreated, preterminal peritonitis, who Hippocrates described as having '...*hollow eyes, collapsed temples; the ears, cold, contracted and their lobes turned out; the skin about the forehead being rough, distended and parched; the color of the whole face being brown, black, livid or lead-colored...*'; these facial features are also described in celiac sprue; Cf Triangular facies

Hippocratic nails Clubbing of fingers, see there

Hippocratic oath The ethical guide for physicians, as timely today as in the 5th century BC; although it has been

---

HIPPOCRATIC OATH

'I swear by Apollo the physician, by Aesculapius, Hygeia and Panacea, and I take to witness all the gods, and all the goddesses, to keep according to my ability and judgement the following Oath:
To consider dear to as my parents him who taught me this art; to live in common with him and if necessary to share my goods with him; to look upon his children as my own brothers, to teach them this art if they so desire without fee or written promise; to impart to my sons and the sons of the master who taught me and the disciples who have enrolled themselves and have agreed to the rules of the profession, but to these alone, the precepts and instructions. I will prescribe regimen for the good of my patients according to my ability and judgment and abstain from whatever is deleterious and mischievous. I will give no deadly medicine to anyone if asked nor give advise which may cause his death. Nor will I give a woman a pessary to procure abortion. I will preserve the purity of my life and practice my art. I will not cut for stone, even for patients in whom the disease is manifest, but will leave this operation to be done by practitioners of this art. Into whatever house where I come, I will enter only for the benefit of the sick, keeping myself far from all intentional mischief and corruption, and especially from the pleasures of love with women or with men, be they free or slaves. All that come to my knowledge in the exercise of my profession or outside of my practice or in daily commerce with men, which ought not to be spoken abroad, I will keep secret and not divulge. If I keep this oath unviolated may I enjoy my life and practice my art, respected by all men and in all times, but should I trespass this oath, may the reverse be my lot'

---

attributed to Hippocrates , the father of medicine and his school, the 'Oath' is of uncertain origin; see Code of Hammurabi

hippus A spasm of the iris, resulting in exaggerated rhythmic contractions and dilatations of the pupil that are not consonant with accommodation and light; see Hiccup

'hired gun' LEGAL MEDICINE 'Whore' A highly colloquial term for a physician whose major source of income derives from his role as the plaintiff's 'expert witness' at court trials for medical malpractice; mercenary 'experts' may have little knowledge of the medical field in which the tort occurred and may have their own fees tied to the monies awarded ('won') in a successful lawsuit; see *Daubert* v *Merrell Dow Pharmaceuticals*, *Frye* rule, Malpractice; Cf Physician expert witness

Note: Most physicians truly welcome the opinion of well-respected peers in their specialty, as such experts may temper the jury's view of the events in medically-related torts with their experience and offer reasons why many acts of alleged negligence are inevitable risks of a diagnostic or therapeutic procedure; occasionally, the so-called experts used by malpractice attorneys may have falsified credentials or may be under criminal investigation (Am Med News 16 March 1992)

hirsutism Excessive growth of body hair, a common complaint in women, divided into 1) Androgen-independent hirsutism in which the entire body is covered with vellous hair evenly distributed over both androgen-dependent and androgen-independent regions ETIOLOGY Congenital disease, eg Cornelia de Lange and Seckel syndromes, drugs,

eg androgen analogs, anti-convulsants, corticosteroids, cyclosporine, minoxidil, phenytoin and progesterone analogs, metabolic disorders, eg anorexia nervosa, porphyria cutanea tarda and 2) Androgen-dependent hirsutism where there is ↑ terminal hair over the 'androgenic' regions of the face and upper chest, which may be

I) NONENDOCRINE HIRSUTISM OF ETHNIC OR RACIAL ORIGIN, with excess hair growth on the face, upper body, chest nipples, or lower abdomen; the intensity and distribution is a function of a person's sensitivity to circulating androgens; a male pattern of hirsutism is more common in southern Europe and distinctly less common in aborigines and Orientals TREATMENT Rule out hormonal dysfunction, then bleach, pluck, and shave; spironolactone or combined spironolactone-progestagen combination therapy

II) HIRSUTISM OF ENDOCRINE (OVARIAN) ORIGIN, either non-neoplastic, eg polycystic ovaries syndrome of Stein-Leventhal (accompanied by hyperthecosis, increased testosterone and variably increased 17-ketosteroids), hyperthecosis, idiopathic, Achard-Thier syndrome or hormonally active neoplasms, eg granulosa cell tumor, gynandroblastoma, gonadoblastoma, Sertoli-Leydig cell tumors (arrhenoblastoma), stromal/pregnancy luteoma, teratoma, hilar cell tumors, lipoid cell tumors

III) HIRSUTISM OF ENDOCRINE (ADRENAL) ORIGIN, either non-neoplastic, eg adrenogenital syndrome (congenital adrenal hyperplasia, deficiency of 11- or 21-hydroxylase), normal testosterone, increased 17-ketosteroids, normal or increased pregnanetriol, Cushing's disease or neoplastic, eg adrenal tumor (carcinoma or virilizing adenoma, with increased 17-ketosteroids)

IV) DRUG-INDUCED HIRSUTISM due to excess of androgens, corticosteroids, contraceptives, menopausal 'cocktails', '19-nor' progestins, cyclosporine, diazoxide, minoxidil, 'stress'; (hyperthecosis and insulin resistance) phenothiazines, phenytoin

V) METABOLIC (AND OTHER CAUSES OF) HIRSUTISM Acromegaly, hypothyroidism, porphyria cutanea tarda

hirsutoid papillomata of the penis Pearly penile papules, see there

hirudin The most potent known inhibitor of thrombin, produced by the medicinal leech, *Hirudo medicinalis*; crystallographic analysis of the hirudin-thrombin complex reveals that 27 of the 65 residues have contacts of less than 4 A, forming 10 ion pairs and 23 hydrogen bonds, explaining hirudin's potency as an anticoagulant, as the affinity is much stronger than that for thrombin's natural inhibitor, anti-thrombin III

Hirudinea A class of segmented annelids, ie leeches, the most well-known of which is *Hirudo medicinalis*, that evolved from earthworms and is found in fresh water and soil in the subtropics and tropics; the genera include *Haemadipsa*, the medicinal leech as well as *Dinobdella*, *Haementeria*, *Helobdella*, *Hirudinaria*, *Hëmopis*, *Limnatis*, *Macrobdella*, *Poecilobdella*, *Pontobdella*; the leech is flat, has two suckers, the cranial sucker houses a mouth (the impression left by a leech bite has been fancifully likened to the Mercedes-Benz insignia); the caudal sucker is involved in crawling; the leech has a highly branched digestive system and a simple nervous system with one neurotransmitter, serotonin, which has made the leech a good model system in neurobiology; leech phlebotomy first began with the Greeks, and is undergoing a limited renaissance for various indications, including removal of excess blood from an operative site, stimulating capillary regrowth into reimplanted, traumatically amputated extremities, in plastic surgery for harvesting hirudin, a potent anticoagulant and in cancer research, as leech saliva inhibits tumor extension; not all leeches are so happily symbiotic; *Limnatis nilotica* (*Hirudo aegyptica*), an aquatic leech of North America, Europe and the Middle East may be ingested with drinking water and attach to the oropharynx and urogenital region, causing blood loss and anemia and, if excessive, asphyxia

HIS Hospital information system, see there

His bundle electrocardiography A relatively recent and sophisticated usage of the bipolar cardiac catheter electrode system for recording His bundle activity, studying the cardiac physiology of a patient with recurrent arrhythmias, optimizing pacemaker implantation and for differentiating true AV blocks from pseudo-AV block

His disease His-Werner disease A louse-borne, rickettsial

(*R quintana*) infection CLINICAL Intermittent fever, generalized myalgia, shin pain, vertigo, malaise and relapses; Cf Her's disease

histamine A bioactive amine produced through the decarboxylation of histidine, stored in mast cells and basophils, and secreted by monocytes, neural and endocrine cells; it is responsible for a wide range of physiologic and pathologic responses in different cells and tissues; it causes smooth muscle contraction, including bronchiolar and small vessel constriction, increased vascular permeability and secretion by nasal and bronchial mucous glands and is responsible for the symptoms of hay fever, urticaria, angioedema and the bronchospasm of anaphylactic reactions; histamine acts via histamine (H_1, H_2, and H_3) receptors, and mediates normal and abnormal (ie allergic) responses to inflammation, eg smooth muscle contraction in the respiratory and GI tracts, inducing release of nitric oxide from vascular endothelium, stimulating guanylate cyclase and increasing levels of cGMP resulting in vasodilation; histamine acts through H_1 and H_2 receptors to cause hypotension, tachycardia, flushing and headache; activation of H_2 receptors alone increases gastric acid secretion (N Engl J Med 1994; 330:1663ʀᴠ)

'histamine' headache see Cluster headache

histamine receptors Cell membrane receptors located on the basolateral membrane of the acid-secreting gastric parietal cell; when histamine is bound to H_2 receptors,

---

HISTIOCYTIC LESIONS-CLINICAL CLASSIFICATION

BENIGN HISTIOCYTIC LESIONS

1) FAMILIAL HISTIOCYTOSIS WITH EOSINOPHILIA A chronic disease of infants with recurring bacterial infections, diarrhea, eczema, alopecia, associated with immunodeficiency

2) SINUS HISTIOCYTOSIS WITH MASSIVE LYMPHADENOPATHY Rosai-Dorfman disease A disease most common in adolescent blacks with massive cervical lymphadenopathy as well as enlargement of extranodal (orbit, skin, bone, salivary gland, testis) lymphoid tissues and

3) VIRUS-ASSOCIATED HEMOPHAGOCYTIC SYNDROME A condition induced by viral infections, often accompanied by abnormal liver function tests, coagulation assays and pancytopenia PATHOLOGY Histiocyte hyperplasia, hemophagocytosis and replacement of native bone marrow elements

INTERMEDIATE HISTIOCYTIC LESIONS

1) Histiocytosis X, increasingly known as Langerhans' cell histiocytosis, see there

2) REACTIVE HEMOPHAGOCYTIC SYNDROME, see there

MALIGNANT HISTIOCYTIC LESIONS

1) HISTIOCYTIC MEDULLARY RETICULOSIS, see there

2) HISTIOCYTIC PROLIFERATIONS, eg acute monocytic leukemia (FAB M3), histiocytic lymphoma (see there), malignant histiocytosis (see there)

---

adenylate cyclase is activated, increasing the intracellular concentration of cAMP, activating the parietal cells' proton pump, an H^+K^+-ATPase which secretes H^+ ion against a large concentration gradient; H_1 and H_2 receptors are expressed on a variety of cells (lymphocytes, monocytes, basophils, eosinophils, smooth muscle cells and gastric parietal cells)

H_1 receptor A histamine receptor present on the surface of some smooth muscle cells that responds to histamine by dilation of arterioles and constriction of veins and bronchioles

H_2 receptor A receptor present on gastric parietal cells that increases the rate of HCl secretion in response to histamine

H_3 receptor A histamine receptor present in the lungs, spleen, skin, brain and on nerve endings surrounding blood vessels

histamine (H_1 and H_2) receptor antagonists A family of therapeutic agents that counter histaminic activity; H_1 receptor mediation of motion sickness can be attenuated by H_1 blockage with diphenhydramine; H_2 receptor-mediated gastritis and benign gastric ulceration usually respond to H_2 blockage by cimetidine and ranitidine, which inhibit gastric acid secretion by blocking the histamine H_2 receptors on the gastric parietal cells; H_2 blocking agents are used to treat recurring duodenal ulcers, gastric

ulcers, gastroesophageal reflux; HRAs are used to treat conditions linked to ↑ histamine release, eg mast cell disease, basophilic leukemia SIDE EFFECTS Antiandrogenic, eg gynecomastia and impotence

Note: H_2 receptor antagonists are used to treat Zollinger-Ellison syndrome as well as erosive esophagitis, reducing parietal cell hydrogen ion output, but require high doses, making omeprazole‡, a viable alternative

histidinemia A common (1:10 000), often asymptomatic AR [MIM 235800] condition characterized by a deficiency of histidase[1], the enzyme that converts histidine to urocanic acid in the liver and skin CLINICAL Variable[2], which when symptomatic, is of neonatal onset with impaired speech, growth and mental retardation LABORATORY Some of the accumulated excess histidine is transaminated to imidazole, the urinary metabolite of which, imidazolepyruvic acid, is detectable by the ferric chloride test or by Phenistix, otherwise used to diagnose phenylketonuria

[1]Histidine ammonia-lyase [EC 4.3.1.3] is the name recommended by the Nomenclature Committee of the IUBMB (International Union of Biochemistry and Molecular Biology) [2]Note: 99% of cases are clinically normal despite having biochemical disease; in the symptomatic 1%, treatment (histidine-free formula) is of little benefit

histiocytic lesions Lesions composed of histiocytes may be benign, indeterminant, or malignant in proliferative potential; in order to reduce the confusion related to these lesions, it has been suggested that histiocytoses be subdivided into different categories (table)

histiocytic lymphoma A very rare lymphoma consisting of discrete mass(es) in lymphoid tissues, skin and bone of histiocytes, which may also have T cell or B cell markers;

HISTIOCYTIC LESIONS-HISTOLOGIC CLASSIFICATION

CLASS I LANGERHANS-CELL HISTIOCYTOSES Histiocytosis X

CLASS II NON-LANGERHANS HISTIOCYTOSES Infection-associated hemophagic disease and familial erythrophagic lymphohistiocytosis

CLASS III HISTIOCYTOSES Rare malignant histiocytic proliferations, eg acute monocytic leukemia (FAB M3), malignant histiocytosis, histiocytic sarcoma

---

many of the lesions first described by Rappaport, now known as 'Rappaport's histiocytic lymphoma', ultimately proved to be comprised of transformed lymphocytes mimicking histiocytes; see Lymphoma

histiocytic medullary reticulosis A systemic proliferation of mature histiocytes with hemophagocytosis, BM necrosis, pancytopenia, hepatitis and coagulopathy; HMR has proven confusing, the combined result of differing criteria used to establish its diagnosis, its relative rarity, regional preferences for different terms for the same condition and misapplication of criteria used to establish the diagnosis; HMR is subdivided into 1) Malignant histiocytosis of Robb-Smith A premalignant neoplasm composed of large atypical circulating histiocytes that actively phagocytose RBCs, WBCs and platelets CLINICAL Aggressive with generalized lymphadenopathy, hepatosplenomegaly, pulmonary involvement and pancytopenia, often fatal DDx Virus-associated hemophagocytic syndrome and reactive histiocytosis of T-cell proliferations 2) 'Regressing atypical histiocytosis' An indolent pre-histiocytic lymphoma accompanied by chromosome defects CLINICAL Vaguely defined heterogenous clinical picture with a peak onset in the third decade of life, commonly with extranodal disease of the GI tract, skin and BM PROGNOSIS Relatively good

histiocytoid angioma A variant of pyogenic granuloma consisting of a heterogeneous group of non-regressing large vascular tumors with increased vascular spaces lined by cuboidal histiocyte-like epithelial cells with large, pale cleaved nuclei

histiocytosis X Langerhans' cell histiocytosis, see there

histocompatibility The degree to which two individuals share similar (nonimmunogenic) antigens; a desirable prerequisite for tissue allograft transplantation is perfect immune compatibility of tissues or a high degree of histocompatibility; in absence of a perfect HLA (human leukocyte antigen) match, recipient lymphocytes are stimulated to reject donor tissue by recognizing its 'non-selfness'; these identification characteristics are encoded by a cluster of genes known as the major histocompatibility complex (located on chromosome 6 in humans and on 17 in mice); see HLA

histogram A bar graph that represents the frequency of sample distribution found between each of many determined values, as in a chronologic histogram, eg the per capita consumption of cigarettes in the US and China

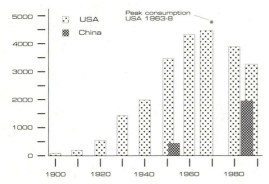

Per capita cigarette consumption (> age 18)

histogram

histologist 1) Anyone who prepares tissues for light and/or electron microscopic examination who is not certified by examination(s) sponsored by the American Society for Clinical Pathologists (ASCP) 2) Any person who studies tissues

histological technician A person who prepares tissue for microscopic examination with one or more years of formal training, designated by the American Society of Clinical Pathologists as HT(ASCP)

histomorphometry Histology, understood by some as cytomorphometry, see there

histone MOLECULAR BIOLOGY Any of a group of five 11–21-kd basic globular proteins of unknown function that interact in a periodic fashion with eukaryotic DNA; every 150-180 base pairs of DNA are bound to one molecule of H1 and two molecules of H2A, H2B, H3, H4; the evolutionary conservation of the histone 'motif' is considerable as there is significant sequence homology between bovine H3 histone and the garden pea; see Spliceosomes

histopathologist Anatomic pathologist A physician who has undergone a formal training period (in the USA, three or more years) in histopathology, who is eligible or certified by the American Board of Pathology and who interprets histologic slides prepared from diseased tissue

historian A person or patient who *PROVIDES* (in contrast to the usual dictionary definition*); the term is used in positive or negative terms, as in a good or poor historian, when the patient is able or unable to provide reliable information (N Engl J Med 1992; 326:1785c)

*One who records history

histotechnologist A histologic technician HT(ASCP) with far more extensive training than a histological technician, designated as HTL(ASCP)

history A timetable (see facing page) of periods in the Earth's development (please indulge the author)

histrionic personality disorder Hysterical personality disorder PSYCHIATRY A state characterized by '...*perva-*

sive and excessive emotionality and attention-seeking behavior', which begins by early adulthood, and is present in various contexts (DSM-IV™); HPD may be regarded as a 'Chinese menu disease' as its diagnosis is established by the finding of five or more of a laundry list of criteria (table)

hit COMPUTERS A 'visit' of a particular service or address on the Internet, the frequency of which reflects the popularity of a particular service; in March 1995, Oncolink, the cancer database/service, now operated by the University

---

HISTRIONIC PERSONALITY DISORDER ≥ 5 criteria

1) Person is uncomfortable unless he/she is center of attention
2) Interactions with others may be sexually inappropriate or provocative
3) Volatile and/or shallow emotions
4) Use of physical appearance to draw attention to self
5) Impressionistic speech pattern
6) Theatricality, exaggerated emotions
7) Suggestible, ie easily influenced by others
8) Regards relationships as more intimate than they are

modified from Diagnostic and Statistical Manual of Mental Disorders, 4th ed, Washington, DC, American Psychiatric Association, 1994

---

of Pennsylvania had 350 000 hits (Nature Medicine 1995; 1:502) SUBSTANCE ABUSE A small dose of any illicit psychotropic drug

hit-and-run accident PUBLIC HEALTH A motor vehicle accident (MVA) often involving a pedestrian, in which the vehicle and/or the vehicle's driver (often DWI at the time of the accident) leaves the scene of the accident (a criminal act) without concern for the safety and welfare of the victim

HITT Heparin-induced thrombocytopenia/thrombosis, see there

hitchhiker Uncertain, '*A gene that has no selective advantage, or may even be harmful, but that nevertheless temporarily becomes widespread because it is closely linked and coupled with a highly advantageous gene that is strongly selected.*' (Stedman's Medical Dictionary, 25th ed, Williams & Wilkins, Baltimore, 1990)

hitch-hiker's thumb A condition characterized by bilateral abduction of the thumbs (proximally placed and hypermobile) associated with deformed and dense carpal and metacarpal bones, seen in diastrophic dwarfism, occasionally Fanconi's anemia and acrocephalosyndactyly

In the US, the traditional way in which a person petitioned strangers for a ride was to stand on the side of a road with the right arm held outward, the fist loosely clenched and the thumb left extended

HIV-1 Human immunodeficiency virus The retrovirus intimately linked to AIDS, formerly, AIDS-related virus (ARV), human T-cell lymphotrophic virus, type III (HTLV-III, R Gallo, National Institutes of Health, USA) and lymphadenopathy-associated virus (LAV, L Montagnier, Pasteur Institute, Paris) **acute HIV infection** Primary symptomatic HIV infection Early HIV infection May be asymptomatic or accompanied by a 'viral syndrome' CLINICAL Fever, severe fatigue, sore throat, myalgia, arthralgia, nausea, vomiting, diarrhea, anorexia, weight loss, headache, photophobia, lymphadenopathy, pruritic maculopapular or urticarial rash, lymphocytic meningoencephalitis and peripheral neuropathy, all of which remit, reappearing as AIDS after a variable latency period of up to several years PATHOGENESIS High titers of cytopathic virus, which form syncytia in the H9 cell line (N Engl J Med 1991; 324:954, 961)

HIV-associated cognitive motor complex AIDS-dementia complex, see there CLINICAL CLASSIFICATION,

HIV-1 infection (table) **dermatology** Skin disease occurs in 79% of HIV-infected subjects includes Seborrheic dermatitis, herpes simplex, herpes zoster, KS, dermatophytosis, cellulitis, skin abscess formation, drug reactions, and others (**N Engl J Med 1993; 328:1670oa**) DIAGNOSIS ELISA is a screening tool that detects the presence of IgM antibodies to HIV Note: Antibodies cross-reactive to HIV-1 core antigen are rare, but may occur in normal subjects or those with autoimmune disease, cutaneous T-cell lymphoma and multiple sclerosis; low-level false positive ELISA occurs in alcoholic hepatopathy, pregnancy, non-HIV infected IV drug abusers and hemodialysis patients; ELISA-positive sera are then subjected to Western immunoblot hybridization (see below), which detects specific antibodies to HIV antigens, including p24 (often the first antibody to appear), p41 and p17 antigens Note: ELISA followed by Western blotting if the serum is positive by ELISA is the standard 'work-up' of blood donors for HIV status; other HIV-1 antigens, eg gp160, gp120, gp50-65 and p31 may evoke antibody production, but are only variably present or less specific; Western blot's rate of false positivity is 1/135,187 ; in terminal AIDS, sero-reversion may occur with loss of antibodies to p24 and p17; HIV-1 antigen titers in the blood may be quantified, levels of 30, 3200 and 3500 tissue culture infective doses are observed in subjects with asymptomatic HIV infection, AIDS-related complex and AIDS, respectively, suggesting a direct effect of HIV-1 in the progression of AIDS; HIV viremia is more indicative of AIDS than p24 antigenemia which is present in only 45% of those with detectable viremia; other AIDS tests include 1) Agglutination reaction between HIV peptides conjugated to red cells or latex particles, an inexpensive test allowing HIV antibody detection in 10 µl of blood in 2 minutes (false negative rate, 2%) 2) HIV culture in cell lines and chloramphenicol acetyltransferase-signal bioassay (low sensitivity, expensive) 3) HIV-Antigen assay (slow, expensive)

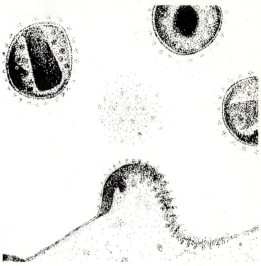

ultrastructural appearance of budding HIV

HIV-ACTIVE DECONTAMINATING AGENTS	
AGENT	MIC (REC CONC)*
Acetone:Ethanol	1:1
Chlorhexidine gluconate:Ethanol	4:25
Ethanol (ethyl alcohol)	25% (50%)
Formalin	2% (4%)
Glutaraldehyde	0.1% (1%)
Hydrogen peroxide	0.3% (1%)
Isopropyl alcohol	30% (50%)
Lysol	0.5% (1%)
NP-40 detergent	1%
Paraformaldehyde	0.5% (1%)
β-Propiolactone	1:400 dilution
Quarternary ammonium chloride	0.08% (1%)
Sodium hypochlorite (bleach)	0.02% (0.5%)
Sodium hydroxide	30mM

*Minimum inhibitory concentration (Recommended concentration, if differ-

DISINFECTION HIV is inactivated by bleach (750 ppm, or 1:10 dilution for 40 minutes) and formaldehyde (2% for 10 hours); high laundry temperatures (90% reduction in viable HIV), eg 25 minutes at 71°C or 10 minutes at 80°C may be effective; low temperature washing without bleach does not remove HIV (**Lab Med 1988; 19:88**) EPIDEMIOLOGY In infant with maternally acquired HIV, the rate of disease progression reflects the severity of HIV-related disease in the mother, where clinical AIDS develops within the first 18 months in 50% of infants of mothers with class IV disease and 14% of those whose mothers are class II or III (**N Engl J Med 1994; 330:308oa**); the median age at the time of HIV infection has declined in the US, from 34 years old (1979) to 25 (1990) (**N Engl J Med 1994; 330:789c**)

HETEROSEXUAL TRANSMISSION Worldwide, the predominant mode of transmission of HIV is heterosexual intercourse; in a longitudinal study of 124 couples in which one partner was infected, use of condoms prevented transmission of HIV to the other partner; in 121 couples, condom use was sporadic, and HIV seroconversion occurred at a rate of 4.8/100 person-years (**N Engl J Med 1994; 331:341oa**) IMMUNE STATUS Evaluation of progression has been based on measurement of the CD4 cell count, although measurement of HIV mRNA in peripheral blood mononuclear cells may be more efficient (**New York Times 1 Februrary 1994; C7**) INFECTIONS HIV-positivity tends to worsen the response to other infections, and T-cell response to infections in HIV-positive subjects may trigger multiplication of dormant HIV; AIDS patients have an increased susceptibility to disseminated vaccinia after immunization, neurosyphilis, TB, herpes and other infections that respond to standard therapy (**N Engl J Med 1991; 324:289**); several viruses may co-infect with HIV-1, transactivating HIV-1's long terminal repeat (LTR) sequence, eg Herpesvirus, HHV-6, papovavirus, adenovirus and HTLV-I LONG-TERM SURVIVORS Nonprogressive HIV-1 infection, see there **Mycoplasma**

CLINICAL CLASSIFICATION, HIV-1 INFECTION
GROUP SYMPTOMS

I Acute HIV-1 infection

II Asymptomatic HIV-1 infection

III Persistent generalized lymphadenopathy with HIV-1 infection

IV HIV-1 infection and either clinical AIDS or other AIDS-related symptoms, eg involuntary weight loss, fever or diarrhea for <\>> one month, dementia, peripheral neuropathy, hairy leukoplakia and oral candidiasis that fall short of the CDC's definition of AIDS

Subgroup A Constitutional symptoms

Subgroup B Neurological symptoms

Subgroup C Infectious disease

MMWR 1987; 36:3S-15S

Simultaneous HIV-1 and *Mycoplasma fermentans* (incognitus strain) infection results in ↑ cytocidal effects on CD4+ T cells (**Science 1991; 251:1074**) PATHOGENESIS HIV-1 infects cells by attaching to susceptible host cells at the extracellular amino acid residues 37-53 of the CD4 receptor, a glycoprotein receptor found on the surface of the helper subset of T cells, most monocytes and macrophages; HIV may also invade cells via IgG's Fc receptor; once inside the cell, HIV uses reverse transcriptase to transcribe its RNA into a DNA provirus, which then integrates itself into the host DNA, either remaining dormant or entering into a 'lytic' cycle forcing host cells to produce retrovirus; see Reverse transcriptase PRECAUTIONS see Universal blood and body and fluid precautions

HIV serology

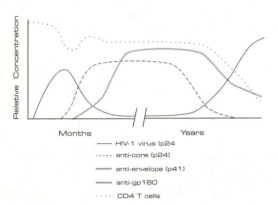

Months   Years

——— HIV-1 virus (p24
····· anti-core (p24)
——— anti-envelope (p41)
——— anti-gp160
····· CD4 T cells

SEROPREVALENCE IN AFRICA Sub-Saharan Africa ♂ 1 in 40 are infected; 1:40, focally up to 1:5; North America ♂ 1:75; 1:700 (**Science 1991; 252:372**) SEROPREVALENCE US 650 000-1 400 000 (0.2-0.5% of the population) are infected with HIV-1 (1990), ranging from 0.1% in rural regions with low 'risk' activities to 7.8% in urban populations; in low-prevalence regions, HIV-1 positivity is more common in men; in high-prevalence regions, the male:female ratio is 2.9:1; 20% of men in high-prevalence regions are HIV-positive; seropositivity is up to 9-fold greater in those refusing to be tested ARMY (US) PERSONNEL Seroconversion rate among soldiers is 0.29 per thousand person-years (**JAMA 1991; 265:1709**) CHILD-BEARING WOMEN (US) Inner-city 8.0/1000, urban (not inner-city) and suburban 2.5/1000 Suburban and rural 0.9/1000; 4.5-5.8/1000 in New York, New Jersey, Washington DC and Florida and 1.5/1000 in the entire US; rate of HIV transmission to the child is 30% (**JAMA 1991; 265:1704**) ER PATIENTS (US, 1987) 3% of all and 16% of 25-34 year-old ER patients are HIV positive, 80% of whom were unsuspected HEALTH CARE WORKERS (HCW) HIV positivity in HCW reflects HIV positivity in the general population; in the US, less than 100 HCW without other known risk behaviors have seroconverted; seroconversion after needle or mucosal exposure to HIV-infected patients is approximately 0.3%; dentists: see Acer cluster NEWBORNS Rural New York 0.16% positivity, New York City 1.25% positivity PRISON POPULATION Prevalence 2.1-7.6% in ♂; 2.5-14.7% in ♀ (**JAMA 1991; 265:1129**) SEXUALLY ACTIVE ADULTS 5% of those with STD are HIV-1 positive, especially those who also had syphilis or a history of genital herpes TESTING Detection of HIV infection in neonates is complicated because of circulating immune complexes composed of passively transferred maternal antibodies and HIV antigens; patient samples were pretreated with glycine hydrochloride to dissociate immune complexes followed by TRIS-HCl neutralization allowing the use of a commercial HIV p24 antigen assay (**N Engl J Med 1993; 328:297OA**) the FDA has approved kits for oral specimens as tests for

the presence of HIV-1, which has a ± 2% false positive and false negaive rate (**Laboratory Medicine 1995; 26:303N&V**) TRANSMISSIBLE FLUIDS AND TISSUES Blood, tissues, breast milk are recognized HIV 'vectors'; casual household contacts, feces, skin, tears and urine are not known to transmit HIV; saliva inhibits the ability of HIV to infect lymphocytes, see Bergalis case TREATMENT All therapy directed against HIV is experimental, and includes soluble CD4 injected into the circulation, of potential use in binding HIV before it invades cells via the CD4 receptor; CD4 linked to an Fc Ig fragment, forms an 'immunoadhesin' that has the theoretical advantage of both combining with HIV and stimulating the immune system by activating cytotoxic T-cells Note: HIV-1 survives despite brisk humoral and cellular immune responses by the host **Western blot** An immune assay that confirms HIV infection when an ELISA screening assay is positive TECHNIQUE Crude HIV is 'sieved' by gel electrophoresis, separating the HIV molecule into distinctive molecular weight protein bands, some of which are considered diagnostic for HIV infection by the CDC: Definitely positive p24 or p31 and gp41 or gp 120/gp 160 Possibly positive gp41 and gp 120/gp 160 or any combination, one from each gene product Indeterminant One HIV-related band; with time, HIV-1 products may disappear from the serum, especially p24, with a concomitant decrease in anti-core antibody; false positivity in the Western blot for HIV occurs in 0.01 to 0.0007% of cases; indeterminant results are 100-fold more common, occurring in 0.3-0.5% of the general population; if the person with indeterminant results is in a high-risk group, they usually convert within one month; low-risk individuals with a persisting indeterminant Western blot at 3 months may be regarded as negative and require no further followup (**J Gen Intern Med 1992; 7:640**) see Western blot WINDOW PERIOD A time span of ≥ 3 months during which an HIV-1-infected person is capable of transmitting the virus, but cannot be undetected by currently available tests Note: Blood is screened by the ELISA, which detects the antibody and not HIV-1 antigen; HIV-antibody-negative but HIV-1 positive donors in the 'window' period may still transmit HIV; see AIDS, Mosquito connection, Monkey connection, Zagury, Zidovudine

HIV conspiracy A broad deception allegedly being committed by the mainstream researchers in the retrovirology community, the majority of whom ascribe to the belief that AIDS is intimately linked to infection by HIV; according to one politician, the US *'federal AIDS effort–based on the conclusioin that HIV causes AIDS–will be seen as the greatest scandal in American history...'* (**Science 1995; 268:191**)

HIV-1 genes *art/trs* gene *rev* gene, see there *env* gene Encodes viral coat proteins gp 120 and gp 41, which mediate CD4 binding and membrane fusion, controlled by tat and rev *gag* gene Encodes nucleocapsid core proteins including p24 **LTR** Long terminal repeat Provides the binding sites for host transcription factors, which regulate HIV replication *nef* gene 3' orf, B gene, ORF-2 gene Encodes a protein of unknown function found in infected patients that may down-regulate viral expression (nef deletion results in a five-fold increase in viral DNA synthesis and replication) *pol* gene Encodes reverse transcriptase, protease, integrase and ribonuclease **R** gene Encodes the TAR (transcription activating response) element, which has a nonspecific immunodeficiency effect *rev* gene *art/trs* gene Encodes a 19-kD post-transcriptional protein regulator required for HIV replication, up-regulating HIV synthesis by transactivating anti-repression, ↑ the levels of envelope RNA by regulating the *env* gene; inactivation of the *rev* gene prevents viral replication (as measured by the successful production of the p24 glycoprotein) by infected monocytes can be massively ↑

by addition of cytokines to the culture medium ***tat*#** **gene** Encodes a potent 14-kD transcription activator that amplifies HIV replication, the inactivation prevents viral replication ***vif*#** **gene** A gene that facilitates infectivity of free HIV ***vpu*#** **gene** A gene unique to HIV-1 that encodes a 16-kD product, which when mutated, has a 5-10-fold reduction in replicative capacity and is critical for efficient budding of virions (N Engl J Med 1991; 324:308rv) see HIV virion

‡ = Gene encoding structural protein

= Gene encoding regulatory protein

HIV-associated nephropathy A group of renal diseases linked to HIV infection, including focal or global glomerulosclerosis with mesangial deposition of C3, IgM, and occasionally IgG CLINICAL HAN is typically characterized by severe nephrotic syndrome of abrupt onset, ↓↓↓ albumin, and rapid progression to end-stage renal disease; other permutations of HAN include the relatively uncommon HIV-associated IgA nephropathy (N Engl J Med 1992; 327:702OA, 729ED)

HIV virion HIV has a 100 nm in diameter lipid envelope surrounding a dense cylindrical nucleoid containing core proteins, reverse transcriptase and a genome with sequence similarity to non-cell-transforming lentiviridae, eg visna and caprine encephalitis viruses; envelope proteins gp41, gp120; nucelocapsid proteins p24, p17, p9, p7

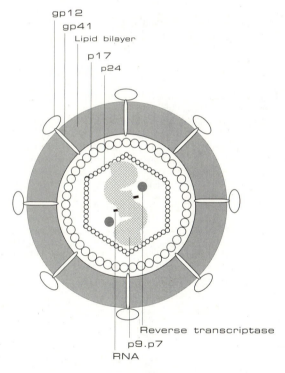

gp12
gp41
Lipid bilayer
p17
p24
Reverse transcriptase
p9.p7
RNA

HIV structure

HIV-vaccine Three facets of the human immunodeficiency virus (HIV) make it a difficult candidate for vaccine production

1) It can hide within normal (but infected) cells, protected from the immune system, cloaked within vesicles made from host membrane (the 'Trojan horse' effect)

2) The gene encoding the envelope glycoprotein, gp120, is highly mutable and the change of but one or two of gp120's amino acids alters the immune response, forcing the immune system into a constant (and losing) battle to produce antibodies against HIV-1's ever-changing proteins in gp120's 'loop' region; gp120's env region contains many such hypervariable regions ('hot spots'); any antibody to such 'hot spots' would be useless, although an antibody 'cocktail' to portions of gp120 is of potential use Note: Recombinant gp120 provides protection against HIV-1 in monkeys, but gp160 does not,

which is possibly related to the constancy of gp120's 'pit' region

3) HIV has marked affinity for the CD4 molecule; for a vaccine to skirt that affinity, it would need a molecular motif similar to the CD4 molecule Disadvantage: When a non-mutating CD4 'look-alike' is introduced, the immune system may recognize the CD4 antigen as foreign, destroying self CD4 T cells and macrophages

4) HIV inserts its genome into the host's genome; development of an anti-HIV vaccine is further hampered by factors extrinsic to the virus

a) in vitro testing of anti-HIV activity cannot prove whether there is adequate in vivo defense

b) Dangers and/or uncertainties of clinical trials with an HIV vaccine, eg paucity of altruistic volunteers for a live attenuated vaccine and

c) Lack of a suitable animal model, although chimpanzees appear to be suitable for testing, given the similarity of HIV to SIV/STLV-III

An effective vaccine must elicit antibodies capable of recognizing HIV before it binds to the CD4 receptor on CD4-bearing T cells and macrophages, which must be very rapid given the high affinity that HIV has for CD4 Recombinant virus expressing a limited number of epitopes ('epitope' vaccines) may result in immune-mediated damage clinical disease by T cells; this family of vaccines, to prevent HIV infection in the early exposure period may elicit unwanted immune destruction (Science 1991; 251:195); potential types of HIV vaccines

1) Live attenuated HIV; the possible danger of this approach is exemplified by the finding that live attenuated polioviruses in vaccines may rarely reactivate and themselves cause polio

2) Whole inactivated (killed) HIV

3) Live recombinant viruses, ie ones containing HIV fragments of sufficient immunogenicity to evoke a protective immune response

4) Synthetic peptides or antigenic subunits, eg gp120 or its C21E subfragment, gp160 Note: Peptides might combine with an inappropriate adjuvant and the tandem molecule may elicit an anomalous and exhuberant immune reaction and

5) Others, eg natural products, recombinant DNA products, anti-idiotype molecules and passive immunization

New strategies in vaccine design that may be of use in HIV-1 vaccines include recombinant viral or bacterial vectors, 'naked' DNA and synthetic immunogens (Science & Medicine 1995; 2/3:38); as of early 1995. there is no effective anti-HIV vaccine

HIV wasting syndrome AIDS A clinical complex associated with chronic renal insufficiency, and caused by poor nutrition, endocrine dysfunction, and catabolic stresses, eg infection, uremia and dialysis; in absence of disease, starvation results in death at 66% of ideal body weight; in AIDS, cell mass at death is 54%; WS is mediated by TNF (as well as by IL-1, IFN-α, IFN-β, and IFN-γ), which ↓ lipoprotein lipase, ↓ synthesis of fatty acids, and ↑ lipolysis in fat cells; wasting is also related to anorexia, and protein catabolism secondary to infections (N Engl J Med 1992; 327:329RV) TREATMENT Recombinant human growth hormone (rhGH) increases lean body mass by ± 3 kg (19%) with an ↑ capacity for physical work (Bio/Technology 1995; 13:206)

HIV-2 Formerly LAV-2, HTLV-IV, SIV/AGM An immunodeficiency virus first identified in West Africans with abnormal reactions to HIV-1 and simian immunodeficiency virus (SIV), HIV-2 is genetically closer to SIV/MAC (70% sequence 'homology') than to HIV-1 (40% sequence 'homology'), with 50% conservation for gag and pol and even less for other genes; HIV-2 has structural antigens p24, gp36 and gp140 CLINICAL Some cases are clinically similar to AIDS; others are essentially 'benign' EPIDEMIOLOGY HIV-2 is largely confined to West Africa and has an AIDS epidemiology pattern II (heterosexual transmission); HIV-2 contains X-ORF (as does SIV/Mne) and vpx, which are unique to HIV-2; HIV-2 appears to be less lethal than HIV-1

HIV-3 A 'third' human immunodeficiency virus has been described by various workers, who are peripheral to mainstream HIV research efforts; if an HIV-3 exists, it is poorly studied

HLA Human leukocyte antigen complex A system of genes unique to each individual human that are statistically shared with one in four of his/her siblings; the HLA regions are found within the major histocompatibility complex (MHC) and were first recognized when the serum from multiply transfused subjects and multiparous females were found to agglutinate leukocytes; multiparous women continue to be the best source for HLA typing antisera, which is harvested from placentas; the MHC is located on the short arm of chromosome 6, 32 centimorgans from the centromere and divided into three classes Class I proteins include HLA-A, HLA-B and HLA-C, have a transmembrane hydrophilic region with two disulfide-linked and one non-disulfide linked extracellular domain bound to β_2-microglobulin, encoded on chromosome 15 and expressed on all nucleated cells; class I antigens are defined serologically by the microcytotoxicity assay, are recognized during graft rejection, are responsible for refractoriness to platelet transfusions and serve as homing targets for HLA-specific cytolysis (efferent limb of virally-infected cells) and may be lysed by killer cells; the class I region also encodes a group of non-polymorphic proteins, HLA-E, F and G; some structural motifs in class I antigens appear in insulin receptors, epidermal growth factors and γ-endorphin Class II proteins, HLA-DR, HLA-DQ and HLA-QP, consist of two similar (α and β) chains with transmembrane hydrophilic regions and two extracellular, disulfide bond-linked domains, are expressed on sperm, B-cells, myeloid cell precursors, activated T-cells and antigen-presenting cells (monocytes, macrophages, Langerhans' and dendritic cells), endothelial cells; class II antigens act in the sensitization phase (afferent limb) of cell-mediated cytotoxicity, coordinating the presentation of antigen to T-cells, facilitating T-helper function, suppression and cooperation, and mediating graft-versus-host disease; class II antigens (HLA-DR and HLA-DQ*) are identified by mixed leukocyte reaction Lymphocytes (responder cells) from a potential organ recipient are incubated with irradiated lymphocytes from a donor that are antigenic, but immunoparalyzed, thus being capable of eliciting proliferation of immune-competent cells, measuring the $\uparrow$ in H_3 uptake in recipient cells b) HLA-DP specificity is determined by primed lymphocyte typing, which identifies differences in antigens among members of a species; primed lymphocyte typing is essentially in vitro immunization, using lymphocytes from any two subjects to prepare reagents that detect antigenic differences in HLA class II

Note: HLA-DQ and HLA-DR are heterodimers composed of a 34-kD α chain and a 29-kD β chain MHC Class III encodes 21-hydroxylase, complement proteins C2, C4 and factor B of the alternate complement pathway

HLA and disease The association of HLA haplotypes with specific diseases is determined by calculating 1) Relative risk Patients with a particular HLA antigen 'X' Number of control subjects without the antigen, divided by Patients without the antigen 'X' Control subjects with the antigen (but not the disease) and 2) Absolute risk Patients with the HLA antigen divided by the control subjects with the antigen X Prevelance of the disease in the population; in certain conditions, virtually all patients have the same HLA antigens, eg HLA-B27 associated with ankylosing spondylitis, HLA-DR4 with pemphigus vulgaris and HLA-DRw52a with primary sclerosing cholangitis; other HLA associations include HLA-B8, chronic active hepatitis, sicca syndrome, dermatitis herpetiformis, coeliac disease, idiopathic Addison's disease, Graves' disease, multiple sclerosis HLA-B27 see there, HLA-DR3 IDDM, Graves' disease, Addison's disease, celiac disease

HLA-B27-related arthropathies A group of joint diseases that more commonly occur in subjects with the HLA-B27 antigen, including ankylosing spondylitis, juvenile rheumatoid arthritis, psoriatic arthritis, Reiter syndrome, *Salmonella*-related arthritis, *Yersinia*-related arthritis

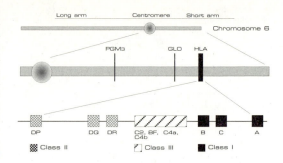

HLA specificities

HLA-DM A critical regulatory molecule of the MHC class II-restricted antigen presentation; HLA-DM may function as an intracellular site promoting MHC II-peptide association (Nature 1994; 368:551OA); HLA-DMA and HLA-DMB are thought to encode subunits of a funtional heterodimer critical in the pathway of MHC class II antigen presentation (Nature 1994; 368:554OA)

HLA-DP A 26–34-kD family of the MHC class II antigens distinct from HLA-DQ and HLA-DR; HLA-DP is present on ± 10% of peripheral lymphocytes, and on 95% of tonsillar B lymphocytes

HLA-DQ A 26–34-kD family of the MHC class II antigens distinct from HLA-DP and HLA-DR; HLA-DQ is present on ± 10% of peripheral lymphocytes, and on 95% tonsillar B lymphocytes

HLA-DR A heterodimeric transmembrane glycoprotein antigen composed of a 36-kD α– and 27-kD β-subunit; HLA-DR is expressed on B cells, activated T and NK cells, monocytes/macrophages, on thymic epithelium, B cell-dependent areas of the spleen and lymph node, as well as B-cell lymphomas

HLA-G An HLA class I antigen expressed on trophoblasts, ie placental cells, and tumors of trophoblastic origin; this unique antigen is not polymorphic and is found only on cells that do not express HLA-A, B and C, eg extravillous cytotrophoblast from the placenta and choriocarcinoma; HLA-G is most prominently expressed in the first trimester of pregnancy; since it is thought that the trophoblast cells at the maternal-fetal interface play a role in the survival of the semiallogenic fetus, HLA-G-positive cells may form a barrier, preventing 'rejection' of the fetus; the high expression of HLA-G implies a global immune tolerance by the mother

---

DISEASES LINKED TO HLA SPECIFICITIES
Addison's disease (B8, DR3, Dw3), ankylosing spondylitis (B27), Behcet's disease (B5), Buerger's disease (B12), celiac disease or gluten-sensitive enteropathy (B8, Dw3), chronic active hepatitis (DR3), deQuervain thyroiditis (Bw35), dermatitis herpetiformis (Dw3), Goodpasture syndrome (DR2), mesangioproliferative glomerulonephritis (DR4), Graves' disease (B8 in caucasians, Bw35 and Dw12 in Japanese, Bw46 in Chinese), hemochromatosis (A3, B7, B14), IDDM (B8. B15, DRw3, DRw4), juvenile rheumatoid arthritis (B27, DR5, DR8), late onset adrenal hyperplasia with hirsutism (Aw33/B14), myasthenia gravis (A1, A3, B8, Dw3, DR3), psoriasis (Cw6), psoriatic arthritis (B27), Reiter syndrome (B27), rheumatoid arthritis (DR4), *Salmonella* arthritis (B27), Sjögren syndrome (DR3, B8), lupus erythematosus (DR2, DR3), Takayasu's disease (B52), *Yersinia* arthritis (B27)

HLA match The number of HLA antigens at the HLA-A, B, and DR loci of the donor and recipient that match, ranging from a maximum of 6 to minimum of 0; in one report, the 1-year graft survival is 84% with no HLA mismatches and 77% for grafts with 4 mismatches; a resource-based allocation system with nation-wide rationing of organs based on HLA matching would ↓ the number of mismatches, theoretically increasing the 5-year graft survival from 58.5% to 63% (N Engl J Med 1994; 331:765OA)

HLH Helix-loop-helix motif, see there

HLHS Hypoplastic left heart syndrome, see Baby Faye heart

HMB-45 SURGICAL PATHOLOGY A monoclonal antibody that can be linked in the avidin-biotin peroxidase immunohistochemical method for identifying the presence of certain antigens in cells and tissues; HMB-45 is classically positive in malignant melanoma and in perivascular smooth muscle cells, eg renal angiomyolipoma and lymphangioleiomyomatosis (Arch Pathol Lab Med 1994; 118:732OA, 846OA)

HMBA Hexamethylene bis-acetamide An agent that is reported to induce termination differentiation in certain malignancies, eg in myelodysplastic syndrome, where complete

HMCK High-molecular-weight cytokeratin

HMG CoA reductase inhibitors A family of drugs that inhibits the activity of 3-hydroxy-3-methylglutaryl coenzyme A, an enzyme involved in an early step of cholesterol synthesis; the first approved agent with this activity permits enough mevalonate to be synthesized so that there is adequate cholesterol for cell membrane function and steroidogenesis; HMG CoA reductase evokes a significant reduction in LDL-cholesterol, the main atherogenic factor in the atherosclerotic process; these agents are used in younger men with total cholesterol levels above 6.47 mmol/L (US: 250 mg/dl), at low doses, eg 20 mg/d lovastatin; 20 mg lovastatin ↓ total cholesterol by an average of 17% and ↑ HDL-C by 7%; in a cost-analysis study, use of HCRIs to ↑ life expectancy is relatively cost-effective (JAMA 1995; 273:1032)

HMwK High-molecular-weight kininogen A 150-kD plasma glycoprotein involved in initiating the intrinsic coagulation pathway

HMO Health maintenance organization A managed system that provides comprehensive prepaid health care that provides or ensures delivery of a set of basic and supplementary health maintenance and treatment services in a defined geographic region to a voluntarily enrolled group of persons, requires that its enrollees use the services of designated physicians, hospitals and other providers of medical care and receives reimbursement through a predetermined, fixed periodic prepayment by or on behalf of each individual or family unit regardless of the amount of services provided; ± 17.3 % (45.1 million) of US citizens are enrolled in an HMO; major HMOs are Blue Cross/Blue Shield (6.9 million), Kaiser Foundation (6.6 million) (Am Med News 10 October 1994 p 7); HMOs are large multi-specialty groups that homogenize medical care by utilizing physicians as interchangeable parts

Note: There is an trend for younger physicians to work for HMOs as the burden of patient billing is eliminated, on-call schedules at night are shared with a larger group of colleagues and there is compelling need to pay medical school debts

HMO model Extrapolation model, see there

HMR Histiocytic medullary reticulosis, see there

HMU 5-Hydroxymethyluracil, see there

hnRNA Heterogeneous nuclear RNA, see there

hobnail A fanciful adjectival descriptor for a 2– or 3-D jutting of mutiple large rounded masses above a flattened surface

hobnail cell A nonspecific term for any of a group of cells that juts above an adjacent epithelial or endothelial surface or lining; the hobnail pattern's significance differs according to the organ, and it can be neoplastic as in mesonephroid-type ovarian cystadenocarcinoma, clear cell carcinoma, endometrial carcinoma, mesotheliomas or reactive, as the jutting of type II pneumocytes above the alveolar lining in lungs with diffuse alveolar damage or the bulging of succulent, secretion-filled, vacuolated, enlarged and pleomorphic cells in the lobules of a lactating breast

hobnail metaplasia A benign transition of endometrial glands into hobnail-like cells that prolapse into the lumen and which may be associated with endometrial hyperplasias or endometrial carcinoma, but alone has no prognostic significance

hobnail pattern LIVER PATHOLOGY Bumpy nodularity separated by broad trabecular scars seen macroscopically on the liver surface in posthepatitis cirrhosis Note: A hobnail has a massive head and short tang and is used to protect soles of heavy boots

Hobson model see Dreams

hockey stick An adjectival descriptor for an elongated cylindrical mass ending in a gentle curve, fancifully likened to a hockey stick

hockey stick cells A descriptive term for cells seen in certain conditions HEMATOPATHOLOGY Unicellular Reed-Sternberg cells with a large vesicular nucleus and peripheral nucleolus Hooked cells NEUROPATHOLOGY Neurofibroblasts in type I neurofibromatosis (von Recklinghausen's disease)

hockey stick deformity ORTHOPEDICS A descriptor for the femoral deformity (figure) that may be seen in Jaffe-Lichtenstein syndrome (monostotic and polyostotic fibrous dysplasia), and if severe, which simulates a hockey stick

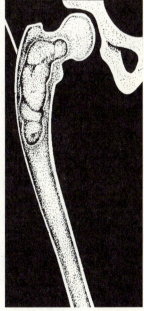

hockey stick deformity

Hodgkin's disease A type of lymphoma that is most common in young adults, which accounts for ± 0.7% of all new cancers in the US (±7500 cases); HD is clinically distinct as it often responds well to chemotherapy, and histologically distinct as its sine qua non diagnosis rests on the finding of the Reed-Sternberg cell ETIOLOGY The ↑ prevalence of HD in 19/187 monozygous twin pairs in contrast to 0/179 dizygous twin pairs (RR for monozygous twins = 99) supports the contention that there is genetic predisposition to HD (N Engl J Med 1995; 332:413OA) see Hematopoietic growth factor receptor STAGING Ann Arbor classification, see there PATHOLOGY HD is characterized by a mixture of eosinophils, lymphocytes, monocytes, plasma cells, and the sine qua non cell required for the diagnosis of HD, the Reed-Sternberg cell; HD is divided into 4 types, lymphocyte predominance, mixed cell, lymphocyte-depletion and nodular sclerosing types TREATMENT Radiotherapy, MOPP (mechlorethamine, vincristine, procarbazine, prednisone); 20% are treatment 'failures' and may respond to various other 'cocktails, eg ABVD (doxorubicin, bleomycin, vinblastine, dacarbazine), salvage therapies, third lines therapies (N Engl J Med 1993; 328:560oA)

hof German, courtyard A focal perinuclear clearing seen at the nuclear concavity in plasma cells and in others, eg lymphoblasts, Reed-Sternberg cells, or osteoblasts with eccentrically placed nuclei; the hof is best seen with Wright-Giemsa or other Romanowsky stain; it may also be seen in the inclusions in chlamydia-infected epithelial cells in trachoma inclusion conjunctivitis, where the 'hof' is created by the nucleus

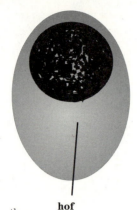

hof

Hogness box TATA box, see there

HOHD syndrome Hair-onychodysplasia, hypohydrosis-deafness syndrome An AR condition characterized by lifelong baldness, microdontia, dysplastic toenails, hypohidrosis, palmo-plantar as well as knee-elbow hyperkeratosis that may be accompanied by sensorineural defects

höhendiurese A physiological reaction to high altitudes, in which there is increased excretion of fluids; in acute mountain sickness, there is increased weight, infrequent urination, peripheral edema and rales on chest examination, ie fluid accumulation possibly related to the loss of this physiological response

holandric GENETICS Passing of chromosomal material exclusively from father to son, as in the passage of the Y chromosome

Hold-Oram syndrome Heart-hand syndrome An AD [MIM 142900] disorder with structural defects of the heart and upper limbs CLINICAL Upper limb defects may be uni- or bilateral and involve structures of the embryonic radial ray causing aplasia, hypoplasia, fusion and anomalous development of the radial, carpal and thenar bones resulting in a wide spectrum of phenotypes including triphalangeal or absent thumbs, foreshortened arms and phocomelia; cardiac abnormalities are variably present and are either structural, eg single or multiple atria, ventricular septal defects, or functional including sinus bradycardia and various degrees of AV block MOLECULAR PATHOLOGY HO syndrome is linked to a mutation of a gene on chromosome segment 12q2 (lod score = 16.8, ie odds favoring linkage to this region of $6 \times 10^{16}:1$) (N Engl J Med 1994; 330:885oA)

'hole-in-the-stomach' man PHYSIOLOGY Alexis St Martin, a French-Canadian fur trapper whose accidental shotgun blast to the stomach in 1822 never properly healed; Wm Beaumont, a US Army surgeon, took the opportunity to study gastric physiology and for the next eight years popped things in and out of Alexis' stomach including Limberger cheese, tripe, inebriants and other comestibles; these crude studies served to identify pepsin and hydrochloric acid

holiday heart Atrial fibrillation or flutter that occurs 1) After binge alcohol abuse (Am J Heart 1978; 95:555) or 2) As a startle response to loud noises, eg firecrackers on July 4th, the US day of Independence (N Engl J Med 1989; 320:402c)

holistic medicine Alternative medicine, see there

Holliday model MOLECULAR BIOLOGY A model that seeks to explain the mechanism of gene conversion during a recombination event, in which there is reciprocal exchange of distinct markers; according to the model delineated by R Holliday, homologous chromosomes I and II are aligned, adjacent chains are nicked at homologous sites, the strands are allowed to cross, then rejoin and the newly exchanged branches migrate back

Hollingshead index SOCIAL MEDICINE A simple scoring system for determining socioeconomic status based on two objective criteria

OCCUPATION The occupation of the head of household, allowing a score of 1 for major professionals (physicians, lawyers, certified public accountants), higher executives, major military or political officials, proprietors of large businesses, to a score of 7 for unskilled laborers and

EDUCATION The amount of formal education, with a score of 1 for those who had completed graduate/professional schooling to 7 for those who had not completed six years of formal education

holly leaf appearance 1) A descriptor for the scalloped regenerative nodules separated by broad bands of fibrosis, typical of the macronodular cirrhosis of well-advanced hemochromatosis 2) A descriptor for the irregularly spiculation of erythrocytes (drepanocytes) due to polymerization of 'sickling' hemoglobins (eg Hb C, D and S, sickle-trait Hb aka HbAS, S-thalassemia, Hb C-Harlem, hemoglobin S-Memphis) when erythrocytes are exposed to low-oxygen environments

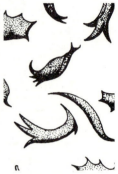

holly leaf pattern

Holocaust The constellation of activities carried out by the Nazis that were specifically directed at the ethnic cleansing of the Aryan 'race' and concomitant mass murder of lebesunwertes Leben (life unworthy of life) and genocide committed against Jews and other undesirables, eg Gypsies (RJ Lifton, The Nazi Doctors, Harper Collins, 1986); the term originated in film produced by NBC and aired in 1978, and has come to represent man's inhumanity to man (NY Newsday 22 Feb 1995; B4) see Nazi Science

holoprosenephaly Midline cleft syndrome EMBRYOLOGY A genetically heterogeneous often AD [MIM 157170] condition linked to defects in at least five (2,3,7,13,18) chromosomes which is characterized by the failure of the forebrain (prosencephalon) to differentiate into two cerebral hemispheres and diencephalon; it may be seen in severe cyclopia and is commonly associated with thirst defects and dehydration (N Engl J Med 1994; 331:432oA)

'Holstein cow pattern' A descriptor for the gross appearance of the patchy midbrain demyelinization typical of multiple sclerosis, seen with myelin stain

Holter monitor A noninvasive electrocardiographic device used to evaluate the efficacy of antiarrhythmic drugs in patients with sustained ventricular tachyarrhythmias; a drug is considered effective if it suppresses 1) Premature ventricular complexes detected by Holter monitoring, or 2) Inducible arrhythmias detected by invasive electrophysiologic studies; both methods for predicting arrhythmic drug efficacy are equally effective (N Engl J Med 1993; 329:445oA)

home access HIV testing* A proposed but (as of mid-May 1995) not yet FDA-approved format for allowing an individual to directly submit blood specimens to identify the presence of HIV in blood, while obtaining the specimen in the privacy of his/her home; the FDA would allow home collection, eg pricking of the finger and blotting of the blood on a filter paper which would be then sent to a laboratory approved to test for HIV, usually by the ELISA method; the specimens would remain anonymous except to the individual submitting the specimen, who would have a special code that would allow access to his/her results by a touch-tone telephone; those specimens that are positive for HIV antibodies, would then be retested by

Western blot to confirm the presence of HIV proteins (N Engl J Med 1995; 332:1296sB, 1308); there has been considerable discussion about the pros and cons of the inpersonal nature of telephone notification of HIV status, which in those who are positive may evoke suicidal behavior

*The more commonly used term, home HIV testing lends to confusion, in that the unsophisticated observer might believe that like other tests (eg home pregnancy tests), the testing occurs within the home, which it does not-Author's note

home-bound syndrome House-bound syndrome, see there

'home brew' product LABORATORY MEDICINE A product that a laboratory develops 'in-house' from existing products or from components already on the market for use within the laboratory or hospital, and not intended for commercial manufacture, sale, or distribution (Nature Medicine 1995; 1:501); the FDA has questioned whether certain unapproved home-brew products, eg monoclonal antibodies are appropriate to use for diagnostic purposes; under the CLIA'88 regulations, such tests are formally designated as 'not commercially available' (see CAP Today Jan 1993 p5)

home health care A segment of the health care industry that provides equipment, eg miniature intensive care units with ventilators, central venous pressure lines, telemetry, health care providers, eg licensed practical nurses, registered nurses and other services including socialization and communication, with the intent of maintaining a person in an environment, eg the patient's home, that is comfortable and cost-effective (JAMA 1991; 265:769rv)

home infusion therapy The IV administration of various therapeutic agents outside of a formal healthcare environment; HIT is used to administer analgesics, antibiotics, chemotherapy, parenteral nutrition; because of liberal reimbursement policies, overbilling and other abuses by HIT providers are alleged to be relatively common (US News & World Report 9 May 1994:63)

homelessness SOCIAL MEDICINE A state of disenfranchisement, in which a person or persons lack a permanent residence, often living on the streets without protection from the environment and/or ready access to sanitation facilities; between 250 000 and 3 million people are homeless in the US, and are often victims of violence, 'disaffiliation', suffer multiple infections, STD, especially AIDS and high levels of substance abuse; 40% are considered mentally disturbed; most deaths in the homeless occur in males under age 60 and are alcohol-related MORTALITY Is 3.5-fold > than the general population; ± 50% of deaths occur in the summer months; mortality is highest in white substance abusers; in others, the mortality is 3-fold > than the general population with an ↑ in death due to injuries, heart and liver diseases, intoxications and others (N Engl J Med 1994; 331:304sA) the long-term homeless may have dental, orthopedic, psychiatric, or respiratory problems and may have untreated infections (Am Med News 4 May 1992 p27); the US vagrancy laws are often abused in dealing with those who are guilty of no other crime than lack of money or a job and/or a place to go; see 'Fourth World', Shelterization

homeobox A lineage-restricted 183-base pair segment of DNA that contains homeotic genes, which control identity, polarity and segmentation of body parts, ie spatial organization and which plays a role in embryogenesis and spermatogenesis; the homeobox is highly conserved, with 75% amino acid homology between frogs, fruitflies and more 'advanced' species; the homeobox is a fairly 'ancient' DNA sequence, which has been found in yeasts, estimated to be 100 milion years old; the homeobox encodes a 61- residue homeo domain, a DNA-binding protein that controls the homeobox by trans-activation, binding by a 'helix-loop-helix' motif to the DNA near the gene's start codon; human homeoboxes are similar to the *Drosophila* boxes, discovered in the 1980s in the *Antennapedia*, fushi tarazu and

engrailed genes; Cf Oct-1, Oct-2 genes

homeopathic Pertaining or referring to homeopathy; because the crux of homeopathy is the seemingly counterintuitive philosophy that smaller concentrations of a particular substance have greater therapeutic effects, the adjective 'homeopathic' has also been used by some mainstream medicos to refer to a dose or therapeutic level of a particular substance that is too low to be of clinical utility

homeopathy A form of alternative medical care, formulated by SF Hahnemann (1755-1843) that was heretical at the time for its opposition to blood-letting, emetics and cathartics; homeopathy is based on the principle of '*similia similibus curantur*' (like cures like), ie a disease caused by a substance, eg arsenic, could be cured by that same substance in infinitely diluted doses; homeopathy has lost support for the lack of reproducibility of reported results; in the current environment, some of its practitioners have been severely criticized; in one report (Nature 1988; 333:816) ultra-low (homeopathic) concentrations of IgE evoked basophil degranulation; there was no plausible explanation of the phenomenon, the results were poorly reproducible (Nature 1988; 335:200); homeopathy thus remains unsubstantiated; see Alternative medicine, Naturopathy

homeotic genes Those genes that establish primitive embryonic structural pathways giving rise to adult structures, the mutation of which causes a transformation of body parts into structures that are appropriate for other positions in the organism; see Homeobox

Homer-Wright rosette Perivascular pseudorosette NEUROPATHOLOGY A spherical or annular cluster of small tumor cells arranged in 'garlands', surrounding a central space filled with pale-staining neurofibrillary material, packed around a delicate fibrovascular core; the tumor cells themselves have scant, poorly-defined cytoplasm, the nuclei are dark, have coarse but evenly dispersed chromatin, may have marked mitotic activity (olfactory neuroblastomas have low mitotic activity) (Am J Surg Pathol 1986; 10:478oA); H-W rosettes are a classic histological feature of neuroblastoma and medulloblastomas, and may be seen in peripheral nerve sheath tumors; see Neuroblastoma

Note: Esthesioneuroblastomas have been subdivided into tumors with true rosettes (neuroepitheliomas), tumors with pseudorosettes (neuroblastomas) and those that don't form rosette-like structures (neurocytomas), the last being a distinction of questionable usefulness

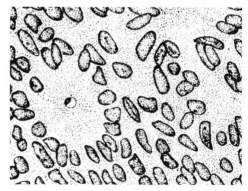

Homer-Wright rosettes

homeric laughter Uncontrolled spasmodic laughter induced by mirthless stimuli, a symptom of organic brain disease that indicates a poor prognosis; mirthless laughter may be seen in multiple sclerosis, pseudobulbar palsy, epilepsy, intracranial hemorrhage, frontal lobotomy and is especially characteristic of Kuru, a disease that causes 'laughing death'

homicide A rare event in civilized nations that reaches epidemic proportions in the US; in ♂ aged 15-24, homicide rate ranges from 0.3-0.5/10⁵ (Austria,) Japan to 5.0/10⁵ (Scotland), and 22/10⁵ (US), 86/10⁵ in blacks and 231/10⁵ in the state of Michigan; 12-40% of homicides in the US are drug-related and the victims often have cocaine metabolites (eg benzoylecgonine) in their body fluids at the time of death (**JAMA 1991; 265:760**) see Manslaughter, Murder; Cf Suicide

homing receptor selectin see Selectins

Hominidae ANTHROPOLOGY The primate family that contains *Homo sapiens* and both the ancestral and collateral (but extinct) species; explanations for the origin of Hominidae is have invoked many different selective pressures, including bioenergetic, migratory, morphological, and thermoregulatory considerations associated with foraging and feeding behavior, as well as aspects of life history patterns and social systems.' (**Science 1994; 264:955OA**); a critical component of these explanations is the assumption* that from 15 million to 5 million years ago, the African rain forest became more restricted, drier and seasonal woodlands and grasslands evolved with ↑ in habitat diversity

*Based on analysis the stable carbon isotope composition, there has been no change in vegetation in the past 15 millions years, weakening this assumption

homocysteine An amino acid not incorporated into proteins that is a critical intermediate in cysteine and methionine metabolism; in the breakdown of methionine, it reacts with serine to form cystathionine, or it can be methylated to form methionine; there is a statistical link between ↑ homocysteine and atherosclerosis–it promotes the growth of smooth muscle cells and inhibits the growth of endothelial cells, possibly by promoting cyclin gene expression (**New York Times 5 July 1994; C8**)

homocystinuria An AR [MIM 236200] condition caused by a defect of cystathionine β–synthase [EC 4.2.1.22] which is characterized by ↑↑↑ levels (> 300 µmol/L) of homocysteine in the blood CLINICAL Overgrowth of long bones, mental retardation, osteoporosis, ectopia lentis and thrombosis; most die before age 30 of arterial and venous occlusive disease; lesser ↑ of homocysteine is seen in heterozygotes (for homocysteinuria) of , and those with low levels of folic acid, vitamin B₁₂, in renal insufficiency and after cardiac transplantation (**Mayo Clin Proc 1995; 70:125OA**) TREATMENT Administration of pyridoxine (vitamin B₆)

homogeneity MRI Uniformity of the static magnetic field being used in MRI, a criterion of the magnet's quality; the requirements for homogeneity in MR imaging are less stringent than for MR spectroscopy, but must be maintained over a larger region; see Magnetic resonance imaging

homologous recombination GENETICS A recombination event that occurs at regions of chromosome homology, through the breakage and union of DNA, an event that has been used in transgenic models, where existing genes are knocked out and replaced with a modified gene; see Recombinant DNA technology

homology EVOLUTIONARY BIOLOGY A term that implies common ancestral origin of DNA and proteins, which has been incorrectly used by molecular biologists for the degree (in percentage) of sequence relatedness either for DNA (nucleotide or DNA 'homology') or proteins (amino acid or protein 'homology'); evolutionary biologists decry this misuse of 'homology' and suggest 'sequence similarity' as a viable substitute

Note: Given the firm entrenchment of the incorrect use of homology in the biological literature, and that evolutionary biologists are a more exotic species in the research food chain, the 'wrong' definition may ultimately prevail

homophobia PSYCHIATRY A term coined in 1967 in reference to an irrationally negative attitude toward those with homosexual orientation; homophobia in the US is linked to heterosexism* and religious fundamentalism, and has

caused many health care professionals to hide their sexual orientation from colleagues and patients (**N Engl J Med 1994; 331:923SA**) see Gay-bashing

*The belief that heterosexual activities and institutions are superior

homosexual behavior Same sex activity Note: The frequency of HB may be underreported because of social stigma that continues to be attached to homosexual orientation (**N Engl J Med 1994; 331:923SA**)

♂–20% have had a homosexual experience resulting in orgasm before age 19, 7% after age 19; 2-6% are exclusive homosexual, ± 3% are bisexual; gay ♂ often become sexually active at an earlier age (12.7 vs 15.7) and are more likely to have had multiple partners

♀–data is scanty; it is estimated that 3% of ♀ are homosexual in orientation

homosexuality The latent or manifest sexual attraction of one person to another of the same sex; the psychoanalytical view of C Socarides in that homosexuality is a sexual deviation arising from a common core disturbance consisting of a partial or complete arrest in the preoedipal phase of development (**N Engl J Med 1992; 327:1765BR**); Kinsey's seminal studies in the 1940s on sexual behavior in the US were based on data from white middle-class ♂; at the time, 4% of US ♂ were exclusively homosexual; data from 1970 and 1988 indicate that 20.3% of adult ♂ had had homosexual contact prior to age 19, 6.7% after the age of 19 and 1.6-2.0% within the last year; never-married ♂ are more likely to be homosexual, but also one-half of the current homosexual group was married Note: Minimum estimates are assumed as under-reporting of homosexual activity is probable; although still controversial, there is data to suggest that homosexuality is at least in part biological in origin, and not strictly driven by environmental cues and factors; a region in the anterior hypothalamus designated INAH3 has been reported to be 2-fold greater in the ♂ heterosexual than in the ♂ homosexual brain; other data supporting biological (ie genetic) factors in homosexuality derive from pooled twin studies, where 13% of brothers (13% of sisters), 24% of ♂ fraternal twins (16% of ♀ fraternal twins) and 57% of ♂ identical twin (50% of ♀ identical twins) were also homosexual (**Sci Am 1994; 270/5:44**) (Note: The case against a genetic component of homosexuality is made in the following article in the same issue, **Sci Am 1994; 270/5:50**); see AIDS, Gay bowel disease, Circumstantial homosexuality, HIV; Cf Sexual deviancy

homosexual panic A form of schizophrenic anxiety in which a person becomes greatly agitated, fearing that he/she is homosexual, will inadvertently commit an act viewed as being homosexual in nature, or will be accused of being homosexual; these anxiety attacks are transient and are often accompanied by delusions, hallucinations, irrational behavior or thought and shallow or inappropriate affect; see Circumstantial homosexuality; Cf 'Don Juan' syndrome

homunculus 'Little man' NEUROANATOMY A diagrammatic representation of the volume of the cerebral cortex dedicated to either motor (precentral or Brodman's areas 4 and 6) or sensory (postcentral or Brodman's area 3) zones with respect to each corporal region; the grotesque little man (facing page) has hands and tongue that are far more prominent than the trunk and extremities, indicating their relative importance

honeybee 'syndrome' A model for experimental teratogenesis, created by adding D-mannose to rat-embryo culture, causing growth retardation and faulty neural tube closure, which is attributed to low-level inhibition of glycolysis (hypoxic glycolysis is a major source of ATP during early rodent development and presumed to be so in humans); the defects are thought to result from aberrant 'fuel mixtures' during critical stages of embryogenesis, explaining some of the defects seen in children of diabetic mothers, in whom increased glucose causes defective glycolysis (**N Engl J Med 1981; 310:223**); the adjective 'honeybee' refers to the deleterious effects of D-mannose that were initially seen only in Apidae (honeybees); other hexoses (fructose, sorbitol, galactose) cause low-level growth retardation; the D-mannose effect can be overcome by increasing the O_2 or glucose in the system, suggesting that mannose and glucose compete with each other for available hexokinase

honeycomb atropy Atrophodermia vermiculata

honeycomb pattern A reticulated or net-like pattern with relative periodicity in a two-dimensional plane BONE RADIOLOGY A honeycomb pattern may be seen in a plain skull film as patchy new bone fills in the underlying osteoporosis circumscripta typical of Paget's disease of the bone GYNECOLOGIC CYTOLOGY 'Honeycombs' are monotonous clusters of benign endometrial cells seen on Papanicolaou-stained cervical smears, seen as monolayers of small epithelial cells with uniform, oval nuclei, bland or slightly granular chromatin PULMONARY DISEASE 'Honeycombing' is a localized or diffuse coarsening of pulmonary parenchyma with partial alveolar wall destruction and incomplete replacement, and alveolar wall thickening by interstitial fibrosis (in contrast, emphysema demonstrates alveolar wall attenuation), a pattern typical of advanced interstitial pneumonia; the radiologic honeycomb pattern is more vague, and may be seen in a plain chest film in interstitial fibrosis, as well as SLE, progressive systemic sclerosis, lymphangiomatosis syndrome, end-stage sarcoidosis and adenocarcinoma; Cf Chicken wire pattern

honey intoxication Infant botulism that may be due to ingestion of *Clostridium botulinum* spores, which germinate in the GI tract, producing toxin, causing constipation, feeding difficulties, floppy baby symptoms, facial grimacing, dysphagia, ↓ sphincter control, reflexes and sudden apnea; an estimated ½ of cases of infant botulism worldwide have been linked to honey, as the same serotype of *C botulinum* is isolated from both the honey and the infant MORTALITY < 3%

honeymoon cystitis A nonspecific urethritis caused by local irritation due to prolonged, frequent or first-time sexual activity in women with a low baseline of sexual traffic; damage to the vesicovaginal wall may evoke cystitis, hematuria, dysuria, increased frequency and urgency; although cultures are often negative, the condition may respond to antibiotics; resolution may be hastened by a rest period

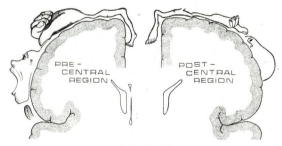

homunculus

honeymoon period A phrase used in various fields of medicine referring to a time period following the diagnosis of a disease, but preceding its full effect or impact, fancifully likened to the period of early marriage when the husband and wife are most cordial and passionate with each other DIABETOLOGY A period of residual β-cell function and insulin secretion in early-onset IDDM that follows stabilization of the patient's hyperglycemic presentation; in the honeymoon period, most children require ½ of the calcu-

lated insulin dose, ie 0.5 U/kg or may even go into temporary 'remission', signaled by recurring hypoglycemia at the initial dose, a time period that is short-lived, usually less than one year in duration NEPHROLOGY A period of optimism and euphoria accompanying the early stage of chronic dialysis by patients in renal failure; the honeymoon period lasts from 6 weeks to 6 months and is followed by a 'mourning period', see there PEDIATRIC SURGERY A postoperative time period in an infant with congenital diaphragmatic hernia characterized by stable vascular resistance, relative ease of ventilation and normalization of blood gases; this deteriorates within hours to days and the infant develops pulmonary hypertension and resultant right-to-left shunting through the ductus arteriosus and foramen ovale; see Extracorporeal membrane oxygenation

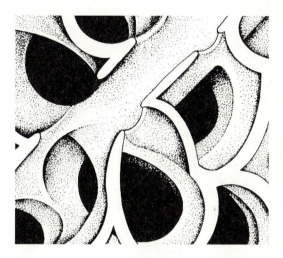

honeycomb pattern

honk PEDIATRICS A widely-transmitted precordial whoop, described as a high-pitched, musical, late systolic murmur in some patients with mitral valve prolapse, a sound attributed to resonation of the valve leaflets and chordae; non-honking patients with mitral valve prolapse may be made to honk by having them stand or lean

Note: 'Honk' is the sound produced by geese or or older automobile horns

H2O syndrome Hypogonadotrophic hypogonadism, muscular hypotonicity and obesity; see HHHO syndrome

honorary chromosome A highly colloquial term for mitochondrial DNA (see there), which contains 16 569 base pairs, and which has been also anointed as the 25th chromosome (X and Y being the 23rd and 24th, respectively)

honorary co-authorship Spurious co-authorship A practice in which the name of senior researchers are added to research reports that are the work of others, eg undergraduates and postdoctoral fellows working in their laboratories, regardless of whether they have participated in the research itself (**Nature 1987; 325:207**); this practice may prove embarassing to the co-author if the research results are not reproducible, or even problematic should the work prove to be problematic to be fraudulent; see Authorship, Baltimore affair, CV-weighing, Darsee affair

HOOD syndrome Hereditary onycho-osteodysplasia, see Nail-patella syndrome

Hoogsten base pairing MOLECULAR BIOLOGY A variant DNA conformation that occurs in a region where proteins interact with the double helix; Hoogsten pairing requires higher energy to maintain the physicochemical conformation by protonation of the cytosine ring; most double helices of DNA are in the classic Watson and Crick conformation

'hook and deliver' technique A recently devised method for removing Norplant contraceptive delivery device, in which one or two vertical incisions are made parallel to the capsules, leaving a 21-gauge needle in place for stabilization; the capsules and stabilizing needle are then hooked and delivered (N Engl J Med 1995; 332:821c)

hook effect IMMUNOPATHOLOGY An artefact occasionally seen in the immunoradiometric assay (IRMA) that appears when the hormone being measured is present in very high concentrations; the detector system will not measure that excess, as it will have reached a theoretical limit; the decreased counts bound with the labeled antibody at high hormone levels results in a spuriously low result being reported; IRMA should not be used for measuring hormones which may be in high concentrations (hCG, prolactin, or gastrin) in clinical samples; the hook effect requires that two different concentrations be measured to establish linearity

hookworm PARASITOLOGY Any hematophagous nematode of the family Ancylostomatidiae, eg Old World hookworm (*Ancylostoma duodenale*) and New World hookworm (*Necator americanus*) that targets the small intestine, resulting in sensitization of the penetration site, eg skin, causing 'ground itch', or lungs, eg Loeffler syndrome as they wiggle therethrough, causing eosinophilia and, due to bloodsucking, anemia LABORATORY Rhabditidiform larvae may be confused with *Strongyloides stercoralis* and the eggs may be confused with those of *Trichostrongylus* and *Meloidogyne* species (Sci Am 1995; 272/6:70)

HOPG Highly ordered pyrolytic graphite The most common substrate used in scanning tunneling microscope studies (SEMs) for analysis of the surface morphology or 'signature' of biomolecules, eg DNA Note: Because HOPG, which is attached electrophoretically to the molecules being studied, has its own 'signature' with features including periodicity and meandering of molecules over steps that were previously attributed to biomolecules, it is unclear whether SEM studies using HOPG are completely valid (Science 1991; 251:641)

hora somni Bedtime

horizontal ray RADIOLOGY A central projection ray that remains horizontal regardless of the patient's position; horizontal rays are of use in determining fluid levels, as these appear as sharply-demarcated lines, delineating two different densities and in films of joints to assess rugosity of an articular surface

horizontal transmission EPIDEMIOLOGY The transmission of an infection in individuals of the same generation; Cf Hereditary transmission, Vertical transmission

hormonal therapy GYNECOLOGY see Estrogen replacement therapy, Hormone replacement therapy ONCOLOGY A therapeutic modality for certain cancers, some of which partially respond to manipulation of hormonal receptors on the surface of the tumor cells BREAST CANCER Hormonal manipulation intends to block membrane receptors for estrogens and, to a lesser extent, progesterone, reducing the aggressiveness of the malignancy LYMPHOPROLIFERATIVE DISORDERS Adjuvant therapy uses corticosteroids in both induction of remissions and maintenance doses PROSTATE CANCER Hormonal therapy attempts to either inhibit gonadotropin at the pituitary by using potent analogs, eg buserelin, leuprolide acetate, blocking gonadotropin-releasing hormone, or block the peripheral action of androgens at the cellular level, eg flutamide, nilutamide; other therapeutic uses of hormones include treatment of deficiency states and use of pharmacologic doses of steroids as an anti-inflammatory agent or an immune suppressant; see Ectopic hormones, Estrogen receptors

hormone family A group of hormones that share consid-

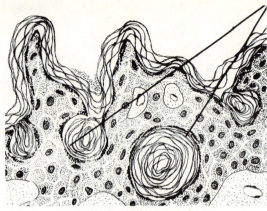

horn pseudocyst

erable sequence similarity ('homology') in terms of peptide motifs, including GI tract hormones and neuropeptides; hormone families are thought to have arisen through gene duplication during evolution and have been divided into

1) Gastrin, cholecystokinin

2) Secretin, glucagon, VIP, gastric inhibitory polypeptide (GIP), growth hormone releasing factor (GRF), glicentin, and oxyntomodulin

3) Pancreatic polypeptide, peptide YY, neuropeptide Y

4) Tachykinin, bombesin, substances K and P, neuromedin B

5) Opioid peptides

6) Proenkephalins, eg met- and leu-enkephalins

7) Pro-opiomelanocortins, including ACTH, α- and β-MSH, β-endorphin

8) Predynorphin group, including β-endorphin, dynorphin, leu-enkephalin, leumorphin

9) Calcitonin, epidermal growth factor (EGF), insulin and somatostatin

hormone-replacement therapy GYNECOLOGY A generic term for the administration of ovarian hormones (estrogen or progestogens) to women to alleviate the symptoms of menopause (eg urogenital atrophy and psychological symptoms), and more recently to slow or reverse osteoporosis and reduce the risk of ischemic heart disease; addition of progestins to estrogen does not ↓ the incidence of breast cancer in ♀ receiving ERT; the RR of breast cancer is 1.46 in ♀ age 50-55 who have received ≥ 5 years of exogenous estrogen, which rises to 1.71 by age 60-64 (N Engl J Med 1995; 332:1591oA)

*Note: As all the treatment regimens (oral or parenteral estrogen or combined estrogen and progestogen) contain estrogen, it is more commonly known as Estrogen replacement therapy, see there

hormone resistance syndrome A generic term for any condition caused by a reduced or absent end-organ responsiveness to a biologically active hormone, that may be caused by a defect in a hormone receptor or a post-receptor defect (N Engl J Med 1995; 332:155oA)

hormone response element Short, circa 20 base pairs in length cis-acting sequences of DNA that are required 'receptor' sites for hormonal activation and transcription; insertion of HREs to otherwise hormone-nonresponsive sites causes a gene to become responsive to a hormone; HREs function in a position- and orientation-independent fashion, thus acting like transcription enhancers, although differing therefrom as HRE activity requires a protein ligand

horn cell Keratocyte A normocytic, normochromic erythrocyte with lateral notches and two pointed ends, which corresponds to ruptured vacuoles; the cells have a semilunar or spindled shape; associated with intravascular protuberances, eg cardiac valve protheses, synthetic intravascular grafts and fibrin in DIC

horn pseudocyst DERMATOPATHOLOGY Laminated, whorls of 'basket-weave' cornified keratin that dip below the epithelial surface, forming pseudocystic spaces, a characteristic histologic finding seen in inflamed ('irritated') seborrheic keratosis; Cf Squamous eddies, Squamous pearls

horror autotoxicus Self tolerance, see there

horse riding stance see 'Plucked chicken' appearance

horseshoe kidney A relatively common (1/700 live births) lesion (♂:♀ ratio, 2:1), seen alone or associated with trisomy 18, characterized by fusion of the renal poles; this developmental anomaly occurs after the metanephric ducts have joined the metanephric blastema, but before the kidney's cephalic ascent, which occurs in the second gestational month; in most cases, the fusion is at the lower pole, the isthmus consists of renal parenchyma, lies anterior to the aorta and often is located in the lower pelvis as ascent is prevented by the inferior mesenteric artery; associated anomalies include urogenital anomalies, eg polycystic kidneys, ureter reduplication, as well as GI, cardiac, and skeletal anomalies and a slight increase in transitional cell carcinoma of the renal pelvis CLINICAL The clinical spectrum is broad, from asymptomatic to advanced renal disease, eg hydronephrosis, infection and concrement formation, which may be accompanied by chronic GI symptoms and pain; the 'classic' Rovsing sign, ie abdominal pain localizing to the kidneys, accompanied by nausea upon spinal retroflexion is rarely of help, but when present is due to the pressure of the isthmus of the kidney on the nerves and vessels and may occur in S-shaped or L-shaped kidneys

horseshoe lung Partial fusion of lungs behind the pericardial sac; one lung is smaller than the other but both have their own bronchial supply; the horseshoe lung is a morphologic anomaly seen in the scimitar lung that may be accompanied by pulmonary dysplasia

hospice An institution expressly intended to provide care and comfort for those who are dying of cancer and, more recently, AIDS; hospice care recognizes that death is inevitable and rather than attempt to cure a disease, alleviates the patient's and family's physical, mental, social and spiritual suffering in the final moments of life, by providing nursing care and relief of pain; an estimated 1700 hospices in the US provide care for ± 200 000 people, ½ of whom receive Medicare benefits

Note: Hospices were created in the Middle Ages as places where the Christian crusaders could receive care and replenishment

hospital-acquired penetration contact A break of skin or mucosal barriers by needle sticks, paper cuts, broken glass, resulting in contact infection by highly infectious, blood-transmitted, usually viral infections, eg HIV-1, hepatitis B, or Jakob-Creutzfeldt agent; the frequency of HIV infection via this route is low, generally regarded as being much < than 1 per 100 infected penetrations; see Sharps

A cardiology resident physician in Baltimore was the first physician to be infected by HIV-1 through an HAPC

hospital autopsy A postmortem examination based on interest in a person's cause of death by a family member or by the clinical staff, and not motivated by forensic concerns*; permission to perform a hospital must be given by the closest living relative (next-of-kin)

*Because such autopsies haved been 'cleared' by the medical examiner's (coroner's) office, as the deaths are not regarded as forensically suspicious, they are also known as non-official autopsies, an unfortunate term that to the less sophisticated connotes an autopsy performed by a physician with lesser training or skills

hospital-based physician A physician who provides 'clinical support' for patient management, performing his medical services within a hospital or medical facility; hospital-based physicians include radiologists (interventional and diagnostic), anesthesiologists, pathologists and emergency room physicians ('RAPERs'), as well as physicians specialized in nuclear medicine, radiation oncology, phys-

ical and rehabilitation medicine, occupational medicine, public health and forensic pathology; see RAPERs; Cf House physician, Medical specialties, Primary care, Surgical specialties

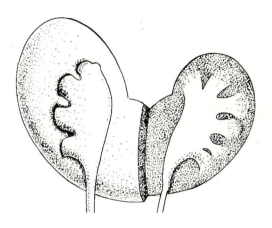

horseshoe kidney

hospital bed 'syndrome' Cot sides 'syndrome' An event with medicolegal implications that occurs in brain-damaged patients (who often are, in addition, elderly and suffer osteoporosis), who have fallen out of a hospital bed with the sides up, which is a fall from a greater height than that which occurs with the sides down PROGNOSIS Poor; coma and death are common

hospital chart A specific type of medical record, which is a legal document open to public examination; hospital charts should be complete (see S.O.A.P.), dated often and the prose should be terse Note: Changing of dates and details in the chart at a later date is unethical and puts the defendant at risk for punitive damages, or loss of the license to practice medicine; a good hospital record should '...contain sufficient information to identify the patient, support the diagnosis, justify the treatment and document the results accurately' (Standard II of the JCAHO Accreditation Manual)

hospital information system The computer hardware and software that processes a hospital's information, including financial, patient and 'strategic' management, including patient accounts, tracking of patients, payroll, reimbursements, taxes and statistics; a complete hospital computer integrates monitoring of medication usage, laboratory results, patient and nurse scheduling, on-line library information, inventory control and food management; budget costs for an HIS average $550 000/year in hospitals of less than 250 beds to $4.1 million in hospitals with more than 500 beds; Cf Laboratory information system

hospitalization The period of confinement in a health care facility that begins with a patient's admission and ends with his discharge; hospitalization also refers to a group health insurance program that pays employees all the expenses incurred during a period of hospitalization, including both the hospital costs per se, the so-called part 'A', as well as a portion or the entirety of the physicians' costs (part 'B'); see Bed, Per diem

hospital mortality rate A parameter used by some federal agencies in the US to measure the quality of medical care; hospital mortality rates: osteopathic facility 129/1000, for-profit facility 121/1000, public facility 120/1000, private non-teaching facility 116/1000, private not for-profit facility 114/1000, private teaching facility

108/1000; see High-mortality outlier

hospital utilization A group of statistics referring to a population's use of hospital services; in the US (1985), hospital utilization was 148 days/1000 persons in a population; average length of stay: 6.5 days and was due to cardiovascular disease (5.5 million admissions), childbirth (4.3 million admissions) and GI disease (3.9 million admissions)

hospitalization hazard A generic term for any risk to health that is inherent in hospitalization, eg medication prescribing errors, normal complications of anesthesia or surgery, and others (JAMA 1990; 263:2329) see July phenomenon

host COMPUTERS The computer that performs centralized functions, eg making program or data files to computers in a network, which may be self-contained or located on Internet; Cf Server IMMUNOLOGY An alternative term for graft recipient INFECTIOUS DISEASE Any organism (animal or plant) that provides sustenance for another organism, usually understood to be a undesired parasite

host defense The protection an organism is afforded against infections, which may be 1) Nonimmunologic, including mucocutaneous (integumental) barriers, cilia, microvilli and mechanical, eg urinary outflow, vascular perfusion of tissues and native flora that are capable of 'outcompeting' and 2) Immunologic, including chemotaxis, phagocytosis, immunoglobulins, complement, cell-mediated (T cell) defense

hostility see 'Toxic core'

hot air balloon sign RADIOLOGY A fanciful descriptor for the radiological appearance of a massively dilated diverticulum of the sigmoid colon, where the point of attachment is the 'gondola'; that occurs in association with a slowly expanding abscess

'hot and heavy' MOLECULAR BIOLOGY A method for examining DNA-protein (histone) interactions, by using two different radioactive labels, one is detected by radioimmunoassay and labeled with ^{3}H ('hot'); the other radioisotope is detected by density separation, and labeled with ^{13}C and ^{15}N which are 'heavy' isotopes

hot antigen suicide IMMUNOLOGY A technique for determining whether antibody-producing cells descend exclusively from the antigen-binding cells; the antigen in the experimental system is labelled with a highly radioactive isotope, eg ^{131}I and if the antigen-binding cell is the ancestor of the antibody-producing cell then no antibody will be produced, since binding of the 'hot' antigen would be tantamount to cellular suicide; the hot antigen suicide theory is considered proof of the clonal selection theory

hot area Hot zone, see there

hot-cold disease system A therapeutic philosophy rooted in classical Greco-Roman and Persian-Arabic medicine that arrived with 'los Conquistadores' and merged with local Mayan medicine; the system is practiced in its waning years by 'curanderos' in Central America; all illness is viewed as either 'hot' and treated with their opposite, ie 'cold' remedies, eg limes, cauliflower and roses or viewed as 'cold', treated with 'hot remedies', eg rue (*Ruta graveolens*), garlic and crude brown sugar

hot comb alopecia A rare condition affecting women who straighten their hair with a 'hot comb', which may cause centrifugal scarring of the scalp

hot cross bun skull Turmschädel, see there

hotdog headache Pulsating cephalgia with facial flushing, caused by sodium nitrite-preserved meat, especially hotdog (frankfurter) meat; in addition to preserving meat, nitrites impart a red tinge that imparts a desirable ('marketable') appearance for displaying meats to shoppers

The hotdog's ancestors began life in Ancient Babylonia circa 1500 BC and evolved in the Middle Ages in the butchers' guilds in various European city-states; the first 'frankfurter was born in the early 1850s in Frankfurt (are you surprised?), which was differed (for better or worse) from the wurst, the 'standard issue' German sausage, as it was streamlined and curved; the name hot dog has been attributed to Tad Dorgan, a syndicated Hearst newspaper cartoonist who couldn't spell dachshund, the alternative name for frankfurter at the time being dachshund sausage (C Panati, Extraordinary Origins of Everyday Things, Harper & Row, New York, 1987)

hot flashes/flushes GYNECOLOGY A symptom afflicting 80-85% of middle-aged women, first occurring during the perimenopause, continuing with decreasing intensity for years, manifesting itself as transient waves of erythema and uncomfortable warmth beginning in the upper chest, face and neck, followed by fine sweating and chills; hot flashes are precipitated by emotional stress, meals and environmental cues, and are more intense when the ovaries are surgically removed than when the decline of ovarian function occurs more gracefully ETIOLOGY Idiopathic, due to the response of the autonomic nervous system to ↓ estrogens; ↓ estrogens are also held responsible for osteoporosis, atrophy of vaginal epithelium, leukorrhea and pruritus; the relation of ↓ estrogen to coronary artery disease is unclear* THERAPY Although hormonal therapy, eg estrogens in ♀ and androgens in ♂ ameliorates the symptoms, these agents may be contraindicated in ♀ with breast cancer, and in ♂ with prostatic cancer; megestrol acetate reduces the incidence of hot flashes by 85% (vs 20% in placebo group) (N Engl J Med 1994; 331:347OA)

*Although estrogen replacement minimizes the complications of menopause, it also 'drives' proliferation of endometrial, which may result in adenomatous hyperplasia and occasionally endometrial carcinoma Note: Hot flashes occur in eunuchs and in most men who have been acutely deprived of testosterone as in castration, a therapeutic modality for advanced prostatic carcinoma; diethylstilbestrol may stop the flashes, but exacerbate cardiovascular disease, which in Europe is treated with cyproterone acetate

'hot' food see Spicy foods

'hotline' A telephone system often manned by volunteers and dedicated to answering questions about a particular disease or group of diseases, eg AIDS 'hotline'; or designed to facilitate access to a particular service, eg Abused women 'hotline'

hot nodule NUCLEAR MEDICINE A focal increase in radioisotope uptake on a ^{123}I scintillation scan; in the thyroid, hot nodule(s) often correspond to toxic nodular or multinodular goiter, in which functional thyroid lesions suppress TSH (thyroid-stimulating hormone) synthesis; Cf Cold nodule, Warm nodule

'hot paper' SCIENTIFIC JOURNALISM A paper or article published in a peer-reviewed journal that receives an increased number of citations (see Citation impact) by other authors, implying that it has presented unique or important data; see 'Fast track' paper, Landmark article; Cf Uncitedness index

hot sauce see Louisiana hot sauce

hot scan RADIOLOGY A rounded region of increased imaging intensity in a solid organ, eg the liver, when viewed by immunoscintigraphy; in one such protocol, anti-CEA monoclonal antibody was labeled with ^{99m}Tc and whole body and SPECT scans performed; the significance of a 'hot' vs 'cold' vs a 'hot' scan is uncertain (Croatian Med J 1994; 35:233)

'hot seat' SURGICAL PATHOLOGY A location in some academic departments of pathology that provides tentative diagnoses for all tissues received from the previous days' surgery and endoscopic procedures; the 'hot seat' allows a patient's attending physician to treat the patient without delaying clinical decisions, waiting for the paper copy of a histologic diagnosis; it is a legacy from Lauren Ackerman, the father of Surgical Pathology

hot spot EPIDEMIOLOGY Any situation in which there is a marked increase of a particular disease, eg HIV infection among disenfranchised inner-city inhabitants (N Engl J Med 1994; 331:1451ED) see Designer antibodies IMMUNOLOGY A hypervariable region present in the DNA segments that encode the variable region of the heavy (V_H) and light (V_L) chains of an immunoglobulin molecule, also known as complementarity-determining regions (CDR); these points provide the necessary specificity for binding antigens and determine an immunoglobulin's idiotype, while the background support regions of the heavy and light chains are known as framework regions FR; the hot spots on the kappa and lambda light chains are located near amino acid residues 30, 50 and 95 MOLECULAR BIOLOGY A region of DNA where mutation and recombination occurs at a much higher than normal rate; HIV has an entire hypermutable region of 'hot spots', the env of the gp120 protein; thus HIV is constantly 'ahead' of the host immune system; similar hotspot regions for mutations occur in the *p53* gene, eg in skin cancer at codons 196, 248, 278-81, and 342 (New York Times 18 January 1994; C1) THERMOGRAPHY A circumscribed increase in skin temperature of the breast, which may be seen in both carcinoma and mastitis; the unacceptable high false positive and false negative rates of thermography caused it to be abandoned

hot start PCR A permutation of PCR in which the reaction chamber is preheated to 82°C prior to adding Taq DNA polymerase, so that the polymerase chain reaction can 'hit the floor running'; while the technique is regarded by some workers as cumbersome, the theoretical advantage is that by heating the reactants, the stringency required for allowable hybridization is increased, thereby decreasing the likelihood that the wrong primer will be amplified (see Diagn Mol Pathol 1992; 1:256) see PCR

hot tub dermatitis A generalized pruritic infection caused by *Pseudomonas aeruginosa* acquired in communal hot tubs and whirlpools CLINICAL Hot tub folliculitis begins hours to days post-ablution with vesiculopustular eruptions over the trunk, buttocks, arms and legs, and may resolve without therapy in a week

hot zone Hot area, hot side EPIDEMIOLOGY A Biosafety Level 4 room or area in which trained personnel are working with highly virulent infectious oragnisms, eg Ebola virus (R Preston, The Hot Zone, Random House, New York, 1994)

hotel services Those services and departments in a hospital or health care facility that pertain to providing the services that overlap those provided by a hotel, eg food services, linen services, and maintenance of relevant inventory of supplies, etc

Hottentot apron Excessive elongation of the labia minora seen in the Hottentot tribe of southern Africa, which when seen elsewhere has been attributed to masturbation

Hounsfield units CT number A unit of tissue density used in computed tomography; Hounsfield units measure the amount of attenuation of a biological material: bone is +1000 H units, water is 0 H units, air is −1000 H units; the units were named in honor of Hounsfield, the British physicist who fathered computed tomographic imaging analysis, while working at EMI, the British recording and engineering firm; the first person 'imaged' was his secretary who had a glioma of the brain

72-hour fast ENDOCRINOLOGY A test performed in a hospital setting that is used to identify the cause(s) of hypoglycemia; the test begins as of the last ingestion of calories; calorie- and caffeine-free beverages are allowed, medications are eliminated or reduced to a minimum; glucose, insulin, C peptide, and proinsulin are measured at 6-hour intervals; the 72-hour fast is of use in identifying insulinoma, factitious hypoglycemia, sulfonylurea-induced hypoglycemia, hypoglycemia mediated by IGF, non-insulin-mediated hypoglycemia, and nonhypoglycemic disorders (N Engl J Med 1995; 332:1144RA)

hourglass A popular adjectival descriptor for any cylindrical mass with a central constriction

hourglass deformity CARDIOLOGY A focal stenotic ring within large arteries, typical of supravalvular aortic stenosis TREATMENT Insert Dacron™ or pericardial patch RADIOLOGY A finding by 'barium swallow' in patients with combined sliding and para-esophageal hernia of the esophagogastric junction, where the 'waist' of the hourglass corresponds to constriction from the hiatal ring UROLOGY A congenital malformation of the urinary bladder in which there is incomplete transverse reduplication of the vesical; most cases occur in men and have no clinical significance

hourglass gallbladder Dumbbell gallbladder A deformity without clinical significance, consisting of transverse septation between the body and fundus; Cf Phyrigian cap

hourglass mark An identifying red spot with a central constriction which is located on the ventral aspect of the female black widow, *Lactrodectus mactans*; see Black widow

hourglass nucleolus An elongated nucleolus with a central constriction that may be seen in the lymphocytes of Burkitt's lymphoma accompanied by coarse chromatin

house-bound syndrome PSYCHIATRY A type of panic disorder that most commonly occurs in women (ratio, 2-4:1), affecting 2-6% of women between ages 18 and 64; house-boundness is characterized by agarophobia, difficulty in functioning in public and generalized anxiety, which evokes cardiovascular symptoms, eg chest pains, tachycardia, arrhythmia, as well as GI distress, headache, vertigo, syncope and paresthesiae; see Panic disorder

Note: In the DSM-IV, neither agoraphobia nor panic attacks are codable disorders, but defined in a specific context; the closest equivalent term is 'panic disorder with agoraphobia' [300.21, DSM-IV]

house dust mite *Dermatophagoides farinae, D pteronyssoides* An organism that feeds on detritus in the house, which is highly allergenic, the degree of exposure to which can be measured by RAST

housekeeping genes MOLECULAR BIOLOGY Those genes that are expressed (or have the potential for being expressed) in all cells, theoretically at all times; constitutive genes encode proteins involved in basic cellular functions, eg glycolysis and electrolyte balance and are thus required by all cells

housemaid's knee Occupation-related traumatic bursitis see 'Beat knee', Genu genuflectum

house officer A resident in residence*

*ie a physician in training who is in house (hospital)

house physician A loosely-defined term referring to physician who 'covers' the medical needs of patients in a hospital; a house physician may not be board-certified, but usually has had a number of years of formal training (ie residency) in clinical medicine in a teaching hospital, and works in a secondary care facility, usually carrying out the wishes of the patient's 'private' physician

house staff The body of physicians and other health care providers who participate in patient management within the confines of a hospital; in teaching hospitals, the house staff includes interns, residents, and fellows who act with an increasing degree of autonomy under the tutelage of licensed, board-certified physicians in an officially accredited graduate medical education program; in non-teaching hospitals, the house staff is comprised of physicians

1) Whose practice is confined to the hospital, eg radiologists, anesthesiologists, pathologists, emergency physicians (RAPERs), critical care specialists, high-risk neonatologists, and others

2) Who do not have private patients, but rather provide service to the patients of other, 'attending' physicians, see House physician and

3) Who are may not be eligible for certification in a specialty of medicine board or received prolonged specialty training; house staff may include dentists, osteopaths and podiatrists; see Hospital-based physician, RAPERs

house-tree-person test PSYCHIATRY A clinical test in which facets of a person's character and internal conflicts are inferred from the manner in which he/she draws a house, a tree, and a person

Howard Hughes Medical Institute A philanthropic institution created in 1953 by American aviator-industrialist-billionaire, Howard Hughes; unlike other research institutes, the HHMI is largely 'de-centralized' and is based in 30 university-hospital complexes throughout the USA; HHMI's stated areas of interest include genetics, immunology, metabolic regulation, neuroscience and structural biology and in 1990 had a budget of $230 million for 180 investigators and 1350 ancillary staff (**HHMI, Bethesda, MM, USA 20817**); Cf Imperial Cancer Research Fund, Wellcome Trust

Howell-Jolly bodies Small (< 0.5 µ in diameter) rounded basophilic intraerythrocytic inclusions; the inclusions represent residual nuclear material, possibly chromosomal material; H-J bodies are 'pitted' from reticulocytes during passage through the interendothelial slits in the splenic sinus; H-J bodies are typically present following splenectomy, and in those with hemolytic anemia, megaloblastic anemia, and hyposplenism

Hox A family of vertebrate genes which, like the homeobox genes first discovered in *Drosophila melanogaster* (with which they share significant sequence homology), are important regulators of vertebrate development, by an as-yet unknown mechanism (**Nature 1991; 350:473, 458**) see Homeobox

Hoxsey method An unproven method of cancer therapy in which a 'brown tonic' containing potassium iodide, licorice, and herbs is administered for internal malignancies or one of three topical escharotic formulations is administered for external malignancy, in conjunction with a 'positive attitude' and special elimination diet; there is no data to support its efficacy; see Unproven method of cancer therapy; Cf Alternative medicine

HPETE Hydroperoxyeicosatetranoic acid The parent molecule for the leukotrienes arising from the 5-lipoxygenase pathway of arachidonic acid metabolism, where HPETE is converted to leukotriene A_4, B_4 and the slow-recting substances of anaphylaxis (leukotrienes C_4, D_4 and E_4); see Arachidonic acid

HPF see High power field

HPFH Hereditary persistence of fetal hemoglobin, see there

HPLC High-pressure (500-1500 pounds/square inch, psi) or high performance liquid chromatography LABORATORY INSTRUMENTATION A highly sensitive analytic method used in pharmacology, toxicology, and hormonal analysis (steroids, catecholamines and small peptides), as well as in industrial and clinical laboratories; HPLC is of use in the clinical area in TDM, toxicology, sports medicine, and in classifying patients (**Am Clin Lab July 1994**) METHOD A microliter volume liquid sample is injected into a moving stream of solvent flowing through a 'column', which separates the sample molecules by adsorption, partition, ion exchange or size exclusion; the molecules are eluted or 'pulled off' the column and detected by an ultraviolet light detector, fluorometer or electrochemical analyzer; HPLC may be used in tandem with various forms of liquid chromatography, eg gel filtration, adsorption, partition and ion exchange

HPRT Hypoxanthine-guanine phosphoribosyl transferase, see there

HPSF Hepatocyte proliferation stimulatory factor A heat-labile trypsin-sensitive protein, the production of which is increased in rodent livers that have suffered toxic insults; a similar factor is presumed to exist in humans

HPV Human papillomavirus A virus with premalignant potential, which is most prevalent in those with the greatest number of sexual partners; 65 genotypes of HPV (a genotype is considered distinct if it has < than 50% DNA sequence similarity or 'homology' with its closest relative) have been described; HPV has been identified by in situ hybridization in epithelial proliferations that are benign, eg condyloma acuminatum, or malignant, eg squamous cell carcinoma of the anus, penis, and uterine cervix, or of uncertain clinical behavior, eg inverted papillomas of the nasopharynx; uterine cervical carcinomas that are negative for HPV sequences have a 2.6-fold ↑ risk of relapse, a 4.5-fold ↑ risk for distal metastases, and have a ↑ incidence of positive regional lymph nodes; anal HPV infection is associated with anal intraepithelial neoplasia; HPV types 6 and 11 are not considered premalignant*, while HPV types 16, 18, 31, 33 and 35 are associated with cervical dysplasia, CIN and anogenital cancer; 78% of ♀ with HPV, especially 16 and 18 develop CIN-2 to CIN-3 (**N Engl J Med 1992; 327:1272oa**); the mechanism for malignant degeneration occurs is unclear, but HPV encodes a viral protein E6 produced by clinically aggressive HPV that binds to the tumor suppressor protein p53 implying that HPV evokes de-repression phenomena; Cf Cervical intraepithelial neoplasia

*Although types 6 and 11 have been identified in Buschke-Löwenstein tumors, which in turn are linked to penile cancer

Also 1) Hemophilus pertussis vaccine 2) High passage virus 3) Hypoxic pulmonary vasconstriction

HRE Hormone response element, see there

HS *hora somni*, bedtime

HSE Heat-shock consensus element CTNGAANNTTCNAG A 14, or possibly 10 base pair segment of DNA that is present in multiple copies and located upstream from all heat-shock genes; single base pair substitutions of the HSE (and of immediately flanking regions) cause considerable variation in the production of heat shock proteins; see Heat shock, Heat shock proteins

HSIL High-grade squamous intraepithelial lesion, see there

hsp Heat shock proteins, see there

hsp65 A gene that encodes a 65-kD heat shock protein expressed in mycobacteria, which is a major target of the host immune system; *hsp65* is present in all known *Mycobacterium* spp, but not in non-*Mycobacterium* species studied thus far; based on RFLP (restriction fragment length polymorphism) analysis, *hsp65* has been found to be highly variable, and thus an ideal target for molecular epidemiologic studies (**Arch Pathol Lab Med 1995; 119:123oa**)

HSR Homogeneously staining region(s) MOLECULAR BIOLOGY Duplicated chromosomal regions present in up to 100 copies that often correspond to oncogenes, eg N-*myc*; HSRs may span a several hundred kilobase segment of DNA and are most prominent in malignant cells; duplicated regions confined to the chromosome, are HSRs; when the same fragments split off as independent particles, they are termed 'double minutes'; Cf Tandem repeats

HSV Herpes simplex virus

HSV Herpes simplex virus, see Herpesvirus, also 1) Head small veins (anatomy) 2) Highly selective vagotomy

HTLA antibody High-titer, low-avidity antibody, see there

HTLV Human T cell leukemia/lymphoma virus A family of enveloped, single-stranded retroviruses, subfamily Oncoviridae that produce a DNA copy from viral RNA by using reverse transcriptase; the HTLV as a group are capable of immortalizing and transforming T cells EPIDEMIOLOGY The HTLV family all appear to be transmitted by blood and mucosal contacts and thus concomitant infections may occur, eg HTLV-I and HIV-1; HTLV-I may be a cofactor facilitating production of large quantities of HIV-1 by infected leukocytes

HTLV-I A retrovirus that immortalizes T cells; it is associated with 1) Adult T-cell lymphoma/leukemia in endemic regions of southern Japan (where up to 40% of leukemic patients are HTLV-I-positive) and the Caribbean 2) Chronic progressive myelopathy (tropical spastic paralysis), a condition endemic to the Caribbean, tropical Africa and South America and 3) HTLV-I-associated neuropathy; HTLV-I, like HIV-1, is a blood-borne infection; the carrier incidence of HTLV-I in the US and Europe ranges from 0.03% to 0.10%; 1% of HTLV-I-infected subjects develop clinical disease, which may reflect host susceptibility and variant strains of the virus; neurological disease is attributed to the presence of high circulating levels of HTLV-I-specific cytotoxic T lymphocytes that are CD8+, HLA class I-restricted, which recognize products encoded in the regulatory pX region

HTLV-II A retrovirus that may transform CD4 T cells, that may rarely be linked to disease, eg hairy cell leukemia; HTLV-I and HTLV-II have a 60% homology with each other, both use the same cell membrane receptor (encoded on chromosome 17cen-qter) to penetrate T cells, evidenced by interference with syncytium formation, have a tax gene encoding the transactivating protein, p37xII required for replication, immortalize T cells, causing malignant transformation by trans-activation, and increase the expression of genes attached to appropriate viral control sequences (these proteins are probably encoded near the 3' end of the viral genome)

HTLV-III HIV-1, see there

HTLV-IV HIV-2, see there

HTLV-V A retrovirus described in a case of CD4+/Tac-mycosis fungoides associated with cutaneous T cell lymphoma

hub Gateway, see there

Huckleberry Finn 'syndrome' Truancy syndrome A psychodynamic complex in which the obligations and responsibilities avoided as a child, eventuate into frequent job changes and absenteeism as an adult, a response that may represent a defense mechanism arising from parental rejection, a deeply-ingrained feeling of inferiority and depression in a relatively intelligent person

Note: Huckleberry Finn is the key character in Mark Twain's book by the same name, who shirked responsibilities

HUGO Human Genome Organization

human adjuvant disease A human correlate to adjuvant disease‡ of animals, which was first described in the mid-1960s in Japanese women who had undergone injections of silicone, paraffin, and other unknown materials into their breasts; as many as ½ of women who have had silicone breasts implants have circulating anti-collagen antibodies; HAD per se appears to be an uncommon complication of systemic leakage of silicone and is characterized by rheumatoid arthritis, systemic sclerosis, malignant hypertension, and other manifestations of chronic connective tissue disease (N Engl J Med 1994; 331:1231c)

human catastrophe see Disaster

human chorionic gonadotropin see hCG

human chorionic sommatomammotropin Placental lactogen A single-chain 21-kD polypeptide hormone produced by the syncytiotrophoblast that is lactogenic, somatotrophic, luteotropic, and mammotropic

Human Frontier Science Project A foundation created by Japan's Ministry of International Trade and Industry (MITI), based in Strasbourg, France that has a primary goal of promoting research on the brain and molecular biology, through multinational collaboration and sharing of the incurred financial burden (Nature 1991; 350:97n)

Human Genome Project A multinational collaborative effort to sequence (map) all 3×10^9 nucleotides of a haploid set of the human genome, begun in 1987 and projected to be completed by the year 2000 at a total cost of US

3×10^9; if the sequencing were carried out by hand it would require 30 000 person-years of labor, at an error rate of circa 1 base per 1000; the newer sequencers substantially reduce the error rate and time required for sequencing; the database created from the Genome Project is less useful than the technological advances engendered by the project itself; in the early stages, the map intends to 'blanket' each of the 23 chromosomes with evenly spaced genetic 'signposts', the more markers (a minimum of 500 to several thousand), the finer the resolution; the strategy proposed by M Olsen is to use short, tagged segments of DNA sequence as landmarks, 'creating an STS map' and relying on the language and techniques of PCR as a standard; the STS (sequence tagged site) approach allows facile integration and cooperation among 'big' and 'little' laboratories; it is hoped by the year 2000, a map and the function of 6000 genes will be developed; another approach is that of creating a complementary DNA (cDNA) map of only those genes that are expressed in cells, thereby by-passing all of the information-poor ('junk') DNA, which comprises circa 95% of the human genome; the advantage to the cDNA map approach is that the genetic information obtained from the genome in terms of enzymes and various proteins could be used immediately; see Sequencers

Note: An argument against such 'big science' projects is that they divert funds and manpower away from researcher-driven ('little science') projects

human granulocyte ehrlichiosis A recently described condition that begins with nonspecific flu-like symptoms, high fever, muscle pain, headache, shaking chills, and coughing, followed by a septic state; HGE is caused by a rickettsia-like organism genetically similar to *Ehrlichia phagocytophila* and *E equi* TREATMENT Doxycycline

human herpes virus see Herpesvirus

human immune globulin A therapeutic agent prepared from a donor pool screened for the presence of HIV-1, both at the time of 'harvesting' and once the plasma is pooled; one form of HIG, Sandoglobulin is produced by the Kistler-Nitschmann method of cold ethanol fractionation at acid pH, a process that completely inactivates viruses; 7.5 million grams of HIG have been infused and no case of HIV, HAV, HBV or non-A, non-B hepatitis has been reported (personal communication, Sandoz Pharmaceuticals) INDICATIONS, HIG Primary immunodeficiencies, eg X-linked agammaglobulinemia, severe combined immune deficiency and combined variable immune deficiency, as well as in acute or chronic ITP

human immunodeficiency virus HIV-1, see there

human placental lactogen Human chorionic somatomammotropin, see there

human replication protein RPA, see there

human shield The use of a person to protect a kidnapper, terrorist, or combatant in a conflict from gunfire

humanized antibody A product created by recombinant DNA technology in order to reduce the immunogenicity of non-human monoclonal antibodies, transferring the hypervariable genes of a rat antibody (which encodes peptide segments capable of recognizing the desired epitope), into the normal human gene; the resulting immunoglobulin is largely human, thereby reducing the 'xenophobic' response or allograft rejection when the hybrid molecule is administered to a human, confining the nonhuman portion to the necessary recognition site; the constant region may be selected for desired effector functions including complement fixation, antibody-dependent cell-mediated cytotoxicity and maximum serum half-life; Cf Designer antibody

'humanized' milk NEONATOLOGY A modified formulation of cow milk, the fat ratio of which closely mimics human milk (40% casein, 60% whey), indicated in infants below 2000 g; see Milk; Cf White beverages

HUMARA The X-linked human androgen receptor gene, which is of use in determining clonality given the high rate (> 90%) of heterozygosity seen at this locus, accompanied by consistent patterns of methylation (**N Engl J Med 1994; 331:1540A**)

humidifier lung A transient condition related to mechanical ventilation of buildings related to the heating and cooling systems, possibly caused by water-borne amoebae, which develops 1-3 days after exposure CLINICAL Malaise, cough, chest tightness, shortness of breath and with time, weight loss; the symptoms appear 4-6 hours after re-exposure to a workplace, often after the weekend, thus the common synonym of 'Monday sickness'; the symptoms resolve spontaneously, regardless of continued exposure RADIOLOGY Negative LABORATORY Antibodies to *Negleria gruberi* and *Acanthamoeba* spp; other humidifier lung organisms include *Aspergillus fumigatus*, *Aureobasium pullulans*, *Micropolyspora faeni*, *Thermoactinomyces vulgaris* and other water-born organisms; see Sick building syndrome

humor A fluid or gel-like substance

humoral doctrine MEDICAL HISTORY The medical philosophy of the ancient Greeks in which the state of health and disease was determined by the four body 'humors', blood, yellow and black bile, and phlegm and the relationship of these with the four humors of air, fire, earth, and water

humoral immune system B cell immunity An arm of the immune system that develops in vascular compartments or extracellular fluid spaces, which is mediated by specific, eg immunoglobulins and nonspecific, eg complement molecules, contrasting with cellular or T cell immunity; Cf Cell-mediated immunity

Note: Subdivision of immune labors into the neat 'B' and 'T' boxes oversimplification as the two systems are intimately linked

hump NEPHROPATHOLOGY A finding (figure, right) in post-streptococcal glomerulonephritis, characterized by deposits of subepithelial immune complexes on Bowman's capsule PATHOLOGY Masses of immunoglobulins attached to the glomerular epithelium that are red by Masson's trichrome stain or blue by toluidine blue stain EM Discrete electron-dense, 'domed' deposits, projecting outward from the epithelial aspect of the glomerular basement membrane at the site of slit pores, separated by an electrolucent zone, often demarcated from the overlying epithelial cell by cytoplasmic condensation IMMUNOFLUORESCENCE Variable deposits of complement C3 and IgG as well as alternate pathway proteins, eg properdin and factor B, implying that complement is being activated; humps may disappear four to eight weeks after infection and when humps are persistent and confluent, may be associated with incomplete clinical resolution Note: Humps also occur in nonstreptococcal infectious glomerulonephritis (with infective endocarditis), Henoch-Schönlein purpura and membranoproliferative glomerulonephritis

hump sign RADIOLOGY A distortion of the gas-fluid levels in a plain abdominal film caused by an intraluminal bolus of *Ascaris lumbricoides* within the intestine, an uncommon finding in massive intestinal involvement by roundworms

Humpty-Dumpty etymology The redefinition of terminology that already has widely accepted definition(s), according to the whims of the lector or writer, arising from Humpty-Dumpty's statement, *'When I use a word, it means just what I choose it to mean, neither more nor less'*; the Humpty-Dumpty conundrum is typified by the problem facing evolutionary biologists, for whom 'homology' refers to common evolutionary origin, while molecular biologists later applied the term to the degree of sequence relatedness; see Homology

Humpty-Dumpty 'syndrome(s)' A group of allegorical

terms derived from the children's nursery rhyme Humpty-Dumpty, who *'...all the king's horses and all the king's men couldn't put together again'*; the term has been applied to 1) A form of disability neurosis in which there is physical recovery from an injury, but the 'scars' of childhood psychological trauma intervene, preventing mental recuperation 2) Borderline psychiatric personalities that cannot be salvaged 3) Polytraumatized patients who require multiple, not fully corrective procedures and 4) Specialty 'fragmentation'; see Frankenstein, Twigging

hunchback A 'trivial' name for angular kyphosis that has retained its popularity in non-medical parlance*; angular kyphosis in children is 1) Congenital, due to a lack of segmentation or lack of formation of one or more vertebral bodies TREATMENT Surgical fusion of vertebrae or 2) Acquired angular kyphosis in children is idiopathic and often accompanied by a compensatory increase in lumbar lordosis; in adults, the hunchback deformity may be due to infections, eg midthoracic TB or neoplastic, eg myeloma or infiltration by an osteophilic carcinoma, eg breast or kidney

*It is difficult to imagine the 'politically correct' revision of Victor Hugo's work as 'The angular kyphotic of Notre Dame'-Author's note

'hungry bones' syndrome Post-parathyroid surgery recalcification tetany Transient hypoparathyroidism secondary to resection of significant portions of a hyperactive parathyroid gland; 'hungry' bones occur in the face of high pre-operative PTH (due to excess PTH secretion as occurs in parathyroid hyperplasia and adenoma), high alkaline phosphatase and extensive bone demineralization, resulting in a rapid 'rebound' recalcification of bones after prolonged hypocalcemia; bone hunger is exacerbated by a pre-existing compromise in renal function RADIOLOGY Mottled zones of bone hypodensity LABORATORY ↑ Calcitriol, ↓↓↓ Ca^{++}, eg 1.5 mmol/L (US: 6 mg/dl) or lower, ↓ phosphorus, ↓ magnesium and a reactive ↑ in PTH (if there is residual secretion); the danger lies in attributing the symptoms to acidosis, which may accompany and exacerbate the complex TREATMENT Vitamin 1,25(OH)D_2

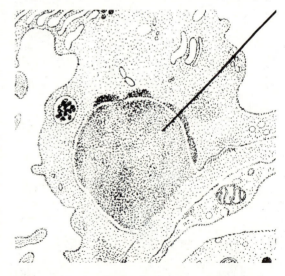

glomerular hump

hunter-gatherer ANTHROPOLOGY A step in the societal evolution of man, that preceded that of the farmer; of the few remaining hunter-gatherer societies, the !Kung San of Botswana have been closely examined, as they are thought to approximate features of the Stone Age foragers (**JAMA 1993; 269:1477MN&P**)

hunter-gatherer diet CLINICAL NUTRITION A diet rich in animal protein, fruits, and plants, with virtually no grains or dairy products, which is thought to be fare of primitive man; consumption of grains and use of dairy products translate as the ability to cultivate and harvest plants and domesticate milk-producing animals, both of which represent relatively anthropologic development of early man and (to be politically correct) early woman; some alternative health care providers posit that the increase (real or perceived) of allergic diseases is caused by changes in dietary consumption

hunting phenomenon PATHOPHYSIOLOGY An auto-thermoregulatory 'maneuver' on the part of a hypothermic body attempting to conserve a cold extremity, where with prolonged corporal exposure to temperatures below 15ºC, blood flow increases intermittently to the extremities; if the hypothermia persists, the limb will lose its blood flow entirely in order to maintain the core temperature

Huntington's disease An AD [MIM 143100] degenerative disease of adult onset (ages 40-50) that leads inexhorably to death CLINICAL Slowly progressive mood and personality changes, loss of coordination, chorea, cognitive decline, chronic fatigue, and apathy PATHOLOGY Degeneration of cerebral cortex and corpus striatum, most prominently in the caudate nucleus MOLECULAR PATHOLOGY CAG trinucleotide expansion (CAG repeat) on chromosome 4p16.3 (N Engl J Med 19934; 330:1401₀ₐ) TREATMENT None; see 'Escapee'

huperzina A A semisynthetic agent derived from *Huperizia serrata* that is reported to improve the memory of patients with Alzheimer's disease; like FDA-approved tacrine, HA ↑ synaptic acetylcholine by inhibiting acetylcholinesterase; HA is also reported to be effective in the loss of memory and in myasthenia gravis

hurricane A natural disaster characterized by highly destructive winds with speeds of 210 km/hour (130 mph) or more, heavy rains, and tidal surges, causing floods that formerly claimed most lives (reduced by early warning systems); hurricanes occurs in the tropical zones of North Atlantic or Pacific Oceans and are classified according to severity on a scale of 1 to 5; Hurricane Andrew (August 1992) was a category 4, and caused $30 **x** 10⁹ in damage, destroyed 30 000 houses or apartments, and caused major structural damage to 60 000 other houses (MMWR 1992; 41:685)

Rogue's gallery of hurricanes: 1900–Galveston, Texas 6000 deaths due to storm surge; 1928–Florida, Puerto Rico 2100 deaths; 1963–Hurricane Flora, Cuba and Hispañola, 7100 deaths; 1974–Hurricane Fifi, Honduras, 8000 deaths; 1988–Hurricane Gilbert, the most powerful hurricane on record, West Indies, Mexico, 300 deaths

Hürthle cell tumor A tumor of the thyroid characterized by granular eosinophilic cytoplasm which may be benign or malignant CYTOLOGY Cells are aggregated in nests, moderate to marked anisocytosis and anisokaryosis, multinucleation, prominent nucleoli (Acta Cytologica 1993; 37:317₀ₐ)

HUS Hemolytic uremic syndrome, see there

HUT78 A cell line established in 1978 from a patient with mycosis fungoides by J Minna's research group; the cell's name was changed to H9 by workers at the US National Institutes of Health, and was successfully infected with HIV-1 and has become the 'workhorse' cell line in HIV-1 research

hut operon Histidine utilization operon An example of autogenous regulation, where a regulatory protein controls its own synthesis; bacterial (*Klebsiella aerogenes* and *Salmonella typhimurium*) degradation of histidine into NH₃, glutamic acid and formamide is dependent upon two (hut) enzymes, which are the gene products encoded by two separate hut operons, each with its own operator and promoter; without histidine in the medium, a single repressor protein binds to both hut operons, preventing transcription; when present, histidine combines with the repressor and transcription is allowed to continue

Hutchinson-Gilford syndrome An AD [MIM 176670] condition first seen in infancy, characterized by poor growth, early onset atherosclerosis, periarticular fibrosis, attenuated subcutaneous fat, dwarfism, small face, beaked nose, baldness, parchment-like skin with brownish discoloration, poor dentition, poor muscle development and early death; Cf Cockayne syndrome

H-V interval CARDIOLOGY A value measured by electrophysiological studies of the heart equal to the time from the beginning of the H deflection to the earliest onset of ventricular depolarization recorded in *any* of the leads; the HVI is relatively constant (30-55 msec) irrespective of the heart rate or autonomic tone, and corresponds to the conduction from the His bundle through the bundle branch-Purkinje system to the time of ventricular muscle depolarization; the HVI can be increased by some Class I antiarrhythmic agents, eg moricizine (N Engl J Med 1992; 327:255₀ₐ); Cf HV interval

hwa-byung *hwa*, Korean, anger, *byung*, disease PSYCHIATRY A term for a Korean culture-bound symptom complex that is attributed to the suppression of anger, characterized by malaise, anorexia, dyspnia, exhaustion, fear of impending doom, generalized aches and pain, insomnia, palpitations, and panic (DSM-IV™, 1994) see Culture-bound syndrome

hyaline arteriosclerosis A degenerative change of aging that most affects the spleen and kidneys, commonly seen in accelerated ('malignant') hypertension, and DM; hyaline changes may occur in the pancreas, adrenal glands, liver, GI tract, brain, choroid and retina PATHOLOGY Glassy eosinophilic hyalinoid material corresponding to iC3b is deposited in the arteriolar walls by slow spontaneous activation of the alternate complement activation pathway and random deposition of the metastable C3b to hyaluronic acid in the arteriolar wall, inactivated by alternate complement pathway factors I and H

hyaline body (skin) Cytoid body, see there, Civatte body

hyaline cell Plasmacytoid cell ORAL PATHOLOGY A myoepithelial cell seen in pleomorphic adenoma that is small, dark, polygonal with an eccentric nucleus and 'glassy' pink cytoplasm, some of which have squamous differentiation

hyaline globules SURGICAL PATHOLOGY Variably sized, rounded PAS-positive, diastase resistant 1–7-mm masses seen intra- and extracellularly in KS, possibly representing effete RBCs

hyaline membrane PULMONARY PATHOLOGY Layered, eosinophilic, pink, glassy membranous material on the alveoli that corresponds to degenerated cells and exudate, constituting a major feature of hyaline membrane disease and DAD ETIOLOGY Any condition or 'insult' that can cause DAD may also evoke hyaline membrane production, eg viral infection, uremia, toxic gas, eg phosgene inhalation, and connective tissue disease, eg rheumatoid arthritis

hyaline membrane disease A morbid process occurring in up to 50% of neonatal deaths in the US, ie 40 000/year CLINICAL Atelectasis, hypoventilation, hypotensive shock, pulmonary vasoconstriction, alveolar hypoperfusion, shutdown of cellular metabolism; 60% of HMD occurs in infants, most are under 28 weeks of age; 5% occur in infants older than 37 weeks PATHOGENESIS Surfactant deficiency, due to the combined effects of prematurity (insufficient phosphatidyl glycerol), intrapartum hypoxia, 'subacute' fetal distress, acidosis, hypoxia familial predisposition; α₁-antitrypsin deficiency, thyroxine, prolactin, cortisol, estrogen; HMD is more frequent in the second twin delivered, twin-to-twin transfusion recipient infant, male infants, children of diabetic mothers and in cesarean sections; a vicious cycle begins where decreased surfactant results in atelectasis, decreased ventilation (↑ pCO₂, ↓ pH, ↓ O₂) and hypoxia exacerbating the lack of surfactant, causing shock and more hypoxia CLINICAL Early onset of tachypnea, prominent grunting, intercostal retractions (air hunger), cyanosis; the infants may not respond to oxygen; blood pressure and corporal temperature fall, asphyxia intervenes and causes death or the symptoms peak at 3 days and the infant recovers DDx Neonatal pneumonia, birth-related asphyxia, group B streptococcal sepsis, cyanotic heart disease TREATMENT Supportive with O₂, correction of acidosis and administration of surfactants

hyalinosis cutis A rare skin disorder causing subcutaneous deposits of amorphous PAS-positive material that corresponds to a mixture of monoclonal kappa light chains, an adhesive 90-kD glycoprotein and type I collagen and high serum levels of IgM antibodies to cytokeratin

hyaluronidase A term loosely used for three different high molecular weight enzymes* with acid phosphatase activity, one or more of which is produced by some strains of streptococci (promoting the spread of microorganisms–spreading factor), pneumococci, bee and snake venoms, sperm and joint fluid (where it may cause ↓ joint fluid viscosity)

*Hyaluronoglucosaminidase [EC 3.2.1.34], hyaluronoglucuronidase [EC 3.2.1.35], hyaluronate lyase [EC 4.2.2.1]

H-Y antigen Histocompatibility-Y antigen A male-specific histocompatibility antigen which was postulated to exist and encode a testis-inducer, a hypothesis (**Nature 1975; 257:235**) that has been abandoned; see Testis-determining factor

hybrid-arrested translation Hybrid-selected translation, see there

Hybrid Capture assay LABORATORY MEDICINE A proprietary detection system that can be used to detect and monitor viral (eg HBV) infections; ↑ HBV in serum indicates ↑ viral replication and potential liver damage; HCA is a 'sandwich' method in which the DNA from a specimen of interest is denatured, and allowed to hybridize with a mixture containing an RNA probe in solution; the solution is then transferred to a tube coated with antibodies to DNA-RNA hybrids; the captured hybrids are then incubated with another antibody conjugate to which alkaline phosphatase is attached; following a wash step, a chemiluminescent substrate is added; the number of photons detected by the luminometer are proportional to the (HBV) DNA present in the specimen (**CAP Today July 1992**)

*Only 40% of HBV-infected patients respond to IFN-α-2b; the decision to treat a patient with IFN-α-2b cannot be capricious, as it is expensive and associated with side effects, including fever, fatigue, headache, and myalgias

hybridization MOLECULAR BIOLOGY The formation of a complex of complementary nucleotides; hybridization methods are a group of techniques for determining the relatedness or sequence 'homology' between two strands of nucleic acids, allowing precise identification of relatively short (up to 20 kilobases) segments or sequences of DNA (Southern blot) or RNA (Northern blot) TECHNIQUE, DNA HYBRIDIZATION A sample of DNA is denatured by a salt, eg NaOH, which causes the double helix to separate into single strands; these single strands are then 'chopped' at specific sites by restriction endonucleases into short (up to 20 kilobases) segments of single-stranded DNA and electrophoresed on a slab of agarose, which separates the DNA fragments by size; the gel is then bathed in a solution containing a probe (an exact base pair 'mirror image' of the single-stranded DNA that now lies at a certain point on the slab of agarose; the probe is labelled by a radioactive isotope, eg ³²P or ³⁵S, or a fluoresceinated or a biotinylated 'tag', each of which is coupled to a detection system); if the probe finds its complementary strand, it 'hybridizes', reforming a double strand; after hybridization, the material on the gel is transferred to a nitrocellulose or nylon membrane (Southern transfer) and either autoradiographed or further manipulated; DNA hybridization under low-stringency conditions, ie not requiring exact complementarity of base pairs may be used to isolate related gene segments, eg identification of the mineralo-

corticoid receptor gene from the known structure of the glucocorticoid receptor gene; see Dot hybridization, Immunoblotting, in situ hybridization, RNA hybridization

hybridoma A 'tumor' cell line (figure) originating from two cells that are interdependent upon one another's metabolic machinery, created by fusing a mouse cell line producing copious amounts of antibody against an antigen of interest, with an immortal mouse myeloma cell line; the broadly applicable hybridoma technique and its authors, Köhler and Milstein were accorded the 1984 Nobel Prize together with Jerne (who provided the theoretical groundwork on idiotypic networks) METHOD Antibody-producing cells that lack the ability to secrete hypoxanthine guanine phosphoribosyl transferase (HGPRT, an enzyme required for DNA nucleotide synthesis) are fused with an immortal myeloma cell line; if the pathway of nucleotide synthesis is blocked, the myeloma cells become HGPRT-dependent and the mutual survival is a symbiotic relation, where the antibody-producing cell line provides the HGPRT and the myeloma cell line provides immortality; the advantages of hybridomas is that one highly specific antibody is produced in unlimited supplies that may be stored permanently

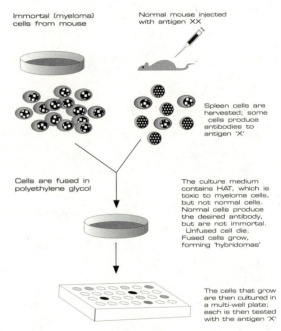

Immortal (myeloma) cells from mouse

Normal mouse injected with antigen XX

Spleen cells are harvested; some cells produce antibodies to antigen 'X'

Cells are fused in polyethylene glycol

The culture medium contains HAT, which is toxic to myeloma cells, but not normal cells. Normal cells produce the desired antibody, but are not immortal. Unfused cell die. Fused cells grow, forming 'hybridomas'

The cells that grow are then cultured in a multi-well plate; each is then tested with the antigen 'X'

hybridoma

hybrid production see Hybridoma

hybrid protein Fusion protein, see there

hybrid-selected translation MOLECULAR BIOLOGY A method for screening the clones from a cDNA (complementary DNA) library, where a sequence of DNA of interest is hybridized to a complementary mRNA strand under 'R-looping' conditions; the two hybrid strands are then separated and the mRNA is allowed to translate the sequence into a polypeptide; hybrid-arrested translation is a permutation of this theme in which the same selection process occurs, but the DNA-mRNA hybrid is deleted from the system and the polypeptide is not translated

hydantoin syndrome Fetal hydantoin syndrome, see there

hydatid cyst disease *Hydatid*, Latin, drop of water A condition caused by cysts of tapeworm larvae,

Echinococcus granulosa, E multilocularis EPIDEMIOLOGY Most common in cattle, especially sheep of the Southern hemisphere DEFINITIVE HOSTS Canine carnivores, eg coyote, wolves INTERMEDIATE HOSTS Sheep, cattle, pigs, and is an accidental 'tourist' in man; once the tainted meat is ingested, the ova hatch, penetrate the intestinal wall, migrate to the liver, proliferate there or pass to the lung, kidney, heart, skeletal muscle and CNS before beginning reproduction; the unilocular hydatid cyst is most often located in the liver, but may also develop in the lungs

WARNING Violation of the thick fibrous capsule liberates protoscolices, causing disseminated disease with significant morbidity; alveolar hydatid disease is caused by the larval stage of the sylvatic, or more rarely, the domestic small animals; the lesions are similar but are often multilocular as the larvae proliferate and spread by budding off from the mother or 'brood' capsule; identification of hydatid cyst is often a fortuitous radiologic finding of a cystic hepatic mass, confirmed by immune assays

hydatid 'sand' Granular mixture of echinococcal scolices and necrotic debris which results in a radiological 'fluid' level with floating sand-like elements

hydatid thrill A vibrating sensation palpated on the portion of the body overlying a hydatid cyst

hydatidiform mole OBSTETRICS A pathologic product of pregnancy or trophoblastic tumor, which occurs in 1:2000 pregnancies in the USA; it is a benign neoplasm or 'allograft' of trophoblastic tissue, characterized by edematous chorionic villi with a varying amount of proliferative trophoblast Moles are divided into

COMPLETE MOLE The chorionic villi are swollen, often accompanied by trophoblastic proliferation but not fetal tissue; CMs are 10-20 times more common in Southeast Asia, and grossly demonstrate innumerable grape-like avascular chorionic villi, the usual fate is passage of the product most CMs have a 46 XX genotype, of which both X chromosomes are of paternal origin, and in 10-15% of the complete moles that are 46 XY, both the X and Y chromosome are of paternal origin; it is thought that complete moles are due to abnormal gametogenesis and fertilization, where in the 46 XX moles, there is fertilization of an empty ovum with no effective genome by a haploid sperm that duplicates without cytokinesis; in the 46 XY complete moles, there may be fertilization of an empty ovum by two haploid sperms with subsequent fusion and replication **PARTIAL MOLE** A mass characterized by a mixture of fetal tissue with normal edematous villi and/or hydropic degeneration; most partial moles are triploid (47 XXY > 47 XXX, > 47 XYY, rarely also trisomy 16), and are thought to be the result of unsuccessful dual fertilization of a single ovum; the conceptus does not die, but remains as a proliferating 'tumor'

INVASIVE MOLE A trophoblastic proliferation that penetrates the myometrium, and may rarely undergo malignant degeneration into a choriocarcinoma

LABORATORY In all moles, human chorionic gonadotropin is ↑↑↑; for the genetics of the mole

Note: Hydropic degeneration of chorionic villi is relatively common and should not be interpreted as being a mole occurs in 20-40% of spontaneous abortions and is associated with chromosome defects and ovarian disease; 20% of moles have theca lutein cysts

hydergine The only drug approved for treating Alzheimer's disease, which consists of a combination of ergoloid mesylates, described as a 'metabolic enhancer', hydergine's efficacy has not been well established; there is no effective drug for Alzheimer's disease, a common diagnosis at the time of death in the US, estimated to cost the US health care system $24-48 x 10^9 per year

hydramnios The presence or ≥ 2 liters of amniotic fluid*; the mechanism of hydramnios is unexplained; 20% of fetal malformations are accompanied by hydramnios, 20% are associated with anencephaly, 10% with multiparity, 5-10% with DM; other conditions associated with hydramnios include esophageal and duodenal atresia, hydrops fetalis, hydrocephalus, spina bifida, achondroplasia, and toxemia; about 50% have no fetal or maternal abnormalities

*At the 38th week, 500 ml/hour is produced by a combination of fetal kidneys, amnion and transudate of maternal serum

hydrocolonic ultrasonography A permutation of transabdominal ultrasongraphy (US) with retrograde instillation of water (≤ 1500 ml) to improve imaging; it is reported that with this method, conventional US detects 31% of colonic carcinomas, hydrocolonic US detects 97% (N Engl J Med 1992; 327:65oA, 327:1459c) range of detection of 83-100% for polyps ≥ 7 mm (smaller polyps are not often associated with colorectal carcinoma) (N Engl J Med 1995; 332:1581c) Note: Up to 40% of carcinomas and 70% of colonic polyps are missed by examination of stool for occult blood; 40% of carcinomas are missed by sigmoidoscopy alone

hydrofluorocarbons HFCs see there

hydrogen peroxide therapy ALTERNATIVE MEDICINE A form of 'oxidative' therapy in which hydrogen peroxide (H_2O_2) is administered parenterally or more commonly topically per rectum to induce oxidative inactivation of various organisms or toxins in the body; HPT is reported by some of its advocates to be of use in treating a wide range of human miseries, including arthritis, cancer, candidiasis, chronic fatigue syndrome, depression, emphysema, fractures, multiple sclerosis, SLE, varicose veins, and others (Alternative Medicine, Future Medicine Pub, Puyallup, Wash, 1994) see AIDS fraud, Alternative medicine, Oxygen therapy; HPT had been promoted as having antiviral (anti-HIV), antimicrobial and antitumoral activity, and determined by the FDA to be fraudulent (Am Med News 21 Nov 1994 p13) see Alternative medicine

hydrogen tunneling BIOCHEMISTRY A quantum mechanical effect that allows the movement of hydrogen to overcome energy barriers, eg as occurs in the conversion of benzyl alcohol into benzyaldehyde, a transformation in which a hydrite (a hydrogen ion with an electron) is cleaved from alcohol by alcohol dehydrogenase of yeast origin

hydrolethalus syndrome Salonen-Herva-Norio syndrome An AR [MIM 236680] condition that is fatal in the early neonatal period, characterized by polydactyly (preaxial of the feet and postaxial of the hands), clubbed feet, small-mandible, poorly formed nose, cardiac malformations (large AV communis), airway stenosis and abnormal pulmonary lobation, massive polyhydramnios, and stillbirth

hydrophobic pocket theory ANESTHESIOLOGY A hypothesis about how anesthetics function, which holds these agents disrupt the oscillation of single electrons in hydrophobic pockets (New York Times 30 August 1994; C1) Cf Lipid theory

hydrops fetalis OBSTETRICS The accumulation of fluid in neonates, resulting in a 'puffy', plethoric or hydropic appearance that may be caused by various etiologies (table) CLINICAL Ascites and edema, due to heart failure, ↓ protein or chronic intrauterine anemia, hepatosplenomegaly, cardiomegaly, extramedullary hematopoiesis, jaundice, pallor COD Heart failure; see Hemolytic disease of the newborn; Rh type can be determined prenatally by PCR of amniotic cells, a procedure of considerable use in the case of RhD-negative mothers who may be carrying RhD-positive fetuses against whose red cell antigens, the mother's immune system may form antibodies, leading in

HYDROPS FETALIS, ETIOLOGIES

IMMUNE Mother produces IgG antibodies against infant antigen(s), often a red cell antigen, most specifically anti-RhD, which then passes into the fetal circulation, causing hemolysis

NON-IMMUNE Hydrops may result from various etiologies including

1) Fetal origin, eg congenital heart disease (premature foramen ovale closure, large atrioventricular septal defect), hematologic (erythroblastosis fetalis, α-thalassemia due to hemoglobin Barts, chronic fetomaternal or twin-twin transfusion), infection (CMV, herpesvirus, rubella, sepsis, toxoplasma), pulmonary (cystic adenomatoid malformation, diaphragmatic hernia, with pulmonary hypoplasia, lymphangiectasia), renal (vein thrombosis, congenital nephrosis) and teratomas, skeletal malformations (achondroplasia, osteogenesis imperfecta, fetal neuroblastomatosis, storage disease, meconium peritonitis, idiopathic)

2) Placental Chorangioma, umbilical or chorionic vein thrombosis

3) Maternal DM, toxemia

extreme cases to hydrops fetalis (**N Engl J Med 1993; 329:607oa**)

hydrotherapy ALTERNATIVE MEDICINE The use of steam, hot or cold water, or ice to maintain and restore health by immersion in baths, saunas, or local hydration either externally in the form of sitz or foot baths or compresses, or internally, eg colonic irrigation or enemas; hydrotherapy is believed by its advocates to be an effective adjunctive therapy for AIDS, cancer, STDs, upper respiratory tract infections, and other diseases (**Alternative Medicine, Future Medicine, Puyallup, WA, 1994**) see Alternative medicine

Note: While various forms of hydrotherapy are popular in Europe, there is little evidence in peer-reviewed journals to establish hydrotherapy as effective therapeutic modality

hydroxamate see Matrix metalloproteinase inhibitor

hydroxyapatite deposition disease RHEUMATOLOGY A crystal-induced arthropathy CLINICAL Mono- or polyarticular periarthritis accompanied by joint erosions and destruction; HADD may be secondary to collagen vascular disease, renal failure and osteoarthritis

hydroxychloroquine sulfate A 4-aminoquinolone agent with antimalarial activity that is indicated for lupus erythematosus (discoid and systemic), and rheumatoid arthritis; the mechanism of activity is unknown WARNING Children have an ↑ sensitivity to this agent, and it has been implicated in a number of fatalities after accidental ingestion

17-hydroxycorticosteroid Any steroid hormone formed in the adrenal gland by action of 17-hydroxylase, which includes cortisol, cortisone, 11-deoxycortisol and tetrahydro derivatives; urinary excretion of 17-OHCSs is a rough guide of both the functional status of the adrenal gland and rate of catabolism; 17-OHCs are ↑ in pregnancy, Cushing's disease, obesity and pancreatitis and ↓ in Addison's disease and hypopituitarism Normal, < age 1, 1.4-2.8 μmol/day (US: < 1 mg/day); Adult 8.2-27.6 μmol/day (US: 3-10 mg/day)

5-hydroxy-indole acetic acid 5-HIAA An oxidative deaminated metabolite of serotonin that is excreted in the urine and accounts for 1% of degraded tryptophan Normal 10.5-42 μmol/d (US: 2-8 mg/day); 5-HIAA may be markedly (25-50-fold normal) elevated in carcinoid tumors, Hartnup's disease, nontropical sprue, and reserpine therapy and ↓ in massive GI tract resection, renal insufficiency, and phenylketonuria

5-hydroxymethyluracil HMU MOLECULAR EVOLUTION A molecule that is related to uracil which is thought by some workers to been a component of ancient RNA; HMU is more reactive with many of the molecules that are postulated to have been in the prebiotic (primordial) soup and would have allowed ancient catalytic RNA to form chemical pathways with greater efficiency and versatility than would modern RNA which contains uracil (**MP Robertson, SL Miller, Science May 5, 1995, in Science News May 6 1995, p279**)

hydroxyproline A hydroxylated proline that is present in high concentrations in collagen and has a major role in cross-linking collagen; urinary hydroxyproline is ↓ by malnutrition ↑ by acromegaly, parathyroid adenoma, Paget's disease of bone, fibrous dysplasia, Marfan's disease

hydroxyurea A non-alkylating, myelosuppressive chemotherapeutic agent of relatively low toxicity that inhibits ribonucleotide reductase, which is used to treat myeloproliferative disorders; HT blocks the synthesis of DNA (by binding to ribonucleotide reductase) and thus differs from other antineoplastic agents; it is the enzyme responsible for the conversion of ribonucleotide diphosphates to deoxyribonucleotides, and is commonly used as a single agent to control blast transformation in CML, to manage polycythemia vera, essential thrombocythemia and, in conjunction with prednisone, to treat idiopathic hypereosinophilic syndrome; long-term therapy may prevent recurrent thrombotic phenomena (**N Engl J Med 1995; 332:1132oa**); hydroxyurea therapy (HT) has also had currency in treating melanoma, and inoperable ovarian cancer; it induces ↑ HbF synthesis in sickle cell anemia, which may comprise 25% of the total Hb (the remainder being HbS), seemingly enough to prevent the formation of HbS polymers, the bête noire of sickle cell anemia (**ibid 332:1372ed**); hydroxyurea may be used to ↑ fetal hemoglobin production (by increasing γ-globulin production) and RBC survival and ↓ bilirubin and LDH in patients with sickle cell anemia; addition of IV recombinant erythropoietin and iron supplementation to hydroxyurea results in a greater ↑ of FH and FH-containing erythrocytes than that seen with hydroxyurea alone; this results in a decrease in intracellular polymerization of hemoglobin S at physiologic O_2 tensions (**N Engl J Med 1993; 328:73oa**); in one report, HT effected a 44% ↓ in the number of painful crises; HT evokes minimal myelotoxicity, but requires ≥ 1 year of HT more for its fullest benefit to take effect (**ibid 332:1317oa**) LONG-TERM EFFECTS Unknown; in the patients with polycythemia vera, the incidence of acute leukemia is 3-fold higher in HT than in those treated with phlebotomy

hygromycin B An aminoglycoside antibiotic that selectively penetrates virally infected cells, inhibiting protein synthesis at the translocation step on 70S ribosomes; it induces misreading of the mRNA template, and has been used to select mutants in broad range of cells, from plant

HYPERCALCEMIA-DIFFERENTIAL DIAGNOSIS

Ca^{++}	PO_4	
↑	↑	Parathyroid carcinoma, adenoma or hyperfunction, tertiary hyperparathyroidism
↑	↓	Multiple myeloma, hypervitaminosis D, bony metastases, sarcoidosis, milk-alkali syndrome
↓	↑	Malabsorption, chronic diarrhea
↓	↓	Status/post parathyroid ablation
N	N	Hypervitaminosis A, healing of fractures, adolescence

to mammalian origin

Hymenolepis A genus of human tapeworms infecting humans that includes *H diminuta* and *H nana*, both of which are global in distribution INTERMEDIATE HOST Rodents, infection occurs by ingesting grains with rodent feces containing eggs; the worms measure up to 60 cm in length; the eggs measure 30-50 μm in diameter by 60-85 μm in length CLINICAL When massive, the tapeworms cause nausea, vomiting, diarrhea and convulsions, otherwise asymptomatic TREATMENT Niclosamide

hymenopterans Insects of the venom-carrying family, including honey bee, yellow jacket, yellow hornet, white-faced hornet, polistes wasp and ants; see Immunotherapy, Killer bees

hyperactivity syndrome Attention deficit-hyperactivity disorder, see there

hyperadrenalism Cushing syndrome

hyperalimentation Total parenteral nutrition, see there

hyperammonemia congenital A heterogeneous group of five AR* inborn errors of metabolism, each of which is deficient in one of the urea cycle enzymes (arginase, argininosuccinase, argininosuccinic acid sythetase, carbamyl phosphate synthetase, ornithine transcarbamylase); all begin in late infancy or childhood, except arginase deficiency, which is neonatal CLINICAL The accumulation of urea precursors, eg ammonia, glutamine causes progressive lethargy, hyperthermia, apnea and marked hyperammonemia NEUROPATHOLOGY Cerebral edema, swollen astrocytes DIAGNOSIS may be established in utero by restriction fragment (RFLP) analysis TREATMENT Restrict dietary protein; activate alternate pathways of waste nitrogen excretion, eg sodium benzoate or dietary supplementation with arginine

*Except ornithine transcarbamylase deficiency, which is X-linked

hyperbaric oxygen The intermittent administration of O_2 in a chamber at greater than sea-level atmospheric pressures (three atmospheres), increasing the dissolved O_2/dl of blood to 6 ml (normally 1.5 g/dl); HO is considered effective therapy for air (or gas) embolism, smoke, inhalation cyanide intoxication, acute carbon monoxide poisoning; traumatic ischemia, as in compartment syndrome(s) and crush injury, decompression, see caisson's disease, to enhance healing of recalcitrant or necrotic wounds, clostridial gangrene (acute tissue hypoxia and myonecrosis), chronic osteomyelitis, extreme blood loss, osteoradionecrosis, compromised skin flaps COMPLICATIONS Barotrauma (air embolism, pneumothorax, tympanic membrane damage), O_2 toxicity (CNS, pulmonary, reversible visual changes), fire or explosion and claustrophobia ALTERNATIVE MEDICINE HO has been administered by some alternative health care providers as a form of 'oxidative' therapy; HO is reported by some of its advocates to be of use in treating a wide range of human miseries, including AIDS, alcohol and drug addiction, multiple sclerosis, strokes and vascular problems (**Alternative Medicine, Future Medicine Pub, Puyallup, WA, 1994**) see Oxygen therapy

hypercalcemia An increase* in calcium levels in the serum ETIOLOGY Hypercalcemia may be due to excess PTH, calcitriol, thyrotoxicosis, drugs, eg corticosteroids, thiazides and may be associated with granulomas, eg berylliosis, sarcoidosis, silicon injection, TB, thyrotoxicosis CLINICAL Nausea, anorexia, vomiting, CNS depression, fatigability, muscular weakness, corneal calcification, peptic ulcers, pancreatitis; a calcium level > 2.95 mmol/L (US: 12 mg/dl) is a medical emergency and when prolonged, causes lytic bone lesions (cystic degeneration of bone or 'brown tumors', osteopenia and 'punched-out' lesions), joint pain, finger clubbing, dystrophic calcification in various tissues, the kidneys may react to these deposits with polyuria EKG Long Q-T intervals LABORATORY Increased alkaline phosphatase, cAMP in urine; Cf Long Q-T syndrome

*Normal levels of (total) calcium 2.10-2.55 mmol/L (US: 8.4-10.2 mg/dl) levels of ionized calcium 1.12-1.23 mmol/L (US: 4.48-4.92 mg/dl)

hypercalcemia of malignancy A clinical complex, 50% of which results from hypersecretion of parathyroid hormone-related protein (PTHRP, also known as parathyroid hormone-related peptide); HCM may result from either direct replacement, eg in lympho– and myeloproliferative malignancies (eg leukemias, adult T cell lymphoma, Burkitt's lymphoma, lymphosarcoma, myeloma) or solid tumors (eg carcinoma of breast, lung, pancreas), or due to factors; normal subjects have low (<2.0 pmol/L) levels of PTHRP, while those with HCM may have plasma levels above 20.9 pmol/L; hypercalcemia may be moderate 10.8-12 mg/dL; or severe >12 mg/dL; HCM is relatively uncommon (± 1%) and occurs in those with more advanced disease, distant metastases, and poor prognoses (**Cancer 1993**;

71:1309) Note: PTHRP is assumed to have a normal function, given its high levels in human breast milk; in HCM, lymphokines stimulate activated macrophages to produce 1,25-dihydroxyvitamin D_3; PTHRP ↑ cAMP and phosphorus, ↓ calcium and may be produced by carcinomas of the lungs, breast, kidney, ovary, leukemia, lymphoma and sarcoma; less common causes of HCM include direct resorption (common in breast carcinoma), ↑ prostaglandin E_2 production, stimulating osteoclast resorption, ↑ cytokine production, eg osteoclast-activating factor, interleukin-1, tumor necrosis factor and lymphotoxin (TNF-β) DIAGNOSIS RIA TREATMENT HCM may respond to bleomycin

hypercalcemia syndrome Williams elfin face syndrome, see there

hypercholesterolemia, primary Familial hypercholesterolemia, see there

hypercholesterolemia, secondary see Hyperlipidemia

hypercoagulability Disseminated intravascular coagulation, see there

hyperdipsia Polydipsia, see there

hyperemesis gravidarum A potentially pernicious condition of early pregnancy that respects no race, parity status or social class, characterized by vomiting in the first trimester (3.5/1000 pregnancies), of a severity that may induce renal failure and require hospitalization; if the patient stabilizes, there is no risk of toxemia during the latter part of gestation, nor is there an increased risk of spontaneous abortion or deformities

hyperendemicity A state of prevalence of active disease, often infectious in nature in a population that surpasses that considered to be endemic for the region, but which falls short of being considered an epidemic

hypereosinophilic syndrome(s) An idiopathic and heterogeneous group of conditions characterized by persistent peripheral eosinophilia with infiltration of eosinophils in the BM, heart, and other organs may represent a form of myeloproliferative disorder (? eosinophilic leukemia) as 1) 25% have chromosomal abnormalities, eg aneuploidy and ↓ vitamin B_{12} with persistent eosinophilia (> 1500 x 10^9/L) for > than 6 months 2) Absence of secondary causes of eosinophilia, despite aggressive workup and 3) Symptoms due to organ involvement or dysfunction PATHOGENESIS The microvasculature stimulated by an ↑ in eosinophilic stem cells or the colony-stimulating factor CLINICAL Age of onset, 20 to 50 with generalized weakness, dyspnea, cough, malaise, myalgia, anorexia, angioedema, rash, low-grade fever, night sweats, weight loss, rhinitis, and symptoms of Loeffler's endocarditis; eosinophils cause organ dysfunction, affecting the heart, BM, liver and spleen, CNS dysfunction, which is either focal, due to emboli or diffuse, causing altered behavior and cognition, psychosis, ataxia, spasticity, peripheral symmetrical polyneuropathy, coma, as well as GI tract symptoms (diarrhea, abdominal pain and malabsorption), lungs (interstitial inflammation with eosinophils) and nonspecific rashes; once the heart is involved (eg endocardial fibrosis, thrombosis and restrictive cardiomyopathy), death occurs within 9 months TREATMENT Some cases respond to corticosteroids

hyperglycinemia Isolated nonketotic hyperglycemia A group of AR conditions* characterized by glycine accumulation due to a catabolic pathway defect in glycine cleavage, which is confined to the mitochondria, and composed of 4 protein components, designated as P-protein (a glycine decarboxylase, defective in type I, the most common form), H-protein, T-protein, and L-protein CLINICAL Presents shortly after birth with marked CNS depression, seizures and convulsions, failure to thrive, mental retardation, and later develop atonia and areflexia

*Type I [MIM 238300], type II [MIM 238310], type III [MIM 238330]

hyperglycinuria Glycine excess with wastage as either

1) Iminoglycinuria, an AR [MIM 242600] renal tube defect that 'spills' imino acids (proline and hydroxyproline) and glycine into the urine or

2) Iminoglycinuria type II, glucoglycinuria, an AD [MIM 138500] increase of glycine in both the urine and serum

hypergonadotropic hypogonadism Primary hypogonadism A condition that results from the lack of target organ response to the pituitary hormones, eg follicle-stimulating hormone and/or luteinizing hormone; see Hypogonadism

hyperhidrosis ↑ sweating, which may be a primary symptom in asymmetric hyperhidrosis, due to a local neural or visceral lesion, gustatory hyperhidrosis, due to surgery to the parotid glands, elicited by spicy foods and 'mental' hyperhidrosis, due to emotional stress or anxiety; in thermoregulatory hyperhidrosis, sweating is merely a symptom of chronic diseases, eg CNS disease (psychiatric stress, cortical lesions, hypothalamus, medulla and spinal cord), dermatopathies (dyskeratosis congenita, pachydermoperiostosis), drugs (anticholinesterase, overdose, eg aspirin, pilocarpine or withdrawal from narcotics), dumping syndrome, endocrinopathy (acromegaly, hypoglycemia, reactive hyperadrenalism, Graves' disease, pheochromocytoma, menopause), familial dysautonomia (Riley-Day syndrome), infections (brucellosis, TB), lymphomas (classically, the Pel-Epstein fever of Hodgkin's lymphoma) and others

hypericin A polyhydroxypolycyclic hydrocarbon extract from the St John's wort plant (*Hypericum* spp), which causes photosensitization in grazing animals, and which has been anecdotally reported to prevent retroviral infection (Am Med News 21 Nov 1994 p13) Cf AIDS fraud

hyperimmune globulin A generic term for a preparation of IV immunoglobulin containing high titers of antibodies against an antigen of interest

hyperimmunoglobulin E syndrome Job syndrome A condition characterized by an early onset of eczema, frequent abscesses of the skin, lungs, sinuses, eyes and ears by *Staphylococcus aureus, Haemophilus influenzae, Streptococci pneumonia*, group A streptococci and *Candida* species LABORATORY ↑ eosinophils, IgE > 5000 IU/mL, ↓ antibody response to vaccines and major histocompatibility antigens, ↓ CD4:CD8 (T cell helper:suppressor) ratio PROGNOSIS Long-term survival is possible

hyper-IgM immunodeficiency syndrome An immunodeficiency characterized by normal to elevated serum IgM with markedly decreased/absent IgG and IgA, associated with frequent infections and neoplasia at an early age; heredity: X-linked, AD, AR, or related to congenital rubella; the defect lies in the inability of T-lymphocytes to provide the 'switch' signal for IgM-secreting cells to become IgG- and IgA-secreting cells CLINICAL Patients present with recurrent bacterial infections, eg otitis media, pneumonia or opportunistic infections, recurrent neutropenia, lymphoid hyperplasia, and autoimmune phenomena LABORATORY: ↓ IgG, IgA, IgE; ↑ IgM, IgD; the CD40 ligand has been identified as the gene defective in X-linked hyper-IgM immunodeficiency (N Engl J Med 1994; 330:969oA)

hyperinfection syndrome Disseminated parasitosis in immunosuppressed, malignant or malnourished hosts, caused by autoinfection with *Strongyloides stercoralis* CLINICAL Abrupt onset of high fever, abdominal pain and distension, intestinal ulcerations, gram-negative sepsis and shock; intense transpulmonary nematodal migration is characterized by dyspnea, cough and hemoptysis TREATMENT Thiabendazole PREVENTION Shoes

hyperkalemic periodic paralysis see Periodic paralysis

hyperkinetic heart Athlete's heart syndrome, see there

hyperlearning INFORMATICS A process of acquiring information that is common in all work tasks and occurs in a multidimensional space formed by a matrix of digitally integrated information technologies with human and non-human components (Forbes ASAP Oct 25, 1993)

hyperlipidemia A generic term for an ↑ of various lipids in the circulation

hyperlipoproteinemia A generic term for any condition with ↑ circulating fatty acids, triglycerides and cholesterol (hyperlipidemia), which is related ↑ carrier lipoproteins (hyperlipoproteinemia) and the presence of degradative enzymes, including lipoprotein lipase; ↑ circulating lipids are responsible for cardiovascular disease, the major cause of morbidity and mortality in older adults in developed nations; secondary hyperlipidemias may be a symptom of an otherwise unrelated condition Note: Only 30-40% of the population is sensitive to dietary cholesterol and thus ↑ dietary cholesterol, ↑ cholesterol in the circulation; ↑ lipids occurs in 1) Secondary hypercholesterolemia, seen in acute intermittent porphyria, cholestasis, hypothyroidism and pregnancy, 2) Secondary hypertriglyceridemia, seen in DM, acute alcohol intoxication, acute pancreatitis, gout, gram-negative sepsis, glycogen storage disease I, and use of oral contraceptives and 3) Combined hypercholesterolemia and hypertriglyceridemia, seen in nephrotic syndrome, chronic renal failure, steroid therapy and immunosuppression

HYPERLIPOPROTEINEMIA

I FAMILIAL LIPOPROTEIN LIPASE DEFICIENCY An AR [MIM 238600] condition characterized by the inability to release triglycerides (TG) from chylomicrons, causing marked hypertriglyceridemia (> 20 g/L) CLINICAL Childhood onset, diarrhea, pancreatitis (potentially fulminant), xanthomata, lipemia retinalis, hepatosplenomegaly, but no ↑ risk of atherosclerosis; this condition is similar to apoC-II deficiency LABORATORY TGs > 4.0 g/L (US: 400 mg/dl), cholesterol normal, ↑ chylomicrons, ↓ post heparin lipolytic activity; this lipoprotein pattern may be mimicked by SLE

II FAMILIAL HYPERCHOLESTEROLEMIA An AD [MIM 144400] condition characterized by tuberous xanthomata of tendons, accelerated coronary atherosclerosis, early myocardial infarcts and ischemic events, onset between ages 20 and 50; it is due to an absence or defect in low-density lipoprotein (LDL) receptors due to mutant alleles Rbo, Rb- and Rtio, resulting in the inability to absorb cholesterol from LDL, which is complicated by increased hepatic production of LDL, a response to the loss of the negative feedback loop LABORATORY Cholesterol 5 to 6 g/L in homozygotes, 3 to 4 g/L in heterozygous

TYPE IIA [MIM 143990] ↑ cholesterol, normal VLDL (normal TGs)*

TYPE IIB [MIM 144010] ↑ cholesterol, ↑ VLDL (↑ TGs)

*This lipoprotein pattern may be mimicked by hepatic tumors

III REMNANT REMOVAL DISEASE Dys-β–lipoproteinemia Broad or fused β band disease An AD [MIM 107741] condition characterized by decreased intermediate-density lipoprotein catabolism CLINICAL Obesity, accelerated atherosclerosis, thromboembolism and strokes, palmo-plantar xanthomas, measuring up to 10 cm, associated with diabetes mellitus, obesity and hypothyroidism LABORATORY Increased triglycerides, cholesterol and abnormal (diabetic) glucose tolerance test; this lipoprotein pattern may be mimicked by myeloma

IV HYPERTRIGLYCERIDEMIA An AD [MIM 145750, 144600] condition that is the most common form of hyperlipoproteinemia CLINICAL Most patients are asymptomatic and rarely suffer peripheral and coronary vascular disease LABORATORY Mildly elevated triglycerides and very-low density lipoprotein TREATMENT Clofibrate, gemfibrozil Acquired causes of hypertriglyceridemia include diabetes mellitus, chronic uremia, dialysis, obesity, estrogen use and alcohol, use of diuretics, glucocorticoids and β-adrenergic agents

V Mixed hyperlipoproteinemia A heterogeneous group of conditions characterized by eruptive xanthomata, pancreatitis, lipemia retinalis, ↑ VLDL and chylomicrons

hyperlysinemia An AR [MIM 238700] condition of childhood onset characterized by increased lysine or metabolites Type I hyperlysinemia is due to a lysine α-ketoglutarate reductase deficiency with increased lysine, homoarginine and NH₃, causing mental retardation, hypotonicity and coma; high-protein diets result in attacks which begin with vomiting TREATMENT ↓ Dietary lysine Type II hyperlysinemia may be due to an as yet undiscovered enzymopathy, with milder symptoms; see Lysinemia

hypermobile joint syndrome Systemic joint laxity A generalized ↑ in joint mobility, which may be seen in various rheumatic conditions, and may be associated with temporomandibular joint dysfunction

hypernatremia, congenital Idiopathic neonatal hypernatremia of Ballard A potentially life-threatening clinical complex of perinatal onset with ↑↑↑ serum sodium, often > than 134-146 mmol/L (US: 310-340 mg/dl) CLINICAL CNS dysfunction, seizures, neuromuscular spasms, production of low volumes of concentrated urine, weight loss, hypotension, ↑ BUN; the symptoms are exacerbated by concomitant sepsis, asphyxia or CNS hemorrhage ETIOLOGY ↑ Na⁺ loss, as in diabetes insipidus, either ↓ ADH secretion or ↓ sensitivity to ADH, osmotic diuresis, diaphoresis, diarrhea; ↓ intake, due to disordered thirst sensation, ↑ salt ingestion without adequate fluid, electrolytic imbalance, ↑ Ca⁺⁺, ↑ K⁺

hypernephroma Obsolete for renal cell carcinoma

hyperornithinemia Ornithinemia, see there

hyperostosis A proliferation of bony matrix

hyperostosis corticalis deformans juvenilis Hyperphosphatasia, see there

hyperostosis corticalis generalisata Generalized cortical hyperostosis, see there

hyperostosis corticalis infantalis Infantile cortical hyperostosis, see there

hyperostosis frontalis interna Morgagni-Stewart-Morell syndrome A form of osteopetrosis that is more common in middle-aged ♀ and associated with obesity, hirsutism, fatigue, hemiplegia and hemiparesis; HFI affects the cranial bones, structurally compromising the hypophysis (causing dysmenorrhea, virilism, hirsutism, diabetes insipidus, and glucose intolerance), and cranial nerve foramina (causing vertigo, tinnitus, anosmia, and visual defects)

hyperoxaluria see Primary hyperoxaluria

hyperparathyroidism Parathyroid gland hypersecretion causes several relatively specific clinical complexes, including a myopathic 'syndrome', a skeletal 'syndrome', a urologic 'syndrome' and a CNS 'syndrome', in addition to the classic findings of peptic ulcer, hypercalcemia and acute pancreatitis **PRIMARY HYPERPARATHYROIDISM** is most commonly due to parathyroid hormone (PTH) hypersecretion secondary to parathyroid adenomas or hyperplasia (parathyroid carcinomas are extremely uncommon), PTH may also be ectopic and occur with MEN I and II syndromes, see there CLINICAL Hypercalcemia symptoms, including nausea, anorexia, vomiting, CNS depression, fatigability, cornea calcification, muscular weakness, peptic ulcers, pancreatitis; levels above 2.9 mmol/L (US: 12 mg/dl) require immediate therapy and when prolonged, cause lytic bone lesions, eg osteitis fibrosa cystica or 'brown' tumors, significant osteopenia with 'punched-out' lesions of the bone, joint pain and finger clubbing as well as ectopic calcium deposits in various tissues, in particu-

lar, the kidney, resulting in polyuria and eventually renal failure EKG Decreased Q-T intervals **SECONDARY HYPERPARATHYROIDISM** is usually due to end-organ defects (renal failure and hemodialysis) or the rare malabsorption syndrome; Cf Hypercalcemia

Note: The histopathological criteria separating parathyroid adenomas from parathyroid hyperplasia differ widely among pathologists

hyperphenylalaninemia A group of eight different congenital enzymopathies characterized by an accumulation of phenylalanine and related metabolites, eg phenylpyruvate, phenyllactate, phenylacetate, phenylacetylglutamine, in addition to a deficiency of tyrosine, an amino acid that forms catecholamines, thyroxine (T₄) and triiodothyronine (T₃), melanin and other proteins; the most common or 'classic' phenylketonuria (PKU or hyperphenylalaninemia, type 1) is an AR [MIM 261600] condition characterized by a deficiency in phenylalanine hydroxylase, which if not recognized early (urine has a 'mousy' odor) and treated by restricting dietary phenylalanine, results in a child with tremors, seizures, eczema, hyperactivity and hypopigmentation and an IQ of < than 50; other hyperphenylalaninemia types, eg types 2, 3 and 7, are relatively benign

hyperphosphatasia Hyperostosis corticalis deformans juvenilis, juvenile Paget's disease An AR [MIM 239000] condition characterized by enlarged and defective bones, and ↑ bone density LABORATORY ↑ phosphatase, normal Ca⁺⁺, PO₄

hyperphosphatemia The elevation of phosphate(s) above 1.5 mmol/L (US: 4.5 mg/dl) ETIOLOGY Increased growth hormone, either physiologic with growth spurts or pathological in gigantism and acromegaly, decreased parathyroid hormone and pseudohypoparathyroidism or in renal failure

hyperprolinemia A condition characterized by a defect in imino acid metabolism **HYPERPROLINEMIA, TYPE I** An AR [MIM 239500] condition characterized by a defect of proline oxidase, which produces pyrroline carboxylate from proline and is associated with renal tube defects, without mental retardation; **HYPERPROLINEMIA, TYPE II** An AR [MIM 239510] condition characterized by a defect of delta'-pyrroline-5-carboxylic acid dehydrogenase with variable mental retardation, seizures and renal tube defects

hypersensitive sites MOLECULAR BIOLOGY Regions of a eukaryotic genome that have an increased sensitivity to DNAse cleavage and which often correspond to regulatory sequences

HYPERSENSITIVITY PNEUMONITIS

SYNDROME	SUSPECTED ANTIGEN
Bagassosis	*Thermoactinomyces vulgaris*
Bird fancier's lung	Bird droppings
Pigeon handler's lung	*Histoplasma capsulatum*
Cheese worker's lung	*Penicillium* spp
Detergent worker's lung	*Bacillus subtilis* enzyme
Fish meal lung	Fish proteins
Farmer's lung	*Micropolyspora faeni, Thermoactinomyces vulgaris*
Humidifier lung	Thermophilic actinomycetes
Malt worker's lung	*Aspergillus clavatus*
Maple bark disease	*Cryptostroma corticale*
Mushroom picker's lung	*Micropolyspora faeni*
Sequoiosis	*Graphium* spp, *Auerobasidium* spp
Suberosis (oak bark)	*Micropolyspora faeni*
Vineyard sprayer's lung	Copper
Wood dust pneumonitis	Oak and mahogany dust
Wood pulp worker's lung	*Alternaria* spp

*See separate heading

hypersensitivity pneumonitis A group of disorders caused by an exuberant pulmonary reaction to aerosolized immunogens (table), that with time may develop interstitial lung disease; the prototypic HP is Farmer's lung, which is accompanied by fever, malaise, cough, chest tightness and myalgias; see Farmer's lung, Humidifier lung

hypersensitivity syndrome A severe idiosyncratic reaction to certain drugs (eg anticonvulsants, sulfonamides, allopurinol) characterized by rash (eg exfoliative dermatitis) and fever, which may be accompanied by arthralgias, carditis, hepatitis, lymphadenopathy LABORATORY Atypical lymphocytes, eosinophilia, abnormal liver function tests (N Engl J Med 1994; 331:1272ᴿᵛ)

hypersexuality A pathologic ↑ in the sexual drive, a phenomenon that is inducible in experimental mammals by bilateral lesions in the limbic region, localized in the piriform cortex overlying the amygdala, causing the animals to mount females that are not in estrus, other males, animals of other species and inanimate objects; non-psychogenic hypersexuality has been reported in some patients with bilateral lesions adjacent to the amygdaloid nucleus; see Temporal lobe syndrome; Cf 'Don Juan' syndrome, Nymphomania, Satyriasis

hypersomnia 1) Primary hypersomnia-bulimia syndrome of Klein-Levine A condition characterized by semiannual bouts of hyperphagia followed by a 2–5-day 'sleep-off' described in young males 2) Hypersomnia-sleep apnea syndrome A condition described in obese and hypertensive middle-aged males characterized by daytime grogginess and loud snoring; these patients are at an increased risk for acute MI and cerebrovascular accidents; see Sleep apnea syndrome 3) Secondary hypersomnia is a symptom caused by focal CNS disease, eg brain tumors, especially those of the posterior hypophysis or diencephalon, encephalopathia lethargica and meningitis or systemic disease, eg hypothyroidism, trypanosomiasis; see Narcolepsy, Sleep disorders; Cf REM sleep

hypersomnolence Excessive sleepiness, which may be defined as excess and/or uncontrollable daytime sleepiness or waking up unrefreshed, regardless of the length of time slept (see N Engl J Med 1993; 328:1230ᴏᴀ)

hypersplenism A pathologic enlargement of the spleen due to any etiology, characterized by splenomegaly, pancytopenia and hyperplasia of the BM precursor cells with clinical improvement upon splenectomy **Congestive hypersplenism** is due to stasis of blood flow and most often secondary to cirrhosis of the liver, as well as thrombosis and other vascular abnormalities; less common causes of hypersplenism include lymphoproliferative disorders, eg lymphoma, leukemia, especially CML, infections, eg infectious mononucleosis, kala azar, TB, and infiltrations, eg Gaucher and Niemann-Pick diseases CLINICAL Isolated hypersplenism is asymptomatic, but the primary diseases may be accompanied by general malaise, fever, fullness, purpura or may present with hematemesis or GI bleeding LABORATORY ↓ RBC survival, reticulocytosis and 'left shift' of the myeloid series; Cf Splenosis

hypertelorism Any excess separation of paired organs, eg the breasts or eyes MAMMARY HYPERTELORISM is relatively uncommon, and is typical of the Turner syndrome OCULAR HYPERTELORISM A not uncommon craniofacial defect seen in various congenital anomalies, many of which have been eponymically dignified, eg Apert syndrome (acrocephalosyndactyly), Crouzon's disease (craniofacial dysostosis), Opitz' syndrome (Hypertelorism-hypospadia or BBB syndrome), and Taybi syndrome (otopalatodigital syndrome)

hypertension An abnormal ↑ in tension or pressure, in the context of medicine, referring exclusively to an ↑ systemic or pulmonary arterial pressure; hypertension affects ± 60 million persons in the US, defined as a systolic blood pressure of greater than 160 mm Hg and/or diastolic blood pressure of 95 mm Hg and graded according to the intensity of increased diastolic blood pressure

Class I (mild) Diastolic pressure 90-104 mm Hg

Class II (moderate) Diastolic pressure 105-119 mm Hg

Class III (severe) Diastolic pressure > than 120 mm Hg Evaluation of hypertension requires clinical history for patient and family history, two blood pressure determinations, fundoscopic examination, identification of bruits in the neck and abdominal aorta, evaluation of peripheral edema, peripheral pulses and residual neurologic defects in stroke victims, chest films to determine cardiac size and laboratory parameters to rule out causes of secondary hypertension (table) PATHOGENESIS The mechanism by which hypertension causes morbidity is not understood; ⅓ of cases have an ↑ cardiac load, the remainder have ↑ peripheral arterial pressure and generalized vasoconstriction due to autonomic nervous system dysfunction and a defective end organ response in the vessels, related to ↑ renal cytochrome P-450 and P-450-induced arachidonic acid metabolites, activation of the renin-angiotensin and kallikrein-kinin systems, with contributions from arginine vasopressin and atrial natriuretic peptides RISK FACTORS Race (blacks more common), males, family history of hypertension, obesity, metabolic defects of lipid metabolism, DM, sedentary lifestyle, cigarette smoking, electrolyte imbalance, including ↑ sodium, phosphorus, ↓ potassium and tin; sodium's link to hypertension is unclear (in one report, administration of sodium chloride, but not sodium citrate, to patients with essential hypertension ↑ systolic and diastolic blood pressure by 16 mm and 8 mm Hg, respectively) TREATMENT Hypertension may respond to diet, eg sodium restriction (see previous caveat), ↓ calories, alcohol and cigarettes (although the weight gain accompanying smoking cessation tends to offset the minimal reduction in blood pressure), calcium supplementation, or lifestyle manipulation, eg biofeedback, ↑ exercise; antihypertensive medications, eg diuretics (benzothiadiazines, loop diuretics, potassium-sparing diuretics), sympatholytic agents (central and peripheral-acting α-adrenergics, β-adrenergics, mixed α- and β-blocking agents), direct vasodilators, converting enzyme inhibitors, calcium channel blockers; Cf Pseudohypertension, 'White coat' hypertension **ESSENTIAL HYPERTENSION** Idiopathic hypertension The major form comprising 90% of all hypertension, see above **MALIGNANT HYPERTENSION** A sustained blood pressure > 200/140 mm Hg, resulting in arteriolar necrosis, most marked in the brain, eg cerebral hemorrhage, infarcts and hypertensive encephalopathy, eyes, eg papilledema and hypertensive retinopathy and kidneys, eg acute renal failure and hypertensive nephropathy; if malignant hypertension is uncorrected or recalcitrant to therapy, the patient may enter into a hypertensive crisis in which prolonged high pressure causes left ventricular hypertrophy and congestive heart failure **PAROXYSMAL HYPERTENSION** Transient or episodic waves of ↑ blood pressure of any etiology, punctuated by periods of normotension, classically described in pheochromocytoma **PORTAL HYPERTENSION** ↑ portal vein pressure caused by a back-flow of blood through the splenic arteries (resulting in splenomegaly) and collateral circulation (the latter of which results in esophageal varices and/or hemorrhoids); PH may be of intra- or extrahepatic origin, and is most commonly caused by hepatic cirrhosis, or rarely portal vein disease, venous thrombosis, tumors or abscesses **PULMONARY HYPERTENSION** A condition defined as a 'wedge' systolic/diastolic pressure > 30/20 mm Hg (Normal: 18-25/12-16 mm Hg), often secondary to stasis of blood in the peripheral circulation, divided into passive, hyperkinetic, vaso-occlusive, vasoconstrictive and secondary forms, see Pulmonary hypertension **RENOVASCULAR HYPERTENSION** see there **SECONDARY HYPERTENSION** (see table)

hypertension panel A battery of 'cost-efficient' serum tests used to evaluate a person with hypertension, which include the most common causes of secondary hypertension, measuring BUN/creatinine, chloride, CO_2 content, free urinary cortisol, potassium, sodium, thyroxine, vanillylmandelic acid, urinalysis and bacterial colony count; Cf Organ panel

hypertensive crisis A rare clinical event characterized by a severe and/or acutely increased diastolic blood pressure above 120-130 mm Hg; it constitutes a medical emergency if there is evidence of rapid or progressive CNS disease (encephalopathy, infarction or hemorrhage), cardiovascular (myocardial ischemia, infarction, aortic dissection, pulmonary edema) and renal deterioration, eclampsia or microangiopathic hemolytic anemia; HCs most commonly occur in pre-existing chronic hypertension, but may be due to renovascular hypertension, parenchymal renal disease, scleroderma and collagen vascular disease, ingestion of sympathomimetic and tricyclic antidepressant drugs or after withdrawal from antihypertensive drugs, use of recreational drugs, eg crack, spinal cord syndromes, and pheochromocytoma CLINICAL Severe headache, transient blindness, vomiting, and rapid deterioration of renal function PATHOLOGY Intravascular fibrin deposition and fibrinoid necrosis of vessels walls COMPLICATIONS Acute end-organ damage, eg myocadial ischemia or infarction, renal failure, aortic dissection, or stage 3 or 4 hypertensive retinopathy (N Engl J Med 1995; 332:1029ED) TREATMENT Therapy must target the organ most affected by the crisis, using calcium channel antagonists, labetalol, asmolol, loop diuretics, nitroglycerin and sodium nitroprusside PREVENTION Stannous chloride has an antihypertensive effect in rats, reducing cytochrome P-450-derived metabolites of arachidonic acid PROGNOSIS Untreated, five-year mortality is 100%

hyperthecosis A condition occurring in ♀ age 20-30, which is characterized by hyperplasia of the theca interna of a maturing ovarian follicle, and may be associated with hirsutism and amenorrhea; see Hirsutism

hyperthermia 1) Heat stress detoxification, see there 2) A clinical condition defined as a corporal temperature of greater than 42°C; as a defense, there is peripheral vasodilation (↓ effective volume), resulting in an ↑ pulse rate, a response to perceived blood loss, ↓ cardiac efficiency, hypoxia, ↑ permeability of cell membranes with ↑ potassium and cardiac failure; see Malignant hyperthermia

hyperthrombocytosis see Essential thrombocythemia, Reactive thrombocytosis

---

SECONDARY HYPERTENSION
AGING
CARDIOVASCULAR Open heart surgery, coarctation of aorta, ↑ cardiac output (anemia, thyrotoxicosis aortic valve insufficiency)
CEREBRAL ↑ Intracranial pressure
ENDOCRINE Mineralocorticoid excess, congenital adrenal hyperplasia, glucocorticoid excess, eg Cushing syndrome, hyperparathyroidism, acromegaly
GYNECOLOGIC Pregnancy, oral contraceptives
NEOPLASIA Renin-secreting tumors, pheochromocytoma
↓ PERIPHERAL VASCULAR RESISTANCE Arteriovenous shunts, Paget's disease of bone, beri-beri
RENAL DISEASE Vascular, parenchymal

---

hyperthyroidism EPIDEMIOLOGY: Affects 2% of all, especially older women; 0.2% of men ETIOLOGY: Common (Graves' disease, iatrogenic illness, toxic nodular goiter, thyroiditis); Rare (Neonatal hyperthyroidism, exogenous iodide, factitious illness, malignancy struma ovarii) CLINICAL: ↑ O_2 consumption, basal metabolic rate, asthenia,

weight loss LABORATORY: ↑ T_3 and/or T_4 TREATMENT: Antithyroid drugs (methimazole, carbimazole, propylthiouracil), radioiodine, surgery (N Engl J Med 1994; 330:1731RV)

hypertrichosis Hirsutism, see there

hypertrichosis lanuginosa The presence of lanugo over a large part of the body, which may be inherited, more commonly AD [MIM 145700] than AR, or acquired, either drug-induced or associated with internal malignancies of breast, ovary, bladder, and other epithelial, as well as nonepithelial malignancies

hypertrophic cardiomyopathy Idiopathic hypertrophic subaortic stenosis A group of diseases characterized by either symmetric (concentric) or asymmetric (eccentric) hypertrophy, the latter with disproportionate thickening beneath the mitral valve, which occurs in the absence of any other cardiac disease; ½ of cases are congenital, with an AD [MIM 192600] pattern CLINICAL Younger patients, ranging from asymptomatic to diastolic dysfunction, dyspnea, fatigue, chest pain and syncope, an ↑ incidence of severe obstruction, congestive heart failure and sudden death, simulating acute MI EKG ↑ QRS complexes, T-wave inversion and Q waves in the inferior and left precordial leads PATHOLOGY Asymmetric septal hypertrophic ventricle, myofiber disarray, thick-walled intramural coronary arteries MOLECULAR PATHOLOGY HC has been linked to a defect in chromosome 14q1 (lod score of 9.4, ie a ratio of 2×10^9:1 TREATMENT Symptomatic, ie relief of dyspnea or chest pain DRUGS β-adrenergic agents are effective short-term; calcium channel blockers, which ↑ diastolic filling of the ventricles SURGERY Recalcitrant cases may require a transaortic ventricular septal myotomy-myectomy

hypertrophic (pulmonary) osteoarthropathy A clinical complex characterized by clubbing of fingers and toes, periostitis of the ends of long bones, arthritis, pain and occasionally, autonomic dysfunction including pallor, flushing and profuse diaphoresis; although it may rarely occur as an idiopathic condition (pachydermoperiostosis), it is classically associated with pulmonary disease, including abscesses, cancer, COPD, emphysema, chronic interstitial pneumonitis; Cf Clubbing

hypertrophic pyloric stenosis A condition of neonates occurring within a few weeks of birth PATHOGENESIS Defect in pyloric relaxation and pylorospasm due to a deficiency of nitric oxide synthase (aka NADPH diaphorase, EC 1.14.13.39) CLINICAL Gastric outlet obstruction, bile-free vomit, metabolic alkalosis, dehydration (N Engl J Med 1992; 327:511OA)

hypertyrosinemia Tyrosine, see there

hypervalinemia Valinemia, see there

hypervariable region see Hot spot

hyperventilation syndrome Tachy-dyspnea 'syndrome' A clinical complex affecting neurotics with anxiety attacks; the hyperventilation, in addition to the characteristic EEG changes (bilateral synchronous theta wave followed by delta activity with spike and slow-wave discharges) causes respiratory alkalosis, tightness in the chest, dizziness without syncope, numbness of hands and feet and tetany TREATMENT Rebreathe air in a paper bag, as the ↑ CO_2 facilitates physiologic compensation

hyperviscosity syndrome A clinical complex evoked by a marked increase in plasma viscosity, which is 18- to 33-fold greater than blood; hyperviscosity is most commonly seen in Waldenström syndrome due to a ↑↑↑ in circulating IgM, less commonly in IgG or IgA plasma cell dyscrasias CLINICAL Findings reflect sluggish blood flow, seen in the CNS (dysarthria, paralysis), retina (engorged 'sausage-link' veins), ear (tinnitus and vertigo), and petechial hemorrhage (due to microcirculatory sluggishness, hypoxia and capillary damage) TREATMENT Plasmapheresis, with removal and washing of 2-3 units of plasma/day until the viscosity normalizes, then repeated as needed

Note: Viscosity is the measurement of a fluid's resistance to flow, a function in biological systems of protein concentration and the intrinsic 'stickiness' of each constituent protein; normal plasma viscosity is about 1.8 x more viscous than water

hypervitaminosis A generic term for any clinical condition attributed to the ingestion of vitamins in great excess of physiologic or pharmacologic levels; see Vitamin

hyphae see Dimorphic fungi

hypnosis A modality that has theoretical currency in behavior modification and biofeedback; its success is difficult to evaluate, as using double-blind studies cannot be performed, given that all studies must evaluate the success (or failure) to achieve the intended effect(s) on a per-case basis; hypnosis is claimed to be useful in speech therapy, smoking cessation, ameliorating panic disorders and in lower back pain

hypnotherapy ALTERNATIVE MEDICINE A form of health care that has some support in mainstream medicine, eg in psychiatry and anesthesiology, with the major recognized effect being that of relaxation, and possibly control of habits; hypnotherapy has been used as an adjunct in controlling acute and chronic pain (and in rare cases, has been used in place of anesthetics); hypnotherapy may also be useful in overcoming the abuse of alcohol, tobacco, and other substances; see Alternative medicine

hypnotics A family of therapeutic CNS depressants, of which benzodiazepines are the drug of choice for 'primary' insomnia; short-acting hypnotics, eg triazolam and oxazolam are used to induce sleep; to maintain sleep throughout the night, longer-acting hypnotics, eg flurazepam, are required

Note: When insomnia is secondary, treatment of the underlying condition, eg Parkinson's disease, also 'treats' the insomnia

hypo-betalipoproteinemia An AD [MIM 107730] condition due to ↓ low-density lipoprotein and ↓ apoB-100 CLINICAL Variable; atherosclerosis is not a major component; longevity is not affected LABORATORY ↓ cholesterol 1.81-3.11 mmol/L (US: 70-120 mg/dl) and acanthocytosis; see Hypolipoproteinemia

hypochlorite Bleach, CLO⁻ and salts

hypochondroplasia An AD [MIM 146000] condition character-

HYPOGAMMAGLOBULINEMIA CONGENITAL

X-LINKED AGAMMAGLOBULINEMIA OF BRUTON An AR condition in which the B cells are arrested at the pre-B cell stage of development and disease becomes manifest as the passively transferred immunoglobulin of maternal origin fall below 200 mg/dl, which occurs at about 6 months of age, given IgG's serum half-life of 20-25 days CLINICAL Recurrent pyogenic organisms with intact T-cell and NK cell-mediated immunity; malabsorption associated with *Giardia* infections COMPLICATIONS Polyarthritis collagen vascular disease and fatal dermatomyositis TREATMENT Immunoglobulins

TRANSIENT HYPOGAMMAGLOBULINEMIA A quasi-physiological state which is similar to Bruton's disease in presentation, but merely represent a normal delay in immunoglobulin production by the infant rather than rather than the inability to produce them

SWISS-TYPE LYMPHOPENIC AGAMMAGLOBULINEMIA, in which there are both B-cell and T-cell defects see Severe combined immunodeficiency

OTHER CONGENITAL HYPOGLOBULINEMIAS include selective deficiencies in the production of IgA, IgM, subclasses of IgG, associated with 5'nucleotidase deficiency or X-linked with lymphoproliferative disorders, eg Duncan syndrome,

COMBINED VARIABLE IMMUNODEFICIENCY B-cell precursors are present but don't differentiate into plasma cells and is associated with T-cell defects; Acquired hypogammaglobulinemia may be associated with drug and protein-losing states

---

ized by short limbs, ↓ height, caudal syringomyelia

hypogammaglobulinemia ↓ Production of proteins, usually Igs migrating in the gamma region of a protein electrophoretic gel; hypogammaglobulinemia may be congenital (table), as in Bruton's disease, or other B cell defects or

acquired, as in CLL, which may be accompanied by monoclonal gammopathies TREATMENT Human immune globulins; see Immunodeficiency, B cell

hypoglycemia A ↓ in circulating glucose which is often a symptom of systemic disease CLINICAL Headache, tremors, sweating, pallor, syncope, ↓ concentration, coma; fasting hypoglycemia occurs in endocrinopathies, including hypopituitarism, Addison's disease, adrenogenital syndrome, islet cell tumors, factitious insulin ingestion, nonpancreatic neoplasms, eg retroperitoneal sarcoma, producing ectopic insulin, hepatic disease, glycogen storage disease; postprandial hypoglycemia may be functional and idiopathic, associated with preclinical DM, status post-gastrectomy or drug-related, by for example sulfonylureas, oral hypoglycemic agents, including chlorpropamide, tolbutamide, tolazamide, acetohexamide, as well as alcohol, aspirin, phenformin and insulin

hypoglycin 2-amino-3-(2-methylenecyclopropyl)propionic acid A toxic amino acid derived from the unripe ackee fruit that evokes hypoglycemia, and inhibits the catabolism of branched-chain amino acids and the other symptoms of Jamaican vomiting sickness, see there

hypogonadism A clinical condition with decreased or absent phenotypic expression of a person's sexual genotype, which may be primary, due to a lack of end organ response to FSH or LH produced normally by an intact pituitary gland (hypergonadotropic hypogonadism), or secondary to defective hypothalamic or pituitary hormonal activity (hypogonadotropic hypogonadism) (table)

HYPOGONADISM

♀ HYPERGONADOTROPIC (1º) HYPOGONADISM Turner syndrome, XX Turner sydrome, XX pure gonadal dysgenesis, mixed gonadal dysgenesis, autoimmune ovarian disease

♀ HYPOGONADOTROPIC (2º) HYPOGONADISM Carpenter syndrome, hypopituitarism, Lawrence-Moon-Biedl, multiple lentigines syndrome, polycystic ovaries

♂ HYPERGONADOTROPIC (1º) HYPOGONADISM Congenital anorchia, rudimentary testes, germ cell hypoplasia (del Castillo syndrome), XY Turner phenotype (Noonan syndrome), Klinefelter syndrome and variants, XX males, XYY males

♂ HYPOGONADOTROPIC (2º) HYPOGONADISM Amyloidosis, Carpenter syndome, fertile eunuch syndrome, Froehlich syndrome, Sheehan syndrome, Kallmann's disease, Laurence-Moon-Biedl disease, Lowe syndrome, Prader-Willi syndrome

---

hypogonadotropic eunuchoidism Kallmann syndrome see there

hypohidrosis Reduced sweat production (table)

hypohidrotic dysplasia An uncommon familial condition characterized by peg-shaped teeth, focal anodontia, facial dysplasia, hyperthermia, decreased sweat glands

hypolipoproteinemia A group of conditions characterized by ↓ lipoproteins, either acquired, eg secondary to malabsorption, anemia(s), hyperthyroidism or congenital

ABETALIPOPROTEINEMIA Bassen-Kornzweig syndrome An AR [MIM 200100] condition chercterized by an absence of apoB and LDL-cholesterol (when homozygous) CLINICAL Fat malabsorption, ataxia, retinitis pigmentosa, neuropathy, acantholysis; in one kindred with the disease, a truncated apo-B results from a four nucleotide deletion, a frameshift mutation and production of a premature stop codon

HYPOBETALIPOPROTEINEMIA An AD [MIM 107730] condition due to ↓ low-density lipoprotein and ↓ apoB-100 CLINICAL Variable; atherosclerosis is not a major component; longevity is not affected LABORATORY ↓ cholesterol 1.81-3.11 mmol/L (US: 70-120 mg/dl) and acanthocytosis

TANGIER DISEASE analphalipoproteinemia An AR [MIM 205400] condition characterized by absent HDL and ↓↓↓ apoA-I and apoA-II, with deposits of cholesteryl esters in the tonsils, other lymphoid tissues and corneal opacifications

hypomagnesemia A condition defined as a serum magnesium ≤ 1.5 mg/dL, which is manifest by muscular hyperirritability; hypomagnesemia present in the first 24 hours after admission to a health care facility is associated with ↓ survival (9.3 vs 17.9 days) in acutely ill patients, independently of the APACHE II scores (**Crit Care Med 1993; 21:203**)

hypomanic episode PSYCHIATRY A discrete period (lasting at least 4 days) of an abnormally and persistently elevated, expansive, or irritated mood that is accompanied by various 'ancillary' symptoms, including ↑ self-esteem, nondelusional grandiosity, flight of ideas, ↑ distractibility, ↓ need for sleep, ↑ in goal-directed activities, or psychomotor agitation (**DSM-IV**); unlike a manic episode, an HE is controllable by its 'host' and does not cause significant impairment of social or occupational functioning

hypoperfusion syndrome A 'prerenal' circulatory disorder that is secondary to 1) Occlusive renal arterial disease with stenosis and ischemia, resulting in ↑ renin, hypertension and azotemia, affecting one or both kidneys 2) ↓ Effective circulatory volume, due to ↑ vascular capacitance, eg induced by sepsis, sequestration of fluids in compartments, eg in the hepatorenal syndrome or ascites, or the inability to effectively transfer fluids from the venous 'compartment' to the arterial 'compartment' due to congestive heart disease or pericardial limitations due to constrictive pericarditis or effusions; the ↓ volume form of hypoperfusion is associated with oliguria, azotemia, ↓ sodium excretion and ↑ renin, but not hypertension

hypophosphatasia A congenital rickets-like metabolic disease, defined by low serum alkaline phosphatase (which is presumed to be due to a defect in the the alkaline phosphatase gene [MIM 171760]) and disease manifestations of variable intensity; clinical forms

CONGENITAL (IN UTERO) An AR [MIM 241500] form of hypophosphatasia characterized by 50% neonatal mortality, often due to respiratory insufficiency due to inadequate thoracic ossification CLINICAL Bone deformities, softened skull and delayed closure of the fontanelles, bowing of legs, irregularity of metaphyseal mineralization, short extremities, blue sclera, failure to thrive, irritability DDx Osteogenesis imperfecta, achondroplasia, cleidocranial dysplasia, campomicromelic dwarfism, skeletal dysplasias

INFANT ONSET (6-24 MONTHS) An AR [MIM 241510] form of hypophosphatasia characterized by less severe bony changes than those seen in the congenital onset form; premature loss of deciduous teeth, metaphyseal defects, growth retardation, craniosynostosis, periostitis, ↑ fractures and infections, anorexia, polyuria DDx Rickets, renal osteodystrophy, metaphyseal dysostosis, cystic fibrosis, phosphate depletion

ADULT ONSET An AD [MIM 146300] form of hypophosphatasia characterized by mild disease, early loss of permanent teeth, radiolucencies, osteoporosis, bone fragility with fractures and pseudofractures

hypophysis The pea-sized powerhouse that orchestrates the endocrine symphony, saddled in the sella turcica and separated into an 1) Anterior lobe, containing cells pro-

---

HYPOHIDROSIS

I INHERITED CONDITIONS, eg hereditary anhydrotic ectodermal dysplasia, ichthyosis, or angiokeratoma corporis diffusum universale

II ADQUIRED CONDITIONS

COLLAGEN VASCULAR DISEASES, eg Sjögren syndrome, progressive systemic sclerosis

DERMATOPATHIES, eg anhidrotic asthenia, miliaria profunda, pemphigus vulgaris, psoriasis

DRUGS Anticholinergics, eg atropine, scopolamine; ganglionic blockers

ENDOCRINOPATHIES Diabetes insipidus, hypothyroidism, hypothalamic lesions

ENVIRONMENTAL STRESS Heat stroke and dehydration

PERIPHERAL NEUROPATHIES Alcohol, amyloidosis, DM, Horner syndrome, leprosy

---

ducing ACTH, FSH, growth hormone (GH or somatotropin), LH and TSH Note: The formerly used division of cells into chromophobes or chromophils (subdividing these into acidophilic or basophilic cells) is obsolete as some cells produce more than one hormone; monoclonal antibodies may be used to identify the predominant hormone produced by each cell type 2) Intermediate lobe, which produces MSH and 3) Posterior lobe Neurohypophysis, which, under the hypothalamic baton, produces antidiuretic hormone (vasopressin) and oxytocin

hypopituitarism A clinical condition characterized by decreased secretions from the pituitary gland (hypophysis) ETIOLOGY Pituitary tumor, hypothalamic or infundibular cyst or tumor, infiltrative, vascular, or other disorders, aor radiotherapy CLINICAL The symptoms and signs of pituitary hormone deficiency are similar to those of a primary defect of the target organ, eg corticotropin deficiency is associated with asthenia, headache, anorexia, nausea, vomiting, abdominal pain, and alteration of mental functions TREATMENT Because cortisol and thyroxine are necessary for life, their prolonged absence is fatal; hormone-replacement is required and is a 'life sentence' (**N Engl J Med 1994; 330:1651**RV)

hypoplastic left heart syndrome A group of congenital cardiac defects that have right ventricular hypoplasia, left ventricular hyperplasia and an atrial right-to-left shunt; right-sided cardiac hypoplasia occurs in tricuspid or pulmonary valve atresias, pulmonary stenosis, or in the rare right ventricular hypoplasia; see Baby Fae heart

hypoplastic right ventricle Right ventricular dysplasia, see there

hypotensive ALTERNATIVE MEDICINE *noun* A medicinal preparation, usually of herbal origin that is reported by some alternative health care practitioners to be of use in reducing blood pressure

hypothalamic fever ↑ temperature due to an alteration in the hypothalamic thermostat, caused by hemorrhage, trauma or tumor Note: Most patients with hypothalamic damage are hypothermic

hypothalamic-pituitary-adrenal axis A tightly linked interdependent endocrine unit, which in concert with the systemic sympathetic and adrenomedullary systems, comprises a major peripheral limb of the stress system, the main function of which is to maintain basal and stress-related homeostasis; the hypothalamus and pituitary (adenohypohysis) form the central part of the HPA axis, and are active even at rest, responding to various blood-borne or neurosensory signals, including cytokines (eg IL-1, IL-6, and TNF-α); at the highest level, corticotropin-releasing hormone (CRH) and noradrenergic neurons innervate and stimulate each other, which is controlled by an autoregulatory, ultrashort negative-feedback loop, in which CRH and noradrenergic collateral fibers inhibit presynaptic CRH and $α_2$-noradrenergic receptors; a key hypothalamic region is the paraventricular nucleus, which has 3 parvicellular divisions that act either locally or project into the hind brain or spinal cord, secreting CRH and arginine vasopressin (AVP); each hour relatively synchronous pulses of CRH and AVP enter the hypophysial portal system, which in part stimulate corticotropin and cortisol secretion (**N Engl J Med 1995; 332:1351**RV)

hypothalamic-pituitary 'axis' A group of feedback systems that co-ordinate the activity of the major peptide hormones, where the hypothalamus synthesizes releasing hormones that act on the pituitary, which in turn evokes end-organ responses; the five axes include the hypothalamic-pituitary (HP) adrenocortical-ACTH-adrenal gland axis, HP-FSH/LH-gonadal axis, HP-TSH-thyroid gland axis, HP-growth hormone-somatotroph axis and the hypothalamic-lactotroph-breast axis

hypothermia CRITICAL CARE MEDICINE A body temperature < 37°C (classically < 98.6°F), which becomes significant < 33°C (classically below 91°F); systemic hypothermia is defined as a reduced core (rectal) body temperature < 35°C (95°F) and may result from long term occupational or recreational exposure to ↓ air or water temperatures CLINICAL ↓ Respiratory rate, metabolic acidosis, ↓ pulse, ↓ blood pressure, ventricular fibrillation, hypo- or hyperglycemia, coagulopathy, hemoconcentration, pneumonia, renal failure, pancreatitis; when extreme and prolonged, drowsiness, delirium, coma PATHOPHYSIOLOGY ↓ Temperature results in ↓ O_2 consumption, slowing of myocardial repolarization, peripheral nerve conduction, GI motility, and respiratory rate; physiologic defenses include superficial vasoconstriction and ↑ production of heat TREATMENT External rewarming, best performed in a warm tub at 40-42°C (104-107.6°F); internal rewarming is recommended for those with severe hypothemia and includes extracorporeal blood warming using a femorofemoral bypass and/or repeated peritoneal dialysis with 2 L of warmed (43°C) K⁺-free dialysate solution

hypothermia A clinical condition defined as a core temperature of 35°C or less that causes 750 annual deaths in the US; those most at risk for hypothermia are the exposed extremes of age, the homeless, alcoholics, those with hypothyroidism and young adults involved in winter sports

hypoxanthine-guanine phosphoribosyltransferase An enzyme encoded on the X chromosome and found in high concentrations in the brain, responsible for transfer of phosphoribosyl groups; deficiency of the HGPRT enzyme results in two syndromes 1) Lesch-Nyhan disease, with hyperproduction of uric acid and CNS abnormalities, including mental retardation, spasticity, choreoathetosis and compulsive self-mutilation and 2) Gout without the neurologic disease; variant forms of the enzyme: HGPRT Toronto, London, Ann Arbor, Munich; HGPRT-deficiency has been established in a mouse embryonal stem cell (transgenic mouse), allowing experimental dissection

HYPP Hyperkalemic periodic paralysis, see Periodic paralysis-hyperkalemic

hysterical amnesia PSYCHOLOGY A state of amnesia which may occur in hysterical ♀ or sociopathic ♂ involved in a crime; in general HA is accompanied by normal outward appearance and behavior

hysterical personality disorder Histrionic personality disorder, see there

hysterectomy The 2nd most common (after cesarean section) operation performed in the US (± 590 000/year); annual cost ± $5 x 10⁹; among developed nations, a 6-fold range in frequency of hysterectomy with the highest in US, where it is higher in blacks 500/10⁵ at a younger age-42 vs 410/10⁵ in whites, average age 46 (New York Times 16 Nov 1993; C1) the rate of hysterectomis is lowest in Sweden, Norway, UK INDICATIONS Uterine leiomyomas (30%), dysfunctional uterine bleeding (20%), endometriosis and adenomyosis (20%), genital prolapse (15%), chronic pelvic pain (10%), pelvic inflammatory disease, endometrial hyperplasia, and others malignancy (eg CIN, endometrial cancer), and other indications (eg massive postpartum hemorrhage, septic endometritis) COMPLICATIONS Fever, infections, major (transfusion-requiring) intra– and postoperative hemorrhage, long-term adverse effects include, urinary symptoms, early ovary failure, retain ovary syndrome, constipation, fatigue, changes in sexual interest and function, depression and psychiatric morbidity MORTALITY 7-20 deaths/10⁵ hysterectomies for cancer, 2.9-3.8 deaths/10⁵ hysterectomies for pregnancy-related indications, 0.6-1.1 deaths/10⁵ hysterectomies for other indications (N Engl J Med 1993; 328:856RV)

hysteresis A phenomenon in which the values or data points in a cyclical or periodic process occur along a different route in one direction as the other, which may be described by a hysteric response curve (figure displays the relationship between lung volume and intrapleural pressure)

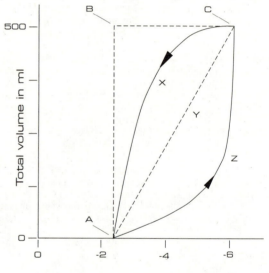

hysteresis curve

I Symbol for: 1) Electric current 2) Hypoxanthine 3) Incisor 4) Inosine 5) Intensity 6) Iodine 7) Ionic strength 8) Isoleucine 9) Luminous intensity

i Symbol for: Isochromosome

IADL Instrumental activities of daily living, see there

Ia antigen Immune-associated antigen Any of the cell surface antigens encoded by the I region genes of the major histocompatibility complex (located on chromosome 17) of the mouse which corresponds to the human HLA-DR (chromosome 6), Class II MHC; Ia antigens are expressed on B cells, monocytes and some subsets of T cells, acting as gene-specific mediators of the immune response

IAPP Islet amyloid polypeptide, see there

IARC International Agency for Research on Cancer

IAT Intra-operative autologous transfusion, see there

iatrogenic illness Any complication related to diagnosis and treatment of disease, regardless whether the condition occurs as a known risk of a procedure or through errors of omission or commission; iatrogenic disease is a major source of morbidity and mortality for hospitalized patients, the most common of which is cardiac arrest, comprising 14% of the in-hospital cardiac arrests, most often related to errors in medication, especially of digoxin (JAMA 1991; 265:2815)

IBD Inflammatory bowel disease, see there

IBM Ideal body mass

IBM 'clone' Any microcomputer that is fully capable of writing and reading software written for the three generations of microcomputers based on Intel's 80C88, 80C286 and 80C386 microprocessors using Microsoft Corp's disk operating system (MS/DOS)

Note: By the time of the release of Intel's 486 microprocessor in the early 1990s, sales of 'clone' PCs (eg Compaq, Dell, etc) had sufficiently challenged IBM's dominance of the microcomputer market that the term IBM-cone was being phased out in the working parlance, and replaced with 'PC' for personal computer, which itself originated in essence from IBM

IBS Irritable bowel syndrome, see there

IBT see Ivy bleeding time

IBW Ideal body weight

ICAM-1 Intercellular adhesion molecule-1 A protein ligand the production of which is induced by γ-interferon and required for neutrophils to migrate into inflamed tissues; in Sézary syndrome, clinical aggression is associated with ↓ ICAM-1 expression, possibly due to ↓ IFN-γ production by the malignant T cells

Icarus complex PSYCHIATRY A constellation of mental conflicts, the degree of which is a function of the dispropor-

tion between a person's desire for success, achievement or material goods and his ability to achieve those goals; the greater the gap between the idealized goal and reality, the greater the likelihood of failure; the Icarus analogy* has been applied to a 'driven' or aggressive 'type A' person who cannot recognize his own limitations; alternately this conflict has been considered an internalization of father-son rivalry; see Type A, 'Toxic core'

Daedalus and Icarus were a father and son in Greek mythology who had been imprisoned by King Minos on Crete to prevent their return home; they fashioned wings of feathers and attached them with wax; Icarus, despite his father's ministrations, flew too close to the sun, melted his wings and fell to his death

ICD-9-CM International Classification of Disease, 9th edition, Clinical Modification A systematic and standardized classification of disease, injuries, and causes of death according to etiology and anatomic localization that allows clinicians, statisticians, politicians, health planners and others to speak a common language at the national and international level; infectious diseases are 001-139, neoplasia 140-239, endocrine 140-279, blood-related 280-289, mental disease 290-319, nervous 320-389, circulatory system 390-459, respiratory system 460-519, GI tract 520-579, genitourinary tract 580-629, pregnancy-related 630-676, skin 680-709, connective tissue disease 710-739, congenital anomalies 740-759, conditions of perinatal origin 760-779, vaguely defined conditions 780-799, injury and poisoning 800-999; other details may be added to the classification, including a V prefix for a virulent or communicable disease and E for external causes of injury

ICE IL-1β-converting enzyme A cysteine protease, the activity of which is critical in the induction of apoptosis mediated by the Fas/APO-1 signal transduction receptor (Nature 1995; 375:78, 81L)

ice

'ice' The 'street' name for the smokable, crystal form of the psychostimulant, (+)- or D-methamphetamine HCl; oral abuse of methamphetamine has occurred in epidemic waves in Japan, Sweden and the US since the 1950s; an inhaled smokable form of the crystalline form, which has an ice-like appearance (hence, 'ice') represents a new form of abuse; ice induces an effect similar to intravenous injection of methamphetamine, ie far more intense than that achieved by oral ingestion; the mechanism of action differs from cocaine, but has a stimulant effect similar and of longer duration (hours versus minutes for cocaine); because methamphetamine is synthetic, an unlimited supply may be manufactured in illicit laboratories as a 'designer drug'; ice is being touted as the 'drug of the 1990s' and in Hawaii has become the most common drug of abuse; the low cost of the raw material (phenylacetic acid, $1300/kg) and the high street value of the finished product, ice ($500 000), make it likely that ice addiction will increase; 1.2% of US high school students have used it, 3% in the Western states; ice, like 'crack' has a prolonged 'high' and is more socially acceptable to upper class; Ice's neurotoxicity is prolonged with severe depression of the caudate dopamine levels, lasting six months or more after last use in animal models (JAMA 1990; 263:2717) COMPLICATIONS Pulmonary edema, dilated cardiomyopathy, acute myocardial infarction, cardiogenic shock and death (JAMA 1991; 265:1152); see 'Designer' drug

'ice ball' method GYNECOLOGY A method for treating

benign lesions of the uterine cervix, in which special probes previously frozen with either liquid nitrogen or freon are placed on the cervix for 2-3 minutes, freezing and then excising a lesion ADVANTAGE Reduced postoperative pain, infection, discharge and better hemostasis DISADVANTAGE Freezing introduces considerable histological artifact that makes the ice-ball technique controversial in treating dysplasia and carcinoma

iceberg sign Thoraco-abdominal sign A sharply-demarcated radiopacity seen in plain films of the chest or abdomen that may be either sub- or supradiaphragmatic and corresponds to a paravertebral tuberculous abscess, aneurysm, esophagogastric lesion or the azygous continuation of the inferior vena cava

iceberg lesion Dumbbell tumor, see there

ice cream headache A migraine headache triggered by oropharyngeal irritation due to cold foods, the ingestion of which causes bifrontal headaches in many patients with migraines

ice hockey see Silo-filler's disease

Iceland disease Epidemic neuromyasthenia, benign myalgic encephalomyelitis An epidemic disease, described in the summer among student nurses, that resembles poliomyelitis ETIOLOGY Unknown, psychosocial dysfunction has been implicated CLINICAL Severe headache, myalgia, fatigue, myasthenia, variable cranial and peripheral nerve dysfunction and depression; recuperation requires up to a year

'ice man' FORENSIC PATHOLOGY A free-lance 'con' artist* who was allegedly linked to an unknown number of murders in the New York metropolitan area in the early 1980s, whose business associates often 'disappeared'; the sobriquet stems from his modus operandi--after incapacitating his victims with cyanide and/or strangling them, he stored the bodies for a year or two in a freezer, as the ice crystals destroyed the evidence for a time of death

*Who dealt in contraband guns and stolen cars

the Iceman of Tyrol ANTHROPOLOGY A 5300-year old man (now known as Otzi) discovered in a melting Tyrolean glacier, whose skull has been reconstructed using a technique known as sterolithography (Biophotonics Intl 1995; 2/2:34)

ice-pick scar DERMATOLOGY A deep punched-out scar that is typical residual lesion of acne vulgaris, which may partially respond to dermabrasion

I-cell disease Type II mucolipidosis An AR [MIM 252500] condition caused by a defect in a protein traffic and sorting factor (N-acetylglucosamine-1-phosphotransferase) which directs correct compartmentalization of catabolic enzymes, by phosphorylating mannose, without which, the lysosomal enzymes are present but 'forget' their final destination in the lysosomes, resulting in massive accumulation of intracellular and extracellular waste products, especially glycolipids CLINICAL Hurler-like disease (type I-H mucopolysaccharidosis) with a gargoyle face, early onset of psychomotor retardation, joint contracture, hepatosplenomegaly and cardiac decompensation which causes death in childhood

Note: The term 'I-cell' derives from the light microscopic finding of numerous dark cytoplasmic inclusions in fibroblasts grown from biopsies of these patients

ICER Inducible early cAMP early repressor The protein product of the CREM gene which is produced in a circadian rhythm in the pineal gland, being high at night and low during the day; the dynamic expression of ICER is thought to be a central player in the neuroendocrine axis (Nature 1993; 365:314)

ichthyosis A group of hereditary diseases characterized by dyskeratosis and non-inflammatory scaling of the skin, subdivided into four major primary forms, including ichthyosis vulgaris, X-linked ichthyosis, epidermolytic hyperkeratosis and lamellar ichthyosis and three minor primary forms, including harlequin ichthyosis, erythrokeratodermia variabilis and ichthyosis linearis circumflexa; the secondary ichthyoses occur in conjunction with neuroectodermal or mesodermal defects, eg Conradi-Hünermann, Netherton, Refsum, Rud, and Sjögren-Larsson syndromes, rhizomelic chondrodysplasia punctata, as well as acquired conditions including Hodgkin's disease, lymphoma, leprosy, hypothyroidism

icon-driven COMPUTERS An adjective referring or pertaining to a system design in microcomputers that enables the user to transfer, copy, open, close, and otherwise manipulate files and software programs while in the computer's 'root directory', by pointing and clicking on an icon (a small schematic, often trademarked representation of a software program, file, directory, or subdirectory); the icon-driven environment may be combined with pull-down menus, both of which may be controlled by 'user-friendly' devices, most commonly, a 'mouse', allowing a non-computer-literate person to use a microcomputer and circumvent the need to memorize arcane disk-operating system commands; see Computers; Cf Menu-driven

ICP-MS Inductively coupled plasma-mass spectrometry (spectroscopy) A powerful analytic technique that is used in research and industry to detect low (parts per trillion) levels of elements, eg calcium, iron, lithium potassium, sodium, and others (Am Lab Feb1995 p48D; 48DD)

ICP47 VIROLOGY A 9-kD immediate early cytoplasmic protein that is expressed by the herpes simplex virus; ICP47 lacks a recognizable signal sequence and blocks the presentation of viral peptides to MHC class I-restricted T cells by binding to TAP, the transporter associated with antigen processing (Nature 1995; 375:411) *Inhibition of peptide translocation by a viral protein indicates a previously undocumented ...mechanism for viral immune evasion* (Nature 1995; 375:415)

ICRF see Imperial Cancer Research Fund

ICRP International Commission on Radiological Protection; see BEIR studies, Chernobyl, Sellafield studies

ICSH Interstitial cell-stimulating hormone, now known as luteinizing hormone, LH

ICU Intensive care unit A ward of a secondary or tertiary health care facility, in which 20% of all patients spend some time during their hospitalization; Criteria for admission and continued stay in the ICU include chest pain and suspected myocardial infarction, pulmonary edema and syncope

id PSYCHIATRY The unconscious source of mental energies and libido, the id corresponds to the first (selfish and supremely egocentric) mind of the neonate, which is driven by the pleasure principle; it is later modified by the ego (the conscious being) and the superego (the parental and social conscience), which impose a sense of reality and control on the id's egocentric drives; Freud created the id concept and felt that repression of the id led to neurosis, inhibition of the id led to sexual deviation and sublimation of the id led to artistic creativity; Cf id reaction

IDDM Insulin-dependent diabetes mellitus, see there

ideational apraxia NEUROLOGY The inability to execute a sequence of movements in an orderly fashion; although individual components of the movement are executed, the entire act remains uncompleted, eg a match may be removed from its cover but not struck

identical twins Monozygotic twins Twins resulting from the division of a single fertilized egg, which usually share a common chorion and placenta, although usually each may have a separate amnion; Cf Fraternal twins

Note: Both terms are in active use, identical is more colloquial, monozygotic more formal

identifier sequence see ID sequence

identity crisis PSYCHOLOGY A conflict in a person's perceived role in society, which may be accompanied by a loss of the sense of self and historical continuity; adolescence is a form of IC in which the adolescent's role changes in terms of what is socially and educationally expected of him, which is accompanied by strengthening of drives and physical capacity

ideokinetic apraxia NEUROLOGY The dissociation of an idea and the motor act, eg a patient cannot whistle when commanded to do so, but may do so spontaneously

idiogenic osmole PHYSIOLOGY Any volume-regulating organic solute (eg *N*-acetylasparatate, choline, glycerophosphoryl choline, *myo*-inositol, taurine) that is generated in the brain as a protection against rapid dehydration (or chronic hypernatremia); the accumulation of IOs allows intracellular osmolarity to ↑ while minimizing the loss of intracellular water (ie shrinkage) in the brain; it is well-recognized that overly rapid correction of hyperosmolarity may be fatal, as replacement of the extracellular fluid increases intracellular water, leading to cerebral edema (N Engl J Med 1994; 331:439oa)

idiopathic CD4+ T-lymphocytopenia A rare, recently described heterogeneous syndrome for which the CDC has published a provisional (laboratory) definition: < 300 CD4+ T cells/mm³, or a CD4+ T cell count < 20% of total T cells on 2 occasions and no evidence of HIV infection*; in one study (N Engl J Med 1993; 328:373oa) of 47 patients with ICT, 29 (62%) had no identified risk factors for HIV infection; 19 (40%) had AIDS-defining conditions (eg cerebral toxoplasmosis, *Pneumocystis carinii* pneumonia, esophageal candidiasis, cryptococcal meningitis, HIV encephalopathy, wasting syndrome, extrapulmonary *Mycobacterium avium* complex, CMV retinitis, and others); 24 (53%) had conditions that were not AIDS-defining, although 11/24 had risk factors for HIV, 6% were asymptomatic, but all 3 were at risk for HIV infection (see also N Engl J Med 1993; 328:380-393oa, 429ED)

*Tests performed and found negative in patients with ICD: 1) Plasma antibodies by ELISA, RIA, and Western blot (anti-HIV-1, anti-HIV-2, anti-HTLV-I/II) 2) Plasma antigens (HIV-1–p24, HIV-2–p27) 3) Viral cultures (HIV-1, HIV-2) 4) PCR HIV-1 (LTR/*gag*, gp120, gp41) HIV-2 (*pol*) HTLV-I/II (*tax/rex*) (N Engl J Med 1993; 328:380oa)

idiopathic cyclical edema Cyclical edema syndrome, see there

idiopathic dilated cardiomyopathy '...*primary myocardial disease of unknown cause characterized by left ventricular or biventricular dilatatation* (sic) *and impaired myocardial contractility.*' (N Engl J Med 1994; 331:1564oa) as the etiology of IDC is rarely known, the adjective idiopathic is commonly deleted; see Dilated cardiomyopathy

idiopathic hypertrophic subaortic stenosis Hypertrophic cardiomyopathy, see there

idiopathic intracranial hypertension A rare (annual incidence 1-2/10⁶) that is far more common in obese ♀ of reproductive age, which may cause reversible loss of vision PATHOGENESIS Vasogenic extracellular brain edema and low conductance of CSF outflow at the arachnoid villi DIAGNOSIS ↑ Intracranial pressure, normal CSF, negative findings by neuroimaging (Mayo Clin Proc 1994; 69:169)

idiopathic midline destructive disease Lethal midline granuloma of Stewart A condition that is a diagnosis of exclusion (criteria, table), which consists of a midline granuloma of unknown etiology, which unlike most granulomas of the midline are secondary manifestations of a primary process, including vasculitis, eg Wegener's granulomatosis, malignancy, eg lymphoma, nasal carcinoma and infections, eg destructive fungal infections in immunocompromised patients TREATMENT Radiotherapy; see Lethal midline granuloma, Midline granuloma

IDIOPATHIC MIDLINE DESTRUCTIVE DISEASE
1) Local destruction of the upper respiratory tract
2) Lack of progression to system disease (average follow-up, 7 years)
3) Acute/chronic inflammation with variable necrosis, without vasculitis, atypia or malignancy
4) No evidence of infection or malignancy

idiopathic interstitial fibrosis of lung A disease more common in middle-aged men, possibly related to collagen vascular disease, with positive 'rheumatoid' serology CLINICAL Aggressive with a rapid onset of dyspnea, orthopnea, hemoptysis, cyanosis, clubbing of the fingers and toes, pulmonary hypertension, bibasilar rales, non-productive cough and death in 3-6 years RADIOLOGY Diffuse reticulonodular infiltrates PATHOLOGY-EARLY Fibrinous edema, RBCs, desquamated macrophages, hyaline membrane disease PATHOLOGY-LATE Bronchial cells undergo columnar or mucinous metaplasia, muscular hyperplasia, later collagenous replacement of the alveolar wall causes compression, collapse and alveolar 'honeycombing' and has a bossellated or 'hobnailed' pleural surface; pulmonary fibrosis is subdivided into usual, desquamative, lymphocytic and giant cell interstitial pneumonitides

idiopathic panarteritis Takayasu's disease

idiopathic postprandial hypoglycemia Idiopathic postprandial syndrome, see there

idiopathic postprandial syndrome ENDOCRINOLOGY A condition characterized by vaguely defined symptoms that follow ingestion of food; initially thought to result from post-cibal hypoglycemia (resulting in the alternative name postprandial hypoglycemia), this is no longer considered correct, as decreased serum glucose is not always present (N Engl J Med 1995; 332:1144oa)

idiopathic (acquired) sideroblastic anemia Acquired refractory sideroblastic anemia A pluripotent stem cell defect characterized by ineffective erythropoiesis with a slight ↓ in red cell survival, mild maturational impairment of all hematopoietic cell lines, coupled with defective iron metabolism and iron accumulation; ISA affects older patients, often related to radio- or chemotherapy, 10-30% of whom later develop acute non-lymphocytic leukemia CLINICAL Pallor, fatigue, weakness, dyspnea and palpitations on exertion LABORATORY 'Dimorphic' anemia with hypochromic-microcytic and macrocytic features; 40% of the erythroblasts are ring sideroblasts, anisocytosis, basophilic stippling, reticulocyte with impaired heme synthesis, ↓ delta ALA synthetase and protease activity TREATMENT Pyridoxine is often administered, usually without therapeutic response PROGNOSIS ISA is usually characterized by chronic stable anemia, and less commonly by evolution to leukemia, or to marrow failure; Cf Refractory anemia with excess blasts

idiopathic thrombocytopenic purpura Werlhof's disease A condition[1] characterized by '...*thrombocytopenia in which apparent exogenous etiologic factors are lacking and in which diseases known to be associated with 'secondary' thrombocytopenia have been excluded...ITP is thus a diagnosis of exclusion, even though in most patients, the disorder is the result of accelerated platelet destruction attributable to an immunologic process.*' (TC Bithell, in GR Lee, et al Eds, Wintrobe's Clinical Hematology, 9th ed, Lea & Febiger, Philadelphia, 1993) Acute ITP is more common in children, causing a self-limited wave of ecchymotic hemorrhage secondary to viral infection or vaccination; chronic ITP is more common in adults and often is autoimmune with mucocutaneous, CNS, cardiac and renal hemorrhage (and potentially infarction), bruisability and transient thrombocytopenia (with normal or increased megakaryocytes in bone marrow); ⅔ of cases have IgG antiplatelet antibodies and hemolysis within the splenic sinusoids PATHOGENESIS: Caused by the removal of autoantibody[2]-coated platelets from the circulation by splenic and hepatic macrophages; ITP may be a complication of SLE or B-cell lymphomas, but most cases are idiopathic CLINICAL ♀:♂ ratio 3:1, microangiopathic hemolytic anemia, fever, transient neurologic defects, renal failure, microthrombolic 'showers' to the brain, heart, lungs, kidneys, adrenal glands, spleen and live (see table) Note: ITP should be differentiated from the microthrombi of TTP of young ♀, microangiopathic hemolytic anemia, neurologic defects and renal failure TREATMENT The efficacy of most therapeutic agents used in ITP is uncertain, especially in view of the possibility of spontaneous remission, the small populations studied, and the wide difference in patient populations; modalities include splenectomy (75% markedly improve with splenectomy according to some authors) prednisone, IV gamma globulin, immunoadsorption apheresis on staphylococcal protein A columns, plasmapheresis; refractory ITP may respond to low-dose corticosteroids or to pulsed high-dose dexamethasone (N Engl J Med 1994; 330:1560oA), or combination chemotherapy (eg azathioprine, cochicine, cyclosporine, danazol, and vincristine) (N Engl J Med 1993; 328:1226oA)

[1]Logic to the contrary, the widely preferred term for this condition, which is often pathogenically linked to immune-mediated destruction of platelets, is idiopathic thrombocytopenic purpura, a highly questionable convention other less commonly used terms are immunologic thrombocytopenic purpura, and autoimmune thrombocytopenic purpura [2]Against platelet membrane proteins, in particular glycoprotein IIb/IIIa and Ib/IX complexes, resulting in platelet destruction by the reticuloendothelial system

TP, CLINICAL FEATURES	ACUTE	CHRONIC
Peak age	Children, age 2-6	Adults, age 20-40
Sex (♀:♂ ratio)	1:1	3:1
History, recent infection	Common	Rare
Onset	Abrupt	Insidious
Hemorrhagic bullae-oral	Present if severe	Rare
Eosinophilia, lymphocytosis	Common	Rare
Platelet count	< 20 x 10⁹/L	30-80 x 10⁹/L
Duration	2-6 weeks	Months, years
Spontaneous remission	Common (± 80%)	Rare (± 20%)

after TC Bithell, in GR Lee, et al Eds, Wintrobe's Clinical Hematology, 9th ed, Lea & Febiger, Philadelphia, 1993

idiot savant Savant syndrome A mentally retarded person who lacks the ability to reason abstractly, but who has a remarkably overdeveloped a skill, eg mathematical or calendar 'calculation', memory, mechanical ability or talent in music and the visual arts; most idiot savants are male and have IQs above 40*; they may be blind and autistic; the savant's talent may appear and disappear virtually overnight; the pathogenesis is unclear but may be related to a dichotomy of function between the right and left brain

*Although the the adjectival modifier 'idiot' is incorrect, as the now obsolete term idiot, referred to those with an IQ less than 25, it is inextractably linked to the term savant, and is unlikely to be deleted from the working parlance in the forseeable future–Author's note

idiotype The specific type of an immunoglobulin, defined by the myriad of possible combinations of the V (variability), D (diversity) and J (joining) exons as elucidated by Tonegawa; idiotypic specificity resides in the variable region of the heavy and light chains and is specific for an epitope, see Immunoglobulin; Cf Mimotope

idiotype suppression IMMUNOLOGY The suppression of idiotype antibody synthesis by suppressor T lymphocytes that have been activated by anti-idiotype antibodies

IDL Intermediate-density lipoprotein A plasma lipoprotein with a density of 1.006-1.019 g/dl, which is formed by VLDL hydrolysis with lipoprotein lipase that is partially depleted of triglycerides; IDL is composed of 15% protein (predominantly apolipoproteins B and E), 25% phospholipid, 30% cholesterol and 30% triglycerides and transports cholesterol from the intestine to the liver, and once in the liver, is delipidated by hepatic lipoprotein lipase to form low-density protein

idling reaction MOLECULAR BIOLOGY The transient binding to a ribosome's 'A' site by a tRNA lacking an attached amino acid, resulting in the temporary halting of the growth of the polypeptide chain and breaking ATP's high-energy phosphate bonds converting GDP to pppGpp; this phenomenon has been fancifully likened to the idling of an automobile motor that is running by not 'in gear'

-id reaction Dermatophytid reaction A localized or generalized rash of sudden onset associated with, but located at a distance from, a site of cutaneous inflammation and/or infection; IRs occur on the hands and arms, as sterile papulovesicular pustules, classically associated with dermatophytosis, eg tinea pedis, tinea capitis and may be associated with stasis dermatitis, eczema and contact dermatitis, which disappear after successful therapy; because the IR is similar to the original lesion, it is thought to represent an immune to circulating antigens; Cf Isomorphic phenomenon

ID sequence Identifier sequence MOLECULAR BIOLOGY Any of circa 80 base pair in length segments of DNA that are transcribed in the brain and thought to control tissue-specific gene expression

IEF Isoelectric focusing, see there

IF 1) Initiation factor 2) Interstitial fluid 3) Intrinsic factor, see there

IFE Immunofixation electrophoresis, see there

IFN Interferon, see there

ifosfamide An antineoplastic agent approved under a treatment investigational new drug (IND) protocol as a third-line chemotherapeutic agent for treating germ-cell testicular malignancy (N Engl J Med 1994; 330:153oA), which is also used to treat cervical cancer, soft tissue sarcomas SIDE EFFECTS Myelosuppression, encephalopathy (confusion and coma), hemorrhagic cystitis TREATMENT Hemorrhagic cystitis may respond to mesna, encephalopathy may respond to methylene blue (N Engl J Med 1995; 332:1239c)

IgA Immunoglobulin A

IgA deficiency Selective immunoglobulin A deficiency An AD [MIM 137100] condition that is the most common (1:600, US) primary disease of the immune system, characterized by a decrease of IgA to less than 50 mg/L (normal 760-3900 mg/L; US 76-390 mg/dl); 40% of patients produce subclass specific anti-IgA antibodies (anti-A1, -A2, -A2m(1), -A2m(2)), deficiency of B cell development, lymphokine deficiency; patients may also have IgG2 and IgG4 deficiencies or an HLA-A1/B8 haplotype CLINICAL Potentially fatal hemolysis occurs if these patients receive blood transfusions due to production of natural anti-IgA antibodies; other features include myotonic dystrophy, intestinal lymphangiectasia, gluten-sensitive enteropathy, allergies, arthritis, 7S IgM antibodies to food, especially to milk, cirrhosis, autoimmune disease and sinopulmonary infections TREATMENT IV immune globulin, eg Gammagard (Baxter), has minimal IgA and thus may be well-suited for boosting the humoral immune system (N Engl J Med 1991; 325:110rv)

IgA nephropathy Berger's disease Idiopathic IgA nephropathy is the most common glomerular disease in the world; in 20-40% of patients, it progresses to renal failure 5-25 years after diagnosis; IgA nephropathy may occur in HIV-infected patients and may contain circulating immune complexes composed of IgA idiotypic antibody reactive with anti-HIV IgG or IgM antibodies (N Engl J Med 1992; 327:702oA) TREATMENT None, anticoagulants, antiplatelet drugs, corticosteroids, cyclosporine, and phenytoin have proven unsuccessful; dietary fish oil‡ is reported to slow the progress of renal failure (**N Engl J Med 1994; 331:1105₀ₐ**) PROGNOSIS More rapidly progressive disease is seen in males, older patients, hypertension, persistent proteinuria, baseline of impaired renal function, glomerulosclerosis or interstitial fibrosis at the time of initial evaluation

IGCN Intratubular germ cell neoplasm, see there

IGF-I Insulin-like growth factor I A 7.6-kD single-chain polypeptide hormone structurally similar to proinsulin that is synthesized in the liver and fibroblasts, giving fibroblasts a paracrine function; IGF-I is considered to be the sole effector of growth hormone (GH) action, ie GH acts indirectly; IGF-I is an age-dependent primary growth regulator; serum levels correlate with the development of secondary sex characteristics in puberty; IGF-I is bound to a carrier-protein and therefore has relatively constant serum levels; because GH fluctuates widely during the day, IGF-I reflects GH activity Normal levels < age 5 < 100 µg/L, peaks during puberty < 225 µg/L, over age 50 < 100 µg/L); IGF-I is ↓ in starvation, anorexia nervosa and African pygmies and ↑ with ↓ somatomedins* in Laron dwarfs, kwashiorkor, and hepatic disease in children

Note: Somatomedins include somatomedins A and B and IGF-I and -II

IGF-II Insulin-like growth factor II A protein structurally homologous to IGF-I that may be produced by tumors, eg leiomyosarcoma, mesotheliomas, and others and cause reactive hypoglycemia; IGF-II receptor is similar, if not identical to the receptor for mannose-6-phosphate

IgD Immunoglobulin D

IgE Immunoglobulin E

IgG Immunoglobulin G

IgG Fc receptor type III CD16, see there

IgG index LABORATORY MEDICINE A value determined by the ratio of production of IgG and albumin in the brain and in the peripheral tissues, which is elevated in a wide range of infectious, inflammatory and neoplastic disorders of the CNS; Cf Oligoclonal bands

IgH Immunoglobulin heavy chain

IgL Immunoglobulin light chain

IgM Immunoglobulin M

IgM deficiency syndrome Immunoglobulin M deficiency syndrome A rare clinical condition usually without clinical consequences that may have ↓ complement activation and an ↑ susceptibility to respiratory infections, fulminant septicemia and various tumors, which may be associated with deficiency in 5-ecto nucleotidase on the B-cell surface

IgM index A measure of the total IgM synthesis in the blood-brain barrier (BBB), which is characteristically ↑ in infectious meningoencephalitis by bacteria or *Borrelia burgdorferi*; IgM may also be ↑ in multiple sclerosis and SLE affecting the CNS

iguana *Iguana iguana* A lizard that has become popular in the US as a household pet, and linked to infection by unusual serotypes of *Salmonella* (*S* Wassenaar, *S*, Rubislaw, *S* serotype IIIa41:z4z23:-(*S* subspp *Arizonae*), *S* Kintambo) and others (**MMWR 1995; 44:347**)

IHSS Idiopathic hypertrophic subaortic stenosis, now known as Hypertrophic cardiomyopathy

Ii antigens A pair of non-allelic antigens present on the surface of hematopoietic, typically red cells and non-hematopoietic cells; the i antigen is immature and present on fetal red cells and red cell precursors; I antigen results from the enzymatic conversion of aliphatic galactose-*N*-acetyl-glucosamine to a complex branched form; therefore two 'alleles' don't exist, merely immature (i) and mature (I) forms; expression of the I antigen indicates red cell maturation, occurring by age 2; in the absence of the I

antigen, only i antigen is expressed; anti-i antibodies cause hemolysis in infectious mononucleosis; anti-I antibodies are uncommon, but when seen are of high titer and have a wide thermal amplitude

IIFL Idiopathic interstitial fibrosis of the lung, see there

I₍KACh₎ MEMBRANE PHYSIOLOGY A G-protein-gated atrial K⁺ (potassium) channel that is a heteromultimer of two inwardly rectifying K⁺ channel proteins, GIRK1 and CIR (**Nature 1995; 374:135**)

IL Interleukin, see there, also 1) *Ilium* [NA6] 2) Incisolingual (dentistry)

Also 1) Intermediate loop 2) Interpolated learning (psychology)

ileal bypass operation A surgical procedure that may be indicated for extreme obesity or high serum cholesterol METHOD The distal ⅓ of the small intestine (± 2 m) is bypassed and bowel continuity is restored by an end-to-side ileocecostomy; ileal bypass surgery improves the lipid profile of those with a previous myocardial infarction (reduction of total and LDL-cholesterol by 23% and 38%, with 5% increase in HDL-cholesterol; post-operative coronary artery disease is reduced but not significant (**N Engl J Med 1990; 323:946**) SIDE EFFECTS The jejuno-ileal bypass procedure is a more extensive variation on the 'morbid obesity surgery' theme, resulting in significant weight loss, although complicated by steatorrhea, diarrhea, hepatic failure, cirrhosis, oxalate deposition, and concrement formation, bile stone formation, electrolyte imbalance (↓ Ca⁺⁺, K⁺, Mg⁺⁺), hypovitaminosis, psychogenic problems, polyarthropathy, hair loss, pancreatitis, colonic pseudo-obstruction, intussusception, pneumatosis cystoides intestinalis, and blind loop syndrome; see Gastric bubble, Jaw wiring, Morbid obesity

Note: Many of these same symptoms occur to a lesser degree with less extensive surgery

ileal loop test Rabbit ileal loop test, see there

ileocecal valve lipohyperplasia A condition condition by excessive adipose tissue at the submucosa of the ileocecal valve with thickening and protrusion into the cecum and obstructive potential

ileus Impairment of the caudad flow of GI contents, which is either 1) Adynamic or paralytic, secondary to electrolyte derangements, mesenteric arterial vascular accidents, peritoneal irritation, surgery, trauma or as a paraneoplastic phenomenon or 2) Obstructive, due to adhesive bands, foreign bodies, hematomas, intussusception or tumors CLINICAL Symptoms are a function of the level of obstruction and the type of ileus; paralytic ileus causes little pain and is first evident through abdominal distension and vomiting; a post-operative paralytic ileus may manifest itself through increased nasogastric secretions or oliguria; mechanical ileus is associated with vomiting, abdominal colic, distension and constipation, that may be episodic with intermittent relief through production of voluminous, watery stools TREATMENT Stabilize, decompress, repair

iliac horn PEDIATRIC RADIOLOGY A feature of the nail-patella (HOOD or hereditary onycho-osteodysplasia) syndrome, seen in early infancy as bilateral chondro-osseous extensions from the iliac wings; iliac horns may also be seen in thanatophoric dwarfism and achondroplasia; bilateral horns without other clinical findings, are known as Fong's disease; unilateral horns have no significance

ILGF Insulin-like growth factor, see IGF-I

Ilizarov technique(s) Transosseous osteosynthesis A group of techniques for bone regeneration developed by GA Ilizarov (1921-1992) of the former Soviet Union, in which a long bone, most often of the lower extremity is gently fractured and held in place for a short period or time, and then slowly distracted with an external fixator; the method has been successfully used to treat a wide range of osseous defects, including discrepancies in leg length, dwarfism, fracture nonunions, osteomyelitis, bone defects, and angular deformities (N Engl J Med 1993; 329:365BR)

illness The state of being unwell, a term used by regulatory agencies, eg the US Food and Drug Administration, which modifies 'illness' with certain adjectives, in order to allow patients to receive experimental drugs that do not have FDA approval; see Life-threatening illness, Severely debilitating illness

ILO International Labor Organization

IM Intramuscular, also 1) Index Medicus 2) Infant mortality 3) Infectious mononucleosis 4) Internal medicine 5) Intramedullary 6) Inverted microscope

Also 1) Immature 2) Immunosuppression method (gynecology) 3) Indomethacin 4) Infantile myofibromatosis 5) Injection mold 6) Institute of Medicine (of the US National Academy of Science, IOM is more commonly used) 7) Intestinal metaplasia 8) Invasive mole

image analysis LABORATORY MEDICINE The evaluation and interpretation of objective or quantifiable parameters of cells or tissues; IA encompasses a constellation of either 'manual', eg imaging cytometry, DNA ploidy analysis or computer-assisted, eg morphometry, and automated microscopy linked to expert systems (currently being used to screen Papanicolaou-stained smears ('Pap' smears) of uterine cervical cells; these techniques are being increasingly used in clinical and research laboratories to analyze neoplasia, immune dysfunctions, and physiopathological mechanisms

imagery PSYCHOLOGY The evoking of a visual, audio, or other internalized mental image that retains the 'flavor' and sensory qualities of the original external stimulus

imaginary pregnancy Pseudocyesis, see there

imaging Production of non-invasive images of body regions through use of ionizing radiation, eg CT or mammography or electromagnetic radiation, eg MRI or ultrasonography, with or without radiocontrast medium; the information obtained may then be analyzed by a computer to produce a 2-D display; the information provided may be anatomic (CT, MRI, mammography, ultrasonography), metabolic (positron emission tomography, SPECT) or data on electrical activity (SQUID) LABORATORY MEDICINE A key component in pathology imaging is the ability to record, transmit, and store images of pathological lesions; applications in varying stages of development or implementation include attaching a photographic image of a lesion on the pathology report, and telepathology, in which a remote and/or unstaffed pathology service can communicate with a larger medical center by transmitting high-resolution video images of a lesion or diagnostic dilemma

imaging center A facility that has the equipment necessary to produce various types of radiologic and electromagnetic images, and the professional staff to interpret the images obtained; in the US, ICs are often free-standing and independent financially from, but may be affiliated with a health care facility or hospital, operated on a fee-for-service basis, and owned by a group of investors, some or all of whom may be radiologists

Note: Because of the wide profit margin and potential for proliferation of ICs as vehicles for profit, some states require that an IC obtain a 'Certificate of Need' prior to reimbursing the services provided

Imanishi-Kari affair Baltimore affair, see there

IMAO Inhibitor of monoamine oxidase, see MAOI

IMDD Idiopathic midline destructive disease, see there

IMG International medical graduate, see there

(familial) iminoglycinuria A benign AR [MIM 242600] condition characterized by defective tubular resorption and urinary spilling of proline, hydroxyproline and glycine; iminoglycinuria is a normal physiologic event that occurs in neonates, whose renal transport mechanisms are immature; iminoglycinuria may also occur in Fanconi syndrome and hyperprolinemia; see Hyperglyinuria

immediate cause of death '...the disease, injury, or complication that directly precedes death', which is the ultimate consequence of the underlying cause of death (Arch Pathol Lab Med 1995; 119:123OA); as an example, fulminant acute peritonitis is the immediate cause of death, which is the end result of a shotgun blast to the abdomen, the underlying (aka primary or proximate) cause of death; Cf Underlying cause of death

immediate early gene Any of a number of genes that are regulated by changes in intracellular Ca^{2+}; IEGs are rapidly induced, do not require the synthesis of new proteins for their transcription, and often encode transcription factors (eg c-Fos, c-Jun) that regulate subsequent waves of gene expression (Science 1995; 268:244) Cf Delayed response gene

immediate-spin crossmatch TRANSFUSION MEDICINE A test that is used as a final serologic check for incompatibility between a donor RBCs and the intended recipient's serum; the 'immediate spin' detects ABO incompatibility in nearly 100% of cases, but fails to detect IgG red cell alloantibodies; the efficiency of this test in detecting ABO incompatibility may be improved by delaying the 'reading' time and resuspending the RBCs in a saline-EDTA solution (Transfusion 1991; 31:197)

immersion foot An affliction of sailors who wear cold and damp rubber sea boots for extended periods; the cold induces peripheral vasoconstriction and ischemia which, when severe, may require amputation; Cf Trench foot

immersion oil An oil with a refractive index of 1.52 that allows high power (from 600x to 1800x) magnification for LM, of particular use in cytopathology, hematology and microbiology

Note: Examination of tissues 'under oil' is of limited use in histopathology, as most diagnoses are rendered between 40x and 400x magnifications

immobilized enzyme An enzyme that has been fixed by physical or chemical means to a solid support, eg a bead or gel to confine a reaction of interest to a particular site

'immortality' enzyme Telomerase, see there

immotile cilia syndrome Kartagener syndrome An uncommon (1:20 000) AR [MIM 242650, 244400] disease of childhood onset due to defective or afunctional cilia in the respiratory tract, resulting in chronic sinusitis, defective mucociliary transport and bronchial clearance, bronchiectasia, chronic otitis media and chronic, potentially incapacitating headaches, related to immotility of ependymal cilia in the walls of cerebral ventricles REPRODUCTION ♂ are infertile, ½ of ♀ are impregnatable, the other ½ sterile; ½ of cases have Kartagener's triad, ie chronic sinusitis, bronchiectasis and situs inversus totalis, the last of which is possibly due to an in utero defect with the cilia beating in the contrary direction EM Cilia lack dynein arms; the related Young syndrome is characterized by sinusitis, bronchiectasis and azoospermia, which may follow a fertile phase; other defects associated with immotile cilia include cardiovascular, renal and ocular defects, and absence of frontal sinuses; see Cilia

immune complex disease A condition caused by circulating antigen-antibody (immune) complexes, which in the face of mild antigen excess, lodge in small vessels and filtering organs of the circulation; ICs are involved in complement activation, phagocytosis, neutrophil, basophil and mast cell degranulation, platelet aggregation, humoral responses and activation of CD8 suppressor T-cells; ICD occurs if the immune system has had sufficient time to develop antibodies against an antigen and is then re-exposed to the antigen; 'immunocytes' with C3 or Fc receptors are attracted to the site of the immune response and attempt to eliminate the ICs; in ICD, size is critical: large ICs are insoluble and are rapidly cleared, small ICs circulate without eliciting a reaction, while intermediately sized ICs activate the complement cascade; immune complex-mediated conditions CLINICAL Fever, enlarged and tender joints, splenic congestion, proteinuria due to glomerular IC deposition, eosinophilia, hypocomplementemia, lymphadenopathy, glomerulonephritis (hypertension, oliguria, hematuria, edema), skin (purpura, urticaria, ulcers), carditis, hepatic inflammation, myositis, and necrotizing vasculitis ASSAYS THAT DETECT ICs C1q binding assay, solid phase C1q assay, Raji cell assay, conglutinin assay, staphylococcal protein assay, polyethylene precipitin assay; ICs appear in connective tissue disease and inflammation (SLE, periarteritis nodosa, mixed connective tissue disease, scleroderma, rheumatoid and juvenile rheumatoid arthritis, temporal arteritis, Behçet's, Reiter's, and Wegener's granulomatosis, Sjögren syndrome, ankylosing spondylitis, eosinophilic fasciitis), bacterial infections (*Neisseria meningococcus*, *N gonorrhoeae*, streptococcus, leprosy, syphilis, salmonellosis), viral infections (HBV, infectious mononucleosis, CMV, subacute sclerosing panencephalitis, dengue), malignancy (carcinoma, melanoma, neuroblastoma, lymphocytic leukemia, lymphoma), inflammation (inflammatory bowel disease, optic neuritis, idiopathic glomerulonephritis, interstitial pneumonitis), neurological conditions (multiple sclerosis, myasthenia gravis, Guillain-Barré disease) and others (bullous pemphigoid, DM, intestinal bypass, pemphigus, primary biliary cirrhosis, Henoch-Schönlein syndrome, sickle cell anemia, TTP)

immune thrombocytopenic purpura   Idiopathic thrombocytopenic purpura, see there

immune tolerance   Immune paralysis, self tolerance The immunologic nonreactivity to specific, usually 'self' antigens in an otherwise immunocompetent organism; IT is an active process by which limits are placed on the responsiveness of lymphocytes to self antigens, through multiple complementary pathways and feedback loops; since autoantibody formation is a common event, the loss of self-tolerance is best considered quantitative; T-cell tolerance is more rapid (inducible in 1 day vs. 10 days for B cells), occurs at lower doses of immunogen (1/100th as much as for B cells) and lasts longer (150 days vs. 50-60 days for B cells); natural tolerance to self antigens is related to suppression of T helper cell activity that may be mediated by T suppressor cells and it is thought that the continued presence of these antigens is necessary for maintaining the tolerant state; B-cell tolerance occurs by several mechanisms

1) Immature B cells at very low doses of antigen are highly susceptible to tolerization, with subsequent clonal 'abortion' (in contrast, T-cell tolerance is not maturation-dependent)

2) Clonal exhaustion All B cells capable of responding to an immunogen are stimulated into cell maturation and short-lived antibody production, 'exhausting' or functionally deleting that portion of the B cell repertoire, seen in T-independent antigens

3) Antibody-forming cell blockade A short-lived form of B-cell intolerance in which antibody-bearing cells are profusely covered with antigens, such that the cell is incapable of response

---

IMMUNE COMPLEX-MEDIATED CONDITIONS

ARTHUS REACTION Acute hemorrhagic necrosis that follows re-exposure to an antigen, which attracts PMNs, activates complement, binds ICs by the Fc receptor, causing phagocytosis, ↑ production of chemotactic factors, especially C5b67 and ↑ anaphylotoxins C3a and C5a, resulting in vasodilation

SERUM SICKNESS A reaction that is milder than the Arthus reaction, occurring 8-12 days after exposure to the antigen, at the time of 'equivalence' (antigen and antibody are in a 1:1 ratio), after injection of a foreign protein mixture, eg horse serum for antitoxin to tetanus

---

immunoadsorbent   Any material, eg a gel or inert solid used to adsorb or purify antibodies from a solution

immunoassay   LABORATORY MEDICINE Any assay that measures an antigen-antibody response, the sensitivity of which varies according to the method; the least sensitive method is immunoelectrophoresis which can detect antigen levels of 5-10 000 ng/ml, agglutination 1-10 000 ng/ml, single agar diffusion 1-10 000 ng/ml, double agar diffusion and nephelometry < 1000 ng/ml, enzyme immunoassay 1-10 ng/ml, complement fixation 5 ng/ml, immunofluorescence, ELISA and RIA, which are sensitive to < .001 ng/ml

immunoaugmentive therapy   An unproven method of cancer therapy being administered in clinics in the Bahamas, Mexico and Germany ; there is little scientific evidence of efficacy nor safety of IAT, an expensive ($50 000) therapy that entails parenteral administration of tumor cell lysates and serum from both cancer patients and normal subjects; the putative active agents include 'blocking' and 'deblocking proteins', tumor antibody and 'complement' (which is not complement as understood by immunologists); independent analysis of some of the sera used in IAT were found to be contaminated with various organisms; see Unproven methods of cancer treatment

immunoblast   Lymphoblast A transformed B or T cell (lymphocyte) that may differentiate into a plasma cell or a committed T cell

immunoblastic lymphadenopathy   Angioimmunoblastic lymphadenopathy, see there

immunoblastic sarcoma   A lymphoma composed of cells with features of immunoblasts (transformed lymphocytes) that is subdivided into B-CELL IMMUNOBLASTIC SARCOMA Malignant lymphoma, large cell, immunoblastic plasmacytoid type The predominant cell is immunoblast-like, mixed with Reed-Sternberg-like and plasmacytoid cells; it is the most common lymphoma arising in a background of natural immunodeficiency, immunosuppression and immunoproliferative states, eg angioimmunoblastic lymphadenopathy and other diseases of the immune system, including Hashimoto's thyroiditis, Sjögren syndrome, α-chain disease and SLE PROGNOSIS Poor; 14-month median survival T-CELL IMMUNOBLASTIC SARCOMA Malignant lymphoma, large cell, immunoblastic clear cell type Less common than the B-cell immunoblastic lymphoma, characterized by cells with a 'water-clear' cytoplasm, round-to-oval nuclei, fine chromatin, 1-3 nucleoli, nuclear folding, lobulation and occasional multinucleation, interspersed with benign histiocytes, plasma cells, delicate fibrous bands; this lymphoma may arise in a background of mycosis fungoides, with generalized lymphadenopathy and polyclonal hypergammaglobulinemia

immunoblot   see Western blot

immunochemistry   The field that studies the complex properties of immune molecules, attempting to resolve the sites that are active in immune responses, formulate the rules that limit antigen and antibody reactions and ultimately, to design newer structures, including catalytic antibodies and other biological catalysts (Science 1991; 252:659)

immunocompromised   Referring or pertaining to a state of impaired or decreased immune responsiveness, which may occur in a background of congenital immunodeficiencies, infection (eg HIV, TB), or following chemotherapy

immunocyte adherence   see Rosetting

immunocytochemistry   The application of immune reactions in analyzing the presence of antigens or antibodies in cells (immunocytochemistry) or tissues (**immunohistochemistry**); IC reactions are based in essence on the 'sandwich' method delineated by Becker and Wilchek (Biophys Acta 1972; 264:165); the system relies on the covalent binding of biotin to biologically active molecules and the high affinity that avidin (or alternatively, streptavidin) has for biotin; the antigens of interest are detected by linking the last antibody in the sandwich to either a fluorescent molecule or to an enzyme, bathing the tissues in the final step with an enzyme-linked chromogen (**Lab Med 1994; 25:502**); see Avidin-biotinylated complex method

immunodeficiency A generic term for any partial or complete defect in the immune reaction **Acquired immunodeficiency** A generalized reduction in the immune response to antigenic stimuli due to a wide variety of conditions including aging, AIDS, Alzheimer's disease, amyotrophic lateral sclerosis, burns, chemotherapy, coeliac disease, corticosteroids, depression and psychologic stress, inflammatory bowel disease, leprosy, NSAIDs, radiation, sarcoidosis, sepsis, hematological and lymphoproliferative disease (Hodgkin's disease, NHL, leukemia, myeloma, Waldenström's macroglobulinemia, aplastic and agranulocytic anemias, sickle cell disease), systemic disease (malnutrition, chronic diarrhea, fulminant mycosis, sepsis, terminal cancer, DM, uremia, and nephrotic syndrome), splenectomy, surgery and trauma **Congenital immunodeficiency** A heterogeneous group of relatively uncommon diseases, that are often accompanied by autoimmune disease, allergy, increased incidence of malignancy, GI abnormalities **Incidence** IgA deficiency 1:500, agammaglobulinemia 1:50 000, severe combined immunodeficiency 1:100 000, see Adenosine deaminase, Combined variable immunodeficiency, Purine nucleoside phosphorylase deficiency, Severe combined immune deficiency

---

CONGENITAL IMMUNE DEFICIENCIES
DEFECTIVE CELL TYPE
STEM CELL Reticular dysgenesis, severe combined immunodeficiency with thymic dysplasia or adenosine deaminiase deficiency, Swiss type, common variable immunodeficiency (CVID) associated with ectodermal dysplasia and dwarfism, X-linked agammaglobulinemia
B-CELL DEFECTS, comprising 50% of congenital immunodeficiencies, including Bruton's disease or other forms of congenital hypogammaglobulinemia variably associated with thymoma, CVID, X-linked hyper-IgM syndrome
T-CELL DEFECTS, comprising 10% of congenital immunodeficiencies, including Nezeloff's disease (thymic hypoplasia), DiGeorge syndrome, nucleoside phosphorylase deficiency, chronic mucocutaneous candidiasis
COMPLEX IMMUNODEFICIENCIES with combined B- and T-cell defects, comprising 30% of congenital immunodeficiencies, including Wiskott-Aldrich syndrome, cartilage-hair hypoplasia, ataxia-telangiectasia, hyper-IgE syndrome
DISORDERS OF MOLECULAR SYSTEMS AND NON-SPECIFIC IMMUNE CELLS
PHAGOCYTIC DEFECTS (6% of total)
    1) Leukocyte disorders, eg neutropenia, Chediak-Higashi, lazy leukocyte syndrome, hyper-IgE syndrome
    2) Defective bactericidal activity, eg chronic granulomatous disease (combined neutrophil and macrophage defect), myeloperoxidase deficiency, Chediak-Higashi disease (neutrophils and macrophages with defective lysosomes, chemotactic defects, defective bactericidal activity) and glucose 6-phosphate dehydrogenase deficiency
COMPLEMENT DEFECTS (4% of total) Defects of the 'early' complement proteins are associated with autoimmune disease, especially SLE; 'late' complement proteins are associated with recurrent infections, especially by *Neisseria* species; complement protein defects may be combined with other immune defects, including
    1) Chemotactic defects
    2) Complement defects, eg C1r, C2, C3, C5 combined with B- and T-cell disorders, including Wiskott-Aldrich disease, chronic mucocutaneous candidiasis, opsonization defects, sickle cell disease, defects in purine metabolism defects

---

immunodiffusion assay A technique for detecting either an antigen or antibody; a serum or fluid presumed to contain the molecule of interest is placed in well A cut in a slab of agar gel; a standardized antigen or antibody is placed in well B; if there is an affinity between the antigen and antibody, precipitation occurs as the two diffuse toward each other; see Radial immune diffusion, Rocket electrophoresis

immune electron microscopy A technique that uses ferritin-labeled antibodies to study the ultrastructure of various intracellular organelles

immunofixation electrophoresis A type of electrophoresis that follows gel electrophoresis, in which the gel is overlaid with monospecific antisera and the precipitation reaction appears at a characteristic site, producing a sharper image than that obtained by simple immunoelectrophoresis; IFE is used for detecting monoclonal light chains or small monoclonal peaks in the face of a polyclonal expansion, which may be otherwise undetectable due to an 'umbrella' effect, detection of immune complexes, borderline Bence-Jones proteinuria, transferrin bands, specific immunoglobulins (measles, rubella, mumps, herpes simplex), separating very close biclonal populations, phenotyping α-1-antitrypsin

immunofluorescence LABORATORY MEDICINE A method in which a fluorochrome dye (eg FITC-fluorescein isothiocyanate, or rhodamine) is linked to a critical participant (ie an antigen or antibody) in an immune reaction; if the component of interest is present, the fluorochrome dye will remain in the reaction milieu, 'tagging' said participant for qualitative (eg immunofluorescence microscopy) or quantitative (eg by flow cytometry) evaluation

immunofluorescence microscopy A technique in which tissues and cells are examined by a fluorescent light microscope to detect the presence or deposition of immunoglobulins, complement and other immune mediators; in direct immunofluorescence, an anti-human antibody, with a fluorescent tag, eg fluoresceinated isothiocyanate (FITC) is incubated directly with an antigen of interest; in the more sensitive indirect method, unlabeled anti-human antibody is first incubated with the antigen, then incubated with an antibody that has a fluorescent tag allowing 'amplification' of the signal; IM is used to study immune deposits in Berger's and Goodpasture's diseases and hemolytic uremic syndrome and to study the epidermal-dermal junction in bullous pemphigoid, pemphigus vulgaris, and dermatitis herpetiformis; standardized tissues may be overlaid with the serum of patients suspected of having circulating autoantibodies, allowing classification of connective tissue diseases; see Antinuclear antibodies; Cf Microscopy

immunogen Antigen

immunogenicity Antigenicity The degree to which a molecule (usually a protein) is capable of evoking an immune response and producing a specific antibody; immunogenicity is influenced by certain characteristics of the antigen itself; other factors affecting immunogenicity include the host's capability for producing antibodies and the manner of antigen presentation, eg a high-dose may overload the system and prevent an immune response; see Immune tolerance

In the working parlance, the molecule itself is termed an antigen, while the process or ability to evoke an immune respone is generally referred to as immunogenicity

immunoglobulin A highly-specific molecule of the immune system produced by mature B cells in response to an antigen; an Ig is composed of two identical light and two identical heavy chains; the light and heavy chains have constant and variable regions, the latter of which which are critical for the recognition of the antigen to which they are capable of binding; the production of an immunoglobulin (Ig) requires previous rearrangement of the variable, diversity and joining gene segments that form part of the enormous potential repertoire of 10^{10}-10^{12} antibody molecules that may be encoded in response to a molecule's surface binding site or epitope; Igs are defined as idiotypes, which are Igs that have been evoked by a particular epitope, isotypes, which are Ig subtypes (IgG, IgA, IgM, IgD, IgE) that all normal individuals have, and allotypes, which are subtypes that are shared by population groups, eg with racial differences; see Hinge

immunoglobulin A deficiency see IgA deficiency

immunoglobulin M deficiency see IgM deficiency

immunoglobulin-like domain MOLECULAR BIOLOGY A structural motif in certain β-sheet-rich proteins that is 100-amino acid residues in length, has intrachain disulfide bonds, associates in pairs by non-covalent bonds, which is present in immunoglobulins, IL-1, IL-6, platelet-derived growth factor and T cell receptor

immunohematology Transfusion medicine, see there

immunohistochemistry see Immunocytochemistry

immunoisolation CLINICAL THERAPEUTICS A generic term for the isolation of a transplanted cell or substance from the host's immune system, usually by enclosing within a semipermeable nonimmunogenic sheath or capsule; immunoisolation is a means of introducing non-self cells or tissues, eg insulin-producing pancreatic islet cells that are capable of responding to small MW stimuli (eg glucose) but which remain isolated (ie protected) from the host immune system; see Biohybrid artificial pancreas, Islet cell transplantation (Science & Medicine July/August 1995, p16); Cf Liposome

immunologic tolerance Immune tolerance, see there

immunomodulation Immunotherapy Manipulation of the immune system with either 1) Non-specific biological response modifiers, including natural molecules, eg lymphokines or synthesized hybrid molecules ('magic bullets'), eg anti-CD5-ricin or 2) Specific molecules that have been generated against a patient's self cells

immunonephelometry LABORATORY MEDICINE A diagnostic modality that detects relatively small antigen-antibody aggregates in a solution by measuring the light scattered at a 90° angle to the light source (a laser, although optional, increases sensitivity), and measured by a spectrophotometer at 340-360 nm; in contrast, turbidimetry detects large clumps and particles in a system based on a drop in light from a direct beam of light, ie by 'forward angle light scatter'

immunopathology 1) The discipline that studies the relationship of immune reactions to the pathogenesis, diagnosis, and treatment of disease 2) A generic term for any defect or lesion induced by the immune system

---

IMMUNOGENICITY (ANTIGENICITY)-REQUIREMENTS

FOREIGN Non-self

LARGE Minimum size 1 kD; most antigens are > 10 kD

CHEMICALLY COMPLEX The more twisted and complex the surface of the antigen, the more immunogenic, eg amino acid homopolymers elicit no antibody, in contrast to heteropolymers of three or more amino acids do

CHEMISTRY OF AMINO ACIDS Aromatic side chains increase antigenicity, where the degree is proportional to the protein's tyrosine

---

immunoperoxidase method LABORATORY MEDICINE A technique that detects antigens in tissue sections by a series (see below) of incubations; see Avidin-biotinylated complex, PAP, Sandwich method

1) A tissue section is bathed with a monoclonal antibody (of mouse origin) solution, followed by a wash step to remove unbound monoclonal antibody

2) The tissue incubated with an anti-mouse antibody which has an attached peroxidase enzyme, followed by another wash step and finally

3) The tissue is incubated (bathed) with an uncolored substrate; if the monoclonal antibody is bound in the first step, the substrate is digested by the peroxidase and a red-brown color develops that may be viewed by light microscopy

immunophilins Cytoplasmic receptor proteins that bind with high affinity to immunosuppressants, including cyclosporin A, tacrolimus (formerly FK 506) and rapamycin and inhibit rotamase activity, inhibiting the interconversion between the cis- and trans-rotamers of the peptidyl-prolylamide bond of peptide and protein substrates; immunosuppressants are thought to act by inhibiting the T cell receptor-mediated signal transduction pathway, preventing the activation of the nuclear factor of activated T cells; immunophilins thus far identified include cyclophilin and FK 506-binding protein (Science 1991; 251:283, Nature 1991; 351:248) see Cyclophilin, FKBP

immunoradiometric assay see IRMA

immunosuppression The suppression or inhibition of the immune response, which be either unintentional and due to concurrent disease (eg AIDS, herpes infection) or exposure to exogenous agents (antimetabolites, radiotherapy), or active, as in immunosuppressive therapy (eg with cyclosporin)

immunosuppressive therapy The use of pharmacologic agents to suppress the immune response, eg to ameliorate allograft rejection; the most effective techniques include destruction of immunocompetent cells prior to transplantation and inhibition of lymphocyte differentiation and proliferation; agents that impair proliferation include antimetabolites, alkylating agents, toxic antibiotics, and ionizing radiation; once begun, rejection phenomena are difficult to reign in

immunotherapy ALLERGY MEDICINE Hyposensitization therapy A treatment modality in which an allergen, eg hymenopteran venom, is administered in increasing doses to subjects with potentially fatal hypersensitivity reactions to the allergen; immunotherapy attempts to elicit production of blocking IgG antibodies, interfering with antigen-Fab (a portion of an Ig molecule) combination, preventing fixation of IgE ('l'enfant terrible' of anaphylaxis), thereby attenuating or eliminating anaphylactic reactions; immunotherapy is of little use if the insect-sting reactions are confined to the skin ONCOLOGY A therapeutic modality that attempts to non-specifically stimulate the immune system to destroy malignant cells; immunotherapies with anecdotal success in treating malignancy include BCG immunotherapy*, which may be effective in treating melanomas, AML, and solid tumors, Coley's toxin and heat-killed formalin-treated *Corynebacterium parvum*, an immunopotentiator and immunomodulator in animals that evokes reticuloendothelial hyperplasia, stimulation of macrophages and B cells and which may enhance T-cell function by increasing its blastogenic response to T-cell mitogens (concanavalin A, PHA and pokeweed mitogen); see BCG, Coley's toxin, Malariotherapy

*BCG is of use in urology for controlling superfical transitional cell carcinomas by instillation in the bladder

immunotoxin A conjugate of a cell-reactive antibody and a toxin or subunit of a toxin; first generation ITs are those in which the antibody is coupled via a cross-linker SPDP (*N*-succinimidyl-3-(2-pyridydithio)propionate) to the A chain of ricin; second-generation ITs are designed to arrive to their target, eg by being smaller using F(ab') fragments; third-generation ITs will be developed using recombinant DNA technology; their use as therapeutic agents for treating malignancy is still on the horizon, and requires further work in basic science, but may be viewed as having potential for synergistic activity with other treatment modalities

Note: ITs are one of the 'magic bullets' envisioned by Paul Ehrlich, which may be designed to be tumor-specific, where a monoclonal antibody or portion thereof is attached to various toxic molecules, including radioactive isotopes, chemotherapeutic agents, bacterial or plant toxins, produced with the hope that these 'bullets' will concentrate in the malignant tumor, destroying it; recombinant DNA techniques allow creation of highly specific hybrid molecules with therapeutic potential, although the immunotoxins thus far created in the laboratory have encountered in vivo difficulties, including accessibility of the immunotoxin to the tumor, instability of the cross-linking protein, rapid metabolism and development of anti-immunotoxin antibodies

immunotyping Immunophenotyping HEMATOPATHOLOGY A method for identifying cell surface or cytoplasmic antigens; the information derived allows determination of clonality and classification of B- or T-cell lineage; immunotyping of chronic lymphocytosis (145 cases) revealed that the majority are malignant and of B-cell origin, lymphocytosis (121 B-CLL, 11 lymphosarcoma), T-cell lymphocytosis (5 cases, 4 indolent), hairy cell leukemia (2), reactive lymphocytosis (6); see CD (cluster of differentiation)

IMP 1) Immunoperoxidase 2) Inosine monophosphate

Also 1) Impulse generator 2) Incomplete male pseudohermaphroditism 3) Integral membrane protein 4) Intermembranous particle 5) Ion moderated partition

impaired Acting under a handicap, see Impairment

impaired health care provider A physician or health care worker whose ability to function in his usual role has been reduced or otherwise compromised by various internal and external forces; see Impairment; Cf 'Handicapped' health care provider, 'Incapacitated' health care provider

impairment A generic term for a handicap, partial disability, loss of function, or functional defect; although 'impairment' implies any physical or mental reduction in capacity (to provide medical care), the term is often used in a pejorative sense, and in some circles, is a euphemism for substance (addictive drugs, alcohol) abuse or acute psychiatric decompensation, both of which potentially place patients at ↑ risk of poor judgement by the care-giver

impedance plethysmography CARDIOVASCULAR DISEASE A noninvasive method that measures the changes in electrical resistance between two probes, which indicates the changes in the volume of different regions of the body, as may be seen in obstruction to venous outflow; IP was the most widely method for the diagnosis of deep vein thrombosis, but has been superseded by B-mode ultrasonography; the positive predictive value (PPV) of an abnormal IP for the presence of deep vein thrombosis is 83%; the PPV for an abnormal compression ultrasonography is 94% (**N Engl J Med 1993; 329:1365OA**)

Imperial Cancer Research Fund A London-based charity that is Europe's largest independent cancer research organization, which employs 1500 staff including researchers, physicians and technicians, funding one-third of all cancer research in the United Kingdom, often working in conjunction with the British Medical Research Council; the income is generated by charity shops, stocks, assets and legacies (estates); ICRF supports basic research (⅔ of budget) and clinical research (⅓ of budget); Cf Howard Hughes Medical Institute

impertinent *adjective* Not pertinent

impingement syndrome A clinical complex caused by the limitation of a space between bones and fascia, compromising the flow of blood and irritating the nerves passing through the space; common impingement syndromes include the carpal tunnel syndrome which affects middle-aged women and that of the shoulders in which the space beneath the coraco-acromial arch for the supraspinatus and biceps tendons is reduced, resulting in a painful arc of movement and paresthesias, common in competitive swimmers MECHANISM Ischemia or osteophyte rubbing the acromium

Although *impingement* implies a lesser degree of neurovascular compromise than *entrapment*, the distinction is both subjective and arbitrary, and thus of little use; it would seem appropriate to delete the former-Author's note

implant DENTISTRY A synthetic device constructed of titanium (eg Brånemark system, Nobelpharma) that is surgically placed in the mandible or maxilla, allowed to 'fuse' (which occurs in 3 to 6 months) to the bone (osseointegration), and then serve as an anchoring point for attaching artificial teeth SURGERY *Noun* Any device that is inserted to preserve or maintain a function, eg a hip or knee prosthesis, or to preserve, enhance or alter a contour, eg a breast or chin implant *Verb* To surgically place such a device in its appropriate site SURGICAL PATHOLOGY A term* for a cluster of epithelial cells seen in the peritoneal cavity in patients with epithelial neoplasms of the ovary that are of either 'borderline' (ie of uncertain malignant potential) or frankly malignant (eg serous, mucinous cystadenocarcinoma) (**Am J Surg Pathol 1994; 18:863OA**)

*The term is semantically problematic as it implies implantation of a primary lesion elsewhere in the peritoneal cavity, usually of the ovary, and ignores the possible origin of such implants from 'renegade' embryonic rests in the peritoneal cavity, and/or a multicentric origin of the lesions

implantable hearing aid ENT A device used to correct hearing loss in as 'physiologic' a manner as possible*; IHAs are believed to improve sound fidelity in individuals with moderate to severe sensorineural hearing loss; the mechanism for signal amplification per se can be either electromagnetic or piezoelectric

*± 20 million (US) are afflicted with hearing loss of a sufficient degree to require an acoustic amplifying device, ie a hearing aid, and in most cases, a conventional device will suffice

implantation recurrence SURGICAL ONCOLOGY A rare phenomenon occurring at the site of a surgical resection for malignancy, where tumor cells, often of epithelial origin, 'spill' from an operative field or are carried by needles or stapling devices, 'seeding' malignancy into previously uninvolved sites; these lesions often appear anecdotally, as recently reported in a patient who had a laparoscopic cholecystectomy and, apparently, implantation seeding in the skin through which the gall bladder (subsequently shown to have adenocarcinoma) was removed (**N Engl J Med 1991; 325:1316c**)

import CELL PHYSIOLOGY *Noun* A product that has been transported into a cell *Verb* To transport a (required) substance into a cell

impotence The inability to achieve or maintain a penile erection adequate for the successful completion of intercourse, terminating in ejaculation; for an erection to achieve a successful outcome, it requires 1) An intact CNS, ie without underlying medical or psychological disease, or central-acting drugs, intact sympathetic and parasympathetic circuitry, ie without spinal trauma or degenerative disease 2) An intact vascular supply to the penis and 3) An intact, anatomically correct penis; 25% of impotence may be psychological or 'partner-specific', 25% has an organic component and 50% of impotence is organic in nature; in organic impotence, nocturnal penile tumescence is not present TREATMENT Microvascular surgery to bypass occluded vessels (most effective in younger men), penile prosthesis and combined therapy with phentolamine and papaverine (self-injected by the patient, wielding an erection of one hour's duration SIDE EFFECTS Priapism, penile plaques or Peyronie's disease) Note: Drugs associated with impotence include antihypertensives, eg methyldopa, guanethidine, reserpine, clonidine, due to decreased blood pressure, antidepressants, eg phenelzine, isocarboxazide, amitriptyline (causing altered moods and decreased libido), tranquilizers, eg chlordiazepoxide and lorazepam and the muscle-relaxing diazepam, cimetidine, which increases prolactin levels, and is associated with impotence and loss of libido

imprinting Genomic imprinting MOLECULAR BIOLOGY The variable phenotypic expression of a gene depending on whether it is of paternal or maternal origin, which is a function of the methylation pattern; imprinted regions are more methylated and less transcriptionally active; the 'imprints' are erased and generated in early embryonic development of mammals; imprinted genes include those for insulin-like growth factor-2 and its receptor, fragile X syndrome, Prader-Willi syndrome, Angelman (happy puppet) syndrome and Wilms' tumors (Science 1991; 252:1250n&v) PSYCHOLOGY Imprinting A form of learning restricted to certain critical or sensitive time periods of life, and which stops when definitive learning occurs or when a critical phase has passed; imprinting may occur before the organism is capable of an appropriate response, is irreversible and is characteristic of the species of organisms being imprinted

IMViC reactions MICROBIOLOGY A mnemonic for the classic 'bench' tests (table), including indole production (I), methyl red production (M), Voges-Proskauer (V) and citrate utilization (C) that are used to differentiate among the major genuses of *Enterobacteriaceae*

IMViC Reaction	I	M	V	C
Arizona spp	-	+	-	+
Edwardsiella spp	+	+	-	-
Enterobacter spp	-	-	+	+
Escherichia coli	+	+	-	-
Klebsiella spp	-	(+)	+	+
Proteus spp	-	+	-	(v)
Providentia spp	+	+	-	+
Salmonella spp	-	+	-	(+)
Shigella spp	(-)	+	-	-
Yersinia spp	(-)	+	(-)	-

IN Intraepithelial neoplasia, see these

in denial see Denial

in house Within the confines of a campus, complex of buildings, health care center, hospital, or other institution; a common usage of the term would be that test is performed 'in house', ie not referred to an independent laboratory

inaccuracy LABORATORY MEDICINE Bias The numerical difference between the mean of a set of repeated measurements and the true value of the analyte; in general inaccuracy is evaluated by comparing a reference method of known accuracy with a new method, usually using a specified number (eg 40) of patient samples (Arch Pathol Lab Med 1992; 116:714oA)

inactivated vaccine Killed vaccine, see there

inactive ingredient Additive, Excipient CLINICAL PHARMACOLOGY Any substance that is regarded by the US Food and Drug Administration as having no effect on a drug's absorption or metabolism, which is added for the manufacturer's expediency; these 'inert' ingredients are added to either 1) Impart satisfactory processing and compression characteristics to the drug formulation, including binders, diluents, glidents or lubricants or 2) Confer desirable physical characteristics to the finished product, including disintegrants, colorants, flavors and sweetening agents; Cf GRAS substances

INAD Investigational new animal drug A therapeutic modality with potential for use in food animals that is under an FDA protocol prior to being approved; see Bovine growth hormone; Cf IND

inadequate care of the elderly 1) Elderly abuse 2) Elderly neglect

INAH3 A region in the anterior hypothalamus is reported to be two-fold greater in the male heterosexual than in the male homosexual brain, and has been held as a part of the 'biological' (versus the environmental) explanation of male homosexuality (Scientific American 1994; 270/5:44)

inappropriate HEALTH CARE An adjective with considerable weight in the clinical practice of medicine, as various parties (insurance companies, peer review organization, hospital administrations, malpractice lawyers) have an interest in both defining the inappropriateness of a diagnostic or therapeutic procedure, and ensuring that inappropriate care or tests are not performed; one analyst, RH Brook stated *'If one could extrapolate from the available literature, then perhaps ¼ of hospital days, ¼ of procedures, and ⅖ of medications could be done without.'* (JAMA 1989; 262:3027)* see Appropriateness, Practice guidelines

*If this estimate is accurate, the US health care budget could be trimmed by $100 billion without public harm-Author's note

inappropriate care According to the RAND corporation is defined as *'...that for which the expected risks or negative effects significantly exceed the expected benefits for the average patient with a specific clinical scenario.'* (JAMA 1993; 269:1503L)

inborn error of metabolism A term coined in 1908 by A Garrod based on his studies of alkaptonuria, in which he anticipated the one-gene, one-enzyme concept; inborn errors of metabolism are an ever-expanding group of inherited metabolic and biochemical disorders, numbering in the hundreds that may be loosely divided into those affecting 1) Small molecules, including simple sugars, amino or organic acids that often have an acute onset in infancy and early childhood and 2) Large molecules, most commonly ↑ in 'storage diseases', eg mucopolysaccharidoses and glycogen storage diseases that usually affect older children

INBORN ERRORS OF METABOLISM (CONSEQUENCES)

LOSS OF CERTAIN MOLECULES, eg albinism (defect of tyrosinase) or Ehlers-Danlos disease (defect of lysyl-hydroxylase) or others of a vast array of enzymes

ACCUMULATION OF NORMAL METABOLITES, eg alkaptonuria (defect of homogentisic acid oxidase) or galactosemia (defect of Galactose-1-phosphate uridyl transferase)

TRANSPORT DEFECTS, eg cystinuria (dibasic amino acids) or intestinal disaccharidase deficiency

DEFECTS IN ERYTHROCYTE METABOLISM, eg glucose-6-phosphate dehydrogenase deficiency NEW PIGMENT DEFECTS, eg acute intermittent porphyria

DEFECTS IN MINERAL METABOLISM, eg Wilson's disease

VITAMIN DEFECTS, eg vitamin D-dependent rickets

DEFECTS IN INTESTINAL ABSORPTION, eg cystic fibrosis

OTHER DEFECTS OF UNKNOWN ORIGIN, eg achondroplasia

inbred strain MOLECULAR BIOLOGY A set of organisms, eg mice that is produced by 20 or more backcrosses or intercrosses to the parents or brother **x** sister, which can be traced back to a single ancestral pair in the 20th or consecutive generation; inbred animals are virtually homogeneous, and thus provides a consistent genotype for analysis (from Science 1994; 264:1725) Cf Congenic strain

inbreeding GENETICS A process in which littermates or siblings are mated to each other over multiple generations, resulting in a strain of animals that is virtually identical genotypically; highly inbred animal lines allow the study of certain traits in a relatively pure form; see Bottlenecks, Consanguinity; Cf Hybrid vigor

'incapacitated' health care provider A physician or health care worker who is acutely impaired in his ability to provide care either for physical or mental reasons; Cf

'Handicapped' health care provider, 'Impaired' health care provider

incarcerated hernia The herniation of a tissue, classically a loop of intestine, into a mesothelial sac, that cannot return to its original position without surgery; Cf Strangulated hernia

incarceration PUBLIC HEALTH The imprisonment or detention of a person for crimes committed or allegedly committed; rates/10⁶ population: Russia 558; US 519, South Africa 368, Singapore 229; Canada 116, Germany 80; Japan 36; India 23 (**US News & World Report 19 September 1994:17**) Cf Capital punishment

incidence PUBLIC HEALTH The number of new cases of a disease that occur in a population divided by a unit of time, usually a year; Cf Prevalence

'incident' HOSPITAL CARE ADMINISTRATION An event that represents a marked negative deviation from the 'standard of care' that occurs in a health care facility; if the incident is regarded as serious and has potential for harming a patient, an 'incident report' is generated and put in the responsible party's employment record for possible disciplinary action or dismissal; incidents include major substitution of medications or leaving a patient unattended for a prolonged period of time; Cf Misadventure

'incidentaloma' An incidentally discovered tumor mass, detected by computed tomography, magnetic resonance imaging or other modality performed for an unrelated reason; the 'classic' incidentaloma is a sellar mass that may be accompanied by visual disturbances and altered pituitary hormone secretion; most subjects with incidentalomas remain asymptomatic, some may have a pituitary adenoma or chemodectoma (**JAMA 1990; 263:2772**) see Pathologist's tumor; Cf Ulysses syndrome

incident report see Incident

incinerator ENVIRONMENT An enclosed device using controlled flame combustion to thermally break down radioactive, biohazardous, or other waste to ash residues with little or no combustible material; see Medical waste incinerator

inclusion body HISTOPATHOLOGY A generic term for any circumscribed mass of foreign (eg metal–lead or mercury or viral particles–herpes or CMV) or metabolically inactive materials (eg ceroid or Mallory bodies), within a cell's cytoplasm or nucleus

inclusion body myositis A type of idiopathic myositis that is not autoimmune and does not respond to immunosuppressive therapy, which is a clinical diagnosis of exclusion, confirmed by characteristic histological features CLINICAL Slowly progressive disease of middle-aged ♂, beginning in the legs, causing atrophy and weakness of the quadriceps, while sparing the facial and oropharyngeal muscles EMG Abnormal electrical 'irritation', slowing of nerve conduction and ↑ wave amplitude PATHOLOGY Rimmed vacuoles within fibers, occasional eosinophilic intranuclear and intracytoplasmic inclusions, scattered atrophic fibers, endomysial inflammation composed of cytotoxic T lymphocytes EM Myelinoid inclusions and virus-like particles (**N Engl J Med 1991; 325:1487rv**)

incompetence A generic term for the inability to perform a task or function, which in medicine can be defined in terms of CLINICAL MEDICINE Organ dysfunction; the use of incompetent is this context is waning in popularity, and being replaced by insufficiency, as in cardiovascular, hepatic, renal, or other insufficiency; notable exceptions include incompetence (competence) of valves, eg cardiac or ileocecal FORENSIC MEDICINE/MALPRACTICE Inability of a health care professional to perform his/her duties; while in the spoken parlance, a physician may be referred to incompetent, the 'politically correct' adjective impaired is

increasingly PSYCHIATRY Inability (of a patient) to enter into legally binding contractural arrangements (ie inability to appropriately exercise free will), as may occur in a person with Alzheimer's disease; incompetence is thus defined within a legal framework, and requires that the person be formally declared incompetent to make his/her own decisions, and that a surrogate decision-maker be appointed as the person's 'advocate'

incompetent A generic adjective referring to the inability (incompetence) to perform a task or function, see Incompetence

incomplete abortion Partial expulsion of fetus and placenta with pain and bleeding, which is potentially fatal for the mother, and treated with curettage

inconclusive data Results from the study of a phenomenon that fall far below that required for statistical significance, eg p > 0.05; alternately, data from multiple studies that consistently reach opposite conclusions of low statistical power; see Data

(population) increment-decrement life tables EPIDEMIOLOGY A life table that integrates opposing time-dependent trends in the size of a cohort; an IDLT is a device developed by demographers to analyze '…population-mobility phenomena, eg migration among regions and changes of marital status (single, married, divorced, widowed, etc) during a lifetime. For these phenomena, complete census data, vital-statistics data, or both usually provide stable age-specific estimates of movement rates or the probability of transition from one category to another. When only sample data is available, as in the estimation of working status life tables, the observed age-specific estimates of rates or transition probabilities are less stable, so that considerable graduation ('smoothing') by means of moving averages or related techniques is required for the application of population-based life-table procedures.' (**N Engl J Med 1993; 329:1100A**)

incremental risk Any potential risk associated with participation in a research protocol relative to the natural consequences of the medical condition, or any potential risk associated with receiving an experimental intervention relative to receiving the standard treatment for the medical condition' (**JAMA 1995; 273:1283**)

incretins A family of insulinotropic substance originating in the GI tract that is released into the circulation by oral glucose, the most well-studied of which is glucose-dependent insulinotropic polypeptide; others include glucagon-like insulinotropic peptide (GLIP), and glucagon-like peptide (GLP-1) (**N Engl J Med 1992; 326:1352sB**); incretins are secreted in response to oral but not parenteral administration of nutrients (taking their signals directly from the GI lumen) gastrin-inhibiting polypeptide (GIP) is the most potent of the incretins; others include gastrin, peptide histidine methionine (PHM), YY peptide and neurotensin, each of which have lesser incretin activity

IND Investigational new drug CLINICAL PHARMACOLOGY A status assigned to a drug by the US Food and Drug Administration (FDA) prior to its study in humans; the first step in this long (up to ten years in duration) process of bringing a drug to the marketplace is 'sponsored' (ie sponsored by a pharmaceutical firm or other interested party) submission of an **IND APPLICATION**, which allows only the 'sponsor' and investigators named in the application to study the drug; without a sponsor, clinical investigation cannot be carried out, since the FDA does not itself investigate new drugs* **COMMERCIAL IND** status allows a drug's sponsor to collect data on its clinical safety and effectiveness, which is required for a new drug application (NDA), permitting a drug to be marketed for specific uses **NONCOMMERCIAL IND** status allows a sponsor to use a drug in research or in early clinical investigation; the **IND**

REWRITE (1987) clearly delineated the phases of clinical trials for an IND and addressed the study's design prior to performing the clinical phases required for an NDA; see Phase 1, 2, 3 studies

*Final approval of an IND requires reviews of earlier animal, and then preclinical studies, in addition to proof of safety and efficacy

indebtedness see Medical student debt

indemnity HEALTH CARE ENVIRONMENT An agreement on the part of an insurer to provide health-related benefits in the form of cash payments to or on the behalf of a beneficiary for the services provided in lieu of the services per se LEGAL MEDICINE Payment for losses including the payment of judgements, costs, and attorneys' fees

independent contractor A distinct category of (non-salaried) employee, eg 'temp' nurse, 'per-diem' physician, clinical consultant, or other, who provides a service at a rate that is higher than that of a salaried full-time employees; independent contractors do not receive health benefits, retirement contributions, paid vacations, and do not have a portion of their salary deducted for taxes; see Per diem

independent practice association HEALTH CARE ADMINISTRATION A format for the practice of medicine in which the physician/health care provider retains his/her traditional practice autonomy, while at the same time integrating them into self-directed groups that solve group-related problems and exert political influence (JAMA 1995; 273:197)

indeterminant syndrome Overlap syndrome, see there

index of inequality SOCIOLOGY A summary measure of the differences in mortality according to the level of education or income status among persons of similar sex, race, and family status, based on mortality ratios; the IoI between whites and blacks (based on education and economic status) has widened in the US from 1960 to 1985 (N Engl J Med 1993; 329:103oA, 110oA)

Index Medicus INFORMATION SCIENCE A database maintained by the US National Library of Medicine that is available in printed form on a monthly and annual basis; the Index catalogs the articles that appear in 3200 biomedical journals, over ½ of which are written in English; an expanded form of the Index Medicus can be retrieved electronically from the Medline database, allowing searches of the biomedical literature and relevant abstracts to its inception in 1966; see GRATEFUL MED, MEDLARS, MEDLINE

index of suspicion A catch-phrase broadly used in various medical fields to indicate how seriously a particular nosology (disease process) is being entertained as a diagnosis; as an example, there would be a high index of suspicion that rapid and unexplained weight loss in an elderly patient would be due to a carcinoma of the pancreas and a low index of suspicion that it would be due to AIDS

India ink cells A descriptive term for the densely hyperchromatic, loosely cohesive cells seen in small (undifferentiated non-keratinizing) cell carcinoma of the lung; see Small ('oat') cell carcinoma

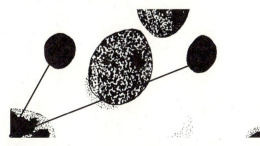

India ink cells

India ink spot nucleus A nucleus with have dark, homogeneous chromatin and a smooth contour, which may be seen in occasional cytological preparations of keratinizing epidermoid carcinoma from endobronchial washings; the nuclei may be surrounded by 'dirty' blue-gray or orange cytoplasm, the latter indicating the cells' partially consummated desire to produce keratin

Note: Similar hyperchromatic nuclei may be seen in mesothelial cells as well in lentigo maligna (Hutchinson's melanotic freckle)

Indian childhood cirrhosis A fatal disease of early childhood onset with familial tendencies that was first described in the middle classes of rural India, which occurs elsewhere in the tropics and subtropics CLINICAL Irritability, fever, anorexia, hepatomegaly, jaundice, fulminant cirrhosis, hepatic failure, coma, death LABORATORY ↑ Immunoglobulins, ↑ serum and hepatic copper levels PATHOGENESIS Idiopathic, copper cookware has been incriminated PATHOLOGY Massive hepatocyte degeneration, global inflammation, Mallory body formation, diffuse fibrosis and 'micro-micronodular' cirrhosis

Indian filing Indians in a file SURGICAL PATHOLOGY Single cell 'cords' that are compressed within a densely hyalinized or desmoplastic stroma, a finding typical of infiltrating lobular (21%) or ductal (36%) breast carcinomas (Cancer 1967; 20:363); single cell 'Indian file' arrangement may also occur without the dense stromal reaction in bronchoalveolar carcinoma, meningioma, medulloblastoma, Spiegler-Fendt's pseudolymphoma of the skin, well-differentiated lymphocytic leukemia of the skin, at the periphery of terminal duct carcinoma of the salivary gland and at the normal mantle zone of lymphocytes in lymph nodes; this pattern may also be seen in both tissues and effusions with pancreatic adenocarcinoma (Acta Cytologica 1993; 37:483oA)

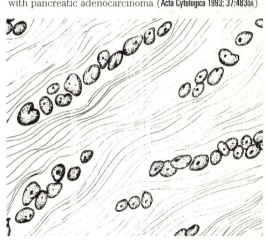

Indian filing

'India rubber man' A fanciful and nonspecific term referring to the hyperlaxity of joints and hyperextensible, fragile and bruisable skin accompanied by cutaneous and vascular friability characteristic of patients with Ehlers-Danlos disease

indication 'A symptom, sign, or circumstance that points to a specific treatment (or sequence of workup modalities) for an illness' (International Dictionary of Medicine, J Wiley & Sons, New York, 1986)

indicator enzyme LABORATORY MEDICINE A generic term for any enzyme (eg alkaline phosphatase, peroxidase) that is of use in detecting the presence of a particular substance, which acts by catalyzing a reaction in which a colorless substrate is digested, yielding a colored material that can be untified or semiuntified spectrophotometer

indirect billing HEALTH CARE FINANCING The submission of bills for services rendered to the physician who ordered the test; indirect (or 'physician') billing promotes the practice of mark-up, increasing the bill for services the physician submits to the patient; in one survey in 1988, the physician mark-up for services performed by a reference laboratory was 139% (**Clin Lab Sci 1994; 7:72F**)

indirect Coombs' test see Coombs' test

indirect costs Overhead costs ACADEMIA The monies required to construct and maintain buildings, including the costs for energy, heating, water and electricity, support costs, library services, and other forms of institutional support, as well as administrative costs and salaries, eg lawyers, bureaucrats, financial office personnel that are levered by a university against the budgets of investigators receiving government grant support; as an example, an indirect cost of 50% for a $100 000 grant requires that an extra $50 000 be included in the grant proposal (**Science 1991; 252:636n&v**) it has been urged that the term indirect costs be replaced by two terms: Research administrative costs and research facilities costs, a separation that would allow comparison among institutions (**Nature Medicine 1995; 1:196**) see Circular A-21; Cf Direct costs

Note: Indirect costs are a normal financial consideration in preparing hospital budgets and differ somewhat from the term as used by grant-giving bodies and grant recipients; in a health care facility, indirect costs include depreciation of equipment or the cost of construction or renovation; direct costs include overhead, employee salaries, disposables, drugs, laboratory reagents and waste disposal

indirect immunofluorescence IMMUNOLOGY A two-step technique that is a modification of the indirect Coombs' (antiglobulin) test, in which the antigen reacts with a primary antibody; the primary complex then reacts with an antibody that has been labeled with a fluorescent tag; because the indirect method eliminates the need to purify and conjugate antibodies to a particular antigen, it is widely preferred to 'direct' methods; Cf Direct immunofluorescence

indolent malignancy A lesion that is malignant by cytological, genetic, histopathological or other criteria, but which rarely displays the classic *sine qua non* criterion that defines a malignant lesion, which is metastasis; indolent malignancies include lymphomatoid papulosis and pagetoid reticulosis (Woringer-Kolopp disease)

indolent myeloma A slowly progressive myeloma with an average survival of 10 years, which contrast to untreated multiple myeloma, 6-month survival and treated myeloma which has a 3 to 5 year survival; stable myeloma comprises 5% of multiple myelomas and is often detected by routine laboratory test for unrelated reasons; most patients have stage I disease and the mitotic activity, as measured by ^{3}H-thymidine labelling index, is low at less than 0.8%; see Monoclonal gammopathy of undetermined significance, Myeloma

indomethacin A therapeutic agent that has antiinflammatory, antipyretic, and analgesic properties, which is used to treat various arthropathies; it has profound effects on platelet and neutrophil function cerebral, mesenteric, and renal hemodynamics, renal tubular function, and O_2 consumption of the GI tract; indomethacin is a potent inhibitor of prostaglandin synthesis and had been used as a tocolytic agent, but its use may increase the risk of serious neonatal complications (eg sepsis, intracranial hemorrhage, renal dysfunction, and necrotizing enterocolitis) in infants born at or before 30 weeks of gestation (**N Engl J Med 1993; 329:1602OA**)

indoor air pollutants CLINICAL TOXICOLOGY Any of a number of usually low-level toxins that may become relatively concentrated in the air of commercial or residential buildings; these pollutants include cigarette smoke, cooking and combustion products, eg natural gas, oil, wood and kerosene, volatilized chemicals, eg solvents, cleaning fluids, paint strippers including methylene chloride, asbestos in old buildings and formaldehyde in new furniture; see Passive smoking, Radon, Sick building syndrome

induced abortion Termination of pregnancy The voluntary elimination of gestational products, a procedure that can be brought about by instruments, eg dilatation and curettage when performed in the first trimester or by saline infusion (saline abortion) when performed later

induced erythrocythemia Blood doping, see there

induced fit model Sequential model BIOCHEMISTRY A model for the interaction of an allosteric enzyme with its substrate, proposed by Koshland, Nemethy, and Filmer (KNF) that holds that an enzyme's active site undergoes a series of sequential changes in conformation that affect the rate of binding of substrate, positive and negative effectors; the 'KNF model' is a modification of Fisher's 'lock-and-key' hypothesis for enzyme action, where instead of a rigid site for the interaction between an enzyme and its substrate, both enzyme and substrate are distorted on binding and the substrate molecule is forced by the enzyme into a 'stressful' conformation that approximates the transition state; see Lock-and-key model

induction OBSTETRICS Induction of labor, see there ONCOLOGY Induction of remission, see there

induction chemotherapy Drug therapy given as a primary treatment for patients who present with an advanced cancer for which no alternative treatment exists; selection of agents is based on the effectiveness of the drugs in rodent models; combinations of agents are usually empirical and based on effectiveness, limiting toxicity and cross-resistance; induction chemotherapy is most successfully used in lymphoproliferative disease, where it comprises a component of standardized protocols, see above; induction chemotherapy with cis-platinum and 5-fluorouracil (5-FU) in combination with radiotherapy is of use in lymph node negative patients with advanced (stage III or IV) squamous cell carcinoma of the larynx, allowing preservation of the vocal cords, improving the quality of life, while reducing the co-morbidity associated with surgery (**N Engl J Med 1991; 324:1685**) see Salvage treatment

induction of labor The use of artifical maneuvers to hasten the onset of labor, including the use of prostaglandin E_2 gel, oxytocin infusion, and amniotomy; in post-term pregnancy, induction of labor results in a lower rate of cesarean section than serial antenatal monitoring (**N Engl J Med 1992; 326:1587OA**)

induction of remission ONCOLOGY The initial phase of a three-step therapeutic chemotherapeutic regimen used in treating acute leukemia; in ALL, prednisone and vincristine induce complete remission in 90% of children and 50% of adults, which may be increased up to 80% by the addition of a third drug, eg L-asparginase, daunorubicin or doxorubicin; in AML, the therapeutic levels of these agents are close to levels that are also toxic to the BM, thus by extension, successful induction of remission may be a pyrrhic victory associated with aplastic anemia; cytosine arabinoside followed by an anthracycline (daunorubicin or doxorubicin) induces remission in 50-85% of those < age 60 and 30-40% of those > age 60; see Consolidation chemotherapy, Maintenance chemotherapy

inductively coupled plasma-mass spectroscopy (or spectrometry) ICP-MS LABORATORY MEDICINE A technology used to identify heavy metals at concentrations lower than previously achievable, of particular interest for lead testing

inductive signaling DEVELOPMENTAL BIOLOGY A type of regulatory signaling that operates between developing nonequivalent cells; in IS, a cell develops based on 1) The restricted expression of particular receptors and ligands and 2) The timing of cell-cell contact (**Science 1995; 268:225**) Cf Lateral specification

industry screening HEALTH CARE ENVIRONMENT Black-listing, see there

indwelling catheter A generic term for any catheter, usually understood to be of the urinary bladder (often a 'Foley') that is left in place for a prolonged period of time

inevitable abortion A 'terminal' and irreverisible stage of threatened abortion where there is dilation of the cervix and rupture of membranes, which is treated with curettage; see Abortion

infanticide FORENSIC MEDICINE The active or semi-passive killing of a viable conceptus that is older than 20 gestational weeks and breathes spontaneously; in differentiating stillbirth from live birth and subsequent death, ie suspected infanticide, 'soft' and 'hard' criteria are examined (table); see Battered child syndrome, Child abuse

---

'INFANTICIDE
'HARD' CRITERIA
COMPARISON OF GASTRIC FLUID COMPOSITION with that of a toilet bowel-active drowning
PEURAL SURFACES WITH PETECHIAE Seen in induced suffocation, most significant when coupled with hematomas and petechiae on the mouth and epiglottis; the lingual frenulum may be torn and the lips bruised, indicating active attempts at suffocation
LUNGS Stillbirth lungs are not aerated and do not float
EDEMATOUS FOAM ON NOSTRILS An indicator of active breathing
MECONIUM Resuscitation of a true stillborn may push meconium into the perianal region, but extensive staining of the placenta and umbilical cord is due to antenatal stress
'SOFT' CRITERIA
DENIAL OF PREGNANCY If the woman is obese or a dullard, she may not know she was pregnant
RIGOR MORTIS A finding that is poorly appreciated in neonates
IMPRESSION OF THE BODY in soil, blood or fomites, requiring diligent and timely scene investigation
MACERATION OF SKIN A finding typical of stillbirth
PUTREFACTION Stillborns do not putrefy as they have sterile bowels
UMBILICAL CORD A cut cord indicates active intervention-time undetermined; an intact cord is consistent with stillbirth
DETERMINATION OF AGE Viability, most fetuses born before 18 weeks' gestation die despite resuscitative efforts, age is determined by skeletal dating, antenatal studies corroborating fetal death, eg Spaulding sign of in utero death characterized by overlapping cranial bones

---

infant mortality EPIDEMIOLOGY A standard indicator of health, defined as the number of infant deaths before age 1, which in the US (1992) was 8.5/1000 live births; in 1990, the US IM rate ranked 24th among countries or geographic areas with a population of > one million (MMWR 1994; 43:905; JAMA 1995; 273:101); main causes of IM include congenital anomalies, short gestation and unspecified low birth weight, pneumonia and influenza, infections specific to the neonatal period, complications of placenta, cord, and membranes, intrauterine hypoxia and birth asphyxia, respiratory distress syndrome, accidents and adverse effects, SIDS; Cf Postneonatal mortality

infantile cortical hyperostosis Caffey disease, Caffey-Silverman syndrome An AD [MIM 114000] complex characterized by early onset of hyperostosis and neo-osteogenesis, affecting the facial and, less commonly, the long bones, accompanied by soft tissue swelling, hyperirritability, dysphagia, fever, pleuritis LABORATORY ↑ ESR, alkaline phosphatase

infantile digital fibromatosis Kissing tumor A tumor of infants of the terminal phalanges of the fingers and toes, which measures < than 2 cm PATHOLOGY Poorly circumscribed fibroblasts with the pathognomonic hyalinoid eosinophilic inclusions seen by PTAH (phosphotungstic acid hematoxylin) or Masson's trichrome stains PROGNOSIS

Benign, although 60% recur locally

infantile genetic agranulocytosis IMMUNOLOGY An AR [MIM 202700] condition of early infant onset, characterized by profound neutropenia (< 0.3 x 10^9/L) (US:< 300/mm³), absolute monocytosis and eosinophilia, recurring pyogenic infections of skin and lungs PATHOLOGY Vacuolation of myeloid precursors with normal colony-stimulating factor and colony-forming units TREATMENT None, universally fatal in childhood

infectious mononucleosis 'syndrome' A generic term for any of a group of often viral agents that acutely induce a marked monocytosis in the peripheral blood and cause symptoms typical of classic EBV-induced infectious mononucleosis, eg CMV, herpes virus, HHV-6, HIV-1 and *Toxoplasma gondii*

inferior petrosal sinus sampling ENDOCRINOLOGY A test used to localize the source of excess ACTH production, based on the drainage routes of pituitary (hypophysis) venous blood, which flows first into the cavernous sinuses and then into the inferior petrosal veins; if the excess ACTH is being produced by the pituitary, ie 'central', then there is a central-to-peripheral gradient, although if the ACTH production is pulsatile, a gradient is not evident; in IPSS, a catheter is inserted via the femoral vein and after a baseline sampling, bovine CRH (corticotropin-releasing hormone) is injected, and samples are taken at timed (2, 5, 10, and 15 minutes) intervals; a 2-fold central-to-peripheral ACTH gradient is usually significant (see N Engl J Med 1994; 331:629OA)

inferior vena caval filter CARDIOLOGY A semipermanent device* placed in the inferior vena cava percutaneously by an interventional angiography in order to prevent recurrent pulmonary thromboembolism due to thrombi arising in the lower part of the body; IVCFs are indicated when anticoagulation is either contraindicated or has been tried and failed, or as prophylaxis for high-risk patients, eg those with cor pulmonale or after surgical pulmonary embolectomy (N Engl J Med 1995; 332:1099c)

*IVCFs include the Mobin-Uddin filter (which was commonly used from 1969 to 1977, but is no longer available in the US), the Greenfield filter, which has an appearance likened to the 'cage' surrounding the cork on a champagne bottle, and the Bird's Nest filter, which when viewed through a patent vessel appears as a fine wire mesh, which is now preferred by the Braunwald group at Brigham and Women's Hospital in Boston

inferior vena caval interruption CARDIOLOGY A generic term for any form of therapy that prevents the free flow of blood (and possibly of emboli from the lower half of the body) through the inferior vena caval; most IVCI is undertaken with inferior vena caval filters (see there), with inferior vena caval ligation and external clips being rarely used

inferiority complex PSYCHIATRY A popular term for a constellation of behaviors, including diffidence, timidity, and others, which may be accompanied by a deep-rooted sense of inadequacy; Cf Superiority complex

infertility The involuntary inability to conceive, which contrasts with sterility, the total inability to reproduce; 8.5% of married couples (US) are infertile (N Engl J Med 1993; 329:1710OA; N Engl J Med 1994; 331:239OA) or inconceivable; successful impregnation requires the production of an adequate number of normal motile spermatozoa that are ejaculated through patent ducts into an unobstructed reproductive tract of an accomodating female who contributes by ovulating at the appropriate time and releasing an ovum that the incoming sperm is capable of fertilizing, which then develops and implants in a well-prepared endometrium; ½ of infertility is due to ♀ factors, eg fallopian tube defects (20-30%), uterine and cervical pathology (10%), vaginal disease (< 5%), amenorrhea and anovulation (15%), nutritional and metabolic defects (5%), immunologic defects (< 5%) and ovulatory defects < 5%); 40% of infertility stems from ♂ factors including decreased production of spermatozoa, abnormal sperm, ductal obstruction, ejaculatory defects (psychogenic or anatomic) or immunologic defects; 10% of cases are idiopathic; see Assisted reproduction, in vitro fertilization

infibulation The practice of stitching or clasping the labia majora in young ♀ or the prepuce of young ♂ as a means of preventing copulation; infibulation is a type of female circumcision that has been divided into

TYPE IV aka Total infibulation, which '...*involves removal of the clitoris and part of the labia minora, plus incision of the labia majora to create raw surfaces that are stitched together to cover the urethra and the entrance to the vagina with a hood of skin, leaving a very small posterior opening for the passage of urine and menstrual blood.*'

TYPE III, a modification of type IV, in which there is a larger posterior opening; like the other forms of female circumcision, these procedures are deeply rooted in the culture of certain African countries and symbolize societal control over the woman's fertility, as infibulation hinders childbirth TREATMENT De-infibulation by central incision and use of hemostatic sutures (N Engl J Med 1994; 331:712SA)

see Female circumcision, Re-infibulation; Cf Clitoridectomy

inflammatory bowel disease A generic term applied to several including Crohn's disease (CD), ulcerative colitis (UC) and idiopathic inflammatory bowel disease, the last of which is a diagnosis of exclusion that mimics and/or overlaps with CD and UC both clinically and pathologically HEREDITY First-degree relatives of those with CD and UC have an 8- to 10-fold increased risk of developing the same form of colitis; the risk of first-degree relatives of UC patients of developing CD or the risk of first-degree relatives of patients with CD of developing UC is 1.7 and 3.8 respectively (N Engl J Med 1991; 324:84; see ibid, 325:928rv, 325:1008rv); intestinal inflammation may also be induced by ischemia, irradiation, uremia, cytotoxic drugs, heavy metal intoxication; IBD patients often have two or more of the following: Visible abdominal distension, relief of pain upon defecation, looser and more frequent bowel movements when the pain occurs; ♂:♀ ratio is 2:1 and is more common in Jews; IBD is associated with mucocutaneous disease (pyoderma gangrenosa, erythema nodosum, oral ulcers, annular erythema, vascular thromboses, epidermolysis bullosa acquisita), ocular disease (uveitis, iridocyclitis), hepatopathy (chronic active hepatitis, cirrhosis, sclerosing cholangitis), arthropathy (ankylosing spondylitis); Cf Irritable bowel syndrome

inflammatory carcinoma Erysipeloides A carcinoma characterized by invasion of the dermal lymphatics by malignant cells, most often of breast origin, less commonly in malignancies of the lung, GI tract, and uterus CLINICAL Diffuse swelling, erythema, pain and edema, simulating acute mastitis or cellulitis, and potentially delaying the diagnosis and therapy PROGNOSIS Poor

inflammatory fibroid polyp A benign presumed reactive gastric, usually antral 'tumor', associated with hypo- or achlorhydria PATHOLOGY Polymorphic inflammatory cell population, predominantly eosinophils with submucosal edema DDx Eosinophilic gastroenteritis

inflammatory oncotaxis The attraction of malignant tumor cells to sites of tissue trauma, inflammation and capillary disruption, as seen after radiation and surgery; cutaneous metastases from colon, kidney and uterine cervix may settle on surgical incisions; Cf Implantation recurrence

inflammatory polyp 'Allergic polyp' ENT A non-neoplastic, reactive, recurrent often bilateral 'tumor' that forms in response to infection, allergy and mucoviscidosis PATHOLOGY Mucous glands covered by respiratory epithelium, a loose myxoid stroma, and when associated with allergy, a marked eosinophilic inflammatory infiltrate

inflammatory polyp GASTROENTEROLOGY Postinflammatory polyposis, 'pseudopolyposis' Any of a number of often bizarre polyps and/or bridges of mucosa, which when single may mimic malignancy, and when multiple mimic a polyposis syndrome; IPs may arise in a back-

ground of inflammatory bowel disease (Crohn's disease, ulcerative colitis), amebic colitis, bacterial dysentery, and chronic schistosomiasis, and are benign, nonspecific sequelae of inflammation of the intestinal mucosa CLINICAL IPs are rarely symptomatic, but pain, obstruction, and if large, intussusception may occur

Note: In the past, the term pseudopolyp has been used (a practice that continues to the present in some circles), they are by definition true polyps

inflammatory pseudotumor A solitary, expansile but resectable tumor, composed of mature lymphocytes, which clinically and pathologically mimics malignancy, located in lungs, ocular orbit, abdominal cavity ETIOLOGY Trauma, surgery, local infection, myocardial infarct, aortic aneurysm, connective tissue disease PATHOLOGY Edema, plasma cells, bizarre fibroblasts and lipid-laden histiocytes; Cf Pseudolymphoma, Pseudosarcoma

inflammatory pseudotumor of liver A relatively uncom-

INFLAMMATORY BOWEL DISEASE		
	ULCERATIVE COLITIS	CROHN'S DISEASE
CLINICAL		
Rectal bleeding	Common	Rare
Abdominal mass	Rare	10-15%
Abdominal pain	Left-sided	Right-sided
Abnormal endoscopy	95%	< 50%
Perforation	12%	4%
Colon carcinoma	5-10%	Rare
Response to steroids	75%	25%
Surgical outcome	Excellent	Fair
Rectal involvement	> 95%	!0%
RADIOLOGY		
Ileal involvement	Rare	Usual
Cross-hatched ulcers	Rare	Occasional
Thumbprinting	Absent	Common
Fissuring	Absent	Common
Skip areas	Absent	Common
Strictures	Absent	Common
PATHOLOGY		
Distribution of lesions	Diffuse	Focal
	Superficial	Transmural
Mucosal atrophy/ regeneration	Marked	Minimal
Hyperemia	Often marked	Minimal
Crypt abscess	Common	Rare
Cytoplasmic mucin	Decreased	Intact
Lymphoid aggregates	Rare	Common
Lymph nodes	Reactive hyperplasia	Granulomas
Edema	Minimal	Marked
Granulomas	Absent	60%

mon benign reactive lesion measuring 1-20 cm in diameter, age range ± 1-83 years (mean 37), ♂:♀ ratio 3:1 PATHOGENESIS Uncertain, possibly bacterial CLINICAL Fever, weight loss, malaise LABORATORY ↑ WBCs, ↑ ESR TREATMENT Surgical resection (Am J Surg Pathol 1993; 17:221OA)

*Synonyms include fibroxanthoma, histiocytoma, plasma cell granuloma, plasmacytoma, pseudolymphoma; IPL is not regarded as a synonym of hepatocellular pseudotumor

inflammatory pseudotumor of urinary bladder An uncommon benign reactive lesion* measuring 1-7 cm in diameter, age range 19-60 years (mean 35) PATHOGENESIS Uncertain, possibly an abnormal reparative response to trauma CLINICAL Hematuria, flank pain, recurrent urinary tract infections PATHOLOGY Spindle-shaped fibroblasts and myofibroblasts immunoreactive for vimentin and actin with granulation tissue formation FLOW CYTOMETRY Diploid, ie benign TREATMENT Transurethral resection, partial cystectomy (Am J Surg Pathol 1993; 17:264OA)

*Synonyms include atypical fibromyxoid tumor, atypical myofibroblastic tumor, nodular fasciitis of the bladder, myofibroblastic tumor, plasma cell granuloma, pseudosarcomatous fibromyxoid tumor, pseudosarcomatous myofibroblastic proliferation

influenza A An avian virus, especially of ducks (which in China live in close proximity to the pig reservoir and 'vector'); periodic mutations of the virus (13 hemagglutination and 9 neuraminidase subtypes) are responsible for 'flu' epidemics and pandemics, the most memorable of which was the 1918 global pandemic that killed 20-30 million; every year, minor random mutations in the virus occur (genetic or antigenic drift); about every 20 years a major mutation occurs resulting in an alteration of the surface hemagglutinin (genetic or antigenic shift); influenza type A (H3N2 immunotype) was the most prevalent cause in the 1989-90 season; see Antigenic drift, Antigenic shift

'influenza syndrome' A clinical complex characterized by fever, headache, malaise, dizziness, ataxia, leukopenia, thrombocytopenia, muscular weakness, gastrointestinal symptoms (nausea, vomiting and diarrhea) and potentially renal failure, a potential side effect of intermittent therapy with rifampin Note: Influenza-like syndromes may occur with virtually any infection, especially of viral origin and are highly non-specific

Infobahn Internet, see there; information superhighway

informant Historian A person or patient who provides a medical history

information overload An excess of information made available to a person in certain situations, causing them either to make wrong decision or resulting in the passing of misinformation 1) Patients must have sufficient information at their disposal to give an informed consent for, eg an elective surgical procedure; this may become problematic when the patient is made aware of certain (usually very rare) complications or side effects of the procedure or the anesthesiology; the information excess may cause the patient to decide against undergoing a diagnostic or therapeutic procedure which in the opinion of the physician is medically indicated 2) Physicians suffer from the information overload because of the amount of material they are required ingest and integrate into daily practice (N Engl J Med 1994; 330:1611sB) see Uninformed consent

information therapy A highly colloquial term for empowerment of patients by encouraging their access to information relevant to their disease, which may itself be therapeutic (JAMA 1992; 267:2592)

information superhighway Internet, see there; Infobahn

'informed' An adjective for an employer, co-worker or family member of a person with an infectious disease that is not spread by casual contact, who is (theoretically) completely at ease with the infected person in the workplace or in a social setting; 'informed' is a euphemism that first appeared in the AIDS epidemic for persons in contact with HIV-positive citizens, which contrasts to an 'uninformed' person, who responds in a hysterical and irrational fashion to the knowledge that a colleague or acquaintance is infected with HIV (Science 1991; 252:1798)

informed consent LEGAL MEDICINE Voluntarily obtained and legally documented agreement by the patient to allow performance of a specific diagnostic or therapeutic procedure or procedures; the doctrine of informed consent has had enormous impact on the provision of health care in the US and has been cited as a major factor in erosion of the 'doctor-patient relation', which was formerly paternalistic in nature); a procedure performed without valid informed consent makes the physician liable for a lawsuit with a formal charge of assault and battery (A&B, for exceptions to the requisite for informed consent, see Emergency doctrine, Therapeutic privilege doctrine) Note: Obtention of informed consent from minors (< 18

years of age) is potentially problematic as, under the US legal system, an 'emancipated' or 'mature' minor may give permission for a procedure, if he understands its nature and outcome, although it may be against the wishes of his parents, who could sue the physician for A&B; alternately, the parent may give permission to perform a procedure which the minor obviously understands and does not want, who could then sue the medical team for A&B; *informed consent is a legal doctrine that requires a physician to obtain consent for treatment rendered, an operation performed, or certain diagnostic procedures, and is a process not a form. The law of informed consent varies significantly from state to state...It is essential that the patient fully understand the procedures to be performed; the courts can view the doctrine of informed consent from the 'reasonable physician' standard or increasingly from the 'patient viewpoint' standard* (*Risk Management Principles & Commentaries for the Medical Office, American Medical Association/Specialty Society Medical Liability Project, 1990, Chicago); the following should be discussed with the patient 1) The risks and benefits of a proposed treatment or procedure 2) The alternative treatments or procedures and their risks and benefits, and 3) The risks and benefits of doing nothing; see Malpractice

infrared lamp Heat lamp A lamp that generates electromagnetic radiation in the near infrared (760-1500 nm) and/or far infrared (1500-15 000 nm) range, which may be used clinically for the deep heating of tissue

infrared spectrometry LABORATORY TECHNOLOGY The analysis of points on the infrared spectrum, which has advantages over other techniques as it is nondestructive to the sample, provides virtually instantaneous results, and can be used for analyzing solids, liquids, or gases; IS-based instruments are used in medical diagnostics, ambient air monitoring, food and beverage analysis, automotive exhaust gas analysis, and others (Am Lab Feb1995 p16)

infrastructure A generic term for the physical plant required before a market can develop in a new technology '...For the PC industry it was motherboards, chips sets, disk drives. For the information highway, it will be the network of switches, fiber and coaxial cable that connects the country.' (Forbes ASAP 27 Feb 1995, p42) see Enabling technology

infusion pump A device designed to deliver various drugs and/or 'biologicals', at low doses and at a constant or controllable rate; increased rates of delivery in such devices may be associated with local hemolysis, compromising the potential benefits of a calibrated delivery system; Cf Pancreatic transplantation

infusion ALTERNATIVE MEDICINE A medicinal preparation of herbal origin in which a ground substance (eg bark, root, nuts, or seeds) is boiled in water to obtain the extract of interest, eg chamomile, peppermint, and rosehips; Cf Decoction

Note: As here defined, the terms herbal tea and infusion are often used interchangeably

---

INFORMED CONSENT requires that the patient understand
The nature of his/her illness/injury
The nature and purpose of the treatment
The risks and potential for death or injury during the procedure and the consequences of the proposed treatment
The probability of success
Other treatment options and their associated risks and benefits
The risks, benefits, and prognosis when treatment does not occur

Ingelfinger rule SCIENTIFIC JOURNALISM A set of guidelines delineated by Franz J Ingelfinger, MD, the late editor of the New England Journal of Medicine, who felt that two criteria were imperative in accepting papers for publication in a scientific journal of high quality: 1) A news embargo on articles scheduled for appearance in the journal and 2) Strict application of the Ingelfinger rule: '*The journal undertakes review with the understanding that neither the substance of the article nor the figures or tables have been published or will be submitted for publication during the period of review. This restriction does not apply to abstracts published in connection with scientific meetings or to news reports based on public presentations at such meetings*'; the Ingelfinger Rule has become the standard of high-quality medical and scientific journalism (**N Engl J Med 1991; 325:1371**) see Authorship, Clinical alert, Vancouver group; Cf Embargo arrangement

inhalation anthrax Woolsorter's disease An occupational form of anthrax caused by inhalation of *Brucella anthracis* spores affecting those exposed to aerosols during the early stages of processing of goat of other infected animal hair CLINICAL IA is biphasic, the early symptoms are influenza-like, lasting 2-3 days, which is followed a period of presumed resolution, and then by severe respiratory distress, hypoxia and dyspnea, mediastinal LN involvement, subcutaneous edema of the upper body, meningeal signs, shock, and in most cases death in 24 hours MORTALITY High; 12/13 documented cases in the US died TREATMENT Penicillin

Note: The high mortality caused by aerosolized *B anthracis* has made it a popular experimental agent for biological warfare, although it has never been deployed; see Sverdlosk

inhalation class RADIATION SAFETY A classification scheme for inhalated materials based on its rate of clearance from the lung, where class D is cleared in ≤ 10 days, class W in 10-100 days, and class Y ≥ 100 days

'inheritance powder' Arsenic A metal available in a powdered form that has enjoyed intermittent popularity as an unsuspected poison that induces slow mental deterioration and vague GI symptoms in its victims, who may have been poisoned by next-of-kin eager to inherit (hence the macabre sobriquet) the victim's worldly possessions

inherited *adjective* Referring or pertaining to a trait or characteristic that is intrinsic to one's genotype; in this context, the synonym hereditary is widely preferred

inherited palmoplantar Hereditary palmoplantar keratoderma, see there

inhibin REPRODUCTIVE PHYSIOLOGY A heterodimeric glycoprotein hormone composed of α and β subunits secreted by the granulosa cells of the ovary and Sertoli cells of the testicles; its major physiologic action is to inhibit the secretion of FSH by the adenohypophysis (anterior pituitary gland); inhibin is secreted through the entire menstrual cycle and during pregnancy; serum inhibin levels are increased in 15-100% of women with ovarian neoplasms, the highest levels being seen in granulosa cell tumors (3/3 cases), mucinous carcinomas and borderline tumors (18/22) and benign diseases of the ovary (11/41) (**N Engl J Med 1993; 329:1539OA**); inhibin peaks at 800 U/L in the follicular phase of the menstrual cycle and forms a negative feedback loop that prevents the maturation of cohort follicles; inhibin is a tumor transforming factor with a reciprocal relation with activin and may be increased in granulosa cell tumors; see Follistatin

inhibitory transmitter NEUROPHYSIOLOGY A generic term for a substance, eg GABA (γ-amino butyric acid), produced by one neuron that attenuates or inhibits the firing of another neuron

iniencephaly sequence A primary neural tube malformation that occurs at the level of the thoracic and cervical vertebrae, which results in a 'sequence' of secondary features including retroflexion of the upper spine, shortened neck and trunk, cervical anomalies, defects of thoracic cage, anterior spina bifida, diaphragmatic defects, with or without hernia, hypoplasia of the lung and/or heart; see Sequence

INIT Initial device COMPUTERS Any small software program that is 'loaded' into the random access memory (RAM) prior to the disk operating system, bypassing the microcomputer's 'resource manager', which is responsible for directing the flow of information through the computer; INITs are not recognized by the resource manager and thus are 'invisible', but may cause problems in an often unpredictable fashion, especially if software has been written for older operating systems; INITs in the MacIntosh environment include Pyro!, RAM doubler, Virex, Suitcase and Adobe's Type Manager; see Computers

initial body see Reticulate body

initiation MOLECULAR BIOLOGY The first step in the synthesis of a polypeptide chain, requiring the formation of a ribosome-mRNA-initiator tRNA complex ONCOLOGY The first 'hit' in a two- or multi-'hit' carcinogenic cascade, which theoretically is due to a short intense exposure of the DNA to a carcinogen, resulting in mutation; for a tumor to develop, subsequent steps are required, and the cell(s) must be acted on by a promoter; see Tumor promoter

initiation codon Start codon, see there

initiation complex see Initiation factor(s)

initiation factor(s) A family of proteins that help the ribosome find an initiation site, which is necessary to induce protein synthesis, without which the 'initiation complex' of mRNA, Met-tRNA, GTP, and the small ribosomal subunits does not form

Initiative 119 A 'landmark' legislation proposed in the state of Washington, and voted upon in late 1991 (it was defeated by 54 to 46), which would have allowed physicians to legally perform active euthanasia without criminal sanction, on a '*conscious and mentally competent, qualified patient*'; under Initiative 119, a candidate for euthanasia would be terminally ill or have an irreversible condition that, in the opinion of two physicians would result in death within six months; under the proposal, the patient would be required to be fully conscious, mentally competent and voluntarily request the service in writing at the time of its being rendered (**Am Med News 7 January 1991**) see Euthanasia, Kevorkian, Physician-assisted suicide, Proposition 161 ,and 'Slippery slope'

Note: Although euthanasia is practiced in the Netherlands, it is technically illegal

injection technique OTOLARYNGOLOGY Any of a number of types of phonosurgery (see there) including vocal fold augmentation with alloplastics and bioimplants, or management of spasmodic dysphonia with transcutaneous or peroral injection of botulinum toxin

Injury Severity Scale EMERGENCY MEDICINE A numerical scoring system for calculating the probability of survival, and seriousness of wounds or trauma sustained; it is mathematically derived from the Abbreviated Injury Scale (see there), calculated as the sum of the squares of the highest abbreviational injury scores in each of the three most severely injured body parts, resulting in scores from 1 (minor injury) to 75 (generally fatal) which correlate well with length of hospitalization, time to death, disability and need for surgery (see **N Engl J Med 1994; 331:1105OA**) an ISS of greater than 20 implies a poor prognosis; see Revised Trauma Score, Trauma Score (**J Trauma 1974; 14:187**)

ink blot test Rorschach test, see there

'inkwell' GI SURGERY A surgically constructed vagination ('intussusception') of a short sleeve of esophagus sewn into the stomach, which as intragastric pressure increases, is compressed, forms a functional valve, for example, the Nissen fundoplication Note: Inkwells are reservoirs for ink pens, designed in such a way as to prevent the glass container from tipping on its side and were replaced by the self-contained (fountain) pen

inlet patch GASTROENTEROLOGY A remnant of heterotopic but normal glandular epithelium, usually gastric, that may be found in the esophagus of otherwise asymptomatic subjects, which is thought to be a embryonic rest (**Sci & Med Nov/Dec 1994 p16**); inlet patches occur in 4-20% of normal subjects in the lower esophagus above the Z-line; since this finding (early embryonic esophagus having been lined by columnar epithelium with secondary ingrowth by squamous epithelium) may be confused with Barrett's esophagus, esophageal biopsies should be well above the Z-line; see Barrett's esophagus

innocent bystander hemolysis A non-immune phenomenon caused by adsorption of carrier protein-bound drugs to the red cell surface; drugs causing innocent bystander hemolysis include sulfonamides, phenothiazines and quinidine, which act as haptens, eliciting drug-specific complement-fixing immune hemolysis of 'innocent' erythrocytes (activated by the alternate complement pathway); the direct antiglobulin test (Coombs' test) reveals only membrane-associated cleavage products, eg C3dg; the indirect antiglobulin test (indirect Coombs' test) is negative

innocent murmur Any cardiac murmur that occurs in a normal person; IMs are divided into six systolic murmurs, eg vibratory systolic murmur (Still's murmur) and the mammary souffle and two diastolic murmurs, eg the venous hum; innocent murmers occur in all normal people at some time in their lives, most commonly occurring during mid-systole; the greatest danger in innocent murmurs lies in their mis-interpretation as representing serious cardiac pathology, resulting in recommendation of restriction of life-style, thereby becoming a cardiac cripple

inoperable *adjective* Referring or pertaining to a disease (usually understood to mean a widely disseminated malignancy) that would not be positively affected by surgical therapy

iNOS Cytokine-inducible nitrogen oxide synthesis A form of NOS that is activated by various immunologic stimuli, leading to an ↑ production of nitric oxide that is cytotoxic; mice lacking iNOS had ↑ susceptibility to *Leishmania major*, ↓ nonspecific response to carrageenin, and are resistant to liposaccharide-induced mortality (**Nature 1995; 375:408**)

inosine prabonex Isoprinosine AIDS A para-acetamidobenzoic salt of N,N-dimethylamino-2-propan-olo:inosine in a 3:1 molar ratio that enhances various immune functions (possibly increasing IL-1 and/or IL-2 production, resulting in T-cell proliferation and increased NK cell activity); in a trial of HIV-positive subjects, < 0.5% of those treated with IP developed AIDS vs. 4% in the placebo group (**N Engl J Med 1990; 322:1757, 322:1807ed**)

inositol A ring-shaped structure formed of 6 linked -CHOH groups, which is present in phospholipids, eg phosphoinositol, the main isomeric form of which, *myo*-inositol; it is a component of breast milk that has been reported to ↓ the complications of prematurity and ↓ death due to respiratory disease, bronchopulmonary dysplasia, and retinopathy of prematurity (**Am Med News 25 May 1992 p35**)

inositol 1,4,5-triphosphate IP$_3$ MEMBRANE PHYSIOLOGY A major and ubiquitous intracellular second messenger involved in signal transduction, which has two forms: *chiro*-inositol and *myo*-inositol that act in part by liberat-

ing calcium ions stored in cells; after an extracellular signal (hormone, neurotransmitter, inflammation, immune modulator) is received at the appropriate receptor and interacts with protein G, membrane phosphatidylinositol 4,5 biphosphate is targeted for signal-dependent hydrolysis, producing 1) IP$_3$, which mediates calcium release in an all-or-nothing fashion from the cytoplasmic membrane and mitochondria and 2) 1-2 Diacylglycerol (DAG), which activates protein kinase C, playing a key role in cell growth; IP$_3$ has high affinity binding sites and directly opens calcium channels in nanomolar concentrations, allowing amplification of signals by minute amounts of calcium; transient changes in intracellular calcium punctuate cell cycle events (eg pronuclear migration, nuclear envelope breakdown, metaphase-anaphase transition of mitosis, and cytokinesis) and appear to be driven by cyclical changes in the intracellular levels of IP$_3$ (**Nature 1994; 368:875L**) see 1,2-Diacylglycerol, Protein kinase C, Second messenger

Note: NIDDM has decreased excretion of chiro-inositol and decreased myo-inositol in the muscle, which may be related to insulin resistance (**N Engl J Med 1990; 323:373**)

inotropic agent Positive inotropic agent A therapeutic agent that increases the strength and/or force of myocardial contraction; there are two major classes of oral positive inotropic agents, those that 1) ↑ intracellular concentration of cAMP by stimulating the β-adrenergic receptor or inhibiting phosphodiesterase, eg milrinone and those that 2) ↑ intracellular sodium, eg digoxin, vesnarinone, see there

Inoue balloon CARDIOLOGY A device for performing percutaneous mitral valve commisurotomy that is becoming the preferred modality for treating mitral valve stenosis, since it is non-invasive and allows resumption of full-time employment within 1 week in contrast to the 6-8 weeks of recuperation required after an open-heart surgical procedure (**Mayo Clin Proc 1991; 66:276, 332**) see Balloon valvoplasty, percutaneous; Cf Percutaneous transluminal coronary angioplasty

inpatient *adjective* Pertaining or referring to that which occurs within a hospital setting *noun* A person who is hospitalized (**PL Fine, The Wards, Little, Brown and Co, Boston, 1994**) Cf Outpatient

INR International normalized ratio, see there

insane *adjective* Pertaining or referring to unsoundness of mind or insanity, see note, Insanity

Synonyms include balmy, bananas, batty, bonkers, chiflado, cuckoo, daffy, deranged, dippy, dotty, foaming (at the mouth), half-baked, in orbit, kooky, loco, loony, mad, mad as a hatter, mad as a March hare, meshuga, missing a few buttons, non compos mentis, not firing on all cylinders, not quite right, nuts, nutty as a fruitcake, off one's rocker, out in left field, out there, potty, raving (mad), screwy, unglued, unhinged, wacko, wacky

insanity FORENSIC PSYCHIATRY A legal and social term for a condition that renders the affected person unfit to enjoy liberty of action because of the unreliability of his behavior with concomitant danger to himself and others, denoting, by extension, a degree of mental illness that negates an individual's legal responsibility or capacity

Note: The term insanity is not sanctioned by the psychiatry community; the closest equivalent is 'psychosis', which is now preferably (per the DSM-IV, 1994) known as psychotic disorder

insanity defense FORENSIC PSYCHIATRY An argument advanced by the defense in a trial of law that seeks to explain the defendant's criminal actions with the claim that at the alleged time that the alleged act was alleged to have been perpetrated, the defendant was insane; the insanity plea is made in less than 1% of criminal trials in the US, rarely results in acquittal, and may be evoked as an act of desperation by the defense attorneys; after its successful use in the 1982 acquittal of the defendant in the assassination attempt on US President Reagan, the insanity defense fell into disfavor in the US legal system; the ID is rarely attempted, only 7% of ± 3 cases per 1000 in New

York State where the ID is used as a legal tack go to trial; the remainder result in plea bargains or are brought before a judge (New York Times 27 Nov 1994; 58) see Long Island Rail Road massacre; Cf 'Black rage' defense, Television intoxication, 'Twinkie' defense

INSERM Institut Nationale de la Santé et de la Recherche Medicale Founded in 1941 as the Institut Nationale d'Hygiene and renamed in 1964; INSERM has nine scientific commissions and is France's major medically-oriented research organization; INSERM laboratories may be freestanding, often closely proximous to affiliated hospitals; many INSERM projects overlap with CNRS, see there; Budget 1990: FF 1830 million employing 1900 researchers in 260 French research units; Cf NIH, Max Planck Institute(s), SERC

insertin An actin-capping protein that allows the barbed end of actin to maintain an equilibrium with the monomer pool, with growth still being allowed

inserting sequence BIOTECHNOLOGY A 500 base-pair segment of DNA with an inverted repeat sequence at each plus end of the DNA; inserting sequences are used in molecular biology to manipulate DNA and under natural conditions, are responsible for transferring antibiotic resistance and thus act as information 'shuttles', but are themselves incapable of autonomous existence; see Transposons

insertion The interposition of one or more nucleotides or base pairs in a chain of DNA or RNA, resulting in a 'frame shift' mutation

insertion sequence A 'jumping gene', or extra piece of DNA which, when inserted in the middle of a gene, causes inactivation of that gene; insertion sequences have been identified in bacteria (six in *Escherichia coli*), the inserted molecule contains at one end, an inverted repeat (of the other end) of several hundred to a few thousand nucleotides; ISs have no known raison d'etre and have thus been called selfish genes; Cf Transposons

insertion vector A type of lambda cloning vector that accepts DNA inserts up to 12 kb in length, which are generally used for construction of cDNA library construction; Cf Replacement vector

insertional mutation MOLECULAR BIOLOGY A generic term for any gene mutation that occurs only after one or more nucleotides has been inserted into the cognate sequence of DNA

in-service In-service training A generic term for any form of on-the-job training; in-service can be used as both a noun and as an adjective, as in, to in-service an employee

in situ carcinoma see Carcinoma in situ

in situ hybridization A method for detecting the presence of a sequence of DNA, mRNA or proteins; ISH is a three-step process in which 1) DNA from the target and the probe are denatured 2) The probe hybridizes to the target DNA 3) The amount of hybridization is measured; cells or tissues are heat- or acid-fixed on a glass slide, denatured with 70% formamide, bathed in a hybridization solution containing a label, eg 2-acetyl-aminofluorene-tagged, biotinylated or radiolabelled DNA or RNA that is complementary to the mRNA in the tissue; if present, the complementary strands hybridize in the cells or tissue, linking to their complementary strand, which may then be detected by autoradiography, then counterstained with a standard histological stain to delineate cellular, tissue or other architectural landmark; the amount of DNA probe hybridized is directly proportional to the amount of DNA complementary to the probe that is present in the specimen; see Hybridization, Immunoblotting; Cf Southern blot

in situ PCR MOLECULAR PATHOLOGY A permutation of PCR* in which the reaction occurs directly on/in a cell or tissue mounted on a glass slide; one method that is thought to enhance the reaction's specificity is the 'nested' PCR, in which there are two rounds of reaction, the first occurring in the outer flanking primers, and the second in the inner flanking primers (Bio/Technology 1995; 13:445)

*Polymerase chain reaction, which is used to amplify a segment of DNA of interest, eg HIV-1 provirus directly in cells (eg peripheral mononuclear cells) or tissues; once the target DNA has been amplified, it can be identified by conventional means, eg by in situ hybridization or immunocytochemistry; this technique is capable of detecting HIV-1-specific nucleic acids in from 1 in 5 to 1 in 100 000 cells (N Engl J Med 1992; 326:1385OA)

in situ transcription MOLECULAR BIOLOGY A technique for reverse transcription in fixed tissue where the mRNA serves as a template for complementary DNA

insomnia The inability, either perceived or actual, to sleep for the accustomed amount of time Note: 2-3% of the population either takes hypnotics or seeks consultation for sleeping disorders; see Circadian rhythm, Jet lag, REM sleep, Sleep disorders

---

INSOMNIA

CHRONOLOGIC CLASSIFICATION

TRANSIENT INSOMNIA, eg 'jet lag', which does not require treatment

SHORT TERM INSOMNIA, < 3 weeks in duration, related to travel to high altitudes, grieving the loss of a loved one, hospitalization, pain

LONG TERM INSOMNIA, > 3 weeks in duration, eg related to medical, neurologic or psychiatric disorders or addiction

ETIOLOGIC CLASSIFICATION

PHARMACOLOGIC INSOMNIA, due to ingestion of coffee, nicotine, alcohol

REBOUND (WITHDRAWAL) INSOMNIA, related to abrupt discontinuation of hypnotic drugs

DELAYED SLEEP PHASE INSOMNIA, due to shift work, chronic pain, sleep apnea and restless leg syndrome

---

InsP$_3$ Inositol 1,4,5-triphosphate, see there

inspection A generic term for an official (ie by a governmental or other regulatory agency) examination or observation of records, tests, surveys, and monitoring of procedures and operations to determine compliance with regulations, requirements, and rules of the agency of interest

inspissated milk syndrome Intestinal obstruction in infants fed either powdered or concentrated milk RADIOLOGY Dense, amorphous intraluminal masses surrounded by halos of gas TREATMENT Hydration, increasing the water in milk products

Institute of Medicine A Washington, DC-based organization founded in 1970 under the auspices of the US National Academy of Science that identifies, studies and reports on the (US) nation's major problems in medicine and the health sciences and recognizes outstanding achievements in the field of medicine

institutional abuse A generic term for physical and/or emotional abuse of an institutionalized person by his/her caregivers; IA can occur to any person in an institution including the mentally incompetent and the elderly; in one survey of nursing home staff members, 40% reported having psychologically, and 10% reported having physically abused the residents; the acts of abuse include unreasonable use of restaints, injudicious use of psychotropic medication, isolation from other nursing home residents, and failure to respect the wishes of an elderly but competent with regard to the use of medication or other intervention (N Engl J Med 1995; 332:437RA)

institutional advertising HEATH CARE MARKETING A generic term for any form of advertising of hospital and health care services to the public by an institution PHARMACEUTICAL INDUSTRY A form of 'Teaser' advertising in which a drug company is linked to a field of research; see Advertising

institutional conflict of interest A generic term for any form of financial conflict of interest in which an institution of higher learning, medical school, or hospital performs clinical research, in particular of interest to human health that has the potential for introducing bias into the results; ICIs include financial interest(s) in the form of licensing agreement(s) and/or patent(s), or an equity interest in a company that is developing a compound, process, or therapy (N Engl J Med 1995; 332:262SB)

'institutional effect' A colloquial term for biases in therapeutic decisions, diagnoses or interpretation of data that are related to guidelines or 'cut-off' values for laboratory parameters promulgated within a health care facility or hospital (JAMA 1991; 265:97) see Referral bias

institutional review board BIOMEDICAL ETHICS A group of physicians and lay persons at a hospital who debate and approve or reject clinical research projects prior to their initiations; the IRB in a university hospital or academic health care facility that is specifically charged with ensuring the safety and well-being of human subjects involved in research projects at the institution; the existence of an IRB is required by US federal regulations operating under the Department of Health and Human Services; research proposals require that

1) The risks to individuals are minimized

2) The risks are reasonable in relation to the anticipated benefits

3) The selection of individuals is equitable

4) Informed consent is obtained and documented from the subject or his legal representative

5) There are provisions for maintaining the individual's privacy and

6) There are safeguards that prevent undue influence on vulnerable subjects by nature of educational or economic disadvantage or by dint of severe illness

see Ethics committee, Helsinki Declaration, Nuremburg code

institutionalization 'syndrome' SOCIAL MEDICINE The constellation of psychological changes that occurs in individuals who have been maintained in segregated communities, eg mental institutions, state-run nursing homes CLINICAL Apathy, dependence, depersonalization and retreat from reality Note: This complex is similar, if not identical, to 'shelterization', described in homeless persons; see Homeless(ness), Shelterization; Cf Survivor syndrome

instrumental activities of daily living A series of life functions necessary for maintaining a person's immediate environment, including obtaining food, cooking, laundering, housecleaning, managing one's own medications, use of the telephone; IADL is a measure of a person's (elderly, mentally handicapped or terminally ill) ability to live independently

instrumental variables estimation An analytical method that addresses the selection bias inherent in observational studies; IV methods have been used in econometrics but are essentially untested in estimating the relationships between medical therapy and outcomes; instrumental variables are observable factors that influence treatment but do not directly affect outcomes, thus mimicking the randomization of patients to the different probabilities of receiving alternative therapies ; the method differs from randomized trials in that the randomization is not deliberate, and because the groups being

compared differ only in probabilities of being treated, the method estimates a marginal or incremental effect only over the range of the variation in treatment across the IV groups (see JAMA 1994; 272:859OA)

insulin A disulfide-linked polypeptide hormone produced by the pancreatic islet β cells that stimulates the expression of genes encoding glyceraldehyde-3-phosphate dehydrogenase, c-Fos, glucokinase and α-amylase and inhibits expression of phosphoenolpyruvate carboxykinase, see PEPCK MECHANISM OF ACTION Unknown; it appears to act via serine protein kinases, eg insulin receptor serine kinase, acetyl CoA carboxylase kinase, microtubule associated protein-2 (MAP-2) kinase, protein kinase C, Raf-1, myelin basic protein kinase; insulin activates type 1 protein phosphatases that control glycogen metabolism, by phosphorylating (or dephosphorylating) specific serine residues

insulin-dependent diabetes mellitus IDDM Juvenile, type I, or 'brittle' diabetes mellitus, which is the more severe form of DM; it is caused by a deficit in endogenous insulin production and comprises about 10% of diabetes mellitus GENETICS IDDM is more common in HLA-DR3, DR4-positive subjects; concordance between identical twins is 55% CLINICAL Extreme hyperglycemia, lability of glucose control and ketosis; IDDM of recent onset may have IgG autoantibodies directed against glucose transport proteins; see Honeymoon period; Cf NIDDM

insulin-like growth factor-I IGF-I, see there

insulin-like growth factor-II IGF-II, see there

insulin pump Insulin infusion device A generic term for any device used to delivery insulin in a timed fashion to a diabetic; the basic components of the artificial 'pancreas' are an insulin reservoir, a pump, a power source, electronic controls, and a glucose sensor; currently available insulin pumps are either portable or implantable; portable pumps weigh < 100 g, deliver 0.7-2.0 U/hour, and have battery lives of 1-4 months; implantable pumps are powered by vapor pressure and are FDA-approved for infusing heparin, and chemotherapeutic agents, and have either a single rate program or are programmable (Lab Med 1992; 23:652) a wait-and-see policy prevails; Cf Biohybrid artificial pancreas, Islet cell transplantation

insulin receptor A heterodimeric membrane receptor composed of α and β chains that has tyrosine kinase activity after binding insulin; receptor deficiency is an uncommon cause of diabetes mellitus and may be due to a gene rearrangement, causing a deletion in the tyrosine kinase domain, a point mutation with a loss of the ATP binding site or other genetic defect

insulin-regulatable glucose transporter A protein expressed in muscle and fat that migrates from the cytoplasm to plasma membrane in response to insulin, resulting in increased intracellular transport of glucose

insulin resistance A suboptimal response hypoglycemic response to physiological levels of insulin, which may be due to local allergic reaction to insulin, acute exacerbation of chronic leukemia, and DKA; insulin resistance (as measured by oral GTT, and hyperinsulinemia) is a risk factor for developing NIDDM (N Engl J Med 1993; 329:1988OA); IR may also be due to increased circulating glucagon or a relative insulin receptor deficiency, where plasma insulin is high relative to glucose; in uremia, IR may be due to non-specific receptor antagonism, as the insulin binds poorly to receptors and hypocalcemia increases proinsulin secretion (table); defects in glycogen synthesis are pivotal in the insulin-resistance of non-insulin-dependent diabetes mellitus (NIDDM), as muscle glycogen synthesis is the main pathway of glucose disposal in normal and diabetic subjects; see Subcutaneous insulin-resistance syndrome; Cf Syndrome X

TYPE A 'PRE-RECEPTOR' PHASE IR, related to defects in synthesis and secretion of insulin, seen in the HAIR-IN syndrome, with hyperandrogenism (to a degree suggesting hyperthecosis, ovarian neoplasia, or polycystic ovaries), which is of pubertal onset, with ↑ levels of endogenous insulin, overt DM and resistance to exogenous insulin, related to anti-insulin antibodies

TYPE B 'RECEPTOR' PHASE IR, related to decreased insulin binding to receptors, ↓ number of receptors, or to marked insulin resistance, which may be associated with acanthosis nigricans, autoimmune disease, and overt DM due to circulating anti-receptor antibodies

TYPE C 'POST-RECEPTOR' PHASE IR, related to defects arising after the insulin-receptor complex has formed, eg a defect in the cascade that follows receptor-ligand interaction

insulin sensitivity The systemic responsiveness to glucose, which can be measured by 1) The insulin sensitivity index, which measures the ability of endogenous insulin to ↓ glucose in extracellular fluids by inhibiting glucose release from the liver and stimulating the peripheral consumption of glucose, and 2) The glucose-clamp technique, which measures the effect of changes in insulin concentration on glucose clearance (glucose uptake rate divided by plasma glucose concentration) per unit of body surface area (N Engl J Med 1994; 331:1188OA)

insulin sensitivity index An index that represents the ability of endogenous insulin to reduce glucose in the extracellular fluid by inhibiting the release of glucose from the liver and stimulating the peripheral consumption of glucose; it is calculated from plasma insulin and glucose values after IV administration of glucose

insulin shock A rarely observed clinical event in which excess insulin is administered, causing profound hypoglycemia to levels below that required for normal brain function, causing anxiety, delirium, convulsions, coma and death

insulinogenic index The ratio of insulin to glucose, a commonly used measure of the impact of meals on subjects with diabetic potential

insult CLINICAL MEDICINE A generic term for any stressful stimulus, which under normal circumstances does not affect the host organism, but which may result in morbidity when it occurs in a background of preexisting compromising conditions; the term most commonly refers to an acute hypoxic episode in a patient with underlying atherosclerosis, who may suffer such 'insults' as a transient ischemic attack of the brain (a 'stroke'), angina or an acute MI

int-1 A recently reclassified proto-oncogene, see *wnt-1*

integral membrane proteins Any transmembrane protein that is so intimately linked to a biological membrane that it cannot be removed without disruption of the phospholipid bilayer membrane itself, eg the Rh antigens of red cells

integrase A bacteriophage enzyme that creates and resolves Holliday junctions, which are present in a form of genetic recombination

integrated circuit COMPUTERS A semiconductor circuit that contains two or more transistors or other electronic devices or components

integration The insertion of a variable number of base pairs (or bases) into a nucleic acid, either DNA (or RNA)

integrin 'RGD superfamily' CELL BIOLOGY The major family of cell surface receptors that mediate attachment to the extracellular marix; some also mediate critical cell-cell adhesive interactions (Science 1995; 268:233); integrins are a family of more than 15 cell surface adhesion receptors composed of heterodimeric (α and β subunits) membrane-spanning glycoproteins that recognize the tripeptide, arginine-glycine-aspartic acid (occasionally serine), known as the RGD sequence on the β subunit, which acts as a receptor recognition signal; integrins mediate cell binding to major components of the extracellular matrix; integrins are subdivided based on differences in the β subunit, which confers specificity, acting as receptors for collagens, fibronectin, fibrinogen, platelet glycoprotein IIb-IIIa, laminin, LFA-1, Mac-1, osteospondin, p150,95, thrombospondin, VLA1-6 (very late antigens 1 to 6), vitronectin and von Willebrand factor; this group and their receptors constitute a recognition system critical in cell anchorage, traction for migration, signals for polarity, position, differentiation, growth, phagocytosis, platelet aggregation and complement binding; the receptors are intracellular and anchored to cytoplasmic proteins (actin, talin, ankyrin, vincullin, fibroconnexin) integrin $\alpha_V\beta_3$ is required for angiogenesis (Science 1994; 264:569R) Cf RGD family

Note: Absence of the β subunit (LFA-1, and Mac-1) results in leukocyte adhesion deficiency syndrome; the $\beta1$ subfamily (VLA proteins) mediates cell binding to collagen (VLA-1, -2, -3), fibronectin (VLA-3, -4 and -5) and laminin (VLA-1, -2, -6)

integrin $\alpha_2\beta_1$ Glycoprotein Ia/IIa

integrin $\alpha_5\beta_1$ Glycoprotein Ic/IIa

integrin $\alpha_{IIb}\beta_3$ Glycoprotein IIb/IIIa

integrin family of leukocyte adhesive proteins see CD11/CD18 family

integrin-mediated adhesive interaction CELL BIOLOGY A generic term for any interaction between integrins (*vide supra*), a major family of cell surface receptors and the proteins of the extracellular matrix; IMAIs mediate critical cell-cell interactions involved in the regulation of embryonic development, tumor cell growth, hemostasis, leukocyte homing (to targets), clot retraction, and the response of cells to mechanical stress (Science 1995; 268:233) see Integrin-mediated adhesive interactions

intellectual property A type of intangible property that cannot be touched as it has no physical evidence of its existence, which includes patents, copyrights, trademarks, registered designs, and trade secrets (Nature 1993; 364:659N)

intelligent terminal 'Smart' terminal, see there

intensity of care An ordinal measure of the number, technical complexity, or technical risk of health care services provided to a patient; in the US, IoC has increased because 1) Fee-for-service form of reimbursement encourages the production of reimbursable services 2) Fear of malpractice claims increases the intensity of care 3) New forms of technology are generally more expensive 4) Intensity of care is a product of an aggressive medical culture 5) Medical standards of practice are heavily weighted toward specialization, which is the result of an oversupply of specialists (N Engl J Med 1992; 327:424SB)

intensification ONCOLOGY A generic term for any strategy for administering chemotherapy that is more aggressive than a previous standard; intensification is thought to be responsible for the improved survival in children with acute lymphoblastic (lymphocytic) leukemia (N Engl J Med 1993; 329:1289OA) and may be of use in acute myeloid (myelocytic) leukemia (ibid 1994; 331:896OA, 941ED)

interactive (digitizing) morphometry The quantification of various cytologic parameters, eg nuclear contour or nuclear area, by inputting data points into a computer via a graphic interface; IM is in a nascent stage of development, and the methods used to collect data (eg zone sampling and the systematic randon sampling) have not been standardized (see Anal Quan Cytol Histol 1993; 15:281)

interactive video see Shared decision program

intercalated duct carcinoma Epithelial-myoepithelial carcinoma, see there

intercalation The interposition of a flat molecule between two adjacent nucleotides in the DNA double helix, eg ethidium bromide, which generates positive superhelical turns in closed circular DNA molecules, or acridine orange, which results in frameshift mutations; see Acridine Orange, Ethidium bromide

intercellular signaling The up– and/or down regulation (ie 'communication') among cells in multicellular organisms, which is mediated by either direct cell-to-cell contact, or by soluble signaling molecules including hormones, eicosanoids, neurotransmitters, and cytokines (Perspect Biol & Med 1993; 36:611) Cf Intracellular signaling

'interesting' disease A generic term for any clinical or pathologic nosology that is rare, difficult to diagnose, challenging to treat, poorly understood pathogenically, or any combination of the above

Note: When a lesion is characterized by pathologists as 'interesting', it often implies a poor prognosis

interface CHEMISTRY A boundary, eg between two phases, as in a solid-liquid COMPUTERS An electronic circuit that controls the connection between two hardware devices allowing them to reliably exchange data

interface driver Gateway, see there

interface engine Gateway, see there

interference Cross-over effect GENETICS The effect that the crossing over of a chromosome at one locus has on the frequency of cross-over at another locus, termed positive interference if the frequency is decreased and negative interference if the frequency is increased

interference microscopy A type of light microscopy that is used to examine unstained, transparent, or reflecting specimens; in IM, the light is affected by the meeting of wavelengths that enhance or attenuate interference; the incident and diffracted waves of light from a single light source are recombined at the image plane, where the interference causes differences in refraction and light transmission becomes visible, as optical path differences in the object being viewed are converted into differences in the intensity of the image; the image produced is similar, but superior to that produced in a phase-contrast microscope; see Microscopy

interferon Any of a family of immune regulatory proteins (immunomodulators) produced by T cells, fibroblasts and other cells in response to double-stranded DNA, viruses, mitogens, antigens or lectins; IFNs increase the bactericidal, viricidal and tumoricidal activities of macrophages (JAMA 1991; 266:1375rv); most of the more than 20 IFNs are alpha type, one beta, one gamma, and recently omega and tau; IFN-α and IFN-β are known as type I interferons as both are growth inhibitory cytokines whose biological activities depend on induced changes in gene expression; type I IFNs are composed of a single chain of amino acids; they induce infected cells to produce proteins that inhibit the proliferation of viruses and cells; virtually any virally infected cell can produce IFN-α; fibroblasts are the main producer of IFN-β; type II IFN (ie IFN-γ) is produced by T lymphocytes and natural killer (NK) cells and consists of a dimer of two identical amino acid chains unrelated to the type I amino acid sequence; IFN-γ promotes activity by components of the immune system that eradicate tumors and infection in culture; (Sci Am 1994; 270/5:68) see MAF and MIF

interferon-alpha IFN-α A family of leukocyte-derived immunomodulating glycoproteins, numbering 13 at last count, which have antiproliferative and antiviral activity, the gene for which is located on the short arm of chromosome 9 and the receptor on the long arm of chromosome 21 THERAPEUTIC INDICATIONS Recombinant IFN-α has been used to treat hairy cell leukemia, CML[1], Kaposi sarcoma, HPV-related epithelial proliferations, eg condyloma acuminatum, respiratory papillomatosis and pulmonary hemangioendotheliosis; IFN-α induces prolonged clinical and histologic remission in ⅓ of patients with chronic hepatitis, eg hepatitis C[2] and may be used to treat renal cell carcinoma, either alone or in combination with vinblastine, yielding a 21% response rate and the osteoclastic lesions may regress (N Engl J Med 1991; 324:633c) and NHL[3]; IFN-α2b 3x/week x 18 months results in significant histologic reversal and serum ALA response in patients with chronic non-A, non-B hepatitis (N Engl J Med 1995; 332:1457oa) SIDE EFFECTS Flu-like symptoms, malaise, fatigue, headache, anxiety, vertigo and depression, increased aminotransferase, bone marrow suppression (granulocyte toxicity), supraventricular tachyarrhythmia with hypotension or hypertension and potentially fatal congestive heart failure, exacerbation of multiple sclerosis; ½ of cases, especially those with cirrhosis and hypersplenism don't tolerate therapy as it causes fatigue, profound thrombocytopenia and neutropenia

[1]Chronic myelocytic leukemia Use of IFN-α-2a combined with donor mononuclear cells may induce remission, offering an alternative to a second bone marrow transplantation in CML (N Engl J Med 1994; 330:100oa); Philadelphia chromosome-positive CML treated with IFN-α-2a has more karyotypic responses, a lower rate of disease progression, and prolonged overall survival than a matched population treated with conventional chemotherapy, ie hydroxyurea or busulfan (N Engl J Med 1994; 330:820oa) [2]Hepatitis C The response of HCV-associated cryoglobulinemia to IFN-α-2a is a function of the titers of HCV (N Engl J Med 1994; 330:51oa) [3]Non-Hodgkin's lymphoma Addition of IFN-α to the COPA (cyclophosphamide, vincristine-Oncovorin, prednisone, doxorubicin-Adriamycin) protocol is reported to ↓ treatment failures (61% in COPA alone, 38% IFN-α-COPA), and ↑ overall and disease-survival (87% and 71% with IFN-α-COPA vs79% and 46% with COPA alone (N Engl J Med 1992; 327:1336oa) Addition of IFN-α-2b to protocol, eg CHVP (cyclophosphamide, doxorubicin, teniposide, prednisone) containing doxorubicin is associated with an ↑ rate of response- and event-free, and overall survival, although some patients were unable to tolerate IFN-α-2b's side effects (N Engl J Med 1993; 329:1608oa)

interferon-beta FIbroblast interferon IFN-β A 20-kD protein with anti-viral activity that has 30% 'homology' with interferon-α, is encoded on chromosome 9 and produced by fibroblasts in response to viruses or polyribonucleotides

interferon-gamma IFN-γ A 21–25-kD glycoprotein lymphokine encoded on chromosome 12q, consisting of a heterodimeric protein with six α helices in each chain (Science 1991; 252:698) that is produced by activated T and NK cells; IFN-γ is antiviral, regulating the expression of class II MHC antigens, Fc receptors and immunoglobulin production and class switching, activates monocyte cytotoxicity and enhances NK cell activity; IFN-γ is ↓ in IgA deficiency, lymphoma, CLL, infections (eg CMV, EBV, rubella, lepromatous leprosy, and TB), SLE, rheumatoid arthritis, sickle cell anemia, post-transplantation THERAPEUTIC INDICATIONS Recombinant IFN-γ is used to treat giant condylomata acuminata, CLL, Hodgkin's disease, mycosis fungoides, rheumatoid arthritis and may be of use in treating leprosy, TB, toxoplasmosis and chronic granulomatous disease (to prevent infections); IFN-γ suppresses collagen synthesis by fibroblasts, reduces the size of keloids, causing a local ↑ in inflammatory cells and mucin production, and may be of use in controlling abnormal fibrosing conditions SIDE EFFECTS Acute renal failure, rash, headache, chills; IFN-γ receptor is encoded on chromosome 6q; may be of use in treating nontuberculous *Mycobacterium* infection (N Engl J Med 1994; 330:1348oa)

interferon-stimulated response element A *cis*-acting DNA element encoded by genes transcribed when interferon-α interacts with its membrane receptor, a signal thought to be mediated through arachidonic acid metabolism (Science 1991; 251:204)

'interim' methadone treatment A form of administration of methadone for heroin addicts, in which the drug is provided with minimal service to the ex-addict; this became necessary given the lack of funds and manpower combined with the finding that effective methadone maintenance is associated with a reduced incidence of HIV infection

interleukin(s) A family of cytokines produced by lymphocytes, monocytes and other cells that induce growth and differentiation of lymphoid cells and primitive hematopoietic stem cells Note: The integration of the 'short' form, IL, is virtually complete, and is only placed in alphabetical order to adhere to lexicographic convention; see Biological response modifiers, Tumor necrosis factor

IL-1 Leukocyte-activating factor An 11-kD cytokine produced by monocytes, B, NK, endothelial, epithelial, microglial, mesangial and antigen-presenting cells, fibroblasts and large granular lymphocytes, as well as by malignancies, eg AML (FAB M3, FAB M4), squamous cell carcinoma, Hodgkin's disease, and melanoma; IL-1 elicits the acute phase response, acts on the CNS as a pyrogen, stimulates fibroblast, B- and T-cell proliferation and differentiation, and ↑ lymphokine, collagenase and prostaglandin production; IL-1 ↑ the activity of NK cells against tumor targets, stimulates myocytolysis (via prostaglandins), elicits hormone release from the pituitary gland (including ACTH, LH, GH and TSH release and prolactin inhibition, via corticotropin-releasing factor), evokes the release of PMNs from the BM, and PMN degranulation, ↑ oxidase activity and hexose monophosphate shunt activity; in synovial cells, IL-1 stimulates proliferation and production of collagen, prostaglandin and plasminogen activator; IL-1 production is stimulated by various agents, eg calcium ionophores, IFN-α, IFN-γ, lipopolysaccharides, muramyl dipeptide, aluminum hydroxide, phorbol myristate acetate, staphylococci, silica and others and inhibited by corticosteroids, prostaglandin E_2 (acting via the cyclooxygenase pathway), suppressor T cells, cyclosporin (which specifically inhibits T cell-induced IL-1 production) IL-1 and disease; IL-1 may have a role in 1) IDDM, increased IL-1 production by macrophages occurs in the early β-cell destructive lesions of IDDM 2) Atherosclerosis (n-3 fish oils reduce circulating IL-1) and 3) Rheumatoid arthritis, where IL-1 acts in conjunction with substance P

IL-1α THERAPEUTIC USES Oncology IL-1α is reportedly effective in accelerating the recovery of the platelet counts after high-dose carboplatin and may be useful in thrombocytopenia induced by other chemotherapeutic agents (N Engl J Med 1993; 328:756OA)

IL-1 receptor IL-1 mediates its action on target cells by high-affinity receptors on fibroblast and T-cell membranes; receptor expression may be ↑ by prostaglandins and glucocorticoids; it binds both IL-1α and IL-1β and has 319 extracellular amino acid residues with 3 immunoglobulin-like domains, a transmembrane region and a 217-residue cytoplasmic 'tail'; other IL receptors (IL-2 β chain, IL-3, IL-4, IL-6) and erythropoietin share a common structural motif

IL-2 T-cell growth factor A 15-kD glycoprotein that is produced at low baseline levels by the CD4 T (helper) cells; after presentation of antigen by antigen-presenting cells, accompanied by IL-1, T cell production of IL-2 and IL-2 receptor (IL-2Rβ) on the membrane increases, peaks at 6 hours and falls to baseline levels; IL-2 is also produced by medullary thymocytes and a subset of large granular lymphocytes, the NK cell activators; IL-2 up-regulates the immune system, causing lymphokine-activated killer (LAK) cells to lyse tumor cells, see IL-2/LAK cells SIDE EFFECTS IL-2 requires weeks of intensive care due to toxic effects, including a 'capillary leakage syndrome', malaise, gastritis, GI symptoms, anemia, thrombocytopenia, rigors,

fever, hypotension, azotemia, jaundice, hyperbilirubinemia, rash (erythroderma globalis), confusion, ascites, fluid retention, pruritus, agitation, respiratory insufficiency, cardiac failure and irreversible demyelinization and hypothyroidism; see IL-2/LAK cells

Note: Cytotoxic T lymphocytes (CTLs), when incubated with certain MHC Class II molecules, eg HLA-DR may down-regulate their lytic activity; IL-2 causes antigen-activated B cells to progress through the cell cycle and differentiate into antibody secreting cells, actions carried out by a receptor-transduction 'complex'

IL-2 receptor A heterodimer of 75-kD β and 55-kD α (aka CD25, or Tac antigen) chains that is transiently expressed on T cells, induced by IL-2, TNF, IL-1, IL-4 and IL-6; IL-2R enhances lymphokine production and protein kinase C activation, and is up to 6-fold ↑ in Kawasaki's disease, a condition causing mucocutaneous erythema, fever and cardiac damage; the critical signal for IL-2R activity is phosphoryation of the IL-2Rβ chain by the *src*-family protein tyrosine kinase p56^{lck}, the activity of which is initiated by IL-2 stimulation of T cells (Science 1991; 252:1523)

IL-2/LAK cells Interleukin-2/Lymphokine-activated killer cells NK cells that have been activated by co-incubating in IL-2 and injected into cancer patients in a therapeutic modality known as adoptive immunotherapy, which may evoke temporary tumor regression in non-Hodgkin's lymphoma, melanoma, colorectal carcinoma, and renal cell carcinoma, and induce regression of hepatic and pulmonary metastases; IL-2/LAK cells are in experimental protocol for treating advanced renal cell carcinoma (partial remission 15%, complete remission 4%) and malignant melanoma COMPLICATIONS The typical transient defect in neutrophil chemotaxis may explain the high morbidity typical of IL-2/LAK therapy ADVERSE EFFECTS Pulmonary edema, congestive heart failure

IL-3 A lymphokine* produced by activated CD4 T (helper) cells and others that bind to high- and low-affinity receptors, inducing tyrosine phosphorylation, promoting colony formation of multiple (erythroid, megakaryocytic, myeloid and lymphoid) hematopoietic lineages, mast cell proliferation and histamine release; IL-3 induces 20-α-hydroxysteroid dehydrogenase, assisting T-cell maturation; the IL-3 gene is on the long arm of chromosome 5

*Synonyms include burst-promoting activity, hematopoietin, mast cell growth factor, multi-CSF, multi-colony stimulating factor, P cell stimulating factor, T-cell stimulating factor, WEH1-3 growth factor

IL-4 A 20-kD cytokine produced by T helper cells and mast cells that is co-mitogenic for B cells and thymocytes, activates macrophages and stimulates hematopoiesis; IL-4 competes with IL-2 at its receptor in the transduction pathway, possibly altering the signal of whether a lymphocyte will mature to synthesize pentameric IgM or monomeric IgG1 or IgE

IL-5 An 18-kD cytokine produced by CD4+ T lymphocytes that co-stimulates B cell proliferation and differentiation and IgA class switching; IL-3 and IL-5 may function in concert to potentiate production of eosinophils via eosinophil-colony stimulating factor

IL-6 IFN-β-2 A 26-kD cytokine* that mediates host response to injury and infection and plays a role in growth and differentiation of B cells, T cells, myeloma-plasmacytomas, hepatocytes, hematopoietic stem cells and nerve cells; the presence of IL-6 in psoriatic plaques suggests a pathogenic role in that condition; IL-6 is critical for the development of IgA-related immunity; targeted disruption of the IL-6 gene in mice (knock-out approach) blunts IgA responsiveness to immunological challenges (Science 1994; 264:561R, 485R); IL-6 is a major mediator of the acute phase response (APR), stimulating hepatic production of APR proteins (Perspect Biol & Med 1993; 36:611)

*Synonyms include B-cell differentiation factor, B-cell stimulatory factor-2, BSF-2, cytotoxic T-cell differentiating factors, hepatocyte stimulating factor,

hybridoma/plasmacytoma growth factor, IFN-β_2, interferon-β_2, 26-kD protein, MGI-2A

IL-6 receptor A membrane receptor that measures 468 amino acid residues and is homologous to an immunoglobulin domain (constant 2) Note: IL-6, nerve growth factor and growth hormone have no tyrosine kinase domains, and thus process extracellular signals by a less well understood mechanism

IL-7 A 152-aa monomeric protein produced by the stromal cells of the BM (and fetal hepatocytes); IL-7 is a lymphopoietic factor, converting stem cells into early pre-T, as well as B cells, and promoting the growth of pre-B and pro-B cells, proliferation of T cells, and the proliferation, cytotoxic activity, and generation of LAK and cytotoxic T cells; it is active in primitive lymphocytic leukemias

IL-8 A dimeric protein[1] with 69, 72, 77, or 79 amino acids, which is produced by most cells[2] that targets T cells, as well as neutrophils, up-regulating the binding activity of leukocyte adhesion receptor CD11b/CD18; IL-8 dynamically regulates its own receptor (CR1) expression on neutrophils, and is chemotactic for basophils, neutrophils, and T cells; it activates neutrophils to release lysosomal enzymes, induces neutrophil-endothelial cell adhesion, and induces neutrophil change in shape change, chemotaxis, granule release, and respiratory burst by binding to receptors of the seven transmembrane segment class[3] (**Science 1994; 264:90oA**); IL-8 is antiviral, antiproliferative and immunomodulatory, inhibiting neutrophil adhesion to cytokine-activated endothelial cells, preventing neutrophil-mediated damage

[1]Synonyms include leukocyte adhesion inhibitor, MDNCF, monocyte-derived neutrophil chemotactic factor, NAF, NAP-1, neutrophil attractant/activating factor, neutrophil attractant/activating protein-1 [2]Chondrocytes, endothelial cells, epithelial cells, fibroblasts, hepatocytes, keratinocytes, monocytes, neutrophils, and T cells [3]A class of molecules best known as 'heptaspans' (see **Nature 1994; 369:270c**)

IL-9 A 126-aa monomeric glycoprotein cytokine produced by T cells and B cells, megakaryocytes, and mast cells that enhances T-cell and mast cell survival, and acts synergistically with erythropoietin to enhance the development of erythroid burst-forming units by the bone marrow; IL-9 has been isolated from a megakaryoblastic leukemia, expressed in several human T cell lines and in mitogen-stimulated peripheral lymphocytes; IL-9 is structurally and functionally related to mast cell growth-enhancing activity, and its gene maps to chromosomes 5 and 13

IL-10 A 160-aa homodimer produced by macrophages, B cells, and keratinocytes that suppresses macrophage functions, eg production of inflammatory cytokines by activated monocytes/macrophages, and enhances B-cell proliferation and immunoglobulin secretion; IL-10 is also produced by TH1 helper T cells and inhibits the synthesis of IFN-γ by activated helper T cells and stimulates mast cell precursors (**J Exp Med 1991; 173:507**); in mice, IL-10 is produced by B-cell lymphomas and normal B cells; first identified in mice, the predicted IL-10 structure has extensive homology with an open reading frame (BCRFI) in the EBV genome and with the EBV virus protein BCRF1

IL-11 A 178-aa monomeric lymphopoietic and hematopoietic cytokine produced by stromal fibroblasts, trophoblastic cells (? also by B cells, megakaryocytes, and mast cells); IL-11 acts synergistically with IL-3 and IL-4 to shorten the G_0 period of early hematopoietic cells, with IL-3 to ↑ the size, number, and ploidy value of megakaryocytic colonies, and stimulates the synthesis of hepatic acute-phase proteins (see **Arch Pathol Lab Med 1994; 118:417RV**)

IL-12 A heterodimeric* cytokine produced by B cells and macrophages that is critical in inducing the Th1 response through the differentiation of uncommitted T cells, and capable of dampening the Th2 response; in absence of T cells, IL-12 stimulates the growth and function of NK and T cells and may have a therapeutic role in enhancing

immune-defenses against parasites, malignancy, and immunodeficiencies, eg AIDS (**Science News 1994; 146:120**, see**Arch Pathol Lab Med 1994; 118:417RV**) IL-12 has potential as a therapeutic agent as in addition to an array of 'usual' immune regulatory activities, IL-12 is antiangiogenic, and thus has potential in treating cancer, as tumors without a blood supply cannot survive (**J Folkman, et al, JNCI, May 1995**)

*Composed of a p35 (197-aa) monomer produced by many cells and a p40 (306-aa) monomer produced by macrophages and B cells

IL-13 A 132-aa monomeric cytokine produced by T cells that enhances B-cell growth and differentiation of inflammatory cytokines by mo/mas

IL-14 A 468 aa monomeric cytokine produced by T cells that induces the proliferation of activated B cells, and inhibits Ig secretion from mitogen-activated B cells

IL-15 A cytokine produced by a wide variety of cells (eg peripheral blood mononuclear cells, epithelial and fibroblast cell lines) and tissues (especially placenta and skeletal muscle, but also heart, kidneys, liver, and lung) stimulates the proliferation of T lymphocytes; IL-15 interacts with the β chain of the IL-2 receptor and has some IL-2-like properties (**Science 1994; 264:965oA**)

interlocking OBSTETRICS A rare (estimated to occur in 1 in 817 twin gestations) complication of vaginal delivery of twins, where the first twin presents in breech and descends 'locking' his head above the head of the second twin in vertex presentation; if the second baby is already in the pelvis, loss of the first baby is almost inevitable and interventional decapitation of the first infant may be necessary to salvage the second infant, an event that virtually never occurs as the vast majority of twin gestations are delivered by cesarean section prior to the spontaneous onset of labor Note: there are rare cases of salvage of both twins by either epidural anesthesia and cesarean section or use of β-sympathomimetic drugs; Cf Selective termination

intermediate body The final stage of the development of *Chlamydia trachomatis* infection, comprised of reticulate bodies that have molded themselves in a perinuclear fashion and become septated; see Elementary bodies

intermediate care facility An institution providing the minimal health care and services required for mental or physically handicapped individuals; Cf Hospice, Nursing home, Shelter, Tertiary care center

intermediate cells Primitive cells described in neonatal and infant intestines, in and adjacent to colonic inflammation and seen in adult small intestinal neoplasia, which stain positively for Paneth cell granules within goblet cells

intermediate density lipoprotein see IDL

intermediate filaments A diverse group of abundant, cell lineage-specific intracellular filaments that are seen by EM, which measure 7-11 nm in diameter, a size intermediate between the 6-nm actin microfilaments and the 25-nm microtubules; IFs have considerable (40-70%) sequence similarity ('homology') with each other and differ according to embryologic origin, which can be determined by the cells with monoclonal antibodies raised against each filament; epithelial cells produce 40–68-kD cytokeratin IF, muscle cells produce 53-kD desmin IF, mesenchymal cells produce 55-kD vimentin IF, glial cells produce 55-kD glial fibrillary acidic (astrocytic) protein IF and neurons produce 68–100-kD neurofilament Note: Primitive cells may be negative for all IFs or may express more than one IF, as malignant cells dedifferentiate and 'forget' their cell lineage; such co-expression of IFs is not uncommon in sarcomas, which may co-express vimentin and desmin, eg mesothelioma, synovial and epithelioid sarcomas; malignant tumors, eg renal cell, ovarian, lung, endometrial, anaplastic, thyroid carcinomas, as well as benign tumors, eg pleomorphic adenomas may co-express vimentin and cytokeratin

intermediate-impact sport Moderate impact sport, see there

intermediate-grade lymphoma Any of a group of lymphomas of intermediate aggression that are classified according to the Working Formulation (Cancer 1982; 49:2112), which have survival periods between the indolent low-grade lymphomas (survival 5 to 7.5 years) and the aggressive high-grade lymphomas (survival less than one year); intermediate lymphomas include the follicular predominantly large cell lymphoma, diffuse small cleaved lymphoma, diffuse mixed large and small cell lymphoma with epithelioid cells (Lennert lymphoma) and diffuse large cell cleaved and non-cleaved cell lymphoma; see Lymphoma, Working Formulation

intermediate lymphocytic lymphoma Mantle-zone lymphoma, see there

intermediate syndrome CLINICAL TOXICOLOGY A clinical complex due to organophosphorus insecticide poisoning, so-called as it is neither acute, which is associated with neurotoxic symptoms nor delayed, ie occurring 2-3 weeks after exposure, which is associated with chronic distal motor polyneuropathy; as the symptoms occur in a 'window period', they are relatively unexpected CLINICAL 10% of those exposed develop paralysis of the cranial motor nerves, proximal limb, cervical flexor and respiratory muscles; onset, 1-4 days after a cholinergic phase PROGNOSIS Less than 5% of those exposed develop the condition, possibly due to a neuromuscular junction defect

intern A term essentially equivalent in context to 'apprentice', used in North America for a graduate of a medical, osteopathic or dental school who is serving his first year (an 'internship') of graduate clinical training, usually in a teaching hospital; following internship, the physician may then enter private practice (a route chosen by few physicians) or enter a period of post-graduate education, ie residency training; see GME; Cf CME, Extern, Fellow, Internist

Note: The term has been widely used in other fields and may refer to virtually any period of training that follows the closure of a period of formal education

internal standard INSTRUMENTATION A standardized, stable and constant substance added to a chromatographic (GLC or HPLC) sample that neither interferes with nor has a molecule 'signature' overlapping that of the molecular species being analyzed, serving as a positive 'control'; see Blanks, Control, Quality control

internal version OBSTETRICS A transvaginal procedure that attempts to convert a difficult fetal presentation to a vaginally deliverable situation by hand-rotating the fetus in utero; Cf External version

Note: In the US, given the high potential for litigation should an internal version 'go sour' and compromise the fetus, most obstetricians prefer to perform an elective cesarean section rather than risk a potentially complicated delivery

international medical graduate Foreign medical graduate A physician (medical doctor, MD) who has graduated from a non-North American (ie Canada or US) medical school; there has been a long tradition of not unjustified (given the generally acknowledged differences in standards of education) discrimination against IMGs; recently Canada has examined measures to limit IMGs access to residency training positions (Am Med News 2 November 1992, p 10); US and Canadian-trained students had a pass rate in the US Medical Licensing Examination of 85%; foreign citizens trained in foreign schools had a pass rate of 37%, and USFMGs had a 23% pass rate (JAMA 1995; 273:1162MN&P); although the hope is that IMGs might add to the pool of generalists, the pattern of specialization among IMGs is similar to that of American medical graduates (JAMA 1995; 273:1521OA) see Off-shore medical school, USFMG

international normalized ratio HEMATOLOGY INR A way to report prothrombin time (PT) results for patients on oral anticoagulant therapy; the INR is defined by the formula $(PT_{Patient}/PT_{MNPT})^{ISI}$* that uses the international sensitivity index to adjust the PT results from thromboplastin of different sources and offers a means of monitoring anticoagulant therapy when using more than one laboratory and of comparing a patient's PT results with published standards for treatment (CAP Today March 1993; Arch Pathol Lab Med 1993; 117:602OA; ibid, 1994; 118:110) see International sensitivity index

*PT_{MNPT} = mean of the PT reference interval; ISI = international sensitivity index

International Classification of Disease, 9th edition, Clinical Modification ICD-9-CM, see there

International Red Cross & Red Crescent Movement Red Cross, see there

international relief organization An organization, often non-governmental, dedicated to the provision of humanitarian (ie nonmilitary) relief, eg CARE (Cooperative for American Relief Everywhere), CONCERN, Save the Children Fund-UK, Médecins Sans Frontières, and others; factors hindering relief in countries with civil conflict may be 1) Political, with the IROs being a pawn in local or tribal battles 2) Medical, including the provision of health care 3) Logistic, eg transport of medicines, supplies, food, and water (JAMA 1992; 268:1986MN&P)

international senstivity index HEMATOLOGY A measure of thromboplastin-activating capacity, or the sensitivity of a thromboplastin reagent to anticoagulation; the ISI can be used to compare the prothrombin times of thromboplastin from different sources to standardize warfarin doses, and is determined by a statistical method known as orthogonal regression analysis, see there (N Engl J Med 1993; 329:696OA; Arch Pathol Lab Med 1993; 117:602OA) see International normalized ratio

International Unit Any arbitrarily defined and internationally sanctioned unit of measurement for a naturally occurring substance, eg hormone, enzyme or vitamin; see SI (Systeme International)

International Workshop classification for chronic lymphocytic leukemia A clinical staging system that blends features of the Rai and Binet classification of CLL

STAGE A No anemia or thrombocytopenia and less than three involved lymphoid regions

STAGE B No anemia or thrombocytopenia and more than three involved lymphoid regions and

STAGE C Anemia and/or thrombocytopenia, regardless of the amount of involved lymphoid tissue

Internet Information superhighway, Infobahn COMPUTERS A global computer network that facilitates the exchange of text-based information, consisting of thousands of networks linking schools and universities, businesses, governmental agencies, libraries, nonprofit organizations, and millions of individual computer users; sending and receiving information on the Internet requires that the user have a PC (Compaq, Dell, IBM, etc), either a Macintosh (Apple Computers), or one supporting Microsoft Windows and a modem capable of ≥ 9 800 bits per second of data transmission (New York Times 5 April 1994; C6, Sci Am 1995; 272/2:30)

Internet is a spin-off of the US Department of Defense computer system, ARPAnet, an experimental network intended to facilitate scientific collaboration in military research; the communication philosophy of ARPAnet was that each computer in the system was a free-standing unit not requiring mediation of a centralized controlling computer; a second key feature was that the system had to be capable of linking computers with different data storage types and operating systems; in a sense ARPAnet design is 'regulated anarchy' Note: Currently little in the way of audio and video data is exchanged on the Internet, as this requires high-speed connections

INTERNIST see Expert systems

internist A practitioner of general medicine who is certified by the American Board of Internal Medicine (ABIM) and who has had three years of formal training in internal medicine; in the US, board eligibility or certification by the ABIM is an implied prerequisite for further training in the form of one or more years of fellowship for various specialties of internal medicine, eg gastroenterology, hematology/oncology, infectious diseases; Cf Family practitioner, Intern

the internist's tumor A colloquial term for renal cell carcinoma which is known for its protean manifestations and ability to mimic (aka the great mimic) other malignancies or benign conditions (**N Engl J Med 1992; 327:1667**CPC) see the Great imitator

interpersonal psychotherapy A specific semistructured treatment in which the patient is educated about depression and depressive symptoms, and the patient's relation to the environment, in particular his/her social functioning; unlike traditional psychotherapy, IP focuses on the present tense and not on the underlying personality structures (see **N Engl J Med 1993; 329:1974**BR)

interphase cytogenetics The analysis of chromosomal abnormalities of terminally differentiated cells or cells in the interphase stage of the cell cycle, the most popular method of which is by FISH (fluorescent in situ hybridization), see there

interpulse time MRI The time period between successive radiofrequency pulses used in pulse sequences; of particular importance are the inversion time (TI) in inversion recovery, a time period between a 180° pulse and the subsequent 90° pulse; the period between repetitions of pulse sequences is known as the repetition time; see Magnetic resonance imaging

intersecting epidemics The linkage of two epidemics, in such way that one impacts or predisposes a population to the risk of suffering a second, epidemic, eg the 'epidemic' of crack* abuse and the epidemic of HIV infection/AIDS, which intersect, as both men and women may perform sexual work to obtain the crack (**N Engl J Med 1994; 331:1422**SA)

*A highly addictive, smokable form of cocaine, see Crack

intersex syndromes A group of clinical complexes that occur in subjects with ambiguous genitalia Note: Testis-determining factor (TDF) is present by the sixth embryologic week and stimulates wolffian duct (♂) development; without TDF, the embryo 'defaults' to müllerian duct (♀) differentiation despite genotypic maleness

Intersex syndromes include TRUE HERMAPHRODITISM Gonads contain both ovarian and testicular tissue, genotypically either 46, XX or 46, XY; 75% are raised as boys; the testicular tissue is dysgenic, doesn't produce sperm and may undergo malignant degeneration (requiring prophylactic removal); ovarian function in those raised as girls may be adequate to produce term pregnancy MALE PSEUDOHERMAPHRODITISM Testicles are present and cryptorchid, but testosterone production is inadequate (due to decreased LH or hCG receptors on the Leydig cells); patients are raised as females (Morris syndrome) and may have defects of the central nervous system, eg defective gonadotropin response, primary gonadal defects, eg idiopathic, defective pregnanediol (3-β 17-α, 17,20 des and 17 β) synthesis, regression of müllerian tubes, Leydig cell agenesis, androgen insensitivity, increased susceptibility to breast cancer, Sertoli adenoma, germinoma in situ, seminoma, Leydig cell tumor FEMALE PSEUDOHERMAPHRODITISM Ovaries are present, but the infant is masculinized by in utero androgen exposure during fetal development (maternal ingestion or the result of congenital adrenal hyperplasia with virilization) GONADAL DYSGENESIS Underdeveloped or imperfectly formed gonads; the prototypic gonadal dysgenesis is Turner syndrome 45, X0, seen in 1/2-7000 female births CLINICAL Short stature, webbed neck, cubitus valgus, micrognathia with high arched palate, epicanthal folds, lymphedema of the hands and feet, aortic coarctation, renal malformation, osteoporosis, diabetes, widely-spaced nipples, sexual infantilism PATHOLOGY Ovaries are small and thin ('streak' ovaries); a variant, mixed gonadal dysgenesis is characterized by a mosaic phenotype 45,X/46,XY, and a streak ovary on one side and a testis or germ cell tumor on the other side, accompanied by intense virilization

interstitial collagenase Matrix metalloproteinase 1, MMP1

interstitial floor HOSPITAL DESIGN An unoccupied floor of minimum ceiling height that is built between occupied floors of a building, eg a hospital; IFs house critical utilities, eg air conditioning units, water and drain pipes, pneumatic tubes, electrical and telephone line conduits;

IFs (or utility corridors) simplify the alteration and servicing of utilities as they minimize the need to tear out walls and ceilings of existing structures (**MLO April 1995, p22**)

interstitial lung disease A generic term for an increase in the volume of pulmonary interstitial tissue, conceptually divided into

1) DISTORTION-TYPE ILD A reversible condition in which the alveolar walls are distended by inflammatory cells without damaging normal structures or the cells lining the alveolar spaces, seen in sarcoidosis and early hypersensitivity pneumonitis and

2) FIBROSIS-TYPE ILD A condition that is either idiopathic or induced by inorganic dusts, eg silica, asbestos, diatomaceous earths, coal dust, metals and rare earths, with fibroblast proliferation in the alveolar walls and deposition of connective tissue; the normally flattened type I pneumocytes are partially replaced by type II pneumocytes; FILD is often progressive and ultimately fatal

interventional neuroradiology A subspecialty of neuroradiology in which minimally invasive therapy can be effected by advancing various devices within a blood vessel to a point of a previously identified lesion, eg an intracranial aneurysm; because of the rapid evolution of the field, it is at present uncertain what role IN will play in treating intracranial aneurysms and when the neuroradiologists' balloons and platinum coils will be preferred to the neurosurgeon's aneurysmal clips (**Mayo Clin Proc 1995; 70:153**RV) Cf Clipping, Trapping

interventional radiology A subspecialty of general radiology that provides either

DIAGNOSTIC INFORMATION, eg CT-guided 'skinny' needle biopsies and dye injection for analysis of various lumina and tracts, eg arteriography, cholangiography, antegrade pyelography or

THERAPEUTIC OPTIONS, eg percutaneous nephrostomy or biliary drainage

intestinal 'angina' Chronic intermittent occlusion of intestinal arteries, analogous to angina pectoris, causing sporadic claudication of the vascular supply to the intestine; ingestion of food results in angina as digestion increases the blood flow through the gut, which is supplied by the celiac axis, superior and inferior mesenteric arteries; postprandial abdominal pain implies major atherosclerotic narrowing of more than one vessel given the rich anastomotic network among these vessels

intestinal flu Epidemic vomiting, see there

intestinal knot syndrome Compound volvulus A clinical condition characterized by torsion of the terminal ileum around the sigmoid colon, which itself is rotated on its own axis CLINICAL Intense abdominal pain, distention-type ileus with rapid progression RADIOLOGY Barium studies demonstrate dilated small intestine, right-sided distended sigmoid

intoxication 1) A generic term for a pathologic state induced by an exogenous or (less commonly) endogenous toxic substance 2) Drunkenness, inebriation

intracardiac electrophysiological studies CARDIOLOGY A study of the state of the cardiac conduction system, performed by introducing multipolar catheter electrodes into the vascular system, and positioning them in various parts of the heart, which allows simultaneous recording of multiple leads; the catheters are used to both record local electrical activity and to stimulate the heart; these studies measure the AV, HA, and PA interval, the last of which, the PA interval, has little clinical value

'intracellular immunization' A coinage of recent vintage to describe a potential use of a dominant negative mutant viral gene to interfere with the replication of wild-type virus; the most attractive potential application of this concept would be to protect cells against HIV-1, as the targets, CD4-bearing peripheral cells, are easily accessible; that goal has been achieved with *gag*, *tat* and *rev* mutant genesand with a CD4 mutant containing the 'KDEL sequence (see there), allowing its retention within the endoplasmic reticulum, preventing transport of HIV envelope proteins to the cell surface

intracellular pathogens Microorganisms that are adept at eluding the host's immune system, residing most often with histiocytes, in particular, *Mycobacterium tuberculosum*, *M lepra*, *Listeria monocytogenes*, *Salmonella typhi*, *Trypanosoma cruzi*, *Toxoplasma gondii*, and *Chlamydia* species

intracellular signaling The up– and/or down-regulation of metabolic pathways within a cell, which involves cAMP, Ca^{2+}, phosphoinositol turnover, activation of protein kinases A and C, and others, and is mediated hormones, eicosanoids, neurotransmitters, and cytokines (**Perspect Biol & Med 1993; 36:611**) Cf Intercellular signaling

intracoronary stent Coronary stent, see there

intraductal papillary-mucinous neoplasm of the pancreas A recently identified low-grade malignancy characterized by dilation of the main pancreatic duct that is filled with mucus-laden villous-papillary tumors and an 'ugly' histologic pattern, which arises in a background of chronic inflamation (**Arch Pathol Lab Med 1995; 119:209**)

intraepithelial neoplasia An in situ carcinoma that is confined to an epithelium that may superficially penetrate adnexal glands, measuring less than either 3 mm or 5 mm depending on the criteria used; intraepithelial neoplasia (IN) is adjectivally modified according to the site of origin (table); see CIN

INTRAEPITHELIAL NEOPLASIA	
AIN	Anal intraepithelial neoplasia
CIN	Cervical intraepithelial neoplasia
OIN	Oral intraepithelial neoplasia
PAIN	Perianal intraepithelial neoplasia
PIN	Penile intraepithelial neoplasia
VAIN	Vaginal intraepithelial neoplasia
VIN	Vulvar intraepithelial neoplasia

intralaminar nuclei NEUROANATOMY *nuclei reticulares (intralaminares thalami)* [NA6] The nuclei in the internal medullary lamina of the thalamus, which encompass the anterior centromedian and parafascicular nuclei, and the more rostral paracentral, lateral central, and medial central nuclei; the afferent connections include fibers from the spinal cord, brainstem, basal ganglia, and cortex; the efferents are broadly distributed; it has been postulated that the function of the interlaminar nuclei, hitherto of uncertain nature, might be to coordinate consciousness, by sending waves of scanning sweeps across the cerebral cortex, reportedly at a rate of 40 cycles/sec (**New York Times 21 March1995, pC1**)

intralobar pulmonary sequestration Bronchopulmonary sequestration, see there

intramural esophageal diverticulosis Pseudodiverticulosis A complex characterized by multiple small diverticuli lined by squamous epithelium present in the superior esophagus or occupying its entire length; apparently arising from the mucous gland ducts; Cf Inlet patches

intraoperative autologous transfusion Intraoperative blood salvage, see there

intraoperative blood salvage TRANSFUSION MEDICINE Intraoperative autologous transfusion A procedure in which the blood shed or otherwise lost into a surgical operative field is collected under sterile conditions, filtered and reinfused as a packed unit of red cells; IAT may be used in 'bloody' procedures, including cardiovascular surgery, eg for aortic aneurysms or coronary artery bypasses or orthopedic surgery, eg hip arthrodesis, reduc-

ing a patient's exposure to multiple donors and may be used in conjunction with pre-deposit autologous donation, in which packed red cell units are collected from the patient before surgery; IBS is reported to reduce the blood usage by 62% (see **Arch Pathol Lab Med 1994; 118:411oa**) Cf Autologous transfusion

intraoperative hemodilution TRANSFUSION MEDICINE A form of perioperative autologous blood transfusion, in which 1-2 units of blood are withdrawn from the patient at the time of surgery and replaced with crystalloid; the blood is stored at room temperature in the operating room, thereby eliminating the need to formally collect, test, and store blood; IH is most useful if the patient is expected to lose two or fewer units of blood during surgery (**N Engl J Med 1995; 332:740ed**) Cf Autologous blood transfusion, Intraoperative blood salvage

intraperitoneal loose bodies Peritoneal 'mice' Any of a number of asymptomatic often indurated structures in the peritoneal cavity formed by torsion or infarction, detached appendices, epiploicae or small detached uterine leiomyomas; Cf Joint mice

intratubular germ cell neoplasm An in situ carcinoma affecting up to 80% of the residual seminiferous tubules in testicles with germ cell tumors; 1% of infertile men have IGCN and many evolve to invasion within 5 years DIAGNOSIS Biopsy of contralateral testis, clinical follow-up and serial serum levels of α-fetoprotein, HCG, and human placental lactogen

intrauterine transfusion The in utero administration of RBCs to a fetus with hemolytic disease of the newborn; the optimal technique is a combination of 1) Intravascular transfusion (IVT) using a fetoscope to direct a needle into the chorionic plate or umbilical venous puncture under ultrasound guidance and 2) Intraperitoneal transfusion (IPT) which acts a reservoir to allow slow absortion of RBCs between IVTs; the IVT/IPT combination results in a more stable fetal hematocrit; early IUT was complicated by fetal movement resulting in injury to the fetal viscera, which is now avoided using the technique of fetal paralysis PROGNOSIS Nonhydropic fetus 90%; hydropic fetus 82% (**Arch Pathol Lab Med 1994; 118:421rv**) see Fetal paralysis

intravenous drug use IVDU* The habitual IV injection of drugs of abuse EPIDEMIOLOGY In the US ± 2.5 million (population ± 235 million) have used IVDs; in 1990, 20 000 died of IVDU, 9000 from AIDS; a hospitalized intravenous drug user costs the US health care system ± $33 000/year INFECTIONS Pyogenic, eg endocarditis, pneumonia, sepsis; usual agents: *Streptococcus pneumoniae*, *Haemophilus influenzae*, hepatitis (HBV, alcoholic) STD, TB (**N Engl J Med 1994; 331:450rv**)

*The term intravenous drug abuse has been essentially retired from the written parlance, possibly because the term abuse is less 'politically correct' than use; while the alternative term injection drug use is more correct as the drug can also be injected either intramuscularly or subcutaneously, it has not been popularized

invasin MICROBIOLOGY Any of a family of proteins present on the outer membane of certain bacteria, eg *Yersinia pseutuberculosis* and *Y enterocolitica*, which mediate invasion into nonphagocytic host cells, by binding to β1 integrins, initiating signal transduction (**Science & Medicine 1995; 2/3:16**) see Virulence factor

intravenous immune globulin A formulation of immune globulins, predominantly IgG, prepared by pooling plasma from approximately 1000 donors, which has a broad spectrum of activity against CMV, HAV, HBV, measles, rubella, tetanus and varicella zoster; IVIG is not regarded as appropriate therapy for replacing plasma proteins in adults with AIDS (as the defect is predominantly cellular) or with CLL, in whom its use costs ± $6 million for every year gained of quality adjusted life (**N Engl J Med 1991; 325:81**); IVIG is indicated in low-birth weight children with repeated infections or in children with major defects in humoral immune responses, eg AIDS, X-linked agammaglobulinemia, common variable immunodeficiency syndrome(s) (ibid, 1991; 325:110rv, 123ed); in children with AIDS and low CD4+ T cells, IVIG ↑ the duration of bacteria-free periods (ibid, 1991; 325:73); IVIG may be of use in ITP, autoimmune phenomena (hemolysis, neutropenia, thrombocytopenia), Kawasaki's disease and pediatric AIDS SIDE EFFECTS Pyrogenic, hypersensitivity, and anaphylactic reactions and minor systemic reactions, including headache, myalgia, fever, vasomotor disease and cardiovascular abnormalities, lability of blood pressure and tachycardia; Cf Human immune globulin

intraventricular neuroblastoma A tumor with a prognosis intermediate between low- and high-grade malignant glial neoplasms, which is thought by some authors to be biologically distinct from hemipheric neuroblastomas, and are clinically less aggresive if neuronal differentiation is present (Arch Pathol Lab Med 1994; 118:897oA)

intravesicular therapy ONCOLOGY The irrigation of urinary bladder with topical agents, eg thiotepa, mitomycin C and BCG, to halt the progression of superficial transitional cell carcinoma; the most widely studied agent is thiotepa; it has little effect on normal bladder epithelium, but destroys established cancers, inhibits tumor reimplantation and retards the development of new lesions; 30% achieve complete and 30% achieve partial remission; other agents include adriamycin, epodyl and 5-FU

intrinsic factor A 45-kD low-affinity vitamin B_{12}-binding glycoprotein secreted by the gastric parietal cell, which closely parallels the secretion of HCl; IF secretion is stimulated by histamine, gastrin and methionine, and usually greatly exceeds that required for B_{12} absorption; IF is reabsorbed by specific receptors in the ileum (the absence of which causes Imerslund syndrome, an AR [MIM 261100] vitamin B_{12}-IF complex malabsorption complex; the high-affinity B_{12} binder, R protein, attaches to vitamin B_{12} in the acidic environment of the stomach, later releasing B_{12} to IF after cleavage by pancreatic enzymes; IF is decreased in patients with low gastric acid production or by agents which reduce gastric acid secretion by blocking parietal cell receptors, eg H_2-blockers, but is unaffected by agents that block H^+/K^+-ATPase-induced gastric acid secretion; see H_2-blockers

intrinsic factor antibodies A family of antibodies directed against either the binding site (known as type I or 'blocking' antibodies) or any other epitope site (type II antibodies) on intrinsic factor, which are present in 75% of patients with pernicious anemia

intrinsic pathway An arm of the coagulation cascade, initiated by negatively charged surfaces (contact factors eg sulfatide micelles, kaolin) which bind factor XII and high molecular weight kininogen (HMWK); HMWK binds prekallikrein and factor XI activating the latter; XIa then activates IX which in turn activates factor X, initiating the common pathway of coagulation: see Common pathway, Extrinsic pathway

introductory advertising Promotional activities for a drug that has not yet been released; see Advertising

intron MOLECULAR BIOLOGY An 'intervening sequence' or segment of mRNA that is spliced out and not part of the primary transcript from which mRNA reads the DNA-derived message, the exon that is ultimately transcribed to become a protein; because introns do not serve a known function, they are considered less interesting biologically, to the point of being considered to have derived from 'junk DNA'; introns have been free to evolve without selective pressure, but are nevertheless felt to have an as yet unknown function as the intron-exon junction is at least 1.7×10^9 years old Note: Introns themselves are

capable of generating split genes, which encode proteins; Cf Exon

intron lariat A loop of mRNA transcribed from intron DNA that is spliced out of the maturing mRNA in the nucleus after transcription and prior to translation into a mature protein product

inulin A plant-derived homopolysaccharide composed of polymeric D-fructose, which is used to measure renal clearance

inv IMMUNOLOGY A group of allotype antigenic sites in the constant region of the kappa light chain of an immunoglobulin

invariant chain An intracellular protein that associates with a class II MHC in the endoplasmic reticulum, preventing the binding of endogenous peptides to the class II molecule, shepherding it to the relevant intracellular compartments; truncation of the invariant chain generates a second targeting signal that may be operative in the trans-Golgi network, preceding the transport of class II molecules to the cell surface

invasion The penetration of a basement membrane by a neoplastic process usually, but not invariably implies a malignancy with metastatic potential; an exception to this rule is the identification of 'foreign' tissues within lymph nodes, eg clusters of melanocytes or thyroid tissue, see Lymph node inclusions, or in the perineurium with breast glands, as may occur in sclerosing adenosis; see Metastasis

invasion of privacy MEDICAL MALPRACTICE An evolving area of tort law defined as '...*public use for profit of personal information about another or some type of intrusion on one's physical solitude...*' a physician's defense for acts alleged to represent IOP may refer to the privileges that exist for publication of information of public interest or concerning public figures (LW Way, Ed Surgical Diagnosis & Treatment, 10th ed, Appletone & Lange, Norwalk, 1994) see Malpractice

invasive Interventional *adjective* Referring or pertaining to any form of therapy in which mucocutaneous barriers are violated, eg invasive cardiology; Cf Non-invasive

invasive *Streptococcus* A Killer bug A variant of *Streptococcus* group A linked to necrotizing fasciitis and myositis; 13 of the first 15 patients died of the disease in the UK where it resulted in a media 'epidemic'(Nature 1994; 369:344o); the CDC believes there are ± 15 000 cases/year of invasive Streptococcus A (US), of which 5-10% are associated with necrosis; nonetheless, the most recent 'epidemic' may be different, the incidence of necrotizing fasciitis more prevalent, and the cases more severe than those reported before the 1980s, possibly due to production of excess amounts of cysteine proteinase (exotoxin B), an enzyme that causes excess tissue necrosis (Science 1994; 264:1665rN; New York Times 14 June 1994; C3)

inversion MRI A nonequilibrium state in which the macroscopic magnetization vector is oriented opposite to the magnetic field; usually produced by adiabatic fast passage or by 180° radiofrequency pulses; see Magnetic resonance imaging

inversion recovery MRI A pulse MR technique that can be incorporated into MRI, where the nuclear magnetization is inverted at a time on the order of T1 before the regular imaging pulse-gradient sequences; the resulting partial relaxation of the spins in the different structures being imaged can be used to produce an image that depends on T1, enhancing the differences in the appearance of structures with different T1 relaxation times; see Magnetic resonance imaging

Note: IR does not produce a direct image of T1, but rather one that is calculated from the change in the MR signal from the region due to the inversion pulse compared with the signal with no inversion pulse or an inversion pulse with a different T1 inversion time

inverted comma sign A radiologic finding seen by a plain chest film in a not uncommon (1/200 subjects) variation of the azygous lobe, which is invested with its own pleural membrane in the medial aspect of the right upper lobe

inverted epidemiology A neologism for the misuse of epidemiologic data, in which the 'investigator' tries to identify statistically significant correlations (**Am Lab July 1994**)

inverted mushroom and stem sign GI RADIOLOGY A cap-like radiopacity surrounded by a 'coiled spring'-like appearance, seen by barium enema in intestinal intussusception

inverted papilloma SURGICAL PATHOLOGY A proliferation characterized by a thin investment of epithelium overlying papillary fronds of epithelium; IPs may occur in either transitional epithelium (renal pelvis, ureters, bladder and urethra) or in stratified cuboidal epithelium (paranasal region, ¾ of patients had concomitant HPV infection, types 6b and 11 and lesions of the upper respiratory tract); IPs tend to recur in the nasopharynx, but not in the urinary tract; the bladder papillomas have been subdivided histologically into glandular and trabecular patterns, a distinction of uncertain clinical utility

inverted repeat see Palindrome

inverted '3' sign of Frostberg RADIOLOGY An acquired deformity of the duodenum and adjacent ampulla of Vater with fixation of the pancreatic and common bile ducts at the ampulla of Vater and associated edema of the medial duodenal wall; first described as characteristic of carcinoma of the head of the pancreas, it occurs in only 10% of these patients and may be seen in acute pancreatitis or duodenal ulcers Note: The adjective 'reversed' is more semantically correct

inverted 'U' sign RADIOLOGY A massively dilated (possibly extending to the diaphragm), redundant loop of sigmoid colon that twists on its mesenteric axis and may be seen in a volvulus of the sigmoid colon; see Hot air balloon sign

inverted umbrella sign of Fleischner A gaping ileocecal valve with immediately proximal stenosis, simulating an umbrella turned inside-out by a gust of wind, seen in barium contrast studies; this sign was first described in tuberculous ileitis, but may also be seen in Crohn's disease

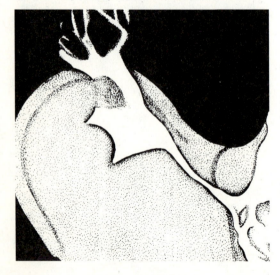

inverted umbrella sign

inverted 'V' sign RADIOLOGY Lateral umbilical ligaments made prominent by gas percolated on either side of the ligaments, characteristic in a plain supine film of pneu-

moperitoneum, when the patients are too sick for erect studies; see also Double wall sign

inverted 'Y' field NUCLEAR MEDICINE A large radiotherapy field for treating contiguous lymph nodes involved in Hodgkin's disease or other lymphomas, which covers the para-aortic, splenic hilar, iliac, inguinal and femoral lymph nodes Note: Less than 3600 cGy (rads) is a prophylactic dose, used when lymphoid tissue is not involved by tumor, 3600-4400 cGy constitutes a tumoricidal dose; see Abdominal bath, Mantle port

investigational drug A generic term for any drug that is experimental in nature when applied to a specific disease, and includes drugs that are not comercially available; see IND

investigational new drug see IND

'invisible' profession Nursing

in vitro fertilization A form of assisted ('artificial') fertilization in which an inseminated egg in early embryogenesis is implanted into the uterus; the success rate (in experienced centers) is 20-25% overall (7.7% success when cryopreserved pre-embryos are used and 24% when fresh embryos are used); IVF bypasses certain causes of infertility ETHICS AND HUMAN IVF The experimental use of human embryos created by IVF has engendered heated debate, resulting in a ban on its use in federally-funded research in the US; in the UK, Parliament allows regulated research on human embryos up to 14 days post-conception LEGAL ISSUES, IVF When gametes are joined in vitro and frozen for future transfer into a mother, 'product' ownership is unclear and may be decided in a court of law, should the couple then get divorced after creation of the pre-embryos, the couple got divorced COST The cost per successful delivery of one or more live births ranges from $50 000 to $72 727 for the 1st through 6th cycles* if the infertility was due to a tubal defect, and $160 000 to $800 000 for the 1st through 6th cycle if the couple was older or the infertility was due to a male factor, eg low spem count (**N Engl J Med 1994; 331:239oA**) Note: 14-20 000 babies have been born by various forms of IVF since its first success in 1978; see Assisted ('artificial') reproduction, Infertility, Surrogate motherhood, Test tube baby

*A complete cycle of in vitro fertilization (cost ranges from $7-11 000) involves 4 steps: 1) Use of fertility drugs to stimulate the development of eggs 2) Retrieval of eggs by an outpatient transcervical procedure 3) The eggs are fertilized in the laboratory with husband's or partner's sperm 4) Fertilized eggs are implanted into the uterus for completion of the pregnancy

involuntary hospitalization FORENSIC PSYCHIATRY A form of civil commitment in which a person is formally confined as a result of mental illness, incompetence, alcoholism, drug addiction, or other, as he/she is regarded as being dangerous to him/herself or others

involuntary infertility Sterility The incapacity of a woman to bear a living child during the span of reproductive years; II may be due to anatomic abnormalities of of the reproductive tract, malfunction of ovulation precluding conception, recurrent intrauterine loss of pregnancy, or specific diseases, eg infections

involuntary smoking Passive smoking, see there

iodine deficiency disorder A generic term for any of a number of conditions (to wit cretinism and varying degrees of brain damage, goiter, and hypothyroidism) attributable to iodine deficiency and correctable by adequate dietary addition (**N Engl J Med 1994; 331:1770eD**)

'iodine mumps' Bilateral swelling of the parotid glands that may accompany administration of organic or inorganic iodine, eg triiodothyronine for treating hypothyroidism

IOM Institute of Medicine, see there

ion channels PHYSIOLOGY A large heterogeneous family of voltage-activated proteins that control the permeability of cells to specific ions (Na+, K+, Ca++, Cl-) by opening or closing in response to differences in potentials across the plasma membrane, an action which in sodium, potassium and calcium channels may be controlled by the S4 sequence of polypeptides; ion channels participate in the generation and transmission of electrical activity in the nervous system and in the hormonal regulation of cellular physiology; all are composed of 4 or 5 homologous domains or subunits, each of which contains numerous membrane-spanning α-helices; the polar faces of the α-helices from neighboring subunits aggregate to form a pore or alternately, are less polar and composed of serine, threonine and cysteine residues; ion channel control of intracellular concentrations of ions, eg calcium, in turn controls such diverse cell functions as secretion and cell division; ion channels are embedded in the cell membrane and are either

LIGAND-GATED, eg nicotinic acetylcholine receptor, GABA receptor and glycine receptors all of which mediate local increase in ion conductance at chemical synapses, thereby either depolarizing or hyperpolarizing the (pre)synaptic region or

VOLTAGE-SENSITIVE, which mediate rapid changes in ion permeability during action potentials in excitable cells and modulate membrane potentials and ion permeability in inexcitable cells; see Ball-and-chain model, Na^+/H^+ antiporter, Na^+/K^+ ATPase, Potassium channel, Voltage-dependent anion-selective channel, Voltage-dependent calcium channel

ionization chamber A sealed, usually cylindrical chamber for measuring the electric currents produced when a gas is bombarded by ionizing radiation (electrons, protons and X-rays); such chambers comprise the detection unit in a Geiger-Müller counter

ionized calcium Free calcium One of the 3 fractions[1] of calcium (comprising 46-52% of the total) in the peripheral circulation; ionized calcium is the most physiologically relevant fraction and is essential for excitation-contraction coupling and conduction in the heart, hormonal regulation, coagulation and energy metabolism; reference range for IC is 1.12-1.30 mmol/L (4.49-5.21 mg/dL)[2], and as IC falls below 1.04 mmol/L, mortality ↑; IC is ↓ in sepsis, hypotension, dysrrhythmias, cardiogenic shock, cardiopulmonary arrest (**Arch Pathol Lab Med 1993; 117:890SA**)

[1]The other fractions are protein-bound calcium (42-47%) which consists mainly of calcium bound to anionic sites on albumin, and complex-bound calcium (4-8%) [2]Critical values are ≤ 0.82 (0.85 children) mmol/L or ≥ 1.55 (1.53 children) mmol/L

ionizing radiation All particles capable of producing ions, including alpha particles, beta particles, gamma rays, X-rays, neutrons, high-speed electrons or protons, and other high energy particles; see Electromagnetic spectrum; Cf Nonionizing radiation

Note: The adjective *ionizing* is often assumed, and thus not used in the working parlance

iontophoresis CLINICAL THERAPEUTICS A specific type of transcutaneous drug delivery in which an electric current is applied to the skin in order to facilitate the movement of a substance through the skin; iontophoresis enhances the absorption of large polar (hydrophilic) molecules and peptides, eg insulin, and incorporates a level of electronic control in the format for delivering the therapeutic agent (**Mayo Clin Proc 1995; 70:581**) see Transcutaneous drug delivery; Cf Phonophoresis

IP Interstitial pneumonia, see Interstitial lung disease

IP₃ Inositol 1,4,5-triphosphate, see there

IPA Independent practice association, see IPO

IPAT equation ENVIRONMENT An acronym referring to the manmade detrimental forces that impact on the environment, where I refers to the impact, which is largely a function of the population P, A is the level of affluence, and T is the technology; in early evaluations of environmental impact of the human on the environment, A and T were ignored; as the developing nations evolve, the levels of affluence rise and the desires become more 'Westernized', an adjective formerly synonymous with wantonly wasteful Note: The IPAT equation is being slowly reversed, with a fall in birth rates, and more efficient use of energy (**sci Am 1994; 271/4:114**)

IPCC Intergovernmental Panel on Climate Control ENVIRONMENT A formal forum of scientists from different countries that are currently assembling data on the potential effect of greenhouse gases (**Nature 1991; 350:219**) see CFCs, Greenhouse effect, Montreal protocol

IPO Independent practice organization A legally defined entity in the US, in which physicians and/or dentists enter an arrangement to provide services through an entity, eg a prepaid health plan, while at the same time maintaining their own private practices; see HMO, PPO

IPPNW International Physicians for the Prevention of Nuclear War An organization of doctor do-gooders that won the 1985 Nobel Prize for Peace; Cf Amnesty International, Red Cross, Medecins sans Frontieres

IPPV Intermittent positive pressure ventilation, see PEEP

IPSID Immunoproliferative small intestinal disease Mediterranean lymphoma α heavy chain disease A heterogeneous group of conditions characterized by monoclonal increases in production of immunoglobulin (usually α) heavy chain, without accompanying light chains, ie 'truncated' immunoglobulins; all or part of the variable region is lost as well as one (usually C_H1) or two constant domains; the mRNA is very short and has mutations, deletions or insertions; IPSID is usually a 'secretory' or α chain proliferation, but may also be a γ or mu chain CLINICAL Malabsorption, diarrhea, weight loss, abdominal pain, due to marked expansion of the proximal small intestine and mesenteric lymphoid tissue, clubbing of fingers and toes TREATMENT Without antibiotic therapy, eg tetracycline, IPSID may evolve to malignant lymphoma (B cell immunoblastic sarcoma)

IR Infrared, also 1) Immune response 2) Index of response 3) Internal rotation (rehabilitation medicine) 4) Inversion recovery (MRI) 5) Inverted repeat (molecular biology)

Also 1) Immunoreactive 2) Incident report 3) Individual referral 4) Inferior rectus (anatomy) 5) Intelligence ratio (intelligence quotient, see IQ) 6) Interim report

IRAP Interleukin-1 receptor antagonist protein A natural inhibitor of IL-1 bioactivity on T lymphocytes and endothelial cells

IRB Institutional review board, see there

IRGT Insulin-regulatable glucose transporter, see there

Irish's node Left anterior axillary lymph node, which is a site of predilection for involvement by metastatic gastric carcinoma; see Sentinel node, Sister Mary Joseph node

iris lesion Target lesion, bull's-eye lesion DERMATOLOGY An erythematous annular macular or papular lesion that develops an inner red-purple ring, papule or macule, a finding characteristic of erythema multiforme

iris pearls A fanciful term for the multiple whitish, opalescent, miliary lepromata seen in the optic fundus in ocular leprosy

IRMA Immunoradiometric assay LABORATORY MEDICINE A quantitative 'sandwich' assay using radioiodinated label to measure certain plasma proteins; IRMA differs from RIA in that the antibody in the detector system is radioactive and not the competing hormone derived from the patient; see Hook effect

iron-chelation therapy The use of an iron-chelating agent, eg deferoxamine, to reduce excess body stores of iron, which cause morbidity either directly, eg hemochromatosis or indirectly, as may occur in cerebral malaria;

iron chelation is reported to hasten clearance of *P falciparum* parasitemia, possibly by reducing iron and enhance recovery from deep coma, possibly related to iron's role as a redox agent in generating free radicals that mediate ischemic tissue damage (**N Engl J Med 1992; 327:1473oa**)

iron-deficiency anemia An anemia that occurs when hemoglobin production ↓ due to insufficient iron; idiopathic IDA 62% have lesions of either the upper (36% most in the form of ulcers, –itis, and –oma), lower (25% most as –omas and –itis) or both (1%) ends of the GI tract that were potentially responsible for the iron deficiency, ie blood loss; the most common lesions of the upper GI tract are ulcers, of the lower GI tract are carcinomas and polyps (**N Engl J Med 1993; 329:1691oa**)

iron hypothesis ENVIRONMENT A proposal that CO_2, the primary major gas responsible for the greenhouse effect could be markedly reduced by stimulating the growth of algae in the Antarctic with iron, fancifully termed the 'Geritol fix' after a proprietary iron supplement (**Science 1991; 253:1490**), the limiting nutrient for algal growth; according to the initial estimate, the reduction would be 150 ppm of CO_2; another model (**Nature 1991; 349:228, 198**) estimates a mere 30 ppm reduction after 100 years of successful iron 'fertilization' and potentially nefarious side effects of algal overgrowth; 1990 CO_2 level: 345 ppm; 2100 (estimated) CO_2 level: 1200 ppm

iron lung A tank ventilator that encases a patient up to his neck, enabling artificial respiration by intermittent applied negative pressure around his/her body, externally expanding the thoracic cavity Note: IPPV has a similar effect internally with positive internal pressure; see Mechanical ventilation, PEEP

iron-responsive element CAGUGX, see there

iron stores HEMATOLOGY The amount of bone marrow iron is a crude indicator of a disease state and is graded on a scale of 0 (no discernable iron) to 4+ (ponderous clumps of hemosiderin); a marked decrease or absence of marrow iron occurs in chronic disease, hemorrhage, ↓ iron intake, hypochromic anemia and polycythemia vera; a marked increase in BM iron may be due to conditions affecting erythrocyte production, eg β-thalassemia, hemolytic anemia and sideroblastic anemia, the liver, eg hemochromatosis, alcoholic cirrhosis, viral hepatitis, and other diseases, eg porphyria cutanea tarda, Gaucher's disease; increased iron stores have been reported to ↑ the risk of acute MI (see **Circulation 1992; 86:803**)

ote: The decalcification step required in the preparation of BM for LM dissolves some of this iron

irritable bowel syndrome Spastic colon A heterogeneous group of chronic functional disorders; there is no complete consensus on the minimum criteria necessary to define the condition, although the presence of symptoms for ≥ is an accepted temporal parameter; 6 symptoms have been identified that are more common in IBS than in organic GI disorders, to wit: Abdominal distension, relief of pain with bowel activity, more frequent stools with the onset of pain, looser stools with the onset of pain, passage of mucus, and a sensation of incomplete evacuation; other features include gastroesophageal reflux, heartburn, dysphagia, globus sensation, urologic dysfunction, fatigue, and gynecologic problems (**N Engl J Med 1994; 329:1940rv**); the IBS is an intestinal dysmotility complex, thought to be related to psychophysiologic stress with maladaptive reinforcement of autonomic visceral responses CLINICAL Most often seen in anxious 20-40 year-old females with colicky abdominal pain and altered bowel habits PATHOPHYSIOLOGY Altered secretory patterns, ↑ sensitivity to cholinergic agents, hyperalgesia with intestinal distension and ↑ secretion of prostaglandin E_2 (altered bowel habits, ↑ transit time, ↓ slow wave activity of the intestinal smooth muscle, ↑ segmenting contractions, delaying gastrocolic

response) PATHOLOGY Although there are no consistent findings, edema, varying degrees of inflammation, hyperemia and subepithelial collagen deposits may be seen TREATMENT None consistently effective; attempted modalities include high-fiber diet, laxatives (with caution), psychotherapy, emotional support, biofeedback, sedatives, tranquilizers and antidepressants, and anticholinergics to relieve pain; Cf Inflammatory bowel disease, 'Unhappy gut'

irritant A generic term for any noncorrosive chemical substance or mixture which on immediate, prolonged, or repeated contact with mucocutaneous surfaces, induces a local inflammatory response

IRPPHS LABORATORY MEDICINE International Reference Preparation for Proteins in Human Serum An international secondary matrix reference matrix released jointly by the the Bureau Communitaire de Réference of the European Economic Community and the College of American Pathologists; the IRPPHS includes 14 plasma proteins: transthyretin (prealbumin), albumin, α_1-acid glycoprotein (orosomucoid), α_1-antitrypsin (α_1-protease inhibitor), ceruloplasmin, haptoglobulin, α_2-macroglobulin, transferrin, C3, C4, IgG, IgA, IgM, and C-reactive protein; the IRPPHS is intended to set a standard for working calibrants and controls for immunoassays of serum proteins (**Arch Pathol Lab Med 1993; 117:22oa**)

IS see Insertion sequence

iscador see Unproven methods of cancer treatment

ischemic colitis A condition characterized by transient and recurring colicky abdominal pain accompanied by nausea, tenesmus, fever, and bloody diarrhea, resulting from atherosclerosis of the mesenteric arteries supplying the intestine, that most intensely affects the descending colon (**N Engl J Med 1995; 332:804cpc**)

ISCOM CLINICAL PHARMACOLOGY A lipid bilayer with a rosette conformation, which has been manipulated to integrate proteins; ISCOMs have potential as drug delivery vehicles or as 'vectors' for viral products in vaccinations

ISI International Sensitivity Index, see there

ISIS 2922 A phosphorotioate antisense oligonuleotide that inihibits mRNA of CMV in humans, which may be of use in treating patients who have become refractory to the standard agents (ganciclovir and foscarnet) used to treat CMV retinitis (**JAMA1995; 273:1458**)

islet amyloid polypeptide A 37-amino acid peptide produced in the pancreatic beta cells; IAPP is the principal component of the amyloid in insulinomas, and is present in 90% of patients with NIDDM, with which it has been pathogenically linked; IAPP has diabetogenic effects (inhibits glucose uptake and glycogen synthesis and impairs glucose tolerance) and may cause insulin resistance; the increased IAPP in the plasma of patients with pancreatic carcinoma may explain the insulin resistance typical of pancreatic carcinoma (**N Engl J Med 1994; 330:313oa**)

islet autograft see Pancreatic-islet transplantation

islet cell transplantation A technique that has had limited success in treating DM; successful transplantation requires 1) An adequate number (800 000+) of functioning islets from at least two cadaveric donors, verified by purification, culturing and assays for insulin production and 2) Adequate immune suppression, the most successful agent is tacrolimus (formerly FK 506) METHOD Islet cells are injected into the portal vein and the liver acts as the 'host organ'; Cf Biohybrid artificial pancreas, Insulin pump, Pancreatic transplantation

islet encapsulation EXPERIMENTAL ENDOCRINOLOGY A generic term for any procedure (eg hollow fiber, microencapsulation, chamber/shunt) in which pancreatic islets are enclosed in a plastic shell to protect them from the wiles of a host immune system; IE is in the early stages of development, but may ultimately prove useful as a therapeutic modality for treating type 1 diabetes (Sci Am July 1995, p50)

ISO 9001 A series of standards developed by the International Organization for Standardization in Geneva, Switzerland, that certifies commercial products and processes, recognizing that they meet or surpass certain rigorous physical and chemical standards of quality

isodisomy Inheritance of two identical copies of an allele, gene, or chromosome from one parent (from glossary, N Engl J Med 1992; 326:1599OA)

isoelectric focusing LABORATORY MEDICINE An electrophoretic technique that separates amphoteric compounds, eg proteins, by charge along a stable pH gradient, allowing them to migrate to an isoelectric point where their overall charge is zero or neutral; IEF is used to detect abnormal hemoglobins, myoglobin and glycohemoglobin and to separate amylase isoenzymes; IEF allows subdivision of alkaline phosphatase into 12 isoforms; the 10 present at the isoelectric point of 4.73, derives from activated T lymphocytes (especially CD4 type) and is a useful surrogate marker for perinatal HIV-1 infection in children (Arch Pathol Lab Med 1994; 118:873OA) see Alkaline phosphatase; Cf Two-dimensional gel electrophoresis

isolated angiitis of the central nervous system Granulomatous angiitis of the central nervous system, see there

isolation INFECTIOUS DISEASE The segregation or 'quarantining' of a patient, his body fluids or fomites to prevent transmission of an infection to other patients or hospital personnel; various terms are used by the CDC for the levels of required: Blood/body fluid isolation or precautions (Creutzfeldt-Jakob disease, HBV, HIV); see Biosafety levels, Disinfection, Precautions, Sterilization; Cf Reverse 'precautions'

isomorphic effect Köbner's phenomenon DERMATOLOGY The induction of skin changes at site 'B', that follows minimal non-specific trauma (heat or light) when identical lesions are already present elsewhere at site A; the IE is characteristic of psoriasis and may be seen in lichen planus, active eczema and in verruca; Cf Id reaction

isoniazid INH A first-line anti-tuberculosis drug YD isoniazid is thought to interfere with the ability of *Mycobacterium tuberculosis* to assemble its waxy external mycolic acid coat, by binding to the product of the **inhA gene**, the enzyme involved in that assembly; the recently-recognized isoniazid-resistance in *M tuberculosis* may be due either a mutation of InhA resulting in an enzyme that does not bind the enzyme, or due to an increased production of enzyme (New York Times 18 January 1994; C3--see Science of same vintage) see Multi-drug-resistant tuberculosis

isoprenoids Terpenes A large and diverse group of lipids, eg steroids and bile acids, lipid-soluble vitamins, coenzyme Q and others that derive from five-carbon isoprene units and which may help anchor proteins to cell membranes

isoprene 2-methyl-1,3-butadiene A hydrocarbon that is a basic unit from which more complex molecules, eg steroids are formed; isoprene gas is emitted from plants, a production estimated at 3×10^{14} g/year (similar to methane); it reacts with hydroxyl radicals and plays an important role in atmospheric chemistry; it is photosynthesis-dependent and accounts for 2% of the carbon produced at 30°C by aspen and oak trees; isoprene production is stopped in a pure N_2 atmosphere, by darkness, and inhibitors of photosynthesis (Nature 1995; 374:769C)

isoretinoin 13-*cis*-retinoic acid A proprietary agent that has been used to treat severe recalcitrant acne; isotetinoin is considered a category X drug (ie teratogenic, and not to be used in pregnant women), as it has been associated with cardiovascular defects (ventricular septal, aortic arch and conotruncal defects), external ear deformity, cleft palate, micrognathia, and CNS malformations; isotretinoin is capable of inducing long-term clinical and laboratory remission in juvenile CML; in a pilot study, 2 of 10 had complete response, and 3 had partial remission of symptoms (N Engl J Med 1994; 331:1680OA) see Vitamin A analogs

isosbestic points LABORATORY MEDICINE The wavelength at which the spectral curve for two substances, eg barbiturates, intersects or has the same absorption

Isospora belli PARASITOLOGY An enteropathogenic sporozoite parasite of unkown prevalence that is more common in the tropics and subtropics of the Western Hemisphere and in Southeast Asia; *I belli* infection is probably underreported, as in uncompromised hosts, it mimics viral gastroenteritis, although when associated with AIDS may cause fulminant disease CLINICAL Watery diarrhea with variable hemorrhage, colicky pain, weight loss, steatorrhea and eosinophilia PATHOLOGY Mucosal atrophy, attenuated villi, crypt hypertrophy and inflammation of the lamina propria TREATMENT Trimethoprim-sulfamethoxazole

isothiocyanate see FITC, Spicy food

isotonic *adjective* 1) Referring or pertaining to maintaining a uniform muscle tone 2) Referring or pertaining to a uniformity of osmotic pressure *noun* A type of sports drink‡ which in addition to replacing water and electrolytes, contains either fructose or glucose polymers allowing a slow-release of carbohydrates for replenishing reserves of energy consumed while exercising

isotope A nuclide of an element that has the same number of protons and atomic number, while differs in the number of neutrons and the atomic mass; isotopes of medical importance include positron emitters

isotretinoin 13-*cis*-retinoic acid An analogue of vitamin A reported to be of use in treating oral leukoplakia with high-dose induction and low-dose maintenance (N Engl J Med 1993; 328:15OA)

isotype IMMUNOLOGY A subtype of an immunoglobulin that is present in all normal individuals, regardless of race, which are differentiated based on the size and number of domains and the number of intra- and interchain disulfide bonds in the constant region; IgG has four isotypes: IgG1, IgG2, IgG3 and IgG4; IgA has two isotypes: IgA1 and IgA2; the remaining heavy chains as well as light chains have only one isotype; Cf Allotype, which differs according to the gene pool and Idiotype, which differs according to epitope

ISS Injury severity score, see there

ISSI-3 Third International Study of Infarct Survival (see N Engl J Med 1992; 327:1OA, 7OA)

itai-itai byo Japanese, 'Ouch-ouch' disease CLINICAL TOXICOLOGY A form of renal osteodystrophy with marked bone pain, described in multiparous Japanese women due to accumulation of cadmium in bone, related to eating fish contaminated by industrial pollutants PATHOGENESIS Its occurrence in multiparous women suggests that the iron, calcium and other divalent cations lost in multiple pregnancies may be replaced by cadmium

ITP Idiopathic thrombocytopenic purpura, see there, immune thrombocytopenic purpura

Also 1) Inferior thalamic peducle (neuroanatomy) 2) Inosine triphosphate 3) Interrupted task paradigm (psychological testing) 4) Intrathoracic pressure

'It's Over, Debbie' ETHICS The title of an anonymous, personal account of the mercy killing of a young woman dying of terminal ovarian cancer, by the author, a young resident in gynecology, written in the 'Piece of my Mind' column of the Journal of the American Medical Association (1988; 259:272); '*it's over, Debbie*' became one of the 'battle cries' of the euthanasia movement; for those who would defend the physician's action, the 'victim' was emaciated, racked with pain and according to the author, wanted to get it (presumably the dying process) over with; the ensuing controversy was enormous and physicians were 4:1 against the act; see DNR, 'Doctor Death', Euthanasia

IUD 1) Intrauterine death 2) Intrauterine (contraceptive) device A contraceptive that is being used with decreasing frequency in the US, given that the wave of litigation initiated by the doomed, deemed defective device, the Dalkon shield, engendered secondary waves of lawsuits that forced the manufacturers of similar contraceptive devices to withdraw from the market in the USA, see Copper-Seven, Dalkon shield, although these IUDs are widely used elsewhere; IUDs are associated with actinomycosis, a fungal infection affecting 85% of women with an IUD in place for more than three years; approximately 20% of ectopic pregnancies occur in wearers of IUDs; pelvic infections are three to seven-fold more frequent in IUD users, often of a polymicrobial nature, including aerobic and anaerobic bacteria, mycoplasma and *Chlamydia* species PATHOLOGY Focal acute and chronic inflammation in 25-40% of IUD users, also, squamous metaplasia, premature predecidual reaction, focal fibrosis and pressure atrophy EM Giant mitochondria are seen in proliferative phase endometrium, premature predecidual changes in secretory phase endometrium; copper IUDs induce increased mitochondria (with vacuolated matrix) and lysosomes; 75% epithelial cells reveal the myelin figures that correspond to the 'wear-and-tear' pigment, lipofuscin Note: Although no IUD-related neoplasia has been reported in humans, stainless steel or polyethylene loops implanted in virgin Wistar rats induce sarcomas and carcinomas; see Dalkon Shield, Pearl index

IUGR Intrauterine growth retardation A phenomenon afflicting high risk infants, associated with perinatal asphyxia, hypoglycemia, hypothermia, pulmonary hemorrhage, meconium aspiration, necrotizing enterocolitis, polycythemia and multiple complications of infections, malformations and syndromes seen in the children; see Low birth weight

IUPAC International Union of Pure and Applied Chemistry

IV Intravenous, also 1) Interventricular (neuroanatomy) 2) Intervertebral 3) Intravascular 10) Intraventricular (cardiology)

Also 1) In vitro 2) In vivo 3) Independent variable 4) Initial velocity (ballistics) 5) Internal velocity 6) Invasive 7) Iodine value (biochemistry)

IVBAT Intravascular bronchiolar and alveolar tumor An uncommon tumor of ♀ presenting as multifocal slowly-growing intrapulmonary nodules that mimic pulmonary metastases; first described as a variant of bronchoalveolar cell carcinoma, IVBAT is a neoplasm a sui generis caused by vascular proliferation CLINICAL Often asymptomatic or minimal shortness of breath, 40% of patients are < 30 years old; 50% of patients die of disease, 25% within the first year; it may be related to endotheliomatosis or identical to epithelioid hemangioendothelioma RADIOLOGY Multiple bilateral pulmonary nodules < 2 cm in diameter PATHOLOGY Tumor nodules with peripheral growth and central coagulative necrosis, dystrophic calcification or ossification; cells have rounded nuclei with overlapping contours, fibrillar, ground-glass, hyalinized, myxomatous or vacuolated cytoplasm IMMUNOPEROXIDASE Vacuoles stain for factor VIII-related antigen, suggesting primitive endothelial differentiation

Ivermectin TROPICAL MEDICINE A single dose antifilarial drug, that is now preferred by many workers to the previous standard, diethylcarbazine, which requires a 12-day course and patient compliance; ivermectin is effective against *Onchocerca volvulus, Wuchereria bancrofti* (**Am A Trop Med Hyg 1994; 50:339**), *Brugia malayi,* requires a lower dose and has fewer side effects; treatment of an entire

community markedly reduces the prevalence of infection and may form the basis of effective eradication of *O volvulus,* the agent of river blindness

IVF In vitro fertilization, see there

IVH Intraventricular hemorrhage

IVIC syndrome An AD [MIM 147750] condition characterized by multiple congenital defects including a defect in the radial 'ray' (an embryologic structure from which the radial bone and related musculoskeletal structures arise), strabismus, deafness, thrombocytopenia Note: The complex was first described in the IVIC (Instituto Venezolano Investigationes Cientificas)

IVIG see Intravenous immunoglobulin

IVLEN Inflammatory verrucous linear epidermal nevus DERMATOLOGY Persistent and pruritic linear lesions composed of erythematous slightly verrucous scaling papules, that may be associated with immune compromise DDx Lichen striatus

ivory tower syndrome A highly colloquial ad hoc term for the blatent disregard that academic physicians have for economic realities when teaching medical students the practice of medicine; in the academic construct, information that is deemed extraneous to learning the foundations of medicine is regarded as unncessary or unworthy of a medical student's time (**Am Med News 24 April 1995 p15**)

ivory vertebrae Osteosclerosis of vertebrae (figure, facing page) most common in osteoblastic metastases, classically seen in adenocarcinoma of the prostate, rarely also in colonic carcinoma, in particular those treated with hormonal or chemotherapy, Hodgkin's disease, sclerotic Paget's disease of the bone and multiple myeloma

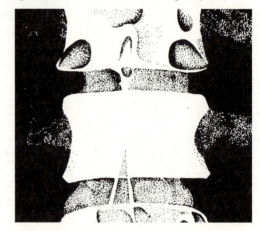

ivory vertebrae

Ivy bleeding time HEMATOLOGY A quantitative coagulation assay based on a standardized skin wound that measures the platelet and vascular response to injury METHOD A sphygmomanometer is placed around the upper arm and inflated to 40 mm Hg pressure, a 5-mm incision is made on the flexor surface of the forearm; the time required to stop bleeding is then measured Normal 1-6 minutes Increased in patients with Bernard-Soulier disease, Glanzmann's thrombasthenia, platelet defects, eg thrombocytopenia, storage pool disease, vascular defects, eg Ehlers-Danlos disease and von Willebrand's disease

Ixodes scapularis Deer tick A tick with a 2-year life cycle and 3 feeding seasons; the cycle begins in the spring with the deposition of fertilized eggs in the soil; by summer the larvae emerge and imbibe a blood meal from a small vertebrate, eg white-footed mouse (*Peromyscus leucopus*) which may be infected with *Borrelia burgdor-*

feri (maintaining the spirochete in the tick population) (*Sci Am 1994; 270/9:34*) see *Borrelia burgdorferi*, Lyme disease

Izumi fever A water-borne scarlatina-like disease endemic to rural Japan, first described in 1929 that may have sporadic epidemic foci; the long form is characterized by a diphasic fever, while the short form has a single febrile peak; ↑ in atypical lymphocytes, is similar or identical to infectious mononucleosis, with EBV antibody titers exceeding those seen in Burkitt's lymphoma

common abbreviations: 2-D Two-dimensional **3-D** Three-dimensional **±** About, approximately, circa **‡** see there **aa** Amino acid **ACE** Angiotensin-converting enzyme **AD** Autosomal dominant **AFB** Acid-fast bacillus **AIDS** Acquired immunodeficiency syndrome **aka** also known as **ALL** Acute lymphocytic (lymphoblastic) leukemia **ALS** Amyotrophic lateral sclerosis **ALT** Alanine aminotransferase (formerly GPT) **AMA** American Medical Association **AML** Acute myelocytic (granulocytic, myeloid, myelogenous) leukemia **ANLL** Acute nonlymphocytic leukemia **apo** Apolipoprotein **aPTT** Activated partial thromboplastin time **AR** Autosomal recessive **ARDS** Acute respiratory distress syndrome or adult respiratory distress syndrome **AST** Aspartate aminotransferase (fomerly GPT) **AV** Atrioventricular **BCC** Basal cell carcinoma **BM** Bone marrow (or basement membrane) **BUN** Blood urea nitrogen **CAD** Coronary artery disease **cAMP** Cyclic adenosine monophosphate **CBC** Complete blood count **CDC** Centers for Disease Control and Prevention **cDNA** Complementary DNA **CEA** Carcinoembryonic antigen **CHF** Congestive heart failure **CIE** Counter-immunoelectrophoresis **CIN** Cervical intraepithelial neoplasia **CK** Creatinine phosphokinase **CML** Chronic myelocytic (granulocytic, myelogenous, myeloid) leukemia **CNS** Central nervous system **COD** Cause of death **COPD** Chronic obstructive pulmonary disease **CPR** Cardiopulmonary resuscitation **CSF** Cerebrospinal fluid **CT** Computed tomography **CVA** Cerebrovascular accident **DAD** Diffuse alveolar damage **DDx** Differential diagnosis **DIC** Disseminated intravascular coagulation **DM** Diabetes mellitus **DNA** Deoxyribonucleic acid **DOA** Dead on arrival **DSM-IV** Diagnostic and Statistical Manual, fourth edition **DWI** Driving while intoxicated *E coli* *Escherichia coli* **EEG** Electroencephalogram, electroencephalographic **eg** *exempli gratia*, for example **EGF** Epidermal growth factor **EKG** Electrocardiography **ELISA** Enzyme-linked immunosorbent assay **EM** Electron microscopy, ultrastructure **EMG** Electromyography **EMT** Emergency medical technician **ENT** Ears, nose, and throat, otorhinolaryngology **EPA** Environmental Protection Agency **ER** Emergency room, emergency ward **ERCP** Endoscopic retrograde cholangiography **ESR** Erythrocyte sedimentation rate **ESRD** End-stage renal disease **FDA** United States Food and Drug Administration **FDP** Fibrinogen degradation product(s) **FISH** Fluorescence in situ hybridization **FNA** Fine-needle aspiration (biopsy or cytology) **FSH** Follicle-stimulating hormone **FUO** Fever of unknown origin **GABA** gamma-aminobutyric acid **GC-MS** Gas chromatography-mass spectroscopy **GFR** Glomerular filtration rate **GGT** Gamma-glutamyl transferase **GI** Gastrointestinal **GM-CSF** Granulocyte-macrophage colony-stimulating factor **GMS** Gomori-methenamine-silver **GN** Glomerulonephritis **GNP** Gross National Product **GVHD** Graft-versus-host disease **HAV** Hepatitis A virus **HBV** Hepatitis B virus **hCG** Human chorionic gonadotropin **HCV** Hepatitis C virus **HDL** High-density lipoprotein **H&E** Hematoxylin & eosin **HHV** Human herpesvirus (HHV-1, HHV-etc) **HIV** Human immunodeficiency virus **HLA** Human leukocyte antigen (the major histocompatibility complex of humans) **HMO** Health maintenance organization **HPLC** High-performance liquid chromatography **HPV** Human papillomavirus **HSV** Herpes simplex virus **HTLV-I** Human T cell leukemia/lymphoma virus **ICU** Intensive care unit **IDDM** Insulin-dependent diabetes mellitus **ie** *id est*, that is (to say) **IFN** Interferon **Ig** Immunoglobulin **IL** Interleukin **IM** Intramuscular **ImPx** Immunoperoxidase **IQ** Intelligence quotient **IR** Infrared **ISH** in situ hybridization **ITP** Idiopathic thrombocytopenic purpura **IUD** Intrauterine (contraceptive) device **IV** Intravenous **IVDU** Intravenous drug use/user **JCAHO** Joint Commission of Accredited Hospitals Organization **K⁺** Potassium **kD** Kilodalton **KS** Kaposi sarcoma **LDH** Lactate dehydrogenase **LDL** Low-density lipoprotein **LGV** Lymphogranuloma venereum **LH** Luteinizing hormone **LM** Light microscopy **LN** Lymph node **MAOI** Monoamine oxidase inhibitor **MEN** Multiple endocrine neoplasia **MHC** Major histocompatibility complex **MI** Myocardial infarction **mo/ma** Monocyte/macrophage (tissue histiocyte) **MPS** Mucopolysaccaride(s), mucopolysaccharidosis **MRI** Magnetic resonance imaging **mRNA** Messenger RNA (ribonucleic acid) **MS** Multiple sclerosis **MVA** Motor vehicle accident **MW** Molecular weight **Na⁺** Sodium **N/C ratio** Nuclear/cytoplasmic ratio **N-CAM** Neuronal-cell adhesion molecule **NGF** Nerve growth factor **NHL** Non-Hodgkin's lymphoma **NIH** National Institutes of Health **NHL** Non-Hodgkin's lymphoma **NIDDM** Non-insulin-dependent diabetes mellitus **NK cell** Natural killer cell **NO** Nitric oxide **NSAID** Nonsteroidal anti-inflammatory drug **OR** Operating room, operating suite **OSHA** Occupational Safety and Health Administration **PAF** Platelet activating factor **PAS** Periodic acid-Schiff **PCBs** Polychlorinated biphenyls **PCP** *Pneumocystis carinii* pneumonia **PCR** Polymerase chain reaction **PDA** Patent ductus arteriosus **PG** Prostaglandin **PID** Pelvic inflammatory disease **PMN(s)** Polymorphonuclear neutrophil(s) or leukocyte(s), segmented neutrophil(s) **ppm** Parts per million *pron* Pronounced **PT** Prothrombin time **PTE** Pulmonary thromboembolism **PTH** Parathyroid hormone **aPTT** (activated) Partial thromboplastin time **QA** Quality assurance **QC** Quality control **RA** Rheumatoid arthritis **RBCs** Red blood cells, erythrocytes **RDS** Respiratory distress syndrome **REM sleep** Rapid eye movement sleep **RFLP** Restriction fragment length polymorphism **RIA** Radioimmunoassay **RR** Relative risk **rRNA** Ribosomal RNA (ribonucleic acid) **RSV** Respiratory syncytial virus **RT** Radiation therapy, reverse transcriptase **SD** Standard deviation **sec** Second (time) **SI** International System (of units), see there **SIDS** Sudden infant death syndrome **SLE** Systemic lupus erythematosus **STD** Sexually-transmitted disease **TAH-BSO** Total abdominal hysterectomy with bilateral salpingo-oophorectomy **TB** Tuberculosis **TDM** Therapeutic drug monitoring **TGF-β** Transforming growth factor-β **TIA** Transient ischemic attack **TIBC** Total iron-binding capacity **TLC** Thin-layer chromatography **TNF** Tumor necrosis factor **tRNA** Transfer RNA (ribonucleic acid) **T-S** Trimethoprim-sulfamethoxazole **TSH** Thyroid-stimulating hormone **TTP** Thrombotic thrombocytopenic purpura **TX** Thromboxane **U** 1) Unit 2) University **UK** United Kingdom **URI** Upper respiratory tract infection **US** United States **UTI** Urinary tract infection **UV** Ultraviolet **VDRL** Venereal disease research laboratory (test) for syphilis **VIP** Vasoactive intestinal polypeptide **VLDL** Very low density lipoprotein **V/Q** Ventilation/perfusion **vs** versus, in contrast to, in comparison with, in contrast to **VSD** Ventricular septal defect **VZV** Varicella-zoster virus **WBCs** White blood cells, leukocytes **WHO** World Health Organization **X-R** X-linked recessive ↓ Decrease, decreased, decreases, decreasing ↑ Increase, increased, increases, increasing ♀ Female, women ♂ Male, men

J Symbol for: Joule

J5 antiserum A polyclonal preparation of antibodies raised against the core glycolipid of Enterobacteriaceae, which is may reduce the mortality of gram-negative infections, except in patients with neutropenia (N Engl J Med 1993; 328:1323ᴏᴛ)

J-chain A 15-kD polypeptide that allows polymerization of immunoglobulins by disulfide bonds between polymeric serum IgA and all secretory IgA, as well as IgM and IgG-secreting glandular tissue; the J-chain has a high content of arginine, aspartic acid and glutamic acid and has 77% 'homology' to the mouse J-chain, formed in the mouse by splicing 4 exons; its synthesis is increased by interleukin-2

J curve phenomenon Epidemiology A relationship (figure) that exists between risk factors for, and the mortality from a particular pathological process, such that as the risk factor (eg alcohol consumption-AC, blood pressure-BP, and total cholesterol-TC) increases, so does the mortality; in diseases with a JCP, there is a critical point below which the AC, BP, TC is too low and there is opposite trend, and decreasing these risk factors below a critical point may be associated with an ↑ risk of morbidity and death of uncertain origin (JAMA 1991; 265:489) alcohol; although there are an estimated excess of 100 000 deaths/year (US) attributed to alcohol, a mean of 81 000 excess coronary heart disease-related deaths are attributed to abstinence (JAMA 1994; 272:967ᴇᴅ), dietary fat, and the incidence of breast cancer (J Nat Cancer Inst 1991; 83:336) Cf U curve

J-1 visa Exchange visitor visa A visa for those who '…*are formally participants in the Exchange Visitor Program (EVP) administered by the US Information Agency, the purpose of which is to enhance educational exchange… visitors must be guaranteed employment by an accredited educational institution, such as a hospital or…other organization such as the National Institutes of Health…(the) sponsorship is for a limited duration, generally not exceeding 7 years. Applicants for J-I visas must obtain ECFMG certification before they are granted the visa. On completion of the EVP, exchange visitors are required to return to their home country for a minimum of 2 years before attempting to return to the US in a permanent immigrant status* (JAMA 1995; 273:1521ᴏᴀ) Cf H1-B visa

While the purpose of the J-1 was to allow foreign national international medical graduates access to the US form of graduate medical education and have them practice in their home countries, it has become a conduit for physicians to emigrate from their countries to the US, resulting in a 'brain drain' effect; the pattern of specialization among IMGs is similar to that of American medical graduates (JAMA 1995; 273:1521ᴏᴀ)

J wave of Osbourne A quasi-pathognomonic EKG change seen in ⅓ of patients with hypothermia, appearing as a positive 'hump' at the end of a QRS complex that disappears on rewarming the patient; other cardiovascular changes include bradyarrhythmia, atrial flutter and fibrillation EKG Prolongation of the P-R and S-T intervals and T-wave inversion

jaagziekte *jaag* Afrikaans, hunted, *ziekte* sickness Pulmonary adenomatosis A disease* first described in sheep in the Republic of South Africa Etiology Caused by a ovine retrovirus Pathology The lungs have microscopic features that are analogous to bronchoalveolar cell carcinoma of humans

*The name derives from the manner in which the animals become dyspneic, perceive themselves pursued and run until they die

jabberer Screamer, see there

jack-knife phenomenon Clasp knife phenomenon, see there

jackknifing technique Statistics A method that examines whether a final logistic regression model from multiple sets of data is unduly influenced or skewed by a particular set of data; in this method, each dataset is deleted in turn, and the regression coefficients are reestimated from the remaining datasets and tested for outliers (JAMA 1994; 272:841ᴏᴄ)

'jackpot' experiment Research An experiment designed in the hope (or with the assumption) that the results of the experimental sequence will corroborate an unusual scientific phenomenon; such goal-oriented research is rarely rewarded with the desired result, ie the 'jackpot'

Note: Most research proceeds with a slow deliberate pace likened to the plodding of the Tortoise in Aesop's fable of '*The Tortoise and the Hare*'

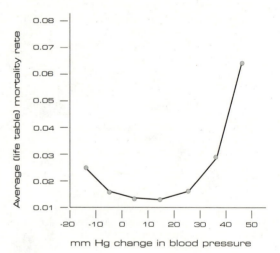

J curve phenomenon

Jackson Hole group Health Care Environment An informal 'think tank' composed of supporters (of health care reform) from academic institutions, private business, publishing and the health care industry that periodically convenes at the home of Dr Paul Ellwood, Jr, in the Grand Teton mountain range in Wyoming (US) to discuss policy and means of implementation of health care reform (N Engl J Med 1993; 328:1208ᴇᴅ); the major 'product' of the Jackson Hole group has been the concept of Managed competition, see there

Jackson Laboratory The world-renowned resource of live genetic material that maintains over 1000 colonies of inbred strains and stocks of mutant mice for sale and distribution to scientists; located in Bar Harbor, Maine, Jackson Laboratory is also a genetic information resource and maintains banks of frozen mouse embryos and a mouse DNA bank; Cf ATCC

'jack-straw' crystals ANATOMIC PATHOLOGY A descriptor for the haphazardly arranged, intracytoplasmic crystals, seen by the phosphotungstic acid-hematoxylin (PTAH) stain and thought to represent Z-band material, which in addition to increased mitochondria and glycogen, is characteristic of rhabdomyomas; see Spiderweb cells

jail bars sign RADIOLOGY Dense osteosclerosis of the ribs, seen on a plain antero-posterior chest film, resulting in horizontal bands fancifully likened to the bars of a prison window, first described as characteristic of agnogenic myeloid metaplasia, it may also be seen in sickle cell anemia and osteopetrosis

jail fever Epidemic louse-born typhus fever

Jak-STAT pathway A molecular pathway that transduces the signals of many cytokines and peptide growth factors; once a ligand is bound to its cognate receptor, the receptor-associated Jak family tyrosine kinases rapidly trigger the tyrosine phosphorylation of STAT proteins, resulting in their activation; activated STATs then dimerize and translocate into the nucleus, where they directly activate target genes by binding to specific promoter-type DNA sequences (Science 1995; 265:1990R); unlike the complex cascade of molecules involved in the RAS pathway, the JSP requires only two families of proteins, the JAKs (Janus kinases) and the STAT (signal transducers and activators of transcription) proteins; in the JSP, a ligand binds to a membrane receptor, which phosphorylates a JAK, after which a DNA-binding STAT protein passes to the nucleus, binds to a cognate region of DNA, and stimulates the transcription of the desired protein; the JAK-STAT pathway is involved in the response to IFN-α, IFN-γ, as well as other growth factors and cytokines (Sci Am 1994; 270/3:18)

Jamaican neuropathy A condition characterized by spasticity and other signs of corticospinal tract disease, which has been divided into 1) An ataxic form, which is thought to be more common in Nigeria, accompanied by sensory ataxia, numbing and burning of the feet, deafness, visual defects with optic atrophy and a central scotoma, spasticity, leg atrophy and footdrop, findings that may be due to subclinical malnutrition and 2) Tropical spastic paraparesis, a subacute neuropathy with predominantly pyramidal tract disease which affects the posterior column, causing paresthesia, loss of sensation, bladder dysfunction and girdling lumbar pain; 80% of patients have antibodies to HTLV-I

Jamaican vomiting sickness An intoxication by 'bush tea' made from unripe fruit of the Jamaican ackee tree (*Blighia sapida*), caused by hypoglycin, a propionic acid derivative that inhibits isovaleryl CoA dehydrogenase, provoking violent vomiting, prostration, drowsiness, convulsions and hypoglycemia as low as 0.56 mmol/L (US: 10 mg/dl) MORTALITY High, often within 24 hours of ingestion, caused by the metabolites of hypoglycin A, an amino acid that is converted to coenzyme A thioesters and carnitine derivatives, which sequester intracellular carnitine, inhibiting fatty acid oxidation, causing accumulation of isovaleric acid with continued fatty acid esterification, resulting in a fine-droplet fatty liver (N Engl J Med 1976; 295:461)

jamais vu French, never seen PSYCHIATRY A group of paramnesias in which there is a complete absence of memory for events known to have been experienced by the subject, each of which has been associated with neurotic depersonalization and temporal lobe epilepsy

JAMAIS ENTENDU Intense feeling of never having previously heard something JAMAIS EPROUVÉ Intense feeling of never having previously experienced something JAMAIS FAIT Intense feeling of never having previously done something JAMAIS PENSÉE Intense feeling of never having previously thought something JAMAIS RACONTÉE Intense feeling of never having previously related something (as in having told someone) JAMAIS VÉCU Intense feeling of never having previously lived through something JAMAIS VOULU Intense feeling of never having previously wished something JAMAIS VU Intense feeling of never having previously seen something; Cf Deja

Jane Doe A term for a generic or nameless female; see John Doe

Japanese cerebrovascular disease Moya-Moya disease, see there

Japanese encephalitis The single most common epidemic form of viral encephalitis, reaching an incidence of $50/10^5$ (in contrast, the peak of the poliomyelitis epidemic did not surpass $10/10^5$); JE is often fatal or crippling, especially in Thailand, where an annual summer peak may affect 2000 people, carrying a 20% mortality; vaccination in Thailand has resulted in a ten-fold ↓ in JE, as well as a ↓ in the incidence and severity of dengue fever (both are flaviviruses, a family that includes yellow fever and St. Louis encephalitis virus) CLINICAL Abrupt onset with fever, headache, meningeal irritation, convulsions, muscular rigidity, mask-like facies, coarse tremor, paresis, hyperactive deep tendon reflexes PATHOLOGY Cortical neuronolysis, chronic perivascular inflammation of the brain, especially affecting the sustantia nigra, thalamus, hypothalamus, cortices, and basal ganglia VECTOR *Culex* mosquito

Japanese illusion NEUROLOGY A clinical test used to elicit right-left confusion in unilateral anesthesia; the patient crosses arms, opposes the palms and clasps fingers; the clasped hands are then rotated inward and the arms extended, making it difficult for the subject to tell the right from the left fingers

Jarvik-7 An artificial heart that was first transplanted into a dentist who survived 620 days; the second patient was transplanted in 1982 and died four months later; other subsequent deaths contributed to the FDA's decision to revoke approval for the Jarvik-7 as a permanent replacement organ, although it had been considered an adequate temporary 'hold-over' or bridge device and 6 of 8 of those for whom it was used for this purpose lived to hospital discharge; see Penn State Heart

jaw winking Marcus-Gunn phenomenon NEUROLOGY Elevation of a ptotic eye by jaw movement, as seen in AD [MIM 178300] congenital ptosis, due to faulty innervation of levator palpebrae; inhibition of the levator muscle of the jaw accompanied by 'winking' is known as the inverse Marcus-Gunn phenomenon

jaw wiring An extreme treatment of morbid obesity that utilizes the same methods and devices as those used for jaw fractures, allowing only the intake of liquids; although this technique is effective while the patient is 'wired', the patients usually regain the weight unless it is combined with another modality, eg ileal bypass surgery; see Gastric bubble, Ileal bypass surgery, Morbid obesity

JCAHO see Joint Commission on Accreditation of Healthcare Organizations

JC virus A polyoma virus, named after the index patient that causes progressive multifocal leukoencephalopathy (a subacute demyelinating infection of oligodendroglia, affecting immunocompromised hosts); during its long latency, the virus is maintained within monocytes and eventually penetrating the glial cells by the Virchow-Robin space; when the virus is injected into rodents and primates, many develop CNS tumors (astrocytomas, ganglioblastomas and retinoneuroblastomas)

Jeep seat An inflammation of a pilonidal cyst and sinus that arises in a congenital malformation of the sacrococcygeal region with focal persistence of the neuroendocrine canal and ingrowth of hair into the cyst/sinus; 'Jeep driver's seat' is often first seen after repeated trauma as may occur in young military recruits who bounce over the countryside in shock absorber-less military vehicles or 'jeeps'

Jeffrey Dahmer FORENSIC PSYCHIATRY A 31-year-old candy factory worker from the midwestern US who is alleged to have murdered 16 young men and boys, dismembered their bodies in his apartment, and performed sexual acts on and/or eaten parts thereof (**CAP Today April 1992**) Dahmer was beaten to death by a fellow prisoner in 1994, while serving multiple life-time sentences; see Serial killer

Jeffries probe DNA fingerprinting, see there

jejuno-ileal bypass see Ileal bypass surgery

'Jekyll-and-Hyde' syndrome A symptom complex described in the elderly who cyclically improve with hospitalization (general stabilization, rehydration, appropriate administration of drugs) and undergo mental and physical deterioration while at home

Note: This reference to the hero/villain of RL Stevenson's short story of Dr Jekyll and Mr Hyde, is inappropriate, as the elderly are not so Janus-faced

Jello™ sign OBSTETRICS A characteristic undulation of the scrotum that occurs with fetal limb movement, a 'soft' but relatively reliable criterion for determining an infant's sex by ultrasonography, which may be seen after the 22nd gestational week; the movement has been fancifully likened to that evoked by a proprietary brand of instant gelatin

jentigo DERMATOLOGY A term for a histologic finding that consists of a combined junctional nevus and simple lentigo, coined by the Ackerman group of dermatopathology; in the natural history of a simple lentigo, increased melanocytes, originally distributed singly in the basal layer, tend to aggregate into nests at the epidermal-dermal junction; differentiating this lesion from a melanoma in situ rests on finding single and nests of melanocytes scattered along a broad front, poor circumscription and larger size in the malignant melanoma

Jerne network theory IMMUNOLOGY A hypothesis born from experimental data suggesting that after production of an antibody, 'Ab-1' to an antigen, 'X', the Ab-1 antibody-producing cells would be down-regulated by a second group of antibodies, 'Ab-2' that are formed against Ab-1, which recognize an epitope near the binding region of Ab-1; this network of interrelated and down-regulating antibodies allows immunologic 'homeostasis', so that endless antibody production to differing 'self' antigens does not occur, preventing uncontrolled antibody production

Jervell and Lange-Nielsen syndrome Long Q-T syndrome, see there

Jessner's solution DERMATOLOGY A cocktail that contains resorcinol, salicylic acid, lactic acid, and ethanol, which may be used in combination with 35% tricholoroacetic acid as a therapy for widespread actinic keratosis of the face (**Arch Dermatol 1995; 131:176**)

jet lag An acute shift in the circadian rhythm, caused by travelling across multiple (usually three or more) time zones CLINICAL Alterations in mood, performance efficiency, temperature rhythms, rapid eye movement and slow-wave sleep; the patterns revert to normal either in a linear or monotonic fashion after several days 'acclimatization' in the new time zone; see Circadian rhythm, Insomnia, Shift work, Sleep disorders

jet lesions CARDIAC PATHOLOGY Vegetations that develop where a regurgitant 'jet' of turbulent blood flow strikes the endocardium, causing fibrosis and roughening of the endocardial wall, typical of anomalies of blood flow from a high-to-low pressure region, eg aortic stenosis or coarctation, mitral stenosis, ventricular septal defect and patent ductus arteriosus, as occurs in rheumatic fever or congenital heart disease; the roughened lesions may give rise to small emboli and produce cerebral thromboembolism

jet phenomenon RADIOLOGY A narrow-shouldered column of barium seen as it gushes past the stenosis caused by an esophageal web, or a dysfunctional cricopharynx

jet sign UROLOGIC RADIOLOGY A thin, obliquely-oriented high-pressure stream of radiocontrast seen in excretory urograms of a normal bladder, the result of peristaltic emptying of the ureters

jet ventilation A technique used during tracheal reconstructive surgery where a catheter tube is passed through the endotracheal tube into the distal main stem bronchus; a small tidal volume is delivered at a high (60-150 'breaths'/minute) frequency which serves to maintain lung expansion, alveolar ventilation and oxygenation

JGA Juxtaglomerular apparatus

jigsaw puzzle cell Poikilocyte, see there

jigsaw-puzzle contours OPHTHALMOLOGY A variegated, mosaic pattern of hyperpigmentation seen in angioid streaks of the retinal fundus, located posterior to the retina itself

jigsaw-puzzle model MOLECULAR BIOLOGY A hypothesis that proteins undergo a random set of folding intermediates before assuming their native or in vivo configuration; the protein folding process in barnase (and presumably others, if not all proteins) appears to follow a defined pathway in which there is one or more distinct intermediate transition states

jigsaw puzzle tumor Cylindroma, see there

Jim Henson's disease Toxic shock-like syndrome, see there

jitter NEUROLOGY A finding in motor neuron disease characterized as instability in subcomponents of motor unit action potentials when measured by single-fiber electromyography and thought to be due to inefficient transmission of impulses in recent neural collaterals or due to abnormal neuromuscular transmission (**Mayo Clin Proc 1991; 66:54**)

jitter phenomenon NEUROPHYSIOLOGY A normally variable interval in the firing of a muscle impulse, attributed to 'chaos' that exists among action potentials of the muscle fibers in the same motor unit, as recorded in single-fiber electromyography; in myasthenia gravis, the jitter time is increased and the impulses may not appear at the appropriate interval ('blockings')

Jo-1 syndrome A clinical complex related to the production of antibodies against the Jo-1 antigen (histidyl-tRNA synthetase), which is associated with myosotis, arthritis and interstitial lung disease

Note: Anti-Jo-1 antibodies are present in 25% of patients with various forms of myositis, including polymyositis, dermatomyositis and the 'overlap' syndrome

job burnout OCCUPATIONAL MEDICINE A generic term for the end-stage of work-related stress, in which the employee functions at a 'ground state'; at greatest risk for JB are those with the lowest income, college education, and single women with children (**Am Med News 25 May 1992 p17**) Cf Compassion fatigue

job lock HEALTH CARE ENVIRONMENT A situation in which a person is in effect (although not in actual fact) forced to remain in one company's employ either through fear of losing health care coverage or because a potential employer's health plan refuses to cover a medical circumstance, eg a pre-existing condition, in the employee or his/her dependent (**Congressional Quarterly, 1993, in Clin Lab Sci 1994; 7:141**); it is estimated that 20% of the US population, in particular the 'working poor' suffer from job lock (**Am Med News 2 November 1992, p 36**) is a hidden cost of the present system; when a person takes a new position, there are long 'pre-existing condition' waiting periods, higher rates than for those who are already in the system, and outright denials (**Am Med News 25 October 1992, p7**)see Pre-existing condition

job stress The work-related combination of high psychological demands and low decision latitude; intuitively, hypertension has been related to job stress and has a relative risk of 3.1 (J Am Med Assoc 1990; 263:1929); see 'Toxic core', Type A personality

Job syndrome An immunodeficiency* characterized by multiple recurring abscesses CLINICAL Multiple episodes of otitis media, sinusitis, severe, life-threatening staphylococcal infections, chronic eczemoid lesions and recurring abscesses of the lungs, skin and joints LABORATORY Defects in neutrophil and monocyte chemotaxis, hyperimmunoglobulin E (see there)

Note: The biblical Job was cursed and covered with boils (abscesses) from head to toe (one of the calamities he suffered to test his faith in God); hyperimmunoglobulin E syndrome is the accepted synonym for Job syndrome because of the characteristic multiple recurring abscesses; however, since the description of his affliction was vague, historians have postulated that Job syndrome was due to syphilis, yaws, leprosy, smallpox, pemphigus, dermatitis herpetiformis, pellagra or scurvy

Jocasta complex PSYCHIATRY 1) The sexual love or desire, usually latent that a mother has for a son or 2) The domineering non-incestuous, quasi-adulatory love that an affect-hungry mother has for an intelligent son, often in the face of an absent or weak father figure

Jocasta of Greek mythology was the mother of Oedipus; while Oedipus' desire for his mother was completely innocent, Jocasta's incestuous act was conscious; see Oedipus complex; Cf Phaedra complex

jodbasedow disease Hyperthyroidism in iodine-(German, Jod) deficient patients that occurs after iodine replacement, resulting in a hypermetabolic goitrous state with exophthalmos, causing an autoimmune disease with antibodies directed against the TSH receptor

Note: von Basedow described the condition in 1840, Graves in 1835

jogger's foot Tarsal tunnel syndrome, see there

John Doe A term for a generic or nameless male, which is of particular use in clinical and forensic medicine, when it acts as a temporary identifier for persons without identification; see Jane Doe

Johnson v Calvert SURROGACY A legal case that arose when the gestational surrogate (ie the gestational, but not the biological mother) changed her mind and wanted to keep the child created by the biological parents; the court held for the biological parents, because they were the genetic and the intended parents, and therefore the legal parents (N Engl J Med 1994; 331:685BR)

Johnson v University of Chicago Hospitals A legal case that involved the routing of a seriously injured infant to another hospital when the University of Chicago's pediatric intensive care unit was 'on bypass', as its 13-bed unit was filled to legal capacity; the infant subsequently died, and the infant's mother sued under the Emergency Medical Treatment and Active Labor Act (popularly known as the COBRA legislation‡), which was intended to minimize patient dumping (the transfer of indigent patients from private hospitals to public hospitals for financial reasons); it has been broadly applied to include patients who were either never admitted to a hospital, or could not be for various reasons (Am Med News 16 Nov 1992 p1)

Johnson Controls decision see Maternal-fetal conflict(s)

'joint' SUBSTANCE ABUSE A colloquial term for a cigarette made from dried marijuana (Cannibas sativa) leaves, which is 'toked' in order to produce a 'high', and if smoked in excess, 'get stoned'; see Hallucinogen, Marijuana, Substance abuse, THC receptor

Joint Commission on Accreditation of Healthcare Organizations JCAHO HEALTH CARE ENVIRONMENT A private, nonprofit organization sponsored by a number of medical associations (American Hospital Association, American Medical Association, American Dental Association and by the American College of Physicians and American College of Surgeons), the purpose of which is to maintain a high standard of institutional care, by both establishing guidelines for the operation of hospitals and other (psychiatric, ambulatory and long-term) health care facilities and by 'policing' those facilities through surveys and periodic inspections; 'accreditation' of a facility is a requirement adopted by health insurers, funding agencies and public programs (CAP Today February 1994)

joint implementation ENVIRONMENT A proposal for reduction in greenhouse gases that would '...allow nations with advanced technology to offset some of their own emissions-reduction quotas by helping less developed nations lower their own emissions.' (Science 1995; 268:284, 204) see Berlin Mandate

joint mice ORTHOPEDICS A fanciful term for free bodies within the synovial cavity, especially of the knee, which are composed of fibrous tissue covered by cartilage and measure 0.5 to 1.5 cm in diameter, classically described in degenerative joint disease; joint mice are a relatively nonspecific finding, since they may also be seen in synovial osteochondromatosis, chondrometaplasia, neuropathic arthropathy, osteoarthritis dissecans, pigmented villonodular synovitis and gout

joint venture HEALTH CARE REIMBURSEMENT An ownership arrangement* which in the context of medical practice, refers to the ownership by physicians of health care facilities to which they refer patients for services, but at which they do not themselves practice medicine VENTURE CAPITOL '...any group of activities, including attempting to make, making, or performing a contract, by two or more persons for the purpose of A) Theoretical analysis, experimentation, or systematic study of phenomena or observable facts B) The development or testing of basic engineering principles C) The extension of investigative findings or theory of a scientific or technical nature into practical application for experimental and demonstrative purposes, including the experimental production and testing of models, prototypes, equipment, materials, and processes D) The collection, exchange, and analysis or research information E) The production of any product, process, or service or F) Any combination of the above, and may include the establishment and operation of facilities for the conducting of research, the conducting of such venture on a protected and proprietary basis, and the prosecuting of applications for patents and the granting of licenses for the results of such venture (American Technology Preeminence Act of 1991 (Pub L 102-245); US Dept Commerce, Technology Administration, National Institute of Standards and Technology, Advanced Technology Program Proposal Preparation Kit, Nove 1994, Appendix A, Subpart C, Sec 5131, Sec 28j1,)

*BACKGROUND Under US Federal law, it is illegal for physicians to recieve 'kickbacks' (see there) for referring patients with Medicaid or Medicare coverage to a particular physician; such laws also exist in 36 states; these laws do not prohibit referral to health care business ventures at which a physician does not actually practice, resulting in the financially abusive practice of disguised kickbacks; such joint ventures lead to overuse of services, ↑ cost to the consumer, ↓ access to the poor and services of reduced quality (N Engl J Med 1992; 327:1497SA) see Kickback,

Jones' criteria CARDIOLOGY/RHEUMATOLOGY A set of criteria for guidance in the diagnosis of acute rheumatic fever first proposed by TD Jones in 1944, and subsequently revised and updated by the American Heart Association; ARF can be diagnosed with reasonable certainty with two (or more) major criteria[1], or one major and two minor[2] criteria (see table), assuming previous evidence of group A streptococcal infection (JAMA 1992; 268:2069CC)

[1]Carditis, erythema marginatum, polyarthritis, Sydenham's chorea and subcutaneous nodules [2]CLINICAL a) Previous rheumatic fever or known rheumatic heart disease, arthralgia or fever b) LABORATORY Acute phase reactants, erythrocyte sedimentation rate, antistreptolysin O, C-reactive protein, ↑ P-R interval on EKG

Joseph complex PSYCHOLOGY An allegorical descriptor for intense sibling rivalry, derived from the favorite and youngest of the twelve sons of Jacob, the Israelite, Joseph, who was cast out by his brothers

journal club A form of graduate (and less commonly, continuing) medical education used by physicians during the residency training period, in which a small group convenes and discusses, analyzes and reviews a limited number of articles from major medical journals, often on a weekly or monthly basis; while there are no rules, the journal club attempts to increase a professional's reading of timely information, presenting it from different vantage points, improving the resident's knowledge of epidemiology and biostatistics with the hope that he/she will be critical in the assimilation of new information, and continue to learn long after the completion of the formal education period

Note: The first journal club was organized by Sir William Osler at McGill University in 1875 (see JAMA 1988; 260:2537)

journaling LABORATORY MEDICINE A type of laboratory information system back-up in which every 'transaction' is recorded on both the primary system files (which can be wiped-out in a system 'crash') and on a special transaction log stored on a separate disk or tape; in the event of a primary system failure ('crash'), the combination of a back-up tape and the transaction file, which was 'journaled' since the last backup was created, would (theoretically) allow the system to recreate all patient files; in practice journaling is often incomplete, and it is recommended that two forms 'minibackup' be used, ie both journaling and mirroring; Cf Mirroring

J pouch COLORECTAL SURGERY A reservoir formed from a J-shaped loop of the terminal ileum where the loops are sectioned, forming a pouch and then anastomosed to a continent anorectum, preserving anal sphincter function; the procedure is used following total proctocolectomy for familial polyposis coli or ulcerative colitis totalis; see S pouch

J-shaped sella A shallow, elongated or 'boot-shaped' sella turcica with an elongated anterior recess, extending below the anterior clinoid process, classically seen in Hurler's mucopolysaccharidosis (due to the accumulation of dermatan and keratan sulfates or glycosaminoglycans); the change may also occur in the orodigitofacial syndrome and mannosidosis

J syndrome Jamaican syndrome A form of DM thought to be identical to the 'Third diabetic syndrome', see there

Judaism, practice of see Haman-Tashen intoxication, Seder syncope, Shmita salmonellosis, Shofar-blowing emphysema, Yom Kippur effect; Cf Hanukkah factor, Harvest Moon phenomenon

judicial bypass LEGAL MEDICINE A form of surrogacy in which a guardian's authority is circumvented and the decision-making autonomy is allowed to pass to the person for whom the guardian had been appointed or designated; a judicial bypass may be evoked to authorize an abortion in a teenage girl who does not want her parents to know, or who wants an abortion against her parents' wishes

jughandle view RADIOLOGY A modified basal view of the skull used to visualize the zygomatic arches, of particular interest in evaluating midfacial fractures

juice therapy ALTERNATIVE MEDICINE The ingestion of fresh raw fruit and vegetable juices to 'replenish' the body and provide nutritional support; JT is believed by its advocates to have anticarcinogenic, suppressive, and detoxifying effects, and is claimed to be an effective adjunctive therapy for AIDS, allergies, cancer, rheumatic diseases, and others, claims that are difficult to refute (or confirm); see Alternative medicine

juicy baby A fanciful term for an infant who produces excess mucus in the early post-partum period; 'juiciness' is a soft criterion for esophageal atresia, which when accompanied by respiratory distress (cyanosis and tachypnea), implies concomitant tracheoesophageal fistula

Jukes family BEHAVIORAL GENETICS An Irish family studied and reported by RL Dugdale in 1874 that appeared to lend support to the controversial concept of hereditary crime; of the 709-member cohort studied, 200 had been on relief (welfare, public assistance), 128 had been prostitutes, 76 were convicted criminals, and 18 kept brothels; despite continued interest in putative 'crime genes'‡, there is no current evidence that they exist (New York Times 15 Sept 1992; C1)

July phenomenon A popular myth in North America holds that the quality of medical care deteriorates and mortality rate increases in teaching hospitals during the month of July (the time when interns, fresh from medical school begin their training period); one study indicated that the length of hospital stay and costs may actually be reduced during July (JAMA 1990; 263:953) see Libby Zion; Cf DRGs, 'Quicker and sicker'

Note: Given the financial pressures in the US to discharge patients as soon as possible, there has been a drive to reduce hospital length of stay, a patients may be discharged 'quicker and sicker'

jumper syndrome Vertical deceleration injury A distinct form of blunt trauma from jumping or falling from heights, usually greater than five stories; the injury severity score is 41 (predicted survival, 50%; actual survival is less); all had multiple fractures, eg 'ring fracture' of the skull base, separating the rim of the foramen magnum from the remainder of the base and compression fractures of the vertebrae, both of which occur when the victim lands on his feet or buttocks; many jumpers may also have coup and/or contrecoup injuries of the brain; over ½ arrive in the emergency ward in shock; most have angiographic evidence of retroperitoneal hemorrhage; see Lover's heels

jumping Chromosome jumping, see there

'Jumping Frenchmen of Maine' syndrome A culture-specific complex that is evoked in the members of a religious sect that originated from Wales and residing in North America, the rites of which includes jumping, rolling on the ground, barking like dogs and so on until a state of ecstasy is achieved, which subsides after the ceremonies, or which may be re-evoked on command; the reflex may be considered an exaggeration of the normal startle reflex (hyperexplexia) seen in 'startle diseases' that may be elicited by any, often auditory stimulus, causing a stiffening of the body, arm flexion, a jump, involuntary shout or fall to the ground; such complexes were thought to be inherited in an AR [MIM 244100] fashion, but are now believed to result from a form of operant conditioning, and must be differentiated from Giles de la Tourette and startle epilepsy

jump position Posture of a spastic child who stands with his knees and hips flexed and the ankles in equinus position, a characteristic stance in spastic paraplegia of cerebral palsy

jumping genes Mobile DNA elements, which were first recognized by B McClintock in maize (*Zea mays*) in 1931, which she viewed as agents capable of moving into and out of (ie, 'jumping') genes, concomitantly alternating the genetic activity of those genes; jumping genes include insertion sequences, transposons, viral and non-viral retroposons

jumping library A cloned 'library' of transposible DNA elements, produced by cloning a locus by reverse genetics, crossing over hundreds of kilobases; here reverse genetics with chromosomal map positions and genetically-linked DNA markers are used to identify and clone DNA sequences 100 or more kilobases away from starting point METHOD Pulsed field electrophoresis (see there); see Library

jumping PCR A PCR reaction that amplifies an incorrect segment of DNA as the specimen of interest has been denatured and therefore broken into smaller amplifiable segments (CAP Today October 1994)

jun An oncogene that induces avian sarcoma and transforms certain avian cell lines in vitro; the viral oncogene, v-*jun* and the related cellular genes c-*jun*, *jun* B and *jun* D encode transactivating or repressing DNA-binding proteins, forming homodimeric (Jun-Jun) or heterodimeric (Jun-Fos) protein complexes that recognize the AP-1 consensus sequence, a response element that makes cells susceptible to the tumor-promoter, phorbol ester TPA, as well as cell growth factors; v-*jun* lacks a nucleotide sequence for 27 amino acids encoded by c-*jun*, has mutations causing amino acid substitutions not seen in c-*jun* and its protein product is highly expressed in v-*jun*-infected cells; the c-*jun* protein product is structurally similar to GCN4, a protein that activates yeast genes by binding to a DNA binding site similar to that of AP-1 a human transcription factor; *jun* binds to *fos* by a leucine zipper, together effecting greater control over gene transcription than either can alone; the jun protein is structurally and functionally similar to the *fos* protein; c-Jun-mediated transactivation may be augmented independently of c-Fos by Ha-Ras, which stimulates phosphorylation of c-Jun's activation domain and possibly explains how oncoproteins participate in the transformation of cells in culture (**Nature 1991; 351:122**) see *fos*, Oncogene, One-hit/two-hit model

Note: *jun* was named by a post-doctoral fellow, as an abbreviation of ju-nana, Japanese for 17, as it was the 17th in a group of 30 avian sarcoma viruses recovered from the tumors encountered in a poultry house by Vogt et al, which causes a fibrosarcoma in chickens

junk DNA Long stretches of non-protein-coding DNA that comprise 95-98% of the human genome, which has been highly conserved over thousands, possibly millions of years; JD is mobile, capable of self-replication, but serves no known function*, thus is also known as selfish DNA; these quasi-autonomous segments include spacer DNA, satellite DNA, and exons that are spliced out when the primary transcript of the RNA becomes mRNA; some JD may act as subtle enhancers of gene expression; other JD provides the message for what is the optimal shape in the form of folds and pleats; some of the junk may act as a reservoir of change, allowing DNA to be more easily shuffled, hastening evolutionary steps; others act as buffers, absorbing genetic shock, eg by heat, viruses, and mutating toxins; see Human Genome Project, LINES, SINES

*The term junk is based on the assumption that anything that is not a gene that encodes a protein is useless, making viruses and bacteria the most efficient of organisms in that there is little intervening noncoding (junk) DNA

junk food A popular term for any food that is low in essential nutrients and high in carbohydrates; junk foods may be highly salted, eg potato chips/crisps, pretzels, high in refined sugar (empty calories), eg cake, candy, soft drinks and high in saturated fats and cholesterol, eg cake and chocolates; see Cafeteria model, 'Couch potato', 'Fast' food

junk science A colloquial term for any study or report that reaches sweeping conclusions, despite weaknesses in the method for the collection and analysis of the data (**N Engl J Med 1995; 332:1307c**)

junkie A US colloquialism for a person, usually an IV narcotic abusing addict, whose life is disorganized in terms of family and societal structure and whose existence revolves around obtention (often through theft, prostitution or other illicit means) of another 'fix' of narcotics, known in some circles as 'junk'; see Cold turkey, Shooting galleries

Note: The term junkie has been further colloquialized to imply anyone with an 'addiction' for a particular food or habit, eg Chocholate junkie, Junk food 'junkie'

Jupiter see MOO

'jury collar' A type of hardened plastic neck brace that may be worn by a plaintiff who claims that an accident or a medical procedure has resulted in neck or cervical spine injuries; the use of such a collar has a graphic effect on a jury, which may reward the plaintiff a large financial settlement for injuries allegedly caused by an automobile accident or by a physician's alleged incompetence

juvenile aponeurotic fibroma Calcifying aponeurotic fibroma, see there, aka Keasbey's tumor

juvenile carcinoma Secretory carcinoma A rare breast carcinoma seen in children, average age 9 PATHOLOGY Small, well-circumscribed, fibroadenoma-like tumor with tubuloalveolar and focal papillary formations lined by vacuolated cells producing eosinophilic, PAS-positive secretions TREATMENT 'Lumpectomy' is usually adequate

juvenile hyaline fibromatosis A rare AR [MIM 228600] condition, characterized by generalized subcutaneous and gingival nodules, which vaguely resembles myofibromatosis, but lacks mature collagen DDx Soft tissue proliferations are not uncommon in childhood and adolescence, most of which are benign, including calcifying aponeurotic fibroma, congenital fibromatoses (solitary or multiple), digital fibromatosis (see Kissing tumor), fibromatosis coli, fibrous hamartoma, infantile (desmoid-type) fibromatosis, infantile myofibromatosis, juvenile angiofibroma, hyaline fibromatosis and giant cell fibroblastoma

juvenile laryngeal papillomatosis A neoplasm in children caused by HPV types 6 and 11 that may also occur in adults in the upper respiratory tract (known as recurrent respiratory papillomatosis); the lesion is analagous to condyloma acuminatum of the genital tract; the tumor rarely undergoes malignant degeneration, although it may be accompanied by severe airway compromise, the major complication of this lesion, a lesion of such recalcitrance that hundreds of surgical resections may be required; although leukocyte interferon significantly reduces the growth rate of the tumors during the first six months of therapy, the effect is not sustained

juvenile 'melanoma' An obsolete misnomer for the spindle and epithelioid cell nevus or Spitz nevus, a benign pigmented nevus that occurs before puberty, commonly presenting as a raised pink or red nodule on the facial skin

juvenile myoclonic epilepsy A seizure disorder that comprises ± 4% of epilepsies CLINICAL Normal IQ, onset in adolescence, affecting the flexor muscles of the head, neck and shoulders; the attacks tend to occur as clonic-tonic-clonic seizures upon awakening EEG 4-6 Hz multi-spike and wave pattern; 40% of relatives, especially female, have myoclonus TREATMENT Valproate

juvenile pemphigoid A pruritic variant of bullous pemphigoid that affects the genitalia and face of children

juvenile periodontitis Early onset periodontitis, affecting adolescents, ♂:♀ ratio 3:1, characterized by an early loss of alveolar bone surrounding permanent teeth; 84% have underlying endocrinopathies and 12% had systemic disease, eg DM, neutropenia, Down and Ehlers-Danlos syndromes, hyperkeratosis palmaris et plantaris, histiocytosis X, and hypophosphatasia ETIOLOGY *Actinobacillus actinomycecomitans* and others; when accompanied by palmo-plantar hyperkeratosis, the disease is called Papillon-Lefèvre syndrome, characterized by loss of alveolar bone, premature dental exfoliation, clinical features of hereditary ectodermal dysplasia and calcifications of the falx and dura

juvenile xanthogranuloma A yellowish tumor of early childhood involving the face, head, neck and extremities PATHOLOGY Abundant dermal histocytes apposing adnexal structures, extending into the subcutis PROGNOSIS Spontaneous involution

juxtacrine interaction A type of cell-mediator interaction, in which a cell produces cytokines that interact directly with receptors of different types of cells, eg the interaction between smooth muscle cells in atheromatous lesions and the immediately adjacent endothelial cells (Arch Pathol Lab Med 1992; 116:1292oa)

juxtaovarian adnexal tumor An adnexal tumor of probable wolffian origin, which is located in the leaves of the broad ligament and often asymptomatic, affecting patients between ages 30 and 60 PATHOLOGY The tumors measure up to 12 cm, from rubbery to friable in consistency, appearing by light microscopy as clusters of epithelial-like mesothelial cells PROGNOSIS Often benign, rarely, these tumors may recur or metastasize

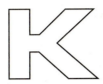

K Symbol for: 1) Equilibrium constant 2) Degrees (kelvin) 3) kilobyte (which is actually 1024 bytes) 4) Lysine 5) Potassium

k Symbol for: kilo- (10^3)

K_a The symbol for the ionization constant of an acid in an equilibrium reaction

K_b The symbol for the ionization constant of a base in an equilibrium reaction

K_{Ca} Calcium-dependent potassium channel

K_d The symbol for dissociation constant in an equilibrium reaction

K562 An immortalized cell line, originally obtained from a patient with CML in blast crisis, which is a 'standard' target for measuring NK cell activity, see NK cells

K antigens German, Kapsul MICROBIOLOGY A group of antigens present on the surface of gram-negative bacteria that are of two types 1) Protein (fimbriae) and 2) Acid polysaccharides, expressed on the surface of *Klebsiella* spp and *Escherichia coli*; K antigens are located external to the somatic 'O' antigen and are heat-labile and cross-react with other encapsulated bacteria (*Haemophilus influenzae*, *Streptococcus pneumoniae*, and *Neisseria meningitidis*); certain K antigens are associated with more virulent urinary tract infections; anti-K antibodies, while protective against the strain of bacteria, are often weak

K cell IMMUNOLOGY see Killer cell PULMONARY MEDICINE see Kulchitsky cell

K complexes NEUROLOGY High amplitude deflections (bursts) of high-voltage diphasic slow waves over the cranial vertex seen by EEG that are either spontaneous or due to sensory stimuli during stage 2 and 3 of the sleep cycle in response to arousal stimuli; K complexes are associated with bursts of sympathetic nerve activity and transient increases in blood pressure; asymmetric K complexes may indicate organic cerebral lesion or may rarely occur in patients with cortical atrophy, eg Alzheimer's disease (see **N Engl J Med 1993; 328:303oA**)

'K Mart model' A highly colloquial term for a state in which the loss of relatively low-paid personnel, eg 'floor' nurses in a hospital is compensated for by increasing the salary of those who remain (**JAMA 1990; 264:3117**)

K region MOLECULAR BIOLOGY A region of benzo(a)pyrene, an aromatic hydrocarbon with potent carcinogenic effects; the metabolic system, cytochrome P-450 can 'choose' two routes of metabolism for this molecule—one that results in a highly electrophilic (ie carcinogenic) diol-epoxide, a reaction centering around the opposite face of the molecule, the 'Bay' region, and the other which acts at the K region, leading to the non-carcinogenic 4,5-dihydrodiol, lending support to the model of carcinogenesis as defective DNA repair

Kabuki mask facies A congenital complex of unknown etiology with a characteristic facial dysmorphia (long palpebral fissures, eversion of the lateral lower eyelids, broad depressed nose, fancifully likened to a mask worn in a Kabuki theater), large ears, a high arched or cleft palate, mental and growth retardation, scoliosis and recurrent otitis (**Clin Genet 1982; 21:315**)

kabure An urticarial skin reaction that occurs 4-8 weeks after penetration of the skin by the burrowing cercariae of *Schistosoma japonicum*, which may be accompanied by fever, purpura, malaise, arthralgia, abdominal cramps, diarrhea, and hepatosplenomegaly

kallikrein A hydrolytic enzyme that cleaves kininogen to produce bradykinin, a nonapeptide that acts on vessels, evoking vasodilation, increasing capillary permeability; kallikrein also acts on smooth muscle, pain receptors and is chemotactic for neutrophils

kallikrein-kinin system An interconnected family of endogenous vasopressive peptides that maintain blood pressure by controlling regional blood flow and electrolyte and water excretion; kallikrein stimulates renin release and kinin production; the kallikrein-kinin and renin-aldosterone-angiotensin (RAA) systems interact to control blood pressure and are closely linked, as evidenced by kininase II that inactivates kinin and converts A-I to A-II; see Kinin, RAA system

Kallmann syndrome Hypogonadotropic eunuchoidism A rare condition with a highly variable hereditary pattern* characterized by secondary hypogonadism (↓ gonadotropin-releasing hormone due to hypothalamic or pituitary dysfunction) with testicular failure, and anosmia (due to hypo– or aplasia of the olfactory bulbs and tracts) in most, ↓ FSH and LH impairs both sperm and androgen production CLINICAL Delayed puberty, micropenis, eunuchoid features, cryptorchidism, midline defects, eg cleft lip and palate, unilateral renal agenesis, horseshoe kidney nerve deafness and hearing loss, color blindness, skeletal abnormalities; synkinesia, spatial attentional defects, spastic paraplegia, cerebellar dysfunction, horizontal nystagmus, pes cavus, mental retardation MOLECULAR PATHOLOGY The cognate gene product may be involved in migration of a specific subgroup of neurons, and possibly a more generalized defect in both neuronal and nonneuronal systems; there is 3.3-kb deletion confined to *KALIG-1*, a gene assigned to chromosome segment Xp22.3 in X-linked forms of KS (**N Engl J Med 1992; 326:1772oA**) TREATMENT Androgens may be used to induce anatomic maturation and gonadotropins or LH-releasing factor for spermatogenesis

*Reported frequency ranges from 1:10-60 000; most cases are X-linked [MIM 308700] and predominantly in ♂; rarely KS may be AR [MIM 244200] or AD [MIM 149750]

Kanagawa phenomenon MICROBIOLOGY A laboratory finding in *Vibrio parahemolyticus*, which becomes hemolytic on a Wagasumi agar, first described in Kanagawa, a prefecture of Japan and is of diagnostic use during epidemics

Kanemi oil intoxication see Yusho

Kane surgery Any surgical procedure performed by the surgeon on himself; Dr E O'Neill Kane operated upon himself for an inguinal hernia, appendicitis and amputated his own finger; one commentator on this form of surgery, noted that '...*an autosurgeon who represents himself for negligence has a fool for a surgeon, a patient, a prosecutor and a defender.*' (**JAMA 1987; 257:825**)

kang cancer Heat-induced squamous cell carcinoma seen in NW China, due to soot (**HT Lagcock Br Med J 1948; i:982**) Cf Kangri cancer

kangri cancer Heat-induced squamous cell carcinoma

seen in natives of Kashmir, occurring on the skin of the inner thighs and umbilicus, caused by the heat and volatile products produced by the kangri, an earthenware charcoal 'hibachi' worn for warmth by Kashmiris (Brit Med J 1923; 2:1255) Cf Kang cancer

kanteserin A serotonin antagonist that acts at the cognate receptors in the arterial wall but not in the endothelium; see Serotonin

Kaposi sarcoma A once rare, indolent malignancy that predominantly affected older Italian or Jewish men or those immunocompromised through the vicissitudes of transplantation, immunosuppression of lymphoproliferation; KS has become extremely common, occurring in 46% of male homosexuals with AIDS, 12% of female intravenous drug-abusers (IVDA) with AIDS and 4% of male IVDA with AIDS; KS is characterized by a proliferation of lymphatic or vascular channels, driven by growth and regulatory factors, including IL-1-β, IL-6 and tat protein PATHOLOGY Jagged blood vessels filled with red cells that percolate into the adjacent tissue, subdivided into inflammatory and polymorphous types TREATMENT Based on the findings that 1) KS is more common in ♂ and 2) when it does occur in ♀, it may regress in pregnancy, one group used β-hCG (human chorionic gonadotropin) to treat KS cell lines, which reportedly died when exposed to hCG (Nature 1995; 375:64oA) see Promontory sign

Note: Kaposi also described lupus erythematosus profundus (Kaposi-Irving syndrome), a variant of xeroderma pigmentosum (Kaposi syndrome, type II) and eczema herpeticum (Kaposi syndrome, type III)

Kaposi sarcoma-related herpesvirus KS330$_{233}$ An as yet-uncharacterized infectious agent, presumed to be a herpesvirus, which is believed to be the cause of both 'classic' and AIDS-associated KS (Science 1995; 267:959RN, N Engl J Med 1995; 332:1181oA) and body cavity-based lymphomas (N Engl J Med 1995; 332:1186oA)

Note: This agent may ultimately be designated human herpesvirus-8 (N Engl J Med 1995; 332:1227ED)

κ (kappa) chain One of the two light immunoglobulin chains; present in a 2:1 ratio with lambda

κ (kappa) rhythm NEUROLOGY An EEG pattern with alpha waves (8-13/sec, 50 µV sinusoidal waves, aka theta frequency), recorded over the temporal regions during normal mental activity

κ (kappa) statistic An index of interrater agreement in terms of peer assessment of quality of care

Karen Ann Quinlan see Persistent vegetative state

Karnovsky scale A scale of objective criteria for the quality of life, which is used for patients with incapacitating diseases; the scale was developed for patients with cancer and of use in AIDS; a KS of 100 indicates that there is no clinical evidence of disease; those with scores above 80 are able to maintain normal activities; a score between 50-70 precludes work and is accompanied by decreasing levels of autonomy; a person with a score between 10-40 is severely ill and requires hospitalization; a person with a score of 0 requires interment

karyotype An organism's chromosome complement, best studied by high-resolution photography in the metaphase of mitosis, the stage of maximum condensation and point when the chromosomes' morphology is most distinct; a haploid number (n) bears one half of a full set of the organism's chromosomes, 23 in humans; a full or euploid set of chromosomes in most mammals is 2n, one n being contributed during meiosis by the male and one n by the female to form a 2n complement of chromosoms; polyploidy refers to full multiples of n, eg 3n, 4n, 5n...; aneuploidy is a lopsided number of chromosomes (n x Y) + Z, where Z is not = n and Y is a whole number

karyotype analysis CLINICAL GENETICS The evaluation of a person's chromosomes for detection of a particular disease

process; KA is indicated for children born with congenital anomalies, mental retardation without due cause, intersex, primary amenorrhea, male or female infertility, habitual abortion without anatomic abnormalities, previous spontaneous abortions, advanced maternal age or family history of chromosome abnormalities; see also Banding, Chromosomes

Kaspar Hauser syndrome Psychosocial dwarfism, see there

katal The SI (International System) unit for measuring enzymatic activity, which is equal to 1 mol/ml of substrate consumed per second under specified conditions; depite the SI's 'blessing' of the katal, the International Unit (U) continues to be a widely preferred unit of measurement

Katayama disease Acute schistosomiasis caused by *S japonicum* and *S mansoni*, and rarely *S hematobium* after a 2-10 week incubation, corresponding to oviposition of juvenile worms; the disease severity is a function of worm load and evokes a serum sickness-like disease due to immune complex deposition INTERMEDIATE HOST Oncomelania snail DEFINITIVE HOST Water buffalo, domestic animals, human CLINICAL Abrupt onset of fever, chills, sweating, headache, cough, hepatosplenomegaly, lymphadenopathy, eosinophilia, potentially fatal if the worm load is heavy

Katskee v. Blue Cross/Blue Shield of Nebraska HEALTH CARE COVERAGE A legal dispute (245 Neb 808, 515 NW 2d 645 (1994)) brought before the Supreme Court of Nebraska regarding what medical services a health insurance company should cover; Ms S Katskee's mother and maternal aunt had both died of ovarian cancer at ages 47 and 48; HT Lynch, a well-respected expert on hereditary cancer, was consulted and estimated that Ms Katskee and her sisters had a 50% probability of developing breast and/or ovarian cancer, for which he recommended TAH-BSO; the Nebraska state 'Blues' refused to pay for the procedure, as the familial breast-ovarian carcinoma syndrome was not an illness at the time of the surgery, and therefore not deemed to be medically necessary (N Engl J Med 1994; 331:1027UM)

katzenellenbogen German, Cat's elbow sign Lichen planus actinicus DERMATOLOGY A variant of lichen planus, seen in the Middle East, on sun-exposed parts, especially the face, characterized by annular lesions with pigmented centers, central thinning of epidermis and well-demarcated pale, raised margins

Kawasaki disease Mucocutaneous lymph node syndrome An endemic and epidemic disease of children under age 5 that often follows a 1-2 week incubation, presenting with fever, cervical lymphadenopathy, palmo-plantar and mucosal erythema and edema, aneurysms of small and medium-sized coronary arteries with arteritis (occasionally causing sudden death; mortality, 1-5%), and may affect peripheral arteries ETIOLOGY Various microorganisms have been implicated, eg *Proprionobacterium acnes* or retroviruses, but none definitively LABORATORY Increased erythrocyte sedimentation rate, C-reactive protein, complement, globulin levels TREATMENT Early gammaglobulin in a single intravenous bolus (N Engl J Med 1991; 324:1633) or aspirin 80 IV cases have been reported in Japan with three epidemics in 1979, 1982 and 1986; fatality rate 0.4% especially in children under age 2 (JAMA 1991; 265:2699rv)

Note: Any of the CDC's criteria (see table) may occur as an isolated finding in toxic shock: Fever refractory to antibiotics, large and medium vessel vasculitis death due to acute myocarditis with CHF, arrhythmia, pericarditis, cardiac tamponade, thrombosis, MI, development of coronary arterial aneurysm

Kb Kilobase, see there

KB cell A cell line in permanent culture that was derived from a carcinoma in 1954; Cf HeLa cell

KCT Kaolin clotting time

kD see Kilodalton

72-kD (type IV) collagenase Matrix metalloproteinase-2, MMP-2

92-kD (type IV) collagenase Matrix metalloproteinase-9, MMP-9

72-kD gelatinase Matrix metalloproteinase-2, MMP-2

92-kD gelatinase Matrix metalloproteinase-9, MMP-9

kDal kilodalton; the term molecular weight (symbol, M_r) is increasingly preferred; a molcule with a mass of 28.0 kDal would be designated 28 000 M_r

KDEL sequence A tetramer of amino acids (Lys-Asp-Glu-Leu, abbreviated as KDEL in the one letter system) that is present at the carboxy-terminus of proteins, eg heavy chain-binding protein, protein disulfide isomerase, calreticulin and glucose-regulating protein 94, which serves as a retention signal for proteins residing in the endoplasmic reticulum, bound by a KDEL receptor; Cf RGD family

k-DNA see DNA

Kelley index of malignancy ALTERNATIVE MEDICINE A questionnaire developed by a researcher in the late 1960s who believed that cancer resulted from a deficiency of pancreatic enzyme(s); the questionnaire was used to allegedly locate and determine the growth rate of tumors, that were then treated with laetrile; see Laetrile, Metabolic therapy, Tijuana, Unproven cancer therapy

keloid Greek, Crab's claw An exuberant skin scar seen most commonly in adults aged 15-45 that is six-fold more common in dark-skinned individuals and in women; keloids may occur in other conditions, eg Rubinstein-Taybi syndrome and be associated with infection, burns, trauma, insect bites PATHOLOGY Rubbery, sharply demarcated, elevated scarred mass with pincer-like extensions, composed of whorled collagen fibers, often located on the seborrheic areas (shoulders and upper chest) and extremities; caused by excessive synthesis of collagen and increased proline hydroxylase activity; unlike hypertrophic scars that flatten with time, keloids are stable TREATMENT Local steroid injection to relieve pruritus or reduce the size in early lesions; post-excisional recurrence is common

Kemp Amendment US legislation passed in 1985 that withdrew governmental funding from any organization supporting abortion or sterilization (Sci Am 1993; 268/4:22)

Kemron A low-dose formulation of IFN-α, reported by some workers in Kenya as a cure or potential cure for AIDS, a claim that has not been substantiated

---

KAWASAKI DISEASE*

1) Fever of > than 5 days

2) Bilateral ocular conjunctival injection

3) One or more changes of oral mucosa, including erythema, fissuring and xerostomia, conjunctival edema, mucosal edema of upper respiratory tract, eg pharyngeal injection, dry, fissured lips and 'strawberry tongue'

4) One or more changes of extremities, including acral erythema or edema, periungual and/or generalized desquamation, polymorphous exanthematous rash, truncal and cervical lymphadenopathy

*CDC definition, requires 4+ of the above

---

keratin pearl Squamous pearl, see there

keratocyte Horn cell An erythrocyte with one or two notches or horns that result from the red cells being squeezed through strands of intravascular fibrin, as seen in DIC, microangiopathic hemolytic anemia, immune complex nephritis or foreign materials within vessels; as a result of this trauma, pseudovacuoles are formed which burst, leaving a horny erythrocyte

keratohyalin granules Dense osmiophilic aggregates of cytokeratin seen within horn cells of the granular cell layer of normal epidermis, eccrine duct cells, rarely also in clear cell type sweat gland tumors

keratosis A condition characterized by an increased production of keratin ACTINIC (SOLAR) KERATOSIS A lesion seen in sun-exposed parts of light-skinned subjects, characterized by hyperkeratosis, parakeratosis, upper dermal atrophy and squamous cell atypia, which may be a precursor of squamous cell carcinoma ARSENIC-INDUCED KERATOSIS A lesion of historic interest seen at a time when arsenic was used to treat arthritis, asthma, psoriasis and syphilis, characterized as warty palmo-plantar excrescences, occasionally evolving to squamous or basal cell carcinomas KERATOSIS PILARIS A lesion associated with ichthyosis vulgaris and atopic dermatitis, often on the extremities (in lichen spinulosus, similar lesions are located on the trunk and buttocks) with pinpoint indurations likened to a nutmeg grater SEBORRHEIC KERATOSIS A lesion common in the face and upper trunk of the middle-aged and elderly, histologically demonstrating hyperkeratosis, acanthosis and papillomatosis

keratolytic agent CLINICAL THERAPEUTICS A generic term for any agent (eg a solution of 2-10% salicylic acid) that is applied topically with the purpose of reducing the thickness of laminated keratin or hyperkeratotic scales, eg of psoriasis (N Engl J Med 1995; 332:581RV)

kerion A severe form of tinea capitis in which well-circumscribed portions of the scalp are transformed into a painful, boggy inflamed and confluent mass with loosening of the hair, purulent folliculitis, crusting, often accompanied by lymphadenopathy, due to a zoophilic superficial mycotic species, *Trichophyton verrucosum* or *T mentagrophytes*; geophilic or anthropophilic fungal infections may abruptly become kerions

Keshan disase CARDIOLOGY A disease of children and young women, first described in the Keshan Province of the mainland China, due to selenium deficiency in that region's water supply, resulting in dilated cardiomyopathy and increased platelet aggregation due to impaired free radical salvage by glutathione peroxidase; selenium deficiency favors selection and replication of a myocarditic form of Coxsakievirus (CVB3) (Nature Medicine 1995; 1:433, 405) PATHOLOGY Focal myocardial necrosis, fibrosis and contraction band formation TREATMENT Selenium

ketoacidosis A syndrome seen in poorly controlled DM, with 'starvation amidst plenty'; despite hyperglycemia, insulin deficiency makes the excess glucose unavailable to the cells, which rely upon lipid metabolites (ketone bodies) for energy, resulting from incomplete lipid metabolism CLINICAL Systemic acidosis, ↓ cardiac contractility and vascular response to catecholamines with thready pulse, hypotension, poor organ perfusion and diabetic ketoacidosis may be the presenting sign in previously undiagnosed DM, accompanied by an acute abdomen and a marked leukocytosis LABORATORY Ketonuria and ketonemia, hyperglycemia, glycosuria, ↓ pH and plasma bicarbonate, ↑ anion gap; hyperlipidemia

ketoconazole An orally administered imidazole used to treat serious fungal infections that acts by inhibiting the cytochrome P450-dependent steroid synthesis in fungi; as this inhibition is nonspecific, adverse endocrinologic effects (eg gynecomastia and azoospermia) may develop during therapy, and the metabolism of certain drugs (eg cyclosporine, erythromycin, nifedipine, and terfenadine) may be significant altered, making the use of these agents in combination with ketoconazole a pharmacologic faux pas (JAMA 1993; 269:1513oc); cytochrome P450 3A4 is responsible for the biotransformation of human sex hormones as well as various drugs, to wit, cyclosporine, erythromycin, nifedipine, and terfenadine (JAMA 1993; 269:1513oc)

ketone body Ketone One of three organic molecules (acetone, acetoacetate, β-hydroxybutyrate) with a carbonyl group, C=O, designated 'oxo-' in formal nomenclature; formation of ketone bodies is a physiological defense in starvation, in diabetes mellitus and in defective carbohydrate metabolism; in DM, the fatty acid levels are very high, as the lack of insulin prevents glucose utilization, metabolic needs are met by fatty acids; glucagon induces ketogenesis by lowering malonyl CoA, markedly increasing carnitine acyl transferase I activity, translocating fatty acids from the hepatic cytosol into the mitochondria converting them into ketone bodies by β-oxidation, providing energy to the nervous system while sparing proteins QUANTIFICATION Sodium nitroferricocyanide reaction; see Ketoacidosis

ketorolac tromethamine A non-opioid anti-inflammatory drug with the analgesic equivalence of morphine that does not depress ventilation at analgesic concentrations

17-ketosteroids 'Male' hormones (androsterone, dehydroepiandrosterone-DHEA, epiandrosterone, etiocholanolone, 11-keto- and 11-β-hydroxyandrosterone, 11-keto- and 11-β-hydroxyetiocholanolone); ♂ urine levels 28-70 µmol/day (US: 8-20 mg/day) reflect adrenocortical and testicular function; ♀ urine levels 21-52 µmol/day (US: 6-15 mg/day) reflect adrenocortical function; 17-ketosteroids are increased in adrenal or testicular tumors or hyperplasias, pregnancy, stress, polycystic ovarian disease and are decreased in primary or secondary adrenal hypofunction, Klinefelter syndrome, castration, hypothyroidism, anorexia nervosa QUANTIFICATION Colorimetry (Zimmerman reaction), GLC

17-ketosteroid reductase Testosterone 17β-dehydrogenase (NADP⁺), see there

17-ketosteroid reductase deficiency Testosterone 17β-dehydrogenase (NADP⁺) deficiency, see there

Kevorkian Dr Jack Kevorkian, a retired pathologist from Detroit, Michigan who has almost single-handedly crystallized the debate in the US about a person's right to die with dignity; Kevorkian is alleged to have been personally responsible for a number of physician-assisted suicides (**US New & World Report 25 April 1994**)

keyhole limpet hemocyanin KLH, see there

keyhole sign RADIOLOGY A pseudolesion of the duodenal bulb in which the radiocontrast in an upper gastrointestinal 'series' is trapped within contiguous parallel folds of the duodenal mucosa, a sign that disappears with peristalsis

key sign TROPICAL MEDICINE Hyperesthesia due to *Trypanosoma brucei gambiense* infection, where the patients are so sensitive to touch that familiar activities, eg locking of doors (which requires the use of keys) are avoided

Khaini cancer A squamous cell carcinoma of the oral cavity seen in men of the Indian states of Uttar Pradesh and Bihar, caused by a non-smoking tobacco habit, where a mixture of slaked lime and tobacco is habitually left in the lower gingivolabial fornix, the site of the malignancy's appearance; see Betel nut chewing

khat SUBSTANCE ABUSE The freshly dried bitter leaves of *Catha edulus*, an evergreen shrub indigenous to eastern Africa, eg Somalia, Ethiopia, and Yemen; khat is chewed for its stimulatory and euphoreffects; it has become regionally popular in the US, but is considered a 'low priority' substance of abuse by the US Drug Enforcement Administration (**New York Times 27 Nov 1994; 58, 14 Dec 1992; B1**)

Ki-1 antigen CD30, see there

Ki-1 lymphoma CD30 lymphoma Large cell anaplastic lymphoma A distinct subtype of lymphoma that affects children and adolescents that usually involves the skin, soft tissue, bone, and GI tract, very rarely the CNS (**Am J Clin Pathol 1995; 103:496₀ₐ**) and pericardium (**Cardiovasc Pathol 1995 4:141**) PATHOLOGY Tumor cells diffusely infiltrate the marginal sinus and parafollicular area of the lymph node; because the tumors commonly express epithelial membrane antigen, they may be misdiagnosed as metastatic undifferentiated carcinoma, amelanotic melanoma, or malignant sinus histiocytosis (**Acta Cytologica 1993; 37:520₀ₐ**)

Ki-67 A monoclonal antibody that is a widely used marker for cell proliferation; Ki-67 reacts with a 345–395-kD nuclear antigen expressed throughout the cell cycle in particular during G_2 and M (**Arch Pathol Lab Med 1994; 118:510₀ₐ**) Ki-67 may indicate a poor prognosis, as it is ↑ in small cell carcinomas of the lung with ↓ survival (**Histopathology 1991; 19:545**)

KIA Kligler iron agar, see Triple iron agar

kickback HEALTH CARE INDUSTRY A practice in which a person or business pays a person who finds new clients (known as referrals) a percentage of the increased transactions resulting from those referrals; in medicine, this is considered an unethical form of fee-splitting and, when performed in an organized fashion with hospitals and multiple health care providers may result in litigation through the US government's 'anti-kickback' law of 1986, which was written with the intent of stopping this practice in the defense industry (**Am Med News 28/Jan/91**); Cf Fee-splitting, Finder's fee

kickback alert A formal warning issued by the US Federal Government (Office of the Inspector General) indicating that certain arrangements by laboratories, eg providing physicians with on-site phlebotomists, discounting prices for a physician's managed care business, or certain services performed for renal dialysis centers could violate federal law (**CAP Today Nov 1994 p1**)

kidney panel A battery of tests that, according to the US form of health care reimbursement (the 'DRGs'), is the most cost-effective in evaluating the kidney's functional status, including albumin, BUN/creatinine, chloride, CO_2 content, creatinine clearance, glucose, potassium, total protein, sodium, 24-hour urinary creatinine and protein; see Organ panel

kidney stone Renal calculus A major cause of morbidity that is thought to be increasing; at any point in time 12% of those developed nations with KS CLINICAL Renal colic, hematuria, ureteral or renal pelvic obstruction, which may lead to hydronephrosis or facilitate infection COMPOSITION Oxalic acid, calcium, uric acid PATHOGENESIS Contrary to previous dogma, an ↑ in dietary calcium is reported to ↓ incidence of KS (RR 0.56); although this finding is somewhat counterintuitive (as 20-40% of ♂ with recurrent KS have idiopathic hypercalciuria and excrete ↑ calcium with ↑ calcium intake) the role of oxalate may have been previously underestimated; with calcium restriction, there is an ↑ absorption of oxalate (a major constituent of KS) from the GI tract OTHER RISK FACTORS ↑ Animal protein intake, ↑ KS (RR 1.33); ↑ in fluid intake, ↓ KS (RR 0.71) ↑ in dietary potassium, ↓ KS (RR 0.49) (**N Engl J Med 1993; 328:833₀ₐ**)

kidney trade see Organ brokerage

KID syndrome PEDIATRICS A non-specific term for a trilogy of symptoms (keratitis, ichthyosis and deafness), which when one is identified, should evoke a search for the remaining two

Kiel classification HEMATOLOGY A classification of non-Hodgkin's lymphomas proposed by K Lennert in 1975 (**Br J Haematol 1975; 31 (suppl):193**) that related cell morphology to lymphocyte lineage; like the Lukes and Collins (L&CC) classification, the KC recognizes follicular nodularity as a marker of B-cell differentiation, but uses the terms centrocyte and centroblast for the cleaved and noncleaved follicle center cells of the L&CC; after 1982, the Working Formulation (for classifying lymphomas) became popular; it is uncertain whether the recently proposed REAL classification will replace this surfeit of classifications; Cf REAL classification, Working Formulation

Kikuchi-Fujimoto disease Histiocytic necrotizing lymphadenitis An idiopathic condition characterized by localized, usually cervical, painful or tender lymphadenopathy that usually resolves spontaneously in 1-4 months; KFD may be accompanied by fever or upper respiratory tract symptoms, ↓ weight, nausea, vomiting, night sweats; 50% of patients have mild ↓ PMNs and ↑ lymphocytes PATHOLOGY Lymph nodes have patchy necrosis, eosinophilic debris and marked karyorrhexis; necrotic zones are punctuated by mononuclear cells, eg cytotoxic T lymphocytes, histiocytes and immunoblasts; granulocytes are absent (Arch Pathol Lab Med 1994; 118:134OA)

killed vaccine A vaccine consisting of dead, but antigenically 'active' viruses or bacteria, which are capable of evoking production of protective antibodies without causing disease; killed viruses may consist of whole inactivated organisms, eg pertussis, exotoxins, either alone or linked to a carrier protein, eg tetanus and diphtheria toxoids, soluble capsular components, eg pneumococcal polysaccharide, extracted material, eg hepatitis B (which is no longer used) or various subunits of the organism; Cf Live attenuated vaccine

killer bee Africanized bee, see there

killer bug Invasive *Streptococcus* A, see there

killer cell K cell IMMUNOLOGY A large granular lymphocyte that mediates antibody-dependent cell cytotoxicity and non-complement-mediated cytolysis of IgG-coated target cells, including virus- or tumor- laden self cells CYTOLYTIC MECHANISM Insertion of a transmembrane protein polymer perforin, perforating the target cell's membrane, similar to the insertion of C9 polymers in complement-mediated cytolysis; perforin is stored in 'small dark organelles' and released under appropriate local conditions, but the K cell's own perforin is prevented from polymerization and autoperforation by the proposed protein protectin SURFACE MARKERS Fc receptors; K cell activity is tested by measuring lytic activity against chicken erythrocytes; Cf Cytotoxic T cells, Natural killer cells

'killer' urine A popular term for the incompletely understood bactericidal effect of urine on bacteria, a function of acid pH, urea and other factors

Killip scale A clinical classification used to stratify the severity of left ventricular dysfunction, thereby determining the clinical status of patients after myocardial infarction Class 1: No rales, no third heart sound Class 2: Rales in ≤ ½ lung field or third heart sound Class 3: Rales in > ½ lung field (pulmonary edema) Class 4: Cardiogenic shock (determined clinically) (Killip T III, et al Am J Cardiol 1967; 20:457)

kilobase MOLECULAR BIOLOGY A reference unit of 1000 nucleotides on a single RNA or DNA strand, which has a molecular mass of approximately 3300 kD on RNA and for a double DNA strand (kilobase pair) of approximately 6 600 kD; Cf Centimorgan

kilobyte Kb A unit of computer memory equal to 1024 bytes (circa one-half page of written text) that is evolving towards obsolescence; the microcomputers of the mid-1970s, had random access memory (RAM) of 16 Kb, floppy diskettes stored 64 Kb of data and hard disks stored 5-10 megabytes (Mb) of data; current microcomputers have 4-512 Mb of RAM, floppy diskettes store 1.4 or more Mb of data, and few hard drives have < than 240 Mb of storage space

kilodalton kD A unit of protein mass, where one dalton or atomic mass unit is equal to one-twelfth the mass of an atom of ^{12}C, weighing 1.661×10^{-24}; a 100 kD protein has approximately 850 amino acids; Cf Kilobase

Kimberly Bergalis see Bergalis

kinase The trivial name for the phosphorylase subclass of transferase enzymes that transfer high-energy phosphates from a donor molecule, eg ATP or GTP to an acceptor molecule (alcohol, carboxyl/acyl, nitrogenous or other phosphate group)

kinase cascade The intracellular signalling pathway that occurs via protein phosphorylations and dephosphorylations, initiated by a hormonal signal at the cell membrane and amplified by adenylate cyclase, cAMP and kinases

kinasing MOLECULAR BIOLOGY The addition of a radiolabeled nucleotide to the 5' end of a hybridization probe, mediated by T4 polynucleotide kinase

kindling NEUROLOGY The tendency of some regions of the brain to react to repeated low-level electrical stimulation by progressively boosting electrical discharges, thereby lowering seizure thresholds; a similar mechanism has been suggested for endogenous depression (Science News 1994; 146:50); kindling consists of a relatively prolonged reduction in the threshold for depolarization for a given impulse or impulses, that can be evoked by repeated administration of an initally subconvulsive electrical stimulus, leading to progressive intensification of seizure activity, culminating in a generalized seizure; kindling can be induced in most regions of the brain; chemical kindling is relatively selective, GABA antagonists kindle the cortex but not the amygdala; muscarinic agonists kindle the amygdala but not the cortex; kindling may be suppressed with phenobarbital and benzodiazepines and variably reduced with other agents; kindling is linked to drugs of abuse (alcohol, cocaine and to a lesser degree, amphetamines and the phenomenon may explain some of the links between partial seizure complexes, eg temporal lobe epilepsy and their psychiatric symptoms; kindling may cause fatal tonic-clonic seizures in chronic cocaine abusers, induced in the limbic system, especially the amygdala by euphoria and an intermittent stimulus, eg procaine or cocaine; see Cocaine

kinectin CELL BIOLOGY An integral membrane protein of the endoplasmic reticulum that binds to and is an essential anchor for kinesin (Science 1995; 267:1834)

kinesin CELL BIOLOGY A ubiquitous 'motor' (mechanico-chemical) molecule that is a microtubule-activated ATPase composed of two heavy and two light chains, converting the chemical energy from ATP hydrolysis into mechanical force to power various forms of intracellular microtubule-based motility in endoplasmic reticulum and for mitosis by a 'stroke-release' mechanism   kinesin's activities include organelle transport, eg plus-end (antero-grade) movement* of vesicles along microtubules and various membrane-trafficking events (Science 1995; 267:1834)

*Minus-end (retrograde) movement of vesicles is directed by dynein

kinetochore A specialized region of the chromosome that overlies the centromere, which is critical in mitosis and has two 'motors', one located at a dividing mitotic pole, the other at the chromosome that is regulated by factors that influence phosphorylation (Nature 1991; 351:206, 187)

kinetoplast A perinuclear accessory body consisting of an enlarged specialized mitochondrial subunit composed of DNA; the high concentration of DNA in the kinetoplast of *Crithidiae luciliae* is used as a substrate for the indirect immunofluorescence test for detecting the presence of anti-DNA antibodies in patients with SLE

Kinetoplastida An order of unicellular flagellated protozoa, which includes Trematosomatidae (*Trypanosoma, Leishmania, Crithidia*), many of which are parasitic to humans; the protozoa are characterized by the presence of kinetoplasts

King Kong gel A three foot in length DNA sequencing gel (which by today's standards is very big; currently used gels are 20-30 centimeters) based on the Sanger sequencing method

King Kong peptide A 27-amino acid toxin produced by the cloth of gold cone snail (*Conus textile*), which was so named (Hillyard et al, 1988) as, when it is injected into lobsters, it causes an otherwise subordinate lobster to assume an exaggerated dominant position with bizarre aggressive behavior, a stance fancifully likened to that of King Kong, the venerated Hollywood behemoth; when the King Kong peptide is injected into snails (the cone snail's prey), the victim snail suffers periodic convulsive undulations instead of the normal reaction of retreating within its shell (EMBO J 1990; 9:1015); the peptide's structure or mechanism of action is as yet poorly characterized

King Lear complex PSYCHIATRY Incestuous libido of a father for his daughter; Cf Electra complex

Note: The term is a misapplication of the persona of Shakespeare's King Lear, as Lear's was a true paternal love for his daughter, Cordelia

king's evil Scrofula The lymphadenopathic form of TB (lymph nodes are the most common extrapulmonary site of tuberculous lesion and are often confined to the cervical region)

The name derives from the popular belief in the Middle Ages that scrofula was curable by the royal touch

King syndrome An AD [MIM 145600] form of malignant hyperthermia characterized by facial dysmorphia (malar hypoplasia, micrognathia, ptosis, antimongolic slant of palpebral fissures), pectus carinatum, delayed motor development and cryporchidism

Note: Malignant hyperthermia may be evoked in these patients by halothane or succinylcholine

Kingella A genus of non-motile gram-negative, facultative anaerobic rods, normally pharyngeal saprobes; *K kingae* is β-hemolytic and occasionally pathogenic; *K dinitrificans* is non-pathogenic but shares many features with *Neisseria gonorrhoeae*, with which it may be confused

kinin A family of potent vasodilators and natriuretics, inhibiting sodium transport in the distal nephrons, altering the osmotic gradient of the renal medulla; in addition kinins interface with the immune system

kinin system Kallikrein-Kinin system, see there

kinky hair disease Menke syndrome Trichopoliodystrophy An X-linked recessive [MIM 309400] condition due to defective copper metabolism with excess copper accumulation in certain tissues, eg fibroblasts, kidneys and intestinal mucosa and a relative deficiency of copper in other tissues, eg brain and liver, accompanied by defective copper enzymes, eg lysyl oxidase, tyrosinase; the defects result in arteriopathy (fragmentation of the elastica, intimal thickening), neuropathology (cerebral degeneration with loss of cortical neurons, gliosis and cystic changes), ↓ of amorphous elastin of the skin (hypopigmented brittle skin), a relative ↑ of aortic and cutaneous myofibrils with tortuous blood vessels and occasional vascular occlusion, ↓ in collagen and elastin cross-linking (osteoporosis); mitochondria from the brain and muscle have ↓ cytochrome oxidase a and a$_3$ activity; the hair is morphologically similar to the wool of copper-deficient sheep CLINICAL Failure to thrive, seizures, hypothermia, ↑ infections, kinky hair (pili torti due to defective disulfide bond formation), seborrheic dermatitis, mental and growth retardation, myoclonic seizures, scurvy-like radiological changes of the long bones, death often occurs in early infancy with progressive neurologic and vascular degeneration; kinky hair also occurs in AD trichodento-osseous syndrome; Cf Giant axonal neuropathy, Uncombable hair syndrome, Woolly hair disease

Kinshasa Highway AIDS Highway The road that links Kinshasa, Zaire, with East Africa, which is thought by some workers to be main route by which HIV traveled in its early evolution from the central African rain forest (R Preston, The Hot Zone, Random House, New York, 1994)

'kissing balloon' coronary angioplasty CARDIOLOGY A technique used in interventional cardiology to treat stenoses of the coronary arteries at bifurcations (which normally have a difficult access); the kissing balloon technique is difficult and unwieldy as it requires two guiding catheters or a single catheter with two long exchange guidewires; the alternate dual probe method allows two balloons to be passed through the same catheter and may improve angioplastic results at bifurcations

kissing bug Reduviid bug A cone-nosed hematophagous insect with various hosts in the tropics and subtropics that measures 1-4 cm, 'autumn-colored', the bite of which elicits papules, painful urticaria, hemorrhagic, bullous lesions, occasionally angioedema, anaphylactoid reaction and shock; the bug is also the vector for trypanosoma (Chaga's disease), causing inflammation, atrophy and fibrosis of Auerbach's plexus ganglion cells, resulting in acquired megacolon

kissing chancre A mirror-image lesion seen in syphilis, caused by autoinoculation due to prolonged apposition ('kissing') of a primary chancre; Cf Kissing ulcer

'kissing' disease A trivial synonym for infectious mononucleosis, which refers to a common mode of transmission of EBV, ie by kissing and salivary exchange; the first contact with EBV occurs in childhood in lower socioeconomic strata and in adolescence whilst osculating in the upper strata; see Epstein-Barr virus, Infectious mononucleosis

kissing sequestra An articular lesion characterized by extensive denudation of cartilage and joint fusion seen in the resolving phase of tuberculous osteoarthritis, classically located in the knee, accompanied by extensive cortical destruction, in the middle of which are two preserved islands of apposed ('kissing') sclerotic bone, seen on a plain film

kissing spine A descriptor for the enlarged facets, arches and spinous processes of vertebral bodies in generalized hypertrophic osteoarthritis, seen on a plain spine film

kissing tumor Infantile digital fibromatosis, see there

kissing ulcer Kissing lesion An ulcer seen on an apposing side of the vulva, due to autoinoculation by *Haemophilus ducreyi*, which may be associated with suppurative lymphadenopathy; see Groove sign; Cf Kissing chancre

'kiss of death' surgery A surgical procedure, which under certain clinical conditions, is relatively contraindicated and associated with an increased mortality, eg abdominal surgery during acute pancreatitis has been considered a kiss of death procedure

'kiss of death' test CRITICAL CARE MEDICINE A sobriquet for any clinical or laboratory test which, when positive, infers a poor prognosis and may presage a patient's demise, eg

1) Lactate levels > 10 mEq/L

2) 'LDH6' An abnormal lactic dehydrogenase band that migrates cathodic to the usual LDH isomers (85% mortality)

3) Delta osmolality, which when greater than 40 mosm/ml indicates a poor prognosis

4) Multifocal atrial tachycardia (43% mortality)

c-kit A proto-oncogene of the tyrosine kinase receptor family that binds to the hematopoietic growth factor SCF, see there

***kit*-ligand** Mast cell growth factor, see there

'kiting' A form of health care fraud in which zeros are added to a physician's prescription for a drug, increasing the quantity of drug or reimbursement; 'kiting' may be performed by a pharmacist who provides the patient with the prescribed quantity of medicine, then 'kites' the bill in order to receive a larger reimbursement from a third party payer, eg Medicaid; 'kiting' by a patient is usually for the purpose of obtaining more of a dependency-type of drug

kittniere *kitt*, German, putty or cement, *niere*, kidney Calcified, contracted scarred and afunctional kidneys filled with encapsulated, mortar-like or stony masses, surrounded by fibrosed renal pelvis, seen as a 'healed' phase of tuberculosis of the kidneys

Kleihauer-Betke test HEMATOLOGY A staining method that identifies the presence of fetal hemoglobin (HbF) in red cells, based on the relative resistance of fetal hemoglobin to alkaline buffer elution; the KBT is most commonly used to establish the presence of fetal cells in the mother's circulation, where fetal RBCs appear as red refractile cells after alkaline buffer treatment and eosin staining, while maternal cells* appear as red cell ghosts lacking hemoglobin

*Assuming the mother does NOT have the rare condition of hereditary persistance of fetal hemoglobin

Klenow fragment The proteolytic fragment of *Escherichia coli* DNA polymerase I, which has DNA polymerizing and 3'→5' exonuclease activities; it is a well-studied DNA-synthesizing enzyme in terms of high-resolution structural information and a good experimental enzyme for analyzing template-directed DNA synthesis; 2 domains are inferred from the crystal structure, corresponding to the larger -COOH terminal domain with polymerase function and the smaller -NH$_2$ terminal domain with 3',5'-exonuclease function

Kligler iron agar MICROBIOLOGY A growth medium used to differentiate Enterobacteriaceae: *Escherichia coli* ferments glucose and lactose, *Proteus mirabilis* ferments glucose and *Pseudomonas aeruginosa* ferments neither

KLH Keyhole limpet hemocyanin An agent used experimentally to test primary sensitization in delayed cutaneous hypersensitivity

kneecapping EMERGENCY MEDICINE The most common (1900 cases recorded) type of 'punishment shooting' (see there) inflicted by sectarian societies, in particular the Irish Republican Army, for transgressions or alleged transgressions against the group's philosophies; Royal Victoria's emergency department in Belfast has become the world's expert in kneecapping, which as implied by the name, may shatter the patellar bone (Am Med News 7 Nov 1994 p14)

KNF model see Induced fit model

knife-and-fork model Kornberg mechanism A fanciful term for an in vitro system used to study DNA replication, which contains DNA ligase, DNA polymerase and endonuclease

knife-blade atrophy Walnut brain Extreme and global thinning of the gyri of the cerebral cortex seen in the frontal and temporal lobes in Pick's disease; Cf Windswept cortex

knob PARASITOLOGY A specialized membrane modification that allows *Plasmodium falciparum*-infected red cells to adhere to vascular epithelium, resulting in relative blood stasis through less-well oxygenated tissues

knob sign RADIOLOGY Decrease or absence of the aortic 'knob' on a plain antero-posterior chest film, a finding typical of secondary atelectasis of the left lower lobe of lung

knock Pericardial knock, see there

knock knees Genu valgum Internal deviation of the knee joint; some degree of 'knock-knee' is present in all children from 2-6 years of age and most autocorrect with time; when marked, the work in walking may fatigue the child, causing pronation, shoe top bulging and medial collapse over the medial longitudinal arch; to compensate for the shift in gravity, the child deviates the foot medially (toe-in) or laterally (toe-out); the degree of knock knee is best

determined by measuring the distance between the medial malleoli (ankles); knock-knee may be a congenital component of Ellis-van Creveld syndrome, due to rickets or may occur as a complication of epiphysiodesis

knock-out drop effect see Mickey Finn

knockout mouse A genetically engineered mouse created by the technique of gene targeting (targeted gene disruption), in which a specific gene of interest is deleted by homologous recombination to study the effects of its absence; if, as a result of knocking out a gene, a part of the cerebellum is defective, then it is assumed that the knocked-out gene is involved in cerebellar development; knock-out mouse models of human disease have been created for atherosclerosis, cancer, and cystic fibrosis (Sci Am 1994; 270/3:52) see Gene targeting

Knodell index SURGICAL PATHOLOGY A numerical scoring system for assessing histologic aggressiveness of asymptomatic chronic viral (formerly active) hepatitis, which ranges from 0 to 22 and evaluates the intensity of fibrosis, portal inflammation, and periportal bridging necrosis (N Engl J Med 1995; 332:1457oA)

knot A popular term for any mass or perceived mass, which is generally used in either of two situations: 1) A knot in muscle, a group of muscles that are in spasm or 2) A knot in the stomach, a manifestation of anxiety, which does not per se represent a palpable mas

knots Umbilical cord knots OBSTETRICS False knots of the umbilical cord result from twisting and meandering of the umbilical vein and are of no clinical significance; the umbilical arteries are relatively linear; true knots require that the umbilical cord be sufficiently long to permit the infant to pass through a loop of cord; since the cord is composed of erectile tissue, irreversible cord knotting is rare

Knudson's theory see One-hit, two-hit model

'Koala bear' syndrome A fanciful synonym for the physiognomy of the AD [MIM 118650] Conradi-Hünermann syndrome in which there is a flat face and nasal bridge, a hypoplastic nose and a mild mongoloid slant that may be accompanied by pulmonary calcifications, mental retardation and right ventricular hypertrophy

Koch's postulates A series of four conditions that must be met to establish an infectious agent as the cause of a particular disease

1) The agent must be present in all cases of the disease

2) The agent must be isolated from someone with the disease and grown in pure culture

3) Inoculation into a susceptible organism of the agent (from a pure culture must produce the disease)

4) The agent must be recovered from the infected (inoculated) organism and grown again in culture

see Molecular Koch's postulates

Koebner's phenomenon Isomorphic reaction The appearance of new lesions of a skin disease (in particular psoriasis, but also lichen planus or eczema) at a site of trauma; see Psoriasis

koilocytosis *koilo-*, Greek, Hollow A cytological abnormality of the superficial epithelial cells (see figure, page 464) of the uterine cervix, less commonly, of the oropharynx and elsewhere, which is characterized by large cells (koilocytes) with cleared cytoplasmic, pyknotic, rugose nuclear membranes with inconspicuous nucleoli; koilocytosis is induced by human papilloma virus (HPV) infection, ie condyloma acuminata, and while not per se a premalignant lesion, it is typically seen in HPV infection and some serotypes of HPV (types 16 and 18), which are premalignant, its presence should alert the clinician about possible future malignancy; koilocytotic changes may occur in atrophy-related vacuolar degeneration of the cervix, as seen in menopause, or occur in non-HPV infections, including trichomoniasis, *Gardnerella vaginalis* and candidiasis

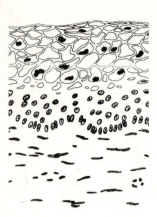
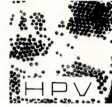
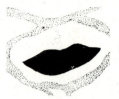

koilocytes

konzo A distinct upper motor neuron spastic paraparesis described in Africa due to cyanide poisoning, related to consumption of high-carbohydrate cassava, which in droughts produces more cyanogenic glycosides and, due to the food shortage, causes the food manufacturers to take short-cuts in the steps designed to remove the cyanide

Korean hemorrhagic fever Hemorrhagic fever with renal syndrome A condition seen in Central and Far Eastern Asia, caused by a Bunyavirus, the Hantavirus, isolated in the Hantaan River, acquired through aerosolized rodent feces and urine (*Rattus rattus, Apodemus agrarius, Clethrionomys glariolus, Microtiae*); in China, 100 000 cases are reported/year and are thought to be increasing in number CLINICAL Fever, flushing, edema, petechiae, conjunctivitis, headache, aches/pains, thrombocytopenia and renal tubular dysfunction, ranging from mild proteinuria to transient anuria; the mortality rate may be determined by the rodent vector itself, *Apodemus*-associated infections (3-7% mortality) appear worse than the so-called nephropathia epidemica, which has a vole (*Clethrionomys*) vector DIAGNOSIS IgM is measured by ELISA, indirect immunofluorescence assay and plaque reduction neutralization assay

koro PSYCHIATRY An unusual culture-bound desomatization complex, described in Malaysia characterized by an intense fear of abrupt onset, that the penis (nipples and vulva in females) will disappear into the body and cause death; the subject may attempt to 'prevent' his penis from shrinking and disappearing within his body by tying the it to the outside of his body with various devices (**DSM-IV™, 1994**) see Culture-bound syndrome; Cf Piblokto

Korotkov sounds CARDIOLOGY Low frequency vibrations (< 200 mHz) originating in vascular walls and heard distal to cuff compression of a peripheral artery, subdivided into: An initial or transient murmur (opening tap) and a compression murmur (rumble); evaluation of Korotkov sounds was a crude and subjective method for determining the severity of occlusive peripheral arterial disease, having had its heyday in the pre-Doppler era

Kostmann's disease (severe) Congenital neutropenia, see there

kpn family A family of intermediate-sized repeated fragments of DNA, measuring less than 6 kilobases in length, so called as they result from kpn I restriction enzyme digestion

Krankenkaße see German-style system

kraurosis vulvae Lichen sclerosis, see there

Krazy glue™ Ethyl-2-cyanoacrylate A commercial 'super-adhesive' that is also used as a surgical adhesive; compared to longer chain cyanoacrylate derivatives, eg butyl-2-cyanoacrylate, Histoacryl, Krazy glue is thought to evoke greater histotoxicity in the form of seromas, acute inflammation, necrosis and foreign-body giant cell reaction

Krebs' carcinoma A transplantable anaplastic carcinoma of mice, probably arising in the mammary gland

'Krimsky index' An informal system delineated by a Dr Krimsky of Tufts University as a measure of an academic department's non-academic ties and potential for 'conflict of interest', calculated as the number of faculty members with commercial ties divided by the total number of faculty members; see CRADA

kringle MOLECULAR BIOLOGY A triple-looped, disulfide-linked protein domain (figure) that is involved in binding membranes, proteins and phospholipids and in regulating proteolysis; the kringle is a common structural motif, so-named for its resemblance to the kringler, a Danish pastry and is present in coagulation-related and fibrinolytic proteins and other plasma proteinases, eg tissue plasminogen activator (t-PA), urokinase and apolipoprotein A (possibly explaining the increased coagulation seen in atherosclerosis) and may be present in multiple copy numbers, eg apolipoprotein-A has up to 37 kringle domains, while t-PA has five

Krüppel A *Drosophila* transcription factor protein that is encoded by a gap gene and '...*required for proper segmentation of the embryo; Krüppel converts from an activator (of RNA polymerase II) to a repressor in a concentration-dependent fashion; ie at low concentrations it is a monomer that activates transcription, while at higher concentrations it is a homodimer that binds to the same DNA sequence, but is a potent transcriptional repressor*'; in humans a number of similar activator-repressor switches exist, eg thyroid hormone, p53, WT1, Rel, YY1, and the binding element of each (**Nature 1995; 375:105**)

KS Kaposi syndrome, also 1) Ketosteroid 2) Klinefelter syndrome

also 1) Katoptric system (optics) 2) Kidney sac 3) Kveim-Seltszback test (sic **Abbreviations, 1994**), now known as the Kveim test

KUB Kidneys ureters bladder UROLOGY A colloquial term for a plain, ie without radiocontrast, antero-posterior film of the abdomen, used as a crude method for detecting nephroliths (kidney stones); the KUB film may be used as a 'scout' examination prior to performing the more definitive intravenous pyelogram

Kulchitsky cell An enterochromaffin cell containing neurosecretory granules that is native to the respiratory tract, produces bombesin, vasoactive intestinal polypeptide and leu-enkephalin, and gives rise to bronchial adenoma, pulmonary carcinoid (tumorlet), oat cell carcinoma (of the lung and elsewhere), APUDomas, sugar tumor; Kulchitsky cell tumors may be subdivided into typical, atypical and small-cell carcinomas; see Carcinoid, Dense core granules

kurtosis STATISTICS A measurement of the degree to which a one-dimension probability curve with a gaussian distribution of data is concentrated in a single peak; if the peak is flat, it is 'platykurtic', if sharp, 'leptokurtic'

kuru New Guinea dialect, Trembling with fear A subacute spongiform encephalopathy, recently recognized as being induced by a prion, see there; kuru was responsible for the deaths of 90% of females in the once cannibalistic Fore tribe of New Guinea (females were most affected as they prepared and ate the infected brains) CLINICAL Cerebellar ataxia, shivering tremors, dysarthria, progressing to complete motor paralysis and death in 3-9 months due to infection or malnutrition; the disease may terminate with uncontrollable, compulsive laughter (aka 'laughing death') PATHOLOGY Spongiform encephalopathy, cytoplasmic vacuolization of neurons, especially of the striatum and cerebellum; the kuru plaques are positive with a PAS/diastase staining reaction Note: Kuru symptoms have been induced in primates after a 20 year latency

Kuskokwim syndrome An AR [MIM 208200] form of arthrogryposis described in Alaskan Eskimos, who due to the early onset of impaired movement and joint contractures, waddle like ducks

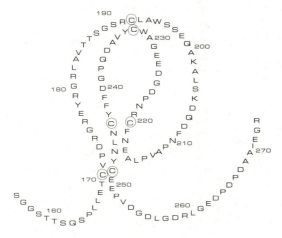

kringle domain

KUTE A recently coined acronym for 'Key User and Training Employee', a person who plays a critical role in implementing a new computer system; it is uncertain if this neologism will take root (CAP Today July 1992)

kwashiorkor Protein malnutrition often associated with marginally adequate caloric intake, occurring in African children weaned from the 'high-octane' protein-rich maternal milk and fed protein-poor cereals, cassava and sweet potatoes CLINICAL Pitting edema, massive ascites, retarded growth, apathy, skin rashes, dry skin with desquamation and ulcers, hepatomegaly, anorexia, diarrhea, decreased size of the heart and kidneys PATHOLOGY Severely flattened, small intestinal villi may be due to coincident infection and not Kwashiorkor per se LABORATORY Anemia, ↓ hematocrit, blood volume, ↓ albumin Treatment Succotash, a dietary mixture that provides all the deficient amino acids

Note: In the Gia dialect of Ghana, kwashiorkor translates as 'deposed child' or *'the sickness older child gets when next child is due'* (as the child's weaning results in the deterioration in the quality of nutrition; in another dialect, kwashiorkor translates as 'red-boy' since the afflicted children often have reddish hair; Marasmus, kwashiorkor's cousin, is a global decrease of proteins and carbohydrates

Kyasanur forest disease A tick-borne flaviviral disease of the Mysore and Karnataka states of India, maintained by infected monkeys and rodents; those living in wooded farmlands are at the highest risk CLINICAL High fever, myalgia, prostration, enteric, uterine or pulmonary hemorrhage, meningismus, leukopenia, thrombocytopenia, albuminuria DIAGNOSIS Isolation of virus from blood, complement fixation PROGNOSIS 5-10% mortality

L Symbol for: 1) Lambert, a unit of luminance or photometric brightness 2) Left 3) Leucine 4) Levorotatory 5) Light chain (of immunoglobulin) 6) Liter (abbreviation as used in US) 7) Lumbar 8) Lung

L- A descriptive prefix to indicate one of two entantiomeric forms of optically active organic compounds (sugars and amino acids), the mirror image is the D-entantiomer

L-shaped curve see U-shaped curve

L735,524 MK-639, see there

l Symbol for: 1) Length 2) Ligament 3) Liter (abbreviation as used in the SI, International System)

'Ls of dermatology, the 5' A group of skin lesions associated with dense patchy infiltrates of upper dermal lymphocytes, including lupus erythematosus, lymphoma, pseudolymphoma of Spiegler-Fendt, polymorphous light eruption of plaque type, Jessner's lymphocytic infiltration; other dermal lymphocytic infiltrates include actinic reticulosis, angioimmunoblastic lymphadenopathy, arthropod bites, lymphomatoid papulosis, phenytoin-induced drug eruption

La Crosse encephalitis The most common form of the mosquito-born California encephalitis Vector *Aedes triseriatus*, which breeds in old tires and small puddles AGENT Bunyavirus CLINICAL Summer-fall epileptiform meningoencephalitis in children under age 15, ♂:♀ ratio, 2:1, mortality less than 1%

La Niña ATMOSPHERIC SCIENCES A cold portion of the atmospheric cycle (the opposite of El Niño), which has been linked to the Bangaladesh floods and the 1988 drought of the UD Midwest; Cf El Niño

'lab rat' A highly colloquial term referring to a graduate student or 'post-doc' dedicated to bench research to the virtual exclusion of a personal and family life, who may be acting out an idealized fantasy or image of a dedicated scientist; because 'lab rats' may be ostracized for their social ineptness and lack of 'political savvy', they are often ill-equipped to address the realities of practicing science in the 1990s, which requires organization, social graces and political skills; see Gentleman scientist, 'New scientist'

label A marker, eg an enzyme or a radioactive isotope of a normal molecule, eg ^{35}P that replaces a non-radioactive ^{32}P, which is used to mark or indicate the presence of a protein or molecule of interest, by one of a variety of identification systems, eg immunoperoxidase staining or RIA

labeling index A measurement of the mitotic activity of a cell population, defined as the number of cells in the S phase of the growth cycle divided by the total cells in the population

labor Parturition OBSTETRICS The process that results in the expulsion of a conceptus and placenta from the uterus via the cervix and vagina; the onset of labor is triggered by oxytocin released from the posterior hypophysis, and it is divided into three stages, the first from the time of the onset of purposeful (ie, 'serious') uterine contractions to complete dilatation of the cervix; the second stage ends with the delivery of the infant, and the third with the delivery of the placenta **PRECIPITATE LABOR** Parturition of less than three hours in duration in a primigravida **PROLONGED LABOR** Parturition of greater than 24 hours in duration in a primigravida **FALSE LABOR** Parturition that results from disordered uterine action where regular painful contractions are not accompanied by effacement or dilatation of the cervix that may either cease or be followed by the onset of true labor

laboratory director LABORATORY MEDICINE A licensed (by the state or other jurisdiction) individual, usually physician (MD or DO), less commonly a PhD, who has a period (two to four years) of formal training in clinical laboratory medicine and science; the on-site presence of pathologist in a commercial laboratory results in an estimated 20% improvement in objective parameters of service quality (see Arch Pathol Lab Med 1992; 116:681oa)

laboratory error A nonspecific term for any error in results or result reporting that can be attributed to a clinical laboratory or its workers; much of the data on the rates, sources and types of laboratory errors was reported in an era when many tests were performed manually, and the results calculated and logged and/or transferred manually; in the current environment, instrument technology has advanced to the point of full automation, and results are transferred and reported by computer; in this setting, it is appropriate to divide the steps at which laboratory error occurs into preanalytical, analytical, and postanalytical components; in one study analytical errors are reported to be the main source of laboratory errors (Arch Pathol Lab Med 1993; 117:714oa)

laboratory information system A 'dedicated' computer, often a minicomputer with connected workstations, that controls the flow of various data through the laboratory; the capacity required of an LIS is a function of

1) The type of instruments the system supports[1]

2) The type of communication the computer must provide with the rest of the hospital in the form of direct communication with the 'floor', patient billing, admitting and discharge and elsewhere

3) The need for long-term information storage and retrieval

4) The needs for statistical analysis in terms of quality control and quality assurance and, perhaps most importantly

5) The number of laboratory sections, eg chemistry, hematology, microbiology and blood bank[2], and the number of instruments being served

The anatomic (cytology and surgical) pathology section is also less commonly integrated in the LIS, as pathology deals with a limited number of the patients admitted to the hospital, requires relative self-containment of information and is 'text-intensive', rather than data intensive; as of late 1992, 44% of laboratories (US) had LIS (Arch Pathol Lab Med 1993; 117:12oa); the largest LIS vendors in the US are Cerner Corp (417 operational contracts), Medical Information Technology, Inc (425), Sunquest Information Systems, Inc (509) (CAP Today Nov 1994 p1) see Computers; Cf Hospital information system

[1] Noting that the computer must convert an instrument's analog data to digital data [2] LISs may not integrate blood bank modules given the potential danger to a patient of lost data regarding, for example, the presence of life-threatening antibodies or rare blood types, or the potential liability to the hospital if a unit of autologous blood donated pre-operatively, is 'lost' and a random packed red cell unit is transfused to the patient during surgery

laboratory test A generic term for the analysis of one or more components of material from a subject (ie a patient's specimen) performed in a site (laboratory) dedicated to assuring accurate and timely results; laboratory tests are performed to: 1) Detect a morbid process (a 'disease')

screen for or diagnose a disease, or to rule out its presence 2) Determine the severity of a disease 3) Monitor the progress of a disease, its response to therapy and determine prognosis 4) Monitor drug toxicity (Arch Pathol Lab Med 1992; 116:704₀ₐ)

labrea hepatitis A form of hepatitis seen in South America characterized by massive hepatic necrosis and steatosis, thought to be caused by either hepatitis delta or by intoxication with rotenone, a toxic plant (*Deris negrensis* and others) found along Amazonian river banks

labs A colloquial 'short form' for laboratory work or other studies of analytes performed in a clinical laboratory

labyrinth *labyrinthus* [NA6] Labyrinth A complex of interconnecting canals and cavities which characterizes the internal ear, the essential organ of hearing and the final destination of the vestibulocochlear nerve, is composed of the membranous labyrinth, a series of communicating membranous sacs and ducts, separated from the bony labyrinth by the perilymph (fluid), both of which lie within the petrous portion of the temporal bone

***lac* operon** A complex of three *Escherichia coli* genes that encode the enzymes involved in lactose metabolism: β-galactosidase, β-galactosidase transport protein and β-galactosidase transacetylase; the *lac* operon has proven to be a useful experimental system for deciphering the mechanisms of gene regulation

lace-like appearance Lacy appearance, see there

Lachman test SPORTS MEDICINE A clinical maneuver used to determine the effects of anterior shear loads applied to the knee as 30° flexion; the LT is preferred to the anterior drawer test for evaluating the integrity of the anterior cruciate ligament (JC DeLee, D Drez, Jr, Eds, Orthopedic Sports Medicine WB Saunders, Philadelphia, 1994)

LACI Lipoprotein-associated coagulation inhibitor, see there

lacquer crack appearance OPHTHALMOLOGY A pattern in the optic fundus characterized by branching clefts in the lamina vitrea with choroidal atrophy seen in progressive myopia

lacquer crack appearance

α-lactalbumin A protein found only in milk which is a component of the enzyme lactose synthase; the amino acid composition of lactalbumin is considered ideal for humans and thus is a 'gold standard' used in evaluating all protein substitutes in the diet

lactase Lactose galactohydrolase An intestinal mucosa enzyme [EC 3.2.1.108] that hydrolyzes lactose to form D-glucose and D-galactose, which is isolated as a complex which also catalyzes the reaction of glucosylceramidase [EC 3.2.1.62], aka phlorizin hydrolase

Note: The term lactase is also an alternative name for β-galactosidase [EC 3.2.1.23], which lends to confusion (Recommendations (1992), Nomenclature Committee, International Union of Biochemistry and Molecular Biology)

lactase deficiency β-D-galactosidase deficiency Lactose intolerance syndrome A condition that is either acquired, or AR [MIM 223000] and common in non-Caucasians, which is due to a deficiency of lactase on the intestinal brush borders CLINICAL Cramps, bloating, flatulence, inability to metabolize disaccharides (resulting in osmotic diuresis, diarrhea and acidic stools) DIAGNOSIS Lactose tolerance test, in conjunction with a glucose tolerance test TREATMENT Symptomatic, lactose restriction

lactate A salt or ester of lactic acid; the time required to clear or normalize lactate is useful prognostic tool in trama

victims, where survival of 100% is reported in those with lactate normalization within 24 hours, 77.8% if normalization occurred in 24-48 hours, and 13.6% if the normalization of lactate required more than 48 hours (J Trauma 1993; 35:584) Cf 'Kiss of death' test

lactate dehydrogenase CARDIOLOGY An oxidoreductase [EC 1.1.1.27] present in the cytoplasm of all cells that catalyzes the reaction lactate + NAD⁺ ↔ pyruvate + NADH + H⁺, the equilibrium of which favors lactate + NAD⁺ at neutral pH LD consists of an enzyme tetramer composed of two different 34-kD subunits, H (heart) and M (muscle), which are separable by electrophoresis; the HHHH tetramer (LD₁) is the most rapidly migrating or anodic fraction and has a mobility similar to α₁ globulin; the slowest migrating or cathodic fraction is composed of the MMMM tetramer (LD₅) and migrates to the gamma (γ) region in a serum protein electrophoretic gel; there are thus five LD isoenzymes; after the total LD is measured as a screen for the presence of non-specific enzyme abnormalities, the serum is then separated by electrophoresis into isoenzyme fractions, localizing the abnormality to a particular tissue; total LD is ↑↑↑ in myocardial infarction (MI), megaloblastic anemia and severe hypoxia, ↑↑ in CML, hemolytic anemia and ↑ in liver disease (hepatitis, obstructive jaundice, cirrhosis, delirium tremens); LD₁ is classically ↑ in MI, peaking by the 4th post-infarct day; abnormal LD bands occur when serum proteins complex with isoenzymes, seen in 25% of tested patients with cirrhosis and these LD-IgG complexes may be associated with shock (cardiogenic, septic or hemorrhagic) and a concomitant increase of LD₅; see Flipped LD, LD₆

lactic acid The product of anaerobic glycolysis of lactose; the D-form is produced by some genera of bacteria, eg *Listeria, Lactobacillus, Erysipelothrix, Streptococcus*; a DL-racemic mix is produced in sour milk and in the stomach; the L-form is an end-product of anaerobic glucose metabolism that is ↑ in congenital, eg glycogen storage disease and acquired conditions, either in physiologic, eg strenuous exercise or pathologic conditions, eg hypoxia with ↓ clearance in hepatic failure, cardiac decompensation, respiratory failure, septicemia, oral hypoglycemic agents, eg phenformin, infarction, neoplasia LABORATORY ↓ Bicarbonate and pH, increased anion gap and PO₄

lactic acidosis A metabolic acidosis characterized by ↑ H⁺, secondary to ↑ lactic acid due to tissue hypoxia or ↓ conversion of lactate to pyruvate, as may occur in exercise, or due to endogenous or exogenous metabolic defects LABORATORY ↑ Anion gap TREATMENT Dichloroacetate treatment of patients with severe lactic acidosis results in statistically significant (but clinically unimportant) changes in the pH and the arterial blood lactate and does not alter the hemodyanimcs or survival (N Engl J Med 1992; 327:1564₀ₐ)

lactoferrin An iron-binding protein that belongs to the transferrin family of iron-binding glycoproteins; it is the second most abundant protein in human milk, and is also present in other external secretions, including intestinal mucus, bile, nasal and genital secretions, saliva, and tears; lactoferrin's binding of iron makes it unavailable to bacteria, and thus has a non-specific immunoprotective role in the primary host defense at the mucosal surface; it is ↑ in inflammatory diarrhea (Am Clin Lab May 1994); lactoferrin is a stable protein that is a marker for leukocytes is produced in the secondary granules of PMNs; it binds to iron and intestinal receptors; in the recombinant DNA form, lactoferrin is a potent broad-spectrum antimicrobial protein (Bio/Technology 1995; 13:498)

lacto-ovo vegetarian A vegetarian who eats non-flesh animal protein including eggs and dairy products; Cf Vegan vegetarian

lactose Milk sugar A reducing disaccharide that is hydrolyzed by β-galactosidase into of D-galactose and D-glucose; lactose is synthesized by mammalian mammaries, and is blamed for intolerance to milk products that occurs in some adults

²H-lactose test A test to detect lactase deficiency METHOD 1.0 g of lactose/kg body weight is given per os; an increase of breath ²H of > 20 ppm above basal levels of ²H indicates lactose malabsorption, the release of which depends on release of the ²H from unabsorbed lactose through bacterial metabolism

lactulose A synthetic disaccharide, used to treat hepatic encephalopathy, administered per os, acting as a laxative, reducing intraluminal NH_3, which via the extracellular fluid, reduces NH_3 in the blood

lacunar amnesia Amnesia only for certain events; Cf Selective memory

lacunar cell An enlarged, 40-50 μm in diameter Reed-Sternberg cell variant, which has a polylobated nucleus, lacy chromatin and one or more variably sized nucleoli, is surrounded by a rim of clear to eosinophilic cytoplasm and is located in clear lacunae that are thought to be an artefact of formalin fixation; lacunar cells were first described in nodular sclerosing Hodgkin's disease, but may occur in aggregates in the other types of Hodgkin's disease; similar cells are seen in undifferentiated nasopharyngeal carcinoma; see Reed-Sternberg cell; Cf Popcorn cell

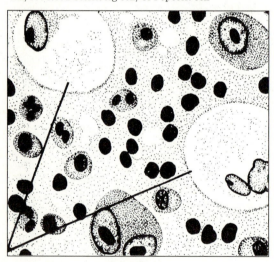

lacunar cell

lacunar infarcts NEUROPATHOLOGY Multiple small cerebral infarcts in the corona radiata, internal capsule, striatum, thalamus, basis pontis, cerebellum, occasionally preceded by transient symptoms, see Lacunar state; the infarcts are due to involvement of the penetrating branches of the middle and posterior cerebral and median branches of the basilar arteries; resolution of infarcts is characterized by residual 1-3 mm cavities or lacunae, characteristic of long-standing hypertension; see Multi-infarct dementia

lacunar skull A skull, the diploë of which is characterized by irregular rarefactions or shadowy depressions and a smooth outer contour, seen radiologically over the fronto-parietal region in 50% of those with meningocele or meningomyelocele, which may be complicated by hydrocephalus; the area is lined by dura and bordered by osseous tissue; the entire bony skull becomes attenuated and the lacunae disappear upon separation of the cranial sutures; Cf 'Punched-out' lesions

Note: This is identical to that of the 'beaten brass' appearance and separation between the two is of dubious utility

lacunar state État lacunaire NEUROLOGY A condition characterized by multiple minute infarcts (lacunes) in the basal ganglia, often seen in severe hypertension; when numerous, LS causes dementia or a lacunar 'syndrome' CLINICAL Loss of recent memory, altered time-space orientation, paranoia, headache, vertigo, giddiness, convulsions; the focal nature of the infarcts explains various neurological defects including homolateral cerebellar ataxia, isolated hemiplegia, pure segmental sensory stroke and dysarthria-clumsy hand syndrome PATHOLOGY Multiple small infarcts associated with fibrinoid degeneration and lipohyalinosis of small penetrating vessels of the basal ganglia, internal capsule, thalamus, and pons

lacy appearance MICROBIOLOGY A descriptor for the delicate, filigreed pattern that contaminating fungi impart on a Thayer-Martin (*Neisseria*) agar plate BONE RADIOLOGY A descriptor for the coarsely trabeculated shadows seen in the long bones in secondary syphilis, corresponding to gumma and syphilitic periostitis*, seen in early hyperparathyroidism or chronic osteomyelitis; when marked, the bony resorption is said to have a 'scooped-out' appearance with trabeculation and radiolucency of the medullary cavity; Cf Ground-glass appearance, Veiled appearance

*A term also referring to subperiosteal bone resorption and loss of cortical definition

LAD Leukocyte adhesion deficiency

laddergram CARDIOLOGY A schematic method used to analyze complex arrhythmias in which a simple rhythm strip from a standard electrocardiogram is subdivided into an A (atrial) line, an A-V (atrio-ventricular junction) line and a V (ventricular) line; the lines representing conduction are diagrammed under the actual tracing and accurately drawn so that the 'A' line begins at the P wave and the 'V' line at the beginning of the QRS; ladder diagrams were first described in 1896 by Engelmann to explain cardiac tracings inscribed by the electrocardiograph

ladder pattern CLINICAL TOXICOLOGY A characteristic linear serrated wheal produced by the adherent tentacles of the box jellyfish (*Chironex fleckeri* and *Chiropsolmus quadrigatus*), coelenterates native to the Pacific basin LABORATORY MEDICINE Light chain ladder A recently recognized phenomenon that may be observed on routine high-resolution agarose gel electrophoresis (AGE) and immunofixation of urine specimens; LCLs may be observed under the same conditions (50-fold concentration) as those used to identify Bence-Jones proteins (BJPs) in the urine (BJPs usually present on AGE as a single narrow band of protein migrating in the γ-globulin zone; BJPs may have two or more charge forms resulting in multiple bands on zonal electrophoresis that cluster in the same region of gammaglobulin zone) LCLs are electrophoretically more homogeneous, are usually kappa (κ) light chains (although occasionally also may be lambda (λ) light chains), and widely distributed over the γ-globulin zone; LCLs have been identified in patients with lymphoproliferative diseases (eg lymphoma, myeloma), monoclonal gammopathy of undetermined significance, various infections, and inflammatory conditions (Arch Pathol Lab Med 1993; 117:707oA) PEDIATRICS A clinical sign seen on the abdominal wall in children with obstruction of the lower GI tract, seen as parallel loops of distended small intestine, causing a 'stepped' pattern

ladder sequencing MOLECULAR BIOLOGY Any method, eg those delineated by Sanger or Maxam and Gilbert, where the sequence of the nucleotides in a nucleic acid is read from the step-like bands in an electrophoretic gel, fancifully likened to a ladder

LADS see Leukocyte adhesion deficiency syndrome

'Lady Godiva syndrome' A fanciful, albeit incorrect synonym for exhibitionism*; see Sexual deviancy

*Which unlike Lady Godiva's threadless equestrian peregrination through Coventry decrying her husband's excess taxes of the citizens, is considered a form of deviant behavior

Laennec's cirrhosis Alcoholic cirrhosis, see there

laetrile 1-Mandelonitrile-β-glucuronic acid A preparation from bitter almonds or apricot or peach pits that is high in cyanide, which had ben claimed to be effective in treating cancer; see Manner cocktail, Tijuana, Unproven forms of cancer therapy

The use of laetrile arises from a modernization of the 'Trophoblastic theory of cancer' espoused by the Scottish zoologist and embryologist, James Beard (1857-1924); laetrile has no proven effect in cancer treatment, and is alleged to have been associated with a number of cancer-related deaths Note: The agent was named by its discover, ET Krebs, as it is levo-rotatory (left-handed) and amygdalin is chemically a mandelonitrile

laetrile

lager syndrome see Concentration camp syndrome

lagging strand see Replication

lag phase BURN PHYSIOLOGY The earliest phase (first 12 hours) of wound healing, which precedes the histopathological changes, a period during which chemical mediators of inflammation, eg arachidonic acid metabolites, cytokines, kinins and edema accumulate in the burn site(s) EMERGENCY MEDICINE The period between the time a person is exposed to a toxic inhalant, eg cadmium fumes, dimethyl sulfate, methyl bromide, ozone, nitrogen oxides, phosgene, phosphorus compounds and others and development of pulmonary edema, a period lasting up to 12 hours MICROBIOLOGY The period prior to the logarithmic growth phase where the bacteria are too busy gearing up their enzymatic machinery (producing macromolecules, eg proteins and ribosomes) to proliferate

lai tai Sudden unexplained nocturnal death, see there

LAK cells Lymphokine-activated killer cells; see IL-2/LAK cells

Lake Nyos ENVIRONMENT A crater lake in the Northwest Province of Cameroon, which in 1986 was the site of a massive natural release of CO_2 gas, causing an estimated 1700 deaths; the lake contains 300 million m^3 of CO_2 gas that is increasing at a rate of 5 million annually, another disaster may occur at any time

Lake Tahoe mystery disease Chronic fatigue syndrome, see there

LAM-1 Leukocyte adhesion molecule A membrane protein with a 'homing' function, related to its lectin-like domain that binds specific glycoconjugates on target cells, regulating leukocyte migration by mediating the binding of lymphocytes to high endothelial venules and binding of neutrophils to endothelium in sites of inflammation (**Nature 1991; 349:691**); see Selectins

Lamarckism A philosophy advanced by French naturalist JP Lamarck in 1809 that holds that phenotypic adaption, eg hypertrophy or atrophy, made during an organism's lifetime could be imprinted on the genome; Lamarckism is diametrically opposed to mendelian genetics; but may in part be supported by the phenomenon of DNA methylation; see Imprinting, Lysenkoism, Methylation

Lamaze technique OBSTETRICS A program of instruction and orientation towards an uncomplicated vaginal delivery with participation of the father or 'significant other'; the LM teaches the mother how to breathe and relax during parturition, thereby ↓ the anxiety associated with childbirth and the amount of anesthesia required for ♀ delivering a child; see Doula, Midwifes, Natural childbirth

LAMB syndrome Carney's complex An AD [MIM 160980] clinical triad of young adult onset, which consists of spotty mucocutaneous lentigenes, cutaneous and cardiac myxomas, endocrine hyperactivity, as well as multifocal myxoidfibroadenomas of the breast, adrenocortical hyperplasia and calcifying Sertoli cell tumors of the testes; Cf NAME syndrome

lambda (λ) Symbol for: 1) Decay constant; 2) Light chain (immunoglobulin) 3) Wavelength

lambda (λ) **bacteriophage** MOLECULAR BIOLOGY A DNA virus with affinity for *Escherichia coli* which, once inside the host, either directs the production of phage particles, causing bacteriolysis or integrates itself into the genome, with the phage dividing in tandem with the host *E coli* genome; the lambda phage has proven a good model for studying protein-DNA interactions; see Bacteriophages, Lambda vector

lambda (λ) **chain** A 22-kD protein that is one of the two immunoglobulin light chains, the normal lambda to kappa light chain ratio is 2:1

lambda (λ) **vector** A type of lambda bacteriophage used to transport DNA into an *Escherichia coli* for the purpose of cloning a particular segment of DNA; there are two classes of lambda cloning vectors: 1) Insertion vectors, which accept DNA inserts up to 12 kb in length, which are generally used for construction of cDNA library construction and 2) Replacement vectors, which accept 9–23-kb inserts, commonly used for genomic library construction

lambda waves Sharp, low-amplitude EEG waves in the occipital region in non-REM sleep and in newborn children; of no known significance

Lambert-Eaton syndrome NEUROLOGY A disorder of neuromuscular transmission characterized by chronic progressive muscular weakness usually of the legs, aching and fatigability, autonomic dysfunction (dry mouth, impotence, constipation, blurred vision, dyshidrosis) and absence of deep tendon reflex PATHOPHYSIOLOGY Defective neuromuscular-junction transmission and interference with the presynaptic release of acetylcholine from the presynaptic motor terminal due to antibody-mediated destruction of the postsynaptic voltage-gated P/Q calcium channel antibodies (**N Engl J Med 1994; 331:528CPC**); LES is often paraneoplastic, and is most commonly linked to primary lung carcinoma, 'classically' small cell type, but also squamous cell carcinoma, and adenocarcinoma (**N Engl J Med 1995; 332:1467OA**)

lamellar body Myelin figure A nonspecific descriptive term for concentrically layered, fingerprint-like, osmiophilic material derived from membranes and organelles, eg the endoplasmic reticulum, seen by electron microscopy DERMATOPATHOLOGY Lamellar or Odland bodies or keratinosomes are seen by electron microscopy in the stratum spinosum and in the intercellular spaces; although their function is not known, they may play a role in keratinization and are increased in lamellar ichthyosis HEMATOPATHOLOGY see Ribosomal lamellar complexes PULMONARY PATHOLOGY Lamellar bodies are membrane-bound layered material seen by EM, corresponding to surfactant, a normal product of type II pneumocytes that is increased in interstitial lung diseases (desquamative interstitial pneumonitis, usual interstitial pneumonitis and diffuse alveolar damage), primary pulmonary proteinosis, pulmonary toxicity (methotrexate, bleomycin, cytoxan, busulfan), type II glycogen storage disease, cystic fibrosis, bronchoalveolar cell carcinoma and diffuse pleural mesothelioma Note: Lamellated structures have been seen by EM in the adrenal cortex related to spironolactone therapy, in the liver secondary to phenobarbital therapy, in the proximal renal tubules in gentamicin- and aminoglycoside-induced nephropathy, in uteri with IUDs, and in normal oocytes and neurons; by LM, lamellar bodies correspond to concentrically laminated lipoprotein- phosphatide complexes with ↑ uptake of H_2O, ceroid, seen in the autophagic vacuoles of Fabry's disease, granular cell tumors, malignant fibrous histiocytoma, and spermatocytic seminoma

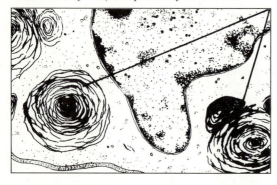

lamellar body

lamifiban Ro 44-9883 A potent nonpeptide inhibitor of ligand binding to the glycoprotein IIb/IIIa (integrin $\alpha_{IIb}\beta_3$) receptor, which is currently in phase 3 clinical trials (**N Engl J Med 1995; 332:1553**RV)

lamifiban

lamin Any of a group of fibrous proteins of the intermediate filament family, which are divided into lamins A, B, and C; lamins form a 2-D network on the inner face of the nuclear membrane, binding DNA in the nucleoplasm; lamin phosphorylation by a kinase triggers disassembly of the nucleus and condensation of chromatin at the time of mitosis; see Intermediate filaments

laminectomy ORTHOPEDIC SURGERY A procedure for treating a herniation of an intervertebral disk; the 'classic' laminectomy entails removal of the entire lamina of a vertebral body; the permutations of the procedure depend on the case and the field of exposure desired by operator

LAMINOTOMY Fenestration Removal of a portion of the superior and inferior aspects of the lamina adjacent to the diseased disk HEMILAMINECTOMY Unilateral excision of the vertebral lamina with removal of variable parts of the adjacent facet LAMINECTOMY Bilateral removal of the lamina as well as varying portions of both facets MICROSURGICAL LAMINECTOMY Diskectomy A technique that avoids vertebral exploration prior to disk surgery, reducing the risk of the feared 'Failed disk syndrome' as there is minimal excision of bone and epidural fat and minimal nerve root adhesion (**JAMA 1990; 264:1469**DATTA)

laminin CELL BIOLOGY An 820-kD basement membrane glycoprotein of the integrin receptor family that has a cruciform structure (deduced by the 'rotary shadowing' method), and has binding sites for Type IV collagen, heparin sulfate proteoglycan and surface receptors of normal and malignant cells; laminin promotes cell attachment and migration, and plays a role in differentiation and metastasis; it is produced by macrophages, endothelial, epithelial and Schwann cells, and appears as early as the morular stage of the embryo, serving as the 'glue' for the primitive endothelium, epithelium, and mesothelium; soluble laminin fragments have theoretic currency in preventing the attachment of malignant cells

s-laminin *pronounced* 'slaminin' Synaptic laminin A ubiquitous extracellular protein on which neurons can grow; data suggest that s-laminin signals regenerating motor neurons that they have arrived at the right site and can drop their synaptic anchor on muscle cells

laminin receptor A heterodimeric membrane-bound protein composed of a large subunit joined by a disulfide bond to a small subunit; laminin receptor functions include cell attachment and neurite outgrowth; structural motifs of the laminin receptor are shared by other integrins, eg fibronectin and vitronectin

laminotomy Fenestration ORTHOPEDIC SURGERY A procedure for treating a herniation of an intervertebral disk, consisting of removal of a portion of the superior and inferior aspects of the lamina adjacent to the diseased disk; see Laminectomy

lamivudine 3TC, see there

lamotrigina 3,5-diamino-6-(2,3-dichlorophenyl)1,2,4-triazine An antiepileptic agent that blocks sodium channels and causes presynaptic inhibition of the excitatory amino acids glutamate and aspartate SIDE EFFECTS Somnolence, exanthema, vomiting, laryngitis, and exacerbation of convulsions (**Medico Interamericano 1995; 14:125**)

lampbrush chromosome A large chromosome with expanded, mitotically paired chromosomes that are transiently expressed in the early prophase (diplotene stage) of meiosis of spermatocytes and oocytes at various philogenic levels, from *Drosophila* to vertebrates; LCs are very active in RNA synthesis, with 'innumerable' very long loops of chromatin covered by newly transcribed RNA packed in dense RNA-protein complexes; these loops, like polytene puffs, correspond to fixed units of folded chromatin that are opened up and transcriptionally active, a transition that requires topo-isomerase II, without which the cell cannot replicate; the lampbrush and supercoiled DNA chromosomal conformations are seen by Dapey stain; Cf Feather pattern

LAN Local area network, see there

'L&D' Labor and Delivery A commonly used colloquialism for the obstetric unit of North American hospitals

land mine GLOBAL VILLAGE/MILITARY MEDICINE An antipersonnel device that is buried in a road, field, and countryside, and intended to maim or kill the enemy du jour; there are ≥ 100 million land mines in 60 countries that cause ± 15 000 casualties/year, most often innocent civilians, inflicting overwhelming social and economic damage on communities struggling to recover from armed conflicts; LMs cause injury by direct tearing of tissues, but also by driving contaminated soil, clothing, metals, plastics, and so on into open wounds, and may be fatal due to hemorrhage, tetanus, or gangrene; countries with many buried LMs include Angola, Cambodia, Nicaragua, Somalia, and the former Yugoslavia (**N Engl J Med 1995; 332:1525BR**)

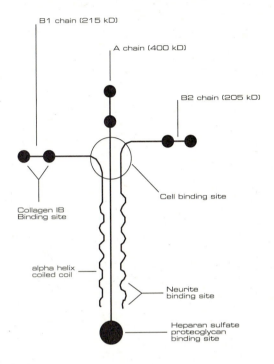

B1 chain (215 kD)

A chain (400 kD)

B2 chain (205 kD)

Cell binding site

Collagen IB Binding site

alpha helix coiled coil

Neurite binding site

Heparan sulfate proteoglycan binding site

laminin

landmark article An article or abstract in a scientific journal that is considered by the workers in a field to have been a seminal study or to have had substantial impact on that area of knowledge, eg Banting and Best's *The Internal Secretions of the Pancreas* (**J Lab Clin Med 1922; 7:251**), JW Conn's *Primary Aldosteronism, a New Clinical Syndrome* (**J Lab Clin Med 1955; 45:3**) and RF Schilling's *Intrinsic factor studies II. The Effect of Gastric Juice on the Urinary Excretion of Radio-activity after the Oral Administration of Radioactive Vitamin B_{12}* (**J Lab Clin Med 1953; 42:860**); like citation classics, landmark articles are benchmarks of original work with potential for a Nobel prize; see Citation classic, 'Hot paper'; Cf Uncitedness index

lane LABORATORY TECHNOLOGY A 'corridor' in an electrophoretic support medium, eg agar gel or paper, at the beginning of which is a well or point on which a fluid containing a molecule of interest is 'spotted', after which the support is subjected to a unidirectional electric current, causing the molecular migration within the lane and separation into 'bands' according to size

Langerhans' cell Dendritic reticulum cell A specialized macrophage (dendritic cell) of the epidermis that presents antigen to lymphocytes in the upper dermis at the suprabasilar layer and sends dendritic processes both to the granular layer and to the basal lamina; LCs by H&E have a clear appearance; they are positive for CD1a, Fc receptor, HLA-DR, S100, and by EM may demonstrate Birbeck granules (see there)

Note: Paul Langerhans (1847-1888) described the cell while a medical student under Virchow in Berlin

Langerhans' granules see Tennis racquet granule

LANGERHANS' CELL HISTIOCYTOSIS (HISTIOCYTOSIS X)
SOLITARY BONE INVOLVEMENT Eosinophilic granuloma A lesion of younger patients that may affect any bone (sparing the hands and feet), most commonly those of the cranial vault, jaw, humerus, rib and femur RADIOLOGY Mimics Ewing sarcoma TREATMENT Simple curettage PROGNOSIS Excellent
MULTIPLE BONE INVOLVEMENT Polyostotic eosinophilic granuloma Hand-Schüller-Christian disease A lesion that variably affects the skin, accompanied by proptosis, diabetes insipidus, or chronic otitis media or combination thereof, marked by a prolonged course with waxing and waning symptoms PROGNOSIS Relatively good
MULTIPLE ORGAN INVOLVEMENT Letter-Siwe disease A lesion that affects bone, lung and skin, which while histologically indistinct, but far is far more aggressive than the other forms PROGNOSIS Poor prognosis if < 18 months at time of diagnosis, hemorrhagic skin lesions, hepatomegaly, anemia, thrombocytopenia, bone marrow involvement

Langerhans' cell histiocytosis Histiocytosis X An autonomous proliferation of a specific cell of the lymphoreticular system, the Langerhans cell (see there) that stains positively with antibodies to ATPase, S-100 and CD1a; aggregates of Langerhans' cells are accompanied by eosinophils, foamy cells, neutrophils, fibrosis; histiocytosis X is commonly divided into three clinical forms (table) (**N Engl J Med 1994; 331:148OA**)

Note: LCH is a recently introduced term for the diseases encompassed under the rubric of histiocytosis X (a term that is likely to reverberate in the literature for the forseeable future); given this transition, it seems most appropriate to refer to the older terms (eosinophilic granuloma, Hand-Shüller-Christian disease, Letterer-Siwe disease) by a hybrid name, eg Langerhans' cell histiocytosis-eosinophilic granuloma type, Langerhans' cell histiocytosis-Hand-Schüller-Christian type, Langerhans' cell histiocytosis-Letterer-Siwe type

Langerhans' islets Nests of endocrine cells* located in the pancreas, which are more numerous in the tail, invested with a well-developed capillary network, composed of 1) α cells, comprising 20% of islet cells, which produce glucagon, 2) β cells, 70% of total, which produce insulin and 3) delta cells, 10% of the cells, which produce somatostatin

*Formally known as pancreatic islets, *insulae pancreaticae* [NH3]

Langhans' giant cell A giant cell (figure, right) composed of fused epithelioid histiocytes, whose multiple (up to 50) nuclei are arranged in a garland-like fashion or horseshoe fashion measuring up to 50 μm in diameter, surrounding glassy cytoplasm; when accompanied by caseating necrosis, the Langhans' giant cell is virtually diagnostic for tuberculosis, but may also be seen in other chronic granulomatous conditions, eg leprosy, schistosomiasis, and secondary syphilis

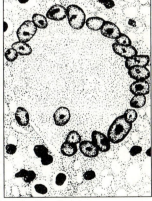

T Langhans, Swiss pathologist 1839-1915

LAP 1) Laboratory Accreditation Program (US Dept of Commerce) 2) Laparoscopy 3) Laparotomy 4) Left atrial pressure 5) Leukocyte alkaline phosphatase A phosphomonoesterase with optimal activity at pH 10.0 that is concentrated in granules of normal neutrophils; LAP is ↓ in CML, paroxysmal nocturnal hemoglobinuria, ITP, infectious mononucleosis and aplastic anemia; LAP is ↑ in CML in remission, polycythemia vera, Hodgkin's disease, myeloid metaplasia, corticosteroid therapy, and pregnancy Also 1) Learning accomplishment profile (psychology) 2) Leucine aminopeptidase 3) Lyophilized anterior pituitary (an obsolete therapeutic substance)

lap traveler PUBLIC HEALTH A child travelling in an automobile seated on an adult's lap and who is not restrained in an infant or car-seat; often the person holding the child will survive as they are cushioned from the dashboard injuries by the child who dies; in older statistics, up to 40% of infants who died in automobile accidents were lap-travellers; see MVA

laparoscopic cholecystectomy A minimally invasive technique for removing the gallbladder, in which the entire procedure is performed through the laparascope, with an average in-hospital stay of 1.2 days, in contrast to the usual 5.6 days; 5% of cases in one series needed conversion to an open cholecystectomy due to anatomic variations Complications 5%, versus 6-21% in conventional cholecystectomy (**N Engl J Med 1991; 324:1073**) there has been a 33% decrease in mortality rate/procedure; overall mortality has not decreased given the ↑ in number of procedures performed (**N Engl J Med 1994; 330:403ʀᴀ**)

LAPAROSCOPIC VS OPEN CHOLECYSTECTOMY

	LAPAROSCOPIC	OPEN
Bile duct injuries	13/1518	1/1200
Hospital stay/recovery time	1 day/<1 week	5 days/4-6 weeks
Source of costs	↑ Surgeon fees/OR time	↑ Inpatient costs

‡Am Med News May 4 1992

laparoscopic surgery An evolving group of minimally invasive procedures in which intra-abdominal surgery is performed via instruments that provide minimal tactile feedback (ie à la Nintendo); LS ↓ post-operative pain, ↓ length of hospital stay and ↓ of disability TECHNIQUE A working field is created by insufflating the abdominal cavity with CO_2 at a pressure of 10-15 mm Hg, followed by insertion of a laparoscope with a video camera and laparoscopic instruments, which are modifications of standard surgical instruments ACCEPTED LAPAROSCOPIC PROCEDURES Diagnostic laparoscopy (evaluation of abdominal pain, trauma, staging of malignancy), and laparoscopic cholecystectomy LAPAROSCOPIC PROCEDURES UNDER DEVELOPEMENT Appendectomy, common bile duct exploration, inguinal hernia repair, colonic resection, gastroesophageal reflux-related procedures, peptic ulcer procedures COMPLICATIONS CO-induced gas embolism, hypercapnia, acidosis, arrhythmias (**N Engl J Med 1994; 330:403ʀᴠ**)

lardaceous spleen A spleen with diffuse amyloidosis, where there is prominent red pulp involvement of a firm enlarged spleen, the cut surface of which is waxy and translucent; Cf Sago spleen

large cell undifferentiated carcinoma of lung A pleomorphic aggressive carcinoma that is considered a poorly differentiated squamous cell carcinoma, adenocarcinoma or small cell carcinoma; the lesions may be associated with marked peripheral eosinophilia or leukocytosis CLINICAL Similar to pulmonary adenocarcinoma in that 50% metastasize to the brain; if more than 40% of the cells are 'giant', it is designated giant cell carcinoma and has a very poor prognosis, with an average survivial of less than one year; Cf Small cell carcinoma

lariat MOLECULAR BIOLOGY An intermediate structural motif arising in the pre-mRNA splicing reaction, consisting of a novel 2"-5' phosphodiester bond that enables one adenosine nucleotide to formphosphodiester links with three other nucleotides rather than the usual two, resulting in a branched intermediate, which is followed by 3' splice-site cleavage (intron excision), ligation of the exons and freeing of the lariat structure

Larmor equation MRI A formula stating that the frequency of precession of the nuclear magnetic moment is proportional to the magnetic field. Equation: $w_o = \gamma B_o$ (radians/sec) or $f_o = \gamma B_o/2\pi$ (hertz), where f_o is frequency, γ is gyromagnetic ratio, and B_o is the magnetic induction field Note: A negative sign (−) indicates the direction of rotation; see Magnetic resonance imaging

Larmor frequency (w_o or f_o) MRI The frequency at which magnetic resonance can be excited, given by the Larmor equation; by varying a magnetic field across the body with a gradient magnetic field, the corresponding variation of the LF can be used to encode position (for protons, the LF is 42.58 MHz/tesla); see Magnetic resonance imaging

larva currens A form of larva migrans due to an infestation by female larva of *Strongyloides stercoralis* that penetrate the skin, causing intense, transient, pruritus, and urticaria; which may be accompanied by systemic symptoms, eg bronchitis, abdominal pain, diarrhea, constipation, nausea, vomiting, anorexia, or weight loss; see Hyperinfection syndrome

larva migrans An infestation by non-human nematodes that penetrate, and migrate through the skin, but which cannot complete their life cycle in man CUTANEOUS LARVA MIGRANS results from the dog and cat hookworm, *Ancylostoma braziliense*, the larvae of which migrate a few millimeters/day, producing pruritic serpiginous tracks in the stratum germinatum that are visible below the skin VISCERAL LARVA MIGRANS is due to the dog (*Toxocara canis*) or cat parasites (*T cati*), the life cycles of which in their usual hosts resemble that of *Ascaris lumbricoides* in humans; in this form, the embryonated eggs are accidentally ingested and hatch in the intestine, penetrating the mucosa, aimlessly wander through the circulation, passing to the hepatic and/or pulmonary vasculature and are potentially fatal if they involve the myocardium or CNS; in the eye, the resulting retinal granuloma mimics retinoblastoma

laryngeal complex The structural elements (strap muscles*, elastic suspensory ligaments, and laryngeal elevators) that determine the position of the larynx in the upper aerodigestive tract; the LC is elevated during expiration and depressed during inspiration, but is most displaced during deglutition; the LC muscles are innervated by the descending hypoglossal portion of the cervical loop (*ansa cervicalis* [NA6], formerly *ansa hypoglossi*), derived from C1 to C3; see Strap muscles

*The infrahyoid group of intrinsic laryngeal muscles, which are antagonistic to the elastic suspensory ligaments and elevators of the larynx

laryngeal electromyography A technique analogous to conventional electromyography that is used to differentiate neurogenic from a myogenic disorder, determine the site of a neurogenic lesion (ie upper vs lower neurons), and to differentiate organic from a functional defects; LEMG is used to evaluate patients with vocal fold dysfunction, including those with tremor, myoclonus, pyramidal and extrapyramidal disorders, and primary muscular disorders, allowing the delineation of specific (superior vs recurrent laryngeal) nerve involvement, and provide prognostic information

laryngeal microsurgery OTOLARYNGOLOGY Any of a number of types of phonosurgery (see there) in which microsurgical techniques are used to manage benign vocal fold pathology, including cysts, edema, nodules, polyps, sulci, and tumors

laryngeal nerve transplant A surgical attempt to repair

damage to the recurrent laryngeal nerve (RLN), which may uni- or bilateral, temporary or permanent and occurs in 0.2% of cases of thyroid surgery for non-malignant conditions and 5% of cases treated for thyroid malignancy; asymptomatic unilateral paralysis requires no treatment; bilateral RLN injury may result in defects of the respiratory toilet and if extreme, airway obstruction; the surgeon usually attempts a direct repair if severance is recognized at the time of surgery or performs a tracheostomy and awaits spontaneous return of nerve function; repair of the recurrent nerve is better than the nerve transplant procedures, eg splitting of the vagus nerve and end-to-end anastomosis to the distal end of the RLN or the Tucker procedure, in which the omohyoid muscle is implanted into the cricothyroid muscle

laryngeal nodule Singer's node, see there

laryngeal web An uncommon congenital laryngeal anomaly resulting from incomplete separation of the fetal mesenchyme between both sides of the larynx, consisting of a fibrovascular lamina at the anterior aspect of the vocal cords, causing respiratory obstruction that may present as a neonatal emergency

laryngismus stridulus Pseudocroup PEDIATRICS A childhood cough with a whooping character that is due to spasmodic laryngeal closure with crowing inspiration, which is a manifestation of tetany CLINICAL Cyanosis accompanied by apnea, paresthesia, tingling of hands and feet; LS is most common at night, often waking its victim LABORATORY ↓↓↓ Serum calcium, normal magnesium; see Latent tetany syndrome; Cf Whooping cough

laryngostroboscopy A technique for examining the vocal fold's vibratory function, and assess the effectiveness of medical, surgical, and speech therapy; it is used to evaluate voice complaints in singers (eg vocal fold paralysis), dysphonia in absence of obvious lesions, laryngeal lesions that result in a pathologic voice (eg subplical vocal fold lesions, depth of involvement in laryngeal carcinoma), assess mucosal hygiene, and provide feedback on the results of phonosurgery

laryngotracheal reconstruction Any of a number of number of methods used to enlarge and stabilize the upper airway

laser Light amplification by stimulated emission of radiation PHYSICS The principle on which lasers are based was postulated by Einstein in 1917; the first working model was built in 1961 at Princeton University PRINCIPLE Atoms of a suitable material are excited to a higher energy level by energy 'pumping'; if during the excitation phase, an additional photon with an appropriate frequency impinges on the excited system, it is forced into resonance and releases identical photons as the system reverts to a lower energy state; the photons 'bounce' back and forth between a highly reflecting and a semitransparent mirror, stimulating the release of more resonant photons, causing an 'avalanche' effect; the beam of laser energy differs from thermal light as the beam is highly coherent, collimated, ie 'focused', and monochromatic; in addition to the thermal effects, lasers may evoke photodissociation of molecules, and generate shock waves by creating an ionized plasma capable of disintegrating mineral deposits, causing a target tissue to fluoresce and to interact with a dye, destroying a target cell or tissue; lasers have been used since the early 1960s in ophthalmology for the destructive effects of the intense heat, and its selective nature; an argon laser that generates a green beam selectively absorbed by the retina's melanin pigment, causes damage without destroying adjacent structures; the argon laser is of use in 'riveting' detached retina and for treating both opened and closed angle glaucomas; lasers are being increasingly used in other areas of health care, dermatology for coagulation-bleaching of tattoos and port-wine nevi (see Selective photothermolysis), endoscopy for coagulating vascular malformations (see Nd-YAG laser), gynecology (see Roller ball technique); in the laboratory lasers may be a critical component of the instrument itself, serving as the light source in flow cytometry and spectrophotometry; short wavelength lasers include argon, krypton, neodymium and ruby; long wavelength lasers include CO_2, erbium-yttrium-aluminum-garnet (YAG) laser (Biophotonics Intl 1995; 2/2:26)

Note: Lasers have been used in dentistry to treat cavities; the data is thought by some workers to be preliminary

(CO_2) laser ablation GYNECOLOGY The excision of a portion of the uterine cervix to treat CIN (cervical intraepithelial neoplasia), circumscribed foci of carcinoma in situ and occasionally, HPV changes (condylomas)

lasers in dentistry Zapping with short low-energy bursts results in annealing that eliminates some of the carbonate impurities in the calcium phosphate that result in an increased susceptibility to decay (Biophotonics Intl 1995; 2/2:49)

laser stapedectomy A surgical procedure using an argon laser to treat hearing loss, which attempts to reduce the conductive deafness to < 10 decibels POSTOP COMPLICATIONS Cochlear deafness (< 1%), prolonged vertigo, facial nerve injury

laser thrombolysis CARDIOVASCULAR MEDICINE A technique under development in which a fiberoptic catheter containing a laser operating at 570 nm is passed through an artery, eg the coronary artery, and the blood clots vaporized using ultrashort bursts of energy; LT is envisioned by some workers as complementing more invasive or traumatic therapies, eg bypass surgery, balloon angioplasty, and thrombolytic drugs (Biophotonics Intl 1995:2:21)

Lassa fever An acute highly communicable arenavirus infection, first described in northeastern Nigeria, which is endemic in western Africa (10% of fever in Sierra Leone is Lassa-related), causing 250 000 annual cases in small epidemic clusters EPIDEMIOLOGY Vector is house rat (*Mastomys natalensis*), transmitted by the oral-fecal route, rarely human-to-human CLINICAL Many cases are mild, subclinical or have an insidious onset of fever, weakness and malaise followed by headache, dry cough, pharyngitis, back pain, myalgia, diarrhea, cough, vomiting, lymphadenopathy, sensorineural deafness and, if severe, hypovolemia, hypotension, pleural effusion, ascites, pulmonary edema, and shock MORTALITY 5-30%

LASERS IN MEDICINE

Type	Wavelength	Power/energy	Specialties
Alexandrite	700-800 nm	to 1 J/pulse	Derm, Urol
Argon	450-515 nm	to 6 W	Dent, Derm, Ophth
CO_2	10.6 µm	to 100 W	Card, Dent, Derm, Gen Surg, Orthoped
Diode	800 nm	to 50W	Gen Surg, Urol
Er:YAG	2.94 µm	to 1 J/pulse	Dent, Ophth
Excimer	193 nm	≤ 0.6 J/pulse	Card, Ophth
Holmium YAG	2.10 µm	to 60 W	Card, Ophth, Orthoped
Nd:YAG, pulsed	532, 1064 nm	to 0.5 J/pulse	Dent, Derm, Ophth
Nd:YAG, CW	532, 1064, 1044 nm	to 125 W	Card, Derm, Gen Surg, Neurol, Orthoped, Urol
Pulsed dye	504-620 nm	to 2 J/pulse	Derm, Ophth, Urol
Ruby	694nm	to 2 J/pulse	Derm

Biophotonics Intl 1995; 2/2:26

latah PSYCHIATRY A psychiatric reaction to a sudden stressful stimulus, resulting in automatisms, command obedience, and uncontrollable motor and verbal responses, eg echolalia, echopraxia, coprolalia, as well as dissociative and trancelike behavior; the term latah is from Malaysia, where it is most common in middle-aged women (DSM-IV™, 1994) see Culture-bound syndrome, Zombies

Other names for the condition in other parts of Asia include amurakh, baah-ji, bah-tschi, bah-tsi, ikota, imu, irkunii, lata, mali-mali, menkeiti, myriachit, olan, silok

'latchkey' child SOCIAL MEDICINE A child who arrives home after school, who lets himself/herself into the house (with a 'latchkey'), and who is unattended until the parents' arrival several hours later; the major concern is for the safety of the younger and lack of supervision of the older children; whether this transient lack of supervision has a negative influence on the child's behavior, socialization or on performance in standardized test scores is controversial; an ongoing study of 5000 children reveals a two-fold ↑ risk of drug and alcohol abuse, feeling of stress and anger, and ↓ school performance for those children who spent ≥ 11 hours/week in self-care (JAMA 1992; 268:2628MN&P). Cf 'Supermom'

late abortion An abortion performed after the 12th week of gestation

late dumping syndrome see Dumping syndrome‡

late gene VIROLOGY A gene produced by the cell long after the integration of a virus into the host genome, which encodes structural proteins of interest to the virus; see Early gene

late luteal phase dysphoric disorder Premenstrual syndrome, see there, aka (in the psychiatric literature) premenstrual dysphoric disorder [DSM-IV]

late-onset immune deficiency An idiopathic condition associated with gastric carcinoma, atrophic gastritis, pernicious anemia, autoimmunity, malabsorption variably accompanied by lactose intolerance, small intestinal atrophy, thymoma and agnogenic myeloid metaplasia with immunoglobulin defects and the Prasad syndrome

late phase reaction A delayed or secondary response in asthmatics after an antigenic challenge, in which neutrophils release histamine, stimulating secondary mast cell and basophil degranulation, in turn evoking bronchial hyperreactivity; LPR differs from the primary response in that prostaglandin PGD2 is not produced; LPRs may also be evoked by irritants, eg cold air, ozone, viruses TREATMENT β-adrenergic aerosols

late potential CARDIOLOGY A high-frequency, low-amplitude signal at the end portion of the QRS complex, which is thought to be due to fragmented and delayed electrical conduction through the borders of a myocardial scar; delayed conduction of LPs allows reentry of electrical impulses and ↑ susceptibility to ventricular arrhythmias; detection of late potentials by SAE correlates well with inducibility of ventricular tachycardia during electrophysiologic testing (Mayo Clin Proc 1995; 70:132OA)

late whiplash syndrome A condition the very existence of which is highly controversial as is it reported to affect 20-40% of the > than one million persons/year (US) who suffer 'garden variety' whiplash injury; while the changes of LWS may be attributed to unresolved injury, there is considerable evidence for psychological factors or the hope of financial gain (see 'jury collar') as evidenced by resolution of muscle and ligament injuries elsewhere in the body (N Engl J Med 1994; 330:1083ED) see Quebec classification, Whiplash

latency NEUROPHYSIOLOGY The time between application of a stimulus and response thereto, which is divided into 1) Sensory latency The time required to process the message of irritation and 2) Motor latency The time between a message's arrival and the corresponding muscle response

latent homosexuality Unconsciously repressed homosexuality; Cf (in the) Closet, Homosexuality

Note: Homosexuality that is consciously repressed or acted upon is regarded as being 'in the closet'

latent tetany syndrome A physiological state of neuromuscular hyperexcitability, delineated by physical examination and electromyography CLINICAL Trousseau and Chvostek signs of hypocalcemia, bowel irritability, laryngismus stridulus, anxiety, asthenia, migraines and mitral valve prolapse

lateral specification DEVELOPMENTAL BIOLOGY An at-present partly hypothetical regulatory process by which initially equivalent developing cells signal to each other, possibly by means of random fluctuations in some signaling activity present in the original population of cells that might be amplified in some cells and inhibited in others (Science 1995; 268:225) Cf Inductive signaling

latex A lactescent gel of molecular homogeneity, obtained from plants and composed of microglobules of natural rubber; latex may be airborne and linked to automobile tires (Science News 1995; 147:244) LABORATORY MEDICINE The term 'latex' has been broadened in scope to include neoprene, polystyrene, polyvinylchloride and synthetic 'rubbers'; latexes are the inert vehicles that may be used to carry antibodies or antigens in latex agglutination immunoassays; or rubber latex-like plastic monomer used to manufacture minute plastic beads usually of polystyrene

latex agglutination test LABORATORY MEDICINE Any assay that uses visible agglutination as an end-point to detect a reaction between derivatized particles and an analyte; the specificity of an LAT is conferred by any of a wide range of binding specificities; in the usual design, an antibody is bound to latex beads in a solution that is placed in contact with material of interest; LATs have been a mainstay in clinical laboratory, eg for detecting rheumatoid factors; they have become increasingly popular as they can be formatted in a one-step process making them ideal for home testing, eg for pregnancy testing by relatively unsophisticated users and may be automated (Am Clin Lab March 1993)

latex allergy The presence of IgE-mediated sensitivity to latex proteins present in latex gloves, dental rubber dams, condoms, barium enema catheters, and other medical rubber devices, which occur in association with symptoms of anaphylaxis, angioedema, asthma, contact urticaria, or rhinitis when a sensitized person comes in contact with latex allergens*; LA is common, affecting ± 17 million in the US (population, 250 million) and ≥ 15% of health care workers; smoking may be related to severity of the allergic reaction (Arch Pathol Lab Med 1993; 117:897OA, 874ED); latex from sources other than the Brazilian rubber plant (*Hevea brasiliensis*), eg guayule (*Parthenium argentatum*), a wild desert shrub found in the southwestern US is reported to be less allergenic (Science News 1995; 147:254)

*Latex allergy is distinguished from allergic contact dermatitis caused by latex

latex glove allergy OCCUPATIONAL MEDICINE A permutation of latex allergy with an estimated prevalence rate of 8.8%, clinically characterized by contact urticaria, (JAMA 1992; 268:2695)

lathyrism A disease of livestock that grazes on *Lathyrus* species of sweet peas, which induces spastic paralysis, skeletal and cardiovascular abnormalities, and collagen defects*; lathyrism in humans is due to excess consumption of fava beans, which contain β-aminopropionitrile, an irreversible inhibitor of the copper-bearing amino oxidase (in blood) and lysyl oxidase (in bone and connective tissue), preventing hydroxylation of proline and lysine, in turn preventing the cross-linking of tropocollagen CLINICAL Spastic paraplegia, pain, paresthesia, ↑↑↑ in urinary excretion of hydroxyproline, skeletal deformities, eg marfanoid habitus, kyphoscoliosis and aortic aneurysms

*Lathyrism is a useful experimental model for studying collagen disease

Latrodectus A genus of highly venomous spiders (Family Theridae, which includes the black widow spider, *Latrodectus mactans*), endemic to the US, with a characteristic orange-red hourglass-shaped marking on the abdomen; the venom is a non-hemolytic neurotoxin CLINICAL Latency period of hours, followed by severe myalgia, myospasm, truncal rigidity, nausea, vomiting, diaphoresis, and shock; most cases resolve spontaneously, small children are at ↑ risk of mortality and morbidity TREATMENT Establish airway, supportive care

LATS Long-acting thyroid stimulator, see there

LATS protector An antibody present in 90% of patients with Graves' disease, which in vitro prevents the inactivation of LATS; the LATS-P assay is a sensitive marker for Graves' disease, but is too cumbersome to utilize as a diagnostic tool

lattice BIOCHEMISTRY An organized three-dimensional scaffold of usually similar molecules; Cf Domain, Motif

lattice dystrophy OPHTHALMOLOGY Localized deposition of amyloid between an irregular epithelium and Bowman's membrane of the cornea

laughing death Kuru, see there

laughing disease Pseudobulbar palsy, see there

laughing gas Nitrous oxide (N₂O), see there

'laundry list' A fanciful term for a long and relatively complete list of symptoms, diseases, or etiologies that share something in common, eg differential diagnosis of acute abdomen

LAV Lymphadenopathy-associated virus; see HIV-1

lavage The washing out of a body cavity or hollow organ to obtain fluids for diagnostic cytology from the pleura and pericardial cavity, to detect hemorrhage in blunt trauma or to remove toxins, eg gastric lavage in overdose; see BAL (bronchoalveolar lavage)

lavender top tube LABORATORY MEDICINE A phlebotomy tube with EDTA anticoagulant, used in 1) Chemistry Measure carcinoembryonic antigen, lead, renin, 2) Hematology Measure parameters that require separated cells, including counts of white and red cells, hemoglobin, hematocrit, mean corpuscular volume (MCV), mean corpuscular hemoglobin (MCH), mean corpuscular hemoglobin concentration (MCHC), differential counts, sedimentation rate, glucose-6-phosphate dehydrogenase, sickle cell preparation, hemoglobin electrophoresis, platelet and reticulocyte counts

law of mass action A universal physicochemical law that states, '*At equilibrium in a reversible chemical reacting system, the rates of forward and reverse reactions, substrate utilization and product formation are constant*'; this law applies to any equilibrium that does not require the input of energy

law of the minimum MICROBIOLOGY The growth and/or development of an organism is limited by whichever essential nutrient is available in the least amount

law of partial pressure A universal law that each gas in a mixture of gases will exert a pressure that is proportionate to the percentage of that gas independently of the other gases in the mixture

lawn plate MICROBIOLOGY A bacterial culture plate in which the organisms are inoculated with a McFarland turbidity standard of 1.0 (circa 10⁸ organisms/ml of a clear fluid) that were previously incubated in a Müller-Hinton broth and are then grown to confluence (a 'lawn') on a nutrient medium, eg blood agar; LPs are used to detect minimum bactericidal concentration of antibiotics (MIC);

see MIC

laxative abuse GASTROENTEROLOGY A phenomenon often accompanied by factitious diarrhea that is found in ± 4% of new patients seen by gastronterologists and up to 20% of those evaluated in a tertiary referral center; laxative abusers are available in five flavors, to wit, those with eating disorders (eg anorexia nervosa, bulimia), hysterical personalities, emotional problems, Munchausen syndrome, and Polle syndrome (child abuse with laxatives) CLINICAL Finger clubbing, skin hyperpigmentation, colonic inflammation, steatorrhea, osteomalacia, protein-losing enteropathy, nephropathy, melanosis coli (sigmoidoscopy), ahaustral right colon (barium enema) LABORATORY ↓ K⁺, uric acid kidney stones; ↓ stool osmolality (eg < 250 mOsm/kg), ↑ stool sulfate and phosphate (**N Engl J Med 1995; 332:725ʀᴠ**)

laxative screen Laxative survey LABORATORY MEDICINE A battery of tests performed in specialized reference laboratories, using an array of diagnostic modalities, eg spectrophotometry and TLC of urine or stool supernatant to identify anthraquinones, bisacodyl, phenophthalein, castor oil, mineral oil, magnesium, phosphate, components of laxatives, which are commonly abused and thus need to be ruled out/in as a cause of chronic diarrhea (**N Engl J Med 1995; 332:725ʀᴠ**)

'layer cake' education The technique for teaching science in the US, where in the final years of secondary education, biology, chemistry and physics are taught in separate academic years, fancifully likened to the 'layers on a cake', as opposed to integrating the disciplines over a period of years, a methodologic philosophy that has been highly criticized as a cause of the deterioration of the quality of secondary education in the US in the 1980s

Lazarus complex Near-death experience, see there

lazy bladder That which occurs in children with a history of infrequent (one-two times per day) voiding and overflow incontinence; because of the bladder decompensation from chronic overdistension, the bladder does not properly empty and the children are prone to urinary tract infection

lazy eye Suppresion amblyopia Subnormal visual acuity in one or more eyes despite appropriate correction of refractive errors, subdivided into **ORGANIC AMBLYOPIA**, in which there is pathologic change affecting the visual pathways including macular scarring seen in chorioretinitis, retrolental fibroplasia, retinoblastoma, optic atrophy, meningoencephalitis and other organic lesions and **FUNCTIONAL AMBLYOPIA**, in which there is no underlying pathology and visual impairment is either sensory deprivation amblyopia, which may be the long-term result of anisometropia (mismatch of the refractive state of the eyes) or due to inhibition of visual sensation, ie misuse

lazy leukocyte syndrome An idiopathic disease due to defective neutrophil chemotaxis after appropriate stimuli, eg endotoxin or epinephrine and inefficient egress of neutrophils from the bone marrow CLINICAL ↑ Pyogenic infections, including gingivitis, abscess formation and pneumonia, mild neutropenia PROGNOSIS Uncertain

LBP Lipopolysaccharide-binding protein, see there

LBW see Low birthweight

LC₅₀ Median lethal concentration, see there

LCA Leukocyte common antigen, see there

LCAM see Leukocyte cell adhesion molecule

LCR 1) Ligase chain reaction, see there 2) Locus control region, see there

LCAT Lecithin:cholesterol acyl transferase, see there

L cells 'Null' or non-T, non-B cells; variant lymphocytes with labile cell surface IgG and high-affinity Fc receptors, which unlike B cells, are resistant to trypsin digestion

LCM Lymphocytic choriomeningitis, see there

LCR Ligase chain reaction, see there

'LD$_6$' An extra lactate dehydrogenase (LD) band seen by electrophoresis in myocardial infarcts and in cardiogenic shock that migrates cathodally to LD$_5$; the LD$_6$ band is associated with a very poor prognosis, in one review 95 of 108 patients died shortly after the appearance of LD$_6$; see 'Kiss of death' tests, Lactate dehydrogenase

LD$_{50}$ Median lethal dose The radiation dose that is lethal to 50% of those exposed (2.5-6.0 Gy), assuming that optimal care, ie transfusions, trauma and nursing care, antibiotics and nutrition is available; given that a nuclear war would destroy hospitals and blood donors, drugs or food would not be available, a lower radiation exposure eg 1.5 Gy to the marrow and 2.2 Gy to the body would be lethal

LDH isoenzymes Lactate dehydrogenase, see there

LDL Low-density lipoprotein, see there

LDL-cholesterol Cholesterol carried by LDL which, when elevated, is a major risk factor for atherosclerosis; until 1993, the only way of determining LDL-cholesterol in the clinical laboratory was indirectly by the Friedenwald calculation‡, a situation that changed with commercial availability of the LDL-DIRECT™ produced by Genzyme Corp (CAP Today Nov 1994 p34)

LDRG Laboratory diagnosis-related groups; see Organ panels

LE-CAM Leukocyte-endothelial cell adhesion molecule; see Selectins

LE cell RHEUMATOLOGY A neutrophil characteristically seen in the synovium or peripheral blood in patients with lupus erythematosus; the cytoplasm is distended by a red-purple homogeneous or 'glassy' inclusion ('hematoxylin' body) with an eccentric nucleus, corresponding to phagocytosed deoxyribonucleoprotein (DNA-histone complex); LE cells are also seen in scleroderma, drug-induced lupus erythematosus and in lupoid hepatitis

hematoxylin bodies

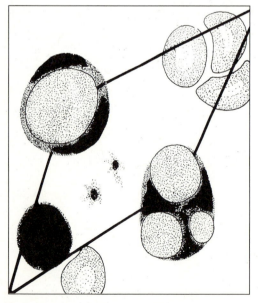

LE cells

LE cell 'prep' RHEUMATOLOGY A test in which heparinized blood is gently agitated with glass beads, releasing neutrophil nuclei which are then incubated with anti-nuclear protein in the serum; the 'glassy' appearance of LE bodies

results from homogenization of the chromatin; these bodies are then phagocytosed by the remaining neutrophils

lead *pronounced* Leed, similar to deed CARDIOLOGY Any of a number of specific sites for the placement of electrodes in electrocardiography (EKG); the standard 12-lead EKG includes three bipolar limb leads (I, II, III), three augmented unipolar limb leads (aV$_R$, aV$_L$ and aV$_F$) and six precordial leads (V$_1$-V$_6$); the EKG is calibrated so that a 1-mV potential results in a 1-cm deflection and the paper moves at 25 mm/sec

lead *pronounced* Lead, similar to dead CLINICAL TOXICOLOGY A heavy metal that paints a broad clinical palette EPIDEMIOLOGY Inorganic lead sources include gasoline, old paints, burning car batteries, 'moonshine' liquor distilled in tubing soldered with lead, foods and beverages served on Mexican ceramic or leaded crystal; lead in canned and packaged foods in the US derives from fossil fuels with lead additives (which were banned from motor vehicles but continue to be used in agriculture and thus find their way to crops, lead-bearing water and equipment in processing the foods and lead in the solder on canned products); lead levels in canned vegetables are 15–30-fold greater than levels in fresh-frozen vegetables (N Engl J Med 1991; 324:416c); drinking water (not soil, food, air, or paint chips) appears to be the main source of lead exposure, with concentrations of up to 160 μg/L (N Engl J Med 1993; 326:1361oA) see Port Pirie Cohort Study; serum levels above 25 mg/dl are considered excessive (MMWR 1991; 40193cr) levels that are considered toxic has dropped from 60 μg/dL (1969) to 10 μg/dL (1991); children with > 10 μg/dL has dropped from 88% in 1969 to 9%; 33% of African-American, 17% of Hispanic, and 6% of white children have levels > 10 μg/dL (New York Times 21 March, 1995, C3) peripheral blood reveals red cells with coarse basophilic stippling, anemia, reticulocytosis, erythroid hyperplasia, autofluorescence of erythrocytes and erythroid precursors CLINICAL Chronic poisoning is characterized by neuromuscular disease with wrist drop and encephalopathy (convulsions, mania, delirium), abdominal pain, Fanconi syndrome (aminoaciduria, glycosuria, fructosuria, phosphaturia) and occasionally protoporphyria-like symptoms PATHOLOGY Lead deposits may be seen in various tissue, eg renal tubules (figure, lead inclusions) and in erythrocytes, see Basophilic stippling TREATMENT Chelation, including dimercaprol, calcium EDTA, D-penicillamine and succimer; see Saturnine gout, Succimer

lead line A horizontal blue-black hyperpigmented line on the gingiva, due to chronic intoxication with lead, mercury or other heavy metal, often accompanied by intranuclear inclusions in renal tubular epithelium and radiodense 'lead lines' in the epiphysis of growing children

lead pipe rigidity A 'smooth' rigidity in flexion and extension that continues through the entire range of the stretching muscle, seen in atherosclerotic parkinsonism; virtually identical to Gegenhalten; Cf Garden hose

lead poisoning A generic term for any form of excess exposure to metallic lead, which may be acute or chronic; in the 1960s, blood levels of lead were considered dangerous if they were ≥ 60 μg/dL; public health officials are now believe that lead levels in children should be ≤ 10 μg/dL (Am Clin Lab September 1994)

Ancient Romans produced ± 60 000 tons of lead for use in vessels for food and drink, and to line aqueducts, and is thought to have been a major factor in the fall of the Roman Empire; nearly two millenia later, thousands of Napoleon's troops fell to lead poisoning related to its use in a major innovation of the era, food in cans ('tins') that were held together by lead-based solder

lead-time bias A bias introduced into a long-term study of the efficacy of a particular therapeutic maneuver, eg radio– or chemotherapy for malignancy; if the disease process is diagnosed early (due to newer or more sensitive diagnostic procedures or techniques), the maneuver is viewed as being effective, when in fact the patient survives 'longer' because his disease was diagnosed earlier (see **N Engl J Med 1994; 331:403c**) see Will Rogers effect

leader sequence MOLECULAR BIOLOGY An untranslated segment of RNA nucleotides located at the 5' end of mRNA preceding the AUG start codon that contains the 'Shine-Delgarno sequence', which pairs with 16S ribosomal RNA, assuring the proper alignment of the mRNA transcript to the ribosome prior to initiation of translation into a protein and may also contain regulatory elements

leading front technique IMMUNOLOGY A technique used to evaluate cell migration (chemotaxis), detecting the differences in the migration of stimulated and nonstimulated cells; the disadvantage is that it assumes that the fastest cells represent the majority of cells capable of migrating

leading strand Replication, see there

leaf appearance Ash leaf appearance, see there

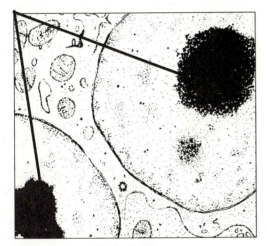

lead inclusions

leafless tree appearance RADIOLOGY The finding of multiple abrupt cut-offs of terminal bronchioles in an air bronchogram, fancifully likened to a leafless deciduous tree in winter; this sign was first described in bronchoalveolar carcinoma, but is relatively non-specific, as it has been seen in chronic bronchitis and bronchiectasis, and in the era of CT is a rarely evoked sign

leaflet PHYSIOLOGY One of the two layers of the phospholipid bilayer of the cell membrane; each sheet is characterized by a hydrophilic head that is oriented either to the exterior or interior of the cell and has hydrophobic residues that are 'buried' within the membrane itself; see Fluid mosaic model

leaky patch A focal ↑ in the permeability of the cell membrane produced by the transmembrane assembly of complement in the phospholipid bilayer, which allows free passage of water and ions; Cf Doughnut model

'leap-frog method' TRANSFUSION MEDICINE A technique for maximizing the amount of autologous blood available for elective surgery (table); because of the shelf life of red cells (up to 42 days), a practical maximum available by this method is four units

---

LEAP-FROG METHOD

WEEK 1 One unit 'A' of red cells is drawn

WEEK 2 One 'A' unit is re-infused-2 'B' units are drawn

WEEK 3 Two 'B' units are re-infused-3 'C' units are drawn

WEEK 4 Three 'C' units are re-infused-4 'D' units are drawn

'Lear complex' King Lear complex, see there

learned helplessness *pronounced* Lerned, similar to burned GERIATRIC MEDICINE A state of overdependency that is discordant with the degree of physical and mental disability seen in nursing homes PSYCHOLOGY A state of apathy or passiveness induced in experimental animals by either classical (respondent) or operant (instrumental) conditioning; the animal is subjected to aversive noxious stimuli, eg electric shock, which it can neither avoid nor escape; when the experimental conditions are changed and appropriate behavioral responses are effective in reducing or avoiding the noxious stimuli, the animal is seemingly too apathetic to attempt to learn the appropriate avoidance behaviors; learned helplessness has been proposed as a laboratory model for clinical depression

'learned profession' *pronounced* Lern–ed, similar to burn-bed BIOMEDICAL ETHICS A calling or vocation requiring specialized knowledge and often long and intense academic preparation; as such, a learned profession entails individual and group self-governance, service to the poor without expectation of compensation, deliverance of quality; high level of learning, autonomy of activity, self-sacrifice, altruism with threadbare nobility, heroism as needed and ethical practice with public accountability; learned professionals are historically distinguished from tradesmen and businessmen and include doctors, lawyers and clergy; according to E Pelligrino (**Kennedy Institute of Ethics**), a fundamental difference between a business and a profession is that '*at some point in a professional relationship, when a difficult decision must be made, the true professional can be relied upon to efface his own self-interest*'; the relationship of the professional with the poor is considered unique; service to the indigent is known as stewardship for the clergy and *pro bono publico* for lawyers

learning curve A negative (lower than expected) deviation in a desired or anticipated outcome or result that rises toward a norm as experience with the activity of interest increases; for heart transplantations, there is an institutional learning curve, where the mortality rate for the first five transplantations of 20% falls to 12% as experience increases; the improved outcomes are more related to the accrual of experience in management of rejection and infection, the domain of transplantation coordinators and cardiologists, than to increased technical skills in performing the procedure, as cardiovascular surgeons are already well-trained in most of the components of the transplantation procedure (**N Engl J Med 1992; 327:1220sa**)

learning disability PSYCHOLOGY A generic term for a suboptimal ability to read, write, perform mathematical operations or other cognitive skills in a child of presumed normal intelligence; ± 2.3 million school children in the US (population ± 250 million) are designated as LD; the formal study of LDs is hindered by a lack of consensus on case definition and on its pathogenesis, which some authors attribute to a deficit in phonological awareness, ie the ability to decode words into individual sound units (**Science 1995; 265:1896n&c**)

learning organization '*An organization skilled at creating, acquiring, and transferring knowledge, and at modifying its behavior to reflect new knowledge and insights*' (**Harv Bus Rev July/August 1993**) see High-power institution, Teaching hospital

least-squares regression STATISTICS A technique used to determine linearity; the dependent variable plotted on the y-axis is the test result (or data point), ie the instument reading; the independent variable plotted on the x-axis may correspond to known concentrations of a control material or may correspond to unitless numbers that reflect the relative concentrations of samples being tested

leather bottle stomach see Linitis plastica

lecithin-cholesterol acyl transferase An enzyme* [EC 2.3.1.43],the gene for which is located on chromosome segment 16q22; LCAT is secreted in the liver and catalyzes the reaction between phosphatidylcholine and a sterol (eg cholesterol), yielding 1-aylglycerophosphocholine (lysoleci-thin) and a steryl ester (eg cholesteryl ester), a critical step in the formation of lipoproteins; LCAT circulates in the plasma complexed with HDL, and is involved in reverse cholesterol transport

*Also known as phosphatidylcholine-sterol *O*-acyltransferase, the term recommended (1992) by the Nomenclature Committee of the IUBMB (International Union of Biochemistry and Molecular Biology) Note: LCAT and lipoprotein lipase are markedly ↓ in a-β–lipoproteinemia (Tangier's disease), resulting in a ↓ rate of cholesterol esterification due to relative lack of cholesterol, causing a pseudo-LCAT deficiency

lecithin-cholesterol acyl transferase deficiency syndrome An AR [MIM 245900] condition of adult onset characterized by corneal opacifications, proteinuria, renal insufficiency with hypertension, premature atherosclerosis, hemolytic anemia, obstructive jaundice and hepatic failure LABORATORY ↑ Ratio of free cholesterol to cholesteryl ester, variably ↑ phospholipids and triglycerides, and presence of lipoprotein X; see Fish eye disease

lecithin:sphingomyelin ratio L:S ratio, see there

lectin Any of a family of simple (ie non-immunogenic) carbohydrate-binding proteins and glycoproteins derived from plant seeds, mollusks and other animals that contain two or more binding sites for animal proteins; lectins are mitogenic and stimulate lymphocyte transformation, cell-cell recognition and agglutination of certain red cell antigens; in the blood bank, lectin specificity may be used to identify blood types (eg *Dolichus biflorus* binds A$_1$ RBCs *Ulex europaeus* reacts with H substance, and *Arachis hypogea* binds anti-T)

Note: Some cytokines, eg IL-1, IL-2, TNF have lectin- and/or carbohydrate-binding sites

lecturer An individual who is primarily (if not entirely) involved in the teaching activities of an academic center, who is not expected to perform research or patient management; in general, lectureships are non-tenured positions

leech *noun* A segmented annelid that evolved from earthworms and is found in either fresh water or soil in the tropics and subtropics; leeches have two suckers, a cranial sucker housing a mouth, the bite mark of which has been fancifully likened to the Mercedes-Benz emblem and a caudal sucker involved in crawling; the classic medicinal leech is *Hirudo medicinalis*, other leeches include *Poecilobdella, Dinobdella, Limnatis, Haemadipsa* and *Macrobdella*; the leech has recently reacquired a modicum of respect in the biomedical sciences; the simplicity of the its nervous system, it has only one neurotransmitter, serotonin, has made it a useful model for neurobiologist, and leech phlebotomy is undergoing a renaissance for 1) Removing excess blood from an operative field 2) Stimulating capillary ingrowth in reimplanted, traumatically amputated extremities and in plastic surgery 3) To obtain hirudin, a potent anticoagulant, and as yet poorly delineated substances in leech saliva that inhibit tumor spread Note: Not all leeches are so happily symbiotic; *Limnatis nilotica*, an aquatic leech of the Northern Hemisphere may be ingested with drinking water and attach to the oropharynx, nasal passage, larynx, and esophagus, causing anemia that may be fatal in children, asphyxia, local wounds, pruritus, hoarseness, dyspnea, hemoptysis, dysphagia and hematemesis; see Hirudin *verb* To treat with a leech, to let blood

Note: The leech has had a time-honored place in medicine and was used by Greek and Moor physicians; its use extended into the late 1700s, when bleeding was the standard of proper medical care; in one session, a leech can ingest up to 17 grams of blood and leeching was a practice that was instrumental in hastening the deaths of George Washington and Louis XIII

LEEP Loop extrasurgical excision procedure GYNECOLOGY A recently introduced therapeutic modality for treating cervical and vulvar lesions that uses a high-frequency, low-voltage, alternating current that minimizes thermal damage while preserving good hemostatic properties; LEEPs are most commonly used to treat condylomas and cervical intraepithelial neoplasia (CIN) and are particularly popular as they can be performed in an office setting with a lower equipement cost, minimal damage to surrounding tissue, and with low comorbidity; Cf Cone biopsy

Le Fort fractures TRAUMA SURGERY Any of three types of midfacial fractures (figure, below) which were defined by R Le Fort in 1901; in the Le Fort I (aka dentoalveolar dysjunction), the lines of fracture are transverse through the pyriform aperature above the alveolar ridge and pass posteriorly to the pterygoid region; the diagnosis is suggested by lip lacerations, patient complaints of malocclusion, and mobility of the fractures bone when the examiner moves the incisor teeth; in the Le Fort II (aka pyramidal fracture), the superior fracture lines are transverse through the nasal bone and/or maxillary articulation; the diagnosis is suggested by the free mobility of the anterior maxilla; in the Le Fort III (aka craniofacial dysjunction), the lines of fracture, the central third of the face is separated from the base of the skull; the diagnosis is suggested by 'big league' facial edema, ecchymosis, and facile mobility of the middle third of the face by the examiner; Le Fort III is the most severe of the midfacial fractures,

Le Fort fractures

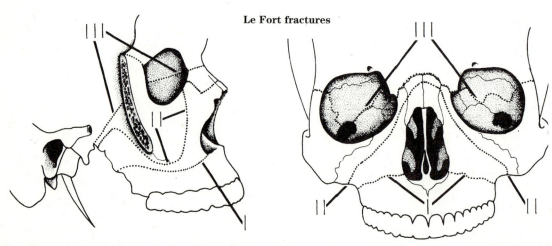

and may require both open reduction and internal fixation (GJ Jurkovich, CJ Carrico, in DC Sabiston, Ed, Textbook of Surgery, 14 th ed, WB Saunders, Philadelphia, 1991)

left axis deviation CARDIOLOGY Any shift in the pattern of the EKG leads; when seen in conjunction with a counter-clockwise loop abnormality in the frontal plane of the vector cardiogram, a left axis deviation is characteristic of the ostium primum type of partial atrioventricular canal defect

left-handed DNA An alternate secondary structure of DNA, which is the reverse of more common right-handed helical form (B-DNA); conformational microheterogeneity or 'left-handedness' is thought to play a role in regulation of major cell processes, including replication andrecombination, mutagenesis and carcinogenesis (and repair thereof), transcription, chromosomal organization and viral packaging; the sites where the right-handed DNA twists to become left handed DNA are mutagenic 'hot-spots' ; see DNA forms

Note: Z-DNA is a type of left-handed DNA, which has been the most extensively studied and is a term often used interchangeably with left-handed DNA

'left shift' CLINICAL CHEMISTRY see Neuroblastoma HEMATOLOGY An increase in the peripheral blood smear consisting of immature granulocytes with decreased nuclear segmentation, ie 'band' forms, due to increased production of the myeloid series in the marrow, caused by acute infection Note: 'right' shifts have not described, although hyperlobation of neutrophils seen in megaloblastic anemia might warrant this designation RESPIRATORY PHYSIOLOGY An ↑ in hemoglobin's affinity for oxygen (as represented by the oxygen dissociation curve), where the P_{50} is ↓ and shifted to the left, as occurs with ↑ pH (Bohr effect) or ↓ temperature; Cf Right shift

left-sided 'appendicitis' A colloquial term used to describe the clinical findings in acute diverticulitis with impending rupture, which is a mirror image mimic of (left-sided) appendicitis

left-sided colon see Malrotation

legal blindness A state defined in the United Kingdom as being '...*so blind as to be unable to perform work for which sight is required.*' (National Insurance Act, 1948), and in the US as 20/200 or less corrected distant visual acuity or 20 degrees or less of visual field

'legend' drug An obsolete term for 'Prescription' drug

Legionella A genus of small, fastidious, facultative intracytoplasmic gram-negative bacilli, comprised of more than 20 species, 14 of which have been implicated in human disease, including *L micdadii* (Pittsburgh pneumonia agent), *L anisa, L bozemanii, L dumoffi, L gormanii, L jordanis, L longbeachae, L oakridgensis, L rubrilucens,* and others; 12 of the 39 serotypes correspond to *L pneumophila* (Legionnaire's disease agent); *Legionella* species are aerobic, motile nonsaccharolytic bacilli, cultured with techniques usually reserved for *Rickettsia* species, ie within embryonal eggs or injection into guinea pigs; *Legionella* also grow on CYE (charcoal yeast extract) agar, supplemented with branched-chain fatty acids; chief energy source is amino acids; although they are gram negative, *Legionella* are best seen with certain stains, eg Gimenez, silver stains, and direct-fluorescent techniques; liposaccharide wall components function as endotoxin, hemolysin, and protease

Legionnaire's disease A dramatic epidemic that occurred in an American Foreign Legion convention in Philadelphia in 1976 (specifically caused by *Legionella pneumophila*); Legionnaire's disease is either sporadic or epidemic with a mortality of up to 15%; depending upon the population, *Legionella* species are thought to cause 1 to 27% of community acquired pneumonias; male:female ratio, 3:1 CLINICAL 2-10 day incubation, followed by an abrupt onset

of malaise, headache, myalgia, a dry initially non-productive, later productive cough; hemoptysis is relatively common; fever to 40°C, rigors are seen in most, associated with bradycardia; less commonly: nausea, diarrhea and confusion, delirium, septicemia, abscess formation, acute myocarditis and pericarditis and rhabdomyolysis RADIOLOGY Patchy interstitial infiltrate, often progressing to nodular condensations LABORATORY ↓ Na⁺, and phosphorus, ↑ liver enzymes, proteinuria, microscopic hematuria, relative leukocytosis (leukopenia is often associated with a poor prognosis) COMPLICATIONS Empyema, shock, DIC, renal failure, neurological sequelae, peripheral neuropathy PATHOLOGY Acute fibrinopurulent, necrotizing pneumonia with macrophages and neutrophils, diffuse alveolar damage and possibly permanent pulmonary fibrosis TREATMENT Erythromycin, T-S PREVENTION Chlorination, and UV irradiation of water supplies; Cf Pontiac disease

legless mutation see Transgenic mice

Leishmania tropica The causative agent of cutaneous leishmaniasis, which has been blamed for a miniepidemic of visceral leishmaniasis reported in a small cohort of veterans of Operation Desert Storm CLINICAL FUO, chronic fatigue, malaise, cough, intermittent diarrhea, abdominal pain, lymphadenopathy, and hepatosplenomegaly, which occurred as long as 7 months after their return to the US LABORATORY Determination of antibody titers by immunofluorescence, detection of amastigotes with an indirect immunofluorescent-monoclonal antibody assay, culture of parasites TREATMENT Sodium stibogluconate (N Engl J Med 1993; 328:1383OA)

LEL Lower explosive limit, see there

LEM Leukocyte endogenous mediator A polypeptide implicated in anemia of chronic disease, which is released by neutrophils and macrophages after stimulation by bacterial toxins

Lemierre's disease Postanginal sepsis

lemon sign OBSTETRICS An ultrasonographic finding seen when a major neural tube defect accompanies the Arnold-Chiari malformation, with herniation of the cerebellar tonsils and midbrain structures into the foramen magnum, causing ventriculomegaly due to compression of the outflow from the third and fourth ventricles; downward traction of the brain causes a reduction in the anterior calvarium, in turn resulting in a triangular-shaped head in the biparietal diameter, fancifully likened to a lemon

Lennert's lymphoma Malignant lymphoma with high content of epithelioid cells A diffuse mixed cell NHL with a large number of benign epithelioid histiocytes (Virch Arch Path Anat 1968; 344:1) that affects older patients CLINICAL Generalized lymphadenopathy, hepatosplenomegaly and 'B' symptoms (fever, night sweats and weight loss), which is often first seen in stage III or IV; see Lymphoma, Working classification; Cf Progressive transformation of germinal centers

Note: The very existence of Lennert's lymphoma was controversial (Cancer 1980; 45:1379), as many of the original cases were later reclassified as Hodgkin's, non-Hodgkin's and immunoblastic lymphomas, as well as histiocytosis X

Lennox-Gastaut syndrome A severe encephalopathic form of epilepsy that constitutes 5% of all childhood epilepsies; it is characterized by an early onset of multiple types (eg absence, atonic, and others) of seizures, slow spike-wave EEG pattern, cerebral atrophy, and mental retardation that is frequently progressive; the seizures are poorly controlled even with multiple anticonvulsant agents; the prognosis for cognitive development is poor; felbamate, an investigational antiepileptic drug is reported to decrease the symptoms of L-G syndrome (N Engl J Med 1993; 328:29OA) see Felbamate

lentigo Freckle A pigmented, flat or slightly elevated macule, with increased melanin, melanocytic hyperplasia, epidermal pigmentation and elongation of the rete ridges **LENTIGO MALIGNA** (Hutchinson's freckle) A pre-melanoma located on sun-exposed aging skin that begins life as an unevenly pigmented macule with an irregular border, which slowly extends peripherally, ⅓ of which progress to melanoma, the transition may require 10-15 years **LENTIGO SENILIS** A pigmented red-brown macular lesion, often multiple, affecting sun-exposed skin, often seen in caucasians, closely mimicking seborrheic keratosis, both of which have been referred to as 'liver spots' and are of merely cosmetic concern **LENTIGO SIMPLEX** A clinical mimic of junctional nevus that has three forms: lentiginosis profusa, mutiple lentigines syndrome (see Leopard syndrome) and speckled lentiginous nevus

Lentiviridae A subfamily of retroviruses first recognized 50 years ago in epidemic pulmonary (maedi) and CNS (visna) infections of sheep in Iceland; lentiviruses are 'slow infections' with prolonged incubation periods, remaining within the host macrophages, disseminating by a 'Trojan horse mechanism' (see there), often persisting in the CNS, where one of the most common manifestations of lentivirus infection is neurologic deterioration; other RNA lentiviruses include HIV, bovine immunodeficiency virus, feline lymphotropic virus (FTLV), simian lymphotropic virus (STLV) and others; see HIV, Retroviruses, STLV; Cf Prions

leonine facies A deeply furrowed 'lumpy' face with prominent superciliary arches, classically seen in lepromatous lepra; a similar facial deformity may occur in hyperimmunoglobulin E syndrome (Job syndrome), chronic granulomatous disease, van Buchem's disease, leontiasis ossium (idiopathic leonine facies); the features may be due to overgrowth of bones, as in Paget's disease or McCune-Albright syndrome, polyostotic fibrous dysplasia or soft tissue, as in hypothyroidism with myxedema of periorbital tissues, epidermoid carcinoma, Sézary syndrome, which is characterized by generalized exfoliative dermatitis, edema, erythema, pachydermia and palmoplantar keratoderma

leopard skin Focal macular hyperpigmentation of the skin in a hypopigmented background, accompanied by scaling, seen in infection by *Onchocerca volvulus*

'leopard spotting' A fanciful descriptor for the postmortem, non-inflammatory and geographic brown-black mottling seen in esophagomalacia due to superficial mucosal autolysis, the result of acid digestion of hemoglobin, seen when the gastric juices flow onto the esophageal mucosa

leopard syndrome Multiple lentigines syndrome An AD [MIM 151100] condition with thousands of 1–5-mm darkly pigmented macules on the skin but on the mucosal surfaces CLINICAL characterized by the mnemonic acronym LEOPARD, for Lentigines, Electrocardiographic (EKG) disturbances, Ocular hypertelorism, Pulmonary stenosis, Abnormalities of genitalia (gonadal or ovarian hypoplasia), Retarded growth and neural Deafness

lepra cells Foamy macrophages replete with clumps (known as 'globi') of *Mycobacterium lepra*; the macrophages are unable to digest the bacteria due to the loss of cell-mediated immunity, typical of lepromatous leprosy; lepra cells are distinctly less common in borderline leprosy and never seen in the tuberculous leprosy; see Intracellular pathogens

leprechaunism Donohue syndrome An AR [MIM 246200] polydysmorphic complex with parental consanguinity that is more common in ♀ (↑ ♂ fetal wastage in utero) and characterized by a coarse gnome-like face with a saddle nose, broad mouth, large, low-set ears, hirsutism, cutis laxa, atrophy of subcutaneous adipose tissue, dwarfism, extreme wasting, mental retardation, dysphagia, enlarged

nipples, breasts, clitoris, penis, kidneys, pancreatic islets and ovaries (with premature follicular maturation), hepatic nodules, insulin receptor dysfunction and early death

lepromin A heat-killed extract of *Mycobacterium lepra* skin nodules that is injected intradermally ('lepra test') and evokes granuloma formation in 3-4 weeks in normal subjects and in those with borderline and tuberculous leprosy, but not in subjects with anergy and lepromatous lepra

leptocyte *leptos*, Greek, thin A wafer-thin erythrocyte with peripheral marginated hemoglobin, which is seen in thalassemia and obstructive liver disease, as well as in iron-deficiency anemia and chronic inflammation

Leptophaeria A genus of fungi causing maduromycosis

Leptopsylla A genus of rodent fleas of the family Leptosyllidae that are a vector of the plague

Leptospira A genus of coiled aerobic spirochetes that belong to the Spirochaetaceae family, which are diagnosed with difficulty (darkfield microscopy and Giemsa stains are unreliable), and cultured on Fletcher and Stuart media, intraperitoneal inoculation of blood or urine into guinea pigs or hamsters, serologically rising titers are most commonly due to *L interrogans* (formerly *L icterohemorrhagiae*) after ingestion of water contaminated with infected livestock or rat urine

LES Lower esophageal sphincter, see there

lesbianism Female homosexuality A sexual preference and/or behavior that is is far less studied from a medical standpoint than the male counterpart; the scanty data available indicates that there is no increased incidence of enteric or other sexually transmitted disease, possibly due to a combination of relative monogamy and sexual practices; see Homosexuality; Cf Sexual reassignment, Transexuality

Lesch-Nyhan syndrome An X-R [MIM 308000] condition caused by a deficiency of 24 kD hypoxanthine-guanine phosphoribosyl transferase* [EC 2.4.2.8], resulting in an accumulation of uric acid crystals in the renal pelvis and bladder, pseudogouty arthritis, erosive changes of fingertips, accompanied by compulsive self-mutilation, choreoathetosis, mental retardation LABORATORY ↑ Oxypurines, hypoxanthine and xanthine in cerebrospinal fluid due to purine overload

*Note: The first transgenic mouse was 'engineered' to be deficient in HGPRT; recently embryonal stem cells without the enzyme were introduced into mouse fibroblast females to produce germline chimeras

'lesionectomy' NEUROSURGERY A colloquial term referring to stereotactic resection of poorly-circumscribed intraaxial (a region often considered inoperable) brain masses including vascular malformations and glial neoplasms, identified by magnetic resonance imaging that may be associated with epileptiform seizure activity; Cf Lumpectomy

let-down reflex OBSTETRICS A physiological response occurring in puerperium that evoked by sucking (or negative mechanical pressure) on the female nipple or by psychological stimuli, causing the release ('let-down') of breast milk in a nursing mother; the reflex is due to myoepithelial cell contraction of the alveolar glands elicited by oxytocin and may be lost if the mother is under stress or fatigue, resulting in milk retention

lethal agranulocytosis IMMUNOLOGY Infantile genetic agranulocytosis, see there

lethal dose A dose of a toxin, virus or any substance that is lethal to all the members of a species within a specified or well-defined time period'; see Poisons

lethal equivalent The sum of 'semilethal' genes (lethal genes present in the heterozygous state, and therefore clinically silent); three to five lethal equivalents are thought to be present in all individuals

lethal gene A mutant gene which, when autosomal dominant, is invariably lethal; when an gene is lethal only when in the homozygous state, the heterozygous state is 'semi-lethal'

lethal hit A critical event caused by an ionizing particle that inactivates a virus or impacts on a genome, resulting in death; Cf 'One-hit, two-hit' model

lethal midline granuloma A condition that is confusing to those who read about it and often to those who write about it; LMD is best considered a clinical syndrome rather than a specific histological entity, consisting of a destructive lesion of the upper respiratory tract (nose, nasopharynx, palate and midface), and is either idiopathic or secondary to

WEGENER'S GRANULOMATOSIS, an ulcerating, necrotizing and osteolytic lesion of the upper respiratory tract and lungs, defined as having systemic necrotizing vasculitis, a ♂:♀ ratio 2:1, hemoptysis, fever, rash, prostration, arthritis, neuropathy, splenomegaly, and progressive glomerulonephritis ending in terminal renal failure

LYMPHOMA of the region, including large cell lymphomas, eg T cell lymphoma or

MALIGNANT HISTIOCYTOSIS, see there; see Idiopathic midline destructive disease, Midline granuloma

lethal mutation Any mutation of a genome, including frameshift mutation, deletion, insertion and others that leads to the premature death of the host

letter E sign E sign, see there

Letterer-Siwe disease A clinical form of Langerhans' cell histiocytosis (histiocytosis X) characterized by an onset in infancy of fever, erythematous eczematoid rash, lymphadenopathy, hepatosplenomegaly, anemia, and death; the histiocytoses X are no longer considered to be reactive but rather clonal neoplasms (N Engl J Med 1994; 331:154OA) see Langerhans' cell histiocytosis

Note: A unifying term that connotes both the interrelation of the various histiocytoses, while recognizing their specificity, eg Langerhans' cell histiocytosis-Letterer-Siwe type represents a viable alternative

leu-CAM Leukocyte-cell adhesion molecules; see CD11/CD18 family

leucine aminopeptidase Leucyl aminopeptidase A zinc-linked enzyme [EC 3.4.11.1] that hydrolyzes N-terminal peptides, especially aliphatic amino acids; it is abundant in the cytosol, most active in the duodenum, liver, and kidney, and ↑ in bile duct obstruction, pancreatitis, pancreatic carcinoma, hepatopathies, and infectious mononucleosis

leucine-rich repeat A recently characterized structural motif that is important in moleculaar recognition processes as diverse as cell adhesion, cell development, DNA repair, RNA processing, and signal transduction; LRRs alternate between 28 and 29 residues in length structural β-α hairpin units, with the β-strand and α-helix being nearly parallel, and the units are nearly parallel to a common axis; the resulting structure has a non-globular horseshoe-like shape, the concave face of which is exposed to the solvent (Nature 1995; 374:177; 1993; 366:751)

leucine zipper MOLECULAR BIOLOGY A structural motif (figure) found in oncogenic proteins and in some DNA-binding proteins consisting of a sequence of approximately 40 amino acids composed of regularly spaced hydrophobic amino acids (leucine) arranged in an α-helix; the LZ contains a periodic array of 4 or 5 leucine residues at every seventh amino acid position ('heptad spacing') along the enhancer regulator protein, over a distance of 8 helical turns (of the DNA); the LZ promotes homo- or heterodimerization through hydrophobic interaction between arrays of leucine residues on participating zippers, intertwined as coiled coils; dimerization through a zipper interaction is a prerequisite for sequence-specific DNA-binding

of oncogenic transforming proteins (Fos, Jun, Myc) and enhancing or regulating transcription factors (C/ERP, CREB, GCN4) and the zipper is required for cell transformation and regulation ; Cf DNA-binding motifs

leucovorin 'rescue' ONCOLOGY A therapeutic modality used to prevent excess 'collateral damage' to normal cells when treating patients with methotrexate (Mtx), an antimetabolic chemotherapeutic agent used to treat lymphoproliferative disorders and other malignancies, causing potentially severe myelosuppression and gastrointestinal symptoms; leukovorin (reduced folate) is a direct Mtx antagonist, and is administered immediately after chemotherapy, 'rescuing' the normal cells; up to 1500 mg/m^2 of Mtx may be given in one session, if it is followed by leucovorin 15-50 mg/m^2 qid x 48 hours, a classic leucovorin 'rescue' protocol, a dose that must be ↑ in the face of renal dysfunction, due to delayed elimination of Mtx

leukapheresis TRANSFUSION MEDICINE A technique that removes circulating white cells (eg activated B and T lymphocytes) from the peripheral circulation of either 1) Healthy subjects to pool and transfuse the cells to immunocompromised and leukopenic patients, which may be effective in short-term therapy of acute infections; long-term, patients become either immunized against the donor antigens or infected with virulent organisms; 10^{10} granulocytes are needed for adequate 'coverage' against infections; to maximize the harvest, the donor receives corticosteroids, or 2) Patients with leukemia in whom excess cells compromise normal circulation and is indicated to temporarily relieve the symptoms of hyperleukemia in excess of $100 \times 10^9/L$; in a typical procedure, ± 6 liters of whole blood are processed with the intent of removing $5-10 \times 10^9$ Note: Leukapheresis for removing lymphocytes (and by extension, the offending lymphokines) does not improve the clinical outcome of idiopathic inflammatory myopathies, eg dermatomyositis, or polymyositis (N Engl J Med 1992; 326:1380OA) Cf Cytapheresis, Hemapheresis

leukemia A relatively uncommon (incidence, US $3.5/10^5$ per year) malignant clonal expansion of myeloid or lymphoid cells that is characterized by an ↑ in circulating leukocytes, which is often first diagnosed either as an incidental finding when evaluating an unrelated clinical problem, or when the expansion compromises BM production of one or more cell lines causing anemia, thrombocytopenia or granulocytopenia; leukemias are divided by chronology (acute or chronic), by cell lineage (lymphoid, myeloid, monocytic or megakaryocytic) and subdivided by stage of maturation or cell size; see FAB classification CLINICAL BM infiltration by leukemic cells, causing anemia, thrombocytopenia, granulocytopenia, immune paralysis, ↓ B cells and helper T cells, ↑ suppressor T cells, infiltration and leukostasis, cranial nerve palsies, meningitis, lymphadenopathy, hepatosplenomegaly, testicular and cutaneous involvement, metabolic derangements, eg ↑ calcium, potassium, lactate dehydrogenase, ammonia, weight loss, less commonly, autoimmune hemolytic anemia, pallor and arthralgia

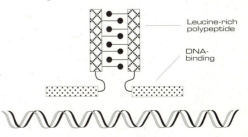

leucine zipper

RISK GROUPS, LEUKEMIA

LYMPHOCYTIC LEUKEMIA

HEMATOLOGIC DISEASE Idiopathic thrombocytopenia, paroxysmal nocturnal hemoglobinuria, refractory sideroblastic anemia, polycythemia vera

MALIGNANCY, eg carcinoma of the breast or ovary, Hodgkin's disease, multiple myeloma

CONGENITAL PREDISPOSITION Twin of leukemic patient, underlying congenital genetic predisposing condition, eg ataxia-telangiectasia, Fanconi's anemia, osteogenesis imperfecta, von Recklinghausen's disease, and syndromes, eg Bloom, Down, fragile X, Klinefelter, and Wiskott-Aldrich

RADIATION EXPOSURE Radiologists, (possibly children of nuclear power plant workers, see Sellafield) or other radiation exposure, see Chernobyl and Goiana

IMMUNOSUPPRESSIVE THERAPY Alkylating agents in chemotherapy for malignancy

TOXIC EXPOSURE Chronic benzene exposure and chloramphenicol, see Secondary malignancy

MYELOID LEUKEMIA

EXPOSURE TO IONIZING RADIATION and in those with HLA-Cw3 and HLA-Cw4; unlike ALL, other genetic factors and exposure to chemotherapeutics or chemicals do not play a major role

CONGENITAL LEUKEMIA Extremely rare (usually myeloid)

ACUTE LEUKEMIA is more common in children, 80% of which are ALL, often occurring before age 10, with a peak between ages 3 to 7 in whites, $\male:\female$ ratio, 1.3:1 Cell types Early pre-B cell 67%; pre-B cell 18%; B cell 1%; T cell 14%; 50-85% are cALLA positive (common acute lymphocytic leukemia antigen, CD10); 5% have Philadelphia chromosome CLINICAL ALL is more abrupt than AML, with petechial hemorrhage, bone and abdominal pain, headache and vomiting due to ↑ intracranial pressure, lymphadenopathy, splenomegaly and hepatomegaly LABORATORY 70% have ↓ lymphocytosis (less $< 20 \times 10^9$) at the time of diagnosis TREATMENT Protocols vary according to standard- or high-risk clinical features, and may include BM transplantation PROGNOSIS Table

CHRONIC LEUKEMIA usually affects adults and older children and is often myelogenous; CML is Philadelphia chromosome positive and may occur < age 5 with myelomonocytosis, anemia, thrombocytopenia, lymphadenopathy; WBC count is $< 50 \times 10^9$, ↑ hemoglobin F, ↑ muraminidase; adult CML comprises 20% of all leukemias CLINICAL Gradual onset of fatigability, anorexia, splenomegaly; lymphadenopathy is uncommon LABORATORY $> 25 \times 10^9/L$ leukemic cells in blood (often with an absolute lymphocytosis of $> 15 \times 10^{10}/L$, < 10% blasts in bone marrow, myeloid:erythroid ratio is 10-30:1, 90% of cases have low-to-absent leukocyte alkaline phosphatase and rarely also, ↑ vitamin B_{12} and B_{12}-binding capacity TREATMENT see

Chemotherapy, Induction PROGNOSIS see Remission

leukemia, chemotherapy-induced A leukemia that is etiologically linked to the previous use of chemotherapeutic agents to treat a malignancy; most commonly inculpated are the alkylating agents, which induce acute nonlymphocytic leukemia (ANLL), often accompanied by mutations of chromosomes 5 and 7; 15 years after chemotherapy-treated Hodgkin's disease, the risk of leukemia is from 5-11% (versus 0.9% when radiotherapy alone is used), ANLL may follow chemotherapy for non-Hodgkin's lymphoma, polycythemia vera, multiple myeloma, breast and ovarian carcinoma, or use of these agents for certain recalcitrant non-neoplastic diseases eg multiple sclerosis, rheumatoid arthritis and Wegener's granulomatosis; see Secondary malignancy

leukemia inhibitory factor A 179-amino acid monomer produced by T cells, Mo/Mas, fibroblasts, stromal cells of the bone marrow, and astrocytes; LIF potentiates IL-3-dependent proliferation of hematopoietic precursors and maintains the pluripotent phenotype of hematopoietic stem cells; LIF is synergistic with and has overlapping functions with IL-6, IL-10, and oncostatin M

*Synonyms include CNDF, DIA, differentiating stimulating factor, differentiation inducing factor, DRF, HILDA, HSF III, MLPLI

leukemic coagulopathy A variant presentation of leukemia, which is accompanied by hemorrhagic diathesis resulting from 1) Abnormalities related to the leukemia

---

PROGNOSISTIC FEATURES, LEUKEMIA

ACUTE LYMPHOCYTIC LEUKEMIA

Good prognostic features Ages 2-10, CD10 positivity, hyperdiploid karyotype

Poor prognostic features Ages < than 2 or > than 10, B-cell phenotype, especially the L2 phenotype by the FAB classification, presence of chromosomal translocations, central nervous system involvement, mediastinal masses and a high initial white cell count

ACUTE MYELOID LEUKEMIA

Good prognostic features, Young age, presence of Auer rods, short time required to objective therapeutic response

Poor prognosis features Older age, prior malignancy, prior therapy, multiple chromosomal defects

---

per se, eg BM infiltration, dysmorphic megakaryocytes, decreased platelet lifespan, qualitative platelet defects (decreased platelet aggregation with ATP and collagen stimulation or defects in ADP release) and DIC due to sepsis or transfusion reactions and coagulopathy due to leukemic therapy 2) BM toxicity due to combination

patterns of leukemia in BM

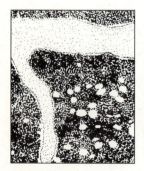

diffuse

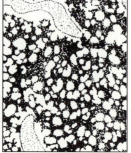

interstitial

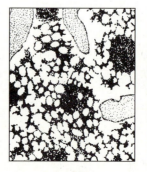

nodular

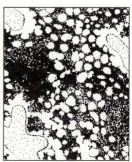

mixed

chemotherapy that may ↓ fibrinogen, factors IX, XI, plasminogen, antithrombin III, ↑ factor V, uric acid nephropathy (due to massive cytolysis of malignant cells), vitamin K deficiency (treatment of infections due to granulocytopenia, reduces the vitamin K-producing intestinal bacteria) and heparin anticoagulation

leukemogenesis A process in which successive transformational events enhance the ability of hematopoietic progenitor cells to proliferate, differentiate, and survive (see N Engl J Med 1993; 328:614oa) see Autonomous proliferation

leukemoid reaction An abnormal polyclonal proliferation of leukocytes, defined as greater than 25 x 10⁹/L; leukemoid reactions reflect a normal marrow response to trauma, stress, metabolic disease, drugs, inflammation, connective tissue disease or malignancy, resulting from secretion of colony-stimulating factor and they are often associated with immaturity of other cell lines; in contrast to leukemia, LRs almost invariably have leukocyte counts of < than 50 x 10⁹/L; often only the granulocytes are ↑ without marked basophilia or eosinophilia LABORATORY ↑ Leukocyte alkaline phosphatase, which is ↓ or absent in leukemia, 'left shift' of myeloid cells (↑ bands, metamyelocytes, myelocytes), plasma cells and plasmacytoid lymphocytes, toxic granulation, Döhle inclusion bodies, vacuolization (which implies intracellular bacterial phagocytosis) **PHYSIOLOGICAL LEUKOCYTOSIS** may be idiopathic or hereditary, neonatal, induced by heat or solar irradiation, diurnal, ↑ in the afternoon, related to stress, eg pain, nausea, vomiting, anxiety, womanhood (↑ during ovulation and near term, ↑↑↑ during labor), ether anesthesia, increased adrenalin, convulsions, paroxysmal tachycardia, pain, nausea, vomiting, anoxia, exercise and convulsions **PATHOLOGICAL LEUKOCYTOSIS** may be related to infections, often bacterial, inflammation, severe burns, post-operative, myocardial infarct, strangulated hernias, intestinal obstruction, gouty attacks, acute glomerulonephritis, serum sickness, rheumatic fever, immune disorders and connective tissue diseases, metabolism (ketoacidosis, uremia, eclampsia), heavy metals (lead, mercury), petrochemicals (benzene, turpentine), drugs (phenacetin, digitalis), black widow spider venom, endotoxin or toxoid injection, Jarisch-Herxheimer reaction, hemorrhage (often into cranial cavity), serosal surfaces (pleural pericardium and peritoneum) or acute hemolysis, malignancy (gastrointestinal tract or hematopoietic) and Cushing syndrome

leukocidin An exotoxin produced by pathogenic staphylococci and streptococci, which induces a profound, albeit transient neutrophilia; leukocidin destroys neutrophils by inserting pores in the membranes of the enzyme-filled lysosomes

leukocyte adhesion deficiency syndrome LFA-1 immunodeficiency syndrome A co-dominant or AR [MIM 116920], often consanguineous immune deficiency due to a defect in lymphocyte function-associated antigen (LFA-1); LFA-1 is a 95 kD β chain that is normally linked by covalent bonds to the CD11a molecule, which facilitates NK binding, cytolytic T-cell mediated killing and helper T cell response CLINICAL Inflammation, delayed separation of the umbilical cord, recurrent pyogenic mucocutaneous infections, pneumonia* and poor wound healing due to abnormal cell adherence, chemotaxis and a reduced respiratory burst; the condition is linked to defects in the integrin family of leukocyte adhesive proteins, aka CD11/CD18 family, specifically in the gene encoding the CD18 protein, located on chromosome segment 21q22.1-qter; a genetically engineered retrovirus with this gene has been successfully inserted into a LADS patient cells and may eventually be inserted into patient stem cells; see CD11, CD18, Leu-CAM

*Recurring staphylococcal or *Pseudomonas* bacteremia

leukocyte alkaline phosphatase Neutrophil alkaline phosphatase A phosphomonoesterase [EC 3.1.3.1] with optimal activity at pH 10.0 that is concentrated in granules of normal neutrophils; LAP is ↓ in CML, paroxysmal nocturnal hemoglobinuria, ITP, infectious mononucleosis and aplastic anemia; LAP is ↑ in CML in remission, polycythemia vera, Hodgkin's disease, myeloid metaplasia, corticosteroid therapy and pregnancy

leukocyte common antigen CD45 A single-chain glycoprotein with five different 180–220-kD forms arising from alternative mRNA splicing; because LCA is present on the membranes of all leukocytes (B and T cells, monocytes, macrophages, and granulocytes), it has been used as an immunoperoxidase marker for differentiating between poorly differentiated carcinoma, which is often positive with antibodies to cytokeratin and/or epithelial membrane antigen and the LCA-positive lymphomas; see CD45

leukocyte depletion0 Leukoreduction, see there

leukocyte inhibitory factor A heat-stable 68-kD protein produced by sensitized lymphocytes that immobilizes neutrophils during early inflammation

leukocyte reduction TRANSFUSION MEDICINE Leukocyte depletion Any of a number of techniques that substantially reduce the number of leukocytes in transfused blood products, eg red cells and platelets; LR to < 5 x 10⁸ virtually eliminates nonhemolytic (immunologic) transfusion reactions*; more stringent LR, eg < 5 x 10⁶ is required to prevent the transmission of leukocyte-associated infections (eg CMV, EBV, HTLV-1) or prevent alloimmunization and refractoriness to platelet therapy (30-50% of those receiving chronic platelet transfusion eventually become refractory to therapy) METHODS The traditional freeze-and-wash method has given way to various types of filters, and a proprietary leukocyte trapping system; for platelets, prestorage leukocyte reduction appears to be the most effect method INDICATIONS FOR LR Prevention of recurrent nonhemolytic febrile transfusion reactions to RBCs, prevention or delaying of alloimmunization to leukocyte antigens, prevention of CMV infection (Arch Pathol Lab Med 1994; 118:350RV, ibid 118:392oa) see Blood filters, Transfusion effect

leukocytoclastic vasculitis Cutaneous necrotizing vasculitis A type III hypersensitivity reaction in which antigen-antibody complexes are deposited in the walls of venules, evoking complement-dependent infiltration by neutrophils which release proteolytic enzymes; LV is less a disease a sui generis than it is a finding seen in various clinical settings, including antigen-induced serum sickness, drug-related hypersensitivity reactions, connective-tissue disease (SLE, rheumatoid arthritis, Sjögren syndrome), infection (bacterial sepsis, candidiasis, hepatitis C, herpes simplex), in patients with circulating immune complexes (Henoch-Schönlein purpura, mixed cryoglobulinemia, Waldenström's macroglobulinemia), and more recently associated with staphylococcal protein A column therapy (N Engl J Med 1994; 331:792cpc)

leukocytosis Any leukocyte count > 11 x 10⁹/L (US: 11 000/mm³), benign or malignant; see Leukemoid reaction, Leukemia

leukodystrophy NEUROPATHOLOGY A heterogeneous group of disorders (see table, page 484) of myelin or its metabolism (eg Krabbe's disease, metachromatic leukodystrophy, 'sphingolipidoses') that share certain pathological features, eg global distribution, bilateral and symmetrical myelin degeneration, relative sparing of arcuate fibers, and eventually, segmental peripheral nerve degeneration CLINICAL 'White matter disease', ie predominantly motor, dominated by progressive paralysis and ataxia rather than dementia

Note: The concept of leukodystrophy was introduced in 1887 by Heubner, expounded upon in 1912 by Schilder, and confused by everyone since then, including Schilder himself, who included under the rubric of leukodystrophy (which he called 'encephalitis periaxialis diffusa'), such diverse conditions as multiple sclerosis, inflammation-induced demyelinization, and hereditary defects of myelin metabolism, the group that comprises the current leukodystrophies, which are separated based on differences in clinical presentation, histopathology and defective enzymes

LEUKODYSTROPHIES

I KRABBE'S DISEASE Globoid cell leukodystrophy A AR [MIM 245200] condition of early (age 4-6 months) onset due to galacto-cerebrosidase deficiency CLINICAL Progressive spastic weakness of extremities, hyperkinesis, tonic fits, hyperkinesia, tonic seizures, dysphagia, polyneuropathy PATHOLOGY Abundant globoid cells in the demyelinated areas; see Globoid cells

II METACHROMATIC LEUKODYSTROPHY An AR [MIM 250100] form of progressive cerebral leukodystrophy of infant to adult onset which is due to sulfatase deficiency and characterized by metachromasia of the demyelinated tissue CLINICAL If the involvement is mild, it may be completely symptomatic

III X-LINKED LEUKODYSTROPHY

a) With adrenal involvement (adrenoleukodystrophy) due to a defective peroxisomal fatty acid oxidation system and accumulation of very long chain fatty acids or
b) Without adrenal involvement (Pelizaeus Merzbacher disease) An X-R [MIM 312080] condition caused by a unknown defect with accumulation of proteolipid protein (aka lipophilin) CLINICAL Early onset, head tremor, nystagmus, athetosis, followed by ataxia, intention tremor, nystagmus, slowed speech, progressive spastic paralysis, initially hyperreflexia, later hyporeflexia

IV OTHERS Leukodystrophies that cannot be further classified are 'lumped' together as 'unclassified leukodystrophy', or sudanophilic leukodystrophy

leukoedema Edema of the oral mucosa of undetermined significance that may clinically mimic early leukoplakia, an often premalignant condition, characterized by acanthosis, intracellular edema and superficial parakeratosis

leukoencephalopathy Progressive multifocal leukoencephalopathy, see there

leukoerythroblastic reaction An ↑ in the peripheral blood of immature RBCs, ie normoblasts, and immature leukocytes, metamyelocytes and bands, which may be associated with metastatic cancer, hematopoietic malignancy, hemolytic anemia, Gaucher's disease, polytraumatized patients, BM infiltration by various processes, including infection (eg fungal, viral, TB), sarcoidosis, histiocytosis, hypoxia; ⅓ of patients with LE have no known underlying disease; Cf Leukemoid reaction

leukokinin Tuftsin, see there

leukoplakia A white patch or plaque seen by gross examination of mucosae characterized by epithelial hyperplasia and keratosis, and clinical diagnosis of chronic irritation; leukoplakia affects the mucosa of oral cavity and upper respiratory tract, vulva and uterine cervix and renal pelvis and urinary bladder; in each site the significance is different ORAL CAVITY Leukoplakia is often tobacco-induced (either smoked or chewed) and is regarded as a premalignant lesion, especially in pipe smokers, 15-20% of which are dysplastic, carcinoma-in-situ or frankly invasive carcinomas at initial evaluation and 15-20% of remainder develop cancer within 10 years of follow-up; other 'white patch' lesions of the oral cavity include lichen planus, syphilis, candidiasis, SLE, chemical burns, alcohol, endocrine dysfunction, ↓ vitamin A, and ↓ vitamin B complex EXTERNAL FEMALE GENITAL Leukoplakia is not per se premalignant, although intraepithelial neoplasia (Bowen's disease, carcinoma-in-situ) and invasive squamous cell carcinoma may produce 'white patches', as does lichen sclerosis UTERINE CERVIX Leukoplakia usually corresponds to hyper-or para-keratosis and may be seen with in-situ or invasive cervical carcinoma as a coincidental finding PROGNOSIS Oral leukoplakia (histologically diagnosed as dysplasia) transforms into cancer in 11 to 36% (depending on the length of followup) TREATMENT Localized lesions—surgical removal, laser ablation; multiple ('field') lesions—high-dose induction and low-dose maintenance with isotretinoin (N Engl J Med 1993; 328:15oA)

*Alloimmunization related to HLA-mismatch and leukocyte antigens (febrile reactions, anti-platelet antibodies, transplant rejection), acute lung injury, GVHD, and immune modulation (Arch Pathol Lab Med 1994; 118:350rv)

leukoreduction Leukocyte reduction, see there

leukorrhea GYNECOLOGY A nonspecific whitish malodorous vaginal discharge accompanied by dyspareunia and intense pruritus, which may be induced by infection, eg *Candida albicans, Gardnerella vaginalis, Trichomonas vaginalis, Neisseria gonorrhoeae*, foreign body-related infections, estrogen depletion, neoplasms and as a postpartum phenomenon

leukotrienes A family of low-weight, biologically active molecules that mediate the inflammatory reaction, which are produced by leukocytes, macrophages, mast and other cells in response to immunologic and non-immunological stimuli; leukotrienes are synthesized by 5-lipoxygenase-induced oxidation of arachidonic acid at C-5, which is subsequently transformed into an unstable epoxide intermediate LTA_4, followed by either hydration to LTB_4 or addition of glutathione to form LTC_4 (elimination of a γ-glutamyl residue yields LTD_4; further removal of a glycine yields LTE_4); LTA_4 is produced in the asthmatic lung, in neutrophils and mast cells, causing smooth muscle contraction and bronchoconstriction; LTB_4 is produced by neutrophils, causing adhesion and chemotaxis, stimulating neutrophil aggregation, enzyme release and superoxide generation within neutrophils; LTC_4, LTD_4, LTE_4 and platelet-activating factor comprise the 'Slow-reacting substances of anaphylaxis' or SRS-A; LTC_4 may have a central neuroendocrine function; 5-lipoxygenase pathway products are linked to ARDS, allergic rhinitis, asthma, gout, inflammatory bowel disease, neonatal pulmonary hypertension, rheumatoid arthritis (N Engl J Med 1990; 323:645rv) see Eicosanoid, Lipoxin

levamisole HCl A L– form of tetramisole which is most commonly used as an anthelmintic to treat roundworm, hookworm, and *Strongyloides* infections; in addition, it has been recommended as a therapy for stage C colorectal carcinoma (N Engl J Med 1990; 322:352oA)

levan DENTISTRY A fructose homopolymer linked by β-2,6 bonds, formed by the partial digestion of sucrose by *Bacillus* and *Streptococcus* spp, which is a component of dental plaque representing the first biochemical event in cariogenesis; see Caries, Plaque; Cf Periodontal disease

level of care The intensity of medical care being provided by the physician or facility

PRIMARY CARE Coordinated, comprehensive and personal care, available on both a first-contact and continuous basis; it incorporates the tasks of medical diagnosis and treatment, psychological assessment and management, personal support, communication of information about illness, prevention and health maintenance; primary care is that provided by the family physician, general practitioner and by physicians in the emergency room

SECONDARY CARE That medical care available in the community hospital, comprising the bulk of in-patient medical care provided in the US; secondary care centers are equipped to provide all but the most specialized of care, surgery and diagnostic modalities

TERTIARY CARE Highly specialized medical care for patients who are usually referred from secondary care centers, which consists in subspecialty expertise in 1) Surgery Organ transplantation, pediatric cardiovascular surgery, stereotactic neurosurgery and others 2) Internal medicine Genetics, hepatology, adolescent psychiatry and others 3) Diagnostic modalities PET (positron emission tomography) and SQUID (superconducting quantum interface device) scanning, color Doppler electrocardiography, electron microscopy, gene rearrangement and molecular analysis and 4) Therapeutic modalities Experimental protocols for treating advanced and/or potentially fatal disease, including AIDS, cancer and inborn errors of metabolism

levels SURGICAL PATHOLOGY Step-sections of paraffin-embedded tissue with the specific intent of confirming the presence of a lesion that has been tentatively identified on an initial section (level) of tissue; the pathologist may request levels when faced with a focal, possibly malignant or microinvasive lesion; unlike recuts, each 4-6 μm in thickness section of tissue must be examined; Cf Recuts

'Leveno method' A design for a clinical study in which the patient's permission is not obtained for entry in either of the two blinded arms of a protocol, since both arms represent widely accepted 'standards of care' (N Engl J Med 1987; 315:615, ibid; 316:480); Cf Zelen design

Levi's Terms of Engagement OCCUPATIONAL MEDICINE GLOBAL VILLAGE Distances in the world are 'shrinking' in terms of international commerce and communication; components of consumer goods originate as raw materials in one place, are manufactured in a second, assembled in a third, and marketed and sold to all; given the interrelation of international economic communities and disintegration of borders, those in the developed nations can no longer ignore the abject misery and plight of workers in less developed nations, especially when purchasing products made by them; the Terms of Engagement by Levi Strauss & Co (an apparel company with $5.2 x 10^9 in world-wide sales) delineates ethical workforce practices required of companies manufacturing its products; the TEs address issues of wages and benefits, working hours, child labor (< 14 years of age), prison or forced labor, discrimination and disciplinary practices; the economic leverage exerted by the Levi codes and other economic pressure may ultimately prove to be a powerful tool for fostering human rights (Fast Company, November 1993)

levonorgestrel Norplant, see there

LEWIS BLOOD GROUP

GENOTYPE	SECRETOR STATUS	PHENOTYPE
Le, H, se	Non-secretor	Le^{a+b-}
Le, H, Se	Secretor	Le^{a-b+}
le, H, Se	Secretor	Le^{a-b-}
le, H, se	Non-secretor	Le^{a-b-}

Lewis system A group of erythrocyte antigens that differs from other red cell antigen groups as 1) The antigen is present in the soluble form in saliva and blood, and red cells acquire their phenotype by adsorbing the antigen from the plasma onto the red cell membrane (table) 2) The Lewis phenotype expressed depends on whether the subject is a 'secretor' or 'non-secretor' of the Lewis gene product and 3) Lewis phenotype expression depends on another blood group, the ABO phenotype; Lewis antigens are carbohydrates and those with the Lewis blood 'secretor' status are at increased risk of urinary tract infections by *Escherichia coli* and other bacteria which attach to carbohydrate residues of glycolipids and glycoproteins on the urothelial cell

Lewis Y antigen Le^Y A member of the Lewis blood group that is thought to function as an oncodevelopmental cancer-associated antigen, which has been used as a clinical marker for the diagnosis, prognosis, and monitoring of various malignancies, in particular of the lower GI tract; Le^Y expression correlates with dedifferentiation and the proliferative activity of hepatocellular carcinoma (Cancer 1995; 75:2827)

LFA Leukocyte function-associated antigen

LFA-1 deficiency Leukocyte adhesion deficiency, see there

L-form MICROBIOLOGY A special slow-growing (transitional phase) variant bacterium, eg streptococcus, that has lost its rigid murein layer, and replicates as small filterable elements in hypertonic media; L-forms arise spontaneously or may be induced, eg using gradients of penicillin in the agar, which inhibits bacterial wall formation and may be recovered in pyelonephritis and endocarditis; may revert to normal either spontaneously or with Mg^{2+}

Note: The 'L' designation honors the Lister Institute of London

LFT Liver function tests, see there

LGC Lymphoid glandular complex, see there

LGL Large granular lymphocyte, null cell A lymphocyte that lacks the usual B- or T-cell markers, but has IgG Fc fragment receptors; LGLs comprise 3.5% of lymphocytes and are thought to be of marrow origin and are further divided into 1) Natural killer (NK) cells, comprising 70% of LGLs and defined by the monoclonal antibodies, B73.1, anti-Leu 11 and N 901, which bind to corresponding antigens on the cell surfaces and 2) Killer cells which mediate antibody-dependent cell-mediated cytotoxicity; see ADCC, Killer cells, Natural killer cells

LGSIL see Low-grade squamous intraepithelial lesion, Cf High-grade squamous intraepithelial lesion

LGV Lymphogranuloma venereum, see there, also large granular vesicle

LH Luteinizing hormone, see there

Also 1) Lateral hypothalamic 2) Learning handicapped 3) Left hand 4) Left hyperphoria (ophthalmology) 5) Lewisite-mustard gas mix 6) Lipid hydrocarbon 7) Lues hereditaria (obsolete for congenital syphilis)

LHRH Luteinizing hormone-releasing hormone A decapeptide synthesized by hypothalamic neurons that stimulates the release of FSH and LH in response to central nervous system stimulation; LHRH may be used to stimulate normal testicular function and to suppress testosterone production in prostatic carcinoma, thus functioning in a similar fashion as estrogen, eg diethylstilbestrol therapy or orchiectomy

LI 1) Labeling index, see there 2) Locomotion index, see there

Li-Fraumeni syndrome SBLA syndrome An AD [MIM 151623] condition with a marked predilection towards multiple malignancies (Ann Med 1969; 71:747), including sarcomas, carcinomas of the adrenal cortex, breast, larynx and lung, brain tumors, leukemia, and lymphomas occurring at any time from infancy to adulthood MOLECULAR BIOLOGY Skin fibroblasts from these patients are resistant to killing by ionizing radiation and have 3-8 times greater than normal expression of the c-*myc* gene product and activation of the c-*raf*-1 gene; LFS is linked to a mutation in the tumor suppressor gene, p53 [MIM 191170] (N Engl J Med 1992; 326:1301OA); the early onset of malignancy may be a confirmation of Knudson's one-hit/two-hit model of carcinogenesis, initially enumerated in retinoblastomas (Medical Hypothesis 1979; 5:15) see One-hit/two-hit model

LIA Lysine iron agar MICROBIOLOGY A growth medium for gram-negative rods that overlaps the characteristics of Kligler iron agar and Triple sugar iron agar, see TSI

liability MEDICAL MALPRACTICE A broad term referring to all character of obligation, amenability, and responsibility for an act before the law; see Malpractice

Libby Zion A young woman who died shortly after admission to the emergency room in a New York hospital in 1984, related to inadequate care provided by overworked and undersupervised medical house officers; based on her medical history, she was diagnosed as having a viral syndrome with hysterical symptoms, but at autopsy had fulminant bilateral bronchopneumonia; the 'Libby Zion case' became a cause célèbre and the catalyst for increasing the supervision of physicians-in-training (residents), especially those who are working in emergency rooms and reducing their work-load to 80 hours/week

Note: The cost of increasing the 'coverage' of a hospital's physician staff to full-time (in order to compensate for the mandated reduction in hours), would add an estimated hundreds to thousands of millions of dollars annually to the cost of health care in the US, if the precedent set in New York State becomes a norm

'liberated' CR1 A truncated complement receptor CR1 that lacks the transmembane and intracytoplasmic domains, which may have a role in limiting the size of myocardial infarcts by reducing complement activation; 'liberated' CR1 may have a therapeutic role in other forms of ischemia, burns, autoimmunity and inflammation, since it is a natural inhibitor of complement activation

library DNA library MOLECULAR BIOLOGY A complete set of genomic clones from an organism or of complementary DNA clones from one cell type; a DNA library is prepared by extracting all of an organism's DNA, derived from cells presumed to have a full set of sequences, eg sperm or embryonal cells; the DNA is then digested using a restriction endonuclease of bacterial origin, eg *Eco*RI, which cleaves the double-stranded DNA into 2 to 20 kilobase pair fragments, each end of which has a short, single-stranded four nucleotide (AATT) segment known as a 'sticky' end; the DNA fragments are then mixed with an equal amount of lambda bacteriophages that have also been subjected to *Eco*RI digestion; *Eco*RI digestion of the lambda phage yields three fragments, a disposible middle segment and two flanking segments; the flanking segments attach to the 'sticky' ends of the previously digested 2-20 kilobase pair fragments of DNA; DNA ligase is then added to the mixture to rejoin the recombinant DNA molecules; the recombinant molecules are then coated with bacteriophage proteins; only the molecules of an appropriate size will be 'packaged' into a coherent and viable recombinant bacteriophage

Note: 'Library' also refers to the full complement of sequence elements that encode the two variable regions on the immunoglobulin light chain or the three variable regions on the immunoglobulin heavy chain

library search Literature search, see there

license A generic term for a certificate of authorization by a governmental or other regulatory agency that allows a person, group of persons, or enterprise to carry out a particular activity

licensed material Radioactive material that is subject to general or specific licensing and regulatory control by a governmental or regulatory agency

licensing factor Replication licensing factor, see there

lichen Greek, tree moss A generic term that may be applied to any skin condition characterized by thickened papular eruptions

lichen sclerosis GYNECOLOGY A pruritic lesion* of the mucosa that is more common in older, often post-menopausal women, more common in whites, that may have a vague genetic component in a background of autoimmunity; the cutaneous lesions consist of flat-topped white macules that coalesce, forming white patches PATHOLOGY Blunting or loss of the rete ridges with homogenization of the upper upper dermal collagen and mid-dermal inflammation and edema, with loss of melanocytes, occasionally hyperkeratosis with follicular plugging and mild epithelial atypia; LS evolves towards malignancy in 5% of men, but it is not considered premalignant in women

*When confined to the genitalia is termed kraurosis vulvae in women (formerly lichen sclerosis et atrophicans) and balanitis xerotica obliterans in men

licorice A preparation from the root of the European legume *Glycyrrhiza glabra*, which has a high content of glycyrrhizic acid (glucuronic acid + glycyrrhetinic acid), which is structurally similar to steroids; excessive ingestion of licorice may cause a syndrome of mineralocorticoid excess, with sodium and water retention, hypokalemia and myopathy with myoglobulinuria, acting not by molecular mimicry, as had been previously postulated, but rather by suppressing both 11 β-hydroxysteroid dehydrogenase and the renin-angiotensin-aldosterone axis (**N Engl J Med 1991; 325:1223**)

LID Late-onset immune deficiency, see there

Liddle syndrome Pseudoaldosteronism, see there

lidocaine $C_{14}H_{22}N_2O$ A water-insoluble, solvent-soluble local anesthetic that is widely used for dental anesthesia and in the treatment of cardiac arrhythmias; some of lidocaine's degradation products 2,6-dimethylaniline (2,6-DMA), 4-hydroxy-DMA, and N-hydroxy-DMA are either clearly carcinogenic, or at least mutagenic by the Ames test (**Scientific American 1994; 270/5:28**)

lie detector test Polygraph test, see there

life event A generic term for major change in person's circumstances (eg divorce, death of spouse, loss of employment etc), that affects interpersonal relationships, work-related, leisure or recreational activities; LEs can be usual, ie not unexpected and therefore not evoking stress or unusual, ie unexpected and commonly associated with stress; see Unusual life event

life extension Gerontology, see there

lifespan The length of person's existance; the period between birth and death in an individual organism

lifestyle A mode of living that is unique to an individual, and which lends a pattern of consistency to the activities, behavior, manners of coping, motivation, and thought processes used by the individual in pursuing the basic goals of life

life support measures The care provided to a person in profoundly obtunded or nearly moribund state that is usually administered in an intensive care unit to maintain the patient in a stable and/or 'compensated' clinical state, requiring 24-hour monitoring and extraordinary therapeutic measures; see Advance directive, DNR orders

life table DEMOGRAPHICS A table that corresponds to the pattern of mortality occurring in each generation of a population, most commonly constructed using the age-specific death rate; LT data '...*describe the mortality experience or survival of a person or a group over a lifetime.*' LT analysis answers the question '*What would be the mortality experience and life expectancy of a group of people who had these probabilities of death at each age for the rest of their lives.*' (**JM Last, RB Wallace, Eds, Public Health and Preventive Medicine, 13th ed, Appleton & Lange, Norwalk, Ct. 1992**); a completed LT shows that for each year of age, the probability of person dying before attaining the next age; LTs provide data on the life expectancy of a person alive at time x, the number of persons dying in a given time period, the number of person-years lived during a particular interval, the person-years lived by survivors to a particular age Actuarial life table, Kaplan-Meier survival estimate PUBLIC HEALTH A table that presents the results of a clinical study in which the subjects enter and leave the trial at different times; each subject has a well-defined point of entry (onset of treatment) and end point (relapse, death or other) and all subjects may be evaluated at determined intervals with respect to the expected survival of an idealized person, based on actuarial analysis of census data and mortality rates

life-threatening illness A morbid condition in which the likelihood of death is high unless the course of disease is interrupted, eg AIDS, high-grade or preterminal cancer, or conditions in which the end-point is mere survival, eg severe cerebrovascular accidents with significant residua;

line HEALTH CARE ADMINISTRATION A funded or paid employee position, regardless of whether the person is full- or part-time SUBSTANCE ABUSE A 'unit' of cocaine consisting in an elongated trail of relatively pure powdered cocaine that is snorted through a tube or drinking straw

lines of Blaschko DERMATOLOGY Alterating stripes of affected and unaffected skin in certain cutaneous diseases; these lines neither correlate with dermatomes, and nor follow the vascular, neural, or lymphatic structures of the skin; the 'mosaic' pattern is thought to result from the clonal proliferation of two genetically distinct groups of cells arising from a postzygotic mutation that occurred during embryogenesis; diseases with clinical mosaism are classically linked to the X chromosome, and include Conradi-Hünermann syndrome, focal dermal hypoplasia, incontinentia pigmenti, and the carrier state for hypohidrotic ectodermal dysplasia, but clinical mosaicism may also occur in non-X-linked diseases, eg McCune-Albright syndrome (N Engl J Med 1994; 331:1408OA)

line CLINICAL MEDICINE A colloquial term for an IV catheter SUBSTANCE ABUSE A format for cocaine abuse, with the pulverized cocaine being placed in a line and 'snorted' using a tube or drinking straw

linear accelerator RADIATION ONCOLOGY A device for accelerating charged particles, which employs electrodes and gaps arranged in a straight line, so proportioned that when the potentials are varied in the proper amplitude and frequency, particles passing through the waveguide receive successive increments of energy, and are therefore accelerated; the device is designed to deliver therapeutic radiation in the range of 4 to 25 million volts, as either radiation or high-energy electron beams (most commonly, ^{60}Co), delivering 2-10 Gy/min (200-1000 rads/min) at the center of an internal malignancy; linear accelerators are used to treat Hodgkin's disease and other lymphoproliferative malignancies, seminomas and localized carcinoma of the breast, in combination with a 'lumpectomy'

linear model CELL PHYSIOLOGY A simple cell's responses reflect a summation (ie linear) of the intensity values in the stimulus; while the linear model is attractive, eg it allows characterization of response with relatively small number of direct measurements, and explains the selectivity of simple cells for position, and direction of motion, it may be oversimplistic; the normalization model (see there) has been proposed to explain the nonlinear aspects of simple cell responses (Science 1994; 264: 1333RR)

linear regression A generic term for statistical methods that are used to 'fit' a straight line to scattered data points of paired values Xi, Yi, where the values of Y (the ordinate or vertical line) are observations of a variable, eg systolic blood pressure and the values of X (the abscissa or horizontal line) increase in a relatively nonrandom fashion, eg age; the crude technique of 'eyeballing' a scattergram of data points is rapid but subjective, inelegant, imprecise and not amenable to statistical analysis; linear regression is a simple way of evaluating the validity of data by determining the trueness of its 'fit' to a straight line and can be used to summarize data or calculate the change between the outcome, response or dependent variable and the main variable known as the predictor variable

FORMULA FOR LINEAR REGRESSION
Predicted outcome
= Intercept + Slope X Predictor value

linear staining IMMUNOLOGY A pattern of immune deposition described as continuous, smooth, thin, delicate and ribbon-like; linear deposits of IgG and C3 are seen in patients with either anti-glomerular basement membrane disease or Goodpasture syndrome, when viewed by immunofluorescent microscopy; weakly staining linear deposits of IgG may occur in diabetes mellitus, celiac disease, human allografts and minimal change nephrotic syndrome; linear staining in the skin corresponds to IgA deposition at the dermal-epidermal junction in bullous dermatosis, which is seen by indirect immunofluorescence; Cf Band test, Lumpy-bumpy pattern

linear transformation The mathematical conversion of an equation into one providing data that can be plotted in a straight line, eg transformation of the Michaelis-Menten equation into Lineweaver-Burk plot

linearity STATISTICS A straight line relation between two quantities, where when a value 'X' is increased or decreased, 'Y' is proportionately increased or decreased; linearity assumes that the relation between X and Y (abscissa and ordinate) can be summarized in a straight line, known as a least-squares regression method; linearity is a requirement for quality control in laboratory medicine and is applicable to most 'chemistries' where the coefficient of variation is less than 10.0; linearity is tested by analyzing dilutions of a specimen, or of graded mixtures of 2 analytes, and evaluated by plotting the results on xy graph paper and

1) Visualizing ('eyeballing') the data, an exercise that requires expert understanding of the method

2) Using least-squares regression procedures

3) Using 'deltas' (slopes between adjacent points on a line), an analytic technique used to simulate the visual assessment of linearity and

4) Comparing the observed values with the expected values (Arch Pathol Lab Med 1992; 116:746OA)

or by formally subjecting the data to linear regression analysis; one of the first indications of the deterioration of a reagent or an instrument problem is a ↓ in linearity (Arch Pathol Lab Med 1992; 116:714OA, 746OA); linearity allows comparison of interlaboratory data, as in the Linearity Surveys sponsored by the College of American Pathologists (CAP Today Jan. 1994)

lingua geographica Geographic tongue, see there

Linguatula A genus of tongueworm, a primitive parasite lacking circulatory and respiratory tracts that invades the respiratory tracts of carnivores; linguatuliasis is the direct human infection by the third-stage larvae, which most commonly affects those of the Middle East who ingest undercooked liver or lymph nodes from sheep or goats, migrating from the stomach to the nasopharynx CLINICAL Pain, itching and irritation in throat with dyspnea, dysphagia and vomiting; with intense infestation, asphyxia; alternatively, the worms may emerge in the intestine and encyst in the liver, spleen, lymph nodes, and lungs

linitis plastica Greek, inen cloth A descriptive term of waning popularity that refers to the appearance of certain hollow viscus organs, consisting of a rigidly thickened wall, classically described in a common variant of gastric carcinoma RADIOLOGY Upper gastrointestinal series demonstrates neither ulcer nor mass but a fixed, non-distensible stomach, absent folds and narrowed lumen, fancifully likened to the Spanish leather wineskin, la bota PATHOLOGY Extensive desmoplastic reaction with numerous scattered signet ring cells and clusters of moderately-differentiated adenocarcinoma; linitis plastica may rarely occur in other hollow epithelial cell-lined organs, eg colon or bladder

link sausage appearance MICROBIOLOGY A descriptor for the light microscopic appearance of the elongated blastospores with focal constrictions typical of *Candida* species; Cf Box-car appearance OPHTHALMOLOGY see Sausage link appearance

linkage analysis GENETICS The formal study of the association between the inheritance of a condition in a family and a particular chromosomal locus; LA is an analytic technique based on certain ground rules of genetics; if a trait of interest, eg diabetes mellitus, is genetically influenced, then the relatives of a cohort who share the trait will share the gene with a frequency greater than that expected by chance alone; for traits affected by only one gene, linkage will precisely locate the gene of interest on a chromosome; for complex traits LA helps determine whether a genetic component is at least plausible

linkage disequilibrium GENETICS The tendency for certain alleles at different loci to occur far more (or less) frequently in the same haplotype than expected based on statistics alone, the result of proximity of those alleles, as occurs on the major histocompatibility complex, located on chromosome 6; in a random population breeding under ideal conditions, the occurrence of individual genes is a product of the frequencies, ie random; thus the relation of one gene to another should be purely statistical; as an example, if HLA-A1 occurs in 16% of a population and HLA-B8 in 10%, an expected 1.6% of the population should have the allelic combination, although the combination actually occurs in 9%; other examples include 1) MNSs blood group, where an association of group N with s is five times more common than the N with S, 2) The extended haplotype HLA A1, Cw7, B8, DR3, Dw3, MB2, MT2 occurs four times more frequently than expected based on chance MECHANISMS OF LINKAGE DISEQUILIBRIUM 1) Selection Linkage may occur via immune response genes, by interaction of HLA gene products with environmental agents or 2) Crossover suppression Crossing-over during meiosis occurs at a significantly lower rate

linkage map A genetic map based on the coinheritance of allele combinations across multiple polymorphic loci; parental combinations usually delineate the locations of chromosomal 'landmarks', measured in centimorgans (the number of crossovers/100 meioses) from the chromosomes centromere; see Human Genome Project, Lod score

linkage number Winding number MOLECULAR BIOLOGY The number of times one strand of the double helix crosses over the other; see DNA topology, Cf Twist, Writhe

linkage study GENETICS A study that identifies the chromosome responsible for a disease, requiring a large family with multiple living relatives who have the disease, high diagnostic reliability and sufficient genetic markers to ensure that at least one is close to the gene; see Lod score

linker DNA A segment of DNA that links adjacent nucleosomes in a chromosome to each other, which is held in place at the H1 histone molecule

linking number Linkage number

linoleic acid An essential 18-carbon fatty acid with 2 unsaturated bonds, derived from plant oils; see Essential fatty acids

linolenic acid An essential 18-carbon fatty acid with 3 unsaturated bonds, derived from either plants (α-linolenic acid) or animals (γ-linolenic acid); see Essential fatty acids

LIP Lymphocytic interstitial pneumonia, see there

lipase Triacylglycerol acylhydrolase* A 45-kD pancreatic esterase [EC 3.1.1.3] that hydrolyses glycerol esters of long chain fatty acids; pancreatic lipase cleaves the outer 1, 3 ester linkages of long chain fatty acids; lipase is elevated only in pancreatitis (markedly so in acute pancreatitis) and pancreatic duct obstruction; a diagnostic sensitivitiy of 100% and a specificity of 97% has been reported for the elevation of serum lipase in acute pancreatitis; see Lipoprotein lipase

*Lipase is the widely preferred trivial name; triacylglycerol acylhydrolase is the name recommended by the International Union of Biochemists and Molecular Biologists

lipid A MICROBIOLOGY A major and highly conserved component of bacterial endotoxins* which is present on the outer membrane of gram-negative bacteria (**Science & Medicine 1995; 2/3:16**) see Virulence factor; Cf Exotoxin

*Which are composed of carbohydrates and a lipid, in contrast to bacterial exotoxins which are composed of proteins

lipid bilayer see Fluid mosaic model

lipid cell tumor Steroid cell tumor, see there

lipid hypothesis CARDIOLOGY A widely accepted postulate that hyperlipidemia in the form of increased cholesterol, and to a lesser degree, other lipids in the circulation is responsible for atherosclerosis, the major cause of death in the US, levels which, when altered by dietary or pharmacologic manipulation, result in a decreased risk of atherosclerosis-related morbidity; the hypothesis appears to be valid, as

1) Atherosclerotic plaques contain lipids, most of which are derived directly from plasma lipoproteins

2) Atherosclerotic lesions may be produced in hypercholesterolemic experimental animals

3) Hyperlipidemia is more prevalent in groups with documented atherosclerosis

4) Atherosclerosis is more prevalent in subjects with certain familial hyperlipidemias and

5) Epidemiologic studies demonstrate a graded increased risk in atherosclerosis-related morbidity and mortality with increasing levels of LDL-cholesterol and decreasing levels of HDL-cholesterol; Cf Lipid theory

lipid panel LABORATORY MEDICINE A standard (CPT-4 code 80061) panel of laboratory tests used to evaluate the baseline lipid status; for Medicare or Medicaid reimbursement, the LP must include total serum cholesterol, directly measured lipoprotein, HDL-cholesterol, and triglycerides (**CAP Today March 1993**)

lipid profile LABORATORY MEDICINE An abbreviated battery of tests performed on an automated multichannel chemical analyzer, including total cholesterol, LDL-cholesterol, HDL-cholesterol and triglycerides, which helps stratify patients according to risk of atherosclerosis-related mortality and morbidity

lipid storage diseases A group of rare conditions, including Fabry's disease, Niemann-Pick disease, and the sea-blue histiocytosis syndrome, which are often fatal in early childhood, usually due to a catabolic defect of lipid metabolism and characterized by the accumulation of lipids in one or more organs, some of which, eg Gaucher disease, GM-1 gangliosidosis type I and fucosidosis demonstrate foamy histiocytes in the BM, while others, eg Tay-Sachs disease, Krabbe and metachromatic leukodystrophy do not; the diagnosis can be established in utero by performing enzymatic studies on cultured amniotic fluid cells, which can be completed by the 20th week of gestation; see Pseudo-Gaucher's disease, Sphingolipidosis

lipid theory ANESTHESIOLOGY A unified hypothesis (which is being discarded) of how anesthetics function, which holds that fat-soluble agents bind to sites in the lipid layer of the cell membrane, swelling the membrane, which disrupts the cells blocking transmissions (**New York Times 30 August 1994; C1**) Cf Hydrophobic pocket theory

lipidation see Protein lipidation

Lipiodol A proprietary iodized oily agent that selectively remains in tumros for prolonged periods of time, which is reported to enhance the antitumor effect of certain chemotherapeutic agents; Lipiodol chemoembolization ↑ the survival of patients with unresectable hepatocellular carcinoma, but is associated with a marked ↑ in liver failure, and the number of days in the hospital was higher in the treated group (**N Engl J Med 1995; 332:1256OA, 1294ED**)

lipoblastoma A rare benign adipose tissue tumor of children under age 3, that is usually well-circumscribed, subcutaneous, and located on the legs PATHOLOGY Lipoblasts, myxoid stroma, spindled and stellate prelipoblasts DDx Myxoid liposarcoma TREATMENT Complete excision (see **Acta Cytologica 1993; 37:563OA**)

lipochrome A generic term for any natural, fat-soluble pigment including lipofuscin, carotenes and lycopenes

lipofuscin A pigmented lipid degradation product thought to derive from peroxidative destruction of the mitochondrial polyunsaturated lipid membrane or the mitochondria itself; the malonaldehyde produced by mitochondrial peroxide damage may block DNA template activity contributing to heart failure; lipofuscin accumulates with age in the heart, muscle, liver, nerve and in lysosomes

lipoid adrenal hyperplasia (congenital) Adrenal hyperplasia I An AR [MIM 201710] subtype of congenital adrenal hyperplasia, which is most common in the Japanese, due to a defective cholesterol side-chain cleavage enzyme P450$_{SCC}$, formerly 20, 22 desmolase; LAH is associated with ↓ peripheral conversion of cholesterol to pregnenolone, accumulation of cholesterol and lipids in the adrenal cortex and, given the lack of testicular hormone production, all infants are phenotypic females PROGNOSIS Death in early infancy in a state of adrenal 'crisis' due to insufficient mineralocorticoid and glucocorticoid production

lipoid cell tumor Steroid cell tumor, see there

lipoid pneumonia Golden pneumonia A pneumonitis caused by exogenous oils that percolate into the lungs through intranasal instillation of mineral oil, forced administration of cod liver, castor or other oils or due to a congenital defect in the oropharyngeal diaphragm, eg cleft palate or an intense gag reflex; the intensity of the response is a function of the oils' irritability, ranging from the least irritating vegetable oils to liquid petrolatum, which may act as a foreign body and animal oils and milk, which may evoke a pneumonitis PATHOLOGY Accumulation of abundant foamy lipid-laden macrophages in the alveolar spaces, and lesions that progress from interstitial proliferation to exudation, with proliferative fibrosis and eventually, miliary paraffinoma-like nodules; see Mineral oil

lipoid proteinosis An AR [MIM 247100] condition of childhood onset characterized by coalescent aggregates of lipid and mucopolysaccharides, resulting in numerous yellowish plaques, papules, nodules and induration of the skin (pachydermia), eyelids, oropharynx and larynx with hoarseness, hyperkeratosis of the knees and elbows, hyalinization of the blood vessels; calcification of the hippocampal gyri, while uncommon, is pathognomonic and held responsible for the associated convulsions

lipoleiomyoma A uterine leiomyoma-like neoplasm of obese, post-menopausal women with cholecystitis that may cause vague abdominal pain, backache, vaginal discharge or hemorrhage

lipomatosis dolorosa Dercum's disease A perimenopausal disease characterized by multiple circumscribed masses of adipose tissue accompanied by local pain at the sites of accumulation CLINICAL Neuroasthenia, headache, depression, ecchymoses and cardiovascular decompensation due to cardiac overload TREATMENT Weight reduction; Cf Lipomatosis dolorosa

lipooxygenase pathway An arachidonic acid metabolic pathway leading to 5-HPETE (5-hydroperoxyeicosatetraenoic acid), that is further metabolized to 5-HETE, lipoxins or leukotrienes (LTC$_4$, LTD$_4$ and LTE$_4$); see SRS-A (slow-reacting substances of anaphylaxis)

lipophilin Proteolipid protein, see there

lipopolysaccharide-binding protein A trace plasma protein that binds to the lipid A moiety of bacterial lipopolysaccharide (LPS) or to endotoxin (a glycolipid present in the outer membrane of all gram-negative bacteria); the complexes formed between LPS and its binding protein may stimulate monocyte release of TNF; LBP binds to CD14 on the surface of monocytes, which leads to monocyte activation; anti-LBP antibodies appear to suppress endotoxin-related shock in mice, which may pave the way to its use in humans (**Sci & Med Nov/Dec 1994 p 28**)

lipoprotein A family of lipid-carrying, water-soluble proteins including chylomicrons, high-, intermediate-, low- and very low-density lipoproteins that are responsible for the transport of cholesterol and cholesterol esters, phospholipids and triglycerides throughout the circulation; lipoprotein composition (table, below); lipoproteins are classified based on the density by ultra-centrifugation; some are subdivided by gel electrophoresis **HDL** High-density (1.063-1.21 kg/L) lipoprotein is synthesized in the liver and intestine and is responsible for cholesterol metabolism; HDL migrates electrophoretically as an α globulin, major protein components are apoA-I and apoA-II; HDL is further subdivided into HDL$_1$ (1.050-1.063 kg/L, which has a density overlapping LDL as well as HDL$_2$ (1.063-1.120 kg/L) and HDL$_3$ (1.120-1.210 kg/L); the higher the HDL-cholesterol level, the lower the risk of myocardial infarct and HDL is used to screen for atherosclerosis, see HDL **IDL** Intermediate-density (1.006-1.019 kg/L) lipoprotein is a β-globulin-migrating metabolic intermediate formed by the action of lipoprotein lipase on chylomicrons and VLDL **LDL** Low-density (1.019-1.063 kg/L) lipoprotein migrates as a β-globulin with apolipoprotein-B being the major protein component and cholesteryl linoleate the major lipid component; increased LDL is a major risk factor for atherosclerosis and coronary artery disease, when LDL is subdivided by gel-electrophoresis, patients with increased small dense LDL subclass are at highest risk for myocardial infarcts **VLDL** Very low-density (< 1.006 kg/L) lipoprotein migrates in the pre-β region of the electrophoretic gel; the main lipid component is triglyceride and the major proteins are apolipoprotein-B, apolipoprotein-C and apolipoprotein-E

lipoprotein(a) A lipoprotein that has a wide range of serum levels 0.05-1.90 mmol/L (US: 20-760 mg/L), which has a lipid content similar to LDL, and binds to the LDL receptor with lesser affinity than LDL; Lp(a) has considerable sequence similarity ('homology') to plasminogen, a finding of unknown significance; although its metabolism and relation to atherosclerosis is unclear, it is increased in those at risk for coronary heart disease in a large (15 000 middle-aged white ♂) nested case-control study, there was no evidence of an association between baseline plasma concentrations of Lp(a) and future risk of thromboembolic stroke (**JAMA 1995; 273:1269**) because Lp(a) is part of the acute-phase response, the previous reports of an ↑ of Lp(a) in acute MI may be flawed and an effect of the general response rather than a marker of ↑ risk (**JAMA 1993; 270:2195**) subjects with Lp(a) levels ≥ 18 mg/dL are reported to have a 21-fold ↑ in the risk for stroke (**New York Times 22 February 1994; C6**)

COMPOSITION OF LIPOPROTEINS

	CHOL	TGS	PROT	PPLS
HDL	20	5	50	25 α$_1$ migration
VLDL	12	60	10	18 α$_2$ migration
LDL	50	10	25	15 β migration
IDL	30	40	10	20
Chylo	1	5	90	5

Chol Cholesterol PPL Phospholipids Prot Protein TG Triglyerides

lipoprotein-associated coagulation inhibitor Tissue factor pathway inhibitor, see there

lipoprotein lipase A hydrolytic enzyme [EC 3.1.1.34] that is bound by glycosaminoglycan to capillary walls, which breaks ester bonds of di- and triglycerides from chylomicrons and low-density lipoprotein to form free fatty acids and glycerol, acting in the capillary endothelium of adipose tissue, skeletal and cardiac muscle

lipoprotein lipase deficiency An AR [MIM 238600] condition characterized by the absence of lipoprotein lipase, resulting in massive hypertriglyceridemia of neonatal onset and recurrent episodes of pancreatitis; in 73% of the well-studied French-Canadian cohort of patients with lipoprotein lipase deficiency, the defect lies in a missense mutation on residue 207 of exon 5 (N Engl J Med 1991; 324:1761), detectable in homozygous and heterozygous subjects by dot-blot analysis CLINICAL Fatty food intolerance, eruptive xanthomas and hepatosplenomegaly that regresses with dietary control; because hydrolysis of triglycerides from chylomicrons and endogenous VLDL requires both LPL and its activator apoC-II, apoC-II deficiency has a similar clinical picture

lipoprotein X An abnormal lipoprotein composed of 65% lecithin, 30% cholesterol and 5% protein (apoC and albumin) that is seen in lecithin-cholesterol acyl-transferase deficiency and in obstructive biliary disease, which is associated with cholestatic jaundice

liposome CHEMISTRY A vesicle composed of phospholipids that forms spontaneously when phospholipidas are placed in water, with the hydrophobic portion of the bimolecular layer is oriented toward the inside, and the hydrophilic portion oriented toward the aqueous phase on the outside CLINICAL THERAPEUTICS A synthetic, relatively uniform bilayer lipid membrane-bound vesicle formed by emulsification of cell membranes in dilute salt solutions; liposomes are being developed as an approach for drug delivery in which relatively toxic drugs, eg amphotericin B, doxorubicin and pentavalent antimony are 'wrapped' inside a liposome and tagged with an organ-specific antibody

liposuction Suction-assisted lipectomy A plastic surgical technique used to remove focal fat deposits; a metal cannula with side holes is connected to a high-pressure vacuum, removing fat from the face, neck, breasts, abdomen, thighs; see Body sculpting

β-lipotropin A 91-residue protein of unknown function produced by the anterior pituitary and co-secreted with ACTH, which has sequence homology to endorphins and enkephalins

lipoxin Any of a group of arachidonic acid-derived products formed by 5- and 15-lipoxygenase and peroxidase that contain a conjugated tetraene structure and three alcohols; lipoxin A (LXA) and lipoxin B (LXB) inhibit natural killer cell-induced cytotoxicity; alone, LXA dilates arterioles, induces glomerular hyperperfusion and hypertension and contracts pulmonary muscle, and when added to neutrophils, stimulates superoxide generation

lip stripping DERMATOLOGY Excision and advancement of oral mucosa, a technique used in plastic surgery when the vermilion border becomes indistinct, due to squamous metaplasia or labial hyperkeratosis, a potentially preneoplastic lesion of light-skinned sun-exposed elderly subjects; Cf Chemical peel

liquefactive degeneration Immune-induced liquefaction at the dermal-epidermal interface, which 'loosens' the basal cells, resulting in coalescing subepidermal vesicles in dermatitis herpetiformis, dermatomyositis, dyskeratosis congenita, erythema multiforme, fixed drug reaction, incontinentia pigmenti, lichen nitidus, lichen planus, lichen sclerosis, lichenoid drug reaction, SLE, pinta, poikiloderma atrophicans vasculare, poikiloderma congenita of Rothman-Thompson, and Riehl's melanosis

liquefaction necrosis A pathological state characterized by fulminant enzymatic hydrolysis of tissue, due to ischemia, resulting in myocardial and cerebral infarction or due to bacterial, often pyogenic, infections which, when associated with gas production, yield cystic spaces; liquefaction is a necrotizing process evoked by hydrolytic enzymes that may be produced by coagulase-positive staphylococci, β-hemolytic streptococci and *Escherichia coli*

liquid diet A very low calorie diet that fulfils the daily fluid requirements and places little functional demand on the GI tract; liquid diets have little fiber and do not provide adequate protein or calories, circa 1000 kcal/day

liquid hybridization A reaction between strands of complementary nucleic acids that occurs in solution

liquid-protein diet A very low-calorie weight-reduction diet that provided 800 calories and protein in the form of hydrolyzed collagen; the quality of protein in collagen is so poor that it is immediately converted to glucose, resulting in a negative nitrogen balance; LPDs were inculpated in a number of sudden cardiac arrests in dieters on this regimen and have been abandoned; see Diet

liquid scintillation counter An instrument that detects low-energy β-particle emissions from ^{14}C and ^{3}H, for immunoassays of substances, eg proteins, of biological interest PRINCIPLE Radioactive samples are dissolved in toluene, a substance that absorbs low-energy β-emissions; the energy is then transferred to a fluor, which emits a photon detectable by a photomultiplier; see POP, POPOP, Quenching, RIA

LIS Laboratory information system, see there

LISS Low-ionic strength saline TRANSFUSION MEDICINE A low-concentration saline solution used in the blood bank to reduce the zeta potential (the electron cloud separating erythrocytes) allowing weak antibodies to agglutinate and be detected by the usual agglutination tests; see Zetacrit

Listeria A genus of small gram-positive motile bacilli with a palisading growth pattern, similar to the Chinese letter appearance of *Corynebacteria* species; *L monocytogenes* is named for its marked affinity for and residence within macrophages EPIDEMIOLOGY Outbreaks may be associated with contaminated milk products and cheese (N Engl J Med 1988; 319:823) MICROBIOLOGY Most cases (US) are caused by serotypes 1/2a, 1/2b, and 4a; the ↓ in incidence in the US has been attributed to industrial, regulatory, and educational efforts MORTALITY 20-40% (JAMA 1995; 273:1118oA) CLINICAL ⅓ of reported cases of listeriosis occur in pregnant women, causing transplacental infection with abortion, stillbirth and premature delivery PERINATAL INFECTION Infants may present with septicemia, diarrhea, vomiting, cardiorespiratory distress and meningoencephalitis Immunocompromised adults may suffer meningoencephalitis, endocarditis, disseminated granulomatosis, lymphadenitis, peritonitis and cholecystitis TREATMENT Ampicillin, gentamicin, erythromycin, chloramphenicol

literature A colloquial 'short form' for information that is written in peer-reviewed journals about a particular subject

literature search Library search A review of the literature that is relevant to a particular subject for the purpose of writing a report, preparing for a conference or guiding patient management; most medicine-related literature searches in the US begin with the venerated Index Medicus and are then carried out by 1200, 2400 or 9600 baud modem, accessioning the US National Library of Medicine; the average cost per search is $2-4 and requires the GRATEFUL MED software, a user identification number and a password

lithium carbonate $LiCO_3$ CLINICAL PHARMACOLOGY An alkali used to treat bipolar I disorder* that blocks neurotransmission at the 'second messenger' phosphoinositide-mediated cholinergic neurons in the hippocampus , inhibiting the release and uptake of norepinephrine at nerve endings by inhibiting receptor-mediated synthesis of cAMP NEUROPHARMACOLOGIC EFFECTS-ANTIMANIC Blocks development of dopamine receptor supersensitivity, ↑ GABA function, ↑ acetylcholine function ANTIDEPRESSANT ↑ 5-HT function, ↓ β-adrenoceptor stimulation of adenylate cyclase, ↓ $α_2$-adrenoceptor function THYMOLEPTIC ↓

Neurotransmitter-coupled adenylate cyclase activity and cAMP formation, ↓ receptor-G protein coupling, ↓ phosphoinositide metabolism, alters kinetics of alkali cations (Na⁺, K⁺, Ca²⁺, Mg²⁺) (N Engl J Med 1994; 331:591ʀᴠ) SIDE EFFECTS Hyperirritability, hyperpyrexia, stupor, coma, gastroenteritis, cardiovascular disease, eg arrhythmia, hypotension, ↓ ST wave, T inversion, osteoporosis ANALYSIS Flame photometry, atomic absorption spectrophotometry TERATOGENESIS Severe cardiac malformations may occur in 10% of infants born to lithium-treated bipolar I (manic-depressive) ♀ TOXICITY Overdose causes death in ¼ of patients TREATMENT Potassium-sparing drugs

*296.0x per DSM-IV, formerly known as manic-depressive disorder

lithostathine Pancreatic stone protein A 14-kD protein secreted by pancreatic acinar cells, which is abundant in pancreatic juice, ductal plugs, and stones; it is precipitated by ↑ H⁺, and changes in the local concentration of salts; in vitro, lithostathine inhibits precipitation of $CaCO_3$ from pancreatic juice (N Engl J Med 1995; 332:1482ʀᴀ)

lithotripsy Shock-wave lithotripsy A non-surgical, non-invasive method for dissolving renal, and more recently biliary tract calculi; the patients lie prone and partially immersed in a large bathtub-like vat; shock waves are generated extracorporally by high-energy underwater spark discharge focused on the patient's ventral aspect by a reflector

litigation cells CYTOLOGY A colloquial term for parakeratotic cells with slight atypia, which when viewed prospectively, fall in the range of reactive and/or reparative changes; when reexamined by a plaintiff's expert, these same cells may be re-classified as clearly abnormal, opening the person(s) who first examined the case to litigation (ASC Bulletin 1995; 32/3:1) see Artifical organ

litogen LEGAL MEDICINE A drug used during pregnancy that is not teratogenic, but which nevertheless results in lawsuits (N Engl J Med 1986; 315:1234); the term was coined by the editor of the journal Teratology in response to the Wells v Ortho case, in which the plaintiff was awarded $5 million for alleged teratogenesis by spermicides, which have not been inculpated in congenital malformation; thus any litigation-generating agent, could be a litogen, regardless of its teratogenic, carcinogenic, or toxic potential

Little Boy RADIATION MEDICINE The bomb that flattened Hiroshima; see IPPNW, Nuclear war

Note: The biggest bomb in the US arsenal, the B-53 (deployable on the B-52 bomber), was built in the 1960s and is currently 'moth-balled' as 'safer' bombs (an interesting oxymoron) are available; the B-53 is equivalent to 9 megatons of TNT, ie 750-fold more destructive than Little Boy and 30 times more destructive than the current MX family of nuclear warheads

little gastrin see Gastrin

Little League elbow PEDIATRIC ORTHOPEDICS A form of medial epicondylitis manifesting as apophyseal tenderness with ulnar nerve irritation, which may require surgery if severe, with potential for lifelong arthralgia due to injury of the physeal cells under the articular cartilage; permanent damage results from repeated and excessive axial loading, which compresses the cells against the osseous matrix; later sequelae include osteochondritis dissecans

Little League shoulder PEDIATRIC ORTHOPEDICS Fracture of the proximal humerus through the epiphyseal growth plate (the weakest point of growing long bones), the result of a growing shoulder articulation chronically insulted by throwing a baseball

Note: Little League is an international organization dedicated to the sportsman-like practice of baseball for children under the age of 12

'little science' A phrase used by US government science policy makers, for investigator-initiated research, which contrasts with 'big science' that is applied in scope and goal-oriented; Cf 'Big science'

Little's disease Bilateral congenital spastic diplegia A variant of cerebral palsy with agenesis of the lower motor neurons in the inferior extremities, which affects ± 300 000 (USA) CLINICAL Spasticity, muscle weakness, mental retardation and ocular defects, due to neonatal hypoxia, mechanical trauma and prematurity; congenital cerebrovascular malformations and immune-related kernicterus account for a low percentage of cases PATHOLOGY Focal cerebral atrophy, microcystic and spongiotic changes of the white matter, potentially associated with basal ganglia atrophy DDx Brain tumors, 'Floppy infant' syndromes, leukodystrophy and muscular dystrophy

'Little Women' syndrome A Laron-type dwarfism* variant seen in a highly inbred population of Spanish descent living in the province of Loja in southern Equador that predominantly affects females as the gene mutation may be linked to a trait lethal in males; features unique to this variant include blue sclera, limited elbow extensibility, shortened extremities, high-pitched voices and hip dysplasia in adults PATHOGENESIS Both forms (see below) result from ↓↓↓ production of growth hormone-binding protein with ↓ insulin-like growth factor I (IGF-1)

*Laron dwarfism is an AR [MIM 262500] condition with a high incidence of consanguinity, small facies, micrognathia, prominent forehead, saddle nose, sparse slow-growing hair, poor dentition, small hands and feet, high-pitched voice in children and hypoglycemia

littoral cells Normal fixed macrophages of the spleen that are involved with sequestration and destruction of effete and/or abnormal RBCs

live attenuated vaccine A vaccine that induces an immunologic response more closely resembling that of a natural infection than that elicited by killed vaccines, as the organisms contained therein actively reproduce until held in check by the recipient's own antibodies, thus often conferring life-long immunity; live attenuated vaccines include measles, mumps, polio and rubella; see Killed vaccine

live birth The '...Complete expulsion or extraction from its mother of a product of conception...which, after such separation, breathes or shows any other evidence of life such as the beating of the heart, pulsation of the umbilical cord, or definite movement of voluntary muscles, whether or not the umbilical cord has been cut or the placenta is attached'—American Public Health Association

liver dialysis CLINICAL THERAPEUTICS The use of hepatocytes either in cartridges, as in an bioartificial liver or via cross-perfusion with another organisms, either human or of animal origin by means of perfusion to provide metabolic support for a person in acute hepatic failure (Science & Medicine 1995; 2/3:73) see Artifical organ

'liver eater' TRANSPLANTATION A highly colloquial term of uncertain usefulness for a patient who has rejected two or more transplanted livers

liver function tests Clinical parlance for a battery of biochemical determinants, that are measured in the serum and reflect the liver's metabolic reserve capacity; thus defined, LFTs include those that

1) Measure hepatic ability to a) Excrete endogenous (bilirubin, bile acids, ammonia) or exogenous (drugs, dyes, galactose) substances and b) Perform metabolic functions including conjugation and synthesis of proteins

2) Measure substances elevated in a) Hepatic disease, inflammation or necrosis (elevation of transferases and other enzymes, vitamin B_{12}, iron and ferritin) or b) Biliary tract obstruction (bilirubin, cholesterol, enzymes and lipoprotein-X)

Note: Other nonfunctional biochemical and immunologic markers of specific hepatic disease include serological markers for hepatitides (HAV, HBV, HCV, HDV, HEV) and HIV, autoimmune diseases (anti-mitochondrial antibodies, primary biliary cirrhosis), malignancy (α-fetoprotein, relatively specific hepatocellular carcinoma) and metabolic diseases (ceruloplasmin in Wilson's disease and transferrin levels in hemochromatosis)

liver panel A battery of tests that is considered to be the most cost-effective in evaluation of the liver's functional status, ie produce proteins and metabolize toxic substances, and detect inflammation, measuring the transferases (AST/GOT, AST/GPT and γ-glutamyl transferase), alkaline phosphatase, total bilirubin, conjugated bilirubin, total protein, albumin, prothrombin time; see Liver function tests, Organ panel

liver 'rounds' A colloquialism for a regular social function in which there is beer and/or other inebrients (hence, 'liver'), and comestibles; liver rounds are usually held at the end of the work-week, often in academic institutions, and are especially popular with physicians-in-training, and house staff (see **N Engl J Med 1992; 327:351sb**)

Note: The mock-serious term derives from the term grand rounds, see there

liver scan Next time and DC with current applicability and relevance

liver-spleen scan A radionuclide imaging technique that uses a scintillation camera to detect metabolically-active potentially malignant masses of ≥ 2 cm diameter that are labeled with radioisotopes, eg ^{99m}Tc and ^{198}Au

Note: For detection of masses, the images obtained by CT and MRI are far superior, which thus limits this technique to highly specific applications

'liver spots' A relatively non-specific lay term for red-brown skin lesions associated with aging, including pigmented seborrheic keratosis and lentigo senilis; see Lentigines

liver tongue A rarely observed blue-red tongue with engorged capillaries seen in advanced cirrhosis, equated to palmar erythema or spider hemangiomas, which may be accompanied by papillary atrophy or hypertrophy

liver transplantation A procedure that replaces a cancer conquered, metabolically defeated, or substance subjugated liver with one that is no longer required by its owner, many of whom 'donate' said organ after a motor vehicle accident; LT is being performed with increasing frequency and impunity; patients with acute liver disease respond better to liver transplantation as the manifestations of chronic liver disease have not yet developed; LTs have been performed for alcoholic cirrhosis, chronic active hepatitis, primary sclerosing cholangitis, primary biliary cirrhosis, HBV, hepatitis D, α_1-antitrypsin deficiency and LDL-receptor deficiency; in high-risk operative candidates for orthotopic liver transplantation, auxiliary heterotopic liver transplantation, leaving the patient's own liver in place, may be compatible with up to 12 years' survival TRANSPORT MEDIUM University of Wisconsin solution OPERATING TIME 6.5 hours; average blood use during transplantation, 13 units of packed RBCs; rejection phenomena occur in 60%, which usually respond to various 'cocktails' containing corticosteroids, OKT3 antibody, cyclosporin, tacrolimus (FK 506), rapamycin and experimental agents EARLY COMPLICATIONS Hypothermia, hyperglycemia LATE COMPLICATIONS Infection, eg CMV, gram-positive bacteremia, renal insufficiency, due in part to cyclosporine nephrotoxicity, hypertension, hypokalemia, metabolic alkalosis, and fever; 1 year survival, 83%; 2 year survival 70%; despite ample indication that alcoholics can survive well with liver transplantation, there is an ethical dilemma of whether a person who is solely responsible for his terminal illness has a 'right' to the procedure (**JAMA 1991; 265:1295, 1299**); 90% of rehabilitated alcoholics who survived transplantation returned to a productive life; 20% required retransplantation

living will A term coined in 1969 to describe an 'advance directive' document in which a mentally competent adult formally expresses his preferences regarding medical treatment in the event of future incapacitation or should he become incompetent to make medical decisions; a liv-ing will is essentially a statement of a person's right to die without what might be considered senseless resuscitation efforts or artificial life support; such a document is 'living' since it is prepared prior to the time of incapacitation and a 'will' as it delineates the person's directions ante incapacitatum (**N Engl J Med 1991; 324:1210ed**); it is statutorily binding in most US states and goes into effect once competence is lost (**JAMA 1990; 263:2365**); the language recommended by the National Conference of Commissioners on Uniform State Laws is, *'If I should have an incurable or irreversible condition that will cause my death within a relatively short time, and I am unable to make decisions regarding my medical treatment, I direct my attending physician to withhold or withdraw procedures that merely prolong the dying process and are not necessary to my comfort or to alleviate pain'*; most older adults prefer that LW discussions be initiated by the physician; those who have LWs tend to be more educated (**Arch Int Med 1992; 152:954**) see Advance directive, DNR, Cf Durable powers of attorney, Euthanasia

lizard skin appearance A fanciful descriptor for the lichenoid changes of the skin, eg drying, scaling, cutaneous atrophy and depigmentation seen in the chronic dermatitis of *Onchocerca volvulus*, which is characterized by layers of keratin that are loosely attached to the epidermis, accompanied by scarring and loss of dermal elastin fibers

LM Light micoscopy, also 1) Laboratory manager 2) Lateral meniscus 3) Licentiate in medicine 4) Light microscope 5) Low molecular 6) Lower motor 7) Lumen, an SI (International System) unit of luminous flux

Also 1) Laboratory microscope 2) Laboratory module 3) Lactose malabsorption 4) Lateral malleolus 5) Left male 6) Legal medicine 7) Leptomeningeal metastases 8) Linguomesial (dentistry) 9) Light minimum 10) *Listeria monocytogenes* (rarely used) 11) local memory 12) Longitudinal muscle 13) Low meaningfulness (psychology)

LMP2, LMP7 GENETICS Two subunits of proteosomes encoded in the MHC (on the short arm of chromosome 6) that are thought to play a role in generating endogenous peptides for presentation by class I molecules to cytotoxic T cells; the LMP genes *LMP2* and *LMP7* may have independent effects on the susceptibility to IDDM (**AM J Hum Genet 1995; 56:528**)

LN Lymph node, also 1) Background noise level 2) Laser nephelometry 4) Lesch-Nyhan syndrome 6) Licensed nurse 7) Lot number

Also 1) Lane 3) Laser nephelometry 3) Lateral neuropil

load LABORATORY MEDICINE *noun* A batch of specimens, the testing on which is to be performed, usually to be performed on a batch analyzer *verb* To place specimen(s) being tested or evaluated, as well as the positive and negative controls at the starting point of a support medium for chromatographic or electrophoretic procedure; alternatively, to position multiple samples in carousel or tray for automated feeding into a a multichannel analyser

loading dose Initial dose CLINICAL PHARMACOLOGY The first dose of a drug that is administered in excess (of the maintenance dose) in order to build therapeutic levels of a drug as quickly as possible; Cf Maintenance dose

lobster claw deformity A deep congenital cleft between the third and fourth digits of the hands or feet, due to an absence of the central embryologic 'ray'; the LCD is more common in the foot, and is often accompanied by syndactyly of varying severity; the deformity classically occurs in ectodermal dysplasia, eg in the EEC syndrome (ectrodactyly, ectodermal dysplasia and cleft palate), which may be associated with a variety of organ defects

local area network A series of computers that are linked over limited distances by telephone lines or direct cabling, allowing them to share hardware, eg a printer, data, software and software applications; each member in a LAN has its own independent central processing unit, in contrast to mini- and mainframe computers which often communicate in unidirectional fashions, where peripheral 'dummy' terminals largely function as input and query devices

local bus COMPUTERS A type of PC (personal computer) architecture in which certain devices communicate with the CPU (central processing unit) using a special data path or bus that is separate from the main computer bus used for other expansion boards and devices (**CAP Today 4/1994**)

localization procedure RADIOLOGY A generic term for any imaging modality intended to identify the location of a particular lesion, eg a breast or lung mass, or foreign body, eg a bullet, shrapnel, pet rocks

lochkern German, hole-ridden nucleus A vacuolated nucleus that is a commonly seen in both mature fat and lipomas, which may simulate lipoblasts; see Brown fat

lock-and-key model BIOCHEMISTRY A model that assumes an enzyme and substrate have a rigid interaction with each other, where a substrate fits in a key-like fashion to its lock, the enzyme, turning on the reaction; while this concept, formulated by Emil Fisher in the 1890s is essentially correct, the 'induced fit model' is more accurate, as the enzyme molds to the substrate before binding and fully activating an enzyme; see Induced fit model; the lock and key model has become a central theme of cell biology and has been applied to the specificity of antibody-antigen, receptor-ligand interactions, and cell recognition based on surface glycopeptides or carbohydrates (**Sci Am 1993; 268/1:82**)

'locked-in' syndrome REHABILITATION MEDICINE Flaccid tetraplegia with facial paresis and complete incapacity of expression (ie anarthric and aphonic); the LIS is the result of damage or dysfunction of descending motor pathways or peripheral nerves, due to bilateral destruction of the basis pontis or medulla and sparing of tegmentum, caused by infarcts or central pontine myelinolysis; the patients are conscious and alert and only capable of communicating by moving their eyes (voluntary eye movement) and eyelids (blinking)

locked knee Trick knee A knee that is limited in its range of movement because of a loose body ('mouse') in the joint, a tear of the meniscus (often the medial meniscus), or a patellofemoral derangement

'locked lung' Paradoxic bronchospasm, Refractory status asthmaticus A clinical state due to excess use of nebulized isoproterenol, resulting in complete loss of response to epinephrine, aminophyllin, corticosteroids and intermitten positive pressure, which requires weaning from isoproterenol

lockjaw Trismus Spasm of the masseter muscles with stiffness of the jaw caused by tetanospasmin, a neurotoxin produced by *Clostridium tetani*, resulting in unrestrained muscle firing and sustained muscular contraction, which when severe, causes dysphagia or acute respiratory insufficiency by causing prolonged diaphragm contraction

LOCM Low-osmolality contrast medium, see there

locomotion index Leukotactic index A measurement of the ability of leukocytes to migrate in response to chemotactic stimuli; neutrophils are used for in vitro assays of chemotaxis, by either the micropore filter technique or the 'under agarose' method; the leukotactin is obtained from the supernatant of *Escherichia coli* in culture, which measures the white cell's ability to move along a chemoattractive gradient, complement C5 is used to test monocyte chemotaxis; locomotion or chemotaxis is decreased in the congenital lazy leukocyte syndrome or in the face of circulating chemotactic factor inactivator, which is increased in cirrhosis, lepromatous leprosy, sarcoidosis, SLE, Hodgkin's disease, and hairy cell leukemia

locum tenens A term that refers either to 1) A person who is filling another's place for a defined temporary period of time, usually in for vacation coverage, or 2) The position being covered; physicians in a locum tenens ('locum') almost invariably have the same qualifications as the person for whom they are covering

locus control region A '...*genetic element* (ie a sequence of DNA) *that directs tissue-specific levels of gene expression in a predictable manner independent of position effects at the site of integration*.'; although the mechanism by which LCRs function is unknown, they depend on enhancer-like activity which determines tissue-specific expression and chromatin opening domain activity which overcomes the positional effects; each cell type has a characteristic LCR that regulates the expression of other genes (**Nature Medicine 1995; 1:502**)

lod score GENETICS A value representing the logarithm ($\log_{10}$) of the odds (probability) of a gene being linked or associated with a disease; linkage analysis calculates the odds for or against the association of a DNA 'marker', ie a segment of DNA, expressed as a 'lod score'; a lod score of +3 or more indicates a significant probability that the DNA marker is linked to a disease, while a lod score of -2 or less indicates a significant probability that there is no linkage

log Logbook A journal or ledger containing data and dates when the data was collected; logs are used to record scheduling information, document patient-physician encounters, to record quality control data in the laboratory and may be used as a legal document; Cf Notebook

log-cell kill (hypothesis) ONCOLOGY A malignant tumor mass exposed one time to a chemotherapeutic drug will undergo under the best of circumstances a maximum of a 2 log-cell kill, ie reduction to 1% of the original 100% or 10^2 tumor volume; since often a tumor mass may be 10^{12} cells in volume, adequate tumor shrinkage depends on multiple log-cell kills by various effective agents

Note: In contrast to bulk tumor destruction, which is the intended goal of chemotherapy, immunotherapy is effective against small tumor masses but useless when a tumor is > 0.1 cm, and thus theoretically of use in the lower 'log kill' range

logic CLINICAL DECISION-MAKING The sum total of education and experience that is integrated into a physician's medical decision-making processes; see Aunt Millie approach, Heuristic logic, Markov process, ROC analysis, Stochastic process

logic board COMPUTERS The electronic circuitry designed to perform logical functions by a series of logical operations, using logical variables following logical instructions, operating on a two-valued (true or false) system

log-rank test STATISTICS A statistical maneuver used for univariate analyses

log-transformed value STATISTICS A numerical value that is transformed into its logarithmic form merely as a device to facilitate calculations or fitting to a curve

logistic-regression analysis STATISTICS See linear regression

loin pain-hematuria syndrome A benign, relatively rare ($<1/10^6$) condition characterized by recurring episodes of uni– or bilateral loin pain (which may be severe enough to require denervation or autotransplantation) accompanied by hematuria of unknown origin; it is more common in ♀ and may be related to hormonal factors, eg use of oral contraceptives, or to defects in renal vasculature PATHOGENESIS Uncertain; it may be related to alternate pathway complement activation (**Arch Pathol Lab Med 1994; 118:1016ᴏᴀ**) CLINICAL Episodic gross hematuria, pelvic pain and mild hypertension that resolves upon discontinuation of contraceptives

'logs in a stream' pattern MICROBIOLOGY A fanciful descriptor for the elongated blastoconidia that readily dissociate from the pseudohyphae, seen by LM in *Candida*

lollipop' appearance MICROBIOLOGY A fanciful descriptor for the microscopic appearance of stalks of varying lengths of *Blastomyces dermatitidis* conidia when cultured at room temperature

lollipop culture A synonym for an experimental technique for isolating mutant forms of the outer dynein arms in *Chlamydomonas reinhardtii*, a biflagellate unicellular alga used to study the functional, genetic and structural aspects of flagella and their assembly; by shearing a population of cells ('lollipops'), relatively pure amounts of flagella may be obtained for study

lollipop follicles HEMATOPATHOLOGY A fanciful descriptor for the histologic appearance of capillaries ensheathed by collagen extending into a germinal center in the hyaline-vascular form of Castleman's disease or angiofollicular lymphoid hyperplasia, figure

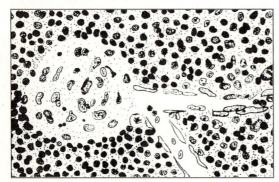

lollipop follicle

lollipop tree appearance A cholangiographic pattern consisting of multiple, variably-sized cystic spaces that freely communicate in and along the intrahepatic biliary ducts in Caroli's disease and congenital hepatic fibrosis

London fog incident A man-made smog (smoke + fog) 'attack' that began on December 5, 1952 when a severe temperature inversion (a blanket of warm air settling over a layer of cooler air, preventing the latter's diffusion) caused a substantial accumulation of air pollutants from fossil fuel combustion, and an abrupt increase in mortality (4000 excess deaths during the five-day period of the inversion), the majority attributed to respiratory diseases; this unique form of London fog '...*left little doubt that air pollution was the cause of the deaths.*' (N Engl J Med 1993; 329:1807ED)

loner PSYCHIATRY A single young man who is estranged from society, who suffers from psychogenic pain, and tends to live 'on the edge', vacillating between aggression and depression; loners often have unrealistic goals, but are unable to work towards those goals PROGNOSIS Guarded; progressive depression, poor functionality, suicidal tendencies

Lone Star tick *Amblyomma americanum* A three-host (wild animal, domestic animal, human) hard tick that is native to the southern US, Central and South America, which is implicated in the transmission of Rocky Mountain spotted fever, and occasionally in the transmission of Lyme disease, see there

long-acting thyroid stimulator LATS A 7S IgG anti-thyroglobulin autoantibody that mimics thyrotropin, which is produced by most patients with Graves' hyperthyroidism, often associated with exophthalmos

Note: The original LATS assay was developed in the mouse; in humans, levels of LATS-related thyroid-stimulating autoantibodies are measured

long interspersed repeated elements LINES, see there

long leg syndrome Short leg syndrome A condition caused by inequity of leg length resulting in mechanical disturbances of gait and posture CLINICAL The first manifestations are back and knee pain, where a persistent deformity causes a compensatory pelvic tilt, lumbar scoliosis, backache and rheumatologic symptoms; the longer leg is held in flexion with excess lateral strain, causing premature degenerative changes and valgus deformity due to a collapse of the lateral compartment

long feedback loop PHYSIOLOGY A self-adjusting circuit in the 'central' endocrine system, where the hypothalamic hormones are schematically represented as an 'axis' consisting of two circuits, the short hypothalamic-adenohypophysis (or pituitary) loop and the long adenohypophysis (or pituitary)-end organ loop; see Loops

long Q-T (interval) syndrome CARDIOLOGY An often underdiagnosed clinical complex defined by Bazett as a prolonged QT interval corrected for heart rate (QT_c) > 0.44 sec, where QT_c is calculated as $^{QT\,observed}/_{(RR)^{1/2}}$ (N Engl J Med 1992; 327:846OA); LQTS is most common in otherwise healthy young females evoked by fright or physical exertion, resulting in episodic syncope, or if the stimulus is extreme, sudden death related to ↑ autonomic tone that occurs during periods of exercise and excitement, eg sudden death while exercising on a hot day due to sudden onset of ventricular arrhythmia; once diagnosed, all related family members should have an EKG, as a prolonged Q-T interval is associated with an ↑ incidence of malignant ventricular arrhythmia, eg 'torsades de pointes' MOLECULAR BIOLOGY LQTS is tightly linked (Lod score: 16.4 = 10^16.4:1 in favor of linkage) to the Harvey ras (H-*ras*-1) oncogene (a gene linked to many different signal transduction pathways) on the short arm of chromosome 11 (Science 1991; 252:704); LQTS may also be induced by drugs, eg antiarrhythmics, phenothiazine, tricyclic antidepressants and lithium, metabolic and electrolyte imbalances, low-energy diets, CNS and autonomic nervous system disease, coronary artery disease and mitral valve prolapse

LQTS also occurs as a symptom in congenital disease, in 1) Jervell-Lange-Nielsen syndrome, an AR [MIM 220400] condition accompanied by deafness and 2) Romano-Ward syndrome, an AD [MIM 192500] condition without deafness

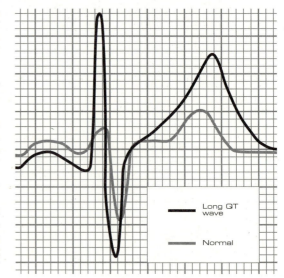

long Q-T syndrome

long-term depression An activity-dependent ↓ in synaptic efficacy that may be an important mechanism* permitting neural networks to store information more effectively; LTD appears to be in part the result of a signalling pathway in which calcineurin dephosphorylates, inactivating inhibitor-1, which in turn ↑ serine/threonine protein phosphatase 1 activity (**Nature 1994; 369:486ₗₜₙ**)

*Similar but opposite that of long-term potentiation

long-term potentiation NEUROPHYSIOLOGY A type of synaptic plasticity that is thought to form the molecular and cellular basis of learning and memory, in which neural connections (synapses) corresponding to new information are strengthened; the LTP model supported by quantal analysis, a technique that determines the physical signal passing across a synapse from one neuron to another, implies that synaptic strengthening is presynaptic and relatively permanent; induction of LTP requires transient activation of the NMDA receptor system; during low-frequency transmission, NMDA activation is prevented by GABA-mediated synaptic inhibition; during high-frequency transmission, the GABA block is reduced by a GABA autoregulatory mechanism, permitting induction of LTP (**Nature 1991; 349:609**); see Long-term depression, Neural network, Synaptic plasticity

long-term survival with HIV infection Non-progressive HIV infection, see there

long terminal repeat see LTR

longevity The condition of having a long life, or having lived a long life; the average life expectancy of adults continues to spiral upward, and it is thought that the upper limit of average human life expeectancy range from 85 to 100 (**N Engl J Med 1995; 332:999sa**) see Lifespan

longitudinal magnetization M$_Z$ MRI The component of the macroscopic magnetization vector along the static magnetic field; after excitation by a radiofrequency pulse, M$_z$ will approach its equilibrium value designated M$_o$, with a characteristic time constant, T1; see Magnetic resonance imaging

longitudinal relaxation MRI The return of longitudinal magnetization to its equilibrium value after excitation, which requires exchange of energy between the nuclear spins and lattice; see Magnetic resonance imaging

longitudinal study EPIDEMIOLOGY A study design that evaluates the effects over time of one or more variables on a process, eg the Port Pirie study, an ongoing analysis of the long-term effects of blood lead levels on IQ (**N Engl J Med 1992; 327:1285oa**)

'look-back' program PUBLIC HEALTH An organized study of subjects exposed to a disease, usually infectious, from whom specimens, eg sera, epidemiologic, demographic or other data is examined retrospectively to determine whether the subjects are currently infected; look-back programs have been developed during the AIDS epidemic to evaluate HIV antibody seroconversion in subjects exposed to potentially contaminated blood products (prior to the availability of serum screening assays) or who were treated by HIV-positive health care providers, from whom the possibility of HIV antibody seroconversion, is considered minimal, but which will have a major impact on the liability industry

loop Feedback loop, see there

loop diuretics NEPHROLOGY A family of therapeutic agents that are the most potent diuretics in clinical use; LDs act on Henle's loop, especially on the thick ascending limb, causing excretion of 20-25% of the filtered Na⁺; these 'high-ceiling' diuretics are most indicated in pulmonary edema, CHF, and renal impairment and include furosemide and ethacrinic acid, which ↑ renin, angiotensin II, and prostaglandins and ↑ natriuresis by inhibiting the sodium-potassium-chloride cotransport system, which is responsible for solute resorption in the thick ascending loop of Henle; since both agents are secreted in the tubular lumen by the organic acid pathway, they are less effective in the presence of endogenous or exogenous organic acids; because loop agents cause marked hypokalemia, they may be used in tandem with other potassium-sparing diuretics

loop extrasurgical excision procedure LEEP, see there

loop-to-loop pattern A fanciful descriptor for the arrangement of clusters of endometrial cells seen in endometrial cytology specimens from patients with IUDs

lop ear A prominent deformity of the external ear resulting from the lack of bending of the cartilage forming the antihelix TREATMENT Cosmetic surgery before age 5, when auricle is more fully developed; Cf Cauliflower ear

Lorenzo's oil A concoction of oleic and erucic acids alleged to be useful in treating adrenoleukodystrophy or adrenomyeloneuropathy SIDE EFFECTS Thrombocytopenia, neutropenia, and lymphocytopenia with immunosuppression and recurrent infections (**N Engl J Med 1993; 329:745c, 1994; 330o:577c**)

Note: The popular term for this mixture of fatty acids originates from a popular movie, *Lorenzo's Oil*, that left the impression with many lay persons and assorted non-cognoscenti that it was therapeutically useful

loss-of-function mutation A gene mutation that results in the loss of a particular function, eg tumor suppressor activity (p53) or production of a particular protein, eg an enzymopathy; Cf Gain-of-function mutation

loss of heterozygosity An 'adjective' referring to a mutation that results in the loss of allelic uniqueness, which is often defined as a ≥ 40% ↑ in signal intensity of allelic signal; LOH of chromosome 17 is linked to mutations of the tumor suppressor gene p53, and in one study occurred in 80% of bladder cancers, and in another report, in ⅓ of colorectal carcinoma genes; LOH is most frequently identified in certain chromosomal regions, including 5q, 17p, and 18q (see **Diagn Mol Pathol 1993; 2:90**)

'loss leader' A business term for an item sold to the public at or below the original cost in order to entice the customer to purchase other, more expensive items; in the health care industry, a 'loss leader' is a service provided below cost, in order to attract (well-insured) patients to return and refer other patients in need of services that produce income above the cost of the 'loss leader'; in hospitals, the emergency room was considered a 'loss leader' that would increase the hospital's census, filling beds and increasing hospital revenues; with the Medicare reforms under TEFRA in 1982, it became apparent that emergency rooms often attracted financially 'undesirable' patients with inadequate insurance coverage; consequently some private hospitals have closed their emergency rooms; see Dumping, Skimming, TEFRA

lossless compression COMPUTERS/TELEMEDICINE An evolving format of data compression that allows both the efficient compression and accurate decompression at the receivin endg; 'lossy' compression is usually adequate for transmission of visual images that have no potential medicolegal liability; in the interpretive fields of telepathology and teleradiology, few physicians are willing to compromise themselves by rendering formal opinions on images from which blocks of diagnostic information is absent (**Am Med News 1995; 17 April 1995 p19**) see Telemedicine; Cf Codec, Modem, T-1; see Data compression

lossy compression see Data compression

lot A batch of a manufactured product, eg chemicals, drugs, reagents, or specimen tubes, which were produced or packaged from one production run, simultaneously subjected to quality control testing; the identification of defects in a lot of a material by number allows rapid localization of the entire run and recall of the product

Lot syndrome Lot's wife syndrome Hypercalcinosis A fanciful descriptor for a rare condition characterized by exuberant 'metastatic' calcification (mineralization) of soft tissues due to 1) Hyperparathyroidism and/or hypervitaminosis D with massive bone resorption or 2) Chronic hypodipsic hypernatremia A condition with normal blood volume and renal function

The condition is named after the biblical Lot and his wife, who turned for one last look at the sinful city of Sodom and turned into a 'pillar of salt'

Lou Gehrig disease Amyotrophic lateral sclerosis, see there

The popular (trivial) name used in the US for amyotrophic lateral sclerosis, named after Lou Gehrig, the 'Iron Horse', a first baseman for the New York Yankees (1925-39), who played 2130 consecutive major league games (a record that remains unbeaten); he died of the disease in 1941, thereby immortalizing the disease Note: Stephen Hawking, cosmologist also suffers from the condition

louse A flat wingless parasitic insect that is divided into

BITING LICE, Order Mallophaga, which rarely affect humans and

SUCKING LICE, Order Anoplua, family Pediculidae, which are global in distribution, and serve as either

1) Disease vectors, eg *Borrelia recurrentis* (*Bhermisi turcatae, B parkeri*) or

2) Are themselves the cause of the disease *Pediculus humanis capitis* head lice, *Pediculus humanis corporis* body lice, *Phthirus pubis* crab or pubic louse

louse-borne fever see Relapsing fever

Louisiana hot sauce A condiment with various formulae (horseradish, lemon, tabasco, ketchup, etc) that has been shown to inhibit the in vivo growth of *Vibrio vulnificus* and other vibrio that often contaminate raw shellfish, eg oysters; the component responsible for the protective effect has not been identified (New York Times 19 Oct 1993; C3)

lovastatin Mevacor® A lipid-lowering drug of the 3-hydroxy-3-methyl-glutaryl coenzyme A (HMG-CoA) reductase inhibitor family; lovastatin is a partial inhibitor of HMG-CoA reductase activity in early cholesterol synthesis, allowing sufficient mevalonate production to provide adequate cholesterol for cell membrane function and steroidogenesis; it is well tolerated, lowering LDL-cholesterol an average of 41%, while raising HDL-cholesterol 10% (Am J Cardiol 1990; 66:Symposium); in healthy volunteers, it ↓ LDL-cholesterol by 35%, apolipoprotein-B by 25%, VLDL-cholesterol and IDL-cholesterol by 30-40%, and ↑ HDL-cholesterol by 10%; clinical 'logic' to the contrary, use of high doses of lovastatin to lower the serum lipid levels prior to percutaneous coronary angioplasty neither prevents nor delays restenosis (N Engl J Med 1994; 331:1331OA) LABORATORY ↓ Total cholesterol, ↓ LDL-cholesterol, ↓ triglycerides, ↑ HDL-cholesterol; lovastatin has an additive effect when combined with a low-fat–low-cholesterol diet on improving the lipid profile (N Engl J Med 1993; 328:1213OA) Cf Cholesterol-lowering drugs, Gemfibrozil; HMG CoA reductase inhibitors

Love Canal ENVIRONMENT A major site of toxic contamination of soil and water, which became one of the first targets for the US Environmental Protection Agency's 'Superfund'; Love Canal was dug in 1892 by William Love for an industrial complex near Niagara Falls, New York and was used from 1947-53 as an industrial dump by a chemical and plastic manufacturer; after a heavy rainfall in 1976, the canal began to leak 82 different chemicals, 11 of which were carcinogens; the local residents whose drinking water was contaminated from the canal had an increased rate of spontaneous abortions, birth defects, cancer, urinary tract and hepatic disease; see Bhopal, Bitterfeld, Haff disease, Minamata disease, Times Beach

the 'love drug' see Ectasy

'love handles' A colloquial term for the bilateral overhangs of adipose and soft tissues on the antero-lateral flank that are relatively common in older men; LHs are refractory to dieting and of little importance, except as occasional barriers to medical communication, causing

accidental detonation of beepers (N Engl J Med 1991; 324:1517c)

love-hate relationship Ambivalence PSYCHIATRY A clinical complex characterized by essential changes in Freudian impulses; love-hate is normal for children passing through the 'anal-sadistic' phase of development, in which there is both love and 'murderous' hatred toward the same object, often occurring simultaneously; in the normal course of personality development, most of this aggression is neutralized and what remains becomes a desire to win out over (rather than destroy) the other person; in obsessive-compulsive disorders, the person consciously expresses both the love and hate components and thus is stuck in repeating cycles of doing and undoing behaviorisms; Cf Passive-aggression

'love' surgery Vulvovaginoplasty A virtually abandoned vaginal operation for treating '*coitally connected inflammation of the bladder and internal pain with intercourse, ie dyspareunia*'; the operation entailed '*rotation of the vaginal axis away from alignment with the internal genitalia and bladder*'; the physician who performed these operations claimed the procedure increased penile-clitoral contact during intercourse, although in some cases, it left the patient with painful sequelae; the 'love surgeon' has retired from practice and is living on Social Security income in Florida (Am Med News 17 October 1994 p32) Cf Female circumcision

lover's heels FORENSIC MEDICINE A comminuted intra-articular fracture of the os calcis with severe crush injury to the bones of the foot with major anatomic distortion, described in 'jilted' lovers who jump from major heights, see Jumper syndrome INFECTIOUS DISEASE A fanciful synonym for gonococcal tenosynovitis of the Achilles tendon

Note: Migratory gonococcal arthritis is usually pauciarticular, affecting the knees, ankles, elbows and wrists and resolves spontaneously

Lovejoy's classification A classification (table) for the severity of neurological disease in Reye syndrome

LOVEJOY'S CLASSIFICATION (COMA STAGES IN REYE SYNDROME)
1) Vomiting, lethargy and sleepiness
2) Combativeness, hyperventilation, hyperreflexia, responsive to noxious stimuli
3) Obtunded, comatose with decorticate activity; intact cranial nerves
4) Deepening coma, decerebrate activity, no cranial nerve response
5) No deep tendon reflexes, respiratory arrest

low back pain Discomfort of the lower lumbar region, which in the US is the second most common cause (after the common cold) for seeking medical care; low back pain affects ± 31 million US citizens at any given time and costs $8 x 10⁹/year DIAGNOSIS MRI examination of lumbosacral spine; in one study, MRI scans from normal subjects were examined by neuroradiologists; 52% had a bulge at one or more levels, 27% had a protrusion, 1% had an extrusion; 38% had an abnormality at more than one level Conclusion: Bulges and protrusions of the disk on MRI examination are common in normal subjects, and appear to be coincidental findings (N Engl J Med 1994; 331:69OA)

'low back syndrome' A generic term for any complaint referable to the lower back, attributable to degenerative, infectious, neoplastic or traumatic origin; the low back syndrome may be acute or chronic, temporary or permanent, congenital or acquired and is quite common in the older, especially female population

low birthweight NEONATOLOGY A 'condition' in a newborn infant that is often a risk factor *a sui generis* for morbidity in early infancy; LBW is defined as an infant who at birth weighs less than 2500 g; moderate LBW is 1500-

OUTCOMES, VERY-LOW-BIRTHWEIGHT CHILDREN			
BIRTHWEIGHT	≤ 750 g	> X <	≥ 1.5 Kg
Sample number	68	65	61
MPC score*	87	93	100
Mental retardation (IQ < 70)	21%	8%	2%
Poor cognitive function	22%	9%	2%
Poor academic skills	27%	9%	2%
Poor gross motor function	27%	9%	0%
Poor adaptive function	25%	14%	2%
Cerebral palsy	9%	6%	0%
Severe visual disability	25%	5%	2%
Hearing disability	24%	13%	3%
< Normal Wt/Ht/HS	22/25/35%	11/5/14%	0/0/2%‰

*Mental Processing Composite score **N Engl J Med 1994; 331:753
Ht Head size HS Head size Wt Weight

2500 g; very low LBW infants weigh less than 1500 g, a group accounting for 50% of neonatal mortality (85-95% survival if more than 1250 g, 65-75% survival if more than 800 g, 2% survival if less than 600 g) WORLD RECORDS The lowest birthweight recorded for a child with normal mental and psychomotor development is 380 g (**N Engl J Med 1990; 322:1753c**), a delivery necessitated by hypertension and coagulopathy; the lowest birthweight recorded for a long-term surviving infant, albeit with a low IQ is 280 g (**ibid, 1991; 324:1599c**); central to neonatal survival is control of fluid balances and modern neonatal 'hardware', including radiant warmers, phototherapy, ventilators, arterial catheters, cardiorespiratory monitors; 6-7% of US neonates have LBW, the rate in blacks is twice that of white infants, an incidence that declined until 1985, followed by reversal (**MMWR 1990; 39:137, 148**) Relevant definitions **APPROPRIATE FOR GESTATIONAL AGE** An adjective applied to an infant whose gestational age and weight are synchronous according to standardized age and growth curves **INTRAUTERINE GROWTH RETARDATION** A generic term for any delay in achieving intrauterine developmental milestones, most commonly related to maternal drug, tobacco and alcohol abuse **SMALL FOR GESTATIONAL AGE** An adjective applied to an infant whose gestational age and weight gain are below that expected for age, most common in infants exposed in utero to drugs of abuse (cocaine 93 g decrease, marijuana 79 g, tobacco 200-400 g; 26% of SGA infants have severe mental impairment, which can be reduced to 4% if they are given daily activities in intensive care unit, massages, and audiotaped conversation from their parents and classical music; weight gain is faster and neurological development improved with increased levels of dopamine, norepinephrine and epinephrine in the urine of premature infants treated with massage, which reduces incubator time and shortens the length of intensive hospital-based care; prophylactic ligation of the patent ductus arteriosus at the time of birth may reduce the incidence of necrotizing enterocolitis, but has no effect on bronchopulmonary dysplasia, retinopathy or intraventricular hemorrhage; SGA infants are at ↑ risk for future developmental disability, which can be reduced by early intervention (including neonatal nursery, home visits, child development centers and parent groups), increasing the average IQ and is associated with fewer behavioral problems in the future; see Prematurity

low cardiac output syndrome Forward failure 'syndrome' A clinical condition in which the cardiac output falls below the tissue needs for oxygen LABORATORY Increased vascular resistance and oxygen consumption, lactic acidosis, decreased cardiac index, and oxygen saturation TREATMENT Digitalis, vasopressors, dopamine, dobutamine, vasodilatation PROGNOSIS Poor if unresponsive to drugs

low-density lipoprotein LDL A plasma lipoprotein with a density of 1.019-1.063 kg/L (SI), which is 23% protein (predominantly apoB-100), 27% phospholipid, 62% cholesterol and cholesterol esters and 11% triglycerides, and transports cholesterol from the intestine to the liver, and is a major transporter of cholesterol that binds to the LDL receptor at apo-B100, inhibiting cellular 3-hydroxy-3-methyl-glutamyl coenzyme A reductase (HMG CoA, which synthesizes cholesterol) and regulating LDL-receptor expression on membranes; defective LDL-receptor is implicated in certain forms of hypercholesterolemia and may be responsible for accelerated atherosclerosis; in early atherosclerotic lesions, fatty streaks and foam cells accumulate in the arterial wall, in a sequence that is mediated by a variant LDL-receptor, the acetyl (or 'scavenger') LDL-receptor, which has a high affinity for oxidized and abnormal LDL, possibly induced by macrophages through lipo-oxygenase and/or generation of oxygen free radicals, changes that can be abolished with antioxidants, eg vitamin E Note: Acetyl LDL-receptor does not recognize normal LDL, but does recognize oxidized LDL, a molecule with other biochemical modifications including conversion of LDL lecithin to lysolecithin, oxidation of cholesterol, increasing negative charge and LDL density, while decreasing polyunsaturated fats (due to oxidation), LDL receptor-mediated uptake, degradation of apoB100 (histidine, lysine and proline); oxidated LDL chemotactically attracts monocytes; this model of atherogenesis may be valid in vivo as probucol (an antioxidant) slows the atherogenic process in rabbits; LDL receptors regulate the amount of circulating ligands (apoB-100 and apoE) by internalizing them BIOCHEMISTRY LDL is subdivided by ultracentrifugation into an LDLA profile composed of large, light LDL molecules, present in 70% of humans and an LDL$_B$ profile composed of small, dense and heavy LDL molecules, a pattern associated with a higher risk for heart disease in a small cohort; studies in a Mormon cohort suggest that a single gene regulates a subject's LDL 'A-ness' or 'B-ness'

Note: The LDL-receptor, which netted the 1984 Nobel prize in medicine and physiology, may not play a major role in the early stages of atherosclerosis, a condition occurring in the animal model for atherosclerosis, the Watanabe rabbit, which lacks LDL receptors

low–fat diet see Diet

low-frequency antigen Private antigen TRANSFUSION MEDICINE A red cell antigen that is uncommon in the general population, and thus rarely associated with antibody production, eg C^x, C^w, He, Lu^{a+b-}, Sw^a, Wr^a

low-grade squamous intraepithelial lesion GYNECOLOGIC CYTOLOGY A lesion defined by an array of cytopathologic findings (cells occur singly or in sheets, nuclear abnormalities in cells with mature cytoplasm, bi- or multinucleation, well-defined optically clear perinuclear halo, distinct cell borders and others) that translate into either HPV infection or mild dysplasia (CIN 1) of the uterine cervix (a diagnosis made on histologic examination of biopsied tissue); in contrast to high-grade squamous intraepithelial lesion, the diagnosis of LSIL does not force the clinician to take further action, and he/she can either follow the patient or excise a portion of the cervix by cone biopsy, or by LEEP (**RJ Kurman, D Solomon, The Bethesda System, Springer-Verlag, New York, 1994**) Cf High-grade squamous intraepithelial lesion

low-grade lymphoma A group of relatively indolent lymphomas classified according to the Working Formulation (**Cancer 1982; 49:2112**) that have a prolonged survival of 5 to 7.5 years, often with minimal therapy; low-grade lymphomas include the small lymphocytic (plasmacytoid) lymphoma, follicular small cleaved cell lymphoma, follicular mixed small cleaved and large cell lymphoma; see Lymphoma, REAL classification, Working Formulation

low-impact sport SPORTS MEDICINE A generic term for any physical activity or sport in which there is minimal wear and trauma to weight bearing joints, in particular of the foot, knee, and hip; LISs include golfing and bowling; participation is LISs is encouraged in those who wish to engage in physical activities after hip and knee arthroplasty (Mayo Clin Proc 1995; 70:342oA) Cf High-impact sport, Moderate impact sport, No-impact sport

low-level laser therapy Cold laser therapy, see there

low-level (radioactive) waste A specific form of (man-made) radioactive waste for which there is reasonable assurance that public exposure (should it occur) presents only a fraction of the current dose limits; LRW is divided into 3 classes based on the time to radionuclide decay and storage requirementsis

CLASS A Decay to harmless levels in < 100 years

CLASS B Decay to harmless levels in < 200 years

CLASS C Decay to harmless levels in < 300 years, or behind concrete barriers with an expected structural integrity of ≥ 500 years

extremely low-level radioactive waste, eg ^{3}H, ^{14}C, and ^{35}S, may in some jurisdictions be released into the sewer system; see Plutonium, Radioactive waste; Cf High-level waste

low-molecular-weight heparin A form of heparin used to treat deep vein thrombosis (DVT); compared to standard heparin, LMW heparin has a higher bioavailability, longer half-life, and does not require monitoring the degree of anticoagulation; in contrast to warfarin therapy for DVT, LMW heparin is more expensive, but easier to monitor; it is associated with a lower incidence of DVT but an increased bleeding intensity (N Engl J Med 1993; 329:1370oA) Ardeparin sodium, like other LMWHs is reported to ↓ the incidence of DVT in patients undergoing prosthetic replacement of the hip or knee (Am J Clin Pathol 1995; 103:642oA)

low-osmolality contrast medium RADIOLOGY Any of a group of radiologic contrast media first used in Europe which are said to have fewer side effects after intravenous injections, but which are more expensive and may cause hypercoagulability

low-output gastrointestinal fistula An external (ie communicates with the skin) gastrointestinal fistula that produces less than 200 ml of fluid, originating from the distal small intestine and large intestine; Cf High-output fistula

low-pass sequencing MOLECULAR BIOLOGY A generic term for the superficial scanning through a genome to identify any useful (ie non-'junk') DNA sequences (Science 1995; 268:1270)

low quality protein CLINICAL NUTRITION A protein usually of plant origin that lacks one or more essential amino acid, eg corn, which is low in lysine, or beans, which are low in tryptophan; the poor quality of protein is a major impediment to progress in developing nations, which responds to a simple expediency of succotash, a gruel containing both foods; low quality protein in the form of the 'liquid diet' had transient currency in the US 'weight loss industry' and resulted in a number of deaths prior to its abandonment; see Liquid diet; Cf Succotash

low-stringency hybridization MOLECULAR BIOLOGY A hybridization between two molecules capable of forming nucleotide base pair dimers, eg DNA with DNA or DNA with RNA under conditions that allow 'sloppy' alignment of bases; the stringency of a hybridization can be controlled by titrating the temperature and salt concentrations

low T$_3$ syndrome Euthyroid sick syndrome, see there

low T$_4$ syndrome A 'laboratory' disease seen in patients undergoing regular hemodialysis or continuous ambulatory peritoneal dialysis, in which 40% have serum T$_4$ (thyroxine) < than 5 µg/dl but who have normal free T$_4$ levels

low-tar cigarettes Cigarettes that are lower than average in nicotines and tars; a 50% reduction in tar is thought to result in a 20% reduction in lung cancer mortality; smokers of 'low-yield' cigarettes do not have a lower incidence of myocardial infarction, possibly due to deeper inhalation of pollutants by these smokers; see Non-smoking tobacco, 'Pack-year', Passive smoking, Smoking

'low-yield' medicine A philosophical posture for practicing medicine that encompasses services that provide minimal patient benefit, the value of which to the patient is less than society's cost in providing them; forms of low-yield medicine include such 'excesses' as an extra test, doctor visit, or day in the hospital; in general if the insurance is there to allow for 'extras', the conscientious physician is likely to order them; like the practice of defensive medicine (see there), the 'low-yield' form of practice is a major factor in the cost-containment debate (JAMA 1993; 269:631oc)

lower esophageal sphincter A 3-5 cm in length zone of increased pressure at the junction of the distal esophagus with the gastric cardia, located at the hiatus, which forms a physical barrier in preventing gastric reflux

lower explosive limit OCCUPATIONAL SAFETY LEL The lowest concentration (% volume in air) of a dust, fume, gas, mist, or vapor that is capable of combustion or explosion if a source of ignition is present

lozenge Troche, see there

L-phase bacteria L-form, see there

LPR Late phase reaction, see there

LPS Lipopolysaccharide

LPSTGE A highly conserved six-residue (Leu-Pro-Ser-Thr-Gly-Glu) oligopeptide that is adjacent to the hydrophobic region of all known surface proteins of gram-positive bacteria and required for their attachment; see M protein

LQT1, LQT2, LQT3 Three distinct genes located on chromosomes 11, 7, and 3 respectively, that have been linked to the long QT syndrome; *LQT2* encodes a K$^+$ ion channel and *LQT3* encodes a Na$^+$ ion channels, either of which when mutated, have increased activity and an ↑ in cardiac excitability and ↑ arrhythmias (Cell in NY Times March 14 1995, C12)

LQTS Long Q-T interval syndrome, see there

LRR Leucine-rich repeat, see there

L/S ratio OBSTETRICS The ratio of lecithin (phosphatidyl choline) to sphingomyelin, a 'bench' parameter used to determine infant lung maturity and predict the infant's ability to survive without developing respiratory distress; surface-active lecithin appears in the amniotic fluid at 24-26 gestational weeks; sphingomyelin is similarly produced but remains relatively constant; before the 32nd week, the L/S ratio is less than 1.5, after the 34th week, the L/S ratio is > than 2.0, which corresponds to an adequate level of surfactant for adequate extra-uterine pulmonary function LABORATORY L/S ratio may be determined by TLC and 2-D chromatography, the latter of which has fewer false negatives; see Biophysical profile, Lung profile, Respiratory distress syndrome

Note: The L/S ratio is plague by problems, which is an impetus to find better tests, including general insensitivity, nonspecificity among diabetic mothers, and interference by blood and meconium staining of the amniotic fluid

LS and A Lichen sclerosis et atrophicus, see Lichen sclerosis

LSD D-Lysergic acid diethylamide A synthetic indole amine with hallucinogenic activity that derives from ergot alkaloids that produces mood elevations, sensory distortion, depersonalization which may provoke panic attacks and flashbacks DOSES LSD is 3000– to 5000-fold more potent that mescaline; in adults, 100-150 µg is enough for a 'trip' CLINICAL-PSYCHOMIMETIC EFFECTS Spatial and temporal distortion, illusions, animation, hyperacusis and background amplification, distortion of body image, sensory hallucinations with the hearing of smells and sights, smelling of images and sounds, seeing smells and sounds and others CLINICAL-SYMPATHOMIMETIC & PARASYMPATHOMIMETIC EFFECTS Dilated pupils, ↑ heart rate, ↑ body temperature, ↑ salivation, ↑ lacrimation, ↑ sweating, nausea, vomiting DIAGNOSIS Physical examination, laboratory methods: GC-MS, HPLC, RIA, TLC ADVERSE EFFECTS Bad trips characterized by fear of insanity, depersonalization; flashbacks, which may occur 5-10 x/day and up to 18 months or more after last use of LSD (Clin Chem News Aug 1993) see Designer drugs, 'Ice'

LSD was first synthesized by A Hoffmann of Sandoz Laboratories in 1938; it was used during the 1950s as an analgesic for the terminally ill, and to treat various 'psychologic' disorders, eg alcoholism, autism, psychoneurosis, sexual disorders, and sociopathy; produced illicitly, it was popularized during the 'hippie' movement of the 1960s for its 'mind-expanding' hallucinogenic and psychedelic properties, but subsequently fell into disuse, although its popularity is thought to be resurging; it is unclear how teratogenic LSD is, as most of the data is anecdotal

LSIL Low-grade squamous intraepithelial lesion, see there

LTD Long-term depression, see there

LTP Long-term potentiation, see there

LTR Long terminal repeats MOLECULAR BIOLOGY The two end segments of 250-1200 base pairs in length double-stranded retroviral DNA that are synthesized by reverse transcriptase of retroviral origin; LTRs contain many of the signals required for retroviral function, including promoter and enhancer sequences, polyadenylation sites, and encode peptides integral to integrating the virus into the host genome; see HIV, HTLV, Retrovirus

LTS see Latent tetany syndrome

lucid interval NEUROLOGY A period of time preceding the loss of consciousness and coma that occurs in subdural and epidural hematomas, and intracranial edema; Cf Window period

luciferase Any of a number of enzymes responsible for the bioluminescent reaction of the certain organisms, in particular the firefly [*Photinus*, EC 1.13.12.7*], but also other photoluminescing organisms, eg bacteria and coelenterates, which catalyzes the oxidation of luciferin, releasing a photon of light; this reaction can be modified to allow detection of molecules present in low levels in both the clinical and research laboratories; see Chemiluminescence

*Known as *Photinus*-luciferin 4-mono-oxygenase (ATP-hydrolysing), the term recommended (1992) by the Nomenclature Committee of the IUBMB (International Union of Biochemistry and Molecular Biology)

Lucy AL 288-1 ANTHROPOLOGY The trivial name given to a female hominid (*Australopithecus afarensis*) skeleton that was discovered in the Afar Triangle of Ethiopia in 1974, the pelvis of which indicates that modern man probably walked erect about 3 million years ago; in contrast to the relatively vertical chimpanzee pelvis, in which babies are delivered without rotation, Lucy's children needed a ¼ turn for delivery, while the relatively flat modern human pelvis, adapted for bipedalism, requires the fetus to make a full turn in order to successfully pass out of the birth canal; see Anthropology, Eve; Cf Mitochondrial Eve, Vole clock

LUF syndrome Luteinized unruptured follicle syndrome A condition characterized by the development of a dominant follicle without disruption and release of the ovum, an abnormality diagnosed by ultrasonography or laparoscopy; LUD is thought to be an extremely rare and sporadic cause of infertility

luftsichel sign German, Air crescent RADIOLOGY A curved often left-sided perihilar opacification seen on a plain antero-posterior chest film that is characteristic of upper lobe atelectasis, due to interposition of the lower lobe apex over the atelectatic upper lobe

Lugol's solution GYNECOLOGY An iodine solution that colors the normal uterine cervix a homogeneous brown color when seen by colposcopy; any alterations in the color may indicate an underlying defect in the glycogen content of the cervical epithelium that may be associated with cervical carcinoma and appear as a whitish discoloration

Lukes-Collins classification HEMATOLOGY A classification of non-Hodgkin's lymphomas proposed by Lukes and Collins in 1974 (Cancer 1974; 34:1488) that related cell morphology to lymphocyte lineage; like the Kiel (KC) classification, the LCC recognizes follicular nodularity as a marker of B cell differentiation, but uses the terms cleaved and noncleaved follicle center cells for the centrocyte and centroblast of the KC; after 1982, the Working Formulation (for classifying lymphomas) became popular; it is uncertain whether the recently proposed REAL classification will replace this surfeit of classifications; Cf REAL classification, Working Formulation

lumone A hormone of the GI lumen; see Incretins

lumpectomy Segmental mastectomy SURGICAL ONCOLOGY A cosmetically acceptable, but variably complete excision of breast carcinoma; lumpectomy of early (< 4.0 cm) breast carcinoma combined with radiotherapy offers a 90% five-year survival* (JAMA 1991; 265:391) the American College of Surgeons has taken no official position regarding the definition or applicability of 'lumpectomy'; some data suggest that a lumpectomy with axillary lymph node dissection may be as effective as a mastectomy in treating carcinoma of the breast; Cf Lesionectomy, Radical mastectomy ONCOLOGY Stage I and II breast cancer treated with breast conserving therapy (lumpectomy, axillary node dissection, and irradiation) and modified radical mastectomy offer similar results at 10 years of followup (N Engl J Med 1995; 332:907oA)

*Recurrence of breast carcinoma is often a late event, thus 10- and 15-year survival statistics are more relevant than five-year survival statistics

lumping Reductionism CLINICAL DECISION-MAKING The practice of aggregating diseases or pathologic nosologies with variably distinct features under a common term; 'lumpers' take a pragmatic approach to the diagnosis and treatment of various diseases, rather than attempt to differentiate among subtle subclassifications, recognizing that these distinctions may be arbitrary and/or artificial; Cf 'Splitting'

lumpy-bumpy pattern RENAL PATHOLOGY A pattern seen by immunofluorescent microscopy, which consists in granular deposits of IgG and C3 along the glomerular basement membrane, caused by a wide variety of conditions, including serum sickness nephritis (exogenous foreign proteins), exogenous antigens (bacterial endocarditis, leprosy, syphilis, hepatitis B, malaria), endogenous antigens (DNA, thyroglobulin, tumor-associated antigens)

lumpy deposits see Humps

lumpy jaw INFECTIOUS DISEASE A jaw characterized by painful, 'wood-hard' fibrotic induration of the parotid and submandibular regions, arising in a background of dental disease (caries, periodontitis or extractions), characteristic of cervicofacial actinomyces, the most common form of actinomyces infection; lumpy jaw in humans is caused by *A israeli*, *A meueri*, *A naeslundi*, *A odontolyticus*, and *Arachnia propionica*; lumpy jaw in cows is caused by *A bovis*; other manifestations of cervicofacial actinomycosis include trismus, multiple draining sinus tracts bearing the classic yellow-white sulfur granules, fever, leukocytosis, extension to the facial soft tissue, bone and if untreated, the CNS TREATMENT Penicillin

lung cancer Lung carcinoma is the most common cause

of cancer death accounting for 30% of the cancer deaths in the USA, the vast majority of which is directly attributed to tobacco abuse; once diagnosed, the average patient survives one to two years, with 5-10% surviving five years after diagnosis; the prognosis of small cell (undifferentiated) carcinoma is slightly better than the more differentiated squamous cell and bronchoalveolar carcinomas, assuming they respond to chemotherapy

LUNG CARCINOMA, CLASSIFICATION

% TOTAL	TYPE I	5-YEAR SURVIVAL II	III
38% SQUAMOUS CELL (EPIDERMOID)	38%	16%	9%
23% ADENOCARCINOMA	32%	7%	3%
a) Papillary adenocarcinoma			
b) Alveolar cell			
c) Bronchiolar carcinoma			
d) Mucinous adenocarcinoma			
e) Adenosquamous carcinoma			
29% UNDIFFERENTIATED SMALL CELL	0%	0%	0%
a) Oat cell carcinoma			
b) Intermediate cell type			
c) Combined oat cell type			
9% UNDIFFERENTIATED LARGE CELL	30%	6%	5%
Rare GIANT CELL CARCINOMA	Highly lethal		

lung profile NEONATOLOGY A 2-D chromatograph prepared on a thin plate of silica gel containing 5% ammonium sulfate from an acetone-precipitated lipid extract of bloody amniotic fluid; the lung profile allows determination of relative amounts of lecithin, sphingomyelin, phosphatidyl glycerol, phosphatidyl inositol and phosphatidyl serine (measured by densitometry after charring) and in experienced hands allows determination of fetal lung maturity; in the presence of phosphatidyl glycerol, respiratory distress syndrome does not occur; see L/S ratio; Cf Organ panels

lung stones Broncholiths Calcification of necrotic and/or infected tissue within bronchioles, secondary to tuberculosis, histoplasmosis, sarcoidosis and papillary carcinoma

lung transplantation The transplantation of a lung allograft into a patient whose lungs are failing; the early days of the procedure were characterized by problems with surgical technique, resolved in part by the use an omental flap, and suboptimal immunosuppression which caused acute and chronic rejection, resolved in part by newer immunosuppressants, eg cyclosporine; approximately 200 patients per year (US) receive lung transplants for various indications, one lung is transplanted in pulmonary fibrosis, both lungs in diffuse pulmonary disease, eg cystic fibrosis, bronchiectasis, emphysema and both the heart and lungs in cases where there is combined pulmonary disease and end-stage heart disease (**N Engl J Med 1990; 322:727, 772**); cost $240 000, $47 000 annual maintenance; Survival 70% at one year, 55% overall; some cases have survived more than five years; see Cyclosporin, Domino-donor transplantation, Tacrolimus (FK506), UNOS

lung volumes PHYSIOLOGY A group of air 'compartments' into which the lung may be functionally divided **EXPIRATORY RESERVE CAPACITY** (ERV) The maximum volume of air that can be voluntarily exhaled **FUNCTIONAL RESIDUAL CAPACITY** (FRV) Volume left in the lungs at the end of a normal breath which is not normally part of the subdivisions **INSPIRATORY CAPACITY** (IC) The maximum volume that can be inhaled **INSPIRATORY RESERVE CAPACITY** (IRC) The maximum volume that can be inhaled above the tidal volume **TIDAL VOLUME** (V_T) The normal to-and-fro respiratory exchange of 500 cc; vital capacity is the maximum amount of exhalable air; after a full inspiration, which added to the residual volume, is the total lung capacity **TOTAL LUNG CAPACITY** (TLC) The entire volume of the lung, circa 5 liters **VITAL CAPACITY** (VC) The maximum volume that can be inhaled and exhaled

lupoid hepatitis An autoimmune hepatitis most common in young women, many of whom produce anti-nuclear, anti-smooth muscle and antimitochondrial antibodies, termed 'lupoid' for the presence of the LE cell phenomenon, which occurs in 15% of cases; the lesion is histologically characterized by chronic active hepatitis, a low incidence of carcinoma and good response to corticosteroids

lupus anticoagulant LABORATORY MEDICINE Lupus inhibitor A generic term for IgG or IgM class antibodies that arise spontaneously in patients with lupus erythematosus[1] (LE) and are directed against various anionic phospholipoproteins or phospholipid components (including phosphatic acid, phosphatidylinositol and phosphatidylserine[2]) of coagulation factors; although these antibodies produce in vitro interference with phospholipid-dependent coagulation, eg activated partial thromboplastin time (aPTT) and kaolin clotting time assays in specimens from patients with LE, they don't produce in vivo coagulopathy in absence of other platelet defects or coagulation defects or the presence of drug-induced antibodies; LAs have been identified in patients with HIV, SLE, deep vein thrombosis, and others LABORATORY ↑ aPTT; LAs also interfere with derivative assays for factor VIII, IX, XI, and XII (**Arch Pathol Lab Med 1993; 117:595OA**) LAs may be present if patient:control clotting time is 1.5 X normal at a dilution of 1:1000 and the altered aPTT is corrected by 1:1 mix with normal plasma; LAs include anticardiolipin and other antiphospholipid antibodies Note: Anticardiolipin antibodies (ACA) are often associated with but are not identical to the LA, ie an elevated ACA titer may not always coexist with a positive LA test; Cf Anticardiolipin antibodies

[1]The adjective 'lupus' is retained for convention, as these antibodies also occur in neoplasia, drug reactions or in normal subjects [2]LAs have greatest affinity for phosphatidylserine, which is the most active lipid in aPTT

lupus erythematosus, drug-induced A lupus erythematosus-like syndrome that may develop in patients taking certain drugs, including procainamide, hydralazine, isoniazid, phenytoin, mesantoin, D-penicillamine and ergot compounds; nearly 50 different agents have been implicated, either idiosyncratically or in a dose-dependent fashion; 80% of drug-induced lupus have anti-nuclear, as well as anti-histone antibodies; only ⅓ have clinical changes of lupus, eg arthralgia, fever, serositis; the renal and CNS changes of classic lupus are distinctly uncommon; many of these patients are 'slow acetylators', resulting in accumulation of non-acetylated metabolites that bind to macromolecules, acting as haptens; by extension, this condition is a situation in which a metabolic abnormality induces autoimmunity

lupus nephritis Any of the nephropathies seen in systemic lupus erythematosus Classification (see table, facing page) PATHOGENESIS Classes II-V are thought to share the same pathgenic mechanism, to wit, the deposition of

lung volumes

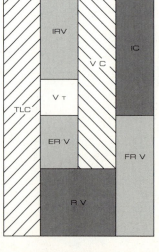

DNA-anti-DNA immune complexes containing Ig and complement, as well as cryoglobulins TREATMENT Prednisone and cyclophosphamide; addition of plasmapheresis to the therapeutic regimen (although seemingly 'logical') does not improve the clinical outcome in lupus nephritis (N Engl J Med 1992; 326:1373OA)

lupus psychosis A clinical complex seen in lupus erythematosus, attributed to an antibody to P protein, a polypeptide present in ribosomal phosphoproteins; lupus patients may have a transient increase in anti-P antibodies during periods of psychotic exacerbation; cerebral lupus may also cause acute vasculitis and immune complex deposits in choroid plexus

lutein CLINICAL NUTRITION A carotenoid that is abundant in broccoli, greens (collard, turnip), spinach, and is linked to a ↓ risk of lung cancer (New York Times 21 Feb 1995; C1) see Carotenoid

luteinizing hormone-releasing hormone LH-RH, see there

luteoma A non-neoplastic yellow-gray mass measuring up to 20 cm in diameter due to hyperplasia of luteinized cells that involutes spontaneously after parturition; this 'luteoma of pregnancy' is most common in young multiparous black women, multiple in ½, and accompanied by virilization or exacerbation of hirsutism in ¼; testosterone levels may be 70-fold greater than normal with transient virilization of the female infants

luxury genes Genes that are not universally expressed, ie those that encode proteins only in specialized cells, eg gastrin production in parietal cells, immunoglobulin production in plasma cells and melanin production in melanocytes; Cf Housekeeping genes

luxury perfusion syndrome A cerebrovascular state in which there is increased blood flow to the brain but decreased oxygen uptake by cerebral tissue, resulting from acute lactic (metabolic) acidosis accompanied by cerebral edema; luxury perfusion is nonspecific and may occur in strokes, trauma, tumors, alcoholism, sickle cell anemia, diabetic ketoacidosis, and meningoencephalitis; Cf Carotid steal syndrome, Robin Hood syndrome

LW antibody An antibody that was thought to be directed against the Rhesus factor (anti-Rh), later recognized as a distinct erythrocyte antigen, which although closely linked to the Rh gene family, is inherited separately; the antigen was designated 'LW' to honor Landsteiner and Wiener's work in the rhesus monkey; anti-LW antibody is very rare

---

LUPUS NEPHRITIS (CLASSIFICATION PER WHO)

CLASS I Normal (rarely recognized)

CLASS II Mesangial lupus GN (10% of SLE patients) Minimal clinical manifestations, mild hematuria, mild proteinuria LM Granular mesangial deposition of Ig and complement

CLASS III Focal proliferative glomerulonephritis (± ⅓ of patients) Moderate clinical manifestations, recurrent hematuria, moderate proteinuria, possible progression to renal failure LM Focal swelling and proliferation of endothelial and mesangial cells, neutrophil infiltration, fibrinoid depoistion

CLASS IV Diffuse proliferative GN (45-50%) Overtly symptomatic, microscopic or gross hematuria, proteinuria ± nephrotic syndrome, ± hypertension, often ↓ GFR LM Global glomerular involvement, proliferation of endothelial and mesangial, and sometimes epithelial cells

CLASS V Membranous GN (10%) Overtly symptomatic, microscopic or gross hematuria, severe proteinuria with nephrotic syndrome, hypertension, ↓ GFR LM Thickening of capillary walls similar to idiopathic membranous GN

GFR Glomerular filtration rate GN Glomerlonephritis LM Light microscopy

---

and can react with Rh+ or Rh-, but not with Rh$_{null}$ cells

lyase A class of enzymes responsible for non-hydrolytic or oxidation-reduction cleavage of carbon-carbon, carbon-oxygen and carbon-nitrogen bonds, resulting in two products, one or both of which have double bonds; lyases include aldolase, deaminase, decarboxylase, dehydratase, hydrase, nucleotide cyclase, synthase

lycopene CLINICAL NUTRITION A carotenoid that is abundant in tomatoes and tomato products, and has potent antioxidant activity; lycopene consumption is linked to a ↓ risk of bladder, and colon cancer and cancer cell growth in vitro; unpublished data suggest that lycopene may be the most cardioprotective of the carotenoids (New York Times 21 Feb 1995; C1) see Carotenoid

LYDMA A membrane antigen expressed by EBV-infected B cells that is a target for activated T cells and may play a role in host defense against infectious mononucleosis

lye injury TOXICOLOGY A condition often secondary to the ingestion of bleach, of suicidal intent in adults and of accidental nature in children; periodic follow-up is obligatory as 5% develop squamous cell carcinoma 20-40 years after the insult CLINICAL, ACUTE Tachycardia, intense retrosternal pain, production of copious frothy mucus, vomiting of blood, sloughing of esophageal mucosa, dysphagia, followed by fibrosing stricture Barium 'swallow' studies demonstrate a pencil-thin esophageal lumen TREATMENT Bougienage is a therapeutic mainstay; given the potential for perforation, it is best begun five or more days post-insult; large-bore nasogastric tubes appear preferable to bougienage, as the strictures formed are of a large and useful diameter; pharmacologic doses of corticosteroids appear to minimize fibrosis

Lyme disease A condition* caused by *Borrelia burgdorferi*, and possibly mediated by IL-1 CLINICAL Lyme disease is divided into Stage I Erythema chronicum migrans Rash stage, associated with wood tick bites and confined to Northern Europe until 1970 when the first US cases were described, presenting as a solitary reddish papule and plaque with centrifugal expansion (up to 20 cm), peripheral induration and central clearing, persisting for months to years; potentially pruritic with IgM and C3 deposition in vessels Stage II Cardiovascular (myocarditis, pericarditis, transient atrioventricular block, ventricular dysfunction); neurological (Bell's palsy, meningoencephalitis, optic atrophy, polyneuritis) symptoms; HLA-DR4 and HLA-DR2 may be more common in chronic Lyme arthritis and resistance to antibiotics Stage III Migratory polyarthritis; Lyme disease may be accompanied by headache, stiff neck, fever, and malaise that is subsequently manifest as migratory polyarthritis, intermittent oligoarthritis, chronic arthritis of the knees, chronic meningoencephalitis, cranial or peripheral neuropathy, migratory musculoskeletal pains, cardiac abnormalities; some workers (WV Adams, Pediatrics, August 1994) believe the neuropsychological changes may be less severe than previously reported DIAGNOSIS ELISA, immunofluourescence assay, solid-phase fluorescence immunoassay; PCR can be used to identify *B burgdorferi* DNA in synovial fluid of untreated patients (N Engl J Med 1994; 330o:229OA) LABORATORY Nonspecific findings include ↑ ESR, IgM and cryoglobulins, decreased C3 and C4, increased IgG and IgM antibody titers to *B burgdorferi*, agreement among laboratories as to whether a subject has Lyme antibodies, when tested by indirect fluorescent antibody (IFA) or ELISA is low and lacks standardization; histologic stains of involved tissue (Warthin-Starry and Dieterle) have a low diagnostic yield; definitive diagnosis requires identification of IgG antibodies to *B recurrentis* by the 'Western' immunoblot EPIDEMIOLOGY 8000 cases were reported in 1993 (US), making it the most common zoonosis in the US, especially along the Eastern 'seaboard; *B burgdorferi* has also been identified in

Northern Europe and Australia Vectors Deer tick (*Ixodes dammini*, Eastern USA, up to 60% of which carry the spirochete), white-footed mouse tick (*I pacificus*, Western USA, about 1% of which carry the organism), wood tick (*I ricinus*, Europe), Lone Star tick (*Amblyomma americanum*), and rarely deerflies and horseflies (**N Engl J Med 1990; 322:1752c**) HOST Deer mice, field mice MOLECULAR BIOLOGY DNA sequences of *B burgdorferi* were identified by PCR in archival specimens of *Ixodes dammini* that had been stored since the 1940s, making Lyme disease older by two decades than previously thought PROGNOSIS 60% of untreated subjects develop recurring bouts of arthritis (chronic Lyme arthritis) lasting up to years after infection TREATMENT One month of doxycycline or amoxicillin or two weeks of IV ceftriaxone or penicillin; based on cost-effectiveness analysis, empirical antibiotic treatment is recommended if the probability of *B burgdorferi* infection after a bite is ≥ 0.036 (ie, ≥3.6%), and not warranted if the probability of infection is ≤ 0.01 (**N Engl J Med 1992; 327:534oa**) even in Lyme disease endemic areas, the risk of *B burgdorferi* infection after a recognized deer-tick bite is so low that prophylactic antibiotic treatment is not routinely indicated(**N Engl J Med 1992; 327:1769oa**) VACCINE Osp A vaccine, see there

*Lyme disease was first seen in Lyme, Connecticut where it presented as an 'epidemic' of juvenile rheumatoid arthritis (Still's disease); one astute mother alerted Yale epidemiologists who then 'discovered' the disease

chronic Lyme disease A predominantly neurologic condition ranging from mild, eg fatigue, paresthesia, arthralgia, memory loss, mood swings, and dysomnia, to severe, eg spastic paraparesis, tetraparesis, ataxia, chorea, cognitive impairment, bladder dysfunction, cranial nerve deficits, myelitis, brainstem encephalitis and demyelination Lyme disease triad: Lymphocytic meningitis, cranial neuritis (especially of the 7th and 8th cranial nerve) and radiculitis DIAGNOSIS Specific IgG antibody ('Western' immunoblotting) to *B burgdorferi* that may disappear with time; persistent, ie treatable infection should be ruled out by a specific T-cell lymphoblastic response assay Note: Chronic neurological abnormalities of encephalopathy, leukoencephalopathy and polyneuritis may improve with antibiotics

Lyme embryopathy A complex of congenital malformations described in infants born to women with Lyme disease while pregnant, which includes syndactyly, cortical blindness, intrauterine fetal death, prematurity and neonatal rash

lymphadenopathy Enlargement of the lymph nodes of virtually any etiology; the differential diagnostic considerations are enormous and have been divided for convenience into reactive patterns; benign lymphadenopathy is characterized by 1) Variability of the follicle (germinal center) size 2) Lack of capsular or fat invasion 3) Mitotic activity that is confined to the germinal center, and 4) Cortical localization and inhomogeneous distribution of the follicles; see Benign lymphadenopathy

lymphangiomatosis Diffuse or multifocal lymphangioma A rare lesion confined to children, characterized by well-demarcated osteolytic lesions variably accompanied by sclerosis, often misdiagnosed as fibrous dysplasia; while the condition is histologically benign, the prognosis is poor if the lesions affect the liver, spleen or thoracic duct as these sites are not amenable to adequate resection; the bone lesions may be stable unless they are in the vertebral body in which case the patients may develop cord compression (**Arch Pathol Lab Med 1994; 118:846oa**)

lymphangiomyomatosis syndrome A rare thoracic duct defect causing chylothorax in women of child-bearing years related to estrogen production or occurring in tuberous sclerosis CLINICAL Exertional dyspnea, hemoptysis, cough, chest pain, pneumothorax, chylothorax and progressive respiratory insufficiency RADIOLOGY Reticulonodular changes, cysts or bullae, effusion and hyperinflation PATHOLOGY Diffuse smooth muscle proliferation within small blood vessels and lymphatics, lymphangiectasia, 'honeycombed' pulmonary parenchyma, lipid pneumonia PROGNOSIS Although this condition was initially thought to have a poor prognosis, most patients survive 8+ years TREATMENT Possible response to hormonal manipulation, eg tamoxifen, medroxyprogesterone acetate

lymphedema A condition characterized by the accumulation of interstitial fluid (lymph) due to interference with lymphatic drainage (eg obstruction of lymphatics, lymph node disease or surgical removal of lymph nodes in the face of cancer), with expansion of the interstitial fluid compartment; lymphedema may be lymphedema is defined clinically as an ↑ in arm circumference of 1-1.5 cm > than the unaffected arm; post-mastectomy lymphedema may be 1) Acute and transient, which occurs in 35%, which resolves spontaneously in 6 weeks or 2) Chronic, which develops 6 weeks to 20 years after surgery, and may be complicated by cellulitis or lymphangiosarcoma (Stewart-Treves syndrome) (**CAP Today May 1995, p51**); according to etiology, lymphedema may be

1) Congenital, eg Milroy's disease, related to poor development of the lymphatic channels

2) Acquired through microfilarial infection or involvement by malignancy or by modalities for treating cancer, eg lymphadenectomy or regional lymphoid irradiation

3) Idiopathic, which affects young ♀ with unremitting swelling in one or more extremities

lymph node inclusions The presence of benign tissues within lymph nodes, a phenomenon that may result in the misdiagnosis of malignancy; benign 'metastases' include salivary gland tissue, thyroid follicles, müllerian epithelium, endometriosis, nevus cell aggregates and breast tissue; other non-neoplastic inclusions with lymph nodes include adipose tissue, ectopic thymus, hyaline and proteinaceous material; Cf Benign lymphadenopathy

lymph node necrosis A nonspecific finding that can be divided into 1) Focal necrosis, usually benign, seen in infection by bacteria, cat-scratch disease, EBV, fungemia, LGV, toxoplasmosis, TB, and tularemia, trauma, vascular compromise, post-vaccination lymphadenitis or autoimmunity, eg lupus erythematosus, mucocutaneous lymph node syndrome (Kawasaki's disease), necrotizing lymphadenitis (Kikuchi's disease) and 2) Global necrosis, 80% of which is associated with lymphoma

lymphocytic choriomeningitis An aseptic meningitis of low morbidity caused by an arenavirus (single-stranded RNA virus containing two glyco- and nucleoproteins) that is transmitted through rodent excretia, affecting adults in winter, when rodents move indoors CLINICAL Biphasic fever with flu symptoms followed by meningitis with fever, headache, lymphocytosis in the cerebrospinal fluid, often associated with leukopenia and thrombocytopenia, this latter may be a hyperimmune response DDx Infectious mononucleosis, enterovirus, herpes zoster

lymphocytic interstitial pneumonia A diffuse pulmonary disease of insidious onset that is most common in middle-aged women and which may be accompanied by Sjögren's disease, hypergammaglobulinemia or hypogammaglobulinemia CLINICAL Progressive shortness of breath, cough RADIOLOGY Reticulonodular infiltrates on a plain chest film, which may be accompanied by Kerley 'B' lines PATHOLOGY Nodular interstitial process of the alveolar and interlobular septae in a perivascular pattern characterized by mature lymphocytes admixed with plasma and other 'round' cells Note: LIP may mimic lymphoma, as it is characterized by cellular monotony with aggregates of small lymphocytes, bronchial mucosal ulceration, parenchymal infiltration and is considered by some authors to be a pre-malignant lesion; with time, many patients progress to end-stage lung disease or develop lymphoma

lymphocytotoxicity assay A complement-mediated assay commonly used in HLA (human leukocyte antigen) typing laboratories, which tests for the presence of cyto-toxic antibodies in the serum of the potential recipient that are capable of reacting with the lymphocytes of the potential donor; see Mixed lymphocyte culture

lymphoepithelioma Undifferentiated nasopharyngeal carcinoma A malignancy with a marked lymphocytic com-ponent, subdivided into 1) SCHMINCKE TYPE Diffuse mixing of epithelial and lymphoid elements, making the lesion dif-ficult to distinguish from lymphoma, since the epithelial cells may mimic lymphoblasts or the lacunar cell variants of Reed-Sternberg cells and 2) REGAUD TYPE Cohesive car-cinoma cell aggregates that are large enough to make the epithelial nature of the tumor obvious DIAGNOSIS Immunoperoxidase stains are positive for cytokeratin

lymphogranuloma venereum A sexually-transmitted dis-ease caused by one of three immunotypes (L_1, L_2 and L_3) of *Chlamydia trachomatis*; LGV is uncommon in USA, regionally endemic in Asia, Africa and South America CLINICAL Papulo-ulcer that forms and spontaneously heals at the inoculation site, followed by matted and painful loco-regional (inguinal and perirectal), lymphadenopathy, described as 'kissing' lesions with a 'groove' sign, sloughing of skin, purulent drainage, hemorrhagic proctocolitis, malaise, fever, headache, aseptic meningitis, anorexia, myalgia, arthralgia, hepatitis, conjunctivitis and erythema nodosum LABORATORY Antibody assays, eg immunofluores-cence, counterimmunoelectrophoresis, complement fixa-tion titers > 1:32 PATHOLOGY Inclusion bodies in Giemsa-stained histiocytes, 'stellate abscesses' in lymph nodes TREATMENT Tetracycline, excision LATE COMPLICATIONS Urethral and rectal strictures, lymphedema, rectovaginal fistulas

lymphoid granular complex A large intestinal microbur-sa that was initially described as a morphological marker for inflammatory bowel disease, but which is recognized as the local recipient site for antigens destined for future immune recognition, forming an integral component of the gastrointestinal-associated lymphoid tissue; see GALT

lymphokines A heterogeneous group of nonspecific hor-mone-like polypeptides that are secreted by various cells of the immune system during anantigen response 'cas-cade', enhancing or suppressing the immune system, hav-ing either paracrine (locally cytostimulatory) or autocrine (self-stimulatory) activities; lymphokines are produced by activated T cells and natural killer cells, promote cell pro-liferation, growth and/or differentiation, regulate cell func-tion by acting on gene transcription and in inflammation; lymphokines include γ-interferon, interleukins IL-2 to IL-6, granulocyte-macrophage colony-stimulating factor and lymphotoxin; see Biological response modifiers, Colony-stimulating factors, Interferons, Interleukins, Tumor necrosis factor

Note: The term cytokine is increasingly preferred as certain 'lymphokines' are also produced by monocytes and macrophages and thus could theoretically be designated as 'monokines'

lymphokine-activated killer cells LAK cells, see there

lymphoma A malignant neoplasm of B or T lymphocytes, arising from a monoclonal, ie derived from a single prog-enitor cell, proliferation of lymphocytes; the proliferative process is considered lymphomatous in the appropriate clinical setting, given that not all monoclonal expansions have a malignant behavior Note: The process of producing and secreting immunoglobulin (B cells) or membrane receptor (T cells) is preceded by a DNA rearrangement, in which the introns are spliced out, ie eliminated and the exons linked together (V/J or V/D/J rearrangement), form-ing a mature messenger RNA molecule that is unique to one individual cell; when a cell produces abundant daugh-ter cells, the monoclonal 'expansion' is detectable by Southern blot hybridization; B- and T-cell malignancies are driven by the common mechanism of translocation and oncogene regulation; the prognosis is favorable in follicu-lar lymphomas, especially those with cleaved, mixed and large non-cleaved cell types, and may also be favorable in certain diffuse lymphomas, eg small lymphocytic, cleaved cell, Burkitt's, non-cleaved cell and convoluted cell types; a distinctly unfavorable prognosis is characteristic of dif-fuse plasmacytoid lymphocye, mixed cell, mixed small noncleaved cell and large noncleaved cell types; advanced age, anemia and high mitotic activity are associated with a poor prognosis **ANGIOTROPIC LYMPHOMA** see there **B-CELL LYMPHOMA** A lymphoma composed of follicular center cells Note: It is unclear whether there is a difference in clinical behavior between B- or T-cell lymphomas that have a sim-ilar morphology by simple light microscopy; the Working Formulation (see there) has been shown to be clinically valid despite the lack of not identification of B- or T-cell lineage; the overall survival and survival by stage are sim-ilar in cutaneous T-cell lymphomas and in histologically favorable B-cell lymphomas **BICLONAL LYMPHOMA** see there **BURKITT'S LYMPHOMA** A lymphoma of children that is 'dri-ven' by the Epstein-Barr virus endemic to certain regions of Africa (see Lymphoma belt), which presents in the young African jaw or in young American abdomen, affects the bone marrow and usually responds well (initially) to chemotherapy; Burkitt's lymphoma is characterized by sheets of monotonous small round cells punctuated by a 'starry sky' pattern, see there **CENTROCYTIC LYMPHOMA** see below, Diffuse small cleaved cell lymphoma **COMPOSITE LYMPHOMA** A rare lymphoma composed of two or more malignant cell lines in the same lymph node **DIFFUSE LYMPHOMA** A lymphoma composed of sheets of cells and lacking all attempts to recapitulate germinal cen-ters, which often spill into the adjacent adipose and other tissues; in general, diffuse lymphomas are more aggressive than follicular lymphomas **DIFFUSE LARGE CELL LYMPHOMA** A complex and heterogeneous group of NHL that corre-sponds to the 'histiocytic' lymphoma and reticulum cell sarcoma of older classifications affecting those circa age 60, which is composed of small round cells with little cyto-plasm that may present in advanced stages, 20% of which may be accompanied by monoclonal gammopathy PROGNOSIS 60% five year survival **DIFFUSE MIXED (SMALL AND LARGE CELL) LYMPHOMA** A clinicopathologically het-erogeneous group of lymphomas, most of which are the diffuse counterparts of follicular lymphoma or peripheral T-cell lymphoma **DIFFUSE SMALL CLEAVED CELL LYMPHOMA** A (usually) B-cell lymphoma composed of follicular center cells with one-half the survival rate of follicular small cleaved cell lymphoma **DISCORDANT LYMPHOMA** A rare lymphoma composed of two or more histological subtypes in separate anatomic locations; therapy is directed at the lineage with the worst prognosis **EXTRANODAL LYMPHOMA** A lymphoma that is often histologically diffuse, appears in the stomach, tonsils, skin, small intestine and salivary glands and which is usually slightly more aggressive than nodal lymphomas **FOLLICULAR LYMPHOMA** A heteroge-neous group of lymphomas arising in follicular center cells, which comprises 50% of all NHL in adults (US), it is more common in the elderly and distinctly uncommon in those under age 20, and in blacks; FLs are usually confined to lymph nodes, often have a 8:14 chromosomal transloca-tion and when accompanied by del 13q32, are more aggressive and may enter a leukemic phase; FLs are histo-logically divided into those with predominantly small cleaved cells (large cells comprise less than 20% of the cells), those with more than 50% large cells, and those with mixed, small cleaved and large cells **GASTRIC LYM-**

PHOMA A diffuse low-grade lymphoma composed of monotonous mature or atypical lymphocytes with 5- and 10-year survivals of 57% and 46%, respectively, in which the histologic subtype, clinical stage, and mode of therapy are of little prognostic value **HISTIOCYTIC LYMPHOMA** A very rare lymphoma consisting of discrete masses of histiocytes in lymphoid tissues, skin and bone, which may also have T-cell or B-cell markers; many of the lesions first described by Rappaport, now known as 'Rappaport's histiocytic lymphoma', ultimately proved to be transformed histiocyte-like lymphocytes **INTERMEDIATE LYMPHOCYTIC LYMPHOMA** An indolent B-cell lymphoma of the middle-aged and elderly, related to small cell follicular lymphoma, composed of cells similar to those of well-differentiated lymphocytic lymphoma **Ki-1 LYMPHOMA** Pleomorphic histiocytic lymphoma A heterogeneous group of childhood lymphomas, the cells of which react against the monoclonal antibody Ki-1, (an antibody that also reacts with Reed-Sternberg cells), leukocyte common antigen and epithelial membrane antigen; despite the anaplastic 'ugly' histology, the tumor may respond to chemotherapy with prolonged remission or complete cure **LARGE CELL LYMPHOMA WITH FILOPODIA** A rare type of large cell lymphoma, characterized by abundant filiform projections on the cell surfaces, a functional variant of dubious distinction **LENNERT'S LYMPHOMA** Lymphoepithelioid lymphoma A lymphoma of large cells that are more pleomorphic than those of large cell lymphoma (with which it was confused in early reports), which have immunocytochemical evidence of monocyte-histiocytic differentiation; these lymphomas are nodally based and tend to involve the skin and bone, carrying a relatively good prognosis **LYMPHOBLASTIC LYMPHOMA** A lymphoma composed of diffuse monomorphous sheets of large cells, punctuated by a focal starry sky pattern; it is most common in children and adolescents, arises in the mediastinum, and without therapy, is highly aggressive, causing rapid multisystem dissemination and death within a year of presentation **MEDITERRANEAN LYMPHOMA** see IPSID (Immunoproliferative small intestinal disease) **MONOCYTOID B-CELL LYMPHOMA** A distinct B cell lymphoma that represents the malignant counterpart, ie a clonal expansion of the monocytoid cells seen in reactive lymphoid hyperplasias that arise in a background of toxoplasmosis and other benign lesions **NODULAR LYMPHOMA** see Follicular lymphoma **NON-HODGKIN'S LYMPHOMA** 60% of all lymphomas are NHLs, of which 55% are diffuse, 45% are nodular; 27 000 new NHLs are diagnosed/year (US) **PEDIATRIC LYMPHOMA** An uncommon lymphoma that is often extranodal, diffuse, and responds well to chemotherapy **PLEOMORPHIC (NON-BURKITT'S) LYMPHOMA** A lymphoma composed of pleomorphic cells, midway in size between small cleaved and large cells, which tends to involve the gastrointestinal tract and the bone marrow and may be more aggressive clinically **PULMONARY LYMPHOMA** see Lymphocytic interstitial pneumonia **RAPPAPORT'S HISTIOCYTIC LYMPHOMA** see above, Histiocytic lymphoma **SIGNET RING CELL LYMPHOMA(S)** A group comprising up to 1% of all B-cell and T-cell lymphomas that share nothing in common beyond having scattered-to-abundant 'signet ring' lymphocytes; the cleared vacuoles are derived from multivesicular bodies, a form of lysosomes, which in some cases, may be filled with immunoglobulins; these lymphomas are otherwise heterogeneous by histological (many are follicular center lymphomas), clinical and immunohistochemical criteria; SCLs thus are curiosities of questionable significance **SMALL LYMPHOCYTIC (WELL DIFFERENTIATED) LYMPHOMA** A relatively indolent lymphoma that affects the middle-aged to elderly with a good prognosis, some cases of which represent the tissue equivalent of chronic lymphocytic leukemia; most are of B-cell type and have monoclonal antibodies on the cell surface; in those cases with T-cell markers, the cells are larger and more aggressive clinically **SMALL INTESTINAL LYMPHOMA** see IPSID **SMALL NON-CLEAVED CELL LYMPHOMA** A high grade B-cell lymphoma composed of B cell markers, which is arbitrarily subdivided into Burkitt's lymphoma and Pleomorphic (non-Burkitt's) lymphoma **T-CELL LYMPHOMA** 90% of all patients with TCL have extracutaneous involvement at the time of diagnosis Note: The overall survival and survival by stage is similar in cutaneous T-cell lymphomas and in histologically favorable B cell lymphomas PATHOLOGY Vascular proliferation, TdT (Terminal deoxynucleotidyl transferase), T helper (CD4) or T suppressor (CD8) cell subsets; pleomorphic nucleus and cleared cytoplasm; see T-cell lymphomas **UNDIFFERENTIATED LYMPHOMA** see Small non-cleaved cell lymphoma; see AIDS, Hodgkin's disease, Monoclonality, Pre-lymphoma, Working classification; Cf Leukemia

lymphoma belt A region of Central Africa between 10 north and 10 south of the equator that has a high incidence of EBV-induced Burkitt's lymphoma (BL); in Uganda, BL is the most common cause of childhood malignancy; similar environmental and climatic conditions are seen in Papua New Guinea, another focus of BL Note: EBV is present in 90% of African BL, but in less than one-half of non-African BL (Br J Med 1962; 2:1019, Nature 1962; 194:232)

lymphomatoid granulomatosis A condition initially thought to be a variant of pulmonary angiitis and granulomatosis, now considered a lymphoproliferative disorder, which presents in middle-aged subjects with well-circumscribed bilateral nodules seen on a plain film of the chest and some cases occur in immunosuppressed renal transplant recipients and in those with Sjögren syndrome CLINICAL 80% of cases have extrapulmonary involvement, eg skin, CNS, kidneys, liver, spleen, adrenal glands, heart, GI tract and other organs PATHOLOGY Vasocentric polymorphic infiltrate comprised of plasma cells, immunoblasts and large atypical lymphocytes PROGNOSIS 64% mortality with a median survival of 14 months, the death being due to pulmonary destruction accompanied by sepsis; the malignant deterioration is associated with severe impairment of the T-cell function possibly explaining the tendency for malignant degeneration; Cf Lymphoid interstitial pneumonia

lymphomatoid papulosis A recurring papular eruption of the skin with a benign clinical course that histologically resembles malignant lymphoma; although most lesions behave in an indolent fashion, gene rearrangement studies demonstrate a clonal expansion of T cells; 10-20% are associated with or evolve toward T-cell lymphoma

lymphostatic verrucosis Lymphedematous keratoderma, mossy foot A manifestation of chronic lymphedema of the lower extremity characterized by a lawn of velvety hyperkeratotic filiform projections

lymphotoxin A heterodimeric glycoprotein cytokine with a 5-D and a 15-kD protein fragment produced by T cells that evokes B-cell proliferation, which also specifically inhibits tumor growth, in vivo and in vitro, inhibiting transformation of cells induced by chemical carcinogens and ultraviolet light

lyonization A normal genetic event described by Mary Lyon, a British geneticist that consists of inactivation of all X chromosomes (although portions of the 'inactivated' chromosome may remain functional) that are in excess of one; lyonization occurs during embryogenesis and results in the formation of 'Barr bodies', present in all nucleated somatic cells, but best visualized in PMNs and scraped squamous cells of the buccal mucosa

lyophilization Freeze drying A method for preserving foods or biologicals, where a substance, eg coagulation factor VIII, is 'snap-frozen' in liquid nitrogen (-70°C) and placed in a high vacuum to remove the water vapor as it sublimes; once the water is removed, the substance is brought to room temperature and stored; Cf Quick-freeze technique

Lysenko, Trofim The infamous president (born 1898, died 1976) of the Lenin (Soviet) Academy of Agricultural Sciences, who largely during the Stalin years (from 1938 until 1956) promoted the concept that characteristics acquired by modifying environmental conditions could be passed on to subsequent generations; this concept contrasts sharply with Mendelian genetics, the widely accepted priniciples on which modern genetics is built, and a number of geneticists during this period were sent to the gulags

Lysenkoism A pseudoscientific doctrine based on Lamarckism that was espoused by the Russian geneticist TD Lysenko, which formed the basis of Soviet genetics from 1932 to 1965; see Lamarckism

lysergic acid diethylamide LSD, see there

lysinemia A heterogeneous group of diseases with increased lysine or its metabolites in the blood, including hyperlysinemia, types I and II, saccharopurinuria, hydroxylysinuria, pipecolic acidemia and α-ketoadipic aciduria

lysogeny The inherited ability of certain strains of bacteria to act as viral vectors, integrating themselves into the bacterial genome itself; lysogenic bacteria may differ from their non-infected comrades, eg *Corynebacterium diphtheriae,* only produce toxin in the presence of lysogenic phages; lysogeny can be stimulated by suboptimal growth conditions or through inhibition of bacterial protein production, eg adding chloramphenicol to a culture

lysosomal storage diseases A generic term for a heterogeneous group of diseases with specific defects in lysosomal enzymes; LSDs include

SPHINGOLIPIDOSES with defects in sulfated mucopolysaccharide catabolism, eg Niemann-Pick, Gaucher's, Krabbe's, Fabry's diseases and others

MUCOPOLYSACCHARIDOSES, with defects in glycosaminoglycans, which can be identified by culturing skin fibroblasts, eg Hurler, Scheie, Hunter, Sanfilippo, and other syndromes and

MULTIPLE STORAGE PRODUCT DISORDERS, including various mucolipidoses; Cf Inborn errors of metabolism

lysosome A membrane-bound cytoplasmic organelle that contains a vast array of digestive enzymes, including ribonuclease, deoxyribonuclease, phosphatase, glycosidase, arylsulfatase, collagenase and cathepsins; once a 'virgin' lysosome or primary granule encounters a substrate for digestion, it becomes known as a secondary lysosome or granule

lysozyme A class of hydrolytic enzymes responsible for hydrolysis of mucopolysaccharides and mucoproteins, found in tears, milk, saliva and serum as well as neutrophils and cells of the monocyte phagocytic system

LysR family MICROBIOLOGY A family of virulence factor regulators present in various pathogenic bacteria that activate transcription (Science & Medicine 1995; 2/3:16) see AraC family, Virulence factor

'lytes *noun* A colloquial term for electrolytes which includes the core of Na^+, K^+, Cl^-, and CO_3^-, and may include Mg^{2+}, Ca^{2+}, and PO_4^-

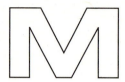

M Symbol for: 1) mega– (10⁶, per SI-International System) 2) Methionine 3) Molar concentration 4) Mitosis, phase of the cell cycle

m Symbol for: 1) Mass 2) Median (statistics) 3) Mean of a sample 4) meta- (organic chemistry, benzene ring position) 5) Messenger (RNA) 6) Meter 7) milli– (10⁻³, per SI-International System) 8) Molal concentration

M chain One of the two protein chains required to form a tetramer of lactate dehydrogenase

M component A narrow peak or 'spike' seen on serum protein electrophoresis which is presumptive evidence of a monoclonal lymphoproliferation of mature B cells producing IgG, IgA, or IgM; the M component may occur in multiple myeloma, Waldenström's disease, heavy chain disease and in lichen myxedematosus (a rare disease of proliferating fibroblasts)

M current NEUROPHYSIOLOGY A time and voltage-dependent potassium current that persists at slightly depolarized membrane potentials; MC is ↓ by muscarinic cholinergic agonists and certain peptides and is partially responsible for the slow excitatory postsynaptic potentials in sympathetic neurons; MC in hippocampal neurons is ↑ by somatostatin, thus indicating that one ion channel has two different regulating receptors, the latter of which are mediated by arachidonic acid metabolites

M protein A term that has been applied to at least three different molecular entities, to wit

1) HEMATOLOGY Monoclonal IgM, myeloma protein

2) MICROBIOLOGY An α-helical fibrillary molecule on the surface of group A streptococcus that confers resistance to phagocytosis; the 80 distinct serotypes of group A streptococci differ according antigenic variation in the M proteins, which share certain common structural motifs, having a coiled-coil rod in the center, flanked by a) A C-terminal anchor constructed of a highly conserved hexapeptide (Leu-Pro-Ser-Thr-Gly-GluA or LPSTGE), which may be the idoneous antigen to use for producing a vaccine and b) An N-terminal anchor, the antigens of which are highly variable; host antibodies against an N-terminal epitope would confer protection against only one of the 80 serotypes (Sci Am 1991: 264:58)

3) PHYSIOLOGY A structural protein found in the M band of striated muscle

M2 protocol ONCOLOGY A widely used chemotherapeutic protocol for treating multiple myeloma, which includes the alkylating agents vincristine, BCNU (carmustine), cyclophosphamide, melphalan and prednisone (VBCMP)

Note: There is little evidence in well-conducted trials that any one multi-agent protocol for multiple myeloma improves survival more than another

M wave NEUROPHYSIOLOGY The tracing of the earliest electromyographic response to the stimulation of a muscle nerve, which corresponds to muscle excitation through the motor axon

MAAC Maximum allowable actual charge HEALTH CARE FINANCING The practical limit on the amount of money that physicians who don't accept Medicare 'assignment' may collect from Medicare patients

MAB Monoclonal antibody, Monoclonal antibodies

mabiki Japanese, thinning out SOCIOLOGY The killing of unwanted offspring, usually female, practiced by rural peasants in old Japan, by suffocation or a blow to the head, where the ideal ratio of progeny was two male children to one female

Female infanticide has also been practiced among the Aborigines, Arabs, Chinese, in India and Oceania; women have been historically weaned earlier, underfed and overworked throughout the world, a practice that continues today in Africa, the Middle and Far East

Mac Macintosh, see there

MAC 1) Mammalian artificial chromosome 2) Maximum allowable concentration 3) Membrane attack complex, see there 4) Minimum alveolar concentration 5) Mitral annular calcification, see there 6) *Mycobacterium avium* complex A common cause of systemic infection of AIDS patients, affecting as many as two-thirds of AIDS patients with CD4-positive T cells in the circulation; MAC responds poorly to combination anti-tuberculous drug 'cocktails', but responds well to clarithromycin (Am Med News 22-29/Apr/91)

MAC program Maximum Allowable Cost program A US federal program that purchases drugs from several commercial sources in order to obtain the lowest possible price and limit reimbursement for prescription drugs under the Medicare and Medicaid programs

MAC regimen GYNECOLOGIC ONCOLOGY A chemotherapeutic regimen used to treat malignant trophoblastic disease (choriocarcinoma) which consists of methotrexate, dactinomycin, and chlorambucil; treatment 'failure' may respond to other chemotherapeutic agents including bleomycin, cisplatin, hydroxyurea, and vinblastine

MacConkey agar MICROBIOLOGY A differential and selective growth medium used to isolate and identify gram-negative bacilli, often enteric pathogens, based on the fermentation or lack of fermentation of a sugar added by the user; MA is peptone-based and contains bile salts and crystal violet (which inhibit the growth of gram-positive organisms) a sugar (usually lactose) and a pH indicator, which allows differentiation of lactose-fermenting (indicated by pink colonies, eg *Escherichia coli*), and non-lactose-fermenting (colorless colonies, eg *Proteus mirabilis*) bacteria

machine error COMPUTERS A hardware error versus a software 'bug'

machine language COMPUTERS A set of instructions written in symbols and graphic representations in the logical language for and understood by a computer ADVANTAGE Flexibility DISADVANTAGE It is error-prone and considerable skill is required to write the programs

machinery murmur A continuous harsh, rasping or rumbling cardiac murmur characteristic of patent ductus arteriosus that begins shortly after the first sound, reaches a maximum at the end of systole and wanes in late diastole; it is best heard in the second left intercostal space, transmits to the chest and neck and may be felt by the patients as a palpable thrill or 'buzz'; it may also be heard in ventricular septal defect, rarely in pulmonary hypertension and in penetrating soft-tissue injury with formation of an arteriovenous fistula

machinist hands RHEUMATOLOGY A descriptive term for

the changes seen in the hands of patients with dermato-myositis; MHs are characterized by periungual erythema, linear erythematous discoloration around the nailbeds, accompanied by scaling, hyper- and hypopigmentation, and eventually brauny induration with darkened or 'dirty' horizontal line across the lateral and palmar aspects of the fingers (from whence the name) and pink to violaceous scaling overjoint flexures, eg the knuckles, elbows, and knees (WN Kelley, et al, Eds, Textbook of Rheumatology, 4th ed, WB Saunders, Philadelphia, 1993); see Polymyositis-Dermatomyositis

Macintosh Mac COMPUTERS A PC (personal computer) manufactured by Apple Computer, Inc (Cupertino, California) that is widely regarded as having revolutionized the computing industry and placed the power of computers in the hands of the general population; the first primitive Mac produced in 1984 had the same basic elements[1] as are now considered standard for all PCs, including software formats such as 'pull-down' menus, 'point-and-shoot' commands, and icons to represent files, programs, and landmarks on the desktop, as well as hardware elements, eg a mouse to navigate through the software and wysiwyg (what you see is what you get) screen displays; Macs and (since the early 1990s with the release of Microsoft's Windows program) also PCs are 'user-friendly' and so that the most unsophisticated and computer-illiterate person is able to use computers without the need to understand them; see Computers; Cf Windows

[1]The Mac's forte has traditionally been in graphics and in producing the printed word, and is the preferred device among design professionals, publishers, and artists Since 1984, Macs, which are built around Motorola's CISC microprocessors, have achieved ever-increasing levels of sophistication and speed that roughly parallel those of Intel's 386, 486, and Pentium; the next generation of microprocessors (chips) for the Mac, based on a RISC design (which is simpler and allows for faster throughput of data), was released in 1994; the Macs with RISC chips (also produced by Motorola and known as the PowerPC chips) are known as PowerMacs

MACOP-B ONCOLOGY A 'third-generation' combination chemotherapy regimen consisting of methotrexate with leucovorin rescue, doxorubicin, cyclophosphamide, vincristine, prednisone, and bleomycin; despite extensive clinical research, CHOP is considered better than MACOP-B for non-Hodgkin's lymphoma as it is less expensive, less complicated to administer, and has fewer fatal toxic side effects (N Engl J Med 1993; 328:1002OA), see CHOP

macroamylase A 200-kD plasma amylase, usually of salivary type that circulates complexed to various high-molecular-weight plasma proteins, eg IgG, IgA, polysaccharides, glycoproteins and α_1-antitrypsin; persistent six-to-eightfold elevation of macroamylase occurs in 1% of older subjects, often accompanied by abdominal pain, associated with alcoholism, pancreatitis, malignancy, diabetes mellitus, cholelithiasis, autoimmune disease

Macrobdella A genus of fresh water leech; see Leech

macrobiotic diet see Macrobiotics

macrobiotics ALTERNATIVE MEDICINE A diet and philosophy taught by G Ohsawa and M Kushi and popularized in the 1960s in the US, based on an idiosyncratic version of the ancient concept of yin and yang, arbitrarily assigning foods as having a 'male' or 'female' quality; the diet consists predominantly of whole grains, vegetables and enough food of animal origin to prevent malnutrition; non-macrobiotic diets have been linked to the development of cancer by the followers of the macrobiotic philosophy, who mistakenly believe that any diet that can prevent cancer is also appropriate in its treatment Note: Kushi himself recognizes that the diet is to be used in conjunction with cancer treatment regimens; see Unproven methods of cancer treatment

macrocephaly Megalocephaly An enlarged head; in the pediatric age group, macrocephaly is defined dynamically and in vivo as an occipitofrontal circumference of greater than three standard deviations above the mean; in the

adult, macrocephaly may be static and is defined in vitro as any brain weighing more than 1800 g, due to the expansion of any subdural component, including cerebral tissue, liquid, blood, tumor or storage disease DDx–NON-HYDRO-CEPHALIC CAUSES A benign familial form in which the sibs also have large heads, achondroplasia, Banayan syndrome, cerebral gigantism (with macrosomia or Sotos syndrome), cutis marmorata telangiectatica congenita, fragile X syndrome, Klippel-Trenauny-Weber syndrome, mucopolysaccharidosis, neurofibromatosis and Weaver syndrome

The largest brain on record weighed 2.1 kg (4 lbs, 8.29 oz); size is no indicator of intellectual prowess

macro-creatine kinase An atypical electrophoretic creatine kinase(CK) band that migrates between CK-MM and CK-MB and consists of either CK-BB or CK-MM complexed to another serum protein, often IgG, rarely IgA or lipoprotein

macrocyte An enlarged (> 100 µm³ volume) red cell with ↑ hemoglobin and ↓ lifespan, which may be secondary to various stresses, eg hemolytic anemia, hyperthyroidism, massive bleeding, erythroblastosis fetalis, which is accompanied by ↑ erythropoietin production, or due to ↓ vitamin B_{12} or folic acid

macroenzyme 1) An obsolete term for aspartate amino-transferase (AST) 2) A normal enzyme or isoenzyme that is complexed with an immunoglobulin, which may result in the persistant false elevation of a serum enzyme; the false increase may result in an aggressive and/or invasive workup to identify a nonexistent condition; macroenzymes include macro-amylase, macro-AST, macro-CK, macro-LD, and are most common in those > age 60, and are identified by serum electrophoresis (CAP Today November 1993) see Ulysses syndrome

macrogamete PARASITOLOGY The larger egg-like ♀ gamete of *Plasmodium* species, which conjugates with the microgamete (♂), forming a zygote that develops into an oocyst, the part of the *Plasmodium* life cycle that occurs in the human; the asexual phase occurs in the mosquito

macroglia An obsolete generic term for all cells in the CNS that are neither neurons nor microglia (tissue-based macrophages), eg astrocytes, oligodendroglia and glioblasts; 'macroglia' provide nutrition, support and synthesize myelin

macroglobulin A generic term for any large serum protein, usually ≥ 400 kD, eg IgM (900 kD), α_2-macroglobulin (820 kD); macroglobulins are detected by sharp peaks on a simple zone electrophoresis, usually in the γ-region Note: Because of the differing charges on the radicals, the electrophoretic mobility, pI, on the agar may shift and monoclonal spikes may occur in the β or, less commonly, the α regions

macroglossia Enlargement of the tongue due to accumulation of various substances, edema, presence of ectopic tissues, tumors and others; macroglossia occurs in amyloidosis, Beckwith-Wiedemann syndrome, congenital hypothyroidism, cystic hygroma, Down syndrome, ectopic thyroid, glycogen storage disease, type II (Pompe), hemangioma (of the tongue), Hurler syndrome, intestinal duplication, lymphangioma, mannosidosis, neurofibromatosis, rhabdomyoma and Sandhoff's disease

macrolide PHARMACOLOGY A natural lactone with a large (14-20 carbon) ring structure that inhibit protein synthesis, eg erythromycin

macrolide antibiotic Any of a group of broad-spectrum antibiotics, eg erythromycin, that are produced by *Streptomyces* species, which contain a lactone ring and inhibit protein synthesis in target bacteria

macronucleolus GYNECOLOGIC CYTOLOGY An enlarged nucleolus seen in cells in both repair and in invasive carcinoma on a Papanicolaou smear, but not generally seen in 'intermediate' (dysplasia, carcinoma in situ) lesions PARASITOLOGY The larger of two nucleoli (the smaller being known as a micronucleolus) seen in ciliated protozoa, which is thought to orchestrate metabolic activities of the vegetative cell SURGICAL PATHOLOGY Macronucleoli are highly characteristic of certain malignancies, eg carcinoma of the kidney, breast and thyroid, malignant melanoma, Hodgkin's disease and immunoblastic lymphoma

macrophage IMMUNOLOGY A nonspecific immune defense cell that interacts with proteins and polysaccharide antigens, internalizing and partially degrading them, and/or presenting the antigens to T cells in a MHC context; macrophages are involved in secretion, immune interaction with T and B cells, provide lymphokine receptors (once activated, macrophages are highly microbicidal and tumoricidal), often closely associated with the blood vessels, epithelium and mesothelium, appropriate sites for nonspecific immunocytes; macrophages can be divided into

1) Monocytes, comprising 3-5% of circulating leukocytes

2) Tissue-bound macrophages, located in the alveoli, central nervous system (designated as microglial cells), liver (Kupffer cells), lymph nodes, peritoneum and skin (Langerhans' cells) and

3) Histiocytes

Substances secreted by macrophages include binding proteins (transferrin, transcobalamin II, fibronectin), chemotactic factors (for neutrophils), complement components (C1-C5, factors B and D, properdin, C3b inactivator, β1H), endogenous pyrogens, enzymes (neutral proteases, plasminogen activator, collagenase, elastase, angiotensin-convertase, acid hydrolase, proteases, lipases, ribonuclease, phosphatase, glycosidase, sulfatase, arginase, lysozyme), enzyme inhibitors (plasmin inhibitor, α_2-macroglobulin, oxygen radicals: H_2O_2, superoxide, hydroxyl radical, singlet oxygen), bioactive lipids (arachidonic acid metabolites, eg prostaglandin E_2 and F_1, thromboxane A_2, leukotriene, HETE, SRS-A and platelet activating factors), mitogens (colony-stimulating factors, lymphocyte activating factors, growth factors for fibroblasts, endothelium, granulocytes, IL-1), nucleosides and metabolites (thymidine, uracil, uric acid), regulatory proteins (haptoglobin, collagenase, elastase)

macrophage activation The array of processes that form part of the up-regulation of macrophage activity, in which there are multiple

1) Structural changes, eg increased size and number of cytoplasmic granules, spreading of cytoplasmic membrane, membrane ruffling, and

2) Functional changes, eg increased amino acid and glucose metabolism and transport, increased enzymatic activity, eg adenylate cyclase, collagenase and lactate dehydrogenase production and increased in plasminogen activator, prostaglandins, cGMP, intracellular calcium ions, pinocytosis, phagocytosis, bacteriolysis and tumorlysis

macrophage activating factor Any of a heterogeneous group of lymphokines secreted by sensitized lymphocytes; the most potent MAF is IFN-γ but other IFNs and molecules have this activity; IFN-activated macrophages have increased bactericidal and tumoricidal activity and morphological evidence of 'maturation', including enlargement, increased spreading, pseudopod formation and vacuolization

macrophage chemotactic factor A generic term for any cytokine that functions in tandem with the macrophages, mediating migration; mutiple factors are involved and include interleukins and interferons, appearing in the supernatant of graft-versus-host disease

macrophage function assay A generic term for a test that determines the functional activity of macrophages, testing 1) Chemotaxis A chemoattractant is placed at one end of a Boyden chamber and macrophages at the other, and the ability of the cells to migrate towards the test substance is evaluated 2) Lysis A chemoattractant is placed in a chamber and the radioactivity of the supernatant is measured after a target (bacteria, tumor cell) has been destroyed and 3) Phagocytosis Active ingestion by macrophages of a radiolabelled target, yields a radioactive macrophage

macrophage inflammatory protein-1-α An endogenous heparin-binding pyrogen (other pyrogens include interleukin-1 and tumor necrosis factor) that is not affected by cyclo-oxygenase inhibition, which is secreted in response to endotoxin; MIP-1 is identical to SCI (stem cell inhibitor), an inhibitor of hematopoietic stem cells and may be a key actor in the growth regulatory network for hematopoietic cell production

macrophage mannose receptor see *Pneumocystis carinii*

macrophage migration inhibition factor Migration inhibition factor, see there

macrophage/monocyte inhibitory factor A 25-kD lymphokine produced by T-cells in response to antigenic stimulus that inhibits macrophage migration MECHANISM ↑ intracellular cAMP, polymerization of microtubules, halting macrophage progression; some interferons have MIF and MAF activity

macroretinal dystrophy 'Spider' dystrophy, see there

macroscopic magnetization vector MRI The net magnetic moment per unit volume (a vector quantity) of a sample in a given region, considered to be the integrated effect of all the individual microscopic nuclear magnetic moments; see Magnetic resonance imaging

macula densa *macula densa* [NH3] HISTOLOGY A short specialized region in the distal renal tubule at which point specialized cells with large and densely packed nuclei converge; the macula densa is part of the juxtaglomerular apparatus, the components of which include the afferent and efferent glomerular arterioles, Lacis cells and nongranular cells

Mad A tumor suppressor protein produced in the cell nucleus that is thought to shut off the *myc* oncogene; Cf Myc

'mad cow' disease Bovine spongiform encephalopathy, see there

mad dog' FORENSIC PSYCHIATRY A colloquial term for a person who may be regarded as so depraved* that he may be likened to a rabid dog (New York Times 19 March 1995; 37)

*eg Jeffrey Dahmer, who killed nearly 20 people, and ate and/or performed sexual acts on various body parts

Mad Hatter syndrome A descriptor for the neurologic component of chronic mercuric nitrate poisoning, which is clinically similar to prolonged exposure to mercury vapor, erethism; exposed persons undergo psychological changes including anxiety, depression, eccentricity, reclusiveness, emotional instability, irritability, as well as circumoral, glossal and limb tremors, gingivitis, arthralgias, headaches and extrapyramidal signs; see Minamata Bay disease

Note: It is uncertain, although often assumed, that the Mad Hatter described by Lewis Carroll in *Through the Looking Glass* (popularly known as Alice in Wonderland) was a victim of mercury poisoning (Br Med J 1984; 288:324); a major labor-related mercury intoxication occurred in a felt hat factory (hence the fanciful trivial name) during World War II in Italy; of 100 affected, 30 had permanent sequelae (Med Lav 1949; 40:65)

mad honey Nectar derived from pollens of certain plants, including rhododendron, western azalea, California rosebay, mountain laurel and sheep laurel containing toxic diterpenes (grayanotoxins); ingestion of 'mad honey' causes an abrupt attack that may simulate acute myocardial infarction CLINICAL Vertigo, weakness, diaphoresis, nausea, vomiting, profound hypotension, bradyarrhythmia, heart block and potentially, convulsions; all victims recover within 24 hours

Madura foot Mycetoma, see there

MAF Macrophage-activating factor, see there

MAFH Multicentric angiofollicular lymphoid hyperplasia,

see there

MAG Myelin-associated glycoprotein

magenstraße German, gastric 'street' *canalis gastricus* [NA6] The pliable, linear rugal folds of the gastric mucosa that follow the lesser curvature and are bound externally by the gastrohepatic ligament, which is the site of most spontaneous gastric rupture, due in part to the lesser distensibility of the lesser curvature

magenta bodies CYTOLOGY A characteristic, variably-sized red-to-purple perinuclear inclusion seen by Romanovsky stains (eg Wright-Giemsa) in breast carcinomas, both primary or metastatic

magenta tongue A deeply red-to-purple, smooth tongue seen in riboflavin deficiency

maggot Larvae (a worm-like feeding state) of flies (order Diptera) that include the green (*Phaenicia sericata*) and black (*Phormia regina*) bottle flies, which were once used to treat osteomyelitis and chronic suppurative infections, as the larva only thrive in necrotic tissue, secreting allantoin, thought to be a stimulant for epithelial growth; pernicious maggots that thrive on live tissues include *Auchmeromyia luteola* (Congo floor maggot) nocturnal blood suckers, *Eristalis*, and *Helophilus* (hover-fly maggots) which frequent stagnant water and have a predilection for the nasopharynx and intestine; Cf Leeches, Roaches

magic bullet IMMUNOLOGY A term coined by Paul Ehrlich, circa 1900, for what he considered would be an ideal therapeutic agent, which would only to a designated cell or target; the higher the organism is phylogenetically, the more difficult it is to achieve this goal, as the metabolism of the target and host cells are similar; antibiotics are a form of 'magic bullet'; for modern immunologists the term refers to any agent that would act with the specificity of an antibody and have the lethal potential of a toxin; monoclonal antibodies linked to a toxin were crude first-generation magic bullets that have fallen short of their intended aim, as the constant region of the monoclonal antibody doesn't support cytocidal activity; later magic bullet candidates linked cytokines or monoclonal antibodies to toxins (*Diphtheria* toxin, *Pseudomonas* toxin A, or ricin); one apparently successful 'magic bullet' therapeutic approach uses monoclonal anti-B cell antibodies, 'raised' against the CD21 and CD24 antigens to suppress the B-cell lymphoproliferative syndrome (**N Engl J Med 1991; 324:1451**) see Orthozyme CD5plus

'magic bullet' theory FORENSIC PATHOLOGY A posit that has been argued *ad infinitum** regarding a bullet (Warren Commission exhibit 399) identified after the assassination of President John F Kennedy that is believed to have struck both JFK and Governor Connally; proponents of the JFK assassination-as-conspiracy theory have suggested that bullet 399 was pristine and could not have performed the seemingly magical feat of entering two men; rifle range simulations firing 6.5-mm Western Cartridge Company bullets from Lee Harvey Oswald's Mannlicher-Carcano firearm at gelatin-filled skulls resulted in slug deformations and projected trajectories similar to that pieced together by forensic experts of the Warren Commission (**JAMA 1993; 269:1507L, 1544sc**)

Note: In the US, the proposal that the John F Kennedy assasination was a government conspiracy, while virtually devoid of scientific facts and supporters in the forensic science community, has become an entertainment 'industry' a sui generis that no longer requires factual information for self-pepetuation (**JAMA 1993; 269:1540sc**)

*et ad absurdum et ad nauseum

magic factor LABORATORY MEDICINE A highly colloquial term for any intangible factor that affects the performance of a particular test, which makes it difficult to obtain consistent results; certain immunoassays, eg tissue staining by immunoperoxidase methods, may yield inconsistent

results in relatively inexperienced hands, due (some might say) to the MF

magic mushrooms see Peyote

magic number BIOCHEMISTRY The number (20) of different amino acids present in proteins of all plants and animals Note: Although other amino acids are present in proteins, these represent minor biochemical modifications of the 'magic 20'; see Degenerate code

magic spot nucleotides A pair of spots (which when first described were of unknown nature, therefore 'magic') seen on thin-layer chromatograms that were later identified as guanosine 5'-diphosphate 3'-diphosphate (ppGpp) and guanosine 5'-triphosphate 3'-diphosphate (pppGpp), two nucleotides that accumulate during the stringent response reaction in bacteria, in which multiple metabolic pathways shut down when one or more amino acids are present in limited quantities

magical thinking A form of deretic thought, similar to a normal phase of childhood development (Piaget's pre-operational phase), in which thoughts, words or actions assume power, ie they can prevent or cause events to happen without a physical action occurring, ie 'by magic'; magical thinking may be unnerving to those with obsessive-compulsive disorders who fear aggressive thoughts; dereism is thought that is not concordant with logic or experience

maginot line pattern Fortification phenomenon A fanciful descriptor for teichotic scotomata, which are jagged, slightly off-center scintillating lines characteristic of the visual aura that often precedes visual migraines

Note: The Maginot Line is a 20-mile stretch of tooth-like concrete 'barriers' built after World War I, by the worried, war-wearied French with the intent of preventing a third German invasion

magnesium A principle cation in living systems that is in part responsible for the electrochemical properties of living systems, and required for the activity of many enzymes PHYSIOLOGY Serum level: 0.65-1.05 mmol/L (US 1.3-2.1 mEq/L); ↓ Mg^{++} is associated with hypertension of various etiologies, eg of pregnancy, headaches and migraines, hypercholesterolemia and atherosclerosis, some complications of DM, eg diabetic retinopathy (**Science & Medicine 1995; 2/3:28**)

magnetic core memory see Computers

magnetic field The region surrounding a magnet (or current carrying conductor); in a magnetic field, a small magnet experiences a torque that tends to align it in a certain direction; magnetic fields are vector quantities, the direction of which are defined as the direction to which the north pole points when in equilibrium; this field produces a magnetizing force on any object within that field, a cause for potential safety concerns given the large magnetic fields used in MRI; formally, the forces experienced by moving charged particles, current carrying wires and small magnets in the vicinity of a magnet are due to magnetic induction (B), including the effects of magnetization, while the magnetic field (H) is defined so as to not include magnetization (in practice, however, both B and H are often used to denote magnetic fields; see Magnetic resonance imaging

magnetic flux Theta The lines of a magnetic field, which indicates the strength of a magnetic field, expressed by the International System (SI) unit, weber, which is equal to one volt-second

magnetic moment A measure of the net magnetic properties of an object or particle; a nucleus with an intrinsic spin will have an associated dipole moment, so that it interacts with a magnetic field, acting as if it were a small bar magnet; see Magnetic resonance imaging

magnetic resonance The absorption or emission of electromagnetic energy by nuclei in a static magnetic field after excitation by a suitable resonance frequency magnetic field; the peak resonance frequency is proportional to the magnetic field and is given by the Larmor equation Note: Only nuclei with a non-zero spin exhibit magnetic resonance

magnetic resonance angiography CARDIOLOGY YD

magnetic resonance imaging The creation of images by the phenomenon of magnetic resonance (MR), which is a function of the distribution of hydrogen nuclei (protons) in the body; the MR image is a computerized interpretation of the physical interaction of unpaired protons with electromagnetic radiation in the presence of a magnetic field; image brightness in a given region depends on

1) Spin density and

2) Relaxation times, the relative importance of which is determined by the imaging technique being employed as well as

3) Motion such as blood flow

It was postulated in 1971 that MR might be clinically useful for analyzing the whole body; the early work was performed by EMI Ltd of England before the MR imaging became a reality; the images derive from analysis of the amplitudes and frequencies of the weak signals produced by MR, allowing deduction of the sample's chemical composition, with protons providing the best images; the strength of a signal reflects the amount of hydrogen modified by the tissue relaxation parameters, T1 (the spin lattice parameter, which depends on the interaction of hydrogen with other molecules) and T2 (the spin-spin parameter, a function of the interaction of the protons with each other); MR signal intensity is influenced by the proton bulk motion effect, which is a function of the 50 msec lag time between signal production and its registering on the detector PRINCIPLE When tissue is placed in an intense magnetic field, the hydrogen nuclei behave like weak magnets, orienting themselves along the lines of flux; if the tissue is then 'zapped' with a pulse of a specific wavelength of radiofrequency electromagnetic energy (measured in tesla, high field strengths being 1-2 tesla, low energy < 0.5 tesla), which changes the alignment of hydrogen nuclei by absorption of that energy; as the nuclei return to their previous state of alignment, they emit a characteristic radiofrequency length signal which, when compared to other signal 'densities' within the sample, allows construction of an image; the magnetic signal is strongest immediately after the tissue has received the radiofrequency impulse and the time to achieve 'relaxation' depends upon differing hydrogen concentration in various tissues, resulting in different decay times T1 and T2; the longitudinal (T1, spin-lattice) relaxation time is that required for the nuclei to return to the pre-RF pulse ground state; the transverse (T2, spin-spin) relaxation time refers to the signal decay, which is a function of the interaction of the nuclei in tissues; signal decay is rapid for rigid molecules (proteins and nucleic acids) and these molecules are not major contributors to the image quality; the MR signal is largely a function of the tissue's water content, with lesser signals contributed by lipids and muscle, allowing excellent soft-tissue differentiation; MR has multiplanar capabilities without the ionizing radiation of computed tomography CLINICAL APPLICATIONS Because conventional MR imaging requires a few minutes to obtain the image, mobile organs, eg heart, GI tract are relatively 'fuzzy', although the image obtention time can be 'gated' to reduce this problem POTENTIAL HAZARDS Patients undergoing MRI are exposed to static magnetic, pulsed, radiofrequency, electromagnetic and gradient (time-varying) fields; gradient fields allow ultrafast imaging, reducing the scan time of 10 minutes in a conventional MR imager to milliseconds, with the disadvantage of potentially triggering cardiac arrhythmias and unwanted electrical activity (Science 1991; 252:1244n&v)

GLOSSARY FOR MRI (modified from JAMA 1987; 258:3422)

ANGULAR MOMENTUM A quantity given by the product of the momentum of a particle and its position vector; in absence of external forces, the AM remains constant, therefore a rotating body tends to maintain the same axis of rotation; when a torque is applied to a rotating body, the resulting change in angular momentum results in precession; atomic nuclei possess an intrinsic angular momentum referred to as spin, measured in multiples of Planck's constant CARR-PURCELL SEQUENCE A sequence of 90° radiofrequency pulses followed by repeated 180° radiofrequency pulses, producing a train of spin echoes that is used to measure T2 CARR-PURCELL-MEIBOON-GILL SEQUENCE A modification of the Carr-Purcell radiofrequency pulse sequence with 90° phase shift in the rotating frames of reference between the 90° pulse and subsequent 180° pulses, reducing the accumulating effects of imperfections in the 180° pulses; suppression of effects of pulse error accumulation can also be achieved by alternating the phases of the 180° pulses by 180° CHEMICAL SHIFT (DELTA) The change in the Larmor frequency of a given nucleus when bound to different sites in a molecule, due to magnetic shielding effects of the electron orbitals; chemical shifts are responsible for the differences among various molecules and different sites within the molecules in high-resolution magnetic resonance spectra; the amount of shift is proportional to strength of the magnetic field strength and is usually specified in parts per million of the resonance frequency relative to a standard ECHO PLANAR IMAGING A technique of planar imaging in which a complete planar image is obtained from one selective excitation pulse FREE INDUCTION DECAY A transient MR signal produced by transverse magnetization of the spins, eg by a 90° pulse, which decays toward zero with a characteristic time constant T2 (or T2*); in practice, the first part of the FID is not observable due to residual effects of the powerful exciting radiofrequency pulse on the electronics of the receiver; FID is observed while periodically switching the y-gradient field in the presence of a static x-gradient field; the Fourier transform of the resulting spin-echo train can be used to produce an image of the excited plane FLIP ANGLE The amount of rotation of the macroscopic magnetization vector produced by an RF pulse with respect to the direction of the static magnetic field FOURIER TRANSFORM A mathematical procedure that separates the frequency component of a signal from its amplitude as a function of time or vice versa; the Fourier transform is used to generate the spectrum from the free induction decay in pulse MRI and is essential to most imaging techniques GRADIENT MAGNETIC FIELD (GMR) A magnetic field that changes in strength in a given direction; such fields are used in MR imaging with excitation that 'selects' a region for imaging and encodes the location of MR signals received from the object being imaged; the GMR is measured in teslas/meter HOMOGENEITY Uniformity of the static magnetic field, a criterion of the magnet's quality; the requirements for homogeneity in MR imaging are less stringent than for MR spectroscopy, but must be maintained over a larger region INTERPULSE TIME The time period between successive RF pulses used in pulse sequences; of particular importance are the inversion time (TI) in inversion recovery, a time period between a 180° pulse and the subsequent 90° pulse; the period between repetitions of pulse sequences is known as the repetition time (TR) INVERSION A nonequilibrium state in which the macroscopic magnetization vector is oriented opposite to the magnetic field; usually produced by adiabatic fast passage or by 180° RF pulses INVERSION RECOVERY A pulse MR technique that can be incorporated into MRI, where the nuclear magnetization is inverted at a time on the order of T1 before the regular imaging pulse-gradient sequences; the resulting partial relaxation of the spins in the different structures being imaged can be used to produce an image that depends on T1, enhancing the differences in the appearance of structures with different T1 relaxation times Note: Inversion recovery does not produce a direct image of T1, but rather one that is calculated from the change in the MR signal from the region due to the inversion pulse compared with the signal with no inversion pulse or an inversion pulse with a different T1 inversion time LARMOR EQUATION A formula stating that the frequency of precession of the nuclear magnetic moment is proportional to the magnetic field. Equation: $w_0 = \gamma B_0$ (radians/sec) or $f_0 = \gamma B_0/2\pi$ (hertz), where f_0 is frequency, γ is gyromagnetic ratio, and B_0 is the magnetic induction field Note: A negative sign (–) indicates the direction of rotation LARMOR FREQUENCY (w_0 or f_0) The frequency at which magnetic resonance can be excited, given by the Larmor equation; by varying a magnetic field across the body with a gradient magnetic field, the corresponding variation of the LF can be used to encode position (for protons, the LF is 42.58 MHz/tesla) **LONGITUDINAL MAGNETIZATION** M_z The component of the macroscopic magnetization vector along the static magnetic field; after excitation by a radiofrequency pulse, M_z will approach its equilibrium value designated M_O, with a characteristic time constant, T1 **LONGITUDINAL RELAXATION** The return of longitudinal magnetization to its equilibrium value after excitation, which requires exchange of energy between the nuclear spins and lattice **MACROSCOPIC MAGNETIZATION VECTOR** Net magnetic moment per unit volume (a vector quantity) of a sample in a given region, considered to be the integrated effect of all the individual microscopic nuclear magnetic moments **MAGNETIC FIELD** (H) The region surrounding a magnet (or current carrying conductor); in a magnetic field, a small magnet experiences a torque that tends to align it in a certain direction; magnetic fields are vector quantities, the direction of which are defined as the direction to which the north pole points when in equilibrium; this field produces a magnetizing force on any object within that field, a cause for potential safety concerns given the large magnetic fields used in MRI; formally, the forces experienced by moving charged particles, current carrying wires and small magnets in the vicinity of a magnet are due to magnetic induction (B), including the effects of magnetization, while the magnetic field (H) is defined so as to not include magnetization (in practice, however, both B and H are often used to denote magnetic fields **MAGNETIC MOMENT** A measure of the net magnetic properties of an object or particle; a nucleus with an intrinsic spin will have an associated dipole moment, so that it interacts with a magnetic field, acting as if it were a tiny bar magnet **MAGNETIC RESONANCE SIGNAL** An electromagnetic signal in the radiofrequency range produced by the precession of the transverse magnetization of the spins; rotation of the magnetization induces a voltage that is amplified and demodulated by the receiver; the signal may refer only to this induced voltage **MAGNETIZATION** The magnetic polarization of a material produced by a magnetic field, ie the magnetic moment per unit volume; Cf Macroscopic magnetization vector **MAGNETIZATION DIPOLE** North and south magnetic poles separated by a finite distance, corresponding to an electric current loop, including the effective current of a spinning nucleon or nucleus, which may create an equivalent magnetic dipole **MULTIPLE PLANE IMAGING** A variation on the sequential plane imaging techniques that can be used with selective excitation techniques and does not affect adjacent planes; adjacent planes are imaged while waiting for relaxation of the first plane toward equilibrium, resulting in decreased imaging time **NUCLEAR SPIN** An intrinsic property of certain nuclei that gives them an associated characteristic angular momentum and magnetic moment; Cf Spin **PARTIAL SATURATION** An 'excitation' technique that consists of administration of repeated radiofrequency pulses in time periods equal to or shorter than T1; in MRI, although partial saturation results in decreased signal amplitude, it is possible to generate images with increased contrast between regions with different relaxation times Cf Saturation recovery **PERMANENT MAGNET** A magnet composed of a permanently magnetized material **PRECESSION** The relatively slow gyration of the axis of a spinning body, allowing it to 'race out a cone'; precession is caused by the application of a torque that tends to change the direction of a rotation axis and continuously directs it at right angles to the plane of the torque; the magnetic moment of a nucleus with spin will experience such a torque when inclined at an angle to the magnetic field, resulting in precession at the Larmor frequency, eg effect of gravity on a gyroscope or spinning top **PULSE, 90° (Π/2 PULSE)** A radiofrequency pulse that is designed to rotate the macroscopic magnetization vector 90° in space as referred to the rotating frame of reference, usually about an axis at right angles to the main magnetic field; if the spins are initially aligned with the magnetic field, the pulse produces transverse magnetization and a free induction delay **PULSE, 180° (Π PULSE)** A radiofrequency pulse that is designed to rotate the macroscopic magnetization vector 180° in space as referred to the rotating frame of reference, usually about an axis at right angles to the main magnetic field; if the spins are initially aligned with the magnetic field, the pi pulse produces inversion **PULSE LENGTH** or width The duration (delta time) of a pulse; for an RF pulse near the Larmor frequency, the longer the pulse length, the greater is the angle of rotation of the macroscopic magnetization vector (> 180° brings the pulse length back to its original orientation) **PULSE SEQUENCES** A set of RF (and/or gradient) magnetic field pulses and time intervals between these pulses; used in conjunction with gradient magnetic fields and MR signal reception to produce MR images; Cf Interpulse time **RADIOFREQUENCY** The frequency on the electromagnetic spectrum that is intermediate between auditory and infrared, which in MRI is in the megaherz range; the principal effect of RF magnetic fields on the body is the deposition of power (heat), usually confined to the corporal surface, being the main safety concern **RADIOFREQUENCY COIL** A component of the MRI hardware that transmits RF pulses and/or receives MR signals; commonly having a solenoid or saddle configuration **RADIOFREQUENCY PULSE** A brief burst of RF magnetic field delivered to the object by the RF transmitter; for an RF near the Larmor frequency, the RF pulse results in rotation of the macroscopic magnetization vector in the rotating frame of reference; the amount of rotation depends on the strength and duration of the RF pulse, most commonly 90° ($\pi/2$) and 180° (π) pulses **RECEIVER** The component of the MRI hardware that detects and amplifies RF signals picked up by the receiver coil, which is comprised of a preamplifier, amplifier and demodulator **RELAXATION TIME** The time period after excitation that is required for spins to return to a ground state or state of equilibrium distribution, in which there is no transverse magnetization and the longitudinal magnetization is at its maximum value and oriented in the direction of the static magnetic field; the transverse magnetization decays toward zero with a characteristic time constant T2; the longitudinal magnetization returns toward the equilibrium value M_O with a characteristic time constant T1 **REPEATED FREE INDUCTION DECAY** A form of MR in which repeated 90° pulses are applied, which results in partial saturation if the interpulse times are equal or less than T1 **RESOLUTION** Spatial resolution The ability of the imaging process to distinguish among adjacent structures within an object being imaged, which is a measure of image quality; the criterion for determining resolution depends on the type of test being used (bar pattern or contrast detail phantom); the ability to separate or discern objects depends on their contrast and different MRI object parameters affect different imaging techniques, thus for example, comparison of resolution phantom tests from different machines may be difficult as the images differ **ROTATING FRAME OF REFERENCE** A point and its corresponding coordinate system that is rotating about the axis of the static magnetic field B_0 (with respect to a stationary or 'laboratory' frame of reference) at a frequency equal to that of the applied RF magnetic field, B_1; although B_1 is a rotating vector, it appears stationary in the rotating frame, and allows simple calculations **SEQUENTIAL PLANE IMAGING** An MRI technique in which an image is built up from successive planes in the imaged object; these planes are selected by oscillating gradient magnetic fields or by selective excitation **SIGNAL-TO-NOISE RATIO** The ratio obtained from the relative contributions of detected true signal to that of random superimposed signals ('noise'); SNR is a function of the electromagnetic properties of the sample or the patient being studied; the higher the SNR, the better the image's resolution; SNR may be improved by 1) Averaging several measurements of a signal since random signals tend to cancel themselves, 2) Sampling large volumes (with corresponding loss of spatial resolution) and 3) Increasing the magnetic field's strength **SPECTRUM** An array of the components of the MR signal according to frequency; nuclei with different resonant frequencies appear as peaks ('lines') at different frequencies in the spectrum **SPIN** The intrinsic angular momentum of an elementary particle (or system of particles such as a nucleus) that is responsible for the magnetic moment; the spins of nuclei have characteristic fixed values and when pairs of neutrons and protons are aligned, they cancel out the values of their spins, so that nuclei with an odd number of neutrons and/or protons will have a net nonzero rotational component characterized by an integer or half-integer quantum 'nuclear spin number' **SPIN DENSITY** The density of resonating spins in a given region, which is a prime determinant of the strength of an MR signal from the region, measured in SI (International system) units (moles/m^3); for water, 0.11 moles of H_2O/m^3; spin density cannot be imaged directly, but is a complex series of calculations received from different pulse times **SPIN ECHO** The reappearance of an MR signal after the free induction decay is complete, due to effective reversal of the dephasing of the spins ('refocusing') by various techniques, eg reversal of a gradient magnetic field, which is a form of 1) 'time reversal' or 2) Specific RF pulse sequences such as the Carr-Purcell sequence (applied in a time shorter than or equal to T2); multiple spin echoes or a series of spin echoes at different times can be used to determine T2 without 'contamination' through the effects of the inhomogeneity of the magnetic field **SPIN-ECHO IMAGING** A type of MRI where the spin-echo signal is measured (in contrast to measuring the FID); spin-echo images are largely a function of T2 **SPIN-LATTICE RELAXATION TIME** see T1 **SPIN-SPIN RELAXATION TIME** see T2 **STATIONARY RECOVERY** A type of partial saturation pulse sequence in which preceding pulses leave the spins in a state of saturation, so that recovery at the time of the next pulse takes place from an initial condition of no magnetization **SUPERCONDUCTING MAGNET** A magnet with a magnetic field originating from current flowing through a superconductor, which is encased in a cryostat **SURFACE COIL MR** A small RF receiver coil placed over a region of interest on the object being imaged which has an effective selectivity for the area of interest, eg the shoulder, knee, brain, spine and elsewhere **T1** Spin-lattice or longitudinal relaxation time A time period after transverse magnetization, the characteristic time (a constant) for spins to align themselves back to the external magnetic field; starting from zero magnetization in the z direction, the z magnetization increases to 63% of its final maximum value in a time T1 **T2** Spin-spin or transverse relaxation time The time period (a constant) for the loss of phase coherence among spins oriented at a right angle to the static magnetic field, a result of interactions between the spins, with the resulting loss of transverse magnetization and MR signal; starting from a non-zero value of magnetization in the xy plane, the xy magnetization decays and loses 63% of its initial value in a time T2 **T2*** The time constant for the loss of phase coherence among the spins oriented at an angle to the static magnetic field due to a combination of magnetic field inhomogeneities, deltaB and spin-spin transverse relaxation, which results in a more rapid loss in transverse magnetization and MR signal **TE** Echo time The time between the middle of the 90° pulse and the middle of the production of the spin-echo, for multiple echoes, TE1, TE2 and others **TESLA** The International System (SI) unit for magnetic flux density, equivalent to 10 000 gauss, the formerly used unit **TI** Inversion time The time period between the middle of the inverting (180°) RF pulse and the middle of the 90° pulse, used to detect longitudinal magnetization **TR** Repetition time The period between the beginning of the pulse sequence and the beginning of the succeeding (virtually identical) pulse sequence **TRANSVERSE MAGNETIZATION** Mxy The component of the macroscopic magnetization vector at right angles to the static magnetic field (B_0); precession of the transverse magnetization at the Larmor frequency is responsible for the detected MR signal; in absence of an externally applied RF energy, the transverse magnetization will decay to zero with a characteristic time constant (T2 or T2*) **VOLUME IMAGING** Simultaneous volume imaging An imaging technique in which the signals are gathered from the whole object at one time, with appropriate encoding of pulse/gradient sequences to encode the positions of the spins; in principle, many sequential plane images can be generalized to volume imaging **ZEUGMATOGRAPHY** A coinage from Greek that dignifies magnetic resonance imaging, translated as '*the spatial relation of the image to a gradient magnetic field*' it is unlikely this ad hoc coinage will prevail (author's note)

magnetic resonance signal An electromagnetic signal in the radiofrequency range produced by the precession of the transverse magnetization of the spins; rotation of the magnetization induces a voltage that is amplified and demodulated by the receiver; the signal may refer only to this induced voltage; see Magnetic resonance imaging

magnetic resonance spectroscopy LABORATORY MEDICINE A technique for determining the structure of organic compounds, the first practical use of the principle of magnetic resonance; MRS has become an indispensable tool in pharmacokinetics, biochemistry and molecular biology

magnetization MRI The magnetic polarization of a material produced by a magnetic field, ie the magnetic moment per unit volume; Cf Macroscopic magnetization vector; see Magnetic resonance imaging

magnetization dipole MRI North and south magnetic poles separated by a finite distance, corresponding to an electric current loop, including the effective current of a spinning nucleon or nucleus, which may create an equivalent magnetic dipole; see Magnetic resonance imaging

magnification see Microscopy

'Magnificent Seven' A highly colloquial synonym for the G protein-coupled membrane receptors, which belong to the same gene family, so named as they all span the cell membrane seven times, see Heptaspan

The term is intended as a play-on-words after the Hollywood film by the same name, although the parochial nature of the sobriquet appears to make preferable the more widely-used (and scientific) term 'G protein receptor', see there, or the term Heptaspan (see there) as suggested by LL Brunton

MAIDS see Murine acquired immuodeficiency syndrome

MAILLARD REACTION

Aldose [ketose] sugar + NH_2-Protein

$\uparrow \downarrow \pm H_2O$

N- substituted ketosylamine [aldosylamine]

$\downarrow$ Amadori (Heyns) rearrangement

1-amino-1-deoxy-2-ketose [2-amino-2-deoxyaldose]

$\downarrow$ Dehydration, condensation, reduction, fragmentation, oxidation, cyclization

Furfurals, reductones, fission products, free radicals

$\downarrow NH_2$-protein

AGEs* (heterogeneous cross-linked protein aggregates

*Advanced glycosylation end-products —from Nature Medicine 1995; 1:189

Maillard reaction CLINICAL NUTRITION A non-enzymatic heat-activated chemical reaction between sugars (especially ribose) and amino acids that occurs in food as it forms glycosylamines and Amadori compounds, which is responsible for 'browning' of baked or cooked foods, eg bread crusts and barbecued steak; browned foods are mutagenic by the Ames assay; it is possible that the age-related changes in collagen are partially mediated through the Maillard reaction; it has been suggested the MR might be involved in certain neurodegenerative diseases, eg Alzheimer's, Creutzfeldt-Jakob, and Parkinson's diseases (Nature Medicine 1995; 1:189) see Browning reaction; Cf Rancidity

'mail order' medicine A derogatory phrase for the basing of therapeutic decisions solely on the results of tests, eg Radioallergosorbent test, sent to a referral laboratory; see RAST

main-en-lorgnette *lorgnette*, French, opera glass RHEUMATOLOGY A classic descriptor for a hand afflicted by arthritis mutilans, accompanied by extensive compressive erosion, collapse of the proximal phalanges with 'telescoping' of bones upon themselves and overriding of the fingers by metacarpophalangeal dislocation, resulting in destroyed contracted hands; although most characteristic of advanced rheumatoid arthritis, 'main-en-lorgnette' may also occur in psoriatic arthritis, erosive osteoarthritis, chronic infection, diabetes and leprosy

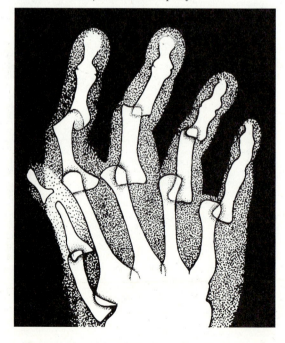

main-en-lorgnette

main-en-trident A short broad hand with a foreshortened middle finger, resulting in equal length of all digits; the characteristic shape of the index and ring finger results in an appearance fancifully likened to Neptune's trident, a finding classically seen in achondroplasia

'mainstreaming' The placement of learning-impaired or otherwise handicapped children in the same classroom as other children, while supplementing their learning with various educational maneuvers, a process that is thought to improve socialization; by extension, mainstreaming refers to any effort to integrate a person with an affliction, eg mental health patients, into society

mainframe computer A really big computer that manipulates large blocks of data by 'multitasking' logical sequences; although only one flow of logic can occur at one time (unless there are multiple sequential processors), the power and speed of a mainframe computer, eg an IBM 3060, is such that the transition from one task to another is virtually 'seamless'; 'dedicated' mainframes are used to process data in CT, MRI, and hospital information systems and have speeds of up to hundreds of MIPS (million instructions/sec); see Computers; Cf Microcomputer, Minicomputer, Parallel processing, Supercomputers

Note: The speed of 'microcomputers' has continued to increase (at an estimated average of 55%/year) since the first IBM-PCs were sold in the early 1980s, and some workers believe that mainframes may be replaced by desktop computers in as little as 5 years

maintenance see Remission

maintenance dose CLINICAL PHARMACOLOGY A dose of a drug that is administered after achieving stable levels of the therapeutic agent of interest in the body, which is intended to maintain the therapeutic status quo; Cf Loading dose

MAIS complex *Mycobacterium avium-intracellulare-scrofulaceum* Three mycobacterial species that are indistinguishable from each other in terms of surface lipids and antigens, pigment production, biochemical reactions, antibiotic susceptibilities, often in the same clinical company INCIDENCE MAIS is relatively uncommon, but affects 5-8% of patients with AIDS, who are increasingly susceptible as the CD4+ T cells fall below 0.1×10^9 (US: 100/mm^3) CLINICAL Persistent fever possibly accompanied by night sweats, chronic diarrhea, abdominal pain, extrahepatic obstruction and potentially, severe anemia TREATMENT Ciproflozacin, clofazimine, ethambutol and rifampicin, to which amikacin is added if the initial therapy is unsuccessful by the fourth week; promising, not-yet-approved agents include rifabutin, clarithromycin and azithromycin (N Engl J Med 1991; 324:1332rv)

MAIS-intermediate A MAIS that differs from other MAISs as it is urease-negative, hydrolyzes Tween, has variable pigmentation and catalase activity

major air pollutants PUBLIC HEALTH Principal pollutants in the ambient air, to wit, carbon monoxide, nitrogen dioxide, ozone, particulate matter, and sulfur dioxide (N Engl J Med 1994; 331:1542oa)

major basic protein An 11-kD (11 000 M_r) protein that is a major component of eosinophilic granules and forms a characteristic crystalloid; the adjectival 'basic' derives from MBP's isoelectric point of greater than pH 10; MBP is capable of killing parasites, as well as host cells; it causes bronchial epithelial damage and a wheal and flare response when injected subcutaneously and has been linked to asthma; MBP has been identified in low concentrations in the granules of other myeloid cells

major breakpoint region A 150-bp region of DNA on chromosomal segment 18q21 located in the 3' untranslated region of bcl-2 exon III; 50-70% of t(14:18) translocations (seen in most follicular lymphomas) are linked to mbr, which can be identified by PCR; see Minor cluster region

major crossmatch TRANSFUSION MEDICINE The testing of a patient's serum against a potential donor's red cells to detect the presence of ABO incompatibility and other major antibodies; see Immediate spin crossmatch, Minor cross-match; Cf Back typing, Front typing

major depressive episode A condition that is defined as '...a period of at least 2 weeks during which there is either depressed mood or the loss of interest or pleasure in nearly all activities...(and) ... experience at least four additional symptoms (including) ... changes in appetitite or weight, sleep, and psychomotor activity; decreased energy; feelings of worthlessness or guilt; difficulty thinking, concentrating, or making decisions; or recurrent thoughts of death, or suicidal ideatin, plans, or attempts.' (DSM-IV)

major diagnostic category DRGs, see there

major groove MOLECULAR BIOLOGY A deep and wide furrow present in Watson-Crick DNA that extends over the entire length of DNA as long as the molecule remains in a normal or right-handed configuration; for the usual B-DNA, the major groove is 22 nm wide; see Minor groove, Z-DNA

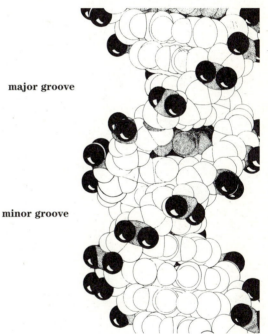

major groove

minor groove

major histocompatibility complex see MHC

major life activities SOCIAL MEDICINE The constellation of human activities that constitutes economic, intellectual and functional self-sufficiency, including the ability to maintain a job, learning, mobility and self-direction; these activities or the inability to perform them are used by governing bodies to determine a person's eligibility for programs offering assistance to people with handicaps, mental retardation and developmental disabilities

'major medical' Major medical expense insurance HEALTH CARE INDUSTRY A health insurance policy or 'rider' (extension) to an insurance policy that finances medical expenses incurred in injuries, catastrophic or prolonged illness, providing benefit payments above the base paid by the insurance company

major surgery A generic term for any hazardous surgical procedure that may be defined as an operation 1) Within or upon the contents of the abdominal (or pelvic), cranial, or thoracic cavities, or 2) A procedure, which given the locality, condition of the patient. level of difficulty of the procedure, or length of time to perform, constitutes a hazard to life or function of an organ or body part; major surgery usually requires general anesthesia, a period of hospitalization of varying length, often less than a week, and may be performed by a general (board-certified) surgeon in a secondary care hospital, but by a surgical subspecialist in a tertiary care hospital setting; Cf Minor surgery

malakoplakia *malakos*, Greek, soft plaque A lesion often seen in the urogenital tract (bladder, renal pelvis, ureter, uterus, broad ligament, endometrium, testes, epididymis and prostate, with female:male ratio of 4:1) and rarely also in the retroperitoneum, colon, stomach, appendix, lymph nodes, lungs, bone and skin, with a ratio of 1:1; malakoplakia is more common in the immunosuppressed transplant recipients PATHOGENESIS Defective macrophage response to coliform bacteria (often *Escherichia coli*, but also *Klebsiella* spp and *Mycobacterium intracellulare*); the condition was described in 1903 by von Hansemann and consists of soft, yellow, elevated and friable 3-4 cm in diameter mucosal plaques PATHOLOGY Swollen submucosal histiocytes (von Hansemann cells) extending into connective tissue replete with Michaelis-Gutmann bodies (spherical cytoplasmic structures layered by calcium/iron salts, contained within phagosomes, figure, page 417, upper right) TREATMENT Long-term antibiotic therapy, ascorbic acid, cholinergic agents; if recalcitrant, surgical excision

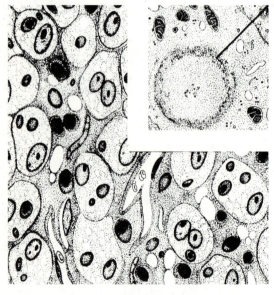

malakoplakia

malarial pigment Black pigment in cerebral white matter composed of hematin and protein, a characteristic postmortem finding in *P falciparum* malaria; the malarial brain is congested and edematous with indurated, flattened gyri and petechiae

malaria prophylaxis Prevention is preferable to treating malaria and prophylaxis is recommended by the CDC for travel to areas of *Plasmodium falciparum* endemicity AGENTS Chloroquine, hydroxychloroquine, mefloquine, quinine sulfate, doxycycline (not recommended during pregnancy), proguanil, pyrimethamine-sulfadoxine, primaquine and more recently, mefloquine, currently the prophylactic agent of choice

malaria vaccine A viable vaccine against malaria is not available; the current 'gold standard' for a *Plasmodium* that is immunogenic but not pathogenic is the radiation-attenuated sporozoite, although a combination of circumsporozoite protein and the 140-kD sporozoite surface protein 2 (SSP-2) may be as effective (Science 1991; 252:715); another candidate is Pfs25, a 25-kD, cysteine-rich sexual stage surface protein of *P falciparum* that has been inserted into a vaccinia virus and elicits transmission-blocking antibodies in, but not restricted to mice (Science 1991; 252:1310); other approaches include eliciting natural antibodies against circumsporozoite (CS) protein, attempting to block the pre-hepatoinvasive stage; *P falciparum* is a highly mutable parasite for which there may never be a viable vaccine, given that 1) The parasite reproduces sexually within the insect host, leading to maintenance and increase of heterozygosity and 2) Natural immunity to the organism requires continued contact with the parasite for constant enrichment of genetic diversity, as opposed to a 'one-shot' exposure of a vaccine

malariotherapy Iatrogenic malaria Intentional inoculation of benign tertian malaria (*Plasmodium vivax*), a modality used in the pre-antibiotic era for treating neurosyphilis; the data from uncontrolled studies suggest that there was little, if any effect on the underlying syphilis, despite the non-specific immune reaction with fever and secretion of TNF and IL-1, as the reports of success were largely clinical without laboratory confirmation; although it was thought that patients with neuroborreliosis (advanced Lyme disease) might respond to malariotherapy, this appears to complicate or exacerbate an already poor clinical situation; Cf BCG, Immunotherapy

malate dehydrogenase An oxidoreductase [EC 1.1.1.37] located in both the mitochondria and cytosol that catalyzes the reversible NAD⁺/NADH reaction in the presence of (*S*)-malate, yielding oxaloacetate, which is a step in the citric acid cycle; MD is ↑ in MI, hepatocellular necrosis, megaloblastic anemia, and malignancy

malathion An anticholinesterase-type organophosphate which is effective against insects (aphids, spiders, mites, houseflies, and other creepy crawlers); see Intermediate syndrome

mal de ojo Spanish, evil eye A term for a culture-bound symptom complex described in certain Mediterranean countries (eg Italian, mal occhio) that is more common in children and if it affects adults, more often women, which characterized by unrest, fitful sleep, fever, diarrhea, vomiting, crying without reason (from DSM-IV); see Culture-bound syndrome

mal de Meleda An AR [MIM 248300] condition causing symmetric palmoplantar hyperkeratosis and acanthosis accompanied by circumscribed hyperkeratosis of the wrists, knees, forearms and ankles, brachydactyly, koilonychia, growth and mental retardation, seen in the highly inbred population of the island of Meleda off the coast of Dalmatia in western Yugoslavia

mal puesto Rootwork, see there

MALDI-TOF system Matrix-assisted laser desorption-ionization time-of-flight mass spectrometer system A newly-developed (ie 'high tech') system used to determine the molecular weight of biopolymers ranging from 100s to 300 000 daltons, at picomolar to femtomolar levels; the MALDI-TOF systme's development was made possible by advances in detectors, fast digitization circuitry, microprocessors, pulsed lasers, and vacuum crystallization (Am Lab Sept 1994 p32c)

male see Anabolic steroids, Circumcision, H-Y chromosome, Testes

male menopause Andropause A popular term for the changes accompanying the ↓ in testicular function with ↑ age, eg ↑ body fat, and ↓ bone and muscle mass, energy, virility, and fertility; while many experts do not believe MM is a valid clinical entity*, the presence of such a male analogue to menopause has been evoked as a excuse for the frivolity and philandering that accompanies the so-called 'midlife crisis'; unlike the ♀ climacteric in which the end of ovarian hormonal function is abrupt, the decline in testicular function occurs at a slower pace, and thus a more analogous situation is that of castration, in which the hormonal deprivation is abrupt (JAMA 1992; 268:2486MN&P) see Midlife crisis; Cf Menopause

*MM has been described by those who believe in its existance as a psychogenic complex characterized by diminished libido, impotence, fatigue, hot flashes, irritability, depression, poor ability to concentrate and insomnia LABORATORY Androgenic hormones are usually within normal limits PATHOLOGY Testes demonstrate variable ↓ in spermatogenesis and tubular atrophy

male pseudohermaphroditism '...a heterogeneous condition in which the gonads are exclusively testes, but the genital ducts and/or external genitalia are incompletely masculinized.'* MP is a type of intersex in which the testes are present and cryptorchid, but testosterone production is inadequate (due to decreased LH or hCG receptors on the Leydig cells); patients are raised as females (Morris syndrome) and may have CNS defects, eg defective gonadotropin response, primary gonadal defects, eg idiopathic, defective pregnanediol (3-β 17-α, 17,20 des and 17 β) synthesis, regression of müllerian tubes, Leydig cell agenesis, androgen insensitivity, increased susceptibility to breast cancer, Sertoli adenoma, germinoma in situ, seminoma, Leydig cell tumor

*MM Grumbach and FA Conte in JD Wilson, and DW Foster, Eds Williams Textbook of Endocrinology, 8th ed, WB Saunders Philadelphia, 1992

malemission Failure to ejaculate during intercourse; Cf Nocturnal emission

malformation see Teratogenesis

malfunction 54 RADIATION ONCOLOGY A software 'bug' that caused a 25-Megaelectron volt (MeV) linear accelerator (used in radiation oncology) to accidentally deliver 25 000 rads of 25 MeVs in one second, resulting in three known fatal radiation overdoses; the computer at fault used 'assembly' language and the software failed to access the appropriate calibration data

malice 'The intentional doing of a wrongful act without just cause or excuse, with an intent to inflict an injury or under circumstances that the law will imply an evil intent.' (Black's Law Dictionary, 6th ed, West Publishing, St Paul, Mn, 1990)

Malice is rarely inferred in cases of medical malpractice, and is here included only as a point of reference-Author's note

malignancy see Cancer, Carcinogens, Congenital malignancy, Multiple primary malignancy syndrome, Metastasis, Oncogenes, Secondary malignancy

malignant Tending to harm, kill, or maim, usually referring to either a neoplasm or a pernicious process such as malignant hypertension; the one absolute criteria for malignancy is the presence of metastasis; to define a tumor as malignant in absence of detectable metastasis, as may occur in malignant brain tumors, requires the use of soft criteria, eg extreme cellular pleomorphism, presence of bizarre (eg tripolar) mitotic figures, aneuploidy detected by flow cytometry, and an increase in S-phase tetraploid nuclei; other neoplasms, eg pleomorphic adenoma of the salivary glands or thymoma may be defined as malignant based on the presence of infiltrative destructive growth (see Arch Pathol Lab Med 1994; 118:252OA)

malignant angioendotheliomatosis Angiotropic lymphoma, see there

malignant blue nevus A rare skin lesion that usually involves the scalp, presenting as a multinodular plaque > 2.0 cm with a history of progressive enlargement, which is often associated with a cellular blue nevus; the behavior of th MBN is unpredictable (N Engl J Med 1995; 332:656RV) see Melanoma

Note: 'Garden variety' cellular blue nevi may give rise to 'benign metastases' to regional LN (± 5% of cases), but differ from true metastases in that the cell are cytologically benign

malignant cell A cell that has undergone 'transformation', ie is in a state of permanent proliferation and is capable of metastasis; MCs are defined by various phenotypic changes, including ↓ intercellular adhesion and electrical repulsion (due to a loss of anchorage dependence), ↓ intracellular K^+ and Ca^{2+}, aneuploidy, loss of response to (control by) the usual cytokines and mitogens, ectopic hormone production, the use of aberrant metabolic pathways, biochemical convergence (cells lose features of differentiation and organ-specific features, eg microvilli, desmosomes, intermediate filaments), cytopathological changes (nucleolar margination, a sign of rapid growth), cytologic atypia, nuclear irregularity, hyperchromasia and high nuclear:cytoplasmic ratio, swelling of mitochondria and flooding of the mitochondrial matrix; other features include alterations in growth parameters and cell behavior, cell-surface alterations, loss of actin myofilaments, increased transforming growth factor release, protease secretion, altered gene transcription, and immortalization of cells

malignant fibrous histiocytoma A pleomorphic mesenchymal malignancy of older adults, which affects deep soft tissues (involving muscle 60% or fascia 20%) of the lower (50%) and upper (20%) extremities, retroperitoneum 15% and abdominal cavity; MFH metastasizes to the lung 80%, lymph nodes 30%, liver, bone PATHOLOGY Storiform pattern with a pleomorphic mixture of primitive fibroblasts (collagen production), myofibroblasts, histiocytes (with phagocytic capacity), xanthoma cells, siderophages, giant cells (bizarre, osteoclast-like), lymphocytes, plasma cells and eosinophils DDx Other sarcomas, pleomorphic or primitive carcinoma, and bizarre melanoma PROGNOSIS 40-65% of resected tumors recur; 25-50% metastasize MFH variants **ANGIOMATOID MFH** A sarcoma of adolescent females, often subcutaneous in the lower extremity CLINICAL Systemic effects are common despite its small size, including fever, chills, weight loss, anemia PATHOLOGY Well-circumscribed mass with a fibrous pseudocapsule rimmed by lymphoid follicles and sheets of relatively monotonous fibroblast- or histiocyte-like cells with 0-3 mitotic figures/high-power field; the cytoplasm is filled with hemosiderin and lesser amounts of lipid, foam cells and rare multinucleated giant cells PROGNOSIS Similar to usual MFH **OSSEOUS MFH** A rare primary MFH, affecting the lower extremity of young adults; male:female ratio, 2:1, which may arise in bone infarction RADIOLOGY Poorly-circumscribed radiolucency PATHOLOGY Histiocytes with phagocytic capacity that may differentiate into fibroblasts, having a storiform pattern; 35% 5-year survival

malignant hepatopathy A paraneoplastic condition characterized by biochemical abnormalities (↑ alkaline phosphatase, ↑ cholesterol, ↑ PT), and hepatosplenomegaly, which is associated with and regresses following successful treatment of, renal cell carcinoma and malignant schwannoma

malignant histiocytoma Histiocytic lymphoma, see there

malignant histiocytosis Histiocytic medullary reticulosis A rapidly fatal disease associated with aggressive proliferation of atypical histiocytes and precursors in lymph nodes, splenic red pulp, BM, skin, GI tract, kidneys, adrenal glands and lungs; although idiopathic, MH is associated with ALL and AML, post-renal transplantation immunosuppressive therapy and EBV viremia CLINICAL ♂:♀ ratio, 2-3:1; MH occurs at any age and presents with fever, weakness, weight loss, diaphoresis, chest and back pain, rashes, lymphadenopathy, hepatosplenomegaly, subcutaneous tumor nodules, pancytopenia, increased bilirubin followed by jaundice and may cause rapid deterioration PATHOLOGY Large pleomorphic or anaplastic, erythrophagocytic cells with hyperchromatic and irregular nuclear membranes and enlarged nucleoli that more commonly infiltrate in a 'leukemic' or diffuse fashion in sinusoids of the reticuloendothelial system and vessels, in contrast to a 'lymphomatoid' or nodular fashion LABORATORY Most patients have ↑ to ↑↑↑ (> 700 µg/L) serum ferritin, a finding that is less common in reactive histiocytosis and Langerhans' cell histiocytosis (aka histiocytosis X) (Br J Haematol 1993; 83:326) IMMUNOPEROXIDASE Muramidase + HISTOCHEMISTRY Acid phosphatase +, nonspecific (α-naphthylacetate or butyrate) esterase + (complete inhibition by sodium fluoride), PAS + EM Langerhans granules are rare; more constant ultrastructural criteria include rudimentary junctional complexes and pseudopodia DDx AML-FAB M5, hairy cell leukemia, 'histiocytic', and Hodgkin's lymphomas, melanoma, anaplastic or 'large cell' carcinoma, virus-associated hemophagocytic syndrome, infectious mononucleosis, sinus histiocytosis with massive lymphadenopathy, familial hemophagocytic reticulosis, Langerhans' cell histiocytosis TREATMENT Multidrug regimens are used with protocols similar to those used in large cell lymphoma, including vincristine, cyclophosphamide, doxorubicin and prednisone achieving a high proportion of long-term remission; see Histiocytosis

malignant hypertension Acclerated hypertension A condition characterized by severe hypertension, retinopathy with or without renal insufficiency, fibrinoid necrosis of renal arterioles, and a rapidly progressive and fatal clinical course (N Engl J Med 1995; 332:1029ED)

malignant hyperthermia syndrome An AD [MIM 180901] condition (of variable penetration) in which the subject when subjected to anesthetic (halothane, diethyl-ether, cyclopropane, enflurane) and certain psychotropic agents develops a potentially fatal (up to 70% mortality in acute episodes) clinical complex, occurring in 1/15 000 administrations of anesthesia in children, 1/50-100 000 adults; ½ of cases had not been previously sensitive to anesthesia CLINICAL Tachycardia, tachypnea, cyanosis, labile blood pressure, muscle rigidity, rapid and marked hyperpyrexia, acidotic, hyperkalemic, possibly DIC, and renal failure; similar reactions may be evoked in these subjects by warm weather, exercise, emotional stress or without known environmental cue and are initiated by muscular hypermetabolism, due to an idiopathic ↑ in sarcoplasmic calcium occurring under general anesthesia PATHOGENESIS MH may be related to a defective calcium channel in the sarcoplasmic reticulum; the genetic markers near the MH susceptibility locus are near the ryanodine receptor gene, which encodes a calcium channel; in MH, the total body O_2 consumption increases 2-3-fold normal, body temperature may spiral upward as rapidly as an increase of 1°C per five minutes peaking at 43°C (109°F) ↑ base excess to > than -10, $PaCO_2$ to 70-110 mmHg, K⁺ to more than > 7 mEq/ml and enzymes, including CPK, LD, AST ↓ Serum pH to below 7.2 DIAGNOSIS Muscle contraction test with halothane or caffeine challenge TREATMENT Hypothermia, hydration, sodium bicarbonate infusion, mechanical hyperventilation, diuretics to increase urine flow, dantrolene (an agent which blocks excitation-contraction coupling between the T tubules and the sarcoplasmic reticulum)

Note: MH may also be a symptom in myotonic disorders, Duchenne dystrophy, brachial hypertrophic myopathy, central core disease and in congenital myopathy with dysmorphic features

malignant lymphoepithelial lesion MLEL, 'eskimoma', lymphoepithelioma-like carcinoma A poorly differentiated squamous cell carcinoma admixed with non-malignant lymphoid stroma, formerly affecting the salivary glands and esophagus of Eskimo women, related to the manner in which they prepare mukluks, ie by chewing sealskins covered by ashes (a source of lye and potential co-carcinogen (Cancer 1964; 17:1187)

malignant lymphoma Lymphoma, see there

malignant melanoma Melanoma, see there

malignant mesenchymoma see Mesenchymoma

malignant mimic A nonspecific term for any lesion that either grossly or microscopically mimics malignancy, which may be induced by inflammation, irradiation and chemotherapy, evoking cytologic features that are similar to malignant lesions; endoscopic lesions mimicking malignancy include 'ragged' well-circumscribed ulcers that histologically appear in an amorphous eosinophilic background, with sheets of closely packed variably-sized acini, cells with swollen granular cytoplasm, variably-sized, often hyperchromatic nuclei, mitotic activity and a lesion that fades into benign regenerative mucosa; other endoscopic malignant look-alikes seen in the esophagus, stomach and rectum, consist of fibrinopurulent exudate, which covers aggregates of bizarre cells with variable amounts of granular cytoplasm, hyperchromatic pleomorphic nuclei PATHOLOGY Various lesions mimic malignancy; classic 'dyads' include chondroma and chondrosarcoma, infarcted fibroadenoma and scirrhous carcinoma of breast; necrotizing sialometaplasia and mucoepidermoid carcinoma of the oral cavity; nodal angiomatosis and KS; keratoacanthoma and squamous cell carcinoma; Spitz nevus and malignant melanoma; see Lymph node inclusions

malignant narcissism PSYCHIATRY A term that defines a range of psychopathic personality disorders characterized by the coexistence of marked narcissistic and antisocial traits; manifestations of this 'inhumanity and propensity toward evil' ranges from modest to extreme, the latter of which may affect notorious murderers, despots and dictators; Cf Serial killers

malignant nephrosclerosis The form of renal disease associated with 'malignant' or accelerated phase hypertension; while the clinical condition may arise virtually de novo, it usually occurs in a background of benign essential hypertension; this condition comprises only 5% of hypertension and has a predilection for young black males PATHOLOGY Grossly, petechial hemorrhages on the renal capsule have been fancifully designated as 'flea-bitten' PATHOLOGY 1) Fibrinoid necrosis of arterioles and necrotizing arteriolitis, causing petechia on the renal cortex and 2) 'Onion-skinning' of the interlobular arteries and arterioles with concentric layering of collagen (hyperplastic arteriolitis), variably accompanied by necrotizing glomerulitis

malignant neuroleptic syndrome A complex which affects less than 1% of those exposed to neuroleptic agents (phenothiazine, butyrophenones) CLINICAL Onset 1-3 days after beginning antidepressant therapy causing hyperthermia, autonomic instability, muscle rigidity and myoglobinuria

malignant osteopetrosis Marble bone disease, see there

malignant osteoporosis Osteolysis secondary to infiltration by malignancy, which is often accompanied by pain; 80% of bone metastases arise from carcinoma of the breast, kidney, lung, prostate and thyroid, and most cause weakening of the bony trabeculae, with the exception of prostatic carcinoma, which classically is an osteoblastic lesion; 70% of bone metastases involve the axial skeleton, while the remainder affect the proximal appendicular skeleton LABORATORY ↑ Acid phosphatase, if extensive, hypercalcemia TREATMENT Remove primary carcinoma, radiotherapy (effective in most cases) and fixation of of unstable bone; see Hypercalcemia of malignancy

malignant schwannoma A malignant tumor presumably of Schwann cells* that is thought to arise from the neural crest; although it is the most common malignancy of peripheral nerves, it is poorly understood and because of the difficulty in establishing the Schwann cell as the schwannoma's cell of origin, there is a justification for the equivalent term 'malignant peripheral nerve sheath tumor'

PATHOLOGY Few intracytoplasmic filaments, abundant cytoplasmic processes, layered basal lamina, numerous granular lysosomes PATHOGENESIS In one schwannoma tumor line, a potent mitogen was isolated that is an epidermal growth factor, an autocrine growth factor as well as a mitogen for astrocytes, Schwann cells and fibroblasts; see Peripheral nerve sheath tumor

*By convention, 'benign schwannomas' are preferably known as neurilemmomas, while the malignant counterpart is known as malignant schwannoma

malignant transformation ONCOLOGY The constellation of changes in the growth properties of cells in culture evoked by various agents, eg radiation, toxins, and viruses that result in development of tumors; although this process is assumed to occur in vivo, direct correlation to tumor induction is difficult to confirm; transformation of cell lines by viruses, eg polyoma virus and cellular oncogenes, eg *ras* plus *myc* oncogenes, requires two proteins, a T protein that immortalizes the cells and another, the mid-T protein, that changes the cells' properties; transformed cells have a characteristic phenotypic 'signature', including altered growth parameters and cell behavior, cell-surface alterations, loss of actin myofilaments, increased transforming growth factor release, protease secretion, altered gene transcription and immortalization of cells

malingering Fraudulant simulation of illness or exaggeration of the symptoms of a minor illness or injury, usually to avoid work or school; permutations of malingering include that which occurs in anticipation of collecting insurance benefits, known as 'goldbricking', and malingering with psychological underpinnings, of either endogenous origin, eg factitial dermatitis or exogenous origin, eg Munchausen syndrome; see Factitious disease(s)

mallet finger ORTHOPEDICS A flexion deformity of the terminal phalanx of a finger that is evoked by striking the dorsal surface of the finger tip; the MF is due to a partial or complete rupture of extensor tendon of the terminal phalanx, or fracture and/or avulsion of a bony fragment of the extensor insertion at the dorsal base of the distal phalanx, which occurs in a background of closed hyperflexion-type blunt trauma; in pre-adolescents, the injury is an open Salter-Harris type I or II injury where the extensor tendon insertion remains undisplaced and the remainder of the phalanx is acutely flexed by the unopposed flexor profundus tendon; in older subjects, hyperflexion injury causes a displaced type III dorsal physeal fracture, representing a 'true' mallet injury

mallet toe A flexion deformity of the distal interphalangeal joint of the lesser toes, affecting one toe or two adjacent toes; the condition is less common than hammer toe (which is a flexion deformity of the proximal interphalangeal joint) and becomes symptomatic in adolescence or adulthood with the development of a painful 'corn' at the tip of the toe; see Hammer toe

Mallophaga An order of biting lice that may affect humans

malnutrition see Kwashiorkor, Marasmus

malocchio PSYCHIATRY Mal de ojo, evil eye A cultural phenomenon of uncertain validity of unknown frequency, most commonly described in children, and characterized by restless sleep, crying for no reason, diarrhea, vomiting, and fever (DSM-IV™, 1994) see Culture-bound syndrome

malocclusion ODONTOLOGY Misalignment of the maxillary and mandibular teeth, causing a 'poor bite', corresponding difficulties in mastication and, with time, periodontal disease

malpractice Professional misconduct or unreasonable lack of skill in the performance of a professional act, a term that may be applied to physicians, lawyers, and accountants; see Medical malpractice

malrotation, intestinal The incorrect rotation of the intestines in utero, which may occur to a greater or lesser degree than normal; coincident with the growth in length, the primitive intestinal loop rotates 270° counterclockwise around an axis formed by the superior mesenteric artery; a counterclockwise rotation of only 90°, results in a left-sided colon; a reverse or clockwise rotation of 90° causes the transverse colon to lie behind the duodenum and superior mesenteric artery, causing a kinking of the arterial supply, potentially resulting in pseudo-obstruction and malabsorption

MALT Mucosa-associated lymphoid tissue IMMUNOLOGY The umbrella term for extranodal aggregates of lymphoid tissue in the bronchus (BALT), gut (GALT) and skin (SALT) as well as breast and uterine cervix; MALT is the arm of the immune defense that is in closest contact with exogenous antigens, thus differing from the compartmentalized peripheral somatic lymphoid tissues which include lymph nodes, thymus and spleen; dimeric IgA or 'secretory' IgA appears to be under MALT's control and MALT may be the sites of origin of extranodal lymphomas

MALT lymphoma A MALT– (mucosa-associated lymphoid tissue) derived B-cell lymphoma that arises from the lymphoid aggregates in the lamina propria; MLs are low-grade and indolent, arising in the stomach, salivary gland, lung and thyroid, and are often CD20-positive and CD5- and CD10-negative; gastric MLs may (**N Engl J Med 1993; 329:149OA, 1994; 330:1265**) or may not (**ibid 1995; 332:1153CPC**) regress with treatment of *Helicobacter pylori* infection

Malta fever Brucellosis caused by *B melitensis*

Maltese cross appearance A descriptor for a microscopic pattern likened to a Maltese cross, which may correspond to granules of talc or cholesterol crystals JOINT Maltese crosses have been described in arthroscopic fluid, associated with traumatic arthritis MICROBIOLOGY The tetrad form of *Babesia* species, including *B canis, B microti* and *B bovis,* has been termed 'Maltese cross' and is an uncommon but characteristic finding within infected red cells in a peripheral blood smear; Cf Rabbit ear appearance PULMONARY PATHOLOGY Maltese crosses measure 5-15 mm in diameter, appear as scintillating granules by polarized light microscopy and correspond to starch and talc granules, which are common in the lungs of IV drug abusers who 'cut' the heroin with various powders; the granules may be accompanied by foreign body-type giant cell reaction and appear in other tissues URINALYSIS 'Maltese crosses' are anisotropic or birefringent cholesterol-rich fat droplets, associated with finely granular renal casts, which have a cruciform appearance when seen by polarized light and are found both within and outside of the cells in the urinary sediment of patients with nephrotic syndrome, eclampsia, renal toxicity, fat embolism, after crush injury and in Fabry's disease (due to aggregates of glycosphingolipids)

malt workers' lung An extrinsic allergic alveolitis due to hypersensitivity to spores from *Aspergillus clavatus* and *A fumigatus* in moldy barley and hay, which are ingredients for malt liquors; see Farmer's lung

MAMA Mid-arm muscle area, see there

mammary dysplasia SURGICAL PATHOLOGY A non-specific term applied to various benign microscopic nosologies in the breast, including periductular fibrosis, ductal dilatation, apocrine metaplasia and others; since the term 'dysplasia' implies premalignancy, the term is invalid and should be deleted from the literature; see Fibrocystic disease

mammary souffle CARDIOLOGY An innocent systolic or continuous cardiac murmur of presumed arterial origin heard during late pregnancy or in the early post-partum period that is differentiated from pathological lesions as it is unaffected by the Valsalva maneuver

mammography Radiologic examinaton of the breast using a specifically designed dedicated device, which is the single best noninvasive screening procedure for detecting breast cancer; mammography yields a false negative rate of 6% and a false positive of 11%; the most characteristic mammographic finding in malignancy is the presence of finely-stippled microcalcifications and suspicious, eg poorly-circumscribed, geographic densities in the mammogram; other findings (as classified by Wolf) are thought to be less reliable; the radiation dose during the usual mammographic study is 25-35 kV; the American Cancer Society and the National Cancer Institute (US) both recommend self examination of the breast after age 20, a baseline mammogram between ages 35-45, and annual or biennial mammograms thereafter, the frequency of which is a function of the subject's relative risk factors for breast cancer (first-degree relative with breast cancer, Caucasian, later pregnancy, etc); after the age of 50, annual screening mammography is recommended; 24% of biopsies of non-palpable breast masses with calcification (more than 15 calcifications or calcifications in a linear or branching fashion) have ductal or lobular carcinoma; VARIABILITY The diagnostic consistency among radiologists is moderate (78%); there was a 74-96% recommendation for immediate workup (with biopsy) in mammograms *with* cancer, and 11-65% in mammograms *without* cancer (N Engl J Med 1994; 331:1493sA) the false negative rate is 10-15% (ibid, 331:1521ED) see Cancer screening; Cf Lumpectomy

Bottom line: The interpretation of the mammography continues to be a subjective science (oxymoron noted) and is thus prey to observer variability, ie differences in interpretation-Author's note

mammoplasty A generic term for any form of surgery to the breast; aside from reconstructive surgery required for breast cancer, mammoplasty is performed because the breasts are

1) Too small, see Augmentation mammoplasty, Breast implants

2) Sagging, see Mastopexy

3) Too big, see Reduction mammoplasty

(the) man on the Clapham bus Reasonable person principle, see there

man-in-the-barrel 'syndrome' NEUROLOGY A fanciful term for a form of reverse paraplegia with severe arm weakness without leg weakness, described in comatose patients who survive an episode of severe hypotension; the location of the lesion is uncertain but may be bilateral and pre-rolandic; the fanciful term derives from the fact that, like a man in a barrel, the patients have full use of their legs while their upper body is paralyzed

manage *verb* To be encharged with a patient's clinical care

managed care HEALTH CARE ENVIRONMENT A format for providing health care services in which there are financial incentives to encourage 1) Physicians and allied health care providers not to order order unnecessary services 2) Clients (or patients) to use the providers within the MC system, and 3) The organization to maintain the clients as healthy as possible (Am Med News 25 October 1992, p7) MC is thus viewed as a health care delivery philosphy based on capitated payments to encourage efficiency and reduce unnecessary costs; it is managed by a number of 'exercises', eg by closely monitoring the battery of tests ordered to establish a disease, or how a disease is treated, or by reducing referrals to costly specialists; in general, MC attempts to control costs by using primary-care physicians or case-workers as 'gatekeepers' to coordinate (ie limit) the consumer's use of health services; MC networks are organized by insurance companies, employers, or hospitals (N Engl J Med 1994; 331:1167) the number of US citizens (population 230 million) enrolled in managed care plans has

risen from 6 million in 1976 to 38.6 million in 1991 (N Engl J Med 1992; 327:742sR)

managed competition HEALTH CARE ENVIRONMENT A health care system that is the 'brainchild' of Jackson Hole group (see there) in which insurance companies and healthcare providers (ie physicians and others) create health plans that compete with other health plans for large groups of consumers; MC is defined by its key architect, Alain Enthoven of Stanford University as a purchasing strategy with empowered (consumer) demand designed to reward cost-efficient quality care; in MC consumers are organized into large health purchasing groups to but insurance; health care providers are organized in a network that would vie for the health purchasing group's business, which would have sufficient clout to bargain with the network to obtain the best value (ie cost) per individual; MC would result in an unprecedented restructuring of the US health care system (N Engl J Med 1993; 328:1208ED; 329:879sB; 885c)

the Manchester sailor* A man who died of an unknown (and presumably immune-related) disease in 1959 (Lancet 1960; ii:951) whose preserved tissues were subsequently examined by PCR; early reports in the literature (Lancet 1990; 336:51) concluded that he was the first known case of AIDS (ie the so-called Patient Zero); his primacy in the AIDS epidemic was questioned by Zhu and Ho, who constructed a phylogenic tree using the neighbor-joining method and believed that the HIV-1 identified in the PCR analysis reported in 1990 was more recent in evolution (see figure, 'B' cluster); the results were subsequently acknowledged to be 'anomalous' (Nature 1995; 375:4N)

*or apprentice printer

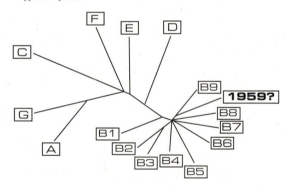

phylogenic tree, Manchester sailor

mandated choice A mechanism suggested by the AMA's Council on Ethical and Judicial Affairs for increasing the number of cadaveric organs available for transplantation; in mandated choice, the individual would be required to choose (to donate or to not donate) while registering for his/her drivers' license, filing income tax form or performing other tasks mandated by the state (JAMA 1994; 272:809cR) see Cadaveric organ transplantation, Presumed consent

mandatory assignment HEALTH CARE FINANCING A format for reimbursing health care services that requires physicians to accept Medicare reimbursement as payment in full; this is to say that MA does not allow balance billing, see there (Am Med News 25 October 1992, p7)

mandatory reporting The obligatory reporting of a particular disease to a 'higher' authority; MR is required for communicable disease and for abuse INFECTIOUS DISEASE A state board of health maintains records and collects data resulting from MR of communicable or other diseases that represent a hazard to the public; see Reportable disease PSYCHIATRY The physician is required to report abuse or suspected abuse of children, spouses, or the elderly; MR statutes grant immunity to physicians who report their suspicions in good faith (N Engl J Med 1995; 332:437RA) see Abuse

Manhattan Project for HIV PUBLIC HEALTH A proposed multidisciplinary approach intended to conquer AIDS; which as currently conceived, refers to the coordination and streamlining of research activities, as well as wide dissemination of research finding as a means of accelerating progress in developing therapeutics and vaccines (JAMA 1995; 273:1143OA)

mania PSYCHIATRY A hyperkinetic psychiatric reaction which may affect 1% of US citizens, either temporarily or on a permanent basis; the term is no longer used by the mainstream psychiatric community; the closest equivalent in the Diagnostic and Statistical Manual of Mental Diseases, 4th edition is the manic episode, see there

manic-depressive illness Bipolar I disorder, see there

manic episode A persistently elevated, expansive or irritable mood, ↑ energy, ↓ sleep, distractibility, impaired judgement, grandiosity, flights of ideas, sexual indiscretions, buying sprees, and unusual business transactions, most often affecting those under age 25; manic episodes are seen in those with primary (idiopathic) affective illness or bipolar I disorder, in which patients vacillate between hypermania and abject depression; specific criteria for a manic episode have been delineated (table)

MANIC EPISODE-CRITERIA

A A distinct period of abnormally or persistently elevated, expansive, or irritable mood of ≥ 1 week or any period of hospitalization

B During the period, ≥ 3 of following symptoms
1) Grandiosity or inflated self-esteem
2) Decreased need for sleep
3) Increased talkativeness
4) Flight of ideas, or impression that thoughts are 'racing'
5) Distractibility
6) Increased goal-oriented activity (socially, work- or school-related) or psychomotor agitation
7) Involvement in various activities with potentially dire consequences, eg buying sprees, sexual indiscretions, inappropriate business transactions

C Symptoms do NOT meet criteria of a mixed episode

D The mood disturbance is sufficient to marekdly impair occupational or social function

E Symptoms are unrelated to the direct physiological effects of a substance (of abuse, medication, or other therapy) or to a general medical condition (eg hyperthyroidism)

DSM-IV™, American Psychiatric Association, Washington, DC, 1994

Manner cocktail A therapeutic modality used as alternate form of cancer therapy, consisting of a mixture containing vitamins A and C, laetrile and dimethylsulfoxide (see DMSO), administered on a daily basis as an unproven form of cancer therapy developed and practiced by a researcher who died in 1988; see DMSO, Tijuana, Mexico, Unproven cancer therapy

manner of death The fashion or circumstances that result in death, which may be designated as either natural or unnatural (Arch Pathol Lab Med 1995; 119:123OA), the latter may be further defined as accidental, homicidal, or suicidal, or in absence of unequivocal accurate determination of the MOD, undetermined; see Natural death, Unnatural death

manpower shortage A dearth of persons with a particular skill, which in a free market economy driven by 'supply-and-demand', may result in increased salaries and difficulty in obtaining their services; certain specialties are recognized as having manpower shortages, either current, eg general surgery, psychiatry, occupational medicine or evolving, eg pathology; Cf Physician 'glut'

manslaughter The unlawful, unjustifiable, and/or inexcusable killing of one human by another under circumstances devoid of premeditation, deliberation, and express or implied malice; manslaughter may be

1) VOLUNTARY MANSLAUGHTER That which is committed voluntarily in a heat of passion

2) INVOLUNTARY MANSLAUGHTER That which occurs when a person commits an unlawful act that is not felonious or tending to cause great bodily harm or when a person is committing a lawful act without due caution or requisite skill (eg a surgeon performing an operation while intoxicated) and inadvertently kills another; Cf Murder

mantle port RADIATION ONCOLOGY A radiotherapy field that covers the axillary, mediastinal, hilar, cervical, supra- and infraclavicular lymph nodes, used to treat multiple contiguous lymphoid regions involved by Hodgkin's lymphoma Dosage 36-44 Gy are tumoricidal, while less than 36 Gy is considered to be prophylactic; see Abdominal bath, Inverted 'Y' field

mantle-zone lymphoma A type of B cell lymphoma that is low-to-intermediate grade by the Working Formulation (Cancer 1982; 49:1429), which accounts for 1-8% of NHLs, and is most common in ♂ ≥ age 55; it is characterized by a proliferation of small lymphocytes in the mantle zone, surrounding benign germinal centers; MZLs may have a higher clinical stage but lower aggression, thus being exceptions to the Lukes and Collins (Br J Cancer, suppl II, 1975; 31:1) proposal that all nodular lymphomas are of follicular center origin; MZLs are often aggressive and involve the spleen, liver, BM, and other sites when diagnosed CLINICAL Massive splenomegaly, generalized lymphadenopathy, ⅓ present with 'type B' symptoms, including fever, weight loss, night sweats PATHOLOGY Cells are of B lineage and range from small to relatively large blasts with round-to-irregular contours with clumped chromatin; MZL usually expresses IgM lambda, pan-B cell antigens (CD19, CD20, and CD22), CD5 and CD43, variable presence of IgG and IgD, Ia, BA1 and Leu-1; CD10 and CD23 are rare MOLECULAR pathology In 73%, a chromosomal translocation t(11;14) (q13;q32) joins the *bcl*-1 region on chromosome 11 to the Ig heavy-chain gene locus on chromosome 14, causing an upregulation of *bcl*-1 mRNA in affected cells (N Engl J Med 1994; 331:1576CPC) and an overexpression of cyclin D1/PRAD1, which is not expressed in normal or reactive lymphoid tissues (Am J Clin Pathol 1995; 103:756) MEDIAN SURVIVAL 31 months; 40% achieve complete remission with chemotherapy; see Lymphoma

manometry The recording of pressure in an inelastic liquid or gas; manometry is the standard for the diagnosis of motor disorders of the body of the esophagus and lower sphincter, and allows intraluminal evaluation of pressure based on perstaltic performance, contraction wave configuration, and the sphincter's basal pressure and relaxation

MAO 1) Maximum acid output A measurement of the maximal secretory capacity of gastric hydrogen ions, defined as the sum of four 15-minute acid outputs (Normal: 5-60 mmol of titratable acid/hr), after either pentagastrin or histamine stimulation; MAO is markedly increased in the Zollinger-Ellison syndrome and conditions of increased gastrin production; see also BAO, PAO 2) Monoamine oxidase

MAOI Monoamine oxidase inhibitor A family of therapeutic drugs, eg phenelzine, that are used to treat atypical depression or when tricyclic agents fail; MAOIs have traditionally been relegated to a secondary role treating depression, given the tendency towards inducing hypertensive crises when MAOI-treated patients ingest tyramine-containing products; MAOIs appear to be most effective when depression is accompanied by anxiety

map A two-dimensional graphic representation of a topology or the location of multiple points in a 'universe' **cDNA**

MAP MOLECULAR BIOLOGY complementary DNA map; see cDNA **'CONTIG' MAP** MOLECULAR BIOLOGY A map of a segment of a gene that is formed by arranging in order a number of contiguous and overlapping cloned segments of DNA **FATE MAP** EMBRYOLOGY A map that is drawn on the surface of a bisected blastoderm of an organism, consisting of physical landmarks of cell clusters that later give rise to mature adult structures; the distance between these sites is measured in 'Sturts', after Alfred Sturtevant's studies in 1929 of *Drosophila simulans* **RESTRICTION MAP** MOLECULAR BIOLOGY A 'map' of a chromosome that is delineated in terms of where a particular restriction endonuclease cleaves the oligomeric sites along the DNA; as there are numerous restriction endonucleases, there are potentially dozens of different restriction maps for a given chromosome **STS-MAP** see Sequence-tagged site map; see Human genome project

MAP Microtubule-associated protein(s) A family of proteins that promotes the assembly and polymerization of α- and β-tubulins and limits the growing and shrinking phases of dynamic microtubules, which are subdivided into

LARGE MAPS > than 200 kD, subdivided into

MAP1, which has 3 subgroups (MAP1A, MAP1B and MAP1C) and MAP2 2 groups of unknown function confined to axonal dendrites

SMALL 'TAU' 30–50-KD PROTEINS; MAP2 and tau proteins share a binding motif and are present in the neurofibrillary tangles typical of Alzheimer's disease

MAP-30 A protein derived from bitter melon, an Asian plant, administered as an extract in tea, capsules or in retention enemas; it is claimed to 'purify' blood, prevent infections, and anecdotally reported to have antiretroviral activity (**Am Med News 21 Nov 1994 p13**) Cf AIDS fraud

map-dot dystrophy Bilateral, symmetric intraepithelial, grayish cystic corneal opacities, thought to be aggregates of basement membrane material which wax and wane; the opacities have no pathological significance, but impart a foreign-body sensation

MAP kinase Mitogen-activated protein kinase A family of proteins that control the proliferation and differentiation of mammalian cells (**Nature 1994; 365:781**) MAP kinases are rapidly stimulated by growth-promoting factors that act on various cell-surface receptors, which in turn phosphorylate, regulating intracellular enzymes and transcription factors that control cell proliferation; Ras-dependent MAP kinase pathway activation is mediated by G-protein βγ subunits (**Nature 1994; 369:341BL**) see Raf/MEK/MAPK cascade

map unit Centimorgan, see there

maple bark stripper's lung Cryptostromosis An extrinsic allergic alveolitis due to hypersensitivity to spores from *Cryptostroma corticale*; see Farmer's lung

maple syrup urine disease Branched chain ketoaciduria A rare AR [MIM 248600] inborn error of metabolism due to ↓ branched-chain α-keto acid dehydrogenase complex activity FREQUENCY General population 1:200 000; in the Pennsylvania Mennonite kindred of German descent 1:176; the defect in oxidative decarboxylation of branched chain amino acids (BCAA, valine, leucine and isoleucine) results in accumulation of BCAA CLINICAL Neonatal onset, ↓ Moro reflex, dyspnea, spasticity, opisthotonos, mental and growth retardation, severe hypotonia, feeding difficulties, hypoglycemia, convulsions, and decorticate rigidity LABORATORY ↑ BCAA, ↓ threonine, serine, alanine in urine and serum, a positive dinitro-phenylhydrazine test for α keto amino acids, which form insoluble hydrazines NEUROPATHOLOGY Gliosis, defective myelinization TREATMENT Dietary ↓ of BCAA, plus dietary overloading (twentyfold excess) of thiamine PROGNOSIS Mortality was formerly 100%, often due to intercurrent infection; with BCAA-free infant formulas, the survival is virtually 100% and mental retardation completely preventable; since acute decom-

pensation by BCAA and BCKA is due to a breakdown of endogenous proteins resulting in metabolic acidosis, ketosis, anorexia, emesis and potentially fatal encephalopathy, patients may respond to parenteral solutions of BCAA-free amino acids (**N Engl J Med 1991; 324:175**)

marantic endocarditis Non-bacterial endocarditis, see there

marasmus A state of severe malnutrition, due to a ↓ ingestion of protein and calories, resulting from an inadequate diet, improper feeding habits or parent-child relations or metabolic disturbances CLINICAL Failure to thrive, weight loss, emaciation, loss of skin turgor, subcutaneous atrophy; afflicted children appear wizened, with a distended abdomen and edema, develop 'starvation stools', become listless with muscular atrophy, hypotonia, hypothermia and reduced rate of metabolism; Cf Kwashiorkor

marble bone disease Albers-Schönberg disease(s) Malignant osteopetrosis An AR form [MIM 259700] of osteopetrosis of early onset with failure to thrive, bone fragility and multiple fractures, osteomyelitis and other infections, as well as proptosis, blindness, deafness and hydrocephalus due to bony overgrowth of cranial foramina; osseous replacement of marrow spaces evokes extramedullary hematopoiesis in the liver and spleen with resultant hepatosplenomegaly LABORATORY ↑ acid and alkaline phosphatases, ↓ Ca²⁺, pancytopenia, defective T-cell functions; see Osteopetrosis

marble brain disease An AR [MIM 259730] condition due to carbonic anhydrase II deficiency CLINICAL Mental and growth retardation, facial dysmorphia, dysodontogenesis, cerebral calcification with a 'veined' pattern, osteopetrosis, renal tubular acidosis, restrictive lung disease due to rib deformity LABORATORY Metabolic acidosis, hyperchloremia, alkaline urine; Cf Etat marbre

marbling CLINICAL NUTRITION/FOOD INDUSTRY The ↑ of intramuscular fat in cattle, which ↑ the tenderness of beef–select beef has 4% fat and choice beef has 5% fat; ultrasonography may replace the 'eyeball' technique traditionally used by meat inspectors for evaluating fat content (**Science News 1994; 145:7**) FORENSIC PATHOLOGY A mosaic of discoloration due to prominent subdermal vessels, seen on the skin surface of a body in the early stages of decomposition, also termed 'venous patterning'

Marburg (virus) disease A rare viral hemorrhagic fever occurring in small clusters in Europe and Africa due to direct contact with monkey tissue, blood or human serum infected with the Marburg virus; the condition was first described in Marburg Germany in 1967, when laboratory workers were exposed to African green monkey (*Cercopithecus aethiops*) virus, a member of a newly designated family, Filoviridae, an elongated filamento-tubular bacilliform rod CLINICAL Incubation 5-9 days; otherwise similar to Argentine or Bolivian hemorrhagic fever with insidious or abrupt onset of headaches, fever, diarrhea, myalgias, rash, pharyngitis, thrombocytopenia, leukopenia, hemorrhage, and renal failure; 7/31 of the Marburg cases died; Cf Ebola virus

march foot A condition characerized by painful swelling of the forefoot, which may be accompanied by stress fracture(s) of a metatarsal bone (aka 'march fracture), which occurs in soldiers on long marches

march fracture A metatarsal stress fracture seen in military recruits who are unaccustomed to the repeated, otherwise trivial trauma to the feet associated with long marches when carrying heavy equipment

march hemoglobinuria Exertional rhabdomyolysis An episodic hemoglobinuria resulting in hemolysis due to repeated mechanical injury to RBCs that travel through small vessels overlying the bones of the hands and feet in long-distance marching (soldiers), marathon running, calisthenics, karate LABORATORY Myoglobinuria, proteinuria, ↑ BUN, ↑ enzymes (creatinine phosphokinase), ↑ lactic acid PATHOLOGY Rhabdomyositis, rhabdomyolysis

'marching' cavity The creeping expanding erosion of the contiguous thick-walled cavities of chronic pulmonary histoplasmosis

'marching in place' NEUROLOGY Repetitive movements of the legs when standing, a clinical finding in tardive dyskinesia, a feared complication of chronic antipsychotic medication, which may be persistent or permanent; tardive dyskinesia may also manifest as body 'rocking', 'flycatching' (darting movements of the tongue) and 'piano playing' (involvement of the digits)

MARCKS Myristoylated alanine-rich (protein) C kinase substrate

'Marcus Welby syndrome' American slang for the desire on the part of patients to be treated as a whole person by one physician*, rather than being treated as an organ or organ system by a specialist (**New York Times 6 Feb 1994; C1**); Cf Mayo Clinic syndrome

*As if by the protagonist of the highly romanticized television series, Marcus Welby, MD, aired during the late 1960s, who was a kindly grandfatherly gentleman, regarded as typical of an earlier era of medicine

Marfan syndrome An AD [MIM 154700] connective tissue disease with a prevalence of 1:10 000; 25% occurs in absence of parental defects, implying de novo mutations in parents; MS is characterized by a wide range of clinical expression that varies according to the family affected CLINICAL Ocular (ectopia lentis, myopia), cardiovascular (eg dissection of ascending aorta, mitral valve prolapse, aortic valve regurgitation), and skeletal (scoliosis, arachnodactyly, abnormally long fingers and extremities) defects, pneumothorax and others MOLECULAR PATHOLOGY MS is caused by a mutation in *FBN1*, a gene located on chromosome segment 15q21.1 that encodes fibrillin, an extracellular matrix glycoprotein; each family appears to have a unique mutation, precluding the routine use of mutation screening for presymptomatic diagnosis of Marfan syndrome (**N Engl J Med 1994; 331:148OA**) see fibrillin, *FBN1* TREATMENT β-Adrenergic blockade (eg with propranolol) reportedly slows pace of aortic dilation and may ↓ aorta-related complications in some patients with Marfan syndrome (**N Engl J Med 1994; 330:1335OA**)

marfanoid habitus A leptosomic body type that is tall and thin with long hands; marfanoid features may be familial in nature or pathological as occurs in homocystinuria and MEN type IIb, mimicking some of the changes of Marfan's disease, but not accompanied by luxation of the lens, funnel chest and dissecting aneurysm of the aorta

margarine disease A condition of historic interest characterized by an erythema multiforme-like disease linked to the use of an emulsifier in oleomargarine, described in Germany and the Netherlands

marginal form see Applique form

marijuana 'Pot', 'Weed' SUBSTANCE ABUSE A substance derived from the hemp plant *Cannabis sativa*, the leaves of which are smoked, producing a hallucinogenic effect due to the neurochemical Δ⁹-tetrahydrocannabinol (THC), which has a cognate THC receptor in the brain IMMUNE SYSTEM THC stops monocyte maturation NERVOUS SYSTEM Impaired motor skills, defective eye tracking and perception; THC receptors are most abundant in the hippocampus, where memory is consolidated, explaining marijuana's detrimental effect on memory and least abundant in the brainstem, explaining why death by overdose is unknown with chronic marijuana abuse RESPIRATORY TRACT Marijuana is inhaled or 'toked' in a fashion that differs from that of tobacco; in order to maximize THC absorption and elicit the desired 'high', the subject prolongs inhalation, markedly increasing carbon monoxide and tar levels, and

thus is comparable to tobacco smoke THERAPEUTIC USES Although marijuana is an analgesic, it cannot be used as such, due to the inseparable hallucinogenic effect; it is of use for 1) Control of nausea and vomiting in terminal cancer patients; two antiemetic cannabinoids are commercially available, nabilone (Cesamet), a synthetic derivative of marijuana and dronabinol (Marinol) the principle psychoactive substance in marijuana; both are designated as second-line therapies, given their psychotomimetic effects and side effects (drowsiness, dizziness, vertigo, loss of ability to concentrate and mood swings) and 2) Control of intraocular pressure in open-angle glaucoma, administered orally, in topical drops or smoked in the crude form Note: The four-to-six marijuana cigarettes required to treat glaucoma, are sufficient to cause chronic marijuana intoxication, impacting on psychosocial development, motivation, memory, motor function and coordination; other possible therapeutic uses of marijuana include improved clinical response to neuroleptics in motor disorders, eg de la Tourette syndrome; marijuana's effects are equivalent to diazepam in torsion dystonia, and may relieve symptoms of Huntington's disease, given its potent effect on the extrapyramidal system through a nicotinic cholinergic mechanism TOXICOLOGY THC and metabolites are detectable in the urine one hour after smoking or later when used as a garnee for cooking, ie 'pot' in the pan; Sensitivity of method 100 ng/ml, urine in RIA and standard EMIT (homogeneous enzyme immunoassay); 50 ng/ml TLC; 5-20 ng/ml enhanced EMIT; 5 ng/ml GC-MS; see Amotivational syndrome, Joint, Substance abuse, THC receptor, Toke

$$CH_3$$

$$OH$$

$$H_3C$$

$$H$$

$$H_3C \quad O \quad C_5H_{11}$$

marijuana (THC Δ⁹-tetrahydrocannibol)

mariner's wheel appearance Pilot's wheel appearance A descriptive term (figure, right) for the yeast form of *Paracoccidioides brasiliensis*, in which there is a large central yeast cell and multiple peripheral budding yeasts, with a double-contoured rim attached to the 'mother' by a base of varying thickness, yielding an morphology fancifully likened to a wheel of a sailing ship

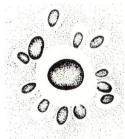

marionette lines COSMETIC SURGERY A fanciful yet accurate term for deep age-related wrinkles that are develop at the nose, corners of the lips and chin, which may be treated by a technique known as facial sculpturing, in which the proprietary material Gore-tex is layered below the skin surface (**NY Newsday 20 March 1995; B15**) see Rhytidectomy

marker gene MOLECULAR BIOLOGY A variant allele used to label a biological structure or process throughout an experiment; these genes are located in a constant genomic position in the studied organism

marker rescue experiment MOLECULAR BIOLOGY Retrieval of a fragment of DNA which has been introduced and incorporated into a lambda phage DNA, by inducing lysis of the carrier bacterium; when different strains of bacteria are used, this technique allows analysis of the marker content of the DNA fractions

marketing see Advertising, Detailing, Yellow professionalism

Markov model Markov decision-making model, state-transition model A framework for evaluating the potential outcomes of a disease process that are defined as specific health states, transitions among which are modeled iteratively; the distribution of a cohort among possible health-state outcomes changes as transitions between states occur based on age, treatment, parameters of the disease process being studied, and so on; markovian models are of particular use in analyzing the effects of conditions involving multiple risks and time-dependent events, which are compared to an idealized 'illness-free life expectancy' and are useful in modeling diseases in which the same event recurs, eg osteoporotic fractures, thromboembolism, recurrence of malignancy in the same patient

Markov process A stochastic process in which the conditional probability distribution for a system's state at any given instant is unaffected by details on that system's previous state; the markovian process is a modeling technique that may be used in medical decision-making analysis for conditions in which the prognosis of a morbid condition is described by a 'natural history' or series of chance events (adverse outcomes) and the value of these outcomes depends on whether and when they occur; to translate a markovian process into comparable units, objective values must be used, eg quality-adjusted life expectancy, abbreviated as QALE (JAMA 1992; 268:2679oa)

markovian analysis The use of the Markov process to project future events in a system with multiple hypothetical components; in MA, the patient's health is represented by a series of 'health states', which over time, move to other states (usually of lesser health, greater morbidity, or death) according to the laws of probability; see Receiver operator characteristic

Note: Markov analysis may be used as part of an algorithm in decision-making by artificial intelligence

markovian texture analysis An algorithm for quantifying nuclear texture or chromatin pattern, based on determining gray-level transition possibilities; the use of selected Markovian textural features, eg chromatin granularity (finely granular vs coarsely clumped), amount of contrast, thickness of peripheral chromatin, and number of nucleoli; MTA would allow a more rational approach to image analysis for cell classification, and may be useful in automating image analysis devices for screening cytological specimens (Anal & Quant Cytol & Histol 1993; 15:227oa)

MARSA Methicillin-aminoglycoside resistant *Staphylococcus aureus*, see there

masculinization Virilization, see there

mask-like face A hypomimic, expressionless physiognomy or complete lack of facial affect, characteristic of Parkinson's disease, a finding that may be seen in depression, facioscapulohumeral-type muscular dystrophy, infantile botulism, Möbius' syndrome, myotonic dystrophy, Prader-Willi disease, and Wilson's disease

mask of pregnancy see Melasma

mask phenomenon Post-emetic purpura that follows prolonged vomiting ('retching'), appearing as evanescent punctate macules on the face and upper neck, thought to be due to abruptly increased intrathoracic pressure; similar lesions occur in violent coughing, the Valsalva maneu-

ver, or in strangulation, and are accompanied by conjunctival petechiae

masked depression A form of adolescent depression in which the young subject deals with despair by denial, somatization (headaches, abdominal or other pain), or 'acting out' (truancy, substance abuse, multiple accidents)

masochism PSYCHIATRY A paraphilia (sexual deviancy) in which there is a need (or preference) for humiliation, physical abuse, or other form of suffering in order to achieve sexual arousal or orgasm; Cf Sadism PSYCHOLOGY Moral masochism A pattern of behavior in which a person seemingly invites abuse and exploitation by others, presumed to originate in unresolved childhood conflicts

masked mRNA Masked message sequence An mRNA sequence present in unfertilized eggs and other eukaryotic cells that is tightly bound by a macroprotein and floats about the nucleus as ribonucleoprotein complexes, which becomes activated and translated only after the egg is fertilized

mass A cohesive aggregate of often similar components, composition, cells or molecules

ATOMIC MASS UNIT Dalton 1.6604×10^{-27} kg

ELECTRONIC MASS The mass of a negative electron (8.999×10^{-28}) when moving at a moderate velocity

ELECTRON MASS UNIT 511 keV The energy required to annihilate an electron

mass extinction A massive (>15%) ↓ in the diversity and number of microbes, algae, fungi, protists, plants, and animals on the planet; 7 mass extinctions have been identified according to the fossil record, the most intense of which occurred in the Early Cambrian period (circa 500 million years ago) when there was ± 68% ↓ in taxa (Science 1995; 268:52)

mass injury claim PUBLIC HEALTH Any demand for compensation often in the form of a class-action lawsuit that is initiated by a large group of plaintiffs who claim to have suffered injury from a commercial product, eg asbestos (defendent Johns-Manville Corporation), Dalkon Shield intrauterine contraceptive device (defendent AH Robins), and breast implants (defendent Dow Corning); after establishing a compensation fund, it is common practice for the defendent corporation to file for bankruptcy (NY Times 16 May 1995, A1)

mass number The number of protons and neutrons in a nuclide, eg 14 in ^{14}C

massacre HUMAN RIGHTS The systematic killing of a population, either in its entirety, or the majority thereof; a massacre may be perpetrated with support within a community or the group in the society in which it occurred, and usually is a single event; Cf Genocide

massive transfusion TRANSFUSION MEDICINE The infusion, within a 24-hour period, of a blood volume that approaches or exceeds the recipient's own calculated blood volume; MTs may be administered in medical or surgical emergencies or in the course of 'bloody' operations, and have a variety of effects on the recipient including depletion of coagulation factors, lowering of core temperature, due to the infusion of cool blood (uncommon in practice), and the inability to properly 'type' red cells, as the majority of the circulating erythrocytes are of donor origin

mass spectroscopy Mass spectrometry An analytical method for measuring molecular mass and structure, in which a specimen is ionized and passed through either an electron beam (for liquid samples) or spark (for solids) PRINCIPLE Ions are accelerated by a variable electrostatic field and deflected along a circular path by a constant magnetic field; the radius of the path is inversely proportional to the ion's velocity and its charge/mass ratio; the system may be coupled with gas chromatography (MS-

GC) to measure a second parameter (dimension) of the specimen, thereby increasing its precision; the GC-MS hybrid is a 'gold-standard' device for confirming the results from screening techniques such as thin-layer chromatography and EMIT, and is used to quantify opiates, cannabinoids and narcotics; Cf EMIT, Gas-liquid chromatography

MAST EMERGENCY MEDICINE 1) Military antishock trousers A pressure device designed to provide life support in patients with external or internal subdiaphragmatic hemorrhage, which acts to stabilize movement of the lower extremities and pelvis as well as treat the hemorrhagic-traumatic shock by producing hemostasis and increasing systemic vascular pressure; Cf Pressure pants 2) Military Assistance to Safety and Traffic A program in the US in which the military contributes helicopters and medical assistance to low-population density areas Note: The major MAST users are high-risk infants in rural settings

mast cell A nonspecific immune cell that stains metachromatically due to its high proteoglycan content and abundant electron-dense granules; like basophils, mast cells are activated by cross-linking of IgE on the cell surface and secrete neutrophil and eosinophil chemotactic factors, histamine, leukotrienes, neutral proteases, peroxidase, serotonin, superoxide dismutase, prostaglandins and platelet-activating factor; the release of these factors may also be evoked in response to various substances including hormones, peptides, proteins, calcium ionophores, narcotics, muscle relaxants, dextran, complement C3a and C5a (anaphylotoxins); the mast cell is detected by measuring serum trypticase (a neutral protease in mast cell secretory granules); levels > 4 ng/ml indicate systemic mast cell activation; see Mastocytosis

mast cell growth factor *kit*-ligand A cytokine that is the ligand for the protein product of the c-*kit* proto-oncogene, which stimulates the growth and differentiation of mast cells in vitro, the accumulation of mast cells in the skin in vivo; and the proliferation of melanocytes and production of melanin; soluble mast cell growth factor is increased in patients with mastocytosis; this finding suggests that some cases of mastocytosis may represent reactive hyperplasia and not neoplasia (N Engl J Med 1993; 328:1302oA)

*Note: The term mast cell growth factor (MCGF) may be suboptimal, given that MCGF is a former synonym of IL-3 (interleukin-3); the alternative terms stem cell factor, c-*kit* ligand, and steel factor are preferred by basic scientists, a lead that their clinical colleagues might well follow

mast cell leukemia A neoplasm that develops in 15% of patients with malignant systemic mastocytosis CLINICAL Fever, anorexia, weight loss, fatigue, abdominal colic, diarrhea, pruritus, bone pain, duodenal ulcer, hepatosplenomegaly, lymphadenopathy; see Mastocytoma

master log LABORATORY MEDICINE A formal and legally required record of all specimens received, processed and/or tested in a licensed laboratory

master-servant doctrine see Respondeat superior

master-slave hypothesis MOLECULAR BIOLOGY A theory that attempts to explain the lower than expected frequency of mutations in tandem arrays of repeated sequences of DNA; according to the master-slave hypothesis, sequence identity is maintained through either frequent unequal meiotic crossovers or gene conversion in which one gene (the master) corrects the other multiple copies (the slaves) that are arranged in an end-to-end fashion

mastocytoma A focal aggregate of mast cells of undetermined significance, common in dogs, occasionally in cats and cows, rare in humans; see Mastocytosis

mastocytosis A heterogeneous group of uncommon, poorly understood lesions characterized by an ↑ number of mast cells in one or more tissues or organs, in particular the skin PATHOGENESIS Some cases may be reactive in nature and due to ↑ soluble mast cell growth factor (*kit*-ligand, possibly due to an ↑ in proteolytic processing), a cytokine that causes mast cell accumulation, melanocyte proliferation and ↑ melanin production (N Engl J Med 1993; 328:1302oA) mastocytosis may be classified according to extent and behavior (table) **REACTIVE MASTOCYTOSIS** A focal increase in mast cells due to immediate or delayed hypersensitivity reactions, which may also occur in lymph nodes draining benign or malignant lesions, eg chronic liver or renal disease, leukemia, lymphoproliferative disorders or Hodgkin's disease; benign mast cell diseases include localized mastocytosis, which may be cutaneous or extracutaneous and urticaria pigmentosa **SYSTEMIC MASTOCYTOSIS** A potentially aggressive condition characterized by a proliferation of mast cells in the skin, liver, lymph nodes, BM, GI tract CLINICAL Excess histamine production with flushing vertigo, palpitations, pruritus, colicky pain, dyspnea, nausea and vomiting, which may be asymptomatic, mild to moderate with intermittent symptoms or severe, disabling and progressive **'MALIGNANT' SYSTEMIC MASTOCYTOSIS** A form of mast cell disease that is fatal within two years of conversion to an aggressive form; see Mast cell leukemia

---

MASTOCYTOSIS

I LOCALIZED MASTOCYTOSIS
   a) Focal Single skin lesion: mast cell 'nevus'
   b) Generalized Urticaria pigmentosa

II SYSTEMIC MASTOCYTOSIS:
   a) Indolent
   b) Progressive
   c) Malignant

III MAST CELL LEUKEMIA

IV MAST CELL SARCOMA

---

mastopexy A surgical procedure for the correction of sagging or ptotic breasts affected by the viscissitudes of aging, atrophy, lactation, pregnancy, and gravity PROCEDURE Correction may be done with simultaneous reduction or augmentation, and usually requires general anesthesia, drains, and hospitalization* COMPLICATIONS Hematoma, infection, breast asymmetry, altered sensation, loss of function in nipple areolar region, scars

*Unlike augmentation mammoplasty, which may be performed on an outpatient basis

matagen Masking tape for gene expression Synthetic, chemically-modified sequence-specific analogs of gene segments composed of non-ionic oligonucleoside methylphosphonates, corresponding to enzyme-resistant RNA and DNA; modifications include methylation or adding sulfur at various points on the phosphate backbone of antisense DNA with the purpose of blocking viral expression

the 'Match' GRADUATE MEDICAL EDUCATION The 'Match' is a system used in North America by which both teaching hospitals rank their preferences for candidates to fill their first year post-graduate training positions, and graduating medical students rank their preferences for those (internship year) positions; some graduate programs allow certain graduate training positions to be filled 'outside of the match'; in 1995, 13 549 medical students participated; Match Day is traditionally held in mid-March (M Aviram et al, Am J Clin Nutrition March, 1995)

matching grant ACADEMIA A form of usually non-peer-reviewed funding in which a foundation or philanthropy contributes a sum of money that 'matches' a financial contribution made by an institution, university or hospital; Cf 'Approved but not granted'

maté *pronounced* Ma-tay A tea-like beverage obtained

from an infusion of the leaves of a South American shrub (*Ilex paraguayensis*), habitually ingested at high temperatures in southeastern South America; high volume drinkers are 2.2-fold more likely to have esophagitis, and have a relative risk of 1.47 for esophageal cancer; ingestion of more than 2.5 liters/day is reported to be associated with a relative risk of 12.2 for esophageal cancer (**Cancer Res 1990; 50:426**)

Material Safety Data Sheet MSDS OCCUPATIONAL SAFETY A document containing information and instructions on hazardous materials present in the workplace; MSDSs contain details about hazards and risks relevant to the substance, requirements for its safe handling, and actions to be taken in the event of fire, spill, or overexposure; MSDSs are used by an employer to help comply with both OSHA standards and with state and local governmental requirements; see Hazardous materials

maternal age effect The impact that ↑ age has on obstetrical events; ↑ age is widely thought to adversely impact on pregnancy as 1) The complication rate is greater in older pregnant women (see Elderly primigravida) and 2) There is an ↑ rate of fetal malformation in older women, possibly the result of an unknown effect of aging on the uterus and eggs (table); ↑ frequency of non-disjunctional events has been associated with advanced maternal age in Down syndrome and other aneuploid conditions, as well as Prader-Willi syndrome, in which there is uniparental disomy of chromosome 15 (**N Engl J Med 1992; 326:1599oa**) Cf Paternal age

MATERNAL AGE & CHROMOSOME DEFECTS		
AGE	TRISOMY 21	OTHERS
<20	1/1900	1/526
25	1/1200	1/476
30	1/885	1/384
35	1/365	1/178
40	1/109	1/63
45	1/32	1/18
49	1/12	1/7

'maternal-fetal conflict' BIOMEDICAL ETHICS A dilemma with considerable medicolegal ramifications that arises when a mother wishes to carry out an activity, eg drinking alcohol or working at a job with an occupational exposure to high levels of lead, that is potentially harmful to the fetus; the current thinking in the US judicial system, as exemplified by the Supreme Court in the *International Union* v *Johnson Controls* ruling, is that protection of the fetus over the mother's personal freedom is both paternalistic and inappropriate and that the ultimate decision-maker must be the woman herself (**N Engl J Med 1991; 325:740**); Cf Emancipated minor

maternal-infant transmission INFECTIOUS DISEASES A generic term* for any of several routes by which an infant may become infected with a pathogen of maternal origin; MIT has been reported for CMV, herpes, HIV, and TB (**N Engl J Med 1994; 330:1051oa**), and may occur in utero (ie transplacentally), perinatally and/or during labor and delivery (eg in the birth canal), or postnatally (eg by breast-feeding); the administration of zidovudine antepartum and intrapartum and to the infant for 6 weeks after birth is reported to ↓ MIT of HIV by ⅔ (**N Engl J Med 1994; 331:1173oa**)

*While maternal-infant transmission is in effect synonymous with vertical transmission, the latter may also refer to the possible (albeit extremely rare) transmission of an infection to the mother from the fetus

maternal milk see Breast milk

matrix-assisted laser desorption/ionization time-of-flight mass spectrometer system see MALDI-TOF system

matrix bias LABORATORY MEDICINE A generic term for any deviation in values for a particular analyte introduced by a matrix effect‡; MB impacts on proficiency testing values and laboratory results in general (**CAP Today Jan 1993 p1**)

matrix effect LABORATORY MEDICINE The difference between the value of an analyte from a fresh patient specimen and from stabilized processed reference materials (PRMs); ideally, PRMs and fresh patient specimens produce the same (or similar) values with routine methods; unfortunately, PRMs used to transfer and assess accuracy among laboratories often have reactive properties that differ from fresh patient specimens; the matrix effect may be due to modification of the solution matrix of source materials by additives, by steps required to stabilize the PRMs, eg lyophilization, or by use of nonhuman source materials; matrix modifications impact on analytical results in a complex fashion through various mechanisms, eg changes in macromolecular structure, (electrical) charge reactivity, solution viscosity, difference in protein isoforms between patient samples and calibration materials, proficiency testing materials or PRMs, the need for completely nonhuman materials (eg fluorocarbons to simulate blood gas specimens), and combinations of analytes at superphysiolgical concentrations (**Arch Pathol Lab Med 1993; 117:343-436oa**) see Reference material

matrix metalloproteinase MMP A class of proteases that is ubiquitous in human disease and development, and critical to tissue remodeling (**Bio/Technology 1995; 13:554**); MMPs are expressed in certain malignancies and are intimately linked to invasion and metastasis, an activity that may be specifically blocked by tissue inhibitors of metalloproteinases (TIMPs); MMPs have considerable amino acid homology and similar activation mechanisms, but have different substrate specificities; neutral MMP-1 (formerly interstitial collagenase) is active on interstital type I collagen; MMP-2 (formerly 72 kD type IV collagenase) hydrolyzes type IV collagen, and nonfibrillar collagens, eg types V, VII, and IX, as well as elastin, fibronectin, and gelatin, and has been linked to a malignant phenotype; MMP-3 and MMP-10 (formerly stromelysin-2) hydrolyze collagen types III, IV, V, and X, as well as fibronectin, gelatins, laminin, and proteoglycans; MMP-7 digests fibronectin and gelatins, MMP-9 digests type IV collage and gelatins; as the net matrix proteolysis depends on the local balance between the MMPs and the natural tissue inhibitors of metalloproteinases (TIMPs), a MMP-TIMP profile is of interest as a potential tool for determining the invasive and metastatic potential of a particular tumor (**Diagn Mol Pathol 1993; 2:74**)

matrix metalloproteinase inhibitor A generic term for any inhibitor of MMPs, which may be native (TIMPs-tissue inhibitors of metalloproteinase) or synthetic in nature; MMPIs have attracted considerable interest in the pharmaceutical industry as potential therapeutic agents as MMPs have been implicated in a vast array of human miseries including arthritis, cancer, connective tissue diseases, and others; although hydroxamates are the most studied class of MMPIs, the issues of oral bioavailability, low long-term toxicity, and 'intellectual property' may prove insurmountable, making the search for alternative agents desirable (**Bio/Technology 1995; 13:554**)

matrolysin Putative metalloproteinase

matt Dull MICROBIOLOGY A standard descriptor for a nonglistening surface seen on culture plates of bacteria that don't produce capsules, characteristic of many Enterobacteriaceae species; cultures of bacteria that produce capsules are described as glistening or 'mucoid'

Matthew effect Halo effect An allegorical term applied to the observation that an eminent scientist, eg Nobel laureate or other person of renown, will receive a disproportionate amount of credit for a discovery, despite a relatively small contribution to the ultimate success of a project; the name derives from Matthew, one of Christ's twelve disciples who said, *'For to every one who has, more shall be given and he shall have in abundance; but from him who has not, even what he has will be taken'*; the term has been borrowed by epidemiologists for tabulating the 'hard' and 'soft' risk factors of a disease, as those subjects with more risk factors will be more likely to suffer from the disease

matting Enlargement and cohesion of lymph nodes, which is classically described in tuberculosis, which may occur in other infections, eg histoplasmosis, or in metastatic carcinoma; see 'Shotty' lymphadenopathy

maturation arrest HEMATOLOGY The presence of relatively mature cytoplasm and an immature nucleus, which occurs in patients with megaloblastic anemia due to a deficiency of vitamin B_{12} and/or folic acid and acute leukemias; the change affects all cells, is most prominent in the bone marrow and is characterized by enlarged cells with delicate, open chromatin and prominent parachromatin; this 'Nuclear:cytoplasmic asynchrony' is due to decreased DNA synthesis and a block in mitosis, attributed to the slowing of cobalamin-dependent pathway of methionine synthesis, which in turn sequesters folate as N^5-methyl FH_4 that cannot be used by thymidylate synthetase to generate dTMP from dUMP

maturation index Squamous cell index GYNECOLOGIC CYTOLOGY A crude evaluation of the female estrogen status, based on the Papanicolaou ('Pap') smear, using three values X, Y and Z, that total 100, corresponding to the percentage of parabasal, intermediate and superficial squames respectively seen in the smear; cells for the MI are taken from the lateral vaginal wall, 100 or more cells are counted

1) PARABASAL CELLS Immature round to oval squames with a large nucleus

2) INTERMEDIATE CELLS Mature, often polygonal squamous cells with a well- or partially lysed vesicular nucleus and

3) SUPERFICIAL CELLS Mature squames with large polygonal borders and pyknotic nucleus

'Typical' MI patterns **0/60/40 MIDCYCLE PATTERN** is seen on the middle day of a normal cycle or an elderly woman with estrogen supplementation **5/35/60 OVULATION PATTERN** is due to an estrogen effect, seen with endometrial hyperplasia or carcinoma, Stein-Leventhal syndrome, ovarian tumors, hepatic insufficiency **100/–/– PRIMARY AMENORRHEA** the 'Pap smear' is composed of immature parabasal cells, due to complete lack of hormonal activity and **–/100/– PROGESTERONE EFFECT**; parabasal cells predominate in early post-partum period, during lactation or in the prepubertal period; the MI has waned in popularity as a means of evaluating hormonal status as serum levels of hormones can be easily measured; the MI is absolutely reliable in only two situations: marked estrogen effect and total absence of estrogen MI cannot be evaluated in cervical inflammation, due to excess cytolysis by Döderlein bacilli, drugs that alter squamous maturation, eg tetracycline, digitalis, thyroid, regional surgery and conization

maturity onset diabetes mellitus of the young see MODY

max An enzyme that interacts with myc, the protein product of *myc* by means of a leucine zipper motif, instructing a cell to mature, divide, or undergo autodestruction or apoptosis (New York Times 5 May 1992; C1)

Maxam-Gilbert sequencing MOLECULAR BIOLOGY A chemical method for determining the sequence of DNA, described by A Maxam and W Gilbert (Proc Nat Acad Sci, USA 1977; 74:560) METHOD The 5' end of a single strand of DNA (derived from a double-stranded segment) is labeled with ^{32}P; the DNA is then cleaved with a restriction endonuclease; one fragment of double helix DNA is isolated in a

relatively pure form and one strand is separated from the other, yielding a population of identical strands that have been radioactively-labeled at one end; the sample is then divided into four samples, each of which is subjected to a chemical reaction that destroys one or two specific nucleotide bases, either cytosine, or guanine, or adenine and guanine or thymine and cytosine; the loss of the bases at this point facilitates the breaking of the deoxyribose-phosphate bond, thus being similar to restriction mapping; the broken pieces are then electrophoresed and arranged on a 'sequencing' gel in order of length; see King-Kong gel

maximum acid output MAO, see there

maximum allowable cost program MAC program, see there

maximum androgen ablation A form of hormonal therapy for prostate cancer using combined therapy to reduce the effects of both gonadal and adrenal androgens, eg the use of a gonadotropin-releasing hormone agonist pluse flutamide; MAA provides a ± 6 month survival advantage and is an option for patients requiring hormonal therapy, but requires further data before it can be recommended for all patients (N Engl J Med 1994; 331:996RA)

maximum containment facility A 'level 3 to 4' research facility that is equipped to, and experienced in handling exotic, dangerous and potentially life-threatening infectious agents, eg HIV-1 and Lassa fever virus; all clothing changed prior to working with the organisms and at the day's end, appropriate decontamination procedures are carried out if warranted; see Biosafety

maximum contaminant level ENVIRONMENT The ceiling of an inorganic chemical that the US Environmental Protection Agency (EPA) will allow in drinking water before declaring it unsafe for human consumption, eg 0.002 mg/L for mercury, 0.05 mg/L for arsenic, cadmium, chromium, lead and silver, 1 mg/L for barium and 10 mg/L for nitrates; in 1977, the EPA determined that 95% of US drinking water was affected by pollution

maximum expiratory flow rate see Lung volumes

maximum tolerated doses The highest dose of a substance that can be given without causing serious weight loss and other signs of toxicity

Max-Planck Institutes Originally founded in 1911 as the Kaiser-Wilhelm Gesellschaft in Berlin, the MPI is comprised of 61 self-administering research institutes of social and natural sciences, including Institutes for Biochemistry, Biology, Biophysics, Biophysical chemistry, Brain research, Cell biology, Coagulation, Developmental biology, Endocrinology, Experimental medicine, Immunology, Molecular biology, Molecular genetics, Multiple sclerosis, Nutrition, Psychiatry and others

Max-Planck Gesellschaft zur Forderung der Wissenschaften eV 8000 Munchen 1 Postfach 647, Rezidenzstr 1A

'Mayo Clinic syndrome' American slang for the treatment of a patient as organ or organ system by a specialist, named after the Mayo Clinic, a 'center of excellence' that dedicates itself to the diagnosis and treatment of 'difficult diseases' (New York Times 6 Feb 1994; C1) see Center of Excellence; Cf Marcus Welby syndrome

Mayo risk score A decision-making model for primary biliary cirrhosis based on five variables: bilirubin levels in the serum, age, albuminemia, prothrombin time, and the severity of edema, which allows determination of prognosis

MB fraction see CPK-MB

M-BACOD A standard multiagent chemotherapeutic regimen used to treat lymphoma, consisting of methotrexate, bleomycin, doxorubicin (Adriamycin), cyclophosphamide, vincristine (Oncovorin) and dexamathasone, which is of use in treating AIDS-related lymphoma (JAMA 1991; 266:84)

MBC see Minimum bactericidal concentration

MBEST A variant of magnetic resonance imaging (MRI) consisting of a heavily-weighted T2 sequence, which is based on the echo-planar technique of MRI, developed by P Mansfield (Nottingham), used for ultra-high-speed imaging of the brain; see BEST, MRI; the advantage of the ultra-high-speed image is to allow rapid screening, functional imaging and analysis of the CSF fluid and blood flow patterns and rapid 'shooting' of restless patients

MBP see Major basic protein, Myelin basic protein

mbr Major breakpoint region, see there

MCAD see Medium-chain acyl-CoA dehydrogenase deficiency

MCAT Medical college admission test An examination administered by the Psychological Corporation, Inc, which is required in the US prior to entrance in the first year of medical school; the MCATs are an objectve evaluation of a candidate's verbal skills and scientific knowledge, which by extension, is assumed to be an adequate measure of the candidate's likelihood to succeed in medical school; see Graduate medical education, Medical student

McArdle's disease Glycogen storage disease V An AR [MIM 232600] condition caused by muscle phosphorylase [EC 2.4.1.1] deficiency CLINICAL Exercise intolerance, premature fatigue, myalgia, and cramping MOLECULAR PATHOLOGY Multiple point mutations have been identified by sequence analysis in the gene encoding muscle phosphorylase located on chromosome 11: T→C at codon 49 in exon 1, changing arginine to a stop codon; A→G at codon 205 in exon 5, changing glycine to serine; C→A at codon 542 in exon 14, changing lysine to threonine (N Engl J Med 1993; 329:241oA)

McCollough effect A phenomenon observed by subjects who have worked for a prolonged period with a computer monitor that displays green lettering on a darkened background, who find that white paper acquires a pink hue; the effect is caused by adaption of cortical neurons to specific combinations of color and form; it may last for several weeks and is of no clinical significance

McCune-Albright disease An AD [MIM 174800] condition possibly related to altered regulation of cAMP CLINICAL Precocious puberty, polyostotic (cystic) fibrous dysplasia (spontaneous fractures at an early age), cafe-au-lait spotting of skin, ovarian cysts and endocrinopathy including hyperthyroidism, hypophosphatemia and cyclical (4-6 week) fluctuations of plasma estrogen; afflicted young girls have decreased gonadotropins and reactivity to luteinizing hormone-releasing factor LABORATORY ↑ Testosterone, ↑ alkaline phosphatase (N Engl J Med 1993; 328:496cPc) TREATMENT Aromatase inhibitor testolactone

Note: Hormonal manipulation is logical use of the presence of estrogen and progesterone receptors on the osteogenic cells of McCune-Albright patients

MCH Mean corpuscular hemoglobin A measurement of the hemoglobin per individual erythrocyte Reference range 26-34 pg/red cell (SI: International System)

MCHC Mean corpuscular hemoglobin concentration A value that is derived on automated (eg Coulter) cell counters from measured parameters Reference range: 31-36 g/dl

McKusick classification A classification of human disease delineated by Victor McKusick, Osler Professor of medicine at Johns Hopkins medical school and 'Linnaeus' of human genetics, who single-handedly organized the congenital diseases of man; his opus magnum, Mendelian Inheritance in Man (11th edition, 1994) forms the basis for international communication in genetic disease; each condition found in the work has been assigned an 'MIM number', subdivided into broad categories depending on whether the conditions are autosomal recessive, autoso-

mal dominant or linked to the X chromosome, eg McKusick 23625 corresponds to 5,10-methylenetetrahydrofolate reductase deficiency; see Human Genome project, MIM number

MCL Maximum contaminant levels, see there

MCLN Mucocutaneous lymph node syndrome, see Kawasaki's disease

MCM family Minichromosome maintenance family CELL BIOLOGY A family of interacting proteins that were first identified in yeasts, which are components of the so-called licensing factor, a complex of proteins that are responsible for a single controlled round of replication of chromosomal DNA in each mitotic cycle (Nature 1995; 375:418, 421, 360)

MCP-1 see Monocyte chemotactic protein-1

mcr Minor cluster region, see there

MCT 1) Medium-chain triglycerides, 2) Medullary carcinoma of the thyroid

MCTD see Mixed connective tissue disease

MCV Mean corpuscular volume A calculated value for the average volume of peripheral red cells Reference range: 80-100 femtoliter/cell

MD 1) Macular degeneration (ophthalmology) 2) Medical department 3) Medical discharge 4) Medical doctor (medicinae doctor) 5) Megadalton 6) Mitral (valve) disease 7) Moderately differentiated (pathology, refers to differentiation of a cancer) 8) Multinomial distribution (statistics) 9) Muscular dystrophy 10) Myotonic dystrophy

Also 1) Magnetic deflection 2) Maintenance dose 3) Malate dehydrogenase (also MDH) 4) Male treated with deoxycorticosterone 5) Malic dehydrogenase 6) Manic-depressive (now known as bipolar I disorder) 7) Mantoux diameter 8) Maternal deprivation 9) Mediodorsal 10) Medium dosage 11) Mentally deficient 12) Mentally disabled 13) Mesiodistal (dentistry) 14) Methyldichloroarsine 15) Methyldopa 16) Middle deltoid 17) Mildly diabetic (rarely used) 18) Minimum dosage 19) Moderate dose 20) Molecular diameter 21) Molecular dynamics 22) Monocular deprivation (ophthalmology) 23) Movement disorder 24) Multiple dissemination (usually widespread dissemination) 25) Myocardial damage 26) Myocardial disease

MDA 3,4-Methylenedioxymethamphetamine, see Ecstasy

MDD Major depressive disorder

MDM 3,4-Methylenedioxymethamphetamine, see Ecstasy

MDF Myocardial depressant factor, see there

MDGC Multidimensional gas chromatography, see Gas chromatography

MDMA 3,4-Methylenedioxymethamphetamine, see Ecstasy

MD/PhD ACADEMIA An individual holding both a degree in medicine and a doctorate of philosophy; the two combined degrees may be obtained either by 1) Completing a four year medical school education (requiring four years in the US, since the prerequisite for entry to medical school is four years or more of university education), which is a relatively standardized experience, followed by the studies required for a doctorate of philosophy (Ph.D.), which can range from several years of a poorly-supervised and/or part-time educational experience in virtually any discipline to five or more years of intense post-graduate education and bench research or 2) Completion of a six-year combined program, in which the medical education is mixed with research activities extending over the entire six years of education, a philosophy that is thought to facilitate a physician's entry into research

MDR Multidrug resistance ONCOLOGY The simultaneous cross-resistance to multiple chemotherapeutic agents, including antitumor antibiotics, eg daunorubicin, vinca alkaloids and epidophyllotoxins; mutants resistant to the effect of drug X occur with a frequency of 10^{-5}-10^{-8}; destruction of drug-sensitive cells 'selects' for resistant cells, explaining the increased efficacy (and necessity) of combination chemotherapy; in malignancy, cell membranes may 'bristle' with P-glycoprotein (P170), the protein encoded by the MDR gene, which ushers toxins to the cell's exterior, related to increased expression of the mdr1 locus, causing gene amplification, with production of up to 60 copies in resistant cells; resistant drugs include colchicine, vincristine, actinomycin, daunorubicin MECHANISM P170-mediated resistance is related to decreased drug accumulation (the P170 permeability glycoprotein pumps drug out of the tumor cells); MDR gene expression is amplified in methotrexate (MTX) resistance (MTX blocks formation of purine precursors), with the resistant cells producing more dihydrofolate reductase; non-P170 mediated resistance in MDR cells is related to an altered glutathione redox cycle Note: Increased expression of P170 may be ameliorated with verapamil, an antiarrhythmic that inactivates the P170 pump

Note: An MDR-related gene is expressed in higher copy numbers in drug-resistant *Plasmodium falciparum*

MDS Myelodysplastic syndrome, see there

'me too' drug CLINICAL PHARMACOLOGY A colloquial term for a generic drug that has an identical formulation and stated indications for use as those agents that have passed the clinical testing phase, the appropriate regulatory hurdles and product safety standards; these drugs are usually approved 'automatically' based on their virtual identity with other previously approved therapeutic formulations; the FDA approves ± 35 new molecular entities per year; techniques used by a drug company to induce physicians to change their prescribing habits from one to another equally efficacious 'me too' agent include seeding trials, unsubstantiated claims of superiority over competing products, and switch campaigns; see Seeding trial, Switch campaign

'Only a minority (offer) a clear clinical advantages over existing therapies. Many of the others are considered 'me too' drugs because they are so similar to brand-name drugs already on the market; the preponderance of 'me too' drugs has created a highly competetive marketplace for prescription drugs. Pharmaceutical companies wage aggressive campaigns to change prescribers' habits and to distinguish their products from competing one, even when the products are virtually indistinguishable. This (occurs) in many therapeutic classes—antiulcer products, ACE inhibitors, calcium channel blockers, selective serotonin-reuptake-inhbitor antidepressants, and NSAIDs, to name a few; victory in these therapeutic class wars can mean millions of dollars for a drug company. But for patients and providers it can mean misleading promotions, conflicts of interest, increased costs of health care and …inappropriate prescribing (N Engl J Med 1994; 331:1350sA)

MEA Multiple endocrine adenomatosis, see Multiple endocrine neoplasia

mean time between failure COMPUTERS The operating time between the beginning of a component's life to its first electronic or mechanical failure; one of the most critical components of a microcomputer is the hard drive which may have MTBFs of 250 000 hours

'meaningful existence' see Futility

meaningful time Quality time, see there

measles vaccine Measles is a condition that kills an estimated two million children/year worldwide; in children hospitalized for treating complicated measles (with pneumonia, croup or diarrhea), treatment with large doses of vitamin A reduces the mortality by 50% and the hospital stay and co-morbid conditions by one-half the Edmonston-Zagreb vaccine may be more immunogenic than the Schwarz vaccine and can be given by 6 months of age (N Engl J Med 1990; 322:580)

measurement The International System (SI) officially sanctions the use of certain prefixes for SI units (table); see SI

mechanical restraint A device used on an individual to restrict free movement, including seatbelts, straitjackets (camisole), and vests, or physical confinement; the US legal system requires documentation of medical conditions that would justify the use of restraints, which include unsteadiness, wandering and disruptive behavior, often secondary to psychiatric conditions and/or dementia, which may, in addition, require pharmacologic restraints (JAMA 1991; 265:469)

mechanical theory of metastases see Seed-and-soil hypothesis

mechanical ventilation Mechanically assisted respiration in which inspiration is driven at a preset frequency or triggered by the patient; although expiration is passive, intra-alveolar pressure may be purposely raised by positive end-expiratory pressure (PEEP) in those suffering from pulmonary edema or increased lung compliance; mechanical ventilation is indicated if the PO_2 is less than 60 mm Hg, despite best non-interventional efforts (mask, bronchodilators, diuretics and physical therapy); the iron lung is a variation on this theme, where negative external pressure is applied to the thoracic wall in patients encased from the neck down in a negative pressure chamber INDICATIONS FOR MECHANICAL VENTILATION Chest wall restriction (kyphoscoliosis, thoracoplasty), chronic obstructive pulmonary disease, CNS and brainstem disease (central apnea, primary alveolar hypertension, tumors, vascular malformation), degenerative disease (Shy-Drager disease, spinocerebellar degeneration), neuromuscular disease (amyotrophic lateral sclerosis, multiple sclerosis, muscular dystrophy, myopathy, phrenic nerve damage, poliomyelitis), spinal cord disease (cervical trauma, quadriplegia, syringomyelia)

'mechanism' A doctrine that holds that all the details of a process, eg evolution, the genetic code or pathogenesis of a disease, can be explained in terms of a limited number of physico-chemical cause-and-effect relations

mechanism of death '*a physiologic derangement or a biochemical disturbance produced by a cause of death. The mechanism, because of its incompatibility with life, is the means by which the cause exerts its lethal effect. (Examples include) cardiorespiratory arrest, asystole, and respiratory arrest. Mechanisms lack etiologic specificity, are unacceptable substitutes for cause of death, and, in general, are not to be included in cause of death statements.*' (Arch Pathol Lab Med 1995; 119:123oA) Cf Immediate cause of death, Underlying cause of death

mechlorethamine An alkylating chemotherapeutic agent of the nitrogen mustard group, used to treat lymphomas and a component of the MOPP regimen SIDE EFFECTS GI symptoms, bone marrow suppression, skin vesication on contact

Meckel's diverticulum A pouch in the small intestine, which corresponds to the omphalomesenteric (vitelline) duct remnant, is located along the antimesenteric border and may contain gastric (and be associated with peptic ulcer disease) or pancreatic tissue; a popular mnemonic is the 'rule of twos', as the diverticulum is two feet (circa 0.65 m) from the ileocecal valve, two inches long (circa 5 cm), two cm in diameter, found in two percent of the population and two-fold more common in males; as Meckel's diverticulum is a favored site for carcinoids, it may be excised prophylactically when the surgeon is in the abdominal cavity for other reasons

meconium Green viscid mucus-like material found in the intestine of all neonates; it is the first stool passed by the newborns and is passed in the first

MEASUREMENT	
googa	100^{100}
exa	10^{18}
peta	10^{15}
tera	10^{12}
giga	10^{9}
mega	10^{6}
kilo	10^{3}
hecto	10^{2}
deka	10^{1}
deci	10^{-1}
centi	10^{-2}
milli	10^{-3}
micro	10^{-6}
nano	10^{-9}
pico	10^{-12}
femto	10^{-15}
atto	10^{-18}
zepto	10^{-21}

Note: 10^{12} corresponds to the British billion; 10^9, the American billion, corresponds to a British millard

24-48 hours of life

meconium aspiration syndrome NEONATOLOGY A symptom complex caused by the aspiration of meconium at the time of delivery CLINICAL Low APGAR scores, tachypnea, dyspnea, and cyanosis, which either resolves in the first three days of life, or if the amount of aspirated meconium was intense, progresses displaying patchy infiltrates on chest films accompanied by atelectasis, emphysema and rales; Cf APGAR

meconium ileus Meconium plug syndrome A condition characterized by obstruction of the neonatal intestine by intensely viscid glue-like meconium that may be confined to the ileus, a finding highly characteristic of cystic fibrosis CLINICAL Non-passage of stool in the first two days of life, accompanied by nausea, vomiting and abdominal distension COMPLICATIONS Volvulus, intestinal infarction PATHOLOGY Goblet cell hyperplasia Note: Meconium 'plugging' of the rectum may also signal the presence of Hirschsprung's disease, which is histologically characterized by segmental aganglionosis

MEDAC syndrome Multiple endocrine deficiency, Addison's disease and candidiasis, see APECED (autoimmune polyendocrinopathy-candidiasis-ectodermal dystrophy)

Medea complex PSYCHIATRY Murderous hatred by a mother for her child or children, arising from a desire for revenge on her husband

Medea of Greek mythology was a sorceress and the wife of Jason, who imprisoned her when she decided to marry Creusa; Medea responded by killing their children

Médecins sans Frontières Doctors Without Borders The world's largest independent medical relief organization that provides short- and long-term medical aid to war zones, sites of natural disasters, and refugee camps, in the form of emergency care, immunization services, food, hygiene, education and training; MSF was begun in 1971, has funded 4500 individual missions and often operates in volatile political environments, resulting in the deaths of some of its workers (Am Med News 18 March 1991); ¼ of MSF's funding is provided by the United Nations, the remainder from private donations; Cf Amnesty International, IPPNW, Red Cross

media 'epidemic' A flurry of interest displayed by the news media (newspapers, television, radio) for an item of medical importance, eg a new therapeutic modality, 'breakthrough', or a new disease, which follows a report in a major medical journal; the 'media' are often less interested in reporting the facts than in exploiting the potential sensationalist impact of the news item in question; this may result in distortion of the details, as journalists are rarely scientifically sophisticated, thus may have difficulty in placing the information they present in an appropriate context; see Embargo arrangement, Ingelfinger rule

medial necrosis see Cystic medial necrosis

medialization thyroplasty A technique for treating vocal fold motion impairment ADVANTAGES Local anesthesia, the patient is positioned anatomically during the procedure, the procedure is potentially reversible, and the given the location of the prosthesis (lateral to the inner perichondrium of the thyroid lamina), and the vocal fold's structural integrity is preserved DISADVANTAGES The procedure is 'open', it is more difficult technically, and the intubation required for the procedure may damage regional structures

median lethal concentration LC$_{50}$ OCCUPATIONAL SAFETY The average concentration of a chemical substance or mixture present in air as a gas, vapor, mist, fume or dust that is capable of killing ½ of a group of test animals exposed to the chemical by inhalation under specific test conditions, LC$_{50}$ is most commonly expressed in ppm or mg/mg^3

median lethal dose LD$_{50}$ OCCUPATIONAL SAFETY The average amount of a drug, toxin, chemical substance or mixture, or microorganism that is capable of killing ½ of a group of test animals under specific test conditions, LD$_{50}$ is most commonly expressed in mg/kg, by oral intake or skin exposure

median rhomboid glossitis A condition first regarded as a developmental abnormality of the tongue, now considered a manifestation of chronic infection by *Candida albicans*, facilitated by the high glucose levels as it is often seen in diabetics CLINICAL Rhomboid or diamond-shaped red plaque or patch on the dorsum of the tongue anterior to the circumvallate papillae PATHOLOGY Loss of papillae, hyperparakeratosis, proliferation of the spinous layer, elongation of the rete ridges, lymphocyte and neutrophil infiltration of connective tissue, increased blood vessels and lymphatics, degeneration and hyaline formation of the underlying tongue TREATMENT Nystatin or amphotericin B may cause regression

mediastinal 'crunch' SPORTS MEDICINE A substernal crepitant sound, often synchronous with the heartbeat, caused by percolation of air into the mediastinum (emphysema) as occurs in esophageal perforation or secondary to expansion of gas in rapid ascent in scuba divers (Caisson's disease)

Medicaid A federally-funded, state-operated and state-administered program of medical assistance in the US that is authorized by Title XIX of the Social Security Act of 1965 and provides medical assistance to certain low-income groups, including the elderly, blind, disabled, single-parent families, and the unemployed, who are eligible for welfare cash programs, eg 'Aid to Families with Dependent Children' and 'Supplementary Security Income' programs, and to those with income sufficient for basic needs, but not for medical care; in 1987, Medicaid paid $45 x 10^9 to 23 million recipients; Medicaid recipients in urban areas have limited access to outpatient health care, and often rely on hospital emergency departments to provide primary (outpatient) care (N Engl J Med 1994; 330:1426OA) which explains the 34% ↑ in emergency room visits by Medicaid recipients from 1985-1990

Note: Some health care providers have found that the cost of processing the paperwork required to be reimbursed for services rendered to Medicaid patients is greater than the reimbursement obtained by the physician and thus Medicaid work may be viewed in a 'pro bono publico' context

Medicaid buy-in HEALTH CARE FINANCING A proposed system that allows those who are not eligible for Medicaid coverage to enroll by paying premiums on a sliding scale; although the concept is supported by the AMA, critics believe it doomed to failure in that there are few inclined to buy into a program stigmatized as 'welfare' in nature (Am Med News 25 October 1992, p7)

Medicaid fraud A type of 'white-collar crime' committed by physicians, most commonly by foreign medical graduate and psychiatrists in which Medicaid was billed for a variety of fraudulent practices; these practices included padding of bills, charging for tests and services that were unnecessary or never performed, illegally prescribing controlled drugs, and charging Medicaid for therapeutic time while having sexual intercourse with patients (N Engl J Med 1993; 329:892BR)

'Medicaid mill' A for-profit organization (in the US) that provides health care, usually on an ambulatory basis in locations where few medical services are available, eg inner city ghettos and rural communities; these 'mills' are characterized by high productivity (as measured by the number of patients seen) and are frequently accused of a variety of abuses of the Medicaid reimbursement system; see also Family 'ganging', 'Ping-ponging'

'Medicaidization' A shift of financial liability for medical care of the financially disadvantaged to the public sector;

in the USA, Medicaid bears the brunt of health care costs for the financially disenfranchised, paying a small fraction of the actual cost of the services provided; many AIDS patients are below poverty levels and there is an increasing tendency to shift the costs of providing care for these patients and indigents from private insurance companies to the agency (Medicaid) that pays the least for services; Cf 'Dumping', 'Safety net' hospital, 'Skimming'

medical 'arms race' A highly colloquial term (derived from the nuclear arms race between the US and the former Soviet Union) referring to escalating health care costs due to proliferation and use of expensive medical technology and devices (N Engl J Med 1993; 328:1356ᴏʀ)

medical center A health care organization that is defined by

1) Structure The physical plant usually includes a hospital and a complex of buildings in which health care, research, staff support, and ancillary services are provided

2) Function The MC provides a range of medical services that is usually more complex than that provided by the traditional community hospital

medical device 'Any article or health care product intended for use in the diagnosis of disease or other condition or for use in the care, treatment, or prevention of disease that does not achieve any of its primary intended purposes by chemical action or by being metabolized. Examples include diagnostic test kits, crutches, electrodes, pacemakers, catheters, and intraocular lens.' (JAMA 1994; 272:955sc); the US FDA regulates 80 000 MDs (produced by > 18 000 companies) and classifies them as being either a significant or a nonsignificant risk device; see Significant risk device, Silicone implant; Cf Nonsignificant risk

medical ethics The moralistic constructs focused on the problems of individual patients and medical practitioners (see N Engl J Med 1993; 328:360ʙʀ) medical ethics is a burgeoning field that attempts to formally address the moral dilemmas affecting broad medical decisions, and may be divided into 1) The broad ethical principles that impact as a society on patients, physicians and health care institutions and 2) The individual code of ethics of health care providers, delineated by the Hippocratic oath Note: A number of landmark cases that have helped delineate the boundaries of medical ethics, in particular those regarding a person's control over his/her body are described in detail elsewhere in this work, see Baby Doe, Brouphy, Conran, Jefferson, Kevorkian, Quinlan, Roe v Wade

medical 'failure' A patient who does not respond to a non-interventional modality used to treat a non-malignant, but potentially pernicious condition, and who, due to this failure, may benefit from surgery; the traditional philosophy is to attempt medical (drugs, change in lifestyle, diet and exercise) therapy when there is no clear benefit of performing surgery for a disease, as in the continuing controversy between coronary artery bypass surgery versus medical treatment to treat symptomatic atherosclerotic heart disease: if the patient does not respond to conservative ('medical') therapy, the patient's physician(s) then recommend bypass surgery or another semi-invasive modality, eg percutaneous transluminal angioplasty

medical futility MF of medical interventions, eg CPR is divided into quantitative futility (low probability of success) and qualitative futility (poor quality of life if CPR is performed); application of the futility rationale in withholding or withdrawing medical interventions (eg DNR orders) requires both practice guideline and a better understanding of the MF concept (JAMA 1995; 273:124ᴏᴀ) see DNR

medical informatics The science that concerns itself with the cognitive processes of medical decision-making and the processing of medical information, which includes the technology and communication tasks of medical practice, education and research; see Artificial intelligence, Computers, Expert system, Electronic journal, Electronic publishing, MEDLINE, Online database

medical IRA Medical savings account, see there

medical laboratory technician MLT A person who is trained to perform most laboratory tests, but who doesn't have the educational background of a medical technologist, and who does not in general have authorization to report on or to perform the most technically demanding tests in the clinical laboratory; Cf Medical technologist

medical malpractice Negligent conduct or unreasonable lack of skill in the performance of a medical task on the part of a physician or a party (eg a health care facility) in which that act or task occurs; most cases of medical malpractice fall under the rubric of civil law, ie a legal action filed by one person against another, rather than criminal law, ie a legal action filed by a state or the federal government against an offending person(s); medical malpractice is based on the theory of negligence, which is conduct that falls below the 'standard of care' recognized by the law for protecting others against unreasonable risk of harm, ie deviation from accepted standards of care, resulting in harm to others; four elements must be alleged and proven in a court of law in order for the complaining party (the plaintiff) to sustain (win) a lawsuit for negligence

DUTY The plaintiff must prove the existence of a legal relationship, ie duty between himself and the defendant

BREACH OF DUTY Once duty is established, the plaintiff must prove that the physician breached that duty by failing to comply with accepted standards of care by malfeasance (an act not conforming to accepted standard of practice) or by non-malfeasance (failure to perform an act expected under the circumstances)

DAMAGES The plaintiff must prove that he has sustained some injury as a result of the alleged negligent act, injury that is translated into a monetary value, either compensatory (tangible, either lost wages, lost earning capacity, medical expenses) or punitive (intangible, often in the form of 'pain and suffering', where multimillion-dollar awards are not uncommon) and

CAUSATION The plaintiff must prove a reasonable connection between the alleged negligent act or omission of the defendant and suffered injury

STATISTICS, US In one 5-year period, 48% of surgeons and surgical specialists, 34% of obstetricians-anesthesiologists and 15% of other physicians had had malpractice claims; 85% of all payments were made on behalf of 3% of the insurance policy holders, and those with previous claims had a greater risk for future claims; in the USA, a physician may be sued for doing too much (the government and reimbursement organizations penalize a physician who orders 'too many' tests) or too little (eg by ordering too few tests, a relatively rare disease may be 'missed'); see Assault and battery, Blood shield laws, Confidentiality, Consent, Countersuit, 'Defensive medicine', 'Difficult patient', DNR (do not resuscitate), Emergency doctrine law, Emergency psychiatric committment, Expert witness, 'Good Samaritan laws, Informed consent, Jehovah's Witness, Medical record, Misdiagnosis, Negligence, Patient-physician relationship, Quinlan case, Respondeat superior, Standard of care, Therapeutic privilege doctrine, Wrongful birth

GLOSSARY **ABANDONMENT** A physician's unilateral severance of a professional relation with a patient, without reasonable notice and at a time when the necessity for continuing medical attention remains; acts of abandonment include refusal, or more commonly, alleged refusal to treat after he has seen a person needing care, refusal to attend to a case in which the physician has already assumed responsibility, eg visit while the patient is in the hospital, failure to provide follow-up attention and failure to arrange for a competent substitute in times of absence **BORROWED SERVANT DOCTRINE** A principle under which the party usually liable for a person's actions, eg the hospital being responsible for a nurse, is absolved of that responsibility when that person is asked to do something, eg by a surgeon, which is outside of the bounds of hospital policy Note: A hospital is only liable if the plaintiff can prove that the hospital was negligent in removing a physician or employee known to be incompetent **BREACH OF CONTRACT** see

Abandonment, above **CAUSATION** The establishment of a cause-and-effect relation between the allegedly negligent act and the purported injuries **CONTRIBUTORY NEGLECT** Conduct on the part of the plaintiff, which occurred after he came under the physician's care that falls below that which a reasonable person would exercise for his own protection, thereby contributing to the alleged act of negligence **DAMAGES, COMPENSATORY** An award that pretends to restore the victim to the state he would have been in had the 'wrong' not occurred, ie lost wages, pain and suffering, permanent disabilities, mental anguish and loss of consortium (conjugal fellowship, exchange of body fluids) **DAMAGES, PUNITIVE** An 'Insult-to-injury' award given by jury in order to castigate the defendant, designed to prevent him from repeating the offense; punitive damage awards are either 1) Special (wages, lost profits, past and future medical fees) and other compensatory awards, the monetary value of which can be reasonably calculated or 2) General (pain and suffering, humiliation, disfigurement) awards that elude standardized formulae **EMOTIONAL DISTRESS** Intentional infliction of emotional distress The 'outrage' tort A legal action initiated against a defendant who allegedly said or did something so completely absurd (medically) or insulting to the plaintiff that he suffered emotional damage **FRIVOLOUS LAWSUIT** A groundless lawsuit in which injury did not occur or which was so negligible that it caused no damage, real or perceived, to the plaintiff; such lawsuits have little prospect for success and are brought with the purpose of annoying or embarrassing a defendant; see de minimus rule **LIABILITY** A broad term referring to all character of obligation, amenability and responsibility for an act **REFERRAL AND CONSULTATION** A physician should always refer difficult cases to competent specialists Note: If the consultant proves to be incompetent, the referring physician may be sued for so advising the patient; consultation should be sought when the diagnosis is difficult, the illness is unfamiliar, complex or fraught with complications, the patient doesn't improve in a reasonable time and at the patient's request **RES IPSA LOQUITOR** *The thing speaks for itself* A doctrine in which the plaintiff's burden to prove negligence is fairly light, not usually requiring expert witnesses, since the details of the incident are clear and understandable to a jury, eg foreign objects left behind in surgical procedures **RESPONDEAT SUPERIOR** *Let the master answer for the servant* A doctrine in which the liability for a negligent act is passed to 'captain of the ship', eg the surgeon, despite the fact that the act is performed by another person, eg an operating room nurse; the hospital may under this doctrine claim that although the hospital is the nurse's employer, at the time of the negligent act, the nurse was under someone else's guidance **STATUTES OF LIMITATIONS** A doctrine that allows the plaintiff two years from the time of alleged malpractice to file a lawsuit, unless the plaintiff is 1) Minor, who has two years after reaching the adulthood to file a lawsuit or 2) Later discovers the act of negligence **TORT** A civil wrong for which the wrongdoer (tortfeasor) may be held liable in damages; negligence is a type of tort equivalent to malpractice

medical record The written documentation of a person's medical history, the diagnostic and therapeutic procedures performed, and the patient's clinical status at the time he was last seen by health care providers; the purpose of the medical record is to serve as the basis for planning and ensuring continuity of care, provide a means of communication among physicians and others contributing to patient management, provide documentation of the patient's course of disease and treatment, serve as a basis for review and evaluation, protect the legal interests of the patient, hospital and responsible physicians and provide data for use in billing, research and education; it is imperative that complete, accurate and timely records be kept, as lawsuits may be initiated years after the alleged occurrence of an event, at which time, independent recollection of the event is unlikely; the medical record should be accurate, timely, objective, specific, concise, consistent, comprehensive, logical, legible*, clear, descriptive, and reflective of rational thought process(es); see Hospital chart

*Although physicians tend to 'write like doctors', nothing erodes credibility in front of a jury more quickly than the inability of the defendant to read his own handwriting

medical saving account HEALTH CARE ENVIRONMENT A proposed means of reducing the costs of the fragmented and expensive US health care system; MSA would give those with health insurance a financial incentive to save money and bring the costs of health care under control; with an MSA, a person eligible for health care (in any form, eg annual check-ups, diagnostic tests, etc) has a certain amount of 'chits' placed in an account that he/she may 'cash in' at his/her discretion, usually at the end of a certain period of time; MSA proposals would allow a person to purchase cheaper catastrophic health insurance policies with high deductibles, and place the savings in personal tax-free accounts to cover routine bills, with a rolling over of unused funds to be used a future time for medical bills, should the need arise; in theory, the MSA concept would force a greater prudence in spending for health care, as the consumer has a vested interest in controlling costs; MSAs are reported to ↓ medical costs, ↑ consumer choice and ↓ administrative interference (**JAMA 1995 273:997**) critics of the MSA concept believe it might exacerbate risk segmentation, undercut the benefits of managed care, ↑ administrative costs, and ↑ spending for uncovered care (**Am Med News 7 Nov 1994 p3**)

Note: Some MSAs have been called Medical IRAs (individual retirement accounts) as they are tax-free and may in part finance a person's retirement

medical school debt see Medical student debt

'medical' specialty A field of medical care that provides specialized patient care, by treating patients in a non-interventional fashion, ie with drugs, or with minimum intervention, eg balloon catheterization; 'medical' specialties include internal medicine (allergy and immunology, cardiology, gastroenterology, hematology and oncology, neurology, infectious and pulmonary diseases), dermatology, pediatrics, psychiatry, preventive medicine, aerospace medicine; Cf Hospital-based physicians, 'Surgical' specialty

medical staff The organized body of licensed physicians and health care providers who are permitted by law and by a hospital to provide medical care within that hospital or health care facility; the medical staff may be 'closed', ie allowing a defined number of specialists to practice, recruiting new members only when vacancies exist or it may be 'open', accepting new members on a continuing basis; the medical staff is encharged with accounting for the quality and appropriateness of patient care rendered by all practitioners authorized to practice in a particular institution; the MS makes recommendations to the chief of staff with respect to appointments, reappointments, and clinical privileges; see House staff, Staff courtesy, Staff privileges

medical student abuse An widely extant practice, in which medical students are psychologically 'abused' by superiors (interns, residents, fellows and attending physicians) in the form of badgering, belittling and being forced to perform menial, degrading tasks; see Pimping, Scut work

Note: The opinion has been privately voiced by some health care workers that abuse is part of the medical student experience, which helps 'harden' them for the realities of practicing medicine

medical student debt The amount of fininacial obligations or monies owed (with interest) to various parties by a medical student; in the USA, higher education is costly and medical students are required to pay an annual university tuition fee (ranging from $10-25 000), in addition to living costs ($15-20 000/year), during the four years of medical school; the average graduating medical student owed $50 000 (1992); less than 20% of the US medical students graduate from medical school debt-free; there are two types of loan repayment: deferment, in which the borrower delays repayment without accrual of interest, and forbearance, in which the borrower delays repayment but interest accrues; to address this issue, one author proposes the institution of a public service plan to reduce or eliminate indebtedness; there is little correlation between the amount of indebtedness and the choice of specialty (N Engl J Med 1993; 328:651SB)

medical superintendent Chief of staff, see there

medical tattooing ANTHROPOLOGY A practice among some primitive cultures which is regarded as a precursor of acupuncture; the oldest known MT has been identified on the Ice Man, 5000-year-old man found mummified in the Tyrolean Alps (Science 1995; 268:33)

medical team The group of physicians and health care workers who are responsible for a patient's medical needs while in the hospital and during a reasonable follow-up period; the 'team approach' has become the prevalent form of patient management in the US, which recognizes that no one person can be expected to diagnose and treat all aspects of a patient's condition

medical technologist LABORATORY MEDICINE A laboratory worker who has received at least four years of formal college or university education (a bachelor of science degree in medical technology) and training in the performance of various techniques in clinical pathology, including hematology, microbiology, chemistry, blood banking, immunology and other areas of the clinical laboratory; MTs are eligible for certification by the American Society of Clinical Pathologists, and upon successful completion of the appropriate examination are titled, MT(ASCP); technologists are empowered to perform and report the results of clinical tests; Cf Medical laboratory technician, Technician

medical underwriting HEALTH CARE FINANCING The process of determining the medical needs of an individual or group prior to providing coverage; MW may have a negative overtone, as it is a process undertaken by the insurer, and may be intended to penalize (if only financially) those who are at high risk for (or already have) certain diseases, by charging them higher premiums or by completely denying coverage (Am Med News 25 October 1992, p7)

medical waste PUBLIC HEALTH A form of biohazardous waste that is generate in the context of a health care setting (eg patient outpatient testing, invasive testing, surgical procedure) and is regarded by regulatory agencies as having the potential for carrying viable human pathogens; MW includes body parts and tissues, blood- or body-fluid-soaked garments, linen, all of which is appropriately placed in the so-called 'red bags' (in the US) that are marked with biohazard emblems and disposed of a fashion that is acceptable according to the law and to regulatory agencies; since the advent of AIDS, concern has heightened for proper disposal of MW, which can be safely released to the environment only after it has been subjected to one of several means of rendering it harmless; the standard method of MW disposal has been incineration, which of late has raised concerns about its environmental impact; other means of safe MW disposal include autoclaving, chemical disinfection, electrothermal deactivation, and microwaving (Laboratory Medicine 1995; 26:323OA)

medical waste incinerator PUBLIC HEALTH A device that eliminates medical waste by incineration; the ± 3700 MWIs in operation in US hospitals are being evaluated by the EPA in terms of environmental impact, as many of the devices are aging, and upgrading to meet the more stingent EPA standards would be difficult to impossible, hospitals and health care facilities with MWIs are exploring alternative methods for disposing of MW (Laboratory Medicine 1995; 26:323OA) see Medical waste

medicalization A neologism referring to the erroneous tendency by society (and often perpetuated by health professionals) to view the effects of socioeconomic disadvantage as purely medical issues; this tendency arises when the terms health care and medical care are

'...used interchangeably, reflecting a cultural view that they are synonymous...'health care' and 'medical care,' however are not synonyms. Health care permeates all aspects of daily life. It centers on the prevention of illness. Health care includes social elements such as good housing and sanitation, a safe work environment, stable interpersonal relationships, sufficient income, and education. Medical care, in contrast is only one aspect of health care. It centers on the diagnosis and treatment of disease *after* (emphasis added) it has developed....By viewing social problems as medical problems, we arrive at the erroneous conclusion that reform of the medical care system is the best route to improved health.' (N Engl J Med 1993; 329:130ED)

medically underserved area A region that has a relative or absolute deficiency of health care resources, including hospital beds, equipment and/or medical personnel and resources

Medicare A federal (US government-administered) program enacted as Title XVIII of the Social Security Act of 1965, providing hospital and medical insurance protection for those aged 65 and older, disabled persons under age 65 who receive cash benefits under Social Security and persons of all ages with chronic kidney disease; aliens and some federal civil service employees have been eligible since 1973; Medicare has 37 million elderly and disabled enrollees (45% males, 55% females); $80 x 10^9 was paid by the US federal government to Medicare enrollees in 1987; > ¾ had income < $25 000; the 1995 out-of-pocket expenses are projected at $3053/beneficiary (Am Med News 15 May 1995, p3) Medicare consists of two parts 1) Compulsory hospitalization insurance, known as 'Part A', which is financed by contributions from employers, employees and participants and 2) Voluntary supplementary medical insurance, known as 'Part B', which is financed in part by monthly premiums paid by those enrolled and partly by the US federal government; insurance companies, Blue Cross and Blue Shield (see there) and several independent organizations act as fiscal intermediaries for the government; 6500 hospitals participate in the Medicare's 'Prospective payment system', the basis for which is the diagnosis-related groups, see DRGs; exceptions to Medicare coverage are health care facilities specialized in psychiatry, pediatrics, long-term care and rehabilitation; see Part A, Part B; Cf Medicaid, Socialized medicine

Note: Medicare does not cover outpatient prescription drugs, hospitalization > 150 days; skilled nursing > 100 days, preventive services (eg physical examinations, colorectal and prostate cancer screenings, routine foot care, immunizations, hearing aids, glasses), and physician balance billing (Am Med News 15 May 1995, p3)

medicine's 'rocking horse' A term coined by GD Lundberg (editor of the Journal of the American Medicl Association) referring to personal philosophies in the practice of medicine, with 'money grubbers' and 'altruistic missionaries' being at either extreme, and in the middle, those physicians who have a balanced view of medicine (JAMA 1995; 273:1539ED)

medicolegal impasse A situation in which the potential for medicolegal liability outweighs all other considerations, resulting in complete inaction; medicolegal impasses are not uncommon in the US, in particular related to drugs and medical devices, the manufacturers of which have endured long and costly legal battles* when one of their products has been linked to death or deformity; medicolegal impasses have been held responsible for loss of interest in developing products for certain areas, in particular contraceptive drugs and devices, the concern being if a 'bad baby' is linked to the product, opening a sluice-gate of lawsuits; similarly the manufacture of HIV immune globulin dropped commercialization plans in view of the potential for enhanced transmission of HIV to an infant (JAMA 1992; 268:1987MN&P)

*The manufacturer of the Dalkon shield (see there) was forced into bankruptcy and set up a $2.5 x 10^9 fund to pay for all relevant product-related lawsuits

Medicus Nursing Classification Score LONG-TERM NURSING A global measure of patient acuity that reflects the amount of nursing care required for a patient (JAMA 1995; 273:865)

medigap HEALTH CARE FINANCING A generic term for

employer-sponsored, individually purchased health insurance that is a supplement to the benefits provided by Medicare (**N Engl J Med 1995; 332:1132₀ₐ**)

MedisGroups Medical illness severity grouping system (**MediQual, Westborough, Massachusetts**) A system for classifying patients admitted to a hospital based on the severity of disease, formulated as an alternative to the diagnosis-related groups (DRGs) under which those hospitals admitting 'sicker' patients with the same DRGs were penalized since these patients had longer stays, thereby encouraging the practice of 'dumping'; under the MedisGroups, those patients admitted in group 0 to 1 (based on a list of key clinical findings) had a 1% mortality rate, while 60% of those in group 4 had imminent organ failure (**JAMA 1988; 260:3159**); see Kiss of death test; Cf DRGs, High mortality outlier

Note: MedisGroups admission severity does not adjust for interhospital case mix differences in outcome studies (**ibid, 1991; 265:2965**)

Mediterranean anemia β-thalassemia, thalassemia major

Mediterranean diet A loosely defined dietary regimen that differs according to the country, and includes an increased consumption of olive oil and complex carbohydrates (**N Engl J Med 1992; 327:52c**) Cf Affluent diet

Mediterranean diet pyramid A creation of the WHO, Harvard School of Public Health, and the Oldways Preservation and Exchange Trust, which, like the US Department of Agriculture's food diet pyramid (FDP), makes recommendations on the amounts of particular foods that should be consumed each day; in contrast to the FDP which lumps high protein foods, eg meat, poultry, fish, and beans in one category, the MDP recommends ↓ red meat, ↑ fish, passes beans into the nuts and legumes category, ↑ olive oil consumption, and categorizes wine as option (**N Y Times 29 March 1995, C1**) Cf Exercise pyramid, Food pyramid

Mediterranean fever 1) Generalized brucellosis 2) Familial Mediterranean fever see there

Mediterranean lymphoma IPSID, Immunoproliferative small intestinal disease

medium MICROBIOLOGY A liquid or solid matrix with nutrient designed to support the growth of microorganisms **DIFFERENTIAL MEDIA** are often solid and contain various chemical and other substances, eg colorants that may be produced by certain microorganisms, aiding in their identification **ENRICHMENT MEDIA** are often liquid and contain specific nutrients giving one or more of the microorganisms a growth advantage **SELECTIVE MEDIA** are those in which nutrients are added to either promote the growth of one or more group of bacteria, or inhibitors, eg nalidixic acid, malachite green and others to slow the growth of certain bacteria, giving the desired organisms a 'selective' growth advantage

medium chain acyl-coenzyme A dehydrogenase deficiency An uncommon (1:6-10 000) AR [MIM 201450] disease of fatty acid oxidation that presents in the first two years of life as either sudden unexplained death at home, or when seen in the hospital, as Reye syndrome; the diagnosis is established by mutation analysis of postmortem tissue obtained from paraffin-embedded blocks of tissue (**N Engl J Med 1991; 325:61c**)

medium chain triglyceride CLINICAL NUTRITION A triacylglycerol dietary substitute for long-chain triglycerides that is administered to very low-birth weight infants who cannot absorb longer chain fatty acids; MCT is derived from coconut oil and is theoretically useful in preventing steatorrhea, as 8-10 carbon triglycerides are more readily hydrolyzed by pancreatic enzymes, they don't require bile acids for absorption of the hydrolytic products and the metabolized products pass directly into the portal circulation; because MCTs provide less energy (8.3 kcal/g vs 9.0

for LCTs, no more than 400 calories of MCT may be used/day)

Note: A small percentage of MCTs undergo omega oxidation, forming the metabolically useless dicarboxylic acid

MEDLARS MEDical Literature and Analysis Retrieval System MEDICAL INFORMATICS The computerized bibliographic retrieval system formed from the Index Medicus that provides access to the biomedical literature, which is maintained by the National Library of Medicine in Washington, DC

MEDLINE MEDICAL INFORMATICS The most heavily-used of the more than 20 electronic (online) databases within MEDLARS, extending from 1966 to the present that is retrievable by a desktop computer using a modem at data-throughput speeds of 300, 1200 or 2400 baud or more

medroxyprogesterone acetate Depo-Provera‡

meds Colloquial for physician-prescribed medications

Medspeak A highly colloquial term for the working medical parlance which has a core of terms based on abbreviations, jargon, acronyms, and neologisms that range in origin from the classic roots of Greek and Latin to video games, movies, and television advertising; the express purpose of Medspeak is to facilitate communication among physicians and is the unofficial language of medicine; few can match the obfuscating elegance of Dr PL Fine's example of MedSpeak's reductio ad quasi-absurdum

Pt's SOB + DOE ↓ed. AF w/ VSS. CXR: LLL ASD /s Δ. WBC 11K; S/B Cx → GPC c/w PC w/o GNR, will d/c cef → PCN

which translates as 'The patient's shortness of breath and dyspnea on exertion are diminished; the patient is afebrile with stable vital signs; a chest film shows left lower lobe air space disease without change (from original film); the patient's white blood cell count is 11 000/dL; because the sputum demonstrates gram-positive cocci (consistent with pneumococcus) without gram-negative rods, cefuroxime therapy with be discontinued and switched to penicillin.' (**PL Fine, The Wards, Little, Brown and Co, Boston, 1994**)

This work is in part an effort to rectify the paucity of information on Medspeak–Author's note

medullary carcinoma, breast A variant of ductal carcinoma affecting women under age 50, described as more common in Japanese women PATHOLOGY Often well-circumscribed, reaching a large size before metastasizing to the axillary lymph nodes PATHOLOGY Prominent lymphohistiocytic inflammation peripheral to the 'pushing' tumor margins PROGNOSIS 84% 10 year survival (ductal carcinoma, 63% 10-year survival)

medullary carcinoma, thyroid A tumor comprising 3-10% of thyroid malignancies, arising in the C (parafollicular) cells of ultimobranchial cleft (neural crest) origin; there are two clinical forms of MCT: **SPORADIC MCT** Comprises 80-90% of cases, mean age of onset 45, presenting as a solitary 'cold' (by thyroid scan) nodule variably accompanied by intractable diarrhea and Cushing's syndrome **FAMILIAL MCT** Comprises 10-20% of cases (in one study with a long-term-average 23.5 years follow-up) 11% were familial (**Mayo Clin Proc 1992; 67:934**), mean age of onset 35, presenting as a multifocal and bilateral mass, accompanied by C-cell hyperplasia of residual thyroid tissue; familial MCT is often AD and associated with multiple endocrine adenomatosis, usually type II (which has a germline abnormality on chromosome 10, an earlier age of onset, and is often bilateral), or occasionally type III (IIb, less common, but more aggressive) and rarely a non-aggressive form of MCT that is not associated with other neural or endocrine lesions CLINICAL MCT presents as induration(s) that may metastasize to cervical lymph nodes, mediastinum, lungs, liver, bone and adrenal glands; the ↑ production of calcitonin by MCT is responsible for the hypercalcemia, hypertension, paraneoplastic syndromes, eg Cushing syndrome and neuromas; MCTs may produce ACTH-like substance, biogenic amines, CEA, corticotropin-releasing factor, nerve growth factor, prolactin-releasing hormone, prostaglandins, melanin-stimulating hormone, histaminase, β-endorphin, 5-hydroxytryptamine, serotonin, somatostatin and thyroglobulin PATHOLOGY Amyloid is a relatively constant feature, as the presence of neuron-specific enolase; microscopic patterns include carcinoid-like nests, trabecular, glandular and pseudopapillary (with psammoma body formation) patterns with variable inflammation EM Abundant 80-400 nm dense-core neurosecretory granules, fibrillary material corresponding to amyloid, mitochondria and aggregates of polyribosomes TREATMENT Total thyroidectomy PROGNOSIS 70-80% 5-year survival; sporadic MCT has a 50% 10-year mortality (10- and 20-year survival is 63% and 44% respectively (Mayo Clin Proc 1992; 67:934); in contrast, papillary thyroid carcinoma has 95% 5- and 10-year survival

medullary cystic disease A group of AD (and less commonly AR) renal diseases characterized by renal cysts located at the corticomedullary junction in a background of scarring; MCD presents as functional tubular defects and Fanconi syndrome associated with azotemia, uremia and renal failure 3-5 years after presentation CLINICAL Retarded growth, renal osteodystrophy, tapetoretinal degeneration LABORATORY Salt wasting, ↓ Na⁺, acidosis with hyperchloremia

medullary sponge kidney Polycystic kidneys, see there

medulloblastoma A relatively common brain tumor of childhood (representing 20-25% of intracranial tumors in this age group) and adolescence CLINICAL Presents with nausea, vomiting, headache, ataxia, papilledema, nystagmus, irritability, lethargy, cranial nerve palsy, dizziness, altered vision; two year-survival after relapse is 46% in those treated with salvage chemotherapy or irradiation and 0% in untreated patients MOLECULAR PATHOLOGY The most common abnormality is isochromosome 17q [i(17q)]; 50% of cases lack chromosome segment 17p, distal to the p53 gene (Diagn Mol Pathol 1993; 2:22); other abnormalities include the presence of double minutes and amplification of c-*myc*, N-*myc*, and EGF receptor PATHOLOGY The tumors are most common at the midline of the cerebellum and on the roof of the 4th ventricle; the lesion is composed of small, sense poorly differentiated cells that forms pseudorosettes SURVEILLANCE The use of CT and MRI allows detection of tumor recurrences, but this does not improve survival (N Engl J Med 1994; 330:892OA)

medulloepithelioma An undifferentiated primitive neuroepithelial tumor of children that may contain bone, cartilage and skeletal muscle, which is highly malignant and tends to metastasize outside of the cranial cavity; when it occurs in the eye, it arises in the ciliary epithelium, and is known as a diktyoma

Medusa head appearance A fanciful descriptor for anything with undulating or serpentine lines radiating from a central mass HEPATOLOGY The Medusa head appearance refers to the engorged veins that radiate from a recanalized falciparum ligament in portal hypertension most often seen in advanced alcoholic cirrhosis MICROBIOLOGY Medusa head is a fanciful descriptor for the gross appearance of colonies of *Bacillus anthracis* (Anthrax agent) when grown on a 48-hour blood agar plate; the adjective 'Medusa head' is also applied to the light microscopic appearance of the serpentine clusters of the gram-positive *Clostridium sporogenes* PSYCHIATRY Freud viewed Medusa's decapitation as an allegory to the fear of castration, where Medusa's locks represent the female genitalia, especially those of the mother; the allegory is carried further, since Medusa's victims turned to stone, which Freud equated to an erect penis RADIOLOGY The Medusa head or whirlpool sign describes a plain abdominal film finding of multiple aggregates of *Ascaris lumbricoides* worms in the intestinal lumen, admixed with gas, simulating the undulations of hair

Note: In Greek mythology, Medusa was one of the three Gorgon sisters, who were so ugly that one look at them turned mortals into stone; Perseus found a loophole in the Mythical Law *'...don't look a Gorgon in the eye...'*, and beheaded Ms Medusa, taking aim through a mirror

mefloquine The prophylactic agent of choice for prevention of malaria in those traveling to areas with drug-resistant *Plasmodium falciparum*; see Malaria prophylaxis

MEFR Maximum expiratory flow rate

mega-author paper SCIENTIFIC JOURNALISM A recently introduced term for a scientific paper with 50+ persons sharing in the glory of authorship; until 1990, 1-2 papers/year in medicine had 100+ authors; by 1994, nearly 40 papers had 100+ authors; 500+ MAPs first appeared in the late 1980s (Science 1995; 268:25)

megacolon A massively distended colon with decreased large intestinal activity, due to defective innervation, intraluminal overgrowth of microorganisms or of psychogenic origin CONGENITAL MEGACOLON Hirschsprung's disease Congenital aganglionosis A disease affecting 1:5000 live births, with a sibling risk of 1% for girls and 5% for boys; Hirschsprung's disease is ten-fold more common in Down syndrome; other anomalies in Hirschsprung's disease include hydrocephalus, ventricular septal defect, cryptorchism, diverticulosis of the urinary bladder, renal cysts and agenesis, polyposis coli and the Laurence-Moon-Biedl syndrome PATHOLOGY In affected regions the colon is narrowed and the intramural ganglion cells are absent in both the submucosal (Meissner's) and myenteric (Auerbach's) plexi TREATMENT Resection of aganglionic colon ACQUIRED MEGACOLON A condition related to narcotics or disruption of ganglionic innervation, including idiopathic hypomotility, neuropathies (parkinsonism, multiple sclerosis, myotonic dystrophy, diabetic neuropathy, Chagas' disease), smooth muscle disorders (amyloidosis and progressive systemic sclerosis) and metabolic disease (hypokalemia, lead poisoning, porphyria, pheochromocytoma, hypothyroidism) and may be due to intraluminal overgrowth of microorganisms in Crohn's disease and ulcerative colitis (toxic megacolon), in the latter of which there is mucosal necrosis, transmural inflammation and systemic 'toxicity' associated with high fever, tachycardia, leukocytosis and diarrhea; in the psychogenic form of megacolon, no radiological or pathological abnormalities are present and the condition may be related to a 'fixation' in Freud's anal retentive stage of psychosexual development, with constipation of later onset than in Hirschsprung's disease, possibly secondary to abuse of the anthracine group of laxatives

megaesophagus A condition classically occurring as a late complication of Chagas' disease, occurring 2-20 years after infection by *Trypanosoma cruzi*, which evoke dysphagia when 50% of the ganglion cells in the esophagus are destroyed and megaesophagus when 90% are destroyed, possibly the combined result of toxic effects of the parasite and the chronic inflammatory and connective tissue response CLINICAL Dysphagia, aspiration pneumonia, pulmonary abscess and rarely esophageal carcinoma

megajoule The internationally-sanctioned 'derived' unit for measuring energy, work or force, defined as the work produced by the force of one newton acting over a distance of one meter, where 4.2 MJ is equal to 100 kcal

megakaryoblastic leukemia Megakaryocytic leukemia An uncommon clonal proliferation of platelet stem cells arising in severe myelofibrosis CLINICAL Pallor, weakness, excess bleeding, anemia and leukopenia DIAGNOSIS Immunocytologic studies of von Willebrand factors and lineage-specific glycoproteins (GPIb, IIb/IIIa or IIIa); relatively mature, PAS-positive leukemic cells

megaloblast An erythrocyte precursor with an enlarged nucleus that arises in a background of vitamin B_{12} and/or folic acid deficiency; such a deficiency causes an alteration in the nuclear:cytoplasm maturation, where cytoplasmic hemoglobinization proceeds normally, while nuclear maturation slows as the maturation-dependent methyl precursors (usually provided by B_{12} and folic acid) are not present; see Maturational arrest

megaloblastic madness The neurologic manifestations of vitamin B_{12} deficiency, including alteration of personality and dementia, spastic weakness and ataxia, due to demyelination of the lateral and posterior columns of the spinal cord (subacute combined degeneration) Note: Folic acid deficiency, the other cause of megaloblastic anemia is less implicated in neurologic disease

megamitochondria Massively enlarged mitochondria that are typically seen in the liver, classically associated with alcoholic liver disease, which also occur in malnutrition, in skeletal muscle in some myopathies and in tumor cells

Megan's law PUBLIC HEALTH A popular term for legislation aimed at registration and community notification of the movements of convicted perpetrators of sexual assault; the law was named after a 7-year-old girl, Megan Kanka from New Jersey who was sexually assaulted and strangled to death by a sexual assailant who had moved across the street from her family's home, but the community was not informed

megarectum A feces-filled rectum in which electrical activity that would otherwise stimulate the external anal sphincter and puborectalis muscle has ceased, most common in the elderly, resulting in constipation; see Megacolon

megaureter A large ureter of any etiology, divided by some urologists into reflux megaureter, obstructed ureter and the non-reflux or idiopathic megaureter

megavitamin therapy The administration of excess or 'hyper-doses' of water soluble vitamins, either physician-guided, usually to treat diseases of the CNS, or self-prescribed by health-food advocates; water-soluble vitamins include niacin (nicotinic acid) and niacinamide (nicotinamide), B_6 (pyridoxine, pyridoxal, pyridoxamine) and vitamin C are the most common components of megavitamin therapy ADVERSE EFFECTS 1) Thiamin excess is associated with CNS responsiveness (convulsions), Parkinson's disease (antagonizes L-DOPA), sensory neuropathy (destruction of dorsal axon roots) 2) Excess niacin and niacinamide are (vitamin B_3) exacerbates asthma (histamine release), cardiac disease (arrhythmias), GI symptoms, eg nausea, vomiting, diarrhea, anorexia, DM (hyperglycemia), gout ($\uparrow$ uric acid), liver disease (enzyme leakage, hepatocellular injury, portal fibrosis or massive necrosis, cholestatic jaundice), peptic ulcer disease (histamine release and $\uparrow$ acidity), skin disease 3) Excess vitamin B_6 causes paresthesia, headaches, asthenia, irritability 4) Excess vitamin C increases iron absorption, possibly causing iron overload, evoking diarrhea, renal calculus formation and possibly inhibiting the bacteriolytic activity of neutrophils, G6PD deficiency ($\uparrow$ RBC lysis), megaloblastic anemia ($\downarrow$ B_{12} absorption), nephrolithiasis (oxaluria) (**Diagn Clin Testing 1990; 28:27**) Cf Decavitamin

megaYAC A very large YAC (yeast artificial chromosome), see there

megestrol acetate A synthetic progestational agent reported to reduce the incidence of hot flashes by 85% in menopausal ♀ and androgen-deprived ♂ vs 20% in placebo group (**N Engl J Med 1994; 331:347DA**)

meiosis-activating sterol Any of a family of C_{29} sterols (eg FF-MAS, T-MAS) that is present in the gonads of different species, both ♂ (mouse and bull testes) and ♀ (humans, in the preovulatory follicular fluid); MASs induce a resumption of meiosis; the MASs thus far identified are nonspecific across sex and species and this family of compounds may be of use in treating infertility (**Nature 1995; 374:559L**)

FF-MAS meiosis-activatingsterol

MEK MAP (mitogen-activated protein) kinase kinase; see Raf/MEK/MAPK cascade

melancholia *melan*, Greek, black; *chole*, bile PSYCHIATRY Psychotic depression, which is similar or identical to the depression of bipolar disease, which is characterized by severe depression with a loss in interest in all activities early morning awakening with intensification of symptoms, marked $\uparrow$ or $\downarrow$ functionality, anorexia with weight loss, and inappropriate feeling of guilt; melancholia contrasts to the 'normal' melancholy of mourning, Freud views melancholia as an 'impoverishment' of the ego itself, as there is an internal loss (in mourning, the loss is external); because of the internal loss, the melancholic ego appears empty and has a shattered self-esteem, due to reproach and attack from the superego; melancholia is more common in women and is accompanied by helplessness, suicidal ideation or attempts; Cf Melancholy

melancholy PSYCHIATRY A temporary or transient depression that follows an external event, eg mourning the loss of a loved one; Cf Melancholia

melanin The body's natural pigment, which is a complex polymer of oxidized tyrosine synthesized from DOPA and dopaquinone in response to actinic stimulation and bound to a carrier protein by melanocytes (in the skin, mucous membrane, pia arachnoid, retina, inner ear and mesentery); melanin is detected in tissue sections by the Fontana-Masson stain; see Albinism, DOPA, Melanoma

melanocyte-stimulating hormone A group of polypeptide hormones derived from the prepro-opiomelanocorticotropin (POMC) molecule and secreted in the middle lobe of the hypophysis; MSHs include 1) α-MSH, which shares the 13 amino acids of the N-terminal end of ACTH and has some corticotropic activity 2) β-MSH, which shares the 17 amino acids at the C-terminal end of γ-lipotropin and γ-MSH; MSH release is stimulated by MRH (an oxytocin-related releasing hormone) and inhibited by MRIH (a tripeptide release inhibitor), both of which are secreted by the hypothalamus; MSH's function in humans is unknown

melanocytic nevus The most common nevus, which is characterized by melanocytes in the dermis or epidermis; MNs are subdivided into

COMPOUND NEVUS Nevus cells and nests are present at the dermal-epidermal interface (the 'junction') and in the dermis

INTRADERMAL NEVUS Nevus cells and nests are confined to the dermis

JUNCTIONAL NEVUS Nevus cells and nests are confined to the dermal-epidermal interface and

SPINDLE AND EPITHELIOID CELL NEVUS OF SPITZ A compound nevus with elongated and/or epithelioid nevus cells and nests present at the dermal-epidermal interface (the 'junction') and in the dermis; it is histologically bizarre but benign

melanogens A group of melanin-related compounds that are excreted in the urine of patients with well-advanced malignant melanoma

melanoma Malignant melanoma A tumor first described by Hippocrates and identified in mummies from the pre-Colombian Peruvian Incas; melanoma comprises 1-3% of all newly diagnosed malignancies (18 000/year) and causes 6500 deaths/year (US), most in age 30 to 50; the incidence of melanoma is increasing more rapidly (± 7%/year) than any other malignancy (Annual statistics, NCI, Wash DC, GPO, 1988; III.B.12-13, Pub # 88-2789); the incidence in Northern US has increased from $3/10^5$ (1950) to $9/10^5$ (current) affecting the head and neck in men and rising from 4.4 to $11.7/10^5$ in females, predominantly affecting the legs CHILDREN 2% of MMs occur in < age 20; 0.3-0.4% in prepubertal children, and may be aggressive (time to recurrence, 6.2 years vs 8.4 years in adults) and metastasize PATHOLOGY Superficial spreading and nodular types RISK FACTORS Giant congenital melanocytic nevus, dysplastic nevus, xeroderma pigmentosum, immunodeficiency (N Engl J Med 1995; 332:656RV) Note: Ocular melanomas are not thought to increase the risk for cutaneous melanoma; melanoma metastasizes to liver, lung, intestine, pancreas, adrenal, heart, kidney, brain, spleen and thyroid MOLECULAR BIOLOGY Abnormalities of chromosomes 7 (site of the c-erbB oncogene) and 11 (site of H-ras and ets-1 oncogenes) have a less favorable prognosis; loss of chromosome 6 (the responsible gene is as yet not known) is associated with melanoma ; an increased relative risk for melanoma is reported in those with persistent pigment changes in moles, especially in those patients older than age 15, in large or irregularly pigmented lesions or dysplastic moles, familial moles, lentigo maligna and congenital moles; Caucasians are at a twelve-fold greater risk for melanoma than blacks; other risk factors include previous melanoma, melanoma in first-degree relative, immunosuppression and solar sensitivity or increased sun exposure TYPES OF MELANOMA (in order of aggressiveness)

PREMALIGNANT MELANOMA ⅓ of lentigo maligna (aka Hutchinson's freckle) progress to malignant melanoma after 10-15 years

THIN MELANOMA Stage I cutaneous melanoma A lesion measuring less than 1 cm in diameter, with virtually 100% survival Note: The prognosis is less favorable if the lesions is greater than 0.73 mm in thickness (73% five-year survival) or greater than 1.5 mm (63% five-year survival)

LENTIGO MALIGNA comprises 10% of melanomas, and affects those older than age 60, appearing as flat, indolent lesions on the face, arising from a premalignant freckle with greater than 90% 5-year survival, etiologically linked to prolonged actinic exposure

SUPERFICIAL SPREADING MELANOMA 70% of cases, affects those from age 30 to 60, especially female in lower legs or trunk, occurring as a flat lesion (radial growth phase) that may be present for months to years, average 5-year survival 75%, etiologically linked to recreational actinic exposure

NODULAR MELANOMA 15% of cases, is similar clinically to superficial spreading melanoma; 50% average 5-year survival

ACRAL LENTIGINOUS MELANOMA is a rare, flat, palmoplantar or subungual lesion that is more common in non-whites, average 5-year survival less than 50%, unrelated to actinic exposure, but possibly related to ectopic pigmentation

AMELANOTIC MELANOMA is rare, poorly differentiated and occurs in those with a previous pigmented melanoma; since the Fontana-Masson stain is rarely positive in amelanotic melanoma, special studies are necessary, including immunoperoxidase staining with antibodies to the S-100 antigen and ultrastructural examination for presence of premelanosomes

Note: Prolonged survival with metastatic melanoma may occur in rare patients, who have been reported to survive up to 20 years after histologically confirmed metastases (Cancer 1969; 24:574)

melanoma-dysplastic nevus syndrome Dysplastic nevus syndrome, see there

melanoma growth stimulatory activity see MGSA

melanosis coli Brown bowel syndrome A benign condition characterized by segmental or global darkening of the colonic mucosa associated with chronic constipation, due to prolonged abuse of the cascara/sagrada family of laxatives, the anthraquinone content of which is converted to a melanin-like or lipofuscin-like (ceroid) pigment within histiocytic lysosomes and intestinal wall, which is positive by PAS (periodic acid-Schiff), Fontana-Masson, modified acid-fast, and oil red-O stains CLINICAL Chronic abdominal pain, pancreatitis, biliary atresia, cirrhosis, peptic ulcer disease and mucoviscidosis

melanotic whitlow A form of malignant melanoma that presents under or adjacent to the fingernail, which may extensively involve the finger; see Whitlow

MELAS NEUROLOGY Mitochondrial Encephalomyopathy with Lactic Acidosis and Stroke-like episodes, a condition that first affects children and is associated with intermittent vomiting, proximal limb weakness and recurrent cerebral insults resulting in hemiparesis, hemianopia or cortical blindness; MELAS is due to an adenine-to-guanine substitution in a highly conserved portion of gene for tRNALeu(UUR), impairing the termination of mitochondrial transcription (Nature 1991; 351:236); the same mutation has been identified in some cases of IDDM and NIDDM (N Engl J Med 1994; 330:962OA) Cf MERRF

melasma Chloasma, mask of pregnancy A darkening of facial and neck skin with 'blotchy' coalescing hyperpigmented macules, seen in pregnancy, in oral contraceptive use, attributed to both estrogens and progesterones, due to oxidation of tyrosine to melanin, often regressing with delivery; a similar mask may appear in normal men without abnormal hormone levels, as well as those treated with phenytoin

melatonin N-acetyl-5-methoxytryptamine Melanocyte-inhibiting factor A hormone formed by methylation and acetylation of serotonin, which is produced in a diurnal cycle by the pineal gland (a tissue with a verisimilitude to the 'third eye' or photosensory organ of lower vertebrates), in response to light; melatonin is synthesized from L-tryptophan → 5-hydroxytryptophan → serotonin → N-acetyl-serotonin-melatonin; its binding sites are concentrated in the suprachiasmatic nucleus of the hypothalamus (directly connected to the eyes and possibly also the biological clock PHYSIOLOGY Melatonin secretion is intimately linked to the light-dark cycle, and peaks ± midnight and are higher/24 hours in winter than in summer; melatonin secretion decreases with age, measuring 1080 pmol/L (250 pg/ml) age 1-3, 520 pmol/L (120 pg/ml) age 8-15, 86 pmol/L (20 pg/ml) age 50-70; daytime levels in all ages is 17-43 pmol/L (4-10 pg/ml) (**N Engl J Med 1992; 327:1378ED**), melatonin profoundly influences the reproductive system in seasonally breeding animals; melatonin may be markedly increased in patients with hypothalamic or hypogonadotropic hypogonadism, or delayed puberty, and may be decreased with precocious puberty (**N Engl J Med 1992; 327:1356A**) see Circadian rhythm, Jet-lag, Shift work

Melbourne chromosome M1 chromosome A chromosome 17 or 18 with deleted short arms that had been in the past associated with an increased risk for Hodgkin's disease and follicular lymphoma

melena The passage of black tarry stools

melioidosis Pseudoglanders A tropical infection primarily of rats by *Pseudomonas pseudomallei*, an aerobic gram-negative bacillus found in wells and stagnant waters; epizootic infection occurs in sheep, goats and pigs; human infection is water-borne, ie not by direct animal contact disease; the infection is transmitted via the skin or by inhalation and is most common in Southeast Asia; in one report *P pseudomallei* was cultured from 23% of patients with sepsis in northern Thailand; the latency period is long, up to 26 years (!); it is estimated that 225 000 veterans of the Vietnam conflict have subclinical melioidosis CLINICAL Ranges from asymptomatic to fulminant sepsis with multiple abscesses developing in the liver, spleen, and lungs, resolving in the form of granulomas (mortality without antibiotics, 90%, with antibiotics 50%), high fever, chills, tachypnea, myalgia; the chronic form has a lower (10%) mortality and is characterized by an intermittent, TB-like pneumonia, pulmonary cavitation and chronic drainage TREATMENT The third-generation cephalosporin ceftazadime appears to be the most effective agent (**N Engl J Med 1992; 327:1081CPC**) tetracycline, chloramphenicol, and aminoglycosides may be effective

melittin A 26-residue polypeptide containing the toxic and hemolytic components of bee venom

melituria A nonspecific generic term for any sugar spilling into the urine, eg fructose, glucose, maltose and pentose

Meloidae Blister beetle, see there, aka Spanish fly

melorheostosis Lèri's disease An idiopathic defect of long bone growth, which is characterized by cortical thickening of the long (tubular) bones, which when stripped of muscle, simulate a candle with wax dribbled down the side; meloheostosis may be accompanied by pain, limitation of movement, contraction and/or fusion of joint spaces, it generally affects only one limb

MELS catalyst Molecularly engineered layered structure MOLECULAR DESIGN Any of a group of catalysts that consist of crystalline layers of zirconium, oxygen, and phosphorous atoms which surround a 'filling' of organic molecules that react with the substrate molecules that diffuse through the substrate

melting temperature T_m MOLECULAR BIOLOGY The point in a hybridization reaction at which 50% of the nucleotides are annealed (linked to their complement, ie are double-stranded), which is a function of the stringency of the hybridizing conditions

membrane attack complex IMMUNOLOGY A complex of complement proteins that assembles at and later inserts into a cell membrane, causing (complement-mediated) lysis; the membranolytic sequence is initiated when complement C5b interacts with C6 and binds to C7, which becomes hydrophobic and inserts into the membrane; C8 binding causes slow cell lysis, although a fully active MAC, with accompanying rapid cell lysis requires the insertion of C9 polymers

membrane potential NEUROPHYSIOLOGY That electrical potential due to the differences in the concentrations of ions on either side of a semipermeable membrane

membrane protein A membrane-related protein that is either peripheral, ie easily stripped from the membrane and soluble in aqueous solutions or intrinsic, the removal of which requires membrane disruption by a detergent; intrinsic membrane proteins have a hydrophilic extracellular peptide segment with an end amine (NH_2) group, a hydrophobic transmembrane portion and an intracellular hydrophilic segment ending in a carboxyl (COOH) group; see Fluid mosaic model, Receptor; Cf Extracellular matrix

membrane transport PHYSIOLOGY The active translocation of a plethora of proteins from the site of production in the cell to the sites of storage or to the cell membrane for eventual release; such transport requires 1) Translocation-competent membranes, eg endoplasmic reticulum, peroxisomal membrane and the mitochondrial inner membrane, 2) Membrane-targeting signals to direct the molecules, often in the form of an NH_2-terminal oligopeptide with peroxisomal target proteins; the transported protein or presequence, has one of two basic structures: either a completely hydrophilic primary sequence or one which is hydrophilic at both the NH_2 and COOH ends, separated in the middle by an apolar hydrophobic core

meme PSYCHOLOGY A thought construction that endows an individual with certainty about his/her fate (**Nature 1993; 365:290**)

memory COMPUTERS The capacity of an electronic data storage device or component; memory is measured in 1) **RANDOM ACCESS MEMORY** (RAM), ie that which is immediately available to the central processing unit, ranging to 256 Megabytes in the microcomputers of the mid-1990s; RAM information is 'labile' and therefore lost when the device is turned off 2) **READ-ONLY MEMORY** (ROM), which is information that is 'hard-wired' in the form of specifically designed circuitry, comprising a form of permanent software; see Computers IMMUNOLOGY The increased ('positive' memory) or decreased ('negative' memory) immune response to an antigen after previous exposure NEUROPHYSIOLOGY The persistence of the effects of learning and experience on an organism's behavior, which is a process that is currently thought to be due to molecular transformation in the incoming neuronal branches (dendritic trees); each neuron may receive as many as 200 000 signals and since the sensory pattern probably stimulates relatively few sites on any 'tree', the numbers of patterns that may be stored are incalculable **LONG-TERM MEMORY** A type of memory in which the information is stored in a permanent or semipermanent fashion; LTM (aka long-term potentiation) is enhanced when mice are fed immediately after learning a task, a cholecystokinin-induced vagal nerve stimulation, possibly representing an evolutionary advantage by reinforcing actions that result in finding food and which should be retained in the memory; equally important to memory (for which long term potentiation—the repeated use of one of the neuron's synapses correlates with the activity of another—is becoming an accepted model) is the ability to forget, which may occur by long term depression, acting at a voltage-dependent threshold at the neuronal membrane **SHORT-TERM MEMORY** A type of memory characterized by minimal retention of information; STM (aka short-term potentiation) is due to a modulation of synaptic strength by neurotransmitters, eg serotonin, acting by second messenger systems and protein kinases, to increase the duration of an action potential; protein phosphorylation decreases the number of potassium S channels causing a greater influx of calcium ions and increases the release of neurotransmitter

memory cell IMMUNOLOGY A B lymphocyte that has processed specific antigenic information, undergone a maturational se-quence, ie the appropriate rearrangement of the V, D and J segments of the immunoglobulin repertoire, and which stands poised for the appropriate immune reaction; see Antigen-presenting cells, Capping, V(D) J recombination; Cf T cells

MEN Multiple endocrine neoplasia Multiple endocrine adenomatosis A group of autosomal dominant, often overlapping diseases characterized by hyperplasia or neoplasia of more than one endocrine gland, many of which are members of the APUD (see there) system

MEN TYPE 1 (I) A complex characterized by pituitary adenoma or hyperplasia, adrenal adenoma or hyperplasia, parathyroid adenoma or hyperplasia, acromegaly, pancreatic islet cell tumors (insulinoma, carcinoid), Zollinger-Ellison syndrome, WDHA syndrome, increased gastrin secretion, peptic ulcer, Note: Nonhereditary factors may influence the expression of MEN I as the condition may be unequally expressed in identical twins; the defective gene is located on chromosome 11q13

MEN TYPE 2A (II/IIA) A complex characterized by medullary carcinoma of the thyroid (bilateral and present in virtually 100% of cases) producing calcitonin, histaminase, prostaglandins, ACTH, potentially causing Cushing syndrome, pheochromocytoma and parathyroid adenoma or hyperplasia DIAGNOSIS Conventional diagnostic modalities (eg radiologic imaging, histopathology, and laboratory values–↑ plasma calcitonin, ↑ urinary catecholamines, and catabolites,) for MEN-2A identifies relevant tumors, but not carriers MOLECULAR PATHOLOGY The *MEN-2A* gene mutation identified by linkage analysis in the *RET* proto-oncogene, specifically at exon 10 or 11, is highly specific (no false positive) and highly sensitive (no false negative), allowing early diagnosis of MEN-2A (N Engl J Med 1994; 331:828oA) see *RET* gene; the defective gene is located near the centromere of chromosome 10 PROGNOSIS Excellent

MEN TYPE 2B (III/IIB) Mucosal neuroma syndrome A complex characterized by bilateral medullary carcinoma of the thyroid (producing calcitonin, histaminase, prostaglandins, ACTH and potentially, Cushing syndrome), pheochromocytoma, parathyroid adenoma or hyperplasia, mucosal (gut) neurofibromas, associated with thickened lips, submucosal oral nodules, intestinal ganglioneurofibromatosis, infantile intestinal dysfunction and cranial nerve hyperplasia) and connective tissue disease (Marfanoid habitus, scoliosis, kyphosis, pectus excavatum) PROGNOSIS 20% mortality

mendelian principles Mendel's laws CLINICAL GENETICS A group of three laws on which current understanding of the

inheritance of single traits is based

PRINCIPLE OF UNIFORMITY IN F_1 In a mating between a parent with a dominant phenotype (due to homozygosity of an allele) and another parent with a homozygous recessive phenotype controlled by a different allele at the same locus, the progeny will all be genetically heterogenous and express the dominant phenotype

PRINCIPLE OF SEGREGATION A principle that holds that alleles separate or segregate at meiosis and are carried in different gametes

LAW (PRINCIPLE) OF SEGREGATION A principle that holds that allelic pairs·of unlinked loci are independently assortedsorted and transmitted to gametes (International Dictionary of Medicine, J Wiley & Sons, New York, 1986)

meningeal melanocytoma A rare benign neoplasm* of the CNS that produces melanin DIAGOSIS Positive for S100 protein, neuron-specific enolase, melanoma-specific antigen DANGER Can be misdiagnosed as melanoma, on frozen section analysis by the inexperienced surgical pathologist (Arch Pathol Lab Med 1995; 119:542)

*Synonyms include cellular blue nevus (meninges), melanotic meningioma, pigmented meningioma

meningioma A tumor of meningeal cells that is most common in middle-aged ♀ CLINICAL Meningiomas are often asymptomatic masses, attached to the dura usually where the arachnoid villi are prominent; the symptoms are related to tumor growth and compression PATHOLOGY Whorled fibroblast-like cells with psammoma body formation; it is divided into fibroblastic, syncytial or meningothelioma-like, psammomatous, transitional (between fibroblastic and syncytial types) and angioblastic (highly vascular) types; the subtyping of meningiomas is an exercise of no predictive value; aggressive meningiomas are characterized by bone destruction, florid mitotic activity and metastases; the hemangioblastic meningioma and hemangiopericytic meningioma variants are usually more aggressive

meningismus A constellation of clinical signs and symptoms (eg headache, neck stiffness) that that are suggestive of meningitis; it is characterized by meningeal irritation without objective findings; it is relatively more common in young patients with systemic infections, eg the 'flu', pneumonia

meningitis belt A region of sub-Saharan Africa in which cyclical epidemics of group A meningococcal infection occur about every 10 years

meniscus sign Air crescent sign RADIOLOGY A semilunar radiolucency peripheral to a pulmonary mass lesion that was initially described as characteristic for echinococcal infection or hydatid cyst disease; the most common cause in the US for an air meniscus is a fungus 'ball', usually due to *Aspergillus fumigatus*, although the meniscus may be seen in lung abscesses, benign and malignant tumors, hematomas, granulomatous infections and Rasmussen's aneurysm

meniscus sign of Carmen RADIOLOGY A large semi-lunar hypodense zone that may be seen in ulcerated gastric adenocarcinomas, where there is a flattened polypoid mass with a broad central ulceration; the gastric mucosa adjacent to the polyp is smooth, forming the smooth inner margin of the meniscus; see Whalebone in a corset; Cf Quarter moon sign

menopause Climacteric, 'time of life' The cessation of menstrual activity due to failure to form ovarian follicles, an event that occurs between ages 45 and 50, characterized by menstrual irregularity, 'hot flashes', irritability or psychosis, ↑ weight, painful breasts, dyspareunia, ↑ or ↓ libido, osteoporosis, atrophy of female tissues (table, p 540); see Hot flashes Note: Menopause under the age of 40 is considered premature; see Premature ovarian failure

MENOPAUSE

FEMALE STRUCTURES

BREASTS	↓ Size, softer consistency, sagging
PELVIC FLOOR	Uterovaginal prolapse
VAGINA	Bloody discharge, dyspareunia, vaginitis
VULVA	Atrophy, dystrophy, pruritus
BLADDER	Cystourethritis, frequency and/or urgency, stress incontinence
CARDIOVASCULAR	Angina, atherosclerosis, coronary artery disease
ENDOCRINE	Hot flashes
MUCOCUTANEOUS	Atrophy, dryness, or pruritus, facial hirsutism, dry mouth
NEUROLOGIC	Psychologic, sleep disturbances
SKELETON	Osteoporosis, fractures, low back pain
VOCAL CORDS	Deepening of voice

menstrual extraction ALTERNATIVE MEDICINE OBSTETRICS Suction extraction of an early (up to eight weeks of gestation) conceptus, performed by lay persons Equipment A sterile syringe, a rubber stopper, a one-way valve plastic tubing and jars; there are pros and cons to this unconventional, do-it-yourself procedure; while not wholly dissimilar to an abortion performed by a physician, the procedure is not without danger and women so treated may not seek timely medical intervention when needed; since the data is anecdotal, the claims for menstrual extraction's success may be bloated and the real or potential complications (uterine perforation, ectopic pregnancy, gram-negative sepsis and continued pregnancy) may be minimized by its advocates

mental abilities PSYCHOLOGY The parameters measured when evaluating cognitive skills, including spatial orientation, inductive reasoning, verbal meaning, mathematical skills, and word ability

mental decline NEUROLOGY The loss of mental abilities with advancing that is thought to be a normal aging process; the sharpest decline in mental abilities occur in mathematical ability, the least in spatial orientation for men, and in inductive reasoning for women (New York Times April 36, 1994; C1)

mental disorder '...a clinically significant behavioral or psychological syndrome or pattern that occurs in an individual and that is associated with present distress (eg a painful symptom) or disability (ie impairment in one or more important areas of functioning) or with significantly increased risk of suffering death, pain, disability, or an important loss of freedom. In addition, this syndrome or pattern must not be merely an expectable and culturally sanctioned response to a particular event, for example, the death of a loved one' (*Diagnostic and Statistical Manual of Mental Disorders, 4th ed, Washington, DC, American Psychiatric Association, 1994)

mental illness Mental disorder, see there

mental retardation Intellectual activity that is significantly below average and associated with impaired social function; MR is defined as two standard deviations below the mean intelligence quotient (IQ) as measured on a psychomimetic test, eg Stanford-Binet scale IQ less than 85, mild 57-67, moderate 36-56, severe 20-35 and profound < 20; formerly used terms indicating severity of mental retardation, eg 50-70 moron (Queen's English, dullard), 25-49 imbecile, less than 25 idiot, have fallen into disuse given their negative and derogatory nature; MR is classified based on ability to function or to be trained; 90% of MR is mild and 50% of those with IQs of 60-80 can func-

tion adequately in society CLASSIFICATION **IDIOPATHIC MENTAL RETARDATION** MR secondary to sociocultural, emotional and/or environmental deprivation **ORGANIC, STATIC MENTAL RETARDATION** MR that does not progress and which is largely attributable to intrauterine or antepartum events, eg hypoxia, infections, chromosomal defects, teratogens, especially alcohol, maternal malnutrition, neurotoxins and others **ORGANIC, PROGRESSIVE MENTAL RETARDATION** MR in which the infant may be normal at birth, but which undergoes inexhorable deterioration with time, eg metabolic as in the 'inborn errors of metabolism', hormonal imbalances, malnutrition, neuroectodermal dysplasia and slow viral infections STATISTICS 3% of any population is mildly retarded; in 15%, a genetic component is found; other causes include maternal substance abuse and exposure to environmental toxins, perinatal trauma and/or hypoxia (implicated in cerebral palsy), neonatal meningitides, metabolic diseases (eg phenylketonuria) and hyperbilirubinemia Quantification of MR: Stanford-Binet, Wechsler scales (WISC and WPPSI); Cf Psychological testing

mentoplasty The reconstruction of the chin by altering the mandibular contour, often in the context of cosmetic surgery

mentor GRADUATE MEDICAL EDUCATION A senior professional who serves as a role model, and gives attention and feedback to a junior colleague; a mentor is a resource for career advancement, graduate clinical, research, and publishing opportunities, funding, credential support, and obtention of tenure-track positions (CAP Today May 1993)

mentoring Those 'noblesse oblige' activities carried out by a mentor, see there

menu COMPUTERS A display on a computer monitor of the activities that the computer is currently capable of performing

menu-driven COMPUTERS A feature of certain software programs that provides a simplified means ('user-friendly') of manipulating data, which for microcomputers is often used in conjunction with a 'mouse', a specialized input device; in the usual menu-driven program, a handheld mouse is pointed to a location on the computer's monitor, a menu is 'pulled down' and a command is selected; menu-driven architectures contrast with more unwieldy and often arcane commands of non-menu driven programs, and are an integral part of all Macintosh (Apple Computer) microcomputer software and any IBM and 'IBM-clone' program that supports Microsoft Corporation's Windows; see Computers, Icon-driven

MEP Mucoid exopolysaccharide, alginate The outer polysaccharide coat of certain bacteria; the inability to produce an opsonizing anti-MEP antibody in patients with cystic fibrosis is inculpated in the increased morbidity in this disease (Science 1990; 249:537)

meprobamate A potentially addictive therapeutic agent with anticonvulsant, anxiolytic, muscle relaxing, sedative, and tranquilizing properties that blocks spinal interneurons THERAPEUTIC LEVELS 5-20 µg/ml TOXIC LEVELS > 50 µg/ml, which may cause hypotension, depressed brainstem functions, coma and death QUANTIFICATION TLC, GLC, colorimetry

M:E ratio Myeloid:erythroid ratio HEMATOLOGY The ratio of maturing myeloid cells to erythroid cells within the bone marrow is normally 3-4:1; in certain conditions, the M:E ratio may be ↓ (eg hemolytic and megaloblastic anemias), ↑ (eg CML, leukemoid reactions), or may be normal and not reflect any change in the bone marrow, as both the myeloid and erythroid series are equally affected, eg aplastic anemia, myelosclerosis, chloramphenicol toxicity

2-mercaptoethanol A reagent containing a thiol group that breaks disulfide bonds, which is used to differentiate between IgM- and IgG-induced agglutination; IgM antibody agglutination doesn't occur after 2-ME treatment, while IgG agglutination remains intact

6-mercaptopurine A chemotherapeutic agent that is a structural analog (the thiol group replaces the 6-hydroxyl) of hypoxanthine, which is activated by hypoxanthine phosphoribosyl transferase and converted in vivo to thioinosinic acid, a competitive inhibitor in purine synthesis, targeting rapidly dividing cells SIDE EFFECTS Myelosuppression, anorexia, nausea, vomiting, and jaundice appear after several cell cycles

Note: The wide variation in 6-MP bioavailability and suboptimal doses during maintenance regimens are attributable causes for the high incidence of relapse in children with ALL in remission

Mercedes-Benz sign RADIOLOGY The finding of gallstones on plain films of the abdomen; gallstones contain intorgen gas which fills the spaces left by cholesterol crystals and appears as stellate (triradiate) translucent areas, fancifully likened to the emblem of a German motor vehicle (**Am J Radiol 1973; 119:63**)

Merkel cell carcinoma Cutaneous neuroendocrine carcinoma A highly malignant tumor of skin, usually of the head and neck, most commonly affecting elderly patients PATHOLOGY MCC has either a nodular or diffuse lymphoma-like pattern of growth or a carcinomatous pattern with cells in nests cords, and trabeculae PROGNOSIS Poor, 3-year survival 68% ♀, 36% ♂ TREATMENT Wide surgical excision, prophylactic LN dissection dissection, radiotherapy, chemotherapy

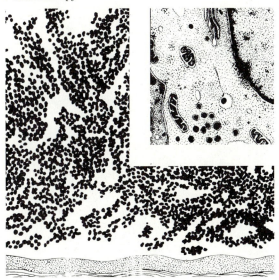

Merkel cell carcinoma

mermaid syndrome Sirenomelia, see there

merozoite A motile, pre- and extra-erythrocytic form of a sporozoan (eg plasmodia), resulting from the asexual division of a schizont during shizogony, which in *Plasmodium* spp occurs in the liver or red cells; merozoites either infect other RBCs or spontaneously develop into sexual forms, ie microgametes (♂) or macrogametes (♀)

***mer*R gene** Mercury-resistant gene The gene that encodes the MerR metalloregulatory DNA-binding protein, which mediates the induction of resistance by bacteria to mercury and other heavy metals

MERRF Myoclonus Epilepsy with Ragged Red Fibers A mitochondrial myopathy clinically characterized by myoclonus, epilepsy and ataxia, maternal inheritance; by light microscopy there are 'ragged red' muscle fibers when stained by the Gomori trichrome EM Increased mitochon-

dria; MERRF is attributed to a point mutation in the gene for tRNALys (**Cell 1990; 61:931**); see Ragged red fibers; Cf MELAS

mesangial ring IMMUNOPATHOLOGY Annular deposition of C3, C4 and properdin in the glomerular mesangium, seen by immunofluorescence in membranoproliferative glomerulonephritis, type II Note: The mesangium is the renal stroma or matrix, in intimate contact with the filtration apparatus (foot processes and fenestrated epithelium) and is the site of immune contact, phagocytosis and immune complex deposition

MESC Ministry of Education, Science and Culture The agency of the Japanese government responsible for administering Japan's universities and funding university research; Cf SERC

mescaline $C_{11}H_{17}NO_3$ A hallucinogen derived from the peyote cactus (genus *Lophophora*); see Hallucinogen

Meselson-Stahl experiment The definitive experiment that proved that DNA replication occurred in a conservative fashion; in the 1950s, it was not known how DNA replicated; three mechanisms had been postulated 1) Conservative replication One daughter DNA double helix was an entirely new duplex and the other was entirely conserved 2) Dispersive replication Both of daughter double helices had dispersed fragments from mother duplex DNA 3) Semiconserved replication Each daughter DNA double helix had a conserved and a newly synthesized chain; Meselson and Stahl grew *Escherichia coli* in a medium containing radioactive and heavy ^{15}N (a 'hot and heavy' experiment) that was incorporated during bacterial growth; based on the flotation levels of the replicated DNA in a cesium chloride gradient, they concluded that DNA was replication in a semiconservative fashion in eukaryotic cells (**Proc Nat Acad Sci 1958; 44:671**)

mesenchymal cystic hamartoma A rare lung lesion associated with hemoptysis, pneumothorax, hemothorax, pleuritic chest pain, dyspnea and combinations thereof PATHOLOGY Primitive mesenchymal mass, associated with papillary excrescences in a subepithelial plexus of small airways lined by unremarkable respiratory epithelium; the masses are solid but undergo cystic degeneration above 1 cm in diameter; the mesenchymal cells are restricted to a subepithelial 'cambium' (see there) layer

mesenchymoma A generic term for any of several benign or malignant tumors that contain two or more mesenchymal elements in addition to fibroblasts; the term carries a specific significance in each affected organ CARTILAGE Mesenchymoma is a synonym for vascular or cartilaginous hamartoma, a benign chest wall tumor of infancy LIVER Hepatic mesenchymoma is a large, aggressive embryonal or 'primitive' sarcoma of the pediatric liver with a median survival of less than one year, characterized by necrosis, hemorrhage and cystic degeneration, histologically characterized by atypical fibroblasts and florid mitotic activity, entrapping hyperplastic bile duct-like structures MUSCLE Ecto-mesenchymoma A variant of embryonal rhabdomyosarcoma in which there is ganglionic differentiation; see Triton tumor

mesenteric artery syndromes A group of clinical complexes pathogenically linked to occlusion of one or more mesenteric arteries, common in older subjects secondary to atherosclerosis, occasionally described in oral contraceptive users, possibly related to vasospasms CLINICAL, EARLY Non-specific GI complaints and abdominal pain LATE Abdominal distension, shock and peritonitis TOO LATE 45% mortality Note: The superior (midgut) mesenteric artery supplies the small intestine below the ligament of Treitz and the large intestine to the transverse colon; the inferior mesenteric artery supplies the remainder of the large intestine and rectum; based on the vascular supply, there is a superior mesenteric artery 'syndrome' and an inferior mesenteric artery 'syndrome'

Mesocestoides A genus of non-human tapeworms that may rarely afflict humans who eat poorly-cooked encysted muscle

mesoderm *mesoderma* [NE3] The primary germ tissue layer that is formed between the ectodermal (outermost) and the endodermal (innermost) layers of the embryo; the mesoderm gives rise to muscle (myotome), cartilage and bone (sclerotome), subcutaneous tissue (dermatome), support tissue and matrix, cardiovascular system, urogenital system (excluding the urinary bladder), serous membranes or mesothelium (pleura, peritoneum and pericardium), spleen, and adrenal glands

mesoderm-inducing factor Any of a group of proteins that are capable of changing the usual fate of an embryonal tissue from its 'programmed' epithelial end-stage to a mesodermal, eg muscle end-stage; MIFs are divided into the fibroblast growth factor family and the transforming growth factor β family which includes XTC-MIF, produced by *Xenopus* XTC cells and activin A, a *Xenopus* analog

mesodermal mixed tumor see Mixed mesodermal tumor

Mesogastropoda An order of snails, one of which, *Oncomelania hupensis*, hosts the parasite, *Schistosoma japonica*

mesoblastic nephroma Fetal hamartoma A rare, usually benign congenital renal neoplasm first seen in early infancy, which consists of an indurated, well-circumscribed yellow-gray leiomyoma-like mass, composed of fascicles of spindled fibroblast-like cells, which may be punctuated by cysts and contain cartilage TREATMENT Early and complete excision appears to prevent the rare cases of recurrence and metastasis

mesonephros EMBRYOLOGY The second stage in renal development (pronephros, mesonephros, metanephros or adult kidney), which first appears after the first month of embryologic development as an oblong mass that codevelops with the embryonal gonads and disappears with fetal maturation; in adults, vestigial residual mesonephric tissue (wolffian duct remnants) are present in adults as efferent ductules in the testis, and tubules of the epiphoron in the female; see Wolffian duct; Cf Müllerian duct

mesothelioma A benign or malignant neoplasm of serosal surfaces, including the pleura, peritoneum, pericardium, tunica vaginalis, and scrotum, occurring in 5-10% of those who were occupationally exposed to asbestos, with a latency period of 20-40 years; the incidence of mesothelioma increases exponentially if the subject is also a smoker; up to 10% of heavily asbestos-exposed workers die of mesothelioma Note: Mesotheliomas may follow radiation exposure and collapse (plombage) therapy for TB PATHOLOGY Fibrous encasement of organs; papillary and tubular clusters of cells with hyperchromatic vesicular nuclei, prominent nucleoli, finely vacuolated cytoplasm, hyaluronic acid stain is positive, mucicarmine stain is negative; mesotheliomas are classified as epithelial, fibrous (sarcomatoid), or mixed, depending on the predominant histological pattern; 50% of mesotheliomas are epithelial and given their tendency to exfoliate, may be diagnosed by a pleural 'wash'; 20% are fibrous with dense sarcoma-like pattern; the remaining 30% have mixed epithelial and fibrous patterns INTERMEDIATE FILAMENTS Epithelial mesotheliomas express both simple epithelial cytokeratins (7, 8, 18, 19), the cytokeratins expressed by pulmonary adenocarcinoma, as well as cytokeratins 4, 6, 14 and 17 and basic polypeptide 5; the fusiform cells of fibrous and biphasic mesotheliomas express vimentin EM Desmosomes, nuclear irregularity, free cell surfaces covered by microvilli, free glycogen bundles of tonofilaments,

dense clusters of perinuclear filaments; see Asbestos

messenger RNA mRNA The 'transcript' of a structural gene that has had the non-polypeptide-encoding intervening sequences of DNA (introns) spliced out, which comprises the template from which a protein is produced; see Exons, Introns, Pre-mRNA

met A gene first identified in murine osteosarcomas that belongs to the protein-tyrosine kinase class of oncogenes, which encodes a receptor for hepatocyte growth factor, transducing signals in a fashion similar to receptor kinases; see Tyrosine kinase receptor

met Metabolic equivalent The resting metabolic rate, which is equivalent to 3.5 ml of O_2 consumption/kg/min; the met unit is of use when planning the rehabilitation of patients who have had a myocardial infarction; Sleeping 1.0 met, desk work 1.5-2.5 met, coitus 2.0-5.0 met, walking 3 mph 3.0 met, medium housework 3.0-5.0 met, bicycling 3.5-15.0 met, shoveling snow 4.0-7.0 met, jogging 6 mph 10.0 met; see Exercise

MET Metabolic equivalents of oxygen consumption A metabolic unit used to quantify the intensity of physical activity, defined as the ratio of the metabolic rate during exercise to the metabolic rate at rest; one MET corresponds to an energy expenditure of approximately 1 kcal/kg of body weight/hour, or an oxygen uptake of 3.5 ml of O_2 consumption/kg/hour (N Engl J Med 1994; 330:1550oA) see Table

---

METABOLIC EQUIVALENTS (MET)

1 Sleeping, reclining, 'couch potatoing'

2 Sitting, eg deskwork, highway driving

3 Very light exertion, eg office work, city driving

4 Light exertion with normal breathing, eg slow walking, mopping, golfing with a cart

5 Moderate exertion with deep breathing, eg normal walking, golfing on foot, calisthenics, raking leaves, downhill skiing, hunting, fishing, slow dancing, interior painting

6 Vigorous exertion with panting; overheating, eg slow jogging, speed-walking, tennis, swimming, cross-country skiing, fast biking, shoveling snow, heavy restaurant work, laying bricks, heavy gardening, heavy household repairs

7 Heavy exertion with gasping and sweating, eg fast jogging, running, continuous racquetball, touch football, moving heavy rocks, mixing cement, using a jackhammer, shoveling deep or heavy snow, hanging drywall

8 Peak or extreme exertion, eg fast running, jogging uphill, aggressive sports with no rest, extreme work, pushing or pulling with one's entire might (strength)

FROM N ENGL J MED 1993; 329:1677

---

meta-analysis An analytical discipline *a sui generis* that critically reviews and combines the results of multiple studies, applying formal statistical methodology to sets of separate but similar experiments in the hope of reaching an unbiased conclusion, thus attempting to improve traditional methods of narrative review by aggregating information and quantifying impact, synthesizing large volumes of relatively recent literature; in being a retrospective discipline, meta-analysis is prone to the biases introduced by the authors of the original works; there is also up to 20% disagreement on what papers are suitable for inclusion (Science 1990; 249:455rv) meta-analysis is the study of studies, which attempt to synthesize the results of many trials; first performed in the early 1980s, the field of meta-analysis is maturing, and the standards for design and formulation of meta-analyses are of necessity as stringent as those for the clinical trials they attempt to study; these standards include criteria for inclusion or exclusion of studies and determination whether the characteristics of the patients, therapies received, and outcomes measured are comparable (**N Engl J Med 1992; 327:273**) as an example of the power of meta-analysis, 13 studies (each with its own intrinsic biases) on the effect of chemotherapy with or without radiotherapy were assembled for subsequent dissection (**ibid; 327:1618₀ₐ**) see Cumulative meta-analysis

R Peto and R Doll, champions of the meta-analytic process was recently awarded the Horten Research Award, an international prize, likened in scope by some to the Nobel prize (**Science 1991; 254:373n**)

metabolic bone disease A generic term for any local or systemic defect in bone absorption or deposition, resulting in an alteration of the parathyroid hormone/calcium-phosphate/vitamin D axis, associated with increased bone fragility; metabolic bone disease occurs in fibrous dysplasia, Langerhans' cell histiocytosis (histiocytosis X), acromegaly, corticosteroid therapy, heparin, hyperparathyroidism, hyperthyroidism, rickets, immobilization syndrome, bone metastases, metabolic disease, congenital (Ehlers-Danlos syndrome, homocystinuria, hypophosphatasia, Marfan syndrome, osteogenesis imperfecta), osteoporosis, Paget's disease of bone (osteitis deformans) DIAGNOSIS 'Workup' of these patients requires a measurement of calcium, phosphate, parathyroid hormone and other hormone levels, bone biopsy, tetracycline test

metabolic equivalents of oxygen consumption see MET

'metabolic' therapy A unconventional and unproven form of cancer therapy that originated with Dr Max Gerson in the 1920s, which consists of bowel enemas to rid the body of unspecified toxins (putatively accumulated by an 'unhealthy' lifestyle, eating unnatural foods, preservatives, pesticides and industrial pollution), as well as dietary modifications, often supplemented with vitamins or minerals; metabolic therapies include the Gerson method, the Kelley treatment and the Manner method; see Tijuana, Unproven methods of cancer therapy

metabolic unit see MET

metachromasia HISTOCHEMISTRY The property of a tissue due to the presence of sulfated polysaccharides, and sialic acid mucins that causes it to stain differently from the surrounding structures, and from the colors used in the dye; the color shift has been attributed to a shift to a shorter wavelength of visible light resulting from the polymerization of the dye(s); metachromatic dyes include methylene and toluidine blues and safranines

metachromatic leukodystrophy NEUROLOGY An AR [MIM 250100] lysosomal storage disease due to arylsulfatase A deficiency, characterized by marked sulfated sphingolipid accumulation and loss of myelin in neural tissue; MD has been loosely subdivided into three clinical forms according to age of onset, with the infantile forms being most severe, the adult form least severe, and the juvenile form intermediate; the alleles designated I and A are defective in ½ of the cases with metachromatic leukodystrophy; early severe forms are homozygous for the I allele (**N Engl J Med 1991; 324:18**) CLINICAL Onset by age 2, death by age 5 with upper and lower motor neuron disease, reduced nerve conduction, spasms, ataxia, oculomotor paralysis, bulbar palsy, blindness, deafness and dementia; see Leukodystrophy

Metagonimus yokogawai A 3 mm in length trematode or fluke found in the Mediterranean rim and in the Far East, which may be ingested with improperly cooked fish, as with sushi

metal fume fever An influenza-like illness due to occupational exposure to copper dust or fumes, usually inhaled by miners as a sulfide ore (CuS, Cu_2S, $CuFeS_2$, Cu_3FS_3) CLINICAL Chills, myalgia, fever, nausea, dry throat and irritation of the upper respiratory tract, cough, weakness, lassitude and a low-grade leukocytosis; most workers develop a tolerance to the fumes that is quickly lost, thus a return to work is accompanied by a resumption of symptoms; MFF may also becaused by zinc ores, or zinc dusts that appear in welding and galvanizing, which may be accompanied by malaise, shivering, fever, myalgia, and destruction of alveolar lining cells; Cf 'Monday death'

metalloelastase Matrix metalloproteinase 12, MMP12

metalloenzyme An enzyme that contains a metal ion, usually held by coordinate-covalent bonds on the amino acid side chains, or bound to a prosthetic group, eg heme; the metal ions have a function similar to coenzymes, imparting activity to the enzyme that is not present in its absence; metalloenzymes include alcohol dehydrogenase (zinc), ascorbic acid oxidase (copper), cytochrome (iron), cytochrome oxidase (copper), glutamate mutase (cobalt), glutathione peroxidase (selenium), urease (nickel), xanthine oxidase (molybdenum)

metallothionein A low molecular weight, cysteine-rich, heavy metal-binding protein present in many tissues from most species; its production is stimulated by heavy metals including cadmium and mercury, and is involved in the transportation, storage and regulation of copper, silver, tin, and zinc; its presence in tissues may have prognostic value, as ↑ metallothionein immunostaining in breast cancer is associated with ↓ rates of disease-free and overall survival, and when present in LN-negative and ER-negative tumors, is reported to be an independent predictor of a poor prognosis (**Virchow Arch A Pathol Anat Histopathol 1993; 423:215**)

metal shadowing Shadow casting RESEARCH A technique used to obtain information about the shape of purified viruses, fibers, enzymes and subcellular particles, where a thin layer of evaporated metal, eg platinum, is sprayed at an angle to the biological specimen; an acid bath then dissolves the biological material leaving the metal replica, which is then examined by transmission electron microscopy

metamyelocyte The M5 stage of a maturing granulocyte, which is morphologically between a myelocyte (M3 or M4) and a polymorphonuclear neutrophil (M6 or M7); metamyelocytes are usually confined to the bone marrow; the nucleus is kidney-shaped, with coarsely clumped chromatin, and no identifiable nucleoli; the cytoplasm is acidophilic and contains both primary and secondary granules

metanephrine Methoxyepinephrine A metabolite of epinephrine that is normally excreted in the urine (normal, adults 0.03-0.69 mmol/mol creatinine), the excretion of which is increased in pheochromocytomas and neuroblastomas, as well as during stress, sepsis, shock or metastatic malignancy

metanephros Definitive kidney The tubular system that is the embryonic precursor of the adult kidney that is caudal to the mesonephos and develops after it; it is formed from mesenchymal tissue arising from fused nephrotomes in the sacral region and from ureteric bud, which is an outgrowth of the mesonephric duct

metaphor SOCIOLOGY '...a high-level similarity between different things or different processes. It can reflect a deep structural resonance or merely a superficial resemblance. Most of our most basic cultural assumptions rest on the foundations of a metaphor. Metaphors are incisive and misleading, valuable and dangerous.' (**Nature 1994; 369:287ᴮᴿ**)

metaphyseal chondrodysplasia-Jansen type A rare form of short-limbed dwarfism associated with asymptomatic but often profound hypercalcemia and hypophosphatemia MOLECULAR PATHOLOGY Mutation in the gene encoding the parathyroid hormone-parathyroid hormone-related peptide receptor (**Science 1995; 268:98**)

metaplasia The conversion of one type of adult tissue and/or cells into another, which most commonly occurs in epithelia Note: As premalignant potential of metaplasia is unknown, there is a tendency among pathologists to consider the term metaplasia as a benign histological transformation of undetermined significance INTESTINAL META-PLASIA occurs in the stomach, and is more common in stomachs that ultimately develop adenocarcinoma PANETH CELL METAPLASIA and ENTEROCHROMAFFIN CELL METAPLASIA occur in the gall bladder, and are associated with adenocarcinoma of same SQUAMOUS METAPLASIA The transformation of a glandular or ciliated epithelium into stratified sqamous epithelium; in SM of the upper respiratory tract, squamous epithelium replaces ciliated columnar epithelium; this event, which is particularly common in smokers, feeds the controversy regarding the possibility that this metaplasia may actually represent a dysplastic process with premalignant potential; squamous metaplasia of the endocervix is not associated with malignancy TUBAL METAPLASIA of the endometrium, ie replacement of the normal endometrial glands with ciliated (fallopian) tubal cells, may occur in endometrial polyps, mild adenomatous hyperplasia and in senile endometrium, but is rarely, and then only coincidentally, associated with malignancy

metarubricyte Orthochromatic normoblast, see there

metastasis The distal spread of a malignant neoplasm, either by penetration of a blood or lymphatic vessel or by spread along a serosal membrane and eventual development into a secondary focus of malignancy; dissemination of lymphoproliferative malignancies is not regarded as metastatic, as they are by nature located within channels that facilitate widespread extension

metastatic sequence A series of steps that occurs in malignant cells, which consists of their extension into surrounding tissues, penetration and subsequent release into body cavities and vessels, with transportation, arrest, implantation, and invasion of secondary sites, accompanied by evasion of local host defense which attempts to inhibit growth of the malignant cells at the new site; in the final step, the malignant cells create a suitable microenvironment; see Invasion

metastatic disease panel LABORATORY MEDICINE A battery of cost-efficient tests that are used to detect, albeit in a crude fashion, the appearance of metastatic malignancy, usually of epithelial origin; the panel measures albumin, alkaline phosphatase, calcium, CEA (carcinoembryonic antigen), lactate dehydrogenase and transaminase (AST/GOT)

metastatic tumor cell A cell that has undergone multiple changes allowing it to invade, disseminate, implant, survive and grow at sites distant from the site of origin

STEPS TO METASTASIS

Degradation of basement membrane collagen, type IV and progression from in situ to invasive carcinoma

1) LOCAL ↓ CA²⁺ causing ↑ adherence of cells to tissues

2) AMEBOID MOVEMENT OF CELLS

3) ↑ PRODUCTION OF CYTOKINES BY MALIGNANT CELLS In the milieu surrounding the cells, there is an ↑ production of 'spreading' factors, eg hyaluronidase, type IV collagenase and autocrine motility factor and a TIMP (Tissue inhibitor of metalloproteinases) mutant which instead of inhibiting basement membrane-degrading enzymes, binds the receptors and leaves them in the 'on' position; *fos* oncogene turns on transin (an enzyme that lyses basement membrane) production

4) CRABTREE EFFECT

Changes in metastatic cells include alterations of the cell surface carbohydrates (↑ sialylation and β1-6-linked branching of complex-type aspariginine-linked oligosaccharides; gp130 (a cell surface glycoprotein that is a major target of ↑ β1-6 branching and the β1-6 expression) is directly related to metastatic potential

metastatic calcification Haphazard calcification occurring in sites other than bone, which may occur in the kidneys, blood vessels (vascular media), lungs, stomach, heart and eyes, usually not associated with malignancy

Note: Given the considerable potential confusion that the adjective 'metastatic' (a term that the noncognoscenti often equate with the secondary spread of malignancy), might engender, the more non-committal, dystrophic calcification may be preferable

meter Metre* The SI unit of length, which is defined as 1 650 763.73 wavelengths of the orange emission band of krypton (the transition between levels $2p_{10}$ and $5d_5$ of ^{86}-Kr (US 39.37 inches)

*British and remainder of civilized world; in the US, meter

metered-dose inhaler CLINICAL PHARMACOLOGY A device used to delivery a specified number (100-300) of doses of a therapeutic inhalant, eg β-agonist for asthma; delivery of the correct amount of medication cannot be assumed after a specified number of inhalations even though the cannister is not empty, and in absence of an adequate system for detecting product consumption, the patient is advised to tally the 'blasts' (JAMA 1993; 269:1506ʟ)

metformin ENDOCRINOLOGY An antidiabetic agent (Glucophage™, Bristol-Myers Squibb) of the biguanide class of drugs used in NIDDM, either alone or in combination with sulfonurea; metformin acts to sensitize certain cells

$$\begin{array}{cc} HN & NH \\ \| & \| \end{array}$$
$$[CH_3]_2NCNHCNH_2$$

to the effects of insulin, lowering both glucose and insulin levels; and also ↓ triglyceride and in some subjects, is an appetite suppressant

methadone A synthetic, relatively long-acting oral opiate (figure) that was developed in Germany in World War II, which is used to detoxify heroin addicts; the L-isomeric form acts by occupying the opiate receptor, allowing methadone-maintained addicts to function in society; rehabilitation is rarely successful, and methadone maintenance is a lifetime proposition, implying a persistent opiate receptor disorder; the clinical features of methadone overdose are similar to that of opiates, causing respiratory depression, stupor, coma ANALYSIS Spectrophotometry, gas chromatography, enzyme-linked immunoassay or radioimmunoassay; Cf Heroin

methadone

methamphetamine SUBSTANCE ABUSE A sympathomimetic amine that is a methylated derivative of amphetamine, which is more potent in its CNS stimulatory effect, and by extension more likely to be abused; methamphetamine has enjoyed intermittent popularity as a recreational drug and its abuse has increased exponentially in the past few years, rising to epidemic proportions ABUSER PROFILE Caucasian, age 20-35, high school education Form of abuse IV 62%, 'snorting' 18%, oral 13% and smoking 7% FETAL EFFECTS Prematurity, low birthweight (JAMA 1991;

265:1968); see Adam, Designer drugs, Eve, 'Ice'

methanol A highly toxic polar alcohol used as an industrial solvent (it is miscible with water, ethanol, ether, and petroleum derivatives, eg gasoline), in canned fuel and in antifreeze, where it may be abused as an inebrient by indigent alcoholics; methanol is metabolized to formaldehyde and formate causing significant metabolic acidosis and damage to the optical nerve and blindness; toxic range 60-250 ml, although as little as 15 ml has caused death TREATMENT Overload the subject with ethanol*, as ethanol competes with methanol for sites on alcohol dehydrogenase, thereby reducing methanol metabolites and toxic effects

*'Oh death! where is thy sting...'-W Shakespeare

methaqualone Quaalude, 'ludes' An addictive hypnotic-sedative of the quinazolone group, which is a 'schedule II' controlled drug that has similar effects to barbiturates which has ben linked to physical or psychological dependence CLINICAL, OVERDOSE Delirium, headache, nausea, pyramidal signs, convulsions, renal and cardiac failure and rarely, aplastic anemia TREATMENT Hemoperfusion to eliminate toxic overload DIAGNOSIS Spectrophotometry, GLC

methenamine Hexamethylenetetramine A disinfectant that at one time had currency as a per os urinary tract antiseptic; in acid urine, methenamine decomposes, generating formaldehyde that is toxic to urinary tract bacteria

methicillin-aminoglycoside resistant *Staphylococcus aureus* An organism with multiple antibiotic resistances, including aminoglycosides, chloramphenicol, clindamycin, erythromycin, rifampin, tetracycline, streptomycin, cephalosporin; in addition, some strains of MARSA have decreased sensitivity to certain antiseptics TREATMENT Vancomycin (N Engl J Med 1991; 324:601IV); see R factor

methionine malabsorption syndrome An AR [MIM 250900] disease characterized by albinism, hyperpnea, convulsions and mental retardation, the synonym 'oasthouse disease', derives from the hops or burnt sugar-like odor of the urine after methionine loading, which is accompanied by increased α-hydroxybutyric acid and causes the smell

Note: An oasthouse is a building for drying hops, used for making beer, hence the alternative terms oasthouse urine disease, oasthouse syndrome

method evaluation CLINICAL CHEMISTRY An early phase of testing in which a series of experiments are performed to estimate the magnitude of analytical error; a manufacturer determines and establishes the performance parameters of a new method during the development phase; the end-user then verifies or validates the performance claims of the manufacturer; method evaluation requires that all aspects of performance be evaluated, including carryover, comparison with reference ('gold standard') imprecision, inaccuracy, interference, linearity, reference range, sensitivity, stability, and other operation properties (Arch Pathol Lab Med 1992; 116:714OA) see Partitioning factor, Reference values

method of least squares STATISTICS A method for drawing a straight line from a set of data points, such that the sum of the squares of the standard deviation from the mean of each point is minimized

methotrexate ONCOLOGY A widely used anti-metabolic chemotherapeutic agent, which may be used alone to cure choriocarcinoma, and in combination with other agents for lymphoproliferative malignancy (acute lymphocytic and non-lymphocytic leukemias, as well as Hodgkin's, non-Hodgkin's, Burkitt's and histiocytic lymphomas, mycosis fungoides, myeloma), head and neck, ovarian and small-

methotrexate

cell carcinomas, osteosarcoma, medulloblastoma Note: Nonmalignant conditions, eg recalcitrant psoriasis, rheumatoid arthritis; in combination with cyclosporine and prednisone, methotrexate (Mtx) reduces the incidence of acute GVH disease from 23% to 9%, without affecting the disease-free survival (N Engl J Med 1993; 329:1225OA); Mtx is a potent folic acid antagonist (anti-folate), competing with dihydrofolate (the natural substrate), for binding sites on dihydrofolate reductase (DHFR), blocking production of tetrahydrofolate (folate is the vitamin co-factor in methyl group transport for purine and thymidilic acid synthesis and DNA synthesis); see Leucovorin rescue and MDR gene STRUCTURE Pteridine ring, para-aminobenzoic acid and a glutamyl residue; it is metabolized to polyglutamate and derivatives Note: Tumor cells may become resistant to Mtx by increasing DFHR synthesis and by decreasing the tumor cell affinity for DHR or Mtx, or by decreasing Mtx transport into cells, polyglutamination and thymidylate synthetase activity; Mtx may interfere with aspirin (by renal tubule competition), sulfonamides, phenytoin, ethanol, anticoagulants, Amphotericin B TOXICITY Nausea, vomiting, anorexia, stomatitis, CNS changes, hypersensitivity, hepatocellular damage, ocular irritation, dose-limiting myelotoxicity may appear 4-7 days after beginning therapy, nephrotoxicity (crystallization within renal tubules) LABORATORY Transient elevation of 'liver function tests' ANALYSIS Mtx is measured by enzyme-linked immunoassay (EMIT), RIA, and HPLC

methoxamine CARDIOLOGY A vasopressor used for hypotension and for paroxysmal atrial tachycardia; it improves performance in patients with chronic left ventricular dysfunction, which may be linked to exercise-induced vasodilation of airway vessels (N Engl J Med 1993; 329:1225OA)

methylation The addition of a methyl group to any molecule; this simple biochemical reaction has acquired a special significance in molecular biology, where it usually refers to the addition of a methyl group to a cytosine residue on double-stranded DNA; methylated genes are inactive and therefore the pattern of methylation is critical in gene expression, eg in the program of B cell maturation; these patterns may be passed from one generation to the next, in a process known as imprinting; genes may be demethylated or methylated de novo in accordance with the cell and/or tissue function or during normal development (Nature 1991; 351:239) Note: Phosphorylation is another form of semi-permanent gene control; see Imprinting, Phosphorylation

methyl bromide CLINICAL TOXICOLOGY A highly toxic insecticide and rodenticide, delivered as a volatile fumigant that is three times more dense than air and absorbed through the skin, producing narcosis, pulmonary edema, renal tubule damage, jacksonian type of convulsions, CNS depression, and peripheral neuropathy; permanent neurological sequelae may follow prolonged exposure

methylene blue A thiazine dye that is used as an indicator for the oxidation-reduction reaction, where an oxidized form is blue and the reduced form is in clinical medicine to reduce methemoglobin and used as a urinary tract antiseptic, in hematology for the 'Romanowsky' stains, eg Wright-Giemsa and in histopathology for delineating connective tissue; Cf Toluidine blue, Trypan blue

3,4-methylenedioxymethamphetamine MDMA, see Ecstasy

5,10-methylenetetrahydrofolate reductase An enzyme [EC 1.7.99.5*] that catalyzes FAD-linked reduction of methylenetetrahydrofolate to methyltetrahydrofolate, providing a methyl group for methylation of homocysteine
*Formerly, EC 1.1.1.68 and 1.1.99.15, per recommendations, Nomenclature Committee, International Union of Biochemistry and Molecular Biology

5,10-methylenetetrahydrofolate reductase (MTHFR) deficiency An AR [MIM 236250] condition that is more common in females, characterized by developmental delay, motor, gait and typical EEG changes and early death LABORATORY ↑ Homocysteine in serum and urine, ↓ methionine

methyl green pyronine stain A variant of the Pappenheim stain that is used to identify RNA present in nucleoli, Nissl bodies and ribosomes

methylphenidate CLINICAL PHARMACOLOGY An agent used to control the attention deficit-hyperactivity disorder (ADHD) and hyperactive mentally retarded children Note: The use of this agent in mentally retarded adults is thought by some workers to be based on unreliable data that was generated by a researcher who is alleged to have committed research fraud; the psychiatry community supports the data generated in pediatric use of methylphenidate for ADHD

methyl-tert-butyl ether see MTBE

'me too' drug see under Me

metoprolol succinate A β_1-selective (cardioselective) adrenoreceptor blocking agent used to treat hypertension and angina

metrizamide RADIOLOGY A water-soluble, iodinated radiopaque contrast medium used for myelography and for enhancing computed tomographic images

metrizoate RADIOLOGY A water-soluble, triiodobenzene-based radiographic contrast medium used for angiography and urography

Metropolitan Life tables A correlative table generated by the Metropolitan Life Insurance Company that compares the weight of subjects to minimums of mortality in actuarial data, ie an obesity/mortality ratio (Stat Bull Metrop Life Insur Co 1983; 64:2-9); Cf Obesity

Metsovo lung Mesothelioma and/or pleural calcification affecting the lungs of inhabitants of a region of Northwest Greece, due to a tremolite type of asbestos contained in the whitewash used on the houses

metyrapone 2-methyl-1,2,-di-3-pyridyl-1-propanone A diagnostic tool for evaluating the hypothalamus-pituitary-adrenal 'axis', in particular abnormalities in pituitary activity; metyrapone inhibits 11-β-hydroxylase, the final enzyme in cortisol synthesis; the inhibition results in accumulation of 11-deoxycortisol in the adrenal cortex, resulting in decreased negative feedback of ACTH synthesis by the pituitary, therefore increased ACTH and increased 11-deoxycortisol, and its metabolite, tetrahydrocortisol, which can be measured in the urine as Porter-Silber compounds

mevalonate 3-methyl-3,5-dihydroxy valerate A molecular precursor of many compounds, including cholesterol and coenzyme Q and carotenoids; mevalonic aciduria is a disease of infant onset characterized by failure to thrive, retarded development, hepatosplenomegaly, anemia, central cataracts, dysmorphias, marked increase in urinary cholesterol and nonsterol isoprene precursor molecules including mevalonic acid

Mexico City policy POPULATION CONTROL A 'white paper' that was released by the Reagan Administration in 1984 at the UN-sponsored International Conference on Population in Mexico City, which stated among other things, '...*the relationship between population growth and economic development is not a negative one*', a philosophy that is so contrary to conventional wisdom and logic that it has been termed 'voodoo demographics' (Science 1991; 252:1247n&v) see Amsterdam strategy, Gag rule, ZPG
Note: The Mexico City policy typified a conservative trend in US (foreign and domestic) policy-making that holds that population growth need not be controlled, a position that explains the US Supreme Court's 'Webster' decision, see there

MFD 1) Minimum featal dose 2) Monostotic fibrous dysplasia, see Fibrous dysplasia

MFO Mixed function oxidase, see there

MG see Myasthenia Gravis

m7GpppX MOLECULAR BIOLOGY A 5' cap structure located on eukaryotic cellular RNA that facilitates binding to ribosomes and which is required for efficient translation; see eIF-4F

MGSA/gro Melanoma growth-stimulatory activity/growth-regulated gene A gene that encodes a protein produced in copious amounts in a melanoma as well as lung, kidney, prostate and skin cancer cell lines, which evokes autostimulation of its own production, inflammatory response, both inhibition and stimulation of cell division; MGSA/gro is a member of the larger family of growth regulators

MGUS Monoclonal gammopathy of unknown significance, see there

MHC Major histocompatibility complex A relatively small region of the genome that is highly conserved in vertebrate evolution, and encodes three classes of polymorphic molecules of the immunologic interest, aka the immune recognition unit; the MHC is located on the short arm of chromosome 6 in man and on chromosome 17 in the mouse, and was first identified in Japanese 'waltzing' mice; the products of the MHC gene complex are membrane-bound receptors for antigens and peptides, which when bound, are displayed to T lymphocytes; if the bound peptides are recognized by the T lymphocytes, an immune response is initiated against those peptides

CLASS I MHC products are transplantation antigens, the heavy chain of which is encoded by the MHC genes; the heavy chain is linked to a β_2-microglobulin light chain (see figure) and together class I antigens restrict the response of T lymphocytes to antigens by requiring that foreign antigens be formally presented to the immune system by a self/native antigen-presenting cell; class I MHC includes the proteins encoded by HLA-A, -B, -C
Note: Chromosome 'walking' with overlapping cosmids has revealed a 435-kilobase segment of DNA that contains the genes for tumor necrosis factors (TNF-α and TNF-β) and HLA-B associated transcripts, abbreviated as BATs centromeric to the HLA-B region

CLASS II MHC genes span an 1100-kilobase region of chromosome 6 and encode the α and β chains (see figure) of a group of membrane glycoproteins (HLA-DP, -DQ, -DR); class II antigens are expressed on the surface of macrophages and B cells that bind antigenic fragments of foreign and self proteins, presenting the bound fragments to T cells; class II is a complex heterodimer with a 33-kD α and 27–30-kD β chain; polymorphism in these genes determines the specificity of an immune response and is related to development of autoimmunity; certain amino acid residues are associated with ↑ susceptibility to IDDM, rheumatoid arthritis, and pemphigus vulgaris

CLASS III MHC region is located between class I and II and the genes include those that encode complement proteins C2, C4 and factor B (alternate pathway of complement activation) as well as the gene encoding 21-hydrolase; see HLA

*Also 1) Mental health course (British) 2) Moisture holding capacity 3) Multiphasic health checkup 4) Myosin heavy chain

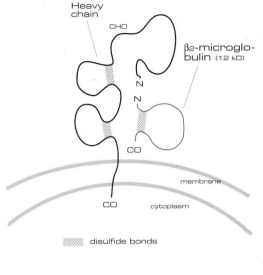

Heavy chain

CHO

β2-microglo-bulin (12 kD)

N

N

CO

membrane

CO   cytoplasm

▨▨ disulfide bonds

MHC I

MHC II

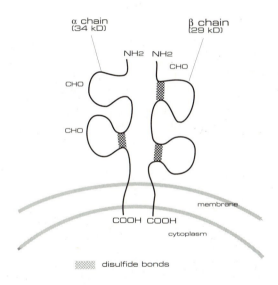

α chain (34 kD)

β chain (29 kD)

NH2 NH2

CHO

CHO

CHO

CHO

membrane

COOH COOH

cytoplasm

▨▨ disulfide bonds

MHC restriction The ability of T cells to recognize antigens when they are associated with the organism's own major histocompatibility complex (MHC) haplotype, providing a dual recognition system critical to T-cell function; this selective process occurs in the thymus before a T lymphocyte becomes a functional antigen-specific cell in the peripheral immune system; the selection process operates on the α/β heterodimer of the T-cell receptor assuring that the T cells will react with the product of the MHC and not with self antigens, ie the process is 'self-tolerant'; see Antigen-presenting cell

MHz Megaherz COMPUTERS A measurement of clock speed for microcomputers, which is related to the efficiency of the circuit design and the microprocessor; the earliest microcomputers introduced in the 1970s, using the venerated Intel 8088 chip, had speeds of 4.77 MHz or less; the current generation of microcomputers from Apple and IBM have speeds up to 100 MHz and because of the increased 'width' of the information pathway and more advanced chips, carry far more information Note: MIPS (milion instructions per minute) and MHz do not translate well, as the systems' architecture and pathways of information flow differ substantially; Cf MIPS

MI Myocardial infarction, see there also 1) Medical inspection 2) Melanophore index 3) Menstrual induction 4) Mental illness 5) Meso-inositol (now known as myo-inositol) 6) Metabolic index 7) Migration inhibition 8) Mitotic index 9) Mitral (valve) insufficiency 10) Motility index (GI tract)

Also 1) Mechanical impedance 2) Meconium ileus 3) Medical Illustrator 4) Medical improvement 5) (Mercaptoethyl)trimethylammonium iodide 6) Mercaptoimidazole 7) Mesioincisal (dentistry) 8) Metastases, inferior (below the head and neck) 9) Methylindole 10) Migration index 11) Mitral (valve) incompetence 12) Morphologic index

MIC Minimum inhibitory concentration, see there

MIC2p[30-32] antigen A 30–32-kD cell surface glycoprotein of unknown function that is increased in the Ewing family of tumors (osseous Ewing sarcoma, atypical Ewing sarcoma, and peripheral primitive neuroendocrine tumors); it is encoded by *MIC2*, a gene located in the homologous (pseudoautosomal) portion of chromosomes X and Y (N Engl J Med 1994; 331:294oA)

mice see Joint mice

micelle An organized component of colloidal suspensions, consisting of spherical or laminar aggregates of polar surface-active molecules (soaps), in which the hydrophilic portion of the molecule interacts with the other members of the aqueous solution, ie are oriented 'outside' in water, and the hydrophobic ends huddle together within the micelle; micelles of the small intestine are composed of bile salts with fatty acids and monoglycerides are released by pancreatic lipase; Cf ISCOMS

Michaelis-Menten equation An equation for evaluating the kinetics in an enzymatic system, which assumes that a rapid equilibrium is reached among the enzyme, its substrate, and the enzyme-substrate complex, and that the initial velocity of the reaction is proportional to the concentration of the enzyme-substrate complex; the equation is defined as $v = V[S]/Km + [S]$, or, as below, as an inverse relation, where v is the initial velocity of the reaction, V the maximum (or limiting) velocity, [S] is the substrate concentration and Km is Michaelis' constant

Michelin tire baby An extremely rare cutaneous malformation, characterized by generalized folding of redundant skin, fancifully likened to the Michelin tire company's mascot; four cases of this condition have been reported; one had no histologic defects; another had hamartomatous smooth muscle; the two remaining cases had diffuse or focal lipomatous hypertrophy, one of whom had microcephaly, mental retardation, hemiparesis and a balanced translocation on chromosome 11

Mickey Finn A mixture of chloral hydrate in whiskey; chloral hydrate causes hypotension, pinpoint pupils, cardiac arrhythmia and in high doses, may evoke gastric irritability with perforation and hepatotoxicity and nephrotoxicity Note: Chlorals are the oldest class of hypnotics; trichlorethanol is the first metabolite of chloral and is responsible for its hypnotic effect

Mickey Finn was barkeeper who operated the Lone Star Saloon and Palm Garden on Chicago's Whiskey Row in the 1890s; his concoction was used to incapacitate any lone clients who would come into his establishment; once they fell into a deep sleep, Finn would relieve them of excess material goods; Mickey Finns were used in THE MALTESE FALCON to produce the alleged 'knock-out drop' effect on Humphrey Bogart, an effect not seen on volunteers (Clin Pharm and Therap 1972; 13:50)

Mickey Mouse appearance A descriptor for the facial appearance of sportsmen wearing combined intraoral and extraoral mouthguards designed to prevent dental trauma, especially in contact sports such as ice hockey and football; the extraoral guards were rejected by the players for esthetic reasons and thus never popularized as they made the players 'look like Mickey Mouse'

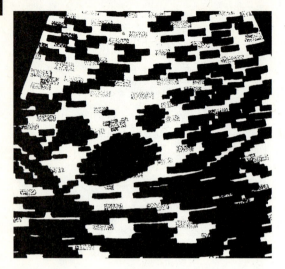

Mickey Mouse appearance

Mickey Mouse ears A fanciful descriptor for the appearance of the large and protruding external ears typical of Cockayne syndrome, an autosomal recessive progeria-like disease, which is accompanied by enlarged, cold and cyanotic hands and feet, dwarfism, microcephaly, mental retardation, photosensitivity, skin atrophy and scarring, retinitis pigmentosa and deafness

Mickey Mouse figure see Mariner's wheel appearance

'Mickey Mouse' medicine A derogatory reference to non-patient-oriented duties that impact on physicians' time, eg paperwork, bureaucracies and committees, all of which are necessary to ensure quality of health care, but which do not utilize the skills for which physicians are trained; 'Mickey Mouse' physicians, an extension of the above, are those who dedicate themselves to 'Mickey Mouse medicine', ie 'medicrats' or practitioners of medical paperwork; 'Mickey Mouse' in this context is an American colloquial synonym for *reductio ad absurdum*, ie anything that is not to be taken seriously, named after the Walt Disney cartoon character

Mickey Mouse sign RADIOLOGY Bilateral hydronephrosis in children seen on a plain film and made more evident by excretory urography, where the 'ears' correspond to the massively dilated ureters and the face to the bladder itself (**JG Rabinowitz, Pediatric Radiology, JB Lippincott 1978**) ULTRASOUND A normal landmark when evaluating the size of the common bile duct; in a transverse plane, the bile duct and hepatic artery correspond to the left and right ears, respectively and the portal vein to the head (**Semin Ultrasound 1980; 1:102**)

Note: This landmark more closely simulates 'Mickey Mouse ears', a hat worn by members of the Mickey Mouse Club, a US television program in the 1950s

miconazole A broad-spectrum antibiotic used primarily as an antifungal, topically for cutaneous candidiasis, IV for systemic mycosis (candida, coccidioides and paracoccidioides) or intrathecally for cryptococcal meningitis SIDE EFFECTS Local pruritus when topical, nausea, vomiting and fever when systemic

microabscess A nonspecific term for a focal aggregate of neutrophils that may appear in a variety of conditions, eg skin conditions, eg mycosis fungoides (Pautrier's microabscess), psoriasis (Munro's microabscess) and bullous pemphigoid (papillary microabscess) or may appear in other sites, eg in the perivascular tissues of the lung in Wegener's disease

microaerophile MICROBIOLOGY A bacterium requiring O_2 only as a terminal electron acceptor; microaerophiles grow poorly at ambient (21%) O_2 levels and therefore do not grow on the surface of culture plates; they also grow poorly in anaerobic conditions; as an example *Campylobacter jejuni* grows optimally at 5% O_2 (10% CO_2 and 85% N_2) see Anaerobes

microaggregate TRANSFUSION MEDICINE A clump of leukocytes, platelets, and fibrin that may cause intravascular sludging and by extension, pulmonary insufficiency, most of which may be removed by 170 µm in diameter micropore filters

microaggregate filter TRANSFUSION MEDICINE Micropore filter A second-generation blood component filter that has a micropore screen (pore size 20-40 µm) which removes 75-90% of leukocytes; MFs are used for transfusing packed red cells (**Arch Pathol Lab Med 1994; 118:392OA**) see Blood filters, Leukocyte reduction

microalbuminuria The excretion of 30-300 mg albumin/day; ↑ albumin excretion is predictive of the hemodynamic and morphologic changes of diabetic nephropathy (**N Eng J Med 1995; 332:1210RV**) the risk of microalbuminuria in IDDM ↑ abruptly when the Hb_{A1} value rises > 10% (**N Eng J Med 1995; 332:1251OA**) see Diabetic nephropathy

microanalysis see Micro methodology

microaneurysm A teensy-weensy aneurysmal dilatation of small arteries, arterioles, or capillaries that is 'classically' seen in the retina of those with long-standing DM, which may be associated with edema and hemorrhage; microaneurysms also occur in other sites in diabetics, and are well-described in other conditions, eg thrombotic thrombocytopenic purpura; see Cherry-red spot

microangiopathy A generic term for any defect of very small blood vessels, usually capillaries, most common in DM; despite thickening of the vascular basement membranes, by a hyaline-like material which corresponds to advanced glycosylation end products (AGEs), the vessels are 'leaky' and allow transvascular passage of plasma proteins; AGEs or advanced diabetic microangiopathy-induced ischemia directly impacts on the retina, the kidney and the peripheral nerves

microcapsule CLINICAL THERAPEUTICS A biohybrid device in which cells of interest (pancreatic islet cells) are encapsulated in alginate poly-L-lysine or in the case of xenografts, simple in alginate; microcapsules circumvent the host's immune system and are the most promising of the biohybrid 'organs' devised to date, as they are easily implanted (requiring simple injection by a 'standard issue' syringe), biocompatible and achieve excellent glucose control (**Science & Medicine July/August 1995, p16**) see Biohybrid organ; Cf Micro-spherule MICROBIOLOGY An invisible virtual layer surrounding some bacteria that contains antigens

microcell hybridization technique A method for introducing a limited number of chromosomes in a hybridization (**Nature 1991; 349:340; Science 1990; 247:568, 707**)

microcephaly Any brain or head that is three or more standard deviations below the mean for the person's age, sex, height, weight and race; microcephaly is associated with many eponymic (Cockayne, Miller-Dieker, Smith-Lemli-Opitz, Rothmund-Thomson, and Wolf-Hirschhorn) syndromes, chromosomal defects (cat-cry or 5p- and trisomy 13 syndromes), in utero infection (CMV, rubella, toxoplasmosis), toxic exposure (fetal alcohol and fetal hydantoin syndromes), radiation or trauma

microchimerism Migration of cells from an allograft into recipient tissue; systemic microchimerism occurs after allotransplantation and appears to be the mechanism by which organ (eg liver, kidney) transplantation is capable of correcting pancellular enzyme deficiencies, eg α-1,4-glucan:α-1,4-glucan 6-glucosyltransferase, absent in type IV glycogen storage disease, or β-glucocerebrosidase, absent in type 1 Gaucher's disease; cell migration after liver transplantation explains why patients with lysosomal storage diseases, Gaucher's disease, Niemann-Pick disease, sea-blue histiocytosis syndrome, and Wolman's disease receive more benefit from liver replacement than simply improved hepatic function (N Engl J Med 1993; 328:745OA)

microcirculation A generic term referring to the circulation of blood at the terminal arterioles, capillaries, and small venules

'microcolon' PEDIATRIC RADIOLOGY The unused portion of the large intestine below a site of small or large intestinal atresia, which demonstrates a pencil-thin column of radiological contrast

microcomputer A computer with the arithmetic logic unit and control unit contained in an integrated circuit known as a microprocessor; the two predominant microcomputer 'environments' in the mid-1990s are 1) IBM-PC and IBM-PC 'clone' family of personal computers that operate with MS/DOS (Microsoft disk operating system), using CISC (complex instruction set computers) architectures, either with a) Intel's microprocessing chips (8088, 80286, 80386, 80486, or b) the Pentium, each with increasing power and speed (ranging from 4.77 Hz to 100 MHz) or 2) the MacIntosh family of computers, based on Motorola's 68000 series of microprocessor with clock speeds of 8 to 80 MHz; in late 1994, Apple and IBM announced plans to merge environments by 1997, a process that was begun with their mutual embracing of RISC (reduced instruction set computers)-type microprocessors; the first microcomputers introduced in the mid-1970s had 16 kilobytes of random access memory (RAM) with little permanent storage capacity, usually on floppy diskettes, and were regarded as toys by computing professionals; the microcomputers available in the mid-1990s have 4 to 256 megabytes of RAM, with larger RAM being required for three-dimensional manipulation of graphics, eg in space-filling models of molecules; the data is stored either on magnetic media where practical ceilings occur at around 2 gigabytes and optical storage devices which have capacities that start in the gigabyte range

Note: The term microcomputer is evolving toward obsolescence, as the memory and speeds of the silicon chips from Hitachi, Intel and Motorola have put minicomputer-, and more recently mainframe-sized computing power on desktop machines; see Computers, Mainframe computer

microconidia The reproductive form of certain fungi

microdeletion syndrome CLINICAL GENETICS A generic term for technique used to measure the DNA

microdensitometry IMAGE ANALYSIS A technique used to measure the DNA content of a population of cells by use of a microdensitometer, yielding results that are similar to those provided by flow cytometry for DNA index, S-phase fraction value, and G_0G_1 population (Anal Quan Cytol Histol 1994; 16:25)

microfibrillar fibers A group of discrete pleomorphic fibers, largely consisting of fibrillin, which is more widely distributed than elastin; by electron microscopy, MFF are linear bundles containing many microfibrils (10^{-12}m in diameter tubular threads) forming long rods, sheets and meshwork, serving as scaffolding for elastin and found in the mature tunica media of the aorta and other blood vessels, dermal-epidermal interface of the reticular dermis, ciliary zonules of the ocular lens, dura mater, cartilage, kidney, muscle, perichondrium, periosteum, pleura, skin and tendon

microfilaments A group of elongated, 5-7 nm in diameter, cytoplasmic fibers composed predominantly of actin, which form a cytoskeletal latticework; Cf Intermediate filaments

microfilaria The prelarval progeny of parasitic nematodes of the superfamily Filarioidea, family Onchocercidae, which measure 200-300 μm in length, 5-7 μm in diameter and inhabit lymphatic channels CLINICAL Lymphatic filariasis may present as asymptomatic microfilaremia, tropical eosinophilia, filarial fever and lymphatic obstruction, which over time causes lymphatic dilatation, pitting edema and brawny edema with induration of subcutaneous tissue, hyperkeratosis, elephantiasis, fissuring of the skin and inflammation; human disease is caused by *Brugia malayi* (vector, mosquito), *Loa loa* (vector, tabanid fly) and *Wuchereria bancrofti* (vector, mosquito), *Mansonella perstans* (formerly *Dipetalonema perstans*) and *M ozzardi* may both circulate in the blood, but being sheathless, are essentially asymptomatic; microfilaria circulate in the peripheral blood with circadian periodicity, *B malayi* and *W bancrofti* at night, *Loa loa* during the day Note: The microfilaria of *Onchocerca volvulus* (vector, blackfly) and *Dracunculiasis medinensis* (vector, copepod—a nematode), are usually confined to serous cavities and do not circulate DIAGNOSIS Microfilaria are distinguished based on the pattern of the nematode's sheathing and arrangement of nuclei HOST DEFENSES Major basic protein and eosinophil peroxidase, stored in eosinophil granules, display in vivo toxicity against *Brugia malayi* microfilaria and are most effective when delivered with a peroxide-generating system and a halide, eg iodide (J Immunology 1990; 144:3166)

microfold cell M cell GASTROENTEROLOGY An intestinal mucosal cell that overlies Peyer's patches and has microfolds instead of microvilli, which allows lymphocytes to approach the intestinal lumen without violating its integrity; M cells are thought to add the secretory piece to immunoglobulins, eg IgA; see MALT

microgamete The smaller (♂), of the two motile conjugating gametes in the sexual cycle of *Plasmodium* species that fertilizes the macrogamete (♀) during the insect phase of the plasmodial life cycle, leading to the formation of a zygote

microglial cell Hortega cell A perivascular cell derived from the bone marrow, that is native to the CNS, belongs to the mononuclear phagocytic system, eg monocytes, macrophages, dendritic cells and granulocytes, and presents antigen in a MHC-class II restricted context

microglobulin A generic term of waning popularity for a low-molecular-weight (< 40 kD) 'globular' protein, eg Bence-Jones protein; see β_2-microglobulin

microinequity A newly proposed term referring to factors which in aggregate reduce the equality of opportunities for job promotions and career advancement, as experienced by minority groups, and by women (Am Med News 19 Sept 1994) see Glass ceiling

microinvasive carcinoma A superficially invasive epithelial malignancy, which has a specific significance in gynecologic pathology UTERINE CERVIX Stage Ia A squamous cell carcinoma that penetrates less than 5 mm from the base of the epithelium or less than 7 mm in horizontal spread; anything larger is Stage Ib; cervical microinvasive carcinoma has a much greater than 95% 5-year survival; lymph nodes are involved in approximately 1% of microinvasive carcinomas VULVA A squamous cell carcinoma that measures less than 2 cm in diameter and with less than 5 mm of invasion into the stroma; 5% of cases have lymph node metastases TREATMENT Vulvectomy and lymph node resection, if involved; see Carcinoma in situ

microlaminectomy see Laminectomy

micromegakaryocyte A small platelet precursor with agranular cytoplasm, hyalinoplasmic zones (pseudopods), a rounded, dense nucleus and 1-3 small nucleoli, which is associated with large atypical platelets; micromegakaryocytes are often indicative of abnormal megakaryopoiesis and associated with myeloproliferative disorders, eg myelofibrosis with myeloid metaplasia* (aka agnogenic myeloid metaplasia), less commonly in a blast crisis of CML; the PAS-positive cytoplasm is either replete with miniplatelets or reduced to a narrow rim

*Also present in MMM are megakaryoblasts with few α granules and a primitive nucleus and 1-2 nucleoli

micromelia Phocomelia

micrometastasis SURGICAL PATHOLOGY An aggregate of metastatic malignant cells that are identified only by histologic examination, the presence of which was detectable by neither physical examination, nor by imaging techniques; micrometastases within lymph nodes can be detected by various immunostains using antibodies to antigens, eg cytokeratin, melanin, thyroglobulin being produced by the primary malignancy; the data on whether micrometastases have clinical significance is unclear, although most reports have minimized their importance (see Arch Int Med 1993; 153:862oA)

micro method Micro methodology LABORATORY MEDICINE The use of smaller than usual samples (100 mg or 100 ul) for analyses, often for very sick patients or premature infants, in whom multiple specimens are required, potentially causing iatrogenic anemia; 'micro' samples may be obtained in early neonates by heel-sticks with capillary tubes

'micro-micronodular' cirrhosis HEPATOLOGY A form of diffuse cirrhosis, which is characteristic of hepatic copper overload, or Indian childhood cirrhosis, in which oligocellular clusters of hepatocytes are surrounded by bands of fibrosis, accompanied by thickening of the hepatic vessels and diffuse ballooning degeneration of hepatocytes

Micromonosporaceae A family of fungi including *Micropolyspora faeni* and *Thermoactinomyces vulgaris*, which are responsible for Farmer's lung, see there

microneurography NEUROPHYSIOLOGY A technique in which tungsten microelectrodes are inserted into sympathetic nerve fascicles, allowing direct recording of peripheral sympathetic nerve traffic to the skeletal muscle vascular bed (see N Engl J Med 1993; 328:303oA)

micropenis A small penis; a normal infantile penis measures 3.9 cm ± 0.8 when stretched; micropenis may be idiopathic, a common finding in obese infants and boys or may be related to decreased activity of the hormonal axis, as in hypogonadotropic hypogonadism (Kallmann, Prader-Willi and Rud syndromes and septo-optic dysplasia), primary hypogonadism (Klinefelter's disease) and in partial androgen insufficiency; microphallus may be a component of a variety of congenital, eg Carpenter, Cornelia de Lange, Down, Fanconi, Hallermann-Streiff, 18q deletion, Noonan, Robinow, Williams syndromes, in hypopituitarism, and X-linked hypogammaglobulinemia

microphthalmia A congenital ↓ in ocular size, with the ocular bulb measuring as little as ½ of the normal volume in the most extreme cases, due to an abnormal development of the optic vesicle in the optic cup, which may be 1) Congenital, as in encephalo-ophthalmic dysplasia, focal dermal hypoplasia, Hallermann-Streiff syndrome, incontinentia pigmenti, Lenz's microphthalmia syndrome, retinopathy of prematurity, trisomy 13-15 or 2) Infectious, eg CMV, rubella, toxoplasmosis

microprocessor COMPUTERS The pivotal hardware component of a microcomputer that contains the central arithmetic unit, a logic board and the associated circuitry which has been reduced in size so that it fits on one or several silicon chips; see Computer, Microcomputer, Silicon chip

micro-protein sequencing A technique for sequencing proteins, based on Edman degradation, where amino acids are removed one at a time and analyzed by HPLC, thereby providing a 'signature' of proteins in a cell

microsatellite A segment of DNA composed of multiple repeats of a few bases

microsatellite instability An abnormality in a sequence of DNA in which a microsatellite is either longer or shorter than normal, which is most commonly due to defective mismatch repair (Science 1995; 268:1336, 1276)

microsatellite marker MOLECULAR PATHOLOGY A short tandemly repeated DNA sequence, often in the form of dinucleotides repeated 20-30 times; there are about 1000 microsatellites distributed relatively evenly over the entire genome and can be used to localize a chromosomal mutation in the genome by means of positional cloning; one allelic form of a microsatellite is inherited from each parent, and there is a ≥ 80% probability that any person is heterozygous for a change in a microsatellite marker, such that a marker is usually informative and useful; a further advantage of microsatellites is that they can be assayed by PCR amplification followed by gel electrophoresis, and when electrophoresed, they migrate to similar regions on the gel; the DNA nucleotides flanking the microsatellites have been sequenced and olinucleotide primers that recognize these sequences are commercially available (N Engl J Med 1994; 331:213oA, Sci & Med Nov/Dec 1994 p48) see Positional cloning

microscopic hematuria Hematuria that can only be detected by light microscopic examination of the urine; in one report of 168 cases of MH detected by dipstick and subsequently biopsied; 78 (47.3%) were abnormal with IgA nephropathy (49/78), mesangial proliferative glomerulonephritis (12/78), and others including focal segmental proliferative glomerulonephritis; cystoscopy contributes little to the diagnosis (Q J Md 1994; 87:329)

microscopy Anton van Leeuwenhoek (1632-1723), is regarded as the father of microscopy, as he made the first practical microscope by placing a series of well-ground lenses in tandem; he discovered sperm, erythrocytes and bacteria; today's laboratory light microscope is binocular and compound, having 10-15x ocular lenses and multiple objectives on a rotating 'nose-piece' ring; histopathologists often use the term 'scanning' power for 25 to 40x (ocular 10x multiplied by a 2.5x to 4.0x nose piece), 'low' power for 100x, 'high' power for 400x, 'high dry' power for 600x and 'oil' of 1000x; see Confocal microscopy, Darkfield microscopy. Electron microscopy, Fluorescent microscopy, Interference microscopy, Microsurgery, Nomarski interference microscopy, Phase-contrast microscopy, Polarization microscopy, Positron microscopy, Scanning electron microscopy, Scanning tunnel microscopy, Slit-lamp microscopy, Transmission electron microscopy

microsomal enzymes A group of enzymes on the smooth endoplasmic reticulum that areare abundant in the liver, are present in the kidneys and GI tract, and are divided into 1) Glucuronyl transferases and 2) Mixed-function oxidases (MFO), which require NADPH and O_2; Microsomal MFOs catabolize endogenous substances, eg corticosteroids by hydroxylation and are the major pathway for catabolizing exogenous substances, eg for detoxification of various drugs, involving many reactions: N-, O- and S-dealkylation, aromatic or aliphatic hydroxylation, N- or S oxidation, deamination or desulfuration and epoxidation (epoxide: a cyclic ether composed of an O_2 molecule bound to 2 different carbons); usually, microsomal enzymes operate by first-order kinetics (catabolism at the first pass through the system) and only rarely by zero-order kinetics, which are reactions limited by substrate kinetics, as would be competition; many substances can induce hyperplasia of the microsomal enzyme system; MFO may be induced by at least two classes of compounds 1) Phenobarbital and related molecules and 2) Polycyclic hydrocarbons, eg 3,4 benzpyrene

microsomes A heterogeneous group of variably sized and variably shaped lipoprotein-rich vesicles formed from ruptured endoplasmic reticulum and large polyribosomes, when a cell is subjected to ultracentrifugation at 100 000 g for 60 minutes; at lower speeds (eg five minutes at 15 000 g) mitochondria, lysosomes and peroxisomes settle to the bottom of the ultracentrifuge tube; at higher speeds (eg 2 hours at 300 000 g) ribosomal subunits and small polyribosomes sediment to the bottom of the ultracentrifuge tube

microsphere CLINICAL THERAPEUTICS A small (10-40 μm in diameter) bead made from poly(lactic-coglycolic) acid which is used to entrap therapeutic agents or vaccines to be delivered in a timed fashion over a period of days to months; microsphere encapsulation is a process currently under development that may become commercially use in 5-7 years and would solve many of the problems inherent in delivering various proteins (eg insulin), hormones (eg growth hormone for patients with dwarfism), or vaccines (cholera, diphtheria, hepatitis B, rabies, and tetanus are under development), which may require multiple daily injections or, in the case of vaccines, booster shots (Science News 1995; 147:262) Cf Microcapsule

microspherocyte HEMATOPATHOLOGY A small, round erythrocyte seen in excess blood loss, burns, hemoglobin C, myelofibrosis, and pernicious anemia

microsporidia PARASITOLOGY A phylum of ubiquitous unicellular obligate intracellular parasitic protozoa that have a long polar filament and a polar cap that serves as a means of extrusion; microsporidia infect insects and vertebrates, which include ≥ 5 genera (*Enterocytozoon**, *Encephalitozoon*, *Nosema*, *Pleistophora*, *Septata**, and the poorly characterized genus *Microsporidium*); they infect humans, most of whom have AIDS (Arch Pathol Lab Med 1993; 117:1208OA)

*Which cause systemic disease; in one report, the prolonged production of intra- and extracellular spores by *Enterocytozoon bieneusi* was not associated with systemic disease (Arch Pathol Lab Med 1995; 119:424OA)

Microsporum A genus of fungi causing tinea capitis, tinea corpus, ringworm, and other dermatophytoses, see Tinea

microsurgery Any surgical procedure that is performed with the aid of a low-power (circa 7x to 15x) microscope using special equipment, surgical thread, clamps, scalpels, to repair either severed blood vessels or nerves

microsurgical laminectomy Diskectomy ORTHOPEDIC SURGERY A procedure for treating a herniation of an intervertebral disk, which avoids vertebral exploration prior to disk surgery, thereby reducing the risk of the feared 'Failed disk syndrome' as there is minimal excision of bone and epidural fat and minimal nerve root adhesion; see Laminectomy

microtome HISTOLOGY A mechanical device used to section tissues for microscopic examination; metal blades are used to cut paraffin-embedded tissues for light microscopy at a thickness of 4 to 9 μm; glass or diamond blades are used in an ultramicrotome for cutting plastic-embedded tissues for electron microscopy at a thickness of 0.05 to 0.10 μm; see Thick sections, Thin sections

microtubule A cylindrical, 24 nm in diameter tubule of variable length composed of α and β tubulin protein subunits that is a major component of the eukaryotic cytoskeleton and has key roles in cell division (the mitotic 'spindle' is a microtubule connecting centrioles with kinetochores during mitosis), motility, determination of cell shape, movement (microtubules are the key component of cilia and flagella), intracellular transport, eg in axons; microtubules facilitate two-way traffic of mitochondria and one-way traffic of other organelles; microtubules extend from the microtubule organizing center (MTOC) and are relatively dynamic, depending on the cell's whims and needs; microtubules may be transiently expressed, appearing as required for the mitotic spindle; others are permanent as are those associated with flagella and cilia; see also MAPs (microtubule-associated proteins); Cf Cilia, Intermediate filaments, MTOC

microtubule organizing center see MTOC

microvascular disease Diabetic microangiopathy, see there

microvascular free toe transfer HAND SURGERY The transfer of the great toe to a hand in which the thumb* has been lost due to trauma; the functional and aesthetic outcome of an MFTT is relatively good; the psychosocial adjustment to operation is a function of how well-adjusted the patient (or his/her parents in the case of a child with MFTTs) is prior to surgery (J Hand Surg 1994; 19B:689)

*The thumb being critical to forming the prehensile grip, a key hand position

microvasculature The system of minute terminal capillaries, the endothelium of which secretes platelet antiaggregates, prostaglandin I_2, procoagulant factor VIII, anticoagulant plasminogen activator, matrix proteins and fibronectin

microvilli Finger-like projections from the surface of specialized epithelial cells, which are constructed of complex plasma membrane folds surrounding an actin microfilament core; microvilli greatly increase the cell surface and by extension, the capacity of absorptive cells; epithelial cells and their microvilli are known as the brush border, are located on the luminal aspect of the small intestine and are covered by glycocalyx, a fibrous network of glycoproteins containing glycosidases and peptidases

microvillus inclusion disease An AR condition characterized by protracted diarrhea of neonatal onset and a high infant mortality PATHOLOGY The enterocytes of the small and large intestine have scant disorganized and short microvilli with cytoplasmic vesicular bodies (inclusions) (N Engl J Med 1994; 330:1580RA)

microwave A 1-100 GigaHerz (10^9) wave on the electromagnetic spectrum with a wavelength of 1-1000 mm; exposure to minimal amounts of microwaves is common with the advent of domestic microwave ovens; leakage of infrared waves ranges from 1 milliWatt/cm² at the time of sale of a microwave oven to 5 mW/cm², measured at a distance of 2 inches; older pacemakers had a tendency to misfire when the wearer was exposed to the earliest microwave ovens available to the consumer; in older literature, the use of microwave ovens was linked to an ↑ incidence in cataracts Note: There is little substantive data to suggest that microwave exposure is associated with increased morbidity SURGICAL PATHOLOGY Microwave treatment of a specimen can be used to improve retrieval or to 'unmask' an antigen (Lab Med 1994; 25:520); microwave ovens are in common use to speed the timing of of certain staining procedures

microwave antigen retrieval SURGICAL PATHOLOGY The use of a microwave oven to enhance the immunoreactivity (ergo the identification) of antigens, eg p53 in formalin-fixed paraffin-embedded tissues (Arch Pathol Lab Med 1995; 119:360OA)

microwave diathermy SPORTS MEDICINE A form of medical diathermy that delivers shorter waves of higher frequency high-frequency electromagnetic waves than that delivered by shortwave diathermy; MD has the advantage of < 10% loss of energy when administered and is of use in treating fibrous muscular contractions, tendinitis, and chronic tenosynovitis; the standard frequencies delivered in the US are 915 MHz and 2456 MHz; lower frequency of MD is more effective in penetrating fat, although if the fat is > 1 cm in thickness, neither form of diathermy is recommended (JC DeLee, D Drez, Jr, Eds, Orthopedic Sports Medicine WB Saunders, Philadelphia, 1994) see Diathermy; Cf Shortwave diathermy

microwaving PUBLIC HEALTH A method for treating medical waste (MW) to render it noninfectious to humans, in which the MW is shredded, moistened with steam and fed by conveyor into a treatment chamber that heats MW to ± 95° C, which is hot enough to kill but not enough to create the emissions that has forced the retirement of many aging medical waste incinerators (Laboratory Medicine 1995; 26:323ₒₐ) see Medical waste

MICU Mobile intensive care unit A vehicle, usually a specially-designed minivan or truck with the capacity for providing emergency care and life support to the severely injured or ill at the scene of an accident or natural disaster and which transports the patients to a medical facility where their treatment may continue; see Air ambulance

MID Multi-infarct dementia, see there

mid-arm muscle area A derived value used to estimate the lean body mass as a function of skeletal muscle; 30% below a standardized value (52-55, males; 31-35, females) from the Health and Nutritional Examination Surveys (HANES) data indicates a depletion of lean body mass, ie malnutrition; Cf Triceps skin fold

middle-aged A nebulous adjective for a person between ages 40 and 65, commonly used in taking a patient's history; 'older' refers to someone between ages 60 and 80-85 and 'elderly' to those above 80

Note: To be accurate (given the average lifespan of 69 in males in developed nations); middle-aged should refer to ages 23 to 46

middle lobe syndrome Chronic atelectasis and collapse of the right middle lobe of the lung due to extrinsic compression of the right middle bronchus by thymoma, hilar lymphadenopathy, eg TB, sarcoidosis, or lymphoma, tumors or obstruction (due to intraluminal tumors or foreign bodies); the compression results in chronic pneumonitis, bronchial obstruction, bronchiectasis and decreased lung capacity; other findings, related to the primary pathology include calcified hilar lymph nodes, granuloma formation and erosion into the bronchopulmonary apparatus

'middle molecule' toxins A group of small, ie 3-3.5 kD molecules which include uric acid, guanidino compounds and metabolic end products, eg phenols, that are not removed during dialysis of patients with chronic renal failure and which are incriminated in the peripheral neuropathy and pericarditis commonly occurring in uremia; middle molecules may include 1–1.5-kD polypeptides; the 'MMT fraction' is also held responsible for inhibition of hemoglobin synthesis, deranged glucose metabolism, lymphoblast transformation, phagocytic activity and defective nerve conduction

Middlebrook media MICROBIOLOGY A group of growth media (Middlebrook and Cohn 7H10, Middlebrook 7H11, Middlebrook selective 7H11, Middlebrook 7H12 medium, Middlebrook 13A medium, Middlebrook 13A enrichment) used for the optimal growth of *Mycobacterium* spp

midge An insect of the Order Diptera, of the families Chironomidae, Ceratopogonidae (eg genus *Culicoides*, which are blood-sucking intermediate hosts for filarial worms, eg *Mansonella perstans* and *M ozzardi*) and others

midlife crisis PSYCHOLOGY A popular term for a 'crisis' that often occurs in a person's 'middle' years (from late-30s to early 50s), in which he/she evaluates his/her life events to date in terms of what has been accomplished and, based on previous trends, what he/she is likely to accomplish before turning in the 'feedbag'

The MC is provoked by dissatisfaction on one or more fronts, eg personal, familial, professional, and sexual, and may provoke immature or reckless behaviors, eg purchasing exotic Italian car, retaining a paramour, engaging in dangerous sports, as the person may wish to return to a point in his/her youth when the choices were perceived as easier and the possibility of success greater

midline granuloma Destruction and necrosis of tissues of the midline* of various etiologies, which may be due to

1) Idiopathic midline destructive disease, see there

2) Wegener's granulomatosis, see there

3) Malignant midline reticulosis, a pleomorphic lymphoma often of T-cell lineage

4) Various infections, see below, and other less common, less necrotizing, diseases including sarcoidosis, relapsing polychondritis and necrotizing sialometaplasia

CLINICAL Progressive, ulcerating lesion of nasopharyngeal and midline facial tissues; the pathogenesis is unclear and the disease may represent a poor immune response to various infections in an immune- or otherwise compromised patient, eg a diabetic ETIOLOGY Infection, bacterial (*Actinomyces*, *Brucella* spp, *Mycobacterium leprae*, *M tuberculosis*, *Klebsiella rhinoscleromatis*, *Treponema pallidum*), fungal (blastomycosis, candidiasis, coccidioidomycosis, histoplasmosis, phycomycosis, rhinosporidiosis), parasitic (leishmaniasis and myiasis) or malignant (squamous cell carcinoma, rhabdomyosarcoma, lymphomatoid granulomatosis and lymphoma); see Lethal midline granuloma

*North of the mediastinum, south of the cranial cavity, aft of the nose and bow-side to the vertebrae

mid-systolic click syndrome see Mitral valve prolapse syndrome

mid-T protein see Malignant transformation

midwife OBSTETRICS A formally trained person, often an adanced practice registered nurse, who assists in childbirth; midwifery is undergoing a renaissance, and provides obstetric services for lower income women, and is a delivery option chosen by some upper income women who desire a greater involvement in childbirth Note: There is an accelerating trend in litigation-oriented societies for obstetrician/gynecologists to shift their practice away from obstetrics, given the high cost of obstetric malpractice insurance and, regionally (eg inner cities, economically depressed rural regions) increased numbers of financially disadvantaged women, making obstetrics a 'loss leader' service; see 'Natural' childbirth; Cf Lamaze technique

MIF 1) Macrophage/monocyte inhibitory factor, see there 2) Mesoderm-inducing factors, see there

mifepristone RU 486, see there

Mighty Mouse CELL BIOLOGY A transgenic mouse being developed by workers at the Whitehead Institute (Boston) that has a mutation in the erythropoietin receptor, resulting in a truncation (shortening) at the end of the receptor that is the attachment site of SH-PTP1; erythrocytes that lack SH-PLP1 are far more sensitive to erythropoietin; there is a 25-50% ↑ in hemoglobin in humans with the mutation, which was first found in a famed family of fleet-footed Finns, one of whose wins in the Olympics prompted investigation of this particular 'experiment of nature' (Science 1995; 268:25)

migraine Hemicrania An idiopathic, episodic, uni– or bilateral, pulsating (vascular) headache of moderate to severe intensity; migraines are exacerbated by physical activity, associated with dilation of branches of the carotid artery, related to the release of vasomotor substances, eg bradykinin, histamine, prostaglandins, serotonin and substance P, which have a noxious effect on nerve endings supplying the artery; migraines are divided into classic, common, complicated and variant forms CLINICAL 'Classic' migraines are most common in ♀, with the first appearing before puberty and remitting at menopause; migraines may be accompanied or preceded by nausea or vomiting, photophobia and other visual phenomena (eg hemianopia, scotomas, fortification spectra), phonophobia TREATMENT-ACUTE Analgesics (eg aspirin, acetaminophen, propoxyphen, codeine), NSAIDs (eg naproxen, ibuprofen, ketorolac), 5-HT agonists (eg ergotamine, sumatryptan), dopamine antagonist (eg chlorpromazine, metoclopramide) PREVENTION Avoidance of precipitating factors; if conservative measures fail and the attacks are more common than once/week, pharmacologic prophylaxis is indicated, which may be 5-HT-influencing (eg amitriptyline, methysergide[1]), β-adrenergic antagonist (eg propranolol[2], metoprolol), calcium channel blocker (eg nifedipine, verapamil), NSAIDs (eg ketoprofen, mefenamic acid, aspirin) (N Engl J Med 1993; 329:1476RV) see Aura

[1]A serotonin antagonist that is regarded as the most effective agent, which has significant side effects, including vascular insufficiency, retroperitoneal and pleural fibrosis and fibrosis of the cardiac valves [2]Regarded as one of the safest agents

migrating testis Elevator testicle A testicle that is highly mobile within the inguinal canal, which may even migrate into the abdominal cavity; such cases require urological surveillance, as they have an increased risk for testicular torsion

migratory thromboembolism Thrombophlebitis occurs in up to 10% of patients with malignancy, classically seen in mucin-secreting gastrointestinal adenocarcinomas, but may also occur in carcinoma of the breast, lung, ovary and prostate Note: Trousseau described this sign in himself, and it presaged his own death by pancreatic adenocarcinoma

mild traumatic brain injury Dinging SPORTS MEDICINE An '... *immediate and transient impairment of neural function such as alteration of consciousness, disturbance of vision, equilibrium, and other similar symptoms.*' features common to MTBI are '...*limited or absent loss of consciousness, limited post-traumatic amnesia, and an initial Glasgow Coma Scale of ≥ 13 of 15.*' (Advance for Dir in Rehab Med June 1995; 4: 31)

miliaria Prickly heat DERMATOLOGY A skin lesion characterized by multiple minute bumps and vesicles caused by the retention of sweat within keratin-plugged eccrine sweat glands and ducts; in the face of increased pressure, retained sweat leaks into the dermis causing erythema and inflammation, variably accompanied by pruritus, appearing as multiple papules on the skin surface, affecting overbundled children in winter, soldiers in the tropics and in fever CLINICAL Pruritus and hypohidrosis may cause irritability and insomnia Note: The clinical variant terms of miliaria crystallina (minute superficial, non-inflamed clear fluid-filled vesicles), miliaria profunda (deep lesions) and miliaria rubra (deeper lesion with papulovesicles and intense erythema, confined to flexures, accompanied by maceration, candidiasis and folliculitis in the diaper region) appear to reflect intensity and have no diagnostic utility; Cf Diaper dermatitis

miliary *adjective* Pertaining or referring to any disseminated process comprised of innumerable millet-seed sized lesions, classically seen in miliary TB in the pre-antibiotic period, where the 'millet seeds' correspond to granulomas; also refers to disseminated histoplasmosis and CMV pneumonitis

milium Whitehead DERMATOLOGY One of multiple, small subepithelial keratin cysts arising in eccrine sweat ducts, often located on the face, which may be present from infancy onwards, and most often occur in young ♀ after sunbathing

milk see Breast milk, Humanized milk, Unpasteurized milk

milk-alkali syndrome A condition characterized by hypercalcemia due to excess consumption of dairy products, overuse of calcium-containing (> 5g/day) antacids (eg CaCO₃) or alkalis (eg sodium bicarbonate for treating peptic ulcer or Sippy antacid diet, of largely historical interest) CLINICAL Lethargy, constipation and renal decompensation LABORATORY Hypercalcemia, severe compensat-

ed metabolic alkalosis, normo- to hyperphosphatemia; long-term metabolic derangement may cause renal insufficiency or failure through a combination of nephrocalcinosis, loss of ability to compensate for the alkalosis and dehydration

milker's nodes Paravaccinia An infection by a bovine parapoxvirus that occurs through direct inoculation while manually milking cows, characterized by red-blue firm and tender nodules that may develop into a papulovesicular eruption of the arms and extremities and disappear in 1-2 weeks

'milking' CARDIOVASCULAR SURGERY The gentle squeezing of any blood vessel, often a distal vein or the extremity itself, 'milking' it in the proximal direction in an attempt to extract a non-adherent thrombus

'milk' leg OBSTETRICS Phlegmasia alba dolens Extensive deep vein or iliofemoral thrombosis due to stasis of uterine blood, accompanied by painful swelling and pallor of the entire extremity, a condition formerly common in parturition (hence, 'milk leg'), more often seen in recent abdominal or pelvic surgery; with progression, all the veins become thrombosed, blood cannot return to the heart and the leg becomes cool, painful and cyanotic, known as phlegmasia cerulea dolens or painful blue leg

milk let-down see Let-down reflex

milkmaid's grip NEUROLOGY A sign of generalized muscle weakness and the inability to maintain tetanic muscle contraction; the subjects, when asked to squeeze the examiner's fingers, do so by a 'milking' motion of contraction and relaxation, a finding typical of Sydenham's chorea, one of Jones' major criteria for the diagnosis of rheumatic fever

Milkman syndrome Generalized osteomalacia A radiologist's disease that is more common in middle-aged ♀; it is characterized by alternating symmetrical radiolucent bands or pseudofractures that corresponds to resorption and mineralization adjacent to arteries, a condition that responds to vitamin D therapy

milk-of-calcium appearance An appearance resulting from minute concrements composed of calcium carbonate, which have a 'sandy' or 'ground-glass' radiological appearance and seemingly float as a suspension, within pyelogenic cysts, simple cortical cysts of arterionephrosclerosis and in the cysts of polycystic kidney disease; the substance is best identified in plain films as a bilayer, with fluid on top and a granular layer on the bottom, separated by the whims of body position and gravity; a similar appearance may be seen in obstructed gall bladders

milk-rejection sign An anecdotal clinical observation that breast-fed infants will not take milk from a breast affected by carcinoma (Cancer 1966; 19:1185); in a similar context, infants tend to suck less when the mother has ingested alcohol prior to breast feeding (N Engl J Med 1991; 325:981), related to objective changes in the quality of the milk

milk spots Large white to gray-white patches on the left ventricular surface of the heart seen by gross examination in idiopathic dilated cardiomyopathy, which corresponds to ischemia-induced fibrosis due to long-standing focal hypoxia; MSs on the right ventricular surface are viewed as an incidental autopsy finding, possibly linked to healed pericarditis

milk stool PEDIATRICS The viscid dark green neonatal feces, ie meconium, gives rise to yellow-green and more liquid stools that later develop into the firm caramel-to-milk chocolate stool of the milk-fed infant

Note: The stool of human milk-fed infants is looser and less malodorous than those fed cow's milk

mill wheel murmur CARDIOLOGY A descriptor for the 'splashing' precordial murmur heard in significant (ie greater than 200 ml) venous air embolism, which is accompanied by ↑ pressure, cyanosis, tachycardia, and syncope

milrinone A positive inotropic phosphodiesterase inhibiting agent that provides short-term benefit; it is reported to have a deleterious effects on chronic heart failure (N Engl J Med 1992; 326:1565c)

Milwaukee Brace Moe brace ORTHOPEDICS A whole body brace that extends into neck and is used in the conservative therapy of scoliosis

Milwaukee shoulder A painful, destructive, bilateral upper girdle dysfunction of the elderly female consisting of capsular calcification, joint effusions (increased collagenase without inflammation), erosion of rotator cuff tendons and glenohumeral joint degeneration on the dominant side; the condition is worse at night or following heavy usage with accumulation of basic calcium phosphate crystals in inflamed joints

MIM number A numerical assignment given to inherited diseases that are listed in VA McCusick's (Wm Osler Professor of Medicine, Johns Hopkins Medical Center, Baltimore, Maryland) comprehensive and monumental catalog, Mendelian Inheritance in Man (11th edition, 1994); each condition is given a five digit number, where 10005-19447 correspond to AD (autosomal dominant), 20010-27900 to AR (autosomal recessive), and 30002-31500 to X-chromosome linked conditions

mimotope A peptide sequence that immunologically mimics an antigen's epitope without having sequence homology to the antigenic site, an effect that is due to mimicry of the three-dimensional conformation of the epitope

Minamata disease ENVIRONMENT A disease that spanned 15 years, first recognized in 1953 in the city of Minamata, a coastal community in southwest Japan, caused by consumption of fish and shellfish contaminated with organic methylmercury (inorganic mercury is not considered to be a major teratogen) discharged into nearby rivers by industrial plants that produced acetaldehyde, which used mercury as a reactive catalyst; by 1972, 704 cases had been confirmed in all age groups in Minamata and 121 in Niigata City, 40 of whom were affected in utero (1200 more cases were unconfirmed) CLINICAL Severe mental and neurological impairment, degenerative changes of the cerebral and cerebellar cortex, paresthesias, blindness, deafness, inability to concentrate, dysarthria, tremors that evolved to persistent vegetative state; a similar epidemic occurred in Iraq when grain treated with a methylmercury fungicide, intended for planting was baked into bread, resulted in 6530 cases of poisoning and 459 deaths; Cf Bhopal, Haff disease, Mad hatter syndrome, Mercury, Toxic oil, and Yusho oil syndromes

mineralization An in vivo precipitation of mineral salts, usually calcium and phosphate due to a focal increase in concentration

minerals, dietary Those metallic elements that are required for optimal functioning of the body; dietary requirements for minerals range from molar to trace amounts/day

MAJOR MINERALS, BONE Calcium, phosphate, magnesium

MAJOR MINERALS, ELECTROLYTES Sodium, potassium, chloride

MINOR MINERALS, METALLOPROTEINS Iron, copper, manganese, iodine, cobalt, molybdenum, selenium, chromium, fluoride and zinc

TRACE MINERALS Nickel, silicon, vanadium and tin

mineral oil A mixture of liquid petroleum-derived hydrocarbons with a specific gravity of 0.818-0.96; mineral oil was formerly used with impunity as a vehicle for drugs applied to the nasal mucosa and internally as a laxative; when applied too liberally, mineral oil may evoke exogenous lipid pneumonia; although mineral oil may be used as a laxative without major adverse effect; excess use of mineral oil as a laxative may cause anorexia, malabsorption of fat-soluble vitamins and absorption of the oil itself; see Lipoid pneumonia

minicomputer An increasingly obsolete term that was defined as a computer with a speed and memory capacity that fell between that of a microcomputer (speed measured in MegaHerz, the first of which had speeds of 4.77 MHz and 16 to 64 kilobytes of memory) and that of a mainframe computer (speed measured in MIPS or million instructions per second and a memory of hundreds to thousands of megabytes of data storage capacity); the current generation of personal (micro-) computers has surpassed many of the features, eg speed and memory capacity of minicomputers; see Computers, Mainframe computer, Microcomputers

minichromosome Artificial chromosomes that have been created by linking restriction endonuclease digested fragments of DNA

minichromosome mainenance proteins MCM family, see there

minifilm RADIOLOGY A 10 cm² film used for producing chest X-rays that requires 2.0 mrad (in contrast to ≥ 9.2 mrad for the 'standard' 35 x 42.5 cm film); the diagnostic quality of images on minifilms are reported to be as good as the normally-sized films and have the advantage of lower costs, and faster screening of large numbers of subjects, eg inmates in a correctional facility to identify pulmonary TB (JAMA 1992; 268:3176MN&P)

minigene A segment of a gene that encodes a variable region of either the heavy or light chain of an immunoglobulin

'minilap' An abbreviated laparotomy used to obtain cells, document intraperitoneal hemorrhage, obtain fluids for determining the presence of bile amylase, bacteria or fecal material by peritoneal lavage

minimal access surgery Minimally invasive surgery, see there

minimal deviation adenocarcinoma of cervix Minimum deviation adenocarcinoma of the uterine cervix, see there

minimal risk FORENSIC MEDICINE '...*the probability and magnitude of harm...anticipated in the research* [is] *not greater...than* [that] *encountered in daily life or during the routine performance of routine physical ...examinations.*' (Sci Am 1995; 272/2:56) The term was introduced into the regulatory lexicon by the National (US) Commission for the Protection of Human Subjects of Biomedical and Behavioral Research to guide recommendations for (US) federal regulations regarding experiments with human subjects; see Helsinki Declaration, Nuremburg Code of Ethics

minimally-invasive surgery A generic term for an evolving 'platform' for the management of surgical disease; MIS has in part been driven by consumer demand, but made possible only by technological advances on a number of fronts; MIS encompasses laparoscopic surgery which began with the gallbladder (laparoscopic cholecystectomy) and has since become popular in other under the analogue that may be administered vaginally in conjunction with mifepristone (RU 486) as an abortifacient (N Engl J Med 1995; 332:983OA) see Abortion, Gemeprost, Mifepristone, Sulprostone

mini-mental test NEUROLOGY A brief clinical evaluation of mental status, where each correct answer in a series of questions is given one point for a total score of 30

ORIENTATION IN TIME Year, season, month, date, day (total 5

points)

ORIENTATION IN SPACE Country, state, county, town, place, hospital ward (5 points)

COGNITION Serial sevens (x 5) or spell world backwards (5 points)

SHORT RECALL Name three objects (total 3 points)

MEMORY Rename three above objects (3 points)

FOLLOW A THREE-PART COMMAND Take a paper, fold it, put it on the floor (3 points)

COMMON OBJECT RECOGNITION Name two familiar objects (2 points)

RECOGNITION OF COMMON PHRASE 'No ifs, ands, or buts' (1 point)

READ AND OBEY 'Close your eyes' (1 point)

WRITE SIMPLE SENTENCE (1 point)

COPY DRAWING Intersecting pentagons (1 point)

A person with a change in mental status and a score of greater than 27 points most often has affective depression; patients who are depressed and have cognitive impairment have scores of about 20 and those with true dementia often have scores of less than 10 (**J Psych Res 1975; 12:189**)

minimum bactericidal concentration MICROBIOLOGY The lowest concentration of an antibiotic that is bactericidal to at least 99.9% of an original inoculum; MBC is a form of antibiotic susceptibility testing in which an antimicrobial agent in broth is serially diluted, or titrated in a standardized (McFarland) suspension of bacteria; tubes in which there is no growth are subcultured in an antibiotic-free growth medium; the MBC may vary as a function of certain intrinsic features of the bacterium; see Persistence phenomenon, Paradoxic effect and Tolerance

Note: It is unclear whether determination of the MBC is indicated for streptococcal endocarditis, staphylococcal endocarditis or osteomyelitis and Enterobacteriaceae or *Pseudomonas* species from patients with meningitis, given the poor correlation between *in vitro* sensitivity and *in vivo* effectiveness

minimum change disease Lipoid nephrosis, nil disease A primary glomerulopathy that is more common in children, and characterized by nephrotic syndrome PATHOLOGY Glomeruli are normal by LM and by immunofluorescence microscopy; by EM, there is fusion of the epithelial cell foot processes TREATMENT Corticosteroids, immunosuppressive therapy (eg cyclophosphamide, chlorambucil) PROGNOSIS Spontaneous remission is common, as are relapses

minimum deviation adenocarcinoma of the uterine cervix Adenoma malignum A rare, very well-differentiated adenocarcinoma arising in the endocervical columnar epithelium that is remarkable for its bland histology; although the prognosis is similar to that of the usual type of endocervical adenocarcinoma when correctly diagnosed, in actuality, this tumor has a relatively poor prognosis given its verisimilitude to benign endocervical glands, and its subsequent underdiagnosis DDx Benign lesions, eg Nabothian cysts, microglandular hyperplasia, mesonephric hyperplasia, and the recently described entity, florid deep endocervical glands (**Am J Clin Pathol 1995; 103:609OA**)

minimum inhibitory concentration CLINICAL MICROBIOLOGY The minimal amount of antibiotic necessary to inhibit bacterial growth from a clinical isolate, which serves as a form of antimicrobial susceptibility testing; the MIC is a laboratory test in which the lowest concentration of an antibiotic to be administered to a patient is extrapolated from various 'bench' tests that determine the amount of inhibition of bacterial growth in culture, including the disk elution test and determination of the diameter of non-growth surrounding a paper disk impregnated with antibiotics (disk diffusion test) METHOD A specimen is grown to confluence or a 'lawn' on a blood agar plate; standardized paper disks, each containing an antibiotic, are dropped on the plate and the amount of growth inhibition is measured in millimeters; antibiotic resistance and sensitivity of an organism obtained by the MIC allows modification of the antibiotic regimen; MIC can also be determined by broth or agar dilutions, but is more time consuming and labor-intensive

Note: in vitro sensitivity to an antibiotic does not guarantee in vivo response to that antibiotic

minimum lethal dose The minimum amount of a toxin, noxious substance or agent, eg bacterium, chemical, drug, ionizing radiation or virus that is lethal to 100% of a test population

'minipill' An oral contraceptive that contains only the progestational agent, norethindrone in very low amounts (0.35 mg), or norethindrone and seemingly 'homeopathic' doses of estrogen; the minipill reduces sperm penetration of the cervical mucus, interfering with luteinization and implantation and decreases gonadotropin secretion; the minipill may be slightly less effective than combined contraceptives and has been associated with dysmenorrhea; Cf Norplant, RU 486

miniprep MOLECULAR BIOLOGY A generic term for a rapid and abbreviated method for identifying the presence of cloned DNA in a culture of host bacteria; steps in minipreps include lysis of host cells, cutting the cloned DNA/vector with a restriction endonuclease, and running the digest on an electrophoretic gel to identify characteristic bands

minisatellite MOLECULAR BIOLOGY A short (1–5-kilobase pair) region of simple sequence DNA comprised of 20-50 repeats of 15-100 nucleotide in length sequences, a size that distinguishes them from DNA satellites, which measure 10^5 to 10^6 bases in length; the small size of minisatellites allows facile Southern blotting and highly specific identification of individual subjects by determination of restriction fragment length polymorphisms (see RFLP), which are often associated with moderately repeated sequences; minisatellites are used for DNA 'fingerprinting', paternity testing, forensic medicine and human genome mapping; as such, minisatellites are unstable repetitive sequences of DNA present throughout the human (and other) genome(s); mutation of minisatellites, eg HRAS1 minisatellite locus, is an attributable risk for nearly 10% of cancers of the breast, colorectum and urinary bladder (**N Engl J Med 1993; 329:517OA**); minisatellites are most common in telomeric regions, and may be intimately associated with genes and gene clusters within chromosomes; α-globin and immunoglobulin heavy chain loci contain minisatellites in intergenic and intronic locations; minisatellites are present in introns of IL-6, myoglobin, retinoblastoma, and von Willebrand factor genes; apolipoprotein B, collagen II and insulin have minisatellites immediately up– or downstream from the coding sequences; in other genes, eg those encoding epithelial mucin, involucrin, and proline-rich proteins, minisatellites contain transcribed and translated minisatellite elements; minisatellite instability is a manifestation of the RER phenotype, may occur in sporadic colorectal carcinomas and in hereditary non-polyposis colorectal carcinoma (**N Engl J Med 1994; 331:213OA**) see Double minutes

'Minnesota experiment' A protocol which determined the physiological consequences of malnutrition; 32 male volunteers were semi-starved for six months, resulting in decreases in body weight (24%), cardiac stroke volume (18%), cardiac index (38%), vital capacity (8%) and tidal volume (19%); other changes of voluntary starvation include decreased enzymatic activity, decrease in organ size, slowing of metabolism, increased transit times, poor wound healing and immune dysfunction; see Kwashiorkor, Marasmus; Cf Nazi 'science'

Minnesota Multiphasic Personality Inventory see MMPI

minor cluster region A 500-bp region of DNA, located 20-30 kb in the 3' direction from the mbr (major breakpoint region) in which 20-30% of the t(14:18) translocations (seen in most follicular lymphomas) occur; mcr can be identified by PCR; see Major breakpoint region

minor crossmatch TRANSFUSION MEDICINE The testing of a patient's cells against a potential donor's serum to detect the presence of ABO incompatibility and other major antibodies; see Immediate spin crossmatch, Major crossmatch; Cf Back typing, Front typing

minor depression Dysthmic disorder (300.4, per DSM-IV) see there

minor groove MOLECULAR BIOLOGY A shallow 'furrow' in a DNA double helix measuring 1.2 nm across, which extends the entire length of DNA as long as the molecule remains in a normal or right-handed DNA conformation; see DNA forms, Major groove

minor histocompatibility peptides H antigens Minor antigens identified include that encoded by the H-3 gene, β_2-microglobulin and the male-specific H-Y antigen; nearly 50 other genes have been mapped but incompletely identified

minor lymphocyte stimulating genes see Mls genes

minor surgery A generic term for any surgical procedure that may be loosely defined as an operation that can be performed in a brief period of time (usually less than an hour) under local anesthesia, does not (under normal circumstances) constitute a major hazard to life or function of organs or body parts; minor surgery does not generally require hospitalization and may be performed as an elective procedure, usually by a general (board-certified) surgeon in a secondary-care hospital setting; Cf Major surgery

minoxidil A drug, which when administered per os, is a direct vasodilator, and first used for severe refractory hypertension; side effects of oral minoxidil include sodium and water retention, pericardial effusion, hypertrichosis and hirsutism; as a 1-5% topical solution, minoxidil evokes terminal hair growth in 8-31% of ♂ with early (< 5 years duration) androgenic (♂ pattern) baldness; normal scalp hair density is 500/cm²; minoxidil increases the thin areas by 83 hairs/cm², yielding satisfactory results for up to 48% of those treated MECHANISM Unknown, although it may be related to local vasodilation; see Hair replacement

minus-minus phenotype see Null phenotype

minus strand A segment of DNA, produced by a single-stranded DNA virus infecting a eukaryotic host cell, which is complementary or antiparallel to the first strand; when such segments are derived from the virus, they are termed 'plus' strands and the complementary strand is designated the 'minus' strand

minutes pronounced min-nutts The record that summarizes the proceedings of a committee meeting and its important points

minutes pronounced mai-'n(y)üts see Double minutes

MIP-1 Macrophage inflammatory protein A heparin-binding protein secreted by macrophages in response to endotoxin; MIP-1 differs from other endogenous pyrogens, eg tumor necrosis factor (TNF) and IL-1, as its effect is not mediated through prostaglandin synthesis (and therefore is not abrogated by cyclooxygenase inhibitors, eg ibuprofen)

MIPS Million instructions per second A measurement of speed for mainframe computers, as used in computed tomography, which process information at speeds of 20 or greater MIPS; the speeds of the Cray and Hitachi supercomputers are giving press to a new acronym, GIPS for a billion (British = Milliard) instructions per second; Cf MHz

mirror image biopsy A biopsy of the contralateral breast when lobular carcinoma-in-situ is found in one breast, a procedure that is necessary to rule out invasive carcinoma Note: Lobular carcinoma-in-situ is associated with a 1% annual risk of malignant degeneration and thus requires close follow-up; Cf Lumpectomy

mirror movement NEUROLOGY The involuntary copying by one extremity of the movement occurring in another

mirror syndrome The maternal mirror syndrome is a poorly understood clinical phenomenon in which the mother displays the same physiopathological conditions, eg hydrops, as her fetus, possibly causing high-output cardiac failure in the mother, which is postulated to be related to the release of hormones or vasoactive substances by the placenta

mirroring LABORATORY MEDICINE A type of laboratory information system back-up in which every 'transaction' is recorded on identical primary system files, where the two hard disks are in exact synchronization; while the use of mirror systems is preferred because of the better security and reliability Note: Mirroring is not perfect and if the motherboard is at fault, both copies of the backup will be corrupted, which can be avoided by a second type of mini-backup, known as journaling, see there

MIS Medical information system, see Hospital information system, Laboratory information system

misadventure An accident or unintentional act, as in an occupation-related 'homicide by misadventure'; in medicine, the term has become an elegant euphemism for a therapeutic error, as in a surgical misadventure, in which the wrong leg was amputated; see Mistake; Cf Miscall

miscall A diagnostic error, as in a pathologist miscalling a benign tumor as malignant, see Misdiagnosis; Cf Misadventure

*¹'Boo-boo' is a widely used American contribution to low-brow lexicography, used for 1) Children who have small cuts, or bruise, as in '...baby has a boo-boo..' and 2) Adults who have commited a blunder, as above, a term of uncertain parentage

misconduct '*Misconduct in science, as in other professions, comes in all shapes and sizes. It ranges from the flagrant and persistent fabrication of data* (J Darsee, Emory and Harvard, 1981) *to proven plagiarism* (J Felig & R Suliman, Yale, 1984) *to the obstinent defense of an indefensible paper* (T Imanishi-Kari & D Baltimore, Tufts and Whitehead Institute, 1986).' (Nature 1994; 369:261ED); the US Public Health Service, whose rules govern the National Institutes of Health, operates under a strict definition of scientific misconduct that includes fabrication, falsification, and plagiarism (Nature 1994; 369:513N) see Fraud in science

misdiagnosis The incorrect diagnosis of a morbid condition; misdiagnosis alone is insufficient to result in a successful lawsuit for malpractice if the physician can support the contention that he exercised reasonable and prudent medical judgement in arriving at a diagnosis in accordance with accepted medical standards; the plaintiff must then prove that the misdiagnosis caused injury; see Overcall, Undercall

misinformed consent see Information overload; Cf Informed consent

mismatch phenomenon NEUROPHYSIOLOGY A ratio of neurotransmitter to neuroreceptor that differs from the expected 1:1; high concentrations of neuroreceptors for substance P are found in the neocortex and hippocampus, although the neurotransmitters themselves are in low concentrations; such a mismatch implies the presence of another system(s) of cell communication, which may have a role in non-synaptic interaction among cells

mismatch repair system MOLECULAR BIOLOGY A set of proteins that detects errors in the nucleotide base sequences of newly synthesized strands of DNA; if the new strand does not complement the template strand on which it is being modeled, the MRS excises the defective segment with a portion of up- and downstream DNA; DNA polymerase then fills in the gaps; the MRS prevents incompatible DNA from existing, ie between even closely related species from cross-breeding (≥ 10% of divergence of DNA is sufficient to prevent cross-breeding), thus erecting a reproductive barrier against 'erroneous' new strand formation; defects in the MRS has been linked to certain forms of malignancy; in one form, there is a mutation in the TGF-β receptor, rendering cells unresponsive to TGF-β's growth inhibitory effects, removing one of the brakes in tumor progression (**Science 1995; 268:1336, 1276**) Cf Patch and cut repair

misoprostol OBSTETRICS A synthetic prostaglandin E_1 analogue that may be administered vaginally in conjunction with mifepristone (RU 486) as an abortifacient (**N Engl J Med 1995; 332:983OA**) it is approved (US) for preventing NSAID-induced peptic ulcer disease; in the UK, misoprostol is also approved for treating both peptic and duodenal ulcers (**N Engl J Med 1992; 327:1575RV**), and as a second-trimester abortifacient; when compared to PGE_2, misoprostol induced complete (passage of fetus and placenta simultaneously) abortion more often (43% vs 32% for PGE_2), was more convenient (insertion of 2 100-µg tablets @ 12 hours vs insertion of 20 mg suppository @ 3 hours + antidiarrheal, antiemetic, and antipyretic medication required for PGE_2 therapy) was associated with fewer side effects, including fever (11% vs 63%), vomiting (4% vs 33%), diarrhea (4% vs 30%), and less expensive ($0.97 vs $315.30) (**N Engl J Med 1994; 331:290OA**); misoprostol may be of use in reducing acute rejection of renal allografts, a phenomenon partially due to ischemic damage of kidneys that occurs between the time of 'harvesting' and re-establishment of the blood flow; see Abortion, Gemeprost, Mifepristone, Sulprostone

mispairing The mismatching of nucleotides or noncomplementary pairing of DNA strands that may occur in low-stringency hybridization studies; see Low stringency; Cf High stringency

MISS Modified Injury Severity Scale A method for quantifying pediatric multi-trauma injuries; MISS is the sum of the squares of the 3 most injured body regions, modified from the American Medical Association's abbreviated injury scale (AIS; burn victims are not included in the analyses), substituting the Glasgow coma scale for neurological evaluation

missed abortion The retention of a fetus known to be dead for four or more weeks; the interventional approach is expectancy as spontaneous delivery occurs usually by the sixth post-mortem week; see Abortion

missense codon Any altered codon (triplet of DNA nucleotides) that encodes an incorrect amino acid or stop signal, resulting in an altered or non-functioning protein product

missense mutation MOLECULAR PATHOLOGY A DNA mutation in which one or more nucleotides in a codon are altered, resulting in a different amino acid being translated from mRNA into a growing protein

mistake Medical mistake An act, omission or error in judgement by a health care provider that has or may have serious consequences for a patient and that would be judged to be wrong by knowledgeable peers; for physicians in residency training, these errors include errors in diagnosis (33%), prescribing (29%), evaluation (21%), procedural complications (11%) and communication (5%); one-half discussed the mistake with superiors and one-fourth discussed it with non-medical peers or with the patients themselves (**JAMA 1991; 265:2089**); Cf Misdiagnosis, 'Overcall', 'Undercall'

Mister The British title for a surgeon

mistreatment of the elderly 1) Elderly abuse 2) Elderly

neglect

mithridatism Tolerance developed against a toxin, which is induced by gradual incrementation of the toxin, a technique likened to tolerization therapy used in allergy medicine

It is named after Mithridates VI (131-63 BC), the king of ancient Pontus; Rasputin, the 'mad monk' was thought to have ingested increasing amounts of strychnine for this purpose

MITI 1) Ministry of International Trade and Industry The central agency of the Japanese government encharged with coordinating research activities with industry; MITI recently opened up the rights to patenting R&D projects (**Nature 1991; 350:102n**) 2) Myocardial Infarction, Triage and Intervention trial

mitmachen German, to do with NEUROLOGY A finding in catatonic patients, who despite instructions to the contrary, allow an extremity to be placed in any position without resistance to light pressure, and then return the body part to the original resting position, once the extremity is released by the examiner

mitochondrion A double-membraned intracellular organelle invested with its own DNA and energy-producing enzymatic machinery, including the electron transport chain complexes of oxidated phosphorylation, which are grouped as complex I, the NADH dehydrogenase system, complex II (succinate dehydrogenase system), complex III (cytochrome b-c complex) and complex IV (cytochrome oxidase C); see Mitochondrial DNA

mitochondrial disease A generic term for any of a clinically heterogeneous group of multisystem diseases characterized by neuromuscular abnormalities of the brain (mitochondrial encephalopathies) and/or muscles (mitochondrial myopathies) due to defects of the protein complexes of the electron transport chain of oxidative phosphorylation; MDs include Alper, Kearn-Sayres, Leigh, Lowe, Menke's kinky hair and Zellweger syndromes, lactic acidosis, Luft disease, MELAS, MERRF, rhizomelic chondrodysplasia punctata, and stroke-like episodes

---

MITOCHONDRIAL DISEASES

GROUP 1 PROGRESSIVE EXTERNAL OPHTHALMOPLEGIA

a) Kearns-Sayre disease (ophthalmoplegia plus syndrome)

b) Ocular myopathy

c) Leber's hereditary optic neuropathy (due to a point mutation)

GROUP 2 MITOCHONDRIAL ENCEPHALOMYOPATHIES

a) Mitochondrial encephalomyopathy with lactic acidosis and stroke-like episodes, see MELAS

b) Myoclonus epilepsy with ragged red fibers see MERRF

c) Leigh syndrome

GROUP 3 UNDEFINED MITOCHONDRIAL ENCEPHALOMYOPATHIES, eg congenital lactic acidosis

GROUP 4 MITOCHONDRIAL MYOPATHIES

a) Luft syndrome

b) Enzyme defects, eg ATPase, cytochrome oxidase

---

mitochondrial DNA Mitochondria have their own DNA that is smaller and different from nuclear DNA; mtDNA measures 16.5 kilobases and is a circular double helix with 13 structural genes encoding respiratory chain elements, 22 tRNA genes and 2 genes that encode the 16S and 12S mitochondrial rRNAs that translate into the proteins responsible for the mitochondrial energy pathway, including NADH dehydrogenase, cytochrome c oxidase, ATP synthase and ubiquinol-cytochrome c oxidoreductase Note: Dogma has held that mitochondrial DNA is transmitted in a non-mendelian fashion from the mother; pater

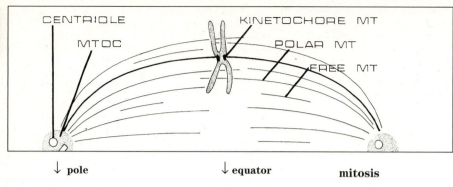

↓ **pole**　　　　　↓ **equator**　　　　**mitosis**

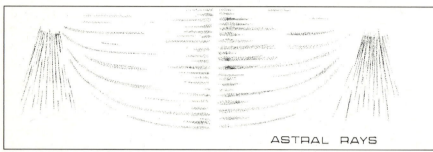

ASTRAL RAYS

Figure: MT: Microtubule; MTOC: Microtulue organizing center

mitotic activity The degree to which a cell population is proliferating, an indicator of tumor aggression, measured as the frequency of cell division; mitotic activity can be semi-quantified by counting of mitotic figures per high-power field, or by flow cytometry; see Flow cytometry, High power fields

mitotic spindle MOLECULAR BIOLOGY A transiently expressed structure consisting of microtubules, which is responsible for the alignment and movement of chromosomes during cell division; the spindle organizes the chromosomes and cytoplasm, and is composed predominantly of relatively labile microtubules, which are too thin to be studied by conventional light microscopy, requiring instead polarization microscopy; three types of microtubules or fibers are present in the spindle 1) Polar fibers extending from one of the spindle poles to the equator, 2) Kinetochore fibers extending from the chromosome's centromere toward the pole and 3) Astral fibers extending from the mitotic pole to the periphery of the cell; see MTOC

nal transmission of mtDNA in mussels, mice and *Drosophila* has been reported (Nature 1994; 368:817sc, 811n&v); mDNA evolves much more rapidly than nuclear DNA

mitochondrial encephalopathies see Mitochondrial diseases

mitochondrial Eve ANTHROPOLOGY A hypothetical 'mother of mankind', who is postulated to have lived in Africa circa 200 000 years ago (Science 1991; 253:1503); the ancestry of this first female *Homo sapiens* is inferred from phylogenetic trees constructed from restriction fragment length polymorphisms of mitochondrial DNA that are passed only by females; analysis of mitochondrial DNA may ultimately identify the female at, or close to the root of, the phylogenetic tree; see Anthropology, Lucy; Cf Urkingdom

mitogenesis theory A model for carcinogenesis that holds that the rate-limiting step in malignant transformation is the induction of increased cell division; the theory is supported by the fact that low-doses of environmental toxins, eg dioxins and others are not genotoxic and contrasts with the more 'mainstream' multistep process theory of carcinogenesis, in which low-level toxic exposures may be one of the 'steps' in malignant transformation

mitosis CELL BIOLOGY The division of a cell's nucleus that results in the production of two daughter nuclei with a genome identical to that of the parent; mitosis is a controlled process that has been divided into four steps

PROPHASE The duplicated chromosomes appear in a species-specific number, initially appearing as long thin paired chromatin threads that shorten and become more compact, which is followed by dissolution of the nuclear envelope

METAPHASE The shortened compact chromatin threads form the mitotic spindle (MS) and move to the metaphase plate, reaching the plate with all centromeres aligned at the MS's equator

ANAPHASE The sister chromatids separate and move to the opposite poles of the MS

TELOPHASE The chromatids arrive at their respective poles, the nuclear envelope is formed and the chromtin uncoils

mitoxantrone ONCOLOGY A synthetic anthracenedione-based DNA intercalating anthracycline analog with 3 planar aromatic rings PHARMACOKINETICS Similar to doxorubicin SIDE EFFECTS Dose-limiting granulocytopenia, as well as thrombocytopenia, nausea and vomiting, mitoxantrone's therapeutic potential is as yet undetermined, early data suggests that it may be of use in breast cancer, and lymphoproliferative malignancies

mitral annular calcification A noninflammatory chronic degenerative process of the fibrous support structure of the mitral valve; MAC is more common in women and in the elderly and is associated with hypertension, obesity, atrial fibrillation and arrhythmias, heart block, congestive heart failure and stroke (N Engl J Med 1992; 327:374oA)

mitral facies CARDIOLOGY A physiognomy characterized by florid malar flushing associated with mitral valve stenosis; other physical findings in mitral valve stenosis include distended jugular veins with an 'a' wave, an accentuated first heart sound at the apex, an opening snap and a diastolic rumble

mitral valve prolapse syndrome Barlow syndrome, Floppy valve syndrome A condition most commonly affecting young females, in which the mitral valve prolapses into the left atrium, a condition that affects up to 5% of the general population, potentially causing sudden death by arrhythmia or rupture of cordae tendinae EKG Inverted T waves in II, III, aV$_F$ leads, prolongation of Q PATHOLOGY Myxoid degeneration of valves with an increase of ground substance

mittelschmerz German, Middle pain GYNECOLOGY Pain of the lower female abdomen at the time of ovulation, due to a ruptured graafian follicle

mitten hand deformity An end-stage lesion in the AR dystrophic epidermolysis bullosa, with fusion of digits, loss of fingernails and dermal fibrosis CLINICAL Failure to thrive, growth retardation, repeated infections, subepidermal blistering and 'weeping' of lesions, involvement of the orogenital mucosae, esophageal fibrosis with malnutrition and flexion contractions of joints

mixed connective tissue disease A connective tissue disease that has features of SLE, dermatomyositis, and rheumatoid arthritis CLINICAL Pleuritis, Raynaud's phenomenon, sclerodactyly and a good response to corticosteroids LABORATORY MCTD is unique as it has a speckled nucleolar pattern due to the presence of a specific circulating antibodies to ribonucleoprotein, absent antibodies to double-stranded DNA and Sm antigen; see Antinuclear antibodies, 'Chinese menu' diseases, Overlap syndrome

mixed episode PSYCHIATRY A period of time of ≥ one week in which the criteria for both manic and depressive episodes are met on nearly every day, with abrupt mood swings from sadness, irritability, and euphoria; the symptoms of an ME may include agitation, insomnia, appetite dysregulation, psychotic features, and suicidal ideation, and are of sufficient severity to cause impairment of social and occupational function and/or require hospitalization (Diagnostic and Statistical Manual of Mental Disorders, 4th ed, Washington, DC, American Psychiatric Association, 1994)

mixed field agglutination TRANSFUSION MEDICINE An in vitro phenomenon, in which two or more different populations of red cells are present in the test tube, resulting in varying intensities of agglutinating reactions, eg one cell population may agglutinate strongly and another weakly or not at all; the most common cause of mixed field agglutination is a recent blood transfusion, other causes include hemolytic disease of the newborn, twin-to-twin in utero transfusion, weak subgroup of A (often A_3) or B, leukemia, Tn polyagglutination, true chimeras; pseudo-mixed field agglutination occurs with rare blood groups, eg Sd(a+) and Lu^a

mixed function oxidase Mono-oxygenase PHYSIOLOGY An enzyme that oxidizes two substrates at once, in which usually one substrate accepts oxygen and the other furnishes two hydrogen ions, eg cytochrome P450, NADPH-cytochrome c reductase plus phosphatidyl choline; p450 is the terminal electron acceptor of the system (absorbs at 450 nm); the activity of MFO may be induced by CCl_4 and bromobenzene

mixed leukemia Biphenotypic leukemia, see there

mixed lymphocyte culture An in vitro assay of cell-mediated immunity that determines antigen specificity of HLA-A, -B, -C, -DR loci in the major histocompatibility complex; the MLC is used in HLA typing in order to obtain the closest immune match between the recipient and host and to minimize organ rejection during transplantation, serving as a predictor of graft-versus-host disease METHOD The donor lymphocytes are 'paralyzed' by irradiation preventing them from dividing, so the only cell capable of proliferation is the recipient's CD4 (helper) T cell, which undergoes blast transformation, indicating immunologic disparity between the two cells, which is more intense as the antigenic disparity between the individuals increases; the intensity of the blast transformation is measured by the degree to which transformed cells incorporate 'hot' (radiolabeled) ^{14}C or ^{3}H; MLC is also used to diagnose T-cell immunodeficiency; Cf Lymphocytotoxicity assay

mixed mesodermal tumor Malignant mixed müllerian tumor A rare carcinosarcoma of the elderly uterus CLINICAL Post-menopausal bleeding and uterine enlargement by a polypoid mass arising from the myometrium PATHOLOGY The tumors are either 'homologous', ie containing stromal cells native to the uterus, eg smooth muscle cells and fibroblasts or 'heterologous', containing stromal tissue not native to the uterus, eg bone, cartilage, fat and striated muscle, the last of which is thought to have a slightly worse prognosis; MMT of the ovary has a 1-year survival with homologous elements and six-month survival with heterologous elements; more important than the tissue of differentiation is staging; those tumors restricted to the inner half of the myometrium do relatively well; extrapelvic, lymphatic and hematogenous spread is relatively common and is associated with a 25% 5-year survival in uterine MMTs

mixed message PSYCHOLOGY A colloquial term for a form of the approach-avoidance conflict, in which a person's projects both a desire and lack of enthusiasm for a particular task, goal, or relationship, leaving the recipient of a mixed message as perplexed as the responsible party is confused

mixed tumor Pleomorphic adenoma A usually benign salivary gland tumor, that may also be seen in the breast and pancreas; mixed tumor comprises 60% of parotid gland tumors, where it is 10 times more common than in the submandibular gland, often affecting younger women PATHOLOGY The tumors may have a 'frightening' appearance, characterized by dense clusters of glandular (epithelial) and myoepithelial cells in a mucoid, myxoid, chondroid stroma; the recurrence rate reflects the adequacy of the initial excision; 2-10% are malignant; mixed tumors of the breast in humans are rare and usually benign; Cf Composite tumor

Note: 20-25% of mammary lesions of dogs are mixed tumors; see Collision tumor

mixed wound infection A skin infection containing many different organisms, including both aerobes, anaerobes and occasionally sabrobic fungi, most commonly associated with soil contamination; some of the organisms cultured by the laboratory are commensal flora and may be considered 'contaminants' by the laboratory personnel as they are uncommon causes of human disease, eg *Corynebacterium* spp, α-hemolytic streptococci, coagulase-negative staphylococci, *Propionibacterium* spp and *Bacillus* spp; other bacteria grown from wounds are best considered potential pathogens, eg *Staphylococcus aureus*, β-hemolytic streptococci, *Escherichia coli*, *Pseudomonas aeruginosa*, other pseudomonads and enterococci; anaerobic culture must be carried out on all mixed wound infections, to rule out *Bacteroides* spp, *Clostridium perfringens* and other rare clostridia, eg *C cava*, and *C liniosa*, as well as *Actinomyces israeli*, *Mycobacterium marinum* and peptostreptococci

mixing study HEMATOLOGY An assay, eg activated partial thromboplastin time, in which a 50:50 ratio of patient:control plasma is used to identify the deficiency of a particular factor or protein (Arch Pathol Lab Med 1993; 117:595OA)

MJ Megajoule, see there

MK-383 Tirofibran, see there

MK-571 A potent synthetic leukotriene D_4-receptor antagonist that inhibits exercise-induced bronchoconstriction in subjects with asthma and causes a 20% decrease in the forced expiratory volume in one second or FEV1 (N Engl J Med 1990; 323:1736)

MK-639 L-735,524 AIDS An inhibitor of HIV-1 protease that has therapeutic potential for treating HIV infection; when first administered, MK-639 results in a rapid and precipitous (up to 1000-fold) drop in HIV replication and a transient recuperation in the CD4 cell counts, but eventually is bested by the emergence of MK-639-resistant HIV-1 variants (Nature 1995; 374:569, 493, Bio/Technology 1995; 13:206) see ABT-538

MK-801 A non-competitive NMDA antagonist that inhibits opiate tolerance and attenuates the development of morphine dependence (Science 1991; 251:85); MK-801 is of potential use for treating neurodegenerative disease as it interferes with excitatory and toxic action of certain amino acids; MK-801 binds to the PCP receptor in rats, eliciting a toxic reaction; see NMDA receptors

MK-CSF Megakaryocyte colony-stimulating factor, now known as thrombopoietin, see there

MLC 1) Minimal lethal concentration, see Minimum bactericidal concentration 2) Mixed lymphocyte culture, see there

MLD 1) Metachromatic leukodystrophy, juvenile type, see there 2) Median lethal dose 3) Minimum lethal dose, see there

MLEL Malignant lymphoepithelial lesion, see there

MLNS Mucocutaneous lymph node syndrome, see Kawasaki's disease

MLO Mycoplasma-like organism(s)

Mls antigens Minor lymphocyte stimulatory antigens A group of cell surface molecules first identified in mice that are immunogenic for unprimed T cells; MAs have limited polymorphism and have two forms (Mls_a and Mls_c); anti-Mls response correlates with expression of T cell receptor Vβ molecule, is a function of intrathymic contact of CD8 T cells and is pivotal in the development of immune tolerance; during maturation of the immune system, autoreactive T cells with the T-cell receptor Vβ chain (encoded by the Mls genes) are clonally eliminated (**Nature 1991; 350:207**) see MMTV, Superantigens

Mls **genes** Minor lymphocyte stimulatory genes A family of genes encoded by mouse mammary tumor (retro)-viruses (MMTV), the protein products of which, known as 'superantigens', are capable of markedly stimulating the proliferation of CD4 T cells in mixed lymphocyte cultures

MLT Medical laboratory technician, see there

MLT(ASCP) A laboratory worker licensed in the US, equivalent to an LPN (licensed practical nurse), who is certified (by examination) by the American Society of Clinical Pathologists to perform certain lab procedures and who must complete a formal two-year-in-duration classroom and on-the-job training program; MLTs may report normal range values to physicians, but not panic values; Cf MT(ASCP)

MMM Myeloid metaplasia with myelofibrosis

MMP Matrix metalloproteinase, see there

MMPI 1) Matrix metalloprotein inhibitor, see there 2) Minnesota Multiphasic Personality Inventory A true-false test for evaluating a subject's psychological and personality 'profile'; the MMPI is used in 124 countries in 46 languages and consists of 550 questions (16 of which are repeated to ensure consistency); it is administered to those over age 15, yielding 14 ranks of personalities from 'social' to schizophrenic; it is imperative to update this fifty-year-old test, as at the time the MMPI was created, the average US citizen was 35 years old, married, lived in a small town, had had 8 years of general schooling and was employed in a skilled or semi-skilled trade; a revision (**Mayo ClinProc 1989; 64:3**) of the test divides it into a four-parameter validity scale (measuring the subjects' willingness to complete the test, inability to read, psychological defensive behavior) and a 10-parameter clinical scale (measuring various abnormal psychological tendencies (depression, sexual orientation, hypochondriasis, hypomania, hysteria, introversion, paranoia, psychasthenia or anxiety, psychopathy and schizophrenia); see Psychological testing

MMPS Medical mortality predictor scale A system used to predict the outcome of certain diseases

MMR vaccine (live) Measles-mumps-rubella vaccine A trivalent vaccine containing an aqueous suspension of live attenuated strains of measles, mumps, and rubella viruses grown in chick or duck embryo cells; the vaccine is supplied in a lyophilized form for reconstitution prior to administration; MMR is usually given at 15 months of age, and repeated at entry to middle school (± 11-12 years old); MMR may be given at 12 months of age in areas of recurrent measles transmission; if given prior to 12 months of age, it should be repeated at 15 months (recommendations per the American Academy of Pediatrics and Centers for Disease Control and Prevention, in **N Engl J Med 1992; 327:1794**) in the 1970s annual incidence of measles was $366/10^5$, of mumps $240/10^5$, and rubella $104/10^5$; use of the MMR vaccine has resulted in coverage of ≥ 95% in Finland and a 99% decrease in the incidence of all three diseases with < 30 cases of each per year; the vaccine 'takes' in the vast majority; failure is due to poor timing of the dose, ie before 15 months of age, due to persistence of residual maternal antibodies or due to poor storage of the vaccine; MMR is contraindicated in pregnancy, immunodeficiency states, therapeutic immunosuppression or in acute febrile disease; see Killed vaccine, Live attenuated vaccine

MMTV Mouse mammary tumor virus A group B oncovirus, the genome of which is integrated in the mouse genome, forming Vβ deletion ligands or minor lymphocyte stimulating genes, which are encoded in MMTV's open reading frame; in the MMTV experimental system, mice are congenitally infected with MMTV, and are immune tolerant to certain antigens common to the virus and to the characteristic tumor; the MMTV may produce suppressor T cells that blunt the T- and B-cell response to the tumor antigens, accelerating tumor growth; see Minor lymphocyte antigens, Superantigen

MMWR Morbidity and Mortality Weekly Report A news bulletin produced by the Centers for Disease Control and Prevention (CDC) in Atlanta, Georgia that provides a vast array of epidemiological information, eg statistics on the incidence of AIDS, rabies, rubella, sexually-transmitted and other communicable diseases, causes of mortality, eg homicide and suicide, divided by region, sex, age and race

M'Naghten rule FORENSIC PSYCHIATRY A ruling promulgated in 1843 by the English House of Lords that holds that a person accused of a crime is not criminally liable thereof if he/she '...*was laboring under such a defect of reason from disease of the mind as not to know the nature and quality of the acts, or, if he did know it, that he did not know that what he was doing was wrong.*'; see Insanity defense, Temporary insanity

Mo1 A member of the adhesive glycoproteins found on neutrophils and monocytes, designated as Leu-CAM, which functions as the receptor for iC3b, a complement component that mediates complement-dependent monocyte functions, possibly by direct release of inflammatory mediator(s); see CD18/CD11 family

mobile domain EVOLUTIONARY BIOLOGY Any of a number of discrete block of amino acids (domains) that were in part preserved and modified only slightly to adjust to an intracellular need; MDs range from 18 residues in length (eg collagen, leucine-rich domains, 'Gla' domains, and others) to 100 or more (eg lectin-like, SH2, SH3 domains) and have been divided into those that contain disulfide bonds (eg complement C9, epidermal growth factor, Fn1, Fn2, and others) and those that do not (eg collagen-binding, Fn3, SH2, and SH3 domains) (**Sci Am 1993; 269/4:53**)

Mobiluncus A recently identified genus of organisms that are gram-positive, curved, which have spinning motility and have been implicated in bacterial vaginosis

Mobin-Uddin filter see Inferior vena caval filter

MOC-31 A monoclonal antibody that identifies a 40-kD membrane glycoprotein reportedly present in epithelial but not in mesothelial cells; MOC-31 is of potential use in differentiating adenocarcinoma cells from their cytologic mimics, reactive mesothelial cells in washings of body cavity fluids (Arch Pathol Lab Med 1994; 118:265OA)

moccasin distribution A pattern of foot involvement in chronic tinea pedis due to *Trichophyton rubrum*, most common in adult males, with Cushing's disease or lymphoproliferative disorders (implicating defective cell-mediated immunity) CLINICAL Asymptomatic, finely scaling diffuse erythematous lesion

Note: Acute tinea pedis, caused by *Trichophyton mentagrophytes*, is an intensely pruritic vesiculo-bullous and macerating lesion

model-fitting analyses An approach that permits estimates of genetic and environmental effects of a process (N Engl J Med 1993; 328:1150OA)

modeling PHYSIOLOGY The process of bone formation that ends with bone maturation; remodeling is a dynamic process of osseous turnover that maintains the structural integrity of bones, a function of the 'stress lines' and stresses that are perpendicular to the bone's long axis PSYCHOLOGY A normal process that occurs as a part of personality development, in which a child learns appropriate social and cognitive behaviors by imitating a significant other who himself/herself is socially accepted; these behaviors are positively reinforced and eventually integrated into the child's personality profile RESEARCH The simulation of an experiment based on hypothetical conditions, considered by some to be a 'third form of science' in addition to theory and experimentation; modeling allows the examination of a problem and the testing of highly complex hypothetical solutions thereto, performing only the experiments with a high probability of success based on predictions; modeling is used in neural networks, molecular dynamics, cell membrane interactions and in biosphere analysis

modem Modulator/demodulator COMPUTERS An acoustic coupling device that converts a computer's digital signals to analog signals, allowing transmission of data through telephone lines, which are most commonly used in the health care setting for accessing electronic databases, the cost of which is a function of the time 'on-line'; the data is transmitted in bauds (equal to one bit/second); the standard speeds of transmission are 300 baud, 1200 baud, 2400 baud and 9600 baud; V.32 bis transmits data at 14.4 kbps; the V.34 transmit data at 28.8–57.0 kbps

moderate-impact sport SPORTS MEDICINE A generic term for any physical activity or sport in which there is relatively intense wear and trauma of weight-bearing joints, in particular the foot, knee, and hip; MISs include aerobics, backpacking, ballet, cross-country skiing, downhill (alpine) skiing, ice-skating, softball, speedwalking, tennis, and volleyball; MIS activities are allowable after hip and knee arthroplasty if the person participating therein uses viscoelastic shoe inserts and sport- and joint-specific therapy (Mayo Clin Proc 1995; 70:342OA) Cf High-impact sport, Moderate-impact sport, No-impact sport

modified neck dissection A subtotal resection of the neck, usually performed for carcinoma of the floor of the mouth; most modifications of the radical neck dissection hinge around preservation of the spinal accessory nerve, internal jugular vein, and the sternocleidomastoid muscle; MND in selected cases is equal to RND for contolling disease and has the obvious advantage of better post-operative function and cosmetics; see Commando operation; Cf Radical neck dissection

modified radical mastectomy The standard surgical procedure for localized carcinoma of the breast, which includes the breast, an ellipse of skin, usually with the nipple and the axillary lymph nodes; the controversy continues to rage, as to whether the more cosmetically acceptable 'lumpectomy', or slightly larger 'quadrantectomy' procedures coupled with radiation represent adequate long-term therapy for breast cancer, see Lumpectomy

Note: Radical mastectomies, which include the pectoral muscle, are rarely performed, given the common complication of extensive lymphedema of the arm on the side of the surgery, the compromise in quality of life and the rarity of post-mastectomy angiosarcoma

Modigliani syndrome Pseudo-goiter Excessive cervical lordosis of the cervical spine in which there is a reversed 'C' or swan-like configuration or a somewhat elongated neck; the four cases in the original report were referred to the clinician for 'goiter'

The gracile neck seen in these patients was fancifully likened to the women drawn by Amedeo Modigliani, eg Lunia Czechowski, 1919 (Cleveland Clin Quart 1975; 42:319)

modulation Regulation of the rate at which a specific gene is transcribed

MODY Maturity onset diabetes mellitus of the young A mild form of NIDDM, with the onset of disease occurring as < than age 25; MODY has been linked to both a diabetes mellitus susceptibility gene on chromosomes 20, the identity of which is unknown, and a defect of the glucokinase gene on chromosome 7 (N Engl J Med 1993; 328:697OA); An AD [MIM 125850] variant of non-insulin-dependent diabetes mellitus (NIDDM), the gene for which is located on the long arm of chromosome 20, probably 20q13 (Proc Natl Acad Sci 1991; 88:1484, N Engl J Med 1993; 328:697OA) see NIDDM

mogul sign Third mogul sign A mogul is a mammillation of packed snow found on a ski slope; in radiology, moguls are sharply demarcated (suggestive of serosal covering, ie extrapulmonary) margins seen on a plain chest film; the left-sided moguls are of interest: the third mogul is an abnormal protuberance located below the left mainstem bronchus and pulmonary artery corresponding to an enlarged or herniated left atrial appendage seen in rheumatic heart disease, a pericardial defect, disease of the chordae tendineae or papillary muscle, papillary muscles, left atrial tumors, cardiomyopathy; alternatively, the left ventricle may be elevated in tetralogy of Fallot, Ebstein anomaly or in a left-sided ascending aorta in corrected transposition of the great vessels; the first mogul is paratracheal in location and corresponds to the aortic arch; the second mogul is left of the carina, located above the left mainstem bronchus and corresponds to the main pulmonary artery; the fourth mogul corresponds to the cardiac apex and lies on the left hemidiaphragm

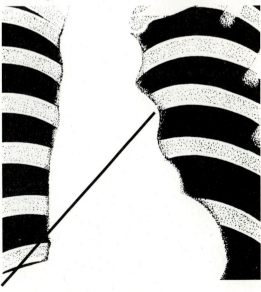

mogul sign

Mohs surgery CANCER CHEMOSURGERY A therapeutic modality for treating broad-based, but shallow basal and squamous cell carcinomas, in particular lesions that are 1-2 cm, recurring or cancer recurring-prone sites (nose, eyes, ears) and aggressive histologic subtypes, eg morphea-like basal cell carcinoma TECHNIQUE The surface of the lesion plus 3–5-mm margin of normal tissue is coagulated with dichloracetic acid, overlaid with a 20% zinc chloride paste and covered with an occlusive dressing; the $ZnCl_2$ fixes the tissue similar to formaldehyde and after 24 to 48 hours, a 'saucer' of tissue is removed and submitted for frozen section analysis to determine sites, if any of deep tumor extension; although tedious in short-term, MS reduces the incidence of recurrent disease, while preserving non-involved tissue

MOHS is also an acroeponym for Microscopically-Oriented Horizontal Section

molality A fraction of a solution that is expressed in moles of solute per kilogram of solvent

molarity The amount of substance of a solution that is expressed in moles of solute per liter of solution (mol/L)

molar tooth appearance MICROBIOLOGY A descriptor for the appearance of colonies of *Actinomyces israeli*, which are rounded, raised and have a glistening, white-yellow pearly bossellated surface, fancifully likened to molars

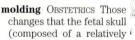

molding OBSTETRICS Those changes that the fetal skull (composed of a relatively rigid face and base and the mobile cranial vault) undergoes to accommodate itself into the birth canal

mole DERMATOLOGY A nonspecific term used by lay persons for any pigmented lesion, benign or malignant OBSTETRICS Hydatidiform mole, see there

molecular anthropology A field of evolutionary biology that analyses the time-dependent changes in the human genome; the rate of change in nucleotides is four times faster in some lower mammals, eg the rat than in humans, raising the question whether the use of a universal molecular clock can be applied in sorting out various species, based on the rate of mutations (Science 1995; 265:1907RN)

molecular biology The newest major discipline of science that marked its birth with the publication of Watson and Crick's seminal report, *'General Implications of the Structure of Deoxyribonucleic Acid'* (Nature 1953; 171:737), which elucidated the double helical nature of DNA; molecular biology seeks to understand the mechanisms controlling gene expression, in physiological and 'disease' states, and will ultimately provide the tools necessary for treating genetic diseases Note: A major new vantage point will be reached in this field when the entire human genome is sequenced, a project projected for completion by the year 2005; see Human genome project

molecular chaperone A generic term for a protein that enhances the proper conformational folding of newly produced proteins within cells and enhances the assembly of proteins into complexes; although some small proteins may be able to fold sans chaperon (sic), many proteins require one or more passes through chaperone complexes for optimal folding; proteins that may be regulated through chaperone interactions include tyrosine kinases (eg v-src, Wee1), serine/threonine kinases (eg v-raf), nuclear receptors (eg steroid receptors), heat shock proteins, and others (Science & Medicine July/August 1995, p41)

molecular clock Evolutionary clock A term referring to the finding that mutations occur at a relatively constant rate in any gene; the more mutations there are in a given segment of DNA, eg that which encodes mitochondrial proteins, the older it is, and this would allow determination of the point of divergence of similar proteins in different species

molecular disease A generic term for any condition that is traceable to a defect in the gene encoding one or a limited number of molecules, eg sickle cell anemia or Gaucher's disease; see Inborn errors of metabolism

molecular dynamics The science of simulating the motion of a system of particles, which provides biologists with the computational and theoretical framework necessary to explore molecular configurations; the complexity of biological macromolecules and their interactions caused the field to remain in its infancy until supercomputers became available, structural data based on NMR and X-ray analyses was refined, newer equations were integrated, which restricted the simulations to specific sites of interest, reducing the computation time by a factor of 10 to 100; the field of molecular dynamics promises to speed development of drugs through rational design, elucidate the role of flexibility in ligand binding, facilitate calculation of free energy changes, and identify causes of genetic mutations

molecular epidemiology A rapidly evolving field that studies the relatedness of microorganisms based on variations in shared gene sequences (eg *hsp65* for *Mycobacterium* spp) using molecular genetic techniques, eg ribotyping, and chromosomal fingerprinting; at its current stage of development, the most viable data in ME is provided by direct sequencing of PCR-amplified gene segments (Arch Pathol Lab Med 1995; 119:131OA); ME is of use in determining the source of a pathogen, and relating it to similar organisms present in the environment (N Engl J Med 1994; 331:98IOA)

molecular evolution The change in the molecular (as opposed to bone) structure of organims as they evolve Note: A second definition for the term molecular evolution has been introduced, to wit, '…the process of selecting random collections of combinatorially synthesized molecules', a practice deplored by W Bains (Bio/Technology 1994; 12:433C), who suggests the term 'Darwinian cloning' for the latter definition

molecular genetic criteria A nonspecific term for parameters used to detect, define or diagnose a disease by analysis of DNA or RNA transcripts, rather than by indirect methods that detect transcriptional products, ie protein, enzymes and other 'processed' molecules; eg lipids and carbohydrates; the role of molecular genetics is expanding and becoming an important adjunct to other diagnostic modalities, eg surgical pathology and laboratory medicine, and in some cases actually (by virtue of increased specificity and sensitivity) replacing traditional diagnostic criteria

molecular Koch's postulates MOLECULAR PATHOLOGY A series of modifications of Koch's original postulates on the pathogenesis of infection diseases, which provide a framework for determining the molecular genetic basis of pathogenicity of infetious diseases (and disease in general)

1) The phenotype or property under investigation should be associated significantly more often with pathogenic members of a genus, species, or strain than with nonpathogenic members

2) Specific inactivation of the gene or genes putatively linked to the pathogenesis of the condition should result in a measurable decrease in virulence

3) Restoration of full pathogenicity should follow replacement of the mutated (attenuated) form of the gene with the original (wild-type) putatively pathogenic gene (GL Mandell, RG Douglas Jr, JE Bennett, Eds, Principles and Practice of Infectious Diseases,

3rd ed, Churchill-Livingstone, New York, 1990) see Koch's postulates

molecular medicine A generic term for the application of the techniques of molecular biology to clinical medicine; MM encompasses 'diagnostic' methods, eg Southern (and other direction) blot hybridizations, DNA signal amplification by PCR, and the use of agents produced by recombinant DNA techniques, eg biological response modifiers and vaccines, and more recently the insertion and manipulation of the genome per se

molecular memory CHEMISTRY A poorly understood phenomenon whereby the functional properties of a substance depends on the sample's history; there is a growing body of spectroscopic evidence that many proteins undergo profound but reversible conformational changes that may be imprinted by the protein's ligand (**Nature 1995; 374:596N&v**)

molecular motor CELL BIOLOGY A generic term for any protein present in the cytoplasm that effects movement, in particular of organelles and macromolecules; MMs include kinesin, which is anchored by kinectin (**Science 1995; 267:1834**), dynein and others

molecular prognostication A generic term for the use of the techniques of molecular biology and immunopathology to determine the prognosis of a malignant, premalignant, or other disease process; a number of techniques and approaches have been used with varying degrees of reliability and reproducibility and it is likely as the nascent 'discipline' of MP matures, tumor- and site-specific MP profiles will include evaluation of total DNA content (by flow cytometry), fractional allelic loss (by Southern blot analysis), microsatellite instability (by PCR amplification followed by gel electrophoresis), activating mutations of proto-oncogenes (eg K-*ras*), and loss of or mutational inactivation of tumor-suppressor genes (eg p53, and *DCC*) (see **N Engl J Med 1994; 331:213OA**)

molecular scissors Ribozymes, see there

molecular sieve chromatography Gel filtration chromatography, see there

molecular tectonics The science of the chemical construction of organized architectures, as the '*ability to construct organized nanoscale... and bulk inorganic materials from molecular compenents is of importance in electronics, catalysis, magnetism, sensory devices, and mechanical design.*' (**Nature 1993; 365:499**)

molecular therapeutics see Recombinant pharmacology

molluscum bodies Intracytoplasmic inclusion bodies seen within the epithelial cells of molluscum contagiosum, composed of aggregates of molluscum contagiosum virus, a member of the poxvirus family; the bodies first appear as minute ovoid eosinophilic structures in the lower stratum Malpighii immediately above the basal cell layer of the epidermis; as the cells mature, the molluscum bodies become larger than their host cell pushing the nucleus to the side; EM reveals a 230 nm in length nucleoid that is rectangular viewed en face, and dumbbell-shaped in profile

MOM Multiple of mean LABORATORY MEDICINE A statistic calculation of use for highly variable analytes, eg α-fetoprotein, which changes with fetal age; MOMs are used to establish a cut-off between normal and abnormal values, eg about 90% of anencephalics and about 80% of spina bifida infants have AFP-MOM values of greater than 2.5; Cf Cut-off values

MOMs Mitochondrial outer membrane proteins

mo/ma Monocyte/macrophage

'Monday death' OCCUPATIONAL MEDICINE An occupation-related phenomenon in the dynamite industry, attributed to exposure to nitroglycerin and ethylene glycol dinitrate; during the week, the workers developed 'tolerance' to these two substances which are known to cause throbbing headaches, tachycardia, palpitations, nausea, vomiting and alcohol intolerance; after a week-end of abstinence the affected workers suffered sudden death on Monday

Monday morning sickness Exertional rhabdomyolysis, see there

Monday sickness Humidifier lung, see there

monellin A carbohydrate-free, 94-residue heterodimeric protein produced by the African fruit, serendipidy, *Dioscoreophyllum cumminsii* Diels, which contains a 45-residue A chain and a 50-residue B chain linked by weak noncovalent bonds; monellin, like thaumatin is a sweet protein with a high affinity for the sweet taste receptors, eliciting a sensation of sweetness that is 10^6 times sweeter than D-glucose on a molar basis (**Bio/Technology 1992; 10:561**) see Sweet protein, Thaumatin; Cf Artificial sweeteners

monensin LABORATORY MEDICINE A naturally occurring antibiotic that can be chemically modified (eg by amide substitution) to serve as a sodium-selctive ionophore (sensor) in the clinical analysis of electrolytes; substituted monensin appear to be less sensitive to interference by various substances (eg drugs) in the urine and in other body than the standard synthetic ionophores, eg Fluka I and Fluka III (**Am Clin Lab Feb 1994**)

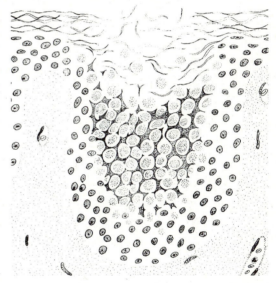

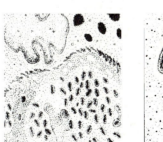
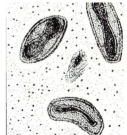

molluscum contagiosum

mongolian heart A complex of cardiac anomalies affecting 40-60% of those with trisomy 21, which includes ventricular septal defect and atrioventricular canal (endocardial cushion defects), less commonly, tetralogy of Fallot, secundum atrial septal defect and patent ductus arteriosus; in adults, aortic regurgitation and mitral valve prolapse may occur; cultured fibroblasts from trisomy 21 patients have an increased adhesiveness, implying an association with septal and cushion defects

Mongolian spot DERMATOLOGY A relatively large macule that are slate-gray in color due to the Tyndall effect, which have variably defined margins, usually over the presacral regions, posterior thighs, legs, back, and shoulders, most common in Blacks and Orientals, less in Caucasians, often fading with age (persisting in 4% of Japanese adolescents); Mongolian spots are of no clinical significance; the lesion is thought to be due to arrested migration of melanocytes from the neural crest to the epidermis; the pigment changes are confined to the dermis, and characterized by slender wavy dendritic cells admixed with melanin

monilethrix Beaded hair disease An AD [MIM 158000] condition characterized by short brittle and beaded hair that may evolve to alopecia, which is accompanied by an ↑ cataract formation

monitor COMPUTERS see Video display terminal HEALTH CARE INDUSTRY Any parameter that is regularly and consistently used to evaluate the quality of care LABORATORY MEDICINE A component of an instrument that detects physical or chemical fluctuations in electromagnetic radiation

monitor pathology PEDIATRICS A colloquial term referring to the constellation of responses (eg anxiety, feelings of helplessness) that the parents of a child presumed to be at risk for SIDS have when an apnea monitor is in place at home (Technology Rev July 1995, p31) see Apnea monitor

monkey see Executive monkey, SAIDS, Silver Spring Monkeys, SIV

(the) 'Monkey' connection A colloquial term for the poorly understood relationship between the simian immunodeficiency virus (SIV_{MAC}) and HIV-1 and HIV-2, which cause similar clinical disease and share an R gene; Cf Africa connection, Mosquito connection

monkey face A fanciful descriptor for the appearance trophoblasts of *Giardia lamblia* which have a semi-piriform shape, bearing two nuclei at the broad end and flagella at the tapered end

monkey juice SPORTS MEDICINE A pituitary extract from the rhesus monkey that is high in growth hormone, which was transiently popular among athletes as a possible performance-enhancing agent; the complete lack of efficacy of the hormone in humans, coupled with the high price of the 'donors' ended this form of monkey business (JC DeLee, D Drez, Jr, Eds, Orthopedic Sports Medicine WB Saunders, Philadelphia, 1994)

monoamine oxidase A flavin-rich catcholamine-metabolizing* enzyme [EC 1.4.3.4] that is located on the outer mitochondrial membrane; the two (or more) forms of MAO, MAO-A and MAO-B, differ in molecular weight and tissue distribution, and are present in varying amounts in the liver, basal ganglia, hippocampus, cerebral cortex, and cerebellum, and are regulated by different genetic and hormonal factors

*Other MAO substrates include MPTP, tryptamine and tyramine

monocle sign A morphological variation seen on a plain chest film of the central pulmonary artery, which when partially calcified and viewed 'on end' simulates a calcified lymph node

monoclonal antibody MAb A highly specific antibody formed either naturally (eg cold hemagglutinin disease, plasma cell dyscrasia) or synthetically by fusing an immortal cell (mouse myeloma) to a cell producing an antibody against a desired antigen; the technique was pioneered by Köhler and Milstein (Nature 1975; 256:495), partially based on Jerne's network hypothesis (all workers shared the 1984 Nobel prize); certain immunogens elicit an inadequate response in mice; to this end, monoclonal antibodies have been produced in rabbits MAbs are of use in diagnostics by radioactively-labelling MAbs to target malignant cells, detecting metastases, differentiating tumor subtypes with batteries of MAbs against intermediate filaments or membrane antigens, screening body fluids for microorganisms or measuring levels of circulating hormones; MAbs had been envisioned as having potential as 'magic bullets', which would destroy malignant cells; B72.3 is a MAb expressed in 50% of breast carcinomas and 90% of endometrial, GI (colon, gastric), lung, ovary and pancreatic carcinomas; when radiolabelled with ^{131}I or ^{90}Yt, primary and metastatic malignancy is detectable in circa 70% of cases by gamma scans; recently monoclonal antibodies have been reported to be of therapeutic use (antibody directed the platelet glycoprotein IIb/IIIa receptor) in preventing ischemic complications of coronary angioplasty (N Engl J Med 1994; 330:956OA) see Hybridoma

monoclonal gammopathy of undetermined significance Benign monoclonal gammopathy CRITERIA Normal hemoglobin, serum albumin less than 20 g/L (US: < 2 g/dl), presence of an M-component, no Bence-Jones proteinuria, < 5% plasma cells in the bone marrow, no osteolytic lesions; with time, 20-40% of MGUS progress to malignant monoclonality Note: Monoclonal 'spikes' are usually malignant when the spike is greater than 20 g/L (US: 2 g/dl), the other immunoglobulins are ↓ and Bence-Jones proteinuria is present (non-secretory monoclonal gammopathies comprise 1-2% of all myelomas); in a long-term (20-35 years) of 241 patients with MGUS, 47% had died of unrelated disease, 19% had stable serum M protein, 10% had ↑ M protein without developing myeloma or related disease; 24% (59 patients) had developed progressive disease in the form of multiple myeloma (39/59), systemic amyloidosis (8/59), macroglobulinemia (7/59) and malignant lymphoproliferative process (5/59) (Mayo Clini Proc 1993; 68:26); in one series of (851) patients with monoclonal gammopathy, 66.9% had MGUS, 13.5% multiple myeloma, 8.9% primary systemic amyloidosis, 5.2% lymphomas and others (see N Engl J Med 1994; 330:920CPC) Note: MGUS differs from myeloma in that the plasma cells in the bone marrow are < 20%, and the ESR and monoclonal component are lower (J Int Med 1993; 234:165)

monoclonal immunoglobulin A protein produced by clonally expanded immunoglobulin-producing cells, and occurs in multiple myeloma, Waldenström's disease, chronic lymphocytic leukemia and other lymphoproliferative disorders; monoclonal immunoglobulin production may be evoked by other malignancies, eg adenocarcinoma and carcinomas of the bladder, cervix and liver, as well as angiosarcoma and Kaposi sarcoma; nonmalignant conditions associated with monoclonality include infections (eg *Acanthocheilonema perstans*, *Endolimax nana*, *Entameba hartmanni*, filariasis, schistosomiasis, septicemia, syphilis, trichuriasis, TB, viral hepatitis), hematologic disorders (anemia, autoimmune hemolytic anemia, hereditary spherocytosis, thalassemia), autoimmune disease (glomerulonephritis, pemphigus vulgaris, scleroderma), and others, eg chronic hepatopathies and nephropathies, amyloidosis, acute porphyria, chronic salpingitis, systemic capillary leak syndrome, Gaucher's disease, uterine fibromas, cerebrovascular disease, atherosclerosis

Note: Although the terms monoclonal antibody and monoclonal immunoglobulin describe the same molecule, the former often refers to the product of an in vitro phenomenon, in which two disparate cells are fused, forming a 'hybridoma'; the term monoclonal immunoglobulin is of use to indicate a protein produced in vivo under natural conditions by a clonally expanded cell under malignant or benign circumstances; see Hybridoma

monoculture AGRICULTURE The cultivation of a single food crop in a confined space or farm; monoculture may result in less sustainable agricultural and land management policies, especially in developing countries; monoculture is equated with 'modernization', ie application of technology and capital; the end result is often specialization of crops, in particular those that have a world market, and economies of scale that favor rich farmers, reducing employment opportunities and economic diversity; monoculture also is responsible for three major problems in conservation: it reduces biodiversity, increases the use of fossil fuels and chemical pesticides and fertilizers, resulting in air and water pollution, and mechanization often hastens soil erosion (Sci Am 1994; 270/7:30) see Polyculture

monocyte A monocytic phagocyte of marrow origin that derives from a common progenitor, CFU-GM (colony-forming unit, granulocyte-monocyte); the monocyte 'daughter' cells circulate in the blood, forming both resident and transient populations in various sites; resident monocytes (histiocytes) include Kupffer cells in the liver, Langerhans cells in the dermis, microglial cells in the brain, pleural, peritoneal, alveolar macrophages and osteoclasts; the circulating monocyte makes up 2-5% of the circulating WBC population, measures 15-25 μm, has a reniform nucleus with lacy chromatin and gray blue cytoplasm containing lysosomal enzymes, including acid phosphatase, arginase, cathepsins, collagenases, deoxyribonuclease, lipases, glycosidases, plasminogen activator and others and surface receptors, eg FcIgG and C3R; monocytes are less efficient in phagocytosis than neutrophils but have a critical role in antigen processing

monocyte chemotactic protein–1 A human homologue of JE, a murine gene cloned from platelet-derived growth factor (PDGF)-stimulated fibroblasts; MCP-1 is a potent macrophage chemoattractant produced by vascular endothelial and smooth muscle cells after activation by oxidized lipoproteins and is present in macrophage-rich atherosclerotic lesions (Arch Pathol Lab Med 1992; 116:1292oa)

monocyte-derived neutrophil chemotactic factor see Interleukin-8

monocyte-phagocytic system The most correct term for nonspecific immune responses which are carried out by the monocyte/macrophage cell line and based in the spleen; the term 'reticuloendothelial system' continues to be the more popular, albeit illogical and incorrect, synonym

monocytosis A relative or absolute ↑ in the number of monocytes, which may be a benign reactive process, premalignant or frankly malignant (non-Hodgkin's or Hodgkin's lymphoma); reactive monocytosis may be due to infections, eg brucellosis, cat-scratch disease, HIV-1, infectious mononucleosis, malaria, Rocky Mountain spotted fever, trypanosomiasis, TB; reactive monocytosis includes histiocytic lymphadenitis, nonspecific lymphoid hyperplasia, and a syndrome which may evolve toward lymphoma

monogamy The state of having only one spouse, or (for animals) one mate; in the UK, 1:20 married ♂ and 1:50 ♀ had had > 1 partner in the previous year (New York Times 1 Februrary 1994; C9) adjective **monogamous**

monokines Cytokines, see there

monopsony HEALTH CARE INDUSTRY The power that a large paying segment of the users of a service, eg health care, have over controlling the price of that service without fear that the providers of the services, eg the physicians, will refuse to render the service for a fair market price (J Am Med Assoc 1990; 263:1981)

monosodium glutamate see MSG

monozygotic twins Identical twins Twins resulting from resulting from the division of a single fertilized egg, which usually share a common chorion and placenta, although usually each may have a separate amnion Note: Both terms are in active use, identical is more colloquial, monozygotic more formal; Cf Fraternal twins

monster adjective Pertaining or referring to anything (eg a cell or entire organism that is strange, bizarre, or extremely unusual noun A popular term of waning popularity for a person with severe external malformations that may (in the politically insensitive) evoke images and reactions reserved for carnival freaks

monster, acardiac A variant form of twinning in which there is circulatory reversal through various interplacental anastomoses in a diamnionic-monochorionic placenta; malformations range from major malformations in the face of normal skeletal and cerebral structures to complete lack of limbs; usually the umbilical artery is single and the twins are of the same sex; four-legged monster (J Bone & Joint Surg 1982; 64:88)

monster cells NEUROPATHOLOGY Large bizarre tumor giant cells, characterized by splayed nucleoplasm, a complex nuclear membrane, often with florid mitotic activity with tri- and quad-polar mitotic figures; the embryologic lineage is often indeterminant; MCs are not necessarily malignant and rarely occur in normal epididymal cells, or in benign fibrous histiocytoma, but are more common in malignant fibrous histiocytoma, undifferentiated sarcomas and in grade III or IV astrocytoma (figure); despite their 'frightening' appearance, tissue cultures of monster cell tumors reveal that these cells have no growth advantage, and may actually represent effete end cells, in contrast to smaller tumor cells which grow aggressively in culture; Cf Giant cells

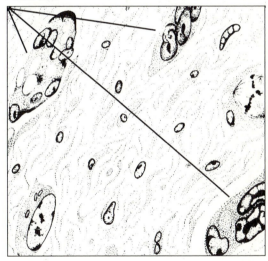

monster cells

monstrocellular astrocytoma A morphologic variant of astrocytoma grade IV, less commonly of grade III, which is characterized by abundant pleomorphic and bizarre tumor giant cells with eosinophilic intra- and extranuclear inclusions, which has a very aggressive clinical course with a poor prognosis

Monte Carlo simulation A mathematical method that evaluates high-dimensional integrals by applying probabalistic sampling, a technique used in analyzing 'queuing' theory (see there) problems, which requires the construction of a model of a process in which the events are not completely predictable; the process is then simulated multiple times, each time assigning the values in a random fashion; each of these values is selected, usually by computer from a distribution of possible values, allowing estimation of the average values and distributions of the simulation; Monte Carlo simulations may be applied to a complex structure, eg a protein, allowing it to arrange in such a way that energy is minimized; in reverse Monte Carlo simulation, the structural model is adjusted so as to minimize the difference between the calculated diffraction pattern and that measured experimentally, so that good agreement is inevitable

Montevideo units OBSTETRICS A graphic portrayal of uterine activity, which corresponds to the product of the uterine contractions in 10 minutes multiplied by the intensity of the contractions (the average intrauterine pressure peaks of all contractions occurring in the same 10 minute span)

The term was coined by Caldeyro-Barcia and Alvarez of Uruguay (capitol Montevideo)

Montezuma's revenge Traveler's diarrhea, see there

Montreal platelet syndrome An AD [MIM 231200] condition characterized by giant platelets, thrombocytopenia, a prolonged bleeding time, spontaneous platelet aggregation in vitro at pH 7.4 and normal platelet aggregation in response to ADP, collagen and ristocetin

Montreal Protocol An international accord signed by 35 countries freezing chlorofluorocarbon (CFC) production at the 1986 level, with further reductions in their use by the end of the century; CFCs (and NO_2) are responsible for depleting the ozone layer that protects the earth from ultraviolet radiation; hydrochlorofluorocarbons (HCFCs) are an interim substitute for CFCs that also deplete the ozone layer but to a lesser extent; the MP did not include dates for elimination of HCFC production; the most recent revision of the protocol cuts CFCs to 50% of its current use by 1995, to be phased out completely by 2000; halons will also be eliminated by 2000 except for their use in fire-fighting; carbon tetrachloride and methylchloroform will be phased out by the year 2000 and 2005 respectively; one 13-nation 'breakaway' group has announced an even more rapid reduction in the use of these chemicals (**Nature 1991; 349:451**) see CFCs, Greenhouse effect, Ozone layer, Ultraviolet light

MOO Multiple-user dimension, Object Oriented A virtual interface also described as a shared customizable environment for day-to-day science and scientific communication that runs on a computer at the Bioinformatics Unit of the Weizmann Institute in Jerusalem*; BioMOO is being used by an increasing number biologists on three continents who are collaborating on the design of electronic tools for doing science; MOOs offer a 'place' to meet other scientists, and 'talk' in real time, share data, research tools, and information, and showcase their research to interested colleagues; in its current incarnation, BioMOO is strictly a text-based environment, where users communicate with each other by typing dialog; researchers at PARC (Xerox's Palo Alto Research Center) are finishing the next generation of MOO, called Jupiter, which will include full-color graphics, windows, audio, and video (**Science 1994; 264;900N&V**)

*To visit BioMOO, telnet to: bioinfo.weizmann.ac.il 8888 or 132.76.55.12 8888; at the BioMOO welcome screen, type 'connect guest'

moon crescent Crescent, see there

moon face A rounded face with a double chin, prominent flushed cheeks, and fat deposition in the temporal fossa and cheeks, which is classically seen in both Cushing's disease and syndrome and in the cri-du-chat (5p-) syndrome; the name has also been applied to a broad, round face with bright-red cheeks in well-developed, broad-chested children with pulmonic stenosis and a right-to-left shunt

moonlighting An American colloquialism, meaning to take a second job after regular working hours, ie to work 'by moonlight'; a resident's salary at a typical US teaching hospital is sufficient to cover living expenses but not to repay medical school loans (average $45 000 per person at the time of graduation from medical school); consequently, many young physicians 'moonlight' on a second job, working up to 110 or more hours per week, and are thus often overworked*; while this 'sink or swim' method of training physicians has long been the standard in the USA and functions with surprisingly few errors, occasionally there are break-downs that result in mismanagement of patients; see Libby Zion, Medical school debt

*Performing secretarial, clerical and phlebotomy duties, colloquially known as 'scut-work', rather than providing patient care

Moon's molars Mulberry molars, see there

'moonshine' An American colloquialism for illicitly distilled whiskey, intended to circumvent the high government taxes on alcoholic beverages; the equipment used for distillation may contain lead solder and be a source of chronic lead poisoning; moonshine is most commonly produced in the Southeastern US; see Saturnine gout

'moon suit' 'Space suit', see there

MOPP Mechlorethamine (nitrogen mustard), vincristine (Oncovorin), Procarbazine and Prednisone A well-studied four-drug combination chemotherapy regimen used to treat stage III Hodgkin's disease; in stage IV, MOPP is given with alternating non-cross-reacting drugs, eg MOPP-ABVD (Adriamycin, bleomycin, vinblastine and DTIC); a slightly less toxic substitute for MOPP is the BCVPP regimen (BCNU, cyclophosphamide, vinblastine, procarbazine and prednisone) TOXIC EFFECTS Sterility in both sexes, nausea, vomiting, subclinical immunosuppression with ↑ infections, and secondary myelosuppression or myelodysplasia or acute nonlymphocytic leukemia; 6-8 months of ABVD (doxorubicin-adriamycin, bleomycin, vinblastine, dacarbazine), an alternate regimen is reportedly as effective as 12 months of MOPP-ABVD and both are reportedly more effective than MOPP alone (**N Engl J Med 1992; 327:1478OA**)

moral masochism PSYCHOLOGY The need by a person to seek verbal abuse or castigation from another through such behaviors as extreme passiveness, complete subservience to the demands of others, or the provocation of negative reactions in others; MM is attributed to unresolved conflicts of early childhood

moral treatment MEDICAL HISTORY An early therapeutic philosophy applied to the treatment of those with mental disorders, based on Wm Tuke's retreat model; MT consisted of removing the afflicted from their homes and placing them in a surrogate 'family' of 250 members or less, often under the guidance of a physician in residence (**JAMA 1995; 273:923ED**)

morbid obesity CLINICAL NUTRITION A condition defined as 45 kilograms over the ideal body weight, 2 **x** greater than the ideal or standard weight, or for children, a triceps skin fold that is greater than the 95th percentile of all children (**National Health Examination Survey, Am J Dis Child 1987; 141:535**) PHYSIOPATHOLOGY Superobese subjects react to the 'stress' of weight loss by increasing lipoprotein lipase, which in the capillaries of adipose tissue, hydrolyzes triglycerides from circulating lipoproteins into free fatty acids that are taken up by adipocytes, enhancing lipid storage, making further weight loss more difficult; non-surgical therapy is rarely successful and some previously used surgical procedures (jejunocolostomy, jejunoileostomy) have been abandoned; despite significant weight loss following jejuno-ileal bypass, the procedure is complicated by steatorrhea, hepatic failure, cirrhosis, oxalate deposition, bile stone formation, electrolyte imbalance: ↓ Ca^{++}, Mg^{++}, K^+, avitaminosis, psychogenic problems, polyarthropathy, hair loss, pancreatitis, colonic pseudo-obstruction, intussusception, pneumatosis cystoides intestinalis, and blind loop syndrome); see Gastric balloon, Obesity, Pickwick syndrome

morbilliform rash *morbilliform* Latin, measles-like An exanthema most commonly due to Echovirus 9 consisting of fine, discrete maculopapules on the head and neck, rarely elsewhere, mimicking the rash of rubella, meningococcal petechiae (Waterhouse-Friderichsen syndrome), and Kawasaki's disease, which with the low-grade fever resolves in a week

Morbillivirus A genus of viruses of the Paramyxoviridae family that includes canine distemper virus, rinderpest virus, measles virus, and equine morbillivirus, the last of which may rarely infect humans (Science 1995; 268:29, 95)

moricizine A phenothiazine derivative approved by the FDA in 1990 for treating life-threatening ventricular arrhythmias, which like other Class I antiarrhythmic agents (encainide, flecainaide), reduces the fast inward sodium current of the action potential; it had been entered clinical trials (CAST-II) to determine its efficacy in suppressing asymptomatic or mildly symptomatic ventricular premature depolarizations in survivors of myocardial infarction; CAST-II was halted when 14-day treatment with moricizine, as delineated by the study protocol was associated with a five-fold increase in mortality (N Engl J Med 1992; 327:227OA)

'morning-after pill' Interception pill A high-dose estrogen given in the early post-ovulatory period to prevent implantation of a potentially fertilized egg following unprotected intercourse; MAPs include: 1) DES (diethylstilbestrol 25-50 mg/day (now contraindicated given its teratogenic potential, see DES) 2) Ethinyl estradiol 1-5 mg/day and conjugated estrogens; the morning-after pill is taken within 72 hours after an isolated midcycle coitus and continued for 5 days; the pregnancy rate is 0.3-4% SIDE EFFECTS Nausea, vomiting, breast tenderness and menstrual irregularities Note: Non-expulsion of gestational products should be followed by interventional termination; see Contraception, Norplant, Pearl index, RU 486

morning dipping PULMONARY MEDICINE A colloquial term for a measurable ↓ in the expiratory air flow rates that most commonly occurs between 2 and 4 AM, resulting in the loss of sleep due to coughing and breathlessness; MD is an indicator that more aggressive therapy is required

morning glory 'syndrome' A predominantly ocular disease complex characterized by mottled peripapillary pigment and an enlarged, funnel-shaped optic disc filled with pale tissue, surrounded by an elevated rim and tortuous radiating vessels (hence the name, morning glory, a flower); the lesion may be bilateral with impaired vision, strabismus and potentially, retinal detachment; other rare associations include cleft lip and palate, agenesis of the corpus callosum and omphalocele

morning sickness Pregnancy-related nausea often accompanied by vomiting upon awakening, thought to be related to hunger; morning sickness occurs in one-half of pregnancies in the first 2-12 weeks of gestation, which if severe, may cause dehydration and acidosis; the only drug approved by the FDA for treating this problem was Bendectin*; less effective control of morning sickness is by frequent small meals of low-fat, high-carbohydrate foods

*Which was withdrawn for this purpose due to mounting litigation for an alleged teratogenic effect, see *Daubert* v. *Merrell Dow Pharmaceuticals*

Moroccan leather skin 1) see Pigskin 2) Thickening and grooving of the skin of the face, neck, axillary folds, antecubital fossa, inguinal and periumbilical regions, a characteristic finding in pseudoxanthoma elasticum

moron see Mental retardation

morphea A disease characterized by subcutaneous sclerosis, divided by some authors into 1) A generalized form: Scleroderma and 2) A localized form, subdivided into a) Circumscribed morphea Characterized by one or more round-to-oval firm reddish plaques measuring up to several centimeters in diameter with a yellow-white center and a lilac telangiectatic border, b) Linear morphea or linear scleroderma and 3) Frontoparietal lesions (en coup de sabre) with or without hemiatrophy of the face

morphine An opium alkaloid with potent analgesic effect that owes its narcotic properties to its particular aromatic ring structure CLINICAL Euphoria, respiratory depression, drowsiness, nausea, vomiting, ↓ GI motility, and an ↑ risk of potential addiction; see Controlled drug substances, Designer drugs, Heroin, Substance abuse

morphogen Any substance, eg retinoic acid, that triggers the growth, proliferation and differentiation of cells and tissues in a concentration-dependent fashion EMBRYOLOGY A generic term for a hypothetical molecule that orchestrates the development of an organism from the stage of a single cell to early embryogenesis; the existence of morphogenic molecules responsible for indicating to a cell its orientation in time and space, was assumed* but unproven until the discovery of hedgehog proteins (New York Times 11 January 1994; C1) see Hedgehog genes

*There was speculation that retinoic acid could act as a universal morphogen, a posit that has been abandoned

mortality Death rate EPIDEMIOLOGY A parameter used in health statistics that corresponds to the total number of deaths in a population divided by the population's total number, resulting in a rate defined as deaths/1000 population; leading causes of mortality, USA: Cardiovas-cular (including arteriosclerosis and aneurysm) disease 39%, cancer 22%, cerebrovascular disease 7.6%, accidents 4.6%, pneumonia or influenza 3%, lung disease 3%, diabetes-related 1.8%, suicide 1.4%, cirrhosis 1.3%, nephritis 1.0%, homicide 1.0%, and others to 100% Mortality rate in viral infections: Rabies 99%, HIV 50+%, Ebola 20-80%, smallpox 1-30%, hepatitis B virus 3-5%, polio circa 0.1% Mortality, under age 19 Fatal injuries for 1986 (MMWR 1990; 39:442) Motor vehicle accidents 47% (33% occupants, 8% pedestrians), homicide 12.8% (usually firearms), suicide 9.6% (male:female ratio 4:1), drowning 9.2% (most common in those under age 4, 90% of which is in residential pools), fire/burns 7.2% (most common under age 4, black:white ratio, 3:1)

Mortality Probabilities Models see MPM II

mort d'amour CARDIOLOGY Death due to coitally induced cardiac overload; in one case, a robust but severely atherosclerotic man died while so engaged; while uncommonly reported, la mort d'amour may occur in anyone with underlying cardiac disease, especially in those with hypertension, arrhythmias, or with cerebral aneurysms

morular cells Spherical to ovoid variant plasma cells measuring 12-20 μm in diameter, containing an eccentric hyperchromatic nucleus and cytoplasm replete with 1-3 μm in diameter acidophilic globules (Russell bodies) filled with immunoglobulins and neurofibrillary material; when the cytoplasmic contour is smooth, the cells are 'morular', when the globules cause superficial bosselations, they are known as mulberry cells; morular cells classically occur in the brains of patients with Western African sleeping sickness (AGENT *Trypanosoma gambiense* VECTOR Tsetse fly), but may also occur in *T brucei rhodesiense* infections

c-mos MOLECULAR BIOLOGY A proto-oncogene that encodes pp39mos, a tubulin-associated serine-threonine protein kinase, aka cytostatic factor; c-mos is responsible for the arrest of meiosis in metaphase II and contributes to the formation of the mitotic spindle (Science 1991; 251:671) linked to control of the early embryonic cell cycle, the critical control point of which is polyadenylation of the cognate mRNA (Nature 1995; 374:511OA)

mosaic *adjective* A patchwork of one sharply demarcated 'jig-saw'-shaped pattern imposed upon another of different color, tissue pattern or radiologic density *noun* GENETICS An individual with two or more genotypically (karyotypically) distinct cell lines, arising from a single zygote by somatic mutation, crossing-over or nondisjunction during mitotic division, an event more common in older mothers; 30-40% of Turner syndromes are mosaics: 45,XO/46,XX; 45,XO/47,XXX and 45,XO/46,XY; 5-10% of Klinefelter patients are mosaics: 46,XY/47,XXY; 46,XY/48,XXYY; 45,X/46,XY/47,XXY; 46,XX/47,XXY; see Chimera, Freemartin

Note: The mosaic is an art form in which a surface design is produced closely inlaying colored pieces of marble, glass, tile or semiprecious stone; in the Roman empire, floors were decorated with mosaics made of large marble slabs in contrasting colors or of small marble cubes (tesserae); mosaics reached their height as an art form in the 6th century in Byzantium

mosaic artifact DERMATOLOGY A mimic of fungal infection of mucocutaneous tissues when dystrophic epithelial tissue is stained with potassium hydroxide; the 'mosaic' consists of an irregular band surrounding epithelial cells which is less translucent than the squamous cells

mosaic bone see Mosaic pattern, bone

mosaic bones Wormian bones, see there

mosaic pattern BONE A variegated pattern with haphazard cement lines (instead of the normal parallel arrangement in trabecular and cortical bone); the marrow space may be devoid of marrow elements or acellular and replaced by collagen, fibroblasts, fibroconnective and vascular tissue; these changes are due to a marked increase in bone turnover with increased osteoclastic and osteoblastic activity, calcification and accumulation of woven bone; this pattern is classically described in Paget's disease of bone and may occur in chronic osteomyelitis, irradiated bone, osteosarcoma and osteoblastoma CERVIX A colposcopic abnormality seen at an atypical transformation zone of the uterine cervix (atypical when the cervix is covered by 3% acetic acid); the fields of the sharply demarcated 'mosaic' are separated by reddish (vascularized) borders; this pattern may signify any epithelial proliferation ranging from mild dysplasia to carcinoma in situ MUSCLE A variegated pattern of distribution of dystrophin seen by immunostaining of muscle tissue from patients with Duchenne's muscular dystrophy SKIN 1) A haphazard arrangement of the minute arthrospores seen ensheathing hairs in tinea capitis caused by *Microsporum*, which differs from tinea capitis caused by *Trichophyton*, as the arthrospores are larger and appear in parallel chains outside or within the hair shafts 2) A pattern of skin involvement in which there are alternating stripes (known as the lines of Blaschko) of affected and unaffected skin; diseases with a MP are often linked to the X chromosome, and include Conradi-Hünnermann syndrome, focal dermal hypoplasia, and incontinentia pigmenti (**N Engl J Med 1994; 331:1408oA**)

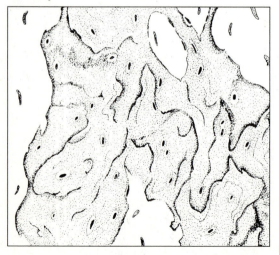

mosaic pattern, Paget's disease of bone

mosaic proteins A group of functionally diverse proteins that have evolved by duplication, insertion and deletion of a common pool of structural units or modules (defined as consensus sequences containing conserved disulfide bonds); mosaic proteins are involved in cell adhesion, migrations, embryogenesis and in the coagulation, fibrinolytic and complement pathways and include fibronectin, coagulation factor XII and tissue plasminogen activator

mosaic wart A large flat verrucoid plaque composed of confluent contiguous plantar warts, thought to be caused by HPV-2 Note: 3-7% of the population has or has had plantar warts, most commonly during early adolescence

Moses 'syndrome' A poetic term of little utility referring to the difficulties that a health care system has in trying to maintain a balance between cost, quality and access to health care, likened to the tribulations of Moses who eventually led his people to the 'Promised Land'; Cf Frankenstein 'syndrome'

mosquito An arthropod of the dipteran family Culicidae, the ♀ of which is a bloodsucker[1]; the eggs are laid on he water (which forms the basis for programs of eradication, where insecticides are spayed on stagnant water[2]), where the larvae feed on debris or occasionally other living organisms; most of the mosquitoes of medical importance in the genera include *Aedes*, *Anopheles*, *Culex*, *Stegomyia*; the mosquito a vector for various blood-borne parasites, eg filariasis (*Brugia malayi*, *Wuchereria bancrofti*), *Plasmodium* spp, *Trypanosoma* spp), and viruses, including alphaviridae, flaviviridae and togaviridae, which cause California, eastern equine, Venezuelan and western equine encephalitides, O'nyong-nyong, dengue fever, Rift valley fever and yellow fever

[1]A biological pattern that some workers believe is repeated in humans [2]Note: *Culex pipiens* are resistant to organophosphate pesticides arising from the overproduction of nonspecific esterases, mediated through amplification of the corresponding structural genes, designated B2 (**Nature 1991; 350:151, 107**)

mosquito connection A postulated relationship between the high incidence of AIDS in a farm community in Florida and the number of mosquitoes, which were thought to act as vectors in blood-to-blood transmission of HIV-1, given that the 'no known risk' group was double the national average; intense epidemiological investigation revealed that all the infected patients were in high-risk groups, eg homosexuals, intravenous drug abusers, Haitians or hemophiliacs; see Belle Glade; Cf Africa connection, Monkey connection

mossy fiber system NEUROPHYSIOLOGY A neural integration system of the cerebellar cortex that originates in various sources and provides (through the granular cells), a massive amount of innervation, up to 200 000 parallel fiber inputs for each Purkinje cell; in conjunction with the climbing fibers, the MFS provides information that is critical for proprioceptive feedback, as well as the status of those movements, and is responsible for the continuous tonic discharge of Purkinje cells (**Nature 1995; 374:450, 405**)

mossy foot Lymphostatic verrucosis, see there

most significant other SOCIAL MEDICINE The person in a patient's universe upon whom the patient most heavily depends, for moral and physical support during periods of crisis and stress; MSOs include parents, spouses, children, lovers, siblings or friends; the help of a patient's MSO may be enlisted by the medical team in patients with terminal disease

Note: In the working parlance, 'most' is being slowly deleted, such that 'significant other' is the term likely to prevail by the end of the 20th Century

moth ball syndrome A colloquial term for a congenital deficiency of glucose-6-phosphate dehydrogenase (see there), which results in hemolytic crises following exposure to naphthalene (moth balls)

Note: Moth balls are a commonly used household fumigant, composed of crystallized coal tar-derived naphthalene, effective against cloth moths and carpet beetles

moth-eaten A common adjective referring or pertaining to lesions or masses in which one radiologic density, color or low-power histological pattern with 'ragged' margins is imposed upon a dark or light background

moth-eaten alopecia Patchy hair-loss characteristic of secondary syphilis, where the hair falls out in small, scattered and irregular patches, commonly affecting the scalp but which may spread to the eyebrows to the beard; similar patchy loss may occur with trichomalacia and trichotillomania

moth-eaten bone A nonspecific descriptor for patchy osteolysis that is seen radiologically in Gaucher's disease, lethal hypophosphatasia (at the ends of the long bones with severe global defects in ossification and shortening of the long bones), leukemia, osteosarcoma, reticulum cell sarcoma and osteolytic metastases

moth-eaten macrophage A nonspecific descriptor for the histiocytes seen in amebiasis, where the ragged histiocytic contour differs from the smooth rounded margins of the *Entamoeba histolytica* trophozoites which are further distinguished from the histiocytes by the presence of ingested erythrocytes within the amoeba and their PAS positivity

moth-eaten mouse A mutant from the inbred C57BL/6J strain of mice characterized by patchy hair loss, increased susceptibility to infection, polyclonal gammopathy, impaired cell-mediated immunity and autoimmunity with immune complex deposition in the glomeruli

moth-eaten pattern LYMPH NODES A histologic morphology characterized by partial architectural effacement, mottling, irregularity of follicles, follicular and paracortical hyperplasia, focal necrosis, capsular and pericapsular infiltration, seen in infectious mononucleosis DDx CMV, EBV, other viral lymphadenitides and poorly differentiated lymphocytic lymphoma RENAL PATHOLOGY A histological descriptor for focal disintegration of the glomerular capillary basement membrane which follows spike deposition in membranous glomerulonephritis SKIN An oozing and encrusted reddish skin erosion with a sharp cutaneous margin with raised borders, characteristic of Paget's disease of the breast; extramammary Paget's disease is similar but often accompanied by pruritus; moth-eaten skin also appears in Bowen's disease and in pagetoid spread of malignant melanoma

moth-eaten skull Patchy variegated defects with a ground-glass center seen by a plain skull film in the diploe in hyperparathyroidism; this same descriptor is occasionally applied to the patchy, skull lesions seen in multiple myeloma, although the bony defects are usually more sharply demarcated and have also be termed 'punched-out'

'mother of us all' hypothesis Out of Africa hypothesis, see there

'Mother Superior' complex PSYCHIATRY A highly colloquial term for a role adopted by a psychotherapist, who injects an excessive amount of authoritarianism in the context of therapy

mother yaw The initial lesion of yaws, which develops after a 3–5-week incubation of *Treponema pallidum pertinue*, which is characterized by papules on the extremities, usually the legs that enlarge to papillomas and eventually ulcerate; see Yaws

motherhood The state of being a mother, which implies giving care to offspring who/that are perceived as belonging to the mother; this tenacious but difficult to study bond that is common to all mammals, and many vertebrates, although distinctly less common in aquatic animals, for obvious logistic reasons; in mammals, maternal touch stimulates the release of β-endorphin, without which the production of growth hormone is minimal; maternal contact also stimulates ornithine decarboxylase activity, directly affecting the synthesis of putrescine, spermadine and spermine, which regulate the synthesis of the nucleic acids in the brain, heart, lungs, spleen and other tissues; see Bonding

motif MOLECULAR BIOLOGY Any recurring design element present in a family of molecules that shares structural and usually functional similarity; eg in proteins, the 'leucine zipper' and the 'zinc finger' are DNA-binding and regulatory motifs; Cf Domain

motilin A 22-residue GI peptide that is released into the small intestine by changes in pH; motilin mediates gallbladder and smooth muscle contraction, stimulating intercibal, but not postprandial motility of the gastric antrum and the upper duodenum by stimulating specific smooth muscle receptors, a response that is lost in severe IDDM; response to motilin may be restored by simple administration of macrolide compounds, eg erythromycin

motion sickness A clinical complex that results from activation of the vestibular system, which may be related to the central triggering zone; the characteristic vomiting is often preceded by nausea, cold sweats, headache, hypersalivation and pallor; motion sickness may be studied by either placing the subjects in a slowly rotating drum, a linear accelerator or 'roller coasters'; electrogastrography is used to detect increased gastric slow wave activity TREATMENT H₁ family of antihistamines

motivational intervention A generic term for any intervention designed to change one's habits (eg the pattern and the frequency of test ordering) by using a well-respected peer to discuss the habit in question (CAP Today June 1995, p20)

motor neuron disease A term for a group of conditions characterized by progressive degeneration with dysfunction of the motor neuron or anterior horn cell, the most common of which is amyotrophic lateral sclerosis (ALS); the terms are difficult to differentiate, and thus used interchangeably and subdivided into 1) The Western Pacific form, seen in the Marianas and on Japan's Kii peninsula, which is associated with a high incidence of parkinsonism and dementia and 2) Classic or sporadic form, with an incidence rate of 2/10⁵, which is characterized by upper limb weakness, atrophy, and focal neurologic signs (Mayo Clin Proc 1991; 66:54rv)

motor oil appearance A fanciful descriptor of the golden-brown greasy fluid present in the cystic spaces of craniopharyngioma, derived from Rathke's pouch, composed of a suspension of cholesterol

motor vehicle accident PUBLIC HEALTH A preventable morbid condition that claims 45 000 lives annually (US), 60% of whom are under age 35; MVAs account for 500 000 hospitalizations and most of the 20 000 spinal cord injuries in the US, at an annual cost of $75 billion; ½ of MVA fatalities in those ages 15-45 have excess blood alcohol levels and ¼ have cocaine metabolites; the higher the population density in a given area, the lower the proportionate incidence of motor vehicular mortality (2.5/10⁵ of Manhattan residents die annually of MVA, the adjusted rate in Nevada is 558/10⁵), due to a combination of poor road conditions, higher speeds, longer time in arriving at a hospital, less use of safety belts and higher use of vehicles with rolling tendencies, eg jeeps and trucks

MOTT Mycobacteria other than *M tuberculosis* An acronym for non-tuberculous mycobacteria (eg *M avium-intercellulare* complex, *M chelonei*, *M kansasii*, *M malmoense*, and *M xenopi*) which are being increasingly recognized due to an increased awareness and by extension, diagnosis of these organisms and decreasing incidence of

M tuberculosis (The incidence of *M tuberculosis* reached its nadir in the US in 1986 and, given its relation with AIDS, has begun to increase); the ratio of MOTT:*M tuberculosis* is a function of the population and is lower in hospitals serving more indigent populations Note: *M avium-intercellulare* is often resistant to the usual antibiotics; see Runyon classification

mottled enamel Dental enamel that is punctuated by patches of white and/or brownish discoloration; ME may be due to infection and/or antibiotic therapy or fluorosis

moulage French, a cast, a mold A descriptive term for the smooth contour of the small intestine, with loss of mucosal folds, a finding that is described as characteristic of radiocontrast studies in sprue-induced atrophy

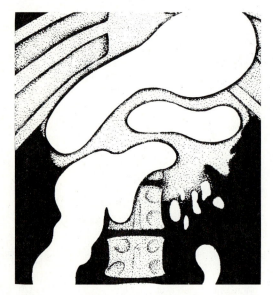

moulage

mountain medicine A subspecialty of wildness medicine that addresses the medical (and technical) aspects of high-altitude adventure travel and mountain sports, which include mountain rescue and resuscitation, high-altitude physiology and pathophysiology, as well as 'mountain diseases' per se, eg frostbite, hypobaric hypoxia, pulmonary edema, solar irradiation (N Engl J Med 1992; 326:1574BR)

mountain sickness, acute A symptom complex of usually less than a week in duration associated with rapid ascent to 2500 meters or higher, occurring in 30% of subjects above 3000 meters and 75% of subjects above 4500; in the first 8-24 hours there is marked frontal throbbing headache (worsened by exercise), nausea, vomiting and insomnia and in 4-40% of subjects, retinal hemorrhage; far less common is life-threatening high-altitude pulmonary, cerebral edema with convulsions and coma PATHOGENESIS The condition is attributed to the combined effect of hypoxia and hypercapnia; Cf Höhendiurese TREATMENT Dexamethasone; in the absence of response to the symptoms of CNS edema and physiological derangements, the subject should descend immediately; subjects who have ascended to ultrahigh (Himalayan) heights have mild but significant residual deterioration of memory, long-term verbal memory, accompanied by aphasia, perhaps the long-term effects of hypercapnia; the condition is diagnosed if a subject has three or more major symptoms including anorexia, dyspnea, fatigue, headache or insomnia; the symptoms may be ameliorated with dexamethasone; see High-altitude pulmonary edema, Höhendiurese

mountain sickness, chronic A clinical complex in which a previously acclimatized person living for prolonged periods at 4000 or more meters loses his/her tolerance to hypoxia CLINICAL Drowsiness, dyspnea, asphyxia, cyanosis, cough, nausea, vomiting, palpitations, muscular weakness, pain in the extremities, headache, giddiness, intermittent stupor and loss of weight PULMONARY FUNCTION TESTS Increased PCO_2, decreased pulmonary ventilation and arterial oxygen saturation and impairment of sensitivity of the respiratory center to hypoxia LABORATORY Intense polycythemia, with hemoglobin at 25 g/dl and hematocrit to 80%

'Mount Everest experiment' RESEARCH An experiment that is 'ludicrously difficult'*

*Performed (as one might say in climbing Mount Everest) *'because it's there'*; such experiments are reserved by the sane for those less so and justified by the investigator, who may perceive himself to be elucidating a greater truth, eg a disease mechanism

mourning reaction A 3–12-month period of depression, disillusionment, and discouragement that follows an initial stage of euphoria in patients on chronic hemodialysis; the patients initially deny illness, then recognize that they have lost their health and independence and have an uncertain future, with difficulties in performing their usual employment and in meeting both familial and financial obligations; the mourning reaction is further characterized by role reversal, marital difficulties and changes in functions; the suicide rate among hemodialysis patients is said to be 300-fold greater than a similar, but healthy population; see Dialysis dementia, Honeymoon period; Cf Melancholia

mouse COMPUTERS A device with one or more control buttons that is used to manipulate files indicated by symbolically represented by icons and to access information and execute commands from pull-down menus; a mouse consists of a weighted ball enclosed in a plastic shell allowing an arrow to be moved to various sites on the monitor's screen so that commands are given in a 'point and shoot' fashion; Cf Trackball

mouse elbow OCCUPATIONAL MEDICINE A repetitive-strain injury produced by the constant lifting and shifting of a computer mouse; ME can be minimized by use of keyboard commands and/or substitution of a trackball input device, which allows the hand and forearm to remain in one position, while the fingers do the working

'mouse incident' A case of apparent scientific misconduct that occurred at a cancer research center in New York City and pivoted around an experiment in which tissue immunogenicity was alleged to have been circumvented merely by incubating that tissue in culture medium for a few weeks; acting under pressure to produce results, the investigator allegedly used a felt-tipped marker and painted on a 'successful' engraftment of tissue from a black mouse onto a white one (JAMA 1974; 229:1391); see Cooking, Fraud in science, Trimming

mouse mammary tumor virus MMTV, see there

Movat pentachrome A five-dye connective tissue stain in which the nuclei are black, elastic fibers are purple, collagen is yellow, ground substance is blue-green and muscle is red

moxibustion A variant form of acupuncture that uses heat, in which the mugwort (*Artemisia vulgaris*) is rolled into a small cone, placed point up, burned almost to the skin, then removed; see Acupuncture, Alternative medicine

moya-moya disease *moya-moya*, Japanese, Hazy, smoky NEUROLOGY An idiopathic condition first described in 1961, the name of which derives from the cerebral angiographic appearance of prominent collateral vessels of the basal ganglia accompanying narrowed and distorted cerebral arteries with thin collateral vessels, appearing to arise in a wispy, net-like fashion from the circle of Willis, caused by slowly progressive occlusion CLINICAL Patients are in a 'fog', related to ischemia in younger patients or subarachnoid hemorrhage and altered mental status in older patients; most cases have occurred among the Japanese and appear as recurrent strokes in otherwise healthy female children and adolescents with a familial tendency, often following a febrile illness with abrupt onset of hemiparesis, transient aphasia, convulsions and spontaneous resolution PATHOLOGY Intimal thickening and defects in the elastic lamina LABORATORY Useless

Note: The 'puff of smoke' pattern may also be seen in intracranial arteriosclerotic occlusive disease, radiation arteritis, intravascular tumor proliferation and tuberculous meningitis

Mozart ear A defect of the auricle in which the crura of the helix and antihelix are joined, resulting in an outward bulge of the upper part of the ear; the ME is so named in honor of Wolfgang Amadeus Mozart, who had the defect

MNGC Multinucleated giant cell, see Giant cells

6-MP 6-Mercaptopurine, see there

MPF M-phase promoting factor A protein kinase composed of p34^{cdc2} and cyclin, which when activated, induces mitosis; the transition of the cell cycle from metaphase to anaphase occurs when cyclin is degraded by ubiquitin-mediated proteolysis, an event that marks the end of cell cycle (Nature 1991; 349:132) see PSTAIR

M-phase promoting factor see MPF

c-Mpl A membrane-bound thrombopoietin receptor; megakaryocytic colony stimulation and platelet elevation are evoked by thrombopoietin-Mpl interaction (see Nature 1994; 369:533A, 565L, 568L, 571L, 519N&V)

c-Mpl ligand Thrombopoietin, see there

MPM Mortality Probabilities Models INTENSIVE CARE A computer-based prognostic scoring system that stratifies patients receiving intensive care according to their risk of hospital death or need for emergency surgery; although MPM is attractive as it doesn't require disease classification and limits its questions to previous health states, it performs less well than APACHE II in statistical analysis of patient outcome

MPM II Mortality Probabilities Models INTENSIVE CARE MEDICINE A 'third-generation' system* for estimating the probability of hospital mortality in adult ICU patients based on logistic regression modeling techniques; MPM II differs from APACHE III and SAPS II in that 1) It collects data on diseases noted at the time of admission, eg acute renal failure, cardiac dysrhythmia, cerebrovascular accidents, and GI bleeding, which may evolve concurrently and 2) It measures fewer variables, but does so at the time of admission MPM$_0$, at 24 hours (MPM$_{24}$), at 48 hours (MPM$_{48}$), and at 72 hours (MPM$_{72}$); SAP II, APACHE III, and MPM II are well-researched systems for collecting ICU-related data, can be used to assess prognosis, and to stratify patients as to severity of disease for clinical trials (JAMA 1994; 272:1049CECC) see Prognostic scoring systems

*The others are APACHE III and SAPS II

MPS Mucopolysaccharide(s), also 1) Member of Pharmaceutical Society (British) 2) Meters per second 3) Mononuclear phagocytic system 4) Mucopolysaccharidosis 5) Myeloma progression score

Also 1) Marriage prediction schedule (psychology) 2) Medical provider survey 3) Movement-produced stimuli (neurology) 4) Multiphasic screening

MPTP 1-Methyl-4-phenyl-1,2,3,6-tetrahydropyridine A potent neurotoxin that acts on neuromelanin, producing the symptoms of Parkinson's disease; MPTP was first identified as a toxic byproduct in an amateur attempt to produce a meperidine analog, for use as a synthetic heroin and was responsible for a number of cases of permanent parkinsonism; pretreatment of monkeys with pargyline (a monoamine oxidase B inhibitor) prevents both the clinical

and pathological evidence of neurotoxicity; see Designer drugs; the selective destruction of the dopamine neurons in the MPTP model is the direct result of its metabolite, MPP+ (1-methyl-4-phenyl-pyridium); the neurotoxic effect on the substantia nigra may be prevented by systemic treatment with N-methyl-D-aspartate (NMDA) antagonists, see MK-801 (Nature 1991; 349:414), or reversed by local treatment with brain-derived neurotrophic factor (BDNF, Nature 1991; 350:230, 195) see BDNF, Parkinson's disease

MPTP

MRA 1) Magnetic resonance angiography, see MR angiography 2) Medical records administrator

MR angiography Magnetic resonance angiography A non-invasive method for evaluating blood vessels that is 1) more sensitive than conventional cerebral contrast angiography* (CCA) and 2) has less morbidity, eg transfemoral angiography complication rate = 8%, intravascular contrast mediums cause severe reactions in 0.22% of patients; MRA is useful for detecting occult runoff arteries in arterial occlusion of the lower extremities as a prelude to limb-salvage procedures (N Engl J Med 1992; 326:1577OA) PRINCIPLE MRA detects the movement of protons in the blood under a magnetic field; the signal is produced as the protons shift from a high-energy state (induced by radiofrequency pulses) to equilibrium, resulting in the production of an electrical signal in a receiver coil, which is transformed into diagnostic images by a computer using a variety of algorithms ADVANTAGES MRA is non-invasive, painless, has no known complications, is much more rapid than CCA and allows construction of images in any plane DISADVANTAGES The signal-to-noise ratio and spatial resolution at present are inferior to the 'gold standard' of CCA and to digital subtraction angiography, as MRA tends to overestimate the degree of arterial stenosis in cerebral (carotid) vessels; due to the effect of turbulence on the magnetization vectors (the current algorithms are primitive,); MRA has been improved by using 'time of flight imaging', although the 'phase projection' techniques are slow; MRA is useful for imaging of atherosclerotic disease and dissecting aneurysms of the neck and intracranial aneurysms '...*in spite of technological shortcomings, MR angiography can provide new diagnostic information about ischemic peripheral vascular disease. This should not be interpreted as indicating that MR angiography will soon replace X-ray angiography...*' (N Engl J Med 1992; 326:1624ED) Cf Spiral computed tomography

*A technique that uses iodinated contrast, causes paresthesia and carries a risk of ischemia, hemorrhage and idiosyncratic reactions

MRC Medical Research Council

MRC scale A system developed by the Medical Research Council (UK) for testing muscle strength, in which the strength of 18 different muscle groups are evaluated and given a value of 1 to 5 for a maximum MRS score of 90 (see N Engl J Med 1993; 329:1993OA)

MRD Mortality rate doubling The time required for an organism's mortality to double, a measure of senescence; MRD parallels the increased incidence of spontaneous degenerative disease; see Gerontology

MRFIT Multiple Risk Factor Intervention Trial A long-term prospective study designed to analyze the effects of modifying the risk factors for heart disease; 'Mr. Fit' achieved notoriety in 1976 when it was found that one of the clinical centers involved had falsified data to include of a group of patients that was not otherwise eligible for inclusion in the study; re-analysis of the 'contaminated' data to exclude the suspect group of 27 patients did not change the study's early conclusions reported in 1982 (**New York Times April 12, 1994; C3**); it is reported that addition of low-dose thiazide with potassium-sparing diuretics reduced the risk of primary cardiac arrest in patients with hypertension (**N Engl J Med 1994; 330:1852OA**)

MRI coronary angiography MRCA A form of MR angiography of use in identifying clinical important coronary artery stenoses; with standard MRI spin-echo and gradient-echo techniques, coronary arterial visualization is suboptimal and limited to the proximal segments, apparently related to respiratory and cardiac movements; in MRCA, the image is obtained while holding the breath, reducing the respiratory 'noise'; cardiac movement is minimized by obtaining the image during mid-diastole (a point of the cardiac cycle with relative diastasis) and the temporal resolution is minimized by using k-space segmentation; while still in the nascent stages of clinical evaluation, MRCA provides a new approach for evaluating coronary artery patency, and may be combined with MR perfusing imaging, anatomic and functional MRI to provide a comprehensive cardiac profile (**N Engl J Med 1993; 328:828OA**)

Note: Other MRI methods for imaging proximal coronary arteries include MRI subtraction methods, 3-D MRI formed by stacking multiple 2-D planar images, and fast spiral MRI

mRNA Messenger ribonucleic acid The reverse template 'message' from DNA that is required for protein synthesis; under most circumstances (and according to the 'Central dogma), the 'message' flows from the DNA to the RNA, which is then translated into protein: DNA is wrapped around proteins (histones) in chromatin; the DNA unwinds, allowing transcription by one of the three RNA polymerases, forming a primary (nuclear) RNA transcript that is then processed by removing the intervening RNA sequences (introns), yielding a mature mRNA molecule which then passes through the nuclear pores into the cytoplasm where translation into proteins occurs; when a particular mRNA is no longer needed it is degraded by ribonucleases; see Central dogma, RNA

MRSA Methicillin-resistant *Staphylococcus aureus,* see MARSA

MRT Magnetic resonance therapy; MRI guided surgery that may reduce the post-operative recuperation

MS 1) Medical student 2) Multiple sclerosis

MS 1) Mass spectrography 2) Mass spectroscopy 3) Mass storage 4) Master of Science 5) Master of Surgery 6) Medical student 7) Mental status 8) Methionine synthase 9) Methyl salicylate 10) Metric system 11) Mitral (valve) stenosis 12) Morphine sulfate 13) Mucosubstance 14) Multiple sclerosis 15) Musculoskeletal

Also 1) Magnetic stirrer 2) Maladjustment score (psychology) 3) Marijuana smoke 4) Marital status 5) Master switch 6) Maximum stress 7) Medical services (British) 8) Medical staff 9) Medical supplies 10) Medical survey 11) Medicine and surgery 12) Mobile surgery (British) 13) Modal sensation 14) Modal sensation 15) Molar solution 16) Molecular sieve 17) Mongolian spot (rarely used) 18) Muscle shortening 19) Muscle strength 20) Musculoactive substance (a nebulous term of waning popularity)

MSBOS Maximum surgical blood order schedule TRANSFUSION MEDICINE A list of commonly performed elective surgical procedures with the maximum number of units of blood to be cross-matched preoperatively; MSBOS's goal is to have a close correlation between the number of units ordered and number of units actually transfused (crossmatch to transfusion ratio), thereby minimizing the wasted labor in the laboratory, a goal best achieved by tying the MSBOS into the hospital computer system; see Cross-match/transfusion ratio

MSDS Material Safety Data Sheets, see there

Mseleni disease A crippling form of idiopathic polyartic-ular osteoarthritis, endemic in Northern Zululand (now KwaZulu) which affects the appendicular joints of 20% of men and 40% of women; in the end-stage disease, most patients walk on their hands and knees

Note: Pathological studies on the bones of Mseleni disease occur after the vultures have stripped the flesh since it is a local custom to leave the dead to be eaten by scavengers

MSG Monosodium glutamate A flavor-enhancing amino acid used in processed, packaged, and fast foods that functions as an excitatory neurotransmitter and neurotoxin, which is most commonly ingested in Chinese food; other sources with up to 40% MSG include autolyzed yeast, calcium caseinate, hydrolyzed protein, and sodium caseinate (**Vitality June 1993**) SENSITIVITY SYMPTOMS Headaches, heart palpitations, skin flushing, tightness of the chest; MSG may cause convulsions when injected into the peritoneal cavity of experimental animals, stimulating neurons until they die, which has been implicated in brain damage in strokes, hypoglycemia, trauma, seizures as well as in Huntington's, Parkinson's and Alzheimer's diseases, and in Guam-type amyotrophic lateral sclerosis; see Chinese restaurant syndrome, Domoic acid

Note: Domoic acid, a potent glutamate analog, may cause toxic envenomation in mussel eaters, in some resulting in an Alzheimer-like disease

hMSH-2 A gene located on chromosome 2 that encodes a protein involved in the repair of mismatched DNA, which is mutated in patients with hereditary nonpolyposis colon cancer‡, which comprise 5-10% of all colorectal cancers (**CAP Today March 1994, p1**) Cf *APC* gene, Familial adenomatous polyposis

MSOF Multisystem organ failure, see there

Mst II MOLECULAR HEMATOLOGY A restriction endonuclease used to detect sickle cell anemia, as the recognition site is abolished by a point mutation on the β globulin gene; Mst II-digested Southern blots of fetal DNA provide the most reliable currently available prenatal diagnosis of sickle cell anemia

MSUD Maple sugar urine disease, see there

MT 1) Medical technologist, see there 2) *membrana tympani* [NAG] tympanic membrane 3) Metatarsal 4) A region of the brain where neurons specialize in detecting movement and in which the neurons are grouped in columns, each of which scans a part of visible space for objects moving in a certain direction

MTBE Methyl-tert-butyl-ether CARDIOLOGY An aliphatic ether that rapidly dissolves cholesterol stones in vivo, which is introduced under local anesthesia via a percutaneous transhepatic cholecystectomy catheter, as a non-invasive method for treating gallstones; after injection, the dissolved 'slurry' is drained from the bladder Complications are rare and minor, including nausea, vomiting, bile leakage, drowsiness, transient elevation of liver enzymes, anorexia and hypotension; MTBE stone dissolution is effective when the patients are selected for cholesterol stones; dissolution of stones is improved and accelerated by adding transcutaneous ultrasound energy (**Invest Radiol 1990; 25:146**) see Lithotripsy ENVIRONMENT An octane-boosting additive used in reformulated gasoline that helps the gas burn cleaner

MTBF Mean time between failure, see there

mtDNA Mitochondrial DNA see there

MTHFR 5,10-Methylenetetrahydrofolate:NADP+ oxidoreductase, see there

MTOC Microtubule organizing center CELL BIOLOGY A subcellular structure adjacent to the nucleus in resting cells, consisting of a centriole from which microtubules emanate, extending to the plasma membrane; see Microtubule

MTP-PE Muramyl tripeptide-phosphatidyl ethanolamine PHARMACOLOGY A synthetic lipophilic analog of a bacterial cell wall component, muramyl dipeptide that is 'bundled' in fat, in a liposomal vesicle and delivered into the pulmonary vasculature, theoretically turning on the tumorilytic machinery of the pulmonary macrophages; MTP-PE is in phase II trials for metastatic osteosarcoma

MTS Mouse thyroid stimulator, see LATS

MTX Methotrexate, see there

mu (μ) Symbol for: linear attenuation coefficient (statistics); mean (statistics); micro- (10^{-6}); heavy chain of IgM

mu chain disease A rare paraproteinemia that affects the middle-aged to elderly, most of whom have or slowly progress to chronic lymphocytic leukemia (CLL) CLINICAL Lymphadenopathy, hepatosplenomegaly and BM infiltration by vacuolated plasma cells, often accompanied by ↑ kappa chain production TREATMENT As with CLL; see Heavy chain disease

mucicarmine HISTOLOGY A common stain used in surgical pathology that contains carmine in combination with aluminum hydroxide and/or aluminum chloride in 50% alcohol; the mucicarmine stain is strongly positive with acid mucins secreted by the GI tract and, with certain fungi, in particular *Cryptococcus neoformans*

mucin A group of hydrated glycoproteins that may be 1) Stromal or dermal ('ground substance') composed of acid mucopolysaccharides, predominantly hyaluronic acid; it is hyaluronidase-labile, PAS-negative, stains with alcian blue at pH 2.5, but not at pH 0.4 and stains metachromatically with methylene and toluidine blues at pH of 3.0 but not at 1.5; with aging, this mucin undergoes basophilic degeneration and 2) Epithelial mucin, produced by glands, containing neutral and acid mucopolysaccharides; when stained, it is hyaluronidase-resistant, PAS-positive, stains with alcian blue at pH 2.5, but not at pH 0.4 and does not stain metachromatically with alcian, methylene and toluidine blues

mucin clot test see String test

mucin lake SURGICAL PATHOLOGY A nonspecific term for 'pools' of mucin-staining material seen by light microscopy in various settings, eg in connective tissue as a component of aging or in degenerative diseases, in the peritoneum in a mucocele of the appendix or in protein-rich, lightly basophilic material admixed with adenocarcinoma cells seen in colloid type adenocarcinomas of the colon and breast

mucocutaneous lymph node syndrome see Kawasaki's disease

mucopolysaccharidosis A heterogeneous group of diseases each of which is due to a specific enzyme deficiency, resulting in an accumulation of substrate mucopolysaccharides (glycosaminoglycans) including dermatan sulfate, heparan sulfate, and keratan sulfates CLINICAL Childhood onset of symptoms that include developmental delay, mental retardation, short stature, skeletal anomalies (dysostosis multiplex), coarse facial features, hepatosplenomegaly DIAGNOSIS Urine screens, consisting of 'spot' tests in which basic dyes (alcian and toluidine blue) stain the acid mucopolysaccharides, modified turbidometric method may be false positive or false negative, modified Dische carbazole reaction, which measures uronic acid Note: Morquio syndrome doesn't excrete uronic acid and is not detected; see Gargoyle face

mucopolysaccharidosis VII Sly syndrome A lysosomal storage disease of mice and men* caused by an inherited deficiency of β-glucuronidase, which results in accumulation of glycosaminogly-

cans in the brain and other tissues, resulting in progressive mental deterioration and death TREATMENT Transplantation of neural progenitor cells into the cerebral ventricles of mice results in correction of the lysosomal storage in neurons and glia (Nature 1995; 374:367)

*And dogs

mucormycosis An opportunistic infection by fungi of the order Mucorales, which are found in decaying organic matter and grow in tissues as hyphae, thus being defined as molds; most grow within 2-5 days in the usual culture media; the most common pathogenic mucormycoses are *Rhizopus* spp and *Rhizomucor* spp; others include *Absidia* spp, *Apophysomyces* spp, *Cunninghamella* spp, *Mucor* spp, and *Saksenaea* spp CLINICAL The fungi enter the respiratory tract and gain a foothold in the nasopharynx, usually in hosts who immunocompromised by AIDS, corticosteroids, DM, malnutrition, terminal cancer, or transplantation Clinical forms Rhinocerebral, pulmonary, cutaneous, GI, cerebral and miscellaneous forms; once the host defense has been circumvented, the hyphae are vasculocentric, explaining the commonly associated necrosis and thrombosis TREATMENT Amphotericin B, azoles (ketoconazole and others) and surgical debridement

mucosa *tunica mucosa* [NH3] Mucous membrane A nonsquamous cell epithelium, that corresponds to the innermost surface of tubular organs and hollow organs, which includes the glandular lining of the nasal and oral cavities, as well as the epithelium of the upper respiratory, and GI tracts and external genitalia

mucous *adjective* Pertaining or referring to either mucosa, eg mucous membrane, or to mucus, eg mucous secretion

mucus A clear viscid fluid that is produced by the various mucosae, which contains mucopolysaccharides, enzymes, IgA and other proteins, desquamated epithelial cells, inorganic salts in a fluid vehicle

muddy complexion A characteristic 'soiled' appearance of patchy hyperpigmentation seen on the face in older malnourished children, accompanied by pallor, lassitude, hypochromic anemia, delay in epiphyseal development, delayed puberty, irregularities in dentition, anorexia and increased susceptibility to infection; see 'Crazy pavement'

muddy lung A descriptor for the lungs of those who have drowned or nearly drowned in stagnant water (and who subsequently die); muddy lungs are characterized by crystalline material, foreign body type giant cell and granulomatous reaction with carnification, massive fibrosis of the pulmonary parenchyma and abundant diatoms

mud fever Leptospirosis caused by *Leptospira interrogans* serovar *grippotyphosa*, which affects those who work in muddy worksites, eg flooded fields

Muerto Canyon virus A hantavirus identified by PCR (see there) (CAP Today May, 1994)

mulberry appearance Any pathological mass or appearance characterized by a rounded mass with multiple superficial bossellations, likened to the appearance of a mulberry or cluster of grapes (unripe) OPHTHALMOLOGY A fanciful descriptor for the fundoscopic appearance of a retinal phakoma or glial hamartoma, consisting of a multinodular or multicystic yellow-white mass, classically seen in patients with tuberous sclerosis

mulberry calculus UROLOGY A descriptor for urinary bladder concrements composed of calcium oxalate that may be of dietary origin, due to intestinal malabsorption or seen in the rare primary hyperoxaluria; Cf Casts

mulberry cell Cluster of grapes appearance

mulberry molar Moon's tooth PEDIATRICS An abnormal lower deciduous (first) molar characterized by a dome-shaped crown, small biting surface and multiple cusps, seen in children with congenital syphilis (other dental anomalies of congenital syphilis include enamel defects causing ↑ caries and the peg teeth of Hutchinson)

mulberry pattern GYNECOLOGIC PATHOLOGY A descriptor of the relatively characteristic pattern of calcification seen in gonadoblastoma

mulberry spots GYNECOLOGY see Powder burn appearance

mulberry stone see Mulberry calculus

Mulibrey nanism An acronym from the organs most commonly affected (muscle, liver, brain and eye) in an AR disease first described in Finland, which is further characterized by constrictive pericarditis with pericardial effusions, yellow dots on the optic fundus, fibrous dysplasia of long bones and abnormalities in the shape of the skull and sella turcica

Mueller-Hinton agar MICROBIOLOGY A starch and beef-infusion bacterial growth substrate that was originally developed for the isolation of pathogenic *Neisseria* spp is the recommended medium for antimicrobial susceptibility testing of commonly encountered anaerobic and aerobic bacteria; see Minimum inhibitory concentration

Muller's ratchet EVOLUTIONARY BIOLOGY A hypothesis that attempts to explain why sex exists; if most mutations are deleterious, a high rate of mutations could account for the evolution of sex; according to Muller, where the mutation rate is high, eventually mutation-free individuals become rare and lost in small populations, due to genetic drift; if the population is asexual, the loss is irreversible, ie occurs in a ratchet wrench-like fashion, and the load of deleterious mutations increases as the mutation-free individuals decrease in the population; according to Muller's ratchet, sexual differentiation increases the fitness of a population, as error-free individuals are created from mutated individuals, effectively stopping the ratchet effect; while the concept is theoretically attractive, it is unproven (**Nature 1993; 364:680sc**); see Hybrid vigor; Cf Bottleneck

müllerian duct *ductus paramesonephricus* [NE3] Para-mesonephric duct EMBRYOLOGY Either of paired structures that appears between the 6th and 7th weeks of embryologic development (during the sexually indifferent period as an invagination of coelomic epithelium, lateral to the cranial portion of the mesonephric duct); in the ♀ fetus the two müllerian ducts fuse during the 9th gestational week, forming the upper vagina, uterus and fallopian tubes, while the remaining degenerates; incomplete fusion of these ducts results in the didelphic uterus; in the ♂ fetus, the müllerian ducts regress at 7th-8th week, portions of which remain as müllerian duct remnants

mullerian duct inhibiting factor A 240-kD glycoprotein encoded on chromosome 19, secreted by the Sertoli cells of the fetal testes (circa 8th week of gestation), which inhibits müllerian duct development, while potentiating wolffian duct development; when the fetal gonads are ovaries, no MDIF is produced and the fetal external genitalia 'default' to female differentiation; a deficit of MDIF is responsible for the persistent müllerian duct syndrome (see **Arch Pathol Lab Med 1994; 118:752oa**)

müllerian mixed tumor see Mixed mesodermal tumor

multiaxial system A generic term for system used to classify a particular psychotic condition based on the assessment of several axes, each of which relates to some aspect of mental function and physical and/or environmental factors that influence mental function (**DSM IV**)

multiband imaging The evaluation of a cell or tissue by fluorescence microscopy (FM) that isolates two (dual band) or more spectral bands*, allowing the viewer to simultaneously examine distinct cellular features by using different fluorochromes; in the near UV range–DAPI and Indo, in the mid-visible range–FITC, Nile Red, Fura, Bodipy, and Snarf, and in the near IR–TRITC, Texas Red, and Cy-5; multiband imaging is of use in FISH, and may be of use in confocal microscopy (**Am Lab Sept 1994 p44**)

*The engineering problems with MI, in particular those related to the design and production of multiband filters have been overcome

multicentric angiofollicular lymphoid hyperplasia Multicentric Castleman's disease

multichannel analyzer LABORATORY MEDICINE An automated laboratory instrument, eg Beckman's 'CX' series, that simultaneously measures multiple analytes including calcium, glucose, phosphorus, lactate dehydrogenase, alkaline phosphatase, and others by separating plasma into minute aliquots and passing each through a separate plastic tube (channel), within which a particular reaction occurs that is measured by a spectrophotometer that is pre-set to measure light at an optimal wavelength

multi-copy prescription forms CLINICAL PHARMACOLOGY A triplicate form used in some states of the US (eg California, Illinois, New York, Texas), to monitor prescriptions of controlled drug substances, where a copy of the prescription is retained by the pharmacist, by the physician and by the state government; see Controlled drug substances

multicystic kidney see Polycystic kidney

multicystic nephroma see Multilocular cyst of the kidney

multidisciplinary approach A generic term referring to the convergence of multiple specialties and/or technologies to establish a diagnosis or effect a therapy

multidrug-resistant bacteria MICROBIOLOGY: A key factor in multidrug resistance (MDR) is the acquisition of antibiotic-resistant genes by most bacterial pathogens; complicating factors include alterations in ecosystems, increase of at-risk populations due to immunocompromise, eg AIDS, increased frequency of interventional medical procedures, and increased survival in those with debilitating disease; MDR has been increasingly reported in both nosocomial and community-acquired pathogens (**N Engl J Med 1994; 330:1247rv**)

multidrug-resistant tuberculosis Infection by *Mycobacterium tuberculosis* that is resistant to at least isoniazid, rifampin, ethambutol, and streptomycin; clusters of TB have been identified by molecular methods, eg RFLP (restriction-fragment-length polymorphism) which yields unique strain-specific banding patterns; the probability of having a 'cluster' of MDR-TB in the San Francisco area was associated with birth in the US, diagnosis of AIDS (or known HIV infection), ethnicity (Hispanic), race (black), and with poor patient compliance (ie patient not taking appropriate doses of anti-TB drugs) (**N Engl J Med 1994; 330:1703oa**); similar epidemiology was reported in the Bronx (**ibid, 330:1710oa**); recently transmitted TB accounts for ± 40% of incident cases and ± ⅔ of drug-resistant cases; isoniazid and rifampin are the most common agents for which resistance develops; see Tuberculosis

multifocal atrial tachycardia A cardiac arrhythmia characterized by irregularity, variable 'P' waves and (in adults) a poor prognosis; MAT is seen in 0.05-0.32% of the EKGs interpreted in general hospitals and is more common in the acutely ill (burns, sepsis, respiratory failure) and elderly TREATMENT Magnesium, potassium, calcium-channel blockers, eg verapamil and β-adrenergic blockers, eg metoprolol PROGNOSIS 43% of patients with MAT died during the hospital stay in which the arrhythmia was documented, but death was usually related to the underlying disease

multi-infarct dementia A condition characterized by global cognitive impairment due to atherosclerosis-induced cerebrovascular disease, which is more common in women and associated with diabetes mellitus, hypertension, smoking and rarely, amyloidosis CLINICAL Gait and motor defects, abnormalities of language, mood, abstract thinking, apraxia, agnosia and urinary incontinence; the repeating 'mini-infarcts' of hypertension mimic the gradual deterioration typical of the more common Alzheimer's disease, which occurs without prominent motor changes and reflexes PATHOLOGY Variably sized infarcts of sensorimotor areas and cortical zones involved with cognitive functions, especially in zones irrigated by the anterior and middle cerebral arteries, imparting a lacunar or 'Swiss cheese' appearance

multileaf collimater RADIATION ONCOLOGY A device that contains 20-40 pairs of thin metal leaves that can be moved independently and rapidly to attenuate the beam of a linear accelerator, allowing the creation of a radiation field of any desired shape (N Engl J Med 1995; 332:371RV)

multi-lineage leukemia A leukemia that is clonally committed to myeloid differentiation and also demonstrates multiple clonal, eg megakaryocytic and/or erythrocytic, expansions, a finding more common when associated with monosomy 7; the finding of multi-lineage expansions, implies that the proliferative signal has occurred at the progenitor-cell stage of differentiation; Cf Biclonality, Composite tumor

multilocular renal cyst A unilateral idiopathic lesion that arises in infancy, producing symptoms by the presence of a mass or by ureteral obstruction, and consisting of multiple cysts ranging from 1 mm to 15 cm, which do not communicate with each other or with the remaining (unremarkable) renal parenchyma; it is unknown whether the cysts are neoplastic (as they may be associated with Wilms' tumor or renal cell carcinoma), segmental dysplasias (as they may occur in Potter type 2 renal dysplasia) or developmental defects (as they may be associated with hamartomas), although absence of other congenital malformations favors an acquired etiology; see Polycystic kidneys

multilocus enzyme electrophoresis A characterization method for determining the genetic relationships among strains of related organisms by indexing polymorphisms (allelic variations) in a sample of genes that encode 'housekeeping' (critical metabolic) genes; isolates with identical allelic profiles, eg bacteria are classified as clones and considered to originate from a common precursor cell; this method can be used to provide real-time epidemiologic analysis of bacterial infections (Arch Pathol Lab Med 1994; 118:1280A)

multimedia COMPUTERS The convergence of different electronic and communication technologies with the integration of audio, photographs, animation, graphics, and video into a 'single' format; as multimedia matures, new tools are being added to the core hardware of the PC environment, including CD-ROM, digital cameras, gigabyte hard-drives, MIDI interfaces, videoboards; multimedia promises to change the format of education, and would allow students in remote areas of the world to benefit from master lecturers

multiorgan donation The best single source of multiple organs from a non-relative for allograft transplantation is a 'brain dead' donor, as the recipient is exposed to only one set of foreign antigens; 56-77% of such donations are from CNS catastrophes (subarachnoid bleeding or CNS tumors); the remaining donations are from cardiopulmonary arrest, anoxia, drug overdose, drowning or burn victims or those with prolonged ventilatory support

Note: Donations from patients with prolonged brain death are less desirable given the potential for infectious complications; for management of multiorgan 'donors' and exclusionary criteria, see JAMA 1989; 261:2222

multiorgan failure Multisystem organ failure, see there

multipayer system HEALTH CARE FINANCING The existance of a pluristic health reimbursement scheme which is a mixture of private and public financial providers (Am Med News 25 October 1992, p7) Cf Nationalized health insurance

multiple-antibiotic-resistant pathogenic bacteria Multidrug-resistant bacteria, see there

multiple autoimmune disorders A pair of conditions, divided into

MAD, TYPE I Defined by at least two of the following: Addison's disease, hypoparathyroidism, mucocutaneous candidiasis and

MAD, TYPE II Schmidt syndrome, characterized by two or more of the following, including Addison's disease, autoimmune thyroid disease, IDDM with or without hypopituitarism and mucocutaneous candidiasis

multiple basal cell nevus syndrome Basal cell nevus syndrome, see there

multiple chemical sensitivity syndrome see Clinical ecology

multiple cholesterol emboli syndrome A clinical complex of subacute onset caused by showers of emboli occurring days to weeks (or months) after coronary artery catheterization or aortic surgery, resulting in ischemia of affected organs (N Engl J Med 1993; 329:1821c)

multiple comparisons method(s) STATISTICS A group of procedures for handling multiple inferences within the same data sets, including Bonferroni technique, Scheffe's contrasts, Duncan multi-range procedures, Newmann-Keuls procedure

multiple hamartoma syndrome Cowden's disease A rare AD [MIM 158350] genodermatosis characterized by an increased susceptibility to hamartomatous neoplasms of ectodermal, mesodermal, and endodermal origin, of the mucocutaneous surfaces as well as malignancy, including papillary or follicular thyroid carcinoma and breast cancer, and osteosarcoma (Arch Pathol Lab Med 1993; 117:1254OA) Cf Chromosomal breakage syndromes, Li-Fraumani syndrome

multiple lentigines syndrome see Leopard syndrome

multiple lymphomatous polyposis A rare lymphoproliferative disorder affecting those > age 50, ♂:♀ ratio, 2:1, and characterized by multiple polypoid tumors involving several segments of the GI mucosa, in particular the duodenum; MLP is high-grade B-cell lymphoma with mantle zone features that is often accompanied by BM, lymph node, and liver involvement and generally has poor prognosis (Cancer 1994; 74:3042)

multiple malformation 'syndromes' PEDIATRICS A group of disorders defined as having developmental anomalies of two or more systems possibly related to chromosomal damage, teratogens and other environmental influences, including the Cornelia de Lange, Prader-Willi, Rubinstein-Taybi, and Williams' syndromes; see Dysmorphology, Sequence

multiple myeloma A neoplastic proliferation of plasma cells characterized by tumor cell aggregates in the bone marrow and in extramedullary sites MM may be characterized by lineage 'infidelity', ie expression of multiple lineages, including megakaryocytic (88%), monocytic-myeloid (65%), lymphocytic (58%) and erythroid (39%) lines, both mature, eg surface immunoglobulins and immature, eg cALLA antigens EPIDEMIOLOGY MM comprises 10% of hematopoietic malignancies, causing 10 000 deaths/year (US); ↑ with age; black:white 2:1 LABORATORY Monoclonal immunoglobulins, often light chains, identified in serum and urine COMPLICATIONS Painful pathological fractures, anemia, hypercalcemia, renal failure, recurrent bacterial infections TREATMENT Primary chemotherapy: Melphalan and prednisone induce a remission (75% ↓ in myeloma proteins, 95% ↓ Bence-Jones protein in urine, and < 5% of plasma cells in marrow) in 40% of patients; VAD (vincristine, doxorubicin-Adriamycin, and dexamethasone) is of use in newly diagnosed myeloma; IFN-α has been used for maintenance; myeloablative therapy may be of use (**N Engl J Med 1994; 330:484**ᴰᵀ) see Myeloma kidney

multiple personality disorder The '*presence of two or more distinct identities or personality states...that recurrently take control of behavior*.' MPD is accompanied by an inability to recall important personal information that is well beyond ordinary forgetfulness; there are estimated 20 000 patients with MPD in the US (**Nature Medicine 1995; 1:490**)

*The term preferred in the Diagnosis and Statistical Manual for Mental Disorders, 4th edition (1994) is 'dissociative identity disorder', which is unlikely to be integrated into the vox populi in the forseeable future-Author's note

multiple plane imaging MRI A variation of the sequential plane imaging techniques that can be used with selective excitation techniques and does not affect adjacent planes; adjacent planes are imaged while waiting for relaxation of the first plane toward equilibrium, resulting in decreased imaging time; see Magnetic resonance imaging

multiple primary malignancy syndrome ONCOLOGY The finding of two primary malignancies in the same patient is not uncommon, although more than two is distinctly unusual and becomes a 'syndrome', defined by Werthamer's criteria 1) The malignancies must be primary in different organs 2) Paired-organ (breast, kidney) malignancies (synchronous or metachronous) are considered to be a single primary 3) Multiple malignant tumors originating in the same organ are considered as a single primary 4) The lower intestine and uterus (with adnexae) are each considered single organs 5) The malignant nature of the lesions must be confirmed histologically 6) The lesion should be histologically proven to be non-metastatic (although this is sometimes impossible) Note: An additional criterion is valid 7) The malignancy should not have been induced by chemo- or radiotherapy (**JAMA 1961; 175:558**); multiple primary malignancies occur in less than 1% of those with malignancy; the maximum recorded number of multiple primary malignancies is six (**Am J Surg 1949; 78:894**)

Multiple Risk Factor Interventional Trial see MRFIT

multiple sclerosis An idiopathic, demyelinating disease in which the infiltrating lymphocytes (predominantly T-cells) and macrophages eat up the myelin, onset in younger, often female adults, affecting 1:2500 in the US, commonly associated with HLA-A3, B7, Dw2 haplotypes; MS is increased in a south-to-north gradient in the northern hemisphere (ie is more commonly in cold-to-temperate climates) PREVENTION Treatment of acute optic neuritis (AON), a common precursor of multiple sclerosis (20% develop MS within two years of AON) with high-dose IV methylprednisolone and prednisone is reported to reduce the incidence of subsequent MS (**N Engl J Med 1993; 329:1764**ᴏᴀ), a finding that will require confirmation CLINICAL Waxing and waning or slowly progressive paresthesias, gait and visual defects, muscular weakness, absent abdominal reflexes, hyperactive tendon reflexes, cerebellar ataxia, retrobulbar neuritis, loss of proprioceptive sense, spastic weakness of legs, vertigo; the 'classic' Charcot's triad of dysarthria, nystagmus, and intention tremor is rare PATHOGENESIS Three major mechanisms have been evoked including autoimmunity, 'innocent bystander' demyelination and immune destruction of persistently infected (more than 20 viruses have been implicated in MS) oligodendrocytes MOLECULAR BIOLOGY Antibodies are present in the cerebrospinal fluid that react with HTLV-I's GAG (p24) protein; gene amplification, cloning and DNA blotting analysis of peripheral monocytes from MS patients revealed HTLV-I sequences; suggesting a retroviral relation to MS DIAGNOSIS

Oligoclonal elevation of IgG in the cerebrospinal fluid is present in 90% of patients, 'evoked potentials' seen by electroencephalography in the visual cortex and brainstem, multiple defects seen by computed tomography and magnetic resonance imaging Note: All of these tests are nonspecific and must be correlated with the clinical findings NEUROPATHOLOGY Demyelinization, inflammation, and glial scarring, ie a 'dying-back gliopathy'; early lesions involve the paraventricular, frontal and temporal regions, later involving the optic tracts, brainstem, cortical white matter with patchy spinal cord lesions TREATMENT ...*no therapy is truly worthless unless it has been tried and failed in multiple sclerosis...*--anonymous; some of the more recent agents that appear to be less than effective include cop-1, a mixture of 14–23-kD polypeptides containing alanine, lysine, glutamic acid and tyrosine in a ratio of 6:4.7:1.9:1, which is similar to that of myelin basic protein; cop-1 suppresses experimental allergic encephalitis, a murine model of MS, and hyperbaric oxygen (**Arch Neurol 1991; 48:195**); see Cop-1, Faroe Islands, Holstein cow pattern, Oligoclonal bands, Shadow plaques

multipotent reserve cell An undifferentiated cell of the adult breast capable of differentiating into myoepithelial, ductal and lobular cells

multiplex PCR The simultaneous amplification of multiple exons in the same reaction tube, which can be used clinically to detect exon deletions in inherited diseases, eg deletions in the dystrophin gene in Duchenne's or Becker's muscular dystrophy (**N Eng J Med 1995; 332:1218**ᴍᴍ)

multiproblem family SOCIAL MEDICINE A family with a high potential for child abuse; these families are often urban and have an income level far below the poverty level; most of these families are headed by a single parent, half of whom have serious psychiatric disorders and a history of substance abuse and/or alcoholism; 81% had four or more episodes of child abuse in the previous three years, accompanied by severe child neglect in 30-80% of cases (**N Engl J Med 1990; 323:1628**); see Child abuse

multirule procedure LABORATORY MEDICINE A set of rules for QC of laboratory data which combines individual QC rules to increase the probability of error detection without increasing the rate of false rejections to unacceptably high levels; one commonly used procedure is Westgard's multirule procedure in which a 'run' of laboratory data is rejected if the control is 1) 3 standard deviations (SD) above or below the mean for that analyte 2) Two consecutive controls are greater than 2 SD in the same direction of the mean 3) Four consecutive controls are greater than 1 SD in the same direction of the mean 4) The range between 2 consecutive controls exceeds four SD 5) 10 consecutive controls are in the same direction of the mean

multistage carcinogenesis The development of cancer through multiple steps; in contrast to the mechanistically correct, but simplistic model delineated by Knudson in the 'one-hit, two-hit' model of malignancy, malignant transformation of most tissues requires that multiple defects accumulate in the genome through various combinations of DNA defects including the loss of tumor suppressor genes, point mutations and juxtaposition of oncogenes with new sites, eg permanently turning on growth factors; recognizing of these early stages may ultimately allow for 'preneoplastic' therapy to be a viable option; see One-hit, two hit model, p53, Tumor

multiple-system atrophy NEUROLOGY A term encompassing a heterogenous group of neurologic syndromes (corticobasal ganglionic degeneration, olivopontine cerebellar atrophy, progressive supranuclear palsy, Shy-Drager syndrome, striatonigral degeneration) that share clinical features caused by lesions affecting interrelated groups of neurons; in the early stages the differential diagnosis among these entities is difficult, and because they are characterized by slow awkward movements suggestive of Parkinson's disease, they are known as parkinsonism, and with the development of additional and more specific signs, as Parkinson's-plus syndromes (**N Engl J Med 1993; 329:1560**CPC)

multistix see Dipsticks

multisystem organ failure A 'physiologic' shut-down of multiple body systems in the face of critical injury or uncontrolled sepsis; several factors are synergistic in producing organ dysfunction and death (average MSOF mortality 60%): shock, intestinal infarction, malnutrition, alcohol abuse and advanced age; MSOF may begin as cardiocirculatory failure and be followed by respiratory and renal shut-down, hepatic decompensation and metabolic derangements with thrombocytopenia occurring at any time; if the progression of MSOF can be stopped before a second organ fails, the mortality is 30%, otherwise death is virtually inevitable

multitasking COMPUTERS The ability of an operating system to run multiple programs (eg graphics, spreadsheets, word processing) or formats of software development (eg coding, compiling, and testing) simultaneously

multivariate analysis STATISTICS A generic term for any of a number of statistical methods (eg multiple regression analysis, multiple logistic functions, factor analysis) that addresses the effects of multiple variables (eg dietary fat, age, sex, serum cholesterol levels) on a dataset

multivesicular body A form of lysosome appearing as a large, cleared, membrane-bound vacuole surrounded by multiple minute vesicles seen by EM; the MB is thought to result from defective membrane cycling and abnormal internalization of surface antigens in Golgi-derived vesicles; it is characteristic of signet ring lymphoma

multivitamin An over-the-counter and often self-prescribed combination tablet containing lipid-soluble vitamins (vitamin A, vitamin D, vitamin E and vitamin K) and water-soluble vitamins (vitamin B_1, vitamin B_2, vitamin B_6, vitamin B_{12}, vitamin C), folic acid, niacin, pantothenic acid and biotin; these dietary 'supplements' may also contain minerals, including calcium, phosphorus, iron, iodine, magnesium, copper and zinc; the use of periconceptual multivitamins is reported to ↓ the first incidence of neural tube defects (**N Engl J Med 1992; 327:1832**OA), an effect that may be attributable to folic acid (**ibid, 327:1875**ED) and may reduce the risk of anencephaly and spina bifida in general; see Decavitamin, Neural tube defects; Cf Megavitamin therapy

multiwavelength see Multiband imaging

mummified cell LIVER A degenerated eosinophilic hepatocyte described in acute hepatitis, preferably known as an apoptotic cell LYMPH NODE A large effete and degenerated cell (figure, right) that may represent an involuting Reed-Sternberg cell, which is most commonly seen in the diffuse subtype of lymphocyte predominance Hodgkin's disease; this form is characterized by diffuse effacement of the nodal architecture by a lympho-histiocytic proliferation, paucity of diagnostic Reed-Sternberg cells, presence of large abnormal polypoid cells without huge nucleoli (L/H cells, which are also seen in lymphocyte-predominant Hodgkin's disease) and abnormal, often ring-shaped mitotic figures

mumps PEDIATRICS An acute generalized infection by a paramyxovirus that is most common in young children CLINICAL Fever, malaise, parotiditis COMPLICATIONS Aseptic meningoencephalitis, pancreatitis, orchitis VACCINE All children without immune compromise, anaphylactic reactions to eggs or other contraindications should receive the live attenuated mumps virus vaccine which confers lifelong protection; adverse reactions, eg orchitis and parotitis, are rare; most of those born before 1957 have natural immunity

Mumps was first described by Hippocrates; the English name refers to the mumbling speech characteristic in these patients

Munchausen syndrome A pseudo-disease complex seen in subjects who create bizarre lesions or fabricate symptoms in order to enjoy the perceived benefits from hospitalization; the chief complaints include those with vague symptoms, requiring numerous often complicated tests; once the charade is discovered, the 'patient' signs out of the hospital only to be admitted to another Statistics ♀:♂ ratio, 2:1; 74% develop the condition by age 24, and on average are diagnosed as having the Munchausen complex by age 32; the patients often have a history of childhood neglect or abuse, linked to illness, where the hospital represents a place with a comforting and nurturing environment; to maintain their state of illness, some 'patients' may feign torsion dystonia, inject feces or perform surgery upon themselves; although less than 400 cases have been described since its initial recognition (**Lancet 1951;1:339**), these persons are very 'expensive', undergoing multiple hospitalizations and diagnostic procedures; their actual cost to the health care system cannot be estimated

The name derives from a fictional character, Baron Munchausen created by a German, RE Raspe (1737-1794) who wrote the original story in English as Baron Munchausen's *Narrative of his Marvelous Travels and Campaigns in Russia*, based on the true tales of a German soldier and raconteur, Freiherr von Münchhausen (1720-1797) of Hannover Note: The fictional character and the person who inspired the fiction should be distinguished, if only for the sake of accuracy (**JAMA 1983; 250:1976**)

Munchausen-by-proxy syndrome Polle syndrome A form of child abuse in which the children, often under the age of 5-6, are victims of factitious illnesses either fabricated by, eg reports of fever and seizure disorders or induced by the parents or guardians, eg administration of laxatives, withholding antibiotics, friction-induced 'rashes'; this condition may satisfy aberrant psychological needs on the part of the parents

The syndrome is misnamed after Polle, Freiherr von Munchhausen's daughter, who was said to have died at the age of one under suspicious circumstances, an assertion that is not supported historically (**Lancet 1984; 1:166**) as he did not have a daughter named Polle (**Pediatrics 1984; 74:554**)

Munchhausen syndrome see Munchausen syndrome

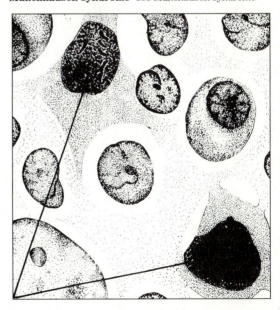

mummified cells

Munro's microabscess Spongiform microabscess An aggregate of neutrophils in a parakeratotic stratum corneum, a classic finding of psoriasis; see Microabscess;

Cf Spongiform pustule

murder FORENSIC MEDICINE The unlawful killing of a human being by another with malice aforethought, either express or implied; see Homicide

MURDER OF THE FIRST DEGREE 'Murder, one' Any homicide perpetrated by means of poison, lying in wait, or other kind of willful, deliberate and premeditated act, or that which is committed while perpetrating a forcible felony, eg arson, rape, robbery or burglary

MURDER OF THE SECOND DEGREE 'Murder, two' A homicide that falls short of criminal or premeditated intent; see Depraved heart murder, Manslaughter, Serial murder

murine acquired immunodeficiency syndrome A condition in mice caused by a defective retrovirus that has similarities to human AIDS, which include abnormal T- and B-cell function, polyclonal B-cell proliferation, lymphadenopathy, splenomegaly, hyperγglobulinemia, ↑ susceptibility to infections, and B-cell lymphomas; MAIDS responds to cyclophosphamide (Science 1991; 251:305)

'murky cell' carcinoma DERMATOPATHOLOGY A droll sobriquet for a primary undifferentiated carcinoma of the skin of undetermined lineage, which has a nonspecific architectural pattern, indistinct cellular features, and vaguely resembles a Merkel cell tumor, a highly aggressive neuroendocrine neoplasm characterized by sheets of small-to-moderately-sized round 'blue' cells

Murray Valley encephalitis A Japanese encephalitis-like disease caused by a flavivirus (group B togavirus) which occurs in small epidemic clusters in Murray Valley and elsewhere in Victoria and New South Wales, Australia, which is maintained by a wild bird and mosquito (*Culex annulirostris*) cycle

muscle *textus muscularis* [NH3] A tissue that has been traditionally divided into three major functional groups, to wit, striated muscle, cardiac muscle, and nonstriated muscle; muscle is of considerable research interest, given that it contains 'motor' proteins; when (skeletal) muscle is being examined for clinical disease, the biopsy should be obtained from a site moderately affected by disease, but not from the (inflamed) site of electromyography

TYPE I MUSCLE (aka slow-twitch or red muscle) is fatigue-resistant, has high mitochondrial oxidative (nicotinamide adenine dinucleotide-tetrazolium reductase or NADH-TR) activity and low glycolytic capacity, which stains lightly with ATPase at pH 9.4 (low myosin) and phosphorylase, and stains darkly with NADH-TR

TYPE II MUSCLE (aka fast twitch or white muscle) is fatigue-sensitive, has high glycolytic activity, displays light staining with NADH-TR and dark staining with ATPase at pH 9.4 (high myosin) and phosphorylase HISTOLOGY Muscle is arranged in a mosaic of type I and type II fibers in a 1:1 ratio; smooth muscle contraction is slower and more energy-efficient than that of skeletal muscle, which is related to the contractile apparatus, where muscle contraction occurs in a corkscrew-like fashion

muscle antibodies Smooth muscle antibodies, see there

muscle biopsy A biopsy intended to evaluate primary (eg dystrophies, myopathies) or secondary (eg drug-related, endocrine, neurologic) muscle disorders, or systemic disease (eg vasculitis); a wide range of special studies can be performed on a properly obtained MB, including biochemistry, EM, histochemistry, immunohistochemistry, and various molecular tests; the site selected for the MB is critical[1], as are the obtention and transportation[2] (Arch Pathol Lab Med 1995; 119:303oA)

[1]The site must be known to be involved, but not so much so that only end-stage changes are seen [2]The preferred method is to use a clamp to stretch the biopsied muscle, and transport the muscle on a saline-soaked gauze at 'refrigerator' temperatures

muscle fiber type grouping see Type grouping

'muscular cirrhosis' A term for the histopathology of end-stage interstitial pulmonary fibrosis, characterized by muscle cell proliferation with fibrosis, differentiating this from pulmonary leiomyomatosis in which the muscular proliferation is accompanied by minimal fibrosis

muscular dystrophy Any of a group of primary degenerative myopathies, which are characterized by selective atrophy and weakness of voluntary muscles, pseudohypertrophy (see Champagne bottle legs), progressive deterioration, and eventually death; usually X-linked, often recessive [MIM 310200], but also AD and AR conditions that affect 1:3500 ♂ children, the most common form of which, Duchenne's muscular dystrophy, often proves fatal by age 20 PATHOGENESIS MDs are related to a defective muscle protein, dystrophin; in those with concomitant mental impairment (30%); which may be due to a defective dystrophin-like molecule is commonly found in the brain; functionally impaired smooth muscle of the GI tract may cause impaired gastric emptying PATHOLOGY Muscle fibers demonstrate longitudinal splitting, ringed fibers, variability in size, juxtaposition of atrophic and hypertrophic cells, regeneration accompanied by endo- and perimysial connective tissue proliferation, fibrosis and fatty infiltration

mushroom appearance PEDIATRIC ORTHOPEDICS The descriptor for a flattened femoral head that is contiguous with a broad neck, accompanied by a widened articular space, premature fusion of the ossification center and trochanteric overgrowth, seen in the re-ossification phase of Perthes disease, ie osteochondrosis of the femoral head, coxa plana; see Sagging rope sign

mushrooming RADIOLOGY A burgeoning of bony excrescences in osteochondromata, often located adjacent to the epiphyseal plate in long bones

mushroom lesion Summit lesion GASTROENTEROLOGY A 'regurgitated' mass of acutely inflamed fibrinocellular exudate seen by low-power LM in early pseudomembranous colitis, consisting of fibrin, mucin, neutrophils, sloughed colonic epithelium and necrotic tips of the glands and abscessed crypts; see Pseudomembranous colitis

mushroom of foam FORENSIC PATHOLOGY A frothy nasolabial 'spume' seen in drowning victims that may be inapparent when the body is first fished out, which appear as pressure is applied to the chest (in either resuscitative attempts or when removing the clothing); the foam is a mixture of air, mucus and water produced in the presence of respiratory movement and is considered proof that the victim was alive at the time of submersion; blood-stained foam is the result of increased intrathoracic pressure, a component of the drowning process; brown and malodorous foam indicates putrefaction; Cf 'Shaving cream' appearance

mushrooms Fifty of the 2000 species of mushrooms are poisonous; the major toxin is the cyclic octapeptide-bearing amanitine, a selective RNA polymerase II inhibitor present in the *Amanita* and *Galerina* species; *Amanita phalloides* causes most mushroom deaths Mortality 40-90% CLINICAL STAGE 1 Abrupt onset, ie within 6-24 hours after ingestion, accompanied by abdominal pain, nausea, vomiting, diarrhea, major fluid and electrolyte imbalances STAGE 2 Apparent resolution, with asymptomatic renal and hepatic deterioration STAGE 3 occurs by days 3-4 and is characterized by complete hepatorenal collapse, cardiomyopathy, disseminated intravascular coagulation, convulsions, coma and death

music The art of making sounds that are beautiful, pleasing, and/or interesting, which is founded in the scientific principles of melody, harmony, rhythm, tempo, and timbre SURGERY Early data suggest that the addition of performance-shaping factors eg surgeon-selected music, is associated with ↓ cardiovascular (autonomic) reactivity and improved performance* of a stressful nonsurgical laboratory task, serial numerical subtraction; investigator-selected (Pachebel's Canon in D) music is less effective than surgeon-selected music, which is more effective than no music (**JAMA 1994; 272:882_{oA}, 1995; 273:1090c**) Music instruction in preschoolers is reported to strengthen cross-communication among brain regions involved in complex mathematics, navigation, sculpting, and others, and ↑ spatial intelligence (**Science News 1994; 146:143**) see Performing arts medicine

*The data may be confounded by the participants personal bias toward or against the use of performance-shaping factors, the potential negative effect such factors might have on other participants in the surgical team, different levels of experience by the surgeons being studied, bodily position, duration of the test, and so on

music therapy Music-facilitated psychoeducational strategy NEUROPHYSIOLOGY The complexity of the production of music and its role in mental development, emotion, language, and intelligence is poorly understood (**NY Times 16 May 1995, C1**) PSYCHOLOGY The use of music as an interventional modality for those who are experiencing symptoms of anxiety, depression, distress, low self-esteem and moodiness; the use of MT in older adults, either with or without a music therapist is reported to be a cost-effective strategy for treating major and minor depression in housebound persons (**J Gerontol 1994; 49:265**)

'musician's wart' A heterogeneous group of calluses, hyperkeratoses and comedonic lesions appearing in regions where a musical instrument contacts or rests on the body, anointed with the highly descriptive terms, 'guitar nipple', 'cello scrotum' and 'fiddler's neck', which are variably accompanied by erythema and papule formation; see Performing arts medicine, Singer's nodule

mustard gas bis(2-chloroethyl)sulfide A potent alkylating agent that loses a chloride ion, forming an unstable 3-member ring with a positively charged sulfur; it is toxic, mutagenic and carcinogenic; at high levels, MG causes vesication and ulceration of skin, pulmonary necrosis, conjunctivitis, nausea and vomiting; it was used in World War I as a chemical weapon and banned in the Geneva Protocol of 1925

mutable gene An unstable gene that is both highly susceptible to mutation and which has a high rate of intrinsic mutation

mutagen Any physical or chemical agent capable of altering an organism's DNA (genome) by inducing mutations that may be passed to subsequent generations

mutation A change in the base pair composition of DNA that differs from either of the parental haploid contributions to the progeny, most of which are not lethal CONFORMATIONAL MUTATION A single nucleotide substitution that alters the three-dimensional shape, ie conformation of the DNA's double helix, changing the mobility of restriction fragments in a polyacrylamide electrophoretic gel MISSENSE MUTATION A genomic mutation in which substitution of one (or more) base(s) encodes a different amino acid resulting in a dysfunctional protein NONSENSE MUTATION A point mutation in which a base pair substitution in transcription of the 'stop' codons UGA, UAA or UAG, which are signals for the mRNA to end translation into a protein POINT MUTATION A mutation that substitutes one base pair for another, but may not cause a restriction fragment length polymorphism; point mutations may be 1) Silent, ie a 'synonymous mutation'; given DNA's 'degeneracy' is a base pair substitution which encodes the same amino acid; see Degenerate code, 2) Yield a different new amino acid, a 'replacement mutation' which results in either a normally functioning protein (the substitution does not adversely impinge on the protein's active site) or a functionally defective protein, 3) Result in the encoding of a missense codon, causing a premature termination of

translation into a protein SPONTANEOUS MUTATION Natural mutation A de novo mutation that comprises 45% of major congenital malformations, which may be subsequently passed to future generations in an autosomal dominant and X-linked fashion TRANSITION MUTATION A type of substitution mutation involving an exchange between purines (adenine and guanine) or pyrimidines (cytidine and thymidine) TRANSVERSION MUTATION A specific base-pair mutation where a purine is substituted for a pyrimidine or vice versa

mutation detection The 'gold standard' for detecting mutagenic activity is the Ames test, an in vitro assay designed to determine an agent's ability to induce mutations in bacteria; while the Ames test is expedient, its relevance to human environmental toxins is unclear; human gene assays are designed to detect mutations of the HGPRT (hypoxanthine guanine phosphoribosyl transferase) gene in T cells, as an indicator of an agent's mutagenic potential; toxins produce characteristic 'fingerprints' of the mutated gene that can be visualized by gradient denaturing gel electrophoresis

mutation repair see SOS repair

mutilating arthritis Arthritis mutilans, see there

mutilating surgery A form of 'heroic'* surgery that consists of massive excision of tissue, usually from a broadly invasive malignancy, with the purpose of removing the tumor and/or metastases, regardless of the 'cost' in terms of deterioration of quality of life, potential infections and other co-morbid conditions; the availability of other modalities, eg chemotherapy, radiotherapy and various 'magic bullet' forms of immunotherapy, have made mutilating surgery a less preferred therapy for neoplasms

* '...another such victory and we are lost...'—Plutarch

muton A generic term of little practical use for the smallest unit of a gene that is capable of undergoing mutation, ranging in size from a single nucleotide substitution, causing point mutations to deletions of large segments of DNA, causing frameshift mutations

mutton fat lesion 'Greasy' rounded, yellow keratic precipitates of lymphocytes, plasma cells, epithelioid histiocytes and pigment adherent to the posterior aspect of the cornea seen in tuberculous iridocyclitis as well as in chronic granulomatous uveitis due to sarcoidosis

MVA Motor vehicular/vehicle accident, see there

M-VAC Methotrexate, vinblastine, Adriamycin (doxorubicin) and cis-platinum A chemotherapeutic regimen for bladder cancer

MVB Multivesicular bodies, see there

MVPS Mitral valve prolapse syndrome, see there

MVPS Medical volume performance standard

Mx protein MOLECULAR BIOLOGY A generic term for any of a family of proteins that are analogues of dynamin, which have been shown to confer resistance to viral infection; like dynamin, Mx proteins are capable of polymerizing into C-shaped and helical molecules (**Nature 1995; 374:186, 190, 116N&V**) see Dynamin, Endocytosis

Mxi-1 A tumor suppressor protein produced in the cell nucleus that is thought to shut off the *myc* oncogene; Cf Myc

myasthenia gravis An autoimmune disorder characterized by weakness and muscular fatigue EPIDEMIOLOGY 5-12.5/10⁵ (± 25 000 active cases, US) peak incidence ♀ 2nd-3rd decade ♂ 6-7th decade PATHOGENESIS Neuromuscular junctions in MG have fewer acetylcholine receptors, simplified synaptic folds, and widened synaptic spaces CLINICAL Ptosis, diplopia, weakness and fatigability of skeletal muscles, generalized in most patients, often of a proximal distribution; gradation is based on severity, ranging from focal disease (grade I) to a life-threatening crisis with impaired respiration (grade IV) DIAGNOSIS Anticholinesterase test (Tensilon test), repetitive nerve stimulation, assay for anti-acetylcholine receptors, single fiber electromyography ASSOCIATED DISEASES Thymoma, thymic hyperplasia, other autoimmune diseases or phenomena, eg thyroiditis, Graves' disease, rheumatoid arthritis, SLE TREATMENT Anticholinesterase agents (pyridostigmine), thymectomy, immunosuppressive therapy (corticosteroids, azathioprine, cyclospirine), short-term immunotherapy (IV immune globulin, plasma exchange) (N Engl J Med 1994; 330:1797RA)

myasthenic crisis Any of a number of clinical complexes characterized by an acute exacerbation of myasthenia gravis symptoms, which are divided into

MYASTHENIC CRISIS An acute increase in requirement for anticholinesterase medication or refractoriness to same, which is diagnosed by a Tensilon test, with transient amelioration of symptoms and 2)

CHOLINERGIC CRISIS An acute decrease in the need for anticholinesterase medication, resulting in 'overmedication' with the customary doses; the Tensilon test exacerbates this form of myasthenic crisis; cholinergic crises may be either

1) MUSCARINIC CRISIS, causing abdominal pain, diarrhea, nausea, vomiting, lacrimation, blurred vision, and bronchial hypersecretion due to over-response to the parasympathetic system or

2) NICOTINIC CRISIS, characterized by muscle weakness, fasciculations, cramping, and dysphagia, due to overdepolarization at the neuromuscular junction; see Tensilon test

c-myb MOLECULAR BIOLOGY A protooncogene that encodes a highly conserved 75–89-kD nuclear phosphoprotein (c-Myb) that is normally expressed in immature hematopoietic cell lines as these cells differentiate; c-Myb is downregulated at the time of terminal differentiation; phosphorylation of Myb by casein kinase II at an N-terminal site prevents Myb from binding DNA and therefore from further activation; oncogenic transformation is associated with loss of this phosphorylation site, allowing Myb to bind to DNA

myc MOLECULAR BIOLOGY An oncogene of cellular (c-myc) or viral (v-myc) origin that was first identified in the genome of a group of acutely transforming retroviruses capable of inducing neoplasia in birds possibly associated with RNA processing; c-myc is present in normal tissues and is dynamically expressed in the mid-gestation mouse embryo in various tissues undergoing expansion and folding of partially differentiated epithelial cells; in humans, translocation of *myc*, designated as t(14;18)(q32;q21) results in the juxtaposition of bcl-2 to an activator of immunoglobulin heavy chains in follicular lymphoma; retroviruses with the *myc* gene inhibit terminal differentiation of myoblasts, locking the cells into continuous cycling (proliferation); c-myc in its normal site on chromosome 8 is transcriptionally silent; in Burkitt's lymphoma, c-*myc* is translocated, and becomes activated due to 1) c-*myc*'s proximity to an immunoglobulin regulator 2) truncation within the gene itself 3) Mutation in the exon I and/or its flanking sequence or 4) Due to a point mutation on the first intron of c-*myc* with a loss of a regulatory protein binding site **N-myc** is amplified (3-300 copies) in stages II-IV of neuroblastomas (but not in stages I and IV-S) 60% of neuroblastomas have a poor prognosis; N-*myc* proto-oncogene amplification identifies a subset of cases with a poor prognosis, less than 5% of whom survive long-term with conventional therapy; with aggressive therapy, the N-*myc* amplified group of neuroblastomas has up to a four-fold increased survival (Diagn Mol Pathol 1992; 1:229); N-*myc* is also amplified in lung cancer and in composite lymphoma, with simultaneous translocation of t(14;18) and t(8;14) **c-myc** MYC A gene that encodes a 439 amino acid nuclear protein that contains domains that mediate oligomerization and sequence-specific DNA binding; it is

involved in regulating cell proliferation and DNA replication, and in the transcription of certain genes; the clinical significance of c-*myc* amplification is uncertain (Diagn Mol Pathol 1993; 2:163) c-*myc* proto-oncogene is amplified in early uterine cervix carcinoma (and may be a better prognostic indicator than lymph node status), lung cancer (more often in small cell carcinoma), promyelocytic leukemia, and is translocated in Burkitt's lymphoma Note: c-*myc* cooperates with H-*ras* in experimental transformation systems and the loss of c-Myc protein binding to DNA in vivo may explain its relation to malignant transformation (Science 1991; 251:186)

Note: The myc gene family has traditionally been written in lowercase either italic (*myc*) or increasing in a non-italicized form (myc, eg N-myc, c-myc, etc) and in many regions continues to be so written; some authors now prefer using uppercase (eg MYCN); for the gene; since this written form is in a state of flux, in this edition of the DMM, the traditional form will be used

myc The protein product of *myc* which acts by means of a leucine zipper motif, instructing a cell to mature, divide, or undergo autodestruction or apoptosis

mycetoma A condition first described by Gill in 1842 in the Madur district of India (hence the synonyms, Madura foot and maduromycosis); mycetoma is a generic term for a slow, relentless, ulcerating fungal (true fungi) infection, which when neglected, may result in osteomyelitis, occurring in a background of impaired host defense AGENTS *Pseudallescheria boydii, Madurella mycetomatis, M grisea, Phialophora jeanselmei,* and others; actinomycetoma is due to aerobic actinomycetes including *Actinomadura madurae, A pelletieri, Streptomyces somaliensis, Nocardia brasiliensis, N asteroides* and others, most common in the feet of young men (5:1) who work in the tropics and subtropics, which may aso be seen in the thigh and shoulders; clinical disease is uncommon unless accompanied by bacterial infection CLINICAL Indurated swelling, multiple draining sinus tracts and location in the foot PATHOLOGY Suppurative granulomas surrounded by an amorphous rim of eosinophilic hyaline material produced as a host defense; the term mycetoma has also been applied to *Acremonium* and *Fusarium* species as well as the actinomycetes (*Actinomadura, Nocardia* and *Streptomyces* species); the most common cause of mycetoma in the US is *Pseudallescheria boydii* TREATMENT Trimethoprim-sulfamethoxazole

Mycobacterium A genus of obligate aerobic bacteria of the family Mycobacteriaceae, order Actinomycetales; all are capable of producing the typical chronic inflammation, Langhans' giant cells and varying amounts of caseating necrosis and are indistinguishable by the acid-fast stain (which is due to the high concentration of lipid in the outer cell wall); the most common portal of entry for non-tuberculous mycobacteria is the skin; see Acid-fast stain, Buruli ulcer, Langhans' giant cells, MOTT, Prosector's wart, Runyon classification, Tuberculosis

Mycoleptodiscus indicus A rarely pathogenic fungus that may occasionally affect gardeners (CAP Today August 1994)

mycophenolate mofetil RS-61443 A mycophenolic ester derivative that may have advantages over azathioprine as an immunosuppressive purine analogue; it appears to inhibit purine metabolism in T and B cells, and inhibits lymphocyte proliferation in vitro

Mycoplasma An incomplete intracellular and extracellular infectious particle that causes 'walking pneumonia' (which resolves in 4-6 weeks) and genitourinary infections; *M pneumonia* produces hydrogen peroxide, may be identified by hemadsorption and complement fixation and infects epithelial cells, without producing leukocytosis, *M hominis* may cause pelvic inflammatory disease, septicemia and urogenital infection MICROBIOLOGY *Mycoplasma* measure 0.25 μm, lack cell wall precursors (N-acetyl glucosamine and N-acetylmuramic acid), divide by binary fusion and fragmentation and have CO_2 and NH_3 as end products of ureaplasma enzymatic hydrolysis; the growth medium requires fresh yeast or fatty acids, sterols and nucleic acids; the 'spherule' seen on culture represents a microcolony and has a 'fried egg' appearance

Mycoplasma-AIDS link A pathogenic mechanism for the development of AIDS, proposed by L Montagnier, in which HIV-1 attaches to cells previously activated by infection with the cell-wall deficient mycoplasma, and associated infection first identified by SC Lo (Science 1991; 251:271n&v)

Mycoplasma pneumoniae A slow growing pathogen that causes primary atypical pneumonia, which most commonly affects older children and young adults in miniepidemics spread by close contact CLINICAL Incubation of ± 3 weeks, followed by an insidious onset of fever, malaise, and headache, and a spectrum of disease that includes rhinitis, pharyngitis, tracheobronchitis, and pneumonia LABORATORY Leukocytosis with a relative ↑ in PMNs, cold hemagglutinins, and a biologic false positive test for syphilis TREATMENT Tetracycline, erythromycin (N Engl J Med 1994; 331:1437CPC) VACCINE In early stages of development

mycosis cells T lymphocytes with scant cytoplasm, irregular hyperchromatic nuclei, a complex cerebriform nuclear membrane and increased mitotic activity, first described in mycosis fungoides and the related Sezary syndrome, which may also (rarely) be seen in lymphomatoid papulosis, psoriasis vulgaris, lichen planus, PLEVA, basal cell carcinoma, actinic keratosis, systemic and discoid lupus erythematosus

mycosis fungoides A rare ($0.3/10^5$/year), malignant neoplasm of paracortical T cells (usually of helper, less commonly, of suppressor subtype) that is two-fold more common in older blacks CLINICAL Skin involvement precedes symptoms by up to 2 years; the leukemic phase (Sezary syndrome) occurs in 80% and is accompanied by fever, weight loss, lymphadenopathy, hepatosplenomegaly, eosinophilia and lymphocytosis, peripheral neuropathy and periarteritis nodosa; MF has been divided into four clinicopathologic stages of increasing aggression: Erythema stage, plaque stage, tumor stage, d'emblee stage TREATMENT Early aggressive radiotherapy and chemotherapy does not alter clinical disease

mycotic aneurysm An intravascular inflammatory response seen in 3-15% of patients with infective endocarditis, which may arise from contiguous infected sites, but more commonly are of hematogenous spread, potentially resulting in thrombosis or rupture of arteries with walls weakened by an inflamed vasa vasorum or by an impaction-necrosis sequence; because the vessels are a poor culture medium for bacteria (commonly, *Staphylococcus aureus*), smaller aneurysms may resolve spontaneously; those larger that 1-2 cm require excision, if surgically accessible; of greatest concern are the cerebral aneurysms; sites of symptomatic mycotic aneurysms include the sinus of Valsalva 25%, visceral arteries 24%, extremities 22% and brain 15%; Cf Berry aneurysm

myelin basic protein A 19-kD protein that is a major component of myelin, a lipoprotein that develops late in embryogenesis; MBP is elevated in multiple sclerosis and may evoke an altered T-cell response to MBP in this condition; many of the T cells responding to MBP have the Vβ17 variant of the T-cell receptor

myelin figure Myelinoid body, see Lamellar body

myeloablative therapy The use of radiation and/or high-dose chemotherapy to eliminate the tumor load, eg of multiple myeloma in bone marrow involvement followed by restitution of the native marrow elements with either allogeneic marrow transplantation or autologous (self) marrow transplantation that is reinfused after purging of the plasma cell using monoclonal antibodies; while MT is attractive in theory, the frequency of relapse appears to be unchanged, it is not suitable for older (> 65) patients, or those in relapse, or with other major medical problems (N Engl J Med 1994; 330:484DT)

myelodysplasia HEMATOLOGY see Myelodysplastic syndrome NEUROLOGY A generic term for a variety of developmental abnormalities of the spinal cord and nerve roots including myelomeningocele, sacral agenesis, spinal dysraphism and caudal regression syndrome; 1/3 of the infants with myelodysplasia develop external urethral sphincter dysfunction, often in the first three years of life, 1/2 of which are permanent

myelodysplastic syndromes HEMATOLOGY A term that may be equated to preleukemia (which is only partially correct as pathologically, 'dysplasia' is neither clonal nor malignant, but may imply a premalignant condition); myelodysplasia is associated with monosomy 7 in granulocytes and monocytes, and may cause defective granulocyte function; see Preleukemia

myelofibrosis An ↑ in the reticulin fibers in the bone marrow, comprising up to 25% of the marrow volume, which may be idiopathic (see Agnogenic myeloid metaplasia) or secondary to CML, ITP, or polycythemia vera PATHOGENESIS MF may be linked to TGF-β, which may deposited by megakaryocytes, and possibly other cells (Am J Clin Pathol 1995; 103:574OA) LABORATORY Thrombocytosis ($1-14 \times 10^{12}$/L) with giant and bizarre forms, hypochromic and microcytic anemia or erythrocytosis, elliptocytosis, Howell-Jolly bodies, target cells, teardrop cells; mild leukocytosis ($15-40 \times 10^{12}$/L) with ↑ 'bands', ie left shift of granulocytes, juvenile metamyelocytes, ± eosinophilia, basophilia, splenic atrophy BONE MARROW Megakaryocytic hyperplasia, ↑ reticulin fibers, giant cells and immature forms, virus-like particles, granulocytic and erythrocytic hyperplasia, chromosomal abnormalities, eg of 21q which may correlate with reverse transcriptase activity LABORATORY ↑ leukocyte alkaline phosphatase, platelet acid phosphatase, uric acid, vitamin B_{12} and low grade disseminated intravascular coagulation

myeloid antigen A generic term for an antigen present on the surface of a leukocyte with myeloid differentiation, eg CD13, CD14, and CD33; the expression of myeloid antigens in acute lymphocytic leukemia carries a poor prognosis and represents the most powerful predictor of survival than any other parameters including initial white cell count, presence of extramedullary disease or T-cell lineage (N Eng J Med 1991; 324:800); see CD antigens; Cf Pan-B cell markers, Pan-T cell markers

myelolipoma A benign tumor of hematopoietic and adipose tissues that is most common in the adrenal gland, less common in the retroperitoneum and pelvis, ie extra-adrenal; MLs are pathological 'exotica', of interest for their potential confusion with other lesions; the 'record' size of an adrenal ML is 5.5 kg, and of an extra-adrenal ML 4.1 kg (Arch Pathol Lab Med 1994; 118:188CR)

myeloma Multiple myeloma, see there

myeloma, IgD type A condition that comprises 1-2% of all cases of myeloma, most common in older men CLINICAL Lymphadenopathy and hepatosplenomegaly, accompanied in 45% of cases by extra-osseous dissemination (which is present in 15% of IgA and IgG myelomas), hyperviscosity, severe anemia, azotemia, marked osteolysis, hypercalcemia and commonly bizarre plasmacytes and plasmablasts; the M component is not markedly elevated

myeloma kidney The combination of structural and functional renal defects that occurs in about 40% of multiple myelomas and includes intraluminal eosinophilic 'blocked pipe' casts composed of PAS-positive homogeneous material and light chains (Bence-Jones proteins) within flattened distal tubules and collecting ducts (pressure atrophy), spilling over of proteinaceous material, eliciting chronic interstitial nephritis, occasionally causing glomerulonephritis; the mesangial widening may mimic diabetic nephropathy; functional abnormalities cause renal failure in 20%, due to hypercalcemia and renal calcinosis, heavy Bence-Jones proteinuria (causing tubular damage), hyperuricemia (increased tumor DNA turnover), proteinuria, amyloidosis and chronic pyelonephritis, acquired Fanconi syndrome, defects in acidification and concentration, acute and chronic renal failure LABORATORY A peak may be seen in the γ-globulin region (usually) of urine electrophoresis or may appear between the α_2 and β regions

myeloperoxidase deficiency A common (1:500-2000) AR [MIM 254600] condition characterized by neutrophil dysfunction, resulting in a prolonged respiratory burst due to defective post-translational processing of an abnormal precursor protein CLINICAL Usually asymptomatic (several cases of *Candida* infections were reported in patients with concomitant DM) TREATMENT Unnecessary

myelosclerosis with myeloid metaplasia Agnogenic myeloid metaplasia, see there

myeloproliferative disorders A generic term for hematopoietic stem cell disease(s) that are divided by chronicity

ACUTE MPD Acute myelogenous leukemia (myeloblastic, promyelocytic, myelomonocytic, monocytic, erythroid, megakaryocytic, eosinophilic, basophilic), acute biphenotypic (with myeloid and lymphoid markers) leukemia, and acute leukemia with lymphoid markers evolving from a prior clonal hemopathy

SUBACUTE MPD Oligoblastic (smoldering) leukemia, refractory anemia with excess blasts (see RAEB), myelomonocytic leukemia

CHRONIC MPD Polycythemia vera, agnogenic myeloid metaplasia, primary thrombocythemia, chronic myelogenous leukemia (Philadelphia chromosome positive or negative), chronic monocytic leukemia, chronic neutrophilic leukemia

myocardial depressant factor An as-yet unidentified molecule(s) that is/are thought to be present in the circulation of patients in shock; since MDF activity closely parallels the blood levels of lysosomal enzymes, MDF is thought to be a small peptide

myocardial infarction Acute necrosis of myocardial tissue; in the early post-insult period, there may be a need to rely on 'soft' data, especially if the 'cardiac' enzymes have yet to increase, or there is a loss of sensation to the pain characteristic of MI, as occurs in circa 10% patients with DM; elderly older women may have normal levels of creatinine phosphokinase during recuperation from a myocardial infarct Risk factors for MI Atherosclerosis, high cholesterol, hypertension, smoking, DM, low selenium and other factors LABORATORY see Cardiac enzymes, 'Flipped' LD PATHOLOGY Chronicle of myocardial changes

GROSS FINDINGS 6-12 hours Pallor by nitrotetrazolium blue test 18-24 hours Pallor by gross examination 2-4 days Yellow with hyperemic borders 4-10 days Yellow-gray to bright yellow with maximum softness 6 weeks Fibrosis and scar formation

LIGHT MICROSCOPY 60 minutes Glycogen depletion 4-6 hours Myofibrillary degeneration 6-24 hours Coagulation necrosis 1-7 days Neutrophils, macrophages, fatty infiltration, nuclear pyknosis 1-6 weeks Scarring, granulation tissue formation

ELECTRON MICROSCOPY 10-15 minutes Glycogen depletion 20-60 minutes Mitochondrial swelling with amorphous densities (tissue recovery is still possible) 3-4 hours Membranes rupture 5-6 hours Fragmentation of myofibrils Potentially fatal complications of MI Shock, cardiac

arrhythmias, rupture of ventricular aneurysms or papillary muscle, acute congestive heart failure, mural thromboembolism

myocardial ischemia Hypoxia of the myocardium, characterized by an increase in tumor necrosis factor (TNF-β), local production of superoxide anions, loss of coronary vasodilation and myocardial necrosis; when given at the time of the ischemic event, recombinant TNF reduces circulating superoxide anions, maintains endothelial-dependent coronary relaxation and reduces the myocardial injury mediated by endogenous TNF

myoclonus Lightning movement Shock-like muscle contraction (or inhibition, 'negative myoclonus', eg asterixis), involving one or multiple muscle groups ranging from a muscle flicker to a synchronous jerk of an entire body segment Types ESSENTIAL MYOCLONUS Idiopathic and non-progressive, eg restless legs syndrome PHYSIOLOGIC MYOCLONUS Associated with sleep jerks and hiccough EPILEPTIC MYOCLONUS Associated with epilepsy and SYMPTOMATIC MYOCLONUS Associated with encephalopathy, spinocerebellar degeneration, metabolic, toxic or viral encephalopathy or trauma

MyoD A sequence-specific DNA-binding protein that can activate muscle-specific gene expression in certain cells in vitro, which requires the interaction with other factors for complete and stable myogenesis (Nature 1990; 347:197)

***MyoD1* gene** A gene that regulates myogenesis, encoding the MyoD1 protein, a nuclear phosphoprotein with partial homology to the *myc* family of oncoproteins, which binds to the enhancer sequences of the muscle-specific creatine phosphokinase gene, inhibiting DNA synthesis and cell proliferation Note: The 20 residue *myc*-like peptide segment converts fibroblasts to myoblasts; an action attributed to the presence of a helix-loop-helix domain in the encoded protein

myoinositol One of the nine isomers of cyclohexane, synthesized from and structurally similar to glucose; these structures are present in most cells and in high concentration in the nervous system in patients with diabetes mellitus; diabetic neuropathy is attributed to 1) ↑ Sorbitol in Schwann cells, which through its osmotic effect, causes intracellular edema, slowing conduction and 2) ↓ MI and its phospholipids within the Schwann cells, impairing Na$^+$-K$^+$-activated transport ATPase; MI is ↓ in the nerves of diabetics during fasting (Mayo Clin Proc 1989; 64:905); Cf Advanced glycosylation endproducts

myophosphorylase deficiency McArdle's disease, see there

myopia Nearsightedness An abnormality of refraction and accommodation in which parallel rays of light come to a focus anterior to the retina; myopic children are usually products of similarly afflicted adults and tend to as a group be more educated and have higher IQs; in addition to the presumed role of genetics in the development of myopia, there is evidence that myopia may have an acquired component, as it is rare in primitive and/or illiterate societies (New York Times 18 May 1993; C3); simple myopia increases through adolescence, and may be associated with degenerative phenomena in the retina; the use of cycloplegic agents and bifocals to retard the progression of myopia is controversial

myosin Any of a functionally divergent family of actin ATPases (mechanicochemical enzymes) involved in a variety of intracellular motile activities; the amino acid structure of myosins is highly conserved in the 130K motor domain (head region), but displays wide differences in the motile and the enzymatic activities, the latter of which correlate with substitutions at the chimeric substitutions at the actin-binding face of myosin (Nature 1994; 368:567OA)

myosin crossbridge model Rowing crossbridge model,

see there

myositis ossificans Bone formed within muscle; the localized form of myositis ossificans is secondary to trauma resulting from a blow or muscle tearing; the generalized form is AD, often accompanied by aplasia of the thumb, great toe, or rarely other digits, in which the first 'tumor' occurs in the paravertebral or cervical region, followed by multiple ossifying tumors, forming calcifying bridges across muscles and joints resulting in massive rigidity and the patient is turned into 'stone' PATHOLOGY A rim of calcification, lucid zone between the lesion and the underlying bone; tends to occur on the arms and legs, along the shaft of bones that are subjected to repeated trauma; it begins as a hematoma, progressing to a benign reactive fibroblastic reaction with peripheral osteoid formation and peripheral lamellar shell of mature calcified bone (**N Engl J Med 1994; 331:1079**CPC); see Zoning phenomenon

myotonia A phenomenon occurring in diseased muscle in which there is delayed relaxation after voluntary contraction (action myotonia) or mechanical stimulation (percussion myotonia); the myotonic muscular disorders (myotonias) can be classified according to molecular genetic defect into chloride channel-related disorders (eg myotonia congenita, Thomsen type), protein kinase-related disease (eg myotonic dystrophy), sodium channel-related disorders (eg hyperkalemic periodic paralysis), and unknown causes (**N Engl J Med 1993; 328:482**RV)

myotonic dystrophy An AD [MIM 160900] condition affecting ± 1:8000, age of onset, age 20-25, impaired intelligence which causes distal myopathy, preferentially affecting certain muscles, eg levator palpebrae, facial, masseter, sternocleidomastoid, forearm, hand and pretibial muscles, resulting in diffuse muscular weakness and atrophy beginning in early adulthood causing the characteristic 'hatchet face'; other changes include lenticular opacities, endocrinopathies (testicular atrophy with androgen insufficiency, ovarian dysfunction which rarely interferes with fertility, diabetes mellitus, hypothyroidism), mild cerebral cortical atrophy, frontoparietal baldness, cardiac and smooth muscle (GI, especially esophageal motility) abnormalities, respiratory dysfunction and hyperostosis frontalis interna; death usually occurs by age 50 PATHOLOGY Variable type I muscle fiber atrophy, with internal nuclei, ringed muscle fibers, increased intrafusal myofibers in the muscle spindles and hypertrophy of type II muscle fibers; internal (centralized) nuclei are characteristic, and occur early, as do sarcoplasmic masses ('pads') and annulets MOLECULAR PATHOLOGY A specific unstable DNA sequence or 'repeat region' (containing the 3 nucleotides, cytosine, thymine, and guanine, CTG) has been identified in MD located in the 3' untranslated region of a protein kinase gene located in chromosome segment 19q13.3; this region can be detected directly by a DNA probe p5B1.4; the repeat is always larger than the normal 9.8 kb allele* (also detected by p5B1.4), and the ↑ in the unstable sequence length correlates with the ↑ in disease severity (**N Engl J Med 1993; 328:471**OA) it has been reported that the reverse mutation (reduced copy numbers) may occur, leading to correction of the phenotypic abnormality (**ibid 1993; 328:476**OA)

*In normal subjects, the number of the repeat units is 5-35, mildly affected patients with MD have ≥ 50 repeats, and severely affected patients have 2000 or more repeats

myotubular (centronuclear) myopathy A myopathy with various patterns of inheritance, which have a common feature of centrally-located nuclei within muscle fibers, which are surrounded by cytoplasmic material with features of maturing myotubules, accompanied by atrophy of type I and hypertrophy of type II muscle fibers; the X-linked form results in neonatal death due to respiratory muscle insufficiency; the AD form is not pernicious

myristate n-Tetradecanoate acid The fatty acid component of glycosyl phosphatidylinositol, an integral membrane component of trypanosomes; see O-11

myristoylated alanine-rich (protein) C kinase substrate see MARCK

myxedema A severe hypothyroid state characterized by yellowish discoloration, nonpitting edema, in particular of the face, which is accompanied by periorbital puffiness, puffy lips and tongue, hoarse voice, and sluggish movement; myxedema elicits several reactions *a sui generis* MYXEDEMA COMA A complication of severe hypothyroidism, in which an additional physiological stress is added to the clinical milieu, eg iatrogenic (sedatives in hypothyroidism are very slowly metabolized), infections, cold exposure or rarely, may occur spontaneously Mortality 20-50% MYXEDEMA MADNESS A condition that is most common in the elderly, characterized by impaired hearing and memory, acalculia, somnolence, psychological withdrawal and paranoia MYXEDEMA MEGACOLON Pseudo-obstruction due to reduced gastrointestinal motility MYXEDEMA WIT Confabulation or use of humorous non-sequiturs by a patient with hypothyroidism in order to draw the interviewer's attention away from the patient's impaired memory

myxoid A non-specific descriptor for any 'loose' pale-to-lightly basophilic by hematoxylin and eosinophilic stroma, the few cells present include fibroblasts and rarely chronic inflammatory cells; myxoid stroma occurs in nodular fasciitis, intramuscular myxoma, ganglion cyst, chordoma, neurofibroma, carcinomas, as well as spindle cell lipoma and lipoblastoma and in myxoid variants of sarcomas, where the distinction is of practical importance, as myxoid differentiation may have a better prognosis, including rhabdomyosarcoma, chondrosarcoma, malignant fibrous histiocytoma, liposarcoma; Cf Mucin lake

myxoma A stromal proliferation of loose connective tissue of unknown histogenesis, and often of uncertain significance which is characterized by a scant amount of stellate and spindled cells swimming in a pool of abundant mucoid material, usually hyaluronic acid, with scant vascularity; common sites that play host to myxomas include the shoulder, thigh, and the left atrium; it is uncertain whether myxomas are neoplastic or reactive; the finding in cardiac myxomas of chromosomal abnormalities (eg telomere-to-telomere translocations, 45, XY) suggests a neoplastic origin; see Atrial myxoma

myxopapillary ependymoma A relatively indolent ependymal cell tumor arising in the conus medullaris and filum terminale of the spinal cord; most cases occur in the 4th decade PATHOLOGY The tumors are composed of clusters of well-defined cuboidal-to-low columnar cells with clear cytoplasm, arranged in a papillary fashion around well-vascularized core of acellular and hyalinized connective tissue with mucinous degeneration; see Ependymoma

myxovirus Any of a group of large single-stranded RNA virus that is divisible into 1) Orthomyxoviruses, eg influenza virus, and 2) Paramyxovirus, eg mumps virus

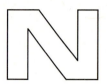

N Shorthand symbol for: 1) Asparagine 2) Avogadro's number (particles in 1 Mole = 6.023 X 10²³) 3) Neutron number 4) Newton 5) Nitrogen 6) Normal solution (equivalents/L) 7) Population size 8) Radiance

n Shorthand symbol for: 1) Haploid number 2) nano- (SI or International System abbreviation for 10⁻⁹) 3) Neutron 4) Refractive index 5) Sample size in data sets

ν Greek nu: 1) Degrees of freedom 2) Frequency, as expressed in hertz 3) Neutrino

N-acetylcysteine A precursor (via cysteine) of glutathione, the principal antioxidant that mops up free radical-induced oxidative damage; N-acetylcysteine deficiency has been linked by some authors to the pathogenesis of AIDS; in one proposed sequence, tumor necrosis factor, a cytokine produced in the early inflammatory response to HIV, enters the T cell, generating free radicals, depleting its intracellular stores of glutathione, ultimately causing T cells to commit suicide; this scenario may explain why T cells are not necessarily HIV-infected but nonetheless die; NAC is in therapeutic trials (New York Times May 3, 1994; C3)

n-3 (polyunsaturated) fatty acids Omega-3 fatty acids A family of long-chain polyunsaturated fatty acids, primarily eicosapentaenoic (C20:5) and docosahexanenoic acid (C22:6)[1]; ↑ in dietary n-3 fatty acids are cardioprotective and have a positive impact on inflammatory conditions, interfering with the production of mediators of inflammation, including leukotrienes, platelet-activating factor, IL-1 and TNF; ↑ consumption of dietary n-3FAs and/or fish[2] are reported to be clinically beneficial in patients with chronic inflammatory conditions, including rheumatoid arthritis, ulcerative colitis and COPD (N Engl J Med 1994; 331:228oA) following ingestion, n3FAs are rapidly incorporated into phospholipids of plasma and blood vessels; n3FAs ↓ plasma levels of VLDL-cholesterol, ↓ platelet aggregation, and ↑ vasodilation (N Engl J Med 1995; 332:977oA) and to protect against coronary artery disease (Arch Pathol Lab Med 1993; 117:102oA) and atherosclerosis[3] see Fish; Cf Olive oil, Tropical oil

[1]Which have a double bond between carbons 3 and 4 [2]fish oils are predominantly n-3 (omega-3) [3]They have also been reported to ↓ plasma LDL, ↑ HDL, ↓ prostaglandin production, and ↓ synthesis of leukotrienes and possibly also IL-1

N protein MOLECULAR BIOLOGY A 25-kD protein of unknown function contained in small nuclear ribonucleic proteins (snRNPs) of neurons, which has been used to understand differences in RNA-processing in cells of different lineages VIROLOGY The major phosphoprotein of the rabies virus, which when it binds to RNA, results in the production of a ribonucleoprotein that is a strong enhancer of oral immunization and is a major target of CD4 (T helper) cells

(Science & Medicine 1995; 2/3:48) Cf G protein

N-telopeptides see under Telopeptides

N-terminal The end of a protein or polypeptide that contains the free amine group, placed by convention at the left of a diagram

NA 1) Nomina Anatomica, see there 2) Numerical aperature (optics)

NAC N-acetylcysteine, see there

NAD⁺/NADH The oxidized/reduced forms of nicotinamide adenine dinucleotide, a redox coenzyme, which is crucial in the intracellular storage (by high-energy phosphate bonds) and exchange of energy; a coenzyme used to transfer hydrogen

NADP⁺/NADPH The oxidized/reduced forms of nicotinamide adenine dinucleotide phosphate; a coenzyme for transfer of hydrogen in the pentose phosphate reaction, which is also a coenzyme for glutathione reductase

Nae I MOLECULAR BIOLOGY A 70-kD dimeric endonuclease that has two binding sites that link it to both the topoisomerase and recombinase families of proteins (Science 1995; 267:1817) see DNA cleavage

Naegleria A genus of free-living flagellated soil-based amoebae of class Rhizopoda that is found in stagnant water, which may cause primary amoebic meningitis, see there

nafamostat mesylate A synthetic serine protease inhibitor that has had currency in Japan as a therapy for acute pancreatitis; NM and its metabolites also reversibly inhibit amiloride-sensitive sodium conductance of renal cortical collecting ducts, thereby impairing urinary potassium excretion (N Engl J Med 1995; 332:687c)

nafarelin A gonadotropin-releasing hormone (GnRH) analogue that is used to treat certain estrogen-driven conditions, eg endometriosis or uterine leiomyomas; the undesired side effect of nafarelin therapy, osteopenia, can be prevented by co-administration of parathyroid hormone in ♀ receiving long-term therapy with GnRH analogues (N Engl J Med 1994; 331:1618oA, Acta Obstet Gynecol, Scand Feb 1994)

nafarelin test A provocative test that can be used to detect functional ovarian hyperandrogenism; 100 μg is administered subcutaneously; a supranormal response, ie elevation of peak plasma concentration of 17-hydroxyprogesterone ≥ 7.8 nmol/L (259 ng/dl) which suggest an ovarian cause of androgen excess (N Engl J Med 1992; 327:157oA)

β-NAG NEPHROLOGY N-acetyl-β-D-glucosaminidase A 150 kD lysosomal enzyme that cannot be filtered through a normal glomerulus, making is an ideal marker of proximal tubular cell damage; an ↑ rate of excretion is associated with renal injury due to drug-related nephrotoxicity or ascending urinary tract infections; β-NAG can be measured by dipstick, or by the chlorophenol red method (AACC poster sessions, 1991)

Na⁺/H⁺ antiporter A 110 kD plasma membrane exchange glycoprotein transporter that regulates intracellular pH, important in signal transduction, which is modified in response to external mitogenic signals (phorbol esters, neurotransmitters, chemotactic peptides, lectins and growth factors) and by oncogenic transformation which induce persistent cytoplasmic alkalinization; antiporter activation is thought to be the result of phosphorylation

Na⁺/K⁺ ATPase PHYSIOLOGY A ubiquitous, integral membrane-bound enzyme that is present in all animal cells, and couples ATP hydrolysis to the countertransport of Na⁺ and K⁺ ions across the plasma membrane; in neurons, dopamine inhibits this pump, providing a mechanism by which neurotransmitters can regulate neuronal excitability; the responsible ATPase is an oligomer with two 90-kD (α) subunits and two 40-kD (β) subunits; cardiac glycosides are thought to act by blocking the receptor's β subunit ; Cf Na⁺/H⁺ antiporter

nail-patella syndrome Hereditary osteo-onychodysplasia, HOOD syndrome An AD [MIM 161200] condition affecting structures of both mesodermal and ectodermal origin with partial-to-complete absence of thumbnails and great toenails, flexion contractions of multiple joints, defective or absent patellae, lordosis, clinodactyly and campylodactyly, conical iliac horns, scapular thickening, radial head subluxation, renal abnormalities (mesangial proliferation, thickened glomerular basement membrane, collagen deposition with proteinuria, microscopic hematuria, glomerulonephritis, pyelonephritis and slowly progressive renal failure), and ocular disease (clover leaf pigmentation of iris, cataracts, microphakia, microcornea, keratoconus, ptosis)

naïve T cell CLINICAL IMMUNOLOGY A poorly understood and characterized cell of the immune system that play a major role in recognizing new antigens in the general circulation; once an antigen is recognized as new by a naïve T cell, it responds by differentiating into an activated memory cell that undergoes clonal expansion; it is thought that depletion of naïve T cells is a more critical clinical event than the reduction of CD4 helper T cells (**New York Times 21 Feb 1995; C3**) see CD4 (helper) T cells

naked DNA A generic term for a sequence of DNA that can effect an immune response by injection of DNA that encodes an immunogen of interest directly into the host; as with live recombinant viral vectors, ND elicits both antibody and CTL (cytotoxic T lymphocyte) reactions, and thus may provide a useful construct for vaccine design (**Science & Medicine 1995; 2/3:38**)

naked granuloma 'Hard' tubercle An epithelioid giant cell response that consists of Langhans' giant cell(s) and chronic, ie mononuclear cell inflammation without necrosis, therefore 'naked', a histologic finding typical of sarcoidosis and granuloma annulare

naked nucleus CYTOLOGY A nucleus in a cytoplasmic preparation that is virtually devoid of cytoplasm, a soft criterion for diagnosing ovarian endometriosis, which may be mixed with slightly elongated, cytoplasm-poor cells with hyperchromatic nuclei Note: Definitive diagnosis of endometriosis requires the presence of endometrial glands, stroma and hemorrhage SURGICAL PATHOLOGY Naked cells are highly characteristic of undifferentiated or small cell carcinomas of any site, most commonly seen in small or 'oat' cell carcinoma of the lung and other sites which have friable ('taffy-pull') nuclei and scant or absent cytoplasm

nalbuphine A narcotic agonist that is chemically related to naloxone with similar action to, but less addictive than morphine

NALC N-acetyl L-cysteine MICROBIOLOGY A mucolytic agent used for collecting sputa destined for TB culture that liquefies the mucus by breaking disulfide bonds

NAME syndrome see LAMB syndrome

NANB see Non-A, non-B hepatitis

Nancy Cruzan see Cruzan

nanotechnology A term that is loosely defined as any process, eg chemical reactions performed on a very small scale; nanotechnology is already integrating itself into the working environment, and ranges from disposible sensors for temperature, pressure and blood chemistries, to the silicon microaccelerators that activate automobile air bags; in varying states of development are nanotechnologies designed to perform micro-PCR (polymerase chain reaction, which will require < 10 μL of reagents), automate leukocyte counting, measure sperm motility (SpermChip, U Pennsylvania that has a complex channel etched on a silicon chip by photolithography), capillary

electrophoresis, and others (**Am Clin Lab July 1994**)

Nantucket disease A blood-borne infection by *Babesia microti*, an intertriginous cyst-forming parasite, named after an island near Massachusetts in the US Northeast coast, occurring along the entire eastern seaboard of the US RESERVOIR White-footed mouse VECTOR *Ixodes dammini* (the 'Lyme disease' tick) In Europe, babesiosis is most common in splenectomized subjects and is often fatal; in the US, it is rarely fatal and the splenectomized subjects comprise ⅓ of cases CLINICAL 1-3 week incubation, malaise, fatigue, anorexia, shaking chills, fever, headache, myalgias, mental depression, and emotional lability DIAGNOSIS Wright-Giemsa-stained smears of peripheral blood, where the ring form resembles that of *Plasmodium falciparum*; indirect immunofluorescent antibody titers > than 1:256 TREATMENT Clindamycin, quinacrine

NAP Neutrophil alkaline phosphatase, see Leukocyte alkaline phosphatase

NAP-1 Neutrophil attractant or activation protein-1, see Interleukin-8

NAP test MICROBIOLOGY A 'rapid' (4-5 days) growth differential test in which an aliquot of bacterial growth medium containing *Mycobacterium* is added to a tube with NAP (*p*-nitro-α-acetylamino-β–hydroxypropiophenone); if the 'bug' is *Mycobacterium tuberculosis* (*M africanis*, or *M bovis*) NAP will inhibit growth; if it is *M avium-intercellulare* complex, its growth in cluture medium increases

naphtha 1) A generic term for any petroleum distillation product 2) Gasoline (British)

naphthalene A crystal formed from 2 benzene rings, used for mothballs and insecticide TOXICITY Headache, nausea, vomiting and hematuria; if severe or prolonged exposure, cataracts, convulsions, hepatocellular necrosis and marked hemolysis, especially in patients with glucose-6-phosphate dehydrogenase deficiency

naphthol A white crystalline phenol derivative intermediate in the synthesis of multiple compounds including pharmaceuticals TOXICITY Abdominal pain, glomerulonephritis, convulsions, circulatory collapse and skin pigmentation

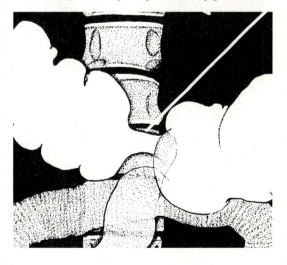

napkin ring lesion

napkin ring lesion Apple core lesion RADIOLOGY A pattern of intestinal constriction caused by mucosal erosion and stenosis with 'shouldering' of the margins, corresponding to an exophytic encircling mass within the large intestinal lumen, usually corresponding to an advanced invasive adenocarcinoma, more often present in the left colon; the mass may obstruct fecal flow, inducing pencil-thin stools and be partially mimicked by concentric amebomas in *Entamoeba histolytica* granulomas, by exuberant submucosal fibrosis in Crohn's disease, in the stenosing fibrotic stages of diverticulosis coli, in a squamous cell carcinoma arising in a dermoid cyst of the ovary with invasion of the muscularis of the rectosigmoid colon (**N Engl J Med 1995; 332:1631sA**) and in small intestinal adenocarcinoma

Napoleon hat sign ORTHOPEDIC RADIOLOGY Marked anteroinferior displacement of the anterior edge of lumbar vertebrum L5, seen as a symmetrical navicular density in a frontal plain film of the lower vertebrae in congenital spondylolisthesis, fancifully likened to an inverted napoleonic hat

narcissistic personality disorder PSYCHIATRY A condition characterized by '...*a pervasive pattern of grandiosity (in fantasy or behavior), need for admiration, and lack of empathy that begins in early adulthood...*' (**DSM-IV**) it is estimated that 1% of the general population, and 2-16% of the clinical population

---

NARCISSISTIC PERSONALITY DISORDER-CRITERIA (5 + OF FOLLOWING)

1) Requires excessive admiration

2) Grandiose sense of self-importance; believes self to be superior

3) Preoccupied with fantasies of unlimited success, power, brilliance

4) Believes that he/she is special and should have only the best

5) Has sense of entitlement, ie deserves special favors or treatment

6) Exploits interpersonal relations, ie takes advantage of others

7) Lacks empathy and concern for others

8) Is envious of others or believes them to be envious of him/her

9) Displays arrogance

Modified from "Diagnostic and Statistical Manual of Mental Disorders, 4th ed, Washington, DC, American Psychiatric Association, 1994

---

narcolepsy A condition characterized by recurring attacks of irresistible desire for sleep and abnormalities of REM sleep; narcolepsy affects 125 000 in the US (prevalence 40/10⁵) and is defined as a daytime mean sleep latency of less than 5 minutes, in conjunction with verification of REM in two of five daytime nap periods; the 'classic' form occurs in 70% of patients with narcolepsy, and is a combination of narcolepsy with cataplexy (abrupt loss of muscle tone, evoked by strong emotion, excitement, anger or laughter), causing them to collapse or fall to the ground, while completely conscious; narcoleptics may have amnesia for the 'absences', have fallen asleep while driving or while at work and prefer shift work as 'drowsiness' is more socially acceptable PREVALENCE From 1:600 (Japan) to 1:500 000 (Israel), ♂:♀ ratio 1:1, onset age 15 to 35, tightly linked to certain class II HLA antigens, eg 98-100% of narcoleptics have HLA-DR2 and/or HLA-DQw1 CLINICAL Narcolepsy tetrad; if accompanied by cataplexy, the patient feels a sense of absolute urgency for sleep in often inappropriate situations (while standing, eating, carrying on conversations) and is accompanied by blurring of vision, diplopia, and ptosis TREATMENT Strategic pre-planned 'catnaps' throughout the day, analeptic drugs, ie long-term stimulants, eg methylphenidate, dextroamphetamine or tricyclic antidepressants that act by inhibiting reuptake of norepinephrine and serotonin; MAOIs may be useful in short term but can cause tardive dyskinesia; see Insomnia(s), Sleep apnea syndrome, Sleep disorders

Note: Despite the common association, cataplexy differs from narcolepsy as it affects cell clusters in the medial medulla distinct from those affected in narcolepsy (**Science 1991; 252:1315**)

narcolepsy tetrad A group of symptoms (cataplexy, hypnagogic hallucinations and sudden paralysis) that is typical of narcolepsy, see there

narcotic A substance causing euphoria and analgesia at the desired abuse levels and physical dependence and CNS depression, stupor, coma and death when administered in excess; narcotics may be 1) Natural products extracted from the poppy plant, yielding morphine and heroin or the coca plant, yielding cocaine and crack 2) Semi-synthetic products with opiate activity, eg meperidine and methadone or synthetics, see MPTP; under the umbrella term of narcotic, alkaloids, eg LSD, mescaline, barbiturates, alcohol, marijuana, cocaine, hallucinogens and stimulants, eg antidepressants and 2) Completely synthetic narcotics, eg fentanyl

'narcs' American slang for narcotics enforcement agents; Cf Narks

'narks' British slang for nitrogen narcosis; see Rapture of the deep

narrow QRS complex tachycardia A relatively rapid (usually > 100 beats/min) cardiac rhythm with a QRS duration of ≤ 100 msec, which while rarely fatal, may be symptomatic MECHANISM Reentry causes > 90% of NQCRs; other mechanisms include triggered activity, and automaticity TREATMENT IV adenosine (**Mayo Clin Proc 1995; 70:365oA**)

NAS 1) National Academy of Science 2) No abnormalities seen

NASA syndrome Not a surgical abdomen syndrome A highly colloquial term for an acute abdomen that has been examined by a surgeon, and deemed not to require surgical therapy, and thus 'punted back' to the nonsurgical attending physicians for a diagnostic workup (**JAMA 1992; 267:2330, 268:2030c**)

nasal airway resistance ENT An objective parameter that determines the state of the nasal passages during breathing, providing a point of reference for determining the degree of nasal obstruction by simultaneously measuring transnasal pressure and airway resistance; NAR is of use in diagnosing and treating nasal obstruction

nasal cycle RESPIRATORY PHYSIOLOGY Alternating congestion and decongestion of the nasal airway that occurs in 70% of the adult population and is controlled by the autonomic nervous system, and may affected by circadian changes in hormone levels, temperature, humidity, posture, and emotion; in the face of a unilateral fixed obstruction, the congestion phase of the side opposite the obstruction may be interpreted as an abnormality of the normal side or 'paradoxical nasal obstruction' (**Mayo Clin Proc 1990; 65:1095**)

nasal packing ENT The filling of the nasal cavities with adaptic gauze impregnated with polysporin ointment, used in treating nasal fractures, reconstructive surgery, after septorhinoplasty and in posterior nosebleeds; with packing the airway improves in 96% of the packing group (versus 64% in the nonpacked group); recurrent deviation occurred in 13% of the packed and 41% of the nonpacked group

NASBA Nucleic acid sequence-based amplification MOLECULAR DIAGNOSTICS An isothermal RNA-based target amplification-type technique for amplifying DNA METHOD

1) A DNA nucleotide primer binds to an RNA target, which may be mRNA, rRNA, or an RNA virus; the DNA nucleotide primer contains the T7 RNA polymerase promoter

2) Reverse transcriptase is used to elongate the primer to make a DNA copy of the RNA target sequence, thus producing an RNA/DNA hybrid

3) RNase H digest the RNA from the hybrid, leaving a single-stranded DNA copy (cDNA) of the target RNA

4) A second DNA primer binds to the cDNA and is extended by RT, producing double-stranded DNA (dsDNA)

5) From the dsDNA, T7 RNA polymerase makes multiple RNA transcripts that corespond to the region flanked by the primers

6) The RNA transcripts are processed by RT and RNase H and become subtrates for further amplification and reaction cycles

NASBA can achieve a 10^9 amplification factor in 90 minutes (CAP Today May1995 p1, Bio/Technology 1995; 13:554)

NASCET North American Symptomatic Carotid Endarterectomy Trial (see JAMA 1992; 268:3120)

nasopharyngeal carcinoma A malignancy endemic to regions of southern China, where it is up to 100-fold more common than in Europe, often associated with HLA-A2, Bw46 and B17; NPC is linked to EBV infection and 65% of NPCs express EBV's latent membrane protein (LMP); when keratinocytes in tissue culture are transfected with the LMP gene, the keratinocytes dedifferentiate, acquiring a 'malignant' morphology

natal teeth A deciduous tooth that is present in 1:2000 neonates, often located in the position of the central mandibular incisors, with minimal gingival attachment, or which less commonly presage early eruption of remaining deciduous teeth CLINICAL If the teeth are loose, they are annoying to the nursing infant; if the teeth are well implanted, they are annoying to the nursing mother COMPLICATION Amputation of the tongue tip (Riga-Fede disease) by the natal teeth at the time of delivery

National Boards Examination A standardized examination that is administered in the US and Canada in lieu of state medical examinations to determine the level of competence of a candidate physician applying for a state's medical license

Note: In the spoken parlance, it is common to refer to it merely as the 'National Boards'

National Bureau of Standards National Institute of Standards and Technology (NIST), see there

National Cancer Institute An organization with a focused interest in cancer research that has provided financial support of many experimental protocols in the US; see Cancer screening

National Formulary One of two (the other is the US Pharmacopeia) official compendia recognized by Federal Pure Food and Drug Act of 1906; in the National Formulary, the approved therapeutic agents used in medical practice in the US are described and defined with respect to source, chemistry, physical properties, tests for identitification and purity, dosage range and class of use

national health care HEALTH CARE INDUSTRY The financing and delivery of health care by the government; while the concept of NHC is virtually synonymous with the Canadian health care system, the Canadian government does not deliver care per se (Am Med News 25 October 1992, p7)

national health insurance HEALTH CARE FINANCING Government-paid insurance for all (Am Med News 25 October 1992, p7) Cf Nationalized health insurance

National Health Federation An organization based in Washington DC with neither medical or scientific affiliations that represents the belief that organized medicine, the pharmaceutical industry and other 'special interest' groups have controlled legislation that does not serve the interests of the American public; see Alternative medicine; Cf Quackery

National Institutes of Health NIH, see there

National Institute for Occupational Safety and Health The research arm and 'scientific conscience' of the US federal health and safety programs; NIOSH responsibilities include

DEVELOPMENT OF 'CRITERIA DOCUMENTS' that recommend exposure limits to hazardous substances

TRAINING AND EDUCATION of occupational health professionals

DEVELOPMENT OF EXPOSURE MEASUREMENT AND SAMPLING METHODS and

PERFORMANCE OF INDUSTRY-WIDE STUDIES to evaluate the health effects of low level long-term exposure to potentially hazardous substances or processes

Exposure to environmental toxins in the workplace is usually measured in parts (1 to 5000 or more, depending upon the substance) per million (ppm) of exposure/8 hours (Publications Division, NIOSH, 4676 Columbia Pkwy, Cincinnati, Ohio 45226)

National Institute of Standards and Technology (formerly National Bureau of Standards) A branch of the US government responsible for maintaining primary reference standards and developing reference methods and reference materials

National Practitioner Data Bank A database established by the US Congress to facilitate professional peer review and restrict the ability of incompetent physicians and dentists to move from state to state, eluding discovery of previous substandard performance or unprofessional conduct; the NPDB is accessible only to authorized persons and there are criminal penalties for misuse of the data or accession by unauthorized parties; the NPDB is overseen by the Health Resources and Services Administration, and has since September 1990 collected data on all malpractice payments and disciplinary actions against physicians, dentists, and other licensed health professionals

The financial 'floor' for reporting information to the NPDB has not yet been set, although one suggested by MJ Astrue, General Counsel of the Health and Human Services is $100 000 for neurosurgeons, obstetricians, and possibly other 'high risk' groups, $50 000 for other physicians, and $20-30 000 for dentists (Am Med News 21 September 1992 p1)

nationalized health insurance HEALTH CARE FINANCING Government as single payer for health insurance (Am Med News 25 October 1992, p7) Cf National health insurance

native *adjective* Pertaining or referring to an unaltered or ground state of a molecular species, in which state in vivo biological systems are presumed to function

natural antibody Normal antibody An antibody present in the circulation, without there being known previous exposure to the antigen; anti-A and anti-B of the ABO blood group are the only naturally-occurring antibodies that are virtually always present in subjects who lack the relevant antigen; NAs in other blood groups are relatively uncommon and include anti-I (Ii system), anti-Le^a and anti-Le^b (Lewis system), anti-Lu^a (Lutheran group), anti-M, anti-N, anti-S, anti-M^g, anti-Vw, and anti-En^a (MNSs system), anti-P, anti-P$_1$ and antiPP$_1$P^k (P system), and others

natural carcinogen A substance that is normally present in foods, which is carcinogenic when tested by standard mutagenic assays in rodents or in bacteria, eg Ames' test; it is unclear whether the 14 parts per million (ppm) of 5-8-methoxypsoralen, present in parsley and parsnips, and carcinogenic to rodents or the 50-200 ppm of caffeic acid, present in apples, carrots, cherries and others, actually present a carcinogenic potential in humans, or as Ames et al have implied (Proc Natl Acad Sci, USA 1990; 87:7777), there is a threshold at which critical mutation occurs (Science 1990; 250:743) see Ames' test, Toxicity testing

natural childbirth A normal vaginal delivery in which the mother is more actively involved in the parturitional mechanics (than in the 'unnatural' birth); the 'natural' mother is awake during delivery often without general anesthesia, has actively 'trained' in the birthing process, and is 'attended' by the father (or 'significant' other) at the time of delivery; see Bonding, Breast milk, Lamaze method

natural death *'A death that is caused solely by disease and/or the aging process...'* (Arch Pathol Lab Med 1995; 119:123OA) Cf Unnatural death

natural disaster see Climatological disaster, Geological disaster; Cf Man-made disaster

'natural experiment' method EPIDEMIOLOGY A 'technique' in epidemiology that seeks to identify two or more naturally occurring cohorts with clear differences in sex, race, religion, occupation, geography and 'exposures', analyzing their risks for suffering certain diseases; 'natural experiment' populations include Mormons (non-smoking, non-drinking); Italians (low incidence of cardiovascular disease); Japanese and Icelanders (high incidence of gastric carcinoma); much of current knowledge about various morbid conditions, eg cancer and cardiovascular disease), their putative etiologies, early detection, and prevention is initially recognized by statistical analysis of 'natural experiments'

natural food movement see Health food movement

natural gas An odorless (odorant is added to the gas as a safety precaution) combustible gas derived from underground petroleum deposits, which are used for cooking and heating, the principal components of which are short-chain hydrocarbons, eg CH_4 (methane), ethane, propane, butane, CO_2, N_2 and H_2S TOXICITY At high ambient levels, the volatile hydrocarbons induce hypoxia by replacing alveolar gas, crossing the alveolar-capillary barrier and causing CNS depression; Cf Flatulence

natural killer cell NK cell A subset of 'null cells' or large granular lymphocytes (LGLs) that comprise 3-5% of peripheral leukocytes, 75% of which are NK cells with a high cytoplasmic:nuclear ratio and an intrinsic non-antibody-mediated ability to kill various cells, including virus-transformed fibroblasts, solid or hematopoietic tumor cells, microorganisms, embryologic, marrow and thymic cells; NK cells are stimulated by IL-2 to release eosinophilic granules (primary lysosomes) and IFN, increasing the number of target-binding NK cells, their cytotoxicity and speed of cytolysis Note: Cytolysis is normally slow (18 hours), triggered by protein kinase C, facilitated by lymphokines, and mediated by perforins that insert transmembrane 'doughnuts' allowing free passage of ions into the cells; NK activity may also be stimulated by K-*ras* oncogenic activation; NK activity decreases with age, malignancy (especially immunoproliferative) and immunodeficiency, eg severe combined immunodeficiency, X-linked and Chediak-Higashi syndromes NK cell surface markers IgG-FcR(2), low affinity T-cell markers (CD3), C3bi, Leu-7, HNK-1, OKM1, Mac 1, CD16 (Leu11) and B67.1 (T cell markers) QUANTIFICATION OF NK CELL ACTIVITY Measurement of lysis of the radioactive K-562 target cells

nature-nurture debate PSYCHOLOGY An ongoing controversy regarding the degree of influence the genome ('nature') has in determining behavior and shaping personality, and to what degree environmental factors ('nurture') determine personality; this issue is unlikely to be resolved as it is not amenable to statistically valid experiments

naturopathy 'Holistic medicine' An unorthodox approach to healing that uses the forces of nature as therapeutic modalities; naturopathy espouses the philosophy that disease results from violation of natural laws of living, ie drugs of any sort are harmful, while 'natural' products and activities are deemed therapeutic; 'naturopaths' are not licensed, but rather meet self-determined criteria; conventional drugs are proscribed and 'therapy' is prescribed, based on the use of natural forces (ie earth, wind, fire, light, heat, cold, air, physical activity) and foods, herbs, teas and massage; see Alternative medicine; Homeopathy

navicular cells CYTOLOGY Glycogen-rich variant of intermediate squamous cells seen in the Papanicolaou-stained cytological preparations of the vagina and cervix; navicu-

lar cells comprise the most abundant cells in pregnancy and are seen in early menopause, hormonal deficiencies and inflammation; see Maturation index

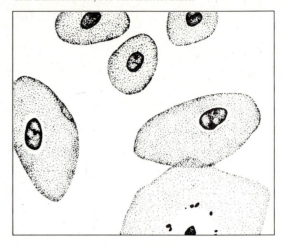

navicular cells

NBE Non-bacterial endocarditis, see Mycotic aneurysm

NBS National Bureau of Standards, now known as National Institute of Standards and Technology, see there

NBQX 2,3-Dihydroxy-6-nitro-7-sulfamoyl-benzo(F)-quinoxaline A non-NMDA (excitatory amino acid) receptor antagonist that has a protective effect against cerebral ischemia; Cf NMDA

NBT test Nitroblue tetrazolium test LABORATORY MEDICINE A quantitative test that measures neutrophil peroxidase activity; if phagocytosis is intact, NBT is converted to blue-black clumps of reduced NBT known as formazan* which occurs via the hexose monophosphate shunt; NBT reduction is defective in chronic granulomatous disease, see there

*Indicating phagocytic capacity, the ability to reduce NBT which precipitates as deep blue granules if superoxide or O_2^- is produced in tested cell

N-cadherin see Cadherins

N-CAM Neural-cell adhesion molecule A glycoprotein present at the interfaces of cell clusters in early developing embryos; N-CAM's sequence, elucidated by cDNA (complementary DNA) analysis, reveals an extracellular region with 5 domains homologous to each other and to the immunoglobulin superfamily (immunoglobulins and T cell receptor); N-CAM modulates extracellular regions resulting in different extracellular signal 'messages' during embryogenesis and mediates post-translational changes in the oligosaccharides on the cell surface; N-CAM also mediates interneuronal and neuromuscular cell adhesions, influencing intercellular events, eg junctional communication and interaxonal associations with pathways, targets and signals altering neurotransmitter levels; low polysialic acid (PSA) levels in N-CAM triggers adhesion and contact-dependent events; high N-CAM PSA content inhibits cell-cell interactions; transition of the N-CAM isoform from 145 kD to 125 kD is associated with maturation from the myoblast to the multinucleated skeletal form

N:C ratio Nuclear:cytoplasmic ratio, see there

NCHGR National Center for Human Genome Research, an agency of the US National Institutes of Health

NCI National Cancer Institute, see there

NDA New drug application PHARMACEUTICAL INDUSTRY A document usually generated by a pharmaceutical company, which is the first step in developing a commercial drug; in the US, many years are required before a drug arrives at the 'marketplace'; after the chemist creates an 'interesting' compound, it is tested on the usual battery of beasts; if it is neither toxic nor teratogenic, the company may submit a commercial IND (investigational new drug) application, passing through phases 1 to 3 of clinical pharmacology; if both the FDA and drug's sponsor are satisfied that the drug has a desirable effect and an acceptable (low) level of toxic effects, an NDA is submitted*; ± ⅔ of the NDAs are returned to the sponsor for more information, often pertaining to issues regarding the drug's chemistry or manufacture; the average time from submission of an NDA until its approval is 32 months, during which time, labeling, indications, dosages, and methods of administration are delineated **(N Engl J Med 1989; 320:281)**; see IND, Phase 1, 2, 3 studies

*While this slow, tedious process is claimed to stifle creativity (as the cost of developing novel agents is financially burdensome), the US was spared the brunt of the thalidomide tragedy, which resulted in 10-15 000 cases of partial or complete phocomelia, largely in Germany

Nd-YAG laser Neodymium-yttrium aluminum garnet laser A photocoagulation unit used to control acute and chronic gastrointestinal hemorrhage, eg an endoscopically guided Nd-YAG laser may be used to control esophageal varices, vascular ectasias, angiodysplasia, radiation-induced telangiectasia, watermelon stomach, telangiectasia of Osler-Weber-Rendu, palliation of malignancy and management of benign and malignant obstructive biliary tract lesions; see Lasers

near-death experience A phenomenon of unclear nature that may occur in patients who have been clinically dead and then resuscitated; the patients report a continuity of subjective experience, remembering visitors and other hospital events despite virtually complete suppression of cortical activity; near-death experiences are considered curiosities with no valid explanation in the context of an acceptable biomedical paradigm; see Harvard criteria

The trivial synonym, Lazarus complex, refers to the biblical Lazarus who was raised from the dead by Jesus of Nazareth

'near miss' sudden infant death syndrome A prolonged, usually nocturnal apneic period in children, in whom the non-fatal outcome of apnea is attributed to continuous monitoring; 'near-miss' SIDS children may have enlarged adenoids or nasopharyngitis which responds to adenoidectomy; see SIDS

'near poor' Working poor SOCIAL MEDICINE A growing segment of the US population with earnings sufficient only for daily needs, who are not qualified for US government assistance programs; the near poor seldom have medical insurance and when ill, are a major burden to the health care system; Cf Engel's phenomenon, 'Fourth World', Homelessness

nebulin A 550-kD protein, located in the A and I bands that constitutes about 3% of skeletal muscle protein, forming long non-distensible filaments extending from the Z disks; nebulin is thought to regulate the number of actin monomers 'allowed' to polymerize into each thin filament during myogenesis and facilitate actin filament organization into its usual hexagonal geometry; nebulin is present in fetuses and infants with Duchenne-type muscular dystrophy, but disappears with disease progression; the locus for which has been assigned to chromosome segment 2q31-q33; Cf Titin, Tropomyosin

NEC Necrotizing enterocolitis, see there

neck face syndrome A transient clinical complex characterized by oropharyngeal spasms, dysarthria, tachycardia and hypertension occurring after beginning chlorpromazine therapy

neck hold FORENSIC MEDICINE A form of restraint used to subdue overactive, unruly, violent or inebriated subjects with the intent of preventing them causing physical harm to themselves and others; NHs are of medico-legal inter-

est, as accidental death may be caused by police, orderlies, or emergency medical technicians trying to restrain a subject undergoing acute psychotic attacks or other excited states; the two major NHs are the 1) Carotid sleeper, in which local compression of the carotid baroreceptor causes asystole or marked slowing of the ventricular rate, a fall in the blood pressure and syncope, usually within 6-10 seconds and 2) Choke hold, in which the upper airway is occluded by compressing the thyroid cartilage and displacing the tongue posteriorly, a hold that is considered more dangerous

necklace pattern CLINICAL MEDICINE A descriptor for a distinct annular distribution of lesions seen in AIDS-related Kaposi sarcoma CYTOLOGY A descriptor for the perinuclear distribution of the PAS-positive granules in Lutzner's small cell variant of Sézary cells

neck-tongue syndrome An acquired condition characterized by sharp pain and tingling of the upper neck and/or occiput upon sudden rotation of the neck, associated with numbness of the ipsilateral half of the tongue, thought to be the result of stretching of the C2 ventral ramus which contains proprioceptive fibers from the lingual nerve to the hypoglossal nerve and on to the second cervical root

necrobiosis Physiologic cell death seen during normal turnover in the bone marrow, endometrium, gastrointestinal tract and skin

necrobiosis lipoidica DERMATOLOGY An inflammatory condition that occurs in 50-80% of DM, most commonly located on the legs; in 10%, NL precedes the onset of DM PATHOLOGY Firm, sharply delineated rounded to oval firm red papules or plaques with yellowish waxy centers; central fat necrosis, lipid-laden macrophages, and foreign body-type giant cells, all confined to the upper dermis

necropsy Autopsy

necrosis The constellation of changes that accompany and follow irreversible cell injury in living organisms **(Arch Pathol Lab Med 1993; 117:1208OA)** or more simply defined as the death of cells or tissue PATHOLOGY Necrotic cells have typical findings in the nucleus (eg karyolysis, karyorrhexis, pyknosis) and cytoplasm (eg eosinophilia, vacuolization, and homogeneity of cytoplasm) **ASEPTIC NECROSIS** Non-infected tissue death, usually related to ischemia **CASEOUS NECROSIS** Tissue death grossly appearing as dry-yellow-white, ricotta cheese-like in consistency material, due to a combination of coagulative and liquefactive necrosis, secondary to autolysis, ischemia and focal bacterial necrosis, forming a proteolipid 'paste', most often seen in the central portions of granulomatous lesions, classically in TB, but also seen in cat-scratch disease, deep fungal infections, LGV, plague, sporotrichosis, syphilis, tularemia; a similar material is seen in gouty lesions **COAGULATION NECROSIS** The most common type of tissue death, in which the cells are converted to pale eosinophilic 'ghosts' due to acute ischemia, affecting the heart, kidney and adrenal glands; the healing phase involves enzymatic liquefaction or neutrophilic phagocytosis of the debris **FAT NECROSIS** A process in which neutral fats of adipocytes are converted into fatty acids and glycerol, as in trauma-induced fat necrosis of the breast or acute pancreatitis attributed to the release of enzymes PATHOLOGY 'Ghosted' fat cells surrounded by calcium, forming 'soaps', which has a chalky-white appearance, see Calcium soap **FIBRINOID NECROSIS** A misnomer for what is not true necrosis but homogeneous, granular eosinophilic material, composed of fibrin, proteins (eg complement and immunoglobulins) and platelets; the process is seen in the various forms of necrotizing vasculitis **GANGRENOUS NECROSIS** see Gangrene **LIQUEFACTIVE NECROSIS** That which occurs during abscess formation, caused by enzymatic degradation **PATHERGIC NECROSIS** Dissolution of tissue without apparent cause, which may be seen at the site of trauma, and accompanied by scattered histiocytes, eg Wegener's granulomatosis; pathergic necrosis must be differentiated from two similar processes: 1) 'Garden variety' necrosis, mediated by neutrophils that actively pour histolytic enzymes into the milieu and 2) Autolysis, due to enzymes released upon cell death, a common finding in the pancreas after death; see Acute tubular necrosis, Bridging necrosis, Cystic medial necrosis, Papillary necrosis, Piecemeal necrosis

necrotizing enterocolitis A disease of premature infants, affecting the terminal ileum 3-10 days after birth, representing 2% of neonatal ICU admissions and 10% of admissions of premature infant or low birth weight neonates and causing significant mortality and morbidity; NEC is usually prevented by either human breast milk or per os IgA-IgG immunoglobulin concentrate prepared from human serum Note: Hyperosmolar solutions used for these infants have been inculpated MECHANISM Intestinal ischemia and breakdown of the mucosa with invasion by gas-forming bacteria causes the pneumatosis intestinalis CLINICAL From banal to fulminant with abdominal distension, vomiting, hematochezia, intestinal gangrene, perforation, sepsis and shock, survival 80%; NEC is less common in breast-fed children, who may be protected by secretory IgA in maternal milk; per os IgA-IgG solution in low-birth-weight infants may afford protection; prophylactic ligation of the patent ductus arteriosus at the time of birth may reduce the incidence of necrotizing enterocolitis, but has no effect on other 'prematurity' lesions; Cf Pigbel

necrotizing fasciitis A rapidly progressive bacterial infection that spreads along fascial planes, which in absence of effective therapy, including debridement results in the breakdown of skin with bleb and bulla formation, accompanied by small vessel thrombosis and secondary necrosis, leading to subcutaneous anesthesia; most cases are due to streptococci, but gram-negative and mixed bacteria may be identified ETIOLOGY (Arch Pathol Lab Med 1993; 117:1208oA)

necrotizing sialometaplasia A benign self-limited reactive inflammatory process of salivary glands, which may clinically and histologically mimic malignant lesions, eg mucoepidermoid carcinoma; most cases occur in the minor salivary glands (SG), but may also occur in SGs of the upper aerodigestive tract, or in one report, the larynx (Am J Clin Pathol 1995; 103:609oA)

needle aspiration cytology A diagnostic preparation of cells, eg smears and/or a 'cell block', see there, which is obtained from a clinically or radiologically identified mass, using a 'skinny' needle to spread the material on a glass; in well-trained hands, aspiration cytology specimens have a 90% sensitivity and 95% specificity for diagnosing thyroid and breast masses, using 21–25-gauge or 'skinny' needles; the procedure is helpful when positive, but when negative, requires further diagnostic procedures; a rare complication with larger bore needles is tumor implantation along the needle tract; the physical 'set-up' includes computerized tomographic guidance, a microscope and staining materials during the procedure in order to establish immediate diagnosis

needle biopsy A diagnostic preparation which in principle is the same as that of aspiration cytology, but the larger bore (19-gauge) needle obtains architecturally intact tissue, yielding a higher diagnostic success rate than with cytology alone; CT-guided transthoracic needle biopsies are used for lesions less than 2.0 cm in diameter, while lesions larger than 2.0 cm are best diagnosed by fibroptic bronchoscopy if accessible; despite the small size of the material obtained, needle biopsies may be analyzed by histochemistry and immunohistochemistry, cell culture and culture for organisms, electron and immunofluorescence microscopy, receptor analysis, in situ hybridization and polymerase chain reaction

needle exchange programs INFECTIOUS DISEASE PUBLIC HEALTH A group of programs intended to slow the spread of AIDS among intravenous drug abusers (IVDAs), in which an agency, either governmental or charitable, exchanges sterile needles for 'dirty', potentially HIV-contaminated needles used by IVDAs when 'shooting' heroin (or less commonly cocaine); the controversy engendered by needle exchange programs is 1) Whether it actually helps stop the spread of AIDS (soft data suggest that it does) and 2) Whether government funds should be used to support an illicit activity EFFECTIVENESS 68% of needles collected before the NEP in New Haven, Connecticut, were HIV-positive; after the NEP was in place, 43% of needles were HIV-positive, suggesting that it is effective (N Engl J Med 1992; 327:1883c) but is hard to 'sell' in the US as an official governmental policy (JAMA 1995 273:978)

needle-stick injury An occupational injury that may affect any health care professionals; needles act as vehicles for at least 20 different microorganisms; most physicians have sustained at least one such injury during their training, $\frac{1}{3}$ of which occurred during recapping; in urban US teaching hospitals, 20% or more of the population is HIV-positive; the risk of HIV transmission through a needle stick is currently estimated at 0.0035; see Hospital-acquired penetration contacts, Sharps

needs model HEALTH CARE POLICY A model for determining the future needs for a particular product or supplier of a service (eg surgeons) that is based on the projected needs for the product or supplier is in a hypothetically 'perfect' world (CAP Today 1995; 9:5) Cf Demand model, Extrapolation model, Supply model

nef An HIV-1 gene that encodes the regulatory protein Nef, which had been thought to have a role in down-regulating viral reproduction, an effect now known to be an isolated phenomenon occurring in one cell line; mutations in the nef gene may be responsible for generating the different HIV-cell tropisms; in one study of subjects with nonprogressive HIV infection, the auxiliary gene *nef*, which is required in simian immunodeficiency virus for the development of AIDS in the rhesus monkey, is defective or absent (N Engl J Med 1995; 332:228oA)

Nef AIDS A regulatory protein that is thought to pave the way for HIV to cause disease, by binding to HIV's protein kinase, which would then signal the molecule NK-κB to scuttle the inhibitor I-κB, allowing NK-κB to migrate into the nucleus and initiate HIV's transcription (Science 1995; 267:959RN)

NEFA Non-esterified fatty acids Fatty acids (straight or branched-chain monocarboxylic acid) that are not bound in the form of lipid esters, ie not esterified to a glycerol; NEFAs are absorbed in the ileum, represent about 5% of the total plasma lipids (0.3-0.95 mmol/L), primarily as straight-chain fatty acids (stearic and palmitic acids) are transported bound to albumin and represent an important source of energy

negative-acting regulatory proteins Those proteins that bind to DNA at or near a promotion site, preventing access of RNA polymerase to the corresponding gene or operon, preventing transcription into mRNA

negative acute phase protein Transthyretin, see there

negative acute phase reactants Those molecules that are produced in reduced amounts during the acute phase reaction, eg albumin, alpha-fetoprotein, α_2-HS glycoprotein, transferrin, and transthyretin, which is also known as negative acute phase protein (Perspect Biol & Med 1993; 36:611)

negative feedback Feedback, see there

negative interference Gene mapping GENETICS A term

referring to an overabundance of double cross-overs; without 'correction' for cross-overs, marker distances are not additive, ie they interfere in a negative fashion with evaluation of distance

negative predictive value STATISTICS The number of true negatives divided by the sum of the number of true negatives (TN) and false negatives (FN), representing the proportion of subjects with a negative test result who do not have a disease; Cf Positive predictive value

negative strand virus An RNA virus (class V virus) with a nucleotide base sequence complementary to that of the virus' mRNA, which requires that the genetic material be first copied by an RNA-dependent RNA polymerase before it is able to translate information into proteins; Cf Positive strand virus

negative symptom Deficit symptom Any of a number of symptoms typical of schizophrenia, depression, as well as other psychological symptoms, including decreased affect, range of emotion, sense of purpose, and social drives, as well as poverty of speech and loss of interests (see N Engl J Med 1994; 330:681RV) see Schizophrenia

negativistic personality disorder Passive-aggressive personality disorder, see there

neglect '...the failure of a caretaker to provide basic shelter, supervision, medical care, or support.', neglect of children (of the elderly), a form of child maltreatment increases with poverty (N Engl J Med 1995; 332:1425RV) see Child abuse, Elderly abuse

negligence LEGAL MEDICINE The failure (usually on the part of a physician, or other health care professional) to exercise ordinary, reasonable, usual, or expected care, prudence, or skill (that would usually and customarily be exercised by other reputable physicians treating similar patients) in the performance of a legally recognized duty, resulting forseeable harm, injury or loss to another; negligence may be an act of omission (ie unintentional) or commission (ie intentional), characterized by inattention, recklessness, inadvertence, thoughtlessness or wantonness*; in health care, negligence implies a substandard deviation from the 'standard of medical practice' that would be exercised by a similarly-trained professional under similar circumstances **CONTRIBUTORY NEGLIGENCE** An act or omission that constitutes the lack of reasonable care on the part of a plaintiff for his own preservation; in a malpractice lawsuit, a patient may have 'contributed' to a significant degree to his own condition by ignoring a physician's well documented advice or requests for the patient to return for follow-up visits **GROSS NEGLIGENCE** Reckless provision of health care without regard for the consequences, an act that is more serious than an inadvertent error, but which does not imply intentional wrong; grossly negligent health care is best described as 'sloppy' **WANTON NEGLIGENCE** Provision of health care without regard for potential injury to the patient without an actual intent to cause injury, ie 'reckless' **WILLFUL NEGLIGENCE** Provision of health care in an intentionally substandard fashion, the most serious form of negligence, which may carry with it criminal charges; the accusation of negligence comprises a major cause for malpractice litigation; see Adverse event, Malpractice

*This definition is a composite from a number of sources, and intended to encompass virtually all parameters by which negligence can be measured-author's note

negotiated fee schedule HEALTH CARE FINANCING Fees for professional services that are set by means of collective bargaining, which may be used to determine global budgets (Am Med News 25 October 1992, p7)

negotiated payment schedule Negotiated fee schedule, see there

negotiated safety STD A term coined by Australian researchers for a stance in which HIV-negative sexual (in particular homosexual) partners abandon the use of condom; because the strategy requires open communication between the partners about emotionally volatile issues, eg admission of liaisons outside of the relationship, either or both the partners in the relationship may have a false sense of security, giving rise to an alternative term, 'negotiated danger' (Village Voice, Jan 31, 1995)

nemaline myopathy nemaline, Greek, rod-shaped A benign AD [MIM 161800] muscular dystrophy affecting 'floppy infants' and characterized by non-progressive muscular weakness, reduced deep tendon reflexes and hypotonicity, causing skeletal abnormalities, a typical facies (oval face, micrognathia, malocclusion and a high arched palate), kyphoscoliosis, dislocation of hips and pes cavus; nemaline myopathy is compatible with a normal lifespan; 'nemaline' refers to the ultrastructural finding of rod-like Z-band material in both type I and type II myocytes; Cf Central core myopathy, Floppy infant syndrome

Negri body VIROLOGY An eosinophilic cytoplasmic inclusion that is virtually pathognomonic for rabies, and found in rabies virus-infected neurons, most prominently seen in Ammon's horn of the hippocampus

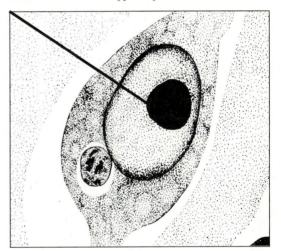

Negri body

N-end rule CELL BIOLOGY The principle that the amino acid at a peptide's NH_2-terminus determines its metabolic stability and how rapidly it will be degraded; eg for β-galactosidase, methionine, alanine, serine, threonine, valine and glycine terminal amino acids are degraded within 20 hours; peptides with other N-end amino acids have shorter half lives; the half-life of an intracellular protein ranges from a few seconds to several days; most damaged or abnormal proteins are metabolically unstable and catabolically eliminated by various regulatory proteins, while other proteins are long-lived and maintained as components of macromolecule complexes such as ribosomes and multimeric proteins; when these proteins are dissociated from these macromolecular complexes, they too are metabolically unstable and catabolized; this selective degradation process is an ATP-dependent and nonlysosomal process in which ubiquitin covalently conjugates with the short-lived proteins 'tagging' them for catabolism; intracellular proteins are recognized as proteolytic substrates by the N-end rule, a phenomenon discovered in yeasts, where any 8 stabilizing amino acids at the N-terminal of the protein are associated with long (> 20 hours) intracellular half-lives while any of 12 destabilizing amino acids at the N-end have a short (3-30 minutes) half-life; in mammalian cells, the rule is more complex; there are three classes of N-end destabilizing residues and the types of proteins degraded as a function of the cell's physiology; the N-end rule requires that in addition to a destabilizing N-end amino acid, there is a lysine in position 15 or 17, the probable site of ubiquination; Cf PEST hypothesis

neoadjuvant chemotherapy Induction chemotherapy, see there

neo-Darwinism A key paradigm of evolutionary biology that synthesizes the concepts of Darwinian natural selection and mendelian genetics, and assumes that the environment is a static force that does not interact with organisms that survive based on their 'fitness' in an adverse environment; Cf Autopoietic Gaia

neomembrane NEUROPATHOLOGY A thin sheet of reactive fibrous tissue overlying a chronic subdural hematoma

neonatal 'hepatitis' A generic term for diseases that affect the newborn hepatic parenchyma, which are commonly associated with ↑ conjugated hyperbilirubinemia; diagnosis of this condition requires three or more of the following: fatty changes, cholestasis, bile duct proliferation, fibrosis, pseudoacini and cirrhosis; neonatal 'hepatitis' is caused by infection (syphilis, listeriosis, HBV, rubella, CMV, echovirus, adenovirus, toxoplasmosis), metabolic disease (α1-antitrypsin deficiency, cystic fibrosis, Wilson's disease, galactosemia, fructosuria, tyrosinemia), mechanical (choledochal cysts, intrahepatic ductal atresia hypoplasia, familial intrahepatic cholestasis) and others (Bylers disease, hemolytic disease of the newborn) PATHOLOGY Lobular disarray, focal hepatocellular necrosis, prominent giant cell 'transformation', mononuclear infiltration in the portal spaces, reactive hyperplasia in the Kupffer cells and cholestasis; Cf Giant cell hepatitis

neonatal intensive care unit A ward in a tertiary care center that provides intensive medical care; an NICU requires trained medical personnel at all levels, 24-hour availability of the appropriate specialists, monitoring devices, alarm systems for continuous assessment of vital functions, equipment for resuscitation and respiratory therapy, drugs and full laboratory coverage; the mortality of the very low birth weight (<1500 g) has fallen from 72% in 1960 to 27% in 1985; the mortality of those with moderate-to-severe residual handicaps (4-10%) was stable for that time period; the proportion of infants who survive in relatively good health has increased from 7.2% to 57%; see Low birth weight

neonatal withdrawal syndrome A condition affecting the infants of mothers who chronically abused CNS-active substances during pregnancy, for which the infant developed an in utero tolerance and who upon delivery, undergoes withdrawal; agents inculpated in NWS include opioids (heroin, methadone, meperidine, codeine, pentazocine, propoxyphene, cocaine and 'crack'), alcohol, clomipramine and sedative-hypnotics (barbiturates, meprobamate, benzodiazepines) CLINICAL Wakefulness, irritability, seizures, tremulousness, lability of temperature, tachypnea, hyperacusis, hyperreflexia, hypertonicity, diarrhea, sweating, respiratory distress and apnea, rhinorrhea, autonomic dysfunction, respiratory alkalosis, lacrimation, yawning and sneezing; the symptoms appear from twelve hours to one week after birth TREATMENT Swaddling (firmly wrapping in blankets), reduction of external stimuli and tincture of opium; see Crack babies

neonate An infant in the first 4 weeks of life

neoplasm Any autonomous proliferation of cells, classified according to

BEHAVIOR Benign, borderline or malignant

DEGREE OF DIFFERENTIATION Well-differentiated, ie the neoplastic cell simulates its parent or progenitor cell or poorly-differentiated, ie the neoplastic cell is bizarre and 'ugly', as defined by pathologic criteria

EMBRYOLOGIC ORIGIN Epithelial, lymphoproliferative, mesenchymal, neural crest, etc and

GROSS APPEARANCE Well-circumscribed or infiltrative; benign neoplasms are in general slow-growing, well-circumscribed, often invested with a fibrous capsule and are often only symptomatic if they compromise a confined space, eg massive meningioma of the cranial cavity, or encirclement of vital blood vessels; malignant neoplasms are often aggressive with increased mitotic activity, bizarre cells, necrosis and invasion of adjacent structures and have metastatic potential; see Cancer, Doubling time, Metastases

neoplasm panel LABORATORY MEDICINE A battery of tests which is considered to be the most cost-efficient means of delineating a malignancy of unknown origin, including measurement of acid phosphatase, alkaline phosphatase, α-fetoprotein, carcinoembryonic antigen (CEA), chorionic gonadotrophic hormone, and lactate dehydrogenase; because of the low yield of these assays, chemical 'cancer screens' have little active role in the early diagnosis of malignancy, and when 'negative', introduce a false sense of security that malignancy is not present; of the tests available PSA and CEA are the most widely used

Note: The only test with a proven 'track record' is prostate-specific antigen (PSA), see there

neopterin A metabolite of guanosine triphosphate, produced by macrophages that have been stimulated by IFN-γ produced from activated T cells; levels of serum and urinary neopterin are elevated in progressing HIV-1 infection; the combination of decreasing CD4+ lymphocytes and increasing levels of either neopterin or β_2-microglobulin, which indicates lymphoid activation are relatively predictive of progression of HIV-1 infection to clinical AIDS

neovascularization The formation of new blood vessels, ie capillary ingrowth and endothelial proliferation in unusal sites, a finding typical of so-called 'angiogenic diseases', which include angiogenesis in tumor growth, diabetic retinopathy, hemangiomas, arthritis and psoriasis

neper A unit of measurement expressing the ratio of two levels of electrical power, eg the ratio of the electricity in a comb charged with static electricity to a bolt of lightning; the neper is the natural logarithm of the square root of that ratio

nephelometric turbidity unit A parameter used to determine the quality of a water supply; an NTU of ≤ 0.1 is ideal and would make the presence of cryptosporidium oocysts and other major pathogens unlikely, but may be difficult to achieve; a typical municipal water supply might have an NTU ≤ 0.3 (N Engl J Med 1994; 331:161oA)

nephelometry LABORATORY MEDICINE A technique that detects the amount of light scattered at 90 degrees to the incident light by particles dispersed in a clear solution; the amount of light scattered is a function of the number and size of the particles; nephelometry is most commonly used to detect immune complexes when the participating antigen or antibody is unknown; Cf Turbidimetry

nephritic syndrome An obsolete and nonspecific term that referred to a renal lesion histologically characterized by inflammation and necrosis of the glomeruli; Cf Nephrosis, Nephrotic syndrome

nephroblastoma Wilms' tumor, see there

nephroblastomatosis A congenital dysontogenic condition that may be bilateral, multifocal, and both confused with and associated with Wilm's tumor, demonstrating a continuum between microscopic foci, termed nephrogenic rests or metanephric hamartomas and massive lesions or nephroblastomatosis, either of which may be surrounded by sclerosis, indicating regressive changes; focal lesions appear in 1% of normal fetal kidneys and 30% of kidneys affected by Wilms' tumor TREATMENT Conservative

nephrogenic diabetes insipidus A form of DI characterized by significant polyuria and polydipsia due to a congenital or acquired (due to lithium or democlocycline toxicity) defect of the collecting tubules, resulting in ↓ responsiveness to vasopressin PATHOGENESIS Aquaporin-2 is essential for vasopressin-dependent concentration of urine and was found defective in a patient with NDI (Science 1994; 264:92OA) see Aquaporins

nephrogenic rests Small foci of persistent primitive blastemic cells that may be found in neonatal kidneys, and present in virtually all children with inherited susceptibility to Wilms' tumor (WT), and is present in 25-40% of children with sporadic WT; nephrogenic rests may represent clonal precurosor lesions that either regress spontaneously or degenerate into WT (N Engl J Med 1994; 331:586OA) see Wilms' tumor

nephronophthisis 1) Medullary cystic disease of kidneys 2) Familial juvenile nephronophthisis

nephropathic cystinosis An AR [MIM 219800] lysosomal storage disease characterized by early-onset renal tubular Fanconi's syndrome, progressive photophobia, and renal failure severe enough to require either hemodialysis or transplantation by age 10, caused by defective trans-lysosomal membrane transport of cystine, resulting in tissue deposition of cystine causing corneal erosions, DM, and neurologic deterioration CLINICAL Dehydration, acidosis, vomiting, electrolyte imbalance, hypophosphatemic rickets and failure to grow TREATMENT β-mercaptoethylamine (aminothiol cysteamine) to deplete intracellular stores and by extension dissolve tissue crystals, oral cysteamine therapy improves growth and delays renal deterioration; see Salla disease

nephrosclerosis A generic term indicating global fibrosis and atrophy of the glomeruli, which is most commonly seen in arteriosclerotic kidneys, divided into

BENIGN NEPHROSCLEROSIS A relatively common, symmetrical and indolent process* causing 'benign' hypertension, average age of onset, 60, 5% of whom die of renal failure PATHOLOGY Hyaline arteriolosclerosis, scarring of glomeruli

*Some authors prefer the term arteriolonephrosclerosis

MALIGNANT NEPHROSCLEROSIS An uncommon process affecting 5% of hypertensives, often beginning under age 45 PATHOLOGY Fibrinoid necrosis of small arteries (necrotizing arteriolitis), intimal hyperplasia of larger interlobular arteries (hyperplastic arteriolitis, 'onion-skinning'), collagen deposition and fibroblastic proliferation with luminal narrowing, thrombosis and necrosis of the glomeruli with atrophy and parenchymal scarring

nephrosis A term used by clinicians as a synonym for nephrotic syndrome, which corresponds to a non-inflammatory derangement of glomerular function, characterized by increased glomerular leakage with loss of albumin and other macromolecules; see Nil disease, Myeloid nephrosis, Myeloma kidney; Cf Nephritis

Note: The term is nonspecific and best used with adjectival modifiers, eg lipoid nephrosis

nephrotic syndrome A condition characterized by the triad of edema, proteinuria (> 3.5 g protein/1.73 m²/24 hours) and hypoalbuminemia (< 30 g/L) LABORATORY ↑ α_2-globulin, ↑ β globulin, ↓ albumin; ↑ cholesterol, ↑ triglycerides, ↑ phospholipids; the increases are confined to lipoproteins containing apoB (chylomicrons and LDL cholesterol), due to ↑ production of apoB; other findings in NS include ↓ HDL₂ and ↑ VLDL URINALYSIS Maltese cross-shaped structures (cholesterol), oval fat bodies, renal tubular casts (fatty, waxy, cellular, granular) PATHOLOGY, CHILDREN Minimum change 65-90%, membranoproliferative 7-10%, focal glomerulosclerosis, membranous, prolif-erative, other glomerulonephritides PATHOLOGY, ADULT Membranous 50%, minimum change 10-20%, focal glomerulosclerosis 10-20%, membranoproliferative proliferative, and other glomerulonephrites; other causes of nephrotic syndrome include amyloidosis, DM, infection, malignancy, SLE, and toxins, eg colloidal gold, 'street' heroin, penicillamine Idiopathic NS is characterized by heavy proteinuria, corticosteroid resistance with focal and segmental glomerulosclerosis, and end-stage renal disease TREATMENT Ex vivo adsorption of plasma on protein A Sephadex columns decreases proteinuria

Note: The adsorbed protein when injected into animals, alters glomerular permeability, implying that the adsorbed factor(s) may have a role in pathogenesis (N Engl J Med 1993; 330:7OA)

nerve conduction studies NEUROLOGY A noninvasive method for assessing a nerve's ability to carry an impulse, providing quantitative data on latency periods and conduction velocities; larger peripheral motor and sensory nerves are electrically stimulated at various intervals along a motor nerve; the maximum (normal) velocity for peripheral nerves requires complete myelination, and is between 40 and 80 m/s; nerve conduction may be ≤ ½ normal in segmental demyelination, as occurs in polyneuropathy, eg in Charcot-Marie-Tooth disease, diabetic neuropathy, Guillain-Barré syndrome, diphtheria, metachromatic leukodystrophy; entrapment syndromes result in localized slowing of conduction; motor nerve conduction studies differentiate between peripheral nerve or muscle disease and anterior horn cells, measuring the resulting muscle twitch/action (M response) is measured; see F wave, H-reflex, Latency period

nerve-derived transglutaminase A fish enzyme that acts in conjunction with IL-2 to repaired damaged nerve by selectively destroying oligodendroglial cells, which are thought to release a factor that is thought to prevent axons from elongating (Sci Am 1994; 271/4:31)

nerve gas see Chemical warfare

nerve growth factor A 118-residue protein encoded on chromosome 1 and synthesized by neurons; NGF has a trophic role in embryogenesis, regulating the proliferation and differentiation of neuronal stem cells in the embryonic brain after they have been stimulated by fibroblast growth factor; NGF increases mitotic activity, enhances differentiation, eg neurite outgrowth, and is required for development and maintenance of sympathetic and sensory peripheral neurons; NGF guides growing or regenerating neurites along a concentration gradient and may have anti-mitogenic activity; cholinergic neurons respond to NGF by increasing production of choline acyltransferase, and NGF's message may be mediated by signal transduction through TRK, a tyrosine kinase receptor NGF induces terminal neuronal differentiation in neuroblastoma cells; deprivation of NGF leads to neuronal cell death and increased proto-oncogene TRK expression (N Engl J Med 1993; 328:847OA) see Nerve growth factor receptor, Neuroblastoma, TRK; Cf Epidermal growth factor

Note: The original NGF work was done on chick embryos engrafted with fragments of mouse sarcoma by R Levi-Montalcini (Nobel Prize, 1986)

nerve growth factor family A group of proteins with various effects on neural tissues; proteins under active study include nerve growth factor, brain-derived neurotrophic factor, see BDNF, neurotropin-3 (NT-3), and ciliary neurotrophic factor, see CNTF; Cf Epidermal growth factor

nerve growth factor receptor A family of receptors for the neurotrophin, NGF; the low affinity NGF-receptor gene encodes a transmembrane protein that is glycosylated, yielding a 75 kD glycoprotein (p75^LNGFR) which is not known to mediate any biological responses; the high-affinity NGF receptor is a heteromeric complex that includes p75^LNGFR and p140^proto-TRK, the product of the proto-oncogene TRK (N Engl J Med 1993; 328:847OA) NGF-Rs are present on cells of neural crest origin, mast cells, cholinergic and adrenergic neurons; see TRK

nerve regeneration NEUROPHYSIOLOGY The ability to form viable and functional neural connections following the transsection, formerly regarded as an irreversible event; neuronal regeneration is increasingly evident, eg sensory cell regeneration after acoustic trauma in chickens (mitosis of support cells) and resynapsis of severed nerves; much of the groundwork has been by F Nottebohm in his seminal work with nerve regeneration and alteration of neural pathways in songbirds

nervine ALTERNATIVE MEDICINE *noun* A medicinal preparation, usually of herbal origin that is alleged by some alternative health care practitioners to stimulate the nervous system, by strengthening and restoring the nervous system (nervine tonic), reducing anxiety and tension (nervine relaxant), or stimulating neural function (nervine stimulant)

nervios PSYCHIATRY A idiom used by Hispanics of the Western Hemisphere referring to both an increased susceptibility to mental stress and the broad palette of symptoms attributed thereto, including nervousness (hence the name nervios), loss of ability to concentrate, emotional distress, headaches, insomnia, gastric discomfort, mareo —a vertigo-like sensation, trembling and so on (from DSM-IV™, 1994); see Culture-bound syndrome

nesidioblastosis Islet cell hyperplasia (and neoformation of islets after birth) with variability of size and shape, vascular dilation, poor demarcation, clustering, abnormal interstitial location, arising from the exocrine ducts; it is associated with DM, affecting infants of diabetic mothers, diabetics with long-term oral hypoglycemic agents (sulfonylurea, tolbutamide) and in endocrinopathies, either congenital, as in the MEN (multiple endocrine neoplasia) syndrome(s) or may be induced by glucagon and corticosteroids (Arch Pathol Lab Med 1994; 118:155oA)

nested deletion A plasmid into which foreign DNA of interest is inserted for cloning designed to facilitate characterization of cloned inserts; plasmid vectors are of use for high-resolution restriction mapping, rescue of single-stranded DNA, RNA transcription, sequencing of single- and double-stranded nucleic acids, generation of nested deletions, site-directed mutagenesis, and both pro– and eukaryotic expression

nested PCR MOLECULAR PATHOLOGY A permutation of PCR (polymerase chain reaction) that is thought to enhance the reaction's specificity; in NP, there are two rounds of reaction, the first occurring in the outer flanking primers, and the second in the inner flanking primers (Bio/Technology 1995; 13:445)

nesting COMPUTERS The inclusion of a block of data or programming subroutine within another subroutine, often in the form of a functional loop of logic, performing the routine a number of times before continuing with the program; see Computers OBSTETRICS Frenetic house cleaning by a woman in late pregnancy, which most often occurs with the first-born child, fancifully likened to birds building a nest

net national product GLOBAL VILLAGE The gross national product minus the value of coal and/or crude petroleum extracted and timber logged (Sci Am 1995; 272/2:44)

net primary product ENVIRONMENT The amount of vegetable mass produced by photosynthesis, ie food and fuel molecules, $\pm$ 225 x 10^9 metric tons/year; 4-5% of this total is consumed by direct human activities, eg feeding people, pets, livestock, or burning of firewood; an additional 13% is consumed indirectly by reducing the amount of land available for photosynthesis, eg clearing forests, marshes and grasslands for human use in the form of parking lots, building sites, landfills, and less productive pastures (AAO-

HNS Bulletin/May 1994)

netrin NEUROEMBRYOLOGY One of a family* of chemicals that guide developing neurons in forming the complex patterns that allow them to relay sensations to the brain; netrin is thought to be secreted by the floor plate of the developing embryo in the 3rd-4th week of life; the tip of the primitive axon, the growth cone senses the netrin and stretches the axon toward the floor plate; once the growth cone has fulfilled its role, it matures to become a synaptic terminal (New York Times 16 August 1994; C1)

*Netrin translates from Sanskrit as 'one who guides'; two have been thus far identified, netrin-1, and netrin-2, and these have $\pm$ 50% homology (which is fairly significant, by molecular biology standards) with unc-6, a nematode protein that guides the migration of sensory axons and neurites

'Nettergram' A color medical illustration rendered by Frank H Netter, MD (1906-1991) that summarizes in a lucid and graphic form the clinical and pathological findings of a disease state; most of these illustrations are found within the 'CIBA collection', a 10-volume set, the first of which was released in 1953 and has helped educate more than three generations of medical students in the US and elsewhere

network Any series of points in a system that is connected by numbered lines and arrows, indicating the flow of materials, personnel, energy, widgets

network analysis A management tool designed to reduce a system's energy or labor expenditure to a minimum, attempting in addition to accurately estimate the amount of time that the growth of interrelated tasks or a 'network' will take by arranging the network in time-dependent routes, where the critical path is the one that requires the most time and which requires input from the previous steps; see Neural networks

network hypothesis IMMUNOLOGY A theory proposed by Jerne (Nobel Prize, 1984) that lymphocytes form a network of cells bearing idiotypes, each potentially capable of eliciting anti-idiotype antibodies; each 'new' antigen disrupts the balance of an immune network by stimulating an antibody response which then elicits an anti-idiotype-antibody response, which is followed by further anti-idiotypes, attenuating, and eventually quenching the response, bringing the system back into balance

network theory The theory advanced by Jerne to explain the ability of the immune response to regulate itself; according to the network theory, each antigen receptor or idiotype (of either a T or B cell) is capable of evoking the production of anti-idiotypic cells, and these cells or their products act to down-regulate the production of the original idiotype

networking PSYCHOLOGY A term of recent vintage referring to the aggressive interaction among those who wish to 'climb' various social and occupational ladders, through various vehicles, eg 'power' meals (eg breakfast, lunch), 'power' sports (eg golf, tennis); networking serves to establish contacts that can be 'tapped' for favors, employment, information and so on

neu A tyrosine kinase oncogene that is turned off by addition of tyrosine phosphatase, and which encodes the NEU protein

Note: Because the gene and its products were studied by a number of different research groups, it acquired a number of synonyms, including c-*erb*B-2, HER-2, MAC 117; ERB-B2 (see there) is preferred by many authors

NEU protein ERBB2, see there

neural crest *crista neuralis* [NH3] Either of longitudinal bands of ectoderm that separate from the dorsolateral border of the primitive neural tube prior to its closure (a process known as neurulation) and separation from the ectodermal goof; the NC appears in the fifth week of development and giving rise to the sensory and autonomic nervous systems and melanocytes; as the embryo develops, NC cells migrate laterally, forming cells of the APUD system, melanoblasts, and pia-arachnoid, odontoblast, Schwann cells and sensory neurons; tumors of NC origin include medullary thyroid carcinoma, derived from the ultimobranchial cleft, pheochromocytoma, medulloblastoma, neuroblastoma), undifferentiated neural crest tumors (**Science 1989; 243:1608**) and the pigmented neuroectodermal tumor of infancy

neural growth factor Nerve growth factor, see there

neural network A computer design in which multiple microprocessors interact simultaneously, modifying each other's output; NNs are inspired by the architecture of the nervous system and are designed to simulate how the brain is thought to function; NNs are composed of units analogous to neurons in that they have multiple connections; the analogy to the brain is further enhanced by integration of the back-prop algorithm, which allows the network to auto-correct errors, avoiding future errors; NNs solve problems by generalizations and approximations, (ie pattern recognition) based on limited data (rather than requiring the exact answers dictated by the 'linear' algorithms of traditional serial processing computer design); NNs are thus best suited for pattern recognition (eg fingerprint classification, handwriting and speech recognition, seismic analysis, document processing, and others) and signal processing, as in noise filtration; newer algorithms have integrated self-correction or back-propagation; the similarities between the nervous system and a computer are considerable (see **Arch Pathol Lab Med 1995; 119:350oA**) a massively parallel supercomputer is likened to the brain, the 'boards' to each of the regions of the brain, the nerve networks to the computer's circuitry, and the neurons themselves to the chips

Note: A true thinking machine based on independent ability to perform artificial intelligence algorithms has thus far proven elusive (**Science 1989; 243:481**)

neural tube defects A group of congenital developmental malformations of the CNS characterized by a defective closure of the neural tube at one or more segments; NTDs include anencephaly and spina bifida cystica that are attributed to multifactorial events and noxious environmental agents; NTDs occur in 1:1000-5000 live births, ♂:♀ ratio 2-3:1, with regional differences (they are reported to be higher in Ireland), and a 2-7% recurrence rate CLINICAL Cinercephaly, cephalocele, spina bifida and myelodysplasia; failure to close neural tube at 4th-5th fetal week LABORATORY ↑ α-fetoprotein, which may be detected in antenatal screening of maternal serum or amniotic fluid PREVENTION The use of multivitamins during early pregnancy may ↓ the risk of NTDs, although the effects of 'healthier' lifestyles or demographics cannot be ruled out NTDs are reported to be 10-fold higher in mainland China, possibly related to malnutrition, and may respond to folic acid supplementation (**New York Times 11 January 1994; C3**)

Synonyms include dysraphia, dysraphism, dysrhaphia, dystectia, rachischisis, schistorachis, spondyloschisis, status dysraphicus

neurally-mediated syncope Neurocardiogenic syncope, see there

neuraminidase Exo-α-sialidase, acylneuraminyl hydrolase An enzyme [EC 3.2.1.18] that breaks the glucoside bonds between sialic acid and hexose and hexosamine, located on the extracellular portion of membrane-bound glycoproteins, glycolipids and proteoglycans; neuraminidase in addition to hemagglutinin is located on the 'spikes' of influenza virus; neuraminidase deficiency occurs in the autosomal recessive mucolipidosis, type I

neuraminidase deficiency with beta-galactosidase deficiency Galactosialidosis, see there

neurapraxia Partial or complete conduction block over a segment of a nerve fiber, producing temporary paralysis

neurasthenia Effort syndrome A chronic nonspecific clinical finding, often associated with depression or anxiety neurosis, characterized by the subjective findings of fatigue and inability to function and accompanied by autonomic changes, including tachycardia, sighing, blushing, dysdiaphoresis; the patients are often convinced there is an organic and not a psychological underpinning to their condition

neuroarthropathy Neuropathic arthropathy, Charcot's joint

neuroblastoma A highly malignant neural crest-derived neoplasm composed of undifferentiated neuroblasts, a tumor that is the second most common neoplasm of children, after leukemia and other lymphoproliferative disease CLINICAL Median age of onset is < age 2; stage I survival is 80-90%, stage IV, 15% Note: Stage IV-S (see there) is an exception; higher stage neuroblastomas metastasize to bone, lymph nodes and liver PATHOLOGY Two cell types are typical of neuroblastomas, either 'blue cell tumors', arranged in Homer-Wright rosettes, or 'small round cell tumors of infancy' EM 100 nm neurosecretory ('dense core') granules, neurofilaments, microtubules, variably-sized glycogen granules ImPx Neuron-specific enolase, S-100 LABORATORY Catecholamines and metabolites are ↑ by TLC, GLC, HPLC, with a 5-fold increase in VMA (vanillylmandelic acid) and HVA (homovanillic acid); a high HVA, the 'early end of catecholamine metabolism' relative to VMA, the 'late end of catecholamine metabolism', which is known as a 'chemical shift to the left', may indicate a poor prognosis; also increased in neuroblastomas are epinephrine, norepinephrine, DOPA, dopamine, 3-methoxytyrosine, vanillactic acid, MHPG, metanephrine and LD PROGNOSIS A better prognosis is associated with stage I, II, or IVa disease, younger age (< 1 year), high level of TRK (the protein product of the proto-oncogene *TRK*) expression (5-year survival with a high level of TRK expression is 86% vs 14%), a normal N-*myc* copy number (5-year survival 84% vs 0%), and low level of N-*myc* expression (**N Engl J Med 1993; 328:847oA**) see Nerve growth factor receptor, 'One-hit, two-hit' model, TRK

Note: Tumors lacking dopamine β-hydroxylase are more primitive and have a worse prognosis than those producing 'differentiated' hormones. eg epinephrine, norepinephrine and VMA

neuroblastoma, IV-S syndrome A type of neuroblastoma (IV-S for special (S) stage IV tumor) comprising 10-20% of all neuroblastomas, where the primary tumor may be small, confined to the adrenal gland, but have widespread disease with massive involvement of the liver and skin; bone may be involved but osteolysis is not present; despite these 'metastases', the tumor regresses spontaneously through a maturation sequence from neuroblastoma, the most immature lesion composed of neuroblasts to ganglioneuroblastoma, and finally ending in ganglioneuroma, which is the most mature of the sequence and is composed of ganglion cells; Knudson postulated (**N Engl J Med 1980; 302:1254**) that the tumor represents a unique form of hyperplasia, as the cell clusters seen occur in sites to which cells of neural crest origin usually migrate, to later differentiate into Schwann cells or melanocytes

neuro-Calvinism see Biological determinism

neurocardiogenic syncope Vasovagal syncope A form of syncope possibly occurring on a psychogenic substrate, in which there is a predisposition to bradycardia and hypotension CLINICAL Abrupt neurogenic loss of vascular tone, accompanied by nausea, diaphoresis, and pallor DIAGNOSIS Tilt test–the patient is placed on a tilt table at a 40° to 80° from horizontal and maintained in a motionless upright position for 10-15 minutes or more MECHANISM Uncertain, probably activation of myocardial mechanoreceptors (C fibers), with ↓ efferent sympathetic tone and ↑ efferent parasympathetic tone, resulting in peripheral vasodilation, hypotension and syncope TREATMENT Beta blockers, eg metoprolol, are the most widely used agents, followed by theophylline, and disopyramide (**Science & Medicine** 1995; 2/3:14, N Engl J Med 1993; 328:1085OA)

neurocutaneous syndromes Phakomatoses A group of multisystem diseases characterized by involvement of the brain, skin, eyes and other organ systems, including neurofibromatosis type I (von Recklinghausen disease), tuberous sclerosis (Pringle-Bourneville disease), von Hippel-Lindau disease (all AD) Sturge-Weber syndrome (for which no hereditary pattern is recognized) and ataxia-telangiectasia

neurocysticercosis Cerebral cysticercosis, see there

'neurodermatitis' An eczematous dermatitis with hereditary (and possibly psychologic) component(s) that is accompanied by pruritus, which when disseminated, is known as atopic neurodermatitis and localized, as lichen simplex chronicus

neuroendocrine bodies Intrabronchial structures that are thought to act as intrapulmonary hypoxia- and hypercapnia-sensitive chemoreceptors, which undergo physiologic hyperplasia in the lungs of those living at high altitudes; NEBs proliferate when exposed to certain nitroso compounds and contain neuron-specific enolase, serotonin, bombesin and calcitonin and may be the point of origin of microcarcinoids and bronchial tumorlets

neuroendocrine cells Isolated neuroendocrine cells are scattered throughout the body and thought to have a paracrine and regulatory function EM Dense core neurosecretory granules ImPx Variable amounts of ACTH, bombesin, calcitonin, neuron-specific enolase, serotonin, leu-enkephalin and somatostatin, contained in the neurosecretory granules; each organ has a neuroendocrine component derived from the primitive neural crest; in the lungs, the neuroendocrine system is comprised of neuroendocrine cells and neuroepithelial bodies; hyperplasia of pulmonary neuroendocrine cells may occur in those living at high altitudes, or in smokers, implying that it is a reponse to hypoxia, and may also be seen in various lung diseases, eg bronchopulmonary hyperplasia, cystic fibrosis, asthma, chronic obstructive pulmonary disease, eosinophilic granuloma; it is thought that neuroendocine cell hyperplasia of lungs may be a primary process causing airway fibrosis (**Engl J Med** 1992; 327:1285OA) see APUD system, Neural crest, Neurosecretory granules

neuroendocrine tumors Neoplasms that share a characteristic morphology, often being composed of clusters and trabecular sheets of round 'blue cells', granular chromatin and an attenuated rim of poorly demarcated cytoplasm Neuroendocrine tumors include carcinoids, small ('oat') cell carcinomas, medullary carcinoma of thyroid, Merkel cell tumor, cutaneous neuroendocrine carcinoma, pancreatic islet cell tumors, pheochromocytoma EM Neurosecretory granules in tumor cells ImPx Tumor cells often stain for pan-endocrine markers, eg neuron-specific enolase, chromogranins, synaptophysin, and opioid receptors, as well as specific tumor cell products, eg calcitonin, bombesin, CEA, and hCG; see Neurosecretory granules

neuroendocrinoimmunology The study of the neuroendocrine influences on the function of immunocompetent cells and the way in these cells in turn influence neural function and endocrine activity (**N Engl J Med** 1993; 329:1246RV)

neuroepithelium The embryonal ectoderm that gives rise to the cerebrospinal axis; in the mature mammal, neuroepithelium corresponds histologically to the simple columnar epithelial cell receptors for external stimuli (as well as the cochlea, olfaction and tongue); see Neural crest

neurofibrillary tangles NEUROPATHOLOGY A characteristic histological finding seen in the perikaryon of large cortical neurons of patients with Alzheimer's disease, the number of which loosely correlates with the severity of dementia; NFTs consist of intensely argyrophilic aggregates of altered neurofilaments with an 800 A periodicity, forming 'twisted tubules' displacing cytoplasmic contents of the neurons; NFTs are also common in Down's syndrome and post-encephalitic parkinsonism, or may be seen in normal adults (confined to the hippocampus); see Granulovacuolar degeneration, Paired helical filaments, Senile plaques

neurofibromatosis, type 1 von Recklinghausen disease An AD [MIM 162200] condition affecting ± 100 000 (US), caused by a mutation of a large (± two million base pair in length) gene on chromosome 17 t(1;17)(p34.3;q11), which has sequence similarity ('homology') to tumor suppressor genes, as well as genes encoding the catalytic region of GAP (GTPase-activating protein), this latter possibly explaining the aberrant proliferation of melanocytes and Schwann cells typical of NF-1, as cAMP triggers division of these cells; NF1 is diagnosed in the presence of two or more of the following 1) Six or more 'cafe-au-lait' macules measuring 5 mm in greatest diameter are identified in a prepubertal or > 15 mm in greatest diameter in postpubertal patients 2) Two or more histologically-confirmed neurofibromas (or one plexiform neurofibroma) 3) Freckling in the axillary or inguinal regions 4) Optic glioma 5) Two or more Lisch nodules (iris hamartomas, the most common feature of NF1 in adults) (**N Engl J Med** 1991; 324:1264) 6) Distinct bone lesions, eg sphenoid dysplasia, cortical thinning of long bones, pseudoarthrosis and 7) The subject has a first-degree relative with NF1

neurofibromatosis, type 2 Central neurofibromatosis Bilateral acoustic neurofibromatosis An AD [MIM 101000] condition that is less common than NF1, which affects several thousand patients in the US, in 95% of whom the gene defect is located on chromosome 22q11.21-q13.1, first seen in late adolescence; NF2 is diagnosed in the presence of either bilateral eighth nerve masses by CT or MRI or when a subject known to have a first-degree relative with NF2 presents with either a unilateral eighth nerve mass or two or more 'neural crest' tumors, eg neurofibroma, meningioma, glioma, spinal neurofibromatosis, schwannoma or juvenile posterior subcapsular lenticular opacity

neurofibromatoses, types (3 and 4) Subtypes of neurofibromatosis of questionable validity, which have varying components of both NF1 and NF2

neurofibromin The protein encoded by *NF1*, a gene with sequence homology for yeast and mammalian GTPase-activating proteins; neurofibromin's GTPase-activating domain binds to Ras and accelerates GTP hydrolysis; see *NF-1*

'Taken together, the strong association of activating RAS mutations with oncogenesis, the increased risk of certain malignant conditions in patients with neurofibromatosis type 1, and the biochemical activity of neurofibromin on Ras proteins suggest that *NF1* belongs to the tumor-suppressor class of recessive cancer genes.' (**N Engl J Med** 1994; 330:597OA)

neurofilament A generic term for any of a number of elongated tubular chains of proteins of variable length that are present in the bodies, axons and dendrites of neurons, which can be seen by EM; see Intermediate filaments

neurogenesis A generic term for the development of the nervous system; see Nerve regeneration

neurogenic bladder A urinary bladder with loss or impairment of voluntary control of micturition, which may be either

SPASTIC, due to lesions of the spinal cord, accompanied by urgency, increased frequency, decreased functional capacity, spastic contractions and poor voluntary control or

FLACCID, due to segmental lesions at S2 to S4, interfering with voluntary and reflex control, loss of the sensation of bladder fullness, causing 'overflow' incontinence, when the bladder contains 2+ liters

neuroimmunomodulation The influence of the nervous

system on the immune response (N Engl J Med 1993; 329:1246ʀᴠ)

storage capacity of the brain

neuroimmunology The study of the effects of the neurologic status on immune function, or the effects of immune function on neurologic status (N Engl J Med 1993; 329:1246ʀᴠ)

neuroleptic malignant syndrome ANESTHESIOLOGY A disorder seen in 1% of those treated with antipsychotic agents (especially haloperidol), major tranquilizers, and other agents (eg phenothiazines, reserpine, and butyrophenone), an effect attributed to antidopaminergic activity; NMS may also be associated with anesthesia, affecting an estimated 1:50 000 patients exposed to inhalation anesthesia, most commonly in young ♂, who have been transiently weakened by exhaustion or dehydration CLINICAL Fever ≥ 41°C, extrapyramidal symptoms (eg rigidity, involuntary movements, facial dyskinesia) skeletal muscle hypertonicity, variable loss of consciousness, autonomic lability (pallor, sweating, tachycardia, arrhythmia, transient hypertension, which if severe may cause renal dysfunction and failure MORTALITY 20-30%, often between days 3-30, usually from renal failure TREATMENT Bromocriptine or dantrolene shorten the clinical disease from 6.8 days to < than 1.2 days (Arch Intern Med 1989; 149:1927)

neuroleukin A 56-kD protein cytokine produced in the brain and in T cells, which has sequence similarity ('homology') to both phosphohexose isomerase and HIV-1's gp120; competitive inhibition by gp120 at the neuroleukin receptor may explain AIDS-related dementia

neurolymphomatosis A rare lymphoma with a predilection for peripheral and cranial nerves, lumbar and brachial plexi and nerve roots, meninges, and vessels in the brain; ½ of cases are accompanied by systemic lymphoma, which may be clinically silent; neurolymphomatosis may present as a painful chronic sensorimotor neuropathy with asymmetric distribution and prominent bulbar involvement, and has been associated with HIV and HTLV-I infections (N Engl J Med 1995; 332:730ᴄᴘᴄ)

Note: The animal model is Marek's disease which is induced by an oncogenic herpesvirus

neuromuscular choristoma Benign Triton tumor, neuromuscular hamartoma A rare well-circumscribed tumor of young children that arises in association with a large nerve trunk PATHOLOGY Hazphazard arrangement of mature skeletal muscle and myelinated nerve TREATMENT Surgical (Am J Clin Pathol 1995; 103:460ᴏᴀ)

neuromuscular junction Motor end-plate The expanded terminal of a motor neuron that corresponds to the region of contact between a motor nerve and the effector striated muscle PHYSIOLOGY A nerve impulse or wave of depolarization arrives via the axon to the junction, releases acetylcholine contained within synaptic vesicles into the synaptic cleft; acetylcholine binds to its receptors located on the post-synaptic membrane resulting in depolarization, the production of an end-plate potential on the muscle; neuromuscular blockade may be due to 1) Reduction of post-synaptic receptors, eg myasthenia gravis, 2) Defective acetylcholine release from storage vesicles, eg botulism, myasthenia, or Eaton-Lambert syndrome and 3) Competition for binding sites, either pharmacologic blockade, eg neostigmine, edrophonium or toxic blockade, eg organophosphate insecticides

neuron neuron [NH3] The principle cell of the central and peripheral nervous system, which consists of a body, containing the nucleus and cytoplasm, as well as radiating processes (the axons and dendrites) of varying size and shape; dogma has long regarded the neuron as the nervous system's smallest unit; it has been shown that a single Purkinje cell may have six or more independently functioning dendritic units

Note: The subdivision of a single cell into multiple quasi-discrete units has broad implications, as it adds an extra 'layer' of complexity to the processing and

neuronal ceroid lipofuscinosis A heterogenous group of progressive, degenerative encephalopathies, which are attributed to an accumulation of lipofuscin and/or ceroid, and accompanied by optic nerve atrophy CLINICAL Seizures, progressive mental retardation, macular degeneration of the retina, retinitis pigmentosa PATHOLOGY The affected tissues are yellow-gray with a waxy consistency and autofluorescent lipopigment in the brain, liver and muscle; NCL is divided into 1) Major forms a) Juvenile type of Batten or Vogt-Spielmeyer b) Late infantile type of Bielschowsky c) Subacute-chronic adult type of Kufs and d) Infantile type of Santavuori-Haltia and 2) Minor forms, including congenital type, acute adult type, acute-subacute variant type, chronic childhood form with pervasiveness, chronic infantile form with autism and chronic juvenile form with ataxia and spasticity; NCL may be classified by chronology Acute a) Infantile or Finnish type Santavuori-Haltia disease [MIM 256730] Onset in early infancy with myoclonus, seizures, blindness, dementia, rapid deterioration, spasticity, rigidity, ataxia, seborrhea and peliosis PATHOLOGY Multinucleated phagocytic histiocytes with granular autofluorescent lipofuscin-like material b) Late infantile form of Jansky-Bielschovsky [MIM 204500] Onset at age 2-3, characterized by minor seizures, myoclonic spasms, squirming ataxia, progressive loss of mental skills and optic atrophy, seborrhea, poliosis and hirsutism PATHOLOGY, as above c) Adult onset form of Zeman-Dyken Onset in early adulthood (20-25 years), characterized by mental retardation PATHOLOGY As above EM Granular and curvilinear bodies Chronic 1) Juvenile form of Batten (aka Vogt-Spielmeyer or Spielmeyer-Sjögren syndrome) [MIM 204200] Onset age 6, characterized by blindness, dementia, late seizures, motor defects EM Granular and fingerprint bodies 2) Adult form of Kufs-Böhme [MIM 204300] Characterized by seizures, ataxia, myoclonus, dementia and hypertension without blindness Atypical variants Subjects with amaurotic idiocy, sea-blue histiocytosis, cherry-red spot-myoclonus syndrome and others

neuron-specific enolase A homodimeric enolase isoenzyme composed of two γ chains; NSE was first regarded as specific for neurons and neuro-endocrine cells and tumors as well as astrocytomas; NSE is also commonly present in medullary carcinoma of the thyroid, pituitary adenomas and endocrine neoplasms of the pancreas and gastrointestinal tract; NSE may also occur in many other benign and/or non-neuronal tissues and tumors (meningioma, fibroadenoma, carcinoma of the breast, kidney and ovary, occasionally lymphoma) and other non-malignant conditions; Cf S-100

neuropathic arthropathy RHEUMATOLOGY The mechanical failure of a joint due to impaired sensory input; NA is a destructive and productive arthropathy with a loss of pain and nociceptive sensation that is thought to be due to the cumulative effect of trauma and joint laxity RADIOLOGY Joint effusion, fragmentation of the articular surface and eburnation of bony surfaces, and eventually complete joint disorganization ETIOLOGY DM, syringomyelia, tabes dorsalis; rarely also congenital indifference to pain, amyloidosis, meningomyelocele and other 'exotica'

*Synonyms include Charcot's joint, nervous arthropathy, neuroarthropathy, neurogenic joint, neurotrophic arthritis

neuropathy A generic and highly nonspecific term referring to virtually any disorder of peripheral nerves, which may be congenital (eg hereditary sensory radicular neuropathy or hypertrophic interstitial neuropathy), traumatic (entrapment, eg carpal tunnel syndrome), metabolic (eg, due to amyloid or DM), toxic (eg, tobacco or alcohol-related amblyopia, cis-platinum, vincristine)

neuropeptides A family of low (less than 5-kD) molecular weight intracellular peptides that transmit information in the CNS, GI tract, and elsewhere; neuropeptides include ACTH, angiotensin II, bombesin, bradykinin, calcitonin gene-related products, carnosine, cholecystokinin, corticotropin-releasing factor, dynorphins, β-endorphin, leu-enkephalin, met-enkephalin, gastric inhibitory polypeptide, gastrin, glucagon, growth hormone, growth hormone releasing factor, insulin, luteinizing hormone-releasing factor, α-melanocyte-stimulating hormone, melanotropin-inhibiting factor, motilin, neurotensin, oxytocin, prolactin, secretin, somatostatin-14 and -28, substance P, thyroglobulin-releasing factor, thyrotropin, vasoactive intestinal peptide, vasopressin

neuropeptide Y A widely distributed 36-residue tyrosine-rich neuropeptide, prominent in the hypothalamus and in limbic regions, that co-exists with other neurotransmitters (epinephrine and norepinephrine, GABA, galanin, somatostatin) in discrete regions of the central, peripheral, and enteric nervous systems; NY has considerable sequence homology with pancreatic polypeptide (PP) and peptide YY, and is involved in a vast array of neuroendocrine activities, including autonomic functions (vasoconstriction and decreased absorption of electrolytes in the GI tract), circadian rhythm, eating, drinking, sexual and motor activity, and stress responses that may be altered by psychotropic drugs and excitatory neurotoxins and is being studied in Alzheimer's and Huntington's diseases, parkinsonism, eating disorders and depression while NY receptors are widely distributed in the brain, NY-like immune reactivity does not always overlap the presumed receptors, see Mismatch phenomenon

neurophysin A carrier protein for oxytocin and vasopressin

neuroprobe REHABILITATION MEDICINE An electrical stimulation device that may be used to identify tender areas or trigger points, to locate points for placing the electrodes of a TENS (transcutaneous electric nerve stimulation) unit, or may itself be used to deliver electrical impulses to treat pain (JC DeLee, D Drez, Jr, Eds, Orthopedic Sports Medicine WB Saunders, Philadelphia, 1994) Cf Shortwave diathermy

neuroprotection An evolving field of neurosciences that attempts to prevent the secondary damage that follows a primary neurologic insult, eg trauma or stroke; neuroprotective agents and methods include N-methyl-D-aspartate receptor antagonists, calcium channel blockers, gangliosides, free-radical scavengers, insulin, hypothermia, lazaroids, self-protection of the brain, and others; while still in the embryonic stages, the field of neuroprotection is likely to be integrated into clinical neurology and neurosurgery in the forseeable future (N Engl J Med 1993; 329:215BR)

neurorecurrence A generic term for the recurrence of any neurologic disease, but more specifically used for neurologic disease that follows (within 6-12 months) inadequate therapy of syphilis; this ultrarare 'early' form of neurosyphilis affects mesodermal tissues and is characterized by acute meningitis, cranial nerve abnormalities, and/or stroke; this contrasts with late ('usual') neurosyphilis in which ectodermal involvement is linked to dementia, psychosis, and/or tabes dorsalis (N Engl J Med 1994; 331:1516ED)

neuroregulator Neurotransmitter, see there

neurosarcoma Malignant schwannoma, see there

neurosecretory granule Dense core granule A small, round, membrane-bound vesicle, which contains norepinephrine, oxytocin, vasopressin, and others; by EM, NGs appears as a dense black spot measuring 50 to 500 nm in diameter, surrounded by a cleared space, in turn surrounded by a dark thin rim; neurosecretory granules contain various hormones, eg calcitonin, gastrin, glucagon, and VIP and are relatively specific for the neuroendocrine system, ie the neural crest and APUD system; these granules have been divided by size

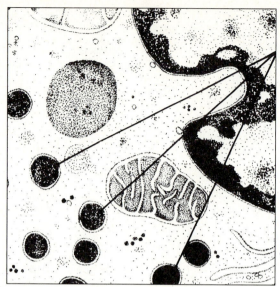

neurosecretory granules

100-200 NM GRANULES seen in the TSH-producing cells of the pituitary gland, PP cells of the pancreas and D_1 endocrine cells of the gastrointestinal tract

500-1500 NM GRANULES seen in somatotrophic cells, prolactin-producing cells and carcinoid tumor cells and

200-600 NM GRANULES that occur in all other cells

Neurosecretory granule shape varies and may contain paracrystalline material with irregular sharp edges as in the α cells of the pancreatic islets; the dense core granule's limiting membrane may be tightly bound and indistinct, as in D cells of the pancreatic islets or have a gray halo, as in A cells of the pancreatic islets; in addition to the neuroendocrine system, dense core granules are seen in several types of neurons, adrenal neuroblastoma, pheochromocytoma, chemodectoma

neurosis PSYCHOLOGY A generic term of waning popularity* for any of a number of disorders characterized by excessive anxiety and prominent avoidance behaviors; as used by psychoanalysts, a neurosis arises from an unresolvable conflict between the id (instinct) and ego (conscious thought); subtypes include anxiety, manic-depressive disorder (bipolar I disorder, per DSM-IV) or pure depression, hysteria, obsessive-compulsive behavior, and phobias

*Note: Because the term neurosis is ill-defined and nebulous, it has fallen into disfavor and is not formally recognized in the Diagnostic and Statistical Manual of Mental Disorders, 4th edition (DSM-IV™) published by the American Psychiatric Association

neurosyphilis Any of a number of uncommon manifestation of tertiary syphilis that may follow secondary syphilis; neurosyphilis may be 1) Asymptomatic with only a positive VDRL in the cerebrospinal fluid, 2) Gummatous, 3) Meningovascular or thromboembolic form with cerebral infarction or cranial nerve defects, 4) Tabetic with degeneration of the posterior columns of the spinal cord and nerve roots, decreased peripheral reflexes and proprioceptive sensation, evoking Charcot's joints and 5) General paresis or chronic meningoencephalitis CLINICAL Personality defects, aphasia, paralysis and seizures PATHOLOGY Diffuse cortical atrophy (see Windswept cortex), neuronal depopulation and microglial proliferation; in patients with early syphilis who are also infected with HIV individuals, high-dose penicillin G benzathine therapy may be ineffective (N Engl J Med 1994; 331:1469DA) see STS-RPR, VDRL; Cf Quaternary syphilis

neurotensin A 13-amino acid neuropeptide secreted in the

GI tract that evokes vasodilation and inhibits gastric secretion and intestinal motility

neurothekeoma *neuron*, Greek, nerve, *theke*, sheath Nerve sheath myxoma A benign neural tumor of childhood, affecting the midline face, arms and shoulders at the dermal-epidermal interface PATHOLOGY Large, mitotically active epithelioid cells with nuclear atypia and scattered spindled schwann cells in a mucinous matrix, divided into lobules by fibrous connective tissue IMPx Tumor cells display variable amounts of S-100 antigen

neurotoxin A nonspecific term for any toxic agent that acts directl;y on neurons; as an example, exotoxins that are present in many plants and animals and either block conduction of the nerve impulse or synaptic transmission, by binding to the voltage-gated Na+ channel protein or evoke increased neuronal activity; neurotoxins are produced by *Corynebacterium diphtheriae*, *Clostridium tetani*, *C botulinum*, *Shigella dysenteriae*; other neurotoxins include conotoxin, saxitoxin, and tetrodotoxin; see Conotoxin, Puffer fish, Red tide

neurotransmitter PHYSIOLOGY Any of a number of small molecules present at synapses or neuromuscular junctions that are capable of transmitting an electrical impulse by binding to their cognate receptor; to be defined as a neurotransmitter

1) The synaptic vesicles in the presynaptic neuron must contain the substance and release it into the space at the time of an impulse

2) Introduction of the substance into the synaptic space must elicit the same response as does stimulation of the presynaptic nerve and

3) The substance must be rapidly degraded in the synaptic space with restoration of the membrane potential

virtually any molecule capable of modifying neural signals may function as a neurotransmitter, including such diverse molecular species as amino acids (aspartic acid, GABA, glutamic acid, glycine), biogenic amines (acetylcholine, bradykinin, dopamine, epinephrine, norepinephrine, melatonin, serotonin or 5-HT), hypothalamic neuropeptides (LH, somatostatin, TSH), opioids (β-endorphin, neuroenkephalin), neuropeptides (angiotensin, cholecystokinin, gastrin, nerve growth factor, neurotensin, substance P, VIP) and others (ACTH, ATP, corticosteroids, estrogens, melanin-stimulating hormone, nitric oxide, oxytocin, prolactin, prostaglandins, testosterone, vasopressin); Cf Neuropeptides

neurotrophic factor A generic term for any of a family of substances with roles in maintenance and survival of neurons, eg secretory proteins, nerve growth factors (see there), brain-derived growth factor and neurotrophin-3

neurotrophin NEUROBIOLOGY Any of a family of homologous proteins which includes brain-derived neurotrophic factor, neurotrophin-3 (NT-3) and neurotrophin-4/5 (NT-4/5), each of which promotes the survival of a specific population of neurons; some populations of neurons express not only neurotrophins but also their cognate receptors (the Trk family of tyrosine kinases), which were once thought to be expressed only by their innervating neurons (Nature 1995; 374:450, 405)

neurotrophin-3 NT-3 A member of the nerve growth factor family that stimulates the growth of a select number of nerves, at present incompletely studied; see BDGF (brain-derived growth factor), Nerve growth factor

neutral collagenase Matrix metalloproteinase 8, MMP8

neutral fats see NEFA

neutral endopeptidase 24.11 see CD10

neutral lipid storage disease Chanarin-Dorfman syndrome An AR [MIM 275630] condition characterized by congenital ichthyosis, hepatosplenomegaly, myopathy, and diffuse accumulation of triglycerides, and vacuolated granulocytes

neutralizing antibody An immunoglobulin produced by the host as a defense against bacteria, reducing its infectivity; neutralization assays are used in the clinical laboratory as serologic tests to demonstrate a subject's previous exposure to the microorganism producing an exo- or endotoxin; alternately, the patient's serum or body fluid can be tested for the presence of an antigen, eg a virus by performing a neutralization assay with a standardized antibody or antitoxin

neutron A non-charged elementary particle with a ½ spin and the approximate* mass of a proton; alone a neutron has a $T_{1/2}$ (half-life) of 12-15 minutes, and decays into a proton, an electron, and an antineutrino, but is stable when bound within an atom; in radiotherapy, neutrons have considerable advantages over γ radiation in that the oxygen enhancement ratio is lower for neutrons than for photons, there is little or no repair of DNA damage with neutrons and the variation in the cell sensitivity with the mitotic phases is less with neutrons than with other radiotherapeutic modalities; see Linear accelerator
*1.0014 times greater than, for those counting

neutron activation analysis LABORATORY MEDICINE A highly sensitive reference method for quantifying elements in nanogram amounts, which is too complex for routine use METHOD The specimen is bombarded with neutrons that interact with the specimen's atoms, thus generating radioactive products that are identified based on the pattern of energy spectrum of the emitted γ rays

neutron capture NUCLEAR MEDICINE A reaction that forms the basis on which radioisotopes of medical interest are produced in a reactor, where a neutron is temporarily absorbed by a nuclide (protons/neutrons comprising an atomic nucleus); once the neutron is absorbed, the radioactive nuclide emits γ rays (8 MeV), lower energy protons (β particles) and neutrons (α particles)

neutropenic colitis with aplastic anemia Mulholland syndrome A clinical condition that affects young adults consisting of right-sided colonic necrosis, profound agranulocytosis, aplastic anemia, fever, watery diarrhea, generalized abdominal pain without inflammation, accompanied by transmural bacterial infiltration often following antibiotic therapy TREATMENT Non-interventional; see Pseudomembranous colitis

neutrophil-activating factor-1 IL-8, interleukin-8, see there

neutrophil dysfunction syndromes A heterogenous group of diseases characterized by qualitative disorders of neutrophils, subdivided into defects of 1) Adhesion, eg cell adhesion deficiency, drug-induced adhesion defects 2) Locomotion, eg lazy leukocyte syndrome, abnormalities of actin polymerization 3) Phagocytosis 4) Microbial killing, eg chronic granulomatous disease, myeloperoxidase deficiency, hyperimmunoglobulin E syndrome, glucose-6-phosphate dehydrogenase deficiency 5) Structure of the nucleus or organelles, eg hereditary macropolycytes, hereditary hypersegmentation, specific granule deficiency, Alder-Reilly, May-Hegglin, and Pelger-Huët anomalies, Chediak-Higashi disease and 6) Multiple or mixed disorders

Nevirapine AIDS A compound that binds to a hydrophobic pocket in HIV's reverse transcriptase-DNA (RT-DNA) complex close to the polymerization active site (Science 1995; 267:988A) see Nonnucleoside reverse transcriptase inhibitor, TIBO

nevoid-basal cell carcinoma syndrome Basal cell nevus syndrome, see there

nevus A congenital circumscribed pigmented tumor of the skin and/or mucosae, which is due to either an excess or deficiency of normal cutaneous structure(s); nevi are considered hamartomas and contain spindle-shaped melanocytes; see Blue nevus, Giant hairy nevus, Halo nevus, Melanocytic nevus; Cf Lymph node inclusions

nevus anemicus White nevus A sharply circumscribed, pale macule on the trunk, neck or limbs, attributed to a functional defect in the superficial dermal vessels, as these are not affected by vasodilators; the white nevus contrasts to achromic or depigmented nevi, eg Ito's nevus is due to a focal loss of melanin pigmentation

nevus of Ota A bluish or gray-brown macular lesion of the periorbital skin innervated by first and second branches of the trigeminal nerve; the NO is a serious cosmetic problem for ± 0.6% of the Japanese population, but is also described in other groups PATHOLOGY Benign dendritic melanocytosis of papillary and upper dermis TREATMENT Selective photothermolysis using a Q-switched ruby laser (N Engl J Med 1994; 331:1745oA); other less successful modalities include surgical removal, skin grafting, dermabrasion, and cryotherapy

nevus spilus Speckled lentiginous nevus, see there

New Age '...a metaphor for the expression of a transformative, creative spirit...for being in the world in a manner that opens us to the presence of God...in the midst of our ordinariness; NA...calls us to live in a delicate balance between tranformation and routine, between metamorphosis and maturation, between the birth of what could be and the care of what is, between surrender, between empowerment and surrender.' (D Spangler in The New Age Catalogue, Island Pub Co, Dolphin, Doubleday, New York, 1988); see Alternative medicine

In the backdrop of this relatively nebulous definition, a vast array of philosophies, activities, belief systems, and concepts have either aligned themselves or been identified with the NA movement, including astral projection, astrology, channeling, graphology, global concerns, mystics, near-death experiences, NA music, transformational travel, visionary art, and others; the NA movement also encompasses various forms of alternative medicine and/or therapy, including acupressure, chiropractic, herbology, homeopathy, massage, nutrition, Oriental medicine, and others

new drug application see NDA

New Jersey vesicular stomatitis virus An enveloped RNA rhabdovirus with a single-stranded negatively coiled genome that replicates in infected host cell cytoplasm, first identified in the 1920s with a reservoir in wild animals, eg swine in Georgia, spider monkeys in Central America CLINICAL 60% of exposed subjects develop disease after a 1-2 day incubation, with fever, chills, malaise, myalgias, nausea, vomiting and pharyngitis; despite the name, oral vesicles are relatively uncommon PROGNOSIS Spontaneous resolution in one week

New Orleans asthma Yokohama asthma, see there

'new scientist' A PhD scientist who has recognized the changing atmosphere in research; the modern scientist is no longer able to sustain a career in research by merely doing benchwork, but must also be part businessman, communicator, and 'grantsman', and must be financially and politically adept, computer-literate and have strong interpersonal skills; Cf 'Lab rat'

New York City medium MICROBIOLOGY A growth medium containing hemolyzed equine erythrocytes, horse serum, yeast extract, vancomycin, colistin, amphotericin and trimethoprim, which is used to identify Neisseria gonorrheae allowing better recovery of organisms than that obtained with the Thayer-Martin medium; NYC medium also supports the growth of mycoplasma and ureaplasma

New York Heart Association classification A functional classification (table) of cardiac failure, that serves to stratify patients accorrding to severity of disease and the need for (and type of) therapeutic intervention (Criteria Committee of the New York Heart Association, Inc: Diseases of the Heart and Blood Vessels, 6th ed, Little Brown, Co, Boston 1964)

NEW YORK HEART ASSOCIATION
I Asymptomatic heart disease
II Comfortable at rest; symptomatic with normal activity
III Comfortable at rest; symptomatic with less than normal activity
IV Symptomatic at rest

New Zealand mice Two strains (New Zealand black NZB and New Zealand white NZW) of inbred mice that are used to study autoimmunity; NZW mice are asymptomatic; NZB mice develop autoimmune hemolytic anemia, extramedullary hematopoiesis, and low titers of antinuclear antibodies, spontaneously activated B cells, defective T cells and defects in DNA repair; when NZW are crossed with NZB, the progeny develop an autoimmune syndrome with severe immune complex disease, glomerulonephritis, lupus cells and high titers of anti-nuclear antibodies; thus the F_1 generation of NZB/NZW mice serves as an animal model for autoimmune disease and lupus erythematosus

Newcastle disease A self-limited unilateral follicular conjunctivitis caused by an avian paramyxovirus which inhibits the oxidative burst in phagocytes, inducing the release of pyrogenic cytokines; spontaneous recovery follows 1-2 weeks of illness; the Newcastle agent causes a fatal pneumoencephalitis in fowl

the Newport Hospital case An infamous situation that occurred in 1992-93, placing a community hospital and its laboratory in the state of Rhode Island under a spotlight, when it was discovered that a woman had invasive squamous cell carcinoma after having four prior (erroneously) normal results on Pap tests performed by four different technicians dating from 1984 (CAP Today March 1994 p26)

news embargo Embargo arrangement, see there

news release SCIENTIFIC JOURNALISM A document of public record that formally announces matters of interest to media 'consumers'; NRs have a clear goal of informing while attracting publicity to the institution where the newsworthy event(s) occurred, and are in general accurate and devoid of 'hype'; NRs can be problematic in that claims made to the public (eg a cure for a 'dreaded disease', eg AIDS or cancer) may not survive scientific scrutiny resulting in a credibility gap (NY Times 10 Jan 1995; C3)

nexin A 150-kD protein that is integral to axonemic structures in cilia and flagella; see Cilia, Dynein

next-of-kin A term that '...is used with two meanings 1) nearest blood relations according to the law of consanguity and 2) those entitled to take under statutory distribution of intestate's estates, and the term is not necessarily confined to relatives by blood, but may include a relationship existing by reason of marriage, and may well embrace persons, who in the natural sense of word, and in contemplation of Roman law, bear no relation of kinship at all.' (Black's Law Dictionary, 6th ed, West Publishing, St Paul, Minn, 1990)

nexus Site of electrical connection between two cells; see Neuromuscular junction; Cf Gap junction

NF National Formulary, see there

NF1 The gene on chromosome 17 that encodes neurofibromin; NF1 may belong to the tumor-suppressor class of recessive cancer genes and is mutated in malignant myeloproliferative diseases of children with neurofibromatosis type 1 (N Engl J Med 1994; 330:597oA) the mutation rate of NF-1 (1 x 10^{-4}) is one of the highest rates in the human genome, and appears to be passed to progeny in the form of germ-line mosaicism (N Engl J Med 1994; 331:1403QA)

NF-AT Nuclear factor of activated T cells A DNA-binding transcription complex that is required for IL-2 gene transcription and for the expression of the proteins that coordinate the immune response; NF-AT has been implicated as a nuclear target of the T-cell receptor, and is responsible for synthesizing some of the early activation cytokines, eg IL-2; the cytoplasmic subunit (NF-AT$_c$) has been cloned (Nature 1994; 369:497L, 443N&v); the 120-kD NF-AT$_p$ subunit is a substrate for calcineurin and interacts with Fos and Jun, providing a unique mechanism for combinatorial regulation of IL-2 gene transcription (Nature 1993; 365:352); NF-AT$_c$ translocates to the nucleus in response to calcium signals that can be inhibited by the immunosuppressants cyclosporin A and FK506; the nuclear subunit (NF-AT$_n$) contains *jun/fos* family products; see Immunophilins

n-3 fatty acids see beginning of letter N

NGF Nerve growth factor, see there

NGU Non-gonococcal urethritis

NHL 1) Non-Hodgkin's lymphoma, see there 2) Nodular histiocytic lymphoma 3) Normal human lymphocyte

NHLBI National Heart, Lung, and Blood Institute, an agency of the National Institutes of Health (US)

NHTSA National Highway Traffic Safety Administration; see MVA

niacin test MICROBIOLOGY Niacin (nicotinic acid) plays a key role in the oxidation-reduction reaction in mycobacterial metabolism; although all *Mycobacterium* species produce nicotinic acid, *M tuberculosa*, *M simiae* and *M szulgai* produce the greatest amount; lesser amounts are produced by *M africanum*, *M bovis*, *M marinum* and *M chelonei*, ss *cheloni* and *M chelonei*, ss *abscessus*; differences in nictonic acid production form the basis of a test allowing speciation of positive mycobacterial cultures

NIAID National Institute of Allergy and Infectious Diseases An agency of the National Institutes of Health Director A Fauci; among its major roles, NIAID coordinates activities related to the therapy of AIDS

NICHHD National Institute of Child Health and Human Development, an agency of the US National Institutes of Health

nick MOLECULAR BIOLOGY *noun* A single-stranded break in double-stranded helix of nucleic acids, usually DNA; 'nicked sites' are characterized by increased mobility and absence of a phosphodiester bond between two adjacent nucleotides on a chain of nucleic acids in a double helical conformation *verb* To effect a nick

nick translation MOLECULAR BIOLOGY A method used to prepare a radioactive 'probe' of a segment of DNA of interest, where the polymerase and 5'→3' exonuclease activities of DNA polymerase I are allowed to occur simultaneously TECHNIQUE *Escherichia coli* DNA polymerase I is added to a solution containing 1) A duplex DNA molecule of interest to be used as a 'probe' and 2) A radioactive or 'hot-labelled' nucleotide containing either a purine or pyrimidine labeled with ³²P; the DNA polymerase both 'nicks' the DNA (acting as a 5'→3' exonuclease and 'mends' the double-stranded DNA (acting as a 3'→5' polymerase) using a ³²P-labelled nucleotide in the repair process; once a probe is radioactive or labelled, it may then be placed in a hybridization fluid containing a Southern-blotted nylon or nitrocellulose membrane containing the DNA segment of interest and allowed to anneal with its 'mirror-image'

nickase A restriction endonuclease that introduces a break in one strand of the double-stranded DNA

'nickel and dime' lesions A fanciful descriptor for the annular, waxing and waning maculopapular lesions seen at the mucocutaneous borders at the mouth and nasolabial folds in protracted untreated secondary syphilis, more common in dark-skinned subjects; these lesions may coincide with anogenital condylomata lata

Note: Nickels are US coins with a value of $.05, dimes are worth $0.10

NICODARD National Information Center for Orphan Drugs and Rare Diseases; see Orphan disease, Orphan drug

nicotine A colorless toxic liquid obtained from tobacco plant; used as a biological insecticide (N Engl J Med 1994; 331:123SB) see Tobacco

nicotine 1-methyl-2-(3-pyridyl) pyrrolidine SUBSTANCE ABUSE A toxic pyridine liquid alkaloid found in cigarette smoke; urine levels of nicotine in smokers 0.616-18.480 μmol/L (US: 0.1-3.0 mg/L) and in nonsmokers < 0.431μmol/L (US: < 0.07 mg/L); nicotine is a highly toxic and rapidly acting natural insecticide, which may cause human intoxication by inhalation, skin absorption or ingestion, either the result of accidental exposure or suicidal ingestion CLINICAL Transient CNS stimulation followed by depression or paralysis, accompanied by nausea, hypersalivation, abdominal pain, vomiting, diarrhea, cold sweats, headache, vertigo, confusion, incoordination, ↓ pulse rate, dyspnea with potentially paralysis of the respiratory musculature and intense vagal stimulation which may cause transient or permanent cardiac arrest; death occurs within 1-4 hours of ingesting a fatal adult dose (> 60 mg) TREATMENT Emesis, gastric lavage, atropine (*Nicotiana tabacum* stimulates the cholinergic receptors); see Conicotine, Nicotine gum, Passive smoking, Smokeless tobacco, Smoking

nicotine gum Nicotine polacrilex A masticant that slowly releases nicotine, ameliorating the effects of tobacco withdrawal and the intensity of relapse factors, eg weight gain

nicotine patch Nicotine transdermal delivery system A device used to help a person stop smoking; NPs produce end-of-treatment smoking cessation of 18-77%, a six-month abstinence of 22-42% (vs 5-28% for placebo patches), and reduce many of symptoms of nicotine withdrawal; available data suggests that 6-8 weeks of NP therapy is adequate in most patients; for success in smoking cessation to be most effective, NPs should be used in conjunction with adjuvant smoking cessation counseling (JAMA 1992; 268:2687)

nicotine replacement therapy SUBSTANCE ABUSE The use of nicotine gum (nicotine polacrilex chewing gum) and transdermal nicotine patches to alleviate or attenuate the symptoms of nicotine withdrawal; non-smoking nicotine replacement must be supplemented by behavioral intervention and training to minimize recidivism; transdermal patches are two-fold more effective than placebos and may be more effective than nicotine gum, currently the only approved replacement therapy in the US; see Nicotine gum, Nicotine patch

NIDA National Institute on Drug Abuse, a division of the National Institutes of Health

NIDDM Non-insulin-dependent diabetes mellitus, see there

nifedipine A calcium-channel-blocking vasodilator that ↓ systolic and diastolic blood pressure, resulting in a ↓ left ventricular volume and mass and ↑ in ejection fraction; nifedipine is the most commonly used drug for hypertension and angina of use in managing severe aortic regurgitation, and delays the need for aortic valve-replacement surgery in patients with aortic regurgitation SIDE EFFECTS Occur in 42%, and include tachycardia, headache, peripheral edema (N Engl J Med 1994; 331:689OA)

night blindness Nyctalopia Defective vision in reduced illumination, often implying defective rod function with delayed dark adaptation and perceptual threshold; it is either congenital and stationary with myopia and degeneration of the disc, eg retinitis pigmentosa, hereditary optic atrophy or progressive and acquired with retinal, choroidal or vitrioretinal degeneration, eg cataract, glaucoma, optic atrophy, retinal degeneration and, the 'classic' cause of nyctalopia, vitamin A deficiency

nightmare A fearful dream that most commonly affects children during REM (rapid eye movement) sleep, which is accompanied by hyperactivity of the autonomic nervous system TREATMENT None

'night soil' Human feces used as a fertilizer for ground crops (tubers, vegetables, berries), which may serve as a vehicle for various parasites, commonly, *Ascaris lumbricoides* in the Western hemisphere, the eggs of which remain viable for long periods, and *Clonorchis sinensis* in the Orient

nightstick fracture FORENSIC MEDICINE A solitary ulnar fracture occurring when the arm is raised to parry the blow of a nightstick, which may be used by some police and security guards

night sweats Nocturnal, often drenching diaphoresis, a clinical finding described as characteristic of terminal Hodgkin's disease, tuberculosis, trypanosomiasis and giant cell (temporal) arteritis

NIHL see Noise-induced hearing loss

NIH National Institutes of Health A group of US governmental agencies located in Bethesda, Maryland that funds and directs government-sponsored medicine-related research activities in the US, directed by Harold Varmus (Nobel laureate, 1989) who delineated a plan for reorganization in the face of certain intra- and extramural controversies (Science 1994; 264;897N&C); the NIH has an annual budget of $8 X 10^9; Cf INSERM

NIH scoring system IMMUNOLOGY A technique for typing the human leukocyte anti-gens HLA-A, -B, -C, -DQ and -DP, devised at the National Institutes of Health, which uses a 150 power inverted microscope, giving a value of 1 for every 10% of cells lysed, detected by active exclusion of a dye, trypan blue (table)

NIH SCORING

SCORE	% LYSIS	INTERPRETATION
1	0-9%	NEGATIVE
2	10-19%	± NEGATIVE
4	20-39%	± POSITIVE
6	40-79%	POSITIVE
8	80-100%	POSITIVE

NIHL see Noise-induced hearing loss

nikethamide A centrally acting CNS stimulant formerly used in emergent situations in cardiovascular and respiratory failure; because of its narrow therapeutic range (slight overdose is associated with convulsions), direct supportive measures, eg mechanical ventilation and maintenance of cardiovascular function have proven more useful, and nikethamide has been abandoned

nilutamide RU 23908 An antiandrogenic agent used to prevent the potentially fatal flare-up reaction that may occur in early treatment of metastatic prostatic carcinoma; see Disease flare-up

NIMH National Institute of Mental Health

nimodipine AIDS therapy An L-type calcium channel antagonist that preferentially binds to the channels when the cells are depolarized, maintaining them in an opened state, theoretically preventing the accumulation of gluta-

mate, which has been pathogenically linked to AIDS dementia complex (N Engl J Med 1995; 332:934RV)

911 EMERGENCY MEDICINE A telephone number that in many areas of the US provides the public with rapid access to communication centers linked to mobile EMS (Emergency Medical Service) units via a radio network, which are in turn linked to an on-line supervising physician at the hospital

9 + 2 pattern Nine plus two arrangement A configuration of microtubules characteristic of eukaryotic cilia and flagella, in which a pair of central tubules is surrounded by nine peripheral doublets of microtubules; see Cilia

NINDS National Institute of Neurological Disorders and Stroke, an agency of the US National Institutes of Health

ninhydrin Triketohydrindene CLINICAL TOXICOLOGY An oxidizing reagent that reacts with tamino acids and proteins, and is used to screen urine specimens for the presence of, and semiquantify α-amino acids, as it yields colored compounds

Nintendo® surgery Laparoscopic surgery, telepresence surgery A generic term* that encompasses new techniques applied to surgery, which are performed at a distance from a highly restricted operating field, using endoscopy and laparoscopy combined with applied video, miniaturization, and computer-based technologies (JAMA 1992; 267:2329L)

*Although laparoscopic is the most commonly used formal adjective applicable to this evolving area of surgery, it does not convey the Gefuhl of Nintendo® video games in which control pads are used to perform tasks at a distance from the operator; the term Nintendo surgery is even more appropos in view of the fact that the Nintendo surgeon may be young enough to have been raised in the 'video age'

NIOSH National Institute for Occupational Safety and Health, see there

nipple appearance CYTOPATHOLOGY A 'succulent' nuclear protrusion of blasts seen in Papanicolaou-stained cerebrospinal fluid, a finding which in combination with prominent nucleoli is characteristic of leukemic involvement of the central nervous system; see Nuclear blebbing; Cf 'Tit' sign

nipple discharge Serous and/or serosanguinous discharge from the breasts that is most common in peri- and postmenopausal women, caused by a variety of lesions, eg benign intraductal Papilloma (nipple adenoma), ductal ectasia and Paget's disease of the breast, as well as advanced ductal carcinoma of the breast

NISH Non-radioactive in situ hybridization, see FISH; Cf NOSH, NIOSH

Nissl substance Aggregates of rough endoplasmic reticulum seen in active neurons which are seen by LM as basophilic cytoplasmic material

NIST National Institute of Standards and Technology, see there

nit An empty louse egg shell, deposited by *Pediculus capitis, P corporis* and *Phthirus pubis* ('crabs')

nitrates NO3-bearing compounds are a major component of explosives and fertilizers; when drinking water is obtained from wells contaminated by runoffs from nitrogen-fertilized fields (EPA standards for well water allow a maximum 10 ppm or 10 mg/L of nitrate), nitrates are converted in vivo to nitrites, and may cause fatal methemoglobinemia in newborn infants and, less commonly, in adults deficient in glucose-phosphate dehydrogenase Note: Nitrates may be converted in the stomach to N-nitrosamines, a potent gastric carcinogen; deionizers, desalination, reverse ionization, ion exchange, and distillation remove nitrates in the drinking water; in-line charcoal filters do not (Nature 1991; 350:223) see Blue people, Monday death, Nitroglycerin

nitric oxide ENVIRONMENT A gas byproduct of high temperature combustion, eg internal combustion engines which upon exposure to light results in NO_2 formation, a highly irritating smog gas and a major contributor to the Greenhouse effect PHYSIOLOGY Nitric oxide (NO) has been recently identified as a neurotransmitter; it is released when glutamate binds to the NMDA receptor, allowing the entry of calcium ions, which combine with calmodulin, activating nitric oxide synthase (NOS), releasing NO into the synaptic space; once in the post-synaptic neuron, NO activates guanylyl cyclase, which generates cGMP, which in turn initiates a phosphorylation cascade; NO (formerly, endothelium-derived relaxing factor) is a potent locally acting vasodilator requiring L-arginine as a substrate that is generated by NOS in blood vessels, cytotoxic macrophages, adrenal gland and brain and other tissues; NO relaxes smooth muscle both indirectly by stimulating guanylate cyclase with resulting accumulation of cGMP and cGMP-dependent modification of intracellular processes, eg activation of potassium channels via cGMP-dependent protein kinase, as well as directly stimulating Ca^{2+}-dependent K^+ channels (**Nature 1994; 368:850L**) in the stomach, it is released by non-adrenergic, non-cholinergic nerves, resulting in a reflex relaxation of the stomach to accommodate increased volume of food and fluids (**Nature 1991; 351:477**); excess NO may be neurotoxic and play a major pathogenic role in neurodegenerative disorders including Huntington's and Alzheimer's diseases; NO inhalation therapy may be of use in treating ARDS, as it causes a ↓ in mean pulmonary artery pressure, ↓ intrapulmonary shunting, and ↑ in the ratio of partial pressure of arterial O_2 to the fraction of inspired O_2 (PaO_2/FiO_2), an index of arterial oxygenation efficiency (**N Engl J Med 1993; 328:399OA**); NO is a free radical implicated in several forms of neuronal plasticity, and in synaptic suppression (**Nature 1995; 374:262L**)

nitric oxide synthase NADPH diaphorase [EC 1.14.13.39] L-Arginine, NADPH:oxygen oxidoreductase (nitric-oxide-forming); a major enzyme of the human economy; NOS has sequence homology with cytochrome P450 reductase, an enzyme intimately involved in the hepatic metabolism of drugs (**Science 1991; 252:1788n&v**) see Nitric oxide

nitroblue tetrazolium test see NBT

nitrogen balance CLINICAL NUTRITION A crude indicator of the adequacy of nutrition is the protein lost during a 24-hour period, calculated by urinary excretion of nitrogen products produced by the urea cycle; usually 0.5 g/day of dietary protein is adequate to maintain an appropriate nitrogen balance; in a negative nitrogen balance, loss exceeds intake, a situation seen in aging, burns and protein-losing enteropathy

Note: In the induction phase of chemotherapy, a 'physiologic' negative balance occurs due to massive lysis of malignant cells; a positive balance is typical of growth periods, ie in the young, in pregnancy and in convalescence from burns

nitrogen mustard(s) ONCOLOGY A family of alkylating agents used primarily to treat malignant lymphoma, in the MOPP regimen for stage III and IV Hodgkin's disease, in acute lymphocytic leukemia, topically for mycosis fungoides; all mustards have a $-N(CH_2CH_2Cl)_2$ group and enter the cells via the choline transport system; tumor cells may develop mustard resistance through enhanced repair of alkylated DNA or thiol-mediated mustard inactivation TOXICITY GI tract (nausea, vomiting), myelosuppression with pancytopenia, alopecia, local tissue injury, diarrhea, diaphoresis

nitrogen narcosis Rapture of the deep A neurological response to ↑ nitrogen gas dissolved in the blood, resulting in causing euphoria, apathy, loss of judgement; NN occurs in scuba divers and is most common at depths below 20 meters PREVENTION Use of helium-oxygen gas; see Caisson's disease

nitrogen washout curve RESPIRATORY PHYSIOLOGY A measurement of the time required to eliminate N_2 gas from the lungs when breathing another gas (usually O_2), a clinical test of use in identifying the presence of poorly ventilated lung regions

nitroglycerin Glycerol trinitrate An organic nitrate that serves as a short-acting agent for the treatment of anginal pain and congestive heart failure SIDE EFFECTS Headache, tachycardia, nausea and hypotension; other organic nitrates, eg ethylene nitrate and trinitrotoluene (TNT) are used to produce explosives

nitrotetrazolium blue test Nitroblue tetrazolium test, see NBT test

NK cell Natural killer cell, see there

NK-mediated lysis EXPERIMENTAL IMMUNOLOGY The destruction of various pathogens (intracellular bacteria, viruses, protozoa, fungi) by natural killer cells; NK cells lyse cells by direct action and influence subsequent T cell responses by secreting mediators of inflammation (lymphokines); if an NK cell's receptor engages self MHC class I molecules, both the lytic machinery and lymphokine production is turned off; recognition of the self MHC class I molecule (the event that differentiates between self and nonself cells) requires a specific self peptide complexed with class I MHC molecules (**Science 1995; 267:976P, 1016R**)

NK receptor(s) A family of receptors for the tachykinin family of peptides, designated NK1 for substance P, NK2 for neurokinin A and NK3 for neurokinin B; see Substance P, Tachykinins

NMDA N-methyl-D-aspartate A chemical used in neurophysiology to probe a group of membrane proteins, designated 'NMDA receptors'

NMDA receptor(s) N-methyl-D-aspartate receptors A family of membrane-bound ion channels that open when NMDA as well as neurotransmitters, eg acetylcholine, glycine, GABA and glutamate are bound, regulating the strength and stability of excitatory synapses, allowing positively charged ions to flow into the neuron; NMDA-Rs mediate the slow component of excitatory post-synaptic potentials and play a key role in neural, synaptic and behavioral plasticity and may be pivotal in the development of opiate tolerance and dependence (**Science 1991; 251:85**); the NMDA receptors can undergo robust synapse-specific long-term potentiation, which is related to learning and memory (**Nature 1991; 349:157**) NMDA-Rs are involved in pathological cerebral processes, in excitotoxic neuronal death due to cerebral ischemia and epilepsy; NMDA-R activation requires glycine acting at an allosteric site tightly coupled to the receptor; NMDA-R-activated ion flow in the hippocampus is inhibited by ethanol (possibly by membrane 'fluidization'), thus explaining the CNS depression associated with intoxication; the NMDA-R is unusual as both chemical transmitters or a change in electric potential can activate the sodium, potassium and calcium ion channels regulated in cultured hippocampal neurons by serotonin/threonine protein phosphatases 1 and 2A (**Nature 1994; 369:231L**), by tyrosine kinases and phophatases in mammalian central neurons (**ibid; 369:233L**), and by Ca^{2+}-dependent phophatases (**ibid; 369:235L**)

NMN Nicotinamide mononucleotide

NMR Nuclear magnetic resonance see Magnetic resonance imaging

NMR spectroscopy A technique that analyzes molecules by studying magnetic structure; the nucleus of each hydrogen atom (other molecules are involved but have a lesser contribution) acts as a magnet and sets up its own field and influences the fields of other, nearby atoms; by perturbing a field and observing the response, data is generated which, with the proper algorithms, allows structur-

604

al analysis, and is a technique used in research to analyze three dimensional protein conformations; the 'dimensions' of NMR spectroscopy do not refer to physical dimensions, but rather how the data is collected and displayed **ONE-DIMENSIONAL NMR** A straight line of data is obtained, where a powerful magnet is used to align all the nuclear spins in the same direction; the sample is then bombarded with radiofrequency radiation turning the nuclear 'magnets' on their sides, rotating them around the axis of the applied magnetic field, causing the rotating (or 'precessing') nuclei to generate their own magnetic fields which are detected by the magnetic coil and analyzed; each molecule 'precesses' at a different 'resonance frequency', due to their bonding to other molecules; 1-D NMR provides enough information to solve the structure of simple molecules; with complex molecules, the NMR spectrum is too 'busy' to solve the structure **TWO-DIMENSIONAL NMR** Analysis of a series of 1-D NMR experiments, typically 1000 'runs', allowing examination of proton interactions; if the amino acid sequence is known, the information obtained in the 2-D NMR can be used to determine how a protein twists upon itself; 2-D NMR has a 'resolution' limit of proteins with 100 or fewer amino acids **THREE-DIMENSIONAL NMR** adds a step in which the spins of the precessing hydrogen ions interact with the spins of the precessing carbon ions, in a series of abbreviated 2-D NMR 'runs'; 3-D NMR has a 'resolution' limit of 150 amino acids **FOUR-DIMENSIONAL NMR** is expected to resolve proteins up to 300 residues in length Note: NMR analysis of protein conformation (ie three-dimensional structure) is preferred to X-ray crystallographic analysis, which requires a pure crystal of a protein that may require months to obtain; the advantage is that it allows the study of proteins in solutions and in non-crystalline states, which more closely simulate physiologic environments METHOD A sample is 'zapped' with a beam of electromagnetic energy, exciting nuclei of certain atoms, especially hydrogen to a higher energy state; when the beam is turned off, the excited molecules return to a ground state; as each of the molecules returns, it has a characteristic relaxation 'signature'; an increase in the relaxation time (normal 0.154 msec) of fat's methylene (NH_2) component may be seen in metastases, but is not statistically significant; NMR spectroscopy and scanning tunnel microscopy offer new insights into the dynamics of protein molecules and protein-folding

NMS Neuroleptic malignant syndrome, see there

NNAL 4-(methylnitrosamino)-1-(3-pyridyl)-1-butanol, see NNK

NNK 4-(methylnitrosamino)-1-(3-pyridyl)-1-butanone A potent pulmonary carcinogen, that induces predominantly adenocarcinoma in rodents regardless of the route of administration; it is extensively metabolized in primates, and while NNK is barely detectable in the urine of passive smokers, up to 25% is excreted as glucuronide conjugates of its carbonyl reduction product, 4-(methylnitrosamino)-1-(3-pyridyl)-1-butanol (NNAL); nonsmokers exposed to sidestream cigarette smoke absorb and metabolize sufficient amounts of NNK to support the the proposal that environmental tobacco smoke can cause lung cancer (**N Engl J Med 1993; 329:1543oa**) see Sidestream cigarette smoke

NNP Net national product, see there

'no code' orders see Do not resuscitate (DNR)

no-impact sport SPORTS MEDICINE A generic term for any physical activity or sport in which there is virtually no wear or trauma to weight-bearing joints; NISs include bicycling, sailing, scuba diving, and swimming (laps); NISs is encouraged after hip and knee arthroplasty for those who wish to participate in physical activities (**Mayo Clin Proc 1995; 70:342oa**) Cf High-impact sport, Low-impact sport,

Moderate-impact sport

Nobelist Nobel laureate A person who has won a Nobel Prize

Nobel prizes Physiology or Medicine (P&M), Chemistry (Chem, if applicable), Physics (Phy, if applicable); in brackets [], the value of the prize in that year **1994** (P&M) AG Gilman and M Rodbell, both American, U Texas, Dallas and Nat Instit Env Health Sciences (ret), for work on G-proteins that convert extracellular signals into intracellular messages [$930 000] **1993** (P&M) P Sharp, American, Massachusetts Institute of Technology, R Roberts, British, New England Biolabs, for independent discovery of split genes, ie that a gene was formed of squences of DNA that are interspersed with intervening segments of nonsense DNA (Chemistry) K Mullis, American, Cetus Corp, for 1985 invention of polymerase chain reaction (PCR), M Smith, British-Canadian, U British Columbia, Vancouver, for development of oligonucleotide-based site-directed mutagenesis [$825 000] **1992** (P&M) EH Fisher, EG Krebs, both American, U Washington, Seattle, for identifying the importance of kinase-induced phosphorylation, which catalyzes the conversion of carbohydrates to energy in muscle [$1.2 million] **1991** (P&M) E Neher and B Sakmann, both German, both Max-Planck Institute; Development of the patch-clamp technique and discovery of ion channels in cell membranes **1990** (P&M) JE Murray and ED Thomas, both American, at Harvard and Fred Hutchinson (Seattle), respectively; Pioneer work in renal and bone marrow transplantation, respectively (Chem) EJ Corey, American, Harvard, Devising methods to synthesize complex molecules found in nature [$710 000] **1989** (P&M) JM Bishop and HE Varmus, both American, both at U California, San Francisco; Cellular and viral oncogenes [$475 000] (Chem) S Altman, Canadian-American, Yale, Connecticut; TR Cech, American U Colorado, Denver; RNA autosplicing [$475 000] **1988** (P&M) GB Elion and GH Hitchings, both Americans, both at Burroughs-Wellcome, North Carolina and Sir J Black, British, U London; Development of drugs essential for treating heart disease, peptic ulcers, gout and leukemia [$390 000] **1987** (P&M) S Tonegawa, Japanese, Massachusetts Institute of Technology; Generation of antibody diversity [$340 000] **1986** (P&M) R Levi-Montalcini, Italian-American and S Cohen, American; Nerve growth factor and Epidermal growth factor respectively (Phy) E Ruska, G Binnig, Germans and H Rohrer, Swiss; Electron microscopy [$290 000] **1985** (P&M) MS Brown, JL Goldstein, both American, both U Texas; Lipoprotein lipase and cholesterol metabolism (Chem) HA Hauptman, J Karle, both Americans; X-ray crystallography for analysis of biological molecules [$225 000] **1984** (P&M) C Milstein, Argentinian at Cambridge, GJF Köhler, Swiss at Basel; Monoclonal antibodies; NF Jerne, Dane at Basel; Theoretical groundwork in immunology (Chem) RB Merrifield, American, Rockefeller Institute; Protein analysis and drug development [$190 000] **1983** (P&M) B McClintock, American, Cold Spring Harbor; 'Jumping genes' [$190 000] **1982** (P&M) S Bergstrom, B Samuelsson, Sweden and JR Vane British; Prostaglandin synthesis (Chem) A Klug, South African, Cambridge; Structural analysis of viruses and subcellular particles [$157 000] **1981** (P&M) RW Sperry, DH Hobel, TN Wiesel, Americans; Brain research [$180 000]

'nocebo' A negative placebo effect that may occur when patients in a clinical trial recognize (or think they recognize) that they are getting a placebo (ie, not receiving therapy), and fare worse due to the effect of negative suggestibility (**Lancet 1991; 338:899**); Cf Placebo

nociceptor Pain receptor Any of a class of sense organs and neural receptors, including reflex loops for reception and response to pain, which are periarticular and mucocutaneous

nocturnal emission Wet dream Semen seeping while sleeping

nocturnal polysomnography A high-cost, labor-intensive procedure that is the current gold standard method for detecting the obstructive sleep apnea syndrome; in NP, the subject is 'wired' to an EEG and evaluated in a controlled environment for one or more nights; it has been suggested that the less expensive and less onerous method of pulse oximetry might provide the same information as NP (Mayo Clin Proc 1995; 70:591) see Obstructive sleep apnea syndrome, Pulse oximetry, Sleep apnea syndrome

NOD mouse Non-obese diabetic mouse A mouse strain with an inherited predisposition toward autoimmune diseases that resembles human insulin-dependent diabetes mellitus (IDDM); both IDDM and NOD mice have similar genetic defects in HLA-DQ (human class II MHC) and I-A (the murine class II homologue); NOD mice lack a large segment of DNA in their MHC I-E region; in transgenic NOD mice, insertion of either I-E or correction of the I-A defect reduces insulinitis and prevents disease progression (Nature 1990; 345:722, 724, 727, 662n&v)

nodal cell P cell, pacemaker cell A specialized ovoid-to-stellate, 5-10 μm in diameter myocyte (*myocytus nodalis* [NH3]) found in clusters in the sinus node of the heart, which has few mitochondria, little sarcoplasmic reticulum and myofibrils, and is thus assumed to be an electrical rather than a contractile cell; Cf T cells

nodes CARDIOLOGY The intrinsic pacemakers of the heart, the nodes are composed of neural tissue; the sinoatrial node (normal rhythm, 70/min) is located at the junction of the superior vena cava with the right atrium and conducts impulses by way of three Purkinje fiber tracts (the anterior internodal tract of Bachman, the middle internodal tract of Wenckebach and the posterior internodal tract of Thorel) to the AV node (normal rhythm, 45/min) located in the right posterior portion of the interatrial septum, which in turn is continuous with the bundle of His (normal rhythm, 35/min)

nodovenous shunt A surgical decompression procedure used to reduce and eliminate the future development of lymphedema caused by lymphatic blockage, classically due to microfilariasis, in those patients who have 'failed' diethylcarbamazine therapy

nodular adenosis A benign, well-circumscribed lesion of the breast that has features of both sclerosing adenosis and blunt duct adenosis

nodular fasciitis A benign rapidly growing proliferation of fibroblasts that involves the upper extremities, trunk, or neck of young adults PATHOLOGY Whorls of fibroblasts often in a loose myxoid stroma

Synonyms include pseudosarcomatous fasciitis, pseudosarcomatous fibromatosis, subcutaneous pseudosarcomatous fibromatosis

no-fault An adjective used in the context of liability for an accident (usually motor-vehicular, as in no-fault insurance) or adverse outcome (as is being proposed by some authors for tort reform in malpractice law); under no-fault rules, no individual or organization is assigned responsibility, regardless of the cause of the adverse outcome, and the victim may be nonetheless be reimbursed (JAMA 1992; 267:2355sc)

noise Random variation in signals of the electromagnetic spectrum that carries no useful information from the source; Poisson noise is statistical fluctuation in the number of information carriers (photons, electrons), which appears as 'snow' in a cathode ray tube, a function of the statistical variation of the rays received by the detector and number of electrons produced by the photomultiplier; see White noise; Cf Chaos

noise-induced hearing loss Reduction in auditory perception induced by loud sounds, inculpated in one-third of the 28 million hearing-impaired adults in the US, occurring with prolonged exposure to sound levels above 85 decibels, although there is a wide range (30-50 dB) of individual susceptibility to sound

noise pollution The presence of noise and sounds in the workplace and environment that is annoying or excessive to the point of causing loss of productivity PREVENTION Active noise control

noma Gangrenous stomatitis, cancrum oris An acute necrotizing, polymicrobial and ulcerating infection of the orofacial tissues seen in malnourished children, which rapidly erodes to deep tissue, exposing bone and teeth MICROBIOLOGY Anaerobic fusospirochetes, eg *Borrelia vincenti* and *Fusobacterium nucleatum*, less commonly, *Bacteroides melaninogenicus* and filiform gram-negative bacteria TREATMENT High doses of IV penicillin; correction of dehydration and malnutrition

'No-Man's land' HAND SURGERY A fanciful synonym for the fibrous sheath of the flexor tendons of the hand, specifically in the zone from the distal palmar crease to the proximal interphalangeal joint; any tendon injury to the distal forearm, wrist of hand could be a 'no-man's land' if 1) The facilities and/or equipment is inadequate 2) The operator is inexperienced or exhausted or 3) The tendon is potentially damaged beyond salvage; see Rule of threes

Note: A 'no-man's land' is a belt of ground between the most advanced elements of opposing armies or an area controlled by neither side of conflict

Nomarski interference microscopy A type of light microscopy, in which the light from a reference beam is used to interfere with the light reflected from a surface, thereby producing a relief image of the reflecting surface that is not affected by variations in the refractive index of the surface; see Microscopy

Nomina Anatomica The vast majority of anatomic terminology is derived from classic roots, with some disagreement on minutiae, more often related to loyalties to tradition, mentors or jingoism than to logic; the first system was established in 1895 by the German Anatomical Society, which held its first meeting in Basel, since known as the Basel Nomina Anatomica (BNA), which gave the names in Latin; the nations adopting the system then translated the terms into their own respective languages; the French were the first to break away from the BNA pack, as they felt that terms based on ancient Gallic tradition served them better; the British left the BNA fold in 1933, as they felt the arbitrary anatomic positions were too rigid and did not reflect human anatomy, and therefore generated the 'Birmingham revision'; the Germans (who started it all) were the next to break away, and in 1936 delivered to the not-so-eagerly-awaiting world, the Jena Nomina Anatomica; oddly, the Americans* remained true to the original BNA; in 1955, the Fifth International Congress of Anatomists approved the Paris Nomina Anatomica, which comprises the 'state of the art' anatomic nomenclature, the details of the 12th Congress of Anatomists held in 1985, 'der letzte Schrei' in the scintillating world of anatomy is summarized in: Nomina Anatomica:Nomina Histologica:Nomina Embryologica (Churchill-Livingstone, New York, 1989)

*Who (one recalls) won the West, popularized the hoola-hoop and chewing gum, and created an internationally envied image of individualism

nominal group technique PSYCHOLOGY A survey technique that elicits the ideas of each individual in a group, allowing the members in the group (regardless of background and socioeconomic status) to build on each others ideas, then as collective cerebroplasm, identify the most important concepts (JAMA 1995; 273:1914)

nomogram An alignment chart in which there are three or more abscissas (see figure, pg 606), each measuring a specific parameter and mathematically or empirically defined as having a relation to each other; the abscissas are placed parallel to each other on an open two-dimensional field; a straight line drawn when two of the parameters are known, allows determination of the value of the third (unknown) parameter

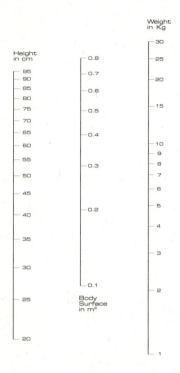

nomogram

non-A, non-B hepatitis The major cause of transfusion-related hepatitis; incidence, $7/10^5$/year, USA NANBH risk factors: 42% intravenous drug abuse, 40% no known risk factors, 6% sexual contact, 6% blood transfusion, 3% household contact, 2% health care professional; of the estimated 150 000 annual cases in the US, 30-50% become chronic carriers and 20% of these develop cirrhosis; NANBH may also rarely be epidemically transmitted; NANBH comprises a group of not fully characterized hepatitides; in general, parenteral NANBH is most commonly hepatitis C and enteric NANBH is hepatitis E; testing blood for antibodies to HCV is part of the battery of tests used in screening of blood to reduce NANBH, since about one-half of transfusion-related NANBH is associated with antibodies to hepatitis C virus, many of the remainder are in 'window' period for hepatitis C; this screen reduces the false positivity due to nonspecific ALT elevation; during the 1970s (US), 7-17% of transfusions resulted in hepatitis; 78-92% due to non-A, non-B hepatitis TREATMENT 3 million units of IFN-α2b 3x/week x 18 months results in more significant histologic reversal and serum ALA response than that seen with lower doses and/or shorter durations of therapy (**N Engl J Med 1995; 332:1457**0A) PROGNOSIS No ↑ in overall mortality with chronic NANBH, but ↑ liver-related deaths (**N Engl J Med 1992; 327:1906**0A) see Hepatitis

nonabsorbable suture see Silk, Synthetic nonabsorbable suture

non-bacterial endocarditis Marantic endocarditis Endocarditis with 1-5 mm sterile vegetations on both faces of the valve leaflets composed of fibrin and clots with possible rupture of the papillary muscles, a condition clinically indistinguishable from infectious endocarditis characterized by petechiae, fever, murmurs and emboli ETIOLOGY

Debilitating diseases, eg terminal malignancy, protracted malnutrition, collagen vascular disease, chronic sepsis, renal failure

noncaseating granuloma Nonnecrotizing granuloma

non-clathrin coated vesicles Golgi-derived coated vesicles, see there

noncompliant patient A patient who does not conform to the prescribed program of medical therapy, as may occur in patients who are being treated with chronic dialysis (**JAMA 1991; 265:1579**) see Patient compliance, Negligence (contributory); Cf 'Good' patient

non-coital sex PUBLIC HEALTH A generic term for any form of safe sexual activity that does not include vaginal penetration, eg masturbation (**Sci Am 1995; 272/2:10**) see Safe sex practices

non compos mentis Not of sound mind, nuts

noncontrollable life-style specialty A field of medical specialization that cannot be scheduled in terms of work hours, NLSs include general surgery, obstetrics, and primary care including family practice, general internal medicine, and pediatrics (**JAMA 1992; 268:2060**SC) Cf Controllable life-style specialty

noncoverage A generic adjective pertaining or referring to the lack of insurance benefits, usually used in the context of limited access to 'covered' medical care

nondiscrimination A philosophical stance formally adopted or inferred for both who has the right to the practice medicine (ie the practitioner), and who has the right to receive medical care (ie the patient), where such rights cannot be denied based on sex, race, creed, color, or national origin; Cf Affirmative action, Reverse discrimination

nondisjunction GENETICS The failure of homologous chromosomes or sister chromatids to separate during mitotic anaphase, an event resulting in one daughter cell receiving both copies of the entire chromosome, eg in Down syndrome, one daughter cell is trisomic for chromosome 21, ie has 47 (2n + 1) chromosomes, while the other daughter cell is monosomic, ie has 45 (2n - 1) chromosomes

nonessential amino acids Any amino acid that can be synthesized by an organism from available substrates; Cf Essential amino acids

nongonococcal urethritis A condition causing dysuria, pyuria and symptoms similar to, but less intense than gonorrhea, most commonly caused by *Chlamydia trachomatis*; NGU is more common in heterosexuals (14% had chlamydial isolates, homosexuals 5%) than gonococcal urethritis (12% versus 25% in homosexuals); other causes of NGU include *Ureaplasma urealytica* and *Mycoplasma genitalium* although NGU, defined as the presence of abundant neutrophils in the urine, often reveals no organisms

non-Hodgkin's lymphoma Any lymphoma that is not Hodgkin's disease EPIDEMIOLOGY Incidence ↑ $8.5/10^5$, 1973; $15/10^5$, 1990, ± 35 000 new cases/year (US) TREATMENT Chemotherapy, especially CHOP (**N Engl J Med 1993; 328:1023**0A) see REAL classification, Working Formulation

non-insulin-dependent diabetes mellitus NIDDM Type II diabetes mellitus A condition comprising 90% of DM; 80% of NIDDM patients are also obese (an association known as 'diabesity'), insulin-deficient and insulin-resistant; NIDDM is diagnosed when 1) Fasting glucose is 7.8 mmol/L (US > 140 mg/dl) on two or more occasions or 2) When in a 75 g glucose tolerance test, the 2-hour and one of the other values (drawn at the 30, 60 or 90 minute intervals) are greater than 11.2 mmol/L (US > 200 mg/dl) PATHOGENESIS A key feature of NIDDM is hepatic and muscular resistance to insulin; in muscle under normal conditions, glucose is either oxidized to CO_2 and H_2O (oxidative pathway) or stored as glycogen (nonoxidative pathway); impaired activation of glycogen synthase occurs in NIDDM and in insulin-resistant first-degree relatives MOLECULAR GENETICS There is strong evidence that NIDDM is a genetic disease with ± 90% concordance in identical twins; lifetime risk for the child of a diabetic parent is 40%; a recent report has identified* an *Xba*I polymorphism of the glycogen synthase gene, the A_2 allele, linked to a subgroup of NIDDM patients with a strong family history of NIDDM, a high prevalence of hypertension, and marked insulin resistance (N Engl J Med 1993; 328:10oA) YD-DM with an onset usually older than 40, decreased incidence of ketoacidosis, may develope microvascular complications TREATMENT NIDDM does not usually require exogenous insulin, although it may be required during 'crises'; see Glucose tolerance curve, MODY; Cf IDDM

*Method: DNA from each of 107 patients with NIDDM, and DNA from each of 164 unrelated nondiabetic subjects with no family history of NIDDM was digested using the restriction enzyme *Xba*I; the digested fragments were then separated by agarose-gel electrophoresis, transferred to nitrocellulose filters (Southern blot), then hybridized to a complementary DNA (cDNA) probe of the human glycogen synthase gene

noninnovative drug 'Me too' drug, see there

non-invasive Non-interventional An adjective referring or pertaining to any form of therapy in which the integrity of mucocutaneous barriers is not violated; Cf Invasive

nonionizing radiation Electromagnetic radiation that does not induce the formation of ions, eg visible light, infrared light, ultraviolet light, microwaves, and radio waves; Cf Ionizing radiation

non-ionizing radiation Electromagnetic radiation, the photons of which have insufficient energy to ionize atoms, including sound, ultraviolet, visible and infrared light, and radiowaves

nonlinear analysis see Chaos

nonnucleoside reverse transcriptase inhibitor AIDS A family of compounds that bind to a hydrophobic pocket in HIV's reverse transcriptase-DNA (RT-DNA) complex close to the polymerization active site; NRTIs eg tetrahydrobenzodiazepine (TIBO) derivatives and the dipyridodiazepinone Nevirapine (figure) inhibit RT at low concentrations and with high specificity, making them candidates for treating AIDS; NRTIs block the chemical reaction involved in DNA polymerization, but do not interfere with nucleotide binding or with nucleotide-induced conformational changes (Science 1995; 267:988A) as with nucleoside analogues, eg zidovudine (AZT) and 2',3'-dideoxycytidine (ddC), forms of RT that are resistant to NRTI have been identified

non-official autopsy Hospital autopsy, see there

non-operative cranioplasty Head shaping, see there

nonoxynol 9 AIDS A spermicide had been in early clinical trials as an anti-HIV agent capable of preventing its transmission (it kills HIV on contact) that was abandoned when it was reported that its use caused irritation and ulceration, and thus could increase HIV transmission; further studies are pending (JAMA 1995 273:979)

nonparametric test STATISTICS A value, eg a median or percentile, or a statistical test, eg a rank-sum test that does not assume a specified mathematical form for the underlying distribution; results from nonparametric analysis have less statistical power but eliminate the need for specifying the mathematical form for the underlying distribution of data

non-'participation' The non-acceptance of a physician of the fees paid by Medicaid, or less commonly in Medicare; nonparticipation is a key factor in lack of access of low-income Americans to adequate health care and is attributable to the low rate of reimbursement by Medicaid for the actual costs of the services rendered, delays in reimburse-

ment and increasing costs of malpractice insurance; see Participation

nonphotochromogen MICROBIOLOGY One of a group of atypical mycobacteria that produce a scant amount of pale yellow pigment; unlike the so-called 'photochromogens', exposure of nonphotochromogens to light does not intensify the color, a feature seen in *Mycobacteria avium-intracellulare*, *M gastri*, *M haemophilum*, *M malmoense*, *M nonchromogenicum*, *M terrae* and *M triviale*; see MAIS, MOTT, Runyon group, Tuberculosis

nonprogressive HIV-1 infection A generic term for any long-term survivor of HIV infection; an estimated 5% of those infected with HIV may survive for prolonged periods of time (eg 10-15+ years) without developing AIDS, a feat that results from a feisty immune response to HIV, preservation of the lymphoid tissue, and attenuation of the virus (N Engl J Med 1995; 332:201oA, 209oA; 1646c); in one study of subjects with NHI, the auxiliary gene *nef*, which is required in simian immunodeficiency virus for the development of AIDS in the rhesus monkey, is defective or absent (N Engl J Med 1995; 332:228oA)

non–Q-wave infarction CARDIOLOGY A subendocardial MI in which the EKG pattern consists of a persistent abnormal ST-segment depression in all but the aVR lead (which shows ST-segment elevation), often accompanied by T-wave changes; most cardiologists diagnose a non-Q-wave MI when the clinical, enzymatic and radionuclear findings are consistent with MI, with or without the above EKG changes; despite their better initial prognosis, non–Q-wave MIs are unstable, have ↑ incidence of extension of the original infarction, re-infarction, and a greater subsequent morbidity (JAMA 1992; 268:1545oc) see Thallium imaging

non-reducing sugar A sugar that does not contain an aldehyde or potential aldehyde and will not reduce inorganic ions in solution

non-repetitive DNA Unique DNA DNA that is known to exist only once in a haploid genome; most structural DNA and introns are thought to be unique DNA sequences; see Single copy DNA Cf Repetitive DNA, Tandem repeats

nonresting energy expenditure PHYSIOLOGY A metabolic value that corresponds to the energy cost of physical activity, which represents approximately 30% of the total energy expenditure, see there (N Engl J Med 1995; 332:621oA)

nonsecretor see Secretor

nonsense codon Stop codon A triplet of nucleotides (UAA, UAG or UGA) of mRNA that cause ribosomes to stop transcription

nonsense mutation MOLECULAR PATHOLOGY A point mutation in the DNA of a 'structural' gene that results in any of three nucleotide triplets (or codons, to wit, ATT, ATC or ACT) that are transcribed as stop codons (UAA, UAG or UGA) of mRNA, which when detected by the translation machinery, terminate protein synthesis*, effectively eliminating the gene's product and its function; another effect of such mutations is a situation where a stop codon is normally present and a nonsense mutation results in an elongated protein product, as the appropriate stop codon no longer exists

*These being known as 'truncated' protein products

nonsense suppressor gene A gene that encodes a tRNA molecule that 'reads through' a nonsense (stop) mutation, resulting in the translation of an amino acid instead of protein chain termination

nonsense syndrome Ganser syndrome PSYCHIATRY A condition in which a person gives 'astonishingly' incorrect answers to simple questions; although this illness is considered to be factitious in nature, the 'nonsense symptom' may occur in hysteria, schizophrenia, or transiently in normal subjects under stress or when fatigued; Cf Factitious 'diseases'

nonsignificant risk device A medical device that does not have the potential for causing significant risk to the health, safety, or welfare of a subject; nonsignificant devices may be divided into those that require FDA clearance* prior to marketing the product, and those that do not eg tongue depressors, cotton swabs (**JAMA 1994; 272:955sc**) see Medical device, Substantial equivalence; Cf Significant medical device

*The FDA determines whether the product is substantially equivalent to a previously marketed predessor, eg surgical staples, eyepatches

non-small cell carcinoma of lung A generic term for any non-undifferentiated carcinoma of the lung MANAGEMENT Use of preoperative chemotherapy (cisplatin, ifosfamide, mitomycin–combined with radiotherapy) increases median survival in advanced stage NSCC (26 vs 8 months) (**N Engl J Med 1994; 330:153oA**)

non-smoking tobacco see Smokeless tobacco

non-specific esterase α-naphthyl butyrate esterase An enzyme on the external face of the plasma membrane of alveolar macrophages and circulating monocytes; NSE is a common monocyte 'marker', the activity of which is inhibited by sodium fluoride, which does not occur in granulocytic esterase and inhibits gastric secretion and intestinal motility

nonsteroidal antiinflammatory drug Any of a family of weak organic acids that 1) Inhibit prostaglandin biosynthesis, by inhibiting cyclooxygenase, and to a lesser degree lipooxygenase and 2) Interfere with membrane-bound reactions, eg NADPH oxidase in neutrophils, phospholipase C in monocytes and G protein-regulated processes; at high therapeutic doses, NSAIDs interfere with proteoglycan synthesis by chondrocytes, transmembrane ion flux, cell-cell interaction, and unmask T-cell suppressor activity (**N Engl J Med 1991; 324:1716rv**); other postulated activities include ↓ production of free radicals and superoxides, which may interact with adenylate cyclase, altering intracellular cAMP levels, reducing vasoactive and nociceptive mediator release from granulocytes, basophils, and mast cells THERAPEUTIC USES Rheumatoid arthritis, gouty arthritis, ankylosing spondylitis, osteoarthritis, serosal inflammation, Bartter syndrome, and other inflammatory conditions CHEMICAL CLASSES Carboxylic acid: Acetylated, eg aspirin (figure) or nonacetylated, eg sodium salicylate Acetic acid analogs, eg indomethacin, tolmetin, sulindac Propionic acid analogs, eg ibuprofen (figure), naproxen Fenamic acid analogs, eg mefanamic acid Enolic acid analogs, eg oxyphenbutazone, phenylbutazone and nonacidic compounds, eg proquazone SIDE EFFECTS Rash, pruritus, edema, vertigo, drowsiness, tinnitus, aseptic meningitis, nausea, vomiting, gastric ulcers and potentially fatal GI hemorrhage, jaundice, Stevens-Johnson syndrome, Henoch-Schönlein syndrome, fatal aplastic anemia, acute renal failure; those who use acetaminophen have an ↑ risk (odd ratio of 2.4) of end-stage renal disease if lifetime number of pills ingested is > 5000 versus a baseline of 1000 (**N Engl J Med 1994; 331:1669oA**) see NSAID enteropathy

Note: Although aspirin is an NSAID, most practitioners equate NSAIDs with the newer non-aspirin agents derived from propionic acid, indoles or pyrazolone or designated as fenamates, pyrrole alkanoid acid or oxicams

nonstochastic effect Deterministic effect A generic term for a dose-related health effect that is linear in severity after a certain threshold of exposure or dosage has been passed, eg radiation-induced cataracts

non-stress test OBSTETRICS An indirect non-invasive monitor of the well-being of a fetus, where the frequency of fetal movement, degree of heart rate acceleration and beat-to-beat variation of the heart rate are monitored to determine the 'health' of the placental vasculature; see Deceleration, Montevideo units; Cf Fetal heart monitoring

non-traditional cancer therapy Unproven method of cancer therapy, see there

non-traditional medicine Alternative medicine, see there

nontuberculous mycobacteria A generic term for a *Mycobacterium*, eg *M avium* complex, *M kansasii*, *M marinum*, *M ulcerans*, and others, which may be effectively treated with IFN-γ (**N Engl J Med 1994; 330:1348oA**)

non-ulcer dyspepsia A condition characterized by ulcer symptoms in the absence of gross ulceration; 30-60% of dyspeptics have no demonstrable macroscopic lesions CLINICAL Symptoms range from that of a classic duodenal ulcer (epigastric burning 1-3 hours after meals, relieved by food or alkali) to functional indigestion (bloating, belching, fullness and nausea, not relieved by antacids and worsened by meals); fat intolerance is common ENDOSCOPY The duodenal mucosa demonstrates edema, erythema, petechial hemorrhage and erosions; Cf Dumping syndrome

non-union ORTHOPEDIC SURGERY A diaphyseal fracture that is 1) Unhealed after more than nine months and 2) Has no synovial pseudoarthrosis (a non-union in which a synovioid membrane forms, filled with synovioid fluid) TREATMENT Non-invasive electrical stimulation of bone; see Ilizarov method

$$[CH_3]_2CHCH_2 \!-\!\!\langle\bigcirc\rangle\!-\!\! \overset{\displaystyle CH_3}{\underset{\displaystyle \;}{CH}}COOH$$

NSAID ibuprofen

NOR Nucleolar organizer region, see there

NORAP Nucleolar organizing region-associated protein A large (± 70) family of proteins that includes RNA polymerase I, nucleolin (C_{23} protein), and numatrin (B_{23} protein) (**J Histotech 1992; 15:185**)

NORD National Organization for Rare Disorders A private non-profit organization* that 1) Acts as a 'clearing house' of information for Orphan diseases (see there) and 2) Facilitates communication among governmental agencies and the research community (eg by locating patients for clinical trials); see NICODARD, Orphan disease, Orphan drug/product

*PO Box 8923; New Fairfield, Connecticut 06812; ☎ 1.203.746.6518

normal distribution STATISTICS A generic term for any member of the parametric family of probability distributions that have symmetric, bell-shaped curves of data points, eg Gaussian (probability) distribution, see there

normality CHEMISTRY An obsolete term that expresses the concentration of a solution as gram-equivalents of substance X per liter of solution; Cf Molality and Molarity

normoblast An immature nucleated erythrocyte; in order of maturation, the erythroid series develop into pronormoblast, followed by (→) mitosis, basophilic normoblast I (E2→mitosis), basophilic normoblast II (E3), polychromatophilic normoblast (E4→mitosis), polychromatophilic normoblast (E5), orthochromatic normoblast, reticulocyte, erythrocyte

Norplant® Levonorgestrel A proprietary implantable contraceptive that prevents pregnancy by inhibiting ovulation and causing thickening of cervical mucus; Norplant consists of six cylinders filled with Levonorgestrel (a progestin) allowing five years of protection against unwanted pregnancy, with a 'failure rate' similar to fallopian tubal ligation and vasectomy; it should not be used in women with liver disease of any nature, a history of breast cancer or thrombotic tendencies SIDE EFFECTS Menstrual irregularities, headache, nervousness, nausea, vertigo and increased size of the ovaries and fallopian tubes, dermatitis, acne, weight gain, breast tenderness and hirsutism; of adolescent Norplant users, 95% continued to be compliant with therapy at one year; 1/48 became pregnant; this contrasts with 33% compliance with oral contraceptive use and 19/50 pregnancies (N Engl J Med 1994; 331:1201SA)

Note: Norplant's 'Achilles' heel' revolves around the issue of removal, which may be required by prolonged or irregular bleeding, weight gain, hair loss, pain at the insertion site, or the desire to become pregnant; while most implants are easily removed, with 19% requiring at least one hour for removal (N Engl J Med 1994; 331:1230OA); Norplant removal may be facilitated by the recently devised 'hook and deliver' technique (N Engl J Med 1995; 332:821c)

North American blastomyocosis Infection with *Blastomyces dermatitidis*, blastomycosis

'North American operation' CANCER SURGERY A term attributed to the pelvic surgery service at Memorial Sloan-Kettering Hospital in New York, for radical surgery of a 'frozen pelvis', consisting of radical en bloc resection of the uterus and urinary bladder; see 'Frozen pelvis'; Cf 'All-American' and 'South American' operations

Northern blotting MOLECULAR BIOLOGY A technique used to detect the presence of specific mRNA molecules; the RNA in a sample is denatured, eg with formaldehyde, to prevent hydrogen bonding between base pairs and ensure that the RNA is unfolded and linear; the sample is separated according to size by gel electrophoresis and transferred or 'blotted' on a nylon or nitrocellulose membrane, placed in a solution containing a labeled DNA 'probe' and then autoradiographed, a procedure similar to Southern blotting; see Blotting, Southern blotting

Norwalk agent(s) Any of a group of 27 nm parvoviruses (single-stranded DNA) that cause 'winter vomiting disease', first described in Norwalk, Ohio, which are inculpated in up to 40% of nonbacterial epidemics of gastroenteritis in the US and a frequent cause of traveler's diarrhea CLINICAL After a 1-2 day incubation, it may present explosively (and keep an entire community on the edge of its seat), often accompanied by nausea, vomiting, abdominal cramping, anorexia, malaise and myalgia, transmitted in an oral-fecal fashion, eg exposure to recreational swimming water or by ingestion of raw shellfish, cake-frosting, stored water on cruise ships, and others; the Norwalk agent is difficult to identify as it doesn't grow in cell culture and there are no animal models; cDNA has been constructed and the amino acid sequence motif of the RNA polymerase has been identified PROGNOSIS Spontaneous resolution without sequelae

Norwegian scabies Crusted scabies A severe variant of scabies most common in institutionalized persons, especially those with Down syndrome or either debilitated or immunosuppressed patients are covered by hosts of mites (*Sarcoptes scabei* var homini) causing a psoriasis-like pachydermia, variably accompanied by thickened nails, generalized hyperpigmentation, eosinophilia and pyoderma with lymphadenopathy; see Seven-year itch

Referral to a particular country by this or other names (eg Norwegian itch), is politically incorrect (N Engl J Med 1995; 332:611c) and future editions of this work will be adjusted accordingly-Author's note

nose coverage MALPRACTICE INSURANCE A component of a medical malpractice insurance policy in which a physician's liability is assumed by the previous malpractice insurance carrier, usually until such time as the physician has a new policy; the 'nose coverage' period is usually brief and may be extended as a courtesy by the insurance carrier when a physician moves to another state in the US; Cf Tail coverage

'nose job' Rhinoplasty, see there

nosocomial AIDS Acquired immunodeficiency syndrome

that may occur in certain disadvantaged nations, where a hypodermic needle may be used and re-used; in the Soviet Union, two outbreaks of HIV-1 seroconversion have been reported (N Engl J Med 1990; 323:1844c), infecting 58 and 23 children respectively; see AIDS-malaria connection

nosocomial infection An infection that begins three or more days after admission to a hospital; the microorganisms that cause nosocomial infection are a function of 1) The underlying disease process, eg burns are associated with *Pseudomonas aeruginosa*, leukemia with enterobacteriaceae due to indwelling vascular accesses, DM with anaerobes, gram-negative bacilli and *S aureus*, and post-operative wounds with *S aureus*) and 2) The organ system involved, often facilitated by an indwelling catheter, tracheostomy or other device; NIs affect 2-4 million patients/year (US) at a cost of $\pm$ $4.5 x 10^9 (MMWR 1992; 41:783) SITES Urinary tract 38.5%, lower respiratory tract 18%, surgical wound 17%, blood 7.5%, other 19%; nosocomial infections occurred in 33.5/1000 hospital discharges (Arch Pathol Lab Med 1994; 118:116OA) Handwashing decreases the incidence of NI; use of chlorhexidine with handwashing decreases NI more than alcohol and soap (N Engl J Med 1992; 327:88OA); NI is not reduced in very low-birth-weight infants with prophylactic immune globulins (N Engl J Med 1994; 330:1107OA)

'notch' HEALTH CARE POLICY A precipitous drop in health care benefits for individuals or families despite a marginal increase in incomes, where those with earnings above the 'notch' will not qualify for the benefits

notch signaling DEVELOPMENTAL BIOLOGY An activation pathway that is thought to play a pivotal role in the differentiation of uncommitted cells, which is thought to involve direct signal transmission from the cell surface to the nucleus, and may play a role in tumorigenesis (Science 1995; 268:225) see Inductive signaling, Lateral specification

Note: The *Notch* gene encodes Notch of *Drosophila melanogaster* and has numerous homologs in other animals, eg *lin-12*, and *glp-1* of *Caenorhabditis elegans* as well as vertebrates, which have virtually identical pathways

notching RADIOLOGY Small grooves on the anterior aspect of ribs seen on a plain chest film of children with post-ductal (ductus arteriosus) coarctation of the aorta, due to the 'tracks' from the pressure of collateral vessels on the ribs, which may be seen on a plain chest film

notched nuclei see Buttock cell

notch sign of Rigler RADIOLOGY A short, straight radiolucency best appreciated by tomography that penetrates a relatively well-circumscribed lung mass, first described as typical of malignancy, where the notch corresponds to the shadow of a feeder vessel penetrating the mass; since the notch sign is also seen in other conditions, eg granulomatous infections, the sign is of questionable usefulness

notebook RESEARCH A book, that is generally bound with sewn pages in which a person performing bench research documents or otherwise records (preferably dated and in ink), the nature of each experiment and all of the data collected from each 'run' of an assay, column chromatogram, gel electrophoretogram or other objective test, either copied from instrument, or the actual tape or hard copy read-out from the instrument; see Raw data; Cf Log(book)

Note: Laboratory notebooks have been scrutinized in at least two cases of alleged fraud in science (see Baltimore affair) and thus may prove to be a research scientist's single most important 'accountability document'

notebook computer A small 'laptop'-type microcomputer that weighs 2-4 kg (4.5-9 lbs), has 2 + megabytes (up to 40 Mb) of random access memory (RAM), uses a CISC-based microprocessor produced by either Intel (80386 or 80486) or Motorola (68030 or 68040), and a hard drive of a least 40 megabytes (up to 500 Mb) of storage capacity; see Microcomputer

notifiable diseases PUBLIC HEALTH A group of communicable diseases that a local, state or federal government wishes to maintain under surveillance in order to control and prevent the spread of infections; the US system of reporting notifiable diseases evolved from the Quarantine Act of 1878, which authorized the US Public Health Service to collect morbidity data on cholera, smallpox and yellow fever; each state in the US has its own list of notifiable infectious diseases and depends largely on reporting by the individual physician, where the completeness of reporting ranges from 6-90%; Infectious diseases that are 'notifiable' in most of the United States include amebiasis, anthrax, botulism, brucellosis, campylobacteriosis, chancroid, chickenpox/H zoster, cholera, diphtheria, encephalitis (unspecified), giardiasis, gonococcosis, invasive *Haemophilus influenzae*, hepatitis (all forms), HIV-1 and HIV-2 infections, legionellosis, leprosy, leptospirosis, lymphogranuloma venereum, malaria, measles, meningitis (aseptic, ie presumed viral, and bacterial), meningococcal disease, mumps, pertussis, plague, poliomyelitis, psittacosis, rabies, Reye syndrome, Rocky Mountain spotted fever, rubella, salmonellosis, shigellosis, syphilis, tetanus, toxic shock syndrome, trichinosis, TB, tularemia, typhoid fever, typhus and yellow fever; see Reportable occupational diseases

notochord *notochorda* [NE3] The rod-shaped body of cells derived from the mesoblast that is located below the primitive groove, which correspnds to the vertebral column of the embryo; it is composed of cartilage and eventually replaced by bone; vestigeal rests of the notochord persist in the adult as nucleii pulposi, which may rarely give rise to chordomas

Novacor A proprietary implantable cardiac ventricular assist device in the protocol stage, which may serve as a mechanical bridge while a patient in terminal cardiac failure is waiting for a heart transplant

novelty diet see Diet, Fad diet

novobiocin MOLECULAR BIOLOGY A toxic antibiotic with a narrow therapeutic range that is not used in clinical medicine but is of use in research; novobiocin interferes with ATP-dependent gyrase (a type II topoisomerase introduces negative supercoils into a relaxed closed circular molecule) by preventing ATP from binding to gyrase's B subunit

noxious thing FORENSICE MEDICINE A generic term for any '...*substance unlawfully administered to another or taken by oneself with a deliberate intent to cause ill effects or death.* (which) *may be a poison or any substance capable of producing injury. The amount administered, the form of administration, and an individual's response must be considered before a substance can be designated a noxious thing.*' (International Dictionary of Medicine, J Wiley & Sons, New York, 1986)

N-proCT N-procalcitonin A protein secreted by the parafollicular (thyroid C) cells, which is highly conserved among diverse species (from salmon to humans) and stimulates osteoblasts and inhibits osteoclasts; N-proCT may have a role in osteoporosis and is related to the calcitonin gene-related peptide; see C cells, CGRP

NPP Net primary product, see there

NPT Nuclear Non-Proliferation Treaty An international accord signed by 120 nations, pledging not to pursue development of nuclear weapons; see IPPNW, London Club, Nuclear war

NRC Nuclear Regulatory Commission NUCLEAR MEDICINE A US government agency that licenses users of radioactive materials, sets limits of worker exposure and regulates the production, use and disposal of radioactive materials; 'NRC units' are used to quantify exposure to radiation, where the maximum allowable exposure is 100 µCi (3700 kilobecquerels) per 3 months or by bioassay

NSABP National Surgical Adjuvant Breast and Bowel Project A series of ongoing multicenter clinical trials that are evaluating the effects of certain chemotherapeutic agents, eg tamoxifen and 5-FU in treating advanced carcinoma of the breast and large intestine

NSAID enteropathy A term that dignifies the intestinal changes induced by nonsteroidal anti-inflammatory drugs, including intestinal inflammation, occult blood loss, protein-losing enteropathy, as well as iron-deficiency that may be due in part to nonspecific small intestinal ulceration (in particular of the jejunum and ileum), with hemorrhage and perforation, intestinal strictures, and ileal stenoses (N Engl J Med 1992; 327:749OA)

NSE 1) Neuron-specific enolase, see there 2) Non-specific esterase α-naphthyl butyrate esterase, see there

NSILA Non-suppressible insulin-like activity An action displayed by acid-dissociable 7.5 kD serum complex with activity of insulin-like growth factor (IGF-I and IGF-II), somatomedins A and C; most NSILA is associated with a high molecular-weight protein (NSILP), which has significant homology with IgG's Fc fragment

NST Non-stress test, see there

5'-NT 5'-Nucleotidase, see there

NT-3 Neurotrophin-3, see there, Nerve growth factor family

'nth' admission A colloquial term for any one of multiple hospital admissions, which is great in number, ie more than the fist, second, or third admission, and therefore can be measured as an 'nth', of the ordinal number, eg fourth, fifth, sixth, seventh, eighth, ninth, tenth, eleventh, etc (JAMA 1992: 268:1872OC)

nuclear blebbing An ultrastructural finding of unknown significance that is typical of malignant lymphocytes as seen in lymphomas, which consists of the loss of coherence of the nuclear membrane with the nucleoplasm; nuclear blebbing has virtually no diagnostic utility, as prognostication and diagnosis of lymphoproliferative diseases are based on light microscopy, immunoperoxidase, flow cytometry and various methods of molecular biology; see Nipple appearance

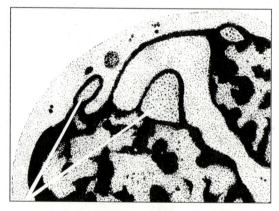

nuclear blebbing

nuclear cardiology The use of nuclear imaging techniques in the noninvasive study of cardiovascular disease, including myocardial perfusion imaging, by either planar imaging, or by SPECT (single-photon-emission computed tomography) (N Engl J Med 1993; 329:775RV)

nuclear contour index IMAGE ANALYSIS A value obtained by measuring the complexity of the nuclear rim with a graphic digitalizer on an electron micrograph, which allows evaluation of the cerebriform cells of mycosis fungoides; see Nuclear blebbing; Cf Nuclear roundness factor

*A value which has no diagnostic, prognostic, or therapeutic utility-Author's note

nuclear crash The economic collapse that would follow a nuclear war; if 1% of the global nuclear arsenal targeted the US liquid fuel production and importation, 8% of the US population would die immediately; 60% would die of starvation in the next two years; it has been projected that post-attack economies would be operating at 40% of pre-attack capacity for up to 25 years after a nuclear exchange; see Nuclear war

nuclear:cytoplasmic asynchrony see Maturational arrest

nuclear:cytoplasmic ratio N:C ratio A crude parameter used in cytology and surgical pathology, where interphase, ie nondividing, nuclei are proportionately larger than their accompanying cytoplasm; the N:C ratio is usually increased in malignant cells

nuclear dust Leukocytoclasis PATHOLOGY Abundant scattered basophilic granularity seen in acutely inflamed and necrotic tissue, which corresponds to karyolytic nuclear debris, and, if infected, bacteria, as may occur in leukocytoclastic vasculitis or a ruptured abscess RENAL PATHOLOGY Rounded fragments of 1-3 mm in diameter basophilic debris derived from partially degraded hematoxylin bodies, classically described in focal proliferative glomerulonephritis seen in SLE (WHO morphologic classification class III)

nuclear envelope A double-membrane envelope that separates the 'noble material' from the cytoplasm, communicating therewith by 70 nm in diameter nuclear pores; the outer nuclear membrane is contiguous with the endoplasmic reticulum

nuclear family SOCIAL MEDICINE The core family unit, classically consisting of heterosexually oriented male and female partners and their direct (usually unmarried) genetic progeny; disintegration of this unit and its central role in society is widely held to be responsible for significant losses of mental equilibrium (see **Science News 1994; 146:106**) Cf Extended family, Single-parent family

nuclear magnetic resonance Magnetic resonance imaging, see there, NMR

nuclear medicine An area of medicine that uses radioisotopes for the diagnosis and treatment of disease, ie radiation oncology; diagnostic nuclear medicine encompasses in vitro assays of clinical specimens, eg immunoassays for various hormones, eg human chorionic gonadotropin (β-HCG), insulin, and thyroid-stimulating hormone (TSH)

Note: RIAs are being increasingly replaced by ELISAs, which are easier to perform, the reagents are more easily stored and do not have the problems inherent in using and disposing of radioactive waste; nuclear medicine also encompasses in vivo diagnostics in the form of scintillation counters to 'scan' various body regions for the presence of increased uptake of radionuclides, which when focal, implies primary neoplasia or metastases

Nuclear Nonproliferation Treaty GLOBAL VILLAGE The global pact that prohibits other nations from 'going nuclear', which was signed in 1970 and negotiated with 170 participating nations; some nations, eg India, Israel, Pakistan have refused to sign the NPT (**US News & World Report 17 April, p39**) see Crypto-powers, Third nuclear age

nuclear pores see Nuclear envelope

nuclear power plant Nuclear reactor; see Chernobyl, Radiation injury, Sellafield study, Three Mile Island; Cf ENVIRONMENT

nuclear receptor Any of a 'superfamily' of soluble (non-membrane-bound) receptors for a constellation of physiologically active compounds (ligands), including retinoids, steroids, thyroid hormone, vitamin D, and hypolipidemic drugs; when nuclear receptors are activated by their cognate ligand, they form dimers, bind DNA, and activate transcription of relevant primary target genes

nuclear roundness factor The degree to which a nucleus in cross section approximates a perfect circle; increased nuclear irregularity is often associated with aggressive cell growth, and may be used to grade epithelial malignancy; like the nuclear contour index, the NRF has little diagnostic, prognostic or therapeutic utility, and thus although the objective nature of the NRF makes it a candidate for computer-based imaging analysis, the wide variability of cell populations in malignancy and the existence of malignant 'bland cell' tumors, make the relatively primitive structural details provided less useful than functional analysis of a tumor's potential for aggression by measuring gene amplification, the loss of tumor suppressor genes, or DNA ploidy

nuclear spin MRI An intrinsic property of certain nuclei that gives them an associated characteristic angular momentum and magnetic moment; Cf Spin; see Magnetic resonance imaging

nuclear terrorism GLOBAL VILLAGE The use or the threat of the use of a nuclear device of any size or form of delivery[1] as a means of 'leverage' to coerce a government or population to submit to a terrorist 'agenda' (**Science 1994; 264:337N&c**); the use of nuclear weapons as a device for extortion has not occurred[2]; various delivery systems are envisioned, ranging from the 'low-tech' so-called 'dirty' bomb, in which a conventional ballistic missile[3] is filled with highly radioactive material, to the formal assembly of a device using high-grade plutonium, to be detonated locally or delivered by a ballistic system

[1]While the NT is at present only the stuff of Hollywood, some 'think tank' workers believe that it is no longer a question of *whether* such a device will be detonated by terrorists, but *when* it will occur [2]the fall of the former Soviet Union with its stockpiles of warheads and plutonium make this a potential with disturbing implications (**Atlantic Monthly June 1994:61**) [3]Readily available to the highest bidder, or wherever 'toys' are sold ('toys' being a bizarre euphemism for weapons of mass destruction

nuclear war A hypothetical exchange and detonation of nuclear warheads between two or more countries with atomic bombs; the potential medical consequences of even a limited nuclear war would have been devastating, (table); see Disaster, Fire winds, LD50, Nuclear crash, TTAPS model; Cf Biological warfare, Chemical warfare

NUCLEAR WAR, BLAST EFFECTS:			
A	B	C	
1.3	140	750	Everything flattened, 'moonscape'
4.8	70	460	Almost everything is flattened
7.0	35	255	Heavy construction is not flattened
9.5	20	150	Building walls blown away
18.6	7	55	Survival possible

A Kilometers from 'ground zero' (blast epicenter)
B Air pressure, Kg/m²
C Wind velocity in Km/hour

nuclear waste A specific form of radioactive waste that is the spent fuel from a nuclear reactor, eg a power plant, the most dangerous product of which is plutonium, which 1) Can be used as a core material for producing atomic bombs and 2) Requires disposal in a 'safe place' (**NY Times March 14 1995, C1**) see Radioactive waste

nuclear winter A prolonged period of cold weather due to massive atmospheric soot injections in a full-scale nuclear 'exchange'; according to the TTAPS model, the midsummer land temperatures would decrease by 10-20°C in northern latitudes, to sub-freezing in the southern hemisphere, disrupt the monsoons, and deplete the ozone layer; see Nuclear war

nuclease A generic term for any hydrolytic enzyme that

cleaves the phosphodiester bonds in the nucleic acids of DNA and RNA, which can be either exonucleases (EC 3.1.11-16) or endonucleases (EC 3.1.21-31); see Restriction endonuclease

nuclease An enzyme that catalyzes the hydrolysis of the phosphodiester bond of polynucleotide chains (ie a nucleic acid), which are produced by most biological systems; the 100s of nucleases are defined by

1) Substrate specificity, ie are DNases or RNases

2) Single- or double-stranded attack

3) Site of attack-exonucleases act on the ends of nucleic acids; endonucleses act inside the chain

4) End-products, ie 3' or 5' hydroxy terminus

(Am Biotech Lab March1995, p60)

nucleation The process of forming a nucleus CHEMISTRY The formation of crystals in a supersaturated inorganic solution PHYSIOLOGY The assembly of G-actin subunits into small oligomers, which is a rate-limiting step in actin polymerization

nucleic acid A polymeric molecule that is either a double-stranded chain of DNA nucleotides (carrying genetic information) or a single-stranded chain of RNA (critical in protein synthesis); the individual units of the nucleic acids are pyrimidine nucleotides (cytosine, which is present in both DNA and RNA, thymine, present in DNA and uracil, present in RNA), purine nucleotides (adenine and guanine, nucleotides shared by DNA and RNA); both nucleotides are linked to another nucleotide base and attached to a sugar (RNA and DNA chains each have a pentose sugar: D-deoxyribose for DNA and D-ribose for RNA), which is attached to the phosphate group; without the phosphate, the sugar and base together are called nucleosides; with one phosphate, it is a mononucleotide, eg AMP, a second phosphate, a dinucleotide, eg ADP, and a third high-energy phosphate, a trinucleotide, eg ATP; see DNA, mRNA, Purines, Pyrimidines, RNA, rRNA, tRNA

nucleic acid hybridization assay A generic term for any test designed to detect the presence of a specific sequence of nucleic acids (usually DNA, but also RNA) by using a labeled (ie radioactive, biotinylated, or chemiluminescent) nucleic acid probe (usually DNA) that is complementary to the bases of the target sequence; NAH requires two steps 1) Removal of the stand of DNA or RNA that is complementary to the region of interst by denaturing it, which exposes the hydrogen bonds for subsequent hybridization, and 2) Reaction with a complementary probe, the non-hybridizing excess of which is removed; NAH techniques include FISH and other forms of in situ hybridization, Southern blot hybridization, and others

nucleic acid sequence-based amplification see NASBA

nucleolar organizing region AgNOR, NOR Any of a number of segments of DNA that encode for ribosomal RNA (known as rRNA cistrons), which in humans are located in the short arms of chromosomes 13, 14, 15, 21, and 22; NORs have constant positions and are used by cytogeneticists as markers for detecting certain trisomies and translocations; in a Giemsa-stained metaphase spread preparation, NORs appear by light microscopy as achromatic gaps; during interphase, they condense to form argyrophilic fibrillar centers, or AgNORs, the number of which in a cell population is an measure of the cell's proliferative status, ie the more the AgNORs, the greater is the mitotic activity, a parameter of use in evaluating malignant lymphomas (J Histotech 1992; 15:185)

*Which is an artefact, as these gaps do not exist when the chromosome is examined by electron micrsocpy

nucleolin 1) A 100-kD protein associated with intranucleolar chromatin and ribosomal particles that is thought to have a role in mRNA transcription and assembly of ribo-

somes 2) An obsolete term referring to the constituents of the nucleolus, in particular DNA, RNA, and proteins

nucleolini Small, spherical clumps of ribonucleoprotein in the nucleolus, which by electron microscopy appear as zones of fibrillar lucency surrounded by granular, electron-opaque rings; the size variability of the nucleolini is greater in malignancy than in benign conditions

nucleolus A dense round RNA-rich region of the eukaryotic nucleus composed of ribosomes, strands of DNA, and enzymes, which is the site of rRNA transcription; cells with small or inconspicuous nucleoli do not as a rule, actively divide or produce proteins, and are in general benign; nucleoli are usually basophilic and may reach considerable size in certain malignancies (breast and renal cell carcinoma, epithelioid sarcomas, immunoblastic and Hodgkin's lymphoma), the nucleolus may be eosinophilic and reach gargantuan proportions

nucleoside analogue A generic term for a molecule that structurally mimics a nucleoside; the dideoxynucleoside family, eg dideoxycytidine, 2',3'-dideoxyinosine and 3'-azido-2',3'-dideoxythymidine, inhibits reverse transcriptase after anabolic phosphorylation and used in altering the clinical course of retroviral infections, eg HIV-1; see Zidovudine (3'-azido-2',3'-dideoxythymidine)

nucleosome A coherent aggregate of highly basic proteins that is associated with chromosomes, originally classified according to the proportion of the content of basic amino acids in each; the H1, H2A, H2B, H3, H4 classes of histones occur in all eukaryotes (H5 is a unique variant in avian erythrocytes); the histone complexes contain a 140 base-pair strand of DNA coiled around double cylinders of histones H2a, H2b, H3 and H4; nucleosomes are separated from each other by 'naked' 25-100 base pairs in length segments of DNA Note: The H1 histone can be removed with impunity and thus is considered extrinsic to the histone complex; histones allow tight organized packing of DNA while limiting DNase cleavage or 'attack'; see Histone

5'-nucleotidase LABORATORY MEDICINE A hydrolytic enzyme [EC 3.1.3.5] that cleaves the phosphate from 5' ribonucleotide; elevation of 5'-NT is more specific than alkaline phosphatase in hepatobiliary disease and is highest in patients with posthepatic jaundice, intrahepatic cholestasis and infiltrative hepatic lesions

nucleotide see Nucleic acid

nucleus HISTOLOGY The cell 'organelle' that contains the genetic material (DNA) and the replicative and transcriptional machinery (RNA and binding proteins) necessary to copy the genomic information and encode the structural and functional proteins required for cell function NEUROANATOMY An aggregate of neuronal cell bodies sharing a common function, eg accessory nucleus, caudate nucleus, nucleus ambiguus ORGANIC CHEMISTRY The portion of a molecule that is the major determinant of chemical behavior, eg benzene ring, β-lactam ring, cyclopentanoperhydrophenanthrene in steroids

nuclide An atom with a specific atomic number, mass number and energy level

NUD Non-ulcer dyspepsia, see there

nude mouse A strain of laboratory mice that is hairless, thymusless (congenital thymic aplasia) and T cell-less, which must be raised in a gnotobiotic environment; nude mice are of greatest use in studying graft-versus-host disease; see Bubble boy

'nuke' A colloquial term for any activity intended to render a population or location devoid of life, eg by incineration, exposure to chemicals, and various forms of irradiation, eg IR or UV light (R Preston, The Hot Zone, Random House, New York, 1994)

Note: The term derives from an abbreviation of nuclear war

null allele A segment of DNA that is not known to produce a protein product

null cell A lymphocyte lacking T-cell and B-cell markers including lineage-specific cluster of differentiation (CD antigens and surface immunoglobulins, formerly known as a 'third population' cell, which comprise up to 20% of peripheral lymphocytes; null cells participate in antibody-dependent cell-mediated cytotoxicity and is the cell phenotype most commonly seen in childhood acute lymphocytic leukemia; null cells are of three types: 1) Undifferentiated stem cells that later mature into T or B cells, 2) Cells with labile IgG and a trypsin resistant high-affinity Fc receptor and 3) Large granular lymphocytes (NK and K cells); see ACDD, Large granular lymphocytes, Pan-B cell markers, Pan-T cell markers

Note: Null cell lymphoproliferative disorders demonstrate heavy and/or light chain rearrangements and thus null cell malignancies are often of B-cell origin

null DNA preparation A method used to determine the overlap of genes in various tissues; the mRNA from the tissue in question is allowed to react with non-repetitive DNA; the DNA that reacts is isolated, constituting the mDNA preparation; the DNA that does not react is the 'null' DNA; the 'null' DNA is then hybridized in excess mRNA from another tissue; the proportion of the mDNA that reacts serves to identify the proportions of genes expressed in the second tissue as well as the first tissue

null hypothesis STATISTICS A hypothesis that assumes that if there are no differences between two populations (or sets of data) being compared, a statement of probabilities (P value) can be made

null mutation Nonsense mutation, see there

null phenotype The non-expression of a protein because its corresponding gene is defective or absent on both inherited haplotypes; most null phenotypes involve the red cell, eg blood group O, M-N-S-s-, Fy(a-b-), Jk(a-b-), Rh null (---/---); although the most common null phenotype is that of the ABO group O, which occurs in 45-to-55% of the population; null phenotypes are relatively uncommon; other null phenotypes include non-red cell proteins, as in non-expression of complement proteins ($C3_o$), transferrin (Tf_o) and haptoglobin (Hp_o); see Bombay phenotype

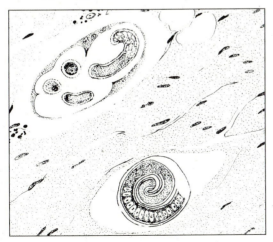

nurse cells

null syndrome Rh/null syndrome, see there

nullisomic gamete A gamete lacking a specific allele, gene, or chromosome; Cf Disomic gamete

'numb chin' sign A rare clinical finding that may be the first sign of carcinoma metastatic to the mandible

numbers see Measurement

number three ('3') sign A finding on a plain anteroposterior chest film which, when seen with rib notching, left ventricular hypertrophy and precordial systolic murmurs is suggestive of coarctation of the aorta

NUREMBURG CODE

The voluntary consent of the human subjects is absolutely essential. This means that the person involved should have legal capacity to give consent; the person should be so situated as to be able to exercise free power of choice, without the element of force, fraud, deceit, duress, over-reaching or other ulterior form of constraint or coercion, and should have sufficient knowledge and comprehension of the elements of the subject matter involved as to enable him to understand and make an enlightened decision. This latter element requires that before the acceptance of an affirmative decision by the experimental subject, it should be made known to him the nature, duration and purpose of the experiment, the method and means by which it is to be conducted, all inconveniences and hazards to be reasonably expected and the effects upon his health or person which may possibly come from his participation in the experiment. The experiment should be such as to yield fruitful results for the good of society, unprocurable by other methods or means of study and not random and unnecessary in nature... The experiment should be conducted so as to avoid all unnecessary physical and mental suffering and injury... The degree of risk to be taken should never exceed that determined by the humanitarian importance of the problem to be solved by the experiment.

Nuremburg code BIOMEDICAL ETHICS An internationally sanctioned code of research ethics that was formulated in response to the revelations of the extent and brutality of the Nazi war crimes that forced experiments of little scientific value on concentration camp victims; the Nuremberg code establishes strict standards for scientific studies on human subjects based on the principles of autonomy and informed consent (see page 503 for wording); the Declaration of Helsinki is an extension of this code that was formulated in 1964 and revised in 1975; see Declaration of Helsinki, Geneva Convention, Institutional review board; Cf Unethical medical research

nurse cells A term that has been used in several different contexts HEMATOLOGY Macrophages of erythroblastic islands in the bone marrow, involved in erythrophagocytosis, iron storage and transfer PARASITOLOGY Histiocytes and other cells that serve as a 'nursery' for the bradyzoites of *Toxoplasma gondii*, affecting the immunocompromised or in infants PATHOLOGY Skeletal muscle cells which the larvae of *Trichinella spiralis* modify to create an intracellular environment suitable for their own survival and later encystation

nursemaid's elbow Subluxation of the head of the radius, caused by a longitudinal 'yank' on the forearm (by a nursemaid, nanny or caregiver), forcing the child's elbow into extension; the child's arm is immobile and the child is in pain; the subluxation is reduced by firm supination at 90° and extension, followed by immobilization with a posterior splint or a sling

nurse endoscopist An advanced practice (ie specialized) nurse who is trained to perform endoscopic examinations, eg of the lower gastrointestinal tract; it is reported that trained nurses can perform flexible sigmoidoscopic examination as accurately and safely as experienced gastroenterologists (N Engl J Med 1994; 330:183sA) see Advanced practice nurse

nursing home HEALTH CARE INDUSTRY A facility that is largely dedicated to the long-term care of the elderly; there are currently about 1.5 million nursing home residents in the USA, estimated to cost $34.7 billion (US); the probability of nursing home use increases sharply with age; 17% of those age 65-74 spend one or more years, as do 60% of those aged 85; 21% spend five or more years in a home and this use is up to two-fold greater in women than in men (**N Engl J Med 1991; 324:595**); see Geriatrics, Home health care; Cf Hospice

nurse practitioner A nurse fulfilling the requirements of, and who is certified in a particular jurisdiction (eg in New York State, section 6902 of the Education Law) to diagnose illness and physical conditions, and perform therapeutic and corrective measures within a designated specialty area of practice; NPs may write orders for routine laboratory and clinical tests, and prescribe routine drugs (ie not controlled substances), devices, and immunizing agents as specified in his/her privileges in a particular health care environment or hospital; all such orders must be countersigned by an attending physician

nutcracker esophagus Corkscrew esophagus, see there

nutcracker phenomenon A clinical finding in hemoglobin SC disease, in which left-sided renal hemorrhage causes infarction of renal papillae, due to increased pressure as the left renal vein passes between the aorta and the superior mesenteric artery; increased pressure causes renal medullary anoxia sufficient to sickle the red cells

nutmeg liver A descriptor for a liver with chronic passive congestion, a hepatopathy due to cardiac decompensation and failure, the gross morphology of which has been fancifully likened to a cut nutmeg; if the congestion is severe, these changes may be accompanied by hemorrhagic necrosis PATHOLOGY Intense congestion with deep red, centrilobular zone, sharply demarcated from the pale tan peripheral zones corresponding to the liver plates due to stasis and fatty degeneration of the liver; the central veins are dilated and congested, the sinusoids are widened by extravasated red cells and thickened arterial walls, and hepatocytic atrophy (shrunken eosinophilic cells with pyknotic nuclei)

nutrient medium MICROBIOLOGY A generic term for any culture medium that provides the physical support and the essential nutrients required for the growth of microorganisms, usually carbohydrates, eg dextrose and protein, eg birdseed or brain-heart infusion

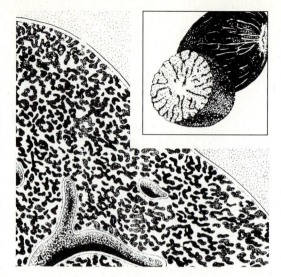

nutmeg liver

nutritional 'mumps' Chronic, asymptomatic bilateral enlargement of the parotid and/or submaxillary salivary glands that occurs endemically in a population suffering from multiple clinical signs of malnutrition including cachexia, hypoproteinemia, anemia, angular cheilosis, pellagroid hyperpigmentation

nymphomania Female hypersexuality A popular term for a ♀ psychosexual disorder characterized by ↑↑↑ in sexual activity and desire, which is viewed in the psychoanalytical context of representing a reponse to an inferiority complex and/or a need for affection

Synonyms include andromania, clitoromania, cytheromania, estromania, female hypersexuality, female satyriasis, furor femininus, furor uterinus, hysteromania, lascivia

NZB/NZW see New Zealand mice

suppressor gene on chromosome 3 TREATMENT Non-surgical; up to 85% respond to combination chemotherapy using CCNU, cyclophosphamide, doxorubicin, vincristine and etopoisde (VP-16); although extensive disease at time of discovery is often fatal within two years, 50% of those with limited metastases respond to therapy and 15-20% survive two years; radiotherapy may control bone pain, spinal cord compression, superior vena cava syndrome and bronchial obstruction; see Small cell carcinoma

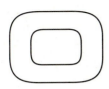

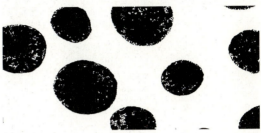

oat cell

O Symbol for: 1) Nonmotile strain of a bacterium (after ohne Hauch, German, without tail) 2) Occiput 3) Oculus 4) Oxygen

o Symbol for: ortho-

O-11 10-(propoxy)decanoic acid) An analogue of myristic acid that is highly toxic to trypanosomes and non-toxic to human cells, which has therapeutic potential in treating trypanosomiasis, for which the only agent available for treating end-stage (meningoencephalitic) disease is melarsoprol, which itself causes death in 5% of patients (Science 1991; 252:1851)

OAF Osteoclast-activating factor(s), see there

oak leaf spots A descriptor for the size and shape of the pigmented cutaneous macules seen in patients with von Recklinghausen's disease and tuberous sclerosis

O antigen MICROBIOLOGY A bacterial lipopolysaccharide-protein antigen which is used in the serological classification of enteric bacteria, including *Proteus* species, forming the basis of the Weil-Felix test (used for classifying *Rickettsia* species) and *Shigella* species for categorization of its 40 serotypes TRANSFUSION MEDICINE An oligosaccharide precursor for the A and B antigens of the ABO blood group, fucose-galactose-N-acetylglucosamine-glucose; see Bombay phenotype

oasthouse urine disease A rare AR [MIM 250900] disorder characterized by increased α-hydroxybutyric acid in the urine and stools, which imparts a characteristic 'oasthouse' odor, described in methionine malabsorption (defective intestinal absorption of methionine and other amino acids); the GI bacteria ferment the excess methionine into α-hydroxybutyric, α-ketobutyric and α-aminobutyric acids which are then absorbed and excreted CLINICAL White hair, failure to thrive, seizures, hypotonia and edema, and mental retardation; α-hydroxybutyric acid may also rarely appear in the urine of patients with phenylketonuria

Note: An oasthouse is a building or kiln for drying hops, which are the ripe, dried pistillate catkins of a hop (*Humulus lupulus*) used especially to impart a bitter flavor to malt liquors

oat cell carcinoma A histologic subtype of small cell carcinoma of the lung, characterized by a dense hyperchromatic oval nucleus, often with a vague central groove and minimal cytoplasm EM Neurosecretory granules, containing hormones (ACTH, ADH, bombesin, calcitonin, CRF, estrogen, FSH, hGH, histaminase, HPL, LH, MSH, PTH, renin, serotonin) CLINICAL Highly aggressive with a 3-month survival without therapy, often accompanied by cerebellar degeneration (80% have metastasis to the brain) MOLECULAR PATHOLOGY Homozygous loss of tumor

ob A gene that sends a hormonal message (a putative satiety hormone) from the fat cells to the brain to stop eating; if mutated or damaged, the message is not sent, failing to make the hormone (Nature 1994; 372:425, N Engl J Med 1995; 332:679) same as the thrifty gene

obesity A state of excess accumulation of body fat, which is regarded by some authors as a premorbid addiction disorder, defined as 10% (or 20%) above an individual's standard weight; the ideal body weight is 21 kg/m^2 (the average American is 20% overweight-30 million Americans are obese and weigh an average excess of 25.5 kg/m^2); the child is father of the man—an obese child is often an obese adult and the patterns may be established as early as three months of age (decreased energy expenditure in infants of obese mothers DIET RESISTANT OBESITY Obesity characterized by an inability to lose weight despite ↓ caloric intake and ↑ exercise; a substantial proportion of diet-resistant obesity is related to underreporting of actual caloric consumption and/or overreporting of physical activity rather due to low energy expenditure (N Engl J Med 1992; 327:1893OA) 33% of US adults are obese (an ↑ of 8% in the last decade, with an average ↑ of 3.5 kg), based on a body mass index of ≥ 27 (JAMA 1994; 20 July) in the past 20 years, there has been a 54% ↑ in obesity and a 98% ↑ in superobesity in children 6 to 9 years of age; obesity is classified according to

ANATOMY 1) Android ('beer-gut') obesity is more common in ♂, more central or truncal in distribution and places the subject at ↑ risk for DM 2) Gynecoid obesity is more common in ♀, the fat is distributed in the lower abdomen and legs and is less commonly associated with atherosclerosis

PSYCHOLOGICAL PROFILE

AGE OF ONSET, eg juvenile, mature, during pregnancy or other

TYPE OF TISSUE CHANGE, eg hyperplastic or hyperplastic-hypertrophic and

PRIMARY OR SECONDARY 1) Primary obesity is associated with HLA-B18 and is a component of Allström, Blount, Cohen, Carpenter, Laurence-Moon-Biedl, Prader-Willi and other eponymically dignified syndromes 2) Secondary or acquired obesity comprises the bulk of obesity

LABORATORY Obesity mimics the findings of NIDDM, including insulin resistance, ↑ glucose, cholesterol and triglyceride levels, ↓ HDL and norepinephrine and depression of the sympathetic and parasympathetic nervous system; CONDITIONS ASSOCIATED WITH OBESITY Cardiovascular disease, thromboembolism, cholecystitis, cholelithiasis, abnormal GI transit, poor wound healing, atelectasis, hepatic steatosis and fibrosis TREATMENT Diet, exercise, behavior modification; Cf Adipsin, Diets, Gastric 'balloon',

Morbid obesity, Superobesity

'obe-tension' A relatively common clinical association of obesity with hypertension; Cf Diabesity

obitiatrist A neologism proposed by Dr Jack Kevorkian for a practitioner of the as-yet highly controversial field of euthanasia and/or physician-assisted suicide; see Euthanasia, Kevorkian, Physician-assisted suicide

object-oriented programming COMPUTERS A format for writing software, in which objects (blocks of a computer program and related methods that describe some way to manipulate data), can be 'plugged' together or pulled apart to make different systems and environments; OOP would allow a relatively unsophisticated user to modify software to his/her particular need (**Sci Am 1993; 268/1:145**)

obligate aerobe Strict aerobe MICROBIOLOGY An aerobe that requires molecular oxygen as a terminal electron acceptor, resulting in the formation of water and does not obtain energy by fermentative pathways, eg *Micococcus* and *Pseudomonas* species

obligate anaerobe Strict anaerobe MICROBIOLOGY Any of a group of anaerobic bacteria that may be either 1) Moderate, ie capable of growth in reduced oxygen (2-8%) environment, eg *Bacteroides fragilis, B melaninogenicus, Fusobacterium nucleatum, Clostridium perfringens* or 2) Strict, ie incapable of growth in $O_2 > 0.5\%$, eg *Clostridium haemolyticum, C novyi B, Selenomonas ruminantium, Treponema denticola*; because obligate anaerobes lack superoxide dismutase, they may be killed with minimal exposure to O_2; see Oxygen toxicity

OBRA 1993 Omnibus Budget Reconciliation Act of 1993, popularly known as Stark II, see there

OBS Organic brain syndrome, see there

obscene phone call see Telephone scatologia

'observation' hip ORTHOPEDICS A condition characterized by transient focal osteolysis of the hip bones that may be accompanied by mild synovitis or osteoarthritis, which is either idiopathic or secondary to minor trauma and infection TREATMENT None, observation (hence the name) usually suffices

obsession PSYCHIATRY A behavior defined as a *Recurrent and persistent thoughts, impulses, or images* (TII, that are perceived) ... *as intrusive and inappropriate and that cause marked anxiety or distress* (**DSM-IV, 1994**)

obsessive-compulsive disorder PSYCHIATRY A condition characterized by either obsessions or compulsion

OBSESSIONS ARE

1) Recurrent and persistent thoughts, impulses, or images (TII), that are perceived as intrusive and inappropriate and cause marked anxiety or distress,

2) That are not excessive reponses to genuine real-life problems

3) Active attempts are made to suppress or neutralize the TIIs by some thought or action and

4) The person recognizes that the TIIs are products of his/her own mind

COMPULSIONS ARE

1) Repetitive behaviors, eg handwashing, double-checking, mental acts (praying, repeating words silently) that a person feels compelled to perform in response to an obsession, or in accord with rules that must be applied strictly

2) Behaviors or mental acts aimed at preventing or reducingdistress or preventing some dreaded event or situation, which are not realistically connected with what they are intended to neutralize or prevent, or behaviors that are clearly excessive (modified from **DSM-IV, 1994**)

OCD was once considered a rare, therapeutically refractory neurosis; OCD affects 1-2% of the US population, has a neurophysiopathological component and may respond to certain tricyclic antidepressants PATHOGENESIS The biological roots of OCD are extrapolated from avian studies by K Lorenz who hypothesized that certain bird behavior, eg nest-building, courtship, and grooming were 'hard-wired' into the brain and, like OCD, repeated in exactly the same sequence TREATMENT Clomipramine is of use in trichotillomania and in other forms of OCD Cf Obsessive-compulsive personality disorder (see note)

obsessive-compulsive personality disorder PSYCHIATRY A condition characterized by *'A pervasive pattern of preoccupation with orderliness, perfectionism, and mental and interpersonal control at the expense of flexibility, openness, and efficiency...'* (**DSM-IV, 1994**); persons with OCPD may be excessively devoted to work to the exclusion of leisure activities, friends, and family; they may be incapable of discarding worn-out or worthless objects ('pack rat' mentality), and are often rigid and/or stubborn; Cf Obsessive-compulsive disorder

Note: Although OCD and OCPD have similar names, the clinical findings are viewed as completely different; OCPD is not characterized by Os or Cs, but rather by a pervasive preoccupation with neatness and order

obstetric hypercoagulability profile A battery of tests for a woman who may be at risk, eg repeated abortions for coagulopathic diatheses, which supplements the details provided by the obstetric screening profile, measuring in addition, proteins C and S, anti-thrombin III, lupus anticoagulant, fibrinogen and plasminogen

Note: Prothrombin and partial thromboplastin times are measured on admission for delivery

obstetric panel LABORATORY MEDICINE A standard (CPT-4 code 80055) panel of laboratory tests used to evaluate a pregnant woman's baseline health status; the OP is used for women not known to have, or to be at risk for, conditions that might complicate labor and delivery; for Medicare or Medicaid reimbursement, the OP must include a CBC with a differential white cell count, hepatitis B surface antigen(HBsAg), rubella antibody, a quantitative test for syphilis (eg VDRL, RPR), an antibody screen, and both ABO and Rh(D) blood typing (see **CAP Today March 1993**)

obstetric (screening) profile Obstetric panel, see there

obstructive airways disease A generic term for lung diseases (asthma, COPD-chronic obstructive pulmonary disease) that share in common the presence of airway obstruction and hyperresponssiveness TREATMENT Inhaled corticosteroid, and maintenance therapy with β_2-agonist, eg terbutaline reduces mortality, airway obstruction and hyperresponssiveness (**N Engl J Med 1992 327:1413oA**)

obstructive hydrocephalus Noncommunicating hydrocephalus PEDIATRICS Hydrocephalus due to interference with the flow of cerebrospinal fluid, resulting in enlarged ventricles; obstructive hydrocephalus may be due to congenital aqueductal stenosis or atresia, eg Dandy-Walker syndrome, a complication of intracranial infection, violent birth trauma or transmitted in an X-linked recessive fashion; Cf Communicating hydrocephalus

obstructive sleep apnea syndrome A clinical complex due to the pathophysiological response to anatomic defects of the nasopharynx, characterized by loud snoring, nocturnal oxyhemoglobin desaturation and disrupted sleep, accompanied by daytime hypersomnolence, related to the loss of the mechanisms designed to prevent death by asphyxiation CLINICAL Many symptoms are cardiovascular, eg apnea-induced arrhythmia, bradycardia, ↑ ventricular ectopic activity and hypertension and are associated with obesity, nasal obstruction, adenoidal and tonsillar hyperplasia, macroglossia, retrognathia, acromegaly, hypothyroidism TREATMENT Therapy should be individualized and may include surgery, eg uvulopalatopharyngoplasty is successful in 50% of cases; Cf Snoring; Cf

Narcolepsy, Sleep disorders

obturator sign RADIOLOGY A unilateral $\uparrow$ in the obturator muscle bulk, seen as a soft tissue bulge on the inner pelvis with medial displacement of the normal fat line, considered characteristic of infectious arthritis, which may be seen in trauma-induced hemorrhage

Occam's razor see Ockham's razor

occipital horn Broad, calcified protrusions (occipital exostoses) that extend caudally from the base of the skull, characteristic of X-linked type IX Ehlers-Danlos syndrome, a morbid process, which like Menke's kinky hair disease is related to defective copper metabolism, resulting in secondary lysyl oxidase deficiency and by extension, collagen defects; other anomalies in type IX Ehlers-Danlos syndrome include hyperextensibility and facile bruisability of skin, a long thin face and neck, atrophic scars, cardiac murmur, medullary sponge kidney and polycystic kidneys, episodic syncope, borderline intelligence, hammer-shaped distal clavicle and saber shins (**Radiology 1984; 152:665**)

occult blood Grossly inapparent blood, usually understood to mean hematochezia, which often presages colonic adenocarcinoma may also be seen in amebiasis, heavy metal poisoning and acute GI ischemia

occult blood testing LABORATORY MEDICINE The testing of stool for the presence of grossly inapparent blood to detect possible malignancy Note: Usually more than 50 cc/L is required to recognize blood in the stools, which is detected by

1) The guaiac method eg, Hemoccult II, a low-cost screening technique that uses a guaiac-impregnated paper to indirectly measure hemoglobin by semi-quantitating hemoglobin's pseudoperoxidase activity; while sensitive, the guaiac method is nonspecific, as peroxidase activity is present in uncooked red meat, fish, uncooked fruits and certain cruciferous vegetables, eg broccoli and cauliflower; false guaiac positivity occurs in GI bleeding at a distance, either 'north' eg gingiva, stomach or 'south', eg hemorrhoids of the rectum and with drug therapy, eg iron therapy, aspirin, nonsteroid anti-inflammatory drugs and topical iodine; false negative results may be due to improper storage of test slides, intermittent bleeding of lesion, hypervitaminosis C and degradation of hemoglobin by colonic bacteria;

2) HemoQuant is more specific as it quantifies the conversion of heme to fluorescent porphyrins

EFFICACY 13-year cumulative mortality was 5.88/1000 in those screened annually for fecal occult blood (reducing mortality by $\pm$ ⅓) vs 8.83/1000 in the control group (**N Engl J Med 1993; 328:1365**oA)

Note: These tests assume that the carcinoma has produced an ulcer and therefore is bleeding; 20-30% of patients with colorectal cancers have a negative fecal occult blood test

occult infection An infection that is first recognized by secondary manifestations, eg elevated polymorphonuclear leukocytes in the circulation or fever of unknown origin, most often caused by a bacterial infection in an obscure site, eg an abscess of the subphrenic or other intraabdominal region

occult primary malignancy Occult cancer, unknown primary A malignancy of unknown primary site or origin that is symptomless, which first manifests itself as metastases or secondary (paraneoplastic) phenomena, and usually has a poor prognosis; OPMs are problematic as appropriate therapy requires that the primary malignancy be eradicated, and many remain obscure despite an aggressive diagnostic work-up; certain malignancies metastasize to certain sites with greater than expected frequency (table), in OPMs affecting the brain, the primary arises in the lungs in up to 85% (**Arch Pathol Lab Med 1993; 117:1165**oA) TREATMENT Up to 30% of patients with metastases arising from an occult primary adenocarcinoma may respond to chemotherapy (using mitomycin C, adriamycin and vincristine); poor therapeutic response is more common in men and in those with hepatic and/or infradiaphragmatic metastases (**Am J Clin Oncol 1990; 13:55**)

OCCULT PRIMARY MALIGNANCIES

BONE Breast, bronchus, prostate, thyroid, kidney

CNS Breast, bronchus, kidney, colon

HEAD & NECK Carcinoma of the oropharynx, nasopharyngeal and thyroid-most are squamous cell carcinoma, others include adenocarcinoma, melanoma, rhabdomyosarcoma, oat cell, salivary gland and thyroid carcinomas

LIVER Stomach, colon, breast, pancreas or bronchus

LUNG Breast, colon, kidney, melanoma, sarcoma, stomach, testis, thyroid

LYMPH NODES

Cervix Naso- and oropharynx, thyroid, larynx, lymphoma

Supraclavicular Bronchi, breast, stomach, esophagus, pancreas, colon, lymphoma

Axillary Breast, melanoma, lymphoma

Inguinal Urogenital tract, anus, melanoma, lymphoma

OVARY Stomach, colon

SEROSAL SURFACES Bronchi, breast, ovary, lymphoma

SKIN Melanoma, breast, bronchus, stomach or kidney

occupational asthma A clinical complex that causes predominantly pulmonary symptoms in previously healthy subjects exposed to a noxious fumes or gases in the working environment; occupational asthma may affect 3% of the US population, many of whom function adequately, despite the symptoms; the causative agent elicits an immediate hypersensitivity reaction, divided into low molecular weight substances, eg isocyanates, anhydrides, soldering metals, metal salts and wood dusts, which act as haptens and high molecular weight substances, eg plant dusts, laboratory animal danders, shellfish and enzymes; see Hypersensitivity pneumonitis, Monday morning sickness, Sick building syndrome

occupational dose RADIATION SAFETY A dose received by an individual during his/her employment in which the assigned duties involve exposure to ionizing radiation and radioactive materials

occupational medicine The medical specialty concerned with disease or dysfunction arising from work-related injuries and/or exposure to noxious agents or stimuli; the most prevalent occupational afflictions include exposure to asbestos (resulting in asbestosis or asbestos-induced pleural plaque formation), noise (causing hearing loss), solvents, welding fumes, fiberglass (causing upper respiratory irritation and bronchitis, solvent intoxication and asthma), musculoskeletal dysfunction due to repetitive trauma, heavy metal intoxication, silicosis, toxic hepatitis, dysfunctional psychologic reactions to the workplace

Note: Dermatoses are under-represented as an occupational disease as patients with work-related dermatopathies are most often seen by dermatologists (**N Engl J Med 1990; 322:594**); in the US, regulations regarding occupational safety are promulgated by the Occupational Safety and Health Administration (see OSHA) and the National Institute of Occupational Safety and Health, see NIOSH

occupational exposure to bloodborne pathogens An event that occurs in a healthcare setting; OEtBP is formally defined by the OSHA as '...*any reasonably anticipated skin, eye, mucous membrane or parenteral contact with blood or other potentially infectious materials that may result from the performance of an employee's duties...*'; the OSHA rulings on OEBP requires that the employer maintain and/or provide an exposure control plan, record keeping, work practices, personal protective equipment, HBV vaccination and follow-up and other provisions (**Advance/Lab May 1994**)

ocher codon One of three mRNA nucleotide codons signaling chain termination (nonsense codons); ocher corresponds to UAA; see Amber, Opal, Nonsense suppressor

Ockham's razor Law of parsimony CLINICAL DECISION-MAK-

ING The simplest expression of scientific truth(s), named after William Ockham, a 14th century (1285c-1349) philosopher who held that '...*a plurality must not be stated without necessity...*' ie theories should be expressed as simply as possible and when two theories exist to explain a similar phenomenon, the most parsimonious should prevail, ie be no more complicated than necessary

OCT see Oxytocin stress test

oct-1, oct-2 Vertebrate homeobox genes with roles in segmentation, anterior-posterior axis determination and cell type specification, which appear after the primitive streak stage of embryological development, and encode the Oct-1, Oct-2 and Oct-3 proteins, which up-regulate transcription by means of an octamer of amino acids known as the OCTA motif

oct-3 A vertebrate gene that encodes a transcription factor containing a POU-specific domain and a homeodomain, expressed in undifferentiated pluripotent cells of the early embryo and in primordial and female germ cells

OCTA motif MOLECULAR BIOLOGY An eight-base-pair regulatory sequence of DNA that is a B-cell-specific promoter of immunoglobulin genes; the transcription control elements (including the TATA box, the OCTA motif and the enhancer) of the immunoglobulin gene chains ensure that these chains will be synthesized within the B lymphocytes but not in other cells

octasanol SPORTS MEDICINE A solid alcohol found in wheat germ and vegetable waxes that can be ingested, which was transiently popular among some atheletes as it was believed to improve stamina, strength, and reaction time (JC DeLee, D Drez, Jr, Orthopedic Sports Medicine WB Saunders, Philadelphia, 1994)

octreotide acetate Sandostatin A somatostatin analog with high affinity for growth hormone (GH) that causes a marked decrease in serum GH and amelioration of symptoms in 70% of patients with acromegaly and is more effective than bromocriptine; octreotide also reduces the effects of TSH-secreting tumors, malignant or metastatic carcinoid, pancreatic endocrine (islet cell) tumors and theoretically, any tumor that has a high concentration of somatostatin receptors; when radiolabelled, octreotide may be used to localize somatostatin receptor-rich tumors (Mayo Clin Proc 1991; 66:283)

ODONTOGENIC CYSTS

PRIMORDIAL CYST
DENTIGEROUS CYST
  Eruption cyst
PERIODONTAL CYST
  1) Apical
  2) Lateral
GINGIVAL CYST
  1) Newborn
  2) Adult
ODONTOGENIC KERATOCYST
  Basal cell nevus-bifid rib syndrome
CALCIFYING ODONTOGENIC CYST

WG Shafer, et al, Eds, Textbook of Oral Pathology, 4th ed, WB Saunders, Philadelphia, 1983

---

ocularist A person who makes ocular prostheses (artificial eyes), which are cosmetic surrogates for eyes that have been removed as a result of tumors, in particular retinoblastoma; see Artificial eye

oculist Obsolete for ophthalmologist

oculocerebrorenal syndrome Lowe syndrome An X-R [MIM 309000] disorder that maps to chromosome Xq24-26

CLINICAL Congenital cataract, corneal ulceration, hydrophthalmia, glaucoma, mental retardation, renal tubular dysfunction (Fanconi syndrome), aminoaciduria, vitamin D-resistant rickets, areflexia, hypotonia, and idiopathic joint swelling LABORATORY Proteinuria, ↑ muscle enzymes, α_2-globulin, HDL-cholesterol, metabolic acidosis TREATMENT Alkalinization of urine, supplemental potassium, phosphate, calcium carnitine (N Engl J Med 1991; 324:1318)

oculocutaneous albinism type I (tyrosinase-negative) An AR [MIM 203100] condition caused by a defect in decreased pigment, amelanic melanocytes in the skin, central fixation, and nystagmus MOLECULAR PATHOLOGY Point mutation in the TYR (tyrosine gene) locus at chromosome segment 11q14-q21, resulting in defective tyrosinase [EC 1.14.18.1], which catalyzes the first two steps in the conversion of tyrosine to melanin

oculocutaneous albinism type II (tyrosinase-positive) An AR [MIM 203200] condition characterized by reduced melanin production in the skin, hair, and eyes; in OCA type II, the cutaneous albinism and visual acuity are not as severely affected as OCA type IA (tyrosinase-negative) MOLECULAR PATHOLOGY Point mutation of *P* gene (located in chromosome segment 15q11-q13) which encodes a transmembrane polypeptide that may transport small molecules, eg tyrosine, the precursor of melanin

Note: *P* gene mutations have also been identified in Prader-Willi syndrome and AR ocular albinism (N Engl J Med 1994; 330α:529α)

OD 1) Optical density 2) Overdose, see there 3) Right eye (*oculus dexter* [NA6])

ODD syndrome Oculodental dysplasia An AD [MIM 164200] condition characterized by hypertelorism, microphthalmia, myopia, hypoplastic teeth, syndactyly, camptodactyly, and visceral malformation, in absece of mental retardation

odds ratio STATISTICS: The ratio of the odds of an event occurring under a set of circumstances p, to the odds of the same event occurring under a set of circumstances P, calculated by the formula

$$OR = \frac{p\,(1-P)}{P(1-p)}$$

The odds ratio is estimated by the ratio of the cross products in a fourfold table; assuming statistical independence, the odds ratio is 1

odontogenic cyst ORAL PATHOLOGY A cyst derived from odontogenic epithelium, which derives from the dental lamina or from the enamel organ; OCs have been classified into 6 broad categories (table)

odor Numerous, relatively uncommon conditions may be associated with typical odors of the urine and/or breath, often occurring in inborn errors of metabolism (table facing page)

Oedipus complex PSYCHIATRY The constellation of consequences (according to Freud) that result from the sublimation of a boy's psychosexual desire for his mother, likened to the Oedipus of Greek mythology who killed his father and married his mother

Note: Oedipus' desire for his mother, Jocasta, was completely innocent, while her incest is regarded by some scholars as having been a conscious act of knowing him to be her son; see Jocasta complex

OFAGE Orthogonal field alternation gel electrophoresis MOLECULAR BIOLOGY A technique that allows separation of large, chromosome-sized, ie 200-3000 kilobase pair segments of DNA, that would be used to compare the homology of related organisms; once the large segments are separated, they may be manipulated by Southern blotting (Nucleic Acids Res 1984; 12:5647); Cf Pulsed field gradient gel electrophoresis

'off campus' The location of an off-site affiliate of a large medical center complex; Cf 'On campus'

'off-ladder' ACADEMIC MEDICINE *adjective* Pertaining or referring to a non-tenure track position (eg lecturer, assistant, associated) or activity (eg raising a family) that hinders a person from climbing a career 'ladder' (Sci Am 1995; 272/6:49) see Glass ceiling, Sticky floor phenomenon

off-shore medical school A medical school that is located in the Caribbean and operated as a for-profit venture (ie expensive); the students at such schools are almost invariably US citizens whose cumulative grade-point average was less than that require to be admitted to North American schools; currently active OMSs include American University of the Caribbean in Montserrat, Ross University in Dominica, St George's University in Grenada, and Spartan Health Sciences University in St Lucia (Am Med News 9 November 1992, p 34), a major concern about OMSs is the inadequate standards, and in some cases the ethical standards by which they operate; one now-defunct OMS, British West Indies Medical College, is alleged to have granted medical degrees after as little as 10 months of medical education (JAMA 1995; 273:1162MN&P) see International medical graduate, USFMG

office The suite of rooms where a physician receives and treats patients, and otherwise practices medicine, commonly known in the UK as 'surgery'

Office of Alternative Medicine A section of the US National Institutes of Health established by the US Congress, the purpose of which is to investigate the claims of efficacy for various forms of alternative therapy, and their possible health benefits; the OAM's first director resigned; projects being funded by pilot projects include acupuncture for unipolar depression, guided imagery for asthma, homeopathy, hypnosis for acclerated fracture healing, massage therapy for HIV, music therapy for psychosocial adjustment after brain injury, prayer intervention for substance abuse (Am Med News 17 October 1994 p13) see Alternative Medicine

Note: Criticism has been leveled that the very existence of such an agency has the potential for legitimizing virtually any form of unproven therapy that claims to be 'alternative' (Sci Am 1993; 269/3:39)

Office of Management and Budget An agency of the US federal government established in 1970 to evaluate, formulate and coordinate management procedures and program objectives within and among Federal departments and agencies, controlling administration of the Federal Budget, routinely providing the president with recommendations regarding budget proposals and relevant legislative enactments

Office of Research Integrity An agency of the US Department of Health and Human Services that succeeds the Office of Scientific Integrity*; the ORI is encharged with ensuring research integrity; the definition of fraud (as of May 1994) included the phrase '...*practices that seriously deviate from those that are commonly accepted within the scientific community for proposing, conducting, or reporting research...,* which has been viewed as being too broad; the ORI has issued a report finding a Boston-based researcher guilty of misconduct (Nature 1994; 372:391N)

*A body organized in 1989 under the auspices of the US National Institutes of Health, which was encharged with investigation of allegations of scientific misconduct and fraud by investigators who are receiving US federal grant monies

Office of Scientific Investigation Office of Research Integrity, see there

Office of Technical Assessment An organization established by the US Congress in 1972 as a nonpartisan analytical support agency, which aids Congress to evaluate the impact of new technologies, anticipate, plan for their consequences on society and coordinate large-scale international research projects

officinal PHARMACOLOGY *adjective* Pertaining or referring to a medication or chemical substance that is regularly carried in a pharmacy's stock, which contrasts with those medicines that are formulated on request, ie by request (prescription)

off-label use CLINICAL PHARMACOLOGY The use of a drug, eg tretinoin, an analog of vitamin A or medical device, eg injectable collagen to treat a condition for which it has not received approval by a regulatory agency, eg the US Food and Drug Administration, the penalty for which may be seizure, injunction and prosecution (JAMA 1991; 266:11)

Odors of Biomedical interest	
Acetone (Russet apples)	Chloroform, ethanol, isopropanol, ketoacidosis, lacquer
Acrid (pear-like)	Chloraldehyde, paraldehyde; *Bacteroides melaninogenicus*
Ammonia	Renal failure, uremia, N-ethyl morpholine
Bitter almonds	Cyanide
Burned chocolate	Infection by *Proteus* species
Cabbage	Methionine (see also Hops)
Campherous	1,8-cineole
Carrots	Circutoxin
Coal gas	Carbon monoxide
Disinfectants	Phenol, creosote
Eggs,rotten	H_2S, mercaptans, disulfuram (Antabuse)
Ether-like	Ethylene chloride
Fecaloid, putrid	Infection by *Clostridium* species
Fishy	Vaginal infection by Gardnerella vaginalis, 'rice-water' choleric stools; di-N-butylamine, diethylamine, hepatic failure
Floral (sweet, fruity)	Diabetes, acetone, ethyl- and isobutyl- acetate, phenyl methylethyl carbinol
Fruity/alcohol	Amyl nitrate, ethanol, isopropanol
Garlic	Arsenic, phosphorous, selenium, tellurium, thallium, malathion, parathion, DMSO (dimethyl-sulfoxide)
Grape juice	Infection by *Pseudomonas* species
Halitosis	Oral infections
Hop-like	Oasthouse disease α-hydroxybutyric acid
Maple syrup	Maple syrup urine disease
Mint	Menthone
Mothballs	Camphor-products
Mousy/musty	Phenylketonuria
Musty basement	Infection by *Streptomyces* and *Nocardia* species
Musty (fish, raw liver)	Hepatic failure, zinc phosphide, pentadecanolacetone
Odorless urine	Acute tubular necrosis
Peanuts	RH-787 (Vacor, see Vacor diabetes)
Pungent	Ethylchlorvynol; formic acid
Putrid	Dimethyldisulfide
Rancid fish	Tyrosinemia
Rotting fish	Trimethylaminuria
Shoe polish	Nitrobenzene
Sour and pungent	Ethyl acrylate, 2-methyl-5-ethyl pyridine, propionic acid, 2,4-pentanedione
Sweaty feet	Glutaric acidemia, type II, isovaleric acidemia
Sweet and musty	Isobutylacrylate
and rancid	2,6 butanol
and sharp	Methylethylketone
Swimming pool	Hawkinsinuria
Tomcat urine	β-Methylcrotonylglycinuria
Violets	Turpentine
Wintergreen	Methylsalicylate

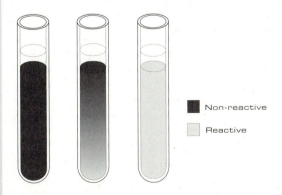

■ Non-reactive
□ Reactive

oxidative-fermentative test

O-F test Oxidative-fermentative test MICROBIOLOGY A test used to characterize the fermentative qualities of gram-negative rods, which detects the acid production by fermentative bacteria; two tubes are partially filled with different concentrations of fermentable sugars and a peptone (Hugh-Leifson medium), one of which is overlayed with sterile mineral oil, creating an anaerobic environment; oxidative bacteria (glucose oxidizer, eg *Pseudomonas aeruginosa*) produce acid only in the open tube exposed to atmospheric oxygen (figure, right); fermenting organisms (glucose fermenter, eg *Escherichia coli*) produce acid in both tubes and nonsaccharolytic bacteria (non-saccharolytic, eg *Moraxella* sp) are inert

OGOD approach MOLECULAR GENETICS The one gene, one disease approach is a philosophical stance that addresses complex traits that lack a simple mendelian pattern of inheritance, and thus unlikely to simple genetic defects; it is therefore often assumed that complex traits consist of an aggregate of several disorders, each caused by a separate gene; the OA assumes that complex traits are composed of several subtraits, each influenced by a single gene; the OA has been successful in dissecting the hereditary pattern of severe mental retardation of phenylketonuria (PKU) which is linked to multiple mutations in the phenylalanine hydroxylase gene (Science 1994; 264:1733A) Cf Quantitative trait locus (QTL) analysis

'oid-oid' disease DERMATOLOGY An uncommonly used colloquialism for the combination of exudative disc*oid* dermatitis and lichen*oid* dermatitis

oil(s) The relative health benefits of the different types of dietary fats is not clear and definitive studies have yet to be performed, although it is known that the more saturated, ie the greater the number of double bonds in the carbon chain of the fatty acid, the greater is the risk for atherosclerosis; see Fatty acids, Fish, Olive oil, Tropical oils; Cf Mineral oil

oil disease Yu-Cheng, see there

'oil droplet' appearance A descriptor of the early lesions of the corneal stroma, often with a refractory rim seen by ocular examination of children with galactosemia, which may develop into opacification within the first few postpartum weeks

oil red O SURGICAL PATHOLOGY A histologic stain for detecting neutral fat (triacylglycerides); optimal results are obtained with frozen tissues, as the paraffin-embedding process requires a fat-dissolving xylene step; oil red O positivity serves to distinguish thecomas from fibromas and supports the diagnosis of renal cell carcinoma, when the surgical pathologist is confronted with a clear cell tumor of unknown origin; fat stains are of little use in distinguishing liposarcoma from other sarcomas as the former may be negative and the latter positive; oil red O positivity may occur in ceroid or lipofuscin-rich tissues, demonstrating a speckled pattern

okadaic acid EXPERIMENTAL NEUROPHYSIOLOGY An inhibitor of protein phosphatases, PP1 and PP2, that prolongs ligand-gated channel openings and inhibits T antigen, mimics the stimulation of glucose transport into adipocytes by insulin and increases macrophage production of prostaglandin E_2

Okazaki fragments MOLECULAR BIOLOGY Segments of DNA that are produced in discontinuous replication BACKGROUND DNA replication (duplication) is a synthetic process that occurs in the 5'→3' direction using the antiparallel strand as a template; while replication of the 3'→5' mother strand forms a continuous 5'→3' daughter strand, replication of the 5'→3' mother strand occurs in the same 5'→3' direction, but only in short (circa 1000 nucleotide) segments known as Okazaki fragments in 'semi-continuous' replication, utilizing short RNA primers to begin the 5'→3' replication; linkage of the Okazaki fragments requires removal of the RNA, filling of the gaps and

nick ligation (figure, right); see Replication

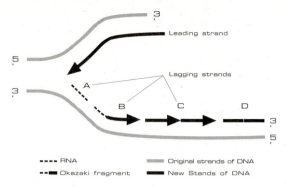

Okazaki fragments

okra sign A normal radiologic finding when the upper duodenal bulb is mildly twisted and filled with air, the cross-sectional view of which is fancifully likened to a transected okra (*Hibiscus esculentus*)

OKT4, **OKT8** see CD4 and CD8

old fluff INFECTIOUS DISASE A descriptive term for degenerated *Pneumoystis carinii* cysts and debris that do not stain with the GMS technique, which by LM have a granular and proteinacous appearance (Arch Pathol Lab Med 1995; 119:142OA)

'old man sleeping after dinner' NEUROLOGY A fanciful descriptor for the image evoked by a full-scale activation of the parasympathetic nervous system, which may be accompanied by bradycardia, bronchoconstriction resulting in noisy respiration, snoring, meiosis and increased salivation (drooling)

old soldier's heart Old sergeant syndrome A descriptive term for the predominantly cardiac symptoms of combat fatigue, seen in war-weary soldiers and consisting of precordial pain, dyspnea, exercise intolerance, mental and physical fatigue, dizziness, giddiness and palpitations, often precipitated by emotional and physical stress; see Combat fatigue

'Old Sparky' A generic (and ghoulishly facetious) term for any electric chair used in capital punishment; the original 'Old Sparky' is in Raiford, Florida, and continues in operation; the sobriquet is also used for the electric chair in New York State (New York Times 27 Nov 1994; p49), and elsewhere and derives from the fact that sparks often emanate from electrical wires when wet; see Capital punishment; Cf Hangman's fracture

oldest old GERIATRICS Individuals who are older than 85, the fastest growing age group in the US* and in developed nations; the expense of caring for the 'graying' population will become an enormous burden that may only begin to plateau in the year 2020; the two most costly non-fatal age-dependent diseases are dementia and osteoporosis, often associated with hip fractures high-resistance exercise training effectively counteracts muscle weakness and physical frailty in the OOs (N Engl J Med 1994; 330:1769OA) MORTALITY 3-year mortality in patients ≥ age 85 (Sweden) with vascular dementia is 67%, vs 23% of 85+-year-olds without dementia (N Engl J Med 1994; 330:164OA)

*Where there 3.5 million people ≥ 85 years of age, an increase of 232% from 1960, ♂:♀ ratio, 1:2.6; the US Census Bureau estimates that by the year 2040, there will be 8-24+ million in the ≥85 age group (for more demographic details and projections, see N Engl J Med 1994; 330:1819ED)

olestra Sucrose polyester A synthetic, no-calorie fat that has an appearance, taste, and texture virtually identical to fat, but unlike the usual dietary fats, is composed of three fatty acids linked to a glycerol, it is composed of eight fatty acids linked to glucose and is too big for digestion by the body's enzymes

O-level An English examination taken at age 16 by the more academically able students, including those who intend to attend university, which has been replaced by the GCSE; see Polytechnic; Cf A-level

olfactory hallucination Phantosmia The illusion of smelling a foul odor that is perceived to be either 1) Extrinsic, ie of non-self origin and which is mildly annoying but not a pervasive problem for the patient or 2) Intrinsic, ie perceived to emanate from the patient's own sweat, flatus or halitosis and which may prove overwhelmingly disconcerting to the patient

olfactory reference syndrome PSYCHIATRY A condition in which a person complains of unpleasant odors emanating from the skin or from a specific body orifice that is unrelated to any physiologic process (JAMA 1995; 273:1171; Acta Pychiatr Scand 1991; 47:484)

'oligo' see Oligonucleotide

oligoanalgesia A generic term for the underuse of analgesic medication in the face of valid indications (eg the intense bone pain typical of terminal cancer) for its use (JAMA 1993; 269:1537oc)

oligoclonal bands LABORATORY MEDICINE Multiple discrete bands in the γ region of cerebrospinal fluid electrophoresed on an agarose gel and stained with Coumassie blue; OBs, while nonspecific, are seen in 90-95% of patients with multiple sclerosis (corroborated by measuring myelin basic protein); OBs may also occur in other encephalopathies, to wit: herpetic encephalitis, bacterial or viral meningitis (40-60% of cases have bands), carcinomatosis, toxoplasmosis, neurosyphilis (60% positive), progressive multifocal leukoencephalopathy, subacute sclerosing panencephalitis (90% have bands), and may appear transiently in Guillain-Barré disease, lupus erythematosus vasculitis, amyotrophic lateral sclerosis, spinal cord compression, DM, cerebrovascular events

oligogene A gene which, when mutated, produces major phenotypic alterations, as it encodes segments of multiple structural genes; Cf Polygene

oligohydramnios A relative deficiency of amniotic fluid which occurs when the fetus swallows more often than usual, secondary to placental insufficiency, donor twin, urinary tract malformation

oligomeganephronia A condition that may be a subtype of renal hypoplasia, which is characterized by a markedly reduced number of nephrons with hypertrophy of the remaining nephrons; the kidneys are often small, the glomeruli are enlarged, as are the tubules, which may become cystic; it is often first identified in early childhood as a cause of polyuria, polydipsia, and growth failure; it is accompanied by a defect in urinary concentration, sodium reabsorption, and acid excretion, often resulting in metabolic acidosis and slow progression to chronic renal failure (N Engl J Med 1994; 33o:1072cPc)

oligonucleotide A short (10-100 bases or nucleotides) of DNA, often shortened by hard core cognoscenti in molecular biology to 'oligo'

olive oil CLINICAL NUTRITION A vegetable oil obtained from ripe fruit of *Olea europae*, which is used in foods, as a demulcent, and laxative; OO contains the highest (77%) level of monounsaturated fatty acids of all cooking oils; some evidence has favored the use of olive oil for reducing cholesterol; in one study of polyunsaturated fat-supplemented diets, HDL_2 was 50% higher, HDL_3 was 7% lower (resulting in a 23.5% total increase in HDL levels) and the apo-B, 5.4% higher than those using predominantly monounsaturated fats, data that contradicts some reports that olive oil is optimal in lowering cholesterol; never-

less, the high olive oil consumption and relatively low incidence of cardiovascular disease in Italians suggests a cause-and-effect relation between the two; Cf Fish oil, Tropical oils

Note: Olive oil is produced in Greece, Italy, Spain and Tunisia and is graded as pure (refined to remove acid), Virgin (a natural olive oil with 1-3.3% acid) and Extra virgin (less than 1% acid); the FDA (US) uses the adjectives Virgin (oil extracted after the first pressing) and Refined (extracted after a second pressing with chemicals added to reduce the acidity)

olive sign see Pyloric olive

olympic brow Marked thickening of the bony prominence of the forehead, due to persistent or recurrent periostitis, a classic manifestation of late congenital syphilis

OMB Office of Management and Budget, see there

omega-3 fatty acids n-3 fatty acids, see there

omega loop GI RADIOLOGY see Bird's beak sign MOLECULAR BIOLOGY A nonregular secondary protein structural motif composed of a segment of continuous polypeptide that traces a looped path in three-dimensional space; initially described as random coils, omega loops are often located on the protein's surface and thus assumed to have key roles in molecular function and biological recognition

omega oxidation A metabolic pathway for short 8-12 carbon fatty acids in which the terminal methyl group is first oxidized to a hydroxyl group then to a carbonyl group, leading to the formation of a dicarboxylic acid; seen-3 fatty acids

omega protein Type I topoisomerase An enzyme first discovered in *Escherichia coli* that relaxes negative supercoils in DNA without leaving nicks in the double helix; see DNA supercoiling, DNA topology

omega sign CLINICAL MEDICINE A sign seen in melancholia in which the patients have a furrowed brow due to sustained contraction of the corrugator muscle, which is often accompanied by Veraguth's folds, which are upward, inward peaking of the upper eyelids, a finding fancifully likened to the Greek letter omega

omental cake Pancake omentum, see there

omeprazole A benzimidazole analog that is effective in treating gastroesophageal reflux disease (GERD) resistant to H_2-receptor antagonists; omeprazole inhibits gastric secretion by altering the activity of the transmembrane proton pump, H+/K+-ATPase, which is the final step in acid secretion in the parietal cells of the stomach; omeprazole appears to be more effective than the H_2-receptor antagonists, eg cimetidine, ranitidine in treating duodenal and gastric ulcers, reflux esophagitis and Zollinger-Ellison syndrome (N Engl J Med 1991; 324:965rv) prolonged omeprazole therapy is associated with persistent ↑ in serum gastrin levels, atrophic gastritis, and micronodular argyrophilic cell hyperplasia (Annals Int Med 1994; 121:161)

–omics A neologistic vehicle popular in some English-speaking regions that allows marriage of the term economics to a particular politician, as in Reagonomics, Clintonomics

While this definition is peripheral to the raison d'être of the current work, the environment in which a physician practices and scientists perform research, are often affected by the finances of the politics 'du jour'-Author's note

OMS Organic brain syndrome, see there

Omsk hemorrhagic fever A tick-borne flavivirus infection occurring in the summer in the steppes of southwestern Siberia causing hemorrhage and encephalitis VECTOR Tick (*Dermacentor pictus*) CLINICAL Abrupt onset with high fever, headache, myalgia and prostration of 1-2 weeks in duration, hemorrhage from all orifices, anemia, leukopenia, thrombocytopenia, and albuminuria; the disease may also be biphasic, with the latter phase being more intense MORTALITY 1-2.5% TREATMENT Supportive, symptomatic, analgesic

'on campus' The on-site location of an area or section of a large medical center complex with multiple buildings; Cf 'Off campus'

onanism Coitus interruptus A term incorrectly equated to masturbation, but Onan's act was to spill his 'seed' on the ground during coitus with his brother's wife

onchocercal dermatopathy TROPICAL MEDICINE A generic term for any of several skin changes caused by infestation with *Onchocerca volvulus* microfilaria (onchocercosis), which is more common in the 'forest' strain than in the 'savanna' strain of *O volvulus* CLINICAL Itching of such severity as to interfere with sleep and work; the lesions may be thickened ('elephant skin'), roughened and shiny ('lizard skin') and discolored, changes that may result in social and occupational isolation TREATMENT Ivermectin (NY Times March 28 1995, C7) see River blindness

onchocerciasis River blindness A disease of littoral regions in tropical Africa and Latin America, caused by *Onchocerca volvulus* affecting ± 30 million people, the earliest immunogenic marker for *O volvulus* infection is designated OV-16 (Science 1991; 251:1603) AGENT *Onchocerca volvulus* VECTOR Blackfly, genus *Simulium* CLINICAL Although the adult may reach 0.5 m in length and travels under the skin causing pruritic bumps and scarring, the microfilaria are the most problematic, as they plug the lymphatic channels, causing elephantiasis, and blindness (punctate keratitis, pannus formation, corneal fibrosis, iridocyclitis, glaucoma and optic atrophy) PREVENTION Pesticides to eliminate blackflies, while impractical, are often used TREATMENT Ivermectin, 1-2 doses/year, which inhibits reproduction of the parasites and paralyzes the microfilaria, appears to be the current first line therapy, alternatively, diethylcarbamazine; see Ivermectin

oncocyte Oxyphilic cell An enlarged, pale eosinophilic epithelial cell filled with granular (mitochondria-laden) cytoplasm, with a high ATPase and oxidative enzyme activity; oncocytes increase with age and starvation, thus implying that oncocytes are associated with degenerative phenomena; oncocytes and benign oncocytomas occur in bronchial, lacrimal, salivary, parathyroid, and thyroid glands (Hürthle cell), the anterior pituitary and kidney; rarely, malignant oncocytomas occur in salivary glands, nasal cavity, paranasal sinuses, mediastinum and thyroid and the kidneys; renal oncocytomas are unique in that, unlike renal cell adenomas, they may become very large without being malignant and are considered by some authors to be renal cell carcinoma variants with a good prognosis (grade I tumors), which when the nuclei are atypical are designated as oncocytic renal cell carcinomas; other proliferations of oncocytes include oncocytic carcinoma of the pancreas, oncocytic carcinoid of the lungs, clinically similar to the 'garden variety' carcinoid and oncocytosis of the salivary gland, considered an age-related hyperplasia

oncofetal antigen ONCOLOGY Any of a number of antigens that are expressed in the fetus during embryogenesis, but which are not produced in significant quantities in adults; oncofetal antigens may re-appear during malignant dedifferentiation and include α-fetoprotein (AFP), which is elevated in 70% of hepatocellular carcinomas) and carcinoembryonic antigen (CEA), which is present in the fetal gut, liver and pancreas, and although it is elevated in many benign or malignant processes in adults, it is commonly used to monitor tumor recurrence in patients with known colonic adenocarcinoma

oncogene(s) A heterogeneous family of 'cancer genes' that are capable of inducing malignant transformation, which are derived from oncogenic RNA (oncorna-) viruses and from normal genes (proto-oncogenes); these genes are highly conserved in evolution and encode proteins vital to regulating gene expression or growth signal transduction; proto-oncogenes may undergo malignant transformation ('activation') by translocation, eg Philadelphia chromosome, gene amplification or by point mutation, eg K-*ras*; oncogenes are elucidated by either using the viruses that cause cancer (viral oncogenes or v-onc) in animals or by isolating tumorigenic genes from malignant cells; the human genome has more than 20 proto-oncogenes and cellular oncogenes (normal genes with tumorigenic potential); the presence of an oncogene is insufficient for carcinogenesis, as malignant transformation is a process that requires multiple genetic events or 'hits'; allelic loss is considered indicative of the presence of an anti-oncogene, eg the loss of 3p, 13q and 17p alleles occurs in various malignancies and may represent early transitional phases on the road to malignancy; oncogenes encode proteins of four types (table); see Proto-oncogene

oncogene theory A theory of carcinogenesis that attributes malignancy to activation of latent retroviral genes that are normally present within cells by radiation or carcinogens; once activated, the oncogenes 'drive' the cancer through synthesis of various hormones or possibly through assembly of a complete oncogenic virus; according to this theory, all cells have written in their genome the potential for malignant degeneration

oncogenic HPV A generic term for any human papillomavirus (HPV) genotype, in particular types 16, 18, and to a lesser extent types 31, 33, and 51, that have been temporally and pathogenically linked to the development of intraepithelial neoplasia, most often of the uterine cervix, commonly designated CIN; see CIN, HPV

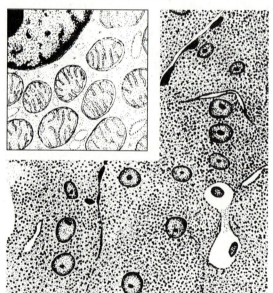

ooncocyte

oncogenic virus Any DNA virus, eg human papillomavirus or RNA virus, eg retrovirus that is capable of causing malignant transformation of cells

OncoLink An online service on the WWW (World Wide Web-address **http://cancer.med.upenn.edu**) that was created in March 1994 by LE Buhle and now operated by the University of Pennsylvania that has a vast array of information on cancer and therapies, and various cancer-related forums and postings; in March 1995 alone (after being in service only one year), OncoLink registered 350 000 'hits' from 100 countries, making it the largest non-government-operated medical Internet service in the world (Nature Medicine 1995; 1:502)

'Oncomouse' A proprietary transgenic mouse produced that carries human genes, which increases the mouse's susceptibility to cancer, serving as a tool for pharmaceutical and medical research; see Transgenic mouse

oncornavirus An obsolete term for oncogenic RNA viruses and retroviruses

oncostatin M A 196-amino acid monomeric cytokine produced by T cells and monocytes/marcophages that inhibits the growth of certain tumors, eg melanoma and solid tumors, and stimulates the growth of fibroblasts and Kaposi sarcoma cells

oncotope TUMOR BIOLOGY An epitope found on gene products that is unique to a tumor, which stimulate a B– and T–cell response during progressive tumor growth in a syngeneic or autochthonous host (**Bio/Technology 1994; 12:432**)

ondansetron A selective antagonist of serotonin S_3 receptors, used to ameliorate chemotherapy*-induced nausea and vomiting; combination with metopimazine (a dopamine D_2 receptor antagonist) may be more antiemetic than ondansetron alone (**N Engl J Med 1993; 328:1076OA**) in breast cancer treated with cyclophosphamide, methotrexate, and fluorouracil, ondansetron may be less effective than dexamethasone and metoclopramide (**N Engl J Med 1993; 329:1081OA**) see Chemotherapy-induced emesis

*eg Cisplatin, a chemotherapeutic (*cis*-dichloro-diamineplatinum) used to treat ovarian, testicular, urinary bladder, and head and neck cancers

Ondine's curse Sleep apnea syndrome, see there

one and one-half syndrome Fischer syndrome NEUROLOGY A unilateral pontine lesion involving both the medial longitudinal fasciculus and the pontine paramedian reticular formation, causing the combination of ipsilateral gaze palsy and internuclear ophthalmoplegia on the contralateral gaze; the only remaining horizontal movement is abduction of the contralateral eye; the eyes are straight or exodeviated ETIOLOGY Focal lesions of the brain stem, eg multiple sclerosis, primary or secondary tumors, eg glioma, hemorrhage or infarction, arteriovenous malformations and basilar artery aneurysm

one bone-two bone sign OBSTETRICS A simple method to differentiate the upper arm or thigh (each of which has one bone) from the forearm or lower legs (two bones) in evaluation of the fetus by ultrasonography

one-dimension gel quantification see Gel electrophoresis, Polyacrylamide gel electrophoresis

one-eyed vertebra RADIOLOGY A descriptor for the unilateral ('one-eyed') destruction of a lumbar vertebral pedicle, fancifully likened to the one-eyed jack of a deck of playing cards, where the 'nose' is contributed by the spinous process; the one-eyed vertebra is a rare finding seen on a plain anteroposterior film in carcinoma metastatic to a vertebral body, 'classically' of breast origin

one gene, one enzyme theory A hypothesis of historic interest that held that one gene encoded a specific enzyme or other protein, a posit now known to be correct in principle, but naïve, in that one gene encodes a polypeptide chain and a complete protein requires the splicing out of intervening sequences (introns) of mRNA, which are derived from 'junk' DNA, prior to the translation of mRNA into a protein

one-hit theory A hypothesis stating that red cell lysis occurs if the damage to only one site on the membrane is sufficient to evoke complement activation

one-hit, two-hit model of Knudson A hypothetical paradigm of mutagenesis that explains the disparity in the hereditary patterns in children with retinoblastoma, where one or two steps are required for cancerization; in brief, a malignancy may require homozygous mutated alleles; one mutated allele (the first 'hit) is inherited from a parent; the second allelic 'hit' may occur through environmentally-induced damage, initiating a tumor 'cascade' (**Proc Natl Acad Sci (USA) 1971; 68:820**); normal genes may also have antioncogenic properties; see Retinoblastoma, Tumor suppressor genes

Note: While the one hit-two hit model of carcinogenesis is being increasingly validated, most tumors are far more complex and require multiple 'hits' before becoming metastatic malignancies; in transgenic mice, the expression of the oncogene v-*jun* is insufficient alone to produce tumors but requires wounding, which provides a second epigenetic 'hit'

one-tail test STATISTICS A test of a null hypothesis* against an alternative hypothesis or hypotheses, which is assumed to be false in a particular direction; OTTs are used to test statistical significance in terms of being either greater or less than a value established by the hypothesis; Cf Two-tail test

*A hypothesis that is tested against an alternative hypothesis, which is nullified in favor of the alternative and subject to a certain level of error

one, two, three sign The finding of massive but discrete lymph nodes in the right paratracheal, right and left hilar regions, which is seen in a plain chest film of sarcoidosis; the sign may be a technical artifact as the same patients seen by tomography demonstrate *bilateral* paratracheal involvement

onion bulb formation Onion skin appearance, see there

onion skin appearance A pattern characterized by concentric laminations of differing radiologic or histologic densities, described in BONE RADIOLOGY Laminated periosteal reaction due to neo-osteogenesis, either benign, eg osteomyelitis, pulmonary hypertrophic osteoarthropathy, rickets or malignant, which may be coarse laminations, eg osteosarcoma or delicate laminations with periosteal layering, eg Ewing sarcoma HEMATOPATHOLOGY Concentric fibrosis of the splenic central and penicilliary arteries, characteristic of lupus erythematosus, most common in those with thrombocytopenic purpura HEPATIC PATHOLOGY Concentric lamellar fibrosis surrounding medium-sized bile ducts in the portal spaces of livers with sclerosing cholangitis, which may be accompanied by aggregates of lymphocytes with germinal centers and granulomas GI PATHOLOGY Concentric perivascular arrangement of fibroblasts and loose collagen seen by the Masson trichrome stain in gastric inflammatory fibroid polyps MALIGNANT HYPERTENSION 'Onion skin' changes are descriptive of concentric arterial thickening with progressive luminal narrowing, due to hyperplasia of the smooth muscle cells and basement membrane reduplication, which may be accompanied by necrosis and fibrinoid deposits (necrotizing arteriolitis) and ischemic damage with renal involvement; similar changes may occur in the gallbladder, periadrenal fat, peripancreatic intestinal arterioles NEUROPATHOLOGY A term referring to the connective fibrous tissue surrounding the periaxon in Dejerine-Sottas disease, a neuropathy due to incomplete spinal cord injury specifically to the trigeminal nerve, characterized by hypalgesia or analgesia that spreads centrifugally in a laminated fashion; alternately in the peripheral nervous system; 'onion skinning' may also be due to repetitive myelination and demyelination, in large peripheral myelinated nerves in Charcot-Marie-Tooth and Roussy-Levy syndromes (onion-bulb formation) OBSTETRICS Laminated pockets of myometrial gas, seen in septic abortions, especially due to *Clostridium perfringens*; despite the severity of clinical disease, hysterectomy may not be necessary, if the uterine cavity is curetted and antibiotic therapy is adequate VASCULAR PATHOLOGY Perivascular collagen deposition as seen in lupus erythematosus, in necrotizing arteriolitis and in any stage of syphilitic obliterative endarteritis with proliferation of the endothelial cells with luminal narrowing

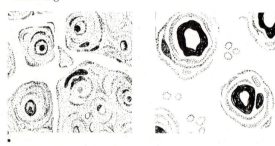

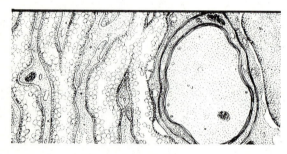

onion bulb appearance

on-line *adjective* Pertaining or referring to a direct connection with a computer, most commonly referring to a successful hookup with a host computer in client server network (B Pfaffenberger, Computer User's Dictionary, 4th ed, Que Corp, Indianapolis)

on-off phenomenon NEUROLOGY An increasing refractoriness to L-dopa's ability to control the smooth movement of skeletal muscle in Parkinson's disease; the phenomenon is characterized by a fluctuating response in which there are periods of excessive abnormal movements ('on') alternating with periods of prolonged immobility or freezing periods ('off') (see N Engl J Med 1992; 327:1549OA) the term 'on-off' also refers to the waxing and waning of the parkinsonism itself

ONPG *o*-nitrophenyl β-D-galactopyranoside MICROBIOLOGY A substance used for determining the presence of β-galactosidase in bacteria (present in *Escherichia coli*) causing the release of the yellow *o*-nitrophenol into the medium; the test may be used to differentiate lactose-delayed organisms from lactose-negative organisms and to differentiate *Pseudomonas cepacia* and *P maltophilia* (positive) from other *Pseudomonas* spp (negative)

'ontogeny recapitulates phylogeny' EVOLUTIONARY BIOLOGY A postulate that holds that some stages in the development of an individual (ontogeny) repeat certain aspects in the evolutionary development of a species of organisms (phylogeny)

onyalai A variant of ITP described in males of the Bantu tribe, possibly related to vitamin C deficiency and characterized by perioral and periorbital hemorrhagic vesicles and bullae

O'nyong-nyong fever A dengue-like alphavirus infection of East Africa VECTOR *Anopheles funestus* CLINICAL

Abrupt onset of fever, frontal or retro-orbital headaches, an early generalized, blanching macular rash, and severe arthralgias EKG Sinus bradycardia, ventricular ectopia, prolonged P-R interval, flattened T waves LABORATORY Pancytopenia, acidosis, hemoconcentration TREATMENT Symptomatic, supportive

OP-1 Osteogenic protein 1 A protein used to pack tooth roots, and may be of use in regenerating dentin (Sci Am 1993; 269/5:106)

OPD syndrome Otopalatodigital syndrome, see there

o, p'-DDD Minotane A therapeutic agent derived from insecticides that selectively destroys (by blocking mitochondrial activity and inhibiting steroid synthesis) both normal and neoplastic adrenal cortex (zona fasciculata and reticularis); o,p'-DDD is used to treat adrenocortical carcinoma; the patients become hormonal 'cripples' requiring supplements of glucocorticoids and mineralocorticoids SIDE EFFECTS Anorexia, nausea, diarrhea, vomiting, skin rashes, gynecomastia, arthralgia, and leukopenia

open architecture COMPUTERS Any computer system with design specifications that are made public so as to allow unrelated companies to develop add-on products that will adapt to the computer

open artery theory Open infarct-related artery theory CARDIOLOGY A widely-accepted theory based on Blumgart et al's work (Am Heart J 1941; 22:374) in dogs subjected to transient ischemia, in which the duration of occlusion affects the extent of infarction; this theory forms the basis for modern therapy for acute MI, and holds that early reperfusion of the infarct-related coronary artery translates into myocardial salvage, improved ventricular function, and survival; the first studies (GISSI-2, ISIS-3) of the effects of reperfusion agents, eg t-PA and streptokinase, found no benefit of attaining early patency in the affected arteries, a finding that shook the cardiology community for its seeming lack of logic (some workers believe there are major flaws in some clinical mega-trials)–a more recent study (GUSTO) may support Blumgart's work—early reperfusion, in particular with t-PA, which may improve survival; a key factor is the rapidity with which thrombolytic therapy is begun (N Engl J Med 1993; 329:1650ED)

open enrollment HEALTH CARE INDUSTRY A stance adopted by some state 'Blues' (Blue Cross/Blue Shield) that accepts all individuals, regardless of their individual medical history, life style, occupation, or potential disease risk factors (Am Med News 25 October 1992, p7)

'open-face sandwich' domain A type of 3-D protein structural motif seen in the enzyme RuBisCO in which one surface is exposed to solvent; the enzyme initiates photosynthesis and is comprised of 8 large and 8 small subunits

open heart surgery A generic term for surgery in which the pericardial cavity is 'violated' in order to gain access and repair, on an elective or emergent basis, conditions directly affecting the heart, great vessels of the heart, coronary arteries, or valves; the most commonly-performed elective open heart procedure is a coronary artery bypass graft, typically performed on an older white male; 15% of these procedures are limited to valvoplasty; factors adversely affecting the outcome of OHS include a subsequent need for reoperation, recent MI, dialysis dependency, DM, congestive heart failure and a low ventricular ejection fraction; see Atherosclerosis, Coronary artery bypass graft; Heart-lung machine

open protocol system CLINICAL PHARMACOLOGY An FDA-approved protocol that allows the use of drugs or other therapeutic agents outside of a controlled trial (and prior to approval of these agents by the FDA); open protocols may be indicated for patients with terminal disease for which there is no known cure or for a condition that has failed to respond to standard therapies; although drug efficacy data cannot be generated, as the cases are single and usually scattered among multiple health care institutions and care-givers, ie 'anecdotal' in nature, side effects and potential complications can be determined, and added to the pool of information weighed in whether to approve a therapeutic agent; see Compassionate IND protocol

open reading frame A long uninterrupted sequence of mRNA that begins with the start codon AUG, and ends with (but does not itself contain) a stop codon (UAG, UGA, UAA); most ORFs have been assigned to proteins, the remainder are called URFs or unassigned reading frames

open set speech AUDIOLOGY Speech without referential cues (N Engl J Med 1993; 328:281ED)

open system architecture COMPUTERS A design of a computerized information system that uses a network manager (a centralized electronic 'clearinghouse') to retrieve data and send it back to the requester; the OSA philosophy circumvents many of the problems inherent in integrating the diverse elements of hospital information systems, since it allows each individual department, eg laboratories, pharmacy, finances, and others to choose the hardware and software most appropriate for its particular needs; see Computer, Hospital information system, LAN

opera glass hand Main-en-lorgnette, see there

operable *adjective* Pertaining or referring to a condition, usually understood to be malignant that is amenable to operation, with an attendent ↑ in survival; Cf Inoperable

operant *adjective* Pertaining or relating to a response or pattern of responses that are contingent or influenced by their impact on the environment or a situation, and/or the ability of the response(s) to achieve reward or reinforcement

operating system COMPUTERS The software that allows a computer to respond to system commands and to run applications programs, eg word-processing, databases and other applications, eg Microsoft™'s MS/DOS is a standard disk operating system in the IBM and IBM 'clone' types of microcomputers

operating team The participants in a sterile surgical operation that is performed under general (less commonly, local) anesthesia, divided into the scrubbed sterile members, including the surgeon, assistants to the surgeon (commonly understood to be licensed physicians, although other persons may fill this role in routine procedures) and a scrub nurse; the nonsterile team members include the anesthesiologist, a circulating nurse, a pathologist, should an intraoperative consultation be required and technical personnel to operate complicated devices, eg heart-lung machine or intraoperative blood salvage devices, used during the procedure

Operation Ranch Hand ENVIRONMENT A herbicide-spraying program carried out during the Vietnam conflict between 1961 and 1971 that used agent Orange (2,3,7,8-tetrachlorodibenzo-p-dioxin, TCDD, intracorporal half-life, seven years); the mean residual TCDD level in non-exposed Vietnam veterans is 5 parts per trillion (ppt), the mean in 'Ranch Handers', 49 ppt and in the highly exposed, 200-2000 ppt (MMWR 1988; 37:309; those exposed have been reported to have a 50% ↑ in skin cancer, predominantly of basal cell carcinoma (JAMA 1995; 273:1494Q&A) see WA Buckingham, Operation Ranch Hand: The Air Force and Herbicides in Southeast Asia, 1961, Washington DC, US Air Force, 1982); see Dioxin

operative microscopy see Microsurgery

operative mortality Percentage of patients who die while hospitalized during or after an operative procedure

operative report A document produced by the physician(s) who have participated in an interventional procedure, which contains a detailed account of the findings, the technical procedure used, the specimens removed, the preoperative and postoperative diagnoses, and the names of the primary performing practitioner and any assistants; the OR report is usually dictated shortly after the procedure and is usually accompanied by summary notes in a patient's chart that summarizes the salient points of the procedure

operator (gene) A segment of DNA adjacent to one or more structural genes, which controls the transcription of the genes by the presence or absence of repressor proteins

operon The functional unit of transcription, which contains an operator, its cognate repressor protein, and the gene that the operator-repressor dyad controls; see Transcription unit

ophthalmia neonatorum Acute neonatal conjunctivitis A condition that in a broad sense could refer to any inflammation of the neonatal conjunctiva, but which commonly refers to conjunctival infection by either *Neisseria gonorrhoeae* or *Chlamydia trachomatis*; ON was the main cause of blindness in 19th-century Europe, and still causes blindness in up to 4000 newborns/year in Africa alone TREATMENT Silver nitrate, erythromycin and other antibiotics; povidone-iodine is reported to be more effective, and less costly and toxic; moreover, its antiviral activity includes HIV and herpes simplex (N Engl J Med 1995; 332:562OA)

ophthalmologist A physician trained in the diagnosis and treatment of diseases of the eye who may prescribe drugs and perform surgery EDUCATION Twelve years (four years each of college or university, medical school, and residency); Cf Orthoptist, Optician, Optometrist

opiate A generic term for any natural (eg opium), semi-synthetic (eg morphine) or synthetic (eg fentanyl), usually alkaloid narcotic agent with opium-like activity

opioid peptides Endogenous opiates A group of natural polypeptide neurotransmitters that are involved in the perception of pain, response to stress, regulation of appetite and sleep, memory and learning, which are derived from three precursor molecules (prodynorphin, proenkephalin A and proopiomelanocortin or POMC), giving rise to more than 20 endogenous opioids, all of which have the same amino terminal tetrapeptide (Tyr-Gly-Gly-Phe); presence of opioids in tumors may indicate neuroendocrine differentiation

Opitz' BBBG syndrome G syndrome, see there

opium A narcotic first used by the Romans, extracted from the unripe seedpod of the poppy, *Papaver somniferum*; morphine was extracted from opium by a German pharmacist Sertuerner; other opiates later derived from opium include heroin and the less potent and less addicting codeine; see Heroin, Narcotics

OPLL Ossification of the posterior longitudinal ligament, see Dagger sign

opportunistic INFECTIOUS DISEASE *adjective* Pertaining or referring to a microorganism[1] that may be part of the normal nonpathogenic flora[2], which causes disease should the opportunity arise, eg through a compromise of the host's immune status

[1]Or the disease/infection it evokes [2]eg of the colon, upper respiratory tract, genitourinary tract, or skin

opportunistic infection An infection caused by a microorganism, usually bacterial that is part of the normal 'flora', which becomes pathogenic when the host's immune system is compromised by an unrelated disease, eg AIDS, chemotherapy, or DM

opsin A transmembrane protein that is the major component in the photoreceptor, rhodopsin, which has seven membrane-spanning helices and interacts with the transducing G proteins; Cf Retinal

opsoclonus-myoclonus Dancing eyes-dancing feet syndrome, see there

opsonin Greek, to make appetizing A generic term for any substance or 'factor' that binds to RBCs, bacteria or other exogenous agents, increasing their susceptibility to phagocytosis, including antibodies, complement proteins and basement membrane components, eg fibronectin; relative strengths of opsonins in humans: IgG3 > IgG1 > IgG2, C3b

optical disk archiving COMPUTERS A format for storing the original image of a paper ('hard') copy of a record, allowing its retrieval for legal purposes, without the need to store the bulkier paper copy (see **CAP Today November 1993**)

optical immunoassay An immunoassay in which a specific immobilized antibody is bound to an optical thin film on a silicon wafer; when a sample is placed on the silicon wafer, the immobilized antibody captures the antigen in the sample, increasing the thickness of the film, altering the path of the reflected light, which is perceived as a color change; OIA allows rapid (ie minutes) detection of group A β-hemolytic streptococcus (Strep A OIA™ test-Biostar Inc), and is of potential use for rapid detection of a wide range of specimens, eg blood, sputum, CSF, and analytes, eg antibodies, antigens, haptens, and other molecules of various size (**Am Clin Lab May 1994**)

optical tweezers A tool in cell biology in which a beam of laser light is used to manipulate subcellular organelles, creating an optical trap or allow measurement of mechanical forces of motor molecules including myosin, kinesin and dynein

optician A health care worker who grinds eyeglasses and fits contact lenses according to a prescription written by optometrists and (less commonly) by ophthalmologists EDUCATION One- to two-year apprenticeship or training program Note: Not all states in the US require licensing of opticians; Cf Ophthalmologist, Optometrist

opticokinetic nystagmus Railroad nystagmus NEUROLOGY A normal bilateral optical response to objects moving slowly across a field of vision, which is thought to result from a combination of pursuit and refixation saccades; this response may be calibrated by varying the size and speed of the moving objects and has been likened to the constant refixation of the eyes that occurs when people view fixed objects while seated in a moving railroad; Cf 'Seesaw' nystagmus

Optochin (disk) test P disc test MICROBIOLOGY Optochin is a quinine derivative with detergent-like activity, causing selective lysis of *Staphylococcus pneumoniae* at low concentrations (< than 5 µg/ml), typically the zone of lysis around a 6 mm paper disc impregnated with optochin is 14 mm; lack of inhibition by optochin implies that the organism on the growth plate is not *S pneumoniae*; Cf MIC (minimum inhibitory concentrations)

optometrist A health care worker qualified to examine the eyes and related structures in order to identify abnormalities; optometrists prescribe eyeglasses and other visual aids, but are not qualified to establish a definitive diagnosis, prescribe drugs, or perform surgery EDUCATION 6 years (2 + years of college education and 4 years of optometry school); Cf Ophthalmologist, Optician

OR Operating room, operating suite; also odds ratio

Also 1) Observed ratio 2) Oil retention 3) Oleoresin (pharmacology) 4) Oligomer restriction (molecular biology) 5) Operation record (often termed OR notes) 6) Organ recovery 7) Orosomucoid 8) Orthopedic 9) Out of range

OR notes A generic term for a document, usually written by the surgeon, that delineates in relative detail, the course of a surgical procedure; ONs variously include reasons for the operation and details about the patient's status prior to the procedure, type of procedure, and means of access into the field of operation, time required for the operation, and patient's status upon completion of the procedure

oral contraceptive A preparation of synthetic hormones intended to render a ♀ inconceivable through inhibition of ovulation; there are two formats of OCs, combined method and sequential method; the sequential method, in which an estrogen pill was taken for each of 15-16 days, has been abandoned (in the US) as it has been linked in epidemiologic studies to an ↑ in endometrial cancer; in the combined method, an estrogen/progestin pill is popped for each of 21 days; recent epidemiologic study of 2203 ♀ with and 2009 ♀ without breast cancer has shown a 2-3 fold ↑ in breast cancer among OC users*, especially those who bagan use at a younger age (**LA Brinton in 7 June JNCI, in Science News 1995; 147:356**) see Contraceptives; Cf Norplant, RU-486

Note: These data are controversial as other studies have reached opposite conclusions

oral rehydration therapy PUBLIC HEALTH A treatment modality directed at correcting dehydration diarrhea; the most accepted form of administration is the 'dry pack' distributed by UNICEF and the WHO, which contains 3.5 g NaCl, 2.5 g $NaHCO_3$, 1.5 g KCl and 20 g of glucose to be dissolved in one liter of water, given per os; despite the relatively low cost, there may be economic barriers to the use of commercial rehydration solutions (**JAMA 1991; 265:1724**) Cf Ringer's lactate

oral tolerization A therapeutic modality in the early stages of development based on ancient Chinese medicine, which is likened to vaccination via the GI tract; OT appears to be effective against a wide range of conditions that develop in a background of autoimmunity, eg multiple sclerosis, and may be effective in treating rheumatoid arthritis, type I diabetes (IDDM), in ameliorating or preventing organ rejection in transplant patients (**New York Times 18 October; C1**)

Orange book CLINICAL PHARMACOLOGY Approved Drug Products with Therapeutic Equivalence Evaluations; a document (**Publication # 917-016-00000-3**) produced by the US Government Printing Office, listing the FDA-approved generic equivalents of brand-name drugs

orange suit Racal space suit, see there

orangeophilia CYTOLOGY A term of waning popularity for a finding by light microscopy that corresponds to a vague attempt to form keratin on the part of some cells of poorly-differentiated epidermoid carcinomas; a peculiar variant is described in which the cytoplasm has a 'pumpkin orange' color, which is held by some to be relatively specific for squamous cell carcinoma of the head and neck region

orange peel skin appearance Peau d'orange appearance, see there

orange person syndrome A rare clinical condition caused by an overdose of rifampin, which colors the skin and body fluids a deep orange, accompanied by altered hepatic function (elevated bilirubin, alkaline phosphatase and transaminase levels) and pruritus

Note: The skin of subjects ingesting excess carotinoids, eg 'carrot diet' may also have a deep orange hue, which is of merely cosmetic interest, as it resolves by appropriate dietary alterations; see Red man syndrome

orcein HISTOLOGY A brownish material containing 14 different substances produced when orcinol is oxidized in ammonia water; orcein is used to stain elastic fiber, chromosomes and, before the availability of immunoperoxidase stains for hepatitis B antigens, to identify hepatitis B surface antigens in the tissue of chronic carriers

Note: Orcein stains for identifying hepatitis has been replaced by in situ hybridization

order see Orders

ordered test A unit of productivity in the hospital laboratory equal to a billable test in the commercial laboratory; see Billable test

orderly *adjective* Neat, organized, when pathologically so, compulsive *noun* An assistant or other health care worker who in general scuttles about (lifting, pushing, pulling, delivering) at the virtual bottom of the medical 'food chain', and who takes orders from virtually everyone in the hospital, except from medical students who in teaching hospitals *ARE* at the food chain; Cf Scut-monkey

orders Any written (or less commonly verbal) 'command' on the part of an attending physician that clearly and specifically delineates how a diagnostic or therapeutic intervention is to be carried out by responsible supporting staff; orders are usually written (and if not, verbally with appropriate documentation of any specific changes) in the patient's chart or active medical record, and most commonly indicate doses of medication(s) specified in the metric system, route of administration, length of treatment, and time of discontinuation

Oregon Plan HEALTH CARE REIMBURSEMENT A legislative modification of the US State of Oregon's Medicaid program that has become a focus of debate on all aspects of the US national health policy, including access to limited services, costs, effectiveness, rationing of services and provision of basic care; the Oregon plan is an attempt to reconcile the finite financial resources with the virtually ceiling-less needs for health care; Oregon will fund a prioritized list of about 600 services, designed as a comprehensive health benefit package for the poor (who are covered under the auspices of the Medicaid program); priority services that are reimbursed include pneumococcal pneumonia, various acute infections and intoxications, heart failure and physical and sexual abuse, including rape; not covered under the plan is artificial insemination, acute tonsillitis, end-stage HIV disease and counseling for obesity (Clin Lab Sci 1994; 7:137F; N Engl J Med 1992; 327:642c)

orf Ecthyma contagiosum A benign self-limited parapoxvirus infection acquired by handling infected sheep and goat skins and flesh, which in young animals causes watery warty lesions of the cornea, mucous membranes, and lips CLINICAL Hypertrophic bullae at the site of inoculation, which in the immunocompromised patient, may be very large AGENT The orf virus is similar to that which causes milker's nodes

ORF Open reading frame, see there

organ bank A repository, usually shared by multiple hospitals for relatively long-term storage of certain tissues destined for transplantation, including acellular bone fragments, bone marrow and corneas; other major organs, eg heart, lung, liver, kidneys and pancreatic islets are not stored in organ banks as their viability is limited to 48-72 hours and require immediate transplantation; Cf UNOS

organ-based specialty A generic term for any specialty (or subspecialty) of medicine or surgery that is focused on the diagnosis and treatment of diseases of a particular organ or organ system, eg neurology, neuropathology, neuroradiology, neurosurgery, etc

organ brokerage TRANSPLANTATION The sale of an organ[1], eg a kidney by a living donor, or any commercial transaction in which an organ for transplantation is obtained through coercion (JAMA 1991; 265:1302) India had been the site of some of the most flagrant OB, which culminated with the break-up of a kidney racket[2] and the arrest of 4 prominent physicians who were charged with removing at least 1000 kidneys in two years; as of February 1995, trading in human organs was outlawed in India (Nature Medicine 1995; 1:190)

[1]In the USA, medical centers involved in organ procurement traditionally rely on altruism as a source for organs, as the National Organ Transplant Act (Public law 98-507, 3 USC) makes it illegal to acquire, receive, or transfer any human organ for valuable consideration [2]Kidney, anyone?

organ cluster transplantation A procedure used in primary upper abdominal malignancy affecting the biliary tract, duodenum or stomach with secondary involvement of the liver; the Pittsburgh group resected all or most of the stomach, liver, pancreas, spleen and major portions of the small and large intestine, filling the structural and functional void with an 'organ cluster graft' comprised of the liver, pancreas, duodenum and a portion of the jejunum; while seemingly 'heroic' in scope, 8 of the 10 were alive at 3 to 9 months with adequate hepatic and pancreatic function; Cf Heroic surgery

organotherapy MEDICAL HISTORY The ingestion of any of a cornucopia of human and nonhuman tissues to cure diseases or improve performance, eg the heart for courage, brain to treat idiocy, and other body parts including bile, blood, bone, feces, feathers, placenta, which were intended to address various evil humors; organotherapy using various forms of testicular tissue or extracts was more therapeutically successful, and through early work by CE Brown-Séquard*, was a founding event of modern endocrinology (Sci Am 1995; 272/2:77)

*Who in 1889 at the age of 72 reported that he had reversed his own aging by using liquid extracts from the testicles of dogs and guinea pigs; modern workers believe the positive effects reported by BS were placebo in nature; however, his principle of hormonal replacement therapy is correct

organ-limited autopsy A generic term for a postmortem examination that is restricted to one organ (or body region); OLAs have the advantages of providing final histologic confirmation of neoplasms identified by imaging modalities (CT, MRI) antemortem, of ensuring high-quality medical care, and are more often permitted by family members who would otherwise refuse permission for a more extensive autopsy that might evoke negative images in the bereavement period (Arch Pathol Lab Med 1995; 119:440oA) see Autopsy

'organ' panel(s) Laboratory diagnosis-related groups A group of diagnostic tests that have been determined to be the most cost-effective, sensitive and specific for evaluation of a particular diseased organ, organ system or disease (JB Henry, CLINICAL DIAGNOSIS AND MANAGEMENT, 18th ed, WB Saunders, 1991) see Anemia panel, Bone/joint panel, Cardiac injury panel, Cardiac risk evaluation panel, Collagen disease and arthritis panel, Collagen disease/lupus erythematosus panel, Coma panel, Diabetic panel, Electrolyte/fluid balance panel, General health panel, Hepatitis (immunopathology) panel, Hypertension panel, Kidney panel, Liver panel, Metastatic disease panel, Neoplasm panel, Pancreatic panel, Parathyroid panel, Pulmonary panel, Thyroid panel, TORCH panel

'organ recital' PSYCHIATRY The listing by a hypochondriac of a litany of complaints from multiple organs and organ systems; the physician may himself naïvely perpetuate the 'illness', as the patient is gratified by a relationship that can only be maintained as long as the subject is perceived to be sick; see Factitious 'disease', Munchausen syndrome; Cf Ulysses syndrome

organ shortage The gap between the amount of organs transplanted and the number needed; the waiting list for kidneys is 24 973 patients as of December 1993; in 1990 the median waiting time was 420 days, and has grown; 935 died while waiting; ± 30-50/10⁶ cadaveric kidneys are potentially available annually; $17/10^6$ are procured (N Engl J Med 1994; 331:365Rv) see UNOS; Cf Organ brokerage

organic acidemia A clinical presentation of 'inborn errors of metabolism', often first seen in infants who present with poor feeding, vomiting, tachypnea, acidosis, hyperammonemia, ketosis, ketonuria, irritability, and convulsions or hypotonia and lethargy, findings that are otherwise suggestive of neonatal sepsis; diseases accompanied by organic acidemia include isovaleric and propionic acidemias, maple syrup urine disease, medium chain acyl dehydrogenase deficiency, glutaric, methylmalonic and formiminoglutamic acidurias

organic brain syndrome NEUROLOGY Cerebral degeneration in the form of cortical atrophy with 'simplification' of myelinated tracts, a process that is usually irreversible, often age-related and associated with atherosclerosis; see Lacunar state, Multi-infarct dementia PSYCHIATRY A generic term for any alteration of the mental status, behaviors, and mood which is caused by organic disease, including alcoholic liver disease (hepatic encephalopathy), infections (AID dementia), renal failure (uremia), and others

organic foods A broadly-defined category of comestibles that in the purest form, are grown without reliance on chemical fertilizers or pesticides; see Health food; Cf Enriched food, Fortified food, Refining

organic mood syndrome, manic type A persistently expansive or elevated mood, caused by nonpsychogenic conditions that may be evident by history, physical examination or laboratory tests, often affecting subjects older than age 35, due to CNS infections, eg viral and cryptococcal meningitides, neurosyphilis, trauma, eg thalamotomy, right hemispherectomy, tumors either primary or metastatic, vascular accidents, eponymic disorders, including Klinefelter syndrome and Huntington's, Kleine-Levin, Parkinson's, Pick's and Wilson's diseases, carcinoid tumor, idiopathic cerebral calcification, hyperbaric oxygen therapy, systemic disease, endocrine, eg hyperthyroidism, hypothyroidism with starvation diet, puerperal and premenstrual psychoses, systemic infections, eg Q fever, infectious mononucleosis, renal failure, eg uremia, hemodialysis, drugs, eg bromide, bromocriptine, cocaine, corticosteroids, H_2-blocking agents, isoniazid, L-dopa, phencyclidine, procainamide, procarbazine, thyroid preparations, hypovitaminosis, including decreased vitamin B_{12} and niacin

Note: The term used in the DSM-IV (*Diagnostic and Statistical Manual of Mental Disorders, 4th ed, Washington, DC, American Psychiatric Association, 1994*) is the relatively cumbersome 'Mood disorder due to general medical condition-with manic features'

organic peroxide An organic compound containing a bivalent –O–O– 'motif' that is a derivative of H_2O_2, in which one or both of the H^+ ions have been replaced by an organic radical

organicism see Alternative medicine

organizer EMBRYOLOGY Any of a number of regions of the early embryo that controls morphologic differentiation and fate of other regions, eg by secreting graded concentrations of a particular growth factor

organoid A synthetic 'organ' that has some properties, eg angiogenic and secretory capacities of an organ; the first generation organoids are composed of Gore-Tex, collagen, heparin-binding growth factor-1 and endothelial cells with an inserted gene and have therapeutic potential as delivery systems for CD4 in the treatment of AIDS, Alzheimer's and other diseases; see Biohybrid artificial pancreas; Cf Liposome

ORI Office of Research Integrity, see there

Oriental flush complex A facial erythema seen in up to 80% of Orientals who drink alcohol, possibly due to an atypical isomer of alcohol dehydrogenase that causes rapid metabolism of ethanol and high acetaldehyde levels

Oriental sore A form of cutaneous leishmaniasis occurring in 1) The Near East Desert rodent HOSTS *Rhombomys opimus, Psammomys obesus* VECTOR Sandfly *Phlebotomus papatasii* or 2) Mediterranean rim and subsaharan Africa HOST *Procavia* species VECTOR *Phlebotomus longipes* CLINICAL OSs begin as erythematous papules on the face or extremities 2-8 weeks after exposure; the papule later vesiculates, pustulates and ulcerates, the dry form is crusted, the wet form, oozing TREATMENT Most lesions spontaneously heal in six months, otherwise pentavalent antimony

ORIF Open reduction of an internal fracture

origin LABORATORY TECHNOLOGY The point of application in a chromatogram or an electrophoretic gel of a specimen or sample MOLECULAR BIOLOGY The point in a sequence of DNA at which replication is initiated

'origin-of-life' experiment An experiment used to clarify the chemical reactions that occurred on primitive (prebiotic) earth; in the original Miller-Urey experiment, a mixture of ammonia, formaldehyde, and hydrogen cyanide in a closed vessel was subjected to continuous electrical discharges (simulating lightning on the primitive planet), resulting in formation of glycine, alanine, valine, and other amino acids (Sci Am 1994; 271/4:77) see Bubble hypothesis

'original antigenic sin' IMMUNOLOGY The tendency to produce antibodies to an epitope or antigenic determinant that resembles a determinant on an antigen encountered previously, thus being similar to a secondary immune response

Note: The term derives from the biblical story of Adam in the Garden of Eden, who fell from God's grace, committing the 'original sin' of eating a forbidden fruit, forever dooming humanity to inherit sin

Ornish regimen A diet consisting of beans, bean curd, grains, maximum of two ounces of alcohol, fruits, vegetables, weekly sessions of 'meditation' and stress management PROHIBITED Meat, poultry, fish, egg yolks, caffeine, dairy products (except one cup of fat-free yogurt); no fat or oil added to foods RESULT Weight loss; 39% ↓ in total cholesterol, 59% ↓ in LDL-cholesterol; see Diet

ornithinemia, type I HHH (hyperornithinemia, hyperammonemia, and homocitrullinuria) syndrome, see there

ornithinemia, type II Gyrate atrophy (with ornithine aminotransferase deficiency), see there

ornithine transcarbamylase A homotrimeric (36-kD subunits) mitochondrial matrix enzyme* [EC 2.1.3.3] that catalyzes the conversion of ornithine and carbamyl phosphate to citrulline in the urea cycle; OTC is expressed in the liver and intestine and its mitochondrial activity is required for ammonia detoxification

*Also known as ornithine carbamoyltransferase, the term recommended (1992) by the Nomenclature Committee of the IUBMB (International Union of Biochemistry and Molecular Biology)

ornithine transcarbamylase deficiency An X-D [MIM 311250] condition characterized by chronic hyperammonemia, with episodic hyperirritability, vomiting, and lethargy, protein avoidance, ataxia, coma, growth and developmental delay, and often mental deterioration caused by a mutation in the ornithine transcarbamylase (OTC) gene MOLECULAR PATHOLOGY The OTC gene maps to Xp21.1; OTC also maps to the X chromosome in mice, which, when mutated (C-to-A transversion) causes the sparse fur phenotype; see Hyperammonemia

Oroya fever An infection by *Bartonella bacilliformis*, the cutaneous or verrucous form was long known in Peru; the acute form was first recognized in 1870 during construction of the railway from Lima to Oroya, the bacterial nature of the condition was established by D Carrion, a medical student who inoculated himself with verrucous material and subsequently died therefrom EPIDEMIOLOGY Most common in northern South America, where the sandfly vector, *Phlebotomus verrucarum* flourishes CLINICAL The onset may be either insidious or abrupt and accompanied by high fever, chills, diaphoresis, headaches, changes in the mental status, brisk hemolysis causing marked anemia (0.5×10^{12}/L; US: 500 000/mm³) and a leukemoid reaction, followed by myalgias, arthralgias, dyspnea, insomnia, angina, delirium (and if extreme, coma and death in 30% of cases), accompanied by thrombocytopenic purpura and lymphadenopathy; the verrucous form may follow Oroya fever or be the only sign of infection TREATMENT Chloramphenicol (to prevent the frequent complications of salmonellosis), blood transfusion PREVENTION DDT

spraying to eliminate sandfly vector

Orphan Annie eye nuclei SURGICAL PATHOLOGY A descriptor for the nuclei characteristic of the follicular variant of papillary carcinoma of the thyroid, which are large, round-to-oval and cleared of chromatin, fancifully likened to the vacuous eyes of Little Orphan Annie

Li'l Orphan Annie is the heroine of a comic strip by the same name created in 1924, in which all the protagonists (including her faithful dog Sandy, who punctuates Annie's diatribes with a sympathetic 'arf-arf', Daddy Warbucks and his man-servant Punjab) have the same pupil-less eyes

Orphan Annie facies A descriptor for certain physiognomic features of the fetal alcohol syndrome, characterized by hypertelorism, rounder and shorter palpebral fissures and exotropia, likened to the round, blank eyes of the 'Little Orphan Annie'

orphan data A generic term for any information that is regarded as peripheral to the clinical decision-making process as it adds no information that can be weighed in a differential diagnosis or which impacts on the treatment of the condition of interest; orphan data includes breast thermography, some types of radionuclide scanning and, possibly because of the low rate of its performance and long turnaround time, the autopsy (see JAMA 1993; 269:1525oc)

'orphan' disease Any morbid condition affecting fewer than 200 000 people in the US, ie affecting less than 1/1000 people; because of the need for public information, a 'hotline' is available for professionals and family members of those with orphan diseases (☎ 1.800.999.6673); orphan diseases include acoustic neuroma, Addison's disease, ankylosing spondylitis, amyotrophic lateral sclerosis, autism, brain tumors, Charcot-Marie-Tooth, chronic fatigue syndrome, chronic granulomatous disease, Cornelia de Lange syndrome, craniofacial deformities, cystinosis, dizziness, dysautonomia, dystonia, epidermolysis bullosa, essential blepharospasm, 5p- syndrome, Friedreich's ataxia, glycogen storage disease, Guillain-Barré disease, graft-versus-host disease, Huntington's disease, ichthyosis, non-AIDS immune deficiencies, Klippel-Trenaunay syndrome, Langerhans' cell histiocytosis (histiocytosis X), leukodystrophy, Lowe syndrome, Lyme disease, malignant hyperthermia, Marfan syndrome, Ménière's disease, multiple sclerosis, mucopolysaccharidoses, narcolepsy, neuroblastoma, neurofibromatosis, Paget's disease, Parkinson's disease, polycystic kidneys, porphyria, Prader-Willi disease, retinitis pigmentosa, Rett syndrome, sarcoidosis, scleroderma, sickle cell disease, Sjögren syndrome, Sturge-Weber disease, TAR syndrome, Tay-Sachs disease(s), (Giles de la) Tourette syndrome, tuberous sclerosis, Turner syndrome, William syndrome, Wilson's disease; see NICODARD, NORD

Orphan Drug Act A US federal law (Public Law 97-414) designed to provide tax incentives, developmental grants and a seven-year marketing monopoly for companies developing drugs for orphan diseases (see there); Some 'orphan drugs' have been very successful (PEG-ADA, for severe combined immunodeficiency, Enzon Corp; erythropoietin, for anemia in chronic dialysis, Amgen Corp; human growth hormone, Genentech), allowing up to $100 million in revenues; Cf Pseudo-orphan drugs

orphan drugs/product Drugs, biologics, medical devices and foods of potential or actual use in treating 'orphan' diseases, which are diseases often considered by the pharmaceutical and therapeutic industries to be too rare for developing commercially viable products; from a practical stand-point, only 1 in 10 000 agents 'screened' for therapeutic potential ever reach the marketplace (Science 1991; 252:1080); the US Orphan Drug Act (see there) enacted in 1983 provided an incentive for such development, resulting in a number of approved agents eg, α erythropoietin (used for anemia of chronic renal failure), anti-thrombin III, botulinum toxin A (strabismus and blepharospasm),

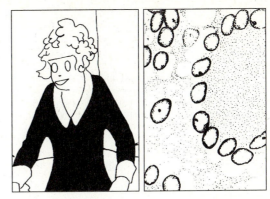

Orphan Annie   **and her nuclei**

cromolyn sodium (mastocytosis), gancyclovir (CMV retinitis), inhalation pentamidine (*Pneumocystis carinii* prophylaxis in 'at risk' subjects), IV mitoxantrone (acute nonlymphocytic leukemia), IV rifampin (TB for those who don't tolerate the drug per os), selegiline (for Parkinson's disease that is refractory to L-dopa or carbidopa), teriparatide (to distinguish pseudohypoparathyroidism and hypoparathyroidism-related hypocalcemia), ucephan (chronic management of patients with uric cycle enzymopathies) Cf Pseudo-orphan drug

Note: NORD (National Organization of Rare Diseases) maintains information on O D/PS ☎ 1.800.999.6673

'orphan patient' A patient with primary hypochondriasis that has its psychodynamic origin in the unconscious gratifications of bodily symptoms and physical suffering that begins when a patient mistakenly assigns serious disease to normal bodily functions or to benign symptoms of trivial illnesses or to the somatic symptoms of emotional arousal; orphan patients are often treated by primary care physicians, because, although they would be better treated by psychiatrists, that would represent acknowledgement of a mental and not a physical disease; see 'Organ recital', Munchausen syndrome, Self-mutilation

ORT Oral rehydration therapy, see there

ortet The single cell that is the precursor for a clone of cells

orthochromatic normoblast Metarubricyte The last cell in erythrocytic development prior to extrusion of the nucleus, which is large, red-orange, has a small nucleus (< ¼ cell volume) with dense chromatin; ONs are usually confined to the BM, but may be seen in the peripheral blood in metastases to the BM, myelofibrosis, anemia of chronic disease; hemolytic anemia (↑ erythropoiesis and 'spill-over' into the peripheral blood) should also be considered in the differential diagnosis

orthodeoxia An unusual finding of ↑ hypoxemia with a change from the supine to the erect position, a finding which may be seen in hepatopulmonary syndrome, see there (N Engl J Med 1994; 331:1098c)

orthogonal regression analysis STATISTICS A method used to determine the ISI (International Sensitivity Index), in which prothrombin times are plotted on a logarithmic scale with the vertical axis corresponds to the time (in seconds) obtained for the reference thromboplastin, and the horizontal axis being results with the working thromboplastin (CAP Today March 1993)

orthophosphate CLNICAL THERAPEUTICS Any anion or salt of orthophosphoric acid (H_3PO_4) or its esters; as a therapeutic modality, orthophosphate reduces urinary supersaturation with calcium oxalate and renal deposition of crystalized calcium oxalate, which in combination with pyridoxine, is reported to be a treatment of choice for primary hyperoxaluria (N Engl J Med 1994; 331:1542oa)

'orthopedic shoes' A term coined by shoe manufacturers, not by the orthopedic community at large; such shoes may cause potential harm to a normal child's foot as they may be too stiff

orthoptist A person who works under the supervision of an ophthalmologist, tests the strength of eye muscles and who teaches exercises designed to strengthen eye muscles and improve eye coordination, eg in patients with 'lazy eye' EDUCATION Three years (two years of college and one to two years apprenticeship); see Ophthalmologist; Cf Orthotist

orthostatic hypotension An abrupt decline in blood pressure which occurs either when one stands up or when one remains in for a prolonged period of time in an erect position; OH is often accompanied by dizziness, dimness of vision, and syncope; patients with OH may be anemic and have a ↓ RBC mass, which may respond to erythropoietin (N Engl J Med 1993; 329:611oa) ETIOLOGY Autonomic failure, which may be primary, or secondary to sympatholytic drugs, or irritation of the sympathetic nervous system, as may occur in DM and late syphilis, where the sympathetic vasoconstrictor fibers attempt to compensate for the effects of gravity; see Autonomic failure

orthotist A person who fabricates, designs and fits orthopedic devices prescribed by a physician; Cf Orthoptist

orthotopic transplantation The transplantation of a donor organ (the so-called orthotopic graft) into the same site as that occupied by the orginal organ that failed; organs that are transplanted orthotopically include the heart, lungs, and liver

orthozyme CD5plus A proprietary anti-T cell immunotoxin composed of the A chain of the castor bean toxin ricin, conjugated to a murine mono clonal antibody, which targets the CD5 antigen present on 95% of peripheral T cells; this agent's ability to selectively deplete T cells, might translate into a therapy for recalcitrant graft-versus-host reactions (JAMA 1991; 265:2041n&v); see Graft-versus-host disease, Magic bullet

γ-oryzonal SPORTS MEDICINE A rice-derived product that was transiently popular among some atheletes as it was believed to stimulate the release of growth hormone, which may also act as an anti-oxidant (JC DeLee, D Drez, Jr, Eds, Orthopedic Sports Medicine WB Saunders, Philadelphia, 1994)

OS/2 COMPUTERS The proprietary operating system used in IBM personal computers, workstations, and mainframes, the most recent version of which is known by its code name, Warp; while OS/2 has been less popular than Microsoft's Windows™ for mainstream PC users, it is very popular with the so-called 'power users', as its strength lies in multitasking, in which product and software developers and accountants can reliably run multiple applications on minicomputers and mainframe computers; OS/2 is also reported to be far less crash-prone than Windows (Forbes ASAP 27 Feb 1995, p42)

OSA Open system architecture, see there

OSHA Occupational Safety and Health Administration An arm of US federal government, created in 1970 by the Williams-Steiger Act, which recommends health and safety procedures and promulgates standards for the work place; OSHA's legislated mission is to '...*assure so far as possible every working man and woman in the Nation safe and healthful working conditions.*' (Occupational Safety and Health Act of 1970. Public Law 91-596) OSHA is not empowered to enforce recommendations but may impose fines of $1-100 000 for non-complying facilities

OSHA citation OSHA violation, see there

OSHA inspection A formal site visit by an OSHA inspector, formally known as compliance health and safety officer (CSHO); contrary to popular opinion, OIs are rarely made without reason; based on carefully formulated standards, OIs are planned (scheduled) for high-hazard industries, or those places that had previously received multiple and/or serious citations (see OSHA violations); low-hazard work sites are visted in a relatively random fashion, such that about 5% of these sites are visited by a CSHO (CAP Today Jan 1993 p28)

OSHA violation A deviation from OSHA standards for workers, which has been identified during the course of an OSHA inspection of a workplace; OVs are divided into four categories:

1) OTHER THAN SERIOUS

2) SERIOUS

3) WILLFUL AND

4) EGREGIOUS; the latter two categories refer to a situation in which an employer knows that a hazard exists, but does nothing about it, thus willfully exposes the employees to the hazard; willful and egregious citations carry fines of up to $70 000 per violation (CAP Today Jan 1993 p28)

OSI Office of Scientific Investigation

OSMED Osteospondylomegaepiphyseal dysplasia An AR form of chondrodystrophy, characterized by dwarfism, deafness and deformities of the external ear, saddle nose, thin hair, leathery skin, soft tissue calcifications, cleft palate and an achondroplasia-like pelvis

osmiophilic Any intracellular substance or organelle that has affinity for the electron-dense osmium tetroxide, reducing it to a black lower oxide

osmium tetraoxide A toxic substance that is used to fix and stain cells for ultrastructural examination; OT is reduced to a lower black oxide by protein- and lipid-rich substances, which explains the osmophilia of certain organelles, eg mitochondria and endoplasmic reticulum

osmolality LABORATORY MEDICINE A measurement of the amount of osmotically effective solute per 1000 grams of solvent; serum osmolality is an often misused clinical test for evaluating hyponatremia, and is a test that is useful to 1) Determine whether the serum water content deviates significantly from the norm and 2) Detect the presence of foreign low-molecular weight substances in the blood, eg ethanol, methanol and isopropanil, sorbitol, mannitol, glycerin and INH; the most common cause of increased osmolality is ethanol (100 mg/dl increases osmolality by 22 mmol/dl) QUANTIFICATION Freezing point depression vs dew-point (based on the colligative property of vapor pressure, equivalent to the total number of particles in a solution which equals the amount by which the dew point is depressed below ambient temperature; the disadvantage is that it doesn't measure ethanol, isopropanol, methanol, since the volatile (alcohol) adds to vapor pressure of the solution while decreasing same due to solute effect, resulting in a lower osmolality measured; contribution of toxic substances to serum osmolality, units in mOsm/kg of water: Methanol 33.7 mOsm/kg H_2O Ethanol 22.8 mOsm/kg H_2O, ethylene glycol 19.0 mOsm/kg H_2O, acetone 18.2 mOsm/kg H_2O, isopropanol 17.6 mOsm/kg H_2O, trichloroethane 9 mOsm/kg H_2O and others

osmolarity The concentration of osmotically active particles in a solution (solute/liter of solution)

osmolar gap The difference between the measured osmolality and the calculated osmolality; the measured osmolality is determined by freezing point depression (osmolality as solute/kilogram of solvent); the calculated osmolality (mOsm) is determined by the formula: $2 Na^+$ (mEq/L) + BUN (mg/dl)/2.8 + glucose (mg/dl)/18

osmole CELL PHYSIOLOGY One of a group of volume-regulating organic solutes that may accumulate in high concentrations within cells without adverse effects on the cell's structure or function; see Idiogenic osmoles FLUID BALANCE A mole of any molecular substance (eg NaClO that exists as separate molecules in solution, je m'explique-one osmole of NaCl is 0.5 mole of NaCl, as 0.5 mle of Na$^+$ and 0.5 mole of Cl$^-$ are equal to 1 osmol of particles, which determines the total osmotic pressure of the solution

osmotic diarrhea Increased volume and frequency of fecal flow caused by ingestion of a poorly absorbable solute (either a carbohydrate or divalent ion) or hypertonic material, resulting in a fecal osmolality higher than plasma osmolality; osmotic diarrhea may occur in antacid therapy, disaccharidase deficiency, magnesium sulfate ingestion and others, lactulose therapy, malabsorption (glucose-galactose, fructose or generalized), mannitol and sorbitol ingestion; see Chewing gum diarrhea

osmotic fragility The susceptibility of erythrocytes to osmotic lysis; in hypotonic solutions, red cells behave as perfect osmometers, where the free water rapidly equilibrates, causing the cells to swell; since the membrane has limits on its extensibility, cells with weaker membranes are more susceptible to osmotic lysis, a susceptibility that is classically increased in hereditary spherocytosis, due to a wide variety of molecular defects, affecting spectrin, ankyrin, protein 4.2 or spectrin-actin interaction, hereditary elliptocytosis and erythrocytic 'senility'; osmotic fragility is decreased in jaundice, iron therapy, thalassemia, sickle cell anemia, following splenectomy and in 'target' erythrocytes; see Spherocytosis

osmotic fragility test HEMATOLOGY A test in which RBCs are incubated in hypotonic saline solutions ranging from 0.9 % (physiologic osmolarity) to 0.0%, incubated for 30 min at room temperature, centrifuged, and the percent hemolysis is plotted on a curve; the OF shifted to the left in hereditary spherocytosis, and to the right for thalassemia

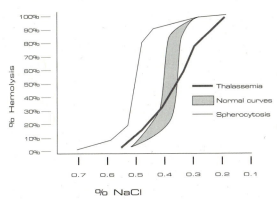

osmotic fragility test

Osp (A, B, etc) Outer surface protein A family of proteins present on the outer surface of *Borrelia burdorferi* that have proven to be immunogenic, and therefore candidates for producing a vaccine against Lyme disease; of the Osps thusfar identified (Osp A-F), only Osp A appears to provide protective immunity; if development procedes without problems, a vaccine may be available by 1996 (**Sci Am** 1994; 270/9:34)

ossicular chain SURGICAL ANATOMY *ossicula auditorius* [NA6] A popular term for the auditory ossicles, the malleus, incus, and stapes; through the interconnectivity of the OC, sound waves are transmitted from the tympanic membrane in which the manubrium of the malleus is embedded to the fenestra vestibuli, which seats the base of the stapes, converting the mechanical vibrations of sound into neural signals

ossicular chain reconstruction ENT A group of surgical procedures for tympanoplasty (see there), using malleus strut, peg-top, and hydroxyapatite cap prostheses, and revision stapedectomy using stapedial tendon reconstruction

osteoarthropathy Hypertropic pulmonary osteoarthropathy, see there

osteoblastic tumor A generic term for any tumor that produces substances with parathyroid hormone-like activity, including metastatic prostate carcinoma, osteoma, osteoblastoma, osteosarcoma, chondrosarcoma; see Hypercalcemia of malignancy

osteocalcin A noncollagenous bone protein, the production of which is stimulated by vitamin D$_3$ and inhibited by glucocorticoids

osteochondritis Combined inflammation of the bone and articular surface (usually aseptic); a legacy of the German school of medicine was eponymic immortalization of each joint, thus Freiberg's disease corresponds to osteochondritis of the metatarsal head, Haglund's disease (osteochondritis of the calcaneus), Köhler's disease (tarsal-navicular bones), Legg-Calve-Perthes disease (epiphyseal femoral head), Osgood-Schlatter disease (tibial tubercle), Panner's disease (humeral head), Sinding-Larsen-Johannson disease (patella), Thiemann's disease (metacarpal and metatarsal bones), Wegner's disease (osteochondritis with epiphyseal separation seen in congenital syphilis)

osteoclast-activating factor(s) A group of lymphokines, eg tumor growth factor α that mobilize calcium and are produced in excess in malignancy and rheumatoid arthritis, causing osteolysis-induced hypercalcemia

osteoclast-like giant cell A multinucleated giant cell with abundant eosinophilic, finely granular or homogeneous cytoplasm containing up to one hundred uniform oval nuclei each measuring 5-7 μm with scattered small nucleoli and peripheral chromatin; osteoclast-like giant cells are often scattered among plump spindled mononuclear cells and may occur in benign and malignant conditions, including fibrous histiocytoma, histiocytosis X, in the mural nodules of mucin-producing ovarian carcinomas, hepatocellular carcinoma, Hodgkin's disease, and tumoral calcinosis (Kikuyu's bursa)

osteogenic osteomalacia A rare syndrome characterized by hypophosphatemia, hyperphosphaturia, low plasma levels of 1,25-dihydroxyvitamin D, and osteomalacia; all biochemical and pathological abnormalities disappear upon removal of the tumor; the 'OO' factor is unknown, but in one report (**N Engl J Med** 1994; 330:1645oA) inhibits sodium-dependent phosphate transport in cultured renal epithelial cells, has PTH-like immunoreactivity, a low molecular weight and is heat-sensitive

osteogenic protein see OP-1

osteogenesis imperfecta A heterogenous group of AD conditions with variable penetration due to a variety of defects, eg deletions, frame shifts, point mutations, rearrangements and substitutions in the genes responsible for collagen production, as well as glycine substitution and exon skipping CLINICAL OIs vary in presentation and may have thin bones, multiple fractures, blue sclera, opalescent teeth, deafness due to middle ear osteosclerosis, scoliosis, thin skin, visceral herniation, dentinogenesis imperfecta, vascular lesions

osteoid *adjective* Bony, bone-like *noun* The collagenous matrix of bone prior to calcification

osteointegration The direct structural and functional connection between living bone and the surface of a load-bearing implant; osteointegrated implants have been used to treat edentulism (see implants) and for head and neck reconstruction to facilitate retention of auricular mandibular, maxillary, nasal, and orbital implants, and for bone-anchored hearing aids

osteomalacia Nutritional rickets Softened bones caused by poor mineralization that occurs in a background of vitamin D deficiency, which may be linked to prematurity, rapid growth, low exposure to sunlight, and renal tube defects CLINICAL Weak, deformed, and deformable bone, which in children may be manifest by craniotabes, bowlegs, and knock-knees, rachitic rosary, compromise of ventilation, which is often accompanied by pneumonia, muscular weakness, loss of appetite, hypocalcemia TREATMENT Vitamin D

osteomeatal complex ENT The area between the middle and the inferior turbinates which is the site of confluence of the drainage from the frontal, ethmoidal, and maxillary sinuses; in several areas of the OMC, two layers of mucosa overlap, creating regions of impaired mucociliary clearance, predisposing to infection even in absence of ostial closure (N Engl J Med 1992; 326:319cc)

osteonecrosis A relatively common condition characterized by in situ death of bone ETIOLOGY Trauma, infection, nontraumatic[1] and associated with childhood diseases[2] MECHANISM 1) Mechanical interruption of vascular supply, eg by fracture or dislocation 2) Thrombosis and embolism 3) Injury to vessel wall 4) Venous occlusion CLINICAL Pain increasing with joint movement DIAGNOSIS Bone scans, MRI MANAGEMENT Prosthetic replacement of larger joints, core decompression, engraftment of vascularized bone (eg fibula), in the elderly—immobilization, nonsteroidal anti-inflammatory drugs, and limitation of joint movement (N Engl J Med 1992; 326:1473RV)

[1]Occurring in a background of aging, alcohol, abuse, arteritis, coagulopathy, connective tissue disease (eg systemic lupus erythematosus), corticosteroid administration, dysbarism, Gaucher's disease, gout, hemoglobinopathy, idiopathic, pancreatitis, pregnancy, radiation, stress fracture [2]Blount's, Köhler's, Larsen's, Legg-Calvé-Perthes, Panner's diseases

osteopathy A school of medicine practiced predominantly in the USA that is based on Dr Andrew Tayor's theory of healing, first delineated in 1874, that holds that a normal body in a state of wellness is in correct adjustment and that disease represents a loss of coherency of structure and/or function and the inability to mount a normal defense against infection, malignancy, inflammation, toxins and other inciting agents; the difference between doctors of medicine (MDs) and doctors of osteopathy (DOs) was formerly greater than in the current environment*, the chief distinction is that osteopaths rely more on 'manipulation' of various body parts; otherwise, DOs prescribe drugs and may train in the same teaching hospitals as MDs; there is a greater tendency for osteopaths to provide primary care as general practitioners of medicine, gynecologists and pediatricians, although there are regional differences

*5% of physicians in the US are DOs, they treat 10% of the US population, as 70% are in private practice (Am Med News 12 October 1992 p32)

osteopenia A generic term for a relative or absolute ↓ of bone which is linked to estrogen deficiency that occurs in ♀ with hypogonadism due to hyperprolactinemia, ↑ exercise, anorexia nervosa, hypothalamic amenorrhea, or in those receiving gonadotropin-releasing hormone (GnRH) analogues; parathyroid hormone prevents bone loss in ♀ receiving long-term therapy with GnRH analogues required to treat certain estrogen-driven conditions, eg endometriosis or uterine leiomyomas (N Engl J Med 1994; 331:1618OA)

osteopetrosis PEDIATRIC ENDOCRINOLOGY Marble bone disease, Albers-Schoenberg disease A heterogeneous group of rare inherited conditions characterized by ↓ osteoclastic activity and ↓ bone resorption, resulting in an accumulation of sclerotic bone compromises the marrow space

TREATMENT Long-term IFN-gamma-1b therapy ↑ the bone resorption, hematopoiesis and improves leukocyte function by ↑ superoxide production by granulocyte-macrophage colonies (N Engl J Med 1995; 332:1591OA) alternatively, BM transplantation—an acceptable donor is found in 40%; 47% of these survive 2 years; 62% of whom are regarded as cured; high-dose calcitriol may ameliorate osteoporosis in 25%

osteopetrosis A heterogeneous group of AD [MIM 166500] and AR [MIM 259700-259720] cortical and trabecular osteosclerotic disorders; the vertebral margins are often rounded, have deep indentations for the anterior and posterior veins and marked osteosclerosis, commonly associated with a central radiolucency, imparting a 'sandwich appearance'; in the long bones, osteopetrosis is characterized by a failure of molding in the metaphysis, a finding also seen in van Buchem's endosteal hyperostosis, dysosteosclerosis and tertiary syphilis; in the murine model, osteopetrosis is AR, has a limited bone remodeling capacity, has a marked decrease in mature macrophages and osteoclasts and is due to a mutation on chromosome 3 in the coding region of the macrophage colony-stimulating factor gene; see Marble bone disease

osteophyte A bony bump

osteopoikilosis An AD [MIM 166700] condition characterized by multiple small foci of osteosclerosis in the spongiosa of the pelvis, metaphysis of long bones, tarsal and carpal bones; often associated with subcutaneous bony nodules

*Synonyms include Buschke-Ollendorff syndrome, osteopathia condensans disseminata, spotted bone disease

osteopontin A protein produced by osteoblasts in response to stimulation by calcitriol, which is involved in anchoring osteoclasts to bone matrix minerals

osteoporosis A condition characterized by attenuation of bone, representing the most common morbid condition of the elderly female STATISTICS Age-related osteoporosis causes more than 10^5 fractures/year in the US (vertebrae 54%, hip 23%, distal forearm or Colles fracture, 17%); 25% of ♀ > 70 have evidence of vertebral fractures, as do 50% of ♀ > 80; 90% of femoral head fractures occur in those > 70; 1/3 of ♀ ≥ 90 have had femoral head fractures, which is a significant risk for long-term institutionalization and in-hospital mortality; the annual cost of osteoporosis is $6 X 10^9, USA CLINICAL FORMS: Primary idiopathic osteoporosis or 'benign' osteoporosis is a rare condition of early onset that is symptomatic in ½ of cases, radiographically mimicking the malignant form, but which is rarely pernicious clinically Primary involutional osteoporosis is divided into

TYPE I ('POSTMENOPAUSAL') OSTEOPOROSIS A relatively common condition with a 6:1 female:male ratio, affecting those aged 50-75, characterized by decreased estrogen, accelerated trabecular bone loss, 'crush' fractures associated with abnormal PTH secretion and age-related decrease in response to vitamin D [$1,25(OH)_2D_2$]; 15-20 years after the onset of menopause, this form of osteoporosis may reach a 'burned-out' phase with no further bone loss

TYPE II ('AGE-RELATED') OSTEOPOROSIS A less common condition with a 2:1 female:male ratio, affects those over age 70 and is characterized by trabecular and cortical bone loss (the elderly female typically suffers a 35% loss of cortical bone and a 50% loss of trabecular bone), affecting vertebral bodies and flat bones, resulting in hip fractures and wedge-type vertebral fractures, due to 1) Decreased osteoblast function (reduced IGF-I, hGH, and local regulators) 2) A marked decrease in calcium absorption (to 50% of 'normal' with reduced vitamin $1,25(OH)_2D_2$, possibly due to decreased activity of renal 1-α hydroxylase) and 3) Other factors, including decreased clearance of parathyroid hormone's carboxyl (COOH) terminals and increased calcium resorption; calcitonin's role in this form of osteoporosis is unclear MORBIDITY Osteoporosis-related fractures occur in1.5 million/year (US) PATHOGENESIS: ♀ lose 50% of cancellous bone and ♂ lose 30% of cancellous bone during their lifetimes; cancellous bone is concentrated in the spinal column and at the ends of the long bones, the sites of most fractures; the skeleton is a reservoir of labile calcium and base (as alkaline calcium salts); age-related osteoporosis may be related to the skeleton's role in acid-base homeostasis, and the effects of lifelong mobilization of skeletal calcium salts to compensate for endogenous acid generated from dietary precursors RISK FACTORS For every 10-pack years of smoking history, bone density ↓ by 1-2% (N Engl J Med 1994; 330:387₀ₐ) Secondary osteoporosis is 'driven' by non-osseous 'axis' factors, which may be iatrogenic, surgical (early oophorectomy, orchiectomy, subtotal gastrectomy), drug-related (corticosteroids, anticonvulsants, heparin, L-thyroxine), endocrinopathic (hypogonadism, increased adrenocortical or thyroid activity), gastrointestinal (alactasia, malabsorption), bone marrow (mastocytosis, metastatic malignancy, multiple myeloma), collagenopathy-related, due to osseous disease (osteogenesis imperfecta, Marfan syndrome, rheumatoid arthritis) and others, eg immobilization, chronic obstructive pulmonary disease RISK FACTORS Caucasian, elderly, ♀ thin habitus, immobilization, space travel (weightlessness), extreme exercise and/or amenorrhea, alcoholism, endocrinopathies (eg acromegaly, Cushing's disease, hypogonadism, hyperthyroidism, hyperparathyroidism) POSSIBLE RISK FACTORS Heredity, dietary calcium deficiency, smoking (which depresses osteoblastic activity), inadequate exercise, alcohol consumption, low calcium intake, exercise, small body frame, levels of serum and urinary calcium and creatinine; patients receiving physiological doses of levothyroxine may have decreased bone density (JAMA 1991; 265:2688); obesity may exert a protective effect against osteoporosis, possibly due to adipose tissue converting androgen to estrogen, increasing osseous resistance to the lytic effects of parathyroid hormone and/or the fact that obesity increases skeletal loading, which by a piezoelectric mechanism, stimulates an osteoblastic response along the lines of stress PATHOPHYSIOLOGY Estrogen acts on osteoblasts by a receptor, modulating the extracellular matrix, increasing procollagen type I and transforming growth factor-β mRNA, playing a key role in mineralization and remodeling Note: The 'classic' exercise-related osteoporosis may be more a function of aymptomatic disturbances of ovulation, ie estrogen-related rather than due physical activity DIAGNOSIS Bone densitometry TREATMENT Osteoporosis is managed by 1) Antiresorptive agents, eg estrogen, calcium, calcitonin, biphosphonates and others eg anabolic steroids, calcitriol; potassium bicarbonate improves calcium and phosphorous balance by ↓ hydroxyproline excretion (a marker of bone resorption), and ↑ osteocalcin (a marker of bone formation) (N Engl J Med 1994; 330:1776₀ₐ) 2) Bone stimulation regimens, eg sodium fluoride, parathyroid hormone, and growth factors, eg IGF-I, IGF-II, transforming growth factor-β (N Engl J Med 1992; 327:620ᴿᵛ) and 3) Calcium supplementation (1000 mg/day), which is reported to slow axial and appendicular bone loss in normal postmenopausal women (N Engl J Med 1993; 328:460₀ₐ) PREVENTION The bone loss in the early post-menopausal period (< 5 years) is not affected by calcium supplementation; the use of estrogen for osteoporosis must be based on objective diagnosis of osteoporosis, eg single and dual photon absorptometry of the radius, lumbar spine and hip, given estrogen's potential for 'driving' proliferative changes of the endometrium; thiazides increase renal conservation of calcium; cyclic etidronate (a diphosphonate agent) reduces bone resorption by inhibiting osteoclast

activity

osteosclerotic myeloma A plasma cell dyscrasia characterized by sclerotic bone lesions and progressive demyelinating polyneuropathy; see Plasma cell dyscrasia with polyneuropathy

OSTP Office of Science and Technology Policy

OTA Office of Technical Assessment, see there

OTC 1) Ornithine transcarbamylase, see there 2) Over-the-counter drugs, see there

Othello syndrome Erotic jealousy, alcoholic paranoia* A delusion of spousal infidelity, a form of psychotic paranoia that is primary or more commonly, a symptom of organic 'psychopathies', which include senile dementia, cortical atrophy in boxers and alcoholics

*The most appropriate current equivalent is alcohol-induced psychotic disorder, with delusions (DSM-IV 291.5) Othello, Shakespeare's tragic hero murdered his wife, Desdemona, when Iago led him to believe her unfaithful

otopalatodigital dysplasia Taybi disease An X-linked [MIM 311300] condition that is completely expressed in males and partially expressed in carrier females, characterized by conduction-type deafness, a distinct facies with prominent supraorbital ridges, a broad nasal root, flattening of the mid-face and a small jaw, digital abnormalities including short broad fingers; bone dysplasia with dislocation of the radial heads and/or hips, dwarfism, mental retardation

otopalatodigital syndrome An X-linked [MIM 311300] condition characterized by craniofacial deformity (frontal and occipital bossing, hypertelorism, small nose and mouth, partial anodontia, cleft palate), short trunk and brachydactyly; the responsible OPD1 gene maps to Xq26

otoplasty A surgical technique for correcting auricular deformities, often using the Mustarde technique combined with conchal setback; symmetry is best achieved by using a standard point of reference, eg the Frankfort line

otorrhea A discharge from the ear through a perforation of the tympanic membrane or through a surgically placed ventilating tube (N Engl J Med 1995; 332:1560ᴿᵛ)

ouch-ouch disease Itai-itai byo, see there

'out of Africa' hypothesis PALEOANTHROPOLOGY A widely accepted posit that the ancestry of all modern humans can be traced to a single population that lived in Africa ± 200 000 years ago; the data is based on studies of mitochondrial DNA and may be traced to a single female, who has been thus called the mitochondrial Eve

outcome node The final point in a clinical decision-making algorithm that was initiated by a chance node, resulting in a cascade of strategic pathways driven by diagnostic or therapeutic interventions, that diverge at each subsequent decision node based on the results of the intervention (eg response, nonresponse); see Chance node, Decision node, Decision tree

outcomes measurement A method for evaluating the success of an activity, eg continuing medical education (CME); OM in CME attempts to evaluate what person actually learned during the educational session and can take the form of challenge examination, or what is more difficult, how that new knowledge will improve a physician's practice activities (Arch Pathol Lab Med 1992; 116:602₀ₐ) Cf Process assessment

outcomes 'movement' HEALTH CARE An increasingly organized trend in the US health care industry that assesses the results or outcome of various therapeutic modalities, analyzing efficacy and assuring quality in patient care; the OM is based on the assumption that statistical analysis of outcomes, calculations, and applications of diagnostic and therapeutic algorithms are superior to a physician's traditional practice of medicine and care of individual patients learned by experience, intuition, deliberation and cause-

and-effect reasoning; the OM champions a fundamental revision of paradigm from which physicians practice medicine, where the examination and application of data generated in clinical research on outcomes (ie what works and what does not) should supplant intuition (visceral or 'gut' knowledge), physiologic rationale, and unsystematic clinical experience; 'Ultimately, the OM justifies, and even advocates, molding physicians' behavior to match as closely as possible, a 'best' form of medical practice by horatory, economic, or regulatory means,' while attempting to eliminate the 'inefficiency' of practice style (N Engl J Med 1993; 329:1268ED) the 'movement' has been driven by

1) The need for cost containment

2) Competition in the medical marketplace for a 'fair' price of high quality services and

3) Regional differences in the use of certain medical procedures, causing unnecessary and excess expense in high-use areas or suboptimal care in low-use areas; see Outcomes research

Note: The developing outcomes 'industry' is predestined to create new bureaucracies and introduce greater inefficiencies without reducing the cost of what is already the world's most expensive health care system (N Engl J Med 1990; 323:266ed)

outcomes research HEALTH CARE The scientific determination of the components of high-quality and cost-effective medical care, based on analysis of policy positions, payment rules, and practice guidelines; OR examines statistically the effectiveness of specific medical interventions and studies medicine as it is practiced in 'real time' rather than in the context of often idealized clinical trials (N Engl J Med 1993; 329:1268ED) see Outcomes movement

outer surface protein see Osp A, Osp B etc

outgrow *verb* To change the relationship with a condition or structure by dint of increased age or size; while children outgrow clothing, and certain behaviors, they rarely outgrow diseases, eg asthma (NY Times 4 Jan, 1994, C1)

'outlier' HEALTH CARE MANAGEMENT Any patient who has either an extremely long length of stay or who has incurred extraordinarily high costs; see High mortality outlier LABORATORY MEDICINE, STATISTICS Any value that lies far outside of the standard deviations of the mean that would encompass the entirety of a population being tested; see Trimming

Note: The inclusion of 'outliers' in calculations and the establishment of a mean introduces small but potentially significant statistical errors

outpatient *adjective* Pertaining or referring to that which occurs, eg therapy outside of a formal health care environment or hospital setting *noun* A person who is undergoing a diagnostic workup, evaluation, or therapeutic procedure outside of a hospital or health care facility; Cf Inpatient

output media Any floppy diskette, form, paper 'printout', 'hard copy' or device that displays in some readable format computer-processed data; see Computers

output unit Billable test, see there, ordered test

outrage tort MALPRACTICE A legal wrong or injury (tort) in which "outrage" (intentional infliction of serious mental distress) is asserted or proven

outstanding ear An auricular deformity characterized by an excess protrusion of the ear from the head, and attributed to a defective or absence of antihelical fold formation and often accompanied by a large conchal bowl TREATMENT Surgical reduction or alteration of the conchal bowl cartilage

ovalocytosis A condition occurring in up to 30% of certain ethnic groups in southeast Asia caused by a defective band 3 protein, in which there is increased affinity of erythrocyte membrane band 3 to ankrin, resulting in a marked increase in red cell rigidity; ovalocytosis may represent a form of evolutionary defense, as ovalocytes are innately resistant to the parasites of *Plasmodium falciparum* (N Engl J Med 1990; 323:1530)

ovarian cancer The 5th most common malignancy in ♀

FIGO STAGING FOR EPITHELIAL CANCER OF THE OVARY

STAGE I Tumor limited to ovary
IA One ovary, no ascites, intact capsule
IB Both ovaries, no ascites, intact capsule
IC Both ovaries, malignant ascites (positive peritoneal washings) rupture capsule (capsular involvement)
STAGE II Tumor extends beyond ovary into pelvis
IIA Pelvic extension to uterus or fallopian tubes
IIB Pelvic extension to other pelvic organs, eg bladder, rectum, vagina
IIC Pelvic extension + IC findings
STAGE III Extrapelvic extension or positive lymph nodes
IIIA Microscopic seeding outside of pelvis
IIIB Gross lesions ≤ 2 cm
IIIC Gross lesions > 2cm and positive lymph nodes
STAGE IV Distant (extraperitoneal) organ involvement, eg liver, pleura

---

(US), 22 000 new cases/year, and 13 300 deaths/year RISK FACTORS ↑ Risk with nulliparity or first birth after age 35; ↓ risk with childbirth before age 25 or use of oral contraceptives; familial ovarian cancer accounts for 5% of ovarian cancers CLINICAL Presentation with abdominal fullness and early satiety due to ascites and omental tumor implants; disease is rarely confined to the pelvis, and early diagnosis is fortuitous STAGING see table MOLECULAR PATHOLOGY Uncertain; some cases, especially the familial forms may be linked to a candidate gene *BRCA-1* on chromosome 17 at 17q12-q23 THERAPY-LIMITED DISEASE (stage I, II) Total abdominal hysterectomy, bilateral salpingo-oophorectomy and omentectomy with careful examination of peritoneal surface THERAPY-ADVANCED DISEASE (stage III, IV) Debulking of peritoneal tumors, followed byplatinum agents, eg cisplatin (or the less toxic carboplatin), or taxol-containing regimens; 'compassionate' protocols which may minimally improve survival survival include intraperitoneal chemotherapy and autologous bone marrow transplantation PROGNOSIS Stage IA, IB = 91-98% 5-year survival; stage IC, II = 80% 5-year survival; stage III and residual tumor implants ≤ 0.5 cm = 40-month survival; residual tumor implants 0.5-2.0 cm = 18-month survival; residual tumor implants ≥ 2.0 cm = 6-12-month survival (N Engl J Med 1993; 329:1550RA)

ovarian small cell carcinoma of the hypercalcemic type A rare usually fatal malignancy of young ♀ that is often refractory to aggressive chemo– and radiotherapy; of those with stage I disease who have survived, flow cytometric data has not proven helpful as all tumors were DNA-diploid (Am J Clin Pathol 1992; 98:579OA) DDx 'Garden variety' small cell carcinoma of the ovary, malignant germ cell tumor, sex-cord tumors

ovarian vein 'syndrome' A clinical complex due to an enlarged and tortuous right ovarian vein with incompetence of the venous valves, typically seen in pregnancy, which is accompanied by hydronephrosis and pyelonephritis CLINICAL Intermittent right flank pain coinciding with menstruation, recurring urinary tract infection and exacerbation with progesterone TREATMENT Surgical

overdose SUBSTANCE ABUSE Consumption of any therapeutic agent, drug or narcotic in excess of the dose required to produce the usually desired effects; overdoses are either accidental or suicidal and many agents have their own relatively characteristic clinical, diagnostic and therapeutic 'fingerprint'; see 'Designer' drugs, Heroin, 'Ice', Withdrawal

overflow diarrhea Secretory diarrhea in which the fluid

produced in the upper intestine exceeds the resorptive capacity of the lower intestine, classically seen in cholera, mediated by adenylate cyclase, which is locked in the 'on' position by the cholera toxin

overflow proteinuria Persistent proteinuria without glomerular disease, characterized by excess production of filterable, low molecular weight proteins, exceeding the resorptive capacities of the renal tubules, eg increased lysozyme in myelomonocytic (M4) leukemia or Bence-Jones proteinuria; the condition is usually asymptomatic if the protein loss is less than 2.0 g/d

overhanging ledge sign RADIOLOGY A descriptor for prominent chondro-osseous overgrowths commonly seen in the distal acral articulations of gouty arthritis, considered to be most common in those with concomitant diffuse idiopathic skeletal hyperostosis; see DISH

overhead costs Indirect costs, see there

overkill The capacity in excess of that needed to destroy a target with nuclear warheads, measured in 'units' of human mortality; an overkill of 10 indicates a destructive capacity that is 10-fold greater than that necessary to destroy the population; because of the image of senseless excess evoked by the word, overkill has become a mainstream colloquial term in medicine, referring to any excessive means used accomplish a particular goal, as in diagnostic overkill or therapeutic overkill; see Nuclear war; Cf Chemical warfare

overlap syndrome GASTROENTEROLOGY The presence of histologic features of both Crohn's disease (granulomas, well-preserved cytoplasmic mucin, lymphoid aggregates and edema) and ulcerative colitis (crypt abscesses, mucosal atrophy and regeneration and marked hyperemia) in the same colon biopsy specimen, precluding a specific diagnosis of either; significant overlap occurs in about 15% of the biopsies of these two conditions and some authors use the term 'indeterminate' syndrome NEUROLOGY see Parkinsonism plus syndromes RHEUMATOLOGY Overlap syndrome(s) are subtypes of connective tissue disease with features of two or more rheumatologic disorders, including lupus erythematosus-mixed connective tissue disease overlap, rheumatoid arthritis-lupus overlap (1% of cases), scleroderma-polymyositis overlap (8-12% of cases) and lupus erythematosus-polymyositis overlap (5-10% of cases) VASCULAR DISEASE A combination of systemic necrotizing vasculitis with features of polyarteritis nodosa and Churg-Strauss disease (allergic angiitis and granulomatosis), involving small and medium muscular arteries of the lung, causing hypertension and hypersensitivity

overread see Underread

over-the-counter drug A therapeutic agent that does not require a physician's prescription, which the FDA feels can be safely self-prescribed by non-physicians; 300 000 OTC medications are available in the USA, which contain 700 different active ingredients and generate $7.4 x 10^9 in annual sales; self-presciding and use of OTCs is an important factor in health care, as examples, in the US there are ≥ 800 OTCs for treating the common cold (for which $2 x 10^9 is spent/year); ± 70% of all illnesses are treated with nonprescribed drugs; most childhood illnesses are first treated with OTCs, especially acetaminophen (Tylenol®) which had been given to ⅔ of children within the 30 days prior to study-related interview (JAMA 1994; 272:1025oc)
The 'opposite' of an over-the-counter drug is a prescription drug; 'under-the-counter' is a colloquial adjective for any illicit product

overuse injury SPORTS MEDICINE A generic term for sports- or occupation-related injuries that often involve repetitive submaximal loading of a particular musculoskeletal unit, resulting in changes due to fatigue of tendons or inflammation of surrounding tissues; OIs include tennis elbow

and golf elbow (JC DeLee, D Drez, Jr, Eds, Orthopedic Sports Medicine WB Saunders, Philadelphia, 1994)

overuse syndrome SPORTS MEDICINE Chronic trauma caused by repetitive forces on the musculotendinous apparatus and chondro-osseous tissues, causing inflammation, pain or dysfunction of the involved joint(s), bones and ligaments, and potentially avulsion fractures

'overvalued procedure' Any of a group of surgical procedures, for treating non-malignant conditions, eg cholecystectomy that the US Congress has considered to be 'too expensive' and has targeted for budget cuts from Medicare reimbursement; see Resource-based relative value scale

overweight A condition defined as ≥ 75th percentile of body-mass index (weight in kg/(height in m)²; overweight in adults is associated with atherosclerosis, arthritis, cardiovascular disease, DM, gallbladder disease, gout, hypertension, and certain malignancies; overweight adolescents are at increased risk for future developement of coronary heart disease, stroke, and colorectal cancer (N Engl J Med 1992; 327:1350oA) see Obesity

ovolacteal vegetarian Lacto-ovo vegetarian, see there

owl eye appearance A 'classic' descriptor for inclusions seen by LM in CMV infection (N Engl J Med 1994; 331:649iCM), in which the markedly enlarged CMV-infected epithelial cells have massive eosinophilic intranuclear inclusions which may be half the size of the nucleus and surrounded by a clear halo (thus mimicking the inclusions of herpes simplex), clearly delineating the inclusions from the nuclear membrane; CMV-infected cells may also have smaller basophilic inclusions in the cytoplasm, which may correspond to viral capsid proteins; CMV-infected tissues often demonstrate necrosis and chronic inflammation

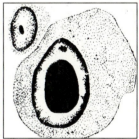

Note: the term 'owl eye nuclei' has also been applied to the caterpillar cell of rheumatic heart disease, when the latter is viewed longitudinally

own side fire Friendly fire, see there

ox eye Buphthalmos A progressively enlarged eye most commonly seen in children with congenital glaucoma; over time, the head of the optic nerve undergoes cupping and atrophy, resulting in blindness

oxalosis Hyperoxaluria, see Primary hyperoxaluria

oxidation-fermentation test OF test, see there

oxidative stress The presence of oxygen free radicals generated by various stressants, eg tobacco, alcohol; the primary antioxidant is glutathione; other antioxidants include vitamins A, C, and E; ↑ oxidative stress is thought to be one of the key factors in the early pathogenesis of AIDS in which the production of TNF increases the production of free radicals within T cells; see Free radicals

oxidation therapy Hydrogen peroxide therapy, see there

oxidizer A non-explosive chemical or substance that initiates or promotes the combustion of other materials, causing fire by itself, or through the release of oxygen or other gases

oximetry see Pulse oximetry

8-oxo-7-hydrodeoguanosine 8-oxod-G GERONTOLOGY A modified guanosine residue formed when DNA suffers oxidative damage, which is a key player in mutagenesis, carcinogenesis and aging; the presence of 8-oxod-G on one strand is permissive to base pairing by either dAMP or dCMP; incorporation of potentially mutagenic dCMP or dAMP nucleotides is followed by transient inhibition of chain extension in the 3' direction of the modified base(s) (**Nature 1991; 349:431**) see 'Garbage can' hypothesis, Oxygen radicals

oxygen dissociation curve   Oxygen saturation curve PHYSIOLOGY   A curve that describes the relationship between hemoglobin oxygen saturation and tension; defined by a sigmoid curve which reflects the interaction of the four hemoglobin molecules involved in oxygen uptake, transport and release; a 'right shift' of the curve indicates ↓ hemoglobin affinity for oxygen, as occurs in ↓ pH, ie acidosis, ↑ temperature, ↑ PCO_2, while a 'left shift' indicates ↑ oxygen affinity with ↑ pH, ↓ temperature, ↓ 2,3 DPG and ↓ PCO_2; see 2,3 DPG

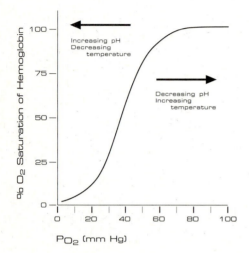

Increasing pH
Decreasing temperature

Decreasing pH
Increasing temperature

oxygen dissociation curve

oxygen free radicals   A family of highly reactive, toxic molecules that appear when electrons are added to oxygen in the presence of hydrogen ions; one electron yields superoxide anion radical, a second electron yields H_2O_2 and a third electron yields hydroxyl radical; free radicals are produced in vascular endothelium and in neutrophils by membrane phospholipid catabolism and are generated in the reperfusion phase after myocardial infarction; the free electrons have reactive affinity for unsaturated fatty acids and sulfhydryl amino acids, attacking cells by breaking protein strands, damaging membrane lipids, destroying lipid cross-links and causing fatty acid oxidation; under normal circumstances, cytochrome oxidase prevents destruction of adjacent molecules; free radicals may be eliminated ('scavenged') by catalase, glutathione reductase, superoxide dismutase, vitamin E; during ischemia, xanthine dehydrogenase (which produces uric acid) is converted into xanthine oxidase producing free radicals from oxygen and hypoxanthine; see Free radicals, Respiratory burst

oxygen paradox   MUSCLE PHYSIOLOGY A phenomenon seen when chronically hypoxic muscle is exposed to normal oxygen levels; the muscle cells 'overdose' on oxygen and die, an effect thought due to oxygen radicals; Cf Calcium paradox

oxygen radical   Reactive oxygen metabolite Any molecule with an unpaired electron in its outer orbital which leads to an unstable and/or short half-life, which are capable of reducing or oxidizing other molecules

(blood) oxygen saturation sO_2 The oxygen concentration of blood expressed as a ratio of its total oxygen-carrying capacity; the OS is a measure of the utilization of oxygen transport capacity

oxygen saturation curve   Oxygen dissociation curve, see

there

oxygen therapy   ALTERNATIVE MEDICINE A generic term for any non-'mainstream' use of oxygen as a therapeutic modality, including (nonconventional) hyperbaric oxygen therapy‡, hydrogen peroxide (oxidation) therapy‡, and ozone therapy‡

oxygen toxicity   Tissue and molecular damage due to the effects of oxygen free radicals in cellular and extracellular micro-environments; oxygen toxicity occurs in older subjects, in shock and in inflammation; the toxic effects of atmospheric oxygen on strict anaerobic bacteria are not fully clarified, possibly related to the lack enzymes, eg superoxide dismutase, catalases and peroxidase, capable of metabolizing free radicals and are incapable of growth in greater than 0.5% ambient oxygen; to reduce the oxidation-reduction or 'redox' potential of a medium, reducing agents such as thioglycolate and L-cysteine may be added to the anaerobic transport medium; see Anaerobes

oxytalan fiber   DENTISTRY A dense connective tissue fiber that is widely and evenly distributed throughout the periodontal tissues under normal circumstances in healthy periodontal tissues; in chronic periodontitis, OFs are fragmented, disintegrated, or disappear (**Chin Med J 1994; 107:785**)

oxytocin stress test   OBSTETRICS A clinical test for evaluating the fetus' ability to 'weather' labor that uses oxytocin, an eight-residue hypothalamic polypeptide released into the posterior pituitary (of both mother and fetus) that induces and stimulates labor; oxytocin is titrated so that three contractions occur in 10 minutes; if three 'decelerations' occur within 10 minutes, the fetus is considered 'at risk' for labor-related complications and should be delivered as soon as possible Note: Because uterine contraction causes ↓ uteroplacental blood flow (see Deceleration), a clinically controlled 'trial of labor' should be performed in women at high risk for uteroplacental insufficiency; such 'at-risk' pregnancies include women with chronic obstructive lung disease, diabetes mellitus, underlying heart disease, hypertension, narcotic addiction, post-term pregnancy, preeclampsia, sickle cell anemia; a positive stress test is characterized by consistent late decelerations and ample indication for an expedient delivery; Cf Fetal heart monitoring, Non-stress test

OZ-12   PUBLIC SAFETY A highly flammable refrigerant containing a mixture of flammable gases including propane and butane that has been marketed as a replacement for the ozone layer-depleting chlorofluorocarbon Freon; OZ-12 might in theory ignite under certain conditions and has been placed on an Environmental Protection Agency preliminary list of unacceptable substances (**US News & World Report 22 November 1994:83**)

ozena   A mucopurulent nasal discharge in chronic atrophic rhinitis, seen in long-standing systemic disease, eg iron-deficiency anemia or chronic local infection, described in southern Europe; the etiologic role of *Klebsiella ozaenae* is speculative as this organism is sensitive to broad-spectrum antibiotics, while ozena is refractory to antibiotic therapy

ozonation   The bubbling of ozone through water as a method of water purification, a process that had been proposed as an alternative to chlorination, which has been linked to an ↑ in cancer; ozone reacts with bromine in drinking water, forming unstable compounds that produce an array of potential carcinogens; these compounds bind to DNA more easily than does chloroform, a potentially carcinogenic byproduct of chlorination, raising the question of whether ozonation is preferable for water purification (**Science 1995; 267:1771**) Cf Chlorination

ozone   The triatomic allotrope of oxygen, which is formed when diatomic oxygen is zapped with an electric discharge ENVIRONMENT There are two types of ozone (O_3); '**GOOD**'

OZONE covers the earth's upper atmosphere and blocks the wavelengths of ultraviolet light (UV-B and UV-C) that cause DNA damage; 'good' ozone is being depleted at a rate of 4-5% per decade, and will result in an extra 200 000 deaths in the next 50 years through sun-induced malignancies (**Science 1991; 252:204n&v**); the recent ↑ incidence of malignant melanoma has been attributed to the destruction of the ozone layer, although atmospheric models have not confirmed this posit; depletion of 'good' ozone is largely attributed to CFC accumulation in the atmosphere after release from air conditioners, spray cans and manufacturing plants that produce electronics and plastics; CFCs break down in the atmosphere, releasing chlorine, catalyzing ozone destruction **'BAD' OZONE** is bluish gas with a slightly pungent odor (which at high levels causes tracheobronchitis, pulmonary edema and hemorrhage) formed in the lower atmosphere through complex photochemical reactions involving volatile organic compounds and nitrogen oxides, internal combustion engine, photocopiers, and laser printers; ozone is used as an oxidizing agent in organic chemical production, as a food disinfectant and as a bleaching agent; the federal guidelines from the EPA, are 0.12 ppm of ozone as an hourly peak, a level which has not been met in 62 US cities, including Denver, Los Angeles, and New York City; ↑ levels at ground levels slows the growth of loblolly pine, an important timber of the US South (**Nature, in New York Times 21 March, 1995, C4**) see Berlin Mandate, CFCs, Greenhouse effect, HCFCs, Montreal protocol

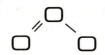

ozone layer ENVIRONMENT An atmospheric zone located 10-50 km above the earth's surface

ozone therapy The administration of ozone ($??O_3$), an oxidizing agent per rectum or intravaginally, which was promoted as having antiviral (anti-HIV), activity, and determined by the FDA to be fraudulent (**Am Med News 21 Nov 1994 p13**) see AIDS fraud

ozone therapy Ozonation ALTERNATIVE MEDICINE A non-conventional therapy that combines 'oxidative' therapy with oxygenation using ozone (O_3), which splits into O$^•$ (which wanders around oxidizing various molecules) and O_2 increasing locoregional O_2 supply; O_3 can be administered parenterally or topically (in a vehicle, eg olive oil or in ozonated water) and is believed by its advocates to accelerate wound healing, inactivate viruses and bacteria, and increase local temperature; OT is reported to be of use in treating AIDS, allergies, asthma, atherosclerosis, cancer, infections, multiple sclerosis, vascular headaches, and others (**Alternative Medicine, Future Medicine Pub, Puyallup, Wash, 1994**) Note: OT does not have FDA approval, and therefore is not administered in the US; see Oxygen therapy

P Symbol for: 1) Para (Obstetrics) 2) Peta– (SI unit for 10^{15}) 3) Phosphate (inorganic) 4) Phosphorus 5) Plasma 6) Polarization 7) Posterior 8) Premolar 9) Pressure 10) Probability (P value) 11) Proline 12) Properdin 13) Pupil

p Symbol for: 1) Atomic orbital with angular momentum 2) Pico- (SI unit for 10^{-12}) 3) Proton 4) Sample proportion (binomial distribution in statistics) 5) Short arm of a chromosome

p– Symbol for *para-* (Chemistry)

Ps The three Ps The association of pituitary adenoma, pancreatic neoplasia and parathyroid adenoma in multiple endocrine neoplasm, type I; see MEN 1

P_{CO_2} Partial pressure of CO_2 in blood, expressed in kilopascals

P_{O_2} Partial pressure of O_2 in blood, expressed in kilopascals

p16 A tumor suppressor protein first identified in a melanoma cell line, that acts as a cell cycle inhibitor, acting on one of the cyclin-dependent kinase inhibitors, CDK4; p16 is encoded by the *p16* gene on chromosome 9p21, a gene that is either deleted or mutated in a wide range of malignancies, eg malignant melanoma, and carcinomas of the bladder, breast and kidney (**Science 1994; 264:436A, 344RN, 1995; 267:963**)

p21 Also known as CIP1, sdi1, WAF1 A protein that is intimately involved in the cell's response to DNA damage or senescence; p21 is capable of direct inhibition of DNA replication (**Nature 1994; 369:574L, 520N&v**) and involved in inhibition of cyclin-dependent kinases; in certain tissues, eg muscle, differentiation induces production of p21, in effect shutting off the cell cycle (**Science 1995; 267:1018, 963**)

p21*ras* **proteins** A family of 21-kD membrane-associated proteins encoded by the c-*ras* gene that bind to guanine nucleotides, which have a low intrinsic GTPase activity and are thought to be involved in the growth-promoting signal transduction pathway

p24 antigen The 24-kD core antigen of HIV-1, which is held responsible for the clinical manifestations of AIDS; p24 is the earliest marker of HIV-1 infection, and is detectable days to weeks before seroconversion to anti-HIV-1 antibody production, as detected by ELISA methods; screening for the p24 antigen does not help identify anti-HIV-1 seronegative or blood donors with 'silent' infections

p24 antigen testing TRANSFUSION MEDICINE The testing of a unit of donated blood for the presence of HIV's p24 antigen, the purpose of which is to increase the safety of blood used for transfusion; the presently available enzyme immunoassays detect HIV as early as 22 days after infection (ie a window period of 22 days); PAT would reduce the window period to 16 days, resulting in a cost of $10 million per case of HIV infection averted (**CAP Today March 1995 p12**)

PAT was briefly introduced in Germany, but abandoned, as it was thought that an increased number of persons at high risk for HIV would donate blood, with the hope of obtaining a free blood test; the US blood banking community is seriously examining the possibility of requiring PAT, if only to minimize the potential lawsuits that would occur when a patient becomes infected during the window period but is undetected as the test was not performed based on cost considerations

p41 PARASITOLOGY A 41 kD polypeptide that is preferentially expressed at the end of maturation in the asexual blood stage of *Plasmodium falciparum*, which has 60% amino acid homology (sequence similarity) with the vertebrate enzyme, aldolase and which has aldolase activity

P_{50} The oxygen tension at which hemoglobin is one-half (50%) saturated, a value equal to 26 torr (mm Hg) in normal red cells; the P_{50} value is obtained from the midpoint of the oxygen dissociation curve and does not reflect the shape of the curve; with increased oxygen affinity, P_{50} decreases, resulting in a 'left shift' (see there) of the dissociation curve; a high P_{50} indicates decreased oxygen affinity of the hemoglobin; see Oxygen dissociation curve

Note: Hemoglobin is almost fully saturated at a partial pressure of oxygen (PO_2) of 85 torr

p53 A nuclear (tumor-suppressing) phosphoprotein encoded by the proto-oncogene *p53*, located on chromosome segment 17p13; in its native or 'wild' form, p53 inhibits cell growth control and transformation[1] and its normal role is in activating the transcription of genes that suppress cell proliferation, thus acting as a tumor suppressor protein; 'wild' p53 is thought to control the entry of the cell into the S phase; p53 suppresses cell division by stimulating synthesis of a cyclin-dependent kinase (Cdk) inhibitor, p2; a *p53* mutation in codon 249 results in a G→T base pair change, and arginine becomes serine in mature p53, acting as a tumor promoter (**New York Times 18 January 1994; C1**); inactivation of the p53 gene by mutation leads to transformation; in clinically aggressive HPV infection, the E6 viral protein binds to p53, preventing its activity; p53 is either low or defective in most lung cancers, colorectal carcinoma and in bladder cancers and may be detected in urine cytology specimens[2] (**Science 1991; 252:706**); loss of p53 is a late event in the multistep process in tumor development and may coincide with the transition from benign to malignant growth; the p53 oncogene is thought to be involved in one-half of colorectal, ⅓ of breast and some small cell carcinomas of the lung and in tumors of the bone and brain, and is mutated in all patients with the Li-Fraumeni syndrome; p53 is an allelic gene that is normally present in pairs, one of which is lost in tumor formation; in most tumors with an allelic deletion, the remaining p53 allele has a missense mutation; a single amino acid substitution in p53 abrogates its tumor suppressive activity, as all mutated p53s thusfar isolated are characterized by a loss of tumor-suppressing activity, increased transforming ability and increased ability to bind to heat shock protein hsp70; p53 mutations differ according to the affected site, including transitions, transversions and base pair mutations, which may reflect differences in etiological contributions of both exogenous and endogenous factors to carcinogenesis (**Science 1991; 253:49**); p53 is the most commonly altered gene in human tumors, identifiable in up to ½ of all malignancies, and an important first step in the tumorigenic process, as exemplified by the Li-Fraumeni cohort in which there is an inherited mutation of the p53 gene, which is followed within 10 to 30 years by various malignancies; p53 immunostaining in needle aspirations of pancreatic malignancies may be of diagnostic value (**Arch Pathol Lab Med 1994; 118:150oA**); p53 accumulation in tumor cell nuclei, detected by immunohistochemistry is associated with a 5–

to 7–fold ↑ rate of recurrence, and ↓ overall survival (**N Engl J Med 1994; 331:1259OA**) STRUCTURE Tumor-suppressor activity requires a tetramer of p53 with a zinc ion (**NP Pavletich, Science July 15 1994**) *p53* mutations occur malignancies of lung ± 56%, colorectum ± 50%, esophagus ± 45%, ovary ± 44%, pancreas ± 44%, skin ± 44%, stomach ± 41%, head & neck ± 37%, bladder ± 34%, sarcoma ± 31%, prostate ± 30%, breast ± 22%, lymphoma ± 12%, melanoma ± 9% (**Science & Medicine Sept/Oct 1994**); p53 overexpression in primary lung adenocarcinoma is associated with cigarette smoking, with p53 overexpression in 10/18 (56%) current smokers, 13/40 (33%) former smokers, and 0/12 of never smokers (**Am J Surg Pathol 1993; 17:213OA**) see Li-Fraumeni syndrome, p21, Tumor suppressor genes, *WAF1*

[1]Tumor production requires that a mutation (deletion, point mutation or rearrangement), commonly affecting a 'CpG island' be present in both alleles, while one wild-type or non-mutated is sufficient to prevent cancer formation [2]Hubert Humphrey (former US vice-president) was diagnosed of borderline malignancy in 1973, invasive bladder cancer in 1976 and died thereof in 1978; PCR performed on his tissue frozen in 1967 reveled a mutation in *p53* (T:A→A:T transversion in codon 227) IMPLICATION Molecular techniques, eg PCR amplification, provide a means by which malignancy can be diagnosed early, in this case nearly 10 years before it was identified by conventional means (**New York Times 16 July 1994; C1**)

p75 A nerve growth factor receptor that has been linked to Alzheimer's disease; in absence of NGF, p75 is reported to allow brain cells to undergo an autodestruct sequence (**New York Times 20 July 1993; C3**)

p95^{vav} Vav, see there

p105 A 105-kD nuclear protein of interchromatin granules that is markedly increased in cells undergoing mitosis; histological identification of p105 overexpression (using a monoclonal antibody) in tissue can be used to confirm increased mitotic activity (**Arch Pathol Lab Med 1994; 118:506OA**)

p105 Proliferating cell nuclear antigen, see there

p107 protein A growth factor-sensitive muscle protein that may be involved in cell cycle regulation of actively proliferating cells that normally does not participate in terminal cell differentiation (**Science 1994; 264; 1467R**)

P170 A 170-kD plasma membrane-bound glycoprotein encoded by the MDR (multidrug resistance) gene, composed of sugar residues and a protein chain that traverses the cell membrane 12 times (a 'dodecaspan', see heptaspan), forming a 'gated' transmembrane pore, using ATP-derived energy to export various drugs from the cytoplasm to the extracellular space; since most of the drugs actively exported are hydrophobic and arrive in the cell by passive diffusion across the membrane, the amount of drug required to reach therapeutic levels in the face of an active exporting system such as P170 may be enormous, reaching levels that are toxic to non-tumorous cells; leukemic blast crises are characterized by increased expression of P-glycoprotein in leukemic cell membranes; see Multidrug resistance gene

P210$^{bcr/abl}$ Philadelphia chromosome, see there

P450 A protein complexed to cytochrome oxidase, which has a peak spectrophotometric absorption at 450 nm and forms the terminal portion of the electron transport system in adrenal mitochondria and hepatic microsomes; P450 is responsible for hydroxylation of phenobarbital, increasing water solubility and hydroxylation of polycyclic aromatic hydrocarbons for conjugation with glucuronate or sulfates

P-450$_{scc}$ side-chain cleaving enzyme (formerly 20,22 desmolase) An enzyme [EC 1.14.15.6] of the mixed function oxidase and cytochrome P-450 systems that removes a hydroxyl side chain from cholesterol yielding Δ^5-pregnenolone

P-450$_{c17}$ hydroxylase/17,20-lyase (formerly 17,20 desmolase) A single enzyme encoded by a gene on chromosome 10 that mediates both the 17-hydroxylation of pregnenolone and progesterone and the conversion of the C_{21}-steroids 17-hydroxypregnenolone and 17-hydroxyprogesterone to the

C_{19}-steroids dehydroepiandrosterone and androstendione

P antigen An antigen linked to the ABH blood group that is located on the red cell surface and composed of three sugars (galactose, N-acetyl-galactosamine and N-acetyl-glucosamine), containing P antigens, P_1, P_2, P^k and p, of which P^k and p are rare; the relatively rare anti-P_1 antibody produced by P_2 individuals may produce clinically significant hemolysis; the anti-P_1 antibody can be neutralized with echinococcal hydatid cyst fluid, serving to identify this IgM molecule; a 'biphasic' autoanti-P antibody occurs in patients with paroxysmal cold hemoglobinuria, fixing complement at 4°C, hemolyzing RBCs at 37°C; the P antigen is present on the surface of RBCs, megakaryocytes, endothelial, placenta, fetal liver and heart cells; it is the receptor for B19 parvovirus and subjects lacking the P antigen are naturally resistant to B19 infection as it has no portal of entry (**N Engl J Med 1994; 330:1192OA**) see B19, P blood group; Cf H antigen

P blood group A group of red cell discovered in 1927 and contains the common antigens P_1 and P (globoside) and the rare P^k antigen (ceramide trihexose); red cells of persons with a blood-group P_1 phenotype have either P_1 or P antigens; P_2 phenotypes have P antigen; P_1^k phenotypes have both P_1 and P^k antigens; those with p phenotype have none of the P group antigens and are at risk for massive hemolysis when given blood with P antigen; see P antigen

P-component CARDIOLOGY One of the two components of amyloid detected by electron microscopy; the major component is fibrillary and has a characteristic periodicity; the minor or P-component, appears as stacks of pentagonal doughnut-like structures with a hollow core, forming short rods, similar to the histiocytosis X body (external diameter, 9 µm, internal, 4 µm); the P-component circulates as a soluble serum protein and is of unknown significance

P gene A gene located in chromosome segment 15q11-q13 that corresponds to the pink-eyed locus of mice; it encodes a transmembrane polypeptide that may transport small molecules, eg tyrosine, the precursor of melanin; *P* gene mutations (frame shift, missense resulting in amino acid substitution, and one affecting mRNA splicing) have been identified in various clinical phenotypes, eg Prader-Willi syndrome, oculocutaneous albinism type II (tyrosinase positive), AR-type ocular albinism (**N Engl J Med 1994; 330:529OA**)

P pilus MICROBIOLOGY A filamentous bacterial structure encoded by the *pap* (pyelonephritis-associated pilus) gene, which promotes the adhesion of *E coli* to the urinary tract epithelium, specifically by various adhesin proteins (**Science & Medicine 1995; 2/3:16**) see Virulence factor

PA interval CARDIOLOGY The interval between the onset of the P wave in the surface tracing of the EKG, which slightly precedes the onset of high right atrial recording, and the low right atrial deflection, measured in the His lead; while the PAI corresponds to the intra-atrial conduction time, it has little clinical value; Cf AH interval, HV interval

PAAC Physicians Association for AIDS Care

PABA para-aminobenzoic acid, see there

PAC Papular acrodermatitis of childhood (Gianotti-Crosti syndrome); political action committee; premature atrial contraction; pulmonary artery catheterization

pacemaker syndrome A relatively common (up to 20%) complication of implanted pacemakers, characterized by vertigo, syncope, dyspnea, weakness, decreased exercise tolerance, postural hypotension, palpable hepatic and jugular vein pulsations ETIOLOGY Alternating AV asynchrony in which the atrium contracts against closed valves, raising venous pressure or the ventricle contracts before the blood has arrived, causing transiently inadequate cardiac output TREATMENT Dual chamber pacing

pacemaker theory CELL BIOLOGY A hypothesis that attempts to explain the aging process, postulating that certain organs have a predetermined lifespan, the functions of which deteriorate with age in the form of immunosenescence (75% ↓ in T-cell activities, ↑ in autoantibody formation and ↑ risk of infection and malignancy) and neuroendocrine changes (altered carbohydrate metabolism and sleep patterns) Cf Garbage can hypothesis

pachydermoperiostosis An AD [MIM 167100] condition characterized by induration of the skin in the natural folds, accentuation of the creases of the face and scalp, clubbing of the fingers and periostosis of the long bones; acquired pachydermoperiostosis appears in later life, is classically associated with bronchogenic carcinoma, and is known as hypertrophic (pulmonary) osteoarthropathy, see there

pachydermy A nonspecific term for leathery subcutaneous induration due to an accumulation of inelastic connective tissue, as in acromegaly or due to accumulation of protein-rich mucin, collagen and fibroblasts, as occurs in myxedema

'pack rat' PSYCHIATRY A person who is incapable of discarding worn-out or worthless objects that have no sentimental value; a PR may reason that discarding is wasteful (*'one never knows when we'll need it'*) and becomes genuinely upset when his/her collection of tennis ball fuzz is 'deep-sixed' by a 'significant other' who may be disturbed about the space occupied by the pack rat's collection of broken parts, appliances, magazines, or newpapers; the PR mentality typical of the obsessive-compulsive personality disorder; Cf Obsessive-compulsive disorder

package insert CLINICAL PHARMACOLOGY A document that accompanies a prescription drug, which contains full product information, including the indications for its use, forms of administration, and side effects; see Advertising

packaging MOLECULAR BIOLOGY The process of folding or compacting and insertion of the long (estimated 3 billion base pairs in length) DNA molecule into a smaller and more efficient space or region, eg formation of chromosomes and nucleosomes; Cf Protein folding

packed unit see Packed red cells

packed red cells TRANSFUSION MEDICINE A concentrated unit of erythrocytes prepared from a unit of whole blood by removing most of the plasma, yielding a volume circa 200 ml, of which 80% of the volume is red cells and 20% plasma; 'packed units' may be stored at 4°C in plastic bags for up to 35 days if collected in CPDA-1 (citrate-phosphate-dextrose-additive) solution, and up to 42 days if additive solutions (containing saline, glucose, adenine, and other approved additives); PRCs are used for active bleeding, excess intraoperative blood loss, low 'pre-op' or 'post-op' hematocrits, chronic anemias, eg sickle cell anemia, thalassemia, chemotherapy for cancer, dialysis, blood exchange; see CPDA-1, Quad pack, Single unit transfusion, Storage lesions, Whole blood

packing ENT Nasal packing, see there LABORATORY TECHNOLOGY *noun* The solid material, usually beads of varying porosities that form the solid (stationary) phase in column chromatography *verb* The process of adding the solid material, eg pouring of the beads, into a chromatographic column

packing ratio MOLECULAR BIOLOGY The length of DNA divided by the length of the unit that contains it, which may be as great as 7000; because of DNA's complexity, it cannot be directly packaged, but rather requires hierarchies of organization, the

FIRST PACKING LEVEL is that of DNA wound into beadlike particles, giving it a packing ratio of 6; the

SECOND PACKING LEVEL is the coiling of the 'beaded strings' into a helical array, constituting a 30 nm fiber found in both interphase chromatin and mitotic chromosomes, yielding a packing ratio of 40, the

THIRD (AND HIGHEST) PACKING HIERARCHY is determined by the packing of the fiber itself, which is modified by accessory proteins and has a ratio of 1000 or more

'pack-years' A crude indicator of a person's cigarette consumption, calculated as the packs of cigarettes smoked per day, multiplied by the length of consumption in years; eg two packs of cigarettes smoked per day for 20 years is 40 pack-years, which is associated with a relative risk (RR value) of 60 for suffering a smoking-related malignancy

paclitaxel Taxol™, see there

'pacmen' A highly colloquial term transiently used by some US legislators for hidden liabilities that the government must pay in the future, eg rising costs of health care, which may rise to hundreds of billions (US) of dollars

Pacman is one of the first video games to be popularized, a game in which little 'mouths' gobbled up dots on the game board

padded dash(board) 'syndrome' A vanishingly rare form of trauma, most commonly affecting the right front seat occupant ('passenger side' in many countries) in an automobile accident when he/she is restrained by a lap-type safety belt; in an abrupt stop, the passenger's body is thrown forward at the waist and the hyperextended neck strikes the dashboard at the level of the thyroid cartilage CLINICAL Respiratory distress due to upper airway obstruction, due to a hematoma, fluid accumulation, aspiration of saliva, fluids, subcutaneous emphysema, fractures of cartilage, accompanied by pain on deglution

Note: Shoulder restraints and air bags in automobiles appear to have virtually eliminated this form of motor vehicle-related trauma

padlock sign RADIOLOGY An uncommon finding by CT in which a mass density is accompanied by adjacent ring enhancement, representing eccentric cavitation in a solid intracranial lesion; while characteristic of higher grade astrocytomas, abscesses and metastases, it is also seen in craniopharyngioma, meningioma, prolactinoma (with cystic changes), and TB and thus has little diagnostic specificity

PAF Platelet-activating factor, see there

Also 1) Peroxisome assembly factor 2) Platelet-aggregating factor 3) Posterior auditory field 4) Preadmission assessment form (required by the Health Care Financing Administration) 5) Pseudoamniotic fluid (gynecology) 6) Pulmonary arteriovenous fistula

PAF acetylhydrolase An enzyme that hydrolyzes PAF's acetyl residue, abolishing PAF's potent pro-inflammatory activity; PAF acetylhydrolase may prove useful as anti-inflammatory agent (Nature 1995; 374:549L)

page 1) To contact a person by voice over a public address system 2) Beep, see there

PAGE Polyacrylamide gel electrophoresis, see there SDS-PAGE

Page syndrome A vasomotor dysfunction characterized by periodic blotchy flushing and sweating of the face, upper chest, abdomen, which may be associated with cold extremities, headache, tachycardia, and hypertension, possibly related to vascular compression of the brain stem (N Engl J Med 1993; 329:1449oA)

Note: This may be related to or a permutation of neurogenic hypertension

Paget's disease of bone Osteitis deformans A bone-remodeling disorder of older Northern European ♂ that is most common in the lumbosacral spine, pelvis and skull, which affects ± 10% of the population by age 80 CLINICAL Often asymptomatic; when symptomatic, pain, deformity, pathologic fracture, neural compression PATHOGENESIS Possibly paramyxovirus infection of osteoblasts causing ↑ production of IL-6 and activation of c-*fos* proto-oncogene, resulting in localized osteoclastic activity RADIOLOGY Moth-eaten destruction of trabecular bone, endosteal scalloping, cortical penetration, formation of soft tissue masses LABORATORY ↑↑↑ Serum alkaline phosphatase PATHOLOGY Low-power LM reveals a classic 'mosaic' pattern of thickened, poorly mineralized and osteoclastic bony trabeculae, later demonstrating abnormal hyperplasia, ↑ vascularity, prominent and scalloped cement lines with osteoblastic rimming; osteoid is not prominent and is poorly mineralized EM Measles virus-like intranuclear inclusions COMPLICATIONS Cardiac failure due to arteriovenous shunting; osteosarcoma and other sarcomas occur in 1-25% TREATMENT Biphosphonate, calcitonin, usually of salmon origin; most of the 25% of cases that develop anti-salmon antibodies respond to human calcitonin; alternate therapies include mitrimycin and surgery for decompressing critical cranial structures, or joint replacement (**N Engl J Med 1993; 328:1836CPC**) see Mosaic bone

Paget's disease of the breast A 'weeping', eczematoid erosive lesion of the nipple first described by Sir James Paget in 1874 that is almost invariably associated with underlying intraductal breast carcinoma (carcinoma in situ, ductal type), and when accompanied by a palpable mass implies an invasive carcinoma PATHOLOGY Large clear epithelial cells with atypical nuclei located in the basal layer, often arranged in oligocellular clusters DDx Bowen's disease, malignant melanoma PROGNOSIS Survival is a function of the aggressiveness of the underlying duct cell carcinoma, or less commonly, lobular carcinoma; Cf Intraepidermal carcinoma

Note: Paget's cells may imbibe melanin granules (a process known as cytocrinia), resulting in the misdiagnosis of melanoma

Paget's disease, extramammary A disease that is similar morphologically to Paget's disease of the breast, but less often associated with underlying malignancy; the condition arises from skin adnexae, visceral malignancy or rarely, de novo, appearing in the scrotum, perineum and labia majora and the cells are more often mucin-positive than in Paget's disease of the breast

PAH Polycyclic aromatic hydrocarbon, see there

PAI Plasminogen activator inhibitor, see there

pain NEUROLOGY '*An unpleasant sensory and emotional experience associated with actual or potential tissue damage or described in terms of such damage*'-definition proposed by the International Association for the Study of Pain (**Pain 1980; 8:249-252**); The sensation of marked discomfort that is either sharp and well-localized (conducted along A-delta fibers) or dull and diffuse (conducted along C nerve fibers; Brodmann's area 24 appears to be a catchment region for pain, and thus the cortex is selectively activated in response to pain; the parietal and limbic regions of the cortex may respond to the location and intensity of the pain and the limbic region regulates the emotional response to pain (**Science 1991; 251:1355**) see Brief Pain Inventory, Gait control theory, Patient controlled analgesia

Note: Therapy for recalcitrant pain (post-surgery, burn and terminal cancer patients) is often inadequate due to the care-givers' fear of opiate addiction, or the physician may underestimate the severity of the pain (**N Engl J Med 1994; 330:592OA**); in those with terminal (recurrent or metastatic) cancer, analgesia may be administered more frequently as opiates are less addicting, possibly due to an alteration in the endorphin receptors or processing of endorphins

'pain and suffering' MEDICAL MALPRACTICE A term for the physical discomfort and distress, as well as mental and emotional trauma, which are recoverable as elements of damage in a lawsuit; in 1975, California set a limit on P&S of $250 000 by enacting the Medical Injury Compensation Recovery Act (**Cal Stats 1975, 2d Ex Sess 1975-1976:3949-4007**); as a consequence, malpractice premiums in California have stabilized, and physicans are more comfortable with the knowledge that a malpractice case would not be pursued for its emotional value alone (**N Engl J Med 1993; 329:1733OA**) see Malpractice, damages

painful bruising syndrome A psychosomatic trauma-induced condition of unknown etiology, described in emotionally-labile women that appears on the legs, face and trunk, characterized by recurring painful ecchymoses with a ladder-like morphology, accompanied by syncope, nausea, vomiting, gastrointestinal and intracranial bleeding

painful crisis Vaso-occlusive crisis One of the 'crises' common in sickle cell anemia where 'sludging' of sickled red cells causes capillary stasis and infarction, resulting in incapacitating musculoskeletal pain or 'referral'-type organ pain, hemoptysis, hematuria, melena and central nervous system symptoms; painful crises occur at a rate of 0.8 episodes/year in sickle cell disease, 1.0/year in sickle-β-thalassemia, and 0.4/year in hemoglobin SC-β thalassemia; this frequency is translated into a 'pain rate', which is a measure of disease severity that correlates with early death in patients with sickling anemias (**N Engl J Med 1991; 325:11**) hemolytic 'crises' consist of rapidly evolving anemia, leukocytosis, jaundice and fever TREATMENT Short course of high-dose methylprednisolone ↓ the duration of painful crises but ↑ rebound attacks with discontinuation of steroid therapy (**N Engl J Med 1994; 330:733OA**)

painful fat syndrome An atypical, chronic and symmetric swelling and tenderness of the legs, more commonly affecting adolescent females; the lipoedema is painful on pressure, is non-pitting and fancifully likened to pigskin; Cf Lipomatosis dolorosa

painful feet syndrome Burning feet syndrome, see there

painful heel An idiopathic affliction of older men causing tenderness of the heel associated with focal edema and in one-half of cases, calcaneal spur formation PROGNOSIS Persistent pain or spontaneous resolution

painful leg syndrome 1) Painful leg and moving toes syndrome 2) Painful red leg syndrome 3) Restless legs syndrome, see there

painful leg and moving toes syndrome A condition characterized by spasms or involuntary movements of the toes and feet, attributed to ectopic discharges in sensory roots, ganglia, or nerves, which evokes both pain and organized movements (**VA Adams, M Victor, Principles of Neurology, 5th ed, McGraw-Hill, New York, 1993**)

painful red leg syndrome Erythromelia A condition characterized by an ↑ sensitivity to skin temperatures above 32°C; individual patients often become symptomatic at an exact temperature, with focal vasodilation and a burning sensation TREATMENT Aspirin; secondary erythromelia may occur in hypertension or polycythemia vera

pain rate see Painful crisis

'paintbrush' hair A descriptor for fragile, beaded and longitudinally split hair shafts seen in trichorrhexis nodosa, a common condition caused by hair dryness resulting from 'excess' hair care (too frequent shampooing, combing and brushing); Cf Flag sign, Pili torti, Woolly hair syndrome

paired helical filaments NEUROPATHOLOGY Structures that are the main constituents of the neurofibrillary tangles of Alzheimer's disease, which are composed of 210-nm filaments of predominantly A68 protein wound into a helix; PHFs are relatively insoluble, may be composed of ubiquitin and occur in Down syndrome, Hallervorden-Spatz disease, lead encephalopathy, lipofuscinosis, subacute sclerosing panencephalitis, tuberous sclerosis, in neurites surrounding amyloid-rich senile plaques, and in neuropil threads; see A68 protein, Neurofibrillary tangles, Senile plaques

PAJAMA experiment(s) A series of experiments* that led to the concept of repressor proteins as regulators of gene expression, which act at specific sites along the DNA, designated as operators

*Carried out by A Pardee, F Jacob and J Monod, hence the fanciful acronym; the innovative work led to a Nobel prize awarded in 1965 (**Science 1988;**

pale body A well-circumscribed, pale eosinophilic cytoplasmic inclusion, thought to be characteristic of fibrolamellar carcinoma of the liver

pale cells A nonspecific descriptor for cells with homogeneous, lightly eosinophilic cytoplasm, occurring in 1) Lung Cells in sclerosing hemangioma which have an appearance midway between type II pneumocytes and stromal connective tissue cells, 2) Liver Hepatocytes with a 'washed-out' appearance caused by hypertrophy of the endoplasmic reticulum, as seen in barbiturate intoxication and 3) Lymph nodes Plasmacytoid CD8-positive T cells that are scattered or arranged in clusters in T cell lymphoproliferative disorders, eg immunoblastic lymphadenopathy (IBL), angioimmunoblastic lymphadenopathy and IBL-like T-cell lymphoma

paleoanthropology The field that formally studies ancient man
This contrasts with geriatrics, the field that formally studies ancient men

palindrome Greek, Reading the same, backward and forward MOLECULAR BIOLOGY A sequence of duplex DNA with dyad symmetry, ie a sequence that is the same when either strand is read in a defined direction, eg the 5' to 3' direction; inverted repeats of double-stranded DNA are located opposite each other on contiguous strands of DNA and the axis of symmetry can be drawn to separate the inverted repeats; this symmetry allows formation of hydrogen-bonded hairpin loops and stem-and-loop structures; experimental denaturation of palindromic regions may lead to the formation of semistable cruciform loops capable of interacting with binding proteins (it is uncertain whether cruciform loops exist in vivo); palindromic DNA renatures rapidly and comprises up to 5% of eukaryotic DNA, representing recognition sites for regulatory proteins, eg the lac operon; restriction endonucleases usually cut double-stranded DNA through segments with dyad symmetry, as shown in the accompanying figure (dashed line indicates the cleavage line of the *Eco*RI)

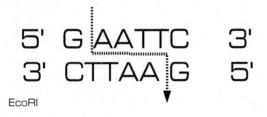

palindrome

palindromic rheumatism A form of monoarthritis that may precede rheumatoid arthritis CLINICAL Intermittent recurring (more than 5 attacks in 2 years) episodes of intense gout-like pain and joint inflammation, more common in middle-aged men, affecting the knee, wrist or dorsum of hand, accompanied by transient subcutaneous nodules; although the condition is distinct between patients, each attack tends to follow the same pattern in the individual patient LABORATORY Nonspecific ↑ ESR and acute phase reactants

Paling scale RISK ASSESSMENT A somewhat facetious albeit potentially useful scale[1] proposed by J Paling[2], that attempts to stratify the risks of daily living based on the likelihood of their occurrence, where 0 is 1 chance in 1 million, the point below which the FDA deems the risk of a potential carcinogen in food to be too small to be a concern over a lifetime (Sci Am 1995; 272/5:20)

[1]Which, like the Richter scale used to determine the magnitude of an earthquake is measured on a logarithmic scale; a Paling value of -6 is one chance in a trillion of an event's occurance; between -4 and -2 is the 'Bobbitt zone', ie the risk of suffering an unscheduled penectomy in the US during a given year; 0 is the risk of drowning in a bathtub, or of a woman being killed by her husband or lover, and so on [2]Formerly of the University of Oxford

palisading Pallisade, picket fence arrangement *palisade*, French, fence made of pales, forming an enclosure or defense A commonly used descriptor for a light microscopic appearance in which elongated and compressed, usually epithelial cells are perpendicular to a surface, eg a basement membrane, an appearance that has been described in chondroblastoma (bone), oligodendroglioma (brain), ulcerative colitis-related dysplasia (colon) due to the vertical arrangement of tall, crowded goblet cells with pseudopalisaded hyperchromatic nuclei, seen lining branched colonic glands, endocervical adenocarcinoma (endocervix), malignant epithelial mesothelioma (lung), rheumatoid pannus (joint), ameloblastoma (oral cavity, also known as a 'tombstone' pattern, which may also be seen in primordial cysts and odontogenic keratocysts), mucinous cystadenoma and mucinous cystadenocarcinoma (ovary) and basal cell carcinoma (skin, see figure); the term also refers to the arrangement of *Corynebacterium* species, more commonly described as having a 'Chinese character' appearance

palliative surgery An operation carried out in the face of hopelessly incurable malignancy, justified to reduce the severity of symptoms and improve the quality of life, relieving pain (cordectomy), hemorrhage (cystectomy for bleeding urinary bladder), obstruction (colostomy or gastroenterostomy) or infection (amputation of a necrotic and malodorous tumor-ridden breast or extremity); see 'Heroic' surgery, Mutilating surgery

palliative therapy Any treatment of a terminally ill patient intended to alleviate pain and suffering, without performing aggressive ('heroic') procedures; palliative therapy recognizes the incurable nature of a pernicious process and seeks, through various modalities, eg surgery and radiotherapy, to reduce or shrink tumor masses compressing vital structures, seeking to ↑ a patient's 'quality time' before death; see 'Band-aid' therapy, Karnovsky scale; 'Heroic' therapy

pallidotomy NEUROSURGERY Incision or partial destruction of the globus pallidum, a technically demanding high-risk procedure that is reportedly useful in Parkinson's disease (PD) patients who are refractory to L-dopa therapy; in pallidotomy, a small probe is inserted through the skull and an electric current is used to produce small lesions in the internal segment of the globus pallidus[*], attenuating those neural signals that cause the classic symptoms of PD, to wit, slowing of reactions, rigidity, tremors, and defects in gait and balance; pallidotomy costs $10-40 000 and may benefit 15-25% of the 1.5 million (US) with PD, especially the younger ones; in two reported small (46 and 18 patient) series, pallidotomy resulted in complete or near-complete relief from rigidity and limitations of movement, gait, and speech COMPLICATIONS Visual defects, loss of speech, seizures, coma, death (Am Med News 24 April 1995 p1)

[*]When the technique was first introduced in the 1940s, the neurosurgical world was underwhelmed, in view of the mixed rate of success, which may have been the result of suboptimal placement of the 'zapping' probe; the ideal location appears to be the most posterior portion of the globus pallidus

PALS Periarteriolar lymphoid sheath, see there

PAM 1) Primary acquired melanosis 2) Primary amoebic meningoencephalitis 3) Pulmonary alveolar macrophage

pamidronate disodium An agent that is administered IV, which is the most potent of the biphosphonates, a family of compounds used to treat the bony complications of malignancy and to stimulate the healing of osteolytic lesions in patients with bony metastases (Cancer 1994; 74:3049)

panagglutination Polyagglutination, see there

pan-B cell marker(s) HEMATOLOGY Surface antigens that are present on all normal B lymphocytes; CD19 is considered the best pan-B cell marker, which may replace identification of surface immunoglobulins as an indicator of B cell lineage; other surface antigens included under the rubric of pan-B markers are CD20 and CD24; see Pan-T cell markers

pancake cell A flattened compressed endothelial cell seen in intravascular fibrous atherosclerotic plaques that stain intensely with actin and which appears to play a role in atherosclerosis

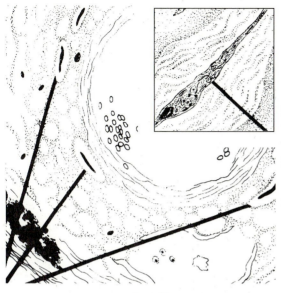

pancake cells

pancake omentum An omentum that has undergone marked thickening and induration secondary to diffuse infiltration by malignancy, usually of epithelial origin, most commonly, by advanced ovarian cystadenocarcinoma, but also by carcinoma of the colon, stomach or pancreas; the omental 'cake' is seen by CT as a flattened layer of tumor separating the small or large intestine from the anterior abdominal wall; Cf 'Policeman of the abdomen'

pancreas divisum A congenital defect of the pancreas that is caused by a failure in the fusion of the dorsal and ventral buds of the pancreas in the embryo, resulting in drainage of the production of the exocrine pancreas though the relatively small duct of Santorini and the accessory papilla; PD is found in 5-10% of autopsy series, and in 2-7% of ERCPs; whether it is responsible for recurrent acute pancreatitis or chronic abdominal pain is uncertain (N Engl J Med 1995; 332:1482RA)

pancreatic cholera syndrome(s) Vipoma syndrome, see there, aka Verner-Morrison or WDHA syndrome

pancreatic endocrine tumors A group of tumors comprising a small proportion of pancreatic neoplasms, including APUDoma, islet cell tumor and nesidioblastoma, most commonly found in the body and tail, the sites of the greater concentration of islets of Langerhans; although PETs appear in 0.5-1.0% of unselected autopsies, the prevalence of functional, hormone-producing tumors is less than $1:10^6$; the tumors are named according to the predominant hormone being produced, eg gastrinoma, glucagonoma, VIPoma, PPoma and others, although most tumors produce more than one hormone PATHOLOGY Patterns include solid, gyriform, glandular and nondescript types PROGNOSIS Most PETs are indolent and a ten-year survival is the norm after initial resection; more aggressive lesions may respond to chemotherapy or streptozocin; see WDHA syndrome, Zollinger-Ellison syndrome

pancreatic islet transplantation The transplantation of a patient's own pancreatic islets (pancreatic islet autograft) into his/her liver via intraportal injection, following pancreatectomy necessitated by severe chronic pancreatitis secondary to such diverse entities as small duct disease and pancreas divisum; the operation has the obvious advantage of being nonimmunogenic as it is of 'self' origin; insulin independence can be obtained with engraftment of as few as 265 000 islets (N Engl J Med 1992; 327:220OA) only 6 of the 22 patients who received islet autografts became insulin-independent in the long term (N Engl J Med 1992; 327:271ED) 800 000 cells (which can be obtained from two cadaveric pancreases) is now considered an optimal number; since 1990, 150 PITs have been performed worldwide with less than scintillating results, most failing within 3 years; reality to the contrary, some workers wax enthusiastic about PIT believing the early failures were due to insufficient number of cells (Sci Am July 1995, p50)

pancreatic panel LABORATORY MEDICINE An abbreviated and cost-effective battery of chemical assays of use in detecting pancreatitis, which includes amylase, lipase, calcium and glucose; Cf Organ panel

pancreatic polypeptide A 36-residue polypeptide of unknown function secreted by the pancreatic islet 'F' cells in various animal species

pancreatic rest A focus or foci of ectopic pancreatic tissue that may have all the histological components of a normal pancreas (including acini, ducts and islets of Langerhans), which remains in the upper GI tract after embryogenic steps including rotation of the ventral anlage and its fusion with the dorsal anlage; pancreatic rests occur in multiple sites in the midgut, eg stomach, small intestine and 'classically' finding in Meckel's diverticulum, and rarely occur in the liver, mesentery and omentum, simulating metastatic adenocarcinoma

pancreatic stone protein Lithostathine, see there

pancreatic sufficiency A term coined in reference to patients with cystic fibrosis (which is equally applicable to DM with adequate insulin production) who have sufficient exocrine pancreatic function to allow normal digestion without enzyme supplements, a finding in patients who have milder disease, are older when diagnosed, who have lower levels of sweat chloride, milder respiratory disease, normal growth and a better prognosis; see Cystic fibrosis

pancreatic transplantation A procedure designed to halt the progression of diabetic neuropathy and achieve complete glycemic control; pancreatic transplantation requires that a large segment or the entire pancreas be harvested, thus donors are often cadaveric; PT is often combined with renal allograft transplantation, necessitated by diabetic nephropathy; because of the limited access to the procedure, recipients must be as 'perfect' (immunologically, as well as clinically, ie stable), as possible; the most common exclusionary criterion is the presence of cardiovascular disease; one-year survival of patients is 93%; one-year graft survival is 50-80%; when a living HLA-matched donor undergoes hemipancreatectomy, the donor's insulin secretion and glucose control deteriorates (whether clinical DM develops in the donor is uncertain, JAMA 1991; 265:510); Cf Biohybrid artificial pancreas, Islet cell transplantation

pancreolauryl test GASTROENTEROLOGY A 'tubeless' pancreatic function test in which fluorescein dilaurate is administered per os, which is cleaved by pancreatic esterases, which release fluorescein that is measured in the urine FALSE POSITIVITY Hepatic disease, renal failure, intestinal malabsorption (N Engl J Med 1995; 332:1482RA) see Bentiromide test, Tubeless test

pancytopenia A global reduction of 'blood cells' characterized by hypoplasia or aplasia of normal hematopoietic precursors in the bone marrow, as seen in hypoplastic myelodysplasia; pancytopenia occurs in aplastic anemia (drug-related, especially common in chemotherapeutic agents used to treat malignancy, radiotherapy, toxins), marrow replacement by hematopoietic, lymphoproliferative and metastatic malignancy, storage diseases, osteopetrosis, myelofibrosis, hypersplenism (congestive splenomegaly, hematopoietic malignancy, storage diseases, sarcoidosis, malaria and kala-azar), infection (fungemia, septicemia, TB), and megaloblastic anemia

pandemic An epidemic affecting a large number of people at the same time and in many different communities; well-described pandemics include

AIDS, first recognized in 1981

CHOLERA Seven pandemics have been described, the most recent of which occurred from 1961 to 1981

INFLUENZA which was uncommon until 1889, after which time (for unknown reasons) influenza pandemics have occurred about every 10 years, where new immunotypes are related to antigenic changes in the surface glycoprotein, hemagglutinin and neuraminidase that protrude from the viral envelope

SYPHILIS The syphilitic or 'great pox' pandemic swept through Europe in the 1500s and is thought to have been more virulent than 'modern' syphilis

PLAGUE (*Yersinia*) pandemics were first described in Egypt, 542 AD, spreading to Turkey and Europe; a second began in Asia minor and Africa in the early 1300s, causing the Black Plague, killing ¼ of Europe; a third occurred in Europe in the pre-industrial age and a fourth pandemic is in progress, which began in China in 1860 and migrated by ship to India, Asia, Brazil, and California

panic attack PSYCHIATRY A discrete period of intense fear, apprehension or discomfort, in which four or more specific symptoms (table) develop abruptly and reach a peak within 10 minutes; PAs are often recurrent, unpredictable, sudden, and intense; while an attack is occurring, the subjects are disinclined to appear in public and thus also suffer from transient agoraphobia; panic attacks affect 3.6% of the adult population in the US (**JAMA 1991; 265:742**), they are transient and fall short of the criteria required to diagnose 'Panic disorder'; according to the DSM-IV, a panic attack is not a codable disorder

---

SYMPTOMS FOR A PANIC ATTACK

1) Palpitations, pounding heart, or ↑ heart rate
2) Sweating
3) Trembling or shaking
4) Sensation of choking, smothering, or suffocation
5) Shortness of breath
6) Chest pain or discomfort
7) Nausea or abdominal discomfort
8) Dizziness, faintness, lightheadedness, or unsteadiness
9) Sensation of unreality or depersonalization
10) Fear of loss of control or going crazy (or being trapped)
11) Fear of dying
12) Paresthesias (numbness, tingling)
13) Chills or hot flashes

From Diagnostic and Statistical Manual of Mental Disorders, 4th ed (DSM-IV™), American Psychiatric Association, Washington, DC 1994

---

panic disorder A psychogenic complex affecting 1.5% of the US population characterized by recurrent and unpredictable episodes (panic attacks) of sudden, intense apprehension, fear and autonomic nervous system hyperactivity CLINICAL Dyspnea, palpitations, chest pain, a sensation of choking, dizziness, loss of reality sense, paresthesias, hot and cold flashes, sweating, faintness, trembling, a fear of dying or of 'going crazy'; the fear of an attack in public may result in functional agoraphobia;

those with panic disorders have an 18-fold greater incidence of suicidal ideation than a mentally 'fit' population; PD is subdivided according to the presence [DSM-IV 300.21] or absence [DSM-IV 300.01] of agoraphobia

Note: Panic attacks and panic disorder differ only in degree and frequency and the potential transient nature of panic attacks

panic values Critical values Laboratory results from patient specimens that must be reported immediately to the clinician, which are often of a nature requiring urgent therapeutic action; other 'critical' values include parameters from

HEMATOLOGY, eg blasts or sickle cells on a peripheral smear, possibly indicating leukemia or sickle cell anemia

MICROBIOLOGY, eg positive gram stain or culture from blood, serosal fluids or cerebrospinal fluid, acid-fast stain or positive mycobacterial culture results

TRANSFUSION MEDICINE Incompatible cross-match and positive serology for VDRL; the panic values differ in each laboratory and the route by which the communication occurs is at the discretion of the laboratory director; see Decision levels

---

PANIC VALUES

ANALYTE	SI UNITS	US UNITS
Calcium	< 1.65 mmol/L	< 6.6 mg/dl
	> 2.22 mmol/L	> 12.9 mg/dl
Glucose	< 2.60 mmol/L	< 46 mg/dl
	> 26.9 mmol/L	> 484 mg/dl
K⁺	< 2.8 mmol/L	< 2.8 mEq/L
	> 6.2 mmol/L	> 6.2 mEq/L
	> 8.0 mmol/L if hemolyzed	
Na⁺	< 120 mmol/L	< 120 mEq/L
	> 158 mmol/L	> 158 mEq/L
CO₂ in	< 11 mmol/L	< 11 mMol
plasma	> 40 mmol/L	> 40 mMol

---

pannus A reticulated membrane of granulation (reactive fibrovascular) tissue that is characteristic of the chronic proliferodestructive phase of rheumatoid arthritis; in the pannus, immune complexes form at the synovial membranes, evoking a nonspecific immune response by macrophages, which produce IL-1, fibroblast-activating factor, prostaglandins, platelet-derived growth factor, substance P, and others, resulting in global destruction of chondro-osseous tissues PATHOLOGY Exuberant synovitis, edema, diffuse swelling, and erythema of the overlying joints with vaguely palisaded histiocytes; with time, the pannus fills the joint space, causing subchondral demineralization and cystic resorption due to the release of enzymes, and fibrous ankylosis Note: Pannus formation also occurs in tuberculous synovitis, and in the fibrovascular proliferative response to *Chlamydia trachomatis* infection of the cornea and conjunctiva, causing blindness

pan-T cell marker(s) A group of cell surface antigens that are present on all normal T lymphocytes, including CD2 (formerly, OKT 11/Leu 5), a 50-kD molecule found only on T cells, corresponding to the sheep erythrocyte rosette marker and CD7, a 41-kD molecule that may also be found in T cell acute leukemias and rare early acute myeloid leukemia; other surface antigens regarded as pan-T markers are CD1 (peripheral T cells and cortical thymocytes), CD3 (mature T cells) and CD5; see Pan-B cell markers

panzerherz German, armored heart A synonym for pericardial calcinosis, a rare complication of chronic pericarditis

PAO Peak acid output, see there

PaO₂/FiO₂ An index of arterial oxygenation efficiency that corresponds to ratio of partial pressure of arterial O₂ to the fraction of inspired O₂ (see **N Engl J Med 1993; 328:399OA**)

PAP 1) Peroxidase-antiperoxidase technique, see there 2) Primary atypical pneumonia, see Interstitial pneumonia 3) Pulmonary alveolar proteinosis

pap 'mill' CYTOLOGY A generic term for any laboratory that encouraged cytotechnologists to screen a virtually unlimited number of Pap smears, by paying them on a per-case basis; PMs became a focus of national attention when evidence mounted that the high volume (200 or more cases/day per screener) being screened resulted in an increased number of 'missed' malignant and premalignant lesions (W Bogdanovitch, Wall Street Journal, Nov 2, 1987); most states have enacted legislation limiting the number of Pap smears that one technologist can screen/day, eg 100 slides/8 hour period in New York State

Pap test Papanicolaou test, Pap smear GYNECOLOGY A cytologic sampling from the uterine cervix and endocervix that is the 'gold standard' method for early detection of HPV, herpes or trichomonad infections, cervical intraepithelial neoplasia (CIN or dysplasia), and squamous cell carcinoma of the cervix; various factors prevent the PT from detecting the theoretical 100% of these lesions, including sampling error, insufficient time devoted to screening and fatigue by the cytotechnologist performing the screening; the PT may suffer from lack of clinical information, inadequate follow-up, and suboptimal reproducibility (JAMA 1989; 261:737); cytologic sampling from the vaginal vault is used to evaluate hormonal status, in one study of 481 ♀ with invasive cervical cancer, 33% had not had a PT within the previous 5 years, 15% did not return for followup after an abnormal or inconclusive diagnosis on a PT, in 7% the laboratory goofed (D Janerich, June 1995 Am J Public Health, in NY Times 7 June 1995; C12) see Bethesda system, Maturation index

The procedure was named after its creator, George Nicholas Papanicolaou (1883-1962), Greek-born US anatomist and cytologist

papain A cysteine proteinase [EC 3.4.22.2] of broad specificity derived from *Carica papaya*, which is used in IMMUNOLOGY, used in early work to delineate immunoglobulin structure, papain digests immunoglobulin into two antibody (Fab) fragments and a crystallizable (Fc) fragment; see Fab fragment, Fc fragment, Pepsin TRANSFUSION MEDICINE Papain, ficin, and other enzymes can be used to modify red cell antigens, enhancing the reactivity of some antigen-antibody systems, eg Rh and Kidd, and abolishing the reactivity of others, eg M, N, Fy^a and Fy^b, thus aiding in the identification of antigens that may cause hemolytic transfusion reactions

Papanicolaou classification GYNECOLOGY A system for stratifying cytologic specimens obtained from the uterine cervix according to presence or absence of malignancy, and the type of optimal followup

CLASS I NEGATIVE FOR MALIGNANCY Absence of atypical or abnormal cells

CLASS II NEGATIVE Nonmalignant but atypical or abnormal cells

CLASS III SUSPICIOUS FOR MALIGNANCY Atypical or abnormal cells are suggestive of malignancy

CLASS IV POSITIVE Atypical or abnormal cells are strongly suggestive of malignancy

CLASS V POSITIVE FOR MALIGNANCY Atypical or abnormal cells are diagnostic of malignancy

The PC has been abandoned for a wide range of reasons for the Bethesda classification, see there, although some physicians continue to feel more comfortable using the class system

paper chromatography A form of partition chromatography that allows separations based on differences in the rate of diffusion, solubility of solute and the nature of the solute, where the stationary phase is a filter paper and the mobile phase is a solvent containing a molecule of interest; paper chromatography was formerly used to fractionate

SUGARS, now separated by column chromatography

AMINO ACIDS, now analyzed by ion-exchange chromatography

BARBITURATES, now analyzed by GLC, TLC, or HPLC

paper money skin A descriptor for the small randomly scattered subcutaneous blood vessels found on the upper arms in hepatic failure as well as the healed lesions of pyoderma gangrenosum, so named as the finding has been fancifully likened to the fine hair-like threads seen in US paper currency, which is so designed to reduce counterfeiting

Papile grading system NEONATOLOGY A system used to stratify peri– and intraventricular hemorrhage into four grades of increasing severity based on findings by cranial ultrasonography (N Engl J Med 1993; 329:1597OA, 1602OA)

papillary SURGICAL PATHOLOGY *adjective* Belonging, pertaining, or referring to a papilla, pathogists' parlance for a morphology characterized by clusters of cells, usually epithelial, that are directly attached to a fibrovascular core; papillary lesions can either benign or malignant, and when malignant (eg papillary carcinoma of the thyroid or papillary urothelial carcinoma of the bladder), tend to be less aggressive than neoplasms with other morphologies

papillary necrosis (of renal papillae) NEPHROLOGY A complication of acute pyelonephritis, consisting of uni- or bilateral lesions of one or more pyramids, with a white-gray discoloration of the pyramid tips, which occurs in a background of acute or chronic renal failure CLINICAL Renal colic, pyuria ETIOLOGY DM, sickle cell anemia, analgesics (aspirin and phenacetin), cyclophosphamide, ischemia, and pyelonephritis related to obstruction PATHOLOGY Coagulation necrosis with preservation of the outlines of the tubules; tissue from the pyramids may slough into the urine

papillary neoplasm (kidney) NEPHROLOGY A neoplasm that was formerly regarded as a variant of renal adenocarcinoma; classification of a renal tumor as a PN requires that at least 50% (or according to some authors, 75%) of the architecture be papillary; PN represents ± 14% of all renal epithelial neoplasms and affects the middle aged population with a ♂ ♀ ratio of 2.5:1 CLINICAL Hematuria, abdominal pain or mass RADIOLOGY Avascular or hypovascular by angiography; tumor calcifications PATHOLOGY CDCs average 8 cm and are usually in a low pathologic stage at presentation; PNs are typically papillary or tubulopapillary formations of cells on fibrovascular stalks; the neoplastic cells are usually of a low cytologic grade and may have abundant macrophages and other inflammatory cells SPECIAL STUDIES Loss of Y chromosome, and trisomy of 7 and 17 are typical findings (Am J Clin Pathol 1995; 103:624OA) see Renal epithelial neoplasms

papillary & solid epithelial neoplasm of the pancreas A low-grade pancreatic carcinoma that is most common in young ♀; the PSENP measures 5-15 cm, and is accompanied by hemorrhage and necrosis; certain histologic features suggest that it may represent a primitive endocrine tumor PATHOLOGY Low mitotic activity, hyaline globules, foam cells PROGNOSIS Excellent with adequate resection

papillary ring A radiologic manifestation of papillary necrosis of the kidneys, seen by contrast studies of the upper urinary tract, in which debris from necrotic medullary tissue and pyramids fills the cup-shaped calices

pa-ping A condition described in mainland China, clinically similar to hypokalemic periodic paralysis (periodic attacks of truncal and limb paralysis) caused by ingestion of barium salts, resulting in hypokalemia by blockage of the potassium channels in skeletal muscle, which prevents the efflux of potassium from the intra- to the extracellular fluid space

papillomavirus see HPV (human papilloma virus)

papovavirus A family of small icosahedral double-stranded DNA viruses*, eg SV40 and polyomavirus, which induce both benign and malignant neoplasms; papovavirus infection may be either 'permissive' or 'non-permissive'; monkey cells are susceptible to permissive infection, within which papovavirus reproduces, causing lysis; rodent cells are 'non-permissive' and early viral proteins (T antigens) cause the cell to undergo transformation, which is permanent if the viral genome becomes integrated into the host's genome or transient if the cell rids itself of the viral genome

*The name is a acronym of pap(illoma), po(yoma), va(cuolating agent)

para-amino benzoic acid A molecule used by certain bacteria to produce folic acid, which is a sulfonamide antagonist; a deficiency state does not exist in human, although its absence rats causes graying of fur

para-Bombay phenotype TRANSFUSION MEDICINE A variant of the Bombay phenotype of the ABO blood group, in which the individuals have an Se (secretor) gene allowing the formation of blood groups A and B and its expression in secretions, but not allowing the formation of A and B red cells, given the absence of the H gene; Cf Bombay phenotype

Note: In Bombay phenotypes, an individual lacks the H gene and its product, fucosyl transferase and thus cannot express blood groups A or B on the red cells or in secretions

paracentesis The withdrawal of fluid from a body cavity for either diagnostic or therapeutic purposes

paracervical block OBSTETRICS Locoregional obstetric anesthesia that is used in the first stage of labor and consists of injecting a local (< 2 hour in duration of action) anesthetic in the lateral paracervical region; ½ of infants experience post-anesthetic bradycardia; paracervical blocks are ill-advised if the placental circulation is already compromised

parachute-related injury Unanticipated complications of jumping out of aircraft for business or pleasure; in the military, the mortality is 1/51 000 jumps and the annual rate of attrition through incapacitation is 0.4%, which has been reduced by modern parachute design and larger canopies; the most common non-fatal injuries are vertebral, lower extremity (see Cavalry fracture), and facial fractures; the amount and intensity of injuries is a function of wind speed, weight of the diver and his state of physical fitness

parachute reaction Anterior propping reaction PEDIATRICS Protective abduction of the arms, extension of the elbows and wrists and spreading of the fingers, which is a normal defense reflex, elicited when an infant is held in ventral suspension and is tilted abruptly forward toward the floor, seen between the 7th and 9th months of age, a response that is asymmetrical in infants with hemiparesis and may be the first manifestation of cerebral palsy

parachute valve complex Shone's complex A cardiac malformation tetrad comprised of a 'parachute' mitral valve (chordae tendinae of both leaflets of the mitral valve inserted into the left ventricular papillary muscle causing obstruction of the blood flow), supravalvular stenosis, subvalvular aortic stenosis and variably present coarctation of the aorta

paracrine interaction A type of cell-mediator interaction, in which a cell produces growth factors and cytokines that interact with receptors of different types of cells, eg the release macrophage colony-stimulating factor by smooth muscle cells in atheromatous lesions (Arch Pathol Lab Med 1992; 116:1292oa)

paradigm An example, hypothesis, model, or pattern; in the usual context, a paradigm refers to a widely accepted explanation for a grouping or constellation of biomedical (or other) phenomena that becomes accepted as data accumulate to corroborate aspects of the paradigm's explanation or theory, as occurred in the 'central dogma' of molecular biology*; see Central dogma, Paradigm shift

*Which held that only DNA could give rise to new strands of DNA and the only way in which proteins could be encoded was by mRNA transcription from DNA and protein translation from the mRNA transcript

paradigm shift A decay or incipient collapse in a paradigm that occurs when new data accumulate, and either partially invalidate the previously-accepted theory (paradigm), or which are completely at odds with the paradigm; a well-described PS occurred when it became evident that RNA could give rise to DNA by way of retroviral reverse transcriptase, which contradicted the tenets of the 'central dogma', see there

paradoxical Paradoxic

paradoxic effect MICROBIOLOGY A biological variable that affects the interpretation of the minimum lethal concentration of an antibiotic, in which the proportion of surviving bacteria increases with an increased concentration of antibiotics, a phenomenon that is most common in cell wall active agents; see Minimum bactericidal concentration

paradoxic embolism Emboli that arise when thrombotic material passes through right-to-left cardiac shunts, circumventing the filtering effect of the pulmonary vessels and passes to the general circulation, potentially causing cerebral abscess CLINICAL Meningeal irritation (stiff neck, drowsiness, fever and headache), focal signs including aphasia, hemiplegia, jacksonian convulsions, ↑ intracranial pressure, coma

paradoxic hypertension A hypertensive episode that develops two to three days following surgery in older patients operated for coarctation of the aorta, and associated with abdominal pain due to increased pressure in visceral arteries that had, prior to the procedure functioned at lower pressure; the 'jolt' of pressure requires intense antihypertensive medication, without which intestinal ischemia is a serious potential consequence

paradoxic incontinence Overflow incontinence A constant or intermittent dribbling of urine due to chronic overdistension of the bladder (volume from 1000 to 3000 ml, normal, circa 500 ml), with attenuation of the muscle; this may be confused (and therefore is paradoxic) with pure stress incontinence

'paradox of the lek' EVOLUTIONARY BIOLOGY A phenomenon described in a vast array of animals (frogs, fish, birds, mammals, man), in which the female selects a mate from a group or 'lek'*, based on elaborate mating displays and other intangible or paradoxical factors (Nature 1991; 350:33)

*Which one author facetiously likened to a 'singles bar'

'paradoxic movement' NEONATOLOGY A misnomer for the respiratory movement of newborns, whose breathing is entirely diaphragmatic; with inspiration, the anterior thorax draws inward and the abdomen protrudes; in the neonate, 'paradoxic breathing' is normal

'paradoxic nasal obstruction' Nasal cycle, see there

paradoxic pulse Pulsus paradoxicus CARDIOLOGY A ↓ of ≥ 10 mm Hg in the systolic blood pressure upon inspiration, a finding which like the Kussmaul sign (an abnormal ↑ instead of a normal fall in jugular venous pressure with inspiration) is strongly suggestive of cardiac tamponade (impaired diastolic filling of the heart due to ↑ intrapericardiac pressure) CLINICAL Air hunger, mild cyanosis and visible distension of neck veins

paraffin bath Wax bath SPORTS MEDICINE The immersion of a hand or foot either by dipping several times in a paraffin/mineral oil solution heated to 126°C for 20-30 minutes, or wrapping after dipping in towels to maintain the temperature (JC DeLee, D Drez, Jr, Eds, Orthopedic Sports Medicine WB Saunders, Philadelphia, 1994); PBs have been used for arthritic complaints, and were once used in the treatment of burns

paraffin section SURGICAL PATHOLOGY A thin (4-7 µm) section of tissue surrounded by paraffin, which is processed by various steps, sliced with a microtome, stained, then mounted on a glass slide and examined by LM; in contrast to the 'frozen section' in which a tissue is examined within minutes of its removal from a patient, 'permanent section' tissues are fixed in formalin and bathed in a series of solutions (in order, formalin, 70% alcohol, 95% alcohol, 100% alcohol, xylene) that dry the tissue and allow its infiltration with paraffin, the optimal embedding material for histologic evaluation of tissue; see Hematoxylin and eosin; Cf Frozen section

paraganglioma A neural crest tumor that is more common in women that occurs in the head and neck; 2-9% of those in the carotid body, vagal body and jugulo-tympanic region are malignant; 25% of laryngeal paragangliomas are malignant CRITERIA FOR MALIGNANCY Central necrosis of zellballen, invasion of vascular spaces and lymph nodes and increased mitotic activity; see Zellballen

parahemophilia Factor V deficiency, see there

parallel interface COMPUTERS A port that transmits or receives byte-sized blocks (8 bits) of data at a time; see Computers, Modem

parallel play CHILD PSYCHOLOGY A form of play typical of very young children, in which the child engages in independent playing essentially without interacting with other children; the PP stage is normal usually until the child toilet-trained, after which associative and interactive play becomes a norm

parallel tracking CLINICAL THERAPEUTICS A mechanism by which promising therapeutic agents are made available in the US at an early stage of the drug development process (without interfering with the necessary research studies) to those who are not eligible to participate in clinical trials because of geographic or entry criteria; the research or clinical trials of the drug proceed on one 'track' while the drug is being used for treatment (outside of trials) on a separate or 'parallel track'; although the treatment IND regulations focus on the early availability of experimental drugs to patients with life-threatening diseases, the parallel tracking plan developed by the combined efforts of the FDA, NIAID, NAPO (National AIDS Program Office), and drug companies, is aimed at speeding clinical testing and marketing approval of potentially useful new drugs

paralogous *adjective* Pertaining or referring to a protein product that is encoded by genes located at multiple separate loci and/or on different chromosomes

paralytic ileus GASTROENTEROLOGY Functional 'obstruction' of intestinal flow, often following abdominal surgery; other causes of 'paralytic' ileus include electrolyte abnormalities, eg hypokalemia, drugs including phenothiazine, narcotics, gram-negative sepsis, circulating catecholamines, diabetic ketoacidosis, mesenteric vascular disease, porphyria, retroperitoneal hemorrhage, spinal and pelvic fractures; see Gastroparesis

paramedic A health professional certified to perform advanced life support procedures, eg intubation, defibrillation and administration of drugs under the direction of a physician; paramedics function in urgent care situations provided from an emergency vehicle or air service; in contrast, an emergency medical technician (EMT) is only certified to perform basic life-support maneuvers; Cf Physicians' assistant

parana hard skin syndrome An AR [MIM260530] form of pachyderma of unknown pathogenesis, described in a small geographic region around Parana, Brazil, characterized by rapidly progressive induration of the skin at all joints, retarding growth and 'freezing' the articulations in semi-flexed positions, later resulting in pulmonary insufficiency due to constriction of the thoracic cage and death, which may be associated with mental retardation

paraneoplastic cerebellar degeneration A rare affliction of patients with 'female' cancers, eg breast, ovary, endometrium, associated with cerebellar symptoms of nystagmus, dysarthria and appendicular and gait ataxia that may precede clinical evidence of cancer by months or years PATHOLOGY Extensive Purkinje cell loss, perivascular and leptomeningeal inflammation PATHOGENESIS Uncertain, possibly an autoimmune reaction to two Purkinje cell antigens, CDR62 and CDR34, by an antibody designated anti-Ro; see Purkinje cell antibodies

paraneoplastic opsoclonus-myoclonus An acquired condition due to antineuronal antibodies, which is characterized by chaotic, omnidirectional, synchronous eye movements accompanied by spontaneous jerks of the extremities, palate, and face, which may be intense enough to prevent functional activities, eg walking, writing, and eating; the condition may respond to immunoadsorption of immune complexes by staphylococcal protein A column therapy (N Engl J Med 1995; 332:192c)

paraneoplastic pemphigus An uncommon autoimmune complex seen in malignancy, especially lymphoproliferative, caused by autoantibodies against desmoplakin I, bullous pemphigoid antigen, and other epithelial antigens CLINICAL Persistent and painful erosions of the oropharynx and vermilion border and severe pseudomembranous conjunctivitis, confluent erythema of the skin of the upper trunk (N Engl J Med 1990; 323:1729)

paraneoplastic syndrome(s) A variegated family of comorbid conditions due to the indirect (remote or 'biologic') effects of malignancy, which may be the first sign of a neoplasm or its recurrence; paraneoplastic syndromes occur in more than 15% of all malignancies, are due to the production of hormones, growth and other as yet unidentified 'factors', often regress with adequate treatment of the primary tumor; the range of expression is broad and includes tumor-related cachexia, hormonal effects, neuromuscular disease, eg peripheral neuropathy, myopathy, CNS and spinal cord degeneration and inflammation, leukemoid reaction, reactive eosinophilia, peripheral 'cytoses or 'cytopenias, hemolysis, DIC, thromboembolism, thrombophlebitis migrans, renal dysfunction, nephrotic syndrome, uric acid nephropathy, GI symptoms (anorexia, vomiting, protein-losing enteropathy, malignant hepatopathy), bullous mucocutaneous lesions, acquired ichthyosis, acanthosis nigricans, dermatomyositis, tylosis, lactic acidosis, hypertrophic pulmonary osteoarthropathy, hyperamylasemia, hyperlipidemia, hypertension, and amyloidosis; see Ectopic hormones

paranoia 1) An evolving or fixed delusional state that is persecutory in nature; the term paranoia per se is not used in the fourth edition of the Diagnostic and Statistical Manual of Mental Disorders (1994, American Psychiatric Association, Washington, DC), although paranoid delusions are an integral component of the paranoid personality disorder and paranoid subtype of schizophrenia 2) Obsolete term for mental disorder

paranormal Pertaining or relating to phenomena that are not explained by natural laws and principles of the physical universe, eg clairvoyance, precognition, telekinesis, telepathy; see Parapsychology

paraphilia Sexual deviancy A mental disorder characterized by '...*recurrent, intense sexually arousing fantasies, sexual urges, or behaviors generally involving 1) nonhuman objects, 2) the suffering or humiliation of oneself or one's partner, or 3) children or other nonconsenting persons, that occur over a period of at least 6 months...*(which) *cause significant distress or impairment in social, occupational, or other important areas of functioning.*' (**Diagnostic and Statistical Manual of Mental**

Disorders, 4th ed, Washington, DC, American Psychiatric Association, 1994); paraphilia is also defined as a sexual excitement to the point of erection and/or orgasm when the object of that excitement is considered abnormal in the context of the practitioner's learned societal norms; the American Psychiatric Association recognizes 8 'formal' types paraphilia, to wit, exhibitionism, fetishism, frotteurism, pedophilia, sexual masochism, sexual sadism, transvestic fetishism, voyeurism, and paraphilia, not otherwise specified, an informal or 'wastepaper basket' category; see Child abuse, Sexual deviancy

Note: The term 'sexual deviancy' is widely preferred in the vox populi; recognizing the dichotomy between the formal written and informal spoken vocabulary of medicine, the author has included a glossary of relevant terms under the entry sexual deviancy

paraphilia-not otherwise specified A 'wastepaper basket' category of paraphilia (see there) that includes the 'really interesting' sexual deviant behaviors, including coprophilia (feces), klismaphilia (enemas), necrophilia (corpses), partialism (focus on one body part only), telephone scatologia (obscene phone calls), urophilia (urine, aka 'water sports'), and zoophilia (animals)

paraprotein A generic term for any immunoglobulin produced in excess quantity, usually in the context of a malignant (eg multiple myeloma, Waldenström's macroglobulinemia), but occasionally in benign (eg monoclonal gammopathy of undetermined significance) clonal proliferations; paraproteins were so named as it was originally thought that they were in some way abnormal, a posit that in the vast majority of cases has proven incorrect, although abnormal paraproteins may be produced in heavy chain disease

parapsychology A field that attempts to apply scientific methods to the study of so-called 'paranormal' phenomena that are not explained by natural laws and principles of the physical universe; these phenomena include clairvoyance, precognition, telekinesis, telepathy

Note: Many of the methods used in parapsychology are regarded by some mainstream scientists as being of uncertain validity

parasitic limbs PEDIATRICS Duplicated extremities seen in arthrogryposis, which are medial, retroflexed, small, immature and have no clinical evidence of innervation; this rare congenital malformation is subdivided into myogenic and neuropathic forms, the latter of which may be associated with spina bifida or the segmental absence of anterior horn cells

paratesticular rhabdomyosarcoma A variant location of childhood rhabdomyosarcoma, the majority of which (97%) are of the embryonal subtype, and when associated with a spindle cell morphology have a better prognosis (Am J Surg Pathol 1993; 17:221₀ₐ)

parathion diethyl-*p*-nitrophenylthiophosphate An acetylcholinesterase-inhibiting organophosphate insecticide and nerve poison that forms a stable covalently bound complex with a serine residue at acetylcholinesterase's active site; acute intoxication is characterized by nicotinic and muscarinic effects which, when severe, may cause respiratory failure within minutes; chronic intoxication may cause demyelinating neuropathy and axonal degeneration TREATMENT Atropine

parathyroid panel LABORATORY MEDICINE A battery of cost-effective tests used to evaluate calcium and phosphate metabolism, including measurement of calcium, phophate, magnesium, alkaline phosphate, total protein levels, albumin, creatinine and urinary calcium; see Organ panel

parathyroid 'squeeze' test ENDOCRINOLOGY A clinical test consisting of massaging or gentle compression (squeezing) of the side of the neck that is thought to harbor a parathyroid adenoma, which will respond by increasing serum parathyroid hormone

paratope IMMUNOLOGY Antibody combining site The sum total of the points of contact between an antigen's epitope and an immunoglobulin's hypervariable regions; whereas most of the 120 amino acid positions of the light and heavy chains in the variable regions have < 10% variability, amino acid positions 29-34, 49-52 and 91-95 on the light chain and positions 30-34, 51-63, 84-90 and 101-110 on the heavy chain are veritable 'hot-spots', having 20-60% variability in the amino acid sequence; this variability confers high specificity, defined as an idiotype, and the ability to recognize the vast number of antigenic epitopes; Cf Epitope, 'Hot spots', Idiotype

parchment heart Right ventricular dysplasia, see there

parental age see Maternal age, Paternal age

parenteral nutrition see Total parenteral nutrition

pareve NUTRITION A food product that completely lacks animal-derived products, often equated to the term 'non-dairy'; see Vegan

parenteral nutrition A generic term for the administration of nutrients in any form in a parenteral fashion, usually intravenous; see Total parenteral nutrition; Cf Forced feeding

parenting The constellation of activities carried out by a parent, eg, supplying physical sustenance and instilling a sense of morality; parenting may be authoritative in which there is both warmth toward the child and high control, authoritarian (little warmth and high control), or permissive (high warmth and little control) (Sci Am 1994; 271/5:78)

parietal cell antibody Anti-parietal cell antibody, see there

Paris Declaration AIDS A political statement signed 2 December 1994 by delegates from 42 nations (21 prime ministers and 21 ministers of health) that named AIDS as a '*serious threat to humanity*', and called for a stronger international commitment to AIDS research and education, and an end to discrimination of people with AIDS (NY Newsday 2 Dec 1994; A19)

parite An intra-arterial fibrous plaque in atherosclerosis, which may display dystrophic calcification

parking-lot crystals A fanciful descriptor for the parallel, herringbone angulated crystalloid material seen by electron microscopy in degenerated mitochondria of 'mitochondrial myopathies'; see Ragged red fiber disease

Parkinson's disease A progressive neurologic disease characterized by tremors and rigidity followed by inhibition of voluntary movement, a shuffling gait due to neuron degeneration in the substantia nigra and corpus striatum, focal loss of dopamine production and, with time, severe mental deterioration CLINICAL Onset in older subjects with static tremor and plastic rigidity of the trunk and extremities, bradykinesia, development of a masklike facies, progressive stoop, slow monotonous voice, slow shuffling gait, often accompanied by autonomic dysfunction in the form of hypersalivation and sweating; MPTP, a toxic contaminant appearing in the production of certain 'designer drugs', causes a clinical picture mimicking Parkinson's disease; the selective destruction of the dopamine neurons is the direct result of its metabolite, MPP⁺ (1-methyl-4-phenylpyridium), an effect reversed by brain-derived neurotrophic factor (Nature 1991; 350:230, 195) TREATMENT L-dopa is effective in early disease, as it is transported to the brain and converted into dopamine, but with time, loses efficacy; 'brain-graft' surgery has proven disappointing in treating parkinsonism, although the related modality, fetal nerve graft (mesencephalic dopamine neurons from 8-9 week fetuses) may be effective, as may be deprenyl, a MAOI that blocks the chemical conversion of MPTP to MPP⁺; see BDNF, MPTP, Fetal-brain tissue grafting

parkinsonism-plus syndromes A generic term for typical Parkinson's disease-like complexes that are accompanied by other neurologic changes, including concomitant impairment of ocular movement, orthostatic hypotension, cerebellar ataxia or dementia; these conditions include olivopontocerebellar degeneration with ataxia, parkinsonism-amyotrophic lateral sclerosis overlap, parkinsonism-dementia (normopressure hydrocephalus, gait disturbance and urinary incontinence), progressive supranuclear palsy with ophthalmoplegia, Shy-Drager syndrome with orthostatic hypotension, striatal degeneration

paroxysmal atrial tachycardia Supraventricular tachycardia, see there

paroxysmal cold hemoglobinuria A disease that is

1) Rarely 'paroxysmal' clinically

2) Not always precipitated by the cold and

3) Not always associated with hemoglobinuria

PCH comprises 2-5% of autoimmune hemolytic anemias and is caused by IgG (Donath-Landsteiner) antibodies that react at < 15°C and are directed against the ubiquitous P antigen on red cells; PCH was first described by Donath and Landsteiner in 1904 in a patient with tertiary syphilis who developed paroxysmal fever, chills, headache and diffuse corporal pain with hemoglobinuria; PCH may be transient and secondary to viral exanthemas of childhood CLINICAL After exposure to the cold, the patient experiences myalgia, abdominal cramping and headaches, hemoglobinuria, Raynaud's phenomenon, cold urticaria and occasionally jaundice LABORATORY Positive direct Coombs test (using anti-C3 antiserum), anemia, hemoglobinuria, ↓ haptoglobin, ↑ LDH, ↑ bilirubin; the antibody is a non-agglutinating IgG that binds to RBCs at cold temperatures and when warmed to 37°C, evokes complement-mediated hemolyses; the Donath-Landsteiner antibody elutes from the red cells in vitro, while the complement remains fixed, and thus is a 'biphasic' hemolysin; anti-P reacts with all normal neutrophil antigens except for p and P^k PREVENTION Keep body warm TREATMENT If PCH is chronic, corticosteroids, immunosuppressive therapy

paroxysmal myoglobinuria 1) Periodic paralysis, see there 2) Idiopathic rhabdomyolysis

paroxysmal nocturnal hemoglobinuria An acquired hemolytic disease due to the proliferation of an abnormal clone(s) of myeloid stem cells, the progeny of which are highly susceptible to complement-mediated membrane damage and hemolysis (CMH), due to a deficiency in the 70 kD delay accelerating factor (DAF, CD55) MOLECULAR PATHOLOGY CMH is the key feature of PNH and is due to a deficiency of cell-surface expression of CD55 and CD59, which protect erythrocytes from complement; *PIG-A,* a mutated gene that encodes molecules responsible for the synthesis of the glycosyl-phosphatidylinositol synthetic pathway is the cause of PNH (**N Engl J Med 1994; 330:249**0A); when susceptible RBCs are exposed to activated (by classic or alternate pathways) complement, the afflicted RBCs bind more C3b than normal; membrane-bound C3b is a positive feedback signal for the alternate complement pathway via factors B and D, resulting in generation of more C3b; C5 convertase and the C5-9 membrane attack complex are activated, resulting in intravascular hemolysis* CLINICAL Thrombotic tendencies, increased susceptibility to infections; PNH may evolve into aplastic or sideroblastic anemia, myelofibrosis or AML LABORATORY Leukopenia, thrombocytopenia, dimorphic RBC population, iron-deficiency, ↓ leukocyte alkaline phosphatase, ↓ erythrocyte acetylcholinesterase, alterations of the properdin (alternate) pathway of complement lysis, hemoglobinuria, hemosiderinuria, positive Ham Crosby test, positive sucrose lysis test; negative direct Coombs' test and ↑ susceptibility of RBCs to CMH

*CD55 is also absent in platelets and myelocytes from these subjects, making them equally sensitive to complement-mediated lysis

parrot beak syndrome of Waardenburg Acrocephalo-

syndactyly type III

parrot fever Psittacosis, see there

parsimony principle see Ockham's razor

part A One of the two components of the Medicare reimbursement system (US), which consists in the compulsory hospital insurance financed by contributions from employers, employees and participants; 'part A' pays for the costs of hospitalization, but does not pay physicians' fees; see Medicare, Part B, TEFRA

part B A component of the Medicare reimbursement system (US) that provides supplementary payments for medical services and supplies that are not covered under part A; part B is voluntary, covers physicians' fees and individual provider services, and is financed in part by monthly premiums paid by the enrollees and in part by the US federal government; see Medicare, Part A, Participation, TEFRA; Cf Medicaid

parthenogenesis A form of nonsexual reproduction in which a genetic ♀ of a species produces offspring in absence of genetic contribution from a genetic ♂

partial saturation MRI An 'excitation' technique that consists of administration of repeated radiofrequency pulses in time periods equal to or shorter than T1; in MRI, although partial saturation results in decreased signal amplitude, it is possible to generate images with increased contrast between regions with different relaxation times; see Magnetic resonance imaging; Cf Saturation recovery

partial thromboplastin time Activated partial thromboplastin time (aPTT) A one-stage coagulation test that is sensitive to defects of the intrinsic pathway of coagulation, which includes the so-called antihemophilic factors; aPTT is prolonged in deficiencies of factors V, VIII, IX, X, XI, XII, Fletcher factor, high-molecular-weight kininogen, lupus anticoagulants (inhibitors) and heparin

partial twinning A group of rare congenital anomalies of cloacally derived structures, including focal doubling of the alimentary tract beginning at Meckel's diverticulum and extending to the anus, doubling of the bladder, vagina, penis, sacrum or lumbar vertebrae

participation HEALTH CARE INDUSTRY A term referring to a formal agreement between Medicare and health care providers, ie hospitals and physicians, in which the provider(s) agree to 'accept assignment', ie accept Medicare's fees as payment in full for any health care services rendered; in 1991, 48% of US physicians participated, ranging from 20% participation in Idaho to 83% in Alabama, differing in specialties from 72% by nephrologists to 37% by anesthesiologists; non-participating providers may charge more for the same services but must submit the bills directly to the patient; participation also refers to the acceptance of an insurance or health plan's established or calculated fee as the maximum amount collectable for the services rendered

particulate air pollution A mixture of solid particles and liquid droplets that vary in size, composition, and origin; inhalable particles have an aerodynamic diameter ≤ 10 μm (PM_{10}); larger inhalable particles of derive from soil and other crustal materials, and are of lesser concern for their detrimental effects; fine (diameter ≤ 2.5 μm) particles are derived primarily from the combustion of fossil fuels in transportation, manufacturing, and power generation, and are mixed with soot, acid condensates, nitrate and sulfate particles, and may pose a greater risk to health as they are generally more toxic and can be inhaled deeply ino the lungs; there is a significant association between fine particulate air pollution and deaths from cardiopulmonary disease, lung cancer, and other causes (**N Engl J Med 1993; 329:1753**0A, 1807ED) see Air pollution

partition chromatography LABORATORY MEDICINE A chromatographic technique in which the distribution of substances in the mobile liquid phase and a stationary liquid phase (which is immobilized on a porous solid, eg a filter paper or on a starch column) is a function of the solubility of the compounds in the two different phases; Cf Reversed phase chromatography

partitioning factor Any objective parameter or criterion that can be used to separate subgroups of a data set or population, which is of use in establishing reference values and/or normal distribution curves; partition factors in humans include age, blood group, diet, ethnic background, exercise, fasting or nonfasting state, geography, race, sex, time of day when sampled, substance use (eg alcohol, illicit drugs, tobacco) (Arch Pathol Lab Med 1992; 116:710OA) see Exclusion criteria, Reference values

partner risk factor Any of a number of risk factors that a sexual partner has for transmitting STD, in particular HIV, which include having sex with a prostitute, or someone with AIDS, or a STD, receptive anal intercourse, or injection of drugs of abuse (MMWR 1992; 41:568) see High risk behavior; Cf Safe sex practices

partner notification program PUBLIC HEALTH A generic term for any formal and systematic means of informing the sexual partner(s) of a person with a sexually-transmitted disease that the person tested is infected with an organism (eg HIV-1, *Neisseria gonorrhoeae*, *Treponema pallidum*) of interest to epidemiologists or public health officials (N Engl J Med 1992; 327:435C)

'partnering' A term coined (Science 1990; 250:1643) in reference to the finding that transcription factors from different classes of molecules, ie those having different structural motifs, can cross-hybridize to form chimeric dimers

'party wall' appearance The apparent but not actual sharing of plasma membranes by distinct and separate cells within glands; the 'party wall' effect is described in canalicular adenoma of the salivary glands and in gastric glands with inflammatory atypia in regeneration and is not thought to have neoplastic potential

parvalbumin A calcium-binding protein involved in Ca^{2+} exchange between sarcoplasmic reticulum and myofibrils that plays a critical role in the contraction and relaxation cycling of vertebrate muscles; the expression of parvalbumin is under neural control, and is present in large amounts in fast-twitch muscles and absent in slow-twitch muscle (Anal Quan Cytol Histol 1993; 15:201) see Fast-twitch muscle

parvovirus Any member of the smallest (*parvo*, Latin, small) known DNA virus family, which measure 5.5 kb in length, 15-28 nm in diameter; the parvovirus is a icosahedral single-stranded DNA (class II) virus that requires either autonomous intracellular replication or that the host cell be co-infected with an adenovirus; a single human strain exists–the designation B19 reflects a laboratory code used to identify the original isolate; parvoviruses have a tropism for erythroid precursors, and parvoviruses depend on actively replicating cells to supply an unknown S-phase function (N Engl J Med 1993; 329:792CPC)

parvus et tardus (pulse) CARDIOLOGY A small arterial pulse with a delayed systolic peak that may be associated with an anacrotic 'shoulder' on the upstroke of the carotid pulse, a pattern seen in older patients with severe aortic stenosis

PAS Periodic acid-Schiff (stain), also 1) Para-aminosalicylic acid 2) Pulmonary artery stenosis

Also 1) Parent attitude scale 2) Patient Administration System (British) 3) Peripheral anterior synechia (ophthalmology) 4) Poly(alkyl sulfone) 5) Polyaminosiloxane 6) Polyarylsulfone 7) Positron annihilation spectroscopy 8) Post abortion syndrome 9) Postacoustic spectroscopy 10) Problem appraisal scales (psychology) 11) Progressive accumulated stress

PASI Psoriasis Area and Severity Index, see there

'passenger or driver' controversy The presence of a particular lesion and a specific microorganism in a host cell or tissue with such regularity that it is unclear whether the microorganism (or lesion) is an epiphenomenon, ie a 'passenger' or whether it is pathogenically linked to the lesion, ie a 'driver'; this debate often arises when analyzing scar cancers, or in the common association of HPV types 16 and 18 with carcinoma of the uterine cervix

passenger leukocyte Any leukocyte that accompanies a transfusion of blood products, eg packed red cells or platelets, or a transplanted organ or tissue; such passengers are capable of causing broad range of responses in the recipient, including graft-versus-host disease, febrile nonhemolytic transfusion reactions due to release of cytokines, eg IL-1β, IL-6, TNFα (endogenous pyrogens) and others (N Engl J Med 1994; 331:6250A, 670ED, Sci Am July 1995, p50)

passivation The coating of a surface of an implanted biomaterial with albumin to reduce the incidence and severity of inflammatory response (Am J Clin Pathol 1995; 103:466BS)

passive-aggressive personality disorder PSYCHIATRY A personality disorder in which the patient expresses personal conflicts through retroflexed anger in the form of covert obstructionism, procrastination, stubbornness and inefficiency; 0.9% or more of the population exhibits passive-aggressive or passive-dependent behavior; the defenses include turning against oneself (a form of sadomasochism), denial, rationalization and hypochondriasis Prognosis for normalization of these individuals is poor*; the term was first used by US military psychiatrists during World War II and is known in Europe as 'passive sociopathy' DIAGNOSTIC CRITERIA see Table Cf 'Anal-retentive'

*Of 73 passive-aggressives followed for 11 years in one series, only 9 were symptom-free, the remainder had persistent psychiatric difficulties, abused alcohol or were clinically depressed

---

PASSIVE-AGGRESSIVE PERSONALITY DISORDER

A A pervasive pattern of negativistic attitudes and passive resistance to demands for adequate performance, beginning by early adulthood and present in various contexts, indicated by at least four of the following
  1) Passive resistance to routine social or occupational obligations
  2) Complains of being misunderstood or underappreciated
  3) Complains of personal misfortune
  4) Sullenness or belligerence (argumentative)
  5) Highly critical of authority
  6) Resents or is envious of those perceived as being more fortunate
  7) Alternates between hostile defiance and contrition
B Not accounted for by dysthymic disorder or occurs exclusively during major depressive episodes

Diagnostic and Statistical Manual of Mental Disorders, DSM-IV, American Psychiatric Press, Washington, DC, 1994

---

passive anaphylaxis A 'borrowed' anaphylactic reaction that occurs when an organism is exposed to antigens after having been injected with preformed antibodies (IgE) to the antigen of interest that were 'raised' in another organism; see P-K test

passive immunity A 'borrowed' and transient immune resistance to various organisms due to the presence of antibodies produced by another organism; PI is either congenital, eg seen in neonates as a result of the passive transplacental transfer of IgG of maternal origin, or active when antibodies of interest are administered to a person with a particular infection that is known to respond to a particular immune globulin

passive learning EDUCATION The acquisition of knowledge without active effort; see Spoon-feeding

passive smoking Involuntary 'smoking' by non-smokers who breathe ambient air containing the same carcinogens inhaled by a cigarette smoker; PS is estimated to cause an estimated 2500-8400 excess annual cases of smoking-related malignancy (US); mere physical space separation allows significant reduction in exposure to 'sidestream' or environmental tobacco smoke (ETS) by non-smokers; 'mainstream' smoke is directly inhaled by the smoker, ETS is produced by the smoker, but absorbed more by non-smokers who don't have the benefit of a filter; passive smokers are exposed to dimethylnitrosamine (a potent carcinogen), benzo(a) pyrene, and carbon monoxide (CO), acrolein, arsenic, benzene, cyanide, formaldehyde, nitrosamines, radionuclides and others); levels of nicotine in unventilated areas may exceed industrial threshold limit levels (> 500 μg/mm³); air zones with CO levels of > than 30 ppm cause a passive smoker to have CO blood levels equivalent to having smoked ≥ 5 cigarettes; prolonged exposure to 30 ppm may cause carboxyhemoglobin levels sufficient to impair visual discrimination and cause psychomotor impairment; ETS ↑ platelet activity, accelerates atherosclerosis, and ↑ tissue damage in ischemia or myocardial infarction; PS ↓ both cardiac delivery of O_2 to the heart and myocardial ability to use O_2 to produce ATP, resulting in ↓ exercise capacity in passive smokers, and ↑ risk of fatal and nonfatal cardiac events (JAMA 1995; 273:1047) it has been suggested that adherence to 'common courtesy' rules by smokers is insufficient to reduce PS and legislation is needed to reduce these risks to PS victims; exposure to three hours/day of PS is associated with an ↑ in cancer of the uterine cervix; in children, neonates and fetuses, PS is inculpated in poor pulmonary function, bronchitis, pneumonia, otitis media and middle ear effusions, asthma, lower birth and adult weights and heights, sudden infant death syndrome (SIDS) and poor lung (and physical) development, and a higher perinatal mortality (related to placental vascular disease including placenta previa and abruptio placentae); these children are themselves more likely to become smokers and are at ↑ risk for developing cancer in a dose-related manner, in all sites 50% higher than expected, and up to two-fold ↑ in NHL, ALL, and Wilm's tumors; PS by children with cystic fibrosis adversely affects growth and health, resulting in ↑ hospital admissions and poor performance in pulmonary function tests; 17% of lung cancer in non-smokers is attributed to high levels of exposure to cigarette smoke during childhood and adolescence; see Conicotine, Environmental tobacco smoke

passive transport The movement of solutes across biological membranes by simple diffusion down a concentration gradient, which requires neither energy expenditure nor carrier molecules

Passover phenomenon Harvest Moon phenomenon, see there

PAS stain SURGICAL PATHOLOGY The periodic acid Schiff reaction results from periodic acid-induced oxidation of hydroxyl groups on hexoses and hexosamines to aldehydes, which then react with a Schiff base, forming a magenta-colored complex; many substances and cells are PAS-positive, including neutral mucosubstances (positive in esophageal, gastric and anal glands), fungi, parasites, ceroid, polysaccharides, glycogen (staining disappears with amylase treatment), glycolipids and glycoproteins; the PAS stain is well-suited for delineating basement membranes and reticulin, for demonstrating the intracytoplasmic crystals in alveolar soft part sarcoma and bacteria-like inclusions in the macrophages of Whipple's disease, as well as Paget's and Gaucher's diseases in which PAS demonstrates glucocerebroside

pass-through phenomenon LABORATORY MEDICINE In the copper reduction test used for glucose determination, when > 11 mmol/24 hour specimen (US: 2.0 gm/24 h) is in the urine, the reagent strip undergoes a rapid transition

through the entire spectrum of color changes and to the unwary, simulates the strip's original color and might be interpreted as being negative, resulting in discontinuation of insulin therapy

pasta loading Carbohydrate loading, see there

Pasteur effect The effect of ↑ O_2 on certain metabolic pathways, with ↑ oxidative phosphorylation and ↑ ATP and ↓ phosphofructokinase activity, resulting in ↓ glycolysis and ↓ lactic acid

Pasteurella multocida A small gram-negative coccobacillus that is part of the normal flora of most domestic animals; human infection with *P multocida* is rare and usually atributed to animal-related trauma or contact with animal secretions, resulting in systemic disease, and rarely endocarditis (Am J Clin Pathol 1992; 98:565oA)

pasteurization Heat 'sterilization' of food products, devised by Louis Pasteur to destroy the bacteria responsible for spoilage of wine and beer, for which it continues to be used; pasteurization of milk requires heating to 62° C for 30 minutes or to 80° C for 15-30 seconds (flash pasteurization), temperatures that destroy all potential pathogens; Cf Ultra-pasteurization

PAT 1) Paroxysmal atrial tachycardia, see there 2) Pre-admission testing, see there

patch-and-cut repair MOLECULAR BIOLOGY A mechanism of DNA repair, in which a damaged segment of DNA is excised by the DNA ligase only after the segment has been repaired by a DNA nuclease

patch-clamp technique Voltage-clamp technique NEUROPHYSIOLOGY A technique in which a micropipette is used to remove by suction, a minuscule (0.5 μm in diameter) patch of plasma membrane that bears one or only a few ion channels; the patch is clamped and the potential of the ions flowing across the patch is measured, thus evaluating the effect on the membrane potential of the closing and opening of single channels and measurement of the different ion compositions of solutions on either side of the membranes; this simple technique resulted in the discovery of ion channels in cell membranes and has provided vast information about the cell and nerve physiology

The technique's co-developers, E Naher and B Sakmann, of the Max-Planck Institute were awarded the 1991 Nobel prize (Science 1991; 254:380n)

patch test An epicutaneous test devised in 1895 by Jadassohn to measure contact-type (delayed) hypersensitivity reactions; the PT consists of applying a patch with a low dose of a potentially allergenic substance to an unexposed body part and observing the site 1-2 days later; the skin of modern man is subjected to numerous organic and inorganic chemicals including toxins, carcinogens, irritants and allergens; up to 5% of the general population has dermatitis and 7% or more of dermatology practice consists in management of allergic contact dermatitis; 50% of occupational absenteeism is related to contact dermatitis the most common sensitizing haptens in North America are poison ivy (*Toxicodendron radicans*), nickel, chromate, paraphenylenediamine (a dye constituent), ethylenediamine (a solvent and emulsifier), local anesthetics, eg benzocaine, rubber, neomycin, and others

patching IMMUNOLOGY Aggregation on the surface of a lymphocyte of membrane receptor proteins that have been cross-linked by lectins and antibodies, a step that precedes 'capping' and internalization of antigen-antibody complex for processing of the antigen and presentation of the antigen in the context of a major histocompatibility complex; see Capping

patency State of openness

patent (*pronounced*, pay-tent) *adjective* Open, not occluded, unobstructed, used in reference to a duct, lumen, or vessel

patent (*pronounced*, pat-tent) *noun* A document that grants an inventor in terms of a determined number of years, the exclusive right to make use of and sell his invention; the duration of US patents is 17 years with an extension for up to eight years (if the product was in the regulatory approval process, eg FDA); when a commercial product is invented in academics, the holder(s) of the patent is required to share income with various departments in the university; at Harvard, the patent holder(s) retain 25-35%, the department where the holder(s) works retains 30-40% (one half for the holder(s)' research activities, one half for the department), the dean and president retain 20% and 15% respectively, for their own technology transfer funds and for use in teaching (re **US Patent and Trademark Office, see Science 1991; 253:20n&v**) see European Patent Office

patent controversy One of the major (and unresolved) controversies in the biotechnology industry has been whether any one individual or a profit-making entity should have the right to seek and be granted patents on DNA sequences, which in effect are thought to belong all individuals; this controversy has centered around one particular worker who left the NIH to become head of a biotechnology venture capital company (see **New York Times 22 February 1994; C1**)

paternalism LEGAL MEDICINE The practice of interacting with a patient as a father to a child, ie carrying out acts intended to benefit the child that may either limit his freedom or be contrary to his wishes; the principle is subdivided into

WEAK PATERNALISM, in which the person is substantially incompetent or very young and

STRONG PATERNALISM, in which the person is competent and may fully realize the impact of a decision made for him; strongly paternalistic acts, eg medicating a dying Christian Scientist (see Christian Science), is an issue with considerable legal impact, as forcing therapy against a patient's wishes may result in the criminal charges of assault-and-battery against the medical team; Cf Doctor-patient interaction

paternity testing FORENSIC MEDICINE A battery of tests required to determine, with reasonable or absolute certainty, a child's genetic parents

DIRECT EXCLUSION OF PATERNITY

1) The child has a genetic marker that is absent in the mother and not present in the father; in complex systems where a child lacks all paternal antigens, the putative father is excluded or 2) The child is an 'amorph', ie does not express a gene present in both mother and father

INDIRECT EXCLUSION OF PATERNITY

1) A gene is present in the child that can be transmitted only by a male, and which the putative father does not have 2) The child is homozygous for markers not seen in a parent or 3) The parent is homozygous for a marker not seen in the child (paternity is excluded); indirect exclusions are accepted when confirmed by a second method by another laboratory Note: Genetic markers are used in 'classic' paternity testing, but those of very high or very low frequencies are of limited value in differentiating among individuals, although very low frequency genetic markers are used to determine statistical likelihood of paternity; genetic markers include red cell antigens (M-N, S-s, Rh-C–c, Rh-E-e, K-k, $Fy^a Fy^b$, $Jk^a Jk^b$), various erythrocyte enzymes (adenosine deaminase, glucose-6-phosphate dehydrogenase) isomers, HLA antigens, immunoglobulin allotypes and non-immunoglobulin serum proteins; since the late 1980s, DNA 'fingerprinting' has become the legally accepted means of establishing or excluding parentage, using the 'Jeffries' probe

paternal age Although ↑ maternal age is classically associated with chromosome defects in the progeny, often occurring in trisomies, there is also an ↑ incidence of certain conditions in children born to older ♂, including achondroplasia, Klinefelter syndrome and Marfan syndrome; paternal chromosomal abnormalities occur in 2.6% of habitual abortions and most are translocations, occur-

ring at a ten-fold greater rate than normal; Cf Maternal age

pathergy see Necrosis

pathfinding mutant see Zebrafish

pathological gambling A persistent and maladaptive behavior disorder which is defined by the presence of multiple symptoms which is not otherwise accounted for by a manic episode

---

PATHOLOGICAL GAMBLING (5+ OF THE FOLLOWING)

1) Preoccupation with gambling, past gambling experiences, and obtaining money for gambling

2) Needs increasing amounts of mony to obtain gambling 'rush' or 'high'

3) Has been incapable of controlling the gambling impulse

4) Becomes irritable when trying to stop gambling

5) Gambles as an escape from problems

6) Returns to scene of previous gambling losses to 'get even'

7) Conceals extent of gambling compulsion from family, friends, therapist

8) Has committed crimes (eg fraud, forgery, theft) to finance gambling

9) Has compromised or lost a significant relationship, job, or educational or career opportunity due to gambling

10) Relies on others to 'bail him out' financially

Diagnostic and Statistical Manual of Mental Disorders, 4th ed, Washington, DC, American Psychiatric Association, 1994

---

pathologists' disease Any lesion that is defined as malignant by histological criteria, identified as an incidental finding, and which in clinical practice is regarded as a nonaggressive lesion, not requiring treatment, eg pancreatic endocrine carcinoma or well-differentiated adenocarcinoma of the prostate

Note: The concept of 'benign malignancy' needs re-evaluation, as 16% of stage A1 carcinomas of the prostate, traditionally regarded as a 'pathologist's tumor', followed for 10 years progress to higher stages and require therapy (**Urology 1990; 36:210**)

pathologize A neologism for diagnosing a normal condition as pathological based on the assumption that it 'should' be, eg adopted children are assumed to develop psychological dysfunction with a higher frequency than their nonadopted counterparts (**Science News 1994; 146:106**)

Patient 'Bill of Rights' (and responsibilities) A statement developed by the American Hospital Association that delineates the treatment that a person has a right to expect while he is a patient in a hospital and the behavior that is expected of the patient with respect to his own therapy, follow-up and conduct while in the hospital

patient compliance The strictness to which the patient adheres to the physician's regimen, diet, treatment and whether the patient returns for re-examination, follow-up or treatment; poor patient compliance with a prescribed plan of therapeutic action may result in complications that are beyond the physician's control and must be documented to prevent legal action by the patient or his estate, should non-compliance prove fatal; noncompliance is common and defies quantification; demographic factors, eg age, sex, race, marital status, education, and socioeconomic status correlate poorly with the degree of compliance to a medical regimen; lack of patient compliance has been implicated in an increased drug resistance and relapse in patients with *Mycobacterium tuberculosis*, which may be minimized by directly observed therapy (**N Engl J Med 1994; 330:1179oa**) see Directly observed therapy

patient-controlled analgesia A method that allows patients to self-administer narcotic-analgesic drugs, usually by a programmable pump; PCA is used for pain related to terminal malignancy (its most widely accepted therapeutic indication), surgical procedures, angina pectoris, and labor and deliver), allowing patients to obtain pulse doses above a baseline level and a degree of autonomy over pain medication; the most commonly used agents include fentanil, meperidine, morphine, sufentanil; most PCA is delivered by IV, more recently also subcutaneously or epidurally; see Pain

patient dumping see Dumping

patient empowerment The provision of information relevant to a particular therapeutic procedure to the patient so that he/she can actively participate in the decision on whether to undergo the procedure and whether there are alternative treatment options; PE by education, eg about therapies for benign prostatic hypertrophy, low back pain, ischemic heart disease, and others, may result in reduced costs for health insurance companies (Am Med News 19 Sept 1994)

patient (medical) record A generic term for all documents that are relevant to the management of a patient, which includes medical history and chief complaint(s), diagnostic and therapeutic procedures performed and current status, usually arranged in a chronological order; because PMR is a document with legal weight, it is advised* that it be periodically reviewed for accuracy, objectivity, legibility, timeliness, comprehensiveness, and rectification or justification for alterations

*Risk Management Principles & Commentaries for the Medical Office, American Medical Association/Specialty Society Medical Liability Project, 1990, Chicago

patient 'mix' The demographics of a patient population being served by a hospital or other health care facility, classified according to disease severity or according to socioeconomic parameters; see Case-mix index

patient-physician relationship A formal relation that exists between the physician and the patient, often equated to medical 'duties' that the physician must perform in a professionally acceptable manner Note: Mere conversation with a patient may be sufficient in the eyes of a court to establish such a relation; in this regard, referral of a patient to a specialist or termination of a relation must be documented, or it may be considered 'abandonment'; see Doctor-patient interaction; Cf Abandonment

patient record see Patient medical record

'patient viewpoint' standard A standard of disclosure of information that is based on what a reasonable person in the patient's position would want to know in similar circumstances; this standard is based on a patient's perception (ie viewpoint) rather than on professional perception of what a patient would want to know; courts increasingly prefer the 'patient viewpoint' standard (Risk Management Principles & Commentaries for the Medical Office, American Medical Association/Specialty Society Medical Liability Project, 1990, Chicago) see *Arato v Avedon*, Cf 'Reasonable physician' standard

'patient zero' A French-Canadian airline steward, whose promiscuity linked him epidemiologically to 40 of the first 248 men to be diagnosed of what had been called gay-related immune deficiency (GRID, now known as AIDS); 'patient zero' died of terminal renal failure, and had had four episodes of *Pneumocystis carinii* pneumonia; see AIDS, HIV, see Manchester seaman

Note: The true 'patient zero' is unknown as earlier cases of AIDS are being discovered from sera that were stored for decades from patients who had died of unusual immunodeficiency syndromes; the earliest case of AIDS in the USA occurred in a 15 year-old male homosexual who died in the St Louis City Hospital in 1968 with florid LGV, culture-confirmed chlamydial infection, lymphopenia, CMV, EBV, HSV (and HIV-1 by Western blot), depletion of the lymphoid tissue, anergy to TB and histoplasmin, a positive Frei test and Kaposi sarcoma (JAMA 1988; 260:2085); an earlier 'patient zero' was an unmarried Manchester seaman who probably acquired the infection in voyages to Africa in 1955-57 and died of a puzzling immunodeficiency (Lancet 1960; 2:951), whose stored serum proved to be HIV-1 positive by PCR (Lancet 1990; 336:51)

PATTY PCR-aided transcript titration assay

pavor nocturnus Nightmare

paxillin A cytoskeletal protein that is tyrosine-phosphorylated and binds in the extracellular matrix to vinculin and

to SH2 and SH3 modular domains (Science 1995; 268:233)

PBC Primary biliary cirrhosis, see there

pBR322 MOLECULAR BIOLOGY A circular plasmid widely used as a cloning vector for amplifying a segment of DNA of interest; pBR322 is itself a recombinant DNA molecule and has unique restriction endonuclease sites (*Eco*RI, *Hin*d III, *Bam* HI, *Sph* I, *Sal* I, *Xma* III) in the tetracycline-resistance gene and restriction endonuclease sites (Pst I, Pvu I) in the ampicillin resistance gene, sites which allow rapid identification (screening) of bacteria bearing these colonies

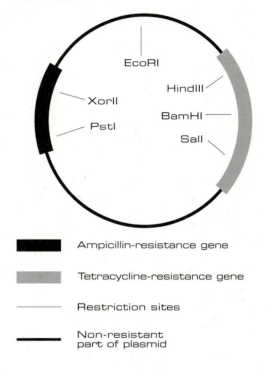

Ampicillin-resistance gene

Tetracycline-resistance gene

Restriction sites

Non-resistant part of plasmid

pBR322

PBS Phosphate-buffered saline

PC 1) Packed cells (RBCs) 2) Paper chromatography 3) Personal computer 4) Phosphatidylcholine (lecithin) 5) Phosphocholine 6) Phosphorylcholine 7) Plasma cell 8) Politically correct, see there 9) Present complaint 10) Professional corporation 11) Pyruvate carboxylase

Also 1) Paracortical hyperplasia 2) Parent care 3) Parent cells 4) Peak capacity 5) Penetrating cell 6) Pentose cycle 7) Pericarditis 8) Pericentral 9) Peripheral cell 10) Phenol coefficient 11) Pheochromocytoma 12) Phobia clinic 13) Phosphate cycle 14) Phosphocreatinine 15) Physocyanin 16) Plasmacytoma 17) Platelet concentrate 18) Platelet count 19) Pneumotaxic center 20) Pocket computer (rarely used, more current is the PDA-personal desk accessory) 21) Polycarbonate 22) Polycarbosilane 23) Population Council 24) Portable computer (rarely used, the term laptop is generally preferred) 25) Portocaval 26) Post-cibum (after meals) 27) Postcoital 28) Posterior chamber (ophthalmology) 29) Posterior commissure (neuroanatomy) 30) Postinflammatory corticosteroid 31) Precaution category (laboratory medicine) 32) Precordia (anatomy) 33) Primary circuit 34) Procarbazine 35) Propylene carbonate 36) Provocative concentration (immunology) 37) Pseudoconditioning control (neurophysiology) 38) Pseudoconditioning control 39) *Pubococcygeus* [NA6] 40) Pulmonary capillary 41) Pulmonic (valve) closure 42) Purkinje cells (neuroanatomy)

PC$_{15}$ A provocation test for evaluating bronchial responsiveness to histamine; PC$_{15}$ measures the concentration of histamine required to produce a 15% reduction in the FEV$_1$ (forced expiratory volume in one second) secondary to bronchoconstriction; **PC$_{20}$** is a permutation of the same theme

PCA Patient-controlled analgesia, see there

PCB Polychlorinated biphenyl(s) ENVIRONMENT Any of a

family of 209 related compounds that were widely used as industrial coolants until the 1970s, but which were banned when they were linked to liver cancer in rats; despite the 20-year moratorium on their manufacture, they remain in the food chain and continue to be inculpated in deleterious effects; PCBs may act as hormones, boosting sperm production and causing hypothyroidism (Science 1995; 267:1770)

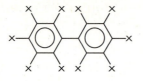

PCB

PCB Family of chemicals that were widely used in industry for fluid-filled capacitors and transformers, hydraulic tanks, plasticizers, resins and carbonless copy paper; the commercial products, known in the US as aroclors are complex mixtures of PCB homologs and isomers and persist for prolonged periods in the environment, and were banned in 1979 due to their toxicity PATHOPHYSIOLOGY PCBs induce ↑ steroid hydroxylase and cytochrome oxidase activity, as well as ↑ drug turnover by inducing endoplasmic reticulum CLINICAL, ACUTE PBC poisoning Chloracne, hyperpigmentation and meibomian gland dilatation; biodegradation of PCBs is limited to molecules with less than five chlorides; see Yucheng disease, Yusho disease

Note; Anaerobic organisms, eg DCB1, have been identified in sediment from the Hudson river (which passes between New York and New Jersey, both active producers of industrial waste including PCBs) that reduce the highly chlorinated PCBs into mono- and dichlorobiphenyls which are then more easily degraded by aerobic bacteria; bacterial dechlorination of PBCs may be accelerated by adding an electron donor, eg vitamin C, exposing PBC to sunlight and maintaining the contaminated soil well hydrated

PCDD Polychlorinated dibenzo-*p*-dioxins, see Dioxin

PCDF Polychlorinated dibenzofuran(s), see Dioxin

P cell Nodal cell, see there

PCH Paroxysmal cold hemoglobinuria, see there

PCNA Proliferating cell nuclear antigen, see there

PCO 1) Patient complains of 2) Physician controlled organization 3) Polycystic ovaries, see there 4) Potassium channel opener

PCP 1) Phencyclidine (phenylcyclohexylpiperidine), see there 2) *Pneumocystis carinii* pneumonia, see there

Also 1) Paired cone pigments 2) Para-chlorophenol 3) Pentachlorophenol 4) Peripheral coronary pressure 5) Polychloroprene 6) Primary care physician 8) Pulse cytophotometer (flow cytometer)

PCR Polymerase chain reaction, see there

Also 1) Physician charge ratio 2) Phosphocreatine 3) Population census report 4) Primary chemotherapy-radiotherapy

PCTA Percutaneous transluminal coronary angioplasty, see there

PDA Patent ductus arteriosus

Also 1) Pediatric allergy 2) Pentadecanoic acid 3) Phenylenediamine 4) Phorboldiacetate 5) Piperidinedicarboxylic acid 6) Pisantin demethylase (?) 7) Polydiacetylene 8) Potato dextrose agar 9) Predialyzed human albumin 10) Prolonged depolarizing afterpotential (neurophysiology) 11) Propanediamine 12) Propylenediamine

PDAPP mouse A transgenic mouse* that has neuropathologic features (eg dystrophic neurites, amyloid deposits, activated glia) of Alzheimer's disease (AD), and may be useful as an experimental model for AD (N Engl J Med 1995; 332:1512)

*PDAPP (platelet-derived growth factor promoter expressing amyloid precursor protein)

PDGF Platelet-derived growth factor, see there

PDGF-B protein Platelet-derived growth factor-B protein A protein with homology to the v-*sis* oncogene product; PDGF-B protein residues 105-144 are responsible for conformational alterations in receptor interaction and may be related to the greater transforming potency of the B protein chain; PDGF-B protein may have a role in atheroscle-rosis, a disease of large and medium-sized arteries characterized by focal thickening of the inner vessel wall; growth-regulatory molecules may be involved in intimal proliferation and accumulation of smooth muscle cells, which in turn is responsible for the vaso-occlusive lesions of atherosclerosis, as the PDGF-B chain is present within macrophages at all phases of atherosclerosis

P-disc see Optochin disc

PDR Physicians Desk Reference A book published annually (Medical Economics Co, Montvale, NJ) that lists the approximately 2500 therapeutic agents that in the USA require a physician prescription; the book is divided into seven color-coded sections

WHITE Manufacturers' index, containing the company addresses and list of products

PINK Product name index, an alphabetical listing of the drugs by brand name

BLUE Product classification, where drugs are subdivided into therapeutic classes

YELLOW Generic and chemical name index

MULTICOLORED Photographs of the most commonly prescribed tablets and capsules

WHITE Product information, a reprint of the manufacturers' product inserts and

GREEN Diagnostic product information, a list of manufacturers of diagnostic tests used in office practice and the hospital; Cf Over-the-counter drugs

peach pit appearance A fanciful descriptor for the 70-85 μm eggs of *Hymenolepis diminuta*, in which the six-hooked oncosphere is surrounded by a membrane separated by a large space from the outer shell, a space likened to the peach flesh itself

'peak' Peak level THERAPEUTIC DRUG MONITORING The maximum serum level of free or unbound drug, a value used to monitor antibiotic therapy where success depends on high levels of antibiotics in the infected site(s), while maintaining the drug below toxic levels, as is required to avoid nephro- and ototoxicity in aminoglycoside therapy; the 'peak' is usually measured ± ½ hour after an oral dose of a drug; Cf Trough levels

peak acid output PHYSIOLOGY A measurement of maximum hydrogen ion (H^+) production by the gastric parietal cells, defined as the sum of the two highest consecutive 15-minute acid outputs after pentagastrin or histamine stimulation, multiplied by 2; PAO indirectly quantifies the number of functional parietal cells and has a normal value of 10-60 mmol/hr, which is similar to MAO; see BAO

'peak E' 1,1'-ethylidenebis[tryptophan] A novel amino acid so designated as it causes a peak (spike) on the paper or 'hard copy' when analyzed by HPLC; the peak E was identified in, and held responsible for eosinophilia-myalgia syndrome, see there

pea soup stool A descriptor for the khaki-green, slimy stools typically seen in the third week of typhoid fever at which point the patients are in a 'toxic state', at greatest risk for intestinal perforation and hemorrhage; similar stools occur in enteropathic *Escherichia coli* infections of infants

Pearl Index OBSTETRICS A formula that facilitates comparison of the efficacy of the method of contraception, calculated as the pregnancy rate in population divided by 100 years of exposure (table); see Condoms, Morning-after pill, Norplant, RU 486

pear-shaped bladder Tear-drop bladder, see there

pearly An adjectival descriptor of the opalescent sheen seen in the colonies of *Bordetella pertussis*

pearly penile papules A localized region of nodularity that represents an anatomic variant of the penile corona that is first seen at ages 20-50 as a verrucous lesion

PATHOLOGY Well-vascularized connective tissue covered by epidermis with central thinning and peripheral acanthosis TREATMENT None required

Synonyms include Hairy penis, hirsutoid papillomata of penis

Pearson correlation coefficient STATISTICS A means by which univariate relations between pairs of variables can be determined, ie a measure of linear association (if the association is nonlinear, the PCC cannot be used); the PCC is calculated by the formula $s_{xy}/s_x s_y$, where s_x and s_y are the standard deviations of x and y, and s_{xy} is the covariance of x and y; as an example PCC can be used to determine whether there is a correlation between the reduction of dietary cholesterol in patients with NIDDM and their lipid profile

*aka Pearson chi-square statistic and Pearson's product moment correlation coefficient

peau d'orange appearance A widely-used descriptive term referring to any bosselated, rugose surface, usually of the skin with deep, pin-point dimpling that was first likened by French authors to the skin of an orange; the 'classic' peau d'orange change occurs in the skin overlying breast cancer OPHTHALMOLOGY A fundoscopic finding corresponding to diffuse, rugose hyperpigmentation of the retinal epithelium in patients with angioid streaks RADIOLOGY One of three radiologic patterns of monostotic fibrous dysplasia, which is described as delicately increased trabeculation with increased opacity and peau d'orange-like mottling of edges of the osseous lesion; monostotic fibrous dysplasia may also appear as a small unilocular radiolucency with sharp borders or as a poorly-circumscribed, radiopacity with innumerable, delicate trabeculations that blend with adjacent normal bone SKIN Peau d'orange-like changes of the skin are classically seen in advanced duct cell carcinoma of breast, in which there is subcutaneous 'puck-ering' accompanied by dermal edema, desmoplastic induration, superficial bossellation, erythema, local tenderness that may be accompanied by ulceration; peau d'orange skin changes

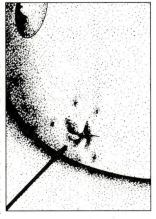

may also be seen in 1) Eosinophilic fasciitis, characterized by diffuse leathery induration of the skin with deep furrows, seen in advanced disease with thickened collagen bundles in the lower **peau d'orange appearance** third of the reticular dermis, entrapment of the eccrine glands, hyalinization, inflammation and induration of the fibrous septae 2) Thrombophlebitis of the superficial veins of the breast (Mondor's disease), in which the skin is dimpled by compressible vessels 3) Erysipelas Group A streptococcal infection, characterized by sharply demarcated, raised

and painful skin lesions, occurring in patients who are very sick and febrile with cellulitis of the lower legs arising in fissures between the toes in tinea pedis 4) Myxedema, appearing as 'doughy' puckering and thickening in the skin due to deposition of glycosaminoglycans with accentuation of the follicular orifices in a background of non-pitting plaques and nodules 5) Traumatic fat necrosis, most common in the breast with minimal trauma and which may present with fixation of the skin to the fascial planes 6) Plaque stage of mycosis fungoides 7) Pyogenic granuloma, characterized by a bosselated mucocutaneous surface overlying a lesion that is neither pyogenic (purulent), nor a granuloma, but rather is a florid proliferation of vessels or a granulation tissue reaction

PECAM Platelet/endothelial cell adhesion molecule, now known as CD31, see there

pectin(s) A heterogeneous family of highly branched, highly hydrated and glucuronic acid-rich polysaccharides derived from fruit and used to produce gelling agents

pediatric AIDS AIDS acquired HIV perinatally or by 'vertical' (maternal-infant) transmission; children with PAIDS may become symptomatic (lymphoid interstitial pneumonia, encephalopathy, recurrent bacterial infection and *Candida* esophagitis) within the first year of life; the five-year mortality is ± 50%; see AIDS

pediatric trauma score EMERGENCY MEDICINE A triage tool that has no advantage over the easier-to-learn Revised Trauma Score (see there); the PTS measures six parameters (weight, airway, systolic pressure, central nervous system status, open wound and skeletal trauma) (N Engl J Med 1991; 324:1477)

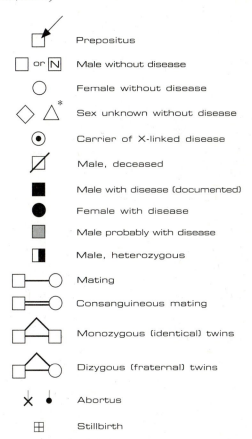

▢↖	Prepositus
▢ or Ⓝ	Male without disease
◯	Female without disease
◇ △*	Sex unknown without disease
⊙	Carrier of X-linked disease
▨	Male, deceased
■	Male with disease (documented)
●	Female with disease
▨	Male probably with disease
▨	Male, heterozygous
▢—◯	Mating
▢=◯	Consanguineous mating
▢⋀◯	Monozygous (identical) twins
▢⋀◯	Dizygous (fraternal) twins
✗ ●	Abortus
⊞	Stillbirth

pedigree symbols

pedigree Clinical genetics An ancestral chart of the blood relatives and mates of a patient (index patient) with a disease or hereditary characteristic of interest (figure)

Note: The name pedigree is of Latin derivation, pes for foot and grus for crane, as a pedigree chart has an appearance likened to that of a crane's foot

PEEP Positive end-expiratory pressure A therapeutic modality that consists in the active (interventional) maintenance of a slightly positive pressure in the tracheobronchial tree during assisted pulmonary ventilation, such that the alveoli are not allowed to completely collapse between breaths; PEEP is of greatest use in adult respiratory distress syndrome (ARDS) and is generated by attaching an airflow threshold resistance device to the expiratory port of the non-rebreathing valve of a manual or mechanical ventilator, allowing a decrease of airway pressure to a plateau level DISADVANTAGES ↑ Intrathoracic pressure results in ↓ cardiac output and may cause alveolar rupture and possible pneumothorax; forms of PEEP PROPHYLACTIC PEEP The pressure is maintained at 1-5 cm H₂O, preventing atelectasis, while increasing the functional residual capacity above closing volume CONVENTIONAL PEEP The pressure is maintained at 5-20 cm H₂O and is indicated where an inhaled oxygen fraction at 0.6 cannot maintain the PaO₂ above 60 Torr HIGH PEEP The pressure is maintained at 20-50 cm H₂O and is of use in marked hypoxia, as may occur in severe pulmonary edema

Peeping Tom 'syndrome' Voyeurism, see there

peer review The objective evaluation of a physician's or scientist's performance by colleagues, which may take the form of either 1) Peer review of articles for publication in official organs of communication, ie journals or 2) Review of the quality, necessity and appropriateness (suitability) of care provided by an individual physician, ie Peer review organizations (PROs), which in the US contract with the Health Care Financing Administration

peer-reviewed journal ACADEMIA A professional journal that only publishes articles that have been subjected to a rigorous peer review process; this process entails submission of a potentially 'interesting' or publishable manuscript received by the journal's editors to physicians or scientists with expertise in an area related to the subject matter in the manuscript; because the 'submission-to-acceptance' ratio may be 5:1 or more, PRJs are rightly regarded as elitist and canonical, ie certifying original thought and medical progress; acceptance of articles in such journals is considered an indicator of appropriate scholarship for an academician seeking career advancement (JAMA 1991; 266:2830c); Cf Throwaway journal

peer review organization PRO, see there

PEFR Peak expiratory flow rate

PEG 1) Percutaneous endoscopic gastrostomy A method for placing an enteric feeding tube that avoids the costs and morbidity of surgical procedure to achieve the same goal (JAMA 1991; 265:1426) 2) Polyethylene glycol CLINICAL THERAPEUTICS An inert long-chain synthetic molecule that may be attached to various proteins making them invisible to the immune system; multiple PEGs have been attached to ADA (adenosine deaminase), one of the enzymes responsible for SCID, allowing long-term survival of the molecule within the body; PEG has been attached to hemoglobin, and has potential as a transport vehicle for artificial blood; in the management of surgical patients, PEG has been used to mechanically purge the large intestine in preparation for surgery

PEG-conjugated IL-2 Polyethylene glycol-conjugated interleukin-2 A formulation of IL-2 that has a 10-fold ↑ in T₁/₂ without loss of efficacy that may be administered parenterally; IL-2 promotes the growth and differentiation of CD4 (helper/inducer), CD8 (suppressor/cytotoxic) T, NK, and lymphokine-activated cells; PEG-conjugated IL-2 reported to be beneficial in cancer, HIV infection, and in

common variable immune deficiency (N Engl J Med 1994; 331:918oA)

peg cells Hobnail cells, see there

peg tooth 1) An incisor* with a barrel-shaped deformity, which when accompanied by a central notch is a 'classic' finding in congenital syphilis; peg teeth may also be seen in 2) Williams (elfinfacies) syndrome, anhidrotic, hipohidrotic, and the Robinson types of ectodermal dysplasia

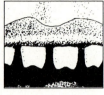
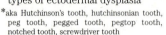

peg teeth

*aka Hutchinson's tooth, hutchinsonian tooth, peg tooth, pegged tooth, pegtop tooth, notched tooth, screwdriver tooth

PEH Pseudoepitheliomatous hyperplasia, see there

PEL Permissible exposure limits, see there

Pelger-Huët anomaly Pince-nez neutrophil HEMATOLOGY A descriptor for PMNs that fail to develop normal nuclear lobes, which are 'arrested' as a bilobed, peanut- or barbell-shaped nucleus with clumped dense (ergo, dark) chromatin, fancifully likened to pince-nez spectacles, a deformity that may also be seen in lymphocytes and monocytes; the condition is either AD [MIM 169400] and asymptomatic, or acquired (pseudo-Pelger-Huët anomaly) and associated with hematopoietic malignancies, eg mycosis fungoides, leukemia, and preleukemia

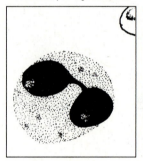
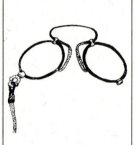

Pelger-Huët anomaly   **pince-nez**

peliosis hepatis An enlarged liver characterized by multiple cavernous blood-filled cysts related to the use of contraceptives and androgenic steroids and occasionally associated with malignancy and TB; a distinct form-bacillary peliosis hepatis has been described in HIV-positive subjects, see Bacillary angiomatosis

pellagrous 'boot' A sharply-demarcated erythema affecting the acral portion of the leg or arm (pellagrous 'glove'), a clinical manifestation of severe niacin deficiency that may be exacerbated by sun exposure; a vesiculo-bullous variant of niacin deficiency known as Casal's necklace occurs in the head and neck PATHOLOGY Dermal edema, superficial collagen degeneration, chronic perivascular inflammation and hyperkeratosis; see Ds (the three Ds)

pellet CLINICAL PHARMACOLOGY A small sterile cylinder measuring 8 mm in length by 3 mm in diameter formed from medicated masses, and used when prolonged (depot-type) absorption of hormones (eg testosterone, estradiol, desoxycorticosterone) is desirable; pellets are administered by implantaion LABORATORY SCIENCE An aggregate of membrane-derived materials, fragmented organelles, and macromolecules , which are found at the bottom on a centrifuge tube; Cf Button

pelvic floor SURGICAL ANATOMY A well-defined region that is bordered anteriorly by the pubis and posteriorly by the sacrum, laterally by the ischial and iliac bones, superiorly by the peritoneum and inferiorly by the levator ani and coccygeus muscles, the last-named forming the pelvic diaphragm; pelvic organs include the uterus and adnexae, anteriorly, the bladder, posteriorly the rectum and neurovascular tissues; see North American operation, Frozen pelvis

pelvic inflammatory disease GYNECOLOGY An imprecise term for the intense pain due to direct extension of a lower genital tract infection (often sexually-transmitted) along the mucosa[1], first causing asymptomatic endometritis, followed by acute salpingitis and increasing symptoms as it spreads into fallopian tubes that become engorged with pus (pyosalpinx) and purulent leakage into the peritoneum; PID is accompanied by leukostasis, fever, chills, nausea and vomiting, extreme tenderness of the uterine cervix and adnexae EPIDEMIOLOGY PID is reported to be 3–4-fold more common in IUD users[2] and in those who douche 3+ times/month; ectopic pregnancy is 7–10-fold more common in PID; 500 000 cases of PID are reported/year (US) ETIOLOGY ½ are due to *N gonorrhoeae*, less commonly, *Chlamydia trachomatis* and others; 15% of those with gonococcal cervicitis develop PID CLINICAL Severe pain, peritonitis, low-grade fever COMPLICATIONS Fallopian tube scarring, and in ¼, infertility EPIDEMIOLOGY PID predominantly affects disadvantaged urban women*, affecting circa 1 million females (US), costing ± $4 billion TREATMENT Cefoxitin, doxocycline, clindamycin, ofloxacin (N Engl J Med 1994; 330:115RV)

[1]Hence the alternative term, salpingo-oophoritis [2]PID is more common in non-white ♀, of low education levels, who begin sexual intercourse earlier and who with ↑ coital activity

pencil-in-cup sign Mortar-and-pestle sign RHEUMATOLOGY A tapering of the convexity and exaggeration of the opposite concavity in the distal phalangeal articulation(s), which is accompanied by osteoporosis and seen in the atrophic neuropathic arthropathy of both severe psoriatic and rheumatoid arthropathy

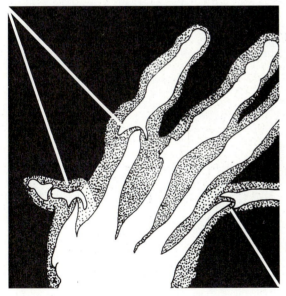

pencil in cup appearance

'penciling' A descriptor for the marked resorption of the distal phalanges (acro-osteolysis), a radiologic finding typical of scleroderma that may be idiopathic or which may also occur in severe burns accompanied by soft tissue contractures, 'black toe' disease (ainhum), hyperparathyroidism, neural leprosy, SLE, neuropathic disease, eg DM, tabes dorsalis, progeria, psoriatic arthritis, exposure to polyvinyl-chloride, Reiter syndrome, and sarcoidosis; Cf Spade deformity

pencil-point thinness Marked attenuation of the cortex

of long bones, seen in advanced scurvy of young children

'pencil pusher' A derogatory colloquialism for any low-level bureaucrat, eg in an academic center, hospital, regulatory or reimbursement agency

pendulous abdomen A loose, fat-filled abdominal wall that hangs over the belt and is accompanied by weakness of the abdominal muscles

penem A member of the β-lactam group of broad-spectrum antibiotics, which acts on the bacterial cell wall and lyses bacteria that are in the resting phase, thus contrasting with penicillins that kill only bacteria in the growth phase by inhibiting cell wall synthesis

penetrance Penetration The disruption of a surface, as in penetrating, eg gunshot wounds, hospital-acquired penetration contact due to infected 'sharps', or forcible penetration in rape GENETICS The degree to which a genotype will be phenotypically expressed when the genes for a condition are present in full complement, which in a single gene trait, requires one allele with the gene of interest in an AD condition or both alleles (homozygosity) in an AR condition

penetrating trauma A generic term for any injury sustained as a result of either 1) Sharp force, which includes injuries from cutting or piercing instruments or objects and nonvenomous bites of animals or humans except arthropods or 2) Firearm injuries from projectiles (JAMA 1993; 269:1525OC) Cf Blunt trauma

penguin gait A fanciful descriptor for the waddling gait of patients with muscular dystrophy in whom there is marked exaggeration of the lumbar lordosis, a rolling of the hips from side to side in the stance phase of each forward step (in order to shift the weight of the body), exaggerated lateral tilting and rotation of the pelvis to compensate for the weakened gluteal muscles accompanied by overuse of the trunk and upper extremities during ambulation

penicillinase-producing *Neisseria gonorrhoeae* Any of a number of strains of *N gonorrhoeae*, many of which have penicillinase-producing plasmids; PPNG are common in non-Caucasian illicit drug abusers, prostitutes and their sexual partners; other penicillinase producers include *Staphylococcus aureus*, which comprise the majority of penicillinase producing organisms, *Haemophilus influenza* and *Escherichia coli* Note: ± 20% of *N gonorrhoeae* isolates are resistant to penicillin, as well as tetracycline, cefoxitin, spectinomycin TREATMENT Ceftriaxone; see Methicillin-resistant *Staphylococcus aureus*

penicillin binding protein An enzyme required for the synthesis of the bacterial cell wall; the PBP gene is mutated in some strains of β-lactam-resistant pneumococci, resulting in excess enzyme production, circumventing penicillin's negative action on cell wall synthesis (JAMA 1991; 265:14n&v)

penile implant An FDA Class 3 medical device composed of silicone polymers, which has been on the market since 1973; ± 30 000 ♂ receive penile implants/year; the FDA receives ± 5000 complaints/year about PIs; most recipients are in their 50s and 60s; PIs have two basic designs: 1) The semirigid PI, which is far less prone to infection, and complications, eg mechanical failure, but has (for some) the disadvantage of always being on the 'flight deck' 2) The inflatable PI has a fluid reservoir that is surgically placed under the abdominal musculature, a pump in the scrotum, and inflatable cylinders in the penis; when 'yellow alert' goes to 'red alert', the patient pumps 'it' up, transferring the fluid (usually saline) into the cylinders; following appropriate use, the cylinders are emptied by means of a deflate button; of 500 reoperations for inflatable PIs, 64% required therapy for mechanical failure of the device, 19% for surgical complications, and 10% for infections (**JAMA 1992; 267:2578**ᴍɴ&ᴘ)

penile reatttachment The surgical reattachment of a penis severed by intentional (eg self-mutilation, criminal acts) or unintentional (eg workplace-related) trauma; recovery of sexual function requires microsurgical techniques that allow the sewing of vessels and nerves of 1 mm or less; chilled on ice, a severed penis is thought to be capable of surviving up to 18 hours prior to reattachment (**New York Times 13 July 1993; C3**) see 'Bobbittize'

peninsula sign A histopathologic finding seen in the patch (early) stage of Kaposi sarcoma, in which pre-existing vessels and/or hair follicles (figure, above) jut into widely dilated, jagged, thin-walled neoplastic vascular spaces, which are lined by attenuated endothelial cells that surround pre-existing superficial and periadnexal vascular plexuses

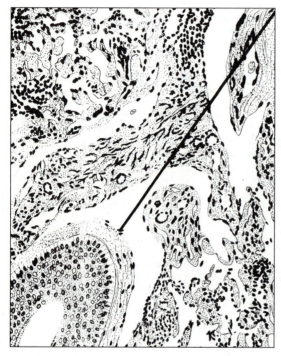

peninsula sign

penis envy Psʏᴄʜɪᴀᴛʀʏ The unconscious desire on the part of females to have a penis, which according to psychoanalysts, corresponds to an unresolved castration complex

Penn State heart An artificial heart that was designed to serve as a 'bridge', prior to transplantation of a permanent heart; the PSH is one of two air-driven models that is approved by the FDA; which continues to be approved (**JAMA 1995; 273:1891**ɴ&ᴠ) the longest survival with this heart was 13 months; see Jarvik-7, Ventricular assist device

pentamidine isoethionate A second-line agent used to treat *Pneumocystis carinii* pneumonia (PCP) in AIDS patients who do not respond to T-S; PI is administered by aerosol, and reduces the episodes of PCP by 65% Aᴅᴠᴇʀsᴇ ʀᴇᴀᴄᴛɪᴏɴs Potentially severe, including arrhythmia, azotemia, hypotension, sterile abscesses at the injection site, pancreatitis, DM and dose-related, potentially life-threatening hypoglycemia

pentafluoropropionyl derivative Cʟɪɴɪᴄᴀʟ ᴛᴏxɪᴄᴏʟᴏɢʏ A generic term for certain cocaine metabolite, eg benzoylecgonine and ecgonine methyl ester, which can be measured in the urine by GC-MS following extraction on a solid phase extraction column (**Arch Pathol Lab Med 1994; 118:988**ᴏᴀ)

penta-X syndrome XXXXX syndrome, see there

pentraxin family A group of circulating glycoproteins with cyclic pentameric symmetry that includes C-reactive protein, complement C1 and serum amyloid P

PEP proteins Priming in exocytosis proteins A family of cytosolic proteins (PEP1, PEP2 , PEP3) that play a key role in the regulated fusion of secretory granules with the plasma membrane; in the rat brain, PEP proteins stimulate the ATP-dependent priming of Ca^{2+}-activated noradrenaline secretion (**Nature 1995; 374:135**)

PEPCK Phosphoenolpyruvate carboxykinase A protein that governs the rate-limiting step in gluconeogenesis; transcription of the PEPCK gene and subsequent gluconeogenesis is increased by glucocorticoids and adenosine 3',5'-monophosphate and decreased by insulin, all three molecules for which the gene has recognition sites

Pepper Commission plan A \$86 x 10^9 health plan* approved by a US Congressional committee, chaired by J Rockefeller, intended to provide 1) either job-based or public health insurance-based access to medical coverage for all Americans, in particular for employees of small businesses and 2) home and community-based care and three months of nursing home care to people of all ages (**Perspect Biol & Med 1993; 36:596**) Cf Catastrophic health insurance

*Named after Representative Claude Pepper who chaired the committee before he died

Pepper syndrome Massive metastatic involvement of liver by neuroblastoma resulting in the 'peppering' of the hepatic parenchyma by innumerable small dark aggregates of tumor cells, described by W Pepper (**Am J Med Sci 1901; 121:287**), giving rise to one form of 'blueberry infant'

peppermint stick candy bones A fanciful descriptor for the radiologic appearance of some cases of osteopetrosis, in which the defect in osteoclastic activity is intermittent, giving rise to radiodense and radiolucent bands, most often in the bony pelvis, paralleling the iliac crest

peptide map Bɪᴏᴄʜᴇᴍɪsᴛʀʏ A 2-D 'fingerprint' of a protein that has been first digested with an enzyme, eg trypsin, followed by thin-layer chromatography in one direction (dimension) and electrophoresis at pH 6.5 in the other direction (**Proc Nat Acad Sci [USA] 1990; 87:26**)

peptide T A short polypeptide present in HIV-1's envelope that had been proposed as having potential for treating AIDS and later discarded prior to reaching the investigational new drug stage fo development

pepT1 A recently described H+-coupled transporter of oligopeptides and peptide-derived antibiotics; PepT1 mRNA has been identified in kidney, liver, brain, and in the intestine, where it may play a key role in the absorption of partially digested proteins (**Nature 1994; 368:563**ᴏᴀ)

peptide YY A 36-amino acid peptide produced in the distal ileum and proximal colon that is released by fatty foods and thought to be involved in secretion of pancreatic enzymes

peptone A variable in length, hydrolyzed mixture of short polypeptide chains that are not precipitated by ammonium sulfate, which may be used in commercial preparations of culture media in microbiology laboratories

per capita consumption A generic term for the average use of consumable items, eg water, food, energy by a population, which is total of the consumable used, divided by the total number of persons in the population; the average American has become more obese, as measured by triceps skin thickness, but is apparently eating better; between 1963-1980, he ↓ his animal fat consumption by 39%, butter by 33%, tobacco by 27%, milk by 24% and eggs by 12%; in addition, he ↑ his consumption of vegetable oils by 58% and fish by 22%, changes that are in part responsible for the 53% ↓ in atherosclerosis-related death and a 38% ↓ in cerebrovascular accidents (both peaked in 1968)

percutaneous balloon valvuloplasty A nonsurgical procedure for treating selected patients with mitral stenosis that is effective both short- and long-term, with marked immediate improvement in hemodynamic parameters and stenosis-related symptoms RESULTS ↑ valve area ± 1.1 cm², ↓ mean transmitral pressure gradient from 14 to 6 mm Hg; 5-year post-valvuloplasty survival ± 76%, and event-free survival 51%; ↓ survival occurs in those with higher New York Heart Association scores, mitral valve deformity, and higher left ventricular end-diastolic pressures (**N Engl J Med 1992; 327:1329OA**); both PBV and open commissurotomy offer comparable results (wedge pressure, mitral pressure gradient, and exercise duration) with low rate of restenosis and provide good functional capacity for 3 years (**N Engl J Med 1994; 331:961OA**) see New York Heart Association classification

percutaneous transluminal coronary angioplasty PCTA CARDIOLOGY A technique of interventional angiography introduced in 1977 for treating coronary arteries stenosed by atherosclerosis and ± 300 000 in 1990 (US) PCTA consists of balloon expansion of one or more stenosed coronary arteries and is indicated for single and multivessel disease, stable and unstable angina and acute myocardial infarction; up to 90% of PCTA procedures are successful under optimal conditions, with re-stenosis occurring in 30%, although it is unclear whether PCTA's long-term outcome is better than coronary artery bypass; when PCTA is compared to tissue plasminogen activator (TPA) combined with heparin and aspirin therapy after an acute MI, PCTA is indicated only in cases with ischemia demonstrable by coronary arteriography; a 60-70% success rate in renovascular hypertension due to atherosclerosis and 90% success in fibromuscular hyperplasia have been reported in renal arteries treated with transluminal angioplasty Note: PCTA is associated with a 3-7% risk of in-hospital coronary closure, a complication that may be prevented by using a balloon-expandable, flexible metallic coil-type coronary artery stent (**Mayo Clin Proc 1991; 66:268**); hospitals that perform more PCTAs have lower short-term mortality rates (**N Engl J Med 1994; 331:1625RA**) MECHANISM OF ACTION Balloon-induced barotrauma causes endothelial denudation; cracking, splitting, and disruption of atherosclerotic plaques; and stretching or tearing of the media and adventitia, with resultant aneurysmal dilatation INDICATIONS Stable angina on exertion, unstable angina, acute MI ('primary' PCTA), post-thrombolytic therapy SUCCESS RATE 90% defined as < 50% stenosis of treated coronary artery AFTER therapy; success is lower with stenoses that are chronic, long, eccentric, angulated, calcified, located at a branch point, or associated with an intraluminal thrombus; the success rate is also lower in patients with unstable angina, advanced age, and may be lower in women (**N Engl J Med 1994; 330:981RA**) Note: The success rate of the two most commonly used revascularization techniques (PCTA vs coronary artery bypass grafting-CABG) is comparable (**N Engl J Med 1994; 331:1044OA**); it is reported that CABG carries a greater risk of acute MI at surgery; PCTA often requires further therapy and antianginal drugs (**N Engl J Med 1994; 331:1037OA**) see Coronary artery bypass surgery, Excimer laser therapy; Cf Balloon valvoplasty

percutaneous transluminal cerebral angioplasty A technique similar to balloon angioplasty of the coronary arteries, designed to reduce the risk of strokes in subjects with atherosclerosis of the cerebral arteries, the procedure consists of the use of an x-ray-guided 2 to 5 (≤ 1 to 3 mm in diameter) French catheter which has a small balloon that is inflated a few times at a site of stenosis (**JAMA 1992; 268:3039MN&P**)

percutaneous umbilical blood sampling PUBS Cordocentesis Ultrasound-guided needle aspiration of umbilical cord blood, a procedure used identify fetal diseases (eg, hemoglobinopathies, hemophilia, autoimmune thrombocytopenia, von Willebrand disease), alloimmunization (Rh disease, Kell and other red cell antigens, alloimmune thrombocytopenia), and to identify metabolic disorders, fetal infection (B19, CMV, rubella, toxoplasmosis, varicella), fetal karyotyping, and for fetal therapy, eg RBC and platelet transfusion (**N Engl J Med 1993; 328:728ED**) COMPLICATIONS Cord hematoma, bradycardia, and fetal wastage ± 2.7% (**Arch Pathol Lab Med 1994; 118:417RV, 118:421RV**)

per diem Latin, by the day *Adjective* Pertaining or referring to the practice by hospitals of charging 'daily' rates, where the expenses incurred on a daily basis are averaged over the entirety of the hospital's census; those who utilize few services will in a sense 'subsidize' those with more expensive and/or extensive and complicated hospital stays *Noun* A temporary employee, eg a nurse, who receives a higher hourly salary but does not get the benefits enjoyed by salaried employee, eg vacation and pension plan

perfluorodecalin see Artificial blood

perforating abscess A generic term for an abscess in which the hydrolytic enzymes (presumed to originate from neutrophils) continue to digest tissue on the surface, causing locoregional necrosis

perforating collagenosis see Reactive perforating collagenosis

perforin HEMATOLOGY A 70-kD monomeric protein present in specific secretory granules of NK cells and cytotoxic T cells which in the presence of calcium, inserts itself into a target cell membrane, forming a self-associating polymer, seen by EM as a 5–20-nm annular transmembrane 'doughnut' which, once inserted into a membrane, is stable, allowing critical ions to diffuse out of a cell, hastening its demise; a knockout mouse model has been created that completely lacks perforin and confirms the existance of nonperforin cytolytic pathways, as yet undefined (**Nature 1994; 369:31OA, 16N&V**) see Membrane attack complex, Porin

performance-enhancing drug Ergogenic drug SPORTS MEDICINE A generic term for any agent that is known or thought to improve performance in particular activity; in large part, the term PED has become a euphemism for anabolic-androgenic steroids which are banned by the Olympic Committee, as well as other official bodies* that oversee amateur and professional athletes (**Sci Am 1995; 272/2:77**); other performance-enhancing agents and modalities include amphetamines, bicarbonate loading, blood doping, caffeine, human growth hormone, and phosphate loading (**JC DeLee, D Drez, Jr, Eds, Orthopedic Sports Medicine WB Saunders, Philadelphia, 1994**)

*eg National Football League, National Collegiate Athletic Association, etc

performance test PSYCHOLOGY A generic term for a non-language based IQ test that focuses on the manipulation of concrete objects, eg blocks, pictures, and printed mazes, rather than relationships that are rooted in linguistics and symbols; Cf Psychologic test

performing arts medicine A developing subspeciality of occupational medicine that formally addresses the medical complaints of those who toot, tickle, trill, or tap for a living, by playing musical instruments, singing, or dancing; in the US, an estimated 200 000 earn their livelihoods from the performing arts (130 000 as instrumentalists, 20 000 as vocalists, 50 000 as 'others'), of whom 50% (more often ♀) have had complaints that threaten or force them to retire from their profession; the most common problems are those of the muscle-tendon unit, which range in severity from mild pain to complete incapacitation, related to a combination of relatively repetitive movements of a limited number of muscles and the awkward position required to hold the instrument and/or weight of the instrument; other clinical disorders include overuse 'syndromes', nerve impingement and facial dystonia TREATMENT Rest; β-adrenergic agents for performance anxiety

perfusion TRANSPLANTATION The intravascular irrigation of an isolated organ with blood, plasma or physiological substance, eg University of Wisconsin solution, for the purpose of either studying its metabolism or physiology under 'normal' conditions or for maintaining the organ as 'fresh' as possible, while transporting the donated organ for transplantation; see Slush preparation

perfusion scan A radionuclide study used to determine the adequacy of the pulmonary blood flow, measured by IV injection of ^{99m}Tc microaggregated albumin, usually as part of a Ventilation-perfusion scan (see there); the early part of the PS is known as the **wash-in**, which is followed by equilibrium and **wash-out** (see N Engl J Med 1992; 327:873OA) Cf Ventilation scan

perfusion shunt CLINICAL THERAPEUTICS A biohybrid device in which cells of interest (pancreatic islet cells) are placed in capillary fibers, housed in a plastic chamber, and anastomosed to a blood vessel; PSs represent the first generation of artificial pancreas, but proved cumbersome given their high displaced volume and difficult (ie surgical) access; further work on encapsulated cell therapy has continued with diffusion chambers, and that which is most promising, the microsphere (Science & Medicine July/August 1995, p16) see Biohybrid organ

perhexilene An antianginal agent that fell into disuse in most countries in the mid-1980s, which was associated with an ↑ frequency of peripheral neuropathy and severe hepatopathy in subjects lacking debrisoquin hydroxylase (P-450 2D6) which is absent in ± 8% of the Caucasian population (JAMA 1993; 269:1550ED)

Periactin Cyproheptadine, see there

periarteriolar lymphoid sheath The layer of lymphocytes surrounding the central arterioles in the spleen (aka white pulp), comprising the bulk of splenic lymphoid tissue; the PALS is composed of T cells surrounding the central arteriole, which are in turn surrounded by B cells; in the unstimulated state, the B-cell zone consists of a primary follicle; following stimulation, a central germinal center is evident

pericardial 'knock' CARDIOLOGY A loud third heart sound occurring when the ventricular filling is abruptly stopped at the end of the early diastolic pressure dip, ie at the end of the rapidly filling phase of the ventricles; classically associated with severe constrictive pericarditis*, or with penetrating trauma to the pericardium, the PK has a relatively high pitch, often ↑ in intensity with inspiration and coincides with the nadir of the 'y' descent of the jugular venous pulse, and resembles a premature third sound; Cf Gallop

*Which is accompanied by increased systemic venous pressure, exertional dyspnea, orthopnea, fatigue, ascites and hepatosplenomegaly

perilipin A hormone-regulated phosphoprotein [MIM 170290] that covers lipid storage droplets in adipocytes, and is major substrate for A-kinase within cells in adipocytes

perinatal substance exposure NEONATOLOGY The contact by a near-term fetus with a substances of abuse (SOA) due to maternal ingestion; PSE is associated with neonatal and obstetric complications in the form of low birth weight, prematurity, abruptio placentae, fetal distress, stillbirth, cerebral infarction, congenital malformations, and neurobehavioral dysfunction; in a study of PSE in California, 29 494 urine samples were screened for SOAs, 11.4% had 1+ SOA* (5.2% had 1+ drugs, 6.7% alcohol, 8.8% tobacco); black ♀ had the highest rates–total PSE was 14.2% (7.8% cocaine, 11.6% alcohol, 20.1% tobacco) (N Engl J Med 1993; 329:850SA)

*It is likely that the estimates of this study are conservative, as urine toxicology can only identify recent exposure to SOAs

perineal pearl NEONATOLOGY A cyst filled with viscid green-white mucoid material, located in the anterior perianal region of a newborn infant, which may extend to the scrotum, a finding pathognomonic for imperforate anus

periodic law A universal law that the properties of elements are periodic function of their atomic weights; if the elements are arranged in order of their weights, each element in the series will share physical properties with the eighth element before or after it

period trend EPIDEMIOLOGY A change in the incidence of a particular condition during a time period, eg epidemics or alcohol-related dementia during the Prohibition (JAMA 1992; 268:3098OC) see Temporal trend

periodic paralyses A group of conditions characterized by centrifugal 'attacks' of paralyzing, focal or systemic weakness of hours to days in duration, accompanied by a loss of deep tendon reflexes, refractoriness of muscle fibers to electrical stimulation, profound changes in potassium levels, variable cardiac arrhythmias and complete recuperation between attacks; rest following vigorous exercise may evoke an attack in a group of muscle fibers without changing the serum K^+ levels **HYPOKALEMIC PERIODIC PARALYSIS** Periodic paralysis I An AD [MIM 170400]] condition of late onset that is more intense in ♂ and occurs following strenuous exercise or carbohydrate meals, affecting the extremities, respiratory and cardiac muscle, potentially causing ventricular tachycardia and premature ventricular contractions TREATMENT KCl, acetazolamide; the severely afflicted may develop persistent weakness and dystrophic changes in muscle DDx Carnitine palmityl transferase deficiency, glycogen storage disease, type V, and all other forms of periodic paralysis **HYPERKALEMIC PERIODIC PARALYSIS** Periodic paralysis II An AD [MIM 170500] variant of muscular dystrophy caused by a defective gene on chromosome 17, which encodes the α subunit of a sodium channel in muscle cell membranes, closely linked to the growth hormone gene GH1 CLINICAL Early onset, most intense in males in whom paralytic attacks follow strenuous exercise, affecting the legs and eyelids; hyperkalemia may be prevented by acetazolamide; with time, severely afflicted subjects develop persistent weakness and dystrophic changes in muscle **NORMOKALEMIC PERIODIC PARALYSIS** Periodic paralysis III 1) Primary or hereditary A condition with attacks of childhood onset that may disappear by middle age; exposure to cold may provoke attacks and over time, result in vacuolar myopathy; the attacks may be provoked by high-carbohydrate, high-sodium diets during periods of excitement and may respond to oral potassium 2) Secondary or acquired A condition associated with thyrotoxicosis, hypokalemia or K^+ wasting by the kidneys or GI tract or due to accidental ingestion of absorbable barium salts that block K^+ channels, reducing the egress of K^+ from the muscles, evoking systemic hypokalemia or hyperkalemia, which may be associated with renal or adrenal insufficiency

periodic acid-Schiff stain PAS stain, see there

periodontal disease DENTISTRY Any disease of the periodontium, which includes chronic gingivitis, extension of infection into the periodontal ligaments and alveolar bone destruction; PD is the most common cause of loss of teeth in adults, the result of combined bacterial infection and impaired host response; 300 different bacterial species occur in healthy mouths, most of which are gram-positive, eg actinomyces and streptococci; in gingivitis, the oral flora changes, streptococci ↓, actinomyces ↑, and other organisms appear including *Fusobacterium nucleatum*, *Lactobacillus*, *Veillonella*, and *Treponema* species; periodontal disease is associated with *Actinobacillus actinomycetemcomitans* in juvenile and *Bacteroides gingivalis* in adult periodontitis (*B gingivalis* implanted subgingivally in primates produces bone loss and periodontitis); other organisms implicated in PD include *B inter-*

medius, B forsythus, Selenomonas sputigena, Eikenella corrodens, and spirochetes DDx Hypophosphatasia, Langerhans' cell histiocytosis (histiocytosis X), leukemia and vitamin C and/or vitamin D deficiencies

Note: Alveolar bone destruction, the bête noire of periodontitis, is the combined result of bacterial products (collagenases, proteases, leukotoxins, low molecular weight metabolites, and bacterial lipopolysaccharide) and a host defense gone awry (alteration of fibroblast response and collagen synthesis, release of lytic enzymes, lymphotoxin, prostaglandins and osteoclast activating factor); leukocyte dysfunction predisposes those with certain conditions to periodontitis, including Chediak-Higashi disease, Crohn's disease, cyclic neutropenia, DM, Down syndrome, and the lazy leukocyte syndrome

perioperative blood salvage Intraoperative blood salvage, see there

peripartum cardiomyopathy A rare but often fatal (50-85% mortality) condition defined as cardiac failure occurring in the last month of pregnancy or within five months of delivery in the absence of an identifiable cause of heart failure, and without demonstrable preexisting or concurrent heart disease; findings include cardiothoracic ratio > 0.55, a left ventricular ejection fraction < 50%, and a diastolic dimension > 95th percentile for age and body-surface area (N Engl J Med 1993; 329:247SA)

peripatry EVOLUTIONARY BIOLOGY A mechanism of speciation that requires geographic separation of a small founding population, a circumstance that has genetic raminifactions that may accelerate the divergence of species (Sci Am 1994; 270/8:25) see Species; Cf Allopatry

peripheral COMPUTERS Any electronic and/or mechanical, non-software component of a computer system that is controled by but external to the computer's critical guts (ie the central processing unit); peripherals include the monitor, disk drive, keyboard, printer, modem, scanning devices, and others

peripheral (reparative) giant cell granuloma ORAL PATHOLOGY A sessile or pedunculated gingival or alveolar growth of the young (age 5-15) mandible, ♀:♂ ratio, 2:1), possibly induced by trauma, eg tooth extration RADIOLOGY Superficial erosion, peripheral cuffing of bone PATHOLOGY Unencapsulated ingrowth of fibrous tissue, capillaries, and osteoclast-like giant cells may arise from a fusion of proliferating endothelial cells DDx Giant cell tumor of bone, hyperparathyroidism-induced 'brown' tumor TREATMENT Curettage, but not (as was occasionally practiced) extraction of the teeth

peripheral nerve sheath tumor Schwannoma Any of a group of tumors thought to arise in the neural sheath; three lesions have received the 'peripheral nerve sheath' adjective

PERIPHERAL NERVE SHEATH GANGLION A rare, tender mass in the nerve, accompanied by pain and/or numbness, most commonly located within the popliteal nerve at the head of the fibula, demonstrating central degenerative myxoid changes, implying a reactive process, rather than a true neoplasm

PERIPHERAL NERVE SHEATH MYXOMA, see Neurothekeoma and

MALIGNANT PERIPHERAL NERVE SHEATH TUMOR Malignant schwannoma (MS), see there Note: Because a direct link to the Schwann cell has proven elusive, the term MS is less appropriate than the non-committal term PNST, but MS is nontheless firmly entrenched in the literature

peripheral neuroepithelioma A primitive neuroectodermal tumor of bone that is closely related (if not biologically identical) to Ewing sarcoma; both share the cytogenetic translocation abnormality, t(11;22)(q24;q12); in both neural markers (eg neuron-specific enolase, S100 protein, neurofilaments triple protein, and HNK-1/Leu-7) can be detected, and ultrastructurally, both have constant pools of glycogen, cytoplasmic processes with neurofilaments and dense core granules (Arch Pathol Lab Med 1994; 118:608DA, 606ED) see Ewing sarcoma

peristalsis GASTROENTEROLOGY A generic term for the progressive waves of contraction that act to propel material through a lumen, almost invariably equated to the smooth-muscle activity of the GI tract

SUBSTANCES FAVORING GI MUSCLE CONTRACTION: Acetylcholine, cholecystokinin, enkephalins, gastrin, gastrin-releasing peptide, histamine (H_1-receptor), motilin, neurokinin A, neurotensin, pancreatic polypeptide, PGs, serotonin (5-HT), substance P

SUBSTANCES FAVORING GI MUSCLE RELAXATION: Adenine nucleotides, calcitonin gene-related peptide, dopamine, GABA, glucagon, histamine (H_3-receptor), neuropeptide Y, NO, peptide YY, secretin, somatostatin, VIP (Sci & Med Nov/Dec 1994 p38)

peristaltic reflex A GI response that is orchestrated by an independent enteric nervous system 'hard-wired' with two layers of intercommunicating neurons in the myenteric and submyenteric plexi which communicate with each other via peptides and neurotransmitters and with the more central components of the nervous system, by fibers, eg via the vagus, projecting to the prevertebral sympathetic ganglia, spinal cord, and the brain (Sci & Med Nov/Dec 1994 p38)

peritoneal dialysis A therapeutic modality used to clear toxic metabolites from patients with terminal renal failure, which may be

INTERMITTENT PERITONEAL DIALYSIS A treatment modality requiring up to eight hours per session, making it only practical for home therapy or

CONTINUOUS AMBULATORY PERITONEAL DIALYSIS A treatment modality in which the patient exchanges 1.5-3.0 liters of sterile dialysate containing hypertonic glucose, 3-5 times/day, requiring 30-40 minutes per session, a therapy that is ideal for diabetics in renal failure who have poor venous access, as insulin may be delivered in the dialysate SIDE EFFECTS CAPD results in hyperlipidemia and obesity due to the high glucose of the dialysate, and sclerosing peritonitis; long-term failure may be due to peritoneal infections, eg candidiasis and phaeohypomycosis (*Fusarium* species)

PD is slower than hemodialysis for clearing low molecular weight solutes (20-25 ml/min vs 150 ml/min for urea), but is better in clearing higher weight substances; see 'Middle molecules'

peritoneal effusion A collection of fluid in the peritoneum which may be benign or malignant; in ♀ malignant ascites is most commonly due to ovarian, gastric, pancreas, and endometrial in ♂ malignant ascites is most commonly due to pleural mesothelioma, gastric, colon and pancreatic carcinoma (Acta Cytologica 1993; 37:483DA)

peritonsillar abscess Quinsy A late stage anaerobic infection that began as an aerobic pharyngitis (Vincent's angina), which consists of marked pharyngeal pain, dysphagia, low-grade fever, inflammation and medial displacement of the tonsil; usually quinsy is unilateral; bilateral lesions may cause partial pharyngeal obstruction MICROBIOLOGY Most intraoral infections are polymicrobial mixtures of aerobes and anaerobes TREATMENT Oral penicillin or a broad-spectrum antibiotic active against *Fusobacterium necrophorum*

perivascular pseudorosette Homer-Wright rosettes, see there

periventricular leukomalacia NEONATOLOGY A clinicopathologic entity that affects extremely premature infant, often arising in a background of subependymal (matrix) hemorrhage; PL is characterized by foci of necrosis deep in the white matter adjacent to the lateral ventricles, in regions that impact on the occipital and sensorimotor radiations of the frontoparietal regions, thereby accounting for the visual, sensory, and motor defects found in older children who were born prematurely PREVENTION Vitamin E, and ethamsylate may reduce periventricular hemorrhage

PERLA Pupils equal, reactive to light and accommodation

A common clinical acronym for normal oculomotor functions

Perlman syndrome An AR [MIM 267000] condition characterized by fetal gigantism, renal hamartomas, nephroblastomatosis which may be accompanied by Wilms' tumor and unusual facies

perlèche Angular cheilitis, see there

permanent magnet A magnet composed of a permanently magnetized material; see Magnetic resonance imaging

permanent section Paraffin section, see there

permanent vegetative state Persistent vegetative state, see there

permissible exposure limits OCCUPATIONAL HEALTH The chemical exposure allowed in the working environment in the US, delineated by the Air Contaminant Standards of 29 CFR 1910; the PEL values are generally provided in ppm (parts per million) but for some chemicals may be expressed in mg/m³*; the hazards associated with various chemicals is rated by the OSHA on a scale of 1 which has the highest PEL > 500 ppm to 6, any substance that is frankly carcinogenic (CAP Today July 1992)

*This can be converted into ppm by multiplying PEL (mg/m³) X 24.45 and dividing the result by the molecular weight of the species

permissive hypercapnia CRITICAL CARE MEDICINE An approach to management of acute respiratory failure in which the tidal volume (V_T) is lower (5-8 mL/kg) than that conventionally used (10-15 mL/kg*), the arterial P_{CO_2} is allowed to rise above the 'normal' of 40 mm Hg, and no attempts are made to compensate for the subsequent changes in blood pH (respiratory acidosis, the deleterious effects of which may have been overestimated); permissive hypercapnia allows physiologic compensation of compromised pulmonary function, and in uncontrolled trials, suggest improved survival with maintenance of lower V_T (JAMA 1994; 272:957CECC)

*Associated with alveolar overdistension and ventilator-induced lung injury (volutrauma)

pernicious vomiting of pregnancy Hyperemesis gravidarum, see there

pernio Chilblains, see there

peroxidase-antiperoxidase technique CLINICAL IMMUNOLOGY A type of immunoperoxidase method used to identify antigens in tissues, using monoclonal antibodies and 'amplification' steps to detect an antigenic 'signal' METHOD The tissue is fixed, eg with formalin, washed with trypsin to block the tissue's endogenous peroxidase, incubated with non-human serum to block nonspecific antibody binding, incubated with a monoclonal antibody raised against the antigen to be tested (which is coupled to an enzyme, eg peroxidase covalently bound to the Fc end of the monoclonal antibody); the tissue is then incubated with a substrate (H_2O_2 and diaminobenzidine); if the antigen is present in the tissue, the substrate will be digested, resulting in a color change that can measured visually or by a spectrophotometer, see ABC

peroxisomal disease Any of a heterogeneous group of diseases in which peroxisomes are either lacking or markedly reduced, resulting in metabolic defects in all major biosynthetic peroxisomal pathways and failure to synthesize lipids or oxidize long-chain fatty acids; these metabolic defects cause a marked ↑ in plasma levels of very long chain fatty acids, especially C26:0 and C26:1 (hexacosanoic acid), ↑ trihydroxycoprostanic acid and ↑ pipecolic acid (an intermediate in lysine catabolism) and ↑ bile acid precursors with defective activity of peroxisomal acyl CoA:dihydroxyacetonephosphate acyltransferase in platelets and fibroblasts; PDs include Zellweger's cerebrohepatorenal syndrome, rhizomelic chondrodysplasia punctata, neonatal adrenoleukodystrophy, infantile Refsum disease, and hyperpipecolic acidemia

peroxisomal proliferators A group of chemicals that evoke a marked proliferation of hepatic peroxisomes and hepatic hyperplasia, including industrial plasticizers, herbicides and hypolipemic drugs that lower triglycerides and cholesterol but which may not have clinical utility given their hepatotoxicity in rodents

peroxisome A membrane-bound cell organelle that contains the enzymes (eg D-amino acid oxidase, catalase, (*S*)-2-hydroxy-acid oxidase-aka glycolate oxidase, and urate oxidase) necessary for synthesizing hydrogen peroxide (H_2O_2)

Persian Gulf syndrome Gulf War syndrome, see there

persistent müllerian duct syndrome A rare form of male pseudohermaphroditism characterized by persistence of müllerian duct structures in a phenotypically normal male CLINICAL First recognized in the pediatric age group, with cryptorchidism, testicular hypoplasia, normal virilization at puberty, and ↑ in testicular tumors and transverse testicular ectopia PATHOGENESIS Uncertain, possibly due to failure of Sertoli cells to secrete müllerian duct inhibiting factor (MIF, also known as antimüllerian hormone), defective timing of AMN release, or failure of end-organ response to AMN (Arch Pathol Lab Med 1994; 118:752OA)

persistent vegetative state '*A clinical condition of complete unawareness of the self and the environment, accompanied by sleep-wake cycles with either complete or partial preservation of hypothalamic and brain-stem functions. The condition may be transient, marking a stage of recovery from severe acute or chronic brain damage, or permanent, as a consequent of the failure to recover from such injuries. The vegetative state can also occur as a result of the relentless progressiion of degenerative or metabolic eurologic disease or from developmental malformations of the nervous system…*(criteria, see table, facing page) PVS is characterized by a prolonged loss of upper cortical function that may follow acute, eg infections, toxins, trauma, or vascular events or chronic, eg degenerative events; in PVS, the patient is bed-ridden and his/her nutritional support is completely passive, either parenteral or via nasogastric tube; PVS patients do not require respiratory support or circulatory assistance for survival and are in a state of chronic wakefulness without awareness, which may be accompanied by spontaneous eye opening, grunts or screams, brief smiles, sporadic movement of facial muscles and limbs; while the eyes blink upon stimulation, they do not do so in response to visual threats; some patients chew or clamp their teeth; urinary and fecal incontinence is universal; recovery generally occurs within the first month if at all, recovery is rare beyond the 3rd month; maintaining the estimated 5-10 000 US patients in a PVS costs $2-10 000/month/person, or a total of $120 to $1200 million/year (US) Note: The US record for longevity in the PVS is since October 1951 (Am Med News, 7 Jan 1991); the ethical and medicolegal issues being raised by these patients are considerable; see Advanced directives, DNR, Harvard criteria, Living will, Quinlan; Cf Procurement

persister phenomenon Persistence phenomenon MICROBIOLOGY A technical artefact that occurs in antibiotic susceptibility testing, where a percentage of organisms persist on the culture plate, simply because they are not in the growth phase at the time of testing, resulting in a 'red herring' that might be misinterpreted as representing bacterial resistance to an antibiotic; if these organisms are subcultured and retested, less than 0.1% of the inoculum persists (Ann Int Med 1982; 97:339)

personal protective equipment OCCUPATIONAL SAFETY Specialized (ie not 'standard issue') clothing or equipment worn by an employee for protection against a hazard, in particular blood-borne pathogens; under the rubric of 'appropriate' PPE, OSHA includes gloves, gown, laboratory coats, face shields or masks and eye protection, mouthpieces, resuscitation bags, pocket masks, or other ventilation devices (Federal Register 29 CFR 1910.1030, pages 64175-64182)

personal risk factors A person's risk factors for STD, in particular HIV, which include having sex with more than one partner, use of IV drugs, receiving money or drugs for sex, having been previously treated for STD, use of drugs or alcohol during sexual episodes, which are associated with nonuse of condoms (MMWR 1992; 41:568) see Sexual work

personality Character The distinctive attributes of a person or characteristic way in which a person behaves, thinks, and feels; there is some consensus that five broad traits or 'super factors' are required to describe personality: 1) Extraversion (positive emotionality) 2) Neuroticism (negative emotionality) 3) Conscientiousness (constraint) 4) Agreeableness (aggression) 5) Openness (absorption) (Science 1994; 264:1700P)

CRITERIA, PERSISTENT VEGETATIVE STATE

1) No evidence of awareness of environment and inability to interact with others

2) No evidence of sustained, reproducible, purposeful, or voluntary behavioral responses to visual, tactile, auditory, or noxious stimuli

3) No evidence of language comprehension or expression

4) Intermittent wakefulness manifested by the presence of sleep-wake cycles

5) Sufficiently preserved hypothalamic and brain-stem autonomic functions to permit survival with medical and nursing care

6) Bowel and bladder incontinence, and

7) Variably preserved cranial nerve reflexes (pupillary, oculocephalic, corneal, vestibulo-ocular, and gag) and spinal reflexes

Multi-society Task Force on Persistent Vegetative State (N Engl J Med 1994; 330:1488BR; 1524ED)

---

personality testing PSYCHOLOGY Any of a number of psychological tests, including the individual Rorschach ink-blot test or the multiple choice California Psychological Inventory that is designed to objectively measure certain facets of an individual's personality and among other claims, to predict his ability to function in the workplace; it is felt by some experts in the field that personality testing is of little benefit and is poorly predictive of future behavior

personal physician A physician who assumes responsibility (or who in a court of law, is held to be responsible) for a patient's care; in the US, this role was formerly carried out by a 'general practitioner' who often had a decades-long relationship with the patient and his/her family; in the current environment of specialization and subspecialization, the personal physician may be in any field, although the role is often carried out by a physician with board certification in family practice or in internal medicine, and who is also board-certified in gastroenterology or cardiology; see Family practitioner, General practitioner, Internist; Cf Private patient

pERT Phenol-enhanced reassociation technique, see there

pertinent *adjective* Pertaining or referring to any datum that is relevant or of use in evaluating a patient's chief complaint

pertussis Whooping cough PEDIATRICS An acute contagious and potentially epidemic bacterial infection caused by *Bordetella pertussis* (less commonly by *B bron-*

choseptica and *B parapertussis*), which most commonly affects children < age 5; it is a major cause of morbidity and mortality causing 600 000 deaths/year in the world CLINICAL (in decreasing order of frequency) Paroxysmal cough, post-tussive emesis, cyanosis, apnea, whoop COMPLICATIONS Pneumonia, atelectasis DIAGNOSIS Culture, direct fluorescent antibody test; it is a common cause of persistent cough in adults that should be considered in the DDx of persistent cough; there is a poor correlation with clinical findings, culture, direct fluorescent antibody, and lymphocytosis (JAMA 1995; 273:1044OA) TREATMENT Erythromycin, trimethoprim-sulfamethoxazole VACCINE Whole cell (DPT) vaccine (N Engl J Med 1994; 331:16OA)

perversion Paraphilia, see there

perversion injuries Traumatic lesions induced by deviant* sexual activities, most commonly involving the anus and rectum or lower urogenital tract, consisting of the tearing of tissues, with resultant infections, caused by various devices ranging from high-pressure hoses per rectum to various objects (sex 'toys') or body parts (see 'Fisting') designed to stimulate or enhance sexual arousal; see Sexual deviancy (paraphilia)

*The formally preferred term in this, the era of 'political correctness' (where no behavior is regarded as deviant) for sexual deviancy is paraphilia; the adjective would therefore be paraphilic—Author's note

Pesaro classification A clinicopathologic classification for patients with β-thalassemia, based on the adequacy of iron chelation therapy, and the presence or absence of hepatomegaly, and portal fibrosis Class 1 None of criteria are present Class 2 One or two criteria are present Class 3 All three criteria are present (N Engl J Med 1993; 329:840OA)

PEST hypothesis A theory of historic interest that held that proteins with a short intracellular half-life (< 2 hours) contained one or more regions rich in proline, glutamic acid, serine and threonine (amino acids abbreviated as P, E, S and T), generally PEST regions are flanked by clusters with positively charged amino acids; it was thought that the PEST amino acids 'marked' proteins for early degradation, a posit that has been replaced by the 'N-end rule', see there

pesticide TOXICOLOGY An agent* for annihilating ambient arachnids, antagonistic arthropods, abominable animals or pugnacious plants, eg fumigants, fungicides, herbicides and insecticides; most pesticides are highly toxic and potentially fatal, given their high arsenical or organophosphate content and store in adipose tissue, given their lipid solubility; a number of pesticides (and industrial compounds, eg PBC) have been reported to disrupt the reproductive cycle from the bottom to the top of the food chain, related in part to hormonal mimicry (New York Times 23 August 1994; C1) see Intermediate syndrome spelling

*Its common usage refers to insects (insecticide), but in a broader sense includes any 'pest', including fungi (fungicide), nematodes, animals, and undesired plants, eg weeds, vines, for which the terms herbicide or defoliant are generally preferred

PET Pancreatic endocrine tumor, see there

pet-associated disease Humans have for millenia domesticated a vast menagerie of animals, usually vertebrate, often mammalian, for companionship or amusement; the human-pet dyad may cause morbidity in man when either

1) The animals act as vectors for various microorganisms, eg dogs (rabies), cats (toxoplasmosis) and parrots (psittacosis) or when

2) The animals attack the owner (popularly known as 'turning'), an event that is relatively common in animals not bred for domestication, eg coyotes, lions, pythons and weasels

Given the often unusual clinical presentations that characterize pet-associated illness, a detailed anamnesis is imperative to establish a diagnosis; see Cats, Dogs, Fishtank granuloma

PET scan Positron emission transaxial tomography NUCLEAR MEDICINE A non-invasive imaging modality that uses radionuclides to detect biochemical and pathological abnormalities in living tissues, most commonly used to evaluate the cerebral cortex PRINCIPLE Decaying radionuclides emit positrons travel a very short distance and collide with electrons and in matter-antimatter interactions, are annihilated, producing a pair of photons (512-keV gamma rays) which are emitted at directions 180° opposite each other; these photons are detected with a PRET camera and a 3-D tomographic image is constructed by computer that corresponds to the spatial distributions of the radionuclides and matter-antimatter annihilations (N Engl J Med 1992; 326:1608RV) PET scans may be used to evaluate AIDS-related neuropathology (response to AZT by local increase of glucose metabolism), dementia (focal neuronal loss, gliosis, allowing differentiation among Alzheimer's disease, Huntington's disease, multi-infarct dementia, tardive dyskinesia), epilepsy (localization of seizure focus, making surgical therapy viable), malignancy (gliomas, residual tumor, pituitary adenomas), Parkinson's disease (decreased dopamine), psychiatric disease (depression, schizophrenia), and analysis of radiopharmaceuticals; PET scanning may be used in cardiology to evaluate coronary arteriosclerosis, regional myocardial blood flow, and ischemia, using oxygen-15-labeled carbon dioxide ($C^{15}O_2$); after an AMI, there is a severely attenuated vasodilator response in the resistance vessels in both the infarcted myocardium and in the myocardium perfused by normal vessels (N Engl J Med 1994; 331:222OA)

Note: Positrons are short-lived particles that do not exist in nature and positron-emitting substances must be generated in a linear accelerator, the β-emitting substance is 'tagged' to a molecule, eg glucose and injected into the blood stream, where it travels to the brain; changes in regional blood flow can be measured in 'real time' for the analysis of various cognitive processes (Science 1990; 248:1556)

PETA People for the Ethical Treatment of Animals, see Animal Rights movement

petaloid globules A descriptor for the serrated flower petal-like degenerated elastic fibers seen by LM in the benign tumor, elastofibroma, best visualized by elastin stains, eg Gomori or Verhoeff stains

Peter Pan and Wendy complex PSYCHIATRY A marital dyad composed of a narcissistic and/or unfaithful husband who devotes considerable time to studies, sports or extra-marital liaisons and a depressed long-suffering wife; see Wendy dilemma

Peter Pan face A descriptor for the wrinkled, dehydrated and hairless facies of a subject with 'classic' hypopituitarism

Peter Pan syndrome(s) Clinical complexes named after the 'boy who would not grow up' ENDOCRINOLOGY Peter Pan syndrome is a state of physical immaturity due to a hypothalamic defect with underdeveloped secondary sexual characteristics occurring in ♂ children with microphalus and ↓ height PSYCHOLOGY A fanciful term referring to a state of unconscious postponement of maturity, characterized by magical thinking, narcissism and chauvinism

petit mal Absence, see there

Petri dish A universal accoutrement of the microbiology laboratory devised by RJ Petri (1852-1921) while he was an assistant to R Koch in Berlin, which consists of two flattened clear glass or plastic plates, one larger than the other, allowing ease of examination of bacterial cultures, while preventing environmental contamination

This simple container was as instrumental as the Gram stain in revolutionizing the field of microbiology and the study of infectious disease; it is increasing written in lower case, thus being an eponymic adjective-Author's note

petrified man syndrome Fibrodysplasia ossificans progressiva, see there

PETT Positron emission transaxial tomography, see PET scan

peyote SUBSTANCE ABUSE A cactus *Lyphophora williamsii*, the flowering heads (mescal buttons) of which have been used as a hallucinogen CLINICAL Minutes after ingestion, euphoria, hallucinations, tachycardia, mydriasis, rarely also fever and seizures

Peyronie's disease Penile fibromatosis A condition characterized by the development of unilateral nodules of fibrosis within the fascial sheath of one or both of the corpora cavernosa, leading to curvature of the penile shaft and painful erection PATHOLOGY Scar tissue formation, dystrophic calcification, and rarely, ossification of the penile shaft; intralesional injection of corticosteroids may ameliorate some symptoms

PF-4 Platelet factor-4, see there

PFGE Pulsed-field gel electrophoresis, see there

PFGE fingerprinting Pulsed-field gel electrophoresis chromosomal fingerprinting MOLECULAR BIOLOGY A genetic assay that detects RFLPs (restriction fragment length polymorphisms) by gel electrophoresis, which is of use in determining relatedness of stains of bacteria, ie molecular epidemiology (see N Engl J Med 1994; 331:981OA) Cf Ribotyping

P-glycoprotein P170, see there

PG Prostaglandin, also 1) Peptidoglycan 2) Phosphatidyl-glycerol 3) Phosphogluconate 4) Postgraduate 5) Pregnanediol glucuronide 6) Proteoglycan

Also 1) Pedal ganglion 2) Pedal groove 3) Pituitary gonadotropin (obsolete) 4) Placebo group 5) Plasma gastrin (rarely used) 6) Plasma glucose (rarely used) 7) Polyethylene glycol (often abreviated as PEG) 8) Polygalacturonase 9) Polyglycine 10) Propyl gallate 11) Propyl glycol 12) Protein granule 13) Pulse generator (pacemaker) 19) Pyoderma gangrenosum

PGO Pontine-geniculate-occipital waves, see there

PGY-1 Postgraduate year 1 The first (second year is PGY-2 and so on) year of post-graduate medical education, usually corresponding to an internship, or a residency in a formal training program in a teaching institution; see Graduate medical education, Residency

PHA Phytohemagglutinin, see there

Phaedra complex The libidinous desire of a stepmother for a stepson; since the two are not genetically related, a sexual liaison would not be regarded as legally incestuous; Cf Electra complex, Jocastra complex, Oedipus complex

Phaedra of Greek mythology married Theseus but was attracted to his son Hippolytus who rejected her advances; the spurned Phaedra then had Theseus kill the son

phage typing A technique that characterizes certain strains of bacteria after initial speciation, in a fashion analogous to DNA 'fingerprinting', using bacteriophages (viruses capable of lysing bacteria) see Bactiophage

phagemid vector A genetically-engineered bacteriophage into which foreign DNA is inserted to facilitate characterization of cloned inserts; PVs are of use for high-resolution restriction mapping, rescue of single-stranded DNA, RNA transcription, sequencing of single- and double-stranded nucleic acids, generation of nested deletions, site-directed mutagenesis, and both pro– and eukaryotic expression

phagocytic diseases A generic term for any of a number of qualitative disorders of phagocytic leukocytes, most of which are rare, many of which are familial, and a good number of which are accompanied by generalized metabolic defects; space only permits the inclusion of a table, modified from Lee et al; Cf Histiocytic diseases

phagocytic index A measurement of nonspecific hyperreactivity of the immune system, manifested by an increased clearance of colloidal carbon, which is accelerated in graft-versus-host disease; see Splenic index

phakomatoses *phakos*, Greek, lens Neurocutaneous syndromes A group of inherited conditions, many of which are AD, that result in the disordered growth of ectodermal tissues, causing distinctive skin lesions and tumors and/or malformations of the nervous system and/or retina **ATAXIA-TELANGIECTASIA** An AR [MIM 208900] disorder characterized by cerebellar ataxia, oculomotor apraxia, telangiectasias of bulbar conjuncta, skin of ears and skin folds (appearing by age three) and sinopulmonary infections; with time, the telangiectasias extend to the butterfly region of the face; most patients die in adolescence **BASAL CELL NEVUS SYNDROME** see Nevoid-basal cell carcinoma syndrome **NEVUS SEBACEOUS OF JADASSOHN** An occasionally AD [MIM 163200] clinical condition characterized by a congenital solitary lesion most often present in the scalp which, when large, may be associated with internal derangements including intracranial masses, seizures, mental retardation, skeletal abnormalities, pigmentary changes, ocular lesions and renal hamartomas; 10% of the skin lesions develop into basal cell carcinoma **STURGE-WEBER DISEASE** Encephalotrigeminal angiomatosis An occasionally AD [MIM 185300] condition characterized by congenital capillary hemangiomas of the head and neck, following normal developmental milestones, mental retardation may ensue, caused in part by the sluggish flow of blood through the pial vessels and venous hemangiomas in the leptomeninges and fronto-parietal cortex with ipsilateral port-wine nevi, 'Tram-track' radiopacities on the skull caused by calcification of the cerebral cortex **TUBEROUS SCLEROSIS** Bourneville-Pringle disease An AD [MIM 191100] disorder (50% arise de novo) CLINICAL Convulsions, seizures, mental retardation, skin lesions (adenoma sebaceum, sebaceous gland atrophy, angiofibromas, dermal fibrosis with dilated capillaries, shagreen patches), cardiac rhabdomyomas, pulmonary fibrosis, bronchiolar hematomas, bilateral tubular adenomas of kidneys, pancreatic cysts, angiomyolipomas, myxedematous glossitis, spina bifida NEUROPATHOLOGY Astrocytic gliosis, which evokes lesions likened to 'candle wax drippings' **VON HIPPEL-LINDAU DISEASE** An AD [MIM 193300] condition with retinal hemangioblastoma, ½ erythropoietin production and cerebellar hemangioblastoma CLINICAL Ataxia, headache, papilledema, angiomas of the liver, kidney, renal adenomas, papillary cystadenomas of the epididymis, pancreatic cysts, adrenal pheochromocytomas Note: ¼ develop renal cell carcinoma **VON RECKLINGHAUSEN DISEASE** A relatively common (1/3500) AD [MIM 162200] condition CLINICAL Neurofibromas, cafe-au-lait spotting of skin, scoliosis, gliosis, glioblastoma multiforme, ependymoma, meningioma and schwannoma, 5-10% sarcomatous degeneration, spina bifida and glaucoma; see Neurofibromatosis

Note: Neurofibromatosis, Tuberous sclerosis, von Hippel disease constitute the 'classic' phakomatoses

---

PHAGOCYTIC DISEASES

STRUCTURAL (AND FUNCTIONAL) DEFECTS
- Alder-Reilly anomaly
- Chédiak-Higashi anomaly
- Familial vacuolization of leukocytes (Jordan's anomaly)
- May-Hegglin anomaly
- Pelger-Huët anomaly
- Pseudo- (or acquired) Pelger-Huët anomaly
- Hereditary giant neutrophilia
- Hereditary hypersegmentation of neutrophilic nuclei

FUNCTIONAL DEFECTS (WITHOUT STRUCTURAL CHANGES)
- Chronic granulomatous disease
- Myeloperoxidase deficiency
- CD11/CD18 adhesive protein deficiency
- Other enzyme defects

GR Lee, TC Bithell, J Foerster, et al, Eds, Wintrobe's Hematology, 9th ed, Lea & Febiger, Philadelphia, 1993

Phalen sign Paresthesia or worsening thereof in the region innervated by the median nerve, by maximum passive flexion of the wrist for one minute, finding typical of entrapment neuropathy; a positive Phalen sign has a sensitivity of 75% and a specificity of 47% for carpal tunnel syndrome (see N Engl J Med 1993; 329:2013cc)

phallotoxin A toxic, heat-stable cyclic heptapeptide derived from poisonous mushrooms, eg *Amanita phylloides, A verna, A virosa, Galerina autumnalis, Cenocybe filaris* and others, which with other cyclopeptides is responsible for 90 to 95% of the 100 annual (US) deaths caused by poisonous mushrooms CLINICAL Stage 1 Abrupt onset of abdominal pain, nausea, cramping, vomiting, diarrhea with blood and mucus Stage 2 Apparent recovery with increasing liver enzymes Stage 3 1-3 days post-ingestion Hepatic, cardiac, and renal failure, coagulopathies, seizures, coma and death TREATMENT None

phantom RADIOLOGY A mass or dummy that approximates tissues in its physical properties that may be used to calibrate or determine the dose of radiation being applied to a tissue; Cf Ballistic jelly

phantom bone disease Disappearing bone disease, see there, vanishing bone disease

phantom limb pain The phenomenon of pain perceived to be present in an absent limb; in one study of 75 pediatric aged amputees, PLP occurred in 32/67 of those who had cancer-related amputations, and 1/8 of those with trauma-related amputations (Mayo Clin Proc 1995; 70:357oa) TREATMENT A recently reported therapy for the sometimes intractable PLP is the use of a mirror in a box that places the intact limb visually in the same site as the missing extremity; with the use of symmetrical movements, the patient 'unlearns' activities that were formerly carried out by the missing limb (NY Times March 28 1995, C3)

phantom limb syndrome Chronic intense pain localized to the site of an amputated or denervated limb; 60-70% of amputees have a phantom limb sensation; 10-15% have phantom limb pain (syndrome); the degree of pain is often a function of the amount of pre-amputation pain; the pain is often refractory to treatments that include excision of amputation neuroma, rubbing, electrical stimulation, peripheral nerve or spinal blocks, narcotics and sympathectomy

Note: Lord Horatio Nelson (1758-1805) lost his lower right arm when his fleet attacked the post Santa Cruz in Tenerife in the Canary Islands and suffered until his death with phantom limb symptoms (Proc Roy Soc Med 1970; 63:299)

phantom tumor A well-circumscribed accumulation of fluid in the interlobular spaces seen on a plain chest film which may occur in congestive heart failure

pharmacist Chemist (British) A person qualified by a graduate degree in pharmacy, who is licensed by the state to prepare, dispense and provide control over controlled drugs, usually having the title of RPh (registered pharmacist); Cf Pharmacologist

pharmacoeconomics *'The measure of a pharmaceutical's cost-effectiveness'* (Bio/Technology 1995; 13:435)

pharmacologic dose CLINICAL PHARMACOLOGY A supraphysiological dose of a substance, eg mineralocorticoids, that is normally present in the body, in order to produce a 'pharmacologic' effect

pharmacologic phlebotomy CRITICAL CARE MEDICINE The use of morphine in pulmonary edema to reduce the fluid load in the pulmonary vessels by pooling the blood into the capacitance vessels

pharmacologic restraint A generic term for any pharmacologic agent (eg anxiolytics, hypnotics, neuroleptics, or sedatives) that may be used to control or restrain an inmate in a sheltered environment, eg mental institution or nursing home; Cf Physical restraint

pharmacologic stress imaging see Thallium stress test

pharmacologist A person with an advanced degree in pharmacology (MA or PhD) who is qualified to conduct research and evaluation of drugs and therapeutic agents, pharmacokinetics and effects; Cf Pharmacist

pharming A colloquial term for the production of pharmaceuticals from transgenic farm animals, including transgenic cows (eg for lactoferrin) pigs (hemoglobin), sheep (alpha-1-antitrypsin), goats, and others; 'farmaceuticals' have major advantages over commercial bioreactors* (CBs); they are more efficient–dairy animals produce tens of grams of useful pharmaceutical proteins per liter of milk, vs milligrams/liter in CBs, less costly to maintain, and make proteins with similar bioreactivity to the desired molecule, eg post-translational glycosylation and gamma carboxylation; farmaceuticals are expected to reach the marketplace by 1997 (Bio/Technology 1992; 10:498)

*Mother Nature is relieved to know that her/his place in the universe is not threatened by progress

pharyngeal arches EMBRYOLOGY A series of primitive structures that appear in the 4th-5th embryologic week, giving rise to major structures of the head and neck; Cf Aortic arches

FIRST PHARYNGEAL ARCH, dorsal aspect gives rise to the maxillary process, incus malleus, muscles: masseter, temporal, pterygoid, anterior digastric, mylohyoid, tensor tympanicus, palatine; the first pharyngeal arch ventral aspect gives rise to the mandibular (Meckel's) process, trigeminal, mucosa of tongue

SECOND PHARYNGEAL ARCH (of Reichert) gives rise to the stapes, styloid, temporal, stylohyoid, stapedius, posterior digastric, auricular, facial 'mimic' musculature

THIRD PHARYNGEAL (HYOID) ARCH gives rise to the stylopharyngeal and glossopharyngeal nerve

FOURTH AND SIXTH PHARYNGEAL (THYROID) ARCH(ES) give rise to the cricothyroid, pharyngeal, laryngeal musculature

FIFTH PHARYNGEAL ARCH never fully develops

pharyngeal clefts EMBRYOLOGY Primitive structures seen in the 5-week embryo, only one of which, the dorsal aspect of the 1st pharyngeal cleft, gives rise to the external auditory canal; the 2nd, 3rd, and 4th pharyngeal clefts undergo atrophy and are covered by the 2nd pharyngeal arch

pharyngeal 'facelift' Palatopharyngoplasty A 'tuck and tighten' surgical procedure for the soft palate and pharynx, which eliminates redundant mucosa in an attempt to reduce the noise level in those who snore; see Obstructive sleep apnea syndrome, Snoring

pharyngeal pouches A series of embryonic structures that appear simultaneously with the pharyngeal arches and clefts consisting of outpouchings along the lateral wall of the pharyngeal gut that have been likened to the gills or branchia of amphibians and fish; this progenitor tissue gives rise to various structures of the pharynx; the 1st pouch gives rise to the middle ear and eustachian tube, the 2nd pouch to the palatine tonsils, the 3rd pouch to the inferior parathyroids and thymus, the 4th pouch to the superior parathyroids and the 5th pouch to the ultimobranchial body in the thyroid gland

pharyngeal structure Any structure including bone, cartilage, lymphoid tissues, muscles, nerves, and spaces that migrates to its respective place during early embryogenesis under the baton of the primitive pharynx (pharyngeal arches, clefts and pouches), each giving rise to specific structures

phase 1, 2, and 3 studies CLINICAL PHARMACOLOGY A series of clinical trials that address the safety and efficacy of an 'investigational new drug' (IND) that is being 'sponsored' by a pharmaceutical company with the purpose of bringing the product to the marketplace

PHASE I-EARLY CLINICAL PHARMACOLOGY STAGE Involves 20-80 subjects and should generate enough data to allow a properly controlled trial; FDA's review at this point ensures that subjects are not exposed to unreasonable risks

PHASE 2 LATER CLINICAL PHARMACOLOGY STAGE Involves several hundred patients with the first controlled clinical studies with the purpose of generating enough data to 1) at least suggest (if not prove) that the drug actually works and 2) demonstrate the most common side effects

PHASE 3 FINAL CLINICAL PHARMACOLOGY STAGE Involves several thousand patients, phase 3 corresponds to the expanded clinical trials which are intended to generate enough information to establish both the drug's effectiveness for specific indications and identify populations at special risk from its use; both phases 2 and 3 are meant to ensure that the scientific design creates the data needed for premarket approval of the drug; NDA (new drug applications) were often rejected because the data from the phase 2 and 3 trials revealed study design flaws, forcing the sponsor to repeat work, which has been largely eliminated by the '1987 rewrite' of the IND status; see Compassionate investigational new drug, IND, NDA, Premarket approval process, Treatment IND

Note: Occasionally, an agent's benefit is so obvious, eg zidovudine (AZT) that the need for phase 3 studies, a stage immediately preceding an official NDA, may be obviated

phase contrast microscope A type of light microscope* that converts the differences in the refractive index as light passes through an object into variations of light intensity, allowing visualization of structural details within unstained living cells; PCM separates the (normally) superimposed diffracted and undiffracted images that are about ¼ wavelength out of phase with each other, allowing in situ observation of intracellular events; see Microscopy; Cf Confocal microscopy

*Designed by Fritz Zernicke, Nobel prize 1932

PHC syndrome Böök syndrome, see there

pheasant hunter's toe A toe affected by an acute attack of podagra (gouty arthritis of the toe), that follows long walks typical of pheasant hunting, a sport of the wealthy, who were most commonly afflicted by gout

phencyclidine PCP, 'angel dust' SUBSTANCE ABUSE A recreational hallucinogen with significant side effects, causing neurologic dysfunction, with schizophrenia-like behavior, analgesia, dysarthria, nystagmus, ataxia, seizures, delirium, coma, as well as GI symptoms, ↑ blood pressure and temperature and depressed pulmonary function; a PCP receptor has been identified and when bound by certain ligands, eg PCP and MK-801, results in neuronal vacuolization and loss of mitochondria in the posterior cingulate and retrosplenial cortices of the rat brain; in utero exposure to PCP results in high levels in the fetus (in experimental rats), due to immaturity of enzyme clearance systems

phenol-enhanced reassociation technique MOLECULAR BIOLOGY A method that identifies seven DNA clones (pERT clones) mapped to band p21 of the X chromosome, one of which, pERT87 is defective in 7% of patients with Duchenne's and Becker's muscular dystrophy, resulting in short protein products of a defective gene

phenotype 1) A generic term for any structural or functional characteristic of an organism that may be observed or identified 2) The sum total of the structural and functional characteristics of an organism that reflect its genetic composition

phenotypic cloning A proposal that animals including humans transmit features of themselves to their progeny without involvement of DNA; according to this hypothetical behavioral Lamarckism, the children in a family unit learn certain behavioral styles that would be selective for the types of mates they chose (NY Times 3 Jan 1995; B13)

phenotypic suppression The suppression of a phenotypic mutation during translation of a DNA sequence into mRNA, or during translation of the mRNA transcript into a protein, eg misreading in the presence of 5-fluorouracil, an agent that inhibits thymidylate synthetase

phenylpropanolamine An 'over-the-counter' sympathomimetic drug used in nasal decongestants, cough medication and diet control aids; there are few side effects, although PPA has been reported to cause short-lived, low-grade increases in systolic and diastolic blood pressure

phenytoin An antiepileptic and anticonvulsant usually administered as a sodium salt; phenytoin inhibits collagenase activity in vitro and had been used in to treat epidermolysis bullosa, for which a randomized double blind study found it to be ineffective (N Engl J Med 1992; 327:1630A)

phenytoin-induced gingival overgrowth Phenytoin-induced gingival overgrowth, see there A hyperplastic process induced by phenytoin's direct stimulatory effect on gingival fibroblasts, resulting in increased collagen synthesis, a phenomenon seen in 10-30% of phenytoin-treated patients; Cf Phenytoin lymphadenopathy

phenytoin lymphadenopathy A phenytoin-induced condition characterized by generalized lymphadenopathy, rashes, and fever PATHOLOGY Effacement of lymphoid follicles, mixed cell infiltrate of immunoblasts, plasma cells, eosinophils, and necrosis; some cases have progressed to malignant lymphoma, although the linkage with phenytoin therapy may be a 'passenger' phenomenon; see Pseudopseudolymphoma

pheochromocytoma 10% tumor A benign paraganglioma of adrenal medulla, 10% of which are associated with systemic disease, including von Recklinghausen's disease, von Hippel-Lindau syndrome, Sturge-Weber disease and MEN IIa and IIb; pheochromocytomas may produce ACTH, calcitonin and VIP CLINICAL The pheochromocytoma triad (headaches, sweating attacks and tachycardia) in a hypertensive patient has a 94% specificity and 91% sensitivity for the diagnosis of pheochromocytoma; absence of all in a hypertensive patient completely excludes pheochromocytoma); other symptoms include nervousness, anxiety, tremor, facial pallor, nausea and/or vomiting, fatigue, chest or abdominal pain, weight loss LABORATORY ↑ Vanillylmandelic acid (VMA), ↑ metanephrine, free catecholamines, MHPG, dopamine and homovanillic acid (HVA) DIAGNOSIS SPECIFICITY OF IMAGING MODALITIES Abdominal ultrasonography 100%; abdominal CT 100%; abdominal MRI 97%; MIBG (metaiodobenzylguanidine) scintigraphy 97% SPECIFICITY OF LABORATORY PARAMETERS, URINE Epinephrine 98%; norepinephrine 95%; VMA (vanilmandelic acid 91%) SPECIFICITY OF LABORATORY PARAMETERS, PLASMA Norepinephrine 97%; chromogranin A 95%; epinephrine 91% (N Engl J Med 1993; 329:1531OA)

pheromone A hormone or other natural scent released by an organism, which is capable of evoking, in a member of the same species, a physiological response that is usually related to mating, eg those that block olfaction in pregnant mice and those that determine sexual orientation of *Saccharomyces cerevisiae*, ♀ insects to attract mates; pheromones have also been used to warn others of the same species of danger and to mark territory; pheromones are highly specific, ie effective against the tomato pinworm, pink bollworm, and coddling moth and may play a role as 'biorational' pesticides (Bio/Technology 1995; 13:219)

Philadelphia chromosome A small acrocentric chromosome from the distal long arm of chromosome 22 that is transferred to the long arm of chromosome 9 [t(9;22)(q34;q11)] in 95% of cases of chronic myelogenous leukemia (CML); the PC is often associated with a better prognosis, yielding a 44-month survival vs 15-months in PC-negative CML (Science 1960; 132:1947); PC may also be present in ALL (5-20% of cases) and ANLL, and is

generated in a pluripotent stem cell (appearing in myeloid, erythroid, megakaryocytic and lymphoid lines) by a reciprocal translocation, resulting in juxtaposition of the c-abl gene on chromosome 9 with a gene of unknown function, with a bcr (breakpoint cluster region) on chromosome 22; the resulting hybrid abl/bcr gene encodes P210^{bcr/abl}, a phosphoprotein unique to CML that resembles v-abl as it has disregulated protein-tyrosine kinase activity; when the hybrid gene is inserted into a retroviral vector, used to infect BM, and then transplanted into irradiated syngeneic mice, CML is induced in the mice; see P210^{bcr/abl}

Philadelphia cream cheese appearance A fanciful descriptor for the caseating necrosis seen in TB, which has a whitish color and 'paste-like' consistency

Phineas P Gage A 25-year-old worker on the New England railroad who in 1848 suffered a blasting powder-related accident in which a tamping rod measuring 3 cm in diameter exploded through his left eye and frontal lobe; he survived the accident but lost his ability to make ethical decisions

PhIP see Heterocyclic amine

phlebodynia Vein pain A hysterical reaction of uncertain validity, which affects women and is accompanied by malaise, headache and mild fever; see Factitious disease(s)

phlebothrombosis Thrombophlebitis

phlebotomy LABORATORY MEDICINE The obtention by venipuncture of blood to be used for diagnostic evaluation; the phelobotomist is at a relatively high risk for certain occupational hazards, eg needlestick injuries which occur ± 9/10⁵/year

phocomelia An intercalary-type of congenital skeletal limb deformity, due to the idiopathic absence of the radial elements of a limb bud; in complete phocomelia, the hand is directly attached to the shoulder or the foot to the pelvis; see Thalidomide

Phoenix plan RESEARCH ADMINISTRATION A proposal for calculating the amount of overhead (indirect) monies to be added to federally funded research grants; the PP would use a national formula to determine the overhead costs for each institution based on federally compiled indices of local wage and construction costs (Nature 1995; 375:3) see Overhead costs

phonophoresis CLINICAL THERAPEUTICS A specific type of transcutaneous drug delivery currently under investigation in which an ultrasonic radiation is applied to the skin in order to facilitate the movement of a therapeutic substance through the skin (Mayo Clin Proc 1995; 70:581) see Transcutaneous drug delivery; Cf Iontophoresis

phonosurgery OTOLARYNGOLOGY A surgical procedure performed on the vocal cords and adjacent tissue with the purpose of improving the timbre, tone and quality of the voice* ASSESSMENT TECHNIQUES Acoustic and aerodynamic measurements, laryngeal stroboscopy, manual compression, and intraoperative monitoring of voice SURGICAL TECHNIQUES Injection technique, laryngeal microsurgery, laryngeal framework modification, see Medialization thyroplasty, and laser techniques; see Injection technique, Laryngeal microsurgery; Cf Uvulopalatopharyngoplasty

*This contrasts with laryngeal conservation surgery in which the primary purpose is control a disease process, eg malignancy

phonotrauma A generic term for any abuse or misuse of the vocal folds, most common in those with professional voices; phonotrauma gives rises to a wide range of lesions, including polyps, nodules, degenerative polyps, cysts, varices, papillomas, and other benign conditions

phorbol ester(s) A family of potent tumor-promoting esters, eg TPA, derived from the alcohol phorbol from croton oil, which evoke various responses in cultured cells including increased cell growth, synthesis of macromolecules and prostaglandins, alteration of cell morphology and membrane permeability; see TPA

phorbol ester

phorbol myristate CLINICAL IMMUNOLOGY A low-molecular-weight ($C_{20}H_{28}O_6$) organic compound used in combination with ionomycin as a nonspecific immune stimulant for in vitro studies of mononuclear cells, and can be used to evaluate cytokine production

phospharamidon A neutral protease inhibitor that prevents the conversion of 'big' endothelin, the pre-pro endothelin into endothelin-1, by inhibiting the action of the endothelin converting enzyme and causes a slow lowering of blood pressure in hypertensive rats; see Endothelin

phosphate loading SPORTS MEDICINE The ingestion of phosphate in order to ↑ O_2 delivery by ↑ production of 2,3-DPG (2,3-diphosphoglyceride); ↑ 2,3-DPG in RBCs shifts the O_2 dissociation curve to the right, facilitating the unloading of O_2 in the tissues, thereby improving oxygenation and (in theory) performance; it is thought that any ↑ in 2,3-DPG is offset by ↓ absorption of O_2 in the lungs, and if PL is indeed effective in enhancing athletic performance, it may be so only at high altitudes (JC DeLee, D Drez, Jr, Eds, Orthopedic Sports Medicine WB Saunders, Philadelphia, 1994) Cf Bicarbonate loading, Carbohydrate loading, Performance-enhancing drug

phosphatidylinositol 4,5 biphosphate An inositol phospholipid present at the cytoplasmic leaflet of the plasma membrane that is hydrolyzed by phospholipase C, yielding 1,2 diacylglycerol and the water soluble inositol 1,4,5-triphosphate (both of which are 'second messengers'), which diffuse to the surface of the endoplasmic reticulum, opening a calcium-specific channel, evoking a specific cell response

phosphatidylinositol-3 kinase One of many enzyme that is stimulated by various growth factors and oncogenes; PK is required for PDGF- (platelet-derived growth factor) mediated mitogenic signaling, and is capable of stimulating various Ras-dependent cell processes, eg oocyte maturation and *fos* transcription (Science 1995; 268:100)

phosphoenolpyruvic acid An intermediate in the Embden-Meyerhof (glycolytic) pathway that donates a high-energy phosphate group to ADP leading to the synthesis of ATP; upon dephosphorylation it degrades to pyruvic acid

phospholipase A_2 Any of a family of enzymes that hydrolyze the 2-ester bond of L-glycerophospholipids; since some forms of PLA_2 catalyze the release of arachidonate, which precipitates the inflammatory 'cascade', it is of interest to produce molecules that mimic PLA_2's active sites, which have been resolved by crystallography

phosphomonoester Any member of a family of phospholipid precursors that form neuronal membranes; phosphomonoesters are ↓ and phosphodiesters are in ↑ schizophrenia, a finding that suggests to some authors that there is an excess 'pruning' of neurons during adolescence, implying that schizophrenia may may be amenable to pharmacologic intervention (Sci Am 1994; 270/3:20)

phosphorus binders A group of orally administered agents, eg calcium acetate that increase GI excretion of phosphorus in patients with chronic renal failure

phosphorylation PHYSIOLOGY The process of adding a phosphate group to a protein, eg phosphorylation of a receptor by a protein kinase, an activity that serves to regulate receptor-mediated transcription of target genes

phossy jaw OCCUPATIONAL MEDICINE A condition caused by chronic occupation-related poisoning by elemental or yellow phosphorus causing mandibular necrosis CLINICAL Early symptoms of toothache and sialorrhea, loosening of the teeth, malodorous discharge, pain and mandibular swelling are followed by bone necrosis and recalcitrant sinus tracts; the current OSHA levels of 0.1 mg/m^3 averaged over an 8-hour shift are below the toxic levels that would cause this complication

phot A CGS (ie non-SI, or International System) unit of light intensity equal to 1 lumen/cm^2; Cf Lux, Photon

photoactivators Ingested substances that enhance reactivity to light, including PUVA, tetracycline, psoralens (celery, parsnips, figs and parsley); see PUVA

photoaging The structural and functional deterioration of sun-exposed regions, resulting in skin wrinkling, altered texture, discoloration, decreased epidermal thickness, basophilic degeneration of the dermis with loss of collagen and dermal vessels and epithelial atypia and dysplasia; most of the changes of photoaging are reversed by retinoin

photobleaching see Fluorescence recovery after photobleaching

photochemical decontamination TRANSFUSION MEDICINE A proprietary process that uses light and photoactive compounds to inactivate blood borne pathogens by inducing an irreversible chemical reaction with the RNA and DNA of the microorganism, rendering it incapable of reproduction (Biophotonics Intl 1995:2:14)

photocurrent deficit ALTERNATIVE MEDICINE A neologism referring to the diminution of neural impulses generated by the eye which is alleged by some alternative health care practitioners to reduce brain activity and lead to anxiety, depression, fatigue, hyperactivity, insomnia, learning disabilities, loss of concentration and coordination, low self-esteem, mood swings, night blindness, seasonal affective disorder, and others, claims that are difficult to substantiate; see Alternative medicine, Light therapy

photodamage DERMATOLOGY Photodamaged skin Skin injury due to exposure to sunlight, which translates into acral lentigines, mottled hyperpigmentation, surface roughness, and wrinkles PATHOPHYSIOLOGY Uncertain, although the ↓ in collagen I (possibly also collagen III) has been closely linked to photodamage TREATMENT Tretinoin (N Engl J Med 1993; 329:530oa)

photodocumentation The use of photography to record and 'document' various aspects of patient management; in certain types of patient care, eg cosmetic surgery, photodocumentation is particularly important as proof that a patient who may not now look like a 'silk purse', was nearly a 'sow's ear' when first seen by the surgeon

photodynamic therapy A therapeutic modality in which tumor cells that concentrate a photosensitizer, eg a hematoporphyrin derivative, are destroyed by exposure to light at an appropriate wavelength, a modality of potential use in treating superficial, low-grade or in situ transitional cell carcinoma of the bladder; in one small study (N Engl J Med 1987; 317:1251), 47% had complete tumor eradication; PDT consists of IV administration of (di)hematoporphyrin ether, a chemosensitizer that is selectively retained by neoplastic and reticuloendothelial tissues; these tissues are then exposed to a 630 nm argon laser resulting in a photochemical reaction that releases oxygen free radicals, the 'agent' that causes cell death and tumor necrosis; PDT may be of therapeutic use in carcinoma of the gastric anastomotic stump (Dtsch Med Wochenschr 1994; 119:951c); PDT has been used in head and neck cancer that has failed conventional (eg surgery, chemo–, radio–, and cryotherapy, and hyperthermia)

photomultiplier tube An electronic tube that amplifies the signal of electrons from incident radiation, which is an integral component of spectrophotometers

photon A quantum of light energy equivalent to hv (h X v), where h is Planck's constant (6.625 x 10^{-27} erg-s) and v is the frequency of light measured in cycles/s; Cf Phot

photon absorptiometry A technique in which the density of an object, eg bone is determined by measuring the absorption of a beam of X-rays or gamma rays passed through the object of interest

photopheresis Photochemotherapy, see there

photoprotection Protection of cells from ultraviolet light-induced damage by exposing the cells to light in the high UV-A and low UV-B (310-370 nm) range, which either inhibits cell synthesis or activates a heat shock protein-like response; Cf Sunscreen

Note: UV-C (200-290 nm) is damaging to DNA and amino acids, UV-B ranges from 290-320 nm and UV-A from 320 to 400 nm

photoreactivation The process of repairing ultraviolet light-induced damage to DNA, which consists of cyclobutyl linkage of thymine residues (dimerization), which is repaired by four enzymes: ultraviolet-activated endonuclease (initiation, responsible for 80% of the defects), exonuclease, DNA polymerase and DNA ligase

photorefractive keratectomy OPHTHALMOLOGY A procedure in which an excimer laser is used to ablate and sculpt the cornea to exact specifications; in myopia, the cornea is flattened by 'shaving' 10-20 microns of corneal tissue from the center and tapering to the edges; in early therapeutic trials, the 20-40 seconds in duration procedure has been most successful in those with myopia of less than 5 diopters; the only reported complication is glare, and preliminary data suggests that PRK will be a better procedure than radial keratotomy, the other method of refractive surgery; PRK s one of two types of refractive surgery (techniques that correct myopia by changing the cornea's conformation); the technique has not yet (early 1995) been granted FDA approval (and is thus viewed as investigational, ie not reimbursed by insurance carriers); it has been conditionally approved by the FDA; in photoreactive keratectomy, an excimer laser (cost of equipment, $300-500 000) cuts concentric circles in the cornea, 'photoshaving' the center of the cornea, imparting a homogenous consistency; in clinical trials, 78% discarded their glasses; 3-7% experienced complications; 250 000 PRKs have been performed in 45 countries; because of the high cost of the procedure ($1200-1500/eye) and the high number (80+% of the 63 million myopes in the US) of potential clients who could be treated with PRK, a battle for 'market turf' is expected to ensue if FDA approves the procedure; it is now unclear who would perform the procedure, optometrists, ophthalmologists, or anyone with experience using a therapeutic laser (Am Med News 7 Nov 1994; p1) see Refractive surgery; Cf radial keratectomy

phrenology An obsolete medical discipline that was popular in the 18th century that held that the configuration of the skull could be used to decipher the intellect, emotions, and instincts that were generated in the region of the brain lying below the surface area being studied

phthisis bulbi A condition characterized by advanced degeneration and disorganization of the ocular globe, accompanied by retinal necrosis, atrophy, softening and shrinkage, thickening of the sclera with permanent scarring and loss of function; phthisis bulbi occurs in retinoblastomas or in untreated purulent endophthalmitis and may be accelerated by intraocular surgery; phthisis bulbi may predispose the retina to malignant melanoma

PHS Pulmonary hemorrhagic syndrome, see there

phycocyanin IMMUNOPATHOLOGY A photosynthetic protein obtained from blue-green algae (cyanobacteria) that contains a bound phycobilin, which is used as a tracer in immunofluorescence asays

phycoerythrin IMMUNOPATHOLOGY A photosynthetic protein obtained from red algae that contains a bound phycobilin, which is an extremely bright fluorescent tracer that is excited at 488 nm, and emits light at 578 nm; phycoerythrin allows the discrimination between the yellow-orange signal of a positive immune reaction and greenish autofluorescent background

phycomycosis Mucormycosis, see there

phyllodes tumor Cystosarcoma phyllodes PATHOLOGY A breast tumor characterized by fleshy, leaf-like papillary projections of epithelial-lined stromal tissue extending into cystic spaces, which is most common in perimenopausal women; phyllodes tumors range from bland, benign and banal, histologically similar to typical fibroadenomas to the aggressive, characterized by florid stromal cellularity that mimics sarcomas; metastases occur in 3-12% of cases, with the stromal component spreading to bone and lung rather than lymph nodes, which is the usual catchment site for epithelial breast malignancies

phylogenetic tree A diagrammatic representation of the evolutionary pathway that is thought to have occurred in the development of a particular species based on criteria from various fields including comparitive zoology, embryology, paleontology, and others; the traditional phylogenic classification is based on differences in an array of physical characteristics, eg feather types, skeletal anatomy, form of reproduction, or for lower organisms, the types of biochemical reactions, pigment production, or metabolic requirements; in the usual PT, the more ancient and often extinct members of the pathway are placed at the bottom, and the recent members at the top; more recent PTs are based on the relatedness of DNA and amino acid sequences of certain proteins, eg those of the respiratory pathway in mitochondria, are more valid, and allow determination of the point in evolution where one species diverged from another; see Urkingdom

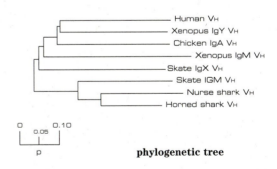

phylogenetic tree

phrygian cap deformity An abnormal angulation or kinking of the distal portion of the gallbladder fundus, due to a transverse fibrous septum of presumed congenital nature, often associated with cholelithiasis

Note: Phrygian caps are conical, bent in front and were called the 'Cap of Liberty' during the French revolution for their symbolic significance, as they were worn in Phrygia, a country of ancient Asia minor by slaves who had won their freedom

physaliferous cells Vacuolated mucin-filled cells, with a soap bubble-like appearance that are arranged in cords, sheets and nests, and divided by thin fibrous trabeculae; physaliferous cells are characteristic of chordomas, which are locally aggressive tumors that arise from remnants of the fetal notochord, most commonly developing in the sacrococcygeal region of women (♂:♀ ratio, 3:1) during the fifth decade of life; the clinical course is marked by frequent recurrences PROGNOSIS 40% develop metastases; many ultimately prove fatal; see Soap bubble

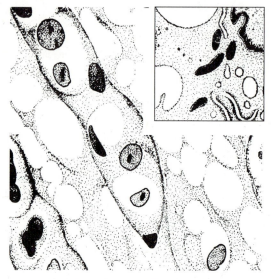

physaliferous cells (EM in inset box)

physical abuse PEDIATRICS '...*involves inflicting bodily injury through excessive force or forcing a child to engage in physically harmful activity, such as excessive exercise*, PA of children, a form of child maltreatment increases with poverty; PA'd children tend to be '...*more aggressive with their peers, have more troubled interpersonal relationships, and more depressive symptoms and affective disorders*.'; when these children become adults they are 2-3 times more likely to have problems with substance abuse (**N Engl J Med 1995; 332:1425RV**)

physical activity A behavioral parameter that can be used to evaluate a subject's cardiovascular 'reserve'; the intensity of physical activity can be quantified using metabolic units (MET); physical activity can take the form of either conditioning physical activity, eg walking 4.2 MET or non-conditioning physical activity, eg walking 3.5 MET; conditioning type physical activity is associated with a reduced risk of myocardial infarction (**N Engl J Med 1994; 330:1550OA**)

physical fitness PUBLIC HEALTH A state of physical well-being and higher-than-average tolerance to increased cardiovascular activity; PF is defined by exercise test tolerance to a standard treadmill protocol, which usually requires a cardiovascular 'reserve'; PF is the degree to which a person meets or exceeds the expected working capacity according to body weight; there is '...*a graded, inverse association between physical fitness and mortality from cardiovascular causes ...that is independent of age and conventional coronary risk factors*.' (**N Engl J Med 1993; 328:533OA**); staying 'in shape' substantially ↓ mortality rates (after adjusting for age, smoking habits, cholesterol, systolic blood pressure, fasting blood glucose and parental history of coronary vascular disease); cardiovascular mortality is 3.5 times ↑ in ♂ and 10 times ↑ in ♀ who are in the least fit quintile of a population; cancer mortality is five-fold ↑ in unfit ♂ and 15-fold ↑ in unfit ♀; in one study, the all-cause and cardiovascular cause death rate was 40/10 000 man-years in physically fit (highest quintile) males and 122/10 000 in physically unfit (lowest quintile) males (**JAMA 1995; 273:1093OA**) see Exercise, Obesity

physical hazard OCCUPATIONAL SAFETY Any agent or activity posing a potential hazard to health; in OSHA parlance,

a PH is any chemical for which there is scientifically valid evidence that it is combustible (liquid), flammable (aerosol, gas, liquid, solid), compressed (gas, explosives, organic peroxide, oxidizing, pyrophoric, unstable, or water-reactive; Cf Health hazard

physical map GENETICS A map of a chromosome or an entire genome in which the distances are measured by methods other than through gene recombination MOLECULAR BIOLOGY A map that locates markers in terms of sequences of DNA with respect to each other, based on distances, measured in thousands of base pairs, between genetic markers; a major difficulty in creating a physical map is the sheer size of the human genome*, a factor requiring an efficient means of both

1) Cloning large fragments of DNA*, now performed using the recently developed YACs (yeast artificial chromosomes) as cloning vectors, which can accept DNA fragments of up to 1 million base pairs–the previous size ceiling for cloning being that provided by cosmids, which can accept a DNA fragment of up to 50 000 base pairs and

2) Separating large fragments of DNA, now performed using pulsed-field gel electrophoresis (PFGE), a technique that allows separation of DNA fragments of > than 1 million base pairs–the previous ceiling for separating DNA fragments by conventional agarose gel electrophoresis is about 50 000 base pairs (**Sci & Med Nov/Dec 1994, p48**)

*Three billion bases, see Human Genome project

physical restraints Restraints, see there

physical setback A popular term for any reversal in progress, usually referring to improvement made in rehabilitation therapy

physical status classification A classification of a subject's physical condition by the American Society of Anesthesiologists that stratifies patients undergoing a surgical procedure into categories of relative risk for suffering complications during an operation or in the immediate post-operative period (table)

PHYSICAL STATUS CLASSIFICATION

CLASS 1 No organic, physiologic, biochemical or psychiatric disturbance; the pathologic process for which the operation is to be performed is localized and does not entail a systemic disturbance, eg inguinal hernia repair in a robust male

CLASS 2 Mild to moderate disturbance caused either by the condition being treated surgically or by a physiopathologic derangement, eg mild cardiac disease, mild diabetes mellitus, chronic bronchitis, essential hypertension

CLASS 3 Severe systemic disease or derangement of any cause, which may defy classification, eg severe cardiac disease, angina or status post-myocardial infarction, severe diabetes with vascular complications, moderate to severe pulmonary compromise

CLASS 4 Severe systemic disease that is already life-threatening, which may not be corrected by surgery, eg organic heart disease with signs of severe cardiac insufficiency, advanced pulmonary, hepatic, renal or endocrine insufficiency

CLASS 5 A moribund patient with little chance of survival who is submitted to an operation in desperation, eg ruptured aortic aneurysm, major cerebral trauma with rapidly increasing intracranial pressure

EMERGENCY OPERATION E A designation for any of the above classes when the operation 'goes sour', eg an incarcerated hernia with strangulation would be a class 1E

(RD Dripps, Introduction to Anesthesia The Principle and Practice, 6th ed, WB Saunders, Philadelphia, 1982 Note: This is found in an abbreviated form in Mayo Clin Proc 1991; 66:155)

physical transfection GENE THERAPY A method of gene insertion in which foreign genes are inserted into a cell of interest by a physical means, eg electroporation or particle acceleration (Bio/Technology 1995; 13:222) Cf Chemical transfection, Viral transduction

physician A generic term for a person trained, qualified, and licensed to practice medicine or dentistry; the term physician can therefore alter according to the jurisdiction, eg in New York State, the term physician includes medical doctors (MD), doctors of osteopathy (DO), as well as dentists (DDS, doctor of dental surgery)

physician assistant An individual who is qualified to perform a wide variety of medically related tasks under a physician's supervision, including taking a patient's history, performing physical examinations and autopsies EDUCATION Two post-graduate years beyond college or university, training as a physician assistant, surgeon assistant, or pathologist assistant*, and designated as PA-Cs; physicians assistants may then subspecialize for a one-to-two year period in various fields including neonatology, pediatrics, emergency medicine, occupational medicine and others; see Pathologist assistant

physician-assisted suicide Any passive intervention on the part of a physician to help a person end his/her own life; PAS is more stringently defined by one group (see below reference) as 'prescription of medication (eg narcotics or barbiturates) or the counseling of an ill patient so he or she may use an overdose to end his or her own life; 53% of physicians believe that PAS should be legal in some circumstances; 50% believe it is ethically justified (39% disagree), only 40% would be willing to actually help a patient commit suicide; hematologists and oncologists are more likely to oppose PAS and euthanasia; psychiatrists are more likely to support these practices (N Engl J Med 1994; 331:89SA; US New & World Report 25 April 1994) see Euthanasia, Initiative 119, Kevorkian, Slippery Slope

physician autonomy The independence or right to determine without uninvited intervention:

1) WHO WILL DO THE WORK OF PHYSICIANS–by establishing criteria for medical school admission, postgraduate training, and licensure

2) WHAT WORK PHYSICIANS WILL DO–by establishing a critical core of knowledge and standards of medical practice

3) WHY THE PROFESSION DOES ITS WORK–by establishing a code of ethics and promoting an orientation toward public service

4) HOW THE PROFESSION WILL ACT–by maintaining professional dominance over other health care providers Note: It is widely recognized that physician autonomy is eroding, both in the US and elsewhere (N Engl J Med 1993; 328:1337CPC)

physician-bashing The verbal persecution of physicians, who are viewed by some as greedy, opportunistic, callous, unprincipled and overpaid entrepeneurs (AAO-HNS Bulletin May 1993ED)

Physician's Desk Reference PDR, see there

physician expert witness A principal actor in the drama of malpractice litigation, defined by an adaption of the Council of Medical Specialty Societies (table)

Note: It is considered unethical to link expert witness fees to the outcome of the case, as there is a potential for introducing bias (Bull, Am Coll Surgeons 1989; 74:6)

physician 'glut' An excess of physicians in a particular geographic region; a PG has been present in some European and South American countries for over a decade, where physicians may supplement their incomes performing various menial tasks; a PG is anticipated in North America*-in 1970 there were 326 000 physicians; 706 000 are projected by 2000 with 271 physicians/10^5 (or 176/10^5 JAMA 1991; 265:2369) Cf Manpower shortage, Physician shortage area

*It is unclear whether a PG will materialize in North America; if it does, it may not cause massive physician unemployment, as new physician roles are being created in a high-technology, litigation-prone society, including new specialties, eg geriatrics, medical informatics and molecular therapy, and the creation of new roles in medicine, eg medical ethicists, quality assurance specialists, physician-bureaucrats, physician-lawyers and others)

'physician invulnerability syndrome' The self-maintained delusion by a physician that he/she is not susceptible to the same diseases as his/her patients; the PIS is the result of a 'contract' having been made with a Higher Being (ie God) that ensures an aura of protection; this delusion results in self-treatment by the physician for potentially pernicious conditions, treatment delays, denial of mental or physical illness, substance (eg alcohol, drugs) abuse, and an unwillingness to bother colleagues who have the expertise necessary to properly treat the illness

physician office laboratory A small laboratory in a physician's office that has an abbreviated menu of tests that can be performed while the patient is still in the office, in order for the physician to make recommendations about the patient's state of health and therapy; there has been an increasing tendency in the US for private physicians to maintain such laboratories, driven by the increased reimbursement (from the 1984 Deficit Reduction Act, supported by the Health Care Financing Agency), convenience and evolving technologies, which allow sophisticated techniques to be performed in a small working space by a staff having little formal laboratory experience; POLs had, because of their small size and the simplicity of methodologies, been exempt from the stringent restrictions imposed on larger laboratories, but have been criticized by some for occasionally producing unreliable results, as POLs may bypass quality control procedures that comprise a large part of the reagent and labor costs borne by larger laboratories; to rectify the situation, the US government formulated the Clinical Laboratories Improvement Act (CLIA), requiring that POLs meet minimum federal certification criteria, including performance of quality control of specimens, maintaining standards for the personnel performing the tests and successful completion of periodic proficiency testing; CLIA regulations exempt those POLs that perform only 'waivered' tests, which either employ methods so simple and accurate as to render the likelihood of error negligible (ie 'idiot-proof'), or tests that pose no reasonable risk of harm to the patient even if performed incorrectly, eg 'dipstick' results, fecal occult blood, microhematocrit, microscopic analysis of pinworms, urinary sediment and vaginal wet mounts, qualitative ovulation tests and urine pregnancy tests; see CLIA

PHYSICIAN EXPERT WITNESS

RECOMMENDED QUALIFICATIONS The physician expert witness should

1) Have a current, valid and unrestricted license to practice medicine in his state of practice

2) Be a diplomate (ie, board-certified) or board-eligible in the specialty deemed relevant to the case

3) Be familiar with the clinical practice of the specialty involved in the case and

4) Be prepared to document the time he spends as an expert witness; see 'Hired gun'

RECOMMENDED BEHAVIOR The physician expert is expected to be impartial and be neither advocate nor partisan in the legal proceedings; he/she should

1) Review the medical information relevant to the case and testify in an unbiased fashion

2) Review the standards of practice prevailing at the time of the event's occurrence

3) Provide the basis from which his testimony is derived, ie testimony based on experience or that derived from the medical literature

4) Receive compensation that is reasonable and reflects the time and effort spent in preparing the case

physician office-to-laboratory link A class of software that allows a physician's office to interface with a laboratory information system, facilitating the ordering of laboratory tests and reporting of results; some states in the US view the providing of computer hardware as an illegal kickback, which may be circumvented by the removal of certain non-data transmitting components (eg hard drive) from the equipment being provided to the POLL client (CAP Today May, 1994)

physician ownership see Conflict-of-interest

physician-patient relationship MEDICAL MALPRACTICE A formal or inferred relationship that exists between a physician and a patient that is established once the physician assumes or undertakes the rendering of medical care or treatment of a patient; the establishment of such a relationship is 'automatic' in certain situations, eg in the physician's private office, but in others, eg physical examination as a health screening procedure, it cannot be assumed to exist; see Doctor-patient interaction

physician profile HEALTH CARE INDUSTRY The list of a physician's fees by procedure, compiled by a 'third-party payer', ie an insurance company or Medicare, by a hospital, or by his own staff in order to control his reimbursements and monitor his income

physician profiling HEALTH CARE FINANCING A method of cost containment that focuses on the patterns of health care provided by a single physician or group, instead of on specific clinical decisions; the resulting profile can then be compared to other norms based on practice (ie other physicians' profiles) or to standards of practice (practice guidelines); profiling takes into account a physician's desire to limit the intrusion of administrative mechanisms in the doctor-patient relation (N Engl J Med 1994; 330:607oA)

Note: Given the flawed and preliminary data generated from physician profiling analysis, New England Journal of Medicine's editor, JP Kassirer comments *'We should resist the argument, fostered largely by the business community, that some data are better than none at all. We do not accept flawed or incomplete data as a basis for medical practice, and we should not accept them for assessing the quality of our care. We should ... insist that all approaches be validated. We should not permit profiling unadjusted for severity of illness and case-mix to be the basis of decisions about quality.'* (N Engl J Med 1994; 330:634oA)

physician self-referral see Self-referral

physician shortage area A region (usually rural and/or of lower income, as in the inner city) where very few physicians practice medicine, in which there may be less than one physician per 5000 population Note: The dialog about physician shortage areas is usually in the context of the US and other developed nations; in some African countries, there may be 1 physician per 10^5 or more people; Cf Manpower shortage, Physician glut

physiognomy The formal study of the human face; for a brief period after C Lombroso's publication of *L'Uomo Delinquente* (1876), certain facial and other physical features was used to classify criminals, eg small restless eyes were thought to be typical of thieves, or bright eyes and cracked voices of sex criminals (New York Times 15 Sept 1992; C1)

phytochemical A compound of plant origin that has no currently known beneficial effect, but for which some evidence exists favoring their use in preventing certain diseases, eg in chemoprevention of malignancy, immune stimulation, and so on; phytochemicals include sulforaphane (obtained from cruciferous vegetables), allium compounds (from garlic and onions), limonene (citrus fruits), isoflavones (beans), ellagic acid (grapes) (P Talalay, PNAS April 12, 1994)

phytochemistry Plant chemistry

phytohemagglutinin PHA CLINICAL IMMUNOLOGY A protein lectin obtained from the red kidney bean (*Phaseolus vulgaris*), which is a tetramer, each subunit of which can bind *N*-acetylgalactosamine; PHA serves as a lymphocyte mitogen that is used in vitro to measure lymphocyte-mediated cytotoxicity, as a nonspecific immune stimulant for in vitro studies of mononuclear cells, and for evaluating cytokine production; it is mitogenic for T cells (lymphocytes), and stimulates CD4 ('helper') T cells more than CD8 ('suppressor') T cells; it is a weaker mitogen for B cells; the degree of response in the respective cells can be measured based on the cell's production of IL-2

phytomedicine Herbal medicine, see there

phytoremediation The removal of toxic chemicals or heavy metals from contaminated soil or dump sites by use of plants that concentrate these substances from the soil; although the mechanism of phytoremediation is unknown, ragwood is reported to concentrate lead 8-fold more than that present in the soil; other metals absorbed from the soil by various plants include cadmium, copper, gold, nickel, uranium, and zinc (New York Times 8 September 1992; C4) Cf Bioremediation

phytotherapy Herbal medicine, see there

pI Isoelectric point CLINICAL CHEMISTRY The pH at which a determined protein has a net charge of zero, the result of a combination of all the different side chains and their degrees of association; the higher the pI, the more cathodic is the protein on an electrophoresis run at a pH of 9.4

PI Principal investigator, see there

PI-3 Phosphatidylinositol-3 kinase

pi granules Lamellations of flattened perinuclear osmiophilic material in benign tumors of the peripheral nervous system, which are of unknown significance; see Myelin figures

PI system see Phosphoinositide system

piano playing NEUROLOGY A fanciful descriptor for the finger movements secondary to the loss of position sensation, in which the patient seeks to discover exactly where his fingers are in space by periodic movement, a feature of Dejerine-Sottas syndrome*; these movement are often accompanied by truncal ataxia and choreic hand movements; 'piano playing' also refers to intermittent flexion and extension of the hands in tardive dyskinesia, a complication of chronic therapy with antipsychotic drugs, eg phenothiazines, butyrophenones

*A severe AR peripheral sensorimotor neuropathy of infantile onset that is accompanied by delayed ambulation and loss of ambulation by early adulthood

pibloktoq PSYCHIATRY, ANTHROPOLOGY A transient hysterical reaction in Eskimo women, in which the subjects rip off their clothes in sub-zero weather, emitting animal and bird sounds, shout obscenities, eat feces, or perform other irrational or dangerous acts, followed by amnesia for the event, a reaction that is postulated to stem from long-standing repression of the personality of the Eskimo female, whose status is that of property (DSM-IV™, 1994) see Culture-bound syndrome; Cf Koro, Zombie

pica The ingestion of unusual substances with no known nutritional value, 'classically' associated with iron-deficiency anemia; the substance ingested may aggravate the iron deficiency, as in geophagy, where the clay eaten acts as a ferro-chelator; other pica ingestants include paint, laundry starch, ice (pagophagia), and newspapers; pica also occurs in zinc, copper and certain vitamin deficiencies, but evidence for a causal relation remains scanty; some cases of pica may be directly explained by the effect of the ingestant, eg coffee grounds (caffeine) and cigarette butts (nicotine); see Geophagy

Pica is a genus of magpies, birds famed for their omnivorous nature; like the magpie, a person or animal with pica craves or eats anything, often indigestibles and non-comestibles

Picasso phone TELEMEDICINE A proprietary device marketed by AT&T that serves as a cost-effective means of communicating diagnostic images of patients and medical conditions among physicians; the Picasso Still-Image Phone connects to a standard camcorder (which can be used to capture images of the eye, wounds, and skin conditions) to either a TV monitor or to a personal computer display; the advantage of Picasso is that it can be used to transmit images over the standard analog telephone lines, currently in operation (Biophotonics Intl 1995:2:14)

pick-up sticks pattern CYTOLOGY A fanciful descriptor for the haphazard arrangement of cells in the cervical and endocervical epithelium in reparative atypia

picket fence fever pattern A descriptor for a saw-tooth pattern of high temperature 'spikes', a finding considered characteristic of pyogenic hepatic abscesses, which is accompanied by chills, sweating, nausea, vomiting, anorexia and pain

picket fence arrangement see Palisading

Pickwick syndrome Cardiopulmonary obesity syndrome A complication of extreme obesity, in which there is marked cardiovascular compromise, with ↓ tidal and expiratory reserve volumes, alveolar hypoventilation, hypoxia, cyanosis (and hypercapnia, if severe and prolonged), dyspnea, polycythemia, cardiac hypertrophy, pulmonary hypertension and edema, congestive heart failure and extreme somnolence; oxygen therapy is potentially fatal as it removes the chemoreceptor drive needed for respiratory movements; Cf Morbid obesity

Note: The condition is named for the fat boy, Joe, in Charles Dickens' *The Pickwick papers*

Picornaviridae A family of small RNA viruses that constitute one of the largest and most important family of human and agricultural pathogens, including aphthovirus (foot-and-mouth disease viruses), enterovirus (including polioviruses, hepatitis A virus, coxsackieviruses, Theiler's murine encephalovirus and others), rhinovirus (agents of the common cold); picornaviral cysteine proteinases share folding homology with serine proteinases (Nature 1994; 369:72L)

picric acid 2,4,6-trinitrophenol A strong (pK 1.0) acid that variably functions as a dye, an antiseptic, and as a fixative; when dry, it is explosive and has been used in the manufacture of explosives and rocket fuels; occupational exposure results in a jaundiced discoloraton of the skin

picrotoxin A plant (*Anamirta cocculin*)-derived convulsant consisting of a 1:1 ratio of picrotoxinin and picrotin, which is a potent GABA antagonist that causes a decrease in mean channel open time

picture frame appearance A descriptor for a type of bone involvement by Paget's disease of the bone where an isolated vertebral body is enlarged, centrally osteoporotic, and surrounded by a rim of osteosclerotic cortex, involving the anterior and posterior margins as well as the vertebral end-plates; despite its increased radiologic density, the bone is more prone to fractures

picture frame area BURN PHYSIOLOGY A limited zone of tissue directly beneath the advancing dermal edge, which contains the 'machinery' necessary for wound contraction and repair; excision of this rim of cells effectively stops epithelialization of burn wounds; the epithelial cells within the 'picture frame' are large, stellate and pale

picture puzzle appearance Jigsaw puzzle appearance (cells, contour, model, tumor), see there

PID Pelvic inflammatory disease, see there

lso 1) Pain intensity differences 2) Phenylindandione (phenindione) 3) Plasma iron disappearance (hematology) 4) Primary immunodeficiency disease 5) Prolapsed intervertebral disk 6) Protruded intervertebral disk

PIE 1) Pulmonary infiltration with eosinophilia 2) Pulmonary interstitial emphysema, a rarely used acronym, given the potential for confusion with the PIE syndrome

piebaldism Partial albinism A rare AD [MIM 164920] condition characterized by patchy amelanotic plaques (focally reduced or absent melanocytes) occurring on the forehead, scalp, thorax, elbows and knees, associated with a white forelock; Woolf syndrome is diagnosed when in addition, the scalp skin changes are accompanied by heterochromic irides, deafness and mental retardation

piecemeal necrosis Necrosis of the liver cell plate in which a chronic inflammatory cell infiltrate is in direct contact with hepatocytes actively undergoing condensation and fragmentation (apoptosis); piecemeal necrosis imparts a 'ragged' low-power appearance to the usually lobular pattern of the limiting plate; PN is a required histologic feature in cirrhosis and chronic active hepatitis and may be seen in primary sclerosing cholangitis

Piedmont fracture An isolated fracture located precisely at the distal third of the radius, named after a case presented by the Piedmont Orthopedic Society of North Carolina; current thinking holds that open reduction and fixation can be performed when only one of the two forearm bones is fractured, as closed reduction results in a high incidence of non-union

PIE syndrome Pulmonary infiltrates with eosinophilia A disease complex characterized by intense, nonspecific symptoms accompanied by chronic relapsing fever, cough and dyspnea, seen in association with chronic eosinophilic pneumonia; PIE has been subdivided into

SIMPLE PIE Löffler syndrome, transient pulmonary infiltrates accompanied by fever, dyspnea, and eosinophilia of the peripheral blood

TROPICAL EOSINOPHILIA, which may be associated with microfilarial infections and parasites, including *Ascaris lumbricoides* and *Toxocara canis* and

SECONDARY CHRONIC PULMONARY EOSINOPHILIA, which is associated with allergic bronchopneumonia related to aspergillosis, bronchocentric granulomatosis, allergic angiitis and granulomatosis (Churg-Strauss syndrome), drugs (nitrofurantoin, sulfonamide), and infections (parasitic, fungal, and bacterial)

piezoelectric sensing BACKGROUND Piezoelectric crystals are those that produce a partial separation of electrical charge when they are deformed, such that equal, but opposite charges arise at the opposite surfaces of the crystal; all known crystals have a natural vibration, known as a resonant or fundamental frequency, which is a function of their chemical composition and each vibration causes the crystal to oscillate; when the crystal is piezoelectric (as is quartz), the resonance results in an oscillating electrical field; the piezoelectric effect has been used to measure antigen-antibody reactions, DNA-RNA interactions, and may be of use in clinical toxicology

PIF Prolactin-inhibiting factor, see there

pig RADIATION SAFETY A whiskey shot glass-sized lead-shielded receptacle used to transport and store radioactive material in clinical or research laboratories, substantially reducing a radioisotope's γ radiation

Note: Origin of the term pig is uncertain, although certain relatives of the word pig are suggestive, eg 1) A pig is ⅛ of an English (250 pounds) ton, a unit of weight of cast iron 2) A pig is an ingot of molten metal (often lead, but also iron and copper) fed from channels called sows, and 3) A derivation from Old English 'pygg' for a crock or jar, that later evolved to pig

PIG-A A gene (named for phosphatidylinositol glycan A) located on X chromosome segment p22.1; *PIG-A* encodes components of the glycosyl-phosphatidylinositol (GPI) pathway, the GPI 'anchors', and is mutated in paroxysmal nocturnal hemoglobinuria (N Engl J Med 1994; 330:249oA)

pigbel The New Guinean name for enteritis necroticans, which is linked to poorly cooked pork infected with type C *Clostridium perfringens*, that may be consumed in orgiastic 3-4 day pork-eating 'marathons'; pigbel is endemic in the New Guinea highlands, affecting in particular those children with a poor immune response to clostridial toxins, low levels of proteases and a protein-poor diet that is high in sweet potatoes, which contain trypsin inhibitors PATHOGENESIS The trypsin-sensitive 'B' toxin of *C perfringens*, type C (an organism isolated from 70% of the villagers) is not degraded given the relative trypsin insufficiency and intestinal parasitosis by *Ascaris lumbricoides*, which secretes a trypsin inhibitor CLINICAL 24-hour incubation followed by intense abdominal pain, vomiting, bloody diarrhea and shock; ½ require resective surgery PATHOLOGY Local infarction, edema, hemorrhage, neutrophil infiltration MORTALITY Up to 40%

pigeon breast deformity Chicken breast deformity An anterior displacement of the sternum, adjacent cartilage and anterior rib cage due to abnormal pulling by respiratory musculature on soft bone, enlargement of the costochondral junctions and flattening of the thorax, a finding characteristic of advanced vitamin D-induced rickets; the deformity is an asymptomatic, asymmetric, and deep depression of the costal cartilage along each side of the sternum, most apparent below the nipple level, involves the 4th to 7-8th costal cartilages, and comprises the most common type of protrusion deformity of the sternum (pectus carinatum) Cf Pouter-pigeon

pigeon breeder's disease A form of extrinsive allergic alveolitis (hypersensitivity pneumonitis) due to inhalation of protein antigens from the sera, excreta, and feathers of parrots, pigeons, and parakeets or budgerigars, which evokes a type III or hypersensitivity reaction that may be followed by a type IV or granulomatous reaction; see Farmer's lung, Hypersensitivity pneumonitis

pigeon toe In-toeing, talipes varus ORTHOPEDICS A deformity of the foot that develops in childhood and is characterized by a medial rotation of the forefoot (metatarsus varus) and medial tibial or femoral torsion, in which the bones are medially rotated; the resulting deformities require orthopedic correction

piggie back device CRITICAL CARE MEDICINE A device used in critically ill patients to optimize the IV delivery of fluids and drugs that need to be infused at different rates; in these devices, the reservoir and the valve controlling the rate of delivery are separate, while the delivery port itself, eg an IV access line may be shared

pigmented neuroectodermal tumor of infancy A tumor* of neural crest origin affecting infants under 6 months of age that may rarely occur in adults, which may be located in the anterior maxilla, oral cavity and skull, and less commonly in the mediastinum, thigh, forearm and epididymis CLINICAL Locally aggressive, 15% recurrence rate, rarely metastatic PATHOLOGY Small pseudoglandular nests of cells and alveolar (cup-like) formations lined by neuroglial cells with abundant cytoplasmic melanin in a dense collagenous matrix LABORATORY ↑ Vanillylmandelic acid in urine; see Pseudonym syndrome

*Synonyms include melanoameloblastoma, melanotic progonoma, pigmented ameloblastoma, retinal anlage tumor

pigmented villonodular synovitis ORTHOPEDICS A lesion usually of the knee (less commonly, the ankle, hip, and shoulder) of young adults characterized by a proliferation of yellow-brown hemosiderin-laden spongy tissue PATHOLOGY Papillary projections in a background of nodular tenosynovitis TREATMENT Excision and if recurrent, re-excision DDx Fibrosarcoma, synovial sarcoma, incontinentia pigmenti

PIGO Phenytoin-induced gingival overgrowth, see there

pigskin appearance Moroccan leather appearance A descriptor for the finely bosselated surface of the renal cortex after removing the capsule, where the papular elevations correspond to sclerotic hyalinized, hypertrophied arterioles, typically seen in benign nephrosclerosis; the 'pigskin' descriptor also refers to the taut, shiny, non-pitting and painful skin of patients with lipemia, usually

affecting the lower extremities; see Painful fat syndrome

'pigtail' 'Spaghetti' TRANSFUSION MEDICINE A regional colloquialism for the plastic tubes clamped off at 5-cm intervals that are connected to transfusion bags, and used for serological testing, in order to determine donor-recipient compatibility prior to transfusion

pigtail catheter A drainage catheter with side holes, used for draining clear non-viscid or coagulable collections of bile, urine or pancreatic fluids; the 'pigtail' is inefficient in draining abscesses from solid organs, but may be used for perihepatic abscesses

PIH see Prolactin-inhibiting hormone

Pilgrim plant A nuclear power station in Massachusetts from which 'soft' epidemiologic data support the controversial conclusions of the Sellafield study, which suggest that there may be an increased incidence of leukemia in those exposed to low levels, ie < 500 mrems/year of radiation; see Sellafield; Cf Three Mile Island

Note: Data from France, a country that derives a great part of its energy from nuclear reactors, does not appear to confirm these studies

pilar sheath acanthoma An uncommon but distinctive skin appendage tumor, presumed to be of hair follicle origin; average age 66 years; ♂:♀ ratio 2:1 TREATMENT Surgical excision (Am J Clin Pathol 1995; 103:508ABSTR)

pili torti A hair shaft defect, most commonly affecting ash-blondes, where the hair is grooved and flattened at varying intervals and twisted on its axis; the defect is usually recognized by age 2-3, the hair having a 'spangled' appearance; pili torti is either an AR [MIM 261900] condition a sui generis or a component of the X-R [MIM 309400] Menke's kinky hair syndrome, associated with mental retardation); Cf Ringed hair, Woolly hair

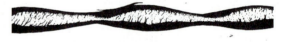

pili torti

the Pill A generic colloquialism for any oral contraceptive

'pill' esophagitis Mucosal injury of the esophagus caused by per os medication, eg aspirin, nonsteroidal anti-inflammatory drugs, anticholinergics, iron-preparations, potassium chloride, tetracycline and quinidine CLINICAL Prolonged 'cancer-like' symptoms including retrosternal pain, progressive stricture, hemorrhage and perforation

'pill hypertension' A form of hypertension affecting women with an intrinsic predisposition for ↑ blood pressure, due to ↑ circulating angiotensinogen induced by estrogens in oral contraceptives

pill-rolling NEUROLOGY *adjective* Pertaining or referring to the tremor characterized by a circular movement of the tips of the index finger and thumb, which is typically seen in Parkinson's disease

pilocarpine HCl A parasympathetic agent that is a muscarinic agonist with mild β-adrenergic activity; topical (conjunctival) pilocarpine is used to ↓ intraocular pressure in glaucoma; pilocarpine causes pharmacologic stimulation of exocrine glands resulting in diaphoresis, salivation, lacrimation (eg and may be used to treat post-radiation xerostomia (N Engl J Med 1993; 329:390OA), gastric and pancreatic secretion

pilot study A generic term for an early clinical trial, usually of a form of therapy, in which a small, highly selected group of patients with a particular disease are treated with the agent of interest; a PS serves to test a hypothesis based on a presumed pathogenesis* (N Engl J Med 1994; 331:1680OA)

*eg That isotretinoin, which is known to attenuate the spontaneous proliferation of leukemic GM-CFUs (granulocyte-macrophage colony-forming units) and decrease the sensitivity of these cells to GM-CSF (granulocyte-macrophage colony-stimulating factor)

pilot's wheel appearance Mariner's wheel appearance, see there

pimping ACADEMIA A practice in which persons in power ask esoteric questions of junior colleagues[1] usually with the sole[2] purpose of publicly demeaning them, which most often occurs on ward rounds with a chief of service in a university hospital; the interrogating 'pimper' is theoretically interested in correct answers[3]; the 'pimpee', usually a medical student, is interested in self-esteem, although correct answers to the questions gain neither recognition for, nor relief from, this form of harassment; pimping serves to establish a 'pecking order' among the medical staff DISADVANTAGE It suppress spontaneous or intellectual questions or pursuits, creates an antagonistic atmosphere and perpetuates medical student abuse (**JAMA 1989; 262:2541-2; 263:1632c**); Cf Pumping

[1]Pimp [2]but unexpressed [3]but in fact is most often interested in proving how erudite he/she is

PIN 1) Penile intraepithelial neoplasia 2) Prostatic intraepithelial neoplasia, see there

pince-nez neutrophil Pelger-Huët anomaly, see there

pincer nail An idiopathic excess tranverse curvature of the nail bed that is associated with intense pain and loss of soft tissue at the fingertips

pine tree appearance see Christmas tree appearance

pineal body *corpus pineale* [NA6], pineal gland A small (100-180 mg) red-gray pedunculated conical structure located between the superior colliculi, attached to epithalamus, and innervated by postganglionic nerve fibers of the cervical sympathetic ganglia; the pineal body's function in humans is unknown as it produces melatonin, as well as a plethora of neurotransmitter (eg norepinephrine, serotonin), hormonal peptides (eg oxytocin, somatostatin); it is believed to have a critical role in resetting the circadian pacemaker, and may be involved in regulating onset of puberty and salt/water metabolism (**Lab Med 1994; 25:372**) see Berry aneurysm

'ping-pong' bone A colloquial term for an attenuated rim of osseous tissue that surrounds a giant cell tumor of bone

'ping-pong' chromatography A variant of affinity chromatography that may be used to purify enzymes capable of forming covalently bonded intermediates METHOD A solution with the enzyme is poured into the chromatography column, allowed to link to its cognate substrate, which has been permanently bonded to the column's stationary phase and, then eluted by breaking the covalent bond, repeated in a simple two-phase, 'ping-pong'-like fashion

'ping-pong' fracture A colloquial term for a depressed skull fracture

'ping pong' infection A descriptor for the epidemiology of sexually transmitted *Trichomonas vaginalis* infection, where a person is treated with antibiotics during the incubation period of his/her sexual partner's infection by the same organism; the partner later becomes symptomatic after the patient has responded to antibiotics, resulting in an infection that 'bounces' back and forth from the treated to the untreated partner, in a fashion likened to a ping-pong ball bouncing back and forth across a net; β-hemolytic streptococci may also have a 'ping-pong ball' pattern of infection

Trichomonas vaginalis affects 3 million women in the USA and is more common in those with multiple partners, affecting at least 70% of prostitutes

ping-pong mechanism BIOCHEMISTRY A sequence of events that may occur in a catalytic reaction, where one substrate molecule is bound and a product molecule is released; a second substrate molecule is bound, releasing the metabolized product that was bound on the previous pass and so on, eg cleavage of polypeptide chains by a ser-

ine protease, or a transaminase-type reaction, where the enzyme transfers an amino group from an amino acid to a ketoacid, yielding a ketoacid where the amino acid was originally and a ketoacid where the amino acid was

'ping-ponging' HEALTH CARE INDUSTRY The unethical practice of repeatedly passing a patient from physician A to physician B and back again for the purpose of overcharging the patient's reimbursement agency, eg Medicaid or less commonly, a private insurance company; see Family ganging, Medicaid mill

pink disease Acrodynia A form of chronic mercury intoxication, now of historic interest, which occurred in infants given teething powder containing elemental mercury CLINICAL Pruritis, red-pink discoloration of cold, clammy skin, especially on the acral parts and on the buttocks, irritability, weight loss, photophobia, conjunctivitis, fever, leukocytosis, albuminuria and hypotonicity; Cf Mercury, Minamata disease

pink noise 1/f Noise, see there

pinkeye Acute contagious conjunctivitis by *Haemophilus aegyptius* or *H ducreyi*; 'pinkeye' has been obfuscated by the lay public, which may use the term for any condition in which the eyes are pink, eg bilateral bacterial or viral conjunctivitis, 'misuse' of the eyes, ie prolonged exposure to smoke-filled rooms, chronic alcoholism, dissipated life style, severe iritis, closed angle glaucoma, and others; see Red eye

pink noise Random variation in an audio signal, ie sound that carries no useful information about the source; pink noise has an equal amount of energy in each octave band; Cf Chaos, White noise

'pink puffer' A descriptor for a patient with COPD and/or severe emphysema, so named as they have a pink complexion and dyspnea; PPs have ↑ residual lung capacity and volume, ↓ elastic recoil, ↓ expiratory flow rate and diffusing capacity and a ventilatory/perfusion (V/Q) mismatch secondary to emphysema-related destruction of blood vessels CLINICAL Hyperventilation, shortness of breath; arterial blood gases (PaO_2 and $PaCO_2$) are usually normal because of the compensatory hyperventilation; see Chronic obstructive pulmonary disease; Cf 'Blue bloater'

Note: 'Pink puffers' may be clinically indistinguishable from 'Blue bloaters', and thus the term is more colorful than useful

the Pink Sheet A specialized weekly report that provides business and US federal regulatory information on prescription pharmaceuticals and the therapeutic biotechnology industry (**FDC Reports, Inc, Chevy Chase, Md**)

pink slip According to the 'classic' colloquial definition used in the US, the 'pink slip' is a note from an employer to the employee saying the latter has been terminated (canned, fired, handed the walking papers, given the boot, sacked)

Note: Pink is also the color most often used in the US for telephone message pads, and thus lends to confusion in some circles (**Am Med News 2 November 1992, p 13**)

pink tag TRANSFUSION MEDICINE A label attached to units of packed red cells in compliance with the California State Blood Labeling Regulations that serves to identify units that are ABO group B Note: Color coding of packed units (group A is yellow, group O is blue and group AB is white) is not required by the FDA, although the 'California system' has been adopted in certain regions in the US

pink tetralogy of Fallot PEDIATRIC CARDIOLOGY A clinical variant of Fallot's tetralogy (ventricular septal defect, dextroposition of the aorta, pulmonary artery stenosis and right ventricular hypertrophy), in which the pulmonary stenosis is moderate and a balanced shunt across the ventricular septum allows a normal pink skin color and adequate oxygenation of hemoglobin, in contrast to the usual patient who is cyanotic and has 'blue' skin due to persistent oxygen desaturation

pink tooth of Mummery Chronic perforating hyperplasia of the pulp A rare lesion consisting in internal resorption of a tooth, initiated by inflammatory hyperplasia of the pulp, usually not associated with caries; the condition may appear as a pinkish area on the crown, and because the lesion is effected by osteoclasts, is known as an osteoclastoma; if detected early, 'root canal' therapy can salvage the tooth, otherwise it must be extracted

Pinkus' tumor Fibroepithelioma A polypoid variant of basal cell carcinoma, commonly located on the back PATHOLOGY Superficial with long, thin branching and anastomosing stands of basal cell carcinoma embedded in a fibrous stroma

Pinkus lymphoma A morphologic variant of T-cell lymphoma, in which the nuclei have a popcorn-like multilobated appearance, but do not differ in clinical behavior

'pinky-printing' see Thumb-printing

pinta A chronic nonvenereal infection by *Treponema carateum* that is virtually identical to syphilis EPIDEMIOLOGY It is endemic to Central and South America and is transmitted by direct mucocutaneous innoculation, resulting in psoriasiform maculopapular lesions, which without treatment over time cause acral cutaneous atrophy and hyperpigmentation; Cf Yaws

pinwheel pattern A low-power LM pattern in which short fascicles of fibroblast-like or endothelial-like cells radiate from a central point bearing a vessel, as seen in sclerosing hemangioma; Cf Cartwheel pattern, Storiform pattern

'pioneer' bacteria The first wave of bacteria to invade dentinal tubules in pre-clinical caries, which is followed by decalcification of the tubules, a process allowing more bacteria to penetrate the tubules, thus forming a true nidus of infection; see Periodontitis, Plaque

pioneer neuron NEUROEMBRYOLOGY Subplate neurons appearing in the mammalian telencephalon, corresponding to the first post-mitotic neurons of the developing brain; these cells form an axonal pathway, facilitating the orientation of axonal projections, forming a neuronal scaffold which traverses the internal capsule and invades the thalamus in early fetal life; once the adult pattern of axonal projections is complete, the subplate cells disappear; pioneer neurons are also required for the formation of embryonic peripheral nerves

PIP Postinflammatory polyposis, see Inflammatory polyps

PIP$_2$ Phosphatidylinositol 4,5-biphosphate, see there

pipestem calcification A fanciful term referring to the tubular mineralization of arteries typical of extensive atherosclerosis, which may cause pseudohypertension as these vessels are relatively nondistensible

pipestem fibrosis A descriptor for the histologic appearance (portal vein fibrosis* with hyaline thickening and tortuosity of vessels) of the portal spaces in chronic hepatic involvement by *Schistosoma mansoni* and *S mekongi*; schistosomal hepatopathy mimics cirrhosis, as there is hepatosplenomegaly, portal and secondary hypertension, and variceal bleeding, but the native architecture is preserved

*aka Symmer's (clay and/or pipestem) fibrosis

pipestem ureter A thickened and fixed, aperistaltic ureter that course in a stiff pencil- or pipestem-like fashion from the kidney to bladder in advanced TB of the urinary tract

PISA Primary idiopathic sideroblastic anemia, see there

'pistol shot' pulse A loud, cracking sound heard by the stethoscope over an artery in which there is distension followed by an abrupt collapse, as classically occurs in large arteries in aortic regurgitation; see Water hammer pulse

***pit*-1 gene** A member of a large family of genes encoding proteins containing a homologous region known as the POU domain; *pit-1* is present early in mammalian embryogenesis and encodes the Pit-1 protein, a pituitary gland-specific factor that activates the transcription of growth hormone and prolactin promoters; mutations in the *pit-1* gene in mice result in a dwarf phenotype and lack of certain pituitary cells (Pit-1 protein is normally detected in somatotrophic, lactotrophic and thyrotrophic cells); see POU-domain family

pitch workers' cancer 3,4-Benzpyrene cancer Squamous cell carcinoma of the head and neck, scrotum and elsewhere, linked to prolonged exposure to 3,4-benzpyrene-rich pitch, shale oil, and tars, differing only from chimney sweeps' cancer in the occupation involved

pitting A splenic function in which intracytoplasmic inclusions, eg Howell-Jolly bodies or siderotic granules are removed from circulating RBCs; coincident with removal of the inclusion, a fragment of erythrocyte membrane is also eliminated

Pittsburgh brain stem score CRITICAL CARE MEDICINE A scale used to determine the clinical status of a victim of cerebral trauma which measures carinal, corneal, 'doll's eye' reflex, eyelash and ice water caloric reflexes, Cf Glasgow scale

Pittsburgh criteria TRANSPLANTATION A democratic multifactorial system used to select recipients of cadaveric kidneys, based on the University of Pittsburgh's transplantation experience; selection of recipients of a limited resource (transplant organs) is based on certain criteria (table); see Procurement, Transplantation; Cf Rationing

PITTSBURGH CRITERIA

WAITING TIME More time yields more points-maximum of 10

QUALITY OF ANTIGEN MATCH Two antigens each at A, B and DR histocompatibility loci, two points are given for each antigen matched-maximum of 12

PRESENCE OF PREFORMED RECIPIENT CYTOTOXIC ANTIGENS, expressed with a panel of reactive antibody number; 10 points is given if the patient is sensitized and forms antibodies to the antigens of most of the human population

MEDICAL URGENCY A rarely used criterion that is awarded when venous access sites for hemodialysis are exhausted

LOGISTIC FACTORS Ease or rapidity of transplantation; points are given if the donor organ was nearing the end of its viable storage, ie > 24 hours post-removal-maximum of 6 points

JAMA 1987; 257:3073

Pittsburgh pneumonia agent *Legionella micdadei* An often intracellular bacteria that is a frequent contaminant of hot and cold water supplies, which may cause bronchopneumonia with consolidation and a fibrinopurulent exudate, fever, pleuritic pain and cough, most often affecting immunosuppressed children; see Legionnaire's disease

pituitary-adrenal axis see Hypothalamus-pituitary-adrenal axis

pituitary apoplexy Acute life-threatening hemorrhagic infarction of the anterior pituitary gland (*adenohypophysis* [NA6]); PA is most commonly associated with an infarcted pituitary adenoma or other tumor, but may occur spontaneously, or secondary to hemorrhage of obstetric origin (Sheehan syndrome), regional radiotherapy, increased intracranial pressure, or systemic anticoagulation CLINICAL The PA 'syndrome' may be transient or permanent, and is characterized by sudden headache, loss of vision, ophthalmoplegia, and if severe, shock LABORATORY ↓ Growth hormone, ↓ gonadotropins, ↓ ACTH, ↓ TSH (with hypothyroidism), abnormal prolactin secretion, and rarely diabetes insipidus TREATMENT Replacement hormones

pituitary dwarfism Growth hormone-deficient dwarfism,

see there

PIXY 321 A formulation of IL-3 and granulocyte macrophage colony-stimulating factor, that had been proposed as a means of 'rescuing' the BM of those treated submyeloablative levels of chemotherapy in various, eg ovarian cancer; early data reveals inefficacy

PiZZ The most common variant allele in α_1-antitrypsin deficiency; the common normal allele is PiMM; see α_1-antitrypsin deficiency

'pizza pie' appearance A descriptor for the fundoscopic appearance of the variegated retinal hemorrhage seen in CMV retinitis, fancifully likened to a pizza pie with 'extra cheese'

P-K test Prausnitz-Küstner's test, see there

PKU Phenylketonuria

placebo An inactive material, often in the form of a capsule, pill, or tablet, which is identical to a drug being tested; the use of placebo controls is a required 'gold standard' component of the FDA's drug approval process, as an agent must be proved to be more effective than a placebo; Cf Nocebo

Note: Questions raised about the ethics of certain uses of placebo controls (N Engl J Med 1994; 331:394sb) are unlikely to be answered in the near future; when a negative or 'placebo' control is required to evaluate the efficacy of a therapeutic maneuver, a de facto placebo may be used, eg sham plasmapheresis

placebo effect The usually beneficial effect that an inactive or inert substance, ie a placebo, has on a patient's clinical course; up to 30% of patients with conditions having psychologic underpinnings may report clinical improvement when medicated with a placebo; diseases that may respond to placebos, eg angina, arthritis, hypertension and post-operative pain, may also respond to biofeedback; the well-described analgesic effect of placebos may be mediated by endorphins; see Biofeedback, 'Halo' effect, Hawthorne effect; Cf 'Nocebo'

placental clock OBSTETRICS A hypothetical 'timer' that is thought by some workers to be intrinsic to the placenta and control the length of gestation; evidence supporting the concept of a PC is the inverse relationship between corticotrophin-releasing hormone (CRH, which rises) and CRH-binding protein (which falls) at the end of pregnancy; the abrupt rise in available CRH is postulated to be the trigger for parturition in humans (Nature Medicine 1995; 1:460, 416)

placental lactogen Chorionic somatomammotropin, human placental lactogen, hPL A hormone that is produced at the time of the implantation of the fertilized egg; the blood levels of hPL increase slowly paralleling the placental mass, reaching a peak production of 1.0 gram/day (!) at the 32nd week of gestation; little hPL enters the fetal circulation and is both lactogenic and somatotrophic; there is indirect evidence implicating hPL in the pathogenesis of gestational diabetes mellitus

placental site trophoblastic tumor GYNECOLOGIC PATHOLOGY A rare uterine neoplasm of gestational tissue occurring in women of reproductive age, presenting as a 'missed' abortion, which ranges from microscopic to massive in size and from 'timid' to highly aggressive that actively secretes hPL (human placental lactogen) PATHOLOGY Proliferation of monomorphic intermediate trophoblast cells that separate myometrial fibers either singly or in sheets PROGNOSIS 10% mortality

placental steroid sulfatase deficiency X-linked ichthyosis, see there

placental transfusion Fetomaternal hemorrhage, see there, aka fetomaternal transfusion

plague An epidemic infection by *Yersinia pestis** spread to humans by fleas that have bitten infected rodents (bubonic or septicemic plague) or by inhalation of highly virulent encapsulated *Y pestis* when in close quarters with those infected (primary pneumonic plague) CLINICAL FORMS Bubonic (90% of cases), septicemic, pneumonic and, as a complication of any of the above, plague meningitis CLINICAL Fever, chills, prostration, headache, vomiting, diarrhea TREATMENT Streptomycin IM, tetracycline, chloramphenicol; see Bubonic plague; during plague epidemics, mortality may approach 100%; the marked aggression of the bacterium is linked to mutations in the genes encoding the proteins Yop-1 and invasin

*Described by Yersin in 1894 in Hong Kong

plaintiff FORENSIC MEDICINE A person, eg a patient who initiates a personal action or lawsuit to obtain restitution for injury or damage incurred as a result of a negligent, or allegedly negligent act

plakoglobin An 85-kD protein of the adhering junctions of epidermal cells that forms part of the antigen complexes in pemphigus foliaceus and pemphigus vulgaris

'plantibodies' Plant-derived antibodies, first produced in tobacco which may have a role in human research and applications, having the theoretical advantage of being less immunogenic than mouse antibodies

plaque CARDIOLOGY An early lesion of atherosclerosis that may be found in subjects of any age in the large to medium-sized vessels DENTISTRY An indurated accumulation of polysaccharides and bacteria eg *Lactobacillus acidophilus* and *Streptococcus mutans*; see Periodontitis DERMATOLOGY A flat, solid, elevated skin nodule ≥ 1.0 cm in diameter that is formed either by extension or coalescence of papules and may be seen in lichen amyloidosis, lichen simplex chronicus, lichen planus and psoriasis; a 'plaque' stage occurs in certain skin tumors, eg the second stages of both Kaposi sarcoma and mycosis fungoides NEUROPATHOLOGY 'Shadow plaques' Multiple, usually well-circumscribed, irregularly shaped and sharply demarcated lesions in both the gray and white matter corresponding to foci of demyelinization, seen in the brain of patients with multiple sclerosis; Cf Senile plaques

plaque-forming assay Plaque technique IMMUNOLOGY One of a group of in vitro methods that semiquantify either 1) The amount of infective particles, ie bacteria or viruses in solution, in the 'plaque assay', in which host cells are mixed with a potential pathogen in a gel and the number of cleared spaces (which represent lysed host cells are counted) or 2) The amount of lymphocytes actively producing antibodies, known as 'Jerne's plaque technique', in which lymphocytes from an animal sensitized to the RBCs of one species are mixed with the RBCs in a gel; addition of complement results in lysis by the antibody-producing lymphocytes, evidenced by a cleared red space on the agar; plaque-forming cell assays may be direct, indirect or 'reversed'

plasma ANALYTICAL CHEMISTRY A misnomer for a specimen (eg inductively coupled plasma, microwave induced plasma) that is in fact a slightly (0.01 to 0.1%) ionized gas with temperatures of 5-10 000°K HISTOLOGY Obsolete for cytoplasm LABORATORY MEDICINE A clear yellow fluid that comprises 50-55% of the blood volume, which is of 92% liquid, 7% protein and less than 1% of inorganic salts, gases, hormones, sugars and lipids; fibrinogen- and coagulation factor-depleted plasma is termed 'serum' PHYSICS A state of matter in which all atoms are ionized, which exists at a temperature of 100 000°K or more, and is colloquially known as the 'fourth state of matter' PHYSIOLOGY The fluid component of lymph

plasma cell dyscrasia Any of a group of lymphoproliferative disorders characterized by the presence of a monoclonal proliferation of plasma cells, which range in clinical behavior from the innocuous extramedullary plasmacytoma and premalignant solitary plasmacytoma of bone to multiple myeloma; Cf Monoclonal gammopathy of undetermined significance, Myeloma

plasma cell dyscrasia with polyneuropathy A rare multisystem disease that often presents with osteosclerotic bone lesions; in an analysis of 2714 plasma cell dyscrasia, 38 patients were identified who also had polyneuropathy; other findings included osteosclerotic bone lesions (82%), skin lesions (58%), lymphadenopathy (42%), papilledema (37%), hepatomegaly (24%), splenomegaly (21%); 33/38 had an abnormal M protein (IgA-λ, or IgG-λ); 5/38 had all the criteria of the POEMS syndrome*; the 5-year survival is reported to be 60% vs 20% for 'garden variety'; the term plasma cell dyscrasia with polyneuropathy encompasses both osteosclerotic myeloma and POEMS syndrome (**N Engl J Med** 1992; 327:1919oA)

*Polyneuropathy, Organomegaly (lymphadenopathy, hepatomegaly, splenomegaly), Endocrinopathy (hypogonadism or hypogonadism), Monoclonal gammopathy, Skin changes

plasma cell leukemia A neoplastic increase in circulating plasma cells; histopathologic criteria: Nuclear vacuolization, monotonous sheets of cells, > 20% leukocytes must be plasma cells or the absolute number of plasma cells in the peripheral blood must be > 2 X 10⁹/L (US: > 2000/mm³) CLINICAL Most cases are well advanced at the time of diagnosis, displaying massive tissue infiltration and marrow replacement at the time of diagnosis with a poor prognosis DDx Reactive plasmacytosis, which may be associated with agranulocytosis, burns, chronic granulomatous disease, collagen vascular disease, exanthematous lesions, hypersensitivity reactions, non-malignant hepatic disease, non-myelomatous malignancy, sarcoidosis, syphilis, subacute bacterial infection, streptococcal sepsis, typhoid, viral infection (especially infectious mononucleosis)

plasma membrane Cell membrane

plasmalemmal vesicle Caveola, see there

Plasmanate A proprietary plasma protein fraction that is approximately 90% albumin by volume; it is of occasional use as a volume expander; see Albumin, Colloid solutions; Cf Crystalloid solutions

plasmapheresis Plasma exchange Removal of plasma from the peripheral circulation, to either remove an undesired substance, eg toxins, medications (in the context of overdosage), antibodies, or other 'noxins', or less commonly, to obtain plasma for donation , resuspended in an appropriate fluid, either albumin or albumin in saline and then readministered to the patient; the removal of one plasma volume (± 2500ml) is sufficient to effect a 65% reduction in the amount of a toxin or deleterious (auto)antibody in the circulation (two volume exchanges reduce the undesired substance by another 20%); plasmapheresis is of therapeutic use in the hyperviscosity syndrome, myasthenia gravis, Eaton-Lambert syndrome, Goodpasture syndrome, post-transfusion purpura, acute Guillain-Barré syndrome, and is of use in reducing the amount of toxins in the circulation, eg paraquat, methylparathion, mushroom (*Amanita phylloides*); see Hemapheresis

Note: Despite the high level of circulating immune complexes, addition of plasma exchange to standard therapeutic regimens in connective tissue diseases does not improve the clinical outcome of either lupus nephritis* (**N Engl J Med** 1992; 326:1373oA) or the idiopathic inflammatory myopathies (**ibid**; 326:1380oA)

*Standard regimen prednisone and cyclophosphamide

plastic pancreas see Islet encapsulation

plasma protein fraction CLINICAL THERAPEUTICS A blood-derived colloid preparation that contains at least 83% albumin, providing volume expansion without risk of hepatitis or HIV-1; PPF, or albumin may be administered in the face of large-scale loss of colloid, eg hypovolemic shock, burns, retroperitoneal surgery; given its high cost, there is little justification for using albumin-based volume expanders when equivalent agents exist; futhermore, albumin infusions may rapidly increase the intravascular

oncotic pressure, drawing large quantities of water from tissues into the vascular space, potentially causing cardiac overload; albumin may also evoke hypotensive episodes by releasing of vasoactive kinins and massive infusions of albumin decrease synthesis of plasma proteins including α, β and γ globulins, fibrinogen and the coagulation factors

plasma R binder protein R binder protein, see there

plasmid EXPERIMENTAL BIOLOGY An extrachromosomal particle of DNA that is present in some bacteria, which consists of a circular segment of double-stranded DNA capable of autonomous replication, ie independently of the bacterium's replicative machinery; plasmids often carry genes that are encode proteins that are useful but not essential for cell growth or survival, eg those that carry antibiotic resistance; plasmids are of great use in recombinant DNA technology, serving as vectors for transporting 'engineered' segments of DNA of interest into bacteria to increase the copy number of the DNA for the purpose of creating radioactive 'probes' or for sequencing, a function that has been partially replaced by the polymerase chain reaction, see pBR322, R plasmid; Cf Cosmid, PCR (polymerase chain reaction), YAC cloning

plasmid vector A plasmid into which foreign DNA of interest is inserted to facilitate characterization of cloned inserts; PVs are of use for high-resolution restriction mapping, rescue of single-stranded DNA, RNA transcription, sequencing of single- and double-stranded nucleic acids, generation of nested deletions, site-directed mutagenesis, and both pro- and eukaryotic expression

plasmin A proteolytic enzyme [EC 3.4.21.7] formed from plasminogen that is responsible for the removal of blood clots; plasmin exists in free and bound (fibrin-adsorbed) forms; the former is destroyed as it is formed by antiplasmins, the latter acts as a serine endopeptidase to solubilize fibrin clots and hydrolyzes lysine and arginine bonds in certain proteins, eg fibrinogen, coagulation factors V and VII; see tPA

plasminogen A 88-kD single-stranded proenzyme (of plasmin) present in the circulation that migrates as a β-globulin contains 5 kringle domains, and is homologous to amino acid sequences in urokinase, tissue-type plasminogen activators, and prothrombin; plasminogen is converted to plasmin by cleavage of the Arg-Val bond, is synthesized in the liver, produced or stored in eosinophils and forms complexes with fibrinogen and fibrin; during coagulation large amounts of the plasminogen is integrated in the fibrin mass or clot

plasminogen activation A critical reaction in diverse biological systems in which plasminogen is converted into plasmin by tissue– or urokinase-type plasminogen activators; because plasminogen activators have been linked to the regulation of angiogenesis, embryogenesis, inflammation, ovulation, and tumor metastasis, the plasminogen-activation system may be an important mediator of tissue remodeling and cell migration

plasminogen activators A group of biologically active proteins that convert plasminogen into plasmin, divided into tissue PAs and urokinase-type PAs; see Tissue plasminogen activator

plasminogen activator inhibitor-1 A 50-kD single-chain glycoprotein member of the serpin superfamily of protease inhibitors, which has structural similarities to angiotensinogen, alpha-1-antitrypsin, and antithrombin III; PAI-1 is present in plasma, platelets, and various tissues, and rapidly forms inactive inhibitor:protease complexes in a 1:1 ratio; intravascular PAI-1 regulates the coagulation-fibrinolysis balance; ↑ plasma PAI-1 is associated with acute MI and DVT, as well as acute inflammation, aging, the dawn phenomenon, hemolytic uremic syndrome (**N Engl J Med** 1992; 327:755oA), insulin-resistance, obesity, pregnancy; PAI-1 undergoes daytime fluctuation-morning samples average 23 ng/mL; afternoon samples average 10 ng/mL (Arch Pathol Lab Med 1993; 117:67OA) extravascular PAI-1 may play a role in certain plasminogen-dependent events, to wit, angiogenesis, lysis of extracellular matrix by malignancies, and rupture of ovarian follicles MOLECULAR PATHOLOGY The PAI-1 gene contains 9 exons on chromosome 7; PAI-1 deficiency may be inherited in an AR [see MIM 173360] fashion, is due to a frame-shift mutation and is associated with major episodes of bleeding (N Engl J Med 1992; 327:1729OA) PAIs are lowest in subjects with high consumption of fruits, vegetable and root vegetables, thus having potential currency as a barometer of health; see Plasminogen activation

plastic bronchitis Fibrinous bronchitis An uncommon condition that may affect any age group, which is characterized by the production of large inspissated casts of the bronchial tree, often associated with allergic bronchopulmonary aspergillosis, bronchiectasis, and cystic fibrosis CLINICAL Dyspnea, wheezing, cough, fever and occasionally, hemoptysis (Mayo Clin Proc 1991; 66:305)

plaster cast lung A lung characterized by extensive pulmonary consolidation, most common in *Klebsiella pneumonia* infection, in which each lung weighs up to 1500 g and is covered with fibrinopurulent exudate and copious slimy, mucoid pus

plastic induration of the penis Peyronie's disease, see there

plasticizer TRANSFUSION MEDICINE Any inert chemical, eg DEHP di-2-(ethylhexylphthalate), which gives the otherwise rigid polyvinyl chloride (PVC) plastic blood collection bags their favorable physical characteristics; because DEHP leaches out from the plastic into the blood and there is some evidence that suggests there may be toxic and potentially carcinogenic effect, it is being replaced by other agents, despite the fact that DEHP increases blood shelf life

plate atelectasis RADIOLOGY Segmental atelectasis that is characterized by linear shadows of increased density at the lung bases that are horizontal, measure 1-3 mm in thickness and a few cm in length, and are typically seen after abdominal surgery or in pulmonary infarction

plateau MICROBIOLOGY A phase in the growth cycle of bacteria in culture, in which the nutrients are sufficient to sustain growth and the cells dying are equal in number to those being produced de novo

plateau development PEDIATRICS A form of disease progression that occurs in infants who reach their normal developmental milestones in the first few months or years of life, later slowing to a 'plateau' and finally begin a slow, inexhorable deterioration until death in early childhood; plateau development is characteristic of children with AIDS, Tay-Sachs disease and certain 'floppy infant' syndromes; see Floppy infant

platelet activating factor A potent pro-inflammatory phospholipid that activates cells involved in inflammation PAF is synthesized by hematopoietic (leukocytes and macrophages) and endothelial cells that causes platelet aggregation, secretion of amines, neutrophil aggregation and enzyme release and increase in vascular permeability; PAF mimics both the physiologic and immunologic effects of some IgE-mediated events of anaphylaxis and cold urticaria, may have a role in endotoxic shock, the pathogenesis of gastric ulcers and a role in ovulation via arachidonic acid metabolism, PAF is inactivated by phospholipases that cleave the substituted glycerides and by PAF acetylhydrolase (Nature 1995; 374:549L)

platelet aggregation studies LABORATORY MEDICINE A battery of assays (table) that measures the response of

PLATELET AGGREGATION					
	ADP	EPI	THROM	COLL	RISTO
B-S syndrome	N	N	N	N	↓
Glanzmann	↓	↓	↓	↓	N
platelet-vWD	Bi	Bi	Mono	Mono	
SPDisease	–	–	–		

Bi Biphasic, Coll Collagen, Epi Epinephrine, Mono Monophasic, Risto Ristocetin, Throm Thrombin
BS Bernard Soulier syndrome platelet vWD Platelet-type von Willebrand disease SPD

platelets to various aggregating substances eg ADP, epinephrine, thrombin, collagen, ristocetin and arachidonic acid, which is determined by an increase in optical density of stirred, platelet-rich plasma; normal platelets exhibit a primary and secondary phase response when exposed to collagen and ADP; platelet aggregation studies are used to diagnose coagulopathies due to platelet membrane defects

platelet antibodies see Platelet antigens

platelet antigens TRANSFUSION MEDICINE A group of antigens found on the surface of platelets that may evoke the production of platelet antibodies and be responsible for neonatal alloimmune thrombocytopenia and post-transfusion purpura, most commonly occurring as a reaction to the P1^{A1} antigen in P1^{A1} antigen-negative recipients; other platelets antigens causing purpura include Pl^{A2}, HLA-A2 and Bak^a

platelet apheresis Plateletpheresis, see there

platelet concentrate TRANSFUSION MEDICINE A blood product prepared from a single donor, which is capable of transiently ↑ the the platelet count by 5-10 x 10^9/L/M^2 body surface area in those patients where thrombocytopenia is not due to an ↑ destruction ADVERSE REACTIONS PC-related febrile transfusion reactions are related to bioreactive substances (IL-1β and IL-6) in the plasma supernatent, which ↑ with ↑ storage time and ↑ number of leukocytes in the stored unit (N Engl J Med 1994; 331:625OA) see Platelet transfusion

platelet-derived growth factor A 32 kD dimeric protein that is a potent connective tissue mitogen, stimulating proliferation of fibroblasts, intimal smooth muscle (PDGF-like substances are autocrine stimulators of smooth muscle cell proliferation in early atherogenesis) and some specialized epithelia, eg lens via tyrosine-specific phosphorylation; other PDGF activities include vasoconstriction, chemotaxis, activation of intracellular enzymes, eg glycogen synthetase and phosphatidylinositol turnover, Ca^{2+} fluxes, increased transcription of certain genes and changes of the cytoskeleton; the PDGF system is involved in atherosclerosis and fibroproliferative pathology, eg pulmonary fibrosis, glomerulonephritis, myelofibrosis, keloid formation and in carcinogenesis; the PDGF dimer is composed of A or B chains, differing in their transforming abilities and has 3 isoforms, AA, AB and BB, recognized by two different PDGF receptors

Note: PDGF's BB homodimer of PDGF has sequence homology with the v-*sis* oncogene

platelet-derived growth factor receptor A 180–190-kD membrane glycoprotein with five Ig-like extracellular domains and a kinase insert in the cytoplasm, which mediates all PDGF's activities; PDGF-R and related receptors (CSF-1 and c-*kit* proto-oncogene) require a conformational change in the receptor protein before signal transduction occurs; a second 120-kD PDGF-R is encoded by a gene on chromosome 4q11; see Immunoglobulin-like domains

platelet factor-1 Obsolete for factor V (coagulation)

platelet factor-2 Fibrinogen-activating factor A poorly characterized protein of unknown physiologic function;

when a crude preparation of PF-2 is incubated with fibrinogen, non-nitrogen protein is released, a finding that suggests that PF-2 is proteolytic; in vitro, it inhibits antithrombin III, induces platelet aggregation, and accelerates the rate of thrombin-fibrinogen interaction

platelet factor-3 Substitute phospholipid A thermostable lipoprotein that has been incompletely characterized; PF-3 is required in two steps of coagulation, to wit: the interaction between factors IXa and VIII (which activates factor X) and the interaction between factors Xa and factor V (which results in the formation of of prothrombinase), and is required for the activation of factor X by Russell's viper venom; current evidence suggests that PF-3 may be no more than platelet membrane that upon 'activation' acquires the ability to bind coagulation factors

platelet factor-4 A platelet-derived heparin-binding protein present in alpha granules and secreted therefrom during platelet aggregation as a high molecular weight tetramer associated with chondroitin sulfate; PF4 is involved in immune modulation, chemotaxis and inhibition of bone resorption and angiogenesis, and with heparin, is an antigenic target for the IgG and IgM antibodies formed in heparin-induced thrombocytopenia (**N Engl J Med 1995; 332:1374oA**)

platelet factor-5 Obsolete for fibrinogen

platelet factor-6 A poorly characterized plasmin inhibitor that may be associated with platelets

platelet factor-7 Cothromboplastin

platelet factor-8 Antithromboplastin

platelet factor-9 Accelerator globulin-stabilizing factor

platelet factor-10 Obsolete for serotonin

plateletpheresis Platelet apheresis A form of exchange transfusion in blood is removed from a patient with an extremely high (> 1-1.5 x 10^9/L) platelet count, which is directly linked to severe thrombotic and hemorrhagic phenomena; to prevent a rebound increase of platelets after the procedure, plateletpheresis must be followed by cytotosic therapy; see Therapeutic apheresis

platelet production rate LABORATORY MEDICINE The speed of turnover of platelets, calculated as platelet count/L x 0.9 divided by platelet survival x initial platelet recovery (**N Engl J Med 1992; 327:1779oA**)

platelet satellitism LABORATORY MEDICINE A relatively uncommon phenomenon characterized by the rosetting of platelets around PMNs, which occurs in EDTA-anticoagulated blood at room temperature; PS is caused by IgG autoantibodies in the serum and is mediated by CD16 (FcgIII) and in automated analyzers may 'flag' low platelet numbers (**Am J Clin Pathol 1995; 103:740**)

platelet transfusion A therapeutic modality for increasing circulating platelets (table); concentrates of platelets are obtained by a low speed ('light') centrifugation of a unit of whole blood, which yields 40-70 ml of platelet-enriched plasma containing 3 to 4 x 10^{11} platelets, a quantity sufficient to raise an 'average' adult patient's platelet levels by 10 x 10^9/L (US: 10 000/mm³); platelets are optimally stored at 20-24°C with gentle agitation and should be transfused within 5 days of harvesting; patients with immunological lability should receive platelets from a single donor; see Platelet antigens

platform Hardware platform COMPUTERS A computer hardware standard designed for a particular family of computers, eg IBM, Macintosh, UNIX, etc; in general, hardware (eg peripheral devices) or software (ie programs) created or written for one platform will not run on another platform; this generalization is rapidly changing as data cannot over long term be confined to the format in which is was created; a hardware device (eg laser printer) that 'crosses the line' is said to be cross-platform compatible

play (or else) Employer mandate, see there

'play or pay' HEALTH CARE ENVIRONMENT A universal health care coverage plan proposed by Presidents Bill and Hillary Clinton in which an employer would either provide his workers with a basic health benefits package ('play'), or pay into a government-managed insurance pool (from **Congressional Quarterly, 1993, in Clin Lab Sci 1994; 7:141**) see Clinton plan HOSPITAL STAFFING A plan begun in California in which physicians may choose either to provide coverage to a department (play) or contribute to a fund for the coverage (pay) (**Am Med News 12 October 1992 p15**)

Playboy Bunny sign A fanciful descriptor for a normal hepatic vein junction, when seen by ultrasonography, where the inferior vena cava forms the bunny's 'head', the middle and lateral hepatic veins the 'ears'; the variably present right vein forms the optional 'pipe'

'playing God' BIOMEDICAL ETHICS The usurping on the part of physicians and the health care system of the role of a 'higher power' or God; certain activities are clearly viewed as playing God, eg the rationing of limited medical resources in underserved areas or underinsured populations, deciding who is entitled to a limited number of organs for transplantation, or terminating life support in those who are terminally ill or in a persistent vegetative state (**Perspect Biol & Med 1993; 36:592**) Cf Physician invicibility syndrome CLINICAL GENETICS A colloquial term referring to the ethical issues relating to the manipulation of the human genome and whether gene therapy represented mortal man's usurping of God's omnipotence (**Nature Medicine 1995; 1:181ED**) see Gene therapy

pleated sheet beta-pleated sheet

pleitrophin A heparin-binding growth factor (formerly, HBGF-8) that is structurally unrelated to the seven members of the HBGF family of polypeptide cytokines; pleiotrophin is mitogenic to fibroblasts in culture, promotes neurite outgrowth, is developmentally expressed and is highly expressed in the brain, uterus and is also found in other sites, including gut, muscle, lung and skin

plenary session A meeting of a governing body of an organization, which may meet in camera claustrum (behind closed doors) for the purpose of discussing in private issues of a delicate or potentially delicate nature

pleomorphic adenoma see Mixed tumor

pleomorphic lobular carcinoma (breast) An aggressive subtype (6/10 dead of disease in 3.5 years of followup; 3/10 had recurrence or developed distal metastasis) of breast cancer with histologic features of lobular carcinoma, eg 'Indian file' pattern of invasion; GCDFP-15, a marker of apocrine differentiation, is positive in all cases (**Hum Pathol 1992; 23:655**)

pleomorphic xanthoastrocytoma NEUROPATHOLOGY A rare variant astrocytoma of the cerebral cortex and leptomeninges, which affects children and young adults

---

PLATELET TRANSFUSION GUIDELINES*

Platelet count < 20 x 10^9/L (US: < 20 000/mm³)

Platelet count < 40 x 10^9/L in active hemorrhage

Platelet count < 50 x 10^9/L in neonates, or patients with documented coagulopathies, recurrent fever, severe infections or patients receiving drugs that may cause platelet dysfunction

Platelet count < 100 x 10^9/L present prior to 'bloody' surgery, eg cardiopulmonary bypass or less than 48 hours after surgery

Bleeding time greater than twice the upper limit of normal

*For transfusing one unit of random-donor platelets/10 kg body weight/24 hours-JAMA 1988; 259:2415

PATHOLOGY Marked cellular pleomorphism, bizarre giant cells, prominent lipid-laden macrophages and mitotic activity without necrosis ImPx Positive for glial fibrillary acidic protein (GFAP) PROGNOSIS Relatively good, despite the tumor's aggressive ('ugly') histologic appearance

pleotypic response The constellation of metabolic processes involved in initiating cell division, including membrane transport, synthesis of DNA, RNA and proteins and protein degradation

plethysmography A technique that measures the changes in the volume of an organ, limb or the body **IMPEDANCE PLETHYSMOGRAPHY** is used to diagnose acute venous obstruction or vascular insufficiency of an extremity by measuring the change in limb volume with each arterial pulse and during cuff occlusion of the venous flow from the limb, the manipulation of which allows evaluation of either the arterial or venous flow **WHOLE BODY PLETHYSMOGRAPHY** measures the volume of gas in the lungs, including that which is trapped in poorly communicating air spaces, which is of particular use in chronic obstructive pulmonary disease and emphysema

pleural effusion A generic term for a collection of fluid in the chest, which may be benign or malignant, and are traditionally divided into transudates (with low concentrations of proteins, due to congestive heart failure, hepatic hydrothorax, nephrotic syndrome, peritoneal dialysis, and others) and exudates with high protein concentrations, due to neoplasia, infection, pulmonary embolization, GI disease, collagen vascular disease, asbestosis, and others; exudative PEs may be caused by CD3 reactivity weakens considerably with stored effusions (Acta Cytologica 1993; 37:267OA)

pleural 'tag' A radiographic 'knob' said to be seen in the periphery of one-fourth of patients with bronchoalveolar carcinoma but not with other pulmonary carcinomas

PLEVA Pityriasis lichenoides et varioliformis acuta DERMATOLOGY An idiopathic papulovesicular disease of acute* onset that is more common in the young, and in males, and characterized by successive waves of lesions of the trunk and extremities; PLEVA has certain features of allergic vasculitis with deposition of immunoglobulin and complement in the vessels, and is thought to be either due to a hypersensitivity response to an infection, eg toxoplasmosis, or in view of the gene rearrangement of the beta chain of the T-cell receptor, a lymphoproliferative disorder PATHOLOGY Spongiosis, dyskeratosis, parakeratosis, extravasation of erythrocytes TREATMENT PUVA, corticosteroids, antibiotics, methotrexate

*The chronic form, pityriasis lichenoides chronica, is more common; the hyperacute ulceronecrotic and hyperthermic form is rare

plexogenic pulmonary arteriopathy An end stage of a process initiated by an ↑ of blood flow through the pulmonary circuit; over time the initial reactive vasoconstriction becomes irreversible with vascular remodeling manifest by concentric intimal fibrosis, fibrinoid necrosis, medial hypertrophy, and the formation of plexiform lesions of the small muscular arteries (N Engl J Med 1992; 326:1682CPC)

ploidy analysis LABORATORY MEDICINE A technique in flow cytometry that evaluates the chromosomal content of cells, a parameter of aggression in malignancy; in general, diploidy, ie the presence of two haploid sets of chromosomes, is a normal or near-normal state; contrast, anaplastic and aggressive tumors are more often aneuploid or hyperdiploid; ploidy analysis is of use in prognosticating cancer of the bone (osteosarcoma), breast, colon, endometrium, lymphoma and ovary; in breast carcinoma with positive lymph nodes, survival is poor in the face of aneuploidy or hypertetraploidy; in osteosarcoma, near-diploid tumors have a low rate of relapse; hyperdiploid tumors have a high relapse rate in the early follow-up peri-

od; the same 'rule' (diploid, good prognosis, aneuploid, poor prognosis) applies to transitional cell carcinoma of the bladder, ovary and endometrium (88% of diploid and 57% of nondiploid tumors undergo progression; see Flow cytometry, S-phase analysis

plowshare-like growth SURGICAL PATHOLOGY A descriptive term for the manner of ingrowth of aggressive dysplasia as it extends laterally beneath benign epithelium; P-LG may also occur when benign epithelium grows beneath regressing dysplasia, a far less common clinical event; Cf Bulldozing pattern, Stabbing pattern

PLP Parathyroid hormone-like protein, see Hypercalcemia of malignancy

'plucked chicken' (skin) appearance DERMATOLOGY A fanciful term referring to the innumerable ('pebbly') 1-3 mm in diameter, yellow-white papules coalescing into patches, a characteristic finding in pseudoxanthoma elasticum; a similar lesion may be acquired in those exposed to Norwegian saltpeter PEDIATRICS An appearance classically described in children with Hutchinson-Gilford progeria, characterized by alopecia, midfacial cyanosis, atrophy of subcutaneous fat, sculptured nose with a 'beaked' tip, a disproportionately large head, prominent eyes and scalp veins, nail and dental dystrophy, micrognathia, xeroderma, pyriform thorax, a horse-riding stance, thin limbs, stiff joints and osteoporosis

plume ENVIRONMENT A 'feather-like' extension of contaminated ground water into an aquifer from the site of the initial in-ground dumping of toxic chemicals, which extends for a variable, usually downgradient distance of up to ten miles; the speed of the spread is a function of the soil's porosity, frequency of rainfall and whether water is being added or removed from the aquifer by human sources; removal of a plume is virtually impossible and it may require decades to centuries before the contaminated soil is washed clean of a pollutant

plump hilus sign Fleischer sign RADIOLOGY An ↑ prominence of the hilar vasculature on the side most affected in acute pulmonary thromboembolism on a plain chest film

pluralistic system HEALTH CARE FINANCING The existence of multiple types of insurance (private and public) and mechanisms (eg fee-for-service, HMOs) for delivery those services (Am Med News 25 October 1992, p7)

plus strand The strand of a nucleic acid (usually RNA) of viral origin (often of bacteriophage origin) that is used as a template for the production of a complementary (minus) strand of RNA; together the plus and minus strands form double-stranded RNA, which is the replicative form of the virus; Cf Minus strand

plutonium Element 94, the isotopic forms of which have mass numbers of 232 to 246; ^{239}Pu has a $T_{1/2}$ of 24 360 years and is produced in quantity from ^{238}U by nuclear power plants; 1-8 kg (2.2-17.6 lbs) of pure plutonium is required to produce a nuclear device (euphemism for bomb); one metric ton (2205 lbs) can produce 125-1000 warheads; there are ± 1200 tons of surplus plutonium in the world, which is becoming an increasing difficult disposal problem, given that there is no place to store it, as the proposed Yucca Mountain site in Nevada has been rejected, in part because of the fear of it reaching 'critical mass' and exploding (NY Times March 14 1995, C1) see High-level waste, Radioactive waste

PM$_{10}$ A generic term for organic particles measuring < 10 µm in diameter, which have been linked to ↑ morbidity and mortality on days of heavy air pollution, which are also found in 'natural' (eg wood) smoke (Science 1995; 267:1771)

PMA Phorbol myristate acetate

PML Progressive multifocal leukoencephalopathy, see there

PMLE Polymorphous light eruption, see there

PMNs Polymorphonuclear leukocytes, Neutrophilic granulocytes

PMP22 A myelin protein gene that maps to chromosome segment 17p11.2-p12; patients with Charcot-Marie-Tooth disease type 1A have a point mutation in *PMP22* with a 1.5 megabase duplication in 17p11.2-p12 which is AD; disease expression may be due to a dosage effect (**N Engl J Med 1993; 329:96**OA)

PMR Proportionate mortality ratio, see there

PMS Premenstrual syndrome(s) Premenstrual dysphoric disorder (per American Psychiatric Association in DSM-IV) A group of disorders characterized by affective, behavioral and somatic symptoms that consistently occur during the luteal (second) phase of the menstrual cycle, resolving with the onset of menstruation and vaguely linked to the fall in estrogen and progesterone from luteal peaks; although PMS was assumed to be a progestational endocrine dysfunction, the use of mifepristone, an antiprogestational agent to induce menses and luteo-lysis, did not affect the severity or duration of a PMS 'attack' (**N Engl J Med 1991; 324:1174, 1208ed**) PATHOGENESIS Uncertain, thought to be linked to serotoninergic dysregulation CLINICAL see Table, premenstrual dysphoric disorder; PMS affects 10-30% of menstruating ♀ and is characterized by several days of mental or physical incapacitation of varying intensity, insomnia, headache, emotional lability (anxiety, depression, irritability, loss of concentration, poor judgement, mood swings and tendency towards violence, evoked by environmental cues), acne, breast enlargement, fullness or tenderness, abdominal bloating with edema, craving for salty, sweet or 'junk' food TREATMENT Fluoxetine (Prozac) is reported to be of use in treating the symptoms of tension, irritability, and dysphoria (**N Engl J Med 1995; 332:1529**OAD) medical or surgical ovariectomy and anxiolytic drugs are reported to be marginally superior to placebos

PMT 1) GYNECOLOGY Pre-menstrual tension see PMS 2) INSTRUMENTATION see Photomultiplier tube

PNA Peptide nucleic acid, see there

PNET Peripheral neuroendocrine or neuroepithelial tumor, see there

pneumatic tube system A system for transporting specimens and drugs in a hospital, which is designed to eliminate bottlenecks of inefficiency that occur with conventional (human) transport; the state-of-the-art PTS is run by computer and supports an extensive network of stations; not all specimens are approved for sending through the PTS; approved items include forms and paperwork, specimens for analysis of blood gases, serum toxicology and hematology, IV or irrigations solutions, blood components, items NOT approved for PTS transportation include body fluids, stool specimens, specimens for viral testing, eg HBV, HIV, investigational drugs, chemotherapeutics, blood derivatives (**Advance/Lab July/August, Sept 1994**)

pneumatosis cystoides intestinalis An uncommon disorder with multiple, variably-sized submucosal blebs of gas in the small intestine, large intestine and stomach that may percolate into the mesentery and omentum; 20% of PCI is related to COPD and respiratory distress, the rest are sporadic and asymptomatic, seen as an incidental radiologic finding on a plain abdominal film; PCI has been described in peptic ulcer disease, intestinal obstruction, GI bypass surgery for morbid obesity, mesenteric vascular occlusion, acute necrotizing enterocolitis, inflammatory bowel disease, perforated diverticulitis, collagen vascular disease, cystic fibrosis, DM, appendicitis, Whipple's disease, abdominal trauma (extrinsic or the result of endoscopy), ingestion of caustics, parasitosis, tuberculosis, lymphoproliferative disease PATHOGENESIS Uncertain;

hypotheses include mechanical percolation of gas pockets into tissue spaces, tissue invasion by bacteria with subsequent gas production and fermentation of carbohydrates in the intestinal lumen

Pneumocystis carinii An opportunistic microorganism[1] causing pneumonia (PCP) in immunocompromised hosts, in particular those with AIDS[2], as well as those with leukemia, lymphoma, organ transplantation, corticosteroid therapy, cytotoxic drugs, and the elderly (**N Engl J Med 1991; 324:246**); the uptake of *P carinii* into macrophages is mediated by a macrophage mannose receptor, a surface glycoprotein of the 'high mannose' type (**Nature 1991; 351:155**); the initial episode of PCP requiring hospitalization carries a 53% mortality; 63% die within a year of the first episode; 75% of those who survive the first hospitalization for PCP survive ≥ 1 year (**JAMA 1991; 266:89**) DIAGNOSIS GMS staining of tissues; *P carinii* also causes otic infection and choroiditis (**Arch Pathol Lab Med 1992; 116:500**OA) PROPHYLAXIS, which is not recieved in ⅔ of patients (**N Engl J Med 1995; 332:786**SA) in patients with advanced HIV infection, aerosolized pentamidine, T-S, and high-dose dapsone are equally effective; the latter two are superior in patients with < 100 CD4+/mm³ (**ibid; 332:693**OA) TREATMENT Anti-pneumocystis chemotherapy: T-S once a day is more effective as primary prophylaxis for PCP than aerosolized pentamidine (**N Engl J Med 1992; 327:1836**OA, **1842**OA), manipulation of the inflammatory response, and immunologic enhancement (**N Engl J Med 1992; 327:1853**RV) pentamidine, atovaquone, trimetrexate glucuronate; in HIV-infected patients with PCP, ↑ CEA (8.8 vs 2.7 ng/mL in normals) is associated with a poor short-term prognosis and a mortality of ± 80% with a CEA > 20 ng/mL (**Scand J Infect Dis 1992; 24:309**)

[1]*P carinii* has been traditionally regarded as a parasite with a thick-walled cyst containing six to eight round sporozoites that develop into trophozoites, it may be related to fungi, given the location of certain major genes and its wall composition (**N Engl J Med 1991; 324:263ed**) [2]PCP is an opportunistic infection that signals the onset of AIDS in children

pneumolysin INFECTIOUS DISEASE An intracellular protein produced by *Streptococcus pneumoniae* and released during bacteriolysis, which is active in pore formation and is cytotoxic to all the cells in the lung (**N Engl J Med 1995; 332:1280**RV)

PNS Peripheral nervous system, see there

pocket DENTISTRY A pathologically altered or enlarged gingival sulcus, which is so defined when the distance from the gingival margin is ≥ 3 mm; in normal and healthy periodontium, gingival tissue is snugly fit around the teeth, and the gingival crevice is essentially zero; in the face of inflammation, the ↑ in the bulk of gingival tissue around the teeth results in an ↑ depth of tissue around the teeth, which if confined to the gingiva is known as a gingival (pseudo-) pocket; if the pocket extends into the periodontium, it is known as a periodontal pocket

pocket dosimeter Pocket chamber RADIOLOGY A small ionization chamber worn by those who are occupationally exposed to ionizing radiation; the PD functions on the condensor-discharge principle and semiquantifies incident X-rays, thus being a means by which a person's radiation exposure can be measured; Cf Air monitor, Film badge

pocket drug A pharmaceutical designed to treat an infection with a virus that has its binding site in a 'canyon', the first one of which was identified in a rhinovirus (agent of the common cold) and measured 2.5 nm x 1.2 nm; PDs would in theory bind in the canyon, deform and stabilize the binding site(s), and prevent viral shedding (**Bio/Technology 1992; 10:502**) see Canyon hypothesis

'pocket shot' SUBSTANCE ABUSE Injection of heroin, cocaine or other substance(s) of abuse into the 'pocket' in the neck located lateral to the sternocleidomastoid muscle and above the clavicle in an attempt to directly inject the internal jugular vein; given the relative lack of dexterity, the abuser may cause an apical pneumothorax or hydrothorax, often left-sided as most people are right-handed, in addition to an abscess related to non-sterile needles; Cf Skin 'Popping'

pocketing DENTISTRY The formation of a pocket, see there

pockmark Pock mark A deep, sharply circumscriped 'icepick'-like scar seen in patients who have recovered from smallpox, a disease now of historic interest

podiatry The field of health care dedicated to the diagnosis and treatment of anatomic or traumatic diseases of the foot; podiatrists (chiropodists) are graduates of a four-year education program that follows a college or university education; podiatrists are examined and licensed by a state's medical board, carry a title of Doctor of Podiatric Medicine (DPM) and treat diseases of the feet by medicine or surgery

POEMS syndrome Crow-Fucase syndrome A multisystem disease characterized by the acronym of POEMS for Polyneuropathy (distal symmetric progressive weakness, paresthesias and ↓ nerve conduction velocity), Organomegaly (hepatosplenomegaly, lymphadenopathy), Endocrinopathy (hirsutism), Monoclonal gammopathy (myeloma and focal osteosclerosis) and Skin lesions (hyperpigmentation, hypertrichosis, pachydermia and Terry-type nails)

poikilocyte Jigsaw puzzle cell Any of a number of bizarre, variably sized and shaped erythrocytes*, fancifully likened to the jagged pieces of a jigsaw puzzle that may be due to mechanical damage, as in severe hereditary spherocytosis or elliptocytosis, denaturation of spectrin, as in in vitro thermal injury to red cells in hereditary pyropoikilocytosis or in Woronet's trait, an asymptomatic genetic curiosity

*Under the rubric of poikilocytes are acanthocytes, dacryocytes, echinocytes, elliptocytes, schizocytes, spherocytes

POISON TOXICITIES	
Minimum lethal dose, mole/kg	
Botulinum toxin A	3.3×10^{-17}
Tetanus toxin	1.0×10^{-15}
Diphtheria toxin	4.2×10^{-12}
Agent Orange	3.1×10^{-9}
Curare	7.2×10^{-7}
Strychnine	1.5×10^{-6}
Cyanide	2.0×10^{-4}

point-of-care option HEALTH CARE REFORM A rider (supplementary policy) that is attached to a health insurance plan that allows an enrollee in an HMO (health maintenance organization) the option to seek care from a particular specialist on a fee-for-service basis, eg an OB/Gyn or psychiatrist with whom the person has a particularly strong relationship; the POC option allows the consumer the freedom of choice at a higher premium cost, and often require co-payments and the meeting of deductibles; it replaces indemnity and preferred provider organizations (Am Med News 19 Sept 1994)

point-of-care testing LABORATORY MEDICINE The analysis* of clinical specimens as close as is possible to the patient, ranging from the bedside to ward (unit), or 'stat' regional response laboratories that service specified areas, including the emergency room or the intensive care unit; while the costs (eg reagents, need to purchase and maintain instruments that duplicate functions of the central laboratory) in POCT are generally much higher than those of similar tests performed in a central laboratory, the total costs may actually be reduced as labor is performed by personnel, eg nurses, physicians' assistants, and others who are already performing different duties at the bedside (CAP Today 1993; 7:1); while POCT would appear to clearly useful, no one has proven that

improved timeliness of test results improves patient care; moreover the implementation of POCT may be hampered by the equipment failure and lack of understanding of rudimentary quality control issues (CAP Today Dec 1993; 7:1, Am Clin Lab Dec/Jan 1994, p6; 11) for further details see Mayo Clin Proceedings 1995; 70:493-4; for pros and cons of POC testing, see Am Clin Lab, July 1994

*Synonyms include '…bedside testing, near-patient testing, decentralized testing, patient-focused testing, ancillary testing, and alternate site testing. This multiplicity of names reflects the wide variety of ways that such a service can be rendered (Mayo Clin Proc 1995; 70:493-4)

point mutation MOLECULAR BIOLOGY A change in one nucleotide on double-stranded DNA; because of the so-called 'degeneracy' of DNA (where 60 different triplets of DNA nucleotides encode only 20 amino acids), there is considerable margin for error, and thus many PMs are 'silent'; PMs can be detected by single-strand conformation polymorphisms and direct sequencing of the DNA after amplifying the sequence with PCR; see Degenerate code, Frame shift mutation

poison A generic term for any substance that adversely affects the metabolism of a cell, tissue or entire organism, evoking biochemical and histologic changes, which may evoke irreversible cell damage and/or death; many toxins are removable by hemodialysis or peritoneal dialysis, eg sedative-hypnotics (chloral hydrate, ethanol, ethylene glycol, methanol, barbiturates, meprobamate), non-narcotic analgesics (acetaminophen, aspirin, phenacetin), amphetamines, heavy metals (arsenic, lead, mercury), metallic salts (eg of calcium or lithium), halides, alkaloids (quinine, strychnine), anilines, carbon tetrachloride, ergotamine, isoniazid, nitrofurantoin, phenytoin, theophylline; other compounds are poorly removed by dialysis, including amitriptyline, anticholinergics, antidepressants, atropine, benzodiazepines, digitalis, hallucinogens, heroin, methaqualone, phenelzine, phenothiazines, propoxyphene

poison ivy 1) A highly allergenic plant that owes this property to the chemical urushiol found in this and other plants, eg mango, japanese lacquer tree and cashews; the most common urushiol-bearing plants in the USA are poison ivy (*Toxicodendron radicans*), located in the eastern US, poison oak (*T diversilobium*), located in the West, and poison sumac (*T vernix*), located in the South Note: Urushiols may be carried by smoke from burning plants, potentially causing tracheitis and pulmonary edema in highly-sensitive individuals; see Urushiol 2) A relative colloquial term for any allergic reaction or dermatopathy caused by 1), above

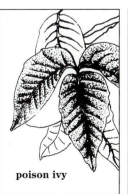

poison ivy

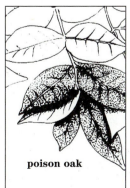

poison oak

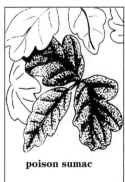

poison sumac

Poisson, R A professor and surgeon at St Luc Hospital in Montreal who was alleged to have falsified and manipulated data on three breast lumpectomy trials (B-06, B-13, B-14) of the NSABP (National Surgical Adjuvant Breast and Bowel Project), that were directed by Bernard Fisher, of Pittsburgh, and compromised the conclusions of some federally funded lumpectomy studies (N Engl J Med 1994; 330:1448ED, 1458C)

pokeweed mitogen A carbohydrate-binding lectin isolated from *Phytolocca americana* that stimulates the growth and proliferation of B cells in culture, resulting in production of cytoplasmic or supernatant immunoglobulin; Cf Concanavalin-A, Lectins, Phytohemagglutinin

pokkuri Sudden unexplained nocturnal death, see there

pol Polymerase, see DNA polymerases

POL Physician office laboratory, see there

pol I RNA polymerase I, see there

pol II RNA polymerase II, see there

pol III RNA polymerase III, see there

pol A structural gene of retroviruses that encodes reverse transcriptase, the other two structural genes are *gag* and *env*; see HIV-1, HIV-2, Retrovirus

Poland syndrome An AD [MIM 173800] condition* characterized by unilateral hypoplasia of skeletal muscle in the shoulder and breast region, affecting the pectoralis major, serratus anterior and latissimus dorsi), which is variably accompanied by hypoplasia of the ribs, hand or entire arm, or ipsilateral syndactyly; as most cases of PS have been sporadic, it is thought that it is largely a nonspecific developmental field defect, ie a sequence (see there)

*Described by A Poland (1820-1872) in 1841

polar anemia Arctic anemia, see there

polar body The non-functional haploid daughter of a reduction division; prior to ovulation, the egg in the graafian follicle undergoes reduction division; one-half of the chromosomal complement, a haploid set is allocated to the mature, or secondary oocyte, the other haploid of 23 chromosomes becomes a small daughter, the first polar body; when the sperm penetrates the egg, a second reduction division occurs, a second polar body is formed which also degenerates; Cf Graafian follicle

polar cap see Capping

polar leprosy A designation for either of the two extreme forms of leprosy; **POLAR LEPROMATOUS LEPROSY** is substantially more aggressive than the polar tuberculous form, with numerous lesions, an intense tissue load of organisms which blatently ignore the effete host defense, progressive papulo-nodular lesions and diffuse cutaneous induration **POLAR TUBERCULOID LEPROSY** has a relatively good prognosis, few organisms are present in the tissue and the body is capable of reacting with granuloma formation; see Borderline disease, Leonine face

polarization SURGICAL PATHOLOGY A technique in which fluids and tissues are analyzed for the presence of crystals or crystalline material with an intrinsic ability to change the direction of light passing through them; when the polarizing lenses are crossed, no light can pass through and the field is black; the '+' and '−' adjectives refer to the change in the pathway of the light when a compensator (prepared from a glass slide with streaks cut in clear cellophane tape) is used; anisotropic crystals appear whitish and are not equal in different directions, thus having 'double' polarizing power or birefringence; anisotropism occurs in urate crystals (birefringence refers to polarization at a refractive index of one); without a compensator, the field is dark except for birefringent crystals of monosodium urate, calcium pyrophosphate, talc, cholesterol, and oval fat bodies; with the compensator added, the field is red and the crystal is either yellow or blue according to the orientation of the crystals; see Microscopy

polarization microscopy A technique used in light microscopy to study the anisotropic properties of various substances, eg crystals; see Microscopy, Polarization

'policeman of the abdomen' A fanciful synonym for the omentum, so designated as it was once thought that the omentum had an intrinsic ability to move within the peritoneal cavity to sites of infection or inflammation; the little movement that does occur with the omentum is due to diaphragmatic excursion, intestinal peristalsis and postural changes (rather than an intrinsic ameboid movement); the omentum's immune role is modest and, at most, acts as a repository for macrophages; Cf Pancake omentum

policy manual LABORATORY MEDICINE A formal document that reflects the philosophy and goals of the laboratory and the hospital, which is approved and dated by the laboratory director and indicates a course of action or standard by which the individual worker will act in various situations

polio(myelitis) vaccine(s) Either of two vaccines available in the US for preventing poliomyelitis; both are highly effective and have a 95% 'take' rate of protection; the per os live attenuated Sabin vaccine is preferred by many workers to the subcutaneous inactivated (killed) Salk vaccine COMPLICATIONS Vaccine-related paralysis occurs in 1 of 2.6 million administrations of vaccines CONTRAINDICATIONS Pregnancy, immunocompromise; see Vaccine

political action committee A 'special interest' group unique to the United States, often based in Washington DC, that distributes literature, lobbies for and makes contributions to politicians in order to influence decisions in the US Congress and Senate; eg a PAC organized by the American Medical Association will lobby for equitable changes in malpractice law, or firearms hobbyists will lobby against gun control; see AMPAC

politically correct Politically sensitive *adjective* Pertaining or referring to language that reflects awareness and sensitivity to another (see table) person's physical, mental, cultural, or other disadvantages[1] or deviations from a norm; 'political correctness' is a stance of recent vintage that has been integrated into the mainstream spoken word, in particular since the Americans with Disabilites Act; , a person is no longer described as mentally retarded, but rather as mentally disabled or challenged; a person is not obese but suffers an eating disorder[2], and so on Note: Some authors believe that 'PC speak' has reached a point of absurdity

[1]PC tries to 'level the playing fields' in human relations; any exercise that attempts to make all men (and women), of all abilities, sizes, shapes, and colors equals is ultimately doomed to failure (eg men have yet to carry an infant to full term) [2]The 'PCness' platform suffers *reductio ad absurdum* when it is applied to those mental or physical features for which it was not originally (see table)

politically sensitive Politically correct, see there

'polka dot' pattern A descriptor for the multiple, small, circular patches involving a few hair shafts, seen in early scalp involvement by the superficial dermatophytic fungus *Trichophyton tonsurans*, which is an endothrix-type infection

POLL Physician office to laboratory link, see there

Polle syndrome Munchausen-by-proxy syndrome, see there

pollen The male gametophyte of flowering plants, which is a major evocateur (sic) of seasonal allergies; although virtually any pollen from grasses (eg Bermuda, blue, orchard, and so on), trees (ash, cedar, juniper, mesquite, etc), and weeds (eg marsh elder, kochia, and others) can trigger an immune response, ragweed (and related henchmen, eg feverfew) has garnered the greatest revulsion among the allergically challenged

Rosy reports in the literature to the contrary, desensitization therapy (shots)

pollen count ALLERGY MEDICINE An estimation of the number of allergenic pollen particles present in a standard volume of air; in the US, pollen counting has been somewhat of a 'cottage industry', and PCs are reported in a haphazard nonstandardized format, a deficiency that the US Academy of Allergy, Asthma, and Immunology, is attempting to rectify, by certifying pollen counting stations (New York Times 5 April 1995, C17)

pollutant A generic term for any unnatural substance released into the environment (air, water, or soil); the majority of pollutants are of industrial origin, and include DDT, dioxins, PCBs, TCE, and petroleum byproducts; some have estrogenic activity and impact on reproduction of animals at all levels of the food chain (Sci Am 1993; 269/3:34)

Pollution Standards Index ENVIRONMENT, PUBLIC HEALTH PSI An index of air quality that converts the daily concentrations of five major pollutants (carbon monoxide, nitrogen dioxide, ozone, particulate matter, and sulfur dioxide) into a single figure representing the worst air quality recorded each day, placed on a scale from 0 to 500, with values of $\geq$ 200 being regarded as an unhealthful (MMWR 1993; 41:967, N Engl J Med 1994; 331:1542OA) see Air pollution, Unhealthful day

Pollyannaism A descriptor for one of the postures in a doctor-patient relationship, in which the doctor (a 'Pollyanna') wears a facade of joviality and exudes unrealistic optimism in the face of terminal illness, disregarding the usual anxiety experienced by the patient, a posture that has been widely criticized; Pollyanna is the key character in Eleanor Porter's novel by the same name, who always looked on the positive side of any situation, however disastrous it might have been

POLITICALLY CORRECT SPEECH–A MICROGLOSSARY	
BLACK	African-American
DEMENTED	Disoriented, severely confused
HOMOPHOBIC	Heterosexually biased
HOUSEBOUND	Domestic
IGNORANCE	Knowledge deficit
(AMERICAN) INDIAN	Native American
MENTALLY RETARDED	Mentally disabled or challenged
MENTALLY SLOW	Educationally challenged
MYOPIC	Visually challenged
OBESE	Large
PHYSICALLY HANDICAPPED	Physically disadvantaged
POORLY EDUCATED	Educationally disadvantaged
RACIST	Culturally insensitive
TALL	Vertically enhanced
SHORT	Vertically compromised
STUPID	Obtunded

poly A Polyadenylation sequence, Poly(A) tail, see there

polyacrylamide gel electrophoresis LABORATORY METHODOLOGY A type of high-resolution zone electrophoresis performed on a cross-linked polyacrylamide gel, which forms a component of the SDS-PAGE and disc gel electrophoretic procedures; see SDS-PAGE

polyadenylation MOLECULAR BIOLOGY The addition of a sequence of polyadenylic acid to the 3' end of mRNA after its transcription from DNA

polyadenylation sequence MOLECULAR BIOLOGY An oligonucleotide segment of DNA that signals RNA polymerase II in ribosomes to terminate mRNA transcription; in thalassemia, poly A (AATAAA) is the signal leading to the premature cleavage of the β globin gene transcript and addition of the poly-A track; in some patients with hemoglobin H disease with a defective α^+ thalassemia gene, a point mutation changes the polyadenylation signal to AATAGA, resulting in an incorrectly processed and prematurely degraded RNA transcript

polyagglutinability The ability to agglutinate with a wide variety of antigen

polyagglutination Panagglutination TRANSFUSION MEDICINE The agglutination of RBCs in the presence of serum containing antibodies, autoagglutinins, or alloagglutinins, which reflects an alteration in the surface antigens; RBCs may have altered membranes and are inappropriately agglutinated by anti-A or anti-B reagent serum, which is related to altered glycoproteins, eg T, Tn and Cad; polyagglutination may also occur with acquired B antigens and in HEMPAS and may be due to contamination of the serum by detergents, silica or metallic cations

poly(A) tail MOLECULAR BIOLOGY A segment of 20-200 adenylic acid residues attached to the 3'-end of eukaryotic mRNA that is thought to increase mRNA's molecular stability by increasing its resistance to nuclease; see Transcription unit

polyarteritis nodosa A generalized arteritis that is classified as a connective tissue disease and is characterized by necrotizing vasculitis of small– to medium-sized arteries, affecting multiple organ systems, including the GI tract, kidneys, liver, muscle, and skin; in > 50%, vasculitis affects peripheral nerves as either mononeuritis multiplex or symmetric sensorimotor polyneuropathy CLINICAL Fever, malaise, myalgia LABORATORY ↑ WBCs, ↑ ESR, 30-50% have HBsAg or HBsAb titers TREATMENT Immunosuppression, eg prednisone and cyclophosphamide yields ± 90% five-year survival (N Engl J Med 1994; 331:93CPC)

Polybrene® Hexadimethrine bromide TRANSFUSION MEDICINE A polyvalent cationic polymer used to reduce the electrostatic repulsion (zeta potential) between erythrocytes, thereby enhancing the detection of weak agglutination when testing red cells for potential donor-recipient transfusion reactions; weak agglutination causes aggregation of normal RBCs that can be dispersed by sodium citrate (in absence of aggregating antibody); if antibodies coat the RBCs, the bridges formed among the RBCs are strong and cannot be broken by sodium citrate; see Zeta potential

$$\left[\ —\ \overset{\overset{\displaystyle CH_3}{|}}{\underset{\underset{\displaystyle CH_3}{|}}{N^+}}\ —\ (CH_3)_6\ —\ \overset{\overset{\displaystyle CH_3}{|}}{\underset{\underset{\displaystyle CH_3}{|}}{N^+}}\ —\ (CH_3)_2\ \right]\ 2Br^-$$

Polybrene®

Polybrene® technique TRANSFUSION MEDICINE A method used to detect the presence of antigens on the surface of RBCs using antiglobulin-reactive antisera and Polybrene®, see there

polychlorinated biphenyls PCBs, see there

polychromatophilia A combination of hemoglobin's affinity for acid stains and RNA's affinity for basic stains, eg Wright-Giemsa stain, a normal finding in young RBCs with residual RNA; polychromatophilia of RBCs may occur in blood loss, hemolysis, anoxia, pulmonary disease, renal cell carcinoma, polycythemia vera and secondary polycythemia, eg living at high altitudes, massive obesity, COPD, ectopic erythropoietin production by tumors, eg hepatomas, pheochromocytomas, and uterine leiomyoma

polyclonal antibodies A bouquet of immunoglobulins produced by multiple, usually non-malignant clones of cells that have been summoned to arms by an antigen, which may evoke multiple clonal expansions, each responding to a different epitope on the antigen; see Epitope, Idiotype; Cf Monoclonal antibodies

polyculture GLOBAL VILLAGE A generic term for the cultivation of multiple food crops in a confined space or farm; polyculture is being increasingly recognized as a more sustainable and economically sound agricultural and land management policy than that of monoculture (Sci Am 1994; 270/7:30) see Monoculture

polycyclic aromatic hydrocarbons Any of a family of compounds (eg benzo[a]pyrene, see figure, Bay region) that are composed of fused benzene rings that are water insoluble but readily absorbed through the lungs or GI tract; PAHs are common byproducts of fossil fuel (coal, wood, diesel) combustion, and as such, common pollutants; they are procarcinogens as their final reaction products are dihydrodiol epoxides that have a strong affinity for DNA, RNA, and proteins, which have a nucleophilic sites and form DNA-carcinogen adducts; PAH exposure has been linked to an ↑ risk of lung and skin cancer

aka Polycyclic and heterocyclic aromatic amines/hydrocarbons

polycystic kidneys A variety of classifications exist for cystic diseases of the kidneys; since none is completely satisfactory or based on either pathogenesis or etiology, a pragmatic approach is to classify these lesions based on gross morphology which correlates reasonably well with clinical presentation and presumed hereditary transmission (table); see Autosomal dominant polycystic kidney disease, Multilocular cyst of the kidney

CYSTIC DISORDERS OF THE KIDNEYS

RENAL DYSPLASIA A relatively common, often acquired condition presenting in infancy as unilateral or bilateral and segmental, focally irregular cystic kidneys, related to mesenchymal immaturity and accompanied by obstruction

INFANTILE POLYCYSTIC KIDNEYS An uncommon autosomal recessive condition first seen in infants with massively enlarged kidneys and aberrant bile duct formation

ADULT POLYCYSTIC KIDNEYS A common (1-2:1000 in the general population) autosomal dominant condition located to a gene on chromosome 16 affecting adults with large bumpy kidneys, cysts in the liver, lung and pancreas and berry aneurysms of the brain

MEDULLARY SPONGE KIDNEYS A relatively common bilateral condition of uncertain pattern of heredity, affecting adults with inability to concentrate urine, hypercalcemia, nephrolithiasis, pyelonephritis, distal renal tubular acidosis and cystic dilation of the collecting ducts; renal function and lifespan may be normal

UREMIC MEDULLARY SPONGE KIDNEY A rare inherited condition first seen in young adults as bilateral corticomedullary junction cysts and functional tubular defects, Fanconi syndrome and uremia

polycystic liver disease A condition characterized by multiple millimeter to centimeter in diameter cysts lined by cuboidal epithelium; the hepatic disease is often obscured by the accompanying adult polycystic renal disease; 40% of the affected livers also contain von Meyenburg's complexes

polycystic ovaries Stein-Leventhal syndrome An idiopathic condition affecting 3.5-7.0% of females that is the most common endocrinopathy causing familial hirsutism CLINICAL Obesity, hirsutism, galactorrhea, secondary amenorrhea following dysmenorrhea, acne vulgaris, and an ↑ risk of endometrial carcinoma due to unopposed estrogenic stimulation; some cases are associated with CNS trauma or injury in childhood DIAGNOSIS Palpation, ultrasonography PATHOGENESIS Uncertain, ↑ in oxidation by 11 β-hydroxysteroid dehydrogenase results in an ↑ ratio of 11-oxo metabolites of cortisol and corticosterone to their 11-hydroxy metabolites in the urine, which may be responsible for the chronic adrenal hyperandrogenism (N Engl J Med 1994; 330:458oa) PATHOLOGY Ovaries are large pale, polycystic with thick fibrous capsules LABORATORY ↑ serum LH (luteinizing hormone) or LH/FSH ratio, ↑ prolactin, ↑ response to nafarelin (a GnRH-gonadotropin hormone-releasing hormone agonist) (N Engl J Med 1992; 327:157oa) that causes a ♂ pattern response, suggesting that PCO has defective regulation of 17-hydroxylase and C-17,20-lyase PCO, sterility, menstrual abnormalities and hyperandrogenism may be associated with valproate therapy for epilepsy (N Engl J Med 1993; 329:1383oa) see HAIR-AN syndrome

polycythemia A generic term for any increase in red cell mass; polycythemia may be 1) Elative, ie above normal but not pathological, see Relative polycythemia 2) Secondary to a various physiopathologic mechanisms, usually hypoxia or ↑ erythropoietin secretion, see Secondary polycythemia 3) Neoplastic, ie polycythemia vera, see there

polycythemia vera HEMATOLOGY A chronic idiopathic myeloproliferative disorder due to the expansion of an abnormal pluripotent stem cell population with ↑ erythropoietin-independent erythropoiesis and megakaryopoiesis LABORATORY ↑ Leukocyte alkaline phosphatase, ↑ platelets, basophils, ↑ vitamin B_{12}, vitamin B_{12} binding capacity (transcobalamin I and III), ↓ erythropoietin and stainable iron in the bone marrow with myelofibrosis and extramedullary hematopoiesis; in PV, erythropoietin is low 2.1 U/L (vs 6.7 U/L), in relative polycythemia, normal (7.0 U/L), and in secondary polycythemia, high (121.7 U/L) (Br J Haematol 1992; 81:603); 15-20% of cases resolve in a so-called 'spent' phase with marrow fibrosis PROGNOSIS 40% die of thrombosis and hemorrhage; others are at ↑ risk of myeloproliferative disease–5-15% of patients develop acute leukemia or myeloid metaplasia, or less comonly, acute leukemia of the FAB-M6 type DIAGNOSIS PV requires that either all of 'A' criteria are present or two 'A' criteria and two 'B' criteria are present (table) TREATMENT Simple phlebotomy yields a 14-year survival; ^{32}P yields a 12 year survival and chlorambucil, a 9 year survival; the latter two may inducer secondary leukemia; hydroxyurea may be used for long-term treatment

POLYCYTHEMIA VERA

A CLINICAL

A1	↑ RBC mass (♂ > 36 ml/kg, ♀ > 32 mg/kg)
A2	Arterial O_2 saturation > 92% (near normal)
A3	Splenomegaly (present in 75%)

B LABORATORY

B1	Thrombocytosis > 400 x 10^9/L (most cases)
B2	Leukocytosis > 12 x 10^9/L, without fever or infection
B3	↑ Alkaline phosphatase
B4	↑ B_{12} > 666 pmol/L (US > 900 pg/ml)

polydactyly with neonatal chondrodystrophy Short-rib polydactyly syndromes, see there

polydrug therapy see Polypharmacy

polyembryoma A rare, highly aggressive ovarian germ cell tumor of young adults characterized by numerous embryoid bodies resembling normal presomite embryos, invariably associated with malignant teratoma; see Embryoid bodies

polyendocrine deficiency syndrome Polyglandular autoimmune syndrome, see there

polyene antibiotic One of a family of antifungal antibiotics produced by *Streptomyces* species that have the broadest spectrum of all antifungal agents; they bind to membrane sterols, in particular ergosterol, causing increased membrane permeability with leakage of cytoplasmic contents and cell death; of the polyenes in use (amphotericin B, nystatin, and pimaricin), amphotericin B is the most widely used despite its substantial toxicity, which may be ameliorated by newer drug delivery systems, eg liposomes, lipid dispersions, and colloidal suspensions, currently being developed (Science 1994; 264:371P)

polygenes A group of genes that controls a phenotypic feature, eg weight, skin pigmentation, or eye color

polyglandular autoimmune syndrome Either of two, often overlapping endocrinopathies characterized by gonadal failure, possibly secondary to hypothalamic defects with vitiligo and autoimmune adrenal insufficiency (80% of cases have autoantibodies); the preferred term for type I, is autoimmune polyendocrinopathy-candidiasis-ectodermal dystrophy, mercifully abbreviated with the acronym APECED; it is an AR [MIM 240300] condition of late childhood onset with hypoparathyroidism, mucocutaneous candidiasis, alopecia, pernicious anemia, malabsorption, and chronic active hepatitis TYPE II or Schmidt syndrome is an AR [MIM 269200] condition of adult onset with Addison's disease, and autoimmune (Hashimoto's) thyroiditis and/or IDDM; these conditions are HLA-linked in an as yet unclear fashion

polygraph Lie detector A device that is designed to detect deception by evaluating the physiologic and emotional responses to various spoken questions; the polygraph measuring and recording the changes in electrical and mechanical impulses that occur in a number of physiologic parameters including blood pressure, respiratory rate, and galvanic skin reflex; the polygraph test

'...purports to offer the same diagnostic accuracy as precise medical tests, such as electrocardiography or serum electrolyte determinations. Such diagnostic confidence is far more difficult to achieve in the complex and often subjective psychological realm of truth and deception...Lie detection by polygraph assumes that telling a lie causes specific and reproducible physiological responses related to the arousal of the autonomic nervous system. In turn, it is assumed that an experienced polygraph examiner can elicit these responses routinely...these critical assumptions remain unproved. Autonomic arousal may be caused by deception, but it may also be caused by myriad potentially confounding factors, ranging from stress, fear and anxiety to anger and embarassment. Deception cannot be measured directly....The typical polygraph instrument simultaneously measures several physiologic indexes that are not primarily under voluntary control, such as blood pressure, pulse, respiration patterns, and the electrodermal response, which is related to skin perspiration....From the relative changes in the measured indexes during the questioning, the examiner forms an opinion about the subject's honesty or dishonesty. The variability in the questions and interpretations distinguishes the polygraph test from (medical or psychological testing standards)...There is

no gold standard with which the results can be compared... There are reports that countermeasures can increases the odds of beating the machine. Such countermeasures includephysical motion or tensing of muscle groups during an examination, drugs, hypnosis, biofeedback, and previous experience in passing a test...(when the same criteria required for evaluating diagnostic medical tests are applied)...polygraph testing was found to have a sensitivity (ie probability of detecting a liar) of 76% and a specificity (ie probability that a truth-teller was declared truthful) of 63%... George Schultze, the former US Secretary of State, threatened to resign if ordered to take a polygraph test..."*it is hardly a scientific instrument*", he said. "*It tends to identify quite a few people who are innocent as guilty, and it misses at least some fraction of people who are guilty of lying.*"...The polygraph appeals to an often simplistic desire for certainty in the face of complexity and a misplaced faith in the power of a machine.' (from R Steinbrook in N Engl J Med 1992; 327:122ED)

polykaryocyte Multinucleated giant cell, see there

polyketide(s) A large class of naturally occurring products including antibiotics, eg erythromycin, pigments, eg tylosin and immunosuppressants (Science 1991; 252:675) that are synthesized by fatty acid synthase-like substances

polylobated lymphoma A morphologic variant of malignant lymphoma, which may be of T- or B-cell lineage; the cellular appearance of which has the colorful descriptor of balloons on a string, is nonspecific; like the 'cerebriform' cells of mycosis fungoides, the 'flower' cells of HTLV-I-associated adult T-cell leukemia/lymphoma or the 'popcorn' cells of Hodgkin's disease may be pathogenically linked to a defect in mitosis which might be exploited therapeutically (Arch Pathol Lab Med 1994; 118:722OA)

polymer fume fever A fever caused by inhalation of fumes from burning polymers, eg polytetrafluoroethylene (Teflon) which contain pyrolytic products released when fluoropolymers are heated CLINICAL Chest tightness, headache, shivering, fever, weakness, shortness of breath; the condition is most common in cigarette smokers; Cf Metal fume fever

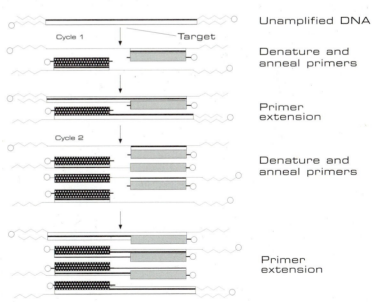

Unamplified DNA

Cycle 1 — Target

Denature and anneal primers

Primer extension

Cycle 2

Denature and anneal primers

Primer extension

polymerase chain reaction PCR MOLECULAR BIOLOGY A molecular technique that uses bacterial DNA polymerases to rapidly amplify (ie increase the number of copies of) a sequence of DNA in a sample; starting from minimal amounts << 1 µg (as little as one copy) PCR exponentially 'amplifies' the target DNA sequence, which has been inserted between two oligonucleotide primers through multiple amplification cycles (figure, above), one step of which occurs at a high temperature, which inactivates DNA polymerase, requiring that this enzyme be added at the beginning of each synthetic (amplification) cycle; PCR allows the synthesis of millions of copies of a DNA segment of interest within hours and can be used to detect deletions, insertions, translocations, and point mutations (Arch Pathol Lab Med 1993; 117:1104rv) PCR has been used for pre-natal diagnosis (sickle cell anemia), detection of HIV-1, gene rearrangements in lymphoproliferative disorders and determination of fetal sex; once a DNA segment has been amplified, it is then evaluated by conventional DNA techniques SENSITIVITY In detecting leukemia in bone marrow, a biopsy has a 65-75% sensitivity, Southern blot analysis of gene rearrangement, 98-99% sensitivity and polymerase chain reaction, 99.999%; the PCR was developed by K Mullis (and colleagues) at Cetus corporation (Science 1985; 230:1350) and was honored with the 1993 Nobel Prize in Physiology and Medicine; the technique promises to revolutionize DNA diagnostics

polymerization The formation of polymer from multiple monomers, eg assembly of G-actin subunits into an F-actin double helical polymer

polymicrobial urine LABORATORY MEDICINE The presence of multiple diff rent bacterial species in urine, which although ususally considered to be contaminants, can be clinically significant if the organism(s) grown in the urine is(are) the same as that(those) grown in blood; suspicion for clinically important (ie requiring treatment) urinary tract infection should be high (even if the urine bacteria concentration is below 10^5/ml) if multiple urine cultures grow the same organisms, and/or the urine is obtained by catheterization (Scand J Infect Dis 1993; 25:85)

polymorphism GENETICS The presence in a population of two or more allelic (or phenotypic) variants appearing as different phenotypes or which result in genetic changes detectable by restriction fragment length polymorphism analysis, eg alleles of α_1-antitrypsin and the Rh blood groups MOLECULAR BIOLOGY see Restriction fragment length polymorphism

polymorphous light eruption DERMATOLOGY An abnormal skin reaction to sunburn range ultraviolet B (290-320 nm) light that is more common in young adults, appearing 4-24 hours after exposure to light as papular, papulovesicular, plaque or diffuse erythematous lesions; the classic PMLE lesion is a plaque in which patchy lymphocytic infiltrates mimic the lesions of early SLE TREATMENT Antimalarial drugs, eg chloroquine

polymyalgia rheumatica RHEUMATOLOGY A relatively common affliction of the middle-aged to older population, ♀:♂ ratio, 2:1, characterized by an abrupt onset of myalgia and arthralgia of the neck and proximal 'girdle' muscles, which is most prominent in the morning and after periods of rest; systemic symptoms are vague and include low-grade fever, anemia, malaise, weight loss and a moderately elevated ESR; PR may be associated with other inflammatory, eg giant cell (temporal) arteritis, connective tissue disorders and malignancy

polymyositis RHEUMATOLOGY An inflammatory myopathy of adult onset that may be acute, subacute, or chronic, the dominant feature of which is symmetric proximal muscle weakness of insidious onset, which is accompanied by electromyographic changes, muscle necrosis, ↑ creatinine phosphokinase, dermal lesions, myalgias, tenderness, and eventually atrophy and fibrosis; the most widely used 'laundry list' of criteria used to define polymyositis (and the related condition dermatomyositis) is that delineated by Bohan and Peter (table) TREATMENT Corticosteroids; if the disease is recalcitrant, methotrexate and radiotherapy may be effective see Polymyositis-dermatomyositis

polymyositis-dermatomyositis RHEUMATOLOGY A form of

polymyositis, which in addition is characterized by the presence of typical dermatologic features (table) and the so-called machinist hands‡ TREATMENT Corticosteroids; see Polymyositis

polymyositis/dermatomyositis complex An 'overlap' syndrome in which polymyositis and dermatomyositis have multiple features incommon, including proximal distribution of muscle weakness, chronic 'round cell' inflammation, presence of an IgM rheumatoid factor, myopathic changes, spontaneous electrical discharges by electromyography and clinical response to corticosteroids

polyol pathway ENDOCRINOLOGY A metabolic pathway implicated in the complications of diabetes mellitus, in which glucose is reduced to sorbitol by aldehyde reductase ([EC 1.1.1.21], alditol:NAD(P)⁺ 1-oxidoreductase, formerly aldose reductase), resulting in damage to the retina (retinopathy), lens (cataracts with sorbitol inhibiting Na⁺,K⁺–ATPase), renal papillae (nephropathy), Schwann cells (neuropathy with *myo*-inositol deficiency and inhibition of Na⁺,K⁺–ATPase), and aorta

polyomavirus A small icosahedral, double-stranded oncogenic DNA virus belonging to the Papovaviridae family, which may be used to induce tumors in mice under experimental conditions; the polyomavirus may be identified in both domestic and wild rodents

polyp A generic term for any elevated 'tumor' mass, commonly understood to be epithelial in nature, which is often neoplastic; polyps are of greatest interest in the colon, female genital tract, nasopharynx and stomach **COLON** Colonic polyps are usually epithelial and either acquired or hereditary **ACQUIRED POLYPS** are adenomatous or tubular (villous) in morphology, ↑ in frequency with age; although often asymptomatic, larger polyps usually announce their presence by bleeding, or cause a change in bowel habits or if large enough, form a leading 'front' of an intussusception; histologic distinction between adenomatous polyps ('tight' round glands) and villous adenomas (finger-like fronds of elongated glands) has little practical importance, as both have malignant potential; periodic colonoscopy and polypectomy yields a three-fold reduction in subsequent cancer; hyperplastic polyps are also acquired but are regarded as having little neoplastic potential **HEREDITARY POLYPS** are often epithelial and may be associated with clinical syndromes that overlap with each other 1) Familial adenomatous polyposis coli (FAP) A premalignant, AD [MIM 175100] condition presenting in early

---

POLYMYOSITIS-DERMATOMYOSITIS, defining criteria

1) Symmetric proximal (limb-girdle) muscle weakness of insidious onset

2) Typical skeletal pathology Necrosis of type I and type II muscle fibers, phagocytosis, regeneration with basophilia, perifascicular atrophy, T-cell inflammation in the muscle fascicles, variation in muscle fiber size, and the presence of 'skip' areas of non-involvement

3) ↑ Serum levels of skeletal muscle enzymes, eg ALA (SGPT), aldolase, AST (SGOT), CPK*, LDH

4) A characteristic electromyographic triad of brief small polyphasic motor unit potentials, fibrillation potentials, positive waves, insertional irritability, and normal conduction velocity

Dermatomyositis is defined by a final criteria

5) Dermatologic findings including a lilac (heliotrope) discoloration the eyelids, with periorbital edema, and a characteristic scaling erythematous rash over the dorsal aspect of the hands (Gottron sign), with involvement of the elbows, knees, medial malleoli and upper body

*Creatinine phosphokinase, MM band

Modified from A Bodan, JB Peter, N Eng J Med 1975; 292:344

adulthood with 100s to 1000s of colonic polyps, related to the loss of the normal repression of DNA synthesis in the entire colonic epithelium; adenocarcinoma occurs in 70-100% of patients, prevented by prophylactic colectomy 2) Gardner syndrome An AD [MIM 175100] condition with premalignant polyps of the entire GI tract, which is identical to FAP, but has in addition extrintestinal tumors; most patients develop colonic carcinoma; other neoplasms occurring in these patients include bile duct carcinoma, osteomas of the mandible, skull, and long bones, soft tissue tumors (fibromas, lipomas), sebaceous cysts and rarely, neoplasia of the thyroid and adrenal glands and 3) Turcott syndrome A rare AR [MIM 276300] condition associated with brain tumors (medulloblastoma, glioblastoma) Other polypoid lesions of the colon include hamartomas, hyperplastic polyps, juvenile and retention polyps, which have little if any neoplastic potential 1) Cronkhite-Canada syndrome A non-hereditary condition characterized by diffuse GI polyposis, accompanied by alopecia, nail atrophy, cutaneous hyperpigmentation, weight loss, protein-losing enteropathy, electrolyte imbalance and malnutrition 2) Peutz-Jeghers syndrome An AD [MIM 175200] condition with hamartomas of the entire GI tract, predominantly of the small intestine, focal Paneth cell hyperplasia, melanin spots in buccal mucosa, lips, and digits, intussusception and bleeding; colonic adenocarcinomas, when seen in these patients arise in adenomatous and not in hamartomatous polyps; some cases of Peutz-Jeghers disease may be associated with Sertoli cell tumor and annular tubules, see SCTAT **FEMALE UROGENITAL TRACT** Endometrial and endocervical polyps represent circumscribed foci of cystic glandular hyperplasia of the mucosa and may cause abnormal bleeding; carcinoma arising is such polyps is distinctly uncommon; when smooth muscle is also present, they are designated as adenomatous polyps DDx Polypoid smooth muscle tumors, benign and malignant; see Müllerian mixed tumor **NASOPHARYNX** Nasal polyps Inflammatory ('allergic') polyps of the nasal cavity are not true neoplasms, but rather a reaction to inflammation or allergy; unlike true polyps, these lesions display edema and chronic inflammation (eosinophils, plasma cells, and lymphocytes), are bilateral, recurrent, and intranasal **SKIN** Squamous polyps and fibroepithelial polyps or 'skin tags' are benign prolapses of upper dermis onto the skin surface, which have no neoplastic potential **STOMACH** Gastric polyps are confusing, as it is often (incorrectly) assumed that the common colonic polyps are analogous to gastric polyps; hyperplastic polyps (designated as type I and II polyps by Japanese authors) comprise 75% of all gastric polyps and are usually benign Note: The occasionally used synonym, hamartomatous polyp is incorrect, as this term is best reserved for Peutz-Jeghers syndrome polyps; neoplastic polyps (Japanese type III and IV polyps) are single large, sessile or pedunculated, often antral tumors with atypical, mitotically active, pseudostratified glands analogous to neoplastic colonic polyps, which are thought to arise in intestinal metaplasia; the incidence of malignant degeneration, although low (3.5%), is twice that of gastric hyperplastic polyps; other gastric polyps are similar to colonic polyps and include hamartomatous polyps and juvenile (retention-type) polyps

polypharmacy CLINICAL PHARMACOLOGY The use of mutiple drugs to treat one or a limited number of conditions, most commonly seen in elderly patients; in the US, very few proprietary and generic drugs are available as 'cocktails' (mixtures of two or more drugs); instead, most drugs are dispensed as single-agent formulations, which is widely thought to allow better titration of dosages and optimal control of each agent while minimizing the toxic effects; reasons to increase the number of drugs to treat a patient

include 1) The patient has multiple conditions 2) The drugs are synergistic with each other and 3) The disease is refractory to an accepted, single-agent therapy; see Therapeutic drug monitoring

polyploidy The presence in a single cell of any multiple of a haploid number of chromosomes; Cf Aneuploidy

polypoid cell see Popcorn cell

polyprotein A large protein, eg pro-opiomelanocortin (POMC) that is translated from a polycistronic mRNA molecule and is a precursor for a number of smaller polypeptides and proteins that are enzymatically cleaved from the mother molecule after translation; see Alternative splicing

polyserositis Inflammation of multiple serosal surfaces as seen in familial Mediterranean fever, or collagen vascular (or connective tissue) diseases

polysomnography A technique for measuring multiple physiologic parameters during sleep; a relatively complete polysomnography includes EEG, EKG, electromyography, electrooculography, and includes noninvasive sensors for nasal airflow (thermocouple), oral airflow (end-tidal CO_2 gauge), tracheal sounds (microphone), thoracic and abdominal respiratory effort (inductance plethysmography), and oxyhemoglobin (finger-pulse oximeter); polysomnography is of greatest use in sleep disorders (**N Engl J Med 1993; 328:1230oA**) *adjective* Polysomnographic

polyspecific anti-human globulin Coomb's reagent TRANSFUSION MEDICINE A reagent containing antibody to human IgG and C3d that may also contain anti-C3b, anti-C4b and anti-C4d; commercially available Coomb's reagent has little activity against IgA and IgM heavy chains, but may react with these immunoglobulins as it may have antibodies reactive against the kappa and lambda light chains; polyspecific Coombs' reagent is used in the blood bank for routine red cell compatibility tests, alloantibody detection and direct antiglobulin test

polytechnic ACADEMIA An institution of higher education created in Britain in the 1960s with the intent of providing vocational education and, more recently, applied research, in contrast to the British universities, which were dedicated to academics and pure research; because the polytechnics had been viewed as low-quality universities, the merging of the two educational systems (**Nature 1991; 351:257n**), resulted in a deletion of the term polytechnic from the British system of higher education; these institutions have been designated as universities since 1992

polytene chromosome MOLECULAR BIOLOGY A specialized form of DNA rearrangement occurring in some the salivary glands of some insects, eg *Drosophila*, in which segments of DNA are amplified (duplicated) up to 1000 copies and arranged into identical parallel arrays of DNA; the molecular basis (and 'logic') for the multiple repeated gene copies within a presumably linear gene is unknown

polyunsaturated fatty acid Any of a number of monobasic aliphatic fatty acids with two or more double-bonded carbons with an alkyl radical linked to a carboxyl group; PFAs of interest to human physiology are broadly divided into

LINOLEIC PFAS 2 double bonds between 9 and 10 ($\Delta 9$) and 12 and 13 ($\Delta 12$), written as C_nH_{2n}-COOH

LINOLENIC PFAS 3 double bonds, $\Delta 9$, 12, 15, written as C_nH_{2n-5}-COOH

4 DOUBLED BOND PFAS 4 double bonds, $\Delta 5$, 8, 11, 14, eg arachidonic acid

PFAs lower the cholesterol, and therefore are 'good for you'; sources rich in PFAs include corn, cottonseed, peanut, safflower, and sunflower oils; see Fatty acids, Fish oil, n-3 fatty acids, Cf Tropical oils

polyvinyl chloride CLINICAL TOXICOLOGY A chemical that

has a boiling point of –13.5°C (ie, is a gas at room temperature); the vinyl chloride monomer ($H_2C\!=\!CHCl$) is converted to polyvinyl chloride (PVC) by heating the liquid form at 40-70°C; in 1980, 2½ million metric tons of PVC were produced (US), 87% of which was consumed by the soft plastics industry; other uses of PVC include colorants, lacquers, lubricants, tubing, packaging and biomedical devices; the acute and chronic interstitial lung disease seen in PVC intoxication is the result of the *bis*(2-ethyhexyl)phthalate (DEHP), an agent for 'plasticizing' vinyl chloride polymers and which has narcotic effects and causes acroosteolysis, PVC-induced hepatitis, soft-tissue changes, Raynaud-like phenomenon, hepatic hemangiosarcoma at doses as low as 250 ppm, brain tumors, poorly differentiated large cell carcinomas and adenocarcinoma of the lungs; the current OSHA limit of this potentially explosive gas is 1 ppm over eight hours; Cf PCBs, Plasticizers, Toxic dumps

POMC see Pro-opiomelanocortin

pompholyx Acute vesicular palmoplantar eczema The presence of bullae on the palmoplantar surfaces, which is accompanied by intense pruritus of possibly psychogenic origin, possibly related to ↑ autonomic nervous system activity; it is more common in warm weather, characterized by crops of vesicles and bullae that may evolve into eczema; see Factitious dermatitis

ponalrestat see Aldose reductase inhibitor

pongid *adjective* Pertaining or relating to the great (or anthropoid) apes of the family Pongidae, which include chimpanzees, gibbons, gorillas, and orangutans

Pontiac fever Pontiac disease A epidemic infection by *Legionella pneumophila* serogroup 6 (and other *Legionella* spp) which is not accompanied by pneumonia, first described in Pontiac, Michigan in 1968 CLINICAL After a 24-48 hour incubation, fever, headaches, myalgia, cough, occasionally diarrhea and neurological signs, with complete resolution within one week (**N Engl J Med 1988; 318:571**) Cf Legionnaire's disease

pontine-geniculate-occipital waves NEUROPHYSIOLOGY An erratic volley of discharges from cholinergic neurons into higher cortical and other regions that only occurs during dreaming; PGO waves stimulate the motor centers in the brainstem which would otherwise cause motor activity, but are inhibited by a signal to the spinal cord preventing actual movement of all muscle groups except the eyelids; PGO waves also impact on emotional circuits, which explains why dreams are accompanied by strong emotions including anxiety, fear, joy, sadness, guilt, and eroticism

Note: It is possible to enter the cholinergic state without being asleep, as occurs in meditation, and drug-induced or schizophrenia-related hallucinations (**New York Times 16 July 1994; C1**)

pool The total quantity of a substance, material or resource in a 'universe', as in a microenvironment, eg metabolic pool, a population group, eg donor pool, or gene pool

popcorn An adjectival descriptor for a radiological or pathological finding that simulates the solitary kernels of 'popped corn'

popcorn calcification Popcorn densities BONE A descriptive term for clusters of small scalloped radiolucencies with sclerotic margins seen predominantly in the epiphysis and metaphysis of the actively growing knee and ankle of children with osteogenesis imperfecta; the popcorn appearance is thought to be due to fragmentation and disordered maturation of the physis with an irregular or defective growth plate, resulting in severe growth retardation LUNG A descriptor for the puffed and lobulated appearance that is typical of a well-circumscribed calcified solitary hamartoma, which is seen on a plain anteroposterior chest film; multiple 'popcorn' nodularities are suggestive of pulmonary histoplasmosis and may be seen on a plain chest film SYNOVIUM The popcorn morphology refers to rounded multilobulated masses seen in the peri-articular region in synovial chondromatosis or in enchondromas, which serve to differentiate these from the radiologically similar low-grade chondrosarcomas

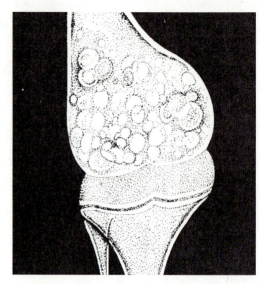

popcorn calcification

popcorn cell Polypoid cell A Reed-Sternberg cell variant with a lobulated 'cloverleaf' nucleus, bubbly nucleoplasm, a small acidophilic nucleolus and a small rim of cytoplasm seen in lymphocyte-predominant Hodgkin's disease; similar 'Reider'-like cells occasionally occur in T-cell lymphoma and Pinkus tumor; see Reed-Sternberg cell

Popeye arm deformity A fanciful descriptor for the clinical changes seen in the Landouzy-Déjérine type of limb-girdle dystrophy (facioscapulohumeral muscle dystrophy), so named for the thinness of the upper arms due to humeral muscle atrophy and pseudohypertrophy or preservation of the forearm musculature, accompanied by involvement of facial muscles, 'winging' of the scapula, incomplete eye closure, inability to whistle or to raise the arms above the head (**N Engl J Med 1994; 330:548CPC**)

'Popeye syndrome' Brachial entrapment syndrome An acquired condition seen in older men who perform heavy work with their arms, resulting in a Popeye-like enlargement of the forearm, which is relatively larger than the upper arm; muscular hypertrophy within fibrous compartments of the forearm results in compression of the brachial artery with ischemia-related forearm fatigue and paresthesias

The 'Popeye' adjective refer to a comic strip sailor whose strength is attributed to the ingestion of spinach

popliteal pterygium syndrome An AD [MIM 119500] condition of neonatal onset and variable penetration and clinical expression CLINICAL A fibrous cord extends from the heel to the ischial tuberosity, limiting leg movement, which is accompanied by syndactyly, bone malformation, club feet, cleft lip and palate, cryptorchidism, and absence of labia majora

POPOP 1,4-Bis-2-(5-phenoxazolyl)benzene and PPO 2,5-diphenyloxazole Two organic liquid scintillation fluids used to detect β radiation in a radioimmunoassay; POPOP, a secondary fluor and PPO, a primary fluor absorb a sample's weak β radiation and emit flashes of light that are amplified 10^6 to 10^8-fold by a photomultiplier, which passes the signal to a scintillation counter; see Quenching, RIA

popsickle panniculitis A rare condition characterized by inflammation of adipose tissue due to localized exposure to the cold, first described in a young child secondary to the ingestion of a 'popsicle', a frozen snack food that is licked; the reaction is attributed to the more saturated nature of fats in children (N Engl J Med 1970; 282:966cr)

population GLOBAL VILLAGE The aggregate of persons in a specified area*; the human population is expected to peak at 9-15 billiion by the end of the next century; futurologists have painted two extremes (and countless intermediate scenarios) that will result from a 2-3-fold ↑ in the world's population, to wit, either 1) Environmental and human catastrophe with deterioration of the planet's ecosystems and mass starvation or 2) Virtually no change of significance (Sci Am 1994; 270/3:37; US News & World Report 12 September1994:54) see Zero population growth STATISTICS The aggregate of data points in a set of data

porcelain doll face The puffy, pale facies described in adults with myxedema, due to accumulation of glycosaminoglycans; in other skin regions, there is a greater amount of anchoring of the deep dermis to the surface, resulting in a 'pitted' appearance, termed 'Peau d'orange' changes

porcelain gallbladder An extensively calcified and indurated gallbladder that appears in a background of acutely exacerbated chronic cholecystitis and cholelithiasis; although extremely rare, the porcelain gallbladder is of interest as up to 20% develop carcinoma

porcelain white appearance Indurated enamel-like fibrous plaques seen on the genitals and trunk with follicular plugging, seen in lichen sclerosis

porin NEUROPHYSIOLOGY A 30–34-kD voltage-gated membrane channel in the outer membrane of gram-negative bacterial walls, mitochondria, and plasma membranes, that is arranged in a lattice of trimers of elliptical cylindrical walls of β protein sheet (Nature 1991; 350:167), serving as a diffusion pathway for molecules that are > 1.0 kD in size, including waste products, nutrients, antibiotics and bacteriophage receptors; porins in the outer membrane of mitochondria, allow passage of 10-kD molecules, especially when positively-charged; see VDAC (voltage-dependent anion-selective channel); Cf Perforin

'pork barrel' funding Earmarking RESEARCH FUNDING The practice by the US Congress of attaching the costs of 'pet projects' to certain government spending packages; the science community opposes bypassing the peer-review process (the usual conduit for obtaining federal funds) in the awarding of grant monies, as a limited number of groups benefit from unfair funding practices, at the cost of many potentially more deserving candidates; universities may, despite the issues of research ethics and fair play, employ lobbyists in order to circumvent peer-review

porphin The parent molecule of porphyrins that is comprised of a tetrapyrrole ring

porphyria A generic term for any of number of inborn errors of metabolism, the most common of which is acute intermittent porphyria, which are characterized by ↑ urinary excretion and circulating levels of porphyrins or their precursors, eg porphobilinogen, δ-aminolevulinec acid

Port Pirie Cohort Study A longitudinal study begun in 1979 that centers around lead-smelting community of Port Pirie, South Australia; the study is designed to determine whether the delayed neuropsychological development attributed to increased lead exposure in early childhood persists into later childhood or adulthood; after controlling for potentially confusing variables (eg socioeconomic status, maternal IQ, parents' level of education, feeding method, duration of breast-feeding, etc), the IQ was 4-5 % lower in children age 7-8 with blood lead concentrations ≥ 1.45 µmol/L (30 µg/dl) than those with levels ≤ 0.48 µmol/L (10 µg/dl) (N Engl J Med 1992; 327:1279OA)

portable *adjective* COMPUTERS Pertaining or relating to a software design in which information can be ported to multiple computer platforms with minimal redesign or program modification (Am Lab March 1995, p46) HEALTH INSURANCE Pertaining or referring to a health insurance policy that can be continued with the same level and format of coverage should a person change employers (Am Med News 25 October 1992, p7)

portable coverage HEALTH CARE FINANCING A type of health care coverage proposed under the Clinton Plan that makes it easier to transfer insurance coverage from one job to another; see Clinton Plan, Job lock

portability see Portable

Port-A-Cath NUTRITION A proprietary (Pharmacia Deltic, St Paul, Minn) indwelling device used to allow long-term IV access for the administration of total parenteral alimentation, blood products, drugs, or high-dose chemotherapy; the distal IV portion is inserted into the superior vena cava or right atrium via either the external jugular or cephalic veins; the extravascular portion has an implanted port that is accessed percutaneously, thereby reducing the incidence of infection (GL Mandell, JE Bennett, R Dolin, Eds, Principles and Practice of Infectious Diseases, 4th ed, Churchill-Livingstone, New York, 1995) Cf Hickman catheter

portacaval shunt A surgical procedure in which the portal vein is anastomosed with the inferior vena cava; the PS diverts blood away from the portal venous system, reducing portal hypertension, the cause of the most feared, and potentially fatal complication of cirrhosis, exsanguination from esophageal varices, although they may themselves cause morbidity due to hepatic failure or hepatic encephalopathy; the PS procedure preferred by many workers is a portacaval H-graft shunt, which facilitates the control of ascites, provides immediate portal decompression, control of variceal bleeding, and the option for future restoration of portal circulation, should hepatic failure or encephalopathy develop

Porter-Silber chromagen Any glucocorticoid detected by the Porter-Silber reaction (phenylhydrazine and sulfuric acid are added to urine), which are 21-carbon molecules with dihydroxyacetone side-chains with a peak absorption at 410 nm, including 11-deoxycortisol, cortisol, cortisone and some 17-hydroxicorticosteroids; the accuracy of the Porter-Silber reaction can be improved by extractions in organic solvents and purifying the urine extracts by chromatography; many drugs, eg chlorpromazine, meprobamate, reserpine and spironolactone interfere with the Porter-Silber reaction, causing a false elevation, while the test may be unreliable in neonates with congenital adrenal hyperplasia due to the production of abnormal (and measured) steroids

port-wine nevus Nevus flammeus Flat hemangioma A common congenital neurovascular malformation, appearing as deep red-purple macular lesions, corresponding to cutaneous angioma(s), often located in the ophthalmic branch of the trigeminal nerve; when located on the meninges, the malformation may be confined to the occipitoparietal pial vessels, where sluggish blood flow predisposes to hypoxia of the underlying cortex CLINICAL 5% of patients with port-wine stains suffer from convulsions, mental retardation, hemiparesis or hemianopsia contralateral to the lesions; port wine nevi may occur in the normal population, eg Mikhail Gorbachev, or may be a component of various syndromes, eg Klippel-Trenaunay, Beckwith-Wiedemann, Cobb, Rubenstein-Taybi and trisomy 13 syndromes PATHOLOGY Densely-packed, dilated capillaries in the dermis and subdermis TREATMENT Flashlamp-pulsed tunable argon dye laser, which is most effective if administered before age seven, often requiring more therapeutic sessions in facial lesions

port-wine urine A descriptor for the transparent, red urine seen in myoglobinuria due to traumatic injury to muscle, intense, prolonged and/or violent exercise, eg marathon-running and karate; in contrast, hemoglobinuria with red cell casts is a turbid red color

port-wine stools Currant jelly stool, see there

positional cloning MOLECULAR BIOLOGY Any of a number of time-consuming molecular methods for cloning a gene, the product of which is unknown; PC entails a series of complex steps to determine the chromosomal location of a mutated gene responsible for a disease; PC begins by mapping the gene of interest to a particular chromosome, by following the pattern of inheritance of markers (short sequences of DNA known as microsatellites) in families in order to identify those markers that are inherited with the disease, and therefore genetically linked to the disease, ie linkage analysis; the 'trick' lies in finding two microsatellite markers that flank the gene of interest; it is then necessary to clone a series of DNA fragments that link the flanking markers; the final step in identifying the gene is the characterization of the cloned DNA fragments, analyzing the coding sequences (ie sequencing) and direct mutational screening of candidate genes against the patient's (defective) DNA (Sci & Med Nov/Dec 1994 p48)

positive feedback Feedback, see there

positive predictive value STATISTICS The number of true positives divided by the sum of true positives (TP) and false positives (FP), a value representing the proportion of subjects with a positive test result who actually have the disease, also known as the 'efficiency' of a clinical assay, defined by the accompanying formula: Note: In predictive values, as with prevalence, as the frequency of a disease decreases, the number of false positive tests increases; Cf Negative predictive value, ROC (receiver operating characteristic)

positron NUCLEAR PHYSICS A short-lived particle emitted by beta decay that is similar to an electron in mass ($\sim \frac{1}{1820}$ amu), spin ($h/2\pi$, h = Planck's constant), and charge ($\sim 4.8 \times 10^{-10}$ esu), except the charge is positive; positrons are antiparticles, which when they unite with an electron, result in mutual annhilation

positron emission (transaxial) tomography PET scan, see there

positron microscopy A technique in development, in which a beam of imaging particles passes through a specimen and the electromagnetic interactions with atoms in the target scatter the beam, producing a characteristic image; see Microscopy

postabortion trauma 'Abortion trauma syndrome', see there

postanginal sepsis A condition that is most common in adolescents and young adults and caused by a parapharyngeal abscess related to tonsillitis, pharyngitis, or dental procedures; the infection spreads regionally by direct extension, lymphatic spread, or into the venous channels, causing thrombophlebitis of the internal jugular vein, giving rise to septic emboli and metastatic abscesses, classically to the lung CLINICAL Local symptoms due to abscess include oral and facial edema, hoarseness, dysphagia; pulmonary involvement is manifest by high fever, rigors, cough, pleuritic chest pain, hemoptysis, and dyspnea MICROBIOLOGY *Fusobacterium necrophorum*, peptostreptococc, bacteroides, *Eikenella corrodens*, *S aureus*, and others LABORATORY Leukocytosis ($\geq$ 30 000/mm³), ↑ liver function tests (see there), ↓ platelets, ↑ urinary sediment TREATMENT High-dose IV antibiotics with coverage for anaerobic organisms (N Engl J Med 1992; 326:2324cpc)

postconcussive syndrome SPORTS MEDICINE A constellation of symptoms (eg anxiety, dizziness, loss of memory or ability to concentrate, fatigability, headaches, sleep distur-

bances, that occurs after mild traumatic brain injury, which when seen in athletes with severe concussion *as alteration of consciousness, disturbance of vision, equilibrium, and other similar symptoms.*' features common to MTBI are '*...limited or absent loss of consciousness, limited post-traumatic amnesia, and an initial Glasgow Coma Scale of $\geq$ 13 of 15.*' (Advance for Dir in Rehab Med June 1995; 4: 31)

post-datism Post-term pregnancy, see there

'post-doc' Post-doctorate fellow A person who has completed the academic and/or research activities required for the completion of his PhD (doctor of philosophy), or less commonly, MD (doctor of medicine), and who is pursuing research (often for a 2-5 year period) in the laboratory of an established scientist

Note: The term may also refer to the activity itself, as in, '*...to do a post-doc*'

postgastrectomy syndrome Dumping syndrome(s) GASTROENTEROLOGY A disease complex seen in about 20% of those subjected to gastric surgery, including resection, gastroenterostomy with total gastric vagotomy and gastric bypass; in particular pyloric ablation and bypass CLINICAL Diaphoresis, palpitations, colicky abdominal pain and diarrhea, due to rapid movement (dumping) of gastric contents into the small intestine; the clinical findings can be loosely divided into those that occur shortly after a meal (early dumping) and several hours after a meal (late dumping)

Early dumping syndrome* A condition affecting 5-10% of those with sub-total gastrectomies, caused by the release of vasoactive substances, eg serotonin, bradykinin, glucagon CLINICAL Onset 20-30 minutes after meals with early satiety, upper GI discomfort and vasomotor phenomena (flushing, diaphoresis, palpitations, tachycardia and hypotension), resolving in one hour, weakness, nausea, diarrhea, cramping and borborygmi, flatulence, aerophagia, vomiting, anemia; when prolonged malabsorption, steatorrhea, weight loss and osteomalacia may ensue LABORATORY ↑ Glucose (worse with high carbohydrate meals), ↑ hematocrit and ↓ blood volume, related to dehydration, decreased serum K^+

Late dumping syndrome A less common condition that is more polymorphous clinically; most symptoms are due to reactive postcibal hypoglycemia, as the rapid entry of glucose releases GIP (gastroactive intestinal polypeptide), inhibiting the hyperglycemic response to glucagon; spontaneous remission may occur 3-12 months after surgery TREATMENT, MEDICAL Smaller meals, ↓ carbohydrate intake, pectin (a dietary fiber), acarbose, anticholinergics, L-dopa and opiates TREATMENT, SURGICAL 2-5% are medical failures, requiring surgical conversion to a Roux-en-Y Note: Other post-gastrectomy syndromes include the small capacity, afferent and efferent loop syndromes, bile gastritis, anemia, postvagotomy diarrhea and metabolic bone disease

Note: Because medical therapy is effective for gastric ulcer disease, gastrectomies are no longer commonly performed, and thus of lesser active interest in the literature

post-mortem Autopsy, see there

postmyocardial infarction syndrome Dressler syndrome A condition of acute onset that develops 2-10 weeks after a myocardial infarction in up to 4% of patients PATHOGENESIS Uncertain, possibly autoimmune in origin (possibly due to antimyocardial antibodies) or leakage of blood into the pericardial space; PMIS has certain features in common with postpericardiotomy syndrome (table) CLINICAL Severe malaise, fever, localized fibrinous pericarditis often with a friction rub, chest pain, and pleuritis since the shift in therapeutic philosophies toward more aggressive use of aspirin and less aggressive anticoagulation, the frequency of the post-MI syndrome has fallen dramatically; Cf Postpericardiotomy syndrome

post-nasal drip ENT The sensation that mucus, secretions, or inflammatory products are passing from the nasopharynx into the oropharynx; PNDs usually occur in a background of chronic sinusitis

postneonatal mortality EPIDEMIOLOGY A standard indicator of health, defined as the number of infant deaths between 28 days of life and 11 months (MMWR 1994; 43:905) Cf Infant mortality

post-operative erythroderma see Post-transfusion graft-versus-host disease

post-operative headache A variably present post-operative complication occurring in the hours after recovery from general anesthesia, which may be due to a caffeine withdrawal state (Anesth Analg 1991; 72:449)

post-operative psychosis A symptom complex said to occur after a surgical procedure, especially those requiring general anesthesia; although this is not considered a true clinical entity, surgery may uncover an underlying psychosis or cause anxiety with psychophysiologic, somatopsychic and psychosocial components

postpartum depression Postpartum 'blues' A stress reaction occurring in women after delivery, characterized by depression, fatigue, irritability, insomnia (from the third to tenth days postpartum) and if extreme in degree, may result in infanticide

postpartum renal failure Postpartum hemolytic uremic syndrome An idiopathic condition with a poor prognosis, characterized by renal failure, microangiopathic hemolytic anemia, thrombocytopenia, and DIC, beginning from several days to ten weeks after a normal pregnancy and delivery; PP-HUS may be preceded by hypertension, proteinuria or preeclampsia CLINICAL Vomiting, diarrhea, flu-like illness may precede the oliguric or anuric phases of acute renal failure accompanied by hemolysis and coagulopathy; complete recuperation of renal function occurs in only 10% PATHOLOGY Fibrinoid necrosis of vessel walls (similar to the changes seen in malignant hypertension), glomerular ischemia, fibrin thrombi in the afferent arterioles and glomeruli and subendothelial deposits of fibrin and C3 TREATMENT No therapy is consistently effective; early diagnosis, control of hypertension and early dialysis may have a role in prevention; see TTP-HUS

postpartum thyrotoxicosis Hyperactivity of the thyroid gland that is temporally linked to delivery, appearing as de novo Graves' hyperthyroidism, recurrent Graves' hyperthyroidism (characterized by high radioiodine uptake) and painless thyroiditis with hyperthyroidism (with low radioiodine uptake); these endocrinopathies are often mild and transient, possibly caused by the unmasking of associated autoimmune phenomena TREATMENT If necessary, propranolol

post-perfusion lung Pump lung A clinical complex seen immediately after cardiovascular surgery CLINICAL Fever, dyspnea, cyanosis, hypotension and pulmonary edema, caused by anoxia, traumatic hemolysis of erythrocytes due to shearing against pump hardware, turbulence and possi-

---

POSTMYOCARDIAL INFARCTION & POSTPERICARDIOTOMY SYNDROMES (FEATURES IN COMMON)

1) Endothelial cell injury and entrance of blood in the pericardial space
2) Delayed clinical response consisting of fever and pericardial inflammation
3) Antimyocardial cell antibodies
4) Dramatic response to antiinflammatory agents, eg aspirin, NSAIDs, corticosteroids
5) Tendency to recur

---

bly anaphylactic reaction against various materials (proteins and other allergens) in the tubing, congestive heart failure, acute renal tubular necrosis and urinary tract infection PATHOLOGY The lungs are dark red, heavy, congested and hemorrhagic TREATMENT Antibiotics, corticosteroids PROGNOSIS Relatively guarded

post-perfusion syndrome A clinical complex* seen in 2% of patients who have undergone cardiac surgery, occurring 3-7 weeks after cardiopulmonary bypass, which resembles infectious mononucleosis or hepatitis and is attributed to viruses transfused with the blood at the time of surgery; although it is characterized by fever, splenomegaly, lymphadenopathy, a maculopapular rash, anemia and atypical lymphocytes, the syndrome is benign and resolves spontaneously without therapy; see Post-perfusion lung; Cf Post-resuscitation syndrome

*aka post-transfusion mononucleosis, post-transfusion syndrome

postpericardiotomy syndrome Postcommissurotomy syndrome A condition of acute onset characterized by fever, pericarditis, and pleuritis that develops two or more weeks after cardiac surgery, in which the pericardium has been 'violated' in the form of wide incision and manipulation* PATHOGENESIS Uncertain, possibly autoimmune in origin (? due to antimyocardial antibodies) possibly triggered by a viral infection; PPS has certain features in common with postmyocardial infarction syndrome (table) CLINICAL Severe malaise, fever, pericarditis often with a friction rub, chest pain, and pleuritis TREATMENT Aspirin, NSAIDs, and if unresponsive, corticosteroids PROGNOSIS PPS is usually self-limited but often recurs and may be disabling; Cf Postmyocardial infarction syndrome

*An identical clinical syndrome may follow other pericardial insults in the form of cardiac perforation, blunt chest trauma, and epicardial pacemakers

post-permanent dentition The appearance of supernumerary teeth after the loss of permanent teeth, which is regarded as a rare event; most teeth that appear after extraction of permanent teeth are due to eruption of previously impacted teeth

post-pill amenorrhea GYNECOLOGY Failure to resume menstruation within three months after discontinuation of oral contraceptives; amenorrhea of greater than 6 months occurs in 0.2% and in 15% is accompanied by galactorrhea; the work-up and treatment is similar to the usual type of amenorrhea, and thus this 'disease' is probably not a distinct entity

post-polio syndrome A progressive late-onset disease occurring years after an attack of acute poliomyelitis, most often affecting previously involved muscles EPIDEMIOLOGY Estimated to affect 500 000 CLINICAL: Fatigue, muscle weakness, fasciculations, and atrophy, difficulty breathing PATHOGENESIS Uncertain, possibly polioviruses, which may become integrated into the host genome, producing symptoms even decades after active infection PATHOLOGY 'Type grouping' of muscles, which is due to a denervation-renervation sequence; PPS is often benign and may reach a plateau phase; see Type grouping (Science 1994; 264:909N&V)

postprandial syndrome Idiopathic postprandial syndrome, see there

post-pump syndrome A severe complication of cardiopulmonary bypass characterized by multiorgan dysfunction in the early post-operative period, a systemic inflammatory response with ↑ capillary permeability, interstitial edema, leukocytosis, fever, renal dysfunction, hemolysis, vasoconstriction and possibly ↑ susceptibility to infection PATHOGENESIS Exposure of blood to nonendothelial surfaces during bypass surgery results in platelet clumping and embolization, protein denaturation, and fat embolization; humoral activation (eg, coagulation complement, fibrinolytic, and kallikrein-bradykinin) systems (N Engl J Med 1992; 327:1740CPC) Cf Post-perfusion syndrome

post-resuscitation syndrome EMERGENCY MEDICINE A clinical complex seen in 'arrested' patients in whom CPR is delayed, characterized by protracted reduction in cardiac output despite normal blood pressure, due to a combination of cardiac pump failure, microthromboembolism (due to intravascular obstruction, causing ↑ systemic vascular resistance and DIC) and vasospasm (multi-organ failure); the pulmonary insufficiency in PRS is due to relative respiratory dysfunction; cerebral ischemia contributes to PRS by triggering dysrhythmia, renal shutdown and pulmonary edema; PRS results from 'autointoxication' occurring when reperfused hypoxic tissues release kinins, bacterial endotoxins, endogenous pyrogens and other toxins; Cf Post-perfusion syndrome

post-splenectomy 'syndrome' A constellation of hematologic findings that follow splenectomy, most prominently affecting the erythroid series, as the spleen is responsible for 'pitting' and 'culling' effete or defective RBCs or those with inclusions LABORATORY ↑ Lifespan of RBCs, codocytes (target cells), schistocytes, Howell-Jolly bodies (nuclear chromatin remnants), and transient thrombocytosis

post-term pregnancy Post-datism OBSTETRICS A gestation that is correctly dated by Naegele's rule and is of greater than 42 weeks in duration; 12% of gestations are undelivered at 42 weeks and 7% at 43 weeks; the longer the delay before delivery, the greater is the mortality (0.7% at 40 weeks, 2.2% > 42 weeks); post-mature infants have ↑ mortality and morbidity as 1) they are bigger and 2) the placenta has planned obsolescence and undergoes fibrosis and infarcts after 40-42 weeks CLINICAL Absent lanugo, attenuated vernix caseosa, long finger- and toenails, abundant scalp hair, pale, parchment-like or desquamating skin and ↑ alertness; Cf Prematurity

Note: Most cases of 'post-datism' represent a miscalculation of the last menstrual period

post-transfusion graft-versus-host disease A condition that is similar or identical to post-operative erythroderma, seen in immunocompetent blood recipients, a condition that may result from engraftment of donor T lymphocytes from blood products, which mount an immune attack against host tissues; PT-GVHD occurs when the donor is homozygous, and the recipient heterozygous for certain HLA antigens CLINICAL High fever, dermatitis, severe diarrhea, hepatic dysfunction and pancytopenia DIAGNOSIS Analysis of RFLPs and/or DNA probes had been used but these methods with either uninformative and/or cumbersome; PCR amplification of polymorphic microsatellite markers followed by gel electrophoresis can be used to identify patients at risk for PT-GVHD (N Engl J Med 1994; 330:398OA) DDx Drug reactions, toxic shock syndrome, viral infections

post-transfusion infection see Transfusion reactions

post-transplantation lymphoproliferative disorder PTLD A complication of 1-10% of organ transplant recipients, which may be poly– or monoclonal; the majority of affected cells contain EBV, usually in a latent stage; post-transplantation patients at risk for PTLD can be identified by detecting expression (in the form of small messenger RNA) of the EBER-1 gene; most cases that occur in solid organ recipients are of host origin (Am J Clin Pathol 1995; 103:748)

post-traumatic stress disorder A psychogenic complex linked to the intense mental stress that follows intense trauma or armed conflict, defined as one or more of the following; symptoms relating to re-experiencing a traumatic event or symptoms related to avoiding the stimuli associated with the trauma or numbing of general responsiveness or symptoms related to ↑ arousal with long-term psychologic 'scars' CLINICAL Nightmares, inability to concentrate, and intrusive thoughts about the traumatic event; PTSD is associated with an ↑ in alcohol dependence (Science News 1994; 146:5) and may arise in a background of child abuse (Am Med News 25 May 1992 p29) PTSD is similar to the 'Vietnam syndrome'*; the 'shell shock' form of PTSD occurs in less than 1% of the general population, 15-35% of Vietnam veterans, 30-50% of those exposed to natural disasters and up to 80% of those exposed to man-made

disasters, eg Bhopal; Cf Battle fatigue

*And for some authors are synonymous; for other authors, however, the stress linked to the Vietnam conflict differs substantially, as moral guilt was placed on the combatants by nonparticipants, which is believed by some to have prevented the ex-soldiers from successfully resolving the stressful issues of 'man's inhumanity to man'

postal worker 'syndrome' FORENSIC PSYCHIATRY A colloquial term for a condition that is alleged* to cause postal workers to 'snap' and kill their colleagues in a bloody rampage by firearm; the most recent alleged case of PWS occurred in New Jersey on 21 March, 1995, and left four persons dead

The PWS is of uncertain validity and of unknown etiology; it could be that the simplest is the most valid, ie there are a lot of kooks in the world, and a lot of people work for the US postal service-Author's note

posterior cord syndrome Posterior column syndrome A neurologic complex* due to the loss of vibration and position sense below a lesion of the posterior spinal cord; the PCS is accompanied by a positive Romberg sign, tingling in the affected regions, sensory ataxia, hypotonia, and preservation of the perception of pain and temperature; as lesions of the posterior cord interrupt the central projections of the dorsal root ganglia cells, they may mimic tabes dorsalis

*Although the term posterior column syndrome is preferred by some neurologists (RD Adams, M Victor, Principles of Neurology, 5th ed, McGraw-Hill, New York, 1993) and is more correct as it refers to the posterior column of the spinal cord, the term posterior cord syndrome is more widely extant in the literature

pot Marijuana, see there

potassium-argon dating PALEOANTHROPOLOGY A method for determining the age of life forms that have died in a relatively distant past, having a limit of less than 300 000 years or older (Science 1990; 247:798N&c) see Carbon-14 dating

potassium ion channels CELL PHYSIOLOGY A group of transmembrane proteins found in both excitable and non-excitable cell types, including thymocytes and T cells, which have a wide range of functional diversity; potassium channels are classified according to differences in biophysical (kinetics, conductance, sensitivity to voltage and second messengers) and pharmacologic properties and whether the channels are homo- or heteromultimeric, ie whether all the transmembrane channels in the complex are formed of the same or of different chains; potassium channels can be activated by intracellular second messengers (eg arachidonic acid in cardiac muscle); see Ball-and-chain model, Voltage-gated channels

'potato chip' desquamation Peripheral elevation of partially desquamated flecks of the superficial keratinized corneal layer of the skin, which follows the resolution of the erythematous lesions in staphylococcal scalded-skin syndrome, morphologically likened to potato chips or potato crisps

'potato chip' operation(s) A highly colloquial term for multiple, increasingly proximal, partial amputations of the lower extremities that are required in the face of dry gangrene, the result of vasculo-stenotic occlusions in peripheral atherosclerosis, most often occurring in elderly patients with DM; since the patients are often disinclined to consent to a full above-the-knee amputation, which is the definitive therapy for occlusive, severely ischemic atherosclerosis, the vascular surgeon is forced to amputate in sequence, one or more toe(s), the mid-foot, the foot, the leg below-the-knee and finally perform an above-the-knee amputation

The sobriquet for these operations derives from an advertisement for potato chips (potato crisps) that claimed that '...one potato chip is never enough.'

potato-dextrose agar MICROBIOLOGY A nonselective growth medium for the growth of yeasts and molds, including *Aspergillus niger*, *Candida albicans*, *Saccharomyces cerevisiae*, and *Trichophyton mentagophytes*; PDA is recommended by the American Public Health Association for plate counts of yeasts and molds in the examination of foods and dairy products, and is used for stimulation of sporulation; in the clinical microbiology laboratory, PDA is less popular than Sabouraud's medium

'potato' liver A fanciful term for a liver punctuated on the surface and in the parenchyma by large indurated nodules of macronodular cirrhosis as seen in Wilson's disease

potato node(s) RADIOLOGY A descriptor for the enlarged nodular hilar and mediastinal lymph nodes seen in sarcoidosis

potato nose A rare deformity inherited in an AD [MIM 164000] fashion characterized by a bulbous proboscis and developmental visual field defect; Cf 'WC Fields' nose

potato tumor A descriptor for a carotid body paraganglioma arising at the angle of the jaw causing a massive tuberoid tumor of young adults PATHOLOGY The tumor is firm, oval, highly vascular and composed of tumor cell nests known as zellballen, see there

potency TRANSFUSION MEDICINE The degree of 'antigenicity' or the intensity of agglutination that may be elicited by different alloantigens; potency is a value that can be calculated by comparing the frequency of an antibody anti-X, in the population to the frequency of the alloantigen, X of interest, multiplied by the opportunity for immunization; the potency of the Kell antigen is equated to 1, Rh D is seven-fold more potent than Kell and Rh e ("little 'e' ") is one-tenth as potent as the Kell

potocytosis MEMBRANE PHYSIOLOGY A mechanism of transport for small molecules that uses caveolae as an uptake vesicle; in the potocytosis, the caveolae open and close periodically, and possibly detach from the cell membrane, creating a temporary compartment that maintains folates at concentrations that are favorable to transmembrane movement of small molecules (Science & Medicine 1995; 2/3:80) see Caveola, Endocytosis

Potomac horse fever Equine ehrlichial colitis

'Potomac fever' A highly colloquial term of uncertain utility for a 'disease' that may affect those* who are temporarily in a position of power in Washington DC, capital of the USA

*eg Elected politicians or appointed health professionals, who bask in the glamor and 'glitz' of Washington and who, when defeated in elections or replaced, are disinclined to return to the 'dreary' hinterlands from whence they came
Note: The Potomac River courses through the middle of Washington

Pott's puffy tumor A fluctuant swelling overlying the frontal bones, when they affected by osteomyelitis, which is accompanied by a subperiosteal (pericranial) abscess, often secondary to chronic frontal sinusitis; the causative organism in children is often hematogenous in origin and in adults due to direct, traumatic origin ORGANISMS *Staphylococcus aureus*, β-hemolytic streptococci, anaerobes DIAGNOSIS Clinical, 'hot' lesion by ^{99m}Tc scanning

Note: The tumor was first described by Sir Perrcivall Pott (1714-1788) in 1760 in association with tuberculosis

povidine-iodine A topically applied solution with used to treat neonatal conjunctivitis (ophthalmia neonatorum) which has certain advantages over the previously standard use of silver nitrate, erythromycin and other antibiotics; PI is reported to be more efficient and has a broader range of bacteria against which it is effective; PI is less costly and toxic; it has moreover, antiviral (eg HIV and herpes simplex) activity (N Engl J Med 1995; 332:562oA)

'pouchitis' Acute inflammation of intestinal mucosa seen in an ileal reservoir that may extend transmurally, occurring as a late complication of restorative proctocolectomy, possibly due to obstruction and stercoral ulceration

POU-domain gene family A family of genes including pit-1, which encode transcription factors, characterized by a 60-amino acid region similar to the classic homeo-domain and a 76-amino acid region or POU-specific domain responsible for regulating cell-specific developmental events; see pit-1, Homeobox, Homeotic genes

POU-domain proteins A family of homeodomain proteins that transcriptionally activate cell-specific genes, participate in cell fate and are thought to act during embryogenesis through either stable activation of genes responsible for specific developmental pathways or for transient activation that occurs during highly specific developmental periods

pour plate MICROBIOLOGY A culture plate that contains both a nutrient agar and an inoculum of bacteria added to the agar while it is cooling, although pour plates had been used in the past to incubate β-hemolytic streptococci and microaerophlic bacteria, most culture plates used in the modern microbiology laboratory are prepared commercially, and thus this relatively unsophisticated test is no longer commonly used

Pouter pigeon breast deformity Chicken breast deformity, see there

poverty SOCIAL MEDICINE A generic term referring to a state that results when a person or family unit has an income level that is insufficient to provide for basic human needs of food, clothing, shelter and health care; in the US, a person at the poverty level is eligible for Medicaid and food assistance programs; 22% of children in US live below the government poverty level of $14 000/year; family income is reported to be the most critical determinant of a child's IQ; poverty is associated with ↑ anxiety, fear, and unhappiness (Science News 1994; 146:24) see Engel's phenomenon, 'Fourth World, Homelessness, Medicaid; Cf Near poor

poverty index A vehicle of convenience for quantifying the level of poverty; there is no 'official' PI; one suggested calculation combines the information on household income and number of people supported by the income, dividing the result by the national poverty level for a particular country in a particular year (JAMA 1994; 272:947oc)

powder-burn spots Mulberry spots A pattern of endometriosis consisting of multiple tiny puckered foci of hemorrhage, surrounded by minute stellate scars and varying fibrosis

powder tattoo FORENSIC PATHOLOGY A geographically shaped lesion caused by a gun fired at close range, where the still-burning gunpowder embeds in the skin and cannot be wiped away, a finding of use in determining whether clothing was worn overlying an entrance wound; Cf 'Stippling'

PowerMac see Macintosh

power stroke Rowboat model, see there

power surge Surge, see there

power 'take-off' lesion OCCUPATIONAL MEDICINE Avulsion of the loose skin of the scrotum and penis caused by moving parts from factory or farm equipment that may engage a trouser leg and twist upward; the skin may be torn from the glans penis (which is spared) and extend to the coronal sulcus

'power user' COMPUTERS A colloquial term for any person who uses the advanced applications of a software program, or one whose need for raw computing power is close to the upper limits or surpasses the capabilities and speed of his hardware, regardless of how advanced the machine

PPD Purified protein derivative (of tuberculin) The antigenic material used to detect previous exposure to TB; all preparations of PPD are compared to a biological standard (PPD-S) that was prepared from a large lot in 1941; A 5 TU dose of PPD is equivalent to 0.0001 mg of PPD-S protein contained in 0.1 ml of solution

PPD test A clinical test for detecting exposure to *Mycobacterium tuberculosis*; 0.1 ml of 5-tuberculin-unit PPD is injected intradermally; an induration of ≥ 10 mm at 48-72 hours is considered a positive; a negative PPD does not necessarily indicate non-TB exposure, but rather loss of reactivity (anergy), as may occur in immunocompromised states, eg AIDS

PPF Plasma protein fraction, see there

PPLO Pleuropneumonia-like organism *Mycoplasma pneumoniae* An organism that induces asymptomatic respiratory infection or inflammation of the upper respiratory tract, including tracheitis and pharyngitis; *M pneumoniae* spreads by aerosol and causes up to ¾ of all 'closed population' (military 'boot' camps, boarding schools, and colleges) pneumonias, affecting ages 5-20 CLINICAL Headache, malaise, myalgia, low-grade fever, cough, chest tenderness COMPLICATIONS Erythema multiforme, Raynaud's phenomenon, cold agglutinin-induced hemolysis; less commonly neurologic, cardiovascular, musculoskeletal defects TREATMENT Erythromycin, tetracycline

PPNG Penicillinase-producing *Neisseria gonorrhoeae*, see there

PPO 1) HEALTH CARE INDUSTRY Preferred provider organization, see there 2) INSTRUMENTATION 2,5-diphenyloxazole A fluor used for liquid scintillation counting; see POPOP

PP-oma A pancreatic polypeptide-producing islet cell tumor, 40% of which are malignant, characterized by hypercalcemia, hyperglycemia, hypomagnesemia and muscular weakness; Cf Gastrinoma, Islet cell tumors, Pancreatic endocrine tumors, WDHA syndrome, Zollinger-Ellison syndrome

PPRC Physician Payment Review Commission

P protein A regulatory protein that reactivates glutamine synthetase after inactivation through adenylation; Cf Protein P

PPS Prospective payment system, see there

'P' pulmonale CARDIOLOGY A sharply peaked P wave in an EKG seen in COPD*, which is most prominent during exacerbation of clinical disease, although it is a relatively non-specific finding

*Other EKG findings in COPD include a right axis shift, early R waves in the precordial leads V_1 and V_2 and net negativity in V_5 and V_6

PQQ Pyrroloquinoline quinone A quinoprotein that may function as a vitamin-like growth factor; mice fed a PQQ-deficient diet grow poorly, do not reproduce, become osteolathyritic, have friable skin and have low quality collagen, with ↓ cross-linking of collagen and elastin and ↓ lysyl oxidase

practice *noun* Surgery (British) The place where a physician practices medicine in a privately managed setting; a practice is 'built' over the space of years and decades and has both tangible value in the physical plant including the office and equipment, and intangible value in the form of patient trust and lists of patients who the physician has treated while practicing medicine; when a physician retires from practice, it is common practice to sell his practice to a younger physician who purchases the tangible assets of the practice, and attempts to transfer its intangible assets (Am Med News 12 October 1992 p15)

practice guidelines A group of clearly defined or delineated parameters for patient management; although there is considerable activity on the part of professional associations, government and accrediting agencies, health care organizations, and the insurance industry to develop PGs, they have not been as yet clearly delineated; once developed and validated, PGs will serve as benchmarks for the care of the individual patient and form the basis for peer review (Arch Pathol Lab Med 1992; 116:602₀ₐ)

PRAD1 Cyclin D1, see there

PRAD1 Cyclin D1 gene, see there

Prader-Willi syndrome A complex developmental and neurobehavioral disease with an AD [MIM 176270] pattern of inheritance, occuring in 1:10⁴ births (US) CLINICAL

Dwarfism with small hands and feet, hypotonia, mental retardation, hyperphagia, obesity, DM, hypogonadism ± cryptorchidism MOLECULAR PATHOLOGY 1) ± 65% are due to a deletion in the chromosome 15 (15q11q13) of paternal origin; ± 20% are due to inheritance of both copies of chromosome 15 from the mother (maternal uniparental disomy)[1] (N Engl J Med 1992; 326:1599₀ₐ) 2) Point mutation of *P* gene[2] (located in chromosome segment 15q11-q13) which encodes a transmembrane polypeptide that may transport small molecules, eg tyrosine, the precursor of melanin; see Angelman syndrome, oculocutaneous albinism type II

[1]This contrasts with the Angelman syndrome in which there is paternal disomy of chromosome 15 (15q11q13) accompanied by maternal deletion of chromosome 15 [2]Note: *P* gene mutations have also been identified in oculocutaneous albinism type II and autosomal recessive ocular albinism (N Engl J Med 1994; 330ₐ:529₀ₐ)

Prausnitz-Küstner's passive transfer test IMMUNOLOGY A clinical assay that measures allergic responsiveness to foreign proteins METHOD Serum from an allergic individual is injected intradermally into a non-allergic subject; the injection site is subsequently re-exposed ('challenged') with serum containing the antigen, which evokes a local anaphylactic reaction due to the release of IgE CLINICAL Urticaria, rhinitis, vasculitis, mononuclear infiltrate

Note: The test originated from Küstner, who was allergic to fish; whose serum caused the passive allergic reaction in his friend Prausnitz's skin, resulting in a typical wheal-and-flare reaction

pravistatin A cholesterol-lowering agent that inhibits HMG-CoA (3-hydroxy-3-methyl coenzyme A) reductase, the rate-limiting enzyme of cholesterol synthesis; pravistatin decreases 1) Lathosterol (a major cholesterol precursor, the level of which reflects the rate of cholesterol synthesis) by 63% 2) LDL-cholesterol by 39% and 3) Total cholesterol by 26%; cholesterol reduction is due to increased LDL receptors on hepatocytes

praziquantel An antiparasitic agent that is the drug of choice for treating schistosomiasis (*S haematobium, S japonicum*), parasitic flukes (*Trematoda*, eg *Clonorchis sinensis, Opisthorchis viverrini, Paragonimus buski, Heterophyes heterophyes, Metagonimus yokogawai*), and tapeworms (*Hymenolepsis nana* and *Taenia solium*) SIDE EFFECTS Drowsiness, headache, nausea, backache, abdominal discomfort

preadmission testing A battery of tests required prior to hospital admission for elective therapy, eg cataract extraction or cholecystectomy, which serve to establish baseline values and parameters; in a community hospital setting, a typical PAT includes a CBC and leukocyte differential count, PT and PTT, a multichannel analysis of blood chemistries, urinalysis, an EKG and a chest film

Note: PAT for ambulatory surgery is of limited usefulness; in one study, 84% of PATs had abnormalities in the biochemical profiles, urinalysis, blood count, coagulation studies, EKG, or chest film; in 3 cases (of 325) abnormalities sufficient to cancel surgery were identified; only 12 of 272 abnormalities were subjected to further evaluation, ie 96% of the abnormalities were ignored (Am J Surg 1992; 163:565) in one study, the hospital charges for finding an abnormality resulting in a change in the treatment costing $7776 (Arch Surg 1992; 127:801)

prealbumin Transthyretin, see there

preapproval advertising 'Teaser' advertising, see there

prebiotic soup Primordial soup, see there

precancer Premalignancy, see there

precancerous *adjective* Pertaining or referring to a lesion (eg actinic keratosis) or condition (eg fragile X syndrome, xeroderma pigmentosum) that develops into cancer in a high percentage of cases

precautions INFECTIOUS DISEASE A generic term for those activities intended to minimize exposure to an infectious agent; the term implies that the isolation of an infected patient is optional but not mandatory; in practice, when a patient is designated as requiring 'precautions', both he and his specimens (body fluids and waste products) are handled with increased circumspection by his care-givers, as the term carries the implication that he is infected with a contagious or dangerous organism, eg hepatitis B or HIV-1; the CDC discourages identifying any specimen with 'precautions' or 'infectious' labels, ostensibly reasoning that all patient specimens should be handled as potentially infected; Cf Isolation; Safe sex practices, Reverse precautions

precession MRI The relatively slow gyration of the axis of a spinning body, allowing it to 'race out a cone'; precession is caused by the application of a torque that tends to change the direction of a rotation axis and continuously directs it at right angles to the plane of the torque; the magnetic moment of a nucleus with spin will experience such a torque when inclined at an angle to the magnetic field, resulting in precession at the Larmor frequency, eg effect of gravity on a gyroscope or spinning top; see Magnetic resonance imaging

precipitate labor Labor of less than three hours in duration in a primigravida, which proceeds so rapidly that there may be an ↑ risk of maternal or fetal harm, which is due either to an ↑ in the force of uterine contractions (eg as caused by administration of oxytocin), or to low birth canal resistance; see Labor

precipitin A term of waning popularity for an antibody that interacts with an antigen to form a precipitate that sediments out of solution

precision LABORATORY MEDICINE A measurement of the reproducibility of a test or assay, ie its capability of producing the same results when the same assay is performed on the same specimen under the same conditions; a set of data with high precision has a low standard deviation and a low coefficient of variation, analogous to a tight cluster of arrows seen in target practice Note: Accuracy is defined as the correctness of results

preclinical medicine Basic sciences That part of the medical school curriculum (2-3 years in duration, depending on the country) that precedes clinical instruction and training; PM provides a core of basic knowledge required for success in the student's rotations though surgery, internal medicine, gynecology, pediatrics, and the other fields of clinical medicine; the basic sciences include anatomy, physiology, biochemistry, molecular biology, pharmacology, microbiology, pathology

precocious puberty ENDOCRINOLOGY The appearance of secondary sexual characteristics before age 8 in girls and age 9 in boys; if the precocity results from activation of the hypothalamic-pituitary axis, it is designated as complete or true precocious puberty; if the precocity is secondary to ectopic production or autonomous secretion of end-organ hormones, it is designated incomplete precocious puberty (table)

predetermination HEALTH CARE FINANCING Prior approval by an insurance carrier to pay for a proposed treatment; while 'standard' therapies are reimbursed by health insurance carriers, payment for costly clinical research trials, eg autologous bone marrow transplantation for breast cancer and experimental regimens by third-party payers is seemingly arbitrary and/or capricious (N Engl J Med 1994; 330:473SA)

predictive value P value LABORATORY MEDICINE A value that predicts the likelihood that a particular result from a clinical test correlates with the presence or absence of a disease process; see Negative predictive value, Positive predictive value; Cf ROC curve

predictive value of a positive test Positive predictive value, see there

predictive value of a negative test Negative predictive value, see there

predisposition Predisposing condition A generic term for an ↑ in susceptibility to a particular condition, eg malignancy or infection

predisposition testing A generic term for the screening of a battery of molecular markers in order to identify inherited mutations that have been linked to malignancies, eg inherited colon cancer (mutations of MSH2 and MSH1), breast cancer (BRCA1), endocrine tumors (RET), melanoma (p16), and Li-Fraumeni syndrome (p53); see BRCA1, p16, p53

preditory pricing HEALTH CARE FINANCING A health insurance pricing structure (of uncertain ethics) in which small groups and individuals who are at low risk for actually using the covered services are charged a low price that rapidly escalates should they begin to use the service and file claims (Am Med News 25 October 1992, p7)

predonation TRANSFUSION MEDICINE The deposition of one or more units of packed red cells for autologous transfusion prior to an anticipated need, eg elective surgery; to virtually eliminate allogeneic blood transfusions, it is recommended that in addition to predonation of two units of blood, that acute preoperative hemodilution can be used to obtain an additional 3-4 units (Arch Pathol Lab Med 1994; 118:333ED) see Autologous donation, Leapfrog method

preeclampsia OBSTETRICS A hypertensive disorder occurring in up 5% of all pregnancies in the third trimester of pregnancy; in addition to hypertension, it is characterized by proteinuria, and usually, dependent edema, vasospasm, and coagulation abnormalities PATHOLOGY XXX TREATMENT Low-dose aspirin ↓ preeclampsia in nulliparas, especially with systolic hypertension; aspirin ↑ risk of abruptio placentae, but does not ↓ perinatal mortality (N Engl J Med 1993; 329:1213OA) RISKS FACTORS < 1 or ≥ 3 glasses of milk/day is associated with an risk of preeclampsia (BE RICHARDSON, DD BAIRD, Am J EPIDEMIOL, APRIL 1995) see Eclampsia

pre-embryo see in vitro fertilization

pre-existing condition Any injury, illness or medical condition, eg cancer, DM, hypertension that a person had prior to issuing a health insurance policy, which might preclude that person from being approved for health insurance; the presence of a PEC may result in 'job lock', a situation where a person cannot leave a place of employment because he/she would not be able obtain health insurance

---

PRECOCIOUS PUBERTY

TRUE OR COMPLETE PRECOCIOUS PUBERTY (affects both sexes)
Idiopathic
Constitutional or familial
CNS disease, eg tumors (hypothalamic and pineal gliomas, craniopharyngiomas, germinomas, hamartomas of the tuber cinereum), as well as encephalitis, abscesses, cysts, sarcoidosis, tuberculosis
McCune-Albright syndrome
Hypothyroidism
Virilizing syndromes, eg congenital adrenal hyperplasia
INCOMPLETE OF PARTIAL PRECOCIOUS PUBERTY
Male Due to gonadotropin-secreting tumors, eg hepatoma, Leydig cell tumor, excessive androgen production or premature Leydig cell and germinal cell maturation
Female Due to ovarian follicle cysts or estrogen-producing neoplasms, eg granulosa cell tumor

at the next place of employment; see Job lock

preferred provider organization HEALTH CARE INDUSTRY A form of managed health care in which a limited number of health providers (physicians, hospitals, and others) provide services to a defined group of clients for a negotiated fee-for-service rate that is below the 'market value' for the service(s); PPOs offer incentives to the clients for using their contracted physicians, where the PPO physicians are paid in full, while the non-PPO physicians are not and the client must pay the difference in the professional fees, usually 10-30% (which allows the client freedom of choice at a price); the number of PPOs has risen from 25 in 1982 to 506 in 1986; physician-sponsored PPOs have an average of 240 physicians; hospital-sponsored PPOs have 430 physicians

pregnancy gingivitis Granuloma gravidarum An exuberant, pyogenic granuloma-like inflammatory response of pregnant gums to an overhanging margin of tooth filling or crown with excess calcium buildup, which was reported to occur in the first trimester in 0.5-2.0% of pregnancies, grow until delivery and regress spontaneously without therapy, although it may re-appear with subsequent pregnancy; regarding this 'condition' Regezi and Sciubba refer to, '...*the infrequently used and inappropriate term 'pregnancy gingivitis'...It is questionable whether significant gingival enlargement during* (pregnancy) *...would be seen in individuals with scrupulous oral hygiene* (Oral Pathology, 2nd ed, WB Saunders, Philedelphia, 1993)

pregnancy-related conditions see Chorea gravidarum, Herpes gestationalis, Melasma, Pregnancy 'tumor', Pruritus gravidarum, PUPPP; Cf Postpartum-related conditions

pregnancy-specific β₁ glycoprotein SP-1 A protein of unknown function produced by the trophoblast that can be detected from the 16th day of pregnancy in the maternal serum and amniotic fluid, which shares sequence homology with the CEA family and contains repeating domains, conserved disulfide bridges and a β-sheet structure typical of proteins produced by the immunoglobulin gene superfamily

pregnancy test A generic term for any of a number of tests used to determine whether a woman is pregnant; the first generation of PTs were bioassays, in which a menagerie of beasts[1] were injected with urine from a possibly pregnant female, and the physiologic response[2] to the urine[3] evaluated; for obvious reasons[4], the bioassay was replaced[5] by other tests in particular, various forms of immunoassays, eg RIA, radioreceptor assays, IRMA, ELISA, and others; do-it-yourself home testing kits[6] are widely used in both the private sector[7] and the clinical setting[8], given their ease of use

[1]Frogs, toads, and rabbits [2]Spermatogenesis [3] Which may or may not contain hCG-human chorionic gonadotropin [4]Cost, space, mess, noise [5]By the 1960s [6]And have been responsible for countless shaving cuts [7]ie the consumer [8]By the gynecologist

preleukemia Myelodysplastic syndrome Any of a heterogeneous group of clonal expansions of BM stem cells, which are characterized by dysmyelopoiesis, a complex of structural and functional abnormalities including abnormal cell morphology, ineffective hemopoiesis and chromosome defects, eg aneuploidy and pseudodiploidy; preleukemic states include acquired idiopathic sideroblastic and non-sideroblastic anemias, pancytopenia with hypercellular marrow and paroxysmal nocturnal hemoglobinuria, which may progress to acute non-lymphocytic leukemia Note: Certain genetic disorders have an ↑ tendency to develop leukemias, including hematologic diseases (Kostmann syndrome, Fanconi syndrome), anomalies of either sex chromosomes (Klinefelter and Turner syndromes) or autosomal chromosomes (ataxia-telangiectasia, Bloom syndrome and Down syndrome); acquired

states predisposed to leukemias include BM injury by drugs, eg chlorambucil, chemicals, eg benzene and radiation, and myeloproliferative disease (agnogenic myeloid metaplasia, CML, ITP, and polycythemia vera)

preliminary diagnosis Working diagnosis, see there, aka provisional diagnosis

prelymphoma A group of conditions characterized by monotonous aggregates of lymphocytes and a known tendency to evolve to lymphoma and thus warrant close clinical follow-up; prelymphomas include pseudolymphoma of the orbit and small intestine, lymphomatoid granulomatosis (an angiocentric lung disease with lymphoma-like extrapulmonary involvement), angioimmunoblastic lymphadenopathy, lymphoid interstitial pneumonitis

Note: Lymphomas may occur in a background of chemotherapy, radiotherapy, connective tissue disease, monoclonality and immunocompromise, both congenital and acquired

premalignancy Precancer Any of a group of lesions with a tendency to undergo malignant degeneration; precancers of epithelial origin may be 1) Glandular, eg adenomatous hyperplasia (endometrium) and adenomatous polyps (colon, stomach) that evolve towards adenocarcinoma of their respective organs or 2) Squamous, eg dysplasia of the uterine cervix or other urogenital mucosae; premalignant lesions of mesenchymal origin include prelymphoma and 'presarcoma' (an ad hoc coinage), the latter of which may be due to a variety of predisposing factors, eg osteosarcoma may arise in Paget's disease of bone, irradiation, hereditary multiple exostoses, polyostotic fibrous dysplasia, enchondroma, and Mafucci's enchondromatosis; osteosarcoma may be induced under experimental conditions by various types of trauma, including chemical, eg turpentine, mechanical, eg local pressure, indwelling foreign bodies and ischemia, eg vessel clamping; Cf Preneoplastic state(s)

Note: Some of the histologic changes of epithelial premalignancy may be reversed by supplementing the diet with vitamin B₁₂ and folate, as well as vitamins C, A and E

premarket approval process A process in which the data generated on the safety and risk to health of a medical device (or drug) intended for clinical use is presented to the FDA, prior to formal FDA approval of the device for marketing; the pre-approval process takes a year or more and is designed to protect the human subjects involved in pre-approval investigations of the device and provide greater certainty on its safety and efficacy (JAMA 1994; 272:955sc) see Premarket notification

premarket notification 501(k) A group of documents that are submitted to the FDA by a manufacturer of a medical device prior to its marketing; the notification assists the FDA in determining whether the device is substantially equivalent to a previously marketed predecessor device (JAMA 1994; 272:955sc) see Premarket approval

premature ejaculation Ejaculatio praecox A manifestation of sexual dysfunction, which is defined in DSM-IV as '*Persistent or recurrent ejaculation with minimal sexual stimulation before, on, or shortly after penetration and before the person wishes it.* (Criterion A), which '*...causes marked distress or interpersonal difficulty.* (Criterion B), and is not substantially associated with the effects of a substance (ie a drug or substance of abuse, Criterion C); in the evaluation of PE, certain factors must be weighed, eg the subject's age, novelty of partner, recent sexual activity, and so on; Cf Nocturnal emission, Onanism

premature ovarian failure Cessation of menses before age 40, accompanied by elevated serum gonadotropin levels, often idiopathic, due to a deletion of a fragment of the long arm of chromosome X (46,XX,del(X)(pter-q21.3:q27-qter), or secondary to known causes including ovarian receptor antibodies, viral infections, cytotoxic drugs and irradiation

premature rupture of membranes OBSTETRICS The leakage of amniotic fluid prior to the onset of labor, an event that occurs in 10% of term pregnancies and 15-20% of pre-term pregnancies; PROM is associated with ↑ mortality and morbidity; the etiology of PROM is unknown, but may be due to the combined action of bacterial or internal enzymes COMPLICATIONS Fetal infections, eg congenital pneumonia or septicemia and fetal wastage TREATMENT Deliver baby within 36 hours

premature ventricular contraction A ventricular discharge characterized by premature, widened, bizarre QRS complexes that are not preceded by a P wave; PVCs are common in young subjects and are of no significance, but may be caused by anxiety, fever, various drugs and stimulants; they require investigation in underlying heart disease, if PVCs increase with exercise, in absence of intervening sinus rhythm, R-on-T phenomenon (see there), and if the patient is aware of the arrhythmia (which may be recognized as a 'skipped beat or 'tickle'); PVCs with a variable contour are considered multifocal; when the PVCs have identical contours, they are classified as unifocal, but may occur in a background of underlying heart disease, increasing the risk for cardiac death; PVCs are associated with drug toxicity (digitalis, quinidine and tricyclic antidepressants) and are an indication for discontinuing therapy

premature infant OBSTETRICS A generic term for an infant who is born significantly before the normal 40 weeks of gestation, which is often understood to also mean of low birth weight; recent data (see chart) suggest that length of gestation is more important than weight (JAMA and New York Times (pC11) of 1 March1995)

prematurity OBSTETRICS The state of being premature, which encompasses a constellation of clinical findings seen in an infant delivered before 37 weeks of gestation (37 weeks from the first day of the last menstrual period) who is often also immature; morbid conditions associated with prematurity include anemia due to low iron and vitamin E, bronchopulmonary dysplasia, intraventricular hemorrhage, especially in the very low birth weight infants, permanent neurological sequelae and retinopathy; the figure below indicates the mortality per thousand infants as the gestational age migrates from the optimal term (0 on abscissa) INTERVENTIONS Weight gain is reported to be faster and neurological development improved, eg ↑ dopamine, norepinephrine and epinephrine in the urine of premature infants treated with stroking, taped messages from parents, soft music, low lighting, reducing incubator time and shortening the length of intensive hospital-based care; see Low birth weight; Cf Post-term pregnancy

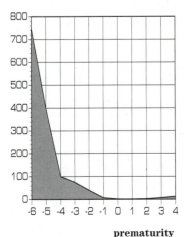

prematurity

premed Premedical *adjective* Pertaining or relating to preparation for a career in medicine *noun* A colloquial term for a student who is studying the core curriculum required or admission to medical school in the US

premelanosome An oval structure with a dense, grainy matrix and 'cross-striations', which comprises a pathognomonic ultrastructural criterion for melanocytes (figure, right, schematically enlarged 100 000 X), which serves to confirm the diagnosis of melanoma; in practice, most melanomas can be diagnosed by simple light microsopy

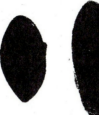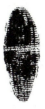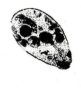

premelanosomes

premelting MOLECULAR BIOLOGY A phenomenon affecting double-stranded nucleic acids, eg DNA and DNA-RNA hybrid molecules, in which the two chains begin to dissociate at temperatures far below that at which complete disassociation occurs; see Breathing

premenstrual dysphoric disorder The 'official' (per American Psychiatric Association in the Diagnosis and Statistical Manual, 4th ed-DSM-IV, 1994) term for Premenstrual syndrome (PMS), see there

PREMENSTRUAL DYSPHORIC DISORDER (RESEARCH CRITERIA)

Five or more of below symptoms occurring in a cyclical fashion, at least one of which is 1-4

1) Depressed mood, self-deprecation, hopelessness

2) Anxiety, tension, feeling 'wired'

3) Emotional lability

4) Marked and/or persistent anger, irritability, or interpersonal conflict

5) Decreased interest in usual activities or relationships

6) Difficulty in concentrating

7) Lethargy

8) Change in appetite

9) Change in sleep habits

10) Subjective sense of loss of control

11) Physical symptoms, eg breast tenderness, headaches, arthralgia, myalgia, bloating, weight gain

(modified from DSM-IV)

premenstrual syndrome Premenstrual dysphoric disorder, see also PMS

pre-mRNA Pre-messenger RNA, nuclear messenger RNA precursor A term that usually refers to the 'primary RNA transcript', a messenger RNA molecule that is the direct transcription product or mirror image of a DNA 'template'; pre-mRNA is an immature mRNA molecule that contains intervening sequences (introns) that are not part of a mature mRNA, which is destined to be translated to form a cognate protein; introns are removed by splicing in a two-step process occurring in the spliceosome, where cleavage occurs at the 5' site and a guanosine residue at the 5' end of the intron is covalently joined to the adenine residue near the 3' splice site in a recognition element, known as the branch point sequence; in the second step, the 3' end of the pre-mRNA is cleaved and joined to the exons forming mature mRNA; some pre-mRNA molecules may be spliced at different sites resulting in the production of different proteins from one pre-mRNA molecule; see Alternative splicing; Cf hnRNA

prenatal tests, fetal OBSTETRICS A generic term for any of the laboratory tests and assays used to detect genetic and/or congenital fetal anomalies that would compromise the infant's well-being and quality of life to such a degree that the parents might prefer an abortion; these tests include measurement of α-fetoprotein levels in the mother's serum or amniotic fluid, chromosomal analysis, ultrasonography, chorionic villus biopsy (performed on or after the 8th-10th gestational weeks, risk of spontaneous abortion or miscarriage-1.0-1.5%), amniocentesis (performed on or after the 16th gestational week-risk of spontaneous abortion or miscarriage, 0.5%), fetoscopy, and embryoscopy; diseases detected include α_1-antitrypsin activity, thalassemias, defects of sex and autosomal chromosomes including trisomies, deletions, mosaicisms, fragile X syndrome, hemophilia, neural tube defects (anencephaly, spina bifida), polycystic renal disease, Tay-Sachs disease; see Embroscopy, Fetoscopy; Cf Wrongful birth

prenatal testing, maternal Obstetric (screening) profile, see there

preneoplastic state(s) A broad group of congenital conditions that predispose to development of malignancy (table); see Fragile X syndrome, Hereditary neoplasms, Premalignancy

---

PRENEOPLASTIC STATES

CHROMOSOME BREAKAGE SYNDROMES Bloom syndrome, Fanconi syndrome

GENODERMATOSES Albinism, dyskeratosis congenita, epidermodysplasia verruciformis, polydysplastic epidermolysis bullosa, Werner syndrome, xeroderma pigmentosa

HAMARTOMATOUS SYNDROMES Multiple exostoses, neurofibromatosis, Peutz-Jegher syndrome, tuberous sclerosis, von Hippel-Lindau syndrome

IMMUNODEFICIENCY SYNDROMES Ataxia-telangiectasia, Wiskott-Aldrich syndrome, X-linked agammaglobulinemia

---

prenylation MOLECULAR BIOLOGY A post-translational modification of protein involving the addition of unit(s) of isoprene (C_5H_8); the function of which is unclear; activation of the Ras protein requires prenylation; isoprenoids may help anchor proteins to cell membranes

pre-op Preoperative *adjective* Pertaining or relating to the preparation for a surgical procedure or other operation *noun* 1) A colloquial term for all forms of care (eg medication) provided to a patient prior to a surgical intervention 2) The ward where patients are held prior to a surgical intervention

preoperative autologous blood donation Autologous blood, see there

'prep' SURGERY The preparation of both the patient and the operative region prior to the first incision, which consists of painting the surface with soap and disposable sponges, shaving of hair, and insertion of a catheter

preproliferative diabetic retinopathy A condition defined as the presence of microaneurysms, retinal hemorrhage(s) and exudates, and intraretinal vascular defects (N Eng J Med 1995; 332:1210RV)

preproprotein An inactive precursor of a secretory protein, which is both a preprotein, ie a secretory protein that still has an attached 'signal sequence' of amino acids, and a proprotein, ie protein that is 'activated' by removing an oligopeptide

prescription benefit management company HEALTH CARE MANAGEMENT A company that acts as a broker for insurance companies, HMOs, large corporations, and others for obtaining the most cost-effective drugs; PBMCs usually obtain the pharmaceuticals at deep discounts provided by the drugs' manufacturers in exchange for bulk purchases and restrictions on competing drugs (Am Med News 24 April 1995 p12)

present (*pronounced* pree sent) *verb intransitive* CLINICAL MEDICINE To be brought to medical attention OBSTETRICS To appear (eg a fetal part) at the opening cervical os during labor *verb transitive* To formally provide information about a case or patient

pressure dressing A misnomer for an occlusive, but pressure-less wound dressing that stabilizes and partially immobilizes a region of skin, used in burns

pressure-generating material OCCUPATIONAL SAFETY A chemical substance or mixture that may 1) Polymerize spontaneously with an increase in pressure (unless protected by the addition of an inhibitor, or by refrigeration or other control) 2) Decompose to release gas in its container, or 3) Comprises the content of a self pressurized container

pressure pants An intermittent pneumatic leg compression device used to reduce the incidence of deep and proximal vein thromboses, which is of use in preventing post-surgical venous thrombosis seen in general, prostatic, orthopedic and neurosurgery; pressure pants may be a viable substitute for pharmacological anticoagulation and is as cost-effective as warfarin which incurs daily laboratory costs for monitoring coagulation parameters; Cf MAST (Military anti-shock trousers)

pressure ulcer Bedsore A decubital ulcer appearing on dependent sites, usually on the lumbosacral region, but also on the heels, knees, or vertebral spine, which is most common in the bed-ridden elderly, seen in up to ¼ of nursing home residents, and associated with an ↑ mortality; PUs are divided into STAGE I Nonresolving erythema with no break in skin STAGE II Erythema with superficial interruption of skin, abrasions or vesiculation STAGE III Full-thickness loss of skin with serosanguinous drainage STAGE IV Full-thickness loss of skin and invasion of deeper tissue RISK FACTORS Nonblanchable erythema, lymphopenia, immobility, dry skin, low body weight, and activity limited to bed or chair (JAMA 1995; 273:865) TREATMENT A 'cocktail' of recombinant platelet-derived growth factor, proteases, and cell-adhesion molecules has been reported to induce healing of wounds that have been recalcitrant to years of therapy (Science 1991; 252:1065n)

presumed consent The assumption that a particular action would have been approved by a person or party had that permission been sought; PC is a mechanism suggested by the American Medical Association's Council on Ethical and Judicial Affairs for increasing the number of cadaveric organs available for transplantation; the stance of PC contrasts sharply with the present system, in which altruism (ie the wish to donate an organ) is not assumed and the potential donor must 'opt in' to be able to donate, and assumes that a person would consent to organ donation, unless specific objections have been formally registered, in which case one must formally 'opt out', rather formally 'opt in' (JAMA 1994; 272:809CR) see Cadaveric organ transplantation, Mandated choice; Cf Informed consent

presyncope Any of the various promonitory signs or symptoms (eg severe weakness or lightheadedness) of imminent syncope (see N Engl J Med 1993; 328:1085OA)

pressured speech PSYCHIATRY A virtually continuous flow of accelerated speech which may be difficult or impossible to interrupt, which may be loud, emphatic, socially uninhibited, and may continue even though no one is listening

(DSM-IV)

prevalence EPIDEMIOLOGY The number of cases of a disease divided by the total number of subjects in the population; Cf Incidence

prevascular phase ONCOLOGY A stable, relatively non-aggressive phase in tumor development that may persist for years, characterized by limited tumor growth; the prevascular phase has been studied in carcinoma of the breast, melanoma, urinary bladder and uterine cervix and may be 'switched' by an unknown mechanism to a 'vascular phase', which is characterized by the presence of angiogenic molecules, rapid tumor growth, bleeding and metastatic potential; semiquantification of the number of vessels (marked by immunoperoxidase staining of tissue with antibodies to factor VIII antigen) in a tumor may serve to identify tumors that have entered a vascular phase (**N Engl J Med 1991; 324:1**) see Metastasis

prevention PUBLIC HEALTH The impedance, avoidance, or hindrance of an adverse effect, disease process or other undesired action; prevention may be

PRIMARY PREVENTION–an intervention made to avert disease or injury, eg vaccination or purification of a potable water supply

SECONDARY PREVENTION–the early detection and treatment of an evolving disease process, eg by screening

TERTIARY PREVENTION–an intervention intended to prevent the progression of a established disease, eg septic abortion or disability, eg spinal cord injury by appropriate therapy

preventive care A generic term for the implementation of services intended to prevent rather than treat a disease state; under the rubric of PC are surveillance and screening activities (eg mammography), immunization (eg measles, mumps, rubella), education on promoting safety (eg use of bicycle helmets) and reducing high-risk (eg smoking) behaviors (**JAMA 1995; 273:1130oa, 1149ed**)

preventive health service PUBLIC HEALTH Any component in the evaluation of a person's health status that attempts to identify or prevent a disease process not known to exist in the patient at the time of initial evaluation, eg genetic counseling, screening for metabolic diseases, eg DM or PKU, immunization/vaccination, or screening for hypercholesterolemia, hypertension, or malignancy (**N Engl J Med 1994; 330:1589ra**) see Screening

preventive medicine The branch of medicine which specializes in the prevention of disease, injury, and disability, and in the promotion of health; PM attempts to identify preventable diseases and risk factors thereof (**JAMA 1995; 273:1403**)

priapism An uncommon condition characterized by prolonged and usually painful penile erection occurring in the absence of sexual excitement or desire; 60% of cases are idiopathic, the rest are due to a vast palette of diseases including leukemia, pelvic infection, pelvic malignancy, sickle cell anemia, substance abuse (alcohol, cocaine, marijuana, methaqualone), scorpion bites, penile or spinal cord trauma, or may be drug-related (anticoagulants, antihypertensives, corticosteroids, neuroleptics, tolbutamide, papaverine) CLINICAL Painful, prolonged erection with a tense and congested corpora cavernosa, constituting a urologic emergency MECHANISM Accumulation of hypoxic blood of high viscosity in the corpora cavernosa, due to a physiologic obstruction of venous blood PROGNOSIS Without surgical decompression, interstitial edema and fibrosis of the penile shaft ensue, causing impotence; priapism may rarely occur in females, eg related to granular cell tumor (**Am J Surg Pathol 1986; 10:497oa**) Cf Bobbittize, Penile prosthesis, Peyronie's disease

Priapus, the Greek god of fertility and procreation, was born of Bacchus and Venus, and has a macrophallus ('well-hung' in the vernacular)

Pribnow box MOLECULAR BIOLOGY A highly-conserved-in-evolution 'consensus' sequence of six DNA nucleotides (TATAAT) that is located about 10 base pairs upstream (in the 5' direction) from bacterial promoter regions and separated by 5-8 base pairs from the initiation site for RNA polymerase

price fixing HEALTH CARE INDUSTRY The reaching of an agreement or understanding with competitors of what a provider of goods or services will charge for those services or goods; it is considered unethical in the free market economy (as it functions in the US) for two physicians to discuss fees for services; in order for a physician to ascertain a 'fair market' price for his services, he may hire a consultant who will use a variety of conversion factors to determine the value of the service provided by the physician in his/her region

PRICE principle SPORTS MEDICINE A general guideline for the steps involved in treating any acute sports injury of a joint, which is conveniently ennumerated by the acronym PRICE: *Protection* of the injured body part by crutches, splints, or an immobilizer, *rest* of injured part, *ice*, *compression*, and *elevation* to ↓ swelling and facilitate early range of motion (**Mayo Clin Proc 1995; 70:549**)

prick test A clinical test for immediate hypersensitivity, in which a diluted allergen is droppered on the skin and a sterile needle is used to 'prick' the epidermal surface; the reaction is then compared to that obtained with standardized mast cell secretogogues, eg compound 48/80, codeine and histamine; in contrast to the intradermal test, in which the very low concentrations of the allergen are allowed to penetrate below the epidermis, the prick test is more rapid, simpler, and causes less discomfort for the patient, can be used to test infants and false positive results are rare, although false negative results are more common; both evoke increased production of IgE antibodies

prickly heat Miliaria, see there

primaquine PARASITOLOGY An oral 8-aminoquinoline antimalarial drug effective in treating relapses of clinical malaria, acting against the hepatic but not intraerythrocytic stages of *Plasmodium vivax* and *P ovale*; it is a potent oxidant, causing hemolysis in glucose-6-phosphate dehydrogenase deficient patients, the so-called 'primaquine sensitivity syndrome' TOXICITY Per os, primaquine is not associated with major systemic effects; parenterally, it may be associated with profound hypotension

$$CH_3$$
$$|$$
$$HNCH(CH_2)_3NH_2$$

primaquine

primary acquired melanosis A condition first seen in the middle-aged population as a unilateral, diffuse brown pigmentation of the conjunctiva which may 1) Remain stationary or regress 2) Slowly enlarge, but remain benign or 3) Undergo malignant degeneration (17% of cases), where melanocytic atypia is a significant predictor of malignancy

Note: Secondary acquired melanosis may be caused by acanthosis nigricans, keratomalacia, metabolic disease (Addison's disease, pregnancy), radiation, toxins (arsenic, thyroxin), trachoma, vernal conjunctivitis, xeroderma pigmentosum

primary amebic meningoencephalitis An intracranial infection caused by free-living amoebae, including *Naegleria* (*N fowleri*, *N grubei*), *Acanthamoeba*,

Hartmanella*, *Entamoeba histolytica* and others CLINICAL PAM may be acute and purulent, causing meningoencephalitis in young healthy persons swimming in stagnant artificial fresh water lakes, typically caused by *Naegleria* species; the inflammation and hemorrhage is most intense along the olfactory tract, inculpating the cribriform plate as the portal of entry via the nose; the prognosis is poor; the few survivors were treated to parenteral amphotericin B, miconazole, and rifampicin, and had major sequelae; PAM may also be subacute with a granulomatous tissue reaction, a finding that is more common in immunocompromised hosts

*'Because of the confusion that existed in the earlier literature with regard to the nomenclature of *Acanthamoeba* and *Hartmannella*, some workers in the field referred to these amebas as belonging to the *Hartmannella-Acanthamoeba* group. Since no true *Hartmennella* species has as yet been found to be pathogenic to humans, all references to *Hartmannella* in human tissues should be corrected to read as *Acanthamoeba...*' (A Balows, et al, Eds, Manual of Clinical Microbiology, 4th ed, American Society for Microbiology, Washington, DC 1991)

primary angiitis of the central nervous system Granulomatous angiitis of the central nervous system, see there

primary antibody A generic term for the first antibody used in a 'sandwich' method, eg ELISA; the PA recognizes the antigen of interest and is raised in a specific animal, eg rabbit, goat, etc; see Sandwich method; Cf Secondary antibody

prior-authorization (requirement) DRUG UTILIZATION Mandatory advance approval for the use of any expensive therapy, eg expensive drugs that are available in a generic form that are regarded as being equally effective; in one study in Tennessee, the simple expediency of requiring P-A for nongeneric NSAIDs resulted in an estimated savings of $12.8 million over a two-year period, a finding which applied on national scale in the US would save an estimated $1 billion/year (N Engl J Med 1995; 332:1612SA, 41SB)

primary autonomic dysfunction A heterogeneous group of autonomic system dysfunctions characterized by hypoadrenergic postural hypotension with blunted vasomotor response to norepinephrine upon standing, decreased sweating, heat intolerance, GI symptoms, impotence, urinary and fecal incontinence PAD type I is characterized by low plasma levels of norepinephrine PAD type II or Shy-Drager disease is further characterized by Parkinson-type cerebral degeneration DDx Postural hypotension may also be due to cerebral and spinal cord lesions, eg degeneration, infection, trauma and tumors and peripheral neuropathy, eg alcohol, amyloidosis, DM, porphyria and toxins

primary biliary cirrhosis A disease of adult ♀ ages 30-65 CLINICAL Fatigue, pruritis, steatorrhea, hepatic osteodystrophy, renal tubular acidosis, and a four-fold increase in hepatocellular and breast carcinoma; 80% of PBC also have autoimmune or connective tissue disease, eg autoimmune thyroiditis, scleroderma, rheumatoid arthritis, and Sjögren or sicca syndrome PATHOLOGY (table) LABORATORY 20-50-fold increase in alkaline phosphatase, IgM and antimitochondrial antibodies (of the 8 known antimitochondrial antibodies, M2 is most commonly associated with PBC); anti-SS-A/Ro antibodies occur in 20% of cases TREATMENT Liver transplantation, colchicine (which is both anti-fibrotic and anti-inflammatory), and ursodiol, a nontoxic bile acid, long-term therapy by which may slow disease progression, reducing the need for liver transplantation (N Engl J Med 1994; 330:1342OA) see Ursodiol

primary care A generic term for basic (ie 'low tech') health care services that are coordinated, comprehensive and personal; PC is available on both a first-contact and continuous basis and incorporates the tasks of medical diagnosis and treatment, psychological assessment and management, personal support, communication of information about illness, prevention and health maintenance;

PC is the least specialized level of medical care, often rendered by a 'primary' physician, who may be a general practitioner, family physician, internist, pediatrician, obstetrician or emergency room physician; primary care includes examination of a patient in a medical, behavioral and social context as well as performing preventive, diagnostic and therapeutic activities; most of a person's need for medical attention may be provided in a primary care situation and it is a point of entry into higher levels of health care; in Canada, primary care is viewed in a more positive light, which may in part be related to the control over specialization in medicine that is exerted by the Royal College of Physicians and Surgeons of Canada (N Engl J Med 1992; 326:1469SA) see General practitioner, Internist; Cf Hospital-based medicine, Medical specialties, RAPERs, Secondary care, Surgical specialties, Tertiary care

primary cause of death Underlying cause of death, see there, aka proximate cause of death

primary fluor LABORATORY MEDICINE An organic compound (or fluor, eg PPO) that is capable of scintillation, which absorbs weak beta radiation, and emits a flash of light in a scintillation device; see POPOP, RIA; Cf Secondary fluor

primary gain PSYCHIATRY The fundamental psychological gain that one obtains from an illness, eg alleviation of anxiety in neurosis by 'converting' emotions into an organic disease, eg hysterical dysphonia; Cf Secondary gain

primary granules Primary lysosomes, see Azurophilic granules

primary hyperoxaluria Oxalosis An AR condition which is divided into

PRIMARY HYPEROXALURIA, TYPE I [MIM 259900], a defect or mistargeting of hepatic alanine-glyoxalate transaminase [EC 2.6.1.44] results in ↑ production of oxalate and glycolate (in the form of glycolic and glyoxylic acids)

PRIMARY HYPEROXALURIA, TYPE II [MIM 260000], caused by deficiencies in glyoxylate reductase and D-glycerate dehydrogenase result in ↑ production of L-glyceric acid and oxalate

CLINICAL In both, the ↑↑↑ calcium oxalate (CO) in the urine results in supersaturation of CO with crystalluria, stone formation, and deposition of CO in the renal parenchyma, which leads to comprise of renal function and CO deposition in multiple organs (oxalosis) TREATMENT Orthophosphate and pyridoxine PROGNOSIS With therapy (*vide sopra*) actuarial ESRD-free survival at 20 years is ± 75%; sans therapy, 80% have ESRD by the 3rd decade of life; renal transplants do not survive well; liver transplantation may be used to correct the enzyme defect (N Engl J Med 1994; 331:1553OA)

primary hypertension Essential hypertension

primary idiopathic sideroblastic anemia Idiopathic (acquired) refractory anemia, see there

---

PRIMARY BILIARY CIRRHOSIS-HISTOPATHOLOGY

STAGE I Ductal hepatitis (triaditis) with florid, asymmetrical destruction of septal and interlobular bile ducts surrounded by a dense infiltrate of CD4 T lymphocytes and granulomas

STAGE II Florid bile duct proliferation, with atypical bile ducts with irregular lumens, diffuse portal fibrosis and mononuclear cells in triads the 'periportal stage'

STAGE III Fibrosis with portal-to-portal 'bridging' and nodule formation

STAGE IV Cirrhosis or end-stage disease which is difficult to distinguish from other cirrhoses, although the absence of bile ducts corroborates the diagnosis

primary intention see Wound healing

primary PCTA Percutaneous transluminal coronary angioplasty that is performed in patients with an evolving Q-wave MI; the 90-96% one year post-MI survival rate with primary PCTA is reportedly better than that of thrombolytic therapy; those undergoing PCTA had fewer adverse effects in the form of reinfarction, fatality, recurrent ischemia (N Engl J Med 1994; 330:981RA) see Per cutaneous transluminal angioplasty

primary response The response that the immune system displays when it is first exposed to an antigen; Cf Secondary response

primary RNA transcript see Pre-mRNA

primary sclerosing cholangitis Sclerosing cholangitis, see there

primary sclerosing cholangitis A chronic idiopathic hepatopathy characterized by inflammation, destruction, and fibrosis of intra- and extrahepatic bile ducts, resulting in cholestasis, cirrhosis, portal hypertension, and hepatic failure; although relatively uncommon (prevalence 1-6/10^5, US), PSC is the 4th most common indication for liver transplantation; 75% of patients with PSC have inflammatory bowel disease; 70% of patients are ♂, with an average of 39 CLINICAL Most patients are asymptomatic until end-stage liver disease has developed; as albumin falls and bilirubin rises, pruritus, fatigue, jaundice, and weight loss dominate the clinical picture, which may be accompanied by fever, chills, night sweats, and right upper quadrant pain PATHOGENESIS Unknown, possibly bacterial products (eg N-formyl L-methionine L-leucine L-tyrosine) acting as toxic proinflammatory agents; other causative factors implicated include ischemia, viral infection, defective immunoregulation; there is an ↑ incidence of PSC in those with HLA-B8, DR3, DR2, and DR4 RADIOLOGY ERCP and transhepatic cholangiography demostrate multiple zones of narrowing and dilatation LABORATORY ↑ Alkaline phosphatase, ↑ aminotransferase, hypergammaglobulinemia, ↑ IgM PATHOLOGY 4 histologic stages have been identified, beginning with inflammation and scarring of the portal triads in stage 1, eventuating in frank cirrhosis in stage 4; the pathognomonic finding is the so-called onionskin lesion (N Engl J Med 1995; 332:924RV) TREATMENT Azacytidine may free patients from the need for transfusion possibly by hypomethylation of fetal globin gene promoters and possibly also enhance fetal globin synthesis (ibid 1993; 329:840a) Butyrate stimulates the fetal hemoglobin gene promoter, leading to ↑ γ-globin gene expression to levels sufficient to ameliorate β-thalassemia symptoms (ibid; 328:81oa) other therapies include iron chelation–early use of deferiprone (ibid 1995; 332:918oa), corticosteroids, penicillamine, ursodiol, methotrexate PROGNOSIS Median survival after diagnosis, 11.9 years

primary structure see Protein structure

primary target gene A gene the expression of which is directly controlled (↑ or ↓) by a nuclear receptor ligand; the promoter region of target genes contain receptor binding sites, and some encode transcription factors that control the expression of secondary target genes

primary tumor A neoplasm that in clinical parlance is regarded as malignant, arising in one site and capable of giving birth to metastatic or secondary tumors; see Metastasis; Cf Tumor of unknown origin

primase A DNA-dependent RNA polymerase that synthesizes RNA 'primers' (4-12 nucleotide segments of RNA), which are required starting points for replicating the lagging antiparallel strands in DNA replication; once the primase adds the primers, DNA polymerase elongates the RNA primers with new DNA

Note: The RNA-DNA complexes (known as Okazaki fragments) on the lagging strand of replicating DNA meet the next RNA primer, DNA polymerase clips out the 5' end RNA and fills in the gap; the last step is carried out by DNA ligase which joins the fragments; see Okazaki fragments

'primed' cell A lymphocyte that has recognized an antigen and represents the theoretical starting point for an immune recognition 'cascade' Note: The 'primed' cell corresponds to the Y cell of the woefully naive 'XYZ cell theory' of immunology

primer A short (18-50 base) sequence of nucleic acid (usually RNA) that is the starting point for the synthesis of the lagging (antiparallel) strand of DNA in DNA replication; a primer is complementary to one strand of DNA, and provides a free 3'–OH at the end, an activity site recognized by DNA polymerase; see Primase

primer walking MOLECULAR BIOLOGY A DNA sequencing technique in which DNA primers are allowed to bind to a unique location on the genome; once the primer is bound, DNA polymerases can be added to the reaction milieu to increase the length of the bound primer by several hundred bases that are complementary to the genomic DNA; the sequence of the far end of the can be used as the next primer after the sequence of the complementary DNA has been determined in a step-wise fashion DISADVANTAGE Primer walking is labor-intensive and each round of walking requires a day (Sci Am 1994; 270/3:22)

priming NEUROLOGY A type of implicit, nonconscious (not procedural, semantic or episodic) form of human memory that acts to improve identification of words and perceptual objects

primordial soup Prebiotic ooze The Gemisch of simple organic molecules that was theoretically present in the primitive (circa four billion years ago) oceans and contained the synthetic building blocks for macromolecules and eventually living cells; the primordial sout contained not only the sugars, amino acids, and other molecules that are the essential substrates for the biochemical reactions that occur in the 'modern' world, but also many other molecules that are now laboratory curiosities; the early reactions in the primordial soup are assumed to have been facilitated by energy stored in phosphate bonds, replenished by a kind of nonmetabolic conversion of solar to chemical energy; see RNA world

primum non nocere One of the guiding ethical principles of the physician, that above all else no harm is to be done to the patient; see Hippocratic oath

'Prince Charles looking to the left' A fanciful descriptor for the eggs of the dwarf tapeworm, *Hymenolepis nana*, which measure 25 x 35 μm, have a smooth shell surrounding an oncosphere with six hooks, and distinctly 'look towards the left'; the oncosphere is contained within a tough inner envelope marked by two auricle-like polar thickenings, from each of which arise four-to-eight thread-like polar filaments; *H nana* is an intestinal cestode of worldwide distribution, but more common in temperate and subtropical regions; heavy intestinal infestations are due to auto-infection TREATMENT Niclosamide

This highly colloquial term is of uncertain origin, and refers to the Prince of Wales' generous auricular endowment

principal investigator The chief 'player' in a grant application, who is often the person with the creative ideas, although he may not do the actual 'bench work', (which explains why the PI is often the last author listed on a publication); the PI is responsible for maintaining the budget, guiding the research team, traveling to symposia and lecturing on his group's research, organizing the publications for the experimental question in the grant proposal and reaching the conclusions based on the obtained data

prion 'Slow spongiform encephalopathy virus' An unconventional infectious particle composed entirely of protein (with attached carbohydrate), which is the smallest known infective particle and is implicated in diseases of man (Creutzfeldt-Jakob disease-CJD, fatal familial insomnia, Gerstmann-Straussler-Scheinker syndrome, kuru, and of animals (scrapie of sheep and goats, bovine spongiform encephalopathy, transmissible mink encephalopathy and chronic wasting disease of captive mule deer and elk); prions do not evoke inflammation or the production of specific antibodies and are resistant to the usual modalities that inactivate viruses, eg formalin, heat, nuclease digestion, radiation and UV light; when co-incubated with abnormal prions, natural (normal) prions convert to abnormal forms (**New York Times 16 August 1994; C1**)) prions contain a unique 28-kD hydrophobic glycoprotein particle, PrP that autopolymerizes into fibrillary amyloid-like (by electron microscopy) structures, existing in 2 isoforms: PrP^C, found in the normal brain and transiently expressed during development and PrP^{Sc} which is associated with cerebral degeneration, including Alzheimer's disease and scrapie, the primary amino acid sequences of both are identical; the gene encoding the PrP proteins is located on the short arm of chromosome 20 and is widely expressed in normal brains and the prions are composed largely of abnormal isoform(s) of the prion protein, generated through point mutations of the prion gene, one of which occurs in Libyan Jews with CJD, suggesting that some cases of CJD may be AD with variable penetration (**N Engl J Med 1991; 324:1091, Science 1991; 252:1515rv**); transfer of a mutated prion gene into transgenic mice evokes a spongiform encephalitis with gliosis, confirming a cause-and-effect association between mutated prions and encephalopathy; see Protein only hypothesis, see there

prior acts coverage Nose coverage, see there

PRISM score Pediatric Risk of Mortality CRITICAL CARE MEDICINE A prognostic scoring system derived from 14 physiologic variables assessed during the first 24 hours of care in an ICU (**Sci Am 1994; 270/9:72**) for pediatric populations that derives from the PSI (physiology stability index); see Prognostic scoring systems

prison overcrowding see Correctional facility

prisoner's dilemma PSYCHOLOGY A type of social dilemma in which there are only two 'players'; the dilemma is worded as follows, a prisoner is given the choice between betraying a fellow prisoner ('defecting') and being freed, or remaining silent ('cooperating'), and risking a harsh punishment if the other prisoner betrays him; the strategies that are successful in the prisoner's dilemma in social interactions are far less useful in larger groups (**Sci Am 1994; 270/3:76**) see Social dilemma, Unethical diner's dilemma

prisoner of war syndrome *'Withdrawal, apathy, and sometimes death occurring as a reaction to capture, imprisonment, and hopelessness about reunion with one's love ones* (**International Dictionary of Medicine, J Wiley & Sons, New York, 1986**) see Torture; Cf Concentration camp (survivor) syndrome

PRIST Paper radioimmunosorbent test An in vitro test that quantifies serum IgE; the range of IgE is broad (0.1-215 IU/mL) and differs with age; Cf RAST

Pritikin diet A diet that is high in complex carbohydrates (which comprise > 90% of caloric intake) and low in protein, fat, and cholesterol, with severely restricted caffeine, salt and sugar; the PD was formulated by a Mr N Pritikin after he was diagnosed of coronary artery disease in 1958; his first total cholesterol was 7.25 mmol/L (**US: 280 mg/dl**) in 1955; at the time of his death (due to complications of a well-differentiated lymphocytic lymphoma) in 1985, his cholesterol was 2.4 mmol/L (**US: 94 mg/dl**); post-mortem examination revealed mild cardiac hypertrophy and widely patent coronary arteries (**N Engl J Med 1985; 313:52c**) see Diet

Privacy Act of 1974 A federal statute (PL 93-579) that reaffirmed a US citizen's fundamental right to privacy, protecting him from misuse and unnecessary transfer of information by the federal government; Cf Megan's law

Note: Such legislation is extremely problematic in tracking persons with fatal communicable infection eg AIDS, as the essence of the Privacy Act is that a citizen's right to privacy overrides the public's rights for safety, an apparent contradiction of the principles of democracy; at least one state has overcome this particular dilemma by declaring AIDS a sexually transmitted disease

private antigen IMMUNOLOGY An HLA antigen that is determined by a single allele, eg HLA-B27 TRANSFUSION MEDICINE An antigen of very low frequency, found on the erythrocytes of less than 0.1% of the population, eg Peters (Pt^a); Wright (Wr^a), Batty (By), Hey, Good, Bishop (Bp^a), Box (Bx); Cf Public antigens

private patient A patient whose care is entrusted to one physician who usually has had a long-term relation with the patient, and who is often directly reimbursed for his services by a 'third party' payer or by the patient; Cf Personal physician

private speech PSYCHOLOGY A verbalized, but internal monologue that accounts for 20-60% of the remarks made by a child under the age of 10; once thought to be abnormal, PS is now recognized as an essential part of cognitive development; types of private speech include egocentric communication, emotional release, fantasy play, reading aloud, self-direction, and inaudible muttering; data suggests that children who engage in private speech learn more rapidly and are more attentive (**Sci Am 1994; 271/5:78**)

privilege Permission granted by a hospital or other health care institution to a physician to render specific diagnostic or therapeutic services; types include admitting privileges (the right to admit patients) and clinical privileges (the right to treat)

PRK Photorefractive keratectomy, see there

prn Latin *pro re nata*, as needed

PRN orders CLINICAL PHARMACOLOGY Any physician-promulgated mandate or regimen ('doctor's orders') for treatment that allows use of the therapy or modality as needed by the patient; in certain situations, eg malignancy or other terminal illnesses, PRN orders, in particular for the control of pain (schedule II through V controlled substances) are more liberal

PRO Peer review organization An independent physician group, often organized in each state of the US that works with the US Federal Government to oversee health care provided to Medicare patients; PRO physicians review a percentage of Medicare patient medical records before, during and after hospitalization to ensure that the care given is medically necessary, provided in the appropriate setting and of a quality that meets accepted professional standards; PROs may review certain procedures prior to hospitalization to assess their necessity, eg carotid endarterectomy, cataract extraction, cholecystectomy, major joint replacement for degenerative joint diseases, coronary artery bypass with graft, peripheral revascularization therapy, hysterectomy, inguinal hernia repair, prostatectomy and pacemaker insertion

proalbumin A protein precursor of mature albumin that has an extra hexapeptide at the amino terminal, which is cleaved as a final step in the Golgi apparatus; defects in proalbumin may be either structural, eg proalbumin Christchurch and proalbumin Lille, or functional, eg proalbumin Pittsburgh; Cf Prealbumin

probability p value STATISTICS The likelihood that an event will occur by chance, which in statistics is given a value between 0 (impossible) and 1 (certainty); ie the higher the p value, the less likely it is that two or more sets of overlapping variables occurred in a random fashion, ie the greater the likelihood that the two events are associated, while the lower the p value, the greater is the likelihood that the events are random associations

In verbal communication, there is a wide difference in interpretation of adjectives used for probability; when health professionals were surveyed, events that were regarded as 'certain' had a 95-99% chance of occurring, 'very likely' events occurred in 85-89%, 'probable' 64-77%, 'likely' 63-73%, 'frequent' 36-63%, 'not unreasonable' 23-47%, 'possible' 21-43%, 'unlikely' 10-20% and 'improbable' 10-13%; these adjectives are thus of little use in scientific communication

proband The first patient of a family or other group with a disease process who comes to medical attention; in general, proband is preferred for 'point man' for an inherited condition, while the term 'index case' is preferred for the first medically identified person with an infectious disease

probandwise concordance CLINICAL RESEARCH The proportion of co-twins of proband twins who are themselves afflicted with a disease of interest (JAMA 1992; 268:1877oc)

probe MOLECULAR BIOLOGY Hybridization probe A generic term for a sequence of DNA or RNA measuring up to several hundred base pairs in length that spans the region of a gene's point mutation or gene rearrangement; probes are labeled with ^{32}P or ^{35}S, or alternately, with a nonradioactive biotinylated tag and hybridize to their 'mirror image', forming dimers of DNA, DNA-RNA and RNA-protein; probes are used in molecular biology to identify the presence of a segment of DNA or RNA of interest in cells and tissues; see *in situ* hybridization SURGERY Explorer A long thin, usually metal instrument that is used to poke around in cavities, fistulae, and wounds

problem-oriented medical record A formally organized medical record in which each of a patient's conditions or complaints are addressed individually, often organized by the acronym of SOAP (subjective criteria, objective criteria, assessment, and plan); see Hospital record, Medical record, SOAP

pro bono (publico) Latin, for the good of the public An adjective referring to a non-reimbursed service (health care, legal) rendered to those who cannot afford to pay professional fees

problem-based learning EDUCATION THEORY, MEDICAL EDUCATION An instructional strategy in which groups of students are presented with clinical problems without prior study or lectures; this popular didactic method is believed by its advocates to be effective in teaching problem-solving skills, as students work through various clinical problems either alone or in interactive groups of various sizes (N Engl J Med 1995; 332:1507ED) PBL is an advanced form of cooperative learning that helps develop independent learning, communication, group interactions, and problem-solving skills (Clin Lab Sci 1994; 7:166F) see Cooperative learning

problem drinker SUBSTANCE ABUSE An individual who meets two of the three criteria in the last 12 months: 1) Having 5+ alcoholic drinks on any one occasion at least once/month ('heavy drinking') 2) One or more alcohol-related social consequences (eg drunk-driving arrests, public drunkenness arrests, other alcohol-related criminal arrests, traffic or other accidents when drinking, confrontations about alcohol-related health problems by a medical practitioner, serious alcohol-related family or on-the-job problems), and 3) One or more symptoms of alcohol dependence, eg having an alcoholic drink upon awakening (an 'eye opener'), shaking hands, awakening not remembering the events that occurred while drinking (JAMA 1992; 268:1872oc) see Alcohol, Binge drinking; Cf Social drinker

proceduralist A generic term for a physician, usually a specialist or subspecialist who performs various diagnostic or therapeutic procedures; there is considerable overlap of this term with that of an interventionist

procedure manual LABORATORY MEDICINE A periodically updated manual that delineates in a step-by-step fashion, each of the diagnostic procedures performed by a clinical laboratory, explained with sufficient detail so that it may be performed by a person unfamiliar with the technique; alternately, a procedure manual may delineate contin-

gency plans in case of an emergency; the procedure manual is often the focus of attention by inspecting and accreditating agencies as they are a mark of the quality of a laboratory's work and its degree of organization; Cf Logbook, Notebook

process assessment A method for evaluating the success of an activity, eg continuing medical education (CME); PA in CME consists of the simple tabulation and documentation of hours devoted to CME; PA thus provides no information on whether a participant in CME actually learned something or is able to apply the new knowledge in practice (Arch Pathol Lab Med 1992; 116:602OA) Cf Outcome measurement

processing BIOCHEMISTRY The synthetic and modification steps that are required for the maturation of various compounds, eg the primary RNA transcript that is processed to form functional mRNA or a protein that is processed by post-translational modifications, including cleavage of peptide bonds, formation of disulfide bonds, hydroxylation, phosphorylation and attachment of prosthetic groups LABORATORY MEDICINE The sum total of the steps that a clinical specimen passes through from the time of its arrival to the laboratory until the generation of a final report, which includes entering the specimen's relevant data in a log-book (usually performed by computer) and actual performance of the requested test

procolipase see Colipase

procollagen suicide MOLECULAR PATHOLOGY An event that occurs in defective collagen synthesis, in which there is a mutation of the collagen I gene, resulting in a protein chain in which there is a substitution of the smallest amino acid glycine* for a larger, bulkier amino acid; this prevents the protein from folding into a triple-helical pattern, resulting in degradation of the abnormal pro-α collagen chain, as well as the normal pro-α chains, hence the name suicide

*Alpha collagen chains are defined as (Gly-X-Y), where Gly is glycine, X is often proline and Y is often hydroxyproline

Proconsul A 16 million-year-old hominoid Miocene ape, the skull and facial bones of which were discovered on Rusinga Island in Lake Victoria by Mary Leakey in 1948; *Proconsul* provided anthropologists with the first cranium from what was thought to be the 'missing link', ie a tree-dwelling monkey with increased cranial capacity (Sci Am 1994; 271/4:37)

proctalgia A pain in the behind

procurement TRANSPLANTATION The process of obtaining organs for transplantation; the ideal donor of multiple organs destined for transplantation is a (recently) brain-dead patient with unimpaired circulation; the procurement process is costly and prior to activation of a 'procurement team', it must be established that the donor meets 1) Physical criteria, eg young age, state of previous excellent health prior to the trauma that left the donor in a persistent vegetative state, absence of history of substance abuse 2) Legal criteria, ie that appropriate permission for organ donation has been obtained from next-of-kin and 3) Laboratory criteria, which consists of a battery of serological tests, including IgG and IgM ELISA tests for HIV-1, HTLV-I, hepatitis A, hepatitis B, hepatitis C, RPR (for *Treponema*); once these criteria are met, the 'team' may charter a small private jet and fly to the donor's hospital; once the donor's thoraco-abdominal cavity is opened, it is packed with a 'slush' preparation (ice and lactated Ringer's solution), which reduces the organs' activities to a metabolic 'ground zero'; the 'team' then organizes itself into 3 to 5 'sections', with each section poised to remove one organ block, eg the liver, pancreas, kidneys (which count as one block), heart-lung block or heart and lungs as separate blocks; there may thus be up to 10 people in the donor's body cavity during the procurement process; once the 'team' is ready, the aorta is cannulated and clamped above the heart; at this critical step (known as 'cross-clamping'), the 'clock' starts, after which time each organ block has an allowed 'cold ischemia time' before it becomes suboptimal for transplantation, which is 4 to 6 hours for the heart-lung block, 20 hours for the liver and pancreas, and 72 hours for the kidneys; after 'cross-clamping', the vena cava is cut and the donor's blood is exsanguinated and a perfusate (the 'Wisconsin solution') is gravity-fed into each organ via the aorta and arteries; the organs are then removed by each 'section' and placed in containers filled with 'slush' preparation, maintained at near 0ºC, and then transported to their respective recipients; see Slush preparation, Wisconsin solution

prodrug CLINICAL PHARMACOLOGY A drug ingested in the inactive form that is transformed into an active form by in vivo metabolic reactions

products of conception OBSTETRICS The aggregate of tissues that are present in a fertilized gestation; in a pregnancy that has been terminated or aborted, the finding of chorionic villi and/or fetal tissue is required to make a definitive diagnosis of intrauterine (as opposed to ectopic) pregnancy, and thus constitute definitive products of conception; decidualized and secretory endometrium may be found in either intrauterine and ectopic pregnancies

Note: Implantation site tissue which is histologically characterized by aggregates of giant cells in theory also constitute a definitive products of conception, although this finding is not an accepted standard criteria

proenkephalin A molecule generated by selective post-translational proteolysis from pro-opiomelanocortin (POMC), yielding met- and leu-enkephalins as well as the opioids, octapeptide and heptapeptide; proenkephalin production is increased in seizures and its gene may be the target of the heterodimeric complex of the proto-oncogenes, c-fos and c-jun

profession An occupation requiring intense preparation in a body of erudite knowledge (eg law, medicine) that is applied in the service of society, has a system of self-governance, and in which success is measured by accomplishments in serving society and/or furtherance of knowledge in the field rather than personal gain; see Learned profession, 'Yellow professionalism'

professional boundaries PROFESSIONAL ETHICS An ill-defined separation that is maintained between a professional and his/her client; PBs in medical practice '... they are the parameters that describe the limits of a fiduciary relationship in which a person (a patient) entrusts his or her welfare to another (a physician), to whom a fee is paid for the provision of a service. Boundaries imply professional distance and respect, which...includes refraining from sexual involvement with patients.' (JAMA1995; 273:1445) although sexual contact is the most extreme form of boundary violation, other behaviors on the part of physicians have potential for exploiting the patient's dependency on the physician and the inherent differential in power, these behaviors include dual relationships (see there), certain gifts, duration of appointments, certain uses of languages, self-disclosure and other behaviors that may be viewed as part of a 'slippery slope' continuum

professional corporation PC A legal entity in which each of the shareholders is a member of the same profession or field, eg accounting, architecture, law, medicine; many individual physicians in the US belong to a PC that has from one individual to a dozen or more professionals; advantages of incorporation and practice in or under the banner of a PC include corporate ownership of equipment, tax and investment advantages, health benefits, leasing of transportation vehicles and limitation of malpractice liability, but does not affect areas of professional responsibility, privilege, or liability

professional courtesy A generic term for the provision of health care to physicians and their families at a reduced rate or free of charge; PC is a time-honored and deeply rooted tradition in medicine, first discussed in the Hippocratic Oath and specifically required by Percival's Medical Ethics, published in 1803; some physicians have expressed concern about the practice of PC, in that it may interfere with an appropriate doctor-patient relationship and may allow physicians to ignore the costs of providing such care; other major changes on the medical panorama that alter PC include the creation of Medicare, nearly universal third-party payment, formation of large group practices, increased malpractice litigation, and the drive to control costs; despite these changes, 96% of all physicians (80% of psychiatrists) in the US offer professional courtesy; 67% believe that PC solidifies bonds among physicians, 62% believe it to be sound business practice (N Engl J Med 1993; 329:1627OA, 1652ED; 1994; 330:1085C)

professional image The constellation of tangible or visible representations and/or perceptions that result from a person's conduct as a professional, which results from ethical behavior and competence

professional liability The obligation that a professional practitioner has to provide care or service that meets the standard of practice for his/her profession, ie reponsibility; when the professional fails to provide the standard of practice, liability refers to his/her obligation to pay for damages incurred by negligent acts; see Liability, Malpractice

professional misconduct A generic term for any behavior on the part of a professional that indicates an intentional compromise of ethical standards; acts of PM include: practicing beyond authorized scope of practice, practicing fraudulently, practicing with gross negligence or incompetence, practicing while impaired by alcohol, drugs, or mental disability, being a habitual abuser of drugs, being convicted of a crime, fee splitting, delegation of duties to an unauthorized person, physical or sexual abuse of a person, filing of false reports, failure to maintain proper records, ordering excessive or unnecessary tests, and others; see Impaired health care provider; Cf Fraud in Science

professional voice PERFORMING ARTS MEDICINE A voice used (ie singing, speaking) to earn a person's major source of income; when people with professional voices, eg actors, news media announcers, singers, have diseases of the speech apparatus, there is a particular need to minimize the changes induced by a particular pathology; the professional voice patient may in addition to medical or surgical therapy, require behavioral therapy and voice retraining PREOPERATIVE EVALUATION Examination of the mucosa, existance of edema or inflammation or superficial lesions, adequacy of glottic closure, use of video endostroboscopy TREATMENT Surgery may include the endoscopic microflap technique

professor A faculty member who has attained the highest possible academic rank at an institution of higher learning, who professes to possess special knowledge in an occupation that requires the acquisition of special skills; in the USA, the 'pecking order' in academic science and medicine is based on 1) Permanence of a position, ie whether it is 'tenured' and 2) Rank, which in increasing order of peer recognition begins at instructor, assistant professor, associate professor and (full) professor, who is at the pinnacle; professors have attained national or international reputation for academic excellence, are among the most accomplished in their field, are eminent researchers, influential and able teachers and, if applicable, outstanding clinicians; see 'Chair'; Cf Chair

professorial rounds A permutation of patient rounds that forms part of the teaching activities at an academic health care facility, in which the clinical, radiological and pathological data from one or a limited number of patients are presented; although the format of these 'rounds' varies, it is intended to be a socratic dialog between the presenter at a podium and his junior and senior colleagues, and serves to evaluate the steps made in arriving at the diagnosis, how to treat the patient(s) and to share the professor's experience; Cf Clinico-pathological conference, Grand rounds, Rounds

proficiency testing LABORATORY MEDICINE The testing of a battery of 'unknown' clinical specimens by a laboratory to determine the laboratory's accuracy and reliability, which is becoming a key factor in determining a laboratory's licensing status; CLIA-88 (Clininal Laboratory Improvements Amendment of 1988) allows various techniques of proficiency testing, eg participant-derived targets (means from a group of participants), targets from a group of reference laboratories, or definitive values from a single source (**Arch Pathol Lab Med 1993; 117:885oA**); performance in PT improves with experience (**ibid 1995; 119:307oA**)

profile EPIDEMIOLOGY A longitudinal or cross-sectional aggregation of health care data applied to any segment of the population being served or the individuals or groups providing the service and the statistics obtained therefrom; there are thus patient, physician and hospital profiles LABORATORY MEDICINE A panel of screening tests used to establish a baseline of normalcy for either a certain population, eg Executive profile, or for a limited group of analytes, eg Lipid profile; see Organ panels

Profile of Mood States A 65-item questionnaire designed to assess mood states, which evaluates vigor, fatigability, confusion or bewilderment, and friendliness (from **N Engl J Med 1992; 327:1041oA**)

profilin PHYSIOLOGY A 15-kD protein present in platelets and neutrophils that regulates the length of actin filaments, and alters cell shape in carcinogenesis and thrombogenesis; profilin may mediate many of the intracellular events that follow binding of growth signal proteins to their cognate extracellular receptors, transferring signals from the cell surface to the nucleus; profilin may prevent phospholipase C (PLC) from catalyzing PIP_2 until PLC is phosphorylated by tyrosine kinase activated by growth factor-receptor interaction (**Science 1991; 251:1231, 1181ed**) profilin also keeps cytoplasmic actin in its place (**Proc Nat Acad Sci (IUS) 1994; 91:15100A**)

progenote The hypothetical precursor organism that is postulated to be ultimate 'stem organism', prior to the divergence of life forms into archaebacteria, prokaryotes, and eukaryotes; see Urkingdom

progeria A group of conditions characterized by markedly premature aging of childhood onset, in which morbid conditions usually seen in the elderly appear during puberty and death from 'old age' occurs by 20; congenital conditions associated with progeria include Cockayne syndrome, and Hutchinson-Gilford syndrome

progestin A generic term for any natural or synthetic compound with progesterone-like activity

progonoma Pigmented neuroectodermal tumor of infancy, see there

prognostic scoring system Any of a number of scoring systems that help predict outcome(s) and identify patients and clinical situations in which the potential value of intensive care is low, while the burden of therapy is high, providing a numerical prediction of patient mortality; see APACHE II, MPS, PRISM, SAPS and TISS

programmed cell death Apoptosis, see there

programmed killing EMBRYOLOGY Selective destruction of the neurons that are overproduced in early brain development; although the neuroembryologic mechanism for this overproduction is unclear, A68 protein may act as a target, marking cells for deletion

progress note A brief summary of a hospitalized patient's current clinical status, which is usually written in sequential order in the patient's chart and reflects information provided by physical examination, laboratory tests, and imaging modalities; PNs serve to communicate perceived changes of the patient's condition among all members of the management team, and serve as a public record of the clinicians' rationale for performing certain procedures, and his/her expectations for outcome; PNs are thus critical 'documents' that may become the legal substrate for determining liability

progressive multifocal leukoencephalopathy A lesion of the CNS characterized by demyelinization in the brain's white matter CLINICAL Dementia, spastic paralysis, blindness, opportunistic infections PATHOLOGY Intranuclear viral inclusions in oligodendrogliocytes, scattered bizarre giant astrocytes, reactive fibrillary astrocytes, patchy cortical loss with scant inflammation; PML occurs in immunocompromised hosts, eg those with leukemia and AIDS and is caused by papova (DNA-type usually JC) virus, rarely also by BK virus associated with AIDS

progressive spinal muscular atrophy Spinal muscular atrophy, see there

progressive systemic sclerosis Sclerodema An idiopathic condition that falls under the rubric of the collagen vascular or connective tissue diseases, in which exuberant fibrosis occurs throughout the body; PSS involves the skin, GI tract, lungs, heart, muscle, and kidney; in some cases, the condition remains confined to the skin for prolonged periods of time, but in most it encroaches on the viscera, causing malabsorption, respiratory insufficiency before death ensues, usually from cardiac or renal failure; two forms are recognized: 1) Diffuse sclerosis, in which there is widespread involvement ab initio accompanied by rapid visceral involvement and clinical deterioration and 2) CREST (acronym for calcinosis, Raynaud's phenomenon, esophageal dysmotility, sclerodactyly, telangiectasia) syndrome, see there

progressive transformation of germinal centers A morphologically distinct lesion of lymphoid tissue characterized by enlarged, reactive germinal centers in a background of follicular hyperplasia and effacement of the relatively sharply defined boundary between the germinal center and the mantle zone; this loss of the usually distinct frontiers between different cell types is accompanied by a 'starry sky' pattern, scattered immunoblasts and epithelioid histiocytes, increased dendritic reticulum cells, mantle zone lymphocytes and increased T cells 'transformed' germinal centers; PTGC is most common in young males, appearing in a single, asymptomatic and enlarged lymph node; although it may occur in patients with nodular lymphocyte-predominant Hodgkin's disease (**Verh Anat Ges 1975; 69:19**); it is thought to be neither neoplastic nor a harbinger for future lymphoid malignancy PTGC is of particular interest as it may be associated with nodular lymphocyte-predominant Hodgkin's disease, but is not itself considered neoplastic; see Germinal centers; Cf Regressively transformed germinal centers

prohormone convertase(s) A family of enzymes that 'clip' functional hormones out of larger parent proteins, eg chopping out hormones at sites of dibasic amino acids

Project 2061 see Project 3000 by 2000

Project 3000 by 2000 An education-reform initiative* by the Association of American Medical Colleges designed to ↑ the ethnic and racial diversity of medical schools, by ↑ the number of unrepresented minorities (UMs, designated as blacks, Mexican Americans, mainland Puerto Ricans, and American Indians); although UMs comprise ± 20% of the general population, they comprise ± 11% of medical school entrants; see Affirmative action, *Bakke* decision, Reverse discrimination, Underrepresented minorities

*The goal is enroll 3000 underrepresented minorities by the year 2000, hence the name; Project 3000 by 2000 is similar to the Goals 2000 program (Clinton Administration) and Project 2061 (American Association for the Advancement of Science)

projectile vomiting Violent and 'explosive' vomiting without antecedent nausea, or vomiting that occurs at the peak of maximum inspiration without the usual rhythmic hyperactivity of the respiratory muscles associated with 'retching' (diaphragmatic spasms that precede vomiting); PV is classically associated with ↑ intracranial pressure, classically occurring in meningitides of young children

prolactin A 23-kD anterior pituitary (adenohypophysis) polypeptide hormone with several molecular forms, eg 'big' and 'little' prolactin; it is under inhibitory control by the hypothalamus; ♂ and ♀ hormone levels are similar (except during pregnancy or lactation, when it is much higher in ♀) ranging from 1-25 ng/ml and have diurnal variation, peaking 4-5 hours after the onset of sleep; prolactin is ↑ in 70% of those with pituitary tumors (57% with > 100 ng/ml and 100% with > 300 ng/ml have pituitary tumors); prolactin is also ↑ by physiologic stimuli (eg exercise, sucking on the nipples by an infant, and hypoglycemia), in cirrhosis, empty sella syndrome, hypothyroidism, renal failure, MEN-I, and in drug therapy (α-methyldopa, L-dopa, ergot alkaloids, cimetidine, phenothiazine, verapamil, hormones, eg estrogen, growth hormone, thyroid-releasing hormone, psychotropic drugs) MEASUREMENT RIA

proliferating cell nuclear antigen Cyclin A 36 kD nuclear protein that is highly conserved in evolution and synthesized in the late G_1 and S phase of the cell cycle, with peak expression in the S phase; PCNA is essential for DNA synthesis as an auxiliary to DNA polymerase-γ (**Arch Pathol Lab Med 1994; 118:510oA**) PCNA positivity correlates with the degree of differentiation and atypia of tumor cells; growth fractions are ↑ in premalignant lesions of the skin and oral cavity: leukoplakia 22.3, senile keratosis 41.2, Bowen's disease 45.2 (normal 9.8) (**Virchows Arch A Pathol Anat Histopathol 1992; 420:377**) optimal identification of PCNA in paraffin-embedded tissue requires that it be fixed in methanol; formalin fixation is reported to cause a four-fold drop in staining intensity (**Arch Pathol Lab Med 1994; 118:1007oA**)

proliferation index FLOW CYTOMETRY The sum of the events occurring in the S and G_2M phases of the cell cycle, expressed as a fraction of the total cell population, calculated by the formula

$$PI = \frac{S + G_2/M}{(G_0/G_1 + S + G_2M)} \times 100$$

(**Anal Quan Cytol Histol 1993; 15:179**) Cf DNA index, Flow cytometry

proliferative breast disease(s) A group of benign breast lesions characterized by proliferation of epithelial cells in the terminal ductal-lobular unit of the breast, which have a two-to-fivefold increased incidence of malignancy; PBD tends to occur in first degree relatives of patients with breast cancer; the susceptibility locus has been located at D17S74; see D17S74, Sclerosing adenosis: Cf Mammary dysplasia

proliferative breast disease SURGICAL PATHOLOGY Epithelial hyperplasia is a risk factor for the development of breast carcinoma; criteria can be used to identify 'risk features' in cytologic specimens (**Am J Clin Pathol 1995; 103:438oA**)

proliferative phase HISTOLOGY The early or preovulation half of the menstrual cycle, initiated by the small peak in follicle-stimulating hormone; this phase, also known as the follicular phase, begins in the late luteal phase of the previous menstrual cycle under the influence of ovarian

estrogen; the endometrium undergoes regeneration in preparation for implantation of an egg, if it becomes fertilized; during proliferation, the cervix becomes more vascularized, the os widens and the cervical mucus increases in volume, elasticity and undergoes arborization; see Ferning; Cf Secretory phase

prolonged labor OBSTETRICS Labor of greater than 24 hours in duration in a primigravida, which may be due to 1) A prolonged latent phase (labor in which the latent phase is greater than 20 hours in a primigravida or greater than 14 hours in a multipara), or 2) Due to a 'protraction disorder' in which there is protracted cervical dilatation in the active phase of labor and protracted descent of the fetus; see Labor

PROM 1) Premature rupture of membranes, see there 2) Programmable read-only memory COMPUTERS A ROM chip that may be updated and altered by special equipment, eg ultraviolet light or electronic signals, which is not ordinarily accessible to the unskilled user, and therefore functions exactly as a ROM chip

ProMACE-cytaBOM ONCOLOGY A 'third-generation' combination chemotherapy regimen consisting of prednisone, doxorubicin, cyclophosphamide, and etoposide, followed by cytarabine, bleomycin, vincristine, and methotrexate with lecovorin rescue; despite extensive clinical research, CHOP is considered better than ProMACE-cytaBOM for non-Hodgkin's lymphoma as it is less expensive, less complicated to administer, and has fewer fatal toxic dose effects (**N Engl J Med 1993; 328:1002oA**), see CHOP

promiscuity MOLECULAR BIOLOGY The ability of a molecule with a conformational specificity, eg a receptor, enzyme or antibody, to bind to various non-specific ligands, substrates or antigens SOCIAL MEDICINE Indiscriminate (ie with multiple partners) sexual relations

promiscuous DNA Segments of DNA that are postulated to have been 'shamelessly' transferred through transpositions between mitochondria, chloroplasts, nuclei and other organelles early in the evolution of primitive life forms

promiscuous rearrangement A second ('inappropriate') clonal gene rearrangement, eg of a T cell receptor-γ chain that occurs in a cell line that has previously undergone clonal differentiation, eg of B-cell ontogeny

promontory sign Peninsula sign, see there

promoter MOLECULAR BIOLOGY A region of the genome or site on the DNA double helix where RNA polymerase attaches and initiates transcription with the synthesis of mRNA; in the classic operon, the promoter is located adjacent (usually upstream) to the operator ONCOLOGY see

PROLIFERATIVE BREAST DISEASE (VS CARCINOMA)

	BENIGN	MALIGNANT
CYTOLOGIC CRITERIA		
Cellularity	+-++	++-+++
Atypia	−	++-+++
Nucleoli	−	+
Single epithelial cells	(−)	+
ARCHITECTURE		
Slit-like lumens	+++	(−)
Rigid lumens	(−)	+++
Intraluminal swirling	+	−
Projections	+	(−)
OTHER		
Myoepithelial cells	+++ (groups)	(−)
Background	Clean	Necrosis, blood

from Am J Clin Pathol 1995; 103:438oA

Tumor promoters

promoter mutation A mutation that affects the promoter region on the DNA, acting to 1) Increase the efficiency of the initiation of transcription, through an increase in RNA polymerase binding to the initiation site, an 'Up' mutation, 2) Decrease transcription, by decreasing RNA polymerase binding to the initiation site, a 'Down' mutation or 3) Create a new promotion site

promoter sequence A sequence of proviral DNA (DNA of retroviral origin that has become integrated into host DNA), which directs the RNA polymerase to a specific initiation site; promoter sequences, like the enhancer sequences are located within the long terminal repeats flanking proviral DNA; see LTR

promotion 1) Oncology Tumor promotion, see there 2) Pharmaceutical industry The act of furthering the sale of a product by advertising or publicity; the purpose of a for-profit enterprise, eg a drug company, is to increase the sales of its product over that of a competitor's; the obligation of the physician, as a prescriber of drugs, is to objectively weigh all information about the advantages/disadvantages of a particular drug or therapy, and prescribed the best, and most cost-efficient agent available; the ethical issues may become clouded when physicians are used to promote (or 'educate') their colleagues about a particular agent, as it places a veneer of legitimacy that the particular educational/promotional activity may not have; RC Noble (U Kentucky) offers a list of criteria of activities that might be regarded as promotional (and less educational) in nature (**N Engl J Med 1992; 327:363c**)

1) The meeting is sponsored by a drug company and the speaker is paid by the company

2) The meeting has a low registration fee, and offers free food, hospitality, or entertainment

3) The program has been repeated at another site, often with some of the same speakers

4) During the presentation, a drug representative is present in the room

5) Attendees are offered gifts

6) The speaker uses slides provided by the company

7) The speaker mentions only one drug; mentions only one by its brand name and the others by generic names, fails to mention that the drug is available as a generic, does not discuss the costs

8) The speaker is a clinical investigator for the drug company

proofreading 1) Journalism see copy-editing 2) Molecular biology see Editing

pro-opiomelanocortin POMC A 31-kD pituitary prohormone gene product released by corticotropin-releasing factor, which by post-translational processing, gives rise to different active peptides in the brain and gut including pituitary hormones (ACTH, α-, β- and γ-MSH), endogenous opiates (β-endorphin and enkephalin), α- and β-lipotropin

pronouncing death The act of monitoring (eg with a stethoscope or an EKG) the condition of a person and determining the point at which a person has actually died (**N Engl J Med 1993; 329:1346sb**) see Harvard criteria; Cf Certifying death

ProPAC Prospective Payment Assessment Commission Health care financing An independent body of experts in the US that recommends adjustments in the 'weight' and classification of the diagnosis-related groups, so that they reflect changes in costs of procedures and changes in technology and diagnosis; see DRGs

propafenone Cardiology A class IC antiarrhythmic agent used to manage severe ventricular and supraventricular arrhythmias, which has β-blocking and weak calcium channel blocking properties, and some negative inotropic activity Complications Ventricular proarrhythmia; conduction defects Side effects Neurologic (headache, dizziness,

paresthesias, and rarely peripheral neuropathy (**Mayo Clin Proc 1995; 70:469**)), GI (eg nausea, vomiting, anorexia)

properdin Immunology A component of the alternative complement pathway that stabilizes C3 convertase, forming a reversible complex therewith; see Alternate pathway

prophylactic *adjective* Preventive *noun* An agent that prevents (whatever)

prophylactic antibiotic therapy The administration of antimicrobials in absence of a known infection, a maneuver that has reduced surgical wound infections, which is a standard practice and one of the most common uses of antibiotics in the hospital setting; the most common surgical wound pathogens are *Staphylococcus aureus*, *Bacteroides fragilis*, *Enterobacter cloacae*; the most commonly used antibiotics are third-generation cephalosporins; PAT is optimal if administered two hours before the surgical incision (**N Engl J Med 1992; 326:281oA**)

proportional-hazards model Cox regression analysis Statistics: A statistical maneuver used for multivariate analyses

proportional-hazards regression analysis Cox regression analysis Statistics A form of multivariant analysis

proportionate mortality ratio Public health A statistic that allows the comparison of two or more populations without requiring knowledge of the population at risk for a morbid condition

Proposition 64 Ballot proposition 64 A proposal made in the early 1980s in a California State legislative referendum that AIDS was a disease of sufficient health risk to warrant quarantining of anyone infected with HIV-1, and prevent AIDS patients from providing health care, teaching in public schools, or handling food; it was not passed; Cf 'Informed'

Proposition 65 Ballot proposition 65 Safe Drinking water and Toxic Enforcement Act of 1986 Clinical toxicology A state law passed in California requiring the government to list all the chemicals known to cause cancer or reproductive toxic effect; 12 months after having been so listed, people may not be exposed (occupational, water and environmental exposures) unless previously warned; 20 months after such listing, the substance may not be discharged into any actual or potential source of drinking water; see 'White-out'

Proposition 99 Ballot proposition 99 Substance abuse A state law passed in California that increases the taxes imposed on tobacco products, 'earmarking' the funds for various anti-smoking activities, including education, treatment, research, and protection of wildlife resources

Proposition 161 An initiative placed before the California voters that addressed the legalization of physician-assisted suicide, addressing specific issues, including witnesses who could determine if the decision was made under duress, the degree of liability for misdiagnosis, who would be best suited to perform the task, whether family members should be notified, or whether counseling, a waiting period, and/or a psychological examination would be required; proposition 161 was defeated in 1992 by the same narrow margin (54 to 46) as a similar proposition (Initiative 119) in the state of Washington; see Initiative 119, Kevorkian, Physician-assisted suicide

proposition 186 The California Health Security Act An initiative placed before the California voters that addresses the issue of health care reform by creating a single-payer system, taking California's system of private, primarily 'managed care' health insurance and placing under state control; the advocates of a single-payer system project savings of $10 x 10^9 which in the current health care system is being spent on administration, advertising, and profit; these monies could then be spent on benefits, eg prescription drugs, long-term and preventive care, dental and chiropractic procedures, mental health services and others; $59 x 10^9 would come from public funds, $46 x 10^9 from new taxes, eg cigarette and payroll taxes (JAMA 1994; 272:991MN&P)

Proposition 187 A state law passed in November 1994 in California that requires publicly funded health care facilities to deny care to illegal aliens and report them to government officials; the proponents of the measure stated that '*While our own citizens and legal residents go wanting, those who choose to enter our country ILLEGALLY get royal treatment at the expense of the California taxpayer*; it has been aregued that P187 would endanger public health as illegal aliens with true medical emergencies or epidemic infections would not seek help until their condition became extremely serious or life-threatening; in addition to compromising the humanitarian role traditionally played by the hospital and the physician, P187 requires that the physician breach the Hippocratic Oath's pledge of confidentiality (N Engl J Med 1995; 332:1095SB)

Proposition 188 An initiative placed before the California voters in 1994 that was sponsored almost in its entirety by a tobacco company, which would weaken nearly 300 anti-smoking laws in California, a state that has the most strict anti-smoking legislation in the United States (Am Med News 19 Sept 1994)

Note: Proposition 188 raises interesting ethical issues regarding the ability of a business to reverse health-promoting policies that have been put into place in democratic system

prosector's wart A clinical form of cutaneous TB that is largely of historic interest, which occurred on the hands of ungloved pathologists (prosectors) who performed autopsies on cases of TB, resulting in hyperkeratotic nodules due to direct tuberculin innoculation

Prospective Payment System The system of reimbursement for hospital and physician services, which is based largely on flat rates per admission calculated for each of 470 diagnosis-related groups that was introduced to force hospitals to become more efficient; see DRGs

Note: Coincident with the introduction of the PPS, the peer review organization system of quality and appropriateness of care was established; early conclusions on the PPS form of reimbursement are that it has not affected the mortality of hospital patients, has provided mechanisms for improving the quality of care, but has increased the likelihood that patients will be discharged from a health care facility with clinical 'instability'

prospective study A study designed so that data is collected as the events being evaluated are actually occurring; prospective studies require precise delineation of the populations' characteristics, of the parameters being measured and of potential outcome(s) being tested; as examples, prospective studies allow testing of hypothesized cause-and-effect relationships, or determination of the effect of a therapy on the progression of disease process; Cf Retrospective study

prostate cancer 106 000 new cases/year of prostatic adenocarcinoma are diagnosed in the US, causing 30 000 annual deaths; 35-50% of men > 70 years of age have PC, although its behavior is difficult to predict, commonly, it remains occult and those with this cancer die of natural deaths; flow cytometry of tumor cells allows partial prediction of tumors most likely to progress, as DNA ploidy analysis reveals that diploid tumors (as elsewhere in the body) have a significantly better prognosis then aneuploid or aneuploid-tetraploid tumors; although early stage A1 prostatic adenocarcinoma is traditionally regarded as a 'pathologist's tumor' not requiring treatment, a 10-year followup indicates that 16% progress to stages requiring therapy Note: PC is more common and aggressive in American blacks than whites SCREENING Screening for PSA, digital rectal examination, and transrectal ultrasonography ↑ the rate of detection but does not ↓ mortal-

ity due to prostate cancer in asymptomatic ♂ (JAMA 1994; 272:773OA) see PSA (prostate-specific antigen)

'prostate years' A colloquial term of little utility for age 60 or older, when men begin to become symptomatic for urinary retention due to prostatic hyperplasia or, less commonly, adenocarcinoma

prostate-specific antigen see PSA

prostatic intraepithelial neoplasia An in situ adenocarcinoma characterized by intraluminal proliferation of cytologically malignant epithelial cells lined by a definite but often attenuated basal layer; PIN is a precursor of invasive prostatic adenocarcinoma, as evidenced by PIN's DNA content, which is less than prostatic adenocarcinoma (Arch Pathol Lab Med 1993; 117:1104RV); cribriform glands may be seen in both high-grade PIN and Gleason's grade III carcinoma; PINs are often positive for antibodies to high molecular weight cytokeratin, while PAs are usually negative (Arch Pathol Lab Med 1994; 118:260OA)

Prospect Hill virus A Bunyavirus related to Hantaan virus; see Korean hemorrhagic fever

prostaglandin-induced abortion GYNECOLOGY A common method for termination of pregnancy (second trimester) in which prostaglandin is administered to induce uterine contractions followed by cervical dilation; PIA allows for delivery of an intact stillborn fetus but has the disadvantage of side effects, eg vomiting and diarrhea in the mother; it is prolonged in duration and uncomfortable; it is contraindicated in those with previous uterine surgery; Cf D&E

prostitution STD The performance of sexual work, ie sexual activity for hire EPIDEMIOLOGY In the US, there are an estimated 500 000 to 2 million prostitutes, age of entry into 'the oldest profession' occurs circa age 14; arrests for prostitution and commercialized vice, 1992 ♀ 47 526 ♂ 24 401; ♂ who have solicited prostitutes 17% (US News & World Report 22 November 1994:11) see Sexual work, Sexually transmitted diseases

protanopia OPHTHALMOLOGY A form of red-green color blindness that is due to a lack of long wavelength (LW, 560 nm) photopigment MOLECULAR PATHOLOGY The genes for both LW and MW (middle wavelength, 530 nm) photopigments are composed of six coding regions (exons); changes resulting in color blindness are attributed to illegitimate pairing between highly homologous genes followed by crossing-over (Science 1995; 267:984A, 1013R)

protein A MICROBIOLOGY A component of the *Staphylococcus aureus* cell wall, which, like protein G, binds to the Fc fragment of all four subclasses of IgG; protein A used to identify immunoglobulins and immune complexes

protein A, B, C MOLECULAR BIOLOGY Three proteins associated with heterogeneous nuclear or nonribosomal RNAs from the HeLa cell line; nuclease treatment releases a 40S particle with these proteins which contain modified amino acids of unknown function, di- and trimethylarginines, located exclusively in nucleus

proteins A, B, C, D HEMATOLOGY Anti-coagulants whose names derive from the immunologic characterization of the vitamin K-dependent clotting proteins into 4 groups (A-D); three of the names are of historic interest, as protein A has become factor IX, protein B has become prothrombin and protein D has become factor X; protein C is in current use

protein B see above

protein blotting Immunoblotting, see there

protein-bound iodine test A thyroid function test in which the iodine in precipitated protein is quantified, serving as a crude indicator of thyroid activity; it has fallen into disuse given the high background of artifact and has been superseded by more specific tests

protein C HEMATOLOGY A 62-kD vitamin K-dependent serine protease with 2 sulfide-bonded glycoprotein chains that is converted to an active serine protease by thrombin and accelerated in this activity by protein S; protein C is a potent anticoagulant; activated protein C (APC) limits clot formation by proteolytic inactivation of factors Va and VIIIa (VIII:C) using protein S as a cofactor, and enhances fibrinolysis (thrombolysis) by neutralizing the major inactivator of tissue plasminogen activator 11, protein C production is orchestrated by the binding of thrombin to thrombomodulin on an endothelial cell receptor, switching it to the activated form

protein C deficiency A condition that is either AD (**N Engl J Med 1994; 330:517OA**) of variable penetration, or acquired, and due to DIC, warfarin therapy, hepatic disease and postoperatively; protein C levels of < 40% normal (4.8 µg/ml) are often symptomatic, causing recurrent venous thromboses; homozygous deficiency (< 1% normal protein C) presents as neonatal purpura fulminans (ischemic necrosis) with massive venous thrombosis and a syndrome mimicked by coumarin-induced skin necrosis; the homozygous form is treated acutely by factor IX and chronically by anticoagulation MOLECULAR PATHOLOGY A missense mutation has been identified in 50% of patients with familial venous thromboses (**Nature 1994; 369:64OA, 14N&V**)

protein D see Proteins A-D (coagulation)

protein diet Liquid-protein diet

protein disulfide-isomerase An enzyme present on the endoplasmic reticulum and on the cell surface that breaks critical disulfide bonds on HIV's gp120 glycoprotein, facilitating its entry into host cells (**Proc Nat Acad Sci (US) 1994; 91:4559OA**)

protein domain see Domain

protein drink Amino acid drink A type of sports drink that often contains whey, a bovine milk product; PDs are commonly used to help recuperate fatigued or overly stressed muscles (**New York Times 7 Dec 1994; C6**) See Sports drink

protein F Fusion protein VIROLOGY A 70-kD glycoprotein that is thought to be integral to the host's ability to mount an appropriate immune response to respiratory syncytial virus; Cf Protein G

protein fingerprint A characteristic pattern of spots that identifies a protein in a relatively specific fashion TECHNIQUE A protease, eg trypsin, digests a relatively pure protein, eg hemoglobin for detecting a β chain of interest; the digestion cuts the protein after every arginine and after every lysine residue; the resulting fragments are electrophoresed, then turned 90° and rechromatographed, producing a 2-D 'fingerprint' that is visualized by spraying with ninhydrin, turning the paper with the polypeptide fragments purple (**Biochim Biophys Acta 1958; 28:543**) Cf DNA fingerprinting, RNA fingerprinting

protein folding The constellation of processes required for a protein to be converted from a simple polypeptide chain to a functional molecule with a three-dimensional configuration; see Protein structure

protein fractionation A generic term for any technique for separating proteins, including centrifugation, chromatography, electrophoresis or precipitation

protein G BACTERIOLOGY A component of the group G streptococcus cell wall that binds to the Fc region of all four subclasses of immunoglobulin G and which may be responsible for successful host defense against this organism VIROLOGY Attachment protein A 90-kD glycoprotein on the surface of and integral to the immune reaction to respiratory syncytitial virus (RSV); antigenic differences in the G protein are responsible for differences in RSV strains; Cf Protein F

protein kinase C A phorbol ester receptor encoded by an α gene on chromosome 17, a β gene on chromosome 16 and a γ gene on chromosome 19; PKC mediates multiple intracellular processes, acting by signal transduction, resulting in hormone secretion (calcitonin, catecholamines, insulin, growth hormone, steroids) and enzymes (amylase, pepsinogen), release of neurotransmitters, mediation of inflammation (release of histamine and serotonin and generation of superoxide) and anabolic effects (lipogenesis and gluconeogenesis); PKC is also involved in cell differentiation and tumor promotion; PKC is an intracellular enzyme with a protein kinase-like domain at the carboxyl terminal that is activated by extracellular signals received at the cell membrane receptors; phospholipase C-dependent hydrolysis of inositol phospholipid (especially phosphoinositol-4,5-bis-phosphate) into two second messengers: diacylglycerol (DAG) and inositol tris-phosphate (IP$_3$, which mobilizes calcium from intracellular stores); DAG activates and lysosphingolipids inhibit protein kinase C

protein lipidation A generic term for any co- or post-translational modification of proteins by specific lipids, which plays a critical role in the proteins' function(s); lipidated proteins are classified based on the attached lipid, which may be N-myristoyl–, S-palmitoyl– (or S-acyl-), S-prenyl, or GPI and are critical in cell signaling (**Science 1995; 268:221**)

protein-losing enteropathy A condition characterized by excess transmucosal efflux of plasma proteins from the intestinal lumen, due to increased permeability related to mucosal cell damage, inflammation-induced ulceration, or leakage from lymphatic vessels secondary to obstruction ETIOLOGY Paraneoplastic syndromes, gastric carcinoma, nontropical sprue, ulcerative colitis, CHF, constrictive pericarditis, superior vena cava thrombosis, pulmonic artery stenosis PATHOLOGY Inflammation, mucosal ulceration TREATMENT Treat underlying cause

protein M M antigen MICROBIOLOGY One of 55 serotypes of a protein located on the fimbriae of group A streptococci which has antiphagocytic properties and contributes to the streptococcal virulence; see LPSTGE

protein-only hypothesis A proposal regarding the nature of prions that states that the prion is identical to PrPSc, a modified form of PrPC, a normal host protein found predominantly on the surface of neurons, PrPSc is a form of PrPC that readily forms protease-resistant aggregates after treatment with detergents; introduction of PrPSc into a cell causes conversion of PrPC into PrPSc, possibly a result of a conformational change; familial forms are thought to be linked to mutations of PrPC that may facilitate spontaneous conversion to PrPSc; sporadic cases are attributed to rare spontaneous conversion of a normal PrPC or to a somatic mutation in the $Prn-p$ gene (from **Science 1994; 264:528P**) see Prions

proteinquake A functionally important movement of proteins, which like an earthquake, relieves the strain at a focus of the chain, with a return to an equilibrium state; see Protein folding, Protein structure

Note: A protein may assume a large number of conformational substates that have the same secondary structures, but different super-secondary structural substates causing a protein to perform its function at different rates; the existence of states and substates in proteins implies that there are two types of motion in proteins, ie equilibrium fluctuations (defined by the mathematics of chaos and equilibrium thermodynamics) and major conformational twists or 'quakes'

protein R GASTROENTEROLOGY A group of related 60-kD cobalamine-binding proteins found in gastric juice, milk, plasma, saliva, so designated as they all are rapid migrants on serum electrophoresis; see R-binding proteins

protein restriction Reduction of dietary protein from its normal level (circa 1.3 g/kg/day), a maneuver that is of use in renal failure (**N Engl J Med 1994; 330:877OA**); extreme protein restriction (very low protein diet, 0.28 g/kg/day) does not significantly slow the progression of renal disease more than moderate protein restriction (low protein diet, eg 0.58 g/kg/day)

protein redistribution diet YD (Arch Neurol 1992; 49:149)

protein S HEMATOLOGY A 69-kD vitamin K-dependent binding protein that is a cofactor for activated protein C (so named as it was discovered in Seattle); protein S exists as an active single chain protein or as an inactive disulfide-linked dimeric protein; when protein S is present with phospholipid, it enhances factor Va inactivation by protein C and binds C4b-binding protein; AD protein S deficiency is clinically and therapeutically similar to heterozygous protein C deficiency and is characterized by pulmonary thrombosis, deep vein thrombosis, thrombophlebitis; protein S is quantified by Laurell rocket electrophoresis, which does not distinguish between the active free protein and the inactive complement C4b-bound protein S; the functional assay is based on protein C's lack of anticoagulant activity in the absence of protein S IMMUNOLOGY see Vitronectin

protein-sparing CLINICAL NUTRITION Pertaining or relating to minimizing the use of proteins; protein-spairing maneuvers include the addition of carbohydrates and fats to a low-protein diet in order to minimize protein catabolism

protein structure The conformation of protein, which is a function of its amino acid sequence and the bonds that are allowed to be formed with itself and other molecules within its sphere of activity **PRIMARY PS** That structure of a protein that is a direct function of the sequence of amino acids **SECONDARY PS** That structure of a protein that results from folding along one axis of the molecule, as in the formation of an α helix, due to the formation of hydrogen bonds along the length of a chain; see Super secondary structure **TERTIARY PS** The 3-D conformation of a polypeptide chain folded upon itself, which may result from the interaction of the side chains of amino acids, and be immediately adjacent to each other or located across a chasm of intramolecular space **QUARTENARY PS** A protein structure that results from the interaction between individual polypeptide chains, or discrete by related proteins **QUINARY PS** Any transient interaction of multiple, unrelated proteins; see Domain

protein 'suicide' Protein inactivation CLINICAL GENETICS A molecular defect seen in a lethal variant of osteogenesis imperfecta, in which one of the three collagen chains (proα$_1$[I]) is markedly shortened, resulting in procollagen molecules incapable of forming a viable triple helix; the concept of protein suicide may help explain the greater than expected effects of certain seemingly innocent genetic defects

protein X pX protein, see there

protein Y Ligandin, see there

protein Z A 44-kD vitamin K-dependent plasma protein of unknown function that is a secondary cytoplasmic bilirubin-binding factor; see Ligandin; Cf Z protein

proteinase K MOLECULAR BIOLOGY A broad-spectrum protease that is a critical reagent for performing PCR on paraffin-embedded tissues, as formalin fixed archival tissue has cross-linked peptide bonds; PK acts by cleaving peptide bonds in which the carbonyl group is contributed by aromatic, hydrophobic, or aliphatic amino terminal; after PK treatment, the solution receptacle is heated to 95°C to inactivate the proteinase K

proteinuria The excretion of an excess amount of protein in the urine; normally, about 150 mg/day of protein is lost in the urine, ⅓ is albumin, ⅓ is Tamm-Horsfall glycoprotein, and the remainder is divided among actively secreted proteins including retinol binding proteins, β$_2$-

microglobulin, immunoglobulin light chains and lysozyme; in absence of disease, large proteins are retained due to their size, while the smaller proteins are actively resorbed proteinuria can be clinically divided into a

GLOMERULAR PATTERN Proteinuria due to a loss of the fixed negative charge on the glomerular capillary wall, allowing albumin and other large (≥ 68 kD) molecules to leak into Bowman's space, seen in glomerulonephritis and nephrotic syndrome Laboratory Decreased albumin, anti-thrombin, transferrin, prealbumin, a$_1$-acid glycoprotein and a$_1$-antitrypsin

HEMODYNAMIC PATTERN Proteinuria due to rheostatic changes elsewhere in the body, causing a loss of variably sized protein (20 to 68 kD) molecules, seen in transient proteinuria, congestive heart failure, fever, seizures, exercise

OVERFLOW PATTERN Proteinuria due to tissue or cell destruction elsewhere in the body, overwhelming the kidney's capacity to excrete certain proteins, as occurs in Bence-Jones proteinuria and myoglobinuria

TUBULAR PATTERN Proteinuria due to renal tubular dysfunction with loss of normally filtered low molecular weight (≤ 40 kD) molecules LABORATORY Decreased β$_2$-microglobulin and lysozyme, as occurs in Fanconi syndrome, Wilson's disease, interstitial nephritis, antibiotic-induced injury and heavy metal intoxication

proteoglycan A high-molecular-weight glycoprotein located on the plasma membranes of mammalian cells and in the extracellular matrix in connective tissue and cartilage; proteoglycans are separated according to differences in the core proteins and the composition of the linear polysaccharide chains or glycosaminoglycans, linked by covalent bonds to serine residues in the core proteins; see Basement membrane, Extracellular matrix; Cf Integrin family, Laminin

Note: Tumorigenesis is in part related to aberrant production of proteoglycans

proteolipid protein Lipophilin One of the two myelin basic proteins, which is major component of myelin encoded on chromosome segment Xq13-q22, which is defective in the X-linked recessive Pelizaeus-Merzbacher disease [MIM 312080], which is clinically characterized by 'jerky' eye movements, spastic weakness of the extremities, ataxia, choreoathetosis, mental deterioration, and death in late adolescence or early adulthood

proteoliposome A vesicular artificial organelle prepared from phospholipids, proteins and enzymes, that may be of use as a pharmacologic delivery system

proteosome A hydrophilic multimeric conglomerate of outer membrane meningococcal proteins that is mitogenic for B cells, a property that makes these structures attractive as possible carriers and adjuvants (nonspecific immune stimulators) for newer generations of vaccines through enhancement of immunogenicity; Cf Liposome

'Proteus inconstans' A group of bacteria placed in a separate genus as two species, *Providentia alcalifaciens* and *P stuartii*

Proteus syndrome A rare AD [MIM 176920] condition characterized by acral gigantism, plantar hyperplasia, hemangiomas, lipomas, varicosities, linear verrucous epidermal nevi, macrocephaly, cranial hyperostosis, pachydermy and hypertrophy of the long bones; see 'Elephant man'

Proteus of Greek mythology tended Neptune's flock of seals and had the gift of prophesy; in order to escape the constant badgering of those interested in the future, he often changed himself into other forms, eg wild animals or raging fire

prothrombin complex concentrate HEMATOLOGY Any of a number of commercial products, eg FEIBA (Factor VIII inhibitor by-passing activity) that contain nonactivated factors IX, in addition to II, XI and X, which may be used to ameliorate the intensity and duration of joint and soft tissue bleeding in hemophiliacs who produce factor VIII inhibitors; PCC are 50% effective in staunching hemorrhage; factor IX concentrates are prepared by adding cold ethanol or ether to citrated plasma, which is then added to either calcium phosphate or ion-exchange resins (eg

DEAE-Sephadex), allowing elution of a protein with therapeutic levels of vitamin K-dependent factors II, IX and X, and factors VII, protein C and protein S

prothrombin F1.2 The amino terminal of native prothrombin, which is released during the conversion of prothrombin to thrombin; prothrombin F1.2 is ↑ in some conditions predisposed to thrombosis, to wit, deficiencies of AT III, protein C, or protein S,and malignancy; normalization of prothrombin F1.2 levels with oral anticoagulants (eg coumadin) or heparin, and the inverse relationship between the levels of prothrombin F1.2 and PT and APTT ratios suggests it may ultimately prove useful in monitoring anticoagulant therapy (**CAP Today March 1993**)

protist see Progenote, Urkingdom

Protocol 076 AIDS An HIV-preventive regimen based on a clinical trial that was begun in April 1991 by the National Institute of Allergy and Infectious Diseases (US); the study's design called for enrollment of 748 HIV-infected pregnant ♀ in the US and France in a placebo-controlled trial of the effect of AZT in preventing the transmission of HIV to their babies; the trial was halted in early 1994, when accumulating data provided compelling evidence that the AZT-treated infants had ⅓ (8.3%) the incidence of HIV transmission as the placebo group (25.5%); in P076 the mothers took AZT five times/day for 11 weeks prior to delivery; AZT was then administered IV during labor; the newborns then received AZT syrup four times/day for 6 weeks; while this is heartening news for those in the developed countries, such a protocol would prove impossible in a developing nation give the costs, logistics, and the fact that virtually all mothers breast-feed, and are encouraged to do so by the WHO and UNICEF (regardless of HIV-status), because breast milk reduces infant morbidity and mortality (**Science 1995; 269:624**)

proton NUCLEAR PHYSICS A nuclear particle that has a single positive electric charge (1.6×10^{-19}) that is equal and opposite to that of an electron, and a mass of 1.67×10^{-24}g, which in solution becomes a hydrogen ion

proton pump CELL PHYSIOLOGY An ATP-dependent H^+ ion transporter presumed to be present in the membranes of lysosomes and vacuoles, which maintains a low pH (4.5-5.0) inside these organelles; proton pumping is also required in the electron transport chain, where an NADH (or FADH) is oxidized to NAD^+ (or FAH^+), releasing two electrons and a proton; Cf Na^+/H^+ antiporter, Na^+/K^+ ATPase

proton 'NMR spectroscopy Water-suppressed proton NMR spectroscopy A laboratory technique that averages the methyl and methylene line widths in the NMR spectra of plasma lipoproteins; this technique was reported to be a valid cancer screen in asymptomatic subjects, a finding not confirmed in subsequent studies (**N Engl J Med 1990; 322:949, 953, 1002**)

proto-oncogene A cellular gene that is homologous to a retroviral oncogene, in that it has latent transforming potential; P-Os include c-erb, c-fos, c-jun, c-myb, c-myc, c-mos, c-raf, c-ras and these act in normal growth and differentiation, as well as in the induction and/or maintenance of malignancy; proto-oncogenes coupled to control elements are capable of transforming normal fibroblasts into tumorigenic cells; slow retroviruses, which themselves lack viral oncogenes become tumorigenic when inserted in DNA adjacent to P-Os; many specific chromosomal translocations seen in human tumors occur at or near the P-O site and some P-Os may be 'amplified' in malignancy; P-Os are thought to become tumorigenic if the gene itself is altered, producing an abnormal gene product, or if there is an ↑ in the amount of the gene product, due to either gene amplification or changes in the control elements, eg there is ↑ expression of P-Os after

cellular insults, or CMV infection results in activation of c-fos, c-jun and c-myc

protoplasmic astrocytoma A rare low-grade astrocytoma that is more common in relatively young men, which most commonly affects the temporal and frontal lobes; complete excision may be beneficial; adjuvant therapy is not (**Am J Clin Pathol 1995; 103:705**)

protothecosis Infection by a ubiquitous, unicellular, alga-like organism that reproduces by endosporulation; human infection is rare, occurs in immunocompromised hosts, and is due to *Prototheca wickerhamii* or *P zopfii*, which cause chronic papulonodular skin lesions, wound infections, disseminated skin infections and lymphadenopathy TREATMENT Amphotericin B

proud flesh A curious term for the exuberant granulation tissue seen in a poorly healed wound, which is characterized by florid, 'geographic' scarring on the skin surface, related to a defect of union of interrupted tissues by 'second intent' healing; see Keloid, Wound healing

pro-urokinase A thrombolyic proenzyme prepared from either urine or by recombinant DNA technology that has a plasma $T_{1/2}$ much longer than that of urokinase; PU is not (as hoped) fibrin specific; PU is nonetheless capable of significant fibrinolysis without causing severe ↓ in fibrinogen, plasminogen, and α_2-antiplasmin (**Laboratory Medicine 1995; 26:323OA**) see Thrombolytic therapy

proverbs test NEUROLOGY A clinical test used to evaluate abstract thinking based on the ability to explain the meaning of a proverb*, which is a facet of intelligence that deteriorates in dementia

*A terse wise saying, eg 'haste makes waste', 'a stitch in time saves nine', etc

provider Health care provider

provirus A latent virus that is a replicative intermediate of an RNA oncogenic virus or bacteriophage, which consists of double-stranded DNA synthesized by reverse transcriptase and stably inserted into a host cell's genome; the proviral DNA is then transmitted vertically to the host's progeny at the time of cell division, and serves as a permanent template for the replication of viral RNA, thus having a 'Trojan Horse' effect

provisional diagnosis Working diagnosis, see there, aka preliminary diagnosis

provost A high level academic or educational administrator in a college or university

proximal carcinogen Ultimate carcinogen A chemical or physical agent that (hypothetically) initiates the first (induction) step of a carcinogenic cascade

proximate cause of death Underlying cause of death, see there

proximity effect The ↑ catalytic response observed when an enzyme's substrate is brought more proximate to the enzyme's reactive sites

Prozac® Fluoxetine HCl An FDA-approved drug for treating clinical depression; during the early 1990s, Prozac has gained popularity for treating other non-FDA-approved conditions, and has been touted by some as being a psychological panacea; 10-15% of users experience anxiety, nervousness, insomnia, and weight loss in underweight individuals; it is countraindicated for those who also are being treated with monoamine oxidase inhibitors (MAOI)

prozone phenomenon IMMUNOLOGY A reduction of, or false-negative antigen-antibody (Ag-Ab) reaction that occurs when antibodies are present in excess, and interfere with Ag-Ab lattice formation and inhibit the precipitation reaction; PP occurs when an Ag-Ab reaction is measured by immune precipitation and immunodiffusion; as immune reactions are optimal at an Ag-Ab ratio of 1:1, if there is strong reason to believe that a sample contains the suspected antibody (and may be displaying a prozone phenomenon), the sample should be serially diluted to prevent the specimen being reported as negative; false-negative serologic test for syphilis occurs in antibody excess; because of the anomalous hyperresponsiveness of B cells to previously 'known' antigens in HIV-infected subjects, negative syphilis serological tests should be diluted and repeated in HIV-positive subjects (Arch Int Med 1993; 153:1496)

PRP antigen Polyribosyl-ribitol capsular polysaccharide A cell wall component of *Haemophilus influenzae* that has intrinsic antiphagocytic activity, thus endowing *H influenzae* with a unique pathogenic mechanism; protective immunity against *H influenzae* requires opsonization with type-specific antibodies; the production of anti-PRP antibodies is poor until children reach age two and thus they may be susceptible to more than one episode; see Hib vaccine

PRP-D Polyribosylribitol-diphtheria toxoid see Hib

prune belly syndrome A condition characterized by complete congenital absence of abdominal musculature, which imparts a rugose, prune-like appearance to the flaccid abdominal wall; 97% occur in males and are accompanied by genitourinary anomalies, eg bilateral cryptorchidism, hypoplastic and dysplastic kidneys; affected females have uterine abnormalities; although considered an X-linked disease, no chromosome defect has been identified, and this disease complex may represent a 'sequence' initiated by in utero urethral obstruction, causing urinary tract anomalies (megaureters, megabladder, patent urachus or urachal cyst); other findings include Potter's facies, talipes, hip dislocation, musculoskeletal and cardiac defects TREATMENT Corsets, excision of redundant tissue PROGNOSIS Oligohydramnios may arise in utero, causing fatal fetal pulmonary hypoplasia, 20% are stillborn, 50% die in infancy

'pruned tree' appearance A descriptor for a pulmonary arteriographic pattern seen in relatively central pulmonary thromboembolism, where embolically enlarged pulmonary arteries are abruptly cut ('pruned') off

'prune juice' discharge A descriptor for the dark brown vaginal discharge characteristic of a hydatidiform mole likened to the juice of stewed prunes (dried plums)

prune juice sputum A descriptor for the watery dark brown hemorrhagic sputum seen in well-developed pneumococcal pneumonia; Cf Rusty sputum

pruritus gravidarum A condition affecting 1:300 pregnancies, beginning in the third trimester, first appearing on the abdomen later extending to the entire corporal surface TREATMENT Antihistamines; see Pregnancy-related conditions; Cf PUPPP

pS2 A 6.2-kD estrogen-inducible protein that is a marker of a functional estrogen regulatory system, which is regarded by some workers as an indicator of potential hormone responsiveness in breast cancer

PSA Prostate-specific antigen A 34-kD 240-amino acid glycoprotein serine protease that has significant homology with other neutral proteases; PSA is secreted exclusively by the prostate epithelium and is responsible for lysis of the seminal coagulum; PSA is increased in 30-50% of patients with benign prostatic hypertrophy and in 25-92% of those with prostate cancer* (PC); PSA is more sensitive than prostatic acid phosphatase (PAP) as a serum marker of PC, and the latter has fallen into disuse; PSA/PAP positivity is 63%/12% in stage A, 71%/22% in stage B, 81%/38% in stage C and 88%/67% in stage D; serum PSA levels (normal = 0.7 ng/mL) can be monitored for recurrent PC, but because PSA is also elevated in acute prostatitis and to a lesser degree, in benign prostatic hypertrophy, serum PSA levels are not a cost-effective screening modality for prostatic cancer; PC is present in 22% of those with PSA levels above 4.0 µg/L, and 60% of those

with levels above 10 µg/L (N Engl J Med 1991; 324:1156); serum PSA is highly variable and the coefficient of variation for patients is ± 55.3%, which contrasts with a mean coefficient of variation for the assay itself of 13.2% (Urology 1993; 42:390)

*Prostate cancer (PC) is the popular term for what is correctly designated prostatic adenocarcinoma

psammoma bodies *psammoma*, Greek, sand Calcospherites, 'corpora amylacea' Round laminated, 20-100 µm in diameter calcified masses that may correspond to degenerated papillary clusters of cellular debris that are especially common in benign prostatic hypertrophy; and may occur in benign and malignant epithelial neoplasms, eg papillary carcinomas of the thyroid, ovary, endometrium, pancreas, and kidney, meningiomas, benign 'sugar tumor' of the lung, mesothelioma, mesothelial cell hyperplasia, bronchoalveolar carcinoma; ovarian serous cystadenoma and dystrophic calcification of matrix vesicles and desmoid tumors

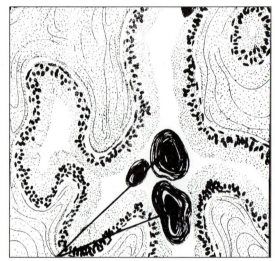

psammoma bodies

Pseudallescheria boydii A perfect (sexual form of) fungus of the class Ascomycetes which is the most common agent of mycetoma; *P boydii* is rarely a human pathogen, but may cause pneumonitis with vascular inflammation, disseminated disease, brain abscesses, and endocarditis, and has been described in AIDS (Arch Pathol Lab Med 1992; 116:535oA)

pseudoacanthosis nigricans A disease of obese darkly pigmented adults, characterized by hyperpigmented patches TREATMENT Weight loss

Note: True acanthosis nigricans occurs in subjects of any size and color in a background of malignancy

pseudoachondroplasia Any of a heterogeneous group of often AD conditions, the most common of which is pseudoachondroplastic spondyloepiphyseal dysplasia CLINICAL Early onset with decreased limb growth (irregular 'mushroomed 'metaphyses, small, irregular and fragmented epiphyses, short bowing diaphyses), flattened vertebrae, lumbar lordosis, scoliosis, kyphosis, 'spatula' ribs, hypermobility of major and acral joints, short hands and feet, contractures of the hips and knees, waddling gait and early onset of osteoarthrosis

True achondroplasia has more prominent truncal shortening, but is otherwise clinically similar

pseudoaldosteronism Pseudohyperaldosteronism, see there

pseudoalleles Two or more closely linked genes that in complementation studies behave as alleles, which may be separated by cross-over studies

pseudoallergy An adverse, nonimmunologic, anaphylaxis-like reaction of sudden onset, that is often associated with food ingestion, which may be due to an anaphylactoid reaction, intolerance, eg psychogenic response, metabolic defect, eg enzymatic deficiency, tyramine, see Cheese reaction, and toxicity, eg tetrodotoxin

True allergies to comestibles are hypersensitivity reactions caused by mast cell release of histamines evoked by IgE, in children, most commonly linked to eggs, milk, peanuts, other nuts, fish, soy beans and shrimp

pseudoanemia A generic term of uncertain utility referring to any clinical parameter (eg pallor and fatigue) that falsely suggests the presence of anemia

pseudoaneurysm False aneurysm, see there

pseudoangina 'Heartburn', see there

pseudoarthrosis ORTHOPEDICS The non-union of two fractured ends of a long bone where the bone is covered by fibrous tissue or fibrocartilage; in the most extreme cases, the false joint is surrounded by a bursal sac containing synovial fluid; congenital pseudoarthroses, while rare, most often occur in von Recklinghausen's disease or in osteogenesis imperfecta; acquired pseudoarthrosis usually follows trauma, far less commonly, tumor-related osteolysis and fibrous dysplasia

pseudoatrophy of brain An apparent ↓ in the volume of cortical tissue, as seen by CT, which is due to changes in CSF production and alterations in the blood-brain barrier with secondary ↓ in cerebral interstitial fluid, resulting from steroid therapy

True cerebral atrophy is irreversible

pseudoautosomal region A small terminal region of homologous DNA sequences that is shared by mammalian sex chromosomes, which pair and recombine during male meiosis; in this region, alleles are freely exchanged between X and Y chromosomes and inherited as if they were autosomal; genes in this region are present in two doses in both males and females, but in the female escape inactivation; two genes are located in the X-Y pseudoautosomal region; MIC2 and encodes a cell-surface antigen and granulocyte-monocyte colony-stimulating factor (GM-CSF); Cf X chromosome inactivation

pseudo-Bartter syndrome Hypokalemic-hypochloremic alkalosis, hyperactivity of renin-angiotensin-aldosterone system with increased aldosterone, normotension, pressor inactivity of angiotensin II, ↑ urinary prostaglandin E and atrionatriuretic peptide, due to furosemide therapy

True Bartter syndrome has a similar laboratory 'signature' but is caused by enlarged juxtaglomerular apparatus

pseudobubo A massively enlarged inguinal lymph node caused by *Calymmatobacterium granulomatis*, the granuloma inguinale agent, characterized by soft subcutaneous fluctuant masses with overlying ulcers

(true) Bubo is a generic term for any massively enlarged lymph node, visible in accessible regions (axillary or inguinal), and thus there is no 'true' bubo; the bubo of *Chlamydia trachomatis* (agent of LGV), has been anointed with various adjectives, including climatic bubo, Frei's bubo, nonvenereal bubo, strumous bubo and tropical bubo; syphilitic bubos have been adjectivally dignified as bullet bubo, primary bubo and venereal bubo; *Haemophilus ducreyi* (chancroid agent) causes the chancroid bubo and virulent bubo; the most famed of all is that of the bubonic plague, the 'malignant' bubo

pseudobulbar palsy Pseudobulbar paralysis, spastic bulbar paralysis A disease of middle age characterized by bilateral spasticity of the facial and deglutitive muscles, resulting in dysarthria, dysphonia, dysphagia, drooling, facial weakness, hyperreflexia of extremities, and shuffling (parkinsonian) gait; PP is remarkable for the highly variable psychiatric component, in which the patients may have a flat affect (simulating apathy or severe depression), or become enmeshed in trivialities, or have inappropriate responses to environmental cues, also known as the 'laughing sickness' for the characteristic pathological (ie inappropriate) laughing (or crying) ETIOLOGY The brains of these patients often demonstrate multifocal infarction, most commonly due to atherosclerosis, but also to hypertension, infections, trauma, and degeneration TREATMENT Antibiotics, if indicated PROGNOSIS Guarded

True bulbar palsy results from weakness or paralysis of the muscles supplied by the lower brainstem motor nuclei (V, VII, IX-XII) and may be of sudden onset, caused by diphtheria and poliomyelitis or more indolent with atrophy of the same muscles

pseudocapsule An investment of fibrous tissue that partially surrounds various neoplasms, especially of mesenchymal origin

True encapsulation implies a benign or at least a proliferating process that is circumscribed enough to allow complete removal; penetration of a tumor capsule is a notorious source of recurrence in otherwise low-grade carcinomas

pseudocarcinomatous hyperplasia Pseudoepitheliomatous hyperplasia, see there

pseudo-Chediak-Higashi anomaly A microscopic finding in Wright-Giemsa-stained peripheral blood smears in occasional patients with acute myelomonocytic and CML, seen as large, round, pink erythrocyte-like inclusions found in myeloblasts and promyelocytes; by ultrastructure, the inclusions correspond to abnormal peroxidase-positive granules that lack azurophilia due to absence of sulfated glycosaminoglycans

True Chediak-Higashi inclusions are present in neutrophils and correspond to giant and abnormal azurophilic granules seen in Chediak-Higashi disease, a condition with increased susceptibility to pyogenic infections, photophobia, albinism, hepatosplenomegaly, lymphadenopathy and early death

pseudocholinesterase An enzyme present in the liver and plasma that rapidly metabolizes succinylcholine, a short-acting (5-10 minutes) neuromuscular blocker used in anesthesia; succinylcholine's duration of action is controlled by its rate of metabolism by PChe; certain subjects have congenital PChe variants with prolonged neuromuscular blockage with 'usual' doses of succinylcholine, which can be identified by the 'dibucaine' number; PChe activity may be decreased in various acquired conditions, including hepatic disease (hepatitis, cirrhosis, metastasis), malnutrition, acute infections, anemia, myocardial infarcts, malignancy, pregnancy, cytotoxic drugs, acetyl-cholinesterase inhibitors and dermatomyositis; see Dibucaine number

True cholinesterase corresponds to acetylcholine cholinesterase

pseudochylous effusion A milky-white pleural effusion mimicking chylothorax, associated with high lipid levels (cholesterol or lecithin-globulin complexes) and seen in chronic pulmonary effusions, as in tuberculosis, rheumatoid arthritis or empyema

True chylous effusions are composed largely of chylomicrons originating from intestinally absorbed triglycerides Note: 1.5-2.5 liters of protein-rich (> 3.0 g/dl) chyle is produced and passes daily through the thoracic duct, which, when interrupted, causes chylothorax; 50% of cases of true chylothorax is due to tumor invasion of the ducts, 75% of which are related to lymphomas; 25% of cases are trauma-related with either open or closed wounds; most of the remaining cases of chylothorax are idiopathic

pseudoclaudication A symptom complex affecting patients with lumbar spondylosis, defined as unilateral or bilateral discomfort or pain, paresthesia and weakness in the lower extremities evoked or exacerbated by walking and relieved by rest, sitting or flexing at the waist; pseudoclaudication is caused by compression of the cauda equina, spinal stenosis, osteoarthritis, or may be due to congenital narrowing of the spinal canal DIAGNOSIS MRI

True claudication is a vascular event that persists despite rest or flexing of the waist and is recognized by the characteristic trophic changes of the extremities and loss of peripheral pulses in the lower extremities

pseudoclue cell A squamous cell seen by the Papanicolaou technique (smear of vaginal and cervical cells) that is overlaid, ie pseudo-infected with Döderlein bacteria (which are normal flora of the external female genitalia)

True clue cells are squamous cells infected by *Gardnerella vaginalis*

pseudocoarctation A kinked and/or dilated blood vessel

that has a radiologic appearance of a coarctation, without significant clinical finding or obstruction

pseudocoma A state mimicking acute unconsciousness with intact self-awareness, occurring in a) Organic disease states, eg 'locked-in syndrome' b) Psychogenic unresponsiveness, due to catatonic states, eg schizophrenia, severe depression, hysterical reactions or in frank malingering or c) Near-death experiences, for which there is no acceptable explanation

True comas are characterized by complete unresponsiveness during a coma state and for complete amnesia of events occurring while comatose

pseudocroup see Laryngismus stridulus

pseudocryptorchidism Retractile testis A testicle characterized by hyperactive cremasteric reflex drawing the organ into the inguinal canal, caused by cold temperature, fear and genital manipulation, occurring most prominently around age 5; Cf Migrating testis DIAGNOSIS The pseudocryptorchid testis can be pushed into the scrotum

True cryptorchidism refers to an undescended testis, which in the absence of spontaneous descent, should be surgically corrected before two years of age, as these patients are at an increased risk for germ cell neoplasm

pseudo-Cushing syndrome A condition defined as one in which there are certain clinical (truncal obesity and purple striae) or biochemical abnormalities ($\uparrow$ urinary cortisol levels that fall short of those typical of Cushing syndrome) that overlap with Cushing syndrome; p-CSs occurs with major depressive disorder, in middle-aged women with obesity (hypertension and DM), and in alcoholics (**N Engl J Med 1995; 332:791RA**) TREATMENT Reduce weight, psychotherapy

True Cushing syndrome has demonstrable increases in hypothalamic, pituitary, or adrenal hormones of either endogenous or exogenous origin

pseudocyesis PSYCHIATRY A symptom complex affecting women with a strong and unfulfilled desire for children, resulting in amenorrhea, morning sickness, induration of breasts and $\uparrow$ abdominal girth; see Pseudopregnancy; Cf Sympathy 'pregnancy'

pseudocyst GASTROENTEROLOGY see Pancreatic pseudocyst PARASITOLOGY A cyst-like 'mass' that corresponds to a macrophage laden with *Toxoplasma gondii* or other sporozoans which is most often seen in the brain, a finding typical of AIDS neuropathy[1] PATHOLOGY A dilated space lined by neither epithelium nor mesothelium, classically seen in the pancreas[2] as unilocular spaces lined by fibrous tissue, often following multiple bouts of acute pancreatitis or in the ultrarare hereditary pancreatitis

[1]True cysts refer to a reproductive 'structure' with daughter cells within the cytoplasm [2]True epithelial cysts of the pancreas include 1) Dysgenic cysts associated with polycystic kidneys 2) Retention cysts, in which tumors, stones or inflammatory strictures cause prolapse of the ductal epithelium with cystic dilatation 3) Dyschylic cysts associated with cystic fibrosis and the most common 4) Cysts arising in pancreatic carcinoma

pseudodementia Dementia-like symptoms due to psychological impairment, eg depression or histrionic episode; pseudodementia is characterized by cognitive impairment of short duration, with preservation of attention and ability to concentrate and variable performance in tests with similar levels of difficulty; it is often transient, common in the elderly and may be due to chronic intoxication by prescribed drugs (anticholinergics, barbiturates, benzodiazepines, butyrophenones, corticosteroids, digitalis, IMAO and tricyclic antidepressants) or due to depression (caused by physical and emotional deprivation, accompanied by apathy, akinesia and anxiety); pseudodementia also occurs in normal pressure hydrocephalus, Creutzfeldt-Jakob, Huntington's, Parkinson's, Pick's, and Wilson's diseases, and endocrinopathy; Cf Pseudoatrophy, cerebral

True dementia is progressive and often demonstrates cortical atrophy by CT and MRI

pseudodiabetes 1) Latent diabetes mellitus 2) A clinical condition characterized by defective carbohydrate metabolism secondary to chronic renal failure (uremia), with reduced glucose tolerance (rapid post-prandial rise and delayed return of glucose to normal), mild baseline hyperglycemia and insulin 'resistance'

pseudo-Du cell TRANSFUSION MEDICINE An erythrocyte that has an Rh blood group that is Du-like in agglutination reactions; testing of the family's red cells reveals an Rh group 'c' allele in the trans position, which suppresses expression of a normal Rh 'D' antigen; see Weak D (formerly Du)

pseudoeosinophilia CYTOLOGY A red color shift in Papanicolaou-stained vaginal and cervical squames, seen when these cells are infected with coccoid bacteria

True eosinophilia of cervical squames is secondary to estrogen effect

pseudoepidemic MICROBIOLOGY A cluster of bacterial 'infections', often by unusual organisms, that are reported as positive by the microbiology laboratory from patients who are not clinically ill; pseudoepidemics are caused by contamination of culture plates, ambient air or other common 'factor' in the environment, eg tap water, and have been described with *Mycobacterium gordonae*, *M avium* complex, *M scrofulaceum*, and *Aeromonas hydrophilus*, each of which may also cause clinical disease, further complicating delineation of the nature of these conditions

pseudoepidermis A membrane prepared in vitro from keratinocytes isolated from full-thickness human or rat skin, which is of potential use to screen chemicals for potential cutaneous toxicity vis-a-vis human response; the characteristics of such a commercial product (eg **In Vitro Technology, Kalamazoo, Mich**) include sensitivity to irritants, reactivity in a dose-dependent fashion, simplicity of assay, ease of transport, ability to be produced in large quantities (**Am Biotech Lab November 1994**)

pseudoepitheliomatous hyperplasia A nonspecific epithelial proliferation corresponding to reactive hyperplasia of stratified mucocutaneous epithelia, seen overlying infections (abscesses, *Blastomyces dermatitidis*, granuloma inguinale), granular cell tumors, inflammation (adjacent to ulcer margins and scars), burns and irritation PATHOLOGY Acanthosis, irregular downgrowth of the rete pegs, pointed epidermal masses, with horn-pearl formation and florid mitotic activity, occasionally extending below the level of the sweat glands

True carcinoma (formerly, malignant epithelioma) usually has prominent cellular atypia and invasive 'fingerlets' of malignant cells that spread beyond subepithelial tissues, although very well-differentiated squamous cell carcinoma, eg verrucous carcinoma spread along a broad base

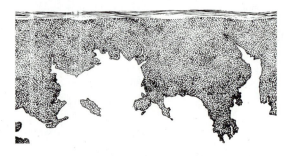

pseudoepitheliomatous hyperplasia

pseudofracture Looser zone A thin radiolucent line that mimics a true fracture and which is quasipathognomonic for osteomalacia in the adult, characterized by complex bony lesions typical of advanced renal failure

pseudofusion beat CARDIOLOGY A finding on the EKG with a cardiac pacemaker that corresponds to the superimposition of an ineffective pacemaker spike on a spontaneous QRS complex originating from a single focus, which is a normal manifestation of VVI (ventricular demand) pacing; the pacemaker stimulus occurs too late to cause true fusion as it falls in the absolutely refractory period of the myocardium previously stimulated by the spontaneous depolarization; Cf Fusion beat

A true fusion beat is usually narrower than a paced impulse and has various morphologies that reflect the relative contributions of the impulse to the ventricular depolarization

pseudo-Gaucher cell A Gaucher-like histiocyte with normal β-glucocerebrosidase activity and abundant, crumpled tissue paper-like linear cytoplasmic deposits of various materials, including cerebroside, seen in conditions where the rate of cell destruction outstrips the macrophages' capacity to phagocytose cerebrosides and other membrane components; pseudo-Gaucher cells occur in CML, ALL, hereditary neutrophilia, Hodgkin's disease, infectious mononucleosis, idiopathic thrombocytopenic purpura (in the spleen), thalassemia, congenital dyserythropoietic anemia, type II aplastic, hemolytic and iron-deficiency anemias, hereditary neutrophilia, post-necrotic cirrhosis, rheumatoid arthritis, and vitamin E deficiency

True Gaucher cells have a crumpled tissue paper-like cytoplasm replete with glucocerebroside, due to glucocerebrosidase deficiency

pseudogene A region of the genome that has a DNA sequence similar to that of a known gene, but which itself is neither transcribed nor encodes a protein or portion thereof, thus also known as 'junk' DNA; pseudogenes may represent vestigial duplicated genes that are no longer active due to a non-functional mutational 'drift' in sequence; pseudogenes may also be defined as a faulty replicate of a normal gene that is found in a genome, and is stable, inherited, but unexpressed, and may lack some of the ancillary structures needed for transcription and translation

pseudoglioma A term introduced in the ophthalmologic literature late in the 19th Century for a heterogeneous group of lesions that may be confused with retinoblastoma (thus the term 'pseudoretinoblastoma' would be more appropriate); pseudogliomatous lesions include 1) Leukokoria Coat's disease, diktyoma, incontinentia pigmenti, metastatic retinitis, Norrie's disease, persistent hyperplastic primary vitreous, retinal dysplasia, retrolental fibroplasia, secondary retinal detachment, toxocara endophthalmitis and 2) Retinal lesions Chorioretinal lesions that are either endophytic, eg retinal hamartomas, myelinated nerve fibers, colobomas, retinochoroiditis or exophytic larval, angiomatous or proliferative conditions

pseudo-goiter Modigliani syndrome, see there

pseudogout Chondrocalcinosis An arthropathy more common in elderly females, characterized by deposition of calcium pyrophosphate dihydrate crystals in large joints (knees, shoulders, hips), due to either local overproduction of pyrophosphate or a deficiency of phosphatase PATHOLOGY Acute synovitis, followed by osteoarthritis; microscopic examination of synovial fluid reveals 'Coffin lid' crystals, which may be seen in other arthritic conditions including gout, osteoarthritis, and rheumatoid arthritis POLARIZED LIGHT MICROSCOPY Crystals with weak positive birefringence

True gout usually affects smaller joints of older men who have increased uric acid levels and urate crystals in the joints; patients may also have DM or hypertension

pseudogynecomastia Enlargement (usually bilateral) of the breast due to excessive adipose tissue deposition with abundant small nerve fibers and occasionally multinucleated fibroblasts, without an increase in the mammary tissue per se, which occurs in young obese ♂ with neurofibromatosis; see Gynecomastia

True gynecomastia is characterized by an ↑ in dense, periductal collagenous connective tissue stroma, and marked hyperplasia of the ductal epithelium with multilayering of cells

pseudohermaphrodite A sex-reversed individual whose genotype is discordant with his/her phenotype; XX pseudohermaphroditic 'males' are first recognized when

they complain of infertility; XY pseudohermaphroditic 'females' are missing a critical fragment of the Y chromosome that would otherwise result in 'maleness'; see X chromosome inactivation

pseudohermaphroditism A state in which an individual has the gonadal tissue of one sex, but the wiring, plumbing, and/or chassis of the opposite sex

FEMALE PSEUDOHERMAPHRODITISM A condition affecting a genotypic (46, XX) female with ovaries, caused by a relative excess of androgen in utero, resulting in equivocal or masculinized genital duct derivatives, ie external genitalia and/or phenotypic male with genital ambiguity and/or virilization ETIOLOGY 1) Adrenogenital syndrome Defects of 21-hydroxylase, 11 β-hydroxylase or 3 β-hydroxysteroid dehydrogenase, or delta 5-4 isomerase deficiency, resulting in increased androgenic intermediates 2) Maternal ingestion of progestins or androgens and 3) Maternal virilizing tumors, eg luteoma of pregnancy; see Hermaphroditism, Intersex, Virilization

MALE PSEUDOHERMAPHRODITISM, A condition affecting a genotypic (46, XY) male with testes, caused by a relative deficiency of androgen in utero, resulting in a phenotypic female with ambiguous genitalia ETIOLOGY 1) Gonadal defects Testicular regression syndrome, persistent müllerian duct origin, Leydig cell agenesis and defects in testosterone synthesis 2) End-organ defects Testicular feminization or androgen insensitivity syndrome, incomplete androgen insensitivity syndrome and 5-α reductase deficiency; see Hermaphroditism, Testicular feminization

pseudo-Hirschsprung's disease Colonic inertia in children of possible psychogenic origin without histologic evidence of defective myoenteric innervation

True Hirschsprung's disease is characterized by the absence of ganglion cells in Auerbach's and Meissner's plexuses

pseudo-Hurler syndrome Mucolipidosis, type III An AR [MIM 252600] dysostotic syndrome of early childhood onset, characterized by a markedly reduced height, coarse, gargoyle-like facies, corneal clouding, mild retinopathy, mild mental retardation, joint stiffness and claw-hand deformity, due to a defect in phosphotransferase activity Note: For other Hurler-like syndromes, see Gargoylism

True Hurler syndrome (mucopolysaccharidosis, type IH) is due to deficient α-L-iduronidase with accumulation of dermatan sulfate and heparan sulfate in various tissues

pseudohyperaldosteronism Liddle syndrome An AD [MIM 177200] aldosteronism-like condition characterized by severe hypertension and spontaneous hypokalemia (potassium wasting, resulting in hypokalemic alkalosis) with ↓ aldosterone secretion PATHOGENESIS Defective sodium resorption in distal renal tubules, ↑ influx of sodium in RBCs PATHOLOGY Atrophy of juxtaglomerular apparatus and loss of renin-secreting granules TREATMENT KCl, amiloride and triamterene to prevent potassium wasting, sodium restriction; renal transplantation (**N Engl J Med 1994; 330:178OA**)

True hyperaldosteronism is due to hyperplasia, an adenoma or rarely, an adrenocortical carcinoma of the adrenal cortex, especially the zona glomerulosa

pseudohyperhypoparathyroidism Pseudohypohyperparathyroidism, see there

pseudohyperkalemia LABORATORY MEDICINE An in vitro phenomenon seen in megakaryocytic hyperplasia, thrombocytosis, leukocytosis, or myeloproliferative disease, where rapid clotting of blood releases potassium from erythrocytes LABORATORY ↑ Serum K+, plasma K+ is normal

pseudohyperparathyroidism Hypercalcemia of malignancy, see there

pseudohypertension Sphygmomanometric cuff pressure that is higher than the actual blood pressure, due to markedly calcified ('pipestem') brachial arteries, most common in the elderly who have extensive atherosclerosis

DIAGNOSIS Osler's maneuver, which is a bedside method for assessing the palpability of the radial or brachial pulse distal to a point of presumed occlusion; Cf Hypertension, Small cuff syndrome, White coat hypertension

pseudohypertrophy A generic term for any ↑ in the size of an organ without an ↑ in the number or size of the organ's native cells; pseudohypertrophy is 'classically' described in Duchenne's muscular dystrophy, where the ↑ in girth of the extremities is due to infiltration of fats cells among bundles of atrophic muscle

pseudohyphae Elongated blastospores with focal constrictions ('link sausage' appearance) that are seen in *Candida* species

True hyphae are 1) Nonseptate and include Zygomycetes, eg *Absidia*, *Mucor* and *Rhizopus* 2) Septate, a) hyaline type Dermatophytes, *Aspergillus*, *Geotrichum*, *Trichosporon* and *Pseudoallescheria boydii* or Septate, b) dematiaceous type *Cladosporium*, *Curvalaria*, *Drechslera*, *Exophila*, *Phialophora* and others

pseudohypoaldosteronism A heterogeneous group of salt wasting syndromes caused by distal renal tubular insensitivity to mineralocorticoids (eg aldosterone) or by a defect in the mineralocortioid receptor in the colonic mucosa, salivary and sweat glands, resulting in salt loss in the face of normal adrenocortical and renal function, which is accompanied by a hyperactive renin-angiotensin system

TYPE I PSEUDOHYPOALDOSTERONISM A rare condition that may be either AD [MIM 177735] or AR [MIM 264350]; it begins in infancy and is characterized by salt wasting, hypotension, ↑ plasma renin, ↑ aldosterone, hyperkalemia, hyponatremia, dehydration and metabolic alkalosis, clinically accompanied by vomiting, failure to thrive and periodic cyanosis when exposed to increased environmental temperatures TREATMENT Salt supplements

TYPE II PSEUDOHYPOALDOSTERONISM An acquired condition due to the so-called 'distal chloride shunt', first seen in older children or adults, characterized by hypertension, hypervolemia, low-to-normal aldosterone, hyperkalemia and metabolic acidosis TREATMENT Salt restriction and diuretics

True hypoaldosteronism is either an isolated event or associated with hypocortisolism; the most common cause is decreased renin secretion (hyporeninemic hypoaldosteronism, seen in the elderly with renal failure, associated with DM, interstitial nephritis or multiple myeloma), deficiency of 18-hydroxylase or focal destruction of the adrenal cortex, resulting in hypereninemic hypoaldosteronism Laboratory Hyperkalemia, metabolic acidosis Treatment Correct primary defect, supplementary mineralocorticoids

pseudohypohyperparathyroidism A clinical condition that is a combination of congenital end-organ resistance to parathormone (pseudohypoparathyroidism) and osteitis fibrosa cystica, seen in hyperparathyroidism, which may be related to differences in the transduction of the bone remodeling response, ie divergence of parathormone secretion and expression of parathyroid hormone receptor; Cf Pseudopseudohypoparathyroidism

Note: Use of the term hyperhypoparathyroidism is discouraged as it lends to confusion

pseudohyponatremia Spuriously low sodium levels due to either 1) Intrinsic properties of a patient sample, as in hyperglycemia or hyperproteinemia (displacement of plasma water or due to the cationic nature of monoclonal proteins which bind sodium), hyperlipidemia or hyperviscosity or 2) Analytic factors, which occur while preparing samples for flame photometry or indirect potentiometry

pseudohypoparathyroidism A hypoparathyroid-like state (hypocalcemia, hyperphosphatemia) due to end-organ resistance to PTH (by both bone and kidney with loss of renal tubule response to PTH) with ↑ PTH secretion and parathyroid gland hyperplasia, despite excess PTH secretion in response to hypocalcemia by a normal or hyperplastic parathyroid gland; the condition is associated with a secondary hypocalcemia-induced ↑ in parathyroid function (administration of pharmacologic doses of PTH normally results in ↑ urinary phosphate excretion and ↑ cAMP, but not in pseudohypoparathyroidism); the pattern of heredity is unclear, ♂:♀ ratio is 2:1; changes include a round face, dental dysplasia, dry course hair, mental retardation **PSEUDOHYPOPARATHYROIDISM, TYPE I** (Albright's hereditary osteodystrophy) is more common, and is almost invariably X-linked [MIM 300100]; AD [MIM 103580] cases (designated type IA) have been reported; there is inadequate cAMP response to parathormone **PSEUDOHYPOPARATHYROIDISM, TYPE II** is due to inadequate end-organ response to increased cAMP levels; children with type II are short and stocky with a round facies, brachydactyly, tetany, foci of bony demineralization, osteitis fibrosa TREATMENT Both forms respond to vitamin 1,25 $(OH)_2D_3$; see Pseudopseudohypoparathyroidism

TRUE HYPOPARATHYROIDISM is most commonly a sequela of thyroidectomy; less commonly, idiopathic or associated with athymia (DiGeorge syndrome) CLINICAL Electrolyte abnormalities (↓ calcium, ↑ phosphorus), which results in neuromuscular hyperexcitability, causing Chvostek sign, Trousseau sign, cramps, convulsions, dyspnea, photophobia, lethargy and ectopic calcification of basal ganglia, cornea. and soft tissue

pseudohypophosphatasia A condition characterized by clinical and radiological features of vitamin D-resistant rickets and phosphoethanolaminuria, with ↑ pyridoxal 5'-phosphate (vitamin B_6 cofactor), caput membraneceum, osteopathy of the skull and long bones, failure to thrive, muscle hypotonicity; in one case, the tissue changes were nonspecific, affecting the liver, bone and kidney, with normal alkaline phosphatase isoenzyme activity accompanied by defective pholytic activity against the usual bone targets

pseudoidiopathic hypoparathyroidism Hypoparathyroidism described in one young adult with the laboratory parameters of idiopathic hypoparathyroidism and normal serum levels of a defective parathyroid hormone, resulting from a defect in peripheral conversion from prohormone or from a defect in peripheral activation of a secreted parathyroid hormone precursor; Cf Pseudohypoparathyroidism

pseudoinclusion An ultrastructural finding in the nuclei of malignant epithelial cells, in which a 'bleb' of cytoplasm prolapses into the nucleus; Cf Nuclear blebbing

pseudoincontinence The inability to retain urine, due to difficulty in reaching the toilet, advanced arthritis, or other physical handicaps, resulting in anger and frustration in the impaired persons

True incontinence only occurs with advanced or sudden spinal cord compression; overflow incontinence is secondary to peripheral (preganglionic or somatic afferent) defects in voiding

pseudoinfarction A Q wave inversion by EKG that mimics the findings of myocardial infarction, which may be seen in Wolff-Parkinson-White syndrome, cardiac amyloidosis, and hypertrophic cardiomyopathy, and is due to elongation and partial stretching of the nerve fibers

True myocardial infarction classically causes abnormalities of the Q wave (an EKG 'marker' for necrosis, often seen at the corresponding cardiac leads), an upward ST-segment displacement (a marker for injury) and an inverted T wave (a marker for ischemia)

pseudoinfectious proctitis Noninfectious inflammation of the rectum secondary to anal-erotic activity including trauma and erosion by inserted body parts, vibrators, bottles, eggs and other objects, allergic response to lubricants used in anal intercourse (cooking oil, suntan lotions, medicinal creams) and reactions due to toxins; see Gay bowel disease; Cf Sexual deviancy

pseudoinsomnia Subjective difficulty in falling asleep that is described in 10% of those who claim to suffer from insomnia, despite objective observations to the contrary; Cf Insomnia, Sleep disorders

pseudoinvasion A histologic finding that mimics the invasion of normal tissue by malignancy, consisting in penetration of nerves by benign processes, eg proliferating ductules in vasitis nodosa, normal and hyperplastic prostate, fibrocystic disease of the breast and normal pancreas; see Lymph node inclusions; Cf Metastasis, Prevascular phase

pseudoisochromic plates Colored plates that are comprised of variably sized dots of different colors and used to classify color blind individuals with protanopsias and deuteranopsias (defective color vision for red and green); standard plates include the Ishihara atlas and Hardy-Rand-Rittler plates

pseudoisoenzyme One of two or more variant conformational forms of an enzyme, all of which have the same primary structure

True isoenzymes differ in primary and secondary structure

pseudo-Kaposi sarcoma Kaposiform dermatitis A condition that clinically mimics Kaposi sarcoma, which is seen in the AV hemangiomas or AV fistulas of Klippel-Trenaunay disease PATHOLOGY Proliferation of capillaries and fibroblasts, extravasation of RBCs and deposition of hemosiderin in dermis True Kaposi sarcoma has, in addition to the above, microscopic features, demonstrates spindling of malignant cells with occasional cellular atypia and formation of slit-like spaces; see Peninsula sign

pseudo-lecithin cholesterol acyl transferase deficiency see Lecithin cholesterol acyl transferase

pseudolymphoma A form of lymphoid hyperplasia which is characterized by a relatively monotonous population of lymphocytes, seen in the breast, GI tract, lung, mediastinum, orbit, salivary gland, skin, soft tissue, thyroid, and other sites; pseudolymphomas are smaller than lymphomas, polyclonal, have well-preserved nodal architecture, intact cortical germinal centers of variable size and shape, little or no infiltration of the capsule or pericapsular fat by lymphocytes, active phagocytosis in the germinal center (nuclear 'dust' within histiocytes), inflammatory cell infiltration between germinal centers, mitotic activity confined to germinal centers, no alteration of the reticular framework; pseudolymphomas occur in a younger population, have been associated with collagen diseases, SLE, Sjögren syndrome, phenytoin therapy, and may present in patients with concomitant lymphoma or in those who later develop lymphoma; see Phenytoin lymphadenopathy; Cf Lymphoma

True lymphomas are monoclonal, partially or completely abolished nodal architecture, germinal centers of uniform size and shape, infiltration of the capsule or pericapsular fat by lymphocytes, mitotic activity that extends beyond germinal centers, no alteration of the reticular framework; lymphomas occur in an older population

pseudomembrane A thin, adherent, gray-white exudative lamination composed of necrotic epithelium, fibrin, bacteria, PMNs, which overlies the mucosa of the 1) Colon, see Pseudomembranous colitis and 2) Oropharynx, which extends from the tonsils to the contiguous soft and hard palates, and pharynx, the removal of which causes hemorrhage; it is composed of necrotic debris and PMNs and is classically seen in diphtheria (due to *Corynebacterium diphtheriae*), causing a bull-like neck; pseudomembranes of the oropharynx may also occur in shigellosis, staphylococcal infections, *Clostridium perfringens*, *C difficile* and less commonly in viral infections of the oropharynx

pseudomembranous bronchitis Plastic bronchitis, see there

pseudomembranous candidiasis Thrush, see there

pseudomembranous colitis An acute illness with often severe diarrhea that follows antibiotic therapy with ampicillin, clindamycin, metronidazole and others, which eliminate the patient's native bacterial flora, resulting in superinfection by *Clostridium difficile*, which is responsible for virtually all cases of PC (**N Engl J Med 1994; 330:257**OA) the condition may occur in 'compromised' hosts or the elderly, in a background of colonic obstruction, leukemia, major surgery, uremia, spinal injury, colonic carcinoma, burns,

infections, shock, heavy metal poisoning, hemolytic-uremic syndrome, cardiovascular ischemia, Crohn's disease, shigellosis, necrotizing enterocolitis, and Hirschsprung's disease CLINICAL Mild diarrhea to fulminant disease with fever, dehydration and shock HISTOLOGIC CLASSIFICATION, STAGE I Early focal and superficial epithelial necrosis that may extend into the lamina propria with increased eosinophils, neutrophils and cytoclastic debris STAGE II Dome-shaped necrotic plaques distended by mucin and neutrophils at the base, covered by a fibrin plaque, necrotic tips of villi, debris and neutrophils ('volcano lesion'); the intervening mucosa is relatively normal STAGE III Little architecture is preserved; mucosal recovery is uncommon; see *Clostidium difficile* colitis

There is no 'membranous' colitis

pseudometabolic acidosis A laboratory artifact seen when vacuum blood collection tubes (eg Vacutainer™) are underfilled with blood, resulting in falsely low bicarbonate value, falsely high anion gap (see table); a crude 'guesstimate' to correct for underfilled tubes would be an $\uparrow$ in bicarbonate by 0.5-0.6 mmol/L and a $\downarrow$ in anion gap by 0.2-0.3 mmol/L (**Ann Emerg Med 1992; 21:177**)

PSEUDOMETABOLIC ACIDOSIS			
Amount of blood in 10 ml tube	1 ml	3 ml	10 ml
Bicarbonate mmol/L, unvented tube	21.7	19.4	16.3
Bicarbonate mmol/L, vented tube	23.3	20.3	17.3
Anion gap mmol/L	16.7	17.5	19.2

[1]Ann Emerg Med 1992; 21:177

Pseudomonas aeruginosa A normal soil inhabitant and human saprophyte that may contaminate various solutions in the hospital environment and cause opportunistic infection in debilitated patients PATHOGENESIS *P aeruginosa* is both invasive and toxicogenic, and infections therewith are viewed as occurring in a three step process: 1) Bacterial attachment and colonization (mediated by pili and defended against host defenses by the antiphagocytic properties of the bug's polysaccharide capsule) 2) Local invasion (mediated by elastase and alkaline protease of bacterial origin) and 3) Dissemination CLINICAL Infective endocarditis in IVDAs, lower respiratory tract infections, UTIs, bacteremia, meningitis, and 'malignant' external otitis TREATMENT Aminoglycosides (eg gentamicin, amikacin, netilmicin, tobramycin, and others) high-dose tobramycin delivered by aerosol is reported to be effective in patients with cystic fibrosis (**N Engl J Med 1993; 328:1740**OA)

Pseudomonas cepacia *Burkholderia cepacia*, see there

pseudomyxoma peritonei A condition characterized by poorly-circumscribed gelatinous masses filled with malignant mucin-secreting cells; 45% of PPs arise from the ovary, usually in a mucinous cystadenocarcinoma, which has prognostic significance, eg mucinous ovarian cystadenocarcinomas of undetermined malignant potential ('borderline' tumors) have a usual 10-year survival of 95%, but when associated with pseudomyxoma, the 10-year survival falls to 40%; 29% of cases of PP are due to the uncommon mucin-producing carcinoma of the appendix; the material must be differentiated from mucinous spillage into the peritoneum by a benign mucocele of the appendix; PP may also be due to various mucin-secreting carcinomas, and rarely to benign lesions, eg ovarian fibroma and teratoma; the appendix is regarded as the primary site of PP in most ♂ and ♀; the associated mucinous ovarin tumors are thought to be secondary neoplasms

pseudoneuritis Pseudopapilledema, see there

'pseudonym' syndrome(s) A disorder with more than five actively used aliases, including 1) Agnogenic myeloid metaplasia (AMM), a disease for which the pathogenesis is poorly understood, the etiology unknown, the prognosis uncertain and the therapy ineffective; synonyms for AMM include myelofibrosis with myeloid metaplasia, splenic myelosis, osteomyeloreticulosis, aleukemic myelosis and primary myelofibrosis Note: Secondary myelofibrosis may occur in acute leukemia, lymphoma, metastases and hairy cell leukemia and 2) Pigmented neuroectodermal tumor of infancy, also known as retinal anlage tumor, benign melanotic progonoma, pigmented epulis of infancy, melanotic adamantinoma, congenital melanocarcinoma and melanoameloblastoma

pseudo-obstruction, acute colonic Ogilvie syndrome, Non-toxic megacolon Massive colonic dilatation without mechanical obstruction, possibly due to a sympathetic nervous system defect, causing chronic peristaltic paralysis, affecting the cecum, right colon, distal small intestine, less commonly, the esophagus and stomach CLINICAL Initially painless abdominal distension with nausea, pain relieved by vomiting and diarrhea and intermittent symptoms extending over years; the condition may be congenital, as in hereditary hollow viscus myopathy, acquired (DM, hypothyroidism, collagen vascular diseases, myotonic dystrophy, parkinsonism, multiple sclerosis, amyloidosis, trauma, surgery, inflammation (pancreatitis), infections, radiation therapy, malignancy, cardiovascular (myocardial infarct), neurologic, respiratory (pneumonia), metabolic (alcoholism, hypokalemia and other electrolyte imbalance, uremia), muscular dystrophy, familial dysautonomia (Riley-Day syndrome), porphyria, dysproteinemia, drug-related (phenothiazines, tricyclic antidepressants, ganglion blockers, clonidine, narcotics, anticholinergics) TREATMENT Decompression of intestine, correction of electrolyte imbalance or cecostomy; see Paralytic ileus

pseudo-orphan drug An orphan drug for which there is active commercial interest in the pharmaceutical industry, as the drug has potentially broader applications than those that fall under its 'orphan drug' status, eg human growth hormone received 11 distinct orphan disease applications from four different manufacturers, and thus would not be considered an 'orphan' product in the spirit of the legislation designed to provide a financial incentive to companies developing therapies for patients with truly rare ('orphan') diseases, eg porphyria; see Ophan disease, Orphan drug

True orphan drugs are those formulated with the specific understanding that the number of potential users is small and will probably always be so, eg cysteamine for treating patients with the very rare nephropathic cystinosis, a true orphan disease (Science 1991; 251:1159ed)

pseudopapilledema OPHTHALMOLOGY A papilledema-like condition that mimics a swollen optic disc, which consists of a 'heaping up' of nerve fibers and glial tissues, associated with hypermetropia or farsightedness (due to axonal crowding at the disc) or drusen (hyaline material in the prelaminar nerve, fancifully known as 'rock' crystals)

True papilledema is progressive and is characterized by dilatation of veins, hemorrhages and exudates

pseudoparaproteinemia An increase of transferrin to two-fold or greater than normal 2-4 g/L (US: 200-400 mg/dl), as a reaction to severe iron-deficiency anemia; because transferrin exists in only one molecular species and migrates as a 'tight' band in the β region in serum electrophoresis, it mimics paraproteinemia

True paraproteinemia is any 'spike' on a gel electrophoresis or serum, which must be 'worked-up' to determine whether it corresponds to a monoclonal gammopathy, either benign or malignant

pseudopelade of Brocq Alopecia cicatrisata A dermatopathy of the scalp characterized by scattered, geographically shaped alopecic patches; early disease is characterized by mild perifollicular erythema, upper dermal mononuclear inflammation and scaling, followed by smooth atrophic atrichous patches, a stage that is indistinguishable from end-stage lichen planopilaris, and mimicking circumscribed scleroderma, discoid lupus erythematosus, and folliculitis decalvans; pseudopelade may be an isolated entity or associated with lichen planus, lichenoid dermatopathies, and Graham-Little syndrome

pseudo-Pelger-Huët anomaly A morphology of granulocyte nuclei in which there is a rounded, hyposegmented pince-nez appearance and coarse chromatin, due to a dissociation between cytoplasmic and nuclear maturation; these cells appear transiently in AML, agnogenic myeloid metaplasia, CML, erythroleukemia, infectious mononucleosis, aplastic and Fanconi anemias, malaria, in response to myelotoxins, and in BM metastases; therapy of the underlying condition causes a regression of the anomaly

True Pelger-Huët anomaly is an AD condition with characteristic bilobed neutrophils; heterozygous subjects with this condition are asymptomatic, although homozygosity for the Pelger-Huët gene may be lethal

pseudoperoxidase see Occult blood

pseudopodagra An intensely painful great toe, due to trauma, degenerative arthritis, psoriatic arthritis, calcium pyrophosphate dihydrate disease ('pseudogout'), rheumatoid arthritis, Reiter syndrome or infection

True podagra corresponds to the classic gouty great toe

pseudopolyp An 'island' of preserved colonic mucosa, surrounded by an ulcerated 'sea' of hemorrhagic mucosa, which is a finding most characteristic of ulcerative colitis that may be seen in nonspecific inflammatory bowel disease, bacterial dysentery, amebiasis due to *Entamoeba histolytica* and schistosomiasis; see Polyps

True polyps in the colon arise from the mucosa, and represent neoplastic proliferations, most commonly designated as adenomatous polyps or villotubular adenomas, which have a tendency, with time to undergo malignant transformation

pseudoprecocity Isosexual pseudoprecocity occurs in female children and consists of signs of sexual maturation induced by functional ovarian tumors, eg juvenile type of granulosa cell tumor, due to increased estrogens and/or androgens CLINICAL Development of breasts, pubic and axillary hair, stimulation and development of the internal and external secondary sex organs, irregular uterine bleeding and a whitish vaginal discharge, acceleration of somatic and skeletal growth, and occasionally clitoromegaly; see Precocity

True precocity is accompanied by progesterone production and ovulation

pseudopregnancy EXPERIMENTAL BIOLOGY A state that may be induced in laboratory rodents by sterile 'coitus' or stimulation of the cervix with a glass rod, which causes a neuroendocrine response, release of prolactin and retention of the corpus luteum, resulting in a pregnancy-like state without carrying a fertilized product(s); see Pseudocyesis; Cf Sympathy pregnancy

pseudopseudolymphoma Paracortical lymphoid hyperplasia with proliferation of immunoblasts, associated with phenytoin therapy, see Phenytoin lymphadenopathy[*]; Cf Lymphoma, Pseudolymphoma

[*]Long-term phenytoin therapy has been associated with a slight increase in the incidence of lymphoma

pseudopseudohypoparathyroidism A rare X-linked [MIM 300800] condition with the skeletal manifestations of pseudohypoparathyroidism, in the face of normal calcium and phosphorous levels; both the 'pseudo-' and the 'pseudopseudo' forms may occur in the same kindred implying that in the latter, a mechanism of an end-organ (renal tubule) resistance to parathyroid hormone is present; Cf Pseudohypoparathyroidism

pseudopuberty The premature development of secondary sexual characteristics while remaining inconceivable, a phenomenon that is caused by ↑ androgen or estrogen secretion in the face of an immature hypothalamic-adenohypophysial-gonadal axis; pseudopuberty in male infants with Leydig cell tumors is associated with growth of pubic hair and penile enlargement \

True puberty requires spermatogenesis in ♂ and menstruation in ♀

pseudorabies Aujeszky's disease VETERINARY MEDICINE A rare acute CNS infection of swine and cattle of global distribution that is caused by an alphaherpesvirus, porcine herpesvirus 1 (herpesvirus suis), which is thought to be spread by direct contact, with some data suggesting airborne transmission of up to several km is distance has occurred CLINICAL Intense pruritus, irritability, bellowing, convulsions, paralysis, coma, and death, usually within days of onset PREVENTION A vaccine is available that reduces losses in infected herds, limits the spread, and decreases the incidence of disease

pseudo-Reed-Sternberg cells Histiocytoid cells mimicking the diagnostic cells of Hodgkin's disease are seen in a variety of benign and malignant lesions, of 1) Epithelial origin Thymoma, carcinoma of the breast and lung, 2) Mesenchymal origin Proliferative myositis, malignant fibrous histiocytoma, 3) Hematopoietic origin Infectious mononucleosis, CMV, rubeola, AIDS, multiple myeloma, megakaryocytic hyperplasia, mycosis fungoides, nodular lymphoma, mixed cell type, and poorly differentiated type lymphoma and 4) Malignant melanoma; see Reed-Sternberg cell

True Reed-Sternberg cells are the sine qua non requirement to establish the diagnosis of Hodgkin's disease; its precise origin has remained elusive

pseudorheumatoid nodule A deep dermal granuloma annulare involving the eyelid, eyebrow, episcleral and orbital tissues; Cf Rheumatoid nodule

True rheumatoid nodules are characterized by palisading histiocytes and a center of degenerated collagen, which is histologically identical to granuloma annulare, but differs therefrom in its periarticular distribution

pseudorosette A gliovascular structure seen by low-power light microscopy in ependymomas, in which blood vessels are surrounded by radiating, tapering processes of tumor cells oriented toward the vessel wall, best demonstrated by cell smears obtained fresh during surgery; pseudorosettes are more common in ependymomas than the 'classic' ependymal rosettes and may also be seen in Merkel cell tumors and Ewing sarcoma; see Flexner-Wintersteiner rosettes, Homer-Wright rosettes

True rosettes form structures in which there is a true central space surrounded by 'petals' in the form of a rim of radiating cells

pseudosarcoma A tumor mimicking a mesenchymal malignancy, the significance of which differs according to the site of origin ORAL CAVITY Pseudosarcoma is preferably known as spindle cell carcinoma, a variant of squamous cell carcinoma SOFT TISSUE Pseudosarcomatous fasciitis is preferably known as nodular fasciitis UROGENITAL TRACT Pseudosarcoma is a small, sessile and/or friable 'tumor' with marked cellularity and mitotic activity that bleeds easily and occurs at the site of recent surgery to the bladder, prostate or in the vagina, representing a florid inflammatory response to a locoregional insult; Cf Inflammatory pseudotumor

True sarcomas are malignant mesenchymal tumors of soft tissues and the musculoskeletal unit, which affect all ages and have a broad range in prognosis

pseudoscience A field described by Nobel Prize laureate Murray Gell-Mann as '*the dissociation of belief from evidence*'

pseudosequestration (lung) A rare acquired condition that mimics bronchopulmonary sequestration in which bronchial arteries undergo systemic arterialization due to inflammation-induced (eg organizing pneumonia) neovascularization; the arterialization may also occur in other vessels, eg intercostal, esophageal, and subdiaphragmatic arteries, and may reverse with resolution of the inflammation (N Engl J Med 1993; 329:1873CPC) Cf Bronchopulmonary sequestration

pseudosilence see Silent ischemia

pseudotabes An uncommon pattern of distal primary sensory neuropathy, in which there is a loss of pain sensation and tendon reflexes; pseudotabes is classically described in long-standing DM and characterized by shooting pains, most prominent at night, cutaneous hyperesthesia, impotence, neurogenic bladder, loss of superficial and deep sensation, painless ulceration of the feet, loss of tendon reflex, causing marked joint deformity, Romberg sign and occasionally Argyll-Robertson pupils

True tabes dorsalis occurs in tertiary syphilis, develops 10-20 years after primary infection and is clinically characterized by impaired vibratory and position sense in the feet and legs, absent knee and ankle reflexes, a Romberg sign, ataxia, urinary incontinence and 'lightning' pains

pseudothrombocytopenia A laboratory phenomenon caused by clumping of platelets in a blood collection tube containing an inappropriate anticoagulant

Note: Specimens for platelet counts should be collected in lavender-topped tubes containing calcium EDTA

pseudotuberculosis CLINICAL MEDICINE An unusual 'condition' described in one young ♀ whose braided hair fell into the field of an antero-posterior chest film, mimicking the radiologic appearance of TB (N Engl J Med 1985; 313:1227c) INFECTIOUS DISEASE Human* infection by *Yersinia* (formerly *Pastreurella*) *pseudotuberculosis* which causes acute mesenteric lymphadenitis, which mimics acute appendicitis, and is characterized by abdominal pain and fever RESEARCH An infection of experimental rodents (mice, rats) by *Corynebacterium pseudotuberculosis* and *C kutscheri*, which causes nonspecific signs of weakness and respiratory distress, possibly progressing to disseminated abscesses or less commonly, granulomas in the lungs, kidneys, myocardium, liver, lymph nodes, and elsewhere; the virulence of this condition is such that once an experimental colony of rodents is infected, it must be destroyed in its entirety

*Y pseudotuberculosis also infects a menagerie of other beasts, to wit, wabbits, wodents, boids, and others

pseudotumor A nonspecific term for any well-circumscribed, nonneoplastic tumor-like mass, including gastric inflammatory fibroid polyps, a bolus of helminths, eg *Strongyloides* species, as seen in Uganda, an 'amyloidoma', an endometrioma or other mass-like lesion

True tumors may be benign or malignant and are invested with a replicative capacity that may ('benign') or may not ('malignant') be under autoregulatory control

pseudotumor cerebri Benign intracranial hypertension A cerebral complex caused by increased intracranial pressure with normal CSF, diagnosed by 1) Presence of bilateral papilledema and objective evidence of increased intracranial pressure 2) Absence of focal neurological symptoms or signs 3) Absence of an extracranial cause of papilledema 4) Normal cerebrospinal fluid CLINICAL Most common in young obese women with dysmenorrhea of ovarian origin, causing visual defects (loss of acuity, diplopia and blind spots), headaches, nausea, vomiting, vertigo and tinnitus ETIOLOGY Anemia, leukemia, hyper- or hypovitaminosis A, lead intoxication, levothyroxine therapy, nalidixic acid, poliomyelitis, Guillain-Barre disease, menarche, pregnancy, galactokinase deficiency, chronic hypoxia, allergies, post-cerebral trauma, corticosteroid therapy for rapid reduction of cerebral edema or withdrawal of steroids, chronic hypocalcemia with hypoparathyroidism with primary adrenal insufficiency, thyroid replacement, endocrinopathies (Addison's or Cushing's diseases), contraceptive use, tetracycline (in infants), intracranial venous occlusion and inflammation

pseudotumor of lung Inflammatory pseudotumor of the lung A generic term for a solitary radiologic lung mass, composed of aggregates of foamy histiocytes, plasma cells, lymphocytes, fibroblasts and collagen that are most often evoked by resective surgery or less commonly, infections; Cf Lymphomatoid granulomatosis

pseudotumor of orbit Inflammatory pseudotumor of the orbit An idiopathic proliferation of the lymphoid tissue surrounding the ocular orbit, which may be autoimmune in nature and related to orbital myositis CLINICAL Pain, exophthalmos, limitation of eye movement, lid erythema, edema, myositis, perineuritis, scleritis, dacryoadenitis; the lesion may be histologically impossible to differentiate from a true lymphoma, and may require molecular studies to determine a lesion's clonality DDx Dacryoadenitis, orbital myositis, vasculitis, sclerosing pseudotumors, lipogranuloma, epithelioid cell granuloma, xanthogranuloma

pseudotumor of soft tissue A nonspecific term for reactive proliferations or repair phenomena that measure < 2 cm in greatest dimension, including hematomas, circumscribed fat necrosis, nodular fasciitis, foreign body granulomas, xanthogranulomas, proliferative myositis, myositis ossificans

pseudo-Turner syndrome Noonan syndrome An AD [MIM 613950] condition with a heterogeneous presentation that mimics some of the clinical findings of Turner syndrome; both are characterized by short stature, webbing of the neck, developmental delays, pectus carinatum or pectus excavatum, and cubitus valgus; Noonan syndrome affects both sexes, and is further characterized by mild mental retardation, congenital heart disease (pulmonary valve stenosis, atrial septal defect and others), a characteristic facies (hypertelorism, epicanthus, antimongoloid palpebral slant, ptosis, low-set ears, and micrognathia) and gonadal defects in ♂ including cryptorchidism, ↓ Leydig cell function, ↓ spermatogenesis

True Turner (45, X0) syndrome affects 1:3000 live ♀ births (95% of fetuses with this anomaly spontaneously abort, 25% of Turner syndromes have 45, X/46, XX mosaicism Clinical Lymphedema of the hands, feet and neck, webbing of the neck, congenital heart disease (Coarctation of the aorta and idiopathic hypertension), gastrointestinal telangiectasia, urogenital malformations and primary amenorrhea due to rudimentary ('streak') ovaries

pseudotype A quasi-distinct type of virus that may result if two viruses reproducing in the same cell exchange coat proteins–coat proteins determine what type of cell a virus can infect (Science 1990; 247:809)

pseudouridine A chemically altered nucleoside found in tRNA

pseudovitamin An organic substance that does not meet the accepted definition (see below) of a required human vitamin; representation of these substances as vitamins is widely regarded as being misleading, as the implication that they have natural curative effects is based on no

PSEUDOVITAMINS

METABOLITES, including

1) Intermediate metabolites, eg orotic acid ('vitamin B₁₃')

2) Substances whose metabolism requires B vitamins (eg choline, inositol, methionine) and

3) Substances which are B vitamins for nonvertebrate organisms (para-aminobenzoic acid, a B vitamin for certain bacteria ('vitamin Bₓ') and carnitine, a B vitamin for mealworms ('vitamin Bₜ')

PHARMACOLOGIC SUBSTANCES, which are allegedly capable of favoring certain metabolic processes in humans, but which produce little (if any) objective improvement, eg bioflavinoids ('vitamin P')

'SNAKE OIL REMEDIES', which meet the legal definition of fraud, which include pangamate ('vitamin B₁₅'), laetrile ('vitamin B₁₇') and gerovital ('vitamin H₃')

True vitamins are organic accessory food factors that usually remain in food after removal of the basic elements including carbohydrates, fats, proteins, minerals, water and fiber, and are 1) Necessary in trace amounts (daily intake in milligram to microgram quantities) and 2) Essential as the body either does not produce them or does so in insufficient quantities

known scientific principles; the US consumer spends an estimated $10⁹/year (US) on pseudovitamins

pseudovitamin D resistant rickets Vitamin D-dependent rickets, see there

pseudo-Whipple's disease A condition that mimics Whipple's disease, which may be seen in *Mycobacterium avium-intracellulare* infection in patients with AIDS, which also occurred in a case report of infection by *Corynebacterium equi*, agent of a suppurative pneumonia in young horses, isolated from the central nervous system of a young homosexual male with AIDS-related complex; Cf Whipple's disease

pseudo-von Willebrand disease Platelet-type von Willebrand disease (vWD) An AD [MIM 177820] condition that is similar to type IIB vWD, with moderately severe symptoms LABORATORY ↑ Bleeding time, ↓ von Willebrand factor (vWF) and factor VIII levels, ↑ ristocetin-induced platelet aggregation, absence of large vWF multimers and presence of those same multimers in platelets; the nature of the defect is unknown but may involve platelet glycoprotein IB TREATMENT Cryoprecipitate

pseudoxanthoma elasticum A rare and progressive condition affecting the connective tissue of the skin, cardiovascular system, joints and eyes CLINICAL An early change is the lax, yellow and redundant 'plucked chicken skin' that coalesces into plaques, becoming thickened, grooved, leathery and inelastic, likened to 'Moroccan leather', involving the head, neck, trunk and upper legs, eye (angioid streaks of the optic fundus, bilateral hemorrhage and exudates into Bruch's membrane, degenerative changes impairing vision, optic pigmentation and chorioretinitis), cardiovascular system (murmurs, hypertension, congestive heart failure, intermittent claudication, angina, vessels with poor peripheral pulses, vascular occlusion*), cerebral visceral and GI hemorrhage; four types of pseudoxanthoma elasticum are described, of which the AR type I is the most common, while the remainder differ according to the severity of skin, vascular and joint involvement

*PXE may be a more common cause of premature cardiovascular degeneration than previously appreciated (N Engl J Med 1993; 329:1237oa)

psittacosis Parrot fever, bird fancier's lung An infection of birds by *Chlamydia psittaci* may cause asymptomatic infection, an influenza-like disease or serious pneumonia in humans who are exposed to feathers, tissues or droppings from a wide variety of psittacine birds (parrots, parakets, and cockatoos), which may be sick or carriers of *C psittaci* CLINICAL Most cases are asymptomatic; symptomatic cases require a 1-2 week incubation, which is followed by chills, moderate to high fever, slow pulse, severe headache and myalgias, anorexia, nausea, vomiting, arthralgia and mental clouding; pneumonic symptoms are less common with production of minimal mucoid sputum mixed with hemorrhage, and if severe, accompanied by hypoxia and cyanosis TREATMENT Tetracyclines

psoas sign RADIOLOGY The loss of the sharp delineation of the psoas muscle border, which is normally seen on a plain erect abdominal film, a finding that may indicate the presence of intra-abdominal or retroperitoneal pathology, eg retroperitoneal hemorrhage in trauma victims or florid acute inflammation in a child with ruptured appendicitis

psoralens A class of furocoumarins that is used as a drug to treat psoriasis and other skin conditions and is used as a nucleic acid probe as it covalently crosslinks nucleic acids between opposing strands of DNA, where the planar psoralen intercalates into the double helix and UV light (320-400 nm) induces a single cyclobutane addition with a pyrimidine base; Cf Photo-reactivation

psoriasis A relatively common (± 3 million, US) chronic hyperproliferative and inflammatory skin disorder of unknown etiology characterized by erythematous papules that coalesce to form plaques with sharply demarcated borders; removal of a 'virgin' yellow-white lesion results in pinpoint hemorrhage (Auspitz' sign); trauma may evoke lesions in new body sites (Koebner's phenomenon); the lesions are more prominent in the scalp, knees, elbows, umbilicus, genitalia PATHOGENESIS Although traditionally regarded as idiopathic, the response of psoriasis to a lymphocyte-selective toxin (eg DAB₃₈₉IL-2) implies that psoriasis is immune-mediated, and that the epithelium is a secondary 'player' (Nature Medicine 1995; 1:442) EXACERBATION Injury (solar, mechanical), infection (beta-hemolytic streptococcus, HIV), drugs (ACE inhibitors, lithium, antimalarials, indomethacin) MOLECULAR PATHOLOGY Psoriasis is linked to certain HLA types, to wit B13, B16, Bw17, Bw37, Cw37; at least one familial form is linked to genetic defects in chromosomal segment 17q TREATMENT Symptomatic (emollients, keratolytics), topical agents (anthralin, corticosteroids, vitamin D analogues), phototherapy, ie UV light exposure (natural sunlight, artificial medium wavelength UVB light, photochemotherapy (methoxsalen + UVA light, PUVA therapy), oral agents (cyclosporine, etretinate, methotrexate) calcipotriene,(N Engl J Med 1995; 332:581RV) dietary supplementation with fish and corn oils is essentially ineffective, although the corn oil-induced ↑ in eicosapentanenoic acid and total n-3 fatty acids may coincide with clinical improvement (ibid 1993; 328:1812OA),

Psoriasis Area and Severity Index An objective scoring system used to determine the severity of psoriasis, based on erythema infiltration, desquamation and area of skin involved (Dermatologia 1978; 157:238 from N Engl J Med 1993; 328:1812OA)

PSS Progressive systemic sclerosis, see there

PSTAIR MOLECULAR BIOLOGY A sixteen-residue polypeptide contained within the maturation promoting factor, which is necessary and sufficient to initiate mitosis by causing a transient surge in intracellular calcium; see Mitotic spindle

PSTT Placental site trophoblastic tumor, see there

psychiatric evaluation A generic term for the assessment of a person's mental, social and psychological functionality; see DSM-IV, table multiaxial assessment, Psychiatric interview

psychiatric history A person's mental profile that includes information about the patient's chief complaint, the present illness, premorbid adjustment, individual and family history of psychiatric or mental disorders, and a developmental history (SC Scheiber, in JA Talbott, et al, Texbook of Psychiatry, American Psychiatric Press, Washington, DC, 1988)

psychiatric interview The central vehicle for assessing a psychiatric patient, during which there is a free exchange of information that forms the basis for therapy; the PI is used to understand how the individual relates with his environment, determine social, religious, and cultural influences on the person's life, conscious and unconscious motivations for behaviors, ego strengths and weaknesses, coping strategies, mental support systems and social networks, points of vulnerability, aptitudes, and achievements (SC Scheiber, in JA Talbott, et al, Texbook of Psychiatry, American Psychiatric Press, Washington, DC, 1988)

'psychic energizers' A colloquial term for antidepressant drugs that elevate mood, increase motivation, and improve the quality of life; see Psychoactive drugs

psychic surgery HEALTH FRAUD A practice associated with 'spirit healing' in rural areas of the Philippines, in which certain persons are alleged to act as mediums for healing forces, allowing them to perform painless surgery using their fingers and unsterile tools without violating the skin surface; psychic surgery is a form of prestidigitation, in which the tissues allegedly removed actually correspond to animal parts, eg chicken intestines or minerals, 'kidney stones' which are pebbles or volcanic rocks; see Unproven cancer therapy; Cf Psychosurgery

psychoactive drugs SUBSTANCE ABUSE Pharmacologic agents that provide pleasure or ameliorate pain, potentially causing physical dependence and tolerance, which is the tendency to increase the drug's dose in order to achieve the same effect; use of non-prescribed psychoactive agents may be 'social'/casual or consist of frank addiction, which in descending order of addictive potential include cocaine and 'crack', amphetamines, opiates, nicotine, alcohol, benzodiazepine, barbiturates, cannabis, hallucinogens and caffeine THERAPEUTICS A group of therapeutic agents that improve a person's ability to functiion in a psychologically appropriate fashion; psychoactive drugs used in a clinical context (eg psychiatric ward, nursing home) are divided into antidepressants (eg desipramine, nortryptyline), antipsychotics (eg haloperidol, thioridazine), benzodiazepines (eg lorazepam, diazepam), and other hypnotics (eg diphenhydramine) (N Engl J Med 1992; 327:163OA)

psychobabble A highly colloquial term for what some experts in human behavior might regard as nebulous, uncertain, or even meaningless phraseology, eg to 'be in touch with one's inner feelings', deep, 'letting go', 'losing touch with oneself', and perhaps the most meaningless adjective, 'meaningful'; Cf New Age

psychodrama see Group psychodrama

psychogenic syndromes Anxiety-related conversion reactions that are caused by various endogenous or exogenous stresses, including hysterical reactions, psychogenic chest pain, psychogenic polydipsia, psychogenic purpura, psychophonasthenia and the 'women who fall' syndrome, a conversion reaction to aggressive or erotic impulses; see Psychosomatic disorder; Cf Factitious disorders

psychological abuse Emotional abuse A form of mistreatment in which there is intention to cause mental or emotional pain or injury, which includes verbal aggression, statements with the intent to humiliate or infantilize, insults, threats of abandonment or institutionalization; PA results in substantial stress and is manifest by social withdrawal, long-term or recalcitrant depression, and anxiety (N Engl J Med 1995; 332:437ra)

psychological autopsy An autopsy that analyzes the cause(s) of death, examining both the body and the circumstances (natural or unnatural) that led to death; in the 'usual' death, a person suffers from a known set of morbid condition(s) and dies as a natural consequence of the terminal progression of those conditions(s); in 'unnatural' death, eg homicide or suicide, determination of nosology is more difficult and requires analysis of circumstances preceding death; the 'psychological autopsy' focuses on the deceased's intentions relating to his own death; data gathered by the investigation team include 1) Life history, eg previous suicide attempts 2) Psychological data, eg indices of depression or agitation, recent loss of appetite or interest in life 3) Communicated information, including indications of morbid thoughts, eg '...I can't go on', '...they'll be sorry...' 4) Nonpsychological details provided by the scene of death indicating attention to details that would ensure death, eg two bottles of the same medication used for overdose (Bull Suicidol July, 1968 pp 39-45) Cf Homicide, Suicide

Note: Psychological autopsies are of interest to both insurance companies and beneficiaries of the deceased, as life insurance policies are often written so that the estate of someone who commits suicide will not collect death benefits

psychological factors affecting medical condition see Psychosomatic disorder

psychological testing A group of tests used to determine a subject's intelligence quotient (IQ), 'normalcy' and future potential (table, page 724)

PSYCHOLOGICAL TESTING

PERCEPTUAL-MOTOR INTEGRITY Designed to rule out an organic (structural or physiologic, ie treatable) cause for the subject's behavior, including the Bender visual-motor Gestalt test, which can be administered from ages 5-adult, evaluating personality conflicts, ego structure and function and organic brain disease

IQ The most commonly used tests in the US have been devised by David Wechsler, including the Wechsler Preschool and Primary Scale of Intelligence (WPPSI, ages 4-6; 1949), Wechsler Intelligence Scale for Children-Revised (WISC-R, ages 5-15; 1974) and the Wechsler Adult Intelligence Scale (WAIS-R, ages 16 to adult; 1981); another commonly used IQ test is the Stanford-Binet that evaluates individuals from age 2 to adult

POTENTIAL ACHIEVEMENT The Vineland Social Maturity Scale evaluates the capacity to function independently, administered to those up to age 25

'PROJECTION' Tests that evaluate the sense of reality, eg the Rorschach ink-blot test, which requires considerable skill in administration, but yields the greatest insight into personality conflicts, ego structure and function, defensive structure and affective integration; other projective tests include the Thematic Apperception Test (TAT), Children's Apperception Test (CAT) and the 'Draw-a-person' and 'Draw-a-family' tests

psychoneuroimmunology The study of the effects of the psychological status on the immune function (N Engl J Med 1993; 329:1246RV); it is an evolving field that is a hybrid of several disciplines, which studies the complex bidirectional interactions between the CNS and the immune systems, where neuroendocrine system modulates immune function and CNS-immune system interactions appear to influence psychosocial dynamics; there are over thirty well-studied overlaps between the 2 systems in terms of shared cells and moderating substances (J Neurosci Res 1987; 18:1rv)

psycho-organic 'syndrome' A petroleum solvent-induced neurological dysfunction characterized by fatigue, memory loss, loss of concentration and emotional lability, occurring after 5-10 years of regular exposure to solvents, eg styrene, toluene, affecting painters, degreasers, plastics and chemical workers (N Engl J Med 1990; 322:675)

psychosis Psychotic disorder, see there

psychosocial dwarfism Kaspar Hauser syndrome, deprivation dwarfism A syndrome of largely irreversible hyposomatotropism that was first personified by Kaspar Hauser, an orphan who was physically and intellectually stunted by abuse and neglect, and found abandoned in 1828 at the Haller Gate in Nuremberg (N Engl J Med 1994; 331:1030BR) see Genie, *The Wild Child*

'psychosocial oncology' A field predominantly peopled by psychologists, which formally attempts to sway the course of advanced and/or metastatic malignancy by helping patients develop a positive' attitude; some 'soft' data suggest that the psyche may have an enhancing effect on the immune defenses; in one study of patients with metastatic breast cancer, those undergoing psychotherapy lived 19 months longer than controls and reported less anxiety and pain than the control group (Lancet 1989; 2:888)

Note: Because of the difficulty in performing formal studies, and the often anecdotal nature of the data, the field is regarded as 'fringe science' by traditional oncologists

psychosocial support Any nontherapeutic intervention that helps a person cope with stressants in his/her home or work environment; one study concluded that ↑ psychosocial support by nurses or social workers for ♀ at high risk (eg ↓ income level, ↓ education, short ≤1.5 m, underweight ≤ 50 kg, previous infant or fetal death) for delivering low-birth-weight infants neither improves maternal health nor ↓ incidence of low-birth-weight infants (N Engl J Med 1992; 327:1266OA)

psychosomatic disorder PSYCHIATRY A clinical complex* in which 1) The individual has a biological predisposition to a particular biomedical disorder, which may have a genetic, trauma-related, or other pathological predisposing component 2) The individual has a vulnerable personality, ie there must be a type or degree of stress with which the individual coping mechanism's and ego structure cannot manage and 3) The individual must experience a significant psychosocial stress in his susceptible personality area (TL Thompsson, II, in A Talbott, et al, Texbook of Psychiatry, American Psychiatric Press, Washington, DC, 1988) see Factitious disorders, Psychogenic 'syndromes'

*The term used for this constellation of disorders in the DSM-III-R was 'psychological factors affecting physical conditions'; in the DSM-IV, an equally verbose alternative, 'psychological factors affecting medical conditions' is preferred; it remains to be seen whether these terms championed by the Ameican Psychiatric Association will be integrated into the vox populi-Author's note

psychosomatic medicine ALTERNATIVE MEDICINE A whole-body or holistic approach to understanding the mind, body, and spirit, which are believed by some workers to intimately affect all disease process (Science & Medicine Nov/Dec 1994) PM differs significantly from mainstream or traditional medicine, and assumes an individual's mental state has a significant impact on the developemment of and response to diseases; see Alternative medicine, Psychoneuroimmunology

psychosurgery A generic term for neurosurgery intended to alleviate psychiatric symptoms, and was first performed in 1890 by G Burckhardt; psychosurgical procedures include topectomy (removal of pieces of cerebral cortex, weighing 20 g for pain to 50 g for fulminant schizophrenia), lobectomy, and leukotomy (popularized by W Freeman during World War II), which consisted of thrusting an icepick-like device through the eye socket and wiggling the handle to rupture myelinated tracts); one author felt that the greatest success was achieved for patients who were older, female, black, and those in simpler occupations; use of the Freeman procedure peaked in the late 1940s, and its decline coincided with the availability of the first generation of psychoactive drugs; tools used in modern psychosurgery to induce selective tract destruction include radioactive ^{90}Yt implants in the substantia innominata, as well as cryoprobes, coagulation, proton beams and ultrasonic waves; psychosurgery is not commonly performed, as it must be established that the patients are unresponsive to all other therapy and that the condition is chronic, ie > than 3 years duration; significant improvement is reported in 60% of carefully selected patients, while in 3%, the symptoms worsen after the procedure; the measurable intelligence quotient may actually increase as there is a better ability to concentrate and memorize, while distraction has been cut to a minimum Complications occur in about 1% and include infections, hemorrhage and seizures; Cf Psychic surgery

psychotic PSYCHIATRY An adjective that may be loosely defined as a behavior resulting in *'impairment that grossly interferes with the capacity to meet the ordinary demands of life.'*, which may be accompanied by the loss of ego boundaries and/or gross impairment of reality testing (Diagnostic and Statistical Manual of Mental Disorders, 4th ed, Washington, DC, Am Psych Ass, 1994)

psychotic disorder Psychosis A generic term for a broad class of mental disorders, which are classified in the DSM-IV under the umbrella term 'schizophrenia and other psychotic disorders', which includes schizophrenia, schizophreniform disorder, schizoaffective disorder, delusional disorder, brief psychotic disorder, shared psychotic disorder (eg folie à deux), psychotic disorder due to a general medical condition, substance-induced psychotic disorder, and psychotic disorder-not otherwise specified; the term psychosis may also refer to delusions, prominent hallucinations, disorganized speech, disorganized or catatonic behavior, severe disturbances of thought including incoherence, and repeated derailment of associations, see Psychotic

psyllium A grain of the plantago family with a high soluble fiber content that provides dietary bulk, acting as both a laxative and an agent to lower cholesterol; because psyllium contains a common aeroallergen, it may evoke an allergic reaction (anaphylaxis, rhinitis and asthma) in health care professionals who handle psyllium-based laxatives and later ingest them in food products

PT 1) Parathyroid 2) Paroxysmal tachycardia 3) Patient 4) Pertussis toxin 5) Phototherapy 6) Physical therapy 7) Pneumothorax 8) Proficiency testing 9) Propylthiouracil 10) Prothrombin time

Also 1) Pain threshold 2) Patellar tendon 3) Performance test 4) Phototoxicity 5) Physiotherapy 6) Pine tar 7) Placebo treated 8) *planum temporale* [NAG] 9) Plastic tube 10) Polythiophene 11) Popliteal tendon 12) Portal tract 13) Posterior tibial 14) Press test (psychology) 15) Pretectal 16) Prior treatment 17) Pulmonary tuberculosis 18) Pulp testing (dentistry) 19) Pyramidal tract

PTAH stain Phosphotungstic acid hematoxylin stain A stain used in histology to delineate various structures, including collagen (colored red), fibrin (blue), muscle (deep purple with well-defined cross-striations) and nuclei (blue); other structures including nerve, mitochondria, bone and elastin are well-visualized by the PTAH method

PTCA Percutaneous transluminal coronary angioplasty, see there

PTE Pulmonary thromboembolism

Also 1) Parathyroid extract (an obsolete therapeutic formulation) 2) Pectin transeliminase (pectate lyase)

PTE Pulmonary thromboembolism

PTGC Progressive transformation of germinal centers, see there

PTH Parathyroid hormone

Also 1) Parathormone (obsolete for parathyroid hormone) 2) Pathology 3) Peak tanning hours 4) Phenylthiohydantoin 5) Post-transfusion hepatitis

PTHrP Human parathyroid hormone-related peptide PTH-like hormone A 453-residue protein first identified in malignancy that is both present in mammalian milk and apparently required for lactation and for transplacental transportation of calcium; see Hypercalcemia of malignancy

PTP laser Potassium-titanyl-phosphate laser A device attached to a flexible endoscope in otorhinolaryngology, which can be adjusted to vaporize, coagulate, or cut; see Lasers

PTP1C Protein tyrosine phosphatase 1C An enzyme that is thought to regulate antibody production by activating B lymphocytes, requiring the presence of FcγRIIB1, the receptor for the constant portion of IgG molecule; PTP1C down-regulates B cell antigen receptor activity in conditions that do not engage FcγRIIB1 (**Science 1995; 268:293, 263**)

PTSD Post-trauma stress disorder, see there

public almshouse MEDICAL HISTORY An institution that evolved in England at the time of Henry VIII when the Catholicism was replaced by the Church of England; the poor and underpriviledged were cared for in the church-controlled abbeys under Catholicism; as the abbeys were dissolved, municipal and county governments became responsible for providing food, shelter, and medical care for the poor, homeless, and sick; the public almshouse was specifically created to care for the aged, alcoholic, chronically ill, feeble-minded, foundlings, insane, for those who had medical or surgical diseases, the poor, permanently disabled, and women before or after childbirth; the almshouse concept was transplanted to the America in the 1600s; the first such institute to evolve into a hospital became the Philadelphia General Hospital in 1731, which functioned as such until 1977, when it suffered the fate of many other inner-city public hospitals, a combination of reduced funding and increased non-paying patients (**Perspect Biol & Med 1993; 36:596**) see Public hospital

public antigen TRANSFUSION MEDICINE An antigen present on the red cell surface of more than 99.9% of a population, the presence of which is determined by an indirect antiglobulin test (Coombs); these 'high frequency' antigens include Js^a, Js^b, Lu^a, Ge, Ve, At^a, Cr^a, En^a, Gy^a, Hy, Jr, Jo^a, Ok^a, Ve, Cellano; common (but not public) antigens are Lewis, P, MNSs, Ii, Kk and Duffy

Note: Antibodies to public antigens are problematic in the blood bank as it is difficult to find a transfusable unit that is negative for these antigens

Public Health Service The bureaucracy responsible for administering all health-related services of the US government, including the Centers for Disease Control, Food and Drug Administration, National Institute of Mental Health and the National Institutes of Health (which includes the National Library of Medicine and the National Cancer Institute)

public hospital A hospital owned by a federal, state, or local government; these institutions evolved indirectly from the English public almshouses; public hospitals have had a significant role in caring for the sick in the US, but are regarded by some as anachronisms, in an increasingly complex and costly health care environment with ↑ operating costs, economic recession, and governmental budgetary restraints; the current problems in the public hospital are

DUMPING, the transfer of uninsured or underinsured patients, resulting in 'free' treatment for the patient and complete financial loss for the hospital

LACK OF CAPITAL (monies), for operations or for modernization of facilities

'INTERNAL' OBSTACLES, eg bureaucracy, political intrigue, application of 'standards of practice' in a suboptimal physical plant

PUBLIC ALMSHOUSE IMAGE, with aging facilities, lack of polish or amenities, evoking Dickensonian image (**Perspect Biol & Med 1993; 36:596**)

public idiotype determinant IMMUNOLOGY A recognition site or paratope present on an immunoglobulin that is shared by multiple other immunoglobulins despite their origin from different clones, also known as cross-reacting idiotypes

public specificity IMMUNOLOGY The property in a human leukocyte antigen (HLA) in which the epitope is identical on multiple HLA molecules; in contrast, a private antigen is a highly-specific epitope recognized by few members of the immunoglobulin superfamily; see also Splits

publication bias SCIENTIFIC JOURNALISM The tendency on the part of investigators to submit, and for some reviewers and editors to accept for publication, manuscripts based on the direction or strength of a study's findings, meaning that negative results (being rather less 'interesting') are less likely to be published (**JAMA 1990; 263:1385**); publication bias is divided into **PRE-PUBLICATION BIAS**, resulting from ignorance, laxity and lack of enterprise (on the part of those who would potentially perform the study) and a double standard created by peer review and informed consent **PUBLICATION BIAS**, as defined above and **POST-PUBLICATION BIAS**, resulting from editorials, reviews and meta-analyses

PUBS Percutaneous umbilical blood sampling, see there

puddle sign A clinical sign used to detect low quantities of ascitic fluid by having the patient on all fours (hands and knees) and bobbing the belly from below; the lower limits of detection of ascites is 1-1.5 liters in the supine patient, in whom a 'blubbery' fluid wave is detectable by striking a flank on one side and palpating the 'splash' on the other

pudendal block (anesthesia) OBSTETRIC ANESTHESIOLOGY Locoregional obstetric anesthesia that is used in the second stage to relieve episiotomy-related pain, by transvaginally injectiong local anesthetics into the pudendal nerve

PUFAs Polyunsaturated fatty acids, see Fatty acids

puff Chromosome puff, see there

puffer fish *Fugu Spheroides* (*Fugu*) *rubripes* Clinical toxicology A Japanese delicacy, some of the tissues (intestine, ovaries, skin) of which contain tetrodotoxin, the most powerful known poison, which blocks the neuromuscular junction, causing numbness, motor weakness, ataxia, and respiratory failure; a similar neuromuscular block can be evoked by the toxins from the blue ringed octopus; see Tetrodotoxin MOLECULAR BIOLOGY The pufferfish is of interest as a potential means of shortening the search for human genes, given that in contrast to the human's 3 billion basepair genome, the puffer fish has a 400 million basepair genome (the smallest genome of any vertebrate), the major difference between the two is that the latter has less so-called junk DNA (New York Times 16 Nov 1993; C1)

puffy tumor of Pott see Pott's puffy tumor

PUGH syndrome OPHTHALMOLOGY A clinical association characterized by the acronym of PUGH: PseudoUveitis, Glaucoma and Hyphema with neovascularization of iris and occlusion of the central retinal vein

pugilistic stance Pugilistic attitude FORENSIC MEDICINE A term for the 'defensive' or fetal position fancifully likened to that adopted by pugilists (boxers, see figure) that is present at post-mortem examination of severely burned bodies; the PS is characterized by flexion of elbows, knees, hip, and neck, and clenching of the hand into a fist; it is caused by the high-temperature of the fire, which causes stiffening and shortening of musculature, and occurs regardless of whether or not the person was alive at the time of the fire

Note: In a court of law, it is of interest to determine if a person died by being burned to death, which for many, is one of the 'ultimate horrors'; in a juried trial, a lawyer attempting to establish that the deceased party died in agony, may show the jury a photograph of the victim's charred body, doubled in a fetal crouch, inferring that the person died in pain; the jury may react by awarding the victim's estate multimillion-dollar settlement, against the party/parties held responsible for the fire; a person who was alive at the time of the fire and died during the fire almost invariably has soot and carbon on the mucosa of tracheobronchial tree

pulmonary alveolar proteinosis A rare disease most common in ages 30-50, ♂:♀ ratio 2.5-4:1; although idiopathic, more than 50% of cases have been exposed to dusts, chemicals, eg busulfan, infections, eg nocardiosis, CMV, *Pneumocystis carinii*, toxins, eg aluminum and antimony; PAP may be idiopathic, associated with immune compromise or thymic aplasia CLINICAL Dyspnea, cough, fever, chest pain RADIOLOGY Symmetric bilateral 'bat wing'-like alveolar infiltrates, less commonly, unilateral patchy infiltrates PATHOLOGY Uniform filling of alveoli by PAS-positive needle-shaped lipid-rich frothy material that may progress to intra-alveolar deposition of granular material (figure), with complete preservation of alveolar architecture EM Surfactant-like laminated material accumulates in necrotic alveolar macrophages PATHOGENESIS Excess phospholipid production by type II pneumocytes or defective pulmonary macrophage clearance of phospholipids TREATMENT Bronchoalveolar lavage (BAL) with saline or heparin and acetylcysteine for removal of phospholipids, is required in more than one-half of patients; without BAL, there is progressive dyspnea and deterioration of pulmonary functions, a higher mortality and the risk of superinfections, especially with *Nocardia*, which may be related to the enhanced growth of certain organisms secondary to the increased content of phospholipids

Note: Some authors prefer the term pulmonary alveolar phospholipoproteinosis

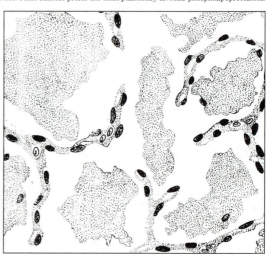

pulmonary alveolar proteinosis

pulmonary alveolitis Inflammation of the alveoli, which can be divided into

CRYPTOGENIC FIBROSING ALVEOLITIS, aka Idiopathic pulmonary fibrosis The most common presentation of interstitial lung disease, which is characterized by an insidious onset of cough and dyspnea over months to years that usually presents in the 6-7th decades RADIOLOGY Patchy subpleural reticular infiltrates, punctuated by cystic spaces TREATMENT Supportive, O_2, high-dose corticosteroids, tapering ASAP to minimum possible dose, immunosuppressives (eg cyclophosphamide, azathioprine); definitive therapy requires heart-lung or single-lung transplantation PROGNOSIS Poor, relentless fibrosis is the rule, average time from diagnosis to death is 4 years

EXTRINSIC ALLERGIC ALVEOLITIS, see Hypersensitivity pneumonitis

Note: Disease activity in both conditions can be monitored by serial measuring of plasma LDH levels, with ↑ of LDH during periods of exacerbation and ↓ during periods of improvement (Eur Respir J 1993; 6:1282)

pulmonary 'burns' Pulmonary parenchymal destruction caused by inhalation of irritating gases, including synthetic nitroso- compounds, eg burning mattresses, polyvinyl chloride containing hydrochloric acid and plastics, which generate toluene di-isothiocyanate: the combination of the toxins and intense heat affects the tracheobronchial tree causing pulmonary edema, congestion, parenchymal hemorrhage, epithelial desquamation and pulmonary necrosis

pulmonary-capillary wedge pressure A key indicator of cardiac function, and of intravascular and pulmonary venous volume; PCWP has been traditionally monitored in acutely ill patients using a balloon-tipped flow-directed catheter wedged in an arteriole of pulmonary circulation, to determine the pressure in the pulmonary capillaries and left atrium; the disadvantage of using a catheter is that is invasive and may cause serious complications; PCWP can be determined by a noninvasive procedure, the pulse-amplitude ratio (N Engl J Med 1992; 327:1715OA)

pulmonary dirofilariasis A benign self-limited disease caused by the lodging of microfilariae of *Dirofilaria immitis* in the peripheral pulmonary artery (see Acta Cytologica 1993; 37:531OA)

pulmonary embolism Pulmonary thromboembolism, see there

pulmonary eosinophilic granuloma An idiopathic localized nonmalignant histiocytosis characterized by pulmonary hemorrhage, pauci-immune crescentic glomerulonephritis, and antineutrophil cytoplamic antibodies ETIOLOGY Uncertain (Arch Pathol Lab Med 1994; 118:523OA)

pulmonary function test A group of maneuvers, eg spirometry, measurement of lung volumes, airway resistance, carbon monoxide diffusing capacity and arterial blood gases that provide objective and quantifiable data of pulmonary function; based on the information they provide, PFTs can be used for

DIAGNOSIS, eg determine the cause of clinical symptoms (cough, dyspnea, wheezing) in smokers or asthmatics

MONITORING, eg determine the value of therapeutic interventions, eg anti-asthmatic therapy

EVALUATION OF DISABILITY, eg vis-à-vis personal injury lawsuits, occupational exposure

PUBLIC HEALTH, for epidemiological surveys (N Engl J Med 1994; 331:25RA) see Pulmonary panel, Lung volumes

pulmonary hemorrhagic syndrome(s) A generic term for nonneoplastic and noninfectious pulmonary pathologies that present with hemoptysis, eg Goodpasture syndrome, idiopathic pulmonary hemosiderosis and hemorrhagic vasculitides including hypersensitivity angiitis and Wegener's granulomatosis

pulmonary hypertension Chronic hypertension of the pulmonary arteries, defined as a mean pulmonary arterial pressure of > than 20 mm Hg, or at altitudes over 5000 meters, above 25 mm Hg, corresponding to 'wedge' systolic/diastolic pressures of > than 30/20 mmHg (normal: 18-25/12-16 mmHg); pulmonary hypertension (PH) is often secondary to stasis of blood in the peripheral circulation and is divided into passive PH and secondary forms (table): the major effect of PH is the increased work required of the right ventricle which, when prolonged, predisposes the patient to right ventricular failure, syncope, precordial pain and sudden death; PH may be idiopathic or secondary to Eisenmenger's complex, the respiratory failure of cystic fibrosis and chronic obstructive lung disease, with inhibition of endothelium-dependent pulmonary arterial relaxation due to depressed synthesis of nitric oxide or endothelium-derived growth factor (N Engl J Med 1991; 324:1539); in contrast to arterial PH is venous PH, which is defined as a pulmonary venous or left atrial pressure above 12 mmHg which, when acutely elevated > 20-30 mmHg, results in pulmonary edema PATHOGENESIS Constriction of small pulmonary arteries and arterioles occurs with focal vascular injury, possibly due to ↑ in thromboxane A_2, a finding suggestive of platelet activation, coupled to ↓ in prostacyclin release (N Engl J Med 1992; 327:70OA); ↑ endothelin-1 may contribute to the vascular abnormalities seen in pulmonary hypertension (N Engl J Med 1993; 328:1732OA) PROGNOSIS Formerly thought to be universal-

ly fatal TREATMENT High-dose calcium channel blockers may induce ↓ pulmonary artery pressure and pulmonary vascular resistance, which may be combined with warfarin (N Engl J Med 1992; 327:76OA)

PULMONARY HYPERTENSION

PASSIVE PULMONARY HYPERTENSION, characterized by systemic congestion due to mitral stenosis, left ventricular failure, left atrial myxoma, anomalous drainage of the pulmonary circulation

HYPERKINETIC PULMONARY HYPERTENSION, where there is increased blood flow through the lungs due to congenital heart defects

VASO-OCCLUSIVE PULMONARY HYPERTENSION, due to recurring vessel obstruction, seen in intravenous drug abuse and pulmonary thromboembolism

Vasoconstrictive pulmonary hypertension, associated with hypoxia, alveolar hypoventilation (mitral stenosis, coarctation of aorta, Eisenmenger's complex, ventricular septal defect and e)

SECONDARY PULMONARY HYPERTENSION, which comprises 10-20% of cases, treated by addressing the underlying disease, including unilateral renal artery stenosis, coarctation of the aorta, primary aldosteronism and pheochromocytoma

pulmonary interstitial fibrosis see Jo-1 syndrome

pulmonary lymphangiomyomatosis A rare and potentially debilitating condition of reproductive-age ♀ characterized by overproduction of pulmonary smooth muscle cells and emphysema

pulmonary panel A battery of cost-effective tests used to evaluate the functional reserve capacity of the lungs in patients who have a clinical diagnosis obstructive or restrictive lung disease; the panel measures CO_2 content, $PaCO_2$, PaO_2, pH, O_2 saturation, a/A ratio; Cf Organ panels

pulmonary renal syndrome An idiopathic condition characterized by pulmonary hemorrhage, immune crescentic glomerulonephritis, and antineutrophil cytoplasmic antibodies (Arch Pathol Lab Med 1994; 118:517OA) the pulmonary-renal 'syndrome' has been also defined as a heterogeneous group of multisystem diseases, eg Goodpasture's and Wegener's diseases that have prominent pulmonary and renal components and microangiopathic vasculitis CLINICAL Asymptomatic pulmonary infiltrates or pulmonary hemorrhage with episodic cough, hemoptysis, dyspnea and widespread alveolar infiltrates on chest films; renal involvement is characterized by microscopic hematuria, red cell casts and increased creatinine PATHOLOGY Segmental necrotizing glomerulonephritis or glomerular crescent formation; rapid clinical deterioration occurs when more than 50% of the glomeruli have crescents

pulmonary sequestration An uncommon (1:1000 adult lobectomy specimens) congenital anomaly characterized by misplaced lung parenchyma, which lacks normal communication with the main tracheobronchial tree that may be intralobar or extralobar (table, page 728)

pulmonary surfactant Surfactant, see there

pulmonary thromboembolism Pulmonary embolism Occlusion of the pulmonary arteries by blood clot, the vast majority of which (± 95%) originate in the leg deep veins; PTE causes ± 4% of all US hospital deaths/year (50 000), and is largely preventable; it is underdiagnosed as the classic signs of dyspnea (seen in 59%), chest pain (17%), and hemoptysis (3%) are absent, or the patient may be unable to communicate as he/she is comatose or sedated (Mayo Clin Proc 1995; 70:417); PTE is found at autopsy in 1% of the general population with no known underlying disease, 10% of those who die acutely in general hospitals, and 30-65% of patients dying with severe burns, trauma, or fractures;

PULMONARY SEQUESTRATION

	INTRALOBAR	EXTRALOBAR
Separate pleura	No	Yes
Location	Posterior basilar	Above or below diaphragm
Age of onset	50% > 20 years	60% < one year
Symptoms	Recurrent pneumonia	Respiratory distress
Laterality	60%, left	90%, left
♂ : ♀ ratio	1:1	4:1
Other defects	Uncommon	> 50%, eg diaphragmatic defects, tuberous sclerosis
Bronchial communication	Uncommon, small	None
Arterial supply	Systemic; single aorta	Systemic; multiple, small
Venous drainage	Inferior pulmonary vein	Systemic; azygous and hemiazygous

when PTE is relatively acute in onset, the classic post-mortem finding is the so-called saddle embolus, which straddles the pulmonary arteries PREVENTION Early post-surgical and postpartum ambulation, or exercise if patient is bed-ridden, anticoagulation in selected cases, or inferior vena caval filters

pulmonary veno-occlusive disease An idiopathic condition of children and young adults that causes progressive fibrous obliteration of veins, resulting in severe, eventually fatal postcapillary pulmonary hypertension ETIOLOGY Uncertain, possibly linked to BM transplantation, chemotherapy, eg carmustine, malignancy, viral infection CLINICAL Nodular zones of congestion, edema, hemorrhage, and hemosiderosis RADIOLOGY Chest films reveal prominent interstitial markings, Kerley B lines, pulmonary artery dilatation PATHOLOGY Obstruction of pulmonary veins and venules by intimal fibrosis with arterialization, medial hypertrophy and hyperplasia TREATMENT Ineffective, temporary response has been reported with vasodilators, nifedipine, α-adrenergic blocker prazosin; ultimately survival hinges (N Engl J Med 1993; 329:1720cPC) PROGNOSIS Poor, most die in 2 years

pulposus Herniated disk 'syndrome', see there

pulsatile tinnitus ENT The perception of abnormal sounds in the ears or head, which occurs in a pulsatile fashion, which are most often caused by conductive hearing loss; PHL may also be caused by a vascular abnormality, eg a glomus tumor, carotid vaso-occlusive disease, AV malformation, or an aneurysm

pulse NUCLEAR MEDICINE 1) A brief exposure to a radioisotope, in order to label a substance and follow its path through a metabolic labyrinth 2) A discharge of electric current produced by radionuclides in an ionization chamber or scintillation counter

pulse, 90° (π/2 pulse) MRI A radiofrequency pulse that is designed to rotate the macroscopic magnetization vector 90° in space as referred to the rotating frame of reference, usually about an axis at right angles to the main magnetic field; if the spins are initially aligned with the magnetic field, the pulse produces transverse magnetization and a free induction delay; see Magnetic resonance imaging

pulse, 180° (π pulse) MRI A radiofrequency pulse that is designed to rotate the macroscopic magnetization vector 180° in space as referred to the rotating frame of reference, usually about an axis at right angles to the main magnetic field; if the spins are initially aligned with the magnetic field, the pi pulse produces inversion; see Magnetic resonance imaging

pulse-chase experiment A technique in cell biology to study a physiologic or metabolic process, in which the incorporation of a radioactive substance and its subsequent metabolism is followed as it moves through various cell compartments and disappears from the system; a 'pulse' of a radiolabeled molecule, eg an amino acid, a nucleoside or a phosphate ion is added to the cell and allowed to incorporate into a molecule of interest, followed several minutes later by flooding the extracellular milieu with 'chase' of unlabelled molecules while measuring the radioactive changes

pulsed field gel electrophoresis MOLECULAR BIOLOGY A technique that is used to separate segments of DNA from several hundred to several thousand kilobase pairs in length, allowing the construction of a full-scale molecular map of *Escherichia coli*, yeasts and the human major histocompatibility complex; pulsed-field electrophoresis fills a resolution gap that had previously existed between molecular cloning experiments that allowed analysis of a relatively small number of DNA base pairs and meiotic linkage allowing analysis of megabase segments of DNA

pulse length Width MRI The duration (delta time) of a pulse; for a radiofrequency pulse near the Larmor frequency, the longer the pulse length, the greater is the angle of rotation of the macroscopic magnetization vector (> 180° brings the pulse length back to its original orientation) see Magnetic resonance imaging

pulse oximetry CRITICAL CARE A method used to determine arterial oxygen saturation (SaO_2) in a continuous fashion, through the noninvasive assessment of arterial hemoglobin-bound oxygen saturation, which is based on the combined techniques of optical plethysmography and spectrophotometry; a pulse oximeter senses the difference in the absorption spectra between oxyhemoglobin and deoxyhemoglobin, detecting differences in the peaks and troughs in the transmission of light caused by the pulatility of tissue (most commonly detected by a probe in the earlobe); these differences are used to calculate SaO_2; PO is reported to be accurate within 5% of a standard co-oximeter when the SaO_2 is in the 70-100% range, but accuracy plummets below 70%; PO is used to detect oxygen desaturation accurately[1], inexpensively[2], quickly[3], and safely[4], and has proven useful in endoscopy, the recovery room, in intensive care units, and may be of use in evaluating the obstructive sleep apnea syndrome, for which the accepted gold standard is nocturnal polysomnography, a costly and onerous procedure (Mayo Clin Proc 1995; 70:591)

[1]Think 'outcomes' [2]Think cost-effectiveness [3]Think DRGs [4]Think lawsuit

pulse sequences MRI A set of RF (and/or gradient) magnetic field pulses and time intervals between these pulses; used in conjunction with gradient magnetic fields and MR signal reception to produce MR images; see Magnetic resonance imaging; Cf Interpulse time

pulse-temperature dissociation BACKGROUND: The pulse rate increases 15 to 20 beats per minute for each degree increase in a fever above 39°C; a lower than normal increase in pulse rate or relative bradycardia is not uncommon and occurs in burns, drug fever, hepatitis, intoxication (eg trinitrotoluene, TNT), legionnaires' disease, malaria (blackwater fever), myocardial infarction, psittacosis, typhoid fever, yellow fever; relative tachycardia is far less common, but is typical of clinically silent pulmonary embolism, diphtheria and clostridial infections

pulseless disease Takayasu arteritis, see there

pulsus alternans CARDIOLOGY A pulse pattern in which the heart beats occur at regular intervals but in which there is rhythmic attenuation of the pulse pressure heights; sustained pulsus alternans may result from severely depressed left ventricular function, accompanied by an altered blood flow in the aorta, left ventricular and systolic pressures and often a third ventricular sound

pulsus paradoxus CARDIOLOGY A marked ↓ in the pulse amplitude during normal quiet inspiration or a ↓ in the systolic pressure by greater than 10 mm Hg, a characteristic finding in cardiac tamponade, but less common in constrictive pericarditis, quantifiable by a sphygmomanometer; PP also occurs in superior vena cava obstruction, asthma, pulmonary embolism, shock, or following thoracotomy

PUMP Putative or punctate metalloproteinase (Bio/Technology 1995; 13:554)

pump lung Postperfusion lung, see there

punch-drunk syndrome Dementia pugilistica, Boxer's encephalopathy NEUROLOGY A complex that was reported to affect up to one-half of all professional boxers in the pre-safety era (JAMA 1928; 91:1103); this condition is currently thought to affect 10-20% of professional boxers, and is regarded as being the cumulative effect of recurrent brain damage and progressive communicating hydrocephalus; the dysfunction is due to extrapyramidal and cerebellar lesions, that translate into dysarthria, ataxia and tremors, as well as pyramidal lesions, which cause mental deterioration and personality changes including rage reaction and morbid jealousy ('Othello syndrome'); early disease is characterized by unsteadiness of gait (with leg dragging), confusion, hand tremors, slowing of movement, head nodding, and eventually, parkinsonism; boxers' brains may demonstrate cortical atrophy that roughly correlates with the severity of dementia, accompanied by enlarged ventricles (normopressure hydrocephaly), a cavum septum pellucidum, loss of Purkinje cells, neuronal degeneration, gliosis of the substantia nigra, neurofibrillary tangles (especially of the medial temporal cortex, the amygdaloid nucleus and the hippocampal gyrus) see Boxing; Cf Alzheimer's disease, Parkinson's disease, Torture, Vascular dementia

Note: Other sports including steeplechasing, soccer, rugby, wrestling are not immune from post-traumatic, or blow-related dementia (JAMA 1984; 251:2676, ibid. 1986; 255:2475) see Boxing

punched-out An adjectival descriptor for rounded, well-circumscribed often multiple lesions that may be seen in various organ sites Note: When 'punched-out' lesions have scalloped borders, some authors prefer the adjective, 'cookie cutter' GASTROENTEROLOGY Punched-out lesions seen in the stomach by endoscopy usually correspond to benign gastric ulcers, which are well-demarcated with a sharply-defined wall and have a smooth base; Cf Heaped-up OPHTHALMOLOGY Single or multiple defects in coloboma of the optic fundus, due to malclosure of the embryonic fissure, leaving a multilayered defect in the retina, retinal pigment epithelium and choroid, exposing the underlying sclera RADIOLOGY Rounded, sharply demarcated, cyst-like spaces without sclerotic margins, characteristic of multiple myeloma of the diploe of the skull, causing sharply demarcated 'holes', resulting from osteoclast-activating factor secretion in the plasma cells; punched-out bony defects also occur in well-circumscribed mutilating sarcoidosis of the small hand bones, chronic gouty arthritis as chondro-osseous lesions that communicate with the urate 'crust' through defects in the cartilage, childhood hypophosphatasia, leukemic foci in the skull and tuberculosis

punctuation 'Punctuation marks' MOLECULAR BIOLOGY Those sequences of nucleic acids that are not themselves part of the structural portion of mature mRNA transcripts, but which provide instructions for the initiation and termination of transcription, likened to the heiroglyphic code of many languages that provide the lector with the 'hinting' for proper understanding of the written word; Cf Editing

punishment shooting A generic term for any shooting (eg 'kneecapping') of a person by a member of one's own group (gang, political cell, terrorist group) for transgressions or alleged transgressions against the group's philosphies (Am Med News 7 Nov 1994 p14) see Kneecapping

punitive damages MEDICAL MALPRACTICE An 'insult-to-injury' award given by jury in order to castigate the defendant who committed a wrong that was determined in a court of law to have been malicious, oppressive, or reckless in nature; punitive damages are designed to prevent an alleged wrong-doer (tort-feasor) from repeating the offense; punitive damage awards are either 1) Special (wages, lost profits, past and future medical fees) and other compensatory awards, the monetary value of which can be reasonably calculated and 2) General (pain and suffering, humiliation, disfigurement) awards that elude applications of standardized formulae (which can thus be very costly); see Damages, Malpractice; Cf Compensatory damages

puppet children A congenital condition due to a reciprocal deletion of imprinted maternal loci at chromosome 15q11-13, resulting in repetitive ataxic seizures, fancifully likened to the jerking movements of marionettes; see Angelman syndrome

PUPPP Pruritic urticarial plaques and papules of pregnancy An erythematous papule and plaque-forming eruption seen late in the third trimester in up to 75% of primigravidas, which does not recur in subsequent pregnancies PATHOLOGY Edema, chronic perivascular inflammation TREATMENT Topical steroids; see Pruritus gravidarum

pure red cell aplasia A type of anemia caused by selective depletion of erythroid cells **ACUTE PRCA** Aplastic crisis A condition often preceded by viral gastroenteritis, pneumonitis, primary atypical pneumonia, mumps, viral hepatitis, pregnancy and drug toxicity CLINICAL General malaise, pallor and other symptoms of a chronic, compensated hemolyzing process TREATMENT The only consistently effective modality is discontinuance of an inculpated drug, if one can be identified **CHRONIC PCRA** may be either 1) CONGENITAL Diamond-Blackfan disease A condition due to a ↓ in erythrocyte stem cells with ↓ colony-forming units and burst-forming units and a poor response to erythropoietin TREATMENT Transfusions, corticosteroids or 2) ACQUIRED 30-50% of chronic acquired PRCA is associated with thymoma, other associations include rheumatoid arthritis, lupus erythematosus, chronic active hepatitis, hemolytic anemia and chronic lymphocytic leukemia

pure white cell aplasia HEMATOLOGY Severe neutropenia, which is analogous to pure red cell aplasia which is either 1) Associated with thymoma and hypogammaglobulinemia, and responds to plasmapheresis or 2) Associated with other immune diseases, eg Goodpasture's disease and responds to antithymocyte globulin or high-dose intravenous immunoglobulin

purge COMPUTERS To remove or delete old or unwanted files or information from a computer system LABORATORY MEDICINE To flush a gas out of a system or replace one atmosphere with another, as in gas-liquid chromatography

purine BIOCHEMISTRY One of 'building block' molecules (adenine and guanine) for ribonucleic acids, which is attached (or 'base pairs') to pyrimidine bases, each of which is separated from its nearest neighbor by a phosphate-sugar backbone, linked to each other with phosphodiester bonds, either with a single strand of ribose, forming ribonucleic acid (RNA), or with a double strand of deoxyribose, forming deoxyribonucleic acid (DNA); under normal conditions, adenine will only form a dimer with thymine (for DNA) or uracil (for hybrid RNA-DNA molecules) and not with a purine; see DNA forms; Cf

adenine   guanine

purines

purine analogue CLINICAL PHARMACOLOGY Any of a family of agents that mimic the chemical structure of purine and therefore act in pathological conditions in which there is increased production of DNA, acting through competitive inhibition with guanine and adenine; purine analogs have a broad range of therapeutic applications, and include aza-thioprine, a potent immunosuppressant, 6-mercaptopurine, a chemotherapeutic used to treat childhood acute lymphocytic leukemia and 6-thioguanine, used to treat the far less common childhood acute myeloid leukemia; other purine analogs include acyclovir and the xanthine oxidase inhibitor, allopurinol; see 6-MP

purine nucleoside phosphorylase deficiency An autosomal co-dominant condition caused by defective purine metabolism and accumulation of deoxyGTP, with resultant immune dysfunction by inhibition of ribonucleotide reductase, and blockage of cell division, causing a predominantly T-cell immune dysfunction CLINICAL Recurring opportunistic infections of the lungs, skin and genitourinary tract, autoimmune hemolytic anemia, BM hypoplasia LABORATORY ↓ T cells, ↑ urine and serum uric acid, ↑ inosine and guanosine; Cf Adenosine deaminase deficiency

purple glove syndrome A clinical complex resulting from IV injection of phenytoin, in which there is discoloration, edema and blister formation of the hand (or acral part distal to an intravenous injection site); the edema evoked may cause ischemic necrosis, necessitating amputation

Note: Phenytoin is alkaline, requires propylene glycol as a stabilizer and tends to crystalize

purple people 'syndrome' A condition affecting psychiatric patients receiving long-term, high dose chlorpromazine therapy, causing purple-gray discoloration of sun-exposed parts (later progressing to a permanent blue-black color), corneal and lenticular opacifications, due to accumulation of a photoactive metabolite of chlorpromazine, an aliphatic phenothiazine once widely used to treat schizophrenia, bipolar disease and psychoses SIDE EFFECTS Pseudodepression, extrapyramidal reaction, eg tardive dyskinesia, autonomic nervous system effects, eg urinary retention, weight gain, amenorrhea-galactorrhea and infertility, agranulocytosis and hypercholesterolemia

purple top tube Lavender top tube, see there

'purple urine bag syndrome' A rare 'condition' in which the urine in a bag from a catheterized patient turns an intense purple hours to days after catheterization, an event most common in elderly women, due to infection of the urine by *Providentia stuartii* which has indoxyl sulfatase-like activity, converting urinary indoxyl sulfate into indigo

'pushing glass' 'Glass pusher', see there

push-pull theory DEMOGRAPHICS A hypothesis that attempts to explain population migrations as a result of the migrating individual responding to negative or 'push' factors at the place of origin, and positive or 'pull' factors at the place of destination (JM Last, RB Wallace, Eds, Public Health and Preventive Medicine, 13th ed, Appleton & Lange, Norwalk, 1992)

putrefaction FORENSIC PATHOLOGY Whole body decomposition, accompanied by autolysis of tissues and gas production, which is the postmortem result of combined bacterial overgrowth and enzymatic digestion, occurring within one week in air, two weeks in water, eight weeks buried in soil or not at all, when buried in the marshes; see Adipocere, Bog bodies, 'Floaters'

PUVA therapy 8-methoxy-psoralen with UVA (320-400 nm) light therapy DERMATOLOGY A therapeutic modality used for treating severe psoriasis; PUVA therapy causes Irregular hyperpigmented macular lesions with increased melanocytes and histological epithelial atypia; those receiving > 260 therapeutic sessions have an 11-fold greater risk of squamous cell carcinoma than those receiving < 160 sessions of PUVA; in one study, invasive squamous cell carcinoma in patients with psoriasis exposed to high levels of PUVA was reported to be over 200 times more common (predominantly of the male genitalia) that the unexposed population; those with low-level PUVA exposure had a greater than ten-fold increase in cancer risk SIDE EFFECTS-SHORT TERM Nausea, burning, pruritus LONG-TERM Wrinkling, irregular hyperpigmentation, lentigines, benign and premalignant keratoses, and skin cancer (N Engl J Med 1995; 332:581RV) see Psoriasis

PV Polycythemia vera, see there

PVC 1) ENVIRONMENT Polyvinyl chloride, see there 2) CARDIOLOGY Premature ventricular contraction, see there

PVS Persistent vegetative state, see there

PWM Pokeweed mitogen, see there

pX protein A 16.5-kD protein encoded by hepatitis B virus (HBV) that indirectly transactivates viral and cellular genes by forming a protein-protein complex with cellular transcriptional factors CREB and ATF-2, subverting their native DNA binding specificities, such that pX-CREB and pX-ATF-2 bind to the HBV enhancer element, thus possibly explaining HBV's role in acute and chronic liver disease as well as hepatocellular carcinoma (Science 1991; 252:842) see Hepatitis

Pygmalion complex PSYCHIATRY The making over of one individual to suit the needs or desires of another; alternatively, high expectations for normal behavior and/or activities in patients with various impairments, eg physically or mentally impaired children, or severely demented elderly subjects

The term derives from GB Shaw's Pygmalion, in which a Cockney flower girl is converted into an elegant woman by a professor of linguistics

pygmies A tribe of Black Africans who are short in stature, partly due to a 50% reduction of high-affinity growth hormone binding protein, the amino acid sequence of which is homologous to the cell membrane's growth hormone receptor, resulting in a primary deficiency of insulin-like growth factor (IGF-I) or somatomedin C

pyloric olive PEDIATRICS An abdominal mass palpated in early infancy that corresponds to a 'knot' of hypertrophied peripyloric smooth muscle and mucosal edema seen in pyloric stenosis, which is most common in first-born male infants, 7 weeks of age CLINICAL Non-bilious projectile vomiting, dehydration ('old man' appearance) LABORATORY Metabolic alkalosis, hypokalemia and hypochloremia TREATMENT Rehydrate, lay open seromuscular layer (Fredet-Ramstedt pyloromyotomy); see Pyloric string sign

pyloric string sign PEDIATRIC RADIOLOGY Elongation and narrowing of the pyloric passage as seen in an upper GI radiocontrast series in a child with hypertrophic pyloric stenosis; Cf Pyloric olive, Tit sign

pylorospasm see Hypertrophic pyloric stenosis

pyrimidine BIOCHEMISTRY One of 'building blocks' for ribonucleic acids, which is attached in chains of other pyrimidine or purine bases, each of which is separated from its nearest neighbor by a phosphate-sugar backbone, either with a single strand of ribose, forming ribonucleic acid (RNA, which integrates uracil and cytosine pyrimidine bases), or with a double strand of deoxyribose, forming deoxyribonucleic acid (DNA, which integrates thymidine and cytosine bases); under normal circumstances, pyrimidines only pair with purines, and not with pyrimidines, ie cytosine only pairs with guanine and thymidine with adenine (DNA) and uracil only pairs with adenine (RNA); see DNA forms; Cf Purines

cytosine　　**thymosine**　　**uracil**

pyrimidines

'pyramid' system GRADUATE MEDICAL EDUCATION A system used in highly competitive and prestigious US teaching hospitals, which limits the number of resident physicians who graduate from highly selective residency programs of post-graduate education, eg neurosurgery, by having a larger number of positions available for the first years of training than in the final years; while this places considerable stress on the resident, it is felt to ensure that only the best possible candidates graduate from the most prestigious programs; see Residency; Cf 'Match'

Pyrococcus furiosus A hyperthermophilic archaeon (archaebacterium) that grows optimally at 100°C, a finding with considerable implications for biology and biotechnology*; one of the key enzymes of *P furiosus* is of the tungsten-containing aldehyde ferredoxin oxidoreductase (AOR); AOR's crystal structure was resolved, revealing a small solvent-exposed surface area and a large amount of ion pairs and buried atoms, which may explain AOR's extreme thermostability (Science 1995; 267:1463OA)

*High-temperature enzymes are critical for PCR (polymerase chain reaction), which is widely regarded as one of the most important reactions in diagnostic and biotech industries, as it rapidly amplifies unidentified target DNA

pyroglobulin A type of myeloma protein that irreversibly precipitates at 56°C, unlike the Bence-Jones protein(s) typical of myeloma that re-dissolve as the temperature is increased above 56°C

pyrophoric material Any chemical substance or mixture that will ignite spontaneously at ≤ 54.4°C (130°F); see Combustible material

pyrroloquinolone quinone PQQ, see there

PZI Protamine zinc insulin

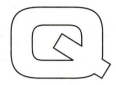

Q Symbol for: 1) Glutamine 2) Metabolic quotient 3) Blood perfusion rate 4) Quantity of electric charge 5) Ubiquinone

q Symbol for: 1) Electric charge 2) Long arm of a chromosome 3) *quaque*, Latin, each, every

QA 1) Quality assessment, see there 2) Quality assurance, see there
Also 1) Quarternary ammonium 2) Quinic acid

QALE Quality-adjusted life expectancy PUBLIC HEALTH A period of time used in models for clinical decision-making, in which each stage of a health-state is correlated with life expectancy, eg in carotid artery disease, a patient may be 1) In his usual state of health 2) Alive with disability or 3) Dead; each stage correlates the risk of instituting a therapeutic modality with the statistical potential for improved quality of life (see JAMA 1992; 268:2678OA) Cf Karnovsky scale

QALY Quality-adjusted life-year An objective parameter that has been advanced as means of ranking the benefits and liabilities of various medical interventions, which allows comparison among seemingly disparate forms of intervention, eg acute care (eg treatment of appendicitis), preventive care (eg cholesterol screening), and long-term care (eg insulin maintenance for DM) (N Engl J Med 1993; 328:1358BR) see QALE

Q band GENETICS A fluorescent band that appears at constant sites when chromosomes are stained with quinacrine, a fluorescent dye that inserts or intercalates into the DNA helix; because the bands fade with time, other chromosome stains are usually preferred; see Banding; Karyotyping (aka chromosome analysis)

QC Quality control, see there, also Quinine-colchicine

Q cycle A 'short loop' of electron transport which occurs on the inner mitochondrial membrane, in which ubiquinone cycles between fully oxidized quinone, fully reduced quinone and the semiquinone intermediate that carries a single electron

Q fever An acute zoonotic rickettsial disease due to the globally distributed *Coxiella burnetii* RESERVOIRS Cattle, sheep, goats and sundry small marsupials VECTOR Ticks, other arthropods Note: *C burnetii* is highly infectious-in theory, a single organism may aggressively multiply and thus be sufficient to cause a clinical infection EPIDEMIOLOGY Pattern 1 Sylvatic Tick 'shuttle' between kangaroos and other marsupials Pattern 2 Human affected by aerosols from asymptomatic cattle, sheep, goats CLINICAL Abrupt onset of high fever, headaches, myalgia, malaise, hepatic dysfunction, patchy interstitial pneumonitis, fibrinous exudate, which may resolve without treatment; Q fever may cause an atypical pneumonia, rapidly progressive pneumonia or be an incidental finding in the background of a systemic febrile illness; the convalescent period may be prolonged but has a low mortality TREATMENT Tetracycline, chloramphenicol

Note: The term 'Q fever' was coined by Derrick, a public health officer in Queensland, Australia, who in 1935 investigated a small outbreak of febrile illness, which he called Q or 'Query' fever

Q-probe Any of a number of studies that help laboratorians identify and evaluate the key factors that influence quality in the laboratory, which are sponsored by the College of American Pathologists to help laboratorians identify and evaluate the key factors influencing the quality in their laboratories (CAP Today September 1994)

Q10 effect PHYSIOLOGY The effect that environmental temperature has on corporal metabolism, such that as the body temperature ↑, there is an ↑ in the rate constant for chemical reactions; for every 10°C ↑ in body temperature, there is a 2–3-fold ↑ in the reaction rate, accounting for a 10-13% ↑ in heat production for each degree Celsius ↑ in body temperature (DW Wilmore, The Metabolic Management of the Critically Ill, Plenum Press, New York 1977) see Pulse-temperature dissociation

Q value NUCLEAR PHYSICS The total energy per atom released in a nuclear reaction, when the radionuclide is reduced to a ground state

Q wave infarction A myocardial infarction affecting the full thickness of the heart, ie transmural; most Q wave infarcts result from thrombotic occlusion of the proximal coronary arteries, often associated with hemorrhage into an ulcerated fibrous plaque; 'non-Q wave infarcts' are due to microthrombosis by platelet 'plugs', associated with low flow and multivessel coronary artery stenoses; EKG findings include prominent and prolonged (greater than 0.04 sec) Q waves, a 30% decrease in the R wave amplitude, prominent peaked T waves (indicating epicardial damage) and a hyperacute ST elevation; Cf Non-Q wave infarction

qi-gong ALTERNATIVE MEDICINE An ancient Chinese exercise that acts to combines movement, meditation, and breath regulation to enhance the flow of qi (the vital life energy) along the acupuncture meridians, which is reported by its advocates to improve circulation and enhance immune function (Alternative Medicine, Future Medicine Publishing, Puyallup, Wash, 1994)

qi-gong reaction PSYCHIATRY An acute self-limited episode of dissociative, paranoid, psychotic, or other symptoms that follows participation in qi-gong ('exercise of vital energy'), a Chinese folk health-enhancing practice (DSM-IV™, 1994) see Culture-bound syndrome

QNS Quantity not sufficient An abbreviation commonly used in the laboratory to indicate that the material (eg blood, urine) submitted for analysis is insufficient for performance of the tests of interest

QNS has 'graduated' from adjectival to nominative status, as indicated by the phrase, '...the specimen is a QNS...', and has on occasion been used as a verb, eg, '...to QNS a specimen.'–Author's note

QRS score A measure of the size of a myocardial infarction based on the evaluation of a 12-lead EKG (N Engl J Med 1993; 329:1442OA)

Q-switched laser pulse DERMATOLOGY A burst of energy obtained from the deep-red wavelength of the ruby laser, where energy is allowed to build up in the laser before discharge, resulting in 'zaps' of high-powered energy that penetrate several millimeters into the dermis and selectively damage melanin, and which have been found to be useful in removing tattoos, especially those with black-blue pigment (colored tattoos respond less well); 72% of amateur tattoos respond with lightening or disappearance, 23% of professional tattoos are effectively treated

Q-switched ruby laser A device used to deliver short (30 nsec) high-energy 6.0 (J/cm²) bursts of deep-red wavelength (694.3 mm) light to effect lective photolysis; the QSRL is the method of first choice in treating the cosmetically disfiguring nevi of Ota, which is due to benign dendritic melanocytosis of papillary and upper dermis (N Engl J Med 1994; 331:1745oa)

QTL analysis Quantitative trait locus analysis, see there

Q-TWiST Quality-of-life-adjusted survival relative to TWiST (time without symptoms of disease or toxicity); a period of time calculated as the number of months preceding the development of a symptom with ≥ grade 3 HIV disease whichever occurred first (N Engl J Med 1994; 330:7380a)

Quaalude Methaqualone, see there

quack Charlatan A person who impersonates a physician; see Quackery, Unproven forms of cancer therapy; Cf Alternative medicine

The term that arrived to English in the 1500s from 'Quacksalver', for one who hawks or 'quacks' about his miraculous cures or 'salves'; the term had currency in the USA during that country's western expansion in the late 1900s, when very little or no training was required to open one's own 'surgery'

'quack buster' A generic term for any person who investigates the claims of efficacy of alternative medicine

quackery False representation of a substance, device or therapeutic system as being beneficial in 1) Treating a medical condition, eg 'Snake oil' remedies 2) Establishing the diagnosis of a disease state, or 3) Maintaining a state of good health; see AIDS fraud, Pseudovitamins, Snake oil remedy, Unproven cancer therapy; Cf Alternative medicine

Note: Unofficial guidelines promulgated by the FDA indicate that it is advisable to avoid: 1) Therapies claiming to cure diseases known to be incurable, or that cure multiple diseases simutaneously 2) Promotions blazoned with superlatives, eg 'foolproof', 'miraculous', 'secret', or which have testimonials only and no scientific evidence, or are administered by practitioners lacking credentials, or with questionable training 3) Experimental treatments that one must pay for, especially if they are extremely costly, administered without a physician's knowledge, or require an interruption of standard therapy (Am Med News 21 Nov 1994 p13)

quad pack Quadruple pack TRANSFUSION MEDICINE A plastic blood collection bag that has three attached 'peripheral' bags allowing the sterile collection and separation of a unit of whole blood (usual volume, 500 ml) into four 125 ml aliquots, which because they are sterile, have a normal shelf life; the host bag may be used to collect plasma (± 220 ml), while each mini-unit bag can be further divided into four microunits; therefore one unit of blood may be used to transfuse up to twelve 20 ml aliquots, as may be required for neonates; see 'Cow method'

quadrantectomy The removal of a quadrant of tissue, usually from the breast which includes both the grossly identifiable malignant tumor and adequate soft-tissue margins; Cf Lumpectomy, Mastectomy

quadrilemmal body A crystalloid structure composed of 4 sets of parallel lines, seen by EM within the abnormal mitochondria of Ragged red fiber disease; QBs may be the same as 'Parking lot' crystals, see there

'quadruple' syndrome A congenital complex characterized by cleft palate, popliteal webbing, lip pitting and genital malformations; see Popliteal pterygium syndrome

qualifying condition A medical condition that requires that a surrogate decision maker be appointed to an incapacitated person: 1) Terminal condition–the condition is irreversible and death is imminent 2) A state of permanent unconsciousness–thought, sensation, purposeful action, social interaction, and awareness of self and the environment are permanently absent (see Persistent vegetative state); a second requirement is that initiation or continuance of life-support treatment would in the context of the patient's status be of minimal benefit 3) An ill-defined collection of states that were delineated to provide a physician with discretionary capacity, including

incurable or irreversible conditions, which must cause severe pain and impose an inhumane burden (N Engl J Med 1992; 327:11350a) see Job lock; Cf Pre-existing condition

quality The capacity to achieve goals (MLO Supplement September 1993)

quality-adjusted life expectancy see QALE

quality assessment LABORATORY MEDICINE A generic term for any mechanism or format for objectively evaluating the quality of a product or service; see Quality assurance, Quality control, Total quality management

quality assurance A process consist of two components, quality assessment and quality control and improvement, which represent measurement and action (Arch Pathol Lab Med 1994; 118:601); QA is a formal and systematic set of activities that provides a continuous audit against an established standard of quality and which provides a vehicle for correcting deviations from that standard so that a product maintains its quality; the four elements of quality assurance are:

1) Verifying process integrity

2) Assessing a product's quality against a standard

3) Accountability and

4) Liability for failure

For health professionals, quality assurance takes the form of continuing medical education, peer review, specialization, state licensing boards, and utilization review; see Peer review organization, Quality control

quality assurance program A generic term for any formal mechanism that evaluates and assures the highest quality of a product, service, or process; with the passage of the CLIA '88 legislation, physician office laboratories (which were formerly exempt from federal oversight regarding the quality and accuracy of their results) must now comply with the same standards and regulations required of other laboratories; the 10 areas included under the regulatory process are technical procedures, proficiency testing, preventive maintenance of equipment, patient management, quality control program, correlation of the diagnostic results, competence of personnel, communications breakdowns, complaint investigations, and safety (Advance/Laboratory May 1994)

quality control LABORATORY MEDICINE A series of mechanism(s) used to determine the accuracy, reliability and consistency of data, assays or tests, often in the context of laboratory medicine, where QC consumes 10-20% of reagent and labor costs; tests performed by accredited clinical laboratories are delineated in their 'procedures manual' which contains the appropriate QC methods, usually requiring standardized solutions containing glucose, cholesterol, electrolytes and other substances that are either commercially available or obtained by pooling specimens from subjects known to be normal for the parameter being measured; see Multirule procedure; Cf QA, Total quality management

quality of life The degree to which a person is able to function at his usual level of activity without, or with minimal compromise of routine activities, which can be objectively measured by the Karnovsky or QWB scales; QOL is one of the most significant factors weighed in the decision of whether or not to aggressively treat a fulminant terminal cancer, as a 3 month prolongation of a poor quality of life may be a Pyrrhic victory; in AIDS, the ↓ in QOL due to the severity of the side effects of early therapy, eg with zidovudine (nausea, headache, anemia, neutropenia, fatigue, fever) equals the ↑ in QOL associated with a delay in the progression of disease (N Engl J Med 1994; 330:7380a) see Karnovsky scale, QALE, Q-TWiST, QWB scale

'quality' time Meaningful time SOCIAL MEDICINE Background: In the 'typical' North American family unit, both parents have full-time (40+ hours/week) jobs and may relegate major tasks in raising their children to babysitters or day-care centers, and thus see their children one to four hours daily, and then, may be too busy with household chores to interact with them; the term stems from the philosophy espoused by some mental health care workers, that this lack of meaningful interaction during a child's critical formative years may be compensated for by assuring that the contact a parent has with his offspring be (high) 'quality' time; see 'Supermom'; Cf Latchkey children

quantal analysis NEUROPHYSIOLOGY A technique used to understand the nature of synaptic transmission at the neuromuscular junction in which 'quanta' or discrete packages of a neurotransmitter, eg acetylcholine are released from a presynaptic site, evoking a post-synaptic response; while the quantal model is largely correct, such a binomial (all-or-nothing) distribution is a gross simplification as synaptic responses are graded along the dendrites and are not identical in all sites (**Nature 1991; 350:344, 271**); see Long-term potentiation

quantitative trait locus analysis A method of potential use in behavioral genetics (as well as other fields that attempt to study single traits controlled by multiple genes) which allows the evaluation of a trait governed by more than one gene; in QTL analysis, organisms with two extremes of expression of a particular trait (eg aggressiveness vs docility in mice) are bred to virtual homogeneity, then backbred to determine effects of the genetic exchange on the expression of the trait of interest; confidence levels fall when a single trait is attributed to an increasing number of gene loci (**Science 1994; 264:1690N, 1715, 1733**) Cf OGOD approach

quarantine EPIDEMIOLOGY Restriction of freedom of movement allowed those with (or presumed to have been exposed to) a highly communicable disease, with the purpose of preventing its further dissemination; see Notifiable disease, Proposition 64

quartan fever The fever pattern characteristic of infection by *Plasmodium malariae* in which fever spikes appear every third day (day one, day four, day seven and so on) in a background of low-grade fever; Cf Tertian fever

quarter moon sign RADIOLOGY A descriptor for a collection of barium seen in an upper 'GI' series, which is relatively typical of benign gastric ulcers, which is produced by an overhanging fold of mucosa surrounding the ulcer mouth; benign ulcers often have a smooth inner margin with the concavity towards the lumen (figure), a finding that contrasts with that of malignant ulcers, which are more commonly characterized by an inner ulcer margin that is rugose with a convexity toward the gastric lumen; see Meniscus sign of Carmen

Note: There has been an accelerating trend in the past decade in the US for gastroenterologists to perform the entire work-up for gastric symptoms, and at the same time as the endoscopic examination of the gastric mucosa, take a biopsy of areas that appear to be abnormal, which is widely regarded as being a more efficient and definitive diagnostic modality than an upper GI series

quasidominance The mimicking of a dominant pattern of inheritance in a simple mendelian trait that occurs when there is a mating of a homozygous recessive with a heterozygous recessive in multiple generations

'Quasimodo syndrome' A clinical complex characterized by severe kyphoscoliosis, dyspnea with associated hypoxia and altered sleep pattern (parasomnia); see Hunchback
Likened to the symptoms suffered by Victor Hugo's Quasimodo, the Hunchback

quasi-species A variant virus eg HIV-1 with a nucleic acid sequence that is somewhat distinct from the usually isolated forms

quaternary syphilis The fourth chronobiological stage of syphilis, which follows tertiary syphilis, and is characterized by necrotizing, spirochete-laden encephalitis, which

may be accompanied by evidence of end-stage HIV-1-induced anergy and/or loss of cell-mediated immunity against treponemal antigens); quaternary syphilis is a rare clinical entity, but may be seen in AIDS patients, who may be more susceptible to neurosyphilis (**N Engl J Med 1987; 316:1569; N Engl J Med 1988; 319:1549c**)

Quebec classification EMERGENCY MEDICINE A classification (table, facing page) that is used to stratify the severity of whiplash-related injury and need for therapy, based on the data from a meta-analysis reported in Spine (1995); see Whiplash

Quellung test MICROBIOLOGY A reaction characterized by the swelling of encapsulated bacteria, eg *Hemophilus influenza*, *Streptococcus pneumonia*, *Neisseria* species, and *Klebsiella* spp, which is caused by antigen-antibody complex formation; the reaction is based on the alteration of the refractory index, when the organisms are with a species-specific antiserum incubated with the patient specimen TECHNIQUE A drop of *H influenzae* type b antiserum is mixed with a drop of the patient's specimen and a small loopful of 0.3% methylene blue; if the patient specimen has the bacterium, the blue-stained organisms are surrounded by a cleared 'halo' (an apparent swelling) which corresponds to antigen-antibody complex formation at the organism's surface

quenching IMMUNOLOGY Suppression of fluorescence, eg by use of molecules that can absorb the fluorescent energy INSTRUMENTATION Any interference with the transfer of energy in a liquid scintillation counter, eg nonspecific absorption of light in a sample 'cocktail' prior to its arrival at the photomultiplier tube, which results in an incorrectly decreased value; quenching may be 1) Chemical-type (due to impurities which absorb energy from the excited solvent) or 2) 'Color'-type (due to photon absorption impurities), corrected for by adjusting the light pulse ratios and by internal or external standardization and occurs in counting β but not γ radiation; see POPOP, RIA

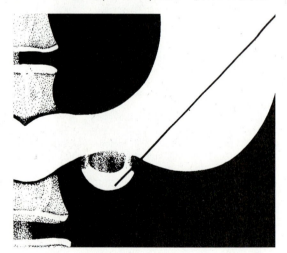

quarter moon sign

questioning mania Folie du pourquoi, Fragesucht An obsessive-compulsive neurosis characterized by the need to ask questions

Quetelet index CLINICAL NUTRITION A parameter used to determine nutritional status, calculated by the formula

$$QI = \frac{\text{Body weight (kg)}}{\text{Height (m}^2)}$$

queuing theory A mathematical model that analyzes the flow of resources (equipment, personnel, widgets, etc)

QUEBEC CLASSIFICATION OF WHIPLASH-ASSOCIATED DISEASE

GRADE	CLINICAL PRESENTATION
0	No complaint about the neck
	No physical signs
I	Neck complaint of pain, stiffness, or tenderness only
	No physical signs
II	Neck complaint AND
	Musculoskeletal signs[a]
III	Neck complaint AND
	Neurological signs[b]
IV	Neck complaint AND
	Fracture or Dislocation

[a]Musculoskeletal signs include ↓ range of motion and point weakness

[b]Neurologic signs include ↓ or absent deep tendon reflexes, weakness, and sensory deficits

Symptoms that may be manifested in all grades include deafness, dizziness, tinnitus, headache, memory loss, dysphagia, and temporomandibular joint pain

Spine 1995; 20/8S:2S-68S

and attempts to optimize their utilization by simulating situations that have characteristics of the resources waiting in a line, ie 'Queuing' (N Engl J Med 1990; 323:604; Worthington DJ J Oper Res Soc 1987; 38:413)

questionable cancer therapy Unproven cancer therapy, see there

'quick and dirty' Crude but effective A colloquial generic term that is applicable to a survey, laboratory procedure, or any type of test using the tools at hand to answer an experimental question in a crude and rough fashion; although 'Q&D' techniques are of inadequate methodologic rigor to allow statistical analysis, they produce results on which reasonable conclusions may be drawn prior to performing a more definitive study with appropriate controls and recording of data

quick-blot MOLECULAR BIOLOGY A generic term for one of the steps in dot-blotting which consists of immobilizing mRNA or DNA from whole cells on nitrocellulose; QBs require tissue lysis, proteinase K treatment, solubilization of nucleic acids in hot NaI, passage through a nitrocellulose filter, and acetylation of residual protein with acetic anhydride (DNA 1983; 2:243) QBs allow rapid quantitative analysis of small volumes of cultured cells; see Dot blot, Slot blot

quickening OBSTETRICS A subjective sensation experienced by the mother during early pregnancy, that occurs around the 16th gestational week, fancifully likened to the 'fluttering of a bird', which corresponds to the mother's first awareness of fetal movement; see Bonding; Cf Lightening

'quicker-and-sicker' HEALTH CARE INDUSTRY A colloquialism that criticizes the prospective payment system (PPS) form of health care reimbursement practiced in the US; under the PPS, the hospital is 'penalized' if a patient is not discharged in a predetermined time period, based on the patient's diagnosis-related group (DRG) disease of admission; the attending physician is more likely to 'efficiently' discharge a patient with clinical instability, ie 'quicker-and-sicker'; since the introduction of the PPS, there has been a 43% increase in patients who have been discharged with unstable conditions, including temperature > 38.3°C, new incontinence, chest pain, dyspnea, tachypnea, confusion, heart rate > 130/min, systolic pressure < 90 mm Hg or diastolic pressure > 105 mm Hg, bradycardia and premature ventricular contractions; see High mortality outlier, July phenomenon

Note: Despite an increase of patients discharged with established parameters of 'instability', there is little reported increase in subsequent mortality

quick-freeze technique ELECTRON MICROSCOPY A method by which subcellular particles, eg the cytoskeleton, can be viewed in a relatively native state; the cells are gently treated with a non-ionic detergent (Triton X-100) which dissolves the plasma and organelle membranes as well as the cytosol; the remainder of the cell contents are frozen within milliseconds with liquid helium (-269°C), allowing no time for the formation of ice crystals or for structural distortion of the cytoskeleton; while the preparation is still frozen, the water vapor is drawn off in a vacuum; the remaining protein fibers are then spray coated with a thin layer of platinum and are ready for conventional electron microscopy; see Lyophilization; Cf Frozen section

quick section Frozen section, see there

quick-stop mutants Temperature-sensitive mutants of *Escherichia coli* that immediately stop replicating once the temperature reaches 42°C; quick-stop mutants are also defective in initiating replication cycles

quiescent smooth muscle cell Contractile smooth muscle cell, see Smooth muscle cell

'quiet zone' PULMONARY PATHOPHYSIOLOGY The terminal airways contribute little to the total airflow resistance (most resistance is contributed by bronchioles > 2 mm in diameter), thus although a disease process may begin in small airways, it may be clinically silent, ie a 'quiet zone' until it affects the larger airways

Quinlan, Karen Ann A young woman who lapsed into a persistent vegetative state in 1975 after ingesting an unknown quantity of tranquilizers and alcohol; this engendered the landmark 'right-to-die' legal case in which her parents received permission by the New Jersey Supreme Court (Re: Quinlan, 70 N.J. 10 (1976)) to remove therapeutic support (a respirator) in 1976; after removal of life support modalities, she 'lived' another nine years, ultimately dying of pneumonia; see Persistent vegetative state; Cf DNR, Euthanasia, It's over Debbie, Right-to-Die movement

The Quinlan decision is widely regarded as the most influential case in the euthanasia controversy, where a person's right to privacy was upheld through her father-Author's note

quinolone Fluoroquinolone Any of a family of antimicrobial agents, including ciprofloxacin, norfloxacin, and ofloxicin that are absorbed orally and are active against a broad spectrum of bacteria; the quinolones target bacterial DNA gyrase (topoisomerase II, an enzyme that introduces negative supercoils in the DNA molecule and separates the interlocked DNA molecule, binding directly to the DNA-gyrase complex, antagonizing virtually all DNA-related activities; bacterial resistance to quinolones is rare and entails mutations of the gyrase itself; quinolones are active against virtually all aerobic bacteria, including bacteria resistant to other antibiotics; these agents are effective in treating genitourinary, GI, prostatic, and respiratory infections, and STD; despite their slightly higher cost, they may be less expensive if they replace parenteral agents SIDE EFFECTS Minimal, GI discomfort, and vague CNS symptoms (N Engl J Med 1991; 264:384rv)

quinoproteins A unique class of bacterial oxidoreductases that utilize pyrroloquinoline quinone (PQQ) as a cofactor; see PQQ

quinsy Peritonsillar abscess, see there

Quintana v United Blood Services TRANSFUSION MEDICINE A lawsuit in which the estate of the plaintiff (a 56-year-old woman) was awarded $6.5 million as she contracted AIDS from a transfusion of blood donated by a homosexual male in 1983; the plaintiff alleged that the blood service in question was negligent in failing to directly ask the donors about their sexual preferences

Note: Many legal experts were disappointed by the Denver Court's decision, as it is viewed as punishing a blood bank despite its having acted responsibly, and in compliance with professional and governmental standards prevailing at the time of the transfusion (CAP Today September 1992)

qui tam lawsuit RESEARCH ETHICS A lawsuit that attempts to recuperate monies paid by the US government to an individual who is convicted of fraudulent use of funds; qui tams originated in the False Claims Act of 1863, written during the US Civil war and were intended to give private citizens, commonly known as 'whistle blowers', a financial incentive for reporting fraud, since in successful lawsuits, the citizen is entitled to 30% of the recuperated monies; see Fraud in science

Note: The existence of qui tams is a powerful disincentive for committing scientific fraud, especially since by law, the damages paid are trebled, thus an NIH grant of $100 000 might prove to be lucrative for the plaintiff, even though in theory the plaintiff is 'altruistically' suing for damages on behalf of the US government; US scientists are concerned that questions of scientific misconduct will be decided in a court of law by a jury of laymen (who would be more swayed by the trial's theatrics than the science being presented before them) rather than by a jury of peers (Science 1990; 249:734ed)

QWB scale Quality of well-being scale (developed by R Kaplan, UCSD) A list of 30 symptoms that determines the value people place on alleviation of those symptoms, quantifying treatment cost per 'quality life year', by examining the age of onset, the number of years of expected remaining life, the frequency of use of a particular procedure for a morbid condition, the efficiency of the treatment for the symptoms and the treatment cost

---

Common Abbreviations

common abbreviations: 2-D Two-dimensional **3-D** Three-dimensional **±** About, approximately, circa **‡** see there **aa** Amino acid **ACE** Angiotensin-converting enzyme **AD** Autosomal dominant **AFB** Acid-fast bacillus **AIDS** Acquired immunodeficiency syndrome **aka** also known as **ALL** Acute lymphocytic (lymphoblastic) leukemia **ALS** Amyotrophic lateral sclerosis **ALT** Alanine aminotransferase (formerly GPT) **AMA** American Medical Association **AML** Acute myelocytic (granulocytic, myeloid, myelogenous) leukemia **ANLL** Acute nonlymphocytic leukemia **apo** Apolipoprotein **aPTT** Activated partial thromboplastin time **AR** Autosomal recessive **ARDS** Acute respiratory distress syndrome or adult respiratory distress syndrome **AST** Aspartate aminotransferase (fomerly GPT) **AV** Atrioventricular **BCC** Basal cell carcinoma **BM** Bone marrow (or basement membrane) **BUN** Blood urea nitrogen **CAD** Coronary artery disease **cAMP** Cyclic adenosine monophosphate **CBC** Complete blood count **CDC** Centers for Disease Control and Prevention **cDNA** Complementary DNA **CEA** Carcinoembryonic antigen **CHF** Congestive heart failure **CIE** Counter-immunoelectrophoresis **CIN** Cervical intraepithelial neoplasia **CK** Creatinine phosphokinase **CML** Chronic myelocytic (granulocytic, myelogenous, myeloid) leukemia **CNS** Central nervous system **COD** Cause of death **COPD** Chronic obstructive pulmonary disease **CPR** Cardiopulmonary resuscitation **CSF** Cerebrospinal fluid **CT** Computed tomography **CVA** Cerebrovascular accident **DAD** Diffuse alveolar damage **DDx** Differential diagnosis **DIC** Disseminated intravascular coagulation **DM** Diabetes mellitus **DNA** Deoxyribonucleic acid **DOA** Dead on arrival **DSM-IV** Diagnostic and Statistical Manual, fourth edition **DWI** Driving while intoxicated *E coli Escherichia coli* **EEG** Electroencephalogram, electroencephalographic **eg** *exempli gratia*, for example **EGF** Epidermal growth factor **EKG** Electrocardiography **ELISA** Enzyme-linked immunosorbent assay **EM** Electron microscopy, ultrastructure **EMG** Electromyography **EMT** Emergency medical technician **ENT** Ears, nose, and throat, otorhinolaryngology **EPA** Environmental Protection Agency **ER** Emergency room, emergency ward **ERCP** Endoscopic retrograde cholangiography **ESR** Erythrocyte sedimentation rate **ESRD** End-stage renal disease **FDA** United States Food and Drug Administration **FDP** Fibrinogen degradation product(s) **FISH** Fluorescence in situ hybridization **FNA** Fine-needle aspiration (biopsy or cytology) **FSH** Follicle-stimulating hormone **FUO** Fever of unknown origin **GABA** gamma-aminobutyric acid **GC-MS** Gas chromatography-mass spectroscopy **GFR** Glomerular filtration rate **GGT** Gamma-glutamyl transferase **GI** Gastrointestinal **GM-CSF** Granulocyte-macrophage colony-stimulating factor **GMS** Gomori-methenamine-silver **GN** Glomerulonephritis **GNP** Gross National Product **GVHD** Graft-versus-host disease **HAV** Hepatitis A virus **HBV** Hepatitis B virus **hCG** Human chorionic gonadotropin **HCV** Hepatitis C virus **HDL** High-density lipoprotein **H&E** Hematoxylin & eosin **HHV** Human herpesvirus (HHV-1, HHV-etc) **HIV** Human immunodeficiency virus **HLA** Human leukocyte antigen (the major histocompatibility complex of humans) **HMO** Health maintenance organization **HPLC** High-performance liquid chromatography **HPV** Human papillomavirus **HSV** Herpes simplex virus **HTLV-I** Human T cell leukemia/lymphoma virus **ICU** Intensive care unit **IDDM** Insulin-dependent diabetes mellitus **ie** *id est*, that is (to say) **IFN** Interferon **Ig** Immunoglobulin **IL** Interleukin **IM** Intramuscular **ImPx** Immunoperoxidase **IQ** Intelligence quotient **IR** Infrared **ISH** in situ hybridization **ITP** Idiopathic thrombocytopenic purpura **IUD** Intrauterine (contraceptive) device **IV** Intravenous **IVDU** Intravenous drug use/user **JCAHO** Joint Commission of Accredited Hospitals Organization **K⁺** Potassium **kD** Kilodalton **KS** Kaposi sarcoma **LDH** Lactate dehydrogenase **LDL** Low-density lipoprotein **LGV** Lymphogranuloma venereum **LH** Luteinizing hormone **LM** Light microscopy **LN** Lymph node **MAOI** Monoamine oxidase inhibitor **MEN** Multiple endocrine neoplasia **MHC** Major histocompatibility complex **MI** Myocardial infarction **mo/ma** Monocyte/macrophage (tissue histiocyte) **MPS** Mucopolysaccaride(s), mucopolysaccharidosis **MRI** Magnetic resonance imaging **mRNA** Messenger RNA (ribonucleic acid) **MS** Multiple sclerosis **MVA** Motor vehicle accident **MW** Molecular weight **Na⁺** Sodium **N/C ratio** Nuclear/cytoplasmic ratio **N-CAM** Neuronal-cell adhesion molecule **NGF** Nerve growth factor **NHL** Non-Hodgkin's lymphoma **NIH** National Institutes of Health **NHL** Non-Hodgkin's lymphoma **NIDDM** Non-insulin-dependent diabetes mellitus **NK cell** Natural killer cell **NO** Nitric oxide **NSAID** Nonsteroidal anti-inflammatory drug **OR** Operating room, operating suite **OSHA** Occupational Safety and Health Administration **PAF** Platelet activating factor **PAS** Periodic acid-Schiff **PCBs** Polychlorinated biphenyls **PCP** *Pneumocystis carinii* pneumonia **PCR** Polymerase chain reaction **PDA** Patent ductus arteriosus **PG** Prostaglandin **PID** Pelvic inflammatory disease **PMN(s)** Polymorphonuclear neutrophil(s) or leukocyte(s), segmented neutrophil(s) **ppm** Parts per million **pron** Pronounced **PT** Prothrombin time **PTE** Pulmonary thromboembolism **PTH** Parathyroid hormone **aPTT** (activated) Partial thromboplastin time **QA** Quality assurance **QC** Quality control **RA** Rheumatoid arthritis **RBCs** Red blood cells, erythrocytes **RDS** Respiratory distress syndrome **REM sleep** Rapid eye movement sleep **RFLP** Restriction fragment length polymorphism **RIA** Radioimmunoassay **RR** Relative risk **rRNA** Ribosomal RNA (ribonucleic acid) **RSV** Respiratory syncytial virus **RT** Radiation therapy, reverse transcriptase **SD** Standard deviation **sec** Second (time) **SI** International System (of units), see there **SIDS** Sudden infant death syndrome **SLE** Systemic lupus erythematosus **STD** Sexually transmitted disease **TAH-BSO** Total abdominal hysterectomy with bilateral salpingo-oophorectomy **TB** Tuberculosis **TDM** Therapeutic drug monitoring **TGF-β** Transforming growth factor-β **TIA** Transient ischemic attack **TIBC** Total iron-binding capacity **TLC** Thin-layer chromatography **TNF** Tumor necrosis factor **tRNA** Transfer RNA (ribonucleic acid) **T-S** Trimethoprim-sulfamethoxazole **TSH** Thyroid-stimulating hormone **TTP** Thrombotic thrombocytopenic purpura **TX** Thromboxane **U** 1) Unit 2) University **UK** United Kingdom **URI** Upper respiratory tract infection **US** United States **UTI** Urinary tract infection **UV** Ultraviolet **VDRL** Venereal disease research laboratory (test) for syphilis **VIP** Vasoactive intestinal polypeptide **VLDL** Very low density lipoportein **V/Q** Ventilation/perfusion **vs** versus, in contrast to, in comparison with, in contrast to **VSD** Ventricular septal defect **VZV** Varicella-zoster virus **WBCs** White blood cells, leukocytes **WHO** World Health Organization **X-R** X-linked recessive **↓** Decrease, decreased, decreases, decreasing **↑** Increase, increased, increases, increasing **♀** Female, women **♂** Male, men

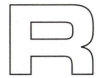

R Symbol for: 1) Arginine 2) Electrical resistance 3) Gas constant 4) Radical 5) Rate 6) Ratio 7) Resistance 8) Respiration 9) Respiratory exchange ratio 10) Rhythm 11) Right 12) Roentgen 13) Rough

Obsolete 1) Behnken unit, an obsolete unit of exposure to radiation, replaced by roentgen units 2) Rankine scale, an obsolete absolute temperature scale based on degrees Fahrenheit 3) Réaumur scale, an obsolete temperature scale devised by René Antoine Feschault de Réaumur (1683-1757) based on a freezing point of 0ºR and a boiling point of 80ºR

r Symbol for: 1) Correlation coefficient 2) Drug resistance 3) Radius 4) Recombinant, see there 5) Reverse 6) Ribose 7) Ribosomal 8) Ring chromosome

R binder protein One of two (the other is transcobalamin II) major extracellular vitamin B_{12} transporters that facilitate the absorption of the vitamin B_{12}/intrinsic factor complex by the intestinal mucosa and its subsequent transport to the liver; RBP may be increased in hepatocellular carcinoma and polycythemia vera; Cf S protein

Note: The 'R' designation refers to the rapid electrophoretic mobility of both transcobalamin I and transcobalamin III; transcobalamin II and RBP are immunologically identical but differ in the carbohydrate composition; congenital deficiency of RBP is extremely rare and may cause a multiple sclerosis-like clinical picture

R factor HEMATOLOGY see R binder protein INFECTIOUS DISEASE Resistance factor An enzyme (chloramphenicol acetyltransferase) that inactivates chloramphenicol by 3-O-acetylation, which is produced by R-plasmids in both gram-negative and gram-positive bacteria, eg *Enterobacteriaceae, Haemophilus influenza, Neisseria gonorrhoeae* and *Streptococcus pyogenes*

Note: Other mechanisms for antibiotic resistance include membrane impermeability, alteration in intracellular target sites, alteration or overproduction of a target enzyme, active pumping out of a substrate and auxotrophic forms which bypass inhibitory steps; see Methicillin-aminoglycoside resistant *Streptococcus aureus*

R plasmid A special type of plasmid that carry genes enabling the host bacterium to resist the otherwise destructive effects of antibiotics, heavy metals, ultraviolet radiation and bacteriophages; see Plasmid

Rs of research The three Rs of research Raw data, Reagents, Responsibility, the triad of 'materials' traditionally shared by scientists; in the current environment, several groups may be actively pursuing the same line of investigation, eg identifying a potentially important gene or protein, selfless cooperation is said to be facing extinction (Science 1990; 248:952)

Note: The phrase derives from nineteenth century rural America when schoolchildren learned the 3 Rs: Reading, 'Riting and 'Rithmetic; Cf 'Safari' research

r value Correlation coefficient A widely used statistical method that determines the relatedness (to a maximum of +1) or unrelatedness (to minimum of −1) of two series of data, allowing calculation of values in a scattergram, so that linearity or degrees of total randomness can be determined

RA 1) Refractory anemia 2) Renin activity 3) Retinoid acid 4) Rheumatoid arthritis 5) Right atrium 6) Risk assessment

Also 1) Radioactive 2) Ragweed antigen 3) Raynaud's phenomenon 4) Rehabilitation Act 5) Relative activity 6) Released action (pharmacology) 7) Renal artery 8) Repeat action 9) Repeated attacks 10) Respiratory allergy 11) Respiratory arrest 12) Retinal anlage 13) Retrograde amnesia 14) Rheumatoid agglutinins 15) Right arm 16) Right auricle 17) Right axilla 18) Rokitansky-Aschoff

RAA system Renin-angiotensin-aldosterone system, see there

Rab3A A small GTP-binding protein that is abundant in brain synaptic vesicles which may play a role in recruiting synaptic vesicles for exocytosis during repetitive stimulation (Nature 1994; 369:493L)

Rab9 A small GTP-binding protein localized to late endosomes, that assists in the transport of mannose-6-phosphate receptors to the *trans*-Golgi network; this localization requires C-terminal prenylation and specific structural determinants; Rab9's membrane target is accompanied by nucleotide exchange (Nature 1994; 369:76L)

Rabbi Bergman see Towers nursing home

rabbit curve R precipitation curve IMMUNOLOGY A symmetrical precipitation curve that is seen when an antigen is tested against its antiserum, the curve is broad and is typical of both rabbit and human antigen-antibody reactions, the latter is an 'H curve'

rabbit ear appearance A descriptor for two elongated, finger-like structures joined at a base CARDIOLOGY A rabbit ear pattern occurs in a variant QRS wave, allowing the differentiation of ventricular tachycardia from the relatively innocent supraventricular tachycardia, in which the left 'ear' spike is higher than the right MICROBIOLOGY An appearance that may be seen in either 1) The characteristic acute angular budding of arthrospores seen by light microscopy in the imperfect fungus *Trichophyton* or 2) The piroplasts of *Babesia microti* (figure) which tend to form packets of twos and threes of intracytoplasmic parasites within circulating erythrocytes

rabbit fever Tularemia

rabbit ileal loop test A technique used to identify enterotoxins produced by serotypes of *Escherichia coli* and *Salmonella* species, in which the supernatant from these organisms in culture is inoculated into a ligated segment of ileum, which responds by 'locking' the intestinal adenylate cyclase into the 'on' position, increasing secretion of fluids into the loop of intestine (Infect Immunol 1973; 7:873)

rabbit nose A descriptor for nose twitching and wrinkling by children with allergic rhinitis, which relieves pruritus or increases air passage; the characteristic upward rubbing of the nose ('allergic salute') may result in a groove formation at the tip of the nose

'rabbit' stool A descriptor for the small rounded, mucus-covered fecal 'pellets' produced in irritable bowel syndrome

rabbit syndrome NEUROLOGY A condition characterized by focal perioral tremors and nose twitching that may be seen in parkinsonism as a late side effect of antipsychotic drug therapy; unlike tardive dyskinesia, the symptoms of RS respond well to antiparkinsonian agents (Clin Neuropharmacol 6 Supplement 1983; 1:S9-S26) see Tardive dyskinesia

rabies A viral infection caused by a bullet-shaped 180 x 80 nm virion containing single-stranded RNA; after intramuscular 'injection' by an animal bite, the virion crosses the neuromuscular junction and infects the nerve, spreading centripetally into the central nervous system and centrifugally into the salivary glands of lower animals Rabies encephalitis in mammals may be either 1) Furious, due to increased irritability of the central nervous system, accompanied by fever, hyperesthesia, anorexia, aggression; immediately prior to death, the afflicted mammal may run for hours until it collapses in complete paralysis or 2) Paralytic, in which sialorrhea is followed by collapse EPIDEMIOLOGY Human rabies is rare--4 cases occurred in the US from 1980-90 (MMWR 1991; 40:132), although a number of other cases occurred outside of the US and developed once the subjects arrived; laboratory-confirmed rabies in mammals is relatively common; of 5606 cases in 1985 (estimated to be 10% of actual number of animals infected), skunks accounted for 46%, raccoons 26%, bats 15%, cattle 4%, foxes 3%, dogs 2%, cats 2%, rabies may be transmitted person-to-person by inhalation or corneal transplant, but not from human bites PATHOLOGY Cerebral edema, congestion, mild perivascular 'round cell' infiltration of the gray matter of the brainstem and spinal cord, marked loss of Purkinje cells, Babe's microglial nodules in the pons and medulla; Negri bodies are present within neurons and are most prominent in the hippocampus, medulla oblongata and cerebellum; a usually fatal viral disease; caused by a single-stranded nonsegmented, negative sense RNA genome that encodes five structural proteins, transcriptase, nucleoprotein, phosphoprotein, matrix protein and glycoprotein; rabies affects wild and domestic animals in particular carnivores EPIDEMIOLOGY 33 000 die/year from rabies in Asia and Africa CLINICAL 18-60 day incubation, followed by nonspecific symptoms including fever, headache, nausea, vomiting, numbness at the site of exposure, and early neurological signs, anxiety, restlesness and depression; the acute nuerological phase is characterized by agitation, confusion, delirium hydrophobia, laryngeal spasms, paralysis and complications (N Engl J Med 1993; 329:1632oa) VACCINATION VRG vaccine, see there; rabies vaccination has been reported to cause false-positive HIV testing (Arch Pathol Lab Med 1994; 118:805oa) see Negri bodies; Cf Pseudo-rabies

RAC Recombinant DNA Advisory Committee A National Institutes of Health (USA) committee involved in approving 'gene therapy', comprised of scientists and members of the public; the first RAC approved recombinant gene experiment involved insertion of a marker gene into terminally ill patients with malignancy to track the progress of tumor-infiltrating lymphocytes (TILs); planned therapies under consideration by the RAC include insertion of therapeutic genes for AIDS, cancer and adenosine deaminase deficiency; see Adenosine deaminase, TIL

Rac1 A critical component in the reorganization of the actin cytoskeleton, which is induced by growth factors or by the oncogene Ras, and which is itself responsible for the transformation of Ras (Nature 1995; 374:457)

RA cell Rheumatoid arthritis cell, see there

Racal space suit Orange suit VIROLOGY A portable positive-pressurized, bright orange space suit with a battery-powered air supply that is used in fieldwork with extreme biohazards (Biosafety Level 4 organisms, eg Ebola virus) that are thought to be airborne; after one or two uses, the entire suit (except the helmet and blowers) is incinerated (R Preston, The Hot Zone, Random House, New York, 1994) Cf Chemturion space suit

raccoon eyes appearance Black eyes A descriptor for bilateral periorbital accumulations of blood or other substances, likened to the nocturnal North American omnivore, *Procyon lotor*; this Panda bear-like appearance is classically described in periorbital hematomas, often associated with anterior-posterior displacement-type automobile accidents or basilar fractures of the skull (N Engl J Med 1992; 327:1507RA); less commonly, the descriptor is applied to the periorbital purpura due to skin infiltration in primary amyloidosis, as a spontaneous event, or after prolonged

eye-strain

Note: Children with rhinitis have an appearance known as allergic shiners

race A subdivision of a species, which although capable of genetic recombination may nonetheless, be divided in part based on biochemical, hematologic, immunologic, morphologic, or serologic differences; for humans race is an ethnic classification, subdivided in the US into five categories, according to origin: 1) White, not Hispanic (Europe, North Africa, Middle East); 2) Black, not Hispanic (Africa); 3) Hispanic; 4) American Native (Indians, Eskimos); 5) Asian and Pacific Islanders; stratification by race is of interest in several areas of medicine for a number of specific reasons CLINICAL MEDICINE Some HLAs are more common in certain racial groups and may be associated with particular diseases, thus helping to diagnose and manage difficult cases PUBLIC POLICY The Civil Rights Act of 1964 mandated equality in employment and educational policy and knowledge of race favors minority candidates; see Equal opportunity TRANSFUSION MEDICINE Certain red cell antigens may be relatively uncommon in a particular race and knowledge of race reduces the labor required to find a suitable unit for transfusion TRANSPLANTATION Human leukocyte antigens (HLA) differ somewhat according to race and may be used to identify potential recipients for organ transplants

racial cleansing CRIMES AGAINST HUMANITY The deliberate and systematic extermination of 'life unworthy of life' (*lebensunwertes Leben*), borrow a phrase used by the Nazis as justification for committing mass murder; RC was practiced in its most 'scientific' form between 1940 and 1945 by doctors, nurses, and orderlies in Nazi Germany and resulted in 200 000 deaths of such 'unworthies' as the mentally ill and retarded, the physically handicapped, those with epilepsy, maladjusted adolescents, those with shell shock, war-wounded soldiers from the eastern front, sick foreign workers, and others (JAMA 1995; 273:1303BR) Cf Ethnic cleansing

racial inequality SOCIAL MEDICINE The disparity in opportunity for socioeconomic advancement or access to goods and services based solely on race; in health care, this disparity translates into excess mortality and morbidity to various diseases, including AIDS, DM, severe hypertension, renal failure, and stroke; in AIDS, blacks were much less likely than whites to receive antiretroviral therapy or *Pneumocystis carnii* pneumonia prophylaxis (N Engl J Med 1994; 330:763SA)

rachitic rosary see Rosary

racquet cells A descriptor for variant 'strap' cells seen in rhabdomyosarcoma, which have a vaguely globose swelling at one end, tapering into elongated wispy cytoplasm, occasionally bearing the diagnostic cross-striations

racquet fingernail An asymptomatic defect of the thumb in which the distal phalanx is shorter and wider than normal, resulting in a shorter and wider than normal nail with a loss of its curvature; racquet nails may occur as an AD 'condition' or in tertiary hypoparathyroidism due to erosion of the underlying bone; Cf 'Clubbing'

rad A quantity of ionizing radiation (X-rays and γ rays) corresponding to an energy absorption of 100 ergs/g of tissue; the rad as a unit was 'retired' in 1985 and has been replaced by the gray (Gy), where 1 Gy equals 100 rads; Cf Roentgen

radial growth phase melanoma DERMATOPATHOLOGY Nontumorigenic melanoma A clinical term for an intraepithelial stage in the evolution of a primary melanoma that is not associated with metastasis, in which the net effect is radial enlargement of the lesion without invasion; the lesions encompassed under the rubric of RGP melanoma differ according to the author, but include melanoma in situ, lentigo maligna, dysplastic nevi (Hum Pathol 1990; 21:1202)

Cf Vertical growth phase melanoma

radial immunodiffusion IMMUNOLOGY A simple method for quantifying antigenic serum proteins (eg apolipoproteins, complement proteins, immunoglobulins, and others) METHOD An agar gel with incorporated antibody has multiple wells cut in it; standard antigens and an unknown are droppered into the wells and the diameter of the precipitation reaction of the unknown is plotted on a curve and compared semiquantitatively with the standards; see Ring test, Spur

radial keratotomy OPHTHALMOLOGY One of two types of refractive surgery (a technique that corrects myopia by changing the cornea's conformation); in RK, a diamond knife (cost of equipment, $2500) is used to make incisions at the edge of the cornea, flattening it, but weakening its overall structure; Cf Photoreactive keratectomy

radial unit model NEUROEMBRYOLOGY A hypothesis explaining how the immense number of neurons in the cerebral cortex arise from progenitors lining the cerebral neocortex, and are then distributed to appropriate layers of distinct cytotechtonic areas; according to this model, the ependymal layer of the embryonic ventricle consists of proliferative units providing a primitive map of the prospective areas; the proliferative units are transported via glial guides to the growing cortex in the form of ontogenetic columns, the final number of neurons dedicated to each column is modified by interacting afferent 'messages'; this model is supported by data provided by ultrastructure, immunocytochemistry, receptor autoradiography and kinetics of cell proliferation

radiation hybrid mapping MOLECULAR BIOLOGY A technique for constructing high-resolution, contiguous maps of chromosomes, consisting of a statistical method that depends on X-ray-induced breakage of chromosomes to determine the distances between DNA markers; Cf Pulsed field electrophoresis

radiation The combined processes of emission, transmission and absorption of highly energetic waves and particles on the electromagnetic spectrum; the depicted symbol is the internationally sanctioned indicator for the presence of radioactivity TYPES **alpha radiation** 2 protons and 2 neutrons, eg plutonium, radon; α radiation travels 15 cm in air and is stopped by a piece of paper; its role in soft tissue malignancy is well-established, see Radium Dial company, although its relation in epithelial malignancy is less certain; it is present in cigarette smoke and may have an additive effect to the known carcinogenic effect of tar; alpha radiation is emitted by radium, thorium, and uranium **beta radiation** Electrons, eg strontium-90, tritium (^{3}H); β radiation travels at the speed of light, is stopped by wood and thin metals and is carcinogenic to skin **gamma radiation** Gamma photon A quantum of electromagnetic radiation of ≤ 1 nm, which is generated by unstable nuclei eg ^{60}Co; γ radiation is stopped by several feet of heavy concrete or 10-40 cm of lead and induces malignancy, inducing mutations at the glycophorin A locus in survivors of atomic blasts; $183/10^5$ excess deaths in survivors of the Hiroshima and Nagasaki blasts, with a 13-fold ↑ in non-lymphocytic leukemia (peaking at 6 years post-blast), thyroid nodules and tumors (peaking at 15-20 years post-blast) and multiple myeloma 6-fold ↑ (peaking 30 years post-blast) CYTOPATHOLOGY Radiation induces marked cellular atypia, elongation or 'spindling', cytoplasmic vacuolization, multi-

nucleation, nuclear hyperchromasia and nuclear membrane wrinkling; the differences in pathology among organs is slight COLON Ulceration, necrosis, bleeding, eosinophilia HEMATOPOIETIC TISSUE Lymphocytopenia, followed by granulocytosis, followed by granulocytopenia, thrombocytopenia, erythroid hypoplasia and aplasia LYMPH NODES Lymphocyte depletion, hemorrhage and fibrosis MUSCLE Fibrosis, Zenker's degeneration PROSTATE Glandular atrophy, squamous metaplasia, cellular and fibromuscular atypia SKIN Atrophy, Epilation, erythema, fibrosis, eventually, soft tissue necrosis; see Acute radiation injury, Nuclear war

Note: After radiation exposure, high-dose potassium iodide may be used to functionally block the effect of thyroid irradiation

radiation pneumonitis Irradiation pneumonitis A condition caused by exposure of lung tissue to radiation, a common complication of therapy for tumors in the mediastinal and thoracic region, including malignant lymphoma, Hodgkin's disease, breast and esophageal carcinomas, the frequency of RP is a function of dose and the amount of tissue exposed to radiation INCIDENCE Radiologic evidence of pneumonitis occurs in 65% of those with irradiated lung fields, although clinically evident pneumonitis occurs in only 6%, 2% of whom die from radiation pneumonitis PATHOLOGY Alveolar septal thickening by collagen and basement membrane material, alveolar proliferation, desquamation of atypical cells within the alveolar septum, hyaline membrane formation and pulmonary vascular changes, protein leakage, interstitial infiltration and reduction of alveolar volume

Note: Other radiation 'syndromes' include radiation arthropathy, radiation carditis, radiation cytitis, radiation dermatitis, radiation enterocolitis, radiation fibromatosis, radiation hepatitis and radiation nephritis

radiation sickness see Acute radiation injury syndrome

radiator theory ANTHROPOLOGY A theory proposed by Dean Falk that attempts to explain how the human brain evolved from a 500-g chimpanzee-like brain of early hominids to the current size of (± 1400 gram) in less than 2 million years (a very short time span in evolutionary biology); Falk argues that the emissary veins are a crucial network that cools the brain in hyperthermia, thus being likened to a radiator, and may have been the crucial preadaption required for the increased size of the brain, given that the substantial differences between the configuration of the vascular systems of humans and non-human primates (Science 1990; 250:1339)

radiation therapy Radio-therapy The administration of ionizing radiation to treat disease, usually malignant, at either low energy levels in locoregional fashion (brachytherapy), with the delivery device located at or near the target lesion*, or at high energy levels at a distance from the lesion (teletherapy), with the energy of the radiation dose being higher, ie in the mediastinum CYTOLOGY Classic cellular alterations (eg bizarreness, vacuolization, cellular degeneration, smudging of nucleolar material, cytomegaly) associated with RT, are not seen consistently in mesothelial cells (Acta Cytologica 1994; 38:10A)

*As in interstitial or intracavitary radiation used to treat gynecologic or head and neck cancer

radical cystectomy A surgical procedure in which there is complete removal of the urinary bladder, pelvic lymph nodes, and adjacent organs with the creation of an ileal conduit or internal reservoir for internal drainage of urine; RC is the standard therapy for muscle-invasive bladder cancer PROS Excellent local control of cancer, although up to 50% develop distant metastatases (usually within 2 year) CONS Morbidity inherent in the loss of a urinary bladder; muscle-invasive bladder can be alternatively treated without RC using a combined modality approach-transurethral surgery, combination chemotherapy (methotrexate, cisplatin, vinblastine), and radiotherapy (4000 cGy); of 53 patients in one study with this regimen (N Engl J Med 1993; 329:1377OA), the rate of bladder preservation was 58%

radical mastectomy A mastectomy that removes the breast in toto, as well as skin, subcutaneous tissue, axillary lymph nodes, and muscle from the anterior thoracic wall; RM was formerly used to treat extensive breast cancer, but has been essentially abandoned in view of the ↑ complications associated therewith and lack of improved survival; Cf Modified radical mastectomy

radical neck dissection The most commonly performed major operation for head and neck malignancies, most of which are squamous cell carcinomas; in a 'radical neck', the neck is opened laterally, the majority of the sternocleidomastoid muscle is removed, as are the regional cervical lymph nodes, the jugular vein, the spinal accessory nerve, the submaxillary gland and most of the parotid gland; a 'radical neck' may be combined with a partial resection of the mandible and tongue, depending on the lesion's topography; the term 'modified radical neck dissection' is ill-defined as there is a spectrum of what can be called 'modified'; some operators merely preserve the spinal accessory nerve, while others spare all functional tissue, including the sternocleidomastoid muscle and the jugular vein; Cf Commando operation, 'Heroic' surgery, Mutilating surgery

radical prostatectomy The complete surgical removal of the prostate, which is the most widely used method for treating prostatic cancer; although the procedure has a prolonged recuperation period, and may be complicated by impotence and urinary incontinence, it is regarded by many workers to be a 'safer' procedure than cryosurgery, which may result in incomplete removal of the cancer (Science News 1994; 146:13) and introduces artefacts which preclude optimal histologic evaluation needed to determine completeness of surgery; see Cryosurgery, Prostate cancer

radical scavenger Free radical scavenger

radical surgery A generic term for any surgical intervention that involves major excision or restructuring of a region of the body; RS is most often used an aggressive and/or high stage (III or IV) malignancy, and includes in 'heroic' operations such as fore- or hindquarter amputation, hemipelvectomy, and the 'Commando' operation (radical neck); see Heroic surgery; Cf Palliative surgery

radioactive decay The spontaneous change in a nucleus of a radioactive isotope, result in the loss of energy with the liberation of neutrons, protons and electrons and a lower energy state

radioactive waste Any unwanted byproduct from the peaceful uses of nuclear energy, which may be low (intermediate) or high level; in 1989, 5% of the volume of RW was contributed by academia, 9% by industry, 24% by medical facilities, and the remainder by the 44%; the most recently proposed long term burial site for radioactive waste in Nevada has been placed on permanent hold (NY Times March 14 1995, C1) see High level waste, Low level waste, Plutonium

radiofrequency MRI The frequency on the electromagnetic spectrum that is intermediate between auditory and infrared, which in MRI is in the megaherz range; the principal effect of radiofrequency magnetic fields on the body is the deposition of power (heat), usually confined to the corporal surface, being the main safety concern; see Magnetic resonance imaging

radiofrequency catheter ablation CARDIOLOGY A technique that selectively destroys foci in the endocardium (and subjacent myocardium) linked to arrhythmias; RCA destroys tissue by means of controlled heat production, avoiding the need for general anesthesia, as pain is minimal, and skeletal muscle contraction does not occur; RCA is widely used to treat refractory supraventricular tachyarrhythmias of adults as well as pediatric patients (N Engl J Med 1994; 330:1481OA, 331:910OA)

radiofrequency coil MRI A component of the MRI hardware that transmits radiofrequency pulses and/or receives MR signals; commonly having a solenoid or saddle configuration; see Magnetic resonance imaging

radiofrequency current CARDIOLOGY A level of electrical energy (31 watts or more), delivered through a large-tip electrode for ablation of the accessory ventricular conduction pathway in the Wolff-Parkinson-White syndrome, a therapeutic modality that produces better results than that of high energy direct current (N Engl J Med 1991; 324:1605, 1612), which generates more than 2000 volts, producing a combination of light, heat, barotrauma and an intense electrical gradient

radiofrequency pulse MRI A brief burst of RF magnetic field delivered to the object by the RF transmitter; for an RF near the Larmor frequency, the RF pulse results in rotation of the macroscopic magnetization vector in the rotating frame of reference; the amount of rotation depends on the strength and duration of the RF pulse, which are most commonly 90° ($\pi/2$) and 180° (π) pulses; see Magnetic resonance imaging

radioimmunoassay see RIA

radioimmunoglobulin therapy Radioimmunotherapy, see there

radioimmunoprecipitation assay A technique that is similar to Western blotting as it identifies antibodies to specific viral components and requires an electrophoretic separation step METHOD Disrupted, purified virus previously grown in culture with a radioactive amino acid is co-incubated with a test sample which may contain an immunoglobulin with specificity against the viral antigen; the immunoglobulins in the test sample are then subjected to polyacrylamide gel electrophoresis

radioimmunotherapy A therapeutic modality in which radiolabeled (monoclonal) antibodies recognizing specific antigens are used to treat a disease; RIT is still in its infancy and it is uncertain whether it will become a permanent tool in the therapeutic armamentarium; in its current incarnation, RIT is experimental and may be best suited for delivering high doses of 'hot' and lethal antibodies to B cell (non-Hodgkin's) lymphomas, which are very radiosensitive; in one myeloablative RIT study, 16/43 patients with stage III or IV disease entered complete remission with ^{131}I-labeled (dose = 234-777 mCi, ie 8.66-28.75 x 10^9Bq) anti-CD20 and anti-CD37 antibody treatment, followed by autologous BM transfusion; when the patients were divided into those with a favorable biodistribution 16/24 entered complete remission; 9 were in remission 3-53 months after treatment; RIT allows delivery of 10-fold higher cytoricidal radiation to tumor sites TOXICITY Myelosuppression, nausea, infections, cardiopulmonary toxicity (N Engl J Med 1993; 329:459OA, 1219OA, 1266ED) Note: Chemoimmunotherapy may be an equally viable therapeutic modality

radiolucent An adjective referring to any material or tissue that allows the facile passage of X rays, ie that which has an air or near air density

radiomimetic drug An immunosuppressive drug, eg an alkylating agent, that is used to treat malignancy, which has effects on nucelic acid, eg DNA mimicking those of ionizing radiation

radionuclide Radioactive isotope, radioisotope An artificial or natural nuclide with an unstable nuclear composition that decomposes spontaneously by emission of electrons (β-particles) or helium nucleus (α-particle and γ-radiation), ultimately achieving nuclear stability; radionuclide are used as in vivo or in vitro labels, for radiation therapy, or as sources of energy

radionuclide scan (lung) Ventilation-perfusion scan, see there

radiosensitivity The relative susceptibility of cells and tissues to irreversible damage by radiation, which either prevents mitosis or the completion of normal metabolic processes; lymphoid, hematopoietic and gonadal tissues are highly susceptible to radiation damage, while terminally differentiated tissues, eg bone, cartilage, muscle and peripheral nerve are relatively radioresistant; some malignancies, eg lymphoproliferative, gonadal malignancies, classically, seminoma and small cell carcinoma of the lung seem to 'melt away' with radiotherapy, whereas others, eg glioma, melanoma, renal cell carcinoma and sarcomas, are notoriously radioresistant

radiotherapy Radiation therapy, see there

Radiothor MEDICAL HISTORY An over-the-counter 'patent' medicine containing radium-226 and radium-228 in water, formulated in 1925 and produced until the early 1930s in the US; radium emits α radiation and can only penetrate short distances, but in that distance produces considerable damage; Radiothor was a self-medication claimed to be an endocrine system 'tonic' and of use in treating impotence and chronic diseases including anemia, rheumatism, multiple sclerosis, gout and others; the 'mild radium therapy' era collapsed when one of its chief proponents and users died of massive radium intoxication (**JAMA 1990; 264:614**) see Health fraud, Quackery

'radish' bacillus A trivial name for *Mycobacterium terrae* and the related *M triviale*, members of Runyon group III (nonphotochromogens) mycobacteria, which are isolated from soil, vegetables (hence, 'radish') and milk and are essentially nonpathogenic

Radium Dial Company A defunct company in Illinois that in the 1920s highlighted clock faces with radium-laced luminescent paint; the workers, mostly women, often licked the tips of their paint brushes to bring them into a point, making their job easier and at the same time ingesting significant doses of radium (a rare radioactive element in the uranium decay series with a $T_{1/2}$ of 1622 years); over time, these women developed severe osteoporosis and mesenchymal tumors including malignant fibrous histiocytoma and osteosarcomas; Cf Radiothor

radon Radon-222 PUBLIC HEALTH A naturally occurring radioactive gas in the decay chain of uranium-238 to lead-206 that has a half-life of 3.8 days, decaying into two solid α particle-emitting daughters; radon exposure is associated with a relative risk of 12.7 due to lung cancer in non-smoking uranium miners and is associated with an ↑ risk of leukemia, childhood malignancy, myeloid leukemia, renal cell carcinoma, melanoma and prostatic carcinoma in adults; 13 000 annual excess cases of lung cancer in the US are attributed to radon gas exposure, an effect that is synergistic with cigarette smoking; long-term exposure to 150 Bq/m³ is held to be equivalent to smoking ½ pack of cigarettes/day; concentrations of radon gas in the home above 4 pCi/L (148 Bq/m³); these data have been re-validated for residential radon exposure in a cohort of 1360 subjects in Sweden; at ≥ 10.8 pCi/L (400 Bq/m³), the relative risk is 1.8; combined radon exposure and smoking exceed an additive and approach a multiplicative effect (**N Engl J Med 1994; 330:159OA**)

radurization PUBLIC HEALTH The use of low levels (eg < 1 mrad) of ionizing radiation to retard spoilage, so named as it has the same effect as pasteurization, ie to improve shelf life and inactivate bacteria that cause food spoilage; see Food irradiation

RAEB Refractory anemia with an excess of (myelo)blasts, see there

raf MOLECULAR BIOLOGY A regulatory proto-oncogene that encodes a ubiquitous cytoplasmic protein kinase, which is a target for multiple growth factors and has a central role in signal transduction; the Raf kinase promotes cell proliferation that depends on growth factor receptors and membrane-associated oncogenes; the *raf* gene is an essential signal transducer that acts downstream of serum growth factors, protein kinase C and the *ras* oncogene (**Nature 1991; 349:426**); with the related *rif*, *raf* modulates hepatic levels of α-fetoprotein (AFP), acting in a 'trans' conformation, regulating AFP production via mRNA; increased expression of *raf* causes radioresistance in human laryngeal carcinoma, while reduced expression of c-*raf*-1 modulates tumorigenicity and radioresistance of squamous cell carcinoma (**Science 1989; 243:1354**)

Raf A protein kinase that is activated by Ras, a GTPase; Raf's activation does not depend on farnesylation or addition of a COOH-terminal sequence, but rather its location in the plasma membrane; Ras recruits Raf to the plasma membrane where a Ras-independent activation of Raf occurs (**Science 1994; 264; 1463R**)

Raf-1 A cytosolic protein kinase that translocates to the plasma membrane in response to the binding of growth factors to their cognate receptors, where it attaches to the cytoskeleton (**Science 1995; 268:247**)

Raf/MEK/MAPK cascade A major pathway for regulating cell proliferation and growth, which also has roles in differentiation, hypertrophy, cell survival, integration of energy through metabolism, changes in cell morphology;

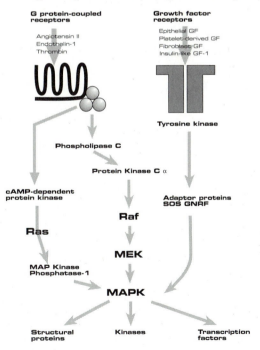

MAPK	MAP kinase kinase
MEK	Mitogen-activated protein kinase
PKC	Protein kinase C alpha
SOS GNRF	'Son of Sevenless' guanine nucleotide releasing factor

the RC often acts by membrane recruitment and activation of Raf serine/threonine kinase, and involves the small GTPase, Ras; as both Ras and Raf are critical transducers of mitogenic signals, inhibition of their activity would in theory provide a means of inhibiting various proliferative event, eg vascular disorders, within the cell, which could be mediated by antibodies, antisense oligonucleotides, or expression of dominant negative mutations; the accompanying figure (simplified from a more complete figure by S Ludwig and UR Rapp) indicates types of interactions and 'players' in this cascade that may ultimately be sites of inteaction with therapeutic agents (Nature Medicine 1995; 1:513)

RAG-1, RAG-2 Recombination-activating genes A pair of adjacent (8 kilobases apart) genes encoding proteins that synergistically activate V(D)J recombination; RAGs are thought by some workers to correspond to V(D)J recombinase

ragged red fiber disease A form of mitochondrial myopathy, defined by histopathology, which consists of extensive cell destruction at the skeletal muscle cell periphery with vacuolated fibers which are 'ragged' under high power, best viewed by the Gomori trichrome stain EM Abnormal enlarged mitochondria with degenerated cristae and unique crystalloid inclusions ('parking-lot crystals'), accompanied by various defects in the mitochondrial electron transport chain, including mitochondrial ATPase, NADH-coenzyme Q reductase, cytochrome oxidase b and cytochrome oxidase c; RRF occurs in the skeletal muscle of mitochondrial encephalomyopathy (see MERRF), AIDS patients treated with AZT as a cytotoxic form of myopathy mediated by MHC Class I-restricted cytotoxic T cells Note: The RRFs may occasionally be more basophilic ('blue') than red, may be seen in other mitochondrial myopathies and in the rare mitochondrial lipid glycogen disease

'Raggedy Ann syndrome' Chronic fatigue syndrome, see there

ragocyte Rheumatoid arthritis cells, see there

ragweed *Ambrosia artemisifolia* An herb of the family Compositae, the pollen from which is highly allergenic, and the most common cause of allergic rhinitis

RAIDS Refrigerator 'AIDS', see there

railroad nystagmus see Optokinetic nystagmus

railroad track appearance A descriptive term for parallel, relatively straight lines, radiopacities or radiolucencies of varying length; when the parallel lines are curved, the adjective 'tramline' or 'tram track' is a more valid descriptor NEPHROPATHOLOGY The railroad track appearance refers to parallel thickening and splitting of the glomerular capillary basement membrane due to subendothelial deposition of immune complexes, mesangial matrix and neutrophilic debris between the glomerular basement membrane and the vascular endothelium causing a double contour by light microscopy, a classic finding in type I and occasionally in type II membranoproliferative glomerulonephritis and cryoglobulinemia, which is best seen by silver and periodic acid-Schiff (PAS)-stains; the outer 'track' of the double contour corresponds to the original basement membrane that is continuous and easily recognized; the inner basement membrane 'track' is discontinuous and of variable thickness; Cf Crescent formation, Tram track appearance

railroad track scars GASTROENTEROLOGY A descriptor for the macroscopic changes seen in the late fibrosing stages of Crohn's disease in which longitudinal mucosal lesions heal in parallel tracks, perpendicular to the length of the colonic lumen PLASTIC SURGERY A scar with obvious cross-hatched stitch marks due to poor repair, excess tension on the skin or to a delay in suture removal, which should be ideally removed on the third to fifth days (except when the sutures overlie highly mobile sites); some body regions, eg trunk, sternum and proximal extremities are more susceptible to cross-hatching

'raining down' DERMATOPATHOLOGY A descriptor applied to 'dropping' of fascicles and individual nevus cells from the epidermis into dermis, a morphological feature of the benign Spitz's nevus, which help differentiate this from malignant melanoma

Raji cell IMMUNOLOGY A B lymphoblastic cell line that was originally obtained from a Burkitt's lymphoma that is used to detect immune complexes; the Raji cell has minimal or no surface immunoglobulin, low avidity Fc receptors and a high density of C3 receptors, making it ideal for detecting levels of background circulating immunoglobulins in serum, of use in diagnosing Waldenström's disease and immune complex disease; see Immune complex

Note: Other methods for detecting immune complexes include the solid phase C1q, conglutination, polyethylene glycol precipitation of high molecular weight immune complexes

rale *râle*, French, to rattle CLINICAL MEDICINE A term for the crackling or bubbling, discontinuous sounds or vibrations, which may be heard by auscultation of various pulmonary diseases, eg bronchitis, pneumonia, atelectasis, pulmonary edema, heart failure, bronchiectasis and tuberculosis

RAM COMPUTERS Random access memory Temporary, immediately available computer memory that disappears upon loss of power, which contrasts to the 1) Permanent 'software memory', stored on magnetic media, eg floppy disks or hard disks and 2) Permanent 'hardware memory', stored on ROM (read-only memory) chips; RAM available to microcomputer users has risen from 16 kilobytes in the 1970s to 250 megabytes in the 1990s, a capacity which allows simulated manipulation of three-dimensional structures, eg for the design and advanced modeling of complex drugs or DNA-protein interactions VETERINARY MEDICINE An uncastrated ♂ sheep

Raman effect That which occurs when a beam of incident light causes rotational and vibrational transitions in molecules, resulting in exiting scattered light that has a different frequency than the in-coming light

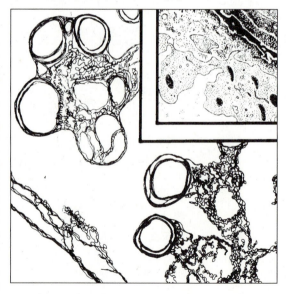

railroad track appearance

Raman spectroscopy A method for studying proteins in their native state by X-ray crystallography that records the spectrum of light scattered by a transparent medium at a right angle to the incident beam of monochromatic light; a peak or 'frequency shift' in the scattered light corresponds to vibration or rotation of the scattering molecules, providing information that is similar and complementary to that provided by infrared spectrophotometry; see X-ray crystallography

RAMI Rate-adjusted mortality index, see there

ram's horn sign Shofar sign, see there

Ran proteins MOLECULAR BIOLOGY A family of Ras-related GTP-binding proteins that function as molecular switches, that cycle between GTP-bound 'on' and GDP-bound 'off' states; Ran is located primarily in the eukaryotic cell nucleus, and is involved in importing proteins into the nucleus, control of DNA synthesis, and cell-cell progression (Nature 1995; 374:378)

Ranch Hand Operation Ranch Hand, see there

rancidity A state characterized by the presence of musty, sharp, sour, or other 'off' or unpalatable (rancid) tastes or odors due to oxidation-related deterioration of unsaturated fatty acids and hydrolysis of triglycerides into mono- and diglycerides, glycerol and free fatty acids; Cf Maillard reaction

R&D Research and development INDUSTRY A term referring to the investment of time and labor into identifying new technologies and bringing to the marketplace products and processes that will generate profit; of the $130 x 10⁹ spent in 1993 on R&D (in % of expenditures), private industry invested more than government, which in turn invested than universities and nonprofit organizations; R&D represents 2-3% of US GNP (Sci Am 1994; 270/9:72)

RAND corporation A nonprofit organization engaged in research and analysis on issues of public welfare and national security, supported by monies from US government, philanthropies and foundations; the publications generated under RAND's aegis include breast feeding in developing nations and issues of cost containment, health care policy and quality assurance

random error STATISTICS The scattering of values in a test system around a point known to be a correct value; random errors in the laboratory can be due to variations in line voltage, lamp output, amount of fluid drawn in pipettors or dispensors; the amount of random error in a system or its precision is measured by its standard deviation and coefficient of variation; Cf Systematic error

random walk THERETICAL MEDICINE The haphazard movement of a particle, eg Brownian movement or fluctuation of a molecule's three-dimensional configuration that is attributable to intrinsic vibration or chaos; see Breathing, Chaos; Cf Fractal analysis

randomization STATISTICS The selection of subjects or samples for each 'arm' of a study or experiment that approximates as far as possible a selection based on chance alone, which is intended to minimize the influence of irrelevant details and selection bias, in order to produce statistically valid data

ranitidine Zantac® An H_2-receptor anatagonist used to treat gastric and duodenal ulcers, esophageal erosions, gastroesophageal reflux, and conditions, eg Zollinger-Ellison disease and systemic mastocytosis in which there is an increased H_2 activity; in patients whose duodenal ulcers heal after severe hemorrhage, long-term maintenance with ranitidine ↓ risk of recurrent bleeding (N Engl J Med 1994; 330:380OA) see H_2 blockers

RANTES A 68-amino acid monomeric cytokine produced by T cells, platelets, renal epithelial and mesangial cells, which is chemoattractive for basophils, eosinophils, monocytes, and T cells, and activates basophils, inducing the release of histamine therefrom

rapamycin Sirolimus, see there

RAPD analysis MOLECULAR BIOLOGY A type of genomic fin-

gerprinting based on the analysis of random amplified polymorphic DNA, which can be used to separate species and subspecies of bacteria (N Engl J Med 1995; 332:819c)

rape FORENSIC MEDICINE 'An unlawful, nonconsensual act of sexual intercourse carried out by force or other forms of duress.' (International Dictionary of Medicine, John Wiley & Sons, New York, 1986) Nonconsent is established by threat of violence, deceit or fraud, impairment of the victim's senses, or other methods to overcome the victim's physical or psychological resistance; rape is an aggressive act that is considered by many workers to be sadistic rather than sexual in nature DIAGNOSIS Detection of choline periodate (Florence test) with its characteristic rhomboid crystal as a marker for ejaculate is still being used in detection of rape, although isolation of DNA fragments with polymerase chain reaction is far more valid, as it serves to identify the perpetrator; because of the legal implications and logistical problems that the 'chain of evidence' may incur, investigation of rape in the US is a costly procedure; sexually transmitted infection occurs in about 40% of rape victims and the agents include *Neisseria gonorrhoeae*, cytomegalic inclusion virus, *Chlamydia trachomatis*, herpes simplex, *Treponema pallidum* and HIV-1 **MALE RAPE** is that of a male by another male, ie anal intercourse **SPOUSAL RAPE** is that by the marital partner, against the partner's will **STATUTORY RAPE** is that where local or state law decrees that one of the partners has not reached adult status, ie is 'underage'; see Rape-trauma syndrome

rape kit FORENSIC MEDICINE A collection of receptacles (cups, envelopes, plastic bags, tubes), disposable items (cotton swabs, napkins, pipettes) and tools (sterile comb for pubic hairs, sheets) used to obtain specimens from a rape victim, which are used establish details in a forensically acceptable fashion about the perpetrator, and manner in which the rape occurrred (N Engl J Med 1995; 332:234RV) see Date rape, Rape

rape trauma syndrome The generic term for the constellation of findings in which the short term phase may last from hours to days and consists of emotional shock disbelief, and despair due the life-threatening events; the external response in this phase varies from emotional instability to a well-controlled behavior pattern; most signs are somatic and include eating and sleeping disturbances, and mood swings, anxiety and depression; the long-term phase during which the victims attempts to restructure her life may last for months to years (N Engl J Med 1995; 332:234RV) see Rape

RAPER(s) A colloquial acronynm for radiologists, anesthesiologists, pathologists and emergency room physicians, a group of board-certified medical specialists who are almost invariably hospital-based; because RAPERs generally do not practice their specialty outside of a medical facility, the health care reimbursement organizations and regulatory agencies in the USA have found it convenient to consider all RAPERs in a category separate from other physicians who 'compete' for patients and have other expenses not incurred by RAPERs

rapeseed oil syndrome see Toxic oil syndrome

rape-trauma syndrome An acute stress reaction to a life-threatening situation in which sexual assault was attempted or successful, divided into psychological phases

PHASE I Disorganization; onset 2-3 weeks post-attack; the victim blames herself for having provoked the attack

PHASE II Long-term reorganization, often the victims are left with residual chronic anxiety, phobias, hypochondriasis, loss of self-esteem or depression

Rappaport classification HEMATOLOGY A classification of non-Hodgkin's lymphomas proposed by H Rappaport in the mid-1950s (Cancer 1956; 9:792) based on pattern of growth (nodular or diffuse) and cell morphology (undifferentiated, poorly differentiated, well-differentiated, histiocytic), which enjoyed enormous popularity given its simplicity and reproducibility that was subsequently superseded by classfications (eg Lukes and Collins, Kiel) that reflected advances in cellular immunology; after 1982, the Working Formulation (for classifying lymphomas) became popular; it is uncertain whether the recently proposed REAL classification will replace this surfeit of classifications; Cf REAL classification, Working Formulation

'rapture of the deep' see Nitrogen narcosis

Rapunzel syndrome A fanciful term for the symptoms of a massive trichobezoar caused by trichotillomania and trichophagia, seen most commonly in mentally retarded or deranged females CLINICAL Epigastric pain, bloating, nausea and vomiting RADIOLOGY A mass lesion, usually gastric with 'strands' of hair extending into the upper small intestine LABORATORY Hypochromic microcytic anemia, the hair acts as an iron chelator TREATMENT Surgery; see Bezoar
Rapunzel was a maiden with long hair in a fairy tale written by Jacob Grimm

RAR Retinoic acid receptor, see there

RAR-α Retinoic acid receptor-alpha A receptor for which the gene is located on chromosome 17q11.2; acute promyelocytic leukemia is associated with a chromosomal translocation (t(15;17)(q22;q12-21)) that fuses the RAR-α gene to an oncogene PML located on chromosome 15; the fusion gene encodes a novel mRNA and protein that is of diagnostic utility (**N Engl J Med 1992; 327:423ED**) see Differentiation therapy

rare disease see Orphan disease

rare earth Any of a group of oxides of widely distributed, but relatively scarce minerals, corresponding to the fifteen elements with atomic numbers from 57 to 71, including erbium, gadolinium, lanthanum, neodymium, some of which have properties making them useful as crystals in lasers; see Lasers; Cf Trace minerals

RARS Refractory anemia with ringed sideroblasts see Idiopathic sideroblastic anemia

ras gene(s) A family of oncogenes and proto-oncogenes, first identified in a rat sarcoma, which encode oncoproteins or proto-oncoproteins; ras genes (c-ras, H-ras, K-ras, N-ras and v-ras) encode 21 kD proteins (p21^{ras}) with roles in the transduction of growth signals, binding guanine triphosphate (GTP) and catalyzing its hydrolysis to guanine diphosphate (GDP); ras proteins acquire cell-transforming potential with 'activating' amino acid substitutions at positions 12, 13 or 61 due to point mutations on the ras gene, located at 11p13; c-ras, the cellular proto-oncogene encodes a highly conserved 21-kD membrane-bound protein with a low GTPase activity; a point mutation in c-ras yields v-ras with impaired GTPase activity and inhibited 'off switch', resulting in sustained activation, possibly of a calcium channel; the ras oncoprotein is an extracellular signal for cell growth received by a transmembrane receptor protein, which induces a GDP-for-GTP exchange with the intracellular ras proteins, resulting in a GTP-ras protein complex required for ras protein function; in neoplasia, this complex is 'locked' in the new conformation and, lacking intrinsic GTP-hydrolytic capacity, is left in the 'turned-on' or neoplastic position; ras is required for the activity of other oncoproteins, including tyrosine kinase and such growth stimulants as the tumor-promoting phorbol ester; ras genes are the most highly conserved oncogenes and are expressed in cancer of the bladder, colon, lung, pancreas, prostate, stomach, in T-cell malignancy, AML, and melanoma; ras expression in the NIH3T3 tumor cell line is associated with an increased intrinsic resistance to ionizing radiation; cell-activating point mutations (at various sites in the DNA) of ras genes are common in some adenocarcinomas, eg pancreatic (90% have a K-ras mutation), colorectal (50% mutated)

and thyroid (50% mutated) carcinomas, but are rare in breast and ovarian malignancy; presence of a point mutation on the K-ras codon 12 in pulmonary adenocarcinoma indicates a relatively poor prognosis, despite a lower clinical stage at time of diagnosis ; see p21^{ras} K-ras point mutations in non-small cell carcinoma of the lung are associated with a poor response to surgical therapy, which is improved by adding preoperative chemotherapy (cisplatin, ifosfamide, mitomycin–combined with radiotherapy, 26 vs 8 months) (**N Engl J Med 1994; 330:153OA**)

Ras A guanosine triphosphatase (GTPase) that is a molecular switch for signal transduction pathways that control growth and differentiation (**Science 1994; 264; 1413P**); like other GTP-binding proteins, Ras cycles between an active (GTP-bound) and an inactive (GDP-bound) conformation; a wide variety of extracellular signals can stimulate the formation of active Ras:GTP; Ras controls a mitogen activated protein (MAP) and functions as a regulated membrane-bound anchor for Raf, which can be activated by epidermal growth factor and other signals (**Nature 1994; 369:411L**)

ras activation A sequence in which there is an ↑ expression of the ras oncogene, which precedes clinical disease; when rats are exposed at birth to a carcinogen, nitrosomethylurea; high resolution restriction fragment length polymorphism analysis of a polymerase chain reaction-amplified ras sequence revealed H-ras and K-ras 2 weeks after the carcinogen treatment but 2 months before the onset of neoplasia; the oncogenes remain latent until the rats are exposed to estrogens, which is then followed by the development of mammary carcinoma; activated ras oncogenes occur in carcinomas of the lung, colon and pancreas as well as in well-defined precancerous lesions, eg adenomas and myelodysplasia; progression to more malignant stages of disease requires activation of other oncogenes or deletion of growth suppressor gene; see Ruffling

ras pathway A major complex and cascade-like pathway by which DNA is turned on and off by a wide range of signals arriving at the cell membrane; although the Ras pathway is not thought to be decisive in transcription signaling, it is critical in growth control; Cf JAK-STAT pathway

Rashkind PDA occluder PEDIATRIC CARDIOVASCULAR SURGERY A device that consists of a double umbrella constructed of foam disks attached to a steel skeleton; the device is considered an investigational (by the US FDA–Food and Drug Administration) alternative to surgical closure of a persistent patent ductus arteriosus (PDA); when compared to surgical closure, occlusion of a PDA with the Rashkind device is more expensive ($11 466 vs 8 838, 1989 US dollars), less 'efficient' (PDA closure with first procedure-77% vs 99.8%) and has more complications (2.7 major and 16.8 moderate complications vs 0.2% major and 11.8% moderate complications) than surgical closure of a PDA (**N Engl J Med 1993; 329:1517OA**) see Patent ductus arteriosus

raspberry tongue A descriptive term for the characteristic enanthema of scarlet fever, in which the tongue is bright red with edematous white papillae; Cf Strawberry tongue

raspberry tumor A fanciful synonym for an intraductal papilloma of the breast, a pink, lobulated and cystic tumor attached to the walls of dilated ducts; the intraductal papilloma may simulate malignancy both clinically, as it often presents with hemorrhage of the nipple and pathologically, due to complexity of the cellular proliferation and loss of the myoepithelial cell layer

RAST Radioallergosorbent test A 'solid phase' radioisotopic method for quantifying specific allergenic IgE antibodies in serum, similar to an agglutination test; the allergen-antigen complex is bound to an insoluble cyanogen-bromide activated paper disk (allergosorbent) and the patient's serum is added; sera containing the antibodies in question will complex to radioactive immunoglobulins, in particular IgE; RAST correlates reasonably well with bronchial provocation testing; rare false positive RAST results from allergies to ragweed/grass, although RAST is neither more sensitive nor specific than skin testing, it avoids the risk of sensitization and anaphylaxis inherent to in vivo testing; see Mail-order medicine

rat The rat, in particular, the Norway rat (*Rattus norvegicus*) has and continues to perform a yeoman's service in experimental medicine and biology; in the mid-19th century, it was used to study physiology and nutrition; in the current experimental environment, rats have been inbred to select for desired feature(s), and strains have been deceloped that are used to study immunogenetics, transplantation, cancer-risk assessment, cardiovascular disease and behavior; 'rat work' is less expensive that working with larger mammals and rats have a shorter breeding time (**Science 1989; 245:269rv**), and are preferred by many to mice (which may be too small); Cf *Caenorhabditis elegans,* Guinea pig, Zebrafish; rats are vectors and/or reservoirs of disease, including Bunyavirus, the black plague and rat-bite fever

rat-bite fever An acute febrile illness usually acquired from a rat bite which inoculates either *Streptobacillus moniliformis*, agent of Streptobacillary rat-bite fever, see Haverhill fever, or *Spirillium minor*, agent of Spirillary rat-bite fever, see Sodoku

'rat-bitten' kidneys A descriptor for kidneys with a renal cortex with one or more small jagged rat-bite-like umbilications on the surface after removing the capsule, which corresponds to one or more infarcts caused by arterionephrosclerosis

rat tail tapering RADIOLOGY HEART A descriptor for a smooth progressive narrowing to a point of maximal stenosis of the left anterior descending coronary artery, seen by angiography; Cf Bridging PANCREAS A descriptor for relatively abrupt narrowing of the pancreatic duct in endoscopic retrograde cholangiopancreatography (ERCP), a finding suggestive of pancreatic adenocarcinoma RESPIRATORY TRACT A descriptor for the abrupt loss* of the normal arborization of the bronchus in bronchography as occurs in intraluminal neoplasms, in particular squamous cell carcinoma

*This sign is rarely evoked in the era of computed tomography

ratchet phenomenon CELL BIOLOGY A term referring to terminal differentiation of cells, as occurs in adipocytes and peripheral neurons, which is a complex structural and functional process representing a point of 'no return'; for normal cells, dedifferentiation or 'simplification' is virtually impossible, while return to a more 'primitive' state is highly characteristic of malignant cells

Note: A ratchet is a wrench that functions in only one direction

rate-adjusted mortality index The expected in-hospital mortality rate based on actual in-hospital rates for diagnoses, grouped by their diagnosis-related group (DRG) code and adjusted for age, race, sex, the presence of co-morbidities and main surgical operative procedure(s); an increased RAMI values imply that the patient is more severely ill ab initio (**JAMA 1991; 265:374**)

rate-limiting step The slowest phase or reaction in a series of reactions, eg the step in a multi-enzyme cascade that sets the pace of the reaction; the presence of a rate-limiting step implies that all other reactions are in equilibrium

rational addiction hypothesis A posit that seeks to explain certain addictive behaviors based on the assumption that 1) Current consumption has a long-lasting, eventually decaying, effect on future tastes and preferences, and 2) Consumers are rational, forward-thinking, and take into account the effect of current consumption on their future propensity to consume the substance in question (**JAMA 1995; 273:1417**)

rational design A generic term for the rational application of knowledge on the structure and function of molecules to the design of molecular structures of interest, eg **rational drug design**; these compounds be 'created' through molecular graphics and manipulated on high-power computers; the complexity of the interactions of larger molecules, eg enzymes, receptors, immunoglobulins, and other macromolecules are such that ball-and-stick modeling is impossible; in rational molecular design, a battery of algorithms are used to calculate conformational energies, molecular orbitals, and various structural interactions

rationalization PSYCHOLOGY An explanation or justification for one's actions, in particular those included under the rubric of psychological defense mechanism

rationing HEALTH CARE POLICY Allocation or distribution of a scarce product, commodity or service; the rationing of medical services is a major issue in the USA, in an era of mounting deficits and limited resources; the US health care system is the costliest in the world, consuming 11.3% of the gross national product and at the same time, is unequally distributed (**JAMA 1991; 265:105**); legislative bodies are becoming increasingly involved in the dialog of how to implement a palatable form of health care rationing; see Health care rationing, Oregon plan

'rave' party A social activity of recent vintage consisting of an all-night dance session at a club or party, often accompanied by the ingestion of a recreational dose (ie not overdose levels) of the 'designer' drug of abuse, ecstasy (MDMA); during ectasy's first wave of popularity in the 1980s, it was generally regarded as safe and used in a relaxed 'mellow' setting; in rave parties, the combination of the heat and poor ventilation in the clubs, sweating and low fluid intake and frenetic pace of the dancing, appear to induce a severe, potentially fatal MDMA-related toxic reaction (**JAMA 1993; 269:1505mn&p**) see Ecstasy

raw data Data that is directly obtained from instrument read-outs, which has not been subjected to calculations, statistical analysis or classification; in research, it is critical to collect raw data consistently, ie in the same place and in a logical and ordered sequence, especially for those receiving US government grant monies, as raw data may be viewed as governmental property, subject to public scrutiny; see Notebook, Rs (three) of Research; Cf Fraud in science

raw milk see Unpasteurized milk

Rb Tumor suppressor retinoblastoma protein The retinoblastoma gene product (which is also the first identified tumor suppressor) that plays a key role in regulating transcription during the cell cycle; Rb suppresses cell growth by inhibiting the activation of transcription by pol I[1] (**Nature 1995; 374:177oa, 114n&v**), and prevent the expression of genes transcribed by pol II[2] that are necessary for proliferation; cell cycle repression can be abrogated by phosphorylation; Rb is a member of the viral oncoprotein-binding pocket protein family that regulates cell cycle progression; Rb regulates transcription in all cells of adults; the active form of Rb represses genes required for cell cycling; inactivation of Rb by phosphorylation inactivates Rb and allows cell division to begin (**N Engl J Med 1994; 330:786ed**); Rb accumulates during embryonic development and cell differentiation and participates in terminal differentiation of various cell lines, eg skeletal myogenesis involves the direct interaction of Rb with muscle-specific basic helix-loop-helix factors of the MyoD family; reversal of this terminal differentiation is mediated by p107 in $Rb^{-/-}$ cells (**Science 1994; 264; 1467r**)

[1]RNA polymerase I [2]RNA polymerase II

RB gene Retinoblastoma gene A tumor suppressor gene located on chromosome 13q14 that encodes a 105-kD nuclear phosphoprotein with DNA-binding activity that regulates cell growth and is expressed in normal tissues and is phosphorylated during the S and G2-M phases of the cell cycle; some RB gene mutations encode in a protein that binds poorly, if at all to the regulatory site; malignancy is facilitated if the defect is homozygous; expression of normal RB protein in tumors is associated with a 60% five-year survival, while heterogeneous or decreased expression of the RB gene product is associated with a less than 30% survival (**N Engl J Med 1990; 323:1467**); RB gene defects are also seen in sarcomas, carcinoma of the breast and bladder and in small cell carcinoma of the lung; RB inactivation is common in parathyroid carcinoma, but not in benign tumors of the parathyroid (**N Engl J Med 1994; 330:757OA**) see Rb, Retinoblastoma, Tumor suppressor genes; Cf Cyclin D1

RBC Red blood cell, erythrocyte

RBE Relative biological effectiveness, see there

RBRVS Resource-based relative value scale, see there

RCA Red cell agglutination

RCF Relative centrifugal force

RDA 1) Recommended daily allowance, see there 2) Respiratory distress syndrome 3) Reticuloendothelial depressing substance (?)

RDW Red blood cell distribution width An estimate of erythrocyte anisocytosis, which is a parameter generated by automated red cell counters, eg Coulter counter, and the Cell-Dyne, which is of use in determining the cause of a given anemia (table); a low RDW in sickle cell anemia indicates milder disease and may be of use in 'working up' such patients (**Clin Lab Haematol 1991; 13:229**)

RED CELL DISTRIBUTION WIDTH

RDW	MCV	DISEASE STATE
N	↓	α– β–thalassemia
↑	↓/N	Iron deficiency, hemoglobin H, S
↑	N	Aplastic anemia
↑	↑	Megaloblastic anemia (folate, vitamin B_{12}
N/↑	↑	Liver disease, myelotoxins, CLL, CML, sickle cell anemia, hemoglobin SC, sideroblastic anemia, myelofibrosis, chemotherapy, mixed iron and vitamin B_{12} deficiency

MCV Mean corpuscular volume

'Re' mutant(s) INFECTIOUS DISEASE A family of mutant gram-negative bacteria that lack all or most of the polysaccharides in the terminal and core regions of the endotoxins; survival in non-immunized patients with gram-negative septicemia correlates with the levels of anti-'Re' lipopolysaccharide antibodies

reactivation A generic term for the restoration of a cell or molecule's functional activity after photochemical, ultraviolet light or ionizing radiation-induced damage

reactive depression PSYCHIATRY A form of depression that is viewed as an exuberant response to stressful life events; in both forms, a stressful life event has occurred in the relatively recent past; see Depression; Cf Endogenous depression

reactive hemophagocytic syndrome A condition with a potentially pernicious clinical course, associated with infections, often viral, eg adenovirus, CMV, EBV, herpes zoster and parainfluenza, gram-negative bacteremia, TB, fungal infection, leishmaniasis, as well as drugs and malignancy, eg ALL, Hodgkin's disease, Lennert's lymphoma and gastric carcinoma PATHOLOGY Dilated subcapsular sinusoids lined by cells with abundant cytoplasm and bland nuclei, erythrophagocytosis and ↑ angiotensin converting enzyme CLINICAL Patients are severely ill with fever, lymphadenopathy, hepatosplenomegaly, and ↑↑↑ mortality

reactive hypoglycemia Plasma glucose measuring < 2.8 mmol/L (**US: < 50 mg/dl**) with symptoms of adrenergic neural activation, eg weakness, palpitations, tremor, sweating and hunger occurring after a meal or following oral glucose loading, caused by compensatory insulin hypersecretion

reactive leukocytosis Leukocytosis, see there

reactive lymphoid hyperplasia An overly exuberant response of lymphoid tissue to various antigens; while true RLH regresses with time, a certain percentage of cases initially diagnosed as RLH are lymphomas; the question of which cases are lymphomas ab initio can only be resolved by molecular markers of early steps in the evolution of malignancy, eg by PCR of the t(14;18) which was reported to be positive in RLH, but only with enhanced PCR techniques (**Arch Pathol Lab Med 1994; 118:791OA**)

reactive marrow A nonspecific descriptor for a polyclonal response of the bone marrow to a local or systemic 'insult', often inflammatory in nature; marrow reactivity may be confined to one cell line, as in reactive granulocytosis, reactive mast cell hyperplasia or reactive thrombocytosis

Note: The polyclonal nature of certain reactive hyperplasias, eg reactive histiocytosis, reactive lymphocytosis and reactive plasmacytosis may be difficult to distinguish from their malignant counterparts

reactive material OCCUPATIONAL SAFETY A chemical substance or mixture that may vigorously condense, decompose, polymerize, or become self-reactive, when exposed to shock, or increased pressure and/or temperature; OSHA categorizes RMs as an explosive material, organic peroxide, pressure-generating material, or water-reactive material

reactive oxygen metabolite Oxygen free radical, see there

reactive perforating collagenosis An AR [MIM 216700] condition of early childhood onset characterized by recurring umbilicated papules due to an ill-defined collagen defect, which is triggered by trauma and exacerbated by cold weather

reactive (hyper)thrombocytosis A platelet count of ≥ 800 x 10^9/L (US = ≥ 800 000/µl), seen in ± 1:200 of hospital patients; 30% of RHT is associated with acute and chronic inflammation, but also occurs in chronic inflammatory conditions (eg RA, SLE), malignancies, neonatal respiratory distress syndrome, and after major hemorrhage, surgery, trauma; in some cases of RHT (eg burns, hypothermia, pre-eclampsia), a lower platelet volume was present (**Lab Med 1992; 23:811**) Cf Essential thrombocytosis

read COMPUTERS To acquire data from an input device, eg an optical scanner, or from storage, eg a floppy drive MOLECULAR BIOLOGY The obtention of specific information from one nucleic acid's 'script' for the production of 1) A complementary strand, as in transcription of mRNA from DNA, 2) A duplicate strand, as in replication of DNA, or 3) A similar message, written in a different 'language', as in the translation of a protein from a mature mRNA transcript

readily achievable PUBLIC HEALTH An ill-defined adjective used in the context of the Americans with Disabilities Act, which refers to the modifications or removal of architectural barriers (to the disabled) in the physical plant of places of public accomodation (hotels, concert halls, museums) that would be required of the owners or operators, if the changes are readily achievable; critics of the law are concerned that the vagueness of the adjective could hinder enforcement of the law (New York Times 24 Oct 1993; 10-1) see Americans with Disabilities Act

reading disability An unexpected difficulty in learning to read despite normal intelligence and the opportunity to learn with competent instruction, occurring in the absence of general health problems, emotional disturbances or sensory defects; RD affects 3-9% of school-aged children, and accounts for 75% of referrals for learning disability; RD is has been attributed to a slowing of the magnicellular visual pathway in the background of a normal visual response (N Engl J Med 1993; 328:989oa)

reading frame A segment of processed and mature mRNA that is capable of being translated into a polypeptide

readmission The admission of a patient to a health care facility for a condition (eg stroke, myocardial infarction, GI bleeding, hip fracture, cancer surgery) that had been the cause of a previous admission; the readmission rate varies widely among regions, and may be a function of the per capita availability of hospital beds*

*In one report, the rate of readmission in Boston was 64% higher (where there are more beds) than the rate in New Haven, Connecticut (N Engl J Med 1994; 331:989sa)

read-through The continuation of either 1) Transcription of DNA by RNA beyond the normal termination signal, due to the inability of the RNA polymerase to recognize the terminator or 2) Translation of a segment of mRNA into a protein beyond the normal stop codon

reagent Any substance or material that is an integral and standardized participant in a reaction or detection method (eg GLC, HPLC, GC-MS) which is used to detect a particular substance of interest

reagent grade chemical LABORATORY MEDICINE Any chemical that meet the specifications of the Committee on Analytical Reagents of the American Chemical Society; RGCs are available as either

1) LOT ANALYZED REAGENTS, for which each indivudual lot is analyzed and the amount of the impurity is reported, eg Cadmium-0.0005%, or as

2) MAXIMUM IMPURITIES REAGENTS, for which maximum impurities are listed, even though the analysis of the substance by the manufacturer may reveal a lower level of a particular impurity than that which is guaranteed by the manufacturer (from NW Tietz, Textbook of Clinical Chemistry, WB Saunders, 1986)

reagent grade water LABORATORY MEDICINE A term for water that meets certain specifications promulgated by the NCCLS (National Committee for Clinical Laboratory Standards); RGW replaces other terms formerly used to indicate water's level of purity, eg deionization and distillation, both of which have been retired, as they refer to the method for purification and not to the quality of the final product; there are three grades of RGW, type I, II, and III, in descending levels of purity, and these are variously defined by microbiological content, pH, resistivity at 25° C, silicates particulate matter, and organics (from NW Tietz, Textbook of Clinical Chemistry, WB Saunders, 1986); in the working parlance, the term 'reagent grade water' refers only to the type 1, the purest form

reagent red cells TRANSFUSION MEDICINE Commercially available erythrocytes that have common antigens (Rh-D, Rh-C, Rh-E, Rh-c, Rh-e, M, N, S, s, P_1, Le^a, Le^b, K, k, Fy^a, Fy^b, Jk^a, Jk^b) on their surfaces; these antigens are the ones most often implicated in potentially fatal hemolytic transfusion reactions, when they are transfused into patients having these antibodies in their serum; the presence of antibodies in the recipient's serum is detected by a 'major cross-match'

reagin An obsolete generic term for IgE, referring to 1) IgE as an initiator of the immediate hypersensitivity reaction and 2) IgE as a nonspecific antibody produced in syphilis that is directed against phosphatidylglycerol (cardiolipin) and measured by the VDRL slide flocculation test and RPR

card agglutination, which may have a high false positive rate, see Biological false positivity

Note: Given its confusing and partially overlapping usages, the term reagin should be 'retired' from the working medical parlance

REAL classification Revised European-American Lymphoma classification The newest[1] of a number of schema[2] used to classify lymphomas, proposed by the International Lymphoma Study group, which is intended to classify tumors that are known clinical entities; unique feature of the REAL classification is the recognition of arbitrary nature of the distinction between lymphocytic leukemias and certain lymphomas; see Lymphoma; Cf Working Formulation

[1]The acronym REAL is not merely an accident as many hematopathologists with a particular interest in lymphomas ('lymphomaniacs') believe that any classification should list the *real* clinical entities seen in practice, rather than fit a lymphoma to an often arbitrary classification [2]eg Kiel Classification, Lukes and Collins Classification, Rappaport Classification, Working Formulation, and others

---

REAL CLASSIFICATION

B CELL NEOPLASMS

Precursor B cell neoplasm: Precursor B lymphoblastic leukemia/lymphoma

Peripheral B cell neoplasms

    B cell CLL/prolymphocytic leukemia/small lymphocytic lymphoma

    Burkitt's lymphoma

    Diffuse large B cell lymphoma (various disease entities)

    Follicle center lymphoma

    Hairy cell leukemia

    Mantle zone lymphoma

    Marginal zone lymphoma

    Lymphoplasmacytoid lymphoma/Immunocytoma

    Plasmacytoma

    Provisional entities: Marginal zone lymphoma of spleen, high-grade B cell lymphoma, Burkitt-like

T CELL AND PUTATIVE NK CELL NEOPLASMS

Precursor T cell neoplasm: Precursor T lymphoblastic leukemia/lymphoma

Peripheral T cell and NK cell neoplasms

    Adult T cell lymphoma/leukemia

    Angiocentric lymphoma

    Angioimmunoblastic T cell lymphoma

    Anaplastic large cell lymphoma

    Intestinal T cell lymphoma

    Large granular lymphocyte leukemia, T cell or NK cell type

    Mycosis fungoides/Sezary syndrome

    Peripheral T cell lymphoma, unspecified (with various provisional entities), eg provisional subtypes, eg hepatosplenic γδ T cell lymphoma, subcutaneous panniculitic T cell lymphoma

    T cell CLL/prolymphocytic leukemia

    Provisional entity: Anaplastic large cell lymphoma, Hodgkin's-like

HODGKIN'S DISEASE

    I Lymphocyte predominance

    II Nodular sclerosis

    III Mixed cellularity

    IV Lymphocyte depletion

    V Provisional entity Lymphocyte-rich Hodgkin's disease

NL Harris, ES Jaffe, H Stein, et al, Blood 1994; 84:1361-1392

'real-time' imaging Visualization of a dynamic process within microseconds after its occurrence, a modality requiring very rapid information processing, ie as the process occurs, as in 'B' mode ultrasound; some ultrafast computers in CT allow quasi-real time imaging

Note: Certain imaging modalities, eg fluoroscopic angiography and other fluoroscopic procedures are intrinsically 'real-time' but are not designated as such

reanneal MOLECULAR BIOLOGY The renaturation of DNA

under experimental conditions, where complementary single strands are of 'self' origin, in contrast to an annealing reaction where the complementary single strands forming the duplex molecule are of different sources, ie hybrid molecules; see High-stringency hybridization, Low-stringency hybridization

rearrangement see Gene rearrangement

reasonable accomodations A standard of providing for a worker's or customer's needs, as mandated by the American with Disabilities Act, which requires that a business make appropriate changes in the environment to accomodate those with mental or physical disabilities as long as such changes do not create an undue (financial) burden (**Advance/Laboratory May 1994**)

'reasonable man (person)' standard MALPRACTICE A standard of behavior that is appropriate and expected for a mentally stable or 'reasonable' person* (also physician or other health care professional) under a particular set of circumstances

*eg The 'man on the Clapham bus' (see **Lancet 1992; 340:1399c**)

'reasonable physician' standard A standard of disclosure of information used in the wording of informed consent documents that is based on what is customary practice or what a reasonable practitioner in the medical community would disclose under the same or similar circumstances; in recent years, courts have increasingly preferred to accept the 'patient viewpoint' standard (***Risk Management Principles & Commentaries for the Medical Office, American Medical Association/Specialty Society Medical Liability Project, 1990, Chicago**) Cf see *Arato* v *Avedon*, 'Patient viewpoint' standard

reasonable prudence MEDICAL MALPRACTICE A legal doctrine expounded upon by Judge Learned Hand in 1932 (**60 F2d737 (2d Cir 1932**) which has become a founding principle of medical malpractice law; the doctrine is based on a maritime case that occurred in 1928; when the tugboats *TJ Hooper* and Northern No. 17 were not provided with radios, their captains were unaware of a brewing storm, and thus could not bring the coal-laden barges they had in tow to safety; the owner was held negligent for the loss of the cargo and barges; the court reasoned that had the information been available to the captains by radio, as reasonably prudent sailors, they would have put to shore (**CAP Today June 1992**)

rebound insomnia Increased insomnia of greater duration than the baseline, which may appear if long-term therapy with hypnotics is abruptly stopped, an effect that is most intense with short-acting agents; see Insomnia

RecA protein(ase) A 38-kD protein with DNA-dependent ATPase activity that is pivotal in gene recombination and SOS repair; see SOS repair

recall NEUROLOGY *noun* (*pronounced*, ree call) An operation that invokes memory of experiences or learned information *verb* (*pronounced*, ricall) To remember experiences or learned information PUBLIC HEALTH *noun* (*pronounced*, ree call) The collection on the part of a manufacturer of a product that has been deemed unsafe, or otherwise unsuitable, which has already been sold to or is intended (ie 'shipped') for sale to the public

recapitulation EMBRYOLOGY The repetition of steps or stages during development that share features with developmental sequences seen in lower animals; recapitulation occurs in the kidney which passes through pronephros and mesonephros stages before arriving at the definitive precursor structure, the metanephros, which gives rise to the adult kidney

recapitulation theory A scientifically naïve theory proposed by Haeckel, now of historic interest which held that an embryologic descendent resembled an ancestral adult

receiver MRI The component of the MRI hardware that detects and amplifies RF signals picked up by the receiver coil, which is comprised of a preamplifier, amplifier and demodulator; see Magnetic resonance imaging

receiver operating characteristic see ROC

receptor CELL BIOLOGY An integral membrane-bound protein with a highly specific recognition or target site; when a ligand, eg an antigen, drug, hormone or virus binds to its respective receptor, the cell responds by activating a membrane-bound enzyme producing 'second messengers'; in the gastrointestinal tract two such activation pathways exist: 1) The adenylate cyclase/protein kinase pathway A pathway that is activated by cholera toxin, secretin and vasoactive intestinal peptide (VIP) and 2) The calcium-inositol-protein kinase C pathway, which is activated by acetylcholine, bombesin, cholecystokinin and substance P; the chief mechanism for down-regulating the number of receptors on a cell surface is endocytosis, ie internalization of the receptor-ligand complex, forming a receptosome; see Cyclic AMP, G proteins, Protein kinase C, Second messengers

Note: Many oncogenes encode proteins with receptor activity, eg *fms* (which encodes colony-stimulating factor), *erb*B (which encodes epidermal growth factor receptor) and *erb*A (which encodes a thyroid hormone receptor in the nucleus)

receptosome A receptor-ligand-laden coated pit that has budded from the cytoplasmic surface; reduction of receptor sites in this fashion serves to down-regulate the activity of a particular substance, eg low-density lipoprotein and lysosomal enzymes

recertification Recredentialing GRADUATE MEDICAL EDUCATION A process that requires a physician or other health care professional to prove periodically that he/she has maintained his/her medical knowledge and skills at a high standard; recertification has been viewed as possibly providing a means of cost containment, although the manner by which it would be implemented is uncertain and might include reexamination by the physician's specialty board* or monitoring of the physician's methods for managing patients (**JAMA 1991; 265:752**)

*17 of 23 specialty boards (US) issue time-limited (7 to 10 years) certificates (**Arch Pathol Lab Med 1992; 116:602OA**) most recently the American Board of Pathology have offered the option for voluntary recertification (**CAP Today April1995 p3**)

recessive dystrophic epidermolysis bullosa An AR [MIM 226600] condition characterized by an abnormal fragility of the skin, in which minor trauma causes blistering below the lamina densa, accompanied by a ↓ in the number of anchoring fibrils CLINICAL Onset in infancy; by adolescence, the scarring has progressed to causing mitten-like contractions of the heands and feet, with involvement of esophageal, laryngeal, upper respiratory, and ocular mucosae that can be life-threatening MOLECULAR PATHOLOGY RDEB is the result of excess collagenase (the gene for which is in the region 11q11-q23) activity, possibly due to a structural abnormality of the enzyme TREATMENT None; because collagenase activity in fibroblasts is ↑ in RDEB, phenytoin (which inhibits collagenase in vitro) had been used, but proved ineffective in double-blinded studies (**N Engl J Med 1992; 327:163OA**)

reciprocal balanced translocation The exchange or relocation of segments of chromosome within the genome in such fashion that genes are expressed without phenotypic abnormality

recognition A highly specific binding interaction that occurs between macromolecules, eg antibody recognition of an antigen or that of tRNA with aminoacyl-tRNA synthetase

recombinant *adjective* Pertaining or referring to the structural rearrangement ('shuffling') of genetic material 1) That occurs normally during meiosis or 2) That is deliberately generated under controlled and/or experimental conditions, as in recombinant DNA *noun* An organism with a combination of alleles from either parent due to crossing over or independent assortment of chromosomes during meiosis

Note: Proteins produced in this manner are often given a prefix of 'r', eg rIL-2 to indicate interleukin-2 produced by recombinant techniques in yeasts or bacteria; because of the potential difficulties in alphabetizing recombinant molecules, in this work these terms are listed by ignoring the letter 'r', the prefix commonly used to indicate recombinant status

recombinant DNA technology MOLECULAR BIOLOGY The constellation of techniques that comprise 'genetic engineering', in which a gene producing a protein of interest from one organism is spliced into the genome of another organism, eg a phage DNA integrated into a plasmid is inserted into a 'carrier' bacterium; recombinant DNA technology entails three general steps: 1) Use of restriction endonucleases to obtain a fragment of DNA of interest 2) Joining or splicing the 'passenger' DNA fragment into a 'vector' DNA and 3) Insertion of the recombinant hybrid molecule into an actively reproducing host cell, which generates multiple copies of the inserted gene per cell; recombinant products are pure and lack the complications of animal-derived proteins, eg severe immune responses or potential mortality from human-derived products, eg human growth hormone that carried the risk of Creutzfeld-Jakob syndrome; see Genetic engineering, pBR322, Polymerase chain reaction

recombinant human colony-stimulating factors Are generally effective in treating granulocytopenia by stimulating granulopoiesis in the face of various clinical situations, eg advanced malignancy, AIDS, aplastic anemia, bone marrow transplantation, chemotherapy for solid tumors or leukemia, congenital agranulocytosis, exposure to radiation, and myelodysplastic syndromes (Arch Pathol Lab Med 1994; 118:624OA)

recombinant human DNAse Dornase alpha A DNAse produced by genetic engineering, which is delivered to the lungs by a nebulizer and is of some use in reducing the high viscosity of pulmonary secretions (which is ± 10% DNA by dry weight) in cystic fibrosis, and results in a slight improvement in pulmonary function SIDE EFFECTS Hoarseness, rash, chest pain, conjunctivitis (N Engl J Med 1994; 331:637OA)

recombinant human erythropoietin Epoietin beta, see erythropoietin

recombinant pharmacology MOLECULAR THERAPEUTICS An emerging field in which recombinant DNA techniques are used to produce DNA-derived biological products for use in treating disease or enhancing a desired biologic function; such products include: IFN-α, IFN-γ, interleukins, tissue plasminogen activator, epidermal, fibroblast, platelet-derived and transforming growth factors, erythropoietin, granulocyte-macrophage colony-stimulating factor, growth hormone, insulin, luteinizing hormone, superoxide dismutase, tumor necrosis factor and factor VIII; see Biological response modifiers

recombinant protein A generic term for any protein encoded by recombinant DNA

Note: It is common practice to preface the abbreviation of a recombinant product with a lowercase r, eg rCG

recombinase A term for the enzyme system responsible for rearrangement (recombination) of the segments (V–variable, D–diversity, J–joining, and C–constant) of antigen receptor genes of immunoglobulins and the T cell receptor; recombinase juxtaposes the gene segments, loops out and excises the intervening DNA, and joins the segments to make a mature template for transcription

recombination A normal meiotic process in which the genes from two genetically distinct individuals are mixed, resulting in progeny that differ from both parents; recombination occurs in the form of crossing-over in humans and conjugation, transduction and transformation in lower

organisms; see Recombinant DNA technology

recombination repair see Sister chromatin exchange analysis

recombination signal sequence A DNA oligomeric 'motif' that is a necessary and sufficient signal for directing the recombination of immunoglobulins, consisting of a dyad-symmetric heptamer, an AT-rich nonamer and a spacing region of either 12 or 23 base pairs; RSSs flank all recombinationally competent V, D and J gene sequences; see RAG-1, V(D)J recombination

recommended daily allowance CLINICAL NUTRITION A guideline of essential nutrients that are recommended by the Food and Nutrition Board of the National Research Council for daily ingestion in an idealized normal person engaged in averge activities in a temperate environment for optimal nutrition, here in a 'standardized' 70 kg man:

VITAMINS Vitamin A 1000 μg; vitamin D 5 μg; vitamin E 10 mg; vitamin C 60 mg; thiamine 1.2 mg; riboflavin 1.4 mg; niacin 16 mg; vitamin B_6 2.2 mg; folacin 400 μg; vitamin B_{12} 3 μg

MINERALS Calcium 800 mg; phosphorus 800 mg; magnesium 350 mg; iodine 150 mg; iron 10 mg; zinc 15 mg

The RDA must be adjusted upward during increased activity, body growth and size, pregnancy, lactation and environmental factors; the RDA are designed for a state of wellness and are poorly applicable in the sick, traumatized and burned

reconstructive surgery A generic term for any surgical procedure that attempts to restore a tissue as closely as possible to its original structure, as in cosmetic reconstructive surgery following a mastectomy or to its original functional state, or in a colostomy 'take-down', restoring a normal fecal flow; see Cosmetic surgery; Cf Mutilating surgery

reconstructive therapy Proliferative therapy ALTERNATIVE MEDICINE The *injection of natural substances* (eg dextrose, glycerine, and phenol) *to stimulate the growth of connective tissue in order to strengthen weak or damaged tendons or ligaments*; RT is reported by its advocates to be beneficial in treating various musculoskeletal disorders including bursitis, carpal tunnel syndrome, degenerative joint disease, migraines, tennis elbow, torn ligaments and cartilage (Alternative Medicine, Future Med Publishing, Puyallup, Wash, 1994) see Alternative medicine

recoverin A 23-kD cyclase protein that is central to the response of the eye to light and dark, which has a key role in the recovery of the dark state; when recoverin is stripped of the calcium that binds at the so-called 'EF hand' sites, it activates guanylate cyclase, promoting the resynthesis of cylic GMP, which in turn opens the cation channels that were closed by light, thus restoring the dark state of the rod or cone (Science 1991; 251:915, 1995; 268:221)

recovery 1) Restoration of health and strength after an illness 2) The state a person is in following a therapeutic intervention; he/she is said to be 'in recovery'

recovery position EMERGENCY MEDICINE A lateral position in which a trauma victim without suspected spinal cord injury is placed

recovery room Recovery unit An area in a hospital that is usually near the surgical suites, in which a recently operated patient is monitored for a period of several hours to ensure recovery from the anesthesia and the physiologic stresses caused by the surgical intervention, prevent post-surgical complications (eg aspiration and suffocation, arrhythmias, hypotension, and others) and/or acute decompensation of pre-existing medical conditions

recreational drug A generic term for any agent (most of which have significant psychotropic effects) that is used without medical indications or prescription in the context of social interactions, eg parties; RDs overlap with the 'classic' drugs of abuse (eg heroin, cocaine) in that their use is illegal, and are described as 'recreational' only if there is no component of addiction; see Gateway drug, Ice, Raves

recruitment DEMOGRAPHICS 1) Addition of a person or persons to a population being studied 2) Addition of a person or persons to a population, through birth or immigration (a less common use of the term) NEUROPHYSIOLOGY The ↑ in the number of active motor units involved in a neuromuscular response, which results from the temporal or spatial summation of a stimulus or through an ↑ in the intensity of the stimulus per se

recurrent laryngeal nerve SURGICAL ANATOMY Section of the recurrent laryngeal nerve had been previous standard therapy for spasmodic dysphonia, but is often complicated by late failure; botulinum toxin injection into laryngeal muscles has become an increasingly popular alternative therapy

recuts SURGICAL PATHOLOGY Sections of paraffin-embedded tissue either to confirm the presence of a lesion tentatively identified on an initial section of tissue or obtained in the context of a second opinion requested by the patient or referring physician; Cf Levels

recycling GLOBAL VILLAGE The re-use of discarded materials (in particular paper, glass, aluminum cans, but also plastics) as raw materials for other products; recycling has a positive environmental effect by reducing the energy cost of manufacturing packaging materials and disposible products, as well as reducing air and water pollution and water use per se; it is of some interest to determine whether examine the logos being used in recycling; when light arrows are over a light background, the material is *recyclable*, but has not been recycled, which according to the views of some might be viewed as a subtle form of subterfuge; light arrows on a dark background means that the material used in manufacturing the present product was recycled (Garbage Sept/Oct 1989, p38); plastics have proven difficult to recycle, in particular given that the differences in the recycling processes and melting temperatures for each major group of plastics, of which there are now at least 7 groups (see table) of plastics; in practice, only the low numbers (ie 1 or 2) are in practice recycled, while the others are added to the landfill

Note: Accidental misplacement of a recyclable plastic (despite similarities in appearance) occurs with some regularity

PLASTIC CONTAINER CODE SYSTEM

1/PETE	Polyethylene terephthalate (PET)
2/HDPE	High-density polyethylene
3/V	Vinyl/Polyvinyl chloride
4/LDPE	Low-density polyethylene
5/PP	Polypropylene
6/PS	Polystyrene
7/OTHER	All other resins

Established by The Society of the Plastics Industry

red bag A red plastic bag that conforms to the standards required for the disposal of non-'sharp' and potentially infectious biohazardous waste by health care facilities; to 'red-bag' has become a verb; see Biohazardous waste

Note: The fouling of beaches, along the Northeastern US coastline in the summer of 1988, with biological waste including blood collection tubes with viable HIV-1, resulted in stringent guidelines for disposal of all human-derived waste, requiring that it be placed in red bags for either 'in-house' incineration or transportation to landfills

red bone A microscopic descriptor for dense, avascular bone seen in advanced otosclerosis which is markedly eosinophilic by the H&E stain

Red Book INFECTIOUS DISEASES Report of the Committee on Infectious Diseases (American Academy of Pediatrics, Elk Grove Village, Ill) see Childhood immunizations PHARMACOLOGY Drug Topics Red Book A reference text[1] used by pharmacies[2] to determine the wholesale price of drugs and other therapeutic agents (N Engl J Med 1995; 332:1418OA) PUBLIC HEALTH A publication generated by the Committee on Infectious Diseases of the American Academy of Pediatrics, which contains the recommendations and immunization schedules for all licensed vaccines, information on hepatitis B control, hemophilus and measles, treatment of tuberculosis, guidelines on AIDS, recommendations and information on sexually transmitted disease and infection control in day-care settings and hopitals, and is updated every 4 to 5 years

[1]DW Sifton, 1993 Red Book, Montvale, NJ, Medical Economics Data, 1993 [2]Chemists to the British

red bugs Chiggers Microscopic chelicerate arthropods that pierce the skin producing intensely pruritic hemorrhagic and papular lesions

red cells A pictionary of erythrocyte shapes for the retentionally challenged 1) Acanthocyte 2) Leptocyte 3) Codocyte 4) Keratocyte 5) Schistocyte 6) Echinocyte 7) Drepanocyte 8) Stomatocyte 9) Spherocyte 10) Drepanocyte 11) Elliptocyte 12) Discocyte

red cell distribution width see RDW

red cell fragmentation syndrome A form of hemolytic anemia which is due to intravascular mechanical trauma with destruction of red cells related to

ABNOMALITIES OF THE HEART AND GREAT VESSELS related to mechanical intravascular defects, eg presence of prosthetic valves, synthetic grafts, valve disease, ruptured chordae tendineae, which may be accompanied by accompanied by low serum haptoglobin, hemosiderinemia and defective red cells, eg schistocytes or

SMALL VESSEL DISEASE AND/OR MICROANGIOGRAPHIC HEMOLYTIC ANEMIA related to disseminated malignancis, chemotherapy, pregnancy, DIC, pregnancy, immune mechanisms (eg SLE, scleroderma, systemic amyloidosis), hemangiomas, malignant hypertension

red cell 'flicker' MEMBRANE PHYSIOLOGY Thermally excited undulation of the red cell membrane that may be seen by phase-contrast microscopy; measurement of these undulations provides an estimate of erythrocytic elasticity, which may be markedly altered by alcohol ingestion, cholesterol loading and cross-linking agents

red cell preservative TRANSFUSION MEDICINE A medium designed to maintain a unit of packed red cells in a fluid state until the time of transfusion; the now-obsolete acid citrate dextrose (ACD) and citrate phosphate dextrose (CPD) allowed the units to be stored for 21 and 28 days respectively; the current generation of blood preservatives, citrate phosphate dextrose with adenine (CPDA) and additive solution (ADSOL) lengthen the viable shelf-life of packed red cells to 35 and 42 days respectively

Red Cross, American A relief agency founded in 1881 under a US congressional charter that fulfills American obligations in certain international treaties, serving members of the armed forces, veterans and families, aiding disaster victims, providing blood services, service opportunities, and training of hospital volunteers Headquarters: Washington DC Budget: $796 million Staff: 20 200

Red Cross, International International Red Cross and Red Crescent Movement An international Geneva-based organization with circa 150 members, which 'endeavors to prevent and alleviate human suffering wherever it may be found, to protect life and health and to ensure respect for the human being; the organization is comprised of the International Committee of the Red Cross and the League of Red Cross (LRC) and Red Crescent Societies; the LRC is similar to that of the American Red Cross, with which it is directly affiliated and plays a major role in coordinating international disaster relief, providing care for refugees outside of conflict areas, health education, blood services and coordinates education efforts and pre-disaster planning; Cf Medecins sans Frontieres

red death An obsolete term for salmon-colored discoloration of the skeletal muscle seen in gas gangrene

red degeneration Carnous degeneration A type of necrosis seen in uterine leiomyomas/fibromas that is thought to occur more commonly in pregnancy PATHOLOGY Aseptic necrosis, autolysis, hemorrhage and acute inflammation

red diaper 'syndrome' A rare form of gastroenteritis of early infancy due to *Serratia marcescens*, which produces a red pigment TREATMENT Sulfasalazine, gentamicin

red eye An inflamed eye caused by conjunctivitis evoked by allergens, bacteria, viruses and air-borne irritants, or which is related to episcleritis, corneal ulcer (infectious or traumatic), uveitis, glaucoma (acute or chronic), cellulitis and others; Cf Pink-eye

red fiber see Red muscle

'red flag' LABORATORY MEDICINE An indicator, eg an asterisk that is usually printed in red and generated in the laboratory when an analyte's value falls 'out of range', ie above or below a laboratory's predetermined values for normal; Cf Decision level, Panic value SCIENTIFIC JOURNALISM An article appearing in a peer-reviewed scientific journal which, when published, reaches startling conclusions that are likely evoke interest and therefore appear in the lay news media, eg Washington Post, New York Times, and others, which may be reported less for their scientific value than for their sensationalist impact; 'red flags' in medical journalism have included articles on the significance of vitamin C and the common cold (**Proc Natl Acad Sci 1971; 68:2678**), pancreatic cancer due to coffee consumption (**N Engl J Med 1981; 304:603**), and validation of the homeopathic principle

(**Nature 1988; 333:816**); while a major component of journalistic excellence is newsworthiness, editors of major legitimate journals dislike 'red flag' papers as any erroneous conclusions reached by the paper's author(s) may compromise the journal's credibility; see 'Media epidemic', Peer-reviewed journal

red gum disease see Erythema toxicum

red 'hepatization' A descriptor for the pathological changes in the lung seen in well-developed lobar pneumonia, which is red (due to extravasation of erythrocytes) and liver-like (firm, carnous and dense due to the accumulation of fibrin), as well as friable due to the incipient necrosis; Cf Gray hepatization

red herring An unusual clinical, radiologic or pathologic finding that should be ignored in the context of a patient's disease presentation; see Sutton's law; Cf 'Zebras'

The herring is a smoke-cured fish (*Clupidae rubis*) with a potent odor that has long had currency for training dogs to follow a scent along the ground; occasionally, the persistent odor may lead the tracking dog astray; by analogy, a 'red herring' is any detail that might side-track the diagnostician, and which should be ignored

'red hot throat' A nonspecific descriptor for an erythematous, acutely inflamed oropharynx that may occur in various infections, including *Streptococcus pyogenes*, *Neisseria gonorrheae*, *Corynebacterium diphtheriae*, *Bordatella pertussis*, and *Haemophilus influenzae* as well as various viral infections

red infarct Focal necrosis that occurs in tissues with dual circulations, eg liver and lung, which is the direct result of venous thrombosis

'red-lining' HEALTH CARE ADMINISTRATION The practice of denying certain services to individuals in a municipality based on geographic differences that have been delineated by red lines on a city map; 'red-lining' is a practice common in real estate and was attempted in an area of San Francisco in a way that would have denied health benefits to AIDS patients; the responsible health maintenance organization was fined $250 000

red man syndrome A centripetal maculopapular erythema of abrupt onset accompanied by hypotension that may occur after rapid intravenous infusion of vancomycin for gram-negative septicemia in neutropenic patients, resulting in a release of histamine causing flushing or cardiac arrest; the rash may involve the head and neck ('red neck' syndrome) or large areas of the body, and affect females ('red person' syndrome, **JAMA 1986; 55:2445c**) and resolves spontaneously in minutes to hours (**N Engl J Med 1988; 319:1053**) Note: The designation 'Red man syndrome' has also been applied to rifampin overdose (**Scot Med J 1975; 20:55**); since this condition causes an orange discoloration, the term Orange person syndrome appears preferable, although both may act by a similar mechanism

red muscle CELL PHYSIOLOGY One of the two main types of skeletal muscle, which corresponds to the 'dark' meat of chickens and contains abundant mitochondria and myoglobin; these fibers, also known as 'slow-twitch' fibers, contract and fatigue more slowly than white fibers and generate ATP by aerobic catabolism of glucose and fats, utilizing myoglobin-bound oxygen; see White muscle

red muscle cell *Myocytus ruber* [NH3] *vide supra*

red neck syndrome see Red man syndrome

red neuron A histopathologic finding in infarcts of the CNS; 6-12 hours after the onset of ischemia, neurons are swollen and display nuclear disintegration, the cell bodies are triangular with a dark blue nucleus and dense bright pink cytoplasm, resulting in myelin sheath disintegration, cell death, loss of astrocytes and oligodendrocytes

'red nose syndrome' WC Fields' nose, see there

red nucleus *Nucleus ruber* [NA6] NEUROANATOMY A prominent egg-shaped region of the tegmentum of the midbrain that extends from the caudal limit of the superior colliculus and receives deep cerebellar fibers from the superior cerebellar peduncle and some fibers from the frontal cortex and projects to the tegmentum, forming the rubroreticular tract, to the caudal region becoming the rubrospinal tract and to the lateral ventral nucleus of the thalamus

'red-out' A homogeneous red-orange color seen by GI endoscopy when the intestinal mucosa is directly covering the endoscope's lens, allowing only the passage of light across the blood vessel-rich mucosa; red-out can be corrected by a puff of air to push the mucosa away from the visual field

red pulp *Pulpa rubra* [NH3] A histologically distinct zone of the spleen that is separated from the white pulp by the marginal zone of lymphocytes; the red pulp is composed of Billroth's cords, a non-endothelialized region of slow passage of circulating red cells, where local hypoxia, low pH and low glucose cause stress on senescent, damaged or otherwise effete erythrocytes (table); Cf White pulp

---

RED PULP FUNCTIONS

CONDITIONING Readying of reticulocytes for the rigors of circulation, ie removal of up to 30% of the membrane and pitting of the last few residual mitochondria

CULLING Macrophage-induced removal of red cells erythrocytes from the microcirculation which have defective membrane proteins, crystallized cytoplasm or other defects

PITTING Removal of erythrocytic inclusions, including Howell-Jolly bodies (residual DNA), Heinz bodies (precipitated hemoglobin) and parasites (malaria, leishmaniasis)

REUTILIZATION OF IRON After hemolysis, iron is stored in the macrophages

---

red pulp disease A generic term for any infiltrative process of the spleen that preferentially affects the red pulp, including CML, heavy chain disease, iron deficiency, hairy cell leukemia, malignant histiocytosis, rheumatoid arthritis; Gaucher's disease completely effaces the splenic architecture and histiocytic lymphoma affects both the red and white pulp; see White pulp diseases

'red tape rationing' Limitation of access to a service through inconvenience ('red tape' is the paperwork generated in a bureaucratic system), which forms a major impediment to efficiency; in the US health care industry, the amount of paperwork and documentation required to justify a person's admission to hospital, treatment or continued hospitalization in the face of complications becomes enormous and has been viewed as a form of health care rationing by 'red tape'; Cf Electronic billing

red tide ENVIRONMENT A body of sea water with high concentrations of dinoflagellates, in which massive algal proliferation imparts a reddish color to the sea surface, described in the gulf of Maine (US); under optimal salinity, temperature and nutrient conditions, the marine algae, *Gonyaulax catanella* and *G tamarensis* proliferate, producing saxitoxin (a potent neuromuscular toxin that blocks voltage-dependent sodium channels in neurons), which is concentrated in clams and shellfish (but not in lobster and finned fish); birds and mammals (and humans) feeding on these shellfish rapidly develop neuromuscular blockade with intense centripetal paresthesias, nausea, vomiting, diarrhea, later vertigo, numbness of the face and scalp, sensory loss, dysphagia, dysarthria and intention tremor; if severe, intoxication may cause flaccid quadriplegia or respiratory paralysis (death); treatment is supportive

Note: Not all red tides are toxic and some outbreaks of 'red tide disease' occur without the red tide; *Gymnodinium breve* causes red tide off Florida and the region surrounding the Gulf of Mexico, but evokes milder neurotoxic reactions, including paresthesias, abnormal temperature sensation, ataxia, nausea, vomiting and diarrhea; Cf 'King-Kong' peptide

'red tide' INFECTIOUS DISEASE A colloquial phrase from the 1950s that died in the 1960s, which referred to the finding that many bacterial infections were gram-negative, ie 'red', an observation attributed to the virtually indiscriminate use of the first widely available antibiotic, penicillin (which is most effective against gram-positive coccal bacteria) for every conceivable infection, resulting in a relative increase in the incidence of infections by gram-negative bacteria, which are pink by the Gram stain, causing a 'red' shift; this imbalance shifted towards equilibrium with the availability of aminoglycosides, agents that are more effective against gram-negative bacteria

red urine disease A generic term for any clinical condition associated with red urine (a term of little diagnostic utility), which include hematuria secondary to glomerulonephritides, bladder tumors, foreign bodies or calculi, infection, inflammation, thrombosis and conditions that may be diagnosed by examining the urinary sediment; less common causes of red urine include trauma-related myoglobinuria or hemoglobinuria, congenital erythropoietic porphyria, porphyria cutanea tarda, acute intermittent porphyria, pyrrolinuria, ingestion of beets, phenol sulfonphthalein, fuchsin, aniline dyes in candy and food, anthraquinolone laxatives if the urine is alkaline, desferroxamine, rifampin, isoniazid and under unusual circumstances, aspirin

redwater fever VETERINARY MEDICINE A term of waning popularity for bovine babesiosis

reducing atmosphere A humid atmosphere rich in oxidizable gases including hydrogen, hydrogen sulfide, nitrogen, ammonia and methane that is thought to have existed on the primitive earth of 4.5 billion BC; see Bubble hypothesis; Cf Primordial soup

reducing substance LABORATORY MEDICINE A generic term for any substance that readily reduces cupric ion in hot alkaline solution; the normal level of RSs in the urine is is 0.5-1.5 mg/dL; an $\uparrow$ of RSs implies a pathological $\uparrow$ in the urine of glucose and galactose; other RSs include sugars (arabinose, fructose, lactose, maltose, ribose, and xylose), endogenous metabolites (ascorbic acid, creatinine, cysteine, glucuronic acid, hippuric acid, homogentisic acid, ketone bodies, oxalaic acid, and uric acid), or exogenous substances (cinchophen, formaldehyde, isoniazid, nalidixic acid, probenecid, salicylates, and sulfanilamide); once an excess of RS is identified in the urine, it can be further characterized by fermentation, optical rotation, specific chemical test, paper chromatography or TLC (assuming it is a sugar), or by chromatography if it is not (**NW Tietz, Textbook of Clinical Chemistry, WB Saunders, Philadelphia, 1986**) see Reducing sugars

reducing sugars Disaccharides that are linked with an

aldehyde or ketone group and the hydroxyl group of another nonreducing sugar, eg galactose, lactose, glucose, maltose, fructose and pentose; reducing sugars are formed by action of amylase on starch and measured by reduction of phosphomolybdate, ferricyanide or 3,5-dinitrosalicylate; the presence of reducing sugars suppresses β hemolysis, therefore should not be used in tests for identifying streptococci; assays for reducing sugars may be false positive by the copper reduction test, in the presence of endogenous or exogenous substances; see Reducing substances

reduction mammoplasty A generic term for a surgical procedure intended to decrease the size of hypertrophied and/or ptotic breasts, which may become a significant disability Procedure Most techniques require a pedicle to carry the nipple areola to the new position, or if the breasts are gigantomastic, the nipple areola is removed and repositioned as a full-thickness graft; general anesthesia is almost invariably required as the blood loss may be significant; Cf Augmentation, Mammoplasty

reductionism A philosophy that higher levels of (often arbitrary) complexity can be understood through reduction to their simplest components; see Lumping; Cf Splitting

redundant publication MEDICAL JOURNALISM An irresponsible practice in which one or more authors try or succeed in getting 'more mileage' from a study than is appropriate, by submitting the same paper to two or more journals; *'The reasons for preventing redundant publication are not arbitrary...multiple reports of the same observations can overemphasize the importance of the findings, overburden busy reviewers, fill the medical literature iwth inconsequential material, and distort the academic reward system.'* (N Engl J Med 1995; 333:449) RP is usually perpetrated by a small group of authors who are attempting to obtain the maximum academic advantages from a relatively small study; this contrasts with 'redundant' publication of 'mega-studies', eg the GUSTO (Global Utilization of Streptokinase and Tissue plasminogen activator for Occluded coronary arteries) trial, the Framingham Heart Study, and others in which the population being studied is enormous and the data of such complexity that splitting the results into multiple soundbites of information is perfectly legitimate; see Salami slicing

Reed-Sternberg cell A large (15-45 µm), binucleated or bilobed, often arranged as a 'mirror image' cell with condensed chromatin at the periphery of the nuclear membrane, large dark 'owl-eyed' nucleoli surrounded by a clear halo; the cytoplasm is abundant and amphophilic; RS cells are the sine qua non requirement for the diagnosis of Hodgkin's disease and are most abundant in the lymphocyte-depleted type; the mononuclear variant cells, while non-diagnostic, may represent an early RS cell and the bi- and multinucleated form may corresponds to RSCs in phases of terminal differentiation EM Large nuclei, dispersed chromatin, large nucleoli, abundant polyribosomes ImPx Classic RS cells express CD30 (Ki-1), CD15 (Leu-M1), Ia-like antigen and peanut lectin receptors; see Hodgkin's disease; Cf Pseudo-Reed-Sternberg cell

reeler An allele, the homozygous mutation of which in mice causes a selective architectonic defect in the cerebellar and cerebral cortex in early embryos and failure of neurons to reach their correct location in the developing brain, resulting in ataxia, incoordination, and tremors in older animals (Nature 1995;374:719, 675)

reelin A 388-kD protein encoded by the *reelin* gene (located in the region of the *reeler* allelic locus on chromosome segment 7q22) that has features of a secreted extracellular protein, and which has homology to F-spondin; reelin is thought to act as a regional 'pathfinder' involved in the primordial organization of the cerebellar and cerebral cortices, and according to this model, is secreted locally by early postmigratory neurons to serve as a neuron-matrix adhesion molecule, and help stabilize early architectonic patterns (Nature 1995;374:719, 675)

re-entry CARDIOLOGY The re-excitation of a region of the heart by a single electrical impulse, which may cause ectopic beats or tachyarrhythmia; re-entry is the common cause of paroxysmal atrial or supraventricular arrhythmia, which is coupled to premature ventricular depolarization; for re-entry to exist, there must be a one-way complete block in conduction, coupled to tissue (eg scar tissue) that responds more slowly to electrical impulses arriving from 'the other end'; once begun, re-entrant arrhythmias are self-sustaining; re-entry may be ordered (ie the circuit for the re-entry is constant) or random (the re-entry circuits are variable in duration and location)

re-entry tear VASCULAR SURGERY The most distal intimal tear seen in a dissecting aortic aneurysm, a point that is presumed to be the site where the blood returns to the circulation

reference LABOR RELATIONS The name of a person that is placed on a resume/CV (curriculum vitae) with whom an applicant for a job or a position (eg professional school) has had a formal relation, and who the applicant believes will speak favorably on his/her behalf; references exist in two often distinct formats, the formally written form, which has greater legal weight but is less often used to select a candidate for a job or position, and the informal verbal form, in which the person being used as a reference is called on the telephone to verify what might have been placed on paper (MLO April 1995, p48) LIBRARY MEDICINE 1) Information that is regarded as authoritative and widely accepted in a particular field, which may be in the form of 'standard' texts (eg Principles and Practice of Infectious Diseases by GL Mandell et al, Churchill-Livingstone) or peer-reviewed journals (eg New England Journal of Medicine) 2) The term reference is also commonly used (albeit incorrectly) as a synonym for citation, as in Nature 1995;374:675

Note: The dichotomy between written and verbal recommendations or references may be extreme, and it is a challenge for a potential employer using the reference as a basis for hiring a candidate to translate what is exactly meant; *'works well with people'* might translate as '...probably works better with animals', *'respected by peers'* might actually mean that the candidate was tried but never convicted for two mafia-related homicides; *'conscientious'* may mean the candidate has a debilitating obsessive-compulsive personality disorder; because of this dichotomy, written references may prove less than reliable

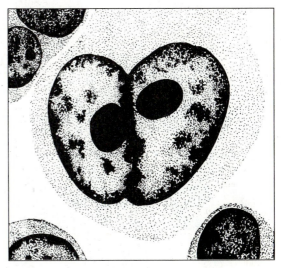

Reed-Sternberg cell

reference interval Reference range, see there

reference laboratory A generic term for any (usually for-profit) laboratory dedicated to performing a broad menu of tests at a distance from the patient, usually outside of the hospital; the referring of clinical specimens is an increasingly common practice in most regions of the world for various reasons

SPACE Certain types of testing, eg virology, mycobacteriology may require large amounts of space that is not available in hospital laboratories

COST, VOLUME, STAFFING The price of performing a wide range of tests are minimal in reference labs as they have the advantages of 'economies of scale' in terms of costs, number of tests performed, and skill of staff performing the tests

TECHNOLOGY The implementation of emerging technologies requires an outlay or monies and expertise until testing methods become automated or standardized

In the the US, there are currently 6000 reference laboratories, which are shrinking in numbers, by either attrition or as a result of buy-outs from the large national laboratories*, which account for 30% of the total reference laboratory testing (**Advance/Laboratory September 1994**) Cf Expert laboratory, Specialized laboratory

*eg The Corning 'family', which includes Metpath, Damon, and Nichols (1992 revenues ± $1.3 x 10⁹), SmithKline/Beecham (± $1.1 x 10⁹), National Health/Allied (± $860 x 10⁶), Roche (± $500 x 10⁶)

reference man A hypothetical male whose anatomic, biochemical, laboratory (chemistry, hematology), and physiologic values represent the norm; the RM is an idealized entity with human physical and physiological characteristics determined by international consensus that serves to standardize experimental results and relate biological insults to a common base

While the concept of an RM if useful in certain areas, eg physiology and anatomy (see Virtual man), the use of references intervals (ranges) for ♂ (and ♀), stratified by age provides far more useful information in the laboratory environment and reduces the risk of placing of a person's values out of range- Author's note

reference manual LABORATORY MEDICINE A test menu produced by a clinical laboratory that includes information on patient and specimen preparation, causes for specimen rejection, and interpretation of results, information on test panels (batteries of tests for a particular disease or organ system), billing information, and name(s) of 'specialized' laboratories to which the laboratory sends (refers) specimens requiring tests not being performed 'in-house' (**CAP Today July 1993**) Cf Procedure manual

reference method LABORATORY MEDICINE Any analytical technique that is highly accurate and used as a 'gold standard' by which other tests that measure the same analyte are compared; in general, the RM has at least one feature (eg too tedious and/or time-consuming; radioactivity in RIA) that prevents it from being used on a routine basis

reference range LABORATORY MEDICINE A set of values established as reasonable maximums or minimums for a given analyte; in order for a laboratory to produce accurate results, ie to control its quality, it must be certain that the normal results are consistent and fall within the range of 'normalcy' and that abnormal results fall outside of this reference interval, which is usually two or more standard deviations above or below a laboratory's mean; most laboratories pool sera from patients who have 'normal' values for the analyte being measured; in establishing the reference range 1) The reference subjects should be normal, healthy and, if indicated, subdivided into various age groups, sex, occupation, ethnic origin or other parameter 2) The laboratory should use a consistent protocol, in which the precision, reliability and accuracy are delineated, preferably on the same instrument; the sample should be obtained under 'standard' conditions, ie pre- or postprandial, similar volume, where each test tube has a standard amount of anticoagulant and thus differences in volume would yield differences in coagulation studies 3) The range for the reference value should be broad enough to encompass the vast majority of normal subjects 4) The statistical methodology and decisions for 'tail cutoffs' must be clearly and logically delineated and 5) The range must allow for updating of patient pool, new clinical data and new methodologies; Cf Decision levels, Panic values

reference technology LABORATORY MEDICINE The constellation of methods and materials that provide a base for assessing analytical accuracy and reproducibility (**Arch Pathol Lab Med 1993; 117:343-436oA**) see Matrix effect

referral A colloquial term for a patient who has been sent (referred) for a second opinion or therapy to a specialist or subspecialist with greater expertise, as the patient has a disease or condition that the primary or referring physician is incapable of or does not wish to treat; see Second opinion

referral center Tertiary care hospital, see there

referral center bias Any skewing in morbidity or mortality statistics based on data generated from referral centers (a term that is often synonymous with tertiary care center, see there), which may not be representative of the population that a hospital of a similar size might service; see 'Institutional effect'

referral and consultation MEDICAL MALPRACTICE The act of sending a patient with disease that is difficult to treat or diagnose to a respected and competent* colleague for a second opinion; consultation should be sought when the diagnosis is difficult, the illness is unfamiliar, complex or fraught with complications, the patient doesn't improve in a reasonable period of time and at the patient's request; see Malpractice, Physician expert

*It is imperative that competent specialists be used for R&C-if the consultant is proven incompetent, the referring physician shares in the liability for negligent acts allegedly performed by the consultant

referred pain Pain that is localized to a region other than the site of disease, eg pain from a myocardial infarct is classically referred to the jaw and upper arm

refining CLINICAL NUTRITION The processing of a food substance to extract a component of interest, usually referring to the refining of sugar; health and natural food advocates are highly critical of this process and tout beet sugar, molasses and honey to be far superior to refined or 'white' sugar, although the nutritive value of the 'virgin' products in terms of trace minerals and vitamins is minimal; see 'Health' food, Organic food

reflectance photometry LABORATORY MEDICINE A form of photometry that measures diffuse reflected light that results when a reaction mixture in a carrier is lighted or from the diffusion of light by a reaction mixture in an illuminated carrier; the intensity of the reflected light from the reagent carrier is compared to the intensity of light reflected from a reference surface; the intensity of the reflected light is not linear with the analyte's concentration; the relation between concentration and reflectance is linearized using certain algorithms (**NW Tietz, Textbook of Clinical Chemistry, WB Saunders, Philadelphia, 1986**)

reflective (eye) protection OCCUPATIONAL SAFETY A generic term for a format of eye protection in which the material (a multilayered film of dielectric material, eg manesium fluoride) used to reduce visible light transmittance (which is necessary when working with lasers) is coated on the lens itself; although their light weight makes them popular in the workplace, REP has the disadvantage that scratches in the lens allow transmission of light (**Biophotonics Intl 1995; 2/2:26**) see Absorptive protection, Eye protection device

reflex diagnostic testing LABORATORY MEDICINE The performance of a test on a patient specimen only after a particular analyte is abnormal or outside of predetermined range; reflex testing is a cost-effective way in which a patient can be further evaluated without the need to draw a second specimen, eliminating the inherent delay in initiating appropriate therapy; reflexes used in clinical laboratories include leukocytes > 20 x 10⁹/L (US > 20 000/mm³) which reflexes into a manual differential cell count, a positive sickle cell screen that reflexes to hemoglobin electrophoresis, an albumin/globulin ratio < 1.0 that reflexes to serum protein electrophoresis, and cholesterol of > 240 mg/dL that reflexes to a coronary artery disease risk profile; Cf Red flag

reflexive ordering see Reflex diagnostic testing

reflexology A form of massage therapy based on the belief that there are nerve endings (up to 72 000, according to one estimate) for most organs and body parts in the feet; there is no proof that reflexology is an effective therapeutic modality; see Alternative medicine, New Age

reflux laryngitis A clinical form of acid reflux characterized by '...*hoarseness, persistent nonproductive cough, a sensation of pressure in the throat and a continual need to clear the throat. The classic symptoms of reflux, such as heartburn and regurgitation are often minimal or absent.*' DIAGNOSIS ± Reflux, and pH abnormalities TREATMENT Omeprazole may be effective (**N Engl J Med 1994; 331:656cc**) see Acid-reflux disorders

reform see Health care reform

refractive surgery OPHTHALMOLOGY A generic term for operative techniques that correct myopia by changing the cornea's conformation; two procedures are currently available, radial keratectomy (a procedure in which incisions are made at the edge of the cornea, flattening it, but weakening its overall structure) and photoreactive keratectomy (a technique that cuts concentric circles in the cornea, 'photoshaving' the center of the cornea, imparting a more homogenous consistency)

refractory anemia with excess blasts HEMATOLOGY A myelodysplastic syndrome of older individuals which is characterized by anemia or pancytopenia and bone marrow hypercellularity CLINICAL Nonspecific findings, including anemia of gradual onset, fatigue, weakness, exacerbation of underlying heart disease if present; 50% of patients are asymptomatic, and the cytopenia is discovered during a 'workup' for other reasons LABORATORY Anisocytosis, megaloblastoid maturation of erythroid precursors, thrombocytopenia; 5-20% of the marrow cells are blasts; less than 5% of the peripheral cells are blasts CYTOGENETIC 50% of patients with MDS have cytogenetic abnormalities, most commonly 5q–, but also monosomy 5 or monosomy 7 PROGNOSIS Guarded, with the average patient surviving less than 1 year; about ¼ undergo leukemic transformation, usually into ANLL TREATMENT Not all patients require therapy; ⅓ die of bleeding or infectious complication linked to pancytopenia; intensive cytotoxic chemotherapy has been used, and may merely substitute one cause of morbidity and mortality for another; cytokines and growth factors may prove effective in the future-stay tuned; see Myelodysplastic syndrome, PISA

refractory hypertension A condition characterized by blood pressure ≥140/90 (≥160/90 if older than 60) in which there is an absence of features of secondary hypertension, maximal dose of at least two* antihypertensive agents is being administered, and adequate time has passed to allow the usual antihypertensive regimen to be effective Note: RH can occur in both essential (primary) and in secondary hypertension DIAGNOSIS & CONTROL Spurious (pseudohypertension) and 'white coat' hypertension must be excluded, as should noncompliance with the antihypertensive regimen, or the presence of exogenous substances that either ↑ the blood pressure (alcohol, anabolic steroids, caffeine, chlorpromazine, cyclosporine, erythro-

poietin, MAOIs, nicotine, sympathomimetic agents, tricyclic antidepressants) and/or interfere with therapy (cocaine, corticosteroids, NSAIDs, sodium chloride); obesity should be controlled (**N Engl J Med 1992; 327:543RV**)

*The term refractory hypertension formerly required nonresponsiveness to three or more agents; given the efficacy of newer agents, 90% of hypertension can be controlled with one or two agents; the remaining 10% are considered refractory

refrigerator 'AIDS' RAIDS A laboratory artifact consisting in an inversion of the ratio of T helper to T suppressor cells (T4:T8 or CD4:CD8 ratio), which occurs when flow cytometric specimens are refrigerated prior to analysis, causing a relative decrease in the CD4+ T cells; see AIDS, Helper:suppressor ratio

refugee GLOBAL VILLAGE A person who, owing to a well-founded fear of being persecuted for reasons of race, religion, nationality, membership in a particular social group or political opinion is compelled to live outside of the country of his nationality; refugees may also include those fleeing from war, civil disturbance, and violence of any kind; a permutation is that of an 'internally displaced' person who moves within the borders of one country for the same, above-mentioned reasons; the mortality rate of refugees is 60-fold greater than that of a similar non-displaced population, is highest in children and is due to measles, diarrhea-related illnesses, acute upper respiratory tract infections, malaria and is in part related to the virtually endemic protein-energy malnutrition and micronutrient deficiencies that characterize the refugee state; there are an estimated 18.5 million refugees worldwide; diarrhea is the most common cause of death; 36 000 children die/day of diarrhea (**JAMA 1991; 266:638, 1992; 268:1986**) see Amnesty International, Red Cross; Cf Disaster, Homeless(ness), Torture

Regan isoenzyme A variant alkaline phosphatase first identified in Patient Regan, a young white male who died from bronchogenic carcinoma metastatic to the lymph nodes, adrenal glands, spleen, kidney, and brain; the Regan isoenzyme is a heat-stable, L-phenylalanine-sensitive carcinoplacental enzyme, similar to placental alkaline phosphatase in electrophoretic mobility which occurs in circa 5% of carcinomas as well as occasionally in normal subjects

regeneration PHYSIOLOGY The sum total of activities leading to regrowth of cells and tissues, eg the healing of a wound; tissues with a high rate or potentially high rate of regeneration, include bone marrow, GI tract, liver and skin; 'stable' populations with a low rate of regeneration include the adrenal gland, kidney, liver, lymph nodes, pancreas, thyroid gland; neural tissue and cartilage are regarded as non-regenerative

regionalization The subdivision of a broadly available service, eg a blood bank, into quasi-autonomous regional centers capable of making decisions and provide better and/or faster service to hospitals and health care facilities that are located the greatest distance from a 'centralized' service's hub

regression CLINICAL MEDICINE The subsiding of disease symptoms or return to a state of health* '*The act of returning to some earlier level of adaptation.*' (**RJ Campbell, Psychiatrc Dictionary, 6th ed, Oxford Univeristy Press, New York, 1989**) Regression is typical of a variety of mental disorders, where there is a conscious or unconscious desire to return (regress) to a state of dependency, as when one was a child STATISTICS Linear regression, see there

In the working medical parlance, it is common practice to use the term *remission* (see there) for regression of symptoms in chronic progressive diseases, eg multiple sclerosis and malignancy, and *resolution* for regression of symptoms of for disease processes that are normally reversible, eg infections-Author's note

regression line STATISTICS A line that defines the amount of change in one variable per unit change in the other; see

regressively transformed germinal centers SURGICAL PATHOLOGY A morphologic finding of uncertain significance seen in lymph nodes characterized by small germinal centers, a marked paucity of lymphocytes, an 'onion-skin' layering of dentritic reticulum cells, fibroblasts, vascular endothelial cells and eosinophilic, hyalinized, PAS-positive intercellular material; see Germinal centers; Cf Progressively transformed germinal centers

regulated waste Waste products that must be handled in a specified fashion in accordance with governmental regulations; regulated waste can be divided into

BIOHAZARDOUS WASTE Potentially dangerous infectious agents, often originating from health care facilities and/or research laboratories; these waste products place a relatively small or confined group of people at risk for infection during the time necessary for the infectious agent to desiccate or otherwise become inactive; see Biohazardous waste, 'Sharps'

RADIOACTIVE BYPRODUCTS from clinical and research laboratories or power stations that emit radiation ranging from low-level and virtually innocuous α particles to high-level γ–radiation emitting products that must be stored decades or centuries in specialized vaults and

NON-BIODEGRADABLE CHEMICALS, including heavy metals, dioxins, halogenated biphenyls, terphenyls, naphthalenes, dibenzodioxins and related products that are toxic to biological systems in very low (parts per million or parts per billion) concentrations, originating from a vast array of manufacturing processes, which unlike biohazardous waste, create problems from the 'cradle to the grave', requiring special precautions during manufacture, storage, shipping, consumption, and disposal; since many of these chemicals are lipid-soluble, they may store for long periods in the adipose tissues of workers handling these products

regulator gene R gene A gene that encodes a DNA-binding protein repressor that controls an operator site on the DNA

regulatory agency A generic term for any agency, organization or body of a federal, state or local government that creates, promulgates, and enforces rules concerning the delivery of a service or product; see Environmental Protectional Agency, OSHA (Occupational Safety and Health Administration)

regulatory proteins MOLECULAR BIOLOGY Proteins that were first discovered in bacteria, which bind to specific regulatory sites in DNA and are crucial in controlling transcription; the structural motifs and chemical modifications that convert the inactive to active forms of regulatory proteins, eg chain cleavage, methylation and phosphorylation, are similar at all levels of phylogenic differentiation

rehydration solution Any fluid that is used to treat severe bacterial (eg *Vibrio cholerae, Escherichia coli*) or viral (eg Rotavirus) diarrhea; these conditions are rarely accompanied by systemic disease other than the severe prostration inherent in massive fluid loss, and are usually the result of intestinal cAMP cyclase having been been locked into an 'on' position, which causes a 'flushing' that responds only to time and appropriate fluid replacement (antibiotics are rarely useful); two types of RSs are available, glucose-based, which ↑ intestinal resorption of fluids and electrolytes, and rice-syrup-based solution, which in addition ↓ the stool output, and therefore may be the agent of choice (N Engl J Med 1991; 324:517)

reimbursement HEALTH CARE FINANCING Payment by a third-party, eg an insurance company, to a hospital, physician, or other health care provider for services rendered to an insured person (beneficiary)

re-infibulation The surgical re-establishment of infibulation, a form of female circumcision after the perineal tissues have been torn by birth-related trauma; infibulation is a form of genital mutilation that is integral to many cultural groups in Africa and symbolizes the society's control

over a woman's fertility; it is being increasingly frowned upon by those in the developed nations; the British Royal College of Obstetrics and Gynecology has made it clear that it regards re-infibulation as illegal (N Engl J Med 1994; 331:712SA) see Female circumcision, Infibulation Cf Clitoridectomy

reinforcement PSYCHOLOGY A generic term for any activity, either a reward (known as positive reinforcement) or punishment (negative reinforcement) that is intended to strengthen or extinguish a particular response or behavior, making its occurrence more probable, intense, or frequent

Reinke space ENT/SURGICAL ANATOMY A potential space located between the internal elastic lamina of the thyroarytenoid (vocalis) muscle and the external elastic lamina; RS is limited on the superior surface of the true vocal cord (TVC) by superior linea arcuata, and extends from the vocal process of the arytenoid muscle to the anterior limit of the TVC; in the presence of lesions of the TVC, eg phonotrauma, the RS fills with fluid (JJ Ballenger, Disease of the Nose, Throat, Ear, Head & Neck, 14th ed, Lea & Febiger, Philadelphia, 1991)

reinsurance pool HEALTH CARE REFORM A common fund that helps insurers mitigate the high financial loss inherent in insuring high-risk groups and individuals (Am Med News 25 October 1992, p7)

rejection An immune reaction evoked by allografted organs; the prototypic rejection occurs in renal transplantation, which is subdivided into three clinicopathologic stages

HYPERACUTE REJECTION Onset within minutes of anastomosis of blood supply, which is caused by circulating immune complexes; the kidneys are soft, cyanotic with stasis of blood in the glomerular capillaries, segmental thrombosis, necrosis, fibrin thrombi in glomerular tufts, interstitial hemorrhage, leukocytosis and sludging of PMNs and platelets, erythrocyte stasis, mesangial cell swelling, deposition of IgG, IgM, C3 in arterial walls

ACUTE REJECTION Onset 2-60 days after transplantation, with interstitial vascular endothelial cell swelling, interstitial accumulation of lymphocytes, plasma cells, immunoblasts, macrophages, neutrophils; tubular separation with edema/necrosis of tubular epithelium; swelling and vacuolization of the endothelial cells, vascular edema, bleeding and inflammation, renal tubular necrosis, sclerosed glomeruli, tubular 'thyroidization' CLINICAL ↓ Creatinine clearance, malaise, fever, hypertension, oliguria

CHRONIC REJECTION Onset is late (often more than 60 days after transplantation), and frequently accompanied by acute changes superimposed, increased mesangial cells with myointimal proliferation and crescent formation; mesangioproliferative glomerulonephritis, and interstitial fibrosis; there is in general a poor response to corticosteroids

see Cyclosporin A, Graft-versus-host disease, Tacrolimus (FK 506)

rejuvenation solution TRANSFUSION MEDICINE A solution that may be used to salvage outdated O-positive and O-negative red cells, which can then be glycerolized and frozen for future use; one such solution, PIPA,contains pyruvate, inosine, phosphate and adenine, which after a one-hour incubation at 37ºC, 'restores' ATP and 2,3-diphosphoglycerate (2,3-DPG) levels to 150% of the levels at the time of donation; see Red cell preservatives, Storage lesion(s)

relapse ONCOLOGY Recrudescence of the manifestations of malignancy, often leukemia; in ALL, the most common sites of relapse are in the BM, testes and central nervous system; aggressive treatment of these sites (eg intrathecal) at the time of initial diagnosis is held responsible for the relatively high cure rate in leukemia; 80% of children and 50% of adults with a relapse of ALL may achieve a second, albeit short-lived remission and some may be cured; the quantity of residual leukemic progenitors (as determined by a combination of flow cytometry and cell sorting with assays of leukemic progenitor cell colonies) is a powerful predictor of relapse following autologous BM transplantation (N Engl J Med 1993; 329:1296OA) see Bone marrow transplantation, Chemotherapy, Cyclophosphamide, Terminal cancer; Cf Remission

relapsing fever Epidemic borreliosis (caused by *B recurrentis*) is louse-borne (*Pediculus humanis*) and transmitted in a person-to-person fashion CLINICAL History of recent outdoor camping, fevers with 'negative' blood cultures, Jarisch-Herxheimer-like hypotensive 'crises' following therapy with antibiotics and thrombocytopenia Endemic borreliosis (*B recurrentis, B hemisi, B turicatae, B parkeri* and others) is transmitted by ticks (*Ornithodoros* spp) that inject borrelia during a blood meal CLINICAL Abrupt onset of high fever, headache, photophobia, nausea, vomiting, myalgias, arthralgias, abdominal pain, productive cough and minimal respiratory distress; late relapses typically involve the central nervous system (meningismus, peripheral neuritis, cranial nerve paralysis) TREATMENT Tetracycline, erythromycin, chloramphenicol

relapsing polychondritis An uncommon condition characterized by inflammation and cartilaginous degeneration, beginning about age 40 CLINICAL Fever, vasculitis and arthropathy DIAGNOSIS 3+ of the following symptoms (in descending order of frequency): auricular chondritis with ear drooping, non-erosive arthritis, nasal chondritis with saddle nose deformity, upper respiratory obstruction, audiovestibular symptoms and cardiovascular disease, eg aortic insufficiency PROGNOSIS 74% five-year and 55% ten-year survival

relative biological effectiveness RADIATION BIOLOGY The ratio of the effect that one form of ionizing radiation has on a biological system to that of an identical dose of a different form of ionizing radiation, a value of interest since equal doses of different types, eg neutrons, γ and X-rays, of ionizing radiation do not produce equal biological effects, eg if 6 Gy of X-rays and 4 Gy of neutrons are lethal to a biological system, then the RBE is 1.5; the former standard used to compare different radiations was 250-kV X-rays, chosen at the time of standardization, as it was the only level widely available

Note: Although RBE is firmly entrenched in the literature, it suffers from problems of comparison

relative bradycardia see Pulse-temperature dissociation

relative polycythemia A spurious ↑ in red cells with a normal red cell mass, and a ↓ in blood volume; RP may occur in a background of mental stress, alcohol abuse, use of diuretics, or in acute nephritis; erythropoietin (EP) levels are normal (± 7 U/L) in contrast to polycythemia vera, in which EP is ↓ (± 2 U/L) or secondary polycythemia, in which the EP is ↑ (± 120 U/L) (Br J Haematol 1992; 81:603) Cf Polycythemia vera

relative tachycardia see Pulse-temperature dissociation

relative value scale Resource-based relative value scale, see there

relative risk see Risk

relative value unit RVU* HEALTH CARE FINANCING A comparative financial unit defined in the context of the resource-based relative value scale used by Medicare (US) for calculating reimbursement; an RVU integrates such disparate factors as the value of the physician's service, practice overhead and malpractice costs; as examples, the RVU for reading a chest film is 0.28, for a routine office visit is 1.0, and for repairing a hernia sac 10.9 (N Engl J Med 1994; 330:607OA)

relaxation MOLECULAR BIOLOGY Any conversion of a system to a state requiring less energy, eg the conversion of a supercoiled DNA molecule to a non-twisted form or the return of muscle to a ground state; Cf Protein folding

relaxation time MRI The time period after excitation that is required for spins to return to a ground state or state of equilibrium distribution, in which there is no transverse magnetization and the longitudinal magnetization is at its maximum value and oriented in the direction of the static magnetic field; the transverse magnetization decays toward zero with a characteristic time constant T2; the longitudinal magnetization returns toward the equilibrium value M_o with a characteristic time constant T1; see Magnetic resonance imaging

relaxed helix A double-stranded circular DNA molecule in which the supercoils have been reduced in number by a topoisomerase

relaxin An insulin-like polypeptide that is produced by the corpus luteum and relaxes parturition-related ligaments at the symphysis pubis and sacroiliac junctions, and softens the uterine cervix during pregnancy

releasing factor Releasing hormone

Relman's criteria see Authorship

'Relman revision' MEDICAL JOURNALISM A modification by former editor (Arnold S Relman, MD) of the New England Journal of Medicine, of the Ingelfinger rule of medical journalism, which requires a news media 'blackout' until the time an article is published in the NEJM; Relman modified the Ingelfinger rule to allow early release of critical information with great potential impact on patient management prior to formal publication in the NEJM (Am Med News 11 March 1991) see Embargo arrangement, Ingelfinger rule; Cf Clinical alert, Media epidemic

rem Roentgen-equivalent in man A unit of absorbed radiation, approximately equal to a rad or 0.01 Seivert; see Gray, Sievert

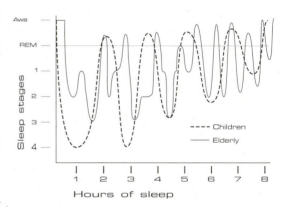

REM sleep Rapid eye movement sleep, desynchronized sleep A 5-20 minutes in duration segment of the normal sleep cycle characterized by irregular heart rate and respiration and blood pressure similar to the awake state; RS is further characterized by involuntary or jerky muscular movement and a higher threshold for arousal; the usual high-amplitude slow brain waves seen by EEG are replaced by rapid eye movement, rapid, low-voltage irregular EEG activity, a pattern similar to that seen in an awake and alert subject, thus also being known as paradoxical or desynchronized sleep; in RS, skeletal muscle tone is lost due to an increase in activity of the reticular inhibiting area of the medulla and clusters of large phasic potentials originating in the pons (pontogeniculo-occipital spikes); dreaming occurs during RS and is the most refreshing form of sleep; in the fetus, RS predominates and may switch to the cyclical pattern as early as two days after birth; RS is characterized by profound sympathetic activation and may be linked to changes in muscle tone;

these changes may play a role in triggering ischemic events, eg myocardial infarction or ischemic stroke (**N Engl J Med 1993; 328:303**OA) see Insomnia, Sleep disorders

REM syndrome Reticulate erythematous mucinosis syndrome in Fitz of dermatology, pg 1671

REM twitch A transient restoration of muscle tone occurring during REM sleep which is associated with cessation of sympathetic discharge and an increase in blood pressure (see **N Engl J Med 1993; 328:303**OA)

remedial advertising Advertising that attempts to rectify a situation in which a company has falsely misrepresented the drug's efficacy or approved uses; see Advertising

remedial profession A generic term for any specialty or area of allied health, eg occupational, physical, recreational, or speech therapy, and rehabilitation psychology that provides assistance or therapy, usually for those with physical handicaps

reminder advertising Advertising that calls attention to a drug's existence in the market; any claims of efficacy in reminder activities requires that the promotional activities meet 'fair balance' and brief summary requirements; see Advertising

remission ONCOLOGY The regression of symptoms or lesions in a malignancy, most commonly referring to the disappearance of a lympho- or myeloproliferative tumor by radio- or chemotherapy and amelioration of clinical symptoms, which may be temporary, partial or complete; a complete remission of long enough duration, eg two years in childhood lymphocytic leukemia, is termed 'permanent remission' or cure, the goal of therapy for all malignancies; see Cure; Cf Relapse

Note: Leukemia therapy hinges on 1) Induction of remission, which is attainable in more than 90% of children and 50% of adults with ALL, using a combination of vincristine, prednisone and doxorubicin 2) CNS prophylaxis The first site of relapse in most children is the CNS, an event largely prevented by 24 grays (2400 rads) of prophylactic radiotherapy, often in combination with intrathecal methotrexate and 3) Maintenance Continuation, consolidation or intensification (of therapy); in ALL, standard maintenance regimens include cycles of methotrexate, 6-mercaptopurine and 'pulses' of remission-inducing agents; when parenteral vincristine and intrathecal methotrexate are administered in the same therapeutic session, there is a real danger of inadvertent switching of syringes and intrathecal administration of vincristine, an error that is well-described in the literature and universally fatal, regardless of how quickly intrathecal 'washout' begins

remodeling CARDIOLOGY The progressive left ventricular dilation that follows a myocardial infarction, a finding that has prognostic import; remodeling can be quantified by measuring the end-systolic and end-diastolic volumes (**N Engl J Med 1992; 327:669**OA)

renal agenesis A rare disease of infants characterized by bilateral renal agenesis, low-set floppy ears, a broad, flat nose and pulmonary hypoplasia; these infants die within hours after birth; infants with unilateral renal agenesis have normal lung development and are asymptomatic in the neonatal period

renal allograft see Renal transplantation

renal epithelial neoplasm An all-encompasing term for any neoplasm of the renal epithelium, which are classified (see table) based is on recent information provided by molecular cytogenetics

'renal' glycosuria A relatively common (1:500) AR condition in which glycosuria occurs without hyperglycemia and is unrelated to diet, the subjects are asymptomatic, have a normal glucose tolerance test and utilization and storage of carbohydrates, but may become transiently ketotic in stress or pregnancy

renal insufficiency A generic term for defects in the kidney's ability to 'clear' waste products, a sign of adequate glomerular filtration

renal panel see Kidney panel

renal transplantation The transplantation of a kidney from a living donor or cadaver to a recipient with end-stage renal disease; in children the most common indications for transplantation in children are congenital malformations of the kidney and urinary tract (42%), and focal segmental glomerulosclerosis (12%); 31% of children were ≤ age 5 years (**N Engl J Med 1992; 326:1727**OA) PROGNOSIS 1-year survival of graft/patient; 43% of grafts came from living relatives with 1– and 3-year survivals of 89%/80%; 57% were of cadaver origin with 1– and 3-year survivals of 74% and 62% ($^{\text{Graft survival\%}}$/$_{\text{Overall survival\%}}$)–Living donor (6482*): HLA identical $^{94.8}$/$_{98.2}$ sibling-1 haplotype match $^{90.9}$/$_{97.9}$ parent-1 haplotype match $^{90.2}$/$_{98.2}$ offspring-1 haplotype match $^{88.6}$/$_{94.2}$ unrelated person, eg spouse $^{86.5}$/$_{95.5}$ Cadaveric (32 932) First transplant $^{79.8}$/$_{94.0}$ Second transplant $^{94.1}$/$_{94.0}$ Subsequent transplants $^{65.5}$/$_{92.1}$ (**N Engl J Med 1994; 331:365**RV) see Organ shortage

Note: The marked race-related disparity in survival of renal allografts is a function of HLA mismatches, and socioeconomic factors (**N Engl J Med 1992; 327:840**OA) *Data are from the US Scientific Registry for Organ Transplantation and the Organ Procurement and Transplantation Network (1990 data)

renal tubular acidosis A condition caused by functional defects in the distal renal tubules, with loss of ability to form ammonia and to exchange hydrogen cations; the glomerular filtration rate is normal with persistent metabolic acidosis and hyperchloremia, there is marked decrease in urinary excretion of acid LABORATORY Acidic urine with acidosis, low bicarbonate excretion, poor ammonium clearance and increased clearance of potassium (table)

renaturation The reforming of a molecule's native configuration after it has been altered by environmental pressures, eg high salt or temperatures MOLECULAR BIOLOGY The reassociation of complementary single strands of nucleic acids into a double-stranded form

renin PHYSIOLOGY A highly specific aspartyl proteinase with one known substrate, angiotensinogen; renin is secreted by the granular cells of the juxtaglomerular apparatus (as well as in the brain and endothelial cells) in response to reduced renal perfusion pressure or decreased kallikrein and cleaves angiotensinogen to yield angiotensin I (a decapeptide), which is the precursor of angiotensin II (an octapeptide) and angiotensin III (a heptapeptide), the latter two of which are potent vasoconstrictors, stimulating thirst and increasing aldosterone production; renin secretion is increased in tumors, malignant hypertension, during increased secretion of CRF (corticotropin-releasing factor), Cushing's disease unlike previously reported, there is no association between plasma renin activity and myocardial infarction (or sudden death from cardiovascular disease) in normotensive males (**N Engl J Med 1993; 329:616**OA) TREATMENT Estrogens and vasodila-

---

RENAL EPITHELIAL NEOPLASMS

ONCOCYTOMA

CHROMOPHOBE CARCINOMA

PAPILLARY NEOPLASM

ADENOCARCINOMA, NOT OTHERWISE SPECIFIED (CLEAR/GRANULAR)

COLLECTING DUCT CARCINOMA

NEUROENDOCRINE TUMORS

   CARCINOID

   SMALL CELL CARCINOMA

Am J Clin Pathol 1995; 103:624OA

BACKGROUND Formerly '...*discussion of renal epithelial neoplasia...was essentially a discussion of renal adenocarcinoma and its cytologic and architectural subtypes.*'

tors; see Hypertension

renin-angiotensin(-aldosterone) system PHYSIOLOGY A biochemical feedback system that plays a key role in regulating blood pressure and vascular tone, and maintaining salt and water homeostasis; renin is a proteolytic enzyme stored in the juxtaglomerular complex (apparatus), the secretion of which is stimulated by sodium depletion, diuretics, hypotension, hemorrhage, etc; renin cleaves angiotensinogen, a glycoprotein formed in the liver forming the decapeptide angiotensin I (A–I); A–I is split by angiotensin I converting enzyme* (ACE) into an octapeptide, angiotensin II (A–II), a potent vasoconstrictor that also stimulates the synthesis and secretion of aldosterone and evokes a dipsogenic esponse in the CNS; further breakdown of A–II results in the heptapeptide A–III which has 40% of the pressor activity of A–II, but 100% of its aldosterone-stimulating activity; the genes encoding components (eg angiotensinogen gene) of the RA system are intimately linked to essential hypertension (**N Engl J Med 1994; 330:1629**OA) the RAA system is activated by congestive heart failure, cirrhosis, edema, nephrosis, protein loss, malignant hypertension, renal artery stenosis; renal vasoconstriction is increased and renin and aldosterone secretion is decreased in those at risk for hypertension

*The formal term for ACE recommended by the Nomenclature Committee of the IUBMB (International Union for Biochemistry and Molecular Biology) is peptidyl-dipeptidase A [EC 3.4.15.1] Note: Minor actors in the control of blood pressure include atrial natriuretic peptide and the kallikrein-kinin system, prostaglandins, (especially PGE_2), arginine and vasopressin

RENAL TUBULAR ACIDOSIS

TYPE I 'Classic' distal RTA, which is due to a selective defect in distal tubule acidification, resulting in a defect in the pH gradient, causing hyperchloremia (with persistent bicarbonate excretion), hypokalemia and mild-to-moderate metabolic acidosis; the urinary pH is inappropriately high (> 6)

TYPE II RTA is accompanied by decreased acidification of the proximal tubule; when the blood pH is decreased, tubular acidification occurs normally; when plasma bicarbonate normalizes, type II RTA wastes bicarbonate, causing metabolic acidosis, as well as hyperchloremia and hypokalemia, which may be accompanied by the Fanconi syndrome; these patients are prone to osteopenia and rickets

'TYPE III' A designation formerly applied to infants with renal bicarbonate wasting that is now considered to be a subtype of type I RTA

TYPE IV RTA Generalized (nonselective) distal RTA, due to aldosterone deficiency or antagonism; hyperchloremia, hyperkalemia, metabolic acidosis and salt wasting

renovascular hypertension Systemic hypertension due to renal artery obstruction by atherosclerosis, fibroplastic disease, aneurysms, and embolism; see Goldblatt kidney; RVH has a wide range of effects, causing hemorrhage in the cerebellum, pons, internal capsule and basal ganglia **ESSENTIAL HYPERTENSION** The kidneys display granularity of cortical surface, and are hisstologically characterized by hyaline atherosclerosis in afferent glomerular capsular arteries, which later become tortuous, thick-walled and narrowed, thus becoming a source of chronic ischemia, which is accompanied by 'piecemeal' necrosis of glomeruli **MALIGNANT HYPERTENSION** The kidneys grossly display 'Rat-bite' scars, and are histologically characterized by arterionephrosclerosis and glomerular capillary necrosis with thrombosis (necrotizing glomerulonephritis), as well as 'flea-bitten' kidneys, with acute glomerular rupture with pinpoint fibrinoid necrosis (hypertensive arteriolitis), petechial hemorrhages on cortical surface, fibrinoid

necrosis of the distal interlobular 'onion-skinned' arteries and afferent arterioles with thrombosis, juxtaglomerular apparatus hyperplasia (also seen in acute and chronic glomerulopathies, hypertension, DM, and polycystic kidney disease) TREATMENT, MEDICAL Empirical, as a function of the severity of disease and a patient's individual response to the available agents, which include diuretics, β-adrenergic blockers, vasodilators, and angiotensin-converting enzyme TREATMENT, INTERVENTIONAL Percutaneous transluminal angioplasty of the renal artery, 60-70% success rate in atherosclerosis; 90% success rate in fibromuscular hyperplasia

'rent-a-doc' A highly colloquial, usually deprecative term that serves as both noun and adjective for, or referring to a physician functioning in a locum tenens position, see there

reovirus A family of naked (non-enveloped), 1-4.0 kilobase double-stranded RNA viruses, which includes orthoreovirus, orbivirus and rotavirus. which are uncommon causes of gastroenteritis, rhinopharyngitis, occasionally hepatitis and rarely, encephalitis, pneumonia and Colorado tick fever; see Rotavirus

repeat Repetitious DNA, see there

repeated free induction decay MRI A form of MR in which repeated 90° pulses are applied, which results in partial saturation if the interpulse times are equal or less than T1; see Magnetic resonance imaging

reperfusion therapy Any of a number of therapeutic maneuvers (eg thrombolytic therapy-tissue thromboplastin activator-tPA, or immediate percutaneous transluminal coronary angioplasty-IPCTA) intended to ensure continued blood flow (and oxygenation) through a vascular bed that has been acutely compromised, by either vasospasm or thrombotic occlusion or stenosis; reperfusion therapy is most common in the coronary vessels of the heart in an acute MI; given the limited success of thrombolysis related to hemorrhage, the virtual impossibility of reperfusing all the occluded coronary arteries, recurrent myocardial ischemia and the relatively low number of appropriate candidates for thrombolysis, IPCTA is superior to t-PA for acute MI, reducing nonfatal reinfarction or death, and has a lower rate of intracranial hemorrhage (**N Engl J Med 1993; 328:673**OA), and is superior to streptokinase, having a higher rate of patency of the infarct-related artery, less residual disease, improved ventricular function, less recurrent myocardial ischemia or MI (**N Engl J Med 1993; 328:680**OA)

repertoire The array of molecules (or capabilities) that are inherent, but not necessarily expressed in a system, a term most commonly used in immunology, referring to the broad responsiveness to specific antigenic signals that both B and T lymphocytes have as a result of the different combinations of genes (variable, diversity, joining) that can be spliced together to create the exquisitely specific immunoglobulins (B cells) or T-cell receptors (T cells)

repetitious DNA Repetitive DNA Any sequence of DNA that is present in multiple copies in a particular genome, a finding common in eukaryotes; 'highly repetitious' segments of DNA, are short (5-10 nucleotides) oligomers, virtually identical in sequence to each other and present in thousands to millions of copies per genome, usually as non-functional or 'spacer' DNA; these short, identical DNA fragments, also known as simple sequence DNA, comprise 10-15% of the genome; 'intermediate repeats' are moderately repetitious segments of DNA comprising 25-40% of the genome, ranging from 150-300 nucleotides to 6000 nucleotides in length, known as SINES (short interspersed elements) or LINES (long interspersed elements) and are present in up to several hundred copies per genome; the RD that encodes rRNA, tRNA and histones is known as Tandem repeat DNA

repetitive motion injury Cumulative trauma disorder OCCUPATIONAL MEDICINE A work-related illness* of the fastest growing health problem in the US, affecting such diverse groups as the textile industry, meat-packers, and keyboard operators

*ie One that develops over time, rather than an injury, which is an abrupt event

replacement analysis LABORATORY MANAGEMENT A relatively simple set of rules used to determine the economics of replacing or updating present equipment 1) Determine actual cash outlay, ie the amount of money needed to replace the equipment, including 'trade-in' value and depreciation on old analyzer, shipping, and start-up costs 2) Compare costs of running the old vs the new piece of equipment (for 5 years, asking such questions as 'does it ↑ the throughput of tests and therefore increase productivity?') 3) Add after-tax salvage value after the device's useful life has ended 4) Add net cash flow in Internal Rate of Return or Net Present Value equation (**Advance/Laboratory July/August 1994**) Cf Breakeven analysis

replacement vector A type of lambda cloning vector that accepts 9–23-kb DNA inserts, which is most commonly used for genomic library construction; Cf Insertion vector

replicating fork MOLECULAR BIOLOGY A Y-shaped region in a replicating DNA molecule in which there is separation of the parent strands of DNA and synthesis of daughter chains; a model system of DNA replication using SV40 was reconstituted using the T antigen (of the SV40 virus) and purified cellular proteins; DNA polymerase–α/primase both synthesizes the RNA-DNA primers for initiating DNA replication at the origin and primes each Okazaki fragment (**Nature 1994; 369:207A**) see Okazaki fragments, Replication, Replication bubble

replication The process of synthesizing a daughter DNA molecule from a parent DNA 'template', which for the double-stranded DNA typical of eukaryotes, occurs during the S phase of the cell cycle in a bidirectional fashion; the DNA is unwound from histones, separated by a helicase into single connected strands of DNA from which a leading and continuous daughter strand of DNA grows in the 3'→5' direction, mediated by DNA polymerase; the lagging and discontinuous daughter strand uses the opposite parent DNA strand as a template, also grows in the 3'→5' direction and requires the action of a DNA polymerase, a primase and a ligase to join the short daughter strands, known as Okazaki fragments; see Lagging strand, Leading strand, Meselson-Stahl experiment, Okazaki fragments

replication bubble Replication eye MOLECULAR BIOLOGY One of multiple transiently expressed bead-like structures that are seen by electron microscopy along a segment of double-stranded DNA, corresponding to multiple sites of simultaneous DNA replication, where each of the bubbles corresponds to growing forks of daughter DNA with replication of double-stranded DNA occurring in both directions simultaneously; see Replicating fork

replication licensing factor CELL BIOLOGY A complex of proteins that is essential for replication of DNA, which gains access to chromosomes during mitosis, and which is inactivated after a single round of replication(**Nature 1995; 375:418, 421, 360**)

replicative antisense MOLECULAR BIOLOGY A technique that radically alters the cellular expression of specific genes, by '...*inserting a gene into the genome in such a way that the RNA transcribed from the gene is opposite, or 'antisense', to the normal, 'sense' RNA. When the cell transcribes both the sense and antisense genes, the antisense RNA can interfere with the translation of the sense RNA by binding to it directly.*' (**Nature Medicine 1995; 1:389**); RA has a wide range of potential DNA-based applications in agriculture, cancer therapy, and the pharmaceutical industry; see Antisense DNA

'report card' HEALTH CARE MANAGEMENT A generic term for a hospital- or physician-specific mortality report* which is updated on an annual basis; one of the first such reports, the Cardiac Surgery Reporting System generated by the New York State Department of Health, indicated that the percentage of patients who died after cardiac surgery differed widely, even after adjusting for differences in patient attributes; while the use of RCs is controversial, the rate-adjusted death rate for coronary artery bypass grafting has declined in New York, suggesting to some workers that provider-specific reporting (ie report cards) may save lives, although according to the US General Accounting Office, '*no evaluative studies have been conducted to determine the report cards validity or reliability.*' (**N Engl J Med 1995; 332:1229SB**)

*A report card is that which school children recieve on a period basis as a formal mechanism to monitor their progress

replicon MOLECULAR BIOLOGY A functional unit of replication, which contains an initiator locus, the site where RNA polymerase binds and produces an RNA primer known as an initiator and a replicator locus, the site of the initiation of replication

reportable occupational disease Reportable event PUBLIC HEALTH A generic term for an occupational or environmentally-related morbid condition that a local, state, or federal government wishes to maintain under surveillance; each of the states in the US has occupational diseases of particular interest, which often overlap, including asbestosis, bronchitis and acute pulmonary edema due to fumes and vapors, byssinosis, caisson's disease, coal worker's and other pneumoconioses, heavy metal, lead, pesticide and radiation poisoning, intoxication with acid, alkali, antimony, benzene, beryllium, cadmium, chlorinated hydrocarbons, chlorine, chromium, Freon™, hydrogen cyanide, manganese, mercury, petroleum products, other solvents and sulfur dioxide), pulmonary fibrosis, silicosis; non-occupational events that require reporting to central health authorities include AIDS, child abuse, drug addiction, venereal disease, (gunshot or stab) wounds; for reportable infectious disease, see Notifiable disease

reporter gene A synthetic gene, the phenotype of which is relatively easy to monitor, as it contains a regulatory (promotor) sequence from one gene coupled to the coding region of another gene, the expression of which can be easily measured (eg by enzymatic or immunologic methods); a reporter gene system allows dissection of promoter functions, eg hormonal sensitivity; RGs may be used to study promoter activity at different points in an organism's development; in recombinant DNA technology, reporter genes may be attached to a promoter region of interest

repressed memory PSYCHOLOGY An event that occurred in a subject's past, the memory of which was actively repressed often because of the psychologically devastating impact of that memory, eg childhood abuse, rape, molestation (**New York Times May3, 1994; C1**); see False memory, Source amnesia

repressor MOLECULAR BIOLOGY A protein that binds to certain (operator) genes at silencer sites, interfering with the function of activators, slowing (or stopping) the transcription rate (**Sci Am 1995; 272/2:56**) see Operator, Transcription activator

reproducibility LABORATORY MEDICINE The degree of agreement among repeated measurements of a particular parameter, which is presented in terms of a standard deviation or coefficient of variation of the results in the set of measurements; reproducibility can be divided into within-run, between-day, and total imprecision-types (**Arch Pathol Lab Med 1992; 116:714OA**); reproducibility is the most critical aspect of any clinical method and is the core criterion for establishing the validity of scientific data

reproductive history OBSTETRICS A set of four numbers that may be used to define a woman's obstetric history, eg 4-3-2-1, would mean four term infants delivered, three preterm infants, two abortions, one child currently living; since this system leads to confusion, it is recommended that only parity and gravidity be used, supplemented with gestational information where relevant

reptation LABORATORY TECHNOLOGY The movement of a substance in a snake-like fashion; reptation occurs in the high-voltage gel electrophoresis of large DNA molecules, and refers to the loss of the sieving effect, which introduces drag to molecules that is proportional to their length, thereby allowing separation of molecules according to size; at a certain length of molecule, the sieving effect falls off, and molecules begin to migrate at similar speeds, regardless of size, and 'reptate' through the gel; see Field inversion electrophoresis

reptilase time HEMATOLOGY The time that reptilase, an enzyme from *Bothrops atrox* venom, requires to cleave fibrinopeptide A, a value that is increased in hypofibrinogenemia < 0.8 g/L (US <80 mg/dl), dysfibrinogenemia and DIC, but not by heparin-induced coagulopathy

res ipsa loquitur Latin, the thing (fact) speak for itself MEDICAL MALPRACTICE A legal doctrine that helps a plaintiff recuperate damages for negligence despite circumstances under which it would be impossible for him/her to prove that negligence occurred; in *res ipsa loquitur*, the plaintiff's burden to prove negligence is fairly light, and often does not require expert witnesses, as the details of the incident are clear and understandable to a jury eg a sponge left behind during surgery; *res ipsa loquitur* is evoked whenever damages would not have occurred in the absence of negligence or had the person in charge (of the patient's management) used 'due' care; see Malpractice

rescue EMERGENCY MEDICINE Any activity that brings a person who is a victim of disaster or accident to safety; Cf Disaster ONCOLOGY Rescue therapy, see Leucovorin rescue

research A generic term for '*scientific inquiry to discover or verify facts, test hypotheses, and confirm theories*' (International Dictionary of Medicine, J Wiley & Sons, New York, 1986) see Notebook, Rs of research; Cf Fraud in science

reserve cell hyperplasia GYNECOLOGIC CYTOLOGY A proliferation of cuboidal subcolumnar cells under the squamo-columnar junction of the uterine cervix; reserve cells appear early in the cervix of infants and are thought to be the cell at risk for malignant degeneration in squamous cell carcinoma of the uterine cervix

residential fire PUBLIC HEALTH A fire occurring in a place of residence; RFs (North Carolina) are often caused by (cigarette) smoking (31% of fatal fires), are more common in mobile homes (odds ratio 1.7), and in those without smoke detectors (odds ratio 3.4); alcohol-impairment was the strongest risk factor for death in RFs (odds ratio 7.5) (N Engl J Med 1992; 327:859oA)

Note: The US statistics for RFs are not easily translated to other parts of world; in the US, most residences are constructed from wood; many citizens live in single-family houses; and the mobile home (the 20th Century version of the nomads' tent) is a common type of residence in certain regions

residency A period of formal graduate medical education that consists of on-the-job training of medical school graduates, which is sponsored by and takes place in a teaching hospital; residencies often follow a one-year internship, are from two to six years in duration, and precede a fellowship; a completed period of residency is required for certification by specialty boards; see Fellowship, GME, Internship; Cf CME (continuing medical education), Extern, Intern

residual bodies Aggregates of undigested granular or coarsely laminated material seen by electron microscopy within lysosomes in a wide variety of clinical conditions, including sea-blue histiocytosis, granular cell myoblastoma and in changes associated with aging, eg lipofuscin deposition

residue Amino acid residue BIOCHEMISTRY The functional portion of a monomeric 'unit' in a polymer (eg an amino acid in a protein or a nucleotide in a sequence of DNA) that lacks the atoms removed during the polymerization process, which is analogous to a building block without the mortar; amino acid residues (–NH–CHR–CO–) in polypeptides include a removed hydrogen atom, a hydroxyl group or a molecule of water, depending on the amino acid's position in the protein

resolution CLINICAL MEDICINE The stage of a disease process (often an infection) that is marked by subsidence of symptoms LABORATORY MEDICINE Definition The minimum distance or degree of separation between two points that can be identified as distinct, defined in terms of light microscopy (aka 'resolving power') or EM, X-ray diffraction patterns, electrophoresis, chromatography or other separation procedures MRI Spatial resolution The ability of the imaging process to distinguish among adjacent structures within an object being image (which is a measure of image's quality); the criterion for determining resolution depends on the type of test being used (bar pattern or contrast detail phantom); the ability to separate or discern objects depends on their contrast and different MRI object parameters affect different imaging techniques, thus for example, comparison of resolution phantom tests from different machines may be difficult as the images differ; see Magnetic resonance imaging

resonance energy transfer assay A fluoresence assay based on quenched fluorogenic substrates, which allows the continuous monitoring of proteolytic activity based on the fluctuations in fluorescence intensity with time (Science 1990; 247:954)

resource(s) The components of a system, eg equipment, space and labor that are available to perform a task of any nature, a term that has currency in the parlance of clinical laboratory bureaucrats HEALTH CARE FINANCING The source of support, eg insurance, personal income

resource-based relative value scale HEALTH CARE ADMINISTRATION A scale that was developed by W Hsaio et al (Harvard U), which ranks physicians' services by the labor required to deliver those services; the RBRVS was sponsored by the Health Care and Financing Administration (HCFA contract 17-C-98795/1-03), in an effort to address the inequalities of physician reimbursement and its data is based on the current procedure codes (CPT codes) for the services paid by Medicare and may be used by Medicare, the major health insurance intermediary in the US to determine which procedures are or are not overpriced; see CPT codes, DRGs, Overrated procedures

resource utilization group HEALTH CARE ADMINISTRATION Any of a number of groups into which a resident in a nursing home is categorized based on the resident's functional status and anticipated use of services and resources; RUGs are similar in concept to DRGs but are calculated on a per-diem rather than a per-case basis as there is a need to provide continuing care in nursing home residents (N Engl J Med 1995; 332:581Rv) see Functional assessment

respirator brain NEUROPATHOLOGY A brain characterized by global necrotic softening* of the cerebral cortex, seen in 'brain dead' bodies that have been kept 'alive' for prolonged period of time by means of mechanical support; Cf Coma dépasse

*With a consistency between custard pudding and egg-drop soup-Author's note

respirator rules An informal set of guidelines for using respirators in an environment potentially contaminated with *Mycobacterium tuberculosis*: Only those trained on the use of and fitted for a respirator should use one; all those present in the potentially contaminated room (PCR) should wear one; the PCR should be at a negative air pressure; respirators should be worn until leaving the PCR; respirators may be reused until they no longer pass spot inspections; respirators should be stored in containers that do not retain moisture (CAP Today Nov 1994 p1) see HEPA respirator

respiratory burst An abrupt ↑ in the consumption of O_2 that is followed by a cascade of metabolic events occurring in neutrophils and mononuclear cells prior to bacteriolysis, which is designed to produce microbicidal oxidants by partial reduction of oxygen; the RB is activated by the same stimuli (contact with ingestible particles or high concentrations of chemotactins) that evoke neutrophil degranulation; the initial event in the respiratory burst is a one electron reduction of O_2 to O_2^- (superoxide) by membrane-bound oxidase; the H^+ liberated in the accompanying hexose monophosphate shunt reaction combines with the oxygen, forming H_2O_2; see Oxygen free radicals

respiratory chain complex(es) A group of proteins encoded by the mitochondrial structural genes that are responsible for the oxidation-reduction reactions in mitochondria Complex I catalyzes the oxidation of NADH by coenzyme Q (ubiquinol) and is composed of seven subunits Complex II catalyzes the oxidation of succinate by coenzyme Q Complex III catalyzes the oxidation of reduced coenzyme Q (ubiquinol) by cytochrome c Complex IV catalyzes the oxidation of reduced cytochrome c by oxygen itself Complex V corresponds to ATP synthase, which consists of two subunits

respiratory distress syndrome see Adult respiratory distress syndrome

respiratory distress syndrome of the newborn see Hyaline membrane disease

respiratory syncytial virus A virus of the family Paramyxoviridae, genus *Pneumovirus,* that measures 100 nm, and encodes at least ten unique 9.5 to 160 kD viral proteins; RSV causes respiratory infection with its morbidity and mortality occurring in infants ≤ two years old, especially those underlying cardiovascular or pulmonary disease TREATMENT High-dose RSV immune globulin (N Engl J Med 1993; 329:1524oA)

'respiratory syndrome' A relatively specific immune response to high-dose rifampin therapy, characterized by a flu-like complex, dyspnea and wheezing, leukopenia and thrombocytopenia; other hypersensitivity reactions caused by rifampin include flushing, fever, pruritus without rash, urticaria, eosinophilia, hemolysis and interstitial nephritis-induced renal failure

respondeat superior Latin, let the master answer for the servant MEDICAL MALPRACTICE A legal doctrine that holds an employer responsible and liable for an employee's wrongful act; thus in *respondeat superior*, the liability for a negligent act is passed to 'captain of the ship', eg the surgeon, despite the fact that the act is performed by another person, eg an operating room nurse; under the doctrine *respondeat superior*, the hospital may claim that although the hospital is the nurse's employer, at the time of the negligent act, the nurse was under someone else's (eg the surgeon's) guidance; application of r*espondeat superior* requires that there be proof of a 'master-servant' or controlling relation; since this doctrine does not absolve the employee of liability, both the injured party and the employer may sue the employee for negligence; see also 'Captain of the ship', 'Deepest pockets', Malpractice

restenosis The reformation of stenosis following otherwise adequate therapy, which may occur in a mitral valve after replacement, or in a coronary artery after angioplasty, an event occurring in 35-45% and 50-60% of those who have undergone single and multivessel procedures; the risk of restenosis is greatest in those patients with activated smooth muscle cells (identified by in situ hybridization for ↑ expression of the B isoform of nonmuscle myosin heavy chain) (N Engl J Med 1993; 328:603oA) see Smooth muscle cell

resting energy expenditure PHYSIOLOGY A metabolic value that corresponds to the energy cost of maintaining transmembrane ion gradients and baseline cardiorespiratory activity; the REE represents approximately 60% of the total energy expenditure (N Engl J Med 1995; 332:621oA) see Total energy expenditure

restless legs syndrome An idiopathic clinical complex characterized by nocturnal cramping of the anterior calf, restlessness, a feeling of heaviness, painful paresthesia and tingling of the legs with uncontrolled twitchings, interfering with sleep; the condition is usually idiopathic, but may occur in uremic polyneuropathy and hypercalcemia or may be associated with sleep disorders TREATMENT Home remedies, eg hot baths, creams and cotton stockings may be as effective as the commonly prescribed clonidine, alternation of chemically unrelated substances (benzodiazepines, opiates, L-DOPA) or transcutaneous electrical nerve stimulation (JAMA 1991; 265:3014o&A)

restraint 1) Control or prevention of an action 2) Any device used to restrict the free movement of patients with behavioral or physical problems, who may cause harm to themselves and others; restraints are most commonly used in the elderly with dementia; physical restraints include chairs with locking lap trays, wrist and ankle cuffs, belts and Posey vests, which are used for from 25 to 85% of nursing home patients; pharmacologic restraints include anxiolytic, neuroleptic, sedative or hypnotic agents, which are used on 11 to 72% of patients, especially if the patients are physically abusive (JAMA 1991; 265:1278)

restricted area OCCUPATIONAL SAFETY An area, the access to which is strictly limited to essential personnel with the purpose of protecting individuals against undue risk from exposure to various materials, eg ionizing radiation, high-level pathogens, toxic chemicals and others

restriction MOLECULAR BIOLOGY The chopping of 'invading' double-stranded DNA (eg of a phage) by any of a number of bacterial endonucleases at short (4-8 nucleotide) highly specific palidromic sites; see Palidrome, Restriction endonuclease

restriction diet A diet intended to reduce the incidence of various conditions, eg

ATHEROSCLEROSIS Goal: Reduction of body weight Method ↓ Saturated fat and cholesterol and ↑ consumption of bran

HYPERTENSION Goal: Reduction of blood pressure Method ↓ Salt-only ½ of patients have a pressor response to salt restriction

CANCER ↑ Dietary fat has been linked to cancer of the breast, colon, prostate and possibly also ovaries; polyunsaturated fats are a substrate for peroxidative reactions and should be reduced; ↑ fiber and cruciferous vegetables in the diet is linked to ↓ colonic carcinoma, an effect thought to be due to ↓ contact of the colonic mucosa with carcinogens; alcohol consumption is associated with hepatoma, oropharyngeal and esophageal cancer with very low cholesterol

RENAL FAILURE Goal: A low protein diet slows the progression of renal failure, see End-stage renal disease

restriction endonuclease A bacterial enzyme that recognizes short (4-6) oligonucleotide sequences, known as 'restriction sites' and cleaves double-DNA wherever such sequences occur; the restriction sites are usually inverted repeats or palindromes, ie they are the same on each chain when they are read in the same direction, leaving a short 4 to 6, single-stranded 'sticky' end of DNA at each site of scission; see *Eco*RI, *Hin*dIII

restriction fragment length polymorphism see RFLP

restriction-minus MOLECULAR BIOLOGY A generic adjective pertaining or referring to a cloning vector that has been specifically designed so that restriction sites that are normally recognized by a host bacterium's native restriction endonucleases do not exist

restrictive cardiomyopathy The least common of the cardiomyopathies (in the US); it is characterized by a 'stiff' ventricle, with diastolic dysfunction, often in the presence of normal systolic function; RC may be due to myocardial hypertrophy, fibrosis, or an infiltrative process, and accompany amyloidosis, collagen-vascular disease, eosinophilia, fibroplastic disorders, hemochromatosis, and neoplasia

RET assay Resonance energy transfer assay, see there

***RET* proto-oncogene** A gene located in the pericentromeric region of chromosome 10 that encodes a transmembrane receptor tyrosine kinase; *MEN-2A* the gene mutated in multiple endocrine neoplasia type 2A, is located at exon 10 or 11 of the *RET* proto-oncogene (N Engl J Med 1994; 331:828OA) see MEN-2A gene

retained acid syndrome A condition occurring in 25% of those treated (time of onset 2nd day to 3rd week of therapy) with all-*trans*-retinoic acid (eg for acute promyelocytic leukemia) CLINICAL Fever, dyspnea, pulmonary infiltrates, pleural effusions PATHOGENESIS Unknown, possibilities include release of vasoactive cytokines, ↑ expression of cell adhesion molecules on myelocytes, acquisition of migratory properties by leukemic cells as they undergo differentiation TREATMENT Immediate therapy with corticosteroids; discontinuation all-*trans*-retinoic acid may be ineffective (N Engl J Med 1993; 329:177RV) see Acute promyelocytic leukemia

retained antrum syndrome A rare complication resulting from the inadequate resection of the distal antrum and pylorus during antrectomy and a Billroth II gastrojejunostomy; in its new location, the retained antrum's pyloric glands are bathed in alkaline secretions, stimulating gastrin release from antral and pyloric cells, resulting in *de novo* peptic ulceration; see Postgastrectomy syndromes

retention time LABORATORY TECHNOLOGY The amount of time that a substance requires to pass through an analytical column, eg in HPLC; the retention time in combination with the amont of absorption at a specific wavelength results in a signature that can be compared to standards and quantify compounds of interest

reticulate (initial) body MICROBIOLOGY A stage of development of *Chlamydia trachomatis*, where multiple perinuclear lobated 2-6 μm gray-brown masses have lost the dense acidophilia characteristic of the preceding elementary body; see Intermediate body

reticulin The loose fibroconnective stromal support tissue of the bone marrow; reticulin increases with age, marrow reticulin ranges from 0-1+ (few discernible fibers) in normal subjects to 4+; a coarsened collagen fiber network is characteristic of myelofibrosis

reticulocyte count The number of immature erythrocytes or reticulocytes in the peripheral blood, which display basophilic reticulum (residual RNA) when stained with a supravital dye, eg brilliant cresyl blue; the RC serves as a simple means of evaluating the rate of red cell production Note: Because of delayed or premature release of erythrocytes from the bone marrow and different rates of cell maturation, correlation of peripheral reticulocytes with erythrocytic hyperplasia is not absolute

retin-A Retinoic acid, see there

retinal 11-*cis*-retinal Vitamin A aldehyde A retinal pigment that absorbs visible light at 400-600 nm, resulting in an isomeric transition of the 11-*cis*-retinal moiety to a trans-retinal conformation causing a G protein-mediated depolarization event

retinal anlage tumor see Pigmented neuroectodermal tumor of infancy

retinal detachment OPHTHALMOLOGY Separation between the neurosensory (rods and cones) retina and the retinal pigment epithelium, opening the vestige of the cavity of the optic vesicle of the embryo; RD is a true ophthalmologic emergency, that requires immediate therapy to prevent blindness; RD affects 18-30 000/year (US) ETIOLOGY 1) Retinal tear, which may be caused by vitreous traction, and results in vitreous fluid accumulation 2) Exudative detachment, in which the neurosensory retina is lifted away from the retinal pigment epithelium by fluids that accumulate in response to local tumors (eg melanoma), local inflammation, or malignant hypertension CLINICAL Progressive loss of visual field, often accompanied by scotomas TREATMENT A silicone oil has been approved by the FDA to treat complicated RTs thar are not correctable with standard therapy (New York Times 8 Nov 1994; C3)

retinal 11-*cis*-retinal Vitamin A aldehyde A retinal pig

(all-*trans-*)retinoic acid Tretinoin The naturally occurring form of the fat soluble vitamin A, which is critical for the transportation of monosaccharides in glycoprotein synthesis as occurs in the turnover of mucosal epithelia of the oral cavity, respiratory and urinary tracts; see Retinal, Retinoic acid receptor, Tretinoin, Vitamin A

Note: According to the most authoritative reference, the Merck Index (of chemicals, drugs, and biologicals), 11th edition, the term preferred for this chemical is retinoic acid, the term tretinoin is more widely used in a therapeutic context, which explains it being listed in two different places in the present work-Author's note

all-*trans*-retinoic acid

retinoic acid receptor RAR One of two receptors for retinoids which has three distinct isoforms (α, β, and γ) which are activated by two bioactive retinoids, all-*trans*-retinoic acid and 9-*cis*-retinoic acid; RARs play a major role in organ development, especially of skin (Nature 1995; 374:159, 118N&V) Cf Retinoid X receptor

retinoid X receptor RXR One of two receptors for retinoids which has three distinct isoforms (α, β, and γ) which are activated by 9-*cis*-retinoic acid; RXRs play a major role in organ development, especially of skin (Nature 1995; 374:159, 118N&V) Cf Retinoic acid receptor

retinol Vitamin A

retinitis pigmentosum A heterogenous group of AR [MIM 268000], less commonly, AD [MIM 180100], and X-linked [MIM 312600]

RESTRICTION ENDONUCLEASES

NAME	CLEAVAGE SITE	ORGANISM
BamHI	G/GATC*C	*Bacillus amyloliquifaciens*
EcoRI	G/AA*TTC	*Escherichia coli* RY13
HindIII	A*/AGCTT	*Haemophilus influenza* Rd
PstI	CTGCA/G	*Providentia stuartii* 164
SmaI	CCC/GGG	*Serratia marcescens* Sb
XhoI	C/TCGAG	*Xanthomonas hocicola*

/ Point of cleavage
* Base modified by a specific methylase
Note: Bacteria do not digest themselves as they have an intrinsic methylase that adds methyl group to one of the nucleotides within the restriction site, preventing autocleavage

forms of retinal degeneration, which affects 1:3500 of the population, which are characterized by nyctalopia and progressive centripetal loss of the visual fields progressing to blindness by middle age, caused by one or more point mutations in the rhodopsin gene located on the long arm of chromosome 3

retinoblastoma A malignant neoplasm usually of children (affecting 1:15-30 000 infants) that arise in retinal cells, which has photoreceptor differentiation; 10-20% are hereditary, most commonly AD; 70% are unilateral and arise *de novo*; bilateral tumors are associated with germ cell neoplasms and occasionally other tumors including osteogenic sarcoma and Ewing sarcoma MOLECULAR PATHOLOGY Retinoblastoma cells lack tumor growth factor-β_1 receptor (a protein that inhibits cell growth); due to a defective retinoblastoma gene identified by RFLP analysis on chromosome 13q14 (which encodes a tumor suppressor protein); the tumor arises when both alleles have been inactivated; mRNA expression of 'retinoblastoma gene' is also absent in 60% of small cell carcinomas of the lung and 75% of pulmonary carcinoids PATHOLOGY Primitive dark blue cells classically arranged in Flexner-Wintersteiner rosettes TREATMENT Radiotherapy; see One-hit, two-hit model, RB gene, Rosettes

retinoblastoma susceptibility gene see RB gene

retinoic acid A morphogenic molecule involved in vertebrate development, which in conjunction with precursor retinoids, is thought to specify positional identity on an axis during embryological development and regeneration in a dose-dependent and graded fashion; RA affects development of chick limb buds, the floor plate of the neural tube and may produce cleft palate in mice; seven retinoic acid receptors have been identified, explaining the broad range of RA effects; RA is used to treat cystic acne, actinic keratosis, psoriasis, photoaging and oral leukoplakia; it is contraindicated in pregnant women, see Retinoic acid embryopathy

retinoic acid embryopathy A teratogenic complex induced by a vitamin A-derived product resulting in a 26-fold increase of congenital malformations, including microtia, anotia, cleft palate, cardiac (conotruncal and aortic arch), neural crest, craniofacial, thymic defects, hyperostoses, retinal and optic nerve abnormalities, central nervous system malformations, premature closure of the epiphyseal plates; an identical embryopathy occurs with 'megadose' ingestion of vitamin A

retirement 'syndrome' PSYCHIATRY Acute or chronic maladjustment to the state of retirement, in which the person no longer works; the 'condition' is most common in those who had no extracurricular activity except their chosen field of labor CLINICAL Irritability, apathy, asthenia, increased alcohol consumption, nonspecific autonomic nervous system complaints

retort tube appearance A descriptor for fallopian tubes affected by acute pelvic inflammatory disease with hyperemia and fibrin deposition; the lumen is filled with pus and the fimbriae are sealed

Note: A retort is a vessel used for distillation with an elongated tapering cone attached to the receptacle containing the fluid to be distilled

retraction balls, axonal NEUROPATHOLOGY Eosinophilic and argentophilic swelling of axons, occasionally seen at the proximal and distal ends of severed nerve fibers undergoing Wallerian degeneration, which is thought to represent extruded axoplasm; retraction balls are seen in the early stages of cerebral hemorrhage or infarcts; retraction balls with brainstem necrosis are characteristic of methotrexate leukoencephalopathy

retroflexion Uterine retroflexion GYNECOLOGY The backward displacement of the uterus, a finding that occurs in the first trimester of ± 10% of pregnancies; despite occasional reports of increased frequency of bleeding in early pregnancy, the retroflexed uterus is not regarded as pathologic condition per se, and only requires therapy in the rare cases where a growing retroflexed uterus becomes incarcerated in the hollow of the sacrum (Williams Obstetrics, 19th ed, Appleton & Lange, 1993)

retroperitoneal fibrosis Ormond's disease A rare condition of unknown etiology that affects younger adults; (ages 30-45, ♂:♀ ratio of 2:1), which is characterized by proliferation of fibrous tissue in the retroperitoneum that encases the ureters, potentially causing renal failure, and which may evoke fibrous proliferation elsewhere, including sclerosing cholangitis and mediastinitis, Riedel's thyroiditis, pseudotumor of the orbit and generalized vasculitis CLINICAL Malaise, vomiting, backache, constipation, hypertension RADIOLOGY Compression of all evaluable intraabdominal structures LABORATORY Oliguria, azotemia, proteinuria, ↑ ESR, anemia PROGNOSIS The behavior of soft tissue sarcomas is a function of histologic aggression, as measured by cellularity, differentiation and pleomorphism, mitotic activity and presence of necrosis

retroposition GYNECOLOGY Retroflexion, see there MOLECULAR BIOLOGY RNA-mediated transposition of genetic material; Cf Transposition

retroposon A mobile segment of genetic information, eg a retrovirus that transposes by way of an RNA intermediate

retrospective analysis Pending good book on statistics

retrospective study CLINICAL EPIDEMIOLOGY A study that analyzes data collected prior to a certain point in time; retrospective studies can be used to identify tentative or hypothetical cause-and-effect relationships or potential risk factors for a disease; such studies are usually followed by prospective studies, see there

retrospectoscope A highly colloquial term used in the context of retrospective analysis through which diagnostic dilemmas are easily resolved when viewed in hindsight (N Engl J Med 1994; 331:11216cps)

Retrovir® Zidovudine, see there

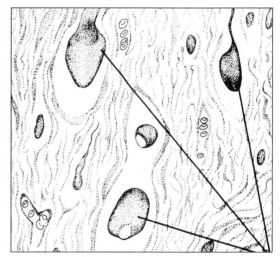

retraction balls

retrovirus An RNA virus with two copies of an 8500 base pair plus-stranded RNA genome that is capable of inserting and efficiently expressing its own genetic information in a host cell's genome, by transcribing its own RNA into DNA that is integrated into the host genome; retroviruses are the focus of major research efforts due to their relation to human T cell lymphotrophic viruses and human immunodeficiency virus (HIV-1, see figure for relatedness among retroviruses); these viruses are widely used in research to introduce foreign DNA into a cell of interest and could theoretically be used to introduce a missing or defective segment of DNA into a cell line or organism for therapeutic purposes; the only approved use of retroviruses in humans is to 'mark' tumor infiltrating lymphocytes in experimental cancer therapy; see HIV, HTLV, Reverse transcriptase, Rous sarcoma virus

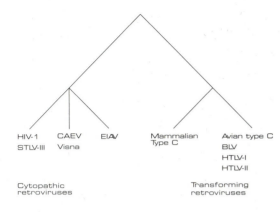

HIV-1   CAEV   EIAV   Mammalian   Avian type C
STLV-III   Visna   Type C   BLV
                                                    HTLV-I
                                                    HTLV-II

Cytopathic   Transforming
retroviruses   retroviruses

relationship among retroviruses

Rev protein An HIV-1 regulatory protein that retrieves unspliced mRNA transcripts from the nucleus that are required for synthesizing structural HIV proteins; Rev deficiency inhibits HIV-1 replication (Proc Nat Acad Sci (US) 1994; 91:5075OA)

reverse CAMP test MICROBIOLOGY An assay that is identical in principle to the CAMP test, which identifies *Clostridium* species, where a known group B β-hemolytic streptococcus is used and if positive, the arrowhead points toward *C perfringens*; Cf CAMP test

reverse cerebral steal Robin Hood syndrome* Reduction of blood flow to relatively well-oxygenated tissue by vasoconstriction, 'freeing' the available blood for ischemic and hypercapneic tissues; in the usual 'steal' syndrome blood flow is robbed from oxygen-poor tissues by oxygen-rich tissues

*The adjectival sobriquet of 'Robin Hood' derives from the legendary English folk hero, who allegedly stole from the rich to give to the poor, allegorically similar to this condition

reverse coarctation see Takayasu's arteritis

reverse psychology The application of an inverted suggestion that would compel a person who is in a 'contrary' state, to perform a desired task

reverse discrimination The denial of employment or admission to a professional or employment position based on the fact that the applicant is not of a minority race; since the US Civil Rights Act of 1964, many organizations have been required to accept applicants from underprivileged socioeconomic strata or previously discriminated-against racial groups; this led to a two-tiered system in which the presumed-to-be-advantaged racial group was often required to meet higher academic standards, while the 'hurdle' was often lowered on behalf of the underprivileged; in the Bakke decision of 1978, a white applicant was allowed admission to medical school after he proved 'reverse discrimination'

reverse '5' sign A finding on a plain antero-posterior film of an infant with hypoplastic left heart syndrome, in which the enlarged right atrium corresponds to the hip of the '5' and the superior vena cava corresponds to the shoulder of the '5'; see Baby Fae heart

reverse genetics MOLECULAR BIOLOGY Any of a number of procedures for identifying mutant genes when a mutant phenotype is known but the responsible gene product(s) or linked markers are not; in 'forward' or traditional genetics, both the gene product, eg a defective protein and the amino acid sequence are often known before the search for the gene itself begins; in 'reverse genetics', identification of the gene is far more difficult, since the gene product is unknown at the time the search for the gene begins; one approach is to create a cDNA library from a cell that does not carry the disease in question, then perform 'subtraction' Southern blots, an extremely arduous technique that was successful in identifying the defective protein in chronic granulomatous disease; RG can also be used to produce mutations by replacing a gene of choice (ie gene to phenotype), allowing the study of development and pattern formation in animal models (Science 1994; 264:1724) see Candidate gene method, Gene scanning

reverse paternity testing FORENSIC MEDICINE The evaluation of a biological specimen alleged to originate from a victim of a crime or a missing person, in order to determine whether that person is the child of parents with known genetic markers; the most commonly used marker is HLA-DQ-α, although any genetic marker, eg GmKm haplotyping, protein polymorphisms and red cell antigens may be used

reverse 'precautions' A group of infection control procedures, including sterilization and isolation used to protect a patient (rather than the care providers or other patients) who is immunocompromised, either as a congenital condition, eg combined variable immunodeficiency syndrome or an acquired condition, eg BM irradiation in preparation for BM transplantation; 'reverse precautions' are required when the absolute neutrophil count falls below 0.5×10^9 (US: 500/mm³); see Gnotobiotic environment; Cf Universal precautions

reverse T₃ 3,3',5'-Triiodothyronine rT₃ LABOARTORY MEDICINE One of the conversion products of T₄ (thyroxine), the level of which reflects the rate of peripheral conversion of thyroid hormones of T₄ to T₃; normal rT₃ levels 0.15-0.77 mmol/L (US: 10-50 ng/dl); most circulating thyroid hormone is T₄; 35% is monodeiodinated to T₃, 15-20% is metabolized to tetraiodothyroacetic acid and the remainder is converted to rT₃; although rT₃ has little or no metabolic activity, an increased rT₃ level in patients with non-thyroidal disease indicates that the patient is not functionally hypothyroid; see Euthyroid sick syndrome

reverse 3 sign Either of a pair of radiologic findings in the GI tract, referring to either 1) Broadening of the duodenal loop with a 'puckering' around the ampulla of Vater, classically associated with pancreatic adenocarcinoma at the head of the pancreas, seen in barium studies of the upper gastrointestinal tract or 2) Indentation of the cecum, which may be seen on a plain abdominal film in acute appendicitis; Cf Figure 3 sign

reverse transcriptase MOLECULAR BIOLOGY An RNA-dependent DNA polymerase* [EC 2.7.7.49] of retroviral origin that is capable of copying genomic RNA into DNA, catalyzing the synthesis of DNA using retroviral RNA as a template; reverse transcriptase has three enzymatic activities; 1) The single-stranded RNA molecule copies itself, 2) The retrovirus then forms a double-stranded DNA-RNA hybrid genome, transcribing a complementary strand of DNA opposite the RNA template, a polymerase activity 3) The strand of RNA is then removed by reverse transcriptase's ribonuclease H function; once the DNA is freed of the RNA, the polymerase portion of the molecule then synthesizes a second strand of DNA (Science 1991; 252:31); RT was first identified in oncogenic retroviruses, and homologous enzymes with similar activities have been found in bacteria, insects, eg *Drosophila*, and mammals; RT is a widely used molecular research tool, and used to make cDNA (complementary DNA) clones from mRNA

*RNA-directed DNA polymerase is the term recommended (1992) by the Nomenclature Committee of the IUBMB (International Union of Biochemistry and Molecular Biology) the scientist who discovered RT, David Baltimore, received the 1975 Nobel Prize

reverse transcription The copying of single-stranded retroviral RNA into double-stranded DNA, which is catalyzed by reverse transcriptase, an enzyme so designated as it is the reverse of the usual direction of tanscription from DNA to RNA, see Central dogma, HIV, Retrovirus

reverse transcription-polymerase chain reaction RT-PCR A type of PCR used to study gene expression by fist converted the identified mRNA into cDNA; RT-PCR is of particular interest as it requires less mRNA than that needed for a Northern blot analysis (Diagn Mol Pathol 1993; 2:120)

reversible ischemic neurological disability A variant of a transient ischemic attack defined as an ischemia-induced focal loss of neurologic function of abrupt onset, the disability from which is greater than 24 hours but less than 3 weeks induration; Cf Multi-infarct dementia, Transient ischemic attack

reversible lymphoma A rarely-described phenomenon[1] in which a lymphoma[2] arises in an immunocompromised[3] background; of interest are these reports 1) Two patients, the maligancies (a large cell lymphoma and Hodgkin's disease) regressed following withdrawal of methotrexate therapy (N Engl J Med 1993; 328:1317OA) 2) A patient with Crohn's disease who developed a B-cell lymphoproliferative disorder with increased production of kappa chain mRNA after azathioprine therapy, which reversed upon discontinuation of azathioprine (N Engl J Med 1994; 331:883OA)

[1]Such reversibility is rarely recognized, but has important implications in understanding the pathogenesis and possible therapeutic approaches to other malignancies being 'driven' by exogenous factors [2]Epstein-Barr virus-associated lymphoproliferative disorders [3]Methotrexate therapy and connective tissue disorders, eg rheumatoid arthritis or dermatomyositis; Azathioprine in Crohn's disease

reversion The change of a mutated nucleic acid to its state prior to mutation

Revici method ALTERNATIVE MEDICINE A form of alternative cancer therapy that is based on Revici's theory that '...*a disease can be dualistic, with a predominance of one group of lipids* (sterols) *or the opposite* (fatty acids), *one anabolic and constructive, the other catabolic and destructive...*'; according to this theoretical framework, the control of disease requires determination of the nature of a biological imbalance and providing the substance that corrects it; the method is alleged to detect catabolic or anabolic processes by urinary pH; catabolic therapeutic agents include fatty acids, magnesium, selenium and sulfur; anabolic agents include caffeine, iron, lipols, lithium, zinc; the method has no demonstrable efficacy and is based on no known or established scientific principle (CA-A Journal for Clinicians 1989; 39:119) see Alternative medicine, Unproven methods of cancer therapy

reviewer SCIENTIFIC JOURNALISM A recognized expert in a field who reviews a manuscript for publication in a major scientific or medical journal and either recommends its acceptance to the journal or advises its rejection based on various criteria; most reviewers rejected an average of 1.5 manuscripts for various reasons, some 'zealots' may find some merit in virtually all the manuscripts they review, while others, the 'assassins', reject most of the manuscripts they recieve (Science 1991; 251:1424n&v) Cf Authorship, Peer-reviewed journal, Publication bias

Revised Trauma Score EMERGENCY MEDICINE A numerical scoring system used to calculate the probability of survival and therefore of use as a trigae tool; the RTS imeasures three parameters to quantitate the physiological severity of injury to wit, the Glasgow Coma Scale, systolic blood pressure, and respiratory rate, with results ranging from 0 (full cardiopulmonary arrest) to 7.84 (essentially normal)

(see N Engl J Med 1994; 331:1105OA) see Injury Severity Score, Triage

revolving door 'syndrome' PSYCHIATRY/SOCIAL MEDICINE A cyclical pattern of short-term readmissions to the psychiatric units of health care centers by young adults with chronic psychiatric disease; this syndrome first appeared in the USA in the 1970s with the implementation of strict(er) criteria for civil commitment of mentally disturbed patients, which arose from a concern about the potential for causing harm to oneself or to others; because more people with major mental illness are no longer hospitalized, and theoretically are well-controlled with drug therapy, eg tricyclic antidepressants, these persons may commit minor crimes and be imprisoned, resulting in 'criminalization' of persons with psychiatric disease Note: 30-40% of the general prison population and homeless people in the USA suffer from psychiatric or addictive disease (Psychiatr J Univ Ottawa 1988; 13:154); see Homeless(ness)

Reye syndrome A potentially fatal condition characterized by acute encephalopathy and fatty degeneration of the liver that is linked in a dose-dependent manner to the use of aspirin in children during viral infections (eg influenza, varicella-zoster) CLINICAL Vomiting, hepatic dysfunction, variable neurological impairment often preceded by viral upper respiratory tract infections or varicella PATHOLOGY 'Fine-droplet' fatty liver; by EM, megamitochondria with distended and fragmented cristae and flocculated matrix LABORATORY ↑ Transaminases, glutamine and ammonia in cerebrospinal fluid, hypoglycemia and metabolic acidosis TREATMENT None is universally accepted; see Lovejoy's classification, Will Rogers phenomenon

'Stage migration' has occurred in Reye syndrome, as milder cases are being diagnosed, and it is increasingly recognized as a relatively 'benign' condition

RF see Rheumatoid factor(s)

RFLP Restriction fragment length polymorphisms, restriction site polymorphism MOLECULAR BIOLOGY Local variations in the DNA sequence of individual humans or animals that may be detected by restriction endonuclease enzymes (which 'cut' the double-stranded DNA whenever they recognize a certain highly-specific oligonucleotide sequence or 'restriction' site); these individual variations or polymorphisms in the DNA sequences occur approximately 1 per 200-500 base pairs and cause the genome to be cut at different sites, yielding fragments of different length that are unique to each individual (the likelihood of two people having the same RFLPs is estimated to be $1/10^9$), but nevertheless normal; these different fragments may then be identified by electrophoresis as larger restriction fragments migrate more slowly; although the differences in fragment lengths may be linked to chromosomal loci for a certain disease, these point 'mutations' rarely translate into functional defects as 1) Not all genes are 'structural', ie do not encode functional protein 2) DNA is 'degenerate', ie obeys the law of DNA conservation, in which 64 different DNA codon sequences encode in only 20 amino acids, 3 stop codons and 1 start codon, thus allowing for multiple 'silent' errors and 3) All individuals carry 5-10 potentially lethal mutations under normal circumstances Note: Single base pair substitutions can either create or abolish restriction endonuclease sites, as will tandem repeats; RFLPs are useful genetic markers as they help identify the inheritance pattern of a gene of interest; if one is able to locate a RFLP that has the same heredity pattern as a genetic condition, then the gene responsible for that disease can be localized, thus one must find a DNA sequence closely associated or linked to a disease of interest; RFLP analysis is of use in identifying genes linked to AD neurologic diseases, including Huntington's disease located on chromosome 4, myotonic dystrophy on chromosome 19 and Duchenne's dystrophy on chromosome X; in allogenic BM transplant recipients, RFLP analysis is of use in documenting chimerism, allograft failure, recurrent leukemia or in identifying a secondary lymphoproliferative malignancy; an alternative method for investigating clonal populations is based on differences in DNA methylation patterns that exist between active and inactive alleles of two X-linked genes

revocation Suspension, eg revocation of a license to practice medicine

RF-S A factor present in human S phase cells that activates DNA replication and contains a homologue of *Schizosaccharomyces pompe* p34*cdc2* kinase that is responsible for control of DNA synthesis; see p34*cdc2*

RGD MOLECULAR BIOLOGY A tripeptide of arginine-glycine-aspartic acid that serves as a recognition site extracellular matrix proteins by cell surface integrins; RGD-directed integrins include certain receptors for fibronectin, fibrinogen, and vitronectin (Bio/Technology 1995; 13:265)

RGD family A group of proteins that are present in the extracellular matrix that have cell adhesion functions, mediated by the 'RGD' tripeptide, Arginine-Glycine-Aspartic acid (designated as RGD by the single letter code for amino acids); RGD proteins include collagens, fibrinogen, fibronectin, glycoprotein IIb and IIIa, LFA-1 with Mac-1 and VLA1-5 on leukocytes, laminin, osteospondin, thrombospondin, vitronectin, von Willebrand factor, together with their respective receptors; the RGD family constitutes a versatile recognition system providing cells with anchorage by interaction of surface receptors with cytoplasmic proteins (talin, ankyrin, actin, vinculin, fibroconnexin) and extracellular proteins (fibronectin, collagen, vitronectin and others), traction for migration and signals for growth, phagocytosis, polarity, position, cell differentiation, platelet aggregation and complement binding; see Integrins

RGD sequence A sequence of three amino acids (Arg-Gly-Asp) that is the adhesive sequence in fibronectin, which is also present in fibrinogen, von Willebrand factor, and vitronectin; peptides containing the RS are potent inhibitors of the interaction between glycoprotein IIb/IIIa receptors and fibrinogen (N Engl J Med 1995; 332:1553RV)

rh Recombinant human

R gene see Regulator gene

Rh OBSTETRICS The Rh system is a group of 7-10 kD erythrocyte membrane-bound antigens that are independent of phosphatides and proteolipids; the Rh system is very complex and much of its genetics and role in red cell structure and function are not understood; Rh$^+$ and Rh$^-$ refer to the presence or absence of the erythrocyte-bound antigen D; Rh 'antigen' is actually a composite of multiple antigens, including Rh-C (c, C, CG, C^w), Rh-D (D, weak D -formerly D^u, D^w), Rh-E (e, E, E^w), Rh-G, Rh-LW, Rh-Ne^a and Rh$_{null}$; Frequency of the Rh antigens in Caucasians: Rh-e, 98%; Rh-D, 85%; Rh-c, 80%; Rh-C, 70%; Rh-E, 30%; unlike the ABO blood group, antibodies against the D antigen are not formed naturally, ie in the absence of exposure, thus an Rh- subject with circulating anti-D antibodies has been exposed to the D antigen by a previous transfusion or pregnancy; exposure to the D antigen is of concern in obstetrics as the mother's anti-D antibody is an IgG, which crosses the placenta, potentially causing hemolytic disease of the newborn (titer > 1:16 at the 8th month usually indicates maternal formation of alloantibodies, evidenced by stomatocytes in the maternal blood) prenatal Rh type can be determined prenatally by polymerase chain reaction in amniotic cells, a procedure of considerable use in the case of RhD-negative mothers who may be carrying RhD-positive fetuses against whose Rh group antigens, the mother's immune system may form antibodies (N Engl J Med 1993; 329:607OA) PROPHYLAXIS 300 µg of anti-D (RhoGAM) immunoglobulin 'neutralizes' a 30 ml

feto-maternal hemorrhage containing 15 ml of Rh-bearing red cells; see Rh immune globulin

Rh antigen Add Any of an allelic system of glycosphingolipids on the RBC membrane that evoke intense antibody response in those with an intact immune system who lack these antigens

Rh immune globulin RhIg RhIg Rh$_o$(D) immune globulin A sterile plasma-based preparation rich in anti-Rh immunoglobulin, used to prevent the production of Rh$_o$(D) antibodies in Rh-negative mothers who may have an Rh-positive infant, thereby avoiding hemolytic disease of the newborn due to Rh-antibody production by the mother; it is used as prophylaxis for unsensitized Rh-negative pregnant ♀; although in early pregnancy, a dose of 50 µg is sufficient, the standard dose of 300 µg is administered to all INDICATIONS RhIg administration may be routine (at 28 weeks of gestation, ≤ 72 hours of delivery if neonate is Rh+), after invasive prenatal diagnostic procedures (eg amniocentesis, chorionic villus biopsy, percutaneous umbilical blood sampling), ectopic pregnancy, spontaneous or therapeutic abortion, antepartum bleeding (eg blunt trauma to abdomen, motor vehicle accidents, threatened abortion, suspected placental abruption, placenta previa) (from Arch Pathol Lab Med 1994; 118:421RV) one commonly used product, RhoGAM, contains 300 mg of antihuman immunoglobulin/vial, sufficient to 'neutralize' a feto-maternal hemorrhage of 15 ml of red cells; RhIg is indicated when the mother is Rh negative or has anti-RhD antibody titer of > 1:4; see Hemolytic disease of the newborn

Rh$_{null}$ (syndrome) TRANSFUSION MEDICINE A rare AR [MIM 268150] Rhesus system phenotype found on erythrocytes in which there is complete non-expression of Rh antigens, resulting from either the more common regulator type defect, consisting in homozygous inheritance of the gene $X^o r$ or inheritance of an amorphic gene (---/---); both Rh$_{null}$ phenotypes are associated with ↓ red cell survival and stomatocytosis due to a membrane defect; Rh$_{null}$ expression is enhanced by concomitant presence on the red cell surface of blood groups M, -N, -En^a and depressed by -S, -s, -U; see Bombay phenotype

rhabdomyosarcoma A malignant tumor of rhabdomyoblasts CLASSIFICATION According to the classic WHO (histological) classification, RMS is divided into alveolar, botryoid, embryonal and pleomorphic types; a newer scheme has been proposed by NCI workers who divide RMS into embryonal, which has a relatively favorable prognosis and the alveolar or solid-alveolar types, which have a poor prognosis PROGNOSIS-FAVORABLE PROGNOSTIC SITES Orbit, GI, and genitourinary tracts POOR PROGNOSTIC SITES Extremities, retroperitoneaum, intrathoracic, head and neck, ear, sinuses (Arch Pathol Lab Med 1992; 116:847OA)

rhabdovirus A family of single-stranded RNA viruses that includes the rabies virus and causes vesicular stomatitis

rheology The formal study of the deformation and flow of materials, whether in solid, melt, or liquid forms; the examination of the response of a material to an applied force helps determine the way in which to best produce, transfer, package, store, and use the material; if the deformation is reversible, the material is said to have elastic behavior; if the deformation is irreversible, the material is said to exhibit viscous behavior or flow; the term viscoelastic refers to materials that have both reversible and irreversible deformation characteristics EVALUATION Flow and deformation properties of materials can be measured by controlled rate or by controlled stress principles APPLICATIONS The rheologic properties of a wide range of fluids and semisolid substances are of broad interest, eg adhesives and sealants, foods, inks and paints, pharmaceuticals and polymers (Am Laboratory, Aug 1993)

rheologic Relating or pertaining to rheology

rheologist A person who studies rheology

rheometer A device for measuring the deformation of materials

rheometry Measurement of the deformation of materials

Rhesus immune globulin RhIg Rh₀(D) immune globulin, see there

rheumatoid arthritis An autoimmune inflammatory and multisystem disease characterized by prolonged inflammation of multiple joints; RA is defined by the 1987 revised criteria (table, 768), which requires that criteria 1-4 be present for > than 6 weeks; the 'revised criteria' yield a 91-94% sensitivity and 89% specificity (**Arthritis Rheum 1988: 31:315**) LABORATORY IgG autoantibodies, aka rheumatoid factors; RA ameliorates in severity during pregnancy when there is a disparity in the HLA classes between the mother and fetus, a finding that suggests that the maternal immune response to paternal antigens may have a role in this amelioration (**N Engl J Med 1993; 329:466₀ₐ**)

RHEUMATOID ARTHRITIS (REVISED CRITERIA)

1) Morning stiffness in and around joints lasting at least one hour before maximum improvement
2) Soft tissue swelling ('arthritis') of three or more joints observed by a physician
3) Swelling (arthritis) of the proximal interphalangeal, metacarpophalangeal or wrist joints
4) Symmetric swelling (arthritis)
5) Rheumatoid nodules
6) Presence of rheumatoid factor
7) Roentgenographic erosions and/or periarticular osteope

---

rheumatoid arthritis cell RA cell An atypical neutrophil containing 1-20 dense, black 0.5-2.0 μm in diameter cytoplasmic inclusions containing IgM rheumatoid factor, IgG, complement and fibrin, which is seen by phase contrast microscopy in wet synovial fluid preparations in patients with rheumatoid arthritis; RA cells comprise 5-100% of the neutrophils of patients with rheumatoid arthritis but are relatively non-specific and may be seen in other connective tissue diseases, including septic arthritis and gout

rheumatoid factors A group of often polyclonal IgM (rarely also IgG or IgA) antibodies that are directed against the Fc portion of denatured IgG; RFs are produced by synovial neutrophils in 80% of patients with rheumatoid arthritis; RFs are non-specific and may be seen in infections (bronchitis, kala azar, leprosy, sub-acute bacterial endocarditis, syphilis, TB, viral), hepatic disease (biliary obstruction, cirrhosis, fatty liver, granulomas, neoplasia and viral hepatitis) and others (DM, idiopathic pulmonary fibrosis, osteoarthritis, paraproteinemia, Raynaud's disease, sarcoidosis, Sjögren syndrome) and are present in 3% of a normal healthy population; RFs may cause immune complex deposits which activate complement and release leukocytic hydrolases from neutrophils, causing tissue injury PATHOLOGY Fibrinoid necrosis in small blood vessels LABORATORY Detection of RFs is not standardized; the tests may be based on erythrocyte agglutination (Rose-Waaler test), latex agglutination (Singer-Plotz test), nephelometry, fluorescence immunoassay and ELISA; RFs have a relatively high specificity (±87%), it has a low sensitivity (±27%) in the diagnosis of RA (**Ann Inten Med 1992; 152:2417**)

rheumatoid nodule A mass on tendons, tendon sheaths, periarticular tissue, serous membranes (pleural, pericardium), meninges, cardiac valves, kidneys, lung parenchyma, skin, spleen, synovium, vessels and viscera, seen in 20% of patients with rheumatoid arthritis, similar nodules occur

in SLE, and rheumatic fever PATHOLOGY Vaguely geographic area of central necrosis (containing collagen, lipids, nucleoproteins, acid mucopolysaccharides, serum proteins and immunoglobulins), surrounded by successive rims of fibrinoid degeneration, fibrosis and palisaded histiocytes

rheumatoid pneumonitis A clinical form of diffuse interstitial pulmonary fibrosis that occurs in 2% of patients with rheumatoid arthritis, which is accompanied by a varying degree of pulmonary compromise; rheumatoid pneumonitis may result from the rare coincidence of two uncommon conditions, ie rheumatoid arthritis and interstitial pneumonia, the latter of which may be induced by gold therapy, exposure to an environmental toxin or related to smoking

rheumatoid vasculitis A necrotizing vasculitis of unknown cause that affects a subset of patients with rheumatoid arthritis CLINICAL Mononeuritis multiplex, GI involvement (infarction, ulceration, perforation, colitis, stricture formation, and hemorrhage) skin infarction, and constitutional symptoms (**Mayo Clin Proc 1995; 70:565**)

RhIg see Rh immune globulin

rhinomanometry ENT A technique for evaluating nasal patency and airflow by simultaneously measuring transnasal pressure and airway resistance; rhinomanometry is used to diagnose and treat nasal obstruction; see Nasal airway resistance

rhinophyma WC Fields nose A nasal nosology occurring only in men, as an end-stage complication of acne rosacea, resulting in a bulbous proboscis PATHOLOGY Diffuse enlargement of sebaceous glands, marked accumulation of connective tissue, vascular ectasia, and lymphocytic infiltrate

rhinoplasty Nose job ENT Rhinoplasty is divided into two basic forms, reconstructive rhinoplasty for defects of the nose cause by trauma or surgery to the region, most often related to extensive locoregional malignancy, and esthetic (cosmetic) rhinoplasty, which constitutes the majority, and for which 25 000 are performed/year (US) 70% in women; 11% under age 18 (**Vitality June 1993**) METHOD A rhinoplasty consists of four interrelated steps, to wit, septoplasty, remodeling of tip wth cephalic rotation, removal of the hump to re-establish the profile, and narrowing of the nose with osteotomies (**JJ Ballenger, Diseases of the Nose, Throat, Ear, Head & Neck, 14th ed, Lea & Febiger, Philadelphia, 1991**) PROGNOSIS Rhinoplasties with a good ultimate outcome include noses with obvious disfigurement, those occupational reasons for correction, and a reasonable desire to appear younger

rho termination factor MOLECULAR BIOLOGY A protein that interacts with a growing mRNA chain in bacteria, terminating transcription of an operon

Rhodococcus equi Add opportunistic pathogen, weakly acid-fast CLINICAL 53 human cases have been reported in the world literature; manifestations of *R equi* infection include pneumonia, pleural effusion, empyema, abscesses of the brain, skin, and elsewhere, osteomyelitis, lymphadenitis, and endophthalmitis (**Am J Clin Pathol 1995; 103:649₀ₐ**)

Rhodococcus equi A pleomorphic gram-positive, non-motile aerobic bacillus that may infect immunocompromised hosts, eg AIDS patients PATHOLOGY Replacement of lung parenchyma by sheets of foamy histiocytes with rounded eccentric nuclei and granular cytoplasm with classic Michaelis-Gutmann bodies, typical of malacoplakia (**Arch Pathol Lab Med 1994; 118:744₀ₐ**)

rhodopsin A member of a family of receptors bearing seven transmembrane helices coupled to G proteins

RhoGAM see Rh immune globulin

rhomboid crystals A descriptive term for 1) The characteristic membrane-bound, rod-shaped crystalloid structures with 10-nm periodicity seen by ultrastructure in the malignant polygonal cells of alveolar soft part sarcoma and 2) The notched cholesterol crystals obtained from joint fluid in patients with diverse chronic inflammatory or chronic degenerative arthropathies

rhythm method GYNECOLOGY The contraceptive method sanctioned by certain religious bodies in which unprotected intercourse is allowed shortly after a menstrual period or before the onset of the next period; the rhythm method is the least effective form of contraception, resulting in 20 pregnancies/100 -years; see Contraceptives, Pearl index

RIA Radioimmunoassay IMMUNOLOGY, LABORATORY MEDICINE A method that measures either an antigen or antibody based on competitive inhibition of labeled antigens on the binding of unlabeled antigens to specific antibodies, the uptake of which displays a characteristic sigmoid curve; RIA allows measurement of minimal amounts of immunogenic substances, including enzymes and hormones and is of great use in research as it is relatively easy to design an assay to detect the analyte(s) of interest; RIAs are being slowly phased out of the clinical laboratory in favor of enzyme assays, which eliminate the regulatory and disposal problems inherent in maintaining radioactive materials on-site; see POPOP, Quenching; Cf ELISA

RIBA Recombinant immunoblot assay

ribavirin 1-β-5-D-ribofuranosyl-1,2,4-triazole-3-carboxamide A synthetic nucleoside analog that restricts the synthesis of viral proteins, interfering with capping of the mRNA of various viruses; ribavirin is FDA-approved for aerosol treatment of influenza A and B in young adults and severe respiratory syncytial virus infection in children, and administered IV reduces the mortality of Lassa fever; it is teratogenic and thus contraindicated in pregnant women

ribbon cell SURGICAL PATHOLOGY An elongated eosinophilic variant of the 'strap' cell seen in pleomorphic rhabdomyosarcoma; see Strap cell

ribbon ribs A descriptor for ribs with marked costal hypoplasia or attenuation, a finding characteristic of trisomy 13-15 and trisomy 18 syndromes, and may be seen in neurofibromatosis, Gorham's angiomatosis, hyperparathyroidism, osteodysplasia, osteogenesis imperfecta, poliomyelitis, rheumatoid arthritis and scleroderma

ribonuclease An endonuclease that catalyzes RNA hydrolysis, cleaving its 3',5' phosphodiester bonds; many of the names have changed in recent years; here the most recent recommendations (1992) of the Nomenclature Committee of the International Union of Biochemistrya and Molecular Biology are used

RIBONUCLEASE A catalyzes RNA yielding mono and oligonucleotides with 3'-pyrimidine termini

RIBONUCLEASE D removes excess tRNA nucleotides from precursor tRNA, forming the 3'-terminus of this molecule

RIBONUCLEASE H removes the RNA molecule that is a template for the first strand of DNA; RNase H is of interest to AIDS researchers as a possible target for a new family of anti-HIV-1 drugs (**Science 1991; 252:88**) see HIV-1, Reverse transcriptase

RIBONUCLEASE I Pancreatic ribonuclease [EC 3.1.27.5]

RIBONUCLEASE II 1) Exoribonuclease II [EC 3.1.13.1] 2) Ribonuclease T_2 [EC 3.1.27.1]

RIBONUCLEASE III [EC 3.1.26.3] hydrolyzes double-stranded RNA

Ribonuclease N_1 Ribonuclease T_1 [EC 3.1.27.3]

Ribonuclease N_2 Ribonuclease T_1 [EC 3.1.27.3]

RIBONUCLEASE P is a ribozyme of bacterial origin that cleaves an oligonucleotide from precursor tRNA at the 5'-end of mature RNA;

Cf RNA polymerase

ribonuclease protection assay MOLECULAR BIOLOGY A test that directly measures the mRNA in a specimen, which more closely reflects DNA transcriptional activity that the less direct measurement of encoded protein; RPA allows in-solution hybridization of single or multiple riboprobes to total RNA after digestion with RNase; because the hybridized fraction is protected from digestion by RNase, the protected probe reflects the amount of target RNA (eg that of CAT mRNA, rather than CAT) present in the total RNA sample (**Am Biotech Lab Sept 1994, p 108**)

ribonucleoprotein A molecule with RNA covalently bound to protein; see snRNPs (small ribonucleoproteins)

ribonucleotide-diphosphate reductase Ribonucleotide reductase A heteromultimeric enzyme [EC 1.17.4.1] that is needed by all proliferating cells for *de novo* synthesis of 2'-deoxyribonucleotide DNA precursors

ribosomal lamellar complex Granulofilamentous body An ultrastructural finding consisting of hollow cylindrical structures composed of ribosome-studded spirals and concentric lamellae; RLCs were first described as pathognomonic for hairy cell leukemia, but also occur in CLL, AML, lymphosarcoma, multiple myeloma, Waldenstrom's macroglobulinemia, adrenocortical adenoma, paraganglioma and other conditions

ribosomal RNA Any of a family of single-stranded nucleic acids ranging from 100-3000 bases in length (ie of relatively high molecular weight), that assemble in heteromultimeric complexes with proteins to form ribosomes, thereby serving as 'docking stations' for mRNA and nascent polypeptide strands

ribosome A complex spherical 15-25 nm in diameter nucleoprotein-rich organelle (the ratio of RNA to proteinsis ± 3:2) that is critical to the translation of a mature mRNA transcript into a protein; ribosomes hold mRNA in place while its message is read, hold the growing protein (peptide chain) in place during chain elongation and serves as a docking station so that tRNA can contribute a cognate amino acid specified by the mRNA; ribosomes either attach to the endoplasmic reticulum or wander freely about the cell

ribotyping MOLECULAR BIOLOGY A genetic assay that detects the RFLPs (restriction fragment length polymorphisms) associated with the multicopy ribosomal RNA operon, which is of use in determining relatedness of stains of bacteria, ie molecular epidemiology (see **N Engl J Med 1994; 331:981oA**) Cf PFGE chromosomal fingerprinting

ribozyme A catalytic RNA that is capable of breaking and forming covalent bonds and functions as an enzyme, cutting and splicing along an 'internal template', acting at restricted 'wobble' base pair sites; T Cech observed that pre-ribosomal RNA could cut and splice itself, thus acting as molecular 'scissors', while S Altman found that transfer RNA could be cut by another separate piece of RNA in conjunction with a protein, observations for which Cech and Altman were awarded the 1989 Nobel prize in Chemistry; the existence of self-splicing RNA molecules raises the question of whether the first inherited molecule in the 'primordial soup' was RNA rather than DNA; modified ribozymes may have potential as anti-HIV-1 therapeutic agents as a ribozyme with a hammerhead structural motif has been isolated that reduces the level of HIV-1 gag RNA expression; ribozymes are also capable of efficiently catalyzing C–N bonds, and of promoting reactions other than those of the RNA sugar-phosphate backbone, confirming a posit that has been popular among proponents of the so-called 'RNA world' (**Nature 1995; 374:777A**)

rib-tip syndrome Intercostal neuralgia accompanied by sharp episodic pain at the costal margin, caused by hypermotility of the anterior end of the costal cartilage of (usually) the tenth rib secondary to trauma

'rib-within-a-rib' appearance A descriptor for the parallel lines seen in the ribs by a plain chest film due to subcortical osteoporosis in pateints with severe chronic thalassemia

rice bodies ORTHOPEDICS Numerous elongated and indurated oval-to-rounded rice-like masses composed of collagen types I, III and V in ratios of 40/40/20 (the same ratio as the synovial membrane), which implies that a common mechanism exists for 'rice body' formation, eg synovial ischemia; rice bodies may occur in the joints of patients with rheumatoid arthritis, lupus erythematosus, septic arthritis, tuberculous bursitis and synovial chondromatosis; Cf Joint 'mice'

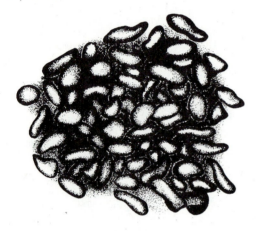

rice bodies

rice water stools Clear and watery diarrhea with a vaguely fishy odor, that is admixed with flecks of mucus, fancifully likened to the appearance of water from boiled rice, an appearance classically seen in cholera; cholera stool is low in protein and isotonic with the plasma, corresponding to a 'secretory' diarrhea in which adenylate cyclase is locked in the 'on' position by enterotoxins produced by *Vibrio cholera* and by some strains of *Escherichia coli*; at early postmortem examination, the intestines are stiff and non-distensible and fancifully likened to 'iron rods, a finding due to the antemortem metabolic acidosis and loss of potassium; see Cholera cot

Richter syndrome The development of a clinically aggressive pleomorphic large (usually) B cell lymphoma in the background of CLL (which occurs in 3-10% of CLLs), or less commonly in background of small lyphocytic leukemia or Waldenström's macroglobulinemia CLINICAL Rapid onset of intractable fever, weight loss, generalized lymphadenopathy, hepatosplenomegaly (**N Engl J Med 1992: 327:1801CPC**)

Richter scale A logarithmic scale that is used to stratify the intensity of earthquakes; the measurements used to calculate the magnitude are based on the records made on a standard seismograph located at a distance 100 km from the earthquake's epicenter (see table)

Rogue's gallery of killer earthquakes: Shaanxi, China (830 000 deaths, 1556), Calcutta (300 000, 1737), Antioch, Syria (250 000, 526 AD), Tangshan, China (242 000, 1976, 6.2 on Richter scale), Yokohama (200 000, 1923, 8.3 on Richter), Nanshan, China (200 000, 1927, 8.3 on Richter)

ricin A toxic vegetable poison from the castor bean plant

(*Ricinus communis*) which causes agglutination and fulminant hemolysis at very high dilutions (1/10⁶) CLINICAL Abdominal pain, nausea, cramps, convulsions, dehydration, hemolysis, cyanosis, renal failure (oliguria, hematuria) and circulatory collapse; see also Magic bullet

Note: Ricin poisoning was implicated in some KGB 'executions' during the Cold War, as with Georgi Markov, a Bulgarian defector

Rickettsia quintana *Bartonella quintana*, see there

rickettsialpox Kew Gardens fever A rickettsial infection caused by *Rickettsia akari* transmitted from rodents to humans by the blood-sucking mouse mite (*Liponyssoides sanguineus*) CLINICAL A typical eschar forms over the initial lesion, followed by fever, malaise, headache, backache, myalgia, conjunctivitis, sore throat, chest pain, cough, regional lymphadenopathy, 5-40 maculopapules and papulovesicules DIAGNOSIS Direct fluorescent antibody testing using *Rickettsia rickettsia* globulin conjugated with FITC (fluorescein isothiocyanate); also serial measurement of *R akari* antibodies TREATMENT Tetracycline, 2-5 days (**N Engl J Med 1994; 331:1612OA**)

RID see Radial immunodiffusion

rider's bone Post-traumatic myositis ossificans (heterotopic bone formation) seen on the upper femur of equestrians in relation to the adductor muscles

rifabutin A semisynthetic rifamycin which when given prophylactically, is reported to ↓ the incidence of disseminated *Mycobacterium avium* complex infection (8-9% vs 17-18% in placebo group) in AIDS patients with CD4 counts ≤ 200/m³; rifabutin therapy ↓ anemia, fatigue, fever, hospitalization, and Karnovsky performance score, and the ↑ in alkaline phosphatase typical of advanced AIDS (**N Engl J Med 1993; 329:828OA, 898SR**)

Rift valley fever A dengue-like viral disease spread by mosquitoes in floods, causing fatal enzootic hepatitis in ruminants (sheep, cattle) and occasional human epidemics, by direct contact; the agent belongs to the phlebovirus genus of the Bunyaviridiae family CLINICAL Abrupt onset with a biphasic fever curve, headaches, prostration, myalgias, anorexia, nausea, vomiting, conjunctivitis, lymphadenopathy; fatalities are related to hemorrhagic fever or encephalitis MORTALITY 5-20%

right middle lobe syndrome Middle lobe syndrome, see there

right shift see Oxygen dissociation curve

right-to-die A philosophical stance that is essentially equivalent to a DNR (do not resuscitate) order, which is to be honored outside of a hospital or health care setting

right-to-die movement A general term for those players who philosophically favor the existance of a choice in death options, including the legalization of euthanasia to DNR (do not resuscitate) orders BACKGROUND The potential for lawsuits in medically 'hopeless' health care situations is enormous and in the US, physicians often feel compelled to attempt what they perceive to be futile resuscitations and other duties in order to maintain the vital functions of an elderly body that is 'rusted beyond

RICHTER SCALE	
MAGNITUDE	INTENSITY
1	Detectable by instruments only
2	Barely perceptible even at epicenter
4.5	Detectable at 30 km
6	Moderate desctruction
7	A major earthquake
8	A great earthquake

van Nostrands Scientific Encyclopedia, 7th ed, New York, 1989

repair'; the 'right to die', and to do so with dignity, is rapidly becoming viewed as a fundamental freedom in the US, and in civilized countries, engendering such organizations as the Hemlock Society; see Advanced directives, 'Doctor Death', DNR, Euthanasia, 'It's over Debbie'; Cf Persistent vegetative state

rigid loop sign One or more non-motile, crescent-shaped segments of edematous small intestine which have been 'paralyzed' in position, ie not changing regardless of whether the film has been taken in the upright and decubitus position, a finding seen in a plain abdominal film in mesenteric venous occlusion

rigid spine syndrome(s) A heterogeneous group of early onset muscle dystrophies, eg X-linked Emery-Dreifuss syndrome, in which muscular atrophy begins by early adolescence, often accompanied by multiple contracture of the spinal musculature and other muscle groups

right ventricular cardiomyopathy Right ventricular dysplasia, see there

right ventricular dysplasia An idiopathic cardiomyopathy* (with strong familial tendency) in which there is a variable amount of infiltration or replacement of the myocardium by adipose and/or fibrous tissue FINDINGS 10% are asymptomatic, others have recurrent ventricular tachycardia with left bundle branch pattern (45%), congestive heart failure (25%), heart murmur (10%), sudden death (5%) DIAGNOSIS Most patients have a T wave inversion in V_1-V_3 of the EKG; 2-D and M mode echocardiography have also been reported to be of diagnostic utility (**Mayo Clin Proc 1995; 70:541**)

*Several entities are included under this general heading, to wit, arrhythmogenic right ventricular dysplasia, parchement heart, right ventricular cardiomyopathy, and Uhl's anomaly

rigor mortis Post-mortem corporal rigidity PATHOLOGY A board-like rigid contraction of skeletal muscles that first appears in the jaw (and other short muscles, eg of the hand) 2-4 hours after death, later appearing on the trunk and extremities, which reaches its peak at 24-48 hours, and disappears in the same order of its development MECHANISM After death, intracellular glycogen is depleted, ATP falls and the pH rises precipitously; rigor begins at ATP levels of 85% normal and disappears as the levels fall below 15%; the rapidity of onset of rigor mortis is related to environmental factors, including temperature, and occurs more rapidly in hot weather, or when accompanied by convulsions, strychnine poisoning, sunstroke and tetanus; rigor also occurs in cardiac and smooth muscle, affecting vessels and the GI and urogenital tracts; RM begins earliest in those muscles with increased activity prior to death, a datum that may provide soft data of potential forensic interest

Riley-Smith syndrome An AD [MIM 153480] condition characterized by benign (ie not associated with hydrocephalus or neurologic defects) macrocephaly, multiple subcutaneous hemangiomas, and pseudopapilledema

riluzole An experimental drug that modulates glutamatergic transmission that is reported in phase 1 trials to slow the progression of amyotrophic lateral sclerosis and possibly improve survival (**N Engl J Med 1994; 330:585oA**)

rimantidine An antiviral agent that is a structural analog of amantadine and estimated to be 75% effective in preventing influenza A disease during community epidemics, although it is only partially effective as therapy and post-exposure prophylaxis for influenza A, as drug-resistant strains rapidly appear; see Canyon region

rim pattern Peripheral rim pattern, shaggy pattern An immunofluorescent pattern that is arranged peripherally along the nuclear membrane, due to the deposition of antibodies directed against double-stranded DNA, deoxyribonucleoprotein and histones; high antibody titers (>

1:200) are often present in the sera of patients with SLE, and may be seen in other connective tissue diseases: see Antinuclear antibodies; Cf Speckled pattern

rim sign GI RADIOLOGY An opacification of the margin of a congenital choledochal cyst seen by a plain abdominal film GYNECOLOGIC RADIOLOGY An attenuated annular radiopacity seen in the pelvis by infusion urography corresponding to cystic pelvic mass(es), usually of ovarian origin; a similar finding may occur in benign unilateral pelvic masses with a smooth serosal contour, eg fibroma-thecoma and cystadenofibroma ORTHOPEDIC RADIOLOGY see Snowcap sign PEDIATRIC RADIOLOGY An annular, attenuated periadrenal radiopacity occurring in the rare cases of neonatal hemorrhage in this region, seen by high-dose excretory urography UROLOGIC RADIOLOGY A series of connected, overlapping physaliferous rims seen in the nephrogram phase of selective renal angiography of advanced hydronephrosis, where the attenuated curved vascular tissue surrounds dilated calices of the renal pelvis

RIND see Reversible ischemic neurological disability

rinderpest Cattle plague VETERINARY MEDICINE A viral infection of cattle that is endemic in parts of Asia and Africa, which is caused by an RNA morbillivirus (Paramyxovirus); it is characterized by high fever, stomatitis, enteritis, profuse bloody diarrhea and a 90-95% mortality; a vaccine is available

ring abscess CARDIOLOGY A descriptive term for the histologic appearance of an abscess seen in infective endocarditis, which consists of a central focus of neutrophils, necrosis and bacteria, surrounded by fibroblasts and fibrosis, frayed cardiac muscle fibers and 'round' inflammatory cells, eg plasma cells and lymphocytes OPHTHALMOLOGY A rounded intracorneal abscess

ring artifact HEMATOLOGY The concentration of hemoglobin at the periphery of erythrocytes, leaving a centrally cleared disk, a finding of undetermined significance

ringbindenfibern see Ringed fibers

ring chromosome CYTOGENETICS An anomalous chromosome in which there is a break near the end of each arm of the chromosome with joining of the broken tips to themselves, such that telomeres are not seen; RCs are defective and meiotically unstable; the phenotypic expression is a function of the amount of lost material; when the X chromosome is involved, r(X), RC's result in a Turner-like syndrome

ring enhancement A finding in the brain by CT imaging, consisting of a radiolucent zone surrounded by a faint radiodense rim, which in turn is surrounded by a second radiolucent zone outside of the rim, where the rings correspond to regional edema, hypervascularity and hypercellularity with early ingrowth of fibroblasts; although ring enhancement per se is nonspecific, it is considered typical of early cerebral abscesses, but may also be seen in various brain tumors, eg cystic astrocytoma, or metastases with central necrosis; intravenous contrast material may be used to enhance faint radiodense 'rings'

ringed fibers Ringbinden Peripheral myofilaments that are reoriented and encircle the other myofibers of the same bundle; there are thus central, longitudinal fibers, surrounded by fibers, which to the German eye, mimic the back of a 'spiral' notebook*; these fibers show no evidence of phagocytosis nor regeneration and are a subtle histological marker for myotonic dystrophy

*Hence the alternative term, Ringbindenfibern

ringed hair Pili annulati A rare AD [MIM 180600] developmental anomaly of the hair shaft with no known clinical significance, which is characterized by alternating bands of light and dark hair due to air cavities within the shafts themselves; Cf Pili torti, Woolly hair disease

ringed sideroblast A pathologic erythroblast characterized by marginated clumps of Prussian blue-staining granules corresponding to iron-loaded mitochondria, seen in the BM or in peripheral smears in red cell maturational disorders accompanied by ineffective erythropoiesis and hyperferremia, eg acquired idiopathic sideroblastic anemia, pyridoxine-responsive anemia, dyserythropoietic anemia, lead intoxication and certain hemoglobinopathies; up to 50% of cases with ringed sideroblasts eventually develop leukemia, including acute monocytic leukemia, myelomonocytic leukemia and erythroleukemia

Ringer's lactate solution A standardized sterile physiologic solution containing calcium chloride, potassium chloride, sodium chloride and sodium lactate, which contains 1.35 mmol/L Ca^{2+}, 4 mmol/L K^+ and 130 mmol/L Na^+ (US: 2.7 mEq/L Ca^{2+}, 4 mEq/L K^+ and 130 mEq/L Na^+), that is used as a topical irrigant and as a crystalloid solution for restitution of fluid volumes

ring form MICROBIOLOGY A characteristic appearance of RBCs infected by *Plasmodium* spp; the trophozoite 'rings' are globose, have a central vacuole, a red chromatin mass and blue cytoplasm; with maturation, the 'rings' evolve to an ameboid form

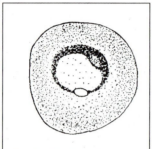

ring formation Ring enhancement, see there

ring granuloma Doughnut granuloma, see there

ring precipin reaction A generic term for a positive immunodiffusion reaction that is performed in a test tube, which in the presence of an antigen and antibody of interest forms a ring of precipitation ('precipitin') at the zone of equivalence

ring-shaped nuclei Nuclei from myeloid cells, eg mature polymorphonuclear granulocytes (neutrophils) in which the lobes of the nuclei are connected by an attenuated bridge composed of nuclear material; ring-shaped nuclei may be a subtle cytologic marker for chronic granulocytic or neutrophilic leukemia

ring shadows A descriptive term for the annular thickening of the bronchial walls seen by a plain chest film in bronchiectasis, which is identical to 'tram-track shadows'

ring sign UROLOGIC RADIOLOGY Annular filling defect(s) seen in the renal calices by intravenous pyelography, which result from necrotic sloughed papilla, see Analgesic abuse, Obstructive uropathy, Papillary necrosis, Sickle cell anemia

ring test IMMUNOLOGY A simple precipitin test, where antigen is layered over an antibody solution and the amount of precipitation at the interface is measured; see Radial immunodiffusion

ringworm Tinea corporis dermatophytosis A superficial fungal infection by *Trichophyton rubrum*, *T mentagrophytes*, *Microsporium canis* and *M gypsum*, rarely also *Epidermophyton*; in children, *T canis* is the most common agent; the trivial name derives from the lesion's characteristic onset as a scaly plaque spreading centrifugally with central clearing DDx Non-fungal dermatopathies, eg erythema annulare, the 'herald patch' of pityriasis rosea, atopic dermatitis, and other dermatitides TREATMENT Most lesions resolve without therapy; otherwise, miconazole, and if severe, griseofulvin

Rio Summit Earth Summit in Rio de Janeiro ENVIRONMENT A conference held in 1992 that provided a forum for addressing the population-related and other man-made changes on the global ecosystem, including tropical deforestation, extinction of species, desertification, declining biodiversity, accumulation of greenhouse gases, air and water pollution, alterations in food production, and others (New York Times 5 May 1992; C1)

RIPA Radioimmunoprecipitation assay, see there

ripple effect see Signal event

rippling effect A descriptor for the layered angiographic appearance of blood vessels in the cortical sulci peripheral to a cerebral abscess through which the blood flows in an undulating pattern; other cerebral lesions differ in that they may be associated with gyral edema or with neovascularization

rippling muscle disease A disorder of adolescent onset that is usually autosomal dominant, occasionally sporadic, which results when local compression of a muscle evokes myoedema, followed by longitudinal contraction of a muscle, moving transversely across the muscle in a 10-20 muscle fascicle wave fancifully likened to 'plucking a chromatic scale on a harp'; while superficially resembling myotonia, the entity is electrically silent and clinically benign

'Rip van Winkle syndrome' Pathologic hypersomnia; see Narcolepsy, Sleep disorders

RISA 1) Radioactive iodinated serum albumin 2) Radioimmunosorbent assay A radioisotopic technique for detecting low levels of IgE; Cf RAST

RISC Reduced instruction set computer COMPUTERS A 'smart' microprocessing chip that uses different algorithms and modern ultramicrocircuitry design to provide greater and more efficient computing power*, while reducing the number of instructions required for each task; RISC chips are used in laser printers and have been incorporated in the next generation of personal computers from Apple Computers and IBM; these use RISC microprocessors produced by Motorola (models 601, 603, 604, and 620), the first of which (the 601) running at 110 MHz is reported in bench tests to outpace Intel Corporation's 100 MHz Pentium

*A RISC processor runs 50 to 75% faster than its CISC (complex instruction set computer) counterpart

RISCC rating CLINICAL NUTRITION Cholesterol-saturated fat index (of Conner et al) The ratio of ingested saturated fat and cholesterol to calories (RISCC), a parameter used in evaluating a diet's fat content, which can be stratified into low– and high-fat diets; the highest RISCC rating in a low-fat diet is 15, and the lowest RISCC in a high-fat diet is 22 (N Engl J Med 1993; 328:1213OA) RISCC rating is calculated by the formula

$$(1.01 \times \text{sat'd fat (g)}) + (0.05 \times \text{cholesterol (mg)})/\text{kcal}/1000$$

risk EPIDEMIOLOGY *'The chance or likelihood that an undesirable event or effect will occur, as a result of use or nonuse, incidence, or influence of a chemical, physical, or biologic agent, especially during a stated period.'* (International Dictionary of Medicine, J Wiley & Sons, New York, 1986); in occupational health, risk is determined by the potential severity of the hazard and the frequency of exposure to the 'risky' substance or activity, usually understood to mean the probability of suffering from a particular disease **ABSOLUTE RISK** The number of persons suffering from a disease when the exposed population is known with certainty **RELATIVE RISK** An estimate of persons suffering from a disease, based on an extrapolation of the persons presumed to be exposed to a predetermined factor; see Epidemiology, see Hazard risk rating

risk assessment TOXICOLOGY The process by which new chemical substances are evaluated for their potential impact on human health, a process that entails determining the substance's toxicity and the number of people exposed to the substance; see Ames' test, Toxicity testing

risk management The constellation of activities (planning, organizing, directing, evaluation and implementation) involved in reducing the risks of injury to patients and employees and reducing property damage or loss within health care facilities; risk management in its various forms, including non-medical liability is estimated to cost 15% of the US federal government budget, ie between $60 and $175 x 10^9 annually

ristocetin A naturally occurring antibiotic obtained from the fermentation of *Nocardia lurida*, which at one time had currency in treating antibiotic-resistant staphylococcal infections, which induces platelet aggregation *in vitro*; the ristocetin cofactor assay quantifies the ability of von Willebrand factor in plasma to agglutinate platelets in the presence of ristocetin; in the absence of ADP, calcium and fibrinogen are required for platelet aggregation, a period designated as 'ristocetin time', which is prolonged in afibrinogenemia, dysfibrinogenemia, heparin therapy, idiopathic thrombocytopenic purpura, infectious mononucleosis, acute leukemia, Glanzmann's disease and storage pool diseases; in Bernard-Soulier disease, there is no aggregation due to the lack of a membrane receptor; in von Willebrand's disease, aggregation does not occur without normal plasma; see Platelet aggregation

risus sardonicus A fixed 'sarcastic' grimace and anxious expression with drawing up of the eyebrows and corners of the mouth due to spasms of the masseter and other facial muscles, accompanied by rigidity of the neck and trunk muscles and arching of the back; the RS is a clinical finding in generalized tetanus, and caused by a neurotoxin produced by *Clostridium tetani*, a soil contaminant with a 7-10 day incubation period, and up to 90% mortality in unvaccinated or susceptible populations, eg urban narcotic addicts; the classic spasms of risus sardonicus (trismus, spasmus caninus) may be elicited by external stimuli and may also be seen in strychnine poisoning, hysteria, catalepsy

Note: The caricature of this grotesque facial expression has been fancifully likened to that seen on Batman's arch enemy, the Joker

Ritalin Methylphenidate, see ther

RITARD model Removable intestinal tie adult rabbit diarrhea model An animal model for studying the pathogenesis of diarrhea induced by *Vibrio cholerae* toxin (Infec Immun 1983; 41:1175)

ritodrine A relatively specific epinephrine-like β-adrenergic agonist, that acts on β $_2$-adrenoreceptors to relax smooth muscle in arterioles, bronchi, and uterus; ritodrine was developed specifically for obstetrical use; it was approved by the FDA in 1980 as a tocolytic agent; despite its wide use for this purpose, it has only marginal benefits in inhibiting preterm labor (N Engl J Med 1992; 327:308OA, 349ED)

ritual PSYCHIATRY A repetitive stereotyped behavior or activity that is a distorted elaboration of some routine of daily life, which is used to relieve stress and anxiety; rituals are a characteristic feature of obsessive-complusive disorder

river blindness 1) Onchocercal dermatopathy, see there 2) Onchocerciasis, see there

RLC Ribosomal lamellar complexes, see there

RLF Replication licensing factor, see there

RNA decoy A synthetic molecule designed to to interfere competitively with normal protein-RNA interactions or that cut viral RNA through RNA-RNA interactions; some authors believe that RNA decoys have therapeutic potential in treating HIV infectiion

RNA editing Any natural alteration of the gene expression that occurs at the level of mRNA, by a variety of mechanisms, including insertion, deletion or substitution of nucleotides in an RNA molecule (Nature 1991; 349:434, 370) RNA editing is induced by guide RNA, which directs the insertion and deletion of nucleotides at 'correct' sites on the unedited RNA; this activity has thus far been identified in *Trypanosoma brucei* and other simple parasites (Science 1991; 253:136RN) see Editing, Guide RNA

RNA fingerprinting A technique used to identify the presence of specific RNA molecules PRINCIPLE RNAse T1 is used to cut RNA at the 3' end of each guanylate residue, resulting in short 2-20 base pair oligonucleotide sequences, allowing a matching of two RNAs by length, without the need to sequence the RNA; Cf DNA fingerprinting, Protein fingerprinting

RNA footprinting A purified fragment of double-stranded DNA is labeled with an isotope at the 5' end of one strand and allowed to interact with RNA polymerase or histones; this same strand (with the attached RNA proteinase) is then subjected to scission by either DNAse I or by the synthetic reagent MPE (methidium propyl-EDTA) causing DNA to be cleaved at every base pair, except at those sites where 'protecting' proteins, ie promoter or regulatory proteins or histones prevent base pair cutting; the sites where DNA remains intact are the sites that are bound by the regulatory proteins and thus these experiments are known as 'DNA protection experiments'

RNA hybridization see Hybridization

RNA ligase An enzyme integral to RNA splicing, which catalyzes the formation of phosphodiester bonds

RNA-recognition motif see RRM

RNA polymerase Any of a family of enzymes* [EC 2.7.7.6] that copies strands of RNA from a DNA template, using nucleoside triphosphates as building blocks and and liberated inorganic pyrophosphate (diphosphate) as a source of energy; RNA polymerase I synthesizes pre-rRNA, is present in the nucleolus and when digested, yields three cleavage products: -28S, 5.8S and 18S; RNA polymerase I is capable of transcribing the DNA from any species, provided that a species-specific transcriptional protein is attached, usually 'upstream' of the gene segment to be transcribed; RNA polymerase III synthesizes RNA outside of the nucleolus, including tRNAs and 5S rRNA; type III RNA polymerase, like type I RNA polymerase requires a species-specific activating protein; Cf Ribonucleases, Ribozymes

*Also known as DNA-directed RNA polymerase, the term recommended (1992) by the Nomenclature Committee of the IUBMB (International Union of Biochemistry and Molecular Biology)

RNA splicing The process in which the non-translating portions or introns from the primary transcript of DNA are removed and the exons are joined together, forming an mRNA transcript from which proteins will be transcribed

RNA world A conceptual time and place in the early evolution of the planet when the Earth was populated by biologically active, self-replicating molecules, that were later assisted by crude polypeptides; the validity of an 'RNA world', albeit brief (lasting less than 100 million years) is supported by the discovery of catalytic activity by RNA, the existance of ribozymes, and vast structural and functional correlations of various types of RNAs and ribonucleoproteins (Science 1994; 264; 1479BR) see Primordial soup

RNAse P MOLECULAR BIOLOGY A generic term for any of a family of catalytic RNA subunits present in all cells studied to date; RNAse P participates in the biosynthesis of tRNA, thus being essential for cell growth; it is present in the nucleus, and may also be active in mitochondria; RNAse P in conjunction with so-called guide sequences may be of use in inactivating genes in mammalian cells and bear fruit in the form of therapies for human disease (Bio/Technology 1995; 13:327)

RO1 (RO-1) The basic grant for the individual researcher, awarded by the National Institute of Health (USA), which averages $200 000; there were 4600 new RO-1s in 1990

RO 24-7429 AIDS A *tat* protein inhibitor that showed early promise as an effective anti-HIV therapy, but which lost financial support by the company (Hoffmann-LaRoche) that produced it (Science 1991; 253:262RN, 254:1715) see AIDS therapy

Ro 44-9883 Lamifibran, see there

roach see Cockroach

robertsonian translocation Centromeric fusion CLINICAL GENETICS A chromosomal rearrangement consisting of a balanced translocation between two acrocentric chromosomes, resulting in a large metacentric or submetacentric chromosome, which is accompanied by loss from the short arm of the 'donating' chromosome; RT is seen in 4% of trisomy (Down syndrome), and occurs between chromosomes 13, 14, 15, 21, and 22, where a segment from the long arm of one chromosome, eg 21 is translocated to another chromosome, most commonly to chromosome 14 t(14q21q); three of the six possible resulting genotypes are viable: One is completely normal, one is genotypically abnormal, but phenotypically normal, ie the chromosomes are translocated but normal and one case expresses Down syndrome, ie both genotypically and phenotypically abnormal; the risk of repetition of a Robertsonian-type Down syndrome is 10-15% for a maternal carrier and 5% for a paternal carrier of the translocation

'Robin Hood syndrome' Reverse cerebral steal, see there

robotics LABORATORY MEDICINE The devices used to automate the production and manufacturing of goods and services; robotic devices minimize the human error inherent in manually operated workstations and instruments, and have been developed to the point where once a specimen is loaded, the robot picks up a sample, injects it into the instrument, analyzes it, and transfers the data back to the technologist at the workstation for evaluation and release of the results to the requesting site or physician

robust STATISTICS Pertaining or referring to any method (or procedure) that is relatively insensitive to violations in the method's required assumptions or rules, or a method that makes few assumptions ab initio

ROC Receiver operating characteristic, relative operator characteristic CLINICAL DECISION MAKING A '...*global measure of of the accuracy of a diagnostic system, independent of the cutoff point used to discriminate 'normal' from 'abnormal' results.'* JR Beck

ROC analysis The formal discipline that addresses the relationship between a true positive fraction and a false positive fraction for a diagnostic procedure that can take on multiple values; as an example of the utility of ROC, RA reveals that measurement of apolipoproteins is not superior to lipid values in discriminating those with or without coronary artery disease (Arch Pathol Lab Med 1994; 118:141OA) Note: RA is a viable alternative to the over-simplistic 4-cell decision matrix, see there

ROC curve A plot of datapoints (figure) in which the horizontal axis represents the false positive fraction and the vertical axis represents the true positive fraction (Semin Nuc Med 1978; 8:299); the curve plots false positives versus false negatives; each point reflects the strategy of calling all results for a given value positive or negative where a binary disease status exists (presence or absence of disease, eg myocardial infarct if CK-MB is elevated, or no myocardial infarction if CK-MB is not elevated)

Rochalimaea spp MICROBIOLOGY A genus of small gram-negative rods that are currently assigned to the Rickettsiaceae (although recent evidence favors reclassification among Bartonellaceae); there are four recognized species *R quintana, R henselae* (which has been associated with cat scratch disease-N Engl J Med 1993; 329:8OA, and bacillary angiomatosis-N Engl J Med 1992; 327:1625RV), *R elizabethae*, and the Canadian vole agent, *R vinsonii*, which has thus far not been associated with human disease (N Engl J Med 1994; 330:1509RA)

Rochalimaea henselae Bartonella henselae, see there

Rochalimaea quintana Bartonella quintana, see there

Rocio encephalitis An epidemic viral infections occurring in Brazil that is similar to Japanese encephalitis and is maintained in wild birds and transmitted by mosquitoes

Rockefeller University Founded in 1901 as the Rockefeller Institute for Medical Research on a 15-acre campus in Manhattan, the 'Rock' supports 600 regular faculty and post-doctoral investigators, 125 graduate students and 975 support staff on an annual budget of $100 million; there are 45 laboratories with a broad range of research, one-third of which concentrate on mechanisms of cancer; other interests include neuroscience, viruses and immunology; 19 Nobel laureates have been associated with the University and two of its students have won the Nobel prize; Cf Howard Hughes Medical Institute, Max Planck Institute, Salk Institute, Whitehead Institute

rocker bottom feet Congenital vertical talus, pes valgus A rigid flatfoot deformity caused by a malpositioned navicular bone at the neck of the talus; the ankle is in severe equinus and the forefoot in dorsiflexion, ie rocker bottom-like, accompanied by contraction of the talonavicular, deltoid and calcaneal cuboidal ligaments, the peroneus brevis and triceps surae muscles Rocker bottom feet occur as isolated deformities or may accompany trisomy 18 and 13 TREATMENT Early manipulation and plaster correction of the forefoot into plantar flexion, inversion and adduction; 'benign neglect' represents malpractice as this deformity requires triple arthrodesis when RBF is ignored by the patent's family or health care providers

rocker bottom shadow A horizontal, broad, curved soft tissue radiodensity that partially overlies the heart, extends into the hilum, corresponding to the thymus, seen in a plain antero-posterior chest film in neonatal pneumomediastinum, and derives its name from old wooden cradles; see Spinnaker sail sign

rocket electrophoresis IMMUNOLOGY A one-dimensional enzyme immune assay in which an antigen-bearing fluid is electrophoresed through agarose containing an antibody to the antigen of interest (figure); rocket electrophoresis is used to quantify von Willebrand factor levels in the blood and derives its name from the sharp projectile-like immunoprecipitin spike

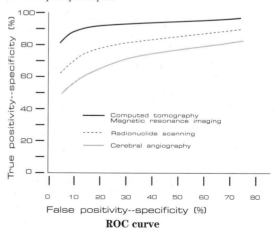

ROC curve

Rocky Mountain spotted fever A exanthematous disease first described in Indian squaws in the Bitterroot Valley, Montana, located in the Rocky Mountains, which is more common in the eastern US from April to October and may occur in large cities, eg, New York (**N Engl J Med 1988; 318:1345**) Agent *Rickettsia rickettsii* Hosts Furry woodland creatures (rodents *et al*) Vectors Wood (*Dermacentor andersoni*) and dog (*D variabilis*) ticks PATHOGENESIS Endo-thelial damage activates platelets, fibrinolysis and the intrinsic and extrinsic coagulation pathways (**N Engl J Med 1988; 318:1021**) CLINICAL 1 week incubation, followed by a discrete pale, blanchable centrifugal maculopapular rash, which may be dusky in color, hence the alias, 'black measles', persistent headache, fever, ± coughs and rales, myalgia, malaise, splenomegaly; nausea, vomiting, abdominal pain, CNS symptoms (delirium, stupor, ataxia, meningismus), myocarditis, EKG abnormalities, thrombocytopenia, multiple coagulopathies, renal failure and shock LABORATORY Weil-Felix test is positive for antibodies to OX-19 and OX-2 TREATMENT Tetracycline, chloramphenicol Mortality 3-10%; ↑ in blacks, ↑ > age 40

rod cell NEUROPATHOLOGY A modified microglial cell that increases in size and number in paretic dementia (tertiary syphilis) as well as in subacute encephalitides, eg encephalitis lethargica, cerebral trypanosomiasis (*T gambiense*); rod cell-like changes are also seen in normal astrocytes after acute toxic insults; the bipolar forms, which are normally perpendicular to the surface, proliferate and increase in size, the nuclei elongated, the cytoplasm loses its trabeculation and is best visualized with a basic aniline dye or Prussian blue, due to rod cells' accumulation of iron NEUROPHYSIOLOGY *epitheliocytus (neurosensorius) bacillifer* [NH3] A retinal visual cell that functions optimally during conditions of reduced light

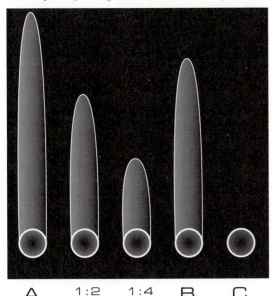

Rocket electrophoresis

A SERIAL DILUTIONS OF A POSITIVE CONTROL AT 1:1, 1:2, AND 1:4

B UNKNOWN OR PATIENT SPECIMEN

C NEGATIVE CONTROL

rodent ulcer A deeply invasive basal cell carcinoma of long duration with induration of ulcerated walls

'Rodney Dangerfield syndrome' A highly colloquial term for the disparaging attitude cast upon primary care specialties, who have traditionally not garnered the same respect as specialists

*Coined by R Petersdorf in reference to US comedian Rodney Dangerfield's trademark line '...I don't get no respect.' (Am Med News 4 May 1992 p26)

Roe* v. *Wade SOCIAL MEDICINE, OBSTETRICS A 'landmark' legal case that was presented before the US Supreme Court in 1973, which has been instrumental in legalizing abortion; the decision was based on the concept that 1) The constitutional right to privacy is broad enough to encompass a woman's right to an abortion if the conceptus is incapable of reasonably functioning outside of the womb, defined as less than 27 weeks of gestation and 2) The state's interest to abridge that constitutional right is related to the stage (in trimesters) of pregnancy; see Mexico City policy, Webster decision; Cf Amsterdam strategy, ZPG

Note: The 1989 US Supreme Court decision in the Webster case‡ is a partial retreat from a legal environment that facilitated abortions, and to some, signals a return to political conservatism

Roemer's law HEALTH CARE POLICY '...*empty beds tend to become filled.*', 'rule' that recognizes that the hospital days per capita increases with the number of hospital beds (**JAMA 1995; 273:1227**)

roentgen A unit of dose exposure to X- and gamma-radiation, corresponding to the amount of radiation capable of producing an electrostatic unit of positive and negative ions when passing through 1 cc of dry air at standard temperature and pressure (2.58×10^{-4} of ions/kg air); Cf Gray, Rad, Rem

roentgen 'hangover' Acute radiation injury syndrome, see there

'roid rage An acute psychotic response of unknown pathogenesis that occurs in subjects who abuse anabolic steroids, usually in the context of body building

role-playing PSYCHOLOGY The voluntary and conscious adoption of a particular role* (eg a child adopting that of a parent) under the guidance of another person, eg a phychotherapist; RP provides 1) Insight on how the person playing the role perceives other person(s) and 2) A window through which the person playing the role may see the other person's vantage

*An integrated behavior and repertoire of responses that is learned and automatic, which reflects a person's function in a situation

rolfing Structural integration ALTERNATIVE MEDICINE A deep massage therapy developed by IP Rolf that seeks to 'realign' the body by altering the tone of myofascial tissues, facilitating 'structural integration'; rolfing is philosophically similar to chiropractic, in that inaccurate or poor posture is thought to be detrimental to a person's health, energy, mental and physical efficiency, and like chiropractic, the claims of therapeutic success are uncertain as large double-blinded studies have not been performed; Cf Alternative medicine

Note: It is probable that the highly individualized nature of these therapies precludes valid statistical studies of their efficacy; see Chiropractic

'roller ball surgery' GYNECOLOGY A colloquial term for laser surgery of uterine leiomyomas, which are benign tumors composed of dense stroma that markedly deform the endometrium, and may make successful pregnancy impossible by preventing normal endometrial expansion; in this technique, the tumors are 'shelled out' by rolling the tumors while cutting with the laser

Rollerblade™ injury EMERGENCY MEDICINE A generic term for any accident that occurs in a person using in-line skates*; in-line skating has been the fastest growing sport in the US for a number of years; there were ± 9.3 million in-line skaters in 1992, ⅔ of whom are < age 17, and 800 000 in-line hockey players; certain aspects of in-line skating (especially for novices) provide an suitable substrate for accidents, to wit high speed, inexperience, and difficulty in braking, which requires that the boot be dorsiflexed to bring the rubber brake in contact with terra firma; the Consumer Product Safety Commission estimated that 83 000 injuries would occur in 1994 ACCIDENT PRO-FILE In a study of 32 injuries seen in an emergency department, the mean age was 17, 78% involved the upper extremity, most commonly fractures of the distal radius; surgical treatment (rod insertion for femoral spiral fracture) was required for one (Mayo Clin Proc 1995; 70:752₀ₐ)

*The author apologizes to the manufacturers of other in-line skates for listing this entry under Rollerblade™ rather than as the more generic term in-line skating injury; the reason was simply that of logistics, as the letter I had already been completed and sent to the publisher; in future editions of this work, this flaw will be corrected

rolling circle replication MOLECULAR BIOLOGY The mechanism by which bacteriophages efficiently reproduce; after injection of the phage chromosome into a host bacterium, the phage directs protein synthesis, using the host's reproductive machinery, first reproducing in the relatively inefficient 'theta' mode; after several rounds of theta reproduction, the phage chromosomes switch to the sigma or 'rolling circle' mode, in which the circle extends a tail; the replication machinery then hooks directly onto the tails, allowing continuous phage production; once the enzyme terminase recognizes the cos sequence of nucleotides at the end of the viral chromosome, it closes the circle and begins another round of replication

roller coaster headache A headache caused by a subdural hematoma occurring in subjects subjected to violent movement of the head as occurs in a roller coaster (N Engl J Med 1995; 332:15815)

ROM 1) Range of motion ORTHOPEDICS The arc of a joint's movement, potentially limited by musculoskeletal defects 2) Read-only memory COMPUTERS A silicon chip that contains permanent instructions, including entire routines or programs that cannot be erased or altered by the microprocessor; Cf PROM, RAM

Roman bridge appearance A descriptor for a histological hallmark of in situ carcinoma of the breast–cribriform type, which consists of curved 'bars' of well-differentiated, bland malignant cells without an intervening fibrovascular core that span two or more points of a duct (figure) Note: This is a 'soft' histopathological criterion for malignancy that is most often confused with intraductal epitheliosis of the breast

The name derives from the histologic mimicking of the voluptuous architecture typical of the water works of the ancient Roman empire, including bridges and aquaducts

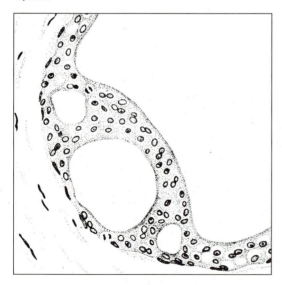

Roman bridge appearance

Roman fever Antiquated for malaria

Romano-Ward syndrome see Long Q-T syndrome

Romanovsky stains PATHOLOGY A group of eosin-methylene blue stains, eg Wright-Giemsa and Leishman that are used for peripheral blood smears; the red cells are stained lilac and bacteria or parasites, platelets, lymphocytes, red to purple

R-on-T phenomenon CARDIOLOGY A premature ventricular depolarization that is so early in the cardiac cycle that it falls on the apex of the preceding T wave, potentially presaging ventricular tachycardia or fibrillation; the EKG finding of an 'R-on-T' is considered an indication for the intensity of anti-arrhythmic therapy eg lidocaine

'room temps' TRANSFUSION MEDICINE Blood bank jargon for antibodies that agglutinate at room temperature, and which have minimal potential for causing transfusion reactions; Cf Cold agglutinin disease

Note: Most antibodies of clinical importance, ie those capable of inducing transfusion reactions, occur with IgG antibodies that agglutinate at 37°C

rooming-in NEONATOLOGY The placing of a newborn in the same room as the mother in the early post-partum period, which is thought to foster maternal-fetal bonding and facilitate breast-feeding (Acta Paediatr Scand 1990; 79:1017); see Bonding, Rooting

'root canal' DENTISTRY A colloquialism for the complete therapy of a tooth with well-advanced decay that is no longer superficial enough for a simple amalgam filling to be adequate permanent therapy; a 'root canal' consists of opening, cleansing and sterilizing the root canal, closing and filling it with an impervious material, eg guttapercha, thereby preventing future infection, and covering the remaining tooth with a porcelain cap

rooting NEONATOLOGY The searching for the mother's nipple by the neonate, which is often accompanied by grunting, opening of the infant's mouth and sucking; this reflex of early infancy is elicited by touching the baby's cheeks and by the smell of milk

rootwork PSYCHIATRY *'A set of cultural interpretations that ascribe illness to hexing, witchcraft, or the evil influence of another person. Symptoms may include generalized anxiety and gastrointestinal complaints (nausea, vomiting, diarrhea), weakness, dizziness...'* and the fear of being poisoned and/or killed; in this context, a 'root' ('spell' or 'hex') must be removed throught the work of a 'specialist' or 'root doctor', who can in turn place a hex on an enemy; the term rootwork is used in the US South and in the Caribbean; among Latinos, it is known as mal puesto or brujeria (DSM-IV™, 1994) see Culture-bound syndrome

rope sign NEUROLOGY An acute angulation between the chin and larynx due to weakness of the hyoid muscles, resulting in posterior displacement of the hyoid bone, and narrowing the hypopharyngeal passage

Rope's test see String test

ROSC Return of spontaneous circulation

'Rorschach proglottid' A descriptor for the broad, short gravid proglottids of *Diphyllobothrium latum*, which have been fancifully likened to the appearance of certain Rorschach ink blots; Cf Zipper proglottid

Rorschach test Rorschach technique of projective assessment Ink blot test A type of personality testing in which 10 ink blots are presented to a subject for his interpretation of what he sees in the 'picture' (figure, facing page) ; the test generates an enormous amount of data, much of which requires subjective interpretation; first used in 1921, the 'ink blot test' reached its peak of popularity in the 1950s but continues to have currency among psychologists; see Psychological testing

rosary An adjectival descriptor of occasional use in medicine, referring to periodic expansions or densities arranged in a linear fashion* **rachitic rosary** Bulbous widening of the costochondral junction due to softened epiphyses seen in infants with vitamin D-deficient rickets; the 'rachitic' rosary may also be seen in congenital neonatal hypophosphatemia, childhood hypophosphatasia and in adenosine deaminase deficiency **scorbutic rosary** Bulbous enlargement of the costochondral junction, similar to the rachitic rosary except that the angulation of the scorbutic 'beads' is sharper than in rickets as it is due to subluxation of the sternal plate

*Likened to a string of beads used to count prayers, especially the Roman Catholic 'Rosary', a devotion consisting of meditation on the five sacred mysteries during recitation of five decades of Ave Marias, each of which begins with a paternoster and ends with a Gloria

rosary bead appearance COLONIC RADIOLOGY A descriptor for the exaggerated haustral contractions that may be seen in barium studies of irritable bowel syndrome, often accompanied by constipation, pain and hardened, dehydrated and pelleted or rabbit-like stools

rosary bead esophagus Corkscrew esophagus, see there

rosebud hands A combination of bony and soft tissue syndactylism seen in Apert's craniocephalosyndactyly syndrome, which may be further accompanied by scaphocephaly, premature closure of the cranial sutures and mental retardation, facial deformities including hypertelorism, a high forehead, bulging eyes, short nose, synostosis of the vertebral bodies and carpotarsal syndactyly or lobster-claw feet

Rosenthal classification A numerical notation system used as an alternative for phenotyping the Rh blood groups Note: although the classification is more logical, it is unlikely to replace the Race-Fisher and Weiner systems that are firmly entrenched in the blood banking literature

Rosenthal fibers NEUROPATHOLOGY Small elongated eosinophilic processes seen by light microscopy in the astrocytes of chronic degenerative neural diseases, eg Alexander's disease, multiple sclerosis and spongioblastoma, as well as in cerebellar astrocytomas

the Rose Sheet A specialized weekly report that provides business and US federal regulatory information in the toiletries, fragrances, skin care industries produced by FDC Reports, Inc Chevy Chase, Md

rose spots INFECTIOUS DISEASE Transient 1-5 mm in diameter reddish macules that blanch on pressure, are located on the lower chest and upper abdomen and are related to bacterial emboli in cutaneous vessels accompanied by focal aggregates of dermal macrophages; rose spots classically occur in *Salmonella typhi*-induced typhoid fever during the first week of disease, coinciding with the onset of splenomegaly

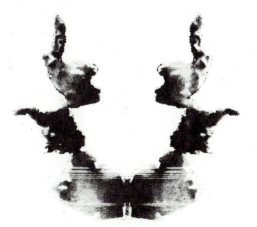

Rorschach inkblot

rosette A term for a garland-like arrangement of structures, cells or bodies around a central point or blood vessel, usually seen by light microscopy HEPATOLOGY Liver cell 'rosettes' correspond to hepatocytes that deviate from their usual trabecular pattern, divided into cholestatic rosettes, a response attributed to biliary obstruction and consequent cholestasis and regenerative rosettes, seen in a background of severe chronic active hepatitis, acute and chronic inflammation

IMMUNOLOGY **E ROSETTES** Nonimmune rosettes The spontaneous clustering of sheep erythrocytes around T-cells; Erythrocyte rosettes are formed by lymphocytes with abundant CD3 receptors, which are 'pan-T' cell markers **EA ROSETTES** Eythrocyte-antibody rosettes Clusters of sheep erythrocytes around monocytes and macrophages sensitized with sheep erythrocyte hemolysin, which occurs when the Fc portion of the hemolysin molecule attaches to the Fc receptor on the surface of the M cell **EAC ROSETTES** Erythrocyte-antibody-complement rosettes Cell clusters formed by B cells, monocyte and macrophages when sheep erythrocytes have been sensitized with a heterophile antibody in the presence of complement NEUROPATHOLOGY **EPENDYMAL ROSETTES** Structures that recapitulate features of the normal ependymal cavity, which have a small central rounded-to-elongated lumina, optional cilia and blepharoplasts (distinct basally oriented granular corpuscles in the cytoplasm) **FLEXNER-WINTERSTEINER ROSETTES** Structures which are virtually pathognomonic for well-differentiated retinoblastomas, consisting of 'bland' nuclei arranged around a fibrillary background of axonal material **HOMER-WRIGHT ROSETTES** Perivascular pseudorosettes A 'classic' finding in neuroblastomas, characterized by a ring of tumor cells arranged in 'garlands', surrounding a central space filled with pale-staining neuro-fibrillary material, packed around a delicate fibrovascular core; the tumor cells themselves have scant, poorly-defined cytoplasm, the nuclei have coarse but evenly dispersed chromatin, may have marked mitotic activity (olfactory neuroblastomas demonstrate low mitotic activity)

rosette blisters DERMATOLOGY Annular arrangement of sausage-shaped bullae around an eschar on the trunk, genitalia and legs in idiopathic linear IgA dermatosis, an eruption with variable pruritus, most commonly seen in infants IMMUNOFLUORESCENCE Liner IgA, occasionally C3 TREATMENT Sulfapyridine or corticosteroids; most cases spontaneously resolve within 2-4 years

rosette test NEONATOLOGY A screening test for detecting significant fetomaternal hemorrhage, where an indicator cell forms easily identified rosettes around individual Rh-D fetal cells that may be present in the Rh-negative mother; this qualitative test can detect a 10 ml or greater fetomaternal hemorrhage and should be followed by a quantitative test, eg the Kleihauer-Betke test

Rose-Waaler test IMMUNOLOGY A specialized passive hemagglutination test for detecting rheumatoid factors, which uses sheep erythrocytes sensitized with a subagglutinating dose of rabbit anti-sheep erythrocyte IgG; when rheumatoid factor is present in test serum, it combines with the membrane-bound IgG, causing agglutination; the Rose-Waaler is not commonly used as most rheumatoid factor tests use latex particles to establish agglutination, which while less specific, are much easier to perform

Rosewater syndrome An X-linked [MIM 306500] form of male pseudohermaphroditism characterized by gynecomastia, sterility, ↑ testosterone, estrogen and gonadotropins; see Pseudohermaphroditism

rose windows Circular pores or fenestrations with wedge-shaped slits covered by a thin diaphragm, located in the capillary walls of endocrine glands, eg pancreatic islet cells, which may be seen by EM and freeze fracturing techniques; the name derives from the circular windows filled with tracery, used in Gothic architecture

rotating crystal technique A method for determining the 3-D conformation of a substance, which consists of analyzing the X-ray diffraction patterns of a single purified crystal of a molecule of interest, which is mounted and rotated around multiple axes, providing multiple diffraction spots that can be used to resolve the molecule's secondary structure

rotating frame of reference MRI A point and its corresponding coordinate system that is rotating about the axis of the static magnetic field B$_o$ (with respect to a stationary or 'laboratory' frame of reference) at a frequency equal to that of the applied radiofrequency magnetic field, B$_1$; although B$_1$ is a rotating vector, it appears stationary in the rotating frame, and allows simple calculations; see Magnetic resonance imaging

rotation Movement around an axis GRADUATE MEDICAL EDUCATION A period of time during which a medical student, or a physician in an early period of his training works in a particular service OBSTETRICS The turning of a fetus around its long axis such that the presenting part changes

rotator cuff SURGICAL ANATOMY The musculotendinous covering of the shoulder joint, which is delineated anteriorly by the subscapularis muscle, superiorly by the supraspinatus muscle and posteriorly by the infraspinatus and teres minor muscles; degenerative changes of the rotator cuff tendons are considered a part of the normal aging process, especially affecting the supraspinatus tendon at the zone of Codman, due to susceptibility of its vascular supply; see Frozen shoulder, Milwaukee shoulder syndrome

rotavirus An encapsulated double-stranded RNA virus with a bilayer 75 nm in diameter capsid that belongs to the reovirus family; it is a major agent of epidemic and endemic gastroenteritis, usually causing mild disease, which may be severe in children under age two due to intense vomiting CLINICAL Diarrhea 2-12 days in otherwise healthy children; in the immunocompromised, disseminated infection with hepatic and renal involvement DIAGNOSIS ELISA, DNA probes, PCR of stool (Sci & Med Nov/Dec 1994 p9) VACCINE The tetravalent reassortment vaccine may be the most effective (JAMA 1995; 273:1191) see Astrovirus, West-to-East phenomenon

rotavirus gastroenteritis see Rotavirus

rough sex A popular term for any sexual activity in which there is a genuine possibility that the participating parties may suffer bodily harm or even death should one or the other(s) lose control; sexual asphyxia in a state of mutual consent (eg bondage) might be regarded as a classic example of RS gone awry, where one party has ligature around the neck and the other party controlling its tightness loses control, resulting in strangulation; see Paraphilia, Sexual asphyxia, Sexual deviancy

roughage Indigestible complex carbohydrates (eg bran and cellulose) of plant origin that form the bulk of the stool; roughage absorbs water, acting as laxatives, and sequesters bile acids and degradation products; ↑ dietary roughage is linked to ↓ diverticulosis and colorectal cancer, and ↓ cholesterol in serum; see Bran

rouleaux Stacks of erythrocytes in groups of 3 to 10 cells, likened to stacked coins; rouleaux formation occurs with increased plasma fibrinogen and globulins, increased sedimentation rate due to dextran and monoclonal gammopathies (multiple myeloma, Waldenström's disease), cryoglobulinemia, sarcoidosis and cirrhosis; rouleaux formation, which interferes with identification of weak antigen-antibody reactions in the blood bank, can be reduced *in vitro* by adding saline or other low-ionic strength solution; see LISS

round *verb* To visit the patients for which a physician is responsible; see Rounds

round cell A generic term referring to a relatively small (10-20 µm) leukocyte with (usually) a single round-to-oval nucleus; RCs include lymphocytes, monocytes, plasma cells and occasionally epithelioid histiocytes

round cell inflammation A nonspecific term for any (usually chronic) inflammatory process histologically characterized by abundant aggregates of 'round' mononuclear cells, eg lymphocytes, monocytes, and plasma cells

'round cell' tumors SURGICAL PATHOLOGY Tumors that are composed of relatively monotonous sheets of cells with bland round-to-oval, relatively basophilic nuclei, clumped chromatin, scanty cytoplasm, and often have a 'primitive' appearance; round cell tumors are often poorly differentiated, defy classification of embryologic lineage by routine histologic examination and may require various special studies including

IMMUNOPEROXIDASE STAINS to detect the presence of intermediate filaments or hormone production

ELECTRON MICROSCOPY to identify dense core granules or premelanosomes and

MOLECULAR STUDIES to detect amplification of genes, as in the T cell receptor's β chain; tumors that may present with a round cell appearance include lymphomas, undifferentiated carcinomas, neuroendocrine tumors, and amelanotic melanomas

round heart disease An idiopathic disease of previously healthy chickens*, which die suddenly, and have postmortem findings of an enlarged round heart

*Raising the question of fowl play

rounds Bedside visits by a physician (or other health professionals) in order to evaluate treatment, assess the current course and to document the patient's progress or recuperation; see Professorial rounds, Round, SOAP; Cf Grand rounds

Rous sarcoma virus A single-stranded type C RNA virus that causes sarcoma in chickens, and which is the prototypic acute transforming retrovirus (ie oncovirus); RSV's genome contains *gag* (which encodes a structural protein in the viral core), *pol* (which encodes reverse transcriptase) and *env* (which encodes envelope glycoprotein) and V-*src* (the viral oncogene responsible for RSV's in vivo and in vitro oncogenic potential); Cf HIV, Retrovirus

routing COMPUTERS The pathway that information travels in a LAN (local area network) in a network of linked computers

Roux-en-Y operation GENERAL SURGERY Any of a group of surgical procedures in which a Y-shaped anastomosis includes the small intestine; the distal resected end is implanted into an organ, eg bile ducts (choledochojejunostomy and portoenterostomy), esophagus (esophagojejunostomy), and pancreas (pancreaticojejunostomy), while the proximal end is implanted into the small intestine further 'downstream' to prevent reflux

rowing crossbridge model PHYSIOLOGY Myosin crossbridge model A proposed mechanism by which actin and myosin filaments interact to produce movement; according to this model, myosin projections transiently bind to actin filaments and rotate about the point of attachment, producing a relative movement of the filament (Nature 1990; 345:398BR)

Royal Malady MEDICAL HISTORY An AD [MIM 176200] condition characterized by attacks of abdominal pain, neuropsychiatric symptoms including psychosis, and ↑ fragility and photosensitivity of the skin; the popular term derives from its presumed presence in King George III (who by most accounts was a tad loopy), and the royal houses of Stuart, Hanover, and Prussia

royal touch Adenochirapsology MEDICAL HISTORY The tapping or touching of a person with scrofula (primary TB of cervical lymph nodes) by a king, which given the lack of therapy, was a practical practice practiced practically during the entire Middle Ages in France and England

R plasmid see Plasmid

sanction A generic term for any penalty or punitive act imposed upon a physician, eg by the medical staff of his/her institution, or imposed against an institution by a regulatory agency, third-party payer, or other

sanctuary sites ONCOLOGY Those regions of the body (eg CNS, testes) where leukemic cells are relatively protected from the cytolytic effects of systemic chemotherapy; before the sanctuary concept was appreciated, more than ½ of patients with leukemia had CNS involvement within 2 years of remission, an event that is usually prevented by prophylactic radiotherapy (1800-2800 cGy) and intrathecal methotrexate; see Remission

sandal keratoderma DERMATOLOGY Lesions of the soles of the feet seen in pityriasis rubra pilaris, which are accompanied by scaly erythematous patches which later become fissured and hyperkeratotic

sanded nuclei A descriptor for globose granular hepatocytic nuclei that are replete with hepatitis B core particles

sandfly Tropical sandfly A small (3 mm), hairy insect with a stinging persistent bite that is a vector for various infectious diseases; the New World sandfly, *Lutzomyia longipalpis*, is a vector for bartonellosis (*B bacilliformis*), and leishmaniasis (*Leishmania mexicana, L braziliensis*) the Old World sandfly, *Phlebotomus papatasi* is the vector for cutaneous leishmaniasis (*Leishmania tropica*), and sandfly fever; New and Old World sandflies may be vectors for kala-azar (*Leishmania donovani*)

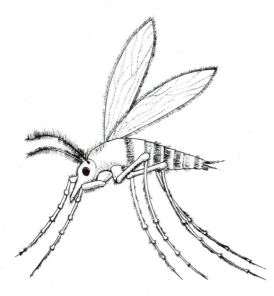

sandfly

sandfly fever Phlebotomus fever An acute, self-limited viral infection caused by five distinct serotypes of Arbovirus, occurring in the Mediterranean rim countries, eastern Africa and Central Asia during dry hot weather CLINICAL Abrupt onset of high fever, headache, ocular pain, photophobia, vomiting, dysgeusia, arthralgia and occasionally aseptic meningitis

sandpaper skin A descriptor for 1) The coarse, bumpy, cool, pale, hypotrichous skin characteristic of hypothyroidism and 2) The skin surface in scarlet fever with indurated hair follicles; sandpaper mucosa refers to the bright bumpy, intraoral erythema of scarlet fever that desquamates with the resolution of infection

'sandwich' method IMMUNOLOGY A generic term for any technique used to identify an antigen or antibody by 'sandwiching' a molecule of interest, X between two other standardized molecules (Y and Y´) that either recognize molecule X immunologically or serve as immune recognition sites PRINCIPLE The first layer is the tissue- (or latex bead-bound) antigen; the second layer corresponds to the first antibody (AB1), raised in (for example) a rabbit against the bound antigen; AB1 is placed in a solution and bathes the bound antigen; if AB1 does not recognize the antigen, it will be washed off; the second antibody, AB2, is an anti-rabbit antibody, the variable end of which recognizes the constant region of AB1; the final layer of the sandwich is an indicator or detector molecule attached to the constant region of AB2, and consists of an enzyme or a radioactive or fluorescent marker; Cf Avidin-biotinylated complex; see Immunoperoxidase method

sandwich vertebrae RADIOLOGY A fanciful term describing radiologic finding of an increased density of the vertebral end-plates with normal bodies and preservation of intervertebral spaces, classically seen in osteopetrosis; Cf Rugger jersey

sandy patch A descriptor for aggregates of calcified submucosal schistosomal (usually *Schistosoma mansoni*) ova, which may be seen in the rectum; see Circumoval bodies, Pipe stem fibrosis

Sanger sequencing Dr F Sanger delineated methods for determining the sequence of DNA and proteins **1)** SANGER (DNA) SEQUENCING dideoxy method is an enzymatic method for sequencing DNA Method: A single strand of DNA to be sequenced is hybridized to a 5'-end-labeled deoxynucleotide 'primer'; four separate radiolabeled (^{32}P) reaction mixtures are prepared in which a 'primer' is elongated using a DNA polymerase; each mixture contains all four possible deoxynucleotide triphosphates, in addition to one of the four possible (^{32}P radiolabeled) dideoxynucleotide triphosphates, in a ratio of 1:100; since the latter have no 3' hydroxyl groups, the chain will not be elongated when these residues are added to the chain, and reactions with these residues end prematurely; each mixture is then denatured and separated by electrophoresis **2)** SANGER (PROTEIN) SEQUENCING A method for determining the amino acid sequence of large polypeptides, in the first step, proteolytic enzymes are used to break the peptide bonds only between selected amino acids, resulting in a number of smaller polypeptide fragments; these fragments are then separated according to their migration speeds in a solvent on chromatographic paper; since the speed of migration differs according to the solvent, 90° rotation and repetition of the electrophoresis produces a characteristic 'fingerprint' for each polypeptide; the fingerprinted spot is then removed and the amino acid sequence of each fragment is then determined by biochemical means; the entire protein's sequence is then determined by fitting together overlapping sequences in a coherent fashion; the latter Sanger sequencing method has been supplanted by Edman's method for sequencing proteins

sangue dormido Portuguese, sleeping blood PSYCHIATRY A culturally linked clinical complex described among Cape Verde Islanders, which has a broad range of neurologic (blindness, convulsions, numbness, pain, paralysis, stroke, tremor); as well as more objective symptoms, including heart attack, infection, and miscarriage (DSM-IV™, 1994) see Culture-bound syndrome

sanitize A euphemism for the mischievous falsification in the form of rewriting and reformatting of various hospital records, in particular those related to peer review (Am Med News 25 May 1992 p3) see Malpractice

San Joaquin valley fever Coccidioidomycosis

S antigen Soluble antigen An incomplete viral form produced in the early stages of some viral infections

SAO Sham feeding-stimulated acid output, see there

Sao Paulo typhus Brazilian form of Rocky Mountain spotted fever

SAP Sphingolipid activator protein Any of a family of small 8–13-kD heat-stable proteins required for sphingolipid hydrolysis; the genes for SAP-1 and SAP-2 are located on chromosome 10 on the same locus **SAP-1** activates hydrolysis of cerebroside sulfate, GM1 ganglioside and globotriaosylceramide by arylsulfatase A, acid β-galactosidase and α galactosidase; SAP-1 deficiency results in accumulation of cerebroside sulfate and other glycolipids, causing a clinical disease with features of metachromatic leukodystrophy **SAP-2** activates hydrolysis of glucosylceramide, galactosylceramide and sphingomyelin by β-glucosylceramidase, galactosylceramide β-galactosidase and sphingomyelinase respectively; SAP-2 deficiency was reported in a case with variant Gaucher's disease **SAP-3** activates hydrolysis of ganglioside GM2 by β-N-acetylgalactosaminidase A and is absent in the AB variant of GM2 gangliosidosis

saponin Any of a group of water-soluble, surface-acting plant glycosides that are detergents at high dilutions and are potent hemolytic agents

SAPS Simplified acute physiology score; see Prognostic scoring systems

SAPS II Simplified Acute Physiology Score INTENSIVE CARE MEDICINE A 'third-generation' system* for estimating in-hospital mortality in adult ICU patients, based on physiological assessments of most severely affected values during the first 24 hours in the ICU and subjecting the results to logistic regression modeling techniques; SAPS II is comparable to APACHE III but contains fewer variables (17 vs 27) in an effort to simplify the collection of data without compromising the score's utility; SAP II, APACHE III, and MPM II are well-researched systems for collecting ICU-related data, can be used to assess prognosis, and to stratify patients as to severity of disease for clinical trials (JAMA 1994; 272:1049CECC) see APACHE III, MPM II

*The others are APACHE III and MPM II

SARA Sexually acquired reactive arthritis, see there

Saranac MEDICAL HISTORY A fresh-air tuberculosis sanatorium, built in 1884 near Lake Saranac in the Adirondack mountains of New York; when effective anti-tuberculosis drugs (streptomycin in 1944, isoniazid in 1951, and others) became available, the raison d'être of this and other anti-tuberculous 'Magic mountains' ceased to exist; see Single disease hospital

sarcoidosis An idiopathic multisystem disease characterized by nonnecrotizing (noncaseating) granulomas*; the initial lesion is alveolitis with an inflammatory infiltrate consisting of CD4+ T cells (activated T lymphocytes of the helper-inducer subset) and macrophages, both of which secrete cytokines believed to be responsible for the granulomas CLINICAL Sarcoidosis is relatively more common in blacks and females; lungs are involved in ≥ 90%, followed by lymph nodes, skin, liver, eye, spleen, bone; lung-function tests show restrictive and, less commonly, obstructive disease IMMUNOLOGY ↓ Cellular immunity (anergy) ↑ humoral immunity (polyclonal ↑ Igs, ↑ IgG in lung lavage fluid) (N Engl J Med 1993; 328:792CPC) TREATMENT Alternate-day prednisone (Mayo Clin Proc 1995; 70:177RV) CAUSE OF DEATH In one series of 38 autopsies; sarcoidosis was suspected or diagnosed antemortem in 45%; it was fatal in ⅔ (28 cases), ¹⁴⁄₂₈ died of cardiac, and ¹²⁄₂₈ from pulmonary sarcoidosis (Arch Pathol Lab Med 1995; 119:167OA, N Engl J Med 1995; 332:1432CPC))

*Which may also be seen in other conditions, eg berylliosis, syphilis, TB

sarcoma A malignant tumor that arises in mesenchymal tissues, including bone (osteosarcoma), cartilage (chondrosarcoma), fat (liposarcoma), fibrous tissue (fibrosarcoma), smooth muscle (leiomyosarcoma), skeletal muscle (rhabdomyosarcoma), stroma (fibrosarcoma), and vascular channels (angiosarcoma*, Kaposi sarcoma); also under the rubric of malignant soft tissue tumors, are those of unknown cellular lineage, which are presumed to be of mesenchymal (connective tissue) origin, eg alveolar soft part sarcoma‡, epithelioid sarcoma‡, Ewing sarcoma‡, malignant fibrous histiocytoma‡, malignant schwannoma‡, synovial sarcoma, and others; the sites of predilection and age of presentation differ according to the tumor; under age 10, lipoblastoma and rhabdomyosarcomas are most common; between ages 15-40, alveolar soft part, epithelioid and synovial sarcomas are common; between ages 25-60, fibrosarcoma and malignant schwannoma are common and after age 45, liposarcoma and malignant fibrous histiocytoma predominate DDx Pseudosarcomas, which are either 1) Mesenchymal and non-malignant soft tissue lesions including fibrous histiocytoma and fibromatoses and 2) Non-mesenchymal and malignant, most commonly spindle cell squamous carcinoma of the oral cavity, anaplastic carcinoma and malignant melanoma; most soft tissue tumors reveal clonal chromosomal aberrations, eg Ewing sarcoma and primitive neuroectodermal tumor are associated with t(11;22) PROGNOSIS The clinical behavior of sarcomas is determined by tumor size (eg > 10 cm is worse), presence of necrosis, and histological grading (which is based on the level of mitotic activity and cellular pleomorphism); sarcomas in men have a worse prognosis; poor prognostic markers in neuroblastoma include 1p- and double minute chromosomes; in mesothelioma 1p-, 3p-, -22, noncomplex karyotype; in synovial sarcoma t(X;18) (N Engl J Med 1991; 324:436) TREATMENT Wide local excision; chemo- and radiotherapy are essentially useless

*Formerly divided into tumors of blood vessels (hemangiosarcoma) or lymphatic vessels (lymphangiosarcoma); there are no markers or immunohistochemical stains that effectively separate the two types; moreover, when such an arbitrary division is made based on morphological features, the prognosis (usually poor) appears to be the same, and there is thus no practical reason for such a division

sarcoma botryoides botrios, Greek, grape A variant of embryonal rhabdomyosarcoma that is most common in young children, 90% of which occur in girls under age five, usually located on the anterior vagina, occasionally in the urinary bladder or nasopharynx PATHOLOGY Superficial grape-like bosselations, with dense superficial cellular ('cambium') layer which overlies loose myxoid stroma TREATMENT Wide local excision Extrapelvic spread may indicate a poor prognosis

sarcomata The correct plural of sarcoma; the incorrect neologism sarcomas is increasingly popular

sarcoplasmic masses 'Smudgy' masses of eosinophilic sarcoplasm devoid of normal striations typically seen by light microscopy in myotonic dystrophy, which is further characterized by cords of nuclei and atrophy of type I muscle fibers

Sargramostim Recombinant GM-CSF IMMUNOLOGY A biological response modifier that accelerates myeloid recovery in patients with lymphomas and ALL whose bone marrow has been suppressed by chemotherapy and/or radiation; because of the limited number of patients who might benefit from sargramostim (estimated 3000 to 5000 autologous bone marrow transplants), it has received an 'orphan' status SIDE EFFECTS Mild rash, diarrhea, asthenia, malaise (JAMA 1991; 265:2315) see G-CSF, GM-CSF

sarin A deadly nerve gas chemically related to certain insecticides (eg malathion) that was developed as a chemical weapon by the Germans in 1936, despite the ban of such weapons under the Geneva Protocol of 1925 MECHANISM OF ACTION Sarin is an anticholinesterase ROUTE OF DELIVERY Aerosol, direct skin contact; one drop may be fatal CLINICAL Pinpoint pupils, severe headache, drooling, nausea, vomiting, convulsions, severe dyspnea and respiratory paralysis TREATMENT Atropine, PAM

Sarin was identified as the cause of a terrorist attack in the Japanese subway system on March 20 1995 that left 10 dead and over 4700 injured, which was allegedly linked to a right-wing anti-American religious cult, Aum Shinri Kyo (NY Newsday 21 March1995; A35)

SART Standard acid reflux test, see there

SAS syndrome Supravalvular aortic stenosis; see Williams (elfin face) syndrome

sashimi see Sushi

satellite A common adjectival descriptor for lesions, masses, patterns or radiologic densities that surround a central point

satellite abscess A characteristic multifocal lesion of nocardiosis, in which there is slow, indolent extension of 'daughter' or satellite abscesses from a central purulent mass, each surrounded by an incomplete fibrotic layer

satellite bags TRANSFUSION MEDICINE A series of plastic bags attached via tubes in a closed system to a 'mother' bag used for the donation, allowing sterile separation of blood components

satellite bodies GENETICS Discrete masses of chromatin attached to the short arm of an acrocentric chromosome, which are not seen in the Y chromosome; Cf Double minutes

satellite cells Cells possibly of histiocytic lineage that are present adjacent to the basement membrane with oval-to-elongated nuclei and a thin rim of cytoplasm containing a few mitochondria, seen in the myocytes of Duchenne's muscular dystrophy PATHOLOGY Oligodendrogliocytes surround neurons in the gray matter

satellite colonies Satellite phenomenon, see there

satellite DNA A segment of highly repeated eukaryotic DNA that differs from the bulk or 'main band' DNA, and may be separated therefrom by ultracentrifugation using a cesium chloride density gradient, resulting in a smaller, 'satellite' band of DNA fragments

satellite infection A 'minigranuloma' that may be seen in atypical mycobacterial infections, eg fish tank granuloma, swimming pool granuloma

satellite nodule DERMATOLOGY A minute tumor cell nest, measuring circa 0.05 mm in diameter that is present in the reticular dermis, panniculus or in vessels in malignant melanoma, which is separated from the melanoma itself; melanomas with satellite nodules are reported to have a four-fold worse prognosis than melanomas of similar thickness without satellites

satellite phenomenon BACTERIOLOGY 1) The growth of colonies of some species of *Haemophilus* (*H influenzae*, *H parainfluenzae*, *H hemolyticus*) in the vicinity of staphylococci, the latter of which produce a growth factor V (NADP); Cf CAMP test, Reverse CAMP test 2) The growth of minute, symbiotic, thiol- or vitamin B_6-dependent mutant bacteria in the vicinity of group A *Streptococcus* 3) The ability to hydrolyze casein and other components of growth media, causing a satellite-like transparency of an otherwise translucent growth medium, allowing differentiation among various aerobic actinomycetes, eg *Actinomadura*, *Nocardia*, and *Streptomyces* species HEMATOLOGY 1) Platelet satellitism The rimming of neutrophils by platelets in the peripheral blood, a phenomenon that may cause spurious thrombocytopenia by automated platelet counters; PS may occur with cryoglobulinemia, hypergammaglobulinemia, immune complexes or result from the use of an EDTA anticoagulant during collection of the blood 2) The rimming of erythrocytes by erythroid siderophages in iron-deficiency anemia

satellite RNA A low-weight (5S to 8S) RNA that may

associate with rRNA in plants

satellite virus A virus that co-infects with a pathogenic virus, eg tobacco necrosis satellite virus, adenovirus-associated virus

satellitism see Satellite phenomenon-Hematology

satiation center Satiety center PHYSIOLOGY A region of the medial hypothalamus in the ventromedial nucleus; stimulation of the SC causes cessation of eating behavior in conscious animals, and its destruction causes hyperphagia; Cf Feeding center

satiety factor A substance as yet (early 1995) unidentified, the existence of which has been postulated as having a pivotal role in controlling body weight

saturated fatty acid A fatty acid lacking double bonds in the alkyl chain; most natural saturated fatty acids contain an even number of double bonds and those with less than ten carbons are liquid at room temperature

saturation A satiated state BIOCHEMISTRY A state in a macromolecule, in which the maximum amount of ligands are bound to recipient sites CHEMISTRY The maximum amount of a solute that can be permanently dissolved in a solution under a defined set of conditions ORGANIC CHEMISTRY Presence of only single bonds on the carbon molecules

saturation mutagenesis DEVELOPMENTAL BIOLOGY A strategy used to identify mutants in a population of interest, in which an adult male of the experimental species, eg fruit fly (*Drosophila melanogaster*) or zebrafish (*Brachydanio rerio*) is treated with a chemical mutagen; this is followed by a search three generations later for embryos that develop abnormally (Science 1994; 264;904N&V) see Zebrafish

Saturday night special FORENSIC MEDICINE A colloquial term attributed to the Detroit* police department, referring to an easily purchased, inexpensive, and often cheaply made 38-caliber (9-mm), revolver that is used for 'crimes of passions', often occurring on Saturday night

*Detroit has dubious distinction of having one of the highest homicide rate in the US, in particular among young unemployed males, such that it was waggishly observed that there were two types of death in Detroit, *'regular, and unleaded'* (personal communication, former trainee in Detroit medical examiner's office)

Saturday night palsy SUBSTANCE ABUSE A group of transient neuromuscular defects affecting a subject who falls in a stuporous state in an unnatural position, classically after an alcoholic 'binge', or overdose of sedatives; the palsies may affect 1) The legs, causing a partial transient deficit known as neurapraxia, affecting the peroneal nerve with a greater motor than sensory loss, with recuperation within six weeks, which may be due to the axon's inability to re-establish a membrane potential rather than actual disruption of the axon or 2) The arms due to compression of the radial nerve against a hard edge or surface; see Alcoholic neuropathy

saturnine gout Chronic lead intoxication A gout-like complex secondary to imbibition of 'moonshine' whiskey distilled in copper tubing joined with lead solder that may present with interstitial nephritis, reduced glomerular filtration rate and hypertension Note: Although in the current environment, excess lead exposure is more common in the lower socioeconomic strata, eg children in inner cities, workers who repair automobile radiators and others; see Moonshine; Cf Pheasant hunter's toe

Note: Gout was historically a disease of the upper class, who continue to be heavily exposed through leaded drinking crystal; fine port contains 89 µg/L of lead before decanting into leaded crystal, rising to 5,331 µg/L after four months of storage and 21,530 µg/L after five years of storage (Lancet 1991; 337;141)

Saturn's ring OPHTHALMOLOGY A whitish ring surrounding the cornea and sclera seen in osteogenesis imperfecta

satyr ear A congenital abnormality of the auricle where the helix lacks the usual rolled contour and the tubercle is unusually prominent, coming to a vague point

Satyrs are minor deities of Greek mythology with pointed ears, horns, a van Dyck beard, a male torso and the body and legs of a goat, who serve Bacchus, the god of fertility, roaming the countryside and having multiple sexual encounters (J Pediatr 1992; 100:250)

satyriasis Male hypersexuality, see Don Juan syndrome

saucerization ORTHOPEDICS A flattened, disciform defect that parallels the shaft of long bones, which may be seen on a plain film, punctuated by microcalcifications; saucerized lesions of bone are typical of fibrosarcoma with bony involvement

saucerization biopsy Deep shave biopsy* A biopsy with a broad rim of epidermis and dermis that is preferred by dermatologists for certain small (< 1 cm) pigmented lesions, eg lentigo senilis, seborrheic keratosis, and dysplastic nevus, for which the clinical diagnosis is benign although malignant melanoma cannot be ruled out; if melanoma is suspected, a full-thickness excisional biopsy with conservative margins is indicated (N Engl J Med 1992; 326:345c)

saucerization

*Note: Both terms are in active use

sausage link pattern OPHTHALMOLOGY A descriptor for the marked dilatation and tortuosity of retinal veins that are focally segmented at arteriovenous crossings, seen in the optic fundus in grade II hypertensive retinopathy, in non-proliferative diabetic retinopathy and, is classically described in Waldenström's macroglobulinemia or hyperviscosity syndrome

sausage link fundus

sausage toes A fanciful descriptor for edematous tenosynovitis of the toes, which may be seen in nonspecific arthritis, as well as in Reiter's syndrome and psoriatic arthritis

'savannah syndrome' A term of uncertain origin that explains the North Americans' mania for maintaining a lawn as a primal human instinct to clear forest and vegetation, imposing his sense of order on the environment

savant Idiot savant, see there

SAVE trial Survival and Ventricular Enlargement trial (N Engl J Med 1992; 327:241, 669)

saw palmetto berry extract A substance that has been claimed to be three-fold more effective than Proscar for ameliorating the symptoms of prostatic hypertrophy

sawfish pattern CARDIOLOGY A descriptor for the jagged systolic narrowing of the left anterior descending coronary artery when seen by angiography, a finding which is considered characteristic of hypertrophic cardiomyopathy; Cf Bridging

sawtooth pattern DERMATOPATHOLOGY An appearance by light microscopy corresponding to a jagged and thickened dermal-epidermal junction, classically described in lichen

planus RADIOLOGY A jagged radiocontrast column seen by barium studies of the colon in ischemic colitis, exudative enteropathy, cathartic colon, necrotizing enterocolitis due to congenital megacolon (Hirschsprung's disease), and rarely in diverticulosis, a pattern attributed to a combination of edema and erosion of the mucosa

saxitoxin A potent paralyzing neurotoxin first isolated from the Alaskan clam (*Saxidomus giganteus*) that binds to the cell membrane's Na^+ channel, blocking depolarization at the neuromuscular junction, which ↑ permeability for Na^+; the toxin is heat-stable, water-soluble and rapidly absorbed from the GI tract; as few as six clams containing saxitoxin may be fatal; see Conotoxin, Red tide

saxitoxin

SBE Subacute bacterial endocarditis

SBLA syndrome Li-Fraumeni syndrome, see there

SBT 1) Serum bactericidal titration see Minimum bactericidal concentration 2) Symplastin bleeding time

SC disease Sickle-hemoglobin C disease A hemoglobinopathy affecting circa 1:800 US blacks, which is characterized by ↑↑↑ in infections, eg bacterial meningitis and *Salmonella* osteomyelitis due to a defect in the alternate (properdin) complement pathway; other effects of SC disease include 1) Osteoporosis, which result in the formation of 'fishmouth vertebrae' 2) Nephropathy*, with poor renal concentration, acidification and ↑ glomerular filtration rate 3) Retinopathy, which occurs in 75% of SC disease in contrast to 15% of patients with the usual form of sickle cell anemia; fundoscopic findings include a 'black sunburst' pattern, due to increased glycolysis in the end-arteriolar system and a 'seafoam' pattern, a proliferative retinopathy LABORATORY ↑ 2,3 DPG, ↑ factor VIII; ↓ osmotic fragility; reticulocytes comprise 5-25% of the peripheral RBCs, which may have a 'holly-leaf' or navicular configuration

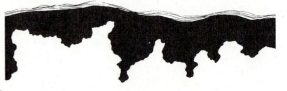

sawtooth pattern

*Note: Juxtamedullary RBCs traverse the hyperosmolar medulla, sickle, and cause papillary necrosis, which is more common in SC disease than in sickle cell anemia

SCAB Single-chain antigen binding protein(s) Unique manufactured polypeptides that link the variable sequence of an antibody's light chain (V_L) to the variable sequence of an antibody's heavy chain (V_H); SCABs can be produced from any monoclonal antibody, have the advantage of smaller size and reduced immunogenity of the heavy chain constant region and are of potential use in chemical separations, biosensors, imaging and in treating malignancy, cardiovascular disease and others; see Abzymes

scabies A condition caused by the 'itch' mite, *Sarcoptes scabei hominis*, which most commonly affects children, is transmitted by direct contact, causes an intensely pruritic linear eruption corresponding to the tracks of the burrowing beasts; the pruritus results in excoriation and secondary pyoderma, often located in the head and neck with sparing of the palmoplantar regions TREATMENT Lindane lotion, benzene hexachloride

scaffold A generic term for any structural matrix that provides the physical support for a functional system, but which participates little in the system's activity

scalable *adjective* COMPUTERS Pertaining or relating to a client-server computer environment in which performance increases in a linear fashion as more servers are added to the system (Am Lab March 1995, p46)

scalded skin syndrome 1) Staphylococcal scalded skin syndrome, see there 2) Toxic epidermal necrolysis, see there

scalenus syndrome see Thoracic outlet syndrome

scaling PERIODONTICS The removal of dental plaque (an early lesion predisposing to periodontitis) and 'tartar' or calculus from the crown of a tooth and root surfaces; see Periodontal disease

scalloping Scallop sign BONE RADIOLOGY A descriptor for a semilunar erosion at the ulnar aspect of the distal radius, seen in patients with advanced rheumatoid arthritis, caused by spontaneous rupture of the digital extensors; the 'scallop' is often more prominent as it may be rimmed by an osteosclerotic margin CHEST RADIOLOGY A descriptor for the tethering of the visceral to parietal pleura, seen in pneumothorax that arises in previous lung disease GI RADIOLOGY A descriptor for the appearance of *Candida* esophagitis, in which there are irregular serrations seen by a barium 'swallow study' PATHOLOGY A descriptive term referring to serration of colloid seen by low-power light microscopy in Hashimoto's disease

SCAN Suspected child abuse or neglect, see there

scanner COMPUTERS A device that measures differences in light absorption, which can be used to input data in the form of printed material or images; scanned print can be processed through optical character recognition software to allow direct entry of written text into a word processing environment; scanners may also be used to input line drawings and photographs that may be subsequently manipulated by graphics or desktop publishing software INSTRUMENTATION A device that measures the differences in chromatic or radioactive intensity on a two-dimensional matrix, eg electropherogram or chromatogram, for the purpose of quantitative analysis of various substances

scanning electron microscopy A type of EM in which the beam of electrons scans over the surface of an object, providing a 3-D image of the object of interest by analyzing the pattern of deflection of primary and secondary electrons; SEM has little use in medicine, given that the image is confined to cell surfaces, although SEM provides some information in renal pathology; SEM is of use in industry as a means of quality control of finely machined

parts and in materials sciences, to detect fragmentaion; see Microscopy; Cf Scanning tunnel microscopy, Transmission electron microscopy

'scanning power' SURGICAL PATHOLOGY The lowest magnification (20x to 25x) power used in diagnostic pathology, which allows surveying of tissues and pattern recognition; see Microscopy; Cf High-power field

scanning probe microscope Any of a class of instruments that are capable of generating 3-D surface profiles of molecular structures with nanometer resolution; SPMs include the scanning tunnel microscope and the atomic force microscope, and these may be used for analysis of biopolymers, cell membranes, chromosomes, DNA and RNA, ligand-receptor complexes, molecular crystals, nucleosomes, peptides, proteins, protein-nucleic acid complexes, and others (Am Biotech Lab March1995, p65) see Scanning tunnel microscope

scanning speech NEUROLOGY A slurring of phonation associated with cerebellar defects, in which there is inappropriate rate, range, force and direction of voluntary movements

scanning tunnel microscope A powerful 'microscope', developed by Binnig and Rohrer (Nobel prize, Physics, 1986) that produces high resolution, 3-D images of atomic and subatomic particles on various surfaces, where the device's tip scans a sample, atom by atom, combining high spatial resolution with spectroscopic analysis; unlike other microscopes, STM uses neither incident light nor radiation, and thus does not require lenses, light or electron sources, but rather uses the electrons from the surface as the only source of radiation TECHNIQUE An ultrafine needle is brought several billionths (10^{-9}) of a centimeter from the surface being analyzed, at which distance, the voltage must be maintained at ultralow levels to prevent electrons from jumping the gap between the needle and the surface being analyzed; because electrons are not in motion, classical physics does not apply; the process is rather explained by the quantum mechanical effect of 'tunnelling', which allows a faint current to pass from the needle to the surface and back as it scans the surface's atomic landscape, producing a 3-D image of organic and inorganic surfaces and biological molecules, including bacteriophage particles, circular DNA and native double-stranded DNA; Cf Scanning electron microscope

scaphoid abdomen A concave or hollowed anterior abdominal wall

scar-cancer A cancer that is often located in the pulmonary apices and associated with pre-existing scars, wounds or inflammation, eg healed TB, infarcts, abscess cavities, bronchiectasis, and metallic foreign bodies, eg bullets; 80% of scar cancers are adenocarcinomas, 15% are squamous cell carcinomas with the rest being of other histopathological types

Note: While it is unclear if scarring is pathogenically linked to cancer, or whether the scar is merely an epiphenomenon, scars have been associated with malignant fibrous histiocytoma; see Passenger/driver controversy

scarlet fever A reaction due to pharyngitis by *Streptococcus* group A (which produces an erythrogenic toxin), consisting of an oral enanthema ('raspberry' tongue, 'strawberry' tongue), generalized blanching erythema (sparing the palmoplantar region and mouth with circumoral pallor) and linear petechiae, known as Pastia's lines

Scarlett O'Hara 'syndrome' A term that refers either to 1) Pretentious eating habits when a person is in the public eye or 2) A peer-group accepted eating 'disorder', due to the 'need' for young ♀ socialites to attend multiple dinners, dances, and parties often in short time periods; the women may self-induce emesis as a form of weight control

The 'syndrome' derives its name from Scarlett O'Hara, the fictional heroine in the American Civil War novel, *Gone with the Wind*, who engorged herself prior to eating meals in public, rather than appear unlady-like; this contrasts with pathological over-eating (the 'binge-purge syndrome') that occurs behind closed doors, and which serves no known social expediency

scar-sarcoidosis Sarcoidosis arising in a scar, a rare condition that may engender a similar controversy to Scar cancer

scatologia The use of obscene language and phraseology with distinctly sexual overtones; see Telephone scatologia; Cf Coprolalia

scatter factor CELL BIOLOGY A 62-kD heterodimeric cytokine joined by disulfide bonds that is secreted by certain fibroblasts, enhancing the movement, dissociation and scattering of epithelial cells; the single-stranded 30-kD peptide has significant sequence homology with hepatocyte growth factor

scattergram A plot of data points in a 2-D coordinate system that is used to determine whether there is a correlation between the two variables on the X and Y axes (figure), is a linear regression of data points correlating the serum levels of calcitriol and physical activity with bone density

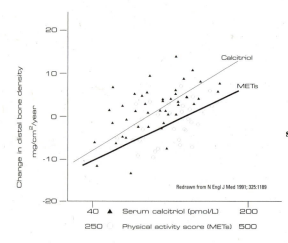

scattergram

SCD Sudden cardiac death

SCEA Sister chromosome exchange analysis , see there

SCF Stem cell factor, see there

'scheduled' drug Controlled drug substance, see there

schistocyte Schizocyte, helmet cell HEMATOLOGY A fragmented erythrocyte that arises from either an intrinsic increase in cell fragility or from intravascular rugosities that traumatize the cells; schistocytes are a nonspecific finding that may be associated with hemolysis, trauma, prosthetic heart valves, megaloblastic and microangiopathic anemias, disseminated intravascular coagulation, hemolytic uremic syndrome and thrombotic thrombocytopenic purpura; Cf Selenoid cells

Schistosoma PARASITOLOGY A genus of elongated sexually dimorphic trematodes, the blood flukes, of the phylum Platyhelminthes, class Trematoda; *Schistosoma* spp infect ± 200 million worldwide, killing 800 000 annually, its morbidity is related to an exuberant tissue reaction to the eggs, as the organisms themselves do not replicate within the host; see Circumoval body, Pipestem fibrosis, Swimmer's itch

schistosome A generic term for a blood fluke, in particular of the genus *Schistosoma*

schizocyte Schistocyte, see there

schizophrenia A heterogenous group of disorders characterized by progressive mental deterioration that may be accompanied by various psychotic symptoms, bizarre behavior, or by negative (deficit) symptoms, including low levels of emotional arousal, mental activity, and social drive; schizophrenia is a diagnosis of exclusion, as none of its clinical, biochemical, neuroradiologic, pathophysiologic, and psychological features are sufficient to establish a definitive diagnosis DSM-IV CRITERIA (table) EPIDEMIOLOGY Worldwide lifetime prevalence is 0.85% across all cultural, geographic, and socioeconomic categories; cost estimated at $33 x 10⁹ (1990, US), ie 2.5% of total health care expenditures DIAGNOSIS MRI neuroimaging with volume measurements and 3-D reconstruction of the brain reportedly demonstrates ↓↓ volume of gray matter of the left anterior hippocampus-amygdala, left parahippocampal gyrus, and left posterior superior temporal gyrus; the degree of loss in the left posterior superior temporal gyrus reportedly correlates with the scores obtained on the thought-disorder index (study population: 15, N Engl J Med 1994; 330:681ᵣᵥ) MOLECULAR PATHOLOGY Some data suggest that a at chromosome 6p had an odds (lod) score of +3.5, which may map to 6p22-pter (Nature Genetics, in Nature 1995; 375:89) TREATMENT Antipsychotic drugs which are used to 1) Reduce hallucinations and delusions, and gradually reduce other thought disturbances and improve symptoms of withdrawal and apathy 2) Control symptoms through maintenance therapy, and 3) Long-term prophylaxis; neuroleptic agents include haloperidol and clozapine (N Engl J Med 1994; 330:681ᵣᵥ) current Medicaid drug-reimbursement benefits are limited to 3 prescriptions/month, which may ↑ the use of acute mental health services in low-income patients with chronic mental disorders (N Engl J Med 1994; 331:650ₛₐ) Cf Schizoid personality disorder

schizoid personality disorder PSYCHIATRY A mental disorder characterized by '...*a pervasive pattern of detachment from social relationships and a restricted range of expression of emotions in interpersonal settings.*' (DSM-IV™) Persons with SPD have a reduced desire for intimacy, sexual relationships, sensory, bodily, or interpersonal experiences, and are viewed as being cold, aloof loners; they often prefer solitary activities, eg mathematical or computer games, and because they respond inappropriately to social cues, they may be viewed as socially inept; see Loner; Cf Schizophrenia

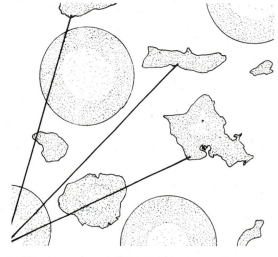

schistocytes

SCID mice A mouse model for AIDS, which may be used to study the interaction of anti-HIV drugs or immune enhancers in an in vivo system, without the ethical dilemma that is posed in human testing of substances with unknown effects; the SCID mouse model is also used to

SCHIZOPHRENIA-diagnostic criteria[1]

A CHARACTERISTIC SYMPTOMS: 2 or more[2] of following, for a significant portion of 1+ months
- Delusions
- Disorganized (or catatonic) behavior
- Disorganized speech
- Hallucinations
- Negative symptoms, eg flattening of affect, loss of volition

B SOCIAL/OCCUPATIONAL DYSFUNCTION

C DURATION 6+ months in duration with 1+ months of 'active' symptoms, defined by criteria A

EXCLUSIONS Symptoms are not better accounted for by

D OTHER MENTAL DISORDERS, eg Schizoaffective disorder or Mood disorder with psychotic features

E OTHER CONDITIONS, eg substance s(medication, substance of abuse) and/or general medical conditions

[1] Modified from Diagnostic and Statistical Manual of Mental Disorders, 4th ed, Washington, DC, American Psychiatric Association, 1994 [2] Only one of criteria A is required if the delusions are bizarre, or the hallucinations include 1 + 'voices in the head'

study tumor interactions in immune compromised hosts

science literacy YD

schlepper German, tugboat, tractor MOLECULAR BIOLOGY A colloquial term for any molecule, eg a carrier protein that combines with a poorly or non-antigenic molecule, eg a hapten, enhancing its immunogenicity and mediating its transporation through the cell or body

Schnitzler syndrome A condition first described in 1974 characterized by chronic urticaria, FUO, disabling bone pain, hyperostosis, ↑ ESR, and macroglobulinemia (Mayo Clin Proc 1995; 70:570CR)

'school of fish' appearance A nonspecific descriptor for a light microscopic pattern characterized by multiple, discrete oval-to-elongated structures arranged in long roughly parallel fascicles SURGICAL PATHOLOGY A variant arrangement of the fascicles of malignant cells in malignant fibrous histiocytoma, more commonly known as a 'storiform pattern' MICROBIOLOGY The light microscopic arrangement of the gram-negative bipolar-staining coccobacillus *Haemophilus ducreyi* (Chancroid agent)

schwannoma A tumor of Schwann cells; by convention, the 'benign schwannoma' is preferably known as neurilemomas, while the malignant counterpart is known as malignant schwannoma; see Malignant schwannoma, Neurilemoma

sciatica NEUROLOGY Lumbosacral pain that radiates down the posterior thigh and lateral leg into the foot, which is caused by compression of the roots of the lumbosacral nerves by injury, prolapse of the intervertebral disk, or locoregional tumors CLINICAL Hyporeflexia, paresthesias, and ↓ muscle strength

SCID Severe combined immune deficiency, see there

Scientology® *"An applied religious philosophy ...defined as the formal study of the spirit in relationship to itself, universes and other life.* L Ron Hubbard, the philosophy's chief architect, further wrote that *'Scientology...improves the health, ability, intelligence, behavior, skill and appearance...*In a message to the public, the Church of Scientology International, it is stated, *'Scientology philosophy and its forerunner, Dianetics® technology, as practiced by the Church, address only the spirit. Although the Church, as are all churches, is free to engage in spiritual healing, it does not...the Church does not wish to accept individuals who desire treatment of physical or mental illness but prefers to refer these to qualified specialists of other organizations who deal in these matters* (Scientology: The Fundamentals of Thought, Bridge Publications, Los Angeles, 1988)

Note: Scientologists are alleged to have mounted a prolonged attack against psychiatry (N Engl J Med 1992; 327:820c) and sued Eli Lilly & Co for $14.7 million in an effort to halt that company's sale of Prozac (Am Med News 18 May 1992 p2)

scimitar syndrome A rare vascular anomaly, more common in women that may present in early childhood, in which some or all of the pulmonary veins drain into the inferior vena cava, often accompanied by hypoplasia of the right lung, dextrocardia, and systemic arterial supply to the right lung from the descending aorta; the name derives from the curvilinear (scimitar-shaped) radiopacity adjacent to the right cardiac border which has been fancifully likened to the Turkish sword, the scimitar CLINICAL Asymptomatic or fever, dyspnea, recurring pneumonia, chest pain, wheezing, and possibly pulmonary hypertension (Br Heart J 1983; 50:182) SURGICAL ANATOMY Right lung and right pulmonary artery hypoplasia, dextrocardia, anomalous origin of pulmonary arteries from the aorta to right lung, anomalous venous drainage of right lung into the inferior vena cava and anomalous right diaphragm TREATMENT Surgical, pneumonectomy or correction of cardiac 'plumbing' defects; Cf Sequestration complex

scintillation The sporadic emission of quanta (flashes) of visible or UV light by fluorescent substances, eg POPOP, after they have been excited by a photon or ionizing (radioactive) particle; scintillation is the process that forms the basis of RIA (radioimmuoassay), as there is one scintillation (flash of light) for each ionizing event, thus allowing for precise quantification of the incident radiation; scintillation is detected using a solid or liquid fluor, which may be mixed in a 'cocktail' to enhance the detection of the flashes of light; see POPOP, Radioimmunoassay

scirrhous *skirrhos*, Greek, gypsum An adjectival descriptor for the dense fibrous stroma of certain carcinomas that produce abundant connective tissue; scirrhous induration (SI) or 'desmoplastic reaction' is characteristic of ductal cell carcinoma of breast, and may be accompanied by microcalcifications; SI may also be seen in pancreatic adenocarcinoma

scirrhous carcinoma A relatively nonspecific term of waning popularity for the gross findings of the 'classic' invasive ductal carcinoma of the breast, in which there is marked induration with 'chalky streaks' due to increased deposition of elastin fibers, often accompanied by microcalcifications detectable on mammography

SCIWORA Spinal cord injury without radiological abnormality Serious spinal cord damage and disruption of tracts in the absence of a fracture, an event that occurs most commonly in children MECHANISMS Flexion, hyperextension, longitudinal distraction and ischemia causing complete and severe partial cord lesions TREATMENT Regional stabilization, neurosurgical exploration

sclerosing adenosis SURGICAL PATHOLOGY A form of hyperplasia of the glandular component (adenosis) of the breast that may be confused with carcinoma, which consists of an indurated, often small multinodular lesion that is more cellular in the center with florid myoepithelial proliferation (immunoperoxidase stain reveals abundant actin); sclerosing adenosis lacks trabecular formations, necrosis and cellular pleomorphism, which are histological findings of carcinoma; malignant degeneration in sclerosing adenosis is rare but well-described; see Fibrocystic disease, Proliferative breast disease(s); Cf Mammary dysplasia

sclerosing cholangitis Idiopathic bile duct inflammation with cholestasis, often associated with other autoimmune diseases, eg Crohn's disease, ulcerative colitis and Addison's disease CLINICAL Jaundice, pruritis, portal hypertension RADIOLOGY ERCP reveals beading and narrowing of the affected biliary tract LABORATORY ↑ Alkaline phosphatase PATHOLOGY Periductal fibrosis and inflammation, portal edema, fibrosis, bile duct dilatation or focal obliteration and loss of bile ducts, copper deposition, cholestasis and with time, evolution into primary biliary cirrhosis (N Engl J Med 1991; 324:186) see Primary biliary cirrhosis

sclerosing epithelial hamartoma Desmoplastic trichoepithelioma A benign hair follicle tumor that is more common on the face of young (< age 30) ♀ PATHOLOGY Compressed epithelial nests, focal calcification, and dermal fibrosis TREATMENT Excision

sclerosing hemangioma 1) PULMONARY PATHOLOGY An often benign lesion of ♀ adults characterized by a well-circumscribed, slowly growing mass of polygonal cells thought to arise from type II pneumocytes with a variably present mesenchymal stroma and 2) DERMATOPATHOLOGY Now known as benign fibrous histiocytoma or less commonly as dermatofibroma and nodular fibrosis

sclerosing lipogranuloma A rare lesion of the penis, scrotum, and vulva, described in adults and thought to be due to autoinjection of exogenous paraffin PATHOLOGY Fat necrosis, histiocytes, foamy macrophages, giant cells, fibrosis, and hyalinization

sclerosing lymphangitis An idiopathic condition characterized by firm cord-like subcutaneous masses encircling the penis at the coronal suture that resolve in 2-6 weeks PATHOLOGY Dilated lymphatics with sprouts of endothelial cells and thickened, fibrotic vessel walls

sclerosing metanephric hamartoma A lesion of children under two years of age that may precede Wilms' tumor, which is histologically characterized by the presence of blastemal and tubular elements in a fibrous stroma; it is subdivided into simple sclerosing hamartoma, simple tubular hamartoma, and sclerosing hamartoma with a central adenoma, which is considered to be an early Wilm's tumor; Cf WAGR syndrome, Wilms' tumor

sclerosing peritonitis Extensive peritoneal fibrosis that occurs in response to asbestos, silica in IV drug abusers, in patients with carcinoid syndrome or those receiving β-blockers PATHOGENESIS Uncertain, possibly related to inhibition of the release of lysosomal enzymes or due to mesenteric panniculitis CLINICAL Intestinal obstruction due to massive peritonial adhesions

sclerosing retroperitonitis Retroperitoneal fibrosis, see there

sclerosteosis syndrome An AR [MIM 269500] condition of children leading to deafness with bony overgrowth and occlusion of cranial foramina, accompanied by an asymmetrically enlarged mandible, syndactyly and onychodysplasia; SS occurs in a highly inbred kinship in Maryland known as the 'We-Sorts', and is thought to be due to osteoblastic hyperactivity

sclerotherapy The use of sclerosing agent to induce fibrous obliteration of pathologic blood vessels, usually to treat hemorrhoids or esophageal varices; see Endoscopic sclerotherapy

sclerotic body MYCOLOGY A thick-walled, 4-12 μm in diameter, round, chestnut-brown structure with a 'copper penny' appearance, which is seen in chromoblastomycosis; the SB is an intermediate fungal form that is midway between yeasts and hyphae, which reproduces under acidic conditions in a muriform (wall-like) fashion, ie multiplying by forming vertical and horizontal septations

scombroid intoxication A histame reaction caused by eating spoiled fish of the Scomberesocidea family (saury, skipjack, maki-maki, dolphin, tuna, bonito, seerfish, butterfly kingfish, mackerel); these fish have free histamine in their muscle that is decarboxylated when infected by *Proteus* spp; if the infection is intense, oral antihistamines or activated charcoal may be needed to ameliorate the sys-

temic effect of the histamine (N Engl J Med 1991; 324:716) see Fish; Cf Ciguatera poisoning

'scoop and run' EMERGENCY MEDICINE A stance taken when a trauma victim's condition is of such severity that there is 1) Insufficient time for the usual format of medical stabilization and 2) The equipment and/or experts needed to save the victim's life are not present in the ambulatory field unit, eg ambulance or helicopter (New York Times 23 October 1994; A32) Cf Stay and play

scope of practice The range of responsibility (eg types of patients or caseload) and practice guidelines that determine the boundaries within which a physician or other professional practices

Scotch™ tape test MICROBIOLOGY A method used in the clinical laboratory for 1) Retrieving eggs from the perianal region in children infected with *Enterobius vermicularis* (pinworm) and 2) Observing fungi in a fashion that is similar to their 'native' conformation in culture; a piece of transparent adhesive tape is touched to a colony of fungi; the tape is then adhered to a glass slide and stained with lactophenol blue

Scotty dog sign RADIOLOGY A descriptive term for the normal appearance of lumbar vertebra when viewed obliquely, where the pedicle, the transverse process, the superior articular process and the inferior articular process form the eye, nose, ear and front legs respectively; spondylolysis will demonstrate a fracture through the dog's neck; Cf Dog ear sign

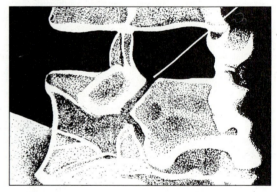

Scotty dog sign

scout films RADIOLOGY Any preliminary film taken of a body region prior to a definitive imaging study, eg a scout chest film prior to performing computed tomography of the chest; 'scouts' serve to establish a baseline and are used prior to angiography, CT, or MRI

sCR1 soluble Complement receptor type 1 A recombinant DNA product that binds activated C3b and C4, promoting their inactivation by complement factor 1; in rats, sCR1 significantly reduces hypoxia-induced myocardial injury, which is in part due to complement activation

'scrambled egg' appearance OPHTHALMOLOGY A fanciful descriptor for the changes of the optic fundus seen in Best's AD vitelliform degeneration; initially, there is a smooth sharply demarcated yellow-orange egg-yolk-like macule with little loss of visual acuity, affecting children and adolescents; later, the lesion degenerates, becoming scrambled-egg-like, resulting in retinal pigmentation, chorioretinal atrophy, and visual impairment

scrapie A prion-induced infection, formerly thought to be due to slow viruses, which causes fatal neurologic degeneration in sheep and goats, who scrape (ergo scrapie) themselves on rocks and other surrogate back-scratchers; the scrapie agent is one of the family of transmissible spongiform encephalopathies, which are thought to integrate themselves into the cell membrane, possibly as replicable glycoproteins; see Bovine spongiform encephalopathy, Kuru, Prion, Slow virus

screamer COMPUTERS A 'rogue' device (eg a PC microcomputer) on a LAN (local area network) that continuously transmits data at a high speed, blocking communication by the other devices in the network; screamers are caused by a defective network card or communication cable (see CAP Today November 1993)

screen PUBLIC HEALTH A generic term for any systematic activity that attempts to identify the presence of a particular disease process in a population

screener CYTOLOGY A generic term for a cytotechnologist, often one who works in a commercial laboratory whose main professional activity is the screening of pap smears for the presence of lesions of the uterine cervix; most states have enacted legislation limiting the number of Pap smears that one technologist can screen/day, eg 100 slides/8 hour period in New York State; see Pap mill

screening MOLECULAR BIOLOGY The use of a low-stringency radiolabeled or biotinylated hybridization probe to detect gene segments of potential interest from genomic or complementary DNA library; see Cloning PUBLIC HEALTH An evaluation of a person's health status that attempts to identify a disease process that is not known to exist in a patient at the time of evaluation, eg hypercholesterolemia, hypertension, or a malignancy (N Engl J Med 1994; 330:1589RA); screening of a population requires measurement of specific clinical parameters, eg blood pressure (to detect hypertension), sigmoidoscopy (colon cancer), radiologic parameters, eg mammography (breast cancer) or laboratory parameters, eg blood cholesterol (coronary artery disease), guaiac-positive stools (colon cancer) or 'Pap' smears of the uterine cervix (cervical cancer); screening tests in general have high sensitivities and low specificities*, allowing detection of most patients with a morbid condition, while having the acceptable disadvantage of a high rate of false positivity; screening strategies are based on whether the screening population is at high or low risk for a particular disease and whether the course of the disease for which screening is being performed will be affected; selection of a cutoff point is a fundamental policy decision required in any screening screening program, eg a risk of ≥ 1:270 is used in the state of Rhode Island for Down syndrome; screening policies by experts:

BREAST examination (♀) by physician-every year > age 40; mammography-every 1-2 years, age 35+ and every year > age 50

CERVICAL CYTOLOGY examination every 1-3 years, starting at age of first intercourse

BLOOD-PRESSURE measurement in normotensive persons-every 2 years, all age groups

CHOLESTEROL measurement-every 5 years, but not in younger subjects; see Cancer screening

*Note: Because screening assays achieve their intended goal in detection, albeit in an inelegant and inefficient manner, they have been fancifully termed 'shotgun' tests as both obtain the desired effect while sacrificing finesse

screwdriver teeth see Peg teeth

screwworm A generic term for any of the flesh-eating larva of various calliphorid or sarcophorid flies; *Cochliomyia hominivorax* is particularly frisky, as it lays eggs in open wounds of live once lively livestock; once hatched, the larvae feed on fresh flesh and may kill a calf via its umbilical cord wound within days; this particular brand of screwworm has recently migrated from its indigenous regions of the Western hemisphere to Libya; other screwworms include *Cochliomyia hominivorax* of the Western Hemisphere, *Chrysomyia bezziana* of the Indian and Pacific Ocean, and *Wohlfahrtia magnifica* of the lower Arctic regions

SCRIMP technique SCRape/IMPrint method PATHOLOGY A method by which a reasonably valid working diagnosis of the findings of a postmortem examination can be rendered in rapid time, consisting of scraping pathological tissues, and imprinting them on a glass slide

Note: The paperwork inherent in a postmortem examination often delays the generation of a final report for up to three or months in the US; hence the potential utility of such a simple technique

script PSYCHOLOGY The verbal component of communication with a patient that recognizes that different phrases may have the same meaning but the order, choice of the words or the manner in which they are said can either stimulate or inhibit communication

scrolls A descriptor for the ultrastructural morphology of mast cell granules, which may also rarely occur in variant CML with basophilia, a structural feature supporting a common origin of mast cells and basophils; the nature of the granular material is unknown

scrotal tongue Grooved tongue Congenital lingual furrows that are a component of Melkerson-Rosenthal syndrome [MIM 155900], or may be seen in Down syndrome, where the furrows are attributed to sucking and mouth breathing; the finding has no pathological significance and is only of interest as food particles get stuck and are later colonized by oral bacteria, evoking halitosis TREATMENT Brush teeth and tongue

(the) scrub *noun* The formal preoperative hand washing ritual that is a *sine qua non* prerequisite for performing an invasive procedure in a body cavity; rules for the scrub are 1) Work from distal (fingertips) to proximal 2) Complete scrubbing before rinsing 3) Let water drain off elbow; Cf Scrubs

scrub *verb* 1) To perform the holy ritual of the scrub, see there 2) To cleanse vigorously as may be required in the emergency room treatment of MVAs in which the wounds are 'dirty', deep, and bloody and studded with gravel, glass, debris, dirt, and other sundry schmutz

scrub nurse A nurse (or technician) who participates in a sterile surgical operation, prepares sterile supplies and passing them to the surgeon, assisting the surgeon during the procedure, accounting for needles, sharps, sponges and other supplies used during the operation, and teaching any new (and qualified) personnel details of operating room protocol; see Circulating nurse, Operating team, Physician assistant

scrub typhus A disease caused by a *Rickettsia tsutsugamushi* VECTOR Chiggers (the larval stage of the mite, *Leptotrombidium deliensis*, or *Trombicula pseudoakamushi*), inhabitants of scrub vegetation that feed on host rodents CLINICAL 1-3 week incubation with prodromal symptoms of headache, malaise, and anorexia; after scarification of the inoculation papule, there is abrupt onset of high fever, with a pulse-temperature dissociation, headache, ocular pain, conjunctivitis, malaise, cardiac dysfunction with minor EKG changes, eg T wave inversion, a pale pink, centrifugal maculopapular rash, lymphadenopathy and interstitial pneumonia DIAGNOSIS *Proteus* OX-K antigen seropositivity TREATMENT Tetracycline, chloramphenicol, ciprofloxin; 10-30% mortality if untreated

scrubs see Surgical scrubs

SCSI Small Computer Systems Interface (pronounced scuzzy) COMPUTERS An interface either integrated into or added as a board onto a microcomputer (PC) that alleviates the data transfer bottleneck between the CPU (central processing unit) and peripheral devices by providing high data transfer rates, performance, flexibility and multitasking I/O* capabilities for PCs and file server; SCSI permits up to 7 devices to to coexist, including various (hard, optical, tape) drives, CD-ROMs, scanners, printers

*Heavy I/O (In/Out) traffic in computers is capable of slowing the fastest of

SCTAT   Sex cord tumor with annular tubules   A rare ovarian tumor with clinicopathologic differences that depend on the tumor's association with Peutz-Jegher syndrome **SCTAT WITH PEUTZ-JEGHER SYNDROME** is a small, bilateral, multifocal and calcified lesion that is rarely functionally active, with some cases being associated with adenoma malignum of the cervix **SCTAT WITHOUT PEUTZ-JEGHER SYNDROME** is often large, unilateral, focal, rarely associated with adenoma malignum; 40% secrete estrogen and 20% of cases behave in a malignant fashion PATHOLOGY Sharply circumscribed, rounded epithelial nests composed of ring-shaped tubules, likened to atrophic testes; also simple and complex ring-shaped tubules with a pattern between a granulosa cell tumor and Sertoli cell tumor

scuba   Self-contained underwater breathing apparatus, formerly written as SCUBA SPORTS MEDICINE A device consisting of one or more tanks of compressed gases ('air') in optimized ratios, a regulator that can be adjusted to regulate the flow of air, and meter to indicate the amount of air remaining in the tanks; a scuba device allows a person to submerge without attachment to an external air supply to depths of 50 or more meters below the water surface; see the Bends, Cf Caisson's disease

sculptured nose   A thinned, sharply chiselled nose with atrophy of the subcutaneous adipose tissue seen in the Hutchinson-Gilford progeria syndrome; see also 'Plucked bird' appearance

scurvy line   White line of scurvy, see there

scut 'monkey'   A highly colloquial and demeaning term that usually refers to a medical student who is usually relegated to the bottom rung of a team involved in patient management team in a university-affilitated health care facility, and performs so-called 'scut' work; see Extern, Medical student abuse, Pimping

scut work   Menial, non-patient care-related activities that are often passed to medical students (externs) or interns, although they are actually the responsibility of other health-care workers; the array of 'scut' details is vast and includes obtaining supplies, performing ward paperwork, going to the pharmacy, laboratory and emergency room with specimens or paperwork, acting as an orderly, cleaning the nurses station, going for pizza and so on; scut duties are often cited as a subtle form of 'medical student abuse'; see Medical student abuse, Pimping

SD   1) Senile dementia 2) Septal defect 3) Serine dehydratase 4) Skin dose 5) Spontaneous delivery 6) Standard deviation 7) Streptodornase 8) Subtotal diskectomy 9) Sudden death

Also 1) Salt depletion 2) Sample data 3) Scientiae doctor 4) Second difference (statistics) 5) Segregation distorter 6) Serologically defined 7) Serologically determined 8) Serum defect 9) Severely diabetic (rarely used) 10) Shoulder disarticulation 11) Shoulder dislocation 12) Skin destruction 13) Splice donator 14) Stone disintegration 15) Strength duration curve 16) Subdural 17) Systolic discharge

SDA   Strand-displacement amplification MOLECULAR DIAGNOSTICS An isothermal technique for amplifying DNA in which a primer containing a restriction site, an exonuclease-deficient fragment of DNA polymerase, and a restriction endonuclease (*Hinc* II) are combined to produce one copy of the DNA target; use of both sense and antisense primers results in an exponential reaction with a 10^7-10^8-fold amplification that is complete in 2 hour; SDA's distinct advantage is its ease of automation (CAP Today May 1995 p1)

SDAT   Senile dementia–Alzheimer type, see there

SDBT   Senile dementia–Binswanger type, see there

SDI1   p21, see there

SDN-POA   Sexually dimorphic nucleus of the preoptic area A group of cells in the rat hypothalamus that is much larger in the male than in the female, that had been implicated in sexual behavior; in one study, the SDN-POA was destroyed bilaterally without impairing sexual behavior (Sci Am 1994; 270/5:50)

SDS-PAGE   Sodium dodecyl sulfate-polyacrylamide gel electrophoresis LABORATORY TECHNOLOGY A technique for determining a polypeptide chain's molecular weight, where short proteins are dissociated with SDS at a neutral pH, minimizing the protein's net charged, in the presence of mercaptoethanol which breaks the protein's disulfide bonds, yielding random coils of polypeptides that have the same charge/mass ratio, which are then separated by the gel's sieving effect as a function of molecular weight; see Polyacrimide gel electrophoresis

seabather's eruption   A pruritic dermatitis that appears on bathing suit-covered areas as an erythematous maculopapular eruption ± urticaria; some cases may be caused by the planula larvae of the sea anemone *Edwardsiella lineata* (N Engl J Med 1993; 329:542OA)

sea blue histiocyte   A histiocyte with abundant light sea blue-staining granular cytoplasm seen when the cells are stained with a 'Romanovsky' stain; the color is due to degradation moieties of complex lipid, seen in lipid storage disease, due to alterations in glycoprotein metabolism or in aging; these cells are often autofluorescent, and are positive with the periodic acid Schiff, Sudan black, and Prussian blue stains; sea blue histiocytes are nonspecific and may be seen in 1) Congenital lipid storage defects, eg Wolman's disease (lipase defect with increased triglycerides and esters), cholesteryl ester storage disease, adult Niemann-Pick disease, Tay-Sachs disease and hyperlipoproteinemia 2) Acquired benign conditions, eg hypochromic anemia, SC disease, post-necrotic cirrhosis, rheumatoid arthritis, vitamin E deficiency, chronic granulomatous disease, ceroid histiocystosis of the spleen in ITP and 3) Acquired malignant conditions, eg Hodgkin's disease, CML, polycythemia vera, erythroleukemia and myelodysplastic disorders

sea blue histiocyte syndrome   An AR [MIM 269500] condition characterized by abundant sea-blue histiocytes causing organomegaly, eg hepatosplenomegaly, thrombocytopenia and masses of histiocytes in the skin, lungs, GI tract and CNS, with compromised function; some authors believe the SBHS is the same as adult, chronic, or B type of Niemann-Pick disease

Seabright bantam   Sebright bantam syndromes, see there

sea fan appearance   OPHTHALMOLOGY A fanciful descriptor for the splayed vessels seen in proliferative retinopathy in sickling hemoglobinopathies (hemoglobin SC and sickle-thalassemia) that may be accompanied by salmon-patch pigmentation, vascular tortuosity and occlusion, and arteriovenous anastomoses

sea foot   Immersion foot, see there

sea gull pattern   Gull wing pattern, see there

seagull wing prosthesis   A molded gull-shaped stainless steel device that is temporarily (removed at 12 months) implanted to facilitate healing of a surgically corrected* pectus excavatum; the SWP is reported to be safe, and relatively easy to implant and remove (Chest 1995; 107:303)

*Surgical technique consists of a double transversal sternotomy at the level of the highest and lowest part of the sternal depression with a longitudinal sternotomy

seal finger   A monoarticular infection of the finger with digital puffiness occurring in coastal Scandinavia and Canada, generally in those working in wildlife and marine-related professions, possibly due to fastidious micrococcal bacterial infection TREATMENT Tetracycline

sealed envelope appearance   A descriptor for the high-power LM appearance of GMS-stained *Pneumocystis carinii*, as seen in lung biopsies and pulmonary cytology specimens; the envelope's 'flap' corresponds to the organism's folded membrane, serving to differentiate these from RBCs and nonspecific debris

seamless COMPUTERS A generic adjective referring any smooth and seemingly uninterrupted transition from one task to another, as may occur in translating simulations into real-world practice

seasickness A form of motion sickness (type C), by a vessel's pitching and rolling

seasonal affective disorder The acronym SAD is so widely used that the author has bowed to the vox populi and listed the term under SAD

seat belt laws PUBLIC HEALTH Legislation that is being increasingly enacted in developed nations, requiring the use of safety belts in motor vehicles; after enactment of these laws, the use of seat belts ↑ to 60%, and fatalities and critical injuries per automobile accident are ↓ by 10-15% (JAMA 1991; 265:1409) see Air bag

seat belt syndrome Contusion of anterior abdominal wall caused by lap seat belts[1], which may produce lumbar spine fractures with horizontal splitting of the vertebral body and posterior arch, trauma to bowel, vessels, spleen and liver; in the US, lap-type safety belts[2] are only found in the front seats of older automobiles, although they continue to be used in the back seats; Cf Dashboard fracture, Padded dash(board) syndrome

[1]Especially if improperly worn, as if they are loose, they allow forward acceleration [2]While over-the-shoulder safety belts are rarely associated with intra-abdominal injury, if loosely worn they may cause severe cervical injuries

the Seattle Committee the 'God committee' BIOMEDICAL ETHICS A group comprised of members of the community of Seattle, Washington that met on a regular basis in the late 1960s to decide the relative 'social worth' (thereby 'playing God') of patients in need of hemodialysis, which at the time was limited in availability; a typical 'God committee' was composed of a clergyman, a banker, two physicians, a housewife, a labor leader; see Health care rationing, 'Rule of rescue', Social worth

Note: The dilemmas inherent in making decisions regarding allocation of limited life-saving resources has become a major ethical and budgetary battleground in the US

SEB *Staphylococcus aureus* enterotoxin B, see there

Sebright bantam 'syndromes' A generic term for clinical complexes caused by defective end-organ responses to structurally and functionally normal hormones, including ADH-resistant DM, growth hormone resistance syndrome of de Morsier, testosterone resistance syndrome (Morris' syndrome), pseudohypothyroidism (parathormone resistance) and Savage's follicle-stimulating hormone resistance syndrome, while the human equivalent of the Sebright bantam rooster is due to an overproduction of estradiol and causes gynecomastia (N Engl J Med 1991; 324:317cr)

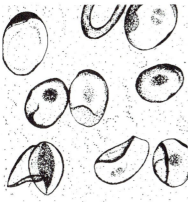

sealed envelope appearance

The Sebright (misspelled in one of the early human-correlation studies as Seabright) bantam rooster has female-in-appearance tail feathers that result from a defective end-organ response to androgenic hormones due to a regulatory mutation that results in a 100-fold ↑ in aromatase (which converts androgens to estrogens) activity; 'Sebright Bantam', then, is a generic adjective for clinical complexes that are caused by defective end-organ responses to structurally and functionally normal hormones

second disease phenomenon The tendency of infection by one pathogen, eg HIV-1 to worsen the response to other infections; AIDS patients have ↑ susceptibility to disseminated vaccinia after immunization, neurosyphilis, tuberculosis, herpes and other infections that usually respond to standard therapy (N Engl J Med 1991; 324:289)

'second genetic code' A term coined (Nature 1988; 333:117) to describe the sites on transfer ribonucleic acid (tRNA) that determine which amino acids will be joined by aminoacyl tRNA synthetase (AAS); the correct attachment of amino acids to specific tRNAs is critical for accurate translation of genetic information from nucleic acid to protein; the 'second genetic code' implies a common set of rules governing tRNA recognition by the various AASs, which appears to be unlikely, and the term 'tRNA identity' better describes the features of the tRNA molecule that make one tRNA recognizable to its cognate AAS and prevents its recognition by other AASs

Note: The 'first' genetic code deciphers the rules governing insertion of specific amino acids in response to the sequence of the mRNA and is the result of alignment of aminoacyl-tRNAs along the mRNA template by base pairing between the tRNA anticodon and the template's codons; because tRNA molecules must interact interchangeably with the protein synthesis apparatus, they all have similar secondary and tertiary structures, but within this framework, variation must exist so that each tRNA is recognizable to its cognate AAS; the 'first' genetic code then, refers to the double helix of DNA that opens temporarily to encode a chain of complementary mRNA and contains the message for the correct order of amino acids to be assembled into proteins; the second step toward protein production requires that tRNA and attached amino acids line up in the order specified by the mRNA; it had been unclear how a particular tRNA and its synthetase (the enzyme which links tRNA to a specific amino acid) recognized each other, as tRNA molecules are virtually identical, a mystery that was partly solved by X-ray crystallography of tRNA and its respective synthetase (Science 1989; 246:1135, 1122)

second-line drug A generic term for any therapeutic agent that is not the drug of choice or the first one used to treat a particular condition; in rheumatoid arthritis, second-line agents* are used when standard 'first-line' therapy, ie anti-inflammatory agents and corticosteroids are regarded as having failed (N Engl J Med 1994; 330:1368DT)

*Gold compounds, antimalarials, penicillamine, methotrexate, azathioprine, sulfasalazine, alkylating agents (cyclophosphamide, chloambucil), and cyclosporine

'second-look' operation A second surgical procedure in the same site as a previous operation, usually in the abdomen, with the intent of continuing therapy that could not be completely performed for various reasons during the first operation GENERAL SURGERY An SLO is performed in the GI tract to re-examine questionably viable segments of small intestine 24-48 hours after an initial massive resection for ischemia, with the hope that sufficient small intestine (at least 30%) remains viable, thereby circumventing the 'short bowel syndrome' GYNECOLOGIC ONCOLOGY A SLO is a laparotomy performed for an ovarian carcinoma that was initially deemed inoperable, and later re-examined to determine whether radio- and/or chemotherapy were successful in reducing the size (or bulk) of the tumor to allow a debulking procedure, or to determine whether therapy may be discontinued or requires modification after 10-12 courses of chemotherapy SURGICAL ONCOLOGY SLOs are performed in colons previously resected for adenocarcinoma and monitored by carcinoembryonic antigen (CEA) levels; an ↑ of CEA > than 35% above the patient's established baseline is suggestive of metastasizing recurrence; at operation, less than ½ prove to be resectable; see Debulking operation

second messenger CELL PHYSIOLOGY A substance released from the cytoplasmic face of a receptor after a ligand interacts with its cognate receptor on the cell's external surface and elicits a response from a G protein; these substances, eg cyclic AMP, inositol 1,4,5-triphosphate (IP_3) and 1,2-diacylglycerol (DAG), in turn mediate various intracellular activities; IP_3 acts on the endoplasmic reticulum, releasing calcium which binds to calcium-binding proteins, troponin and calmodulin, the latter of which undergoes an activating conformational change; the calcium-calmodulin complex then activates: adenylate cyclase, cAMP phophodiesterase, $Ca^{++}-Mg^{++}$-dependent ATPase, glycogen phosphorylase and myosin kinase, resulting in various physiologic effects; DAG acts on protein kinase C, increasing the secretion or production of hormones, enzymes, neurotransmitters, vasoactive compounds and other molecules; see 1,2-Diacylglycerol, G Proteins, PIP_2, Protein kinase C

second opinion Formal or informal advice sought from a second health professional as to the correctness of a diagnosis and/or the appropriateness of a recommended therapy; SOs are sought 1) By the beneficiary of a health insurance policy; SOs are often encouraged by insurance companies, especially when a surgical procedure is recommended, as a second physician may not recommend the procedure, thus reducing the insurance company's costs and 2) By the patient, who may either not trust the rendered diagnosis or proposed therapy or who prefers to corroborate the first opinion for his own peace of mind; see Consultation

second order reaction LABORATORY MEDICINE A chemical reaction, the velocity of which is proportional to either the product of the concentrations of the reactants or to the square of the concentration of one of the reactants

second-set rejection IMMUNOLOGY An accelerated allograft rejection that occurs in a primed (ie previously exposed to the antigen(s) of interest) which is seen in patients who have already rejected one transplanted organ, as are patients who have been fancifully termed 'liver eaters'

'second-wind' phenomenon INBORN ERRORS OF METABOLISM A substrate-dependent variation of exercise tolerance, in which previously fatiguing exercise can be performed with relative ease, after a period of rest; in muscle phosphofructokinase deficiency (Tarui's disease), the 'first' wind is extraordinarily short, as muscle glycolysis is impaired due to an inability to generate pyruvate, the oxidative fuel required to provide normal aerobic power; in these patients, exercise capacity depends on availability of alternate fuels, eg free fatty acids to meet requirements for oxidation in muscle during exercise; high carbohydrate meals in these patients exacerbate their exercise intolerance by inhibiting lipolysis, depriving muscle of its energy source (**N Engl J Med 1991; 324:364**) RHEUMATOLOGY A surge of subjective 'energy' that occurs after a short rest period, typical of the mid-afternoon fatigue seen in rheumatoid arthritis

secondary antibody A generic term for the second antibody used in a 'sandwich' method, eg ELISA, or immunoperoxidase method; the SA is 'raised' against the species of animal, eg rabbit, goat, etc, used to make the primary antibody; see Sandwich method; Cf Primary antibody

secondary binge effect PSYCHOLOGY Any of the constellation of findings and changes that occur external to, and as a result of binge-type consumption of alcohol, eg the negative emotions evoked in those who are non-participants in the baccanalian revelry (**JAMA 1995; 273:1903**)

secondary care Health care provided by a specialist in a non-high technology situation, eg in a private office, or specialty care that is provided in a community hospital, to a patient who has been referred by a primary care physician, for special studies, eg cardiac stress test, CT or special procedures, eg cholecystectomy, endoscopic polypectomy; Cf Primary care, Tertiary care

secondary care center Secondary care facility A community (or 'voluntary') hospital that is equipped to provide all but the most specialized forms of health care, surgery and diagnostic modalities; SCCs include general acute care hospitals or specialized outpatient facilities that treat 'garden variety' diseases, for which the risks of therapy are minimal, well-defined, and the length of hospitalization expected to be short and uncomplicated; Cf Primary care, Tertiary care

secondary deficiency A nutritional deficiency state that is not due to the lack of ingestion of an essential nutrient, ie a primary deficiency, but rather the result of either an ↑ requirement for that substance, eg iron in pregnancy, or ↓ availability or 'wastage' of the nutrient, as in proteinuria in nephrotic syndrome

secondary diabetes Diabetes mellitus that is an epiphenomenon of known pathogenesis, ie occurs other than by type I (IDDM) and type II (NIDDM) mechanisms; secondary DM may result from pancreatitis, pancreatic carcinoma, pheochromocytoma, hemochromatosis, acromegaly or by use of drugs known to impair glucose metabolism, eg corticosteroids

secondary fluor A fluor, eg POPOP, that is used in a scintillation device to shift the wavelength of light emitted by the primary fluor to a longer wavelength, for which the photomultiplier has a greater sensitivity; see Primary fluor, Quenching, RIA

secondary gain PSYCHIATRY The secondary psychological advantages that one obtains from an illness or symptom's thereof, eg increased attention, sympathy, social interaction; Cf Primary gain

secondary granule see Lysosome; Cf Primary granule

secondary intention see Wound healing

secondary lysosome CELL BIOLOGY A lysosome that has fused with a phagocytic vesicle

secondary malignancy A malignant neoplasm that arises in the background of another malignancy treated by radio- or chemotherapy; SM has also be defined as one attributed to environmental toxins, physical agents and radiation; the most common post-therapeutic SMs are ANLL, including acute myelogenous leukemia, acute promyelocytic leukemia, acute monocytic leukemia, erythroleukemia and myelodysplastic disorders (preleukemia); chromosomal changes in secondary leukemias include loss of the entire (or long arms of) chromosomes 5 (-5 or -5q) and 7 (-7 and -7q); survival in spontaneous ANLL is 30% at 12 months, survival in post-therapeutic (secondary) ANLL at 12 months is 10% (**JAMA 1990; 264:1006**); the peak incidence of SM occurs 5 years after chemotherapy is first administered; in ovarian carcinoma, there is a 12-fold ↑ risk for future malignancy in those treated with chemotherapy; radiotherapy does not produce an additive effect; the most leukemogenic chemotherapeutic agents in one study were chlorambucil and melphalan, and as combined therapies, doxorubicin and cis-platin; in Hodgkin's disease, there is a 9-fold ↑ in secondary leukemia in those treated with chemotherapy compared to radiotherapy; after six cycles of chemotherapy the risk increases to 14, the incidence peaks 5-8 years after initiating chemotherapy; the most inculpated agents are procarbazine and mechlorethamine, the risk doubled in those with splenectomy; children treated with alkylating agents have relative risk of 4.7 for future bone sarcomas, while those treated radiotherapy have a 2.7-fold ↑ risk for bone sarcoma, increasing to a 40-fold risk when doses to the bone exceed 6000 rad PRIMARY-SECONDARY MALIGNANCY DYADS include 1) BREAST CARCINOMA Removal of the axillary 'tail' lymph nodes, begets angioedema that may induce angiosarcoma 2) GERM CELL NEOPLASIA Radiotherapy or chemotherapy to sensitive tissue in teratomas may 'activate' non-germ line tissue, giving rise to sarcomas, as well as other tumors, including nephroblastoma, neuroblastoma and adenosquamous carcinoma 3) RETINOBLASTOMA Fatal secondary sarcomas occur in 10% of hereditary retinoblastomas treated with chemotherapy and radiotherapy, but not in non-hereditary retinoblastoma Physical agents causing secondary malignancy include 1) Radiation (actinic or radiotherapeutic) to the head and neck causing secondary basal cell carcinomas; latency period to secondary neoplasm 3-65 years 2) Chronic irritation (Marjolin's ulcer) causing skin cancer or chronic injury, eg heat-induced squamous cell carcinoma (Kairo cancer, Japan; Kang cancer, China; Kangri cancer, Kashmir; 'peat moss' cancer, Ireland) 3) Scar-induced malignancy, eg malignant fibrous histiocytoma arising in sites with metal objects or shrapnel or malignancy induced by mechanical trauma, a relation which in humans is anecdotal and 4) Ischemia and squamous cell carcinoma adjacent to varicose veins

secondary malignant fibrous histiocytosis A tumor of mesenchymal tissues that is the most common malignancy inducible by physical agents; malignant fibrous histiocytoma is associated with other tumors, eg chordoma, or may be induced by radiation, eg to the cervix for cancer, long term foreign bodies, eg shrapnel in bone or induced in rats by chemical, eg injections of 4-hydroxyamino-quinolone-1-oxide

secondary obesity Obesity that is a symptom of other conditions including CNS disease (defects of the hypophyseal-hypothalamic axis, intracranial leukemia and other lesions), congenital (Alström-Hallgren, Bloumant, Carpenter, Cohen, Lawrence-Moon-Biedl, Prader-Willi and Vasquez) syndromes and endocrinopathies (hypothyroidism, insulinoma, Cushing syndrome, polycystic ovary disease, pituitary dwarfism); see Morbid obesity, Obesity,

secondary polycythemia An ↑ in red cell mass in response to a physiologic insult, eg hypoxia due to pulmonary disease, cardiomyopathy, vena cava thrombosis, or in response to excess erythropoietin production in renal cell carcinoma or cystic kidneys; in secondary polycythemia, erythropoietin (EP) may be ↑ (± 120 U/L); in relative polycythemia EP is normal (± 7 U/L) and in polycythemia vera, EP is ↓ (± 2 U/L) (**Br J Haematol 1992; 81:603**) see Polycythemia vera

secondary (immune) response The enhanced immune response of an organism when it is re-exposed to an antigen, after it has had sufficient time to generate an immune recognition 'cascade'

secondary structure see Protein structure

secretin A 27-amino acid helical peptide that is structurally similar to gastric inhibitory polypeptide (GIP), vasoactive inhibitory polypeptide (VIP), and glucagon, which is produced by S cells in the upper small intestine and brain; secretin is released by acid, bile or fat into the intestinal lumen, and stimulates the release of water and bicarbonate from the pancreas, neutralizing gastric acid, stimulating intestinal motility and the release of bile and gastric acid and inhibiting gastrin; since secretin releases gastrin from gastrinomas, secretin stimulation tests are of diagnostic utility in the Zollinger-Ellison syndrome

secretin injection test GASTROENTEROLOGY A provocative test in which porcine (or other) secretin is injected IV and the gastrin levels are monitored; gastrin levels are ↓ in antral G-cell hyperplasia and duodenal ulcers, and ↑↑↑ in gastrinomas and Zollinger-Ellison syndrome (**MH Sleisenger, JS Fordtran, Eds, Gastrointestinal Disease, 5th ed, WB Saunders, Philadelphia, 1993**); the SIT is also used to evaluate exocrine pancreatic function; after secretin injection, the normal pancreas increases volume of secretions and bicarbonate production, which does not occur in a pancreas compromised by cystic fibrosis, chronic pancreatitis, or carcinoma

secretogogue An agent that ↑ GI electrolyte and fluid secretion by ↑ adenylate cyclase activity or by ↑ calcium in the cytosol; secretogogues include bacterial endotoxins

(cholera exotoxins, shiga toxins and others), hormones (calcitonin, glucagon, secretin, vasoactive inhibitory polypeptide and others), detergents (bile acids, fatty acids and hydroxy fatty acids), laxatives and others (eg food allergies and resultant mast cell degranulation)

secretors TRANSFUSION MEDICINE Background: ABO blood group antigens, Le[a] and Le[b] are not intrinsic to erythrocytes but are produced in other tissues, possibly in the intestinal epithelium and adsorbed from the plasma onto red cell glycosphingolipids; the presence of Lewis antigens on red cells depends on whether the subject has inherited one Le or two le genes, which encode fucosyl transferase, adding a fucose to the ABO blood group type I oligosaccharides; those subjects who also inherit the dominant Se(H) gene, producing an antigen, Le[b]; subjects with ABO blood groups, A_x and B_x who don't secrete A or B substance; 80% of the normal subjects are 'secretors', ie ABH antigens are present in their secretions; see Lewis system

secretory carcinoma (breast) Juvenile carcinoma, see there

secretory carcinoma (endometrial) A well-differentiated variant of endometrial carcinoma in which the cells have vacuolated or clear cytoplasm, thus resembling normal secretory endometrium PROGNOSIS Similar to well differentiated endometrial carcinoma DDx Clear cell carcinoma, Arias-Stella reaction, and endometrial hyperplasia with ↑ secretion

secretory component Secretory piece, see there

secretory leukocyte protease inhibitor SLPI, see there

secretory phase Luteal phase The second half (days 15-28) of the uterine cycle following ovulation, in which the endometrial glands secrete a clear mucus, and the stroma becomes vascularized and edematous in response to estrogens and progesterones produced by the corpus luteum; Cf Proliferative phase

secretory piece Secretory component A short polypeptide chain carried by dimeric IgA that serves as a receptor; SP is added to IgA when it is secreted by the intestinal luminal cells, and is thought to confer protection against proteolytic digestion

secure *adjective* COMPUTERS Pertaining or relating to a computer system in which the data is protected from unauthorized access (**Am Lab March 1995, p46**)

SED Spondyloepiphyseal dysplasia, see there

Seder syncope A vasovagal collapse induced by the horseradish (active ingredient, isothiocyanate) used in the celebration of Seder (**JAMA 1988; 259:1943**) see Judiasm-practice of, Spicy food, Sushi syncope

*A symbolic meal that commemorates the bitterness of Jewish slavery in ancient Egypt, which is partaken during the Jewish high holiday of Passover

sedimentation equilibrium A laboratory method used for separating a substance and calculating its molecular weight, which consists of sedimentation by ultracentrifugation, allowing the centrifuge to spin at speeds slow enough and for a long enough period of time to establish an equilibrium for the solute between sedimentation and diffusion; see Ultracentrifugation

'see one, do one, teach one' MEDICAL EDUCATION A time-honored format for acquiring medical skills based on a three-step process of visualization, performance, and didactics (**N Engl J Med 1995; 332:1507ED**)

seed calculi Innumerable small oval concrements that may form in a markedly hydronephrotic renal pelvis in ureteropelvic obstruction

'seed and soil' hypothesis A theory based on Sir James Paget's study of women dying of breast cancer, in whom metastases were relatively common to the liver and brain and uncommon in other organs; Paget postulated that certain tumors were predisposed to spread to certain sites based on the host's ability to support the growth of those particular tumor cells; another facet of the hypothesis is the 'seed' itself, in which there is structural and functional tumor cell heterogeneity that allows the cells to work synergistically to create an environment for distant spread of malignancy, eg tumors implanted in nude mice will not metastasize unless implanted in the appropriate organ; tumors appear to lodge in sites with a high capacity for thrombaxane synthesis, eg lung, liver, and adrenal glands (N Engl J Med 1993; 329:138c) see Metastasis

Paget's theory contrasts with Ewing's 'mechanical theory' of tumor spread, in which tumor colonization is held to be related to the pattern of blood flow away from a malignancy; both theories are partially correct and not mutually exclusive; in terms of 'soil', the host tissue may produce mitogenic factors, eg acid-fibroblast growth factor and hematopoietic factors, general inhibitors that encourage the cells to stay and grow, eg transforming growth factor-β, TNF-α or organ-specific inhibitors; support for the mechanical theory lies in nonspecific production of angiogenesis factors, and specific routes of metastases, eg Batson's plexus which is the route of prostatic metastases to the bone (N Engl J Med 1990; 322:605, Paget, Lancet 1889; 1:571)

seeding trial A drug company-sponsored trial of an FDA-approved drug which has little or no scientifically valid purpose; an ST is often a thinly disguised marketing ploy by a drug company to entice physicians to prescribe a new drug, usually of the 'me too' type; features that distinguish STs from scientifically rigorous studies include the use of study designs that would not support the stated research goals; recruitment of clinical 'investigators' based not on their expertise, but rather on their high volume prescribing practices; inappropriately high payment given to the investigator; minimum requirements for data; collection of data that has little potential use and the lack of double blinding or control groups (N Engl J Med 1994; 331:1350sa) see 'Me too' drug, Switch campaign

SEER program Surveillance, Epidemiology and End Results program A database maintained by the National Cancer Institute, Bethesda, Maryland, which is comprised of 11 population-based registries throughout the US, and represents about 10% of the US population; the SEER database is used to evaluate trends in malignancies and other morbid conditions; the age-adjusted incidence rates for all cancers (from periods 1975-1979 to 1987-1991) has ↑ by 18.6% in ♂ (largely due to prostate cancer), and 12.4% in ♀ (due to breast and lung cancers); mortality in the same period ↑ by 3% in ♂ and 6% in ♀ (J Natl ICancer Inst 1995; 87:175)

'seesaw' nystagmus Torsional-vertical ocular oscillation NEUROLOGY A clinical finding in which one eye moves up while the other moves down, seen in bitemporal hemianopia due to sellar or parasellar mass lesions, a movement that is fancifully likened to the up and down bobbing of a children's seesaw; Cf 'Railroad' nystagmus

SEIR equations A standard epidemiological model for infectious diseases, based on the acronym, Susceptible-Exposed-Infectious-Recovery, representing categories into which a susceptible population is divided; the SEIR model may be an over-idealization of epidemiology while more realistic models demonstrate chaos

Seldane-D® An antihistamine-decongestant (terfenadine + pseudoephedrine-HCl) COUNTRAINDICATIONS Coronary artery disease, severe hypertension, underlying hepatic dysfunction; therapy with erythromycin, itraconazole, ketoconazole, MAOIs

selectin Any of a family of cell adhesion molecules (CAMs) or glycoproteins that are critical to interactions between endothelium and cells in the circulation (Nature 1991; 349:196n&v) the so-called homing receptor selectin gp90mel, LAM-1, LEC-CAM-1 A glycoprotein expressed on leukocytes that facilitates their binding to endothelium during lymphocyte recirculation through peripheral lymph nodes and neutrophil egress from the circulation to sites of inflammation; selectins are asymmetrical composite pro-

teins with a mosaic architecture and 3 distinct (anchoring, transmembrane, and extracellular) domains (Sci Am 1993; 268/1:82) see Adhesion receptors, CD62

selective amnesia PSYCHOLOGY A colloquial term for amnesia for certain events, which as commonly used, may refer to the deliberate inability to remember details about an event

selection bias Any bias introduced into a set of data that may be introduced by the investigator, which demonstrates a directional deviation from randomness

selective molecule Any of a large family of molecules that provides specificity to the involved 'reactants', including cadherins, enzymes, immunoglobulins, integrins and selectins

selective serotonin re-uptake inhibitor CLINICAL PHARMACOLOGY SSRI Any of a family (fluoxetine, fluvoxamine, paroxetine, sertraline) of antidepressants that are thought to be a substantial improvement over the tricyclic antidepressants; SSRIs 1) Have little effect on norepinephrine reuptake 2) Lack anticholinergic properties 3) Do not cause postural hypotension, delay cardiac conduction or have a major effect on seizure activity and are not associated with weight gain CLINICAL UTILITY Dysthymia (minor chronic depression), atypical depression, possibly antipanic therapy SIDE EFFECTS Insomnia, agitation, headache, nausea, diarrhea, and adverse pharmacologic interactions with other agents, especially with fluoxetine (Science & Medicine Sept/Oct 1994)

selective termination of pregnancy OBSTETRICS Selective abortion of one or more products of a 'higher multiple' gestation for various indications, eg chromosomal or physical abnormalities; see Interlocking

selective thermophotolysis A therapeutic modality in dermatology that 'bleaches' certain skin lesions, eg port-wine nevi and tattoos (lesions with preferential light absorption) by using a short-pulsed CO_2 laser that delivers ultrashort 'zaps' of laser energy; see Lasers

selegiline L-Deprenyl A selective monoamine oxidase type B inhibitor, which in combination with L-dopa, is reported to be useful for early symptomatic treatment of parkinsonism (Arch Neurol 1991; 48:31)

selenium A nonmetallic element (with 6 natural and stable isotopes, and 14 radioactive isotopes), trace amounts of which are required for hepatic and cardiac function; selenium is thought to act via glutathione peroxidase to protect the heart against diastolic dysfunction by preventing hydrogen peroxide damage i

Note: Selenium has photoelectric properties, and is used in xerography and in solar cells

selenium deficiency CARDIOLOGY An absence of selenium in the diet, which leads to an ↑ binding of hepatic nucleoproteins to DNA regulatory sequences that activate transcription in response to oxidative stress; SD favors selection and replication of a myocarditic form of Coxsackievirus (CVB3) (Nature Medicine 1995; 1:433, 405), and has been implicated in endemic cardiomyopathy and Keshan disease, which is attributed to a defect in the function of glutathione peroxidase, without which there is ↑ platelet aggregation due to impaired free radical salvage or in the catalytic function of type I deiodinizing thyroxine-activating enzyme (Nature 1991; 349:438) see Keshan disease

selenoid 'cell' Half moon cell An erythrocyte ghost caused by mechanical shearing which occurs when RBCs are abnormal and/or young or the plasma hyperlipemic

self-bougienage A therapeutic modality in which the patient auto-introduces a 44-46-F Maloney dilator tube to treat benign recurrent esophageal strictures; most of one small cohort of subjects with dysphagia prior to the initiation of self-bougienage were asymptomatic during the 3-

year follow-up period

self-disclosure PROFESSIONAL ETHICS A form of boundary violation by a professional, in which areas of personal problems and vulnerabilities are disclosed to a patient; SD is often the first step taken on the road to sexual misconduct, and even if such expression does not evolve in the direction of impropriety, it inappropriately reverses the traditional role in the physician/healer to patient/healer relationship (JAMA1995; 273:1445) see Professional boundaries, Sexual misconduct

self-esteem Self-worth PSYCHOLOGY The internalized sense of one's own worth, which, if it approximates the value or respect from other people in the person's circle(and reflects the person's 'value' in terms of societal norms) is known as 'good self-esteem'; an inappropriately high sense of personal worth, ie views not shared by others and/or society is termed simply high self-esteem, and its opposite, low self-esteem

self-fulfilling prophecy PSYCHIATRY A distorted prediction or statement about a person in a certain setting, that forms a substrate that ultimately leads the person to behave in the predicted manner; as an example, if a child is regularly told about his/her misbehavior and poor performance in school he/she may become the 'prophesized' sociopath

self-help group PSYCHOLOGY Any group of similarly-minded persons who share a problem that is stressful and/or may cause personal, familial, or occupational difficulties; SHGs provide a social network and support that may no longer be readily available from natural (ie family) or professional support systems; SHGs include those for people suffering from mental or physical illness and reform groups for substance abuse and addictions, and may by formed within advocacy groups for certain minorities

self-hypnosis The hypnosis of oneself, an interventional modality for which a person can be trained; SH may be of use in controlling certain habits or behaviors (eg pain control, smoking cessation, weight control) or it can be used to evoke repressed memories and experiences (Freud's 'abreaction') see Hypnosis

self-insured HEALTH INSURANCE *adjective* Pertaining or referring to a practice in which a person carries an individual health insurance policy for him/herself; in general, self insurance is far more expensive than group insurance

self-limited disease A disorder which by its very nature cannot progress, and which usually reverses itself without therapeutic intervention

self-mutilation PSYCHIATRY Any of a number of physically auto-destructive acts that is perpetuated in various guises by an estimated 1:1500 population; most SM is psychogenic in origin, and may be related to physical confinement, deprivation, depression, often related to childhood experiences; the acts may be performed as a form of 'self-cleansing' to cauterize the 'pain of living'; SM is also an integral component of certain hereditary conditions, eg Lesch-Nyhan syndrome and Cornelia de Lange syndrome and is attributed to imbalances of neurotransmitters

self-neglect A generic term for the status of any person, eg elderly who lives alone in the community and is unable to provide for him/herself and maintain physical and/or mental health (N Engl J Med 1995; 332:437RA)

selfness IMMUNOLOGY A generic term referring to the state of immunologic individuality, as defined by the human leukocyte antigens (ie HLA-A, -B, -C, etc) in the major histocompatibility complex (MHC)

self-referral HEALTH CARE INDUSTRY Physician self-referral A generic term for the referral by a physician to an outside health care facility, eg radiologic imaging center at which he/she has a financial interest but no professional respon-

sibility; self-referral has two major impacts on medical care, 1) Ethical Conflict of interest, ie whether the diagnostic procedure ordered is appropriate and 2) Financial, which increases the cost of health care delivery; physician self-referral increases health care costs without improving the quality of care, when such disparate areas of medical practice as magnetic resonance imaging (38% of requests in the self-referral group were inappropriate vs 28% of requests at independent-referral facilities), physical therapy (physical therapy was initiated 2.3 **x** more often in self-referral group than by those in the independent-referral group), psychiatric services (cost of psychiatric evaluation $1165 in the self-referral group vs $870 in the independent-referral group), and radiation therapy (radiation physicists spend 18% less time with patients at joint ventures than at non-joint venture free-standing facilities) were examined (N Engl J Med 1992; 327:1497SA, 1502SA, 1522ED; 1993; 328:1277C); the mean cost of imaging per episode of care is 4.4 to 7.5-fold higher for self-referring physicians; see Fee-splitting, Joint venture, Kickback, 'Safe harbor' rules; Cf Referral, Second opinion

self restriction see MHC restriction

self-sustaining sequence replication 3SR* MOLECULAR BIOLOGY A type of nucleic acid amplification that was developed primarily to amplify RNA, but which may be used to replicate DNA targets; the 3SR reaction is the result of three enzymatic reactions carried out by two enzymes: Reverse transcriptase converts RNA to a DNA copy while degrading the original RNA; the result is single-stranded DNA molecule that is made double-stranded by reverse transcriptase; the double-stranded DNA is then continuously transcribed by the RNA polymerase of the bacteriophage T7; 3SR is 1) Isothermal, and unlike PCR does not require thermal cycling and repeated denaturation of target DNA, 2) RNA-specific, and is targeted to RNA even in the presence of DNA, and 3) A transcription reaction, and thus is more rapid than PCR in which there is only a doubling of DNA per cycle; because the 3SR reaction occurs in one tube, it is amenable to automation; 3SR may ultimately compete with PCR over which it has many clear advantages; see Ligase chain reaction, PCR

self tolerance IMMUNOLOGY Immunologic tolerance to self antigens, despite their proven immunogenicity; loss of ST results in autoimmune diseases

The formerly used term, horror autotoxicus (fear of self-poisoning) was coined by Paul Ehrlich as an explanation for why an individual does not (usually) produce autoantibodies, despite the proven immunogenicity of his/or antigens

'selfish' DNA Junk DNA, see there

selfish replication MOLECULAR GENETICS An anthropomorphic conceptualization of the 'behavior' of genes that guarantees self-perpetuation; in this construct, a defective gene would eventually be eliminated from a species by selective pressure against the expression of a deleterious trait, and only 'robust' genes would be transmitted to subsequent generations (N Engl J Med 1994; 331:1585ED)

Sellafield study An epidemiologic study that attempted to address the finding of a statistically ↑ incidence of childhood leukemia in the region of the Sellafield nuclear reprocessing plant in the UK; four children of fathers exposed to more than 100 mSv (1 rad = 10 milliSieverts) developed leukemia, inculpating a genetic event (the so-called 'Gardner effect') below the legally acceptable exposure level of 50 milliSieverts/year that passed to the fetus via the sperm (Br Med J 1990; 300:423); see Pilgrim plant

Note: While meticulously performed, the statistical power of the study is weak and in mice, the offspring produced with irradiated spermatogonia had no increase in leukemia; furthermore, in France, where 75% of electricity is produced by nuclear power plants, there is no increase in leukemia; in those occupationally exposed to low levels of radioactivity (Oak Ridge National Laboratory, US), the radiation-cancer dose response is ten-fold higher than previous estimates and the incidence of leukemia two-fold greater (JAMA 1991; 265:1397); living near such facilities does not appear to increase mortality (JAMA 1991; 265:1403) SUMMARY The data is complex, the levels of secondary exposure are unknown and the effects of low-level exposure to radiation uncertain (**New York Times 8 March 1994; C1**)

semen The viscid whitish secretion of ♂ reproductive organs (bulbourethral glands, prostate, seminal vesicles, and testis) which contains spermatozoa; see Nocturnal emision

semen analysis A laboratory procedure for evaluating possible ♂ causes of infertility (**Lab Med 1994; 25:509**); one of the major parameters of measured in semen analysis is sperm count which is reported to be decreasing in the 20th century from 113 million/mL in 1940 to 66 million in 1990, a decline believed by some workers to be related to environmental pollutants which have estrogenic activity (**Sci Am 1993; 269/3:34**)

semiconservative replication Meselson-Stahl experiment, see there

semilethal gene A mutant gene that is lethal if it is present in the homozygous state, or a mutation that when present at full 'genomic strength' is lethal to less than 100% of a population with the mutation

semi-starvation neurosis PSYCHIATRY A pre-anorexia nervosa state that most commonly affects ♀ subjects who, as children had been described as being 'good girls', who have perfectionist tendencies and who demonstrate effects of long-term caloric restriction including fatigue, weakness, apathy, passivity, withdrawal and regression; see Anorexia nervosa, Binge-purge syndrome; Cf Starvation

semisynthetic compound A chemical derived from a natural substance that is subjected to one or more synthetic steps to impart desired qualities, eg natural penicillin has a β-lactam ring and a thiazolidine ring; one derivative of the parent molecule, 6-aminopenicillanic acid, when obtained from *Penicillium crysogenum* grown in a side chain-depleted medium yields semisynthetic penicillins, which incorporate specific precursors in culture that have desired properties

senescence CLINICAL MEDICINE see Geriatrics, Gerontology MOLECULAR BIOLOGY A generic term for the constellation of processes that define an aging cell; normal cells, eg human diploid fibroblasts and others have a finite proliferative lifespan, at the end of which the cells remain alive in an arrested state, known as replication senescence, which occurs after about 60 cell divisions, with the cell being arrested at the G_1/S boundary of the cycle; senescent arrest is similar to terminal differentiation as it involves repression of proliferation-promoting genes, through either expression of antiproliferative genes or through activity of post-transcriptional factors, eg loss of telomere sequences; 'escape' of cells from biological aging is rare and occurs in immortal cell lines and in neoplasia; senescent cells are larger and less motile, have an enlarged nucleus and an ↑ content of RNA, protein, glycogen, lipids and lysosomes; senescence is a state due to the presence of inhibitor(s) preventing entry into the S phase; one such inhibitor is p110^{Rb}, a retinoblastoma protein that is non-phosphorylated in quiescent and senescent diploid fibroblasts; fusion of these cells with cells bearing oncogenes (SV40 T antigen, adenovirus E1A and HPV) results in phosphorylation of p110^{Rb} and initiating the S phase in quiescent cells; see Garbage can hypothesis

Note: Quiescent cells cease proliferation, enlarge, senesce and die; senescence is postulated to occur via either 1) An error catastrophe model, with accumulation of random damage and mutations of DNA with loss of proliferative capacity, accompanied by intracellular build-up of poorly metabolized detritus ('garbage'), in particular lipofucsin and/or 2) A genetically programmed model ('pacemaker' theory), in which immortality is, almost by definition, a characteristic of malignant cells; senescence may be driven by a gene on chromosome 1

Sengstaken-Blakemore tube A triple-lumen rubber tube used to quench the bleeding in esophageal varices; the central lumen allows communication of the oral cavity with the stomach; a second tube communicates with a rounded 'bladder' that is inflated to anchor the device in the upper body of the stomach; the last tube communicates with a long inflatable balloon that places gentle pressure on the esophageal lumen, usually quenching the bleeding

senile dementia Progressive neurodegenerative disease(s) that may be divided into two groups of approximately equal size 1) Primary neuronal degeneration or what has become known as Alzheimer's disease* and 2) Vascular degeneration due to atherosclerosis, resulting in a lacunar state; CT and MRI studies indicate that ischemia of the periventricular white matter may be responsible for a significant proportion of senile dementia, which disconnects the relatively intact cerebral cortex, resulting in true subcortical dementia or Binswanger type dementia; Cf Alzheimer's disease, Lacunar state, Multi-infarct dementia, Pseudodementia

Note: The widely extant practice of equating dementia occurring at any age (an event that is common in those older than seventy) with Alzheimer's disease is incorrect, in that Alzheimer's original description referred to PRE-senile dementia, which occurred in the fourth and fifth decades

senile osteoporosis see Osteoporosis

senile plaque Neuritic plaque NEUROPATHOLOGY A histologic finding consisting of a core of extracellular amyloid surrounded by a tangled spherical mass of argyrophilic cholinergic, neurites (axons/dendrites), confined to the grey matter (neocortex, hippocampus, amygdala, less commonly, the basal ganglia and elsewhere; SPs are seen in the brains of older persons, but are ↑↑↑ in Alzheimer's disease; see Paired helical filaments

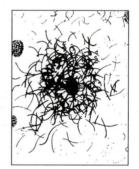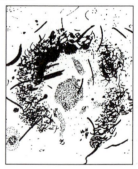

| immature plaque | mature plaque |

senile plaque

'senseless' immune response CpG effect, see there

sensitivity LABORATORY MEDICINE The degree to which a test or clinical assay is capable of confirming (or at least supporting) the diagnosis of a disease X, ie the analyte is appropriately abnormal in a subject with the disease; sensitivity is determined by the simple ratio of those who have a positive test result and the disease (true positives), divided by the sum of those with positive test results and the disease (true positives) and those with negative results who have the disease (false negatives), multiplied by 100 to yield a percentage; sensitivity then, represents the proportion of subjects with a disease which a test is capable of detecting; see Predictive value

sensitivity test Antimicrobial susceptibility test, see there

sensitization IMMUNOLOGY The process in which an individual acquires the ability to react to an antigen, usually of nonself origin

sensitizer PHYSIOLOGY A substance that increases the susceptibility to a stimulus including light, eg a photosensitizer IMMUNOLOGY An immunogenic molecule that is capable of evoking immune responsiveness, eg allergen or adjuvant molecule; Cf Antigen

sentinel animal PUBLIC HEALTH An animal that is susceptible or sensitive to a particular component (eg a toxin, pathogen, radiation) in the environment; the classic SA is the canary which was used in coal mines as an early warning system for cave-ins; a variety of monkeys have been used as SAs for the detection of 'hot' (Biosafety Level 4) agents (R Preston, The Hot Zone, Random House, New York, 1994)

sentinel clot An adherent blood clot or prominent blood vessel, seen by upper GI endoscopy in ⅔ of peptic ulcers that have previously hemorrhaged, occurring when a lateral defect in the arterial wall protrudes as a plug of fibrin above the ulcer base

sentinel loop RADIOLOGY A dilated segment of jejunum seen in the left upper quadrant in an upper GI radiocontrast 'series', which although nonspecific, is considered characteristic of acute pancreatitis; Cf Colonic cut-off sign

sentinel node Signal node of Virchow An isolated, enlarged often left-sided supraclavicular lymph node, classically associated with metastatic gastric carcinoma, which when found, indicates that the malignancy is non-resectable; Cf Mary Joseph nodule

sentinel pile The swelling at the lower end of a chronic anal fissure, palpable as an anal mass, which may be the first or most prominent manifestation of a fissure, hence, a 'sentinel'

separation anxiety PEDIATRICS A state of apprehension, uncertainty and discomfort that may be seen in a child when faced with the anticipated or actual separation from the mother or parent-surrogate; SA, which is often accompanied by irritability and crying is viewed as a normal reaction, which only becomes pathologic when it is excessive or when it continues into an older age

Sephadex® A proprietary group of cross-linking dextrans, available in beads of various diameters, which is used in gel filtration electrophoresis

Sepharose® A proprietary group of agarose gels used in electrophoresis

sepsis Sepsis has been recently redefined* by clinical parameters as '*SIRS (systemic inflammatory response syndrome) plus a documented (ie 'culture-positive') infection*', and is part of a continuum of a biologic inflammatory response to infection that evolves toward septic shock (JAMA 1995; 273:117QA) see Septic shock, Severe sepsis, SIRS

*American College of Chest Physicians-Society of Critical Care Medicine Consensus Conference. Definitions for sepsis and organ failure and guidelines for the use of innovative therapies in sepsis (Crit Care Med 1992; 20:864)

septic shock A condition that has been formally (see Sepsis for reference) defined by clinical parameters as '*Sepsis-induced hypotension despite fluid resuscitation plus hypoperfusion abnormalities...*', which include lactic acidosis, oliguria, or an acute alteration in mental status; SS is end-stage of a continuum of a biologic inflammatory response to infection (JAMA 1995; 273:117QA) see Sepsis, Severe sepsis, SIRS

sepsis syndrome A constellation of signs, symptoms, and systemic responses caused by a wide range of microorganisms that may eventuate into septic shock (N Engl J Med 1992; 326:324CPC); SS is a systemic response to infection, defined as hypothermia < 35°C (96°F) or hyperthermia > 39°C (101°F), tachycardia (> 90/minute), tachypnea (20 breaths/minute), a clinically evident focus of infection or positive blood cultures, one or more end organs with either dysfunction or inadequate perfusion, cerebral dysfunction, hypoxemia (PaO_2 < 75 mmHg), ↑ plasma lactate or unexplained metabolic acidosis, oliguria (< 30 mL/hour) and a leukocyte count of < 2.0 x 10^9/L or > 12.0 x 10^9/L (US: < 2000/mm³ or > 12 000/mm³); SS is one of the most common causes of adult respiratory distress syndrome

Note: The confusing semantics of the terms sepsis, sepsis/septic syndrome, and septic shock are unlikely to be resolved in the forseeable future; the terms sepsis and septic syndrome are essentially interchangeable and would in part overlap with septicemia, ie the early components of a pernicious infectious cascade that has spilled into the circulation; the term septic shock is used when the process becomes virtually irreversible

septic abortion An abortion associated with infection and complicated by fever endometritis, and parametritis; 62% of deaths from illegal abortions are due to infection; in Romania in the 1960s, abortions were outlawed, and the abortion-related mortality ↑ 10-fold, costing an estimated 10 000 lives until it was once again legalized; the WHO estimates that 25-50% of the ½ million maternal deaths/year are related to illegal abortion PREVENTION OF SEPTIC ABORTION-PRIMARY Requires an effective and acceptable means of contraception, provision of safe and legal abortion services in case of contraceptive failure and appropriate medical mangement of abortion SECONDARY Entails prompt diagnosis and treatment of endometritis to prevent more serous complications TERTIARY An extension of secondary prevention as the stage has been set for serious complications requiring hysterectomy or resulting in death (N Engl J Med 1994; 331:310CC)

Note: Fetal loss due to a bacterial infection of the uterus is 50 times more common in intrauterine device users; bacteria implicated include the native vaginal flora, including *Clostridium perfringens*, aerobic and anaerobic streptococci and gram-negative bacilli

septic shock A clinical condition identical to the sepsis syndrome with an added component of hypotension (systolic blood pressure < 90 mm Hg or loss in the baseline systolic pressure of greater than 40 mmHg) EPIDEMIOLOGY SS kills 100-175 000 people/year (US), 13th major cause of death in the US CLINICAL Clinical features either reflect the response to infection, ie tachycardia, tachypnea, changes in temperature, and leukocytosis, or reflect the organ system(s) involved, eg cardiovascular, hematologic, hepatic, renal, respiratory, and is regarded as severe if there is hypoperfusion, lactic acidosis, hypotension, or altered mental status (N Engl J Med 1993; 328:1471RV) PATHOGENESIS SS is induced by a systemic infection with gram-negative bacteria that have a complex glycolipid lipopolysaccharide (LPS, endotoxin) on the outer membrane that overstimulates the host immune system (possibly by binding to the macrophage CD14, activating the cognate protein tyrosine kinase), in particular the macrophages, to generate TNF, IL-1, IL-6, leukotrienes, prostanoids, and nitric oxide; the end result is hypotension, multiorgan failure and death; tyrosine kinase inhibitors of the tyrphostin family AG 126 may prevent lethal toxicity in mice (Science 1994; 264:1319RR)

septic syndrome Sepsis syndrome, see there

septicemia Sepsis syndrome, see there

septo-optic dysplasia sequence of de Morsier An idiopathic condition characterized by incomplete early morphogenesis of the anterior midline brain, causing hypothalamic defects, hypoplasia of the optic chiasma and absence of septum pellucidum CLINICAL Pendular nystagmus, visual impairment, secondary hypopituitarism, sexual precocity and aberrant retinal vasculature TREATMENT Growth hormone replacement

septoplasty Reconstruction of the nasal septum ENT A generic term for any operation that alters the shape (eg deviation) of the nasal septum, which is usually performed in conjunction with rhinoplasty

sequenase MOLECULAR BIOLOGY A proprietary enzyme preparation used in DNA sequencing, which derives from the bacteriophage T7 DNA polymerase that has been modified to optimize the properties for sequencing

sequence MOLECULAR BIOLOGY *noun* A heteromeric chain of similar, but not identical molecules, eg nucleotides or amino acids *verb* to determine the sequence (order of arrangement) of a sequence; see Chromosome walking PEDIATRICS Anomalad A pattern of multiple congenital anomalies arising from a single early primary defect followed by a 'cascade' of secondary and tertiary defects; the Pierre-Robin sequence is caused by primary mandibular hypoplasia, which results in a tongue that is too small for the oral cavity and which drops back (glossoptosis), blocking closure of the posterior palatal shelf, resulting in a high arched U-shaped cleft palate; a sequence then, is a set of clinicopathologic consequences of the aberrant formation of one or more early embryologic structures; sequences are divided into

MALFORMATION SEQUENCES due to poor formation of tissues

DEFORMATION SEQUENCES due to unusual forces acting on normal tissues and

DISRUPTION SEQUENCES in which there is a breakdown of normal tissue

Examples of sequences include athyroidotic hypothyroidism sequence, DiGeorge sequence, early urethral obstruction sequence, bladder exstrophy sequence, cloacal extrophy sequence, holoprosencephaly sequence, jugular lymphatic obstruction sequence, Kartagener syndrome sequence, Klippel-Feil sequence, laterality sequence, meningomyelocele, anencephaly, iniencephaly sequence, occult spinal dysraphism sequence, oligohydramnios sequence, Rokitansky sequence, septo-optic dysplasia (de Morsier) sequence, sirenomelia sequence

sequence homology Homology The relatedness or similarity between (among) two (or more) segments of nucleic acid (DNA or RNA) or amino acids (proteins)

Note: It has been noted that the term as above defined is more properly known as sequence similarity, while the term homology should be reserved for evolutionary biology

sequence tag MOLECULAR BIOLOGY A short region from a complementary DNA (cDNA) library (**Bio/Technology 1995; 13:239**)

sequence tagged site map STS map, see there

sequencer DNA sequencer An instrument* for the semi-automated or automated determination of a sequence of amino acids in a protein (Edman sequencing) or nucleotides in a segment of DNA (Sanger sequencing), the latter of which is known as a 'gene machine'; see Human genome project

The current devices are fully automated; one such device, HUGA (Human genome analyzer), produced by a Japanese consortium that contributed various technologies; because of the need to duplicate sequences for damaged genomic fragments, and as a form of quality control, HUGA's raw speed of 108 000 base pairs/day is reduced to 20-30 000 base pairs (**Nature 1991; 351:593n&v**)

sequencing MOLECULAR BIOLOGY The act of determining the primary order of nucleotides (DNA sequencing), eg Maxam-Gilbert method or amino acids (protein sequencing), eg Edman or Sanger techniques; see Maxam-Gilbert sequencing, mini-protein (Edman) sequencing, Sanger sequencing

sequencing by hybridization MOLECULAR BIOLOGY A technique in which a single-stranded preparation of DNA is presented to an array of oligonucleotide probes and the sequence of the DNA is determined by the pattern of hybridization; SBH may be used to resequence DNA to identify sequence variations and (although it is not methodically robust) for *de novo* sequencing (**Bio/Technology 1995; 13:232**)

sequential model Induced fit model, see there

sequential plane imaging MRI An MRI technique in which an image is built up from successive planes in the imaged object; these planes are selected by oscillating gradient magnetic fields or by selective excitation; see Magnetic resonance imaging

sequestration 1) The development of a sequester; see Pulmonary sequestration 2) The removal or isolation of a chemical, molecule, cell, or tissue from general access, eg binding of certain proteins, eg profilin, thymosin $\beta4$, and Gc protein to G-actin to prevent polymerization

sequestration complex A pulmonary abnormality in which an aberrant pulmonary lobe is separated from the pulmonary parenchyma by its own pleura and own vascular supply arising directly from the aorta; the venous drainage is by the azygous or hemiazygous veins; the complex is frequently associated with diaphragmatic hernias and gastrointestinal malformations; the lung tissue may be normal or chronically inflamed PATHOGENESIS Defective embryogenesis in an abnormal accessory tracheobronchial bud from the primitive foregut; see Pulmonary sequestration; Cf Folded lung, Scimitar syndrome, Trapped lung

Note: Early closure of the normal lung bud would give rise to an intralobar lesion

SERC Science and Engineering Research Council The principal source of funds for academic research in Britain Budget 1991: £400 million; see MERC; Cf INSERM, NIH

serial interface COMPUTERS A connection port to a computer that transfers information in bits, which is slower than transfer of information in bytes; Cf Modem, Parallel interface

serial killer A psychopathic individual who commits serial murders; the prototypic SK is a white δ age 30; 97% of SKs are δ; 80% are diagnosed as sociopaths (**US News & World Report 2 May 1994:12**); SKs share various historical and behavioral patterns, including arsonal tendencies, compulsivity, drug- and/or alcohol-abusing parents, evidence of biochemical and/or genetic abnormalities, history of sexual assault, drug or alcohol abuse, cruelty to animals, interrupted or absence of 'bliss of childhood', pathological lying, sexual deviancy and suicidal tendencies; they may wear masks of sanity, display ritualistic behavior, search for help and have feelings of powerlessness (to prevent the killing), and have a history of perinatal head trauma, severe memory disorders, or neurological impairment; SKs are often the victims of cruel parenting and products of difficult or unwanted pregnancy (**J Norris, Serial Killers, Doubleday, New York, 1988**)

Serial killers of note: Jack the Ripper (circa 1888, 6 or 7 victims); Albert DeSalvo, the Boston Strangler (1962-64, 13 victims); David Berkowitz, Son of Sam (1975-77, 6 victims); John Wayne Gacy (mid-1970s, 33 victims); Ted Bundy (1974-79, 23 victims); Jeffrey Dahmer (1978-1991, 17 victims); Andrei Chikatilo (Russia, 1978-1990, 53 victims)

serial murder FORENSIC PSYCHIATRY Any of a series of homicides in which a single person (or a small group) selects victims based on a common characteristic or, less commonly, at random; the estimated deaths/year in US by serial killers 240 (<1% of all homicides); most victims are prostitutes; only 1% of victims are killed by firearms (from **US News & World Report 2 May 1994:12**)

serial passage MICROBIOLOGY The repeated transfer or inoculation of subpopulations of a pathogenic organism, eg the BCG strain of *Mycobacterium tuberculosis*, through a series of animals, tissue culture cells or growth media, with the purpose of attenuating the pathogen's aggression while maintaining its immunogenicity

serine protease Any of a family of proteolytic enzymes that have a similar 3-D conformation and an active site with a serine residue, forming an ester between the serine's hydroxyl group and the carboxyl group of a catalyzed peptide bond; serine proteases include coagulation cascade enzymes (vitamin K-dependent factors II, VII, IX and X, and factors XI and XII) as well as trypsin, chymotrypsin

'serious misconduct' A euphemism used in the science community for overt and/or intentional act(s) of fraud or fabrication of research data; misconduct in science includes simple 'correction' of data points in an assay, eg trimming, but becomes 'serious' when there is a deliberate attempt to deceive colleagues, as truth-telling is expected of scientists; see Fraud in science

seroconversion CLINICAL IMMUNOLOGY The development of antibodies detectable in the serum following exposure to a particular organism or antigen, in a person who was previously immunologically 'naive' for (ie previously unexposed to) an antigen; seroconversion is often an indicator of current infection (and transmissibility) of an infectious agent, eg HIV-1 (seroconversion to p24 and/or p41 antibody production) or HBV (seroconversion to surface antibody–HBsAb or e antibody–HBeAb production)

serologic crossmatch see Crossmatch

seronegative CLINICAL IMMUNOLOGY The lack of antibodies or other immune markers in the serum that would indicate exposure to a particular organism or antigen; in an immunocompetent person, exposure to an immunogenic antigen results in a seroconversion and the subject is said to then be seropositive; seronegativity therefore implies the capacity for immune responsiveness or seroreactivity; 'seronegativity' in an immunocompromised subject, eg with AIDS is usually termed anergy

seronegativity The state of being seronegative

seropositive CLINICAL IMMUNOLOGY The presence of antibodies or other immune markers in the serum that would indicate prior exposure to a particular organism or antigen; Cf Seronegative

seropositivity The state of being seropositive

serotonin 5-hydroxytryptamine, 5-HT PHYSIOLOGY A vasoactive substance formed by decarboxylation of 5-hydroxytryptophan that is both a neurotransmitter and a hormone; serotonin is contained in dense core granules, released by activated platelets, and has a vasodilating effect on human coronary arteries; it is also released during angioplasty and may contribute to vasoconstriction distal to the site of an angioplasty-induced dilation (**N Engl J Med 1994; 330o:517oA**) damage to the vascular endothelium, as occurs in coronary artery disease results in an unopposed serotogenic vasoconstriction and ischemia; serotonin may be a major actor in acute coronary artery disease, MI, and angina (N Engl J Med 1991; 324:641, 648)

serotonin hypothesis A posit that held that schizophrenia and many of its related symptoms are due to multiple defects in serotonin metabolism; although various agents (eg neurotransmitters) or mechanisms (eg metabolism of biogenic amines) have linked to the development of schizophrenia, none have proven valid

serotonin syndrome A clinical condition consisting of neuromuscular, autonomic, and behavioral changes due to increased activity of serotonin in the CNS PATHOGENESIS Related to the concurrent use of two serotonergic medications, usually a MAOI and either tryptophan or an inhibitor of serotonin reuptake, eg fluoxetine (Prozac®) or sertraline CLINICAL Confusion, diaphoresis, ataxia, fever, hyperreflexia, and myoclonus TREATMENT SS usually resolves within 24 hours after discontinuation of offending medications; if not cyproheptadine may be of use (N Engl J Med 1994; 331:1021c)

serpentine cords A descriptor for the end-to-end arrangement of certain mycobacteria, eg *M tuberculosis* and *M bovis*, which, with the acid-fast stain, have a beaded appearance by high-power light microscopy

serpentine receptor Heptaspan, see there

serpiginous tract The descriptor for a twisted, vermiform radiolucency surrounded by a sclerotic rim, seen in long bones in pyogenic osteomyelitis (organisms include streptococci, staphylococci and *Brucella* species) or in infarction accompanied by intramedullary calcification

serpiginous ulcer INFECTIOUS DISEASE A relatively uncommon clinical variant of the transient genital ulcer seen in chancroid (*Hemophilus ducreyi*), characterized as a single large rapidly-spreading shallow ulcer of the inguinal region; psoriatic lesions have also been described as having a serpiginous pattern of extension; a similar lesion may be seen in late syphilis OPHTHALMOLOGY A necrotizing ulcer of the cornea that occurs 24-48 hours after inoculation with *Streptococcus pneumoniae*, which is characterized by active ulceration at the leading edge and healing at the trailing border; it is often accompanied by hypopyon and dacrocystitis TREATMENT Cefazolin, penicillin G

serpin family A group of 52–65-kD serine protease inhibitor proteins (antithrombins), which are present in low (< 20 mg/dl) levels in the serum (table) serpins regulate a number of key biological processes, eg coagulation, fertilization, and viral inhibitiion of inflammation, acting by means of a short 15-residue reactive peptide loop, which forms a stable covalent complex with the proteinase; the proteinase is then either removed from circulation by specific cell receptors, or cleaved, inactivated and removed from the complex; serpin dysfunction has been associated

---

SERPINS

ALPHA-2-ANTIPLASMIN

ANTITHROMBIN III, which inhibits activated serine protease enzymes including thrombin, IXa, Xa and XIa

HEPARIN COFACTOR II, a protein having significant homology with antithrombin III and which in the presence of heparin (and dermatan sulfate) forms a 1:1 complex with thrombin, inactivating it

PLASMINOGEN ACTIVATOR INHIBITOR-I (PAI-I), which inactivates tissue plasminogen activator

---

with pulmonary emphysema, cirrhosis of the liver, thrombosis and pulmonary thromboembolism (**Nature Struc Biol 1994; 1:48, 250, 201oa**), raising interesting questions in terms of the evolution of the primordial soup

serum 1) The fluid component of blood from which the coagulation factors have been removed; Cf Plasma 2) A protein-rich fluid that contains a high concentration of antibodies to a particular antigen of interest; convalescent sera (from an individual who has recuperated from a particular infection, eg scarlet fever) may be of use in treating an individual who is suffering from the same infection

serum amyloid A protein Amyloid A protein, see there

serum-free media MOLECULAR BIOLOGY A well-defined and controlled culture media that has been processed in some form (eg filtration) to remove inhibitors and/or growth factors; SFMs are not necessarily protein-free or chemically defined; most are optimized for the growth requirements of various cell-specific applications (**Bio/Technology 1995; 13:341**)

serum protein electrophoresis A screening method for determining protein 'homeostasis'; serum proteins are

---

SERUM PROTEIN ELECTROPHORESIS

ABNORMALITY	(PROTEIN INVOLVED) CLINICAL CONDITIONS
↓ Prealbumin	↓ Functional hepatic mass, inflammation, malnutrition
↓ Albumin	Inflammation, malnutrition, malignancy, ↑ extracellular volume, burns
α_1 ↑	(antitrypsin) Inflammation, hepatocellular injury
↓	(antitrypsin) Deficient allele
±	(antitrypsin) Polymorphism of $\alpha_1$antitrypsin
α_2 ↑	(macroglobulin) Selective proteinuria in age extremes
↑	(haptoglobulin) Inflammation
↓	(haptoglobulin) Hemolysis, hepatosplenic sequestration
β_1 ↑	(transferrin) Iron deficiency, estrogens
↓	(transferrin) Malnutrition, burns, inflammation
↓	(lipoprotein) Hypercholesterolemia
±	(transferrin) Polymorphisms of transferrin
β_2 ↑	(complement C3) Chronic inflammation, bile obstruction
↑	(IgA) Malignancy, infection of mucosal surfaces, rheumatoid arthritis, ethanol, cirrhosis
↓	(complement C3) Complement activation
±	(complement C3) Polymorphism of C3
γ ↑	(Immunoglobulin) Monoclonal antibody, polyclonal stimulation

divided into prealbumin/albumin, α1 and α2, β, and γ zones; regions of the protein electrophoresis are ↑ or ↓ in certain conditions, or variable in the presence of gene polymorphism (table)

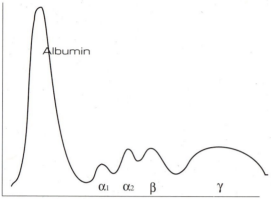

serum protein electrophoresis

serum response element A small regulatory element flanking the c-*fos* gene that is a primary nuclear target and the site of action for two signal transduction pathways, one of which activates protein kinase C (PKC), and the other which transmits signals in a PKC-independent pathway; SRE function requires binding of a protein designated as a serum response factor that acts at two different sites, explaining the specificity of the two signal transduction pathways (Science 1991; 251:189)

serum sickness An immune response seen after re-exposure to an antigen to which an organism had been previously sensitized; immediately after exposure, there is antigen excess; from days 5-14, small antigen-antibody complexes accumulate in the vessels, causing the lesions of serum sickness; by the second week, antibodies predominate, forming larger antigen-antibody complexes that are catabolized by the reticuloendothelial system CLINICAL The soluble circulating immune-complexes result in urticaria, fever, adenopathy, occasionally arthritis and glomerulonephritis; see Immune complex disease, Zone of equivalence

serum spreading factor Either of two serum glycoproteins, weighing 65 kD (vitronectin) and 75 kD, respectively that mediate the attachment, spreading and differentiation of various cells, and which are inculpated in metastases; see Vitronectin

servant see *Respondeat superior*

server COMPUTERS A device, eg a PC-type microcomputer that acts as a central repository for information in a local area network (LAN) and services peripheral clients, including workstations, managing the requests in an orderly sequential fashion; all devices in the LAN communicate with each other via the server (see CAP Today November 1993) Cf Host

service 1) A group of physicians in a particular discipline in a hospital 2) A group of patients for which a particular physician is providing care

service patient Public patient SOCIAL MEDICINE A patient who has become the ward of a health care facility, often by default as he/she has no insurance and a medical condition that requires long-term surveillance or care; SPs are generally cared for by house staff physicians; reimbursement for such patients is often relegated to those programs, eg Medicaid, that pay nominal amounts for the various services provided; see Homeless(ness), 'Safety net' hospitals; Cf Private patient

sestamibi ⁹⁹ᵐTc (technicium-99m) sestamibi A myocardial perfusion agent preferred for assessing the 'at-risk' myocardium, used in conjunction with tomography to determine the final size of a myocardial infarct (N Engl J Med 1993; 328:685₀A)

setting sun sign PEDIATRICS A clinical finding consisting of inferior ocular deviation, characteristically seen in severe infantile hydrocephalus (occasionally also occurring in subdural hematomas) that is often accompanied by the 'cracked-pot' sign, prominence of the scalp veins, thinned and shiny skin, a high-pitched cry and optic nerve atrophy due to nerve and chiasm compression

Seurat spleen A fanciful and rarely used term referring to the punctate pattern of extravasation of radiologic contrast material seen in a ruptured spleen

The term derives its name from the pointillism, the painting technique devised by the French neo-impressionist, Georges Seurat (1859-1891) who used tiny dots of pure color

seven countries study CARDIOLOGY A prospective epidemiological study conducted in Finland, Greece, Italy, Japan, the Netherlands, the US, and in Yugoslavia; the SCS examined the relation of dietary fats with coronary heart disease (CHD), and linked CHD to an excess consumption of saturated fats (Circulation 1991; 83:2154)

seven-day fever A rodent-born infection by the spirochete, *Leptospira heptomadis* that has been reported in Japan and Europe and causes jaundice and fever; Cf Five-day fever

seven transmembrane spanning receptor Heptaspan, see there

seventh day disease Neonatal infection by *Clostridium tetani*, which is most common in the developing nations where contaminated instruments are used to cut the umbilical cord and dress the wound; by the end of the first week (the usual incubation period), the infant becomes irritable, spastic and tetanic MORTALITY Untreated *C tetani* infection carries up to a 70% mortality

70s, the rule(s) of A mnemonic for CNS tumors: 70% are primary CNS neoplasms, 70% of primary neoplasms are glial, 70% of primary glial tumors are astrocytomas and 70% of these are high grade

CHILDREN 70% of tumors arise in the posterior fossa, 70% of those occurring before age 2 are medulloblastomas and 70% of supratentorial tumors are craniopharyngiomas

ADULTS 70% are in the hemispheres, 70% of those in the pineal region are germinomas, 70% of those in the pituitary gland are adenomas, of which 70% are chromophobe

seven-year itch MEDICAL HISTORY An obsolete term for scabies, which afflicted Napoleon's troops in epidemic proportions during the Russian campaign; see Scabies

severe combined immune deficiency A heterogeneous X-linked [MIM 300400, 312863] or less commonly AR [MIM 202500] condition that is more common in blacks with onset in the first few months of life; SCIDs are characterized by dysfunctional T- and B-lymphocytes CLINICAL Morbiliform rash, hyperpigmentation, severe recurring infections (*Candida, Pneumocystis carinii*, CMV, EBV, HBV, and varicella), failure to thrive, and early death IMMUNOLOGY Combined humoral (hypo- or agammaglobulinemia) and cellular immune defects (absent response to T-cell mitogens, eg phytohemagglutinin), T- and B- cell lymphopenia, ↓ IL-2 production; SCID is subdivided according to defects in adenosine deaminase (ADA) and purine nucleoside phosphorylase (PNP, also considered a variant of Nezelof's disease) enzymes and a defect in a DNA-binding protein required for the expression of HLA genes TREATMENT Bone marrow transplant; gene therapy and enzyme replacement in ADA deficiency are in the experimental protocol stage; see Adenosine deaminase deficiency, 'Bubble boy', Gnotobiotic, Purine nucleoside phosphorylase, SCID mice

severe and complicated malaria A generic term for severe malarial disease, which according to WHO criteria is separated into

1) Defining criteria: Coma, respiratory distress (pulmonary edema), hypoglycemia, circulatory collapse (clinical shock), repeated convulsions, severe anemia (< 5g/dL and > 10 000 parasites mm³), acidosis (plasma bicarbonate < 15 mmol/L), hemoglobinuria, renal failure, spontaneous bleeding

2) Supporting criteria: Jaundice, prostration, hyperpyrexia, impaired consciousness, hyperparasitemia (> 500 000 parasites mm³) (N Engl J Med 1995; 332:1399₀A, 1441ED)

severe congenital neutropenia Congenital neutropenia, see there, also known as Kostmann's disease

severe sepsis Sepsis syndrome A condition that has been recently defined (see Sepsis for reference) by clinical parameters as *'Sepsis associated with organ dysfunction, hypotension, or hypoperfusion abnormalities (which include) …lactic acidosis, oliguria, or an acute alteration in mental status*; SS is part of a continuum of a biologic inflammatory response to infection that evolves toward septic shock (JAMA 1995; 273:117₀A) see Sepsis, Septic shock, SIRS

severely debilitating illness A generic term for any condition in which there is major irreversible morbidity, eg Alzheimer's disease, blindness, advanced diabetic nephropathy, neurological degeneration, Parkinson's disease, terminal cancer, and others; see Illness, Life-threatening illness

severity-adjusted death rate A calculated rate of mortality based on the severity of a morbid condition, a statistic of use in determining the appropriate reimbursement from Medicare; see Case-mix index, DRGs, Medicare

Note: In the current economic environment in the US health care industry, a patient's 'allowable', ie reimbursed length of stay in a hospital is determined by the severity of the disease

Seveso Directive ENVIRONMENT A legislative act passed in the European Community aimed at reducing the risks of chemical accidents, which was inspired by an explosion that occurred at a chemical factory in Seveso, Italy in 1976, resulting in a release into the environment of up to 3 kg of the highly toxic compound TCDD (Nature 1995; 375:353)

sex chromosomes The human sex chromosome is composed of a pseudoautosomal region, corresponding to the site of recombination between the X and Y chromosomes and the sex chromosome specific regions; between these two regions, ie in the boundary zone, the sex chromosomes differ, with the Y chromosome having an Alu sequence; see H-Y antigen, Testis-determining factor, X-chromosome inactivation, XIST

sex club A location where sexual activities, usually anonymous, are sanctioned and freely exchanged between two (or more) consenting adults (without exchange of goods or services); in general, various drugs of abuse (eg cocaine, heroin, marijuana, amphetamines, barbiturates) are readily available; while the term sex club refers to social centers with either heterosexual or homosexual orientation, for the latter, the term 'bath-house' is more widely integrated in the working argot; see Anonymous sex, Bath-house

sex cord-stromal tumor SURGICAL PATHOLOGY OVARY A tumor that comprises 5% of all ovarian neoplasms (½ of which are fibroma-thecomas), and differentiate toward sex cords and/or specialized ovarian tissue, in the form of 'female' (ie, granulosa and theca) cells, male (ie, Sertoli and Leydig) cells or indifferent elements; classification of ovarian sex cord-stromal tumors (table) is based on morphology rather than hormonal status and ancillary studies, eg immunoperoxidase and immunohistochemistry) TESTES Tumors of Leydig and Sertoli cells comprise ± 5% of all

testicular neoplasms, 10% of which behave in a malignant fashion; Cf Germ cell tumors

sex determination see Sex selection

sex differential The ♂ to ♀ difference in mortality or morbidity rate; in general, when all causes of death are considered, the mortality rate is lower, the likelihood of survival greater, and life expectancy longer in ♀; Cf Sex ratio

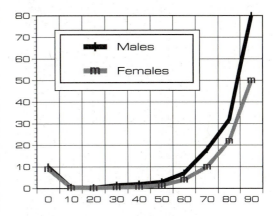

sex differential, mortality

sex guidelines see Safe sexual activities

sex 'industry' Any of a group of activities related to the sale or purchase of sex-related services, especially involving direct contact of orogenital mucosae, which also includes the pornographic end of the entertainment arts; the SI has always functioned with a 'tolerable' baseline of sexually transmitted disease, which has drastically changed since the advent of the AIDS epidemic; in certain underdeveloped countries, the sex industry is intimately linked to tourism and the monies paid for the use of a young teenager's body may provide sustenance for his/her entire family, usually at a salary far below the cost of an adequate supply of the condoms necessary to prevent the transmission of HIV; see AIDS, Condoms, HIV, Safe sexual activities, Sex tourism, Sex work, Sexual deviancy, Sexually-transmitted diseases

sex life A colloquial term which refers to a person's sexual relationships and the level of sexual activity; Cf Sexual life

*Presumed to derive from more encompassing term, sexual life

sex-linked disease Inherited chromosome X-linked con-

SEX CORD TUMORS
GRANULOSA-STROMAL CELL TUMORS
Granulosa cell tumor, adult and juvenile types
Thecoma-fibroma group: Thecomas (typical and luteinized), fibromas, cellular fibromas and fibrosarcomas
Stromal tumors with a minor sex cord component
Sclerosing stromal tumor
Unclassified
SERTOLI-STROMAL CELL TUMORS
Sertoli cell tumors
Leydig cell tumors
Sertoli-Leydig cell tumors Well-, intermediate or poorly-differentiated, or with heterologous elements
GYNANDROBLASTOMA
SEX CORD TUMOR WITH ANNULAR TUBULES
UNCLASSIFIED
Int J Gynecol Pathol 1982; 1:101

ditions, which are carried by the mother and expressed by the son, eg Fabry's disease, pyruvate kinase deficiency, G6PD deficiency, Xg[a] blood group, factor VIII and factor IX deficiencies; see Testis-determining factor

sex ratio The number of ♂ to ♀ in a population, which is slightly higher in females; Cf Sex differential

sex-reversed individuals see Pseudohermaphroditism, Sexual reassignment

sex selection DEMOGRAPHY A generic term for any maneuver intended to increase the likehood of giving birth or raising a child of a chosen sex; SS ranges from sex preselection, prenatal sex determination, and sex-selective abortion, but in less sophisticated cultures also encompasses the 'darker' practices of child marriages, abduction, forced polyandry, and infanticide (**Nature; 1994; 372:503N&V**)

sex tourism GLOBAL VILLAGE Travel to a location for the express purpose of engaging in sexual activities and/or perversions; Southeast Asia, in particular Thailand, but also India and the Philippines have been traditional Reiseziehe; the era of AIDS has made sex tourism an especially disturbing practice, as the desire to engage in such activities with no or minimal risk of transmitting HIV to the purchaser of these services requires that increasingly younger prostitutes (both boys and girls) be pressed into service and has spiraled downward to children age 10 or younger; the practice is deplored by the WHO, the UN Human Rights Commission, and many others (**Am Med News 16 March 1992**)

sexist behavior Actions or language that are discriminatory on the basis of sex (see **N Engl J Med 1993; 328:351ED**) see Sexual harassment

sexual abuse PEDIATRICS '...*inappropriate exposure of a child to sexual acts or materials, the passive use of children as sexual stimuli for adults, and actual sexual contact between children and older people. Sexually abused children, in addition to their depressive and aggressive symptoms, have an increased frequency of anxiety disorders and problems with sex role and sexual functioning.*' (**N Engl J Med 1995; 332:1425RV**) see Child sexual abuse

Note: CSA is not limited to any particular country or region (see Sex tourism) a pedophile ring was uncovered in Londonderry Northern Ireland involving 100 children as young as 3 years of age, masterminded by 20 adults, acts included sodomy, rape, group sex (**NY Newsday 29 Nov 1994; A14**)

sexual anhedonia A form of sexual dysfunction* in which there is a loss of desire (or libido) to engage in sexual activity; SA is most common in males, and is characterized by normal erection and ejaculation occurring without pleasure during orgasm; SA may be psychogenic or due to drug abuse, eg cocaine TREATMENT Detoxification, psychotherapy; see Sexual dysfunction

*Sexual dysfunction is the term preferred by the American Psychiatric Association, formally delineated in the Diagnosis and Statistical Manual, 4th ed (DSM-IV), and the clinical forms are designated as Sexual Dysfunction due to a General Medical Condition, Substance-Induced Sexual Dysfunction, or others depending on the etiology

sexual apartheid A colloquial term referring to the selection of a sexual partner based on the whether he/she has a sexually-transmitted disease, in particular HIV (**Village Voice, Jan 31, 1995**)

sexual asphyxia FORENSIC MEDICINE The intentional restriction of the flow of air to the upper respiratory tract as part of 'rough sex', as hypoxia is alleged to enhance the experience of orgasm; an estimated 500-1000 deaths/year (US) are linked to sexual asphyxia, most often of males who may have various forms of ligatures around the neck while engaged in solitary sex (eg masturbation) and who are unable to free themselves at the moment of climax, a point at which voluntary control is temporarily at a minimum; SA-related deaths may be labeled as accidental if the victim is alone; if a partner is involved and strangled,

the death can be ruled as a homicide or inadvertent strangulation during consensual sex (**J Kuransky, NY Newsday 14 March 1995; B17**)

sexual assault FORENSIC MEDICINE '...*any sexual act performed by one person on another without that person's permission...components* (of sexual assault) *include the use or threat of force, the inability of the victim to give proper consent or both.*'; the incidence of SA is 80/10[5] population/year, accounting for 7% of violent crimes reported in the US, but is vastly underreported due to '...*humiliation, feelings of guilt, fear of retribution, lack of knowledge of legal rights, and disillusionment with the criminal justice system*'; up to 5% of rape victims sustain major nongenital injuries; 1% have moderate to severe genital injury that requires surgical intervention; 0.1% sustain injuries that are ultimately fatal (**N Engl J Med 1995; 332:234RV**) see Rape, Rape trauma syndrome

sexual boundaries see Professional boundaries

sexual bribery A legally recognized form of quid pro quo harassment in which a sexual relationship with an employer or superor is made an explicit or implied condition for obtaining or retaining employment or benefits of employment (**N Engl J Med 1993; 328:322SA**) see Sexual harassment

sexual deviancy Paraphilia Sexual excitement to the point of erection and/or orgasm when the object of that excitement is considered abnormal in the context of the practitioner's learned societal norms; there are 8 'formal' types of paraphilia, to wit, exhibitionism, fetishism, frotteurism, pedophilia, sexual masochism, sexual sadism, transvestic fetishism, voyeurism, and paraphilia, not otherwise specified, an informal or 'wastepaper basket' category; see Child abuse, Paraphilia

sexual deviancy Paraphilia PSYCHIATRY A popular and widely used term for sexual activities that are considered a bit 'out there'

Miniglossary (for those with pedestrian taste) ANAL INTERCOURSE Sodomy Insertion of the penis, other parts of the anatomy, or sex toys per rectum, practiced by 14.3% of men and 18.6% of women ANILINGUS Application of the tongue (and/or lips) to the anal region of a sexual partner BESTIALITY Sexual intercourse with animals BONDAGE AND DOMINANCE A form of sado-masochism in which one partner is tied, hand-cuffed or otherwise restrained in one position while the other partner assumes castigatory and/or authoritative roles and performs a variety of 'punitive' erotic acts CALAMITE A child victim of male homosexuality COPROPHILIA Sexual arousal obtained by manipulating fecal material CROSS DRESSING Wearing of clothes that are designed to be worn by those of the opposite phenotypic sex, an activity that is regarded as mildly deviant, and then, only when it becomes the person's dominant costume; see Transvestic fetishism CRUISING Engaging in multiple anonymous sexual encounters with multiple partners, usually in a male homosexual context EXHIBITIONISM Lady Godiva syndrome Public display of genitalia FISTING Insertion of the fisted hand into the rectum of a sexual, usually male partner FROTTAGE Full body contact between partners without sexual penetration (a non-deviant activity that contrasts with the following entry) FROTTEURISM 'Bakerloo' syndrome[2] Sexual arousal from rubbing against those of the opposite sex in crowds 'GERBILING' The insertion of live gerbils or other small rodents in the anus as a form of eroticism, given that the hypoxia causes the animals to suffer preterminal convulsions which is perceived as pleasurable 'GOLDEN SHOWER' Urination on the sexual partner(s) prior to engaging in sexual activities, most often homosexual PÆDERASTY Homosexual child molestation PÆDOPHILIA Pedophilia (US), see there PARAPHILIA[1] Recurrent intense sexual urges and fantasies in response to sexual objects or situations which are not part of normative arousal patterns, eg clothing fetishes PEDOPHILIA 1) Pædophilia (British) Heterosexual child molestation, defined as a six-month or longer period of recurrent, intense sexual urges and sexually arousing fantasies involving sexual activity with prepubescent(s) (younger than age13); the pedophile must in addition have acted on the urges or be markedly distressed by them; 2) Sexual arousal with feet, now known as partialism PEEPING TOMISM Voyeurism, see there SADOMASOCHISM A form of erotic deviancy[3] in which the sexual dyad is composed of a partner who is sexually aroused while inflicting pain and another who is aroused while receiving pain[3] **SCOPTOPHILIA** Voyeurism, see there **'SHRIMPING'** The sipping of ejaculate following anal intercourse **VOYEURISM** Intense sexually arousing fantasies involving the act of observing unsuspecting person(s) who are naked or engaged in sexual activity **WATER 'SPORTS'** A generic term for the use of urine, eg urinating on a sexual partner, as a component of eroticism[4]; see 'Golden shower'

[1]Paraphilia is the term preferred by the American Psychiatric Association, formally delineated in the Diagnosis and Statistical Manual, 4th ed (DSM-IV) [2]Bakerloo is a subway line in London [3]The term derives from the French novelist, Count Donatien-Alphonse-Francois de Sade who inflicted pain and wrote about it and Leopold von Sacher-Masoch, a German novelist who enjoyed pain and wrote about it [4]aka Urophilia

sexual differentiation see Hermaphroditism, Hirsutism, Müllerian ducts, Precocious puberty, Pseudoprecocious puberty, Testis-determining factor, Virilization, Wolffian ducts, XXX, XXY, XXXY, XYY syndromes

sexual dysfunction PSYCHIATRY An 'umbrella' term that encompasses disturbances in sexual desire, as well as psychophysiologic changes in the sexual response cycle, which may be accompanied by marked distress and interpersonal difficulty; under the rubric of SDs are disorders in sexual arousal, sexual desire (aversive and hypoactive types), orgasm, sexual pain disorders (dyspareunia, vaginismus), and SDs due to general medical conditions or related to substances (**DSM-IV**) see Sexual anhedonia, Sexual response cycle

sexual exploitation see Sex tourism, Sexual harassment, Sexual misconduct

sexual fantasy PSYCHOLOGY An individual's private psychological imagery that is associated with feelings that are explicitly erotic and accompanied by physiologic response to sexual arousal (**N Engl J Med 1994; 331:923SA**); an SF may be defined as an erotic yearning or constellation of mental images that evoke sexual arousal; ♂ SFs are more impersonal and sexually graphic, with a focus on sexual images and explicit acts, often with a variety of partners, and occur an average of 7.2 **x**/day; ♀ SFs are more likely to involve someone the woman knows, and tend to focus on personal details of the partner; ♀ SFs are slower in pace and involve more caressing and nongenital touching, and occur 4.5 **x**/day (**NY Times 14 June 1995; C14**) Cf Paraphilia

sexual favor A generic term for a sexual act that may occur in an employee-employer relationship where the favor is provided in exchange for privileged treatment in a workplace, increased salary, or career advancement; Cf Sexual harassment

sexual harassment A form of socially inappropriate behavior defined by the Equal Empoloyment Opportunity Commission (EEOC, US) as '...*unwelcome sexual advances, requests for sexual favors, and other conduct of a sexual nature.*'; it may also be defined as '...*the creation of a hostile atmosphere or abuse of a position of power in a relationship through sexual behavior or language.*' (**N Engl J Med 1994; 330:1388C**) SH in the workplace, previously considered an unpleasant inevitability, is defined as harassment in civil and human rights' codes and in labor legislation in the US and Canada and has been the focus of media attention and litigation; 25-75% of women have been subjected to SH in all work settings; women in medicine are not immune to SH, and are affected regardless of 'pecking order', from nurses to medical students (**N Engl J Med 1993; 328:322SA**) to physicians (**N Engl J Med 1993; 329:1936OA**) Cf Sexual bribery

sexual history PSYCHIATRY A critical component of a person's psychiatric history, in which information is obtained about the individual's sexual development, orientation, sexual attitudes and behaviors, and presence of sexual conflict or dysfunction; in an SH, the interviewer asks questions about childhood sexual play experiences (eg

doctor and nurse games), how he/she learned about 'the birds and the bees', whether sexual abuse occurred, timeframe of first sexual experiences, content of sexual fantasies, and a plethora of other with whoms, whats, whens, wheres, hows, and how manies

sexual impropriety A form of sexual misconduct* defined by the Medical Council of New Zealand as expressions or gestures that are disrespectful to the privacy and sexually demeaning to the patient; the term overlaps considerably with what is termed sexual harassment in the US, and could be regarded as a synonym thereof (**JAMA1995; 273:1445**) see Note, Sexual misconduct

*Which might be viewed as the least pernicious form of sexual misconduct

sexual life An imprecise term defined as '*The directions and manifestations of the sexual drive that contribute to a person's life-style, sometimes confined to genital activity and sometimes referring to all of the manifestations of libidinal energy in the subject's personality and relationships*' (**International Dictionary of Medicine, J Wiley & Sons, New York, 1986**) see Sex life

sexual maturity rating Tanner staging, see there

sexual misconduct PROFESSIONAL ETHICS Any of a number of behaviors that violate a health professional's ethics through sexual contact of physician and his/her patient; the true prevalence of SM is unknown; in an analysis of six such sex studies, up to 12% of ♂ and 4% of ♀ physicians admitted to SM; 20% involved same sex dyads; regarding SM, the AMA's Council of Ethical and Judicial Affairs includes

1) Predatory physicians who systematically attempt to seduce patients

2) Those who claim to use sex for therapeutic purposes

3) Abuse of the physical examination, in particular when it is not indicated according to his/her standard of care

4) Situations in which the physician asks for a date on the first visit or on a seeing the patient in an emergency department

5) Situations in which a long-term professional relationship evolves into an infatuation

6) Raping or fondling a patient while either awake or under anesthesia

7) Cases of sexual harassment in which the physician makes erotic or suggestive comments to the patient

Note: The Medical Council of New Zealand has proposed a classification of sexual misconduct that is of use in determing the severity of the infraction, and possibly the degree or severity of the sanction levied against the perpetrator; the MCNZ divides SM into sexual impropriety, sexual transgression, and the most severe form, sexual violation (**JAMA1995; 273:1445**) see Professional boundaries

sexual orientation An individual's potential for responding with sexual arousal to persons of the opposite sex, same sex, or both (**N Engl J Med 1994; 331:923SA**)

sexual reassignment The surgical conversion of a person's external (secondary) sexual characteristics to those of the opposite sex

MALE-TO-FEMALE CONVERSION entails bilateral orchiectomy, penectomy, vaginoplasty, and estrogen therapy

FEMALE-TO-MALE CONVERSION is only partially successful and entails mastectomy, hysterectomy and androgenic hormone therapy Note: The male:female ratio of reassignment procedures is estimated at 3 to 7:1 Complications of reassignment are in part a function of whether therapy occurs in a legitimate medical environment, eg breast carcinoma associated with excess estrogen supplementation or whether reassignment is self-performed, eg illicit silicon injections, which may cause high fever, dyspnea, thoracic pain, acute respiratory failure with bilateral pulmonary interstitial infiltrates, airspace consolidation and Swiss cheese-like vacuolization of the dermis and macrophages

sexual response cycle PHYSIOLOGY A term that encompasses the phases of a sexual act from prearousal to denouement; the SRC is divided into four phases (table); Cf Sexual dysfunction

---

SEXUAL RESPONSE CYCLE

DESIRE, which consists of fantasies about sexual activity and the desire to engage in sexual activity

EXCITEMENT, in which the subjective component of sexual excitement is accompanied by physiologic changes, in ♂, penile tumescence and erection, in ♀ pelvic vasocongestion, vaginal lubrication, and swelling of external genitalia

ORGASM, the peaking of sexual pleasure with release of sexual tension, rhythmic contraction of perineal muscles, in ♂, ejaculation, in ♀, contractions of the outer ⅓ of the vagina; in both the anal sphincter contracts rhythmically

RESOLUTION, the final phase in which there is muscle relaxation, and a sense of well-being; during resolution, ♂ are unerectable for a variable period of time; ♀ remain on 'red alert'

---

sexual stimulant A generic term for any drug alleged to enhance sexual performance or libido; no drug has proven effective in increasing libido and sexual performance, although several agents are believed by some authors to have this effect; see Aphrodisiac, Yohimbine

sexual work Any form of sexual traffic (anal, oral, or vaginal) that is performed or allowed by men or women in exchange for drugs or money (see N Engl J Med 1994; 331:1422sa)

sexuality The human sexual response, which is a function of external cues for heterosexual or homosexual orientation and the ability to produce and respond to gonadotropin-releasing hormone, which when disrupted leads to infertility; by age 13, 7.6% of US whites and 15.3% of US blacks have had sexual relations; by age 20, 65% and 85%; see Homosexuality, Transsexuality

sexual traffic Orifice-related sexual activity

sexual transgression A form of sexual misconduct defined by the Medical Council of New Zealand as inappropriate and sexualized touching of a patient that stops short of overt sexual relations, which includes sexualized kissing, touching of breast or genitals when not appropriate for the physical examination, or performing a pelvic examination without gloves (JAMA1995; 273:1445) see Note, Sexual misconduct

sexual violation A form of sexual misconduct* defined by the Medical Council of New Zealand as physician-patient sexual relations, regardless of who initiated the relationship, and would include genital intercourse, oral sexual relations, anal intercourse, and mutual masturbation (JAMA1995; 273:1445) see Note, Sexual misconduct

*Which is viewed as the most pernicious form of sexual misconduct

sexually acquired reactive arthritis A polyarthritic complex of uncertain clinical importance that was reported in HLA-B27-positive subjects and thought to have been triggered by sexually transmitted *Chlamydia trachomatis* (Br Med J 1978; 1:605)

sexually dangerous A constellation of known behaviors and previously committed acts (eg rape and sodomy) by a person that are regarded as having the potential for being repeated in the form of physical injury (Am Med News 24 April 1995 p21) see Megan's law, Rape, Sex tourism

sexually transmitted disease A generic term for any infection or tumor that is acquired by direct genital and orogenital contact; most common sexually-transmitted agents in US: *Chlamydia trachomatis* 3-5 million cases (1990, MMWR 1990; 39:53); HSV-2 2-3 million (1990); *Neisseria gonorrhoeae*, 720 000/25 300 penicillin-resis-

tant (1988); *Treponema pallidum*/secondary syphilis, 40 117 (1988) 357 congenital cases (New York City) STD AGENTS-BACTERIAL *C trachomatis, T pallidum, Mycoplasma hominis, N gonorrhoeae*, streptococcal species, *Ureaplasma urealyticum* STD AGENTS-VIRAL EBV, HBV, HIV-1, HIV-2, HPV, HSV STD OTHERS *Trichomonas vaginalis*, pubic lice, scabies SEXUALLY-TRANSMITTED NEOPLASMS Dysplasia and squamous cell carcinoma of the uterine cervix, penis and anus often arise in a setting of previous HPV infection; HPV types 16 and 33 are implicated in penile intraepithelial neoplasm; HPV types 6, 11 and 42 are implicated in condyloma acuminata, but are unrelated to malignancy; ♂ sexual partners of ♀ with CIN, cervical flat condylomas, condyloma acuminatum or variants of intraepithelial neoplasia

Note: The sexual transmission efficacy of hepatitis B virus is 8.6-fold greater than HIV-1 in insertive anal intercourse in homosexuals (N Engl J Med 1990; 264:230)

Sezary cell syndrome Mycosis fungoides, see there

SGA Small for gestational age; see Low birth weight

SH2 region, SH3 region Src homology regions A group of highly conserved non-catalytic domains typical of proteins with intracytoplasmic tyrosine kinase activity, present in Abl, Fps, Src and tensin (Science 1991; 252:668)

shadow casting RESEARCH A technique of electron microscopy for studying the surfaces of cells and intracytoplasmic regions, which may be carried out after freeze fracturing the region of interest, the fractured surface is sprayed with metal ions at a fixed angle, resulting in the decreased deposition of metal ions on sites that are at obtuse angles from the spray

shadow cell A pale lightly pink cell, often devoid of a nucleus DERMATOPATHOLOGY A pale, lightly eosinophilic anuclear keratinocyte with distinct cytoplasm and borders due to an accumulation of keratin fibrils, and a central cleared ('shadow') zone remaining in the center of the cell where the nucleus was; SCs retain a cohesive 3-D cuboidal form and indicate immature hair matrix differentiation; they are seen in tumors of skin adnexae (eg pilomatricomas, aka calcifying epitheliooma of Malherbe, more commonly in older lesions where the characteristic basaloid cell component may be absent), cutaneous mixed tumors, proliferating trichilemmal tumors, rare basal cell carcinomas, alopecia areata, onychomycosis, epidermoid cysts in Gardner syndrome, and recently, in a dermoid cyst (Arch Pathol Lab Med 1995; 119:371oa) HEMATOPATHOLOGY A descriptor that may be applied to any cell that doesn't stain, ie is negative by the immunoperoxidase stain in tissues or in cytologic specimens, serving as vague tissue landmarks

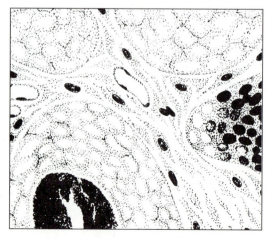

shadow cell

shadow plaque NEUROPATHOLOGY A 'classic' finding in the CNS of patients affected by multiple sclerosis, which corresponds to an area of vague demyelination, which may be seen by gross examination; other histological features of multiple sclerosis include myelin-axonal dissociation, where there are preserved axons without myelin, and accumulation of sudanophilic lipids resulting from myelin catabolism; see Multiple sclerosis

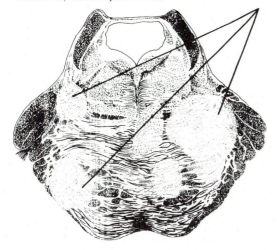

shadow plaques

shaggy heart sign A descriptor for the 'ragged' appearance of the cardiac contour seen in a plain chest film in occasional patients with *Bordetella pertussis* (whooping cough) infection; when seen during the paroxysmal stage; the shagginess is due to densities that obscure the cardiac borders and correspond to peribronchial thickening and infiltration of the basal triangle extending laterally from the hilum to the flattened and lowered diaphragm

shagreen patch An indurated flesh-colored cluster of closely-set papules likened to shagreen that are present on the back and lumbosacral region, seen in tuberous sclerosis and other mucocutaneous lesions, including adenoma sebaceum in a 'butterfly' pattern, hypopigmented macules, gingival and periungual fibromas; Cf Butterfly rash

Note: Shagreen is an untanned leather prepared from the skin of horses, camels and others, covered with round granulations by pressing small seeds into the grain or hair side, scraping off the rugosity when the hide dries and soaking it to cause the compressed or indented portions of the skin to swell in relief and then dyed a bright color, often green

shake test Foam stability index, see there

shaken baby 'syndrome' see Whiplash-shaken baby syndrome

(whiplash) shaken infant syndrome FORENSIC MEDICINE A form of severe child abuse that may be either fatal or leave its victim with permanent neurological sequelae; severe shaking of an infant who has virtually no neck muscle tone may cause bilateral subdural hematomas (resulting from laceration of the veins bridging the dura mater and cerebral cortex caused by rapid acceleration and deceleration as the chin strikes the chest and the occipital bone strikes the back), subarachnoid and retinal hemorrhage, cerebral edema and cortical contusions without signs of external cranial trauma PEDIATRICS '*...acute brain injuries (cerebral contusions or subdural or subarachnoid hemorrhages) in infants who have no discernible evidence of blunt head trauma. Associated findings, especially metaphyseal long-bone fractures and evidence of injury to the cervical spinal cord, suggest that the condition is the result of the child's having been held by the torso and shaken violently, with sub-* *sequent whiplash injury to the head, neck, and limbs.*' (N Engl J Med· 1995; 332:1425RV) see Battered child syndrome, Bucket handle fracture; Cf Infanticide

Notes: 1) Skull fractures are uncommon given the relative softness of neonatal bone; the whiplash shaken infant injury occurs when an adult (often in a state of uncontrolled anger) holds the child by the upper body and violently shakes him 2) Similar lesions may occur when a parent 'rough-house' plays with the child and swings him in a circle or tosses him up and down; thus other signs of child abuse must be investigated (Am Fam Prac 1990; 41:1145)

shaker PHYSIOLOGY A *Drosophila melanogaster* mutant that shakes under ether anesthesia; the shaker gene encodes a structural component of a voltage-dependent potassium channel protein; see Potassium ion channels

shallow dose equivalent H$_s$ RADIATION PHYSICS The dose equivalent at a tissue depth of 0.007 cm (7 mg/cm^2) averaged over an area of 1.0 cm^2, as applied to external radiation to the skin or an extremity

sham feeding A clinical method for determining the completeness of vagotomy; food is smelled, seen and chewed, but not swallowed; acid output is measured by aspirating acid secretions via a nasogastric tube; acid production induced by sham feeding of greater than 10% of pentagastrin-stimulated peak acid output (PAO) implies intact vagal innervation

sham rage NEUROPHYSIOLOGY Outbursts of motor activity that resemble rage (eg in cats, hissing, spitting, defensive posturing, piloerection, and dilation of pupils), which may be seen in decorticate or diencephalic animals, or which may be induced by electrical stimulation of fornix of the hippocampus

shaman A 'medicine man' from an aboriginal society whose healing ability derives from trance-like or 'supernatural' states; see Ethnomedicine, Healer; Cf Alternative medicine, Quack

Shandall classification A system for classifying female circumcision (see there), which is regarded by some authors as inaccurate

shark skin appearance Shagreen patch, see there

shared-decision program CLINICAL DECISION-MAKING A video-based system that provides patients with information relevant to various therapeutic options for a particular disease process (eg benign prostatic hypertrophy, lower back pain, mild hypertension, breast cancer) in an interactive touch-screen format; SDPs are thought to improve the delivery of health care services, as patients 1) have an increased understanding of the types of procedures available, and their chances of success, 2) have an increased confidence that he/she made the right decision (thus reducing the likelihood of a lawsuit, and 3) often choose less invasive (ie less expensive) procedures (Am Med News 16 Nov 1992 p11)

shared psychotic disorder The term preferred by the American Psychiatric Association for the more widely used term, folie à deux, see there

shark cartilage ALTERNATIVE MEDICINE A preparation of elastic tissue of shark origin that has been reported by various practitioners of alternative health care to be of use in treating various types of malignancy; the alleged active component is an as yet unidentified anti-angiogenesis factor (Sci Am 1993; 269/4:24) Note: There are no reports in peer-reviewed journals of successful therapy of cancer using shark cartilage; see Alternative medicine

'sharps' Any sharp object, eg syringe needles, scalpel blades, broken test tubes and glass that may contain human blood, fluids and tissues with pathogenic organism; 'sharps' are a form of biohazardous waste that requires special handling given their ability to penetrate plastic and cardboard receptacles designed for the disposal of human wastes and tissue; see Biohazardous waste, Needle-stick injuries, Regulated waste

'shaving cream' appearance FORENSIC PATHOLOGY A descriptor for the bubbly or foamy material that oozes from the nostrils and mouth of narcotic addicts who have overdosed and died in frank pulmonary edema; Cf Mushroom of foam

SHBG Sex hormone binding globulin ENDOCRINOLOGY A β-globulin synthesized in the liver that binds testosterone, estradiol and other steroids containing a 17-β hydroxy substitution; natural sex hormones may be displaced from their binding site on SHBG by synthetic steroids, eg methyltestosterone and norgestrol, either by intent or inadvertently

sheaf appearance Wheat sheaf appearance, see there

shear stress The frictional force acting tangentially in the direction of flow, which is directly related to fluid viscosity; in blood vessels, shear stress acts on endothelium and is the mechanical force responsible for the acute changes in luminal diameter (Arch Pathol Lab Med 1992; 116:1301oA)

sheath A tubular covering, shell or protective layer that may be formed around 1) Axons sheathed by Schwann cells (it is unknown how many cells a Schwann cell sheathes) 2) Bacteria, either individually or when arranged in chains or 3) Cells when being examined by flow cytometry, the sheath being a 'sleeve' of fluid that surrounds the individual cells; see Flow cytometry

shed mediastinal blood salvage TRANSFUSION MEDICINE A technique in which blood lost into the mediastinal field of operation is reinfused during coronary revascularization surgery, reducing the required allogeneic blood by 50%; despite the theoretical concern that reinfusing SMB ↑ the body load of unwanted activated coagulation factors, FDPs, plasmin, and free hemoglobin, neither renal nor pulmonary compromise has been reported with this technique; SMB is transfused with micropore (microaggregate) filters (Arch Pathol Lab Med 1994; 118:411oA)

shelf life A term borrowed from the food industry, which in the hospital environment refers to the length of time that a blood product or therapeutic agent may be stored under appropriate conditions before it must be discarded by law, which in transfusion medicine ranges from 24 hours for washed red cells to ten years (or more) for frozen red cells

'shelf' sign RADIOLOGY A flattened horizontal mass often accompanied by mucosal irregularity that may be seen by barium enema in colonic adenocarcinoma

shell nail Spoon nail, see there

'shell shock' Post-trauma stress disorder, see there

shelter A building that often has a barracks-like atmosphere that houses abused women and their children, homeless persons or other disenfranchised population, providing them a place to sleep, food and clothing but little privacy; see Institutionalization 'syndrome'; Cf Hospice

'sheltered environment A generic term for an environment that provides protection and custodial care to those who cannot fend for themselves, which would include nursing homes, institutions for the mentally challenged, 'safe houses' for abused women, and halfway houses for former drug addicts

shelterization' SOCIAL MEDICINE An adaptive response by those living in shelters for the homeless in the US, characterized by increased passive behavior and a decrease in personal hygiene; see Homeless(ness), Institutionalization 'syndrome'

shenjing shuairuo PSYCHIATRY A form of neurasthenia described in mainland China, characterized by physical and mental fatigue, inability to concentrate, loss of memory, insomnia, irritability, sexual dysfunction and GI distress (DSM-IV™, 1994) see Culture-bound syndrome

shenkui PSYCHIATRY A clinical form of anxiety of unknown etiology described in China, which is accompanied by backache, fatigability, insomnia, vertigo, and weakness; the condition is attributed to excess loss of semen (the vital force of life) or passage of whitish urine and occurs in background of sexual dysfunction, with frequent masturbation and/or intercourse, and nocturnal emissions (DSM-IV™, 1994) see Culture-bound syndrome

shepherd's crook deformity A rarely observed prominent curving of the proximal femoral shaft, likened to the hooked staff used by the shepherds of yore, described in polyostotic fibrous dysplasia, chondrosarcoma, in Paget's disease of the bone, and in McCune-Albright syndrome (N Engl J Med 1993; 328:496cPc) characterized as a marked softening of femoral neck, associated with cortical thickening, accentuated trabeculation and unilateral shortening of the leg

'Sherlock Holmes' test A test for occult blood that removes iron from heme yielding fluorescing porphorins

Note: The sobriquet derives from Arthur Conan Doyle's fictional character Sherlock Holmes who used a test of uncertain nature to confirm a reddish stain as being blood

Sherman paradox MOLECULAR PATHOLOGY The risk of a person being phenotypically abnormal in a fragile X family is dependent on the position of the individual in the pedigree, which may be similar to phenomenon of genetic anticipation (Arch Pathol Lab Med 1993; 117:1121oA)

shiatsu Acupressure ALTERNATIVE MEDICINE A form of deep massage in which pressure is applied with the fingertips, and held in a position for 3-10 seconds on the same points that are used in acupuncture, see there

shift reticulocytes The finding of reticulocytes in the peripheral circulation longer than the usual 24 hours after their release from the marrow, resulting in a false elevation of the reticulocyte count, which is a common finding in severe anemia

shift syndrome GERIATRICS The mental decline that may occur in an elderly person who has shifted from his/her domicile to a nursing home or long-term care facility

shift work maladaptation syndrome OCCUPATIONAL MEDICINE A generic term for the long-term inability to adapt to shift work, resulting from the stress of desynchronized circadian systems, sleep deprivation, domestic and social dysharmony, relevant health problems, and ↓ work performance (JAMA 1992; 268:3047oTA); the circadian rhythm may be 'switched' by exposure to bright light at night and darkness during the day, possibly related to endogenous melatonin acitivity; see Shift work

shift work OCCUPATIONAL MEDICINE A job in a hospital, company, factory, eg automobile, petrochemical or textile factory, or other business that is open, and often operating at full staff 24 hours per day[1]; 20% of US employees work in a non-diurnal pattern, ie evening and night shifts and because of the relative unpopularity of the 'off' hours, are constantly being 'rotated', such that the workers must continually readjust their sleep/wake schedules; 20% of the population is relatively intolerant of shift work, as it requires abrupt changes of the circadian rhythm; DM and epilepsy are exacerbated by shift work and autonomic dysfunction is common; shift workers suffer an ↑ in fatigue-related accidents,[2] ↑ risk of GI and coronary heart (cardiovascular) disease[3], infertility and long-term poor adjustment (insomnia); see Circadian rhythm, Insomnia, Jet lag, Melatonin, Shift work maladaptation syndrome

[1]The first 8-hour (day) shift begins at 0600-0900; the second (evening) shift begins at 1400-1700 and the third (night or 'graveyard') begins at 2200-0100 [2]On-the-job fatigue and drowsiness in shift workers has been held responsible for the explosion of the Challenger space shuttle, and countless terrestrian tragedies (JAMA 1993; 269:1548c) [3]Possibly related to an ↑ in TGs, 1.26 mmol/L (112 mg/dL) vs 1.03 mmol/L (91 mg/dL) in normal controls; the cause of this ↑ is uncertain, but may be related to stress, the disturbance of the circadian rhythm, or the result of night snacking with less efficient removal of

Shiga neurotoxin An exotoxin produced by *Shigella dysenteriae* type 1 that causes neurotoxicity, enterotoxicity, and cytotoxicity that is structurally similar to the cholera toxin and to ricin (a toxin of higher plants); the A subunit inhibits protein synthesis by enzymatic inactivation of the 60S ribosomes in a fashion analogous to that of ricin's protein inhibition; Shiga-like toxins(formerly designated as 'vero' toxins) are produced by *Shigella* species and *Escherichia coli* and are inculpated in enteropathogenic *E coli* and enterohemorrhagic *E coli* infections as well as in the hemolytic-uremic syndrome; see EHEC, EPEC

Shiley heart valve Björk-Shiley 60 degree Converso-Concave prosthetic heart valve An artificial heart valve manufactured until 1985, when it was withdrawn from the market for valve failure due to strut fractures; 85 000 Shiley valves had been sold worldwide, transplanted into an estimated 23 000 patients in the US and Canada; strut fractures of the valve, first noted in 1976, are associated with a 0.02-0.3% annual death rate, with 800 deaths apparently related to valve failure

Note: Physicians who implanted the valves have been advised to tell their patients, or they too become legally liable should valve failure occur; the manufacturer has begun an aggressive program for identifying and warning the valve recipients of their potential risk

shin-byung PSYCHIATRY A clinical form of anxiety described in Korea characterized by anorexia, fear, GI problems, malaise, and vertigo, and attributed to possession by spirits (DSM-IV™, 1994) see Culture-bound syndrome

Shine-Delgarno sequence MOLECULAR BIOLOGY A segment of mRNA that includes part or all of the 5'-AGGAGGU-3' leader sequence, which pairs with the 16S ribosomal RNA, ensuring the proper alignment of the AUG start codon for the initiation of translation of proteins

shingles Herpes zoster from *cingulum*, Latin, girdle, related to the band-like involvement of neurocutaneous tissues seen in this condition

shin 'splints' Innocuous pain over the antero-lateral aspects of the tibial bone that is relieved by rest, elevation and exposure to cold temperatures

shiny coin appearance A fanciful descriptor for aggregates of basic calcium phosphate crystals seen by phase contrast microscopy; Cf Copper penny appearance, Snow ball appearance

'shiny Schultz' OBSTETRICS A form of placental 'delivery' that follows delivery of the infant, in which the placenta slips through the vagina with the (shiny) fetal surface showing; the blood and clots are within the pocket formed by the placenta; Cf 'Dirty Duncan'

SHIP Steroid hydroxylase inducer protein, see there

shipyard conjunctivitis Epidemic keratoconjunctivitis described in shipyard factory workers during World War II, which was thought to be caused by adenoviruses and spread by the exchange of infected welders' goggles

shivering The involuntary contraction of skeletal muscle as a result of exposure to cold or fright, or which is temporally related to the onset of fever

Shmita-salmonellosis Shmita is the Judaic practice of letting the land lay fallow every seventh year (biblical injunction, Exodus 23:10, Leviticus 25:1, 18, Deuteronomy 15:1); since the land is not being farmed on the 7th year, food is purchased from gentiles; one report (JAMA 1983: 250:2470c) implicated the use of human fertilizer ('night soil') in the salmonellosis due to this religious practice; see Judaism, practice of

SHML Sinus histiocytosis with massive lymphadenopathy, see there

shmoos A descriptor for *Saccharomyces cerevisiae* yeast forms that are inhibited in cell division by an α factor present in the culture medium; in contrast, the α yeast forms of *S cerevisae* are not inhibited in cell division when exposed to α factor, due to a nonrandom gene rearrangement that allows the yeasts to change from 'male' to 'female' mating phenotypes

The term was coined by yeast geneticists who likened the yeasts' appearance to that of minor characters in the 'Li'l Abner' comic strip by Al Capp

shock A condition characterized by clinical signs and symptoms caused by a cardiac output below that required to fill the arterial tree with blood of sufficient pressure to provide organs and tissue with adequate blood flow (after Simeone, 1964); cardinal features of shock include hypotension, poor peripheral perfusion, oliguria, and mental clouding; the most common causes of shock are trauma with major multiorgan system injury, septicemia, fluid losses (major losses of blood or intractible diarrhea), burns, contact with high voltage electric current, abrupt loss of myocardial activity; shock is classified based on separate but related mechanisms of cardiac dysfunction (pump failure), ↓ volume (loss of blood or extracellular fluid) or changes in arterial resistance or venous capacity

shock lung Post-traumatic respiratory insufficiency, traumatic 'wet lung' CRITICAL CARE MEDICINE A condition affecting the lungs, in which a change in pulmonary compliance and oxygenating capacity, results in an adult respiratory distress syndrome-like (ARDS-type) picture with defective aeration of the lungs, due to multiple factors, including aspiration of gastric contents, atelectasis, cerebral injury (affecting respiratory rate), interstitial edema, microembolism, oxygen toxicity, sepsis, oxygen toxicity or fulminant meningococcemia; see Adult respiratory distress syndrome

Shofar-blowing emphysema Painful interstitial emphysema of the head and neck, caused by blowing the Shofar, a difficult wind instrument that requires considerable intraoral pressure (the 'embouchure' of wind instrument players), made more difficult by the blower's lack of practice and underdeveloped buccal musculature, resulting in percolation of the air into the neck; see Judaism-practice of, Shofar sign

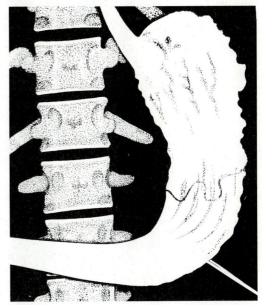

Shofar sign RADIOLOGY A descriptive term for a stomach that has been deformed by chronic Crohn's disease, in which a relatively normal gastric fundus and body funnel into a gastric antrum that has been converted into a stiffened tube with superficial rugosities and sluggish peristalsis; by 'upper GI' radiocontrast studies, the stomach has an appearance fancifully likened to the sacramental Shofar of Jewish high holidays, a finding identical in import to the far more common Crohn's disease of the terminal ileum, where the small intestinal stiffening has been likened to a garden hose Note: Transverse line in figure indicates the usual length of a shofar

Note: The Shofar is a ram's horn trumpet that was blown by the ancient Hebrews in battle and still blown at the time of 'high' Jewish holidays, ie before and during Rosh Hashanah and at the end of Yom Kippur or Yom Teruah, the 'Day of blowing'

shooter bone Myositis ossificans of the deltoid muscle of soldiers evoked by repeated trauma caused by the recoil of a rifle's butt against the upper anterior arm

'shooting gallery' SUBSTANCE ABUSE A location, often an abandoned building in an economically depressed urban area, where intravenous drug abusers congregate, purchase and inject ('shoot') heroin and cocaine; shooting galleries are unique to the US and are places of relative camaraderie in which addicts may share needles, often contaminated by HIV; see Needle exchange programs, 'Pocket shot', 'Skin popping'

shoring effect Buttressing effect, see there

short bowel syndrome A post-surgical syndrome that follows large segmental resections of the small intestine, (eg for ischemia or inflammation) causing complex nutritional imbalances and/or malnutrition; massive small intestinal resection may be required in 1) Multiple congenital atresias or stenoses of the neonatal intestine; when the loss is significant, diarrhea and malabsorption may appear shortly after birth; barium studies reveal a malrotated colon and markedly shortened small bowel; if the infant survives the first few months, intestinal function improves and 2) Massive resection of gangrenous small intestine due to mesenteric arterial occlusion (see 'Second look' operation), traumatic interruption, volvulus, or Crohn's disease; excess resection results in inadequate small intestinal digestion and absorption of nutrients, minerals and vitamins, causing hypovitaminosis and malnutrition, anemia (both hypochromic and megaloblastic anemias), diarrhea, electrolyte imbalances and marked increase in oxalates (derived from bile salt detergents that pass into the circulation, inundating the kidneys with oxalates that crystallize in the renal tubules, causing renal failure, which is not uncommon in the short bowel syndrome), lactic acidosis, osteopenia and steatorrhea; up to 70% of the absorptive surface may be lost and tolerated; if the patient survives the surgery, the residual tissue undergoes adaptive hyperplasia of the absorptive villi, an increase in absorptive cells and an increase in small intestinal caliber; after stabilization and temporary parenteral nutritional support, oral feeding must be initiated as soon as possible to stimulate the adaptive response TREATMENT High in 'quality' (ie essential amino acids) low protein diet, middle chain triglycerides, vitamins and minerals

short draw LABORATORY MEDICINE A generic term for a tube of blood drawn for analysis of chemistries or cells that has less than the recommended volume; SDs are problematic as 1) The amount of anticoagulant in certain tubes, eg 'purple tops' (ie lavender topped test tubes) may be proportionately highly, skewing the results of coagulation tests, and 2) The specimen may be insufficient for performing the necessary tests, a problem that is less common in the current environment, as most state of the art laboratory analyzers require minute samples

shorting A form of health care fraud committed by a pharmacy in which fewer pills or lesser amounts of a drug are dispensed than is specified on the physician's prescription form; Cf 'Kiting'

short interspersed repeated element SINE Any of a family of short, 70 to 300 base pair, repeated segments of DNA that includes the Alu sequence family, which are pre-sent in up to 100 000 copies in the human genome, and which have no known function; Cf Junk DNA, LINE

short leg syndrome Long leg syndrome, see there

short-loop feedback loop PHYSIOLOGY A self-adjusting circuit in the 'central' endocrine system, where the hypothalamic hormones are schematically represented as an 'axis' consisting of two circuits, the short hypothalamic-adenohypophysis (or pituitary) loop and the long adenohypophysis (or pituitary)-end organ loop; see Loops

short PR syndrome Lown-Ganong Levine syndrome A condition comprising a short PR interval, a normal QRS complex, and tachycardia presumed to be related to atriohisian bypass; it is uncertain whether SPS is a disease a sui generis (BE Braunwald, Heart Disease, 4th ed, WB Saunders, Philadelphia, 1992)

short rib-polydactyly syndrome A disease complex characterized by short stature and horizontal ribs, divided into SRPS, SALDINO-NOONAN TYPE (SRPS, TYPE I) An AR [MIM 263530] condition characterizd by hydrops, postaxial polydactyly, defective ossification of the calvaria, vertebrae, pelvis, bones of hands and feet, metaphyseal irregularities of long bones, small iliac bones, transposition of great vessels, and pulmonary hypoplasia; it is lethal in the neonatal period SRPS, MAJEWSKI TYPE (SRPS, TYPE II) An AR [MIM 263520] condition characterized by a narrow thorax, polysyndactyly, cleft lip, malformed ears, ambiguous genitalia, epiglottic and laryngeal hypoplasia, glomerular cysts and absent gallbladder; the most distinctive feature is the disproportionate shortening of the tibia; all die in perinatal period SRPS, VERMA-NAUMOFF TYPE (SRPS, TYPE III) An AR [MIM 263530] condition which characterized by the presence of a short cranial base, bulging forehead, depressed nasal bridge, flat occiput, and defects of the long bones, and anomalous sexual development; all die in perinatal period

shortwave diathermy SPORTS MEDICINE A form of medical diathermy that delivers shortwave frequency electromagnetic waves, which is use in treating various chronic inflammatory conditions including bursitis, neuritis, osteoarthrosis, rheumatoid arthritis, strains, tendinitis and others; SD is contraindicated in the presence of atherosclerosis, hemorrhage, metal implants, infections, malignancy, pacemakers, phlebitis, pregnancy, and wet dressings (JC DeLee, D Drez, Jr, Eds, Orthopedic Sports Medicine WB Saunders, Philadelphia, 1994) see Diathermy; Cf Microwave diathermy

shoshin beri-beri A fulminant form of beri-beri (thiamine deficiency), now of largely historic interest CLINICAL Cardiac dilatation, cardiomegaly, tachypnea, shallow breathing, cyanosis and, due to pyruvate accumulation, cardiovascular collapse, hepatomegaly and mydriasis Note: Thiamine is responsible for oxidative decarboxylation, in its absence, the orange-colored methyl glyoxal and pyruvate accumulate, resulting in myocardial toxicity

shotgun FORENSIC PATHOLOGY A sports weapon, popularized by water fowl hunters, which is widely regarded as the most efficient 'execution' weapon when the hit-man is faced with a moving target; in the US, homicide and suicide by shotgun is not uncommon, while it is exceedingly rare in civilized countries, given the strict gun control laws; the shot or pellets spread out in a relatively consistent fashion, such that the distance from the muzzle in meters is approximately equal to three times the diameter of the target, thus a 60-70 cm in diameter spread of shot pellets corresponds to a muzzle range of two meters, a value of some use in determining the proximity of an alleged perpetrator of a crime; while short-term, a victim might survive certain shotgun wounds, massive infection secondary to multiple perforations in an abdominal blast entails prolonged recuperation, if the surgeon is successful in salvaging the intestine; see Ballistics, Cookie cutter wounds, Drive-by shootings, Execution wounds, Gauge

Note: When new, shotguns have a full 'choke', a narrowing at the end of the barrel to ensure that the shot (pellets) remain closely clustered in their trajectory; when the barrel is shortened by cutting, creating a 'sawed-off' shot-gun, the trajectory of the pellets is shorter, the spread of the shot much wider, and the devastation to the body more complete

'shotgun approach' A diagnostic method or technique in which every conceivable parameter is measured in order to detect all possible clinical or laboratory nosologies, however remote the possibility a rare disease is present; in the US, not considering a potentially treatable disease in a difficult case may result in potentially costly litigation and thus physicians may in the face of such cases resort to the 'shot-gun method', an often-criticized result of practicing 'defensive medicine', increasing the cost of health care without improving patient management; Cf Screening

shotgun experiment 'Shotgunning' MOLECULAR BIOLOGY A crude but effective method used to identify a specific gene associated with a disease, which consists in nonspecifically cloning all the fragments that result from a restriction endonuclease digest of the entire genome of an organism known to contain a gene of interest, yielding a constellation of fragments known as a gene bank or gene library, which is followed by an identification step, consisting in screening for the desired gene; Cf Jackpot experiment, 'Quick and dirty'

shotty lymphadenopathy A nonspecific descriptor for clusters of multiple small*, contiguous and indurated lymph nodes that may be palpated in the inguinal, cervical and other regions in children with viral infections, which, when palpated in adults is characteristic of syphilis, and may be seen in carcinoma metastatic to lymph nodes

*Likened to shot from a shotgun cartridge

'shoulder' OBSTETRICS A descriptor for the gently-sloped acceleration rhythm seen on a paper printout of the fetal heart monitor that either precedes or follows a typical deceleration, in contrast to the usual 'acceleration' (a short-term increase in the heart rate above baseline) occurring in response to fetal movement; see Deceleration

shoulder-hand syndrome NEUROLOGY A clinical complex characterized by shoulder pain, swelling, stiffness, vasomotor symptoms of the arm and hand, cutaneous edema and induration, affecting those over age 50 as a complication of myocardial infarction, or less commonly, a cerebrovascular accident or head trauma, a condition that is thought due to reflex sympathetic stimulation; some patients later develop adhesive capsulitis, sclerodactyly and limitation of motion of the extremity with patchy regional demineralization; see Rotator cuff

Synonyms include algodystrophy, coronary scapulary syndrome, hand-shoulder syndrome, postinfarctional sclerodactylia, posttraumatic osteoporosis of the upper extremity, reflex dystrophy of the upper extremity, reflex sympathetic dystrophy, Steinbrocker syndrome, sympathetic reflex dystrophy

shoulder pad sign Enlargement of the glenohumeral joint due to peri-articular accumulation of amyloid in primary or secondary (multiple myeloma) amyloidosis, appearing as a regional soft tissue density

shoulder pointer 'syndrome' SPORTS MEDICINE A simple separation or 'sprain' of the acromioclavicular joint is commonly associated with contact sports (eg football, wrestling, karate, hockey) as well as non-contact sports due to dislocations or strain (eg swimming, gymnastics without joint instability)

shredded appearance A descriptive term for the light microscopic morphology of skeletal muscle that has been exposed to extreme heat or cold, resulting in necrosis with irregular transverse bands of dense material separated by lighter areas MECHANISM Sudden over-contraction of muscle Note: A shredded appearance may also be seen in myotonic dystrophy or as an artefact of fixation; see

Contraction band necrosis, Wavy changes

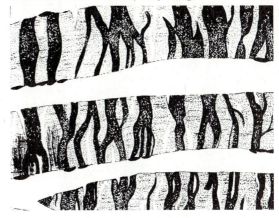

shredded appearance

shredded cassette appearance A descriptor for the morphology of colonies of *Erysipelothrix rhusiopathiae* (erysipeloid agent), likened to the 'confused' tangled strands of a broken audiocassette

shrewmouse profile A fanciful descriptor for the facies of children seen after ankylosis of the jaw following scarlet fever, an extremely uncommon clinical event

shrink *noun* A highly colloquial term for a psychiatrist

'shrinking field' technique RADIATION ONCOLOGY A method used in radiotherapy for treating a large mediastinal lymphoid malignancy, in which the treatment field is decreased in size (shrunken) as the tumor responds or 'melts'; see Mantle port

shrinking lungs Elevation of the diaphragm due to pleural adhesions, plate-like atelectases and chronic fibrosis, a finding described as typical of SLE; shrinking lungs are radiological and pathological findings that may not translate into clinical disease; Cf Pulmonary sequestration

shrinking pleuritis with rounded atelectasis Folded-lung syndrome, see there

shunt The diversion of the flow of a fluid, which may be accidental, as in a traumatic AV aneurysm, or occur by design, eg portocaval shunt or ventriculoperitoneal shunt PEDIATRIC CARDIOLOGY While bypass of the pulmonary circulation (shunting) is a normal physiological process in utero, it becomes abnormal upon delivery of the infant; shunts are of two types 1) Those in which already oxygenated blood in the left heart passes back into the right heart (left-to-right) and 2) Those which partially bypass the lungs, with venous blood directly entering the systemic circulation (right-to-left shunt) **LEFT-TO-RIGHT SHUNT** ACYANOTIC SHUNT The right and left sides of the heart communicate by an atrial or ventricular septal defect and patent ductus arteriosus; the blood flows from the region of highest (left heart) to lowest (right heart and systemic circulation) pressure, as occurs in ventricular septal defects and corrected L-transposition of the great arteries; since the blood does not bypass the pulmonary circulation, it is well oxygenated CLINICAL The plethora of blood causes pulmonary congestion and hypertension that becomes significant when the pulmonary blood flow is 1.5-2.0-fold greater than the systemic flow with diastolic overloading and cardiac dilatation, which without correction results in cardiac failure, a late complication is bacterial pneumonia related to stasis within the pulmonary circulation; left-to-right shunts may also be created surgically, eg in the Blalock procedure **RIGHT-TO-LEFT SHUNT** CYANOTIC SHUNT There is a variable degree of pulmonary circulation bypass accompanied by obstruction of blood flow into the pulmonary circulation; right-to-left shunts include Fallot's tetralogy (ventricular septal defect, pulmonary valve stenosis, overriding or dextroposed aorta and secondary right ventricular hypertrophy), transposition of the great vessels, tricuspid valve atresia, truncus arteriosus and total anomalous return of pulmonary veins; the pulmonary blood flow is less than in left-to-right shunts CLINICAL Cyanosis with limited exercise tolerance, neurological damage and compensatory polycythemia; as children, these patients are often very sick and by adolescence, may suffer acquired coagulopathies

shunt nephritis A form of glomerulonephritis that is thought to be linked to the formation of immune complexes, which is seen in ± 4% of infants with an infected ventriculoatrial (as well as ventriculojugular or ventriculoperitoneal) shunt CLINICAL Weight loss, lethargy, fever, hypertension, arthralgia, lymphadenopathy, hepatosplenomegaly, nephrotic syndrome, often complicated by a delayed recognition of the infection LABORATORY Anemia, (micro)hematuria, proteinuria, azotemia; ↓ C3, rheumatoid factors and cryoglobulins may be present; the most commonly isolated bacteria are *Staphylococcus epidermidis* and *S albus* TREATMENT Antibiotics, possibly also high-dose prednisone PROGNOSIS ½ resolve with therapy, ¼ have persistent urine abnormalities; ¼ die of the neurologic defects that necessitated the ventricular shunt

shuttle A short cyclical metabolic pathway in which reducing elements are passed from the cytoplasmic NADH to the electron transport system within the mitochondria by way of molecular intermediates

shuttle hypothesis PHYSIOLOGY A posit that explains the rapid increase in permeability of collecting ducts of the kidney in response to vasopressin as a result of the movement of a water channel protein (eg aquaporin-2) to the apical plasma membrane (N Engl J Med 1995; 332:1540ₐ)

'shuttle' science The carrying out of research projects by preparing research materials in smaller (often poorly equipped) laboratories, eg in the former Soviet Union, and then conduct the 'expensive' parts of the actual experiment, eg magnetic resonance spectroscopy, or X-ray crystallography, in a well-endowed laboratory (Science 1994; 264; 1267) Cf 'Safari research'

shuttle vector MOLECULAR BIOLOGY A self-sufficient DNA molecule that is capable of replicating in a variety of hosts, including yeasts and bacteria

shy bladder A psychoneurologic reflex, more common in men, characterized by difficulty or inability to initiate urinary flow in public places

SI International System, see SI 1) Sacroiliac 2) Saline injection 3) Saturation index 4) School inventory (psychological test) 5) Sex inventory (psychological evaluation) 6) Solubility index

Also 1) Self-incompatible 2) Self-inflicted 3) Sensation intuition 4) Septic inflammation 5) Serum iron 6) Sexual intercourse 7) Small intestine 8) Soluble insulin 9) Special intervention 10) Speech intelligibility

SI Systeme International d'unites LABORATORY MEDICINE The international system for standardization of units of measurement, which is a refinement and extension of the metric system, which is based on

BASIC UNITS: m meter (length), kg kilogram (mass), s second (time), A ampere (electric current), K Kelvin (thermodynamic temperature), cd candela (luminous intensity), mol mole (amount of a substance) and

DERIVED UNITS that derived from the first group: N newton (force), J joule (energy) and L liter (volume)[1]; the US is the only country that has not yet converted to the SI system of reporting laboratory values[2] for most analytes, the conversion is simple; in hematology, the number of cells (red cells, white cells, and platelets) in a cubic millimeter (mm³) are converted to those present in one liter,

multiplied by 10⁶; in chemistry, the units are converted from milligrams/deciliter to millimoles/liter and most analytes have a 1:1 ratio with SI units; some values are transformed into SI units by using a conversion factor, with appropriate adjustment for the types of units (table)

[1]The SI sanctions l for liter; because this may be confused with number 1, L is often substituted in the USA, a convention adopted by the author [2]In 1992; two premier American medical journals, the Journal of the American Medical Association and the New England Journal of Medicine (N Engl J Med 1992; 327:49ₑ, 50c) reversed their support of SI units and reported laboratory values in conventional (US) units (CAP Today March 1993); this resulted in an outcry by international medical community, which likened this backward step as akin to the World Health Organization deciding that the eradication of polio would be just too tiring (this same provincialism has prevented the US from converting to the metric system); in the author's view, a language of global communication (as is English) is not the 'property' of those who use it as natives; medical English belongs to a larger body that should have the right to decide on certain universally applicable rules and standards, such as is the SI system of units; SI units <u>are</u> used in this work

SIADH Syndrome of inappropriate antidiuretic hormone secretion A clinical complex characterized by excess vasopressin (ADH) secretion despite low plasma osmolarity, water retention and dilutional hyponatremia ETIOLOGY SIADH is due to an excess of vasopressin in the face of normal renal and adrenocortical function, and occurs in untreated Addison's disease, ACTH deficiency, hypopituitarism, ectopic hormone production in carcinomas (small cell, bronchogenic, pancreatic, uterine, bladder and prostatic), lymphoproliferative disorders, mesothelioma, thymoma, CNS disease (trauma, infection, chromophobe adenoma, metastases), pulmonary disease (pneumonia, tuberculosis, use of positive end-expiratory pressure (PEEP) ventilatory support, drugs (chlorpropamide, vincristine), and others, eg porphyria and AIDS LABORATORY Hypervolemia, hypouricemia, often ↓ creatinine, hyponatremia, natriuresis (urinary sodium > 20 mEq/L with ↓ BUN), absence of clinical symptoms of volume depletion, ↓ maximum urinary dilution, normal renal and adrenal function TREATMENT Corticosteroids as they suppress vasopressin secretion

sialadenoma papilliferum A rare, benign exophytic tumor of major and minor salivary gland origin, also seen on the buccal mucosa and palate PATHOLOGY Papillary exophytic overgrowth of both the intercalated duct epithelium and surface squamous epithelium TREATMENT Conservative resection

sialidase Neuraminidase, see there

sialidoses A group of four partially overlapping lysosomal storage diseases; by tradition, type I is also known as the cherry-red spot myoclonus syndrome[1]; as all share a defi-

SI-SYSTEME INTERNATIONAL D'UNITES[1]		
Common US to SI conversions		
	CF[2]	Final units
Acetone	172.2	mmol/L
Albumin	10.0	mmol/L
Alanine aminotransferase	0.482 U/L Karmen units	
Bilirubin	17.10	µmol/L
Calcium	0.2495	mmol/L
Cholesterol	0.0258	mmol/L
Creatinine	88.40	µmol/L
Glucose	0.0555	mmol/L
Hemoglobin	10.0	g/L
Iron	0.1791	µmol/L
Lipoproteins (LDL)	0.2586	mmol/L
Lipoproteins (HDFL)	0.2586	mmol/L
Magnesium	0.4114	mmol/L
Phosphate	0.3229	mmol/L
Potassium levels, mg	0.2558	mmol/L
Protein	10.0	g/L
Trioiodothyronin (T3)	0.1536	nmol/L
Triglycerides	0.0113	mmol/L
Urea nitrogen	0.3570	mmol/L, urine

[1]International System [2]CF Conversion factor

ciency in alpha-N-acetylneuraminidase, it is likely that an encompassing term, eg neuraminidase deficiency[2] with the appropriate qualifying modifiers would eliminate the confusion in terminology

[1]J Spranger has suggested this be designated as sialidosis type IV; according to his schema, sialidosis type I would corrspond to nephrosialidosis, type II to mucolipidosis type I, and type III to neur(-)gal(-)-sialidosis [2]as suggested by VA McKusick in the Mendelian Inheritance in Man catalogs

sialidosis type I Cherry-red spot myoclonus syndrome, see there

sialidosis type II An AR [MIM 256550] condition characterized by coarse facies and dysostosis multiplex which has been divided into a congenital form with ascites, hydrops fetalis, gargoyle-like facies, visceromegaly, mental retardation, myoclonus, tonic-clonic seizures, cherry-red spots, hearing loss, deficiency of alpha-N-acetylneuraminidase, usually with a partial defect of β-galactosidase; the infantile and juvenile forms may be less severe PATHOLOGY PAS-positive inclusions in lymphocytes, bone marrow, neurons and Kupffer cells

sialyl-Lewis X A molecular determinant present on myeloid cells and on some tumor cells, which serves to explain the vasculotropism of some invasive tumors; see ELAM-1

'Siamese' twin(s) Conjoined equal twins A joined gestational product resulting from a failure in division of the yolk sac or due to delayed monovular separation, an event estimated to occur in 1:200 000 term deliveries, most of which are joined at the chest (thoracopagus), the prognosis is a function of adequacy of surgical separation

Note: The most famous Siamese twins, Chang and Eng Bunker, were of the xiphopagus type and born in Siam (now Thailand) in 1811, married the Yates sisters in North Carolina in 1843, respectively fathered 10 and 12 children (whoa!) and died at age 62, within hours of each other

sibling rivalry PSYCHOLOGY The intense, emotionally-charged competition among siblings (brothers and/or sisters) that pits one against the other to obtain parental affection, approval, attention, and love; SR is widely regarded as being a normal (albeit maddening) part of the process of psychological maturation of the individual; the relationships that siblings have as adults are thought to reflect in part unresolved rivalries in their childhood (New York Times & September 1993; C9; US News & World Report 10 January1994:8) Cf Only child, Sibling relational problem

The study may not have been an accurate reflection of the ability of outdoor airflow to correct SBS as this lower limit used in this study was 1.5 **x** > than the American Society of Heating, Refrigeration, and Air Conditioning Engineers recommendation of the minimal supply of outdoor air, promulgated in 1989 (N Engl J Med 1993; 329:503c)

sibling relational problem PSYCHIATRY A term referring to the long-term consequences of the unresolved conflicts of sibling rivalries, which may be associated with clinically significant impairment of functioning; Cf Sibling rivalry

sicca complex Symptoms related to generalized drying of mucosae, affecting 1) Eyes, causing xeroconjunctivitis due to ↓ tears, thick, 'ropy' secretions on the inner canthus, foreign body (tired, itchy and sandy) sensation and ↓ visual acuity and 2) Mouth Xerostomia with ↓ salivation due to lymphocyte infiltration and duct obstruction, with soreness, adhesion of food to mucosa, 'cracker' sign, angular cheilitis, lingual fissuring and acceleration of caries; the sicca complex is most often associated with Sjögren syndrome and may also occur in amyloidosis, hemochromatosis, hyperlipoproteinemia types IV and V, sarcoidosis, vitamin C and/or A deficiency, scleroderma, and other collagen vascular diseases

sick building syndrome Tight building syndrome PUBLIC HEALTH A condition defined by the WHO as an excess of work-related irritations of the skin and mucous membranes and other symptoms, including headache, fatigue, and difficulty concentrating, reported by workers in modern office buildings; 'sick building' symptoms are two to three-fold more common in those who work in large, energy-efficient office buildings Clinical manifestations fall in a number of categories (table) in ¼ of investigations of such 'outbreaks', a specific cause has been identified, eg bacterial contamination of humidification systems, or exhaust of motor vehicles or incineration of waste; the others are classified as SBS; an ↑ in outdoor airflow from 0.85-1.8 m³ (30-64 ft³) is not reported to ↓ symptoms of SBS* (N Engl J Med 1993; 328:821oa; 329:503c) CHEMICALS Off-gassing from construction materials, eg adhesives, varnishes, volatile organic solvents (CAP Today March 1992)

sick cell 'syndrome' A condition characterized by the redistribution of sodium between the intracellular and extracellular compartments without changes in the total body sodium, which occurs in severely ill patients and thought to be due to the inefficiency of the Na^+/H^+ antiporter

sick Santa 'syndrome' OCCUPATIONAL MEDICINE The sum of the infectious diseases afflicting those who seasonally don St Nicholas garb, exposing themselves to infected aerosols; other Santa-related symptoms include frostbite (Salvation army Santas), psychological (repressed anger), neuromuscular symptoms (prolonged periods in uncomfortable positions, eg holding children on the knees)

sick sinus syndrome CARDIOLOGY A diffuse cardiac conduction system disease characterized by a pathologically slow or erratic rate of sinus depolarization due to impaired automaticity; a 'sick sinus' is more common in the elderly and, if severe, may be symptomatic with dizziness, palpitations, exercise intolerance, syncopes and cerebral dysfunction associated with a combination of persistent sinus bradycardia (30-60/min) and supraventricular tachyarrhythmia, thus the trivial synonym, 'brady-tachy' syndrome TREATMENT Verapamil, diltiazem or pacemaker

sickle cell Drepanocyte The fragmented scythe-shaped cells that result from the formation of 'tactoids' within erythrocytes of 'sickling' hemoglobins; hemoglobin exists in two conformations, the 'R', relaxed or oxygenated form and the 'T'*, tense or deoxygenated form, which readily transform, one to the other, depending on the oxygen conditions; deoxygenation of hemoglobin S causes it to polymerize into rigid, rod-like fibers (tense form), which upon curvilinear alignment, give rise to the classic sickle cell shapes; see Spectrin, Tactoid

Note: The SC is in part related to the uncoupling of the spectrin-based membrane skeleton from the lipid bilayer (Science 1991; 252:574)

sickle cell anemia Sickle cell disease, homozygous hemoglobin S disease A congenital hemoglobinopathy that

---

SICK BUILDING SYNDROME (clinical manifestations)

HYPERSENSITIVITY Hypersensitivity pneumonitis and allergic alveolitis in response to various microorganisms including water-borne amoeba, known as Humidifier lung

ALLERGIES Allergic rhinitis and asthma, related to dust mites

INFECTIONS Miniepidemics, eg Legionnaire's disease, Pontiac fever, by airborne organisms of low pathogenic potential that thrive in stagnate water and are disseminated through poorly maintained air conditioning systems

MUCOCUTANEOUS IRRITATION Skin eruptions, due to fiberglass, mineral wool or other particles; contact lens wearers may suffer corneal abrasions

MUCOSAL IRRITATION Dry throat, cough, tightness in chest, sinus congestion and sneezing (formerly due to tobacco smoke), janitorial solvents and cleaning materials, eg chlorine, reactions to photochemical or other toxins, eg in laser printers due to the styrene-butadiene toners (N Engl J Med 1990; 322:1323c) and ozone production by photocopiers

PSEUDOEPIDEMICS related to 'mass hysteria'

affects 0.15% of black children in the US, which is caused by a point mutation on the gene that encodes β hemoglobin, resulting in a defective functioning of hemoglobin, causing erythrocytes to 'sickle' in the face of ↓ O₂; PATHOGENESIS Homozygotes with the sickle gene from each parent produce abnormal (Glu → Val substitution at β6, the sixth amino acid of the β-globin peptide) hemoglobin S, but no normal hemoglobin A; this amino acid substitution creates a hydrophobic patch on the surface of hemoglobin S molecules, enabling them to polymerize when deoxygenated, resulting in rigid RBCs that cause severe hemolytic anemia and intermittent vaso-occlusive episodes.' (N Engl J Med 1993; 328:129ED) TREATMENT Pain is very intense and may respond to dexamethasone; some agents stimulate the human fetal globin gene promoter increasing the expression of the γ-globin gene, eg hydroxyurea or butyrate (N Engl J Med 1993; 328:73OA, 81OA)

Note: Sickle cell anemia was first described in a West Indian student (Arch Int Med 1910; 6:517), and most cases in blacks have been traced to a family in the Krobo tribe in 1670; other sickle cell anemias occur in Greece, Italy, Israel, Saudi Arabia and subcontinental India, and in addition to hemoglobin S, which causes the classic sickle cell anemia, are due to other hemoglobin defects, in which sickling plays a key role in producing clinical disease, including hemoglobin SC disease, hemoglobin SD disease and β thalassemia

sickle cell 'prep' A laboratory test used to screen for sickle cell anemia, where sodium metabisulfite is used to desolubilize hemoglobin S to the crystallized deoxygenated form, causing the cells to sickle

sickle cell trait Heterozygosity for hemoglobin S which occurs in ± 8% of the US black population, and up to 30% of some African populations; SCT is rarely associated with clinical disease; there is no anemia and the RBC morphology is normal; growth, development, an lifespan of individuals with SCT is normal; nonetheless SCT has been linked to a slight, but statistically significant ↑ in sudden unexplained death, and both hematuria and splenic infarction are more common in those with SCT

sickle chest syndrome A complication of sickle cell anemia caused by intravascular 'sludging' of circulating cells CLINICAL Chest pain, dyspnea and fever due to thromboses in the terminal pulmonary arteries PROGNOSIS Guarded

sickle particles A descriptor for the curved bacteria seen by high-power LM in the macrophages of Whipple's disease in the myocardium, lung, spleen, liver, pancreas, mesentery, retroperitoneum, soft tissue, lymph nodes, adrenal glands and brain; see Whipple's disease

Sickness Impact Profile A scale used to assess quality of life in patients being treated for a potentially fatal condition (N Engl J Med 1993; 329:149OA) see Karnovsky scale, QWB scale

SIDA Syndrome d'immunodeficience acquise, French for AIDS Note: The other Romance languages, ie Italian, Portuguese and Brazilian and Spanish use an equivalent acronym for AIDS

siderophilins A family of 80-kD monomeric non-heme iron-binding glycoproteins, eg transferrin and lactoferrin that bind two iron ions in conjunction with two carbonate ions

sidestream cigarette smoke The smoke originating from the smoldering end of a cigarette between puffs, the principal component of environmental tobacco smoke; sidestream cigarette smoke contains nicotine, a noncarcinogenic constituent of tobacco, as well as 4-aminobiphenyl and 4-(methyl-nitrosoamino)-1-(3-pyridyl)-1-butanone (NNK), tobacco-specific lung carcinogens that are held responsible for ↑ in lung cancer, especially adenocarcinoma seen in passive smokers (N Engl J Med 1993; 329:1543OA) see Environmental tobacco smoke, NNK, Passive smoking

sidewalk consultation Curbside consultation, see there

SIDS Sudden infant death syndrome Definition from 2nd Intl Conf on SIDS, World Health Organization 'Sudden

and unexpected death of an infant who was well or almost well prior to death which remains unexplained after an adequate autopsy' Frequency of SIDS in different ethnic groups, US Asian 0.5/1000; white 1.3/1000; black 2.9/1000; American Indian 5.9/1000; SIDS is more common in premature male infants under six months of age; the parents are more commonly in lower socioeconomic strata, narcotic addicts, cigarette smokers, or unwed mothers PATHOLOGY Nonspecific, possibly related to a preterminal asphyxiating event, as petechiae occur on the thymus, epicardium and pleura; one fatal event misinterpreted as SIDS is involuntary smothering (see The Ballad of Moll Magee, WB Yeats) by an exhausted mother who 'co-sleeps' with the infant LABORATORY No consistent defects or changes are known PATHOGENESIS Sleeping in a prone position may be a risk factor (N Engl J Med 1994; 330:63c, ibid 1993; 329:377OA, New York Times 15 March 1995; C11); other possible risk factors include the use of natural fiber (soft) mattresses, swaddling, recent illness in which there was nasal congestion, cough, fever, vomiting, or diarrhea immediately before or on the day of death,and overheating the room (Arch Pathol Lab Med 1993; 117:1246ED); a possible cause of SIDS is the fungus *Scopulariopsis brevicaulis* that grows well on the plastic covering of baby mattresses, producing toxic heavier-than-air trihydride gases (phosphine, arsine, stibine) that may concentrate at the child's head; since they don't move well at this age, the infants may 'smother' from the gas; in some cases reported as SIDS, the infants are found lying face down in soft polystyrene foam-filled cushions, apparently dying of rebreathing type suffocation (N Engl J Med 1991; 324:1858); SIDS increases with prone sleeping position, and is further increased by recent illness, swaddling, use of heat in bedrooms and use of natural fiber (kapok fibers or ti-tree bark, Australia) mattresses (N Engl J Med 1993; 329:377OA)

siemens S The SI (International System) name for the reciprocal ohm, a unit of conductivity that measures the quantity of electricity transferred across a unit area per unit of potential gradient in a unit of time, specifically, 1.0 ampere/volt

sievert Sv The SI (International System) name for the unit of radioactive biological effectiveness (dose equivalence); 1.0 Sv = 1.0 joule/kilogram or 100 rem; see Gray, Rad; Roentgen

'sieving' GASTRIC PHYSIOLOGY A theory that attempted to explain the manner in which food passed from the stomach to the duodenum; it had been assumed by some workers that lighter, partially digested particles would flow as the central portion of a parabolic 'column' into the duodenum; the theory that was later modified to include mechanical and size factors, where particle transit time is directly related to fluid viscosity and velocity and inversely related to particle density and diameter MOLECULAR BIOLOGY Molecular sieving; see Gel filtration chromatography, Reptation

sigma factor MOLECULAR BIOLOGY Any of a number of accessory proteins that help RNA polymerase recognize specific DNA 'promoter' sites to be transcribed, which results in a 'bind-release-bind' sequence fancifully likened to Tarzan swinging from the vines; once the RNA polymerase hits a sigma factor (by analogy, a tree trunk), transcription begins

'sigmoid' esophagus see Bird's beak sign

sigmoid kinetics The rate behavior of an enzymatic reaction that yields a sigmoid (S-shaped) curve for a plot of reaction velocity versus substrate concentration, a curve typical of allosteric enzyme-substrate systems, which demonstrate cooperative interaction

sigmoidoscope A device for examining the sigmoid colonic mucosa, divided into rigid and flexible sigmoidoscopy; because of its simplicity, the rigid sigmoidoscope is of use in examining the anorectum and distal sigmoid; for higher lesions, the flexible sigmoidoscope reduces patient discomfort, has a two to four-fold greater diagnostic yield than rigid sigmoidoscopy and has a useful 'reach' of 60-70 cm, allowing rapid evaluation, photography and biopsies of the large intestine; as the bowel preparation is minimal, electrocoagulation polypectomies are ill-advised, given the danger of explosion due to the various gases in this region; see Endoscopy

sigmoid septum An angulated deformity of the aorta seen in idiopathic hypertrophic subaortic stenosis

signal averaged electrocardiography CARDIOLOGY A technique that amplifies late potentials (high-frequency, low-amplitude signals at the terminal portion of the QRS complex), which are thought to be due to fragmented and delayed electrical conduction through the borders of a myocardial scar; the delayed conduction of late potentials allows re-entry of electrical impulses and ↑ susceptibility to ventricular arrhythmias; detection of late potentials by SAE correlates well with inducibility of ventricular tachycardia, and is useful noninvasive test for identifying ↑ risk of ventricular tachycardia, but is of little use for those patients with conduction defects (Mayo Clin Proc 1995; 70:132OA)

signal event An event, usually man-made, in which there is a tremendous 'signal', often in the form of a 'disaster', eg Love canal‡ or the Libby Zion case‡, which engenders multiple 'ripple' effects of legislation and 'landmark' legal cases, due in part to a popular outcry against prevailing policies that were inadequate or incapable of addressing the event

Note: Such events may result in legislative overreaction and the 'solution' may spawn a host of unanticipated ethical dilemmas

signal hypothesis The theory explaining the mechanism by which secretory proteins are selected for export by the rough endoplasmic reticulum (RER), according to which, the mRNA encoding the secretory protein contains a 'signal sequence' immediately downstream from the start codon; the mRNA's translation is initiated by free ribosomes in the cytosol, which synthesize a hydrophobic N-terminal oligomeric 'signal peptide'; once the signal peptide leaves the ribosome, it binds to a receptor on the RER, around which a transmembrane pore develops, through which the nascent protein extrudes and becomes glycosylated; finally the mature protein is transported via the Golgi apparatus to its final intra- or extracellular destination

signal peptide Signal sequence, see there

signal-to-noise ratio A generic term for the ability to detect a measurable parameter (ie signal) above a background (ie noise), where a high SNR corresponds to a distinct signal, and a low SNR results in an indistinct signal MRI The ratio obtained from the relative contributions of detected true signal to that of random superimposed signals ('noise'); SNR is a function of the electromagnetic properties of the sample or the patient being studied; the higher the SNR, the better the image's resolution; SNR may be improved by 1) Averaging several measurements of a signal since random signals tend to cancel themselves, 2) Sampling large volumes (with corresponding loss of spatial resolution) and 3) Increasing the magnetic field's strength; see Magnetic resonance imaging

signal recognition particle MOLECULAR BIOLOGY A multi-unit 11S cytoplasmic protein with a key role in exporting nascent proteins from the cytoplasm of mammalian cells; SRP is constructed of six discrete polypeptides (P9, P14, P19, P54, P68 and P72) linked to a 300-nucleotide RNA sequence that recognizes a secretory protein's 'signal sequence', allowing transportation of the protein from the site of production at the tRNA into the lumen of the endo-

plasmic reticulum for future extracellular secretion; termination of SRP action requires its dissociation from its receptor, the energy contributed by GTP hydrolysis (Science 1991; 252:1171)

signal sequence MOLECULAR BIOLOGY A prehormone's NH_2 terminal amino acids that are critical for the transfer from its site of synthesis in the cytoplasm to the endoplasmic reticulum; the signal peptide binds the polyribosome complex (mRNA, ribosomes and nascent proteins) to the endoplasmic reticulum; after cleavage of the signal peptide, the protein becomes either a prohormone or a hormone; although there is no homology among the different signal sequences, they have one or more positively charged amino acids near the N-terminus, followed by 6-12 hydrophobic residues; since the signal sequences are not found in the mature proteins, they are thought to be cleaved from the protein while it is being translated

signal transduction A cascade of biochemical interactions initiated by phosphorylation of enzymes, eg protein-tyrosine kinases, and protein-tyrosine phosphatases that transmits a signal to the nucleus; this signal is translated by second messengers that induce specific arrays of genes, altering the processes related to target cell function

signal void MRI An abrupt cessation of signal which, when seen in MRI angiography, indicates a stenotic area of the vessel; see Magnetic resonance imaging

signature 1) A person's name written in script by the person him/herself, which when placed on document, eg patient's chart, prescription for patient therapy, or consent form becomes legally binding 2) A highly specific pattern that defines a substance of interest as being unique, a term that is often used interchangeably with fingerprint

signature-pattern analysis MOLECULAR BIOLOGY A method used to evaluate the evolutionary relatedness of a sequence of DNA to other sequences; in SPA, the DNA sequence of interest is first compared with a set of reference sequences to identify distinctive nucleotides, which correspond to signature patterns (N Engl J Med 1993; 329:1835OA)

signet ring cell An almost invariably malignant cell in which there is copious clear cytoplasm that flattens a hyperchromatic nucleus to one side, having an appearance fancifully likened to that of a signet ring; malignancies composed predominantly of signet ring cells often carry a worse prognosis; the 'classic' (and most common) signet ring cell (adeno)carcinoma occurs in the stomach, but is also well described in carcinomas of the breast[1], colon, gall bladder, lung, nasal cavity, prostate, thyroid (medullary carcinoma), urinary bladder, malignant signet ring cells may also be seen in non-epithelial malignancies, eg mesothelioma, rhabdomyosarcoma, balloon cell melanoma, oligodendrogliomas, myxoid angio-blastomatosis, myxoid liposarcoma, lymphoma[2] and is a morphology typical of normal fat cells and oligodendrogliocytes

[1]Signet ring cell variant of lobular carcinoma of breast (Mod Pathol 1993; 6:516; Arch Pathol Lab Med 1994; 118:245OA) [2]eg Signet ring cell lymphoma, see there

signet ring form A morphologic descriptor for the trophozoite form of *Plasmodium falciparum*, seen by light microscopy in a peripheral blood smear, which are often accompanied by Schüffner's dots

signet ring melanoma A histologic variant of malignant melanoma, which is interest given the potential for confusing this lesion with the far more common signet ring carcinoma; the material accumulated is the signet ring cells is vimentin and not melanin (Acta Cytologica 1993; 37:559OA)

signet ring sign RADIOLOGY Any of a number of hypodense 'rings' corresponding to the thickened bronchioles in bronchiectasia, which may be seen by high-resolution computed tomography of the lungs, corresponding to the ring sign and tramtrack sign of bronchiectasia seen on plain films of the chest

significance STATISTICS A measure of the deviation of data from a statistical mean, defined by a probability (p) value, where a p of 0.05 indicates a 5% possibility or 1 chance in 20 that a data set will differ from a mean and 19 chances in 20 that the data set will not

significant financial interest A term defined by the NIH as \$5000 (or more) in stock or other remuneration, or 5% ownership in a business; this level of 'financial interest' is thought by some to be a point at which investigators with federal grants might compromise their research ethics and slant data that would favor a commercial venture in which the researcher has financial interest (**Sci Am 1994; 271/5:90**)

significant other Most significant other, see there

significant risk device A medical device that has the potential for causing significant risk to the health, safety, or welfare of a subject and is intended for use 1) As an implant and/or 2) To sustain or support human life and/or 3) To diagnose, cure, mitigate, or treat disease or otherwise prevent impairment of human health; FDA-approval is required for investigation of significant risk devices, which include artificial skin, catheters, extended-wear contact lenses, prosthetic heart valves, and ventilators (**JAMA 1994; 272:955sc**) see Medical device Cf Nonsignificant medical device

SIL Squamous intraepithelial lesion, see there

silencer motif MOLECULAR BIOLOGY A 6-12 base pair segment of DNA present within the immunoglobulin light chain that binds to enhancer proteins, preventing upregulation (enhancer activity) of non-B cells

silent angina Silent ischemia, see there

silent carrier state The presence of a genotypic abnormality that is not detected in the phenotype, eg silent carrier state in α-thalassemia in which the defect in globin chain synthesis is so mild that it is inapparent Note: Crossing of a silent carrier with a person bearing the α thalassemia trait results in hemoglobin H

silent (myocardial) ischemia CARDIOLOGY Myocardial hypoxia that is not associated with the usual manifestations of crushing precordial anginal pain, which occurs in 15-30% of acute myocardial infarctions that have objective evidence of myocardial ischemia by EKG (ST-segment depression), radionuclide angiography or echocardiography, associated with coronary artery spasm (which may cause fatal arrhythmias even in absence of structural coronary artery lesions (**N Engl J Med 1992; 326:1451oa**) or atherosclerosis; ischemic silence has potentially grave consequences, as future hypoxia cannot be prevented TYPES OF 'SILENCE' **TRUE SILENT ISCHEMIA** The nociceptive pathways have a marked decrease in sensitivity to pain*, as occurs in DM, present in 10-20% of patients with both coronary artery disease and DM resulting in significant coronary artery spasms **PSEUDOSILENT ISCHEMIA** The patient either 1) Denies the pain, recognizing both its import, and that myocardial ischemia would have an immediate impact on his lifestyle or 2) Recognizes the pain but attributes it to something else, ie heartburn; patients with 'silent' ischemia have more significant three-vessel disease, more severe stenosis of the left anterior descending coronary artery and lower ventricular ejection fractions; they require coronary artery bypass or percutaneous transluminal coronary angioplasty (see PCTA) therapy 3-fold more often and have a 6-fold greater incidence of MI than those with typical ischemia; Cf Angina, Total ischemic burden

*Also known by the 'silent angina', a misnomer as 'angina' refers to pain

silent lesion 'Silent killer' A medical condition that may progress to very advanced stages prior to manifesting itself in the form of clinical disease or at the time of diagnosis; most silent killers are malignant, so named for their vague symptoms, and have often metastatized by the time of diagnosis; silent killers include ovarian cancer, in which there is a slow $\uparrow$ in abdominal girth, lower abdominal malaise and dyspepsia, carcinoma of the tail of the pancreas, brain tumors, especially of the frontal lobe and malignant melanoma, which may involute at the primary site using the best available screening tests (serum CA-125, and transvaginal sonography, TVS) for ovarian cancer (OC) produces a minimal $\uparrow$ of life expectancy, due to OC's $\downarrow$ prevalence in young $\female$ and $\uparrow$ laparotomy-related mortality and $\downarrow$ life expectancy in elderly $\female$ (**Ann Int Med 1993; 118:838oa**)

silent mutation Any mutation that does not cause a detectable phenotypic effect; since 95% of the DNA thus far sequenced does not encode proteins (commonly known as 'junk' DNA), silent mutations are 20-fold more common than those with detectable effects; as a further means of ensuring phenotypic fidelity, the 'degeneracy' of nucleic acid codons is such that point mutations may impact on multiple different codons, and may still be transcribed and translated into a correct amino acid; see Degenerate code, Same-sense mutation

silica SiO_2 The highly fibrogenic mineral form of silicon

silicon A gray-black semiconducting metal that is naturally present in silicates and which is used as 'doped' crystals in electronic semiconducting devices, eg COMPUTERS

silicon chip Chip COMPUTERS A wafer of silicon with electronic microcircuitry etched on its surface, comprising the 'highway' upon which information travels in a microprocessor, see Computers, Microprocessor

silicone A polymer composed of a repeating unit $-R_2Si-O-$ in which $-R$ is a simple alkyl group (a hydrocarbon); silicones can be produced in various forms, eg adhesives, sponges, solid blocks, and gels, and are widely used in medicine given their stability, water repellency, and inert nature; one formerly popular silicone, polydimethylsiloxane was enclosed in plastic bags of various sizes and shapes for use in plastic surgery to impart cosmetically acceptable contours to soft tissues, most commonly used in $\female$ for breast augmentation and in $\male$ for chin augmentation; the complications of such implants in trained hands are minimal and are confined to rupture of the bags and/or fibrosis; subcutaneous, often illicit, injection of silicone for breast enlargement without the enclosing bag (which may be performed in transsexual $\male$) may be associated with high fever, diffuse arthritis, renal failure, dry cough, hemoptysis, diffuse bilateral pulmonary infiltrates with patchy ill-defined airspace consolidaton, acute pneumonitis, hypoxemia, alveolitis (alveolar macrophages with silicone inclusions, neutrophils, eosinophils), $\downarrow$ pulmonary function ($\downarrow$ total lung and ventilatory capacities, forced expiratory volume and PO_2) and granuloma formation; see Breast implants, Human adjuvant disease

silicone arthroplasty The implantation of prosthetic articulations contructed of silicone* to replace joints damaged by arthritis, avascular necrosis, trauma, or used as spacers in certain procedures, eg Keller's bunionectomy; since the first reports of clinical success (**AB Swanson Surg Clin North Am 1968; 48:1113**), hundreds of thousands of silicone implants have restored function to hands, wrists, shoulders, feet, and temporomandibular joints LOCAL COMPLICATIONS Breakage and breakdown, dendritic synovitis or osteolysis, infection, loosening, multinucleated giant cell reaction, and erosion through soft tissues and skin SYSTEMIC COMPLICATIONS Acute pneumonitis, delirium, fever, granulomatous hepatitis, ITP, lymphadenopathy, malaise, progressive systemic sclerosis, renal and respiratory failure, scleroderma, SLE (**Am J Clin Pathol 1992; 98:594oa**)

*Silicone rubber (polydimethylsiloxane) is a polymer of carbon, oxygen, hydrogen, and silica, the polymer chain length is directly proportional to viscosity of liquid silicone; polymer chain cross-linking results in rubber-like solids; the earliest prosthetic devices were relatively inflexible and are subject to fractures with pathological lesions developing in the periarticular tissues; high-performance silicone implants have more bounce to the ounce, and are susceptible to breakdown

silicone elastomer Silastic™ A solid but frangible material that is shed from various implanted materials (eg breast implant, prosthetic joint) or indwelling devices (eg hemodialysis tubing) which are composed in part or entirely of silicone (Am J Clin Pathol 1995; 103:466oA)

silicone implant A generic term for a FDA class 3 medical device composed primarily of silicone or silicone gel, including gel– and saline filled breast implants, and gel-filled chin prostheses, testicular implants, and Angelchik reflux valves, as well as penile implants (JAMA 1992; 267:2578MN&P) see Breast implant, Human adjuvant disease, Medical device

silicone liquid Silicone oil A material used as an antifoaming agent used in cardiopulmonary bypass surgery, which may undergo hematogenous spread to virtually any organ, the long term consequences of which are unknown (Am J Clin Pathol 1995; 103:466oA)

siliconoma A colloquial term for relatively circumscribed tissue response to extravasated silicone, which is accompanied by a foreign body-type giant cell reaction, histiocytes, and bright refractile silicone crystals

silicosis OCCUPATIONAL MEDICINE A form of pneumoconiosis caused by exposure to silica dust (potteries, foundries, sand pits, construction sites, and so on) from quartz and flint; it is associated with emphysema, compromised respiratory function and pulmonary fibrosis; it is thought that silicosis ↑ susceptibility to TB RADIOLOGY Bilateral symmetrical interstitial fibrosis, hilar lymphadenopathy with 'eggshell' calcification; unlike asbestos, it is a non-manufactured product, has received less media attention than asbestos and its workers less financial compensation for undue exposure PATHOLOGY Lymph nodes demonstrate an onion skin-like layering of collagen

silk SURGERY An animal (silkworm) protein-based absorbable suture material, which is favored by many surgeons due to its superior handling characteristics; with time silk loses its strength and thus is not used in for prosthetic devices, eg Teflon vascular grafts or prosthetic heart valves which require permanent sutures; as silk is multifilament, it may serve as a 'sanctuary' for bacteria, which may 'spit' to the skin surface; Cf Catgut

silo-filler's disease Silo-filler's lung OCCUPATIONAL MEDICINE A toxic gas-induced pneumonitis and bronchiolitis caused by inhalation of nitrogen oxides in freshly filled grain silos, often coupled to asphyxia; once grains are in storage, plant nitrates are fermented by microbes to NO_2 and N_2O_4, peaking 1-5 days after storage; nitrogen dioxide reaches the terminal airways, forming highly irritating nitrous and nitric acids, causing a chemical pneumonitis and massive pulmonary edema CLINICAL Cough, light headedness, dyspnea, cyanosis, hemoptysis, choking; forms of presentation include 1) Collapse and sudden death 2) Acute alveolar damage with pulmonary edema 3) Early and reversible bronchiolitis obliterans and 4) Late and irreversible bronchiolitis obliterans DDx Mycotoxicosis, an allergic reaction, see 'Animal House' fever, Farmer's lung TREATMENT High doses of corticosteroids may prevent the bronchiolitis obliterans common in heavily exposed survivors

Note: A similar condition occurs in ice hockey players (JAMA 1990; 263:3024c)

Silver Spring monkeys A colony of primates used by a grant-funded psychologist for research related to rehabilitation of stroke victims, which required total denervation, performed on the monkeys by dorsal rhizotomy; because animals treat their own deafferented limbs as foreign, they chewed off fingers and/or removed bandages; after allegations of cruelty to the monkeys and unsanitary conditions

(Nature 1991; 351:93c), the local police removed the animals to protective custody; the monkeys became a rallying point for animals' rights activism; although the researcher had his animals returned and all the charges against him were dismissed, the research was suspended

Note: As of 1991, the last two monkeys of the original 17 Silver Spring monkeys seized by the police were aging, alive and still providing data on renervation phenomena (Science 1991; 252:1857, 1789n&v)

Silver-Russell dwarfism Russell-Silver syndrome A clinical complex of unknown pattern of inheritance, which is attributed by some authors to an absence of insulin-like growth factor II, causing intrauterine growth retardation, hemihypertrophy, low birth weight and height, increased urinary gonadotropins (with resultant precocious puberty), occasional cafe au lait-type pigmentary changes, incurved fifth finger, syndactyly of toes, triangular face and pouting mouth; 10% develop Wilms' tumor TREATMENT Growth hormone

silver wire appearance A descriptor for the fundoscopic appearance of the arteries in grade IV arteriosclerotic retinopathy, in which the arterial wall becomes completely opaque so the blood column is not seen and the light is completely reflected, yielding a white 'line', likened to a silver wire, regardless of whether the lumen is occluded; patency of the vessel is best determined by fluorescein angiography; Cf Copper wire appearance

simian crease Simian fold A dermatoglyphic pattern seen as a single deep transpalmar crease formed by the fusion of the proximal and distal palmar creases, classically seen in trisomy 21, that may also occur in trisomies 13 and 9, and fetal trimethadione syndrome; see Dermatoglyphics; Cf Triradius

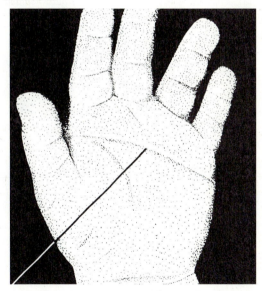

simian crease

simian immunodeficiency virus see SIV

simian virus 40 see SV-40

SIMM Single in-line memory module COMPUTERS An add-on memory board used in the Macintosh family of microcomputers to increase the random access memory (RAM), up to 128 megabytes or more, an amount required for complex molecular modeling; see Computers, RAM

Simplified Acute Physiology Score see SAPS II

simulator sickness Cybersickness, see there

simvastatin Zocor™ An HMG-CoA reductase inhibitor used to treat patients with primary hypercholesterolemia LABORATORY ↓ Total cholesterol, ↓ LDL-cholesterol, ↓

triglycerides, ↑ HDL-cholesterol; see Cholesterol-lowering drugs, Gemfibrozil, HMG-CoA reductase inhibitors

simvastatin

'sin' tax A colloquial term for any direct or indirect tax levied on 'pleasure poisons'*, eg alcohol and tobacco (**Am Med News 12 October 1992 p41**)

*After the German, Genüßgifte

Sindbis virus A mosquito-borne enveloped alphavirus that has a single-stranded RNA genome that is widely distributed in the native form in Africa, Asia, and Eastern Europe, and which can be engineered to express the bacterial protein CAT (chloramphenicol transferase) in various cultured animal cells

SINE Short interspersed repeated elements, see there

sine wave Sinusoidal waveform A waveform of periodic oscillations (eg in alternating current) in which the amplitude of each point in the wave is proportional to the sine of the time from the initiation point CARDIOLOGY An EKG finding described in severe hyperkalemia where the 'P' wave disappears and the QRS complex and 'T' wave merge in an oscillating pattern; a sine wave therefore constitutes a medical emergency, requiring immediate therapy, both short-term (calcium gluconate, sodium bicarbonate and glucose infusion) and long-term (cation-exchange retention enema)

Singer-Nicholson model Fluid-mosaic model, see there

singer's node Laryngeal polyp A non-inflammatory stromal reaction common on the anterior to middle third of the vocal cord, which is caused by phontrauma, and seen in those who misuse their voices, eg singers, disk jockeys, often in the exercise of their profession PATHOLOGY Edema and myxoid degeneration of subepithelial tissue Note: The lesion has no premalignant potential; Cf Noise-induced hearing loss

single breath imaging see Spiral computed tomography

single copy DNA Non-repetitive DNA A unique sequence of DNA that occurs only once in a haploid genome, which correspond to structural genes and introns

single disease hospital A health care facility serving patients suffering from a disease with no known therapy; single-disease hospitals had been built for leprosy, tuberculosis (for which the number of sanatoriums and hospitals in the US peaked in 1925 at 536 facilities) and mental illness (from 1880 to 1950); as therapy becomes available, single disease hospitals lose their raison d'etre and close; in AIDS, 4% of all US hospitals provide care for 32% of all AIDS patients, raising the question of whether 'AIDS-only' hospitals may serve a function; historically, patients in single-disease facilities receive sub-optimal care since often the only change in their status was death; see Saranac

single donor transfusion(s) A form of 'directed donation' consisting of the repeated administration of a particular blood component (eg plasma, platelets) from the same donor to a specific recipient who may have a special need, eg formation of antibodies to a 'public' antigen; see Directed donation; Cf Single unit donation

single gene disorder A genetic disease caused by a mutation in one gene, eg autosomal dominant polycystic kidney disease, familial polyposis coli, Huntington's disease (for ethical issues see **JAMA 1994; 272:875OA**)

single letter designation A simplified coding system for amino acids, that is an expediency to minimize the printed space dedicated to amino acid sequences in journal articles; see Amino acids

AMINO ACID ABBREVIATIONS	
A	Alanine
B	Arginine/Aspartic acid
C	Cysteine
D	Aspartic acid
E	Glutamic acid
F	Phenylalanine
G	Glycine
H	Histidine
I	Isoleucine
K	Lysine
L	Leucine
M	Methionine
N	Asparganine
P	Proline
Q	Glutamine
R	Arginine
S	Serine
T	Threonine
V	Valine
W	Tryptophan
Y	Tyrosine
Z	Glutamine/Glutamic acid

single-parent family SOCIAL MEDICINE A family unit containing the mother or father and unmarried children; accumulating data appear to support a widely held belief that progeny of SPFs have disadvantages in terms of education, future earning potential, and success in marital relationships; see Latchkey children, Quality time; Supermom; Cf Extended family, Nuclear family, Two parent advantage

single-payer system HEALTH CARE REFORM A generic term for any system in which all the costs of health care are reimbursed by a monolithic entity, eg the government; consumers typically pay a uniform tax rather than a premium and the money goes toward a health care trust fund that is used only for health-related expenditures (**JAMA 1994; 272:1101C**) an SPS is a key component of socialized medicine

single photon emission computed tomography see SPECT

single-strand conformation polymorphism analysis MOLECULAR DIAGNOSTICS A screening method that can be combined with PCR for rapid non-radioactive detection of point mutations in p53 (tumor-suppressing gene), *ras* (an oncogene), and others and can be used for direct typing of HPV genotypes

single unit transfusion TRANSFUSION MEDICINE A therapeutic 'agent' that has long been controversial, since if a single unit of packed cells suffices as therapy, it is thought by some workers that the transfusion may not have been indicated at all; SUTs were once popular as 'tonics' for older patients with low-grade anemias, most of whom respond to iron supplements and vitamins; transfusion services generally frown upon SUTs, and without justification, an SUT represents malpractice; see Transfusion 'trigger'; Cf Single donor transfusion

sink-or-float test CLINICAL PHARMACOLOGY A crude and probably ineffective means for determining whether a metered-dose inhaler (MDI) continues to delivery its specified therapeutic inhalant; the SOFT consists of placing the MDI in water; if it floats after a blast, it works, if it doesn't, it doesn't (**JAMA 1993; 269:1506L**) see Metered-dose equivalent

sink testing LABORATORY MEDICINE The illegal and unethical practice of providing falsified analytical results on clinical specimens, eg vials of blood, urine specimens that were deliberately thrown away, ie down the sink

sinobronchial syndrome Kartagener syndrome; see Cilia

sinus histiocytosis A nonspecific term for an ↑ in the number of (benign) histiocytes in the peripheral and medullary sinuses of lymph nodes; Cf Sinus histiocytosis and massive lymphadenopathy

sinus histiocytosis with massive lymphadenopathy

Rosai-Dorfman disease A clinical condition most common in young blacks, characterized by massive bilateral cervical lymphadenopathy (¼ of cases of SMHL are extranodal, affecting periorbital tissues, upper respiratory tract, skin, and CNS, but do not involve the bone marrow or spleen), fever, leukocytosis, ↑ ESR, polyclonal hyperimmunoglobulinemia PATHOLOGY The lymph nodes are matted, yellow with effaced architecture and display florid sinusoidal infiltration by histiocytes that are positive by the immunoperoxidase stain for S-100 PROGNOSIS Uncertain; most cases resolve spontaneously; some cases may be aggressive, and ultimately fatal; Cf Sinus histiocytosis

sinus of Morgagni syndrome Trotter syndrome, see there

sips/chips NURSING A colloquial term for the first ingestibles that are allowed either after a surgical procedure under general anesthesia, or before and after surgery 'under local', where the recuperee is allowed to sip water and other clear liquids or chew on chips of ice (MLO April 1995)

SIR Silent information repressor MOLECULAR BIOLOGY A protein that suppresses transcription of silent DNA copies at the mating locus of a haploid yeast gene

sirenomelia Mermaid syndrome A heterogeneous dysplastic complex that may be inherited (caudal regression syndrome) or teratogenic in nature, which is characterized by fusion (symmelia) of the lower extremities with external leg rotation, musculoskeletal atrophy and clubfoot, as well as other anomalies, including imperforate anus, unilateral or bilateral agenesis of the kidneys and/or genitalia, focal agenesis of the lumbosacral spine and various viscera Note: Some anomalies may be incompatible with life

sirolimus Rapamycin* A macrolide agent with immunosuppressive activity; it is structurally similar to tacrolimus (FK506) but has different properties, acting to suppress B and T cell proliferation, lymphokine synthesis and T cell response to IL-2; the desired immunosuppressive response with rapamycin is achieved at levels ⅛ of the levels required of tacrolimus and 1/100 the levels of cyclosporine; it may work well in combination with cyclosporine, but not with tacrolimus, as both bind to the same protein isomerase (N Engl J Med 1994; 331:1154oA) see Cyclosporine, Tacrolimus

*Isolated from a soil fungus on Rapa Nui on the Easter Islands

SIRS 1) Soluble immune response suppressor 2) Subcutaneous insulin-resistance syndrome, see there

SIRS Systemic inflammatory response syndrome A term that *'was developed to imply a clinical response arising from a nonspecific insult and includes two or more of the following:*

1) Temperature > 38°C or < 36°C

2) Heart rate > 90 beats/min

3) Respiratory rate > 20 breaths/min or a pCO_2 < 32 mm Hg

4) WBC count > 12 x 10^9 or < 4 x 10^9, or the presence of > 0.10 immature neutrophils

Based on the conclusions of a consensus conference (see table), SIRS is regarded as part of a continuum of a biologic inflammatory response to infection which evolves toward sepsis, severe sepsis (sepsis syndrome), and sep-

tic shock; as SIRS progresses through the continuum increasing proportions had ARDS, DIC, acute renal failure, and shock (JAMA 1995; 273:117oA) see Sepsis, Septic shock, Severe sepsis

sis An oncogene isolated from the simian sarcoma virus, which is present in human cells as a proto-oncogene, and encodes platelet-derived growth factor-like protein, SIS, which evokes proliferation of smooth muscle cells, epithelial cells and fibroblasts, providing a link between normal growth-controlling pathways and the unregulated growth of cancer cells

sister Nurse (British), in particular a head nurse

The term derives from the traditional role played by nuns (sisters) of the Catholic (and other) churches as caregivers to the dying and infirm; once used in the entire English-speaking world, this particular non-religious use of the term sister is waning in popularity

sister chromatid(s) A pair of metaphase chromosomes or nucleoproteins that are joined at a centromere

sister chromosome exchange analysis GENETICS A technique used to monitor environmental damage resulting from increased exposure to chemicals, toxins and ultraviolet light, which consists in a dark repair of thymine dimers, where undamaged segments are exchanged for damaged segments between homologous duplex molecules; sister chromatid exchanges are increased in chromosome breakage syndromes, eg Bloom syndrome and in cells from normal individuals when exposed to chromosome damaging conditions; Cf Ames test, Chromosome breakage syndromes

Sister Mary Joseph nodule A non-ulcerating periumbilical nodule that is metastatic from an adenocarcinoma of the stomach, colon, ovary or pancreas, which may be the first mass detected in gastric carcinoma, and is a marker for a poor prognosis; 20% remain of unknown origin at the time of autopsy

Sister Mary Joseph was the superintendent of St Mary's Hospital in Rochester, Minnesota and as Dr WJ Mayo's surgical assistant was credited with recognizing the poor prognosis of this lesion

Sisyphus 'syndrome' PSYCHIATRY A mental characteristic of a stress-driven type 'A' person, who obtains no gratification from accomplishing the difficult goals he places upon himself; see 'Anal-retentive', 'Toxic core', Type A personality

The complex is named after Sisyphus of Greek mythology who angered Zeus and was made to continuously roll a boulder up a hill; each time he came close, but never quite made it to the top

SIT Serum inhibition titration test Schlichter test A serial dilution assay for determining both the optimal antibiotic and its proper dose in treating certain bacterial infections; see MIC (minimum inhibitory concentration)

site-directed mutagenesis CELL PHYSIOLOGY An experimental technique in which amino acids are substituted in a protein of known function to determine the location of a particular activity, eg receptor binding or ion channel activity

sitophobia Fear of eating due to the unpleasant symptoms of nausea, vomiting and abdominal pain that occur after eating; sitophobia is characteristic of chemotherapy-induced anorexia, and may occur in Crohn's disease and chronic mesenteric artery insufficiency, and differs from anorexia nervosa as there is an appetite, but it is curtailed by the anticipated emesis and nausea

situational depression Reactive depression

SIV Simian immunodeficiency virus A primate lentivirus that is morphologically and biologically related to HIV-1 and HIV-2; SIV and HIVs have a lentiviral morphology, tropism for CD4 lymphocytes and macrophages and use the CD4 molecule for a receptor, extra genes (*tat, rev, vip, vpr* and *nef*) that are not found in other retroviruses, typical cytopathologic changes and

SIRS (Systemic Inflammatory Response Syndrome)

	SEPSIS	SEVERE SEPSIS	SEPTIC SHOCK
Progression from SIRS	26%	18%	4%
Positive blood cultures	17%	25%	69%
Mortality (SIRS = 7%)	16%	20%	46%

American College of Chest Physicians-Society of Critical Care Medicine Consensus Conference. Definitions for sepsis and organ failure and guidelines for the use of innovative therapies in sepsis (Crit Care Med 1992; 20:864)

the ability to cause chronic disease after a long latency period; the study of AIDS may be facilitated by the recently identified clone SIV_{MAC239}, which produces an AIDS-like disease in monkeys; SIVs naturally infect some nonhuman primates, eg African green monkeys, and sooty mangabeys with causing immunodeficiency, while in others, eg macaques, SIV causes an AIDS-like chronic wasting syndrome; SIV from captive macaques (SIV_{MAC}) is most closely related to HIV-2, and may transiently infect laboratory workers (designated SIV_{HU}) (**N Engl J Med 1994; 330:172oA**) see Retroviruses, SAIDS; Cf HIV-1, HIV-2

Six Cities Study ENVIRONMENT A study that links exposure to fine particulate (≤ 10 μm) pollutants and particles from the combustion of fossil fuels (including carbon, hydrocarbons, dust, acid aerosols, and sulfates) to an ↑ in mortality due to COPD, asthma, and cardiovascular disease, estimated to cause an excess of 60 000 deaths/year (**Sci Am 1993; 269/5:23**)

sixth disease Exanthem subitum, aka roseola infantum; Cf Fifth disease, Seven-day disease

sixth venereal disease Lymphogranuloma venereum, see there

size acceptance Pertaining or relating to a philosophical stance in which a person's increased girth or berth is accepted or even sought; those who seek bulky friends or partners have been colloquially designated as FAs (fat admirers) or chubby chasers (**NY Newsday 29 Nov 1994, A53**) see Politically correct

ska The gene that encodes streptokinase, a virulence factor that enhances the spread of bacteria; *ska* contains 2 variable regions, V1 and V2 (**Arch Pathol Lab Med 1994; 118:1160A**)

skeletal repair system see Bone paste, Dahllite

skewed lyonization A nonrandom pattern of X-chromosome inactivation (lyonization) that may occur in up to 25% of female subjects (**N Engl J Med 1994; 331:154oA**) see Lyonization

'skimming' HEALTH CARE INDUSTRY A form of 'reverse dumping', in which insurance companies actively enroll, and hospitals actively seek the healthiest, wealthiest, and best-insured segment of the population, since healthy people are less likely to use the services for which they are paying, and the wealthy usually pay their bills; skimming thus ↑ profits for insurance companies and health care facilities (**N Engl J Med 1988; 319:1086**) Cf Dumping, Red-lining

'skimping' HEALTH CARE INDUSTRY Delaying or denial of services to members of a prepaid or 'capped' health plan as a means of controlling costs (since the monies received by the health plan remain constant, providing 'extra' services is more costly to the plan), eg delaying cataract surgery or reducing the frequency of costly procedures to levels below those considered appropriate by other practitioners and health care facilities; see Capitation

skin adnexal tumor Skin appendage tumor SURGICAL PATHOLOGY A family of tumors derived from the primitive ectoderm, which develops into eccrine and apocrine sweat glands, sebaceous glands and hair follicles; most SATs are benign, eg eccrine cylindroma, keratoacanthoma syringoma, trichoepithelioma, although malignant SATs are not uncommon and include extramammary Paget's disease, sweat gland carcinoma PROGNOSIS Most SATs are adequately treated with wide local excision

skin-associated lymphoid tissue SALT The lymphoid tissues of the skin in which the Langerhans' cell, responsible for processing antigens, plays a key role; see Bronchiole–, Gut–, and Mucosa–associated lymphoid tissue; Cf MALT lymphoma

skin cancer A generic term for any malignancy of the skin, which is often divided into non-melanoma SCs (usually basal cell carcinoma, which comprises the majority, and

squamous cell carcinoma), which are common (from 400 000 to one million new cases/year) but relatively innocuous (± 2700 deaths/year) and melanomas, which are relatively rare (± 34 000 new cases/year) but highly aggressive (± 7000 deaths/year)

skin graft Autologous skin, donated skin or surrogate skin that is removed from one body site and used to cover skin surfaces with third-degree burns, which may originate from another site on the 'donor' (ie autograft), from another member of the same species (ie autograft), or from a different species (xenograft); one innovation in covering burn wounds is culturing of the patient's own cells into confluent sheets of keratinocytes to cover exposed areas; despite the theoretical advantages, autologous skin may not 'take', due to the lack of type IV collagen 7-S basement membrane binding sites and anchoring fibrils; see Split thickness graft; Cf Artificcial skin, 'Spray-on' skin

skin 'popping' SUBSTANCE ABUSE Lubrication of needles with oral secretions prior to intradermal injection of narcotics; the resultant subcutaneous abscesses may be infected with *Eikenella corrodens*, an inhabitant of the oral cavity; Cf 'Pocket shot'

skin tag Acrocordon Fibroepithelial polyp DERMATOLOGY A benign polypoid skin tumor that is more common in adults, may first appear as multiple lesions during pregnancy or as an epiphenomenon of malignancy of undetermined significance

skin window of Rebuck IMMUNOLOGY An in vivo method for studying host response to antigenic stimuli, in which a sterile glass coverslip is placed over superficially abraded skin; after 3-4 hours, most of the cells picked up on the coverslip are neutrophils; at 12 hours, 'round' cells, eg lymphocytes, plasma cells and monocytes and at 24 hours, monocytes and macrophages

'skinny' needle A 22-gauge needle used for percutaneous, often radiologically guided biopsies or aspiration cytology specimens obtained from radiologically-identified masses of the breast, lung and sites of difficult access; when positive, skinny needle biopsies avoid the co-morbidity associated with open biopsies; contrarily, negative results may result from sampling errors and should be followed by open biopsy if the lesion is suspected as potentially malignant

Note: Small-bore needles are 20-22-gauge; large-bore needles are 14-18-gauge; see Interventional radiology

'skip' lesion Any lesion in which normal, ie pathologically not involved, tissue is interspersed with tissue affected by the pathological condition; skip lesions are described in 1) Metastatic malignancy, see below 2) Polyarteritis nodosa, referring to the interspersed 'skipping' or sparing of vessels and 3) Crohn's disease, referring to the interposition of the involved (and uninvolved) segments of the terminal ileum that are separated from segments of relatively normal small or large intestine, seen both radiologically and by gross examination Note: The 'characteristic' skip lesions occur in only 20-25% of Crohn's disease

skip metastases The metastatic spread of a malignancy in which contiguous regions are skipped, while distant foci of malignant tumor are present, a finding that carries a poor prognosis; skipping is typical of lymphatic permeation of a lymphoproliferative disease, eg Hodgkin's disease; skipping is also described in rare cases of osteosarcomas with multiple discrete and separate tumor nodules in the same bone, but located at a distance; transarticular skipping of osteosarcoma may occur via the periarticular venous anastomoses

slab A block of gel used for an electrophoretic separation of proteins or nucleic acids

'slam bang' technology A colloquial term for any diagnostic or therapeutic modality with effects that are so dramatic in early clinical trials on small cohorts that the technology is readily accepted (eg renal lithotrypsy) without waiting for the usual lag period required to accumulate data from large cohorts

s-laminin NEUROPHYSIOLOGY A laminin-like protein present in the extracellular sheath surrounding myocytes that is thought to act as a homing signal for the ingrowth of regenerating motor neurons (s for synapse) it is synthesized by muscle cells, is concentrated in the synaptic basal lamina, and regulates the formation of motor nerve terminals (**Nature 1995; 374:258L**) see Laminin

the 'Slammer' US military slang for a Biosafety Level 4 containment hospital located at the Medical Research Institute of Infectious Diseases located at Fort Detrick, Frederick, Maryland; the facility is protected by air locks under negative pressure, double steel doors; the person who has been exposed to a BL4 pathogen (eg Ebola virus) is tended by nurses and physicians in space suits who closely monitor signs that the exposed person may 'crash'; the psychological impact of such enforced long-term 'isolation' may be considerable (**R Preston, The Hot Zone, Random House, New York, 1994**)

slant culture MICROBIOLOGY A bacterial culture that is grown on a solid (ie, agar-based) growth medium that has been poured in a test tube and allowed to solidify at a slanted angle; slant cultures are prepared with various chemical substrates, eg triple iron agar for the purpose of providing both aerobic (when the inoculum is 'streaked' on the agar surface) and anaerobic (when the inoculum is 'stabbed' deep into the agar) environments, allowing identification of specific reactions that are characteristic of a particular bacterial species

slanted palpebral fissures A characteristic facial anomaly seen in various congenital conditions, including Aarskog, Apert, Coffin-Lowry, Cohen, Conradi-Hünermann, DiGeorge, femoral hypoplasia-unusual facies, 5p-, Jarcho-Levin, Miller, Miller-Diker, Nager, Opitz-Frias, partial trisomy 10q, Pfeiffer, rhizomelic chondrodysplasia punctata, Rubenstein-Taybi, Säthre-Chotzen, Sotos, Treacher-Collins, trisomy 9 mosaic, trisomy 9p, trisomy 20p, XXXXX, and XXXXY syndromes

slapped cheek appearance A well-circumscribed, intense facial erythema of sudden onset that is followed by an erythematous maculopapular rash of the entire body, characteristic of 'fifth disease' (erythema infectiosum), due to parvovirus B19 (**N Engl J Med 1994; 331:1062ICM**); see Fifth disease, B19

Slavic type of Wilson disease A predominantly neurologic form of Wilson's disease of late (adolescent) onset with normal ceruloplasmin levels

SLE 1) St Louis encephalitis 2) Systemic lupus erythematosus; see Lupus erythematosus

sleep apnea syndrome Ondine's curse A condition clinically defined by frequent episodes of sleep apnea, hypopnea, and symptoms of functional respiratory impairment; it is potentially life-threatening, and has been associated with daytime hypersomnolence, motor vehicle accidents, and cardiovascular morbidity and mortality in the form of hypertension, stroke, and MI; it is more common in the obese and in heavy snorers; 2% of middle-aged ♀ and 4% of middle-aged ♂ meet the minimal criteria for sleep apnea syndrome (**N Engl J Med 1993; 328:1230OA**) PATHOGENESIS Marked alveolar hypoventilation during sleep (despite normal blood-gas levels while awake) due to a failure of autonomic ventilation, resulting in sleep apnea, as well as ↑ cardiac arrhythmias and hypertension; the condition most often affects the severely obese (due to tonsillar hyperplasia, relative micrognathia and central apnea, with loss of the ventilatory drive in the medulla), but may follow bilateral cordotomy in the cervical region, used to control intense midline or perineal cancer-related pain (through severance of the spinothalamic tract through a ventrolateral incision into the second cervical segment) or may rarely occur in infants; primary hypoventilation is secondary to a loss of CNS chemoreceptor response, which affects men, age 20-60; see Narcolepsy, REM sleep

Note: Ondine was a mythological water nymph who exhausted her human lovers; according to one victim, '...*all of the things my body once did by itself, it does now only by special command...I have to supervise five senses, two hundred bones, a thousand muscles...a single moment of inattention, and I forget to breathe...he died, they will say, because it was a nuisance to breathe*'—J Giraudoux, *Ondine*, 1939

sleep disorders A somewhat unwieldy term commonly being used for the field of 'dyssomnology', which is becoming a medical subspecialty practiced by 'clinical polysomnographers', who have divided sleep disorders into 1) Insomnias Disorders in initiating and maintaining sleep 2) Hypersomnias Disorders of excessive somnolence, eg narcolepsy, sleep deprivation and obstructive sleep apnea 3) Disorders of the sleep-wake schedule, eg jet lag and shift work and 4) Dysfunctions associated with sleep, sleep stages or partial arousals, eg night terrors and enuresis; see Insomnia, Pseudoinsomnia; Cf Shift work

sleep drunkenness A form of hypersomnia in which full alertness is not achieved for a prolonged period of time after awakening; SD is characterized by automatic behaviors, disorientation, drowsiness, and unsteadiness (**Mayo Clin Proc 1995; 70:591**) see Sleep apnea syndrome

sleep paralysis NEUROLOGY An odd paralytic phenomenon that occurs during the transition from the sleeping to the waking state in some otherwise healthy individuals, which is characterized by an inability to 'kickstart' their voluntary muscles, resulting in a transient 'locked in' syndrome; SP may be associated with narcolepsy, the pickwickian syndrome, or various forms of sleep apnea TREATMENT Most cases are isolated events and self-limited; if frequent and uncontrollable, clonipramine, desipramine, and may serve a prophylactic role

sleeping disease Narcolepsy

sleeping sickness Trypanosomiasis

slice RADIOLOGY Colloquial for a collimation scan interval in CT or equivalent in MRI

sliding filament model A model that explains muscle contraction as a telescope-like action, mediated by the hydrolysis of ATP, with the sliding of thick myosin filaments by means of pivoting (myosin) heads past the thin actin filaments; when viewed by electron microscopy, the muscle's A band decreases in thickness

sliding hernia One of two types of hiatal hernias of the esophagus, which is characterized by axial displacement of the esophago-gastric junction into the thoracic cavity through the esophageal hiatus, which, invested with its own peritoneal cloak, slides in and out of the thoracic cavity in response to changes in intra-abdominal and intrathoracic pressures

In contrast, the paraesophageal hiatal hernia is partially fixed at the fundus and the stomach 'rolls' into the chest, and when extreme, becomes an 'upside-down' stomach

slim disease The name for AIDS in Uganda, where clinical disease is characterized by extreme weight loss (hence, 'slim' disease), fever, a pruritic maculopapular rash, malaise, chronic diarrhea, respiratory infections and oral candidiasis; Kaposi sarcoma and lymphadenopathy are relatively less common than in the AIDS described in developed nations

'slip, slap, slop' DERMATOLOGY An abbreviated health care advisory of Australian origin for reducing the risk of ultraviolet light-induced skin damage and malignancy, where patients are advised to slip on a tee-shirt, slap on a hat and slop on some sunscreen

'slippery slope' A generic term for a trivial violation of a boundary (eg overt killing of a terminally ill patient or sexually inappropriate behavior by a physician) which would be regarded as far more serious when viewed in the context of a continuum (ie a 'slope') (JAMA 1995; 273:1445); SS has also been used as an adjective (eg slippery slope abuse) for an extreme boundary of an issue, the ethical impact of which has been incompletely explored, and which itself raises moral questions that are even more on the ethical 'edge' than the original issue; such a slippery slope occurs in the issue of physician-assisted suicide, where once one form of euthanasia were to become sanctioned or acceptable, society would be entering on a slippery slope of allowing the previously unthinkable, ie a healer to become killer

slit lamp OPHTHALMOLOGY A low-power microscope fitted with a specialized illuminating system for generating collimated light, which is used to examine the anterior segment of the eye, allowing visualization of transparent and nearly transparent ocular fluids; the slit lamp is of particular use in dendritic keratitis, foreign bodies of the cornea and in tumors of the iris

Sloan-Kettering affair 'Mouse incident', see there

slot blot analysis MOLECULAR BIOLOGY A rapid method for semiquantitating DNA (eg for detecting gene amplification) in a solution by electrophoresis, which differs from 'dot' blot analysis only in that the well in the agar is a 'slot' rather than a punched-out hole, a 'dot'; see 'Quick and dirty' method

'slow channel' calcium antagonists CLINICAL PHARMACOLOGY A family of drugs used to manage angina, which attenuate vascular contractility and resistance by reducing the entry of calcium into myocardial and vascular smooth muscle cells; SCCAs, eg verapamil, are most effective for Prinzmetal's vasospastic angina, but are also of use in angina pectoris; as some SCCAs may decrease myocardial contractility or AV conduction, these agents cannot be used with impunity in patients with concomitant congestive heart failure, bradycardia, or AV blocks

slow channel syndrome A neuromuscular dysfunction of early onset, characterized by weakness and atrophy of the proximal, cervical and shoulder girdle muscle groups, due to slow closure of acetylcholine receptor ion channels, resulting in prolongation of the end plate potential and accumulation of calcium in the post-synaptic region, where the excess calcium is 'toxic', destroying junctional folds and acetylcholine receptors

'slow code' BIOMEDICAL ETHICS A response to a call for emergency CPR (a 'code') in which the usual celerity in not exercised and the full therapeutic armamentarium is not utilized; 'slow codes' have emerged as a form by which a physician may bypass the paperwork required for a legally acceptable 'Do not resuscitate' order, when the patient is in a hopelessly terminal state and the physician believes that aggressive CPR efforts would be futile; see Advance directives, DNR, Euthanasia, Living will

slow-fast form of AVNRT Atrioventricular nodal reentrant tachycardia, see there

slow pathway CARDIOLOGY An anomalous conduction pathway in the heart that under normal circumstances has no known functions; the slow pathway provides the antegrade limb of the reentrant circuit in atrioventricular nodal reentrant tachycardia (AVNRT)–the fast pathway provides the retrograde limb ; this is thus known as the 'slow-fast' or common form of AVNRT; selective catheter ablation of the atrial end of the slow pathway eliminates AVNRT with little risk of AV block (N Engl J Med 1992; 327:313oA)

slow reactive substance(s) of anaphylaxis SRS-A, see there

slow-stroke syndrome Progressive ischemic stroke, see there

slow twitch fibers Red muscle, see there

slow virus Any of a group of viruses that may cause fatal infectious encephalitides after prolonged latency periods; slow viruses were formerly divided into conventional and unconventional viruses, a division that is no longer valid*; conventional slow viruses include measles, a paramyxovirus, which causes subacute sclerosing panencephalitis, rubella, which causes the rare progressive rubella panencephalitis and papovavirus, which causes progressive multifocal leukoencephalopathy; some soft data have implicated slow viruses in the pathogenesis of insulin-dependent (type I) DM and Paget's disease of the bone; slow viruses are usually inactivated by sodium hypochlorite (bleach), ethanol iodine and autoclaving; see Prions

*As unconventional 'viruses' are now recognized as a group of organisms composed entirely of subverted cell proteins known as prions

slow wave GI PHYSIOLOGY A spontaneous cyclical fluctuation in the transmembrane potential of smooth muscle, which is a function of the site, eg there are 3 slow waves/minute in the stomach and 14/min in the duodenum; the pacemaker for the cyclic activity appears to be the interstitial cells of Cajal; the wave is initiated by an influx of Ca^{2+}, resulting in a rapid depolarization of cells, followed by an efflux of K^+, giving rise to a partial repolarization and plateau stage; the repolarization of the cell becomes complete when C^{2+} reenters the smooth muscle cells (Sci & Med Nov/Dec 1994 p38)

SLPI Secretory leukocyte protease inhibitor *pronounced* Slippy A small protein found in saliva that by an unknown mechanism blocks the attachment of HIV's gp120 to the CD4 on the surface of monocytes; the possibility that SLPI may ultimately become part of the anti-HIV armamentarium is being actively pursued by Amgen Inc, Thousand Oaks, California (New York Times 7 Feb 1995; C3)

Note: The existence of some salivary factor had been long suspected as there are few documented cases of transmission of HIV via saliva

slush preparation TRANSPLANTATION An isotonic medium consisting of sterile saline solution crushed in ice, combined with lactated Ringer's solution; slush preparations are used to maintain the heart, lungs, kidneys, liver and other large organs destined for transplantation at the lowest possible metabolic rate (ie, the lowest possible temperature above freezing), while transporting them from the donor to the recipient; in the earliest stages of procurement, the icy slush is poured into the donor site (of a 'brain-dead' patient), cooling the organs to the maximum at the time of 'cross-clamping', at which time the organs are perfused with the so-called 'Wisconsin' solution; the slush solution is then transported with the organ to the recipient; see Procurement, UNOS, Wisconsin solution

Slutsky affair RESEARCH ETHICS Alleged misrepresentation of data that were published in a series of articles in peer-reviewed journals by a cardiologist in California; it has been suggested that at least 10% of the alleged perpetrator's publications were based on completely unreliable information (JAMA 1990; 263:1416) and ½ of the remainder were possibly invalid; see 'CV-weighing', 'Serious misconduct'; Cf Darsee affair

Sm antigen A non-histone protein which when stained by Sm antibodies has speckled pattern that is relatively specific for SLE

Sm antibodies Anti-Smith antibodies A family of antibodies that are relatively specific for SLE that react with polypeptides found in U1, U2 and U4/6 small nuclear ribonucleoproteins (snRNPs), which have a critical role in the splicing of pre-mRNA; Sm antibodies are present in 29% of cases of SLE and unlike antibodies to double-stranded DNA, do not increase with clinical exacerbation

of SLE; see Antinuclear antibodies

SMA Spinal muscle atrophy, see there

small airways disease A condition in which the airway obstruction is more attributed to the reduced luminal dimension than to inflammation (Arch Pathol Lab Med 1994; 118:969oa, 975oa) of infection; SAD is largely confined to the small airways or bronchioles (< 2 mm in diameter), initiated by inhaled irritants and thus is most common in smokers; it is accompanied by inflammation, hypersecretion, and lesions of the small airways, including fibrosis, ulceration, metaplasia and proliferation of smooth muscle fibers

Note: The functional changes of COPD may be due to small airways disease rather than chronic bronchitis

small 'blues' IMMUNOLOGY A technical artifact due to incomplete mixing of the specimens in histocompatibility testing, seen as acellular debris in the HLA test wells due to excess trypan blue mixed with protein, producing blue 'blobs'

small capacity syndrome One of the post-gastrectomy syndromes characterized by early satiation, which may result in significant weight loss and malnutrition; see Dumping

'small' cell A cell measuring 9-14 μm in diameter with a faint or indistinct rim of cytoplasm and an oval-to-elongated nucleus with relatively dense chromatin, thought to be of neuroendocrine origin, due to the presence of cytokeratin and secretory granules; when a vague 'crease' in the nucleus is also present, the descriptor 'oat cell' may be used; small cells are classically described in the small cell carcinoma of the lung, and may be seen in the bladder, breast, cervix, endometrium, nasopharynx, and elsewhere

Note: Non-epithelial lesions with small cells include sarcomas (Ewing sarcoma, rhabdomyosarcoma of alveolar and embryonal types, granulocytic sarcoma, reticulum cell sarcoma and liposarcoma), Wilms' tumor, neuroblastoma, lymphoma, plasmacytoma

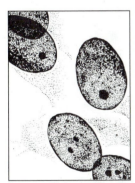 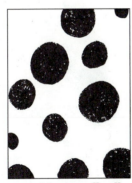

intermediate small cell   **oat-type small cell**
small cell carcinoma

small cell carcinoma A highly aggressive malignancy, usually of the lung that arises in the proximal bronchus and spreads early to the hilum and mediastinal lymph nodes MOLECULAR BIOLOGY Small cell carcinoma, like all malignancy, is a multigene event, in which recessive tumor suppressor genes are lost and oncogenes are activated and the chromosome defects include multiple genomic 'hits' including a 3p deletion* (3p(14-23) and/or translocations to chromosomes 17 and 8), a defective retinoblastoma gene (located in 13q14) and 17p deletions PATHOLOGY Small cell carcinoma of the lung is subdivided into intermediate cell and mixed cell (58%) types and lymphocyte-like (oat) cell type, which comprises the remaining 42%; these cells are 'decorated' by the immunoperoxidase method with antibodies to Leu-7, HNL-1 antigens, neuron-specific enolase and chromogranin TREATMENT

Combination chemotherapy (eg etoposide, cisplatin, cyclophosphamide, doxorubicin, vincristine) with chest irradiation results in 12-16 month median survival with limited disease; 5-year survival = 6-12% (N Engl J Med 1992 327:1435rv) higher initial doses of cyclophosphamide and cisplatin may improve survival (N Engl J Med 1993; 329:1848oa) radiotherapy evokes an objective reduction in tumor bulk in 80-90% of cases PROGNOSIS Without treatment, 3 month survival

Note: 3p changes also occur in 25% of non-small cell carcinomas

small cuff syndrome A form of pseudohypertension in which the cuff used to measure the blood pressure is disproportionately small and both the systolic and diastolic pressures are 'hypertensive'; Cf Pseudohypertension, White coat hypertension

small duct disease A severe painful form of chronic pancreatitis that may require subtotal (± 95%) pancreatectomy

small group reform HEALTH CARE REFORM A generic term for a set of regulations applied to insurers that sell policies to groups of 25-100 workers (ie small businesses) which are designed to make insurance available and affordable (Am Med News 25 October 1992, p7)

small left colon syndrome A rare cause of distal colonic obstruction, described in infants with abdominal distension, 40% of whom are offspring of type I diabetic mothers; the large intestine is small from the anus to the splenic flexure with normal ganglion cells, due to a transient delay in development

small meal syndrome A relatively constant clinical feature of chronic mesenteric ischemia in which dull, gnawing, or cramping periumbilical abdominal pain develops 10-30 minutes after eating; the pain gradually increases in severity, reaches a plateau and subsides within 1-3 hours; initially the pain only occurs with large meals and the patients may obtain some relief by assuming a prone position or squatting, but with increasing severity of the ischemia, becomes unbearable; it may be accompanied by bloating, flatulence, constipation, and diarrhea, and ultimately force its victims to eat minimalist rations (hence the name, small meal syndrome), resulting in significant weight loss

small nuclear ribonucleoprotein snRNP, see there

small parts standard PUBLIC HEALTH A series of mandates by the US Consumer Product Safety Commission, requiring that toys marketed to children under the age of three be free of small parts and other potential hazards, given the tendency of this age group to 'taste test' virtually all non-comestibles (JAMA 1991; 265:2848)

small vessel vasculitis An adverse cutaneous reaction to drugs characterized by palpable purpura, nodules, ulceration, and urticaria, 30-50% of which involve the GI tract, and may be accompanied by fever, neuritis, and glomerulonephritis (N Engl J Med 1994; 331:1272rv)

small round cell tumors of infancy A group of tumors* with overlapping histologic features that may require special studies, eg immunoperoxidase, ultrastructure, and in situ hybridization to delineate the cell of origin and the optimal therapeutic modality; see Ewing family of tumors, Ewing sarcoma

*Ewing sarcoma, neuroblastoma, rhabdomyosarcoma, NHL, and peripheral neuroepithelioma ('Askin tumor')

small stomach syndrome Early dumping syndrome, see Postgatrectomy syndrome

Small syndrome An AR [MIM 216350] variant of Coat's disease characterized by loss of visual acuity, nerve deafness, hypomimia, muscular dystrophy and mild mental retardation; it is thought by some authors that this represents a variant of facioscapulohumeral dystrophy with sensorineural hearing loss [MIM 227340]

smallpox MEDICAL HISTORY A 'conquered' disease of now historic interest; the variola virus probably appeared in the first agricultural settlements (10 000 BC) and typical lesions are present on the mummy of Ramses V (1160 BC); smallpox was well-established in post-Roman Europe and sailed with 'los conquistadores' to the New World, devastating native populations; E Jenner used vaccination, a technique of Turkish origin, to reduce smallpox's then-prevalent mortality of 20% to less than 1%; before vaccination, smallpox killed 500 000/year in Europe and caused ⅓ of acquired blindness; the last case occurred in Somalia in 1977 and the smallpox battle was declared as won by WHO Resolution 33.3 in 1980

Note: The remaining stock of the smallpox virus (held at the Centers for Disease Control in Atlanta and at the Research Institution for Viral Preparation in Moscow) has been scheduled (and re-scheduled) to be destroyed a number of times, most recently by Dec 31 1995 after the virus has been completely sequenced; (it had not been destroyed previously as both superpowers were concerned that the other might use the agent for biological warfare, **Nature 1991; 348:666**)

'smart' card MEDICAL RECORDS An identification card, often of credit card size, containing patient information ranging from 250 bytes of information (a 'dumb' card), allowing only simple identification to 2 megabytes of information, with large files; 'smart' cards are in the early implementation stage in some Japanese hospitals and will solve many of the problems inherent in the paper form of medical records

'smart chip' RISC chip, see there

'smart' terminal A computer terminal with its own central processing unit, allowing both input and output of data, thus having the capacity for free-standing operation; Cf 'Dumb' terminal

smiling face appearance Monkey face appearance A fanciful descriptor for the characteristic morphology of the trophozoite form of *Giardia lamblia*, in which the 'eyes' correspond to the nuclei

Smith-Lemli-Opitz syndrome A rare (1:20-40 000) AR [MIM 270400] condition characterized by severe multiorgan birth defects, with microcephaly, hypotonia, dysmorphic facies (short nose with anteverted nares, ptosis of eyelids, micrognathia), poly- and/or syndactyly, ♂ genital disorders (cryporchidism, hypospadias), endocrine defects, cataracts, cardiac and renal malformations, profound mental retardation, failure to thrive, and high infant mortality LABORATORY ↓↓↓ Cholesterol (< 5th percentile), ↑↑↑ (2000 x normal) cholesterol precursor 7-dehydrocholesterol (detected by gas chromatography) which may be incorporated into cell membranes, interfering with proper functioning thereof (**N Engl J Med 1994; 330:107OA**)

SML see Smoldering myeloid leukemia

smog Photochemical smog ENVIRONMENT An acronym of smoke and fog; smog has little in common with fog as smog results from the combustion of various, often synthetic materials with the production of noxious volatile byproducts; smog mortality ↑ substantially when smoke and sulfur dioxide (SO_2) levels exceed 750 µg/m³ CLINICAL Dyspnea, acute exacerbation of COPD; subjects exposed to smog may present with asthmatiform symptoms (wheezing and markedly ↑ respiratory effort) or if it is intense, marked cyanosis (PaO_2 < 50 mm Hg; $PaCO_2$ 50-100 mm Hg), congestive heart failure, COPD, and hypoxic cor pulmonale; see Air pollution, Bhopal, Clean Air Act, Pollution, Yokohama asthma

Note: Air pollution was first described in 1661 and elevated to an art-form by industrialization; the first major smog 'attack' occurred in the 1930s in Belgium's Meuse valley (63 inhalation deaths), caused by high concentrations of sulfur dioxide, sulfuric acid and fluorides; the December 1952 smog attack of London caused an ± 4000 excess deaths, attributed to sulfur dioxide; the most smog-laden cities in the world are Mexico City and Athens, in the US, Denver and Los Angeles

'smoke' ULTRASONOGRAPHY A haziness occasionally seen by transesophageal echocardiography in the left atrium, sign of blood stasis, fancifully likened to smoke, which correspond to the spontaneous presence of contrast; 'smoke' is associated with an ↑ in thromboembolism (**N Engl J Med 1992; 327:1570OA, ibid 1994; 331:1517ED**) Cf Atrial systolic failure, Moya-moya disease

smokeless cigarette A nicotine delivery product (Eclipse™) being tested by the RJ Reynolds tobacco company; the consumer lights a charcoal tip (rather than tobacco), eliminating the ashes and odor; heated air then passes through a cylinder containing processed tobacco and glycine; the SC is controversial as the tobacco industry argues that it is a cigarette and therefore exempt from FDA regulation, while health advocates regard it as a nicotine-providing device that would fall under the FDA's purview (**NY Newsday 29 Nov 1994, A17**) RJ Reynolds has had an unanticipated secondary problem with the SC which stems from the unwillingness of companies to supply components[1] for the device, in the fear that these companies might be named as co-defendants in lawsuits filed on the part of various plaintiffs[2] seeking restitution for the long term effects of cigarette smoking (**Business Week March 27, 1995, p39**)

[1] eg Glass fibers by Manville Inc.'s subsidiary, Schuller International Inc [2] eg The State of West Virginia, which is seeking to recover Medicaid money spent on treating smokers

SMOKELESS CIGARETTE

KEY TO COMPONENTS → Direction of air flow

A A layer of glass fibers insulate an activated charcoal heating element B Air passes through an aluminum foil-lined chamber packed with reconstituted tobacco to acquire nicotine C The heated air picks up tobacco flavor in a section

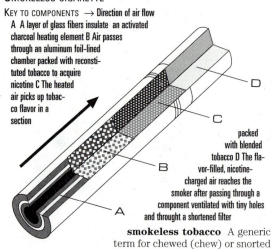

packed with blended tobacco D The flavor-filled, nicotine-charged air reaches the smoker after passing through a component ventilated with tiny holes and throught a shortened filter

smokeless tobacco A generic term for chewed (chew) or snorted (snuff) tobacco products that are regionally popular among athletes, the indigent, Native Americans, and tragically among children (up to 17% of 5 year-olds in certain regions have tried smokeless tobacco); 'chew' is used by an estimated 12 million Americans and is directly linked to oral cancer; 30 000 new cases of oral cancer occur annually in the US with 40% mortality

smoker A person who smokes tobacco, almost always understood to be a cigarette smoker Prevalence of smokers (1990) in various countries: Philippines, 64% of ♂ and 19% of ♀ were smokers, China 61/7, Saudi Arabia 53/2, Russia 50/12, Argentina 45/30, US 28/23; physician smokers are especially problematic, given their high visibility; in Canada, the UK and the US, ± 10% of physicians smoke; in contrast, in Beijing in China, 67.5% of ♂ physicians are smokers (from **Am Med News 3 October 1994**)

smoker profile The number of smokers internationally has increased by 75% in the last 20 years; 10^9 smokers consume ± 10^{12} cigarettes/year (**JAMA 1990; 263:3312**); the US per capita cigarette consumption rose from 54 in 1900 to 4500/year in 1968 and declined to 3200/year in 1988; the tobacco-industry 'loses' up to 2.5 million smokers/year, 2.1 million to health-related 'attrition', ie quitting, and 400 000 to smoking-related deaths; the peak age of initiation of habitual smoking is 16; in mainland China, 400/year were consumed in 1953 and 1900/year by 1988, a trend that has continued to increase, see Histogram EDUCATION 8.3% of physicians smoke (national average, 30%), under age 30, 4.5% of US physicians smoke; 18.4% of college-educated people are smokers, in contrast to 34.2% of high school drop-outs; smoking adolescents have a higher absentee rate, lower grade-point average and lower achievement test scores; the education-addiction disproportion is expected to accelerate; by the year 2000, 40% of high school dropouts will smoke versus 5% of college graduates RACE 34% of adult blacks are smokers, 28% of whites, 27% of hispanics (US)

smoker 'syndrome' see Smoking

smoking An addictive habit causing the most preventable form of cancer, lung carcinoma, which accounts for 25% of all cancer deaths; the annual lung cancer death rate has risen from $2/10^5$ in the 1930s to nearly $50/10^5$/year in 1985, translating into 152 000 new cases in 1988 and 139 000 deaths (US) ECONOMIC COSTS Direct costs due to smoking are ± $16 x 10^9/year, due to hospitalization, and the indirect costs, ± $35 x 10^9, due to lost productivity, earnings, disability, prematurity; the cost of smoking to the entire population is $200 per capita and by an arcane calculation, it has been estimated that one cigarette reduces life span by 5 minutes; smoking-related fires kill 1500/year and injure 4000/year (US); smokers suffer an excess mortality of ± 350-400 000/year

MALIGNANCY In addition to lung cancer, smokers have a 5-fold ↑ in laryngeal, oral and esophageal cancer; 30% of bladder cancer and 30% of pancreatic carcinoma may be smoke-related; there is a 1.5-fold ↑ in gastric, hepatobiliary, and renal cancers, and leukemias; there is a persistant ↑ in the risk of leukemia and myeloma for those who quit smoking later in life, implying the occurrence of a permanent malignant change in the stem cells HEART DISEASE Coronary artery disease, atherosclerosis, aortic aneurysm, cor pulmonale, strokes and infarcts

Note: The relative risk of MI of 3.6 in smoking ♀ declines and plateaus to 1.2 within 3 years of smoking cessation

NON-MALIGNANT DISEASE LUNG, eg emphysema, chronic bronchitis and ↑↑↑ (10-15-fold) incidence of interstitial fibrosis; other derangements seen in smokers include ALTERED DRUG METABOLISM and delayed absorption of alcohol GI TRACT Peptic ulcer, esophageal reflux, cirrhosis (which is possibly a statistical artefact, as smokers may also be alcoholics) Note: Some anecdotal reports imply that ulcerative colitis may be ameliorated by smoking HEMATOLOGY 4.8% of smokers have hematologic parameters that fall in a range of anemia, while 8.5% of non-smokers fall in the same range INFECTIONS The higher incidence of bacterial infection in smokers may be due to increased mucosal adherence of bacteria OBESITY Heavy smokers are more often obese than lighter smokers and in the face of abrupt smoking cessation, experience more intense cravings, implying that there may be a physiological difference in heavy smokers OSTEOPOROSIS and fractures of the wrist, hip and vertebrae, possibly related to reduced endogenous estrogens that occur in menopause, early lower levels of all estrogens in the luteal phase may explain why some series report a reduced incidence of breast cancer in smokers; for every 10-pack years of smoking history, bone density ↓ by 1-2% (**N Engl J Med 1994; 330:387OA**); smoking is also associated with osteonecrosis, ↓ estrogen (due to earlier menopause), ↑ serum sex-hormone-binding globulin (**N Engl J Med 1994; 330:430ED**) TOXINS Tobacco contains hundreds of toxins that act in concert to induce malignancy, with nicotine and tars being the most stongly implicated carcinogens, although ^{210}Polonium and α-radiation may play supporting roles LABORATORY Smokers have ↑ hematocrit, ↑

conicotine, ↑ albuminuria in type I diabetic smokers (**JAMA 1991; 265:614**), and ↓ HDL-cholesterol in children exposed to passive cigarette smoke LABORATORY ↑ FSH, ↑ LH, ↓ PTH, ↑ pyridinoline excretion, ↑ urinary hydroxyproline HEALTH BENEFITS Smoking has been paradoxically associated with a ↓ risk of idiopathic Parkinson's disease (**Science News 1994; 146:15**) by an unknown (possibly related to ↑ production of dopamine in the brain) mechanism, as well as an equally paradoxical ↓ risk of ulcerative colitis; despite 22 Surgeon General reports on the health consequences of tobacco dependence, thousands of research articles documenting the dangers of cigarettes, and more than 6 million deaths attributable to smoking since 1964, 50 million Americans continue to smoke; 70% want to quit, and 35% try each year (**JAMA 1992; 268:2687**) TOBACCO PROMOTION EXPENDITURES 1975 $491 x 10^6; 1981 $1547 x 10^6; 1988 $3274 x 10^6

smoking TEENAGERS Smoking has dropped in black teenagers from 25% (1979) to 4% (1993), in Hispanics from 22% to 12%, and in whites from 29% to 23% (stupid honkies) (**New York Times 19 April 1995, pC10**)

smoking cessation Cessation of cigarette smoking is followed by an average weight gain of 2.8 kg in men and 3.8 kg in women; 10-15% of ex-smokers gain 13 or more kg (**N Engl J Med 1991; 324:739**); most withdrawal therapies, eg hypnosis, psychotherapy, group counseling, exposing smokers to patients with terminal lung cancer and nicotine chewing gum are consistent only in their relative inefficacy; 10% of depressed and 18% of non-depressed subjects are able to quit and cessation in the severely depressed exacerbates the depression (**JAMA 1990; 264:1546**); see Chronic obstructive lung disease, Emphysema, Passive smoking, Smokeless tobacco

'smoking gun' A metaphor referring to the definitive confirmation of a cause-and-effect relation; in the legal system, the act of homicide can only be absolutely confirmed if the perpetrator is found alone with the victim(s), holding a 'smoking gun', a phrase adopted in medicine for determining the etiology of a disease, where the statistical strength and design of a study produces evidence so compelling, that the cause-and-effect relation is likened to that of a 'smoking gun'

'Smoky' The US Army code name for the test detonation of a thermonuclear device in August 1957 in which soldiers were intentionally exposed to radioactive fallout; two decades later, the participants were found to have a significant increase in the incidence of leukemia; the relation of radiation to polycythemia vera remains controversial; see Bravo; Cf Operation Ranch Hand

smoldering myeloid leukemia An indolent form of multiple myeloma that meets all the criteria of myeloma without producing significant anemia; a case may 'smolder' for 20 years, eventuating into osteolytic lesions, hypercalcemia and renal insufficiency, potentially with a survival of five or more years; smoldering leukemic conditions include preleukemia, refractory anemia with excess blasts (RAEB), and subacute myeloid leukemia; most cases arise from an established malignant clone and are accompanied by refractory 'cytopenias, and cellular dysfunction; 'smoldering' states have an indolent course with infections, hemorrhage and occasionally blast transformation; see Preleukemia

smooth muscle cell *Myocytus nonstriatus* **[NH3]** A muscle cell of certain viscera, eg GI tract, which is under the control of the autonomic nervous system; the actin and myosin filaments of SMCs are not organized in the same 'formal' fashion as striated (cardiac, skeletal) muscle, ie to form cross-striations; they are divided into two forms (see table), the activated (synthetic) and the contractile (quiescent) types; the activated form has been pathogenically linked to the restenosis of atheromatous coronary arteries

SMOOTH MUSCLE CELLS	ACTIVATED	CONTRACTILE
Smooth muscle myosin, α-actin	↓↓↓	↑↑↑
Thick filaments	Poorly-developed	Well-developed
Contractility in response to chemical or mechanical stimuli	Absent	Present
Cytokinesis	Present	Absent
Synthetic/proliferative capacity	Marked	Attenuated

from N Engl J Med 1993; 328:6080A

treated with angioplasty, identified by in situ hybridization using antisense probes complementary to the mRNA of the B isoform of nonmuscle myosin heavy chain (**N Engl J Med 1993; 328:603**0A)

smooth muscle antibodies IMMUNOLOGY IgM or IgG autoantibodies present in the serum of ± 60% of patients with chronic active (autoimmune) hepatitis, 30% of patients with primary biliary cirrhosis, and which may be transiently elevated in low titers in various viral hepatitides

SMR 1) Standardized mortality ratio 2) Sexual maturity rating, see Tanner stages

smudge cell HEMATOLOGY Red-purple nuclear debris with clumped chromatin and rounded nucleolar remnants, representing degenerated lymphocytes and nucleated erythrocytes (figure); Cf Basket cells; similar cells are characteristic of the karyorrhectic lymphocytes of acute and chronic lymphocytic leukemia LIVER PATHOLOGY A smudge cell is an enlarged basophilic hepatocyte replete with adenoviral particles PULMONARY PATHOLOGY Smudge cells are diffusely basophilic, streaked cytomegalovirus-infected alveolar and bronchial cells with an indistinct nuclear:cytoplasmic 'frontier' due to vacuolization of the nuclear membrane

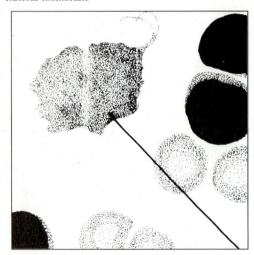

smudge cell

'snake oil' remedy HEALTH FRAUD Any of a group of substances that are claimed (without substantive evidence) to be effective in treating a wide variety of medical conditions; in the classic sense, these therapies were sold by 'quacks' in the late 1800s in the 'wild' western United States, prior to the stringent control of the pharmaceutical industry, which is currently operates under laws and regulations promulgated by the US Food and Drug Administration, and contained alcohol, herbs, narcotics and various other, often inactive, ingredients; see Food and Drug Administration, Pseudovitamins, Quackery,

Unproven cancer therapies

snake skin appearance see Cathartic bowel

snap PSYCHIATRY *verb* To suffer an abrupt decompensation in social or interpersonal coping mechanisms (colloquial)

sneaky mating ANIMAL BEHAVIOR The coupling of a low-ranking ♂ with a ♀ in a group of animals that differs fromt the typical hierarchal pecking order (high-ranking ♂ get the food, the attention, and sexual access to the ♀), which usually occurs in brief time-periods out the view of the highest ranking ♂; SMs are thought to have a survival advantage for the group, as they most commonly occur between a ♂ that is new to the group and a ♀ in the group (**Sci Am 1995; 272/6:29**)

Sneddon syndrome A condition characterized by the presence of fixed patchy livido reticularis and cerebral ischemia LABORATORY Phospholipid antibodies PATHOLOGY Leukocytoclastic vasculitis (**N Engl J Med 1994; 331:792**CPC)

sneeze An abrupt and involutary explosive expulsion of air from the lungs through the opened glottis into the nose and mouth which occurs in response to various irritants

sneezing gas A generic term for any substance that evokes sternutation

sniffer program COMPUTERS A program introduced in an electronic network, eg Internet that is capable of 'sniffing out' fixed passwords allowing an 'infothief' to bypass the only security measure that most computer users (of the PC genre) employ, ie the password

Sn-MP Tin-mesoporphyrin, see there

SNOMED Systematized nomenclature of medicine A nomenclature system used primarily by pathologists to describe, index, retrieve, and analyze disease-related information (**CAP Today March 1992**)

SNOP Systematized nomenclature in pathology

snore Snoring A harsh buzzing noise evoked in a sleeping person attributed to the vibration of a redundant or loose soft palate; snoring ↑ with age, and affects 60% of ♂ and 40% of ♀; it has been associated with a two-fold ↑ risk for high blood pressure, coronary ischemia and stroke, as well as alcoholism, arthritis, asthma, daytime drowsiness, depression, DM, insomnia, and obesity, but as an isolated symptom does not require treatment; snoring may be reduced by using a nasal dilating agent (**Arch Otolaryngol, Head Neck Surg 1990; 116:462**); see Obstructive sleep anpea syndrome; Cf Sleep disorders, Uvulopalatopharyngoplasty

Note: The loudest recorded snore is 88 dB

'snorting' SUBSTANCE ABUSE The preferred method for consumption of cocaine; the powder is placed in a spoon or on a horizontal surface, one nostril is held closed and the cocaine is 'sniffed', often with a drinking straw; with prolonged use, the nasal cartilage may perforate due to repeated ischemic episodes related to the intense vasoconstriction evoked by cocaine; Cf Cocaine, Crack

snowblindness The transient loss of vision caused by UV-light-induced damage to the cornea CLINICAL Tearing, conjunctival hyperemia, corneal clouding, superficial punctate keratitis TREATMENT Topical anesthetic, administered in the ER, homatropine drops, gentamicin, systemic analgesics

snow ball appearance A descriptor for the scanning electron micrographic appearance of the crystalloids seen in the synovial sediment of arthritic joints afflicted with basic calcium phosphate crystal disease(s); Cf Shiny coin appearance

'snowcap' sign ORTHOPEDICS A descriptor for a broad radiopaque band covering up to two-thirds of the articular surface in ischemic necrosis of the femoral head due to various conditions that compromise the epiphyseal vascular supply; after the initial structural failure causing a sclerotic 'snowcap', a thin subchondral fracture 'rim' appears as this portion of the femoral head collapses, giving rise to a 'step' formation; the snowcap is nonspecific and may occur in prolonged ischemia of the femoral head due to anemia, hemophilia, endocrinopathy, congenital disease, and malignancy

snowflake cataract A fanciful descriptor for punctate subcapsular lenticular opacifications that may rapidly evolve to a cataract in young patients with DM

snowman sign PEDIATRIC CARDIOLOGY A rounded, figure-of-eight-like cardiac contour seen on a plain anteroposterior chest film of infants with total anomalous drainage of the pulmonary veins accompanied by dilatation of the common pulmonary vein and supracardiac drainage; the unique contour is produced by the dilated left ventricle and superior vena cavae and left innominate vein; a similar appearance may be secondary to a prominent thymic shadow

Snow Mountain agent A Norwalk agent-like virus that evoked an acute shellfish-related miniepidemic of gastroenteritis that occurred at a ski resort, characterized by a 1-4 day duration, watery diarrhea, vomiting, and abdominal cramping (Am J Epidemiol 1987; 126:516)

snRNPs Small nuclear ribonucleoproteins A family of 100-300 nucleotide in length RNA molecules that form RNA-protein complexes in the eukaryotic nucleus, some of which are involved in RNA processing; the U series of snRNPs contains 2 classes of proteins; one class ('shared proteins') is found in all snRNPs, regardless of the U RNA species and consists of proteins designated as B, B', D, E, F and G; the second class, U ('unique') proteins are unique to snRNPs, and contain specific RNA, eg U1-U7 that may be autoantibody targets in lupus erythematosus

snuff A form of nonsmoking tobacco that is ingested by 'snorting' and delivers the same amount of nicotine; according to one estimate, a universal change in the form of tobacco consumed in the US (from cigarettes to snuff) could result in a drop from 400 000 tobacco-related deaths/year to 6000 (Science News 1994; 146:30 from JAMA 1 July 1994) see Smokeless tobacco, smoking

snuffbox Anatomic snuffbox, see there

snuffles PEDIATRICS Noisy breathing through a partially obstructed nasopharynx accompanied by profuse, mucopurulent and hemorrhagic nasal discharge containing viable *Treponema pallidum*, seen in infants with early congenital syphilis manifest as syphilitic rhinitis; snuffles have also been described with trisomy 21 (Down syndrome)

'snurposome' Spliceosome, see there

snurps see snRNPs

SNX-111 NEUROPHARMACOLOGY A formulation of omega-conotoxin (which is produced by some marine cone snails) that blocks the cascade of secondary neurochemical reactions, in particular the overproduction of glutamate and other neurotransmitters that follow acute cerebral ischemia; SNX-111 is reported to reduce the damage usually seen in animal models of head trauma, cardiac arrest, and stroke (NY Newsday 3 Jan 1995; B24) and has recently had currency in treating the pain of terminal malignancy; see Substance P

SOAP A mnemonic for the data that should be included in a problem-oriented medical record and in each entry in a patient's progress notes during hospitalization, including

SUBJECTIVE DATA, supplied by the patient or family

OBJECTIVE DATA, ie physical examination and laboratory data

ASSESSMENT, a summary of significant (if any) new data and

PLAN of diagnostic or therapeutic action

see Hospital chart, Medical record

soap bubble A commonly used adjective pertaining or referring to dilated smoothly-contoured cyst-like or ballooned, occasionally loculated space(s); see Physaliferous BONE RADIOLOGY An expansile, often eccentric, vaguely trabeculated space with a thin, sclerotic, sharply defined margin, characteristic of an aneurysmal bone cyst (lesions that are neither aneurysmal, nor true cysts, but rather are filled with blood and not invested with a coherent membranous lining); other bone lesions with soap bubble-like expansions include giant cell tumor, osteosarcoma, solitary bone cyst, non-ossifying fibroma, fibrous dysplasia, metastatic carcinoma, chondromyxoid fibroma, the 'combined' stage of Paget's disease of the bone, expansile mandibular lesions of cherubism, and metastatic renal cell carcinoma; the radiological finding of multiple 'punched-out' lytic lesions of bone, including multiple myeloma, angiosarcoma and ameloblastoma have also been described as soap bubble-like GI RADIOLOGY A descriptor for the physaliferous air spaces seen in an abdominal plain film in gas-producing bacterial abscesses MICROBIOLOGY A morphologic descriptor of *Pneumocystis carinii*; see 'Sealed envelope' appearance NEUROPATHOLOGY A descriptor for the microscopic appearance of *Cryptococcus neoformans* when stained with India ink, most prominent in the Virchow-Robin space

soap, calcium Calcium soap, see there

soap colitis Chemical colitis, see there

SOB Shortness of breath

SOB medium A bacterial growth medium designed to quantify bacteria in water, waste water, dairy products and foods, composed of NaCl, KOH and $MgSO_4$, bacto-tryptone and yeast extract

social anxiety disorder Social phobia, see there

social dilemma A situation in which a relatively small group of people attempt to provide themselves with the greatest common good in absence of central authority, the parameters of which can be formulated within the framework of game theory; the decisions made in a social dilemma may be quantifiable, often economic, where the parties involved act rationally, choosing the action that yields the highest payoff, or nonquantifiable, and less amenable to logical analysis, where human dynamics become critical, as in adversarial situations, or 'defection' from group cooperation (Sci Am 1994; 270/3:76) see Prisoner's dilemma, Unscrupulous diner dilemma

'social disease' A euphemism of waning popularity for sexually-transmitted disease, see there

social drinker A person who consumes alcoholic beverages in moderation, ie two or less 'standard drinks', often in a socially acceptable situation; see Alcohol; Cf Binge drinker, Problem drinker

social history A summary of life-style practices (eg diet, exercise, sexual orientation), occupation, and habits (eg smoking, abuse of alcohol or other substance) that may have a direct or indirect effect on a person's health; Cf Family history

social medicine A field of medicine that studies the impact of the collective behavior of organized society on individuals belonging to various, often disadvantaged subgroups within the society; see Engel's phenomenon, Homeless(ness), Latchkey children, Supermom; Cf Socialized medicine

Social & Occupational Functioning Assessment Scale PSYCHIATRY A scale derived from the Global Assessment of Functioning Scale, which focuses on a person's level of social and occupational functioning, but differs from the GAF as it is not directly influenced by severity of his/her psychological symptoms; a SOFAS score of 100 is given if there is superior functioning in a wide range of activities, 70 is given if there is some difficulty in social, occupational, school functioning

social phobia Social anxiety disorder PSYCHIATRY *'A marked and persistent fear of social and performance situations in which embarassment may occur ...(and)...take the form of a situationally bound or ...predisposed Panic Attack*; while social anxiety is normal in children, in adults, this fear is excessive or unreasonable; the social or performance situation is avoided, or endured with dread; see Panic attack

Social Security Amendments of 1983 The federal legislation that provided for the implementation of the current US health care reimbursement system in which payments are based on diagnosis-related groups (DRGs); the reimbursement is divided into a 'service' component, ie hospital-related costs, known as 'part A' and a 'professional' or physician component, known as 'part B', controlled by peer and utilization review; see DRGs, Part A, Part B

'social worth' MEDICAL ETHICS The value of a person's life to society; although the criteria for a person's 'social worth' are nebulous, there is an increasing need for society to delineate objective criteria that facilitate decisions on who is entitled to receive limited (ie, less than infinite), potentially life-saving medical resources; any system of rules that determines the relative value of one person's life versus another's depends on 1) The criteria used for selection and 2) Who is empowered to make these decisions, ie has the right to 'play God'; see Pittsburgh criteria, Seattle committee

A particular patient may be excluded based on 1) Constituency factors, including geography, age and ability to pay for a life-saving procedure 2) Progress of science, ie if the therapy is experimental, then the patient should not have other underlying disease and 3) Prospect of success, ie the treatment should be reserved for those patients most likely to benefit from the therapy

socialized medicine A health care system in which 1) The entire population's health care needs are met without charge or at a nominal fee and 2) The organization and provision of all medical services are under direct governmental control; by extension, physicians and other health care providers are government employees; under SM, there is little private practice; Cf Social medicine

sociodemographic factor A generic term for any facet of a population being studied that might confound the study's conclusion if not considered; SFs include marital status, level of education, adequacy of health care

socioeconomic status A mix of factors that shape a person's relative social position, which is gauged by income, profession, education, or a combination of these three factors (N Engl J Med 1993; 329:126ED)

socioeconomic inequality A disparity based on one's social class, often a reflection of highest level of education attained, and wealth; those in the lowest socioeconomic strata (SS) have a 3-7-fold greater (depending on race and sex) death rate than those in the highest strata; morbidity is also affected by SS, where 7% of those in the lowest SS report themselves to be sick, and are 8 times more likely to be hospitalized for various diseases otherwise amenable to management outside of a hospital, eg asthma, DM, and often have more severe disease when hospitalized (N Engl J Med 1993; 329:103OA, 110OA, 126ED)

Socratic method MEDICAL EDUCATION An 'alternative' curriculum or philosophy for teaching medical students that differs from the traditional format in that instruction is in the form of problem-solving and testing of hypotheses; students taught by the Socratic method score lower in standardized examinations, which test fact-based knowledge, and higher in oral examinations, which test the ability to reason and logically analyze patient management scenarios (JAMA 1991; 265:2373)

SOD Superoxide dismutase, see there

SOD1 Copper-zinc superoxide dismutase, an enzyme that detoxifies the superoxide anion, a ubiquitous byproduct of anaerobic metabolism, which as a free[1] radical[2] is a highly reactive compound capable of damaging most cellular components; some cases of familial ALS are due to mutations of the gene encoding the cytosolic form of SOD1 (N Engl J Med 1994; 331:1091) see Amyotrophic lateral sclerosis

[1]ie, Free to diffuse through the cell [2]ie, Possesses an unpaired electron

sodium azide NaN_3 MICROBIOLOGY A toxic salt added (at a concentration of 0.01%) to a transport medium of laboratory specimens, eg urine for the culturing of bacteria that prevents oxidative phosphorylation and bacterial overgrowth

sodium-calcium exchanger A membrane protein with a critical role in myocardial contractility, which regulates free cytosolic calcium ions; the exchanger depends on an electrochemical sodium gradient for its energy and undergoes conformational changes as it moves ions (Nature 1991; 349:621) Cf Na^+/H^+ antiporter

sodium pump Na^+/K^+-ATPase, see there

sodoku Rat-bite fever A disease caused by *Spirillum minor*, a gram-negative flagellated microaerophilic bacterium found in the saliva of 10% of healthy laboratory and wild rats; 2-3 weeks after exposure, the inoculation site becomes ulcerated, purulent and scarred, accompanied by lymphadenitis, fever that may recur cyclically for months and then spontaneously resolve, myalgias and a purple maculopapular rash, which spreads from the inoculation site to the entire body TREATMENT Penicillin, tetracycline; Cf Haverhill fever

sodomy Anal intercourse, see there

'sofa pillow' liver Hepar lobatum, see there

soft A colloquial adjective for 1) That which does not have statistical significance, ie the statistical 'p' value is not < 0.05, as in 'soft' data or 'soft' risk factors; Cf Fragile data 2) That which is socially regarded as relatively innocuous, as in 'soft' drugs, eg nicotine or alcohol where dependence is often considered psychological or 3) That which is not based on objective data, as in the 'soft' sciences of psychology or sociology

soft data Those results from a study or series of studies that demonstrate a consistent trend, eg the risk of suffering a morbid condition, but which falls short of statistical significance

soft laser therapy Cold laser therapy, see there

'soft' risk factors Those risk factors that place a subject at increased risk for suffering a morbid condition, but which do not reach statistical significance, eg 'soft' risks for atherosclerosis, including sedentary life style, obesity, type A personality, use of oral contraceptives, hyperuricemia, high carbohydrate intake; see 'Soft'

'soft' sciences A term applied to fields of study in which accrual of objective and reproducible ('hard') data is virtually impossible as these fields examine societal phenomena and dynamics that are most amenable to philosophical interpretation; the major soft sciences are anthropology, economics, psychology, sociology, and more recently, social medicine

soft tissue sarcoma Sarcoma, see there

software The sequence of programmed instructions that is used to operate a computer, which includes assemblers, compilers, programs, programming languages, routines, translators, and documentation; software is commonly understood to be any program that is available commercially or through networks that can be used to perform certain tasks; in the PC (microcomputer) environment, software includes word processing programs, databases, spreadsheets, graphics, and desktop publishing programs; see Computer; Cf Hardware

soft water Water with a minimal amount of calcium and magnesium salts (carbonates and sulfates); Cf Hard water

soft X-rays Long-wavelength, low-frequency X-rays of low penetrance, eg Grenz radiation

sol A liquid of colloidal solution that flows in response to stress; the movement of crawling cells (eg neutrophils and platelets) results from the cyclical transition from gel and sol states (Sci Am 1994; 270/9:54) see Cell crawling, Gel, Modulus of rigidity, Sol-gel transformation

sol-gel A liquid-crystal cytoskeleton composed of hollow microtubules oriented toward the cell's center, with microfilaments located in the cell periphery; 'sol-gel movement' is a characteristic ameboid locomotion by unicellular eukaryotes and tissue macrophages, which move by extension and retraction of long pseudopods changing constantly from a fluid-like sol to a semisolid gel state

sol-gel transformation The mechanical fluctuation between a sol, a liquid that flows in response to applied stress and a gel, an elastic material that is primarily liquid but which has solid properties state with concentrated in the cortex of 'crawling' cells) derives from the water-soluble polymers in the cell cytoplasm, which also serve as scaffolding needed to support contractile forces (Sci Am 1994; 270/9:54) see Cell crawling, Gel, Modulus of rigidity, Sol

solar elastosis Degeneration of the subdermal elastic tissue by prolonged actinic exposure, causing wrinkled 'sailor's skin', predisposing the skin to various skin-based malignancies including basal and squamous cell carcinomas, and malignant melanoma; see Actinic (solar) keratosis

solar keratosis Actinic (solar) keratosis, see there

soldier's heart Old soldier's heart, see there

soldier's plaque A descriptor for the pearly white, thickened, non-adherent, epicardial 'plate' that occurs in healed chronic pericarditis

solenoid structure MOLECULAR BIOLOGY A configuration of DNA formed during DNA condensation in the eukaryotic nucleus; the solenoid structure consists of histones wrapped with supercoiled DNA, known as nucleosomes, connected to each other by linker DNA, having an ultrastructural appearance likened to beads on a string; see Histone

solid-state tumorigenesis A phenomenon, in which inert material, eg plastic elicits soft tissue sarcomas, in experimental rodents that have been previously rendered susceptible to malignancies (BS Oppenheimer et al, Further Studies of Polymers as Carcinogenic Agents in Animals. Cancer Res 1955; 15:333); these tumors occur with a characteristic frequency, latency period and histopathologic type; given the broad experience with artificial silicone breast implants, biomechanical prostheses, and other long-term indwelling devices, the phenomenon is not thought to occur frequently in humans

solid waste management ENVIRONMENT The constellation of methods used to eliminate civilization's 'detritus', including burial in landfills, recycling, ie reuse, with the refuse serving as raw material for newly manufactured products, and incineration, the heat from which may be used as a source of energy; Cf Biohazardous waste, Hazardous waste, Regulated waste

solitary congenital nodular calcification DERMATOLOGY A skin lesion seen on the extremities or head and neck region in which the epidermis is acanthotic and hyperkeratotic, with calcified subcutaneous masses of unknown significance

solitary hunter 'syndrome' 'Loner', see there

solitary myeloma HEMATOLOGY A single focus of neoplastic myeloma cells that is responsible for 3-5% of monoclonal gammopathies, SMs may be intraosseous or extramedullary, the latter being most often located in the lungs

or the oronasopharyngeal region; most osseous SMs progress to classic myeloma, while extramedullary SMs are relatively indolent, remain regionally confined and usually treated adequately with local excision

solitary plasmacytoma Solitary myeloma, see there

solitary rectal ulcer(s) syndrome A disease of young adults, more common in females with irregular bowel habits, thought to be related to an internal rectal prolapse associated with an abnormal perineal descent ETIOLOGY Idiopathic or related to laxative abuse or anal intercourse CLINICAL Hematochezia, variably accompanied by anal or abdominal pain, passage of mucus per rectum, excess straining on defecation, with a 'flap valve' effect where the puborectalis muscle fails to completely relax, creating a high-pressure zone, potentially resulting in rectal prolapse; the ulcers average 2 cm in diameter and are close to the anal verge TREATMENT Stool softeners; when SRUS is accompanied by rectal prolapse, rectopexy may be required

solitary thyroid nodule A palpably discrete, enlargement of an otherwise apparently normal thyroid gland EPIDEMIOLOGY ♀:♂ 4:1; the majority of cases are incidental findings during autopsy or surgical exploration for other reasons DDx Colloid (adenomatous) nodule (42-77% of STNs), follicular adenoma (15-40%), carcinoma (8-17%) DIAGNOSIS FNA biopsy*, radionuclide scanning (^{131}I, ^{99m}Tc), ultrasonography TREATMENT Malignant and indeterminant lesions are treated by surgery (N Engl J Med 1993; 328:553cc)

*In a meta-analysis of 9 studies with 9119 patients, 74% of FNA biopsie results were benign, 11% inadequate, 11% indeterminant, 4% malignant (Endocrinologist 1991; 1:194)

solo practice The practice of medicine by a single physician known as a solo practioner; SPs are slowly becoming an anachronism in the health care marketplace, in view of the unshared overhead costs and one-visit expertise limited to a single physician (Am Med News 1995; 17 April 1995 p1) Cf Group practice

soluble antigen A generic term for an antigen present in solution

soluble fiber Water-soluble fiber CLINICAL NUTRITION Any of a number of indigestible fibers that are concentrated in certain foods, eg fruits, dried beans, legumes, guar gums, barley, psyllium and oat cereals, and ↑ the stool bulk and lower LDL-cholesterol; a 5-10 g ↑ in SF in the diet translates into ± 5% ↓ in serum cholesterol; dietary supplementation with soluble fiber results in a statistically significant ↓ in plasma LDL cholesterol and apolipoprotein B, and lesser reductions of HDL cholesterol and apolipoprotein AI (N Engl J Med 1993; 329:80a) see Bran, Dietary fiber

SOLVD Studies of Left Ventricular Dysfunction (see N Engl J Med 1992; 327:685oa) see Consensus II, Enalapril

solve rate FORENSIC MEDICINE The percentage of homicides for which the killer is identified with reasonable certainty, a value that differs according to country, availability of effective homicidal weapons, permissiveness for crimes of passion, substrate of violence, abuse substance subculture, size of community, social inequities and other intangibles; in the US, the solve rate ranges from 55% to 85%

solvent abuse CLINICAL TOXICOLOGY A generic term for the recreational use by inhalation of various chemical solvents in model glue, paint thinner, nail polish remover, the active ingredients of which include acetone, benzene, carbon tetrachloride, naphtha, toluene, xylene; adults at risk include dry cleaners, shoemakers, hairdressers; adolescents (up to 15% have experimente with solvents) at risk tend to come from lower socioeconomic strata and subjected to less parental supervision CLINICAL At low concentrations, solvents induce a pleasant 'buzz', with euphoria and exhilaration; with increasing levels, tinnitus, diplopia, hallucinations, and confusion ensue; further increases in blood levels of solvents are accompanied by muscular incoordination, ataxia, slurred speech, hyperreflexia, nystagmus, and unconsciousness; long term SA may cause hematopoietic (eg aplastic anemia), hepatic (eg hepatocellular necrosis, liver cell carcinoma), renal (renal tubule acidosis), pulmonary, and CNS dysfunction, the last of which may result in irreversible damage in the form of cerebellar degeneration, cognitive impairment, dementia, distal sensory polyneuropathy, and others

solvent mapping A method for identifying drugs of potential interest ('leads') based on the pattern of bound organic solvents in active sites and specificity pockets of proteins, ie functional binding sites; SM '*…can be used to map the binding surface of any crystalline macromolecule, including those of nonenzymatic regulatory molecules interacting with receptors. It brings together observations about water, organic solvents, and protein structure, 'double-sited' solutions, to the inhibitor problem, and computational methods in one neat package.*' (Bio/Technology 1995; 13:199)

Somalia 'factor' GLOBAL VILLAGE The increasing reluctance of Western nations to become embroiled in the ethnic (ie internal) conflicts of African nations (**US News & World Report 18 April 1994:18**) see Burnt-out 'syndrome' (compassion fatigue)

somatization disorder A chronic fluctuating disorder in which an individual on a regularly seks some form of medical attention for unexplained somatic complaint (table); SD is characterized by symptoms suggesting organ dysfunction(s) that are not supported by laboratory or clinical parameters; the symptoms are often vague, do not appear to be under voluntary control and may fulfill some psychological need CLINICAL The patients are sickly (or believe themselves to be), have pseudoneuralgias (visual defects, dysphagia, loss of voice, urinary retention, convulsion, seizures), gastrointestinal symptoms (colicky pain, nausea, vomiting), dysmenorrhea, loss of libido, pain

---

SOMATIZATION DISORDER-DIAGNOSTIC CRITERIA, 300.81 DSM-IV

A History of multiple somatic complaints occurring before age 30, and over a period of years, that resulted in treatment being sought, or in significant social or occupational impairment

B Each of criteria 1-4 are met
1) History of pain in at least four regions (eg abdomen, back, chest, extremities head, joints, rectum) and/or during activities (eg during menstruation, sexual activity urination)
2) History of at least two GI symptoms unrelated to pain, eg bloating, diarrhea, food intolerance, nausea
3) History of one or more sexual symptom, eg sexual indifference, erectile or ejaculatory dysfunction, dysmenorrhea
4) History of one or more pseudoneurologic symptom, eg conversion symptoms (aphonia, blindness, deafness, dysphagia, impaired coordination, paralysis and others) dissociative symptoms (eg amnesia), or loss of consciousness unrelated to fainting

C Either
1) The symptoms of Criterion B (above) are unexplained after a full workup for known medical conditions or effects of substances OR
2) The symptoms of Criterion B (above) and resulting social and occupational impairment are in excess of those expected for an individual with a known medical condition

D The symptoms are unrelated to factitious conditions or malingering

Diagnostic and Statistical Manual of Mental Disorders, 4th ed, Washington, DC, American Psychiatric Association, 1994

(back, genitalia and joints), cardiopulmonary symptoms, including dyspnea, palpitations and chest pains; Cf Factitious diseases

somatomammotropin Any of a family of hormones, eg growth hormone 21.8 kD, prolactin 22.5 kD and placental lactogen 21.8 kD that share intrinsic lactogenic and growth-promoting activity, despite a wide difference in sequence similarity or 'homology' (growth hormone and prolactin have 16% 'homology', while growth hormone and placental lactogen have 83% 'homology')

somatomedin ENDOCRINOLOGY A generic term* for any of a group of low (7-10 kD) molecular weight growth factors (eg IGF-I, IGF-II-insulin-like growth factors) that are released from the liver and kidney by growth hormone and have insulin-like effects on target tissues, leading to ↑ incorporation of sulfate in collagen and ↑ protein synthesis; somatomedin activity is found in epidermal growth factor, fibroblast growth factor, sex steroids, thyroid hormones, erythropoietin, tropic hormones and 'factors' with multiplication-stimulating activity and non-suppressible insulin-like activity; see IGF-I, IGF-II

*There is now a consensus that the term somatomedin should be used only when referring to these peptides in a generic sense, and that IGF I and IGF II should be used when referring to specific peptides (LE Underwood and JJ van Wyk, in JD Wilson, DW Foster, Textbook of Endocrinology, 8th ed, WB Saunders, Philadelphia, 1992)

somatomedin A Insulin-like growth factor-II, see there

somatomedin C Insulin-like growth factor-I, see there

somatostatin NEUROPHYSIOLOGY A 14-residue neuropeptide secreted by the brain that inhibits the secretion of growth hormone, thyroid releasing hormone and insulin, and stimulates glucagon secretion, as well as the delta cells of pancreatic islets and GI tract cells, inhibiting secretogue-mediated changes in ion transport, gastrin and gastric acid secretion, increasing intestinal transit time and stimulating sodium and chloride absorption in the ileum and colon; somatostatin is a paracrine hormone that acts as an 'off' switch in the GI tract, and has a 'yin-yang' relation with bombesin, which acts as an 'on' switch; see Bombesin

somatostatinoma Delta cell tumor A somatostatin-producing tumor of the pancreatic islet delta cells that is characterized by ↓ gastric acid secretion and metastasis to liver and bone; it is associated with DM, cholelithiasis, steatorrhea, and hypochlorhydria, and is most common in the head and tail of the pancreas, but may rarely arise in the duodenum

somatostatinoma syndrome A paraneoplastic syndrome caused by ectopic somatostatin secretion CLINICAL Vomiting, hypochlorhydria, abdominal pain, diarrhea, malabsorption, weight loss, cholelithiasis and defective glucose control, causing secondary DM LABORATORY ↑ somatostatin (which being an inhibitory hormone, evokes 'reactive' decrease in insulin and glucagon), ↓ gastrin, steatorrhea, anemia

somatostatinoma triad A trilogy of symptoms regarded as typical of patients with gallstones, DM and diarrhea

somatostatin-receptor imaging A unique technique for localizing and semiquantifying endocrine and neuroendocrine tumors, eg carcinoids, chemodectomas and pancreatic endocrine tumors, including gastrinomas and insulinomas, by using a radiolabeled analogue of somatostatin (octreotide) and detecting the uptake with either a gamma-camera or by single photon emission computed tomography (SPECT)

somatotrophin Growth hormone, see there

somatotropin Growth hormone, see there

somatotropin release-inhibiting hormone A hormone produced and released from the anterior hypothalamus in response to various stimulants, eg high circulating glucocorticosteroids, which inhibits the release of both growth hormone and thyroid stimulating hormone

somnogen Any of a number of compounds, eg cytokines, eg IL-1α, IL-1β, TNFα, and INFα2, that are intrinsically somnogenic, which injected in the lateral ventricle of rabbits, enhancing non-REM sleep and inhibiting REM sleep, typically in a background of an acute phase response (Perspect Biol & Med 1993; 36:611) Cf Intracellular signaling

Somogyi effect Rebound hyperglycemia A phenomenon described in diabetics in whom hyperglycemia occurs as a counter-regulatory overcompensation to nocturnal hypoglycemia (Bull St Louis Med Soc 1938; 32:498); the Somogyi effect may cause the clinician to ↑ the dose of insulin (in order to compensate for the 'physiological' nocturnal hyperglycemia), which exacerbates the rebound hypoglycemia, when in fact, the insulin dose should be lowered; see Dawn phenomenon, Glucose tolerance test, Subcutaneous insulin-resistance syndrome

Son of Sam David Berkowitz, see Serial killer

Sonic (the) Hedgehog® see Hedgehog genes

SOP Standard operating procedure, see there

sorbinil see Aldose reductase inhibitor

sorbitol A polyhydroxyl alcohol or polyol synthesized from glucose by aldose reductase in nerve tissue, produced in excess in diabetics; sorbitol may be further metabolized to fructose, which together cause ↑ osmotic pressure, intracellular edema, schwann cell swelling, anoxia and nerve demyelination; sorbitol has been implicated in diabetic neuropathy, and has had some currency as a sweetening agent; Cf Advanced glycosylation end products

Sorbonne MEDICAL HISTORY The University of Paris (formerly, the Sorbonne) began as a theological school attached to the cathedral of Notre Dame du Paris and was founded by 1253 by Robert de Sorbon; the Sorbonne had a stormy history, often taking the 'wrong' side in delicate political issues, and was closed by convention in 1790 and as such no longer exists; of the 13 campuses of the University of Paris, Paris I, III, and IV may be considered 'the Sorbonne' as they are housed in the original Sorbonne site in the Latin Quarter (Nature 1990; 346:136n&v)

sorting signals MOLECULAR BIOLOGY Amino acid sequences that are encoded in a polypeptide or which are added after translation to indicate the direction of a protein's flow through the cell

SOS box A 20-base-pair operator sequence present in *Escherichia coli*, that binds the LexA repressor, activating many genes involved in repair of ultraviolet light-induced damage

SOS repair Mutation repair MOLECULAR BIOLOGY An error-prone repair system that functions when *Escherichia coli*'s DNA is damaged by bond-breaking physical agents or toxins; after the 'insult', a group of genes are activated, including the *recA* gene, which encodes RecA protein, lysing certain DNA-binding proteins including the LexA repressor; the LexA repressor binds to the repressor site, activating transcription of proteins involved in repair; although SOS repair is 'sloppy', it restores DNA damaged by thymine starvation, chemicals, eg mitomycin C and ultraviolet light, preventing cell death, hence SOS*, after the international Morse code signal for maritime distress; see Thymine dimer

*In Morse code, the letters SOS (···/---/···) are an international maritime call of distress

sotalol A potent noncardioselective β-adrenergic blocker that ↑ the duration of action potentials in cardiac muscle, ↑ cardiac refractory period, and lengthens the QT interval; it is used as an antiarrhythmic and antifibrillatory agent; it is approved in the US for life-threatening ventricular tach-

yarrhythmias SIDE EFFECTS The ↑ β-adrenergic-receptor blockade may aggravate pre-existing arrhythmias, eg sinus bradycardia, provoke new arrhythmias, eg torsade de points, exacerbate congestive heart failure and hypotension, exacerbate bronchospasm, fatigue, dizziness, dyspnea, headache (N Engl J Med 1994; 331:31RV)

$$CH_3SO_2NH-\bigcirc-\overset{\overset{OH}{|}}{C}HCH_2NHCH(CH_3)_2$$

sotalol

Sotos syndrome Cerebral gigantism An AD [MIM 117550] condition with rapid early somatic growth of neonatal onset, not accompanied by endocrinopathy, accelerated bone maturation, or precocious puberty MOLECULAR PATHOLOGY A balanced translocation was reported in one case; the defective gene may be located at either 3p21 or 6p21 CLINICAL Macrosomia, where growth is accelerated for the first 4-5 years of life, followed by a normal growth pattern, enlarged acral parts (hands and feet), thickened subcutaneous tissues, macrocephaly, mild mental retardation and perceptual defects; EEG abnormalities, dilated ventricles, dolichocephaly, antimongolic slanting of palpebral fissures, macrognathy, hypertelorism, convulsions, poor coordination, and ↑ risk for malignancy, including Wilms' tumor, hepatic, parotid, and ovarian carcinomas

(artificial) sound generator ENT A device used to produced by some form of artificial sound generator, as required by patients with laryngectomies for cancer; SGs have two basic designs, based on the type of force (either breath stream or electromechanical) used to drive them; the breath-driven devices have three basic elements in common: 1) A flexible tube that conveys the breath from the tracheal stoma to a hand-held capsule, 2) A capsule with a reed or membrane that vibrates to generate the sound per se, and 3) A second smaller tube that carries the sound from the capsule into the mouth, where sound is articulated into speech; although the breath-driven devices have the advantages of lower cost, and ease of use, they require one free hand (ie interfere with two-handed activities), they clog regularly and are esthetically suboptimal, as saliva, mucus, and other gooey things seep from the stoma, and few are in current use; electrical devices are hand held and come is two flavors, to wit, 1) A hearing-aid-sized battery-powered buzzer from which the sound travels via a tube into the mouth, and 2) A device that picks up vibrations through the neck tissues; on the plus side, the electrical devices are inexpensive, easily learned and used, and are more hygienically and esthetically acceptable (no goo); the 'down side' of the mechanical devices is that they tie up one hand, interfering with two-handed activities, and produce a constant buzzing field noise that competes with the generated speech (JJ Ballenger, Diseases of the Nose, Throat, Ear, Head, and Neck, 14th ed, Lea & Febiger, Philadelphia, 1991)

sound therapy ALTERNATIVE MEDICINE The use of sound and music (S&M) as a therapeutic modality a sui generis based on the physiologic changes in the breathing and heart rate, blood pressure, neuromuscular tone, and the release of hormones which are induced by S&M; ST is reported to be beneficial in Alzheimer's disease, hospice environments for the terminally ill, and in childbirth, dentistry, and psychotherapy (Alternative Medicine, Future Medicine Pub, Puyallup, WA, 1994)

source amnesia PSYCHOLOGY *'The inability to recall the origin of the memory of a given event. Once the origin* *of the memory is forgotten...people can confuse an event that was imagined or suggested with a true one. This result is a memory that* (al)*though false, carries a feeling of authenticity.*' (New York Times May 3, 1994; C1) Source memory occurs in the frontal lobe; one of the most labile components of memory is the source–the time, place, or way in which a memory originated; see False memory, Repressed memory

South African porphyria Porphyria variegata, see there

'South American' operation A radical surgical procedure for a 'frozen' pelvis, consisting of en bloc resection of the uterus and rectum; Cf 'All-American' and 'North American' operations

'southern blindness' see SC disease

Southern blot A method for detecting the presence of and optimally manipulating specific DNA sequences previously separated by gel electrophoresis delineated by EM Southern (J Mol Biol 1975; 98:503) Southern blot hybridization technique 1) DNA is extracted from cells 2) DNA is digested with a restriction endonuclease, cutting the DNA into fragments several hundred to thousand base pairs in length 3) The fragmented DNA is separated by size with agar gel electrophoresis 4) A nitrocellulose or nylon membrane is placed on the gel 'slab' and bathed in an alkaline buffer solution, which denatures the DNA, separating it into single strands 5) A layer of dry blotting material, often paper towels is placed on top of the membrane, creating an osmotic pressure gradient sufficient to transfer the separated DNA fragments from the delicate gel 'slab' onto the membrane; this step is the 'Southern transfer' per se Note: The transfer may also be effected by vacuum 6) The presence of DNA fragments of interest is then determined by bathing the membrane in a 'hybridization' fluid continuing either a ^{35}S- or ^{32}P-radiolabeled or biotinylated 'probe' (figure); if the DNA fragment of interest is present, the probe binds to the single strand of DNA and is detected by autoradiography, or by substrate digestion if the probe is biotinylated (illustration)

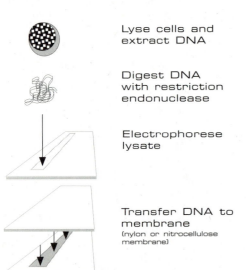

Lyse cells and extract DNA

Digest DNA with restriction endonuclease

Electrophorese lysate

Transfer DNA to membrane
(nylon or nitrocellulose membrane)

Incubate membrane with probe
(Radioactive or biotinylated)

Wash, perform autoradiography

Southern blot hybridization

Southwestern blot A technique that combines the principle of Southern hybridization, which identifies DNA fragments, with 'Western' immunoblotting, which identifies proteins of interest; a protein is hybridized to its cognate membrane-bound single-stranded DNA molecule, usually the gene that encodes the protein, eg an enhancer or regulatory factor (J Biol Chem 1990; 265:8725); the SB is of greatest use for identifying transcription-related proteins located in the nucleus

SP-1 Pregnancy-specific β-1 glycoprotein, see there

SP1 Stimulatory protein 1 An RNA polymerase II transcription factor that contains a zinc-finger domain required for DNA binding; SP1 binds to a guanine and cytosine-rich sequence of DNA lying 200 base pairs or less upstream of the start sites for RNA synthesis and may be a general promoter-binding factor required for activating various genes

SP-A A 28–36-kD glycosylated protein synthesized by type II alveolar cells, which in the native form is a ± 650-kD multimer aggregate; SP-A interacts with other surfactant proteins and lipids to improve surface properties and regulate surfactant cycling pathways via receptors on type II cells and macrophages; SP-A may also have an as yet undefined immune defense role (see N Engl J Med 1993; 328:861RV)

spa A health resort where one bathes in the water of a particular natural spring

space adaption syndrome Space sickness The constellation of the effects of space travel on human physiology include motion sickness, which occurs in 67% of astronauts, in 13% of whom it is severe (which is thought to be due to temporary labyrinthine dysfunction in a background of weightlessness) CLINICAL The condition begins in the vestibular system of the inner ear, causing 'sensory confusion', resulting in vertigo, which is accompanied by nausea, vomiting, gastrointestinal dysmotility, malaise, diaphoresis, sialorrhea, yawning, anorexia, hyperventilation (resulting in hypocapnia with vasodilation of the lower extremities and pooling of blood), causing postural hypotension and syncope; prolonged space flight is associated with osteoporosis and disuse atrophy of muscle and may be punctuated with various inconveniences, eg the in-flight waste management systems fail on most space flights

space crystal Any of a number of protein crystals grown in space; elastase are larger, more uniform in structure, and have better internal order than those grown on earth, which suffer from gravity-related, density-driven convective flow and sedimentation

space medicine A branch of aerospace medicine that addresses the stresses and changes imposed on man by traveling through and beyond the earth's atmosphere and flight in space; SM evaluates the stresses of weightlessness, space adaption syndrome, cardiovascular deconditioning, radiation exposure, the effects of isolation, loss of red cell mass, and bone mineral loss

space motion sickness Space adaption syndrome, see there

space sickness Space adaption syndrome, see there

'space suit' A fluid-resistant disposable garment that covers the arms and legs that is used in combination with gloves (doubled), shoe and head covering, and face mask and/or shield; SS's are used in a health care setting by a person who is involved in direct management of a patient with a highly infectious disease, or when handling biohazardous waste

spade deformity CARDIOLOGY A finding by contrast ventricular angiography, likened to a playing card spade, appearing in focal concentric apical left cardiac ventricular hypertrophy, confined to the ventricular apex, seen at end-diastole in the right anterior oblique ventriculogram and in two-dimensional echocardiography; the deformity may be accompanied by 'giant' negative T waves on electrocardiography

spade hand A descriptor for the progressive cylindrical carpal thickening seen in pachydermoperiostosis; Cf Rosebud hand

spade-like configuration A descriptor for the radiologic appearance of enlarged terminal tufts of the distal phalanges typical of acromegaly; Cf Penciling

'spaghetti' 'Pigtail', see there

'spaghetti tumor' SURGICAL PATHOLOGY A descriptor for the growth pattern of the relatively indolent endolymphatic stromal myosis, a uterine stromal tumor that is clinically characterized by abnormal uterine bleeding, pelvic pain and uterine enlargement PATHOLOGY The cut surface is yellow-orange with bulging polypoid projections, fancifully likened to rigatoni in a melted cheese sauce; mitotic activity is a marker for aggressiveness in uterine stromal tumors; at one end of the spectrum is the mitotically inactive uterine stromal nodule, at the other, stromal sarcomas, which may have more than ten mitotic figures/ten high-power fields; the spaghetti tumor usually has < 5 mitotic figures/10 high power fields PROGNOSIS Up to 85% 15-year survival, despite metastases

Spanish fly Blister beetle, see there

sparse fur mutation A murine model for ornithine decarboxylase deficiency, characterized by abnormal skin and hair and ornithine decarboxylase deficiency, which is due to a single point mutation

spasmodic dysphonia A clinical complex characterized by a strained and strangled speech with multiple breaks in rhythm, which may be accompanied by other dystonias, eg blepharospasm, oromandibular dystonia, torticollis, writers' cramp TREATMENT The previous standard therapy, sectioning of the recurrent laryngeal nerve, is often complicated by late failure; botulinum toxin injection into laryngeal muscles has become an increasingly popular alternative therapy

spasmodic torticollis Wry neck, see there

spasmus caninus Risus sardonicus, see there

spastic colitis Irritable bowel syndrome, see there

spastic pelvic floor syndrome Anismus, see there

spasticity A velocity-dependent increase in tonic stretch reflexes; the severity of spasticity is difficult to measure and can be extremely variable; it is most common in patients with spinal cord lesions above the conus medullarisis, and develops months after spinal cord injury TREATMENT Baclofen which potentiates the inhibitory effect of GABA (gamma-aminobutyric acid) on reflexes (see N Engl J Med 1994; 330:553RV)

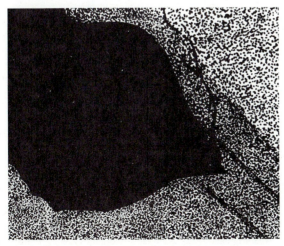

spade deformity

spatula ribs Broad flattened ribs typical of pseudoachondroplasia, see there

Spätzle activity MOLECULAR BIOLOGY A signaling molecule found in the perivitelline fluid around the developing *Drosophila* embryo; the Spätzle signal is transduced across the egg cell membrane, resulting in a gradient of activity of the transcription factor, Dorsal, differing regional concentrations of which activate or inhibit various patterning genes along the dorsoventral axis (Nature; 1994; 372:500N&V) see there); SA's putative receptor, Toll, has significant sequence similarity to the vertebrate IL-1 receptor

SP-B, SP-C Highly lipophilic 8 (SP-B) and 4 kd (SP-C) proteins that facilitate the adsorption and spreading of lipids to form a monolayre of surfactant on the alveolar surface (see N Engl J Med 1993; 328:861RV) see SP-A, Surfactant

Spearman's rank (order) correlation coefficient STATISTICS A calculated value that indicates the relationship between two dependent nonparametric variables or sets of ranks; the coefficient ranges from +1 to -1, where +1 indicates a perfect agreement between ranks, 0 indicates no relationship on ranks, and –1 indicates a complete inverse relationship

speB The gene that encodes streptococcal pyrogenic exotoxin B, an extracellular cysteine protease that cleaves IL-1β precursor to form the mature biologically active IL-1β; 39 distinct alleles of *speB* have been identified in *S pyogenes*; distinct strains have different allelic 'signatures', a feature that can be used in multilocus enzyme electrophoresis (see there), a method for identifying the strain responsible for an epidemic bacterial infection (Arch Pathol Lab Med 1994; 118:128OA)

special fire fighting procedure OCCUPATIONAL SAFETY A generic term for any means of extinguishing a fire that requires special equipment (eg self-contained breathing apparatus, protective clothing or eyewear) or special procedures (eg sodium-potassium alloy); SFFPs are of interest to OSHA, which requires such listings in its Materials Safety Data Sheets‡

special weapons A US Pentagon term for weapons of mass destruction, to wit, biological, chemical, and nuclear

specialist A person who has a recognized expertise in something; in the usual medical context, a specialist is board-eligible or board-certified in a recognized area of medicine, eg pathology, psychiatry, radiology, has undergone a formal residency training program of three or more years and is entitled to sit for the closure ('specialty board') examination in that field; an estimated ⅔ of physicians in the US are specialized, more than any other country in the world; the income ranges from $175-250 000, ± double that of those in primary care ('general') medicine (internal medicine, family practice, pediatrics) type; for ± 15 years there have been warning signs that there are too many* high-priced procedure-oriented specialists in the US, and after the years of skyrocketing, the income pendulum for specialists may swing in the opposite direction, as some generalists take over specialist work, and specialists are barred from managed care networks; as an example the average cardiovascular surgeon's income declined in 1993 to $447 000 from $499 000 in 1992; in the same period, generalists' income rose ± 7% (Am Med News 3 October 1994) Cf Subspecialty

*A study published by the American Society of Plastic and Reconstructive Surgery reported that five times more plastic surgeons were beginning to practice than were retiring

specialization CONTINUING MEDICAL EDUCATION A period of acquisition of special skills or specialty knowledge, often in a formal educational setting, which may be closed with an examination by a specialty board and the awarding of a certificate of special expertise, a process known as board certification

specialized laboratory A type of reference laboratory dedicated to a particular type of 'esoteric' testing, eg allergy, coagulation, drugs (in particular drugs of abuse), endocrinology, genetics, paternity, virology, and others; a reference laboratory may send out its specimens to a specialized laboratory for some of the same reasons that reference labs are used, ie to control costs of performing rare, low-volume tests that require 'expensive' experts (Advance/Laboratory Sept 1994) Cf Reference laboratory

specialty board An organization, recognized and approved by the American Board of Medical Specialists in conjunction with the American Medical Association's Council on Medical Education and the American Dental Association, that certifies, through standardized examinations that a physician has achieved a sufficient knowledge base to practice his chosen specialty; there are 24 specialties governed by 24 specialty boards (☎ 1.800.776.2378, US); see Board certification, Peer review, Residency; Cf State board

species Biologic species A taxonomically distinct group of interbreeding organisms that are reproductively isolated from others; a species is (according to Ernst Mayr, evolutionary biologist extraordinaire) a set of interbreeding populations that is reproductively isolated by behavior and physiology from other groups; new species can only occur through one of two mechanisms, either by allopatry–geographic separation from the rest of its kind or by peripatry–geographic separation of a small founding population, a circumstance that has genetic ramifications that may accelerate the divergence of species (Sci Am 1994; 270/8:25)

species-ism A neologism coined by animal rights activists, for some of whom the use of animals in research is a crime akin to sexism and racism, implying that animals are equivalent to humans as sentient beings; see Animal rights activism, Animal Welfare Act

specific gravity NEPHROLOGY A measure of the solutes in a fluid, a value that reflects the kidney's ability to concentrate urine: if a random urine specimen has specific gravity greater than 1.023, the kidney's ability to concentrate is assumed to be normal; specific gravity is tested by refractometry, which measures the ratio of the velocity of light in air to the velocity of light in a solution; specific gravity increases in the syndrome of inappropriate secretion of antidiuretic hormone (SIADH), uncontrolled DM, proteinuria, eclampsia and obstructive uropathy and decreases in renal tubular damage, chronic renal insufficiency, diabetes insipidus, and malignant hypertension OCCUPATIONAL SAFETY A physical parameter of a liquid that indicates how heavy it is in relation to air (≤ 1.0 = lighter than water; ≥ 1.0 = heavier than water) a datum of interest to OSHA, which requires listing of SGs in its Materials Safety Data Sheets, see there PHYSICAL CHEMISTRY Relative density The ratio of a substance's density to that of a standard substance (usually water) under specified conditions (usually 4°C), or for a gas under standard pressure and temperature

specificity BIOCHEMISTRY The degree of an enzyme's selectivity for a substrate IMMUNOLOGY The avidity of an antibody for an antigen PHYSIOLOGY The degree of a ligand's affinity for a receptor STATISTICS The number of true negatives in a series of data (usually in the context of laboratory tests designed to detect the presence of a disease), divided by the sum of the number of true negatives and false positives, representing the proportion of subjects without a condition that a test will correctly identify as negative; see Efficiency

specificity spillover syndrome ENDOCRINOLOGY A clinical complex caused by the low-affinity binding of peptide hormone to a receptor other than its own, resulting in low levels of hormonal signal transduction, ie stimulation; SSSs include galactorrhea in a background of acromegaly (due to binding of growth hormone to prolactin receptors), hyperthyroidism in a background of trophoblastic tumors (due to high affinity of hCG to TSH receptors), and hyperandrogenism with insulin resistance (due to cross-reactivity of insulin with IGF-I receptors in the ovary)

speckled lentiginous nevus Nevus spilus DERMATOLOGY A form of lentigo simplex that presents at birth, arising secondary to a junctional nevus with maturation of the cells in the dermis

speckled oral leukoplakia A generic term any white flecked or nodular lesion on an erythematous (usually atrophic) base that may be seen in a background of erythroplasia, thus corresponding to a combination of leukoplakia and erythroplasia

speckled pattern RHEUMATOLOGY An immunofluorescence pattern that may be seen when the human epithelial cell line HEp-2 is stained with serum from patients with various connective tissue diseases; speckled patterns are most common in SLE, but may also be seen in mixed connective tissue disease, sicca syndrome, Sjögren syndromes, polymyositis, rheumatoid arthritis and drug-induced immune reactions; the 'speckled' pattern is the least specific, most common and variable of immunofluorescent patterns and is subdivided into 1) Fine or true 'speckles', due to anti-centromere staining, most commonly seen in mixed connective tissue disease 2) Coarse 'speckles', most commonly due to antibodies to nonhistone nuclear proteins: nRNP, Sm, SS-B/La and Scl-70 and c) Large 'speckles', 3-10/nucleus, which occur in IgM antibody to class H3 histones, typical of the undifferentiated connective tissue disease; see Antinuclear antibodies

SPECT Single photon emission computed tomography A non-invasive technique for reconstructing cross-sectional images of the distribution of radiotracers, used to evaluate the central nervous system (acute ischemic episodes, epileptic foci, vascular dementia and Alzheimer's dementia), myocardial perfusion and detect subtle changes in bone metabolism; although SPECT was reported before computed tomography and magnetic resonance imaging (Radiology 1963; 80:653), its clinical application was delayed until the development of suitable radiopharmaceuticals, eg ^{82}Rb, ^{123}I, ^{99m}Tc, ^{201}Th, and instrumentation, ie adaption of the Anger (scintillation) camera to rotate around the patient; SPECT analysis of thallium distribution in dynamic studies of cardiac function reduces the subjectivity inherent in interpretation of thallium scans; ^{201}Th SPECT is less sensitive, specific and accurate than ^{82}Rb PET in imaging myocardial perfusion for those with coronary artery disease; the most commonly used radiotracer is ^{99m}Tc-HMPAO, which is injected IV; SPECT is superior to EEG in detecting focal defects in blood flow which correlate with seizure activity (Medico Interamericano 1995; 14:125)

Note: Positron emission tomography provides similar information as SPECT at the higher cost of positron decay radionuclides

specimen A small sample of something (cells, organ, organism, plasma, tissue, whatever) that represents a whole, from which a diagnosis is rendered or other determination of said object's nature is delineated

'spectacle' sign A well-circumscribed osteosclerotic rim at the sphenoids, which imparts a bespectacled appearance to the skull on a plain film in patients with idiopathic hypercalcemia

spectrin A fibrous protein arranged in a filamentous network, which is composed of α and β subunits, existing either in a 250-kD dimeric or 500-kD tetrameric form; it is anchored to the cytoplasmic face of the erythrocyte membrane and is responsible for both the RBC's shape and its deformability; it is defective in spherocytosis; see Band 3.1, Ghost, Spherocytosis

spectrum Any continuum of values, units, qualities, or other entities that can be arranged in an objective fashion MRI An array of the components of the MR signal according to frequency; nuclei with different resonant frequencies appear as peaks ('lines') at different frequencies in the spectrum; see Magnetic resonance imaging

speech pathology A field of allied health care that evaluates abnormalities of language, speech, and voice, which may be developmental or acquired in nature; SP is encharged with 1) Identifying the nature of the disorder, ie whether the defect(s) relate to speech perception and verbal comprehension, or whether the disorder is structural or neurologic in origin, either of which impair the expression of speech and language, and 2) Correcting the abnormal speech through rehabilitation; among the conditions addressed by the speech pathologist are aphasia, defects in articulation, delayed language development, stuttering, and other voice defects

'speedballing' SUBSTANCE ABUSE A form of IV drug abuse in which cocaine and heroin are injected either sequentially or in tandem to enhance the 'high'

spell Any period during which an individual is in a particular state, eg spell of hospitalization (hospital stay is currently preferred), spell (bout or period) of sickness LINICAL MEDICINE A condition that has no specific definition, which is best described as '*a sudden onset of a symptom or symptoms that are recurrent, self-limited, and stereotypic…*'; in the 19th Century, spells were thought to be psychogenic in naure, and were termed 'vapors'; in the current environment, spells occur in six broad categories of diseases, including endocrine (eg hypoglycemia, thyrotoxicosis, carbohydrate intolerance), cardiovascular (essential hypertension, angina, pulmonary edema), psychologic (eg panic and anxiety disorders), pharmacologic (eg MAOI therapy and cheese, illicit drugs), neurologic (seizure disorders, migraine headaches), and others (eg mastocytosis, carcinoid syndrome, polycythemia vera, POEM syndrome) hyperventilation CLINICAL Facial flushing attributed to vasodilation, which is accompanied by one of various spell phenotypes, eg pheochromocytoma, carcinoid syndrome, or mast cell disease, which may be manifest in the form of diaphoresis, a sensation of numbness, shortness of breath, headaches, chest tightness, increased blood pressure, and others (Mayo Clin Proc 1995; 70:757ᴏᴀ) PSYCHIATRY A trance-like state in which a person allegedly communicates with dead persons, or various (non-mineral, non-grain) spirits, most often in a culture-specific context, most common among African Americans and/or those from the southern US; the importance lies in its misconstruence as a psychotic episode (DSM-IV™, 1994) see Culture-bound syndrome

SPENP Solid and papillary epithelial neoplasm of the pancreas; see Papillary and solid epithelial neoplasm

SPEP Serum protein electrophoresis, see there

sperm antibody An antibody directed against the sperm heads or tails; sperm antibodies were initially reported to occur in 15-20% of infertile women; newer methods using higher titers as 'cut-offs' for positivity have shown that 3% of infertile males and 2-9% of infertile ♀ produce antibodies to sperm Note: The higher the titer of SAs, the more likely the couple will remain inconceivable without some form of intervention, which includes intercourse with a condom so that the woman's immunologic memory is allowed to 'decay', sperm washing and insemination (SWIM method), and corticosteroid therapy

spermatocytic seminoma A distinct variant of seminoma that comprises 5% of all seminomas, which occurs in old men and old dogs PATHOLOGY Gelatinous masses with highly pleomorphic, bizarre and mitotically active cells that are not associated with teratomas PROGNOSIS Excellent, some tumors have a sarcomatous component, which is often

characterized by an aggressive clinical course with metastases TREATMENT Orchiectomy

sperm-binding assay Mannose-binding assay A test that evaluates the ability of an enzyme on the sperm's surface to bind with mannose receptors on the ovum; for a cohort of 80 ♂, the specificity and sensitivity of the assay for the predicting fertilization was reported to be 98% and 44% respectively (Clin Lab News August 1994)

spermicide A contraceptive agent with a high failure rate (11.9/100 woman-years); the forms of administration include foams, creams and sponges; most contain the surfactant nonoxynol 9, an agent that reduces the risk of STDs as it is also bactericidal and viricidal; the incidence of toxic shock syndrome is slightly increased in sponge users ($0.5/10^6$ sponges); spermicides are not associated with teratogenesis or trisomies , although some 'soft' data suggest possible limb reduction defects; see Contraceptives, IUDs, Litogens, Pearl index, RU 486

spermidine $NH_2(CH_2)_4NH(CH_2)_3NH_2$ A polyamine that was first identified in semen, which exists in virtually all tissues as a triply-charged cation, which stabilizes DNA; the addition of spermidine to restriction endonuclease reactions improve the digestion

SPF S-phase fraction, see there

SPF rating Sunburn protection factor rating PUBLIC SAFETY A system promulgated by the FDA that provides a ratio ('X'/1) between the length of time that a person may be exposed to solar radiation covered with a particular sunscreen than without the agent, which corresponds to a multiplication factor ranging up to 30 or 40; the SPF rating suffers from a number of flaws, including the lack of experimental model and that solar radiation is at a peak for circa four hours/day, and it is widely felt that any SPF rating above 15 is of little use; see Malignant melanoma, Sunscreen, Tanning salons, Ultraviolet radiation

SPf66 An erythrocytic stage vaccine for *Plasmodium falciparum* (Science 1995; 267:1577c)

sphenoethmoidectomy OTORHINOLARYNGOLOGY A technique for removing the ethmoid labyrinth in patients with chronic hyperplastic rhinosinusitis (CHR); elimination of the mucosal and bony changes associated with severe CHR usually requires marsupialization of the ethmoid labyrinth and sacrifice of the middle turbinate

spherical 'pneumonia' A rounded radiologic focus of often streptococcal pneumonia that may mimic a pulmonary or mediastinal mass

spherocytosis HEMATOLOGY A condition characterized by an ↑ in osmotic fragility and autohemolysis of globose red cells due to various defects in erythrocyte membrane proteins Hereditary spherocytosis is an uncommon (1:5000) AD [MIM 182900] condition CLINICAL Anemia, intermittent jaundice, splenomegaly, gallstones, which is due to leg ulcers, acquired spherocytosis, etc. Acquired spherocytosis may be the first manifestation of a delayed hemolytic reaction (eg transfusion of ABO incompatible blood, severe burns, or autoimmune hemolytic anemia) or seen in hypersplenism secondary to cirrhosis or chronic infections

spheroid NEUROPATHOLOGY A local axonal dilatation filled with degenerated organelles, seen by light microscopy as a rounded, eosinophilic and granular mass at the edges of infarcts, in axonal dystrophies and in degenerating or regenerating axons

spheroid body myopathy A rare, slowly progressive, AD [MIM 182920] neuromuscular disease affecting type I muscle fibers, which by electron microscopy displays spherical heterogeneous bodies with fine fibrillar and amorphous granularity

spherophakia-brachymorphia Weill-Marchesani syndrome, see there

sphingolipidoses A group of inborn errors of sphingolipid metabolism in which lysosphingolipids accumulate, inhibiting protein kinase C activity in signal transduction, cellular differentiation and in tumor promotion; sphingolipidoses include Fabry's disease (↑ globotriaosylsphingosine, ↑ galabiosylsphingosine), Gaucher's disease (↑ glucosylsphingosine), Krabbe's disease (↑ galactosylsphingosine), metachromatic leukodystrophy (↑ sulfogalactosylsphingosine, sulfolactosylsphingosine), Niemann-Pick disease (↑ sphingosylphosphorylcholine), as well as GM1 gangliosidosis, GM2 gangliosidoses, which includes Tay-Sachs and Sandhoff diseases and GM3 gangliosidosis or sphingolipodystrophy

DEFECTS IN RBC MEMBRANE SKELETON Due to a spectrin deficiency, or due to defective spectrin and protein 4.1 binding

ALTERED MEMBRANE PROPERTIES

↓ Surface area

Changed membrane lipids

Changed calcium content

Changed membrane proteins, eg ↑ membrane-bound catalase, hemoglobin, defective protein aggregation, altered protein phosphorylation

ALTERED CELL METABOLISM

↑ ATP turnover

↑ Glycolysis

↑ Sodium permeability

↓ Phosphoenolpyruvate transportation

Modified from GR Lee, TC Bithell, J Foerster, et al, Eds, Wintrobe's Hematology, 9th ed, Lea & Febiger, Philadelphia, 1993

Note: For many 'inborn errors of metabolism', the defective chromosomal region has been identified, eg the defect in Tay-Sachs disease maps to chromosome (C) 15q, the defect in Sandhoff's disease maps to 5q and metachromatic leukodystrophy maps to 22q

sphinx neck appearance Webbed neck, see there

spicy food Comestibles that are marinated in and/or contain chili peppers, mustards with horseradishes, curry or other spices that evoke a desired intraoral sensation that crosses pain with pleasure, which, when intense may elicit an autonomic nervous system response, including diaphoresis; the most commonly used 'spicy' condiment is hot pepper containing capsinoids, which in mild hot (chili) sauce contains nordihydrocapsaicin and N-nonanoic acid (synthetic vanillylamide); moderate hot sauce contains homodihydrocapsaicin; very hot sauce is high in capsaicin and dihydrocapsaicin, which is effective to dilutions of 1:100 000; 'hot' mustards owe their gustatory effects to horseradish, the active ingredient of which is isothiocyanate, a component of wasabe, a mustard used to season Japanese food (see Sushi syncope), and in religious ceremony (see Seder syncope); it is unclear whether hot foods are carcinogenic, as capsaicin is mutagenic by the Ames assay (a bacterial screen for carcinogens) and may cause colon cancer in rats; on the other hand, capsaicin is also an anti-oxidant, and therefore also has anti-carcinogenic properties; oxidized capsaicin also binds to and inactivates the 'j' form of cytochrome P-450 enzyme, which is thought to activate certain mutagens, including nitrosamine and polycyclic aromatic hydrocarbons; spicy foods have been traditionally denied to gastric ulcer-prone individuals, although jalapeños placed in direct contact with the gastric mucosa cause neither ulcers nor hemorrhage

spider angioma A superficial spider-like cluster of capillaries composed of a central 'feeder' vessel and multiple minute tortuous and dilated radiating vessels with a peripheral erythema; when the involved vessel is large, it may pulsate and blanch on pressure; while classically due to ↑ circulating estrogens as seen in pregnancy and alcoholic cirrhosis, spider angiomas may occur in chronic hepatic congestion secondary to constrictive pericarditis and may be a normal birthmark in children

Synonyms include arterial spider, nevus arachnoideus, nevus araneus, nevus araneosus, spider hemangioma, spider nevus, spider telangiectasia, spider telangiectasis, stellar nevus, stellate angioma, stellate telangiectasia, stellate telangiectasis, vascular spider

spider cell Spiderweb cell GYNECOLOGIC CYTOLOGY A rare variant epithelial cell seen in cervical metaplasia in papanicolaou-stained smears, morphologically similar to those described in rhabdomyomas (see below) and in 'sugar' tumors PULMONARY PATHOLOGY see Sugar tumor SURGICAL PATHOLOGY A variably-sized undifferentiated mesenchymal cell with a small central, acidophilic and stellate mass connected by thin striations to the cell periphery, containing vacuolated cytoplasm and fibers radiating toward the nucleus

Note: Although the larger 'spider' cells are typical of myxomas and myxoid liposarcoma and 'spiderweb' cells are typical of rhabdomyomas and pleomorphic rhabdomyosarcomas, in practice the distinction is arbitrary and of little utility as immunoperoxidase stains and ancillary studies are used to determine the tumor's cell of origin

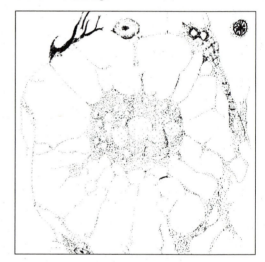

spider cell

spider(-like) colonies MICROBIOLOGY A descriptor for the morphology of the colonies of *Actinomyces israeli* seen under low power LM; Cf Medusa head colonies

'spider' dystrophy Macroreticular dystrophy A branching arachnoid pigmentary pattern seen in an AR form of retinal pigment dystrophy of the epithelium, appearing as bilateral, symmetrical lesions that do not affect vision

spiderweb cell see Spider cell

spiderweb membrane Pseudomembrane, see there

spike INFECTIOUS DISEASE *noun* A colloquial term for a sharply defined febrile peak *verb* To develop a sharp febrile peak LABORATORY MEDICINE A sharp peak seen in the β- or γ-region of a serum or urine protein electrophoresis, most commonly seen in malignant lymphoproliferative disorders, eg multiple myeloma or Waldenström's disease, as well as in a monoclonal gammopathy of undetermined significance and indicate monoclonality unless proven otherwise; spikes may not be seen if the immunoglobulin production is normally very low, as in IgD and IgE myelomas, as the spike may be obscured by the curves corresponding to more abundant IgG, IgA and IgM; see Umbrella effect NEUROLOGY A sharply-defined depolarization on an electroencephalogram RENAL PATHOLOGY Needle-like deposition of basement membrane material* within the mesangial matrix, seen in early membranous glomerulonephropathy, best visualized by the PAS stain VIROLOGY A projection on the surface of the virus that may be seen by electron microscopy, corresponding to either hemagglutinin or neuraminidase, present on the coat of influenza viruses

*Note: Membrane deposition is usually idiopathic but may be secondary to drugs, eg gold therapy, infections, eg syphilis, connective tissue disease, eg SLE, renal vein thrombosis and malignancy

spike-and-dome contour CARDIOLOGY A descriptor for the carotid arterial pulse curve seen in hypertrophic cardiomyopathy (HC), which rises abruptly and falls during midsystole (spike), later rising a second time at a slower rate during late systole (dome); the jugular pulse in HC is characterized by a prominent a (atrial) wave; see Hypertrophic cardiomyopathy, Spade deformity

'spike-and-wave' pattern An EEG pattern seen in absences (absence, formerly petit mal epilepsy), occurring as symmetric and synchronous, ≥ 3 discharges/sec with an abrupt beginning and end Note: Slower spike-and-wave pattern occurring at ≤ 2.5 discharges/sec is more common in the Lennox-Gestaut syndrome

spike potential ELECTROMYOGRAPHY A single rapid (100-200 msec) voltage 'transient' that occurs spontaneously in smooth muscle cells, when the cells have resting membrane potentials above the spike potential threshold, as occurs in the lower esophageal sphincter

spill radioactive/chemical

spillover syndrome Specificity spillover syndrome, see there

spin MRI The intrinsic angular momentum of an elementary particle (or system of particles such as a nucleus) that is responsible for the magnetic moment; the spins of nuclei have characteristic fixed values and when pairs of neutrons and protons are aligned, they cancel out the values of their spins, so that nuclei with an odd number of neutrons and/or protons will have a net nonzero rotational component characterized by an integer or half-integer quantum 'nuclear spin number'; see Magnetic resonance imaging

spin density MRI The density of resonating spins in a given region, which is a prime determinant of the strength of an MR signal from the region, measured in SI (International system) units (moles/m^3); for water, 0.11 moles of H_2O/m^3; spin density cannot be imaged directly, but is a complex series of calculations received from different pulse times; see Magnetic resonance imaging

spin doctor *'A representative for a person, especially a politician who publicizes favorable interpretations of that person's words or actions.'* (The American Heritage Dictionary of the English Language, 3rd ed, Houghton Mifflin Co, New York, 1992) An SD has come to mean any person who soothes any and everyone in a particular situation, trying to make them feel better by putting the correct 'spin' on the truth; pharmaceutical firms may commission spin doctors to approach well-respected health professionals to provide positive 'press', eg writing editorials, or 'ghostwriting' advertising copy that casts a particular drug company's products in a positive light (New York Times 4 October 1994; C3)

spin echo MRI The reappearance of an MR signal after the free induction decay is complete, due to effective reversal of the dephasing of the spins ('refocusing') by various techniques, eg reversal of a gradient magnetic field, which is a form of 1) 'time reversal' or 2) Specific RF pulse sequences such as the Carr-Purcell sequence (applied in a time shorter than or equal to T2); multiple spin echoes or a series of spin echoes at different times can be used to determine T2 without 'contamination' through the effects of the inhomogeneity of the magnetic field; see Magnetic resonance imaging

spin-echo imaging MRI A type of MRI where the spin-echo signal is measured (in contrast to measuring the free

induction decay); spin-echo images are largely a function of T2; see Magnetic resonance imaging

spin-lattice relaxation time T1, see there

spin-spin relaxation time T2, see there

spina bifida A large group of lesions caused by a defective fusion of the vertebral arch and a number of contiguous vertebrae, which normally occurs at the 21-29 somite stage in the fifth fetal week; in SB, the spinal mennges and subcutaneous tissue may herniate through the defect, but remain covered by the skin and subcutaneous tissue LABORATORY ↑ Alpha-fetoprotein; occult spina bifida affects up to 10% of adults seen at tertiary care centers; see Alpha-fetoprotein; Multivitamins

spinal block ANESTHESIOLOGY Locoregional anesthesia that is rapid and complete with very low doses; spinal block is not commonly used in obstetrics as it abolishes the bearing-down reflex and the mother cannot cooperate in expulsion of the infant

spinal cord injury A trauma to the vertebral column and spinal cord, resulting in a significant or complete loss of voluntary control of extremities or autonomic nervous system EPIDEMIOLOGY 10 000 new cases/year; 200 000 currently with chronic SCI (US); motor vehicles cause 45%, falls 22%, acts of violence 16%, sports 13%; ♂:♀ ratio 4:1; mean age = 31; 59% occur in 16-30 age group COMPLICATIONS-2ND YEAR Urinary tract infection 59%, spasticity 38%, chills and fever 19%, pressure sore 16%, autonomic hyperreflexia, contractures COMPLICATIONS-≥ 30 YEARS Pressure sores 17%, muscle and joint pain 16%, gastrointestinal or cardiocirculatory problems, urinary tract infection or other infections (N Engl J Med 1994; 330o:550RV)

spinal fusion Spondylosyndesis ORTHOPEDIC SURGERY A procedure in which multiple vertebrae are operatively fused, usually with diskectomy or laminectomy; while SF increases spinal stability and virtually eliminates pain, the fusion of multiple vertebrae results in significant loss of function, which can be resolved by fusing only two vertebrae, eg by use of JL Margulies' M-frame device

spinal muscle atrophy A heterogeneous group of conditions that are the second most common fatal autosomal recessive diseases after cystic fibrosis, affecting 1:6000-20 000 newborns; SMAs selectively affect the α motor neuron, characterized by degeneration of the α anterior horn cells with associated muscle weakness, atrophy, progressive symmetrical limb and trunk paralysis; SMAs have been arbitrarily subdivided into type I Acute or infantile onset form of Werdig-Hoffman, type II Intermediate form (onset in childhood), type III Juvenile onset form of Kugelberg-Welander, and type IV Adult onset form; despite their clinical heterogeneity, all types have a mutation of chromosome 5q11.2-13.3 (Science 1994; 264; 1474R)

spinal shock CRITICAL CARE MEDICINE A clinical complex caused by trauma to the vertebral column and spinal cord, appearing as a transient (3-6 week in duration) loss of reflex activity due to functional or anatomic interruption of the corticospinal tracts, occurring into two phases

ARREFLEXIA, characterized by complete 'failure' below the lesion, including tetraplegia, paraplegia, overflow incontinence, paralytic ileus, gastric atony and depression of cremasteric reflex, followed several weeks later by

HYPERREFLEXIA, in which there is exaggeration of reflexes with flexor spasms and autonomic dysreflexia, bladder distention, diaphoresis, hypertension, and bradycardia; certain reflexes, eg anal 'wink', bulbocavernosus and cremasteric reflexes, full penile erection, reflex leg withdrawal and Babinski sign, are retained after complete spinal cord transection since these reflexes don't require higher levels of control OBSTETRICS The term 'spinal shock' refers to an idiopathic postpartum vasomotor collapse that follows spinal anesthesia, secondary to various stressants of delivery, including acute blood loss, electrolytic imbalance, adrenocortical insufficiency, pre-eclampsia, anesthesia itself and amniotic fluid embolism

spinal vasculature steal syndrome A clinical complex characterized by arteriovenous malformation of the spinal cord, causing spinal cord compression, that may respond to ligation of the 'offending' artery

spina ventosa A form of dactylitis characterized by fusiform expansion of short diaphyseal bones, especially phalangeal bones with cortical and trabecular destruction and 'ballooning' of the cortex without a sclerotic reaction; spina ventosa was first described in TB, but also occurs in congenital syphilis (spina ventosa luetica)

spindle Mitotic spindle, see there

spindle cell carcinoma An often aggressive and undifferentiated carcinoma composed of sweeping fascicles of elongated epithelial cells of transitional, squamous, undifferentiated or rarely glandular origin that mimics a sarcoma both clinically[1] and pathologically[2]; SCCs have received the confusing synonyms of pseudosarcoma and carcinosarcoma and are most commonly seen in the oral cavity (♂:♀ ratio, 10:1), as a variant of the squamous cell carcinoma; the SCC is well-described in the larynx, upper respiratory and upper GI tracts, thyroid gland, and rarely in the female genital tract; ¼ of these patients have had regional radiotherapy EM Aggregates of keratohyaline, bundles of tonofilaments, scant and poorly developed desmosomes and rare premelanosomes TREATMENT Surgery

[1]Presents as a soft tissue mass [2]Has bizarre fibroblast-like cells with atypical mitotic figures

spindle cell lipoma A benign tumor of adipose tissue, most common in the neck and shoulders of adults, of interest as these tumors may be confused with myxoid liposarcomas by the novice and can be distinguished therefrom by the absence of a plexiform vascular pattern and lipoblasts

spindle and/or epithelioid cell nevus Spitz nevus, see there, aka Juvenile 'melanoma'

'spinnaker sail' sign A descriptor for a displaced thymic shadow seen by a plain chest film in a neonate with a unilateral pneumomediastinum, fancifully likened to a fully-blown spinnaker sail; bilateral pneumomediastinum in the neonate is fancifully designated as the 'angel wings' sign; see Rocker bottom sign

spinnbarkeit German, stretchability The 'stretchability' of cervical mucus, or the length that strands of cervical mucus reach before breaking (at least 6 cm), a reaction that parallels the 'ferning' reaction, peaking on the 14th day (ovulation) of the menstrual cycle; see Ferning; Cf String test

spiral annulets Ringed fibers, see there

spiral computed tomography Helical scanning A permutation of CT imaging based on 'slip-ring' technology, in which a large image volume is acquired by continuous rotation of the detector, scanning images at a speed of 10 mm/second, allowing the acquisition of a 25-cm 3-D 'gapless' block of radiologic information in a single breath; it has been predicted that spiral CT will have a major impact on radiocontrast studies of cerebral vasculature and the GI tract, body regions that are less well studies because of the 2-D nature of the images and the prolonged acquisition time; the information obtained with spiral CT scanning is markedly superior to the single 'slice' images from the current generation of CT imagers and, in the future, the latter machines may be relegated for use only in patients who cannot hold their breath (Diag Imaging 1991; 13:98) the image is made by injecting an iodine-labeled compound into the blood and then recording a series of 30-60

ultrathin slices, and translating the 2-D images into 3-D by volume rendering (Biophotonics Intl 1995; 2/2:26) with SC, up to 500 images can be taken in 30-40 seconds, and the technique may be of use as a partial replacement for certain endoscopic procedures, eg where malignancy is strongly suspected and otherwise requires confirmation by endoscopy (NY Times March 28 1995, C10) Cf High-resolution computed tomography

spirit A solution containing a volatile substance, usually understood to be alcohol

spirometer A device used to measure volumes of inhaled (and exhaled) air; see Lung volumes

spirometry The measurement of the movement of air in and out of the lung during various breathing maneuvers, the most important of the pulmonary function tests, see there (N Engl J Med 1994; 331:25RA)

spironolactone bodies Rounded, eosinophilic intracytoplasmic inclusions that may be observed in the zona glomerulosa of the adrenal cortex of patients receiving spironolactone EM Whorls of endoplasmic reticulum or myelinoid figures with central lipid core; similar inclusions have been identified in adrenal adenoma, adrenogenital syndrome, Conn's disease, pheochromocytoma, and paraganglioma (Arch Pathol Lab Med 1975; 99:416) see Lamellar bodies

Spitz nevus Epithelioid and/or spindle-cell (nevomelanocytic) nevus*, EC-SC nevus A relatively common benign compound nevus occurring on the face of children, adolescents, and young adults; there is no predilection for sex or race CLINICAL EC-SC nevi average 8 mm in diameter and present in various guises, eg a smooth elastic, pink-tan papule that flattens with external pressure, a lightly pigmented papule, single or multiple nevi arising in a large congenital nevomelanocytic nevus, in lesional clusters, and others PATHOLOGY Bizarre mononuclear and multinucleated giant cells, maturation with increasing depth of tumor, eosinophilic globules TREATMENT Excision

*This is the preferred 'written' term for this lesion (in contrast to the 'spoken' form, which continues to be Spitz nevus), and in future eiditions, will be so listed; other synonyms include benign juvenile melanoma, compound melanocytoma, epithelial and/or spindle-cell melanoma, juvenile melanoma, nevus of large spindled and/or epithelioid cells, nevus prominens et pigmentosum, prepubertal melanoma, pseudomelanoma, spindle cell and/or epithelioid nevus, spindle and epithelioid cell nevus, Spitz' juvenile melanoma, and Spitz tumor

'splashback' FORENSIC PATHOLOGY Protrusion of tissue from a bullet's entrance wound, resulting from the kinetic energy imparted by the bullet; although the tissue surrounding the entrance wound closes over behind the bullet, the gases expanding after the bullet find the path of least resistance for escape, leaving via the entrance wound, pushing out fragments of subcutaneous tissue

splenic flexure syndrome A condition caused by swallowed gas that passes often only as far as the transverse colon, producing abdominal distension and discomfort that is relieved by defecation or passing of flatus

splenic index A parameter used to evaluate the extent of experimental GVHD; the ratio of the spleen-to-body weight is relatively constant and ↑ in GVHD; the index is not suitable for humans; see Phagocytic index

splenomegaly Enlargement of the spleen of any etiology, which is almost invariably a manifestation of underlying disease; the only specific finding in splenomegaly is dragging sensation in the upper right quadrant; megalic spleens may reach 4.0 kg or more, eg in agnogenic myeloid metaplasia (table)

splenosis The autotransplantation of splenic tissue to unusual sites after open splenic trauma, eg automobile accidents, gunshot, or stab wounds; the splenic pulp implants appear as red-blue nodules on the peritoneum, omentum, and mesentery, morphologically similar to multifocal pelvic endometriosis; Cf Hypersplenism

splice MOLECULAR BIOLOGY *noun* A generic term for any construct formed from spliced nucleic acids *verb* To join two or more segments of nucleic acid in an end-to-end fashion, often to form a circle

splice junction MOLECULAR BIOLOGY A segment of DNA involved in RNA splicing, defined by the GU dinucleotide at the 5' end of the intron, known as the donor or left junction and an AG dinucleotide at the 3' acceptor or right junction of the intron

spliceosome MOLECULAR BIOLOGY A nuclear structure that folds pre-mRNA into a substrate and splices out the intervening sequences or introns of RNA (which are not translated into proteins) from mRNA precursors and splices together the exons (which are translated into proteins),

---

SPLENOMEGALY

CONGESTION Cirrhosis, congestive heart failure, thrombosis of portal or splenic veins

INFECTION

Bacterial Brucellosis, infective carditis agents, syphilis, TB, typhoid fever

Fungal Histoplasmosis

Parasitic Echinococcosis, leishmaniasis, malaria, schistosomiasis, toxoplasmosis, trypanosomiasis

Viral CMV, EBV

INFLAMMATORY/IMMUNE-RELATED Rheumatoid arthritis, SLE

HEMATOPOIETIC DISEASE/LYMPHOID FUNCTION

Malignant Leukemias, eg ALL, CLL, myeloproliferative disorders (eg agnogenic myeloid metaplasia, CML, multiple myeloma, polycythemia vera); lymphomas (Hodgkin's disease, NHL)

Nonmalignant Hemolytic anemia, histiocytosis, thrombocytopenic purpura

STORAGE DISEASES Gaucher's disease, mucopolysaccharidosis, Niemann-Pick disease

UND SO WEITER Amyloidosis, cysts, hypersplenism, metastatic malignancy, primary tumors

---

forming a mature mRNA molecule; because eukaryotes are rich in nonprotein-encoding introns, the spliceosome function is essential to gene expression in eukaryotic cells; by affinity chromatography, it appears that the minimum components of a spliceosome are four small nuclear ribonucleoproteins (snRNPs U1, U2, U5, and U4/6), which are required for the proper folding of the RNA, splicing it into a mature mRNA; snRNPs aggregate together on the chromosomes as particles ranging from 1 to 20 μm in diameter, designated as 'snurposomes' (Science 1991; 252:1499); other spliceosome components as well as a number of different proteins that have been designated as PRPs (for pre-RNA processing); the release of mRNA from the spliceosome requires the presence of an RNA helicase-like protein PRP22 (Nature 1991; 349:487); other proteins, eg PRP16 an RNA-dependent ATPase are transient in their interaction with the spliceosome (ibid; 349:495); see DEAD-box proteins Note: U6 is widely conserved across species from yeast to human and may be the most critical component of a spliceosome, as experimentally induced U6 mutations either prevent spliceosome formation or interfere with the splicing process; see Transcription unit

splicing MOLECULAR BIOLOGY The cutting and rejoining of strands of a linear molecule, eg DNA, RNA or protein; in the native state, splicing is the process in which the transcribed introns of immature mRNA are removed, and the exons joined to become mature mRNA that is transcribed into a protein; see Alternative splicing **GENE SPLICING** is an experimental procedure in which a segment of DNA is covalently inserted into a 'host' molecule or vector, creat-

ing a 'recombinant' DNA molecule **PRE-mRNA SPLICING** A vital cell process that is intrinsic to eukaryotic cells, consisting in a two-step phosphotransferase reaction requiring ATP hydrolysis, in which segments of template-derived RNA known as introns (intervening sequences that do not encode proteins) are excised and the exons (sequences of RNA that encode proteins) are joined, by action of a 'spliceosome'; the mature mRNA is then translated into a protein; pre-mRNA splicing is site-specific and requires precise sequence recognition at the intron boundaries or splice junction **PROTEIN SPLICING** A phenomenon by which two or more proteins can be generated from a single primary translation product, by a process known as alternative splicing, while a second product is formed upon rejoining of the two ends

splinter hemorrhage A small linear subungual hemorrhage that is red when fresh and brown when aged, located at the distal third of the nailbed PATHOGENESIS The blood 'leaks' into the avascular squames under the fingernails due to microemboli and/or increased capillary fragility; although splinter hemorrhages are characteristic of acute and subacute bacterial endocarditis, they are more commonly due to trauma, occur in up to 10% of normal subjects and in 40% of patients with mitral stenosis; splinter hemorrhages are also described in the retinal disk in papilledema, most commonly due to retinal vein occlusion or subarachnoid hemorrhage, as well as in trichinosis

split gene A gene composed of two or more segments of DNA that encodes polypeptides (exons), separated by segments of non-polypeptide encoding DNA (introns), which are excised or spliced out, forming a transcript from which a cognate protein is transcribed; see Exon, Intron, Spliceosome, Splicing

split hand/foot Lobster claw deformity, see there

split papule A skin nodule with a central linear erosion seen adjacent to the mouth or nose in secondary syphilis

'splits' IMMUNOLOGY A designation for HLA antigens that were first described as private antigens and subsequently shown to be public antigens; the new status is indicated by a parenthesis enclosing its old status; see Private antigen, Public antigen

split thickness graft A 'thin' skin graft (0.25-0.35 mm in thickness) that includes the epidermis and a minimal amount of dermis; STGs have the advantage of more rapid availability of donor sites for further engraftment, more rapid vascularization, longer post-transplantation survival in the recipient site and are of greatest use in contaminated skin sites, burn sites and sites with poor intrinsic vasculature; thick STGs are more resistant to trauma, result in less contraction and allow some degree of sensation but survive poorly in the recipient site; see Skin graft; Cf Artificial skin, Spray-on skin

'splitting' Hair-splitting ACADEMIA The division of a well-defined morbid condition, lesion, or other entity into ever smaller subtypes, eg subdividing Laurence-Moon-Biedl-Bardet syndrome into the Laurence-Moon and Bardet-Biedl syndromes, a practice known as 'hair-splitting'*; Cf 'Lumping' RENAL PATHOLOGY see Railroad track appearance

*Although ostensibly the purpose of splitting is to identify subgroups of patients with a better or worse prognosis or response to therapy, the real (and rarely admitted) purpose may be to generate publications of greater volume than value, which increases the bulk of writer's curriculum vitae without adding substantively to scientific knowledge

spoked wheel pattern A pattern of chromatin clumping seen at the periphery of the nucleus in basophilic normoblast (pre-erythrocyte) and plasma cells

spondee words AUDIOLOGY Two-syllable words that have equal stress on each syllable, eg baseball, toothbrush, which can be used to evaluate baseline hearing (N Engl J Med 1993; 328:233oa)

spondyloepiphyseal dysplasia A heterologous group of inherited conditions characterized by short trunk and short limbed dwarfism, due to a defect in ossification of the epiphyseal growth plates of the vertebral bodies and proximal centers of the long bones, affecting the shoulder and pelvic girdles

sponge kidney Polycystic kidney, see there

spongialization ORTHOPEDIC SURGERY Abrasion arthroplasty Excision of patellar cartilage and subchondral bone, leaving well-vascularized cancellous bone exposed (N Engl J Med 1994; 331:889OA) see Autologous chondrocyte transplantation

spongiform microabscess Munro's microabscess, see there

spongiform pustule Kogoj's microabscess A subcorneal aggregate of neutrophils, which is accompanied by a lymphohistiocytic infiltrate and perivascular round cell inflammation in the upper dermis; SP is characteristic of psoriasis, and may be seen in acrodermatitis continua and infantile acropustulosis; Cf Munro's microabscess

spongy degeneration of infancy Canavan-Van Bogaert-Bertrand disease An AR [MIM 271900] condition characterized by diffuse vacuolization of the deep cerebral cortex, predominantly affecting the white matter, but also the gray matter, caused by hydropic degeneration of the glial cells and myelin CLINICAL Onset in early infancy with hypotonia and poor head control, hyperextension of legs and flexion of arms, optic atrophy and blindness, severe mental retardation, rigidity, hyperreflexia, seizures and progressive macrocephaly; death occurs by 18 months PATHOLOGY Cortical and subcortical vacuolation which produces the spongy appearance; Cf Leukodystrophy

Note: Degenerative and spongiform gliotic reactions may in some cases be due to an abortive retroviral infection, as in defective production of the viral env (envelope) protein

sponsored symposium A collection of papers published as a separate issue or as a special section (eg an appendix) in a regular issue of a peer-reviewed medical or scientific journal, see details under Background

'...data suggest that industry-sponsored symposium are promotional in nature (especially when sponsored by a single drug company and/or on a single agent) and that journals often abandon the peer-review process when they publish symposiums....Financial pressures on journals appear to contribute to increasing publication of symposiums....The acceptance of symposium publications could distort the medical literature and ultimately alter physicians' prescribing practices' (N Engl J Med 1992; 327:1135OA)

BACKGROUND In the US, pharmaceutical companies are severely limited in the types of promotional activities, materials and 'gifts' they may by law give to physicians; these restrictions tend to minimize 'conflict-of-interest' drug prescribing practices, which were common when substantive gifts, eg vacations, were given by drug companies to high volume physician-prescribers (N Engl J Med 1992; 327:1135OA); $100 is the usual ceiling of monetary value for gifts given to physicians

spontaneous abortion A term equivalent to 'miscarriage' as used by the lay; spontaneous abortions occur at any time and for a wide variety of reasons; it is estimated that 20-50% of all conceptuses spontaneously abort, half of which are attributed to aneuploidy, especially loss of a sex chromosome and trisomy, especially of chromosome 16

spontaneous bacterial peritonitis A relatively common[1] condition that accompanies end-stage liver disease and ascites CLINICAL Abdominal pain, ascites, encephalopathy, fever, rebound tenderness LABORATORY Ascitic fluid has > 500 (often 10 000+) PMNs/mm³, protein > 1.0 g/dL, monomicrobials[2] TREATMENT Third-generation cephalosporins, eg cefotaxime MORTALITY 30-40%, less when treated early, worse if accompanied by signs of poor liver function, eg upper GI bleeding, bilirubin > 8 mg/dL, serum albumin < 2.5 g/dL, hepatic encephalopathy, hepatorenal

syndrome (Mayo Clin Proc 1995; 70:365OA)

[1]Estimated prevalence in those with ascites is 7-15% [2]92% are monomicrobials, in particular gram-negative rods (Escherichia coli comprises nearly ½ of cases, followed by Klebsiella spp; gram-positive organisms comprise ± 25%, most commonly, streptococcal spp

spontaneous generation of life Historic interest

spontaneous pneumothorax A condition affecting an estimated 17 000/year (US), which may be idiopathic or secondary to underlying pulmonary disease, eg COPD, most commonly occurring in previously healthy ♂, age 20-40, secondary to rupture of subpleural blebs CLINICAL Sudden onset of chest pain, with dyspnea proportionate to the size of the pneumothorax; tension pneumothorax, while rare, may compromise the circulation by a ball-valve mechanism TREATMENT Suction followed by water seal drainage PROGNOSIS 30% recur on the same side, a tendency that may be reduced by intrapleural tetracycline; 10% occur de novo on the opposite side

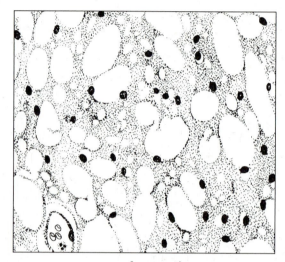

spongy degeneration

spontaneous remission of malignancy A rare clinical event; Everson and Cole catalogued 241 cases as of 1966 (Spontaneous Regression of Cancer, WB Saunders, Philadelphia, 1966), and defined spontaneous regression of cancer as the partial or complete disappearance of a histologically confirmed malignancy in absence of treatment or with treatment deemed inadequate to sufficiently alter its natural course; malignant melanoma comprises 10% of the cases of spontaneous regression of malignancy, with the caveat that in melanoma the primary lesion may involute or completely disappear only to resurface as a fulminant and aggressive malignancy after the reporting of a complete cure

spooning A descriptor for a hand deformity in patients with chorea, in which the outstretched hands, slightly flexed wrists and metacarpophalangeal joints slightly hyperextended demonstrate a distinct concavity

spoon nail Koilonychia A rare acquired nail dystrophy seen in bronchiectasia in which the nail bed is atrophic and the nail has a 'hollowed' appearance or central concave; see Clubbing

sporadic GENETICS Pertaining or referring to an event attributable to changes in somatic DNA, which may be inherited, but not in a predictable fashion

sporotrichoid infection Swimming pool granuloma, see there

sporotrichosis A chronic infection by Sporothrix schenckii which spreads by the lymphatics CLINICAL It may remain localized as a fixed cutaneous or plaque lesion or spread into the lymphatics PATHOLOGY Pyogranulomatous inflammation, PMNs, multinucleated giant cells, epithelioid histiocytes, and lymphocytes TREATMENT Supersaturated potassium iodide, itraconazole (N Engl J Med 1994; 331:181cₚc)

sporozoite surface protein-2 see Malaria vaccine

sport A generic term for any individual who/that differs substantially from the stock, strain, subspecies, species (whatever) from whence he/she/it came CLINICAL GENETICS A phenotypic trait that appears de novo in an individual and is subsequently inherited by his progeny, which is thought to be related to a spontaneous mutation or an environmental mutagen acting on the egg or sperm; Cf Lysenkoism

sports 'anemia' A red cell mass that falls in the mild anemic range, which is typical of 'endurance' athletes; this relative increase in plasma volume appears to be a physiological response to the repeated and transient dehydration that occurs in long races; a 'normal' hematocrit would be detrimental to muscle action and predispose the athletes to life-threatening thrombotic events, thus making 'blood doping' a potentially dangerous practice

sports dermatology The formal study of dermatopathies that affect athletes, which may be traumatic[1], environmental[2], infectious[3], or exacerbations of pre-existing dermatopathies

[1]eg Black heel-better known as talon noir, black palm, friction blister, jazz ballet bottom, jogger's nipples, jogger's (climber's, hiker's, skier's, tennis) toe, runner's rump, turf toe [2]Solar damage, cold injury, water-induced damage-eg green hair, contact dermatitis [3]eg Herpes gladiatorum

sports drink A generic term for a beverage used to quench thirst while participating in various sports-related activities, and which provides a boost in energy and/or build muscle mass; water, sugar, salt, and potassium are core constituents common to all SDs, of which there are three types: isotonics, carbohydrate drinks, and protein drinks; isotonics are used to simply replace fluid and electrolytes during lengthy exercise; carbohydrate drinks contain glucose polymers and are intended to replenish the reserves of energy during and after exercise; protein drinks (aka amino acid drinks) are commonly made of whey, a bovine milk product, and are used to help recuperate fatigued or overly stressed muscles (New York Times 7 Dec 1994; C6)

sports injury A generic term for any injury sustained practicing or competing in a particular sport SITES OF SIs* (Descending frequency-DF) Thigh, foot, knee, lower leg, ankle, heat exhaustion, hip, finger, and others TYPES OF SIs (DF) Contusion, strain, sprain, heat exhaustion, lacerations and others SPORTS WITH SIs Martial arts (judo, Tae Kwon Do), wrestling, gymnastics, power lifting, track and field, soccer, and others (Mayo Clin Proc 1995; 70:549)

*Study of an amateur Olympic-type 'Games event' for those ages 8-59

sports medicine A subspecialty of occupational medicine that is usually practiced by orthopedic surgeons or by rehabilitation medicine physicians, which is involved in the care of those who spring, sprint, splash, bash or bogey, for play or pay; see Anabolic steroids, Boxing, Exercise, Exercise-associated amenorrhea, Running, Sports dermatology; Cf Performing arts medicine

spot *noun* A focus on a chromatogram or electrophoretic gel containing a substance of interest *verb* To apply a minute amount of material to a chromatographic or electrophoretic support prior to performing an electrophoretic procedure

spotted bone disease Osteopoikilosis, see there, also known as Buschke-Ollendorff syndrome

spotted leg 'syndrome' A condition characterized by patches of subdermal atrophy secondary to diabetic vasculitis, most common below the knee in older diabetics; the affected skin is smooth, shiny and hyperpigmented

due to hemosiderin deposition and increased melanin

spotted pigmenti nevi A variant of intradermal nevi that is located adjacent to eccrine ducts and enveloped by nevus cells

spousal benefits SOCIAL MEDICINE Those benefits, including health care insurance and life insurance that are provided to the spouse (ie husband or wife) of an employee; in the US and other developed nations, these benefits are being extended to unmarried partners, including those of the same sex (Am Med News 15 April 1991)

spousal rape A specific form of rape committed by the husband or common law partner, which is regarded as a violent crime; SR is a critical component of the battered wife syndrome, but is less commonly reported to authorities than other forms of rape given the wife's state of economic dependency and sense of personal failure should she seek a divorce (N Engl J Med 1995; 332:234ᵣᵥ) see Date rape, Rape

'spray-on' skin A polymeric material for covering superficial second-degree burn wounds; it is no longer used as it is contraindicated in deep second- and third-degree burns, where it would have been most useful, due to increased superficial infections and non-adherence; see Artificial skin, Split-thickness graft

spreadsheet COMPUTERS An electronic matrix of rows and columns that allows for user-defined entry of data in either an alphabetical or numerical fashion and its simultaneous manipulation

Note: The most popular spreadsheet program in the IBM-PC microcomputer environment has been Lotus 1-2-3

SPROM Spontaneous premature rupture of membranes; see PROM

sprue syndrome 1) Celiac (nontropical) sprue, see there 2) Tropical sprue, see there

spun-glass hair disease Uncombable hair syndrome, see there

spur IMMUNOLOGY A sharply curved projection from a precipitation line that is characteristic of 'partial identity' between two antigens when examined by Ouchterlony's 2-D-double immunodiffusion technique, which indicates that there is cross-reactivity of antigens with a cognate antibody (figure, double immunodiffusion)

spurious authorship Honorary co-authorship A term referring to the widely extant practice of including as coauthors the name(s) of persons who have had little to do with the actual work involved in publishing original research reports; as noted by Nature's Maddox, *'The benefits of authorship are so great that potential authors of manuscripts awaiting publication would probably...sign formal declarations that they had been full members of the group responsible.'* (Nature 1994; 369:353ₙ&ᵥ) see Authorship

SQL Structured query language, see there

squamocolumnar junction The zone of transition from squamous epithelium to secretory and glandular epithelium; squamocolumnar junctions occur in the nasopharynx, esophagogastric junction and anus, as well as the uterine cervix where it may be the site of origin of cervical squamous cell carcinoma; the junction migrates external to the os after vaginal delivery and migrates internally in the postmenopausal endocervix

squamocolumnar Z-line ENDOSCOPIC ANATOMY A zig-zag border seen by upper GI endoscopy related to the abrupt transition from stratified squamous (esophageal) epithelium to columnar (gastric) epithelium; the Z-line's appearance is thought to be due to the change from the multi-celled layer of the esophagus, to the single cell layer of gastric mucosa that is in intimate contact with blood vessels; in patients with Barrett's esophagus, the Z-line is displaced proximally from 1 to 15 cm (Sci & Med Nov/Dec 1994 p16RV)

squamous eddies DERMATOPATHOLOGY Whorls and 'waves' of eosinophilic, flattened squamous cells arranged in an onion-peel fashion, typical of inflammed ('irritated') seborrheic keratosis, simulating either the keratinization of the follicular infundibulum, seen in the proliferating trichilemmal cyst/tumor or the squamous pearls of well-differentiated squamous cell carcinoma; Cf Horn pseudocyst, Squamous pearl

squamous intraepithelial lesion GYNECOLOGIC CYTOLOGY A term that '...*encompasseses a spectrum of noninvasive cervical epithelial abnormalities traditionally classified as flat condyloma, dyaplasia/carcinoma in situ, and CIN. In the Bethesda Classification, the spectrum is divided into low-grade and high-grade lesions. Low-grade lesions encompass the cellular changes associated with HPV cytopathic effect (so-called koilocytotic atypia) and mild dysplasia. High-grade lesions encompass moderate dysplasia, severe dysplasia, and carcinoma in situ/CIN2, 3.*' defined by an array of cytopathologic findings (cells occur singly or in sheets) (RJ Kurman, D Solonmon, The Bethesda System, Springer-Verlag, New York, 1994) see High-grade squamous intraepithelial lesion, low-grade squamous intraepithelial lesion

squamous odontogenic tumor A relatively uncommon oral lesion composed of nests of benign squamous epithelium lying in a fibrous stroma, with a round-to-triangular radiolucency at the neck of the tooth's root, most often first appearing in the adolescent female, causing pain and loosening of the teeth TREATMENT Simple excision

squamous pearl Keratin pearl A compact round cluster of curved and flattened keratinocytes (figure) that have glassy, pale pink laminations, which are most characteristic of well-differentiated squamous cell carcinoma; SPs may also be seen in keratoacanthoma and in synovial sarcoma; when seen in Papanicolaou-stained smears of the cervix and vagina, keratin pearls are indicative of estrogenic effect; Cf Horn pseudocyst, Squamous eddies

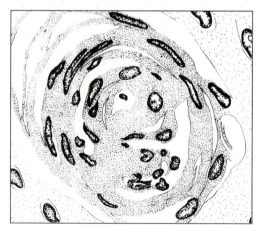

squamous pearl

square root sign CARDIOLOGY A pressure contour seen by cardiac catheterization, which consists of an elevation of the right ventricular diastolic pressure with early filling and a subsequent plateau, a finding suggestive of chronic constrictive pericarditis

square wave CARDIOLOGY An abnormal blood pressure response to the Valsalva maneuver (VM)*, seen in left ventricular failure, where the blood pressure increases at the onset of the VM, remains elevated until the VM is released after which the blood pressure abruptly drops to baseline without 'overshooting' the baseline pressure, accompanied by little change in the pulse pressure and without tachycardia Note: Normal subjects respond to VM with a slow decrease in blood and pulse pressure and increase in heart rate; when VM is stopped, the return to normal is accompanied by an 'overshooting' of the baseline

*↑ Diaphragmatic pressure against a closed glottis, with an ↑ of intrathoracic pressure to 40 mm Hg

square wave jerk NEUROLOGY A brief, intermittent and horizontal ocular oscillation, arising from the defects in the primary gaze position, which is most common in cerebellar disease

'squaring' RADIOLOGY A descriptor for the sharp demarcation of the lower patella, with the conversion of the contour from a voluptuous curve to a virtually teutonic right angle, which is seen after multiple hemarthroses in hemophiliacs

squash drinking syndrome PEDIATRICS A condition recently reported in toddlers which is characterized by poor appetite, poor weight gain, and loose stools, which has been linked to the intake of high energy foods (Arch Dis Child 1995; 72: 141)

'Squash It!' PUBLIC HEALTH A phrase that is being integrated into the African-American street culture, which verbalizes an increasingly popular concept, ie that it is socially acceptable to back down from violence or a fight and defuse a volatile situation; used as a complement to stricter gun control laws, job creation, and welfare reform, public health officials hope to use the 'squash it!' concept to reduce street violence, and achieve the same success that has been reported with the 'designated driver' (see there) campaign (Am Med News 19 Sept 1994)

squash prep see Crush preparation

squat jump 'syndrome' SPORTS MEDICINE A transient clinical complex caused by intense and violent exercise, first described secondary to the 'squat-jump', a form of calisthenic, resulting in myoglobinuria with swelling of the quadriceps, proteinuria, hematuria and hemoglobinuria

squatting PEDIATRICS A position adopted by a child with cyanotic congenital heart disease, classically in Fallot's tetralogy, in the face of acute hypoxia; squatting relieves the exertion-induced dyspnea by decreasing the right-to-left shunt and increasing the systemic vascular resistance and pulmonary blood flow; adults with Fallot's do not squat as they know their exercise tolerance level

'squeaky wheel' effect The effect of placing a problem, complaint, or 'injustice' in an appropriate forum or advertising it in such a way as to produce the greatest stridency, causing it to garner enough sympathy and support to be addressed, regardless of the principle of fair play; this principle resulted in the US government-sponsored reimbursement of experimental autologous bone marrow transplantation for patients with advanced breast cancer (cost $125 000 per patient), which equals the cost of 2000 screening mammograms; since (as the phrase goes) '...*the squeaky wheel gets the oil...*', decisions may be made for a small but vocal minority rather than for the broader interests of society, addressing private patient concerns rather than public health needs and short-term expenditures rather than long-term savings (JAMA 1991; 265:3300) see Rule of rescue; Cf Signal event

SQUID imaging Superconducting quantum interference device imaging SQUIDs are the most highly sensitive (detecting magnetic fields $1/10^9$ that of the earth's gravity) low-'noise' amplifiers in existence; SQUIDs are used in biomagnetic imaging to measure the magnetic flux created when electrical energy flows through neurons; SQUIDs may be connected to a network of superconducting antenna coils designed to measure magnetic flux and housed in a helium-filled dewar (a metal container with an evacuated space between the walls that may be silver coated to prevent the transfer of heat) to maintain a low (-269°C) temperature; optimal imaging requires a room that shields out all radio and sound waves and placement of the sensor as close as possible to the body; the magnetic signals are detected, amplified, filtered, processed and displayed on a computer; SQUIDs cost $2-3 million and may be useful for diagnosing epilepsy, stroke, migraines, language disorders, schizophrenia, motor and sensory defects, and cardiac arrhythmias (Sci Am 1994; 270/8:46) see Imaging

squiggle Tilde A symbol ($\sim$) used to designate a high-energy (usually phosphate) bond

squiggly cells HEMATOPATHOLOGY A colloquial term for a variant cell of no known diagnostic or prognostic significance seen in Lennert's diffuse mixed cell lymphoma and occasionally in T-cell lymphomas

squirting papilla DERMATOPATHOLOGY A histopathologic feature of psoriasiform lesions, characterized by intermittent 'regurgitation' of fluid and leukocytes at the head of the papilla, seen in psoriasis and pityriasis rubra pilaris

3SR Self-sustaining sequence replication, see there

SR 4233 An agent with anti-neoplastic potential, ingested in a non-toxic form and metabolized into a selectively tumoritoxic form, releasing DNA-damaging oxygen free radicals into the oxygen-depleted environment typically inhabited by tumor cells that have outgrown their blood supply and survive in low-oxygen conditions

src The Rous sarcoma virus-derived oncogene that provided the first evidence that cancer could be induced by introducing a gene into a normal cell; *c-src* is a proto-oncogene encoding a 60-kD tyrosine-kinase protein kinase (pp60^{c-src}) that is located in the plasma membrane, has tyrosine kinase activity, and phosphorylates the tyrosine residues of other proteins, thus being a generalized growth-promoting signal; *src*-family proteins interact with cellular proteins via an N-terminal unique region or by a conserved SH2 region; see SH2

Src c-Src protein Src's tyrosine kinase activity is increased during cell-cycle stage G1 and in the G2/M transition by the dephosphorylation of its regulatory tyrosine residue; c-Src protein appears to act on a 68-kD protein (p68), and may regulate the processing, trafficking, or transition of RNA in a cell-cycle dependent fashion (Nature 1994; 368:867, 871L)

Src homology-2 SH2, see there

Src homology-3 SH3, see there

Src homology regions see SH2/SH3 regions

SRIF Somatotropin release-inhibiting hormone, see there

SRP Signal recognition particle, see there

SRS-A Slow reacting substance of anaphylaxis IMMUNOLOGY The group of cysteinyl leukotrienes, LTC$_4$ and LTD$_4$ (LTE$_4$ is also involved but is a lesser actor), polyunsaturated 20-carbon fatty acids derived from arachidonic acid and platelet-activating factor, which are released from mast cells during anaphylaxis; SRS-As cause slow sustained and potent smooth muscle contraction, bronchoconstriction (1000-fold more potent than prostaglandins or histamine) and increased capillary permeability, platelet aggregation, proteolysis of the basement membrane components, providing chemotaxis for eosinophils and neutrophils; are potent bronchoconstrictors, stimulate mucus secretion and increase the permeability of postcapillary venules; SRS-As (especially LTC$_4$ and LTD$_4$) are increased in asthmatics and involved in immediate hypersensitivity, with bronchoconstriction, and cardiac depression

SRUS Solitary rectal ulcer syndrome, see there

SRV-1 A type D simian AIDS virus that infected a macaque colony in California, the genome of which has little in common with HIV-1, although the genes per se are similar, and include an LTR (long terminal repeat), *gag* (inner shell protein), *pol* (polymerase), *env* (envelope) and an *orf* (open reading frame) between the *gag* and *pol* that encodes a viral protease; see SAIDS, SIV, Retrovirus

SRY A gene of the human Y chromosome that is required for induction of male sex determination; *SRY* encodes a protein (SRY) with a high mobility group domain (HMG box) (Nature 1993; 364:685; 675N&V)

SRY The protein encoded by the 14-kilobase *sry* (sex-determining region of the Y chromosome) gene in humans that corresponds to the long-elusive testis-determining gene on the Y chromosome (Tdy); the homologous mouse protein is designated Sry; the *sry* gene is sufficient to assign 'maleness', as corroborated by its insertion into female transgenic mice, which develop into phenotypic males (Nature 1991; 251:117, 96); see X chromosome inactivation

S/S Staples and sutures

SS-A Ro A cytoplasmic antigen against which 25% of patients with SLE and 40% of those with Sjögren syndrome have circulating antibodies; Cf Antinuclear antibodies

SS-B La A cytoplasmic antigen against which patients with SLE and Sjögren's syndrome have circulating antibodies; anti-SS-B antibodies are thought to be associated with a better prognosis in lupus and lower anti-nuclear antibodies, see there

SS disease Sickle cell anemia due to homozygous hemoglobin S

SS syndrome Streptococcal-sex syndrome, see there

SSB protein Single-stranded (DNA) binding protein A heterotrimeric polypeptide protein that binds single strands of DNA, which is involved in constructing an active growing fork in DNA replication in bacteria; SSB acts on the T antigen and topoisomerases to unwind DNA, facilitating access of replication proteins, stimulates the activity of polymerases and has a critical role in DNA excision repair (Nature 1991; 349:539)

SSCP Single-strand conformation polymorphism, see there

Ssc1p, Ssc2p, Ssc3p, Ssc4p Heat shock proteins in yeasts

SSPE Subacute sclerosing panencephalitis, see there

SSRI Selective serotonin re-uptake inhibitor, see there

SSSS Staphylococcus scalded skin syndrome, see there

stab MICROBIOLOGY *noun* Stab culture, see there *verb* To inoculate a semisolid bacterial growth medium, usually in a 'slant' tube by using a jabbing motion, usually performed in conjunction with streaking, which combines anaerobic ('stab') and aerobic ('streak') conditions in the same test tube, as used by the triple sugar iron agar tubes; Cf Streak

stab cells Band neutrophils HEMATOPATHOLOGY Immature, bilobed or not yet fully segmented PMNs that are increased in the peripheral blood in acute infection; see Left shift

stab culture MICROBIOLOGY A culture of bacteria that has been inoculated in an agar tube with a needle that reaches the deep portion of the tube, allowing comparison of aerobic and anaerobic conditions; see Oxidative-fermentative test

'stabbing' invasion SURGICAL PATHOLOGY A pattern of tumor infiltration in which jagged, finger-like strands of malignant epithelial cells invade subepithelial tissue (figure, page 848), classically seen in the 'garden variety' of squamous cell carcinoma, which may be accompanied by a brisk inflammatory reaction; Cf 'Bulldozing' invasion

stabilizing selection Adaptive gridlock, see there

stacked coin appearance GI RADIOLOGY A descriptor for the incomplete filling and parallel spiculation of the plical folds seen in radiocontrast studies of the small intestine

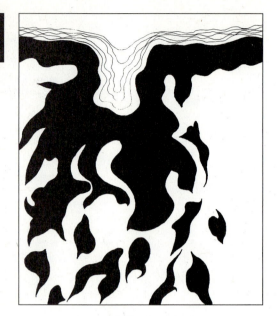

stabbing invasion

(most striking in the jejunum, given the prominence of plical folds), corresponding to thickening of the wall by either intramural hemorrhage or hematoma formation, related to anticoagulants, blood dyscrasia, trauma, Meckel's diverticulum, endometriosis, or infiltration of the intestinal wall, as in lymphoma; Cf Rouleaux

stacking SPORTS MEDICINE The illicit administration of various 'cocktails' of oral and injectable anabolic steroids by athletes, almost invariably body builders, at levels that may reach 40-100 times the therapeutic dose (JC DeLee, D Drez, Jr, Eds, Orthopedic Sports Medicine WB Saunders, Philadelphia, 1994)

staff privileges Admitting privileges The rights that a health professional has as a member of a hospital's medical staff, including hospitalization of his private patients, a seat on committees in the hospital, and participation in decisions relevant to the hospital's future; physicians receive staff privileges when they meet certain standards set by the medical staff and board of trustees, eg board certification, experience and subspecialty expertise, in exchange for which the physician performs certain duties without pay, including teaching, providing emergency care or clinic services; Cf Hospital-based physician, RAPERs

Note: Most physicians in the US are private practitioners who may have staff privileges in more than one hospital

stage migration Will Rogers phenomenon, see there

staggered cut MOLECULAR BIOLOGY A type of scission of the DNA double helix, classically produced by restriction endonucleases, in which there is an overhanging single-stranded tail of four to six nucleotides comprising the 'sticky' ends; see Restriction endonuclease, 'Sticky' ends

staghorn calculus A concrement with broad arborescence that fills (and forms a radiologically visible 'cast' of) the renal pelvicaliceal system (figure) often composed of magnesium ammonium phosphate, concentrated in the urine by urea-splitting bacteria, eg *Proteus* species and some staphylococci, inducing urine alkalinization and mineral precipitation; staghorn calculi may also occur in hyperparathyroidism

staghorn pattern ANATOMIC PATHOLOGY A pattern seen by low-power LM, which consists of multiple sharply-branched and jagged vessels, classically seen in hemangiopericytoma, which may also be seen in Kaposi sarcoma, as well as synovial sarcoma, mesenchymal chondrosarco-

ma, leiomyosarcoma, leiomyoma and myofibromatosis; see Promontory sign

staging ONCOLOGY An evaluation or 'work-up' of a patient to determine the severity and extent of a disease in order to guide therapy, a process that is required as each stage has a relatively standard treatment; as an example, stage I carcinomas often respond to simple resection, but usually require other modalities including radiotherapy and/or chemotherapy in higher stages; staging is performed for malignancy and occasionally, other conditions eg AIDS; for most malignancies, there are four stages, ranging from the early and well-circumscribed stage I to the aggressive, metastatic and preterminal stage IV; epithelial malignancies are staged according to a tumor's direct extension or depth of invasion, lymph node involvement by tumor and presence of metastases; staging in lymphoid neoplasia requires determination of lymphoid region and bone marrow involvement, presence of transdiaphragmatic spread and presence of clinical symptoms, eg night sweats; see B symptoms, Cotswolds staging, Dukes classification, FIGO, TNM classification

stagnant loop syndrome Blind loop syndrome, see there

stain HISTOLOGY A series of dyes used to selectively color tissues or cells for microscopic examination*; hematoxylin and eosin colors the nuclei blue (basophilic) and the stromal or support tissue a light pink (acidophilic or eosinophilic) and is by far the most commonly used stain for examination of tissues removed during surgery; other stains used in diagnostic pathology include acid-fast stain for mycobacteria, Bodian stain for myelin, Congo red for amyloid, Fontana-Masson stain for melanin, Gomori-methenamine-silver (GMS) stain for fungi, Gram stain for bacteria, Grimelius stain for tumors of neural crest origin, eg APUDoma and carcinoid, Masson's trichrome stain to differentiate between muscle and collagen, periodic acid Schiff stain for complex carbohydrate and mucosubstances, Prussian blue stain of iron, and reticulin stain for reticulin

*Special stains are widely used in diagnostic pathology, although it has been waggishly observed, '...*special stains make what you don't know a different color...*'–anonymous

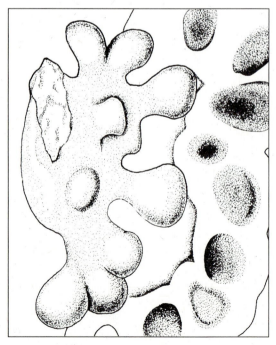

staghorn calculus

staircase pattern LABORATORY MEDICINE A descriptor for a pattern seen when a multimeric protein is separated into lanes in an electrophoretic gel, where each step corresponds to a different length of proteins, as seen in von Willebrand factor multimers; see Rocket electrophoresis

staircase ventilation A form of delivery of positive end-expiratory pressure (PEEP) used in early cardiac arrest, where the lungs are prevented from full collapse (exhalation) in order to 'recruit' collapsed or fluid-filled alveoli, thereby increasing arterial PO_2; since a prolonged ↑ in intrathoracic pressure can both stop a weakly beating heart and (by distending the stomach) predispose to regurgitation, PEEP is 'stepped-down' as quickly as possible; see PEEP, Step-down therapy

staircase vertebra A broad, flattened vertebral body with prominent articular facets and spinal processes, seen on a plain antero-posterior film in spondylometaphyseal dysplasia, an AD condition with short trunk, short stature, and osseous defects

standard acid reflux test GASTROENTEROLOGY An assay that evaluates esophageal pH for reflux esophagitis, utilizing standard stress maneuvers; Cf BAO, MAO

standard of care A level of competence in performing medical tasks that is accepted as reasonable and reflective of a skilled and diligent health care provider, which obliges a physician to confine his practice of medicine only to those areas of his expertise; such standards may be delineated by a hospital's medical staff bylaws or the standards published by a specialty college, eg the American College of Obstetricians and Gynecologists; the term has legal ramifications, as any deviation from a 'standard' may be considered to be an act of negligence; since a jury of laypersons cannot be expected to evaluate these standards; in a court of law, the defendant and plaintiff may call upon 'expert witness(es)' specialized in the appropriate field or involved in a germane area of research, who may quote extensively from the literature, defending or refuting the claim that the 'standard' has been adhered to; see Malpractice, Practice guidelines; Cf Reasonable person standards

standard conditions Standard temperature and pressure, see there

standard deviation Square root of the variance A statistical measure of the dispersion of a set of values about a mean, where a graphic representation of the data points is described by a curve with Gaussian distribution, ie bell-shaped; in a Gaussian distribution curve, ± 1 SD includes 68% of the data points, ± 2 SD includes 95.45% of the data and ± 3 SD includes 99.73% Note: SD cannot be determined when two (or more) relatively distinct populations are mixed, eg glucose values of normal subjects and diabetics, as each population can be accurately defined under a single peaked distribution curve

Note: WS Gosset published his observations and statistical methods under the nom de plume of 'Student'; his methods were delineated in the seminal paper, *The Probable Error of a Mean*, which has been designated as the Student 't' test

standard deviation index LABORATORY MEDICINE An index that is a function of external quality control, allowing the comparison of laboratory A's results with laboratory B, using the same QC material, providing a check of a laboratory's internal QC program; the SDI is a measure of the differences between a specific mean and the unweighted group mean derived for all the laboratories in a specific comparison group

$$SDI = \frac{x - x'}{SD_{(x)}}$$

where x = Mean from laboratory A, x' = Unweighted group mean, and $SD_{(x)}$ = Mean standard deviation

'standard drink' A unit used in clinical medicine to evaluate alcohol consumption; one standard drink is equal to 44 ml (a 'shot') of 40% alcohol by volume, also known as 'hard' liquor (gin, rum, vodka, whiskey) or 150 ml of 12% alcohol by volume, eg wine, or 360 ml of 5% alcohol by volume, eg beer

standard filter TRANSFUSION MEDICINE A first-generation blood component filter that has a screen (pore size 170-260 μm) to remove gross debris and sludge which can be used with all blood components (Arch Pathol Lab Med 1994; 118:392OA) see Blood filters, Leukocyte reduction

standard gamble DECISION ANALYSIS A maneuver that allows incorporation of patient preferences into the medical decision-making process; in a standard gamble, the patients quantify the strength of their preferences with respect to specific outcomes; the patient is asked to choose between a a certainty of a particular outcome, eg postphlebitic syndrome that is intermediate in desirability between the best (ie perfect health) and worst (ie death) possible outcomes and a number of gambles, each with a different probability of having the best and worst outcomes (N Engl J Med 1994; 330:1864OA--explanation of method; ibid 330:1895ED) Cf QALE, QALY

standard gamble metric CLINICAL MEDICINE A tool used in outcomes management that quantifies preferences for a specific health state, '...*by determining what chance of death the patient would be willing to take to be freed from symptoms. The patient imagines a treatment that will completely cure his or her symptoms but involves a risk of immediate death. The standard gamble utility is defined as one minus the risk of death at the point of indifference.*'; as an example if a patient is willing to risk a 5% mortality for a treatment that would completely eliminate symptoms, the standard gamble utility is 100%-5% (JAMA 1995; 273:1185) see Utility; Cf Time trade-off metric

standard operating procedure A technique, method or therapeutic modality that is performed 'by the book', using a standard protocol that has met a set of internally or externally defined criteria; see Procedures manual

standard state A thermodynamic 'reference' state—temperature 25°C; pressure 760 mm Hg; system components present in a defined reference state, ie at neutral pH and 1.0 molar concentration; see Standard conditions

standard temperature and pressure Standard conditions A temperature of 0°C and a pressure of 1 atmosphere (760 mm Hg); Cf Standard state

standardized meal A generic term for a meal that has a specified quantity of carbohydrates, fats, and proteins, which is used to evaluate absorption and digestion

standing order HEALTH CARE BUSINESS A purchase agreement between a supplier of a particular product, usually a 'disposible', eg syringes, gauzes, xylene, oxygen, and its consumer or purchaser, who uses the product regularly in relatively large quantities; these quantities can be anticipated and projected in advance such that the supplier ships a predetermined amount on a regular basis (often at a discount) without the purchaser needing to repeatedly fill out single-unit purchase orders; Cf Standing orders

standing orders CLINICAL MEDICINE Instructions for patient management that are to be followed (usually by the nursing staff) on a regular and consistent basis, unless instructed to the contrary, eg standing orders for medications or changing of wound dressings; Cf Standing order

'Stanford syndrome' see Indirect costs

staphylococcal scalded skin syndrome Ritter syndrome A vesiculo-bullous dermatopathy of low mortality affecting infants in hospital nurseries that resembles a second-degree burn, which is characterized in the early stages by erythema, followed by exfoliation CLINICAL Prodrome of malaise, fever, irritability, generalized erythema and tenderness of skin surface, followed by midepidermal bullae formation, variably accompanied by painful movement of involved areas, anorexia, nausea, diarrhea and vomiting; SSSS/TEN in infants is due to exfoliatin, an epidermolytic toxin produced by staphylococci (*Staphylococcus aureus*, phage group 2, often phage types 71 and 55) which evokes an enzymatic degradation of the upper granular layer of the epidermis and initially has a high mortality that drops to 5%; SSSS/TEN in adults may be due to exposure to drugs, eg sulfonamide, phenylbutazone, salicylate, penicillin and barbiturates or chemical, eg acrylonitrile exposure, and has a mortality rate of 30-40%; Cf Stevens-Johnson syndrome, Toxic epidermal necrolysis, Toxic shock syndrome

*Synonyms include dermatitis erysipelatosa, dermatitis exfoliativa infantum, dermatitis exfoliativa neonatorum, epidemic exfoliative dermatitis, exfoliative dermatitis of the newborn, keratolysis neonatorum, Lyell syndrome, (G RITTER VON RITTERSHAIN) Ritter's disease, Ritter syndrome, scalded skin syndrome, staphylococcal Lyell syndrome, staphylogenic Lyell syndrome

staphylococcal protein A A 42 kD glycoprotein isolated from strains of *Staphylococcus aureus* that binds to the Fc portion of IgG1, IgG2, and IgG4

staphylococcal protein A column A therapeutic device consisting of 200 mg of purified staphylococcal protein A (SPA) covalently bound to a solid silica-matrix support packed in a sterile disposable plastic cannister; the columns are used to treat various thrombocytopenias*, in particular those presumed to be of immune origin; the patient's plasma is percolated over the SPA and the circulating immune complexes and the IgG, both normal and pathological are adsorbed on the columns; the remaining plasma is returned to the patients SIDE EFFECTS 1) Acute allergic reactions occur in up to 75% with fever, nausea, vomiting, musculoskeletal pain, pulmonary reactions and hypotension, and are thought to be due to complement activation (↑ C3a and C5a ≥ 25-fold baseline levels) and release of inflammatory cytokines 2) Cutaneous leukocytoclastic vasculitis occurs in 10% of column-treated patients and is accompanied by fever, arthralgias, and purpura over the lower extremities 3) Thrombosis, due to thrombin activation, evidenced by ↑ prothrombin fragment 1.2, thrombin-antithrombin complexes, and fibrinopeptide A, as well as ↑ ATP release, β-thromboglobulin, and ↑ platelet aggregation and activation (N Engl J Med 1994; 331:792CPC)

*Including autoimmune thrombocytopenia, acute and chronic immune thrombocytopenic purpura, HIV-related thrombocytopenia, and thrombocytopenia associated with chemotherapy

***Staphylococcus aureus* enterotoxin B** A bacterial superantigen that causes food poisoning and is capable of inducing shock; see Superantigen

staple SURGERY A fastening device composed of steel-tantalum alloys used to close operative wounds, especially of the skin , which minimizes infection by not introducing a foreign body that would connect external and internal regions of the body; when compared, there is no difference between staples and sutures in the rate or 'quality' of wound healing; see Surgical closure

star MOLECULAR BIOLOGY A restriction endonuclease blot that is way off in left field

StAR Steroidogenic acute regulatory protein A recently identified acutely regulated, mitochondrial protein that activates steroidognesis in heterologous systems; StAR is intimately linked to the mobilization of cholesterol from lipid stores to the vicinity of the side chain cleavage enzyme P450scc in the inner mitochondrial membrane and, when defective, is believed to be responsible for congenital lipoid adrenal hyperplasia (Science 1995; 267:1828, 1780)

'starch blocker' A crude bean-derived amylase inhibitor that was marketed as a means of allowing one to eat in excess without gaining weight, a claim not corroborated by well-designed studies; the purified amylase inhibitor

may be effective in improving glucose tolerance in DM

starch gel electrophoresis LABORATORY MEDICINE A high-resolution zone electrophoresis in which a charged material migrates through a hydrolyzed starch (agaR0 support matrix

starch granuloma Talc granuloma, see there

Stark II Omnibus Budget Reconciliation Act of 1993 A law authored by Congressman Pete Stark (Democrat, California) and passed by the US Congress in 1994 that prohibits physicians from self-referral for certain 'designated health services', ie from benefiting from referrals of services to organizations where the physician has a vested financial interest or compensation arrangement; Stark II prohibits referrals to self-owned clinical laboratories, home health care, occupational, physical, and radiation therapy, imaging centers, in– and outpatient hospital services, ambulances, parenteral and enteric nutrients, ambulances, and durable medical equipment, and outpatient prescription drugs (Am Med News 19 Sept 1994) as well as equipment and supplies, and prosthetic and orthotic devices (ibid 21 Nov 1994 p5)

Starling forces The sum of the positive intravascular oncotic pressure and the negative pressure provided by the venous flow, which act to maintain fluid in the vessels, minus the oncotic pressure in the interstitial space and the forward pressures of the blood as it is 'driven' into the capillaries, both of which act to pull fluid from the intravascular space; see Third space

'Starry Night' sign A descriptor for the capillary phase pattern in arteriography of a traumatized spleen that demonstrates focal or diffuse small rounded shadows corresponding to stasis of contrast material in the marginal splenic sinusoidal circulation

The appearance has been fancifully likened to the sky seen in Vincent van Gogh's 'Starry Night', painted in 1889 at St Remy-de-Provence

starry sky pattern HEMATOLOGY A descriptor for a pattern seen in lymph nodes by low-power light microscopy consisting of multiple holes corresponding to lymphoblasts or phagocytosing histiocytes lying within a sheet of relatively monotonous lymphocytes (figure), an appearance likened to stars in the sky, a pattern classically in Burkitt's lymphoma, less commonly in other immature lymphomas, granulocytic sarcoma, Mediterranean lymphoma, lymphoblastic leukemia, as well as in benign conditions eg ITP and lymphoid hyperplasia MICROBIOLOGY A 'starry sky' pattern is described in the cytoplasm of infected cells with abundant immunostained *Chlamydia trachomatis* NEPHROLOGY A 'starry sky' pattern may be seen by immunofluorescence in acute post-infectious glomerulonephritis due to the finely granular deposition of C3 and immunoglobulin in the capillary walls and mesangium

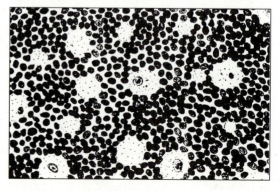

starry sky pattern

start codon MOLECULAR BIOLOGY Initiator codon An mRNA trinucleotide, to wit AUG (which specifies the amino acid methionine) which is the signal for initiating protein synthesis, recognized by methyonyl-tRNA; in some chains, methionine is encoded by GUG, which can also function as a start codon; the function of the SC is to set the frame for reading the entire translated message; Cf Stop codons

starvation CLINICAL NUTRITION A condition resulting from prolonged global deprivation of food, occurring in abnormal environmental conditions, eg during war or famine, or in normal society through wilful neglect of others, eg children, the handicapped or elderly by parents, family, caregivers or guardians or by self-neglect in the elderly, mentally feeble or those who irrespective of means, choose to live in apparent poverty; without food and water, the body loses 4-5% of its total weight/day and few survive beyond 10 days; when water is provided, a starving person may survive up to 60 days CLINICAL Hypovitaminoses, malnutrition, ↓ subcutaneous fat with thin, dry and hyperpigmented skin stretched over bone prominences, atrophy of organs, marked attenuation of the gastrointestinal tract, with an enlarged concrement-laden gall bladder; see Minnesota experiment MICROBIOLOGY A state in bacterial colonies, in which either nutrients are actively withheld for experimental expediency or there is depletion of nutrients through consumption

starvation diabetes (mellitus) Transient glucose intolerance accompanied by glycosuria that occurs when a person ingests carbohydrates after prolonged starvation, an effect attributed to suboptimal glycogen synthesis and storage

starvation diet Very low calorie diet A potentially dangerous permutation of crash diet that provides 300-700 kcal/day, which must be supplemented with high quality protein; given the risk of death through intractable cardiac arrhythmias, SDs should be limited to 3-6 months SIDE EFFECTS Orthostatic hypotension due to loss of sodium and ↓ norepinephrine secretion, fatigue, hypothermia and cold intolerance, xeroderma, hair loss, dysmenorrhea; see Diet

starvation stools Watery green feces that develop when a subject is maintained on a clear-liquid starvation-type diet; see Diet (starvation)

Starzl's criteria Pittsburgh criteria, see there

'stat' CLINICAL MEDICINE *adverb* Immediately LABORATORY MEDICINE *noun* A specimen, often from the critical care unit or emergency room, that is given priority in the clinical laboratory in order to measure various analytes with immediate potential impact on patient management; 'stats' may include, requests for blood glucose levels, hematocrit, electronic leukocyte differential count, certain enzyme levels, prothrombin time, partial thromboplastin time, BUN and creatinine; Cf 'Stats'

STAT Signal transduction and activation of transcription, see STAT proteins

stat lab LABORATOR MEDICINE A free-standing laboratory that is capable of performing an abbreviated battery of tests and serves as a receiving 'node' for the larger laboratory to which the SL is ultimately responsible; the purposes for setting up stat lab include reduced patient length of stay (in a hospital), shortened turnaround time, patient convenience, physician (client) satisfaction, and cost savings (Advance/Laboratory March 1995 p29)

STAT proteins STATs A family of latent cytoplasmic proteins involved in signal transduction and activation of transcription; STATs are activated by the Jaks (Janus kinases) through phosphorylation of tyrosine residues; the activated STAT proteins are then translocated to the cell nucleus where they bind to specific sequences (response elements), stimulating transcription (Science 1994; 264:1415R); the differential activation of different STATs (at least four have been described) in response to different ligands may explain specificity in nuclear signaling from the cell surface (Science 1994; 264:95R)

state board An organized body in a sovereign state of the US that oversees the activities of the licensed physicians and health care professionals in that state, assuring that a high standard of practice by the physicians (and others) is maintained and that the use of controlled drug substances is appropriate and without impropriety; Cf Specialty board

state boards Examinations administered by a (US) state board of medical examiners in order to license a physician in a particular state; these examinations play an ever-decreasing role in state medical licensure, as these bodies now rely on standardized national examinations for assessing a physician's knowledge of medicine; see FLEX exam

state mandate HEALTH CARE REFORM A generic term for any state law that requires private insurers to cover various add-on health-related services eg well baby care, herbal medicine, hair transplants (?), and others, all at an increased cost to the purchaser of the services (Am Med News 25 October 1992, p7)

State-Trait Anxiety Inventory A 40-item questionnaire for measuring anxiety (from N Engl J Med 1992; 327:1041oA)

station OBSTETRICS The position or level of descent of the presenting part in the pelvis in a vaginal delivery; full engagement of the presenting part at the iliac spines is considered station 'zero'; two methods are used to determine fetal station; the more traditional determination of station divides the long axis of the birth canal above and below the ischial spine, where -3 corresponds to a presenting part at the pelvic inlet and +3 corresponds to a presenting part that has reached the perineum; an alternate system starts above and below the ischial spine, measuring five levels, each being one centimeter

Note: Given the potential for confusion, the two systems for classifying obstetric stations are not interchangeable during a delivery (and two different systems probably should not be used in the same health care facility)

'stats' Colloquial for statistics; Cf 'Stat'

State v Schwartz FORENSIC MOLECULAR BIOLOGY An early court case (447 NW 2d 422 (Minn 1989)) that used molecular techniques (which add several magnitudes of accuracy to evidence) to link an alleged perpetrator of a crime to the crime's location; in this case, the court opined that future court considerations would hinge on adherence to technical standards and quality assurance (CAP Today July 1992) see *People* v *Castro*

static resistance SPORTS MEDICINE A constant unchanging resistance that occurs through a range of motion when an isotomic contraction is used to move a load (JC DeLee, D Drez, Jr, Eds, Orthopedic Sports Medicine WB Saunders, Philadelphia, 1994) Cf Variable resistance

'statin' A colloquial term for any (eg pravistatin) of a family of cholesterol-lowering drugs, which some workers believe may be useful in lowering the risk of coronary artery disease, even in the absence of increased cholesterol levels (JAMA 1995; 273:1894)

statistic A generic term for any numerical value that defines some specified characteristic of a population or dataset, eg mean, percentage, rate of reaction, standard deviation, coefficient of variation, or other datum

statistical interaction An interaction among multiple possible relationships in a database, where the frequency of one factor depends on another factor in the study base

stationary recovery MRI A type of partial saturation pulse sequence in which preceding pulses leave the spins in a state of saturation, so that recovery at the time of the next pulse takes place from an initial condition of no magnetization; see Magnetic resonance imaging

'Statue of Liberty' position ORTHOPEDICS The mandatory position for the hand (when standing) after reconstructive and corrective hand surgery or after traumatic injury; while sitting, the hand may be rested with the elbow on the table, as long as the hand is above the level of the heart, in order to prevent accumulation of edema that might compromise the arm's blood supply

status asthmaticus An imprecisely-defined clinical entity of prolonged duration in which there is decreased response by asthmatics to drugs for which they had previously been sensitive; urgent care specialists consider status asthmaticus as the failure to respond to three therapeutic interventions with adrenergic bronchodilators in the emergency department; patients in status asthmaticus are invariably hypoxemic and require hospital admission for monitoring of arterial blood gases and pH TREATMENT Hypercapneic patients should be rehydrated, given oxygen, large doses of aminophylline and methylprednisone; high-dose intramuscular triamcinolone is more effective than low-dose prednisone (N Engl J Med 1991; 324:585); steroids prevent early relapse of acute asthma as long as they are continued (ibid 1991; 324:788)

status fibrosus 1) Fibrous transition of muscle caused by pressure from an adjacent compressing tumor, a reactive process that is distinct from muscle fibrosis, which may be either congenital, affecting the vastus intermedius of the quadriceps in children or acquired in adults, related to intradermal injections of penicillin, pentazocine, or other drugs that cause local irritation 2) An intracranial defect of neonates that affects the basal nuclei, which is characterized by a ↓ in neurons accompanied by gliosis and crowding of myelinated nerve fibers

status/post *adjective* Pertaining or referring to a state that follows a previous condition, as in S/P myocardial infarction or procedure, as in S/P cholecystectomy

status thymolymphaticus A 'condition' described in the late 1940s and 1950s as pathological thymic hypertrophy, which was treated with radiotherapy; it later became apparent that the thymus undergoes normal physiological hypertrophy, reaching a maximum of 15-25 grams at puberty, involuting thereafter; those who received radiotherapy for status thymolymphaticus are at an increased risk for thyroid and breast malignancy; 36 years after irradiation, the incidence of breast cancer was two-fold that of age-matched siblings, with an adjusted rate ratio of 3.6

Note: Radiotherapy was at one time used for a vast array of conditions, eg hypertrophy of tonsils, acne, eustachian tube dysfunction, facial hemangiomas, pertussis, tinea capitis and others

statutes of limitations MEDICAL MALPRACTICE A doctrine that allows the plaintiff two to three years (depending upon the state in the US) from the time of the alleged malpractice or negligence (by a physician or hospital) to file a lawsuit, unless the plaintiff is 1) Minor, who has two years after reaching the adulthood to file a lawsuit or 2) Later discovers the alleged act of negligence; the time period begins either from the moment the alleged act occurred or from the moment the plaintiff discovered that the act was negligent; for children, this period usually begins after he/she reaches age 21 or 18 (or younger if they are considered 'emancipated minors', by virtue of marriage or financial independence) see Malpractice

statutory rape An unlawful act of sexual intercourse that is defined by the statutes of the state or country as being illegal based on the age (in most places, under 18) of the person who was raped, and not on the issue of consent; see Date rape, Rape, Spousal rape

*Rape is defined as 'a nonconsensual act of sexual intercourse carried out by force or other means of duress.' (International Dictionary of Medicine, J Wiley & Sons, New York, 1986)

stavudine see d4T

stay and play EMERGENCY MEDICINE A stance in which a person's injuries are believed to be of such severity as to require some form of treatment and/or stabilization on the scene prior to transporting the patient to a trauma center; Cf Scoop and run

STD 1) Sexually transmitted disease, see there 2) Standard test dose

Also 1) Skin test dose 2) Skin to tumor distance

steakhouse syndrome A clinical complex caused by plugging of the lower esophagogastric sphincter with a large, poorly chewed bolus of food, usually meat, often steak, accompanied by intense epigastric pain that resolves spontaneously if the food passes into the stomach Predisposing factors Alcohol imbibition, edentulousness; Cf Cafe coronary, Sushi syncope

steal Vascular steal syndrome Any of a number of symptom complexes that appear when there are extensive anastomoses between two vascular beds, and the arterial supply to one is stenosed or completely occluded, resulting in the diversion of blood to the other; steals reduce regional oxygenation, as compromised organs and tissues 'steal' blood from adjacent regions; steal syndromes are adjectively designated by the affected artery, eg aortico-celiac steal syndrome or subclavian steal syndrome and may involve the mesenteric, pulmonary, subclavian, renal-splanchnic, spinal, subclavian and thyroid-cervical arterial systems; vascular steal syndromes are most commonly due to 1) Atherosclerosis 2) Therapy, eg coronary artery steal syndrome, a potential side effect of vasoactive agents used for chronic anginal pain, which cause an ↑ of blood flow to well-vascularized regions with normal oxygenation and a ↓ of blood flow to the stenosed and nonreactive vessels or 3) Malformations, eg intracranial steal syndrome, in which increased blood flow into a cerebrovascular malformation is accompanied by progressive neurological disability due either to compression or flow of the blood away from the underlying cerebral cortex; Cf 'Robin hood' syndrome

stealth virus A generic term for a recently described class of cytopathic viruses, so designated as they evoke cellular pathology in absence of an inflammatory response; based on PCR and cross-hybridization studies, stealth viruses have considerable molecular heterogeneity, but all appear to induce a typical foamy cytopathic effect (CAP Today October 1994; 67)

steely hair disease Menkes' kinky hair syndrome, see there

steeple sign Gothic arch sign, see there

steering wheel 'syndrome' A blunt chest injury affecting an automobile driver in a 'head-on' collision, which may result in myocardial infarction-like signs and symptoms; the heart bears the brunt of the injury with contusion of the anterior epicardium and myocardium, compression of the heart between the sternum and vertebral column and sudden increases in intrathoracic pressure, potentially rupturing cardiac structures, including the ventricular septum, chordae or the free wall; Cf Air bags, Dashboard fracture, Padded dash(board) syndrome, Seatbelt injury, Whiplash

Note: Only 20% of major blunt chest injury victims have elevated creatinine phosphokinase and thus the index of suspicion should be high

stefin Any of a number (eg stefin A, stefin B) of cysteine proteinase inhibitors of the cystatin superfamily, which are thought to protect the cell from frisky proteinases that may leak from lysosomes

stem cell HEMATOLOGY A primitive cell that is capable of dividing and giving rise to both primitive daughter cells like itself and cells capable of undergoing differentiation; in adults, the stem cell capability of the early embryo is lost except in the bone marrow where it is retained by the hematolymphoid precursors; SCs are divided into the most primitive and undifferentiated (pluripotent) cells and the partially differentiated (unipotent) cells; in mice, the 'ultimate' stem cell (ie the most primitive cell capable of reconstituting the entire hemato-lymphoid system) subset is negative for lineage differentiation (eg granulocyte, macrophage and others) markers and bears the cell surface differentiation antigen, Thy-1 and an antigen designated as the stem cell antigen-1 or Sca-1

Note: Mature blood cells require cytokines that induce growth or division, eg IL-3 and colony-stimulating factors and differentiation, eg macrophage-granulocyte inducer-type 2; these cytokines act in a programmed fashion, where the interactions determine the balance of mature and immature cells in normal hematopoietic development

stem cell factor A hematopoietic growth factor that is a product of the SI gene in mice and which is a ligand for c-*kit*, a proto-oncogene of the tyrosine kinase receptor family, expressed during embryogenesis in those cells associated with the migratory pathways and targets of melanoblasts, germ cells, hematopoietic stem cells and possibly also the brain and spinal cord (Nature; 1990; 347:667)

stem cell transplantation Bone marrow transplantation; the administration of primitive cells of the hematopoeitic system into a person whose native red or white cells have lost their ability to function; an increasing number of hematologic diseases are being treated by SCT (table)

STEM CELL TRANSPLANTATION 5-YEAR SURVIVAL
LEUKEMIA
CML CHRONIC PHASE 60-85%; BLAST CRISIS 10-20%
AML FIRST REMISSION 50-70%; OTHER REMISSIONS 20-50%
ALL 30-50%
MYELOMA 10-25%
LYMPHOMA
FIRST THERAPY AFTER STANDARD REGIMENS 40-70%
ADVANCED DISEASE 15-30%
MYELODYSPLASIA 20-60%
APLASTIC ANEMIA 60-90%
FANCONI'S ANEMIA 50-70%
SICKLE CELL ANEMIA 50-90%
THALASSEMIA 60-95%
modified from Science & Medicine 1995; 2:38

stent see Intracononary stent

stent-graft Endovascular stent graft, see there

step 1 diet CARDIOLOGY An abbreviation of a series of 9 dietary recommendations from the Nutrition Committee of the American Heart Association which states that the total fat consumption should be less than 30%; the S1D is regarded by some authors as being an ineffective means of reducing cardiovascular disease (New York Times 25 April 1995, pC1)

step-down therapy CARDIOLOGY Downward 'titration' or reduction by stages of the doses and agents used to control blood pressure; the 'steps' in the control of blood pressure range from thiazide diuretics, β blockers or converting enzyme inhibitor (mild hypertension, diastolic < 100 mm Hg) to hydralazine, prazosine, minoxidil, guanethidine or furosemide (severe hypertension, diastolic pressure > 120 mm Hg); Cf 'Staircase' ventilation

step formation Snowcap appearance, see there

stepladder configuration GI RADIOLOGY A pattern seen on a barium enema of the ascending colon, in which rigid fibrosis causes transverse linear fissures intersecting with gullies of contrast material lying in deep longitudinal ulcers, a finding described in regional enteritis (Crohn's disease), when radiocontrast 'spills' past the constricted

and narrowed terminal ileum, imparting a 'railroad track' appearance on gross examination; see Garden hose appearance, String sign RHEUMATOLOGY A descriptor for the consecutive subluxations in the cervical spine seen in rheumatoid arthritis, variably accompanied by narrowing of the intervertebral disk space

stercoral ulcer A colonic ulcer that develops in elderly or mentally retarded patients with intractable constipation secondary to pressure of impacted fecal material and sluggish mesenteric arterial circulation; with time fistula may form subjacent to the ulcer

stercoroma A tumor-like fecal mass in the rectum

stereo drawing BACKGROUND Three-dimensional analysis of complex molecules allows determination of their 'signature' in terms of reactive or binding sites and is having an increasing impact on the design of new therapeutic agents; stereo (3-dimensional) images appear with relative frequency in major scientific journals; to view the image in stereo, either: 1) Hold the figure 10 cm from the eyes without glasses, focus on a distant object, lower the eyes to the drawing and re-focus on the middle image, giving the right-handed (correct) form or 2) Hold the page at about 20 cm, allow the eyes to 'cross', then re-focus on the middle image for the exotic left-handed stereoisomer

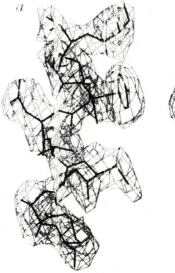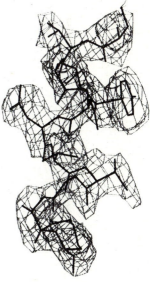

(Science 1986; 233:623c); the stereoform in the figure corresponds to the electron-density map of the zeta isoform of the 14-3-3 protein, which is a regulatory element in intracellular signaling pathways (Nature 1995; 376:191) see Protein structure

stereotactic radiotherapy A therapeutic modality using heavy charged particles (protons or helium ions), photons (γ radiation) or a linear-accelerator to treat intracranial lesions that are inaccessible to conventional neurosurgery; the intent of stereotactic radiotherapy is to induce local endothelial proliferation with vascular wall thickening, occluding the malformation, while sparing adjacent cerebral tissue; a beam of mono-energetic heavy particles such as helium has the advantage of 1) Delivering a very high dose of radiation to a tissue depth known as the 'Bragg ionization peak' 2) A sharper lateral edge and 3) Minimal amounts of secondarily excited, ie radioactive particles; stereotactic radiotherapy effectively reduces symptoms in inaccessible arteriovenous malformations, but has a long latency between therapy and response and suffers a 12%

risk of serious neurologic sequelae; see Gamma knife

steric hindrance A physicochemical barrier that prevents or attenuates a reaction or a conformational response

sterile field SURGERY A 'clean' environment that surrounds an incision, which is relatively free of microorganisms, in particular bacteria; the SF is inhabited by the surgeon(s), scrub nurses, and occasionally, physicians in training

sterility Involuntary infertility, see there

sterilization A process that destroys pathogens, by 1) Autoclaving Pressurized moist heat, 121.5°C x 30 minutes 2) Dry heat sterilization at 129.8°C x 2 hours and 3) Gas sterilization with ethylene oxide (used for equipment that cannot withstand high temperatures, which has the disadvantage of being carcinogenic, expensive, explosive and irritating to mucosal membranes; see Disinfection

steroid cell tumor Lipid cell tumor*, lipoid tumor Any of a group of steroid hormone-producing tumors of the ovary CLINICAL Most cases are associated with virilization, less commonly with Cushing's syndrome, 20% are malignant and those which are malignant are often greater than 8 cm in diameter PATHOLOGY The tumors are yellow-brown, unilateral, composed of cells with theca-lutein, Leydig or hilar cell and/or adrenal cortical cell features including pale pink cytoplasm in polyhedral rounded cell clusters, positive fat stains, and well-developed smooth endoplasmic reticulum and mitochondria with tubulo-vesicular cristae, features typical of cells that produce steroid hormones

*A term less preferred by RE Scully, the most widely read scholar of ovarian pathology, as lipid in various other, non-steroid cell type ovarian tumors is not uncommon

---

STEROID CELL TUMOR CLASSIFICATION

STROMAL LUTEOMA Benign tumors that produce estrogen, rarely androgens

LEYDIG CELL TUMOR Most (82%) are benign, one-half produce excess androgens and they are subdivided into i) Hilus cell tumor and ii) Non-hilus cell tumor

STEROID CELL TUMOR of adrenal cortical type, a tumor that may cause Cushing syndrome

STEROID CELL TUMOR, NOT OTHERWISE SPECIFIED, the most common group, no age predilection, cell of origin unclear; one-fourth are clinically malignant (greater than 7 cm in diameter, with cystic degeneration and necrosis)

---

steroid hydroxylase inducer protein A labile, as yet uncharacterized protein that is thought to regulate some of ACTH's long-term effects by stimulating the transcription of the P450 enzymes involved in cortisol synthesis

steroid receptor superfamily CELL PHYSIOLOGY A group of structurally similar hormone receptors located adjacent to the nucleus that are involved in signal transduction; the binding of a ligand to the receptor is thought to induce an allosteric change allowing the receptor-hormone complex to bind to a DNA response element in the promoter region of a target gene, modulating gene expression; these receptors have a critical role in neuroendocrine and signal transduction leading to growth, morphogenesis, homeostasis, and proliferation; steroid receptor superfamily ligands include glucocorticoids, mineralocorticoids, progesterones, estrogens, estrogen-related 1 hormone, estrogen-related 2 hormone, androgens, ecdysone, retinoic acid, vitamin D_3 and thyroid hormone, as well as the viral oncogene product, v-erbA, and a protein implicated in hepatocellular carcinoma

Stevens-Johnson syndrome A clinical permutation of the erythema multiforme 'motif', in which there are dusky purpuric macules or atypical targetoid lesions with focal confluence and detachment of epithelium of ≤ 10% of body surface; ½ of cases are linked to reactions to drugs (eg sulfonamides, anticonvulsants, allopurinol, and others) 10-30% of cases are accompanied by systemic symptoms CLINICAL Fever, erosive stomatitis, lesions of anogenital mucosae, conjunctivae (keratitis, corneal erosions), and respiratory tract; less than 5% are fatal TREATMENT Withdrawal of offending drug (N Engl J Med 1994; 331:1272RV)

Stewart-Treves syndrome An angiosarcoma* arising in a background of chronic lymphedema; most cases arise in the upper extremity in ♀ after mastectomy and lymphadenectomy, but may occur in extremities affected by congenital, idiopathic, or traumatic lymphedema (N Engl J Med 1993; 328:1337CPC)

*Although the term lymphangioma has been traditionally used for this lesion, differentiation from a hemangiosarcoma is difficult (if not impossible) and serves no practical importance

stick-man syndrome A variant of congenital muscular dystrophy characterized by toe walking in early childhood, contractures, and variable weakness, generalized muscle atrophy and extremely thin (ie stick-like) limbs (N Engl J Med 1994; 330:548CPC)

sticky end Cohesive end MOLECULAR BIOLOGY A single-stranded oligomer of complementary COOH- and NH_2- terminals from the opposite ends of a segment of double-stranded DNA; SEs result from a 'staggered cut', usually by a restriction endonuclease, and may be used as points of insertion of DNA into various cloning vectors; see Restriction endonuclease, Staggered cut

'sticky floor' phenomenon A recently identified permutation* of the issue of the inequality of career advancements of ♂ and ♀ in medicine; despite a similar degree of preparation of candidates for academic careers in terms of board certification, advanced degrees, research during fellowship training, ♀ had fewer alloted resources, less office and allocated laboratory space, less grant support, and less 'protected' time for research (JAMA 1995 273:1022) see Glass ceiling phenomenon

*The choice of terminology by the authors who first described the phenomenon is particularly appropos, in that a 'sticky floor' refers to handicaps that occur ab initio, while a 'glass ceiling' refers to handicaps that are present only at the end ot the advancement process

stiff baby syndrome Hereditary stiff-man syndrome An AD [MIM 184850] complex of variable penetration characterized by ↑ startle reflex and virtually continuous motor activity by EMG, choking, vomiting and dysphagia, which may improve with age; Cf Floppy infant syndrome(s), Stiff man syndrome

stiff heart 'syndrome' CARDIOLOGY A nonspecific term for ventricular pump failure due to restrictive heart disease CLINICAL Chest pain, exertional dyspnea, increased venous pressure, extra-diastolic murmurs, hepatomegaly, ascites and edema ETIOLOGY Idiopathic or related to amyloidosis, constrictive pericarditis (irradiation, mycosis, trauma and tuberculosis), hemochromatosis and myocardiopathies of various etiologies; Cf 'Stone' heart

stiff lung syndrome Adult respiratory distress syndrome, see there

stiff man syndrome A rare GABAergic autoimmune motor dysfunction with a 2:1 ♂:♀ ratio CLINICAL Stiffness of axial and appendicular muscles with intermittent superimposed painful muscle spasms precipitated by emotional or physical stress, accompanied by lower back pain, hyperlordosis, motor and gait abnormalities, diaphoresis and tachycardia ETIOLOGY Probably autoimmune, given the presence of antibodies against glutamic acid decarboxylase and pancreatic islet cells; autoantigenic heterogeneity, anti-glutamate decarboxylase autoantibodies in 60%; in the remaining 40% there are other autoantibodies; in some cases of malignancy-associated SM syndrome there are autoantibodies directed against a 128-kD synaptic protein; it is associated with epilepsy, IDDM and other organ specific autoimmune disorders, eg myasthenia gravis, thyroiditis and adrenalitis DIAGNOSIS Simultaneous video-electroencephalographic surface EMG demonstrates continuous motor unit activity in the afflicted muscles even at rest and abnormal activity of small gamma motor neurons TREATMENT Cortisol if there is adrenocortical dysfunction, benzodiazepines, plasma exchange; Cf Stiff-baby syndrome

stiff neck syndrome Wry neck, see there

stiff skin syndrome A non-progressive AD [MIM 184900] condition of uncertain origin characterized by accumulation of hyaluronidase-digestible material, possibly a variant of mucopolysaccharidosis, with focal indurations of the skin, renal concrement formation, joint enlargement and stiffness, DM and duodenal ulcers

'still' syndrome GERIATRICS A facetious term that may be of broad utility when interacting with the oldest old (> 85), who may accept their physical and mental decline with resignation, but who find the 'still' questions* offensive (N Engl J Med 1994; 331:484BR)

'Are you still interested in politics; still writing, still walking etc

stillbirth Death in utero OBSTETRIC Fetal death prior to complete extraction or expulsion from the mother of a product of conception, irrespective of the duration of pregnancy; death is indicated by the lack of evidence of life or movement once the separation occurs

stimulation test A generic term for any clinical assay that evaluates the synthetic reserve capacity of a substance of interest, providing information on whether the production of the hormone is maximal; stimulation tests include the metapyrone test for adrenal hypofunction and the maximum acid output (MAO) assay in Zollinger-Ellison syndrome; Cf Suppression test

stinging insect Any member of the order Hymenoptera that sting, which are divided into the apids, eg honeybee and bumblebee, and vespids, eg hornet, yellow jacket, and wasp; the stinging apparatus consists of a venom-filled sac attached to a barbed stinger; the multiple barbs on the honeybee's stinger causes it to detach, resulting in the honeybee's death; the vespid stinger has fewer barbs, allowing it to sting many times; see venom (N Engl J Med 1994; 331:523RV)

stippling An adjectival descriptor for a punctate appearance or, in radiology, white granularity in a radiolucent background, which, parenthetically is a term that is similar, if not identical to the more graphic adjectival descriptor of 'salt-and-pepper' BONE RADIOLOGY Punctate calcifications in epiphyseal ossification centers, which may occur in congenital calcific chondrodystrophy, cretinism, ischemic necrosis (osteochondrosis), multiple epiphyseal dysplasia, pituitary gigantism, sclerotic osteopetrosis and sclerotic osteopoikilosis COLONIC ENDOSCOPY A pattern of fine granularity of the mucosa described as being most characteristic of early ulcerative colitis ESOPHAGEAL ENDOSCOPY A pattern seen in esophagitides due to corrosive agents, reflux, infections, eg candidiasis and radiation HEMATOLOGY see Basophilic stippling RENAL RADIOLOGY A pattern seen in papillary transitional cell carcinomas with incomplete filling of the pelvi-caliceal system due to tumoral replacement in the intravenous pyelogram

stitch 1) A popular term for suture, as in the wound required 14 stiches 2) A subjective term for a sharp pain of moderate intensity*

*Lying midway between an ouch! and an expletive-Author's note

stochastic effect Probabalistic effect A generic term for a health effect that is random in nature, and for which the probability (rather than the severity) of the effect occurring is assumed to be a function of dose without a threshold; the effects of heredity and incidence of cancer are sto-

chastic in nature; Cf Nonstochastic effect

stochastic process CLINICAL DECISION-MAKING A method for problem solving that is defined by the laws of probability, ie randomness, where every step is uncertain and the solution is by trial and error; Cf Aunt Millie approach, Heuristic process

stoichiometry The branch of physical chemistry that formally studies the quantitative (mass, volume, moles) relations that chemical compounds (ie products and reactants) in reacting systems have with each other

stocking-and-glove distribution NEUROLOGY A pattern of peripheral nerve disease characterized by a relatively sharply demarcated loss of pain, touch, temperature, position and vibration sensation, accompanied by weakness, muscular atrophy and loss of tendon reflexes, eg the 'stocking' pattern of distal diabetic polyneuropathy is characterized by waxing and waning paresthesias that worsen at night

'stomach virus' A colloquial lay term for any gastroenteritis of presumed viral origin that may be accompanied by diarrhea, fever and possibly also nausea, vomiting and abdominal pain; viral gastroenteritis is commonly caused by enteroviruses, rotavirus and possibly also astroviruses

stomatocyte stomos, Greek, Mouth An erythrocyte with a central fish mouth-like area of clearing that is prominent in Rh_{null} disease, which may be seen in acute alcoholism, hepatopathies, an artefact seen in red cells stored in a hypotonic solution, or related to various red cell membrane defects, ameliorated with splenomegaly

stomatocytosis An AD [MIM 185000] condition characterized by ↑ osmotic fragility of red cells, autohemolysis, splenomegaly and mild anemia that is partially corrected by splenectomy; hereditary spherocytosis has been linked to a defect in a 28-kD RBC membrane protein

'stoned' 'Wasted' SUBSTANCE ABUSE A colloquial expression for a state of quasi-stupor of varying intensity that may be induced with various psychoactive substances of abuse, eg heroin, marijuana and alcohol

Note: Those who abuse sustances generally prefer to stay in a state of pleasant euphoria, or 'high'; a commonly used hierarchy of 'street' terms (in the USA) for the subjective sensations that occur during a session of substance abuse begins with a low-level 'buzz', followed by a 'high', as the intensity of the drug's effect increases, after which the abuser is 'stoned' which when extreme, is referred to as being 'wasted'; see 'High'; Cf 'Bad trip'

'stone' heart CARDIOLOGY Irreversible ischemia-induced cardiac rigor mortis, in which the heart undergoes global spastic contraction in systole; the anoxia rapidly depletes glycogen and ATP, causing death; a heart of stone is exceptionally rare and is most common in severe heart disease (New York Heart Association class IV); see Rigor mortis; Cf Stiff heart 'syndrome'

'stones, bones and groans' A mnemonic used to recall the clinical triad seen in hyperparathyroidism, where prolonged elevation of parathyroid hormone and end-organ response thereto results in disseminated calcium deposition (stones), osteoporosis (bones) and GI symptoms including nausea, vomiting, anorexia, weight, loss and recalcitrant peptic ulcers (groans)

stool Old English, chair Feces; one stool examination may be insufficient for detecting ova and/or parasites (O/P), in one report ± 58% of cases ultimately shown to have O/P were detected with the first stool specimen, ± 21% of cases each were detected with the second and third stool specimens (Br J Gen Pract 1993; 47:76)

stop codon Terminator codon Any one of the three triplets (UAA, UGA and UAG) of nucleotides on a messenger RNA molecule, which when translated, stops the elongation of the chain of polypeptides; see Codon; Cf Degenerate code, Start codon

storage disease Any of a group of diseases often designated 'Inborn errors of metabolism', in which a defective or functionally absent enzyme causes organ dysfunction through accumulation of precursor substances derived from metabolism of glycogen, amino acids, often contained within lysosomes; each has a relatively distinct pattern of organ involvement, eg in glycogen storage disease, the overload substrates compromises the liver, skeletal muscle and cardiac muscle; see Brancher and Debrancher disease

storage lesion TRANSFUSION MEDICINE The constellation of changes occurring in a unit of packed red cells during storage; from the time of collection to the time of transfusion, the following are

↑ **ammonium** to 470 µmol/L (US: 800 µg/dl)

↑ **free hemoglobin** in plasma from 82 to 6580 mg/L (US: 8.2 to 658 mg/dl)

↑ **K⁺** from 4.2 to 78.5 mmol/L (US: 4.2 to 78.5 mEq/L)

↓ **ATP** from 100% to 45%

↓ **2,3 DPG** to less than 10% of original levels (replenished within 24 hours of transfusion)

↓ **labile proteins**, eg complement, fibronectin and coagulation factors ↓ to negligible

↓ **Na⁺** from 169 to 111 mmol/L (US: 169 to 111 mEq/L)

↓ **pH** from 7.6 to 6.7

The physiologic effects of storage lesions are negligible in the absence of a previous compromise of the patient's (recipient's) status; see Red cell preservatives

storage pool disease(s) A group of platelet disorders due to deficiencies of platelet granules, divided into 1) α granule storage pool disease, see Gray platelet syndrome and 2) Dense granule deficiency or delta-storage pool disease CLINICAL Moderate bleeding LABORATORY ↑ Bleeding time, ↓ platelet ADP content, ↓ serotonin levels

Note: Dense granules are also deficient in Chediak-Higashi, Hermansky-Pudlak, TAR and Wiskott-Aldrich syndromes TREATMENT Hemostasis with platelet transfusions, cryoprecipitate and desmopressin acetate (DDAVP), which release von Willebrand factor from storage sites, the first-line treatment of choice

storiform pattern *storia*, Latin, woven hemp, mat A pattern seen by low-power LM, characterized by loosely-arranged whorls of elongated, spindled fibroblast-like cells; although highly non-specific, the pattern is most often seen in fibrohistiocytic lesions and may appear in benign tumors, eg dermatofibroma, giant cell tumor of tendon sheath, in tumors of low malignant potential, eg atypical fibroxanthoma, dermatofibrosarcoma protuberans and in frankly malignant tumors, eg malignant fibrous histiocytoma; the storiform pattern may also be seen in non-histiocytic lesions, including nodular fasciitis, leiomyoma, leiomyosarcoma, Schwann cell tumors and spindle cell carcinoma; see Cartwheel pattern, Pinwheel pattern

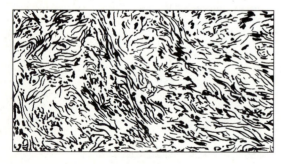

storiform pattern

stork legs Champagne bottle legs, see there

stork marks NEONATOLOGY Capillary 'nevi' seen as focal 'spots' on the face and neck; the lesions usually fade within the first year or two of life, but which may persist on the neck

stormy fermentation MICROBIOLOGY The descriptor for a turbid reaction of *Clostridium* spp in litmus milk with coagulation and gas production, in which the milk is converted into a coagulum with entrapped bubbles of gas

straddle lesion A complex injury of the perineum, usually due to a fall in which the point of impact is between the legs (as in falling on a fence), usually accompanied by major trauma to the posterior urethra, extravasation of blood and urine through Buck's fascia, often extending into the scrotum, perineum, central tensor and anterior abdominal wall under Scarpa's fascia Note: Straddle-type bicycle injuries in young females may mimic the changes seen in sexual assault

straight back (and flat chest) syndrome A physiologic variation of the body due to a loss of the normal thoracic kyphosis, which reduces the anteroposterior chest diameter, making the pulmonary artery and right hilum more prominent, displacing the heart to the left, giving the false impression of cardiomegaly; a straight back is associated with atrial septal defects and scoliosis and may cause mild pulmonary vein obstruction and dilatation evoking a harsh late systolic ejection murmur, which is asymptomatic unless the findings are misinterpreted by the examiner, in which situation, an otherwise healthy individual may become a cardiac 'cripple'

straitjacket Camisole A form of physical restraint that consists of a canvas jacket with overly long sleeves topped with leather straps that buckle in the jacket's back, preventing an unruly or violent subject from hurting him/herself or others

strand-displacement amplification see SDA

strangulated hernia The prolapse of a loop of intestine into a hernia sac with vascular compromise and with time, infarction of the entire prolapsed loop; Cf Incarcerated hernia

strap cell SURGICAL PATHOLOGY An elongated eosinophilic cell with vague cross-striations classically seen in rhabdomyosarcomas of intermediate differentiation, as well as in triton tumors; 'strap' cells may also be seen in teratomas with rhabdomyosarcomatous differentiation Note: The 'strap cell' described in inflammatory pseudotumors lacks cross-striations

strap muscles A colloquial term for the infrahyoid group of intrinsic laryngeal muscles; SMs are small, flat muscles* inferior to the hyoid bone that connect therewith, as they do with the thyroid cartilage; SMs are antagonistic to the elastic suspensory ligaments and elevators of the larynx; Cf Laryngeal complex

*The SMs correspond to the omohyoid (*M omohyoideus* [NA6]), sternohyoid (*M sternohyoideus* [NA6]), sternothyroid (*M sternothyoideus* [NA6]), thyrohyoid (*M thyrohyoideus* [NA6]), and the elevator of the thyroid glands (*M levator glandulae thyroideus* [NA6]) muscles

stratified log-rank test STATISTICS: A statistical maneuver used for univariate analyses

strawberry An adjectival descriptor referring or pertaining to any relatively round, dark red or occasionally dark green mass or lesion, punctuated by light-colored dots, mimicking the fruit, *Euonymus americanus*

strawberry angioma A nasopharyngeal hemangioma, which when it affects children, may cause airway obstruction; rarely, if the blood volume flowing into a hemangioma is large, arteriovenous shunting may cause cardiac decompensation; Cf Strawberry hemangioma

Note: Giant angiomas with thrombocytopenia, are eponymically dignified as the Kassabach-Merritt syndrome

strawberry cell A morula-type plasma cell with red-purple cytoplasm, punctuated by minivacuoles of polyclonal immunoglobulins, seen in the perivascular cuff of 'round cells' in chronic African trypanosomiasis

strawberry cervix A descriptive term for the quasi-pathognomonic colposcopic appearance of subepithelial punctate petechiae seen in the uterine cervix infected by the sexually transmissible *Trichomonas vaginalis*, variably accompanied by 'double hairpin' capillaries; see Strawberry mucosa

strawberry cream blood A highly colloquial term of uncertain clinical utility for blood that has a visibly prominent increase in lipids, inparting an appearance fancifully likened to strawberries whipped in cream

strawberry gallbladder A descriptor for the appearance of the mucosa seen in the relatively common cholesterosis of the gallbladder, where aggregates of cholesterol/lipid-laden histiocytes overlie an erythematous or verdant mucosa, occasionally causing a giant cell reaction

strawberry hemangioma Strawberry mark Strawberry nevus A raised irregular, bright-red capillary hemangioma or reactive proliferation of small subdermal vessels first seen in infancy, that expands aggressively for several years then involutes or disappears (90% are no longer visible by age seven) PATHOLOGY Abundant closely packed and mitotically active spindled cells in spaces with relatively little blood TREATMENT Excision if necessary or high-dose prednisone; Cf Strawberry angioma

strawberry mucosa GYNECOLOGY A lesion identical to the strawberry cervix, characterized by edema, erythema and spotting of tiny blisters, due to infection of the female genital mucosa, vaginal wall, portio and urethral meatus, usually caused by *Trichomonas vaginalis* and seen by colposcopy in up to 92% of women infected with *T vaginalis*, often accompanied by yellowish and/or purulent discharge, vulvar itching and a fish-like odor PATHOLOGY Intense superficial polymorphous cell infiltration by neutrophils, lymphocytes, plasma cells

strawberry spots Small erythematous spots seen by endoscopy of a large intestine infected with *Entamoeba histolytica*

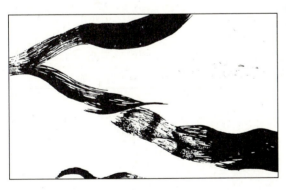

strap cell

strawberry tongue A characteristic enanthema of the tongue, characterized by hypertrophy of the fungiform papillae, accompanied by changes of the filiform papillae in a bright red background; the tongue is classically seen in scarlet fever, but also occurs in Kawasaki's disease (mucocutaneous lymph node syndrome), toxic shock syndrome and in the early stages of yellow fever

straw consumer A term that is a variant of 'straw man', ie an imaginary person who has been created to serve a particular purpose (in its original form, a straw man was made by farmers to scare away crows, ie a 'scarecrow'), or alternately, a propositon or hypothesis created for the sake of argument; a straw consumer, then, is an imaginary consumer of health care (or other) services, who would have opinions on potentially controversial issues, eg the practice of HIV-infected dentists or surgeons

straw Peter syndrome A neurologic complex affecting children, more commonly boys, who are purposelessly hyperactive, impulsive, aggressive and have a short attention span with minimal cortical dysfunction TREATMENT Methylphenidate Note: This syndrome may be the same as the Attention-deficit hyperactivity syndrome, see there

Note: Struwwelpeter was a character in a poem about a frenetic, unruly and unkempt boy

streak MICROBIOLOGY *verb* To inoculate a semisolid bacterial growth plate by running a culture loop across the medium in three different directions or in a 'slant' tube performed in conjunction with stabbing, which provides anaerobic ('stab') and aerobic ('streak') conditions in the same test tube; Cf Stab

'streaked' tonsils Striated yellow-orange discoloration caused by aggregates of lipid-laden macrophages in tonsils, as well as in the thymus, lymph nodes, BM, and GI tract; streaked tonsils occur in most patients with Tangier's disease, which is accompanied by peripheral neuropathy and hepatosplenomegaly LABORATORY ↓↓↓ Cholesterol, ↓↓↓ HDL, both due to a virtually complete deficiency of apoA-I and II

streak ovaries CLINICAL GENETICS Thin, rounded fibrous gonads with an attenuated cortex, medulla and hilum typical of the histologically infantile ovaries of Turner (45, XO) syndrome; oocytes are invariably absent in adult streak ovaries as their development requires granulosa cell activity that doesn't occur in absence of a second X chromosome; primary ovarian tumors in streak ovaries are rare given the virtual absence of germ cells

Note: Turner syndrome patients are at an increased risk for endometrial carcinoma, a complication attributed to neoplasia 'driven' by replacement estrogen, rather than the chromosomal defect

stream see Downstream, Upstream

street virus A virulent virus, eg rabies, that is in its natural or genetically unmodified form, and which may be obtained from domestic and wild animals

'strep throat' A generic term that may be applied to virtually any infectious erythema of the oropharynx and tonsils; although the name implies a bacterial origin (streptococcal throat) and is usually treated with antibiotics, it is most commonly due to viruses, eg EBV and CMV, and less commonly due to streptococci, diphtheria, tularemia, toxoplasmosis, brucellosis, salmonellosis, and TB; true streptococcal pharyngitis has a 2-4 day incubation period, pain on swallowing, headache, malaise, fever, anorexia; children may also suffer nausea, vomiting and abdominal pain EPIDEMIOLOGY (true step throat) Spread by droplets or direct contact PHYSICAL EXAMINATION Extreme hyperemia covered by punctate or confluent yellow-gray exudate with edema, lymphoid hyperplasia, causing an estimated 30 million cases annually; the organism's virulence is related to the M protein, against which a vaccine is under development

streptavidin An avidin analogue produced by bacteria that may be used as a substitute for avidin as it is thought to provide a 'cleaner' signal

streptococcal sex syndrome A rare recurrent erythroderma resulting from post-coital *Streptococcus agalactiae* bacteremia, related to poor lymphatic drainage in women who have had perineal radiotherapy or lymph node excision for malignancy

Streptococcus agalactiae see Group B streptococci

streptokinase A fibrinolytic enzyme that converts plasminogen to plasmin, which is used therapeutically to lyse thrombi in early myocardial infarction, with the purpose of minimizing or reducing the size of the infarct in arterial occlusions and in pulmonary thromboembolism; streptokinase has an efficacy similar to that of tissue plasminogen activator and urokinase; see tPA

stimulated acid output SAO GASTROENTEROLOGY A stimulatory test used to evaluate the adequacy of vagotomy in patients requiring the same for gastric ulcer disease (normal: SAO ranges from 10 to 0% of the peak acid output); see BAO, MAO, PAO

stress fracture A fracture resulting from repeated, unidirectional stress or strain on a particular zone of the musculoskeletal system, or due to repeated relatively trivial trauma to the bone; SFs may affect runners and ballet dancers (fibula or tibia), soldiers (metatarsal bones), jackhammer or pneumatic drill operators (metacarpal bones), and office workers (coccyx)

stress system A tightly linked interdependent endocrine system formed from the systemic sympathetic and adrenomedullary systems and the hypothalamic-pituitary-adrenal axis; the main function of the SS is to maintain basal and stress-related homeostasis and is active at rest, responding to various blood-borne, neurosensory, circadian and limbic signals, in particular from the cytokines (eg IL-1, IL-6, and TNF-α); '*Activation of the stress system heightens arousal, accelerates motor reflexes, improves attention and cognition, decreases appetite and sexual arousal, and increases tolerance of pain...*(and) *changes cardiovascular function and intermediary metabolism and inhibits immune-mediated inflammation.*' (**N Engl J Med 1995; 332:1351**RV) see Hypothalamic-pituitary-adrenal axis

stress test Treadmill exercise (stress) test, see there

stress ulcer An erosion or ulcer of the gastric mucosa, which has been attributed to some form of physical or mental stress; stress-driven individuals are thought to be susceptible to peptic ulceration, a posit supported by animal models; SUs are an important complication in the critically ill; because bleeding from stress ulcers is relatively rare, but has a high mortality (in one report, 48.5% vs 9% without hemorrhage), the use of prophylactic measures, eg neutralization of gastric acid, ↓ gastric acid secretion and cytoprotection is commonly recommended; prophylaxis is best administered to those at highest risk (respiratory failure-odds ratio 15.6, coagulopathy-odds ratio 4.3) for GI bleeding and can be safely withheld from other patients (**N Engl J Med 1994; 330:377**OA) these ulcers have been subdivided according to presumed etiology **ACTIVITY ULCER** A type of gastric erosion that is produced when rats are placed in a running wheel with access to food for only one hourper day **EXERTION ULCER** Gastric ulceration that is associated with excessive and unexpected food activity, eg a rotating cage keeps the rodents constantly running and the gastric juices flowing to the maximum **RESTRAINT ULCER** An ulcer that appears in rats within hours of being placed in a very confined spaces, especially when the ambient temperature is lowered **SHOCK ULCER** Gastric ulceration in humans that is related to burns, eg Curling's ulcer, ischemia, neurologic injury, eg Cushing's ulcer, sepsis or trauma; see Executive monkey, 'Toxic core', Type A personality

*Given the known association with of gastric ulcers with *Helicobacter pylori*, many respond to antibiotic therapy

stress ulceration Stress ulcer, see there

'stretch mark' A purplish 'stripe'* seen on the lower abdomen, thighs, on the iliac crests and breasts in pregnancy and in corticosteroid excess, which become whitish after birth but do not disappear

*The formal (ie written) form is variously designated as pregnancy striae, striae distensae, striae gravidarum

stretching SPORTS MEDICINE An activity that is usually a prelude to exercise and is intended to keep the muscles supple and to improve the range of motion of the joints; in some forms of exercise, eg yoga, stretching constitutes the exercise itself; Cf Aerobic exercise

striction The reduction of the total volume of two substances when mixed, due to solute-solvent interaction

stridor ENT A harsh medium- to high-pitched crowing noise heard when breathing, in particular on inspiration, which is due to an airway obstruction in the larynx or trachea; in children stidor may occur 1) In a background of congenital laryngeal stridor (laryngomalacia), which usually improves with age, and 2) As a persistent or recurrent phenomenon due to allergies, upper respiratory tract infections, papillomas, foreign bodies, mediastinal masses, various cysts

stringent factor An enzyme that synthesizes ppGpp and pppGpp, which regulate the rate of RNA synthesis in the stringent response, a decrease in RNA synthesis that occurs in wild bacteria after removal of an essential amino acid

stringency MOLECULAR BIOLOGY The exactness of the 'fit' required for two strands of nucleic acid to bind in a complementary fashion; the higher the stringency of the hybridization conditions, the fewer the mismatches allowed between the bases in the complementary strands for hybridization to occur; factors affecting stringency include concentrations of salt and formamide, temperature of the reaction, length and GC content of the probe

string of beads sign GI RADIOLOGY A descriptor for radiologic findings in small intestine obstruction, where the 'beads' correspond to pockets of gas oriented in an oblique line, a function of the amount of fluid and the intensity of peristalsis; although characteristic of mechanical obstruction, this sign may also be seen in adynamic ileus due to inflammation PULMONARY RADIOLOGY A descriptive term referring to distribution of sarcoid granulomata along the pulmonary septae

string of pearls sign RADIOLOGY A descriptor for the multiple arterial dilatations and strictures seen in fibromuscular dysplasia, a condition affecting small and medium-sized arteries including the renal and extracranial cephalic vessels

string sign GI RADIOLOGY COLON A linear fraying of the barium column with luminal stenosis, spasm, ulceration and scarring, seen in the terminal ileum in long-standing Crohn's disease that is rarely also seen in ulcerative colitis; grossly, the affected intestine is thickened, rigid and has been fancifully likened to a 'garden hose' ESOPHAGUS An elongated, narrowed and straight single, occasionally dual channel(s) of contrast as seen in well-developed hypertrophic pyloric stenosis

string test Rope's test RHEUMATOLOGY A bedside test for determining the viscosity of synovial fluid, or 'quality' of the mucin clot in synovial fluid, which is a reflection of hyaluronidate polymerization; the further a drop of synovial fluid falls before separating ('stringing effect'), the greater the fluid's viscosity, the more normal it is; a few drops of synovial fluid are added to 10 ml of diluted (2-5%) acetic acid and the length of the 'strand' formed between drops of fluid is measured; a decrease in the strand length implies chemical deterioration due to inflammatory (sepsis, gout, rheumatoid arthritis), but not degenerative joint disease; see Spinnbarkeit UROLOGY A macroscopic method for determining active spermatogenesis; the testicle is bisected, forceps are used to grasp the parenchyma and visually note the separation of the strands of fibers

stripping BIOCHEMISTRY Hydrolysis of amino acid from an aminoacyl-tRNA MOLECULAR BIOLOGY Separation of ribosomal proteins from ribosomes PATHOLOGY Removal of the renal capsule at the autopsy table in order to evaluate the renal surface, which may demonstrate lesions of hypertension; see Flea-bitten kidneys, Rat-bitten kidneys SURGERY Removal of the renal capsule from the kidney and pedicles in order to interrupt the lymphaticorenal fistulas, thereby treating the intractable chyluria induced by *Wuchereria bancrofti*

stroke Cerebrovascular accident A sudden focal neurologic defect lasting more than 24 hours, which is characterized by abrupt loss of consciousness due to either hemorrhage or vascular occlusion of cerebral blood vessels, leading to immediate paralysis, weakness and speech defects; strokes are a leading cause of disability in developed countries (500 000 new victims/year, US, 20-30% of whom are left with severe residua; they are the third leading cause of death (20-30% early mortality) CLINICAL Paralysis, weakness, sensory loss and speech defects ETIOLOGY (of ischemic stroke) Embolism (59%), small-vessel (27%) and large-vessel atherothrombosis (14%), in the last of which, the greatest risk for stroke is seen when the lesion is ≥ 4 mm in thickness (N Engl J Med 1994; 331:1517ED) the predisposing factors of cigarette smoking and hypertension are more predictive of carotid atherosclerosis than are serum lipid and lipoprotein levels (Mayo Clin Proc 1991; 66:259); the residua of a stroke may be either temporary, see Transient ischemic attack or permanent, causing an Alzheimer's dementia-like complex due to a 'shower' of small infarctions (see Multi-infarct dementia) or with large losses of cerebral tissue, may result in a lacunar state, see État lacunaire PATHOGENESIS After ↓ blood flow in the brain due to an arterial occlusion by thromboembolism or vasospasm (or less commonly, spontaneous cerebral hemorrhage), infarction of the cerebral tissue (core region) irrigated by the occluded vessel is inevitable, unless the clot is lysed immediately; an adjacent or penumbral region surrounding the core region may be salvaged if the collateral circulation is adequate; the ischemia-induced damage is explained by the glutamate cascade model, which may be 'dissected' for examining treatment options TREATMENT Warfarin ↓ the risk of stroke in those atrial fibrillation and/or previous MI; in poor candidates for warfarin therapy, aspirin (which is less protective) ± ticlopidine may be used; carotid endarterectomy (CE) is useful if there is 70+% stenosis; CE's role in asymptomatic patients is uncertain; dipyridamole and sulfinpyrazone are useless (N Engl J Med 1995; 332:238RV) PREVENTION Systolic hypertension is a major cause of strokes; low-dose chlorthalidone therapy reduces the incidence (5-year absolute benefit) of strokes by 30 events/1000 participants and major cardiovascular events by 55 events/1000 (JAMA 1991; 265:3255)

'stroke belt' A colloquial term for the southeastern USA, a region with a high incidence of hypertension in the black population, among whom the blood pressure is 10 mm Hg systolic and 6 mm Hg diastolic higher than in similar subjects in Colorado (JAMA 1991; 265:2957c); the 'stroke belt' phenomenon remains an epidemiologic conundrum of uncertain origin variously attributed to differences in geography, intensity of skin color, diet or other factors

stroke in evolution Progressive stroke An incompletely developed stoke

stromal 'crumbling' Fragmentation dense stromal cellularity, a nonspecific histologic feature of dysfunctional uterine bleeding, seen in a specimen from an endometrial curettage

stromelysin family A family of metalloproteinases that are thought to be involved in regulating collagenase activation; stromelysins act on a wide range of substrates, including collagens IV, IX, and XI, elastin, fibronectin, gelatin, laminin, and proteoglycans; see Metalloproteinase

stromelysin-1 Matrix metalloproteinase 3, MMP3

stromelysin-2 Matrix metalloproteinase 10, MMP10

stromalysin-3 A member of the secreted matrix metalloproteinase family, which degrades the extracellular matrix and has been identified in the (desmoplastic) stroma of invasive, but not in situ carcinoma of the female breast; such stromal factors are thought to be responsible for invasion in epithelial malignancy: gene expression, ie transcription of this and other matrix metalloproteinases may be induced by diffusible factors, eg platelet-derived growth factor, fibroblast growth factor, transforming growth factor-α and cytokines, providing a mechanism by which malignant cells may effect the next step in their progression; S3 may play a major role in the destruction of the basement membrane and extracellular matrix in invasive basal cell carcinoma (Diagn Mol Pathol 1992; 1:200)

strontium-89 RADIATION ONCOLOGY A beta-emitting bone-seeking radioisotope ($T_{1/2}$ 50.4 days) that is of use in patients with diffuse bony metastase, eg those with end-stage breast cancer for whom pain medication is often ineffective (N Engl J Med 1995; 332:371RV)

strontium-90 RADIATION ONCOLOGY A beta-emitting bone-seeking radioisotope (physical $T_{1/2}$ 28 years) produced by the fission of ^{235}U fission, which is a dangerous component of radioactive fallout because of its long biological $T_{1/2}$ (7 years) half-life

STRP Short tandem repeat polymorphism

structural biology The field of biology that deals with the relationships between primary stucture (ie the primary sequences of nucleic acids and amino acids), as well as secondary, tertiary, and quarternary structures of biologically active macromolecules; many strucutral, computational and theoretical complexities are being resolved for the purposes of drug design and protein, DNA and RNA simulations; research in structural biology will requires the continued use of old as well as new tools, eg X-ray crystallography, nuclear magnetic responance spectroscopy, electron microscopy, and confocal microsopy (from Nature 1994; 369:11N)

structural gene Any sequence of DNA that is transcribed into mRNA and translated into a polypeptide or protein

structural protein A protein that is critical for the structural integrity of a cell, eg collagen, intermediate filaments and microtubules, rather than a functional component

Structured Query Language SQL A concise query language that is increasingly popular in database management; SQL has only 30 commands, eg SELECT to retrieve data, UPDATE to modify data, DELETE, INSERT, and so on, and was originally developed for use in mini– and mainframe computers; because it is both data– and device independent, it is particularly useful for allowing PCs to communicate with larger computers and with themselves (CAP Today November 1993)

struma ovarii The presence of mature thyroid tissue as the predominant tissue in an ovarian teratoma, potentially causing clinical hyperthyroidism; 5-10% of struma ovarii become malignant, the only absolute criterion for which is the presence of metastasis

struvite stones Triple phosphate calculi, see there

strychnine A highly toxic alkaloid most commonly used as a rodenticide (that is less than effective in this regard as rats avoid its bitter taste), that elicits CNS hyperactivity, causing painful, recurrent tonic motor seizures, muscle tightness and cramping, risus sardonicus, followed by marked flaccidity, decorticate posturing and death; strychnine may be ingested by humans with suicidal or homicidal intent; symptoms appear at doses as low as 15 mg, death occurs with doses above 60 mg, through Renshaw cell inhibition and terminal respiratory paralysis TREATMENT Control seizures with diazepam and phenobarbital; for muscle relaxation, curare and succinylcholine

STS Serological tests for syphilis, see there

ST-segment depression see Silent ischemia

STS-map Sequence-tagged site map MOLECULAR BIOLOGY A means for standardizing communication among the research groups involved in constructing the 3 billion base pair human genome map; the STS proposal is not an alternative to the current strategies for mapping the human genome, but rather redefines the end product; since all DNA mapping strategies use cloned segments of DNA as landmarks, regardless of whether they are 'contig' maps, restriction maps, polymorphism maps or whether the landmarks are sequences that hybridize in situ to a particular chromosomal band, the STS protocol calls for all mapping groups, regardless of whether they are searching for a gene or sequencing an entire chromosome, to also sequence a short tract of DNA from the clone that defines the landmark; this then allows both 'little science' and 'big science' laboratories, to participate in the Human Genome project; the goal is to construct an STS map with landmarks every 10^5 bases within the first five years of the Human genome project; see cDNA library, Human Genome project

stucco keratosis A form of seborrheic keratoses, which is gray-white and symmetrical, measuring 1-3 mm in diameter, seen on distal extremities; SKs are most commonly found on the feet of elderly ♂ PATHOLOGY Hyperkeratosis with church-spire-like extensione of papillae TREATMENT Removal by scraping

student's elbow Bursitis of the olecranon related to prolonged resting of the elbows on table tops, classically seen in students

student loan Medical student debt, see there

student's 't' test A statistical test that determines whether the mean value of 'set A' data differs significantly from that of 'set B' data; the t-test may be performed after an 'F test'

Note: WS Gosset, ex of Oxford, was employed by a brewery in Dublin in 1899 and was responsible for interpreting barley data; his employer preferred that his statistical methods be published under a pseudonym and he chose 'student'; see Standard deviation

STUMP Smooth muscle tumor of undetermined malignant potential; see Borderline tumors

stump 'blowout' Leakage of the blind end (the 'stump') of a duodenum that has been partially resected for ulcer; the leak may be due to technical error or suture line failure, especially in a previously scarred or edematous duodenum; complications of leakage include peritonitis, hepatic bed abscess, pancreatitis and external fistula formation with electrolyte derangement

stump carcinoma A carcinoma arising at the gastric 'stump' that remains after a subtotal (Billroth I or II) gastrectomy; it is unclear whether patients with gastric resection are at ↑ risk for future carcinoma of the stomach; the reported incidence of gastric stump carcinoma ranges from no ↑ in some studies to a 2–3-fold ↑ in others; if the association is real, the incidence of carcinoma accelerates 15-20 years after surgery and may be related to reflux gastritis, which induces dysplasia and cancer, bile reflux or hypochlorhydria which facilitates the colonization of bacteria that release carcinogen(s); the incidence of stump carcinoma may be related to the bile reflux seen in Billroth II resections, or due to chronic infection by *Helicobacter pylori* (N Engl J Med 1991; 325:1127, 1132, 1170ed)

Note: It is possible that there is an increased incidence of gastric carcinoma in patients with gastric ulcers, even in the absence of surgery

'stunned' myocardium Transient (hours to days in duration) postischemic contractile abnormalities seen after myocardial reperfusion begins in acute myocardial infarction (JAMA 1990; 264:455c) Cf Hibernating myocardium

stuttering CLINICAL MEDICINE *adjective* Pertaining or relating to an intermittent progression of a disease state, characterized by a staccato pattern of deterioration, as classically occurs in multiple sclerosis or in a stroke in evolution SPEECH PATHOLOGY *noun* A defective speech pattern that is more common in ♂ and characterized by irregular repetition of syllables, words, or phrases, hesitation and interruption of fluent speech; the most form is that of a staccato repetition of the first phoneme of a spoken phrase; it may be accompanied by facial grimacing, postural gestures, involuntary grunts or loss of airway control; it is thought to be of environmental origin (ie related to the individual's relationship with others), although a vague genetic component may be present; stuttering may coexist with cluttering, see there TREATMENT Bethanechol may be beneficial (N Engl J Med 1993; 329:753oA)

Note: Stutterers in history have reportedly included Moses the Prophet, Aristotle, Lewis Carroll, Winston Churchill, Charles Darwin, Marilyn Monroe, and Jimmy Stewart

styrene Ethenylbenzene A hydrocarbon that is polymerized (polystyrene) by various chemical processes in the manufacture of plastics, synthetic rubbers, resins, and insulation

subacute myelo-optic neuropathy A neuron dysfunction complex that begins with diarrhea and abdominal pain and is followed by sensory and motor disturbances of the lower limbs, ataxia, impaired vision, convulsion and coma

subacute necrotizing encephalomyelopathy Leigh's disease An AR [MIM 256000] condition of neonatal onset CLINICAL Swallowing and feeding difficulties, hypotonia, hyperreflexia, weakness, ataxia, peripheral neuropathy, external ophthalmoplegia, impaired hearing and vision, seizures, and convulsions PATHOGENESIS Defective mitochondrial membrane-bound electron transfer system (respiratory chain) proteins, specifically in the mitochondrial electron transport complex IV, eg cytochrome C oxidase, resulting in lactic acidosis PATHOLOGY Similar to Wernicke's encephalopathy eith focal necrosis, vascular proliferation, and gliosis of the brainstem

subacute sclerosing panencephalitis A slow virus-induced inflammation evoked by the measles virus or by measles vaccines; the long latency period of months to years may be due to the slow development of hypersensitivity or autoimmune response CLINICAL Onset may occur in childhood, with mental dysfunction, dyskinesia, myoclonus, hypotonia and emotional lability; it is usually fatal within 1-3 years PATHOLOGY Perivascular mononuclear and plasma call infiltration in gray and white matter, neuronal degeneration, intranuclear and intracytoplasmic inclusions in neurons and glial cells EM Tubular intranuclear and cytoplasmic inclusions of Dawson EEG Suppression of the normal rhythm, punctuated by bursts of high-voltage slow and sharp waves LABORATORY Paretic gold curve with ↑↑↑ immunoglobulins in the cerebrospinal fluid TREATMENT None; Cf Prion

subclavian steal syndrome Cerebrovascular insufficiency caused by stenosing or occlusive atherosclerosis of the left subclavian artery, proximal to the origin of the vertebral artery, which reverses the blood flow to the vertebral artery, supplying the brainstem, 'stealing' the blood from the brain by the posterior cerebral circulation to supply collateral circulation in the arm causing both cerebral and brachial ischemia, ↓ peripheral pulse and a bruit over the stenotic vessel; the SSS may also occur in congenital vascular malformations, after neurosurgery, and in Takayasu's arteritis, thrombosis, trauma, and tumors, and is exacerbated by exercise of the upper extremity; see Steal; Cf 'Robin Hood syndrome'

subclavian vein catheterization Subclavian venipuncture A common clinical procedure in which the subclavian vein is entered and a catheter placed to enable administration of chemotherapy, total parenteral nutrition, long-term antibiotics, or to maintain fluids during a surgical procedure; SV requires identification of the deep vein based on surface landmarks, and thus in inexperienced hands is prone to complications[1], including failure to locate or cannulate the vein[2], puncture of the subclavian artery, misplacement of the catheter (eg placement of the catheter tip in the contralateral subclavian vein or in either jugular vein), pneumothorax, hemothorax, mediastinal hematoma, and injury to regional nerves (eg brachial or phrenic nerves), cerebral air embolism, and embolism of fragments of the catheter by the insertion needle; ultrasonographic guidance had been recommended as a means of improving catheter guidance, but has proven useless (**N Engl J Med 1994; 331:1735oa**) see Central venous catheterization

[1]Failed attempts at SVC are two times more common in patients who are very thin or very obese, or have had previous major surgery, or regional catheterization [2]As the vast majority of central venous catheters are placed in the subclavian vein, the terms central venous catheter and subclavian vein catheter, and related terms have been used interchangeably

subclinical hyperthyroidism A low serum thyrotropin (TSH) concentration in an asymptomatic person with normal serum thyroid hormone concentrations; SH is more common in older (> age 60) people, and is detected by measuring serum TSH ETIOLOGY Solitary thyroid adenoma, multinodular goiter, subclinical Graves' disease CLINICAL Atrial fibrillation, atrial premature contractions, ↑ pulse rate, ↑ left ventricular mass and contractility, osteoporosis and bone loss TREATMENT It is uncertain whether treatment is appropriate (**N Engl J Med 1994; 331:1249oa, 1302ed**)

subclinical hypothyroidism An ↑ TSH (thyrotropin) before or after administration of TRH (thyrotropin-releasing hormone) in the face of normal T_3 and T_4; SH affects 6-7% of ♀ and 2-3 of ♂, with 5-10% annual rate of progression to overt hypothyroidism (**Am J Med 1992; 92:631**)

subcloning MOLECULAR BIOLOGY A type of cloning in which a segment of DNA of interest that has already been cloned, isolated and 'chopped' with a restriction endonuclease, is subjected to a second round of cloning in an appropriate receptor

subcutaneous insulin-resistance syndrome Insulin-resistance in IDDM that is attributed to an insulin-specific protease present in the subcutaneous tissue, the existence of which is increasingly controversial; if SIRS does exist, it is very rare; see Dawn phenomenon, Somogyi effect

suberosis A form of hypersensitivity pneumonitis (extrinsic allergic alveolitis) caused by exposure to moldy cork dust and fungi, eg *Penicillium frequentans*; see Farmer's lung; Hypersensitivity pneumonitis

subfertility A term referring to a male condition in which semen parameters are below the lower limits of normal on two or more occasions; criteria used include: volume < 1.5 ml, sperm density < 20 million/ml, sperm viability < 60%, motility < 2 (on a scale of 1 to 4), and > 60% abnormal forms; subfertile semen may also demonstrate hyperviscosity, sperm agglutination, polyspermia and/or hematospermia; Cf Anti-sperm antibodies, Infertility

subglottic webs Laryngeal web, see there

subimmunogenic *adjective* Pertaining or relating to a lower than expected immune immune response, usually referring to a vaccine of suboptimal immunogenicity (**JAMA 1995; 273:888ed**)

subinternship A training period for a senior medical student in which he/she assumes the role of an intern as he/she rotates through various services (eg internal medicine, surgery, pediatrics); the subintern is closely supervised by a resident or an attending physician; Cf Extern, Intern, Scut monkey

subluxation An incomplete joint dislocation such than portions of the articular surfaces remain in contact

el 'submarino' see Torture

submersion syndrome Near drowning A symptom complex due to prolonged submersion without death CLINICAL Tachypnea, mild hyperthermia, restlessness, vertigo, confusion, nausea, vomiting, shock, accompanied by pulmonary congestion and edema and depending on the water temperature, hypothermia; see Drowning; Cf Muddy lung

subphrenic interposition syndrome Chilaiditi syndrome A condition caused by the interposition of the colon between the liver and diaphragm, which is most commonly symptomatic in children, and improves with age CLINICAL Abdominal pain, vomiting, anorexia, constipation, abdominal distention (bloating) TREATMENT Avoidance of 'gassy' foods

subroutine COMPUTERS A programming sequence that is be used two or more times in a programming routine

subspecialty A field of sub-specialized expertise, eg interventional radiology in a specialty of medicine, eg radiology that requires one or two years of a fellowship training period beyond residency in an officially recognized training program, at the end of which an examination may be required; some subspecialties may be approached from different fields, pediatric oncologists are usually pediatricians, but may also be oncologists; in the US, there are 59 subspecialties governed by 24 specialty boards, some of which can be shared among specialties, eg hand surgery is a subspecialty of (general) surgery, orthopedic surgery, and plastic surgery; see Fellowship; Cf Specialty

substance 1) A term that is less commonly used than the equally nebulous term, 'factor', which refers to any poorly characterized molecule or group of molecules of plant or animal origin that have some discernible effect either in vivo or in an in vitro system 2) A euphemism for any agent (eg cocaine, heroin, marijuana, but also solvents), usually illicit, than has potential for abuse

Note: Since by the above definition, virtually any molecule or class of agents could be regarded as a 'substance', it has become a less preferred term in scientific parlance

substance abuse An activity that may be defined as 1) The use of illicit, potentially addicting drugs, eg cocaine 2) The misuse of prescribed drugs with stimulatory or depressant activities on the nervous system, eg amphetamines or barbiturates or 3) The habitual use of commercially-available substances that are known to have a wide variety of deleterious effects in addition to the desired effects, eg alcohol and tobacco STATISTICS (National Institute on Drug Abuse, USA, 1988 household survey) two million teenagers had tried illicit drugs, 600 000 used cocaine in the survey year; habitual use of cocaine in most developed nations has increased exponentially; 12% of employed 20-40 year-olds and 5 000 000 women of child-bearing age regularly use illicit drugs (US, 1986): 18 200 000 used marijuana at least once/month, 5 800 000 used cocaine at least once/month Substance abuse among resident physicians (**JAMA 1991; 265:2069**) and medical students (**JAMA 1991; 265:2074**) REHABILITATION Self-help organizations include Alcoholics Anonymous, Cocaine Anonymous, Narcotics Anonymous, many of which have local offices ('chapters') in the US; see Alcohol, Cocaine, Crack, Ice, Marijuana

substance P An 11-residue neuropeptide belonging to the tachykinin family, which is produced by alternative splicing of mRNA, stored in secretory vesicles of the brain and gastrointestinal tract that binds to a receptor designated NK1; SP conveys the sensation of pain and noxious stimuli (heat, pressure, caustic chemicals) to the central and peripheral nervous system, causing nonmyelinated or thinly myelinated fibers to discharge; SP closes potassium channels, increases cell polarizability, responses to all stimuli and cell sensitivity to endogenous opioids (enkephalins and adenosine-mediated neurotransmitters); SP bridges the nervous and immune system, as it promotes inflammatory responses, activating macrophages, recruiting inflammatory cells, increasing the expression of SP receptors in the endothelial cells in the sites of inflammation, eg large intestine in colitis, joints in rheumatoid arthritis, lungs in asthma, skin in psoriasis and nervous system in nerve trauma; SP also causes smooth muscle contraction, vasodilation, stimulation of salivary gland secretion, extravasation of plasma, secretion of prostaglandins, oxygen-free radicals and IL-1, potentiating IL-1-induced fibroblast proliferation; prevention of SP release may help explain the benefits of corticoids in attenuating immune reactions; see CP-96345, SNX-111, Tachykinin

substantia nigra NEUROANATOMY A broad bilateral band of gray matter that contains darkly pigmented nerve cells and is located over the entire length of the mesencephalon, between the crus cerebri and the midbrain tegmentum of the cerebral peduncle; the SN consists of a dorsal compact black area (pars compacta) containing melanin-laden neurons and a ventral diffuse red-brown reticular zone containing iron-laden neurons (pars reticularis); it recieves afferent fibers from the caudate nucleus and putamen, its efferent fibers project to the striateum and thalamic nuclei, and its major neurotransmitter is dopamine; the attenuation of the SN seen in older subjects and in those with Parkinson's disease is linked to a decline in motor performance (Arch Neurol 1992; 49:1119)

substantial pain Pain of a severity sufficient to impair function; see Brief Pain Inventory, Pain

subtype O HIV-1-O (outlier) One of the subtypes (30 thus far identified) of HIV-1; the major problem with the O subtypes is that they evoke anti-HIV-1 antibodies that are undetectable with the tests used to screen blood for transfusion; O subtypes had not been identified in the US as of mid-1994 (New York Times 9 August 1994; C11)

subungual exostosis Subungual or periungual trabecular bone formation appearing as a solitary mass on the dorsal aspect of the distal phalanx of the great toe, most common in young females

'subway chart' A complex set of data generated from positron emission tomography (PET) scanning of the macaque brain which has multiple centers for a specific function and a far greater number of circuits connecting the centers; van Essen of the California Institute of Technology found 32 cortical areas involved in some aspect of vision and 305 circuits connecting these areas Note: As the technique of PET scanning matures subway charts may be developed for humans

succimer A safe and effective water-soluble chelating agent that may be administered per os for heavy metal poisoning, eg to treat severe lead poisoning in children above 2.17 µmol/L (US: 45 µg/dl) (JAMA 1991; 265:1802) or adults with lead poisoning secondary to gunshot wounds (J Toxicol Clin Toxicol 1994; 32:377) see Lead, Saturnine gout

succinylacetone A natural substance that is a potent inhibitor of both antibody-mediated (humoral) and the cellular immune response, which acts by blocking T-cell activity; succinylacetone is of interest as it may be active in preventing GVHD and in treating autoimmune uveitis

succotash CLINICAL NUTRITION A vegetable preparation containing corn (low in lysine, an essential amino acid) and beans (low in tryptophan, another essential amino acid), which in combination provide adequate dietary protein, a food of use in developing nations

sucrose density gradient A gradient prepared with vari-

ous concentrations of sucrose ranging from 5% to 25%, used to separate particles and molecules by mass or chain length of the molecule

Note: 'Density' is a misnomer retained by convention, as the technique is more properly known as zonal centrifugation, see there

suction curettage Vacuum curettage or termination GYNECOLOGY The removal of uterine contents after cervical dilation using a hollow-tipped device through which suction is applied; SC is a commonly used method for performing first trimester abortion

SUD Sudden unexpected death; see Sudden unexplained nocturnal death

Sudan Black B stain A stain with affinity for phospholipids and sterols, used in histology to identify fat; in hematology, both specific and azurophilic granules in cells of the myeloid series are positive, as are the leukemic cells in some acute myeloid leukemias (AML), which by the French-American-British classification, includes AML M1 (promyeloblastic leukemia, 3% of blasts stain with Sudan Black B—SBB, as well as with peroxidase—Px and ASD chloroacetate esterase—CAE), AML M2 (myeloblastic leukemia with maturation, > 85% of blasts stain with SBB/Px/CAE), AML M3 (promyelocytic leukemia, > 85% of blasts stain with SBB/Px/CAE), AML M4 (myelomonocytic leukemia, 20% of blasts stain with SBB/Px/CAE)

sudden cardiac death A clinical term defined as death of cardiac disease ≤ 1 hour after onset of symptoms

sudden death FORENSIC MEDICINE Precipitous demise of any type, most commonly due to cardiovascular disease, caused by ischemia, arrhythmia, shock (aortic dissection), congestive heart failure, accompanied by hypoxia, polycystic disease of the heart, familial endocardial fibroelastosis, and Kawasaki's disease, the latter of which is more common in children; other causes of SD include anaphylaxis and 'cafe coronary', poisons (carbon monoxide, hydrogen sulfide, cyanide, nicotine, organophosphate pesticides), gastric rupture due to Mallory-Weiss syndrome, ulcers, septicemia, obstruction, bezoars, cardiovascular and cerebrovascular lesions; SD is more common in alcoholics, nulliparous women and in those with major psychiatric disease; the most common autopsy finding in SD is pulmonary edema

sudden infant death syndrome SIDS, see there

sudden unexplained nocturnal death An idiopathic condition occurring in young, previously healthy, Southeastern Asian males (Bangungut in Filipinos, Lai tai in Thais, Pokkuri in the Japanese) PATHOLOGY Patchy intense loss of myoglobin from myocardium, with interstitial myoglobin deposition; the condition is thought to be due to an anomaly in the conduction system coupled with 'culture shock' and relocation-related stress in emigrants, as the peak incidence (25 reported cases/year) of SUND coincided with the peak influx of refugees from Southeast Asia; in Thailand, SUND is associated with endemic distal renal tubular acidosis (Lancet 1991; 338:930)

sugar cane workers lung Bagassosis, see there

sugar coating A descriptor for the gray-pink plaque-like elevations of the cerebellar folia, characteristically seen with medulloblastoma

sugar hypothesis A view that refined sugars, eg sucrose, further stimulates hyperactive children, as a result of which physicians may recommend restriction of sugar in a child's diet; '...it appears that any adverse effect of sugar is by no means as severe or as prevalent as uncontrolled observation and opinion would suggest. Specifically, there is no evidence that sugar alone can turn a child with normal attention into a hyperactive child. The same applies to aspartame, which has also been suspected of causing behavior disorders in some children. Several studies reveal no systemic differ-

ences in blood glucose levels after ingestion of sucrose in children with attention deficit-hyperactivity disorder or those reported to be sensitive to sugar.' (**N Engl J Med 1994; 330:355ED**) NEWSFLASH: Recent data has linked the consumption of ↑↑↑ sugar on an empty stomach to an ↑ of adrenalin, resulting in a ↓ in ability to concentrate; based on these findings (**S Boulware et al, Pediatrics Feb 1995**), sweet desserts after meals are thought to be preferable to the consumption of sweet snacks between meals (**New York Times 15 March 1995; C11**)

sugar icing appearance Zuckerguß appearance, see there

sugar substitutes CLINICAL NUTRITION A group of carbohydrates, eg fructose, sorbitol and xylitol, of potential use as replacements of the usual dietary sugars (glucose and sucrose) in diabetics, as these molecules do not require insulin for certain steps in their metabolism; the potential advantage is less than optimal, in that the diabetic liver converts a significant portion of fructose and its metabolites into glucose; see Artificial sweeteners

sugar tumor A benign, sharply defined, but nonencapsulated lung tumor (figure, below) characterized by exuberant vascularity and round, polygonal glycogen-filled clear cells with well-defined borders, which are surrounded by hyalinized boundaries with focal calcifications and 'spider' cell formation; the sugar tumor is thought to be of neuroendocrine origin, given the presence of neurosecretory granules and ultrastructural appearance of the endoplasmic reticulum

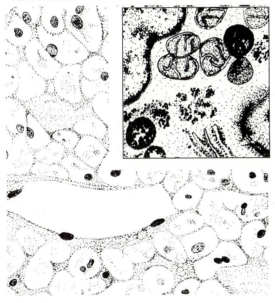

sugar tumor

suicidal behavior PSYCHIATRY Any of a number of covert or completed acts indicating that suicide is being or has been considered; these behaviors include suicidal ideation, attempted suicide or inappropriate euphoria in a person who had previously suffered severe depression PHYSICAL EXAMINATION Often non-contributory, although transverse linear scarring at the wrists may indicate previous suicidal attempts or unusual scars suggestive of self-mutilation may be associated with depression; see Psychological autopsy

suicidal gesture A generic term for any of a number of behaviors or actions that might be* interpreted as indicating a person's desire or intent to commit suicide

*Or might have been, in the case of success completion thereof

suicide A form of death that is illegal in most societies; an estimated one in one hundred people think about suicide annually; many consult a non-psychiatric physician in the six months prior to the act; 29 000/year; it is the 8th leading cause of death in US AGE The rate rises with age, with peaks in adolescence and college (age 15-25), later increasing in older subjects; suicide is more frequent in adolescents who abuse psychoactive drugs MANNER OF DEATH Most successful suicides (US) are by firearms ♂ Firearms 46%, hanging 22%, gas 16%, poison 10% ♀ Poison 41%, strangulation 17%, gas 15%, drowning 10%, firearms 8.5%; in 1970 45% of females died by poison, 32% by firearms; In 1980 poisoning decreased to 20%, firearms increased to 55%, with regional differences Physician suicide rate is the highest of any professional; ♀ physicians are thought by some workers to be three times more likely to autodestruct than other ♀ professionals PREDISPOSING CONDITIONS Mental illness, especially depression, but also schizophrenia; 15% of those with affective disorders die by suicide; 10-15% of alcoholics kill themselves, accounting for ¼ of all suicides (the suicide rate in alcoholics is 500-fold greater than in the general population, and most often occurs by firearm); alcohol abuse and depression are associated with 79-85% of suicides; 90% of those who commit suicide have a psychiatric illness at the time of death; other 'at-risk' conditions include AIDS, cancer, spinal cord injuries, seizure disorders and Huntington's disease; ½ of suicide victims are unmarried, whites commit suicide twice as frequently as blacks ANNUAL INCIDENCE 28 000 (US), 12/10⁵; from 1950 to 1980, the ♂ rate ↑ 305%; ♀ ↑ 67%; from 1955-77, suicides jumped 230% in the 15-24 age group; suicide is attempted more often in ♀, but more often successful in ♂ (♂:♀ ratio, 4:1); 1980, young white ♂, 20.2/10⁵, white ♀, 5/10⁵ SUCCESS RATE Suicide attempt:success ratio is 5:1; in North America, there are seasonal peaks in suicides in March and September; most occur at home; the bodies are often discovered by family or friends; ready access to firearms increases the risk of suicide (**N Engl J Med 1992; 327:467SA, 1878C**), a finding supported by an increase of 36% of suicide by firearms while the rate by other methods remained the same, and a two-fold increase of suicide by firearms among adolescents and young adults (1968-1985)

suicide substrate BIOCHEMISTRY A substrate that is not normally recognized by an enzyme, which has become altered so that it reacts with an adjacent site on the enzyme, covalently linking to an active site on the enzyme, inactivating it

'suits and suites' syndrome A highly colloquial term for the proliferation of well-clad ('suits') administrators ensconced in well-apppointed office spaces ('suites') in health care facilities of all types (**N Engl J Med 1993; 329:428ED**) see Administrative costs, Indirect costs

While not itself the cause of the breakdown of the health care system in the US (and elsewhere), the S&S syndrome increases physicians' growing demoralization and resentment over the oppressive and dysfunctional health care environment-Author's note

sulfadiazine PHARMACOLOGY An antimicrobial sulfonamide that is used in combination with pyrimethamine to treat toxoplasmosis in AIDS patients (**MMWR 1994; 43:671**)

$$H_2N-\text{⬡}-SO_2NH-\text{⬡}$$

sulfadiazine

sulfated polysaccharide AIDS Any (eg carrageenan, isolated from red seaweed) of a family of compounds that may be of use in treating HIV infection, which prevent the interaction of epithelial cells and the release of virus from HIV-infected lymphocytes, possibly by coating the cells and virus with a negative charge, making all players mutually repulsive (**JAMA 1995 273:979**)

sulfites Sulfiting agents (sulfur dioxide, sodium sulfite, sodium or potassium bisulfite or metabisulfite) have been used to prevent discoloration of fruits and vegetables, eg coleslaw, potatoes and avocados served in public places, as in salad bars or are added to packaged foods, eg canned seafood, grapefruit juice, beer and wines; although well-tolerated by most people, up to 5% of asthmatics may be sensitive to sulfites (possibly related to low levels of sulfite oxidase), and respond to exposure with nausea, diarrhea, bronchospasm, pruritus, edema, hives, potentially anaphylactic shock and death; some drugs used for asthma may contain sulfiting agents, potentially exacerbating the problem

sulfite Add used to preserve foods, eg shrimp and frozen potatoes

sulforaphane Sulphoraphane A phytochemical of the isothiocyanate family present in cruciferous vegetables, (eg broccoli), which is thought to stimulate the production of phase 2 enzymes that play a role in detoxifying carcinogens; in one rat study, sulforaphane reduced the incidence of mammary tumors induced by dimethylbenzanthracene (DMBA) (**Proc Nat Acad Sci (US) 12 April 1994**)

'sulfur' granule A descriptive term for the 1–2-mm firm yellow-white nodules lying within a partially encapsulated suppurative mass that may be punctuated by sinus tracts extending to the skin from the tonsils, uterine cervix, peripelvic tissue and lungs in infection by *Actinomyces israeli* PATHOLOGY Basophilic clumps of filamentous, branching actinomycotic bacteria, acute inflammation and necrosis; the yellow color is due to foamy macrophages and tissue response to invasion; in actinomycosis (figure, below), the bacteria are within macrophages; in nocardiosis, the bacteria are extracellular; cultures often reveal mixed organisms including streptococci and fusiform bacteria

Note: Up to 85% of pelvic actinomycosis in females is related to an intrauterine device that has been in place for three or more years

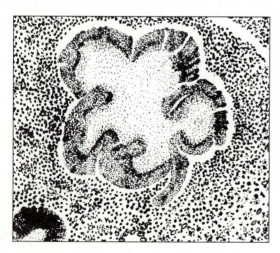

sulfur granule

sulindac An NSAID that has been reported to ↓ the number and size of colorectal adenomas in patients with familial adenomatous polyposis; as this effect is incomplete, sulindac is unlikely to replace colectomy as a primary therapy in FAP (**N Engl J Med 1993; 328:1313OA**)

sulprostone OBSTETRICS A prostaglandin analogue administered intramuscularly that had been widely used in continental Europe in conjunction with mifepristone (RU 486) as an abortifacient; it was withdrawn from the market after it was linked to three cases of MI, one of which was fatal (**N Engl J Med 1995; 332:983OA**) see Abortion, Gemeprost, Mifepristone, Misoprostol

sumatriptan An agonist of serotonin (5-HT) that binds to the 5-HY1D receptor, causing vasoconstriction of the cranial vessels, as well as blocking the extravasation of plasma; sumatriptan is reported to be effective in treating acute migraine, a condition that has been pathogenically linked to intracranial vasodilation, resulting in a reduction in headaches, clinical disability, nausea and photophobia SIDE EFFECTS Tingling, dizziness, hot flashes (**JAMA 1991; 265:2831**)

$$H_3CNHSO_2CH_2 \quad\quad CH_2CH_2N(CH_3)_2$$

sumatriptan

summer itch Hydroa aestivale Hutchinson's prurigo DERMATOLOGY A rare variant of polymorphous light eruption (PMLE) that appears before puberty on covered areas of the skin, characterized by small papules topped by a vesicle, which with time undergo lichenification and scarring; phototesting with ultraviolet-B light may elicit a PMLE-like reaction; see Polymorphous light eruption

summit lesions see Mushroom lesions

sump syndrome Biliary obstruction and food reflux in patients with previous choledocoenteric anastomosis, a condition fancifully likened to a sump pump

sunblock An opaque substance, usually formulated from zinc or titanium oxides, which is designed to completely prevent solar radiation from reaching the skin; Cf Sunscreen

sunburn protection factor rating SPF rating, see there

sunburst pattern RADIOLOGY A descriptive term referring to the appearance of a periosteal reaction, in which dense filiform spiculations are perpendicular to the periosteum, classically seen in osseous infiltration by the common or 'garden variety' osteosarcoma, but which may also be seen in parosteal osteosarcoma, as this latter tumor evokes a minimal periosteal reaction; the adjective 'sunburst' also refers to the irradiating spiculation of the ileal bone around the acetabulum in Voorhoeve syndrome (osteopathia striata)

SUND Sudden unexplained nocturnal death, see there

Sunday morning palsy Saturday night palsy, see there

'Sunday neurosis' PSYCHIATRY The constellation of symptoms described in those who function well in the context of a planned and organized work setting, as the scheduled activities tend to 'bind' their anxieties; when presented with the lack of structure inherent in a weekend and periods of 'relaxation', the usual defense mechanisms are not functioning, and these individuals may manifest symptoms of anxiety, conversion reactions, dissociative states, obsessions, compulsions, and phobias

sundowning PSYCHIATRY Mild to moderate disorientation that occurs with nightfall in elderly subjects and/or those with mild dementia, which is attributed to the loss of visual cues on which they depend for orientation or to compensate for sensorineural defects

sunflower cataract Chalcosis lentis A descriptive term for the radiating orange-tinted anterior capsular and subcapsular opacities in the lens due to copper deposition, seen in adolescents with Wilson's disease; the vision is not affected; see Kayser-Fleischer ring

sunglasses A tinted pair of glasses used to reduce the light arriving to the eye, which in the US are labeled according to the amount of sun blocked; nonprescription glasses are classified according to use and amount of UV radiation blocked **COSMETIC SUNGLASSES** block 70% of UVB and 20% of UVA; they are designed for 'around town' use and 'looking cool' **GENERAL PURPOSE SUNGLASSES** block 95% of UVB and 60% of UVA; they are designed for most outdoor activities **SPECIAL PURPOSE SUNGLASSES** block 99% of UVB and 60% of UVA; they are designed for very bright environments; prescription sunglasses are constructed of plastic or glass, eg CR-39, polycarbonate, polychromic glass; the solar radiation-protecting chemical is allyl diglycol carbonate (New York Times 16 Nov 1993; C5)

sunscreen A transparent substance, eg oxybenzone, and dioxybenzone, that absorbs or scatters UVB (ultraviolet B) light (JAMA 1991; 265:3217); these products may be combined with 5% para-aminobenzoic acid to yield commercial products that maximize UVA absorption, which induces the desired browning effect due to increased melanine production, while minimizing UVB absorption; the ability to block UV light is rated on the poorly standardized SPF (sunshine protection factor) scale, which ranges up to a maximum of 40; contrary to previous assumptions, while sunscreens protect against sunburn and against nonmelanoma skin cancers in experimental animals, they may not protect against melanomas (New York Times 25 January 1994; C3) Cf Melanoma, Sunblock, Tanning salon, Ultraviolet light

sunstroke SPORTS MEDICINE *'The outdated term "sunstroke:" should not be used for heat intolerance conditions because these conditions may occur in absence of sun and have been known to occur indoors... with high heat and excessive humidity.'* (JC DeLee, D Drez, Jr, Eds, Orthopedic Sports Medicine WB Saunders, Philadelphia, 1994) see Heat intolerance

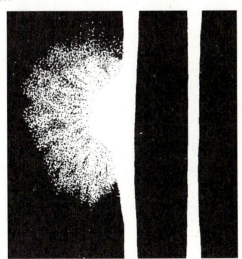

sunburst pattern

'sunk' costs LABORATORY MEDICINE Costs in equipment, reagents and dedicated supplies that have already been incurred, and which should not be included in future budget or financial considerations; in general, sunk costs are monies lost when a certain technique is no longer used or becomes obsolete

Sunna circumcision A type of female circumcision in which the entire or part of the clitoris is removed; see Female circumcision

SUN/PUN Serum urea nitrogen/plasma urea nitrogen; see BUN

superantigen IMMUNOLOGY A protein which in association with class II major histocompatibility complex (MHC)-bearing cells can stimulate any T cell expressing certain classes of the variable β-domain of the T-cell receptor; this circumvents the usual requirement for peptide-specific MHC recognition; the superantigen *Staphylococcus aureus* enterotoxin B can also form complexes with the T-cell receptor in the absence of class II MHC, which may explain the ability of superantigens to induce anergy (Nature 1994; 369:324oA); the p30 superantigen encoded by the *gag* gene from the murine leukemia virus causes the mouse acquired immunodeficiency syndrome for peptide-specific (Science 1991; 252:424) see Mls antigens 2) An antigen that is capable of stimulating the immune system at very low concentration

'superbug' MICROBIOLOGY An organism which, when ingested by macrophages, is either not digested or is resistant to phagocytosis; superbugs include *Mycobacterium leprae, Leishmania* species (which reproduce within the endocytic vesicles) and *Legionella* species (which inhibit intravesicular phagosomal acidification, turning off the system designed to destroy it)

supercoiling Superhelix, see there

supercompensation Carbohydrate loading, see there

supercomputer A generic term for a 'high-end' (± 1 000 billion floating-point operations/sec) computer used for complex calculations, eg for molecular or weather modeling; the traditional supercomputers, the prototype of which includes the Cray family of devices, are designed around a proprietary vector-type architecture; newer supercomputers function by parallel processing in which high-powered RISC* (Reduced instruction set computing)-type microprocessors are linked in series, resulting in a 10-fold drop in price with ↑ throughput of data; massively parallel processing in some machines, eg Silicon Graphics' Power Challenge claim a peak performance of 5.4 billion floating-point operations per second; some industry insiders are predicting that, like the minicomputers and mainframe computers, vector-type supercomputers will be extinct by the 21st century

superconducting magnet MRI A magnet with a magnetic field originating from current flowing through a superconductor, which is encased in a cryostat; see Magnetic resonance imaging

superconductivity A physical phenomenon destined to have broad applications in medicine, especially in information systems, once a superconductor becomes available that operates closer to room temperature; optimized 'high-temperature' superconductors contain a combination of yttrium oxide, barium carbonate and copper oxide; superconductivity is characterized by 1) Zero resistivity (sharp drop in electrical resistance by several orders of magnitude) and 2) Meissner effect (a metal in a constant magnetic field cooled below its superconductivity transitional temperature has zero magnetism filed in its interior, seen as a large negative magnetic susceptibility below the transitional temperature); the physics of superconductivity is poorly understood

Note: The temperature at which superconductivity could be induced had been stagnant at 20° Kelvin until the mid-1980s; it is currently obtained in liquid nitrogen

superfecundation OBSTETRICS Fertilization of a second ovum by sperm from a different act of coitus, after a first ovum has been fertilized; this process serves as an explanation for the rare cases in which twins have different fathers; see Higher multiples, Twin; Cf Superfetation

superfemale see XXX syndrome

superfetation OBSTETRICS Fertilization and subsequent development of a second ovum after the first has already been implanted in the uterus; serving as a theoretical explanation for the difference in times of delivery of fraternal 'twins'; Cf Superfecundation

Superfund ENVIRONMENT A $1.6 x 10^9$ fund created by the US Congress in 1980, begun in 1981 and administered by the Environmental Protection Agency (EPA) that was to have taken 10 years at a cost of $10 x 10^9$; it is estimated to require 40 years and cost > $100 x 10^9$ (NY Newsday, 1 February, 1994); the Superfund was intended to be a 'crash' program to clean up thousands of leaking toxic dump sites in the US; during the first five-year plan, very little was achieved beyond the realization that the magnitude of the environmental contamination had been vastly underestimated, and that many US citizens were living near dumps contaminated with dioxin, PCBs, heavy metals (lead, mercury and arsenic) and other toxic chemicals; in 1986, the Superfund program was renewed under the Superfund Amendments and Reauthorization Act that provided $8.6 x 10^9$ and gave the EPA the 'muscle' to enforce regulations and to fine those who criminally release toxins; see Environmental Protection Agency, Toxic dump site

supergene A segment of DNA containing linked genes that are protected from cross-over exchanging of DNA and are thus transmitted intact from one generation to the next

superhelix MOLECULAR BIOLOGY A structure that results when a circular double-stranded DNA, eg SV40 virus or polyomavirus is twisted on its axis, converting it into a figure of eight or multiple looped chains; a twist in the opposite direction of that of the DNA's double helix is designated as left-handed, negative or underwound, a twist in the same direction as the double helix is termed right-handed, positive or overwound; replication and packaging of DNA in all organisms requires supercoiling, which is described by three parameters: 1) Linking number, which corresponds to the number of times the double helix crosses over on itself 2) Twist, which is related to the frequency and periodicity of the winding of one strand around the other, which under normal physiological conditions occurs every 10.6 bases for right-handed DNA and 3) Writhe, which relates to the pathway in space of the axis of the double helix

superinfection An infection that occurs in the background of a prior infection that occurs when the native flora of a body region are substantially reduced, often by antibiotic therapy, allowing invasion by opportunistic organisms, as occurs in pseudomembranous colitis or vaginal candidiasis

superinfection 'immunity' The finding that two related organisms, eg plasmids, cannot successfully invade a host cell simultaneously

superiority complex PSYCHIATRY A popular term for a constellation of behaviors, including aggressiveness, assertiveness, self-aggrandization, and others, which may represent overcompensation for a deep-rooted sense of inadequacy; Cf Inferiority complex

'supermom' SOCIAL MEDICINE A colloquial term of recent vintage, but uncertain origin, for a woman who raises children, performs the household duties expected of a 'domestic engineer' or housewife, and works a full-time job; the supermom 'syndrome' is poorly studied, but appears to be very common, as 60-70% of US women of child-bearing age are in the workforce, a significant minority of whom are single-parent heads of household; supermoms suffer from a combination of external and largely uncontrollable stresses related to motherhood, as well as internal and self-induced stresses of attempting to perform their regular jobs well or even advance in a career, coupled to the tedium of household tasks; see Latchkey children, 'Quality' time

superobesity Morbid obesity, see there

superovulation therapy The use of clomiphene citrate or human menopausal gonadotropins, which may be of use in treating endometriosis-associated infertility (Mayo Clin Proc 1995; 70:453), which has the disadvantage of increasing the incidence of twinning and multiple births

superoxide anion $O_2\cdot^-$ A highly-reactive free radical that forms when a molecule of oxygen gains an electron, as occurs in inflammation or ionizing radiation; $O_2\cdot^-$ readily combines with protons, other superoxide anions and hydrogen peroxide, forming various toxic and reactive species; $O_2\cdot^-$-induced damage is implicated in age-related degenerative phenomena ('garbage can hypothesis'); $O_2\cdot^-$, is mutagenic and may have a major role in the carcinogenic 'cascade'; see Free radicals

superoxide dismutase An enzyme [EC 1.15.1.1] present in all aerobes that catalyzes the reaction $O_2\cdot^- + O_2\cdot^- + 2H^+ = H_2O_2 + O_2$, which serves to protect the organism against the havoc wreaked by oxygen free radicals; see Antioxidant therapy

super-secondary structure A protein structural motif, eg a β barrel or β meander, which lies between a formal secondary structure, ie α-helix or β-pleated sheet and a formal tertiary structure, ie a domain; see Protein structure

superserver COMPUTERS A network server (see there) that connects 10 to 25 or more PC-type computers, contains two or more microprocessors, up to 256 megabytes of main memory, and is capable of transferring data at a rate of 10-40 megabytes/sec

supertaster SENSORY SCIENCE A person with a high concentration of taste buds who is extremely sensitive to certain taste sensations; supertasters (1100 tastebuds/cm²) comprise about ¼ of the population, ¼ are nontasters (circa 10 tastebuds/cm²), and the remaining are intermediate in the number of tastebuds found on the tongue; male supertasters prefer foods high in sugars, while female supertasters dislike sweeter foods (New York Times 7 Dec 1994; C1)

supervaccine A hypothetical single-dose vaccine for children that would protect against diphtheria, pertussis, tetanus (DPT), polio, *Haemophilus influenzae* type B, measles and others; it is thought that a supervaccine could be developed in as little as 5 years at a cost of $500 million (New York Times 29 March 1994; C3)

'Superwoman' syndrome(s) A clinical complex that may affect any female with more than two X chromosomes, which tends to be more pronounced with more X chromosomes; see XXX, XXXX and XXXXX syndromes

superior mesenteric artery syndrome An uncommon condition caused by compression of the superior mesenteric artery, resulting in the obstruction of the third portion of the duodenum ETIOLOGY Loss of cushioning regional adipose tissues (that maintain an appropriate arterial angle), seen in excess weight loss, rapid growth in children without corresponding gain of weight, in those with an asthenic habitus or in patients fixed in a hyperextended position by spinal injury or surgery CLINICAL Postprandial epigastric pain, distension, nausea, abdominal cramps, weight loss DIAGNOSIS Distention of the proximal duodenum by barium studies and narrowing of the angle between the aorta and the superior mesenteric artery as seen by aortography or sonography TREATMENT The syndrome is a diagnosis of exclusion that often responds to conservative therapy including adoption of a postprandial knee-chest position while prone, smaller meals, and an elemental diet

supplier-induced demand HEALTH CARE POLICY A phenomenon in which the quantity of services provided correlates with the supply of physicians, eg the greater the number of surgeons in given geographic area, the greater the number of operations performed in the region (JAMA 1995; 273:1227)

supply model HEALTH CARE POLICY A simplistic model for the existance of units in a system (eg radiologists) that is based on a simple calculation of those in the system minus those who are projected to leave the system (eg by retirement or other form of attrition) (CAP Today 1995; 9:5) Cf Demand model, HMO (extrapolation) model, Needs model

support group A generic term for a group of people who share a similar problem (eg overeating, marital problems, substance abuse) and meet regularly to provide mental and moral support and who may contact each other in times of stress

suppression test A clinical test or assay, eg dexamethasone suppression test, that is used to determine whether a substance (hormone or protein) being produced in excess is under the control of regulating or releasing factor(s), and therefore responsive to a feedback loop or whether the excess production is autonomous, and not under feedback control; Cf Stimulation test

suppressor gene Tumor suppression, see there

suppressor T cells A complex group of $CD8^+$ T lymphocytes that suppress the immune response by decreasing the activity of the T helper (CD4) cells against both endogenous (self) antigens and exogenous antigens; see Cytotoxic T cells, Helper cells, T cells, T-cell receptor

suppressor tRNA A transfer RNA molecule that is transcribed from a suppressor gene, which cancels the effect of a mis-sense or nonsense mutation by pairing directly with a nonsense (stop) codon, leading to the incorporation of a 'correct' amino acid

supratypic antigen Public antigen, see there

supraventicular tachycardia Formerly, paroxysmal atrial tachycardia* A cardiac arrhythmia initiated by a premature atrial beat conducted through a tract initiated in the AV node; once the ventricle contracts, an echo atrial beat is stimulated via a retrograde tract, resulting in a reverberating re-entry phenomenon, which results in an atrial rate of 180-300 beats/minute; PATs in infants may be life-threatening and result in fatal congestive heart failure; PATs in older children may be secondary to fever, are usually less than 24 hours in duration and relatively benign TREATMENT Simple vagal stimulation, eg carotid sinus massage, an ice bag, breath-holding; if intense, cardioversion or prolonged digoxin therapy (N Engl J Med 1995; 332:162RV)

*Note: The term was deemed obsolete when it was recognized that the arrhythmias being considered arise in the atrioventricular junction and not in atrial muscle per se

supravital stain A stain, eg Janus green B, neutral red, and thioflavin T, eg that is used to examine living cells by light microscopy, allowing visualization of various dynamic processes in situ; supravital stains may be injected into a cell and metabolized in a particular site, then removed, fixed and further evaluated, and are of use in detecting phagocytosis within macrophages and in examining mitochondria

Surat outbreak An epidemic of pneumonic plague (caused by *Yersinia pestis*) that occurred in September 1994 in Surat, India, resulting in 1026 infected individuals, of whom only 50 died; many of the 300 000 who fled the city were given tetracycline, which prevented the disease from spreading (NY Times March 14 1995, C10) see Plague

surface coil MR MRI A small radiofrequency receiver coil placed over a region of interest on the object being imaged which has an effective selectivity for the area of interest, eg the shoulder, knee, brain, spine and elsewhere; see Magnetic resonance imaging

surfactant A mixture of lipids and proteins lining the alveoli (without which they would collapse upon expiration–in accordance with the laws of Laplace) that allows optimal gas (CO_2, O_2) exchange; surfactant is produced by type II pneumocytes and secreted as lamellar bodies into the amniotic fluid; fetal surfactant production begins by the 20th week of gestation, but is only adequate to consistently ward off respiratory distress syndrome on or after the 35th week; see L/S ratio COMPOSITION-NATURAL SURFACTANT 80% phospholipids*, 8% neutral lipids, 12% proteins (½ of which are surfactant-specific proteins, SP-A, SP-B, SP-C) COMPOSITION-REPLACEMENT SURFACTANT Two types 1) Surfactant of mammalian origin Phospholipid profile is similar to the natural profile; some SP-B and SP-C is present, but not SP-A 2) Synthetic surfactant Major component is dipalmitoylphosphatidylcholine; minor constituents, eg hexadecanol, tyloxapol facilitate surface adsorption (N Engl J Med 1993; 328:861RV) see SP-A, SP-B, SP-C, Respiratory distress syndrome, Surfactant replacement therapy

*60% saturated phosphatidylcholine compounds, in particular dipalmitoylphosphatidylcholine, 25% unsaturated phosphatidylcholine compounds, 15% phosphatidylglycerol and phosphatidylinositol

surfactant replacement therapy Intratracheally administered bronchoalveolar fluid derived from calves (98% lipids, comprised of 90% phospholipid, especially dipalmitoyl-phosphatidylcholine and 2% apoproteins), which elicits a marked improvement of gas exchange when used in premature infants; in very low-birth-weight infants, the improvements in pulmonary function are not statistically significant; prophylactic bovine surfactant administered intratracheally decreases the need for neonatal respiratory support and improves the survival rates of premature infants, especially in thosse under 30 weeks; SRT improves early respiratory status, ↓ neonatal mortality, the incidence of pneumothorax, and pulmonary interstitial emphysema; it uncertain whether it is of benefit in intraventricular hemorrhage, bronchopulmonary dysplasia, necrotizing enterocolitis, and patent ductus arteriosus; SRT ↓ both the morbidity, mortality and cost of caring for very low birth weight infants (N Engl J Med 1994; 330:1476OA) and administered as a single dose ↓ the need for mechanical ventilation in infants with moderate-severe respiratory distress (ibid 1994; 331:1051OA)

surfactin An oligopeptide linked to a fatty acid with detergent properties that is released by *Bacillus subtilis* and causes hemolysis

surfer's nodule SPORTS MEDICINE One of often multiple symmetric and usually asymptomatic, flesh-colored fibrous nodules that measure up to 4.0 cm in diameter; SNs are seen along the anterior tibial prominence, less commonly in the middorsum of the foot, and arise in response to repeated trauma against the surfboard

surfer's rib A sports injury caused by the 'lay-back' maneuver in surfing, which results in an avulsion of the first rib at its muscular attachments CLINICAL Pleural hemorrhage, brachial plexus injury (potentially, syncope and sudden death), decreased arm pulses seen by arteriography

surge Power surge* Any increase in the flow of a substance above a relatively constant baseline COMPUTERS A sudden increase in amperage (flow of electrons), that has potential for damaging current-sensitive electronic equipment; surges are rare and most often occur when a power station temporarily shuts down, and another takes over; lightning-related surges are distinctly uncommon REPRODUCTIVE PHYSIOLOGY An abrupt ↑ in luteinizing hormone (LH) secretion Background: LHRL (luteinizing hormone-releasing hormone) is normally secreted in episodic bursts resulting in cyclical peaks of LH; LHRH bursts are ↑ by estrogens and ↓ by progesterone and testosterone and ↑ in frequency until the end of the follicular phase, at which time a surge of LH signals the onset of endometrial secretion in preparation for a fertilized egg

*Both terms are in active use, surge is more colloquial, power surge is more formal and easily understood by the non-cognoscenti, but like the alternative term spike, is disappearing from the working parlance

surgerize (pronounced sur-jur-ize) A highly colloquial verb of recent vintage for surgical therapy, as in '*...the patient was surgerized*'

surgical abdomen A generic term for an acute abdomen (AA) that requires surgical intervention, eg acute appendicitis, acute cholecystitis, acute diverticulitis with bowel obstruction, cancer, and acute vascular disease (eg infarction, abdominal aneurysm) DDx Medical conditions that cause AA include acute intermittent porphyria, addisonian crisis, black widow spider poisoning, herpes zoster, lead poisoning, myocardial infarction, pneumonia, pulmonary embolus, sickle cell crisis, uremia, and others; see Acute abdomen; Cf NASA

Although acute abdomen (AA) and surgical abdomen are listed as synonyms in a number of medical dictionaries, not all AAs are appropriately treated by surgery, as above indicated-author's note

surgical closure see Absorbable sutures, Catgut, Nonabsorbable sutures, Silk, Staples, Tape

surgical oncology The operative ablation of a tumor

surgical review committee Tissue review committee, see there

surgical scrubs A set of cotton or cotton/polyester wearing apparel consisting of a short-sleeved shirt and drawstring pants, which is the universal uniform of those daring men[1] of action, the surgeons; SSs are usually a faded Kelly green color[2] (hence the commonly used synonym, greens), but may also be beige, blue, magenta, purple, und so weiter; Cf Whites

[1]Yes, *and* women [2]The more faded, the more intimidating SSs represent the ultra-chic hospital garb, and although worn throughout the hospital, should be reserved for the OR, use during bloody procedures, and for sleeping while in the hospital–Author's note

'surgical' specialty A specialty of health care in which interventional procedures constitute a significant component of patient management; surgical specialties include obstetrics and gynecology, ophthalmology, otorhinolaryngology, surgery (cardiothoracic, colorectal, general, neurologic, orthopedic, plastic) and urology; Cf Hospital-based medicine, 'Medical' specialty, Primary care

surgical sterilization A generic term for any form of sterilization that prevents the passage of a fertilized egg to the uterus, almost invariably tubal ligation; it is the most common contraceptive method used by ♀ > 30 years in the US; 28% of those age 15-44 have been surgically sterilized (MMWR 1992; 41:568)

surgicenter HEALTH CARE INDUSTRY A generic term for an ambulatory surgical facility in the US, in which minor or 'same day' surgical procedures, eg removal of cysts or skin lesions, are performed Note: The term Surgicenter is proprietary

'surplus lines' company MALPRACTICE INSURANCE A medical malpractice insurance carrier that insures physicians at premium rates several times higher than the rates charged by the 'standard lines' malpractice insurance carriers, which routinely impose large deductibles; they do not advertize their 'products' nor have fixed premium rates; a physician applies to surplus-lines carriers if he has been denied coverage by other carriers, often after having lost his standard coverage due to various reasons including unfavorable claim and 'pay-out' history, governmental or hospital disciplinary action, or after allegations of drug abuse, sexual harassment or Medicare fraud; the typical surplus-line applicant is age 45-55 and is board-certified in neurosurgery, plastic surgery, obstetrics and gynecology, orthopedic surgery, family practice, otorhinolaryngology

or general surgery; non-board certified physicians and international (foreign) medical graduates are no more likely to require 'surplus-lines' coverage than board-certified and US medical graduates

surrogate marker LABORATORY MEDICINE A generic term for a parameter or group of parameters measured in order to detect a pathologic condition when a more specific test doesn't exist, is impractical or is not cost-effective; surrogate testing is used for 1) Non-A, non-B hepatitis, measuring alanine aminotransferase and antibodies to hepatitis B core antigen (anti-HBc) and 2) HIV-1 infection, using p24 antigen levels in serum in pg/ml (< 31 pg/ml is considered negative), level of CD4 T cells/mm^3 (N Engl J Med 1991;324:137) and the helper:suppressor (CD4:CD8) ratio of T lymphocytes

surrogate motherhood True surrogate motherhood is that in which a woman carries a gestational product that is not her own genetically, where one haploid set of genes is contributed by the genetic or natural father and the second haploid is contributed by the genetic mother (who for various reasons, eg hysterectomy, uterus didelphys or other reasons, cannot carry fertilized ovum); in the usual scenario, the diploid product is fertilized in vitro and implanted in the uterus of the surrogate mother; legal issues regarding true surrogacy are relatively simple, at least theoretically, since the gestational mother is performing a service (usual fee, $10 000, early 1990s) in carrying an egg that is not her own genetically; a permutation of this theme, with vastly distinct legal implications, is 'partial surrogacy' in which a genetic father's haploid chromosome complement, ie the sperm is used to artificially inseminate the egg of a woman (the genetic father's wife may be infertile for various reasons) who is both the gestational mother and the genetic or natural mother and who agrees to carry the conceptus to term, at which time the genetic father and his infertile wife retain the newborn infant; the difficulty arises if at the time of delivery the woman carrying the fetus wishes to retain the child, which is, in a sense ½ 'hers'; see Artificial reproduction, Baby M

surrogate parent A person who plays the role of a child's parent while the child is in the hospital

surrogate parenting Artificial reproduction, see there

surrogate testing see Surrogate markers

surveillance EPIDEMIOLOGY The monitoring of diseases that have a certain prevalence in a population; infectious disease (ID) surveillance methods include identifying contaminated food or other products, determining the current strains of influenza virus in the community, and monitoring of the safety of the blood supply; there have been recent indications that ID surveillance systems are deteriorating both in the US and globally (Science 1994; 264:368)

surveillance scanning A generic term for the use of various imaging modalities, eg CT and MRI to detect and follow patients with certain diseases, in particular brain tumors; the practice of SS is based on the assumption that tumors may recur either without symptoms or long before symptoms appear, be managed and improve survival; in medulloblastomas of children, tumor recurrences were detected earlier, but this detection did not improve survival (N Engl J Med 1994; 330:892oA)

survival analysis STATISTICS A component required for critical interpretation of data from clinical trials that uses life-tables with cumulative survival rates, forming a distribution or set of probabilities of a person under a therapeutic protocol of surviving certain time intervals

survivor syndrome Concentration camp syndrome, see there

susceptibility test Antimicrobial susceptibility test, see there

susceptibility theory An attempt to explain the nonrandom ('skipping') lymph node involvement at the time of diagnosis in Hodgkin's disease, postulating that Hodgkin's disease is multifocal ab initio, but only some lymphoid regions are susceptible, ie provide suitable environments for the maintenance of malignant cells; Cf Skip metastasis

sushi A Japanese delicacy prepared from raw fish that may be a vector for parasites, eg *Anasakis* (most commonly, *A simplex*, subfamily Anisakinae, order Ascaridida), Contracecum and Phocanema (*Pseudoterranova decipiens*), which often affect sushi made from mackerel caught in early spring ENDOSCOPY Edema, gastritis, erosion CLINICAL Myalgia, abdominal pain RADIOLOGY Thread-like larvae may be seen in radiocontrast studies TREATMENT Endoscopic removal PREVENTION Cooking to 60ºC for 10 minutes, or blast-freezing to -35ºC for 15 hours or to -23ºC for 7 days FREEZING FOR **24** HOURS, SALTING, SMOKING AND PICKLING DO NOT CONSISTENTLY KILL PARASITES; irradiation is not FDA approved

Notes: 1) Fishes used for preparing sushi that commonly harbor parasites include ceviche or South American cod, green herring (Netherlands), Pacific pollack, Pacific red snapper and squid 2) Other raw fish dishes of parasitic potential include sashimi, gravlax, pickled herring, lomi lomi and lox (cold-smoked salmon) 3) Other organisms present in sushi include *Dioctophyma renale*, *Heterophytes*, *Strongyloides*, trematodes (paragonimiasis, *Nanophyetus salminicola*), *Metagonimus yokogawai*, cestodes (*Diphyllobothrium latum*) and *Vibrio parahemolyticus*

sushi syncope A transient condition caused by ingesting a bolus of wasabe, a very 'hot' mustard (active ingredient: isothiocyanate) used to flavor sushi; the index case had a transient myocardial infarct-like attack with diaphoresis, pallor, confusion and vasomotor collapse (**JAMA 1987; 258:218c**) see Seder syncope, Spicy food

suspected child abuse or neglect SCAN PEDIATRICS A potential case of child abuse, which in the US is a delicate issue, as a false accusation of child abuse opens the physician to the charges of 'defamation of character', while ignoring signs of abuse is moral malpractice; strong indicators of abuse include trauma of any type in a child under one year of age and an infant who arrives dead to a health care facility; see Battered child syndrome, Infanticide

suspended heart 'syndrome' A radiologic finding in which the heart appears as if suspended in the mid-thorax, ie cardio-thoracic 'separation', when viewed in a left oblique and occasionally in the right oblique position; the 'syndrome' is accompanied by low T waves in the II lead and a prominent S-T depression in the III lead and has no known clinical significance

suspicious An adjective pertaining or referring to the consideration of cancer as a diagnostic possibility, as in 'suspicious for malignancy'

sustainable development ENVIRONMENT, GLOBAL VILLAGE The development and utilization of natural resources (eg forests, protected species) in a fashion that does not destroy or deplete them, thereby preventing their use in the future; the intent of the philosophy of SD is that regional biodiversity (with its commercial potential) is maintained and deforestation prevented or minimized (**Sci Am 1995; 272/6:52**) SD represents a philosophical shift in the concept of national economic growth, in which resources are not viewed as expendable but rather as renewable and therefore necessary for future prosperity (**New York Times 15 June 1993; C4**)

susto Fright PSYCHIATRY A folk illness that affects some Latinos of the Western Hemisphere, which develops from days to years after an event frightening enough to (as goes the tradition) cause the soul to leave the body (hence the alternative term, 'perdida de alma'); susto is allegedly linked to wide of symptoms, including loss of appetite, disturbances in sleep, melancholy, sleep disturbances, lack of motivation, low self-esteem and somatic complaints, eg aches, pains, and GI disturbances; treatment may require

the intervention of a healer and rituals to restore the body's balance (**DSM-IV™, 1994**) see Culture-bound syndrome

Sutton's law MEDICAL DECISION-MAKING A guideline evoked to temper the enthusiasm of externs (US medical students in their third and fourth years of school) and other novices in clinical medicine who want to 'work up' a disease, an acute abdomen for porphyria, metastatic medulloblastoma or other esoterica, while ignoring a particular disease's most common causes; see Hoofbeats; Cf Red herring, 'Zebras'

The 'law' is attributed to the noted bank robber, Willie Sutton, who, when asked why he robbed banks, reportedly replied, '...*that's where the money is*'; to apply Sutton's law then, is to search for the most likely cause of a symptom, ie to go where the 'money' is

SV-40 Simian virus 40 A small icosahedral, double-stranded DNA papovavirus, which, like the JC virus, may cause progressive multifocal leukoencephalopathy; SV-40 is of interest as it was the first molecule in which DNA superhelicity was identified and it may be used to transform cells in vitro as a form of 'permissive' infection, eventually leading to host cell lysis

svedberg S An obsolete (CGS system) unit of sedimentation coefficiency or 'buoyancy', equal to 10^{-13} centimeters per second (rate of dispersion), determined by ultracentrifugation; S provides an estimate of a substance's molecular weight, and was named after Svedberg, who won the 1926 Nobel prize for inventing the ultracentrifuge

Sverdlovsk An industrial city (now Ekaterinburg) in the Ural mountains of the former Soviet Union that became a focus of international interest in 1979 through an epidemic of anthrax, which was alleged by some US officials to have been due to a leak in a secret military lab involved in the testing and/or manufacture of biological warfare (prohibited by a treaty signed by the Superpowers in 1975); although cutaneous anthrax responds well to high-dose penicillin, if the spores are inhaled or ingested, the mortality reaches 75%, making anthrax a theoretically ideal biological weapon; of the 96 victims, 64 died during the outbreak; the official Soviet explanation, formerly accepted by American epidemiologists, was that the outbreak was related to tainted spore-infected meat sold by private butchers; more recent official 'reinterpretation' of the incident suggest that biological weapons were at fault; see Biological warfare

swainsonine A plant alkaloid with anti-tumor growth activity, inhibiting synthesis of β 1-6-branched carbohydrate, which serves as a recognition site for endothelial receptors, facilitating retention of tumor cells in the microvasculature; swainsonine is being studied for potential use in human malignancy

swamp fever Synonym for 1) Equine infectious anemia, a viral infection of horses, transmitted by hematophagous arthopods, causing weakness, recurrent fever, marked anemia and muscular atrophy 2) Malaria 3) Marsh fever A water-born infection (VECTOR *Rattus rattus*) by the spirochete, *Leptospira grippotyphosa*, which causes fever, general malaise and aseptic meningitis

Swan-Ganz catheter CARDIOLOGY A balloon-floatation device that is advanced through the inferior vena cava, first into the superior vena cava to measure O_2 saturation, then withdrawn to the right atrium, where the pressure is recorded; the balloon is then inflated with air (or CO_2 if an intracardiac shunt is suspected) and the pressure is measured as the catheter is advanced to the right ventricle, the pulmonary arteries, and in the pulmonary capillary 'wedge' (**W Grossman, in E Braunwald, Ed, Heart Disease, 4th ed, WB Saundrs, Philadelphia, 1992**)

swan neck A descriptor for a thin curved neck, resulting from muscular atrophy characteristic of myotonia dystrophica, which may be accompanied by 'myopathic facies' (see 'Hatchet' face), myotonia, dysphagia, frontal baldness, testicular atrophy and cataracts; a variant of the gracile swan neck is described in the Modigliani syndrome

swan neck deformity RENAL PATHOLOGY A descriptor for the shortened and attenuated initial segment of a dissected proximal convoluted renal tubule seen by light microscopy in patients with De Toni-Fanconi syndrome RHEUMATOLOGY A descriptor for the hyperextended proximal interphalangeal joint and compensatory flexion of the distal interphalangeal joints caused by shortening of the extensor tendon, classically seen in rheumatoid arthritis, which may also be seen in SLE, Jaccoud's (post-rheumatic fever), psoriatic arthritis, scleroderma and camptodactyly; Cf Boutonniere deformity

swan syndrome see Blind spot 'syndrome'

swarming CLINICAL TOXICOLOGY A mass of hymenopteran insects, usually bees that are in transit with a queen, which may sting a person by the hundreds, causing a toxic overdose of yellow jacket venom resulting in GI symptoms, headache, fever, syncope, and less commonly, seizures, renal failure, vasomotor collapse, and death MICROBIOLOGY A descriptor for a light overgrowth of *Proteus mirabilis* or *P vulgaris* on MacConkey agar, that is likened to ocean waves (figure), resulting from *Proteus* motility

swarming

sweat chloride test A diagnostic test for cystic fibrosis; the Gibson-Cooke method is performed preferably after the age of two months; normal subjects have < 50 mEq/L (mean, 18 mEq/L) and those with cystic fibrosis have > 60 mEq/L (average, 100 mEq/L) of chloride in the sweat; the test is also positive in Addison's disease, adrenogenital syndrome, diabetes insipidus (nephrogenic type), fucosidosis, glucose-6-phosphatase deficiency type of glycogen storage disease, malnutrition, nephrotic syndrome, or may be incorrectly positive through a technical error

sweat gland tumor see Skin adnexal tumors

sweatshop PUBLIC HEALTH A generic term for a place of employment, eg in the garment industry, that regularly violates laws designed to protect workers, ignores health and safety codes and pays substandard wages; the workers are often illegal aliens or completely unskilled workers (and often include children) who accept the often appalling working conditions as a price to pay for their illegal status (Sci Am 1993; 269/4:14) Cf Terms of Engagement

sweat testing Of those laboratories that perform sweat testing in the US, 71% test for chloride, 40% for conductivity, 9.5% for sodium, and 8% for osmolality (Arch Pathol Lab Med 1994; 118:865oA) see Cystic fibrosis

sweet protein A protein, eg monellin or thaumatin that binds specifically with taste receptors, eliciting a sensation of sweetness that is 100 000 times sweeter than sugar on a molar basis; breeding of plants to increase their sweetness has traditionally been empirical and based on increasing the sugar content, an approach that is at best difficult given the complexity of carbohydrate metabolism and the limited genetic palette of the plants being bred; the use of SPs through genetic engineering offer an alternative strategy for improving the flavor of edible plant products (Bio/Technology 1992; 10:561) see Monellin, Thaumatin; Cf Artificial sweeteners

swimmer's ear Acute diffuse external otitis media The most common form of external otitis, which occurs primarily in the summer PATHOGENESIS The heat and humidity cause a swelling of the skin's stratum corneum, which blocks the follicular canals; the constant exposure of swimmers to water results in maceration of the skin of the external auditory canal, creating a milieu favorable to bacterial (especially *Pseudomonas aeruginosa*) growth; with time, hyperemia and edema of the canal evoke intense itching, exacerbating the situation, resulting in diffuse swelling of the canal and tenderness of the auricle to movement; the discharge is initially serous but becomes seropurulent TREATMENT Hospitalization, long-term high-dose antibiotics, targeting the usual casuative organism *P aeruginosa*), hitting the infection with a combination of aminoglycosides and synthetic penicillin (for 6 weeks)

swimmer's itch Cercarial dermatitis caused by exposure to nonhuman schistosomes present in the sediment of fresh water lakes frequented by ducks; although the organism cannot complete its life cycle in the human, repeated cutaneous exposure elicits a hypersensitivity reaction consisting of papular erythematous rash with edema and pruritus; a similar eruption may also occur with non-infective contact exposure to human schistosomes, including *S haematobium* and *S mansoni*

swimmer's view RADIOLOGY A patient position that allows optimal visualization of the lower cervical spine

swimming pool granuloma An indolent skin infection clinically mimicking spirotrichosis with cellulitis, lymphadenitis and joint infections, caused by atypical mycobacteria, *M marinum* or *M kansasii* after percutaneous inoculation with contaminated fresh or salt water, developing into a solitary nodule at sites of abrasion (elbows, knees and feet), later becoming indurated and ulcerated, resembling cutaneous tuberculosis, occasionally developing satellite lesions; Cf Fish tank granuloma

swimming suit distribution Bathing trunk distribution, see there

swine influenza vaccine 'affair' PUBLIC HEALTH A misadventure that occurred in the USA in 1976 as an over-reaction to the fear of a major human epidemic; the incident began with a 'signal event' in which two unusual viruses were identified in pigs in New Jersey, with a related mini-epidemic among military recruits; in response, the CDC recommended the manufacture and administration of vaccine before the onset of the 'flu season' the following winter; 50 million received the vaccine, 1000 people suffered vaccine-related Guillain-Barré syndrome; the anticipated epidemic did not materialize and virtually no cases of swine influenza occurred in humans; the unused vaccine was destroyed and $84 million was paid in claims to the Guillain-Barré victims; see CDC

The affair caused a transient erosion in the public's confidence in the CDC, which has played a pivotal role in major epidemics, and in worldwide epidemiology in general

swinging crossbridge model Rowing crossbridge model, see there

swinging flashlight test OPHTHALMOLOGY A clinical test for comparing direct and consensual reactions of each pupil, used to identify an afferent pupillary defect TECHNIQUE A flashlight (more commonly a penlight) is swung back and forth between the two pupils; usually the direct reaction is stonger than the consensual; if the afferent pathway is impaired by disease, the direct response will be weakened, and the consensual efferent response unchanged; as the light is shined on the eye with the affected afferent defect, the pupil will paradoxically dilate*, a phenomenon known as the Marcus Gunn pupil or the afferent pupillary defect

*As the abnormal direct response is weaker than the consensual response initiated by the right optic nerve

'swinging heart' CARDIOLOGY A fanciful synonym for the EKG findings in electrical alternans, in which there is a regular alteration in the direction and/or amplitude of one or more components of the EKG reading, eg simultaneous oscillation of the P waves, QRS complexes and T waves (total electrical alternans); these features are highly characteristic of cardiac tamponade

Swiss agammaglobulinemia IMMUNOLOGY An AR [MIM 202500] form of severe combined immunodeficiency, which has a high mortality in early infancy due to a combination of severe diarrhea, malabsorption with disaccharidase deficiency and villar atrophy; the defective cellular and humoral immunity makes these patients susceptible to a menagerie of opportunistic pathogens, including *Candida albicans*, CMV, measles, *Pneumocystis carinii* and varicella, as well as GVH disease PATHOGENESIS ↓ T and B cells at the stem cell level LABORATORY Lymphocytopenia, anemia, ↑ liver enzymes, electrolyte imbalance secondary to chronic diarrhea TREATMENT Aggressive antibiotic therapy, gammaglobulins; HLA-matched bone marrow transplantation may effect permanent remission; see Adenosine deaminase deficiency

Swiss cheese A popular adjectival descriptor used in various medical specialties for a gross appearance, microscopic pattern or radiologic field punctuated by multiple variably sized, sharply demarcated cystic spaces

'Swiss cheese' brain An artefact that may be seen in brains that have been inadequately infiltrated with formalin, coupled with invasion of the not-quite-fixed brain by gas-forming *Clostridium* spp

'Swiss cheese' breast A nonspecific term for multiple, variably sized spaces lined by ductal epithelium, which may be seen in various benign breast diseases, including blunt duct adenosis, fibrocystic disease and epitheliosis (papillomatosis)

'Swiss cheese' endometrium A colloquial descriptor for the histopathological changes of cystic glandular hyperplasia, which may be seen in the menopausal endometrium, in association with ↑ estrogen from persistent follicles, granulosa-theca cell tumors of the ovaries, adrenocortical hormones or from exogenous estrogen therapy; these endometria may present with postmenopausal bleeding; by light microscopy

there are ↑ epithelial and stromal elements with large dilated Swiss cheese-like glands lined by a one-cell layer of epithelium (figure, below middle)

'Swiss cheese' hemangioma A descriptor for the radiological pattern of ossification described as typical musculoskeletal hemangiomas

'Swiss cheese' histiocytes Mononuclear-phagocytic cells seen in mucopolysaccharidosis type VIII, characterized by granular cytoplasm filled with variably sized, well-circumscribed storage vacuoles

'Swiss cheese' liver A descriptor for the liver in peliosis hepatis, which is punctuated by multiple ≤ 0.2 mm in diameter blood-filled lacunae, which are often devoid of endothelial lining, and thought to represent distended sinusoids or central or portal veins

'Swiss cheese' lung A descriptor for the multicystic appearance of a plain chest film in an infant with cystic adenomatoid malformation, where the involved area is overexpanded and the mediastinum is shifted towards the normal lung; the infant presents with respiratory distress of the newborn and may require an emergency lobectomy or pneumonectomy depending on the extent of the lesion

'Swiss cheese' polyp GASTROENTEROLOGY A descriptor for the low-power LM findings in the juvenile retention polyp, a hamartomatous (not precancerous) lesion of the colon, where the polyp's dilated glands are filled with mucus; retention polyps may be first recognized by rectal bleeding and treated by simple excision

'Swiss cheese' skin A descriptor for the histology of paraffinoma or oil granuloma due to cutaneous injection of lipid-rich substances, resulting in variably sized, swiss cheese-like fibrotic cavities (figure) filled with lipids, scattered foamy histiocytes and a foreign body-type giant cell reaction, without birefringence; this condition may be seen in factitial panniculitis induced by autoinjection of mineral, cotton seed oil and other oils or in illicit injection of silicone; see Silicone, Transsexuals

'Swiss cheese' ventricular septal defect A variant of ventricular septal defect in which there are multiple serpentine defects in the ventricular muscle, making surgical closure difficult

'Swiss roll' technique SURGICAL PATHOLOGY A method for examining the maximum amount of tissue from a flat organ; the tissue is rolled 'a la burrito' and then sectioned perpendicular to the length of the specimen; the technique is of greatest use for examining the stomach and placenta, and derives its name from a popular pastry

Swiss type of hereditary persistence of fetal hemoglobin A laboratory finding without clinical significance characterized by an inherited increase in red cells containing

Swiss cheese

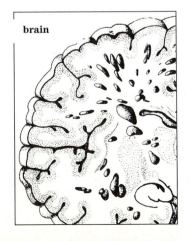

brain

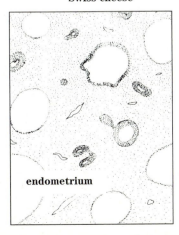

endometrium

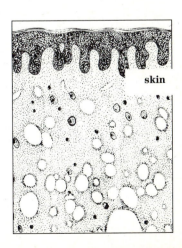

skin

hemoglobin F, first identified in Swiss army personnel

switch campaign An effort on the part of a drug company or third-party provider to change a physician's pattern of prescribing 'me too' drugs, which are essentially equivalent; when appropriate, switching can improve the quality of and/or lower the costs of health care; with less-than-altruistic intentions, SCs are mounted on an on-going basis by drug companies, some formats (eg claims of increased efficacy, payment to the pharmacy of record a fee for finding and 'helping' a physician switched to an alternative 'me too') of which are questionable, if not frankly unethical practices (N Engl J Med 1994; 331:1350SA) see 'Me too' drug

switch defect disease see Hyperimmunoglobulin-M disease

switching HEMATOLOGY The change in expression of the β-like hemoglobin genes during the transition from the embryonic to the fetal and adult stages in erythrocytes; activation and high-level expression of these genes is directed by a locus control region located 5' to the ε gene; expression of the adult β gene requires progressive silencing of early (ε, γG, γA and δ) genes, which is probably mediated by stage-specific factors binding to sequences flanking the genes (Nature 1991; 350:252) IMMUNOLOGY Class switching see V(D)J recombination

SWOG Southwestern Oncology Group

sword of Damocles' syndrome Damocles' syndrome, see there

SWOT analysis An acronym (strengths, weaknesses, opportunities, and threats) for components to be evaluated in conflict resolution

Sydenham's chorea NEUROLOGY Rapid, involuntary movement of the face (causing grins, grimaces, contortions, and tics), extremities (causing erratic flailing and if unilateral, hemichorea), hands (causing repeated partial fisting of the hands or a 'milkmaid's grip'), and the tongue (in which the muscular fasciculation is likened to a 'bag of worms'); SC is most common in children and adolescents, and is a major criterion for the diagnosis of rheumatic fever (status/post untreated streptococal infection) by the Jones' criteria; SC develops after a latency period of weeks to months and may be accompanied by emotional lability and rheumatic heart disease NUEROPATHOLOGY Pathological changes are remarkably sparse and consist of mild inflammation and neuron loss in the corpus striatum

symbiotic psychosis A psychological disorder of questionable validity that may affect young children after a normal infancy and following a precipitating event, eg birth of a sibling; characterized by attacks of panic-like anxiety accompanied by marked regression of social behavior and intellectual development; in the most extreme form, the symbiotic child physically clings to the mother and others in an almost indiscriminate fashion; speech regression may occur and become garbled or jargonistic, ultimately leading to a state of secondary autism that may respond to therapy

sympathy pregnancy Couvade A 'condition' in which a man simulates some of the features of pregnancy, predominantly GI symptoms of anorexia, morning sickness, constipation, diarrhea, toothaches and mood swings, either as a cultural phenomenon, eg practiced by primitive tribes, eg the Tchambulis of New Guinea, in an attempt to symbolically share the suffering(s) of a pregnant woman; in 'civilization', couvade is not a formally practiced custom, and thus 'male pseudopregnancy' is regarded as a benign, self-limited neurosis occurring in the husband of a pregnant woman; see Pseudocyesis; Cf Pseudopregnancy

symport A transmembrane carrier protein that simultaneously binds and transports two substances in the same direction, eg the transport of sodium and glucose into the cell; in contrast, antiport systems are characterized by simultaneous transport of two compounds to the opposite face of a membrane

synapsins NEUROPHYSIOLOGY A group of neuron-specific phosphoproteins that regulate the release of neurotransmitters, and are involved in the formation of nerve terminals; the synapsins interact with actin and other cytoskeletal components in vitro; synapsin II may participate in cytoskeletal organization during the early stages of neuron development (Science 1994; 264:955OA)

synaptic plasticity NEUROPHYSIOLOGY Malleability present in most neurons in various forms, including presynaptic inhibition, homosynaptic depression, presynaptic facilitation and modulation of transmitter release by tonic depolarization of the sensory neuron; activation of a neuron receptor, eg NMDA receptor may directly alter synapse plasticity (Nature 1991; 349:154); endogenous nitric oxide is responsible for synaptic plasticity in the cerebellum (ibid 1991; 349:326); see Nitric oxide

synaptophysin A 38-kD transmembrane glycoprotein isolated from neurons, which spans the synaptic vesicular membrane four times, the carboxy terminal of which is the binding site for various cell factors; synaptophysin is a marker for neuroendocrine differentiation and is produced in neuroblastoma, ganglioneuroblastoma, ganglioneuroma, pheochromocytoma, paraganglioma, as well as carcinoids, medullary thyroid carcinoma and pancreatic endocrine tumors

synchrotron A circular subatomic particle accelerator that produces a beam of positrons at 7 GeV (billion electron volts); the phenomenon of synchrotron radiation is useful for visualizing important biological molecules (DNA, RNA, proteins), most of the previous structural information about which has come X-ray diffraction studies; synchrotron-generated data on structures on the position and movement of individual molecules will allow analysis of the binding of regulatory proteins to DNA, receptor-ligand interactions, toxin penetration of cells, and a plethora of other interactions occurring on a molecular level (JAMA 1994; 272:837MN&P)

synchrotron radiation A phenomenon that occurs when electrons and other charged particles moving at nearly the speed of light are deflected by the magnets (in a synchrotron) that keep them in a circular path; the wavelength of synchrotron radiation depends on the velocity of charged particles and tightness of the bend (JAMA 1994; 272:837MN&P)

syncope A transient loss of consciousness not compatible with other altered states of consciousness in the history of the patient (N Engl J Med 1993; 328:1085OA), a phenomenon usually linked to cerebral ischemia

syncytial giant cell hepatitis An acute and chronic hepatitis described in adults characterized by multinucleated giant cells arranged in a syncytial or rosette pattern, bridging fibrosis and cholestasis, containing viral particles by ultrastructural examination, thought to be induced by paramyxovirus (N Engl J Med 1991; 324:455) see Giant cell hepatitis

syncytiotrophoblast The outermost cell of the trophoblast; syncytiotrophoblasts are large, with basophilic or eosinophilic cytoplasm and multiple nuclei with irregular nuclear contours and finely granular chromatin; the nuclear morphology differs from herpes simplex, which are glassy in appearance and are more pyknotic and atypical that multinucleated histiocytes (Acta Cytologica 1993; 37:451OA)

Note: Syncytiotrophoblasts in a cervicovaginal smear are rare in a normal pregnancy and are commonly assocated with threatened abortion

syndactyly Fusion of the fingers, which may be cutaneous, due to bridging soft tissues, or osseous, due to bone fusion of varying severity; in general, only soft tissue syndactylism is treated, without which ostosis develops at the articulations with loss of function; syndactyly is seen in congenital syndromes including Apert, Bloom, Carpenter, cryptophthalmus, Cohen, Conradi-Hünermann, Cornelia de Lange, EEC, Escobar, Goltz, Holt-Oran, Jarcho-Levin, Langer-Giedion, Meckel-Gruber, Miller, oculodentodigital, oral-facial-digital, partial trisomy 10q, Pfeiffer, Poland sequence, popliteal web, Robert, Saethre-Chotzen, Smith-Lemli-Opitz, and triploidy syndromes; Rosebud hands

syndrome X CARDIOLOGY Microvascular angina A condition characterized by anginal pain without detectable atherosclerotic lesions within the coronary arteries, a condition thought to represent 1 to 15% of patients with anginal pain Note: Atherosclerosis of a degree sufficient to explain angina is seen in 85% of angiograms ENDOCRINOLOGY A clinical complex in older adults with truncal (upper body or central) obesity, characterized by glucose intolerance, and insulin resistance, primary hypertension, dyslipidemia, NIDDM, ovarian androgen hyperproduction LABORATORY ↓ HDL-cholesterol and ↑ triglycerides (**N Engl J Med 1993; 329:1740c**) Cf Diabesity

Note: Because of the confusing terminology for the syndrome(s) X, it has been suggested that alternatives be substituted for the cardiac-type syndrome X (eg coronary microvascular dysfunction syndrome), for the endocrine-type syndrome X (eg dyslipidemic arterial disease), and for those in which symptoms of the two overlap (eg hyperinsulinemia syndrome)

synergism Cooperative interaction between two or more components in a system, such that the combined effect is greater than the sum of each individual constituent ANATOMY The combined action of muscle groups resulting in a force that is greater than that which could be generated by the individual muscles MICROBIOLOGY Bacterial synergism An effect inferred but unproven in anaerobic infections, where there are three or more different species of both aerobic and anaerobic bacteria in an infected site, and the virulence of the lesion is a function of the number of species involved; examples of bacterial synergism include Meleny's cutaneous ulcer (*Staphylococcus aureus* and microaerophilic streptococci), Ludwig's angina and Vincent's angina; see Anaerobes PHARMACOLOGY Pharmacologic synergism An approach to recalcitrant bacterial infections or virulent malignancies in which the therapeutic agents each affect different pathways or steps in a metabolic pathway, making the treatment more efficient, eg penicillin and an aminoglycoside; see Combination chemotherapy

synergistic necrotizing cellulitis A form of necrotizing fasciitis characterized by involvement of skin, subcutaneous tissue, fascia and muscle, where the lesions are usually located on the legs or the perineum, arising in a perirectal abscess PREDISPOSING FACTORS DM, obesity, advancing age and cardiorenal disease CLINICAL Small skin ulcers that ooze a red-brown fetid liquid fancifully termed 'dishwater pus', surrounded by gangrenous patches punctuated by preserved islands of normal-appearing skin, pain, tenderness, tissue gas, systemic toxicity and bacteremia; Fournier's disease is a special form of SNC arising in the scrotum

synexin A protein that causes calcium-dependent aggregation of chromaffin granules and promotes the fusion of these granules during exocytosis

synonym codon Synonymous codon Any of a number of triplets of adjacent RNA nucleotides (codons) that are translated into the same amino acid, eg the messenger RNA codons UUA, UUG, CUU, CUC, CUA and CUG all are translated into the same amino acid, leucine; this redundancy of codons, also known as 'degeneracy', allows point mutations to occur in the genome or during transcription without the host cell being penalized by the loss of a critical structural protein; see Codon, Degenerate code, Samesense mutation, Silent mutation

synonym syndromes see Pseudonym syndrome

synovial sarcoma SURGICAL PATHOLOGY A mesenchymal malignancy that comprises up to 10% of all soft tissue tumors, most common in young (age 20-40) males, occurring in the knee, ankle, foot or other joints PATHOLOGY The tumor ranges from firm and calcified to friable and necrotic, and has a 'biphasic' histologic pattern, characterized by variable interspersed bands of spindled and epithelioid cells; the material within the gland-like spaces is mucicarmine-positive, PAS (periodic acid Schiff)-positive/diastase-resistant tumor that is strongly reactive for keratin stains, thus causing the uninitiated to misdiagnose these lesions as adenocarcinomas; monophasic synovial sarcoma mimics fibrosarcoma, malignant schwannoma and leiomyosarcoma PROGNOSIS 50% five-year survival; extensively calcified tumors have a higher (84%) five-year survival; see Sarcoma

synthetic absorbable suture SURGERY Any of a number of suture materials* with a predictable loss of tensile strength, which evoke minimal inflammatory response in tissue; SASs are of greatest use in GI, urologic, and gynecologic surgery; see Surgical closure; Cf Synthetic nonabsorbable suture

*Composed of polydioxanone sulfate, polygalactin, or polyglycolic acid

synthetic nonabsorbable suture SURGERY An inert suture material that is stronger than wire, that minimizes 'spitting'[1], but which does not 'handle'[2] as well as silk; NSs are required for cardiovascular surgery as they must function indefinitely; vascular anastomoses using prothetic grafts and NSs may lead to aneurysm formation; see Surgical closure; Cf Absorbable suture

[1]The oozing of purulent material via suture tracks [2]Nylon monofilament is the least reactive in terms of spitting, but handles the worst, requiring at least four knots; monofilament polypropylene is intermediate in these properties; plastic monofilaments and multifilaments spits more, but has better handling properties

synthetic smooth muscle cell Activated smooth muscle cell, see Smooth muscle cell

SYR Sex-determining region of the Y chromosome, see Testis-determining factor

syringe exchange program Needle exchange program, see there

syringocystadenoma papilliferum An almost invariably benign skin tumor usually of the scalp or neck with either apocrine or eccrine differentiation PATHOLOGY Cystic or tubular spaces and projecting lumina lined by two rows of cells, an outer cuboidal and an inner row of high columnar cells that display decapitation secretion (**Acta Cytologica 1993; 37:535oA**)

syringoma A sweat gland tumor that is most common in pubertal females, located on the eyelids, neck, upper anterior chest and vulva appearing as multiple flesh-colored to yellowish papulonodules PATHOLOGY The dermis is replete with small ducts, cysts and solid comma-shaped cords or strands of epithelial cells; Cf Cylindroma

systematic error An error on a test system or method; unlike random errors, systematic errors in a test system occur in one direction away from a true value, and can be due to assigned values of calibrators, reagent composition, dispensed volume, electronic signals (**MLO Supplement September 1993**) Cf Random error

systemic angioendotheliomatosis see Angiotrophic lymphoma

systemic idiopathic fibrosis A condition characterized by retroperitoneal fibrosis of unknown etiology that may extend to the anterior chest wall CLINICAL Backache, fever, nausea, vomiting, constipation, anemia, oliguria, anuria, peripheral vascular insufficiency; fibrosis-induced ureteral compression may lead to urinary retention and renal failure

systemic immunoblastic proliferation A recently described condition caused by proliferation of immature lymphocytes CLINICAL Dyspnea, rash, hepatosplenomegaly, lymphadenopathy and a tendency to develop into immunoblastic lymphoma; molecular analysis reveals gene translocations

systemic inflammatory response syndrome SIRS, see there

systemic lupus erythematosus An idiopathic multisystem collagen vascular disease EPIDEMIOLOGY Affects ± 40/10⁵ (North America, Europe), blacks/Hispanics > whites, ♀:♂ ratio = 3:1; 80% onset during childbearing years DIAGNOSIS (see table) CLINICAL Vasculitis, serositis, synovitis, cerebral, renal, and cutaneous involvement PATHOGENESIS Autoantibodies, especially antinuclear antibodies, eg anti-double stranded DNA (**N Engl J Med 1994; 330:1871ᴿⱽ**) see ANA

systemic mastocytosis see Mast cell

system manager The person encharged with coordinating the electronic flow of data from various departments in a hospital or laboratory information system, who often serves as a first rung 'trouble shooter' should any problems arise in the system

systems analysis The formal evaluation of an activity, method, procedure, or technique in which the entirety of the problem is examined in an attempt to improve the workflow

syzygy Fusion of two organs, each of which retains a clear histological distinction, eg Splenogonadal fusion

---

SYSTEMIC LUPUS ERYTHEMATOSUS (1982 revised criteria)

1. MALAR RASH Fixed erythema, in particular over the malar eminences
2. DISCOID RASH Raised erythematous patches with adherent hyperkeratotic scaling; atrophic scarring in some old lesions
3. PHOTOSENSITIVITY Unusual skin rashes in response to sunlight
4. ORAL ULCERS Oral or nasopharyngeal ulcers
5. ARTHRITIS Nonerosive arthritis of two or more joints, accompanied by tenderness, swelling, or effusions
6. SEROSITIS
   a. Pleuritis OR
   b. Pericarditis
7. RENAL DISEASE
   a. Persistent proteinuria > 0.5 g/day OR
   b. Cellular casts
8. NEUROLOGIC DISORDER
   a. Seizures without substance use or medical disease OR
   b. Psychosis in absence of substance use or medical disease
9. HEMATOLOGIC DISORDER
   a. Hemolytic anemia OR
   b. Leukopenia OR
   c. Lymphocytopenia
   d. Thrombocytopenia
10. IMMUNOLOGIC DISORDER
    a. Positive LE cell prep
    b. Anti-DNA antibody
    c. Anti-Sm antibody
    d. False positive srological test for syphilis
11. ANTINUCLEAR ANTIBODY Abnormal titers of ANA in absence of drugs known to be associated with drug-induced lupus erythematosus

T Symbol for: 1) Absolute temperature 2) tera-, SI (International System) abbreviation for 10^{12} 3) Tesla, the SI (International System) derived unit of magnetiflux density 4) Threonine 5) Thymidine 6) Thymine 7) Time 8) Tocopherol 9) Translocation 10) Tritium 11) Twisting number

t Symbol for: 1) Transfer (RNA) 2) A variable (statistics)

T_{max} CLINICAL PHARMACOLOGY The time necessary to reach the maximum concentration of a therapeutic agent

T1 CLINICAL IMMUNOLOGY A murine monoclonal antibody, which in conjunction with a fluorescent label may be used in flow cytometry or fluorescent microscopy to identify CD5-bearing cells, eg medullary thymocytes, and peripheral T lymphocytes (T cells); T1 positivity is common in ALL, CLL, lymphoblastic lymphoma, and Sezary syndrome; see CD5 IMAGING Spin-lattice or longitudinal relaxation time MRI A time period after transverse magnetization, the characteristic time (a constant) for spins to align themselves back to the external magnetic field; starting from zero magnetization in the **z** direction, the **z** magnetization ↑ to 63% of its final maximum value in a time T1; see Magnetic resonance imaging

T-1 COMPUTERS/TELEMEDICINE A telephone line that carries 24 telephone channels, which is a current standard for the high-speed transmission of information, usually in a network (Am Med News 1995; 17 April 1995 p19) see Asynchronous transfer mode switching, Codec, Telemedicine

T2 Spin-spin or transverse relaxation time MRI The time period (a constant) for the loss of phase coherence among spins oriented at a right angle to the static magnetic field, a result of interactions between the spins, with the resulting loss of transverse magnetization and MR signal; starting from a non-zero value of magnetization in the **xy** plane, the **xy** magnetization decays and loses 63% of its initial value in a time T2; see Magnetic resonance imaging

T2* MRI The time constant for the loss of phase coherence among the spins oriented at an angle to the static magnetic field due to a combination of magnetic field inhomogeneities, deltaB and spin-spin transverse relaxation, which results in a more rapid loss in transverse magnetization and MR signal; see Magnetic resonance imaging

T3 CLINICAL IMMUNOLOGY A murine monoclonal antibody used in conjunction with a fluorescent label in flow cytometry or fluorescent microscopy to identify CD3-bearing cells; see CD3

T4 CLINICAL IMMUNOLOGY A murine monoclonal antibody linked to a fluorescent label, which is used in flow cytometry or fluorescent microscopy for identifying CD4-bearing T helper cells; see CD4

T-200 CD45, see there, aka Leukocyte common antigen

T activation TRANSFUSION MEDICINE Removal of an N-acetyl residue (sialic acid) by bacterial neuraminidase, which exposes hidden antigenic epitopes, against which there are natural antibodies in the circulation of most adults, resulting in polyagglutination; T activation can be detected by using aged blood, cord sera or by treating the cells with 2 mercaptoethanol (2-ME) to destroy the IgM antibodies

T1 antigen CD5, see there

T3 antigen see CD3

T4 antigen CD4, see there

T7 assay Free thyroxine index, see there

T8 antigen CD8, see there

T12 assay Free thyroxine index, see there

t(14;18) Chromosomal translocation t(8;14)(q24;q11), see T cell lymphoma

T cell CARDIOLOGY Transitional cell A specialized myocyte that is found in clusters in the sinus node; T cells are intermediate in size, structure and organization between the P cells (see there) and normal atrial myocytes and connect with either of these cells; perinodal T cells surround the sinus tract and are thought to 'bundle' impulses leaving the sinus node and to filter premature ectopic atrial impulses; see P cells IMMUNOLOGY T lymphocyte The T (thymus-drived) cell is the most complex cell of the immune system, given

1) The diversity of T-cell types, including T cells with activator, cytotoxic, delayed hypersensitivity and suppressor activities

2) The wide range of cytokines, growth factors and immune modulators produced by activated T cells; see Biological response modifiers

3) The complexity of T-cell interaction with exogenous and endogenous antigens, eg mediation of delayed hypersensitivity, graft-versus-host disease and

4) The complexity of T-cell maturation in the thymus

50-70% of circulating leukocytes are myeloid; the rest are lymphocytes, of which T cells (defined as having 'pan T cell' markers, CD2 and CD7 and other T-cell markers including CD1, CD3 and CD5) comprise 70-85%, while the B cells comprise 15-30%; T cells respond to an antigen via an antigen-presenting cell, which engulfs and processes extracellular antigen (bacterial, viral or other); the antigen is then transported to the antigen-presenting cell's surface and becomes complexed with the 'self' MHC class II molecules, a process known as MHC restriction

T cell immunodeficiency syndrome Any of a group of immunodeficiency states arising from partial or absolute defects in T-cell function; TCIS are generally more severe than B-cell defects, have no effective therapy and are characterized by recurrent opportunistic infections, eg by *Pneumocystis carinii*, cutaneous anergy, growth retardation, a decreased life span, wasting or 'runting', diarrhea, increased susceptibility to GVHD, potentially fatal reactions to live viral or BCG vaccinations and an increased incidence in malignancy; TCISs include DiGeorge syndrome (thymic hypoplasia), Nezeloff syndrome (cellular immunodeficiency with immunoglobulins) and T-cell defects, eg absence of inosine phosphorylase or purine nucleoside phosphorylase

T-cell lymphoma A malignant proliferation of T cells that is diagnosed by detecting rearrangement of the T-cell receptor's β chain, which may be 'driven' by EBV and other viral infections (table, below) MOLECULAR BIOLOGY TCLs have a characteristic chromosomal translocation t(8;14)(q24;q11), with a chromosome 8 breakpoint 3 kilobases in the 3' direction from the c-*myc*, a cellular proto-oncogene, and a chromosome 14 breakpoint, 36 kilobases in the 5' direction from the constant region gene of the T-cell receptor α-chain, resulting in a gene rearrangement on chromosome 8 and the functional Jα segment on chromosome 14, suggesting that the translocation is simultaneous with the T-cell receptor rearrangement, catalyzed by the same systems involved in joining V-J, this is thus similar to the c-*myc* translocations linked to immunoglobulin loci in B-cell malignancies; 18% of one series of 303 lymphomas were T-cell lymphomas, 73.% were B cell lymphomas and 8% were indeterminant lymphomas Note: The clinical presentation, histology and immunology of TCL is heterogeneous and ½ are extranodal at the time of presentation (table)

T-cell maturation The thymic microenvironment is required for early T-cell differentiation and most migrations of thymic precursor cells occur in the embryonic and early postnatal period; the cells are processed, become competent and are exported to peripheral lymphoid compartments, divided into a conceptual stages

STAGE I The earliest T cells (10% of thymic lymphocytes) have a CD2 (T11) rosetting marker and non-T stem-cell markers, including CD38 (T10) and transferrin (T9); the cells then acquire a thymocyte antigen, CD1a (T6) that reacts with Langerhans' cells and CD4 (the 62-kD MHC class II-restricted antigen) and CD8 (the 76-kD MHC class I-restricted antigen)

STAGE II 70% of thymocytes express CD4, CD8, CD1a and CD38; with maturation CD1a is lost and cells acquire antigens defined by pan-T markers (CD3 and CD11) and segregate into CD4 (helper phenotype) and CD8 (suppressor phenotype) T cells

STAGE III Immunocompetence is acquired in the thymus, as defined by the CD3-associated antigen Ti, maturing with exportation; the CD4 and CD8 cells lose CD38 and express increased CD5 and CD3; CD4 T cells represent 55-70% and CD8 T cells represent 20-35% of circulating T lymphocytes

T-cell receptor A disulfide-linked heteropolymeric membrane-bound protein that is non-covalently complexed to five or more CD3 polypeptides (figure, right in simplefied form); the average TCR-bearing cell has a relatively low (20-40 000/cell) receptor density; TCR specificity is conferred by rearrangement of VDJC (V Variable, D Diversity, J Joining, and C Constant) genes, in a fashion analogous to that of the variable heavy and light immunoglobulin chains in B cells, see Gene rearrangement, which serves as a marker for clonality; the residues present at the V/αJ/α junction are critical to the early selection process, and as the stem cell matures, V, D, J and C exons are spliced together; TCR's α, β and γ genes are variable, while the delta and epsilon genes are constant, and are identified by complementary DNA techniques; TCR regulates signal transduction via 1) The phosphatidylinositol pathway, inducing increased inositol phosphates and diacylglycerol, mobilizing cytoplasmic free calcium and activating protein kinase C, which then activates the 2) tyrosine kinase pathway; TCR responds differently as a function of the ligand, allowing a 'fine-tuning' of T-cell response to antigens (Science 1991; 2552:1308) see CD (cluster of differentiation); T cells express one of 2 receptor heterodimers

αβ **chains** (the majority of T cells), which recognize peptide antigens bound by MHC

γδ **chains**, which recognize naturally occurring small non-peptide antigen (Nature1995; 2375:155)

Note: The β chain has a 3-D molecular structure (resolved by X-ray crystallography) similar to that of immunoglobulins (Igs) and has an Ig-like fold (Science 1995; 265:1984oa 1906n&c)

T-cell-rich large B-cell lymphoma HEMATOPATHOLOGY A heterogeneous group of lymphoproliferative disorders characterized by a polymorphic mixture of small and large (CD20) neoplastic B (lymphoid) cells and reactive T cells; ♂:♀ = 2:1; with aggressive chemotherapy, TBL has a good prognosis and 84% were alive and well at followup (Am J Surg Pathol 1994; 18:455)

T-cell specificity see MHC restriction

T-cell tolerance IMMUNOLOGY The deletion of T-helper, T-delayed hypersensitivity and cytotoxic T-cell subsets under certain circumstances, which leads to tolerance of the suppressor T cells, which are, in turn, responsible for deleting either B or other T cells, directly suppressing cells that have been 'turned on' by T cells, thus being transferred, as a form of 'infectious' tolerance; high zone tolerance refers to the requirement by B-cells for high affinity B-cell receptors to multivalent antigens; low-zone tolerance is required for weakly immunogenic antigens that are not destroyed by T-suppressor cells, which are triggered at lower doses than T-helper, low zone tolerance is partial and only affects some lymphocytes

T helper cells see CD4+ cells T helper cells are divided into two subtypes, TH1 and TH2, see there

T$_H$1 (-type) immunity CLINICAL IMMUNOLOGY One of two types of immune responses that occur after the immune system is activated by antigens interacting with CD4+ T (helper/inducer) cells (lymphocytes); the T$_H$1 immune cascade results in the production of cytokines in particular, IFN-γ, IL-2, and TNF-β and induction of cellular immunity; T$_H$1 type immunity to trophoblastic antigens is associated with unexplained recurrent abortion and embryotoxicity (JAMA 1995; 273:1933)

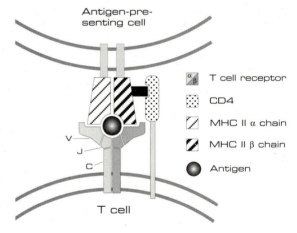

T-cell receptor

T$_H$2 (-type) immunity CLINICAL IMMUNOLOGY One of two types of immune responses that occur after the immune system is activated by antigens interacting with CD4+ T (helper/inducer) cells (lymphocytes); the T$_H$2 immune cascade results in the production of cytokines in particular, IL-4, but also IL-5, and IL-10, and down-regulate cellular immunity, while playing a major role in inducing antibody responses mediated by plasma cells; T$_H$2 type immunity to trophoblast may be a natural response to trophoblast and contribute to successful pregnancy (JAMA 1995; 273:1933)

T ratio STATISTICS A statistical test used when a set of data (or study) has few data points (or subjects); the T ratio is of use in determining whether the results obtained are due to chance alone

T₃ receptor A member of a structurally and functionally similar family of hormone-responsive nuclear transcription factors; T_3 receptor (T_3R) has a carboxy-terminal domain, critical for ligand binding and receptor-receptor interaction, a zinc-finger type DNA-binding domain, and an amino-terminal domain of unknown function; there are two T_3R genes α, and β located on chromosomes 17 and 3, respectively, for each of which there are at least two alternative mRNA splice products, α1, α2, and β1 and β2, which are expressed in developmental and tissue-specific patterns (N Engl J Med 1994; 331:847RA) Cf T cell receptor

T-shaped fracture Y-shaped fracture ORTHOPEDICS A type of intercondylar fracture of the distal femur that occurs in falls from a height with the feet extended, resulting in a violent impact of the femur on the tibial plateau; similar fall-related fractures may occur as the distal tibia impacts on the ankle or as an intercondylar fall-related fracture to the distal humerus; Cf Lover's heels

T-strain A mycoplasma that grows 'tiny' colonies (hence, 'T'), which had been assigned to a separate genus, *Ureaplasma* with one species, *U urealyticum*, an organism confined to humans that causes nongonococcal urethritis and is capable of metabolizing urea

T₃ thyrotoxicosis Hyperthyroidism in which T_3 (triiodothyronine) but not T_4 is elevated; these patients are clinically heterogeneous and lack distinctive signs and symptoms, comprising about 4% of those with hyperthyroidism due to Graves' disease, toxic nodular goiter and thyroid adenomas and a higher percentage of hyperthyroidism in regions with lower levels of iodine

T₄ thyrotoxicosis Hyperthyroidism in which T_4 (thyroxine) but not T_3 is elevated, which occurs in patients with iodine-induced thyrotoxicosis and in euthyroid patients who are sick for other reasons; see Euthyroid sick syndrome

TA-AB Techoic acid antibody assay, see there

tabby A mutant gene that is responsible for a form of ectodermal dysplasia with anhidrosis in ♂ mice, an animal model for the X-linked human disease, hypohidrotic ectodermal dysplasia, which causes hyperpyretic crises in children; post-natal injection of epidermal growth factor in tabby mice elicits growth of dermal ridges and functional sweat glands and may have the same effect in some humans with ectodermal dysplasia; Cf EEC syndrome

tabby cat pattern see Thrush breast appearance

taboo A culture-specific ban or prohibition (eg incest) that is placed on certain actions, behaviors, and thoughts, the abrogation of which results in reproof, persecution, or exile by members of the culture

tabun Dimethyl-phosphoramidocyanidic acid A potent cholinesterase inhibitor that phosphorylates a reactive serine residue of acetyl cholinesterase, which is responsible for its lethal activity (lethal dose, 0.01 mg/kg) that had currency during the first World War as a chemical weapon; Tabun and the use of related 'nerve gases' was banned by the Geneva protocol of 1925; see Chemical warfare; Cf Sarin, Zyklon B

Tac antigen CD25, see there

T-ACE SUBSTANCE ABUSE An abbreviated four-question test that '…circumvents the problems of denial and underreporting that historically make self-reporting (of alcohol abuse during pregnancy)…of limited value…(it) has the further advantage of not seeming to pry into current drinking habits, which might prompt untruthful answers. The key question concerns **T**olerance, one of the best predictors of continued drinking during pregnancy: 'How many drinks does it take to make you feel high?'…more than two …is…enough alcohol to bear a child with ARBD (alcohol-related birth defects). That risk is amplified by positive responses to one of T-ACE's other queries about whether she has been **A**nnoyed by criticism of her drinking, has felt she should **C**ut down, and has ever had an **E**ye-opener (a drink first thing in the morning to steady herself or get rid of a hangover) (JAMA 1992; 268:3183NIH)*

tâche blanche *tache*, French, spot INFECTIOUS DISEASE A small whitish hepatic abscess that may be seen in bacteremia PATHOLOGY A focal fibrotic spot on the epicardium of the elderly, which is of no known significance

tâche noire 1) A blackened cutaneous ulcer at the site of a tick bite, the initial lesion of boutonneuse fever (*Rickettsia conorii*) and scrub typhus (*R tsutsugamushi*) 2) Black palm, see there

tachykinin Any of a family of widely distributed biopeptides that shares the COOH-terminal sequence Phe-X-Gly-Leu-Met-NH_2 and includes substance P, neurokinins A and B, neuropeptide K and neuropeptide-γ; tachykinins cause vasodilation, GI and urogenital smooth muscle contraction and stimulation of salivary gland secretion; tachykinin receptors are designated as NK1, NK2 and NK3; see Substance P

tacrine An aminoacridine-type cholinesterase inhibitor reported to improve (slightly) the cognitive status of patients with Alzheimer's disease; high dose tacrine therapy is limited by potential hepatotoxicity, with ± 45% of tacrine-treated patients having elevated alanine aminotransferase, and in 25%, the ↑ was 3 **x** greater than the upper limit of normal (N Engl J Med 1993; 328:808C; ibid 1992; 327:1253OA)

tacrolimus FK506 An immunosuppressive agent (figure) produced by *Streptomyces tsukubaensis* (Fujisawa, Osaka), developed to counteract transplant rejection; tacrolimus inhibits interleukin-2 (IL-2) synthesis and binding and is both similar to, and synergistic with cyclosporine, but is reported to be 50-fold more immunosuppressive than cyclosporine; it is used in kidney and liver transplantation and is of potential use in lung transplantation SIDE EFFECTS Nephrotoxicity (not dose limiting), neurotoxicity, possible induction of diabetes (effects similar to cyclosporine), as well as headache, nausea, paresthesiae of hands and feet and insomnia; tacrolimus is associated with significantly fewer episodes of acute, corticosteroid-resistant, or refractory organ rejection, but substantially more adverse events (eg GI, nephro–, and neurotoxicity) that may require discontinuation of therapy (N Engl J Med 1994; 331:1110OA)

tacrolimus

tactile agnosia NEUROLOGY An impairment of tactile object recognition, which is a subtle, nondisabling disorder caused by unilateral damage to parietotemporal cortices that may be severe in left cerebral infarctions; tactile agnosia should be distinguished from astereognosis, a complex somatosensory disorder and tactile aphasia (Mayo Clin Proc 1991; 66:129)

tactoid HEMATOLOGY A birefringent fluid crystalloid structure composed of 21 nm in diameter fibers of deoxygenated hemoglobin that distort and decrease the deformability of erythrocytes in sickle cell anemia; these structures consist of seven intertwined double-stranded molecules that form both tactoids and spherulites by a 'double nucleation' model Note: Tactoids are not true crystals since they are arranged in one-dimensional stacks; see Sickle cells, Spectrin

tactoid bodies NEUROANATOMY Rudimentary structures of sensory nerve differentiation, seen as oligocellular whorls of flattened cells, which may be recapitulated by malignant schwannomas

tadpole cell CYTOLOGY An uncommon cell seen in epidermoid carcinoma of the uterine cervix that is elongated and club-shaped with one broad end that tapers to a narrow end, and has an eccentric, rounded hyperchromatic nucleus or nuclei within often keratinized cytoplasm; the related 'spindly' cell, which is tapered at both ends, may also be seen in epidermoid carcinomas of the cervix, as well as of the lungs; tadpole-like cells have also been described in a case of multiple myeloma (Am J Clin Pathol 1992; 98:630oA)

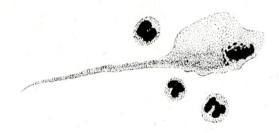

tadpole cell

tadpole sign ULTRASONOGRAPHY A comma-shaped 'shadow' seen under a tumor, which is of lesser sonographic density directly beneath the center of a mass than at the edges; 'tadpoles' appear in malignant masses and have ragged margins, related to necrotic tissue, which is a poor conductor of ultrasonic waves; Cf Tennis racquet sign

taffy candy 'syndrome' CARDIOLOGY A fanciful descriptor for the clinical symptoms that result from elongation of the anterior leaflet of the mitral valve, which may be idiopathic or be associated with rheumatic fever and myocardial infarction

taffy pulling effect Marked elongation of a structure, likened to stretched taffy candy or chewing gum CARDIOLOGY Marked elongation and thinning of the anterior mitral leaflet's chordae associated with mitral valve regurgitation, which may later rupture SURGICAL PATHOLOGY Spindled, darkly basophilic streaks and strands due to the extreme delicacy of the nuclear chromatin; although this 'crush artefact' is highly characteristic of pulmonary small (oat) cell carcinomas, it may also be seen in lymphomas and chronic inflammation

TAG-72 Tumor-associated glycoprotein-72 An antigen present on 97% of ovarian and 83% of colonic carcinomas; TAG-72 can be detected with a proprietary FDA-approved radiolabeled murine antibody, B72.3 (Oncoscint), which can be used to detect recurrent cancer of the ovaries and colon

TAH Transfusion-associated hepatitis, see there

TAH-BSO Total abdominal hysterectomy-bilateral salpingo-oophorectomy

Tai Chi A form of exercise (likened by some authors to a slow ballet) that is rooted in ancient Chinese philosophy and martial arts; TC may be used for training subjects in dynamic balance, and is reported to be useful in reducing the risk of falls in the elderly (JAMA 1995; 273:1341oc) see Falls, FICSIT; Cf Alternative medicine, Vigorous exercise

taijin kyofusho PSYCHIATRY A unique form of social phobia described among the Japanese that corresponds to an intense fear that his/her body, body parts, or functions may prove offensive to another individual (DSM-IV™, 1994) see Culture-bound syndrome

tail An adjective pertaining or referring to an elongated, usually terminal component of an organism, cell, molecule, statistic or other component in a system that slowly arrives to a baseline

tail coverage MALPRACTICE INSURANCE An umbrella of malpractice insurance protection that a physician is obliged to retain until the 'statute of limitations' (a period of two to three years) has been completed, which covers malpractice claims that may be initiated after a physician has moved to another state or retired (the so-called tail period); the cost of 'tail coverage' is equal to at least one year of malpractice premium coverage and may be multiples thereof; see Malpractice, Statutes of limitations Cf 'Going bare', Nose coverage

Note: In the US, malpractice insurance costs from $2000 to $200 000/year, a fee that is a function of location (Florida, California, and New York State are highest) and the relative risk for lawsuit in a specialty (neurosurgery, orthopedic surgery, and obstetrics are often the most expensive); the standard 'claims-made' malpractice insurance policies are less expensive, but do not cover tail periods

tail sign see Comet tail sign

tailing LABORATORY TECHNOLOGY The diffusion of a 'spot' of a substance of interest at the trailing edge in a chromatogram or electrophoretic gel, which contrasts to the sharply-demarcated leading edge MOLECULAR BIOLOGY The addition of a labeled nucleotide to the 3' end of a hybridization probe mediated by TdT (terminal deoxynucleotidyl transferase)

tailings ENVIRONMENT The residual sandy waste remaining after extraction of uranium from mined ore; tailings were used as landfill in one site in the Western US under homes and public buildings, resulting in high gamma-radiation exposure to inhabitants and required removal by the Environmental Protection Agency

Takayasu's arteritis Pulseless disease An idiopathic segmental inflammation of the aorta and major branches, with narrowing of ostia (with 'tree-barking' of the vascular intima) of innominate, left carotid and subclavian arteries, visual disturbances, a 'reverse' coarctation with a thick-walled aorta, adventitial fibrosis, perivascular lymphocyte and plasma cell aggregates, possibly causing thrombosis PATHOGENESIS Unknown, possibly allergic; the disease affects young women, especially of Africa and Asia, causing weak acral pulses of the upper extremities, renovascular ischemia with hypertension, fever, arthritis, myalgia, pleuritis, pericarditis and rashes LABORATORY Increased erythrocyte sedimentation rate and gammaglobulins PATHOLOGY Chronic inflammation and fibrosis of the arterial wall, in particular affecting the branches of the aorta, causing a loss of pulse in the upper extremities (Acta Soc Ophthalmol Jap 1908; 12:554)

'take' TRANSPLANTATION IMMUNOLOGY The adherence of a free skin graft occurring between days three and five of the transfer of skin; if the graft 'takes', it is pink indicating neovascularization; the thinner the graft, the more likely it will 'take', as long as it contains dermis; 'take' also refers to the prolonged survival of any transplanted organ that passes the hyperacute (vascular) and chronic (immune-mediated) phases of rejection

talc A dry lubricant used in a wide range of products in contact with mucocutaneous surfaces, eg condoms, dental dams, and non-surgical latex gloves; talc was banned from surgical gloves in 1991 by the FDA (JAMA 1995; 273:846c)

talc granuloma A foreign body giant cell reaction seen in 1) The peritoneum, body cavities or tissues or elsewhere, due to contamination by surgical glove lubricants, eg talc, lycopodium, mineral oil rice, or corn starch, or by cellulose fibers from disposable gauze pads, drapes, gowns and other paper products 2) Various organs, commonly the lungs of intravenous drug abusers, where the substance of abuse, usually a white powder, has been 'cut' with starch or talcum powder; the granulomas measure 14-50 µm in diameter and are located in eccentric patches of connective tissue and fibrous septae; the lungs show mild medial hypertrophy of the pulmonary arteries, but are not associated with pulmonary hypertension and 3) In patients using talc in the subepithelial tissues of external genitalia, causing talc granulomata of the vagina, cervix, uterus, tubes, urethra and bladder

talc insufflation Topical aerosolized administration of talc as a sclerosing agent, effecting pleurodesis; TI has been reported to be an effective means of controlling pleural effusions due to breast cancer (Cancer 1995; 75:2688)

talin A 235-kD cytoskeletal protein that comprises 3-8% of the platelet's protein, which with vinculin, attaches actin filaments to the platelet's plasma membrane; talin binds to the cytoplasmic face of integrin, vinculin, and phospholipids (Science 1995; 268:233)

talk and die 'syndrome' TRAUMATOLOGY A form of presentation in acceleration-deceleration brain injury which, like a progressive subdural hematoma, has a latency period (here, 48-72 hours) until death; the condition is no longer invariably fatal as early treatment of cerebral edema reduces mortality

talon noir Black heel A condition affecting athletic adolescents who engage in sports requiring major 'footwork', eg lacrosse, tennis, football, tennis; the lesion is the result of a shear-stress rupture of papillary capillaries during violent sports in which there are sudden stops and twists on the heels, resulting in skin that is punctuated by black spots corresponding to calcaneal petechia; see Black palm, Sports dermatology; Cf Tâche noire

TAME Tosyl-L-arginine methyl esterase

TAMI studies Thrombolysis and angioplasty in myocardial infarction studies A series of multi-center clinical trials designed to examine the role of angioplasty, urokinase, heparin and prostacyclin in the management of acute myocardial infarction; see CASS, TIMI studies

tamoxifen ONCOLOGY A widely used agent for treating early estrogen receptor-positive breast carcinoma; meta-analysis indicates that tamoxifen reduces breast cancer mortality by 20% in women over the age of 50, while conventional chemotherapy reduces mortality by 25% in those under age 50; estrogen receptor-negative patients may respond to 5-fluorouracil and methotrexate with leucovorin rescue; prophylactic tamoxifen may be of use in postmenopausal women at high risk for breast carcinoma

T&A Tonsillectomy and adenoidectomy, see there

Ts and Blues SUBSTANCE ABUSE A pair of drugs with some currency as recreational drugs of abuse, which produce a euphoric state likened to that evoked by heroin at a lower cost; pentazocine ('T'), a narcotic analgesic, is mixed with pyribenzamine, an antihistamine dispensed as blue tablets (Blues), which together are heated and injected in mutiple 'sets'; when used during pregnancy, 35% of the infants

suffer neonatal withdrawal syndrome and growth retardation

T&S Type and screen, see there

the Tan Sheet A specialized weekly publication that provides business and US federal regulatory information on nonprescription pharmaceuticals and nutritionals produced by FDC Reports, Inc Chevy Chase, Md

tandem repeat MOLECULAR BIOLOGY A sequence of oligonucleotides present in native DNA in multiple copies and adjacent to each other, ie in tandem; tandem repeats include the genes for 45S pre-rRNA, 5S rRNA, various tRNAs and the histone family of DNA-related proteins; the repeated segments are virtually identical to each other, are arranged in a head-to-tail fashion and are separated by 'spacer' segments of varying lengths of DNA; see Repetitive DNA, Telomere; Cf Junk DNA

Tangier disease Analphalipoproteinemia A rare AR [MIM 205400] condition caused by a deficiency in α-lipoprotein, first described on Tangier Island (Chesapeake Bay, Maryland) CLINICAL Generalized deposits of cholesteryl esters in the tonsils, other lymphoid tissues, lymphadenopathy, hepatosplenomegaly, mild proximal peripheral neuropathy, intermittent diarrhea, corneal opacification LABORATORY Absent HDL, ↓ cholesterol (< 120 mg/dl), ↓ phospholipids, ↓↓↓ apoA-I and apoA-II, ± ↑ triglycerides PATHOLOGY Enlarged yellow-orange tonsils, lymphoid tissues and rectal mucosa due to massive storage of cholesteryl esters in foamy macrophages in the BM, lymph nodes, thymus, spleen, liver, skin, jejunum, Schwann cells and tonsils PROGNOSIS Usually benign, rarely coronary artery disease

'tango and cash' SUBSTANCE ABUSE A form of heroin that is 'cut' with fentanyl, providing its users with more 'bang for the buck', resulting in a number of fatal overdoses; since fentanyl is relatively inexpensive to produce and results in a greater 'high', this combination may increase in popularity (JAMA 1991; 265:2962c)

'tanned' red cells IMMUNOLOGY RBCs that have been treated with a 1:20-40 000 dilution of tannic acid, which allows them to act as antigen carriers, and enhances the visualization of antigen-antibody reactions, eg hemagglutination; protein binding to RBCs is strengthened by adding a covalent binder eg toluene di-isocyanate

Tanner staging Sexual maturity rating A system for objectively determining sexual maturity, correlating chronologic age with a group of anatomic parameters, determining the degree of adolescent maturation; the most commonly used system was delineated by Tanner (Growth at Adolescence, Blackwell, Oxford, 1962); in females, five stages of maturation are recorded for pubic hair and breast development; in males, five stages are recorded for pubic hair, growth of the penis and testicles (Arch Dis Children 1966; 41:454)

tamoxifen

tanning A sedentary activity in which a person bastes him/herself in a beached whale-like fashion under a UVA tanning lamp in 15-30 minute dollops to achieve a natural look (oxymoron noted); heuristically 'logical' evidence that the sleek and well-tanned jet-set wannabes' enviable 'look to die for' might indeed prove ultimately fatal has been lacking; nonetheless, occasional case reports of benign (eg keratoacanthoma), pre- (eg actinic keratosis) or frankly malignant lesions (to wit, basal cell and squamous cell carcinomas, and Bowen's disease) linked to 'recreational' tanning (due to UVA light) occasionally burrow their way into the literature (N Engl J Med 1995; 332:1450c)

tanning devices PUBLIC HEALTH Beds or booths fitted with ultraviolet (UV) light bulbs that emit ultraviolet-A, and lesser amounts of ultraviolet-B radiation, homogeneously delivering maximal light in the minimum time; the desire for a 'healthy' tan' has spawned an industry in the US that is serviced by poorly regulated tanning salons; 58% of subjects in one study reported injury at commercial tanning facilities; 37% were injured at home, with 1) Damage to the eyes Corneal injury 85%, unspecified 13% and combined corneal and retinal injury 3% 2) Damage to the skin Photoaging, first- and second-degree burns 3) Degeneration of dermal blood vessels and 4) Nonspecific dysfunction of the immune system

T antigen MOLECULAR BIOLOGY Any of a group of 90-kD proteins present in the nucleus that bind tightly to DNA, playing a pivotal role in viral DNA transcription and replication during the lytic cycle; the T antigen is involved in the transition from early to late transcription, as occurs when the SV 40 virus invades the cell; the three sites binding T antigen are close to the initiation site for RNA synthesis and a local increase in T antigen decreases the transcription of T antigen's gene; see T proteins; Cf T cell antigens TRANSFUSION MEDICINE 1) An antigen present on the surface of all red cells that is 'hidden' (thus known as a cryptantigen) from the immune system by an N-acetyl neuraminic acid residue; when this residue is removed by a bacterial infection, polyagglutination may occur, as all subjects except infants intrinsically produce antibodies that react with the exposed T antigen, although the hemolytic potential of the antigen is unclear; see T activation 2) Thomsen-Friedenreich antigen A tumor-associated glycoprotein, the antigenic determinant of which, D-galactose-β-(1→3)-N-acetyl-D-galactosamine can be detected using a specific anti-T antibody or the PNA lectin

t antigen 'Little t' An antigen related to the T antigen of the SV40 virus, with which it shares N-terminal sequence homology

TAP Transporter associated with antigen processing A heterodimeric protein consisting of subunits TAP1 and TAP2; TAP delivers cytosolic peptides to the endoplasmic reticulum, where they bind with nascent class I histocompatibility (MHC I) molecules; the class I-cytosolic peptide complexes are then displayed on the cell surface for recognition by cytotoxic T lymphocytes (Science 1994; 264: 1322RR; NATURE 1994; 368:864L), which results in an 'MHC-restricted' T cell response to foreign antigens (Nature 1995; 375:411, 415)

tape SURGERY A fastening modality used to close clean (or contaminated) wounds, which minimizes the likelihood of infection by not introducing a foreign body that would connect external and internal regions of the body; Cf Catgut, Staples

taper To reduce the dose, usually of a therapeutic agent that has a certain amount of undesirable side effects

tapioca pudding appearance Sago spleen appearance, see there

tapir mouth NEUROLOGY A fanciful descriptor for the 'pouting' expression seen in protruding lips due to weakening of the orbicularis oris muscles facioscapulohumeral muscular dystrophy (of Landouzy-Déjerine)

tapir nose A descriptor for a collapsed nose with a 'reversed ski jump' appearance caused by ulceration and destruction of the nasal septum, a classic finding in espundia, an infection caused by *Leishmania braziliensis*; tapirs are nocturnal ungulates of tropical America, Sumatra and Malaya, related to horses and rhinoceri

tap water infection An infection by an organism contaminating drinking water, which causes either true enteral

infections or pseudoepidemics, in which the tap water contaminates a step in the culture of bacteria; tap water organisms include bacteria, eg *Aeromonas hydrophilus* (often associated with GI tract and wound infections), *Legionella pneumophila*, *L dumoffi* (N Engl J Med 1991; 324:109) and other *Legionella* species, *Mycobacterium chelonae*, amebae (eg *Acanthamoeba hatchetti*, *Filamoeba nolandi*, and *Hartmanella* species), *Giardia lamblia*, a diplomonad flagellate, Pittsburgh pneumonia agent (*Tatlockia micdadei*), *Pseudomonas pickettii* (JAMA 1991; 265:981), *Rhodococcus* (*Gordona*) *bronchialis* (N Engl J Med 1991; 324:104) and others of undetermined clinical significance

Note: Some organisms are thermophilic, and colonize hot water supplies, eg *Legionella pneumophila*, *M xenopi*, *M kansasii*, while others are cryophilic, eg *Mycobacterium avium*, *M chelonae abscessus*

Taq polymerase *Thermus aquaticus* polymerase MOLECULAR BIOLOGY An enzyme that extends primers of DNA between two fixed points on the DNA molecule at 'low' (72°C) temperatures; when a round of DNA synthesis is complete, the reaction mixture is heated to 95°C, to melt the newly formed DNA duplexes, which become in turn primers for the next round of synthesis; TP is critical enzyme in the polymerase chain reaction (PCR), a technique that has revolutionized retrieval of minute amounts of DNA from a specimen, see PCR, Thermocycler

TAR Transactivation response protein The HIV-1 tat gene product that transactivates viral gene expression and is essential for HIV-1 replication; TAR inhibits the production of an interferon-induced 68-kD protein kinase (Science 1990; 247:1216)

TARA Tskuba Advanced Research Alliance A university-based research organization that will have more than 200 faculty members on contract, largely temporary; TARA's raison d'être is to foment interactions between government, industry and academia; TARA's focus will be on nanotechnology, biological sciences (eg gene regulation, cell-cell interactions, and neural functions), multimedia and information management, research management and technology transfer (Nature 1994; 369:268N)

Tarasoff v Regents of the University of California FORENSIC PSYCHIATRY A landmark legal case regarding patient-psychotherapist confidentiality that was initiated by the estate of Tatiana Tarasoff who was murdered by a P Podder, a psychiatric outpatient who had previously informed one of his therapists of his intent to kill Tarasoff; her estate claimed that the physician had a duty to warn all concerned of his homicidal intentions (N Engl J Med 1995; 332:1451BR) Cf Anne Sexton

tardive dyskinesia NEUROLOGY A late complication seen in 20% of young adults receiving long-term neuroleptic therapy, consisting of abnormal and irreversible involuntary movements of the face, trunk and extremities; tardive dyskinesia paradoxically disappears with resumption of therapy; see 'Piano playing', Rabbit syndrome

target An adjectival descriptor for any lesion or radiologic finding in which there are three or more relatively well-circumscribed, concentrically arranged annular patterns or radiodensities

target amplification MOLECULAR BIOLOGY A generic term for any method used to identify the molecular (or organism's) species, including 1) Hybridization to species-specific probes that are immobilized on membranes, microtiter plates, or that are in solution 2) Analysis of restriction fragment length polymorphisms of amplified target genes 3) Direct sequencing of PCR-amplified gene segments (Arch Pathol Lab Med 1995; 119:131QA)

target cell CYTOLOGY A metaplastic endocervical cells seen in Papanicolaou-stained smears containing inclusions within vacuoles, characteristic of cells infected with

Chlamydia trachomatis HEMATOLOGY Codocyte An RBC with peripheral and central distribution of hemoglobin related to 1) A relative ↓ in hemoglobin (Hb C or S or thalassemia, the first of which are accompanied by crystal formation or rarely, deficiency anemia, post-splenectomy and acute blood loss 2) A relative ↑ in the membrane itself as occurs in lecithin-cholesterol acyl transferase deficiency or obstructive jaundice or 3) Related to a transient change in pH

target fibers Transversely sectioned muscle cells stained with nicotinamide adenine dinucleotide-tetrazolium reductase (NADH-TR) which have a central inactive zone devoid of membrane-bound organelles surrounded by a dense reactive rim, in turn surrounded by a zone of normal sarcoplasm; target cells occur in 20-30% of denervated muscle, often affecting type I muscle fibers

target follicle HEMATOPATHOLOGY A descriptor for the concentric layering of mature lymphocytes in the mantle zone around germinal centers, seen by low-power light microscopy in the hyaline-vascular form of Castleman's disease (angiofollicular lymphoid hyperplasia)

target lesion DERMATOLOGY A lesion typical of erythema multiforme (EM) in which a vesicle is surrounded by an often hemorrhagic maculo-papule; EM is often a self-limited dermatosis of acute onset that resolves within 3-6 weeks, and has a cyclical pattern; EM lesions are 'multiform' and include macules, papules, vesicles and bullae, and may be idiopathic or follow infections, drug therapy or occur in immunocompromised hosts

target sign GI RADIOLOGY A smoothly-contoured radiopacity with both central and peripheral radiolucency, seen in pedunculated colonic polyps, when viewed en face by double contrast (air-contrast) barium studies; the 'eccentric' target sign is seen in GI diverticuli where a small amount of radiocontrast enters the pouch and is surrounded by the radiopaque body of the diverticulum PULMONARY RADIOLOGY A finding in circumscribed pulmonary aspergillomas or foci of necrotizing bronchopneumonia seen in a plain chest film; Cf Coin lesions

target sequence A short segment of recipient DNA that is the target for transposon insertion; the sequence undergoes self-replication and the transposon is inserted between the two target sequences; see Transposon

targett A low frequency antigen of the Rh system, the presence of which may cause a depression in D antigen expression

TAR RNA Transactivation response RNA A segment of RNA located at the 5' end of the untranslated leader region of all viral messenger RNAs; inversion of TAR RNA eliminates transactivation and point mutation of the segment reduces its activity; HIV-1's Tat protein binds the TAR region and may be involved in HIV's pathogenicity

TAR syndrome An AR [MIM 274000] condition of perinatal onset characterized by thrombocytopenia with absent radius CLINICAL Profound thrombocytopenia, purpura with amegakaryocytosis in bone marrow and bilateral aplasia of the radii and thumbs; up to two-thirds of patients have leukemoid reactions, occasionally anemia and eosinophilia, cardiovascular disease, eg atrial septal defect, Fallot's tetralogy, cutaneous and renal anomalies PROGNOSIS 50% die in the first year of life due to intracranial hemorrhage

tarsal tunnel syndrome A carpal tunnel syndrome-like complex caused by post-traumatic fibrosis, abductor hallucis hypertrophy, tenosynovitis or fascial band entrapment by the posterior tibial nerve CLINICAL Pronounced plantar surface and toe causalgia that may irradiate to the calf, resulting in paresthesias, cyanosis, sensation of coldness, and numbness TREATMENT Massage, steroid injection, weight reduction or surgical decompression of the compartment

tart cell A segmented neutrophil that has retained some nuclear fragments in its evolution towards becoming a full-fledged LE (lupus erythematosus) cell; tart cells retain the chromatin clumps, nucleoli and nuclear membrane; macrophages have also been so designated

TAT LABORATORY MEDICINE Turn-around time, see there MOLECULAR BIOLOGY TAT protein, see *tat* gene PSYCHOLOGY Thematic Apperception Test A projection-type psychological test that evaluates a child's sense of reality and personality traits and gives insight into his fantasies; see Psychological testing

***tat* gene** A gene present in retroviruses, eg HTLV-I, HIV-1, that encodes the Tat transactivating protein, which enters the nucleus, stimulates viral proliferation, possibly via a viral promoter, and in turn activates other retroviral genes; the *tat* gene is oncogenic and induces mesenchymal tumors in experimental systems Note: Tat alone is capable of activating cells, suggesting the existence of an as yet unidentified cellular analog of an activating protein

TATA Tumor-associated transplantation antigen, see there

TATA box MOLECULAR BIOLOGY A highly conserved oligonucleotide (thymidine-adenine-thymidine-adenine) DNA sequence that is present in many frequently and/or rapidly transcribed genes, eg hemoglobin, histone, U6 and 7SK genes, and required for efficient transcription; the TATA sequence is located in a fixed site 25-35 nucleotides upstream (5' direction) from the TATA box and is recognized by and responsible for positioning of RNA polymerase II (RpII), which in turn is responsible for processing and transcribing mRNA; Cf CCAAT box, Pribnow box

TATA protein see TFIID

tat protein A HIV-1 protein that activates HIV-1 gene expression and is essential for viral replication in vitro; Tat inhibits antigen-induced lymphocyte proliferation and may directly contribute to the immunosuppression typical of HIV infection

Tatlockia micdadei An alternative designation proposed for *Legionella micdadei*, aka Pittsburgh pneumonia agent and TATLOCK strain

tattoo An intentionally placed, relatively permanent form of cutaneous decoration that may range from simple, often small dark-colored insignias, messages or symbols that may be performed by amateurs in prison to elaborate multi-colored animals, objects or scenes performed by more skilled workers under relatively sterile conditions; tattooing in the US has been heretofore unregulated, and in many states have neither regulations for infection control, nor mechanism for verifying the tattoo artist's training; although HBV has been transmitted with tattoo needles, no case of HIV transmission from tattooing has been documented (**JAMA 1995; 273:1894**); tattoo pigment is dermal and periadnexal in distribution, similar to argyrosis; the pigments are either 1) Permanent, eg carbon, vermillion, India ink and Prussian blue, some of which may be removed by laser surgery or 2) Nonpermanent, eg cinnabar and aniline; see Laser surgery

tattooing TRAUMATOLOGY The complex skin abrasions and wounds filled with debris, glass and dirt, that result from being dragged along a road, often occurring in pedestrian victims of automobile accidents; treatment requires adequate debridement and often wound healing by second intent

tau Kendall's tau STATISTICS A non-parametric measure of correlation between a known fact and a set of variables, ranging from +1.00 to -1.00, which is used where parametric statistical distortions arise from data distributed in a non-normal fashion or in the presence of extreme outliers of data points

Tau protein(s) Any of a group of 55–62-kD microtubule-associated phosphoproteins (MAPs), first isolated from the brain that have major sequence homology with MAP2; the different sequences of the MAP family are generated by alternative splicing of transcripts; tau proteins migrate in the β-γ region in an electrophoretic gel, are induced during neurite outgrowth, and regulate microtubule assembly, limiting growth and shrinkage of dynamic microtubules, co-localizing with the microtubules, increasing tubulin polymerization, decreasing the rate of microtubular depolymerization, possibly facilitating generation of spirals from the α-β dimer in microtubules, are prominent in Alzheimer's neurofibrillary tangles and are the main antigen of the paired helical filaments that accumulate in the degenerating neurons of Alzheimer's disease

Note: Tau 69 protein may correspond to A68; see A68

tau gene A gene located on chromosome 21 that encodes a protein Tau, which is critical in stabilizing and organizing microtubules in certain axon types, but not in axonal elongation (Nature 1994; 369:487ᴸᵀᴺ)

tautomerism An equilibrium between two or more distinct isomeric forms of a molecule, eg an enzyme

tautomycin A potent cell-permeable protein phosphatase inhibitor obtained from *Streptomyces spiroverticillatus*, which is useful for studying protein phosphorylation

taxol A chemotherapeutic agent that acts on microtubules, inducing tubulin polymerization and formation of stable and non-functional microtubules (vinca alkaloids and colchicine cause microtubule depolymerization); taxol evokes a response in some refractory neoplasms, evoking a positive response in one-third of cisplatin-resistant ovarian carcinoma, as well as malignant melanoma and non-small cell carcinoma of the lung; taxol is a complex molecule obtained from the bark of the yew tree, a native of old-growth forests in the Northwest US, which has antineoplastic potential, taxol is controversial as an enormous amount of ancient forest trees are required to both complete clinical trials and if successful, to market the drug (Science 1991; 252:1780n&v) the earliest taxol was derived directly from the Pacific yew, but that was not the only yew*; the Himalaya yew proved to be a better source for harvesting the raw material, as it could be extracted from the needles and twigs, rather than the bark, which kills the Pacific yew (New York Times 13 Dec 1994; C3); taxol blocks mitosis by stabilizing microtubules and promoting the polymerization of tubulin; taxol is FDA approved for treating therapy-resistant ovarian and metastatic breast cancer (Nature 1995; 375:414, 361)

*To borrow from the song

taxon The group or category of an organism, which is classified according to characteristics that it has in common with other similar organisms; classic taxonomy is based on phenotypic differences between organisms and divided according to a hierarchy of kingdom, phylum, class, order, family, genus, species and, if applicable, subspecies and/or strain, with subdivisions between categories, eg suborder and superfamily; Cf Urkingdom

Note: It is being increasingly recognized that taxonomy must be based on features that are more scientifically valid than the subjectiveness inherent in phenotyping, eg comparison of DNA sequence similarity ('homology')

Tay-Sachs disease GM2-gangliosidosis A rare AR [MIM 272800] lipid storage disease most common in Ashkenazi Jews (carrier frequency 1:30), in which the deficiency of hexosaminidase A causes the accumulation of gangliosides in the neurons, cerebellum, and axons CLINICAL Onset at 4-6 months with arrest and decline of psychomotor activities, irritibility, hyperacusis, convulsions, chorioathetosis, spasticity, decerebrate rigidity and death by age 3

TB 1) Toluidine blue 2) Total bilirubin 3) Tryptone broth 4) Tuberculin 5) Tuberculosis, see there

Also 1) Terabyte 2) Terminal bronchiole 3) Thromboxane 4) Thymol blue 5) Tracheobronchiolar 6) Tracheobronchitis 7) Trapezoid body 8) Tubercle bacillus 9) Tumor-bearing

TBG Thyroxine-binding globulin, see there

TBI Total body irradiation

TBT Transcervical balloon tuboplasty

3TC (-)-β-L-2',3'-dideoxy-3'-thiacytidine AIDS An inhibitor of HIV reverse transcriptase, which when administered in combination with AZT (zidovudine) results in a 1.0 log ↓ in viral load and (in phase II/III studies) an ↑ in CD4+ T cells, unlike combined AZT/ddC therapy in which the CD4+ T-cell counts are ↓ (Bio/Technology 1995; 13:208)

TCA suicide Tricyclic antidepressants, see there

TCBS agar Thiosulfate-citrate-bile salts-sucrose agar MICROBIOLOGY A bacterial culture medium with a high salt concentration and alkaline pH that is the preferred 'recovery' medium for vibrios, eg *Vibrio cholera* and *V parahaemolyticus*; other organisms that grow on TCBS agar are *Enterococcus faecalis*, *Escherichia coli*, and *Pseudomonas aeruginosa*

TCDD 2,3,7,8-Tetrachlorodibenzo-*p*-dioxin, see Agent Orange, Dioxin

TCE 1,1,1-Trichloroethylene $CHCl=CCl_2$ ENVIRONMENT A volatile chlorinated hydrocarbon that boils at 88°C and is highly soluble (1000 ppm) in water; TCE was formerly used as a degreasing agent and disposed of by pouring directly into the ground, and thus has become a major ground water contaminant that is detectable in 'plumes' up to 10 km from its original dump site and is often pre-

taxol

sent in 'Superfund' toxic dumps; some microorganisms co-metabolize TCE when using methane, propane or toluene as sources of oxygen TOXICITY Peripheral neuropathy, carcinogenic in rat; see Bioremediation, Plumes, Superfund, Toxic dumps, 'White-out'; Cf Dioxin, PCBs

Note: Chloral hydrate, a TCE metabolite is used as a sedative, a questionable practice given its known toxicity (Science 1990; 250:359c)

TCID Tissue culture infective dose VIROLOGY An objective measurement of a body fluid's infective potential, where serially-diluted aliquots of a fluid, eg plasma, are placed in cell cultures to detect growth and measured in units of TCID/ml plasma; the $TCID_{50}$ is that dose of virus that produces a toxic effect in 50% of test animals over a specified period of time

TCR T-cell receptor, see there 2) Tetraclororesorcinol 3) Thalamocortical relay

Also 1) T-cell reactivity 2) T-cell recovery column 3) Telemetry compression routine 4) Temperature and coefficient of resistance

TDF Testis-determining factor, see there

TDM 1) Telemetric data monitor 2) Therapeutic drug monitoring, see there

TDO syndrome Tricho-dento-osseous syndrome, see there

TdT Terminal deoxyribonucleotidyl transferase* An intracellular DNA polymerase [EC 2.7.7.31] that catalyzes the irreversible addition of 5'-deoxynucleotides to the 3' hydroxy-ends of DNA; TdT is a marker for human T-cell differentiation from the stem cell to the prothymocytic stages in the thymic cortex and medulla; TdT is detected by indirect immunofluorescence in immature T and B cells, in 1-5% of marrow cells, 60-90% of cortical thymocytes, various leukemias, eg T-cell leukemia, in 90% of common ALL, 50% of acute undifferentiated leukemia, 30% of CML in blast crisis, occasionally in pre-B ALL but rarely in CLL

*Also known as DNA nucleotidylexotransferase, the term recommended (1992) by the Nomenclature Committee of the International Union of Biochemistry and Molecular Biology (IUBMB)

TE MRI Echo time The time between the middle of the 90° pulse and the middle of the production of the spin-echo, for multiple echoes, TE1, TE2 and others; see Magnetic resonance imaging

TEA Tetraethylammonium chloride An experimental K⁺ channel blocker used to study action potentials

teabag HISTOLOGY A small bag originally produced from a porous paper (currently from a plastic mesh) similar to that used for tea; teabags are used to contain fragments of tissue (eg products of conception, which are notoriously prone to floating into other tissues) during the processing of specimens for histologic examination

teaching hospital A hospital, health care center, or institute that has two or more residency training programs approved by the Accreditation Council for Graduate Medical Education

tea-drinker's disease Theism A caffeine-induced nervous condition that is uncommonly reported in the current environment, clinically characterized by congestion of cephalic vessels, excitement, and/or depression, pallor, cardiac dysrhythmia, hallucinations and insomnia (JAMA 1887; 7:410)

team approach see Medical team

teardrop bladder TRAUMATOLOGY A descriptive term for a markedly distended urinary bladder in which a trauma-induced hematoma surrounds the bladder base, lifting it out of the pelvis; external pressure narrows the bladder neck into an attenuated 'stem', while a broad base at the bladder's apex imparts a piriform configuration by excretory urography; other causes of a teardrop bladder include extensive pelvic lipomatosis, inferior vena cava occlusion, psoas muscle hypertrophy, and rarely pelvic lymphadenopathy

teardrop cell Dacrocyte A deformed red cell that has squeezed through a reticuloendothelial system bearing increased connective tissue, seen in agnogenic myeloid metaplasia, myelofibrosis, and other reticuloendothelial replacement disorders that compromise marrow space, causing splenic overload or loss of functional splenic tissue, including megaloblastic anemia, bone metastases, hereditary elliptocytosis and sickle cell anemia; see Red cell glossary; see Red cells

teardrop fracture A fracture-dislocation type of compression fracture of the anterior aspect of the body of a cervical vertebra, caused by hyperflexive compressive forces that burst the vertebral body, separating and displacing a wedge-shaped fragment of bone from the antero-inferior margin of the vertebral body; the potential danger in these fractures is posterior displacement into the spinal canal causing cord compression; Cf Wedge fracture

teardrop sign A clinical finding in which an elongated soft-tissue mass prolapses into the maxillary antrum, which may be seen in a plain film of the face in blunt trauma to the anterior rim of the orbit, causing a 'blowout' fracture to the orbital floor

teaser' advertising Advertising for a product that has not yet come to market; under US regulations, a drug company must choose between either 'Institutional' or 'Coming soon' forms of 'teaser' advertising (JAMA 1990; 264:2409RV)

teat and udder sign RENAL RADIOLOGY A fanciful descriptor for an appearance that may be seen in an excretory urogram when the kidney is affected by a mass lesion located at the cortico-medullary junction, where the papillae and short-stemmed calyces ('teats') are associated with a large displacing mass ('udder')

technologist Medical technologist, see there

technician LABORATORY MEDICINE A person with at least two years of formal college or university education in a wide range of laboratory techniques, who upon passing the appropriate examination written and administered by the American Society of Clinical Pathologists, carries the title of MLT(ASCP); technicians are empowered to perform clinical tests, but not to report the results without the approval of a medical technologist, see there

technicium-99m sestamibi see Sestamibi

technology transfer The conveying of a concept or process from a theoretical realm (usually borne in the womb of the academented) to a commerically viable product; successful TT requires that the players at the academic end understand its importance in the current fiscal environment, that the product or product be marketable, and that it be properly managed to point of financial fruition (Bio/Technology 1995; 13:410); TT encompasses a range of activities including the transfer of information, expertise, intellectual property, materials, potential products and processes from academia to industry; technology transfer is viewed as successful in the US, eg Stanford University and Massachusetts Institute of Technology, earned $13 million and $6.5 million (respectively) in licensing fees in 1989 compared to R&D (research & development) expeditures of less than $1.9 million and $1.3 million (respectively) (Nature 1993; 364:659N) see NIST, R&D

techoic acid antibody assay TA-AB MICROBIOLOGY A test that measures the titers of antibody to techoic acid, a constituent of the staphylococcal cell wall; 90% of patients with *S aureus*-induced endocarditis have increased TA-AB levels and the assay is used to diagnose *S aureus* osteomyelitis, culture-negative endocarditis, to determine response to therapy, and to detect possible relapse

teenage pregnancy Pregnancy in adolescence PUBLIC HEALTH A phenomenon of broad societal concern; 10% of those ages 15-19 (teenagers) become pregnant; this age group accounts for 13% of all live births (US); in one study, when potentially confounding sociodemographic factors* were eliminated from statistical analysis, a younger age independently confers an ↑ risk of adverse pregnancy in the form of low birthweight, prematurity, and ↑ first year infant mortality (N Engl J Med 1995; 332:1113OA) most other studies of TP have reached opposite conclusions, ie that the decreased age was far less a critical factor than suboptimal socioeconomic factors in determining an adverse outcome on the pregnancy, see graph, page 884 (N Engl J Med 1995; 332:1161ED)

*Adequacy of level of education, marital status, and prenatal care

Teflon Polytetrafluoroethylene A proprietary name for a polymeric molecule that is resistant to organic solvents, has a melting temperature of 225°C, which has diverse medical applications including use in prosthetic articulations, vascular grafts and in low-temperature chemical reactions

Teflon injection therapy ENT The injection of a Teflon-based paste lateral to the conus elasticus in order to 'medialize' a unilaterally paralyzed vocal cord (*plica vocalis* [NA6]); TIT is well-suited for unilaterally paralyzed recurrent laryngeal nerve, minimal atrophy of the vocal cord, and a mobile cricoarytenoid, but is contraindicated if the cord is not completely paralyzed as the Teflon may migrate; TIT may also be used abductor spasmodic dysphonia, abnormal patency of the eustachian tube, and cricoarytenoid

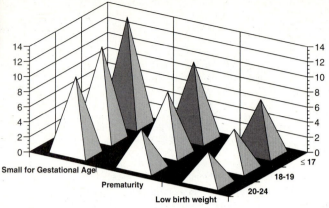

outcomes of teenage pregnancy

joint ankylosis

TEFRA Tax Equity and Fiscal Responsibility Act of 1982 (Public Law 97-248) A US federal law that provided for key health care expenditure reforms, including risk-sharing contracts with health maintenance organizations and revision of reimbursement arrangements with hospital-based physicians, where the hospital's reimbursement from Medicare ('part A') is clearly separated from the professional component (or physician's services, 'part B'); TEFRA placed a ceiling or 'cap' on the annual operating revenues per inpatient Medicare case at each hospital; see DRGs, RBRVS

tegafur 1-[2-tetrahydrofuranyl]-5-fluorouracil A prodrug that is absorbed from the small intestine and metabolized in vivo to 5-fluorouracil (5-FU); administration of tegafur in combination with 5-FU and cisplatin is reported to improve the survival of patients with inoperable non-small cell lung cancer (Cancer 1995; 75:2677)

telecanthus-hypospadias syndrome G syndrome, see there

telecytometry see Telemedicine

teleconsultation A generic term for the obtention of a medical consultation by either a non-medical consumer or by a health care professional from a collegue on an electronic network (usually Internet); the format and legal issues on teleconsultation is evolving rapidly, and it is unclear what licenses are required of a physician who lives in one state and provides legally binding medical opinions in another state (Am Med News 24 April 1995 p1) s

telediagnosis see Teleconsultation, Telepathology, Teleradiology

el 'telefono' see Torture

telekinesis The movement of an object through space without physically apparent cause, a phenomenon that some persons claimed to have done by thought alone

Note: The author is unaware of documented confirmation of the telekinetic phenomenon

telemedicine A generic term for any form of medical practice in which the diagnostic information, eg telecytometry, (cardiac) telemetry, telemicroscopy, telepathology, or teleradiology, are transmitted to the physician for analysis; in its current state, telemedicine requires ± $125 000 investment per facility for the purchase and installation of computers, specialized cameras and video equipment etc A major impediment to implementing telemedicine is the speed of transmission of data; the most primitive format and vehicle is that of the modem, which can only be used for transmitting images and information that is not urgent; an advance that can be used without upgrading copper

telephones lines is the codec (coder/decoder) which compresses data from 10 to 100 fold; one of the standards is the T-1 line that carries 24 telephone channels; the most advanced format is asynchronous transfer mode switching, which is a fiber-optic protocol that merges voice, data, and video communications in a common format, allowing extremely rapid transmission and processing of information (Am Med News 1995; 17 April 1995 p19)

telemicroscopy see Telemedicine, Telepathology

teleology A view of the physical universe that holds that all structures and functions in an organism have a purpose and confer an evolutionary advantage to the organism; according to Aristotle, the purpose of each component was invoked by a supernatural being

Note: In order to dignify the heuristically logical argument that nothing evolves without a raison d'être, while circumventing the mystical import of the concept, the ersatz term 'teleonomy' has been suggested, although teleology continues to be widely preferred

telepathology An embryonic field that may eliminate the need for small rural hospitals to have an on-site surgical pathologist, which utilizes high-resolution video cameras and robotic microscopes to transmit images of tissues specimens over phone lines or fibro-optic cables to a distant center with multiple pathologist experts

telepathy The alleged communication of thoughts and/or mental images by means other than those that can be measured by physical senses and energy transmission

Note: The existance of telepathic phenomena has proven difficult to document

telephone counseling The provision of advice and verbalized moral support to a person with a particular need by a group of either volunteers or a paid staff with some level of experience and/or expertise in the area of interest; TC may include crisis intervention, eg for suicide, HIV infection, or acute or chronic addiction disorders (N Engl J Med 1995; 332:1296sв)

'telephone receiver' deformity ENT A colloquial term for a deformity of the ear, fancifully likened to that of the hand-set of a telephone, which is an undesired end-result of poorly healed trauma to the ear PEDIATRIC RADIOLOGY A descriptor for the long tubular bones of infants with thanatophoric dwarfism; the bones are short, broad with metaphyseal flaring, occasionally display 'cupping' of the end-plates; afflicted bones have a rhizomelic distribution and are markedly curved at the ends; other bone anomalies in this condition include the cloverleaf skull deformity, frontal bossing and H- or U-shaped vertebral bodies (discussed elsewhere)

telephone scatologia PSYCHIATRY A form of paraphilia (sexual deviancy) in which the individual, almost invariably a male, derives erotic pleasure from making obscene telephone calls; TS is classified in the DSM-IV as a paraphilia, not otherwise specified (302.9)

teleradiology A form of delivering expert radiology services by transmitting a digitalized image obtained by angiography, CT, MRI, PET scanning, sonography, thermography and other imaging devices via satellite or telephone cabling to radiologists who may be located hundreds of kilometers away; the major disadvantage currently is the amount of time required to transmit the image, which will be largely resolved by fibro-optic cables; high-resolution teleradiology systems cost $40-60 000 at the sending site, and $85 000 at the receiving site (Am Med News 1995; 17 April 1995 p19)

telescoped fingers Doigt-en-lorgnette A finger in which there is concentric osteolysis and bony collapse, classically seen in yaws-induced osteitis; see Yaws

'telescoped' urine casts LABORATORY MEDICINE Molded proteinaceous material found in the urine sediment that contains all the possible elements found in renal disease, including RBCs, WBCs, hyaline, cellular and granular casts, fat and lipid; these casts are typical of lupus nephropathy, but may also be seen in other collagen vascular diseases and renal disease (eg acute and chronic glomerulonephritis, nephrotic syndrome, and transplant rejection), subacute bacterial endocarditis, hyperviscosity syndrome, malignant hypertension, toxemia, heavy metal poisoning, multiple myeloma, amyloidosis, and sickle cell disease; see Casts

'telescoping' The 'compression' or overlapping of clinical or pathological features of a disease or lesion that is normally subdivided into chronological stages of progression

telescoping fractures Those fractures seen in osteogenesis imperfecta where marked osteoporosis facilitates an axial compaction fracture with collapse, shortening and thickening of the long bones

'television intoxication syndrome' A term that arose from a legal case in which a 'depraved heart' murder was attributed to the alleged perpetrator's suggestibility and loss of reality sense, resulting from his excess television viewing ('intoxication'); see 'Couch potato'

Note: While the term has not been legitimized in the medical literature, it is possible that viewing 40-50 hours of television per week by impressionable young children in the form of passive entertainment may result in unanticipated side effects

telomerase An enzyme that is needed to maintain the genetic integrity of both the germ and somatic cells during the rapid growth that occurs in early fetal development; the genes that encode telomerase are turned off around the time of birth; however in most cancer cell lines, telomerase has been reactivated, allowing malignant cells to circumvent the normal senescence 'program' and become immortal (JAMA 1995; 273:1247MN&P; Science 1995; 268:29); normal human cells carry the telomerase gene, but except in sperm it is not expressed; telomerase is expressed in ovarian malignancies but not in nonmalignant ovarian lesions (Proc Nat Acad Sci April 12, 1994) telomerase therefore qualifies as a new type of tumor suppressor gene; see Telomere

telomere MOLECULAR BIOLOGY A 3–5-kilobase pair segment of DNA composed of variable (in number) tandem 'repeats' of the oligonucleotide sequence TTAGGG, which is added to the end of linear chromosomes by a nontemplate mechanism involving a multifunctional telomerase; the TTAGGG repeats were first described as 'junk' DNA, but are present in high copy numbers in the centromere and demonstrate marked evolutionary conservation among species, possibly preventing incomplete replication and chromosomal instability; telomeres are elongated in immortalized cells and increasingly shortened in normal cells undergoing senescence ; the telomere has been fancifully likened to the plastic caps on shoelaces; when a strand of DNA is duplicated during mitosis, a few of the subunits at one end are lost; with each tick of the mitotic 'clock', pieces of telomere are whittled away, and the telomere shrinks with age; it is hypothesized that the cell' losess its ability to replicate when the telemore falls below a critical length

N-telopeptides A family of cross-linked peptides which are direct degradation products of collagen type I that are generated by osteoclasts during osteoporosis; urinary levels of N-telopeptides are reported to directly reflect the amount of bone collagen being absorbed (advertisement from Ostex International, Inc, in JAMA 1995; 273:1479)

template A mold or pattern used as a guide to form a copy of the original, as is the use of a DNA 'template' to produce a copy of itself or, through transcription into RNA, which subsequently matures into messenger RNA, which is a template for translation into proteins

temporal arteritis Giant cell arteritis A self-limited disease of middle-aged women that evolves to systemic arteritis in 10-15% of cases, with blindness as a potential late complication PATHOLOGY Nodular transmural swelling of arteries, infiltration by neutrophils, eosinophils, mononuclear cells and giant cell granulomas

Note: Although the term giant cell arteritis is more correct from a pathological (and often a clinical) standpoint, temporal arteritis is widely preferred

temporal lobe syndrome The functional loss of major portions of the temporal lobes and rhinencephalon (amygdala, hippocampus, uncus and hippocampal gyrus); this can be reproduced experimentally in monkeys by bilateral temporal lobectomy CLINICAL Visual agnosia, tendency to examine all objects orally and examine immediately all objects seen, loss of emotion, hypersexuality in the form of heterosexual, autosexual and homosexual activity, and increased consumption of meat PATHOLOGY Degeneration of myelinated fiber tracts in most communicating and projecting tracts in the face of minimal retrograde cellular degeneration; see Hypersexuality

temporal trend EPIDEMIOLOGY A variation in the incidence of a particular condition over time, which may be based on age, cohort, or period (JAMA 1992; 268:3098oc) see Age trend, Cohort trend, Period trend

temporary insanity A colloquial term referring to a transient loss of control over one's normal mental and/or judgmental faculties and sense of reason; when applied to commission of a crime, TI is generally not an accepted term vis-á-vis forensic psychiatry, although it is often encompassed by facets of the so-called insanity defense; see M'Naghten rule, Insanity defense

temporomandibular joint syndrome TMJ syndrome, see there

TEN Toxic epidermal necrolysis, see there

tenascin A extracellular matrix protein formed from six identical 210-kD proteins, which is synthesized by the mesenchymal cells of the developing embryo and responsible for differentiation of epithelial tissues

tenase complex HEMATOLOGY A term for the proteins in the circulation that are required to activate coagulation factor X, ie factor IXa, phospholipid, and activated factor VIII after its release from von Willebrand factor

'tender years doctrine' A gender-specific philosophy that prevailed in the American court system that favored placement of young children with the mother in a divorce or separation; this has been replaced by gender-neutral language based on the 'best interests of the child' (NY Newsday 23 March 1995; B4)

tendon sheath (adherence) syndrome OPHTHALMOLOGY A condition characterized by limited elevation of the eye in adduction due to fibrosis and shortening of the tendon of the superior oblique ocular muscle

tennis elbow Lateral epicondylitis SPORTS MEDICINE A condition with no limitation of movement, swelling or pain when the articulation is moved passively, but which is painful when actively moved DIAGNOSIS Active dorsiflexion of the wrist against resistance or firm fingertip pressure over the lateral humeral epicondyle produces sharp pain TREATMENT Rest, splinting and if necessary, local injection of corticosteroids; see Golf elbow

tennis leg Exercise-induced rupture of calf muscles that may occur following any violent exercise in which the rapidly moving body abruptly changes directions, including tennis, soccer, downhill skiing CLINICAL An audible snap may be heard in the popliteal space, accompanied by severe calf pain and hematoma, due to a rupture of the gastrocnemius muscle TREATMENT Immobilization in plantar flexion and physical therapy

tennis racquet An adjectival descriptor for a relatively elongated cell, lesion, structure or radiological density that is globose at one end and elongated at the other, likened to the popular recreational device used in tennis

'tennis racquet' appearance A descriptive term for the ping-pong paddle-like thickening of the mesangium in glomeruli affected by in Kimmelstiel-Wilson disease

'tennis racquet' cell A tennis-racquet-shaped variant of rhabdomyoblast seen in sarcoma botryoides, a form of rhabdomyosarcoma affecting children

'tennis racquet' granule Birbeck granule Langerhans' granule A subcellular particle with a pentalaminar 'handle' and bulbous terminal dilatation of uncertain significance that is seen by electron microscopy in the antigen-presenting Langerhans' cell and in histiocytes (figure)

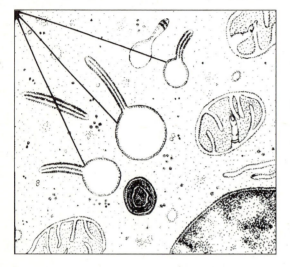

tennis racquet granules

'tennis racquet' sign RADIOLOGY The descriptor for a finding in a 'blighted ovum' in which the ultrasonically empty gestational sac is compressed (the racquet's 'handle') and adjacent to a surrounding decidual reaction (the 'paddle'); Cf Tadpole sign

'tennis racquet' spore MICROBIOLOGY A descriptive term for the morphology of the subterminal spores in the gram-positive *Clostridium tetani*, as well as in *C diphtheriae*

teniposide An investigational drug for ALL in early relapse, while the patient is still in the consolidation phase of chemotherapy, or used to attempt induction in patients who fail a first induction

'ten percent' tumor A mnemonic for pheochromocytomas, as 10% are malignant, 10% are bilateral, 10% are extra-adrenal, 10% occur in children and 10% are associated with other systemic disease, including von Recklinghausen's disease, von Hippel-Lindau syndrome, Sturge-Weber disease and multiple endocrine neoplasia (MEN) IIa and IIb

TENS Transcutaneous electrical nerve stimulation, see there

Tensilon® test A clinical test used in patients with known myasthenia gravis to distinguish between a myasthenic and cholinergic crisis; the short-acting cholinesterase inhibitor, Tensilon (edrophonium chloride), is administered with a syringe containing 10 mg; if one minute after 2 mg is injected, there is no change in muscle strength, then the remainder is injected; in a cholinergic crisis, the weakness will worsen and be accompanied by colicky pain and fasciculation of the eyelids; see Myasthenic crisis

tensin(s) A pair of 150-kD and 200-kD actin-binding proteins that have phosphotyrosine-binding activity and mediate signal transduction pathways in the cytoskeleton; tensins have a SH2 domain and bind in the extracellular matrix to actin and vinculin (Science 1995; 268:233)

tension headache Cephalgia related to prolonged muscle contraction, which beginning as an occipital non-pulsatile, vise-like pain extending fronto-temporally, with 'tight' posterior cervical, temporalis or masseter muscles; tension headaches are most common in women who also suffer migraines and are related to postures requiring sustained contraction of the above muscles, exacerbated by stress

ten/thirty (10/30) rule TRANSFUSION MEDICINE A clinical guideline (transfusion 'trigger') for when to transfuse packed red cells, ie when the hemoglobin is below 100 g/L (US: 10 g/dl) and/or when the hematocrit is below 30%; with the advent of AIDS, clinical decisions to transfuse blood have become more conservative, and unless a patient is actively bleeding, hospital transfusion committees may sanction the lower '9/27' or '8/24' rules, as clinically stable patients often tolerate very low red cell masses without co-morbidity; see Single unit transfusion, Transfusion 'trigger'

tenting CARDIOLOGY A term for the symmetrical 'peaking' of the 'T' wave on the EKG, which is associated with a lengthening of the P-R interval, typically seen in early hyperkalemia; with further ↑ of K⁺, the P wave disappears and a sine wave appears INTERNAL MEDICINE A clinical sign consisting in light pinching of a patient's skin, which under usual conditions, springs back to a flattened position; a delay in flattening ('tenting') is characteristic of relatively severe dehydration and in the elderly whose dermal collagen and elastin have undergone age-related cross-linking

tenure ACADEMIA A status granted to a person with a 'terminal' degree, eg doctor of medicine (MD) or doctor of philosophy (PhD), after a trial period, which protects him/her from summary dismissal; individuals in academia who hold positions on the 'tenure track' are expected to assume major duties in research, teaching and, if applicable, patient care, fostering through their activities, the academic 'agenda' of their respective departments; see Endowed chair, Lecturer, Professor; Cf 'Chair'

teratogen Any agent that acts on a developing fetus, inducing structural abnormalities; maternal medications with known teratogenic effects include aminopterin (abortion, malformations), anticoagulants, anticonvulsants, cytotoxic drugs, mepivacaine (bradycardia, death), methimazole and propylthiouracil (goiter), ¹³¹I (destruction of fetal thyroid), male sex hormones (methyltestosterone, 17-α-ethinyl-testosterone, and 17-α-ethinyl-19-nortestosterone, which is masculinizing to female infants), tetracycline (hypoplasia and pigmentation of tooth enamel) and trimethadione (abortion, multiple malformations, mental retardation); female sex hormones act on genital structures causing masculinization with defective external female genitalia, transplacental carcinogenesis by DES; see Fetal warfarin syndrome, Fetal hydantoin syndrome, Thalidomide; Cf 'Litogen'

teratogenesis The generation of malformations during the early development of the fetus, presumed to be due to any of a number of environmental toxins; major congenital malformations occur in 1:10 000 infants, 45% of which are de novo AD or X-linked mutations that cannot be predicted; 'soft' data implies that some occupations are at an increased risk for fetal malformations, eg nursing (exposure to chemotherapy, hexachlorophene, anesthetics, eg NO₂, halothane), cosmetologists (hair spray, fingernail adhesives), chemical manufacturing and processing (various agents, especially petrochemicals), those in the petrochemical industry; see Bendectin, Crack babies, DES, Fetal syndromes, Sellafield studies, Thalidomide

teratoma A tumor derived from the multipotent cells of one or more of the primitive embryologic layers (ectoderm, endoderm, mesoderm), which differs in prognosis according to the organ involved and degree of maturation of the tissues; teratomas are most common in the mediastinum, ovary and testicle, but may occur in the urogenital tract and various parenchymal organs **MEDIASTINAL TERATOMA** A tumor that may occur in both sexes, which are most commonly composed of mature epithelium, as well as neural, gastrointestinal, chondral and respiratory tissues and are almost invariably benign; mediastinal teratomas composed of immature elements are too rare for valid prediction of their future behavior **OVARIAN TERATOMA** A tumor that includes the common (20% of all ovarian neoplasms) mature teratoma, 98% of which are benign and the uncommon immature (malignant) teratoma, which is graded according to the amount of immature neuroepithelial tissue present (the greater the amount the worse the prognosis) and treated by surgery and multiagent chemotherapy **TESTICULAR TERATOMA** A tumor that is classified as 1) Adult teratoma, if all the cellular elements are mature 2) Immature teratoma, if areas reminiscent of the primitive tissues seen in Wilms' tumor (a 'prototypic' primitive tumor) are present or 3) Teratoma with malignant transformation, if a malignancy, usually a squamous cell carcinoma or adenocarcinoma, arises in an adult teratoma

terbinafine An antifungal agent that is reported to be more effective than griseofulvin in treating fingernail dermatophytosis (**J Am Acad Dermatol 1995; 32:72**)

terfenadine Seldane® A non-sedating antihistamine prescribed[1] for allergy and viral upper respiratory tract infections; it is metabolized in the first pass through the liver by the hepatic cytochrome P450 enzyme CYP3A4, which converts it to the active form terfenadine carboxylate; it has been associated with serious ventricular arrhythmias, eg torsades de pointes[2] should not be used in combination with ketoconazole, an oral antifungal agent that alters terfenadine metabolism, resulting in the accumulation of the parent compound, which blocks a potassium channel, and prolongs the QT interval (**JAMA 1993; 269:1513oc, 1532oc**)

[1]Available in Canada, the UK, and in some other countries without a prescription [2]Which is thought to be due to delayed repolarization with marked QT prolongation, and bizarre T wave changes

terminal COMPUTERS A peripheral component of a computer network that has a monitor, an input device, eg a keyboard and often an output device, eg a printer; a 'dummy' terminal allows simple accession of information; a 'smart' terminal is used for data entry and some forms of data manipulation MOLECULAR BIOLOGY The end of 1) A protein, either the N-terminal or the COOH-terminal or 2) A segment of a polynucleotide chain, either the 3' (upstream) end or the 5' (downstream) end of the molecule

terminal bar CYTOLOGY The portion of the cell below and perpendicular to the cilia seen in Papanicolaou-stained smears of the ciliated columnar cells, which corresponds to the sum of the belt desmosomes, actin filaments and other proteins aggregated at the apical end of the cells; TBs are seen in the normal respiratory epithelium, adenomas, adenocarcinoma, APUDomas, transitional and papillary carcinomas of the urinary bladder, synovial sarcomas, and mesotheliomas

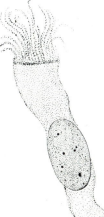

terminal bar

terminal cancer A malignancy that is expected to cause the patient's death within a short period of time, ie weeks to several months; patients with TCs have one or more of the following features: no response to any form of therapy, tumor-related

cachexia and marked weight loss, florid metastases to multiple sites or 'secondary' metastases, ie those arising from an already metastatic focus, marked jaundice (due to liver replacement by malignancy), a need for constant pain medication, and compression of vital stuctures of 'impossible' surgical access; terminal cancer patients are best treated with compassion and moral support administered by 'significant other(s)' in a hospice environment, although some patients may seek 'miracle' cures and undergo 'heroic' forms of surgery or actively seek unproven therapies for cancer; see 'Heroic' surgery, Hospice, Most significant other; Cf Spontaneous remission of cancer, Unproven therapies for cancer

terminal differentiation An event which in mammalian cells consists of two interdependent and (usually) irreversible biological phenomena: 1) Withdrawal from the cell cycle and 2) phenotypic differentiation; this event requires the tumor suppressor retinoblastoma protein Rb; reversal of terminal differentiation is mediated by p107 in Rb[-/-] cells (**Science 1994; 264; 1467R**) TD can be induced, eg by tretinoin as a therapeutic strategy in malignancies of immature cells, eg to 'drive' acute promyelocytic leukemia into a mature nonproliferative state of remission (**N Engl J Med 1992; 327:385oA**)

terminal duct carcinoma A low-grade malignant salivary gland tumor that is most common in the palate, which despite a uniform cell type, has a wide range of architectural configurations, including tubular, cribriform, solid and fascicular patterns PROGNOSIS Recurrence 12%; locoregional lymphoid metastases 10% TREATMENT Excision, post-operative radiation

terminal illness syndrome A condition which includes one or more of the following: A causative illness with a progressive evolution, eg AIDS, cancer, survival defined in days or weeks, Karnovsky score of < 40%, single– or multiorgan failure, failure of conventional or proven treatment measures, absence of other potential proven or experimental therapy, irreversible progressive complications; see Karnovsky scale

terminal repeat MOLECULAR BIOLOGY A segment of redundant oligonucleotides present at one or both ends of DNA; see Long terminal repeat; Cf Telomeres

terminal reservoir 'syndrome' GASTROENTEROLOGY A potentially massive dilation of the descending and sigmoid colon, particularly common in the elderly, which is initially caused by voluntary suppression of defecatory urge; as the rectal stretch receptors degenerate, a vicious cycle of overextension and fecal impaction develops

termination MOLECULAR BIOLOGY The final step in 1) Polypeptide synthesis, after which it is released by the ribosome or 2) The transcription of mRNA from the DNA template by RNA polymerase, which ends with a termination or stop (UAA, UAG, UGA) codon; see Translation

termination mutant see Zebrafish

termination of pregancy* Induced abortion

'Termite' A highly colloquial term for any of the participants in the long-term 'genius' studies initiated by Dr LM Terman in 1921, who selected 1521 children with IQs above 135 using his then-new intelligence yardstick, the Stanford-Binet test (**New York Times 7 March 1995; C1**) the Terman genius study is the longest longitudinal study known and has collected data from people who are now in their 80s

terpene(s) Isoprenoid(s), see there

Terry-Thomas sign An increased space between the navicular and lunate bones seen in a frontal film of a wrist with subluxation of the carpal navicular bone, in which there is backward rotation of the proximal pole and forward rotation of the distal pole; this increased gap has been fancifully likened to the dental diastema of the late British comic actor, Terry-Thomas

tertian fever A fever characterized by febrile paroxysms occurring every third day, as in the 48-hour febrile peaks in *Plasmodium vivax* malaria, also known as benign tertian malaria; malignant tertian fever is caused by the more virulent *P falciparum*, which in its most intense form may be fatal within days; Cf Quartan fever

tertian malaria Tertian fever, see there

tertiary care HEALTH CARE INDUSTRY The most specialized level of health care, which is administered to patients who have complex diseases and/or who may require high-risk pharmacologic regimens or surgical procedures; patients who receive tertiary care are usually referred by either a primary care giver or by a specialist who recognizes that the therapy appropriate for a patient is beyond his ability or expertise to perform in his own environment; such care is provided in 'tertiary care centers', often university hospitals, as it requires sophisticated technology, a team of specialists and often subspecialists, a diagnostic support group and intensive care facilities; Cf Primary care, Secondary care

tertiary care center A hospital or medical center for patients who are usually referred from secondary care centers, and provides subspecialty expertise in

SURGERY Organ transplantation, pediatric cardiovascular surgery, stereotactic neurosurgery and others

INTERNAL MEDICINE Genetics, hepatology, adolescent psychiatry and others

DIAGNOSTIC MODALITIES PET (positron emission tomography) and SQUID (superconducting quantum interface device) scanning, color Doppler electrocardiography, electron microscopy, gene rearrangement, and molecular analysis and

THERAPEUTIC MODALITIES Experimental protocols for treating advanced and/or potentially fatal disease, including AIDS, cancer, and inborn errors of metabolism

tertiary center bias Referral center bias, see there

tertiary structure see Protein structure

tesla MRI The International System (SI) unit for magnetic flux density, equivalent to 10 000 gauss, the formerly used unit; see Magnetic resonance imaging

test of healing A therapeutic trial of H_2-blockers, eg cimetidine, ranitidine that is used in patients with a gastric ulcer, in whom a decrease in ulcer-type of pain is equated with therapeutic success; non-resolution of symptoms after 3-6 weeks of H_2-blocking therapy is considered an indication for endoscopy and endoscopic biopsy as the possibility of a gastric carcinoma must be ruled out

'test-tube' baby A full-term gestational product resulting from in vitro fertilization of an egg that was implanted in a uterus and carried to term by either the genetic mother or by a surrogate (gestational) mother; see Artificial reproduction, Baby M, in vitro reproduction, Surrogate motherhood

Note: The first successful test-tube baby was baby girl Brown born in 1978 (Lancet 1978; 2:366)

test tube rete pegs DERMATOPATHOLOGY A descriptor for the uniformly elongated rete pegs that are accompanied by edema and vascular congestion of the papillae, findings characteristic of psoriasis; see 'Squirting papillae'

testicular feminization syndrome Morris syndrome An X-linked [MIM 313700] pseudohermaphroditic state occurring in genotypic XY males who have a female phenotype; there is normal secretion of and response to müllerian inhibiting hormone, resulting in a phenotypic female with adequate secondary sex characteristics PATHOGENESIS X-linked testosterone receptor deficiency, causing a poor end-organ response to androgens CLINICAL Feminine habitus, sexual behavior and secondary sex characteristics, associated with a blind vaginal pouch without uterine tissue, scanty pubic and axillary hair, and internally, undescended testicles; although the gonads often harbor Sertoli cell adenomas, malignancy occurs in only 4% of cases of testicular feminization; therefore, unlike mixed gonadal dysgenesis in which malignancy is common in younger patients, in testicular feminization, it is better to preserve the gonads until after the pubertal growth spurt LABORATORY Testosterone levels are normal in the face of defective end-organ response; see Male pseudohermaphroditism

testicular malignancy Germ cell tumors, see there

testicular regression syndrome Embryonic testicular regression syndrome, see there Note: It is likely that with time, the adjective embryonic will be deleted in the working parlance, resulting in the simpler term, testicular regression syndrome, as already used in the Mendelian Inheritance in Man catalogs

testis-determining factor A protein encoded by a gene in the SYR region on the short arm of the Y chromosome, which is responsible for development of primary male organs; see X-chromosome inactivation

testotoxicosis A state of male precocious puberty characterized by an autonomous production of androgens of testicular origin, which requires both antiandrogens and aromatase inhibitors to slow the skeletal growth to a prepubertal rate (N Engl J Med 1994; 331:1056oa)

tetanospasmin A 150-kD neurotoxin produced by *Clostridium tetani* that is the most toxic substance known to man, causing profound muscle spasms due to tetanospasmin's blockage of the release of glycine (a neurotransmitter for group 1A inhibitory afferent motor neurons), resulting in unrestrained muscle firing and sustained muscular contraction, potentially causing lockjaw, dysphagia, or acute respiratory failure by tetany of the diaphragm; see Poisons

tetanus Lockjaw An acute infection by the anaerobic spore-forming bacillus *Clostridium tetani*, which is manifest by uncontrolled muscle spasms due to the action of the tetanospasmin; it is frequently fatal, especially at the extremes of age, and preventable by immunization EPIDEMIOLOGY *C tetani* is ubiquitous, and may infect virtually any open wound; no longer a major health problem in the US (incidence has stabilized at ± 0.035/10⁵), in developing nations, it is among the ten top killers (accounting for an estimated 1 million deaths) which develop in a menagerie of mishaps from simple wounds to sloppy abortions, female circumcisions, and the like, therewith packaging the romanticism of the rural in a reality sandwich CLINICAL ± 2 week incubation, followed by localized or generalized weakness, cramping, dysphagia, trismus (lockjaw), ↑ muscle rigidity (eg risus sardonicus), opisthotonus, laryngospasm, and possibly death TREATMENT Benzodiazepines (↓ anxiety, sedation, anticonvulsant, and induce muscle relazation by facilitating GABA-inhibitory transmission in the brain stem and spinal cord), ventilatory support, tetanus immune globulin VACCINE The tetanus vaccine is 96% effective; in the US rates of immunity to tetanus ranges from 79% in white males to less than 20% in Mexican-American females; the rates are higher in those with a higher education and income (N Engl J Med 1995; 332:761oa)

tetanus toxoid A small peptide fragment that selectively elicits helper immune response but not immune suppression; the tetanus vaccine is highly effective for *Clostridium tetani*; most of the US population has received tetanus toxoid at 2, 4, 6 and 15 months (the 'primary' series), a 'booster' between ages 4-6 and (theoretically) should receive another 'booster' every ten years; in open 'dirty' wounds, booster shots are often given, as well as 250 units of tetanus immune globulin to 'cover' for possible clostridial contamination

tethered (spinal) cord syndrome NEUROLOGY An occult spinal dysraphism resulting from a defect in dorsal induction, the earliest major embryologic process in the formation of the brain and spinal cord; during secondary neurulation, the neural tubes atrophies and the ventral remnant persists as the filum terminale; as the vertebral column grows, the filum terminale and nerve roots lengthen; tethering results if the primitive sacral cord does not degenerate or the filum terminale and nerve roots do not lengthen properly; mechanical traction is thought to be the major cause of the condition, accompanied by other defects, eg impaired oxidative mitochondrial metabolism CLINICAL-CHILDREN Static sensorimotor defects, deformities of the spine and feet, skin changes in the lumbosacral region including hypertrichosis, hemangiomas, dimples; pain is rarely prominent in children with TCS CLINICAL-ADULTS Gait defects, upper and lower motor neuron signs, and either a spastic small-capacity bladder or less commonly, a hypotonic large-capacity bladder DIAGNOSIS MRI provides the best resolution; CT with intrathecal contrast, plain films and ultrasonography are also of use TREATMENT Laminectomy at the appropriate lumbosacral level (N Engl J Med 1992; 327:1581CPC)

tethering MOLECULAR BIOLOGY A strategy for preventing insertional mutagenesis that commonly occurs when retroviral vectors are used to transfer sequences of DNA in gene therapy*; *The current models for the mechanism of integration* (of exogenous DNA) *invoke tethering of Ty3 integration machinery to the target DNA by protein-protein contacts with polymerase* (Pol) *III transcription apparatus*; tethering can thus be used to control integration; tethering an integrase to a target DNA can direct localized integration of the gene sequence of interest (Science 1995; 267:1443P)

*While retrovirus integration systems precisely link therapeutic sequences of interest to a host chromosome, they have little target site specificity; haphazard insertion may occur near proto-oncogenes leading to ectopic gene activation and possibly cancer

tetralogy of Fallot A cyanotic congenital heart disease affecting 2700 infants/year in US defined by obstruction of the right ventricular outflow, ventricular septal defect, right ventricular hypertrophy, and an overriding aorta; in a long-term study, the 32 year actuarial survival of patients with a TOF was 86% (who had a Blalock-Taussig palliative shunt prior to repair) compared with an expected rate of 96% in an age– and sex–matched population (N Engl J Med 1993; 329:593OA)

tetra-X syndrome XXXX·syndrome, see there

TFIIA, TFIIB, TFIID, TFIIE, TFIIF MOLECULAR BIOLOGY A group of initiation factors required for RNA polymerase II (RpII) to initiate transcription at promoter sites, which are assembled in a defined sequence; TFIID binds to the TATA box, an oligonucleotide sequence present in most promoters that is transcribed by RpII; after TFIID and TFIIA are bound to the promoter, TFIIB, RpII and TFIIE/TFIIF can be incorporated into the initiation complex; TFIID is a highly-conserved 37.7-kD polypeptide that is probably the polypeptide most central to the initiation of eukaryotic mRNA synthesis, binding to the TATA box promoter element, regulating the expression of most genes transcribed by RNA polymerase II; the C-terminal 181 amino acids of human TFIID have an 80% amino acid sequence similarity ('homology') with a similar protein in the yeast *Saccharomyces cerevisiae* and are functionally interchangeable in vitro

TGF Transforming growth factor(s) A group of distinct polypeptides that have been isolated from virus-transformed rodent cells, capable of altering cell phenotype, causing fibroblasts to lose anchorage-dependence and stimulating angiogenesis; see Transformation

TGF-α Transforming growth factor-α A 50-residue polypeptide synthesized by transformed cells, which has a 35% amino acid sequence similarity ('homology') with epidermal growth factor (EGF); both are angiogenic, but TGF-α is ten times more potent than EGF in stimulating cell growth; see Transformation

TGF-β Transforming growth factor-β A 25-kD homodimeric, regulatory peptide produced by various normal and neoplastic cells bearing TGF-β receptors; TGF-β is thus both autocrine and paracrine, opposing the action of endogenous cytokine, tumor necrosis factor, balancing the immune system; in epithelial and connective tissue, TGF-β recruits macrophages and fibroblasts, evoking collagen production and angiogenesis (capillary formation), forming granulation tissue, playing a role in wound healing; TGF-β inhibits cell proliferation and differentiation, inhibits neutrophil adherence, regulates other cytokines, stimulates extracellular matrix production (ECM) and is down-regulated by decorin ; the inability to produce TGF-β or to respond to its inhibitory effect has a role in carcinogenesis; recombinant TGF-β (Genentech) may be of use in myocardial infarction Note: Because TGF-β1 elicits ECM production, anti-TGF may be useful in treating mesangial proliferative glomerulonephritis; TGF-β1 induces collagen I and III production in cirrhosis, corresponding to the elusive cirrhosis transforming growth factor, causing fibrosis; TGF-α production is increased in cirrhosis with regeneration (N Engl J Med 1994; 331:1286RV) see Transformation

TGF-β receptors A group of receptors (type I–53-kD, type II–75-kD) that are indispensible for signal transduction that form heteromeric complexes on ligand binding

THA 1) Tetrahydroaminoacridine A long-acting acetylcholinesterase co-inhibitor administered with lecithin that was reported to ameliorate the symptoms of Alzheimer's disease, a claim that has not been substantiated 2) Total hip arthroplasty see there

TH1 One of two T helper cell* types, TH1 stimulation results in the cell-mediated **TH1 response** in which there is ↑ the production of IL-2 and IFN-gamma, preparing cytotoxic T cells for their ultimate targets, usually bacteria (Science News 1994; 146:120) see CD4+ T cells

*Also known as CD4+ T cells, initially discovered in mice

TH2 One of two types of T helper cells, which when stimulated, give rise to the **TH2 response** with ↑ production of IL-4, IL-5, and IL-10, initiating the humoral immunity and preparing cytotoxic T cells for their ultimate targets, usually parasites (Science News 1994; 146:120) see CD4+ T cells

TH1-TH2 balance A state of immunologic equilibrium between the cell-mediated TH1 response and the humoral TH2 response; the development of AIDS in HIV-positive subjects may be due in part to a TH1-TH2 imbalance which some workers postulate might be restored with the cytokine IL-12 (Science News 1994; 146:120) see CD4+ T cells, IL-12; see T_H1 (-type) immunity, T_H2 (-type) immunity

thalamus A mass of cerebral gray matter that lies on either side of the third ventricle, which is divided by layers (laminae) into anterior, medial, lateral, and posterior nuclei composed of neurons that 1) Relay incoming signals to specific target cortical areas; these nuclei receive a feedback loop from the sensory cortical region to which the relay projections connect and 2) Synchronize the responses of cells from the cortex*, first identified in the visual cortex (Nature 1994; 369:479L, 444N&V), but presumed to also occur in other regions, eg spinal cord, and midbrain

β-thalassemia Thalassemia major For other details refer

to standard texts TREATMENT Azacytidine may free patients from the need for transfusion possibly by hypomethylation of fetal globin gene promoters and possibly also enhance fetal globin synthesis (N Engl J Med 1993; 329:844OA) butyrate stimulates the fetal Hb gene promoter, leading to ↑ γ-globin gene expression to levels sufficient to ameliorate β-thalassemia symptoms (ibid; 328:810A) other therapies include iron chelation–early use of deferiprone (ibid 1995; 332:918OA) deferoxamine in thalassemia major ↓ the transfusion-related iron overload and helps protect against DM, cardiac disease, and early death (ibid 1994; 331:567OA, 574OA) a serum ferritin of ≤ 2500 ng/mL is reported to provide an optimal result as may BM transplantation with HLA-identical donors, or reconstitution with cord-blood stem cells (ibid 1995; 332:367OA)

thalidomide 2,6-dioxo-3-phthalimido-piperidine A drug that was first marketed as a sedative and sleeping aid, which was held responsible for 12-15 000 cases of embryopathy that impacted on the embryo between days 45 to 55 of gestation, with one dose being enough to cause birth defects, often in the form of phocomelia or 'flipper' extremities; the thalidomide tragedy is a chilling example of the effects of stereochemistry; L-thalidomide is a powerful tranquilizer; the D- form is teratogenic (see Chirality), possibly acting by causing lysosomal defects, as occurs in the Japanese quails, the animal model of thalidomide embryopathy; thalidomide has a new generation of indications, including the treatment of rheumatoid arthritis, photodermatitis, Behçet's disease, SL, and GVH disease; it is also of use in treating the skin lesions of lepromatous leprosy (erythema nodosum leprosum, available in the US as an investigational drug; other leprosy agents include clofazimine, rifampin and dapsone or diaminodiphenyl sulfone)

thalidomide neuropathy A severe polyneuropathy that occurs in up 25% of those treated with thalidomide as a sedative, or higher in those for whom it is used to treat GVHD, as the doses of the thalidomide are much higher; in 50% the loss of sensation is permanent (N Engl J Med 1992; 326:1055OA, 327:735C)

thallium stress test Pharmacologic stress imaging CARDIOLOGY A myocardial perfusion technique in which the radionuclide thallium-201 (^{201}Tl), is injected as a diagnostic adjunct to cardiac stress tests, with the purpose of detecting regional ischemia or infarcts; TST is an increasingly popular alternative to the exercise stress test for evaluating patients with coronary artery disease who cannot perform an adequate exercise stress test, and allows risk stratification; in TST, dipyridamole is infused IV producing marked coronary arteriolar vasodilation, leaving the peripheral arterioles relatively intact; dipyridamole also prevents cell uptake of adenosine, potentiating the agent's vasodilatory effect; in the myocardial regions perfused by normal coronary arteries, blood flow ↑ in the endocardium and epicardium, indicating normal coronary artery reserve; in coronary artery stenosis, there is diminished uptake and clearance of intravenously administered ^{201}Tl, resulting in an initial ^{201}Tl defect that is followed by a delayed redistribution in images viewed 2-4 hours after injection; the side effects induced by dipyridamole are immediately reversible with aminophylline (JAMA 1991; 265:633rv) TYPES STRESS IMAGING Images that identify perfusion defects during exercise REDISTRIBUTION IMAGING Images obtained after a 3-4 hour rest period to identify 'redistribution' of the isotope; Cf Treadmill stress test

Note: In many regions of viable 'hibernating' myocardium, there are defects that appear during stress imaging and which do not disappear upon redistribution imaging, thus falsely simulating irreversible lesions; a minibolus of thallium-

201 at 3-4 hours ('REINJECTION IMAGING') delineates areas that might have otherwise been considered non-viable (N Engl J Med 1990; 323:141); see Treadmill exercise test

THAM Tris(hydroxymethyl)aminomethane Tris buffer EMERGENCY MEDICINE An amine proton donor that is administered IV during early CPR to treat lactic acidosis; THAM is regarded by some to be a completely interchangeable substitute for sodium bicarbonate at the same dosages (in mEq), acting to neutralize fixed acids in tissues ADVANTAGES THAM is not a CO_2 donor, thus hyperventilation of an already compromised patient is not required in order to 'blow off' the CO_2 and it easily enters the intracellular spaces DISADVANTAGES THAM causes apnea, hypoglycemia, venous irritation, and because it is a powder requiring mixture, it is difficult to use in a true emergency

thanatophoric dwarfism *thanatos*, Greek, death, *phoric*, bearing Chondrodysplasia punctata dwarfism of Conradi-Hünermann An AD [MIM 187600] form of dwarfism with a 2:1 ♂:♀ ratio, in which the infants are stillborn or die in the early neonatal period; it is the most common form of lethal congenital skeletal dysplasia CLINICAL Hydrocephaly, megalocephaly with frontal bossing, chondrodystrophy, narrow thorax with respiratory difficulties, congenital heart disease, hypotonia and hyporeflexia (floppy infant), hypertelorism, 'cloverleaf' skull, saddle nose, marked skeletal abnormalities with shortened deformed 'telephone receiver' long bones, affecting the epiphysis, causing micromelia, alteration of the foot, lenticular opacity, shortened extremities with curved fingers, H- or U-shaped vertebrae and pulmonary hypoplasia resulting in short postnatal survival

thaumatin A 207 amino acid heterodimeric protein produced by the African fruit katemfe, *Thaumatococcus danielli* Benth, which like monellin is a sweet protein that binds specifically with taste receptors, eliciting a sensation of sweetness that is 100 000 times sweeter than sugar on a molar basis, given that thaumatin has a greater affinity than dextrose for the sweet taste receptor (Bio/Technology 1992; 10:561) see Monellin, Sweet protein; Cf Artificial sweeteners

Thayer-Martin agar MICROBIOLOGY An enriched chocholate agar-based growth medium, which incorporates antibiotics (colistin, nystatin, trimethoprim lactate, vancomycin); TMA is used to selectively identify *Neisseria* spp, including *N gonorrhoeae*, *N meningitidis*, *N lactamina*, *N flavescens*, and some strains of *Branhamella catarrhalis*; growth of *N sicca*, *Candida albicans*, *Escherichia coli*, and *Staphylococcus epidermidis* are inhibited

THBR Thyroid hormone binding ratio, see there

THC Tetrahydrocannabinol(s) Any of a family of compounds present in *Cannabis sativa* var *indica*, the major constituent of which is the Δ^1-3,4-*trans* isomer, also known as $^9\Delta$-THC; (figure) the only FDA-sanctioned use of $^9\Delta$-THC is as an anti-emetic, and then is only of use in a highly selected group of patients, given this compound's well-known hallucinogenic properties; see Marijuana

THC receptor A receptor that is specific for tetrahydrocannabinol; the once elusive TR, aka cannabinoid (marijuana) receptor has been identified and has characteristics of a G protein-coupled receptor found in the brain and neural cell lines which inhibits adenylate cyclase activity in a dose-dependent, stereoselective fashion; see Marijuana

THCA Trihydroxycoprostanoic acid syndrome, see there

theca cell tumor A sex cord-stromal tumor of the post-menopausal ovary that is yellow, large and unilateral, composed of fascicles of lipid-rich spindle cells interspersed with collagen, reticulin fibers and hyaline plaques; thecomas and other estrogen-producing tumors, eg granulosa cell tumors may induce adenomatous hyperplasia of the endometrium or well-differentiated endometrial carcinoma in 3-20% of cases; see Sex cord-stromal tumors

theophylline Used for asthma Action Smooth muscle relaxation, diuretic and CNS stimulant WARNING Associated with seizures and cardiac arrhythmias etc

therapeutic apheresis A form of exchange transfusion in which blood is removed from a patient, and

1) Plasma is replaced (plasmapheresis‡) with a volume of albumin or various crystalloid solutions, or

2) Cells are removed (cell apheresis) to either prevent or reduce leukostasis (leukapheresis‡) in the brain and renal arteries, or to reduce thrombotic phenomena (platelet apheresis‡)

Note: In the working parlance, the adjective *therapeutic* is usually deleted

therapeutic crisis PSYCHIATRY A generic term for any abrupt and extreme change in the course of therapy in either the positive or negative direction

therapeutic drug monitoring CLINICAL PHARMACOLOGY The regular measurement of the serum levels of those drugs (common drugs monitored include carbamazepine, digoxin, gentamycin, NAPA/procainamide, phenobarbital, phenytoin, theophylline, tobramycin, valproic acid, vancomycin) that require close 'titration' of doses in order to ensure that there are sufficient levels in the blood to be therapeutically effective, while avoiding potentially toxic excess; drug concentration in vivo is a function of multiple factors (table)

therapeutic index CLINICAL PHARMACOLOGY The ratio of a drug's toxic level to its therapeutic level, calculated as the toxic concentration (TC) of a drug divided by the effective concentration, expressed as TC_{50}/EC_{50}, a point at which 50% of patients have a toxic reaction to the drug being monitored; the lower the therapeutic index, the more difficult it is to titrate a drug's dose in a patient and the more imperative it is that the drug be monitored; see Apparent volume of distribution, First-order kinetics, Peak levels, Trough levels, Volume of distribution, Zero-order kinetics

therapeutic misadventure An unintentional (or 'functional') overdose of a therapeutic agent due to unanticipated effects of extraneous factor (s), eg acetaminophen hepatotoxicity in alcoholics, due to cytochrome P-450 induction (N Engl J Med 1993; 329:1862ʀᴠ)

therapeutic privilege MEDICAL ETHICS A paternalistic principle under which the truth is withheld from a patient owing to concern that if the details of a therapeutic procedure are fully delineated, the patient may choose to forego an operation that the physician believes to be in the patient's best interest or his only option for improved quality of life and/or survival; since therapeutic privilege assumes in part that the patient is something less than an autonomous, self-directed person, 'therapeutic privilege' is rarely invoked in the US as a justification for surrogate decision-making, given the fear of litigation on the part of physicians; in the US, a physician's moral duty is to tell the truth, regardless of the potential harm that may result from a patient receiving too much information that he may be incapable of understanding; see *Arato* v *Avedon*, Doctor-patient interaction, Paternalism

'therapeutic privilege' doctrine LEGAL MEDICINE A doctrine with legal weight that protects the physician when faced with a patient who may be too emotional or apprehensive to fully and logically assess his needs for a thera-

THERAPEUTIC DRUG LEVELS IN VIVO (factors involved)

PATIENT COMPLIANCE Ingestion of drug in the doses prescribed

BIOAVAILABILITY Access to circulation, interaction with cognate receptor(s); ionized and 'free', or bound to a carrier molecule, often albumin

PHARMACOKINETICS Drug equilibrium requires 4-6 half-lives of drug clearance (a period of time for ½ of the drug to 'clear', either through metabolism or excretion, multiplied by 4-6); the drug is affected by

1) Interaction with foods or other drugs at the site of absorption, eg tetracycline binding to cations or chelation with binding resins, eg bile acid-binding cholestyramine that also sequesters warfarin, thyroxine and digitoxin or interactions of various drugs with each other, eg digitalis with quinidine resulting in a 3-fold decrease in digitalis clearance

2) Absorption may be changed by GI hypermotility or large molecule size

3) Lipid solubility, which affects the volume of distribution; highly lipid-soluble substances have high affinity for adipose tissue and a low tendency to remain in the vascular compartment, see Volume of distribution

4) Biotransformation, with 'first pass' elimination by hepatic metabolism, in which polar groups are introduced into relatively insoluble molecules by oxidation, reduction or hydrolysis; for elimination, lipid-soluble drugs require the 'solubility' steps of glucuronidation or sulfatation in the liver; water-soluble molecules are eliminated directly via the kidneys, weak acidic drugs are eliminated by active tubular secretion that may be altered by therapy with methotrexate, penicillin, probenecid, salicylates, phenylbutazone and thiazide diuretics Kinetics i) First order kinetics The elimination of a drug is proportional to its concentration ii) Zero order kinetics Drug elimination is independent of the drug's concentration

PHYSIOLOGICAL FACTORS

1) Age Lower doses are required in both infants and the elderly, in the former because the metabolic machinery is not fully operational, in the latter because the machinery is decaying, with decreased cardiac and renal function, enzyme activity, density of receptors on the cell surfaces and decreased albumin, the major drug transporting molecule

2) Enzyme induction, which is involved in a drug's metabolism may reduce the drug's activity; enzyme-inducing drugs include barbiturates, carbamazepine, glutethimide, phenytoin, primidone, rifampicin

2) Enzyme inhibition, which is involved in drug metabolism, resulting in enhanced drug activity, prolonging the action of various drugs, including chloramphenicol, cimetidine, disulfiram (Antabuse), isoniazid, methyldopa, metronidazole, phenylbutazone and sulfonamides

GENETIC FACTORS play an as yet poorly defined role in therapeutic drug monitoring, as is the case of the poor ability of some racial groups to acetylate drugs

CONCOMITANT DISEASE, ie whether there are underlying conditions that may affect drug distribution or metabolism, eg renal disease with ↓ clearance and ↑ drug levels, or hepatic disease, in which there is ↓ albumin production and ↓ enzyme activity result in a functional ↑ in drug levels, due to ↓ availability of drug-carrying proteins; therapeutic drug monitoring requires that

1) The method measures what it is designed to measure, and not bioinactive metabolites and has a turn-around time short enough to allow adjustment of doses

2) The method encompasses a well-defined therapeutic range, and the toxic and therapeutic ranges are close enough to require monitoring, and tolerance to the drug does not develop

3) The concentration of the drug in the serum is proportional to the concentration at the site of action (ie at the receptor) and there is a correlation between the concentration in the serum and the therapeutic effect

peutic intervention; such situations may arise in emergencies, advanced age, and dementia; when possible, the physician should obtain permission from the nearest relative; see Good Samaritan laws; Cf Doctor-patient interaction, Informed consent, Paternalism

therapeutic rating CLINICAL PHARMACOLOGY A rating assigned by the US Food and Drug Administration (FDA) to drugs based on therapeutic efficacy, where an A-rated drug presents an important therapeutic gain, a B-rated agent has a moderate therapeutic gain, and a C-rated agent is viewed as having little or no therapeutic value (N Engl J Med 1992; 327:1135sa)

therapeutic turnaround time LABORATORY MEDICINE The time elapsed between the point at which a decision is made to measure a parameter (eg glucose levels) on which a therapeutic decision is to be made and the point at which the values of interest are available (MLO Today September 1994) see Turnaround time

therapeutic vaccine see Vaccine therapy

therapeutic window The range of a drug's concentration in which the desired effect occurs, below which there is little desired effect and above which toxic effects appear; the therapeutic window differs among patients and may be determined empirically; see Therapeutic drug monitoring; Cf Window

thermic energy of feeding PHYSIOLOGY A metabolic value that corresponds to the energy cost of feeding, which includes the energy expended in the digestion, transportation, and storage of nutrients and metabolic products; the TEF represents approximately 10% of the total energy expenditure (N Engl J Med 1995; 332:621oa) see Total energy expenditure

thermocycler MOLECULAR BIOLOGY A device used in polymerase chain reaction that cycles between a low (72°C) temperature in which a round of DNA synthesis occurs, and a high temperature of 95°C, during which the newly formed DNA duplexes are melted to prepare for another round of synthesis of DNA; the thermocycler is a critical component of efficient PCR, a technique that has revolutionized retrieval of minute amounts of DNA from a specimen, see PCR, Taq polymerase

thermography A transiently popular method for diagnosing breast cancer which is based on the ↑ warmth of skin overlying malignancy, a relatively nonspecific finding that also occurs in mastitis; the technique was abandoned due to the unacceptably high rates of false positivity and false negativity; Cf Mammography, Xeroradiography

thermoluminescence PALEOANTHROPOLOGY A dating method borrowed from solid-state physics that measures time by testing for minute radiation-induced damage to crystals, which ↑ with age; in TL the sample is heated (and therefore can only measure a sample once) to excite the electrons, which leave the crystal lattice, giving off a flash of light that is directly proportional to the stored energy, whih can be measured with a photomultiplier; determination of the age of a specimen is based on correlation with samples of known age; TL has been instrumental in providing the oldest dates for anatomically modern human beings in the Near East and Africa, as it is accurate in the periods that cannot be measured by standard dating methods (Science 1990; 247:798n&c) Cf Electron-spin resonance

*Carbon-14 dating methods reach only 40 000 years in the past, and potassium-argon dating begins counting at 300 000 years

thermoreversible gel AIDS A generic term for a temperature-sensitive gel which acting alone or in consort with anti-HIV agents may be capable of blocking entry of HIV to vaginal, cervical, or anal mucosa; TGs are at early (ie prehuman) stages of development; if successful in animal studies, TGs might be used to coat said mucosa prior to copulatory activity, providing a modicum of protection against STDs (JAMA 1995 273:979)

thesaurocytes Flame cells, see there

thiazolidinedione Any of a family of tyrosine kinase inhibitors that inhibit epidermal growth factor receptor and Src in vitro, that are bisubstrate inhibitors that compete with both protein substrate and ATP (Science 1995; 267:1782)

'thick' section A hardened epoxy resin-embedded section of a tissue measuring 0.5-1.5 µm in thickness that is cut from the same block of tissue as the 'thin' sections to be examined by transmission electron microscopy; examination of 'thick' toluidine blue-stained sections by light microscopy allows rapid selection of the optimal tissue for ultrastructural studies; Cf Thin section

Note: Sections for routine histologic examination by light microscopy are 4-6 µm in thickness and are embedded in paraffin

thin-layer chromatography LABORATORY MEDICINE A technique in which a thin layer of alumina, polyacrylamide gel, silica gel, or starch gel is bonded to a glass or plastic plate and then bathed for 30-90 minutes in a solvent containing a substance of interest, allowing the substance to migrate by capillary action; if further identification of the substance is required, the 'spot' of drug may be scraped off for further analysis by gas-liquid chromatography; TLC is often used to 'screen' for the presence of drugs of abuse; see Therapeutic drug monitoring

thin section A 0.05 µm in thickness section of epoxy resin-embedded tissue that is stained with a heavy metal, eg lead or uranium for examination by transmission electron microscopy; Cf Thick section

think tank An institution or organization composed of similarly minded individuals (often from diverse backgrouns) that evaluates data in an area of broad and proposes theoretical solutions to a particular problem of society or technology; see Rand corporation

thioredoxin A ubiquitous 12-kD protein that donates electrons to ribonucleotide reductase, which also has disulfide isomerase activity, as determined by its ability to catalyze the reactivation of reduced and denatured ribonuclease (rRNase) and ribnuclease (RNase)

thiosulfate-citrate-bile salts-sucrose agar see TCBS agar

third-day blues Postpartum 'blues', see there

third disease Rubella, see there

'third diabetic syndrome' A form of DM described in young black patients that is thought to differ from type I (insulin-dependent/juvenile onset) diabetes in that 1) 30-40% have HLA-DR3 or HLA-DR4 antigen, in contrast to whites, 95% of whom express HLA-DR3 or -DR4 2) 40% have islet cell antibodies, versus 70-80% of whites 3) Most patients are easily controlled by diet or oral anti-diabetes agents and 4) the inheritance pattern appears to be autosomal dominant

third generation cephalosporins A group of broad-spectrum antibiotics including cefatoxime, ceftazidime, ceftriaxone and moxalactam that are structurally related to penicillins and used against penicillinase-producing bacteria; third-generation agents have increased activity against enteric bacteria, are stable against the β-lactamases of *Haemophilus influenzae* and *Neisseria gonorrhoeae*, have a longer serum half-life than the first generation cephalosporins and thus can be administered twice per day, successfully cross the blood-brain barrier and are thus effective against gram-negative central nervous system infections

FIRST GENERATION CEPHALOSPORINS, eg cephalothin, cephaloridine and cefazolin are effective against penicillinase-producing streptococci, pneumococci and staphylococci and active against important gram-negative pathogens, eg *Escherichia coli, Klebsiella* and *Proteus*, having prophylactic currency in intra-abdominal surgical procedures and is of use in treating penicillinase-binding *Staphylococcus aureus* SECOND GENERATION CEPHALOSPORINS, eg cefamandole, cefoxitin and cefuroxime offer only minimal improvement over the first generation, although cefoxitin is of use in treating *Bacteroides fragilis* infections; 'serious' systemic infections are usually treated by third generation cephalosporins FOURTH GENERATION CEPHALOSPORINS do not exist and would need to be active against methicillin-resistant staphylococci and enterococci

third-generation TSH (thyrotropin) assay LABORATORY MEDICINE A term referring to the sensitivity of the current genereration of immunometric assays for thyrotropin (TSH), ie ± 0.01 mIU/L*; the earlier TSH assays were sensitive enough to dtect hyperthyroidism in patients with nonthyroid diseases (Am Clin Lab Dec 1994/Jan 1995, p18)

*The first generation is sensitive to 1 mIU/L; the second-generation is sensitive to 0.07 mIU/L

third generation vaccine DNA vaccine, see there

third heart sound S_3 gallop A heart sound that has been traditionally regarded as a sign of left ventricular systolic dysfunction (heart failure); its significance differs according to the valve involved and the type of underlying defect; prevalence of third heart sounds: Mitral regurgitation 46%; aortic regurgitation 28%; aortic stenosis 11%; mitral stenosis 8% (N Engl J Med 1992; 327:458OA)

third-line therapy Any alternative to conventional (surgery, chemo– or radiotherapy) treatment for malignancy; such therapies are highly experimental, rarely successful, may be accompanied by significant morbidity, and often represent acts of therapeutic desperation on the part of the clinician and/or patient; Cf Unproven forms of cancer therapy

third nuclear age GLOBAL VILLAGE An evolving period of world history, the prelude of which coincided with the collapse of the former Soviet Union; in the second nuclear age, nuclear arms were controlled through compliance with the Nuclear Nonproliferation Treaty (NPT), the global pact that prohibits other nations from 'going nuclear', which was signed in 1970; the playing field has changed considerably, as 1) Nuclear scientists from the former Soviet Union have made their expertise available to governments that wish to have a 'bomb', 2) A number of nations are known or presumed to have the 'bomb', eg India, Israel, Pakistan, and North Korea, and 3) Other nations may develop the capacity within ten years; these factors all contribute to the belief by many experts that a nuclear skirmish is a real possibility within the foreseeable future (US News & World Report 17 April, p39)

The first nuclear age began in 1949, when the Soviet Union expoded an atomic bomb, ending the US monopoly on nuclear weapons; the second nuclear age followed, where the 'Nuclear Club' of five nuclear powers (US, Russia, UK, China, and France) managed to survive the 'cold war' with strategies that followed well-defined rules of deterrence and crisis management

third party HEALTH CARE INDUSTRY A person or organization ancillary to the doctor-patient 'dyad', who/that participates in financing the services rendered, eg a health insurance carrier, or who acts as an administrative agent for processing and paying claims or for health care services provided, eg Blue Cross/Blue Shield, Medicare

third sector Voluntary sector, see there

third space A non-physiologic space into which fluids may pass in emergency clinical situations, the actual size of which is calculated with difficulty; the intracellular space comprises 65-80% of the body fluid volume, and the extracellular space comprises the remaining 20-35%, of which 25-35% is plasma volume and 65-75% is interstitial volume; the 'third space phenomenon' is an emergency situation in which a derangement of 'Starling' forces* allows sequestration of fluids into relatively nonfunctional extracellular 'compartments', eg within the lumen in intestinal obstruction, to the skin in burns, to the pleura or peritoneum in vascular rupture or ascites, or elsewhere; fluid replacement calculations are based on the first and second spaces, and are of little use in determining internal redistribution or 'parasitic losses' of fluid into third spaces; third space losses are treated with saline solutions or crystalloids and 'titration' with blood pressure; see Starling forces

*Starling forces are the sum of the positive intravascular oncotic pressure and the negative pressure provided by the venous flow, which act to maintain fluid in the vessels, minus the oncotic pressure in the interstitial space and the for-

ward pressures of the blood as it is 'driven' into the capillaries, both of which act to pull fluid from the intravascular space

'third spacing' A colloquial term for hemorrhage or other accumulation of fluids into the so-called third physiologic compartment, the interstitial space between the skin and fascia (R Preston, The Hot Zone, Random House, New York, 1994)

thirteen-day fever Shanghai fever A typhoid-like *Pseudomonas* infection described in the tropics, characterized by fever, myalgia and diarrhea that resolves spontaneously without residua

thomsonism ALTERNATIVE MEDICINE A health care philosophy of largely historic interest that was espoused by S Thomson (1769-1843), a farmer and 'endowed healer' from New Hampshire, who qualified the ancient Greek doctrine of disease being the imbalance of the four 'bodily fluids' (blood, phlegm, yellow bile and black bile) with the modifiers of hot and cold, wet and dry; Thomson concluded that cold was the ultimate pathologic state and sought to cleanse the body, adding to the body's heat by using *Lobelia inflata*, as an emetic and in enemas; see Alternative medicine, Homeopathy, Hot-cold syndrome, Naturopathy

thoracic duct *Ductus thoracicus* [NA6] A large lymphatic channel that extends from the upper chylous cistern opposite the upper lumbar vertebrae, passing through the aortic orifice of the diaphragm, anterior to the thoracic vertebrae, reaching the root of the neck to the left of the esophagus, arching downward to empty into the junction between the left internal jugular and subclavian veins; the TD is of considerable functional importance as it drains all the lymph below the diaphragm, and from the left side above the diaphragm, which is rich in mature T cells; at one time chronic thoracic duct drainage was proposed as a method of immunosuppression

thoracic inlet *Apertura thoracis superior* [NA6] The opening of the thoracic cavity which is bound anteriorly by the manubrium of the sternum, posteriorly by the 1st thoracic vertebra and on the sides by the first ribs

thoracic inlet injury Traumatic injury to the base of the neck involving the superior mediastinal vessels (innominate, subclavian, proximal common carotid arteries and veins); damaged vessels in the thoracic inlet are surgically problematic as facile access is blocked by the clavicosternal 'shield'; although the correlation of anatomic defects with clinical symptoms is poor, adequate regional exploration and hemostasis in this region results in reduced mortality

thoracic outlet *Apertura thoracis inferior* [NA6] A tight anatomic compartment that extends from the 12th thoracic vertebrae posteriorly along the arch of the rib to the intrasternal angle anteriorly; the sides are formed by the 11th and 12th ribs and is closed by the diaphragm; the TO contains vessels and nerves that are either resident, in or traverse through the space

thoracic outlet syndrome Scalenus syndrome Any of a group of conditions characterized by compression of the inner branches of the brachial plexus and/or subclavian artery, related among other factors, to kinking of vessels over a cervical rib, fibrous bands passing from a prominent transverse process of the 7th cervical vertebra to the first rib, or edge of the scalenus anterior or medius muscle(s) CLINICAL Pain, unilateral paresthesiae along the medial border of the arm, forearm, and little finger, ischemia, atrophy of the small hand muscles, especially of the thenar eminence, myalgia, myasthenia, with vasomotor disorders, edema and thromboses; TOS most commonly affects women with osteoporosis, and may also occur in pregnancy, trauma or overstretching; compromise of this space causes specific 'syndromes', including cervical rib syndrome, scalenus anticus syndrome, costoclavicular syndrome, pectoralis minor syndrome, and the first rib syndrome; although vascular compromise occurs in 90% of these syndromes, the symptoms are predominantly neurogenic (N Engl J Med 1993; 329:2013cc)

Thorburn's position FORENSIC PATHOLOGY A peculiar reflex position assumed by the elbows immediately after injury to the spinal cord in the lower cervical region; the reflex is of broad popular interest as the Thorburn position was assumed by John F Kennedy at the time of his assassination in Dallas (22 November 1963) and is regarded as evidence *against* the popular (but widely regarded as invalid) 'JFK assassination conspiracy' theory (JAMA 1993; 269:1544sc) see 'Magic bullet' theory

'thorn apple' appearance A descriptor for the yellow-brown spherical ammonium biurate crystals with long irregular spikes, found in normal alkaline urinary sediment, structures that have been likened to thorn apples, the fruit of the jimsonweed, *Datura stramonium*

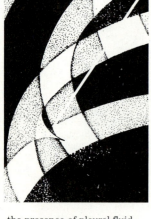

thorn sign RADIOLOGY A vaguely defined spicular radiologic shadow (figure, here enhanced for didactic purposes) that tapers medially from the lateral chest wall, which corresponds to a thickening of the minor fissure, most commonly seen in a right-sided pleural effusion; since the finding appears in most positions, the thorn sign should prompt a lateral decubitus film and ultrasonography to confirm the presence of pleural fluid

Thorotrast Thorium dioxide $^{232}ThO_2$ A radiocontrast medium that emits α particles, has a $T_{1/2}$ of 400 years and is stored in the reticuloendothelial system; Thorotrast was first used in 1928, and was abandoned in 1947 with reports of Thorotrast-induced tumors (TITs); the prototypic TIT is hepatic angiosarcoma, but cholangiocarcinoma and hepatocellular carcinomas are also related to throrotrast (rarely, all three tumors may occur in the same patient, Cancer 1982; 49:2161), as can be leukemias, lymphomas, carcinoma of the lung, kidney and bladder, head and neck sarcomas, mesothelioma and malignant fibrous histiocytoma; see Radiothor, Radium Dial Company

threatened abortion OBSTETRICS Vaginal bleeding at any time within the first 20 weeks of pregnancy, accompanied by colicky pain, backache and a bright red to brownish discharge, occurring in up to 20% of early pregnancies of which one-half progress to inevitable abortion, no therapy is consistently effective, although bed rest, analgesics and sedatives are advised

3/B translocation syndrome A congenital complex due to translocation of a chromosomal fragment from chromosome 3 to a 'B' chromosome (chromosome number 4 or 5), which affects 40% of the progeny of ♀ carriers, causing craniofacial and cardiac anomalies, cleft lip and palate; 15% of the children born to ♂ carriers have the disease, but all are stillborn

three-day fever Pappataci fever A dengue-like infectious disease described in the Balkans and elsewhere in Southern Europe, resulting from the injection of an unidentified virus by the sandfly, *Phlebotomus papatasi*

Three Mile Island ENVIRONMENT A nuclear power plant near Pittsburgh, Pennsylvania that approached core meltdown in 1979 due to delayed recognition of equipment malfunction; no injuries occurred, but the incident resulted in a costly cleanup; see Chernobyl, Goiania; Cf Sellafield

'three-piece suits' A colloquial and nonspecific term for any businessman, which in the health care industry, includes 'medicrats' (MD/MPHs, ie physicians with a master's degree in public health, hospital administrators), pharmaceutical representatives ('detail men'), and 'bean counters' (financial officers), who function in a medical center's bureacracy; see Medicrats, Pencil-pushers, Suits and suites 'syndrome'

threshold The limit at which point a physiological effect takes place, eg threshold of the renal tubules for the absorption of solutes and threshold of photoreceptors for light

threshold limit value OCCUPATIONAL MEDICINE The concentration of an airborne chemical or potentially toxic (measured in ppm/L/hour exposure) or radioactive substance (measured in microcuries) below which employees may work over an eight-hour period without known adverse effect

thrifty genotype hypothesis A hypothesis ascribing survival advantages to a certain degree of insulin resistance in conditions of caloric deprivation that might prove diabetogenic in conditions of caloric adequacy or affluence; the increases in obesity and NIDDM among Native Americans as they move to a more affluent lifestyle and diet favor the hypothesis, while it is challenged by the finding of somewhat opposite effects in those with a thrifty phenotype (N Engl J Med 1994; 331:1226oa)

thrifty phenotype An 'anemic' morphotype that results from malnutrition during fetal and early postnatal life, leading to metabolic dysfunction as adults and insulin resistance; Cf Thrifty genotype hypothesis

thrill CARDIOLOGY A palpable murmur that correlates with zones of maximum intensity of auscultated sounds; rough lower sternal border thrills occur in ventricular septal defect, apical systolic thrills are associated with mitral valve insufficiency; diastolic thrills may be palpated in atrioventricular valvular stenosis

thrombolysis The dissolution of a blood clot or thrombus

thrombolytic therapy A generic term for any therapy, usually understood to mean the use of enzymes (see below, agents), intended to promote the dissolution of intravascular blood clots and/or fibrin thrombi and the digestion of fibrinogen and other proteins, and effect immediate recanalization of occluded vessels (usually arteries) with immediate improvement of circulatory flow; in acute MI, the efficacy of TT hinges on the time elapsed between the onset of symptoms and the administration of therapy; prehospital administration of TT is thought to reduce mortality of cardiac origin (N Engl J Med 1993; 329:383oa; 703rv) INDICATIONS PTE, eg acute massive pulmonary embolus, deep venous thrombosis, acute myocardial infarction, and peripheral artery disease in the form of arterial thrombi LABORATORY TT results in

1) ↓ $α_2$-antiplasmin, coagulation factors (V, VIII:C, IX, XI, XII), fibrinogen, and plasminogen, see there

2) Prolonged aPTT, PT, and thrombin time

3) ↑ FDPs (eg D-dimer), plasmin, 15-42 kD β-related peptides

AGENTS Urokinase, streptokinase, and newer agents, eg acylated plasminogen streptokinase complex (APSAC), pro-urokinase, tPA (tissue plasminogen activator) CONTRAINDICATIONS Active internal bleeding or hemorrhagic diathesis; intracranial hemorrhage, neoplasia, or surgery, recent CVA, or intraspinal surgery (**Laboratory Medicine 1995; 26:330OA**) see Reperfusion therapy

thrombomodulin A 68-kD endothelial cell membrane receptor that mediates anticoagulation, binding thrombin and catalyzing its transformation into protein C activator Pro-C(a), which in the presence of calcium, causes a 30 000-fold increase in activated protein C; thrombomodulin and coumadin both inactivate protein C and in coumadin-induced necrosis, protein C is reduced; Pro-C(a) is constantly inactivating factors Va and VIIIa prior to indiscriminate intravascular coagulation

thromboplastin Tissue factor, see there

thrombopoietin Any of a group of proteins produced in a variety of tissues that regulate the quantity of megakaryocyte-committed stem cells, modulating the maturation and development of platelets; the prototypic thrombopoietin is a 35 000 M_r polypeptide cytokine with a two domain structure with an amino-terminal domain homologous to erythropoietin and a carboxy-terminal domain rich in serine, threonine, and proline; megakaryocytic colony stimulation and platelet elevation are evoked by thrombopoietin-Mpl interaction (**Nature 1994; 369:533A, 565L, 568L, 571L, 519N&V**)

thrombospondin A glycoprotein composed of three 145-kD subunits each of which has several globular domains with different binding specificities; it is stored in the α granules of platelets and secreted at the site of vascular injury, binding to the arginine-glycine-aspartic acid oligopeptide or RGD sequence; thrombospondin mediates interactions of adhesive proteins with integrin receptors, binding platelets to cells at the glycoprotein-IV (CD36) receptor; it is present in platelets, fibroblasts, endothelial cells and in the extracellular matrix, where it binds to collagen V, fibrinogen and fibronectin and is ↑ in inflammation, wounding and stress Note: It may also bind erythroid stem cells to stromal regulatory cells in the formation of erythroblast islands; see Integrin family
Synonyms include thrombin-sensitive protein, endogenous platelet lectin, glycoprotein G

thrombosthenin Platelet actomyosin A contractile protein that acs for 15-20% of the platelet's total protein, which is comprised of platelet actin (thrombosthenin A) and platelet myosin (thrombosthenin M); platelet actin is a 43–55-kD globular protein that polymerizes to form elongated 6 nm in thickness filaments with a 35-nm axial periodicity; platelet myosin is an asymmetric 460-kD molecule that is dissociable into 4 subunits; thrombosthenin functions in a manner similar to the actinomysin system of muscle, forming a sarcomere-like contractile unit, and appears to be regulated by ancillary proteins, including tropomyosin, troponin, α-actinin, gelsolin, profilin, spectrin, and others in an as yet undefined fashion

thrombotic thrombocytopenic purpura A rare (1:10⁶/year) disorder of the microcirculation most common in ♀ age 20-50 CLINICAL Moschcowitz's pentad: Thrombocytopenia, splenomegaly, varying neurological signs, DIC, and fever, as well as pallor, jaundice, thrombosis, fibrin thrombi in renal vessels, heart, liver and spleen, epistaxis, cerebral, retinal and vaginal hemorrhage, neurologic defects, eg headache, confusion, aphasia, transient paresis, ataxia, sensory disturbances and coma, cardiac dysfunction, hepatomegaly and pancreatitis; TTP may be associated with SLE, rheumatoid arthritis and Sjögren syndrome LABORATORY ↓ platelets, usually < 50 000/mm³, normal coagulation factors, ↓ complement proteins, Coomb's-negative microangiopathic hemolytic anemia (often severe, 30% have ↓ hemoglobin < 55g/L, US: < 5.5 g/dl) and reticulocytosis), schistocytes, burr cells, helmet-shaped erythrocytes, normoblasts, and reticulocytosis, ↑ unconjugated bilirubin, ↑ plasma hemoglobin, ↑ hemosiderin, ↓ haptoglobin, proteinuria PATHOGENESIS Platelet-

aggregating factor and/or multimers of factor VIII:vWF (von Willebrand factor) induce TTP-related platelet agglutination, a phenomenon reversed by immunoglobulin therapy, implying absence of antibodies normally responsible for inhibiting platelet aggregation and ↓ endothelial ability to stimulate prostaglandin G synthesis TREATMENT Corticosteroids, aspirin, dipyridamole; if no response, plasmapheresis Note: TTP has been recently recognized to be a polar form of a condition, at the other end of which is hemolytic-uremic syndrome, see there, TTP-HUS

thromboxane Any of a family of substances produced from arachidonic acid by cyclo-oxygenase, which generates prostaglandin G₂ that is subsequently converted by thromboxane (Tx) synthetase into the most biologically important product, TxA₂, which increases after vascular injury, eliciting a primary hemostatic response, inducing platelet aggregation and vasoconstriction; TxA₂ also inhibits platelet adenylate cyclase, reducing cAMP and mobilizing calcium; see Arachidonic acid

throughput LABORATORY MEDICINE An adjective pertaining or referring to the volume of specimens that are processed in a given period of time, usually per hour or per 24-hour period, which is a critical parameter considered in instrument purchases, and for commercial laboratories; in the rapidly evolving commercial diagnostic environment, enterprises (eg MetPATH, Smith-Kline, and others) grow by merger measure profit based on 'economy-of-scale' which hinges on throughput; see Turnaround time

'throw-away journal' A medical journal that is received gratis or by non-paid subscription, which contains (in general) non-peer-reviewed articles, often in the form of reviews; 'throw-aways' are in large part supported by advertising, and have an advertisement/article ratio that is significantly higher than that of their academic counterpart, the 'peer-reviewed journal' (**JAMA 1991; 266:2830c**); 'throw-aways' are broad in the scope of material covered, may provide adequate reviews of emerging areas and relevant updates, have abbreviated bibliographies; a major criticism of 'throw-aways' is that their significant sponsorship by commercial entities with vested interest, eg the pharmaceutical industry, may bias the medical care provided by health professionals; Cf Peer-reviewed journal

thrush Pseudomembranous candidiasis A term of waning popularity first used by Pepys in 1665, that refers to an erythematous intraoral lesion overlaid by white, creamy patches, which correspond to necrotic debris, squames, fibrin, inflammatory cells, abundant fungal hyphae and bacteria

thrush breast appearance A descriptor for the patchy lesions of fatty metamorphosis of the endocardium and papillary muscle, which is most prominent in the left ventricle, caused by prolonged hypoxia, where red-brown myocardium alternates with yellow bands of fatty degeneration; a similar lesion may be caused by diphtheria, see Flabby heart

Thucydides 'syndrome' MEDICAL HISTORY The Plague of Athens (430 to 427 BC) decimated Athens' population of 300 000 and probably signaled the end of Greek civilization, which had in two generations created or nurtured the basic pursuits of philosophy, history, tragedy, comedy and democracy; the Greek general, Thucydides, recorded the plague's clinical features, which are variously postulated to have been due to smallpox, bubonic plague, scarlet fever, typhus, measles, typhoid fever, ergotism or an influenza virus complicated by a toxin-producing noninvasive staphylococci, ie a form of toxic shock syndrome

'thumb' and 'little finger' signs A pair of radiologic findings seen on plain lateral films of the neck; the 'thumb' occurs in acute epiglottitis and corresponds to an edematous aryepiglottic fold (epiglottic shadow) with near-complete obliteration of the valleculae and pyriform sinuses, likened to an adult's thumb; the 'little finger' is used for comparison, where the epiglottic shadow is svelte, resembling an adult's little finger

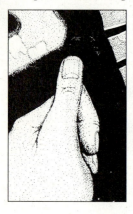 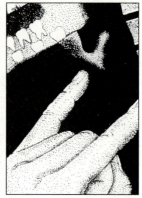

thumb sign   **little finger sign**

thumb ANTHROPOLOGY see Rule of thumb HAND SURGERY The first digit which opposes the remaining five digits; maintenance of viable thumb action is a highly desirable result of any major reconstructive surgery to the hand

thumbprinting A finding in a barium study of the colon, which consists of multiple broad, sharply defined short and rounded often symmetric indentations in the contrast column; although it is described in both 1) Mesenteric artery ischemia or ischemic 'colitis' with infarction and intramural hematoma formation (often at the splenic flexure and descending colon) and 2) Ulcerative colitis, 'thumbprinting' is nonspecific and may be seen in pneumatosis cystoides intestinalis (due to indentation of the barium column by the mucosa-covered gas), pseudomembranous colitis, *Entamoeba histolytica* amebiasis, *Escherichia coli* O157:H7 enterocolitis (due to submucosal edema) and other infectious colitides, hemorrhage, Crohn's disease, endometriosis, hereditary angioneurotic edema, amyloidosis and malignancy (lymphoma, metastases); when the edema affects the mucosal folds of the small intestine, it is called 'Pinky printing'; thumbprinting in the markedly thickened folds of the gastric fundus and body in an upper GI tract may occur in Menetrier's disease (giant hypertrophic gastritis); Cf Collar button lesion

thumpversion Precordial thump CARDIOLOGY The administration of a blow or blows to the anterior chest in a person who has undergone cardiac arrest; despite the American Heart Association's current recommendation that precordial thumps be used only when the patient is being monitored (given the concern that ventricular tachycardia might convert to ventricular fibrillation), some authors urge its continued use, in particular 'in the field', where monitors might not be available

thymic wave sign A subtle radiopaque undulation caused by the costochondral junctions of adjacent ribs, seen by a plain antero-posterior chest film in a normal thymus

Thymic tumors are firm and thus are not indented by the ribs

thymine dimer A focal defect in DNA formed after exposure to ultraviolet light, which consists of pairing of the thymine pyrimidines across the double helix, preventing DNA replication; it is not the dimer itself that is mutagenic, but rather the 'sloppy' repair mechanism, which is carried by the SOS repair system; ultraviolet light may also induce direct mutations into the DNA by base pair substitution (transversion) and 'frame shift' mutations in the form of duplications and deletions; see SOS repair

thymoma A thymic epithelial cell neoplasm located in the

anterior mediastinum, which is often first seen as an incidental finding on a plain antero-posterior chest film CLINICAL Thymomas may be associated with connective tissue disease (giant cell polymyositis, rheumatoid arthritis, SLE, Sjögren syndrome, dermatomyositis, polymyositis and scleroderma) skin disease (pemphigus vulgaris, lichen planus, alopecia areata), hematopoietic disease (erythrocytosis, erythroid hypoplasia, pernicious anemia, aplastic anemia), multiple myeloma, angioimmunoblastic lymphadenopathy, inflammation, eg granulomatous myocarditis, meningoencephalitis, thyroiditis, immunologic disorders (hypogammaglobulinemia, IgA deficiency, monoclonal gammopathy, mucocutaneous candidiasis), malignancy (internal malignancy, which occurs in up to 17% of cases and others including myasthenia gravis, adrenal atrophy, Cushing's disease, ulcerative colitis and Crohn's disease; the prognosis is a function of capsular invasion, mitotic activity, cytologic atypia, nuclear hyperchromasia PATHOLOGY Solid to cystic, yellow-gray, well-encapsulated and separated into lobules by connective tissue PATHOLOGY Aggregates of plump-to-spindled epithelial cells, separated by fascicles of mature, activated lymphocytes DDx Lymphoma

thymosin alpha-1 Thymopoietin A thymic hormone that induces T-cell helper function, stimulating lymphokine production, eg IFN, macrophage inhibiting factor, increasing the expression of Thy-1.2 and Lyt-1,-2,-3 markers on T cells, modulating TdT levels in thymocytes Normal levels: 1250-2250 pg/ml in newborns; 580 pg/ml in adults

thymotaxin β_2-microglobulin, see there

thyroid crisis Thyrotoxic storm, see there

thyroid hormone binding ratio T_3 and T_4 uptake test A laboratory technique that analyzes the distribution of radiolabelled T_3 and T_4 in a serum sample, providing an indirect estimate of the free fraction of T_3 and T_4; the method entails addition of charcoal or a resin to a specimen, then quantifying the radiolabeled ('hot') T_3 bound to the matrix, expressed as a ratio of matrix-bound RIA value to the serum protein-bound RIA value, usually 33-50%; see Free thyroxine index

thyroid hormone receptor A dimeric transcription factor with a binding domain for DNA and one for thyroid hormones, in particular T_3; a hereditary defect in the hormone binding domain is linked to goiter, impaired growth, mental retardation, and cretinism (Sci & Med Nov/Dec 1994 p15)

thyroid panel LABORATORY MEDICINE A standard (CPT-4 code 80092) panel of laboratory tests used to evaluate the baseline thyroid status; for Medicare or Medicaid reimbursement, it must include total thyroxine (T_4), total T_3 resin uptake, and TSH (see CAP Today March 1993) see Organ panel

'thyroidization' see Tubular thyroidization

thyrotoxicosis see Thyrotoxic crisis CARDIOVASCULAR High-output cardiac failure due to 1) Circulatory factors ($\uparrow$ total blood volume, $\downarrow$ systemic vascular resistance) and 2) Cardiac factors ($\uparrow$ contractility, $\uparrow$ heart rate, $\uparrow$ diastolic relaxation), which translate into volume overload, $\downarrow$ myocardial contractile reserve, $\downarrow$ diastolic filling time, tachyarrhythmia MANAGEMENT Inorganic iodine abruptly inhibits T_3 and T_4 secretion, but should be preceded by methimazole or propyluracil to prevent oxidation and organification of the iodine; this should be followed by definitive treatment of 1) Thyrotoxicosis (radioactive iodine, surgical resection) 2) Cardiac disease, eg furosemide (diuretic for volume), beta-adrenergic blocking agents (β-blockers, eg propranolol) in absence of congestive heart failure, and anticoagulant therapy for possible arterial thromboembolism due to atrial fibrillation (N Engl J Med 1992; 327:94RV) see T_3 thyrotoxicosis, T_4 thyrotoxicosis; Cf Thyroid crisis

*Synonyms include thyrotropic hormone, thyroid stimulating hormone, thyrotrophin

thyrotoxic crisis A hypermetabolic state superimposed

on hyperthyroidism, often occurring in Grave's disease, less common in toxic multinodular goiter and rarely in Hashimoto's disease ('Hashitoxicosis'); the symptoms of hyperthyroidism, eg weight loss, heat intolerance, myasthenia, poor mental concentration, diarrhea, diaphoresis and cardiac palpitations, may be triggered by infection (eg streptococcal pharyngitis), thromboembolism, surgery, physical or psychological trauma, parturition or withdrawal from thyroid-blocking drugs, into becoming a life-threatening hypermetabolic state, characterized by hyperthermia, tachycardia and cardiac, hepatic and cerebral dysfunction LABORATORY ↑ Thyroxine (T_4) and tri-iodothyronine (T_3), ↓ cholesterol TREATMENT Reduce hypermetabolic state, inhibiting thyroid hormone release with iodine, blocking thyroid hormone synthesis with propylthiouracil and other anti-thyroid agents, blocking adrenergic neurotransmission with β-adrenergic antagonists and glucocorticoids to 'cover' for functional hypoadrenalism; see Euthyroid sick syndrome, Hashimoto's disease, Hashitoxicosis

thyrotoxic storm Thyrotoxic crisis, see there

thyrotropin TSH (Thyroid-stimulating hormone) A 28-kD glycopeptide hormone produced by the adenohypophysis (anterior hypophysis) that controls thyroid growth, development, and secretion; the α subunit of TSH is structurally identical to that of FSH, LH and hCG; its molecular uniqueness is conferred by the β subunit, and its production is regulated by thyroid-releasing hormone; a low serum level in older (> age 60) people is associated with certain manifestations of subclinical hyperthyroidism, eg atrial fibrillation (**N Engl J Med 1994; 331:1249OA**)

thyrotropin receptor A heptaspan member of the superfamily of G protein-coupled transmembrane receptors, which controls both the function and growth of thyroid cells by stimulating adenylate cyclase and phospholipase C; the TR gene may be alterd by a gain-of-function mutation, resulting in persistent congenital hyperthyroidism (**N Engl J Med 1995; 332:1500A**) or a loss-of-function mutation, resulting in thyrotropin resistance and subclinical hypthyroidism (**ibid 1995; 332:1550A, 332:183ED**) see Heptaspan

*A receptor that spans the cell membrane seven times, also known as a serpentine receptor

thyroxine 3,5,3',5'-Tetraiodo-thyronine T_4 MECHANISM OF ACTION Stimulate O_2 consumption and metabolism THERAPEUTIC UTILITY Replacement therapy for overt, subclinical, transient, or neonatal hypothyroidism, suppressive therapy, as required in thyroid cancer, as well-differentiated thyroid carcinoma may dependent on thyrotropin (**N Engl J Med 1994; 331:174RV**)

thyroxine-binding prealbumin Transthyretin

TI 1) Inversion time The timespan between the middle of the inverting (180°) RF pulse and the middle of the 90° pulse, used to detect longitudinal magnetization; see Magnetic resonance imaging 2) Therapeutic index

TIA 1) Transient ischemic attack, see there 2) Tumor-induced angiogenesis

Also 1) Thallium acetate 2) Thin-layer immunoassay 3) Trypsin inhibitor activity 4) Turbidometric immunoassay

TIBC Total iron-binding capacity LABORATORY MEDICINE A quantitative measurement of transferrin's ability to transport iron; in normal subjects, 33% of transferrin's sites are

occupied by iron; in iron deficiency, pregnancy and viral hepatitis, 15% of transferrin's binding sites are occupied, therefore transferrin's capacity to bind iron or TIBC is increased; in iron-overload syndromes, eg hemochromatosis and hemosiderosis, transferrin has few sites available to bind iron and therefore the TIBC is decreased

TIBO Tetrahydroimidazobenzodiazopinone(s) A class of benzodiazepine-related compounds with anti-HIV activity that at low doses, reduce in vitro viral replication by inhibiting reverse transcriptase; TIBO's inhibition of reverse transcriptase is reported to be five times more potent than that of zidovudine AIDS A family of compounds that bind to a hydrophobic pocket in HIV's reverse transcriptase-DNA (RT-DNA) complex close to the polymerization active site (**Science 1995; 267:988A**) see Nonnucleoside reverse transcriptase inhibitor

tic Habit spasm A complex of multiple abrupt, coordinated involuntary movements, including eye blinking, facial gestures, shoulder shrugging, which the patients feel compelled to complete, which when controlled, may be followed by more intense and frequent 'rebound' contractions; tics are exacerbated by stressants and ameliorated by psychotherapy; Giles de la Tourette syndrome causes a severe form of tics affecting young ♂, age 2-15, characterized by explosive vocalizations and movements (sniffing, barking, obscenities or obscene gestures) that may become more controlled with age; while no consistent anatomic abnormalities have been identified, the constancy of the presentation implies an organic nature of the condition; Cf Jumping Frenchmen of Maine syndrome

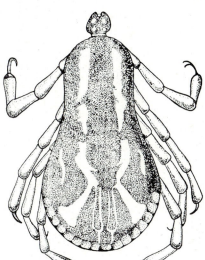

tick A hematophagous ectoparasitic arthropod of the superfamily Ixodoidea, which are divided into hard ticks (family Ixodidae) and soft ticks (family Argasidae); ticks are common vectors of bacterial and viral infections, *Dermacentor andersoni* North America Vector for Rocky Mountain spotted fever, Colorado tick fever, tularemia and tick paralysis, *D marginatus* Asia Vector for Russian spring-summer fever, tick-borne encephalitis virus, possibly also Congo-Crimean hemorrhagic fever virus and *Babesia* Reservoir for Omsk hemorrhagic fever virus, *D occidentalis* Pacific Coast North America Vector (presumed) for RMSF, Colorado tick fever, *D parumapertus* Southwestern USA Vector for RMSF, Colorado tick fever, *D variabilis* Eastern USA Vector for RMSF, tularemia, Colorado tick fever and tick paralysis; Asian and African ticks, vectors of Rickettsialpox *Ixodes dammini* Northern deer tick, vector of *Babesia microti*; see Lyme disease

tick-borne fever Relapsing fever, see there

tick-borne hemorrhagic fever A generic term for a group of diseases in which ticks are incriminated as vectors: CONGO-CRIMEAN HEMORRHAGIC FEVER Vector *Hyaloma marginatum*; KYASANUR FOREST DISEASE Vector *Haemaphysalis turturis, H spinigera*; OMSK HEMORRHAGIC FEVER Vector *Dermacentor pictus, D marginatus*

tick paralysis Ascending tick paralysis A flaccid ascending quadriplegia that resembles Guillain-Barré syndrome, produced by the bite of certain pregnant ticks, eg Rocky mountain wood tick (*Dermatocentor andersoni*) and dog ticks, thought to be due to an unidentified toxin

TREATMENT Tick removal

ticlopidine CLINICAL THERAPEUTICS A thienopridine derivative which (like aspirin) is a platelet aggregation inhibitor, the action of which is maximum at 24-48 hours and irreversible; unlike aspirin, it inhibits platelet aggregation induced by adenosine diphosphate and other agonists by altering the platelet membrane, interfering with membrane-fibrinogen interaction by blocking platelet glycoprotein IIb/IIIa receptor; ticlopidine is FDA-approved as long-term prophylaxis to reduce the incidence of stroke used in patients at high risk for stroke, or who have suffered a previous stroke to minimize stroke progression, cerebral ischemia, and the progression of diabetic retinopathy SIDE EFFECTS BM suppression with severe reversible neutropenia*, diarrhea, rash (N Engl J Med 1995; 332:238RV), gastritis or gastric ulcers (nausea, dyspepsia), hemorrhage, thrombocytopenia, and a slight ↑ in cholesterol; see TIA

*2.4% of those treated suffer moderate (< 1200/mm³) to severe (< 400/mm³) neutropenia

'tiger' substance A striated material of unknown significance, which is occasionally seen by LM in the stroma of dysgerminomas and seminomas (Eur J Cancer 1965; 1:253)

'tiger-top' tubes LABORATORY MEDICINE A sterile blood collection tube with a swirled or variegated red and black or red and green rubber stopper that is coated with silicone, has a gel on the bottom, can be directly centrifuged to separate red and white cells and, like yellow top tubes, are used to collect specimens for HIV, retroviruses (eg HTLV-I and others), acetone, alcohol, urea nitrogen and creatinine

tight junction CELL BIOLOGY A region that completely encircles a cell, in which the contributing plasma membranes of adjacent cells are directly apposed with virtually no intervening space; TJs are typical ultrastructural findings in epithelial cells, and are seen in adenomas, adenocarcinoma, APUDomas, transitional and papillary carcinoma of the urinary bladder, synovial sarcoma and mesothelioma; Cf Gap junction

tigroid nucleus A morphology of the striated muscle cell nucleus due to the resynthesis of contractile proteins, associated with denervation, target fiber formation and type group atrophy

Tijuana A city in Mexico that has occasionally served as a destination (as have other cities) for patients hoping to be cured of terminal malignancy by unproven cancer therapies offered in some 'clinicas' of self-proclaimed cancer specialists, who often describe their therapies as 'alternative', 'holistic' or 'natural', which are based on some form of 'metabolic therapy' (Questionable methods of cancer management, Special communication, 13 June 1990, American Cancer Society); see 'Metabolic therapy', Unproven methods of cancer therapy

TIL Tumor-infiltrating lymphocytes IMMUNOLOGY T lymphocytes with antitumoral activity that are isolated from a patient with cancer, tagged (for later identification) with neomycin-resistance gene and grown by culturing single cell suspensions obtained from tumors in tissue culture media

TIL therapy An experimental therapeutic modality in which antigen-specific tumor-infiltrating T lymphocytes (TILs) are isolated from biopsies of patients with malignancy and co-administered with IL-2; a 30% response rate in high-grade melanoma was reported by one group in 1990 (N Engl J Med 1990; 323:570); Cf LAK/IL-2 therapy

tilt test Upright tilt test CARDIOLOGY A clinical maneuver in which a person is placed in a head-up position placed on a tilt table at a 40° to 80° from horizontal and maintained in a motionless upright position for 10-15 minutes or more, the intent being to provoke syncope, bradycardia, or hypotension; the resulting gravitaional pooling of blood volume evokes a decline in central venous pressure, stroke volume, and blood pressure; the TT is of particular use in detecting neurocardiogenic syncope (Science & Medicine 1995; 2/3:14)

time of flight mass spectrometry TOF-MS LABORATORY MEDICINE A technique that measures the time required by an ion to travel from its source to a detector; at the start of the 'flight', all ions have the same kinetic energy, but separate according to their mass, such that the ions arrive at different times; TOF-MS can be used for measuring the mass and structure of ionized substances, especially for the identification of drugs and their metabolites; see Mass spectrometry

Times Beach ENVIRONMENT A city in Missouri that was abandoned by order of the US Environental Protection Agency in 1983, when dangerously high levels of dioxins were identified in the water and soil, which were the result of the spraying of dioxin-tainted oils (to control dust) on the roads and highways (Arch Environ Contam Toxicol 1988; 17:139) see Agent Orange, Chemical pollutants, Dioxin

time bomb COMPUTERS A software subroutine that automatically disables an information system after an internally specified date, which can be periodically 'reset'; a time bomb can be an information system vendor's 'insurance' that the purchaser of their services and maintenance contracts, eg a laboratory, will comply with the vendor's terms (CAP Today March 1992)

time trade-off metric CLINICAL MEDICINE A tool used in outcomes management that quantifies preferences for a specific health state, '...by assessing how much time a patient would be willing to give up to be freed from a reduced health state. The time trade-off utility is defined as the number of symptoms-free years divided by the number of years with symptoms, at the point of indifference.'; as an example if a patient is willing to sacrifice 4 years of life with symptoms for a total of 16 years of life to be without those symptoms for 12 years, the utility is 12/16 or 0.75 (JAMA 1995; 273:1185) see Utility; Cf Standard gamble metric

TIMI studies Thrombolysis in myocardial infarction CARDIOLOGY A series of long-term multi-center, multi-national, multi-agent studies designed to determine which of a number of early interventions would provide the best survival for myocardial infarctions; the TIMI trials have examined the effects of early thrombolytic therapy in recanalizing occluded coronary arteries, in limiting the size of the infarct and residual cardiac dysfunction, and reduction of mortality, analyzing various combinations of tissue plasminogen activator (tPA), heparin, aspirin and coronary arteriography followed by prophylactic percutaneous transluminal angioplasty; one study concluded that IV β-blockade with recombinant tPA is adequate therapy in uncomplicated myocardial infarcts; in one TIMI trial, mortality was reportedly reduced by 47% if tPA was used within one hour, 17% if the therapy was delayed 3-6 hours and was reported to offer little advantage if therapy began six or more hours after the ischemic insult; see CAST, TAMI studies, tPA

timolol maleate A β-adrenergic antagonist used as a topical solution, which causes a worsening of lipid profiles with ↑ triglycerides and ↑ LDL and ↓ HDL

TIMPs Tissue inhibitor of metalloproteinases A substance which under normal circumstances, inhibit collagenases; a TIMP has been identified in certain tumor cell lines that binds type IV collagenase, but does not inhibit it, possibly leaving it in a fully activated position; there are two types,

TIMP-1 and TIMP-2, which block metalloproteinases (MPs hydrolyze multiple components in the extracellular matrix), which are necessary for normal tissue remodeling; under normal circumstances, TIMPs and MPs coexist in state of equlibrium, a balance that is lost in tumor cell invasion (Diagn Mol Pathol 1993; 2:74, 81)

tin-mesoporphyrin Sn-MP A recently developed drug that may be useful in treating neonatal jaundice, which is characterized by ↑↑↑ bilirubin; because Sn-MP blocks heme oxygen as heme is excreted intact without being converted to bilirubin (New York Times 18 January 1994; C3)

tinea gladiatorum Infection with *Trichophyton tonsurans* transmitted by wrestling (N Engl J Med 1992; 327:821c) Cf Herpes gladiatorum

Tinel sign NEUROLOGY Paresthesia that is evoked by tapping on a nerve, a finding typical of entrapment neuropathy; a positive Tinel sign has a sensitivity of 60% and a specificity of 67% for carpal tunnel syndrome (N Engl J Med 1993; 329:2013cc)

tingible bodies HEMATOPATHOLOGY Karyorrhectic nuclear debris of various sizes present in and adjacent to macrophages in benign lymphadenopathies, often located in the germinal centers in toxoplasmosis, infectious mononucleosis, varicella and herpes zoster lymphadenopathy, cat-scratch disease, and brucellosis

tinted spectacles sign PSYCHIATRY The wearing of dark-colored glasses under normal lighting conditions, in absence of photophobia or photosensitivity; 'soft' data suggests that this sign may sometimes be associated with an underlying psychoneuroses, as the scores for the symptom dimensions measured (anxiety and phobic anxiety, depression, global psychological distress, obsession-compulsion, paranoid ideation, psychotic behavior and somatization) were significantly higher in subjects who don 'shades'

A rose-colored spectacles sign has not been described

TIPS Transjugular intrahepatic portosystemic stent-shunt procedure, see there

tincture A medicinal preparation often of herbal origin in which the ground substrate (eg bark, root, nuts, or seeds) is soaked in alcohol to extract oils or other substances of interest

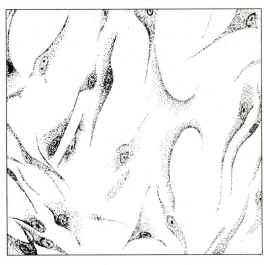

tirofiban MK-383 A potent nonpeptide inhibitor of ligand binding to the glycoprotein IIb/IIIa (integrin $\alpha_{IIb}\beta_3$) receptor, which is currently in phase 3 clinical trials (N Engl J Med 1995; 332:1553RV)

tissue bank A repository of cadaveric tissues ultimately destined for transplantation; banked tissues include bone (an estimated 250 000 bone grafts are performed/year in US), corneas (36 000 transplants), skin (5000), heart valves (2000), cartilage (1100), tendon, fascia, dura, vein, pericardium (each < 500); tissue banking has its roots as a 'cottage industry' and had suffered from lack of standards in terms of data collected at the time of tissue procurement, testing for pathogens, and tracking of the specimens before and after transplantation (CAP Today May 1992 p1) see the Lifenet case

tissue committee Tissue review committee, see there

'tissue culture' appearance SURGICAL PATHOLOGY A loose, haphazard arrangement of plump, spindled cells, usually fibroblasts that may have elongated cytoplasmic processes, typically seen in nodular fasciitis, a 'storiform' pattern

that has been fancifully likened to that seen when normal fibroblasts are grown in culture media

tissue culture appearance

tissue culture infective dose TCID, see there

tissue factor HEMATOLOGY A particulate complex of phosphatides[1], lipoproteins, and cholesterol with molecular weights from 53 to 1500 kD that accelerates coagulation; it may be obtained from homogenates of virtually any normal human (TF is species-specific) tissue, although the most potent TF is obtained from the lungs, brain, and placenta

[1]Phosphatidylcholine, phosphatidylethanolamine, phosphatidylinositol, phosphatidylserine, sphingosine [2]In humans a 52-kD apoprotein has been identified

tissue factor pathway inhibitor Extrinsic pathway inhibitor, lipoprotein-associated coagulation inhibitor '*A multivalent Kunitz-type protease inhibitor that binds to and inactivates Factor Xa directly; In a Factor Xa-dependent fashion, TFPI inhibits the tissue factor-Factor VIIa catalytic complex.*'; serum levels are ↑ in chronic liver disease, in patients with unexplained thrombosis, and those receiving heparin; the clinical relevance of TFPI is at present uncertain (Am J Clin Pathol 1995; 103:391OA)

tissue paper appearance Crumpled tissue paper appearance, see there

tissue plasminogen activator tPA A thrombolytic protease the natural form of which is the physiologic activator of the fibrinolytic system and is released from vascular endothelium by epinephrine, exertion, adherent thrombi, or vascular compression; tPA is commercially available in a recombinant form, r-tPA; tPA has currency in reducing the mortality of myocardial infarction in the immediate post-ischemic period, although it may offer no advantage over other less expensive agents, with a patency rate of the infarct-related artery of 76% in the streptokinase-treated group and 75% in the tPA-treated group; thrombolytic therapy given in the first post-infarct hour reduces mortality by 47% and reduces mortality in PTE PHYSIOLOGY Plasminogen activation elicits formation of plasmin (a proteolytic enzyme that degrades fibrin, the main protein of the thrombus scaffold), modifying platelet function, degrading circulating fibrinogen and coagulation factors V and VIII, lowering the hemorrhagic 'threshold', which is potentially fatal in patients with central nervous system hemorrhage

Note: Other thrombolytic agents include urokinase, streptokinase and APSAC (anisoylated streptokinase plasminogen activatory complex)

tissue processor SURGICAL PATHOLOGY A laboratory instrument used to prepare formaldehyde-fixed tissues for embedding in paraffin (which are subsequently sectioned with a microtome, and stained on a glass slide for examination by light microscopy); the current TPs are controlled by a microprocessor and automatically change the fluids bathing the tissues, passing them from an aqueous phase (formaldehyde) to a lipid-soluble phase (xylene), the final step prior to embedding the tissues in paraffin

tissue (review) committee QUALITY ASSURANCE A committee in a hospital that reviews the appropriateness of all surgical procedures performed in the institution, correlating the pre- and post-operative diagnoses established by the surgeon, and the diagnosis rendered by the pathologist; an active TRC is required for hospital accreditation in the US and serves as a mechanism to ensure that tissues are not removed unnecessarily, ie in the absence of a well-defined pathology

'tit' sign Pyloric tit sign A radiologic finding in an upper GI series of films of a child with hypertrophic pyloric stenosis, in which the completely obstructed antrum and adjoining pyloric canal simulate the voluptuous curves of a breast and nipple; the nipple becomes pronounced as the pyloric muscle unsuccessfully attempts to contract and push the barium beyond the markedly stenosed canal; rarely a normal peristaltic pouch may transiently increase in size, temporarily simulating the tit sign

titer IMMUNOLOGY The amount of a substance that can be detected by serial dilution, ie the reciprocal of highst dilution that evokes a raction; determination of 'titers' is of clinical use in determining a present infection or past exposure to an antigen or virus, where rising titers, ie presence of an antigen-antibody reaction at high dilutions of an antigen, indicate a developing disease (eg 1:32→1:128) while falling titers (eg 1:128→1:64) indicate a resolving condition; see Antibody titers

titin Connectin A large (3000-kD, the largest known polypeptide) myofibrillar protein, the locus for which has been assigned to chromosome segment 2q13-q33; it is abundant in muscle, especially in the M and Z lines as well as in the A and I bands, and helps align myosin thick filaments during contraction; Cf Nebulin, Tropomyosin

'Title X' project POPULATION CONTROL A US federal government-sponsored program for family planning clinics that was initiated under the Reagan Administration; under the recent 'Gag rule' resulting from a US Supreme Court decision, physicians had been interdicted from fully counseling women who are unintentionally pregnant; the wording of the Court's decision has been interpreted as preventing physicians from offering these women nondirective counseling on pregnancy termination, as well as prenatal care, infant and foster care, and adoption, thereby representing governmental interference of the patient-doctor relationship; see 'Gag rule', Mexico policy

TJ Hooper decision 'Reasonable prudence' doctrine, see there

TKO selection GENETICS A tool for rapidly identifying genes that inhibit proliferation in a specific restrictive environment; this assumes that specific inhibition of a growth inhibitory gene conveys growth advantage, 'forward selecting' a desired inactivation event; TKO (technical knock-out) selection identifies thioredoxin as the mediator of a growth inhibitory signal in tumor suppression (Science 1991; 252:117)

TLC 1) Thin-layer chromatography, see there 2) Total lung capacity

Also 1) T lymphocyte clones 2) Total lung compliance 3) Total lymphocyte count 4) Transient late curvature

TLF Trypanosome lytic factor, see there

TLV Threshold limit value, see there

T lymphocyte T cell, see there

T_m 1) Melting temperature 2) Tubular maximum The maximum reabsorptive capacity for glucose in the renal tubules, which is 11.2-13.2 mmol/L (US: 200-240 mg/dl); under usual circumstances, slightly before reaching the T_m, incomplete glucose reabsorption occurs, causing a 'splaying' in the response, a value designated as K_m

TMA Transcription-mediated amplification MOLECULAR DIAGNOSTICS An isothermal target amplification-type technique for amplifying DNA METHOD

1) rRNA is transcribed into an RNA-DNA hybrid by reverse transcriptase and the hybrid becomes a transcriptionally active template, from which RNA is made by T7 RNA polymerase, which generates 100-1000 copies/template

2) The RNA amplicon from the first phase is annealed to a second DNA primer and step 1) is repeated; the reaction becomes autocatalytic

TMA can achieve a 10^9 amplification factor in 90 minutes (CAP Today May 1995 p1)

T-max CLINICAL MEDICINE A colloquial term for the maximum temperature recorded in a 24-hour period

TMJ Temporomandibular joint

TMJ syndrome Temporomandibular joint-myofascial dysfunction syndrome A complex neuromuscular disorder related to dental malocclusion, possibly exacerbated by trauma, psychological stress and grinding of teeth CLINICAL Nonspecific unilateral facial pain and spasms of the masseter muscle TREATMENT No therapy is consistently effective; modalities used with varying degrees of failure have included physical (moist heat) therapy, analgesics, soft diet and surgery, eg high intracapsular condylectomy

TMP-SMX Trimethoprim-sulfamethoxazole, see there

TNF Tumor necrosis factor, see there

TNF-α MAb Anti-tumor necrosis factor-α monoclonal antibody, see there

TNM classification An internationally sanctioned system for staging malignacy, formulated by the UICC (Union International Contre Cancrum) that measures three major parameters: T for size or extent of the primary tumor, as determined by clinical exam, endoscopy, laparoscopy, biopsy or resective procedures, N for number of involved lymph nodes and M for presence or absence of metastases; TNM classification forms the basis of treating malignancy; lower case letters may precede the TNM formulation as a means of providing supplementary staging information, including aTNM (autopsy staging, for cancer diagnosed at advanced stage), cTNM (clinical-diagnostic staging), pTNM (post-surgical resection-pathologic staging), rTNM (retreatment staging), sTNM (surgical-evaluative staging)

Tn syndrome HEMATOLOGY A chronic acquired myeloid dysplasia associated with polyagglutination of erythrocytes, characterized by severe thrombocytopenia, hemolytic anemia and leukopenia; red cells and platelets are deficient in T-transferase (UDPGal:GalNAc-β-3-D-galactosyltransferase), resulting in the inability to express the GPIb glycoprotein and expression of the cryptantigen, Tn, which reacts with naturally occurring antibodies, causing global hemolysis and coagulation

TNTC Too numerous to count MICROBIOLOGY A colloquial abbreviation for a confluent 'lawn' of bacteria on a culture plate that may be seen in urinary tract infections, where confluent growth is approximately equal to 10^5 colonies

toad fish Puffer fish, see there

toad skin appearance see Cathartic colon

toadstool motility Umbrella motility, see there

toad test Male frog test A bioassay of historical interest that used the South African clawed toad, *Xenopis laevis*, to detect increased production of human chorionic gonadotropin; injection of plasma from pregnant human females induces the release of sperm in the toads

tobacco PUBLIC HEALTH A generic term for any consumable product prepared from the dried leaves of *Nicotiana tabacum*, which is rich in the addictive alkaloid, nicotine; tobacco is responsible for enormous mortality (US) ± 425 000/year; cardiovascular deaths ± 180 000/year; lung cancer deaths ± 120 000/year; second-hand smoke deaths 9000/year; number of smokers (x 10^6) $^{1965}/_{1994}$: ♂ $^{28.9}/_{24}$; ♀ $^{21.1}/_{22.3}$ TOBACCO ECONOMICS Annual revenues $ 48 x 10^9; $12 x 10^9 in goverment taxes; 47 000 people employed by tobacco industry; per capita consumption 3488 (1983); 2539 (1993); tobacco produces a trade surplus of $4 x 10^9 (cigarettes exported to Japan 55.5 x 10^9, to Belgium-Luxembourg 51.2 x 10^9) (**US News & World Report 18 April 1994**) see Nicotine, Smoking

tobacco dependence The psychological and physiologic components of addiction to nicotine, which has three addictive components, to wit, habit (smoking is cued by daily activities), pleasure (nicotine produces euphoria

---

TNM CLASSIFICATION FOR STAGING MALIGNANCY

T TUMOR
T-is Carcinoma in situ
T-a Non-invasive
T-x Cannot be evaluated for non-specified reasons
T-0 Localized tumor
T-1 Lesion extends to muscle (bladder, colon, breast)
    T-1a < 0.5 cm in greatest dimension
    T-1b < 1.0 cm in greatest dimension
    T-1c < 2.0 cm in greatest dimension
T-2 Invasion into muscle
T-3 Persistent induration of organ following resection
    T-3a Invasion to deep muscle
    T-3b Invasion through the organ
T-4 Tumor invasion or fixation
    T-4a Adjacent organ invasion
    T-4b Fixation to bladder or colonic wall; in breast, edema

N NODES
N-0 No lymph node metastasis
N-1 One regional lymph node metastasis
N-2 Multiple, mobile regional lymph node metastases
N-3 Fixed regional lymph node metastaseis
N-4 Beyond regional lymph node involvement
N-X Lymph nodes, not evaluable

M METASTASIS
M-0 No evidence of metastases
M-1 Distant metastases are present
M-X Distant metastases, not evaluable

LESS USED COMPONENTS OF THE TNM CLASSIFICATION :
R RESECTIVE SUCCESS
R-0 No residual tumor exists after resection
R-1 Microscopic residual tumor exists
R-2 Gross residual tumor is present after surgery
P PATHOLOGIC STAGING (POST-SURGERY HISTOLOGY)
P   Surgical specimen with histopathological changes
P-is Malignancy in situ
P-0 No tumor in specimen, or completely excised
    in situ malignancy
P-1 Malignancy confined to the lamina propria
P-2 Malignancy extends to < half of muscle layer
P-3 Malignancy extends to > half of muscle layer
P-4 Malignancy extends to > half of muscle layer
    with infiltration of adjacent organs
P-X Malignancy, not evaluable
G HISTOPATHOLOGICAL GRADING
G-0 No anaplasia seen
G-1 Low amount of anaplasia
G-2 Moderate amount of anaplasia
G-3 High amount of anaplasia
G-X Presence of anaplasia, not evaluable

---

similar to other addictive psychomotor stimulants), and self-medication (nicotine use reduces negative affect and physical symptoms) (**JAMA 1992; 268:2687**)

tobacco epidemic PUBLIC HEALTH A generic term for the widespread consumption of tobacco in its various forms, which is intimately linked to disease, disability and death; the TE is becoming more manageable in developed nations with empowerment of the population, a result of enforced smoke-free public places, decreased tobacco consumption, banning of tobacco advertising in media of public access, and successful lawsuits against tobacco companies; the TE has ↑ logarithmically in developing nations, stimulated in part by drive to find 'replacement markets' due to the loss of tobacco-related revenues in developed nations (**Prev Med 1994; 23:535**) the consumption of tobacco in 1977 at 12 854 cigarettes/year for smokers (**Sci Am 1995; 272:44**) see Cigarette marketing

'tobacco nodules' A descriptive term for the appearance of organized perifollicular hemorrhages, ie Gamna-Gandy bodies that are seen in passive splenic hyperemia due to portal hypertension; these structures consist of iron- and calcium-encrusted collagen and fibrosis surrounding atrophic malpighian follicles

tobacco withdrawal syndrome A condition characterized by irritability, sleep disorders, GI disturbances, increased appetite and weight gain; the use of nicotine replacement therapy, eg nicotine patches ameliorate some of the components of TWS, but the impact is modest and selective (**JAMA 1992; 268:2687**) see Nicotine replacement therapy

TOC Total organic carbon A measurable parameter recommended by the EPA to be used in biodegradability testing

tocol A generic term for a group of eight naturally occurring fat-soluble compounds with a 6-chromanol nucleus bearing two methyl groups and a branched isoprenoid chain with vitamin E activity, the most biologically active of the tocol family is D-α-tocopherol; see Vitamin E

tocolytic OBSTETRICS An agent used to stop labor, usually premature; see Ritodrine

toddler's diarrhea PEDIATRICS A condition that is defined as the presence of unresolved diarrhea with mild malabsorption that persists after the resolution of acute gastroenteritis; toddler's diarrhea is considered by some workers to be a possible prelude to the irritable bowel syndrome CLINICAL Abdominal pain, vomiting, loose, malodorous stool, highly irritating rash of the buttocks, dysuria and urinary urgency; the onset of illness may coincide with death, illness, family crisis or environmental stress

todeserwartung German, awaiting death SOCIAL MEDICINE A symptom complex affecting elderly persons who have been relegated to nursing homes by society or progeny CLINICAL Hypochondriasis, hysteria, impulsiveness, loss of self-esteem, withdrawal from reality, and obsession with death THERAPY Displays of affection, household pets, involvement in child care; associated cortical atrophy and mental lassitude may be controlled by using video games for mental stimulation; see Geriatrics; Cf Elderly abuse, Melanocholia, 'Shelterization'

toe-walking ORTHOPEDICS A defective gait, in which the patients walk on 'tip-toes' due to force of habit, congenital tight heel cords or cerebral palsy with mild spasticity

tog A unit of measure reflecting the amount of heat trapping (see **N Engl J Med 1993; 329:425ED; Arch Dis Child 1992; 67:171**)

'toke' SUBSTANCE ABUSE To inhale a large air volume while smoking a substance of abuse, eg marijuana or 'crack', maintaining the lungs expanded with a slight Valsalva maneuver, in order to maximize the substance's absorption; Cf 'Snort'

token ring network COMPUTERS A LAN (local area network) architecture that combines token* passing with a star/ring topology

*A bit configuration that is circulated among workstations

Tokyo-Yokohama asthma see Yokohama asthma

tolerance IMMUNOLOGY see Immune tolerance INSTRUMENTATION The accepted or standardized limit of allowable error in an analytical instrument or procedure MICROBIOLOGY A poorly understood phenomenon in which the minimum concentration of penicillin required to kill staphylococci is up to 30-fold greater than the concentration required to inhibit its growth, values that are normally close to each other; see Methicillin-aminoglycoside resistant *Staphylococcus aureus*, Persister phenomenon MOLECULAR BIOLOGY The ability to accept substitutions of amino acids (related to the 'degeneracy' of DNA) in a protein without loss of function or significant alteration of structure PHARMACOLOGY An increase in dosage of a drug required to achieve the same effect, which is a function of increased metabolism, eg by hypertrophy of the endoplasmic reticulum or increased expulsion of the drug from a cell, eg by amplification of the multidrug resistant gene by a malignant cell; see MDR

tolrestat see Aldose reductase inhibitor

tool-making ANTHROPOLOGY The ability to make and use tools in hominids occurred ± 2.5 million years ago, is regarded as a marker for direct human ancestry, and long thought to be related to the size of the brain; this posit has been challenged by the so-called 'rule of thumb' (see there) which holds that tool-making required an adequate thumb for grasping objects with greater precision and force (New York Times 13 September 1994; C1)

toluidine blue PATHOLOGY A metachromatic thiazin stain used for 'thick' sections in ultrastructural studies; it is toxic by inhalation, ingestion and absorption, may cause hematuria secondary to hemorrhagic cystitis and methemoglobulinuria and thus should be avoided by those with glucose-6-phosphate deficiency

toluidine method LABORATORY MEDICINE A technique in which *o*-toluidine, an aromatic amine, reacts with glucose in a hot acetic acid solution to produce colored derivatives, allowing the quantification of glucose, which gives similar results to those generated by the enzymatic methodology used in multichannel analyzers

'tomato catsup' fundus A fanciful descriptor for the fundoscopic findings in cerebral lipidosis, Prader-Willi syndrome (characterized by hypertonicity, hyperphagia, neonatal obesity, small stature, hands and feet, mental retardation), Sturge-Weber's disease and Zellweger's cerebrohepatorenal syndrome (an AR condition characterized by dysmorphia, hepatomegaly and ↑ long chain fatty acids) (Arch Opthalmol 1974; 92:69)

tomato effect CLINICAL DECISION-MAKING Rejection of an effective treatment for a disease for illogical reasons, as may occur when conventional logic dictates that a drug should have no therapeutic value or is toxic, eg colchicine and aspirin (JAMA 1984; 251:2387)

Note: When the tomato (*Lycopersicon esculentum*), a New World plant from Peru was brought back by Spanish explorers, it was an instant culinary success with the Spaniards and both the Italians (*pommo d'oro*, golden apple) and the French, who thought it an aphrodisiac (*pomme d'amour*, apple of love), but was relatively unpopular in the rest of Europe, as 'logic' held that the tomato was poisonous as it belongs to the deadly nightshade family of plants, which includes belladonna and mandrake; this belief persisted until a tomato was eaten publicly in Massachusetts in 1820; the only known ill effect from tomatoes lies in herbal teas prepared from its leaves; see Herbal teas

'tombstone' advertisement An advertising layout format in which the 'copy' is a white field with text surrounded by a black border, often carrying a message with a potentially negative impact; because of tobacco's adverse effect on health, it has been proposed that the tobacco industry could exercise their right to advertise their products (a right guaranteed by the US Constitution), by using an ironic variant of tombstone advertising, which would carry only the product and its picture, eliminating the implication, through symbols or slogans, that the user's life would be improved through use of the product

tombstone appearance DERMATOPATHOLOGY A fanciful descriptor for the multiple hobnail-like cells (figure) which have lost their intercellular bridges above and lateral to the basal layer of residual epithelial cells in pemphigus vulgaris VASCULAR PATHOLOGY A descriptor for the bulging of epithelial-like endothelial cells into the vascular lumen in Kimura's disease; Cf Hobnail appearance

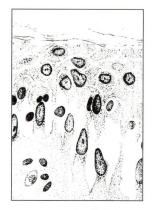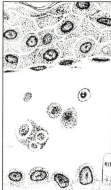

tombstone appearance

tongue worm Pentastomid A blood-sucking parasite that infests the nasal cavity of carnivores; human disease is caused by *Armillifer armillatus* (usual host, snakes) and *Linguatula serrata* (usual host, sheep and goats); pentastomiasis is global in distribution; linguliasis or Halzoun's disease is more common in the Middle East and results from eating poorly-cooked meat; the larvae cause pain, itching, sneezing due to transnasal migration, dysphagia, vomiting and lymphadenopathy; a large bolus of worms may cause fatal obstruction

tonic ALTERNATIVE MEDICINE *noun* A medicinal preparation, usually of herbal origin (eg ginseng) that is most commonly used in traditional Chinese medicine and Ayurvedic medicine, which is claimed by some practitioners of alternative health care to be of use in building vital energy known as qi

toning ALTERNATIVE MEDICINE A form of sound therapy, which consists of making elongated vowel sounds and allowing them to resonate (eg *'ommmmmmmmm'*) through the body, which is believed by its advocates to reduce stress, balance the mind/body, and improve hearing and speech (Alternative Medicine, Future Medicine Publishing, Inc, Puyallup, Washington, 1994)

tonometer A device that measures the tension or partial pressure of a gas in a liquid, used in a clinical setting to standardize arterial blood gas measurement, equilibrating the blood with a known mixture of gas at 37°C, serving as a form of quality control in determining the levels of CO_2 and O_2 in patient specimens

T-on-P phenomenon CARDIOLOGY An EKG finding consisting of sinus tachycardia with prolongation of Q-T and a delayed T wave followed or overlapped by the succeeding P wave; a 'T on P' is suggestive of alkalosis

tonsillectomy and adenoidectomy A simple surgical procedure that was commonly performed in the US in the 1950s by non-specialists for a wide variety of indications, including prophylaxis, a trend that has completely reversed; in the current environment, the two procedures are often performed as separate procedures for different indications, tonsillectomy for recurrent pharyngitis or peritonsillar abscesses and adenoidectomy for chronic or recurrent otitis media MICROBIOLOGY Potential pathogens may be cultured from 80% of pediatric T&As and include α-hemolytic streptococci, *Haemophilus* species, *Staphylococcus aureus* and *Streptococcus pneumoniae*; the relative risk for Hodgkin's disease in elderly subjects who had T&As as children may be as high as 3.0, although the data is sparse

toolmaking ANTHROPOLOGY The ability to alter a material present in the environment to address a particular need, eg killing or skinning an animal, cracking nuts, scraping or grinding basic foods; the oldest artifacts (ie tools) created by early hominids (eg australopithecines), have been dated at 2.6 million years old, which means that toolmaking preceded the genus *Homo* by ± 500 000 years (New York Times 25 April 1995, pC1)

tooth sign Asymptomatic, vaguely dentate ossifications that are perpendicular to the patellar surface seen on an axial ('skyline') view of the patello-femoral joint, which, while associated with degenerative changes, are of themselves of no clinical significance DDx Paget's disease of bone, reactive sclerosis due to chronic osteomyelitis

'toothache in the bones' A fanciful descriptor for the intense aching pain described in the diabetic foot with peripheral symmetric polyneuropathy

toothpaste artefact NEUROPATHOLOGY An artefact seen in the spinal cord, which results from its suboptimal removal from the vertebral column, resulting in a 'telescoping' prolase of spinal cord white matter, which may be interpreted by the neophyte as a spinal cord infarct, which is a rare autopsy finding

toothpaste sign A descriptor for a column of dense radio-contrast that has passed through a narrowed ureteral opening at the trigone and lies in a toothpaste-like fashion on the bladder floor; this finding may be caused by post-operative contraction of the vesical neck, as may occur in transureteral resections of the prostate, as well as in suprapubic and perineal surgery

top-hat function IMAGE ANALYSIS A method of mathematical morphology used to select the particulate structural elements of a gray-scale image for their size and optical density; it is an analytical transformation that '...*corresponds to the thresholded difference between initial and opened images–, ie, transformed by erosion (of image) followed by dilation...(a) top-hat function can be applied to the gray-level initial image to detect light spots on the cytoplasmic background.*' (Anal Quan Cytol Histol 1993; 15:220, ibid 1994; 16:11)

tophus The pathognomonic lesion of gout, which appears grossly as white chalky, pasty material composed of crystalline and amorphous urates, eg monosodium urate monohydrates, surrounded by mononuclear cells, fibroblasts and a foreign body-type giant cell reaction with epithelioid histiocytes; when preserved in alcohol or other non-aqueous solution; LM reveals bright an isotropic negatively birefringent crystals in compensated polarized light; tophi are most often periarticular but also occur in the tendon sheath, epiphyseal bone, subcutis, at the helix and antihelix of the external ear, in the renal pelvis and interstitium; with time, bony ankylosis may ensue, due to cartilaginous destruction, by local collagenase and prostaglandin E_2, synovial proliferation, pannus formation, subchondral osteolysis, bony overgrowth and fibrosis, demonstrating 'punched-out' lesions by radiology; see Gouty toe

topoisomerase An enzyme that alters the topology of DNA, catalyzing the interconversion of one topoisomer to another, changes the amount of superhelicity and forma-

tion of DNA knots and catenations, requiring transient breaking and rejoining of the strands of DNA's double helix; see DNA supercoiling, DNA topology, Superhelicity

TYPE I TOPOISOMERASE Omega protein, swivelase, untwistase An enzyme [EC 5.99.1.2] first found in *Escherichia coli* that introduces a transient single break in the double helix, causing a relaxation of twisted, negative supercoiled DNA helices without leaving nicks in the double helix

TYPE II TOPOISOMERASE An ATP-hydrolyzing enzyme [EC 5.99.1.3] that increases the double helix's winding number and superhelicity while decreasing its stability

topotecan A compound derived from a Chinese tree (*Camptotheca accuminata*) which has potential as a chemotherapeutic agent (Sci Am 1993; 268/1:142)

TOPV Trivalent oral polio vaccine

TORCH(eS) PEDIATRICS Toxoplasma, other, rubella, CMV, herpes simplex (and syphilis) An acronym for a group of in utero infections that may induce major malformation in the fetus and cause prominent neurologic defects, eg seizures, hydrocephalus or microcephaly

TORCH agents **TOXOPLASMOSIS** may cause periventricular microglial nodules, thrombosis and necrosis; obstruction of cerebral foramina causes hydrocephalus; with prolonged survival, there is intracranial calcification, hepatocellular, adrenal, pulmonary, cardiac necrosis and extramedullary hematopoiesis **RUBELLA** may cause low birth weight, hepatosplenomegaly, petechiae and purpura, congenital heart disease, cataracts, micro-ophthalmia and microcephaly; CNS symptoms include lethargy, irritability, dystonia, bulging fontanelles and seizures; see Congenital rubella syndrome **CYTOMEGALOVIRUS** may cause hepatosplenomegaly, hyperbilirubinemia, neonatal thrombocytopenia, microcephaly and a mortality of 20-30%; later manifestations include mental retardation, deafness, psychomotor delays, dysodontogenesis, chorioretinitis, learning disabilities; an ± 33 000 congenital cases/year (US), of which 10% are symptomatic **HERPES SIMPLEX** may cause prematurity, and becomes symptomatic after the first week of life; CNS symptoms include irritability, seizures, chorioretinitis, hydrocephalus, flaccid or spastic paralysis, opisthotonos, decerebrate rigidity and coma; in neonatal HSV infection, no deaths occur in those with localized disease, 15% die if encephalitis is present and 57% die if HSV is disseminated, potentially evoking DIC (N Engl J Med 1991; 324:450) **SYPHILIS** (an optional 'TORCH') Congenital syphilis has ↑ to epidemic rates in the urban US since the mid-1980s; the clinical findings are nonspecific and include fever, lethargy, failure to thrive, and irritability

TORCH antibody panel LABORATORY MEDICINE A standard (CPT-4 code 80061) panel of laboratory tests used to evaluate the possible presence of prenatal infection in a newborn; for Medicare or Medicaid reimbursement, it must measure antibodies to toxoplasma, rubella, CMV, and herpes simplex (CAP Today March 1993)

TORCH panel PEDIATRICS A 'shotgun' serologic screen for diagnosing prenatal infection; the finding of increased IgM in the neonate implies in utero infection, which should be further characterized by measuring the IgM levels for specific organisms Note: The quantitative TORCH screen has a high rate of false positive and negativity

tori palati Benign osseous 'tumors' of the oral cavity that may be associated with malignancy, eg squamous cell carcinoma of overlying epithelium; Cf Pseudoepitheliomatous hyperplasia

torpedo NEUROPATHOLOGY A focal fusiform swelling of the axon of Purkinje cells, located in the first portion of the axis cylinder prior to the origin of collateral branches, often accompanied by swollen dendritic ramifications and patchy displacement of Purkinje cells, a typical pathologic finding in olivopontocerebellar atrophy of the granular layer of the cerebellum

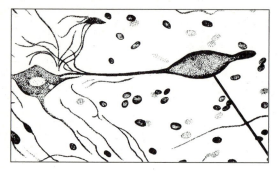

torpedo

torr A non-SI (International System) unit of pressure corresponding to 1/760 atm or a pressure of 1.0 mm Hg (133.3224 pascal)

Note: Although the pascal is the unit for pressure sanctioned offically accepted by the International System, torr continues to be widely used by clinical workers who often measure blood pressures

torsade de pointes *torsade*, French, twist CARDIOLOGY A form of polymorphic ventricular tachycardia with prolonged Q-T intervals that are initiated by a premature ventricular depolarization striking near the apex of a delayed T wave; torsades have irregular rates of 200-250/min with marked variability in amplitude and direction of a QRS wave that seems to twist around an isoelectric baseline; torsades may spontaneously resolve or evolve to ventricular tachyarrhythmia and may be non-specific or due to drugs, eg adrenergics, antihistamine, phenothiazine, procainamide, quinines, sotalol (**N Engl J Med 1994; 331:31ᴿᵛ**) and tricyclic antidepressants, electrolyte imbalance, eg hypokalemia, hypomagnesemia, CNS hemorrhage or trauma, long Q-T wave syndrome, liquid diet and underlying heart disease TREATMENT Isoproterenol

torso The part of the body that is delineated superiorly by the upper neck, anteroinferiorly by the inguinal ligaments and the symphysis pubis, and posteroinferiorly by the gluteal folds

tort MEDICAL MALPRACTICE *noun* A wrongful or allegedly wrongful act that is capable of initiating a civil action, ie a lawsuit; in a tort, the alleged wrongdoer (tortfeasor) may be held liable in damages; negligence is a type of tort equivalent to malpractice; see Malpractice OPTHALMOLOGY *verb* To rotate an eye on its anteroposterior axis

tort reform MEDICAL MALPRACTICE A long-debated series of proposals on details of how to best reduce the high costs of both the medical liability insurance and the costs of practicing medicine; the most critical component of TF is the capping of non-economic damages (the so-called 'pain and suffering' damages) paid to an allegedly injured party to $250 000, a move vehemently opposed by some malpractice lawyers (**Am Med News 1995; 17 April 1995 p1**)

tort reform bill A legislative package that was proposed by the Bush Administration, with the purpose of reducing the health care costs inherent in an advanced free-market system and litigation-prone society, eg US, addressing in particular the excess medical costs related to medical malpractice-related lawsuits; the proposal called for a $250 000 'cap' on non-economic ('pain and suffering') awards, and an end of lump sum payments and duplicate awards; see 'Defensive medicine', Malpractice

tort system A legal system in which wrongful acts may be tried by jury and awards given for (real or peceived) dam-

ages to a plaintiff, which is a key facet of American judicial system; it has been estimated that up to 2.6% ($117 x 10⁹) of the US gross national product (GNP), is consumed by some form of direct or indirect legal fees, including payment of claims, administrative costs and attorney's fees; in contrast, Switzerland spends 0.8% of GNP on its legal system; Canada, Austria, France, 0.6%; West Germany, Italy 0.5%; Japan, Spain, Denmark 0.4%; see Malpractice

Note: There are 14 times more lawyers in the US than in Japan

torticollis 1) Congenital torticollis 2) Wryneck, see there

tortoise shell nucleus Checkerboard nucleus A fanciful descriptor for polychromatophilic normoblast nuclei that are round with dark, coarse and eccentric chromatin and distinct parachromatin, a feature of use in differentiating these cells from lymphocytes in the bone marrow; the cytoplasm is pink and relatively abundant

torture HUMAN RIGHTS The deliberate, systematic or wanton infliction of physical or mental suffering by one or more persons acting alone or on the order of any authority to force another person to yield information, to make a confession, or for any other reason; methods of torture range from verbal threats and humiliation to bizarre displays of man's inhumanity to man including beating the soles of the feet (falanga), suspension from a rod by the hands and feet (la 'bandera'), submersion of the head in water (often soiled by excreta, el 'submarino'), striking blows at the victim's head and ears (el 'telefono'), food and water deprivation, mutilation, forcing the victims to watch others being tortured or killed; the 'torture syndrome' is characterized by a wide range of residual effects, including extreme anxiety, insomnia, nightmares, phobias and suspicion; the long-term effects of torture have been termed 'post-traumatic cerebral syndrome', and are characterized by three or more of the following symptoms: impaired memory, headaches, intolerance of alcohol, sleep disorders, marital and emotional disturbances; it is unclear whether the cerebral atrophy described as a terminal effect of torture is the result of multiple blows to the head; see Amnesty International, Refugee, Unethical medical research; Cf Boxing

Torulopsis glabrata A yeast-like mucosal saprobic fungus, with features of *Candida* and *Cryptococcus*; *T glabrata* may rarely cause an opportunistic infection in immunocompromised hosts CLINICAL Spiking fever, hypotension, urinary tract infection and fungemia Note: *Torulopsis* is closely related to *Candida* and may ultimately be integrated within the genus *Candida*, although *T glabrata* has only a yeast form

torus fracture An incomplete fracture of the diaphysis of long bones with buckling of the cortex on the side opposite the fracture; in contrast, the 'greenstick fracture', is ruptured on the convex aspect of the bone

total effective dose equivalent RADIATION SAFETY The sum of external (deep-dose equivalent) and internal (committed effective dose equivalent) exposure to ionizing radiation

total energy expenditure PHYSIOLOGY A metabolic 'unit' which is the sum of the

1) RESTING ENERGY EXPENDITURE (which is 60% of the TEE)

2) THERMIC ENERGY OF FEEDING (10% of TEE) and

3) NONRESTING ENERGY EXPENDITURE (30% of TEE)

maintenance of a reduced or elevated body weight is linked to compensatory changes in energy expenditures that oppose any body weight that differs from the person's usual weight; these compensatory changes may explain the difficulty that obese subject have in maintaining lower weights (**N Engl J Med 1995; 332:621ᴰᴬ**)

total fertility rate PUBLIC HEALTH The total number of live infants a woman would normally have if she survived through her child-bearing years; the TFR differs according to the country, eg in sub-Saharan Africa, it is 6-8, in Japan and industrialized democracies, it is 1.5-1.8; the higher the TFR, the greater is the region's level of poverty, population growth and environmental degradation (**Sci Am 1995; 272/2:41**)

total hip replacement A procedure that replaces the femoral head and its articular surface with a completely synthetic device, thus being a biomechanical solution for a biological failure; the first 'total hip' was replaced in 1962; in the US ± 120 000 are replaced/year (data from 1990), each costing $8500 INDICATIONS Advanced osteoarthritis and rheumatoid arthritis with disabling pain; according to a consensus conference sponsored by the NIH, THR '...*is an option for nearly all patients with disease of the hip that cause chronic discomfort and significant functional impairment. Most patients have an excellent prognosis for long-term improvement in symptoms and physical function. At this time, a cemented femoral component using modern cementing techniques, paired with a porous-coated acetabular component, can give excellent long-term results.*' revision of THR is required in the face of failure, and continued follow-up is necessary to identify impending failure (**JAMA 1995; 273:197**) COMPLICATIONS Loosening of one or more of the synthetic components, dislocation, femoral head fracture, deep vein thrombosis, nerve damage and (rarely) infection (**N Engl J Med 1990; 323:725rv**)

total ischemic burden CARDIOLOGY The sum total of all episodes of symptomatic and asymptomatic or 'silent' myocardial ischemia

total knee replacement A procedure that substitutes a painful arthritic knee and its articular surface with a synthetic device; the first 'total knee' was replaced in the 1950s but the hinge design was primitive, resulting in high failure rates; these problems were solved by the 1970s by using an unlinked (non-hinged) knee articulation; the excess rigidity problem was solved by retaining and inserting the posterior cruciate ligament into the articular apparatus; ± 120 000 'total knees' are performed/year (US), at a cost of $25-30 000 each INDICATIONS Advanced osteoarthritis and rheumatoid arthritis with disabling pain; in assessing the surgical candidates, the patient's age, weight and physical activity must be considered COMPLICATIONS Loosening of one or more of the synthetic components, dislocation, femoral head fracture, infection (very rare), deep vein thrombosis, nerve damage

total lymphoid irradiation ONCOLOGY Sequential radiation therapy to the 'mantle' and 'inverted Y' lymphoid regions, a combination of fields that may be used in extensive stage IV Hodgkin's and non-Hodgkin's lymphomas

total parenteral nutrition TPN, see there

total pelvic exenteration Bruschwig procedure GYNECOLOGIC SURGERY A form of 'heroic' surgery for extensive carcinoma of the uterine cervix that persists after regional radiotherapy and/or previous total hysterectomy; TPE consists of complete surgical removal of pelvic 'plumbing', including the bladder (with ureters and urethra), rectum, regional lymph nodes, and pelvic peritoneum, and creation of conduits for urinary diversion and a sigmoid colostomy for passage of feces*; because of its high morbidity and mortality, TPE is reserved for 1) Biopsy-proven recurrences of tumor that is believed to be confined to the central portion of the pelvis and completely removable, IF 2) The patient is believed capable of psychologically and physically coping with the stomas necessitated by the operation

*The patient may be candidate for a continent urostomy and a lower rectal reanastomosis

total quality management HEALTH CARE MANAGEMENT The application of management theory of quality, a concept*

that focuses on the quality of a product as a means of increasing sales and saving money; TQM is based on the posit that it is not employees' work that leads to poor quality, but rather poor design of systems and procedures; in TQM, quality goals are examined by scientific methods and a team approach is used to build quality into the various steps of a manufacturing process (process improvement), resulting in products with fewer defects; by minimizing expenditures required to inspect, retest, and reject the manufactured goods, productivity increases; TQM is a customer-driven philosophy, the tenets of which are being embraced by advanced thinkers in the field of health care (**Acta Cytologica 1993; 37:2610A; MLO September 1993**)

*Delineated by industrial engineers WE Deming and J Duran, whose philosophies found little mainstream support in the US when first introduced; TQM is believed to be responsible for the Japanese economic 'miracle' in the past three decades

totipotency The ability of a usually primitive cell to express the entire range of its genetic information and to give rise to a completely differentiated adult organism, adjective, totipotent; Cf Stem cell

'touchdown' PCR MOLECULAR BIOLOGY A technique used to prevent spurious priming gene amplification (**Nucleic Acids Res1991; 19:4008; Diagn Mol Pathol 1993; 2:94**)

tourniquet A cord or constrictive band used to reduce the blood flow to one or more extremity; because tourniquets, especially those using thin or narrow devices, worsen distal ischemia and may increase venous bleeding, direct compression of bleeding vessels is preferable to 'encirclement' for hemostasis; tourniquets continue to have some clinical currency in reducing the centripetal flow of toxins in snake and scorpion bites, and in reducing the cardiac load in acute congestive heart failure, as may occur in an acute myocardial infarct, where the tourniquets are rotated, simultaneously with other emergency measures, including oxygen, lasix, nitroprusside and nitroglycerine; when used, a tourniquet should be confined to the proximal portion of the extremity

tourniquet paralysis A virtually extinct clinical complex caused by prolonged tourniquet compression of an extremity, resulting in loss of touch, light pressure, vibration and position sensation Note: Complete recuperation is usual within three months

tourniquet test Capillary fragility test A clinical sign elicited when the sphygmomanometer cuff is left inflated for 15 minutes on the arm at a pressure midway between the systolic and diastolic pressures; 10 or more petechiae within a circle 2.5 cm in diameter is considered a positive result and may occur with thrombocytopenia of less than 70×10^9/L (US: 70 000/mm³), nonthrombocytopenic purpura or scurvy Note: In practice the tourniquet test is of little use

Tourette syndrome Gilles de Tourette syndrome A condition with an onset between age 2 and 15, characterized by involuntary muscle movement, fast eye blinking, head jerking, facial grimaces, uncontrollable noises (eg grunting, snorting, throat clearing, barking, sniffing, other unusual sounds and involuntary profanity); the pattern of symptoms may change with time, and invariably disappear during sleep; in many cases the disease may only be recognized late in life (**New York Times 1 March1995; C11**)

Touretter A person with Tourette syndrome, see there

Towers nursing home A nursing home in New York that was the focal point of US Federal investigations for possible Medicaid fraud, and alleged physical abuse and starvation of elderly patients during the late 1960s and early 1970s (**Facts on File, Vol 35:1028E1, Vol 38:232F1**)

'towns' ACADEMIA A colloquial term for the clinical faculty of a medical school, who are in relatively close contact with the community, ie work in the 'town', actively practice medicine, see patients and are less (if at all) involved in research activities; *'To practice medicine without books is to sail the seas without charts...'* Sir William Osler; Cf 'Gowns'

toxic OCCUPATIONAL MEDICINE An adjective referring to a chemical or sunstance that 1) Has a median lethal dose (LD_{50}) of 50-500 mg/kg when administered orally to 200-300 g albino rats 2) Has an LD_{50} of 200-1000 mg/kg when administered by continuous contact for 24 hours on the shaved skin of 2.0-3.0 kg albino rabbits 3) Has an LD_{50} of 200-2000 ppm of volume of gas or vapor, or 2-20 mg/L of mist or dust, when adminstered by continuous inhalation to 200-300 g albino rats; Cf Highly toxic

'toxic core' PSYCHIATRY A component or 'factor' hypothesized to cause increased cardiovascular mortality in type A personalities; coronary artery disease-prone type A individuals have a cynical mistrust of others, are angry and repress marked hostility towards others; clinical data suggests that over time, the cardiovascular mortality is up to 4-to-7-fold greater in subjects with a 'toxic core' personality; see Type A personality

toxic dump ENVIRONMENT Any site that is (or was) a repository for chemical pollutants, often placed there illegally, either in standard 50-gallon (± 200 liter) drums or poured directly into the ground; of greatest concern with the thousands of identified toxic dump sites is the slow leaching of toxic chemicals (known as 'plumes') into the water table and aquifers, thereby contaminating drinking water; see Chemical pollutants, Environmental Protection Agency, Plumes, Superfund; Cf Regulated waste

toxic epidermal necrolysis Lyell syndrome An acute life-threatening mucocutaneous reaction often to drugs (80% of cases) characterized by widespread and/or confluent erythema, necrosis, and bulla formation; TEN is thought to represent an extreme form of erythema multiforme, as it is associated with the same etiological factors as EM, including drug hypersensitivity, eg to allopurinol, anticonvulsants, barbiturates, carbamazepine, NSAIDs (eg phenylbutazone, oxicam derivatives) and sulfonamides (eg T-S), infections, vaccination, radiotherapy and malignancy CLINICAL After a prodrome of fever, malaise, and erythema, subepidermal bullae develop, leading to epidemal sloughing COMPLICATIONS Dehydration, electrolyte imbalance or 'third space phenomenon', abscess formation, sepsis, renal failure, heart failure, GI hemorrhage, and shock acute skin failure, erosive stomatitis, lesions of anogenital mucosae, conjunctivae (keratitis, corneal erosions), and respiratory tract; ± 30% are fatal TREATMENT Symptomatic therapy, as with second degree burns, withdrawal of offending drug (N Engl J Med 1994; 331:1272ʀᴠ) see Stevens-Johnson syndrome; Cf Staphylococcus scalded skin syndrome

*Synonyms include Brocq-Debré-Lyell syndrome, Debré-Lamy-Lyell syndrome, epidermolysis acuta toxica, epidermolysis combustiformis, epidermolysis necroticans combustiformis, epidermolysis toxica, erythrodermia bullosa with epidermolysis, Lyell's disease, toxic bullous epidermolysis, toxico-allergic epidermal necrolysis

toxic granulation HEMATOLOGY Any of a number of large, irregular granules that are a dark blue-violet by 'Romanovsky'-type stains, eg Wright-Giemsa stain and variably positive by the periodic acid-Schiff stain; these granules correspond to secondary autolysosomes with an increased membrane permeability, are seen in metamyelocytes, band or segmented neutrophils and lymphocytes and may be induced by rapid turnover of cell products and may be seen in leukemoid reactions and in infections, related to bacterial products; toxic granulations may also be seen in eclampsia, irradiation, hepatic disease and terminal cancer

Note: Also seen in peripheral blood smears of patients with acute infections are 'toxic' cytoplasmic vacuolization, Döhle bodies and a 'left shift' of the myeloid series

toxicity index see Toxicity testing

toxicity risk rating Hazard risk rating, see there

toxicity testing ENVIRONMENT A component of risk assessment that is required by law in the USA for all new chemicals, for new purposes of old chemicals or for combinations of new and old chemicals; toxicity testing attempts to identify hazards, including adverse effects, cancer, nephrotoxicity and teratogenesis and to quantitate exposure-response relation (measured by LD_{50}, the chemical 'dose' that is lethal in 50% of the test animals, and ED_{50}, the 'effective dose' that causes a consistent change in 50% of tested animals); standard 'whole animal toxicity tests' determine acute, subacute, chronic, reproductive and developmental toxicity, and study ocular and skin irritation (Draize test), hypersensitivity, phototoxicity, toxicokinetics and behavioral changes; conventional animal testing for one agent costs \$0.5-1.5 million (US) and may require the sacrifice of thousands of animals to put a chemical into production; the less expensive in vitro assays include the mutagenic bacterial or genotoxicity screen devised by Ames, cytotoxicity (total cellular-protein assay and the neutral red dye test), which measures inhibition of protein production (IC_{50}) and the chorioallantoic membrane test (CAM test), in which the shell of a fertilized chicken egg is removed, revealing a veined chorioallantoic membrane, the site of application of the test chemical (Sci Am 1989; 261/2:24) see Ames test, Risk assessment

toxic megacolon An acute colitis with partial or complete colonic dilatation, which represents a severe life-threatening complication, and occasionally the presenting sign of ulcerative colitis and Crohn's disease CLINICAL High fever, abdominal pain, tachycardia and leukostasis TREATMENT Resection of diseased colon, salvaging rectal sphincter if possible; Cf Megacolon

toxic oil syndrome An epidemic that centered around Avila, Spain, occurring from mid-1981 until mid-1983, resulting from the ingestion of olive oil contaminated with rapeseed oil, the latter of which was intended for industrial use and contained aniline; clandestine factories attempted to chemically remove the aniline and sold the product as olive oil to low-income families CLINICAL Fever, pneumonia-like illness, followed by gastrointestinal disease, eosinophilia and a prolonged rash; late neurological sequelae included myalgias, motor deficits, major muscle group atrophy, carpal tunnel syndrome, contractures of the jaw and extremities; of the estimated 20 000 cases, 340 people died; see Yusho disease

toxic shock-like syndrome 'Jim Henson's' disease An epidemic infection caused by a highly virulent, antibiotic-resistant strain of group A streptococcus, which begins as a mild skin infection or 'strep throat' and rapidly progresses to high fever, hypotension, focal vasodilatation and soft-tissue cellulitis of an intensity that may require amputation; most cases have occurred in patients lacking predisposing factors, and it is unknown whether TSLS is due to a new strain of bacteria or represents the reappearance of streptococcal toxin A, the toxin responsible for scarlet fever that has not been produced in streptococci since the 1940s)

Note: TSLS was first identified by a group of infectious disease specialists, the 'Rocky Mountain Pus Club'and was responsible for the death of Jim Henson of the Sesame Street Muppets

toxic shock syndrome A disease caused by *Staphylococcus aureus* strains that produce the toxin, TSST-1*, formerly, enterotoxin F or exotoxin C is a superantigen; these strains of *S aureus* exhibit lysogeny (presence of a temperate bacteriophage, the production of which is enhanced in Mg^{++}-depleted medium); superabsorbent tampons are divalent cation chelators and thus the intravaginal microbiological milieu favors growth of lysogenic strains; the early cases of TSS occurred in tampon users and most began as vaginal lesions; TSS may also arise in foreign bodies, eg sutures CLINICAL Abrupt onset of high fever (> 40°C), nausea, vomiting, watery diarrhea, which may occur during menstruation, followed by an intense blanching mucocutaneous erythema, desquamative palmo-plantar rash and cleavage of the basal layer of the epidermis; without therapy, the patients deteriorate, become lethargic and confused, develop capillary leakage, hypotension, adult respiratory distress syndrome, renal and multiorgan failure and frank shock; even with appropriate therapy (non-β-lactam containing antibiotics), mortality is 5-10%; 88% of genital and 53% of non-genital TSS have been linked to a single strain of *Staphylococcus aureus*; see Superantigen

*Toxic shock syndrome toxin-1, designated 1 in anticipation of a 2, which has not been identified

'toxic' staring Fixed staring, abnormal behavior, altered mental status, delirium, aphonia and coma, classically described in typhoid fever; see Rose spots

toxic state INFECTIOUS DISEASE A condition typically seen in the third week of typhoid fever at which point the patients are sickest, mentally disoriented and at greatest risk for intestinal perforation and hemorrhage; see Pea soup stool

'toxic tort' A lawsuit that centers around a drug, chemical, or other substance in the environment, that is either incriminated in a disease process, eg DES and thalidomide, or implicated by vague and/or 'soft' circumstantial evidence, eg Agent Orange, electromagnetic radiation, video display terminals; a criticism of the jury process in toxic tort' cases is that they require that the judges, lawyers and juries (who generally are not trained to interpret statistical data of any nature) evaluate the validity of scientific evidence and understand the limits of the techniques used and by extension, the statistical method used; see Bendectin, *Frye* rule, Litogen

toxic vacuolization HEMATOLOGY Rounded 'empty' cytoplasmic spaces within neutrophils seen in gram-negative bacteremia and endotoxemia; see Toxic granulation

toxoid IMMUNOLOGY A bacterial toxin or other antigen that has been treated with formaldehyde in order to decrease the substance's toxicity while preserving antigenicity; toxoids are used to prepare diphtheria and tetanus vaccines

toxoplasmosis An infection by *Toxoplasma gondii* which is usually seen in two distinct clinical contexts: 1) Congenital toxoplasmosis, acquired transplacentally, often accompanied by major neurological residua and 2) Acquired, discussed here EPIDEMIOLOGY Ingestion of inadequately cooked meats with cysts, or due to exposure to infected feline feces CLINICAL In the immunocompetent, infection is benign with transient lymphadenopathy; in the immunocompromised, *T gondii* infection may be accompanied by necrotizing encephalitis, myocarditis, pneumonitis, with CNS involvement in ≥ 50% of cases; in one study focal neurological defects were present in 69% and 91% had enhancing lesions on CT (N Engl J Med 1992; 327:1643QA) TREATMENT Clindamycin, pyrimethamine, and in a case of AIDS, azithromycin (N Engl J Med 1994; 330:575c) see Congenital toxoplasmosis

toxoplasmosis triad A trilogy of typical histopathologic findings seen in lymph nodes infected with *Toxoplasma gondii* consisting of 1) Monocytoid cells in the sinusoides 2) Florid follicular hyperplasia 3) Aggregates of epithelioid histiocytes

toy balloon appearance A fanciful descriptor for the globular red-yellow retinal hemangioblastoma (balloon-like) seen by fundoscopic exam which has paired vessels (corresponding to the balloon's strings) to and from the lesion; Cf Balloon, Hot air balloon appearance

TPA 12-O-tetradecanoylphorbol-13-acetate A potent tumor promoter of the phorbol ester family that mimics diacylglycerol, which locks protein kinase C into the 'on' position; see Phorbol ester

tPA Tissue-plasminogen activator, see there

TPH Transplacental hemorrhage

TPN Total parenteral nutrition IV hyperalimentation CLINICAL NUTRITION A modality that attempts to provide all the body's need for nutrition without using the GI tract; TPN is used for 1) Correction of nutritional depletion in the face of inadequate oral intake and/or intestinal absorption, as in Crohn's disease, malignancy, pseudo-obstruction, radiation enteritis, short bowel syndrome, sprue and 2) Conditions requiring bowel rest and nutritional restitution, eg nonspecific colitides and associated growth retardation, enterocutaneous fistulas and pancreatitis; a typical TPN formulation provides 40 kcal/kg with 1-1.5 g/kg of calories provided by protein, two-thirds of the remainder by carbohydrates, one-third by lipids; 30 ml/kg of H_2O and appropriate electrolytes, trace elements and vitamins; TPN is used in children with diaphragmatic hernia, malrotation, esophageal atresia, tracheo-esophageal fistula, gastroschisis, volvulus, meconium ileus and omphalocele COMPLICATIONS (see table)

COMPLICATIONS OF TPN

HEPATIC DYSFUNCTION Cholestasis, cholelithiasis, hepatic dysfunction, jaundice, hepatomegaly, micronodular cirrhosis, lipofuscinosis and steatosis (most common in premature infants)

RELATED TO INDWELLING INTRAVENOUS LINE Misplacement of line, infections, eg *Candida* spp, aspergillosis

METABOLIC DEFECTS Hyperglycemia (osmotic diuresis, hyperosmolarity), post-infusion hypoglycemia, hyperosmolar coma, ketoacidosis and other metabolic derangements, excess or deficiency of electrolytes, including Na^+, K^+, Cl^-, eg hyperchloremic acidosis and mineral imbalances, affecting Mg^{++}, PO_4, and Ca^{++} with hypercalcemia and accompanying pancreatitis, hypercalciuria and metabolic bone disease

NUTRITIONAL IMBALANCES Generalized decrease in essential fatty acids, trace minerals (required copper, chromium, molybdenum, tin, zinc) and vitamins and increased triglycerides and cholesterol

---

TPR 1) Temperature, pulse and respiration 2) Third-party reimbursement

TQM Total quality managment, see there

TQM/CQI Total quality managment/continuous quality information

TR Repetition time MRI The period between the beginning of the pulse sequence and the beginning of the succeeding (virtually identical) pulse sequence; see Magnetic resonance imaging

TRAb Thyroid-stimulating hormone receptor antibodies Antibodies that are pathogenically linked to Graves' disease, which may be quantified by 1) Bioassays that measure the ability of a patient's immunoglobulins to stimulate thyroid activity, eg increasing cAMP production in Fisher rat thyroid cells (FRTL-5), assays that are less sensitive than 2) Radioreceptor assays that measure inhibition of binding of labelled TSH to its receptor; both assays confirm the diagnosis of euthyroid Graves' disease with ophthalmopathy and atypical hyperthyroid Graves' disease

trabecular bar SURGICAL PATHOLOGY A rigid row of malignant epithelial cells with its long axis perpendicular to the long axis of a 'bar', a histologic criterion supporting the diagnosis of ductal carcinoma in situ of the breast; see 'Roman bridges'

trabeculation of the bladder A forme fruste of bladder diverticulosis caused by partial urinary obstruction at the bladder neck, which is often secondary to prostatic hypertrophy; the increased intravesicular pressure results in mucosal herniation and fibrous cords spread haphazardly across the bladder, histologically characterized by squamous metaplasia, epithelial hyperplasia, chronic inflammation and occasionally transitional or less commonly, squamous cell carcinoma

trace mineral Any of a group of metal ions that are essential for life, functioning as enzyme co-factors and playing critical roles in the organization of molecules, membranes and mitochondria; they are present in milligram or microgram amounts and maintained in a delicate balance between the Scylla of toxic excess and the Charybdis of deficiency, which may induce metabolic failure, an event most common in total parenteral nutrition; trace elements include arsenic*, chromium, cobalt, copper, fluorine, iodine, iron, manganese, nickel, selenium, silicon, tin, vanadium, zinc

*The only one of the group that is not only not essential for life, but is toxic

track SUBSTANCE ABUSE A punctate, erythematous linear scar on the skin of the extremities, neck, and groin, and on mucocutaneous surfaces that may be accompanied by intense venous sclerosis and edema of the extremities, a characteristic finding in long-term heroin addicts; Cf Skin 'popping'

trackball COMPUTERS A type of input device that is similar in principle to a mouse, in that it accesses programs and files symbolized as icons, and is used to execute commands from 'pull-down' menus; the trackball, unlike the mouse, is fixed in one position, and thus requires less desktop 'real estate', making it ideally suited for confined spaces; see Mouse

track sign BONE RADIOLOGY An abnormal anatomic variant of the femur in which the linea aspera or pilaster (site of attachment of the major adductor and extensor muscles) is more prominent than usual and is located on the posterior midshaft, thus having a radiodense 'tube-within-a-tube' appearance that should not be confused with the Blade of grass sign of Paget's disease of the bone

tracking PUBLIC HEALTH The monitoring of a person's status in terms of health-related activities, eg return to primary care-giver for followup visits; when compared with manual tracking, computerized tracking systems increased provider compliance with the health maintenance protocol (Arch FamMed 1993; 3:581)

traditional Chinese medicine ALTERNATIVE MEDICINE A generic term for an ancient method of health care which is preventive in nature and based on the balance of opposing yet complementary forces, yin and yang, which are driven by the life force known as qi, which flow through the body following pathways known as meridians; the tools of TCM are acupuncture, food therapy, massage therapy, and medicinal herbs, eg astragalus, dong quai, ginseng, and others; TCM is reportedly most beneficial in treating chronic conditions including allergies, asthma, DM, gallbladder disease, gynecologic disorders, headaches, hypertension, SLE, and others (Alternative Medicine, Future Medicine Publishing, Inc, Puyallup, Washington, 1994)

traffic 1) see Motor vehicles 2) Sexual traffic, see there

traffic accident Motor vehicle accident, see there

'traffic light' diet A dietary regimen designed to reduce atherosclerosis and weight; see Diet

trailer sequence MOLECULAR BIOLOGY An untranslated segment of mRNA nucleotides that follows the termination signal (stop codon) at the 3' end, which does not include the poly(A) tail

trail-making test Reitan's test A two-part psychomotor test for assessing motor speed and integration, in which multiple dots are connected to form various objects; like the Bender-Gestalt test, the 'Trail-maker' serves as a screening test to detect gross organic defects; see Psychological testing

train track appearance Railroad track appearance; Cf Tram tracks

training A generic term for deliberate goal-oriented practice in a mental or physical activity, usually with the intent of bettering one's performance in competition PHYSIOLOGY Training results in physiologic muscular hypertrophy in particular of the heart, ↑ in skeletal muscle blood supply due to an ↑ in capillaries, and change in the proportion of slow- or fast-twitch muscle, depending on the type of training activity; the neurologic changes that result from practice are less well defined (New York Times 11 October 1994; C1)

TRAM flap Transverse rectus abdominus musculocutaneous flap GENERAL SURGERY A rotated piece of tissue used as an alternative to a prosthesis in post-radical mastectomy reconstructive breast surgery; the operating time and the recovery period is longer, but the cosmetic result is often better

tramtrack appearance Tramline calcification A descriptive term for parallel, curved lines, radio-opacities or radiolucencies of varying length (when the parallel lines are straight, 'railroad track' may be a more valid adjectival descriptor) NEURORADIOLOGY A descriptor for the parallel calcified enhancement of cortical vessels seen in tuberous sclerosis (Sturge-Weber syndrome), due to calcium and iron deposition seen on a plain skull film RADIOLOGY, BONE A descriptor for the split cortical thickening with parallel neo-osteogenesis (endosteal splitting), seen in infarctions of long bones in sickle cell anemia RADIOLOGY, LUNG A descriptor for the parallel, thickened bronchial walls seen on a plain chest film in bronchiectasis; Cf Railroad track, Ring shadow

trans-acting locus MOLECULAR BIOLOGY A region of DNA that responds to a (trans-acting) protein factor that activates transcription by binding to cis-acting DNA sequences, which are required for gene regulation; Cf cis-activation

transactivation VIROLOGY The upregulation of DNA transcription by the products of genes that are immediately translated after infection by a virus, eg Herpes simplex

transactivator Transcription activator, see there

transaminase-type mechanism Ping-pong mechanism, see there

transbronchial needle (aspiration) biopsy An endoscopic technique used to obtain a cytologic specimen from a submucosal endobronchial lesion or an accessible extrabronchial mass, if there is evidence of extrinsic compression; TNAB is of use in establishing the diagnosis of both diagnosing bronchogenic carcinoma, carcinoid, bronchogenic cyst, lymphoma, sarcoid, pneumonia and abscesses COMPLICATIONS Pneumothorax, hemomediastinum, hemorrhage, bacteremia and rarely, false-positive diagnosis of malignancy; up to 37% of malignancy can be diagnosed by TBNA; see Bronchoalveolar lavage, 'Skinny needle' biopsy

transcervical balloon tuboplasty GYNECOLOGY The use of a balloon catheter inserted via the uterine cervix to dilate and re-establish the patency of fallopian tubes, stenosed by the vicissitudes of endometriosis and salpingitis, a procedure that is similar in principle to balloon angioplasty; tubal patency was re-established in one or both tubes in 92% of the 77 ♀ in one study, 22 of whom became pregnant; balloon tuboplasty offers an alternative to microsurgery or to in vitro fertilization for ♀ with 'mechanical' infertility, which is responsible for 25-30% of ♀ infertility

transcranial Doppler ultrasonography A non-invasive modality of bedside imaging of the intracranial cerebral circulation in critically ill hospitalized patients and outpatients, used to diagnosis vasospasm, assess collateral circulation and stenoses, to confirm brain death and to monitor circulation in neurosurgical patients

transcription MOLECULAR BIOLOGY The copying of a strand of DNA to generate a complementary strand of RNA; usually only one of the strands of DNA's double helix is capable of providing information which, when transcribed into RNA is translatable into a cognate polypeptide chain; in eukaryotes, three different RNA polymerases are responsible for producing RNAs: RNA polymerase I (RP-I), which generates ribosomal RNA (rRNA), RP-II, which synthesizes messenger RNA (mRNA) and RP-III which generates transfer RNA (tRNA)

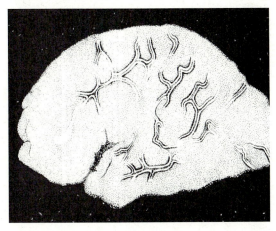

treamtrack appearance

transcription activator A protein that binds to DNA, activating its transcription machinery; in eukaryotes, there are multiple 15- to 20-DNA base pair transcription activator-binding sites; once the activator is bound, a conformational change occurs, forming a pre-initiation complex (containing RNA polymerase, TFIIA, TFIIB, TFIID,

TFIIE and TFIIF) at the transcription start site; DNA transcription activators are either 'universal' or activators that only function in some cells; see TFIID

Note: Transcription requires a transcription activating protein in addition to RNA polymerase II, the TATA box and TATA factor

transcription apparatus MOLECULAR BIOLOGY A group of at least 50 proteins that must assemble in a tight complex on DNA before RNA polymerase can copy (transcribe) DNA into mRNA; the TA consists of 4 different components

1) BASAL FACTORS, which respond to signals from activators and position RNA polymerase at the beginning of a protein-coding region of a gene, sending the RNA polymerase on its mission; basal factors include the *TATA* binding protein and factors A, B, E, F, H

2) ACTIVATORS, which bind to genes at enhancer sites, helping to determine which genes will be transcribed, speeding the rate of transcription

3) REPRESSORS, which bind to certain genes at silencer sites, interfering with the function of activators, slowing the rate of transcription

4) COACTIVATORS, a poorly understood family of 'adaptive' molecules that integrate signals from activators and possibly also repressors, relaying the results to the basal factors (Sci Am 1995; 272/2:56)

transcription-mediated amplification see TMA

transcription factor A protein of the transcription-initiation complex which participates in determining sites of mRNA synthesis and controlling the efficiency of mRNA transcription; TFs are DNA-binding proteins that are necessary for gene activity, but don't themselves participate directly in the regulation of gene activity; most of these factors have a positive effect on gene regulation and are involved in the organism's development

transcription unit MOLECULAR BIOLOGY A DNA sequence that is transcribed into a coherent peptide, which is demarcated by flanking sequences; promoter elements are present -500 to -1000 nucleotides upstream (ie, in the 5' direction) of the transcription unit; closer to the beginning of the exon is the TATA box, located at -30 nucleotides, followed by the cap or initiation site (standardized as +1); from the cap to the ATG (start codon) is an untranslated portion of DNA; the exons are separated by introns, which are removed at the time the primary RNA transcript is processed, yielding mature mRNA; after the final exon is transcribed, there follows an untranslated sequence, containing AATAAA separated 10-20 nucleotides from the poly(A) tail, followed by the termination site at the 3' downstream end and finally the flanking sequence

transcutaneous cardiac pacemaker A device used to

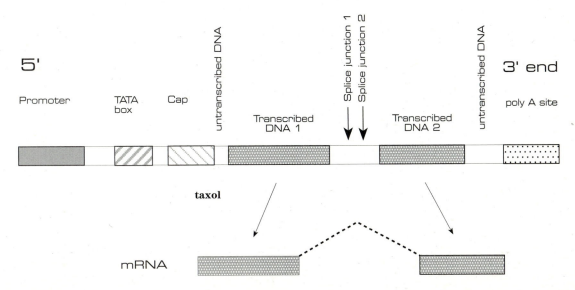

generate electrical stimuli that pace the heart via external electrodes adherent to the chest wall; transcutaneous pacing is of use in some patients with bradycardia; it is reported to offer no benefit in patients with asystolic cardiac arrest (or primary asystole or post-defibrillation asystole), even when performed by emergency medical technicians in the field (N Engl J Med 1993; 328:1377oa)

transcutaneous drug delivery CLINICAL THERAPEUTICS The administration of therapeutic agents across the skin; transcutaneous penetration of a drug requires that it not only traverse the intercellular lipid layer surrounding the cells of the stratum corneum (rather than through the cells themselves), but also the aqueous environment of the more basal cells of the epidermis and the dermis* ADVANTAGES OF TCDD Bypass of GI tract and first-pass hepatic biotransformation and metabolism, control of absorption, mutiple potential 'delivery' sites are available, patient compliance may be improved DISADVANTAGES OF TCDD Local irritation and possible allergic skin reactions, systemic toxicity, long time to therapeutic levels MOST ABSORPTIVE SITES (in descending order) Scrotum, jaw, forehead, scalp, axilla, arm, leg DRUGS/AGENTS APPROVED FOR TCDD Clonidine HCl, Estradiol, fentanyl citrate, nicotine, nitroglycerin, scopolamine POSSIBLE AGENTS FOR TCDD Antiaddictives, antiarthritics, antiasthmatics, antiemetics, antiretrovirals, β-blockers, calcium channel antagonists, centrally acting cholinergics, hormones, and tranquilizers (Mayo Clin Proc 1995; 70:581)

*This is to say that the drug must be both lipophilic and hydrophilic

transcutaneous electrical nerve stimulation A modality for controlling pain that utilizes low-level electric shocks to the skin; TENS effect is explained by the 'gate' theory of pain and is used to relieve pain of the lower back and neck, 'phantom' limb syndrome and amputation stump pain; in lower back pain, TENS may be no more effective than a placebo; Cf Biofeedback

transdermal therapy CLINICAL PHARMACOLOGY A generic term for the use of topical prolonged-release forms of drugs, eg nitroglycerin patches or testosterone replacement therapy

transducer INSTRUMENTATION Any device that transforms one form of energy to another, eg a photocell that converts light into electrical energy; the transducer is the major component in ultrasonographic devices, containing both an emitting and receiving piezoelectric crystal

transducin An 83-kD heterotrimeric G protein composed of Tα, Tβ and Tγ subunits that transduces a light signal into cells, mediating the light activation signal from photolyzed rhodopsin to cGMP phosphodiesterase; for GTP to bind to transducin, the Tγ subunit must have an attached farnesyl moiety

transducin family A family of eleven or more rhodopsin-related proteins that have sensory, neurotransmitter, and hormone receptor functions, which includes β-adrenergic and muscarinic acetylcholine receptors; the transucin family members are membrane-bound, allowing the cell to communicate with the external environment, have significant amino acid sequence homology and similarities in secondary and tertiary structures, including the presence of several transmembrane segments and share a common mechanism of action in that the intracellular signal occurs via G protein activation (Science 1991; 251:558)

transduction The acquisition and transfer of cellular DNA by a virus or other vector; transduction is type of genetic recombination that occurs in bacteria, in which DNA is donated from one cell to another by means of a phage (a virus); the most efficient transducing vectors are retroviruses

transesophageal echocardiography Two-dimensional transesophageal color-flow Doppler echocardiography

CARDIOLOGY An ultrasonographic imaging modality used to examine cardiac structures (valves, chambers and inflow and outflow tracts) and function in which a transducer is placed immediately behind the heart in the esophagus and stomach; because there are no interfering air spaces or bone, the image is superior to that obtained with transthoracic echocardiography and is of particular use in evaluating the status of the endocardium, eg to identify vegetations on the cardiac valves (N Engl J Med 1991; 324:795); the current generation* of TEE is a noninvasive imaging technique for analyzing abnormalities of locoregional fluid distribution or blood flow patterns, and is as sensitive (97.7%) as MRI (98.3%), but less specific (77%) than CT (87%) or MRI (98%) for the identification of thoracic aortic aneurysms (ibid 1993; 328:1oa) although aortography is the current 'gold standard' in the diagnosis of traumatic rupture of the thoracic aorta (N Eng J Med 1995; 332:389ed), it may be displaced by TEE as the modality of first choice (ibid 1995; 332:356oa) INDICATIONS for TEE Identifying cardiac source of embolism (35%), prosthetic heart valve malfunction (20%), endocarditis (16%), aortic dissection (8%), cardiac tumor (6%), valvular disease (5%), and others (11%), based on a series of 5000 patients (ibid 1995; 332:1268rv) see Biplane (intraoperative) transesophageal echocardiography, Echocardiography

*Early devices were one-dimensional, and used a horizontal plane beam, which made it difficult to visualize anterior and posterior structures and to depict contiguous long-axis and off-axis spatial relationships; this problem was resolved with the introduction of two (biplanar) and three (multiplanar) dimensional devices

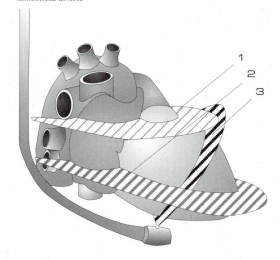

transesophageal echocardiography

IMAGING PLANES IN TEE (see figure)
I UPPER ESOPHAGEAL POSITION Imaging of basal 'short axis' of heart, including the ascending aorta, main pulmonary artery, right and left atria, atrial appendages, pulmonary veins, aortic and pumonary valves
II MIDESOPHAGEAL POSITION Imaging of all four chambers of the heart and the mitral and tricuspid valves
III TRANSGASTRIC POSITION: Imaging of 'short axis' of ventricles

'trans' fatty acid CLINICAL NUTRITION An unsaturated fat in which the carbon moieties on the two sides of the double bond point in opposite directions; minimal TFAs are present in animal fats; TFAs are abundant in margarines, frying fats and shortenings and are formed when polyunsaturated fat-rich vegetable and marine oils and vegetable shortenings are 'hardened' by partial hydrogenation, producing fats with a firmness and consistency desired by both food manufacturers and consumers; TFAs comprise 6-8% of the 120 g fat/day consumed per capita in developed nations; the recent trend away from consumption of tropical oils has resulted in an ↑ TFA consumption; the most abundant TFA is elaidic acid and its isomers, which are 18-carbon molecules with one double bond; , ↑ dietary TFA results in ↑ total cholesterol and LDL-cholesterol and ↓ HDL-cholesterol; the intensity of the lipid changes seen in a high TFA diet are as unfavorable as in a diet rich in saturated fatty acids; a high intake of TFAs is associated with ↑ incidence of coronary artery disease (**N Engl J Med 1993; 329:1970c**); Cf Fish, Olive oil, Polyunsaturated fatty acid, Tropical oils, Unsaturated fatty acid

Note: Oleic acid is a monounsaturated fatty acid with a cis configuration (carbon moieties lie on the same side of the double bond); most natural fats and oils contain only *cis* double bond

transfection EXPERIMENTAL ONCOLOGY The extraction of double-stranded DNA from tumor cells to induce the phenotypic changes of malignancy in a second population of cells, which when performed in non-mammalian cells has been termed transformation MOLECULAR BIOLOGY A procedure in which DNA is introduced (usually by vector) into a cell to express a protein or evaluate a promoter function

transfer *noun* A colloquial term for a patient whose care has been passed from one service to another *verb* To pass the care of a patient from one service forward to another

transfer factor of Lawrence IMMUNOLOGY A substance derived from leukocyte lysates that is dialyzable (ie has a molecular weight of < than 10 kD), is produced by most mammals, elicits a delayed hypersensitivity reaction and stimulates lymphokine production; transfer factor may have some therapeutic currency in selected patients with Wiskott-Aldrich syndrome and mucocutaneous candidiasis and was once used with equivocal results to treat TB and leprosy

transfer RNA A 70–80-residue RNA molecule that is encoded by tandem repeat DNA and has a cloverleaf structure that binds an amino acid, transferring it to a growing polypeptide chain, and releasing the amino acid at the time the tRNA is transiently 'docked' to a ribosome via the complementary anticodon on the messenger RNA; the normal planar representation of transfer RNA folds back upon itself to allow the maximum stability through formation of multiple hydrogen intrachain bonds at the 'arms' of the cloverleaf; segments of RNA that are not hydrogen-bonded are termed 'loops'; Cf Messenger RNA, Ribosomal RNA, 'Second genetic code'

transference PSYCHIATRY The projection of attitudes, wishes, desires, libidinous and aggressive thoughts to another party, usually understood to mean a psychoanalyst; transference is viewed as an unconscious need for the patient to relive past experiences who may endow the analyst with the magical powers and omniscience that the patient's parents had when he/she was a child; transference can be positive (affectinate) or negative (hostile)

transferrin Siderophilin An 80–90-kD iron-transporting β-globulin that binds up to 2 atoms of Fe(III) with bicarbonate; serum concentration: 2-4 g/L

transformation EXPERIMENTAL ONCOLOGY Malignant transformation The conversion of a cell to one with a malignant phenotype, either due to infection with an oncogenic virus or due to environmental factors HEMATOLOGY see Blast transformation MOLECULAR BIOLOGY The alteration of an organism's genome by insertion of DNA from another species, eg bacterial transformation, which follows recombination with an isolated fragment of DNA from a genetically distinct organism; plasmid DNA is most common DNA used to transforma bacteria; Cf Transfection

transforming growth factor(s) A group of distinct polypeptides that have been isolated from virus-transformed rodent cells, capable of altering cell phenotype, causing fibroblasts to lose anchorage-dependence and

TRANSFUSION REACTIONS

I IMMUNE, NON-INFECTIOUS TRANSFUSION REACTIONS

Allergic urticaria with immediate hypersensitivity

Anaphylaxis Spontaneous anti-IgA antibody formation, described in approximately 1:30 of subjects with immunoglobulin A deficiency, which occurs in circa 1:600 of the general population (total frequency: 1/30 X 500-700 = 1/15 000-21 000) Antibodies to red cell antigens, eg antibodies to ABH, Ii, MNSs, P1, HLA

Serum sickness Antibodies to the donor's immunoglobulins and other proteins

II NON-IMMUNE, NON-INFECTIOUS TRANSFUSION REACTIONS

Air embolism A problem of historic interest that occurred when air vents were included in the transfusion sets

Anticoagulant Citrate anticoagulant may cause muscle tremor and electrocardiographic changes

Coagulation defects Depletion of factors VIII and V, a dilutional effect that requires massive transfusion of 10 or more units before becoming significant

Cold blood In ultra-emergent situations, blood stored at 4º C may be tranfused prior to reaching body temperature at 37º C; warming of blood from 4 to 37º C requires 30 kcal/liter of energy, consumed as glucose; cold blood slows metabolism, exacerbates lactic acidosis, decreases available calcium, ↑ hemoglobin's affinity for oxygen and causes potassium leakage, a major concern in cold hemoglobinuria

Hemolysis A phenomenon due to blood collection trauma, a clinically insignificant problem

Hyperammonemia and increased lactic acid Both molecules accumulate during packed red cell storage and when transfused, require hepatorenal clearance, of concern in patients with hepatic or renal dysfunction, who should receive the freshest units possible

Hyperkalemia Hemolysis causes an increase of 1 mmol/L/day of potassium in a unit of stored blood, of concern in patients with poor renal function, potentially causing arrhythmia Iron overload Each unit of packed red cells has 250 mg iron, potentially causing hemosiderosis in multi-transfused patients

Microaggregates Sludged debris in the pulmonary vasculature causing adult respiratory distress syndrome may be removed with micropore filters

Pseudoreaction Various mimics that simulate a transfusion reaction, eg patient anxiety, anaphylaxis related to a drug being administered at the same time as the transfusion

III INFECTIONS TRANSMITTED BY BLOOD TRANSFUSION

Viruses B19, CMV, EBV, hepatitis A-D (hepatitis non-A, non-B, non-C), Creutzfeldt-Jakob agent, Colorado tick fever, tropical viruses (eg Rift Valley fever, Ebola, Lassa, dengue), HHV 6 (**Arch Pathol Lab Med 1994; 118:333-46**), HIV-1, HIV-2, HTLV-I, HTLV-II

Bacteria Transmission of bacterial infections from an infected donor is uncommon and includes brucellosis and syphilis in older reports, while more recent reports include, Lyme disease and *Yersinia enterocolitica* (**MMWR 1991; 40:176**) Note: Although virtually any bacteria could (in theory) be transmitted in blood, it is usually due to contamination during processing rather than transmission from an infected donor

Parasites Babesiosis, leishmania (*L donovani, L tropica*), malaria, microfilaria (*Brugia malayi, Loa loa, Mansonella perstans, Mansonella ozzardi* (**Arch Pathol Lab Med 1994; 118:336oA**), toxoplasmosis (*Toxoplasma gondii, Trypanosoma cruzi*)

stimulating angiogenesis

transforming growth factor-beta TGF-β, see there

transfusion-associated graft-versus-host disease A variant of graft-versus-host disease in which immunocompetent T lymphocytes are transfused to a recipient by a blood transfusion and attack the recipient's immune system; the risk factors for TAGVHD are poorly defined, but may include those bone marrow graft recipients and those who have been otherwise immunocompromised by chemotherapy or malignancy CLINICAL Fever, skin rash, diarrhea and hepatic dysfunction (abnormal liver function tests) and severe pancytopenia; in contrast to the 'garden variety' GVHD, the onset of TAGVHD is earlier (10-12 days), often accompanied by bone marrow aplasia, rarely responds to immunosuppressive therapy and is usually fatal (mortality of 84% within 21 days of transfusion); some underlying diseases, eg leukemia have a lower mortality than others PREVENTION (gamma) Irradiation of blood products with 15-25 Gy (1500 rad); up to 50 Gy can be used for most blood-derived products (**N Engl J Med 1993; 328:766ᴏᴀ, Arch Pathol Lab Med 1994; 118:371ᴏᴀ**)

transfusion effect Immune modulation induced by the transfusion of allogeneic blood products (packed red cells, and platelets) resulting in reduced allograft rejection; although the mechanism and the components responsible for this effect are unknown, a role for leukocytes is suspected; the optimal transfusion effect requires ≤ 2-3 units and HLA-DR mismatch; the magnitude of improvement of heart and kidney allograft survival is less than that acheivable with addition of cyclosporine to the immunosuppressive armamentarium; other immune modulation-related transfusion effects are more controversial and include postulated effects on cancer recurrence and development, postoperative bacterial infection and activation of latent viruses (**Arch Pathol Lab Med 1994; 118:392ᴏᴀ**) see Leukocyte reduction

transfusion medicine Blood banking A field of subspecialization in either clinical pathology or internal medicine that is involved in patient management through administration of blood cells and blood products including fresh-frozen plasma and cryoprecipitate; TM specialists wear many hats and must be versant in relevant areas of hematology, immunology, and infectious disease, both clinically and from a laboratory standpoint, participate in establishing standards for use of these products in a health care facility, and address the legal aspects of transfusions; the major legal issues of transfusion medicine pivot around 1) Whether the product being transfused is safe, ie not infected, especially with HIV, see Blood shield laws and 2) Whether a person has the right to refuse a medically appropriate and potentially life-saving blood transfusion; in the US, the doctrines that protect personal freedoms regard blood transfusions as an 'assault' if the medical team administers blood against the will of a mentally-competent person, who is not pregnant, has no children and refuses transfusion on religious grounds; in the USA, the US Food and Drug Administration and the American Association of Blood Banks (AABB) set standards and provide guidelines in transfusion medicine; see AABB

Note: The transfusion of blood products is problematic when the recipient is a minor and the parent refuses to allow a transfusion (the courts can override this dilemma by intervening in the child's interest); the courts may also oblige a transfusion when the patient is a parent of minor children who would become wards of the state upon the patient's death through exsanguination

transfusion reaction Any of a number of clinical complexes related to the transfusion of blood or blood products; the term may be simplistically viewed as any untoward response to non-self blood products, which elicit febrile reactions that are either minor, occurring in 1:40 transfusions, attributed to nonspecific leukocyte-derived pyrogens, or major, occurring in 1:3000 transfusions, due to a true immune reaction, which are graded according to the presence of urticaria, itching, chills, fever and, if the reaction is intense, collapse, cyanosis, chest and/or back pain and diffuse hemorrhage Note: If any of these signs appear, or if the temperature rises more than 1°C, the transfusion must be stopped; most patients survive if less than 200 ml has been transfused in cases of red cell incompatibility-induced transfusion reaction; over 50% die when 500 ml or more has been transfused; TF mortality is approximately $1.13/10^5$ transfusions Types (table)

transfusion 'trigger' TRANSFUSION MEDICINE The hematocrit (Hct) and hemoglobin (Hb) values at or below which packed red cells are usually ordered for transfusion by a clinician; in the current environment of potentially fatal transfusion-transmitted infections, the formerly used transfusion trigger of 10g Hb and 30% Hct (the '10/30 rule') is no longer acceptable as most patients, especially the elderly, may be stable and asymptomatic with Hb far below 10 g and often respond to iron supplementation, as one of the most common cause of anemia in this age group is iron deficiency; the most widely used current TT is a hemoglobin of 70 g/L, following a NIH consensus development conference Note: Any numerical TT is inappropriate if the patient's clinical status is not taken into account 'PROPHYLACTIC' PLATELET TT Stable patients $< 5 \times 10^9$, patients with recent hemorrhage and/or temperature $\geq 38.5°$ C $< 10 \times 10^9$, patients with significant coagulopathy, anatomic lesion(s), or heparin therapy $< 20 \times 10^9$ 'THERAPEUTIC' PLATELET TT Active hemorrhage or scheduled invasive procedure $< 50 \times 10^9$, hemorrhage and/or thrombocytopenia, as needed (**Arch Pathol Lab Med 1994; 118:380ʀᴠ**); the critical hematocrit at which anemia compromises tissue repair is 15% (**ibid 118:429ʀᴠ**)

transgenic animal Transgenic organism, see there

transgenic chicken An animal of value for both research and the poultry industry, in which genes are inserted using a replication-defective reticuloendotheliosis virus vector

transgenic mice A mouse 'created' in vitro by transferring genes into the mouse embryo, serving as a useful model for studying autoimmune phenomena, oncogenesis, embryology and physiology; insertion of foreign genes may have consequences for the host, eg when PHT1-1 transgenic mice are homozygous for a transgene insertion, eg heat shock protein, hsp 70, the 'legless' mutation appears, in which the hindlimbs are shortened and the forelimbs have bone defects, accompanied by cerebral and craniofacial defects, which are not seen in heterozygotes; transgenic mouse models have been produced for hypoxanthine guanine phosphoribosyl transferase deficiency, sickle hemoglobin, which express the disease and others transgenic mice have been developed that express IgM, IgG, and Igκ in absence of mouse IgM or Igκ (**Nature 1994; 368:856L**)

Note: It had been reported that transgenic mice could be produced by simply fertilizing eggs with sperm mixed in a DNA-containing milieu, a finding that could not be reproduced by other groups

transgenic organism An animal or plant that has been modified by insertion of foreign genes that express proteins of interest; transgenic technology is currently limited by the inability to direct the site of gene insertion, since a gene may be inserted in a position that results in activation of one of the host's structural genes

transgenics A therapeutic modality in which genes of interest are inserted into an organism, compelling it to produce a protein that is either missing or desired; transgenics is in advanced planning stages for treating human disease and is already in use for treating conditions in commercial plants and animals

transgenic sheep A transgenic organism that serves as a factory for coagulation factor IX and α_1-antitrypsin; ABRO* sheep produce higher volumes of useful protein than transgenic mice; in ABRO's protocol, engineered stem cells are first grown in culture to determine whether the DNA of interest is successfully integrated before producing the whole animal

*Edinburgh's Animal Breeding and Research Organization

transient ischemic attack NEUROLOGY A focal, abrupt ischemia-induced loss of neurologic function, accompanied by disability of < than 24 hours in duration*; symptomatic TIAs often precede cerebral infarcts or strokes, more common in older patients with marked cerebrovascular atherosclerosis, potentially affecting any cerebral vessel; despite clinical resolution, CT demonstrates residual anatomic lesions in 15% of RINDs and TIAs PREVENTION Low-dose (eg 30 mg) aspirin, a level at which inhibition of aggregation due to ↓ production of platelet thromboxane A_2 is still complete, but the production of prostacyclin, which has an antiaggregation effect is unaffected in endothelial cells; prostacyclin production is inhibited by higher doses of aspirin (N Engl J Med 1991; 325:1261)

*When the disability is > than 24 hours, it is known as reversible ischemic neurologic disability or RIND

transition MOLECULAR BIOLOGY Any point mutation of DNA in which either a purine is substituted for another or a pyrimidine is substituted for another; Cf Degenerate code

transitional panel Metastatic disease panel, see there

transjugular intrahepatic portosystemic stent-shunt TIPS* A type of portosystemic shunt for treating portal hypertension and hemorrhage of esophageal hemorrhage TECHNIQUE A puncture needle is advanced in a catheter through the inferior vena cava into a hepatic vein, after which an intrahepatic branch of the portal vein is punctured and a metallic mesh stent is expanded to establish a shunt RESULTS Technical success in 93%; ↓ portal venous pressure in 57% COMPLICATIONS Hemorrhage stenosis or occlusion 31%; intra-abdominal, biliary, subcapsular) in 13%; stent migration in 2% OUTCOME Hepatic encephalopathy in 25%; 18% rebleeding at one year; 85% one-year survival (N Engl J Med 1994; 330:165OA) in one uncontrolled study of 62 patients, 74% had complete responses, but mortality from the underlying disease is significant (ibid 1995; 332;1192A)

TRANSPLANTATION STATISTICS, US			
SITE	NUMBER*	COST/CASE‡	#CENTERS
Middle ear	100 000 (1986)	$2 000	Most ENT
Cornea	28 000 (1986)	$6 800	400
Kidney	9 340	$36 000	237
Heart	1988	$110 000	154
Bone marrow	1322 (1986)	$95 000	72
Liver	2524	$238 000	58
Pancreas	528	$35 000	86
Heart/lung	52/185	$165 000	82/77

*1990, except where noted ‡1986

transkaryotic implantation The alteration of the nuclei of implanted cells, eg fibroblasts by adding DNA sequences through stable or transient transfection, a technique that enhances the potential of gene therapy since 1) The transfected cell line can be well-characterized prior to definitive transplantation 2) Different anatomic sites may be used for the transplantation and 3) regulated expression of the gene of interest can be obtained

translation MOLECULAR BIOLOGY The process whereby the genetic information on messenger RNA (mRNA) is 'decoded' and converted into a coherent protein, during which transfer RNA (tRNA) converges on ribosomes packaged as rRNA and, at the behest of mRNA, dispenses amino acids to a growing polypeptide chain; protein synthesis is divided into initiation, elongation and termination steps

translocase A ribosomal enzyme that catalyzes the GTP-dependent translocation reaction in protein synthesis, shifting the tRNA-amino acid complex from the ribosome's A site to its P site, where it proffers the next amino acid to the growing polypeptide

translocation 1) The activity of the translocase, see there 2) The in vivo transfer of a chromosomal segment to another, non-homologous chromosome; such a transfer may link two segments of otherwise silent DNA, resulting

in a 'renegade' gene encoding a hybrid protein, eg P210$^{bcr/abl}$, a phosphoprotein unique to CML, which has deregulated tyrosine kinase activity, thus acting to 'drive' the neoplasm

transluminal angioplasty Percutaneous transluminal angioplasty, see there

transmembrane protein A protein that is fully integrated in the plasma membrane, characterized by a hydrophilic COOH extracellular domain, a hydrophobic 25–30-residue transmembrane region and a hydrophilic NH_2 intracellular domain; see Fluid mosaic model

transmission electron microscope The most commonly used type of electron microscope, which has a resolution of up to 200 000 magnifications; TEM is used clinically to study glomerulonephritides and for classifying tumors, eg identifying cell junctions in poorly differentiated carcinoma, neurosecretory granules in tumors of neural crest origin and for identifying premelanosomes in malignant melanoma TECHNIQUE A beam of electrons passes through the specimen, providing a magnified image of an object on a fluorescent screen; see Microscopy; Cf Scanning electron microscopy, Scanning tunnel microscopy

transmogrification SURGICAL PATHOLOGY A neologism (of uncertain origin) for a change or alteration of tissue into one with a grotesque appearance; placental transmogrification of the lung has been described as a rare histologic variant of giant bullous emphysema (Am J Surg Pathol 1995; 19:563)

transosseous osteosynthesis Ilizarov method, see there

transplantation The use of usually non-self tissue or organs to replace a malfunctioning organ or organ system; solid organ and hematopoietic precursor transplantations are performed with increasing immunologic impunity in bone marrow, bone matrix, cardiac valves, heart, heart-lung, kidney, liver, pancreas, skin and intestine, largely due to the availability of agents, eg cyclosporin A and tacrolimus (FK 506), which effectively battle the otherwise limiting complications of graft-versus-host disease Annual transplantations performed in the US; see Graft-versus-host disease, Liver transplantation, Lung transplantation, Pancreas transplantation, Procurement, Skin graft, UNOS

transplantation antigens see MHC (Major histocompatibility complex)

transplantation rejection The constellation of host immune responses evoked when an allograft tissue is transplanted into a recipient; the rejection phenomena may be reduced by best possible matching of MHC antigens and ABO blood group and ameliorated with various immunosuppressive agents, including cyclosporin, tacrolimus (FK 506) and rapamycin; see Graft-versus-host disease

transporter associated with antigen processing TAP, see there

transposition MOLECULAR BIOLOGY The movement of a sequence of DNA within a genome, eg as occurs with gene jumping; Cf Retroposition PEDIATRICS A generic term that encompasses any malposition of an organ or tissues that occurs during embryogenesis SURGERY Any plastic procedure in which a flap of tissue is moved from one site to another and allowed sufficient time to establish a new blood supply prior to severing the connection with the donor site.

transposon Transposable element A type of 'jumping gene' or segment of DNA that is capable of inserting itself into or excising itself out of a gene locus, an ability that is regulated by genetic, environmental and developmental factors; the tissue specificity and timing of transposon activity is pivotal in ontogeny; in maize (where transposons were first discovered by Nobel laureate Barbara

McClintock) and by extension, in other organisms, the excision of transposons during development is controlled by the host; see 'Jumping genes'

transsexualism Gender identity disorder, see there

transspecies transplants The transplantation of an organ from a lower mammal (eg baboon, pig) to a (putatively) higher mammal (eg human); thus far TTs have been unsuccessful, almost invariably due to the complement-mediated hyperacute rejection; one strategy that may theoretically circumvent hyperacute rejection is breeding of transgenic animals, eg pigs that are bred to incorporate humanized complement and otherwise immunogenic antigens, tricking the recipient's immune system into overlooking the 'foreignness' of transplanted organs of non-self (eg porcine) origin (**New York Times 19 Oct 1993; C3**)

transthoracic echocardiography Two-dimensional transthoracic color-flow Doppler echocardiography TTE A noninvasive imaging technique that can be used as a screening method for analyzing abnormalities of locoregional fluid distribution or blood flow patterns, eg pericardial effusion or aortic regurgitation; TTE is less sensitive than transesophagel color-flow Doppler echocardiography or spin-echo MRI in detecting thoracic aneurysms because of anatomic and technical drawbacks, eg limited field of view (**N Engl J Med 1993; 328:10A**)

transthyretin A 55-kD homotetrameric protein composed of four 127-residue polypeptide chains that binds both thyroxine and retinol Serum levels: 0.15-0.36 g/L (US: 20-40 mg/dl); transthyretin is markedly decreased in malnutrition and in acute and chronic inflammation, and thus is considered a 'negative acute phase protein', which may be defective in autosomal dominant amyloidosis; because transthyretin migrates in front of albumin on a serum electrophoresis, it had been formerly termed 'prealbumin'; since the protein is 1) Structurally distinct from albumin 2) In murine systems, is a term that refers to other proteins migrating in the same electrophoretic regions, eg α_1-antitrypsin and 3) Potentially causes confusion with the term proalbumin, the more informative term, transthyretin has been substituted (**Nomenclature committee of IUB, J Biol Chem 1988; 256:12**) Cf Proalbumin

transverse lie Shoulder presentation OBSTETRICS A non-cephalic, non-breech position, in which the fetus' long axis is perpendicular to that of the mother's, an event occurring in 1:300 births, due to lower uterine obstruction, eg placenta previa, intrauterine leiomyomas or an ovarian tumor in the cul-de-sac, or may occur in a multiparous uterus with a lax wall; TLs are managed by cesarean section or, less commonly, gentle external version if the membranes have not ruptured; the risks of an internal version are unacceptably high and it is rarely performed

transverse magnetization MRI The component of the macroscopic magnetization vector at right angles to the static magnetic field (B_o); precession of the transverse magnetization at the Larmor frequency is responsible for the detected MR signal; in absence of an externally applied radiofrequency energy, the transverse magnetization will decay to zero with a characteristic time constant (T2 or T2*); see Magnetic resonance imaging

transvestic fetishism A type of paraphilia (the politically correct term for what was formerly known as a sexual

---

TRANSVESTIC FETISHISM (DIAGNOSTIC CRITERIA)

A Over a period of ≥ 6 monthsin a heterosexual male, recurrent, intense sexually arousing fantasies, sexual urges, or behaviors involving cross-dressing

B Above causes significant distress or impairment in social, occupational, or other areas of functioning

Diagnostic and Statistical Manual of Mental Disorders, 4th ed, Washington, DC, American Psychiatric Association,

---

deviancy) that focuses on cross-dressing (table); it is necessary to determine whether the TF is accompanied by gender dysphoria (persistent discomfort with present gender role or identity), which, if extreme may eventuate in the individual seeking sexual reassignment

transvestism (DSM-III) Transvestic fetishism [DSM-IV]

TRAP HEMTOLOGY Tartrate-resistant acid phosphatase A 60 kD acid phosphatase isoenzyme that migrates in band 5, which is present in and relatively specific for the leukemic cells of hairy cell leukemia; weak TRAP staining occurs in infectious mononucleosis, CLL, lymphosarcoma, Sézary cells, osteoclastic bone tumors, and Gaucher cells; the hydrolytic activity of some protein phosphatases towards certain phosphoproteins such as casein and histone is resistant to tartrate inhibition; see Hairy cell leukemia MOLECULAR BIOLOGY *trp* RNA-binding attenuation protein (**Nature 1995;374:7693**)

TRAP sequence see Twin reversed arterial-perfusion sequence

trapdoor scar PLASTIC SURGERY A descriptor for an unesthetic scar that puckers above the skin surface in a large healing 'horseshoe' avulsion flap, most commonly seen in automobile windshield injuries

trapped lung A sequestered segment of lung seen in empyema, where a portion of a bacterially infected lobe and visceral pleura 'fix' the affected lung in a partially collapsed position; Cf Folded lung, Scimitar syndrome, Sequestration complex

Note: Hippocrates was the first to recognize and drain an empyema, now a rare complication of bacterial pneumonia due to staphylococci, streptococci and gram-negative bacilli

trapping NEUROSURGERY A definitive therapy for those intracranial aneurysms that are suboptimal candidates for clipping, ie where the aneurysmal neck is poorly defined; trapping of the aneurysm may fail if collateral circulation is present (**Mayo Clin Proc 1995; 70:153RV**)

trash foot Blue toe syndrome, see there

trauma score EMERGENCY MEDICINE A physiologic index measuring systolic blood pressure, respiratory rate and expansion, capillary refill, eye opening and verbal and motor responses, placing them on a scale of 2 to 16; the trauma score is a predictor of injury severity and the probability of survival; below a score of 12, a patient would benefit from transfer to a trauma center; Cf Injury Severity Score

traumatic aortic rupture TRAUMA SURGERY '*Traumatic rupture of the thoracic aorta is a common and often fatal* injury resulting from sudden deceleration in high-speed motor vehicle accidents,*' or falls from height DIAGNOSIS Transesophageal echocardiography may be the diagnostic modality of first choice (**N Eng J Med 1995; 332:356OA**) followed by arch aortography, CT, MRI, and standard films; in one report MRI was superior (95% detection) to TEE (86%) in detecting thoracic aorta dissection (**Radiology 1995; 194:331**)

*TAR accounts for ± 18% of fatalities in MVAs

traumatic tap A diagnostic lumbar puncture in which there is incidental hemorrhage due to violent movement by the patient or tearing of vessels, a risk inherent in the procedure, and thus not a true pathology in the cerebrospinal fluid; a TT is differentiated from subarachnoid hemorrhage by the absence of xanthochromia, decreasing erythrocytes in serial tubes and rapid coagulation of blood

trauma X A euphemism for the physical signs of child abuse; see Battered child syndrome, Child abuse

traveler's diarrhea Montezuma's revenge, Aztec two-step, Turkey trot, Dehli belly A condition defined (**N Eng J Med 1993; 328:1821RV**) as '... *the passage of at least three unformed stools in a 24-hour period ... with nausea,* *vomiting, abdominal pain, or cramps, fecal urgency, tenesmus, or the passage of bloody or mucoid stools ...traveler's diarrhea occurs in a person who normally resides in an industrialized region and who travels to a developing or semitropical country...Diarrhea lasts longer than 1 week in 10% of patients, and longer than one month in 2%. Approximately 20% of patients are confined to bed for one or two days.* 'Most diarrhea in travelers is acquired orally and caused by the heat-stable and heat-labile toxins of *Escherichia coli* and *Shigella*; the intensity of infection depends on the quality of the water supply, previous host exposure and susceptibility; pathogens on cruise ships include *Shigella*, and *Salmonella* (the latter of which is an uncommon cause of traveler's diarrhea in developing nations as it grows best in animal protein, eg mayonnaise-based egg and macaroni salads), *Vibrio parahemolyticus*, less commonly, *Aeromonas hydrophila*, *Campylobacter jejuni*, *Plesiomonas shigelloides*, *V cholerae* (non-01), *V fluvialis*, and *Yersinia enterocolitica*; parasites causing traveler's diarrhea include *Giardia lamblia*, *Entamoeba histolytica*, *Balantidium coli*, *Cryptosporidium* spp, *Dientamoeba fragilis*, *Isospora belli*, and *Strongyloides stercoralis*; viruses are less commonly implicated in traveler's diarrhea, but include Norwalk-like agents and rotavirus TREATMENT Rehydration, bismuth subsalicylate, narcotic analogs to slow the motility and trimethoprim-sulfamethoxazole if antibiotics are required PREVENTION Boil it, cook it, peel it, or forget it (**HH publication no. (CDC) 93-8280**)

Note: Prophylactic antibiotics are rarely indicated, and unless one travels to areas at high risk for a certain infection, most subjects are advised to 'sit it out'

'trawling' MOLECULAR BIOLOGY 1) Traditional DNA sequencing, which like the North Sea fishing technique from whence the analogy, catches everything within range of the 'trawl'; chromosomal 'trawling' contrasts with Chromosome walking and Chromosome jumping, see there, in that there is no 'skipping' from one to another DNA segment 2) An activity of the endocytic microtubule network that constantly 'trawls' allowing certain receptors, eg transferrin to pass through the 'fishnet' while other receptors, eg epidermal growth factor receptor are trapped, forming a multi-vesicular body filled with a specific receptor 'cargo'

treadmill exercise test CARDIOLOGY The most commonly used clinical test for accurately assessing a person's risk of death from cardiovascular events; the treadmill exercise score is calculated as the duration of exercise in minutes – (5 x the maximal ST-segment deviation in millimeters during or after exercise) – (4 x the treadmill angina index, ie no angina during exercise = 0, nonlimiting angina = 1, exercise-limiting angina = 2); the results range from a score of 15 for a normal person at no known increased risk to – 25 for those at highest risk (**N Engl J Med 1991; 325:849**) see Thallium imaging

treadmilling PHYSIOLOGY An equilibrium state in muscle, in which the length of actin and microtubular polymers remain constant, as the rate of addition of monomers of actin or tubulin (which form microtubules) at one end of the molecule is equal to the rate of loss or degradation at the other end

'treated' wood CLINICAL TOXICOLOGY Wood impregnated with preservatives, eg chromium-copper-arsenate, creosote, inorganic arsenicals, and pentachlorophenol, to increase its useful life, preventing attack by insects, fungi and other organisms; chronic exposure to the fumes of burning wood or skin contact therewith may produce a combined heavy metal intoxication syndrome

treatment-investigational new drug A drug that is made available to patients who are very ill with life-threatening diseases, prior to the drug's official approval by the FDA; 1987 IND 'rewrite' makes a limited number of INDs

available if there is a gap in the therapeutic arsenal, ie if there is no known and/or effective therapy for a particular disease which the TIND appears to effectively treat[1]; the prolonged period of time required for the approval of new therapeutic agents is problematic in AIDS, as these patients may clamor for therapy, regardless of how minimal the positive effect; '...*primum, non nocerum*...'[2] ; life-threatening diseases for which TINDs are used include AIDS, advanced congestive heart failure and refractory malignancy; agents that have been under TIND protocols include CMV immunoglobulin for transplanting a CMV-positive donor kidney into a seronegative individual, pentostatin (deoxycoformin) for hairy cell leukemia patients refractory to IFN-α; trimetrexate glucuronate, indicated for *Pneumocystis carinii* as it is reported to have a 1500-fold greater affinity for *Pneumocystis carinii*'s dihydrofolate reductase than does trimethoprim; see Compassionate IND, IND

[1]If a candidate TIND agent is very early in the testing process and the data available is scant, approval for TIND usage is unlikely and one turns to the 'compassionate use' clause (driven by the often desperate plight of AIDS patients) to allow the very ill to at least import their own therapeutics, however ineffective [2]First of all do no harm, from the Hippocratic oath

treatment-related malignancy Secondary malignancy, see there

treatment window HEMATOLOGY A 4–6-day period during which a patient with factor VIII inhibitor-producing hemophilia A may respond to a bolus of factor VIII, which by complexing with the inhibitors may reduce their level to the point to allow hemostasis

tree bark appearance A descriptor for intimal and subintimal plaques that encase the mouth of small aortic branches, due to obliterative endarteritis of vasa vasorum with ischemic destruction of the vascular media causing inflammation, neo-vascularization and fibrous scarring, leading to aneurysms and surface irregularities; although the appearance is typical of late syphilis, it may also be seen in Takayasu's disease, Reiter's disease and rheumatic heart disease

treefrog hand appearance A fanciful descriptor for the broadened distal digits with elongated fingers seen in the otopalatodigital syndrome (Taybi syndrome), an X chromosome-linked disease characterized by a short stature, variable mental deficiency, cleft soft palate, microstomia, and conduction-type deafness; Cf clubbing

tree-structured survival analysis STATISTICS Multi-variate recursive partitioning A method in which the

'...entire patient population is divided into two groups based on the feature that maximizes differences in prognosis according to a log-rank statistic. This process is repeated for each subgroup, creating a tree structure, until further subdivision is not (statistically) significant or the terminal node (subgroup) has no less than 10 cases. Missing values (of which there are very few) are handled by an interpolation algorithm that uses the cases values for another parameter, which most similarly ranks the cases. Cross-validation, which estimates how well a tree will do on future data, is then performed. This procedure deletes a random group of cases from the data, constructs a tree from the remaining data, and uses the group left out as 'new data' on which to test the tree. After a number of iterations, a common, 'pruned-back' tree emerges. This procedure minimizes the risk of overfitting the data to a model and thus overinterpreting the results.' (**Am J Surg Pathol 1993; 17:275OA**)

trembler mice A strain of mice that produces virtually no peripheral nervous system myelin when homozygous for the Tr mutation, despite which they have a normal lifespan

trench diarrhea MEDICAL HISTORY A generic term for any contagious enteropathy (eg cholera) acquired as a result of the living conditions extant in the trenches of WW I

trench fever Werner-His disease A rickettsia-like disease caused by *Bartonella quintana* (formerly *Rochalimaea quintana* and previously *Rickettsia quintana*) transmitted by the feces of the body louse (*Pediculus humanus*) under crowded conditions of poor hygiene, well described in the trenches in World War I and in endemic form in developing nations CLINICAL Abrupt onset of paroxysmal fever, asthenia, chills, vertigo, headache, backache, characteristic shin pain, truncal rash, transient maculopapules and moderate leukocytosis; febrile relapse(s), see Saddleback curve TREATMENT Tetracyclines, broad-spectrum antibiotics, eradicate lice

trench foot A condition first described in World War I in soldiers in the trenches whose feet were damp and exposed to near-freezing temperatures in wet trenches for prolonged periods, causing acral vasoconstriction and heat loss; the resulting ischemia unchains a vicious circle of necrosis, endothelial damage, intravascular 'sludging' of cells, extravasation of protein and fluid, resulting in more ischemia; the prolonged cold is followed by vasodilation, burning pain and paresthesiae with the formation of hemorrhagic blebs or gangrene, accompanied by cellulitis, lymphangitis, swelling, thrombophlebitis, and persistent hypersensitivity to cold with secondary Raynaud's phenomenon PATHOLOGY Perivascular fibrosis, muscular hyperplasia, and necrotizing vasculitis TREATMENT Slow warming of foot; if the tissue is warmed too rapidly, reactive hyperthermia, blistering and possibly thrombosis occur

Note: It may be clinically useful to separate trench foot from the virtually identical 'immersion foot', see there

trench mouth Acute necrotizing ulcerative gingivitis, see there

treponemal tests Serological tests for syphilis, see there

TRIAGE PRIORITIES

HIGHEST PRIORITY Respiratory, facial, neck, chest, cardiovascular, hemorrhage, neck injuries

VERY HIGH PRIORITY Shock, retroperitoneal or intraperitoneal hemorrhage

HIGH PRIORITY Cranial, cerebral, spinal cord, burns

LOW PRIORITY Lower genitourinary tract, peripheral nerves and vessels, splinted fractures, soft tissue lesions

tretinoin all-*trans*-retinoic acid A topically applied cream that reverses some of the effects of photoaging, both clinically (↓ skin wrinkling, improved skin texture and color) and microscopically (↑ epidermal thickness, ↑ collagen and dermal vessels and 'erasing' epithelial atypia and dysplasia); tretinoin is reported to restore the production of collagen I in photodamaged skin (N Engl J Med 1993; 329:530oa), lighten postinflammatory hyperpigmentation (N Engl J Med 1993; 328:1438oa) or induce terminal differentiation of acute promyelocytic leukemia, driving it into a mature nonproliferative state of remission MECHANISM Unknown, possibly related to tretinoin's inhibition of collagenase, which degrades the anchoring fibril collagen; tretinoin therapy doubles the number of anchoring fibrils at the dermoepidermal junction; see Retinoic acid receptor, Vitamin A SIDE EFFECTS Dry skin, bone pain, hyperaminotransferasemia, and hyperhistaminemia (N Engl J Med 1992; 327:385oa) see Retinoic acid

The astute observer would have noted that partially overlapping information and illustration appear under Retinoic acid, the formally preferred term for this substance

TRH Thyrotropin-releasing hormone A tripeptide (pyroglutamic acid-histidine-proline) of hypothalamic origin that releases thyrotropin (TSH) after receptor attachment and activation of the cAMPase

triad A trilogy of clinical or pathological findings, which are first described as typical for a particular disease, but which may over time prove to be relatively nonspecific ASTHMA TRIAD ASA triad Nasal polyps, asthma and aspirin intolerance; variously considered to be inherited or due to environmental factors, related to aspirin's inhibition of cyclooxygenase in prostaglandin production CHRISTIAN'S TRIAD Lytic bony lesions, diabetes insipidus and exophthalmos A classically described, but observed trilogy of symptoms described in histiocytosis X CHARCOT'S TRIAD Nystagmus, 'scanning' speech, and intention tremor A trilogy of clinical signs described as typical of multiple sclerosis; the CT is relatively nonspecific and only occurs in advanced cases HEMOCHROMATOSIS TRIAD Hepatomegaly, DM and bronze cutaneous pigmentation LENNOX'S TRIAD Petit mal epilepsy, akinetic seizures and myoclonic jerks PETIT'S TRIAD Mydriasis, increased intraocular pressure and alteration of the retinal vessels due to autonomic nervous system activity RENAL CELL CARCINOMA TRIAD Pain, palpable mass and hematuria; seen in 10% of patients with renal cell carinoma SAINT'S TRIAD Hiatal hernia, cholelithiasis and diverticulosis TOXOPLASMOSIS TRIAD Marked follicular hyperplasia with active mitosis and phagocytosis, small granulomas composed of epithelioid histiocytes and distension of marginal and cortical sinuses by monocytoid B cells TROTTER'S TRIAD Hypoacusia, impaired soft palate movement, and mandibular neuralgia, described as typical of eustachian tube malignancy WILSON'S TRIAD Chronic active hepatitis, Kayser-Fleischer rings of iris, degeneration of the lenticular nucleus WATERHOUSE-FRIDERICHSEN TRIAD Meningococcemia, multiple petechial cutaneous hemorrhages and bilateral adrenal hemorrhages

triaditis A generic and nonspecific term for chronic inflammation of the hepatic portal triad

triage EMERGENCY MEDICINE *triage*, French, sorting A method first used on the battlefield, in which the most extremely wounded were placed in an 'expectant' category, ie expected to die, and therefore not treated, while the limited medical personnel could attend to those most likely to survive; triaging, then is assessment of injury intensity and the immediacy or urgency for medical attention (table) RESEARCH FINANCING A new method for evaluating potentially fundable research proposals, which is intended to speed the peer-review process by the NIH (US); the goal is to reduce the amount of time spent on proposals that are clearly not grant-worthy, and to increase the time spent evaluating borderline cases (Nature 1994; 369:269N)

trial and error method Stochastic method, see there

trial of therapy The application of a particular therapy, eg edrophonium (Tensilon) to a person who is suspected of having a particular disease, eg myasthenia gravis; response of the condition to the TOT, confirms the diagnosis

triangle of Codman Codman's triangle, see there

triangular face A hypoplastic face with prominent zygomatic arches, sunken cheeks, down-turned mouth and brownish facial discoloration, characteristic of Mulibrey nanism, which has also been described in the Russell-Silver and Turner syndromes; Cf Hippocratic facies

triangular test STATISTICS A group-sequential method used to monitor the progressive accumulation of data while controlling for type I and type II errors (see N Engl J Med 1993; 329:1848oa)

TRIC Trachoma-induced interstitial conjunctivitis

triceps skin-fold thickness A value used to estimate corporal fat, which is measured on the right arm halfway between the olecranon process of the elbow and the acromial process of the scapula; normal, ♂ 12 mm; ♀ 23 mm; Cf Mid-arm muscle mass

tricho-dento-osseous syndrome TDO syndrome An AD [MIM 190320] condition characterized by kinky, curly hair, small defective teeth with enamel hypoplasia and hypocalcification that slough by late adolescence, osteosclerosis and craniosynostosis

α-trichosanthin A possibly anti-AIDS agent--mas cosas, which is normally produced by the Chinese cucumber plant

trichrome stain A stain used in histopathology that colors collagen green, muscle red-purple and myelin brown; the stain is of particular use in determining the presence of muscle invasion in certain carcinomas, eg transitional cell carcinoma of the urinary bladder

Trichosporon beigelii An organism that is widely distributed in soil, stagnant and fresh water and animal excreta that has been isolated from normal skin, urine, respiratory, and GI tracts; although *T beigelii* is rarely pathogenic, it causes white piedra and a summer-type hypersensitivity pneumonia; disseminated infection is more common in those with immunosuppressive diseases, or malignancy TREATMENT Amphotericin B (Arch Pathol Lab Med 1994; 118:191CR)

trick knee Locked knee, see there

'trick' movements HAND SURGERY A series of movements that an active and highly-motivated person will perform to circumvent the limitations of musculoskeletal paralysis; these movements would never be performed under normal circumstances and thus are often bizarre and uncoordinated; the disadvantage is that prolonged 'trick'-type compensation may stretch various hand structures and may persist as a habit once the tendons have been surgically rerouted

tricyclic antidepressant Any of a widely prescribed family of psychoactive drugs that have three central rings and a short linear chain attached to the terminal nitrogen and are thus tertiary amines; TAs were introduced in the late 1950s to treat endogenous depression and have revolutionized the treatment of patients with severe ('decompensated') mental illness, allowing many patients to be deinstitutionalized; TAs are thought to act by central inhibition of the re-uptake of biogenic amines; they inhibit the prejunctional uptake of norepinephrine and serotonin and may be responsible for their antidepressant effect; TAs block muscarinergic, H_1 histamine, and α_1-adrenergic receptors explaining their side effects of mouth dryness, sedation, and hypotension (see N Engl J Med 1994; 331:1354RV) LABORATORY TA levels correlate poorly with the clinical status as circulating levels of the highly lipid-soluble TCA represent a minute portion of the body load, and TCA metabolites with similar clinical effects are not measured CLINICAL, OVERDOSE Parasympathetic disease with anticholinergic effects, including mydriasis, xerostomia, urinary retention, decreased peristalsis, cardiac disease (intractable myocardial depression, hypotension, ventricular tachycardia, fibrillation, or heart block) and CNS disease (confusion, agitation, hallucinations, myoclonus and seizures, lethargy that may progress to coma and respiratory arrest); Cf Fluoxetine

tricyclic antidepressant suicide A term of uncertain validity for a suicide linked to the therapeutic use of tri-

tricyclic antidepressant

$$CH_2CH_2CH_2N(CH_3)_2$$

cyclic antidepressants (TA); TAs are widely prescribed and are the most common drug involved in suicide attempts by single, young females without previous histo-

ry of autodestructive thoughts; the reported TA overdose mortality of less than 15% includes the elderly and children (including accidental TA overdoses) may in fact underestimate the true incidence, as up to 70% of TA suicides are successful and never reach the hospital

trident hand Main en trident, see there

trident sign PEDIATRICS A clinical finding in Turner syndrome, consisting of a low hairline that extends in three vaguely defined vertical bands down the characteristically webbed neck, fancifully likened to a King Neptune's trident, a three-pronged spear

trigeminal neuralgia Tic douloureux NEUROLOGY A condition characterized by stabbing paroxysmal neuropathic pain in absence of sensory or motor paralysis, of the 2nd and 3rd divisions of the fifth cranial (trigeminal) nerve; TN is most common in middle-aged adults and is evoked by touching trigger points, yawning, smiling, chewing, etc, or by oral pathology, or regional tumors, eg acoustic neuroma (which should be ruled out in therapeutically refractory cases) TREATMENT Carbamazepine, phenytoin, alcohol injection

trigeminy CARDIOLOGY A form of arrhythmia in which every third QRS wave is a ventricular premature depolarization or contraction; see PVCs

trigger finger RHEUMATOLOGY A digit in which the flexor tendon passes through a fibro-osseous tunnel*, in which there is a fusiform swelling (congenital, edema or tenosynovitis) of the tendon or tendon sheath causing a painful lock-snap sensation, leaving the finger or thumb in flexion or extension; TF is most common in ♀ in their sixth decade, associated with de Quervain's disease and carpal tunnel syndrome as well as rheumatoid arthritis and collagen vascular disease; trigger digits in children may be idiopathic or associated with chromosomal defects; trigger or locked fingers may also be caused by a variety of fractures, tendinous or ligamentous lesions

*The tendon sheath extends from the distal palm to the distal finger joint

trigger point NEUROLOGY Trigger zone, see there RHEUMATOLOGY A local region of increased tenderness that may occur in fibrositis, often located around the vertebrae medial to the scapula

trigger thumb A congenital fixed flexion deformity of the thumb, related to a narrow flexor pollicus longus tendon sheath in the region of the metacarpophalangeal joint, a condition that may be present at birth or acquired later in life; if severe, TTs may require surgical correction

trigger zone NEUROLOGY A relatively circumscribed region adjacent to nerves, often in the head and neck, which when stimulated even with light touch, may elicit marked neuralgia accompanied by lightning pain; TZs include the lips and buccal cavity (evoking trigeminal neuralgia and tic douloureux), tonsillar or posterior pharynx (glossopharyngeal neuralgia) and in the muscles involved in the myofascial pain syndrome

triglyceride Triacylglycerol A long chain fatty acid ester of glycerol, which constitutes 95% of adipose tissue by weight, and is the major lipid storage form; TGs in serum: 0.11-2.15 mmol/L (US: 10-190 mg/dL); clinical 'logic' to the contrary, serum TG levels do not appear to play an independent role in predicting coronary artery disease mortality (Am J Cardiol 1994; 73:29; N Engl J Med 1993; 328:1220OA)

trihydroxycoprostanic acid syndrome THCA syndrome An AR [MIM 214950] condition of neonatal onset characterized by hepatosplenomegaly, growth retardation, rickets, elevated THCA in serum and bile, histologically characterized by cholestasis, ↓ number of interlobular bile ducts, portal fibrosis and cirrhosis

'trilateral' retinoblastoma The rare (an estimated 1:10⁸ cases occur annually) association of a bilateral retinoblastoma with a tumor of the pineal gland, a region known as the 'third eye' in lower animals, given the presence of afunctional photoreceptors CLINICAL Onset between 3 months and 15 years of age; most are fatal PATHOGENESIS Local inactivation of the retinoblastoma binding protein in the face of an intact retinoblastoma gene locus; see Retinoblastoma

trimetrexate glucuronate Neutrexin™ A lipophilic dihydrofolate reductase inhibitor (ie antifolate) that is structurally related to methotrexate, and which has both anti-neoplastic and antimicrobial activity; TG was recently approved to treat PCP in AIDS patients COST Circa $2624* for a 21-day course of therapy

*Ouch–Author's note

trimetrexate gluconate

trimethoprim-sulfamethoxazole One of the few effective, commercially-produced combination antibacterial available in the US, formulated as a 1:20 ratio of T to S; this broad-spectrum oral agent is effective in genitourinary, GI, and respiratory tract infections and is the antibiotic of choice in treating *Pneumocystis carinii* pneumonia (PCP) for which there is a failure rate of 5-20%; T-S is relatively non-toxic in non-immunocompromised patients, although up to 60% of AIDS patients have adverse side effects, eg ↑ liver function tests, neutropenia, thrombocytopenia, erythematous maculo-papular rash, rarely Stevens-Johnson syndrome, exfoliative dermatitis, nausea, and vomiting; T-S once a day is more effective as a primary prophylaxis for PCP than aerosolized pentamidine; unlike pentamidine, T-S may protect against other infectious agents, including *Salmonella, Shigella, Nocardia* spp, *Haemophilus influenzae, Listeria monocytogenes, Streptococcus pneumoniae, Isospora belli*, and possibly *Toxoplasma gondii*; T-S has a higher incidence of adverse side effects than pentamidine (25% vs 3%) (**N Engl J Med 1992; 327:1836**OA, 1842OA)

Note: Trimethoprim-dapsone may have fewer side effects of an intensity requiring a change to pentamidine therapy (**N Engl J Med 1990; 323:776**) in HIV-infected subjects

'trimming' RESEARCH ETHICS A method used in science to 'correct' experimental data, eliminating the high and low values most in excess of the mean in an experimental 'run'; while these values are within the confines of statistical probability, they make the assay look sloppy on paper, and thus are 'trimmed'; trimming has long been considered a form of scientific misrepresentation (**C Babbage, REFLECTIONS ON THE DECLINE OF SCIENCE, London, 1830**) Cf 'Cooking, Fraud in science

trinucleotide repeat disease A clinically heterogenous group of diseases that share in common the amplification or expansion of specific trinucleotides, including CAG (Huntington's disease, Kennedy's disease), CGG (fragile X syndrome), and GCT (myotonic dystrophy (**Arch Pathol Lab Med 1993; 117:1121**RV)

triple airway maneuver EMERGENCY MEDICINE A procedure used to clear the air passages of those with upper airway obstruction, where the mandible is moved forward and rescue breathing is performed through the mouth and the nose

triple apical pulse CARDIOLOGY A double systolic pulse that is coupled with presystolic distension, an uncommon but characteristic finding by precordial palpation in hyper-

trophic cardiomyopathy

triple-blinded study CLINICAL THERAPEUTICS A study in which the patients and researchers are unaware of whether a treatment (experimental drug) or placebo is being administered (ie 'double-blinded'); in addition, the team analyzing the data is unaware of which group's data they are evaluating, ie from the placebo or treatment arm of the protocol; although triple-blinding ensures that there are no post-trial bias(es) introduced into the study, it is rarely performed in practice; see Blinding, Double blinding

triple bypass surgery Coronary arterial bypass graft, see there

triple helix DNA MOLECULAR BIOLOGY An artificially produced conformation of DNA that has a third strand of antisense DNA, designed to bind at specific oligonucleotide sequences on DNA's double helix; triple helix DNA is of considerable interest experimentally, and has therapeutic potential, given that in a properly designed triple strand, a site otherwise bound by a protein promoter or suppressor can be blocked and the corresponding gene either turned on or off; see Antisense DNA and RNA; Cf Achilles heel cleavage

triple helix protein A polyprotein with a quaternary structural motif composed of three intertwined left-handed α helical proteins, wound in a right-handed helix, a conformation typical of collagen, which owes its strength and resistance to proteolytic digestion to the high number of covalent cross-linking bonds between adjacent tropocollagen molecules

triple iron agar MICROBIOLOGY A nutritionally rich bacterial growth medium that may be used to direct the initial identification of gram-negative bacteria, especially *Enterobacteriaceae*; a bacterium's growth on TIA and the related KIA (Kligler iron agar), can be used to detect three characteristics of bacteria: The ability to produce gas by the fermentation of sugar, the generation of H_2S, which appears as a black precipitate and the fermentation of sucrose (TIA) or lactose (KIA)

triple-marker screen A colloquial term for the use of three specific laboratory tests (alpha-fetoprotein, chorionic gonadotropin, and unconjugated estriol) that are increased in Down syndrome; the screen has been reported to ↑ the rate of detection of Down syndrome, and ↓ the false positive rate (which may cause the parents to opt for abortion), from 6.6% to 3.8%; the triple screen is not a definitive test, and must be followed ultrasound and possible amniocentesis with chromosomal studies; the cost per Down syndrome detected is $150-200 000, which some view as socially acceptable (see **CAP Today Jan 1993**)

triple phosphate calculi Struvite stones Renal concrements composed of ammonium magnesium phosphate, $Mg(NH_4)(PO_4)\cdot6H_2O$, which are formed in the renal pelvis, that may give rise to a staghorn calculus, and in the urinary bladder by action of urea-splitting bacteria, eg *Proteus, Pseudomonas, Klebsiella* and *Staphylocccus* species; TPC appear as coffin-lid crystals in alkaline urine

triple response of Lewis A triad of transient skin changes seen in immediate hypersensitivity when the skin is firmly stroked by a pointed object, characterized as 1) Stroke or immediate response due to the local release of prostaglandin, histamine, serotonin and bradykinin 2) Flare appearing as a red halo, due to vasodilation and 3) Wheal in which there is swelling and blanching of the stroke due to histamine release from mast cells, edema of intercellular junctions with protein and fluid accumulation

triple stones Triple phosphate calculi, see there

triple test A colloquial term for the use of three diagnostic modalities, eg clinical, radiographic, and cytopathologic data to arrive at a diagnosis; a positive triple test is critical in those areas where each method being used is less than 100% specific; as an example, in breast cancer, each component of the triple test is may be consistent with malignancy, but is not of its own enough to make a definitive diagnosis (Acta Cytologica 1994; 38:90A)

'triple threat' physician A rare (and claimed by some to be a vanishing) breed of physician who is 1) A world-class researcher or of a caliber sufficient to obtain self-supporting grants 2) A teacher with the skill of Socrates and 3) A clinician with active patient contact; see Professor, Socratic method

triple X syndrome XXX syndrome, see there

triplet see Codon

triplet repeat mutation A novel form of DNA mutation in which a triplet of nucleotides (eg CAG) is repeated up to 200 times; TRMs have been thus far identified in both hereditary (eg fragile X syndrome, Huntington's disease, myotonic dystrophy and spinal and bulbar muscle atrophy) and in malignancy and in some forms of colorectal cancer (New York Times 11 May 1993; C3)

triploidy syndrome XXX and XXY syndromes, see there

tripod fracture TRAUMATOLOGY A complex maxillofacial fracture that affects the zygoma, orbit and maxilla (N Engl J Med 1994; 330:69c)

tripod sign NEUROLOGY A nuchal-spinal sign in which the sitting position requires a rigid spine and both arms extended towards the back for support, typically seen in children with non-paralytic poliomyelitis

triradius DERMATOGLYPHICS A pattern of whorls (figure, right) seen on the palms of children with trisomy 13 and 21, a finding of itself without pathological significance, which serves merely to support the usually obvious diagnosis of these trisomies

tris Tris(hydroxymethyl) aminomethane LABORATORY TECHNOLOGY A substance used to prepare buffers (tris buffer) for biological systems at a 'physiologic' pH range of 7.2 to 9.2

triskelion see Clathrin

trisomy 12 A chromosomal duplication that has been identified by FISH or by classic cytogenetic analysis in benign ♀ genital tract tumors, the significance of which is uncertain (Diagn Mol Pathol 1993; 2:94)

triton 1) ³H Tritium nucleus, a radionuclide consisting of one proton and two neutrons, which is a weak β-emitter with a physical half-life of 12.26 years 2) A family of proprietary nonionic, surface-active agents

Triton tumor An uncommon peripheral nerve tumor with muscular differentiation that is either benign, usually designated as neuromuscular hamartoma, or malignant; Triton tumors are most common in the head, neck and trunk, with a peak incidence at 35 years of age, often associated with von Recklinghausen's disease; the symptoms are typically neurologic and related to enlarging tumor masses PATHOLOGY Scattered rhabdomyoblasts that may have cross-striations within malignant schwannoma-like stroma (figure); desmin and myoglobin may be seen by immunoperoxidase staining FIVE-YEAR SURVIVAL 12%

Note: The name derives from a group of newts (Genus, *Amblystoma*) or small salamanders (Genus, *Triturus*), trivially known as tritons, in which there is an intimate relation between limb degeneration and innervation, a phenomenon first described by JT Todd in 1823; although the presence of nerves is not an absolute prerequisite for limb regeneration (J Exp Zoo 1959; 140:101), the name triton was retained by pathologists as a tribute to the theory that motor nerves could induce endoneural cell differentiation into muscle cells; the salamanders in turn received their name from Triton, the son of Poseidon and Amphitrite, an inferior sea-deity who had the head and torso of a man and the tail of a dolphin

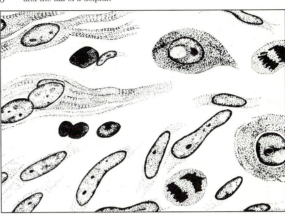

Triton tumor

Triton X-100 A proprietary quaternary ammonium surface-active salt, iso-octyl phenoxy polyethoxy ethanol; in low concentrations, Triton X-100 removes most of the plasma membrane except regions with a hexagonal arrangement; Triton X-100 is used as a surfactant, detergent, wetting agent, and emulsifier

trivial complaint A symptom, sign or lesion, usually identified by the patient, which is regarded as having no impact on the patient's well-being or the management of an unrelated medical condition

Note: Given the litigious environment of medical practice in the US, all investigations of 'trivial complaints' must be documented in writing

trivial name A popular, working, or common name for a disease, organ, eg Bauchspeicheldrüse, German, pancreas, structure, or molecule that is not standard nomenclature or based on 'official' rules delineated by internationally recognized agencies or organizations, eg American Psychiatric Association, Enzyme Commission, the International System, Nomina Anatomica

trk An oncogene that was first identified in colonic carcinoma, which encodes the 140-kD Trk protein, which structurally resembles those of tyrosine kinase receptors, probably corresponding to the high-molecular-weight nerve growth factor receptor; the Trk protein appears to process the intracellular signal after nerve growth factor binds to the extracellular receptor; trk is relatively specific and most prominently expressed on neurons of neural crest origin (Science 1991; 252:554); activation of the trk tyrosine kinase receptor may provide a mechanism for signal transduction by nerve growth factor (Nature 1991; 350:158)

TRK A proto-oncogene that encodes p140^proteo-TRK, a tyrosine kinase-type transmembrane glycoprotein expressed selectively in the developing nervous system; the biologic response to nerve growth factor (NGF) depends on the interactions with p140^proteo-TRK, but it is uncertain whether p140^proteo-TRK is solely responsible for NGF's action; TRK is expressed in many primary neuroblastomas and is inversely associated with amplification of the N-*myc* proto-oncogene; in neuroblastomas, ↑ expression of TRK is strongly correlated with a favorable tumor stage (I, II, or IVa disease, younger age (< 1 year), normal N-*myc* copy number, and low level of N-*myc* expression; 5-year survival with a high level of TRK expression is 86% vs 14% (N Engl J Med 1993; 328:847₀ₐ)

troche Lozenge[1] A form of oral medication that is formulated as a discoid solid containing a therapeutic agent in a flavored base[2]; a troche is placed in the mouth and allowed to slowly dissolve, releasing its active ingredient, eg analgesic, antibiotic, antihistaminic, antiseptic, antitussive, decongestant, or local anesthetic

[1]Lozenge is more popular among the nonmedical rabble [2]Which may be a hard sugar candy, glycereinated gelatin, or sugar with enough mucilage to give the material its form

troglitazone A member of the thiazolidinedione class of antidiabetic drugs that improve insulin resistance MECHANISM OF ACTION Uncertain; it is thought to directly enhance insulin activity in the liver, skeletal muscle, and adipose tissue; in patients with NIDDM, troglitazone improves both fasting and postprandial hyperglycemia and hyperinsulinemia; it also decreases insulin resistance and improves glucose tolerance in obese subjects with normal or impaired glucose tolerance (N Engl J Med 1994; 331:1188₀ₐ)

Trojan horse 'effect' Any disastrous result of an anticipated gain; or, the masking of a dangerous agent within an innocent garb EPIDEMIOLOGY Any unanticipated vector of an organism or potential route of disease transmission, as Hagnaya wreathes as vectors for parasites or used rubber tire casings that provide ideal breeding sites for the northern Asian mosquito, *Aedes albopictus* a potential vector for Bunyaviridae and LaCrosse viruses (Science 1990; 250:1738) INFECTIOUS DISEASE HIV-1 causes a 'Trojan horse' type of infection, in which HIV-1 binds to the CD4 receptor, enters the cell and integrates itself into the host genome as a provirus, thus remaining hidden from the immune system, similar to the Trojan horse; upon lysis of the CD4 receptor-positive cells (helper T cells and macrophages), the virus is liberated and HIV-1 either re-enters the circulation or continues infecting other cells via the CD4 receptor

Trojan horse inhibitor LABORATORY METHODOLOGY A molecule that is introduced by affinity labeling into the active site of an enzyme, or other protein, with the purpose of delineating the enzyme's active site, as the 'Trojan horse' molecular mimic prevents the target protein from performing its usual function

'trolley car' policy An insurance policy that has multiple restrictive riders and clauses that essentially prevent the insured party from collecting benefits except under the most extraordinary circumstances, ie the policy-holder's being hit by a trolley car

*A mode of public transportation which while once common, now exists only in a few cities in the US; such an insurance policy has also been called an 'elephant policy for the same reason

trophoblast cells see Cytotrophoblast, Syncytiotrophoblast

Trophyrema whippelii The proposed causative bacillus of Whipple's disease (N Engl J Med 1994; 331:1343₀ₐ) *T whippelii* may also cause uveitis; the diagnosis of which is suspected based on 'damning' evidnce with EM, is confirmed by PCR which detection of 16S ribosomal RNA gene (rDNA) sequences corresponding to *T whippelii* (ibid 1995; 332:363₀ₐ)

tropical (pulmonary) eosinophilia A clinical complex that primarily affects the lungs of those living in the Near and Far East and caused by a hypersensitivity response to filarial worms, eg *Brugia malayi* and *Wuchereria bancrofti* CLINICAL Malaise, wasting, wheezing, bronchospasm, chronic productive cough with bilateral rales PATHOLOGY Polymorphous cell infiltrate in lungs, composed of eosinophils, 'round' cells, fibroblasts and eventually fibrosis TREATMENT Diethylcarbamazine, Ivermectin

tropical oils A family of cooking oils derived from palm and coconut trees that differ from other vegetable oils in that like animal fats, they have a high content of saturated fatty acids and thus are thought to have significant atherogenic potential; see Fish (oil), Olive oil, Trans fatty acids

tropical spastic paraparesis A form of HTLV-I infection causing progressive lower extremity weakness, sparing the upper extremities and mental faculties; TSP occurs in the Caribbean, West Africa, the Seychelles Islands, and Colombia and is thought to be identical to the HTLV-I-associated myelopathy described in the Japanese, a form of progressive leg paralysis; some cases of 'multiple sclerosis' may correspond to TSP; see HTLV-I

tropical splenomegaly syndrome An idiopathic splenomegaly affecting malnourished children and adult females in malaria-endemic regions, eg New Guinea and Africa, which is thought to be a defective immune response to *Plasmodium malariae* CLINICAL Massive splenomegaly, asthenia, fatigue LABORATORY ↑↑↑ IgM antibodies against *P vivax*, ↓ T-helper cells ↓ CD4:CD8 (helper:suppressor) ratio TREATMENT Chloroquine *P vivax or malariae*

tropical sprue An idiopathic malabsorption complex, described in the tropics, occurring either in miniepidemics or in Caucasians who have recently arrived to the region; it has been related to either subclinical deficiencies of certain nutrients (protein, folate, vitamin B_{12}, fats and sugars) or an as yet unidentified pathogen, resulting in diarrhea-induced weakness that favors the overgrowth of coliform bacteria indigenous to the tropics CLINICAL Malaise, fever, anorexia, intermittent diarrhea, chronic malabsorption, which in the epidemic form first affects adults; prolonged malabsorption causes vitamin deficiencies, muscle wasting, mucocutaneous pigmentation and edema PATHOLOGY Lengthening of crypts, broadening and shortening of villi, chronic inflammation and nonspecific ↑ in lipids, seen in biopsies of the small intestine TREATMENT Folic acid, vitamin B_{12} and broad-spectrum antibiotics, eg tetracycline, intraluminal sulfonamides

tropicamide OPHTHALMOLOGY An antichoinergic agent that blocks the action of acetylcholine, dilating the pupils in Alzheimer's disease (AD) patients in a highly diluted concentrations, a finding that some authors believe may be of use as a clinical test for AD (Sci Am 1995; 272/2:12)

tropocollagen The basic polymeric structural unit of collagen, which is a triple helix of α collagens, which forms larger units of collagen fibrils and fibers

tropoelastin A 68-kD polypeptide composed of nonpolar amino acids

α-tropomyosin A I band muscle protein encoded on chromosome 15 that inhibits contraction in absence of troponin, which when present allows myosin to make contact with actin; α-tropomyosin mutations may result in familial hypertrophic cardiomyopathy (N Engl J Med 1995; 332:1058₀ₐ)

troponin A 76-kD heterotrimeric contractile protein present in low concentrations in the thin filaments of striated muscle, which has the combined functions of binding calcium and tropomyosin, inhibiting actomyosin ATPase and regulating muscle contraction; troponin has three isoforms, C, I, and T

troponin I A regulatory contractile protein that is increased in the serum following myocardial necrosis, and is regarded as a sensitive and specific marker of perioperative MI (N Engl J Med 1994; 330:670₀ₐ)

troponin T A regulatory contractile protein not normally present in the blood, which when detected in the circulation indicates myocardial cell damage and cardiac necrosis; in one study, TT was ↑ in 33/84 patients with unstable angina (vs ↑ CK-MB in 3/84); of the 33, 10 had MIs, of whom 5 died during hospitalization; laboratory measurement of TT appears to be a more sensitive indicator of myocardial injury, and may have prognostic value (N Engl J Med 1992; 327:141₀ₐ) Add encoded on chromosome 1; various mutation in the troponin gene may result in familial hypertrophic cardiomyopathy (**N Engl J Med 1995; 332:1058**OA); there is 6-fold ↑ in the odds of an MI if TnT is ↑ within 2 hours of the onset of chest pain; there is 6-fold ↓ in the odds of an MI if TnT is negative within 8 hours of the onset of chest pain (**JAMA 1995; 273:1279**)

Note: It is as yet unknown whether assays of serum levels of CK-MB subunits (see there) are superior to assays for troponin I and troponin T

Trotter syndrome Sinus of Morgagni syndrome A clinical complex characterized by triad consisting of homolateral deafness, pain in the sensory zone of the mandibular division of the trigeminal nerve, immobility of the ipsilateral palate, and trismus, due to invasion by a malignancy, often a squamous cell carcinoma arising in the lateral nasopharynx, specifically in the region of the sinus of Morgagni

troubleshoot LABORATORY MEDICINE *verb* To determine the source of a systematic error and correct it

'trough' THERAPEUTIC DRUG MONITORING The minimum serum concentration of a drug being administered for a prolonged period, the levels of which are measured immediately prior to administration of the next dose; 'peaks' and 'troughs' are measured for drugs that have a low therapeutic index and potentially serious side effects, eg aminoglycoside antibiotics, which have well-known ototoxic and nephrotoxic effects; trough levels should be above the extrapolated minimum inhibitory concentration of the infecting bacteria; see MBC, MIC, Therapeutic drug monitoring, therapeutic index; Cf Peak levels

true hermaphroditism Gonads contain both ovarian and testicular tissue, genotypically either 46, XX or 46, XY; 75% are raised as boys; the testicular tissue is dysgenic, doesn't produce sperm and may undergo malignant degeneration (requiring prophylactic removal); ovarian function in those raised as girls may be adequate to produce term pregnancy; see Hermaphroditism

trümmerfeldzone White line of scurvy, see there

truncate *verb* To cut short

truncated *adjective* Shortened

TRUS Transrectal ultrasonography, see there

trustworthiness MEDICAL ETHICS A moral principle in which a person both deserves the trust of others and does not violate that trust; trustworthiness is expected of physicians and the trustworthy physician has a duty to fulfil all voluntary commitments and responsibilities of an office or role, eg that of 'healer'; the physician is further expected to neither deceive or cheat another

'truth serum' Sodium amytal A short-acting barbiturate that induces intoxication during which a subject tends to talk with fewer inhibitions; this with visualization and hypnosis is a prime method for introducing false memories, see there

truth-telling Therapeutic privilege, see there

trypan blue dye exclusion test CELL CULTURE A rapid laboratory test that determines the viability of cultured cells or determines the percent of cell lysis as a measure of cytotoxic activity of a tissue culture supernatant fluid; the trypan blue stain is excluded from cells by active transport and thus blue cells are dead cells

trypanosome lytic factor TLF PARASITOLOGY A factor present in human blood, which contains two apolipoproteins (haptoglobin-related protein and paraoxonase-arylesterase), each of which is capable of causing lysis of *Trypanosoma brucei brucei* (a nonhuman trypanosome) in vitro; TLF protects against nonhuman trypanosomes, possibly the result of its peroxidase activity (**Science 1995; 268:284, 204**)

trypanosomiasis-African The genus *Trypanosoma* causes African sleeping sickness, which cripples both the livestock in the region, and an estimated 50 million people are at risk for this hematogenous parasitemia 1) *Trypanosoma brucei rhodesiense* VECTOR Tsetse fly LOCATION East Africa CLINICAL Acute febrile syndrome, rapidly progressing to death 2) *T brucei gambiense* VECTOR Tsetse fly LOCATION West Africa CLINICAL Chronic with CNS depression (sleeping sickness)

trypanosomiasis-American The genus *Trypanosoma* also causes American sleeping sickness, agent *T cruzi* (Chagas' disease) VECTOR Reduviid (kissing) bug CLINICAL The acute form most commonly affects infants, causing malaise, fever, hepatosplenomegaly; the chronic (or asymptomatic) form is more subtle and is accompanied by altered cardiac conduction (the most common cause of congestive heart failure in South America), megaesophagus and megacolon TREATMENT Melarsoprol, a toxic agent used for end-stage meningoencephalitix disease or O-11 10-(propoxy)decanoic acid, a myristic acid analog that is highly toxic to and specific for trypanosomes (**Science 1991; 252:1851**)

tryptophan-associated eosinophilic connective-tissue disease Eosinophilic-myalgia syndrome, see there

tryptophan malabsorption syndrome Blue diaper syndrome An AR [MIM 211000] condition characterized by ↓ growth, hypercalcemia, nephrocalcinosis, recurrent infections, renal defects, and indicanuria; the blue color is due to oxidation of indican to indican blue upon exposure to air; Cf Black urine disease

TSI Triple sugar iron, see there

TSLS Toxic shock-like syndrome, see there

TSP Tropical spastic paraparesis, see there

tsutsugamushi disease *tsutsuga*, dangerous, Japanese, *mushi*, bug see Scrub typhus

TTAPS model A 'nuclear winter' model[1] that concluded that the consequences of even a limited nuclear exchange would result in a 'no-win' situation for any belligerent nation; their manuscript, which became known as the 'Blue book'[2]; the conclusions the TTAPS model have been partially supported by data generated from the burning oil fields in Kuwait; see IPPNW, Nuclear war

[1]Generated by Drs Turco, Toon, Ackerman, Pollack and Sagan [2]It was never published, as one of the authors felt it had created so much dialog that multiple revisions were incapable of salvaging it in the original form

t-test Student's t-test, see there

TTP-HUS The combination of thrombotic thrombocytopenic purpura (TTP) and hemolytic-uremic syndrome (HUS), which are polar expressions of the same disease defined by a pentad consisting of features of TTP described by Moschcowitz, ie thrombocytopenia, microangiopathic hemolytic anemia, neurological abnormalities and fever as well as renal disease (**JAMA 1991; 265:91**cr) CLINICAL Abrupt onset in children following a viral upper respiratory tract infection or may be associated with a verotoxin in *Escherichia coli*-induced gastroenteritis; the hemolytic-uremic component is less common in adults, but may occur in pregnancy, at parturition, or during chemotherapy; spontaneously resolving renal failure occurs in 60% (10% progress to chronic renal failure); renal failure may be more common in *Escherichia coli* O157:H7 infections, and these organisms were inculpated in 16% of those with HUS LABORATORY Reticulocytosis, increased bilirubin and fibrin split products (without DIC), reduced haptoglobin TREATMENT Most cases resolve spontaneously, others require high-dose corticosteroids (**N Engl J Med 1994; 331:661**CPC)

Note: A higher neutrophil count and/or bloody diarrhea on admission may indicate a poor prognosis

T$_H$1-type immunity T$_H$1 immunity, see there

T$_H$2-type immunity T$_H$2 immunity, see there

TU complex CARDIOLOGY see (**JAMA 1993; 269:1513**OC)

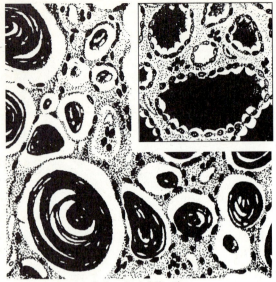

tubular thyroidization

tubeless test GASTROENTEROLOGY A generic term for any pancreatic function test in which various substrate molecules for pancreatic enzymes are administered per os (ie without intubating the patient), followed by measurement of the digestion products; the most popular TTs are the bentiromide and the pancreolauryl tests; other TTs include fecal chymotrypsin, trypsin RIA, serum pancreatic polypeptide, dual-label Schilling, and quantitative stool fat tests (N Engl J Med 1995; 332:1482RA) see Bentiromide test, Pancreolauryl test

tuberculid A non-infectious skin lesion due to hypersensitivity to *Mycobacterium* species, divided into papulonecrotic tuberculid, which consists in symmetrical waves of sterile papules with central ulceration and obliterative vasculitis and lichen scrofulosorum, which consists of groups of tiny, sarcoid-like red papules

tuberculosis A disease first known to the ancients;* one million new cases of *Mycobacterium tuberculosis* develop per year worldwide, of which an estimated 10% of those in underdeveloped nations eventually die; 'smear'-positive cases in Africa (165/10[5]), are more often clinically inactive than those in Asia where the rate is 110/10[5] US incidence: 9.3 cases/10[5] (white/hispanic 5.7/10[5], black 26.7/10[5], Asian 49.6/10[5]); in 1984, the previous trend of a decreasing incidence of TB in the US reversed itself in the mid-1980s, due to increases of *M tuberculosis* and *M avium-intercellulare* in AIDS patients; up to 10 million in the US have latent TB, many of whom are poor, aged, malnourished; homeless or IV drug abusers (N Engl J Med 1991; 324:1644) Unique growth characteristics include arylsulfatase positivity in *M cheloni* and growth inhibition by thiophene-2-carboxylic acid hydrazide in *M bovis*; optimal growth temperature 32ºC in *M marinum*, *M ulcerans*, *M haemophilum*, and 42ºC in *M xenopi*; all *Mycobacterium* species produce nicotinic acid, *M tuberculosis*, *M simiae* and *M szulgai* produce the greatest amount; lesser amounts are produced by *M africanum*, *M bovis*, *M marinum*, and *M chelonei cheloni* and *M chelonei abscessus* Nitrate reduction *M tuberculosis*, *M kansasii*, *M szulgai*, *M flavescens*, *triviale*, *M fortuitum*, *M smegmatis*; *M szulgai* is a scotochrome at 37ºC and photochrome at 25ºC Growth media Lowenstein-Jensen, Middlebrook 7H10 TREATMENT-PRIMARY DRUGS Isoniazid, ethambutol, rifampicin, streptomycin SECONDARY DRUGS Ethionamide, capreomycin, kanamycin, cycloserine, pyrazinamide, para-aminosalicylic acid DIAGNOSIS Ziehl-Neelsen or Kinyoun stains, viewed by light microscopy; auramine-rhodamine stain with fluorescent microscopy; NAP test, nucleic acid probe; see MOTT, Multidrug resistant tuberculosis, Runyon classification

*It was called the 'King of diseases' in Sanskrit, and has been discovered in pre-Columbian mummies in Peru (New York Times 15 March 1994; C1)

tuberculostearic acid assay A test used to detect the presence of *Mycobacterium tuberculosis* (Q J Med 1992; 297:15)

tubular complex Tubuloreticular structure An intracellular inclusion of undetermined nature and significance, seen by EM, which consists of 800-1500 x 20-40-nm cytoplasmic masses of twisted, haphazardly arranged, undulating tubules contiguous with the cisternae of the adjacent endoplasmic reticulum; these structures are focally positive for acid phosphatase and terminal deoxynucleotidyl transferase (TdT) and occur in lymphocytes and endothelium in AIDS and other viral infections, Chediak-Higashi disease, collagen vascular disease, immunodeficiencies, B- and T-cell lymphoproliferative disorders, melanoma and sarcomas, and can be induced in vitro by a variety of tissue culture toxins; Cf Vesicular rosettes

tubular 'thyroidization' RENAL PATHOLOGY The filling of the renal tubules, especially the proximal convoluted tubules, with homogenous pale eosinophilic proteinaceous casts, an appearance likened to colloid in thyroid acini, a typical histologic feature of chronic pyelonephritis, less commonly seen in amyloidosis and ischemia; in the accompanying figure, scalloping of colloid is seen in the inset box in the upper right; Cf 'Blocked pipe' appearance

tubulin A heterodimeric protein composed of a 50-kD α and a 50-kD β chain arranged in repeating head-to-tail units, which form microtubules when warmed to 37ºC in the presence of GTP; see Cilia, Flagella, MAPs, Microtubules, MTOC

tufts Tufting SURGICAL PATHOLOGY A histologic finding consisting of microscopic papillary projections that rise from the epithelial lining in serous carcinomas of low malignant potential, which in addition demonstrate nuclear atypia, increased mitotic activity and absence of stromal invasion; see Borderline tumor

tuftsin Leukocidin A phagocytosis-promoting tetrapeptide (Thr-Lys-Pro-Arg) derived from a leukokinin globulin, which represents residues 289-292 of the immunoglobulin Fc receptor; tuftsin is produced in the spleen and is chemotactic for neutrophils and macrophages, it stimulates phagocytic motility, enhances antigen processing and aids in oxidative metabolism

tumbling motility MICROBIOLOGY A descriptor for the end-over-end motility characteristic of *Listeria monocytogenes*, when these organisms are incubated in nutrient broth at room temperature; when an inoculum of *L monocytogenes* is 'stabbed' in a test tube filled with semisolid medium, its mobility is restricted and it displays an 'umbrella' pattern of growth; see Umbrella growth

tummy tuck Abdominoplasty, see there

tumor-associated antigen IMMUNOLOGY, ONCOLOGY A generic term for any of a number of molecules such as CA 19-9, CA-125 and CA-195 that may be associated with specific tumors, including lymphomas, carcinomas, sarcomas, and melanomas; although the epitopes of these antigens may elicit cellular and/or humoral immune response against the tumor, this response is rarely adequate to defend the host against the tumor; tumor-associated antigens have been subdivided into CLASS 1 ANTIGENS are highly specific to a particular tumor and present in one or only a few individuals and not found in normal cells, eg Tumor specific transplantation antigen CLASS 2 ANTIGENS and are present on a number of related tumors from different patients and CLASS 3 ANTIGENS which present on both normal and malignant cells but which are expressed in increased amounts in malignant cells Note: Class 2 antigens are of greatest potential use in developing clinically useful assays since they are present in many tumors and are rarely observed in normal subjects

tumor doubling time ONCOLOGY A value of clinical interest that allows a relatively accurate prediction of tumor aggressiveness; although tumor doubling is less elegant than evaluating genomic events (recombination, point mutations and gene amplification) in determining tumor aggression, for specific tumor types, it is of prognostic value in determining growth of untreated tumors; tumor doubling times range from 8 to 600 days, depending on the cell and tumor type; see Gompertzian growth

tumor initiator A carcinogen that interacts directly with a susceptible cell's DNA, evoking the first step in a theoretical two-step carcinogenic cascade, which may then be followed by the action of a tumor promoter

tumor lysis syndrome Acute tumor lysis syndrome A constellation of biochemical derangements seen at the onset of cytotoxic therapy for malignancy, where rapid cell death causes hyperkalemia, hyperphosphatemia, hyperuricemia and hypocalcemia Note: Cytolysis of large, mitotically active tumors causes metabolic imbalances themselves severe enough to cause death by renal failure; the serum level of lactate dehydrogenase (LD, especially isoenzymes LD_3 and LD_4) provides a crude estimate of tumor-load; by extension, an elevated LD may indicate an increased risk for ATLS; ATLS occurs in breast and oat cell carcinoma (of the lungs), metastatic adenocarcinoma, lymphosarcoma, NHL, eg lymphoblastic and Burkitt's lymphomas, CML, ALL, multiple myeloma and metastatic medulloblastoma; massive tumor lysis is usually confined to histologically aggressive neoplasms, but has been described in CLL related to 2-chlorodeoxyadenosine therapy (N Engl J Med 1993; 329:1547oa)

tumor markers There is no circulating protein or metabolite that is consistently elevated in, or specific for any malignancy; at best, 'tumor markers' are relatively nonspecific and cannot be used as screening tools, but may, under certain circumstances, be used to detect recurrence (through rising serum levels, eg carcino-embryonic antigen, CEA) in patients with known and treated malignancy; in clinical parlance, tumor markers include oncofetal proteins (α-fetoprotein, CEA) and tumor-associated antigens (CA-125, CA 19-9); several highly nonspecific circulating molecules have been erroneously called 'tumor markers' including enzymes (CK-BB, acid phosphatase, alkaline phosphatase, galactosyltransferase, LDH, lysozyme, neuron-specific enolase), hormones (bombesin, calcitonin, β-hCG, HPL), metabolites (catecholamines, polyamines and sialic acid), proteins (binding proteins, ferritin and hormone receptors) and others (chromogranin A immunoglobulins, polyanions)

tumor necrosis factor Either of two molecules that mediate shock and tumor-related cachexia, divided into TNF-α and TNF-β; TNF-α (cachexin) is a 17-kD pluripotent protein cytokine produced primarily by monocytes and mast cells, the 3' end of which has sequence homology with other biological response mediators, including lymphotoxin, IFNs, IL-1, and GM-CSF; TNF-α production is increased in a broad palette of clinical conditions including inflammation, sepsis, lipid and protein metabolism, hematopoiesis, angiogenesis, collagen vascular disease, terminal chronic heart failure (with activated renin-angiotensin system), host resistance to viruses and parasites, eg severe falciparum malaria, in children dying of severe infectious purpura and in malignancy; corticosteroids inhibit TNF-α biosynthesis SIDE EFFECTS, SHORT-TERM Fever, headache and hypotension LONG-TERM Cachexia, chills, fatigue, anorexia and thrombocytopenia; in rodents, high TNF levels cause piloerection, diarrhea, and a poorly groomed appearance; endotoxemia is a TNF-

induced event with a shock-like clinical picture with interstitial pneumonia, vascular plugging by neutrophils, acute tubular necrosis, GI tract, adrenal and pancreatic ischemia and hemorrhage LABORATORY Hemoconcentration, metabolic acidosis, hypoglycemia and hyperkalemia

tumor necrosis factor receptor A 461-amino acid receptor protein with a cysteine-rich extracellular domain that shares sequence similarity to neural growth factor receptor and to an open reading frame from the Shope fibroma virus

---

TUMOR LYSIS SYNDROME (METABOLIC DERANGEMENTS IN)

HYPERURICEMIA Release of uric and nucleic acid precursors (by massive cytolysis), aggrevated by acid urine, renal dysfunction, dehydration and edema, possibly causing renal shutdown through massive tubular precipitation of uric acid crystals

HYPERKALEMIA Release of intracellular potassium, worsened by acidosis, renal dysfunction, potassium-sparing diuretics, adrenal insufficiency, diabetes mellitus, hypocalcemia or hyponatremia appearing as muscular weakness and cardiac arrhythmias, including atrioventricular block, tachyarrhythmia or cardiac arrest

HYPERPHOSPHATEMIA/HYPOCALCEMIA Minerals released by lysing cells cause soft tissue mineralization, exacerbating renal failure by intratubular crystallization and may cause neuromuscular irritability, with tetany, convulsions

---

tumor promoter Cocarcinogen A substance, often lipid-soluble, that has no intrinsic carcinogenic potential, but which when applied repeatedly, is capable of amplifying the cancer-inducing effects of other substances, ie initiators; the classic tumor promoter is phorbol ester and its derivatives isolated from *Croton flavens*, which is a potent and specific activator of protein kinase C; high-fat diets are 'promotional', eg linoleic acid-rich corn, safflower and sunflower oils are promoters, but olive oil is not; see Antipromoter

tumor promotion The theoretical second stage in a two- or multi-step carcinogenic sequence, which follows an 'initiation' step and requires that the tumor promoting substance(s) be applied in a repeated or continuous fashion

tumor seeding The spillage of tumor cells and their subsequent growth into tumor 'colonies'; tumor seeding is of greater theoretical than actual importance, but has been described in malignant cell spillage from an operative field, and along needle biopsy tracts, as potential complications of diagnostic or therapeutic procedures

tumor suppressor gene Anti-oncogene A growth-regulatory gene that encodes a protein capable of suppressing malignant transformation; in most malignancies, multiple steps are necessary before these genes are either inactivated by mutation or lost; the p53 gene on chromosome 17p13 is mutated or inactivated in all histologic types of lung cancer (Science 1989; 246:491); other tumor suppressor genes include RB, DCC, NM23, ras and tyrosine kinase gene on chromosome 3; see DCC gene, One-hit-two-hit model, p53, Promoter, RB gene, TKO selection

tumorlet A nodular hyperplasia of spindled cells related to Kulchitsky-type neuroendocrine cells, seen in the bronchial wall in patients with bronchiectasia or occasionally associated with carcinoid tumors

tunnel clusters Nodular aggregates of uniform, round open glands seen in the Kurman of the AFIP on cervix

tunnel effect GASTROENTEROLOGY Visualization of only the open end of the stainless steel tube used in rigid sigmoidoscopy, see Sigmoidoscopy

tunneling MEDICAL PHYSICS The transfer of a particle, eg an electron, across a potential energy barrier without the particle passing the barrier; see Scanning tunneling microscopy PARASITOLOGY The quasi-linear subcutaneous burrowing that is typical of scabies

tunnel vision NEUROLOGY Concentric constriction of the visual fields, which is thought to be secondary to degeneration of the cells of the calcarine cortex, a symptom characteristic of chronic methylmercury poisoning, that may also be accompanied by multiple scotomata, diminished auditory acuity and changes in mental status; another organic cause of tunnel vision occurs in infarction of the sensory relay nuclei of the thalamus with relative sparing of the occipital lobes; see Mercury

'tunnel vision' PSYCHIATRY A concentric constriction of both visual fields, where the absolute size of the visual fields tends to be the same regardless of the distance from object being viewed, a finding typical of hysterical reactions or hypersuggestibility states

Note to speakers of English as a second language: the phrase 'tunnel vision' is widely used as an adjective referring or pertaining to an individual lacking a Weltanschauung or any myopic perspective adopted by a person, group, or organization

turban tumor DERMATOPATHOLOGY A variant form of cylindroma (a sweat gland tumor common on the scalp), that appears as a large red-pink, usually hairless tumor with a bosselated surface that has been fancifully likened to a turban, which may grow to 50 cm in maximum size PATHOLOGY The tumor cells are arranged in a pattern fancifully likened to a child's jigsaw-puzzle, see Cylindroma

turbidity test A test for sickle cell anemia based on the decreased solubility of hemoglobin S in dithionate, which is less accurate than the sodium bisulfate or sickle cell test; see Sickle cell test

turbidimetry A laboratory technique that semiquantifies a substance in suspension, based on the decrease in forward light transmission by the suspension; Cf Nephelometry

turf *darbha*, Sanskrit, tuft of grass *noun* The upper stratum of soil bound by grass and plant roots into a thick mat; in medical practice, turf refers to one's range and type of practice and patients for which one is responsible, eg *'Physicians have long opposed giving nurse practitioners a larger role in primary care, but they have often been motivated by considerations of turf.'* (ie territory) (N Engl J Med 1994; 330:204ED) *verb* A highly colloquial verb referring to the placement of a patient in another service's (ef from medical to surgical) ward

turf toe SPORTS MEDICINE A condition affecting athletes who play various sports (baseball, football, soccer) on artificial turf CLINICAL The most common presentation is similar to that of an acute gouty toe (ie painful, swollen, and red), and is accompanied by acute flexor and extensor tendonitis TREATMENT Rest, footwear designed for artificial turf; see Sports dermatology

turmschädel Hot cross bun skull, towerhead, Thickened and prominent frontal bones caused by periostitis of the superciliary arches, hence also known as the Olympian 'brow'; this skull deformity is often accompanied by mild hydrocephalus and although classically described in late congenital syphilis, may be seen in homozygous β-thalassemia and craniosynostosis

turnaround time LABORATORY MEDICINE A parameter of a clinical laboratory's efficiency in reporting test results; the TAT may be defined as the time between the ordering of a test and the reporting of results*; the rapidity of the TAT required is largely a function of the needs of the patient and the ordering physician, where a short TAT (eg 10 minutes) for Po$_2$ is required by emergency department physicians, and for surgeons short TATs are required for glucose, hemoglobin, and potassium (Arch Pathol Lab Med 1993;

117:22OA; MLO SEPTEMBER 1993) Cf Turnover time

*This definition is often used by clinicians and is more difficult to achieve that the laboratorians' definition of TAT as the time between phlebotomy and reporting of results, a subtle but often significant difference

turnkey A generic adjective referring or pertaining to any system or device in which the time and effort required to become fully operational is minimal after installation and setup, ie the implementation is said to require only the turn of a key

turnover time The time needed for a metabolite, nutrient, therapeutic agent, toxin, or other substance to be either completely removed from the system or replaced by more of the same substance, in the case of a therapeutic agent or metabolite; Cf Turnaround time

TURP Transurethral resection of the prostate

Tuskegee Study BIOMEDICAL ETHICS A prospective study of 431 black males in Tuskeegee, Alabama, with seropositive latent syphilis of greater than three years' duration that was begun in 1932 to examine the long-term effects of untreated syphilis; although the study provided information on the ultimate fate of syphilis, ie hypertension and cardiovascular disease were more common than CNS disease, the latter affecting 4% of survivors, a figure far lower than previously reported, a public outcry was raised against nontreatment of a disadvantaged minority solely on the basis of 'scientific curiosity' and the study was stopped in 1972, decades after penicillin had become available; see Nazi 'science', Unethical medical research

TWAR agent MICROBIOLOGY A fastidious strain of *Chlamydia psittaci* (the name derives from the first two isolates, which had been designated TW-183 and AR-39); TWAR may cause outbreaks of community-acquired pneumonia and is thought to be a relatively common cause of upper and lower respiratory tract infections, as the TWAR antibody occurs in 20-45% of normal adults, it is assumed to be transmitted person-to-person and may be fatal in the elderly CLINICAL Acute pneumonia in young adults, pharyngitis, and laryngitis TREATMENT Tetracycline

T wave alternans CARDIOLOGY A series of fluctuations in the overall length of the T wave that are consistently increased in a wide variety of conditions, including coronary artery occlusion, hypothermia, Prinzmetal's angina and the long Q-T syndrome; T wave alternans is predictive of the risk for ventricular fibrillation and is preferable to assessing the potential for fibrillation by provocative tests (Science 1991; 252:437)

Tweedledee and Tweedledum syndrome Folie à deux, see there

Tween A generic term for a proprietary family of non-ionic detergents consisting of fatty acid esters of polyoxyethylene sorbitan

20th Century science A generic term of recent vintage referring to fields of study that came into existance only as a result of technical and scientific advances; these include a vast array of fields including computer science, gerontology, health care management, immunology, molecular biology, neurosurgery, transplant surgery, virology, and others (JAMA 1995; 273:1319MN&P)

'Twentieth Century disease' Environmental hypersensitivity syndrome, see there

twenty nail dystrophy A very rare disease of the finger- and toenails characterized by longitudinal ridging, fragility, notching and opalescent discoloration, associated with spongiosus and keratosis of the adjacent skin or as a variant of lichen planus

'twigging' ACADEMIA Hyperspecialization in active branches of science as in computers and molecular biology or the fragmentation of specialties and subspecialties of medicine and natural sciences into subspecialties and sub-subspecialties, known as 'twigging', as the specialties themselves are 'branches' of the tree of knowledge

twilight sleep A dream-like state of 'conscious sedation' induced by Versed, a drug that allows patients to undergo minimally invasive surgical procedures, eg colonoscopy or minor oral procedures, to be performed without subjecting a patient to general anesthesia, the agent recently associated by with a number of sudden deaths, possibly related to 'overshooting' of the therapeutic levels, and causing the patients to lapse into unconsciousness

'twilight zone' MOLECULAR BIOLOGY A 'gray zone' that exists when base pairs of different DNA molecules, or amino acids from different proteins are compared to determine the degree of sequence similarity ('homology'); in the 'twilight zone', it cannot be said with certainty whether the molecules being compared are or are not related; the zone is broad and is a function of the length of the molecules being compared; molecules that share less than 5 to 10% of nucleotides or amino acids are usually regarded as devoid of sequence similarity, while a similarity of greater than 20 to 25% implies conservation of genomic motifs, among (seemingly unrelated) organisms, ie evolutionary homology, or conservation of structural motifs in proteins; the higher the number of matches between nucleotides in the DNA or amino acids in the proteins being compared, the greater is the likelihood that the sequences being compared are related; a 'match' of greater than 50% virtually confirms a relationship between two or more molecules and match of 80% or more percent are regarded as 'highly conserved'

twin One of two gestational products that develop during a single intrauterine gestational period; monozygotic twins reared apart (MZA) are remarkably similar in temperament, personality, occupation, leisure-time interests and social attitutes; MZAs are as similar to each other as those reared together and these similarities are attributed to genetics on IQ, as the constraints in Western society are relatively loose and do not prevent the development of individual traits; the similarity of psychological traits due to their identical genomes make their effective environments similar; see Higher multiples; Cf Siamese twins

twin reversed arterial-perfusion sequence OBSTETRICS A serious complication of zygotic multiple gestations, affecting ± 1% of monozygotic twins (1/35 000 births); interruption of the vascular communication with the acardiac twin is required to salvage the pump (normal) twin but is difficult to achieve as 1) Removal of the anomalous twin by hysterotomy has the disadvantage of maternal mortality and 2) Ultrasound-directed thrombosis of umbilical circulation of perfused twin is unreliable TREATMENT Ligation of the acardiac twin's umbilical cord by fetoscopy (N Engl J Med 1994; 330:468CR) Cf Twin-to-twin transfusion syndrome

'It has been hypothesized that in the presence of artery-to-artery and vein-to-vein anastomoses in a monozygotic placenta, blood is perfused by the hemodynamically advantaged ('pump') twin to the other ('recipient') twin by means of retrograde flow. Inadequate perfusion of the recipient twin is responsible for the developement of a...lethal set of anomalies, including acardia and acephaly. Typically, the pump twin is structurally normal, but is at risk for in utero cardiac failure and without treatment dies in 50-75% of cases, particularly if the recipient twin weighs more than half as much as the pump twin.' (N Engl J Med 1994; 330:468CR)

twin study EPIDEMIOLOGY A study using twins to determine the interplay of nature (genetic) and nurture (environment) on the etiology of a disease and its treatment; the interpretation of twin study data is often easier as there are exact genetic matches, ie identical (monozygotic) and partial genetic matches, ie fraternal (dizygotic) twins which are used as controls; a moderate genetic influence has been reported on lifetime smoking practices (see N Engl J Med 1992; 327:829OA)

Note: Twin studies were undertaken in a pseudoscientific fashion by Josef

Mengele, the infamous Auschwitz physician, whose paradoxical brutality in performing twin studies cannot be adequately summarized in this abbreviated forum; the reader is directed to Chapter 17 of The Nazi Doctors, RJ Lifton, Harper-Collins, New York, 1986

twin-to-twin transfusion syndrome OBSTETRICS Intrauterine growth retardation in one twin due to an artery-to-artery vascular shunting, which may occur in a diamnionic-dichorionic placenta and be accompanied by hydramnios; the 'donor' twin is anemic, pale, lighter and smaller with organ hypoplasia; the recipient twin is plethoric, polycythemic and macrosomic

'Twinkie® defense' FORENSIC PSYCHIATRY A legal tack that was used by the defense and supported by the defendant's psychiatric experts in the trial of a San Francisco supervisor, who in 1979 allegedly killed Mayor G Moscone and Harvey Milk; the contention was that the emotionally-strained defendant became unbalanced by eating 'junk food', citing the consumption of various carbohydrate-rich food products, including doughnuts, candy bars, soft drinks and a proprietary snack cake (Twinkies®) for his irrational behavior; the ploy reduced the defendant's conviction from that of first-degree murder to voluntary manslaughter, which carries a lesser sentence; see Black rage defense, Insanity defense, Television intoxication syndrome

'twinkling star' sign A fanciful descriptor for the short linear radiations that extend from pulmonary vessels that parallel the long axis of the body on computed tomographic scans, most prominently seen at a 100-200HU window width; 'twinkling stars' help distinguish normal vessels from tumor masses that may have the same tomographic density

twinning ORAL PATHOLOGY A dental malformation characterized by the adjoining of two teeth, most often seen in the mandibular incisors of the primary dentition, due to the processes of germination, fusion or concrescence

twist MOLECULAR BIOLOGY The periodicity of winding of one strand around another, ideally, one per 10.4 base pairs, intracellularly however, probably much less due to protein binding and crowding; see DNA topology, Cf Linking number, Writhe

TWiST Time without symptoms of disease or toxicity AIDS A period of time calculated as the number of months preceding the development of a symptom with ≥ grade 3 HIV disease, whichever occurred first (N Engl J Med 1994; 330:738OA) see Q-TWiST

twisting INSURANCE The convincing of a consumer to buy more life insurance with the promise that it would be paid for with built-up values in their old policies

twisting number MOLECULAR BIOLOGY A value that corresponds to the 'pitch' of the DNA molecule, or the number (T) of turns in its double helix, which is added to the writhe number (W) to yield a linking number (L); see Superhelicity

two-dimensional echocardiography A technique for identifying end-diastolic intraventricular dimensions, septal and free wall thicknesses and depressed ventricular function

two-dimensional gel electrophoresis LABORATORY TECHNOLOGY A technique for characterizing a protein; in the first dimension, a protein is separated according to charge by isoelectric focusing, in which a solution containing protein(s) that has not been denatured is placed in a gradient of pH and subjected to an electric charge, whereupon the protein migrates to the pH at which its total surface charge is neutral; the second dimension consists in rotating the gel 90°, layering it on a SDS-soaked gel and then electrophoretically separating the proteins based on size; the resulting pattern or 'fingerprint' is highly specific and constant

two-dimensional transesophageal color-flow Doppler echocardiography Transesophageal echocardiography, see there

two-dimensional transthoracic color-flow Doppler echocardiography Transthoracic echocardiography, see there

two foot-one hand syndrome A clinical form of tinea pedis with diffuse, dry scaling and mild erythema of the plantar surface, extending to the sides of the feet, in a moccasin-like pattern, associated with dry scaling of one palm, an association of uncertain significance

two-hit hypothesis One-hit/two-hit model, see there

two parent advantage PSYCHOLOGY A psychosocial edge that a child or children from a two parent household have when compared to children raised in a single-parent household; 'soft' data suggest that children with two parents are more socially adept and confident, more adaptable to new situations, independent, and responsible, and score higher on aptitude and intelligence tests (**NY Newsday 3 Jan 1995; B13**) see Father factor, Nuclear family

*Understood in this context to be two parents of the opposite sex

two-state receptor model PHARMACOLOGY A theoretical construct that seeks to explain the manner in which G protein receptors are activated; in contrast to the traditional view, which holds that receptors are or are not activated by a cognate ligand (agonist) and blocked by an antagonist, in the TSRM, the effect of ligands is governed by their differential binding for two receptor states and by the number and ratio of these states in a particular tissue (**Nature 1995; 374:272, 215N&v**)

two-tail test STATISTICS A test of a null hypothesis* against an alternative hypothesis or hypotheses, which is assumed to be false, regardless of the direction; OTTs are used to test statistical significance in terms of being greater or less than a value established by the hypothesis; Cf One-tail test

*A hypothesis that is tested against an alternative hypothesis, which is nullified in favor of the alternative and subject to a certain level of error

two-tiered billing HEALTH CARE INDUSTRY The charging of a larger fee for the same service, when the fee is expected to be paid by a 'third party' insurance carrier or by the settlement in a litigation; two-tiered billing is illegal in the US

two-tiered system SOCIAL MEDICINE The existence of two levels of benefits and care, depending on whether the patient can afford to pay or not, an unfortunate reality that exists in the 'free market' form of medical reimbursement that is practiced in the US

TX 1) Thromboxane 2) Treatment 3) Traction

Ty gene A retrotransposon; 'retro', ie like a retrovirus, it can reproduce itself via an RNA intermediary, using the enzyme reverse transcriptase; 'transposon', ie a piece of DNA that can insert itself in many different sites in a host genome

tylectomy The 'formal' synonym for lumpectomy, see there

tylosis Hereditary palmoplantar keratoderma, see there

tympanoplasty OTORHINOLARYNGOLOGY A technique of middle ear reconstruction intended to restore hearing, which consists of two components 1) Tympanic membrane engraftment, using various materials including canal skin, fascia, and homografts (eg dura, periosteum, knee cartilage, ossicles) and ossicular replacement with hydroxyapatite prostheses 2) Ossicular chain reconstruction, see there

tympanoplasty failure A generic term for an unsuccessful tympanoplasty; therapeutic failures may be due to recurrent perforations, persistent drainage, conductive hearing loss, malleus handle pull-away, anterior sulcus blunting, cholesteatoma and graft material breakdown; 'problem ears' can be repaired in most cases or prevented, requiring removal of offending residual mastoid and middle ear disease and reconstruction with modern techniques

tympanostomy tube OTORHINOLARYNGOLOGY A small metal tube or grommet inserted in the tympanic membrane of patients (often young children) with recurring, antibiotic refractory otitis media; while the ventilating tube is in place, there is a significant decrease in episodes of otitis media; once removed, the surgically treated ear has worse auditory discrimination, more otitis, tympanosclerosis, retraction and atrophy (**Pediatr Infect Dis J 1991; 10:2**)

Tyndall effect DERMATOLOGY The change that light undergoes as it passes through a turbid medium, eg skin, causing the colors of the spectrum to scatter; those colors with the longer wavelength (red, orange and yellow) tend to continue traveling forward while those with the shorter wavelength (blue, indigo and violet) scatter to the side and backward; thus explaining why a subcutaneous lesion that should have a red-brown hue due to hemorrhage or melanin deposition, has a blue tinge

type A simple way of classifying practically anything is to divide it into two (or more) 'types'; in general, typing keeps the number of subgroups to a minimum, while satisfying those with obsessive-compulsive neuroses who are driven to classify diseases, objects, people and mechanisms; see Splitting, Twigging

type 1 diabetes mellitus Insulin-dependent diabetes mellitus, see there, IDDM

type 2 diabetes mellitus Non-insulin-dependent diabetes mellitus, see there, NIDDM

type I error α error STATISTICS Rejection of the null hypothesis when it is correct, or the error of falsely stating that two proportions are significantly different when they are the same; type I errors may occur when a sample is too small for true statistical power; the probability of such an error occurring is a value, designated α, set by the investigator, usually at .05; if the two proportions are significantly different, regardless of whether positive or negative, the α value is nondirectional or 'two-tailed', designated as $\alpha 2$; a difference displayed in one direction, or one-tailed test is designated as $\alpha 1$

type II error β error STATISTICS Acceptance of the null hypothesis when it is incorrect, or the error of falsely stating that two proportions are not significantly different when they actually are; type II errors may occur when conclusions are based on the study of a small number of outcome events, ie misleading due to lack of statistical power; the probability of this occurring is designated as β and it is always unidirectional

type A personality A relatively distinct set of character traits (**JAMA 1959; 169:1286; ibid, 252:1385**) that are commonly observed in individuals who are aggressive, hard-driving, 'work-aholics'; although 'type As' have been traditionally regarded as being at an increased risk for cardiovascular morbidity; it has been more recently postulated that a second component is required to place these people at risk for cardiovascular disease, which consists of of repressed hostilities towards others or hopelessly frustrating situations, inducing induce a 'toxic core' nidus, increasing the susceptibility for heart disease in type A persons; see 'Toxic core'

type B personality A characteristic set of personality traits described in individuals who tend to be relaxed and inclined to do things 'mañana')

type 'C' and 'D' personalities A proposed addendum to the simplistic classification of personality traits into only two types, which adds a cancer-prone type C personality and an anxiety and immunosuppression-prone type D personality

type IV pilus MICROBIOLOGY A filamentous bacterial structure found in a wide range of gram-negative bacteria, eg *Neisseria* spp, *Pseudomonas aeruginosa*, and *Vibrio cholerae*, which mediate attachment to the host cell by a structural component, pilin (Science & Medicine 1995; 2/3:16) see Virulence factor; Cf P pilus

type grouping A descriptor for the histopathologic changes in muscles affected by neurogenic atrophy, where the normal mosaic interspersion of light and dark (type I and II) muscle fibers is transformed into large fascicles of light or dark fibers with similar histochemistry (figure, above), due to limited reinnervation due to ingrowth of collateral sprouts from undamaged healthy axons; type grouping also refers to the presence of two populations of muscle cells: one atrophic and another relatively well-preserved and/or hyperplastic

type-and-screen TRANSFUSION MEDICINE A protocol that consists of determining the ABO and Rh of the red cells, (major crossmatch) and screening the serum for the presence of potentially hemolyzing antibodies; it is performed by using 'reagent' red cells, which have major blood group surface antigens; many transfusion services have a 'type and screen' policy for surgical procedures that are unlikely to require a transfusion; according to the AABB* standards, the type and screen should be repeated every two days in pregnancy and if the subject has received any blood products or immunizing products within the last three months, given the potential for rapid formation of potentially harmful antibodies; see Cross-match, Immediate spin cross-match

*American Association of Blood Banks

type 1-to-type 2 shift AIDS A putative change in the predominant cytokines produced in patients as they develop certain diseases, eg clinical AIDS; type 1 cytokines (eg IL2 and IL12) are responsible for the cellular immune response by stimulating killer cells; type 2 cytokines are responsible for the humoral immune response in the form of antibody production (Technology Rev July 1995, p23)

'Typhoid Mary' EPIDEMIOLOGY A colloquial term for any person who is a carrier for a virulent strain of bacteria, eg salmonella or diphtheria or virus, eg hepatitis or HIV-1; see High disseminator

Typhoid Mary Mallon (1870-1938), the 'most dangerous woman in America' was an itinerant cook and asymptomatic carrier of a highly virulent strain of *Salmonella typhi*; she was held to be responsible for countless deaths in more than a dozen outbreaks of typhoid fever, one of which was the epidemic of Ithaca (1400 cases); she was temporarily quarantined in New York City (1906-1910), and released when she promised authorities she would find another occupation; when the epidemic in 1915 at Sloan Hospital for Women was traced to her, officials permanently retired her pots to Brother Island until her death

typhoid nodule A lesion seen in systemic dissemination of *Salmonella typhi*, classically located in the liver, which corresponds to scattered foci of trabecular necrosis with parenchymal replacement by phagocytosing mononuclear cell aggregates

typhus nodule A lesion of small blood vessels of the cerebral gray matter seen in Rocky Mountain spotted fever, characterized by focal microglial proliferation, admixed with leukocytes (figure, above)

tyramine hypertension Cheese disease A complication of monoamine oxidase inhibiting (MAOI) agents that are used to treat depression and panic disorders; MAOIs inhibit the metabolism of tyramines and catecholamines; ingestion of tyramine-rich food and/or beverages, eg Chianti wine, cheddar cheese, naturally fermented beer, chicken liver or drugs, eg ephedrine and amphetamines) evokes an acute hypertensive crisis due to the release of tissue catecholamines, which may be accompanied by

sweating, tachycardia or arrhythmia

tyrosine kinase An enzyme that is intimately linked to signal transduction (ST), either as a receptor-type TK, which participates in transmembrane signaling, or as an intracellular TK, participating in ST to the nucleus; ↑ or ↓ TK activity is associated with various diseases, and alteration of TK activity at various points in its signaling pathway is of potential therapeutic interest; ↑ TK activity has been implicated in many cancers and other malignant and nonmalignant proliferative diseases, atherosclerosis, psoriasis, and a vast array of inflammatory conditions; ↓ TK activity has been linked to various types of diabetes, or X-linked agammaglobulinemia (Science 1995; 267:1782)

tyrosine kinase inhibitor Any of a number of natural (eg erbstatin, genistein, herbimycin A, lavendustin A, quercetin) or synthetic compounds (derived from the natural compounds, eg tyrphostins) that act at some point in signal transduction either at receptor-type TKs, which participates in transmembrane signaling, or as at intracellular TKs, blocking ST to the nucleus (Science 1995; 267:1782)

tyrosine kinase receptor A family of receptors that phosphorylate tyrosine residues of proteins, leading to various cell responses; TKRs may be integral transmembrane receptors, constituting a signal recognition site for growth factors, eg epidermal growth factor or platelet-derived growth factor, thereby regulating cellular proliferation and differentiation; TRKs may also be intracytoplasmic, including Abl, Fps and Src, the protein products of proto-oncogenes (Science 1991; 252:668)

tyrosine phosphatase Any of a family of down-regulatory enzymes that have an inverse relation to the growth-promoting tyrosine kinases, acting to remove phosphates from tyrosine residues; tyrosine phosphatase closely resembles CD45, aka leukocyte common antigen (Science 1991; 251:744)

tyrosine phosphorylation The phosphorylation of proteins on tyrosine residues, which accounts for < 0.01% of the total intracellular phosphorylation, but may be the primary, if not the exclusive indicator of signal transduction in multicelled organisms (Science 1995; 267:1782)

tyrosinemia type I A rare AR [MIM 276700] condition due to fumarylacetoacetate hydrolase (FAH) deficiency, which is common in the Saguenay-Lac-St Jean area of Quebec, (incidence 1:1850, carrier status 1:16-1:22) CLINICAL Progressive liver dysfunction, cirrhosis, and hepatocellular carcinoma of childhood onset, renal tubular damage, acute porphyria-like neurologic crises MOLECULAR PATHOLOGY Splice, missense, and nonsense mutations in the FAH gene, which maps to chromosome segment 15q23-25 DIAGNOSIS ↑ Succinylacetone in prenatal testing, allele-specific oligonucleotide hybridization TREATMENT Liver transplantation, NTBC (2-(2-nitro-4-trifluoromenthylbenzoyl)-1,3-cyclo-hexanedione) may be effective in 'clearing' toxic metabolites (N Engl J Med 1994; 331:353oA)

tyrphostin Any of a number of synthetic compounds derived from natural tyrosine kinase inhibitors that act at some point in signal transduction either at receptor-type TKs, participating in transmembrane signaling, or as at intracellular TKs, blocking ST to the nucleus; tyrphostins may be of use in treating such diverse diseases as atherosclerosis (acting on platelet-derived growth factor), cancer and psoriasis (acting to inhibit the TK epidermal growth factor), sepsis (acting on LPS, and TNF-α), and many others (Science 1995; 267:1782)

Tzanck smear CYTOLOGY Tzanck test A rapid method for identifying cells in blistering diseases (eg herpetic lesions, pemphigus vulgaris) of the skin, performed by scraping the base of a 'virgin' blister or vesicle[1], spreading the adherent cells on a glass slide and staining with Giemsa, Wright's, or other Romanovsky-type stain; cytologic evidence for HSV and VZV include atypical keratinized cells with large nuclei, ground-glass cytoplasm, multinucleated giant cells, nuclear molding, and peripheral margination of chromatin; in contrast, the epithelial cells of pemphigus vulgaris are rounded and acantholytic; theoretically, viral isolation by culture would allow such a distinction, and has reported sensitivities ranging from 26 to 78%[2]; PCR performed on TSs has a higher diagnostic yield than viral cultures–in one study VZV DNA was detected in 97% of PCR-TS vs 44% for viral culture; HSV DNA was detected in corresponding lesion in 83% by PCR-TS, and 83% by viral culture (JAMA 1992; 268:2541oc)

[1]While virtually 'idiot-proof' in its performance, proper interpretation of a TS is an art-form a sui generis; under optimal conditions and in the hands of an experienced observer, TSs are positive in 50-80% of HSV and VZV–the operational adjectives being optimal and experienced; even when positive, the TS is nonspecific and do not distinguish twixt HSV-1 and HSV-2, and VZV, a distinction that has clinical impact and therapeutic import [2]In the 'real world' of clinical practice, inexperienced persons obtain these specimens, and send the fluids in suboptimal transport media, often to laboratories that rarely handle such specimens, usually on 'long' weekends, the viral cultures are virtually useless

common abbreviations: 2-D Two-dimensional **3-D** Three-dimensional **±** About, approximately, circa **‡** see there **aa** Amino acid **ACE** Angiotensin-converting enzyme **AD** Autosomal dominant **AFB** Acid-fast bacillus **AIDS** Acquired immunodeficiency syndrome **aka** also known as **ALL** Acute lymphocytic (lymphoblastic) leukemia **ALS** Amyotrophic lateral sclerosis **ALT** Alanine aminotransferase (formerly GPT) **AMA** American Medical Association **AML** Acute myelocytic (granulocytic, myeloid, myelogenous) leukemia **ANLL** Acute nonlymphocytic leukemia **apo** Apolipoprotein **aPTT** Activated partial thromboplastin time **AR** Autosomal recessive **ARDS** Acute respiratory distress syndrome or adult respiratory distress syndrome **AST** Aspartate aminotransferase (fomerly GPT) **AV** Atrioventricular **BCC** Basal cell carcinoma **BM** Bone marrow (or basement membrane) **BUN** Blood urea nitrogen **CAD** Coronary artery disease **cAMP** Cyclic adenosine monophosphate **CBC** Complete blood count **CDC** Centers for Disease Control and Prevention **cDNA** Complementary DNA **CEA** Carcinoembryonic antigen **CHF** Congestive heart failure **CIE** Counter-immunoelectrophoresis **CIN** Cervical intraepithelial neoplasia **CK** Creatinine phosphokinase **CML** Chronic myelocytic (granulocytic, myelogenous, myeloid) leukemia **CNS** Central nervous system **COD** Cause of death **COPD** Chronic obstructive pulmonary disease **CPR** Cardiopulmonary resuscitation **CSF** Cerebrospinal fluid **CT** Computed tomography **CVA** Cerebrovascular accident **DAD** Diffuse alveolar damage **DDx** Differential diagnosis **DIC** Disseminated intravascular coagulation **DM** Diabetes mellitus **DNA** Deoxyribonucleic acid **DOA** Dead on arrival **DSM-IV** Diagnostic and Statistical Manual, fourth edition **DWI** Driving while intoxicated *E coli* *Escherichia coli* **EEG** Electroencephalogram, electroencephalographic **eg** *exempli gratia*, for example **EGF** Epidermal growth factor **EKG** Electrocardiography **ELISA** Enzyme-linked immunosorbent assay **EM** Electron microscopy, ultrastructure **EMG** Electromyography **EMT** Emergency medical technician **ENT** Ears, nose, and throat, otorhinolaryngology **EPA** Environmental Protection Agency **ER** Emergency room, emergency ward **ERCP** Endoscopic retrograde cholangiography **ESR** Erythrocyte sedimentation rate **ESRD** End-stage renal disease **FDA** United States Food and Drug Administration **FDP** Fibrinogen degradation product(s) **FISH** Fluorescence in situ hybridization **FNA** Fine-needle aspiration (biopsy or cytology) **FSH** Follicle-stimulating hormone **FUO** Fever of unknown origin **GABA** gamma-aminobutyric acid **GC-MS** Gas chromatography-mass spectroscopy **GFR** Glomerular filtration rate **GGT** Gamma-glutamyl transferase **GI** Gastrointestinal **GM-CSF** Granulocyte-macrophage colony-stimulating factor **GMS** Gomori-methenamine-silver **GN** Glomerulonephritis **GNP** Gross National Product **GVHD** Graft-versus-host disease **HAV** Hepatitis A virus **HBV** Hepatitis B virus **hCG** Human chorionic gonadotropin **HCV** Hepatitis C virus **HDL** High-density lipoprotein **H&E** Hematoxylin & eosin **HHV** Human herpesvirus (HHV-1, HHV-etc) **HIV** Human immunodeficiency virus **HLA** Human leukocyte antigen (the major histocompatibility complex of humans) **HMO** Health maintenance organization **HPLC** High-performance liquid chromatography **HPV** Human papillomavirus **HSV** Herpes simplex virus **HTLV-I** Human T cell leukemia/lymphoma virus **ICU** Intensive care unit **IDDM** Insulin-dependent diabetes mellitus **ie** *id est*, that is (to say) **IFN** Interferon **Ig** Immunoglobulin **IL** Interleukin **IM** Intramuscular **ImPx** Immunoperoxidase **IQ** Intelligence quotient **IR** Infrared **ISH** in situ hybridization **ITP** Idiopathic thrombocytopenic purpura **IUD** Intrauterine (contraceptive) device **IV** Intravenous **IVDU** Intravenous drug use/user **JCAHO** Joint Commission of Accredited Hospitals Organization **K+** Potassium **kD** Kilodalton **KS** Kaposi sarcoma **LDH** Lactate dehydrogenase **LDL** Low-density lipoprotein **LGV** Lymphogranuloma venereum **LH** Luteinizing hormone **LM** Light micoscopy **LN** Lymph node **MAOI** Monoamine oxidase inhibitor **MEN** Multiple endocrine neoplasia **MHC** Major histocompatibility complex **MI** Myocardial infarction **mo/ma** Monocyte/macrophage (tissue histiocyte) **MPS** Mucopolysaccaride(s), mucopolysaccharidosis **MRI** Magnetic resonance imaging **mRNA** Messenger RNA (ribonucleic acid) **MS** Multiple sclerosis **MVA** Motor vehicle accident **MW** Molecular weight **Na+** Sodium **N/C ratio** Nuclear/cytoplasmic ratio **N-CAM** Neuronal-cell adhesion molecule **NGF** Nerve growth factor **NHL** Non-Hodgkin's lymphoma **NIH** National Institutes of Health **NIDDM** Non-insulin-dependent diabetes mellitus **NK cell** Natural killer cell **NO** Nitric oxide **NSAID** Nonsteroidal anti-inflammatory drug **OR** Operating room, operating suite **OSHA** Occupational Safety and Health Administration **PAF** Platelet-activating factor **PAS** Periodic acid-Schiff **PCBs** Polychlorinated biphenyls **PCP** *Pneumocystis carinii* pneumonia **PCR** Polymerase chain reaction **PDA** Patent ductus arteriosus **PG** Prostaglandin **PID** Pelvic inflammatory disease **PMN(s)** Polymorphonuclear neutrophil(s) or leukocyte(s), segmented neutrophil(s) **ppm** Parts per million **pron** Pronounced **PT** Prothrombin time **PTE** Pulmonary thromboembolism **PTH** Parathyroid hormone **aPTT** (activated) Partial thromboplastin time **QA** Quality assurance **QC** Quality control **RA** Rheumatoid arthritis **RBCs** Red blood cells, erythrocytes **RDS** Respiratory distress syndrome **REM sleep** Rapid eye movement sleep **RFLP** Restriction fragment length polymorphism **RIA** Radioimmunoassay **RR** Relative risk **rRNA** Ribosomal RNA (ribonucleic acid) **RSV** Respiratory syncytial virus **RT** Radiation therapy, reverse transcriptase **SD** Standard deviation **sec** Second (time) **SI** International System (of units), see there **SIDS** Sudden infant death syndrome **SLE** Systemic lupus erythematosus **STD** Sexually transmitted disease **TAH-BSO** Total abdominal hysterectomy with bilateral salpingo-oophorectomy **TB** Tuberculosis **TDM** Therapeutic drug monitoring **TGF-β** Transforming growth factor-β **TIA** Transient ischemic attack **TIBC** Total iron-binding capacity **TLC** Thin-layer chromatography **TNF** Tumor necrosis factor **tRNA** Transfer RNA (ribonucleic acid) **T-S** Trimethoprim-sulfamethoxazole **TSH** Thyroid-stimulating hormone **TTP** Thrombotic thrombocytopenic purpura **TX** Thromboxane **U** 1) Unit 2) University **UK** United Kingdom **URI** Upper respiratory tract infection **US** United States **UTI** Urinary tract infection **UV** Ultraviolet **VDRL** Venereal disease research laboratory (test) for syphilis **VIP** Vasoactive intestinal polypeptide **VLDL** Very low density lipoportein **V/Q** Ventilation/perfusion **vs** versus, in contrast to, in comparison with, in contrast to **VSD** Ventricular septal defect **VZV** Varicella-zoster virus **WBCs** White blood cells, leukocytes **WHO** World Health Organization **X-R** X-linked recessive ↓ Decrease, decreased, decreases, decreasing ↑ Increase, increased, increases, increasing ♀ Female, women ♂ Male, men

Common Abbreviations

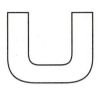

U Symbol for: 1) International Unit of enzyme activity 2) Uracil 3) Uranium 4) Uridine

u Symbol for: Atomic mass unit

U1-U6 A group of uridine-rich small nuclear ribonucleoproteins that has an essential role in processing pre-messenger RNA, splicing out the unwanted introns, which is involved in polyadenylation

U antigen TRANSFUSION MEDICINE A rare antigen of the MNSs red blood cell antigen group present on the erythrocytes of less than 1% of blacks and never in caucasians, which requires membrane sialoglycoproteins, glycophorin A and glycophorin B; in the absence of a U antigen, the s antigen is not expressed

UAS Upstream activating sequence, see there

UBF Upstream binding factor MOLECULAR BIOLOGY An auxiliary RNA polymerase I transcription factor, which is not required for, but stimulates the transcription of ribosomal DNA; UBF's activity is blocked by the *Rb* gene product Rb; the interaction between UBF and Rb indicate that Rb is capable of suppressing cell growth by directly repressing the transcription of rRNA genes (**Nature 1995; 374:177**)

ubiquinone CoQ A protein that acts as a hydrogen carrier, which is intimately linked to the intramitochondrial electron transport cascade; the oxidized form, quinone accepts a single electron, forming semiquinone; acceptance of a second electron and two protons forms the fully reduced dihydroubiquinone

ubiquitin A ubiquitous and highly conserved 7-kD protein found either free in the circulation or bound (through its –COOH terminal glycine residue) to various cytoplasmic, nuclear or integral membrane proteins, linked by isopeptide bonds to multiple lysine residues; it is highly conserved among plants and animals; ubiquitin is linked by ATP to proteins, tagging them for degradation; immunocytochemical staining for ubiquitin can be used to quantify diffuse axonal injury (**Arch Pathol Lab Med 1994; 118:168OA**) see Cyclin

'U-boat lesion' A fanciful synonym for an abdominal aortic aneurysm which, like the Unterseeboot, is silent, deep, detected by reflecting sound waves, ie sonar or ultrasound and must be neutralized before it proves fatal; see Einstein sign

UCR system HEALTH CARE FINANCING An approach to reimbursing physicians by private insurers, Medicaid and Medicare, based on Usual, Customary, and Reasonable fees; as cost containment has become an increasing priority, the UCR system has been largely supplanted by payer-determined fee schedules, or by a resource-based relative-value scale (RBRVS), which sets a fee that varies according to the geographic region for each service by incorporating estimates of the time, clinical and technical skills, physical and stress related to that providing the service (see **JAMA 1994; 272:971HCP**) see RBRVS

UCTS Undifferentiated connective tissue disease, see there

uE3 Unconjugated estriol, see Triple-marker screen

UGH syndrome see PUGH 'syndrome'

'ugly' A colloquial adjective for an aggressive disease or lesion INFECTIOUS DISEASE An 'ugly' infection is one that responds poorly to aggressive antibiotic therapy, most commonly seen in immunocompromised patients or those with terminal cancer ONCOLOGY An 'ugly' malignancy is characterized by fulminant deterioration, multiorgan failure, infection and poor response to therapy SURGICAL PATHOLOGY 'Ugly' usually refers to a malignancy with bizarre, poorly differentiated cells with marked nuclear atypia, pleomorphism and florid mitotic activity, eg giant cell tumor of the lung; the lineage of 'ugly' cells is often unclear, and may require the use of ancillary studies, eg special stains including immunoperoxidase staining for the presence of various intermediate filaments or molecular studies; 'ugly' tumors may be so anaplastic that even these studies do not elucidate the tumor's cell of origin

Uhl's anomaly Right ventricular dysplasia, see there

UIP Usual interstitial pneumonia, see there

ulcer-carcinoma sequence Stump carcinoma, see there

ulcerative colitis A chronic inflammatory bowel disease that most prominently affects the colon and rectum, characterized by bloody diarrhea and abdominal pain EPIDEMIOLOGY Worldwide distribution; high incidence in US, UK, Australia, Northern Europe, 3-15/10⁶/year in whites; Jews (13/10⁵) more than non-Jews (3.8/10⁵); peak age of onset 20-40; smaller peak in elderly CLINICAL Diarrhea, rectal bleeding, passage of mucus, colicky abdominal pain; if severe fever, tachycardia, anemia, ↑ ESR PATHOGENESIS Uncertain; hypotheses include bacterial antigens, allergens in diet, autoimmunity, psychosomatic factors, on a substrate of intestinal cell defect(s) DIAGNOSIS Sigmoidoscopy, colonoscopy, radiology (distention and dilation, collar-stud ulcers, and if long-standing, loss of haustration) PATHOLOGY Lesions are confined to colon and rectum in ±½; in 20% the lesions cover the entire colon; the mucosa is hyperemic, edematous, and punctuated by punctate ulcers that enlarge, coalesce, extend to the lamina propria, and, in severe cases, carpet the colon in a 'bearskin rug'-like fashion; by LM, edema, inflammation of biblical proportions, and the 'classic' finding of crypt abcesses TREATMENT IV corticosteroids; in non-responders, sulfasalazine, mesalazine, IV cyclosporine; if refractory to cyclosporine, colectomy (**N Engl J Med 1994; 330:1841OA**) transdermal nicotine may induce complete remission in acute UC, improving the clinical status, as well as histologic grade, ↓ the stool frequency and sense of urgency, at a cost of nausea, lightheadedness, headache and sleep disturbances (**ibid; 330:811OA**) nicotine is of no use in maintaining remission (**ibid, 1995; 332:988OA**)

ulnar tunnel syndrome(s) A group of clinical complexes caused by ulnar nerve compression, most often due to a ganglion 'cyst', but which may also be occupation- or hobby-related or due to laceration, arteritis, fractures and inflammation CLINICAL Symptoms differ according to the site of nerve compression, and display varying degrees of motor defects and sensory loss of the medial aspect of the hand TREATMENT Physical therapy, occasionally surgery

ultimate carcinogen A hypothetical molecule that reacts with DNA, causing the final step in the carcinogenic process; this agent is postulated to have an electrophilic component, eg a free radical, epoxide or carbonium ion, which reacts with susceptible electron-rich sites in theDNA; Cf Tumor initiator, Tumor promoter

ultracentrifugation RESEARCH The spinning of cells, organelles and various molecules at high speeds (up to 60 000 rpm) with high gravitational force (up to 500 000 g), which allows separation of cell components, as in rate-zonal (differential velocity) centrifugation, in which the gravitational force is increased in a stepped fashion to allow removal of desired components; after filtration of a homogenate of tissue or cells from a culture medium, the sample is spun at 600 g for 10 minutes, which 'sediments' the nuclei; the fluid is then re-spun at 15 000 g for 5 minutes, which sediments cell organelles (mitochondria, lysosomes, peroxisomes); the fluid is then re-spun at 100 000 g for 1 hour, which sediments the plasma membrane, microsomal fraction, fragments of the endoplasmic reticulum and large polyribosomes; the fluid is re-spun at 300 000 g for 2 hours, which sediments the ribosomal subunits and small polyribosomes; the remaining fluid contains the soluble portion of the cytoplasm, the cytosol, which may be morphologically analyzed by the 'quick-freeze technique'; subcellular particles and molecules can also be separated by 'layering' the sample on a sucrose gradient, applying ultracentrifugation, then removing the desired 'zone' by pipette; ultracentrifugation also separates DNA fragments, as in equilibrium centrifugation; the DNA, RNA or proteins are radioactively labeled with either a lighter (eg ^{3}H) or a heavier (^{14}C) isotope, allowing the molecules to separate according to density; the sample may be then mixed with cesium chloride, which when combined with the molecules of interest, establishes a slight density gradient, allowing the molecules to migrate to a particular density equivalent; upon removal of the labeled molecules, a radioassay or electrophoretic gel pattern can be used to identify the fractions

ultrafast Papanicolaou stain CYTOLOGY A recently developed stain for cytology specimens that improves the quality of preparation, and facilitates the interpretation of specimens obtained by fine-needle aspiration; in UPS, the cells are smeared on a glass slide, allowed to dry and washed with hypertonic saline solution (ie salty water), which causes the cells of interest to swell, and the obscuring RBCs to lyse (February 1995 Acta Cytologica in New York Times 25 April 1995, pC3)

ultrasonography An imaging modality that generates diagnostic images based on the differences in the acoustic impedance of various tissues; electricity applied to a piezoelectric crystal or ceramic in the transducer, causes high-frequency (2.25-5.0 MHz/s) mechanical vibration, which emits ultrasound in the form of 'pressure waves'; these waves are transferred into tissues and organs, and at each tissue interface, a portion of the ultrasound wave is reflected, generating echoes; as the echoes return, there is a slight distortion or deformity of a piezoelectric crystal in the transducer, producing minute voltage pulses, which are then amplified and displayed in one of several 'modes' (the transducer is used to both generate the ultrasound beam and detect the returning echo; the number of pulses that may be generated in a second or pulse repetition frequency is inversely related to the tissue depth); the amplitude of the signal is recorded in scales of gray, where the whitest shades reflect the strongest signal, B-mode ultrasonography yields 2-D tissue 'slices' that are produced using different types of transducers, capable of scanning sequentially across a limited region or finite space Types **A-MODE DISPLAY ULTRASONOGRAPHY** An ultrasonographic modality that provides simple displays that are plotted as a series of peaks, the height of which represents the depth of the echoing structure from the transducer **B-MODE DISPLAY ULTRASONOGRAPHY** Brightness-modulated display An ultrasonographic modality with a wide range of applications including imaging of the fetus, kidneys, liver, gallbladder, uterus, cardiovascular structures, breast, prostate, in screening for early ovarian cancer, in evaluating liver transplant recipients both preoperatively (a narrow or thrombosed portal vein precludes transplant) and postoperatively (used to assess various complications—rejection, infection thrombosis and patency of biliary tracts and identifying gallbladder calculi Note: The most common clinical use of B-mode ultrasonography is to evaluate fetal status, providing real-time two-dimensional evaluation of the fetus, presenting the images in rapid succession, likened to a motion picture; the 'biophysical profile' has a B-mode display, and measures the head (cephalometry), thorax, abdomen, estimates fetal maturation and identifies growth retardation and major congenital anomalies, including anencephaly, hydrocephaly, meningocele, congenital heart disease, dextrocardia, fetal tumors, diaphragmatic hernia, gastroschisis, omphalocele, polycystic kidneys, hydrops fetalis, gastrointestinal obstruction and death; B-mode helps localize the amniocentesis needle and is of use in identifying placental anomalies including hydatidiform mole or anomalous implantation, eg placenta previa; the side effects of ultrasonography are minimal as the energy levels for diagnostic imaging are regarded as being too low to produce tissue destruction; leukocytes subjected to ultrasound demonstrate chromosomal defects, a finding of unknown clinical relevance **DUPLEX ULTRASONOGRAPHY** An ultrasonographic modality that combines the standard real-time B-mode display with pulsed Doppler signals, allowing analysis of frequency shifts in an ultrasonographic signal, reflecting motion within a tissue, eg blood flow and is thus useful in evaluating atherosclerosis of the carotid arteries, arteriovenous malformations and circulatory disturbances in the neonatal brain **M-MODE DISPLAY ULTRASONOGRAPHY** Time-motion display A modality in which the echo signal is recorded on a continuously moving strip of paper, with the transducer held in a fixed position over the aortic or mitral valves; each dot represents a moving structure has a sinewy path, while stationary structures are represented as straight lines; M-mode was the first display used and continues to be useful for precise timing of cardiac valve opening and correlating valve motion with EKG, phonocardiography and Doppler echocardiography (JAMA 1991; 265:1155)

ultrasonography angiographic catheterization A technique that uses a unique probe (1 mm diameter, 20-30 MHz energy emission versus the 10 cm diameter probe operating at 5 MHz used for fetal ultrasonography) to analyze the intensity of atherosclerotic plaque deposition (JAMA 1990; 264:2046n)

ultrastructure The sum total of organelles, structures, eg membranes, microtubules, microfilaments and molecules that are beyond the resolution of light microscopy; ultrastructural studies include scanning electron microscopy, of use for studying the surfaces of membranes and cells (magnifications of 2000x to 20 000x), transmission electron microscopy (resolution of structures from 2000x to 150 000x) and scanning tunnel electron microscopy, which has a magnification ceiling of up to 2 million-fold magnification); see Electron microscopy, Microscopy

ultraviolet (light, radiation) The segment of the electromagnetic spectrum between 200 and 400 nm, including photons emitted during electronic transition states; UV-C (200-290 nm) is damaging to DNA and amino acids, but is blocked by the stratospheric ozone layer, UV-B (290-320 nm) is partially blocked by the ozone layer; UV-A (320 to 400 nm) is the least dangerous but may be hazardous with photosensitizing medications (tetracyclines, thiazides), lupus erythematosus and light sensitivity disorders; UV-A suppresses delayed cutaneous hypersensitivity, causes photoaging and ↓ serum carotenoid by 30%; the accelerating depletion of the stratospheric ozone is implicated in the ↑ incidence of cataracts and malignant melanoma, and UV light causes a relative ↓ in CD4 or helper T cells and an increase in CD8 (suppressor) T cells; pyrimidine dimer formation is a major consequence of UV light, affecting the DNA chain where adjacent thymine residues are joined by a cyclobutyl linkage; in bacteria and in yeasts, photolyase directly removes the cyclobutyl linkage in the presence of visible light (photoreactivation); in higher eukaryotes, UV light-induced damage to DNA is repaired by a helicase-like enzyme; UV light may also damage the less-sensitive purines, causing spontaneous depurination, leaving a 'naked' deoxyribose residue in the DNA (apurinic sites); repair of UV light-induced DNA damage is defective in some 'chromosomal breakage syndromes', eg in xeroderma pigmentosa and Bloom syndrome Note: The mutational effect of UV light is not due to direct DNA damage, but rather occurs during the error-prone process of DNA repair; see CFCs, Greenhouse effect, Ozone layer, SOS repair, SPF rating

Note: UVB considered by some workers to be a thousand-fold more carcinogenic than UVA; UVA increases free radical production, causing cell membrane damage and cross-linking of dermal proteins

Ulysses syndrome A complication of false-positive diagnostic tests[1] or clinical observations that is responsible for a complete and aggressive diagnostic work-up to elucidate the nature of what is, in actual fact, a non-disease, before the patient is allowed to return to his original state of health (Can Med Assoc Journal 1973; 106:122) various events may initiate a Ulysses[2] syndrome or sequence of events, including

MISCHIEVOUS (UNNECESSARY) INVESTIGATION That which is motivated by mass screening, eg 'blanket coverage' to pay for testing by an insurance company, house-staff 'overkill' to avoid criticism, laboratory request forms bearing the laboratory's entire menu

2) UNCRITICAL EXAMINATION Lack of familiarity with a body region may mislead the examiner, especially if he encounters trivial anatomic variations of normal structures

3) SERPENTINO 'COMPLEX' Two snakes consuming each other tail first A neurotic patient may succeed in making himself ill when there is unexpected interest in an otherwise trivial complaint

4) INVERTED SERENDIPITY While Marie Curie's serendipitous dropping of a key on a pile of photographic film near radium was the founding event of radiology, 'discoveries' made while using an unfamiliar technique are usually 'red herrings'

5) NON-INVESTIGATIONAL INVESTIGATION When a laboratory request form has a new test on it, the new box is checked off with disproportionate frequency

[1]A review of statistical principles in laboratory medicine makes it surprising that the Ulysses syndrome doesn't occur with greater frequency, since results of certain laboratory tests are placed on a standard Gaussian curve of distribution and any value greater than two standard deviations (SD) above or below a mean is considered statistically abnormal (not biologically abnormal); this verification process is a function of daily fluctuations of machinery and other non-disease factors; thus 5%, ie, one in twenty of any normal population will be greater than two SD from the mean of a value, and therefore, abnormal; one in four hundred normal subjects will be statistically abnormal in two tests and so on [2]Ulysses, who fought in the Trojan war, required 20 years for the return leg of the journey, and all of the harrowing detours were unnecessary

unawareness of hypoglycemia ENDOCRINOLOGY A lack of appropriate warning symptoms prior to developing neuroglycopenia, a common feature of IDDM which prevents patients from taking steps (eg ingestion of sugar); the phenomenon is of uncertain pathogenesis but is associated with intensive insulin therapy, prolonged duration of DM, impaired glucose counterregulation, frequent episodes of hypoglycemia, and may be induced hypoglycemia itself in patients with insulinomas (N Engl J Med 1993; 329:834OA)

umber codon UGA One of the three 'stop' codons that terminates protein production; an umber mutation is one in which a point mutation on DNA results in a nucleotide triplet ACT that is transcribed into a UGA stop codon

umbrella CARDIOVASCULAR SURGERY The Mobin-Uddin umbrella was a stainless steel sieve placed IV below the renal arteries via the jugular vein that was designed to trap deep vein thrombi in the inferior vena cava; the device is of historic interest as it induced inferior vena cava thrombosis in 70% of cases, which occasionally detached, causing fatal PTE

umbrella cells CYTOLOGY A fanciful term for the multinucleated superficial cells of the bladder epithelium with vacuolated cytoplasm, which are thin but cover multiple underlying transitional cells in a parasol-like fashion

umbrella effect IMMUNOLOGY The masking of low levels of immunoglobulin light chains in early clonal expansions of IgM macroglobulinemia and IgA myeloma, by the greater bulk of IgG, as seen in immunoelectrophoresis; this masking effect can be resolved by using immunofixation electrophoresis, which uses specific fluorescently-tagged anti-immunoglobulins

umbrella growth pattern MICROBIOLOGY The characteristic growth pattern seen when *Listeria monocytogenes* is 'stab'-inoculated at 25°C in a tube filled with semisolid culture medium, fulfilling the organism's micro-aerophilic growth requirement, displaying a 'head-over-heels' or tumbling pattern motility

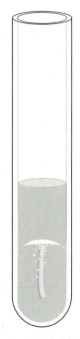

umbrella growth pattern

unassigned reading frame A large segment of DNA present in mitochondrial DNA that has an initiation codon and is not interrupted by stop codons; some URFs are within introns and may be involved in encoding intron-splicing proteins

'unbundling' HEALTH CARE INDUSTRY The separation of a group of health care services that are usually billed as one fee into separate components, resulting in a higher overall fee for those services, eg the 'unbundling' of a TAH-BSO with scar removal and the repair of a hernial sac into three separately billed procedures

uncinate fits NEUROLOGY Partial epileptic seizures that may begin with a patient's perception of an unpleasant odor, later generalizing into a clonic or tonic-clonic seizure, often the first manifestation of a temporal lobe tumor

uncitedness index SCIENTIFIC JOURNALISM A measure of a manuscript's relative 'unworthiness'; if a publication in science is referred to in the bibliography of any subsequent publication, it has been 'cited', thus inferring that the first paper was thought to be of some merit and provide new information; 'uncitedness' implies that a paper was not considered important enough to be referred to by subsequent authors (and possibly had no merit in the first place); according to data collected by the Institute for Scientific Information, less than 20% of publications in physics are uncited, while 90% of papers in political science are uncited, with medicine and biological sciences falling between these extremes (Science 1991; 251:25) see

Citation impact, CV-weighing

unclear disease picture Fehldiagnose, see there

uncoded amino acid An amino acid for which there is no codon; such amino acids arise from post-translational modification of an amino acid after it has been incorporated into a polypeptide chain, eg proline yielding hydroxyproline or lysine giving rise to hydroxylysine

uncombable hair syndrome An AD [MIM 191480] condition characterized by the growth of scalp hair in directional 'anarchy', which may be idiopathic or associated with ectodermal dysplasia, progressive alopecia, atopic eczema, dental dysplasia, and ichthyosis vulgaris PATHOLOGY The hair shaft displays unilateral longitudinal canalicular depression; see Kinky hair syndrome, Woolly hair syndrome

uncompensated care Medical treatment of a patient provided in the US by a physician or other health care professional that is not paid by the patient, the government or an insurance carrier, divided into charity care, bad debt and discounted Medicaid care (**JAMA 1991; 265:2982**) see Medicaid, 'Service' patient; Cf Pro bono

unconventional cancer therapy Unproven therapies for cancer, see there

unconventional 'virus' A group of infectious agents, formerly thought to be a type of slow virus, now known as prions, a small infectious particle, consisting entirely of subverted cell protein; prions cause degenerative encephalopathies in sheep and goats (scapie), cows (bovine spongiform encephalopathy) and humans (kuru and Creutzfeldt-Jakob disease); see Kuru, Prions, Slow viruses

uncoupling PHYSIOLOGY 1) The separation of a metabolic process, eg the uncoupling of oxidative phosphorylation, so that one or more components, eg ATP synthesis, is dissociated from the electron transport chain at one or more phosphorylation sites in mitochondria 2) The separation of activities in receptor-ligand interactions, such that a ligand may bind its cognate receptor, but does not activate the usually coupled receptor

undercall Underread A noun and a verb for an error in which a benign diagnosis was rendered on what later proves to be a malignant lesion; misinterpretation of this type may occur at any stage of patient evaluation, from the time of physical examination of a mass or complaint by a clinician to the endpoint of imaging analysis by the radiologist and microscopic examination by the pathologist; see Misadventure, Overread

Note: There is a tendency to use 'undercall' for errors made in the early stages of patient evaluation, and 'underread' for errors made in the later stages of evaluation, since the radiologist and pathologist are trained in pattern recognition and must interpret or 'read' a pattern

'under general' A colloquial adverb for a surgical procedure performed under general anesthesia

undergraduate education Background: In the US, a four-year (or more) college or university education leading to a bacchalaureate degree is the minimum educational level required for admission to medical school; undergraduate medical education refers to the four years of medical school; graduate medical education refers to formal training programs, eg internship, residency and fellowship that follow completion of medical school, which are multiples of one year in duration and sponsored by teaching hospitals, many of which are affiliated with a university or medical school hospital; Cf CME (continuing medical education)

underimmunization PUBLIC HEALTH A level of immunization that is suboptimal for the person or population; personal and structural barriers to immunization include financial factors, the mother's age, race, education, socioeconomic status, as well as the birth order and receipt of prenatal care (**JAMA 1994; 272:1105oa**)

underinsurance A generic term for insurance policies that require large out-of-pocket payments; underinsurance includes the lack of coverage for catastrophic medical expenses, pre-exisiting condition clauses, benefits not provided clauses, deductibles and coinsurance (**N Engl J Med 1992; 327:275**)

underinsured HEALTH CARE ENVIRONMENT An adjective referring to an ill-defined term for a group of people in the US (an estimated 15 million out of a population of 240 million) whose health insurance is inadequate because 1) High deductibles discourage people from obtaining preventive care 2) Policies don't cover needs such as substance abuse rehabilitation or mental health care, or those that impose a waiting period before coverage begins 3) Those who are 'officially' covered by Medicaid, who cannot find a physician willing to treat clients with Medicaid coverage (**Congressional Quarterly, 1993, in Clin Lab Sci 1994; 7:141**)

'under local' A colloquial adverb for a surgical procedure performed under local anesthesia

underlying cause of death Primary (or proximate) cause of death '…*the disease or injury that initiated the train of morbid events leading directly to death, or the circumstances or violence that produced the fatal injury.*' (**Arch Pathol Lab Med 1995; 119:123oa**) As an example, fulminant acute peritonitis is the immediate cause of death, which is the end result of a shotgun blast to the abdomen, the underlying (aka primary or proximate) cause of death; Cf Immediate cause of death

underrepresented minority A term that encompasses ethnic minority groups* that are underrepresented in professional schools; although UMs comprise ± 20% of the general population, they comprise ± 11% of medical school entrants; to rectify previous inequities, affirmitive action was introduced in the late 1960s-1970s as a balancing mechanism, but was persued less aggressively after the Supreme Court decision in the *Bakke* case, which proved reverse discrimination had occurred, where a minority quota (ie a political agenda) had been given priority over a student's academic standing; it is now obvious that barriers to admission into medical school is not the cause of the underrepresentation, but rather the inability of the institutions of higher learning (colleges, universities) to produce enough well-prepared minority group applicants; to address this issue the AAMC created Project 3000 by 2000 (**N Engl J Med 1994; 331:472sb**) see Affirmative action, Bakke decision, Project 3000 by 2000, Reverse discrimination

*Designated by the Association of American Medical Colleges (AAMC) as blacks, Mexican Americans, mainland Puerto Ricans, and American Indians

undifferentiated carcinoma A group that includes anaplastic carcinomas, 'monstrocellular' carcinomas, oat cell and small cell carcinomas, which may arise in the lungs, larynx, bronchus, esophagus, colon, urinary bladder, uterine cervix and salivary glands and lack epithelial differentiation; the epithelial nature may be subjectively inferred by the tumor pattern or confirmed by special studies including immunoperoxidase studies for cytokeratin and epithelial membrane antigen and ultrastructural studies for desmosomes; see Anaplastic carcinoma

undifferentiated connective tissue disease An early stage of collagen vascular disease in which the predominant organ of involvement or clinical form has yet to manifest itself; Cf Overlap syndrome, Palindromic rheumatism

unethical medical research BIOMEDICAL ETHICS The performance of medical experiments on human subjectss against their will or knowledge of therapeutic options; these experiments range from the Nazi war-crimes including the Dachau hypothermia 'experiments' and other more bizarre pseudoscience projects in which many of the participants died, to the withholding of therapy in order to determine the natural course of an infection as in the Tuskegee study of the evolution of untreated syphilis; there are viable arguments both for, but predominantly against the use of such data, not only regarding the ethical issues, but also that much of the data are flawed and the statistical methods inadequate (**NY State J Med 1991; 91:54**) see Helsinki Declaration, Nazi 'science', Nuremberg Code of Ethics

UNFPA United Nations Fund for Population Activities

'unhappy gut' Functional colitis A term that was introduced because 'irritable gut' had lost its specificity; 'unhappy gut' refers to dysfunctional GI smooth muscle that is not 'in the mood' to function properly, while 'irritable gut' refers to colonic changes attributed to unidentified intraluminal irritants (**personal communication, RW McCullum**) Cf Irritable bowel syndrome

unhealthful day PUBLIC HEALTH Any day in which the air quality for any of the five ambient air pollutants (carbon monoxide, nitrogen dioxide, ozone, particulate matter*, and sulfur dioxide) exceeds an established air quality standard (**N Engl J Med 1994; 331:1542oA**) see Pollution Standards Index

*Air-borne particles measuring < 10μm in diameter

unified health care system HEALTH CARE REFORM A proposed health care system that would include health insurance, workers' compensation, and health-related automobile insurance under one umbrella; advocates of a UHCS believe that it would cut administrative costs (**Am Med News 25 October 1992, p7**)

uniform deceleration OBSTETRICS A fetal heart rate response to uterine contractions that is symmetrical and has a uniform temporal relation thereto; uniform decelerations are DIVIDED INTO A) EARLY DECELERATION TYPE I DIP Due to vagal stimulation elicited in the first stage of labor by fetal head compression and B) LATE DECELERATION TYPE II DIP Due to uteroplacental insufficiency, potentially associated with a less favorable outcome and may signal early vasomotor lability; Cf Variable deceleration

Uniform Anatomical Gift Act A legislative act adopted by 1972 in all of the states in the US that allows an individual to make an anatomical 'gift' at the time of death by providing for such a gift in a signed document, eg in a will or driver's license; the UAGA also freed all persons (physicians, technicians, family members) involved in the organ (anatomical 'gift') procurement process from civil or criminal liability if they attempt to comply with the law in 'good faith' (**CAP Today March 1992**) see *Brotherton* v. *Cleveland*, Cadaver organ, Organ procurement

uninsured HEALTH CARE ENVIRONMENT An adjective referring to anyone lacking any form of health insurance, ± 35 million (US population 240 million); the percentage of uninsured depends on the state ranging from 10 to 22%; Cf Underinsured

uniparental disomy Inheritance of two copies of a specific allele, gene, or chromosome from one parent (from glossary, **N Engl J Med 1992; 326:1599oA**)

unique DNA Non-repetitive DNA, see there

unique sequence probe CYTOGENETICS A FISH probe with a specific DNA fragment from one chromosome, which is used to detect microdeletion syndromes, eg Prader-Willi syndrome, which has a microdeletion in chromosome 15 or the DiGeorge syndrome, which has a microdeletion in chromosome 22; see FISH probes

universal ancestor A phylogenetic term for organisms at or below the branching between progenotes (having rudimentary translation machinery) and genotes (modern translation machinery), based on the 'evolutionary clock', by which organisms are classified according to the evolution of the ribosomal RNA molecule; see Urkingdom; Cf Genote, Progenote

universal code Degenerate code, see there

universal coverage HEALTH CARE REFORM The inclusion of an entire group, eg a nation, under the umbrella of a health care plan, which provides for preventive care (eg vaccines, screening), outpatient visits to a generalist or specialist, hospitalization for basic and catastrophic needs; UC is a critical feature of any proposed national health plan, and was at the core of failed but well-intentioned 'Clinton Plan', directed toward the 37 million uninsured (and countless tens of millions of other underinsured) individuals living in which is regarded as a developed nation (**Am Med News 25 October 1992, p7**)

universal design A generic term for any form of industrial, mechanical or architectural design of a device, physical plant or workplace environment which is intended to be used by all (ie 'universal'), ie does not represent an impediment for individuals with disabilities

universal donor TRANSFUSION MEDICINE A person with blood group O, whose red cells have neither A nor B antigens on the surface and therefore will not elicit a hemolytic transfusion reaction when the blood is transfused to a person with blood group A, B, AB or O; Cf Universal recipient

Notes: 1) The production of anti-A, anti-B or anti-A,B antibodies occurs in everyone except those with blood group AB; this phenomenon that is poorly understood, and, being unrelated to previous exposure to specific antigens, is regarded as a 'natural' antibody 2) The term 'universal donor' requires the caveat that it is always preferable to transfuse type-specific blood, ie transfusion of group A blood to a group A recipient, since packed units of group O blood contains plasma with anti-A,B antibody, which may react with the recipient's blood 3) A 'universal donor' may have other blood group antigens on his/her red cells that are capable of causing hemolysis

universal nucleoside MOLE-CULAR BIOLOGY A non-discriminatory base analogue (1-(2'-deoxy-β-D-ribofuranosyl)-3-nitropyrrole, designated as M, figure, left) which is of potential use in oligonucleotide probes and primers; such a structure is of use in solving DNA design problems related to the degeneracy of the genetic code, or when fragmentary peptide sequence data are available (**Nature 1994; 369:492L**)

universal precautions INFECTIOUS DISEASE A method of infection control in which all human blood, certain body fluids (to wit, amniotic fluid, CSF, pericardial, peritoneal, pleural, and synovial fluids, saliva in dental procedures, semen, vaginal secretions, and any fluid grossly contaminated with blood-see below note), as well as unfixed organs or tissues of human origin, and HIV-containing cell or tissue cultures, or HBV-containing culture medium or other solutions are treated as if known to be infected with HIV, HBV, and/or other blood-borne pathogens (**Federal Register Dec 6, 1991, p 64107, col 2**); in absence of knowledge of the nature of the fluid, it should be treated as if potentially infectious; UPs consists of the constellation of safeguards for handling materials, tissues and fluids that may contain human pathogens; exposure to blood and body fluids is minimized by using isolation materials and removable and disposible barriers (latex and vinyl gloves, protective eyewear, masks and gowns and 'disposable sharps' containers), whenever there is contact or anticipated contact with hazardous body fluids or tissues that may be infected with HBV, HIV (**MMWR 1987; 36(suppl 2S)1S-18S**), Jakob-Creutzfeldt, or any other highly virulent agent; these precautions serve to both protect the health care worker and prevent him/her from acting as an inadvertent vector for these pathogens; body fluids that require 'universal precautions' include blood (serum and plasma) and all body fluids containing visible blood, as well as maternal milk, semen, vaginal secretions and cerebrospinal, synovial, peritoneal, pleural, pericardial, and amniotic fluids; see Precautions, Reverse precautions; Cf Body substance isolation

Note: Fluids that are thought by some experts to not require 'precautions' include feces, nasal secretions, saliva, sputum, sweat, urine and vomitus, unless they contain visible blood; the risk of transmission of HBV and HIV from these fluids is thought to be extremely low or nonexistent (**Lab Med 1988; 19:667**); implementation of 'universal precautions' is estimated to cost at least $336 X 10⁶/year in the US, largely attributed to the increased use of disposable gloves (**JAMA 1990; 264:2083**); universal precautions are reported to be effective in reducing contact with blood and body fluids (**JAMA 1991; 265:1123**)

universal recipient TRANSFUSION MEDICINE A person with blood group AB, whose serum has no anti-A, anti-B and therefore can receive any ABO transfusion without suffering a hemolytic transfusion reaction when blood is transfused from a person with blood group A, B, AB or O; Cf Universal donor

Notes: 1) Although the term 'universal recipient' was coined in reference to the ABO blood group, such a recipient should ideally also be Rh-positive, ie have the Rh-D antigen (the so-called Rh factor) on the red cells, since the absense thereof, potentially sets the stage for development of a hemolyzing 2) It is critical to note that a group O ('universal recipient') may still have other blood group antigens on his red cells that are capable of causing hemolysis

UNIX™ COMPUTERS A workstation-based operating system that is widely used by minicomputers, eg Sun Microsystems, and has the advantage of virtual (ie limitless) random access memory

unknown primary malignancy see Occult primary malignancy

unknown risk A new and/or unfamiliar risk (eg of HIV infection from transfused blood) with delayed consequences (**N Engl J Med 1995; 332:740ED**) Cf Dread risk

unlabeled indication Unlabeled use, see there

unlabeled use CLINICAL PHARMACOLOGY The use of a drug to treat any condition for which the drug does not have FDA approval; eg topical tretinoin, which is approved for treating acne, but not for photoaging, its far more widely marketed 'indication' (**N Engl J Med 1994; 331:1348SA**)

unmasking BIOCHEMISTRY The conversion of a non-reactive site on a protein to a reactive one that is accessible to specific reagents capable of reacting with molecules of interest, eg an enzyme; unmasking reactions include conformational changes or proteolytic removal of a blocking molecule, that might bind nonspecifically to the reactive site

unnatural death A death that is '...*caused by external causes (injury or poisoning)... which includes death... due to intentional injury such as homicide or suicide, and death caused by unintentional injury in an accidental manner.*' (**Arch Pathol Lab Med 1995; 119:123OA**) Cf Natural death

UNOS United Network for Organ Sharing An organization dedicated to optimizing the use of transplantable organs; according to UNOS statistics, 4000 major organ transplantations are performed/year (US), while 1500 to 2000 patients die waiting for organs; since successful survival of transplanted tissue is a function of the degree of histocompatibility matches, the larger the pool of donor and recipient haplotypes, the better the long-term survival of these organs (**JAMA 1994; 272:848c.N Engl J Med 1992; 327:834OA**) see Transplantation

UNOS Telephone 1.800.243.6667 (US) Telephone 1.804.330.8500 (Intl) 3001 Hungary Spring Rd, Richmond, Virginia 23228 USA

UNOS STAT A now obsolete system for prioritizing organ recipients that circumvented the more equitable allocation system (**JAMA 1994; 272:848c**) see Pittsburgh criteria

unpasteurized milk A product reported by self-proclaimed 'health advocates' to have a greater nutritive value than pasteurized cow's milk, which is alleged to reduce the incidence of caries, enhancing resistance to disease and containing beneficial enzymes and antibodies; no significant differences have been substantiated; unpasteurized milk is associated with bacterial infection by *Campylobacter jejuni, Salmonella* species (*S dublin*, uncommon but serious, *S typhimurium* and *S derby*), *Brucella* species, *Escherichia coli, Listeria monocytogenes, Mycobacterium bovis, M tuberculosis, Corynebacterium pseudotuberculosis, Staphylococcus aureus, Streptococcus* spp, *Streptobacillus moniliformis,* and *Yersinia enterocolitica,* toxoplasmosis (goat's milk), and tick-borne encephalitis (sheep's milk); see Holistic medicine; Cf Milk, White beverages

unproven care A generic term for therapies that have no proven* efficacy; unproven therapies have been categorized into those with bioelectromagnetic applications, lifestyle changes, mind/body control, biological therapies, energy therapies, and ethnomedicine or traditional medicine (see table) (**Am Med News 21 Nov 1994 p13**) see Unproven cancer therapy

*As currently known to the NIH Office of Alternative Medicine

unproven therapies for cancer ALTERNATIVE MEDICINE A generic term for a wide variety of unorthodox therapeutic modalities of questionable benefit that are offered by some self-proclaimed cancer specialists (who often have no or little formal medical training); in a comparison study at similar stages of terminal malignancy between patients treated with conventional and unproven cancer therapies, those receiving convential therapy had better survival and quality-of-life scores than those receiving an unproven regimen, which consisted in a combination of autogenous immune-enhancing vaccines, bacille Calmette-Guérin (bCG), vegetarian diets and coffee enemas, although the difference does not reach statistical significance (**N Engl J Med 1991; 324:1180**); at least $4 x 10⁹ are spent annually by US citizens on unproven cancer therapies

unsaturated fatty acid An alkyl chain fatty acid that contains one or more double bonds between carbons; these fatty acids have lower melting points and most are liquid at room temperature; Cf Monounsaturated fatty acids, Polyunsaturated fatty acid

unscrupulous diner dilemma A type of social dilemma in which one person 'defects' from the constraints (usually present but rarely voiced) on group cooperation; the descriptive adjectival modifier refers to a situation in which a small group of diners of varying financial means go to a relatively expensive restaurant; since it is common practice to split the bill evenly, the unscrupulous diner who has the most costly meal would have a superb meal at a bargain price; this dilemma represents a problem that is pervasive in society, and is central to a range of issues beyond those of mere alimentary import, to wit environmental protection, conservation of natural resources, eliciting contributions to charity, containing the global population, and others (**Sci Am 1994; 270/3:76**) see Prisoner's dilemma, Social dilemma

unstable An adjective referring to a chemical or other substance which, in the pure state, or as produced or transported, will vigorously condense, decompose, polymerize, or become self-reactive when subjected to conditions of shock, increased pressure, or temperature

unstable angina A phase of ischemic heart disease that is associated with a high risk of myocardial infarction and sudden death; UA is acute (less than 6 months in duration) coronary insufficiency in which the anginal symptoms are intermediate in severity between those of stable angina pectoris (intense chest pain) and myocardial infarction (crushing chest pain), which is subdivided into: 1) Severe, frequent angina pectoris of new onset, 1-2 months in duration and anginal pain occurring at low or no workload 2) **Crescendo angina** Confirmed coronary artery disease and a well-established pattern of stable angina with recent diminution of exercise tolerance and blunting of response to sublingual nitroglycerin and 3) **Angina at rest** The group at greatest risk for subsequent myocardial infarction with frequent and prolonged at-rest anginal attacks; see Angina, Silent ischemia

unusual life event A life event that is capable of evoking emotional stress, including death in family or among friends, disease in subject, change of job or emotional stress at work, change of relationship, divorce

---

METHODS OF UNPROVEN CARE

BIOELECTROMAGNETIC APPLICATIONS Electromagnetic fields, electrostimulation and neurostimulation devices, magnetoresonance spectroscopy, blue light treatment, artificial light therapy

LIFESTYLE CHANGES Changes in habits and lifestyle, diet, nutrition, megavitamins, macrobiotics, nutritional supplements

MIND/BODY CONTROL Various forms of external or internal therapy (art, humor, hypnosis, music, prayer), relaxation techniques (biofeedback, yoga/meditation), and counseling

PHARMACOLOGICAL AND BIOLOGICAL TREATMENTS Antioxidizing agents (eg vitamin A and E), oxidizing agents (eg hydrogen peroxide, ozone, both identified by the FDA as fraudulent), cell treatment, chelation therapy (other than that normally indicated for accepted medical conditions, eg desferroxamine for hemochromatosis, author's note), naturopathy, metabolic therapy

STRUCTURAL AND ENERGETIC THERAPIES Accupressure, aromatherapy, chiropractic medicine, massage therapy, reflexology, shiatsu

TRADITIONAL AND ETHNOMEDICINE Acupuncture, Ayurveda, herbs, homeopathy, Native American, traditional Chinese, folk medicine

¹Am Med News 21 Nov 1994 p13

---

unwinding protein A protein that binds to the single strands of DNA at the 'Y-fork' during DNA replication, maintaining the strands in an open position, preventing the unwound strands from reannealing before replication is completed; see Okazaki fragments

l'Uomo Delinquente see Physiognomy

UPDRS Unified Parkinson's Disease Rating Scale A scale used to quantify the neurologic defects in Parkinson's disease that measures its motor, mental, and activities of daily living components (N Engl J Med 1993; 328:176oA) see Parkinson's disease

uphill reaction BIOCHEMISTRY An endergonic reaction, ie one that requires energy for completion, eg the breaking of high-energy phosphate bonds in in vivo reactions

UPIN Unique physician identification number A numbering system sed by the (US) Health Care Financing Administration's database, the National Claims History File for physicians, allowing them to be used as a unit of analysis (see N Engl J Med 1994; 330:607oA)

'upper GI' A colloquial term for radiocontrast studies of the upper gastrointestinal tract, which allows examination of the esophagus, stomach and duodenum

upregulate GENETICS To increase the activity of a gene's transcriptional machinery usually by a protein that acts on a promoter region

upright tilt test Tilt test, see there

upset stomach A popular term for a transient gastralgia that may be accompanied by nausea and vomiting, which is often attributed something its victim ingested; Cf

Stomach virus

upside-down films Wangensteen-Rice technique A series of radiologic studies that are performed on a child with a suspected imperforate anus, in which plain films are taken with the child's anus in the most superior position, in order to identify the level of atresia (Ann Surg 1930; 92:77)

upside-down stomach A rare and extreme form of paraesophageal hiatal hernia, in which the entire stomach is within the thoracic cavity, having rotated on the organoaxial axis or cardiopyloric line CLINICAL Chronic occult blood loss with hypochromic anemia; in infants, recurrent vomiting and distended epigastrium RADIOLOGY Globular shadow with an air-fluid level superimposed on the cardiac shadow, seen in a plain chest film TREATMENT Reduction, gastropexy

'upstairs-downstairs heart' Crisscross heart, see there

upstream MOLECULAR BIOLOGY An adjective for a location or sequence of units that lies behind or previous to a reaction site, which is a function of the molecule or process being studied; Cf Downstream

PROTEIN Upstream refers to the sequence of amino acids from the COOH-terminal to the NH$_2$-terminal

REPLICATION Upstream refers to a location opposite that of the movement of the replicating fork

TRANSLATION Upstream refers to a location or sequence of mRNA from the 3' to 5'-end

TRANSCRIPTION Upstream refers to a location or sequence of DNA on the transcribed strand from the 5' to the 3' end

upstream activating sequence An oligonucleotide segment of DNA, located 50 to 300 base pairs in the 5' direction ('upstream') from the promoter site of a gene to be transcribed; the UAS is required for most, if not all transcriptional events and serves as a binding site for transcription factors

upstream binding factor UBF, see there

urate milk Tophus, see there

urease Urea amidohydrolase An enzyme [EC 3.5.1.5] that hydrolyzes the urea to carbon dioxide and ammonia

$$H_2NCONH_2 \text{ (urea)} + H_2O = CO_2 + 2 NH_3$$

uremia A constellation of symptoms caused by advanced renal insufficiency CLINICAL Nausea, vomiting, pruritus, uremic frost, mental clouding, peripheral neuropathies, osteodystrophy, hypertension, pericarditis, pulmonary edema LABORATORY Acidosis, anemia, azotemia, ↓ Ca^{2+}, ↑ PO$_4$

uremic cardiopathy Congestive heart failure due to fluid retention by the kidney in advanced renal failure (uremic state), which may be accompanied by moderate to severe hypertension

uremic frost A clinical finding in severe renal failure of long duration where the concentration of urea is markedly increased in the sweat, causing cutaneous precipitation of crystallized urea

uremic neuromyopathy Fatigue related to electrolytic imbalance with renal wasting of sodium and calcium, and retention of potassium and phosphate related to advanced renal failure, ie uremia

URF Unassigned reading frame, see there

urgent care center HEALTH CARE INDUSTRY A (usually) free-standing mini-emergency center that is equipped to manage either non-life-threatening conditions requiring immediate primary care, or conditions that cannot be treated outside of hospital, but which require stabilization prior to being transferred; such facilities are usually staffed by salaried physicians, often have a 'stat' laboratory and on-site radiology equipment and are operated on a for-profit basis

'urgent need' A philosophical stance that might be taken by a governmental agency when a medical device or therapeutic procedure is under review for efficacy or safety; an 'urgent need' policy has been adopted by the FDA in the face of the mounting controversy about the safety of silicone breast implants, allowing their implantation into women with breast cancer for whom saline-type implants are viewed by their physicians as being unsuitable (**Am Med News 18 May 1992 p4**)

URI Upper respiratory infection

uric acid 'infarct(s)' Yellowish streaks seen in young children at the tips of the renal papillae, corresponding to normal collections of uric acid crystals in the terminal collecting tubules CLINICAL Asymptomatic

urinary ascites The free flow of urine into the peritoneal cavity, in congenital urethral obstruction

urinary tract infection A condition affecting ± 7 million/year (US); UTIs can for therapeutic purposes be categorized into UTIs affecting young women with acute uncomplicated pyelonephritis or cystitis, or recurrent cystitis, and adults with asymptomatic bacteruria or with complicated UTI CLINICAL Dysuria, burning, ↑ frequency, urgency LABORATORY Leukocyte esterase dipstick, 10^2 or $\geq 10^5$ colony-forming units/ml MICROBIOLOGY *Escherichia coli* (± 80%), *Staphylococcus saprophyticus*, *Proteus mirabilis*, *Klebsiella pneumoniae* TREATMENT Oral T-S, norfloxacin, ciprofloxacin (**N Engl J Med 1993; 329:1328cc**)

urinoma PEDIATRIC UROLOGY A tumor-like urine-filled cyst seen in the renal capsule of children, which arises secondary to congenital urethral obstruction, in which urine percolates into the subcapsular or perirenal spaces through ruptured calyceal fornices

urkingdom EVOLUTIONARY BIOLOGY A conceptual 'superkingdom' lying at the root of the divergence between primitive organisms and bacteria from plants and animals, in which the mother organism, recently graduated from the primordial ooze had a minimal complement of 'ur' genes essential for all organisms, including those genes encoding ribosomal RNA, ribosomal protein, enzymes and proteins required for DNA replication, DNA transcription and RNA translation; see Progenote

urogastrone Epidermal growth factor, see there

urogenital diaphragm A triangular fibromuscular membrane that spans the ischiopubic rami lying superficial to the pelvic diaphragm; it consists of the perineal membrane, the spincter of the urethra, and the deep transverse perineal muscles; the membrane is, and is perforated by regional ducts, nerves and vessels and the vagina

urokinase A heterodimeric fibrinolytic enzyme composed of a 22- and 33-kD chain that derives from the prourokinase molecule; urokinase is involved in extracellular proteolysis and has increased activity during cell migration or tissue remodeling, cleaving fibronectin; urokinase has a connecting peptide, a kringle domain, a protease domain and a growth factor-like domain at the amino acid terminus, at which point urokinase binds to its receptor; see Kringle domain; Cf Streptokinase, tPA

urolagnia A paraphilia (sexual deviancy) in which the subject is sexually aroused and or has erotic thoughts linked to various urinary functions, including urinating on partner, drinking urine, and so on

'Water sports' is a currently used term that might be regarded as equivalent to urolagnia-Author's note

uromodulin Tamm-Horsfall protein, orosomucoid An 85-kD α_1 acid glycoprotein that is secreted by epithelial cells in Henle's ascending loop and distal convoluted tube; the kidneys produce up to 150 mg/d of protein of which 30-50 mg is uromodulin; it was first isolated from the urine of pregnant women and has potent immunosuppressive properties attributed to the N-linked carbohydrate residues, acting to inhibit antigen-induced T-cell proliferation and monocyte cytotoxicity Note: Since this 'activity' occurs only when the cytokines are denatured, the immunosuppression may be an artefact (FEBS Lett 1988; 226:314); uromodulin is a specific ligand for interleukins IL-1α, IL-1β and TNF, regulating the activity and the levels of these cytokines in the circulation; uromodulin has sequence similarity ('homology') with the lipoprotein lipase receptor and epithelial growth factor

uropod *uro*, tail, Greek, *podos*, stalk, foot A distinct cytoplasmic process of lymphocytes that attaches to other cells and debris, which appears to play a role in lymphocyte function; see Hand mirror cell

ursodiol Ursodeoxycholic acid A dihydroxy stereoisomer of chenodiol (chenodeoxycholic acid), a non-toxic hydrophilic bile acid that modifies the composition of the endogenous bile acid pool, ameliorating, or even partially reversing the clinicopathologic changes of cholestasis by 1) Reducing the toxicity of cholic and chenodeoxycholic acid and their glycine and taurine conjugates 2) Decreasing the usual elevation of serum alkaline phosphatase and alanine aminotransferase, possibly by stabilizing hepatocyte membranes and 3) Displaces endogenous bile acids by inhibiting absorption of endogenous bile acids, apparently reversing their suspected cytotoxicity on the liver; long-term ursodiol therapy is reported to slow the progression of primary biliary cirrhosis, reducing the need for liver transplantation (**N Engl J Med 1994; 330:1342oa, 1386ed**); ursodiol is used to treat primary biliary cirrhosis (PBC), a condition thought to be due to the toxic effects of bile acids (**N Engl J Med 1991; 324:1548**); PBC patients treated with ursodiol had statistically significant improvements in serum levels of bilirubin, alkaline phosphatase, cholesterol, IgM, alanine and aspartate aminotransferases, γ-glutamyl transferase, antimitochondrial antibodies and the Mayo risk score; see Primary biliary cirrhosis; ursodiol may be used alone or in combination with chenodiol to dissolve gallstones by extracorporeal shock-wave lithotripsy

ursodiol

urushiol The generic name given to the four catechols in the *Rhus* (*Toxicodendron*) genus that differ only in the saturation of their pentadecyl side chain, which induce delayed hypersensitivity; these 'poisonous' plants includes poison oak (*R diversiloba*), poison sumac (*R toxicodendron*) and poison ivy (*R radicans*); urushiol may remain active on unwashed clothing, causing reactions months to years after exposure TREATMENT Varying success is reported with desensitization therapy; see Poison ivy

user-friendly *adjective* 1) Pertaining or referring to complete ease of use 2) Idiot-proof

USFMG United States foreign medical graduate A North American who, for various reasons, often had a less than outstanding academic performance in college or university, and by extension, unable to obtain a seat in an American medical school, graduated from a foreign medical school; in general, USFMGs suffer from a wide array of discrimination and are often considered 'third-class' physicians in terms of abilities and knowledge; USFMGs taking the ECFMG (in descending order) Dominican Republic (1105), Mexico (828), the Philippines (340), Montserrat (204), Dominica (170), and Italy (118)-data from 1991 (JAMA 1995; 273:1162MN&P) see Foreign medical graduate

Note: Malpractice lawsuits, used by some parties as a benchmark for determination of competence are no more common in foreign medical graduates than graduates of North American medical schools

U-shaped curve A curve that describes the dose-response relation between alcohol intake and the risk of myocardial infarction; when viewed vis-á-vis coronary-related fatalities, the relation appears to be more of an L-shaped curve* (N Engl J Med 1994; 330:1241c), where once a threshold of ↓ risk has been reached, there is essentially no further change in cardiovascular fatality, ie a 'saturation' effect; a similar effect has been found for ♀ and alcohol consumption (N Engl J Med 1995; 332:1245oA); Cf J curve phenomenon; the U curve phenomenon also occurs in relation to both weight loss and weight gain, where those subjects with the most stable weight had the lowest mortality for all (nonmalignant) causes and for coronary heart disease; the mortality increases for weight cycling (JAMA 1992; 268:2045oc)

*It is appropriate to underscore the U shape, as morbidity increases for other reasons as alcohol ingestion increases

U-shaped scar A deep fibrotic depression on the cortical surface of the kidney, which is associated with arteriosclerosis and chronicpyelonephritis

U-shaped vertebrum An inverted U-shaped vertebrum (on an antero-posterior film), with marked flattening and central narrowing (lateral film), a characteristic deformity of the lumbar vertebra in thanatophoric dysplasia; see Cloverleaf skull, 'Telephone receiver' deformity

U1 snRNP U1 small nuclear ribonuclear protein A 165-nucleotide RNA that is the most abundant member of the snRNP family, which is intimately involved in the splicing reaction of pre-mRNA molecules by recognizing the 5' spice site, which may be potentiated by U1-specific protein C (Science 1994; 247:69)

Usher syndrome An AR [MIM 276900] condition characterized by retinitis pigmentosa (RP) and sensorineural deafness; US has been divided into 4 clinical forms* MOLECULAR PATHOLOGY Mutations in various loci, to wit 1q, 11p, 11q, and 14q

*Type I-profound congenital deafness with RP by age 10, type II-moderate to severe deafness with RP by adolescence, type III-progessive hearing loss and RP of pubertal onset, type IV-possibly an X-linked form

USMLE United States Medical Licensing Examination A single three-step examination required for medical licensure in the US, which is sanctioned by both the National Board of Medical Examiners and the Federation of State Medical Boards; US and Canadian-trained medical students had a pass rate in the USMLE of 85%; foreign citizens trained in foreign schools had a pass rate of 37%, and USFMGs had a 23% pass rate (JAMA 1995; 273:1162MN&P) see Off-shore medical school, USFMG

USOH Usual state of health

USP United States Pharmacopeia A compendium of drug standards that includes assays and tests for determining drug strength, purity and quality; the compendium is recognized by US federal law and published by the authorities of the United States Pharmacopeia convention; see National Formulary

usual interstitial pneumonia A disease that occurs in the middle-aged, often associated with connective tissue disease, characterized by insidious deterioration of respiratory function with dyspnea and tachypnea, right-sided cardiac failure, loss of lung capacity and decreased residual volume RADIOLOGY Early, 'ground-glass', linear or nodular markings, followed by coarsened shadows and cyst formation; the elevation of the diaphragm in end-stage UIP reflects the amount of tissue loss PATHOLOGY The lungs are heavy, rubbery, firm, accompanied by alveolar and septal breakdown is followed by 'hobnailing' of type II pneumocytes, loss of the flat type I alveolar lining cells and squamous metaplasia of the distal air spaces; end-stage UIP demonstrates chronic inflammation, hyaline membrane formation, 'honey-combing' with macroscopic cysts with a knobby pleural surface due to fibrosis, septal thickening and smooth muscle hyperplasia ('muscular cirrhosis') TREATMENT None has proven effective, although corticosteroids may be used to 'treat the physician'

uterine apoplexy A uterus in which myometrial vessels have been stipped of protective endometrium, and are actively bleeding as occurs in abruptio placentae (Couvelaire uterus, uteroplacental apoplexy), or in placenta acreta or in massive cardiovascular collapse (apoplexia uteri)

uterotonin OBSTETRICS A generic term for any of a number of substances, eg oxytocin, prostaglandins (which is also a uterotropin), and endothelin-1, which act directly on responsive myometrial smooth muscle cells to evoke myometrial contraction; uterotonins can be produced locally, acting in an autocrine or paracrine fashion, or may be produced outside of the uterus, arrive via the circulation, and act in an endocrine fashion; Cf Uterotropin

uterotropin OBSTETRICS A generic term for any substance that acts on the myometrium and cervix to enable the synthesis of functional components needed for labor, accompanied by suspension of phase 0 of parturition (in which the uterus is refractory to contractility); Cf Uterotonin

UTI Urinary tract infection

utility CLINICAL MEDICINE A tool used in outcomes management defined as a quantified expression of a person's preference for a specific health state, where 1 usually corresponds to the best possible outcome of a disease state or therapeutic intervention, and 0 corresponds to the worst outcome, usually defined as death (JAMA 1995; 273:1185) see Standard gamble metric, Time trade-off metric COMPUTERS Utility program, see there

utility program COMPUTERS A program that optimizes the function and efficiency of a computer; although in theory, the disk operating system, eg MS/DOS, should contain all those programming routines that are required to function in the 'environment, they rarely do; UPs include file compression programs (eg Stuffit), shells, undelete programs (eg Norton Utilities), vaccines (anti-virus programs) and others

utilization gap The underutilization of an appropriate therapy, as in the inadvertent non-administration of Rh immune globulin in an Rh-negative woman, which may be required after abortion, ectopic pregnancy or in fetal death; Cf 'Skimping'

utilization review Evaluation of the necessity (eg for surgery or other therapy), appropriateness (of admissions or of services ordered), and efficiency of the use of health care services, procedures, and facilities, cost-containment process used in US health care in hospitals, health maintenance organizations and preferred provider organizations that includes pre-admission reviews, concurrent (while the patient is in the hospital) reviews, and reviews of procedures, levels of care and medical necessity (after the patient's discharge); the utilization review committee assesses the appropriateness of therapy and the efficiency of use of medical services, procedures and facilities

utrophin A dystrophin-related protein encoded on chromosome 6 that is homologous to dystrophin and is located in normal adult muscle exclusively at neuromuscular junctions; it appears to be up-regulated in the face of dystrophin deficiency; utrophin measurement may prove useful in diagnosing Duchenne-type muscular dystrophy (N Engl J Med 1994; 331:1162c)

UV index PUBLIC HEALTH A 'device' created by the joint efforts National Weather Service, the EPA, and the CDC, which consists of a daily computerized forecast of UV exposure based on the geographic location and cloud cover; with a minimal to low (0-4) UI a person with fair skin will burn in 45 to 60 minutes and should wear sunblock and sunglasses; with a high (7+) UI a person with fair skin will burn in 10-15 minutes and should wear sunblock, sunglasses, a hat, and on the beach, should sit under an umbrella (NY Times 14 June 1995; C14) see Sun Protection Factor

UV light see Ultraviolet radiation

uvulopalatopharyngoplasty A procedure for treating obstructive sleep apnea that consists of resection of the uvula, the distal margin of the soft palate, palatine tonsils and any excessive lateral pharyngeal tissue; the procedure is successful in two-thirds of selected cases with obstructive sleep apnea in which there is focal airway collapse, which may cause the patients to snore; see Snore

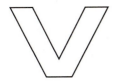

V Symbol for: 1) Valine 2) Vanadium 3) Vector 4) Velocity 5) Volt 6) Volume

v Symbol for: 1) Reaction rate 2) Specific volume 3) Velocity

V factor Nicotinamide adenine dinucleotide MICROBIOLOGY A growth requirement for *Haemophilus* species (*H influenza, H parainfluenza, H aegyptiae*) that may be supplied by yeast extracts, *Staphylococcus*, *Pneumococcus* and *Neisseria* spp; X factor is any of a group of tetrapyrrole compounds that are provided by iron-containing pigments, eg heme, used in the synthesis of catalases, peroxidases and in the cytochrome electron transport system

V gene Variability gene Two segments (exons) of DNA that encode the first 95-100 amino acids (the variable portion) of a light or heavy chain of immunoglobulin or β chain of the T-cell receptor; the proteins encoded have the most extensive amino acid variability of the entire human genome allowing highly specific immune recognition, thus the greater the diversity of the recognition site, the more specific is the potential immune defense; see Variable region, 'Hot spot'

V3 loop Principal neutralizing determinant AIDS VIROLOGY Hypervariable 36-residue disulfide-linked polypeptide loop in HIV-1's envelope protein; monoclonal antibodies raised against the V3 loop, bind to it and neutralize HIV-1 infectivity; V3 elicits the formation of HIV-neutralizing antibodies in vitro but not in vivo; when the peptide fragment is further dissected, a six-peptide subunit (Gly-Pro-Gly-Arg-Ala-Phe, abbreviated as GPGRAF) is sufficient to neutralize the divergent HIV-1 serotypes; V3's large sequence variability has frustrated attempts to use the V3 loop as a vaccine target (**Science & Medicine 1995; 2/3:38**) see HIV vaccines

V statistic STATISTICS A data set in a trial that approximately represents the number of patients in a therapeutic trial with an extremely low number of participants (**N Engl J Med 1995; 332:1256oA**) Cf z statistic

v wave CARDIOLOGY The wave in the normal jugular phlebogram corresponding to the atrial diastole

VA Veterans Administration, Department of Veteran Affairs The hospital system sponsored by the US government for providing medical care directly to civilians, most of whom are related to veterans of the US military; before a 1989 US government budget cut, all 30 million American veterans were eligible for VA benefits; the current rule allows benefits only for those with service-connected disabilities or veterans earning below the poverty levels (< $18 000 annual income); the 171 hospitals in the VA system are scattered throughout the US, the locations having been dictated by historical precedent, political influence, demographic need and educational pressure BUDGET $11 x 10⁹

vaccination see Supervaccine

vaccine A mixture of live, live-attenuated, killed, complete or incomplete microorganisms or products derived therefrom that contains antigens capable of stimulating the production of specific protective antibodies against a microorganism; see Killed vaccine, Live attenuated vaccine

According to G Ada (**Lancet 1990; 335:523**), a vaccine should meet certain immunological criteria; it should 1) Contain a sufficient number of different T-cell epitopes that T-cell responses will be achieved in all members of a genetically diverse outbred population 2) Generate a large pool of memory T (and B) cells; the greater the size of the pool, the more rapid is the appearance of effector T cell activity from the memory cells and 3) Generate persistent high titers of neutralizing antibodies, such that the bulk of a challenge virus is prevented from infecting susceptible cells (**Nature 1991; 349:369n&v**)

vaccine therapy A therapeutic strategy currently in its infancy that attempts to boost the immune response to a particular pathogen to such a degree that the vaccine alone is enough to treat the patient; to date, no therapeutic vaccine has been proven successful, although to some workers, the rabies vaccine, being a post-exposure vaccine, qualifies as a therapeutic vaccine; vaccine therapies are in various stages of development for hepatitis B, herpes, leishmaniasis, leprosy, and TB (**Science 1994; 264:503**)

vaccinia rabies glycoprotein vaccine VRG vaccine, see there

vaccinology A recently coined term for a nascent field of expertise, which has 'borrowed' major components from epidemiology, immunology, infectious disease, pediatrics, preventive medicine, public health, and virology (**N Engl J Med 1995; 332:476BR**)

Vacor diabetes TOXICOLOGY A special form of 'brittle' DM, which is due to accidental or suicidal ingestion of the rodenticide Vacor (N-3-pyridyl-methyl-N'-nitrophenyl urea), a molecule that is structurally related to alloxan and streptozotocin, both of which induce experimental DM in laboratory animals TREATMENT Immediate gastric lavage and hyperdoses of nicotinamide

VACTERYL association Formerly, VATER or VACTER A clinical complex characterized by a multisystem association of vertebral defects, eg hemivertebra and scoliosis, anorectal atresia, cardiac malformations, eg ventricular septal defect, tracheoesophageal fistula, renal anomalies including agenesis, ureteropelvic junction obstruction, vesicoureteral reflux and crossed fused ectopia and radial upper limb anomalies, eg polydactyly

vacuolar myelopathy A heterogeneous group of conditions characterized by spinal cord degeneration PATHOLOGY Vacuolization of the white matter, accompanied by lipid-laden macrophages (resembling somewhat vitamin B$_{12}$ and folic acid-related subacute combined degeneration of the spinal cord), which occurs in up to 20% of AIDS patients, which is most extensive in the lateral columns of the middle and lower thoracic segments; Cf Spongy degeneration

vacuolar myopathy Cleared spaces within muscle cells are not uncommon True vacuoles are bound by membranes derived from the T tubules, sarcoplasmic reticulum or from the Golgi apparatus and perinuclear membranes; non-membrane-bound vacuoles are often mutiple and designated as 'hydropic degeneration'; necrotic vacuolated muscle may occur in anaerobic infections, eg *Clostridium* spp; in absence of infection, polymyositis may be a toxic effect of long-term chloroquine therapy for malaria, amebiasis, acid maltase deficiency, primary or secondary periodic paralysis or nemaline myopathy due to myophosphorylase deficiency

vacuolization Vacuolation The presence in a cell of one or more cleared spaces of vacuoles; cytoplasmic vacuolization is a nonspecific finding described under various conditions CYTOLOGY 'Pap smears' of endocervical cells may be vacuolated in squamous metaplasia or when infected with *Chlamydia* or human papilloma virus HEMATOLOGY Vacuolization of lymphocytes occurs in either 1) Inborn errors of metabolism, including types II, III, V, and VII glycogen storage diseases, GM1 gangliosidosis, Hurler-Hunter syndrome, neuronal ceroid lipofuscinosis (Batten's disease), Niemann-Pick disease, sea blue histiocytosis, Tay-Sachs disease, Wolman's disease or 2) Secondary to acquired conditions, eg Burkitt's lymphoma, chronic lymphocytic leukemia, infectious mononucleosis, as an in vitro artefact of EDTA anticoagulation in an aging specimen, normal lymphocytes and in Sézary lymphocytes HEPATOLOGY Vacuolization may affect circulating red cell normoblasts in alcoholic liver disease ONCOLOGY Vacuolization of plasma cells may occur in BM afflicted by mu heavy chain disease RENAL PATHOLOGY Vacuolization of the glomerular basement membrane may be seen in the resolving phases of mild membranous glomerulonephritis

vacuum phenomenon A linear or oval radiolucency corresponding to gas in the intervertebral space, most often seen in degenerative disk disease, which may also occur in vertebral osteomyelitis, Schmorl's nodes, spondylosis deformans and necrosis-induced vertebral collapse, often accompanied by loss of height and reactive osteosclerosis

vacuum sign A normal radiologic finding seen when traction is applied to a joint, causing coalescence of gas within a joint, a sign that disappears in effusions

vade mecum A fancy generic term for a book, manual, handbook or guidebook

vaginal pouch Female condom, see there

vaginal ring An annular contraceptive device that has been undergoing clinical trials, which is inserted by the woman at/prior to the time of coitus that slowly releases levonorgestrel or progesterone; despite its obvious advantages, it is not approved for use in the US; see Norplant, Pearl index; Cf Female condom

vaginismus '...*recurrent or persistent involuntary contraction of the perineal muscles surrounding the outer third of the vagina when penetration with penis, finger, tampon, or speculum is attempted*...(which causes) ...*marked distress or interpersonal difficulty*...(and) *is not better accounted for by another...disorder* (306.51 DSM-IV, American Psychiatric Association, Washington, DC, 1994)

vaginosis A vaginal infection without leukocyte infiltration; bacterial vaginosis is the most common vaginal infection of reproductive-aged women ETIOLOGY *Mobiluncus* species CLINICAL Range from asymptomatic to having a copious and malodorous milky discharge, which when mixed with 10% potassium hydroxide has a fishy odor

vagrant's disease Parasitic melanoderma

VAHS Virus-associated hemophagocytic syndrome, see there

validation STATISTICS Definition

valley fever A clinical form of primary coccidioidomycosis, first described in San Joaquin Valley, California, most common in white ♀ CLINICAL Fever, cough, pleuritic pain, arthralgia, and erythema multiforme or nodosum DIAGNOSIS Serologic detection of IgM antibody to the mycelial phase antigen, coccidioidin, ↑ complement-fixing antibody, ↑ latex agglutination TREATMENT Ketoconazole (agent of choice), amphotericin B, miconazole

valproate Divalproex sodium NEUROLOGY An antiepileptic drug approved for treating absence seizures, which is as effective as carbamazepine for generalized tonic-clonic seizures SIDE EFFECTS Weight gain, hair loss, tremor (N Engl J Med 1992; 327:765oA) Cf Carbamazepine

Valsalva maneuver Forced expiration against a closed glottis following full inspiration, described by Valsalva in 1704 to expulse pus from the middle ear; the 'Valsalva' increases the intrathoracic pressure for about ten sec-

onds, eliciting a complex series of changes in the pulse rate and blood pressure involving both vagal and sympathetic responses

valvular vegetation CARDIOLOGY Any of the variably sized excrescences that may be present on heart valves, aka vegetative endocarditis (table)

CARDIAC VALVE VEGETATIONS

BACTERIAL VEGETATIONS Friable, necrotic lesions measuring up to 1 cm in diameter that may perforate the underlying valve

LUPUS ERYTHEMATOSUS VEGETATIONS of Libmann-Sacks Lesions consisting of mucoid pools, fibrinoid degeneration and collagenous fibrosis occurring on both sides of the tricuspid and mitral valves

NON-BACTERIAL THROMBOTIC VEGETATIONS Relatively small foci of organizing thrombi occur singly or multiply along the line of the leaflet's closure, or on either side of the ventricle

RHEUMATIC VEGETATIONS Small (1-2 mm) foci of friable fibrinoid necrosis located in the cardiac valve cusps along the lines of closure

---

vampirism CLINICAL MEDICINE A 'vampire' is a clinician who requests excessive blood tests, potentially causing iatrogenic anemia, an event that is most common in young children with chronic, unusual or 'interesting' diseases PSYCHIATRY A form of deviancy in which blood is ingested, variably accompanied by necrophilic activity, occurring in a background of schizophrenia, psychosis, sadomasochism, cult, eg voodoo rituals, cannibalism, fetishism or drug intoxication

Vancouver group International Committee of Medical Journal Editors (JAMA 1991; 265:2697) see Authorship

van Gogh 'syndrome' PSYCHIATRY Self-mutilation, eg amputation of an extremity, enucleation of an eye or castration, which may be associated with dysmorphic delusions, disturbances of the body image or psychosis, or a component of the congenital Lesch-Nyhan syndrome; see Self-mutilation

vanishing bile duct syndrome A poorly understood early complication of liver transplantation, in which there is irreversible destructive cholangitis and loss of bile ducts

vanishing bone syndrome Disappearing bone disease, see there

vanishing diabets mellitus syndrome Houssay phenomenon A marked reduction in the requirement for exogenous insulin that occurs secondary to complete destruction of the pituitary gland, especially the anterior lobe; the phenomenon may rarely occur spontaneously in DM, since infarcts of the hypophysis are three times more common in diabetics; during the 1960s, hypophysectomies were performed to take advantage of this phenomenon, reducing the insulin requirements in these patients, at the considerable cost of making them hormonal 'cripples'; Cf Dawn phenomenon, 'Honeymoon period', Somogyi effect

vanishing lung syndrome Giant bullous emphysema A disease affecting an estimated 1:1000 young, especially ♂ subjects, which is characterized by multiple bullae of the apical portions of one or both lungs CLINICAL ↑ Resonance to percussion with radiologic disappearance of lung markings, hence, the term 'vanishing'; in absence of concomitant emphysema, the vital capacity is relatively normal; with extensive lesions, severe impairment of pulmonary function may occur TREATMENT Surgical excision of the afunctional bullae results in expansion of normally functioning pulmonary tissue and clinical improvement

vanishing testes syndrome Embryonic testicular regression syndrome, see there

'vanishing twin' The spontaneous regression of a second

gestational product, which occurs in 20% of twin pregnancies, detected by ultrasonography in the first trimester; Cf Twins

vapor density OCCUPATIONAL SAFETY The mass of a gas divided by its volume, a quantity that is proportional to the mean mass of its molecules; VD is a physical parameter of a liquid that indicates how heavy the pure gaseous phase is in relation to air ($\leq$ 1.0 = lighter than air; $\geq$ 1.0 = heavier than air); VD is of interest to OSHA, which requires listing of VDs at ambient temperatures in its Materials Safety Data Sheets‡; high VDs may be problematic in certain confined spaces, eg storage tanks, as the vapors collect in the bottom and may cause both the worker and his would-be rescuer(s) to succumb to the effects of the gas

vapor pressure OCCUPATIONAL SAFETY The pressure exerted by the gaseous phase of a liquid, which is a function of the amount of vapor given off by a chemical; a high VP indicates a liquid that evaporates easily, a parameter of interest to OSHA, which requires listing of VPs at ambient pressure in its Materials Safety Data Sheets, which document the use of chemicals in the workplace

variable cost LABORATORY MEDICINE A cost that is a direct function of volume of service, ie supplies and reagents (Advance/Laboratory July/August 1994) Cf Fixed cost

variable deceleration OBSTETRICS A fetal heart response that is asynchronous with respect to uterine contractions; the curves on the fetal heart monitor are more angulated and saw-toothed and may be related to compromise in placental blood flow, eg umbilical cord compression, and like late decelerations may signify parturition-related difficulties; see Fetal heart monitor; Cf Uniform deceleration

variable number of tandem repeat MOLECULAR BIOLOGY Any of a family of DNA repeat elements that arise from head-to-tail concatenation of short-(10-100 bp in length) sequence motifs; VNTRs, through a mutational process that ↑ or ↓ the number of repeat motifs in a given allele, are often unstable and produce highly polymorphic loci that may contain dozens of alleles; VNTRs or hypervariable minisatellites are of considerable use in linkage analysis and as DNA fingerprint probes in forensic analysis (N Engl J Med 1993; 329:1517OA)

variable region The portion of an immunoglobulin (antibody) that is shared by the variable domain of a (kappa or lambda) light chain and the variable domain of a (α, γ, μ, δ or ϵ) heavy chain; the variable region confers specificity to an antibody and is encoded by the V gene region(s); see Hot spot, Monoclonal antibody; Cf Constant region

variable resistance SPORTS MEDICINE A resistance that changes through a range of motion when an isotomic contraction is used to move a load (JC DeLee, D Drez, Jr, Eds, Orthopedic Sports Medicine WB Saunders, Philadelphia, 1994) Cf Static resistance

variance STATISTICS σ^2 *'The average squared deviation of a set of values from their mean…(which) …is determined by dividing the sum of squared deviations by one less than the by number of observations.'* (Intl Dict Med, J Wiley & Sons, New York, 1986); variance corresponds to the variability in a Gaussian distribution of data that is markedly influenced by large outliers; the variance measures the dispersion of data about a mean of X

variant angina Prinzmetal's angina Chest pain at rest that is associated with an ST segment deviation (usually an elevation) without a preceding increase in heart rate or blood pressure; this form of angina is caused by vasospasms of large caliber coronary arteries that oxygenate the entire thickness of myocardium TREATMENT Nitrates, nifedipine, or diltiazem with aspirin; slow calcium channel antagonists, eg verapamil are of use but may contribute to the atrioventricular block

variation phenomenon The differences in the patterns of treatment and diagnostic workups of similar patients in various health care settings; the VP is widespread and may be responsible for a marked regional variation in the costs of medical care without improving the outcomes (N Engl J Med 1994; 331:1017ED)

varicella embryopathy A rare constellation of malformations occurring sporadically in a fetus when the mother contracts varicella before the 20th week of gestation; abnormalities include intrauterine growth retardation, motor and sensory defects, chorioretinitis, cerebral dysgenesis, zosteriform skin lesions, and limb defects PATHOGENESIS Possibly related to cytotoxic anti-varicella zoster virus immune defect (Arch Pathol Lab Med 1992; 116:181OA)

variceal bleeding Hemorrhage from dilated (variceal) veins, most commonly understood to mean esophageal varices related to end-stage liver failure MANAGEMENT-SURGICAL Surgical shunting, endoscopic sclerotherapy, esophageal variceal ligation, transjugular intrahepatic portosystemic stent-shunt (TIPS) procedure‡ (N Engl J Med 1994; 330:165OA) MANAGEMENT-MEDICAL Vasopressin, nitroglycerin, somatostatin, beta-adrenergic blockers, long-acting nitrates

vascular dementia A potentially preventable form of dementia in which cerebral atrophy is caused by various types of cerebrovascular insults; in one study 74% of cases of vascular dementia were of the multi-infarct type, 9% were related to cerebral hypoperfusion, and the remainder a mixture of the two types; the 3-year mortality in patients $\geq$ age 85 (Sweden) with vascular dementia is 67%, vs 23% of 85+-year-olds without dementia (N Engl J Med 1993 328:153OA) see Multi-infarct dementia; Cf Alzheimer's disease

vascular endothelial growth factor *An endothelial cell-specific angiogenic and vasopermeability factor that binds to high-affinity, membrane-bound receptors with tyrosine kinase activity; VEGF's expression is induced by hypoxia in tumors'* (N Engl J Med 1994; 331:1480OA) VEGF is a homodimeric cytokine with at least four (121, 165, 189, 206 amino acid) monomeric variants, which is produced by vascular smooth muscle cells, epithelial cells, macrophages, and various tumor cell lines; inhibition of VEGF activity suppresses tumor growth produced by various cells and stimulates tissues to produce blood vessels, and appears to play a major role in mediating active intraocular neovascularization in the face of retinal ischemia as occurs in DM and in retinal artery occlusion; VEGF is an experimental gene therapy for patients with 'major league' blockage of peripheral arteries, and may prove to someday be useful in the treatment of coronary artery stenosis, in an effort to stimulate neovascularization around blocked vessels (New York Times 13 Dec 1994; C1)

vascular integrity factor A generic term for a putative molecule or protein that is postulated to be produced by platelets, which are presumed to prevent spontaneous hemorrhage; no candidate molecule has been identified

vascular phase Prevascular phase, see there

vascular sling A rare congenital malformation in which the left pulmonary artery arises from the right pulmonary artery, crossing to the left side, and insinuates itself between the trachea and esophagus, forming a 'sling' around the trachea CLINICAL Tracheal stenosis (stridor, wheezing and choking) TREATMENT Surgery

vasectomy Ligation or other form of interruption of (usually) both vas deferens, a form of permanent contraception chosen by up to 500 000 US ♂/year; 10-20 ejaculates are required after the operation before there are no viable sperm; vasectomized subjects may experience long-term scrotal pain, possibly related to sperm granuloma formation, an event seen in 1-10% of cases with congestive epididymitis; ⅔ of subjects develop circulating antibodies PATHOLOGY Post-vasectomy testicles may demonstrate dysspermatogenesis, thickening of the tunica propria and seminiferous tubules, interstitial fibrosis, ↓ Sertoli cells and spermatids, focal interstitial fibrosis (a predictor of reversal infertility) RELATIONSHIP WITH OTHER DISEASES One long-term study of vasectomized ♂ revealed a ↓ in mortality (RR 0.85), ↓ in mortality from cardiovascular disease (RR 0.76); after 20 years of follow-up, there was an ↑ in cancer-related mortality (RR 1.44) (N Engl J Med 1992; 326:1392oA)the 4-fold ↑ in testicular malignancy may be an epidemiologic artefact related to ↑ testicular examination; there is also a reported increased incidence of prostate carcinoma FAILURES In a large single-author series, 1.8% were failures-0.60% early overt, 1.14% technical and 0.08% late overt failures resulting in pregnancy REVERSAL Vasectomies are difficult and expensive to reverse, but may be successful if done within 10 years of the operation; 40-70% fertility is achieved with reversal operations (normal fertility is 85%); pregnancy rate in banked frozen sperm, 5%, see in vitro fertilization

vasoactive intestinal peptide VIP, see there

vasoactive substances A group of circulating substances that regulate the vascular tone, causing either vasodilation (atrial natriuretic peptide, kinins and vasoactive intestinal peptide) or vasoconstriction (angiotensin II, epinephrine and norepinephrine and vasopressin)

vasopermeability reaction PHYSIOLOGY An inflammatory response to a local increase in substances with vasomotor activity which are responsible for the egress of fluids and cells from the vascular compartment during inflamation, a response subdivided into

IMMEDIATE-TRANSIENT RESPONSE mediated by histamine, as well as leukotriene E₄, serotonin, bradykinin and others, a reaction affecting small (< 100 μm in diameter) venules, but not capillaries; during this phase, the endothelial cells contract, widening the interendothelial cell gaps

IMMEDIATE-SUSTAINED RESPONSE follows severe injury, eg burns and is associated with endothelial cell necrosis, affecting the small arterioles, capillaries and venules and

DELAYED-PROLONGED LEAKAGE begins after a delay of hours to days, representing a response to a vast array of environmental 'toxins', eg burns, bacterial toxins, UV light, and X-rays and delayed hypersensitivity reactions, which affect venules and capillaries

see Slow-reactive substances of anaphylaxis, Triple response

'vasopressin resistance' A therapeutic artefact seen in the treatment of diabetes insipidus with pitressin, due to inadequate mixing of the drug and injection only of the oily vehicle

vasospasm An abrupt and/or excess local or regional contraction of the smooth muscle of the vessels, which is implicated as a mechanism underlying amaurosis fugax, coronary artery thrombosis-negative myocardial infarction, migraine, Prinzmetal's angina, Raynaud's phenomenon, subarachnoid hematoma-related cerebral artery ischemia; occlusive vasospasm may be prevented and vasomotor tone stabilized by use of calcium-channel blockers, eg nifedipine (see N Engl J Med 1993; 329:396oA)

vasovagal syncope Neurocardiogenic syncope, see there

Note: Although the adjective vasovagal continues to be widely used, cognoscenti increasing favor the more correct term neurogenic shock; both are included for cross-reference

VATER complex VACTERYL, see there

Vav p95ᵛᵃᵛ IMMUNOLOGY A protein product of the *vav* proto-oncogene that is expressed in hematopoietic cells and contains an array of structural motifs including Src homology domains SH2/SH3 and regions of homology to protein kinase C and others; in absence of Vav, the antigen receptor-mediated proliferative responses of B and T cells in vitro is markedly attenuated (Nature 1995; 374:467, 470, 474)

VBAC Vaginal birth after cesarean section

VBPAC Vaccines and Biological Products Advisory Committee

Vd Volume of distribution, see there

VDAC Voltage-dependent anion-selective channel, see there

VDCC Voltage-dependent calcium channels, see there

V(D)J recombinase MOLECULAR BIOLOGY An enzyme that has yet to be identified, which is capable of recognizing and splicing the V (variable), J (joining) and occasionally D (diversity) gene segments responsible for antibody diversity; one contender for V(D)J recombinase gene is RAG-1 (recombinase activating gene)

V(D)J recombination Class switching A process of exon combination by which developing lymphocytes are able to generate a vast array of binding specificities from a relatively limited 'palette' of genetic information comprised of gene segments designated as variable (V), joining (J) and sometimes diversity (D) gene segments at seven different loci (μ, κ and λ for the immuno-globulin genes of B cells and α, β, γ and δ genes for T cell receptors); this tightly regulated process occurs in chronologic sequence, mediated by recombination signal sequences that are conserved among different loci and species, suggesting the existence of a single 'V(D)J recombinase'; see RAG-1

Note: The experimental work that led to the understanding of V, D, and J gene splicing to produce antibody diversity netted S Tonegawa the 1987 Nobel prize

VDRL Venereal Disease Research Laboratory test A reaginic screening test for syphilis METHOD Heat-inactivated serum is added to the VDRL antigen (a mixture of cardiolipin, lecithin, alcohol, and cholesterol) and agglutination is viewed by light microscopy at 4 minutes (the RPR or rapid plasma reagin test is a variant of the VDRL that is interpreted macroscopically at 8 minutes); reaginic tests are useful screens in early syphilis, and are virtually always positive in secondary syphilis; VDRL test is highly variable in tertiary syphilis and is negative in 40-50% of cases of neurosyphilis; FTA-ABS is positive in the serum of 95% of those with late syphilis; reaginic tests may be biological false positives in malaria (up to 90% positive), acute infections (10-30%), SLE (10-20%, the classic cause of a biological false positive VDRL test), viral hepatitis (10%), infectious mononucleosis (20%), rheumatoid arthritis (5-10%), and others including pneumococcal pneumonia, drug addiction and pregnancy

VDT Video display terminal, see there

vector An 'inactive' vehicle of transport of an agent of disease EPIDEMIOLOGY Vectors include any arthropod capable of transporting an infectous agent, in particular viruses and parasites MOLECULAR BIOLOGY A cloning vector is a segment of DNA capable of self-replication, which contains a selective marker, eg antibiotic resistance, and a site allowing cleavage by a restriction endonuclease; vectors into which DNA can be inserted for cloning are of four broad types, the choice being based on the size of DNA fragment being cloned; DNA fragments of up to 5000 base pairs in length can be inserted into bacterial plasmids; up to 20 000 bps can be inserted into bacteriophages, up to 50 000 bps (longer than the usual human gene) can be inserted into cosmids, and DNA fragments of up to 1 million bps can be inserted into YACs (yeast artificial chromosomes), which require separation by PFGE (pulsed field gel electrophoresis) (Sci & Med Nov/Dec 1994 p48) see Cosmid, Plasmid

vegan CLINICAL NUTRITION A strict vegetarian who ingests no proteins of animal origin, including meat, fish and dairy products; all vegans are at risk for vitamin B₁₂ deficiency; in addition, vegan adolescents are unlikely to meet energy requirements during the growth spurt and, in addition, may become deficient in vitamin B₆ and riboflavin; the high-fiber vegan diet may furthermore chelate calcium, zinc and iron, reducing the absorption of essential cations and trace minerals; see Pareve; Cf Lacto-ovo vegetarian

'vegetable' cell SURGICAL PATHOLOGY An enlarged cell with clear, lipid- and glycogen-laden cytoplasm, angulated borders and a small, hyperchromatic nucleus arranged in bundles and fascicles, which is highly characteristic of typical renal cell carcinomas (RCC), fancifully likened to the light microscopic appearance of vegetable cells; the other main cell type seen in RCCs is a granular, organelle-rich cell with lesser amounts of glycogen and lipid, and is often arranged in papillary clusters; a variant cell, the mitochondria-rich oncocyte, is seen in very well-differentiated RCC, which have a relatively good prognosis; Cf Clear cell (multiple entries), Hobnail cells

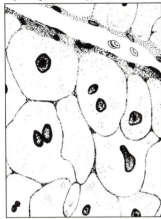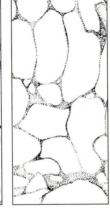

vegetable cell

vegetative state CLINICAL MEDICINE A state in which an individual is incapable of reacting to outside stimuli, which has been divided into permanent VS and persistent VS; because of the sense of hopelessness implicit in the term permanent, the latter term may be confined to use in a strictly medicolegal context (for discussion, see **N Engl J Med 1994; 330:1499**) VIROLOGY A phage phase in which various components are multiplying with the host cell, but reproduction has not begun

vehicle MOLECULAR BIOLOGY A self-replicating DNA molecule, eg a virus, plasmid, or phage that serves as a vector for insertion of a segment of DNA into a host genome PHARMACOLOGY An inert carrier for a therapeutic agent, eg water, alcohol-containing elixirs or a sweetened syrup that solubilizes a drug, facilitating its deglution; Cf Carrier, Schlepper, Vector

veiled appearance A wispy, often punctate linear radiodensity that parallels the shaft and cortex of long bones, described as typical in myositis ossificans

veiled cell IMMUNOLOGY An antigen-presenting cell of the mononuclear phagocytic system that is located in the marginal sinus of afferent lymphatics, which display IL-2 receptor when co-incubated with GM-CSF (**Immunol 1989; 68:108**) see Antigen-presenting cells, Dendritic reticular cells

velocity The rate of a body's motion with respect to time FORENSIC BALLISTICS The speed that a projectile (bullet) attains while in flight; the difference in tissue destruction between high or low velocity projectiles is likely caused by the fragmentation of the bullet itself (as in the M-16 semi-automatic weapon); see Ballistics

vena cava filter Inferior vena caval filter, see there

'venetian blind' artefact SURGICAL PATHOLOGY Parallel ridging and cracking with separation of tissues seen by light microscopy due to tissue brittleness; this artefact may be seen on frozen sections; making the differentiation

between lymphoma and lymphoid hyperplasia by light microscopy a difficult task; Cf 'Cracking' artefact

Venezuelan equine encephalitis An alphavirus infection first identified in a sick horse in Venezuela in 1938 that occurs as an epizootic infection in Central and northern South America; the equine mortality reaches 40%; most exposed humans develop flu-like symptoms; up to 4%, especially adolescents develop encephalitis with a mortality of up to 35% in younger subjects, in adults, less than 10% TREATMENT Supportive VACCINE Under development

venipuncture The puncture of a vein with a needle with the intent to either obtain blood or administer a therapeutic substance; Cf Cut-down

venom A poisonous substance produced by an insect or animal that is produced and stored in specific sites, released by biting or stinging and which is a means by which the animal defends itself or captures prey STINGING INSECTS 1) Honeybee Hyaluronidase, phospholipase A_2, melitten 2) Vespids Hyaluronidase, phospholipase A_2, antigen 5 (**N Engl J Med 1994; 331:523RV**)

venom immunotherapy A type of allergic desensitization therapy for those who are highly susceptible to hymenopteran venom; VI is begun with small doses and increased until a recommended maintenance dose is reached; the therapy may be stopped when a previously positive skin test converts to negative or when the serum venom-specific IgE is undetectable, usually after 3-5 years of therapy (**N Engl J Med 1994; 331:523RV**)

veno-occlusive disease LIVER Obliteration of the small hepatic venules, which may be linked to portal hypertension and progression to cirrhosis, which has been linked to the ingestion of herbal teas LUNG see Pulmonary veno-occlusive disease

venous hum A low-pitched hum auscultated in the neck related to jugular vein turbulence, due to an altered or more intense flow pattern mimicking the machinery murmur of patent ductus arteriosus; the venous hum may be abolished by light lateral neck pressure and may be innocent or heard in younger patients with hyperthyroidism

ventilating tubes Tympanostomy tubes, see there

ventilation scan A radionuclide study of pulmonary ventilation; in a commonly used protocol, the scan is performed after inhalation of ^{133}Xe; see Ventilation-perfusion scan

ventilation-perfusion scan Radionuclide scan of lung A radionuclide study of the ratio of pulmonary ventilation (V) to pulmonary blood flow (perfusion, Q) through the lungs; in a commonly used protocol, the scan is performed after inhalation of ^{133}Xe and IV injection of ^{99m}Tc microaggregated albumin which allows evaluation of inspiratory airflow, lung volume, presence of air trapping and adequacy of perfusion; the V/QS is used to detect pulmonary embolism; quantitative V/Q may be obtained after inhalation of ^{133}Xe and intravenous injection of ^{99m}Tc; a V/Q 'mismatch' indicates preservation of ventilation with a defect in perfusion, a finding commonly associated with pulmonary embolism Note: it is false negative in up to 12% of 'low-probability' scans (PIOPED studies; see Lung volumes, Pulmonary panel)

Note: Both terms are in active use; radionuclide scanning of the lung is more formal and generally the 'written' form; ventilation-perfusion scan is more colloquial and generally the 'spoken' form; ventilation and perfusion studies are complementary to each other and may be performed simultaneously, making the use of the terms **perfusion scan** and **ventilation scan** somewhat confusing

ventilator-induced lung injury Volutrauma* A generic term for the findings related to ventilatory support of patients with acute respiratory failure and/or ARDS, which may exacerbate already compromised pulmonary function PATHOGENESIS Ventilator-driven alveolar distention PATHOLOGY Interstitial alveolar edema, possibly related to loss of surfactant, hypoxia, ↓ lung compliance Treatment Permissive hypercapnia, see there (JAMA 1994; 272:957cecc)

*Although this term is etymologically preferable, as it 'matches' barotrauma, it appears unlikely to be integrated in the medical lexicon, given the continuing shift away from classic terminology-Author's note

ventricular assist device Cardiovascular surgery A portable, battery-powered device that assists the flow of blood while a patient is awaiting heart transplantation; the device is connected at the apex of the left ventricle and pumps the blood past the effete ventricle and aortic valve directly into the aortic arch (JAMA 1991; 265:2930n&v) Cf Artificial heart, Jarvik-7

ventricular premature beat Cardiology An electrical discharge of ventricular origin that occurs prior to the usual sinuatrial beat; simple VPBs are extremely common, and occur in ½ of normal adults monitored by EKG for 24 hours; complex VPBs, eg bigeminy, multiformity, repetitive activity, or ectopic beats early in the cycle, occur in 0.5% of normal adults, and are commonly associated with ischemia Treatment IV lidocaine, IV quinidine, propranolol, amiodarone

vernix caseosa peritonitis An infrequent complication of cesarean section that is presumed to be due to a granulomatous response to amniotic fluid that has spilled into abdominal cavity Pathology Aggregates of anucleated squames (Am J Clin Pathol 1995; 103:681)

verocytotoxin VTEC, see there

'vero' toxin Shiga neurotoxin, see there

verrucous carcinoma A variant of well-differentiated epidermoid carcinoma that is most common in the oral cavity, but also occurs in the larynx, nasal cavity, esophagus, penis, anorectal region, vulva, vagina, uterine cervix and skin, especially on the sole of the foot; most intraoral cases occur in elderly male abusers of 'smokeless' tobacco Pathology Exophytic and well-differentiated Treatment Surgical resection; radiotherapy is not indicated, as up to 30% of verrucous carcinomas treated with radiation become highly aggressive within six months; anorectal verrucous carcinoma may be similar to giant condyloma acuminatum of the penis, which is induced by HPV and comprises 5% of all penile carcinomas

vertical growth phase melanoma Dermatopathology Tumorigenic melanoma A stage in the evolution of a primary melanoma in which a cell population is 'selected' during intraepithelial growth for its capacity to grow into the dermis and form a tumor in the mesenchyma; melanoma cells in the VGP can be defined biologically, as they form permanent cell lines, produce platelet-derived growth factor, are often aneuploid, and require epidermal growth factor and insulin; see Radial growth phase melanoma

vertical integration A merger between two closely related industries that have a potentially vested interest in doing business with each, eg a merger between a manufacturer and a distributer of pharmaceuticals, as was recently approved by Eli Lilly & Co and PCS Health Systems, Inc (Am Med News 21 Nov 1994 p3)

vertical transmission Epidemiology The transmission of an infection through the placenta to the fetus, as occurs in the 'TORCH' infections, including toxoplasmosis, rubella, CMV, herpes, syphilis, as well as HIV Note: 30% of infants born to HIV-positive mothers are also infected, which can be reduced by maternal zidovudine therapy; see Horizontal transmission; Cf Hereditary transmission Genetics A virtually extinct term for the inheritance of a particular phenotype from a parent Microbiology The transovarial passage of a microorganism, eg plasmodia

vertigo A distortion of perception in which there is a sensation of movement, in particular rotational, either of the individual or of his/her surroundings; vertigo is normal in certain settings, eg on a roller coaster, but in absence of an appropriate stimulus, is a symptom strongly suggestive of a defect of the peripheral vestibular apparatus (eg Menière's disease), or an intracranial defect (eg acoustic neuroma); vertigo is often accompanied by nystagmus, and when severe nausea and vomiting Treatment—Medical If acute, diazepam, if recurrent, scopolamine, if accompanied by nausea, an antiemetic; if severe, bed rest, if recurrent, exercise Treatment-Interventional Transmastoid labyrinthectomy, vestibular nerve section, middle ear endoscopy, semicircular canal ablation, streptomycin infusion

very-high-density lipoprotein VHDL A plasma lipoprotein with a density of greater that 1.210 kg/L (US: 1.210 g/dl); VHDL is 57% protein (predominantly apoA-I and apoA-II), 21% phospholipid, 17% cholesterol and 5% triglycerides and transports cholesterol from the intestine to the liver; the larger the HDL molecule, the more efficient the lipid transport and by extension, lipolysis

Note: HDL levels are the single most important predictor of atherosclerosis-induced disease and are inversely related thereto; Cf HDL

very-low-birth-weight infant An infant weighing between 500-1500 g; these children are at extremely high risk for for neurobehavioral dysfunction and poor school performance, see table (N Engl J Med 1994; 331:753oa) see Low birth weight

VERY-LOW-BIRTHWEIGHT CHILDREN (OUTCOMES)			
BIRTHWEIGHT	≤ 750 g	750-1.5 Kg	≥ 1.5 Kg
Sample number	68	65	61
MPC score*	87	93	100
Mental retardation (IQ < 70)	21%	8%	2%
Poor cognitive function	22%	9%	2%
Poor academic skills	27%	9%	2%
Poor gross motor function	27%	9%	0%
Poor adaptive function	25%	14%	2%
Cerebral palsy	9%	6%	0%
Severe visual disability	25%	5%	2%
Hearing disability	24%	13%	3%
↓ Weight/height/head size	22/25/35%	11/5/14%	0/0/2%

*Mental Processing Composite score **N Engl J Med 1994; 331:753

very-low-density lipoprotein see VLDL

vesicular rosettes A nonspecific ultrastructural finding seen within lymphocytes, which consists of circular clusters of vesicles of undetermined significance, possibly originating from the endoplasmic reticulum, first described as characteristic of AIDS, which has subsequently been seen in Hodgkin's disease, other lymphoproliferative disorders and various benign conditions; Cf Tubular complexes

vesicular stomatitis virus An enveloped rhabdovirus with a bullet-shaped morphology and a single-stranded negative sense RNA genome that replicates in the cytoplasm of infected cells; most of those infected with VSV have been in direct contact with the oral secretions of infected livestock Clinical Fever, chills, malaise, myalgia, nausea, vomiting, pharyngitis; see Foot and mouth disease

vesicular transport A process used by eukaryotic cells to transport material from one organelle to another; a subset of components of a donor organelle is packaged into a smaller carrier vesicle that fuses with the target organelle, completing the transfer of product (Nature 1994; 369:31oa, 16n&v) see Clathrin

vesnarinone A quinolinone derivative used as an oral inotropic agent, it ↑ myocardial contractility with little effect on either myocardial oxygen consumption, or heart rate MECHANISM OF ACTION Slowing of potassium currents, ↑ intracellular sodium due to prolonged opening of sodium channels, ↑ intracellular calcium current due to mild inhibition of phosphodiesterase; vesnarinone (60 mg/day) is reported to ↓ morbidity and mortality and improve quality of life in patients with congestive heart failure; vesnarinone appears to have a narrow therapeutic range as higher doses (120 mg/day) are associated with an ↑ in mortality (N Engl J Med 1993; 329:149oA)

vest CPR Cardiopulmonary resuscitation performed using a proprietary vest to ↑ intrathoracic pressure; the vest is pneumatically cycled and applies pressure in a circumferential fashion, which contrasts to the point (sternal) pressure applied in manual CPR; vest CPR is reported to ↑ short-term survival (which may be accompanied by spontaneous return of circulation by an unknown mechanism), possibly due to ↑ aortic pressure and coronary perfusion pressure (N Engl J Med 1993; 329:762oA)

'vest-over-pants' repair A method used in surgical correction of inguinal hernias, where the fascia above the hernia is brought down over the fascia from below, effecting a two-layer closure; there is little evidence that this repair is more effective than well-apposed approximation of the fascial margins

vestibulo-ocular reflex NEUROLOGY A reflex in which a movement of the eyes is produced that is equal and opposite to the movement of the head; loss of the VOR implies vestibular disease that may occur in aminoglycoside toxicity

veto cell An immune cell that suppresses the activity of T cells capable of reacting against self MHC antigens, which derive from Thy lineage; these cells may 'veto' the activity of virtually any T cell that reacts to self surface determinants; veto activity can be found in the normal bone marrow, spleen, thymus and fetal liver, as well as in athymic nude mice; these cells provide specific suppressor activity, depressing host rejection; incubation of T-cell-depleted bone marrow with IL-2 increases veto cell activity and enhances engraftment of MHC-mismatched T-cell-depleted marrow

V_{max}FRC PULMONARY MEDICINE Length-adjusted maximum expiratory flow at functional residual capacity, a value that is believed to reflect the size of the intrapulmonary airways (N Engl J Med 1995; 332:133oA)

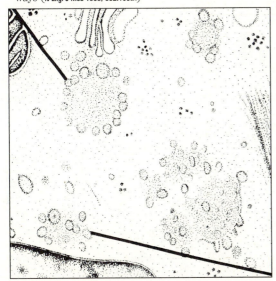

veicula rosettes

Vi antigen The capsular antigen of *Salmonella* species, especially *S typhi*, which is specifically associated with *Salmonella* virulence and which interferes with the serotyping of the 'O' antigen, the heat-stable lipopolysaccharide common to enterobacteriaceae

viability NEONATOLOGY Survival capability, see Limit of viability

viable NEONATOLOGY Capable of (extrauterine) survival, said of a fetus

vibration white finger syndrome An occupation-related, musculoskeletal disorder, in which vibrating hand-held tools, eg electric drills, jackhammers and grinders, evoke ischemia-inducing vasospasms that are virtually indistinguishable from Raynaud's phenomenon; plethysmographic studies reveal temperature-sensitive changes in blood flow, even in the absence of symptoms; with time, these subjects develop pain and numbness of the upper extremities suggestive of cervical, ulnar and median nerve entrapment

vicarious menstruation Cyclical bleeding from various sites, eg the lungs, which occurs in ♀ of reproductive age, usually from endometriosis

Victor the Wild child, see there

video consultation A facet of telemedicine in which video images are transmitted to an expert (consultant) located at a distance from the patient; see Telemedicine

video display terminal Video display unit, see there

video display unit A device containing a cathode ray tube generating a visual display, which emits both extremely- low-frequency (ELF, 45-60 Hz) and very-low-frequency (15 kHz) electromagnetic fields, the latter of which had been associated by some (very) 'soft' data with spontaneous abortion, which is either a statistical canard or due to another factor unrelated to VDTs (N Engl J Med 1991; 324:728)15% of the US workforce spends a large part of its day in front of a VDT; the potential adverse effects of VDTs are related to: 1) Irradiation by ultraviolet light and very low and extremely-low-frequency electromagnetic ELF radiation; four potential associations have been studied and not found to be significantly increased, including cataracts, reproductive disorders, facial dermatitis and epileptic reactions; for leukemia, see ELF 2) Ergonomic effects Visual (see McCullough effect) and musculoskeletal, due to posture required for typing Note: The 'Balans' type of backless chair is reported to significantly reduce lower back strain 3) Stress The psychological stress related to VDT use is thought by some workers to be more a function of the job per se than the VDT itself

Note: The effects from prolonged exposure to liquid crystal display screens as used for laptop computers have not been formerly studied

videodefecography GASTROENTEROLOGY A dynamic technique for evaluating rectoanal function in which barium is injected into the rectum and the changes that occur in response to relaxing, coughing, or straining are evaluated in 'real time' by videofluoroscopy; Cf Defecography

video electroencephalography A method for evaluating a person with a seizure disorder in which the EEG signal is amplified and and encoded by an analog system and transmitted via cable to a central station, at the same time as an analog or digital video image of the patient; video EEG allows precise analysis of seizure phenomena and provides a definitive diagnosis in 82% and can be performed in the hospital or as an ambulatory procedure at a lower cost (Medico Interamericano 1995; 14:125)

videolaryngoscopy OTOLARYNGOLOGY A procedure in which a video camera is attached to an flexible fibroendoscope to record images; the **videolaryngoscope** is used to diagnose and document (medicolegally) pathologic lesions of the larynx

'Vietnam syndrome' The psychosocial consequences of active participation in the Vietnam conflict; when compared with non-Vietnam veterans, active participants in the conflict were reported to have more depression-related complaints (4.5% vs 2.3%), anxiety (4.9% vs 3.2%) and alcohol-related problems (13.7% vs 9.2%); 15% had combat-related post-traumatic stress (2.2% had an 'event' in the month before examination), medical complaints including hearing loss, and low sperm count; see Burned-out syndrome, Post-traumatic stress disorder; Cf Gulf War syndrome

vigabatrin gamma-vinyl GABA An antiepileptic agent that is an irreversible inhibitor of GABA-transaminase A second-line antiepileptic agent that is used for convulsions or seizures that are refractory to other agents SIDE EFFECTS Somnolence, stupor, hyperkinesia, insomnia, ↑ weight, and facial edema (Medico Interamericano 1995; 14:125)

vigilance NEUROLOGY The conscious and semiconscious focusing and sustained attention to subtle sensory signals within a determined modality (eg auditory or visual), while eliminating distracting internal and external stimuli; positron emission tomography studies of humans localize the 'attention center' to the prefrontal and superior parietal cortex primarily in the right hemisphere, regardless of the modality or laterality of the stimulus (Nature 1991; 349:61)

vigorous exercise A form of exercise that is intense enough to cause sweating and/or heavy breathing/ and/or increase of heart rate to near maximum; VE is formally defined as that which requires > 6 METs* and includes brisk walking (rate of 6.5-8 km/hour or 4-5 mph) 45 minutes 5x/wk, rollerblading (2-3 hours/wk), running (rate of 9.5-11 km/hour or 6-7 mph), 3 hours/wk, swimming (laps 3 hours/wk), tennis (singles 3 hours/wk), shoveling snow; there is a graded inverse relationship between total physical activity (in particular vigorous exercise) and mortality (JAMA 1995; 273:1179) see Exercise; Cf the Zone

*MET is the resting rate of metabolism; numeric prefixes correspond to multiples thereof

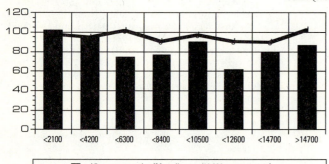

vigorous exercise

- Vigorous exercise (Mortality rate/10 000 person years)
- Non-vigorous exercise (Mortality rate/10 000 person years)

villin A 95-kD actin-binding protein of the microvilli of the small intestine, which in low calcium concentrations, cross-links actin filaments into bundles, forming a 'nucleation' center to accelerate actin polymerization

vimentin A 55-kD protein that is one of the five major intermediate filaments, which is produced by normal mesenchymal cells, including vascular endothelial and smooth muscle cells, fibroblasts, histiocytes, lymphocytes, melanocytes, chondrocytes, osteocytes, astrocytes, rarely ependymal and glomerular cells; malignant cells tend to 'forget' their lineage and thus may display more than one intermediate filament, thus co-expression of cytokeratin

and vimentin, as detected by immunoperoxidase staining, may occur in adenocarcinomas of the breast, lung, kidney, adrenal, endometrium and epithelioid sarcoma; see Brown stains, Intermediate filaments

VIN Vulvar intraepithelial neoplasm An umbrella term encompassing two clinically distinct, but histologically similar lesions 1) Carcinoma in situ (Bowen's disease) is an erythematous plaque-like lesion that may extend to the perineum and anus; most cases demonstrate HPV type 16 by in situ hybridization, 10% of which evolve toward invasive carcinoma when untreated 2) Bowenoid papulosis (bowenoid dysplasia) is characterized by solitary or multiple, often pigmented papules affecting young women, which clinically simulate verrucae and have cytologic atypia approaching that of Bowen's disease; although this lesion is also associated with HPV 16, it tends to resolve spontaneously or respond to therapies that might be considered 'homeopathic'; see Carcinoma in situ, CIN, Intraepithelial neoplasia

vinblastine A chemotherapeutic alkaloid used to treat Hodgkin's disease, leukemia, other lymphoproliferative disorders and malignancies, which specifically binds to unpolymerized tubulin, preventing the formation of microtubules of the mitotic spindle, causing the lysis of rapidly dividing cells

vinclozolin ENVIRONMENT A fungicide (figure, page 947) used to protect fruits, vegetables, and ornamental plants that blocks androgenic receptors in rats, resulting in combined demasculinization and feminization; some of vinclozolin's metabolites are 10-100-fold more potent in blocking androgen receptors (Science News 1994; 146:15)

vincristine A chemotherapeutic alkaloid used to treat leukemia and other malignancies, which like vinblastine, interrupts the mitotic spindle, causing lysis of proliferating cells

vinculin A 130-kD phosphorylated fibrous cytoskeletal protein that is present in the intercalated disks of cardiac muscle and membrane-associated plaques of smooth muscle, which binds α-actinin, paxillin, talin, tensin, and vinculin (Science 1995; 268:233) in the extracellular matrix, uniting the actin cytoskeleton and plasma membrane at the adhesion plaques; increased vinculin production is associated with ↑ phosphotyrosine levels in transformed (malignant) cells, which may explain the hallmarks of these cells, eg altered morphology, reduced actin microfilaments, loss of anchorage dependence for growth, changed mobility of cell surface, changes that may be driven by the *src* and *abl* oncogenes; see Malignancy

vinyl chloride PVC (polyvinyl chloride), see there

violin band mark ENTOMOLOGY A distinct 'spot' on the dorsal cephalothorax of *Loxosceles reclusa*, a spider of the southern US, the bite of which contains a cytotoxin causing painful blistering, necrosis and when severe, residual scarred ulcer; systemic manifestations of recluse spider bites include fever, nausea, vomiting, arthralgia and renal failure (hemoglobinuria and proteinuria), hemolysis and thrombocytopenia, which may be fatal in the very young

violin string adhesions A descriptor for the taut fibrous bands present between the anterior parietal peritoneum and the anterior aspect of the liver, typically seen in *Neisseria gonorrhoeae*-induced perihepatitis, which may be accompanied by upper right quadrant pain, fever and a hepatic friction rub; violin string adhesions may also occur in the uterine adnexae in pelvic inflammatory disease due to *Chlamydia trachomatis* as well as in fibrinous mesothelial inflammation of the pericardium, pleura and peritoneum

VIP Vasoactive intestinal polypeptide A 28-residue neuropeptide of the secretin-glucagon family that is present in the nerve fibers of smooth muscle, blood vessels and in the glands of the GI and upper respiratory tract; VIP stimulates adenylate cyclase, evoking potent vasodilation, pancreatic and intestinal secretion, inhibition of gastric acid secretion, $\uparrow$ cardiac output, glycogenolysis, bronchodilation and inhibition of macromolecule release from mucus-secreting glands; VIP deficiency may contribute to bronchial asthma, given its virtual absent in asthmatics; VIP is $\uparrow\uparrow\uparrow$ in VIPoma, a pancreatic islet G-cell tumor that is morphologically identical to other G-cell tumors; see Watery diarrhea, hypokalemia, achlorhydria (WDHA) syndrome

VIP-receptor scanning A radioisotope-based diagnostic modality based on the finding that certain tumors (GI adenocarcinomas and endocrine tumors) have high-affinity VIP (vasoactive intestinal polypeptide) receptors; after an IV bolus injection of radiolabeled (^{123}I) VIP, its distribution is evaluated using a gamma camera for planar acquisitions; VRS appears to have a greater diagnostic yield than the octreotide (^{123}I-labeled Tyr^3-octreotide) scan (N Engl J Med 1994; 331:1116OA)

vinclozin

VIPoma Pancreatic cholera syndrome(s), Verner-Morrison or WDHA syndrome A group of clinical complexes characterized by diarrhea caused by endocrine tumors of the pancreas, most commonly VIPoma (vasoactive intestinal peptide-producing pancreatic tumor); see WDHA

Note: VIPoma-induced diarrhea is a diagnosis of exclusion, given its incidence of one case/10^6/year, but should be considered when diarrhea of unknown origin with a volume of $\geq$ 1 liter/day is > than four weeks in duration and causes hypokalemia, salt and water depletion

V.I.P. 'syndrome' A very important person (V.I.P.) is anyone whose presence in a hospital, by virtue of fame, position or claim on the public interest, may substantially disrupt the normal course of patient care; often the V.I.P. wants to be treated as any other patient, but may in fact receive less than optimal emergency and critical care, as the patient management team may inappropriately alter its standard operating procedures (N Engl J Med 1988; 319:1421) see Chief 'syndrome'

viral gastroenteritis Intestinal flu A generic term for GE induced by viruses, which can take one of two clinical forms: 1) Epidemic VGE, most often caused by the Norwalk agent or Norwalk-like viruses CLINICAL Nausea, vomiting, diarrhea, abdominal discomfort, anorexia, headache, malaise, low-grade fever; it is rarely requires hospitalization, but may be contribute to death in the elderly 2) Sporadic VGE, is often caused by rotaviruses and differs from the epidemic form of VGE in that it most commonly affects children under the age of two, and evokes a wide range of responses, ranging from subclinical infection to a mild form of the GE, as with the epidemic form, to a severe, potentially life-threatening dehydrating disease (JAMA 1993; 269:627GR-NIH)

viral hemorrhagic fever syndrome(s) A group of clinical complexes caused by various viruses, including Filoviridae, eg Ebola and Marburg agents, Arenaviridae, eg Junin and Lassa agents, Togaviridae, including Flaviviridae, eg Dengue, Omsk and yellow fever agents, and Bunyaviridae, Congo-Crimean, Hantaan virus and Rift Valley fever agents Vectors Arthropods, either ticks or mosquitoes, eg Dengue and Rift Valley and yellow fevers and environmental contaminants, eg Argentine, Bolivian, Ebola, Lassa and Marburg hemorrhagic fevers and hemorrhagic fever with renal syndrome CLINICAL Incubation 3 days to 3 weeks, followed by headache, myalgias, dysphagia, vomiting, diarrhea, abdominal and/or chest pain, pharyngitis, conjunctivitis, cervical lymphadenopathy, macular rashes and shock LABORATORY Leukopenia and/or thrombocytopenia, proteinuria, disseminated intravascular coagulation

viral transduction GENE THERAPY A method of gene insertion in which modified virus infects a cell of interest, introducing viral genome containing the foreign genes (Bio/Technology 1995; 13:222) Cf Physical transfection

virally induced cancer A generic term for a malignancy induced by either DNA or RNA viruses, which include HBV (liver cell carcinoma), human papilloma virus (squamous cell carcinoma of the uterine cervix), HTLV-I (adult T-cell leukemia), and EBV (Burkitt's lymphoma-Africa, nasopharyngeal carcinoma-China); vaccines, eg hepatitis B vaccine are of interest in efforts to prevent these malignancies, but are as yet unproven or unavailable (Nature 1994; 368:495N&V)

'virgin birth' A term referring to a child who is born out of wedlock to a woman through artificial insemination by an often anonymous donor (Nature 1991; 350:96ed) see Artificial reproduction

virgin's disease Iron-deficiency anemia, formerly chlorosis

virilism The presence of $\male$ secondary sexual characteristics in a $\female$, including hirsutism, receding frontal hairline, masculine body habitus, deepening of the voice, $\uparrow$ sebaceous gland secretion, and clitoral enlargement

virilization Physical changes in the female resulting from androgen excess which include hirsutism, temporal balding, deepened voice, acne, enlarged clitoris and clitoral index (the ratio between the sagittal and transverse diameters of the clitoris) The androgen excess may be 1) Adrenal, due to Cushing's syndrome, congenital enzyme deficiency, eg 11– or 21–hydroxylase deficiency or neoplasia, either benign or malignant or 2) Ovarian, due to hyperplasia, eg polycystic ovaries or tumors, eg arrhenoblastoma, steroid cell tumors or gynandroblastoma; Cf Hermaphroditism, Intersex, Precocious puberty

virion A complete virus, the genome of which is encapsulated in a protein coat

virocytes Turk cells Atypical, enlarged lymphocytes with foamy cytoplasm filled with scattered small vacuoles in a moderately to deeply basophilic cytoplasm; the nuclear chromatin is coarse but less so than that of normal lymphocytes, with a sharp chromatin and parachromatin distinction and accelerated DNA synthesis; the term virocyte is appropriate when lymphocytes are reacting to viral infections (hepatitis, herpes zoster, herpes simplex, infectious mononucleosis, mumps, roseola infantum, rubeola, rubella and others)

Note: Morphologically identical 'reactive' lymphocytes occur in other infections (diphtheria, malaria, rickettsial infections, scarlet fever, syphilis, tuberculosis, typhus), as a result of drugs and toxins (phenytoin, barbiturates, butazolidine, lead intoxication) and other causes (post-surgery, exposure to ionizing radiation, serum sickness, agranulocytosis, acute MI, ulcerative colitis, dermatitis herpetiformis, pemphigus vulgaris)

viroid Infectious RNA A 100-kD ($\pm$ 300 base pairs) subviral infectious particle composed of a small circular segment of single-stranded RNA that causes disease in higher plants; viroids are postulated to represent 'escaped' introns, with which they bear a degree of sequence 'homology'; Cf Prion

virokine Any of a family of virally encoded proteins that actively mediate the evasion of the host immune defenses; virokines are structurally similar to complement control proteins, or to cytokine-binding in conjunction with brightfield, fluorescence and other optical techniques

virosome A semisynthetic complex homogenate derived from nucleic acid-free viral particles including membrane proteins and lipids that is prepared with lecithin and diacetyl phosphate and dialyzed

virosome vaccine A 'designer' vaccine for influenza in which hemagglutinin is extracted from the influenza virus and incorporated into the membrane of liposomes composed of phosphatidylcholine and phosphatidylethanolamine; the vaccine appears to be as effective as the commercial whole-virus vaccine (Lancet 1994; 344:160)

virtual critter COMPUTERS A small mobile piece of computer software that can send itself across a computer network and perform a task on a remote machine; unlike an 'agent', which is a passive, ie performs only those tasks for which it has been specifically instructed, a virtual animal can initiate its own action within guidelines written by the programmer (Sci Am 1995; 272/2:28) Cf Agent

VCs being designed include the virtual cockroach (that 'scurries' across a hard disk disposing of old files), virtual bee (that 'buzzes' around the network looking for rich sources of information), the virtual Doberman (that 'nabs' electronic intruders)

virtual memory A programming technique that allows the programmer to use memory external to the CPU (eg the hard drive) as as an extension of RAM (random access memory)

virtual physician A nebulous and at present hypothetical inhabitant of the world of 'cybermedicine', who 'lives' in the Information Superhighway as an entity that provides

---

VIRULENCE FACTORS-BACTERIA

EXOTOXINS

Enzymatic toxins, eg proteases

Pore-forming toxins, eg RTX family

ADHESION MOLECULES

P pilus, eg in *Escherichia coli*

Type IV pili, eg in *Vibrio cholera*

Non-pilus adhesins, eg in streptococci

OTHERS

Invasins, eg in *Yersinia enterocolitica*

'Host-avoidance' factors, eg capsule, enzymes

Immune avoidance factors, eg antigenic variation

Science & Medicine 1995; 2/3:16

---

at any time of the day information on a person's disease, types, cost-effectiveness, and outcomes of various diagnostic modalities and therapeutic options (N Engl J Med 1995; 332:1099c)

Note: There is legitimate concern by physicians that the VP reduces the practice of medicine to the crass role of a consumer-provider relationship

virulence factor MICROBIOLOGY A generic term for those factors produced by microorganisms (usually understood to be bacteria) that help the 'bug' to successfully evade host defenses (Science & Medicine 1995; 2/3:16)

virulence gene MOLECULAR BIOLOGY A generic term for a gene that appears to coordinate the expression of many other genes in response to environmental conditions (temperatures, osmolarity, and pH), eg the *toxR* gene of *Vibrio cholerae* (which controls 14 other *V cholerae* genes); the agr gene of *Staphylococcus aureus* (which controls expression of 12 different proteins) and the phoP regulatory locus in *Salmonella typhi*

virus A small obligatorily intracellular, potentially infec-

tious agent that ranges in size from 10^6 daltons for the small Parvoviridae to 200×10^6 for Poxviridae; viral nucleic acid is single- or double-stranded, either DNA or RNA (classification, table) and is closed in a circle or opened and linear; viral nucleic acid is packaged within a protein coat (capsid) composed of a few distinct types of protein, and most have a helical or icosahedral symmetry; some viruses have a lipid envelope which, as in the case of the influenzae virus may be 'studded' with viral proteins, including hemagglutinin and neuraminidase; viruses may be specifically identified by incubating them within specific 'host' cells and identifying the chacteristic cytopathic effects that each virus induces in the host cells; these cells include diploid fibroblasts (CMV, varicella-zoster, rhinoviridae), rhesus monkey kidney (influenza, parainfluenza, mumps, coxsackievirus and echovirus), human embryonic kidney (herpesvirus, varicella), human foreskin (CMV, HIV) and African green monkey kidney (for detecting rubella-induced 'interference' of cytopathic effects); inclusion bodies may occur in virally-infected cells; DNA

CLASSIFICATION OF VIRUSES

CLASS I Double-stranded DNA is transcribed into plus-stranded mRNA, then translated into a protein, a flow of genetic information identical to Watson and Crick's 'central dogma'

CLASS II Single, plus-stranded DNA generates double-stranded DNA, then transcribed into plus-stranded mRNA and translated into a protein

CLASS III Double-stranded RNA is transcribed into a plus-stranded mRNA, then translated into a protein

CLASS IV Single, plus-stranded RNA is transcribed into minus-stranded RNA, then transcribed into plus-stranded mRNA and translated into a protein

CLASS V Single, minus-stranded RNA is transcribed into a plus-stranded mRNA, then translated into a protein

CLASS VI Single, plus-stranded RNA is transcribed into minus-stranded DNA, which is transcribed to form a double-stranded DNA molecule that transcribes into a plus-stranded mRNA, then translated into a protein

---

viruses often induce cytoplasmic, while those of RNA viruses are often intranuclear MODE OF ACTION Viruses penetrate the host cells by using specific host receptors, including CMV binding to β_2-microglobulin, EBV binding to C3d receptor (CR2), rabies to the acetylcholine receptor, vaccinia virus to the epidermal growth factor receptor and HIV-1 to CD4 with its gp120 glycoprotein; see Cytomegalovirus, Cytopathic effect, Epstein-Barr virus, Herpesvirus, HIV-1, HIV-2, HTLV-I, HTLV-II, Retrovirus; Cf Prion

virus-associated hemophagocytic syndrome A florid reactive hemophagocytic condition described in both immunocompromised (♂:♀ ratio, 1:1) and non-immunocompromised (♂:♀ ratio, 4:1) subjects, most common in a background of herpetic infections, including CMV, EBV and herpesvirus that may occur in infections by adenovirus, rubella, as well as brucellosis, candidiasis, leishmaniasis, tuberculosis, salmonellosis, and has been described in graft-versus-host disease and hemolytic anemia CLINICAL Hepatosplenomegaly, lymphadenopathy, pulmonary infiltrates, pancytopenia (with a depleted bone marrow), skin rash DDx Lymphoma, malignant histiocytosis, sinus histiocytosis with massive lymphadenopathy, lymphomatoid granulomatosis

virus-like particle CLINICAL THERAPEUTICS A drug delivery system composed of self-assembling proteins encoded by the Ty gene of yeasts; when another gene is fused into the

Ty gene, the transfected yeasts produce a hybrid protein that assembles itself into VLPs, bearing antigens on the surface that are encoded by the inserted gene; VLPs have potential for vaccine delivery and are in protocol for delivering HIV's p24 protein with the hope of eliciting protective anti-HIV antibodies

vis-a-tergo CARDIOLOGY A term referring to the force driving the venous return of peripheral, which is supplied by the left ventricle; by the time the blood has passed through the capillary bed, its pressure, the vis-a-tergo, has been reduced to 15mm Hg

visible light transmittance OCCUPATIONAL SAFETY The amount of light that is allowed to pass though an eye protection device to the retina; in humans, the perception of light occurs between 400 and 780 nm; the peak sensitivity to light occurs at 550-620 and the peak shifts according to whether the eye light or dark adapted; the greater the amount of light that the protective device allows, the greater is the VLT; eyewear that reduces the light at the region of peak sensitivity reduces the visual acuity and has a low VLT (Biophotonics Intl 1995; 2/2:26)

the Visible Man A 3-D computer-generated 'cadaver' that was created from thousands of images of a human body donated to science, collected with state-of-the-art photographic and imaging (CT, MRI) techniques; the VM project was sponsored by the US National Library of Medicine at a cost of $4 million* and consists of 15 gigabytes of information derived from 1800 one mm in thickness physical 'slices' of the cadaver; VM's data can be reconstructed and rotated in space, viewed in any plane and 'dissected' (RT Image 30 Jan 1995) Cf VOXEL-MAN

*Which includes VM's wife, the Visible Woman, to be completed in 1996

visual analogue scale PSYCHOLOGY A device used to evaluate changes over time when treating the symptoms of a mood disturbance; the VAS consists of a simple 100 mm scale on which the subject indicates his/her symptoms, eg for tension, irritability, and dysphoria, where 0 mm indicates no symptoms and 100 mm corresponds to the 'max' (N Engl J Med 1995; 332:1529QAD)

visual display terminal Video display terminal, see there

vitalism A philosophical stance, which is unprovable by currently available techniques, that animal functions are dependent on a certain vital force that is distinct from physically measurable forces

vitamin Any of a number of organic accessory factors present in foods in addition to the basic components of carbohydrates, fats, proteins, minerals, water and fiber, which are necessary in minimal or trace amounts (daily requirements of individual vitamins are measured in milligram to microgram quantities), as the body either does not produce them or does so in minute quantities; vitamins are the most commonly abused substances among the lay, vying with laxatives as a form of inappropriate self-medication; water-soluble vitamins are reasonably well-tolerated as they are easily excreted, while the lipid soluble vitamins accumulate in adipose tissue and have significant hepatotoxic potential Note: Lipid-soluble vitamins A, D, E and K and water-soluble vitamins B_1, B_2, B_6, B_{12} and C are valid and accepted terms; in contrast, a vast array of pseudovitamins have appeared on the shelves of 'health food' emporia that are delineated in this work under 'Vitamins'; Cf Chemoprevention, Pseudo-vitamin

'vitamins' A family of substances or pseudovitamins that may be obtained in some 'natural food' stores, which are 1) True vitamins, but not in humans 2) Substances that were first described as vitamins, but no longer widely regarded as such and 3) 'Factors' in the blood, exotic vegetables and fruits, or minerals that have been termed 'vitamins' by various persons Glossary (table); see also Pseudovitamins

vitamin A Retinol, carotene A generic term for all β-

VITAMINS'

VITAMIN B_3 Obsolete for pantothenic acid

VITAMIN B_4 An ill-defined 'factor', of dubious validity, isolated from yeast or liver, described as alleviating myasthenia in experimental animals; vitamin B_4 'deficiency' responds to a variety of agents, including adenine, arginine, cystine, glycine and thiamine

VITAMIN B_5 Obsolete for nicotinic acid (niacin) and nicotinamide

VITAMIN B_7 Carnitine (permeability factor)

VITAMIN B_8 Adenylic acid (a nucleotide)

VITAMIN B_{10} A growth and feathering promoter in chickens, considered a pseudovitamin, corresponding to a mixture of folic acid and vitamin B_{12}

VITAMIN B_{11} A growth and feathering promotor of chickens, similar or identical to Vitamin B_{10} factor see Pseudovitamin

VITAMIN B_{13} Orotic acid, an intermediate in pyrimidine metabolism and considered a pseudovitamin

VITAMIN B_{15} Pangamate, a pseudovitamin with no known effects

VITAMIN B_{17} A toxic substance claimed without evidence to be effective in treating malignancy; see Amygdalin, Laetrile

VITAMIN B_c Folic acid

VITAMIN B_p A factor that treats perosis in chicks that respond to a mixture of choline and manganese

VITAMIN B_t A substance promoting insect growth corresponding to carnitine

VITAMIN B_w Biotin

VITAMIN B_x para-aminobenzoic acid

VITAMIN C_2 Bioflavinoids, substances with activities that partially overlap those of true vitamin C

VITAMIN F Obsolete for linoleic acid, an essential fatty acid

VITAMIN G Obsolete for riboflavin

VITAMIN GH_3 see Gerovital

VITAMIN H Biotin A water-soluble factor with an uncertain role as a vitamin, which is a co-factor in enzymes catalyzing carboxylation reactions, eg pyruvate carboxylase and acetyl CoA carboxylase; biotin-deficiency is uncommon

VITAMIN H_3 see Gerovital

VITAMIN I Synonym for carnitine or vitamin B_7

VITAMIN J Synonym for bioflavinoids or vitamin C_2

VITAMIN L_1 Anthranilic acid, a liver 'factor' thought to be necessary for lactation

VITAMIN L_2 Adenylthiomethylpentose, a yeast 'factor' thought to be necessary for lactation

VITAMIN M Folic acid

VITAMIN N A preparation from the brain or stomach, which was described as being anticarcinogenic

VITAMIN P Synonym for bioflavinoids or vitamin C_2

VITAMIN PP Obsolete for nicotinic acid

VITAMIN P_4 Troxerutin see Pseudovitamins

VITAMIN R A folic acid-related compound that promotes growth in bacteria

VITAMIN S A streptogenin-related protein that promotes growth in chicks

VITAMIN T A mixture of amino acids, DNA nucleotides, folacin and vitamin B_{12} that promotes growth and wound-healing in yeasts and insects

VITAMIN U Methylsulfonium salts of methionine, derived from cabbage juice, claimed to heal peptic ulceration

VITAMIN V A tissue 'factor' composed of NAD+ and NADH, which promotes bacterial growth

ionone derivatives that exhibit the biological activity of trans-retinol; these fat-soluble molecules are required for monosaccharide transport in glycoprotein synthesis, and for maintaining mucosal epithelium (of oral cavity, respiratory and urinary tracts; vitamin A is stored in the stellate cells of the liver, as well as the intestine, kidney, heart, blood vessels and gonads; after oxidation to retinoic acid, it diffuses into the nucleus, binds to a specific nuclear receptor and interacts with a 'responsive element', a DNA sequence that regulates the target genes; vitamin A is critical for fetal development, differentiation, cell proliferation and vision; empirical therapy in asymptomatic children results in two-fold ↓ in childhood mortality from diarrhea, convulsions and infection-related symptoms; vitamin A is also critical in the production of rhodopsin; *'the term vitamin A refers to a combination of preformed vitamin A (retinol, retinyl esters, and related compounds) and carotenoids with provitamin activity'*; it is thought that vitamin A supplements reduce the risk of breast cancer only in those women whose diets are low in vitamin A ab initio; vitamins C and E are not protective against breast cancer (**N Engl J Med 1993; 329:234OA**)

vitamin A deficiency Night blindness, keratomalacia, ↑ in genitourinary tract and nasopharyngeal infections, xerophthalmia

vitamin A embryopathy A condition induced by in utero exposure to vitamin A analogs, which may be associated with cardiovascular (ventricular septal, aortic arch and conotruncal) defects, external ear deformity, cleft palate, micrognathia and CNS malformations; see Category X drugs, Isoretinoin

vitamin B$_6$-dependency syndromes A group of functional or structural enzyme defects that respond to a massive excess (50-100-fold greater than minimum daily requirements) of pyridoxine; the vitamin B$_6$-dependency syndromes are heterogeneous in nature, and include vitamin B$_6$-dependent convulsions, vitamin B$_6$-responsive anemia, xanthurenic aciduria, cystathioninuria, homocystinuria and may be due to a defective structure of the apoenzyme, its coenzyme binding site or some aspect of coenzyme synthesis CLINICAL Predominantly neurological disease including mental retardation, psychiatric symptoms, seizures, convulsions, ataxia, spasticity and peripheral neuropathy TREATMENT Neonates respond well to early therapy

vitamin B$_6$-dependent streptococci MICROBIOLOGY Thiol-dependent, satelliting or nutritionally variant streptococci, which comprise 5-6% of all streptococci that may cause 'culture-negative' bacterial endocarditis; culture media supplemented with pyridoxal or L-cysteine support growth of these organisms and such special media when culturing blood from patients suspected of having a streptococcal endocarditis

vitamin D-dependent rickets Pseudovitamin D resistant rickets An AR [MIM 264700] disorder of bone and calcium metabolism characterized by the signs and symptoms of rickets, hypocalcemia, low-to-normal plasma phosphate, and increased parathyroid hormone; the disease is subdivided into type I Defective (25-hydroxy-cholecalciferol 1-α-hydroxylase) that converts 25-(OH)- to 1,25-(OH)$_2$ vitamin D, and which responds to exogenous 1,25-(OH)$_2$ vitamin D therapy and type II Associated with end organ defects of renal tubules, intestinal mucosa and bone, which is refractory to therapy on page 2497 of IDM

to reduce the risk (RR ± 0.61 after relevent adjustments) of coronary heart disease (**N Engl J Med 1993; 328:1444OA, 1450OA**)

vitamin E deficiency A condition that may result from chronic fat malabsorption, as occurs in cystic fibrosis, but rarely causes clinical disease in humans, including spinocerebellar degeneration, progressive gait ataxia, loss of proprioception, incoordination, dysarthria, ophthalmoplegia, pigmentary retinopathy, generalized muscle weakness, superficial sensory loss, accompanied by chronic liver disease; pharmacologic doses of vitamin E in the elderly are reported to boost the immune system, increasing lymphokine and antibody production, mitogenic response and suppress prostaglandin production; dietary vitamin E supplementation is thought by some workers to reduce the risk for coronary artery disease, cancer and stress Note: Vitamin E deficiency was first associated with testicular atrophy in the male rat, leading to its intermittent abuse as a male 'sexual tonic'

vitamin K

vitamin K A generic term for the fat-soluble vitamins (K$_1$, K$_2$, K$_3$) that are required for the hepatic synthesis of prothrombin and coagulant factors VII, IX, and X) 2-methyl-1,4 naphthoquinone and its derivatives, which have anti-hemorrhagic activity

vitamin K-dependent proteins A group of coagulation factor proenzymes (factors II, VII, IX and X) that are produced in the liver, which contain multiple residues of γ-carboxyglutamic acid, an amino acid produced by the post-translational action of a vitamin K-dependent γ-carboxylase on certain glutamyl residues; four other proteins bear γ-carboxyglutamic acid and have been designated proteins C, S, Z and M; while M is poorly characterized, proteins C, S, and Z have amino-terminal homology with prothrombin; VKDPs also have another unusual amino acid, β aspartic acid, currently of unknown function

vitronectin Epibolin, protein S, serum spreading factor A 65-kD glycoprotein with serum levels of 20 mg/L that mediates cell adhesion and interacts with proteins of the complement, coagulation and fibrinolytic cascade; vitronectin colocalizes with fibronectin in the basement membrane in proliferative vitreoretinopathy and may be etiologically linked thereto

vivisection RESEARCH The cutting open of a living animal for the purposes of experimentation; see Autopsy; Cf Animal rights activism, Sacrifice

VLA proteins Integrins, see there

VLA receptors A group of cell-surface receptors which belong to the integrin receptor superfamily, characterized by heterodimeric α and β transmembrane chains with a VLA-binding region at the arginine-glycine-aspartamine binding region; the VLA receptors are found predominantly on T cells and bind to laminin and fibronectin

VLCD Very-low-calorie diet, see Diet

VLDL Very-low-density lipoprotein A plasma lipoprotein that has a density of 0.950-1.006 kg/L (US: 0.950-1.006 g/dl); VLDL is 6-10% protein (apoB-100 and apoC, with

vitamin E

vitamin E α-Tocopherol A family (basic structure, figure, above) of antioxidant that stabilizes unsaturated lipids, preventing autoxidation, eg peroxidative decomposition of membrane lipids and enzyme inactivation, as well as protecting against chemical toxins; vitamin E is a potent lipid-soluble antioxidant carried in LDL which inhibits smooth muscle proliferation in vitro, and in vivo increases the resistance to oxidation; source vegetable oil; reported

some apoE), 15-20% phospholipid, 20-30% cholesterol and 45-65% triglycerides; VLDL is composed of endogenous triglycerides of hepatic origin

VLIA Virus-like infectious agent A mycoplasma identified at the Armed Forces Institute of Pathology that may be synergistic with HIV-1, exacerbate immunodeficiency; all four monkeys inoculated with VLIA developed low-grade fever and died in 9 months; the agent has been designated '*Mycoplasma incognitus*', although it is probably a strain of *M fermentans*; if the early work survives the scrutiny of research in progress, it is possible that a percentage of AIDS patients may partially respond to antibiotics, a therapy that is effective for treating *Mycoplasma* infections

VLP Virus-like particles

VLT Visible light transmittance, see there

VNTR Variable number of tandem repeats MOLECULAR BIOLOGY Most of the 400 thus far identified polymorphic DNA markers have only two alleles and are thus uninformative for analysis of genetic linkage in families; some of these markers have loci that respond to restriction endonuclease cleavage by producing fragments of different lengths (restriction fragment length polymorphism, see RFLP); this polymorphism is due to tandem repeated segments of oligonucleotide sequences; Cf Lod score analysis

vog A regional term for smog of volcanic origin, which in the Hawaiian islands is the result of sulfur compounds (in particular SO_2) produced by the active volcano, Kilauea (Science News May 6 1995, p282)

Vogt-Koyanagi-Harada syndrome An autoimmune condition characterized by posterior uveitis with a choroidal infiltrate, and exudative serous retinopathy, which is often associated with meningeal irritation and cranial neuropathy, tinnitus, deafness (N Engl J Med 1992; 326:1762CPC)

voice mail A telephone communication system with magnetic storage 'space' that allows one to leave spoken messages; Cf E-mail

voice recognition ANCILLARY MEDICAL SERVICES The identification and processing of voice-dictated material, eg radiology and pathology reports, made possible by advanced software design and a phonetic acoustic analyzer card on a workstation in a computer network; as the still-evolving VR technology matures, human-based dictating services will be used less frequently (MLO April 1995)

void volume Outer volume INSTRUMENTATION The first passage of fluid obtained in protein separation by gel filtration; the VV contains the early 'wash' through the column, usually containing the larger proteins that are not retained by the agarose beads

Note: In gel filtration chromatography, a column is packed with Sephadex or agarose beads that are rated according to pore size, which determines the size of the molecule that will pass through or be retained by a column

volatile organic compounds A family of toxic air pollutants that are of public health concern given their widespread presence in the atmosphere; VOCs, eg dichloromethane, tetrachloroethylene, trichloroethane, and others are released from chemical dumps, landfills, industry, chemical spills, automobile and rocket exhausts, and can be identified in the 50-400 ppb (parts per billion) range by FTIR (Fourier transform infrared) spectroscopy, which can be ued for on-site air pollution analysis (American Laboratory, August 1993)

volcano lesion Mushroom lesion, see there

vole 'clock' PALEOANTHROPOLOGY A signal evolutional change in watervoles that occurred an estimated 500 000 years ago from the early *Mimomys savini*, whose molars have roots and the extant *Arvicola terrestris*, whose molars do not; the vole clock serves as a chronological landmark for dating paleoanthropologic findings (Nature 1994;

369:275N&V) see Boxgrove

volitional collapse Loss of the 'will to live' or volition; Cf Todeserwartung

voltage clamp experiment Patch-clamp experiment, see there

voltage-dependent anion-selective channel A class of transmembrane proteins that form aqueous pores in cell membranes that open or close in response to changes in transmembrane voltage, changing the ionic permeability of the membrane; VDACs are present in membranes of neurons, muscle and other cells (Science 1990; 247:1233); see Porins

voltage-dependent calcium channels PHYSIOLOGY Transmembrane proteins that act as ion channels and are present in all excitable cell membranes, which are closed at normal negative resting membrane potentials (completely closed at -70mV) and 'gated' by small changes in membrane potential (membrane depolarization) into open (completely opened at +20mV), calcium-permeable states of varying duration, a transition requiring 1-2 milliseconds that can be examined with the patch-clamp technique; VDCCs demonstrate tissue variability and different responses to ligands, eg conotoxins and nifedipine (Nature 1991; 350:398); VDCCs modulate synaptic plasticity, oscillatory behavior, and rhythmic firing in certain brain regions, eg hippocampus, and are immobile as determined by photobleaching technique; selective regulation of VDCC immobilization may be critical in determining neuronal firing patterns; see Ion channel

volume of distribution V_d CLINICAL PHARMACOLOGY A calculated value used to estimate the 'pull' that a storage tissue has on drugs in the circulation; lipotropic drugs have V_d of many liters, while high-molecular-weight substances stay within the blood vessels; the V_d is decreased with valproic acid, normal with lithium, phenobarbital and chloramphenicol and increased with lidocaine, procainamide and thiopental; see Apparent volume of distribution, Therapeutic drug monitoring

volume imaging MRI Simultaneous volume imaging An imaging technique in which the signals are gathered from the whole object at one time, with appropriate encoding of pulse/gradient sequences to encode the positions of the spins; in principle, many sequential plane images can be generalized to volume imaging ADVANTAGE Improvement of signal-to-noise ratio by including the signal from the whole object at once and any plane may be subsequently generated, including any oblique projection desired DISADVANTAGE The image reconstruction takes longer and the computations are more complex; see Magnetic resonance imaging

volume learning A model that explains memory based on the diffusion of nitric oxide (and presumably other diffusion 'messengers') over neural connections, contributing to memory formation and the spatial organization of the brain during embryonic development; these effects from nitric oxide's ability to dilate blood vessels and enhance neural connections (Sci Am 1994; 270/5:16); Cf Hebbian model of learning

volume-outcome analysis The analysis of a procedure's success rate based on the number of procedures performed (N Engl J Med 1992; 327:1220SA)

volume rendering BIOCOMPUTING The conversion of a series of two dimensional images, eg those produced in spiral CT into 3-D by means of software extrapolation that fills in the spaces between the slices; VR allows the viewer to manipulation the image of a lesion by 'subtracting' the nonrelevant 'noise', and is of particular use in evaluating intracranial masses or vascular lesions, eg berry aneurysms, which are currently identified by angiography

(Biophotonics Intl 1995; 2/2:26)

voluntary abortion Elective abortion‡

voluntary sector The sum of all the organizations and agencies that are neither private (for profit) nor public (government-sponsored) sectors; this 'third' sector is comprised of non-profit and charitable organizations and philanthropies; see Howard Hughes Medical Institute, Imperial Cancer Research Fund

voluntary hospital Community hospital, see there

von Economo encephalitis Encephalitis lethargica A disease of historical interest, which caused a major global pandemic after World War I, most prominently affecting young adults, of presumed viral origin CLINICAL Ophthalmoplegia, headache, dizziness, fatigue, confusional psychosis, reversed sleep-wake pattern, hypersomnolence (a small subgroup experienced hyperactivity), focal rigidity evolving to complete parkinsonism PATHOLOGY Congestion, perivascular mononuclear cell cuffing, and degeneration of the CNS

von Hippel-Lindau disease A congenital AD [MIM 193300] congenital condition characterized by the presence of retinal angioma, hemangioblastoma of the CNS, renal cysts and carcinoma, pheochromocytoma, pancreatic cysts, polycythemia secondary to increased production of erythropoietin, epididymal cystadenoma (N Engl J Med 1993; 329:1531oa)

von Willebrand factor A large (> 20 x 10^6 daltons) multimeric molecule composed of multiple circa 200-kD monomers, which is synthesized by vascular endothelium, megakaryocytes and platelets; hemostatic efficiency is related to the size of the multimers

FACTOR VIII:C The classic hemophilia A protein

FACTOR VIII:AG The antigen expressed in hemophilia A protein

FACTOR VIII R:AG The antigenic expression of vW protein

FACTOR VIII R:RCo The ristocetin cofactor

Note: von Willebrand's disease is an AD condition, the defective proteins of which are defined by SDS gel electrophoresis; the relative rarity of von Willebrand's disease and the variability of the many multimeric proteins that may be deranged in this condition led one author to query whether this was merely a 'tempest in a teapot', with little clinical significance; see Rocket electrophoresis

voodoo death A precipitous death related to acute psychogenic stress, possibly due to an exaggerated autonomic nervous response to a frightening culturally ingrained event(s), triggering a fatal dysrhythmia; the voodoo cult is practiced in Africa, Brazil, and Haiti and a typical ceremony has two or more hours of pounding rhythms and incantations by the priests; this, in concert with the relevant cultural associations of the participant, act to produce hysterical trances, seizures or twilight states and chronic psychosomatic symptoms which may trigger fatal cardiac dysrhythmia; see Culture-bound syndrome, SUND

VOR Vestibulo-ocular reflex, see there

VOXEL-MAN A 3-D computer-generated 'cadaver' that was created from thousands of images of a human body donated to science, collected with state-of-the-art photographic and imaging (CT, MRI) techniques; the VM project was sponsored by the US National Library of Medicine at a cost of $4 million* and consists of 15 gigabytes of informa-

tion derived from 1800 one mm in thickness physical 'slices' of the cadaver; VM's data can be reconstructed and rotated in space, viewed in any plane and 'dissected' (RT Image 30 Jan 1995) Cf Visual Man

voyeurism Scoptophilia, Peeping Tom syndrome PSYCHIATRY Intense sexually arousing fantasies involving the act of observing unsuspecting person(s) who are naked or engaged in sexual activity 532 in DSM-IV; see Paraphilia, Sexual deviancy

VP16 A HSV-1 protein that is a specific and potent activator of transcription of intermediate-to-early viral genes (Science 1991; 251:87); see Etoposide

VPB hypothesis CARDIOLOGY A widely held posit that the presence of advanced grades[1] of ventricular premature beats[2] (VPBs) are predictors of increased risk of sudden cardiac death

[1]Grade 4 = Repetitive VPBs (salvos of 3+ or ventricular tachycardia) Grade 5 = Early cycle VPBs (R-on-T phenomenon) [2]see there

Vpr An HIV gene that encodes a protein that stimulates latent HIV-infected cells to proliferate; anti-Vpr protein antibodies may be of use to maintain HIV-infected cells in a latent (ie nonproliferating) state (New York Times 8 Nov 1994; C3)

V/Q scan Ventilation/perfusion scan, see there

VRG vaccine Vaccinia rabies glycoprotein vaccine An oral antirabies vaccine produced by recombinant DNA that is currently being used in Europe to rid wild animals, in particular red foxes, of rabies; the route of administration is via air-dropped vaccinated meat (New York Times 5 July 1994; C1) see Negri bodies, Rabies

VSD Ventricular septal defect, also virtually safe dose

V-shaped scar A sharply angulated fibrotic scar on the renal cortical surface, often due to bacterial infection and cortical abscess formation; Cf Rat-bitten kidneys

VTEC Verocytotoxin-producing *Escherichia coli* A serotype of *E coli* that produces verocytotoxin, a toxin similar to that produced by *Shigella dysenteriae* type 1; VTECs include *E coli* O157:H7, O4, O5, O26, O111, O125 and O145; two types of verocytotoxin have been isolated from *E coli* O157:H7, both of which are protein inhibitors; VT1 is homologous to the Shiga toxin except for a single acid substitution in the A subunit; VT2 is 60% homologous to Shiga toxin and shares the same intestinal cell receptor, globotriosylceramide

Vulcan nerve pinch OCCUPATIONAL MEDICINE An ill-conceived keyboard command, the execution of which requires the user to contort the hands in an uncomfortale position (B Pfaffenberger, Computer User's Dictionary, 4th ed, Que Corp, Indianapolis)

The term derives from the first Star Trek television series in which a Vulcan (Mr Spock, played by L Nimoy) would immobilize a person by pinching the neurovascular bundle in the neck

VX-478 AIDS An inhibitor of HIV-1 protease that is in phase I* trials and may ↓ viral load when administered to HIV-infected individuals (Bio/Technology 1995; 13:206)

*Which determine drug safety and pharmacokinetics

V-Y advance PLASTIC SURGERY A type of surgical advancement incision that allows lengthening of a contracted scar, where a 'Y'-shape is sewn into a V-shaped incision

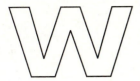

W Symbol for: 1) Tryptophan 2) Tungsten 3) Watt 4) Work 5) Writhing number

w Symbol for: workshop (see there)

Waardenburg syndrome An AD [MIM 193500] condition characterized by a wide nasal bridge due to the lateral displacement of the inner canthi, pigment abnormalities (eg white forelock, heterochromia iris, leukoderma) and (usually) sensorineural deafness MOLECULAR PATHOLOGY WS has mutations in the *PAX3* gene (on chromosome 2q37.3), which encodes proteins involved in embryological development; the defect is similar to the murine 'Splotch' mutation which is also characterized by patchy pigmentation and deafness; hamster data suggest that the variability of expression of WS is due to modifier genes

WAF1 p21, see there

WAF1 A gene that is thought to be a transcriptional target of p53, which is upregulated by the gene product of the wild-type (ie normal) but not by the mutated *p53*

waffle CLINICAL DECISION MAKING A highly colloquial synonym for indecision, which has nominative (eg the diagnosis is a complete waffle) or verbal (eg he/she decided to waffle) status

wagon wheel fracture MEDICAL HISTORY A fracture characterized by a separation of the distal femoral epiphysis, which was most common in children, whose legs were inadvertently caught in the western-bound wagon wheels

WAGR syndrome An AD [MIM 194070] clinical complex characterized by Wilm's tumor, aniridia, genitourinary abnormalities (renal agenesis, gonadoblastoma) and mental retardation; the association between Wilms' tumor (frequency: 1:10 000) and aniridia (frequency: 1:65-100 000) is strong; 1:50 of Wilm's children have aniridia; 1:3 of those with aniridia have Wilm's tumor; the defective gene complex has been localized to chromosome 11p13, near the H-*ras* 1 locus and flanked by the genes encoding catalase and the β subunit of FSH; the gene has a deletion with a balanced translocation which normally encodes a 'zinc-finger' protein; mRNA in situ hybridization analysis of the gene indicates it is well-expressed in developing human urogenital tissues, has a specific role in renal development and a wider role in mesenchymal-epithelial transitions, explaining the multi-system defects of the WAGR syndrome

Note: A WAGR murine model was generated by an interspecies backcross between *Mus musculus* and *M spretus*

waist-to-hip ratio The circumference of the waist divided by that of the hips, a value that is ↑ in ♀ at ↑ risk for the familial form of breast cancer (N Engl J Med 1992; 326:1323oa)

'waiter accepting a tip' sign PEDIATRICS A deformity in which the arm hangs loosely at the side and the partially paralyzed hand is deviated posteriorly, a position fancifully likened to a waiter subtly accepting a pourboir, that may occur in the vaginal delivery of the after-coming head in breech delivery or by extreme lateral flexion of the infant's head in an effort to treat shoulder dystocia, which stretches the upper roots of the brachial plexus, especially C5 and C6 (Erb's palsy), either temporarily or permanently; the lower roots of the brachial plexus are less commonly involved, affecting the small hand muscles and the palmar grasp reflex, causing Klumpke's palsy

waived test LABORATORY MEDICINE A test that is regarded as being of such simplicity that it would require a special talent NOT to perform it correctly (ie to borrow from the vernacular, 'idiot-proof'); WTs include dipstick urinalysis (for bilirubin, glucose, hemoglobin, ketones, leukocytes, nitrite, pH, protein, specific gravity, and urobilirubinogen), visual color tests for ovulation and pregnancy, nonautomated ESR, hemoglobin by copper sulfate method, fecal occult blood, spun microhematocrit, glucose by FDA-approved home-monitoring devices; the adjectival 'waived' refers to the CLIA rules regarding the complexity of tests and the federally mandated standards regarding the quality of clinical laboratory test results; see CLIA-88, Physician office laboratory

waiver HEALTH CARE MANAGEMENT An official permission to circumvent Medicaid, Medicare, and ERISA rules for reimbursement of services, which has been regarded by some as being critical to formulating a plan of comprehensive health care reform (Am Med News 25 October 1992, p7)

walk-in clinic Ambulatory clinic, see there

walking Chromosome walking, see there

'walking' pneumonia A colloquial term for the clinical symptoms typical of the atypical pneumonia caused by *Mycoplasma pneumoniae* CLINICAL Usually mild with an insidious onset of malaise, headache and occasionally fever that is followed several days later by an intense, usually nonproductive cough, mixed with scant mucopurulent or hemorrhagic sputum. accompanied by chest tenderness on inspiration; auscultation may reveal wheezes, rhonchi and occasional moist râles; clinical and radiologic improvement of 'walking' bronchopneumonia with pleural effusions may require 2-6 weeks TREATMENT Tetracycline, erythromycin; a live attenuated vaccine is being developed

walking-through phenomenon CARDIOLOGY Anginal pain that appears while the patient is walking and disappears if he 'walks through' the pain MECHANISM Unknown

wall effect LABORATORY MEDICINE The advanced movement of a substance adjacent to the wall of a chromatographic column, due to the increased rate of solvent migration; in contrast, a solvent migrates more slowly in the column's center as it interacts with the column's 'packing' material

walled abscess A generic term for an abscess that is surrounded by a thickened 'capsule' of fibrosis

wallerian degeneration NEUROPATHOLOGY A histologic rsponse to transection of a peripheral nerve, in which there is axonal and myelin sheath disintegration and digestion by Schwann cells (which are facultative phagocytes) distal to the interruption, while proximal to the transection, the nerve degenerates to the nearest node of Ranvier; if the transection is very proximal, the neuronal cell body undergoes chromatolysis; wallerian degeneration occurs in the ophthalmic and spinocerebellar tracts and posterior columns

walling-off reaction A tissue response to acute and subacute inflammation, in which the focus of infection or inflammation is 'isolated' and surrounded by fibrosis, serving to seal off the lesion, as occurs in the 'maturation' of an abscess

wall sign Halo sign GYNECOLOGY A vague radiolucency imparted by the dense fibrous capsule of an ovarian dermoid cyst (mature teratoma), separating different sharply circumscribed tissue densities, often recognized by plain films of the lower abdomen

walnuts CLINICAL NUTRITION A source of dietary fat* that is reported to ↓ risk of ischemic heart disease, by ↓ cholesterol (total, LDL and HDL), favorably modifying the lipoprotein profile in normal males BIOCHEMISTRY 81% of the total calories from walnuts derive from fat; the polyunsaturated fat:saturated fat ratio is 7.1:1 (one of the highest found in naturally occurring foods); 12% of walnut fat (7g/100g edible content) is n-3 linolenic acid (**N Engl J Med 1993; 328:603oA**, for critiques of report's conclusions, see **ibid; 329:359c**)

*Other nuts, eg almonds, hazelnuts are thought to have similar effects, although the content of a-linolenic acid in walnuts (6.3g/100g) is much higher (< 0.7g/100g)

walnut brain Narrowed cerebral gyri with widened sulci that occur in extreme atrophy of the frontal and temporal lobes, with relative sparing of the posterior brain, characteristic of Pick's disease; Alzheimer's disease is more globally atrophied, and is said to also affect the parietal lobe, and has been called 'knife blade atrophy'; as atrophy evolves, there is compensatory ventricular enlargement (hydrocephalus ex vacuo)

'Walt Disney' dwarfism Geroderma osteodysplastica, see there

Walter Reed Staging System A system (table) for clinical staging of AIDS, which requires that the symptoms persist for > than 3 months in the form of constitutional symptoms (B), CNS involvement (C), Kaposi's sarcoma (K), neoplasia (N), and thrombocytopenia (T) (**N Engl J Med 1986; 314:131; ibid, 315:1357**)

WALTER REED STAGING			
Stage	CD4+T cells*	HIV-1	Clinical findings
WR 0	> 0.4 x 10⁹/L	−	
WR 1	> 0.4 x 10⁹/L	+	No CL[†]
WR 2	> 0.4 x 10⁹/L	+	± CL[†]
WR 3	< 0.4 x 10⁹/L	+	± CL[†]
WR 4	< 0.4 x 10⁹/L	+	± CL[†]; partial CA[‡]
WR 5	< 0.4 x 10⁹/L	+	± CL[†]; complete CA[‡]
WR 6	< 0.4 x 10⁹/L	+	± CL[†]; complete CA[‡], thrush
*CD4 lymphocytes (US: 400/mm³) [†]Chronic lymphadenopathy [‡]Cutaneous anergy			

WAN COMPUTERS Wide-area network A mainstream extension to LANs (local area networks) which is used for electronic mail, file transfers or keyboard/terminal traffic; the data transferred in WANs is a function of the bandwidth and the device being used to transmit the data

wanderer A person, usually with some form of mental disorder, who gains admission to one hospital[1] after another[2] (defined as four or more in one year) who are designated as a **wandering patient** (WP) if the wandering is accompanied by a treatable illness, and a **habitually wandering patient** (HWP) if the behavior extended over a period of five years; in one report, in 1991, 810 WPs were identified who averaged 8 admissions/year and 100 days of inpatient care, for substance abuse and/or mental disease for a total cost of $26.5 million; 35 HWPs were identified who totaled 2268 admissions and 7832 outpatient visits for a total cost of $6.5 million (**N Engl J Med 1994; 331:1752oA, 1771ED**)

[1]The wandering appears to be a phenomenon unique to the US Veterans Affairs hospitals, which offer free medical care and/or hospital admission for prolonged periods of time to any person who is a veteran of military service
[2]While such behavior has features overlapping those of factitious disorders, Munchausen syndrome, and drug-seeking behaviors, it is considered to be a 'pathology' a sui generis

wandering gallbladder Mobile gallbladder A GB that is not attached to the ventral surface of the liver, flopping around its pedicle of attachment, the cystic duct

wandering pacemaker CARDIOLOGY An intermittent shift (or suppression) of one cardiac pacemaker, usually the sinus node to another, often the atrioventricular node; the contraction gradually increases in length of the cycle, most commonly occurring as an innocuous finding in infants, thought to reflect fluctuations in vagal tone; physical findings in a wandering pacemaker include bradycardia, variability of the first heart sound and size and shape of the 'P' wave

wandering spot technique MOLECULAR BIOLOGY A technique for sequencing synthetic nucleotides, in which the 5'-end of the oligonucleotides is labeled with ^{32}P and then partially digested by phosphodiesterase; the resulting fragments are fractionated by cellulose acetate electrophoresis, then chromatography and the sequence is determined by the patterns of mobility shift of the labeled fragments

wanderlust PSYCHOLOGY The desire to leave one's home, originally in search of adventure; in the context of behavioral pathology, wanderlust may refer to the desire to leave one's responsibilities

Wangiella dermatidis A rarely pathogenic fungus that may occasionally affect gardeners (**CAP Today August 1994**)

war on drugs An initiative declared under the Reagan administration that intended to eliminate (or at very least markedly reduce) drug abuse; as indicated in the following editorial comment (**N Engl J Med 1994; 330:355ED**), it failed

'After nearly 10 years of escalation, the government assault on illicit drugs has proved to be a costly failure. We have all been paying the price in misdirected resources, social tension, violent crime, ill health, compromised civil liberties and international conflict. The war on drugs is, in effect if not by intention, a war on drug users. The federal budget for the control of illicit drugs has increased more than eightfold since 1981...These laws needlessly make criminals of at least 20 million Americans (the estimated number of US citizen who abuse drugs on a regular basis). Of the 1 million drug arrests each year, about 225 000 are for simple possession of marijuana....Largely because we imprison so many drug users and petty drug dealers, the United States has a higher proportion of its population incarcerated than any other in the world for which statistics are available....Present drug policies also have disastrous effects on health and health care...a new epidemic of tuberculosis is incubating in ... prisons crowded with drug-law offenders. Infection with HIV is spreading rapidly among intravenous drug users who cannot legally exchange contaminated for sterile needles.'

ward A unit of inpatient beds (usually from 10-40) designated for a particular type of service or care, eg pediatric ward, obstetrics ward, CCU (coronary care unit), ICU (intensive care unit), oncology unit, are referred collectively to as wards

Ward's triangle A radiolucent and fracture-prone area of reduced bone density located on the boss of the head of the femur, bordered by the trabeculae; WT is one of the regions evaluated when measuring bone density

ward X A colloquial euphemism for a morgue (**Appendix IV, M Crichton, A Case of Need, Penguin 1968**), as in '...to be discharged to ward X...'

warfarin An anticoagulant of the coumarin family that inhibits the synthesis of liver-dependent coagulation factors (the prothrombin complex, factors II, VII, IX and X that are formed by γ-carboxylation of the precursor proteins); warfarin is used for long-term prevention of uncomplicated distal deep vein thrombosis, prophylaxis and prevention of cardiogenic thromboemboli and for survivors of acute MI; in one study, warfarin-treated patients had a 24% ↓ in mortality, cerebrovascular accidents and re-infarction; warfarin therapy is monitored by serial evaluation of PT (2-4-fold > the normal of 12-16 seconds); its activity is ↑ by phenylbutazone, clofibrate (by out-competing with warfarin for plasma protein binding sites) and ↓ by barbiturates, which stimulate hepatic metabolism; low-intensity anticoagulation with warfarin

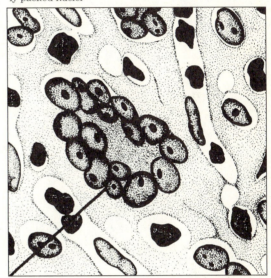

prevents cerebral infarction in older patients with atrial fibrillation without producing an excessive hemorrhage (N Engl J Med 1992 327:1406OA)

warfarin

Note: The agent's development was funded by the Wisconsin Alumni Research Foundation (WARF) in the 1940s (N Engl J Med 1991; 324:1865rv), hence the name; coumarins are also effective rodenticides, and have had intermittent currency as suicidal vehicles

warm agglutinin disease An autoimmune hemolytic syndrome caused by IgG antibodies, 40% of which are secondary to underlying conditions, including neoplasia, eg CLL, ovarian teratoma, collagen vascular disease, eg SLE, progressive systemic sclerosis, rheumatoid arthritis, ulcerative colitis and others CLINICAL Brisk hemolysis is associated with symptoms of anemia, ie pallor, fatigue, exertional dyspnea, dizziness and palpitations with mild jaundice and splenomegaly LABORATORY Moderate to severe anemia with a positive antiglobin (Coombs') test, spherocytes, schistocytes, erythrophagocytosis; bone marrow demonstrates erythroid hyperplasia and may reveal an underlying lymphoproliferative disorder TREATMENT Blood transfusions; glucocorticoids may ameliorate the hemolysis in ⅔ of patients; 20% achieve complete remission when maintained with doses above 15-20 mg/day; ⅔ respond to splenectomy, but may relapse; other modalities with varying degrees of failure include immunosuppressive agents and plasmapheresis PROGNOSIS 73% 10-year survival; Cf Cold agglutinin disease

'warm antibody' TRANSFUSION MEDICINE An antibody or agglutinin (usually IgG) that reacts optimally at 37°C and has an affinity for certain red cell antigens, eg Duffy, Kell, Kidd. MNSs and Rh, and if produced by a blood cell recipient, may cause an immune hemolytic response

'warm' nodule NUCLEAR MEDICINE A relatively circumscribed increase in radioisotope concentration seen by radionuclide imaging of the thyroid ('thyroid scan') in which functional thyroid lesions suppress TSH synthesis, but do not cause hyperthyroidism, the latter of which evokes 'hot' nodules; Cf Cold nodule

warm shock syndrome A clinical complex seen in early septic shock CLINICAL Normal cardiac activity, no fluid losses, enhanced peripheral perfusion and minimal catecholamine effect

warning leak NEUROSURGERY A minor early hemorrhage that occurs in an evolving subarachnoid hematoma or hemorrhage, which is followed by the abrupt onset of an often severe headache, variably accompanied by nuchal stiffness; since significant subarachnoid hemorrhage is fatal if untreated; WLs must be recognized early, treated aggressively, and the underlying pathology (angiomatous malformations, neoplasia, trauma) addressed

wart Verruca Any of a number of verruciform lesions of mucocutaneous surfaces induced by papovaviruses; warts are the single most common reason for dermatologic consultation, most often affect children and adolescents and include the well-described benign 'usual' types, eg the common wart (verruca vulgaris), filiform wart, plantar wart and juvenile flat wart; the clinical course of warts ranges from spontaneous involution, not uncommon in flat warts to extreme recalcitrance, typical of periungual and moist plantar warts PATHOLOGY Hyperplastic epithelium, koilocytosis, basophilic intranuclear inclusions (viral particles), parakeratosis, papillomatosis and eosinophilic cytoplasmic inclusions (keratohyalin) TREATMENT 'Benign neglect' and 'abracadabra therapy' are most effective in young children (implying a component of biofeedback control of the immune system), chemocautery (5-20% for-

malin, phenol-nitric acid-salicylic acid and podophyllin), electrodissection, X-ray (narrow field, low dose, rarely used), and DCNB immunotherapy

Note: The HPV-induced and premalignant giant condyloma acuminatum of Buschke-Loewenstein are located on 'sexual' mucosae, most common on the uncircumcised penis and transmissible to sexual partners

Warthin's tumor Papillary cystadenoma lymphomatosum A benign salivary gland tumor (SGT) that most commonly affects the parotid gland, which represents 0.3-10% of all SGTs and has a ♂:♀ ratio of 5:1 PATHOLOGY Glandular and cystic structures in papillary fronds; the cells have a highly characteristic two cell arrangement with eosinophilic cytoplasm and abundant lymphocytes in the stroma TREATMENT Excision

Warthin-Finkeldey cell Measles giant cell A large multinucleated giant cell (figure) seen in lymphoid tissues (eg lymph nodes, appendix), lungs, and elsewhere in patients in the early stages of the development of measles; the WFC is characterized by abundant (less than 100) densely packed nuclei

Warthin-Finkeldey cell

washboard scalp Cutis verticis gyrata, see there

washed red cells TRANSFUSION MEDICINE Erythrocytes that have been washed in sterile saline (first with a 'light' spin to remove and/or salvage plasma, followed if desired, by 3 to 5 'heavy' spins) prior to transfusion, a process that removes most leukocytes, lytic mediators and non-self antigens; washed cells are most useful in IgA-deficient patients who have circulating anti-IgA antibodies, reducing the incidence of febrile, urticarial and anaphylactic reactions; see Blood filters

Note: Although washing of red cells reduces febrile, non-hemolytic transfusion reactions, it is labor-intensive, and exposes the unit to air and pathogens (if the unit is not transfused within 24 hours, it must be discarded, ie use it or lose), cells are only routinely washed in patients who have previously had a non-hemolytic transfusion reaction, an event that occurs in approximately 1:40 transfusions, which does not respond to the use of blood filters

'washerwoman' skin Superficial cutaneous rugosity, likened to those who have their hands immersed in water for prolonged periods, which later become dry and chapped, these latter known as 'dish-pan hands' FORENSIC PATHOLOGY Markedly rugose skin of the hands and feet seen in bodies recovered from water ('floaters'), the intensity of which is a function of the time immersed and water temperature, occurring as quickly as ½ hour at 15-20°C; the relatively loose skin may slough off in 'gloves' PEDIATRICS The skin of post-term infants that is loose and dry, has been likened to parchment or washer-woman's skin; alternatively, the loss of skin turgor caused by prolonged diarrhea of cholera may cause a similar appearance

Washington Monument crystals A descriptor for the opaque red-brown, tetragonal rod-like hemoglobin crystals with rigid, parallel sides and tapered ends seen inside and outside of red cells in homozygous hemoglobinopathy C, best seen on a Wright-Giemsa-stained peripheral blood smear; similar crystals may also occur in heterozygous hemoglobin C, eg hemoglobin C-S, hemoglobin C-thalassemia, and in hereditary persistence of hemoglobin F

wasp waist A descriptor for the body of a person affected by Löwenthal's disease, a familial condition with a thin waist, relatively enlarged pelvic and shoulder girdles, hyperextended and atonic extremities, muscular sclerosis and rhizomelic contractions

wasserhellezellen Water clear cells, see there

wastage Fetal wastage, see there

waste A generic term that functions as an adjective (eg waste water), a noun (see Biohazardous waste, Hazardous waste, Regulated waste), and a verb, in both medical (as occurs in terminal stages of progressive disease, eg AIDS or cancer) and nonmedical* contexts

*A colloquial verb that has had some currency as a synonym for 'execute' among shadowy creatures of the underworld, as in 'Louie wasted Vinnie'

wasting disease 1) Kwashiorkor, see there 2) Runt disease, see there 3) Wasting syndrome, see there

wasting syndrome A nonspecific generic term for a clinical complex associated with chronic renal insufficiency, attributed to a combination of poor nutrition, endocrine dysfunction and catabolic stresses, including infection, uremia and dialysis; in absence of disease, starvation results in death at 66% of ideal body weight; in AIDS, cell mass at death is 54%; WS is mediated by TNF (as well as by IL-1, IFN-α, IFN-β, and IFN-γ), which ↓ lipoprotein lipase, ↓ synthesis of fatty acids, and ↑ lipolysis in fat cells; wasting is also related to anorexia, and protein catabolism secondary to infections (**N Engl J Med 1992; 327:329**ᴿⱽ) see Starvation

watchful waiting A clinical stance that is the medical equivalent of 'yellow alert' in which no action is taken in terms of therapy for a particular disease process although the potential for recurrence or recrudescence is strictly monitored; WW is appropriate for conditions in which there is low (≤ 10 years) life expectancy, eg in elderly patients, and the lesion being watched has minimal aggression; WW has resulted in low rates of death in elderly patients with localized, low-grade cancer of the prostate (**N Engl J Med 1994; 331:996**ᴿᴬ) other conditions for which WW is regarded as appropriate include aortic aneurysms (< 4.0 cm in diameter), cataracts, gallstones, cardiomyopathy, and uterine fibroids; see Benign neglect

water balance A state of equilibrium in which the fluid intake equals the fluid 'losses'

water bath A water-filled vessel, usually large enough to hold one or more racks of test tubes, the temperature of which is stringently controlled by a thermostat, often set at a physiological temperature, eg 37°C for a biological system

waterbed A bed with a water-filled mattress that has some therapeutic currency ɢᴀsᴛʀᴏᴇɴᴛᴇʀᴏʟᴏɢʏ Waterbed users are reported to be either five times more likely to suffer from reflux esophagitis (**JAMA 1987; 257:2033**), or at no increased risk for reflux, measured by pH monitors (**Dig Dis Sci 1989; 34:1585**) ɴᴇᴏɴᴀᴛᴏʟᴏɢʏ Oscillating waterbeds in preterm infants provide compensatory movement stimulation, reducing uncomplicated apnea of prematurity, with ↑ periods of quiet sleep, ↓ periods of crying/fussiness and enhanced growth; non-oscillating waterbeds are of use in treating narcotic-exposed neonates, one studied group

had significantly lower CNS subscores, required less medication to control withdrawal symptoms and had an earlier onset of consistent weight gain

water-borne infection see Tapwater infection

water-borne pathogen A generic term for any pathogenic organism, usually bacterial; the virulence ranges widely, with many organisms, eg enterotoxigenic *Escherichia coli*, *Campylobacter jejuni*, and nontyphoid *Salmonella* rarely causing death; others are highly virulent and may result in death, eg *Vibrio cholerae*, with ± 15% mortality, or *Salmonella typhi* and *Shigella dysenteriae* type, each of which has 5-10% mortality (**Sci Am 1993; 268/4:86**)

water bottle heart A descriptor for the globose cardiac shadow typical of large pericardial effusions (effusions of less than 250 ml are radiologically 'silent'); pericardial effusions may be serous (due to congestive heart failure or decreased proteins in nephrotic syndrome, hepatic failure, malnutrition), sero-sanguinous (blunt chest trauma, CPR), chylous (lymphatic obstruction, ½ of which are caused by malignancy) and cholesterol ('pseudochylous' effusion, either idiopathic or related to myxedema)

water brash Foam at the mouth Hypersalivation characteristic of reflux esophagitis (variably accompanied by chronic blood loss, anemia, aspiration, regurgitation and recurrent pneumonitis)

water-clear cells Wasserhellezellen A variant, glycogen-rich* parathyroid chief cell (figure) that is clear, large and may form distinct tubules

*The glycogen may be lost in tissue processing

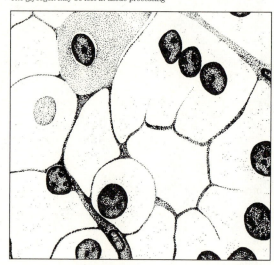

water-clear cells

water-clear cell hyperplasia A parathyroid gland lesion that has been reported with less frequency in recent years which, unlike chief cell hyperplasia, is neither familial nor associated with multiple endocrine adenomatosis; WCCH is characterized by marked parathyroid gland enlargement, up to 100 g, associated with hyperparathyroidism and hypercalciuric hypercalcemia ᴘᴀᴛʜᴏʟᴏɢʏ Combined hypertrophy and hyperplasia, coalescence of glands which form large brown cystic and hemorrhagic masses, and cells with 'water-clear' cytoplasm, minute scattered eosinophilic granules arranged in an 'alveolar' pattern

waterfall hypothesis ʜᴇᴍᴀᴛᴏʟᴏɢʏ A postulated framework* on which current understanding of the coagulation cascade hinges; the WF explains the interactions of the various coagulation factors as a sequence of interconnected reactions that begin with an active surface, usually due to trauma, follows the so-called intrinsic (major players, factors XII, XI, IX, and VIII) and/or extrinsic pathways (factors VII, tissue factor) continues through a common pathway (factors X, V, and XIII), and ends with mature blood clot, which is characterized by stabilized fibrin

*That is believed to approach the physiologic reality

waterfall phenomenon CLINICAL TOXICOLOGY The paralysis of a complex chain of enzymatic events at the beginning of the 'cascade' of reactions, eg intoxication of the cytochrome oxidase system by cyanide; by the time the respiratory paralysis first manifests itself, as occurs in nitroprusside poisoning, therapeutic attempts at removing the cyanide are fruitless

water hammer pulse Collapsing pulse A booming, bounding or pistol-shot-like sound auscultated in aortic regurgitation or in a large patent ductus arteriosus (PDA)*; the so-called 'small water hammer pulse' is due to a brisk rise in systemic arterial pressure in the face of normal pulse pressure

*Smaller PDAs may be asymptomatic or have a 'machinery murmur'

water of hydration Bound water Molecules of water that are buried in a macromolecule, which are thought to stabilize internal structure by acting as bridges between protein hydrogen bond donors and acceptors; in contrast, water molecules located at an active site participate in catalysis and ligand recognition; NMR analysis has identified in addition to the surface water molecules and ordered internal water molecules, water molecules of hydration in hydrophobic pockets that have extremely short (1-2 nanoseconds) residency times (Science 1995; 267:1813)

water intoxication Acute or chronic hyperhydration due to excess ingestion of water, causing dilutional hyponatremia; the condition is most common in patients with psychiatric or neurologic disease, and may be accompanied by impaired renal fluid excretion and increased secretion of antidiuretic hormone; acute WI may also occur in normal subjects attempting to produce urine to elevate the bladder for pelvic ultrasonography or for drug testing (JAMA 1991; 265:84cr); acute WI may be due to a rapid decline in serum Na+ to ≤ 125 mEq/L caused by an acute overload of solute-free water; alterations in mental status, irritability, seizures, somnolence, hypothermia, edema; it is particularly common in infants of parents living in poverty (MMWR 1994; 43:641)

water lily sign Camelot sign RADIOLOGY A rare radiologic finding most often due to a cyst in the lung or liver with a laminated collapsed capsule and floating scolices outlined by air within the cyst, which is typical of echinococcal (hydatid) disease; see Hydatid sand

watermelon stomach A pattern of tortuous vessels along the longitudinal folds of the stomach, radiating from the pylorus toward the antrum, fancifully likened to a watermelon's stripes, a finding characteristic of angiodysplasia of the gastric antrum, Cf 'Emperor's new clothes' syndrome

water-reactive OCCUPATIONAL SAFETY *adjective* Pertaining or referring to any chemical that reacts with water to release a gas that is a physical or health hazard, a datum of interest to OSHA, which requires listing of WR substances in its Materials Safety Data Sheets‡

water-reactive material OCCUPATIONAL SAFETY A chemical substance or mixture that reacts with water to release heat or form a gas that is flammable, highly toxic, or toxic

watershed infarction NEUROLOGY An infarction of a region that is peripheral to two arteries and susceptible to ischemia; WIs occur in the brain after internal carotid artery occlusion, causing vascular 'steal' phenomena, or between the anterior and middle cerebral arteries that are compromised in circle of Willis occlusions, often in a background of generalized atherosclerosis and as a possible complication of directed therapeutic embolization; the cerebral perfusion may be impaired due to cardiac arrest, pericardial tamponade and exsanguination; WIs are often hemorrhagic, as restoration of the circulation allows blood to flow into damaged capillaries and 'leak' into cerebral tissue; WI may also occur in the large intestine at either the splenic flexure, the site of anastomosis between the inferior and superior mesenteric arteries, or at the rectum, a region supplied by peripheral irrigation from the inferior mesenteric artery and the hypogastric artery

water softening The conversion of 'hard' (mineral-laden) water to soft water by ion exchange chromatography, which may be required for certain chemical reactions and for the optimal function of laboratory instruments

water solubility The solubility of a material in water; WS is of greatest interest to OSHA at ambient temperatures, which defines WS as negligible (< 0.1% solubility), slight (0.1-1.0%), moderate (1.0-10%), appreciable (≥ 10%) and complete (100%); see Materials Safety Data Sheets‡

water-soluble fiber Soluble fiber, see there

water treatment PUBLIC HEALTH The processing of water to make it safely potable or otherwise suitable for consumption; if the natural source of the water is not of a desired quality, one or more purification processes must be engineered in the WT plant; the methods in use include adsorption, coagulation, disinfection, distillation, filtration, flocculation, gas exchange, ion exchange, and sedimentation (JM Last, RB Wallace, Eds, Public Health and Preventive Medicine, 13th ed, Appletone & Lange, Norwalk, 1992); one common method for treating drinking water is a multistep process; chlorine and polyaluminum chloride (a coagulant to enhance the formation of larger particles) are added to the water, followed by rapid mixing, mechanical flocculation (which promotes aggregation of particles), sedimentation, and rapid sand filtration (N Engl J Med 1994; 331:161oA)

watered silk appearance PATHOLOGY A pattern of wavy, glistening fascicles seen by gross examination of the surface of granulosa cell tumors of the ovary and uterine leiomyomata

Waterhouse-Friderichsen syndrome A clinical crisis characterized by acute adrenal insufficiency*, often accompanied by septicemia; WFS is most often caused by *Neisseria meningitidis*, but may occur with *Haemophilus influenzae, Streptococcus pneumoniae*, staphylococci, or less commonly, result from hypoxia during a difficult labor and delivery and acute adrenal insufficiency EPIDEMIOLOGY Most common in hot, dry climates, in particular in West Africa CLINICAL Generalized purpuric rash, shock, hypotension

*With massive hemorrhagic necrosis of the adrenal glands that may be confined to the zona reticularis or zona medularis, or affect the entire gland

watering-pot perineum UROLOGY A fanciful descriptor for a complication of trauma to the urethra and covering structures (as may occur in urethral surgery), in which multiple fistulas associated with inflammatory strictures and diverticuli develop parallel to the urethra and penetrate tissues of the perineum and scrotum, forming draining sinuses; as the patient voids, infected urine is forced into these tracts, and the urine dribbles from multiple, watering-pot-like pores

Waters' position RADIOLOGY A position used to visualize the facio-maxillary bones and maxillary sinuses and determine the patency of the maxillary sinuses, in which the patient is placed at a 37° angle with the orbito-meatal line, perpendicular to the mid-sagittal plane

watery diarrhea-hypokalemia-achlorhydria syndrome WDHA syndrome, see there

Watson-Crick DNA B-DNA The model of DNA, now known as B-DNA, proposed by James Watson and Francis Crick in their seminal paper, '*General Implications of the*

Structure of Deoxyribonucleic Acid' (**Nature** i953; 171:737), which is widely regarded as the founding event of molecular biology; see Central dogma, DNA, Human Genome Project

wavefront phenomenon CARDIOLOGY The finding that prolonged coronary artery occlusion results in the expansion of a small subendocardial infarct into a larger transmural myocardial infarct, seemingly spreading in waves

wavelet theory A mathematical model of universal phenomena in the physical universe, which (unlike Fourier analysis* which is conceptually based on a sine/cosine wave stretching into infinity) uses a building block known as a 'mother wavelet', concentrated in an interval between 0 and 1; the daughter wavelets are created by moving the mother wavelet left or right in unit steps and dilating or compressing it by repeated factors of 2, an analogy that is extremely similar to musical notation; wavelet analysis, although in its infancy, is considered a theoretical advancement over the Fourier transform, potentially having applications for data compression of digitalized images, artificial intelligence, synthesis of speech and music and in improving CT images; Cf Chaos, Fourier analysis, Fractal analysis

Background: Fourier analysis, the current paradigm of data analysis, assumes that all data sets in the universe can be defined as sine and cosine curves, stretching to infinity and all subsets of data are miniature versions of the original sine/cosine curve; Fourier analysis is widely used to address such broadly divergent areas as weather prediction and CT imaging; there are two major disadvantages of Fourier transforms: 1) 'Peaks' and 'dips' of data (a normal event in an imperfect and chaotic universe), require that the entire data set be re-analyzed whenever these 'imperfections' are encountered and 2) Gaps in data cause the analytic algorithm to screech to a halt, requiring educated 'guesswork' to fill in the gaps;

wavy change Contraction band CARDIAC PATHOLOGY The undulent kinking of cardiac muscle (figure) typical of early myocardial infarction, often seen within one hour of myocardial ischemia, involving random, focal individual myocytes, patches or extensive areas of the myocardium, usually at the border of the infarct, thought to be due to pulling of noncontracting dead fibers by adjacent viable myocytes; infarct borders are further characterized by vacuolar degeneration or myocytolysis, consisting of fine lipid droplets or large rounded cytoplasmic spaces (filled with water, scant glycogen and lipid) with a peripheral rim of sarcoplasm, seen in viable myocytes

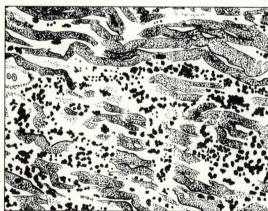

wavy changes

wax doll appearance Porcelain doll appearance, see there

wax epilation DERMATOLOGY A procedure for removing ill-placed and/or undesired hair, in particular on the legs, which consists of pouring of a hot paraffin-like material on the skin and, once cooled, removing the 'cast' en bloc*; because it 'synchronizes' the growth cycle, WE appears to increase hair growth; Cf Electrolysis
*Ouch-Author's note

waxing Wax epilation, see there

waxy casts NEPHROLOGY Homogeneous cylindrical structures seen in the urine by low-power light microscopy, which have a high refractile index (hyaline casts are morphologically similar but are not refractile) and correspond to the degenerated cellular casts typical of long-term oliguria and obstruction of the tubules, as occurs in chronic renal failure, acute and chronic renal rejection and amyloidosis; very broad waxy casts or 'renal failure' casts are typical of end-stage renal failure

waxy degeneration Zenker's degeneration Acidophilic hyalinization of muscle, seen by light microscopy and considered the first step in segmental muscular necrosis; WD may be induced by ischemia, trauma, temperature extremes, infections (scarlet fever, smallpox, typhoid fever, diphtheria, leptospirosis) and dehydration

waxy exudates Retinitis pigmentosa Tapetoretinal degeneration OPHTHALMOLOGY A descriptor for the 'hard', yellow-white macular aggregates of fatty and proteinaceous material that leak into the retina through thinned and atrophied capillaries, seen in DM, causing ↓ visual acuity

WC Fields nose A fanciful descriptor for end-stage acne rosacea, which affects middle-aged adults, characterized by proliferation of sebaceous glands and fibrous tissue, edema, erythema, telangiectasias, follicular and parafollicular abscessification, and eventually rhinophyma; it is cosmetically unesthetic with unpredictable flushing, which becomes especially prominent when eating spicy foods, coffee or when overindulging in alcohol (with which acne rosacea is classically associated) TREATMENT Topical metronidazole, tetracycline, CO_2 laser, which in the defocused mode, bloodlessly vaporizes the skin

Note: WC Fields was a vaudevillian artist cum legendary Hollywood comic actor of the 1930s and 1940s, famed for his inebriation and bulbous, pustular, bright pink bibulous proboscis

WCH-CD Aquaporin-2, see there

WDHA syndrome Watery diarrhea-hypokalemia-achlorhydria syndrome Verner-Morrison syndrome, pancreatic 'cholera' A disease complex due to increased serum VIP (vasoactive intestinal polypeptide), caused by a VIPoma, a pancreatic islet cell tumor, ½ of which are malignant, composed of clusters of insulinogenic B cells, glucagon-producing A-cells, somatostatin-producing D cells and pancreatic polypeptide-producing PP cells CLINICAL Profuse watery diarrhea, dehydration, hypotension, and shock, episodic flushing LABORATORY Achlorhydria, ↑ or ↓ glucose, ↓↓↓ K⁺, ↑ Ca⁺⁺; WDHA in children is associated with ganglioneuromas

Note: 12% of VIPomas cause WDHA, an association that is not uncommon in the context of multiple endocrine neoplasia (MEN) type I

weak D Formerly Dᵘ TRANSFUSION MEDICINE A weakened expression of the Rh D antigen (**CAP Today Jan, 1994**)

wean *wean*, Old English, to accustom CRITICAL CARE MEDICINE The transferral of a patient's dependence on mechanical ventilation to spontaneous auto-regulated breathing, which requires that the indications for the use of mechanical ventilation no longer exist and the patient responds to verbal commands, is stable (circulation, normal chest films, no abdominal distension) and not be receiving muscle relaxants; the single best predictor of successful 'wean-ability' is a low ratio of respiratory frequency to tidal volume (f/V_t); rapid shallow breathing after removal from mechanical supports accurately predicts failure (**N Engl J Med** 1991; 324:1445); once-daily or multiple daily trials of weaning lead to extubation 3 times faster than intermittent mandatory ventilation and 2 times faster than pressure-support ventilation (**N Eng J Med** 1995; 332:345oA) see Pulmonary function tests, V/Q ratio PEDIATRICS The transferral of dependence of an infant on maternal (ie breast milk) to milk from other sources or other forms of sustenance

weaning diarrhea PEDIATRICS A condition occurring in a background of poor sanitation, commonly occurring in children in developing nations, affecting infants between 6-24 months of age, and a major cause of infant mortality in developing nations; weaning from maternal milk results in exposure of the infant to new organisms, deterioration of nutrition (a mechanism similar to kwashiorkor) and loss of the passively transferred IgA CLINICAL Acute, sporadic and watery diarrhea, low-grade fever and variable vomiting, most common in the summer months; in a well-nourished child, the process resolves in 2-3 days with adequate hydration, in the malnourished child, the diarrhea persists and may be associated with comorbidity AGENTS Enterotoxic *Escherichia coli*, rotavirus, occasionally *Shigella* DIAGNOSIS CIE, ELISA, EM of stool

web see Esophageal web

webbed neck Pterygium colli A sphinx-like neck characterized by a thick web or fold of skin that extends from behind the ears to the distal clavicle and to the acromial process, classically described in Turner gonadal dysgenesis syndrome, but which is also seen in the fetal hydantoin, Noonan and trisomy 18 syndromes

Webster decision SOCIAL MEDICINE, OBSTETRICS A legal decision rendered in 1989 by the US Supreme Court (Webster vs Reproductive Health Services, 109 S Ct 3040, 1989) that represented a change in the 'official position on a woman's right to have an abortion; the Court ruled on an abortion in the State of Missouri, and concluded that a state could constitutionally prohibit state-employed physicians from performing an abortion that is not necessary to save the mother's life, could prohibit the abortion from being performed in state-owned facilities, and could require that the physicians attempt to determine fetal viability on or after the 20th week of gestation; see 'Gag rule', Mexico City policy, Title X; Cf *Roe* v *Wade*

'wedding ring' appearance CARDIAC PATHOLOGY A fanciful term for a regurgitating mitral valve deformity, where the valve ring and commissures are calcified, and 'frozen' in an opened position

wedge fracture A sharply angulated post-traumatic fracture of the spine, most common in the thoracic vertebrae, usually with anterior wedging seen in a background of osteoporosis; Cf Teardrop fracture

wedge pressure CARDIOLOGY An intravascular pressure recording obtained when the recording catheter is wedged (ie occludes) in the vessel, which is a means of assessing cardiopulmonary pressure gradients METHOD A Swan-Ganz catheter is inserted into a large systemic vein, 'threaded' through the right atrium under continuous pressure monitoring; the tip is then inflated and carried by the blood flow through the right ventricle and 'wedges' into a pulmonary arteriole, with the vessel being occluded by the balloon at the catheter tip, yielding close approximations of the left arterial or left ventricular filling pressures; the Swan-Ganz catheter also permits serial evaluation of cardiac output and access to the central oxygen supply

wedge resection Any triangular piece of tissue removed in surgery, which is most commonly obtained in two clinical distinct contexts 1) GYNECOLOGIC SURGERY A cuneiform section from an ovary which, by an unknown mechanism, may induce ovulation in polycystic ovaries, usually being performed after clomiphene and gonadotropic therapy have failed to correct infertility in women with polycystic ovaries, aka Stein-Leventhal syndrome 2) SURGICAL ONCOLOGY A wedge of lung, often subpleural, that contains a small radiologically identified lesion, which is thought to harbor a single focus of malignancy

wedge shadow RADIOLOGY A vaguely defined radiopacity extending from the pulmonary hilum, which is thought to be characteristic of pulmonary edema

WEE Western equine encephalitis, see there

Wegener's granulomatosis An idiopathic condition that is first manifest in the middle aged population, which is characterized by necrotizing sinusitis and pneumonia, granulomas of the oral cavity and periorbital regions, systemic vasculitis with fibrinoid necrosis of vascular walls, and renal involvement in the form of glomerulonephritis LABORATORY Antineutrophil cytoplasmic antibodies which are directed against a serine protease found in azurophilic granules of neutrophils TREATMENT Corticosteroids, methotrexate (JAMA 1995; 273:1288GR) cyclophosphamide induces remission in 75%

weight cycling Fluctuation in corporal weight; some data suggest that broad fluctuations in weight on either side of an individual's normal weight is associated with an ↑ in mortality from all causes (except cancer) and from coronary heart disease (JAMA 1992; 268:2045oc)

weight-cycling hypothesis METABOLISM A hypothesis that holds that fluctuations in body weight have negative health consequences, including increased total mortality and increased mortality from coronary heart disease, independent of obesity and the trend of body weight over time (N Engl J Med 1991; 324:1839, 1887ed)

weight-lifter's headache Severe headache and neck pain due to wrenching or tearing of cervical ligaments during the strain of exertion

Weil-Felix test LABORATORY MEDICINE A test in which agglutinins from non-motile strains (OX-19, OX-2 and OX-K) of *Proteus vulgaris* are used to serologically identify rickettsial organisms, by determining cross-reactivity; W-F reactions vary in sensitivity and are relatively non-specific; false positivity is common and occurs in other infections, eg urinary tract infections, leptospirosis, borreliosis, hepatic or biliary tract; W-F agglutination occurs with the OX-2 and OX-19 strains in the spotted fever group (*R rickettsii, R conorii, R siberica, R australis*); the typhus group (*R prowasecki, R typhi*) agglutinates with OX-19 alone; *R tsutsugamushi* reacts with the OK-X antigen; *Rickettsia akari, Coxiella burnetii*, and *Bartonella* (formerly *Rochalimaea*) *quintana* do not react with any OX antigens

Weill-Marchesani syndrome Spheroplakia-brachymorphia An AR [MIM 277600] disorder of connective tissues characterized by short stature, joint stiffness, myopia, subluxation of small, rounded lens (microspherophakia), ectopia lentis, glaucoma, brachydactyly, brachycephaly

welding bodies OCCUPATIONAL MEDICINE Structures associated with asbestosis that are more common than asbestos bodies, and have a golden-brown, iron-rich coating and a central opaque core particle(s) composed of metal of carbon; unlike asbestos bodies, the iron coating is probably of exogenous origin, and is seen in digested samples of lung from welders; see Asbestos bodies

well LABORATORY TECHNOLOGY A hole with sharp vertical margins that is cut into a 'slab' of gel, and into which an aliquot of a specimen, eg DNA, RNA or protein is placed at the beginning of electrophoresis

Wellcome Trust Britain's largest medical research charity; awarded circa £150 million (US $225 million) in fiscal 1993 A philanthropic foundation based in the UK that has a 4.7% stake in the Glaxo-Wellcome drug company (the world's largest pharmaceutical firm), which provides £250-300 million/year in income, making it the richest charity in the world; these monies are used by the WT for biomedical research, especially in the UK, where it supports ± 4000 scientists (Nature Medicine 1995; 1:394)

Wells v Ortho decision Litogen, see there

the 'Wendy dilemma' PSYCHIATRY A marital situation in which a wife is trapped into acting as a mother to her husband, although it reinforces his immature behavior (Aust NZ J Psychiatr 1982; 16:23)

Note: The term derives from the children's story, *Peter Pan* (JM Barrie, Hodder & Stroughton, London, 1911) in which Wendy is the surrogate mother to the Lost Boys in the magical kingdom of Neverland; see Peter Pan and Wendy syndrome

Werther effect PUBLIC HEALTH An increased suicide rate that is alleged to occur after media coverage of suicide(s), or in individuals 'inspired' by reading about or having had a close personal relationship with a 'successful' suicide; the effect, if real, is most common in young males (suicide rate, ages 15-19, $14/10^5$ versus female $3.2/10^5$)

The term derives from Goethe's *The Sorrows of Young Werther*, a story about a sentimental and daydreaming young man who fatally shoots himself; the story was blamed, when it was published in 1774 for a rash of young adult suicides and was banned in Milan, Leipzig and Copenhagen (N Engl J Med 1986; 315:705)

Westergren method A method for determining ESR in which the blood is placed in EDTA in a tube measuring 30 cm in length X 2.5 cm in diameter Normal rate: 0-10 mm/hour in men; 0-20 mm/hour in women; since the Westergren method is inaccurate in renal failure and the values are increased in anemia, the zetacrit has become the ESR method of choice; see Zetacrit

Westermark sign An abrupt radiologic 'cutoff' in pulmonary vessels seen in a standard antero-posterior chest film in pulmonary embolism without infarction, often accompanied by dilation of vessels before the cutoff, eg the right descending pulmonary artery; the sign is also seen in other intravascular occlusions, most commonly in bronchogenic carcinoma, as well as in interstitial pulmonary fibrosis, histoplasmosis, pulmonary arteritis, parasitic embolism (*Schistosoma haematobium, S mansoni*), Swyer-Jones disease, or intravascular sarcoma (Acta Radiol 1938; 19:357)

Western blot Immunoblot AIDS An immune assay that confirms HIV infection, used when an ELISA screening assay is positive TECHNIQUE Crude HIV is 'sieved' by gel electrophoresis, separating the HIV molecule into distinctive molecular weight protein bands that are then blotted onto a nitrocellulose strip, some bands are considered diagnostic by the CDC: Definitely positive p24 and p31 and gp41 or gp 120/gp 160 Possibly positive gp41 and gp 120/gp 160 or any combination, one from each gene product Indeterminant One HIV-related band; with time, HIV-1 products may disappear from the serum, especially p24, with a concomitant decrease in anti-core antibody; false positivity in the Western blot for HIV occurs in 0.01 to 0.0007% of cases; indeterminant results are 100-fold more common, occurring in 0.3-0.5% of the general population; if an individual with indeterminant results is in a high-risk group, he/she usually convert within one month; low-risk individuals with a persisting indeterminant

gp160
gp120
p66
p55
p51
p41
p31
p24

■ Positive

▨ p17

▨ Indeterminant

Western blot at 3 months may be regarded as negative and require no further followup (J Gen Intern Med 1992; 7:640) MOLECULAR BIOLOGY A technique that identifies antibodies to proteins of specific molecular weights, of particular use for confirming HIV-1 antibody screening assays (see above) performed by the ELISA technique (Anal Biochem 1981; 112:195) TECHNIQUE The proteins are separated by one- or two-dimensional electrophoresis, then transferred (blotted) to a nitrocellulose or nylon membrane that is then exposed to radioactively labeled or biotinylated antibody; the antigen of interest is detected either by autoradiography or directly, by using a biotinylated antibody (Proc Natl Acad Sci 1979; 76:4350) see Blots; Cf Northern blot, Southern blot

Western equine encephalomyelitis An uncommon alphavirus infection first identified in a horse with encephalitis in California, seen primarily in the western regions of North America; small epidemics occur in early summer to mid-summer when melted snow or heavy rains favor breeding of the mosquito (*Culex tarsalis* and *C melanura*) vectors; most exposed infants are symptomatic; less than 1% of adolescents develop symptoms; the case-fatality rate is 3-7% RESERVOIR Wild birds; Cf California encephalitis, Eastern equine encephalitis, Japanese B encephalitis, St Louis encephalitis

Westgard's multirule LABORATORY MEDICINE A set of quality control guidelines for the clinical laboratory that act to ensure consistent and accurate results for analytes; see Multirule procedure, Quality control

West Indies ataxic syndrome Tropical spastic paraparesis, see there

West Nile fever An acute, mosquito-borne* flaviviral infection that is endemic (occasionally, epidemic) in regions of the Near East, Africa, the former Soviet Union, and India CLINICAL After a 3-6 day incubation, children present with a nonspecific febrile illness; older patients develop a mild dengue-like disease with fever, rash that clears without desquamation, frontal headaches, orbital pain, backaches, myalgia, anorexia, lymphadenopathy and leukopenia, sore throat and potentially meningoencephalitis in the elderly; usually it is self-limited, resolving in a week

Culex, as well as *Anopheles*, and *Mansonia* spp, less commonly by ticks, eg *Orthodoros* spp

West syndrome Massive myoclonus An occasionally X-linked [MIM 308350] condition characterized by infantile spasms (seizures and secondary generalized epilepsy), hypsarrhythmia, encephalopathy with mental retardation and arrest of psychomotor development, which may be accompanied by immune dysfunction and death at an early age due to bronchopneumonia; see Salaam convulsions

'west-to-east' phenomenon EPIDEMIOLOGY A poorly understood difference in the seasonal peaks in the annual rotavirus epidemic in North America; the epidemic reaches a maximum in Mexico and the Southwestern US in late fall; the Midwestern US peaks in mid-winter and the incidence of rotavirus infections in Eastern US and Canada peaks in early spring

wet cerumen Earwax Cerumen may be 'dry' or 'wet', and the differences may be inherited; ↑ WC production is associated with breast carcinoma, and both are modified apocrine glands; in one series, Oriental women with wet cerumen are two-to-three times more likely to have proliferative breast disease or atypical hyperplasia, possibly related to an as yet unidentified polymorphous trait that influences susceptibility (Breast Cancer Res 1990; 16:279)

wet dream Nocturnal emission

wet drowning The usual form of drowning* or near-drowning, in which the victim aspirates water, as seen at the time of resuscitive efforts or at post-mortem examination MECHANISM Submersion is linked to voluntary apnea, until a certain breaking point, after which the victim voluntarily inspires, and water enters the lungs with accelerating decompensation, gasping, further aspiration, swallowing of water, emesis, aspiration of gastric contents, secondary apnea, neural and cardiac dysfunction, hypoxia, and metabolic acidosis and death; see Drowning; Cf Wet drowning

*Defined as death from suffocation by submersion in water

wet gangrene A condition caused by relatively acute vascular occlusion, eg burns, freezing, crush injuries and thromboembolism, resulting in liquefactive necrosis, causing bleb and bullae formation with violaceous discoloration; see Gangrene

wet lung see Adult respiratory distress syndrome

'wetshop' A 'hands-on' workshop designed to demonstrate a technique, eg immunoperoxidase, in situ hybridization, polymerase chain reaction, with which a person needs to be familiar for research or diagnostic purposes; wetshops are sponsored by either academic institutions or companies interested in selling products related to the technique; Cf Workshop

whalebone in a corset sign An arched configuration seen by barium studies in a semirigid, indurated superficial gastric carcinoma as it partially yields to outside pressure; in contrast, the classic ulcerating adenocarcinoma is rigid; see Meniscus sign of Carmen; Cf Quarter moon sign

wheal-and-flare reaction Triple response of Lewis IMMUNOLOGY A series of three sequential responses that occur in skin that has been subjected to minor trauma, which is caused by tissue release of histamine; the WFR tests for immediate hypersensitivity ('reaginic' or allergic reaction) to an antigen, and can be transferred to a nonallergic person; the skin is scratched with the antigen and if reactive, reveals a characteristic erythema ('flare') and edema (wheal), a phenomenon seen in atopic individuals due to formation and release of IgE, a Gell and Coombs type I hypersensivity reaction; see P-K test

wheat sheaf appearance A descriptor for the crystals seen in acid urine (pH < 5.0), which is most commonly associated with dehydration, and concomitant sulfonamide, eg acetylsulfisoxazole, sulfadiazine, or less commonly, ampicillin therapy; the presence of sulfonamides is confirmed by diazotization of the free amino group, yielding a magenta color; a similar appearance is associated with hypertyrosinemia, in which there are fine silky needles, which may also form rosette or arrowhead structures

wheezing PULMONARY MEDICINE An audible hissing sound that accompanies breathing, which is classically associated with asthma; most wheezing in infants is due to transient conditions, eg viral respiratory infection, which causes reduced airway function at birth but rarely evolves to asthma (N Engl J Med 1995; 332:133oA)

whey The watery fluid that is separated from a clot of casein and fat in making curds from milk, which contains most of the lactose, as well as the water-soluble minerals, and minerals found in milk; in cow's milk; the casein:whey ratio may have an effect on an individual's cholesterol levels as an adult (Science News 1994; 146:137)

WHHL rabbit Watanabe hereditable hyperlipidemic rabbit An animal model for the study of atherosclerosis described by Watanabe (Kobe University, 1978); see Atherosclerosis, Cholesterol, LDL, Lipoprotein

lipase

whiff test GYNECOLOGY A clinical test in which vaginal secretions are mixed with 10% KOH, resulting in a fishy odor highly suggestive of bacterial vaginosis; see Vaginosis

whiplash An abrupt to-and-fro movement that has been appropriately likened to the cracking of a whip, which almost invariably refers to whiplash injury, see there

whiplash injury EMERGENCY MEDICINE Hyperextension injury to the neck, often the result of being struck from behind by a fast-moving vehicle, in an automobile accident; whiplash injuries have been markedly reduced by the high-backed headrests now standard in automobiles in the US; WIs occur in more than one million people/year (US); although most become asymptomatic within a few weeks, 20-40% develop the so-called late whiplash syndrome‡; cervical zygapophyseal joint pain is common in whiplash injury, and was formerly treated with corticosteroids, a modality now reported to be ineffective (N Engl J Med 1994; 330:1047oA) affects ± 120 000/year (US); 90% of such injuries are self-limited, and require neither radiology nor treatment; whiplash has been treated by a wide range of unproven therapies including acupuncture, cervical neck pillows for sleeping, electrical stimulation, epidural (and other) injections, heat, ice, laser, massage, rest, shortwave diathermy, traction, and ultrasound MANAGEMENT (Based on the conclusions of the Quebec Task Force on Whiplash-Associated Disorders (WO Spitzer, in Spine 15 April 1995) see Quebec classification; see Steering wheel syndrome

whiplash decision tree

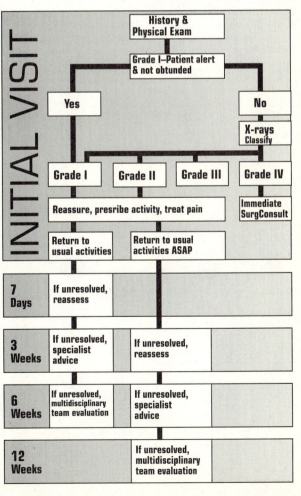

whiplash-shaken infant syndrome Shaken baby syndrome, see there

Whipple's bacillus *Tropheryma whippelii*, see there

(George Hoyt) Whipple's disease Lipodystrophy A systemic malabsorption syndrome characterized by diffuse tissue infiltration by glycoprotein-rich macrophages with abundant bacillary forms CLINICAL Most common in middle-aged ♂ (♂:♀ ratio, 10:1), and accompanied by acropachyia digestiva, cutaneous hyperpigmentation, malabsorption, diarrhea, steatorrhea, arthritis, lymphadenopathy, endocarditis, fever, pleuritis CNS alterations (eg demyelination of posterior columns); the bacilliform inclusions occur in the skin, nervous system, joints, heart, vessels, kidney, lung, serosal membranes, lymph nodes spleen and liver PATHOGENESIS The causative organism has been identified (by amplification of a 16S rRNA sequence) as a gram-positive actinomycete, tentatively designated as *Tropheryma whippelii* gen nov sp nov (**N Engl J Med 1992; 327:293**oa**, 331:1343**oa**)** PATHOLOGY Histiocytes in WD are similar to Gaucher's disease; definitive confirmation of the WD particles requires high-power PAS-stained light microscopy or low-power electron microscopy TREATMENT Penicillin + streptomycin for two weeks, followed by tetracycline for one year; Cf Pseudo-Whipple's disease

(Allen Oldenfield) Whipple procedure Pancreatico-duodenectomy SURGERY An extensive operation consisting of the removal of part or all of the pancreas, the duodenum, proximal jejunum, as well as the distal stomach and common bile duct; the 'Whipple' is considered the therapy of choice for periampullary carcinoma of the pancreas, and in experiences hands has an operative mortality of < 5%; in the recently popularized modified Whipple, the pylorus is spared with no decline in overall survival and multiple mechanical[1], procedural[2], and functional[3] advantages

[1]The 2 cm portion of spared duodenum is more easily anastomosed to the jejunum [2]The operative time is slightly shorter [3]Postgastrectomy complications (eg dumping) and ulceration are lessened; pylorus sparing also has the advantages of preserving the postprandial secretion of gastrin and secretin

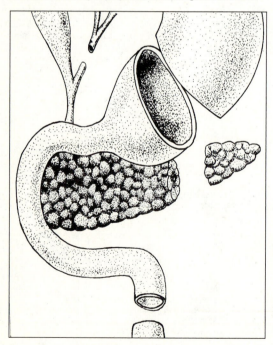

Whipple procedure

whipworm *Trichuris trichiura* The nematode that is the world's most common parasitic infection; it is transmitted by the oral-fecal route, and occurs in a background of poor hygiene CLINICAL Abdominal malaise, colic, abdominal distension and when massive, mild anemia, bloody diarrhea and rectal prolapse TREATMENT Mebendazol

whisker hair Short dark hair of the scalp that resembles pubic hair, first seen during puberty, often later developing into severe androgenic alopecia; whisker hair is a variant of acquired progressive kinky hair; see Kinky hair (Menke's) syndrome, Pili torti, Woolly hair syndrome

whiskering appearance Short, linear spiculation seen by plain films of bone at the sites of muscle insertion and osseous stress, variably accompanied by osteosclerosis, cystic changes and dystrophic calcification, most common in the iliac, ischial and calcaneus bones, due to ankylosing spondylitis, DISH in renal osteodystrophy

whiskey test ENDOCRINOLOGY A stimulation test of historic interest for determining calcitonin levels; 50 ml of 'Scotch' was administered per os to patients with medullary thyroid carcinoma; within 15 minutes, calcitonin increases to levels comparable to those produced by calcium infusions; false negativity is uncommon SIDE EFFECTS Diarrhea and flushing, due to stimulation of hormonal release by alcohol

'whistle-blowing' RESEARCH ETHICS The act of informing authorities of a person's alleged wrong-doings; 'whistle-blowing' in science is used in the context of research fraud, alleged fraud or blatant misinterpretation of data; the whistle-blower may take several levels of action ranging from the mere mention of an 'incident' to a colleague to the reporting of the improprieties to the individual's superiors, granting agency, academic institution or to a major peer-reviewed journal; junior people, eg post-doctorate fellows and graduate students in the academic hierarchy are in a position to recognize data manipulation at the 'bench' level (they also have the most to lose should they 'blow the whistle' on their superiors); a number of scientists at the National Institutes of Health (US) have shifted their research interests and are actively examining cases of alleged fraud, embarking on so-called 'witch-hunts'; see Baltimore affair, 'Dingellization', Fraud in science, Qui tam suits

whistling face syndrome Freeman-Sheldon syndrome Craniocarpotarsal syndrome An AD [MIM 193700] condition with a typical mask-like physiognomy (small 'pursed' lips, deep-set (sunken) eyes, epicanthus, hypoplastic nasal alae, strabismus, blepharophimosis, and ptosis), accompanied by failure to thrive, normal intelligence, short stature, scoliosis, camptodactyly with ulnar deviation ('windmill hands'), and talipes equinovarus or clubfoot

white atrophy Milian syndrome Whitish scleroderma-like plaque(s) with ulceration present on the skin of the lower extremities of females, secondary to venous stasis

'white beverage' CLINICAL NUTRITION A generic term for imitation milks and nondairy milk substitutes (eg soy milk), which are used in developed nations for children who are allergic to milk and milk products and are used in developing economies where animal fats are in short supply; see Breast milk, Unpasteurized milk

white blood cell differential (count) see 'Diff'

White's classification A system for categorizing gestational DM, designed to predict the maternal and fetal mortality and morbidity (table)

white coat A highly colloquial term referring to any health care professional who in the performance of his/her duties dons a white coat; to answer the often thought, rarely expressed question, '...just how clean is that white coat?', D Wong and colleagues (**BMJ 1991; 303:1602**) cultured impressions of the cuffs, front pockets, and other parts of the WC from 100 physicians from various specialties who changed their coats every week, every 2 weeks, 2-4 weeks,

4-8 weeks, and ≥ 8 weeks (!); 42 isolates of *Staphylococcus aureus* were found on the WCs of 29 physicians, in particular nonmedical specialists, eg 9/16 coats from general surgeons, 4/7 from orthopedic surgeons, and 4/6 ER physicians

white coat hyperglycemia The spurious elevation of glucose levels related to the psychological stress of being examined by 'white coats' in the setting of a clinic (**Br Med J 1992; 305:1194**)

white coat hypertension A transient increase in blood pressure that occurs in apprehensive patients when faced with the 'white coat' of the physician, especially when the patient is female and the doctor male, possibly resulting in inappropriate anti-hypertensive therapy; this form of pseudohypertension may be prevented by either having a nurse or technician measure the pressure or by measuring the pressure after a physical examination; Cf Pseudohypertension, Small cuff syndrome

White's disease Generalized familial hyperkeratosis involving face, trunk, scalp and axilla crusted with warty excrescences

white eye reflex Cat's eye reflex, see there

white fat Usual ('garden variety') adipose tissue, which contrasts with brown fat

white forelock Piebaldism A striking focal depigmentation of hair affecting the anterior scalp margin, which has no clinical significance of its own, but is typical of Waardenburg syndrome (an autosomal dominant condition characterized by leukoderma, a flattened nasal bridge and cochlear deafness, see there), and may also be seen in tuberous sclerosis and Vogt-Koyanagi syndrome

Note: Piebaldism is a form of poliosis, localized depigmentation of the hair, especially of the scalp that may be due to alopecia areata, radiotherapy, severe localized dermatitis and vitiligo

'white' graft An anemic, ie 'white', transplantation tissue, eg skin or renal graft that is undergoing hyperacute rejection with overwhelming anoxia; vascularization is prevented from occurring since, although the host and graft vessels are successfully anastomosed, the arteries are immediately occluded by preformed antibodies, causing immediate infarction, necessitating a nephrectomy; see Rejection

white hat POLITICS & MEDICINE A highly colloquial Washington organization which in the 20-question questionnaire that serves as a primary screening tool that is reported to have a 83-97% sensitivity and 63-82% specificity for depression (**JAMA 1995; 273:197**)

whitehead Closed comedo, milium Papular, millet seed-sized skin lesions in the 'sebaceous zones', characterized by aggregates of impacted keratin and sebaceous material, which may rupture 'spontaneously' when infected by *Propionibacterium acnes*

Whitehead Institute RESEARCH A non-profit independent research and teaching affiliate of the Massachusetts Institute of Technology that was founded in 1982 by a gift from EC Whitehead RESEARCH ACTIVITIES at 'the Whitehead' encompass RNA polymerase II, protein folding, myosin,

viral oncogenesis, sex chromosomes, adult DM, AIDS pathogenesis, AIDS vaccine, and others DIRECTOR GR Fink BUDGET (1990) $18.7 million; see Citation impact; Cf Howard Hughes Medical Institute

Note: Research performed as the Whitehead Institute has had an enviably high citation impact on the biomedical sciences, and thus is considered a 'high-power' institution

white infarct Anemic infarct, see there

white leg Phlegmasia alba dolens

white dermographism White line response A 5–20-minute-in-duration pallid line that is seen when the skin surface is firmly stroked with a blunt object, which corresponds to focal vasoconstriction or edema; initially regarded as typical of atopic dermatitis, WD is thought by some authors to be an anomalous response to cutaneous inflammation

white line response White dermographism, see there

white line of scurvy A radiolucent band seen in the primary spongiosa of the metaphysis, corresponding to a zone of complete osseous disintegration susceptible to fractures PATHOLOGY Immature fibroblasts, hyalinoid material and hemosiderin-laden macrophages; below this zone is an area completely free of hematopoietic cells, the 'gerüstmark', composed of connective tissue

white line sign A flat white line seen by ultrasonography corresponding to mucosal thickening in the renal collecting system of renal transplant victims; this finding is not seen in the clinically similar minimal nephrosis

white liver disease Fatty metamorphosis of viscera, see there

white lung The macroscopic morphology of a lung that has suffered repeated bouts of rheumatic pneumonitis, in which the anemic lung is scarred and pale in the lower lobes

white muscle (cell) *Myocytus albus* [NH3] A type of striated muscle that generates ATP by anaerobic metabolism of glucose and glycogen; white muscle or 'fast twitch' muscle, is capable of short and rapid activity that cannot be sustained over time; it has abundant sarcoplasmic reticulum, phosphorylase that utilizes intrinsic glycogen for energy, low oxidative enzyme activity and relatively fewer mitochondria than red muscle fibers; see Red muscle

white muscle disease Nutritional myopathy VETERINARY MEDICINE A disease of young livestock (sheep, cattle) characterized by chalky degeneration of muscle that most prominently affects cardiac and 'fast twitch' muscle; it has been linked to various vitamin and nutritional deficiencies, eg of vitamin E and/or selenium

white nevus Nevus anemicus, see there

white noise That sound that has equal energy at every frequency and can be eliminated by raising the 'cut-off' of the detection device; Cf Chaos

Note: Most early neonates fall asleep within 5 minutes in a background of white noise; ¼ of neonates fall asleep in the same time interval without white noise

'white-out' SUBSTANCE ABUSE A generic term for commercial products, that are used to correct typed or written errors on paper documents by painting over the errors with an opaque white, rapidly-drying liquid; in their original formulations, these products contained trichloroethylene (TCE) and methylchloroform (1,1,1-trichloroethane); the latter substance has had some currency among pre-adolescents as a 'gateway' abuse substance, which is sniffed to induce a transient sensation of euphoria; the State of California's Proposition 65 regulations regarding human exposure to carcinogens forced a reformulation of 'white-outs', eliminating TCE; at the about the same time, allyl isothiocyanate (oil of mustard) was added to these products, the pungency of which discourages most casual abuse; see 'Gateway' drugs, Proposition 65, TCE; Cf Glue-

WHITE'S CLASSIFICATION (MODIFIED)			
CLASS	DURATION	LESIONS	THERAPY
A	Any	None	Diet only
B	< 10 Yrs	None	Insulin
C	10-19 Yrs	None	Insulin
D	> 20 Yrs	Benign retinopathy	Insulin
F	Any	Nephropathy	Insulin
H	Any	Heart disease	Insulin
R	Any	Proliferative retinopathy	Insulin

sniffing WILDNESS MEDICINE A condition that occurs in arctic regions in which no objects are discernible as there is bright sunlight reflecting off snow-covered objects, often resulting in snow blindness, see there

white phosphorus Yellow or elemental phosphorus A reactive and toxic allotrope of phosphorus that reacts spontaneously at room temperature with ambient oxygen, and is highly susceptible to combustion (in particular, above > 30° C); WP formerly had currency in the manufacture of matches, and in treating rickets, scrofula, and other conditions; WP is a waxy solid used in fertilizers, water treatment, food products, beverages and in the synthesis of pesticides, eg rat and roach poisons; the vapors are highly irritating to the eyes and respiratory tract and cause deep thermal burns at sites of skin contact; prolonged exposure is associated with facial bone necrosis, abdominal pain, jaundice, 'garlic breath', anemia, cachexia, blepharospasm and photophobia PATHOLOGY Liver is most severely affected with extensive 'large vacuole' fatty infiltration and necrosis (early periportal necrosis; late massive lobular necrosis); central zone demonstrate 'fine vacuole' fatty infiltration, mid-zone demonstrates coagulation necrosis

white plague Tuberculosis MEDICAL HISTORY A human infection by *Mycobacterium tuberculosis*, the 'robber of youth' has followed man through history, has been identified in the spine of Neolithic man and was first formally described by Homer in 900 BC; modern epidemics of TB began with the industrial revolution-related urban overcrowding in Britain, peaking in the mid-1800s, emigrated with the Europeans to the US and traveled with the settlers as they moved south and west, decimating the American aborigine; the incidence of TB reached a nadir in 1986 and has been increasing since due to its association with AIDS; Cf Black plague SUBSTANCE ABUSE A colloquial term for the epidemic of cocaine abuse

white pulp *Pulpa alba* [NH3] A histologically distinct zone of normal splenic architecture, composed of peri-arteriolar lymphatic sheaths, surrounded by a mantle of small lymphocytes (predominantly T cell) surrounding germinal centers composed of B lymphocytes and B lymphoblasts; blood-born antigens contact the immune responsive cells in the germinal centers and within 24 hours, a primary response (IgM) occurs with immunoblastic proliferation and enlargement of germinal centers; Cf Red pulp

white pulp disease Lymphoproliferative disorders that most prominently affect the white pulp of the spleen, including poorly differentiated lymphocytic leukemia, well-differentiated lymphocytic leukemia, histiocytic lymphoma and Hodgkin's disease

white 'spider' FORENSIC PATHOLOGY An arachnoid skin lesion characterized by concentric geographic scarring and ulceration caused by fibrosis emanating centrifugally from the site of injection of illicit drugs, which is a typical post-mortem sign of subcutaneous heroin injection (skin 'popping')

white sponge nevus DERMATOLOGY An AD [MIM 193900] lesion characterized by variably-sized, painless, albescent plaques, which by LM display a 'basket-weave' epithelium, hyperparakeratosis and acanthosis of mucosae, especially of the nasopharynx (oral, nasal, esophagus, larynx), as well as vaginal and anal mucosae; the waxing and waning nature of the lesions may cause confusion with more serious white intralesions of the mouth, including leukoedema, leukoplakia, irritation, chewing tobacco dysplasia, lichen planus, Darier's disease, dyskeratosis congenita; although usually non-infectious, the skin lesions of white sponge nevus may respond to penicillin

white spot A generic term for any hypopigmented cutaneous macule that may appear in Addison's disease, alope-

cia areata, DM, halo nevus, hypomelanosis of Ito, amelanotic malignant melanoma, piebaldism, thyroid disease, tuberous sclerosis, vitamin B_{12} deficiency, vitiligo and Vogt-Koyanagi-Harada syndrome

white spot fundus Fundus albipunctatus An inherited condition of uncertain genetics* characterized by multiple macular lesions of the optic fundus which, with time, may progress to blindness

*Either AD [MIM 136880] or AR

white strawberry tongue PEDIATRICS Red congested and edematous fungiform papillae in a whitish background of filiform papillae, a coating present between the second and fifth day of scarlet fever, which may also be seen in measles and in other febrile viral enanthemas

whites A popular term for the white 'uniform' worn by medicos the world over, which changes in length according to rank; the lower echelon[1] Herberts (and Berthas) sport a short smock-like sartorial insult with Captain Kangaroo-like pockets, while the elder medical tribesmen[2] are garbed in robes hemmed twixt hip and knee; Cf Scrubs

[1]ie Medical students and interns [2]Higher ranking physicians, ie residents and attendings

whitlow A painful infectious dermatitis of the finger, seeded by contact exposure; see Herpetic whitlow, Melanotic whitlow

Note: Felon and whitlow are regarded as synonyms by standard medical dictionaries; in some surgical texts, felon connotes a deep, often purulent-ab-initio infection of a digit that may require active drainage

whole blood TRANSFUSION MEDICINE A unit of blood that contains all the components (erythrocytes, leukocytes, platelets, plasma proteins and fluid); whole blood still has currency as a transfusion product as 1) It is the raw material from which other products are prepared and 2) It may, under certain circucumstances, have some utility as a stand-alone product; under the usual circumstances, whole blood is almost invariably separated into components as this allows for more specific therapy while reducing the potential for infections and eliciting an immune response in the recipient to the extraneous transfused component; whole blood transfusion is acceptable (albeit not ideal) practice in the face of symptomatic anemia and hypovolemia, although packed red cells and 0.9% NaCl solution causes the patient less immune 'stress'; since patients may be asymptomatic despite a very low hematocrit, it is considered poor policy to transfuse blood products without addressing the underlying condition (Technical Manual, American Association of Blood Banks, Arlington, Virginia 1990)

whole blood tonometry LABORATORY MEDICINE The process of equilibrating fresh whole blood at a given temperature with known concentrations of O_2, CO_2 and nitrogen gases; because the dissolved gas partial pressure is known, the resulting medium has features of the patient's specimen; WBT is useful for measuring the inaccuracy of blood gas analyzers (Am Clin Lab July 1994)

whole genome shotgun sequencing A technique devised by C Venter et al for determining the entire sequence (*verb*, sequence) of a particular organism that was first used to sequence *Haemophilus influenzae* and *Mycoplasma genitalium*; in WGSS, an organism is disrupted with ultrasound, followed by sequencing of relatively short segments of DNA, and arranging them in the proper order by a computer, which identifies overlapping sequences (Science 1995; 268:1273)

whole gut scintigraphy GASTROENTEROLOGY A technique in which two radiolabeled markers are used to evaluate colonic transit ($^{111}InCl_3$-labeled capsules that disintegrate in the terminal ileum and proximal colon) and gastric emptying and small bowel transit (^{99m}Tc mixed in a test meal); by WGS, patients complaining of constipation have a slowed GI transit time, while those with diarrhea had an increased transit time (Mayo Clin Proc 1995; 70:113oa)

whooping cough The characteristic cough of pertussis, which infects ± 60 million and kills 1 million/year (worldwide), caused by the gram-negative nonmotile *Bordatella pertussis*; the 'whoop' occurs during the paroxysmal stage of infection (1-2 weeks after the onset, lasting for 2-4 weeks); a 'paroxysm' consists of 10-20 coughs of increasing intensity, a deep inspiration (the 'whoop') after which a thick, viscid plug of mucus is expelled, occasionally accompanied by vomiting; the paroxysms may occur every ½ hour, often accompanied by ↑ venous pressure, plethoric conjunctivae, periorbital edema, petechiae and epistaxis, infants may be cyanotic until relieved of the obstructing plug of mucus; see DTP; other 'whooping' infections of early infancy include adenovirus, *Bordatella parapertussis*, *B bronchoseptica*

'whore' 'Hired gun', see there

wicking INFECTIOUS DISEASE Enhanced penetration of liquids, and small infectious agents, through minute holes in latex membranes, eg surgical gloves that may occur when washed with surfactants, an effect that militates against the re-use of certain materials

widow-maker lesion CARDIOLOGY Severe stenosis of the left anterior descending coronary artery, so named as it is classically associated with sudden death (N Engl J Med 1994; 331:601cps)

wiggle Squiggle, see there

Wilcoxon's rank-sum test STATISTICS: A nonparametric maneuver that allows analysis of matched pairs of observations, and evaluation of variables in a series, eg differences in patient characteristics, allowing them to be placed in rank order; the WRST is an alternative to the paired t test when the population being studied does not have a normal (gaussian) distribution

The Wild Child A film by François Truffaut about a 'wild child' (subsequently named Victor) who was found in a French forest about 150 years ago (see N Engl J Med 1994; 331:1030br) see Genie, Psychosocial dwarfism

wild woman archetype ETHNO-CLINICAL PSYCHOLOGY A poetic conceptualization of the female psyche and soul as rooted in the 'wilds' of instinct and uncivilized energy (CP Estés, Women WHo Run with the Wolves, Ballantine Books, New York, 1992)

wild Pertaining or referring to that which has been neither intentionally inbred or genetically engineered

wild-type *adjective* Pertaining or relating to an organism or gene locus that predominates in natural or normal populations

wild-type allele GENETICS The allele for an inherited trait that is most frequent in a natural (wild) population

wilderness medicine An evolving specialty of sports medicine that studies the effects of environmental extremes (eg high mountains, glaciers, deserts) on health and disease (Ann Emerg Med 1992; 21:853)

wilding FORENSIC PSYCHIATRY A slang term for a phenomenon of recent vintage described in the US, which is virtually unknown in civilized regions; a 'wilding' consists of an unprovoked and motiveless attack on strangers, merely for the sake of violence, and may include gang rape, stabbing, shooting, and homicide

will 1) Desire, volition, as in 'will to live' 2) '*The legal expression or declaration of a person's mind or wishes as to the disposition of his property, to be performed or take effect after his death*' (Black's Law DIctionary, 6th ed, West Publishing, St Paul, Mn, 1990)

will to live PSYCHOLOGY The sense of self-preservation, usually coupled to a 'future sense', ie dreams, and aspirations, and expectations for future improvement in one's state in life

Will Rogers phenomenon Stage migration EPIDEMIOLOGY The improved survival of patients with cancer (or other disease) due to either reclassification of patients into different prognostic groups by recognizing more subtle disease manifestations, or by using newer diagnostic modalities that allow the disease to be diagnosed at an earlier stage; this results in a 'zero-time shift' and 'improved' prognosis for a given disease; however when classified with symptom stages without new diagnostic procedures, survival for the same cancer has not changed (Ann Int Med 1983; 99:843, N Engl J Med 1985; 312:1604; ibid, 313:1291c); it is believed by some authors that the advances in diagnostic technology has blinded the medical community to the lack of progress in treating cancer

The eponym is dedicated to the American cowboy-philosopher, Will Rogers (1879-1935), who observed that truth was relative to one's vantage point

Williams syndrome Elfin face syndrome A rare (1:20 000) AD [MIM 194050] condition characterized by profound mental retardation coupled with intact or even enhanced verbal abilities, and extreme sociability; with a characteristic elf-like face (small mandible, prominent maxilla, an upturned nose, depressed nasal bridge, anteverted nares, wide mouth, full lips, a 'Cupid's bow' upper lip, small chin, medial eyebrow flare, periorbital puffiness, short palpebral fissures), carious peg teeth, as well as feeding difficulties, failure to thrive, cardiac defects in the form of stenoses of the great vessels supravalvular aortic stenosis and septal defects CLINICAL Angina, syncope and occasionally sudden death, onychodysplasia, statural defects, dental defects, mild mental retardation, classically linked to an adeptness at vacuous 'cocktail party chatter', nephrosclerosis and bony sclerosis induced by hypercalcemia MOLECULAR PATHOLOGY Deletion of elastin gene and adjacent gene(s) on chromosome 7 (New York Times 2 August 1994:C1)

Williams-Campbell syndrome Bronchomalacia An AR [MIM 211450] deficiency of bronchial cartilage resulting in obstruction, cough, wheezing, dyspnea, and recurrent infections of early onset (N Engl J Med 1993; 329:1484cpc)

Willowbrook State School BIOMEDICAL ETHICS An extended-care facility in the US, in which a group of mentally-retarded children were allegedly inoculated with live hepatitis B virus during the 1950s; the case ultimately led to the Willowbrook Consent doctrine (1972), that ruled that the mentally retarded have a right to protection from harm; see Unethical medical research

Wilm's nephritis A term of uncertain specific utility referring to nephrotic syndrome seen in Wilm's tumor

Wilms tumor An embryonal renal tumor that arises in aberrant mesenchymal renal stem cell lines, coupled with the loss of functioning tumor suppressor genes; Wilms' tumor comprises 92% of primary childhood renal malignancies (frequency: 1:10 000); the rest are sarcomas of various subtypes ETIOLOGY 4-8-fold ↑ incidence if the father was an automobile mechanic, welder or auto body repairman, possibly related to occupational exposure to leaded gasoline or due to fumes from repairing automobile radiators with lead PATHOLOGY Blastemal components, including epithelial cells, stroma, tubular differentiation, and glomeruloid differentiation (Acta Cytologica 1993; 37:209oa) MOLECULAR PATHOLOGY Mutation of the *WT1* gene, located on chromosome segment 11p13, converts it from a tumor-suppressor gene into a dominant negative oncogene, disrupting the normal gene products (N Engl J Med 1994; 331:586rv) the mutation abolishes the DNA-binding activity of a zinc finger domain that binds to a site of a growth factor inducible gene, suggesting that the loss of binding may be the critical tumorigenic event in Wilms' tumor formation (Science 1991; 250:1259) CLINICAL Wilms' tumor presents as a mass, often with hypertension 60%, hematuria 24%, nephritis (Wilms' nephritis) and serosal effusions (ascites, pleural effusions); 5% are bilateral and anaplasia connotes a poor prognosis Note: 20% of aniridia is associated with Wilms' tumor (see WAGR syndrome) DDx Infants under 6 months of age may have a congenital mesoblastic nephroma, a histological mimic of Wilms' tumor that usually regresses spontaneously

Wilson's disease An AR [MIM 277900] disorder of copper metabolism characterized by accumulation of copper in the brain, liver, and other organs CLINICAL Hepatic cirrhosis, degeneration of basal ganglia of the brain and neurologic deterioration with involuntary movement, tremors, muscular rigidity, spastic contractures, psychiatric defects, dysphagia, Kayser-Fleischer ring MOLECULAR PATHOLOGY The defective gene is located on chromosome segment 13q14; RFLP analysis can identify carriers and presymptomatic patients; early diagnosis can be performed by chorionic villus biopsy in the fetus (**N Engl J Med 1992; 327:57c**)

wimp allele MOLECULAR BIOLOGY A dominant maternal effect allele that reduces transcription of subsets of segmentation genes in *Drosophila* (**Genes Dev 1991; 5:341**) and has weak tyrosine phosphokinase activity

windblown appearance A descriptor for the enlarged, crowded and hyperchromatic and irregular nuclei in the epithelium of Bowen's disease and bowenoid papulosis of the genitalia; the cells are pleomorphic, dyskeratotic and multinucleated with atypical mitotic figures, acanthosis and parakeratosis

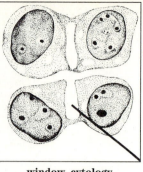

window, cytology

'articulations' PHYSIOLOGY An opening in a biological membrane, through which solutes may be transported RADIOLOGY An interval of photon energies used in a scintillation counter (gamma-ray detector); the so-called 'pulse height analyzer' rejects any photon energy falling outside of the window (and is therefore not counted) SURGERY A region of an abscess in closest contact with the abdominal wall (or any accessible skin surface) without an intervening visceral organ, which can be opened for relatively safe drainage

window period IMMUNOLOGY An interval between the time of inoculation or exposure to a microorganism, usually viral and the ability to detect its presence by serological assays, ie by antigen-antibody reactions, occurring in 1) HBV The hepatitis B 'core window' represents active but undetected HBV infection, in which the circulating HBV surface antigen (HBsAg) has fallen to undetectable levels and antibody to the HBV surface antigen (anti-HB$_S$) has yet to rise to detectable levels; during the core window, the IgM antibodies to the HBV core antigen (anti-HBc) are positive but not always included in the usual hepatitis screening battery 2) HIV-1 window A time interval between the initial infection with human immunodeficiency virus that can be detected by the polymerase chain reaction or detection of the p24 antigen) and production of the anti-p24 and anti-p41 antibodies in quantities sufficient to be measured by the ELISA technique, the method most commonly used to screen for the presence of anti-HIV-1 antibodies; although the HIV-1 window period is thought to be no longer than 45 days under most circumstances ranges from 3-9 months, it may be up to 36 months in duration Note: All units of blood donated in the US are screened for anti-HIV-1 p24 antibody and thus potentially in the 'window period' for HIV-1 infection TOXICOLOGY The 'window period' corresponds to the time interval between ingestion of lethal quantities of a drug or toxin and the production of irreversible organ damage, eg 1) Acetaminophen overdose in which there is a 2-3 day latency or window period, which precedes irreversible liver damage 2) Paraquat poisoning in which irreversible interstitial lung damage follows a 3-5 day window interval 3) Phyllotoxin (*Amanita phylloides*) poisoning in which cardiac, renal and hepatic failure follows a 1-3 day latency period

WIND CHILL EQUIVALENTS IN ºC /ºF FOR REFERENCE WIND SPEEDS OF 2.5 KPH (4MPH)						
TEMP	2.5 (4)	6 (10)	12 (20)	19 (30)	25 (40)	30 (50)
4.5ºC/+40ºF	4.5ºC/+40ºF	-2ºC/+28ºF	-8ºC/+18ºF	-10.5ºC/+13ºF	-12ºC/+10ºF	-13ºC/+9ºF
-1ºC/30ºF	-1ºC/30ºF	-9ºC/+16ºF	-16ºC/+4ºF	-19ºC/-2ºF	-21ºC/-6ºF	-22ºC/-7ºF
-7ºC/20ºF	-7ºC/20ºF	-16ºC/+4ºF	-23ºC/-10ºF	-28ºC/-18ºF	-30ºC/-22ºF	-30ºC/-23ºF
-12ºC/10ºF	-12ºC/10ºF	-23ºC/-9ºF	-32ºC/-25ºF	-36ºC/-33ºF	-38ºC/-37ºF	-39ºC/-39ºF
-18ºC/0ºF	-18ºC/0ºF	-29ºC/-21ºF	-39ºC/-39ºF	-44ºC/-48ºF	-47ºC/-53ºF	-49ºC/-55ºF
-23ºC/-10ºF	-23ºC/-10ºF	-36ºC/-33ºF	-47ºC/-53ºF	-53ºC/-64ºF	-56ºC/-69ºF	-57ºC/-71ºF
-29ºC/-20ºF	-29ºC/-20ºF	-43ºC/-46ºF	-55ºC/-67ºF	-62ºC/-79ºF	-65ºC/-85ºF	-66ºC/-87ºF

JM Last, RB Wallace, Eds, Public Health and Preventive Medicine, 13th ed, Appletone & Lange, Norwalk, 1992

windchill factor WILDERNESS MEDICINE An index[1] used to adjust the actual air temperature to express the intensity of cooling expected from a cold environment as a function of the ambient temperature and wind speed[2], calculated by the formula:

$$H = (10.45 + 10s^{1/2} - s)(33-t)$$

where H is the wind chill expressed in kcal m^{-2}h^{-1}, s is the wind speed in m s^{-1}, and t is the ambient temperature in degrees Celsius; H allows comparison of the cooling effect of various temperatures and wind speed combinations

[1]The correct term is windchill index but is unlikely to prevail in the forseeable future-Author's note [2]Humidity and radiant heat energy tend to be less important in cold environments

winding number Linkage number MOLECULAR BIOLOGY The number of times that the two strands of DNA cross through each other, an event requiring that the strands be nicked and rejoined; see Superhelix, Topoisomerase

windmill hand A fanciful descriptor for a hand with ulnar deviation and induration of the flexor surface of the proximal phalanges, described in the whistling face syndrome

window A common adjective used in various medical specialties referring or pertaining to a place in time (eg window period, see there) or space CYTOLOGY A 'window' is a narrow, slit-like clear space between two or more molded mesothelial cells, which may be joined to each other by

Windows NT COMPUTERS A 32-bit multitasking, multithreaded operating system released in 1993 from Microsoft Corporation that supports the Windows graphic user interface

Windows 95 COMPUTERS The current disk operating system for microcomputers, released 24 August 1995 by Microsoft Corporation, which contains an improved graphic user interface, and integrated on-line software; W95 increases the speed and efficiency with which PCs perform their tasks, but requires significantly more RAM (14 is considered a 'safe' minimum), and a larger hard drive; W95 architecture may be suited for modernizing the aging operating systems used in laboratory and hospital information systems (**NY Times, 24 August 1995, A1, D6**)

The 'launch' of W95 cost circa $200 million in various forms of advertisement and marketing expenditures, and transiently dominated the news, stealing 'thunder' from the other sound-bite favorites du jour, from the momentous (eg the West Bank, Bosnia) to the moronic (eg OJ trial)-Author's note

windsock deformity CARDIOLOGY A descriptor for an aneurysm of the sinus of Valsalva, as seen by aortography, in which there is a wide base at the aortic origin and a nipple-like apex projecting into the right atrium, the usual site of rupture; the aneurysm is characterized by attenuation and separation of the aortic media within the sinus from the common fibrous junction of the aorta, the left ventricle and the aortic valve PEDIATRIC SURGERY A descriptive term for the characteristic balloon-like dilatation seen on a barium enema in neonates with membranous atresia of the colon, ileum or jejunum; when the deformity is colonic, the barium column reaches the membrane but is forced back by the fecal flow in the transverse colon, forming a cup-shaped or windsock-like radiolucency UROLOGY A descriptor for the soft redundant membrane that prolapses into the bulbous urethra, as seen on voiding urethrography in the rare, complete urethral obstruction, which affects boys, and is located in the urethra distal to the verumontanum, presenting in the neonatal period with severe obstruction and dysplastic kidneys; if the 'obstruction' is mild, the condition may present in later childhood with persistent nighttime bet-wetting and incontinence

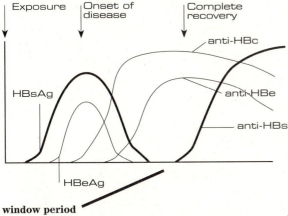

window period

wind-swept cortex A fanciful descriptor for extreme gyral atrophy resulting from florid neurosyphilis that is accompanied by marked necrosis of cortical neurons, microglial (rod) cell proliferation and gliosis; Cf Knife-blade atrophy

'wing beating' A descriptive term for the rhythmic oscillating tremor of the upper extremities as they are outstretched, a characteristic neurologic sign of Wilson's disease, which is often accompanied by cerebellar ataxia and intention tremor

winging of the scapula Elevation of the scapulae, fancifully likened to an angel's wing, which is seen when the arm is abducted, a finding characteristic of limb-girdle dystrophy, due to paralysis of the long thoracic nerve (fifth, sixth and seventh nerve roots), but which also occurs in wrinkly skin syndrome and in heavy manual labor, especially affecting those who carry heavy, sharp-cornered objects on the shoulders, eg 'hod carrier's palsy

'wintering tree' pattern A fanciful descriptor for the angiographic appearance of panacinar pulmonary emphysema, in which the vessels have an arborescent skeleton-like pattern, serving as a 'soft criterion' to differentiate this from bullous emphysema

winter vomiting disease A 1-3 day, often parvovirus-induced intestinal 'flu' that is most common in the winter in temperate climates CLINICAL either mild, afebrile watery diarrhea or more severe, febrile with vomiting, headache and systemic complaints

winter vomiting disease Epidemic vomiting, see there

wire loop lesion RENAL PATHOLOGY A lesion characterized by capillary walls thickened with subendothelial immune complex deposits, located between the glomerular basement membrane and capillary endothelium, which are associated with proliferative glomerulonephritis; wire loops are typical of class IV lupus (diffuse proliferative) nephritis, and may be seen in progressive systemic sclerosis and because they are often accompanied by necrosis, crescent formation and scarring, signal a poor prognosis

WISC Wechsler Intelligence Scale for Children A 10-category test that measures both verbal and performance intelligence quotient; see Psychological testing

Wisconsin solution Viaspan™ TRANSPLANTATION A hypothermic perfusate that contains pentafraction, lactobionic acid, raffinose, glutathione, adenosine and other substances, which is gravity-fed into the vessels of organs destined for transplantation, after draining the blood from 'brain-dead' donors; see Procurement, Slush preparation, Transplantation

wisdom teeth DENTISTRY A colloquial term for the third molars that usually erupt during late adolescence and which, given the physical confines of the jaw, often become impacted
Wisdom teeth are so-called as their appearance coincides with the development in later adolescence of some semblance of wisdom

wish bias A systemic error that is due to the tendency on either the part of a patient, eg to underreport exposure to fatty foods, or the part of an investigator, eg to report only those trials with positive findings or to report results that support a particular vantage point (J Clin Epidemiol 1990; 43:619); see Placebo effect, Publication bias

witch's milk PEDIATRICS A clear-to-lactescent discharge from the nipples of male and female neonates accompanied by breast hypertrophy, the result of transplacental hormonal effects, most commonly occurring in term infants

'witch-hunting' 'Whistleblowing', see there

withdrawal Substance abuse need definition

withdrawal emergent syndrome A tardive dyskinesia-like clinical complex that affects children and adolescents upon abrupt discontinuation of neuroleptic (antipsychotic) drugs, attributed to hypersensitivity of dopamine receptors, characterized by choreoathetosis and myoclonus TREATMENT Reintroduce the drug, taper the dose more slowly or await spontaneous resolution

'withhold' HEALTH CARE INDUSTRY *noun* A device used in some HMOs to give a physician a financial incentive to minimize the costs of his/her style of practice by withholding 5-15% of his/her capitated payment, which the physician receives if the total costs of tests, referrals, or hospital care incurred by his patients meets or falls below a certain level; withholds have fallen into disfavor as they tend to encourage physicians to undertreat patients (Am Med News 4 May 1992 p13)

within-subject biological variation LABORATORY MEDICINE The between-day or between-'draw' variability or imprecision of a measurable laboratory parameter in a particular subject; this imprecision can be expressed as a coefficient of variation and has been identified in hemoglobin concentration, and erythrocyte concentration (Arch Pathol Lab Med 1992; 116:825oA) as well as other laboratory values

witzelsucht German, Joke addiction Moria NEUROLOGY A manifestation of organic brain disease, eg tumors or atherosclerosis-induced lesions of the frontal cortex, in which the person compulsively tells puns, or relates silly jokes, often accompanied by childish behavior, as a defense mechanism to deflect attention from the individual's memory defects

WLU Workload units, see there

***wnt*-1** Formerly, *int*-1 A proto-oncogene that may determine embryonic patterns through an unknown mechanism, encoding a 44 kD protein for which there are multiple receptors, that associates with the cell surface and extracellular matrix after secretion (Science 1991; 252:1173); when *wnt*-1 is activated by insertion into the mouse mammary tumor virus (MMTV), it evokes histologic changes of malignant transformation in mammary epithelial cells

wobble MOLECULAR BIOLOGY An instability in tRNA's affinity for the third base in a codon (at the 5'-end); this looseness allows the base of the anticodon to pair with an anticodon other than that which would normally correspond to it; if perfect Watson-Crick base pairing were required between codon and anti-codon, 61 different transfer RNA (tRNA) species would be required; wobble (nonstandard) base pairing at the third nucleotide position of the codon allows most tRNAs to recognize more than one of the codons specifying for a given amino acid, serving to accelerate protein synthesis Note: The 'GU-wobble' may be responsible for the difference in tRNAs; the ability to recognize more than one codon is such that while the first and second nucleotides of the codon and their partners, the second and third of the anticodon bind by standard pairing, the binding of the third nucleotide of the codon and the first nucleotide of the anticodon is less restrictive and accepts a nonstandard pair, in this the so-called 'wobble' position, eg a single tRNA may bind to multiple codons, eg CUU, CUC, CUA and CUG; see Degenerate code, 'Second genetic code', tRNA

wobbles Enzootic incoordination, equine sensory ataxia VETERINARY MEDICINE Any of a number of conditions that affect the cervical spinal cord ETIOLOGY Equine degenerative myeloencephalopathy (which is idiopathic), locoregional injury, coccidial infection CLINICAL Chronic incoordination with gait clumsiness TREATMENT Decompression in selected cases, most animals must be shot (destroyed)

Wohlfahrtia A genus of flesh-eating flies, *Sarcophagidae,* that are associated with myiasis in living flesh

Wolff-Chaikoff effect ENDOCRINOLOGY An acute adaptive response to administration of high levels of iodine, in which increased intracellular levels of iodide block both the organic-binding and coupling reactions in the thyroid functionally 'turning off' the thyroid, an effect used to advantage in preparing the thyroid for surgery

Wolfe Classification A schema of four putatively distinct mammographic patterns (Am J Radiol 1976; 126:1130), which were reported to allow detection of 'dysplastic' breasts at an increased risk for cancer; subsequent studies revealed that the initially reported features were merely suggestive of malignancy

Wolffian duct Mesonephric duct An embryonal duct that forms from the 25-30th days of gestation in association with the rudimentary pronephros, later becoming the mesonephric excretory duct, the 'second embryonal kidney', giving rise to the male reproductive system (epididymis, vas deferens and seminal vesicles), largely regressing in the female at 10-11th week, a portion of which remains as embryonal 'rests' (Gartner's duct cysts, epoophoron and paroophoron); Cf Müllerian duct

Wolff-Parkinson-White syndrome Pre-excitation syndrome CARDIOLOGY A conduction disorder with ↑ susceptibility to supraventricular paroxysmal tachyarrhythmias, in which the sinoatrial impulse travels directly to the AV node or anomalously via the bundle of Kent which is more rapid, resulting in premature ventricular contraction EKG FINDINGS Short PR interval (< than 0.1 sec), a slur on the upstroke of the R or on the downstroke of an S wave

(known as a delta wave), prolonged QRS complex, and often ST-T changes (figure); common WPW arrhythmias include atrial tachycardia, atrial flutter, and atrial fibrillation; the impulse may 'choose' either the normal route of conduction to the AV node (making the diagnosis of WPW difficult) or it may travel via an anomalous route, detected by a broader QRS with a delta wave; in the latter scenario, the 'physiologic' delay at the AV node is circumvented and the ventricular rate may exceed 200/min; WPW may occur in a normal heart (reverting to a normal rhythm with exercise or atropine) or be associated with premature atrial tachyarrhythmia, Ebstein anomaly, and corrected transposition (ventricular 'reversal') and cardiomyopathy TREATMENT Cardioversion, IV procainamide, lidocaine or radiofrequency current ablation of accessory AV pathway (N Engl J Med 1991; 324:1605, 1612)

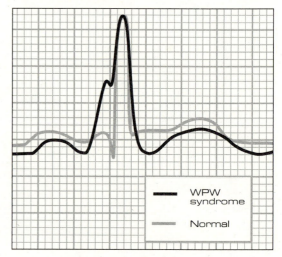

Wolff-Parkinson-White syndrome

Wolf-Hirschhorn syndrome 4p⁻ syndrome CLINICAL GENETICS An AD [MIM 194190] chromosomal deletion complex characterized by low birth weight, microcephaly, 'Greek helmet' facies (micrognathia, hypertelorism, epicanthus, beaked nose, redundant lateral nasal folds), cleft palate, inguinal hernia, cryptorchism, hypospadias and death before age three MOLECULAR PATHOLOGY WHS is caused by de novo deletion or rearrangement of 4p, within 4p16.3

wolfman syndrome Congenital generalized hypertrichosis, see there

Wolfram syndrome DIDMOAD syndrome, see there

wombstone GYNECOLOGY A leiomyoma (fibroid) that has undergone marked calcification OBSTETRICS Stone mole A hydatidiform mole that has undergone extensive dystrophic calcification (an extremely rare finding)

women and disease Disease is unfair; in general, men die earlier and more often through the vicissitudes of war, homicide, and suicide, and die earlier from AIDS, alcohol, drugs of abuse, tobacco and most cancers; ♀ live longer, better, and more disease-free; cancer mortality before age 20 is 22% lower in ♀ and in certain tumors, eg sarcomas and carcinomas, ♀ have longer survival; ♀:♂ ratio SLE-10:1; Sjögren syndrome, chronic active hepatitis, primary biliary cirrhosis-9:1; ITP-4:1; scleroderma, rheumatoid arthritis, myasthenia gravis, chronic fatigue syndrome-3:1

'women who fall' see Factitious 'diseases', Psychogenic syndromes

Wood's lamp DERMATOLOGY A UV lamp with a 365 nm filter that passes through nickel glass, which is of use in evaluating dermatophytosis; hair infected with *Microsporum* spp has a bright green fluoresence; erythrasma is a bright pink, pityriasis versicolor is bright yellow, and *Pseudomonas* spp infection is bright green; hair infected with *Trichophyton tonsurans* may not fluoresce

wood smoke Particulate material (PM_{10}) and chemicals (aldehydes, carbon monoxide, polycyclic aromatic hydrocarbons) from partial combustion of wood are reported to suppress the immune system and ↑ susceptibility to lung infections (Science 1995; 267:1771)

'wooden' sensation NEUROLOGY Tactile numbness of ten or more years' duration, associated with limited cutaneous sclerosis, secondary to occupational use of vibrating machines; see Vibration white finger syndrome

Wood lamp DERMATOLOGY A lamp that transmits filtered ultraviolet light at 365 nm, which is used in darkened rooms by dermatologists to detect and evaluate autofluorescence of superficial fungal (dermatophytic) infections

ERYTHRASMA AGENT *Nocardia minutissima* Color (if present, bright coral-red)

FAVUS AGENT *Trichophyton schoenleinii* Color Dull olive-gray green

MICROSPOROSIS AGENT *Microsporum audoni, M canis* Color Bright green 'black dot'

TINEA CAPITIS AGENT *Trichophyton violaceum*, Color Dull white

TINEA VERSICOLOR AGENT *Malassezia furfur* Color Yellow to gold-en-brown Note: Some bacteria are also autofluorescent, eg *Pseudomonas aeruginosa* Color Blue

Woodruff's 'laws' A group of humorous variations of 'Murphy's law' broadly applicable to (laboratory) medicine

1) A specimen (or hospital chart) is lost only if it is important to a physician's credibility, if there is a lawsuit pending on the specimen, or if not lost, it will be switched with a specimen from a critically ill patient

2) Intense preparation for a conference ensures its cancellation

3) Problems arise a) When the only person who can solve them is on vacation or b) When the party held responsible is due for contract renewal

woolly hair disease Tight curly hair seen at birth in caucasians that is 1) Sporadic, associated with the woolly hair nevus 2) AR [MIM 278150], in which the scalp hair is ash-white and the body hair is short and kinky or 3) AD [MIM 194300], in which the scalp hair is also ash-white, but with normal body hair; Cf Kinky hair disease, Uncombable hair syndrome

woolsorter's disease Inhalation anthrax, see there

word COMPUTERS A unit of data, consisting of two bytes of 8 bits (16 binary bits); one kilobyte is equal to 1024 (210 in binary computation); 1.0 megabyte of memory is approximately equal to 400 typewritten pages of manuscript MOLECULAR BIOLOGY Obsolete for codon

word salad PSYCHIATRY A string of neologisms, words, and phrases in which there is a loosening of associations, shifting of topics that may progress to near incoherence, with a complete lack of logical connection; word salads are characteristic of disordered thought processes, typical of psychosis, eg schizophrenia; Cf Witzelsucht

workers' compensation OCCUPATIONAL MEDICINE Workmans' compensation The benefits provided to employees for injuries suffered in the workplace EPIDEMIOLOGY Work-related injuries affect 8 million employees/year (US) resulting in the loss of 73 million work days and 10 000 lives BENEFITS Compensation benefits attempt to cover a worker's financial loss due to injury or occupational disease, including lost wages (workmans' 'comp' is usually ⅔ of a person's normal wages), medical and rehabilitation expenses, and disability benefits (Advance/Laboratory Sept 1994)

workflow analysis LABORATORY MEDICINE '...*a study of all individual actions involved in requesting, performing and reporting a test.* (it can be divided) *into three parts: preanalytical, which includes test requisition, sample collection, etc; analytical; and post-analytical,*

ie data transport and results interpretation...' (Am Clin Lab May 1994)

working diagnosis CLINICAL DECISION-MAKING A diagnosis based on experience, clinical epidemiology and some confirmatory evidence provided by ancillary studies, eg radiologic findings; working diagnoses allow early treatment of a disease while awaiting special or more definitive studies, eg immunoperoxidase stains or results from a reference laboratory

Working Formulation A classification system for non-Hodgkin's lymphomas, created to facilitate communication among various lymphoma experts[1] which was made difficult by the plethora of then-extant classifications[2]; the WF had a period of transient popularity as it was easily applied by pathologists and relatively predictive of the lymphomas future behavior; in low-grade lymphomas, the affected lymph nodes are rubbery, mobile, not fixed to the skin, enlarge very slowly, may cause lymphedema, nerve compression or ureteral obstruction, but are painless; asymptomatic hepatosplenomegaly is common as are liver, spleen, and BM infiltration; extranodal disease may occur, but CNS and testicular involvement is relatively uncommon; intermediate and high-grade lymphomas share certain clinical and pathological features, eg abrupt enlargement and 'matting' of lymph nodes, induration, fixation to skin with overlying erythema; bulky internal and midline lymph nodes may cause obstructive phenomena, including lymphedema, spinal cord compression, ureteral obstruction, thrombophlebitis, superior vena cava syndrome, hepatosplenomegaly, hepatic dysfunction and intrahepatic obstruction; BM involvement is less common (table); a growing dissatisfaction with the WF[3] resulted in a new schema, the REAL classification, see there

WORKING FORMULATION

LOW-GRADE
Small lymphocytic (plasmacytoid, or CLL)
Follicular small cleaved cell, with diffuse zones (D) and sclerosis (S)
Follicular mixed, small cleaved + large cell + D & S
INTERMEDIATE-GRADE
Follicular, predominantly large cell + D & S
Diffuse, small cleaved + S
Diffuse, mixed large and small cell + S + epithelioid cells (Lennert's lymphoma)
Diffuse large cell, cleaved and non-cleaved + S
HIGH-GRADE
Diffuse, large cell immunoblastic, with various predominating features
Plasmacytoid cells, usually of B cell lineage
Clear cells, usually of T cell lineage
Polymorphous with epithelioid cells
Lymphoblastic Convoluted or non-convoluted cells
Small non-cleaved, Burkitt's or follicular (non-Burkitt's) type
OTHERS
Composite, Sezary syndrome/mycosis fungoides, true histiocytic, extramedullary plasmacytoma
(Cancer 1982; 49:2112)
[1]Somewhat drolly known as 'lymphomaniacs', ie those dedicated to creating new therapeutic modalities for lymphomas [2]Background: By the late 1970s, six different histopathologic classifications of lymphomas were common use, which correlated poorly with clinical disease and did not translate well among pathologists; a group of experts convened and created a new system, the Working formulation (Cancer 1982; 49:2112) [3]Thought by experts at the time of its creation to be the 'classification to end all classifications'

working poor Near poor, see there

workload recording unit LABORATORY MEDICINE A measure of productivity based on the amount of labor necessary to complete a procedure in a given time period–if the procedure is completed in less time, the 'efficiency' increases; WRUs were proposed as a means of determining a laboratory's cost-effectiveness, and while WRU recording system is a useful system for evaluating staffing needs, it does not allow national and international comparisons of efficiency in the clinical laboratory (CAP Today May, 1994) and in 1992, the College of American Pathologists discontinued the method as it did not meet the needs of laboratory managers (ibid, August 1993); the currently preferred unit of laboratory productivity is the billable test unit*, which requires neither expensive and/or lengthy studies nor complex calculations to account for 'nonproductive' time

*In hospitals where the test is not a billable service, the term 'ordered test unit' is preferred

workplace stress OCCUPATIONAL MEDICINE A generic term for work-related psychologic tension causing exhaustion, insomnia, muscle pain, depression, and eventually job burnout; stress in the workplace translates into excess overtime and increased sick leave (Am Med News 25 May 1992 p17)

work practice controls OCCUPATIONAL SAFETY A term defined by OSHA in reference to blood-borne pathogens as controls that are intended to reduce the likelihood of exposure (to blood-borne pathogens) by altering the manner in which a task is performed, eg prohibition of two-handed needle recapping, mouth pipetting and other high-risk practices (Federal Register Dec 6, 1991, p 64175)

workshop ACADEMIA A specialized conference in which experts in a particular area of science or medicine, convene in order to compare data and establish or standardize criteria for a substance, disease or phenomenon; immunologists meet periodically to share information on newly identified human leukocyte antigen (HLA) groups and clusters of differentiation (CD) antigens on cell surfaces; those molecules that remain poorly characterized at the close of the workshop receive a 'w' prefix, eg HLA-DRw52, HLA-DRw53, CDw65, CDw70, to indicate that the experts have yet to fully establish the nature of the antigens; Cf 'Wetshop'

worksite OCCUPATIONAL MEDICINE A setting '...*in which one or more individuals engage in work-related tasks, including offices, factories, warehouses, and other facilities controlled by organizations, vehicles operated by employees (eg trucks, buses, taxis), and residential offices of home workers.*' (JAMA 1995; 273:1136oA)

workstation COMPUTERS A type of computer design loosely defined around UNIX-based desktop products (DEC, Hewlett-Packard, Silicon Graphics, and others), in which applications software bases are linked to certain operating systems; a workstation can also be defined as a desktop or 'personal' computer ('PC') in a local area network (LAN) that runs applications programs and acts as an access point for shared network resources (B Pfaffenberger, Computer User's Dictionary, 4th ed, Que Corp, Indianapolis, 1993); workstations are used by engineers, scientists, software, document, and commercial developers ('power users') who need graphics and powerful central processing units (CPUs); as the speed and power in microcomputers (PCs) increases and the CPU design changes from the less efficient CISC design to the RISC design, the domain of the workstation is being encroached on by PC-based operating sytems* and hardware, former regarded as the 'low-end' of computing; workstations are of particular use in molecular modeling for rational drug design, and for evaluation of receptor-ligand and antigen-antibody interactions

*According to J Durbetaki '*We own both (workstation and 486-based PC) platforms and don't see one having any advantage over the other in terms of comput(ing) power.*' (Computer Design March 1993)

'work-up' *noun* The constellation of procedures, including the taking of a person's medical history, performing a physical examination, and ordering and evaluating laboratory tests and imaging procedures, upon which a person's diagnosis and therapy is based *verb* To evaluate a patient, ie to work him/her up; see Fehldiagnose

Note: During the formative years of residency training, young physicians sail between 1) The Scylla of an excess 'work-up', in which they may establish the presence of 'disease(s)' that the patient may not have; see Diagnostic 'overkill', Ulysses syndrome and 2) The less common Charybdis of paucity, in which a diagnosis is not achieved; 0.5-1.0% of those admitted to a hospital, leave or die without ever having a firmly established diagnosis

World Health Organization GLOBAL MEDICINE An agency of the United Nations, the primary purpose of which is '...*the attainment by all peoples of the highest possible level of health...*' (Article 1 of UN Constitution) the WHO promulgates international standards for biologicals and water, establishes acceptable levels for toxic substances (eg pesticides), maintains an international pharmacopeia, collects epidemiological data on AIDS, cancer, cardiovascular disease, and infectious diseases, and promotes child and maternal care, dental and mental health, education of health professionals, and maintains active research programs, eg in AIDS

world's most expensive drug Alglucerase (Ceredase®), see there

worm Computer worm, see there; Cf Computer virus

WORM Write-once/read-many COMPUTERS A form of permanent computer memory, eg CD/ROM, which allows the efficient permanent storage of data (600 megabyte to 1 gigabyte (CAP Today October 1993), including medical and laboratory records

'worm project' *Caenorhabditis elegans*, see there

wormian bone *Ossa suturalia* [NA6] Sutural bones Any of a number of small irregular bones located between the 'major' bones of the skull, along the lines of suture, in particular the lambdoid suture, and at the fontanelles; these bony mosaics represent detached centers of embryological ossification in the skull), and are classically seen in idiopathic osteolysis, hypothyroidism, progeria, cerebro-hepatorenal (Zellweger) syndrome, pycnodysostosis, Prader-Willi syndrome, cleidocranial dysostosis, otopalatodigital syndrome

'worn tennisball' appearance A fanciful descriptor for the 'fuzzy' margins surrounding a well-circumscribed peripheral adenocarcinoma of the lung seen in a plain chest film, an appearance that contrasts with the smooth margin considered by some to be more typical of a peripheral squamous cell carcinoma

the 'worried well' A colloquial term for a segment of the population that is at an extremely low risk for developing a particular disease[1] that is nonetheless concerned that an occasional pecadillo[2] has evoked a dread disease (N Engl J Med 1995; 332:1296sB)

[1]eg HIV infection, cardiovascular disease, lung cancer [2]eg A 'zesty' liaison with one of ill repute, a clandestine canoli, a surreptitious cigarette

wound healing Repair of incisive insults to tissues may occur in one of two fashions; simple or 'clean' wounds with little loss of tissue heal by 'primary intention', while 'dirty' wounds heal by 'secondary intention'

WOUND HEALING BY PRIMARY INTENTION (time required for each event) Filling-in of wound defects with inflammatory cells (24 hours) Epithelial response, basal cell proliferation (3 days) Infiltration by macrophages and deposition of collagen (5-7 days) Ingrowth of granulation tissue, maximum neo-vascularization, epidermal 'bridging' (2 weeks) Increased collagenization and proliferation of fibroblasts (2 months)

WOUND HEALING BY SECONDARY INTENTION occurs when there is a massive tissue defect with an increase in fibrin, debris, more intense inflammation, large amounts of granulation tissue; massive wounds are prone to re-epithelialization defects and collagen deposition, including 'proud flesh' and/or keloid, which are more common in blacks; the wound-healing process is the result of a delicate interplay between a variety of growth factors, eg basic fibroblast growth factor, transforming growth factor-β and platelet-derived growth factor, cells, eg keratinocytes and extracellular matrix, which contains various proteins, eg integrins, collagen, fibrinogen, fibronectin, heparin and others (Science 1991; 252:1064n)

Note: Topical application of epidermal growth factor stimulates regeneration of proliferation and migration of keratinocytes, binding and activating a tyrosine kinase receptor, although it is believed that proper wound healing requires a 'cocktail' of growth factors to optimize the process

woven bone Bone that contains extensive intervascular connections surrounded by immature bone and collagenous fibers in an irregular nonlamellated network, punctuated by scattered lacunae; woven bone is typical of immature prenatal bone and forms the scaffolding on which mature bone is built; it is present in adults only in certain regions, to wit, tooth sockets, the bony labyrinth, and at the cranial sutures; WB develops following fractures and in rapidly growing bone tumors

WPW syndrome Wolff-Parkinson-White syndrome, see there

wrap-around policy HEALTH CARE INDUSTRY A 'major medical' health insurance policy available in the US at a relatively high cost that provides full payment for any fees charged by a hospital and/or physician(s) that are in excess of the amount of monies reimbursed by the 'basic carriers', eg Blue cross (for hospitals), and Blue shield (for physicians); Cf Blue Cross/Blue Shield, 'Major medical'

wrap-around procedure SURGERY Any of the 'anti-reflux' operations, eg the Nissen, Belsey, and Hill procedures that restore the sphincter function to the lower esophagus; the Nissen procedure may afford the greatest long-term success; see 'Inkwell'

WRAT Wide Range Achievement Test An achievement-type of psychologic test that evaluates a child or adolescent's level in subject areas including reading, spelling and mathematics; see Psychological testing

wreathed nucleus An annular, peripherally placed nucleus lying in pale eosinophilic cytoplasm that may be seen in the giant tumor cells of alveolar rhabdomyosarcoma, which lack the cross-striations required for the definitive diagnosis of rhabdomyosarcoma

'wrecking ball' effect CARDIOLOGY That 'tethered ball'-like effect of a pedunculated tumor in the atrial or ventricular chambers, often due to a calcified myxoma, which may damage the mitral valve, rupture the chordae tendineae or cause severe mitral regurgitation, as it pounds against endocardial structures

wringer injury An uncommon lesion formerly seen in children who, while feeding clothes into (or playing with) an electrically driven laundry wringer, literally got 'caught up' in their work; the injuries associated therewith include crushing of the hand and upper extremity, friction burns at points of increasing diameters, eg metacarpophalangeal joints, thenar and base of hand, elbow and shoulder, neurapraxia, edema, lacerations, hematoma formation, fractures and potentially complete avulsion of a hand or arm; similar injuries may occur in industrial accidents (eg in the hot rollers in a printing press) or in rotating farm equipment; in addition to the above morbidity, these accidents may add components of thermal injury, extensive crushing and soil-related infection, including *Clostridium* species contamination

wrinkly skin syndrome A rare AR [MIM 278250] condition characterized by decreased elasticity and wrinkling of the palmo-plantar and corporal skin, dwarfism, kyphosis, 'winging' of the scapulae, mental retardation, muscle hypotonia, myalgia and decreased visual acuity

wristband An identifying label attached to a patient's wrist at the time of admission to a health care institution, which is the usually the only identifier used throughout a person's stay in a hospital

In one study, wristbands were checked by phlebotomists 2 463 727 times; 67 289 errors (2.2% of total) were identified; of these, the wristband was missing in 49.5%, had erroneous data in 8.6%, there were multiple wristbands with different information in 8.3%, incomplete data in 7.5%, illegible data in 5.7%; 0.5% had data from another patient; possibly the most serious potential complication of improper wristband information is the administration of incompatible or hemolytic transfusion reaction (Arch Pathol Lab Med 1993; 117:573DA)

wristdrop NEUROLOGY Partial or complete paralysis of the extensor muscles of the wrist*, a manifestation of peripheral neuropathy accompanied by a loss of acral motor activity; wristdrop may be seen in various conditions, including amyloidosis, Charcot-Marie-Tooth syndrome, collagen vascular diseases, diabetic mononeuropathy, lead poisoning and severe vitamin B_{12} deficiency; see Footdrop
*Resulting in a fey flopping of the foreflipper

writer's block PSYCHIATRY An occupational neurosis described in fiction authors, in which the creative juices are temporarily or permanently frustrated

writer's cramp Conscious immobility PSYCHIATRY A transient occupational neurosis in which there is temporary loss of highly skilled motor sequences, considered to be a psychogenic conversion reaction

write-up *noun* A document written about a patient, often by a medical student or physician-in-training *verb* To write a patient's history, as in to write him/her up

writhe MOLECULAR BIOLOGY The supercoiling of the overall helical structure in space; see DNA topology, Cf Linking number, Twist

writhe number MOLECULAR BIOLOGY The number of superhelical turns or times a double helix of DNA crosses over itself, corresponding to the concept of supercoiling, but which does not have the exact same value; in a completely relaxed molecule, the writhing number value is zero; see Superhelicity

wrongful FORENSIC MEDICINE An adjective with considerable medico-legal currency that is used in several contexts WRONGFUL BIRTH An event resulting from the failure of a contraceptive or sterilization procedure, eg fallopian tube ligation, failure to diagnose pregnancy, or an unsuccessful attempt to abort a conceptus, see below, Wrongful life WRONGFUL DEATH An event usually falling under the rubric of negligence, see Negligence WRONGFUL LIFE An event in which legal action may be taken by (or on behalf of) the baby suffering from a hereditary or congenital defect, eg Down syndrome or other disease, eg rubella, who would not have been born had the parents had the knowledge to opt for an abortion; wrongful life represents either the failure to 1) Diagnose in utero a condition that would lead to a major life-long handicap or 2) Recognize such a condition in a sibling, allowing a second, similarly afflicted child to be born; the child is the defendant named in a lawsuit initiated to defray the incurred and anticipated medical, nursing and related health expenses; in both wrongful birth and wrongful life, the defendent may be liable for support and care of the infant from 'cradle to grave'

wryneck Congenital torticollis A defect consisting of one-sided contracture and palpable induration of the sternocleidomastoid muscle, causing the chin to turn towards the opposite side and the head to rotate towards the lesion; the wry neck deformity is accompanied by dysplasia of the facial muscles; the etiology of the congenital form is unclear, but may be due to in utero or peripartum trauma to the venous drainage, which may eventuate in asymmetrical development of the face and skull; the later it is recognized, the more likely surgical intervention is required

W syndrome An X-linked [MIM 311450] condition characterized by frontal bossing, hypertelorism, antimongolic palpebral fissures, broad flat nose, camptodactyly, mental retardation and seizures (Pallister PD, Birth Defects Orig Art Ser X 1974; 51-60)

WSXWS An abbreviation for a tryptophan-serine-X-tryptophan-serine 'motif' which with 4 conserved cysteine residues is typical of the cytokine receptor superfamily of cell surface molecules; the WSXWS motif is critical for proper folding of the extracellular region and for hormone binding (N Engl J Med 1994; 330:839RV) see Hematopoietic growth factor (cytokine) receptor superfamily

WT1 A tumor-suppressor gene located on chromosome segment 11p13 that may be tissue-specific or transiently expressed during development; *WT1* is encoded by 10 exons yielding an mRNA subject to a complex pattern of alternative splicing; the gene product **WT1**, which is a 45-49-kD transcription factor that is critical in normal renal and gonadal development; transient elevation of WT1 is associated with suppression of certain growth-inducing genes, including those encoding early growth response, insulin-like growth factor II and platelet-derived growth factor A; dominant negative mutations in *WT1* have been identified in the Denys-Drash syndrome, mesangial sclerosis, and in Wilms' tumor; *WT1* is completely absent in the WAGR syndrome (N Engl J Med 1994; 331:586rv)

WT2 A tumor-suppressor gene located on chromosome segment 11p15 that is defective (genomic imprinting with duplication of the relevant paternal genes) in Wilms' tumors and Beckwith-Wiedemann syndrome (N Engl J Med 1994; 331:586rv)

WT syndrome A rare AD [MIM 194350] condition first described in two families with surnames of W and T, characterized by severe hypoplastic anemia, congenital anomalies (eg hand and arm malformations, irregular hyperpigmentation, sensorineural hearing loss), and leukemia

WYSIWYG What you see is what you get (pronounced, wissy-wig) COMPUTERS A 'hard' or paper copy that corresponds exactly to what is viewed on a computer's visual display, the cathode ray tube; a wysiwyg display on a microcomputer requires a high-resolution monitor, the appropriate graphics card and newer generation of microprocessor

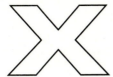

X growth factor MICROBIOLOGY Any of a group of heat-stable tetrapyrrole compounds that are provided by several iron-containing pigments, eg hemin and hematin, used in the synthesis of catalases, peroxidases and enzymes of the cytochrome electron transport system; organisms that depend on exogenous X factors for growth are incapable of synthesizing protoporphyrin from Δ-aminolevulinic acid; X factor is required by certain species of *Haemophilus* (*H influenza, H aegyptiae, H ducreyi, H aphrophilus*)

***X* terminal** COMPUTERS A GUI (graphic users interface) environment design that is emerging as consensus standard, which allows the user to interact with the information system in the same way (eg pull-down menus, mouse-driven input, point-and-shoot commands), regardless of the hardware (eg IBM or DEC) or software (eg UNIX or VMS) being used

xanthelasma A condition characterized by multiple xanthomas of the inner eyelid that are most commonly seen in normocholesterolemic elderly or hypercholesterolemic younger subjects PATHOLOGY Multiple soft, yellow plaques, seen by LM as lipid-laden histiocytes surrounding blood vessels

xanthogranulomatous pyelonephritis A malakoplakia-like lesion of the kidneys, that arises a background of *Escherichia coli* and *Proteus* spp infections PATHOLOGY Gross: Yellowish lobulated masses replacing renal architecture LM: Nodular aggregates of lipid-laden macrophages, giant cells COMPLICATIONS Hydronephrosis, nephrolithiasis (**N Engl J Med 1995; 332:174CPC**)

xanthoma A yellow-orange lipid-filled papule or plaque located on the skin or tendons, which is not uncommon in the general population; xanthomas are ↑↑↑ in various 'lipid' diseases, including lipoprotein lipase deficiency, abetalipoproteinemia, hypercholesterolemia, hypertriglyceridemia

xanthomatosis Generalized, nonspecific ↑ in xanthomas that may occur in malignancy, eg lymphoma, multiple myeloma, or be a component of other disease, eg familial hypercholesterolemia syndrome, Langerhans' cell histiocytosis-Hand-Schüller-Christian type and Wolman's disease

xenobiotics *xeno*, Greek, foreign IMMUNOLOGY Any compound that is foreign to a living system; alternatively, any natural or synthetic toxic, non-self substance, that may stimulate an immune or other form of defensive response

xenodiagnosis PARASITOLOGY A method for diagnosing a disease in one animal by inoculating the putative causative organism in a second animal of a different species; xenodiagnosis allows detection of blood-borne hemoflagellates (*Trypanosoma cruzi* and *T spiralis*) when the peripheral blood smears are negative; insects are fed blood that is presumed to be positive for the hemoflagellate and 'incubated' for 10-30 days, after which the insects' feces are examined for the parasites

xenograft Heterologous graft A graft from an individual of one species to an individual of a different species

Xenopsylla Rat flea A genus of fleas of the family Pulicidae that is a vector for dwarf and rat tapeworms (*Xenopsylla cheopis*), murine typhus (*X cheopis*) and plague (*X astia, X brasiliense, X cheopis*)

xenotransplantation TRANSPLANTATION BIOLOGY The transplantation of cells or tissues from one species to another BACKGROUND Although the technique was first described in 1902, XT was unsuccessful for various reasons, in particular because of hyperacute rejection, which is due to 'natural' antibodies that one species forms against another (even absence of exposure); when the vasculature of a xenograft is connected to a host from a different species, the natural antibodies attach to the graft's endothelium

---

X Symbol for: 1) Any unknown amino acid 2) Any unknown quantity 3) Kienböck's unit, an obsolete unit of radiation dosage 4) Reactance 5) Xanthine 6) Xanthosine

x Symbol for: 1) Abscissa 2) Mean (statistics)

X^2 STATISTICS A maneuver used to define categorical variables

X-body A morphological variant of Birbeck granules that is seen by EM in Langerhans' cell histiocytosis (histiocytosis X); X-bodies represent incomplete 'tennis-racquet' forms lacking a terminal bulge, which have a constant thickness and vague internal striation

X chromosome inactivation A chromosomal event that occurs during embryologic development of females; in a normal XX female, an inactive and active X chromosome is maintained in each somatic cell; determination of which X chromosome is active in peripheral B cells is based on three facets of the Lyon hypothesis 1) Only one X chromosome is active in a normal female somatic cell and that X chromosome is stably transferred to the progeny cells 2) The DNA methylation pattern differs on active cells (and can be monitored by using restriction endonucleases) and 3) Restriction fragment length polymorphisms (RFLPs) of the paternal and maternal genes allow identification of the parent of origin for each chromosome; X chromosome inactivation is thus the functional elimination of all but one X chromosome in mammals and is a unique developmental regulatory event, proposed by Mary Lyon (**Nature 1961; 190:372**), which affects the expression of an entire chromosome (150 million base pairs of DNA and thousands of genes) in a *cis*-limited fashion, resulting in dosage equivalence between females who have two X chromosomes and males who have one X chromosome; the gene responsible for random inactivation of the X chromosome in females is designated XIST (X inactive-specific transcript) and is located to Xq13, within a larger 'X-inactivation center' region; XIST is only expressed in cell lines containing one or more inactive X chromosomes, ie it is female-specific in karyotypically normal individuals (**Nature 1991; 349:38, 82, 15**) and may play a role in establishing the phenotype of Klinefelter and Turner syndromes; see Methylation, Testis-determining factor

X disease 1) Aflatoxicosis 2) (bovine) Hyperkeratosis, a disease of cattle caused by exposure to chlorinated hydrocarbons 3) Uncertain, a condition described by Sir James Mackenzie (1853-1925) which he characterized as ill-defined general malaise, increased cold sensitivity, dyspepsia, GI discomfort, and cardiorespiratory dysfunction; Cf Syndrome(s) X

and stimulate the classic complement pathway, and cause rejection in an hour; the most viable means of blocking the hyperacute rejection reaction is to produce a transgenic species, eg the pig, which carries human complement inhibitors on the vascular endothelial cells; other barriers (eg MHC class I and II incompatibility) of lesser significance have yet to be surmounted before realizing the goal of XT (Nature Medicine 1995; 1:423, 403)

xeroderma pigmentosa An AR [MIM 278700] condition characterized by the inability to repair UV light-induced damage to pyrimidine nucleotide (cytosine, thymidine) dimers due to lack of one or more multigene products or complementation groups; XP may result from the absence of a nuclear factor responsible for binding and recognizing damaged DNA MOLECULAR PATHOLOGY Of 9 genetic complementation groups (groups A-H and a variant group), a defect of group A occurs on chromosome 9q34.1 and encodes a 273-residue protein with a zinc finger domain, which indicates that it has DNA-binding activity, possibly forming part of the enzyme complex making the excision near the damaged sites; the repair defect may occur in fibroblasts, epithelial cells and lymphocytes in XP and in de Sanctis-Caccione syndrome (which also has microcephaly, mental retardation, dwarfism, hypogonadism, deafness, choreoathetosis and ataxia) CLINICAL Incidence 2/10⁶; the patients are normal at birth, freckling and xeroderma occur by age three, accompanied by telangiectasia, keratoacanthomas, keratoses, scarring and eventually cutaneous malignancy, in particular, basal cell carcinoma, as well as squamous cell carcinoma and malignant melanoma and internal malignancy (fibrosarcoma and angiosarcoma); see Photoactivation

xerophthalmia Dry eye syndrome A generic term for dryness of eyes of any etiology, classically associated with vitamin A deficiency, a vanishingly rare condition in populations with adequate nutrition CLINICAL Dry, greasy, thickened and focally denuded cornea which may progress to keratomalacia, corneal ulceration, necrosis and secondary infections; xerophthalmia may also occur in Sjögren syndrome, various autoimmune disorders, and in periorbital lymphoproliferative disorders

Use of the 'classic' linguistic roots of medical terminology is decreasing at an ever-accelerating pace; while the term xerophthalmia continues to have active currency, the synonym dry eye is increasingly preferred; it is to be anticipated that by the end of the 20th Century, this shift will be complete-Author's note

xeroradiography A radiologic imaging technique in which aluminum plates coated with a semiconductor, eg selenium are used to record a latent image as a pattern of varying electrical charges, which is converted into a 'positive' image by a dry (xero-, Greek, dry) photoelectric process; xeromammography provides a relatively good image, since the entire breast is viewed at once and clearly delineates variability in tissue density, blood vessels, calcification and tumors; xeroradiography is on the decline as a major supplier of the technique withdrew from the market, the radiation dose is slightly higher that that used in modern high-resolution mammography, the equipment is prone to breakdown and the boundary between two differently charged areas is distorted, making potentially malignant ('borderline') lesions difficult to interpret

xerostomia Dry mouth A clinical manifestation of salivary gland dysfunction with ↓ secretion, resulting in discomfort accompanied by dry, atrophic and/or inflammed oropharyngeal mucosa; xerostomia is typical of Sjögren syndrome and autoimmune disorders; the salivary glands become inflamed and are eventually replaced by fibrosis ETIOLOGY Irradiation, usually ≥ 4000 cGy, drugs, eg atropine, antihistamine, mechanical, eg calculus blocking salivary duct, others, eg vitamin A deficiency, HIV-1 and Candida spp infections, malignancy and systemic sclerosis TREATMENT Pilocarpine (N Engl J Med 1993; 329:390oa)

XIST X-inactivation-specific transcript see X chromosome inactivation

Xist X inactive-specific transcript gene *Xist* produces very large RNA transcripts, which unlike most RNA transcripts, does not leave the nucleus to encode proteins, but rather binds tightly to the inactive X chromosome in the nucleus that produced it, and may itself be responsible for its inactivation (Sci Am 1993; 268/4:30)

XLD agar Xylose-Lysine-Deoxycholate agar MICROBIOLOGY A highly selective bacterial growth medium used to isolate gastroenteric pathogens, which like the Salmonella-Shigella and Hektoen enteric agars contain substances that inhibit the growth of native coliform flora, allowing identification of *Enterobacteriaceae* (enteric gram-negative rods); 'lysine positive' XLD agar's normal pink color is converted to yellow by acid-producing bacteria, eg *Escherichia coli* and *Salmonella typhi*, the latter of which, in addition produces H₂S, as do some *Proteus* species, resulting in a black color on the culture plate

X-linked adrenoleukodystrophy A X-R [MIM 300100] peroxisomal disease due to a defective gene on chromosome Xq28, in which there is impaired degradation of saturated very long chain fatty acids that accumulate with the cholesterol ester and gangliosides in the CNS, adrenal glands, plasma cells and leukocytes, causing progressive multifocal demyelination MOLECULAR PATHOLOGY The gene defect located on chromosome segment Xq28 encodes an ATP-binding transporter CLINICAL The phenotypic range of expression is broad and it is often first seen in childhood with major neurologic deterioration and death following in a few years TREATMENT Modifications in the lipid intake may normalize the serum levels of VLCFA, the long-term effects of which are unknown, BM transplantation

Note: It had been reported that a concoction of oleic and erucic acids (glycerol trioleate and trierucic acids, popularly known as 'Lorenzo's oil') was of use in treating adrenoleukodystrophy or adrenomyeloneuropathy (N Engl J Med 1993; 329:745c, 1994; 330o:577c) see Lorenzo's oil

X-linked agammaglobulinemia An X-linked [MIM 300300] disease* with defective humoral immunity due to an intrinsic B-cell gene defect that 'maps' to chromosome Xq21.3-22 CLINICAL Recurrent pyogenic infections, affecting boys by 5-6 months of life, coincident with the fall IgG acquired in utero MOLECULAR PATHOLOGY A point mutation on the gene (*Btk*) encoding Btk (the protein product of the gene, Bruton's protein kinase) has been identified that encodes a protein with decreased stability that may block intracellular signaling in one pathway while others continue to function (N Engl J Med 1994; 330:1488br) LABORATORY ↓↓↓ B lymphocytes, ↓↓↓ immunoglobulins, intact T-cell function TREATMENT Antibiotics, monthly injections of gammaglobulins PROGNOSIS Death is inevitable in early childhood, often secondary to fulminant pulmonary infection

*aka X-linked hypogammaglobulinemia, Bruton's disease

X-linked centronuclear (myotubular) myopathy An often fatal, X-R form [MIM 310400] of myopathy that causes severe hypotonia; adult survivors have minimal residual functional incapacity; the associated proliferation of sarcotubular organelles may be caused by impaired innervation; PATHOLOGY Marked cellular hypertrophy, especially of type I fibers, centrally located nuclei with perinuclear halos, and an ultrastructural appearance similar to that of fetal myotubules

X-linked ichthyosis Placental steroid sulfatase deficiency An X-linked [MIM 308100] form of ichthyosis characterized by scaling over the abdomen and points of flexure and a deficiency of placental steroid sulfatase* [EC 3.1.6.2] MOLECULAR PATHOLOGY 80% of XLI is associated with large deletions of the steroid sulfatase gene (located on Xp223-pter) and adjacent regions of the short arm of the X chromosome; the remainder are due to point mutations PATHOLOGY XLI is hypertrophic; ichthyosis vulgaris is atrophic (Am J Clin Pathol

1995; 103:400oA)

*aka Steryl-sulfatase, the term recommended (1992) by the Nomenclature Committee of the International Union of Biochemistry and Molecular Biology

X-linked lymphoproliferative disease An X-R [MIM 368240] condition characterized by fatal or chronic infectious mononucleosis, aplastic anemia, agammaglobulinemia, and NHL following EBV infection, caused by a failure to make the heavy chain class switch from IgM and IgG after a second exposure to antigens MOLECULAR PATHOLOGY XLPD is linked to DXS42, which maps to Xq24-27 PROGNOSIS It is often fatal before age 40 TREATMENT Umbilical cord blood stem cell transplantation from an HLA-identical sibling (N Engl J Med 1993; 329:1623oA)

Synonyms: Duncan's (kindred name) disease, Duncan syndrome, Epstein-Barr immunodeficiency syndrome, X-linked immunoproliferative disease

X-linked myotubular myopathy X-linked centronuclear (myotubular) myopathy, see there

x-rays A portion of the electromagnetic spectrum (wavelength 10^{-10} to 2.5×10^{-6}) named by Roentgen, which corresponds to ionizing radiation resulting from high-energy (1 keV to 1 MeV or more) particles, eg electrons, colliding with target electrons, an event that raises the latter to higher energy levels, releasing high energy photons and a spectrum of characteristic radiation (X-rays) as the target electrons fall back to lower excitation levels; patient exposure levels to X-rays are divided into those that are an undesired side effect of a diagnostic procedure and those that are a necessary component of a therapeutic procedure Diagnostic X-rays impart 30-150 keV of energy and rare reports in the literature infer a possible relationship between exposure to low- (diagnostic-) level X-rays and a slight ↑ incidence of myeloproliferative disorders, recently associated (RR 1.14) with minimal ↑ risk for developing multiple myeloma (JAMA 1991; 265:1290) Therapeutic X-rays can be in the form of 1) Low level radiation, eg 5-10 keV or 'grenz' radiation, which may be used to treat various recalcitrant skin conditions, eg psoriasis or 2) High level, eg megaelectron-volt (MeV) radiation, used to treat internal malignancy; X-rays may be detected by wavelength-dispersive spectrometry, energy-dispersive spectrometry and energy loss spectrometry; X-ray production requires 1) X-ray tube A vacuum tube with a cathode (tungsten filament, which when heated produces an electron cloud) and an anode (containing an angulated deflecting target), mounted within an electrically and radioactively insulated housing, the beam exits via an adjustable aperture (collimator) 2) High-voltage generator A device that generates power in the form of pulsating direct (or 'rectified' alternating) current, the X-rays hit the angulated tungsten target on the anode and useful wavelengths are emitted (90% of the energy is dissipated as heat) through the collimator 3) Control console The electronics which control the voltage, amperage and exposure time

X-ray crystallography X-ray diffraction A technique in which a beam of X-rays is focused on a crystal, diffracted by the molecule(s) of interest and then recorded on film; the pattern of diffraction provides information on the amplitude of the crystal's Fourier transform; the phase information is deduced by comparing the diffraction patterns from related chemicals; X-ray crystallographic images may be resolved by isomorphic replacement, solvent-flattening, model-building and various refinement methods

Note: Watson and Crick's model of DNA as a double-stranded molecule was deduced by X-ray crystallographic analysis of data via the Fourier transform

XTE syndrome A rare AD condition characterized by xeroderma, talipes and enamel defect, accompanied by cleft palate, hypohidrosis and cutaneous bullae

XX male syndrome A rare AR [MIM 278850] sex chromosome anomaly that clinically mimics Klinefelter syndrome, characterized by ♂ psychosexual orientation, masculine appearance, weak secondary sexual characteristics, azoospermia, low androgen levels and small testes MOLECULAR PATHOLOGY 70% of patients have a portion of the short arm of the Y chromosome translocated to the short arm of the X chromosome

XXX syndrome 47, XXX The most common (1:1000) chromosomal abnormality of ♀ CLINICAL Clinodactyly, epicanthal folds, ocular hypertelorism and an ↑ incidence of congenital defects in their children; most subjects with XXX syndrome have a normal IQ, they tend to be emotionally labile, have speech and learning defects

XXXX syndrome 48, XXXX Superwoman A chromosomal defect associated with moderate mental retardation, behavioral problems, midfacial hypoplasia, clinodactyly, radial synostosis, hypertelorism, micrognathia, web neck and menstrual irregularity

XXXXX syndrome 49, XXXXX Penta-X syndrome Females who may present in infancy with patent ductus arteriosus, mental and growth retardation, upward slanting of the eyes, carpal hypoplasia and clinodactyly of the fifth finger

XXY syndrome 47, XXY Klinefelter syndrome

XXXY syndrome (48, XXXY) and XXXXY syndrome (49, XXXXY) A group of chromosomal defects characterized by multiple X chromosomes accompanied by one Y chromosome; the wide range of somatic defects overlap many of the somatic features of Klinefelter syndrome CLINICAL Small testes, hypoplastic penis, gynecomastia, mental retardation, wide-set eyes, ulnar and radial abnormalities; more than one-half of those with the 49, XXXXY syndrome present with low birth weight, muscle hypotonicity, profound mental and growth retardation, malformed ears, a short neck, hypertelorism with a mongoloid slant, a flattened nose, small undescended testes, hypoplastic external male genitalia, clinodactyly, radioulnar synostoses, coxa vara, genu varum, pes planus TREATMENT None, testosterone may improve secondary sexual characteristics

XY gonadal agenesis syndrome Embryonic testicular regression syndrome, see there

xylose absorption test GASTROENTEROLOGY The administration of a pentose per os to determine intestinal absorptive capacity; 25 g of D-xylose is given orally and later measured in the urine; excretion of less than three grams in a five hour period is suggestive of enterogenous malabsorption, since pancreatic enzymes are not required for the absorption of D-xylose; high blood levels of D-xylose with low levels in the urine are typical of renal failure, and thus the test should not be used for patients with renal disease

xylose-lysine-deoxycholate agar see XLD agar

¹⁴C-xylose test A test for general malabsorption METHOD 1.0 g (5-10 µCi) of 'hot' xylose is administered per os; increased breath radioactivity at 30 min indicates overgrowth in the small intestine by gram-negative anaerobes

XYY syndrome YY syndrome A syndrome that became the focus of popular interest when some scientific data suggested that males with an extra Y chromosome (47, XYY) tended to be more aggressive, antisocial and display criminal behavior; other components of this 'syndrome' included facial asymmetry, long ears, teeth and fingers, poor musculoskeletal development, cranial synostosis and a prolonged P-R interval on the electrocardiogram; it was subsequently shown that only a small percentage of subjects with XYY defects have the described anomalies

XYY hypothesis see Crime genes

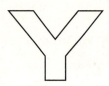

Y Symbol for: 1) Pyrimidine 2) Tyrosine 3) Yttrium

Y-1 PUBLIC HEALTH A tobacco that contains > 6% nicotine (more than double that of comparable tobacco), which was produced by a biotechnology firm* working for Brown and Williamson Tobacco Corp; Y-1 seeds were shipped to Brazil where Y-1 was planted, harvested, and shipped back to the US Note: Deliberate manipulation of the nicotine content of tobacco (eg by breeding special high-nicotine tobacco or by adding ammonia to the cigarettes which increases nicotine transfer efficiency or bioavailability) may open a legal loophole that would allow public health officials to regulate an industry that has long been viewed as 'above the law'

'…cigarette makers have known for decades not only that nicotine is addictive, but also that it possesses other pharmacologic (tranquilizing) properties. Such data help establish the manufacturers' 'intent' in controlling nicotine…Intent is important because (US) federal law defines a drug as anything that 'intended to affect the structure or function of the body.' Deliberately manipulating cigarette recipes to provide smokers with what manufacturers knew to be a pharmacologically active, addictive substance would amount to selling a drug…(this would then make the FDA–Food and Drug Administration) responsible for regulating this drug (Science News 1994; 146:7, 30)

*Using various breeding techniques including anther and tissue culture, hybrid sorting and protoplast fusion

Y body CYTOGENETICS A rounded mass corresponding to the Y chromosome, which is seen in fluorescently-stained metaphase and interphase nuclei of genotypic male (XY) cells—buccal mucosa epithelium, fibroblasts, amniotic cells and spermatozoa

Y cartilage A finding which when accompanied by stippled scimitar-shaped calcification of the inferior margin of the patella is characteristic of cerebrohepatorenal (Zellweger) syndrome that may be accompanied by calcification of the hyoid bone and thyroid cartilage, dolichocephaly, wormian bones, hand and foot deformities and bone immaturity, associated with seizures, flaccidity, facial dysmorphia, cataracts, flexion contractures, renal cortical cysts, liver fibrosis and death in early infancy

Y fork Replicating fork, see there

Y protein Ligandin, see there

YAC cloning Yeast artificial chromosome cloning MOLECULAR BIOLOGY A cloning system based on the propagation of large 60-650 kilobase pair DNA molecules as linear, artificial chromosomes in the yeast *Saccharomyces cerevisiae*; YAC cloning is preferred to conventional closed-end cosmid cloning, since the DNA segments that can be manipulated by YAC cloning are up to ten-fold longer than segments cloned in cosmids, the yeast is a eukaryote (providing a different host environment for the DNA propagation) and the chromosomal DNA is more eas-

ily manipulated, offering the possibility of making specific changes in the large DNA molecules being YAC cloned

YAG laser Laser, see there, Nd:YAG (neodymium:yttrium-aluminum-garnet) laser

yaw FORENSIC PATHOLOGY The angle between the line of flight and the bullet's long axis; bullets enter tissue and tumble once they are inside, rotating 180°, exiting with the base forward, explaining the large size of some exit wound; see Ballistics TROPICAL MEDICINE see Yaws

yaws TROPICAL MEDICINE An infection by a non-venereal spirochete (other non-venereal spirochetal diseases include bejel and pinta), *Treponema pertenue*, which is virtually identical to *T pallidum*, affecting rural children in the southern hemisphere, transmitted by direct contact, facilitated by poor personal hygiene and overcrowding; after a several week incubation, a primary granulomatous lesion, the 'mother yaw' appears at the site of inoculation, consisting of a maculopapular rash, usually on the leg, overlying a cluster of exudative nodules, later ulcerating and healing spontaneously; this is followed by secondary yaws (Yaws II), analogous to secondary syphilis and characterized by generalized granulomatous papulomaculo-squamous coalescing eruptions that become purulent and are accompanied by malaise, lymphadenopathy and osteitis Note: Forest yaws, a localized leishmanial lesion of South America, characterized as a hyperkeratotic papillary lesion, mimics the second stage of yaws; after the second stage, yaws enters a long latency period, reappearing as a tertiary yaws (Yaws III) with painful noduloulcerative papillomas of the hands and feet, gumma of the skin and bones, palmo-plantar hyperkeratosis and depigmentation TREATMENT Penicillin

yeast A unicellular spherical-to-oval organism measuring 3-5 μm, most of which reproduce by budding (some by binary fission), and which when adherent in end-to-end rows are termed pseudohyphae; most fungi are saprobes and used in the commercial production and fermentation of foods and beverages; seven genera of yeasts of the class Deuteromycetes (imperfect fungi) are pathogenic to humans, eg *Candida, Crytococcus, Geotrichum, Pityrosporum, Rhodotorula, Torulopsis, Trichosporon*; the non-pathogenic 'beer-maker's yeast', *Saccharomyces cerevisiae* is of considerable use as a research organism in molecular biology, as like all fungi, it is a eukaryote, contains mitochondria, endoplasmic reticulum, and a wide variety of structural and functional motifs of DNA and proteins; *S cerevisiae* is also of use in studying large segments of genes from other species, see YAC cloning

the yeast connection Candida hypersensitivity syndrome, see there

yellow advertising Yellow professionalism, see there

yellow albinism Oculocutaneous albinism, type IB An AR [MIM 203100.0006] condition that most commonly occurs among the Amish, a genetically isolated population of German descent, living in Pennsylvania, US (rare cases of OCA, type IB have been reported elsewhere in the US, Sri Lanka, and Africa) with white hair which later becomes yellow-red, hypopigmented skin, increased susceptibility for cutaneous malignancy, 'cartwheel' pigmentation in the ocular fundus; these patients do not form eumelanin, but rather a yellowish pigment (pheomelanin); pheomelanosomes mature to stage III melanosomes

yellow beeswax CLINICAL PHARMACOLOGY The purified wax from the honeycomb of the honeybee, *Apis mellifera*, which is a mixture of myricin, cerin, and cerolein YB is used as a stiffening agent in various pharmaceutical preparations and as an ingredient of many polishes; see Inert ingredients

'yellow blood' TRANSFUSION MEDICINE A unit of packed red blood cells with a milky yellow-white discoloration, which almost invariably translates into bacterial contamination of the unit, which must, therefore be discarded

Yellow Creek ENVIRONMENT A river in Kentucky that was used for illegal dumping of toxic chemicals (tannin and chromium) from a local factory; exposure to waters from the YC was linked by some workers to a local epidemic of spontaneous abortions, nausea, rashes, diarrhea and glomerular disease; Cf Love canal

Yellow disease XANTHODROMIA A generic term for yellow skin of any etiology

Yellow Dye 6 FD&C Yellow No. 6, see there

yellow fat disease A vitamin E deficiency syndrome affecting various mammals fed excess n-3 polyunsaturated fatty acids, derived from fish oils; see Fish oil

Note: in humans, excess fish-oils cause increased bleeding time, especially after aspirin ingestion, may play a role in cardiac necrosis and in increasing susceptibility to catecholamine-induced stress

yellow fever An acute mosquito (*Aedes aegypti*)-borne infection of tropical Africa and South America, by a flavivirus (a group B single-stranded 'negative'-sense RNA virus) of the Togavirus family CLINICAL YF may range from benign with a nonspecific 'flu' syndrome to a pernicious disease characterized by an abrupt onset of high fever (with bradycardia, the Faget sign), headache, anorexia, myalgia, lumbosacral pain, nausea, vomiting that becomes blood-tinged up to 7-10 days post-onset, photophobia, flushing of face, a 'strawberry' tongue, insomnia, constipation, hypotension, jaundice ('yellow' fever) ± day 4, generalized petechial hemorrhages and hematemesis, coagulation factor depletion, dilated cardiomyopathy, possibly coma; this is followed by a period of 'remission' of hours to several days in duration, after which the patient deteriorates and dies (up to 50% mortality) LABORATORY Leukopenia, occasionally pronounced, DIC, ↑ bilirubin, proteinuria, albuminuria with renal failure, rising titers in neutralizing antibodies, increased transaminase PATHOLOGY Mid-zonal to complete lobular liver necrosis in a background of fatty degeneration

yellow jacket venom A substance produced by hymenopteran insects, eg bees, wasps, ants that may prove fatal via a type I anaphylactic reaction with the release of vasoactive substances (leukotrienes, ECF-A and histamine), causing generalized urticaria, throat and chest tightness, stridor, fever, chills and cardiovascular collapse; toxic overload of hymenopteran venom may also be fatal to victims of 'swarmings'; see Swarming

yellow krypton laser OPHTHALMOLOGY A device used to treat exudative macular degeneration; in contrast to the YKL, the heat given off by the absorption of red or green light produced by convention lasers may result in scarring and visual loss; see Lasers

yellow nail syndrome A clinical complex characterized by a combination of slow-growing indurated flavescence of all or the distal part of the nail with the loss of the lunula, onycholysis, primary lymphedema of the extremities, idiopathic pleural effusions, lymphedema of the face and extremities, chronic bronchitis and chronic sinusitis; the nails are thickened without visible lunulae and have an exaggerated lateral curvature, in addition to slowed growth, which is thought to be due to primary stromal sclerosis, leading to lymphatic obstruction; although yellow nails are most commonly seen under 'physiologic' conditions on the fingers of heavy cigarette smokers with lung disease, eg chronic obstructive lung disease, the nails may also occur in malignancy, tetracycline therapy, thyroid disease, rheumatoid arthritis, diabetes mellitus, immunodeficiency, eg AIDS; see Harlequin nail

Note: Although the YNS is relatively more common in smokers, it is not the same as the 'nicotine' nail of smokers

yellow ovary 'disease' An asymptomatic finding in which the ovary demonstrates global luteinization, imparting a bright yellow-orange tinge to the organ

yellow phosphorus see White phosphorus

'yellow' professionalism Commercial advertising by health maintenance organizations, and to a lesser extent, by private physicians in the Yellow Pages of telephone directories; competition for patients has traditionally been considered inappropriate in the medical profession; aside from the ethical dilemma, some physicians may not be certified specialists in the area of claimed expertise; the American Board of Medical Specialists maintains a list of physicians certified in one or more of 24 recognized medical and surgical specialties Tel 1.800.776.2378

yellow rain ENVIRONMENT A fungal toxin (trichothecene T-2, produced by the mold, *Fusarium*) that has had some currency as an agent of biological warfare, so named for the yellow cloud that results from the exploding shells when 'delivered' to its target; the weapon was allegedly supplied for use by the Communist troops in Kampuchea and Laos against the Hmong people of Thailand; the yellow 'rain' saga proved rather unclear as a similar cloud is said to be related to digested bee (*Apis dorsata*) pollen (**Nature 1985; 315:284**) CLINICAL Tricothecene, a major radiomimetic substance destroys bone marrow, causing immune compromise and GI disease

yellow salt OCCUPATIONAL MEDICINE A precipitated platinum salt, ammonium hexachloroplatinate that is the crude product from which highly purified platinum is produced; exposure to platinum fumes elicits a type IV hypersensitivity reaction in over half of the exposed workers, who complain of sneezing, runny nose, chest tightness, dyspnea, dry coughing and eventually interstitial pulmonary fibrosis

yellow tag TRANSFUSION MEDICINE The color of the label used for blood group A (California standards); ABO blood group coding is not required by the US Food and Drug Administration

yellow top tube LABORATORY MEDICINE A blood collection tube that may contain sodium polyanethol-sulfonate, used in microbiology for blood cultures, or thrombin for 'stat' chemistries, ACD solution for processing specimens in the blood bank, or may contain no additives

yellow urine A yellow-tinged urine, which in an acid pH urine, may be due to excretion of picric acid, dinitrophenol, phenacetin or chrysarobin or in alkaline pH urine, due to increased secretion of anthocyanin, or associated with ingestioin of beets or blackberries; pure yellow urine is associated with increased acriflavine and has a green fluorescence; yellow-orange urine may be highly concentrated or contain increased bilirubin-biliverdin

Yentl 'syndrome' A phenomenon in which once a ♀ shows herself to be equal to a ♂ (in terms of risk factors), she receives equal medical treatment; the term was coined in an editorial regarding studies that revealed that ♀, despite similar risk factors for coronary artery disease and symptomatic disease, were far less likely to receive the same diagnostic battery as ♂; once cardiovascular disease was demonstrated, the ♀ received the same treatment (**N Engl J Med 1991; 325:274ed**) see Women and disease; Cf Glass ceiling phenomenon, Sticky floor

Yentl is the 19th century heroine of Bashevis' story by the same name, who had to disguise herself as a man to be treated as one; Cf 'Yenta', a gossipy, scandal-spreading woman who cannot keep quiet

Yerkes Regional Primate Research Center The oldest scientific institute dedicated to primate research in the US, which was established in 1930 by R Yerkes of Yale; the center currently operates at Emory University in Atlanta, has a collection of 15 species of apes (2754 monkeys, and 315 greater and lesser apes), and conducts basic research on AIDS and other infectious diseases, cardiovascular disease, congenital vision defects, drug addiction, fertility,

Parkinson's disease, social behavior and other areas; like many research facilities, the Yerkes center has been a target for animal rights' activists (JAMA 1994; 272:907MN&P) Cf Silver Spring monkeys

YIGSR A synthetic pentapeptide (Tyr-Ile-Gly-Ser-Arg) corresponding to the amino acids involved in binding native laminin by metastatic malignant cells; YIGSR inhibits tumor invasiveness when co-injected with malignant cells into mouse recipients and may have some currency in early therapy of cancer

yin-yang hypothesis PHYSIOLOGY A postulate that links cAMP and cyclic GMP as opposing arms of a bidirectional intracellular control system, where an ↑ concentration of one is linked to a ↓ concentration of the other, thus having a balanced relationship, likened to the Chinese yin and yang philosophy of universal balance

'yin-yang tumor' Gynandroblastoma, see there

yoga ALTERNATIVE MEDICINE A system of health care and maintainance that is widely practiced throughout the world, which is believed by its advocates to reduce stress, heart rate, and blood pressure, and even retard the aging process*; yoga is '...organized into eight "limbs" that provide a complete system of physical, mental, and spiritual health ...these limbs ...outline specific lifestyle, hygiene, and detoxification regimens, as well as physical and psychological practices that can lead to a more integrated personal development' (Alternative Medicine, Future Medicine Publishing, Inc, Puyallup, WA, 1994); central to yoga are a series of exercises known as yogic postures (asana) which are divided into meditative and therapeutic asana, and which are ideally performed with breath control

*Other conditions reported to be benefitted by yoga include alcoholism, arthritis, asthma or bronchitis, cancer, DM, duodenal ulcers, gynecologic conditions (dysmenorrhea, PMS, post-menopausal syndromes), heart disease, hemorrhoids, hypertension, insomnia, migraines, neuro- and/or neuromuscular disease, obesity, tobacco addiction, and others

yogurt Yoghurt A smooth semisolid dairy product produced by through the fermentation of milk with *Lactobacillus acidophilus* and other bacteria that convert lactose into lactic acid, the latter of which causes a thickening of milk; consumption of yogurt is associated with a 3-fold ↓ in vaginal candidiasis (Ann Int Med 1992; 116:353)

Note: Yogurt has long had currency among promoters of alternative medicine, and for some has a mystical portent, given its alleged consumption in 'industrial' quantities by very old individuals living in the mountains of Eastern Europe; the argument that the actual age of these allegedly ancient people remains unconfirmed has done little to weaken the conviction on the part of 'health nuts' that yogurt (and other fermented foods, eg buttermilk, sauerkraut, beer) holds one of the keys to the fountain of youth

yohimbine An indoalkylamine alkaloid used to treat impotence that is obtained from the bark of the West African corynan (yohimbine) tree (*Corynanthe johimbe*, and others, eg *Rauwolfia serpentina*); it is chemically similar to reserpine, and blocks presynaptic alpha₂-adrenergic blocking activity resulting in ↑ cholinergic activity (↑ neuronal release of norepinephrine from the central and peripheral nervous systems), while ↓ sympathetic or adrenergic activity; yohimbine may be of use in treating 1) Orthostatic hypotension and ischemic vascular disease caused by autonomonic dysfunction in DM (Hypertension 1990; 15:877) 2) Narcotic overdose, possibly acting to ↑ release of dopamine (Neuropharmacology 1990; 29:25) 3) Psychogenic and organic impotence(Lancet 1987; 2:421), possibly acting to ↑ the inflow and/or ↓ the outflow of blood to the penis, with ↑ erection without ↑ sexual desire

yohimbine

H_3COOC

OH

Note: Yohimbine increases activity of the locus ceruleus, the site of the fear response in animals; low dose yohimbine has been used as a provocative test in those suffering from panic attacks

Yokohama asthma Tokyo asthma ENVIRONMENT A smog-induced asthmatiform complex described in Yokohama (Tokyo's port city), where nocturnal atmospheric conditions favor a dense buildup of industrial pollutants, eliciting wheezing and dyspnea in those with hyperirritable airways; the symptoms are worse when accompanied by chronic obstructive pulmonary disease; see Bhopal, Smog

yolk sac tumor Endodermal sinus tumor A germ cell tumor of the testis, ovary, other genitourinary regions, the mediastinum and sacrococcygeal region LM Tubular, solid and papillary structures, vacuolated cytoplasm, intra– and extracellular deposits of pink homogeneous basement membrane-like material (Acta Cytologica 1993; 37:209OA) FEMALE YST A large (± 15 cm in diameter) tumor of adolescents and young adults, which is associated with ↑ circulating α-fetoprotein levels and reticulated or microcystic areas formed by a loose meshwork of pseudopapillary processes with a central vessel (Schiller-Duval bodies) TREATMENT Combination chemotherapy achieves 50% remission rate in a formerly fatal lesion MALE YST A unilateral teratoma that mimics embryonal yolk sac tissue, that presents as 1) Pure YST A tumor of male children under age two with an organoid cellular arrangement and an excellent prognosis or 2) Mixed germ cell tumor of adults with poor differentiation, increased circulating α-fetoprotein and a poor prognosis similar to that of teratocarcinoma; Cf Sex cord-stroma tumors

Yom Kippur effect Spontaneous premature induction of labor occurring in pregnant Jewish women who observe Yom Kippur, the annual 24-hour religious fast of Judaism, in which there is total abstinence from food and water (JAMA 1983;250:1317cr; JAMA 1983, 250:2469, ibid, 1984; 251:2348c) the YKE appears to be a relatively universal theme, possibly linked to dehydration, as premature labor is more common in the 'dog days' of summer among women with a decidedly distinct demographic pattern serviced by workers at SUNY-Downstate in Brooklyn (S LAJNIAN IN SCIENCE NEWS 20 MAY 1995, p315); Cf Judaism, practice of

Youden plot LABORATORY MEDICINE A plot that graphically represents the paired responses with respect to the mean and standard deviation of the data in each of a series of studies; it is a visual representation of the standard deviation interval‡; Youden analysis can be used to compare the results of proficiency testing among various laboratories, eg of flow cytometry, and help identify causes of nonlinearity (Arch Pathol Lab Med 1994; 118:681OA)

yo-yo dieting CLINICAL NUTRITION Undesirable dietary cycling in which there is a rapid loss of weight followed by its regain;

yo-yo effect UROLOGY A fanciful descriptor for an appearance caused by the disturbed peristalsis in an obstructed megaureter, where a bolus of contrast material cyclically regurgitates into the upper ureter after reaching the bottom of the dilated segment, with only a minute portion passing into the bladder

yo-yo liver A liver characterized by an abrupt waxing and waning hepatomegaly, resulting from intermittent storage of a metabolic product, described in carnitine deficiency states (George Hug, U of Cincinnati, personal communication) distinguishing this from other forms of nonregressing metabolic hepatomegaly

YPLL Years of potential life lost PUBLIC HEALTH A statistic that is a measure of 'premature' death, ie that which occurs before age 65, calculated from the mortality data generated from the CDC's National Center for Health

Statistics CAUSES OF YPLL (1988) Accidents 19%, cancer, any site 15% (respiratory 279/10⁵, breast 206/10⁵, gastrointestinal tract 182/10⁵, oropharynx 28/10⁵), suicide and homicide 11% (black males 1669/10⁵; white females 99/10⁵), congenital anomalies 5.5%; in 1988, AIDS became the sixth most common cause of YPLL, causing a 1.7% increase in the total YPLL (**MMWR 1990; 39:2**0); magnitude of YPLL Cardiovascular disease 325/10⁵, malignancy 192/10⁵, cerebrovascular 64/10⁵; chronic obstructive pulmonary disease, 31/10⁵; pneumonia, 28/10⁵; suicide/homicide 20/10⁵, chronic liver disease, 11/10⁵ YPLL is increasing in AIDS (82%), DM (7%) and others; YPLL is decreasing in SIDS, cerebrovascular disease and prematurity; see 'Healthy people 2000'; Cf QALY

Ypt1 protein A highly conserved 23-kD GTP-binding protein that is required for attachment and/or fusion of secretory vesicles from the endoplasmic reticulum with the acceptor compartment (the Golgi complex) during protein secretion (**Science 1991; 252:1553**)

Yu-Cheng oil disease TOXICOLOGY An epidemic of congenital poisoning that occurred in Taiwan in 1979 due to the ingestion of cooking oil contaminated by polychlorinated biphenyls (PCBs) and dibenzofurans, eg 2,3,4,7,8-pentachlorodibenzofuran; congenital exposure resulted in lower birth weight, delayed growth, physical and mental retardation; defects in gingiva, skin, nails, teeth and lungs imply that the embryonal ectoderm is the most susceptible to the wiles of PCBs (**JAMA 1992; 268:3213oc**) see PCBs, Toxic oil syndrome, Yusho disease

yuppie disease Chronic fatigue syndrome, see there

yusho Kanemi oil intoxication TOXICOLOGY A major episode of food poisoning that occurred in 1968 in Japan due to exposure to polychlorinated biphenyls (PCBs), eg 2,3,4,7,8-pentachlorodibenzofuran, which contaminated cooking oil, allegedly through faulty processing of rice bran oil; yusho afflicted an estimated 13 000 (official figure, 1614; 54 deaths) CLINICAL Nausea, vomiting, persistent ARDS, meibomian gland hyperplasia, chloroacne, cardiovascular and CNS disease, petechial and erythematous rashes with pulmonary hypertension (the latter features were not seen in the clinically similar Toxic-oil syndrome (**N Engl J Med 1984; 310:1261c**) see PCBs, Toxic oil syndrome, Yucheng disease

YY1 A mammalian sequence-specific DNA-binding protein that has some homology with the *Drosophila* transcription factor protein Krüppel, see there

YY syndrome see XYY syndrome

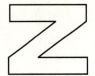

Z Symbol for: 1) Atomic number 2) Electrical impedance 3) (total) Glutamic acid and glutamine 4) Ionic number 5) Net charge 6) Proton number

Z-plasty SURGERY A surgical incision that lengthens a zone of skin or a muscle, 'breaking up' a linear scar or repositioning an incision to a line of least tension; the classic 'Z' incision consists of two triangular incisions with equilateral sides and a 60° angle

Z protein A protein that is normally present in the Z band of striated muscle, which may be positive in rhabdomyosarcoma but, like α-actinin, titin and tropomyosin, is too non-specific a muscle 'marker' to have significant diagnostic utility; Cf Protein Z

z score LABORATORY MEDICINE A value that is the absolute numerical difference between a laboratory's result and the 'true' result divided by the 'true' result; the z score is measure of the overall proficiency testing score for the laboratory (**Arch Pathol Lab Med 1992; 116:681**0A)

Z score Derived standardized score STATISTICS A measure of the deviation from the expected population mean, adjusted for the covariates on a scale where zero = mean, and 1 = standard deviation; assuming a standard gaussian distribution, 95% of a population will have a Z score between +2 and –2; conversion of raw data to Z scores allows comparison of two groups with varying physical characteristics, eg differences in height, weight, menopausal status, and so on (**N Engl J Med 1989; 320:554**0A)

z statistic STATISTICS A data set in a trial that approximately represents the effect of a therapeutic intervention on overall survival when compared to that of conservative management (**N Engl J Med 1995; 332:1256**0A) Cf V statistic

Z value STATISTICS A statistical test for the hypothesis that a population's mean does not differ from the target value, ie assumes no inaccuracy; see One-tailed test, Two-tailed test

Zagury, D An immunologist* in Paris who developed a research protocol using a vaccinia virus that had been genetically engineered to express HIV on its surface (**Science 1991; 252:1608n&v**)

*Whose 15 minutes of fame hinged on his public offer to act as the vaccine's guinea pig

zalcitabine ddC A nucleoside analogue that inhibits HIV reverse transcriptase; zalcitabine and didanosine are similar in survival, disease progression, CD4 count, adverse effects and efficacy (**N Engl J Med 1994; 330:657**0A)

zar PSYCHIATRY A term used in North African and in the Middle Eastern societies for being under the influence of spirits*, which may evoke various emotions or dissociative episodes, but is not regarded as a pathological state by the person's society (**DSM-IV™, 1994**) see Culture-bound syndrome

Z-band material An ultrastructural finding consisting of patches of disorganized myofilaments (figure), which is typical of rhabdomyosarcomas; other sarcomere-related structures seen by electron microscopy that support a diagnosis of rhabdomyosarcoma include thick and thin filaments in a hexagonal array, an A band with thick filaments and H and M bands or leptomeric structures; Z bands also occur in extracardiac rhabdomyoma, variably flanked by I bands

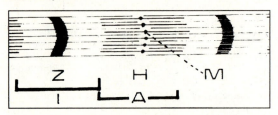

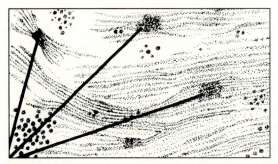

Z band material

Z-DNA A variant configuration of DNA that is 'left-handed', 'antiparallel', has a deep single major groove with a zig-zag configuration, dinucleotide repeating units resulting from the alteration in the strand of sugar 'puckering' and torsional angles about a glycosidic bond; Z-DNA is a dramatic example of sequence-specific conformational change, where the major groove is more extreme and the minor groove is smaller than the 'usual' right-handed B-DNA; the base pairs are the same in each form; segments of Z-DNA occur in native DNA, require higher energy for maintenance than B-DNA, have a high content of guanine and cytosine and may have a role in signal recognition, possibly by initiating replication; see DNA

'zebra' CLINICAL DECISION-MAKING A somewhat hackneyed aphorism often quoted to wide-eyed medical students during their clinical rotations is, *'when you hear hoofbeats, don't think of zebras'*; this variation of 'Sutton's law' is designed to teach students a logical approach to achieving a diagnosis, since common things occur commonly and when one hears hoofbeats, one usually thinks of horses; see Sutton's law; Cf 'Red herring'

Note: In the Republic of South Africa, zebras are more abundant and the word 'canary' is substituted

zebra body A descriptor for a lysosome that contains broad transversely-stacked myelinoid membranes (figure), an ultrastructural finding typical of certain lysosomal storage diseases, found within neurons, Schwann cells, macrophages, smooth muscle cells, endothelial cells, pericytes, glomerular epithelial cells, hepatocytes and other cells; zebra bodies are classically seen in Fabry's disease, but are also well-described in Niemann-Pick, Landing's, and Sandhoff's disease, some mucopolysaccharidoses, eg Hurler syndrome, myelinopathy, phenylketonuria and Tay-Sachs disease

Note: 'Myelinosome' is the most correct term for any layered material within a lysosome; electron microscopists separate the myelinosomes into those with thick layering (zebra bodies) and thin layering, known as lamellar bodies ('myelin figures'), as each type is associated with certain diseases

zebra body myopathy A congenital, non-progressive form of myopathy in which variably-sized muscle fibers have characteristic striped and rod-shaped bodies by electron microscopy (J Neurol Sci 1975; 24:437)

zebrafish DEVELOPMENTAL BIOLOGY An experimental animal (*Brachydanio rerio*) that is useful in studying vertebrate development, which has transparent embryos, short (3 months) generation time and prolific egg production; the zebrafish has proven to be an extremely useful model system for studying vertebrate embryology; using a strategy known as saturation mutagenesis; Nüsslein-Volhard of the Max Planck Institute of Tübingen and co-workers screened 1.2×10^6 zebrafish and have identified 1300 mutants with a vast array of abnormal phenotypes, eg 'pathfinding' mutants in which axons get lost on the developmental pathway, 'termination' mutants in which the axons follow the correct pathway, but innervate the wrong target site (Science 1994; 264:904N&v) see Saturation mutagenesis

For other biological model systems, see *Caenorhabditis elegans*, *Drosophila melanogaster*, Guinea pig, Rat, *Saccharomyces cerevisiae*

ZEBRA gene A gene in the Epstein-Barr virus (EBV) genome that must be activated for the virus to replicate, thus serving as a switch between latency and replication; the gene is termed 'ZEBRA' as it is localized on the EBV Bam HI **Z** fragment that corresponds to the **EB**V **R**eplication **A**ctivator; the protein product of the ZEBRA gene is a transcriptional transactivator (G Miller, Yale)

zebra pattern Alternating light and dark bands of the hair shaft seen by polarizing LM in trichoschisis, an AR condition due to ↓ sulfur content of the hair shaft CLINICAL Mental and growth retardation, ichthyosis and ectodermal dysplasia affecting the eyes, nails, and teeth

zeiosis A variant form of lymphocyte-mediated cytolysis, characterized by nuclear blebbing, disintegration of the nucleus and mitochondrial swelling

zeitgeber *Zeit*, German, time, *geber*, keeper Any factor in the environment with periodicity, capable of synchronizing the endogenous circadian rhythm into a 24-hour cycle; without zeitgebers, the free-running human clock is 25.3 hours; see Circadian rhythm, Jet lag, Shift work; Cf REM sleep

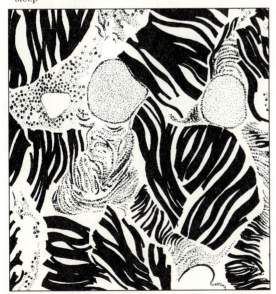

zebra body

Zelen design CLINICAL TRIALS A design for a double-blinded study of experimental cancer chemotherapeutic agents that requires permission only from those patients receiving experimental drugs or therapy (N Engl J Med 1979; 300:1242); the patients are randomly assigned to one of two groups: the first receives the standard treatment, while the second group is allocated to the experimental group and then asked if they will participate; if they decline, they stay in the second group and are treated with the same protocol as the first group; any loss of statistical efficiency is compensated by increased numbers; the advantage is that the trial is truly randomized and the patients know whether they are being treated with an experimental regimen; see Leveno design (N Engl J Med 1986; 315:615)

zellballen SURGICAL PATHOLOGY Nest-like clusters of uniform round-to-polygonal chief cells that are surrounded by delicate richly vascular tissue and sustentacular cells, a pattern characteristic of paraganglioma EM 100-200 nm in diameter dense core granules, which are sites of norepinephrine production

zero-order kinetics THERAPEUTIC DRUG MONITORING The in vivo dynamics related to the rate of drug elimination, which is linear with time, and proportional to the concentration of the enzyme responsible for catabolism and independent of substrate concentration; see Michaelis-Menten equation; Cf First order kinetics

zero population growth POPULATION The birth rate at which there is no net increase in a population (a goal targeted by birth control programs) and the number of births is equal to the number of deaths; the world population will stabilize at 8-14 billion by the middle of next century, but some modellers think that by the time stabilization occurs, it may be 'too late'; already, 15% of the world's population (800 million), live in a constant state of near-starvation; see Amsterdam protocol, Birth control, Greenhouse effect, Mexico City policy, Webster decision; Cf Title X

zero tolerance policy A stance taken by the US government agencies, that any type of drug abuse is punishable by incarceration (JAMA 1992; 268:3176MN&P) see Correctional facility, War on Drugs

zetacrit Zeta sedimentation rate A method for determining erythrocyte sedimentation rate, which is thought to be better than the Winthrobe or Westergren methods as it is not affected by hematocrit, it is linear with respect to fibrinogen and γ-globulin and has no ♂:♀ differences

zeta potential TRANSFUSION MEDICINE The sum total of negative charges on red cell surfaces separating erythrocytes in a cationic medium; the cations in a medium can be divided into those that are firmly attached to the erythrocyte, moving as it moves and cations that are free in the medium; the boundary between these two planes of cations is known as the boundary of shear, a point at which the zeta potential may be measured as ⁻mV; the optimal zeta potential for IgM antibodies is ⁻22 to ⁻17 mV and for IgG, ⁻11 to ⁻4.5 mV; the smaller the absolute mV values, the shorter the distance between cells; an increase of asymmetric proteins in the medium decreases the zeta potential, thereby increasing the erythrocyte sedimentation rate; the zeta potential can be artificially reduced by enzymes, albumin, LISS, and polybrene

zeugmatography MRI A coinage from Greek that dignifies magnetic resonance imaging*, which translated as '*the spatial relation of the image to a gradient magnetic field*'; see Magnetic resonance imaging

Note: It is unlikely that this neologism will prevail over the more widely used term MRI

zidovudine AZT 3'-azido-3'-deoxythimidine A thymidine analogue that slows the progression of AIDS, which act as an HIV-1 antimetabolite, terminating its DNA chain growth; zidovudine is used in AIDS patients with

Pneumocystis carinii and/or CD4+ T-helper cells less than 200/mm³ and in HIV-1 infected children with neurodevelopmental abnormalities; zidovudine therapy benefits patients with CD4+ cell counts > 400/ml (**N Engl J Med 1993; 329:297oa**) and improves the survival of those with AIDS, 190 days without zidovudine, 770 days with zidovudineTHERAPEUTIC EFFECT Improved sense of well-being, ↑ CD4+ T cells, fewer AIDS-related complications; patients may become refractory to AZT after 12-18 months due to development of multiple (three or more) mutations in HIV-1's reverse transcriptase that are less susceptible to AZT, although the strains do not affect clinical disease LONG-TERM COMPLICATIONS Mitochondrial myopathy, see Ragged red fiber disease; AIDS patients with profoundly decreased (< 100/mm³) T cells who survive for long periods owing to AZT therapy, are at ↑ risk for high-grade B cell extranodal lymphoma, estimated to occur in 46% after 36 months of zidovudine therapy; the risk of NHL is ± 1.6/100 patient years of zidovudine therapy (**JAMA 1991; 265:2208**)

SIDE EFFECTS Dose-limiting myelosuppression with granulocytopenia that may respond to lithium, anemia, headache, insomnia, mania, seizures, nausea, myalgia Note: Ribavirin antagonizes AZT's effect on HIV-1's replication; see AIDS therapy TREATMENT GUIDELINES PROPHYLACTIC (500 mg/d) as CD4+ T cells fall below 0.5 x 10⁹/L (US: 500/mm³); in asymptomatic HIV patients with CD4+ T cells < 0.5 x 10⁹/L (US: < 500/mm³), 33/428 of the placebo group followed for one year developed clinical AIDS versus 11/453 of those receiving 500 mg/day of zidovudine COMBINATION THERAPY Zidovudine + 2', 3'-dideoxycitidine may prevent HIV replication within macrophages, and require ⅕ usual AZT dose; alternatively AZT + amphotericin methyl ester (which increases the porosity of HIV's protein coat) thrombocytopenia in AIDS may be due to HIV infection of megakaryocytes and may respond to zidovudine (**ibid 1992; 327:1779oa**)

zidovudine failure A form of drug failure in that is defined as the development of opportunistic infection despite adequate zidovudine therapy, due to infection with zidovudine-resistant HIV-1 (**N Engl J Med 1993; 328:1163oa**)

'zigzag' QRS waves Sinusoidal QRS complexes seen by electrocardiography in ventricular flutter (240-280/min)

zinc A trace metal that is essential* for growth and development, and is required for more than 200 metalloenzymes including DNA– and RNA-polymerases, and reverse transcriptase, as well as for zinc-finger proteins involved in gene expression; zinc is stored in synaptic vesicles and has a role as a synaptic neuromodulator, acting in the hippocampus to induce depolarizing synaptic potentials (**Nature 1991; 349:521**) ~20% of dietary zinc is absorbed; absorption is enhanced by protein-rich foods; ~90% is excreted in feces DISTRIBUTION 50-60% of total is in muscle, 28% in bone (**Clinical Chemistry News August 1993**)

*RDA–recomended daily allowance, 5-15 mg/day; normal range 70-120 µg/dL

zinc deficiency A condition characterized by dermatitis, diarrhea, delayed hypersensitivyt response, poor outcome of pregnancy, retarded growth, hypogonadism and others (**Clinical Chemistry News August 1993**)

zinc finger MOLECULAR BIOLOGY A tertiary protein structural motif found in higher organisms in which parts of a protein fold around a zinc molecule, acting as a hook to attach activator proteins to DNA (**Sci Am 1995; 272/2:56**) some ZFs bind to DNA-RNA hybrids in a sequence-specific manner and with greater affinity that to DNA alone; because these hybids occur during replication and transcription, ZF hybrids may perform a biological function (**Science 1995; 268:282**) ZFs consists of a 28-30 residue polypeptide containing tandemly repeated cysteine or histidine residues that forms a protein loop (a consensus motif, see figure) held together at both ends by a zinc ion; the ZF is tetrahedrically coordinated by cysteine or lysine residues for proper folding and DNA binding (**Science 1991; 252:809**) ZFs are involved in DNA binding or protein-protein contacts and are present in transcription factors (DNA-binding proteins that regulate gene expression by either suppressing or enhancing gene transcription) the DNA-interacting 'fingertip' itself is composed of Lysine, His, Asn, Gln, Thr and Arg and contains an antiparallel β ribbon and an α helix; the ZF motif is present in many proteins that regulate the expression of eukaryotic genes, including proto-oncogenes, Wilms' tumor gene, and growth signal receptors

zidovudine

zinc finger proteins A superfamily of transactivating protein receptors that mediate the actions of steroids and steroid-like hormones; after a zinc finger receptor binds a hormone, it influences gene expression by associating with specific DNA elements, the HREs (hormone-responsive elements; zinc finger domains occur in the Wilms' gene product, protein kinase C proteins, glucocorticoid receptor DNA-binding domain, HTLV-I and HTLV-II transformed cells and the ZPY gene, which encodes a zinc-finger protein once considered a candidate for the testis-determining factor

zinc-α₂-glycoprotein Gross cystic disease fluid protein 44 A component of normal serum that is present in higher concentrations in gross cystic fluids (of the breast), prostate, apocrine cells, serous cells of the parotid gland, and in ± 55% of breast carcinomas; anti-ZPG antibodies with the immunoperoxidase method are reported ly useful in identifying the breast as the site of origin in tumor metastases (**Arch Pathol Lab Med 1992; 116:1181oa**)

'zinc sandwich' A polypeptide hormone-receptor complex in which a hormone, eg growth hormone (hGH) binds to a another, not cognate receptor, eg prolactin receptor, forming a bridge between histidine and glycine residues and zinc, but not other divalent metal ions; a 'zinc sandwich' motif provides a molecular explanation of the broader effects of zinc deficiency (**Science 1990; 250:1709**)

Zinjanthropus boisei ANTHROPOLOGY A 1.8 million year old east African lower Pleistocene hominid skull discovered in the Olduvai Gorge by Mary Leakey in 1959; the skull is characterized by robust posterior dentition, a small cranial cavity, and cresting of the cranium, and is regarded as the first of the group *Australopithecus boisei* (**Sci Am 1994; 271/4:37**)

zippering MOLECULAR BIOLOGY Rapid annealment of two fully complementary strands of RNA and DNA into a double helix, which follows a short nucleation step PHYSIOLOGY The highly organized process of internalization of phagocytosed particles, which requires that the receptor ligands being internalized by the macrophage have multiple contacts with their cognate 'receptor'

zipper-like junction An ultrastructural particle formed in vitro in hairy cell leukemia, as well as in monocytic leukemia grown in tissue culture when these cells phagocytose material from the surrounding culture medium

zipper motif see Leucine zipper

zipper proglottid A descriptor for the proglottid of *Taenia saginata* which have 15-20 lateral zipper-like branches, best seen when injected with safranin dye and India ink; in contrast, the proglottids of *T solium* have fewer than 13 lateral branches and have been fancifully likened to Rorschach bodies

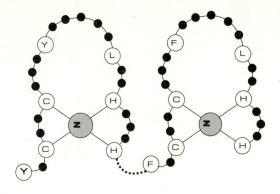

zinc finger

Zodiac FORENSIC PSYCHIATRY A prolific serial killer who is believed to have been responsible for up to 40 murders that occurred during the late 1960s in four Western states, most in California; indicative of Zodiac's disordered thought processes was his reasons for committing the murders was that he was '...*collecting slaves for my afterlife...*'; he (or she, to be politically correct) is believed to be no longer to be active, either through death or confinement to a mental institution (Encyclopedia of American Crime, Facts on File, New York, 1982, Smithmark, New York, 1992)

Zollinger-Ellison syndrome A condition characterized by multiple duodenal ulcers and gastrin-secreting tumors, which causes recurrent and refractory upper gastrointestinal ulceration, diarrhea, steatorrhea and hypoglycemia due to 'little' gastrin, as well as pyrosis and dysphagia due to gastroesophageal reflux and increased gastric acid; 25% of cases have concomitant multiple endocrine neoplasm (MEN-I); malignant gastric carcinoid may be related to chronic gastrin hypersecretion DIAGNOSIS CT, when positive, is reliable in the face of typical clinical findings PATHOLOGY Marked variation in tumor size, 60% are malignant, despite a 'bland' appearance LABORATORY Hypergastrinemia, increased basal acid output (>15 mmol/hour), ↑ post-histamine stimulation acid production, a high ratio of basal acid output to maximum acid output (stimulation testing reveals fasting gastrin levels greater than 1000 pg/mL) and hypercalcemia DDx-HYPERGASTRINEMIA Antral hyperplasia, retained antrum syndrome, chronic atrophic gastritis, pernicious anemia, short bowel syndrome, gastric outlet syndrome, gastric outlet obstruction, gastric carcinoma, pheochromocytoma, chronic renal failure TREATMENT Medical treatment with H_2 receptor antagonists, which with higher doses may be coadministered with antimuscarinic drugs that enhance the inhibition of gastric secretion by H_2 blockage; nonresponse to medical treatment may require total gastrectomy and or vagotomy

zombie One of the 'living dead' of Haitian voodoo folklore; there is no scientific data to support their existence, although one ethnobiologist claimed to have identified Zombie powder from voodoo sorcerers (bokors) and concluded that the active ingredient was tetrodotoxin, which further required that the victim actually believed in zombies, a 'set and setting' event; see Culture-bound syndrome; Cf Ethnomedicine, Voodoo death

zombie effect A descriptor for the personality changes reported to be secondary to haloperidol's extrapyramidal effects, resulting in a syndrome virtually identical to idiopathic Parkinson's disease, with hypomimia, bradykinesia and flat affect

zonal centrifugation MOLECULAR BIOLOGY A method for separating molecules by size, as a function of the time of centrifugation and the mass of the molecule; the level at which the molecules come to rest in an ultracentrifuge (60 000 rpm) is based on sedimentation velocities of the molecules of interest which separate in different zones based on a density gradient which differs from the top to the bottom of the centrifugation tube, and can be stabilized by adding a fluid, eg sucrose solution; see Ultracentrifugation

the 'zone' SPORTS MEDICINE A highly colloqial term used by some amateur athletes for heart rates (zones) that reflect the intensity of a workout or exercise routine; 60-70% of maximum heart rate (MHR) is known as the weight management zone; 70-80% MHR as the aerobic performance zone, 80-90% MHR as the peak performance zone, and 90-100% MHR as the red line zone; as the heart rate increases, metabolism is increasingly anaerobic, and the higher 'zones' are not recommended for prolonged periods of times for the 'weekend warrior' type of athlete (NY Newsday June 12, 1995, pB15)

zone electrophoresis A generic term for any electrophoretic technique in which components are separated into zones or bands in a buffer, and stabilized in solid, porous or any other support medium, including filter paper, agar gel or polyacrylamide gel

zone of equivalence IMMUNOLOGY A region in an antigen-antibody reacting system where the ratio of antigen to antibody is equivalent; the in vivo correlate of a dynamic zone of equivalence is serum sickness, where antigen is excess in the first one to two weeks, and the patient is asymptomatic, as antibody production increases to a 1:1 ratio, immune complexes form, causing clinical disease, which resolves as the balance is tipped toward antibody excess

zoning phenomenon HEMATOLOGY Layering of atypical platelets in the bone marrow in myelofibrosis SURGICAL PATHOLOGY Changes seen by low-power light microscopy in myositis ossificans, in which there are three zones of osteochondroma-like growth, the most immature of which has a fibroblast appearance, demarcating the lesion from the normal tissue

zoo blot A technique used to determine DNA sequence homology among different species, in which a labeled probe of a gene of interest is allowed to hybridize with Southern blots from other organisms

zoonoses Infections in which the microbe's infectious cycle is completed between man and mammal

zosteriform An adjective pertaining or referring to a band-like unilateral skin lesion located along the cutaneous distribution of a spinal or a branch of the trigeminal nerves, usually seen in the recrudescence of herpes zoster but also (rarely) seen in metastatic breast carcinoma and hemangiomas of Sturge-Weber disease

ZPA Zone of polarizing activity EMBRYOLOGY A group of mesenchymal cells in developing vertebrates that is responsible for forming the limb bud, which is aided in its orientation by retinoic acid (Nature 1991; 350:81, 83, 15)

ZPG Zero population growth, see there

zuckergußdarm *Zuckerguß*, German, sugar-icing, *darm*, bowel Whitish induration of the serosal surface of the intestine in chronic fibrosing peritonitis, which may be accompanied by hyalinization

zuckergußleber German, sugar-icing liver A markedly thickened and whitish hepatic capsule, which may be seen in chronic perihepatitis or in cardiac 'cirrhosis', due to congestive heart failure HISTOPATHOLOGY Portal zone fibrosis and bile duct proliferation

zuckerguß spleen German, sugar-icing spleen Perisplenitis, as above

Zung (depression) scale PSYCHIATRY An objective rating instrument that evaluates depression, anxiety, hostility, phobia, paranoid ideation, obsessive compulsiveness and others; use of this scale is declining as it is relatively insensitive to clinical improvement; the ZS consists of a item questionnaire that serves as a primary screening tool that is reported to have a 83-97% sensitivity and 63-82% specificity for depression (JAMA 1995; 273:197)

Zyklon B The cyanide-tear gas combination formulated by the scientists of the Third Reich, and used for the 'efficient' genocide of the Jews and other 'undesirables' in concentration camps; see Chemical warfare, Genocide; Cf Massacre, Tabun, Unethical medical research

zygomycetes A generic term for a group of fungi which grow in compromised hosts including *Absidia, Cunninghamella, Mortierella, Mucor, Rhizopus*, which are pathogenic to humans; other organisms, eg *Basiobolus, Conidiobolus* and *Rhizomucor*, which proliferate but are not regarded as pathogenic

zymotyping MICROBIOLOGY The determination of an organism's specific subtype based on its isoenzyme profile using multilocus enzyme electrophoresis

ZZAP reagent TRANSFUSION MEDICINE A reagent used to dissociate IgG and C3d from the erythrocyte membrane, eliminating spontaneous agglutination and allowing for reliable typing of ABO, Rh-hr and Kidd blood groups; ZZAP is of use in detecting alloantibodies, which are potentially capable of causing a hemolytic transfusion reaction in the face of nonspecific binding of autoantibody to erythrocytes, or for evaluation of patients with acquired immune hemolytic anemia

Note: The name was originally SSAP, indicating a mixture of a sulfhydryl reagent (dithiothreitol, which reduces disulfide bonds, S-S) and the proteolytic enzyme, papain which dissociates IgG and C3d from red blood cells; ZZAP was substituted for euphony